D0144329

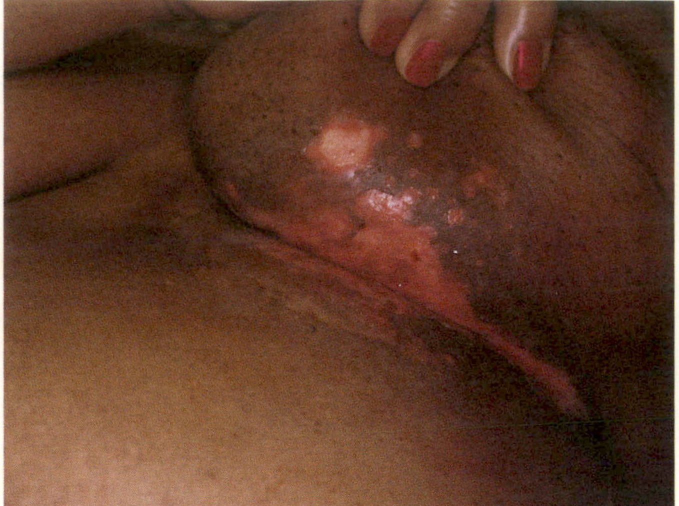

PLATE 1 Moist desquamation with radiation therapy and concomitant Methotrexate, 5-Fluorouracil and Leucovorin (Figure 33-2).

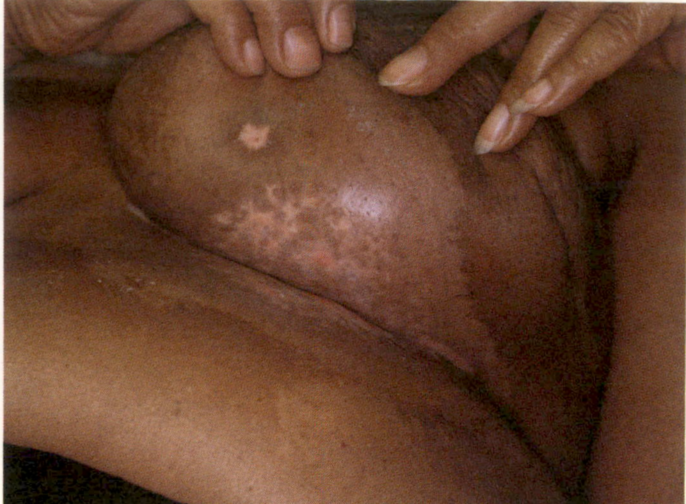

PLATE 2 Two weeks after completion and treatment three times daily with domeboro soaks, wound cleanser, and epithelial stimulating wound gel (Figure 33-3).

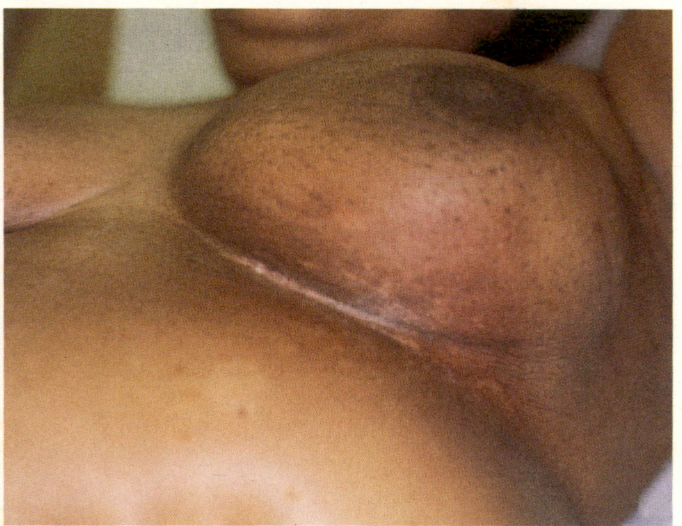

PLATE 3 Three months after completing radiation (Figure 33-4).

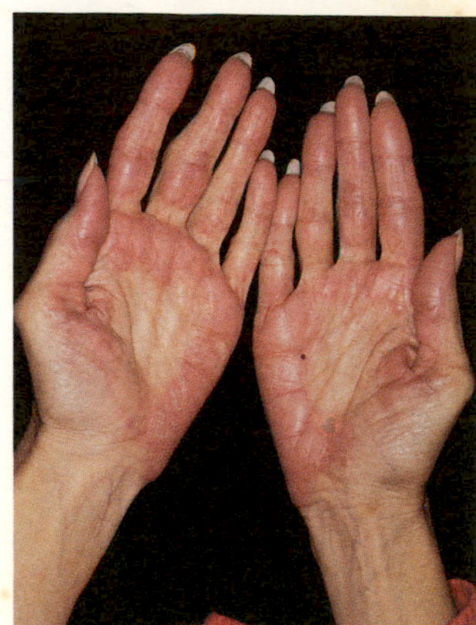

PLATE 4 Acral erythema following Floxuridine infusion (Figure 33-9).

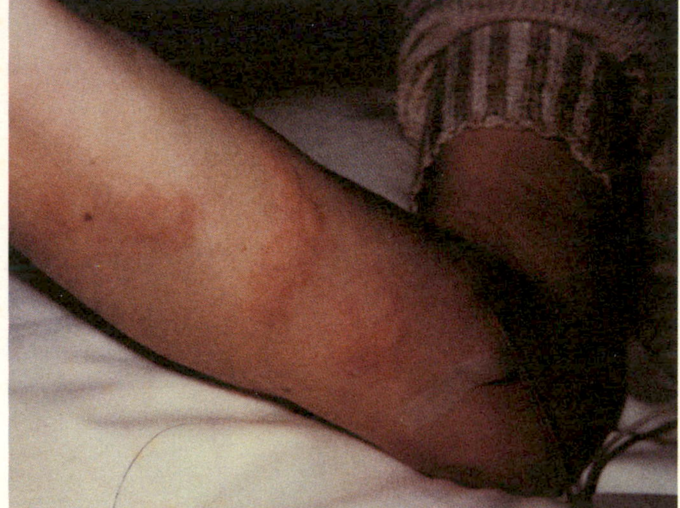

PLATE 5 Venous flare (Doxorubicin) (Figure 33-10).

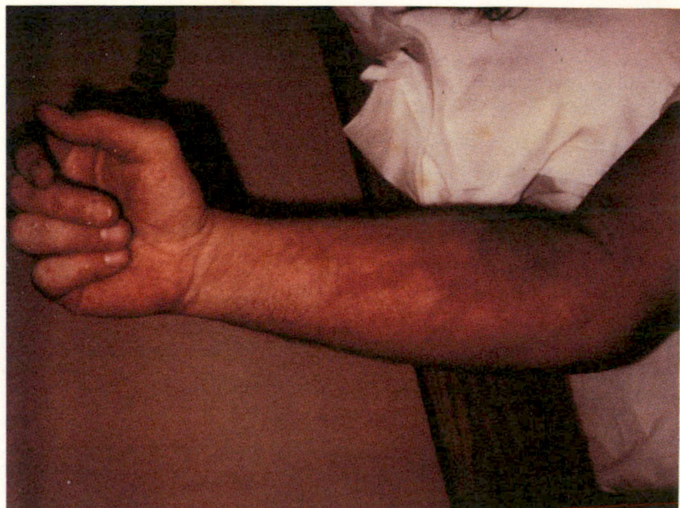

PLATE 6 Venous extravasation $2\frac{1}{2}$ weeks after doxorubicin extravasation (Figure 33-11).

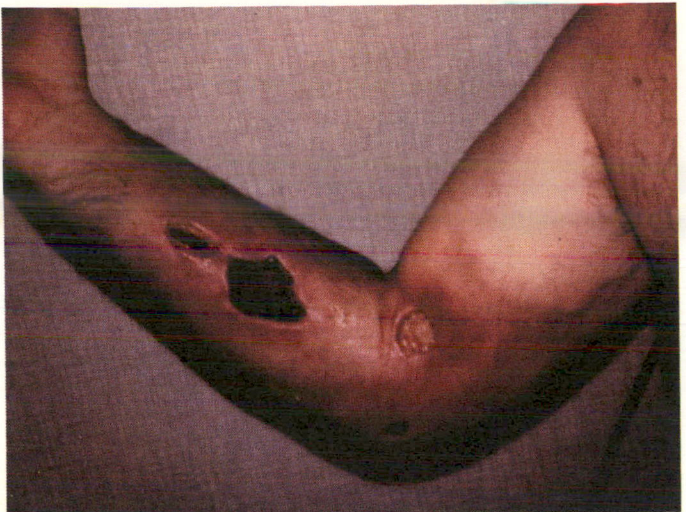

PLATE 7 Same patient $4\frac{1}{2}$ months after doxorubicin extravasation (Figure 33-12).

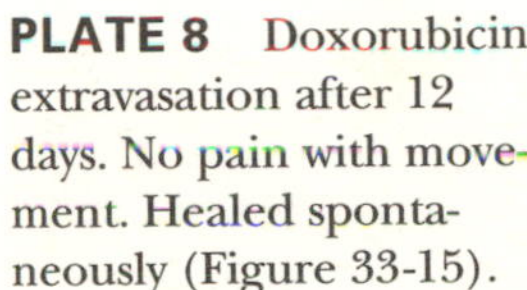

PLATE 8 Doxorubicin extravasation after 12 days. No pain with movement. Healed spontaneously (Figure 33-15).

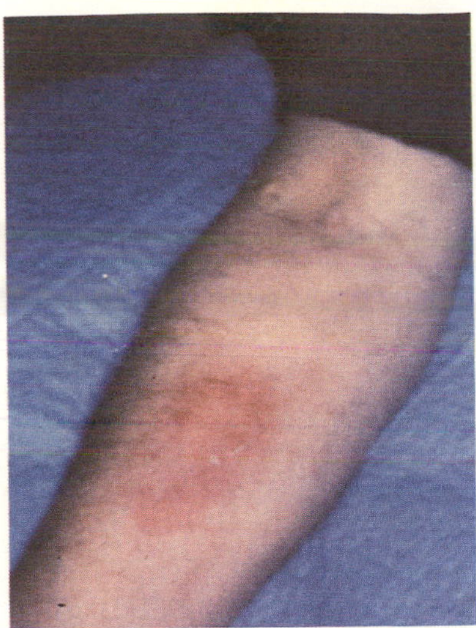

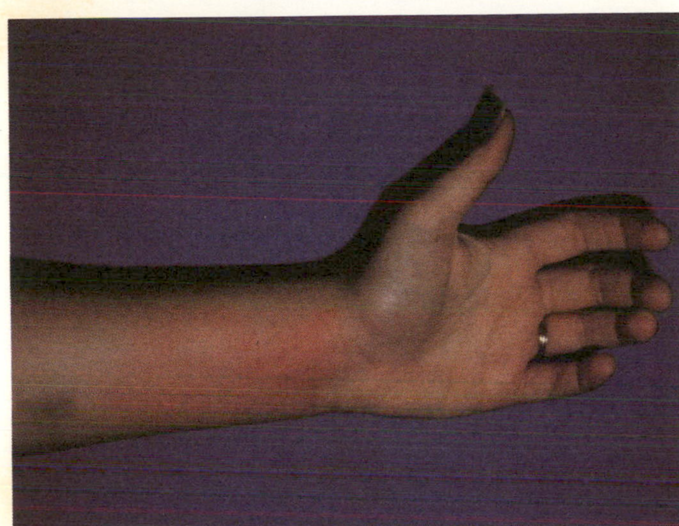

PLATE 9 Erythema and edema at injection site one week after doxorubicin administration (Figure 33-16).

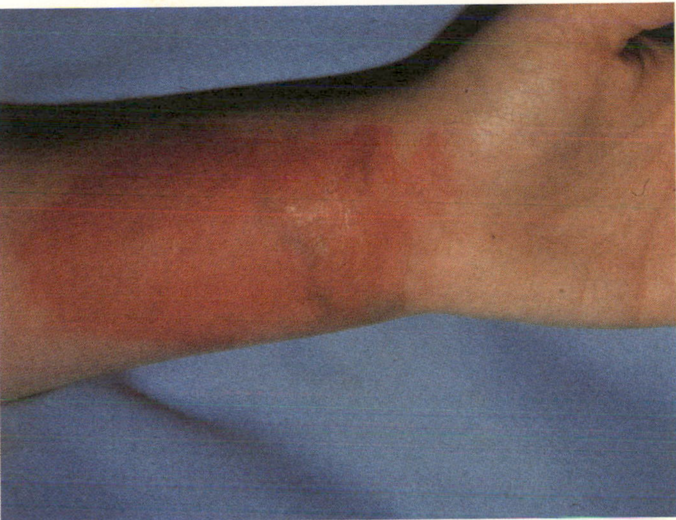

PLATE 10 At three weeks, blister formation and demarcation are present (Figure 33-17).

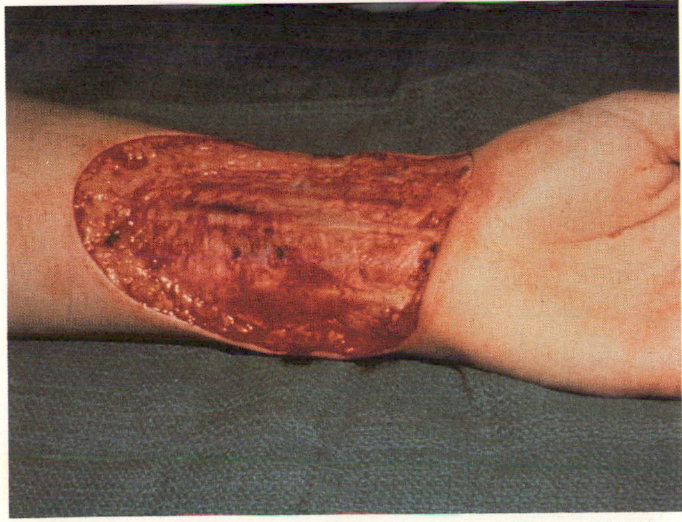

PLATE 11 Damaged tissue surgically excised (Figure 33-18).

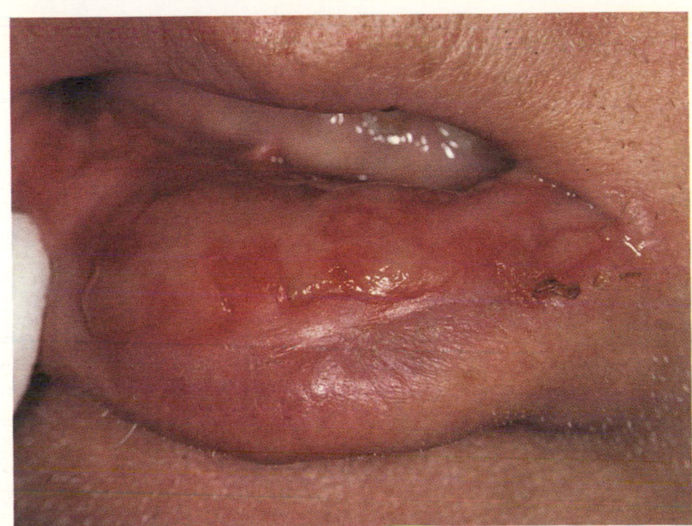

PLATE 12 Methotrexate-induced stomatitis. Grade 3 (Figure 33-23).

CANCER NURSING

The Jones and Bartlett Series in Nursing

Adult Emergency Nursing Procedures, Proehl

Basic Steps in Planning Nursing Research, Third Edition, Brink/Wood

Bloodborne Pathogens, National Safety Council

Bone Marrow Transplantation, Whedon

Breastfeeding and Human Lactation, Riordan/Auerbach

Study Guide for Breastfeeding and Human Lactation, Auerbach/Riordan

Cancer Chemotherapy: A Nursing Process Approach, Barton Burke et al.

Cancer Nursing: Principles and Practice, Third Edition, Groenwald et al.

Chemotherapy Care Plans, Barton Burke et al.

Children's Nutrition, Lifshitz et al.

Chronic Illness: Impact and Intervention, Second Edition, Lubkin

Comprehensive Cancer Nursing Review, Groenwald et al.

A Comprehensive Curriculum for Trauma Nursing, Bayley/Turcke

Desk Reference for Critical Care Nursing, Wright/Shelton

Drugs and Protocols Common to Prehospital and Emergency Care, Cummings

Emergency Care of Children, Thompson

Essential Medical Terminology, Stanfield

Essentials of Oxygenation, Ahrens/Rutherford

Family Life: Process and Practice, Janosik/Green

Handbook of Oncology Nursing, Johnson/Gross

Health Assessment in Nursing Practice, Third Edition, Grimes/Burns

Health and Wellness, Fourth Edition, Edlin/Golanty

Healthy Children 2000, U.S. Department of Health and Human Services

Healthy People 2000, U.S. Department of Health and Human Services

Human Development: A Life-Span Approach, Fourth Edition, Frieberg

Introductory Management and Leadership for Clinical Nurses, Swansburg

Intravenous Therapy, Nentwich

Introduction to the Health Professions, Stanfield

Introduction to Human Disease, Third Edition, Crowley

Journal of Perinatal Education, ASPO/Lamaze

Management and Leadership for Nurse Managers, Swansburg

Management of Spinal Cord Injury, Second Edition, Zejdlik

Math for Health Professionals, Third Edition, Whisler

Medical Terminology, Stanfield

Memory Bank for Chemotherapy, Second Edition, Preston/Wilfinger

Memory Bank for Critical Care: EKGs and Cardiac Drugs, Second Edition, Ervin

Memory Bank for Hemodynamic Monitoring: The Pulmonary Artery Catheter, Second Edition, Ervin/Long

Memory Bank for Intravenous Therapy, Second Edition, Weinstein

Memory Bank for Medications, Second Edition, Kostin/Sieloff

Mental Health and Psychiatric Nursing: A Caring Approach, Davies/Janosik

The Nation's Health, Third Edition, Lee/Estes

Nursing and the Disabled: Across the Lifespan, Fraley

Nursing Assessment and Diagnosis, Second Edition, Bellack/Edlund

Nursing Diagnosis Care Plans for Diagnosis-Related Groups, Neal/Paquette/Mirch

Nursing Pharmacology, Second Edition, Wallace/Wardell

Nursing Research: A Quantitative and Qualitative Approach, Roberts/Burke

Nursing Research with Basic Statistical Applications, Dempsey/Dempsey

Nutrition and Diet Therapy: Self-Instructional Modules, Second Edition, Stanfield

Oncology Nursing in the Ambulatory Setting, Buchsel/Yarbro

Oncology Nursing Drug Handbook, Wilkes et al.

Oncology Nursing Homecare Handbook, Barton Burke

Oncology Nursing Society's Instruments for Clinical Nursing Research, Frank-Stromborg

Pediatric Emergency Nursing Procedures, Bernardo/Bove

Perioperative Nursing: Principles and Practice, Fairchild

Perioperative Nursing Review, Fairchild et al.

Perioperative Patient Care, Second Edition, Kneedler/Dodge

Policy Manual for Bloodborne Pathogens, Wetle

A Practical Guide to Breastfeeding, Riordan

Psychiatric Nursing Diagnosis Care Plans for DSM-III-R, Paquette et al.

Ready Reference for Critical Care, Strawn/Stewart

Understanding/Responding, Second Edition, Long

Women's Health: A Global Perspective, McElmurry/Noit

CANCER NURSING
Principles and Practice

THIRD EDITION

EDITED BY

Susan L. Groenwald, RN, MS
Assistant Professor of Nursing—Complemental
Department of Medical Nursing
Rush University College of Nursing
Rush-Presbyterian-St. Luke's Medical Center
Chicago, Illinois

Michelle Goodman, RN, MS, OCN
Assistant Professor of Nursing
Rush University College of Nursing
Oncology Clinical Nurse Specialist
Section of Medical Oncology
Rush Cancer Institute
Rush-Presbyterian-St. Luke's Medical Center
Chicago, Illinois

Margaret Hansen Frogge, RN, MS
Executive Vice President, Administration
Coordinator, Community Cancer Program
Riverside Medical Center
Kankakee, Illinois

Connie Henke Yarbro, RN, BSN
Editor, *Seminars in Oncology Nursing*
Director, Nursing Resource Development
The Regional Cancer Center
Memorial Medical Center
Springfield, Illinois

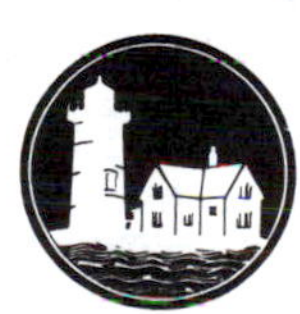

JONES AND BARTLETT PUBLISHERS
Boston London

Editorial, Sales, and Customer Service Offices

Jones and Bartlett Publishers
One Exeter Plaza
Boston, MA 02116
617-859-3900
1-800-832-0034

Jones and Bartlett Publishers International
7 Melrose Terrace
London W6 7RL
England

Library of Congress Cataloging-in-Publication Data

Cancer nursing: principles and practice / edited by Susan L.
Groenwald . . . [et al.].—3rd ed.
p. cm.
Includes bibliographical references and index.
ISBN 0-86720-640-3
1. Cancer—Nursing. I. Groenwald, Susan L.
[DNLM: 1. Neoplasms—nursing. WY 156 C2197 1993]
RC266.C356 1993
610.73'698—dc20
DNLM/DLC
for Library of Congress
93-20419
CIP

The selection and dosage of drugs presented in this book are in accord with standards accepted at the time of publication. The authors and publisher have made every effort to provide accurate information. However, research, clinical practice, and government regulations often change the accepted standard in this field. Before administering any drug, the reader is advised to check the manufacturer's product information sheet for the most up-to-date recommendations on dosage, precautions, and contraindications. This is especially important in the case of drugs that are new or seldom used.

Production Services: Michael Bass & Associates
Production Editor: Natasha Sabath
Cover Design: Rafael Millan

Printed in the United States of America
97 96 95 94 10 9 8 7 6 5 4 3 2

"Any one cell, embodying as it does the record of a billion years of evolution, represents more an historical than a physical event. You cannot expect to explain such a wise old bird in a few simple words."

MAX DELBRUGHT
California Institute of Technology

DEDICATION

To our colleagues in cancer nursing . . .
Who strive to meet the challenges imposed by the manifestations of wayward cells, and . . .
Who care for the complex human beings who live with those manifestations

SLG, MHF, MG, CHY

Contributors

Barbara Barhamand, RN, MS, OCN
Oncology Clinical Nurse Specialist/Manager
Hematology-Oncology Consultants, Ltd.
Naperville, Illinois

Connie Yuska Bildstein, RN, MS
Director of Medical/Oncology Nursing
Northwestern Memorial Hospital
Chicago, Illinois

Barbara D. Blumberg, ScM
Director of Education
Baylor-Susan G. Komen Breast Center
Dallas, Texas

Deborah McCaffrey Boyle, RN, MSN, OCN
Oncology Clinical Nurse Specialist
Arlington, Virginia

Donald P. Braun, PhD
Associate Director, Section of Medical Oncology
Rush-Presbyterian-St. Luke's Medical Center
Associate Professor of Medicine and Immunology/Microbiology
Rush Medical College
Chicago, Illinois

Patricia C. Buchsel, RN, MSN
Senior Research Associate
University of Washington
School of Nursing
Seattle, Washington
Bone Marrow Transplant Consultant
Critical Care of America
Westborough, Massachusetts

Dawn Camp-Sorrell, RN, MSN, OCN
Oncology Nurse Consultant, Private Practice
Adjunct Faculty/Staff Nurses
Vanderbilt University
Nashville, Tennessee

Brenda Cartmel, PhD
Research Instructor
Department of Family and Community Medicine
University of Arizona and
The Arizona Cancer Center
Tucson, Arizona

David F. Cella, PhD
Associate Professor of Psychology
Rush Medical College
Director, Division of Psychosocial Oncology
Rush Cancer Institute
Chicago, Illinois

Diane D. Chapman, RN, MS
Coordinator, Comprehensive Breast Center
Rush Cancer Institute
Rush-Presbyterian-St. Luke's Medical Center
Faculty (Complemental)
Rush University
Chicago, Illinois

Jane C. Clark, RN, MN, OCN
Clinical Nurse Specialist, Oncology
Emory University Hospital
Atlanta, Georgia

Rebecca F. Cohen, RN, EdD, MPA, CPHQ
Assistant Professor, Department of Nursing
Rockford College
Rockford, Illinois

Mary Cunningham, RN, MS
Clinical Nurse Specialist
Department of Neuro-Oncology
Pain and Symptom Management Section
M.D. Anderson Cancer Center
Houston, Texas

Vincent T. DeVita, Jr., MD
Attending Physician and Member
Program of Molecular Pharmacology and Therapeutics
Benno C. Schmidt Chair in Clinical Oncology
Memorial Sloan-Kettering Cancer Center
New York, New York

Kathleen A. Dietz, RN, MA, MS
Clinical Nurse Specialist
Memorial Sloan-Kettering Cancer Center
Associate, Columbia University School of Nursing
New York, New York

Michele Girard Donehower, RN, MSN
Adult Nurse Practitioner
University of Maryland Cancer Center
Baltimore, Maryland

Diane Scott Dorsett, RN, PhD, FAAN
Director
Comprehensive Support Services for Persons with Cancer
Associate Clinical Professor
University of California
San Francisco, California

Susan Dudas, RN, MSN
Associate Professor
College of Nursing
University of Illinois at Chicago
Chicago, Illinois

Henry J. Durivage, PharmD
Associate Director
Clinical Affairs
Theradex
Princeton, New Jersey

Jan M. Ellerhorst-Ryan, RN, MSN, CS
Nurse Clinician
Critical Care America
Cincinnati, Ohio

Ellen Heid Elpern, RN, MSN
Clinical Nurse Specialist
Section of Pulmonary Medicine
Assistant Professor of Nursing
Rush University
Rush-Presbyterian-St. Luke's Medical Center
Chicago, Illinois

Jayne I. Fernsler, RN, DSN
Associate Professor
College of Nursing
University of Delaware
Newark, Delaware

Betty R. Ferrell, RN, PhD, FAAN
Associate Research Scientist, Nursing Research
City of Hope National Medical Center
Duarte, California

Anne Marie Flaherty, RN, MS
Clinical Nurse III
Urgent Care Center
Memorial Sloan-Kettering Cancer Center
New York, New York

Arlene E. Fleck, RN, MNEd
Clinical Specialist Oncology Nursing
Hahnemann University Hospital
Philadelphia, Pennsylvania

Marilyn Frank-Stromborg, RN, EdD, NP, FAAN
Professor, Oncology Nursing
School of Nursing
Northern Illinois University
DeKalb, Illinois

Margaret Hansen Frogge, RN, MS
Executive Vice President, Administration
Coordinator, Community Cancer Program
Riverside Medical Center
Kankakee, Illinois

Sue L. Frymark, RN, BS
Manager, Cancer Rehabilitation
Comprehensive Cancer Program
Good Samaritan Hospital and Medical Center
Legacy Health Care System
Portland, Oregon

Barbara Holmes Gobel, RN, MS
Oncology Clinical Specialist
Lake Forest Hospital
Lake Forest, Illinois
Instructor (Complemental)
Rush University College of Nursing
Chicago, Illinois

Michelle Goodman, RN, MS, OCN
Oncology Clinical Nurse Specialist
Section of Medical Oncology
Rush Cancer Institute
Assistant Professor of Nursing
Rush University College of Nursing
Rush-Presbyterian-St. Luke's Medical Center
Chicago, Illinois

Marcia Grant, RN, DNSc, FAAN, OCN
Director of Nursing Research
City of Hope National Medical Center
Duarte, California

Betty Greig, RN, CETN
Enterostomal Therapist
University of Southern California
Kenneth Norris Jr. Cancer Hospital and Research Institute
Los Angeles, California

Susan L. Groenwald, RN, MS
Assistant Professor of Nursing, Complemental
Rush University College of Nursing
Rush-Presbyterian-St. Luke's Medical Center
Chicago, Illinois

Robin R. Gwin, RN, MN, OCN
Coordinator, Bone Marrow Transplant Program
Emory University Clinic
Atlanta, Georgia

Gloria Hagopian, RN, EdD
Associate Professor of Oncological Nursing
University of Pennsylvania School of Nursing
Clinician Educator
Department of Radiation Oncology
Hospital of the University of Pennsylvania
Philadelphia, Pennsylvania

Beverly Hampton, RN, MS, ET
Department of Nursing Staff Development
Division of Nursing
M.D. Anderson Cancer Hospital
Houston, Texas

Laura J. Hilderley, RN, MS
Oncology Clinical Nurse Specialist
Private Practice of Philip G. Maddock, MD
Radiation Oncology
Warwick, Rhode Island

Barbara Hoffman, JD
Private Consultant: Cancer Survivorship and Discrimination
Princeton, New Jersey

Patricia F. Jassak, RN, MS, CS, OCN
Oncology Clinical Nurse Specialist
Loyola University Medical Center
Maywood, Illinois

Judith (Judi) L. Bond Johnson, RN, PhD, FAAN
Nursing Director, Special Projects
North Memorial Medical Center
Minneapolis, Minnesota

Barbara Kalinowski, RN, MSN, OCN
Oncology Clinical Nurse Specialist
Faulkner Breast Centre
Boston, Massachusetts

Marsha Ketchum, RN, OCN
Clinical Research Nurse, Hematology and Oncology
Arizona Cancer Center
University of Arizona
Tucson, Arizona

Paula R. Klemm, RN, DNSc, OCN
Assistant Professor
University of Delaware
College of Nursing
Newark, Delaware

M. Tish Knobf, RN, MSN, FAAN
Assistant Professor
Yale University School of Nursing
Oncology Clinical Nurse Specialist
Yale-New Haven Hospital
New Haven, Connecticut

Kathy Kravitz, RN, MS
Oncology Nurse Specialist
North Colorado Medical Center
Greeley, Colorado

Linda U. Krebs, RN, MS, OCN
Oncology Nursing Program Leader
University of Colorado Cancer Center
Denver, Colorado

Lori A. Ladd, RN, MSN
Oncology Clinical Nurse Specialist
Department of Therapeutic Radiology
Rush Cancer Institute
Complemental Faculty
Rush University College of Nursing
Rush-Presbyterian-St. Luke's Medical Center
Chicago, Illinois

Luana Lamkin, RN, MPH, OCN
Executive Director
The Queen's Medical Center Cancer Institute
Honolulu, Hawaii

Jennifer M. Lang-Kummer RN, MN
Clinical Assistant Professor
School of Nursing
East Carolina University
Greenville, North Carolina

Susan Leigh, RN, BSN
Cancer Survivorship Consultant
Tucson, Arizona

Julena Lind, RN, MN, PhD cand.
Interim Chair
Department of Nursing
University of Southern California
Los Angeles, California

Ada M. Lindsey, RN, PhD
Dean and Professor
School of Nursing
University of California
Los Angeles, California

Lois J. Loescher, RN, MS
Director, Cancer Control Education Research
Cancer Prevention and Control
Arizona Cancer Center
University of Arizona
Tucson, Arizona

Jeanne Martinez, RN, MPH
Clinical Nurse Manager
Northwestern Memorial Hospice Program
Chicago, Illinois

Mary B. Maxwell, RN, CS, PhD
Oncology Clinical Nurse Specialist
Nurse Practitioner
Veterans' Administration Medical Center
Adjunct Assistant Professor of Nursing
Oregon Health Sciences University
Portland, Oregon

Deborah K. Mayer, RN, MSN, OCN
Assistant Professor
Graduate Program in Nursing
Massachusetts General Hospital Institute of Health Professions
Boston, Massachusetts

Mary Ellen McFadden, RN, MLA, OCN
Clinical Coordinator
The Johns Hopkins Oncology Center
Baltimore, Maryland

Rose F. McGee, RN, PhD
Professor
Nell Hodgson Woodruff School of Nursing
Emory University
Atlanta, Georgia

Deborah B. McGuire, RN, PhD, FAAN
Assistant Professor
The Johns Hopkins Univerity School of Nursing
Director of Nursing Research
The Johns Hopkins Oncology Center Department of Nursing
Baltimore, Maryland

Joan C. McNally, RN, MSN, OCN
Director, Health Care Services
Michigan Cancer Foundation
Detroit, Michigan

Mary Ann Miller, RN, PhD
Associate Professor
College of Nursing
University of Delaware
Newark, Delaware

Ida Marie (Ki) Moore, RN, DNSc
Assistant Professor
College of Nursing
University of Arizona
Tucson, Arizona

Theresa A. Moran, RN, MS
AIDS/Oncology Clinical Nursing Specialist
University of California, San Francisco/San Francisco General Hospital
Assistant Clinical Professor
Department of Physiological Nursing
University of California
San Francisco, California

Marion E. Morra, MA, ScD
Associate Director, Yale Comprehensive Cancer Center
Associate Clinical Professor, Yale University School of Nursing
Associate Research Scientist, Yale University School of Medicine
New Haven, Connecticut

Lillian M. Nail, RN, PhD
Associate Dean for Research/Associate Professor
University of Utah College of Nursing
Salt Lake City, Utah

Sharon Saldin O'Mary, RN, MN
Cancer Care Coordinator
Stevens Cancer Center
Scripps Memorial Hospital
LaJolla, California

Edith O'Neil-Page, RN, BS
Nursing Supervisor
Hoag Memorial Hospital Presbyterian
Newport, California

Diane M. Otte, RN, MS, ET
Administrative Director
St. Luke's Hospital Cancer Center
Davenport, Iowa

Geraldine V. Padilla, PhD
Associate Professor
Associate Dean for Research
School of Nursing
University of California
Los Angeles, California

Patricia A. Piasecki, RN, MS
Clinical Coordinator
Orthopaedic Oncology and Tissue Bank
Rush-Presbyterian-St. Luke's Medical Center and Regional Organ Bank of Illinois
Chicago, Illinois

Sandra Purl, RN, MS, OCN
Oncology Clinical Nurse Specialist
Section of Medical Oncology
Rush Cancer Institute
Complemental Faculty
Rush University College of Nursing
Rush-Presbyterian-St. Luke's Medical Center
Chicago, Illinois

Mary Reid, RN, MPH
Research Specialist
Department of Family and Community Medicine
University of Arizona
Tuscon, Arizona

Patricia E. Reymann, RN, MSN, OCN
Director, Gordon L. Ross Cancer Center
Princeton Baptist Medical Center
Birmingham, Alabama

Kathleen S. Ruccione, RN, MPH
Division of Hematology/Oncology
Children's Hospital of Los Angeles
Los Angeles, California

Vivian R. Sheidler, RN, MS
Clinical Nurse Specialist in Neuro-Oncology
The Johns Hopkins Oncology Center Department of Nursing
Baltimore, Maryland

Carol A. Sheridan, RN, MSN, OCN
Albert Einstein Cancer Center
Montefiore Medical Center
Bronx, New York

Annalynn Skipper, RD, MS, CNSD
Coordinator, Nutrition Consultation Service
Instructor, Department of Clinical Nutrition
Rush University College of Health Sciences
Rush-Presbyterian-St. Luke's Medical Center
Chicago, Illinois

Debra J. Szeluga, RD, PhD
Co-Director, Nutrition Consultation Service
Assistant Professor, Department of Clinical Nutrition
Rush University College of Health Sciences
Rush-Presbyterian-St. Luke's Medical Center
Chicago, Illinois

David C. Thomasma, PhD
The Fr. Michael I. English, S.J. Professor of Medical Ethics
Director, Medical Humanities Program
Loyola University of Chicago Medical Center
Maywood, Illinois

Steven Wagner, RN, BSN
Nurse Clinician
Northwestern Memorial Hospice Program
Chicago, Illinois

Janet Ruth Walczak, RN, MSN
Clinical Nurse Specialist
The Johns Hopkins Oncology Center
Clinical Associate
The Johns Hopkins University School of Nursing
Baltimore, Maryland

Jo Ann Wegmann, RN, PhD
Associate Professor
Graduate Coordinator
Statewide Nursing Program
California State University
Dominques Hills
Carsen, California

Maryl L. Winningham, RN, PhD, FACSM
Assistant Professor
University of Utah College of Nursing
Salt Lake City, Utah

Debra Wujcik, RN, MSN, OCN
Clinical Nurse Specialist
Oncology/Bone Marrow Transplant
Vanderbilt University Hospital
Adjunct Instructor of Nursing
Vanderbilt University School of Nursing
Nashville, Tennessee

Connie Henke Yarbro, RN, BSN
Director, Nursing Resource Development
The Regional Cancer Center
Memorial Medical Center
Springfield, Illinois
Editor, *Seminars in Oncology Nursing*

John W. Yarbro, MD, PhD
Director, The Regional Cancer Center
Memorial Medical Center
Springfield, Illinois

Foreword

The pace of new knowledge continues to require that editors of major textbooks provide fresh, pertinent material to serve their reading audience. In the short span of six years, we have seen three editions of *Cancer Nursing: Principles and Practice*. This publishing feat has provided nurses, for the first time, with access, in a convenient package, to the most modern information on the entire range of problems that anyone in the cancer field must face these days.

Since the last edition, there have been relevant changes that have an impact on cancer nursing. Prevention has become more of a reality and touches nurses in the form of participation in prevention clinical trials, many of which involve normal, healthy people at some special risk. The major limitations of cancer diagnosis and treatment, which have been apparent for decades, such as the inability to detect minimal residual disease to guide intensifying treatment, have come under a more focused attack, thanks to the availability of new molecular probes and tests like the polymerase and ligase chain reactions, to detect minimal amounts of tumor. Intensification of treatment has become an everyday phenomenon due to the availability of biologicals to support these approaches, and a new approach, gene therapy, has entered the clinics, just to mention a few. In short, life in the cancer clinic has become more complicated, but in a scientifically gratifying way.

The promise of all the investment in cancer research appears to be paying off for the patient, or is it? While all these advances are intellectually very satisfying, it will come as no surprise to readers of this text that there appears to be an interminable slowness in the march of these advances to the bedside. Patients are having a difficult time in accessing these new approaches, and medical professionals have an increasingly high level of frustration in piecing together these "promising" packages. Nurses bear the brunt of this frustration because they are on the firing line and often have to mediate between the patient, the doctor, and "the system." I'm referring, of course, to our system of medical care that has become a roadblock to cancer care never anticipated by the framers of the National Cancer Act. Now, at a time of a healthy national debate on the future shape of our health care system, it seems appropriate to warn our collective communities that if we are not careful, the rate-limiting step in the drive to reduce cancer incidence, morbidity, and mortality will become the totally nonscientific trappings of the delivery of medical care. Changes must take the special needs of cancer patients into consideration because cancer care, unlike many other areas of medicine, is still perched between, as Lewis Thomas called it, "halfway technology and the refined technology it promises to be." Parts VII and VIII of this text touch on many of these issues as they relate to nursing. Who can deliver the newest cancer treatment, and also, who pays for it, changes more frequently than in most other fields, and as such the economics of medicine now accounts for a good deal of the slowness in the transfer of technology.

The following needs to be said, and it is appropriate to say it here because nurses have an increasing voice in such matters. As I pointed out in the Foreword to the second edition, the framers of the Cancer Act knew there would be many nonscientific obstacles to the war on cancer, and not only anticipated many of them but also provided protection for them in the Cancer Act, such as a line item budget for prevention and control, which they correctly felt would be most vulnerable to attack. Their concern, however, was primarily at the interface between academia and the research enterprise represented by the NIH. I don't believe that even those wise people could have anticipated the obstacles presented by our current health care system.

So, this text appears at a critical time in the national debate over changes in the health care system toward the direction of more HMOs and managed competition. These changes do not always take into consideration the needs of cancer patients for access to special programs and universal coverage, which would be good for all patients. Thus, the changes that are coming will have impact on the care of cancer patients in different ways, some good, some bad. How the cancer patient is treated in these changed systems will depend in large part on the breadth of understanding of professionals, such as doctors and nurses, who can gain an appreciation of the pace of the changing technology in the cancer field from the contents of this book, and how they communicate this appreciation to policymakers.

Vincent T. DeVita, Jr., MD
Attending Physician and Member
Program of Molecular Pharmacology
and Therapeutics
Memorial Sloan-Kettering Cancer Center
New York, New York

Preface to the Third Edition

By its third edition, a textbook will have established its purpose and focus. Ours is no exception. Everything stated in the two prefaces to the prior editions remains true today.

We are grateful for the opportunity and challenge provided by our enthusiastic readership to provide the most comprehensive and up-to-date information possible to the ever-developing nurses who are our readership, in a field that is not standing still. It is a formidable challenge, but one that we, as editors, and the authors who write the content have taken seriously and have met with vigor. We believe that the product accomplishes and maintains the goals and standards set forth in the first edition.

The exponential increase in knowledge about the biology of cancer and the challenges imposed on the individuals who must apply that knowledge to clinical practice caused us to review thoroughly the second edition to determine what changes needed to be made in the third edition to meet the needs of nurses who are in constantly expanding roles within this complex clinical arena. Our review of the second edition and suggestions from our readers caused us to make substantive changes in this third edition that we believe enhance its usability and value.

Part I: The Cancer Problem has been reordered and the content expanded to be more interesting and relevant to clinical practice. Chapter 1 has new content on cancer control, and Dr. John Yarbro's engaging and interesting Chapter 2, "Milestones in Our Understanding of the Causes of Cancer," chronicles the research findings that have contributed to our current understanding of the biology of cancer. Chapters 3–5 build on Chapter 2 by presenting current knowledge of the biology of cancer and its application to clinical practice.

Part III: Treatment has been enhanced by several changes and additions in content. Dr. David Cella's chapter, "Quality of Life as an Outcome of Cancer Treatment," assists us to establish quality of life of the individual with cancer as an important consideration in cancer treatment rather than just the clinical efficacy of treatment regimens. In addition, the important topic of chemotherapy has been expanded and divided into three chapters: "Principles of Therapy," "Principles of Administration," and "Toxicity Management." All three chapters have authors new to this text—Tish Knobf, Patricia Reymann, and Dawn Camp-Sorrell—who are well known for their expertise in this area. These changes make this the most comprehensive information available on the topic of chemotherapy in any general oncology nursing text.

In *Part VI: The Care of Individuals with Cancer,* content about soft tissue sarcomas was added to the chapter on bone cancer.

The topic of cancer program development, written by Luana Lamkin, was added to *Part VII: Delivery Systems for Cancer Care.* This content was added at the suggestion of some of our readers, as nurses increasingly find themselves called upon to develop cancer programs but feel unprepared for this task because of a lack of nursing education and a lack of resources on the subject. Luana Lamkin has done an excellent job in presenting practical and comprehensive information on the subject.

In *Part VIII: Professional Issues for the Cancer Nurse,* a chapter was added called "Thriving as an Oncology Nurse," written by Mary Cunningham, to address the challenging yet rewarding job of an oncology nurse, the stressors imposed, and suggestions for dealing with those stressors.

A new feature of this edition is the appearance of patient teaching guides where appropriate. The guides are printed in such a way that they can be photocopied and used in clinical practice.

Each chapter that is carried forward from the second edition has been thoroughly reviewed and updated. Many authors are new and bring a fresh perspective to the chapter content.

As in any project of this scope, there are many to thank for its execution. We are especially thankful to our families on whose time most of our work was done. We are appreciative of our employers and colleagues who value our participation in this ongoing project and provide resources and support for its development. We appreciate the staff at Jones and Bartlett who contribute to the success of this text, and the timely and difficult work done by Michael Bass & Associates to get the book produced.

Finally, it is to the cancer nurses who are our readership and the cancer patients for whom they care that this book is dedicated. We hope that this text meets your complex and ever-expanding learning needs.

SUSAN L. GROENWALD
MARGARET HANSEN FROGGE
MICHELLE GOODMAN
CONNIE HENKE YARBRO

Preface to the Second Edition

Our goal in the second edition of *Cancer Nursing: Principles and Practice* is to provide the reader with the most comprehensive information about cancer nursing available in the 1990s. Each of the original 44 chapters in the first edition was thoroughly reviewed and updated. Twenty-five new content areas were added, including Relation of the Immune System to Cancer, Cancer Risk and Assessment, Biotherapy, Bone Marrow Transplantation, AIDS-Related Malignancies, Late Effects of Cancer Treatment, Psychosocial Dimensions: Issues in Survivorship, Sexual and Reproductive Dysfunction, Oncologic Emergencies, Delivery Systems of Cancer Care, Economics of Cancer, Teaching Strategies: The Public, and Teaching Strategies: The Patient. This edition contains 60 comprehensive chapters representing the contributions of over 75 recognized oncology nursing experts.

The exponential increase in information about oncogenes resulting from a massive research effort has provided a greater understanding of the nature of carcinogenesis. This improved understanding is reflected in this second edition and will continue to have a significant impact on the nature of clinical care. Even with this research effort and greater understanding of the nature of carcinogenesis, however, it is unlikely that a magic cure or vaccine for cancer will be available in the near future. There will continue to emerge new approaches to early diagnosis of cancer, new techniques to treat cancer, new measures to ameliorate distressing manifestations of cancer and its treatment, and new approaches to improve the quality of life for cancer survivors. Cancer nurses are integral to these developments. It is to these nurses that this text is dedicated.

The editors wish to gratefully acknowledge the tremendous effort of the contributors who enthusiastically shared their knowledge and expertise and gave their time and energy to this endeavor. We wish to especially acknowledge our husbands Keith, Jim, Larry, and John for their assistance, support, and patience during this mammouth project.

The editors have developed this text to be a comprehensive resource for nurses who provide or manage care for patients in the home, hospital, or community, who teach patients and nurses, and who conduct research to find better approaches to patient care—all of whom contribute to our steady gains in providing quality care to individuals with cancer.

Susan L. Groenwald
Margaret Hansen Frogge
Michelle Goodman
Connie Henke Yarbro

Preface to the First Edition

This text is one I always wished to have. As a graduate student of oncology nursing, and later as an oncology clinical nurse specialist and educator at Rush-Presbyterian St. Luke's Medical Center. I became frustrated by the dearth of texts written at the level of the oncology graduate student or oncology nurse specialist. Oncology nursing texts lack the depth and breadth of scientific information that I believe is an essential element in the armamentarium of the professional nurse; medical literature, while it contains the necessary scientific information, lacks application of scientific principles to the nursing care arena.

In this text, the contributors and I committed ourselves to presenting the reader with the most comprehensive information about oncology nursing available, including relevant science and clinical practice content that addresses both the whys and hows of oncology nursing practice. All chapters cite original published research as the scientific foundation for the application of these findings to clinical practice. All students of oncology nursing—beginning or advanced—will find this book valuable as a text and as a reference for clinical practice.

The disease of cancer in the adult is approached from many angles to address the complex learning needs of the oncology nurse specialist. Part I includes cancer epidemiology and deals with individual and societal attitudes toward cancer and the impact of attitudes on health behaviors. Part II provides the foundation of scientific information about the malignant cell on which all subsequent chapters are built. Concepts such as carcinogenesis, oncogenesis, metastasis, invasion, and contact inhibition are included in Part II, and thorough attention is given to changes that occur in a normal cell and its behavior as it transforms to a malignant cell.

In Part III, the psychosocial dimensions of cancer are approached according to critical phases through which patients, families, and caregivers may pass as they cope with the stressors induced by cancer. Part IV presents a conceptual approach to the most common manifestations of cancer and their effects on the individual with cancer. Each chapter includes pathophysiology, assessment, and medical and nursing therapies. Part V describes each of the major cancer treatment methods, their uses, adverse effects, and nursing care considerations for individuals receiving cancer therapy. Included in this part is a chapter on unproven methods of treatment. Part VI is a comprehensive review of most of the major cancers by body system and the problems experienced by people who live with cancer. (Information pertaining to pediatric malignancies and nursing care of the child with cancer has been omitted. Although pediatric oncology is a critical area of interest for many nurses, it could not be covered in sufficient depth within this text.) Part VII presents continuing-care options for the individual living with the problems imposed by cancer. Part VIII analyzes several issues relevant to the oncology nurse: consumerism, ethics, cancer nursing education, and cancer nursing research. Part IX, which lists oncology resources of many types, is a handy reference tool.

Some of the information presented in this text is out of date even as it is written because of ever-expanding knowledge about cancer and its treatment. As Dr. Vincent DeVita remarked at his swearing-in as Director of the National Cancer Institute (*The Cancer Letter,* 1980:4), "What we now know of the cancerous process and what we do to prevent, diagnose, and treat it will be outmoded and radically different by the end of the 80s." This book is our best effort to put down in writing the science and art of cancer nursing in the 1980s.

Susan L. Groenwald

Contents

PART I

The Cancer Problem

Chapter 1

Cancer Control and Epidemiology

Brenda Cartmel, PhD

Mary Reid, RN, MPH

INTRODUCTION

Epidemiology is "the study of the distribution and determinants of disease frequency."[1] Cancer epidemiology examines the frequency of cancer in populations, the role of certain risk factors that contribute to cancer rates, and the interrelationships or associations that exist between the host, the environment, and the other conditions that may contribute to the development or inhibition of cancer.

The first section of this chapter will review basic epidemiologic concepts. These will help the reader to understand current clinical research better; to identify groups at higher risk for cancer development; to review current medical literature; and to develop relevant research hypotheses related to the field of cancer epidemiology. This information should serve as a basis for understanding the major issues involved in cancer research design, assessment, and estimation of cancer risks. A brief glossary of fundamental terms used in the field of epidemiology is given in Table 1-1. These definitions will be helpful in understanding discussions found later

TABLE 1-1 Glossary of Epidemiologic Terms

Association	*Statistical association* refers to the strength of the relationship between two variables. In epidemiologic terms, association imitates the degree to which the rate of disease in persons with a specific exposure is either higher or lower than the rate of disease in persons without the exposure. The strength of this dependence is greater than what would be expected by chance.
	Causal association is a biologic association, between the occurrence of an exposure and presence of a disease. The available evidence indicates that the presence of the exposure increases the probability of the presence of the disease. Changes in the frequency or quality of an exposure or characteristic would result in a corresponding change in the frequency of the disease or outcome of interest.
Bias	*Selection bias* results from a systematic difference in the manner by which the case and the comparison groups are selected for participation in the study. This bias may produce spurious associations due to the differential inclusion or exclusion of subjects from the disease or exposure groups.
	Misclassification bias is a systematic error that occurs when the measurement of either the exposure (risk factor) or the disease condition is systematically different for the groups being compared (eg, the disease outcome between the exposed and unexposed groups were evaluated by separate physicians using different criteria).
Confounding	The systematic overestimation or underestimation of the effect of an exposure because the influence of a disease risk factor has not been taken into account. A *confounding variable* is a risk factor for the disease being studied that has a chance association with the exposure of interest (eg, smoking status, age, gender).
Epidemiology	A field in medical science concerned with the study of the frequency and distribution of disease in the population, and which also explores the relationship between exposures and development of diseases.
Incidence	The number of *new* events or cases of disease that occur in a defined population at risk within a specified period of time. Incidence rates can be used to evaluate the changing patterns of disease frequency within a population and to assess the effectiveness of screening programs and treatment modalities on disease development.
Population	The number of persons in a defined group who are capable of developing the disease. Can also refer to the general population; a population specifically defined by geographic, physical or social characteristics, or risk; the sampling population; and the study population.
Power	The probability that a study will have the statistical strength to detect relationships that exist between exposures and disease. The power of a study can be maximized by controlling factors such as sample sizes, measurement error, and bias.
Prevalence	The number of *new and existing* cases of a given disease or condition in a defined population within a specified period of time. *Point prevalence* refers to prevalence at one point in time. *Period prevalence* refers to prevalence between two points in time. Prevalence rates can be used to compare disease frequencies across populations and to assess the magnitude of effect of certain diseases on the health status of a population.
Rates and ratios	These calculations are used to compare the frequencies of diseases in a population. Commonly used rates and ratios are given in Table 1-2, which lists the rate names, the numerator and denominator values, and the population factor used to express the rate in a standard format.
Risk measures	*Attributable risk* is the arithmetic or absolute difference between the exposed group and the nonexposed group in the incidence rates or the death rates. It estimates the number of disease cases that can be attributed to or explained by the exposure (eg, the majority of lung cancer cases can be attributed to exposure to cigarette smoking).

TABLE 1-1 Glossary of Epidemiologic Terms (continued)

Term	Definition
Risk measures (continued)	The remaining risk measures, the relative risk and the odds ratio, are calculated using a standard 2 × 2 table that separates the exposed and nonexposed groups by disease status (see Table 1-3). *Relative risk (RR)* is a ratio comparing the rates of a disease among the exposed group and the nonexposed group that serves as a measure of the association between the disease and the exposure. The RR is generally used in cohort studies. The formula for calculating it is: $\frac{a/(a + b)}{c/(c + d)}$ *Odds ratio (OR)* approximates the relative risk by comparing the rates of disease among the exposed and nonexposed groups. The OR is generally used in case-control studies with smaller sample sizes. The formula for calculating it is: $\frac{ad}{cb}$ Both the RR and the OR are expressed as ratios (eg, an OR of 1.0 means the rate of disease among the exposed group equals that of the nonexposed group).
Sensitivity	Measures the probability that a screening test will correctly classify an individual as *positive* for a disease when they actually do have the disease.
Specificity	Measures the probability that a screening test will correctly classify an individual as *negative* for a disease when they actually do not have the disease.
Validity	*Internal validity* is the extent to which the subjects in an epidemiologic study are truly comparable with respect to general characteristics (eg, if most of the cases are from an urban setting and the controls are mainly from a rural setting, the two groups are not comparable; evaluation of the exposure–disease relationship may be affected by these differences). Internal validity is essential for the interpretability and reliability of a study. *External validity,* or generalizability, is the extent to which the study population can be compared to a larger population (eg, the general population). External validity must be assessed before study results can be applied to a broader population (eg, a study that uses as its population a specific profession, such as nurses, may yield results that are not relevant to all women in that general population; while the study may have strong internal validity, the participating nurses may not be representative of the women in the general population or in the nursing profession).

in the chapter on research study considerations and cancer risk factors. Table 1-2 provides the rates and ratios commonly used in epidemiology, and Table 1-3 shows the 2 × 2 table used in calculating relative risks and odds ratio.

Subsequent sections of this chapter will discuss causes of cancer and host characteristics that influence cancer susceptibility, cancer control and related issues, and, finally, the application of epidemiologic principles and cancer prevention and control issues in nursing practice.

BASIC CONSIDERATIONS IN EPIDEMIOLOGIC RESEARCH

Five primary components are considered in evaluating the design of an epidemiologic research project:

- study design
- definition of the population of patients or subjects to be used in the study
- eligibility criteria used to select study participants
- definitions of the disease and exposures related to the research hypothesis
- statistical plan measuring the association between the exposure and the disease
- identification of potential sources of bias and confounding

While it is important that these issues be resolved before a protocol is initiated, it is equally important that the entire research team understand these issues and that there be constant evaluation during the course of data collection.

Study Designs

Several standard study designs are used in epidemiologic research. Although the general features of all of these designs will be covered, the primary emphasis of this section is on those designs most commonly used in clinical cancer research: the case-control and clinical

TABLE 1-2 Rates and Ratios Commonly Used in Epidemiology

Rate Name	Rate Description	Population Factor
Crude birth rate	Number of live births / Average or midyear population	per 1000
Fertility rate	Number of live births / 15–44-year-old women at midyear	per 1000
Crude mortality rate	Total number of deaths / Total population at midyear	per 1000
Age-specific mortality rate	Deaths in specific age group / Midyear population in age group	per 100,000
Cause-specific mortality rate	Deaths from a specific cause / Total midyear population	per 100,000
Infant mortality rate	Deaths of children less than 1 year of age / Number of live births	per 1000
Neonatal mortality rate	Deaths in infants younger than 28 days / Number of live births	per 1000
Case fatality rate	Number of deaths from a disease in a given period of follow-up / Number of diagnosed cases of disease at start of follow-up period	per 1000
Proportional mortality rate	Number of deaths from a given cause / Number of deaths from all causes	per 1000
Morbidity rate	Number of cases of the disease that develop in a given period / Total population at midperiod	per 100,000

trial study designs. The major study designs are experimental, ecologic, cross-sectional, case-control, cohort, and clinical trials studies.

In selecting the appropriate study design, certain factors must be considered. These include the frequency of the disease or condition in the general population and the defined population to be studied, the length of time the disease takes to develop, and the anticipated size of the study sample. The size of the study sample is often affected by the monies available to complete the project, the time allowed for subject recruitment, the diagnostic characteristics of the disease, and the qualities of the exposure that is being tested.

TABLE 1-3 2 × 2 Table Used in Calculating Relative Risks (RR) and Odds Ratios (OR)

	Diseased	Not Diseased
Exposed	a	b
Nonexposed	c	d

Experimental studies

An experimental study design tests a research hypothesis. It attempts to control the variability of all factors except for the exposure of interest. These studies typically use animal models in laboratory settings, and are conducted when a research hypothesis is being developed. They generally determine the biological plausibility of the hypothesis. Once substantial, consistent evidence has accumulated from experimental studies, other study designs may be employed to further investigate the hypothesis in free-living human populations.

Ecologic studies

The next step in investigating a hypothesis may be conducting ecologic or correlational studies. In this design, trends are examined in disease distribution among humans across ecologic or geographic areas. Each geographic area may represent differences in exposures. For example, cancer rates are often evaluated across different countries, or regions of a country, to investigate the effects of nutrient or natural environmental exposures, such as soil selenium or radon, on disease rates.

Cross-sectional studies

The cross-sectional study is another design that allows an investigator to assess the rates of disease and exposure in a population. In this study design a one-time view of a population is taken, and the rates of existing (prevalent) cases of the disease, the degree of exposure, and other demographic characteristics of interest are measured. While cross-sectional studies cannot establish a causal relationship between the exposure and the disease, they do provide descriptive statistics for the population, that is, the prevalence rates for the disease in that population, and are often used as the preliminary step in planning cohort studies.

Case-control studies

The case-control study design should be considered if at least one of the following criteria is met:

- The disease is rare in the general or source population (such as most forms of cancer).
- The investigation is preliminary.
- Time and funding limitations prohibit the use of other, larger, more expensive study designs.

The information gained from case-control studies does not establish a causal relationship between the disease and the exposure, but it does explore the concurrent association between the two. If the strength of this association is significant and is supported by other studies, this information can be used to justify the use of larger cohort studies or clinical trials that can establish causative relationships.

Subjects in case-control studies are recruited on the basis of disease status. Cases of the disease in question, either preexisting or newly developed, are compared to noncases, or control subjects, on the basis of the exposure being investigated. *Control subjects* are defined as persons who do not have the disease at present but who, if the disease did develop, would have the same opportunity to be diagnosed as the case subjects. The selection of an appropriate control group is the major challenge of case-control studies and is often the source of selection bias introduced into the study.[2]

An example of the use of the case-control study design is a study examining the association between malignant melanoma and the use of sunbeds and sunlamps.[3] The case group consisted of 583 individuals diagnosed with melanoma; the control group was comprised of 608 subjects who did not have melanoma. The control subjects were randomly selected from property tax rolls. Each group was evaluated for the exposure, which in this case was the use of sunbeds or sunlamps. The calculated odds ratio, comparing the rate of exposure among the diseased group to that among the nondiseased, found that the exposed subjects, i.e., those who reported using sunbeds or sunlamps, had a 1.45–1.88-fold increase in the risk of developing melanoma. This difference was seen in both the male and the female subjects.

Demographic differences between cases and controls are minimized. To make the two groups comparable, some investigators have used a technique called *matching,* in which certain demographic characteristics of the cases are matched to those of the controls. For example, if a case subject is female, 45 years old, white, and from a low-income household, a control subject would be selected with basically the same characteristics. The advantage of matching, and analyzing the data in pairs of subjects, is that fewer subjects are required in each group to see a relationship between the exposure and the disease, if such a relationship exists. This is useful in situations where there are small numbers of cases of the disease available for study and efficiency is a major issue. Matching is also a means for controlling potential confounding introduced by the selection of the control group. The major disadvantage of matching is that any variable used in matching cannot be studied in relation to the disease. If little is actually known about the relationship between disease and exposure, the investigator may not want to limit the opportunities to study all possible variables. The melanoma study[3] used matching to control the potential confounding variables of age, sex, and residence municipality. The resulting groups contained similar proportions of each variable.

A commonly used alternative to matching is the recruitment of more than one control subject per case subject. For example, two to four control subjects may be recruited for each case subject. This technique affords an increase in statistical power without limiting the variables that can be investigated. In this scenario, the baseline characteristics of both groups would be assessed for comparability. Ideally, the age ranges, racial differences, socioeconomic status (SES), and other known potential confounding variables should not be significantly different between the groups. The association seen between an exposure and the disease can be clouded by extraneous variables that are poorly distributed between the case and control groups.

Another classic example of the case-control design is a study of endometrial cancer and the use of postmenopausal estrogens[4]. In this study, women with endometrial cancer comprised the case group, while women with other gynecologic ailments from the same hospital were recruited into the control group. Matching was not implemented. The increase in risk of cancer related to exposure to the postmenopausal estrogens was dramatic (OR = 11.28). Critics of the study stated that the two subject groups did not have comparable SES and that selection bias explained the elevated risk. The study was redesigned and a new control group recruited. The resulting odds ratios, after an attempt to control the selection bias, still showed that estrogens significantly increased a woman's risk of developing endometrial cancer (OR = 2.30–2.69).

Cohort studies

Once an association between a disease and an exposure has been established, a cohort study may be initiated to test the research hypothesis. The cohort, or group of subjects, that is included in this type of study design represents individuals that do not have the disease of interest. An initial cross-sectional study or assessment of a population can identify and eliminate all active cases of the disease. Once the cohort is selected, the exposures of interest are assessed and the subjects monitored for a designated period of time to record development of the disease.

Cohort studies can be retrospective, prospective, or ambidirectional. *Retrospective* studies use a previously defined cohort, and, through the review of records, individuals that developed the disease are identified and the level of the exposure is assessed. While retrospective studies are often less time-consuming and less expensive than the other cohort designs, the quality of the information collected on the disease and exposure is constrained by the quality of the records available. Many occupational cohort studies are conducted retrospectively.

In *prospective* studies, a current population of disease-free individuals is selected and the exposure(s) measured. This study population is then followed into the future and evaluated for development of the disease. The rate of new cases is compared between levels of exposure to establish the disease–exposure relationship. While prospective studies often require several years of subject follow-up and are generally expensive to complete, they offer the opportunity to establish definitively a causative relationship between the exposure and the disease. In addition, the effect of multiple risk factors on disease development may be investigated.

The Framingham Heart Study[5] is one of the best-known examples of this type of cohort design. The residents of Framingham, Mass., were selected for this prospective study, which examined the risk factors for cardiovascular disease. All eligible subjects were examined extensively for presence of heart disease, and potential risk factors were evaluated, such as family history, nutrition, exercise, smoking status, and alcohol consumption. Monitoring of these subjects for the development of heart disease and/or a cardiovascular-related event has continued to date and now includes a cohort of offspring of the original participants. Significant information on the multiple risk factors and treatment modalities of heart disease have been produced by this study.

The last type of cohort study is the *ambidirectional* cohort study, which starts with a previously established cohort and continues subject follow-up into the future. This design carries the same advantages and disadvantages as the retrospective and prospective designs combined.

The study of the Vietnam veteran's postservice mortality is an example of the ambidirectional cohort design.[6] A cohort of Vietnam veterans was identified retrospectively from service records. The subjects were then followed prospectively through 1983 to determine the vital status and causes of deaths of the cohort. These rates were compared to mortality rates of the veterans from World War II and the Korean War. While the death rates for Vietnam veterans were slightly elevated in the first five years following the end of active service, the overall death rates were not significantly different.

Clinical trials and intervention studies

The final study design to be discussed here is the clinical trial or intervention study. This design tests the effect of an intervention on the rates of disease development. Two groups of subjects are created within the study population, a treatment group (receiving the treatment) and a control group (receiving the placebo or the current therapy). For example, to test the effect of a drug or nutritional supplement on the rates of cancer development, subjects are randomly assigned to one of the two groups and monitored over the time period of the study for the development or recurrence of the cancer. The design is called *double-blind* when the assignment of the treatment group is kept from the subject and the immediate clinical personnel. This controls the potential biasing effects on subject participation, disease diagnosis, and monitoring that can occur when participants and/or clinical staff know the group assignments.

A major benefit of a double-blind, placebo controlled clinical trial is that the random assignment of treatment groups helps to distribute potential confounding variables evenly between the two groups, thus minimizing their effects on the measurement of the association between the exposure and the disease. If this control of confounding is successful and the primary difference between the two treatment groups is the intervention, then a clinical trial can definitively evaluate the efficacy of the intervention.

A current example of a clinical trial is the Physicians' Health Study,[7] which has randomized 22,071 licensed physicians into an expanded design to test the effectiveness of aspirin on decreasing the rates of heart attacks and the effect of beta-carotene on inhibiting the development of cancer. After five years, the aspirin arm of the trial was stopped because a significantly lower risk of heart attack was observed among the subjects receiving aspirin. The beta-carotene arm of the trial is still continuing.

A major limitation of the clinical trial design is that several years of subject follow-up may be required before significant changes in the rate of disease development are observed among treatment groups. The length of follow-up will depend on several factors, one of which is the strength of the effect the treatment has on the risk of the disease. Long-term studies raise patient management issues, such as keeping subjects actively participating, monitoring subject deaths, and tracking subjects who move from the study area. These factors, if unevenly distributed among the treatment groups, may confound the results of the project.

Defining the Population

In addition to defining the type of study design appropriate for testing a research hypothesis, it is also important to define the source population for study subjects and the actual study population. This clarifies to whom the research results can be generalized (external validity), whether the study population represents the general population and source population, and the overall characteristics of eligible subjects.

The *source population* for the study is the larger group or population from which the study subjects are recruited. This could include, for instance, residents in a certain city or neighborhood, university students, or all subjects attending a particular hospital. The source population is usually a subgroup of the general population.

The study population is the group of subjects actually recruited into the project from the source population. Recruitment into the study population, based on the defined eligibility criteria, is planned to access all potential subjects within the source population. In reviewing sources of bias that may have been introduced into the study, it is important to review the type of subjects who were part of the source population but were not eligible or not approached for recruitment. For example, if subjects were recruited from phone interviews, one could conclude that only subjects with telephones were eligible. Since the presence of a telephone in the household could be related to socioeconomic status, the study population could be biased toward recruiting subjects with a higher SES. Because of this selection bias, and the recruitment of a homogeneous group of subjects with respect to SES, the relationship of SES to the disease may be impossible to evaluate and may affect the results of the study.

Eligibility criteria

The selection of the study population is based on established eligibility criteria. These are designed to create a population of subjects with a sufficient prevalence of the disease to test the hypothesis efficiently, and for whom the intervention is considered safe. Examples of commonly used eligibility criteria in cancer research are age, race, gender, disease stage, life expectancy, absence of other cancers or chronic diseases, exposure to certain drugs or treatments, and current health status.

Defining the disease and the exposure

The disease should be defined as specifically as possible, including pathologic criteria, specific blood chemistries, histologic characteristics, specific test results, and physical symptoms according to current medical practice. Clear disease definition helps to control potential misclassification bias. Even with a definition, disease status may need to be confirmed by an external reviewer, further controlling bias.

Equally as important as defining the disease, is clarifying the definition of the exposure used in the study. An *exposure* is considered as a contact that a subject has had with the variable of interest that may influence the development of or improvement in disease status. Exposures can include a broad range of variables, from environmental conditions, medications, nutrients, genetic influences, and health care accessibility to types of exercise. The characteristics of the exposure that are most important to clarify are the *dose* of the exposure, the *duration,* or length of time, of the exposure, and *characteristics* that are specific to the exposure, such as latency effects and effects synergistic with other exposures.

Dose refers to a standardized, measured amount of exposure issued, e.g., standard milligrams (as in the case of drugs), GRAY (GY) for radiation, number of packs of cigarettes per year, drinks of alcohol per day, etc. It is important to assess whether the dose is constant throughout the exposure, or if certain variables, or conditions, have affected the dose over time.

Statistical Plan

In addition to calculating the rates and ratios of a disease as it develops in a population, epidemiological research affords the investigator the ability to examine the relationships of the disease to defined exposures. A major goal of epidemiologic research is to make inferences to the larger population based on information obtained from the study population.[2] The validity of these inferences relies on the assumption that the study population is a representative sample of the larger group.

While risk estimates are useful, other statistical tests afford the opportunity to examine more closely the disease–exposure association. A t-test will evaluate whether the means or averages between two groups are significantly different. The chi-square test will evaluate the differences between the proportions observed and expected between groups.

Potential Sources of Bias and Confounding

The potential sources of bias and confounding in a study are examined to determine if the differences seen between the two groups can be explained by influences other than the research hypothesis. If both of these issues have been well controlled in the study design, and the role of chance is sufficiently small, then the possibility that the hypothesis is correct increases.

Data Sources

There are several data sources and systems in the United States relating to cancer and risk factors for cancer that can be accessed by investigators (Table 1-4). These sources are frequently useful to gain preliminary data to formulate or support a hypothesis, as well as to provide a means of examining national, regional, or temporal differences in cancer or risk factors for cancer.

ENVIRONMENTAL FACTORS ASSOCIATED WITH CANCER CAUSATION

How Do We Decide What Causes Cancer?

It is important to recognize that inference regarding causality cannot be made from a single study. Information from many sources must be drawn on to infer causality. The criteria to be considered are:

- the magnitude of association between the exposure and the disease
- consistency of findings from all studies
- biological credibility
- temporal association between the risk factor and the disease

Tobacco

Tobacco use is still the most important known cause of cancer in the United States. Tobacco causes about 30% of cancer deaths, and cigarette smoking causes 90% of lung cancers.[8]

Active tobacco use has been linked to many cancer types: lung, oropharyngeal, bladder, pancreatic, cervical, and kidney,[9,10] and a clear linear relationship exists

TABLE 1-4 Data Sources for Epidemiologic Research

Source	Description
National Health Interview Survey (NHIS)	Annual survey started in 1957. Household interviews are conducted in approximately 50,000 households representative of the civilian noninstitutionalized population. Provides data on the incidence of illness and accidental injuries, prevalence of chronic diseases and impairments, disability, physician visits, hospitalizations, and other health topics, and on the relationship between demographic and socioeconomic characteristics and health characteristics. The questionnaires change with time to focus on current health topics.
National Health and Nutrition Examination Survey (NHANES)	NHANES III was begun in 1988. Ultimately, 45,000 persons representative of the U.S. population will be selected to participate. Persons undergo physical examinations and clinical and laboratory testing. Eg, data are collected on blood pressure, serum cholesterol, and body measurements. Dietary assessment is also conducted as part of the survey.
Behavioral Risk Factor Surveillance System	Started in 1984, this system is coordinated by the Centers for Disease Control and Prevention (CDC), but the telephone interviews used as the survey methodology are conducted by the participating states—currently, 45 states and the District of Columbia. The survey's purpose is to collect information regarding the prevalence of self-reported health behaviors that relate to the ten leading causes of death, including: cigarette smoking, hypertension, obesity, seat belt use, physical inactivity, and alcohol use. Several of these behaviors are risk factors for cancer. This system provides a means of assessing change in these behaviors over time or in response to an intervention.
National Vital Statistics System	This system provides data on births, deaths, marriages, and divorces. Annual data are produced for the United States, the individual states, counties, and other local areas. Cause of death is included in this system, eg, breast cancer mortality rates can be compared for differing counties within a state, or over time within a specific location.
Surveillance, Epidemiology, and End Results (SEER) Program	This is the principal source of cancer incidence and survival data for the United States. The participating areas are Seattle (Puget Sound), Utah, San Francisco, New Mexico, Hawaii, Iowa, Detroit, Connecticut, and Atlanta (including ten rural counties), which include approximately 9.6% of the U.S. population. For each newly diagnosed cancer case, data collected include: selected patient demographics, primary site, morphology, diagnostic confirmation, extent of disease, and first course of cancer-directed therapy. Active follow-up of all living patients is conducted to help ascertain survival time.
National Death Index	This system aids investigators in ascertaining mortality. A computerized database contains identifying information on all deaths reported by the state vital statistics offices. An investigator can determine if a study subject has died and, if relevant, on where and how to obtain a copy of the death certificate.
Decennial census	The goal of the 10-yearly census conducted in the United States is to count each person according to "usual place of residence." A limited amount of information is requested from each person; a sample of persons is then asked to complete a more detailed questionnaire. Detailed population numbers by age, sex, and ethnicity are important to the epidemiologist, since they are used in the denominator of calculations of population rates. The demographic data from the census can be used to give a population profile of areas of research interest.

between the number of cigarettes smoked and the risk of lung and oropharyngeal cancers.

There is a gradual decrease in the exsmoker's risk of dying from lung cancer; eventually the risk is almost equivalent to that of a nonsmoker's.[11] The rate of decline of the risk after cessation of smoking is determined by the cumulative smoking exposure prior to cessation, the age when smoking began, and the degree of inhalation.[12]

Study results regarding passive smoking as a risk factor for lung cancer are inconsistent, with some studies showing a positive relationship between lung cancer and exposure to sidestream smoke[13,14] and others showing no relationship.[15] Blot and Fraumeni[16] combined data from existing studies and estimated an overall increase in risk for lung cancer of 30% for nonsmoking women married to smokers, and an increased risk of 70% associated with heavy passive smoking. An updated analysis including more recent studies has not changed these estimates.[17]

The use of smokeless tobacco (chewing tobacco and snuff) is a practice that is increasing among U.S. male youth, especially among whites.[18] Its use has been linked to both oral cancer and cancer of the tongue.[19]

The overall smoking prevalence is decreasing in the United States,[20] and this is reflected in declining lung cancer rates among young men and women.[21] However, the decrease in smoking prevalence is not uniform among all groups within society. For the period 1974–1987, smoking prevalence in women aged 20 and over declined more slowly (31.5% to 26.8%) than for men (43.4% to 31.7%), with the smoking prevalence for women aged 20–24 not changing significantly. Smoking prevalence has declined much less rapidly among those who are high school graduates or less. In poorly educated young women, smoking prevalence actually increased from 1974 to 1985. Education now appears to be one of the strongest predictors of smoking status.[22]

It is believed that the lung cancer mortality rate for white men in the United States has now peaked, but the projected peak for mortality rates in women will not occur until the year 2010.[23,24] Similarly, lung cancer mortality for African Americans is not expected to fall until after the year 2000.[24] However, even with the predicted declines in mortality rates, the absolute number of lung cancer deaths will continue to rise[25] because of the increasing size of the population.

Prevention of smoking has an impact not only on cancer rates but also on the prevalence of other common diseases, such as heart and respiratory disease. It was estimated that in 1988, twice as many deaths from heart disease and respiratory disease were caused by smoking as there were deaths from cancers caused by smoking.[26] Therefore, prevention and cessation of smoking in the United States is a major public health goal.

Diet

Interest and research in the role of diet in cancer has flourished in recent years, with many micronutrients and some macronutrients being investigated for adverse or protective effects against cancer, in both human and animal studies. The impetus for many of these studies came from the results of ecologic studies; for example, a high correlation was found between national per capita daily meat consumption and the country-specific colon cancer incidence rates.[27]

Case-control and cohort studies of diet and cancer present several methodologic problems:

1. Accurate assessment of dietary intake is very difficult, especially in large epidemiologic studies. In epidemiology, the two most frequently used methods of dietary assessment are single or multiple 24-hour recalls of dietary intake and the food frequency questionnaire. In the latter method, subjects are asked how many times they ate numerous foods with reference to a given time period, for example, the last year. The validity of these instruments varies with the nutrient of interest. Dietary assessment, including the above methods, has been thoroughly described by Willett.[28]

2. Individual nutrients are often highly correlated because they are strongly related to calorie intake. This makes the assessment of the role of a single nutrient problematic. Statistical methods have been developed to adjust for calorie intake in an attempt to address this problem.[29]

3. Frequently, the range of nutrient intake within the study population is narrow, making it less likely that a nutrient effect will be observed. For example, this problem has been suggested as a possible reason for the lack of association between fat and breast cancer in the large Nurses' Health Study.[30]

4. Recall bias may be present if dietary assessment is being conducted after the presentation of the disease, as in a case-control study. This means that the individual's recall of their past diet might be affected by their knowledge that they have the disease.

To avoid the problems associated with self-reported dietary intake methods, direct assessment of some micronutrients has been developed, involving measuring the serum micronutrient levels.[31] However, this type of measurement has disadvantages; for example, in a case-control study the disease may affect blood micronutrient levels. Serum markers of intake of most macronutrients are not currently available, thus limiting this methodology.

Diet is of great importance in cancer prevention, for it has been proposed as a contributing factor in 20%–70% of cancer deaths[8, 32] and is a modifiable risk factor.

Some current issues regarding diet and cancer are discussed next.

Colon cancer and fat intake Ecologic studies comparing many countries have shown a strong association between per capita meat consumption[27] or dietary fat[33] and incidence of colorectal cancer. However, a causal association cannot be assumed from such studies. Results from case-control and cohort studies generally have supported high fat intake as a risk factor for colon cancer.[34,35,36,37] Difficulties can arise in the interpretation of such results because it is often difficult to separate the effects of fat, protein, and total calories,[36,37] dietary factors that are generally highly correlated.

Colon cancer and fiber intake A majority of studies of differing epidemiologic designs supports the hypothesis that high fiber intake is protective for colon cancer,[38] although not all studies are supportive. Vegetables as well as cereals are sources of fiber; in studies where the source of fiber has been examined, fiber from vegetables appears protective against colon cancer, whereas the data for cereal fiber are less supportive of a protective effect. These differences may be due to the difference in composition of fiber in cereals and vegetables or to the lack of a large range in cereal fiber intake, or these results may indicate that it is some other chemical or nutrient in vegetables that is protective against colon cancer.[38]

Colon cancer and calcium intake A protective role of high calcium intake against colon cancer has been reported in several studies[39,40,41] but not in all.[35,42] Data from supportive studies suggest that to reduce risk of colon cancer, calcium intake for females should be 1500 mg and for males 1800 mg.[43] These recommended intakes are similar to those suggested to prevent other disease states, such as osteoporosis and hypertension.

Breast cancer and fat intake Ecologic studies that use data from many countries show a strong positive relationship between per capita fat intake and breast cancer mortality rates.[27] However, case-control and cohort studies give conflicting results. In a combined analysis of 12 case-control studies of dietary factors and breast cancer, Howe[44] reported an association between high fat intake and breast cancer in postmenopausal women.

Two of the largest cohort studies, the Nurses' Health Study[30,45] and the Iowa Women's Study,[46] show no relationship between dietary fat intake and breast cancer risk; however, some researchers suggest this may be because the range of fat intake in such studies was too small. Current dietary recommendations are for women to reduce fat intake to less than 30% of calories. In Willett's study[45] the range of fat intake was 32%–44% of calories.

Cancer, micronutrients, and intake of fruits and vegetables One of the most consistent dietary findings in analytical epidemiologic studies with regard to cancer is a protective effect of fruits and vegetables.[47] What particular nutrient, nonnutrient, or combination in fruits and vegetables is protective against cancer is still under investigation. Nonnutrient compounds that may have a protective effect, such as ellagic acid, indoles, and dithiolethiones, have been summarized by Wattenberg.[48] The role of several micronutrients in cancer prevention, including the carotenoid, beta-carotene, vitamin A, vitamin E, and selenium, has been extensively investigated. Relatively high levels of these four micronutrients have been found to be associated with lower cancer risk in many studies, although again not all study results are in agreement. The role of micronutrients in cancer prevention has been reviewed by Moon and Micozzi.[49] Micronutrients in the diet generally are correlated with other micronutrients or nonnutrients; therefore, until results of current chemoprevention studies using individual micronutrients are known, the effect of a single micronutrient will not be clear.

The National Cancer Institute Chemoprevention Program began as a result of the promising research from animal and epidemiologic studies concerning the role of certain micronutrients in cancer prevention.[50] In this program, which focuses on micronutrients, populations at high risk for cancer are given certain vitamins or other chemicals that previously have been shown to prevent cancers in animal models. These populations are followed, and the effect of the agent on cancer incidence is assessed. A listing of ongoing human chemoprevention trials funded by the National Cancer Institute is shown in Table 1-5.[50]

Dietary intake has an impact not only on cancer but on many other chronic diseases as well, such as heart disease and diabetes, where its role is more fully understood. Even without proof of the role of a specific nutrient in cancer causation, there may be sufficient knowledge from a public health perspective to recommend that Americans change some aspect of their diet. For example, the role of fat in breast cancer is still controversial, but there exists sufficient knowledge concerning the role of fat in obesity, heart disease, and colon cancer that recommendations to reduce fat intake have been made to the American public.

Several groups, such as the National Research Council, have published recommendations for an optimal diet. Their recommendations include eating at least five servings of fruit and vegetables a day, reducing fat intake to 30% or less of calories, maintaining protein intake at moderate levels, and balancing food intake and physical activity to maintain appropriate body weight.[51] The role of health professionals is to encourage their patients to follow such guidelines and to help them avoid being influenced by the results of isolated studies of diet and its relationship to cancer.

Alcohol

Alcohol has been causally linked to cancers of the oral cavity, pharynx, larynx, esophagus, and liver, and may be linked to cancers of the breast and rectum.[52,53] It is estimated that 3% of cancer deaths are attributable to alcohol.[8] For most cancer sites, alcohol appears to act synergistically with smoking.

Cancers at most sites do not appear to be associated with any particular type of alcohol. Rectal cancer is the exception, for it appears to be associated specifically with beer consumption.[54]

Studies regarding the relationship between alcohol

TABLE 1-5 Chemoprevention Intervention Studies

Target Site Organ	Target/Risk Group	Inhibitory Agents
Cervix	Cervical dysplasia	*Trans*-retinoic acid
Cervix	Cervical dysplasia	Folic acid
Colon	Familial polyposis	Vitamins C and E and fiber
Colon	Familial polyposis	Calcium
Colon	Adenomatous polyps	Beta-carotene and vitamins C and E
Colon	Adenomatous polyps	Piroxicam
Lung	Chronic smokers	Folic acid and vitamin B_{12}
Lung	Asbestosis	Beta-carotene and retinol
Lung	Cigarette smokers	Beta-carotene and retinol
Lung	Smoking males	Beta-carotene
Lung	Asbestos	Beta-carotene
Skin	Albino	Beta-carotene
Skin	Basal cell carcinoma	Beta-carotene and vitamins C and E
Skin	Basal cell carcinoma	Beta-carotene
Skin	Actinic keratoses	Retinol
Skin	Basal cell carcinoma	Retinol and 13-*cis*-retinoic acid
Breast	Adenocarcinoma	4-HPR
All sites	American physicians	Beta-carotene

Reprinted with permission from Boone CW, Kelloff GJ, and Malone WE: Identification of candidate cancer chemopreventive agents and their evaluation in animal models and human clinical trials: A review. *Cancer Res* 50:7, 1990, Table 3.

and breast cancer are suggestive of a positive association, although the level of alcohol consumption required to significantly increase breast cancer risk is unclear.[52] If a causal association is shown, it will be of great importance. The attributable risk could be high, because a large percentage of the population drinks alcohol,[55] and alcohol would present one of the only known avoidable causes of breast cancer.

Little effort has been made to reduce or eliminate alcohol consumption to prevent cancer, possibly because alcohol has only been associated with cancers for which the primary risk factor is smoking. Therefore, the emphasis for prevention has been on smoking cessation. However, if the proposed relationship between alcohol and breast cancer is confirmed, lowering or eliminating alcohol intake may become an important public health goal for breast cancer prevention.

Physical activity

As with dietary assessment, accurate measurement of physical activity in epidemiologic studies has proved to be difficult, and many questionnaires have been developed in an attempt to improve assessment.[56] The close interrelationship of physical activity with obesity and diet, two factors associated with many cancers, also make its role in relation to cancer risk more difficult to assess.

Increased physical activity consistently has been found to be protective for colon cancer[57,58,59] and precancerous colon polyps.[60] Increased physical activity also may be protective for breast cancer.[61] Intense physical activity at the age of usual menarche may be especially important, since it can cause a delay in onset of menarche. Late onset of menarche is known to be protective against breast cancer. Risk of prostate cancer may also be reduced in those who are or were physically active.[62]

Increased physical activity is known to be protective against heart disease, and a general increase in physical activity throughout the population would be beneficial for health.

Occupational exposures

It is estimated that 4%–9% of cancer deaths can be attributed to exposure to occupational carcinogens. The lung is the most commonly affected site.[8]

Reasons for conducting epidemiologic studies of industrial populations include:

- surveillance of groups to identify unusual disease patterns that might indicate exposure to previously unidentified hazards
- to monitor and reevaluate "safe" levels of identified hazards
- to monitor human exposure to complex mixtures of different chemicals or materials that probably have not been tested in animal experiments in the laboratory

A summary of substances that are thought to cause cancer, and occupations in which they are used, is found in Table 1-6.[63]

Pollution

Pollution accounts for less than 1%–5% of cancer deaths in the United States.[8] It can affect the air we breathe, the water we drink, and the food we eat. Epidemiologic studies of pollution present a difficult methodological problem, that is, the assessment of exposure, specifically, assessment of both how long a subject has been exposed and the level of exposure.

Air pollution has been studied primarily in relation to risk for lung cancer. It seems probable that in heavily polluted areas air pollution may contribute to lung cancer mortality; however, insufficient data are available to quantify the risk.[64] Evidence is much stronger for

TABLE 1-6 Known and Suspected Occupational Carcinogens

Carcinogen	Occupation	Cancer
Polynuclear aromatic compounds in soots, tars, some mineral oils	Various, including sweeps, tar workers, cotton spinners, roofers, boat-builders and repairers, fishermen, tool setters	Scrotum, other skin
2-naphthylamine, 4-aminobiphenyl	Chemicals, rubber, cable-making	Bladder
Benzidine	Chemicals, dyestuffs, laboratory reagent	Bladder
? Michler's ketone	Auramine manufacture	Bladder
Mustard gas	Chemicals, warfare	Lung, larynx
bis(Chloromethyl)ether, technical chloromethyl methyl ether	Chemicals	Lung
? Diisopropyl sulphate	Isopropanol manufacture by strong acid process	Nasal sinuses
? Benzotrichloride	Manufacture of benzoyl chloride, etc.	Lung
Vinyl chloride (monomer)	Polyvinyl chloride manufacture	Liver angiosarcoma, ? other sites
Benzene	Chemicals, solvent	Leukaemia
Unknown ? via immunosuppression	Professional chemists	Lymphoma, ? brain
Arsenic compounds	Manufacture, use of arsenical pesticides, mining, smelting of various metals	Lung, skin
Nickel subsulfide, oxide, etc.	Nickel refining	Nasal sinuses, lung
Zinc chromate, other Cr(VI) compounds	Production and use of chromates	Lung
Beryllium compounds	Mining and various uses	Lung
Cadmium oxide, etc.	Battery manufacture, alloying, plating, etc.	? Prostate, ? lung
Radon + ?	Underground mining of haematite and other ores	Lung
Asbestos dust	Mining, multiple uses	Lung (synergism with smoking), mesothelioma of pleura, peritoneum
Wood dusts	Furniture manufacture	Nasal sinuses
Leather dusts	Shoe-making	Nasal sinuses

Reprinted with permission from Searle CE, Teale OJ: Occupational carcinogens. In Cooper CS, Grover PL (eds.): *Chemical Carcinogenesis and Mutagenesis 1: Handbook of Experimental Pharmacology* (vol. 94/1). Berlin: Springer-Verlag, 1990, Table 1, p. 105.

the association of air pollution and increased mortality from respiratory diseases, showing the importance of air pollution as a health risk.

Associations between water pollution and site-specific cancer risk are also unproven. Arsenic in drinking water appeared to be associated with an increase of skin cancer in Taiwan[65] but not in the United States.[66] This observed difference may be due to a higher intensity of exposure in Taiwan.

A type of pollution that may indirectly increase cancer risk is that of chlorofluorocarbons (CFCs). CFCs are destroying the ozone layer in the stratosphere.[67] It is predicted that this destruction will increase the amount of ultraviolet light reaching the earth's surface, thereby increasing the risk for nonmelanoma and melanoma skin cancer. The Environmental Protection Agency (EPA) reports that for every 1% decrease in stratospheric ozone, there results a 2% increase in ultraviolet-B intensity, potentially increasing the incidence of skin cancer by 1%–3% each year that the condition of the deteriorating ozone exists.[68]

Reproductive factors and sexual behavior

Risk factors related to reproduction and sexual behavior have been identified only for cancers in women; these are summarized in Table 1-7. The risk factor patterns are similar for breast, endometrial, and ovarian cancers. Pike[69] discusses the reasons for these observed similarities, such as exposure to unopposed estrogen. In contrast, cervical cancer has a very different risk factor pattern, with only multiple sexual partners being identified as a sexual behavioral risk factor. The number of sexual partners is a measure of the likelihood that an individual has been exposed to the

TABLE 1-7 Reproductive and Sexual Factors Associated with Female Cancers

Risk Factor	Breast	Cervical	Endometrial	Ovarian
Early menarche	X		X	X
Late menopause	X		X	X
Nulliparity	X		X	X
Late first pregnancy, > 35 years old	X			
Obesity	X*		X	
Multiple sexual partners		X		

*Postmenopausal women only.

human papilloma virus, which has been implicated as a cause of cervical dysplasia.[70]

In general, the reproductive risk factors associated with breast, endometrial, and ovarian cancer are unavoidable. Furthermore, there are no other proven risk factors for these cancers that can be avoided. Thus, early detection of these cancers is very important. Unfortunately, only breast cancer screening is available, although screening methods for ovarian cancer are being investigated. Nurses can play a strong role in encouraging all women to obtain mammography and in educating women regarding early signs of endometrial and ovarian cancer. For further information on screening refer to Chapter 7.

Viruses and other biological agents

Zur Hausen[71] suggests that 15% of worldwide cancer incidence is due to viruses. Listed in Table 1-8 are several putative human cancer viruses and their associated cancers. Epidemiologic evidence for their role in cancer causation is relatively strong. Hepatitis B virus and Human T-Lymphotropic virus type 1 may be sufficient alone to cause cancer, whereas Epstein-Barr virus alone is insufficient, and requires the host to be immunodeficient.[72] Burkitt's lymphoma, which is associated with the Epstein-Barr virus, is seen primarily in Africa, where malarial infection causes the required immunodeficiency state.

Growing evidence suggests a role for human papilloma virus (HPV) in the development of cervical cancer,[73] with subtypes HPV16 and HPV18 being most strongly associated with the disease.

Schistosoma haematobium is a parasitic flatworm common in Iraq, Egypt, and southeast Africa; strong epidemiologic evidence exists of a causative role of schistosoma in bladder cancer in these regions.

TABLE 1-8 Cancer Types Associated with a Virus or Other Biological Agent

Virus or Biological Agent	Cancer
Hepatitis B virus	Hepatocellular carcinoma
Human papillomavirus (types 16 and 18)	Cervical cancer
Epstein-Barr virus	Burkitt's lymphoma
Human T-lymphotropic virus type 1	Adult T-cell leukemia-lymphoma (ALT)
Human immunodeficiency* virus	Kaposi's sarcoma; non-Hodgkins lymphoma
Schistosoma	Bladder cancer

*The association may be due to immunosuppression, caused by HIV, which places the individual at increased risk. But even HIV-seropositive patients with no measurable immunosuppression appear to be at higher risk.

Radiation

Doll and Peto[8] estimate that 3% of cancer deaths are due to natural sources of radiation, excluding occupational exposure.

Ionizing radiation For most of the earth's population, over 80% of exposure to ionizing radiation is from natural sources, such as the food chain, air, water, minerals on or near the earth's crust, and cosmic rays. Man-made sources are X rays (80% of exposure to man-made sources in the United States),[74] fallout from nuclear explosions, and emissions and waste from nuclear power stations.

Several populations have been studied to assess the cancer risk of ionizing radiation. These include the survivors from Nagasaki and Hiroshima, people who received radiation therapy for medical reasons, and underground miners who were exposed to radon gas and decay products. There is no doubt that ionizing radiation causes many different cancer types, with the breast, thyroid, and bone marrow being particularly sensitive sites.[75] However, determining the effect of low-dose exposure, the level at which most such exposure occurs, is difficult. Dose extrapolation has many problems. For example, attempting to extrapolate from the cancer risk of the high radon dose that miners received to the relatively low dose that individuals living in a radon-contaminated house receive requires many assumptions regarding exposure to both the miners and the householder.[76] It has been estimated, however, that in the United States 5000–20,000 lung cancer deaths annually may be due to exposure to radon in the home,[77] thus making it of great public health concern.

Occupational exposure to ionizing radiation is highest among underground uranium miners, commercial nuclear power plant workers, fuel fabricators, physicians, flight crews and attendants, industrial radiographers, and well loggers.[78]

Ultraviolet radiation Ultraviolet radiation (UVR) is the major cause of nonmelanoma skin cancer, with cumulative exposure being predictive of risk.[79] The relationship of UVR to melanoma skin cancer is not as clear, because the site of melanoma does not mimic the site of UV exposure, as happens in nonmelanoma skin cancer. However, it is thought that intense intermittent exposure to ultraviolet radiation, especially in childhood, is a risk factor for melanoma.[80] UVR also has been shown to act synergistically with pipe smoking as a risk factor for lip cancer.[8]

Individual exposure to UVR is dependent on latitude, altitude, humidity, and personal behaviors, such as wearing protective clothing, using sunscreens, and staying out of the sun as much as possible.

Nonionizing radiation Nonionizing electromagnetic fields (EMF) are generated from a variety of electrical power, radar, and microwave sources[81] and have only recently been suspected of increasing cancer risk. Both occupational and residential exposures have been studied, and the results suggest that exposure to EMF is associated with increased cancer risk.[82] Evidence suggests that residential exposure is associated with an increased risk of leukemia in children and occupational exposure is associated with increased leukemia risk in adults.[83]

The ubiquitous nature of exposure to EMF makes its measurement difficult. In addition, measurement of quantitative exposure to EMF is generally based on assumptions regarding the relationship of EMF to the electrical wiring configuration of the home, which may not always be correct. More recent technology allows measurement of personal exposure to EMF and may improve dose measurement in future studies.

Drugs

The mechanism of action of many antineoplastic drugs is to damage cellular DNA, thereby killing the cell. However, since these drugs currently cannot be targeted to act specifically on tumor cells, normal cells also are damaged. A late effect of this damage can be the development of a second malignancy. Second tumors most frequently involve hematopoietic and lymphatic systems, but solid tumors also can occur. Single or combinations of antineoplastic drugs that have been implicated in the cause of second malignancies are listed in Table 1-9.[64]

Other drugs that have been associated with malignancies include:

TABLE 1-9 Antineoplastic Agents That Have Been Evaluated by IARC* Working Groups as Carcinogenic, Probably Carcinogenic, or Possibly Carcinogenic to Humans

Agent	Status
Adriamycin	Probably carcinogenic
Azacitidine	Probably carcinogenic
Azaserine	Possibly carcinogenic
N,N-Bis(2-cholor-ethyl)-2-naphthylamine (chlornaphthazine)	Carcinogenic
Bischloroethyl nitrosourea (BCNU)	Probably carcinogenic
1,4-Butanediol dimethylsulphonate (Myleran)	Carcinogenic
Chlorambucil	Carcinogenic
1-(2-Chloroethyl)-3-cyclohexyl-1-nitrosourea (CCNU)	Probably carcinogenic
1-(2-Chloroethyl)-3-(4-methylcyclohexyl)-1-nitrosourea (Methyl-CCNU)	Carcinogenic
Chlorozotocin	Probably carcinogenic
Cisplatin	Probably carcinogenic
Cyclophosphamide	Carcinogenic
Dacarbazine	Possibly carcinogenic
Daunomycin	Possibly carcinogenic
Melphalan	Carcinogenic
Merphalan	Possibly carcinogenic
Mitomycin C	Possibly carcinogenic
MOPP and other combined chemotherapy, including alkylating agents	Carcinogenic
Nitrogen mustard	Probably carcinogenic
Nitrogen mustard N-oxide	Possibly carcinogenic
Procarbazine hydrochloride	Probably carcinogenic
Streptozotocin	Possibly carcinogenic
Tris(1-aziridinyl) phosphine sulphate (Thiotepa)	Carcinogenic
Treosulphan	Carcinogenic
Trichlormethine	Possibly carcinogenic
Uracil mustard	Possibly carcinogenic

*International Agency for Research on Cancer.
Reprinted with permission from Tomatis.[64]

- phenacetin: associated with lower urinary tract cancers
- the immunosuppressive drugs azathioprine and cyclosporine: the former associated with an increase in non-Hodgkin's lymphoma and squamous cell

cancer of the skin, the latter with an increased risk of lymphoma[84]

- 8-methoxypsoralen combined with UV radiation, used for the treatment of psoriasis and vitiligo: associated with an increased risk of squamous cell cancer of the skin[85]

Exogenous hormones

Exogenous hormones are prescribed most commonly for women, either as a contraceptive or as replacement therapy following natural or induced menopause. They are also utilized for disorders of the menstrual cycle and to control abnormal uterine bleeding. Progestins have been used in obstetrics to prevent premature labor and in the management of threatened abortions.

Diethylstilbestrol, a synthetic estrogen used in the past for the treatment of threatened abortions, has been associated with vaginal and cervical cancers in the daughters of treated women.[86] This is the only known carcinogen to act transplacentally.[84] The cancers occur 10–30 years after treatment.

In contrast, use of combined oral contraceptives has been associated with a decreased risk of endometrial and ovarian cancer. Five years of usage is associated with a 55% reduction of endometrial cancer and a 40% reduction of ovarian cancer, compared with nonusers.[87]

An increased risk of liver cancer in young women also has been associated with oral contraceptive use; but as this is a rare tumor, so the absolute number of cases is low.[88] The effect, if any, of oral contraceptive use on breast cancer risk is still under investigation.

An increase in breast cancer risk has been associated with long-term use of estrogen replacement therapy. Key and Pike[89] estimate that five years of estrogen replacement therapy is associated with a 10% increase in breast cancer when users are compared with nonusers.

HOST CHARACTERISTICS INFLUENCING CANCER SUSCEPTIBILITY

Age

Although cancer can occur at any age, it is very much a disease of the elderly, with those over age 65 being ten times more likely (incidence rate 1983.3 per 100,000) than those under 65 (incidence rate 189.8 per 100,000) to develop cancer.[90] Cancer is most common in the elderly because with time the chance of prolonged exposure to cancer-inducing agents increases, and in addition the ability of the immune system to prevent cancer declines.[91]

Increasing cancer incidence is not, however, uniform with advancing age for all cancer sites (Figure 1-1),[89] and the leading cause of cancer deaths changes with age (Table 1-10).[92] Leukemia is the leading cause of death for children under 15 years of age, but is no longer among the five leading causes of cancer death after the age of 35; in contrast, lung cancer is rarely a cause of death under the age of 30, but is the leading cause of death over the age of 35.

Because age is such an important determinant of cancer risk, it is important in epidemiologic studies to make adjustments for age in the statistical analysis unless comparison groups have the same age distribution.

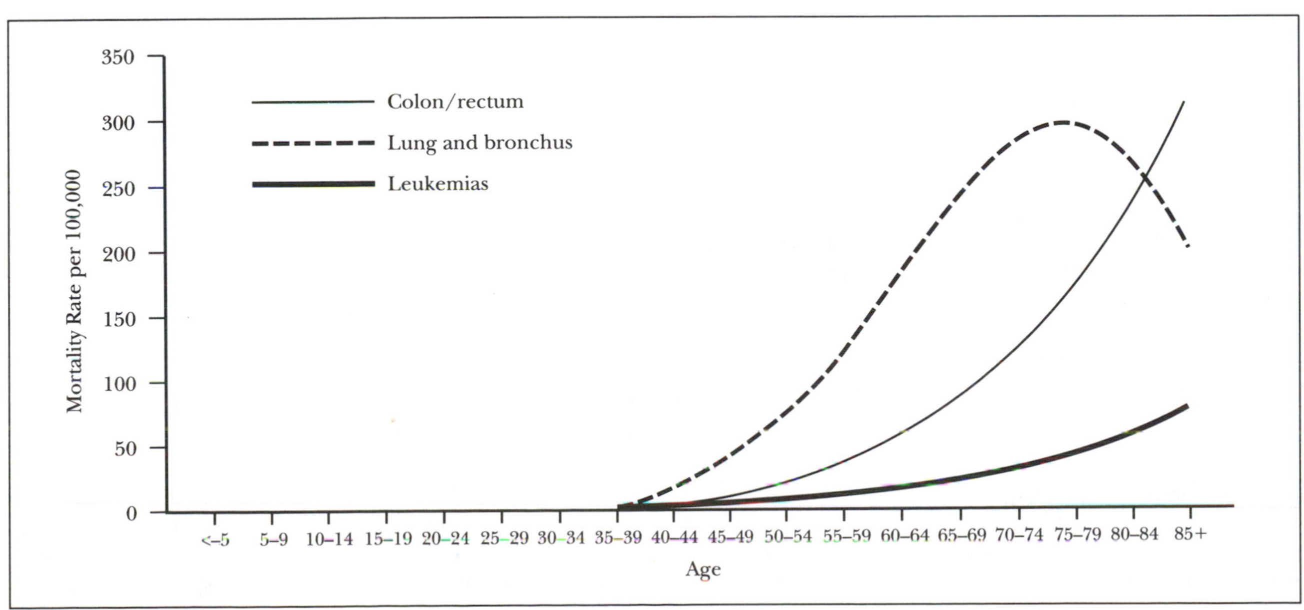

FIGURE 1-1 Changing cancer mortality with age for three cancer sites. (Data from Gloeckler Ries, Hankey, Edwards.[90])

TABLE 1-10 Mortality for the Five Leading Cancer Sites, by Age Group, United States, 1988

MALES					
All Ages	Under 15	15–34	35–54	55–74	75+
All Cancer 258.088	**All Cancer 971**	**All Cancer 3671**	**All Cancer 26.458**	**All Cancer 139.417**	**All Cancer 87.555**
Lung 88.059	Leukemia 362	Leukemia 685	Lung 8.903	Lung 55.092	Lung 23.877
Prostate 28.982	Brain and CNS 234	Non-Hodgkin's lymphomas 459	Colon and rectum 2.369	Colon and rectum 14.451	Prostate 17.303
Colon and rectum 28.111	Endocrine 114	Brain and CNS 438	Brain and CNS 1.360	Prostate 11.339	Colon and rectum 11.086
Pancreas 11.722	Non-Hodgkin's lymphomas 76	Skin 250	Non-Hodgkin's lymphomas 1.354	Pancreas 6.558	Pancreas 3.845
Leukemia 9.724	Connective tissue 38	Hodgkin's disease 241	Pancreas 1.269	Esophagus 4.299	Leukemia 3.483
FEMALES					
All Ages	Under 15	15–34	35–54	55–74	75+
All Cancer 226.960	**All Cancer 756**	**All Cancer 3434**	**All Cancer 27.889**	**All Cancer 109.063**	**All Cancer 85.808**
Lung 45.225	Leukemia 262	Breast 675	Breast 8.757	Lung 27.473	Colon and rectum 15.021
Breast 42.172	Brain and CNS 200	Leukemia 413	Lung 5.216	Breast 20.333	Lung 12.409
Colon and rectum 28.997	Endocrine 88	Uterus 340	Colon and rectum 1.969	Colon and rectum 11.852	Breast 12.403
Ovary 12.397	Connective tissue 46	Brain and CNS 313	Uterus 1.819	Ovary 6.677	Pancreas 5.833
Pancreas 12.126	Kidney 33	Non-Hodgkin's lymphomas 205	Ovary 1,641	Pancreas 5.579	Ovary 3.914

Reprinted with permission from Boring CC, Squires TS, Tong T: Cancer statistics, 1992. CA 42:19–38, 1992.

Sex

The incidence of cancers that are not sex specific (e.g., prostate and cervix) are generally lower in females (Table 1-11).[90] The distributions of cancer types in each sex are shown in Figure 1-2.[92] In part this is due to the differences in lifestyles between the sexes that are associated with cancer; e.g., smoking prevalence historically has been lower in females, therefore smoking-related cancers are less common in females.

Genetic Predisposition

Epidemiologic investigation of genetic predisposition to cancer is growing as developments in molecular biology make it possible to study genetic markers in large populations. The ongoing Human Genome Project[93] is almost certain to accelerate this work by the discovery of new genes or gene markers associated with increased genetic predisposition for cancer.

In the past it has been recognized that individuals with some rare autosomal recessive and X-linked recessive syndromes are at higher risk for certain cancers. Examples of these are summarized in Table 1-12.

Familial polyposis of the colon is an example of an autosomal dominant syndrome, where those with the syndrome develop colon cancer at a young age, in their 30s or 40s, and have a very high number of adenomatous polyps in the colon. The genetic steps required for the development of colon cancer have been studied in subjects with familial polyposis as well as in unaffected individuals who have adenomas or colon cancer. Vogelstein and colleagues[94] reported that the steps in-

TABLE 1-11 Age-Adjusted Cancer Incidence for Males and Females, 1973–1987 (per 100,000)

	Males		Females	
Site	<65	65+	<65	65+
Oral and pharynx	10.7	77.6	4.1	28.9
Esophagus	3.2	34.1	0.9	10.8
Stomach	4.7	79.6	2.1	35.9
Colon/rectum	22.1	417.5	16.6	288.0
Liver and intrahepatic	1.9	22.2	0.8	8.5
Pancreas	4.5	72.8	3.1	55.8
Larynx	4.9	40.7	1.1	6.2
Lung and bronchus	38.4	502.2	20.5	173.7
Melanoma of skin	8.5	39.8	7.7	19.5
Urinary bladder	11.1	197.4	3.0	47.5
Kidney and renal pelvis	6.2	57.8	3.0	26.0
Brain and nervous system	5.4	22.8	3.8	16.5
Thyroid gland	2.0	6.5	5.7	8.8
Hodgkin's disease	3.1	5.1	2.2	3.0
Non-Hodgkin's lymphoma	8.9	73.1	5.5	55.0
Multiple myeloma	2.0	33.8	1.4	22.3
Leukemia	6.6	72.0	4.4	37.4

Reprinted from Gloeckler Ries, Hankey, Edwards.[90]

TABLE 1-12 Examples of Autosomal Recessive and X-Linked Recessive Syndromes That Are Linked to an Increased Risk of Cancer

Syndrome	Associated Cancer
Autosomal Recessive	
Ataxia telangiectasia	Lymphocytic lymphoma Histiocytic lymphoma Acute lymphocytic leukemia Hodgkin's disease Ovarian cancer Gastric carcinoma Tumors of CNS
Fanconi anemia	Acute leukemia
Xeroderma pigmentosum	Skin cancer
Bloom syndrome	Various solid tumors Leukemia
Werner syndrome	Sarcoma
X-Linked Recessive	
Wiskott-Aldrich syndrome	Lymphoma
X-linked agammaglobulinemia	Lymphoma Leukemia
X-linked severe combined immunodeficiency	Lymphoma Leukemia
Dyskeratosis congenita	Carcinomas of the mucous membrane

clude mutational activation of an oncogene, coupled with the loss of several genes that normally suppress tumorigenesis. The mutation affecting individuals with familial polyposis, located on chromosome 5, represents one of these steps.

It has been observed for many years that cancer aggregates in some families. Such familial aggregation could be due to an inherited susceptibility or to common familial exposure(s), for example, diet. The majority of studies of this phenomenon have identified cancer familial aggregation for one cancer type, for example, colon cancer in relatives of colon cancer cases. However, Li and Fraumeni have identified an autosomal dominant syndrome from studying the kindred of children with rhabdomyosarcoma[95] in which the kindred have increased cancer risk of cancers other than rhabdomyosarcoma. The genetic defect in these families may be a mutation in the suppressor gene p53.[96]

Some gene defects may increase a person's risk for cancer because they have an impact on carcinogen metabolism. It has been found that subjects who have slow acetylator status (that is, the metabolism of aromatic amines by acetyltransferase is comparatively slow) are at higher risk for bladder cancer in certain occupational settings.[97] Acetylator status is genetically determined. Similarly, subjects who are slow metabolizers of the probe drug debrisoquine, due to a recessive mendelian trait, appear to be at lower risk for lung cancer.[98]

Ethnicity and Race

Ethnicity and race can be important issues to assess in epidemiologic research. However, several factors must be borne in mind when considering these points. First, ethnicity and race are both prone to misclassification. There is no accepted scientific definition for race. An individual may have grandparents from two or more ethnic or racial backgrounds, and could be classified in many ways. Frost and Shy, in a study of childhood deaths,[99] found that race at birth and race at death were different for 12% of African Americans and 34% of Native Americans, indicating the complexity of this problem.

Second, ethnicity and race are often highly correlated with socioeconomic status. African Americans, American Hispanics, and Native Americans generally have a lower socioeconomic status than white non-Hispanics. Distinguishing an ethnic or racial effect from a socioeconomic effect may be difficult.

However, assessing biological or genetic differences, along with cultural differences, that may make an ethnic or racial group at increased or decreased risk of a specific cancer is important, so special attention can be

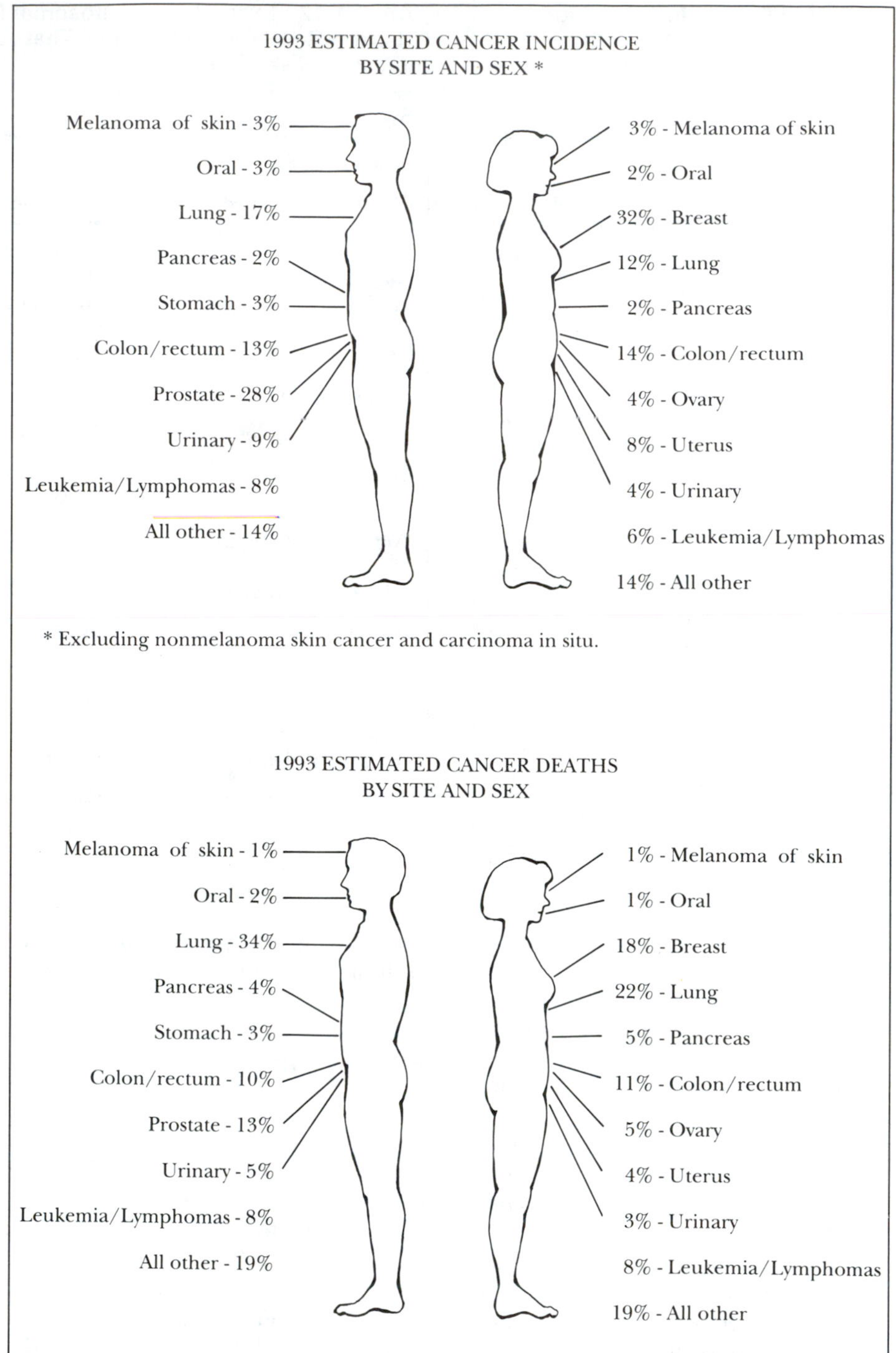

FIGURE 1-2 Estimated cancer incidence and deaths, by site and sex, for 1992. (Reprinted with permission from Boring CC, Squires TS, Tong T: Cancer statistics, 1992. *CA* 42:19–38, 1992.)

given to high-risk groups. Racial or ethnic groups may also differ in attitudes to illness, care seeking, and prevention. It is important to identify such differences so approaches can be tailored to each group to increase preventive health behavior.

There are four main racial/ethnic groups in the United States: African Americans (blacks), Hispanic Americans, Asian/Pacific Islanders, and Native Americans. For most cancer sites, African Americans have higher incidence rates than non-Hispanic Caucasians; in contrast, Hispanics and Native Americans have, overall, lower incidence rates.[100] A comparison of cancer incidence and mortality rates for African Americans and non-Hispanic whites is shown in Figure 1-3.[90]

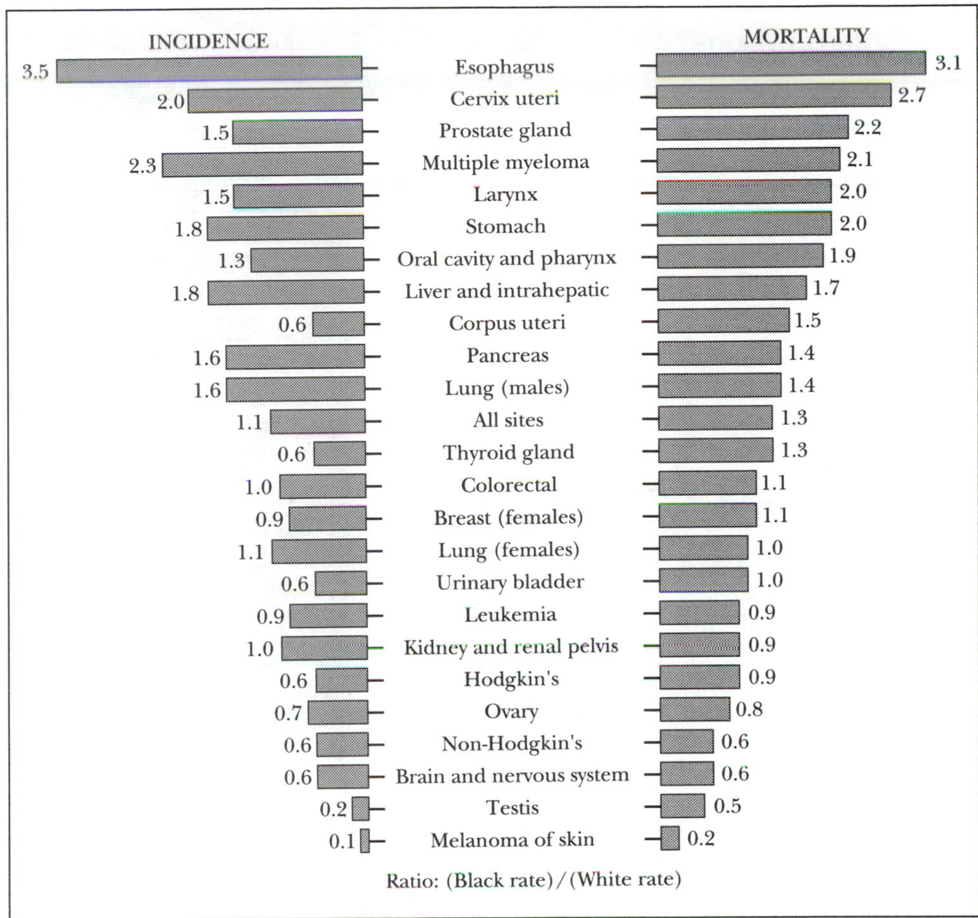

FIGURE 1-3 SEER cancer incidence and U.S. mortality rates, 1983–1987: Ratio of African American rate to white rate for all ages. (Reprinted from Gloeckler Ries, Hankey, Edwards.[90])

Socioeconomic Factors

Socioeconomic status is usually assessed by data on income, education, or percent below the poverty level, and has been found to be associated with some cancers, independent of race.[101] Clearly, SES is not a cause of cancer but is a proxy measure for lifestyle characteristics that differ for cancer type and the particular situation under study. For example, cervical cancer has been associated with lower SES. In this case SES may be a proxy for the number of partners the individual or her male spouse or partners have; the larger the number, the greater the chance of the female partner's being HPV positive. Alternatively, SES may be a proxy for PAP test frequency.

SES is now strongly associated with smoking prevalence, with low-income earners being more likely to smoke cigarettes.[102] Therefore, higher lung cancer rates in the lower SES group are likely to be due to this association.

OTHER APPLICATIONS OF EPIDEMIOLOGY IN ONCOLOGY

Survival

Survival analysis is the calculation of the probability that an individual with a specific disease will be alive at a particular time point after diagnosis; five years is commonly used as this time point. For most cancers the survival rate is greatly affected by the stage of cancer at diagnosis. For example, the five-year survival rate for melanoma diagnosed as local disease is 87%; in comparison, the equivalent survival rate for metastatic melanoma is 11%. The histology of the cancer also affects survival time. For example, men with oat cell lung cancer have a five-year survival rate of 4%, in comparison to other lung histologies, where the five-year survival is 13%. African Americans have a lower

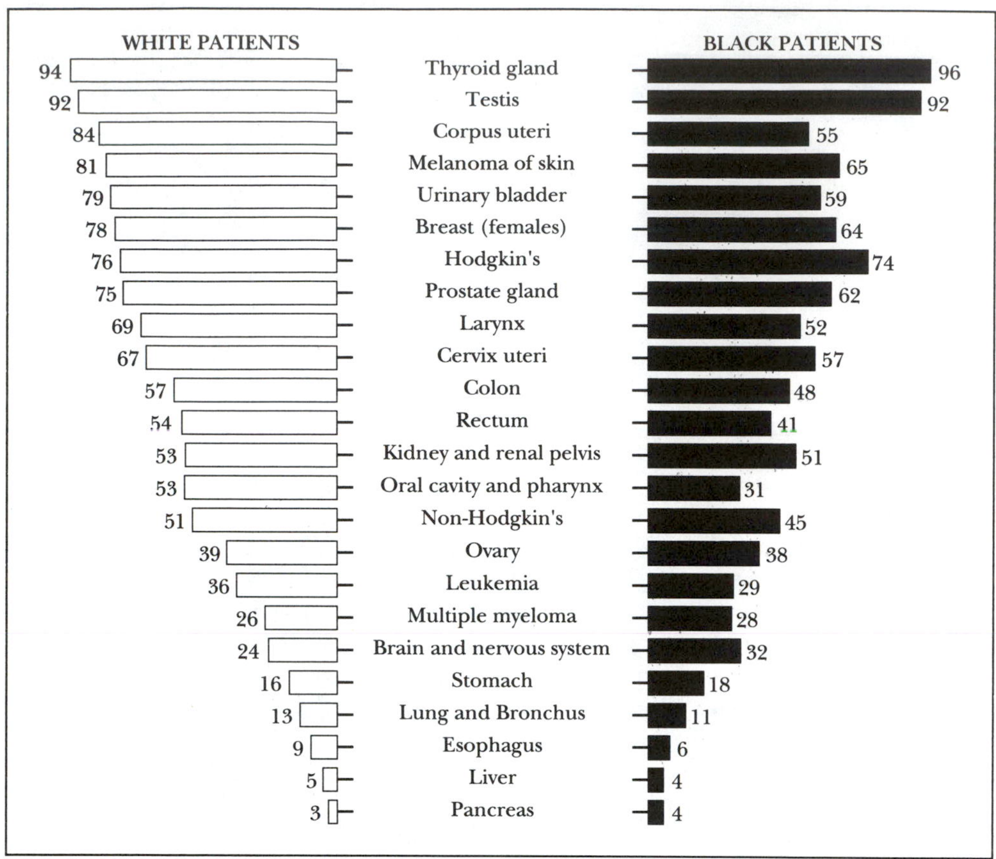

FIGURE 1-4 Five-year relative survival rates for African American and white patients: SEER Program, 1981–1986. (Reprinted from Gloeckler Ries, Hankey, Edwards.[90])

survival rate for most cancer sites as compared with whites (Figure 1-4),[90] due in part to the distribution of stage at diagnosis for the two groups. In turn, stage at diagnosis may be influenced by knowledge or attitudes about cancer (e.g., the importance of early diagnosis). Lack of access to care may also cause a delay in diagnosis.

Survival analysis is also used to assess the effectiveness of new treatment modalities for cancer, where survival following the new treatment is compared with survival following the standard treatment.

CANCER CONTROL

Cancer control has been defined as "the reduction of cancer incidence, morbidity, and mortality through an orderly sequence, from research on interventions and their impact in defined populations to the broad, systematic application of the research results."[103] In this definition the term *cancer control* encompasses both cancer prevention and control. The term will be used similarly in this chapter.

In 1985 Greenwald and Cullen[103] pointed out the need for a national strategy for cancer control so the results of research efforts of the National Cancer Program could be translated into a nationwide reduction in cancer incidence and mortality. To help improve cancer control, a model for cancer control research was developed, the phases of which are shown in Figure 1-5.[103] In Phase I, hypotheses are developed from basic biomedical research, for example, from the results of epidemiologic research. In Phase II, the necessary methods are then developed; for example, the feasibility of an intervention is examined. In Phase III, the efficacy of the intervention is being determined in a group of subjects. In Phase IV, the impact of the intervention is tested using a sample representative of a large target population. In Phase V, an intervention that has been proven effective in Phase IV is applied to a larger population, and the effect of the intervention in the population is evaluated.

In the Healthy People 2000 Study,[104] high-priority research needs for cancer control science in the United States were identified. These needs reflect the numerous disciplines and areas of research involved in the field of cancer control. Some of the main areas of research involved in cancer control are discussed next.

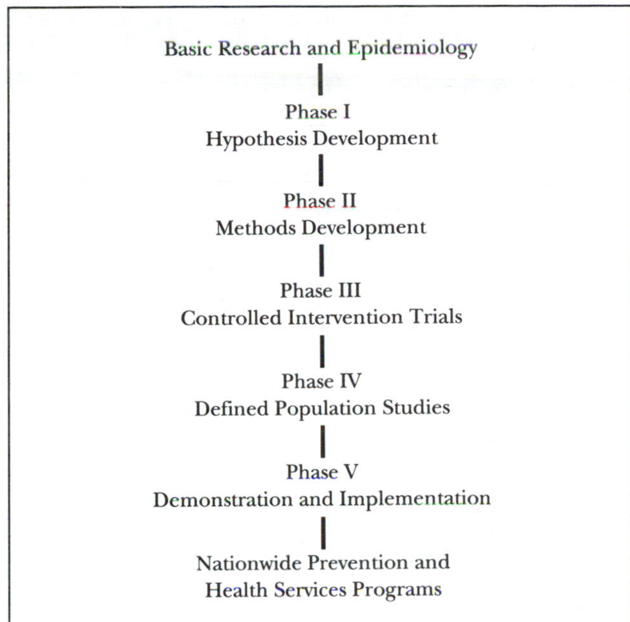

FIGURE 1-5 Phases of cancer control research. (Reprinted with permission from Greenwald, Cullen.[103])

Screening

Screening refers to the detection of disease by use of tests, examinations, or other procedures prior to the development of symptoms. Additional test(s) must follow a positive screening test to diagnose the disease. Epidemiology is an important aspect of developing and evaluating screening programs. During development, data must be available on the incidence, prevalence, distribution, and natural history of the disease. The distribution of the disease may influence the target population for screening and so improve the cost/benefit ratio of the screening program. Evaluation requires following an intervention (screened) population and a nonintervention (unscreened) population to assess the impact of screening on mortality. An implicit assumption regarding screening is that early detection will lead to a more favorable prognosis because treatment begun early in the disease course will be more effective than later treatment. This has shown to be the case for mammography and breast cancer mortality;[105] however, early detection of lung cancer using cytology or X rays has proved to have no effect in reducing lung cancer mortality.[106]

Barriers to Participation in Screening Programs

General barriers to participation in screening programs have been reviewed by Melnyk[107] and include cost, availability, discrimination, time, and patient characteristics such as culture and knowledge. These factors can prevent individuals from benefiting from early detection of cancer. Several studies show that females from minority groups or of low socioeconomic status are less likely to seek mammography or PAP tests for screening.[108,109] In the study of Stein and colleagues,[109] specific barriers to receiving mammography included lack of knowledge, cost, embarrassment, and fear of radiation. Interventions to increase screening compliance, especially among low-utilizer groups, must continue to be developed.

Behavioral change

Public knowledge regarding a risk factor for cancer does not automatically result in behavioral change by the public. For example, it is well known by the American public that smoking causes lung and other cancers, yet a significant proportion of the population of the United States still smokes. Programs that attempt to reduce smoking rates must therefore incorporate several intervention strategies, not education alone. An example of such an experimental program is the Community Intervention Trial for Smoking Cessation (COMMIT).[110] This program incorporates many interventions that have been shown to be individually successful. Within the target communities, several task forces are formed, each of which has several goals. For example, some of the goals of the Public Education Task Force are to promote social action that leads to a smoke-free community, to maintain quality and quantity of tobacco education in local schools, and to reduce adolescent exposure to tobacco products by encouraging endorsement of approved restrictions. In this trial, 22 communities have been randomized to receive the interventions or to receive no intervention.

Government policy

National, state, and local government have an impact on cancer control through legislation. Such legislation may directly affect cancer control. For example, in 1990 legislative action made screening mammography a covered benefit under Medicare.[111] Legislation may also indirectly affect cancer control. For example, under active consideration is legislation to mandate food labeling and to address the issue of health claims made by food companies.[112] Such legislation would provide the public with information with which to select a healthier diet. Many state and local governments have restricted smoking in public places, effectively reducing the public's exposure to side-stream smoke.

Cancer control efforts are affected by the monies specifically appropriated to cancer control in the National Institutes of Health budget by the government. The government can influence advancement in this area by setting national goals for cancer control, such as those in the Healthy People 2000 document.

THE APPLICATION OF EPIDEMIOLOGY TO NURSING PRACTICE

Nursing professionals play integral roles in all aspects of cancer prevention and cancer control. These involve the planning and implementation of cancer screening and educational programs, the design and coordination of cancer-related research projects, and clinical application of cancer control treatments. These roles involve much more than data collection: nurses function as principal investigators, as program directors, as educators, and as patient managers.

Within their roles in cancer prevention and control, nurses apply epidemiologic data and research principles to three main phases of their work:[113]

1. *The development phase.* The epidemiologic statistics of cancer incidence and mortality assist nursing professionals to identify high-risk groups and individuals within their patient community. Changes in incidence and mortality rates over time, demographic characteristics of cancer patients, health-related behaviors, and environmental conditions associated with cancer promotion can be obtained through epidemiologic data. These data can provide a basis for the development of research hypotheses and the theoretical foundation for program planning.

2. *The planning phases of research and prevention programs.* By using appropriate epidemiologic research principles, nurses can design studies that are focused, valid, and ultimately important in the scientific and clinical communities. Program development, short- and long-term goals for cancer prevention and control can be based on epidemiologic evidence from previous projects and new surveys that highlight changing cancer trends.

3. *The evaluation phase.* Via appropriate statistical methods, changes in cancer incidence and mortality rates, in stage of disease at diagnosis, in behavioral changes, and in survival time can be used to evaluate program effectiveness.

In all of these areas, in which nurses are full participants, epidemiology supplies important information and the methodological foundation for the development, planning, and evaluation of cancer prevention and control programs.

REFERENCES

1. MacMahon B, Pugh TF: *Epidemiology: Principles and Methods.* Boston: Little, Brown, 1970.
2. Hennekens CH, Buring JE: *Epidemiology in Medicine.* Boston: Little, Brown, 1987.
3. Walter SD, Marrett LD, From L, et al: The association of cutaneous malignant melanoma with the use of sunbeds and sunlamps. *Am J Epidemiol* 131:232–243, 1990.
4. Horowitz RL, Feinstein AR: Alternative analytic methods for case-control studies of estrogens and endometrial cancer. *N Engl J Med* 299:1089–1094, 1978.
5. Dawber TR: *The Framingham Study: The Epidemiology of Atherosclerotic Disease.* Cambridge, Mass: Harvard University Press, 1980.
6. Postservice Mortality Among Vietnam Veterans. The Centers for Disease Control Vietnam Experience Study. *JAMA* 257:790–795, 1987.
7. The Steering Committee of the Physicians' Health Study Research Group. Preliminary Report: Findings from the aspirin component of the ongoing physicians' health study. *N Engl J Med* 318:262–263, 1988.
8. Doll R, Peto R: The causes of cancer: Quantitative estimates of avoidable risks of cancer in the United States today. *J Natl Cancer Inst* 66:1193–1308, 1981.
9. IARC monographs on the evaluation of carcinogenic risks of chemicals to humans: *Tobacco Smoking,* vol. 38. Lyon, France: International Agency for Research on Cancer, 1986.
10. Wynder EL, Hoffman D: Tobacco. In Schottenfeld D, Fraumeni JF Jr (eds.): *Cancer Epidemiology and Prevention.* Philadelphia: Saunders, 1982, pp. 277–292.
11. U.S. Department of Health and Human Services, Office on Smoking and Health: *The Health Consequences of Smoking: Cancer.* A Report of the Surgeon General. DHHS[PHS] 82-50179. Washington, DC: U.S. Government Printing Office, 1982.
12. Rogot E: Smoking and mortality among U.S. veterans. *J Chronic Dis* 27:189–203, 1974.
13. Janerich DT, Thompson WD, Varela LR, et al: Lung cancer and exposure to tobacco smoke in the household. *N Engl J Med* 323:632–636, 1990.
14. Fielding JE, Phenow KJ: Health effects of involuntary smoking. *N Engl J Med* 319:1452–1460, 1988.
15. Ives JC, Buffler PA, Selwyn BJ, et al: Lung cancer mortality among women employed in high-risk industries and occupations in Harris County, Texas, 1977–1980, *Am J Epidemiol* 127:65–74, 1988.
16. Blot WJ, Fraumeni JF: Passive smoking and lung cancer. *J Natl Cancer Inst* 77:993–1000, 1986.
17. Blot WJ, Fraumeni JF: Passive smoking and cancer. In DeVita VT Jr, Hellman S, Rosenberg, SA (eds): *Cancer Prevention.* Philadelphia: Lippincott, 1989, pp 1–10.
18. Rouse BA: Epidemiology of smokeless tobacco use: A national study. *NCI Monogr* 8:29–33, 1989.
19. Mattson ME, Winn DM: Smokeless tobacco: Association with increased cancer risk. NCI Monogr 8:13–16, 1989.
20. Fiore MC, Novotny TE, Pierce JP: Trends in cigarette smoking in the United States: The changing influence of gender and race. *JAMA* 261:49–55, 1989.
21. Devasa SS, Blot WJ, Fraumeni JF: Declining lung cancer rates among young men and women in the United States: A cohort analysis. *J Natl Cancer Inst* 81:1568–1571, 1989.
22. Pierce JP, Fiore MC, Novotny TE, et al: Trends in cigarette smoking in the United States: Educational differences are increasing. *JAMA* 261:56–60, 1989.
23. Brown CC, Kessler LG: Projections of lung cancer mortality in the U.S. 1985–2025. *J Natl Cancer Inst* 80:43–51, 1988.
24. Mahaney FX Jr: Lung cancer rates in white males leveling off. *J Natl Cancer Inst* 84:83–84, 1992.

25. Novotny TE, Fiore MC, Hatziandreu EJ, et al: Trends in smoking by age and sex, United States, 1974–1987: The implications for disease impact. *Prev Med* 19:552–561, 1990.
26. Centers for Disease Control (CDC). Smoking-attributable mortality and years of potential life lost—United States, 1988. *MMWR* 40:62–63, 69–71, 1991.
27. Armstrong B, Doll R: Environmental factors and cancer incidence and mortality in different countries, with special reference to dietary practices. *Int J Cancer* 15:617–631, 1975.
28. Willett WC (ed.): *Nutritional Epidemiology.* New York: Oxford University Press, 1990.
29. Willett WC: Implications of total energy intake for epidemiologic analyses. In Willet W (ed.): *Nutritional Epidemiology.* New York: Oxford University Press, 1990, pp. 245–271.
30. Willett WC, Stampfer MJ, Colditz GA, et al: Dietary fat and the risk of breast cancer. *N Engl J Med* 316:22–28, 1987.
31. Hunter D: Biochemical indicators of dietary intake. In Willett W (ed.): *Nutritional Epidemiology.* New York: Oxford University Press, 1990, pp. 143–216.
32. Doll R: Lifestyle. An overview. *Cancer Detect Prev* 14:589–594, 1990.
33. Wynder EL, Shigermatsu T: Environmental factors of cancer of the colon and rectum. *Cancer* 20:1520–1561, 1967.
34. Whittemore AS, Wu-Williams AH, Lee M, et al: Diet, physical activity and colorectal cancer among Chinese in North America and China. *J Natl Cancer Inst* 82:915–926, 1990.
35. Jain M, Cook GM, Davis FG, et al: A case-control study of diet and colo-rectal cancer. *Int J Cancer* 26:757–768, 1980.
36. Lyon JL, Mahoney AW, West DW, et al: Energy intake: Its relationship to colon cancer risk. *J Natl Cancer Inst* 78:853–861, 1987.
37. Potter JD, McMichael AJ: Diet and cancer of the colon and rectum: A case-control study. *J Natl Cancer Inst* 76:557–569, 1986.
38. Trock B, Lanza E, Greenwald P: Dietary fiber, vegetables, and colon cancer: Critical review and meta-analyses of the epidemiologic evidence. *J Natl Cancer Inst* 82:650–651, 1990.
39. Slattery ML, Sorenson AW, Ford MH: Dietary calcium intake as a mitigating factor in colon cancer. *Am J Epidemiol* 128:504–514, 1988.
40. Garland C, Shekell RB, Barrett-Connor E, et al: Dietary vitamin D and calcium, and risk of colorectal cancer: A 19-year prospective study in men. *Lancet* 1:307–309, 1985.
41. Sorenson AW, Slattery ML, Ford MH: Calcium and colon cancer: A review. *Nutr Cancer* 11:135–145, 1988.
42. Kune S, Kune GA, Watson LF: Case-control study of dietary etiological factors: The Melbourne Colorectal Cancer Study. *Nutr Cancer* 9:21–42, 1987.
43. Newmark HL, Lipkin M: Calcium, vitamin D and colon cancer. *Cancer Res* 52:2067s–2070s, 1992.
44. Howe GR, Hirohata T, Hislop TG, et al: Dietary factors and risk of breast cancer: Combined analysis of 12 case-control studies. *J Natl Cancer Inst* 82:561–569, 1990.
45. Willett W, Hunter D, Stampfer MJ, et al: Dietary fat and breast cancer: Eight-year follow-up. Program and abstracts of the 15th Annual Meeting of the American Society of Preventive Oncology, 1991.
46. Kushi L, Sellers T, Potter J, et al: Dietary fat and breast cancer: Preliminary results from the Iowa Women's Health Study. Program and abstracts of the 15th Annual Meeting of the American Society of Preventive Oncology, 1991.
47. Steinmetz KA, Potter JD: Vegetables, fruit and cancer I. Epidemiology. *Cancer Causes Control* 2:325–327, 1991.
48. Wattenberg LW: Inhibition of carcinogenesis by minor dietary constituents. *Cancer Res* 52:2085s–2091s, 1992.
49. Moon TE, Micozzi MS: Nutrition and cancer prevention: Investigating the role of micronutrients (ed. 1). New York: Marcel Dekker, 1989.
50. Boone CW, Kelloff GJ, Malone WE: Identification of candidate cancer chemopreventive agents and their evaluation in animal models and human clinical trials: A review. *Cancer Res* 50:2–9, 1990.
51. *The Executive Summary in Diet and Health: Implications for Reducing Chronic Disease.* Washington, DC: National Academy Press, 1989, pp. 3–22.
52. Blot WJ: Alcohol and Cancer. *Cancer Res* 52:2119s–2123s, 1992.
53. *IARC monographs on the evaluation of carcinogenic risks of chemicals to humans: Alcohol drinking,* vol. 44. Lyon, France: International Agency for Research on Cancer, 1988.
54. McMichael AJ, Potter, JD, Hetzel BC: Time trends in colorectal cancer mortality in relation to food and alcohol consumption: United States, United Kingdom, Australia and New Zealand. In Greenwald MD, Ershow AG, Novelli WD, Benton CM (eds.): *Cancer, Diet and Nutrition. A Comprehensive Sourcebook.* Chicago: Marquis Who's Who, 1985, pp. 361–369.
55. National Institute on Alcohol Abuse and Alcoholism: The Sixth Special Report to the U.S. Congress on Alcohol and Health from the Secretary of Health and Human Services (DHHS Publication No. ADM87-1519). U.S. Department of Health and Human Services, Public Health Service, Alcohol, Drug Abuse, and Mental Health Administration, Washington, DC: U.S. Government Printing Office, 1987.
56. Washburn RA, Montoye HJ: The assessment of physical activity by questionnaire. *Am J Epidemiol* 123:563–576, 1986.
57. Slattery ML, Abd-Elghany N, Derber R, et al: Physical activity and colon cancer: A comparison of various indicators of physical activity to evaluate the association. *Epidemiology* 1:481–485, 1990.
58. Gerhardsson De Verdier M, Steinbeck G, Hagman U, et al: Physical activity and colon cancer: A case-referent study in Stockholm. *Int J Cancer* 46:985–989, 1990.
59. Albanes D, Blair A, Taylor PR: Physical activity and risk of cancer in NHANES 1 population. *Am J Public Health* 79:744–750, 1989.
60. Kono S, Shinchi K, Ikeda N, et al: Physical activity, dietary habits and adenomatous polyps of the sigmoid colon: A study of self-defense officials in Japan. *J Clin Epidemiol* 44:1255–1261, 1991.
61. Bernstein L, Ross RK, Henderson B: Prospects for the primary prevention of breast cancer. *Am J Epidemiol* 135:142–152, 1992.
62. Lee IM, Paffenbarger RS, Hsieh C: Physical activity and risk of prostatic cancer among college alumni. *Am J Epidemiol* 135:169–179, 1992.
63. Searle CE, Teale OJ: Occupational carcinogens. In

Cooper CS, Grover PL (eds.): *Chemical Carcinogenesis and Mutagenesis 1: Handbook of Experimental Pharmacology* (vol. 94/1). Berlin: Springer-Verlag, 1990, pp. 103–151.
64. Tomatis L: Pollution. In *Cancer: Causes, Occurrence and Control.* Lyon, France: International Agency for Research on Cancer Scientific Publications, 1990, pp. 229–239.
65. Tseng WP: Effects and dose-response relationships of skin cancer and blackfoot disease with arsenic. *Environ Health Perspect* 19:109–119, 1977.
66. Morton W, Starr G, Pohl D, et al: Skin cancer and water arsenic in Lane Country, Oregon. *Cancer* 37:2523–2532, 1976.
67. McFarland M, Kaye J. Chlorofluorocarbons and ozone. *Photochem Photobiol* 55:911–929, 1992.
68. National Institutes of Health Consensus Development Conference Statement: *Sunlight, Ultraviolet Radiation, and the Skin.* Bethesda, MD: U.S. Department of Health and Human Services, Public Health Service, National Institutes of Health, Office of Medical Applications of Research, 1989.
69. Pike M: The prevention of breast, endometrial and ovarian cancer. In Fortner JG, Rhoads JE (eds.): *Accomplishments in Cancer Research.* Philadelphia: Lippincott, 1989, pp. 327–356.
70. Ley C, Bauer HM, Reingold A, et al: Determinants of genital human papillomavirus infection in young women. *J Natl Cancer Inst* 83:997–1003, 1991.
71. Zur Hausen H: Viruses in human cancers. *Science* 254:1167–1173, 1991.
72. Henderson BE: Establishment of an association between a virus and a human cancer. *J Natl Cancer Inst* 81:320–321, 1989.
73. Koutsky LA, Galloway DA, Holmes KK: Epidemiology of genital human papillomavirus infection. *Epidemiol Rev* 10:122–163, 1988.
74. Henderson BE, Ross RK, Pike MC. Toward the primary prevention of cancer. *Science* 254:1131–1138, 1991.
75. BEIR III, Committee on the biological effects of ionizing radiation: *The Effects on Populations of Exposure to Low Levels of Ionizing Radiation.* Washington DC: National Academy Press, 1980.
76. Abelson PH: Mineral dusts and radon in uranium mines. *Science* 254: 777, 1991 (editorial).
77. Samet JM, Nero AV: Indoor radon and lung cancer. *N Engl J Med* 320:591–593, 1989.
78. NCRP Report No 101. Exposure of the U.S. population to occupational radiation. National Council on Radiation Protection and Measurements. June 1, 1989.
79. Strickland PT, Vitasa BC, West SK, et al: Quantitative carcinogenesis in man: Solar Ultraviolet B dose dependence of skin cancer in Maryland watermen. *J Natl Cancer Inst* 81:1910–1913, 1989.
80. Armstrong BK, English DR: Epidemiologic studies. In Balch CM, Houghton AN, Milton GW, Sober AG, Soong S-J (eds.): *Cutaneous Melanoma* (ed. 2). Philadelphia: Lippincott, 1992, pp. 12–20.
81. Adey WR: Joint actions of environmental nonionizing electromagnetic fields and chemical pollution in cancer promotion. *Environ Health Perspect* 86:297–305, 1990.
82. Savitz DA, Pearce NE, Poole C: Methodological issues in the epidemiology of electromagnetic fields and cancer. *Epidemiol Rev* 131:763–773, 1990.
83. Steverson RK, Davis S: Are there cancer risks associated with electrical power lines? *Cancer Prev* April: 1–11, 1991.
84. Tomatis L: Drugs and exogenous sex hormones. In *Cancer: Causes, Occurrence and Control.* Lyon, France: International Association for Research on Cancer Scientific Publications, 1990, pp. 148–154.
85. Stern RS, Thibodeau LA, Kleinerman RA, et al: Risk of cutaneous carcinoma in patients treated with oral methoxsalen photochemotherapy for psoriasis. *N Engl J Med* 300:809–813, 1979.
86. Herbst AL, Ulfelder H, Poskanzer DC: Adenocarcinoma of the vagina: Association of maternal stilbestrol therapy with tumor appearance in young women. *N Engl J Med* 284:878–881, 1971.
87. The WHO collaborative study of neoplasia and steroid contraceptives: Endometrial cancer and combined oral contraceptives. *Int J Epidemiol* 17:263–269, 1988.
88. Henderson BE, Preston-Martin S, Edmondson HA, et al: Hepatocellular carcinoma and oral contraceptives. *Br J Cancer* 48:437–440, 1983.
89. Key TJA, Pike MC. The role of oestrogens and progestagens in the epidemiology and prevention of breast cancer. *Eur J Cancer Clin Oncol* 24:29–43, 1988.
90. Gloeckler Ries LA, Hankey BF, Edwards BK (eds.): *Cancer Statistics Review 1973–1987.* U.S. Department of Health and Human Services, NIH Publication No. 90-2789, 1991.
91. Holmes FF: *Aging and Cancer.* New York: Springer-Verlag, 1983.
92. Boring CC, Squires TS, Tong, T. Cancer statistics, 1992. *CA* 42:19–38, 1992.
93. The Human Genome Project: Implications for human genetics. *Am J Hum Genet* 49:687–691, 1991.
94. Vogelstein B, Fearon ER, Hamilton SR, et al: Genetic alterations during colorectal-tumor development. *N Engl J Med* 319:525–532, 1988.
95. Li FP, Fraumeni JF, Jr: Rhabdomyosarcoma in children: Epidemiologic study and identification of a familial cancer syndrome. *J Natl Cancer Inst* 43:1365–1373, 1969.
96. Li FP, Fraumeni JF Jr, Mulvihill JJ, et al: A cancer family syndrome in twenty-four kindreds. *Cancer Res* 48:5358–5362, 1988.
97. Cartwright RA, Glashan RW, Rogers HJ, et al: Role of N-acetyltransferase phenotypes in bladder carcinogenesis: A pharmacogenetic epidemiological approach to bladder cancer. *Lancet* 2:842–845, 1982.
98. Ayesh R, Idle JR, Ritchie JC, et al: Metabolic oxidation phenotypes as markers for susceptibility to lung cancer. *Nature* 312:169–172, 1984.
99. Frost F, Shy KK: Racial differences between linked birth and infant deaths records in Washington State. *Am J Public Health* 70:974–976, 1980.
100. Jones LA, Newell GR: Introduction to Section 1. In Jones LA (ed.): *Minorities and Cancer.* New York: Springer-Verlag, 1989, pp. 3–4.
101. Baquet CR, Horm JW, Gibbs T, et al: Socioeconomic factors and cancer incidence among blacks and whites. *J Natl Cancer Inst* 83:551–557, 1991.
102. Centers for Disease Control, Center for Chronic Disease Prevention and Health Promotion, Office on Smoking and Health: *Tobacco Use in 1986. Methods and Basic Tabulations from Adult Use of Tobacco Survey.* DHHS Publ No. OM-90-2004. Rockville, MD: CDC, 1990.
103. Greenwald P, Cullen JW. The new emphasis in cancer control. *J Natl Cancer Inst* 74:543–551, 1985.
104. Healthy People 2000. National Health Promotion and Disease Prevention Objectives. DHHS Publication No. (PHS) 91-50212, 1991.

105. Feig SA: Follow-up studies of the health insurance plan study and the breast cancer detection demonstration project screening trials in the U.S.A. *Recent Results Cancer Res* 119:39–52, 1988.
106. Fontana RS, Sanderson DR, Woolner LB, et al: Screening for lung cancer. A critique of the Mayo Lung Project. *Cancer* 67:1155–1164, 1991.
107. Melnyk KAM: Barriers: A critical review of recent literature. *Nurs Res* 37:196–201, 1988.
108. Peters RK, Moraye BB, Thomas D: Barriers to screening for cancer of the cervix. *Prev Med* 18:133–146, 1989.
109. Stein JA, Fox SA, Murata PJ: The influence of ethnicity, socioeconomic status, and psychological barriers on use of mammography. *J Health Soc Behav* 32:101–113, 1991.
110. COMMIT Research Group: Community Intervention Trial for Smoking Cessation (COMMIT): Summary of design and intervention. *J Natl Cancer Inst* 83:1620–1628, 1991.
111. Oakar MR: Legislative effect of the 102nd congress. Cancer prevention, detection, treatment, and research. *Cancer* 69:154–156, 1992.
112. Chalmers E: Legislative influences on cancer care. *Cancer* 67:1732–1735, 1991.
113. Rempusheski VF: Ask an expert. *Appl Nurs Res* 4:96–98, 1991.

Chapter 2

Milestones in Our Understanding of the Causes of Cancer

John W. Yarbro, MD, PhD

INTRODUCTION

Carcinogenesis, the process by which cancer develops, requires *clonal selection.* By accident, a mutation in a cell may confer a survival advantage. If one of the descendants of that cell is hit by a second mutation that also confers a survival advantage, the next clone grows even more vigorously. A sequence of such events leads to the selection of a clone with the characteristics of a neoplasm and later allows subclones to progress to ever greater stages of virulence characterized by invasion, metastatic spread, drug resistance, and other characteristics that ultimately lead to the death of the host. The number of mutations required to develop cancer indicates that genetic instability (an increased mutation rate) is an early event in the evolving cancer cell. Carcinogenesis is Darwinian evolutionary natural selection on a clonal basis within a single organism. This process is a perversion of the normal growth and repair mechanisms.

Animals have evolved an elaborate set of controls regulating cellular growth and repair. There are signals to turn growth on and off as needed. There are complex fail-safe mechanisms to prevent the overgrowth of a mutant clone. However, cancer escapes this regulation. Step by step—that is, mutation by mutation—cancer overcomes this protection against uncontrolled growth. This happens because the mutations that lead to cancer are mutations of the very same genes that regulate normal growth. Indeed, many of the genes that regulate normal growth were discovered, almost by accident, during the search for cancer genes in oncogenic viruses.

Two types of growth-control genes have been identified. The first, called *oncogenes* or *proto-oncogenes,* are dominant genes that code for proteins that stimulate growth. The second, called *anti-oncogenes* or cancer-suppressor genes, are recessive genes that code for proteins that block the action of growth-promoting factors.

Two types of cancer-causing mutations have been identified: (1) *somatic mutations* are mutations of the ordinary cells of the various organs that are acquired throughout a lifetime due to various carcinogens; (2) *germ cell mutations* are mutations that are transmitted to the next generation at birth and are responsible for hereditary (familial) cancer. Many, perhaps most, human cancers result from a combination of acquired and inherited mutations with alterations of both oncogenes and anti-oncogenes.

Carcinogenesis may result from exposure to chemicals, such as those in tobacco; radiation, such as cosmic rays or radon from natural sources; asbestos; or various types of viruses. In all cases the final common path of action of such agents is through oncogenes and cancer-suppressor genes. Specifically, oncogenes must be mutated so as to be activated, and cancer-suppressor genes must be mutated so as to be inactivated. Many times (exactly how frequently is uncertain), an individual may have inherited a defective cancer-suppressor gene from a parent. Oncogenes usually act as dominant genes; that is, only one gene of each pair needs to be mutated to have an effect. Cancer-suppressor genes usually act as recessive genes; that is, both genes of a pair must be mutated to lose the cancer-suppressive effect.

Our new understanding of the biology of cancer has allowed the development of strategies for prevention and detection as well as for enlightened therapeutic interventions. These include, among many other modern approaches, breast conservation surgery, less radical procedures for melanoma, limb conservation in osteogenic sarcoma, adjuvant therapy, prevention using pharmacological agents such as tamoxifen, enlightened public health measures, and prognosis based on genetic probes.

This sophisticated level of knowledge about the biology and behavior of malignant disease is relatively recent. It has been attained with great effort and suffering over many centuries as physicians and nurses have struggled to heal and learn at the same time. This chapter will present some of the milestones of that heroic struggle.

"THERE IS NO TREATMENT"

The earliest description of cancer appears in the Edwin Smith Papyrus from Egypt in the seventeenth century B.C. After providing the oldest written description of a patient with cancer, the physician advises, "Thou should say concerning him . . . 'There is no treatment.' "[1,p.21]

A thousand years later, Hippocrates, the Father of Medicine, formulated his rules for medical practice in a series of Aphorisms. His cardinal Aphorism, "Primum non nocere" (First, do no harm), is as valid today as it was in the fifth century B.C. It is widely believed that the Greek word for crab, *karkinos,* was first applied to cancer by Hippocrates. Aphorism number 38 states, "It is better not to apply any treatment in cases of occult cancer; for if treated, the patients die quickly; but if not treated they hold out for a long time."[1,p.23] More times than we like to admit, this Aphorism is forgotten today.

Celsus, the great first century Roman physician, compiled an encyclopedia of medicine, *De medicina,* containing many accurate clinical descriptions of cancer. Careful distinctions were made between benign and malignant disease along with treatment recommendations. His treatment was like that of Hippocrates. He noted:

> After excision, even when a scar has formed, none the less the disease has returned, and caused death; while at the same time the majority of patients, though no violent measures are applied in the attempt to remove the tumor but only mild applications in order to soothe it, attain a ripe old age in spite of it.[1,p.26]

Galen, the second-century Roman physician, was the central medical authority for over a thousand years because the church preserved hundreds of his writings and endorsed his views. His effect on the practice of medicine was immense long after the medieval period. He viewed cancer much as Hippocrates did, and his views set the pattern for cancer management for centuries.

The Middle Ages saw little progress in Europe, although medicine flourished in Byzantium and Arabia, where civilization persisted after the fall of Rome. The approach to cancer treatment remained Hippocratic (or Galenic) for the most part. There are, however, descriptions of attempts at radical surgery, as, for example, the following Byzantine procedure cited by Shimkin:

> I personally am in the habit of operating for cancer arising in the breast thusly: I make the patient lie down; then I incise the healthy part of the breast beyond the cancerous area and I cauterize the incised parts until the blood ceases by the formation of a coating. Then I again incise and excise the breast from its depth and I again cauterize the incised areas. And I repeat this procedure often, first cutting then cauterizing until bleeding stops.[1,p.33]

There was, of course, no mention of anesthesia.

"THERE IS NO IMPROPRIETY IN REMOVING IT"

The advent of the Renaissance signaled the beginning of medical progress in Europe. With Galileo and Newton in the seventeenth century, there began what can legitimately be called the scientific method. Harvey's *De Mortu Cordis* in 1628, describing the circulation of the blood, provides the beginning of scientific cardiology. In 1761, Giovanni Morgagni of Padua was the first to correlate the clinical course of cancer to the gross pathological findings at autopsy, laying the foundation for scientific oncology.

Finally, in the eighteenth century, John Hunter, the great Scot surgeon, provided descriptions of the surgery of cancer that would bring nods of approval from modern surgeons:

> Great attention should be paid to the tumor, whether it is moveable or not, for as the disease is further extended so the parts are more united to the tumor. If the tumor is not only moveable but the part naturally so, then there is no impropriety in removing it. . . . [I]f any consequent cancers easy of extirpation are found, they may be safely removed also. But it requires very great caution to know if any of these consequent tumors are within proper reach for we are apt to be deceived in regard to the lymphatic glands, which often appear moveable when, on extirpation, a chain of them is found to run far beyond out of our reach which renders the operation unsuccessful.[1,p.85]

A century was to pass before the development of anesthesia allowed the great surgeons of the nineteenth century to develop cancer operations such as the classic radical mastectomy. But still, the principles of radical surgery can be recognized in the lectures of John Hunter.

"CAUTIONS AGAINST THE IMMODERATE USE OF SNUFF"

The Egyptians blamed cancers on various gods. Hippocrates explained all diseases as resulting from an imbalance of the four humors, in the case of cancer an excess of black bile. Galen and others for over a thousand years echoed Hippocrates. Then, as Europe entered the Age of Reason, Bernardino Ramazzini, an Italian physician, noted the high incidence of breast cancer in nuns and hypothesized that this was in some way related to their celibate lifestyle.[1] The age of cancer epidemiology had begun.

John Hill of London was the first to recognize the dangers of tobacco.[1,2] In 1761, only a few decades after tobacco had become popular in London, he published a description of his observations entitled *Cautions Against the Immoderate Use of Snuff,* which was subtitled "Founded on the known Qualities of the Tobacco Plant and the Effects it must produce when this Way taken into the Body and Enforced by Instances of Persons who have perished miserably of Diseases, occasioned, or rendered incurable by its Use."[2,p.19]

The oft-cited description of scrotal cancer in chimney sweeps by Percivall Pott of St. Bartholomew's Hospital in London[3] was, according to Shimkin,[1] the third in a series of reports that launched the field of cancer epidemiology. Pott's report is the most frequently cited and has influenced our views, but as we shall see it is the "immoderate use of snuff" that is our major cancer problem today.

"WE MIGHT SUPPRESS IT COMPLETELY IN AN EARLY STAGE"

At the beginning of the nineteenth century, a committee of English physicians and surgeons formed to investigate the nature of cancer formulated thirteen questions whose research significance would be instantly recognized by any cancer scientist today.[4] Many of these questions were quite profound:

> Are there premalignant lesions? If so, "though we are unable to cure cancer in an advanced stage, we might extinguish the disposition to it or suppress it completely in an early stage."

"Are there any proofs of cancer being an hereditary disease?"

Is cancer infectious? Do some diseases degenerate into cancer?

"May cancer be regarded at any period or under any circumstances as merely a local disease?"

"Are brute creatures subject to any disease resembling cancer in the human body?" If so, investigation of cancer in animals "may lead to much philosophical amusement and useful information; particularly it may teach us how far the prevalence or frequency of cancer may depend upon the manners and habits of life."

This systematic approach to cancer biology laid a foundation for scientific progress in the nineteenth century. For those of us who watched the National Cancer Plan evolve after the passage of the National Cancer Act in 1971, such a systematic set of questions strikes a familiar chord, especially in view of the fact that some of the questions asked in 1800 were the same ones being asked again after nearly two centuries.

The nineteenth century saw the birth of scientific oncology as science shifted from anatomy to pathology. Early in the century a microscope of sufficient quality for research on tissues became available. Johannes Muller, the German genius, applied this instrument to cancer research and began to correlate cellular pathology with clinical symptoms. He established a *cellular* basis for tumor description. Subsequently, this work was carried on by the man usually described as the founder of cellular pathology, Rudolph Virchow of Berlin, who provided the scientific basis for the modern pathological study of cancer. As Morgagni had correlated the gross autopsy findings with the clinical history of illness, so now the microscopic findings were similarly correlated.

Rudolph Virchow established the microscopic basis for the characterization of cancer. But even Virchow failed to recognize the cellular nature of metastases. He felt that circulating cancer cells in the blood would be trapped by the lungs, and concluded:

> The manner in which the metastatic diffusion takes place seems, on the contrary, to render it probable that the transference takes place by means of certain fluids, and that these possess the power of producing an infection which disposes different parts to a reproduction of a mass of the same nature as that which originally existed. . . . There are, however, many facts, which speak but little in favor of the infection's taking place by means of really detached cells, for example, the circumstances that certain processes advance in a direction contrary to that of the current of lymph, so that after cancer of the breast, disease of the liver takes place whilst the lung remains unaffected. Here it seems pretty probable that juices are taken up, which occasion a further propagation.[5,pp.219,460]

Wilhelm Waldeyer of Berlin did not agree that cancer metastases resulted from some kind of noncellular infectious substance; he felt *embolic* transfer through the blood or lymph channels was the mechanism.[6] The pathological basis of malignancy began to be understood, and pathology began to replace anatomy as the key basic science.

"THIS IS NO HUMBUG!"

Soporific and narcotic agents had been used for centuries to control the pain of surgery. The effect of nitrous oxide (laughing gas) had been noted and led to its social use at parties in the nineteenth century. The suggestion that it might reduce surgical pain was not followed up. Hypnotism had been used to control pain, but this had not been accepted by the medical profession. In 1842, Dr. Crawford Long of Georgia used sulfuric ether, but he did not report this work. Horace Wells, a dentist, attempted to demonstrate laughing gas as an anesthetic before a medical school class at Harvard, but the patient cried out and the dentist was booed and hissed.[7]

Finally, in 1846 anesthesia was shown to work. John C. Warren, a Boston surgeon, had trained under Astley Cooper in London, and Cooper had been a student of the great Scot surgeon John Hunter, who had studied with Percivall Pott. In 1846 Warren performed the first reported operation under anesthesia on a patient anesthetized with ether by a dentist, William Thomas Morton. The absence of pain in his patient led Warren to observe, "Gentlemen, this is no humbug!"[7]

Oliver Wendell Holmes coined the term *anesthesia.* Prior to this time, the notion of anesthesia had bordered on quackery, and it was not immediately accepted. The Calvinist church fathers in England decried its use for childbirth, citing the biblical admonition that women must bring forth children in pain. But Queen Victoria elected to use chloroform anesthesia during the birth of one of her many children, and this brought about general public acceptance.[7] Anesthesia allowed the rapid progress in surgery that caused the next one hundred years to be called "the century of the surgeon."[8]

"THERE IS NO SUCH THING AS AN INEVITABLE INFECTION"[9,p.51]

Eight years after John Warren concluded that anesthesia was "no humbug," Florence Nightingale led a party of 38 nurses on a mission of mercy to the Crimean War. After she returned to England in 1856, the care of the sick and the operation of hospitals would never again be the same. She described nursing as the "finest of the fine arts";[9,p.68] she noted its uniqueness by observing that "nursing and medicine should never be mixed up. It spoils both";[9,p.51] she demanded influence for nurses: "[D]octors are very liable to imagine they must have the control of the whole staff";[9,p.54] she echoed Hippocrates' cardinal Aphorism, relating it to hospitals: "[A] first requirement is that a hospital should do the sick no harm";[9,p.49] and she advocated preventive medicine policies far ahead of her time when she said she wanted to "inoculate the country with the view of preventing instead of cure."[9,p.39]

Nursing is, of course, older than Florence Nightingale. There were many unnamed and unrecognized women (can we doubt that they were women?) who, from the beginning, gave to the sick that solicitude, understanding, and attention to the *human* response to illness that is the essence of nursing. But Florence Nightingale gave the hospital the *professional* nurse and began the tradition of scholarship and dedication that continues today in oncology nursing. She identified the uniqueness in the practice of nursing that was not the same as the practice of medicine, and she based the professionalism of nursing on that uniqueness.

"AMPUTATION OF THE SHOULDER JOINT MIGHT ERADICATE THE DISEASE"

There were great surgeons before the discovery of anesthesia. Such names as John Hunter, Astley Cooper, and John Warren come to mind. But when anesthesia became available at mid-century, there emerged the giants whose work so rapidly advanced the art that the next hundred years became known as "the century of the surgeon."[8] Three surgeons stand out because of their contributions to the art of cancer surgery: Bilroth in Germany, Handy in London, and Halsted at Johns Hopkins. Their work led to the "cancer operation" designed to remove all of the tumor *en bloc* as well as the lymph nodes that normally drained the region where the tumor was located.

William Stewart Halsted, professor of surgery at Johns Hopkins University, developed the radical mastectomy during the last decade of the nineteenth century. His work was based in part on that of W. Sampson Handley, the London surgeon who believed that cancer spread centrifugally through the lymphatics in continuity with the original growth.[10] Halsted's concept of the natural history and biology of cancer and its treatment are best described in his own words:

> We believe with Handley that cancer of the breast in spreading centrifugally preserves in the main continuity with the original growth. . . . Although it undoubtedly occurs, I am not sure that I have observed from breast cancer, metastasis which seemed definitely to have been conveyed by way of the blood vessels. . . . [T]here comes to the surgeon an encouragement to greater endeavor. . . . [W]e must remove not only a very large amount of skin and a much larger area of subcutaneous fat and fascia, but also strip the sheaths from the upper part of the rectus, the serratus magnus, the subscapularis, and at times from parts of the latissimus dorsi and teres major. Both pectoral muscles are, of course, removed. . . . It must be our endeavor to trace more definitely the routes traveled in metastasis to bone, particularly the humerus, for it is even possible in cases of involvement of this bone that amputation of the shoulder joint plus a proper removal of the soft parts might eradicate the disease. So too it is conceivable that ultimately, when our knowledge of the lymphatics traversed in cases of femur involvement becomes sufficiently exact, amputation at the hip joint may seem indicated.[11,p.4]

The Halsted and Handley doctrine stated simply that cancer is contained within anatomical compartments and can be cured by radical resection *en bloc* of these compartments. This became the basis of the "cancer operation" for almost a century, until it was called into question by the work of two twentieth century surgeons.

"THE SEED AND THE SOIL"

At the same time Halsted and Handley were developing their radical operations based on their interpretation of the spread of breast cancer, another surgeon was asking "What is it that decides which organs shall suffer in a case of disseminated cancer?" Stephen Paget wrote, "I have collected 735 fatal cases of cancer of the breast in each of which a necropsy was made and recorded," and he concluded that cancer cells spread by way of the blood stream and further that the disproportion of metastases to certain organs "cannot be due to chance."[12,p.572] In a brilliant leap of logic he drew an analogy between cancer metastasis and seeds that "are carried in all directions, but they can only live and grow if they fall on congenial soil."[12,p.572]

Paget had concluded that cells from a primary tumor are able to grow in only certain other organs—not in any organ in which they happen to come to rest. This accurate but highly sophisticated hypothesis was confirmed by the techniques of modern molecular biology almost a hundred years later.[13] Paget, on the basis of careful pathological examination at hundreds of autopsies, drew the correct conclusion, whereas others viewing the same autopsy material, including Virchow and Halsted, drew the wrong conclusion. The implications for the treatment of cancer are substantially different—indeed, in some ways quite the opposite—because this is the element in the new biological understanding of cancer that is integral to the breast conservation surgery introduced in recent years.

"ALL VESTIGES OF HER PREVIOUS CANCEROUS DISEASE HAD DISAPPEARED"

The end of the nineteenth century saw publication of a second seminal but neglected paper. Thomas Beatson graduated from the University of Edinburgh in 1874 and developed an interest in lactation and ovarian function, because he lived near a large sheep farm in rural Scotland. In 1878 he investigated the effect on the breasts of removing the ovaries of rabbits and found that lactation continued so long as the young were suckling but that the breasts atrophied and became fatty after suckling ceased. Here is the way he described his thoughts in a lecture to the Edinburgh Medico-Chirurgical Society in 1896:

> This fact seemed to me of great interest, for it pointed to one organ holding control over the secretion of another and separate organ. . . . I was struck by the local proliferation of epithelium seen in lactation. Here was the very thing characteristic of carcinoma of the breast, and indeed, of the cancerous process everywhere, but differing from it in that it was held in control by another organ.[14,p.105]

Because the breast was "held in control" by the ovaries, he decided to test oophorectomy in advanced breast cancer. The first patient he treated presented with a massive local recurrence. Regression of the recurrent tumor began five weeks after the operation, and by eight months "all vestiges of her previous cancerous disease had disappeared."[14,p.106] His second case had a far-advanced inoperable primary breast cancer, and oophorectomy led to a good partial remission. His third case, also a woman with an advanced inoperable primary tumor, showed continued progression after oophorectomy.

These cases led him to speculate that "the ovaries may be the exciting cause of carcinoma"[14,p.106] in women with breast cancer, an observation of particular note in view of our present, large trials of tamoxifen as a preventive in breast cancer. Here, for the first time, was an experimental observation that illustrated the potential for *systemic* treatment of cancer.

A half century after Beatson, Charles Huggins, a urologist at the University of Chicago, reported dramatic regression of metastatic prostate cancer following castration.[15,16] In 1966 Huggins received the Nobel Prize.

"A NEW KIND OF RAY" ("UBER EINE NEUE ART VON STRAHLEN")

In 1896, exactly half way through the century of the surgeon, a remarkable lecture was presented by Wilhelm Conrad Roentgen, a German physics professor from Wurzberg. This lecture was to provide the clinician with a second modality of cancer therapy. Actually, the lecture was published before it was delivered because the editor of the journal recognized its major importance and rushed it into print. The paper was entitled "Uber eine neue Art von Strahlen" ("Concerning a new kind of ray"), which Roentgen called the *X ray*, "*X*" being an algebraic symbol for the unknown.[17]

There was immediate worldwide excitement. Roentgen's experiments were confirmed and their significance immediately recognized. Within months systems were being devised to use X rays for diagnosis. This was not surprising, but what was remarkable was that within three years radiation was used in the treatment of cancer. In 1901 Roentgen received the first Nobel Prize awarded in physics.

Radiation therapy began as brachytherapy with radium and as external beam therapy with relatively low-voltage diagnostic machines. It was in France that the major breakthrough took place when it was discovered that delivering radiation over a protracted period of time by use of daily fractions would greatly improve therapeutic response.[18]

"FROM A BIT INOCULATED INTO BREAST MUSCLE OF A SUSCEPTIBLE FOWL"

The nineteenth century had begun with thirteen questions. The twentieth century opened with three important answers: In the short span of 13 years, radiation, viral, and chemical carcinogenesis were clearly demonstrated. These three discoveries changed the entire focus of cancer research.

Radiation was recognized as a carcinogen only seven years after Roentgen's discovery of X rays,[19] and a few years later a relationship to leukemia was recognized.[20] Early workers must have received massive doses of radiation to make the clinical association between radiation and cancer so obvious that it was noticed in such a short time. By comparison, the excess cancer deaths in the Hiroshima and Nagasaki populations were only about 8%, and leukemia was seen at an incidence of only about 1.5 cases per million people per year per rad of dose.[21]

In 1911 Peyton Rous, at the Rockefeller Institute, described a sarcoma in chickens caused by what later became known as the Rous sarcoma virus.[22] He ground up a tumor of chickens and passed it through a paper filter to remove the cells. He then injected this cell-free filtrate into chickens. "From a bit inoculated into the breast muscle of a susceptible fowl there develops rapidly a large firm growth; metastasis takes place to the viscera; and within four weeks the host dies."[22,p.1445] Since neither bacteria nor cells could pass through the filter, the idea that cancer might be caused by a virus was given firm experimental support. A half century later, Rous' virus was the source of the first well-characterized oncogene.

In 1915 cancer was induced in laboratory animals for the first time by coal tar applied to rabbit skin, at Tokyo University by Yamagiwa and Ichikawa.[23] The field of chemical carcinogenesis was launched with a firm scientific foundation and a research technique. This was a century and a half after the most destructive chemical carcinogen known to man, tobacco, was first identified by John Hill, an astute clinician. The aniline dyes had been found to be related epidemiologically to bladder cancer in humans.[24] The first potent synthetic laboratory carcinogen, dibenzanthracene, was discovered in 1930.[25] It was to be many years until we "rediscovered" tobacco as a carcinogen.[26,27,28]

"WE GOT IT ALL"

For the second half of the century of the surgeon, cancer surgery was synonymous with the Halsted radical resection of a cancer and its draining lymph node groups, in the hope of removing the tumor before it spread. The most welcome words a patient could hear after an operation were "We got it all." Radiation therapy was viewed as a means of eradicating local and regional disease that was not resectable by the surgeon. Systemic therapy was virtually nonexistent. The "seed and soil" concept of Paget was forgotten.

Based on several good experiments, cancer was thought to be caused by chemicals or radiation. But the idea was widely held that a single change in the cell somehow transformed it into malignant growth, and this clouded the thinking. Lymph nodes were thought to trap cancer cells, and the notion of regional spread and anatomical containment formed the basis for therapeutic strategy. The clinical behavior of cancer was well understood, but not in modern terms. Progress was held back by the failure to understand multistage carcinogenesis and to grasp the relationship of clonal selection during progression to the metastasis of cancer. A key discovery was made by Peyton Rous.

"THESE TEND TOWARD MALIGNANCY FROM THE BEGINNING AND ATTAIN IT BY A CONTINUOUS SERIES OF ALTERATIONS"

In 1935 Peyton Rous, still at the Rockefeller Institute, was studying the manner in which a benign neoplasm, virus-induced rabbit papilloma, transformed into a malignant lesion. He reported:

> The early stages of the cancerous change cannot be comprehensively described without inclusion of the entire course of events in vigorous papillomas. These tend toward malignancy from the beginning and attain it by a continuous series of alterations. . . . Often the alterations which lead to carcinosis do not stop when malignancy has been achieved, but go further until a state of great anaplasia has been attained. The postcancerous changes appear to be no separate course of events, but only a continuation of what was long since begun. These facts might be taken to indicate that the virus is the immediate cause for the carcinosis; yet they are compatible with the assumption that it merely provides an essential, preliminary cell disturbance.[29,p.537]

In a subsequent paper Rous reported his research with another model of carcinogenesis, the induction of skin cancers by the application of coal tar. It was in this paper that he most clearly defined the difference between what he termed initiation and promotion:

> Tarring provides them with the conditions needed for growth, but after it is discontinued the tumors all more or less gradually disappear unless some other aid is forthcoming. . . . Chloroform has a marked effect to cause latent neoplastic cells to form tumors, as we discovered by accident. Occasionally the external auditory canal of ears long previously painted with methylcholanthrene and still carrying growths became infested with mites. To kill them chloroform was dropped into the canal and in several instances, through a technician's error, it was used for nearly two months and allowed to spread to the surface of the ear. There the skin became swollen and pink and many additional tumors arose and grew rapidly. . . . It seems certain that many agents and influences which have no actual carcinogenicity will be found to stimulate the multiplication of latent neoplastic cells. . . . this is distinct from carcinogenic power.[30,p.111]

These classic experiments, confirmed by Berenblum and Shubik[31] using croton oil as the promoter, formed the prototype for the way carcinogenesis was conceptualized. This led to the concept of *initiation* by one agent followed by *promotion* by another and finally *progression* of the tumor to a more malignant form. The initiator was viewed as able to cause cancer but only after a prolonged time. The promoter was viewed as not capable alone of causing cancer but able to potentiate the effects of the initiator. The term *progression* was said by Rous to designate "the process by which tumors go from bad to worse."[32]

Foulds codified and expanded the concept of multistage carcinogenesis.[33] Progression to the metastatic phenotype has subsequently been well elucidated in modern biological terms by Fidler.[34] Evidence was obtained twenty years after Rous' work indicating that the first stage, *initiation,* is characterized by damage to DNA while the second stage, *promotion,* usually does not involve damage to DNA but, rather, stimulation of cellular proliferation. Promotion is reversible and exhibits a distinct dose-response and measurable threshold, which may be important to smokers who are able to quit. The third stage, *progression,* leads to morphologic change and increased grades of malignant behavior, such as invasion, metastasis, and drug resistance. The highly malignant character that the cancer has attained at the time of diagnosis is the result of progression. In 1966, 55 years after his 1911 paper, Peyton Rous received the Nobel Prize.

"THE CLINICAL RESULTS WERE SOMETIMES DRAMATIC"

The century of the surgeon began in 1846. Fifty years later Roentgen presented his famous lecture on the X ray. Exactly 100 years after the beginning of the century of the surgeon, the first anticancer activity of a chemical was reported. Paul Erlich, the German scientist who discovered Salvarsan for the treatment of syphilis, is called the "father of chemotherapy," but today the term *chemotherapy* is usually applied to cytotoxic agents used in the treatment of cancer. Nitrogen mustard was the first such agent.

Nitrogen mustard was developed by the chemical warfare research division of the U.S. Army in the course of a search for agents more effective than the mustard gas used in World War I. It proved to have remarkable activity against the lymphomas. "Indeed, the results were sometimes dramatic."[35] This agent served as the model for a long series of alkylating agents that killed rapidly proliferating cancer cells by damaging their DNA.

Two years later Sidney Farber of Boston reported the efficacy of aminopterin (the predecessor of methotrexate).[36] Subsequently, Hitchings and Elion developed the antimetabolite 6-mercaptopurine[37] and Charles Heidelberger developed 5-fluorouracil.[38] The era of chemotherapy had begun. The first cure of metastatic cancer was obtained in 1956 by the use of methotrexate in choriocarcinoma.[39] In 1988 Hitchings and Elion received the Nobel Prize.

"CARCINOGENS ARE MUTAGENS"

It was not until 1944 that DNA was demonstrated to be the chemical mediator of heredity.[40] The Nobel Prize-winning discovery of the helical structure of DNA by Watson and Crick followed.[41] Classic work by the Millers had led to the understanding that covalent binding within the cell was essential for carcinogenic activity; and, the active metabolites of carcinogens were later identified as electrophilic reactants that bound to DNA.[42] Carcinogens were found to be converted by a series of metabolic steps into free radicals, that is, compounds with a single unpaired electron that are highly reactive with molecules rich in electrons, such as DNA. Compounds called antioxidants inhibit carcinogenesis because they react with free radicals before the free radicals damage DNA.

A key discovery was made by Ames, who developed a classic assay system to measure carcinogens. The assay, which employs bacteria, is based on the fact that most carcinogens are mutagens, that is, that they damage DNA. The Ames system requires the addition of liver enzymes in order to convert the chemicals to be tested into their active form. The metabolism of a carcinogen leads to the final active chemical, called the proximate carcinogen, that reacts with the DNA.

The Ames assay, of course, identifies only mutagens. And whereas "carcinogens are mutagens,"[43,p.2281] not *all* carcinogens are mutagens and not all mutagens are carcinogens. To prove carcinogenicity, substantially more than merely a positive Ames assay is required. In smokers, for instance, it is possible to directly identify the carcinogen bound to DNA, the so-called hydrocarbon adducts.[44] The proximate carcinogen exerts its effect by mutating DNA directly or by causing errors to be made when the host cell tries to repair the damaged DNA. However, most of the lesions produced by carcinogens are repaired. The best evidence for this is the extraordinary incidence of skin cancer in patients with xeroderma pigmentosum, a disease in which cells are unable to repair DNA damage from ultraviolet light.[45]

Cancer biology was beginning to take form, but, as we shall see, the problems were exceedingly complex. An important next step was to correct the idea of anatomical containment, and this was done in the clinic rather than in the laboratory.

"I'M NOT SAYING IT. THE DATA ARE SAYING IT"

Our recognition of the futility of radical surgery in the management of cancer began with randomized trials in breast cancer and malignant melanoma. Two surgeons, Fisher[46,47] and Veronesi,[48–50] led the way to the overthrow of the classic "cancer operation" by their demonstration that survival in breast cancer and melanoma is independent of the extent of radical resection. The Halsted radical mastectomy was relegated to the ash heap of history and the whole question of the "cancer operation" was thrown open to experimental trial. This not only forced a recognition that our treatment methods must change but, of greater importance, led to the reevaluation of our notion of the anatomical containment of cancer and to an understanding that it is our *biology,* not our anatomy, that restricts cancer spread.

This revolution was not easily accepted. I will always recall Dr. Bernard Fisher's calm response from the podium at a surgical society meeting when an irate questioner challenged his data by almost shouting "You're saying we don't have to remove the lymph nodes to cure the cancer!" Dr. Fisher's answer: "I'm not saying it. The data are saying it."

What was not understood by those for whom anatomy was central to cancer spread was that the cancer cells had spread throughout the body from the time that the first capillaries had been attracted into the growing tumor by angiogenesis factor secreted by the tumor cells. The initial capillary membranes growing into minute tumors are incomplete. Tumor cells spread into the bloodstream from the very beginning, but are unable to establish metastatic deposits because the cells have not yet evolved the capacity to proliferate outside the site of the primary tumor. The most dramatic modern clinical example of this principle occurs when ovarian carcinomatosis is treated by shunting the ascitic fluid and cancer cells into the jugular vein: there are no systemic metastases, even though ovarian cancer cells flow throughout the body in huge numbers.[51]

Rous had observed experimental tumor cells "going from bad to worse," and it is this change that makes metastasis possible, not the breakdown of some anatomical barrier. Time is indeed a factor, as simple clinical experience has long indicated; but the time is required, not to overcome some anatomical containment, but to allow evolution of the cells of the primary tumor into subclones capable of metastatic growth. This is an important distinction because it has implications for alternate therapeutic strategies. Establishing the genetic basis of this biological behavior, however, required the elucidation of the genes that cause cancer, the oncogenes.

"CARCINOGENS, IRRADIATION, AND THE NORMAL AGING PROCESS ALL FAVOR THE PARTIAL OR COMPLETE ACTIVATION OF THESE GENES"

Researchers in chemical carcinogenesis were identifying mutagens, but the target genes of the mutagens were unknown. Virologists were identifying cancer-causing viruses, but the mechanisms of carcinogenesis were obscure. These two separate lines of research were to intersect dramatically.

Increasing numbers of oncogenic viruses were discovered in animal systems. They were originally called *type C viruses* and later *retroviruses,* the latter term applied because they were RNA viruses that were converted to DNA by the enzyme reverse transcriptase. Retroviral DNA is then incorporated into the chromosomes of the infected cell; thus, retroviruses add their genes to the cell and in this way influence the cell's behavior.

Heubner and Todaro focused attention on the word *oncogene* in 1969 when they proposed that RNA viruses somehow placed viral genes in the human genome that were then genetically transmitted:

> It is postulated that the viral information (the virogene), including that portion responsible for transforming a normal cell into a tumor cell (the oncogene), is most commonly transmitted from animal to progeny animal and from cell to progeny cell in a covert form. Carcinogens, irradiation, and the normal aging process all favor the partial or complete activation of these genes.[52]

This was an attempt to identify the targets of carcinogens as retroviral genes inserted into the genome. Their theory was incorrect except in the isolated cell systems, but their notion of the *oncogene* as the target of mutagens persisted.

The basic experiments in retroviral carcinogenesis used animal systems and cell culture systems to demonstrate that the intact virus and isolated genes were able to induce malignant transformation. This allowed the identification of the specific genes of oncogenic viruses that were capable of causing cancer. These genes were called *oncogenes.* A host of retroviruses that caused animal cancers and transformed cells in culture were identified, and each was found to contain an essential cancer-causing gene, which was named after the virus.

Genes are usually designated by a three-letter code in lowercase italics, sometimes preceded by a *v-*, for a viral gene, or a *c-*, for a cellular gene. The abbreviation for the gene often relates to the system in which it was first discovered. Thus, *ras* was discovered in a rat sarcoma, and *sis* was discovered in a simian sarcoma. Some genes, such as *erbB* and Ha-*ras,* have names that do not fit this system exactly. Some authors designate human genes using uppercase italic letters; for example, the human homolog of the animal gene *myc* is sometimes written as *MYC.* Genes are also designated by letters describing the disease in which they were discovered: *RB* for *r*etino*b*lastoma gene, *WT* for *W*ilms' *t*umor gene, *DDC* for *d*eleted in *c*olon *c*ancer, etc. Some writers use the term *proto-oncogene* for a normal gene before it is modified (mutated) to become an oncogene. Other writers use the term *oncogene* as a general term for both the normal and the mutated gene.

Two discoveries led to an understanding of how oncogenes relate to growth factors. It was found that the gene *v-sis* of the simian sarcoma virus coded for a protein that was very similar to platelet-derived growth factor (PDGF),[53,54] which is released by blood platelets in a clot to stimulate scar formation. Second, the gene *v-erbB* of the chicken erythroblastosis virus was found to be very similar to the gene coding for the epidermal growth factor receptor.[55] This provided strong support for the hypothesis that the oncogenes found in retroviruses were the same as the growth factor and growth factor receptor genes found in normal cells.

It is now known that the experimental retroviruses obtain their oncogenes by capture of normal genes from the host cell. The retroviral carcinogenesis experiments did not lead, as was first hoped, to identification of a large number of retroviruses that caused human cancer. Among the human retroviruses, HTLV-1 has been clearly implicated in adult T-cell leukemia/lymphoma

(ATLL), which is a malignancy of mature T4 lymphocytes endemic in Japan, the Caribbean, parts of Africa, and the southeastern United States.[56] Transmission of the virus is by sexual contact or through contaminated blood. The story on the retrovirus HIV in AIDS-related tumors is interesting but not yet complete.[57]

Retroviral oncogene research did, however, allow the identification of many human oncogenes that code for normal growth-promoting substances and improved our understanding of the way in which oncogenes promote normal and neoplastic growth. Oncogenes have been identified for many cell signals in addition to growth factors and growth factor receptors. These include signal amplification and transmission within the cell and signal reception within the nucleus.[58]

We now know that it is the human growth-control genes, first identified as oncogenes in retroviruses, that are the long-sought-after targets of the mutating chemicals and radiation that contribute certain critical lesions leading to human cancer. But mutated oncogenes alone are not sufficient to cause human cancers. Fusing a cancer cell with a normal cell will lead to suppression of malignant growth,[59] indicating that there are genes that suppress growth. These suppressor genes were first demonstrated as the targets of the oncogene products of the DNA viruses.

"THE FIRST DEMONSTRATION OF A PHYSICAL LINK BETWEEN AN ONCOGENE AND AN ANTI-ONCOGENE"[60]

The DNA viruses are involved in several tumors. Unlike the retroviruses, the oncogenes of DNA viruses are not recently captured cellular genes, but their products do react with the products of human genes. The first demonstration of this was the interaction of a protein of adenovirus with the *RB* gene product.[60]

The mechanisms of carcinogenesis by the DNA viruses are more complex than is the case for the retroviruses. Three examples illustrate this complexity. The polyoma virus produces an oncogenic protein that binds to a cellular oncogene protein product (*c-src*). This binding alters the *c-src* protein so that it resembles that of the abnormal protein produced by the retroviral *v-src* of the Rous sarcoma virus. It would seem that the polyoma virus achieves the same end point as the Rous sarcoma virus, but by a different mechanism.

A second example is illustrated by the herpes virus Epstein-Barr (EBV). A characteristic chromosomal translocation is seen in patients with Burkitt's lymphoma that activates the *c-myc* gene located on chromosome 8. This is the same proto-oncogene activated by the chicken myeloid leukemia retrovirus, but the mechanism of activation by the DNA virus is different from that of the retrovirus.

The third example involves three viruses (simian virus 40, papilloma, and adenovirus) all of which transform cells by producing oncogenic proteins that bind to normal cellular proteins and block their function. The function of the affected cellular proteins is to "turn off" cellular proliferation, and they are of very special interest because they are the products of anti-oncogenes (cancer-suppressor genes). It is these cancer-suppressor genes that have recently produced the greatest research excitement.

Work with the oncogenes of the DNA viruses led to discovery of several viruses causing human cancer (as described later) and to a better understanding of normal cellular control mechanisms because the products of DNA oncogenes interacted with and blocked the action of normal growth-regulating cellular proteins.

"GENES I HAVE CALLED ANTI-ONCOGENES"[61]

Oncogenes code for proteins that induce malignant growth by "turning on" cell division. There are proteins with an opposite function, to "turn off" cell growth. These suppressor proteins were discovered because the oncogenic DNA viruses had oncogenes whose products bound to and inactivated them. Since the genes coding for these proteins had a function opposite to that of oncogenes, they were called anti-oncogenes; and because they suppressed malignant growth, they were also called cancer-suppressor genes. The absence of the protein product of one of these genes leads to a cell in which the effect of a growth-promoting factor goes unopposed. It is thought that most human cancers result from a combination of genetic changes that must include both the absence of the protein products of cancer-suppressor genes and the presence of abnormal products of oncogenes.

It is likely that for each "up-regulating" function coded by an oncogene there is a balancing "down-regulating" function coded by a cancer-suppressor gene. For example, to balance the protein kinases that activate molecules by phosphorylation, there exists a set of protein phosphorylases that inactivate the same molecule by dephosphorylation.[62–64] This down-regulating anti-oncogene system is at least as complicated as the up-regulating oncogene system, and it is only beginning to be understood.

The scientific basis for our understanding of this mechanism was laid in 1971 when Alfred Knudson argued, on the basis of a statistical model, that one of the two mutations required for the development of familial retinoblastoma was inherited and the second occurred in the retinal cells of the affected eye. In the nonheritable form, both mutations occurred in the same cell after birth, with neither mutation being inherited.[65] The gene has been identified on chromosome 13 and named the retinoblastoma gene (*RB*). The inheritance is dominant, but both copies of the gene must be absent or damaged for a cell to be transformed, so we know that the function of the gene is to *prevent* malignant growth. Proof of this is that when the retinoblastoma gene is introduced into cultured retinoblastoma cells, the malignant growth pattern is suppressed.[66]

Transcription factors are proteins that bind specifically to DNA and initiate expression of a set of genes controlled by the binding site. The *myc* oncogene produces a transcription factor that stimulates cell division. The *RB* anti-oncogene product binds to the *myc* oncogene product and blocks its action, which is presumed to be a normal physiological control function since mutant *RB* protein does *not* bind *myc* protein.[67] The conclusion is that the protein product of the *RB* anti-oncogene down-regulates cell division by binding to a growth-stimulating normal cellular protein.[68–70] In tumor cells, presumably, the failure of the mutant *RB* protein to bind the *myc* or another transcription factor contributes to transformation.

RB protein is regulated by the master cell cycle control enzyme cdc2 kinase.[71] As a suppressor of cell division, the *RB* gene product competes with stimulating factors, such as cyclin A, for the same transcription factors.[72] When the *RB* gene is mutated, its normal suppression of cell division is absent, thus allowing neoplastic growth.[73] *RB* is commonly mutated in several human cancers, although it was first discovered in retinoblastoma.

"THERE ARE TOO MANY MUTATIONS IN HUMAN CANCERS"

As human cancers were being studied for mutations of the oncogenes and cancer-suppressor genes, it became clear that the number of such mutations was exceedingly large in all human tumors—too large, in fact, to be explained by the simple action of carcinogens on human cells:

> The dilemma is that there are too many mutations in human tumors. . . . The spontaneous mutation rate in somatic cells is not sufficient to account for these multiple mutations. If the multiple mutations in tumors are causally associated with and not just an accompaniment of cancer, then I argue that an early step in tumor progression is one that induces a mutator phenotype.[74,p.3075]

How is this mutator phenotype produced? One of the most important of the cancer-suppressor genes, and the one that appears to be the most commonly altered in human cancer, is the gene located at chromosome 17p13 coding for a protein designated p53.[75] The p53 gene is the most frequently mutated gene in human cancer, being altered in as many as half of the common neoplasms.[76–78] This gene codes for a transcription factor that, in the form of a dimer or tetramer, binds specifically[79] to DNA and mediates RNA synthesis. Originally identified in cells transformed by simian virus 40 and thought to be an oncogene product because mutant forms exerted a dominant transforming effect on cells, p53 has finally been recognized as a cancer-suppressor gene product. Addition of the p53 gene to cultures of prostate cancer suppresses malignant growth.[80]

"THE GUARDIAN OF THE GENOME"

The p53 cancer-suppressor gene is the most important one so far discovered. Not only is it the most frequently mutated, but when it is not mutated, as is the case in some sarcomas, there is another abnormal gene activated that blocks the p53 protein.[81]

What is the normal function of p53? Several observations provide clues. When cellular DNA is damaged by radiation or chemotherapeutic drugs, p53 protein accumulates and the cells are arrested in G1 so that they do not enter mitosis until the DNA is repaired.[82,83] When normal p53 genes are inserted into cancer cells, they may induce programmed cell death (apoptosis).[84,85] There is a cancer family syndrome, the Li-Fraumini syndrome, in which p53 is inherited in mutant form, and a cancer-prone strain of mice has been developed with a mutated p53 gene. Such patients and such mice develop normally, suggesting that p53 has no role in normal cell development; but these patients and mice are at high risk of developing many different forms of cancer, and fibroblasts from patients with the Li-Fraumini syndrome are genetically unstable.[86,87] These observations suggest that the protein product of p53 is the "guardian of the genome."[88,p.15] Its normal function may be to detect the presence of damaged DNA and arrest the cell cycle in G1 until the damage is repaired, or if not repaired to induce cell suicide (apoptosis).

This hypothesis is consistent with the known observations regarding p53. DNA viruses must knock out p53 in order to move the cell into S phase, which they need for their own replication; thus, DNA viruses produce proteins that inactivate the p53 protein. It explains why inherited mutant p53 allows normal development but predisposes to an increased risk of malignancy. It explains the very high rate of mutation of cancer cells that seems to be essential to the evolution of enough abnormal clones to promote transformation. Finally, it explains the susceptibility of cancer cells to radiation and chemotherapy, because since cancer cells often have mutant p53 they are unable to arrest in G1 to repair DNA damage done by treatment.

EXAMPLES OF HUMAN TUMOR CARCINOGENESIS

Our understanding of human carcinogenesis is far from complete, yet it is possible to identify several carcinogenic mechanisms in man. Human carcinogenesis is usually classified as familial, viral, physical, and chemical, but most common human tumors probably result from a combination of these factors rather than from just one. Cancer results when there are enough injuries to the delicate and complex genetic machinery regulating cell proliferation so that a rapidly growing clone emerges with the high mutation rate necessary to allow progression to invasion and metastasis. We understand some of these principles and have identified some of the mutagens and genes involved.

Tobacco, of course, is our principle mutagen, and is responsible for over a third of all cancer deaths. In adenocarcinoma of the lung the *K-RAS* proto-oncogene is mutated.[89] There is evidence of inheritance of a susceptibility to lung cancer accounting for as many as half of cases before age 60 and up to a fifth of all lung cancers.[90] Asbestos exposure greatly multiplies the effect of smoking,[91] and radon in the home contributes to a degree yet to be determined because the level of exposure is not yet known.[92] Many commonly mutated genes have been identified in lung cancer: Mutations of p53 are seen early in half of non–small-cell cancer; all small-cell cancers lose the *RB* gene; *L-MYC* is commonly amplified in small-cell cancer; and, many other gene changes are seen.[93,94] Thus, carcinogenesis in this common cancer results from mutations of oncogenes and cancer-suppressor genes by chemical agents (in tobacco smoke), physical agents (radon and asbestos), and familial factors.

In the case of colon cancer we have a better knowledge of the sequential genetic changes that take place than for lung cancer, but our understanding of the mutagens is far less precise. The work of Vogelstein at Johns Hopkins has provided the best insight so far into the pathogenesis of colon cancer. A sequence of events is required for carcinogenesis and progression. The complete sequence involves more than five steps. A gene at 5q21 called mutated in colorectal cancer (*MCC*) is mutated in a substantial number of colorectal cancers.[95] A second gene in the same location, adenomatous polyposis coli (*APC*), is mutated in a substantial number of spontaneous colorectal cancers and in all individuals with familial polyposis.[96] One of these genes is altered as the first step in colorectal carcinogenesis, leading to increased cell proliferation and polyp formation. The next step is presumed to involve demethylation of DNA, a nongenetic change that alters DNA function. The third step is mutation of the *K-RAS* gene on 12p. Next there is a loss of a gene called deleted in colorectal cancer (*DCC*), located on 18q.[97] Finally, there is a mutation of the gene for p53 located at 17p, leading to genetic instability and progression to frank malignancy with invasion and metastasis.[98] Addition of normal chromosomes 5 and 18 to colon cancer cell cultures reverses malignant growth.[99] The mutagens responsible for these changes are unknown but may be related to diet.

Familial Cancer

Sometimes defective genes are inherited. Hereditary retinoblastoma results when a child inherits a defective retinoblastoma gene and analysis of chromosome 13 has revealed that the chromosome lost during tumorigenesis is the one from the nonaffected parent, whereas the one retained is from the affected parent,[100] proving dominant inheritance. Both the proliferative disease predisposing to breast cancer and early-onset breast cancer are inherited.[101,102] There is a familial aggregation in 13% of breast cancers.[103] Breast cancer seems to segregate as an autosomal dominant. A familial syndrome of multiple cancers, the Li-Fraumini syndrome, results from inheritance of a defective p53 gene.[104]

Ample evidence for a heritable predisposition to cancer is provided by Fanconi's anemia, ataxia-telangiectasia, xeroderma pigmentosum, Wilms' tumor, neurofibromatosis, the dysplastic nevus syndrome, familial polyposis coli (FPC), the cancer family syndrome (CFS), multiple endocrine neoplasia syndromes (MEN I, MEN II, MEN III), and several other heritable cancers.[105] Most inherited cancer syndromes behave as autosomal dominants. These syndromes are, however, rather rare. Colon cancer, to a lesser degree, provides evidence of a familial pattern.

Viral Carcinogenesis

The one clearly established human tumor due to a retrovirus is human T lymphoma/leukemia due to the HTLV-1. A small proportion of patients with Sezary syndrome and mycosis fungoides also have evidence of HTLV-1. Hairy cell leukemia is a disease of B-lymphocytes for the most part. But a small portion of the cases involve T-lymphocytes, and here HTLV-2 has been isolated.

There are several tumors associated with DNA viruses. Human papillomaviruses (HPV) infect squamous epithelium. There are many strains, some of which cause the common human wart. A transforming oncogene protein has been shown to bind specifically to the product of the retinoblastoma gene.[106] HPV causes genital warts, which are, like cervical cancer, associated with promiscuity. DNA from strain HPV-16 or HPV-18 is found in 70% of all cervical carcinomas. Thus, there are strong data supporting an etiological role for some strains of HPV in cervical cancer. To a lesser extent there are associations with all genital cancer, including cancers of the anus, the penis, and the prostate.

Hepatitis B virus (HBV) is endemic in Asia and Africa and is etiological in hepatocellular carcinoma (HCC).[107] In China alone almost a million cases of HCC occur annually. There may be other factors that increase risk, such as aflatoxin, to which there are heavy exposures. Aflatoxin is mutagenic for the p53 cancer-suppressor gene, and in Africa and Asia most of the hepatomas show p53 mutations of codon 249.[108,109]

The Epstein-Barr virus (EBV) causes infectious mononucleosis in the United States and Burkitt's lymphoma (BL) in Africa. It infects B-lymphocytes and stimulates their proliferation. If host immunity is intact, a T-lymphocyte response is generated against an EBV protein expressed on the B-cell membrane and the proliferating B-cells are brought under control. In Africa, for some reason, perhaps because of the effect of chronic malaria on the immune system, a B-cell clone may emerge uncontrolled, leading to BL. The mechanism involves the *c-myc* oncogene, which is activated by a transposition with genes necessary for antibody synthesis. An inherited immune deficiency has been described that is X-linked in which EBV induces a polyclonal lymphoma.[110] Patients with AIDS and patients immunosuppressed for organ transplantation are also at risk for BL associated with EBV in about half the cases. Hodgkin's disease is also associated with EBV in about half of the cases.[111,112]

The Chinese, no matter where they live, are at increased risk for nasopharyngeal carcinoma. Their tumors are associated in 100% of cases with the EBV genome within the tumor cell. There are other causes of this tumor in other races, but the Chinese seem to have a unique association with EBV. The EBV genome is actively transcribed in these tumors in the same way as in latently infected lymphocytes,[113] providing strong evidence for an etiological role.

Physical Carcinogens

Physical carcinogens exert their action on genes by physical rather than chemical means. In some cases the nature of the reaction is known, as, for example, with ionizing radiation, which releases sufficient energy to alter DNA. In other cases the mechanism is obscure, as, for example, with asbestos, which may act as a promoter by an as-yet-unknown method.

Ultraviolet radiation (UV) from the sun damages DNA, causing pyrimidine dimer formation that if not properly repaired leads to mutations. Basal cell and squamous cell carcinomas of the exposed areas of the skin are the result, and these tumors are very common—nearly a half million cases each year. Melanoma, also, is linked to ultraviolet exposure, though not as tightly linked as basal and squamous cancers. The most dramatic example of UV carcinogenesis is seen in patients with xeroderma pigmentosum, an autosomal recessive disease in which DNA repair of UV damage is defective.[114] These patients have a very high incidence of skin cancer, including melanoma. In basal cell carcinomas the p53 gene is often mutated, suggesting that this is a target for UV.[115]

In the United States, an individual's average annual exposure to radiation from all sources is 360 mrem, 82% of this from natural sources.[116] It is estimated that about 3% of all cancer deaths are due to natural radiation (excluding radon). Recent interest has focused on radon, for which the home seems to be the major exposure site. There appear to be substantial geographic variations influencing radon dose. Too little is known about radon doses at present to draw firm conclusions or to make useful recommendations as to prevention, but estimates are that radiation from natural radon contributes about 10% of the lung cancer deaths, bringing total cancer deaths due to natural radiation to approximately 5%.[117]

The risk of medical radiation exposure has probably been exaggerated. Mammography has raised particular public concern. The new techniques provide very low exposures to the breast. Present recommendations of the American Cancer Society for mammography seem reasonable, and are likely to save many more lives than are placed at risk by the very low level of radiation.

Asbestos, a carcinogenic fiber, is thought to be related in the United States to about 2000 cases of mesothelioma annually. Although identified with this rare tumor, asbestos actually causes more bronchogenic cancers, perhaps 6000, because of the synergism between tobacco smoke and asbestos. Lung cancer is rare in asbestos workers who do not smoke.[118] Physical properties such as crystal type and particle size play a major role in the physical carcinogenic properties of asbestos, and only certain forms of asbestos increase the risk of mesothelioma.

Chemical Carcinogens

In spite of the vast array of chemicals discovered to cause cancer in animals, there still remain very few chemicals (other than tobacco) for which there is strong evidence of cancer causation in man. Occasional industrial chemicals have been documented, such as 2-naphthylamine, vinyl chloride, metals, and benzene. But after extensive study, the best estimate is that only 4% of all cancer deaths in America are due to occupational causes.[119]

Aflatoxin is a mutagen for p53, and it is assumed, though not clearly established, that certain bile salts metabolized by colonic bacteria are associated with the mutations leading to colon cancer. Chemotherapeutic agents, of course, are mutagenic and are clearly associated with subsequent development of cancer, especially leukemia and myeloproliferative syndromes. Cyclophosphamide is associated with an increase in bladder cancer.

CONTROVERSIES IN CARCINOGENESIS

Estrogens and Carcinogenesis

One of the most controversial topics in carcinogenesis is the role of estrogens. Animal models and human studies have clearly shown that estrogen is necessary for breast cancer development. There are two practical questions. First, does postmenopausal estrogen replacement therapy increase breast cancer risk? And second, does oral contraceptive use increase breast cancer risk?

A host of case control studies have provided copious data to support either a yes or no answer to the first question. The only controlled randomized trial, however, showed that after ten years the placebo group had more breast cancer than the group treated with hormone replacement.[120] In view of the known benefits of postmenopausal estrogen in the prevention of osteoporosis and reduction of cardiovascular risk by up to half,[121] any decision as to a contraindication of estrogen based on a theoretical or poorly documented breast cancer risk must be carefully evaluated. It is likely that replacement therapy has a weak effect, if any, and does not substantially alter breast cancer incidence, although an association with endometrial cancer seems well established.[122]

The effect of contraceptives in breast cancer risk, likewise, is controversial and not clearly established, with most of the studies showing no relationship.[121,122] It is possible that long-term use before the first pregnancy may increase risk,[123] and this is obviously an important question to answer because this is a frequent pattern of use. At present the issue is unresolved, although the preponderant opinion is that contraceptives are safe.

Involuntary (Passive) Smoking

Cullen reviews the evidence for passive, or involuntary, smoking as etiological in lung cancer.[124] There are insufficient data to allow a firm conclusion, but spousal exposure provides some information. Lung cancer mortality may be about one-third higher in spouses of smokers than in spouses of nonsmokers. This has served as the basis for estimates that exposure of nonsmokers in proximity to smokers may account for up to 20% of nonsmoker lung cancer deaths each year, or about 2400 deaths. The sex of the spouse may be a factor, since, according to a report by the Surgeon General,[125] one-half pack of cigarettes per day increases mortality ratios for women by about 30%–80% and for men about fourfold to ninefold, indicating that males seem to be more sensitive.

Environmental Carcinogenesis

Perhaps the most popular subject for the lay press is environmental carcinogenesis. The term *environmental* is subject to a great deal of confusion. Its original use was intended to include all cancers that were not hereditary, that is, all cancers due to viruses, lifestyle, tobacco, diet, and a host of other causes. It is often stated that 85% of cancer is environmental; this has been misinterpreted by the layperson to mean contaminated air, water, and food. Often it has been further limited in the media to exclude natural carcinogens in our environment so that the focus has been on man-made chemicals. This has led to the mistaken notion that we can virtually eliminate cancer if we identify man-made cancer-causing chemicals in the air we breathe, the water we drink, and the food we eat, and rid our environment of them.

Such a notion is incorrect. Ames has described what he believes are the mistaken assumptions made by those who argue that environmental pollutants represent our highest priority in cancer prevention.[126] He points out the danger of focusing our attention on trivial or nonexistent dangers at the cost of diverting our attention from very real dangers. There are over a half a million deaths each year from tobacco and alcohol, a statistic that dwarfs the insignificant number of deaths resulting from the pollutants we see emphasized so much in the media.

A preferred interpretation of *environmental* would refer to our *personal* environment or, in popular terminology, to our lifestyle. It is the food we eat, the alcohol we drink, the tobacco we smoke that, more than all other factors, have increased our risk of cancer. The enemy is not the chemical plant down the street, but ourselves. Tobacco is directly related to over a third of the cancer deaths. If tobacco-caused cancers are excluded, the death rate from cancer is not increasing; it is, in fact, decreasing.

Diet and Carcinogenesis

In Japan, stomach cancer is common and cancers of the colon and the breast uncommon. When Japanese move to the United States they rapidly develop our pattern of common colon cancer and uncommon stomach cancer. Several generations later they develop our pattern of common breast cancer. This has become a classic epidemiologic observation, and most investigators assume the explanation is diet. There is a striking correlation between the amount of fat a nation consumes and the incidence of colon cancer and breast cancer and a similar correlation between meat consumption and colon cancer.[127] There has been an inability to provide individual, as compared to national, statistics relating breast cancer to fat intake. This has led to a wide acceptance that the relationship is not to fat but to total calories, and especially to total calories consumed early in life. The delay of several generations in the rise of breast cancer incidence among Japanese migrants suggests that the issue is more complex than diet alone.

The role of fat in colon cancer is supported by both the rapid change in incidence with dietary change and the potential relationship of fat consumption to bile acids, which are known to be mutagenic. The improved diet in Japan since 1945 has been associated with an increase in colon cancer but not yet an increase in breast cancer. The well-documented relationship of meat to colon cancer likely reflects animal fat consumption. The role of fiber in colon cancer has been postulated to relate to altered transit time, altered bacterial flora in the colon, and altered exposure of the colonic mucosa to carcinogenic bacterially modified bile acids. Epidemiological studies have suggested an inverse relationship between dietary fiber and colon cancer, and animal studies suggest that the type of fiber may be important.[128] Human studies have shown that wheat bran and cellulose, but not oat bran, are associated with lower stool mutagens by the Ames assay and reduced secondary bile acids.[129]

Stomach cancer has been suggested to be related to the intake of food that is cured, smoked, pickled, salted, or otherwise preserved, but not refrigerated. Some special methods of food preparation have also been incriminated. Lifelong use of refrigeration seems particularly important in reducing the incidence of stomach cancer.[130]

The nature of the effect of fruits and vegetables is unclear. There has been speculation that the antioxidant effect of vitamin C might play a role, but this has not been well established. Many food preservatives have an antioxidant effect and may actually antagonize possible carcinogens, such as nitrites. Alcohol has been well documented as a risk factor in head and neck cancer and more recently incriminated in breast cancer,[131] although this observation is controversial.

Doll and Peto have suggested that perhaps a third of all cancers could be explained by dietary factors.[132] They suggest that up to 50% of breast cancer and 90% of colon cancer in the United States could be prevented by a change in diet. However, these are gross estimates with a very wide range. While there may be a strong dietary relationship, radical dietary changes would be required early in life to effect substantial reductions in cancer incidence. It is difficult to prescribe a reasonable diet that is certain to reduce cancer incidence. Nonetheless, a diet rich in fruits, fiber, and cruciferous vegetables and low in animal fat is desirable for many health reasons and may perhaps reduce the risk of cancer.

SUMMARY

In the process of carcinogenesis, mutant clones progress by natural selection through ever-greater stages of virulence. Carcinogens mutate two types of genes that regulate growth: oncogenes that code for growth factors that cause proliferation, and cancer-suppressor genes that code for growth suppressors that suppress proliferation. Although it is customary to divide carcinogenesis into stages, these stages are hard to distinguish in humans, and carcinogenesis is best viewed as a process involving many steps, each of which activates an oncogene or inactivates a cancer-suppressor gene.

The carcinogens that damage genes are ordinarily classified as chemical, viral, or physical, but inherited factors must also be considered. Human carcinogenesis for the common cancers involves combinations of all mechanisms. Most precise data come from animals but cannot be directly extrapolated to humans, because different metabolic systems cause chemicals carcinogenic for one species to be noncarcinogenic for another. Epidemiology provides a better guide for humans, but is less precise.

In spite of the vast array of chemicals discovered to cause cancer in animals, there remain very few chemicals (other than tobacco) for which there is strong evidence of cancer causation in humans. Occupational exposures probably account for only 4% of cancers in America. A number of inherited cancer syndromes have been identified. But most are rare, and for the common cancers (lung, colon, and breast), the syndromes are not distinct.

Physical carcinogens damage the same genes that chemicals attack. Skin cancers of sun-exposed areas are the result of ultraviolet radiation. In the United States most exposure to ionizing radiation is from natural sources. Asbestos, the major carcinogenic fiber, is related to about 2000 cases of mesothelioma annually and lung cancers in smokers. The potential for prevention of cancer induced by physical agents is actually greatest for stopping smoking, since asbestos acts synergistically with tobacco smoke.

A small number of cancers are viral in origin. There is strong evidence for an etiological relationship of hepatitis B virus with hepatoma, for HTLV-I with T-cell lymphoma, and for human papillomavirus with cervical and anal cancer. The Epstein-Barr virus is probably etiological in Burkitt's lymphoma, lymphoma in Western countries in the presence of an immunodeficiency state, nasopharyngeal carcinoma among Chinese, and Hodgkin's disease.

Carcinogenesis is a controversial topic, especially in regard to estrogens, passive smoking, medical X ray exposure, radon, and diet. The data are conflicting, but the preponderance of opinion is that estrogens, as currently used, are safe. The data on passive smoking and lung cancer are insufficient to allow a firm conclusion, but some investigators believe that spousal exposure may account for up to 20% of nonsmoker lung cancer deaths. Radon levels in the home have become a major public concern, but presently too little is known to draw firm conclusions.

Diet is undoubtedly related to cancer, as demonstrated by differences between incidence rates in different countries, but radical dietary changes would be required early in life to effect substantial reductions in incidence. Nonetheless, a diet rich in fruits, fiber, and cruciferous vegetables and low in animal fat is desirable for many health reasons and may modestly reduce the risk of cancer.

Perhaps the most popular subject for the lay press is "environmental" carcinogenesis. The term *environmental* is confusing, because it leads to the notion that we can prevent cancer by eliminating a few chemicals from the environment. A preferred interpretation would refer to our *personal* environment, that is, our lifestyle. It is the food we eat, the alcohol we drink, and the tobacco we smoke that, more than anything else, increase our risk of cancer. The enemy is not the chemical plant down the street, but our own habits. Tobacco is the cause of a third of all cancer deaths. The paradox of carcinogenesis is simply this: Lung cancer is the most common, the most deadly, and the most *preventable* of all cancers in the United States.

REFERENCES

1. Shimkin MB: *Contrary to Nature,* DHEW Publication No. (NIH) 76-720, Washington, DC, 1977.
2. Redmond DE Jr: Hill cautions against snuff in 1761. *N Engl J Med* 282:18–23, 1970.
3. Pott P: Chirurgical Observations Relative to the Cataract, ye Polypus of the Nose, the Cancer of the Scrotum, the Different Kinds of Ruptures, and the Mortification of the Toes and Feet. London: Hawkes, Clarke, and Collins, 1775.
4. Shimkin MB: Thirteen questions: Some historical outlines for cancer research. *J Natl Cancer Inst* 19:295–328, 1957.
5. Virchow R: *Cellular Pathology.* Translated from the second edition by Frank Chance. London: John Churchill, 1860.
6. Triolo VA: Nineteenth century foundations of cancer research. Advances in tumor pathology, nomenclature, and theories of oncogenesis. *Cancer Res* 25:75–106, 1965.
7. Lyons AS, Petrucelli RJ: *Medicine, An Illustrated History.* New York: H.N. Abrams Publishers, 1978, pp. 527–532.
8. Thorwald J: *The Century of the Surgeon.* New York: Pantheon, 1956.
9. Baly M: *As Miss Nightingale Said.* London: Scutari Press, 1991.
10. Handley WS: The pathology of melanotic growths in relation to their operative treatment. *Lancet* 1:927–933, 1907.
11. Halsted WS: The results of radical operations for the cure of carcinoma of the breast. *Ann Surg* 46:1–19, 1907.
12. Paget S: The distribution of the secondary growths in cancer of the breast. *Lancet* 1:571–573, 1889.
13. Fiddler IJ, Hart IR: Biological diversity in metastatic neoplasms: Origins and implications. *Science* 217:998–1003, 1982.
14. Beatson GT: On the treatment of inoperable cases of carcinoma of the mamma: Suggestions for a new method of treatment with illustrative cases. *Lancet* 2:104–107, 1896.
15. Huggins CB, Hodges CV: Studies on prostatic cancer, I: The effect of castration, of estrogen, and of androgen injection on serum phosphatase in metastatic carcinoma of the prostate. *Cancer Res* 1:293–297, 1941.
16. Huggins CB: Endocrine-induced regression of cancers. *Science* 156:1050–1054, 1967.
17. Roentgen WC: Uber eine neue Art von Strahlen. *Sitzungsber. phys.-med, Gesellsch. Wurzb* 132–141j, 1895.
18. Coutard H: Roentgen therapy of epitheliomas of the tonsillar region, hypopharynx, and larynx from 1920 to 1926. *Am J Roentgenol* 28:313–331, 1932.
19. Frieben A: Demonstration lines cancroids des rechten Handruckens, das sich nach langdauernder Einwirkung von Roentgenstrahlen entwichelt hatte. *Fortschr Geb Roentgenstr* 6:106, 1902.
20. von Jagic N, Scwarz G, von Siebenrock L: Blutbefunde bei Roentgenologon. *Berl Klin Wochenschr* 48:1220–1222, 1911.
21. Preston DL, Kato H, Kopecky KJ, et al: Studies on the mortality of A-bomb survivors: 8. Cancer mortality, 1950–1982. *Radiat Res* 111:151–178, 1987.
22. Rous P. Transmission of a malignant new growth by means of a cell-free filtrate. *JAMA* 56:198, 1911. (Reprinted *JAMA* 250:1445–1446, 1983.)
23. Yamagiwa K, Ichikawa K: Experimentelle Studie uber die Pathogenese der Epitheliageschwulste. *Mitteilungen Med Facultat Kaiserl Univ Tokyo* 15:295, 1915.
24. Rehn L; Blasengeschwulste bei Fuchsin-Arbeitern. *Arch Klin Chir* 50:588, 1895.
25. Kennaway EL, Hieger I: Carcinogenic substances and their fluorescence spectra. *Br J Med* 1:1044, 1930.
26. Wynder EL, Graham EA: Tobacco smoking as a possible etiologic factor in bronchiogenic carcinoma: A study of 684 proved cases. *JAMA* 143:329–336, 1950.
27. Doll R, Hill AB: Smoking and carcinoma of the lung: Preliminary report. *Br Med J* 2:739–748, 1950.
28. Levin ML, Goldstein H, Gerhardt PR: Cancer and tobacco smoking: A preliminary report. *JAMA* 143:336–338, 1950.
29. Rous P, Beard JW: The progression to carcinoma of virus-induced rabbit papillomas (Shope). *J Exptl Med* 62:523–548, 1935.
30. Friedewald WF, Rous P: The initiating and promoting elements in tumor production: An analysis of the effects of tar, benzpyrene, and methylcholanthrene on rabbit skin. *J Exptl Med* 80:101–125, 1944.
31. Berenblum I, Shubik P: The role of croton oil applications associated with a single painting of a carcinogen in tumor induction of the mouse's skin. *Br J Cancer* 1:379–382, 1947.
32. Rous P, Kidd JG: Conditional neoplasms and subthreshold neoplastic states. *J Exp Med* 73:365–389, 1941.
33. Foulds L: The experimental study of tumor progression. A review. *Cancer Res* 14:327–339, 1954.
34. Fidler IJ: The evolution of biological heterogeneity in metastatic neoplasms. In Nicolson GL and Milas L, eds. *Cancer Invasion and Metastasis: Biologic and Therapeutic Aspects.* New York: Raven Press, 1984.
35. Goodman LS, Wintrobe MW, Dameshek W, et al: Nitrogen mustard therapy. *JAMA* 132:126–132, 1946. (Reprinted *JAMA* 251:2255–2261, 1984.)
36. Farber S, Diamond LK, Mercer RD, et al: Temporary remissions in acute leukemia in children produced by

folic acid antagonist 4-aminopteroylglutamic acid (aminopterin). *N Eng J Med* 238:787–793, 1948.
37. Elion GB: The purine path to chemotherapy. *Science* 244:41–47, 1989.
38. Heidelberger C: Fluorinated pyrimidines, a new class of tumor inhibitory compounds. *Nature* 179:663–666, 1957.
39. Li MC, Hertz R, Spencer DB: Effect of methotrexate therapy upon choriocarcinoma and chorioadenoma. *Proc Soc Exptl Biol Med* 93:361–366, 1956.
40. Avery OT, McCarty M, MacLeod CM: Studies on the chemical nature of the substance inducing transformation of pneumococcal types; induction of transformation by desoxyribonucleic acid fraction from pneumococcus type III. *J Exper Med* 79:137–158, 1944.
41. Watson JD, Crick FHC: Molecular structure of nucleic acids. A structure for desoxyribose nucleic acid. *Nature* 171:737–738, 1953.
42. Miller EC: Some current perspectives on chemical carcinogenesis in humans and experimental animals: Presidential Address. *Cancer Res* 38: 1479–1496, 1978.
43. Ames BN, Durston WE, Yamasaki E, et al: Carcinogens are mutagens: A simple test system combining liver homogenates for activation and bacteria for detection. *Proc Natl Acad Sci USA* 70:2281, 1973.
44. Perera FP, Weinstein IB: Molecular epidemiology and carcinogen-DNA adduct detection: New approaches to studies of human cancer causation. *J Chronic Dis* 35: 581–600, 1982.
45. Fry RJM: Principles of carcinogenesis: Physical. In DeVita VT Jr, Hellman S, and Rosenberg SA (eds). *Cancer: Principles and Practice of Oncology.* Philadelphia: Lippincott, 1989.
46. Fisher B, Redmond C, Fisher ER, et al: Ten-year results of a randomized clinical trial comparing radical mastectomy and total mastectomy with or without radiation. *N Engl J Med* 312:674–681, 1985.
47. Fisher B, Bauer M, Margolese R, et al: Five-year results of a randomized clinical trial comparing total mastectomy and segmental mastectomy with or without radiation in the treatment of breast cancer. *N Engl J Med* 312:665–673, 1985.
48. Veronesi U, Valagussa P: Inefficacy of internal mammary node dissection in breast cancer surgery. *Cancer* 47:170–175, 1981.
49. Veronesi U, Adamus J, Bandiera DC, et al: Inefficacy of immediate node dissection in stage 1 melanoma of the limbs. *N Engl J Med* 297:627–630, 1977.
50. Veronesi U, Cascinelli N, Adamus J, et al: Thin stage I primary cutaneous malignant melanoma: Comparison of excision with margins of 1 or 3 cm. *N Engl J Med* 318:1159–1162, 1988.
51. Tarin D, Vass AC, Kettlewell MG, et al: Absence of metastatic sequelae during long-term treatment of malignant ascites by peritoneo-venous shunting. *Invasion Metastas* 4:1–12, 1984.
52. Huebner RJ, Todaro GJ. Oncogenes of RNA tumor viruses as determinants of cancer. *Proc Natl Acad Sci USA* 64:1087–1094, 1969.
53. Waterfield MD, Scrace GT, Whittle N, et al: Platelet-derived growth factor is structurally related to the putative transforming protein p28-sis of simian sarcoma virus. *Nature* 304:35–39, 1983.
54. Doolittle RF, Hunkapiller MW, Hood LE, et al: Simian sarcoma virus onc gene v-sis is derived from the gene (or genes) encoding a platelet-derived growth factor. *Science* 221:275–276, 1983.
55. Xu YH, Ishii AJ, Clark M, et al. Human epidermal growth factor receptor cDNA is homologous to a variety of RNAs overproduced in A431 carcinoma cells. *Nature* 309:806–810, 1984.
56. Poiesz BJ, Ruscetti FW, Gazdar AF, et al. Detection and isolation of type C retrovirus particles from fresh and cultured lymphocytes of a patient with cutaneous T-cell lymphoma. *Proc Natl Acad Sci USA* 77:7415–7419, 1980.
57. Blattner WA: Human retroviruses and malignancy. In Brugge J, Curran T, Harlow E, McCormick F (eds.): *Origins of Human Cancer.* Cold Spring Harbor, NY: Laboratory Press, 1991.
58. Weinberg RA: Oncogenes, tumor-suppressor genes, and cell transformation: Trying to put it all together. In Brugge J, Curran T, Harlow E, McCormick F, (eds.): *Origins of Human Cancer.* Cold Spring Harbor, NY: Laboratory Press, 1991.
59. Pereira-Smith OM, Smith JR. Evidence for the recessive nature of cellular immortality. *Science* 221:964–966, 1983.
60. Whyte P, Buchkovich KJ, Horowitz JM, et al: Association between an oncogene and an anti-oncogene: The adenovirus E1A proteins bind to the retinoblastoma gene product. *Nature* 334:124–129, 1988.
61. Knudson AG: Hereditary cancer: Oncogenes and antioncogenes. *Cancer Res* 45:1437–1443, 1985.
62. Hunter T: Protein-tyrosine phosphatases: The other side of the coin. *Cell* 58:1013–1016, 1989.
63. Marx J: Biologists turn on to "off-enzymes." *Science* 251:744–746, 1991.
64. Shen SH, Bastien L, Posner BI, Chretien P: A protein tyrosine phosphatase with sequence similarity to the SH2 domain of the protein tyrosine kinases. *Nature* 352:736–739, 1991.
65. Knudson A: Mutation and cancer: Statistical study of retinoblastoma. *Proc Natl Acad Sci USA* 68:820, 1971.
66. Huang HJS, Yee JK, Shew JY, et al: Suppression of the neoplastic phenotype by replacement of the RB gene in human cancer cells. *Science* 242:1563–1566, 1988.
67. Rustgi AK, Dyson N, Bernards R: Amino-terminal domains of c-*myc* and N-*myc* proteins mediate binding to the retinoblastoma gene product. *Nature* 352:541–544, 1991.
68. Mihara K, Cao XR, Yen A, et al: Cell-cycle-dependent regulation of phosphorylation of the human retinoblastoma gene product. *Science* 246:1300–1303, 1989.
69. Huang S, Lee WH, Lee EY: A cellular protein that competes with SV40 T antigen for binding to the retinoblastoma gene product. *Nature* 350:160–162, 1991.
70. Bandara LR, La Thangue NB: Adenovirus E1a prevents the retinoblastoma gene product from complexing with a cellular transcription factor. *Nature* 351:494–497, 1991.
71. Wagner S, Green MR: A transcriptional tryst. *Nature* 352:189–190, 1991.
72. Bandara LR, Adamczewski JP, Hunt T, La Thangue NB: Cyclin A and the retinoblastoma gene product complex with a common transcription factor. *Nature* 352:249–251, 1991.
73. Marx J: The cell cycle: Spinning further afield. *Science* 252:1490–1492, 1991.
74. Loeb LA; Mutator phenotype may be required for multistage carcinogenesis. *Cancer Res* 51:3075–3079, 1991.
75. Levine AJ, Momand J, Finlay CA: The p53 tumour-suppressor gene. *Nature* 351:453–456, 1991.
76. Vogelstein B: Cancer. A deadly inheritance. *Nature* 348:681–682, 1990.

77. Hollstein M, Sidransky D, Vogelstein B, Harris CC: p53 mutations in human cancers. *Science* 253:49–53, 1991.
78. Chiba I, Takahashi T, Nau MM, D'Amico D, et al: Mutations in the p53 gene are frequent in primary, resected non-small cell lung cancer. Lung Cancer Study Group. *Oncogene* 5:1603–1610, 1990.
79. Kern SE, Kinzler KW, Bruskin, et al: Identification of p53 as a sequence-specific DNA binding protein. *Science* 252:1708–1711, 1991.
80. Isaacs WB, Carter BS, Ewing CM: Wild-type p53 suppresses growth of human prostate cancer cells containing mutant p53 alleles. *Cancer Res* 51:4716–4720, 1991.
81. Oliner JD, Kinzler KW, Meltzer PS, et al: Amplification of a gene encoding a p53-associated protein in human sarcomas. *Nature* 358:80–83, 1992.
82. Maltzman W, Czyzyk L: UV irradiation stimulates levels of p53 cellular tumor antigen in nontransformed mouse cells. *Mol Cell Biol* 4(9):1689–1694, 1984.
83. Kastan MB, Onyekwere O, Sidransky D, et al: Participation of p53 protein in the cellular response to DNA damage. *Cancer Res* 51(23 Pt 1):6304–6311, 1991.
84. Shaw P, Bovey R, Tardy S, et al: Induction of apoptosis by wild-type p53 in a human colon tumor-derived cell line. *Proc Natl Acad Sci USA* 89(10):4495–4499, 1992.
85. Yonish-Rouach E, Resnitzky D, Lotem J, et al: Wild-type p53 induces apoptosis of myeloid leukaemic cells that is inhibited by interleukin-6. *Nature* 352(6333):345–347, 1991.
86. Donehower LA, Harvey M, Slagle BL, et al: Mice deficient for p53 are developmentally normal but susceptible to spontaneous tumours. *Nature* 356(6366):215–221, 1992.
87. Bischoff FZ, Yim SO, Pathak, S, et al: Spontaneous abnormalities in normal fibroblasts from patients with Li-Fraumeni cancer syndrome: Aneuploidy and immortalization. *Cancer Res* 50(24):7979–7984, 1990.
88. Lane DP: p53, guardian of the genome. *Science* 358:15–16, 1992.
89. Slebos RJC, Hruban RH, Dalesio O, et al. Relationship between K-*ras* oncogene activation and smoking in adenocarcinoma of the human lung. *J Natl Cancer Inst* 83:1024–1027, 1991.
90. Sellers TA, Bailey-Wilson JE, Elston RC, et al: Evidence for mendelian inheritance in the pathogenesis of lung cancer. *J Natl Cancer Inst* 82:1272–1279, 1990.
91. Nicholson WJ, Perbep G, Selikoff IJ: Occupational exposure to asbestos: Population at risk and projected mortality. *Am J Ind Med* 3:258–311, 1987.
92. Perera F, Santella R, Brandt-Rauf P, et al: Molecular epidemiology of lung cancer. In Brugge J, Curran T, Harlow E, and McCormick F, eds. *Origins of Human Cancer.* Cold Spring Harbor, N.Y.: Laboratory Press, 1991.
93. Ihde DC, Minna JD: Non-small cell lung cancer: Part I: Biology, diagnosis, and staging. *Current Problems in Cancer* 15:83–104, 1991.
94. Minna J, Maneckjee R, D'Amico D, et al: Mutations in dominant and recessive oncogenes and the expression of opioid and nicotine receptors in the pathogenesis of lung cancer. In Brugge J, Curran T, Harlow E, McCormick F (eds.): *Origins of Human Cancer.* Cold Spring Harbor, NY: Laboratory Press, 1991.
95. Kinzler KW, Nilbert MC, Vogelstein B, et al: Identification of a gene located at chromosome 5q21 that is mutated in colorectal cancers. *Science* 251:1366–1370, 1991.
96. Nishisho I, Nakamura Y, Miyoshi Y, et al: Mutations of chromosome 5q21 in FAP and colorectal cancer patients. 253:665–669, 1991.
97. Fearon ER, Cho KR, Nigro JM, et al: Identification of a chromosome 18q gene that is altered in colorectal cancers. Science 247:49–56, 1990.
98. Kern SE, Vogelstein B: Genetic alterations in colorectal tumors. In Brugge J, Curran T, Harlow E, McCormick F (eds.): *Origins of Human Cancer.* Cold Spring Harbor, NY: Laboratory Press, 1991.
99. Tanaka K, Oshimura M, Kikuchi R, et al: Suppression of tumorigenicity in human colon carcinoma cells by introduction of normal chromosome 5 or 18. *Nature* 349:340–342, 1991.
100. Cavenee WK, Hansen MF, Nordenskold M, et al: Genetic origin of mutations predisposing to retinoblastoma. *Science* 228:501–503, 1985.
101. Skolnick MH, Cannon-Albright LA, Goldgar DE, et al: Inheritance of proliferative breast disease in breast cancer kindreds. *Science* 250:1715–1720, 1990.
102. Hall JM, Lee MK, Newman B, et al. Linkage of early-onset familial breast cancer to chromosome 17q21. *Science* 250:1684–1689, 1990.
103. Lynch HT, Albano WA, Heieck JJ: Genetics biomarkers and the control of breast cancer. *Cancer Genet Cytogenet* 13:43–92, 1984.
104. Malkin D, Li FP, Strong LC, et al: Germ line p53 mutations in a familial syndrome of breast cancer, sarcomas, and other neoplasms. *Science* 250:1233–1238, 1990.
105. Levine EG, King RA, Bloomfield CD: The role of heredity in cancer. *J Clin Oncol* 7:527–540, 1989.
106. Dyson N, Howley PM, Munger K, Harlow E: The human papilloma virus-16 E7 oncoprotein is able to bind to the retinoblastoma gene product. *Science* 243:934–936, 1989.
107. Beasly RP, Linn CC, Hwang L, et al: Hepatocellular carcinoma and hepatitis B virus: A prospective study of 22,707 men in Taiwan. *Lancet* 2:1129–1133, 1981.
108. Hsu IC, Metcalf RA, Sun T, Welsh JA, et al: Mutational hotspot in the p53 gene in human hepatocellular carcinomas. *Nature* 350:427–428, 1991.
109. Bressac B, Kew M, Wands J, Ozturk M: Selective G-to-T mutations of p53 gene in hepatocellular carcinoma from southern Africa. *Nature* 350:429–431, 1991.
110. Purtilo DT, Sakamoto K, Barnabai V, et al: Epstein-Barr virus induced diseases in boys with the X-linked lymphoproliferative syndrome (XLP): Updates on studies of the registry. *Am J Med* 73:49–56, 1982.
111. Klein G: Epstein-Barr virus-carrying cells in Hodgkin's disease. *Blood* 80:299–301, 1992.
112. Mueller N, Evans A, Harris NL, et al: Hodgkin's disease and Epstein-Barr virus: Altered antibody pattern before diagnosis. *N Eng J Med* 320:689–695, 1989.
113. Pagano JS: Epstein-Barr virus transcription in nasopharyngeal carcinoma. *J Virol* 48:580–590, 1983.
114. Cleaver JE: Defective repair replication of DNA in xeroderma pigmentosum. *Nature* 218:652–656, 1968.
115. Rady, P, Scinicariello F, Wagner R, Tyring SK: p53 mutations in basal cell carcinomas. *Cancer Res* 52:3804–3806, 1992.
116. National Council on Radiation Protection Measurements (NRCP): Ionizing radiation exposure of the population of the United States. NCRP Report No. 93. Bethesda, MD, NCRP, 1987.
117. Darby S: Contribution of natural ionizing radiation to cancer mortality in the United States. In Brugge J, Cur-

ran T, Harlow E, McCormick F (eds.): *Origins of Human Cancer.* Cold Spring Harbor, NY: Laboratory Press, 1991.

118. Mossman BT, Gee JBL: Asbestos-related diseases. *N Engl J Med* 320:1721–1730, 1989.
119. Doll R, Peto R: *The Causes of Cancer.* New York; Oxford University Press, 1981.
120. Nachtigall LE, Nachtigall RD, Beckman EM: Estrogen replacement therapy II. A prospective trial on the relationship of breast cancer and cardiovascular and metabolic problems. *Obstet Gynecol* 54:74–79, 1979.
121. Barrett-Connor E: Postmenopausal estrogen replacement and breast cancer. *N Eng J Med* 321:319–320, 1989.
122. Thomas DB: Do hormones cause breast cancer? *Cancer* 53:595–604, 1984.
123. Pike MC, Henderson BE, Casagrande JT, et al: Oral contraceptive use and early abortion as risk factors for breast cancer in young women. *Br J Cancer* 43:72–76, 1981.
124. Cullen JW: Principles of cancer prevention: Tobacco. In DeVita VT Jr, Hellman S, and Rosenberg SA, (eds.): *Cancer: Principles and Practice of Oncology.* Philadelphia: Lippincott, 1989.
125. US Department of Health and Human Services, Office of Smoking and Health: The Health Consequences of Smoking: Cancer. A Report of the Surgeon General, DHHS Pub No (PHS) 82-50179, 1982.
126. Ames BN: What are the major carcinogens in the etiology of human cancer? Environmental pollution, natural carcinogens, and the causes of human cancer: Six errors. In DeVita VT, Hellman S, Rosenberg SA (eds.): *Important Advances in Oncology 1989.* Philadelphia: Lippincott, 1989.
127. Willett W: The search for the causes of breast and colon cancer. *Nature* 338:389–394, 1989.
128. Wynder EL, Reddy BS: Dietary fat and fiber and colon cancer. *Semin Oncol* 10:264–272, 1983.
129. Reddy B, Engle A, Katsifis S, et al: Biochemical epidemiology of colon cancer: Effect of types of dietary fiber on fecal mutagens, acid, and neutral sterols in healthy subjects. *Cancer Res* 49:4629–4635, 1989.
130. Caggon D, Barker DJP, Cole RB, Nelson M: Stomach cancer and food storage. *JNCI* 81:1178–1182, 1989.
131. Willett WC, Stampfer MJ, Colditz GA, et al: Moderate alcohol consumption and the risk of breast cancer. *N Eng J Med* 314:1174–1180, 1987.
132. Doll R, Peto R: The causes of cancer: Quantitative estimates of available risks of cancer in the United States today. *J Natl Cancer Inst* 66:1191–1308, 1981.

Chapter 3

Differences Between Normal and Cancer Cells

Susan L. Groenwald, RN, MS

INTRODUCTION

The fundamental goals of cancer research are to learn about what factors or events cause a cell to become a cancer cell, how cancer cells differ in appearance and behavior from normal cells, and, ultimately, how that information can be used to prevent and cure cancer. In Chapter 2 a detailed history of scientific inquiry chronicles our understanding of these issues. This chapter is a review of what is known about the features of cancer cells.

RESEARCH MODELS

Limitations of Study of Human Tissues

A technical problem in studying the differences between normal and cancer cells is that researchers cannot be sure in their identification of the normal cell counterparts of human cancer cells. Human tissues are made up of a heterogeneous population of cells, and when the cells in the tissues have been altered by carcinogens, the tissue will represent cells in various stages of differentiation and appearance, making the identification of the cancer cell precursor very difficult. Comparing cancer tissue to the host tissue from which it derived is not the same as comparing a cancer cell to the normal cell from which it came. Therefore, for most human cancers, the normal cellular precursors are not known.

Transformed Cell Models

Because of these limitations, researchers have had to rely on cell culture models. Stable cell lines derived from a variety of animal species are used as the "normal" cell prototypes. For the cancer cell prototype, normal cells derived from normal tissue are established in culture under controlled conditions. The cells all derive from a single cell and are therefore fairly uniform. Further, the environment of these cells can be defined and manipulated. These "cell lines" become permanent or continuous cell lines when they acquire the ability to be propagated indefinitely in tissue culture (see Figure 3-1). These cells can be transformed into cells that behave like malignant cells when they are exposed to

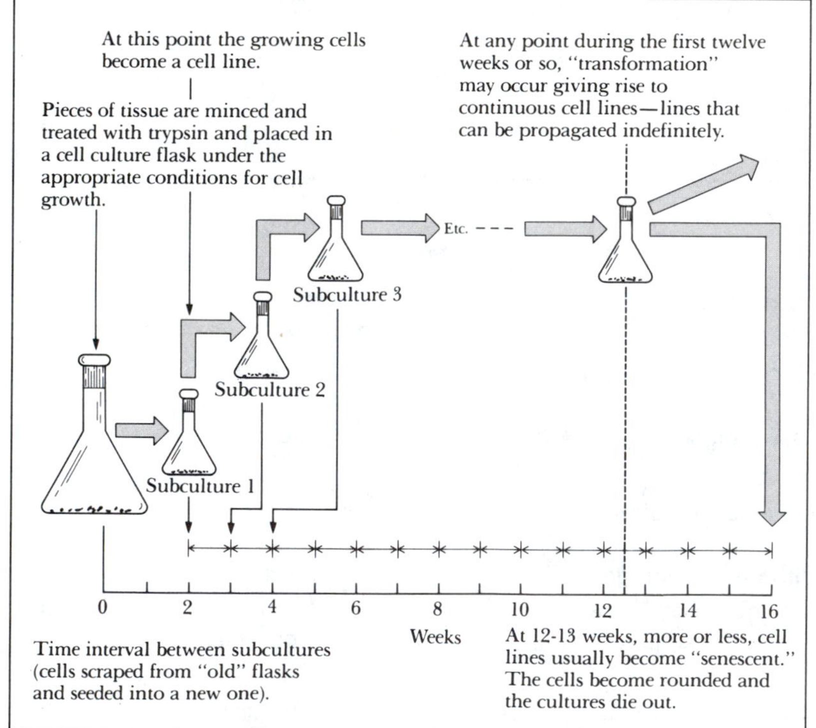

FIGURE 3-1 How cell lines and continuous cell lines are derived. Continuous cell lines arise from normal cells by some kind of spontaneous change or "transformation." Except for their immortality, continuous cell lines behave like normal cells in culture. Transformed cells derive from continuous cell lines that have been exposed to radiation, chemical carcinogens, or oncogenic viruses and subsequently behave like cancer cells. (Source: Kupchells CE: *Dimensions of Cancer.* Belmont, CA: Wadsworth, 1987. Copyright 1987 by Wadsworth, Inc. Used by permission of publisher.)

chemical, viral, or radiation carcinogens.[1] The process is called *transformation,* and the cell lines are called *transformed cells.* Transformed cells are used in research to study differences between normal and cancer cell behavior.

When studying transformation in culture, criteria are required to determine if transformation actually has occurred. The ultimate criterion is whether the cells form a tumor when injected into an animal.[2] Other criteria include reduced requirements for certain nutrients, diminished contact inhibition, altered antigenicity, and the ability to grow unattached to a solid substratum.[3] Not all transformed cell lines exhibit all the characteristics generally found in transformed cells. Two factors—uncontrolled growth and immortality—are observed in all cancer cells.[2]

While transformed cells provide the best model for the study of the differences between normal and malignant cells, the model is not a perfect duplication of what actually occurs in a human being. Thus, problems still arise when experimental models are applied to human cancer. However, for purposes of research and for the discussion that ensues in the following pages, the assumption is made that transformed cells and actual cancer cells share many identical features and that what we have learned about transformed cells can be applied to human cancer.

DIFFERENCES IN GROWTH OF NORMAL AND CANCER CELLS

The primary feature of a cancer cell is its uncontrolled growth. Normal cells are carefully regulated; the number of new cells formed in tissues equals the number lost by cell death or injury. In cancer, cells continue to divide, not necessarily at a faster rate, but continuously and without regard to the needs of the host. In addition, the cancer tissues that develop as a result of the continual replication of cancer cells are without structure and organization.

The average human neoplasm doubles every 2 months. Since the cell cycle time of cancer cells is generally not much different from that of normal cells, this rate of doubling indicates that only a fraction of the cells in a tumor are dividing at any one time. However, the fraction of cells dividing provides a net increase in cells, so in contrast to the balance maintained in normal tissues, in cancer tissues the number of new cells is greater than the number of cells lost, resulting in a tumor mass.

The uncontrolled growth of tumors occurs as a result of several properties of cancer cells: cancer cell immortality, loss of cell-to-cell contact inhibition, diminished serum requirements of cancer cells, the ability of a cancer cell to multiply without being in contact with a surface, and loss of the restriction point.

Immortality of Cancer Cells

Most normal cells are limited to approximately 50–60 generations or divisions before they die. This programmed death is called *senescence,* and its mechanism is unknown. In contrast, cells obtained from cancer tissue do not exhibit this limitation of division and are considered to be immortal. It is thought that cancer cells may lack both the biochemical substances that control cell division and/or the ability to respond to the substances.[4]

Loss of Contact Inhibition

When normal cells are placed in a culture dish containing liquid growth medium, the cells fall to the bottom of the vessel, attach to the surface, and begin to divide, spreading out as they divide. Division continues until the cells reach the sides of the dish and all cells are in one layer, each in contact with other cells. Once the surface of the dish has been covered in a monolayer of cells, cell division stops. If a cut is made in the layer of cells, cells damaged by the cut disintegrate and cell division begins again until the cut area is filled in. It was thought that cell contact was the signal for the turning off of cell division, and the phenomenon was named *contact inhibition of growth*[5] (Figure 3-2).

Recent experiments have shown that when cells crowd each other, their access to nutrients necessary for cell division is inhibited. This phenomenon may explain why normal cells cease division when a contained area is filled with a monolayer of cells. Thus, the term *density-dependent growth* is gradually replacing the term *contact inhibition.*[1]

In contrast to normal cells, when cancer cells are placed in the same culture medium, they continue to divide, crowding the space they occupy until the cells are piled on each other in an unorganized mass. There are several reasons for this lack of contact inhibition in transformed cells. Transformed cells are held less firmly to adjacent cells than are normal cells and seem to move about with more frequency than do normal cells. In addition, cancer cells require lower concentrations of many necessary substances, so their growth may be less affected than normal cells' growth by contact (their growth is less density-dependent than normal cells').[6]

In addition to contact inhibition of growth, normal cells exhibit contact inhibition of movement. Normal cells move freely about until they come in contact with another cell. Once contact occurs, normal cells cease movement and adhere to one another, lining up in an orderly manner. This contact inhibition of movement is regulated by cell-to-cell interactions.

In contrast, the movement of cancer cells is not inhibited by contact with other cells. Cancer cells move on their own course, without regard to adjacent cells, growing in disorderly, multilayered patterns. Normal cell-to-cell interactions are disrupted, altered, or missing. (See Figure 3-3.)

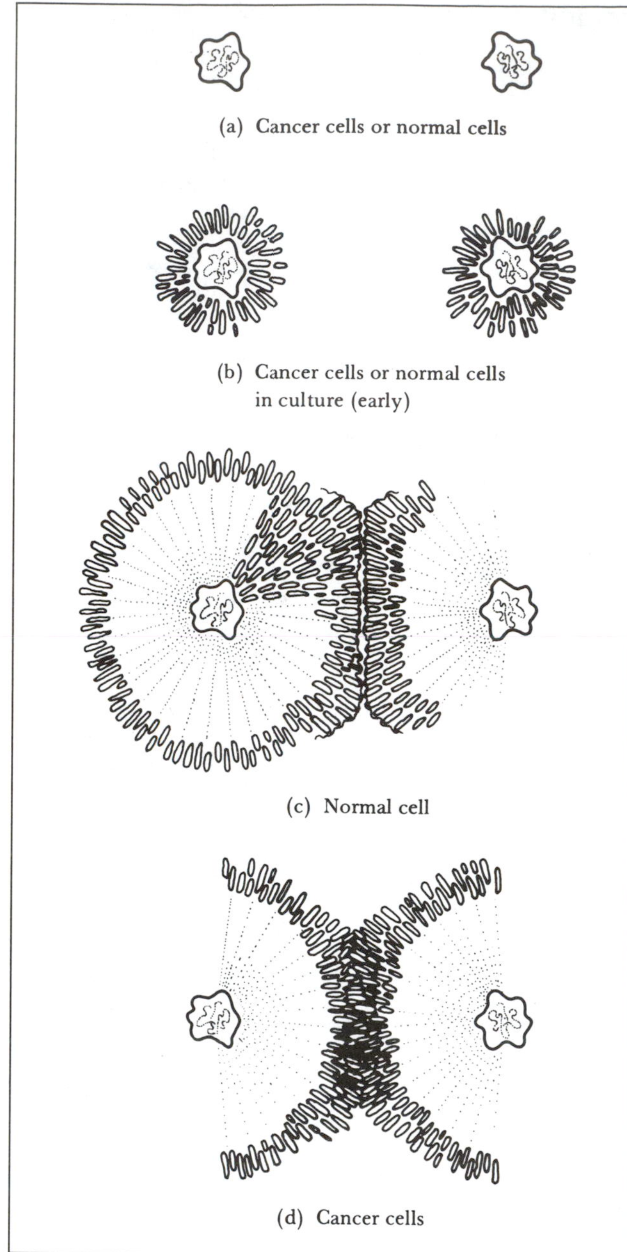

FIGURE 3-2 Impaired contact inhibition of cancer cells.

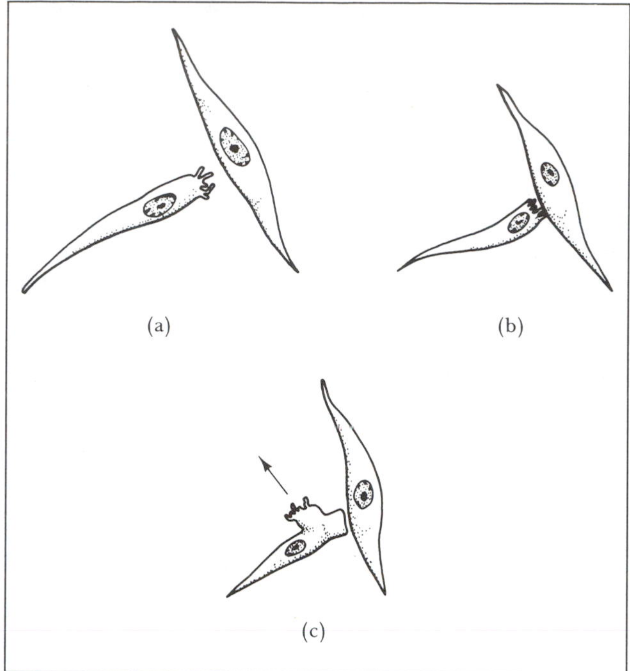

FIGURE 3-3 Contact inhibition of movement.

Diminished Growth Factor Requirements of Cancer Cells

Research has provided an understanding of some of the conditions necessary for cell growth. Substances found in the serum known as *growth factors* have been identified as necessary for the growth of normal cells in culture. Cancer cells and transformed cells are able to multiply in medium containing about one-tenth the usual concentration of serum.[7] Some cancer and transformed cell lines will even grow in the absence of serum; these transformed cells seem to make their own growth factors.[8] Growth factors will be discussed in more detail later in this chapter.

Ability to Divide Without Anchorage

Most normal cells will not divide when placed in suspension in a liquid medium or when embedded in a gel such as agar. The cells find a surface to which they can attach, then spread out and multiply. This type of growth is called *anchorage-dependent growth.* In contrast, cancer cells or transformed cells are able to grow in suspension or gel, and this property is most closely associated with the ability to form tumors.[2]

Loss of Restriction Point in Cell Cycle

Cellular proliferation occurs as a result of two coordinated events: the duplication of DNA within the cell and mitosis, the division of the cell into two daughter cells with identical complements of DNA. The two events combined make up what is known as the *cell cycle* (see Figure 3-4). The G_0 phase in a cell cycle is the resting (quiescent) state; G_1 is the phase during which protein synthesis takes place in preparation for the S phase of DNA synthesis; G_2 is where further protein synthesis takes place in preparation for the M phase where mitosis takes place. Most differentiated cells in the adult body are in a resting or G_0 phase unless called to divide because of cell death or injury. Blood cells, liver cells, and epithelial cells that make up mucous membrane and that line the gastrointestinal tract are rarely in the resting phase because of the constant demand for their replacement.

The decision by the cell to enter G_0 or to continue in G_1 occurs at a point in G_1 called the *restriction point.*

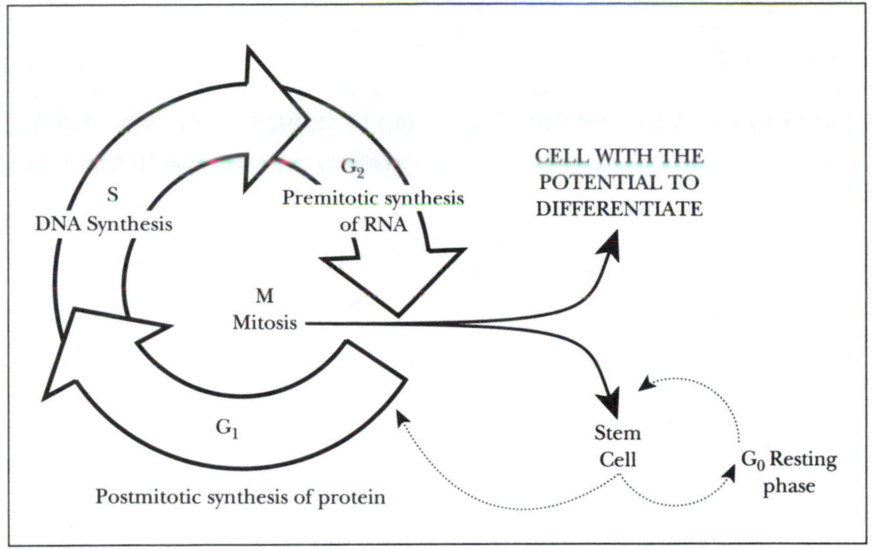

FIGURE 3-4 The cell cycle. (Source: Maxwell MB, Maner KE: Chemotherapy-induced myelosuppression. *Semin Oncol Nurs* 8:113–123, 1992. Copyright 1992, W.B. Saunders, Inc. Used by permission of publisher.)

Once a cell passes this point, it must continue through all phases of the cell cycle and return to G_1.[9]

Neither the biochemical events that regulate the normal cell cycle nor the nature of the transition to G_0 are known. Limitation of nutrients or growth factors may cause the normal cell to leave the cycle at the restriction point and enter the G_0 state as a protective device. Cancer cells lack this control, which is a potential weakness believed to be the reason for the killing effect of anticancer drugs that block cells in the S, G_2, and M phases of the cell cycle.[10]

It is likely that transformation of normal cells to cancer cells involves a recruitment of cells from G_0 into G_1. A large research effort is devoted to understanding the controls of the cell cycle.

DIFFERENCES IN THE APPEARANCE OF NORMAL AND CANCER CELLS

Normal cells have a well-organized and extensive cytoskeleton consisting of bundles of microfilaments and microtubules. These bundles consist of polymerized subunits of proteins that provide the structure and shape of the cell (Figure 3-5a). Transformed cells contain the subunits of proteins, but the proteins are not polymerized, causing transformed cells to have variable sizes and shapes *(pleomorphism)* (Figure 3-5b).

Other important differences in the appearance of cancer cells and normal cells are: The nuclei of cancer cells stain darker *(hyperchromaticism)* (Figure 3-5c) and are disproportionately larger (Figure 3-5d); cancer cells exhibit a variety of abnormal mitotic figures (Figure 3-5e).

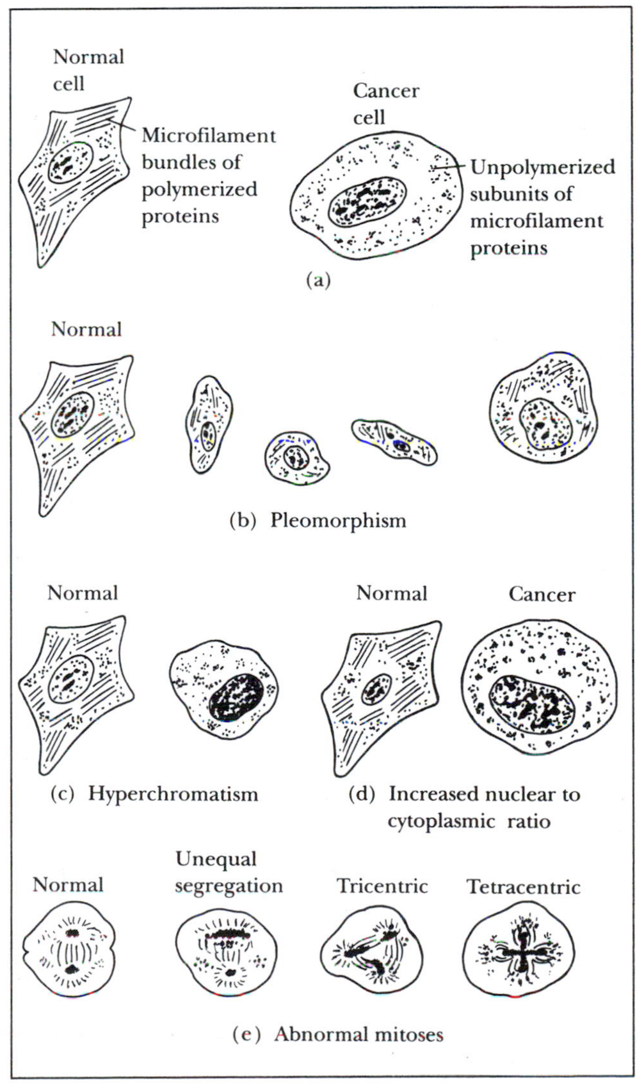

FIGURE 3-5 Differences in appearance of normal cells and cancer cells.

DIFFERENCES IN DIFFERENTIATION OF NORMAL AND CANCER CELLS

As the human organism develops from the fertilized egg into an adult person, all cells derive from the one fertilized egg and carry the identical DNA molecules and hence the same genes. However, as the organism develops, cells become different and specialized for various structural and functional purposes. This process is called *differentiation.* Differentiation occurs because in no cell are all genes active, and in certain cells only particular genes are activated. How this "turning on and off" of genes is accomplished is a major area of research that is only beginning to be understood. It is now understood that one reason cells differ is that different messenger RNA molecules are made, causing cells to have different types of proteins (e.g., blood cells contain the protein hemoglobin; muscle cells contain myosin).[2] The more differentiated a cell becomes, the more its potential is restricted. Fully differentiated cells are often incapable of replicating and are committed to performing the functions of the particular tissues that they compose.[6]

It was once believed that all cancer cells emerged from fully differentiated cells that had somehow reverted toward embryological cell forms as a result of transformation. It is now understood that cancer cells may arise at any point during differentiation. In addition, it is known that genes (oncogenes) that were active in embryos but suppressed during differentiation can be reactivated by carcinogenic agents.[11]

Cancer cells tend to be less differentiated than cells from surrounding normal tissue. Some cancer cells are so poorly differentiated *(anaplastic)* that the tissue of origin cannot be identified. The change from normal cells to neoplastic tissue is a process during which a sequence of tissue alterations occur. These tissue alterations are known as *metaplasia, dysplasia, carcinoma in situ,* and finally *invasive carcinoma*[12] (see Figure 3-6).

DIFFERENCES IN THE CELL SURFACES OF NORMAL AND CANCER CELLS

The cell membrane is the complex covering of animal cells that determines what molecules can enter and leave the cell. It is the element of both cell contact and cell adhesion. The most elementary cell membrane consists of two layers of lipid molecules (called a *lipid bilayer*). Various proteins and *glycoproteins* (proteins with sugars attached) are embedded in the lipid bilayer. Some of the proteins reside exclusively on the membrane surface (peripheral proteins); others are found partly or completely embedded in the membrane (integral proteins). The cell membrane is a loose structure, with many fluidlike properties, and proteins and glycoproteins move both laterally and between the layers, albeit slowly. The fluid nature of the membrane and the existence of mobile proteins within the membrane and on the surface was described by Nicolson and Singer[13] as the *fluid mosaic model.*

The cell surface and membrane are particularly important in cancer biology because they seem to be involved in anchorage dependence, cell adhesion, and invasiveness, not to mention literally hundreds of biochemical interactions. Research has shown that a variety of changes occurs in the surface of a cancer cell. Some new molecules appear, some molecules that normally appear are lost, and other molecules are changed.[14,15] Figure 3-7 summarizes these changes, and the more significant changes are described in the following subsections.

Glycoprotein Alterations

Cell transformation is almost always associated with profound changes in cell-surface glycoproteins. Most of the changes are related to a lower protein content. The glycoproteins that remain are altered, mostly by becoming simpler. Evidence shows that the mechanism

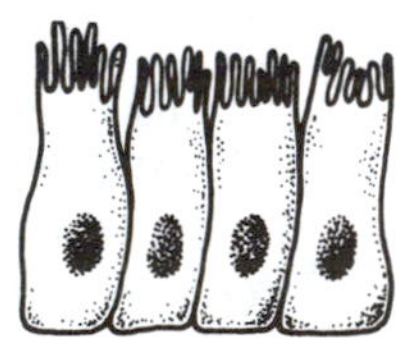

Normal. Highly differentiated columnar ciliated epithelium

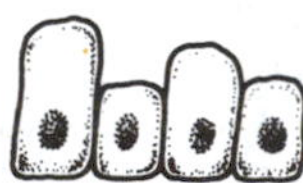

Dysplasia. Deranged cell growth leading to tissue made up of cells of variable size, shape, and appearance

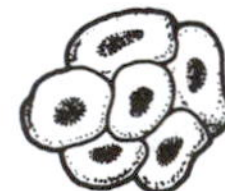

Anaplasia. Primitive-looking, undifferentiated cells

FIGURE 3-6 The transition from normal cell to neoplastic tissue.

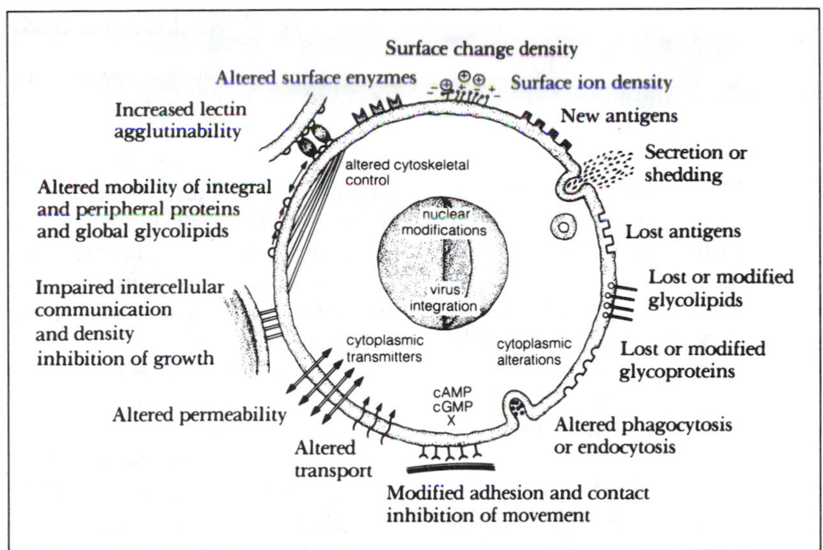

FIGURE 3-7 Summary of the cell surfaces and cell surface–related alterations generally seen in cancer cells. (Source: Adapted from Nicolson GL: Transmembrane control of the receptors on normal and tumor cells. II. Surface changes associated with transformation and malignancy. *Biochim Biophys Acta* 458:16, 1976.)

by which polysaccharides are made and attached to proteins is deranged in transformed cells.[16] Fibronectin and protease glycoproteins are affected.

Fibronectin

Fibronectin is a large glycoprotein found on normal cell surfaces. Together with various proteoglycans, collagen, and elastin, fibronectin forms the matrix in which cells are embedded and that anchors cells in place within tissues. It also serves as an organizing grid for the integral proteins of the cell surface.[17] For many cell types to grow in culture, fibronectin must be present in the serum. Some cell types make their own fibronectin.

Cancer cells and transformed cells have low levels of fibronectin, causing them to attach poorly to the surface of the culture vessel; however, they continue to grow. Hynes[17] suggests that the reason cancer cells have low levels of fibronectin is that they either stop making it or make a defective form of it. Addition of fibronectin to cultures of some tumor cells causes normalization of cell adhesion, flattens cells, and restores contact inhibition of cell movement. However, it does not restore growth control.[1] Since fibronectin plays important roles in cellular organization, cell-to-cell adhesion, and cytoskeletal structure, the lack of fibronectin in cancer cells is an important factor in cancer metastasis. The role of fibronectin in metastasis will be discussed in detail in Chapter 4.

Proteases

Transformed cells have been shown to secrete a variety of protein-degrading enzymes. Research suggests that the proteases are involved in metastasis through local invasion of the extracellular matrices of surrounding tissue rather than in transformation itself.[18,19] The proteolytic enzymes may degrade both the attachment proteins as well as the components of the extracellular matrix.[20] In addition to producing their own proteolytic enzymes, tumor cells may also induce adjacent host cells to secrete enzymes.

Since the quantity and interactions of extracellular matrices differ, it is likely that a variety of proteolytic enzymes are involved in the degradation of extracellular matrices. Proteolytic enzymes that have been shown to contribute to matrix degradation include collagenases, plasminogen activators, stromelysin, cathepsin D, and procoagulants.[21–26] See Chapter 4 for more information on the role of proteases in cancer metastasis.

Glycolipid Alterations

Cell-surface changes in glycolipids are another attribute of transformation. In general, the content and complexity of glycolipids is reduced in transformed cell membranes. In particular, it has been shown that the glycolipid glycosphingolipid interacts with receptor proteins on the surface of normal cells to inhibit their responsiveness to growth factors.[27] Transformed cells have less and/or altered glycosphingolipids on their cell surfaces, increasing the responsiveness of the transformed cells to growth factors. In addition, glycosphingolipids have been shown to serve as components of surface markers involved in cell–cell recognition.

Cell-Surface Antigens

Many of the proteins and glycoproteins on the surface of the cell can be detected by immunological assay and therefore are referred to as *surface antigens.* When cells are transformed, new molecules form on the surface. When the cell is transformed by a virus, the antigens that result are usually determined by the virus in that the same antigen is found in different cell types transformed by the same virus. When the cells are transformed by radiation or chemical carcinogens, the tumor antigens formed in these cells do not depend upon the agent used, but vary with cell type.

In animals and transformed cells, antigens have been identified that are not found on any normal cell; these antigens are *tumor-specific antigens.* In humans, however, antigens do not show this specificity. The great majority of antigens identified in human tumors are *tumor-associated antigens* that have relative rather than absolute specificity for cancer cells.

Tumor-associated antigens are of two basic types: *Tumor-associated transplantation antigens (TATAs)* are antigens that appear on the surfaces of cells transformed by viral, chemical, or radiation carcinogens; *oncofetal antigens (embryonic antigens)* are antigens normally found only on embryonic cells that are re-expressed on certain tumors. Examples of oncofetal antigens are alpha-fetoprotein (AFP), found in liver cancers and some testicular, pancreatic, and gastrointestinal tract tumors; and carcinoembryonic antigen (CEA), found in cancers of the gastrointestinal tract, pancreas, liver, and lung.

Tumor-associated antigens are used clinically as tumor markers for detection of tumors, monitoring of patient prognosis, and evaluation of treatment measures.[28]

Altered Permeability and Membrane Transport

Transformed cells transport materials across the cell membrane at higher rates than do normal cells. Materials that show enhanced uptake include glucose, other sugars, and some amino acids. The mechanism of increased glucose transport has been shown to be production of a glucose transporter protein in transformed cells.[29]

BIOCHEMICAL DIFFERENCES BETWEEN NORMAL AND CANCER CELLS

A number of biochemical substances that are altered, missing, abnormally secreted, or secreted in increased amounts by tumor cells affect cell growth and how cells interact with each other. Following are some of the more important biochemical differences between normal and cancer cells.

Cyclic AMP and Cyclic GMP

Cyclic adenosine monophosphate (cAMP) participates in the regulation of a large number of intracellular biochemical reactions. Research has shown that cAMP levels are generally high in resting normal cells and are low in dividing cells, including cancer cells.[30] In addition, cAMP reduces the rate of division of some normal and some transformed cells in culture. Some of the traits of transformation such as roundedness and diminished adhesiveness can be restored to normal when transformed cells are prevented from degrading cAMP, causing the level of cAMP to rise toward normal.[31] Since cAMP regulates the transport of nutrients such as glucose, amino acids, and phosphate into cells, it could act by controlling the availability of these substances to the cell. Because cAMP is a key in cell regulation it is especially interesting to cancer researchers, as it may prove to be a key to autonomous cell growth.

A related substance, *cyclic guanosine monophosphate (cGMP)* also restricts growth. cGMP varies opposite cAMP; that is, cell division is associated with low cAMP and high cGMP levels.[6]

Nutrients

Cancer cells in culture have been shown to take up nutrients such as amino acids and sugars at rates that are greatly increased over those exhibited by untransformed cells of the same type. This increased transport may be associated with alteration of transport sites on or within the surface membrane of cancer cells. As mentioned above, cAMP may also be important in the differences in utilization of nutrients between normal and cancer cells.

Chalones

Chalones are proteins that inhibit multiplication of normal cells in the skin, lung, liver, bone marrow, lymph nodes, kidney, and uterine lining. The chalones are synthesized by the cells in the specific tissue, and inhibition of mitosis is tissue-specific. Chalones are thought to be responsible for the fact that organs grow to only a certain size.

As may be predicted, cancer tissues have a lower concentration of chalones than do normal tissues. Cancer cells have a defect in their ability either to manufacture chalones or to respond to them.[1]

Growth Factors

In normal cells, growth factors produced by one cell type bind to membrane receptors on another cell type to initiate a cascade of metabolic events leading to cell division. Malignant and transformed cells have been shown to have receptors for growth factors on their cell surfaces, as well as the ability to synthesize growth factors.[32] Research has shown that cancer cells develop an independence from growth factors, probably as a result of release of autocrine growth factors as well as a lack of response to inhibitory controls.[8,33]

Transformed cells are able to proliferate in culture when concentrations of growth factors are much lower than those required by normal cells. In addition, when the concentration of growth-control substances falls below a certain threshold level, normal cells go into quiescence, whereas transformed cells lack this ability to cease proliferation.[7]

A number of growth factors have been isolated that are of interest in cancer biology.

Epidermal growth factor

Epidermal growth factor (EGF) stimulates a wide variety of cell types and is involved in a variety of physiologic interactions unrelated to cell growth. It binds to specific receptors on the cell surface of most epithelial cells. Cells grown in the presence of EGF lack density-dependent growth, suggesting that EGF may play a role in excessive growth of tumors of epithelial cell origin.[34]

Transforming growth factor-α (TGF-α)

TGF-α is produced by human tumor cells of diverse origin and binds to the same receptors as EGF. TGF-α is angiogenic and stimulates the proliferation of endothelial cells.[35,36]

Transforming growth factor-β (TGF-β)

TGF-β is produced by tumor cells of various tissue origins. TGF-β stimulates the growth of fibroblasts and inhibits the growth of a wide variety of cell types of mesenchymal, myeloid, epithelial, lymphoid, and endothelial origin. TGF-β has multiple effects on cell functions such as secretion of proteolytic enzymes and extracellular matrix proteins.[37]

Although the biochemical nature of individual growth factors produced by tumor cells does not differ significantly from that of normal cells, the regulation of their expression differs widely between normal and cancer cells.

Platelet-derived growth factor (PDGF)

PDGF is a protein released into the serum from blood platelets during the coagulation cascade. It promotes growth, though its activity is limited to fibroblasts and smooth muscle cells of arteries.[38,39] PDGF seems to play a role in the development and support of brain tumors such as astrocytomas.[40]

Basic fibroblast growth factors (bFGF)

In contrast to other growth factors, bFGF is not secreted via conventional secretory pathways. It is primarily intracellular but is also present in the extracellular matrix.[41] This growth factor is produced by both normal and malignant cells of mesodermal and neuroectodermal origin. It has strong angiogenic properties and is important in neoangiogenesis.[42]

Insulinlike growth factors (IGF) I and II

IGF-I and IGF-II have autocrine functions in human colon carcinoma, lung carcinoma, pancreatic carcinoma, and neuroblastoma cell lines.[43,44] IGF-I stimulates growth of tumor cells and normal cells and is a motility factor for melanoma cells.[45]

GENETIC DIFFERENCES BETWEEN NORMAL AND CANCER CELLS

Considerable evidence indicates that most neoplasms arise from a single altered cell that acquires a heritable and selective growth advantage over other cells.[46] The initial change in the cell is the alteration of a regulatory gene by a carcinogen that provides the cell with a growth advantage. As the cell divides and produces offspring, each daughter cell inherits the genetic defect that provides it with the capacity to invade, metastasize, grow without regard to inhibitory growth controls, lose responsiveness to hormones, and so on.

In addition to the heritable genetic alteration, tumor cells are genetically unstable when compared to normal cells. This genetic liability may contribute to the sequential acquisition of genetic changes during tumor development and contribute to tumor progression.[47]

Tumor progression results from additional mutations in cells within the clone, involving either growth-regulatory genes or genes responsible for other characteristics of the tumor cells. The result is the sequential appearance within the tumor of subpopulations of heterogeneous cells. Tumor heterogeneity has been identified as the most significant cause of cancer treatment failure.[48–50]

CONCLUSION

As normal cells transform to malignant cells, a vast array of changes takes place in the cell's appearance, function, behavior, and interactions with other cells. Research is directed toward identifying the key factors that cause cancer and cause the differences between normal and cancer cells. To date, most of the differences between normal and cancer cells are not key features of malignancy; that is, many of the differences are the same as those between dividing and nondividing normal cells. When key factors are found that provide information on the distinctive nature of cancer cells, methods can be developed to block or influence these factors to effect improved survival and quality of life for individuals with cancer.

REFERENCES

1. Pitot HC: *Fundamentals of Oncology* (3 ed). New York: Dekker, 1986.
2. Oppenheimer SB: *Cancer: A Biological and Clinical Introduction* (2 ed). Boston: Jones and Bartlett, 1985.
3. Ruddon RW: *Cancer Biology*. New York: Oxford University Press, 1981.
4. Wyke JA, Green AR: Suppression of the neoplastic phenotype. In Kahn P, Graf T (eds), *Oncogenes and Growth Control*. New York: Springer-Verlag, 1986, pp. 341–345.
5. Abercrombie M: The contact behavior of invading cells. In *Cellular Membranes and Tumor-Cell Behavior*. Baltimore, MD: Williams & Wilkins, 1975, pp. 21–37.
6. Watson JD, Hopkins NH, Roberts JW: *Molecular Biology of the Gene: Vol II. Specialized Aspects* (4th ed). Menlo Park, CA: Benjamin/Cummings, 1987, pp. 747–1163.
7. Waterfield MD: The role of growth factors in cancer. In Frank LM, Teich NM (eds), *Introduction to the Cellular and Molecular Biology of Cancer*. Oxford, Eng.: Oxford University Press, 1986, pp. 27–39.
8. Sporn MB, Roberts AB: Autocrine growth factors and cancer. *Nature* 313:745–747, 1985.
9. Tannock IF: Tumor growth and cell kinetics. In Tannock IF, Hill RP (eds), *The Basic Science of Oncology*. New York: Pergamon Press, 1987, pp. 140–159.
10. Tannock IF: Biologic properties of anticancer drugs. In Tannock IF, Hill RP (eds), *The Basic Science of Oncology*. New York: Pergamon Press, 1987, pp. 278–291.
11. Schwab M: Amplification of proto-oncogenes and tumor progression. In Kahn P, Graf T (eds), *Oncogenes and Growth Control*. New York: Springer-Verlag, pp. 332–339.
12. Correa P: Morphology and natural history of precursor lesions. In Schottenfeld D, Fraumeni JF (eds), *Cancer Epidemiology and Prevention*. Philadelphia: Saunders, 1982, pp. 90–118.
13. Singer SJ, Nicolson GL: The fluid mosiac structure of cell membranes. *Science* 175(23):720–731, 1972.
14. Nicolson GL: Transmembrane control of the receptors in normal and tumor cells II. Surface changes associated with transformation and malignancy. *Biochim Biophys Acta* 458:1–72, 1976.
15. Nicolson GL, Poste G: The cancer cell: Dynamic aspects and modifications in cell-surface organization. Parts 1 and 2. *N Engl J Med* 295:197–203, 253–258, 1974.
16. Smets LA, Van Beek WP: Carbohydrates of the tumor cell surface. *Biochim Biophys Acta* 738:237–249, 1984.
17. Hynes RO: Fibronectins. *Sci Am* 254:42–51, 1986.
18. Quigley JP: Proteolytic enzymes of normal and malignant cells. In Hynes RO (ed), *Surfaces of Normal and Malignant Cells*. Chichester, Eng.: Wiley, 1979, pp. 247–285.
19. Sloane BF, Robinson D, Honn KD: Role for cathepsin B and cystatins in tumor growth and progression. *Biol Chem Happe Seyler* 371:193–198, 1990 (suppl.).
20. Liotta LA: Tumor invasion and metastases—role of the extracellular matrix: Rhoads Memorial Award Lecture. *Cancer Res* 46:1–7, 1986.
21. Goldfarb RH: Proteolytic enzymes in tumor invasion and degradation of host extracellular matrices. In Honn KV, Powers WE, Sloane BF (eds), *Mechanisms of Cancer Metastasis. Potential Therapeutic Implications*. Boston: Martinus Nijhoff, 1986, pp. 341–375.
22. Goldfarb RH: Plasminogen activators. *Ann Rep Med Chem* 18:257–264, 1983.
23. Testa JE, Quigley JP: The role of urokinase-type plasminogen activator in aggressive tumor cell behavior. *Cancer Metastasis Rev* 9:353–367, 1990.
24. Sloane BF, Rozhin J, Ryan RE, et al: Cathepsin B-like cysteine proteinases and metastasis. In Honn KV, Powers WE, Sloane BF (eds), *Mechanisms of Cancer Metastasis. Potential Therapeutic Implications*. Boston: Martinus Nijhoff, 1986, pp. 377–398.
25. Rochefort H, Capony F, Garcia M: Cathepsin D: A protease involved in breast cancer metastasis. *Cancer Metastasis Rev* 9:321–331, 1990.
26. Gordon SG: Cancer cell procoagulants and their possible role in metastasis. In Honn KV, Powers WE, Sloane BF (eds), *Mechanisms of Cancer Metastasis. Potential Therapeutic Implications*. Boston: Martinus Nijhoff, 1986, pp. 159–172.
27. Hakomori S: Glycosphingolipids. *Sci Am* 254:44–53, 1986.
28. Herlyn M, Menrad A, Koprowski H: Structure, function and clinical significance of human tumor antigens. *J Natl Cancer Inst* 82:1883–1890, 1990.
29. Birnbaum MJ, Haspel HC, Rosen OM: Transformation of rat fibroblasts by FSV rapidly increases glucose transporter gene transcription. *Science* 235:1495–1497, 1987.
30. Pastan IH, Johnson GS, Anderson WB: Role of cyclic nucleotides in growth control. *Ann Rev Biochem* 44:491–522, 1975.
31. Levitzki A: From epinephrine to cyclic AMP. *Science* 241:800–806, 1988.
32. Todaro GJ, DeLarco E: Growth factors produced by sarcoma virus-transformed cells. *Cancer Res* 38:4147–4153, 1978.
33. Kimchi A, Wang X-F, Weinbery RA, et al: Absence of TGF-B receptors and growth inhibitory responses in retinoblastoma cells. *Science* 240:196–198, 1988.
34. Bennett C, Paterson IM, Corbishley CM, et al: Expression of growth factor and epidermal growth factor receptor encoded transcripts in human gastric tissues. *Cancer Res* 49:2104–2107, 1989.
35. Schreiber AB, Winkler ME, Derynck R: TGF-alpha: A more potent angiogenic mediator than EGF. *Science* (Washington) 232:1250–1254, 1986.
36. Chakrabarty S, Fan D, Varani J: Modulation of differentiation and proliferation in human colon carcinoma cells by transforming growth factor beta 1 and beta 2. *Int J Cancer* 46:493–496, 1990.
37. Barnard JA, Lyons RM, Moses HL: The cell biology of transforming growth factor beta. *Biochim Biophys Acta* 1032:79–83, 1990.
38. Bronzert DA, Pantazis P, Antoniades HN, et al: Synthesis and secretion of platelet-derived growth factor by human breast cancer cell lines. *Proc Natl Acad Sci USA* 84:5763–5768, 1987.
39. Usaki K, Heldin N-E, Miyazono K, et al: Production of platelet-derived endothelial cell growth factor by normal and transformed human cells in culture. *Proc Natl Acad Sci USA* 86:7427–7434, 1989.
40. Maxwell M, Naber SP, Wolfe HJ, et al: Coexpression of platelet-derived growth factor (PDGF) and PDGF-receptor genes by primary human astrocytomas may contribute to their development and maintenance. *J Clin Invest* 86:131–135, 1990.

41. Vlodavsky I, Folkman R, Sullivan R, et al: Endothelial cell-derived basic fibroblast growth factor: Synthesis and deposition into subendothelial extracellular matrix. *Proc Natl Acad Sci USA* 84:2292–2295, 1987.
42. Jaye M, Howk R, Burgess W, et al: Human endothelial cell growth factor: cloning, nucleotide sequence, and chromosome localization. *Science* (Washington) 233:541–547, 1986.
43. Arteaga CL, Osborne CK: Growth inhibition of human breast cancer cells *in vitro* with an antibody against the type I somatomedin receptor. *Cancer Res* 49:6237–6239, 1989.
44. Cullen KJ, Yee D, Sly WS, et al: Insulin-like growth factor receptor expression and function in human breast cancer. *Cancer Res* 50:48–53, 1990.
45. Herlyn M, Kath R, Williams N: Growth regulatory factors for normal, premalignant, and malignant human cells. *Adv Cancer Res* 54:213–224, 1990.
46. Nowell P: The clonal evolution of tumor cell populations. *Science* 194:23–28, 1976.
47. Nicolson GL: Tumor cell instability, diversification, and progression to the metastatic phenotype: From oncogene to oncofetal expression. *Cancer Res* 47:1473–1487, 1987.
48. Schilsky RL: Tumor cell heterogeneity: Implications for clinical practice. *Semin Oncol* 12:203–206, 1985.
49. Heppner GH: Tumor heterogeneity. *Cancer Res* 44:2259–2265, 1984.
50. Heppner GH, Miller BE: Therapeutic implications of tumor heterogeneity. *Semin Oncol* 16:91–105, 1989.

Chapter 4

Invasion and Metastasis

Susan L. Groenwald, RN, MS

THE CLINICAL PROBLEM OF METASTASIS

Although many tumors are now treated successfully by surgery alone, or in combination with chemotherapy, radiotherapy, or immunotherapy, metastasis is the most frequent cause of cancer treatment failure. It is estimated that up to 60% of individuals with solid tumors have metastases at the time of their initial diagnosis, even though many of the metastases are microscopic lesions that remain undetected until later in the individual's disease course.[1]

Knowledge about cancer metastasis has lagged behind other scientific developments in the cancer field because of the complexity of the interactions involved. To tackle this complicated process, researchers have separated invasion and metastasis into a series of defined, sequential steps and have studied the cellular processes and interactions responsible for each step. An effort combining the disciplines of cell biology, biochemistry, and molecular genetics has caused an explosion of information about metastasis, and has yielded new strategies for treatment of metastatic cancer.

This chapter will discuss factors that contribute to metastasis in cancer, describe the cascade of events that leads to metastases, and present suggested strategies for prevention and treatment of cancer metastasis.

FACTORS CONTRIBUTING TO METASTATIC POTENTIAL

Only a very small percentage (<0.01%) of cells in a primary tumor ultimately are able to initiate a successful metastatic deposit.[2,3] Cancer metastasis is a highly selective competition, favoring the survival of a subpopulation of tumor cells that already exist within a heterogeneous primary tumor.[2,4]

In cancer, genetic changes result in an imbalance of growth regulation that leads to uncontrolled proliferation. However, unrestrained growth does not, by itself, result in invasion and metastasis. In fact, tumorigenicity and metastasis have both overlapping and separate features. For invasion and metastasis to occur, an imbalance in the regulation of motility and proteolysis is required, in addition to loss of growth control.[5] At every stage of the metastatic process, cancer cells must avoid host immune mechanisms. Finally, angiogenesis is required for expansion of the primary tumor, as well as for establishment of a metastatic colony.

Following is a discussion of tumor cell and host factors that contribute to the metastatic potential of a tumor.

Tumor Cell Factors

Oncogenes

Progression of tumors from benign to malignant is exemplified by structural alterations in genes and by changes in gene expression that cause proteins to function abnormally, inappropriately, or at improper concentrations, resulting in circumvention of normal controls that regulate cell division and differentiation.[6,7] A growing list of transforming genes or oncogenes has been identified that may be involved in the genetic alterations leading to tumor growth, invasion, and metastasis (see Chapter 2). In addition, suppressor genes have been identified that normally suppress tumor growth and proliferation. These suppressor genes have been shown to be underexpressed in certain types of cancer.[8]

It has been shown that transfection of certain oncogenes into an appropriate recipient cell can induce the complete phenotype of invasion and metastasis,[9] although much research remains to be done linking specific oncogenes and suppressor genes with the metastatic state. While oncogene expression has been found to be correlated with the metastatic behavior in certain classes of human tumors studied to date,[10] the specific family of genes necessary for metastasis appears to be different for each histologic type of tumor. Aberrant gene expression and genetic alterations of the *ras* and *myc* gene families have been shown to be important in the progression of human cancers[11,12] and may be useful as prognostic indicators.[13]

Heterogeneity

That tumors consist of heterogeneous populations of malignant cells was first demonstrated by Fidler and Kripke[14] in the B16 melanoma system, and has since been corroborated.[15] Clones of cells isolated from tumors have been shown to differ in a wide variety of cell characteristics, including karyotype, hormone receptors, cell surface enzymes, morphology, growth properties, response to therapy, and metastatic potential.[16,17] Tumor cells are heterogeneous within a tumor, among different cancers of different histologic origins, and among tumors of the same histologic origin but in different individuals.

Not all cells of the primary tumor are metastatic, and varying degrees of metastatic potential exist among the cells of a primary tumor.[14,18,19] However, recent research with genetic markers has shown that the metastatic subpopulation of cells dominates the primary tumor mass early in its growth.[20] This finding has important clinical implications, in that a measure of the metastatic propensity of cells extrapolated from a sample of the primary tumor can be correlated with clinical parameters of metastasis and recurrence.[21,22]

Tumor cell heterogeneity has other important clinical implications. For example, even if a 99.9% cell kill is achieved in treatment of a 1-cm^3 lesion consisting of 1 billion cells, a significant number (10^6) of nonresponsive cells will remain to continue growing and developing further diverse populations of cells.[15] Additionally, tumor cell heterogeneity explains why one person's tumor may disseminate at a very early stage of growth while another person's tumor of similar size and histologic appearance may continue to grow to a large size without metastasizing. Because of these complexities, the only effective therapeutic modalities against cancer will be developed from an understanding of and regulation of tumor cell heterogeneity.

Production of growth factors

Specific peptide growth factors have been identified as participants in the neoplastic transformation of cells. These peptide growth factors are found in platelets, macrophages, and lymphocytes and are also produced by transformed cells (autocrine growth factors). Platelet-derived growth factor (PDGF) was the first peptide growth factor to be directly implicated in oncogenesis.[23] Peptides resembling PDGF have been found in many different types of cancer cells.[24] Other growth factors known to exert an autocrine action in cancer cells are transforming growth factor-alpha (TGF-alpha), also called epithelial growth factor, transforming growth factor-beta (TGF-beta), granulocyte-monocyte colony stimulating factor (G-MCSF), and fibroblast growth factors (FGFs).[25] Aberrant synthesis of growth factors by the tumor may be a source of signals that stimulate subpopulations of metastatic cells to proliferate and diversify. Some growth factors, such as FGFs, may promote angiogenesis as well as tumor growth.[26] Lack of response of tumor cells to inhibitory peptides potentiates these responses.

Production of angiogenic factors

Once a tumor has been initiated, any subsequent increase in tumor cell population must be preceded by an increase in new capillaries that converge on the tumor.[27,28] The growth and development of these new capillaries is initiated and supported by a group of peptide proteins called *angiogenic factors*. Since the mid-1980s several angiogenic factors have been purified and their genes clones. These polypeptides include FGF, angiogenin, TGF, and tumor necrosis factor.[29,30,31] Angiogenic factors seem to stimulate directly locomotion or mitosis of vascular endothelium, and to release endothelial growth factors,[30] stimulating capillary blood vessel growth (see upcoming section on "Tumor Growth and Neovascularization" for a more detailed discussion of angiogenesis).

Motility

Tumor cell motility is necessary for many phases in the complex metastatic cascade. Once tumor cells detach from the primary tumor, they must infiltrate into adjacent tissue and migrate though the vascular wall into the circulation and out again into the tissue at a secondary site. The movement of cells through biologic barriers such as the basement membrane is probably related to chemotactic mechanisms, such as complement-derived materials, collagen peptides, and certain connective tissue components.[32,33] However, these substances can only account for the directional aspects of a motile response; they are not sufficient to initiate the intrinsic locomotion of tumor cells. Rather, motility factors produced by tumor cells and normal cells influence the tumor cells to move out into the surrounding host tissue.[34]

Motility factors are produced by tumor cells in humans, as demonstrated in an experiment in which the concentration of motility factor in urine was measured by 24-hour urine collection in individuals with transitional cell cancer of the bladder.[35] The higher the pathologic grade of bladder cancer in an individual, the higher was the level of motility factors found in the urine.

Specific cell surface receptors

It has been shown that cells express specific cell surface receptors that recognize a vast array of proteins, including extracellular matrix proteins. One family of cell surface receptors, the integrins, are the proteins that serve as receptors for fibronectin and other components of the extracellular matrix.[36,37] Integrins appear to be crucial for the binding of fibronectin and in laminin. This process is altered in malignant cells. For example, the laminin receptor, which binds to laminin on the basement membrane, has been shown to be augmented in actively invading tumor cells, and may play an important role in tumor cell interaction with the basement membrane.[38] Other receptors for proteins, such as fibronectin, collagen type I, and vitronectin, may also play a role in tumor cell invasion and migration.

Invasiveness

Metastasizing tumor cells meet a variety of host connective tissue barriers as they make their way through various tissue compartments. In normal tissue, the various compartments are separated from each other by two types of extracellular matrix: a series of basement membranes, and interstitial stroma.[39] The matrix determines tissue architecture, performs important biologic functions, and provides a mechanical barrier to invasion. Normal, healthy basement membranes are intact, continuous, and impervious to even small particles. Research has shown that through a series of complex biochemical interactions, tumor cells have the ability to penetrate epithelial basement membrane and enter the underlying interstitial stroma, where they gain access to lymphatics and blood vessels for further dissemination.[39] This ability of tumor cells to invade epithelial basement membrane is central to the basic mechanisms of cancer invasion and metastasis.[40]

Host Factors

Deficient immune response

Throughout the metastatic sequence, tumor cells are subject to attack by the host immune system. It is thought that some defect in the immune system—its components or its functioning—may contribute to the development of cancer and metastases. The roles of natural killer (NK) cells and macrophages in limiting tumor growth and metastatic spread have been shown to be important;[41,42] they are discussed in detail in Chapter 5. Methods for treating micrometastases by amplifying NK- and macrophage-mediated tumor cell destruction are presently being studied in many laboratories and have created considerable interest among scientists.

Intact hemostatic system

Normal platelet function is required for tumor cell metastasis. In 1968 platelets were first shown to play an important role in tumor cell metastasis through the work of Gasic et al.,[43] who demonstrated that a reduction in platelet number correlates with reduction in experimentally induced tumor cell metastases. Since that time, it has been documented that platelets play a central role in the metastatic process,[44,45] though their exact role is unknown. Since during metastasis, tumor cells enter the circulation and come in contact with platelets, it may be that platelets secrete proteins that encourage tumor cell adhesion to vessel walls and subsequent destruction of the basement membrane.[46] Some studies have shown that tumor cells directly activate platelets.[47] There is further testimony to the role of platelets in promoting metastasis. Research has shown that antiplatelet drugs greatly inhibit experimentally induced cell metastases in mice.[47–49] Finally, studies have shown that the platelet-secreted protein thrombospondin potentiates tumor cell metastasis by encouraging tumor cell adhesion to vessel walls.[46]

Favorable target organ environment

It has long been postulated that secondary tumor growth in certain organs is the result of a favorable environment afforded by such tissues ("seed and soil" theory).[50] Hart and Fidler[51,52] demonstrated that those tissues exert growth-promoting or growth-inhibiting effects on cancer cells that make the microenvironment within certain organs more or less conducive to neoplastic growth than in other tissues.

THE METASTATIC SEQUENCE

Metastasis is a series of sequential but interwoven steps involving complex tumor cell–host interactions, and ending in the establishment of one or more secondary tumors at a site apart from the primary tumor. For purposes of examination, the sequence of metastasis is discussed in terms of six steps[4]:

1. tumor growth and neovascularization
2. tumor cell invasion of the basement membrane and other extracellular matrices
3. detachment and embolism of tumor cell aggregates
4. arrest in distant organ capillary beds
5. extravasation
6. proliferation within the organ parenchyma

Tumor Neovascularization and Growth

Neovascularization

Scientific evidence has shown that cancer originates from the genetic transformation of a single target cell.[53,54] Subsequent alterations in the cellular DNA initiate a series of processes that lead to autonomy from normal growth regulatory mechanisms, uncontrolled proliferation, and growth advantages over adjacent host tissues. A growing tumor requires an adequate blood supply to provide nutrients to support cellular proliferation. Folkman demonstrated that tumor cells are capable of releasing angiogenic factors that stimulate growth of new blood vessels *(angiogenesis)*, establishing a capillary network from the surrounding host tissue.[30,55] In addition, growth factors such as TGF-alpha and epidermal growth factor (EGF) have been found to contribute to tumor-induced angiogenesis.[56]

Folkman and co-workers[28] showed that the onset of angiogenic activity precedes tumor formation and correlates with the transition from hyperplasia to neoplasia. Angiogenesis is an invasive process that represents a sequence of events performed by vascular endothelial cells in response to angiogenic stimuli.[57] The same sequence of events takes place whether the angiogenic stimulus is physiological, immunological, or tumor-derived.

New capillaries arise from pre-existing capillaries or venules, never from arteries, arterioles, or veins. In response to the angiogenic stimulus, the parent vessel engorges, increases its permeability, and loses the integrity of its basement membrane. Protrusion of pseudopodial processes through gaps in the basement membrane begins the movement of a column of cells into the stroma toward the stimulus, and subsequent establishment of a lumen and the onset of bloodflow.[58,59]

At the onset of tumor angiogenesis, local shedding of cancer cells into the tumor venous drainage can begin. This extravasation of tumor cells into the circulation is quantitatively related to the surface area of new tumor vessels and may be facilitated by the immature nature of the newly formed vessels.[5]

Tumor growth

As a tumor grows, necrotic areas of the tumor release chemotactic products that attract host cells and cellular enzymes that help degradate surrounding structures, alter immune responses, and in general contribute to the emergence of specialized tumor cells capable of surviving in a hostile growth environment.

Despite the compelling growth advantages that a tumor has over surrounding tissues, an expanding tumor growing in one site would soon expand beyond its space, either becoming necrotic or differentiating and ceasing growth. It is the ability of cancer cells to break away and establish secondary sites that perpetuates the neoplastic continuum.

Tumor invasion and metastasis involves some cellular functions that are quite distinct from those involved in tumor growth. Although high growth rate is not sufficient by itself to make tumor cells metastasize, it may provide opportunities for gene alterations to occur that enable the cell to achieve full metastatic potential.

Invasion of the Basement Membrane and Other Extracellular Matrices

Metastasis begins with the local invasion of the surrounding host tissue by cells from the primary tumor. Invasion can be by single cells or groups of cells. Much speculation has been made about the mechanism of tumor cell invasion. Researchers now know that destruction of the basement membrane is a critical element at this stage in the sequence of metastasis, as well as at later points in the sequence.

The main structural components of the basement membrane are type IV collagen, laminin (a noncollagenous glycoprotein), fibronectin, entactin, and proteoglycan.[60] Of these, type IV collagen and laminin are the most important, because they are the main components of the basement membrane and because they are found only in basement membrane.

A number of distinct changes occurs in the organization, distribution, and quantity of the epithelial basement membrane during the transition from benign to invasive carcinoma.[61] Research has shown that the basement membranes of invasive tumors are lost uniformly because they are actively dissolved by the proteolytic enzymes secreted by and/or potentiated by the invading tumor cells.[41] In contrast, noninvasive and benign tumors retain their basement membranes. Loss of basement membranes in human carcinomas significantly correlates with an increased incidence of metastases and poor 5-year survival.[10]

A collagenase specific for type IV collagen was purified from a highly metastatic murine sarcoma.[62,63] Other proteolytic enzymes, including plasminogen activator, cathepsins, stromelysin, Type I collagenase, and heparanase, have been similarly implicated in the loss of basement membrane associated with tumor invasion.[64] These proteolytic enzymes overcome natural protease inhibitors, such as the tissue inhibitors of metalloproteinases (TIMP), or plasminogen activator inhibitors (PAI). Synthesis and secretion of proteolytic enzymes and their inhibitors are regulated by growth factors and cytokines.

The process of invasion and penetration of basement membranes has been described in terms of three distinct biochemical events:[37] (1) attachment, (2) degradation of the basement membrane, and (3) locomotion.

Attachment

It has been demonstrated that invasive tumor cells possess specific cell surface receptors that facilitate their attachment to vascular basement membrane.[40] Normal epithelial cells have the same cell surface receptors; but since they are in constant contact with the basement membrane, the receptors are permanently occupied. Since invasive tumors have lost their basement membrane, cell surface receptors are exposed, facilitating their attachment to vascular basement membrane.

A number of substances has been shown to enhance tumor cell attachment to epithelial basement membrane. Laminin has been shown to potentiate tumor cell metastasis by increasing cell adhesion to the capillary wall.[38] It is thought that the laminin molecule acts like a bridge: One end of the molecule binds cell surface laminin receptors, and the other end interacts with type IV collagen of the basement membrane of the capillary bed.[65]

Degradation

Once attached to laminin or type IV collagen, the tumor cell either secretes or causes the secretion by the host of proteases and other hydrolytic enzymes such as type IV collagenase that mediate penetration of the basement membrane by the tumor cells.[1,10,66] Tumor cells also produce chemoattractants for inflammatory cells such as monocytes and lymphocytes. The interaction of monocytes and tumor cells produces growth factors, interleukins, interferons, and tumor necrosis factor-alpha for initiation of angiogenesis and invasion.[33] The host responds to the invasive tumor by forming a dense and hard fibrous reaction called *desmoplasia,* which is responsible for the clinically appreciable hard lump that leads to the presentation of many cancers.

Locomotion

The third step in tumor cell invasion is movement by the tumor cell into the area of the matrix altered by proteolysis. Early movement of the tumor cell is by pseudopodia protrusion. The stimulation for pseudopodia locomotion and the direction taken by the tumor cells may be mediated by chemotactic factors released through cell degradation.[10] Pseudopodia act as "sense organs" to determine which direction the cell should take, physically move the cell, and induce local matrix proteolysis to assist the tumor cell in the penetration of the matrix.[67]

Random tumor cell motility and dispersion from the primary site are regulated by the cytokines "autocrine motility factors"[34] and "scatter factors."[68] In addition, the direction of the tumor cells is influenced by host chemoattractants produced by the organ to which the tumor cell subsequently travels. These chemoattractants may play a role in the organ-selective homing of metastasis.[5]

Dissemination

Once tumor cells penetrate the vascular or lymphatic channels, they either grow at the site of penetration or detach and circulate as emboli of individual cells or cell aggregates.[69]

Direct extension

Rapid proliferation of cells within a circumscribed space will cause pressure within the space, forcing fingerlike projections of cells into nearby body cavities and tissues. Local damage from the pressure of an expanding tumor can result in pain, bleeding, bone fractures, loss of function—depending on the tissues involved and the extent of damage.

When malignant cells invade a serous cavity such as the peritoneal, pleural, or pericardial spaces, tumor cells can break off and spread over the serous membranes. This tumor "seeding" in body cavities is a major clinical problem that may lead to ascites or to pericardial and pleural effusions. Tumors of the ovary, prostate, pancreas, uterus, and kidney can disseminate into the peritoneal cavity, resulting in multiple tumor growths at sites of implantations. Tumor cells implanted into serous membranes can proliferate and invade into the subjacent tissues.

Lymphatic dissemination

Tumor cells that enter the lymphatic system are transported passively from the site of detachment from the primary tumor to the first draining lymph node. Some tumor cells pass quickly through the lymph node to distant lymph nodes; others remain in the lymph node, and either proliferate, die, remain dormant, or enter the bloodstream.[70] Tumors with moderate metastatic potentials, such as squamous cell carcinomas of the head and neck, generally spread initially to regional lymphatic sites rather than to distant sites. A mass at the site of the regional lymph nodes draining a tumor may be the first clinical sign of a metastasis.

Hematogenous dissemination

Because of the numerous connections between the lymphatics and the vascular system, most tumor cells that enter the lymphatic system eventually find their way into the vascular system; thus lymphatic and hematogenous metastasis are not separate and distinct processes. In the circulatory system, the tumor cells face many threats, including the mechanical forces of blood turbulence and immune defenses such as lymphocytes, monocytes, and natural killer cells. Subsequent to their release into the circulation, tumor cells frequently adhere both to other tumor cells and to blood cells, especially platelets. These adhesions help protect the tumor cell from circulating immune cells, and produce enlarged emboli that increase the likelihood that tumor cells will arrest in the target organ.

Eventually the tumor cells arrest in capillaries and attach to endothelial cells and/or vascular basement membrane by the same attachment process described earlier in the section describing invasion. Tumor cells probably produce fibronectin to enhance attachment.[60]

Arrest

The factors underlying metastatic colonization of particular organs by certain cancers have intrigued scientists for many years. Experiments have shown that tumor cells reach many organs.[71] Some tumors spread randomly to the first organ linked anatomically to the site of the primary tumor. It is estimated that 50%–60% of metastatic distribution can be predicted from the anatomic route followed by the disseminating tumor cell.[1] Many metastatic deposits occur in the first capillary or nodal bed encountered after the tumor cells leave the primary tumor.

In approximately 40% of tumors, however, the distribution of metastases to various organs cannot be predicted by anatomic considerations alone. The site of arrest of metastatic cells in the parenchyma of organs seems to be selective and to depend on a match between the tumor and the organ. Paget[50] postulated that metastasis distribution was a consequence of specialized tumor cells ("seeds") finding a suitable environment ("soil") in which to grow and develop. Since Paget's time, other researchers have corroborated Paget's hypothesis that metastasis cannot be explained on the basis of mechanical considerations alone.[50,52,72,73] Laboratory experiments and clinical observations have shown that certain tumors have a predilection for metastasis to specific organs, independent of vascular anatomy, rate of bloodflow, or number of tumor cells delivered to each organ.[71] In fact, experiments in animals have shown that melanoma cells can be selected by organ adhesion, invasion, and even pigmentation.[74,75]

The distribution of metastases is probably determined by a combination of several mechanisms: selective target tissue adhesion, selective and directed chemotaxis mediated by tissue-specific chemotactic factors, responses of metastatic cells to growth factors differentially expressed in different organs and tissues.[73]

Recent investigations have shown that differences in the adhesive properties of the basement membranes of certain organs may be a factor in organ preference of metastasis.[76] For example, malignant cells that have higher relative affinities for laminin over fibronectin, such as certain mammary carcinoma cells, tend to metastasize predominantly to the lung, whereas those that have a lower relative affinity for laminin and higher relative affinity for fibronectin, such as many lymphoma cells, tend to metastasize to the liver. Laminin is a prominent component of lung basement membranes but is significantly less prominent in liver tissue basement membranes.[73]

Specific chemotactic factors have also been isolated from various organ sources, such as bone, brain, liver, and lung tissue. In these studies, brain-colonizing melanoma cells responded best to brain-derived chemotactic factors, lung-colonizing fibrosarcoma cells to lung-derived factors, and so on.[77]

Certain cancers (such as some breast cancers) are dependent on specific paracrine growth factors for their growth and development. These factors, preferentially expressed in different organs may be a determinant of organ preference of metastatic cell growth.[78]

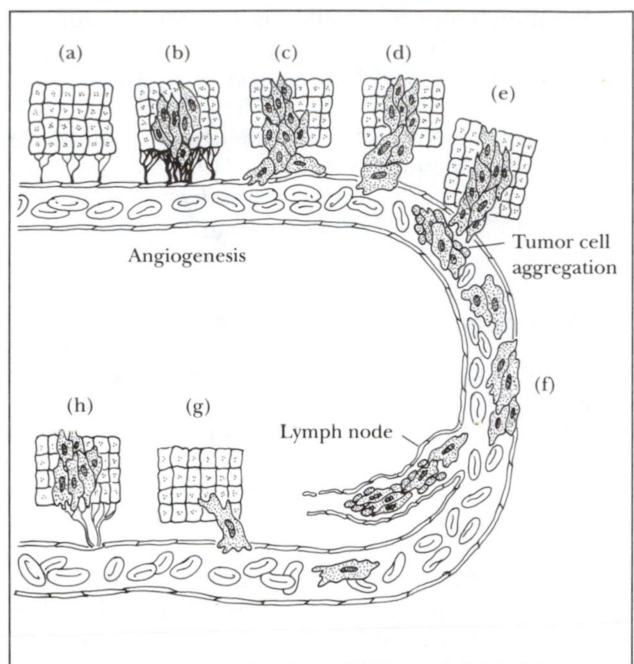

FIGURE 4-1 The metastatic sequence. (a) Normal tissue; (b) angiogenesis and growth of tumor; (c) attachment of tumor cells to epithelial basement membrane; (d) invasion of the basement membrane by tumor cells; (e) tumor cell dissemination into lymphatic and circulatory systems; (f) arrest of tumor cells on capillary wall or in lymph node; (g) extravasation of tumor cells from capillary into target tissue; (h) angiogenesis and growth of the secondary tumor into a clinically detectable mass.

Extravasation

Once the tumor cell arrests in the capillary bed of the target organ, it must find its way to the organ parenchyma by extravasating through the capillary wall. The process of extravasation is the same as the process of invasion that began the metastatic process. Degradative enzymes are produced by the tumor cells that break down the capillary basement membrane, allowing the tumor cell to penetrate through the capillary into the organ tissue.

Neovascularization and Growth of Metastasis

As in the growth and development of the primary tumor, any increase in cell population in the metastatic deposit is dependent first on establishment of a blood supply. The metastatic tumor accomplishes this by the process of angiogenesis in the same manner as did the primary tumor. Subsequent proliferation of the tumor within the organ parenchyma completes the metastatic process. The cycle can begin again with the cells invading host basement membrane, penetrating blood vessels, and entering the circulation to produce secondary metastases.

Figure 4-1 depicts the metastatic sequence.

ANTIMETASTASIS THERAPY

With a basic understanding of the pathophysiology of metastasis comes hope for ways to prevent and treat metastases. Separating invasion and metastasis into a series of defined sequential steps and then studying one step at a time has caused general themes to emerge to researchers that are yielding viable new possibilities for the treatment of cancer.

Failure of any step in the metastatic cascade completely abrogates the metastatic continuum. Therefore, it may appear that the prevention of metastasis lies in our ability to interrupt one or more steps in the metastatic process. However, "prevention" presumes that metastasis has not yet occurred. Unfortunately, for most individuals with cancer, metastasis has already occurred by the time the tumor is first diagnosed.

The only real prevention of metastasis will be the total destruction of all tumor cells with adjuvant therapy.[17] All therapeutic approaches designed to inhibit steps in the metastatic cascade will likely be unsuccessful unless used in combination with standard cytotoxic protocols. Some of these adjuvant antimetastatic treatment possibilities will be discussed in relation to their effect on specific steps of the metastatic process.

Prevention of Tumor Invasion

Tumor cell invasion occurs at least twice during the metastatic cascade. It occurs first at the site of the primary tumor, when tumor cells invade the surrounding tissue, eventually penetrating blood and lymph vessels for their dissemination to distant sites. Invasion occurs a second time after tumor cells arrest at distant sites and extravasate from the blood vessels into the target organ parenchyma.

Proteolytic enzymes capable of degrading basement membranes or extracellular matrix molecules are key factors in the process of invasion. Several in vivo and in vitro studies have documented that significant reduction in tumor metastasis can be achieved by systemic administration of protease inhibitors.[79–81]

Razoxane (ICRF-159) is considered the model antimetastatic drug, but its mechanism of action is still not well defined. Research has shown that razoxane inhibits tumor cell invasion.[82,83]

Antiadhesive Therapy

Based on the premise that binding of malignant cells to the glycoproteins fibronectin and laminin in the basement membranes promotes their invasiveness, substances have been studied for their ability to inhibit the interaction of fibronectin and laminin with specific tumor cell surface receptors.[84] The penetration of human melanoma cell lines and a glioblastoma cell line through the human amniotic basement membrane has been shown to be inhibited by the synthetic peptide Arg-Gly-Asp (RGD).[85]

Monoclonal Antibodies

Monoclonal antibodies against tumor cell surface receptors responsible for tumor adhesion and invasion have been studied.[86–88] These studies have shown a diminished ability of tumor cells to form metastases after the use of monoclonal antibodies, presumably because the antibodies bind to the tumor cell surface receptors for which they are specific, preventing the tumor cell from binding to and invading the basement membrane.

Antibodies to type IV collagenase may also serve as markers for metastasis of the tumor cell and may be useful in development of new diagnostic procedures for identifying occult metastases.[1]

Monoclonal antibodies against growth factors may also be included in the list of potentially active future therapeutic agents. These compounds could inhibit the uncontrolled proliferation of malignant cells.

Finally, antibodies may be developed to bring cytotoxic agents directly to tumor cells that express high levels of the receptor for which the antibody is specific.

Modulation of Tumor Vascularization

Since growth and development of both the primary tumor and metastatic deposit depend on the development of an adequate blood supply, it follows that prevention of angiogenesis would abrogate this process. Researchers have shown that neovascularization can be inhibited by a combination of heparin and cortisone in several tumors, including B16 melanoma, Lewis lung carcinoma, reticulum cell sarcoma, and bladder carcinoma in animal models.[89]

The antimetastasis drug razoxane (ICRF-159) appears to be restorative to the structure and integrity of capillary vessels within cancer, leading to a reduced rate of escape of malignant cells into the bloodstream. Systemic administration of razoxane to mice bearing Lewis lung carcinomas led to a significant decrease in the subsequent incidence of pulmonary metastases.[90]

Anticoagulation Therapy

As described earlier, hemostatic mechanisms and the metastatic cascade are intricately related. The metastatic cascade requires the presence of hemostatic components, especially platelets, for its successful completion. Tumor cell aggregation with platelets assists the tumor cells in their arrest and extravasation into distant organ parenchyma, and helps protect them from immune cells as they disseminate throughout the circulatory system. This relationship provides the rationale for the use of antiplatelet or anticoagulation drugs in the prevention of cancer metastasis. Olden et al. summarize research findings in this area[91]:

- Agents that inhibit platelet aggregation decrease cancer metastasis in some experimental tumors.
- Intravenous injection of intact tumor cells induces a decrease in platelet count.
- Emboli containing fibrin, platelets, and tumor cells can be detected in the circulation shortly after release of tumor cells into the circulation.

Heparin is known to exhibit a variety of biological properties, such as inhibition of blood coagulation, potentiation of angiogenesis,[92] interaction with fibroblast growth factors,[93] and modulation of cell growth.[94] In addition, heparin can bind to adhesion molecules such as fibronectin, laminin, and type IV collagen that promote the adhesion, spreading, and migration of tumor cells.[95] Based on those features, researchers have attempted to inhibit tumor metastasis experimentally by using heparin and its related compounds.[96] Antiplatelet drugs, such as prostacyclin[47] and forskolin,[48] not only prevent platelet activation and secretion but also greatly inhibit experimentally induced cell metastases in mice.

Over the past several decades, a number of clinical trials have demonstrated improved survival for individuals with cancer receiving anticoagulant warfarin therapy, especially in conjunction with standard chemotherapy. Small-cell carcinoma of the lung, ovarian cancer, breast cancer, and lymphosarcoma were shown to be especially responsive.[97,98]

Genetic Manipulation

An understanding of what genes regulate tumor cell growth and metastasis may provide important directions for treating and for monitoring prognosis of cancer. Research has demonstrated that in human breast cancer, loss of function of the suppressor gene nm23 is associated with rapid patient death, as compared to patients with high levels of nm23, who survive much longer.[99,100] Knowledge of how nm23 and other suppressor genes function in the cell could potentially lead to new anticancer drugs that mimic the effect of the suppressor genes. In addition, the suppressor genes could be used as prognostic markers to identify metastases that are clinically undetectable.

Understanding not only what genes are involved in cellular transformation and metastasis but what biochemical processes those genes initiate is important in developing new approaches to therapy. By blocking pathways that regulate the response of cancer cells to control signals, it may be possible to stop or reverse the growth of tumors with little or no toxicity.

Biotherapeutics

As described throughout this chapter, the development of cancer and subsequent metastases is a result of a series of complex interactions between the host and the tumor. The relatively new field of biotherapeutics, which addresses these complex host–tumor interactions, offers potentially the most promising approach to the treatment of cancer.[17] Altering the microenvironment in which the tumor thrives may deprive the tumor of the factors that stimulate and support its growth. For example, as described earlier, it has been demonstrated that a number of naturally occurring growth factors in the host may enhance the development of autonomous populations of tumor cells that have selective advantages over other cells for continued growth and diversification. Therapies that remove growth factors from the vicinity of the tumor, or somehow block the receptors on tumor cells that stimulate cell division and diversification in response to growth factors, may inhibit tumor growth.

Nonspecific and specific immunomodulators have been studied for their efficacy in reducing metastases and prolonging survival in cancer. Phase II and III clinical trials of active specific immunization with viral oncolysates have been encouraging.[101,102]

Lymphokine activation of macrophages leads to macrophage recognition and selective destruction of tumor cells.[103] In addition, the adoptive transfer of lymphokine-activated immune effector cells (LAK) has shown therapeutic promise. Monocytes are incubated with recombinant interleukin-2 (IL-2), activating them to a tumoricidal state. The activated monocytes stimulate and enhance proliferation of cytotoxic T-lymphocytes, helper T-cells, and natural killer (NK) cells. The adoptive transfer of these activated cells causes significant regression of established metastases in both animal and human trials.[104] Finally, interferon has been shown to enhance the expression of the class I major histocompatibility complex antigens and tumor-associated transplantation antigens, leading to enhanced tumor cell recognition and destruction by T-lymphocytes.[105]

Chapter 17 presents a thorough discussion of biotherapeutic approaches to the treatment of cancer.

CLINICAL APPLICATION

While research has shown that promise exists for therapies that interrupt the metastatic process, we unfortunately do not yet know enough about the specific biochemical processes in each step of the metastatic cascade to justify widespread use of such therapies. In addition, the fact that most individuals with cancer have metastases at the time of initial diagnosis makes prevention of metastasis a moot issue. Because of the problems of tumor cell heterogeneity and the complexity of the metastatic process, multiple antimetastatic agents used in combination with conventional cytotoxic therapies will be required for maximum clinical efficacy.[106] Additional research into the specific steps of the metastatic process and how this cascade of events can be blocked must be forthcoming before antimetastatic approaches will be clinically practical.

In the meantime, the clinical challenges that the problem of cancer metastatis puts before us include:

1. accurate identification of the metastatic potential of a primary tumor
2. diagnosis and localization of clinically silent micrometastases at the time of initial diagnosis of cancer
3. complete eradication of all tumor cells in a heterogeneous tumor with primary tumor treatment
4. selective eradication of metastases during treatment of a primary tumor
5. prevention of invasion and metastasis

Our ability to meet these clinical challenges, as always, will depend on advances in knowledge gleaned from the coordinated research efforts of basic scientists and clinicians.

REFERENCES

1. Liotta LA, Kohn E: Cancer invasion and metastases. *JAMA* 263:1123–1126, 1990.
2. Fidler IJ, Hart IR: Biological diversity in metastatic neoplasms: Origins and implications. *Science* 217:998–1003, 1982.
3. Weiss L: Metastatic inefficiency: Causes and consequences. *Cancer Rev* 3:1–24, 1986.
4. Fidler IJ: Critical factors in the biology of human metastasis: Twenty-eighth G.H.A. Clowes Memorial Award Lecture. *Cancer Res* 50:6130–6138, 1990.

5. Liotta LA, Steeg PS, Stetler-Stevenson WG: Cancer metastasis and angiogenesis: An imbalance of positive and negative regulation. *Cell* 64:327–336, 1991.
6. Klein G, Klein E: Conditioned tumorigenicity of activated oncogenes. *Cancer Res* 46:3211–3224, 1986.
7. Nicolson GL: Tumor cell instability, diversification and progression to the metastatic phenotype: From oncogene to oncofetal expression. *Cancer Res* 47:1473–1487, 1987.
8. Sobel ME: Metastasis suppressor genes. *J Natl Cancer Inst* 82:267–272, 1990.
9. Muschel R, Liotta LA: Role of oncogenes in metastases. *Carcinogenesis* 9:705–710, 1988.
10. Liotta LA: Gene products which play a role in cancer invasion and metastasis. *Breast Cancer Res and Treatment* 11:113–124, 1988.
11. Seeger RC, Broudeur GM, Sather H, et al: Association of multiple copies of the N-*myc* oncogene with rapid progression of neuroblastomas. *N Engl J Med* 313:1111–1116, 1985.
12. Clair T, Miller WR, Cho-Chung YS: Prognostic significance of the expression of a *ras* protein with a molecular weight of 21,000 by human breast cancer. *Cancer Res* 47:5290–5293, 1987.
13. Field JK, Spandido DA: The role of *ras* and *myc* oncogenes in human solid tumours and their relevance in diagnosis and prognosis. *Anticancer Res* 10:1–22, 1990.
14. Fidler IJ, Kripke ML: Metastasis results from pre-existing variant cells within a malignant tumor. *Science* 197:893–895, 1977.
15. Heppner GH: Tumor heterogeneity. *Cancer Res* 44:2259–2265, 1984.
16. Fidler IJ, Balch CM: The biology of cancer metastasis and implications for therapy. *Curr Probl Surg* 24:131–209, 1987.
17. Killion JJ, Fidler IJ: The biology of tumor metastasis. *Sem in Oncology* 16:106–115, 1989.
18. Poste G, Doll H, Fidler IJ: Interactions among clonal subpopulations affect stability of the metastatic phenotype in polyclonal populations of B16 melanoma cells. *Proc Natl Acad Sci USA* 78:6226–6230, 1981.
19. Kerbel RS, Waghorne C, Korczak B, et al: Clonal dominance of primary tumors by metastatic cells: Genetic analysis and biological implications. *Cancer Surv* 7:597–629.
20. Kerbel RS: Growth dominance of the metastatic cancer cell: Cellular and molecular aspects. *Adv Cancer Res* 55:87–131, 1990.
21. McGuire WL, Tandon AK, Allred DC, et al: How to use prognostic factors in axillary node-negative breast cancer patients. *J Natl Cancer Inst* 82:1006–1015, 1990.
22. Tandon AK, Clark GM, Chamness GC, et al: Cathepsin D and prognosis in breast cancer. *New Engl J Med* 322:297–302, 1990.
23. Goustin AS, Leof EB, Shipley GD, et al: Growth factors and cancer. *Cancer Res* 46:1015–1029, 1986.
24. Waterfield MD, Scrace GT, Whittle N, et al: Platelet-derived growth factor is structurally related to the putative transforming protein p28 of Simian sarcoma virus. *Nature* 304:35–39, 1983.
25. Stiles CD: The biological role of oncogenes: Insights from platelet-derived growth factor. *Cancer Res* 45:5215–5218, 1985.
26. Killion JJ: Modern views of metastasis. *Cancer Cells.* Cold Springs, NY: Cold Springs Harbor Press, 1989.
27. Folkman J: Tumor angiogenesis: Therapeutic implications. *New Engl J Med* 285:1182–1186, 1971.
28. Folkman J, Watson K, Ingber D, et al: Induction of angiogenesis during the transition from hyperplasia to neoplasia. *Nature* 339:58–61, 1989.
29. Jaye M, Hawk R, Burgess W, et al: Human endothelial growth factors: Cloning nucleotide sequence and chromosome localization. *Science* 233:541–545, 1986.
30. Folkman J, Klagsburn M: Angiogenic factors. *Science* 235:444–447, 1987.
31. Schroder MF, Risau W, Hallmann R, et al: Tumor necrosis factor type, a potent inhibitor of endothelial cell growth *in vitro,* is angiogenic *in vivo. Proc Natl Acad Sci* 84:5277–5281, 1987.
32. Lam WC, Delikatny JE, Orr FW, et al: The chemotactic response of tumor cells: A model for cancer metastasis. *Am J Pathol* 104:69–76, 1981.
33. Graves DT, Jiang YL, Williamson MJ, et al: Identification of monocyte chemotactic activity produced by malignant cells. *Science* 245:1490–1495, 1989.
34. Liotta LA, Mandler R, Murano G, et al: Tumor cell autocrine motility factor. *Proc Natl Acad Sci USA* 83:3302–3306, 1986.
35. Guirguis R, Schiffmann E, Liu B., et al: Detection of autocrine motility factor(s) in urine as markers of bladder cancer. *J Natl Cancer Inst* 80:1203–1211, 1988.
36. Hynes RO: Integrins: A family of cell surface receptors. *Cell* 48:549–554, 1987.
37. Ruoslahti E, Giancotti FG: Integrins and tumor cell dissemination. *Cancer Cells* 1:119–126, 1989.
38. Rao CN, Margulies LMK, Trakla S, et al: Isolation of a subunit of laminin and its role in molecular structure and tumor cell attachment. *J Biol Chem* 257:9740–9744, 1982.
39. Liotta LA: Tumor invasion: Role of the extracellular matrix. *Cancer Res* 46:1–7, 1986.
40. Barsky SH: The metastatic phenotype. *Disease Markers* 6:71–80, 1988.
41. Frost P, Kerbel RS: Immunology of metastasis. Can the immune response cope with disseminating tumor? *Cancer Met Rev* 2:239–256, 1983.
42. Fidler JJ: Macrophages and metastasis—A biological approach to cancer therapy: Presidential Address. *Cancer Res* 45:4714–4726, 1985.
43. Gasic GJ, Gasic T, Stewart, CC: Antimetastatic effects associated with platelet reduction. *Proc Natl Acad Sci USA* 61:46–52, 1968.
44. Gasic GJ: Role of plasma, platelets and endothelial cells in tumor metastasis. *Cancer Met Rev* 3:99–114, 1984.
45. Gasic GJ, Tuszynski GP, Gorelik E: Interation of the hemostatic and immune systems in the metastatic spread of tumor cells. *Int Rev Exp Pathol* 29:173–208, 1984.
46. Tuszynski GP, Gasic TB, Rothman VL, et al: Thrombospondin, a potentiator of tumor cell metastasis. *Cancer Res* 47:4130–4133, 1987.
47. Honn, KV, Cicone B, Skoff, A: Prostaglandin: A potent antimetastatic agent. *Science* 212:1270–1272, 1981.
48. Agarwal KC, Parks RE: Forskolin: A potential antimetastatic agent. *Int J Cancer* 32:801–804, 1983.
49. Gorelik E., Wiltrout RH, Okumura K, et al: Role of NK cells in the control of metastatic spread and growth of tumor cells in mice. *Int J Cancer* 30:107–112, 1982.
50. Paget S: The distribution of secondary growth in cancer of the breast. *Lancet* i:571–573, 1889.

51. Hart IR, Fidler IJ: Role of organ selectivity in determination of metastatic patterns of B16 melanoma. *Cancer Res* 41:1281–1287, 1981.
52. Hart IR: "Seed and soil" revisited: Mechanisms of site-specific metastasis. *Cancer Metastasis Rev* 1:5–17, 1982.
53. Fialkow PJ: Clonal origin of human tumors. *Annu Rev Med* 30:135–176, 1979.
54. Vogelstein B, Fearon ER, Hamilton SR, et al: Use of restriction fragment length polymorphisms to determine the clonal origin of human tumors. *Science* 227:642–645, 1985.
55. Folkman J: Angiogenesis: Initiation and modulation. In Nicolson GL, Milas L (eds.): *Cancer Invasion and Metastasis: Biologic and Therapeutic Aspects.* New York: Raven Press, 1984, pp, 201–209.
56. Schreiber AB, Winkler ME, Derynck R: Transforming growth factor-α: A more potent angiogenic mediator than epidermal growth factor. *Science* 232:1250–1253, 1986.
57. Furcht LT: Critical factors controlling angiogenesis: Cell products, cell matrix, and growth factors. *Lab Invest* 55:505–509, 1986.
58. Ausprunk DH, Folkman J: Migration and proliferation of endothelial cells in preformed and newly formed blood vessels during tumor angiogenesis. *Microvasc Res* 14:53–65, 1977.
59. Mahadevan V, Hart IR: Metastasis and angiogenesis. *Acta Oncologica* 29:97–103, 1990.
60. Martinez-Hernandez A, Amenta PA: The basement membrane in pathology. *Lab Invest* 48:656–677, 1983.
61. Barsky SH, Siegal GP, Jannotta F, et al: Loss of basement membrane components by invasive tumors but not their benign counterparts. *Lab Invest* 49:140–148, 1983.
62. Liotta LA, Abe S, Gehron-Robey P, et al: Preferential digestion of basement membrane collagen by an enzyme derived from a metastatic murine tumor. *Proc Natl Acad Sci USA* 76:2268–2272, 1979.
63. Stetler-Stevenson WG, Krutzsch HC, Wacher MP, et al: The activation of human type IV collagenase proenzyme: Sequence identification of the major conversion product following organomercurial activation. *J Biol Chem* 264:1353–1356, 1989.
64. Herlyn M, Malkowicz SB: Biology of disease: Regulatory pathways in tumor growth and invasion. *Lab Invest* 65:262–271, 1991.
65. Barsky SH, Rao CN, Williams JE, et al: Laminin molecular domains which alter metastasis in a murine model. *J Clin Invest* 74:843–848, 1984.
66. Liotta LA, Thorgeirsson UP, Garbisa S: Role of collagenases in tumor cell invasion. *Cancer Metast Rev* 1:277–283, 1982.
67. Guirguis R, Margulies IMK, Taraboletti G, et al: Cytokine-induced pseudopodial protrusion coupled to tumor cell migration. *Nature* 329:261–265, 1987.
68. Gherardi E, Gray J, Stoker M, et al: Purification of scatter factor, a fibroblast-derived basic protein that modulates epithelial interactions and movement. *Proc Natl Acad Sci USA* 86:5844–5848, 1989.
69. Hu F, Wang RY, Hsu TC: Clonal origin of metastasis in B16 melanoma: A cytogenetic study. *J Natl Cancer Inst* 78:155–163, 1987.
70. Nicolson GL, Poste G: Tumor implantation and invasion at metastatic sites. *Intl Rev Exp Path* 25:77–181, 1983.
71. Price JE, Aukerman SL, Fidler IJ: Evidence that the process of murine melanoma metastases is sequential and selective and contains stochastic elements. *Cancer Res* 46:5172–5178, 1986.
72. Nicolson GL: Organ specificity of tumor metastasis: Role of preferential adhesion, invasion and growth of malignant cells at specific secondary sites. *Cancer Metastasis Rev* 7:143–188, 1988.
73. Nicolson GL: Molecular mechanisms of cancer metastasis: Tumor and host properties and the role of oncogenes and suppressor genes. *Current Opinion in Oncology* 3:75–92, 1991.
74. Nicolson GL, Dulski K, Basson C, et al: Preferential organ attachment and invasion *in vitro* by B16 melanoma cells selected for differing metastatic colonization and invasive properties. *Invasion Metastasis* 5:144–158, 1985.
75. Price JE, Tarin D, Fidler IJ: Influence of organ microenvironment on pigmentation of a metastatic murine melanoma. *Cancer Res* 48:2258–2264, 1988.
76. Pauli BU, Augustin-Voss HG, El-Sabban ME, et al: Organ preference of metastasis. The role of endothelial cell adhesion molecules. *Cancer Metastasis Rev* 9:175–189, 1990.
77. Hujanen ES, Terranova VP: Migration of tumor cells to organ-derived chemoattractants. *Cancer Res* 45:3517–3521, 1985.
78. Naito SR, Giavazzi R, Fidler IJ: Correlation between the *in vitro* interaction of tumor cells with an organ environment and metastatic behavior *in vivo. Invasion Metastasis* 7:16–29, 1987.
79. Stein-Werblowsky R: On the prevention of hematogenous tumor metastases in rats. The role of the protease inhibitor "Trasylol." *J Cancer Res Clin Oncol* 97:129–135, 1980.
80. Thorgeirssen UP, Liotta LA, Kalebic IM, et al: Effect of natural protease inhibitors and a chemoattractant on tumor cell invasion *in vitro. J Natl Cancer Inst* 69:1049–1054, 1982.
81. Sloane BF, Honn KV: Cystine proteinases and metastasis. *Cancer Met Rev* 3:249–263, 1984.
82. Hellman K: Antimetastic drugs: Function and value. *Prog Clin Biol Res* 212:1–16, 1986.
83. Welch DR, Lobl TJ, Seftor EA, et al: Use of the Membrane Invasion Culture System (MICS) as a screen for anti-invasive agents. *Int J Cancer* 43:449–457, 1989.
84. Humphries MJ, Olden K, Yamada KM: A synthetic peptide from fibronectin inhibits experimental metastasis of murine melanoma cells. *Science* 233:467–470, 1986.
85. Gehlsen K, Argraves WS, Pierschbacher MD, et al: Inhibition of *in vitro* tumor cell invasion by Arg-Cly-Asp-containing synthetic peptides. *J Cell Biol* 106:925–930, 1988.
86. Ossowski L, Reich E: Antibodies to plasminogen activator inhibit human tumor metastasis. *Cell* 35:611–619, 1983.
87. Vollmers HP, Birchmeier W: Cell adhesion and metastasis: A monoclonal antibody approach. *Trend Biochem Sci* 5:452–455, 1983.
88. Raz A, Lotan R: Endogenous galactoside-binding lectins: A new class of functional tumor cell surface molecules related to metastasis. *Cancer Met Rev* 6:433–452, 1987.
89. Folkman J, Langer R, Lindhardt RJ, et al: Angiogenesis inhibition and tumor regression caused by heparin or a heparin fragment in the presence of cortisone. *Science* 221:719–725, 1983.
90. James SE, Salsbury AJ: Effect of ICRF 159 on tumor

blood vessels and its relationship to the antimetastatic effect in the Lewis lung carcinoma. *Cancer Res* 34:839–842, 1974.

91. Olden K, White SL, Mohla S, et al: Experimental approaches for the prevention of hematogenous metastasis. *Oncology* 3:83–91, 1989.
92. Taylor S, Folkman J: Protamine is an inhibitor of angiogenesis. *Nature* 297:307–312, 1982.
93. Baird A, Schubert D, Ling N, et al: Receptor- and heparin-binding domains of basic fibroblast growth factor. *Proc Natl Acad Sci USA* 85:2324–2328, 1988.
94. Wright TC, Jr, Castellot JJ, Jr, Petitou M, et al: Structural determinants of heparin's growth inhibitor activity. *J Biol Chem* 264:1534–1524, 1989.
95. Charonis AS, Skubitz APN, Koliakos GG, et al: A novel synthetic peptide from the B1 chain of laminin with heparin-binding and cell adhesion promoting activities. *J Cell Biol* 107:1253–1260, 1988.
96. Villaneuva GB, Nakajima M, Nicolson GL: Heparin derivatives as inhibitors of heparanase from metastatic melanoma cells. *Ann NY Acad Sci* 556:496–498, 1989.
97. Zacharski LR, Henderson WG, Rickles FR, et al: Effect of warfarin anticoagulation on survival in carcinoma of the lung, colon, head and neck and prostate. *Cancer* 53:2046–2052, 1984.
98. Chahinian AP, Ware JH, Zimmer B, et al: Update on anticoagulation with warfarin and on alternating chemotherapy in extensive small cell carcinoma of the lung (SCCL). *Proc Am Soc Clin Oncol* 4:191, 1985.
99. Bevilacqua G, Sobel ME, Liotta LA, et al: Association of low nm23 RNA levels in human primary infiltrating ductal breast carcinomas with lymph node involvement and other histopathological indicators of high metastatic potential. *Cancer Res* 49:5185–5190, 1989.
100. Hennessy C, Henry JA, May FEB, et al: Expression of the anti-metastatic gene nm23 in human breast cancer: An association with a good prognosis. *J Natl Cancer Inst* 83:281–285, 1991.
101. Cassel WA, Murray DR, Phillips HS: A phase II study on the postsurgical management of stage II malignant melanoma with a Newcastle disease virus oncolysate. *Cancer* 52:856–860, 1983.
102. Hoover HC, Surdyke M, Dangel R, et al: Prospectively randomized trial of adjuvant active specific immunotherapy for human colorectal cancer. *Cancer* 55:1236–1244, 1985.
103. Fidler IJ, Poste G: Macrophage-mediated distribution of malignant tumor cells and new strategies for the therapy of metastatic disease. *Springer Semin Immunopath* 5:161–174, 1982.
104. Longo DL: Biological therapy of cancer. In Fortner JG, Rhoads JE (eds.): *Accomplishments in Cancer Research.* Philadelphia: Lippincott, 1986, pp. 233–257.
105. Gorelik E, Gunji Y, Goldfarb RH: Interaction of tumor cells and immune system in metastatic process. *Biochem Cell Biol* 66:617–625, 1988.
106. Nicolson GL: The article reviewed. *Oncology* 3:95–98, 1989.

Chapter 5

Relation of the Immune System to Cancer

Donald P. Braun, PhD

Susan L. Groenwald, RN, MS

INTRODUCTION

That the immune system is capable of responding to the presence of malignant disease has been appreciated for close to a century. The earliest evidence for this contention was based on the histopathologic presentation of tumors, many of which were highly infiltrated with round mononuclear cells. The presence of such infiltrates was found to be associated with a more favorable prognosis than when infiltration was absent. However, the identification of these tumor-infiltrating cells as cells of the immune system was not made until the 1950s, and only recently have modern immunological techniques been applied to study immune cells associated with tumors in humans.

Once the immune response was recognized as a discrete physiologic system, its role in the development and progression of malignant disease was investigated. The earliest definitive studies relied on animal tumor models. As a result of these studies, the presence of tumor-associated antigens was demonstrated and an inverse relationship between immune competence and the development of malignant disease was inferred. Furthermore, the belief that cell-mediated immunity was responsible for tumor resistance while humoral immunity was either irrelevant or even inhibitory to tumor immunity emerged. Although many of these early contentions have since been modified, the ideas that resulted from these initial investigations have dominated and guided much of the thinking about the relationship between immunity and cancer during the past half century. Investigation in the 1970s and 1980s produced a substantial increase in knowledge and understanding of both the immune system and of neoplasia. These separate bodies of information come together topically in the field of modern tumor immunology.

The emphasis and intent of this chapter are to describe what is known currently about the interaction of the immune system and malignant disease. The approach taken is intended to be conceptual, with relevant examples being given to support concepts. Fundamental knowledge of the immune response is assumed; the reader is referred to any modern immunology textbook for a review of the immunologic principles underlying the information in this chapter. Given the growing application of immunologic techniques to cancer patient management and the use of different immunologic products for cancer patient therapy, the information contained in this chapter is fundamental to anyone interested in cancer.

TUMOR-ASSOCIATED ANTIGENS

Tumor cells are capable of provoking immune reactions in immunocompetent hosts because of the expression of different antigenic determinants on the surface of the malignant cells. Several decades ago, researchers demonstrated that animals immunized with a chemically induced tumor could reject a subsequent graft of that tumor.[1–3] The antigens responsible for the tumor rejections observed were referred to as *tumor-specific transplantation antigens (TSTAs)*. Subsequent studies showed that tumors induced by oncogenic viruses also express TSTAs.[4,5] Unfortunately, the antigens that can be identified on malignant cells in humans do not show the same specificity as do most of the TSTAs in animals. The great majority of human antigens known today that are capable of provoking immune reactions against tumor tissue are called *tumor-associated differentiation antigens (TADAs)*. These antigens have relative rather than absolute specificity for cancer cells.[6] These tumor-associated antigens are used clinically as tumor markers for diagnostic purposes and, in some cases, for cancer patient management by monitoring prognosis and response to therapy. In general, these antigens are detected by immunohistologic techniques (tissues) or immunochemical techniques (serum). There are several different types of human tumor-associated antigens, as discussed in the following subsections.

Normal Tissue Antigens Associated with Differentiation

The expression of normal cellular differentiation antigens by tumors permits a definitive identification of their tissue of origin, information that is often fundamental to selection of an appropriate treatment plan. These antigens may include the production of a specific hormone (e.g., human chorionic gonadotropin for placental tumors), a specific enzyme (e.g., prostatic acid phosphatase for prostatic cancers), or a specific cell-surface protein (e.g., immunoglobulin molecules for tumors of B-cell origin).

One of the best examples of the use of a differentiation-associated antigen for cancer patient management is the application of monoclonal antibodies to lymphocyte markers for B- and T-lymphocytes, resulting in extensive reclassification of leukemias and lymphomas. For example, the expression of common antigens or receptor peptides is used to identify specific lymphoreticular tumors.[8] The expression of immunoglobulin molecules on the surface of lymphoreticular tumors is one method that is used to classify the cells as being of B-lymphocyte or T-lymphocyte origin. Similarly, the expression of the common T-lymphocyte antigen (CD3) is used to identify T-lymphocyte lymphoreticular tumors. Many of the markers identified by monoclonal antibodies are called *cluster designations (CDs)*.[7] A given CD number (such as CD3) represents a group of peptide markers of differentiation of a common subpopulation of B- or T-lymphocytes. These markers also appear on leukemia and lymphoma cells. Since many B-cell tumors secrete immunoglobulin peptides or fragments into the circulation, levels of these proteins can be used to monitor total tumor burden and responsiveness to therapy. Newer techniques rely on the expression of different growth factors or cytokine receptors on lymphoreticular tumors to further classify the lineage and differentiation state of a particular lymphoreticular malignancy.[9]

Another example of antigens that arise by modification of normal antigens are the antigens expressed on melanoma cells. Apart from different melanocyte-associated antigens, the melanomas also express different gangliosides, growth factor receptors, cellular adhesion/cellular interaction molecules, histocompatibility antigens, and differentiation antigens. These antigens expressed at variable levels by most melanomas are also expressed on different normal tissues. Thus, it can be appreciated that the immunogenicity of these antigen systems in melanoma patients is related not to their "foreignness" but rather to their altered or modified expression.

Viral-Associated Antigens

The expression of antigens specified by either RNA or DNA virus genetic material is common on many different animal and human tumors. In some systems, immunization with the attachment protein of a particular tumorigenic virus is capable of blocking the induction of tumor by that virus in a subsequent challenge. Similarly, immunization with killed tumor cells induced by a particular virus can protect susceptible hosts against different tumors induced by the same virus, suggesting the existence of one or more common tumor-associated viral antigens.[5]

A role for viruses in the induction of certain tumors in humans is suggested by histopathologic and epidemiologic evidence. This evidence was presented in a 1989 review by Henderson[10] and is also reviewed in Chapter 2. A strong association between the development of tumors and viral infections has been found in the following cases:

- hepatitis B virus and hepatocellular carcinoma
- Epstein-Barr virus and certain B-cell lymphomas (e.g., Burkitt's lymphoma)
- human papillomaviruses and cervical carcinoma
- HTLV-1 and acute T-cell leukemias

These associations have led to the development of vaccines aimed at conferring protective antiviral immunity or antitumor immunity in humans.[11] However, it should be stated that the existence of tumor-associated viral antigens in humans does not directly implicate that virus in the development of a particular malignant disease. Furthermore, the genetic mechanism(s) by which viruses can induce tumors in humans are poorly understood, and the effects produced by a virus can be either direct (as in the case of viral activation of a particular oncogene) or indirect (as in the case of the human immunodeficiency virus).

Oncofetal Antigens

Oncofetal antigens are proteins that are present normally during fetal development but are then suppressed to low but still detectable levels in the adult. These proteins are expressed on tumor tissues and reappear in the circulation of patients with malignant disease. In animal models, preimmunization with oncofetal antigens can protect susceptible hosts against a subsequent lethal tumor challenge. In humans, the expression of oncofetal antigens has been used most frequently as a monitoring tool but more recently has also been used to image tumors using monoclonal antibodies conjugated to radioisotopes.[12]

The most familiar examples of oncofetal antigens include the carcinoembryonic antigen (CEA) and alpha-fetoprotein (AFP). CEA is a glycoprotein expressed in adults at low levels by tissues of the GI tract; AFP is an alpha-globulin similar in structure and function to albumin that is expressed at low levels primarily in the liver. Increased levels of CEA in the circulation are associated with a variety of epithelial tumors (e.g., breast cancers, lung tumors, colorectal tumors). Increased levels of AFP in the circulation are associated with hepatocellular carcinomas and certain germ cell tumors. However, increases in CEA and AFP are also seen in nonmalignant diseases (e.g., cirrhosis, obstructive pulmonary diseases) and can also be elevated in cigarette smokers. Oncofetal antigen levels have been most useful in clinical situations as markers for following the development of tumors. In general, the level of oncofetal antigens in the circulation in patients with diseases associated with the expression of these antigens broadly correlates with the clinical course of the disease.[9]

IMMUNOLOGIC REACTIONS AGAINST TUMOR CELLS

Virtually all of the immune effector cells that have been described can participate in the response to malignant disease. The principal kinds of reactions that are thought to have a significant impact on tumor development and progression are discussed here. In subsequent sections the role played by these immune reactions during specific phases of malignant disease progression will be considered.

T-Lymphocyte Responses

T-lymphocytes account for approximately 80% of all circulating lymphocytes. T-lymphocytes are derived from bone marrow lymphocyte progenitors that migrate to the thymus and differentiate into cells that express a complex polypeptide surface structure known as the CD3 complex. Expression of the CD3 complex marks a cell as having passed through the thymus, making it a T-lymphocyte. The antigenic specificity of the T-lymphocyte is also determined in the thymic environment and is reflected by the expression of antigen-specific receptors. The T-lymphocyte receptor is found in close association with the CD3 complex, which stabilizes the interaction between the receptor and its specific antigen. Each T-lymphocyte receptor is made up of two peptides that are disulfide-linked; each of these peptides is the product of one variable region gene and one constant region gene. There are multiple variable region genes for each chain of the T-lymphocyte receptor and one constant region gene for each chain of the T-lymphocyte receptor. Thus, T-lymphocyte receptors are capable of enormous diversity in antigen recognition.

Further differentiation of T-cells in the thymus leads to cells that express either the CD4 antigen or the CD8 antigen. CD4+ T-lymphocytes are the first T-lymphocytes to become activated when antigen (including tumor-associated antigen) is encountered. Their principal role is to function as helper/inducer T-lymphocytes responsible for activating and amplifying the production of other immune cells, including CD8+ T-lymphocytes. The CD4 complex on these helper/inducer cells functions as a receptor for membrane determinants (class II molecules) on the surface of antigen-presenting cells such as macrophages or dendritic cells. The class II molecules (which are designated HLA-DR determinants in humans) expressed on antigen-presenting cells are encoded by the genes of the major histocompatibility complex (MHC). Thus, helper T-lymphocytes are said to be *MHC-restricted* in their ability to become activated by the need to recognize *both* specific antigen and "self" class II molecules on the surface of the antigen-presenting cell. When a macrophage degrades an antigen such as a tumor cell, peptides from that tumor cell (tumor-associated antigens) become complexed with class II molecules and are then displayed on the macrophage surface. The helper/inducer T-lymphocytes become activated when they engage *both* the tumor-associated antigen (via their specific T-lymphocyte receptors) and the class II molecules (via the CD4 complex) on the surface of the antigen-presenting cells. If either of these recognition events is disturbed, T-lymphocyte activation is aborted. The principal outcome of a successful activation event by the CD4+ T-lymphocytes is the production and secretion of numerous peptides with potent biological effects known collectively as *lymphokines*. Lymphokines are largely responsible for immune cell activation, proliferation, and regulation.

One of the principal targets of the lymphokines made by activated CD4+ T-lymphocytes is the CD8+ T-lymphocyte. CD8+ T-lymphocytes can be further subdivided into functionally distinct cytolytic killer T-lymphocytes or immunoregulatory suppressor T-lymphocytes. Cytolytic or killer T-lymphocytes can interact with tumor-associated antigens on the surface of antigen-presenting cells or directly with tumor-associated antigens on tumor cell surfaces and can secrete different cytolytic peptides (e.g., perforin) that are capable of mediating tumor cell lysis. Once again, however, the activation of this class of T-lymphocytes requires both engagement of tumor-associated antigen (via the T-lymphocyte receptor) and engagement of a gene product derived from the MHC genes (via the CD8 complex). In this case, however, the MHC product that is recognized by the CD8 molecules on cytolytic T-lymphocytes is known as the class I molecule. Virtually all differentiated tissues in the body express class I molecules. Indeed, it is the expression of class I molecules that restricts the tolerance of the immune system to "self." Tumor cells, being derived from self tissues, also express class I molecules. Thus, in the presence of activated antigen-specific, CD8+ T-lymphocytes, tumor-associated antigens on the surface of tumor cells that express class I molecules are engaged by T-lymphocyte receptors and CD8 complexes respectively on the surface of activated cytolytic T-lymphocytes. The outcome of this interaction is the lysis of the tumor cell. Because this interaction is also dependent on recognition of an MHC-derived gene product (i.e., the class I molecules), the lysis of tumor cells by cytolytic T-lymphocytes is said to be MHC-restricted. If the expression of either the tumor-associated antigens or the class I molecules on the surface of tumor cells is abnormal, cytolytic T-lymphocyte function will be impaired.

The other class of T-lymphocytes relevant to tumor immunology is the CD8+ suppressor T-lymphocyte. This class of T-lymphocyte functions to attenuate or suppress the development of immune cell activation. Like the other classes of T-lymphocytes discussed, the suppressor T-lymphocytes also bear antigen-specific T-cell receptors. And, like the CD8+ cytolytic T-lymphocytes, the suppressor T cells are restricted by the need to recognize tumor-associated antigens together with class I molecules and thus are MHC-restricted. However, the antigens recognized by suppressor T-lymphocytes are thought to be different from those recognized by either the helper/inducer T-lymphocytes or the cytolytic T-cells. When the suppressor T-lymphocytes recognize a different class of tumor-associated antigens on the surface of a tumor cell, the outcome of that event is suppression of immune cell activation. The target of the action of the suppressor T-lymphocytes is the CD4+ helper/inducer T-lymphocytes. The mediators of this suppression can be either antigen-specific (i.e., they shut off only those T-lymphocytes that are being driven by the recognition of tumor-associated antigens) or nonspecific (i.e., they shut off other immunologic reactions to antigens unrelated to the tumor cells). These nonantigen-specific suppressor T-lymphocyte events are responsible for much of the immune deficiency seen in patients with cancer, as will be considered later in this chapter.

Natural Killer Cells

Natural killer (NK) cells are large granular lymphocytes that account for between 10%–15% of the total circulating lymphocytes. Because NK cells differ morphologically from the more typical small agranular lymphocytes, and because they do not express either the CD3 antigen of T-lymphocytes or surface immunoglobulins of B-lymphocytes, the NK cells are thought to represent a distinct lymphocyte lineage. The predominant surface structure that typifies all large granular lymphocytes (including those with NK activity) is a glycoprotein designated CD16 that functions as a receptor for IgG immunoglobulin. This surface receptor allows NK cells to interact with IgG antibodies in a mechanism known as *antibody-dependent cellular cytotoxicity*. NK cells have azurophilic granules that contain esterase and other enzymes that participate in the cytolysis of target cells. NK cells, like cytolytic T-lymphocytes, are capable of lysing a broad range of tumor cells. However, unlike T-lymphocytes, NK cells do not require sensitization by prior exposure to tumor antigens to exert their cytolytic effects against tumor cells. In fact, NK cells were discovered originally by demonstrating that lymphoid cells from normal healthy individuals were capable of spontaneously destroying certain cultured tumor cell lines without any prior or deliberate exposure to those cells.[13, 14]

Not surprisingly, NK cells do not rely on the same recognition structures as do T-lymphocytes, although the manner in which NK cells recognize potential target cells has not been elucidated completely as yet. Based on in vitro studies, it appears that at least one receptor on NK cells recognizes glycoprotein structures on tumor cells and that this can be blocked by simple sugars.[15] Whatever the mechanism of recognition, it is clear that NK cells are capable of conjugating to tumor cells and lysing susceptible tumors within 4 hours after conjugation. Furthermore, if conjugation is disrupted after 30 minutes, the lysis of the tumor cells can still proceed normally, indicating that a "lethal hit" can be delivered by the NK cell during the first 30 minutes of target cell binding. The fact that human NK cells can lyse tumor cells from different individuals and even from different species without previous exposure to those tumors shows that NK cells, unlike T-cells, are not MHC-restricted.

Apart from their cytolytic function, NK cells are also active secretors of lymphokines with potent biologic effects, including interleukin-1 (IL-1), IL-2, tumor necrosis factor-α, interferon-α, and several different hematopoietic colony stimulating factors. These secretory products of NK cells can participate in inhibiting the growth of some tumor cells directly and also participate in promoting and regulating the development of antitumor immunity by other cells. It is important to recognize that almost all cells capable of mediating tumor killing have receptors on their surface for lymphokines. Interaction of these cells with the appropriate lymphokine can activate the tumor cytolytic function of these cells, as discussed below.

Lymphokine-Activated Tumor Cell Killing

In the early 1980s it was found that incubation of mononuclear cells from the peripheral blood of healthy individuals with the lymphokine interleukin-2 (IL-2) elicited a potent tumor killing response.[16] This antitumor response has since come to be called *lymphokine-activated killing (LAK)*. The ability to mediate LAK function has been shown for both NK cells and for T-cells. When purified NK cells are incubated with IL-2, the mechanism for their killing effect is identical to what is seen with normal NK-mediated cytolysis; however, the range of tumor target cells that can be killed is increased greatly.[17] Of considerable importance is the fact that NK cells incubated in IL-2 can kill virtually all fresh human tumor cells and not merely established tumor cell lines. When purified T-lymphocytes are incubated with IL-2, the LAK exhibited differs from that of classic cytolytic T-lymphocytes in that the tumor killing effects are *not* restricted to MHC-matched tumor cells. Furthermore, this form of T-lymphocyte-mediated tumor killing does not require prior exposure to tumor antigens. As previously discussed for classical NK function, LAK function depends on recognition structures on tumor cells that have not been identified and characterized as yet. The recognition that lymphokines can greatly increase the tumor killing capacity of NK cells and T-lymphocytes has prompted the development of several different approaches to tumor immunotherapy relying on either or both immune cells and specific lymphokines.

Macrophage-Mediated Tumor Cell Killing

Of all the immune cells capable of participating in tumor immunity, cells of the mononuclear phagocyte series, generally known as *macrophages*, show the greatest diversity in effects. Although macrophages can be made to exhibit a wide variety of functions, many of these complex functions are attributed to the "activated" macrophage. Of the more complex macrophage functions described, some of the most important for tumor immunology are the processes of tumor antigen presentation, regulation of other immune cell types, and the capacity to destroy tumor cells,[18, 19] The process of activating macrophages to the point where they can kill tumor cells depends, once again, upon lymphokines. The prototypical macrophage activator is interferon-gamma. When macrophages are incubated with interferon-gamma, they undergo a complex series of biochemical changes that culminates in the ability of the macrophages to destroy a wide variety of tumor cells. However, it is important to appreciate that these activated, tumoricidal macrophages are extremely specific for tumor cells and normal tissues are not affected. As is the case with NK function and LAK function, macrophage-mediated tumor cell killing is *not* restricted to MHC-matched tumor cells.

The mechanism for macrophage-mediated tumor cell killing involves binding of the macrophage to the tumor cells by a recognition system that has not yet been identified or characterized. It appears, however, that macrophages may recognize a common structure on the surface of all neoplastic cells that apparently is not recognized by sensitized lymphocytes.

Following tumor cell conjugation, the destruction of the target tumor cells occurs via secretion of various effector molecules from the macrophage into the tumor cells.[20,21] These events occur over a more extended period of time than in the case of T-cell–mediated or NK cell-mediated killing,[22] with cell death occurring within 24 hours of initial contact.

A number of discrete effector molecules have been isolated from activated macrophages that mediate the cytotoxic effects on tumor cells. One of these molecules is a neutral serine protease termed *cytotoxic factor (CF)* that is extremely potent against susceptible tumor cells.[23,24] Another factor isolated from activated macrophages with the capacity to mediate tumor killing is tumor necrosis factor-α (TNF-α).[25,26] This molecule is also produced by inflammatory macrophages and has been shown to contribute to the cachexia that is often seen in individuals with cancer.

Apart from mediating the lysis of tumor cells, activated macrophages have a remarkable capacity to mediate tumor cell cytostasis events. In this phenomenon, which may depend on the nitric oxide molecule, activated macrophages that are either conjugated to tumor cells or in the proximity of tumor cells induce a state in which there is no evidence of cell division or DNA synthesis.[27] Unlike macrophage-mediated tumor cell killing, however, the cytostasis can be produced in both normal and malignant cells. Activated macrophages often induce cytostasis in neoplastic cells prior to tumor cell death. This can come about through the macrophages causing tumor cells to undergo a "reductive division" where the tumor cell continues to divide in the absence of DNA synthesis, ultimately resulting in cell death.[28] In contrast, normal cells are not killed by this cytostasis mechanism even though they may stop dividing. The explanation for the resistance of normal cells to macrophage-mediated cytotoxicity or cytostasis remains to be determined.

Antibody-Dependent Tumor Cell Cytotoxicity

The binding of antibodies to tumor-associated antigens on tumor cell membranes usually does not lead to the destruction of the tumor cell, even in situations where the lytic mediators of the complement cascade are deposited on the tumor cell surface. The observation of this fact has led most investigators to conclude that tumor cells, like most nucleated mammalian cells, are relatively resistant to complement-dependent cellular cytotoxicity.[29] In murine systems where comparative studies are possible, it appears that lymphoreticular tumors are somewhat sensitive to antibody and complement-mediated cytotoxicity, whereas carcinomas and sarcomas are essentially resistant to this mechanism of cytotoxicity. With lymphoreticular tumors, both IgM antibodies and IgG antibodies can participate in complement-dependent tumor cell killing. The exquisite recognition capabilities of antibodies facilitate tumor cell destruction in collaboration with different immune effector cells. This sort of mechanism is referred to generally as *antibody-dependent cellular cytotoxicity* and is mediated almost exclusively by antibodies of the IgG class. Of the cells discussed previously, both NK cells (large granular lymphocytes) and macrophages have the capacity to interact with IgG antibody-coated tumor cells leading to tumor cell lysis. The basis for this interaction is through membrane receptors for the Fc portion of IgG molecules on both NK cells and macrophages. NK cells express one such receptor, designated Fc-RIII, and macrophages express two such receptors, known as Fc-RI and Fc-RII.

The ability of antibodies coated on tumor cell surfaces to increase tumor cell lysis in collaboration with NK cells or macrophages is based on two factors. First, antibodies on tumor cells increase the possibility of immune cell–tumor cell binding and the affinity of this interaction. Thus, the range of tumor cells that can be recognized by NK cells or macrophages is increased when antitumor antibodies are present and the interaction between the cells is stabilized. Second, the binding of the Fc portion of antibodies to the receptors on NK cells or macrophages provides an activation signal to these immune effector cells. This activation signal leads to increased killing function on the part of the immune cells in a manner analogous to the action of lymphokines on NK cells or macrophages. Thus, antibodies serve to focus more immune cells to the surface of tumor cells and also further activate the lytic activity of these immune cells beyond the levels achieved by the immune cells alone.

HOW TUMOR CELLS EVADE THE IMMUNE SYSTEM

The outcome of the neoplastic process is determined, at least in part, by the balance between the capacity of the immune system to destroy tumor cells and the capacity of tumor cells to evade immune-mediated destruction. This contention is supported by observations in experimental models of carcinogenesis that demonstrate that immune stimulants reduce the incidence of neoplasia and immune suppressants increase the incidence of neoplasia.[30,31] Further support for this idea in humans comes from epidemiological studies that demonstrate a strong correlation between age, immune competence, and cancer incidence.[32,33,34] In addition, immune deficiency resulting from genetic predisposition or acquired as a result of drug treatment or viral infection is associated with an increased incidence of malignancy.[35,36] But apart from these considerations, it is also clear that tumors do arise in immunocompetent individuals and that immune stimulation that leads to significantly increased antitumor immunity is not sufficient to destroy the vast majority of spontaneous tumors in humans. For this reason, it is important to recognize that tumor cell escape from immunological destruction is a fundamental property of most human malignant diseases. The manner in which this comes about constitutes a major area of investigation in tumor immunology.

The most important tumor escape mechanisms can be subdivided into mechanisms that distort tumor cell recognition and mechanisms that suppress antitumor immunity.

Mechanisms That Distort Tumor Cell Recognition

Tumor cells evade recognition in two ways. The first such mechanism is termed *antigenic modulation.* Tumor cell antigen modulation includes both the loss of membrane-associated tumor antigens and the modulation of membrane-associated antigenic structures. The loss of tumor-associated antigens on tumor cells is thought to come about as a result of increased membrane biosynthesis and turnover by tumor cells.[37] This produces a relatively unstable membrane on many tumor cells and often results in membrane proteins being shed from tumor cell surfaces into the circulation. In addition, tumor cells can modify the expression of certain membrane-associated structures that are critical for immune cell interaction. An important example of this is seen in the case of the altered expression of histocompatibility antigens on tumor cell membranes.[7] Thus, changes in tumor cell class I and class II MHC expression have been observed in human melanomas resulting in aborted tumor cell recognition on the part of MHC-restricted cytolytic T-cells.

Tumor cell recognition can also be distorted by factors that sterically block or mask tumor-associated antigens. Such "blocking factors" hinder sensitized immune effector cells from recognizing and conjugating to tumor cell surfaces. The most important blocking factors are antibodies.[38,39] Thus, antibodies can play opposing roles in tumor cell recognition, either facilitating recognition and destruction by immune cells or aborting such recognition. This suggests that a lethal immune cell–tumor cell conjugation mediated through antibodies is qualitatively distinct from one that is protective. However, it is still unclear what determines the outcome of the interaction of tumor cells with antibody.

Mechanisms That Suppress Antitumor Immunity

The other way in which tumors escape immunological destruction is by suppression of antitumor immunity. Suppression of antitumor immunity appears to come about through two principal mechanisms: (1) the secretion of suppressor factors from tumors and (2) the hyperactivation of suppressor T-cells and suppressor macrophages during progressive tumor growth.

The production of nonimmunoglobulin immunosuppressive factors from tumors that can be isolated from both serum and malignant effusions in individuals has been described for a wide variety of lymphoreticular and nonlymphoreticular solid tumors.[40,41] In almost all cases where such factors have been demonstrated, however, the relevance of that factor to the in vivo level of antitumor immunity and thus to tumor progression has never been critically analyzed. Almost all of these sorts of studies have concentrated on isolating and characterizing the factor(s) that have immunosuppressive activity without attempting to eliminate that factor in vivo.

The activation of suppressor T-cells by tumors is thought to reflect immunological responses to "suppressogenic" epitopes on tumors.[42] Evidence for such suppressogenic antigenic moieties has been provided in animal models for UV-induced tumors,[43] virally induced tumors,[44] and chemically induced tumors.[45] The importance of suppressor T-cells in inhibiting tumor cell killing in vivo in animal tumor models has been convincingly demonstrated in a series of elegant studies in plasmacytomatous mice by Mokyr's group.[46] There is no convincing evidence for the existence of suppressogenic epitopes on human tumors as yet, but there is an extensive literature that demonstrates that suppressor T-cells are activated during the course of tumor growth in humans.[47] Furthermore, the potential importance of suppressor T-cells in human cancer patients has been inferred by the results of studies showing improvement in in vitro tumor cell killing following elimination of suppressor T-cells[48] and by the demonstration of improved tumor regression in response to tumor cell vaccines when suppressor T-cells are selectively eliminated by low-dose cyclophosphamide therapy.[49–51]

Suppressor macrophages have also been shown to be hyperactivated during progressive tumor growth in animal systems and in humans.[47] Abnormal macrophage-mediated suppression was first described in patients with Hodgkin's disease[52] and has since been demonstrated for essentially all of the major lymphoreticular and nonlymphoreticular solid tumors that have been investigated.[47] The principal way in which cancer is thought to affect macrophage suppressor function is by altering macrophage cellular arachidonic acid (AA) metabolism.[53] AA is metabolized in most cells including macrophages via the cyclooxygenase and lipoxygenase enzyme systems. The metabolites produced are known collectively as *eicosanoids* and include prostaglandins (PGs), thromboxane (TBx), leukotrienes (LTs), and hydroxyeicosatetraenoic acids (HETEs).[54] In patients with cancer, increased levels of eicosanoids in the circulation and in extravascular secretions have been documented[55] and implicated in essentially all of the immunologic abnormalities associated with tumor progression.[56,57] Apart from secretion by suppressor monocytes, increases in eicosanoids in individuals with cancer have also been attributed to active secretion by tumor tissues, and as a result of the attendant activation of the coagulation and inflammation pathways that occurs in individuals with disseminated malignant disease.[58–61] For this reason, attempts to modify hyperactive macrophage-mediated suppressor function have been undertaken in humans, with preliminary results demonstrating that improved immune function and clinical tumor responses can be achieved when individuals are treated with prostaglandin synthesis inhibitors.[62]

THE IMPORTANCE OF THE IMMUNE SYSTEM FOR SPECIFIC ASPECTS OF NEOPLASIA

Having described some basic principles of the immune response to cancer, it is now necessary to turn attention to the importance of these interactions for the neoplastic process itself in human malignant disease. In this section the impact of the immune system on the carcinogenic process, the clinical course of malignant disease, and the problem of cancer-associated immunodeficiency will be considered.

The Role of the Immune Response in Carcinogenesis

The concept that cancer develops by a multistage process arose originally from early studies of virally induced tumors and from the cocarcinogenic effects of croton oil (see Chapter 2). The terms *initiation, promotion,* and *progression* are now used to describe the discrete phases of the carcinogenic process.

Initiation

The initiation phase of carcinogenesis requires the production of a mutation in the genetic material of a cell. This mutation results in a permanent alteration of the cell's growth characteristics. The mutation or mutations in question must be nonlethal, heritable from generation to generation of cells, and must also confer on the cell the characteristics of malignant cell growth. There is no evidence to suggest that the immune system plays any role in initiation events responsible for the carcinogenic process.

Promotion

Neoplastic cell promotion represents the phase of the carcinogenic process in which initiated clones of cells become adapted to a particular microenvironment producing a malignantly transformed clone of cells capable of growing in that microenvironment. Thus, the outcome of the promotion event is the production of a malignant tumor (as opposed to the outcome of the initiation event, which is, in fact, the production of a clone of cells that is capable of producing a tumor). In experimental systems the promotion phase of the carcinogenic process is facilitated by using different promoting agents that are understood to be unable to act as initiating agents but which greatly increase the efficiency of the development or incidence of tumors. Most promoting agents are known to stimulate cell division and to modulate cellular differentiation processes. Not surprisingly, therefore, most promoting agents are known to affect the immune system and to suppress natural immunity to varying degrees. In contrast, it is also important to note that the promotion phase of the carcinogenic process can be retarded by agents that stimulate certain kinds of immunologic events.

The antitumor immune functions of large granular lymphocytes (NK cells and LAK cells) and macrophages during the promotion phase of the carcinogenic event are most responsible for any immune surveillance against developing cancers. It is the existence of these cells that explains why animals or humans that lack T-cells do not demonstrate a greater than normal incidence of nonlymphoreticular solid tumors (e.g., breast cancer, lung cancer) but do develop greater numbers of lymphoreticular malignancies. Specific T-cell immunity against tumor-associated antigens is probably also triggered at some time during the promotion phase of the carcinogenic event and probably plays a role in selecting against the most antigenic or immunogenic forms of tumor. Thus, what arises at the end of the promotion event is a weakly immunogenic, weakly antigenic tumor.

Progression

The final phase of the neoplastic process is the progression phase. In the progression phase a tumor that arose during the promotion phase behaves in a malignant, uncontrolled fashion. The progression phase includes the expansion of the tumor as well as the spread of this tumor by different means. The role of the immune system in the metastatic behavior of tumors is discussed later. In general, continued clonal selection can occur during the progression phase by the elimination of susceptible sublines of neoplastic cells; one of the major physiologic selection processes that operates during this phase is the immune response. During the progression phase the potential for further modification of tumor cell biologic characteristics as a result of immunostimulation or immunosuppression is great. By modifying the existing host environment with antineoplastic therapies, progression may be modulated. Thus, the progression phase of malignant disease can be greatly influenced by immune reactions, but this influence can be both positive (i.e., can retard tumor growth) or negative (i.e., can facilitate tumor growth and metastasis). In general, it appears that strong immunological reactions or immune stimulation during the progression phase of malignant disease serve to retard tumor growth, whereas weak immunological reactions or weak immunostimulation serve to subvert antitumor immunity and facilitate progression of tumor growth.

The Role of the Immune System in Metastasis

A fundamental property that distinguishes *most* tumor cells from *most* benign cells is the capacity of these cells to metastasize (see Chapter 4). However, this is not a comprehensive distinction, since certain malignant tumors (e.g., brain tumors) do not readily metastasize and certain nonmalignant growths (e.g., endometriotic lesions in women who have endometriosis) are capable of spreading and growing in distant sites. Nevertheless, the metastatic process is the most significant biologic behavior of most malignant tumors since it is metastasis that kills the host in the overwhelming majority of instances. The immune system can influence several phases of the metastatic process. Unfortunately, these sorts of immunologic reactions can actually facilitate metastasis.

Invasion of vessels

The first step in the metastatic process involves tumor cells gaining access to the lymphatics or the bloodstream. For this to happen, a number of different structural barriers inherent in blood or lymph vessels must be breached. These include the parenchymal cells (epithelium and endothelium), basement membranes to which parenchymal cells are attached, and interstitial connective tissue barriers. In metastatic tumors, invasion comes about through a combination of increased tissue pressure exerted by local tumor growth and by the production of different degradative enzymes. These enzymes are produced both by tumors and by inflammatory cells of the immune system. Thus, inflammatory macrophages that are activated in response to local tumor growth produce enzymes such as collagenase, hyaluronidase, and cathepsin B that participate in the destruction of vessel barriers.

Arrest from circulation

Once the bloodstream or lymphatics has been breached, tumor cells are capable of spreading to distant sites. Before that can occur, however, these cells must survive the circulatory environment and must leave the circulation. The question of tumor cell survival within the circulatory environment is not insignificant since cells in the circulation are subjected to shear forces exerted by the passage of different cells within the rapidly moving bloodstream that are capable of disrupting tumor cell membranes. To facilitate survival within these fluids and to facilitate trapping in capillary beds at distant sites, tumor cells have the capacity to form emboli in collaboration with platelets, polymorphonuclear leukocytes, and macrophages. Products of these activated inflammatory cells that facilitate tumor embolization include prostaglandins, procoagulants, and proteins of the complement pathway.

Intravasation to the tissues

Once tumor cell emboli are trapped in the capillary system, intravasation through the capillaries needs to occur. This can occur by direct intravasation through thin-walled capillaries or by the production of enzymes that cleave the proteoglycans of basement membranes. Certain tumor cells show a preference for attachment to different constituents of basement membranes, particularly type IV collagen. This is generally associated with the capacity of tumor cells to specifically decompose type IV collagen. Once again, however, host immunological responses to tumor trapped in capillary systems can produce local inflammatory reactions, causing white blood cells to accumulate in the area, leading to the release of hydrolytic enzymes that facilitate tumor cell invasion and/or intravasation through the capillary beds.

IMMUNODEFICIENCY IN CANCER

The capacity of the immune system to produce immune deficiency has been one of the central areas of study of tumor immunology for the past 50 years. This is due, in large part, to an early recognition that the degree of immune deficiency in patients is often correlated with the clinical stage of the disease. Also, in certain individuals, immune deficiency is responsible for the development of difficult infections that contribute significantly to morbidity.

In general, there is a hierarchy of immune deficiency development with advancing stage of disease. The first sort of immunological function to be eliminated, often very early in the tumor's development, is the capacity to develop T-cell immunity to a novel (never-before-encountered) antigen. This is typically tested by painting a chemical (dinitrochlorobenzene) on the skin of an individual and watching for the development upon rechallenge of delayed cutaneous hypersensitivity (DCH). In individuals with Hodgkin's disease, the loss of the capacity to develop DCH to dinitrochlorobenzene has been associated with a poorer prognosis and less likelihood of surgically resectable disease than in individuals who maintain this reactivity.

The next form of immune function that is eliminated with advancing disease is the capacity to develop a primary antibody response against novel antigens. This is followed by the loss of memory antibody synthesis, generally tested by rechallenging an individual with tetanus toxoid and looking for rises in antibody titer.

The last immunological function that is eliminated—generally only in patients with widespread, disseminated disease—is recall T-cell immunity to ubiquitous environmental fungal or mycobacterial pathogens. This is typically tested by injecting streptokinase/streptodornase into the skin of an individual to determine recall antigen DCH.

The investigation of immune competence in individuals with cancer can also be used to gauge the results of attempted definitive therapy. In Hodgkin's disease, individuals who following surgical resection of their disease reacquire the ability to mount primary T-cell or antibody immunity are, in general, individuals who have had definitive surgical resections. Individuals who fail to regain that immunity generally have residual disease.

Although it is difficult to make specific statements about clinical parameters and patterns of immune deficiency in individual cancer patients, when groups of patients are analyzed statistically, immune deficiency is found to correlate with both the clinical stage of disease and the histopathological tumor cell grade.[63,64] The most common patterns of immunological deficiency that have been associated with tumor stage and grade include the following:

1. decreased lymphocyte counts in association with relative monocytosis
2. decreased inflammatory cell chemotaxis
3. decreased antigen processing and presentation
4. decreased proliferative responses to antigen and nonspecific stimulants
5. decreased NK function
6. decreased helper and cytotoxic T-cell function
7. increased suppressor T-cell function
8. variable macrophage-mediated cytotoxicity
9. increased macrophage suppressor function
10. variable effects on cytokine synthesis

More recently, it has also become apparent that the response of patients to cytotoxic chemotherapy may be influenced by immune deficiency.[65,66] The mechanism whereby this occurs is thought to result from a need for synergy between antitumor immunity and cytotoxic drug therapy. In chemotherapy regimens that permit or even potentiate the development of antitumor immunity (e.g., by the selective elimination of suppressor cells), the patient's clinical response to the tumor may be significantly greater than in patients where the chemotherapy does not produce such an immunomodulatory effect. Similarly, drug treatment regimens that are profoundly immunosuppressive have been shown, in animal model systems, to be less effective than the same drug treatment regimen given by a dose and schedule that is not so immunosuppressive.[67] The capacity to combine cytotoxic chemotherapy with specific immunological manipulations is currently under intense investigation.

Finally, the capacity of individuals to respond to different immunotherapeutic manipulations such as the interferons, interleukin-2, monoclonal antibodies, and tumor cell vaccines is directly influenced by the level of immune competence in the patient. For all of these reasons, the immunodeficiency produced by malignant disease has been a major area of investigation. It appears that the most important mechanisms for immune deficiency are a combination of leukocyte depletion and the elicitation of immunosuppressive factors by tumors or by cells of the immune system themselves, the suppressor cell network.

PATTERNS OF ANTITUMOR IMMUNITY AND CLINICAL COURSE

Apart from the changes in general immunocompetence that have been observed in individuals with cancer, recent studies have also addressed the relationship between the presence or absence of specific antitumor immunity and the clinical course of the disease. In certain diseases such as melanoma, the loss of cytotoxic T-lymphocytes against the tumor from the circulation occurs only in very advanced stages of the disease. In other tumor systems such as transitional cell carcinoma of the bladder, the predominant pattern of antitumor immune reactivity that has been observed is an initial decline in antitumor reactivity following surgical resection or cytotoxic therapy followed by the reappearance of antitumor reactivity coincident with disease recurrence.[68] Such studies demonstrate that individuals with bladder cancer generally have detectable antitumor cytotoxicity prior to surgery. Following surgery, most patients lose reactivity. Individuals who relapse do not demonstrate reactivity for extended periods of time, up to 1 year, but then regain reactivity at or about the time of clinical detection of recurrent disease. Individuals who achieve tumor control lose reactivity following therapy also, but they rapidly regain and maintain that reactivity. Similar results have been reported for individuals with breast cancer,[69] in which most patients lose reactivity to tumor antigen preparations following mastectomy but regain reactivity upon relapse. The other major pattern of antitumor reactivity that has been found in serial studies of individuals with solid tumors is a loss of reactivity prior to or coincident with disease relapse, as in some studies of individuals with surgically resected stage I or stage II breast cancer or individuals with lung cancer.[70]

In general, it is still not possible to utilize specific immunological assays to make clinical decisions about patient management in conventional oncologic settings. This may not be true, however, for patients receiving experimental immunotherapy. In that situation, patient immunocompetence is a critical determinant of a patient's capacity to respond to the immunotherapy and, therefore, should be determined prior to entering patients on such therapies.

CRITICAL ISSUES FOR THE FUTURE OF TUMOR IMMUNOLOGY

As previously discussed, numerous studies have provided ample demonstration that immune function is affected in patients with solid tumors and that such effects are often associated with prognosis. In certain situations, immunocompetence may also correlate with or even be a determinant of the response of individuals to cytotoxic cancer therapies.[71,72] For these reasons, a wide array of immunological functions will continue to be assessed in diverse oncologic settings, and the results of these investigations will be used to guide the development of therapies aimed at stimulating specific kinds of immune function in cancer patients. To date, however, the results have been at best provocative but for the most part disappointing. One possible explanation for the failure of these efforts to produce significant improvement in cancer patient management or treatment is the fact that most studies have been restricted to assessments of systemic immunity in the peripheral blood.

Recent studies in individuals with cancer have focused on extending immunologic investigations into microenvironments that are more intimately associated with tumor tissues than the peripheral blood, and these need to be continued. In general, the results of these sorts of studies to date have demonstrated that the immune function of cells found in proximity to tumor tissues differs significantly from that of the peripheral blood cells. This has been found to be true for virtually all recognized forms of tumor immunity, including NK cell function, T-cell immunity, LAK function, and macrophage function.[73,74] Thus, although the capacity of tumoricidal immune cells to arise in patients during tumor growth is well documented, what is less clear is whether such cells actually mediate useful and beneficial antitumor immune reactions in situ. For example, research has demonstrated that many of the cells that infiltrate tumors are T-cells whose phenotype corresponds to the cytotoxic subset of T-lymphocytes. Furthermore, most of these cells have rearranged T-cell receptor gene products on their surfaces, indicating that they are capable of recognizing tumor-associated antigens and localizing to tumor tissues in vivo. Nevertheless, most studies have demonstrated that the T-cells taken from tumors are immunologically crippled compared to phenotypically identical cells taken from the circulation of cancer patients. Studies evaluating the function of macrophages and NK cells in tumor microenvironments are also just beginning in humans; not surprisingly, the results have been inconsistent and controversial. For example, several investigators have reported that alveolar macrophages from lung cancer patients have a normal or even an increased capacity to develop antitumor cytotoxicity compared to the peripheral blood monocytes from the same patients.[75,76] On the other hand, others have observed just the opposite.[77,78] Comparable sets of conflicting results exist for peritoneal macrophages from women with gynecological malignancies[79,80] and for macrophages from patients with malignant ascites.[81] It may be that immune cells that infiltrate tumors become shut off once they are in the tumor microenvironment. This local immunological impairment is perhaps the most important issue that needs to be addressed in future studies of human tumor immunology.

It is important to emphasize once again that not all immunologic reactions to malignant cells contribute to tumor control. As already described in this review, numerous studies have demonstrated that different immunologic reactions actually facilitate tumor growth and progression. It is imperative, therefore, to define which immunological reactions are most beneficial and, contrarily, which are least beneficial or even undesirable for specific clinical cancer settings. But in this situation and depending on the information derived from such studies, there is good reason to expect that application of that information to cancer patient management could be rapid. This is because the past decade of investigation has seen a considerable increase in the basic understanding of how the immune system functions. Central to this understanding has been the identification and characterization of numerous cytokines that are elaborated by immune cells during various phases of cellular development and activation and that are largely responsible for most of the recognized antitumor effects and immunomodulatory effects of the immune system. Also, the technology exists and has already been utilized to produce virtually unlimited quantities of these molecules in highly purified form. Therefore, it is quite possible that these cytokines can be used to affect cancer patient immunity and, ultimately, to provide the means for specifically manipulating the function of immune cells both in the circulation and in tumor microenvironments with resultant therapeutic benefits. This will only come about, however, through careful and critical laboratory and clinical investigations aimed at extending our basic knowledge of tumor immunology. Clearly, a great deal remains to be learned about the complex interaction between malignant disease and the immune system in humans.

REFERENCES

1. Gross L: Interdermal immunization of C3H mice against a sarcoma that originated in an animal of the same line. *Cancer Res* 3:326–336, 1943.
2. Foley EJ: Antigenic properties of methylcholanthrene-induced tumors in mice of the strain origin. *Cancer Res* 13:835–837, 1953.
3. Prehn RT, Main JM: Immunity to methylcholanthrene-induced sarcomas. *J Natl Cancer Inst* 18:769–778, 1957.
4. Sjogren HO, Hellstrom I, Klein G: Transplantation of polyoma virus-induced tumor in mice. *Cancer Res* 21:329–337, 1961.
5. Habel K: Immunological determinants of polyoma virus oncogenesis. *J Exp Med* 115:181–186, 1962.
6. Roth JA (ed): *Monoclonal antibodies for the diagnosis and therapy of cancer.* Mount Kisco, NY: Futura, 1986.
7. Sell S: Cancer markers. In Moossa AR, Schimpff SC, Robson MC (eds), *Comprehensive Textbook of Oncology* (2d ed). Baltimore, MD: Williams & Wilkins, 1991, pp. 225–238.
8. Foon KA, Todd RF III: Immunologic classification of leukemia and lymphoma. *Blood* 68(1):1–31, 1986.
9. Pohl AL: Surveillance of cancer patients with tumor markers. *J Tumor Marker Oncol* 2(1):1–14, 1987.
10. Henderson BE: Establishment of an association between a virus and a human cancer. *J Natl Cancer Inst* 81:320–321, 1989.
11. Szmuness W, Stevens CE, Harley EJ, et al: Hepatitis B vaccine: Demonstration of efficacy in a controlled clinical trial in a high-risk population in the United States. *N Eng J Med* 303:833–841, 1980.
12. Cimino F, Birkmayer GD, Klavins JV, et al (eds): *Human tumor markers. Biology and clinical applications.* New York: de Gruyter, 1987.
13. Lotze MT, Grimm E, Mazumder A, et al: *In vitro* growth of cytotoxic human lymphocytes IV: Lysis of fresh and cultured autologous tumor by lymphocytes cultured in T cell growth factor (TCGF). *Cancer Res* 41:4420–4425, 1981.
14. Rayner AA, Grimm EA, Lotze MT, et al: Lymphokine-activated killer (LAK) cell phenomenon: Analysis of factors relevant to the immunotherapy of human cancer. *Cancer* 55: 1327–1333, 1985.
15. Lotzova E: Immunobiology of natural killer cells. Boca Raton, FL: CRC Press, 1986.
16. Ettinghausen SE, Lipford EH III, Mule JJ, et al: Systemic administration of recombinant interleukin-2 stimulates *in vivo* lymphoid cell proliferation in tissues. *J Immunol* 135:1488–1497, 1985.
17. Rosenberg SA, Lotze MT, Muul LM, et al: A progress report on the treatment of 157 patients with advanced cancer using lymphokine-activated killer cells and interleukin-2 or high-dose interleukin-2 alone. *N Engl J Med* 316:889–897, 1987.
18. Nathan CF, Cohn ZA: Cellular components of inflammation: Monocytes and macrophages, In Kelley WN, Harris ED Jr, Ruddy S, et al (eds): *Textbook of Rheumatology.* Philadelphia: Saunders 1985, pp. 144–169.
19. Fidler IJ, Schroit AJ: Recognition and destruction of neoplastic cells by activated macrophages: Discrimination of altered self. *Biochim Biophys Acta* 948:151–173, 1988.
20. Nathan CF: Secretory products of macrophages. *J Clin Invest* 79:319–326, 1987.
21. Drysdale BE, Agarwal S, Shin HS: Macrophage-mediated tumor injury: Mechanisms of activation and cytotoxicity. *Prog Allergy* 40:111–116, 1988.
22. Rosenberg SA, Longo DL, Lotze MT: Principles and applications of biologic therapy. In DeVita VT Jr, Hellman S, Rosenberg SA (eds), *Cancer: Principles and Practice of Oncology.* Philadelphia: Lippincott, 1989, pp. 301–347.
23. Adams DO, Nathan CF: Molecular mechanisms in tumor-cell killing by activated macrophages. *Immunol Today* 4:166–170, 1983.
24. Somers SD, Johnson WJ, Adams DO: Destruction of tumor cells by macrophages: Mechanisms of recognition and lysis, and their regulation. In Herberman RB (ed), *Cancer Immunology: Innovative Approaches to Therapy.* Boston: Martinus Mijhoff, 1986, pp. 69–123.
25. Urban JL, Shepard, HM, Rothstein JL, et al: Tumor necrosis factor: A potent effector molecule for tumor cell killing by activated macrophages. *Proc Natl Acad Sci USA* 83:5233–5237, 1986.
26. Watanabe N, Umetasu T, Sone H, et al: Stimulation of antitumorigenic cytotoxicity in macrophages by tumor necrosis factor. *Cancer J* 2(5): 165, 168, 1988.
27. Harris JE, Braun DP: Abnormal immunoregulation and the tumor dormant state in human cancer. In Stewart THM, Wheelock EF (eds), *Cellular Immune Mechanisms and Tumor Dormancy.* Boca Raton, FL: CRC Press, 1992, pp. 261–280.
28. Evans R: Macrophages and neoplasms: New insights and their implication in tumor immunobiology. *Cancer Metastasis Rev* 1:227–239, 1982.
29. Ortaldo JR, Woodhouse C, Morgan AC, et al: Analysis of effector cells in human antibody-dependent cellular cytotoxicity with murine monoclonal antibodies of the IgG3 subclass. *J Immunol* 138:3556–3572, 1987.
30. Old LJ, Benacerraf B, Clarke DA, et al: The role of the reticuloendothelial system in the host reaction to neoplasia. *Cancer Res* 21: 1281–1300, 1961.
31. Woodruff M, Speedy G: Inhibition of chemical carcinogenesis by *Corynebacterium parvum. Proc R Soc Lond* 201: 209–215, 1978.
32. Devesa SS, Silverman DT, Young JL Jr et al: Cancer incidence and mortality trends among whites in the United States, 1947–84. *JNCI* 79:701–770, 1987.
33. Weigle WO: Effects of aging on the immune system. *Hosp Prac* December 15, 1989, 112–119.
34. Mason TJ: Age-specific cancer mortality in the United States among persons over 55 years of age. In Balducci L, Lyman GH, Erschler WB (eds), *Geriatric Oncology.* Philadelphia: Lippincott, 1992, pp. 35–41.
35. Filipovich AH, Spector BD, Kersey J, et al: Immunodeficiency in humans as a risk factor in the development of malignancy. *Prev Med* 9:252–259, 1980.
36. Penn I: Principles of tumor immunity: Immunocompetence and cancer. In DeVita VT Jr, Hellman S, Rosenberg SA (eds), *Biologic Therapy of Cancer.* Philadelphia: Lippincott, 1991, pp. 53–67.
37. Nicolson GL, Poste G: The cancer cell: Dynamic aspects and modification in cell surface organization. *N Engl J Med* 295:197–203, 253–257, 1976.
38. Messerschmidt GL, Henry DH, Snyder HW Jr, et al: Protein and immunoadsorption in the treatment of malignant disease. *J Clin Oncol* 6(2):203–212, 1988.
39. Stevenson HC: Adoptive cellular immunotherapy of cancer: An overview. *Immunol Ser* 48:1–18, 1989.

40. Ebert EC, Roberts AI, Devereux D, et al: Selective immunosuppressive action of a factor produced by colon cancer cells. *Cancer Res* 50(19): 6158–6161, 1990.
41. Somers SS, Dye JF, Guillon PJ: Immunosuppressive tumor cell products. *Br J Cancer* 62:17, 1990 (suppl 11).
42. Naor D, Klein BY, Tarcic N, et al: Antigenic entities of the tumor that induce suppressor cells. In Naor D, et al (eds), *Immunosuppression and Human Malignancy.* Clifton, NJ: Humana Press, 1989, pp. 41–55.
43. Kripke ML: Immunologic mechanisms in UV radiation carcinogenesis. *Adv Cancer Res* 34:69–106, 1981.
44. Yamamoto H: Isolation of immunogenic and suppressogenic glycoproteins from adenovirus type 12 hamster tumor cells. *Microbiol Immunol* 28:339–348, 1984.
45. Jesup JM, LeGrue SJ, Kahan BD, Pellis NR: Induction of suppressor cells by a tumor-derived suppressor factor. *Cell Immunol* 93:9–25, 1985.
46. Mokyr MB, Dray S: Some of the advantages of curing mice bearing a large MOPC-315 tumor with a low dose rather than a high dose of cyclophosphamide. *Cancer Res* 43:3112–3118, 1983.
47. Von Roenn JV. Harris JE, Braun DP: Suppressor cell function in solid tumor cancer patients. *J Clin Oncol* 5:150–159, 1987.
48. Yu A, Watts H, Jaffe N, et al: Concommitant presence of tumor specific cytotoxic and inhibitor lymphocytes in patients with osteogenic sarcoma. *N Engl J Med* 297:121–127, 1977.
49. Berd D, Mastrangelo MJ: Depletion of suppressor-cytotoxic T-lymphocytes by administration of a murine monoclonal antibody. *Cancer Res* 47:2727–2732, 1987.
50. Berd D: Low doses of chemotherapy to inhibit suppressor T cells. *Prog Clin Biol Res* 288:449–458, 1989.
51. Berd D, Maguire HC Jr, McCue P, et al: Treatment of metastatic melanoma with an autologous tumor-cell vaccine: Clinical and immunologic results in 64 patients. *J Clin Oncol* 8(11):1858–1867, 1990.
52. Twomey JJ, Laughter AH, Farrow S, et al: Hodgkin's disease. An immunodepleting and immunosuppressive disorder. *J Clin Invest* 56:467, 1975.
53. Braun DP, Harris JE, Rubenstein M: Relationship of arachidonic acid metabolism to indomethacin-sensitive immunoregulatory and lymphocyte PGE sensitivity in peripheral blood mononuclear cells of disseminated solid tumor cancer patients. *J Immunopharmacol* 6:227, 1984.
54. Kuda T, Yasumoto K, Yano T, et al: Role of antitumor activity of alveolar macrophages in lung cancer patients. *Cancer Res* 47:2199–2202, 1987.
55. Thomassen MJ, Wiedemann HP, Barna BP, et al: Induction of in vitro tumoricidal activity in alveolar macrophages and monocytes from patients with lung cancer. *Cancer Res* 48:3949–3953, 1988.
56. Goodwin JS, Messner RP, Bankhurst AD, et al: Prostaglandin-producing suppressor cells in Hodgkin's disease. *N Engl J Med* 297:963, 1977.
57. Braun DP, Cobleigh MA, Harris JE: Multiple concurrent immunoregulatory defects in cancer patients whose peripheral blood leukocytes exhibit depressed PHA-induced lymphoblastogenesis. *Clin Immunol Immunopathol* 17:89, 1980.
58. Droller MJ, Lindgren JA, Claessein HA, et al: Production of prostaglandin E_2 by bladder tumor cells in tissue culture and a possible mechanism of lymphocyte inhibition. *Cell Immunol* 47:261, 1979.
59. Honn KV, Cicone B, Skoff A, et al: Thromboxane synthetase inhibitors and prostacyclin can control tumor cell metastasis. *J Cell Biol* 87:64, 1980.
60. Erickson KL, Somers SK, Chapkin RS: Mechanisms of dietary fat involvement in tumorigenesis: Role of fatty acids and eicosanoids in macrophage function. *Prostaglandins Leukotrienes Cancer.* 6:377–395, 1989.
61. Kort WJ, Bijma AM: Tumor metastasis: The possible role of eicosanoids. *Prostaglandins Leukotrienes Cancer.* 6:199–218, 1989.
62. Braun DP, Taylor SG, Harris JE: Modulation of immunity in cancer patients by prostaglandin antagonists. In Mitchell M (ed), *Immunity to Cancer II.* New York: Liss, 1989, pp. 439–448.
63. Haskill S (ed): *Tumor immunity in prognosis. The Role of Mononuclear Cell Infiltration.* New York: Dekker, 1982.
64. Krieder JW, Bartlett GL, Butkiewicz BL: Relationship of tumor leucocytic infiltration to host defense mechanisms and prognosis. *Cancer Metastasis Rev* 3:53–74, 1987.
65. Creaven PJ, Mihich E: The clinical toxicity of anticancer drugs and its prediction. *Semin Oncol* 4:147–161, 1977.
66. Morton DL, Economou J: Cancer immunology and immunotherapy. In Haskell CM (ed), *Cancer Treatment* (3d ed) Philadelphia: Saunders, 1990, pp, 102–119.
67. Braun DP, Harris JE: Cancer chemotherapy and its impact on the immune system. In Carter SK, Hellman K (eds), *Fundamentals of Cancer Chemotherapy.* New York: McGraw-Hill, 1987, pp. 77–97.
68. O'Toole C: A-51CR release assay for detecting cytotoxicity to human bladder carcinoma. *Int J Cancer* 19:324, 1977.
69. Rieche K, Arndt A, Pasternak G: Cellular immunity in mammary cancer patients as measured by the leukocyte migration test (LMT). A follow-up study. *Int J Cancer* 17:212, 1976.
70. McCoy JL, Jerome LF, Cannon GB, et al: Reactivity of lung cancer patients and leukocyte migration inhibition assays to 3 M NaCl extracts of fresh tumor in tissue cultured cells derived from lung cancer. *J Natl Cancer Inst* 59:1413, 1977.
71. Kleinerman EG, Howser D, Young RC, et al: Defective monocyte killing in patients with malignancies and restoration of function during chemotherapy. *Lancet* 2:1102–1105, 1980.
72. Braun DP, Harris JE: Effect of chemotherapy on NK function in the peripheral blood of cancer patients. *Cancer Immunol Immunother* 21:240–245, 1986.
73. Braun DP, Harris JE: Serial immune function testing to predict clinical disease release in patients with solid tumors. *Cancer Immunol Immunother* 15:165, 1983.
74. Weissler JC, Nicod LP, Toews GB: Pulmonary NK cell activity is reduced in patients with bronchogenic carcinoma. *Am Rev Respir Dis* 135:1353–1357, 1987.
75. Gangemi JD, Olsen GN, Fechtez C, et al: Phagocytic activity of alveolar macrophages in patients with bronchogenic carcinoma. *Cancer Immunol Immunother* 20:158, 1985.
76. Thomassen MJ, Wiedemann HP, Barna BP, et al: Induction of in vitro tumoricidal activity in alveolar macrophages and monocytes from patients with lung cancer. *Cancer Res* 48:3949–3953, 1988.
77. Weissler JC, Lipscomb MF, Lem VM, et al: Tumor killing by human alveolar macrophages and blood monocytes: Decreased cytotoxicity of human alveolar macrophages. *Am Rev Respir Dis* 134:532, 1986.

78. Siziopikou KP, Harris JE, Casey LC. et al: Impaired tumoricidal function of alveolar macrophages from patients with non–small cell lung cancer. *Cancer* 68:1035–1044, 1991.
79. Mantovani A, Ming WJ, Balotta C, et al: Origin and regulation of tumor associated macrophages: The role of tumor-derived chemotactic factor. *Biochem Biophys Acta* 865:59–67, 1986.
80. Tay SK, Jenkins D, Maddox P: Tissue macrophage response in human papillomavirus infection and cervical intraepithelial neoplasia. *Br J Obstet Gynaecol* 94:1094, 1987.
81. Hammerstrom J: Structure and function of human effusion macrophages from patients with malignant and benign disease. *Acta Path Microbiol Scand,* Section C 88:191, 1980.

PART II

Prevention, Detection, and Diagnosis

Chapter 6

Factors Affecting Health Behavior

Jayne I. Fernsler, DSN, RN

Mary Ann Miller, PhD, RN

INTRODUCTION

Promotion of positive health behavior has become a national initiative. The knowledge that unhealthful personal lifestyle choices account for a large proportion of both morbidity and mortality in the United States and the subsequent cost of these choices to society have been the impetus for major policy and program development.

The health behavior initiative is an important component of cancer care. Personal choices with regard to diet, tobacco use, alcohol consumption, and sun exposure can have a powerful impact on cancer prevention. In addition, personal decisions about learning and performing routine self-examinations, participating in cancer screening activities, and seeking appropriate help when cancer signs and symptoms are noted are pivotal to the early detection and potential cure of cancer. Also, behavior with regard to following a recommended treatment regimen and maintaining a healthful lifestyle while experiencing cancer may enhance both quantity and quality of life. Consequently, individual health behavior is a concern of health care professionals who interact with people at any phase of the cancer continuum.

The purpose of this chapter is to define *health behavior* and related terms, to identify national initiatives, and to describe factors that influence health behavior. Selected models and theories of health behavior are explained, and their applications in research on cancer care are described. Nursing practice implications of health behavior theory and research are discussed in the conclusion of the chapter.

NATIONAL INITIATIVES

The evolving body of knowledge about the association between personal behavior and cancer control has spurred activity in both the public and the private sectors. Major initiatives are the National Cancer Institute (NCI) objectives for 1985–2000,[1] the American Cancer Society's (ACS) priorities for the 1990s,[2] and the U.S. Department of Health and Human Services (USDHHS) objectives for health promotion and disease prevention.[3] The NCI's goal of reducing cancer mortality by 50% by the year 2000, as well as the ACS's stated priority on cancer prevention and detection, and the USDHHS objectives for cancer control all focus strongly on efforts to influence people's health behavior. The behaviors of people who are disadvantaged and/or at high risk for cancer are a major target of these efforts.

DEFINITIONS

Health Behavior

Generally, *behavior* involves something that people do or refrain from doing, consciously or unconsciously, voluntarily or involuntarily.[4] A number of definitions of health behavior have been advanced by experts in the field. Gochman defines *health behavior* as "those personal attributes, such as beliefs, expectations, motives, values, perceptions, and other cognitive elements; personality characteristics, including affective and emotional states and traits; and overt behavior patterns, actions and habits that relate to health maintenance, to health restoration and to health improvement." Such "personal attributes are influenced by, and otherwise reflect family structure and processes, peer group and social factors, and societal, institutional, and cultural determinants."[5,p.169]

Health behavior involves actions taken by persons who believe they are healthy, and who have not been experiencing any signs or symptoms of illness, in order to remain disease free.[6,7] According to this definition, health behavior is confined to preventive actions. In 1979 Harris and Guten[8] introduced the broader term *health protective behavior* to include both preventive and health-promoting activities. They define it as "any behavior performed by a person, regardless of his or her perceived or actual health status, in order to protect, promote or maintain his or her health, whether or not such behavior is objectively effective toward that end."[8,p.18]

Pender[9] differentiates between the concepts of *health promotion* and *disease prevention.* She defines *health promotion activities* as those directed toward increasing the level of well-being that already exists, thus actualizing the health potential of individuals. Primary prevention activities decrease the probability of specific illnesses; secondary prevention activities focus on early diagnosis and intervention; tertiary prevention activities involve rehabilitation and restoration to optimal level of functioning. Whereas prevention is disease specific, health promotion is not. Prevention represents avoidance behavior, whereas health promotion activities aim to increase one's positive potential for health.

Illness Behavior

Kasl and Cobb define *illness behavior* as "any activity, undertaken by a person who feels ill, to define the state of his health and to discover a suitable remedy."[6,p.246] Thus, illness behavior refers to a person's perceptions and actions resulting from the recognition of bodily signs or symptoms, recognition of the need for advice, the decision whether to seek it, and the choice of advisor, whether it be relatives, friends, and/or lay or professional health care practitioners.[10–12] Illness behaviors are undertaken to clarify the meaning of certain signs and symptoms. This may mean waiting to see if the symptoms will disappear without therapy.

Sick Role Behavior

Sick role behavior is the activity taken by individuals who believe themselves (or whom others believe) to be ill in order to get well. It usually involves a range of dependent behaviors, includes accepting treatment, and leads to some neglect of one's usual duties.[6]

The distinctions made among these various types of health behaviors (Figure 6-1) and their determinants should not be minimized.[4] Although their apparently common relationship to "health" unites them, more research is needed to confirm underlying commonalities among the categories or to uncover the variety of determinants to which each category is specifically related.[4]

MODELS AND THEORIES OF HEALTH BEHAVIOR

A number of theories and models to explain health behavior have been developed during the past 20 years. Their evolution has emphasized the complexities of health behavior and its determinants.

To determine similarities and differences among the explanatory approaches to health and illness behavior, Cummings, Becker, and Maile[13] reviewed 14 such models, all drawn from a variety of theoretical constructs and chosen because of their predictive ability and frequency of citation. The authors found the general classes of explanatory variables to be quite similar. A set of six categories emerged from the original 109 variables described in the models. These include attitudes toward health care benefits and health care quality, perception of symptoms and beliefs about susceptibility to illness, accessibility of health services, knowledge about the disease/condition, social support characteristics, and demographic variables (particularly social status, income, and education). Because there is not a single unifying theory on which the models are based, health care practitioners have had to choose the model that best fits a specific health behavior in order to determine appropriate interventions to stimulate behavior change. Some of the predominant theories and models used to explain health behavior and their application to cancer care are presented in the following sections.

Social Learning Theory

Bandura's social cognitive theory currently represents one of the most formally developed theories of behavior.[14] It provides an umbrella framework for analyzing health behavior in terms of a continuous, mutual interaction among cognitive, behavioral, and environmental determinants (reciprocal determinism). According to Bandura, "the primary determinants of adoptive behavior are the influences closely tied to it—the stimulus inducements, the anticipated satisfactions, the observed benefits, the experienced functional value, the perceived risks, the self-evaluative derivatives, and the various social barriers and economic constraints."[15,p.54]

The environment is the source of social supports that provide cues for reinforcement of behavior. The environment also provides the social and physical situation within which a person must function. In so doing, it provides the incentives and disincentives for the performance of behavior (expectancies). People have the potential for self-control over their actions. In order to do this, they must have a certain amount of knowledge

Behavior	Health		Illness		Sick role	
Identity	Healthy		Feel sick		Am sick	
Role performance	Usual social roles		Diminished function	Preparing to enter sick role	Being in sick role	Leaving sick role
Health	Health	Asymptomatic disease	Symptoms	Diagnosis	Treatment	Outcome

FIGURE 6-1 Continuum from health to disease, related to behavior, identity, and role performance. (Source: Kasl S, Cobb S: Health behavior, illness behavior, and sick role behavior: I. Health and illness behavior. *Arch Environ Health* 12:246–266, 1966. Reprinted with permission of the Helen Dwight Reid Educational Foundation. Published by Heldref Publications, 1319 18th Street, N.W., Washington, D.C. 20036-1802. Copyright 1966.)

and skill. They can anticipate certain events and outcomes and respond to them, based on their own past experiences or the experiences of others whom they have observed. If all other things are equal, people will choose to perform an activity that maximizes a positive outcome or minimizes a negative one (principle of maximization).[14]

Sources of influence

Bandura[15] views human behavior in terms of three interdependent sources of influence: antecedent determinants, consequent outcomes, and cognitive determinants of behavior. Antecedent determinants stem from objects or events that precede behavior change. Cognitive factors partly determine which external events will be observed, how they will be perceived, and how information they convey will be organized for future use. In order to function effectively, individuals must anticipate the probable consequences of these different events and courses of action. They then regulate their behavior on the basis of such predictive antecedent events.

The more individuals believe that influences of past events remain viable, and the more severe the outcome they expect (e.g., their perceived susceptibility to ill effects due to a particular behavior), the stronger their anticipatory reaction will be. The failure of anticipated risks to materialize reinforces the expectation that the subsequent behaviors prevented their occurrence. Thus, most behavior is maintained by anticipated rather than by immediate consequences.[15]

Rewarding experiences are repeatedly associated with expressions of the interest and approval of others (their social support) and unrewarding experiences with their disapproval. These social reactions themselves become influential predictors of consequences and become incentives. Thus, the impact of rewards or punishments can be explained in terms of motivation. By representing foreseeable outcomes symbolically, individuals can convert future consequences into current motivations of behavior.[15]

Efficacy and outcome expectations

Bandura[15] proposes that behavioral changes are generated from the common mechanisms of personal efficacy and outcome expectations. An *outcome expectation* is defined as a personal belief that a given behavior will lead to certain outcomes.[16] An *efficacy expectation* is the conviction that one can successfully execute a specific behavior required to produce a specific outcome.[17,18] Outcome and efficacy expectations are differentiated because individuals can believe that a certain course of action will produce certain outcomes but question whether they can perform those actions. Both outcome and efficacy expectations reflect individuals' beliefs about their capabilities and behavior-outcome links. Although self-efficacy and outcome expectations are conceptually distinct, the types of outcomes that people anticipate are strongly influenced by efficacy expectations, the most important prerequisite for behavior change.[14,19]

The strength of people's convictions in their own effectiveness determines whether they will even try to cope with difficult situations. Bandura[16] speculates that perceived efficacy forms a mediating link between knowledge and behavior. Efficacy expectations determine how much effort people will expend and how long they will persist in the face of barriers and aversive experiences. In general, stronger efficacy expectations will produce more active and sustained efforts.[18]

Perceptions of efficacy usually are acquired through direct environmental interaction or through social experiences.[18] The most dependable and powerful source of efficacy expectations is personal experience.[15] Another source is vicarious experience, i.e., live or symbolic modeling or seeing what happens to others who perform activities with certain consequences. Of the numerous cues that influence behavior, none is more common than the actions of others.[15,16,20]

A third source of information about efficacy expectations is verbal persuasion. The efficacy expectations that it generates, however, are likely to be weak, and short in duration. The fourth source is one's own physiological state or emotional arousal (anxiety, agitation, fatigue) in threatening situations.[20]

Efficacy expectations vary greatly, depending on a particular task that confronts the person. Individuals with low self-efficacy about a particular task may concentrate on personal deficiencies rather than thinking about accomplishing the task at hand. This can impede successful performance of the task.[21]

Application of beliefs about self-efficacy to cancer care

In the application of social learning theory to analysis of health behavior, a major task becomes trying to learn what beliefs a person has developed about targeted health problems or behaviors. Taking the theoretical application one step further, one might conclude that, when strong beliefs about health risks are combined with a strong sense of efficacy for avoiding them and a belief in the value of the avoidance behaviors, healthier outcomes can result.

The influence of self-efficacy has been studied in relation to general cancer prevention practices,[22] smoking cessation,[23–26] testicular self-examination (TSE),[27,28] breast self-examination (BSE),[29–33] and compliance with screening for fecal occult blood.[34] Generally, a strong belief in one's ability to carry out a required activity was a powerful influence in the decision to engage in healthy behavior. Self-efficacy has been shown to be particularly influential in promoting positive action among smokers who have contemplated quitting.[24–26] In a study on general health promotion, subjects who smoked had the lowest self-efficacy scores.[35]

Summary

Social learning theory as an umbrella framework addresses many of the constructs that will be discussed in the models and theories that follow. Along with the Health Belief Model (HBM) and the Theory of Reasoned Action, it contains constructs that can be viewed as belonging to the larger family of expectancy-value theories. Outcome value has been a traditional component of these theories. While the HBM explicitly sets forth outcome benefits/barriers as a variable, Bandura[15] suggests the construct of outcome value by emphasizing the role of rewarding outcomes in determining behavior. The Theory of Reasoned Action includes evaluation of outcomes as a specific determinant of attitude toward behavior. This is another variable that is made explicit in the HBM. There is already a body of research to support the utility of both the concept of self-efficacy, as explained by Bandura,[15] and the variables of the HBM in studies of preventive health behavior.[36,37]

Another influential variable, social support, is alluded to in the reciprocal determinism of social learning theory, the environmental influence proposed by the HBM, and the variable of social norms in the Theory of Reasoned Action. Janis[38] asserts that social support is especially important for individuals who find it difficult to sustain a high level of motivation when pursuing a stressful course of action, such as trying to abstain from smoking. A high level of motivation is often contingent on the presence of "personal assets" or resources, including the presence of "important others" for emotional support.

Early social learning theory also provided the foundation for current behavioral theories that include the variable of personal control. These include locus of control and health locus of control. Control also appears as a variable in attribution theory.

Health Belief Model

The Health Belief Model (HBM) was originally developed in the 1950s by Rosenstock and Hochbaum to explain preventive health behavior, using psychosocial variables and psychological theories of decision making.[39] It evolved from a central tenet of Lewin's theory of goal setting: that behavior depends on the value that individuals attach to a given outcome and their expectation that a particular action will result in that outcome.[40] Translated to health behavior, the value becomes the desire to avoid illness or to get well, and the expectancy is the belief that a particular personal action will prevent or lessen the threat of illness. People will usually choose the behavior that they think will produce the maximum number of good outcomes and the minimum number of bad ones (principle of maximization).[14]

The HBM is based on the assumption that an individual's subjective perception of the environment determines behavior.[41] Variables tested in current applications of the model are susceptibility, severity, benefits, barriers, and self-efficacy. See Table 6-1. Research has shown that the variable *perceived barriers* is the most powerful single predictor of behavior, although *perceived susceptibility* and *benefits* are strong also. *Perceived severity* is the weakest predictor, but appears to be strongly related to sick role behaviors.[37,42]

The stimulus or cue to action may be internal, such as the perception of a symptom, or external, such as interaction with others or mass media communications.[39] The true role of such stimuli has been difficult to study because they may be only barely perceptible in the individual's consciousness.[42]

It is now believed that self-efficacy must be added to the HBM in order to increase its explanatory power.[36] Efficacy expectations, or the belief that one can successfully execute the behavior required to produce the outcome, are crucial in lifestyle behaviors requiring long-term changes, such as smoking. They affect how much effort a person puts into a given task and what levels of performance are attained. Repetition builds self-efficacy, which affects task persistence and endurance, and thus promotes behavior change.[42]

TABLE 6-1 Health Belief Model

Variable	Definition
Perceived susceptibility	Perception of vulnerability to a condition
Perceived severity	Perception of the seriousness of the consequences of developing a condition
Together the two variables above constitute a perceived **Threat** and provide the individual with a psychological readiness to take action.	
Benefits	Effectiveness of the action in reducing threat
Barriers	Psychological and other costs or negative aspects associated with the proposed action
Cue to action	Stimulus to behave in a certain manner
Self-efficacy	Conviction that one can successfully behave in the manner required to achieve a specific outcome
Modifying variables	
Demographic	Age, gender, etc.
Structural	Access
Attitudinal	Satisfaction
Interactional	Patient/practitioner relationship
Enabling	Social pressure

Source: Compiled from Strecher, DeVellis, Becker, et al;[36] Rosenstock;[41,42] Becker, Maiman.[43]

Application of the Health Belief Model to health behavior

The HBM has been applied to all preventive health actions, illness behaviors, and sick role behaviors. The model has been one of the most influential and widely used psychosocial approaches to explaining health-related behavior, and, in fact, is one of the few psychosocial models developed expressly to promote understanding of health behavior.[42]

Underlying the ability of the model to explain health behavior is the assumption that people can accept the possibility that they may have a serious illness in the complete absence of symptoms. This may provide the rationale for many decisions to seek screening for health related reasons. For example, the failure to believe in the possibility of asymptomatic illness may help to explain less-than-desirable responses to cancer screening programs.[42,44]

The HBM is based on the premise that health is a valued goal for most individuals. As such, it can only account for as much of the variation in individuals' health-related behaviors as can be explained by attitudes and beliefs.[37] It is recognized that other forces also influence behavior. There is a habitual component to some behavior (e.g., smoking); some behaviors occur for nonhealth reasons (e.g., dieting to appear more attractive); and, in some cases, economic or environmental factors prevent an individual from taking a preferred mode of action (e.g., residing in a city with high air pollution).[21,42]

Another limitation of the HBM is its lack of quantification beyond an ordinal scale. One of the advantages of the model, its ability to measure beliefs specific to a given condition, is also one of its limitations. There is not a generic instrument with proven reliability and validity that can be used by all researchers. Instead, a multitude of measures exist, each with different behaviors as targets.

Application of the Health Belief Model to cancer care

The Health Belief Model has been used extensively as a framework for the identification of individuals who engage in behaviors relevant to primary and secondary cancer prevention. The HBM has been used to identify health beliefs of individuals who practice BSE,[30,33,45–54] TSE,[55–58] skin cancer prevention,[59–61] cancer risk reduction and early detection,[62] smoking cessation,[63] and general health promotion.[35] In addition, health beliefs have been studied in relation to participation in mammographic screening for breast cancer,[64,65] Pap smear screening for cervical cancer,[66,67] and fecal occult blood screening for colorectal cancer.[34]

In general, health motivation and perceived barriers are strong predictors of people's intentions and behaviors related to cancer prevention and screening activities.[30,35,44,48,59,65] Perceived susceptibility was found to be associated positively with frequency of BSE[51,52] and having a Pap test when perceived benefits were high.[67] The relationship between beliefs about severity of a potential illness and health behavior has not been supported in the cancer literature.[45,65,68] In fact, women at high risk for breast cancer were found to practice BSE less frequently as their perceptions of the severity of breast cancer increased.[45] In another study, women without breast cancer perceived the disease to be more severe and practiced BSE less often than women who had a mastectomy for breast cancer.[69] For patients who had hematologic malignancies, perceived severity was a strong predictor of depression and was related to reported levels of pain, discomfort, and activity.[70] The influence of beliefs about barriers was supported in a study of the use of unorthodox therapies by patients with advanced cancer.[71] Patients who used these methods had negative attitudes toward barriers to standard treatment.

The influence of health beliefs alone on people's behaviors with regard to cancer prevention and screening activities is equivocal and, as discussed later in this chapter, may be modified by other factors, such as age,[34,66,68] past experience,[59] and confidence in one's ability to perform a task.[30,33–35] Consequently, several researchers have used the HBM in conjunction with other concepts and theories in an attempt to predict health behaviors.[22,30,33,35,53]

Theory of Reasoned Action

Ajzen and Fishbein's Theory of Reasoned Action,[72] like the HBM, is also a value-expectancy theory. It has been used to predict a person's intention to perform a behavior in a specific situation. The model is based on the assumption that intention to perform (or not to perform) a specific behavior is the immediate determinant of that behavior. For intention to predict behavior, the behavior must be under voluntary control, and the intention must be assessed close to the time of the behavior. The longer the time interval between statement of intention and the behavior, the more likely events will occur that may change the intention.[73]

Two factors contribute to the strength of the intention to perform a specific behavior: attitude toward the behavior, and the influence of the social environment or general subjective norms on the behavior. See Figure 6-2. Attitude is determined by an individual's belief that a specific outcome will occur if he or she performs the behavior (similar to outcome expectation) and by an evaluation of the outcome (cost/benefit analysis). The influence of norms stems from a person's belief about what significant others believe that he/she should do, weighted by the individual's motivation to comply with their wishes (social pressure to perform).[74] The model also emphasizes normative influences that might affect intention for *any* reason, health-related or otherwise, thus adding a cultural component to the prediction of behavior.[21]

1. *Behavior* is determined by *behavioral intention.*
2. Strength of *behavioral intention* depends on *attitude toward the behavior* and influence of the social environment or social norms.
   A. Attitude toward the behavior is determined by:
      1. Belief that a specific outcome will occur if the behavior is performed
      2. Evaluation of the outcome as positive or negative
   B. Social norm is determined by:
      1. The person's belief about what significant others think should be done
      2. The person's motivation to do what others wish

FIGURE 6-2 Theory of reasoned action. (Source: Compiled from Ajzen, Fishbein.[72])

Variables other than attitude or subjective norm can influence intention and behavior indirectly. For example, variables such as personality traits and demographic characteristics affect intention and behavior through their influence on the attitudinal or subjective normative components.[73]

When this theory is used to explain health behavior, the effectiveness of interventions to encourage people to change behavior is greatly determined by the professional's ability to identify major concerns and barriers that the person confronts in making the decision to change. Data generated through interviews and open-ended questions with selected individuals ultimately result in the development of a questionnaire that can be used to identify beliefs that can be changed. Although this method provides for a systematic identification of those issues that are most salient to the person's decisions about performing a specific behavior, it is possible that not all important variables will be discovered in the interview process. The method also involves a measurement technique that can be complicated, cumbersome, and time-consuming. Although the model is very well developed theoretically, there is not yet a large body of data on which to judge its predictive validity.[74]

Application of the Theory of Reasoned Action to cancer care

The Theory of Reasoned Action has been used in research on BSE,[47,49] women's beliefs, attitudes, and behaviors regarding Pap tests,[66] and seeking care for symptoms of breast cancer.[73] Both studies of women's behavior with regard to BSE behavior and the one on cervical screening used the Health Belief Model also. In one study, normative beliefs were not significantly related to BSE practice.[49] In the other study, behavioral intention, as measured in the model, was predictive of BSE frequency and, to a lesser extent, BSE proficiency.[47] Hennig and Knowles[66] found that the oldest group of women in their study (ages 60–82) had the lowest intention to have a Pap test. They suggested that subjective norm referents may not be available to older women, because of widowhood or loss of close associates.

Timko[73] found that in women with a breast cancer symptom, intention to delay seeking medical care was associated with having a positive attitude toward delay and perceiving social pressure to delay. Women who delayed did not foresee a negative health outcome.

Social Support

The field of relationships that individuals have with others in daily living has been called their social or personal network. It depends on the existence of people on whom individuals can rely, who will let them know that they care about, value, or love them.[75] Conceptual definitions of social support abound. The definition proposed by Kahn is "interpersonal transactions that include one or more of the following: the expression of positive affect of one person toward another, the affirmation or endorsement of another person's behaviors, perceptions, or expressed views; the giving of symbolic or material aid to another."[76,p.85] Thus Kahn proposes affect, affirmation, and aid as the three components of supportive transactions.

The precise mechanism of action linking social support and health is not known. Researchers have advanced three hypotheses.[77] The first is that social ties provide a buffer against the effects of high stress. The second is that social ties increase the development of coping strategies, thereby facilitating adaptation to change. The third hypothesis is that a perceived sense of support from others leads to a person's more generalized sense of control and responsibility.

Langlie[78] points to two other considerations in how social support may influence health status. One is that social groups differ in terms of both their norms regarding preventive health behavior and their ability to exert pressure to conform to those norms. The other is that interaction with others may provide specific practical information, such as how to prevent disease and where to go for health services.

It is unfortunate that none of the hypotheses concerning the mechanism of action whereby social support contributes to health maintenance or disease prevention can be strongly supported or refuted on the basis of existing evidence.[79] One can, however, infer from the evidence that affective (emotional) support may have a more significant relationship with well-being than instrumental (tangible) support.[80]

Relevance of social support to health behavior

Becker and Maiman[81] found increasing evidence that social support, particularly that provided by the patient's family, has a positive influence on compliance with medical advice. They emphasize that the patient's family remains a largely untapped means for reminding, assisting, encouraging, and reinforcing the patient with regard to following therapeutic directions.

Gottlieb[82] and McKinlay[83] elaborate on this association. They state that members of the help seeker's social network perform two functions prior to their mobilization as a support system. Initially they engage in formal and informal diagnostic functions. Through the former, they help to shape the definition of the help seeker's problem and judge its significance for well-being. Through the latter, they control the direction of help seeking and condition expectations about how help will be given. For example, a woman in a new town seeking health care will consult other women she has met either at work or in the community, trying to identify medical resources that are best suited to her health beliefs and special needs.

The lay network controls flow of clients to practitioners. By conditioning accurate expectations about the type of help given by health professionals, the lay network can decrease the likelihood of the help seeker's dropping out of treatment. It can speed or delay use of professional services by involving the help seeker in long or short periods of informal referral. It can contradict or concur with professionals' diagnoses of problems and attributions about their causes and improve or interfere with the patient's ability to follow the prescribed regimen.

Application of social support to cancer care

Rutledge[54] examined social support as well as health beliefs and other variables in relation to BSE practice in upper-middle-class women. She found no relationship between the women's perceived social support and their frequency of BSE practice.

Other applications of the theory of social support in the area of cancer-related health behavior were in the study of smoking behavior.[84–87] In all cases, support and/or smoking behavior of either family members or close associates was related to the smoking behavior of the subjects. Those subjects whose close social contacts were either nonsmokers or former smokers were likely to be nonsmokers or successful abstainers also. Consequently, social support may be more influential with preventive than with detective behavior.[54]

Locus of Control/Health Locus of Control

Locus of control

When Rotter[88] applied early social learning principles to clinical psychology in 1954, he developed the concepts of *internal* and *external locus of control.* They refer to the degree to which individuals perceive events in their lives as being a consequence of their own actions, and thereby controllable (internal control), or as being unrelated to their own behavior, and therefore beyond personal control (external control). Rotter proposed that persons who were more internally controlled were more likely to self-initiate change. Those who were externally controlled were more likely to be influenced by others.[89]

Health locus of control

In 1978 Wallston and Wallston[90] developed a new construct, the *health locus of control,* a generalized expectation about whether health is controllable by one's own behavior or by forces external to oneself. The Wallstons saw this construct as more useful in health-related research because an individual's sense of control often varies according to health-related experiences. Their model includes the concepts of internal and external locus of control. External locus of control is represented by two constructs, that of *chance* (health determined by fate) and *powerful others* (health determined by externals such as health professionals).

The conviction that outcomes (good health) are determined by one's own actions can have a number of effects on behavior. People who view health as personally determined but who believe they lack the skills needed to carry out the behaviors that would result in good health (low self-efficacy) would approach those activities with a sense of futility.[21]

Beliefs about internal locus of control, in combination with a high value placed on health, should predict preventive health behaviors. However, there is no theoretical reason for people with such beliefs who do *not* value health highly to perform health-relevant behaviors. Thus, if these constructs are used to study health behavior, the interaction between health value and health locus of control should be examined. The fact that many investigators have not done this may explain why beliefs about health locus of control have not been linked consistently to the performance of a variety of preventive health behaviors.[91]

Application of health locus of control to cancer care

The influence of beliefs about health locus of control has been examined in relation to BSE behavior,[52,92,93] seeking medical care for breast symptoms,[73] and adjustment to cancer.[70] Among a sample of southern African American hospital employees, BSE was practiced less frequently by women who believed that powerful others (health professionals) had control over their health.[93] In a sample of young Caucasian women, BSE was practiced more frequently by women who perceived an internal locus of control in combination with beliefs in high susceptibility and benefits.[52] In an earlier study, internal health locus of control in women was not related to their proficiency in BSE technique.[92] In another study, on the other hand, patients with hematologic malignancies who believed that physicians controlled their health were likely to expect a positive outcome from having treatment.[70] The authors speculated that patients' beliefs about control change throughout the duration of the disease.

Attribution Theory

Attribution Theory involves the explanations that individuals use to make sense of their world and the behavioral and emotional consequences of those explanations. The assumption is made that people are motivated to engage spontaneously in attributional activities; they ask "why?" or "why me?" This search for information is ultimately connected to the broader concept of personal or cognitive control.[94]

Ascribing causes can be especially relevant when one's health is threatened, when symptoms or tensions are heightened, or when a catastrophic event takes place. If one can assign a cause, one can manage the situation more effectively and can plan future action.

Attributions can be used to predict behavior, feelings, and expectancies, and can serve to maintain self-esteem and reduce anxiety.[94] Attributions may be conscious and deliberate, or preconscious. There are four dimensions of causal attributions. Each of them is associated with certain consequents. See Table 6-2.

Attributions that people generate have significant implications for their subsequent thoughts, feelings, and actions. Lewis and Daltroy[94] speculate that there is some optimal set of attributions that best predict a person's exercise of health behaviors. Attributions of success are usually related to stable, global, and internal causes. In general, the goal of the health professional is to encourage attribution of failure (e.g., failure to stop smoking) to unstable, specific, uncontrollable, and external causes. The person can then act on the belief that the health behavior in question was not potentially achievable at that time, and that it was not a personal deficiency that resulted in the failure. It becomes possible, therefore, for the individual to try again in the future. By obtaining information on the individual's attributions, the health professional can begin to understand the motivations behind the behaviors and can tailor health behavior interventions appropriately.[94] Research in the area of causal attributions is still limited, and much more needs to be done in order to determine whether the dimensions of attributions can be manipulated, in what manner, and by what method.

TABLE 6-2 Attribution Theory

Dimensions of Attributions (Causes)	Consequents
Locus of Cause	
Internal to the person (*Example:* innate ability)	Can be associated with low self-esteem or depression or taking responsibility for one's treatment
External to the person (*Example:* chance, luck, environmental pollutants)	Can be associated with poorer long-term morbidity or better coping and adjustment
Controllability	
Controllable (*Example:* level of effort)	Usually results in increased effort, enhanced performance
Uncontrollable (*Example:* innate ability, task difficulty)	Offers little hope of influencing future outcomes
Stability	
Stable (*Example:* personal ability) Unstable (*Example:* attention span, mood)	Both stability and instability are important determinants of goal expectations and can be used to predict cognitive and motivational deficits
Globality	
Global (*Example:* innate intelligence)	Affects a wide variety of outcomes; can result in extensive performance deficits
Specific (*Example:* test anxiety)	Affects a limited set of outcomes in a given situation

Source: Compiled from Lewis, Daltroy;[94] Weiner.[95,96]

Application of Attribution Theory to cancer care

The influence of beliefs about attribution has been examined in relation to adjustment or response to cancer.[97–105] Lewis et al.[101] found that patients with late-stage cancer used several processes, such as monitoring progress to maintain control over their lives, despite their terminal illness. Other researchers have attempted to relate patients' attributions of the cause of their cancer to adjustment behaviors.[99,100,103–105] Timko and Janoff-Bulman[105] found that adjustment of women with nonmetastatic breast cancer was associated positively with attributions to an individual's own behavior and negatively with attributions to other people or to the individual's personality. Although no clear association has been validated consistently, Gotay[99] has suggested that not making strong causal attributions may be a positive factor in patients' adjustment.

RELATED FACTORS

Sociodemographics

The influence of sociodemographics on health behavior is variable. In a relatively homogeneous sample of rural women, Gray[48] found that practicing BSE was not significantly related to sociodemographic variables. Reno[56] found similar results with regard to TSE practice among college males.

Knowledge and educational level

Because knowledge is often related to educational level, both factors are discussed in this section. Being knowledgeable about a specific cancer or cancer detection or screening measure has been found to relate positively to health behaviors such as skin protective behavior,[59,61] having a mammogram,[65,106] having a Pap test,[107,108] practicing BSE,[46,109] and practicing TSE.[56] Likewise, educational level has been found to relate positively to having a mammogram,[65,106,110,111] practicing BSE,[53] and having a Pap test.[107,108] In a large sample of adolescents, nutrition education was associated with both increased knowledge and positive nutritional practices.[112]

On the other hand, being knowledgeable and/or having a high level of education is not associated consistently with positive health behaviors.[44] Portnoy and Christenson[112] reported that many adolescents were unable to choose appropriate foods, despite their knowledge of the risk associated with eating a diet that is high in saturated fats. Gould[113] found that education was associated negatively with monitoring one's own health and that consciousness about health in general was unrelated to demographic variables. Newell and colleagues[71] found that patients who used unorthodox cancer therapies were both more knowledgeable and more educated than nonusers of these methods. In relation to cancer detection, women at high risk for breast cancer were found to be more knowledgeable about BSE than low-risk women but did not practice it more frequently.[45] Similarly, women who had personal knowledge about breast cancer did not necessarily report their symptoms of breast cancer promptly.[114]

In one study, an educational intervention was found to increase men's knowledge about TSE, but other factors such as attitude and perceived self-efficacy were better predictors of TSE behavior.[28] In another study of TSE behavior, the educational intervention did not increase men's knowledge about testicular cancer, but did increase their practice of TSE.[57] Both knowledge and practice of TSE increased as a result of an educational intervention in another study.[115] With regard to mammography screening for breast cancer, an educational intervention was found to increase levels of knowledge and perceived benefits among women, but did not increase their use of mammography.[64]

Knowledge and educational level apparently influence health behavior both positively and negatively. Other factors, such as fear,[107] may override the positive influence of knowledge on behavior. On the other hand, fear messages can have a positive effect if they are used with a person whose fear level about a disease is not already overwhelming, and who believes that certain health behaviors would be helpful. If fear messages are used, they are likely to be most influential if they are given in the initial attempt to change behavior and if they contain advice that can be quickly and easily followed.[21]

Socioeconomic status

Educational level is sometimes used as an indicator of socioeconomic status (SES), another factor that has a strong association with health behavior. People of low SES have been found to be less likely than people of high SES to report symptoms of colorectal cancer,[116] participate in screening for cervical cancer,[107] and participate in screening for breast cancer.[117] In addition, individuals of low SES are less likely to be successful with smoking cessation,[26] more fearful of getting cancer,[58] more likely to believe that physicians have control over their health,[70] and more likely to respond to a physician's encouragement than to printed media regarding mammography screening.[110]

Age

Like educational level and SES, age is an important influence on health behavior. Age modifies the influence of health beliefs, and confidence in one's ability to carry out a task is influential regardless of age.[34] Although several researchers found that older women were more likely than younger women to practice BSE[50,93] and have a Pap test,[50] others have found the reverse, especially in regard to the Pap test.[66,67,118,119] Older women tend to believe that they no longer require Pap tests because they are no longer sexually active or bearing children.[67] Also, they tend to have fewer close associates, such as spouses and friends, who would encourage them to have the test.[66] Older women have been found to delay seeing a health care provider for evaluation of symptoms of breast cancer.[114] In addition, older adults (over age 65) were found to be significantly less compliant than younger people (ages 20–35) with skin protective measures, after an educational intervention following removal of a skin cancer.[120]

Race

Differences in cancer incidence, mortality, and survival rates among people of different races have stimulated researchers to examine the health behaviors of these groups. The influence of race, exclusive of SES and educational level, is not evaluated easily. In Bloom and colleagues'[118] study of African Americans, most of the women had had breast examinations and Pap tests, and knew the warning signs of cancer but not the predisposing factors. Many believed that cancer was spread by air, and women were more likely than men to harbor cancer myths. Vaz and associates[58] found no difference between African American and white adolescent males' knowledge about TSE or testicular cancer, although the African American adolescents were more afraid of getting testicular cancer, less likely to consult a physician, and less optimistic about the prognosis.

Secondary analysis of data from the 1987 National Health Interview Survey[121] revealed that race was not a predictor of health behavior when knowledge was considered as a factor. One exception to this finding was that African American women were found to smoke less than white women. Nevertheless, Guillory[122] cautioned that African Americans are not a homogeneous group with regard to health behavior, and health care professionals should avoid stereotyping them.

The causal attributions, values, and traditional remedies of Native Americans can influence their health behaviors.[98,123] They may attribute cancer to exposure to lightening,[98] to witchcraft, or to breaking a taboo,[98,123] and may not seek prompt help in the health care system. Navajos are reluctant to address the potential fatality of an illness and are more interested in finding out why they contracted the disease.[98] Interestingly, Navajos have a low rate of cigarette smoking and a low rate of lung cancer.[98]

In a study of 600 elderly Hispanic women, Richardson and colleagues[109] found no differences in their breast cancer screening behaviors in comparison to the general population. However, 10% of the Hispanic women refused to touch the breast model. Mexican American adolescents with cancer were similar to their Anglo counterparts in their psychological responses, except that their illness had a greater impact on their families. The Mexican American group's refusal to participate in a behavioral intervention study in one setting was attributed to the responsiveness of the health care providers rather than to the ethnicity of the group.[124] Similarly, in another study the fatalistic beliefs and lack of value in early diagnosis expressed by Mexican American subjects were attributed to lack of education rather than to cultural factors.[125]

Family Factors

Families in the child-bearing years are likely to access the health care system for obstetrical and child care services and may be more likely than older families to hear health-related messages directly from providers. These messages can influence health behaviors positively.[108,110,119]

Family ethnicity can be a powerful influence on health behavior. Some ethnic groups, such as Native Americans,[123] Japanese Americans, and Hispanic Americans,[126] place great value on family involvement in decisions and care and do not value individualism. In one study, Arab women with breast cancer were found to seek support from the matriarchal family rather than from their husbands.[127] In another study, a large sample of predominantly rural, Caucasian women ranked encouragement from the family and from husbands as important factors in their decisions to have a mammogram.[110]

Social Factors

Social support, social roles, and social stigma all influence health behavior of individuals with regard to cancer prevention, detection, and treatment. Social support has been found to have a positive influence on people's smoking cessation efforts.[84–87] Social roles may influence health behavior either positively or negatively. As alluded to previously, women in childbearing and childrearing roles who may have more contact with the health care system are more likely than older women to practice BSE and participate in cancer screening programs. Older women, on the other hand, who are no longer wives and/or engaged in childbearing often perceive that they do not need Pap tests. In addition, fear of embarrassment at having to expose certain body parts may negatively influence a woman's participation in cancer screening.[107]

Cultural factors have been found to influence people's decisions both to participate in screening and to delay seeking help from symptoms of cancer. In Moslem culture, delay in seeking care is associated with the belief that disease is not present unless it is accompanied by noticeable signs.[127] Also, reluctance to talk about one's cancer is related to the belief that this disclosure inhibits recovery.[127] Jewish Israeli women with breast cancer who had a Western orientation were found to be active in seeking medical help, whereas those with an oriental orientation were passive and submissive.[97] In Native American culture, delay in seeking care may be related to the use of Native American remedies rather than to denial of illness.[123]

Cancer is discussed relatively freely in the dominant culture of the United States. Media coverage of the diagnosis and treatment of cancer in both President[128] and Mrs. Reagan[129, 130] had a positive influence on the information-seeking and cancer screening behaviors of the public.

Institutional Factors

The organization of the health care delivery system influences people's health behavior. Services organized around care for the sick often include barriers for those people who seek prevention or screening services. Social priorities and, to some extent, the political system determine the allocation of resources to various health services. In the United States, women at high risk for cervical cancer often do not participate in screening, whereas in Sweden all women are screened.[131] The Swedish system eliminates barriers such as cost, and provides reminders to women as a cue to initiate healthy behavior. Cost and reminders are two areas that have been identified as a focus for interventions to increase women's participation in cervical screening[53,66] as well as breast cancer screening[65,110,132–135] in the United States. Current availability of at least some level of Medicaid reimbursement for Pap tests in most states, and mammography in many states,[136] should reduce the cost barrier for many disadvantaged women.

Health care providers influence people's health behavior in a number of ways. Women have reported that a physician's recommendation or reminder to have a Pap test was important in their decision to do so.[66,108,110,119] Also, women have reported lack of physician referral as a major reason for not getting a mammogram.[137] In a sample of elderly women, frequency of the practice of BSE was associated with having been taught BSE by a nurse.[68] One would hope that the positive influence of the nurses' teaching was due to the modification of the teaching to accommodate the elderly women's physical changes.[138] Among a large group of elderly Hispanic women, knowledge, recency, and frequency of BSE practice were associated with having been taught BSE by a physician.[109] Prompt, courteous, and competent examinations by health care providers were associated with women's continuation in a national breast screening study.[139] In a cancer prevention clinic for high-risk families, staff helped clients to deal with emotions that could negatively influence their health behaviors.[140]

Health care providers tend to respond to patients with cancer according to their perceptions of them. Providers may actually foster negative emotional states and behaviors in patients, if they perceive patients as having these qualities.[141] Similarly, providers' responses to patients of various ethnic backgrounds may influence patients' behaviors with regard to compliance with treatment or participation in studies.[124]

IMPLICATIONS FOR NURSING PRACTICE

People's health behaviors are influenced by multiple interacting factors. Theories and models have been developed to identify and describe the interaction of these variables and to predict and prescribe health behavior. Nevertheless, human behavior is not totally predictable, and the totality of its complexity has not yet been described.

Nurses can apply some of the empirically validated concepts and propositions of health behavior by incorporating them into the nursing process. The models provide guidelines for assessment, nursing diagnosis, intervention, and evaluation. For example, health beliefs, self-efficacy, and beliefs about control can be incorporated into both assessment and evaluation. The concept of self-efficacy should be included in interventions with patients and families as well as the public, particularly in education programs where mastery of a skill is important.[31,142]

Considering the association between health behavior and demographics,[143] nurses need to examine this aspect of the community. A thorough assessment of people's cultural beliefs and practices[122] and the use of developmental and communication principles[144] are crucial to nurses' success in influencing people's health behaviors positively.

REFERENCES

1. Greenwald P, Sondik EJ: Cancer control objectives for the nation: 1985–2000. *NCI Monographs* 2:3–11, 1986.
2. American Cancer Society: *American Cancer Society Priorities for the 1990s.* Atlanta: Author, 1990.
3. U.S. Department of Health and Human Services: *Healthy People 2000.* National Health Promotion and Disease Prevention Objectives (DHHS Publication No. (PHS) 91-50212). Washington, DC: U.S. Government Printing Office, 1991.
4. Gochman D: Health behavior: Plural perspectives. In Gochman D (ed.): *Health Behavior: Emerging Research Perspectives.* New York: Plenum, 1988, pp. 3–17.
5. Gochman D: Labels, systems and motives: Some perspectives for future research. *Health Educ Q* 9:167–174, 1982.
6. Kasl S, Cobb S: Health behavior, illness behavior, and sick role behavior: I. Health and illness behavior. *Arch Environ Health* 12:246–266, 1966.
7. Rosenstock I: Why people use health services. *Milbank Mem Fund Q* 44:94–124, 1966.
8. Harris D, Guten S: Health protective behavior: An exploratory study. *J Health Soc Behav* 20:17–29, 1979.
9. Pender N: *Health Promotion in Nursing Practice* (ed. 2). Norwalk, CT: Appleton and Lange, 1987.
10. Mechanic D: *Medical Sociology* (ed. 2). New York: Free Press, 1978.
11. Steele J, McBroom W: Conceptual and empirical dimensions of health behavior. *J Health Soc Behav* 13:382–392, 1972.
12. Mechanic D: Response factors in illness: The study of illness behavior. In Jaco E (ed.): *Patients, Physicians and Illness: A Sourcebook in Behavioral Science and Health* (ed. 2). New York: Free Press, 1972, pp. 118–130.
13. Cummings K, Becker M, Maile M: Bringing the models together: An empirical approach to combining variables used to explain health actions. *J Behav Med* 3:123–145, 1980.
14. Perry C, Baranowski T, Parcel G: How individuals, environments, and health behavior interact: Social learning theory. In Glanz K, Lewis F, Rimer B (eds.): *Health Behavior and Health Education.* San Francisco: Jossey-Bass, 1990, pp. 161–186.
15. Bandura A: *Social Learning Theory.* Englewood Cliffs, NJ: Prentice-Hall, 1977.
16. Bandura A; Self-efficacy: Toward a unifying theory of behavioral change. *Psychol Rev* 84:191–215, 1977.
17. Bandura A: The self system in reciprocal determinism. *Am Psychologist* 33:344–358, 1978.
18. Bandura A: Self-referent thought: A developmental analysis of self-efficacy. In Flavell J, Ross L (eds.): *Social Cognitive Development: Frontiers and Possible Futures.* Cambridge, Eng.: Cambridge University Press, 1981, pp. 200–239.
19. Bandura A: Recycling misconceptions of perceived self-efficacy. *Cog Ther Res* 8:231–255, 1984.
20. Bandura A: Self-efficacy mechanism in human agency. *Am Psychologist* 37:122–147, 1982.
21. Becker M: Theoretical models of adherence and strategies for improving adherence. In Shumaker S, Schron E, Ockene J (eds.): *The Handbook of Health Behavior Change.* New York: Springer-Verlag, 1990, pp. 5–43.
22. Seydel E, Taal E, Wiegman O: Risk-appraisal, outcome and self-efficacy expectancies: Cognitive factors in preventive behavior related to cancer. *Psychol Health* 4:99–109, 1990.
23. DiClemente C, Prochaska J, Gibertini M: Self-efficacy and the stages of self-change of smoking. *Cog Ther Res* 9:181–200, 1985.
24. Godding P, Glasgow R: Self-efficacy and outcome expectations as predictors of controlled smoking status. *Cog Ther Res* 9:583–590, 1985.
25. Strecher V, Becker M, Kirscht J, et al: Psychosocial aspects of changes in cigarette smoking behavior. *Patient Educ Counsel* 7:249–262, 1985.

26. Wilcox NS, Prochaska JO, Velicer WF, et al: Subject characteristics as predictors of self-change in smoking. *Addict Behav* 10:407–412, 1985.
27. Brubaker RG, Fowler C: Encouraging college males to perform testicular self-examination: Evaluation of a persuasive message based on the revised Theory of Reasoned Action. *J Appl Soc Psychol* 20:1411–1422, 1990.
28. Brubaker RG, Wickersham D: Encouraging the practice of testicular self-examination: A field application of the Theory of Reasoned Action. *Health Psychol* 9:154–163, 1990.
29. Baker J: Breast self-examination among older women. *Health Educ Res* 3:181–189, 1988.
30. Champion VL: Breast self-examination in women 35 and older: A prospective study. *J Behav Med* 13:523–538, 1990.
31. Olson R, Mitchell E: Self-confidence as a critical factor in breast self-examination. *J Obstet Gynecol Neonatal Nurs* 18:476–481, 1989.
32. Rippetoe PA, Rogers RW: Effects of components of Protection-Motivation Theory on adaptive and maladaptive coping with a health threat. *J Pers Soc Psychol* 52:596–604, 1987.
33. Rutledge DN, Davis GT: Breast self-examination compliance and the Health Belief Model. *Oncol Nurs Forum* 15:175–179, 1988.
34. Hoogewerf, PE, Hislop G, Morrison BJ, et al: Health belief and compliance with screening for fecal occult blood. *Soc Sci Med* 30:721–726, 1990.
35. Kelly RB, Zyzanski SJ, Alemagno SA: Prediction of motivation and behavior change following health promotion: Role of health beliefs, social support, and self-efficacy. *Soc Sci Med* 32:311–320, 1991.
36. Strecher V, DeVellis B, Becker M, et al: The role of self-efficacy in achieving health behavior change. *Health Educ Q* 13:73–91, 1986.
37. Janz N, Becker M: The Health Belief Model: A decade later. *Health Educ Q* 11:1–47, 1984.
38. Janis I: The role of social support in adherence to stressful decisions. *Am Psychologist* 38:143–160, 1983.
39. Maiman L, Becker M: The Health Belief Model: Origins and correlates in psychological theory. In Becker M (ed.): *The Health Belief Model and Personal Health Behavior.* Thorofare, NJ: Slack, 1974, pp. 9–26.
40. Lewin K: *A Dynamic Theory of Personality: Selected Papers.* New York: McGraw-Hill, 1935.
41. Rosenstock I: Historical origins of the Health Belief Model. In Becker M (ed.): *The Health Belief Model and Personal Health Behavior.* Thorofare, NJ: Slack, 1974, pp. 1–8.
42. Rosenstock I: The Health Belief Model: Explaining health behavior through expectancies. In Glanz K, Lewis F, Rimer B (eds.): *Health Behavior and Health Education.* San Francisco: Jossey-Bass, 1990, pp. 39–61.
43. Becker M. Maiman L: Sociobehavioral determinants of compliance with health and medical care recommendations. *Med Care* 13:10–24, 1975.
44. Rimer B, Keintz M, Kessler H, et al: Why women resist screening mammography: Patient-related barriers. *Radiology* 172:243–246, 1989.
45. Alagna SW, Morokoff PJ, Bevett JM, et al: Performance of breast self-examination by women at high risk for breast cancer. *Women and Health* 12:29–46, 1987.
46. Bottimore AH, Hailey BJ: Promotion of breast self-exam behavior: An attempt to modify health beliefs. *Int Q Community Health Educ* 9:273–282, 1988–89.
47. Chrvala C, Iverson D: Predictive models for frequency and proficiency of BSE performance. *Prog Clin Biol Res* 293:159–173, 1989.
48. Gray ME: Factors related to practice of breast self-examination in rural women. *Cancer Nurs* 13:100–107, 1990.
49. Hill D, Shugg D: Breast self-examination practices and attitudes among breast cancer, benign breast disease and general practice patients. *Health Educ Res* 4:193–203, 1989.
50. Hill D, Gardner G, Rassaby J: Factors predisposing women to take precautions against breast and cervix cancer. *J Appl Soc Psychol* 15:59–79, 1985.
51. Massey V: Perceived susceptibility to breast cancer and practice of breast self-examination. *Nurs Res* 35:183–185, 1986.
52. Redeker N: Health beliefs, health locus of control, and the frequency of practice of breast self-examination in women. *J Obstet Gynecol Neonatal Nurs* 18:45–51, 1989.
53. Ronis DL, Harel Y: Health beliefs and breast examination behaviors: Analyses of linear structural relations. *Psychol Health* 3:259–285, 1989.
54. Rutledge D: Factors related to women's practice of breast self-examination. *Nurs Res* 36:117–121, 1987.
55. Blesch K: Health beliefs about testicular cancer and self-examination among professional men. *Oncol Nurs Forum* 13:29–33, 1986.
56. Reno DR: Men's knowledge and health beliefs about testicular cancer and testicular self-examination. *Cancer Nurs* 11:112–117, 1988.
57. Rudolf VM, Quinn KL: The practice of TSE among college men: Effectiveness of an educational program. *Oncol Nurs Forum* 15:45–48, 1988.
58. Vaz RM, Best DL, Davis SW: Testicular cancer. Adolescent knowledge and attitudes. *J Adolesc Health Care* 9:474–479, 1988.
59. Cody R, Lee C: Behaviors, beliefs, and intentions in skin cancer prevention. *J Behav Med* 13:373–389, 1990.
60. Cockburn J, Hennrikus D, Scott R, et al: Adolescent use of sun protection measures. *Med J Aust* 151:136–140, 1989.
61. Keesling B, Friedman H: Psychosocial factors in sunbathing and sunscreen use. *Health Psychol* 6:477–493, 1987.
62. Millon-Underwood S, Sanders E: Factors contributing to health promotion behaviors among African-American men. *Oncol Nurs Forum* 17:707–712, 1990.
63. Pederson L, Wanklin J, Baskerville J: The role of health beliefs in compliance with physician advice to quit smoking. *Soc Sci Med* 19:573–580, 1984.
64. Reynolds K, West, S, Aiken L: Increasing the use of mammography: A pilot program. *Health Educ Q* 17:429–441, 1990.
65. Rutledge DN, Hartmann WH, Kinman PO, et al: Exploration of factors affecting mammography behaviors. *Prev Med* 17:412–422, 1988.
66. Hennig P, Knowles A: Factors influencing women over 40 years to take precautions against cervical cancer. *J Appl Soc Psychol* 20:1612–1621, 1990.
67. Lerman C, Caputo C, Brody D: Factors associated with inadequate cervical cancer screening among lower-income primary care patients. *J Am Board Fam Pract* 3:151–156, 1990.
68. Williams RD: Factors affecting the practice of breast self-

examination in older women. *Oncol Nurs Forum* 15:611–616, 1988.

69. Strauss L, Solomon L, Costanza M, et al: Breast self-examination practices and attitudes of women with and without a history of breast cancer. *J Behav Med* 10:337–350, 1987.
70. Marks G, Richardson JL, Graham JW: Role of health locus of control beliefs and expectations of treatment efficacy in adjustment to cancer. *J Pers Soc Psychol* 51:443–450, 1986.
71. Newell SM, Price JH, Roberts SM, et al: Utility of the modified Health Belief Model in predicting compliance with treatment by adult patients with advanced cancer. *Psychol Rep* 59:783–791, 1986.
72. Ajzen I, Fishbein M: *Understanding Attitudes and Predicting Social Behavior*. Englewood Cliffs, NJ: Prentice-Hall, 1980.
73. Timko C: Seeking medical care for a breast cancer symptom: Determinants of intentions to engage in prompt or delay behavior. *Health Psychol* 6:305–328, 1987.
74. Carter W: Health behavior as a rational process: Theory of Reasoned Action and Multiattribute Utility Theory. In Glanz K, Lewis F, Rimer B (eds.): *Health Behavior and Health Education*. San Francisco: Jossey-Bass, 1990, pp. 63–91.
75. Sarason I, Levine H, Basham R, et al: Assessing social support. *J Pers Soc Psychol* 44:127–139, 1983.
76. Kahn R: Aging and social support. In Riley M (ed.): *Aging from Birth to Death: Interdisciplinary Perspectives*. Boulder, CO: Westview Press, 1979, pp. 77–91.
77. Hamburg B, Killilea M: Relation of social support, stress, illness, and use of health services. In *Public Health Service: Healthy People: The Surgeon General's Report on Health Promotion and Disease Prevention—Background Papers* (DHEW Publication No. (PHS) 79-55071A). Washington, DC: U.S. Government Printing Office, 1979, pp. 253–256.
78. Langlie J: Social networks, health beliefs, and preventive health behavior. *J Health Soc Behav* 18:244–260, 1977.
79. Minkler M: Applications of social support theory to health education: Implications for work with the elderly. *Health Educ Q* 8:147–165, 1981.
80. Israel B: Social networks and health status: Linking theory, research, and practice. *Patient Counsel Health Educ* 4:65–79, 1982.
81. Becker M, Maiman L: Strategies for enhancing patient compliance. *J Community Health* 6:113–135, 1980.
82. Gottlieb B: *Social Support Strategies*. Beverly Hills, CA: Sage, 1983.
83. McKinlay J: Social networks, lay consultation, and help-seeking behavior. *Soc Forces* 51:275–292, 1973.
84. Eisinger R: Psychosocial predictors of smoking recidivism. *J Health Soc Behav* 12:355–362, 1971.
85. Graham S, Gibson R: Cessation of patterned behavior: Withdrawal from smoking. *Soc Sci Med* 5:319–337, 1971.
86. Lauer R, Akers R, Massey J, et al: Evaluation of cigarette smoking among adolescents: The Muscatine Study. *Prev Med* 11:417–428, 1982.
87. Mermelstein R, Lichtenstein E, McIntyre K: Partner support and relapse in smoking cessation programs. *J Consult Clin Psychol* 51:465–466, 1983.
88. Rotter J: *Social Learning and Clinical Psychology*. Englewood Cliffs: N.J.: Prentice-Hall, 1954.
89. Rotter J: Generalized expectancies for internal versus external control of reinforcement. *Psychol Monogr* 80:1–28, 1966.
90. Wallston K, Wallston B: Locus of control and health. *Health Educ Monogr* 6:107–117, 1978.
91. Lau R: Beliefs about control and health behavior. In Gochman D (ed.): *Health Behavior: Emerging Research Perspectives*. New York: Plenum, 1988, pp. 43–63.
92. Alagna S, Reddy D: Predictors of proficient technique and successful lesion detection in breast self-examination. *Health Psychol* 3:113–127, 1984.
93. Nemcek MA: Factors influencing black women's breast self-examination practice. *Cancer Nurs* 12:339–343, 1989.
94. Lewis F, Daltroy L: How causal explanations influence health behavior: Attribution Theory. In Glanz K, Lewis F, Rimer B (eds.): *Health Behavior and Health Education*. San Francisco: Jossey-Bass, 1990, pp. 92–114.
95. Weiner B: A theory of motivation for some classroom experiences. *J Educ Psychol* 71:3–25, 1979.
96. Weiner B: A theory of motivation for some classroom experiences. In Gorlitz D (ed.): *Perspectives on Attribution Research and Theory, The Bielefeld Symposium*. Cambridge, MA: Ballinger, 1980, pp. 39–74.
97. Baider L, Sarell M: Perceptions and causal attributions of Israeli women with breast cancer concerning their illness: The effects of ethnicity and religiosity. *Psychother Psychosom* 39:136–143, 1983.
98. Csordas TJ: The sore that does not heal: Cause and concept in the Navajo experience of cancer. *J Anthrop Res* 45:457–485, 1989.
99. Gotay CC: Why me? Attributions and adjustment by cancer patients and their mates at two stages in the disease process. *Soc Sci Med* 20:825–831, 1985.
100. Kroode H, Oosterwijk M, Steverink N: Three conflicts as a result of causal attributions. *Soc Sci Med* 28:93–97, 1989.
101. Lewis FM, Haberman MR, Wallhagen MI: How adults with late-stage cancer experience personal control. *J Psychosoc Oncol* 4:27–42, 1986.
102. Mumma C, McCorkle R: Causal attribution and life-threatening disease. *Int J Psychiatry Med* 12:311–319, 1982–83.
103. Taylor SE: Social cognition and health. *Pers Soc Psychol Bull* 8:549–562, 1982.
104. Taylor SE, Lichtman RR, Wood JV: Attributions, beliefs about control, and adjustment to breast cancer. *J Pers Soc Psychol* 46:489–502, 1984.
105. Timko C, Jannoff-Bulman R: Attributions, vulnerability, and psychological adjustment: The case of breast cancer. *Health Psychol* 4:521–544, 1985.
106. Champion VL: The relationship of selected variables to breast cancer detection behaviors in women 35 and older. *Oncol Nurs Forum* 18:733–739, 1991.
107. Peters RK, Bear MB, Thomas D: Barriers to screening for cancer of the cervix. *Prev Med* 18:133–146, 1989.
108. Mamon JA, Shediac MC, Crosby CB, et al: Inner-city women at risk for cervical cancer: Behavioral and utilization factors related to inadequate screening. *Prev Med* 19:363–376, 1990.
109. Richardson JL, Marks G, Solis JM, et al: Frequency and adequacy of breast cancer screening among elderly Hispanic women. *Prev Med* 16:761–774, 1987.
110. Kruse J, Phillips DM: Factors influencing women's decision to undergo mammography. *Obstet Gynecol* 70:744–748, 1987.
111. Anda RF, Sienko DG, Remington PL, et al: Screening mammography for women 50 years of age and older: Practices and trends. *Am J Prev Med* 6:123–129, 1990.

112. Portnoy B, Christenson GM: Cancer knowledge and related practices: Results from the National Adolescent Student Health Survey. *J Sch Health* 59:218–224, 1989.
113. Gould SJ: Health consciousness and health behavior. The application of a new health consciousness scale. *Am J Prev Med* 6:228–237, 1990.
114. Lierman LM: Discovery of breast changes. Women's responses and nursing implications. *Cancer Nurs* 11:352–361, 1988.
115. Ostwald S, Rothenberger J: Development of a testicular self-examination program for college men. *J Am Coll Health* 33:234–239, 1985.
116. Funch DP: Predictors and consequences of symptom-reporting behaviors in colorectal cancer patients. *Med Care* 26:1000–1008, 1988.
117. Fink R, Shapiro S: Significance of increased efforts to gain participation in screening for breast cancer. *Am J Prev Med* 6:34–41, 1990.
118. Bloom JR, Hayes WA, Saunders F, et al: Cancer awareness and secondary prevention practices in Black Americans: Implications for intervention. *Fam Community Health* 10:19–30, 1987.
119. Paskett ED, Carter WB, Chu J, et al: Compliance behavior in women with abnormal pap smears. *Med Care* 28:643–656, 1990.
120. Robinson J: Behavior modification obtained by sun protection education coupled with removal of a skin cancer. *Arch Dermatol* 126:477–481, 1990.
121. Jepson C, Kessler LG, Portnoy B, et al: Black-white differences in cancer prevention knowledge and behavior. *Am J Public Health* 81:501–504, 1991.
122. Guillory J: Ethnic perspectives of cancer nursing: The black American. *Oncol Nurs Forum* 14:66–69, 1987.
123. Antle A: Ethnic perspectives of cancer nursing: The American Indian. *Oncol Nurs Forum* 14:70–73, 1987.
124. Zeltzer LK, Lebaron S: Does ethnicity constitute a risk factor in the psychological distress of adolescents with cancer? *J Adolesc Health Care* 6:8–11, 1985.
125. Sugarek NJ, Deyo RN, Holmes BC: Locus of control and beliefs about cancer in a multi-ethnic clinic population. *Oncol Nurs Forum* 15:481–486, 1988.
126. Kagawa-Singer M: Ethnic perspectives of cancer nursing: Hispanics and Japanese Americans. *Oncol Nurs Forum* 14:59–65, 1987.
127. Baider L, De-Nour AK: The meaning of a disease: An exploratory study of Moslem Arab women after a mastectomy. *J Psychosoc Oncol* 4:1–13, 1986.
128. Brown ML, Potosky AL: The presidential effect: The public health response to media coverage about Ronald Reagan's colon cancer episode. *Public Opin Q* 54:317–329, 1990.
129. Lane DS, Polednak AP, Burg MA: The impact of media coverage of Nancy Reagan's experience on breast cancer screening. *Am J Public Health* 79:1551–1554, 1989.
130. Stoddard A, Zapka J, Schoenfield S, et al: Effects of a news event on breast cancer screening survey responses. *Prog Clin Biol Res* 339:259–268, 1990.
131. Howard J: "Avoidable mortality" from cervical cancer: Exploring the concept. *Soc Sci Med* 24:507–514, 1987.
132. Baines CJ, Christen A, Simard A, et al: The National Breast Screening Study: Pre-recruitment sources of awareness in participants. *Can J Public Health* 80:221–225, 1989.
133. Lane DS, Polednak AP, Burg MA: Breast cancer screening practices among users of county-funded health centers vs women in the entire community. *Am J Public Health* 82:199–203, 1992.
134. Mayer JA, Dubbert PM, Scott RR, et al: Breast self-examination: The effects of personalized prompts on practice frequency. *Behav Ther* 2:135–146, 1987.
135. Mayer JA, Kellogg MC: Promoting mammography appointment making. *J Behav Med* 12:605–611, 1989.
136. Boss LP, Guckes FH: Medicaid coverage of screening tests for breast and cervical cancer. *Am J Public Health* 82:252–253, 1992.
137. Vogel V, Graves D, Vernon S, et al: Mammographic screening of women with increased risk of breast cancer. *Cancer* 66:1613–1620, 1990.
138. Ludwick R: Breast examination in the older adult. *Cancer Nurs* 11:99–102, 1988.
139. Baines C, To T, Wall C: Women's attitudes to screening after participation in the National Breast Screening Study. *Cancer* 65:1663–1669, 1990.
140. Josten DM, Evans AM, Love RR: The cancer prevention clinic: A service for cancer-prone families. *J Psychosoc Oncol* 3:5–20, 1985.
141. Katz I, Hass RG, Parisi N, et al: Lay people's and health care personnel's perceptions of cancer, AIDS, cardiac, and diabetic patients. *Psychological Rep* 60:615–629, 1987.
142. Redman BK: Strengthening patient education programs in oncology. *J Psychosoc Oncol* 3:75–81, 1985/86.
143. Fink D, Sheehan H: Cancer prevention and detection: An overview of variables influencing adoption and practice. *Cancer* 61:2391–2395, 1988.
144. Buller DB, Buller MK: Approaches to communicating preventive behaviors. *Semin Oncol Nurs* 7:53–63, 1991.

Chapter 7

Cancer Risk and Assessment

Rebecca F. Cohen, RN, EdD, MPA, CPHQ

Marilyn Frank-Stromborg, RN, EdD, NP, FAAN

INTRODUCTION

Health risk appraisal has been credited to Dr. Lewis C. Robbins, who worked extensively on the prevention of cervical cancer and heart disease during the 1940s. He developed a "health hazard chart" to give the medical examination a more prospective orientation toward preventive efforts. By the end of the 1960s life insurance actuarial principles were being applied to risk assessment, and risk multipliers were quantified for patient characteristics that affect mortality risk. The presence of these necessary elements thus led the way to quantitative risk appraisal. In 1970 Robbins and Hall[1] published a manual entitled *How to Practice Prospective Medicine,* which provided a complete health risk assessment (HRA) package, including questionnaire, risk computations, and feedback strategy.

When HRAs were first presented for use, the medical profession generally ignored their presence. However, the potential for computerization of the risk-estimation procedure, commercial interest, and the involvement of government agencies led to a proliferation of HRA programs. As of 1985, there were approximately 52 HRAs identified by the Office of Disease Prevention and Health Promotion in the U.S. Department of Health and Human Services. While questions have been raised concerning the validity of the databases and procedures used in HRA risk estimation, few empirical evaluations of the adequacy of the HRA procedures have been reported.[2]

Precise prediction of disease or mortality by any means is currently an attainable goal because of incomplete knowledge of the total set of risk factors, their time-dose levels, and the true functional form of their contribution to risk. Similar risk models are successful in differentiating high-, medium-, and low-risk persons and in estimating relative risk, but are much less successful in estimating absolute risk in individuals or across populations. In contrast, measurements applied to individuals should attain higher levels of accuracy than measurements used only in correlational studies, where there is opportunity for random errors to offset one another.[2]

HRA as a vehicle for what might be termed "prospective health assessment" potentially has a number of very desirable qualities for clinicians and health educators: preventive orientation, systematic approach, ability to emphasize modifiable factors, and a scientific knowledge base. However, a major concern is the value of quantitative estimates of absolute risk. Would the use of relative risk, risk scores, health scores, and other less quantitative measures, given the limitations in scientific knowledge and risk-estimation methods, be more helpful than the dependence on absolute risk assessment? Schoenbach[2] suggests that while HRAs may have valuable purposes, sophistication and precision in risk estimation are not necessarily the measure of their quality.

DEFINITIONS OF RISK

Risk is the potential realization of unwanted consequences of an event. Both a probability of occurrence of an event and the magnitude of its consequences are involved.[3,4] According to Rowe,[5] *hazard* implies the existence of some threat, whereas *risk* implies both the existence of a threat and its potential for occurrence. Since a risk can occur only if a potential pathway for exposure exists, a hazard may exist without implying risk. For example, there are toxic chemicals that are hazardous, but until the chemical actually exists in some form with a potential pathway to man or the environment there is no risk. A risk estimate in this case involves both potency of the substance and exposure to a population in terms of the number of persons who might receive specified dose levels. This definition of risk does, however, imply that risk is always negative. A more general definition of risk, which would not be in conflict with other definitions, is that risk "is the downside of a gamble."[5] This definition implies that (1) living itself involves gambles, (2) some gambles are involuntary, (3) tradeoffs are often required between quality and quantity of life, and (4) there is no such thing as zero risk, only involuntary and voluntary gambles for which minimum risk for acceptable gain is one criterion for decision making.[5]

A person's "cancer risk" would generally mean a factual estimate of the likelihood and severity of adverse effect, or the odds of incurring cancer. The estimation of health risks is an empirical problem filled with many uncertainties. After risks are estimated, decisions must be made about whether to bear the risks or to minimize them by reducing their source or taking protective actions. These decisions, often referred to as *risk evaluation,* are based on personal and social value judgments.[3,4] As Rowe[5] has stressed, the issue is really whether a particular risk is "acceptable" or is similar to risks already accepted or to the risks of alternatives.

Two approaches that can be used to calculate risk are relative risk and attributable risk. *Relative risk* is a ratio that compares the rate of the disease among exposed persons with the rate of the disease among unexposed persons. Although relative risk does not reveal the probability that the exposed person will have the disease, it does measure the strength of the association between a factor and the outcome.[6] The *attributable risk* is the difference in the disease rates between the group exposed to the factor and unexposed groups. Attributable risk is used to calculate the magnitude of change when a particular factor is added or subtracted.[6]

CANCER RISK FACTORS

Cancer prevention strategies can be divided into two major areas: (1) identification of the contributors to the cause(s) of cancer, and (2) the action taken in response to this knowledge. Identification is the function of the researcher, and action is usually enacted by legislative control or preferably by voluntary actions taken on the part of concerned individuals. It is, according to Newell,[7] very possible that we could know the cause of every cancer and not be able to prevent any of them. Cancer prevention depends, therefore, on what individuals do with this knowledge and how they perceive, accept, and act on it. What really counts is behavior modification, or agent change, whether in the environment, the medical care system, or the individual.

Cancer risk factors are specific risk factors or individual characteristics that are associated with an increased cancer risk: personal behavior, genetic makeup or familial traits, and exposure to a known cancer-causing agent.[3–10] Breslow[9] divides the factors that cause cancer into two groups: those that are under a person's control (personal habits, such as cigarette smoking), and those outside a person's control (age; hereditary characteristics such as familial polyposis). Risk factors have also been divided according to whether they are unique to an individual or shared by a group of persons. Individual risk factors include the individual's lifestyle, nutritional habits, medical conditions, and exposure to radiation or drugs. Group risk factors are those shared by persons from the same geographic residence or the same occupation.[10] Eventually the role of such factors may be describable in terms of chemical or metabolic mechanisms that might relate to multistage or cocarcinogenesis in humans.[3]

One important function of categorizing risk factors is to provide a database from which to develop an individual's cancer risk profile, to make recommendations about risk factors, and to plan specific interventions for risk reduction. The two biggest challenges for the cancer research establishment are (1) the implementation of interventions to prevent cancers from known or proven causes, and (2) the verification of highly suspected causes of major types of cancer.[10]

Another function of categorization is to emphasize the many causative factors and the complex etiology of cancer. For example, some cancers, such as skin cancer, appear to have one factor that is especially important (i.e., ultraviolet radiation). For most types of cancer, however, it appears that an interaction of multiple factors is probably necessary.[3,11–15]

In general, the predominant carcinogenic risk factors believed to be responsible for 70%–90% of cancers in humans in Western industrial societies can be put into the following categories:

A. Environmental
    1. Nonoccupational
        a. Habits
            i. Smoking
            ii. Alcohol consumption
            iii. Sunbathing
            iv. Dietary factors
        b. Customs (e.g., noncircumcision)
        c. Air and water pollution
    2. Occupational
        a. Chemical (e.g., asbestos)
        b. Physical (e.g., radiation)
B. Sex differences (e.g., hormones)
C. Virus
D. Racial differences
E. Habitat: urban vs. rural environment
F. Genetic factors
G. Marital status
H. Socioeconomic class
I. Psychologic
    1. Personality profile theory
    2. Stressful life events
J. Medical-therapy-related cancers

CANCER RISK FACTORS IN MINORITY POPULATIONS

Multifactorial Aspects

Chinese American women experience lower rates of breast cancer incidence (55.2 per 100,000) than the general population (106.1 per 100,000), but their survival rates (64% at 5 years) are comparable to those of Caucasian women (71% at 5 years).[16] African Americans have an 11% greater risk of developing cancer and a 25% lower 5-year survival rate than the general population.[17–19] The cancer death rate among African Americans is 27% higher than for the general population and has increased by approximately 50% in the past 30 years. This presents a 10% increase among African American women and a 77% increase among African American men. The higher cancer prevalence, higher mortality, and lower survival rates for African American men place them at greater risk than other ethnic groups. Orientals and Hispanics within the United States have a lower cancer incidence rate per 100,000 than either whites or blacks and a survival rate that is higher than that of blacks but similar to the rate for whites.[18] High-incidence cancers for specific ethnic groups are identified by site in Table 7-1.[20]

These aggregate data may, however, mask the fact that subgroups within an ethnic minority may be at increased risk of cancer incidence or mortality. These subgroups include immigrants, the elderly, the non-English speaker, the illiterate, and the economically disadvantaged. Members of these subgroups may not attend screening programs, due to real or perceived barriers, such as language difficulties, negative cancer beliefs, fear of cancer, and cost of services.[16] In addition, most of the rate differences among ethnic groups may be attributable to behavioral, social, and environmental factors rather than to biological or genetic characteristics. In particular, differences in dietary patterns have been suggested as the major contributor to rate differences among blacks and Hispanics, whereas delayed diagnosis is believed to contribute most to mortality differences.[21,22]

TABLE 7-1 High-Incidence Cancers, by Site, for Specific Ethnic Groups

Ethnic Group	Cancers of Highest Incidence
Hispanic	
Men and women	Gallbladder, liver, stomach, pancreas
Men	Prostate
Women	Cervical
Black	
Men	Prostate, lung, bronchial, pancreas
Women	Cervical, breast
Men and women	Multiple myeloma
Hawaiian	
Men and women	Lung, stomach, rectal, esophageal
Women	Uterine, cervical, breast
Men	Liver, pancreas
Alaskan Natives	
Men	Lung, nasopharyngeal
Eskimo men	Liver
Women	Renal cell, gallbladder, thyroid, colorectal
Men and women	Gallbladder
Navajo	
Children	Retinoblastoma
Men and women	Melanoma, gallbladder
Men	Lung
Pueblos	
Men and women	Mesothelioma
Other Tribes	
Chippewa	Gallbladder
Sioux	
Arapaho	
Shoshone	
Pima	
Apache	
Chinese	Nasopharyngeal, liver, esophageal, lung, stomach
Japanese	Stomach, esophageal, liver, gallbladder
Korean	Liver, biliary, lymphoma, thyroid
Philippino	Liver, biliary, lymphoma, thyroid

Source: Reprinted with permission from Frank-Stromberg M, Olsen S: *Cancer Prevention in Minority Populations: Cultural Implications for Health Care Professionals.* St. Louis: Mosby Year-Book, 1993.

Socioeconomic/Educational Factors

Studies have been done that consider income and education in relation to the incidence of cancer. For example, Devesa and Diamond[23] found a significant inverse trend between lung cancer incidence and both income and education among white and black males, and the effect of income exceeded that of education. Poor Americans, regardless of race, are at a disproportionate risk of dying of cancer. Americans living below the poverty level have a 5-year cancer survival rate that is 10%–15% lower than that for other Americans.[24,25] In addition, by the time a diagnosis is made among poor people, the disease is usually terminal.[25] Four critical issues involving cancer and the poor are[25]:

1. The poor face substantial obstacles in obtaining and using health insurance and often do not seek needed care if they cannot pay for it.
2. Poor people and their families must make personal sacrifices to obtain and pay for health care, and often have to choose between food or shelter and paying for care.
3. Cancer education and outreach efforts are insensitive and irrelevant to many poor people, whose primary concern is survival.
4. The poor often have a fatalistic attitude about cancer, despite advances in both diagnosis and treatment.

Racial Factors

Racial differences in cancer incidence rates have also been demonstrated in both men and women when cancer is diagnosed at ages 20–44 and 45–54. In contrast, little racial difference is seen when cancer is diagnosed among people over 65 years of age.[26]

According to Freeman,[24] a basic profile of the nation's poor has emerged, based on Bureau of Census findings. The aspects of poverty that affect the problems of early detection, treatment, and survival of cancer include:

- unemployment
- inadequate education
- substandard housing
- chronic malnutrition
- diminished access to medical care

As a result of these findings, the American Cancer Society Special Report made several recommendations to reduce the disproportionate effect of cancer in the socioeconomically disadvantaged. Some examples of those recommendations related to cancer risk assessment are[24,pp.22–23]:

1. Efforts should be made to improve the cost-effectiveness of cancer screening, with the ultimate goal of providing all Americans at risk with this preventive measure, through advocacy and/or direct involvement.

2. Funding mechanisms, both direct and indirect, should be developed to screen indigent populations at high risk for specific cancer sites.

3. Emergency rooms and clinics should have outreach programs, including mobile vans, for screening persons in high-risk categories presenting themselves for treatment of other illnesses at primary care clinics, and emergency rooms should be encouraged to avail themselves of cancer screening.

4. Studies should be performed to evaluate factors that affect prognosis and survival for the socioeconomically disadvantaged, such as compliance, nutrition, and home environment.

5. Studies should be performed to determine the most effective strategies for smoking cessation among the socioeconomically disadvantaged.

6. Profiles of each community to be served should be developed, with the principles based on encouraging people to modify their behavior to help reduce the risk of cancer.

7. Emphasis should be placed on encouraging lifestyle and behavior changes that might help reduce the risk of developing cancer.

8. A major effort should be made to educate health professionals about the important role of socioeconomic factors in the incidence and mortality of cancer, particularly cervical, prostate, lung, esophageal, laryngeal, and oral cancers, since many of these sites lend themselves to risk reduction through altering lifestyle factors such as smoking and drinking.

9. Strategies should be developed to enlist and train the socioeconomically disadvantaged to serve as volunteers in their own communities.

10. Innovative communication strategies should be devised to reach the socioeconomically disadvantaged with specific messages about cancer control.

11. Additional research is needed on the factors affecting the cancer incidence and survival of Hispanic, Asian, and other populations.

Cardwell and Collier[27] believe it is vital that the cancer prevention needs of the black community in particular be considered, because black Americans are slightly more likely than white Americans to get cancer and much more likely to die from it. In 1985 it was estimated that 6.6 million of America's 26.5 million black people would develop cancer at some time during their lives. Thirty percent of these individuals would survive the disease compared to a 41% survival rate among whites. Cardwell and Collier[27] have offered suggestions for educating blacks about cancer but caution that specific information and how best to communicate it to a given locality will depend on local needs and resources.

RISK FACTORS FOR SPECIFIC CANCERS

When assessing risk factors for specific cancers, it is important to recognize that risk factors can replace each other. A very high blood pressure and normal serum cholesterol may have the same effect as a moderate blood pressure and hypercholesteremia. It appears that the actual risk from a single factor depends on: (1) the number and intensity of other coexisting factors in a given individual, and (2) the intensity of the factor itself. It is possible for a client with only one risk factor to be placed in a "high-risk" level because of the potency of that factor. Also, as age advances, more factors accumulate and come into play, thus potentiating each other. This makes risk appraisal of the elderly an important nursing concern. Risk factors for specific cancers are summarized in Table 7-2. The risk factors presented are those for which there is strong evidence from laboratory, epidemiological, or clinical research of being linked to the development of cancer.[28,29]

Bladder Cancer

The strongest risk factors for bladder cancer involve occupational exposures and lifestyle practices. In developing countries, bladder infection with the parasite

TABLE 7-2 Risk Factors for Selected Cancers

BLADDER CANCER	
Personal risk factors	Male White Infection with schistosomiasis
Lifestyle	Cigarette smoking Coffee drinking? Drinking liquids with artificial sweeteners?
Occupation	Occupations working with benzidine, aniline dye, and 2-naphthylamine—apparel, textile, and leather workers, workers in dye industry, rubber workers, metal workers, painters
Drugs	Cyclophosphamide (alkylating drug)
BREAST CANCER	
Personal risk factor	History of benign breast disease Being Jewish Being single Some researchers believe that all women should be treated as being at risk
Lifestyle	Alcohol consumption Higher socioeconomic status Diet high in fat
Reproductive history	Early menarche Nulliparity Late menopause Late age at birth of first child
Family history	Family history of breast cancer
CERVICAL CANCER	
Personal risk factors	Black women Dysplasia Infection with herpes genitalis and condyloma accuminatum
Reproductive history	Early age at first marriage or coitus Multiple marriages or sexual partners Use of nonbarrier contraceptives

TABLE 7-2 Risk Factors for Selected Cancers (continued)

COLORECTAL CANCER	
Personal risk factors	Increasing age Family history of colon cancer Disease with hereditary predisposition—Gardner's syndrome, Turcot syndrome, Peutz-Jeghers syndrome, familial polyposis of colon Ulcerative colitis Crohn's disease History of colon cancer, female genital cancer, bladder cancer, breast cancer Sporadic colorectal adenomas
Lifestyle	A diet high in fat, low in fiber, and low in fruits and vegetables containing vitamins A and C Obesity Sedentary lifestyle
Geographic location	Living in highly developed countries
LIVER CANCER	
Personal risk factors	Men between the third and fifth decades of life Cirrhosis Infection with hepatitis B virus Infection with hepatitis C virus
Lifestyle	Living in non-Western countries, eg, China, Asia, Africa Homosexual and bisexual men, who are at increased risk for hepatitis B virus
Medical treatments	Hemodialysis patients, who are at increased risk for hepatitis B virus
Chemicals	Vinyl chloride
LUNG CANCER	
Personal risk factors	Cigarette smoking Family history of lung cancer
Lifestyle	Exposure to smokers over a period of time Exposure to high levels of indoor radon
Occupation	Working with iron oxide, nickel, arsenic, chromium, asbestos, petroleum-related products, mustard gas, chloromethyl ether; occupations involved: iron ore miners, nickel smelters, miners, chromium producers, millers, textile workers, insulation workers, shipyard workers, mustard gas workers, chemical workers, diesel jet testers, iron foundry workers, oil refiners, vintners
Geographic location	Living in an urban area or coastal community

TABLE 7-2 Risk Factors for Selected Cancers (continued)

ORAL CANCER	
Personal risk factors	Tobacco use Heavy alcohol use Nutritional deficiencies Poor dentition and oral hygiene Plummer-Vinson syndrome
Occupation	Long-term exposure to the sun (lip cancer)
OVARIAN CANCER	
Personal risk factors	White upper-income groups in the Western hemisphere Cancer of the breast Family history of ovarian cancer
Reproductive history	Delayed age at first pregnancy Nulliparity
Medical treatments	Radiation to the pelvic area
Occupations	Occupations involving asbestos
PROSTATE CANCER	
Personal risk factors	Increasing age Black males—highest incidence in the world
Lifestyle	Diet high in fats, oils, sugar, eggs, milk, animal protein (under investigation) Sexual activity? History of venereal disease?
Occupation	Occupations related to use of cadmium
SKIN CANCER	
Personal risk factors	Light-skinned, fair-haired, freckles, burns easily History of severe sunburn under the age of 20 Increasing age Presence of congenital moles Personal history of dysplastic nevi, cutaneous melanoma History of excessive sunbathing Xeroderma pigmentosum (a progressive sun-sensitive disease that develops in early childhood) Albinism Epidermodysplasia verruciformis (multiple virus-induced warty lesions that develop in early childhood) History of tropical ulcers, burns, and scars related to squamous cell carcinoma and increased incidence
Family history	History of melanoma in children, siblings, and parents
Occupation	Outdoor work—farming, ranching Uranium miners, radiologists

(continued)

TABLE 7-2 Risk Factors for Selected Cancers (continued)

SKIN CANCER	
Drugs	Treatment for psoriasis known as PUVA
Precursor lesions	Solar (actinic) keratosis Bowen's disease
Chemicals	Polycyclic aromatic hydrocarbons
Immunologic factors	Organ transplant recipients
TESTICULAR CANCER	
Personal risk factors	White males Family history Younger men (ages 20–40) Cryptorchidism Higher socioeconomic status
ENDOMETRIAL (UTERINE CORPUS) CANCER	
Personal risk factors	Obesity Hypertension Diabetes mellitus
Lifestyle	Higher socioeconomic class
Reproductive history	History of menstrual irregularities Nulliparity Infertility through anovulation
Drugs	Long-term use of conjugated estrogens
VAGINAL CANCER	
Personal risk factors	Mother's use of DES during pregnancy Radiation of cervix for cancer Elderly

Schistisoma haematobium has been linked to the development of bladder cancer.[30] In the United States, however, risk factors for bladder cancer involve primarily occupational exposures and tobacco use. Workers exposed to aromatic amines (2-naphthylamine, benzidine) have a fourfold greater risk of bladder cancer.[31,32] Persons in high-risk occupations include apparel, textile, and leather workers, workers in the dye industry, rubber workers, metal workers, and painters.

Cigarette smoking is the most important known risk factor for bladder cancer. Smokers develop bladder cancer two to three times more often than nonsmokers.[33] Drug use has also been found to increase the risk of bladder cancer. Cyclophosphamide can cause bladder cancer.[34] In addition, long-term use of analgesics containing phenacetin may contribute to the development of transitional cell carcinoma of the renal pelvis, urethra, or bladder.[33] It has been reported that there is a latency period of as much as 18 years before bladder tumors develop after exposure to carcinogens.[35]

There is conflicting information concerning the role of coffee drinking and the use of artificial sweeteners and the risk of bladder cancer. Further research is needed to determine the association between these two substances and the incidence of bladder cancer.[33,36]

Breast Cancer

The primary risk factors for breast cancer are a family history of breast cancer, history of benign breast disease, late age at first live birth, nulliparity, early age at menarche, late age at menopause, higher socioeconomic status, being Jewish, estrogen-replacement therapy, exposure of the female breast to ionizing radiation in infancy, mammographic parenchymal patterns that are dense (P2 and DY), and being single.[37–40] However, several authors stress that all women 35 or older should be treated as being at risk for breast cancer.[41,42]

There are conflicting data on the relationship between consumption of alcohol and risk of breast cancer. One study reported that moderate alcohol consumption is associated with an elevation in the risk of breast cancer of 50%–100%. Several other reports found no association between alcohol and breast cancer.[43–45] The same type of debate has revolved around the use of birth control pills and increased risk of breast cancer.[46] A study by the Centers for Disease Control and the National Institute of Child Health and Human Development found that use of birth control pills did not increase the risk of breast cancer in women. However, use of oral contraceptives around menopause and onset of puberty may increase the risk of breast cancer.[47]

There is considerable debate about the influence of diet on the development of breast cancer. Since the worldwide distribution of breast cancer is very similar to that of colorectal cancer, it is believed by many researchers that a high fat intake is a causative factor in breast cancer, especially in older women.[48] Additional evidence of this association comes from clinical and laboratory animal studies.[49] How much reduction in fat intake is necessary to lower the risk of cancer is also unknown at this time. Willett et al.[50] reported from their study of 85,538 U.S. nurses that a moderate reduction in fat intake by women is unlikely to result in a substantial reduction in the incidence of breast cancer.

Table 7-3 shows the various known risk factors for breast cancer and the approximate degree of increased risk. This table compares the increased-risk group (e.g., women in North America) with a comparison group known to be at low risk for breast cancer (e.g., women in Asia) and gives the approximate degree of increased risk.[51]

Cervical Cancer

Race, personal factors, and venereal disease are the major risk factors associated with cervical cancer. Personal risk factors include early age at first coitus, multiple marriages or sexual partners, and use of nonbarrier contraceptives.[52,53] Venereal infections associated with

TABLE 7-3 Risk Factors in Human Breast Cancer

	Risk Group		
Factors*	**Increased-Risk Group**	**Comparison Group**	**Approximate Degree of Increased Risk**
Sex	Female	Male	High
Geography	North America	Asia	High
Age (years)	>50	<35	High
Personal history of cancer	Breast Endometrium, ovary	Negative Negative	High Moderate
Personal history of:			
Atypical hyperplasia (ductal, lobular)	Positive	Negative	Moderate
Carcinoma in situ	Positive	Negative	High
Mammographic parenchymal pattern	Extremely dense, dysplastic (Dy)	Negative	Moderate-high
Family history of breast cancer	Any first-degree relative Premenopausal bilateral breast cancer in first-degree relative	Negative Negative	Mild-high Moderate-high
Reproductive status:			
First full-term pregnancy at age (years)	>30	<20	Moderate
Parity	Nulliparous	Multiparous	Moderate
Menopause	Late	Early	Moderate
Menarche	Early	Late	Moderate
Alcohol	Consumers of >3 drinks/week	Abstainers	Mild–moderate
Radiation	Heavily exposed	None	Mild–moderate

*Additional factors with risk ≤2 or not presently conclusively quantified include (high-risk group first): Jewish vs. gentile; high vs. low socioeconomic status; obesity vs. leanness (postmenopausal); high vs. low fat consumption; use of birth control pills or menopausal hormone vs. no use.

Source: Reprinted with permission from Stefanek ME: Counseling women at high risk for breast cancer. *Oncology* 4:27–38, 1990, Table 1.

increased risk are herpes genitalis and condyloma acuminatum caused by human papillomaviruses (HPV).[54] With the existence of major new sexually transmitted infectious diseases (i.e., HIV infection, Chlamydia trachomatis, genital herpesvirus), health professionals anticipated that sexual practices would markedly change to reflect a desire on the part of women to avoid infection. A study of women who consulted gynecologists at a university student health service in 1975, 1986, and 1989 found that sexual practices among college women did not change markedly in 14 years.[55] Although the use of condoms increased, the majority of sexually active women did not report their regular use.

Incidence rates for cervical cancer are approximately two times higher for blacks, Hispanics, and Native Americans than for whites. The rates for orientals and whites are similar.[56] Certain religious groups in the United States have been noted to have low incidence rates of cervical cancer: Jews, Mormons, and Seventh-Day Adventists.[57]

Recent information supports an association between smoking and the incidence of cervical cancer. It has been reported that smokers have about a 50% higher risk than nonsmokers for developing squamous cell cancer of the cervix.[58]

Colorectal Cancer

High rates of colorectal cancer are found in highly developed countries (e.g., North America, northern and western Europe, New Zealand), and low rates are found in Asia, Africa, and most countries of Latin America. There is substantial evidence that differences between nations in the incidence of colorectal cancer are due at least in part to environmental factors, such as diet.[59] Obesity, high fat intake, low fiber content, and a dearth of fruits and vegetables containing vitamins A and C have been identified as risk factors.[60–63] A sedentary lifestyle has also been implicated as a risk factor for colorectal cancer.

Age is considered a significant risk factor for colorectal cancer. Risk begins to increase at age 40, increases rapidly above age 55, and roughly doubles with each successive decade, reaching a peak at age 75.

Familial and hereditary factors are another significant risk, believed to account for at least 20% of colorectal cancers.[64,65] The specific diseases with a hereditary predisposition are Gardner's syndrome, Turcot syndrome, Peutz-Jeghers syndrome, and familial polyposis of the colon.[66]

Having ulcerative colitis is another significant risk factor for colorectal cancer. The risk of carcinoma of the large intestine is 20 times greater than in the general population among individuals with extensive ulcerative colitis for 10 years or more. Because of the strong association of ulcerative colitis and colorectal cancer, it has been recommended that in "patients with ulcerative colitis that is diagnosed before the age of 15 prophylactic proctocolectomy might be an alternative to close surveillance in reducing mortality from colorectal cancer."[67,p.1233] Crohn's disease also places individuals at higher risk of colorectal cancer. Persons with a past history of colon cancer and adenomatous intestinal polyps are also at increased risk.

Liver Cancer

The incidence of hepatocellular carcinoma (HCC) increases with age, predominantly affects men, and occurs most often between the third and fifth decades of life.[68,69] There is a pronounced geographic variation in its incidence throughout the world. In the United States and Western countries, HCC is rare, ranking twenty-fifth among cancers in the United States and occurring at a rate of four to five per 100,000 population in North America, the United Kingdom, and Australia. In contrast, HCC is probably the most common cancer in the world among men. The risk factors for HCC include: hepatitis B virus, cirrhosis, hepatitis C virus, and the chemical vinyl chloride.[70–74]

Groups at high risk for hepatitis B infection in the United States include institutionally developmentally disabled, intravenous drug users, homosexual and bisexual men, and hemodialysis patients.[75,76] It is generally believed that "chronic hepatitis B virus infection is probably the leading cause of HCC throughout the world, accounting for 75%–90% of the world's cases."[77,p.1956] Epidemiological evidence has shown that at least in some high-risk populations the chance of developing HCC is more than 160 times greater in hepatitis B virus carriers than in HBV-free individuals.[77,78]

Although rare, oral contraceptives taken for more than 8–9 years have been associated with HCC.[79] The etiologic relationship between liver disease and subsequent HCC has long been debated and remains controversial.[79]

Lung Cancer

The major risk factors for lung cancer are geographic location, social class, occupation, and tobacco use. Cigarette smoking increases the risk of lung cancer to a greater degree than any other risk factor. It is estimated that in the United States cigarette smoking may contribute to at least 80% of all lung cancer in males and 40% in females.[80,81] In 1990, an estimated 89.9 million (50.1%) U.S. adults had smoked at least 100 cigarettes in their life, and 45.8 million (25.5%) were current smokers. Approximately 44.1 million (49.1% of all ever-smokers) were former smokers in 1990.[82] Studies have also found an elevated risk of lung cancer as well as heart disease among individuals who have never smoked but are living with a spouse who smokes cigarettes.[83] There is a wide body of evidence that points to the likelihood that the involuntary inhalation of tobacco smoke has a causal effect on the risk of lung cancer in nonsmokers. It is estimated that approximately 17% of lung cancers among nonsmokers can be attributed to high levels of exposure to cigarette smoke during childhood and adolescence.[84]

Another environmental risk factor for lung cancer is indoor radon exposure. "Radon exposure may be the most significant risk factor for the nonsmoker that can be readily reduced."[85,p.274] Radon exposure may be responsible for about 10,000 lung cancer deaths per year, while smoking accounts for 85% of the lung cancer deaths annually. Much of the increased risk seems to occur in smokers. There has been some suggestion that radon acts synergistically with cigarette smoking to enhance the risk of lung cancer.

High-risk occupations are those in which persons work with asbestos, polycyclic hydrocarbons, chromium, mustard gas, chloromethyl ethers, radon, nickel, and inorganic arsenic. Included in this group are welders, gas workers, roofers, uranium miners, workers in the chrome pigment industry, nickel refinery workers, copper smelter workers, vineyard workers, and insulation workers.

International studies of geographic variation have shown that lung cancer is most common in urban and coastal communities.

Oral Cancer

Tobacco is a major risk factor for oral cancer. The habitual smoking of cigarettes, cigars, and pipes and the use of chewing tobacco or snuff has long been associated with oral cancer.[86,87] In other countries, different tobacco-chewing habits place users at increased risk of oral cancer. In India, betel nut, or "pan," is chewed; in Bombay, "bidi" is chewed; "keeyo" is chewed in Thailand; and "nass" is chewed in central Asia. Mixing tobacco with these other products increases the risk of oral cancer.[88] Another significant risk factor for oral cancer is excessive alcohol intake. The risk of oral cancer among heavy drinkers and smokers is approximately six to fifteen times greater than among nonsmokers and nondrinkers.[86,89] Alcohol appears to act chiefly by augmenting the effects of tobacco.

Other risk factors are nutritional deficiencies and poor dentition. Plummer-Vinson syndrome has a positive association with oral cancer. However, other nutritional deficiencies linked with an increased risk of oral cancer may be related to heavy use of alcohol, which influences dietary intake.[90] A relationship between infrequent vegetable intake and ingestion of hot infusions (maté) has been linked to cancer of the tongue in men in Uruguay.[91]

Evidence indicates that physical irritation (e.g., from dentures, irregular or sharp teeth, hot or spicy foods) plays little or no part in the natural history of oral carcinoma.[89] Occupations related to long-term exposure to the sun have been associated with cancer of the lip.

Ovarian Cancer

The risk factors for ovarian cancer are less well known than those of the other major gynecologic cancers.[92] Women who have two or more first-degree relatives with a history of ovarian cancer have a significantly increased risk for this cancer.[93] Ovarian cancer tends to be more common among white upper-income groups in highly industrialized countries.[94] The risk of ovarian cancer is associated with delayed age at first pregnancy and with a smaller number of pregnancies. These risk factors suggest an abnormality of endocrine secretion as an important component of ovarian carcinogenesis.[95] Present information suggests that oral contraceptive use might protect against ovarian cancer.[96] Other risk factors are radiation to the pelvic area, cancer of the breast, and occupations involving asbestos.

Endometrial (Uterine Corpus) Cancer

The risk factors for cancer of the uterus are well known. Obesity, hypertension, and diabetes mellitus have been correlated with the development of endometrial cancer.[97] Women who have a history of menstrual irregularities and infertility through anovulation are also at increased risk. Long-term use of conjugated estrogens is an iatrogenic risk factor for this cancer.[98] On the other hand, the use of oral contraceptives (containing both estrogen and progesterone in each pill) for at least 1 year has a protective effect against endometrial cancer.[99,100] In addition, women of high socioeconomic status are at increased risk.

Prostate Cancer

Age and race are significant risk factors for prostate cancer. Black Americans have the highest prostate cancer incidence rate in the United States, and Japanese American men have the lowest incidence rate.[101,102] Prostate cancer affects the elderly more than the young to a greater extent than any other cancer.[103] Average age at diagnosis of prostate cancer is 70, and 80% of cases are found in men over 65.[104]

Other risk factors for prostate cancer are tentative at this time and require more research. A positive relationship has been found between the consumption of fats, oils, sugar, animal protein, eggs, and milk ("over nutrition") and mortality rates among men with prostate cancers.[105,106] There may be a familial tendency toward the development of prostate cancer. If a man has a first-degree relative (i.e., father or brother) with prostate cancer, he has a 2.5 relative risk for developing prostate cancer.[107] However, whether it is due to environmental or genetic factors has not been determined. An increased risk of prostate cancer in association with an increasing number of sexual partners, prior history of venereal disease, frequency of sexual intercourse, and an early onset of sexual activity has been suggested.[103] Occupations that have been linked to increased risk of prostate cancer are those in which workers are exposed to cadmium (e.g., welding, electroplating, alkaline battery production). However, other studies have linked the development of prostate cancer with a multitude of other occupations that have no common carcinogenic exposure. At this time the evidence relating occupation and increased risk of prostate cancer is weak and needs further study.

Skin Cancer

The chief risk factor for the development of basal cell and squamous cell carcinomas of the skin is exposure to ultraviolet radiation (UVR). Exposure to UVR in a tanning booth may also increase the risk of skin cancer.[108,109] Melanoma is also related to ultraviolet radiation, but there are several other influential risk factors: familial predisposition, hormonal factors, dysplastic nevus syndrome, and nearness to the equator.[110] The risk in the general population for developing malignant melanoma is approximately 0.53%, while the risk in a dysplastic nevus syndrome patient population is 10% (20 times greater), and even greater is the risk for a dysplastic nevus family member who has already developed malignant melanoma.[111]

Overall, those at greatest risk of skin cancer are fair-skinned white persons, particularly those with reddish or blond hair, blue or light eyes, those with a tendency to freckle or burn easily, and individuals who have spent considerable time in the sun.[112] Non-Europeans with various skin pigmentations have a substantial incidence of melanomas of the volar surface of the feet, but Africans seem to be notably less pigmented in that area and certainly have, for the same area of skin, particularly increased rates of occurrence of melanoma.[113] Other risk factors for skin cancer are occupation, personal risk factors, family history, drugs, precursor lesions, chemicals, and immunologic factors.[114]

Testicular Cancer

A significant risk factor for testicular cancer involves race and age. This cancer occurs about 4.5 times more frequently in whites than in blacks and in men between the ages of 20 and 40 years. Another significant risk factor is undescended testicles, especially in men who have a testicle that descended after the age of 6 or a testicle that never descended (cryptorchidism).[115] During the past few decades, several case reports and series of familial testicular cancers have been described in the literature supporting the possibility of familial testicular cancer.[116] Other possible risk factors are trauma, hormonal drugs, and socioeconomic status.

The possibility that intrascrotal temperature is involved in the etiology of testicular cancer was investigated by Karagas et al.[117] They interviewed 323 men with germ cell tumors of the testis diagnosed between 1977 and 1984, and 658 randomly selected controls were interviewed with regard to type of shorts worn, use of long underwear, heat-resistant clothing, and hot tubs or saunas, and a history of varicocele. Their results provided little or no support for the hypothesis that intermittent intrascrotal temperature elevation plays a role in the etiology of germ cell testicular cancer.

Vaginal Cancer

A risk factor for vaginal cancer that has received much attention is diethylstilbestrol (DES). Adenosis of the vagina has been identified in the offspring of women who received DES during pregnancy. This agent is no longer given to women to prevent threatened miscarriages. Another risk factor is radiation of the cervix for cancer of this organ. Postradiation carcinoma in situ of the vagina is of the epidermoid type and may occur one or more years after apparently successful treatment of cancer of the cervix.[118] Brinton et al.[119] conducted a study of 41 patients with carcinoma in situ or invasive cancer of the vagina and compared them to 97 community controls in an effort to identify potential risk factors for vaginal cancer. They report that some risk factors for vaginal cancer are similar to those for cervical cancer and include: low education and family income, history of genital warts, history of previous abnormal Pap smear, and vaginal discharge or irritation.

CANCER RISK ASSESSMENT

The purposes of a cancer risk assessment include:

1. providing an individual with information about his or her health-related behavior that may increase cancer risk
2. serving as an effective aid for educating patients about the relationship between risk factors and the likelihood of cancer
3. stimulating a person to participate in activities aimed at changing lifestyle and improving health.[9,120]

In addition, analysis of cancer risk may help patients identify their options so that they can make realistic decisions about their health care. Physicians have also found that risk analyses help in the development of health regimens that are tailored to each individual's risk and tolerance for living with that risk.[119]

Before information is provided about an individual's specific risks, however, it is important that there be an understanding of the risk to an average person in the population.[119] This average risk serves as a baseline against which individuals can measure the magnitude of their increased risk, if any. Also, tables that show risks to various ages are useful because they indicate that cancer risk in the general population usually increases with certain activities (i.e., smoking) and with age.

One of the problems that exists in assessment of cancer risks is that some persons are unwilling to seriously consider what their risks might be. If a relative has had cancer, they may assume that their risk is "high" but fear that an examination of this assumption might in some way further increase their risk. They may also be dealing with various emotions, such as low self-esteem, denial, fear, anger, guilt, embarrassment, and insecurity, which are often seen in persons who come from families with a history of cancer. These emotions act as barriers to effective communication and can result in an inability to face a risk analysis. Other individuals may believe that as long as they suffer by worrying about their high risk, their worry will act as a shield, and they will be spared the suffering of cancer itself. Finally, there often is the belief that if one worries about risks, one is engaging in "negative thinking that can cause cancer." Through the process of learning to understand one's fears, learning that such ideas are perfectly normal, and taking positive action to reduce the risks, an individual can be helped to understand the importance of risk assessment. Those who have received information about risk are more likely to schedule regular checkups and undergo necessary diagnostic procedures than are those who hold unrealistic health beliefs.[121]

It is also extremely important that a clear definition of the meaning of risk be provided when a health risk analysis is conducted. Many believe that when one's cancer risk is considered to be "high," it means that their risk of dying is high. This, of course, is inaccurate because risk implies occurrence of disease and complications, not just mortality rate. Therefore, health professionals need to make sure the health care consumer understands such concepts as "carcinogen," "risk," "cancer risk," "carcinogenic risk factors," and "cancer risk assessment" so that they will know exactly what the assessment can and cannot do for them and how to use the data obtained.

When a cancer risk assessment is done, the carcinogenic risk of exposure of individuals or populations to a particular risk factor is quantified.[122] However, assessment is only one aspect of a complete risk analysis. A comprehensive risk analysis should include: (a) the identification of risks and the estimation of the likelihood and magnitude of risk occurring, and (b) an evaluation that measures risk acceptance (the acceptable levels of societal risk) and risk management (the control of risks, including methods of reducing and avoiding risk).[5]

Constanza et al.[123] point out that risk assessment is not only a part of cancer prevention but must also be included in detection procedures to maximize the chance that one can discover cancer at its smallest or earliest possible stage.

Evaluation

The assessment of every patient should start with the history. The history format should include information on the following factors[4]:

- demographic data
- current past medical problems
- family medical history
- surgical and (if appropriate) obstetric history
- childhood illnesses
- allergies
- current medications
- psychologic status
- social history
- environmental background
- review of systems

In most cases this information, excluding the review of systems, can be supplied by the patient on one of the many questionnaire forms available (see Table 7-4). It is important to remember that there is an element of fear of the diagnostic implications of admitting

TABLE 7-4 Health Risk Assessment Instruments

Instrument	Description	Source
	COMPUTER-SCORED HRAs	
COSTPREDICT AND HEALTHPREDICT	It calculates costs and savings related to 51 health-related conditions and 44 risk factors. Reports give predicted costs and savings related to risks, absenteeism, and hospitalization. (200-item questionnaire re: habits, stress, medical history, and women's health)	CompuHealth Associates (also available for IBM-PC)
HEALTH AND LIFESTYLE QUESTIONNAIRE	It emphasizes current quality of life over long-term risks. Report assigns scores ranging from "excellent" to "immediate attention" and discusses the individual's risks. (54-item questionnaire re: health habits, psychological and job attitudes, and social relationships)	Health Enhancement Systems
HEALTH HAZARD APPRAISAL	Computer analysis provides a 4- to 5-page report that is a combination of bar graph, narrative, and tabulated data, including summaries of health age, projected health cost, and stress. (80-item questionnaire re: medical history, family history, lifestyle, stress, and women's health)	Prospective Medicine Center
HEALTHLINE	A 4-page report discusses leading probable causes of death and alterable risk factors. A 15-page report shows specific risks such as frustrations, satisfactions, and stresses. (44-item questionnaire re: medical history, lifestyle, women's health, stress, social and psychological factors, exercise, and nutrition)	Health Logics
HEALTHLOGIC	20-page report focuses on impact of lifestyle changes on health, fitness, and risk of chronic disease. (17-page booklet with questions on health history, men's and women's health, stress, and motor vehicle safety)	HMC Software Inc.

(continued)

TABLE 7-4 Health Risk Assessment Instruments (continued)

Instrument	Description	Source
	COMPUTER-SCORED HRAs	
HEALTHPATH	14-page report scores participants in 11 health habit areas. (72-item questionnaire covers 13 risk/lifestyle areas. Physical measurements and laboratory data are optional.) Helps to serve cost-containment objectives of a corporation.	Control Data Corp.
HEALTH WRAP	Both a standard risk profile and a "wellness index" are provided. (93-item questionnaire)	Lifestyle and Health Promotion
LIFE	Report lists 20 major risk indicators (mostly physical measurements), patient's values for these, and recommended values. Also lists 20 leading causes of death for patient's age and sex, making recommendations to reduce risks where appropriate. A nutrition profile, stress profile and appraisal, and achievable ages are included. (16-page questionnaire re: personal and family medical histories, habits, and lifestyle, attitudes about health, physical measurements, diet, exercise, and other health habits)	Wellsource
LIFESCORE PLUS	Report projects lifespan and identifies risks. (62-item questionnaire: biomedical measurements, lifestyle habits, health history) Booklet suggests guidelines to reduce or eliminate health risks.	Center for Corporate Health Promotion
LIFESTYLE ASSESSMENT QUESTIONNAIRE (LAQ)	Printout suggests specific resources on topics selected and compares level of wellness with average of others who have taken the LAQ. The top 10 risk factors are listed, as well as ways to reduce them. (270-item questionnaire re: "Wellness inventory" section with six dimensions of wellness and "Personal Growth" section to identify preferred topics for further information)	National Wellness Institute
LIFESTYLE DIRECTIONS	Short, 30-question instrument, which covers diet, exercise, and health. Report presents graphic information on risks for five major diseases.	Lifestyle Directions, Inc.
PERSONAL STRESS PROFILE	12-page booklet aimed at employees in a workplace environment contains explanations on stress and specific recommendations for behavior change. (167-item questionnaire re: personal and family medical history, lifestyle behaviors, socioeconomic status, and stress)	General Health, Inc.
HEALTHPLAN AND HEALTHPLAN PLUS	12-page booklet provides narrative and graphic information on 8 health areas, current risk as compared to average and achievable risk, and specific recommendations for behavior change. Individual's 5 leading health problems in order of importance are included. HealthPlan Plus has a longer and more detailed pro-	General Health, Inc.

(continued)

TABLE 7-4 Health Risk Assessment Instruments (continued)

Instrument	Description	Source
	COMPUTER-SCORED HRAs	
	file. (111-item questionnaire re: personal and family medical history, behavior habits, socioeconomic status, and women's health)	
HEALTH RISK APPRAISAL	4-page report tabulates risks for 5 leading causes of death, recommends ways to reduce risks, and gives a 20-year future projection. (50-item questionnaire re: health habits and medical status) A wider-ranging Lifestyle Development Questionnaire is available.	University of Michigan (also available for IBM-PC)
HEALTH RISK APPRAISAL QUESTIONNAIRE	2-page report explains patient's risk factors for the 12 leading causes of death as percentages by which he or she deviates from the average; appraisal and achievable ages are given as behavioral changes that could reduce risks. (39-item questionnaire re: personal and family medical history, health habits, and women's health)	St. Louis County Health Dept.
HEALTH RISK ASSESSMENT	Report recommends ways to reduce risks and compares the client's risk factors with those of others of the same age, sex, and race. (85-item questionnaire re: personal and family medical history, alcohol, smoking, and driving habits, and women's health)	University of California
HEALTH RISK ASSESSMENT QUESTIONNAIRE	3-page report describes risks and gives information on health age, achievable age, and top 10 mortality causes and risk factors sorted into 4 categories: ideal, average, risky, and nonmodifiable. (96-item questionnaire re: medical history, physical examination, family history, women's health, and personal health habits)	Wisconsin Center for Health Risk Research
HEALTH RISK QUESTIONNAIRE	Report discusses risk factors for 15 major diseases with an emphasis on cancer.* (39-item questionnaire re: lifestyle, medical history, and physical and laboratory measurements)	Health Enhancement Systems (also available for IBM-PC)
RHRC HEALTH RISK APPRAISAL	In addition to assessing individual risks, this instrument estimates the impact of workplace wellness programs. 5-page report includes 10-year mortality estimates for the 12 leading causes of death, estimated annual hospital days, and advice on reducing risks. A group profile includes the estimated reduction in work force mortality and hospitalization achievable through specific wellness programs. (39-item questionnaire re: lifestyle, medical history, frequency of medical screening, optional laboratory data, and women's health. An additional "General Well-Being Questionnaire" measures stress)	Regional Health Resource Center (also available for IBM-PC)

(continued)

TABLE 7-4 Health Risk Assessment Instruments (continued)

Instrument	Description	Source
	COMPUTER-SCORED HRAs	
WELL AWARE HEALTH RISK APPRAISAL	Emphasis is on quality of life and current risks. 16-page report includes mortality predictions and stresses practical measures to improve health. (Questionnaire includes health habits, lifestyle, health knowledge, stress, women's health, diet, motor vehicle safety, alcohol use, sociability, and physical and laboratory data)	Well Aware About Health
	MICROCOMPUTER-BASED HRAs	
AVIVA	Provides an overall risk score adjusted for age and sex, the contribution of each risk factor to the score, and suggestions for modifying risks. This instrument assesses hospitalization risks, but concerns only those risks that an individual can modify. (5- to 10-minute or 15- to 20-minute versions available. Screens users to ensure that the interview is appropriate; questions cover alcohol use, driving habits, weight, blood pressure, cholesterol levels, depression, and smoking. User can ask why certain information is requested and receive explanations.)	Center for Research in Medical Education and Health Care, Jefferson Medical College
HEALTH AWARENESS GAMES	This is a set of 5 microcomputer programs that draw on statistics about lifestyle and health as they relate to life expectancy. Appropriate for junior high school through college and is suitable for home use. (5 programs include Coronary Risk, Why Do You Smoke? Exercise and Weight, Life Expectancy, and Life-Style.)	Queue Inc.
HEALTH RISK APPRAISAL	Profile displays the user's risks for 10 leading causes of death and provides a 1-page summary printout. (40-item questionnaire re: lifestyle and physiologic indicators. For Apple II, II+, IIe, and IBM-PC)	University of Minnesota Media Distribution
LIFESCAN	Each individual receives a printout listing his or her top 10 risk factors and suggested methods to reduce those risks. Special feature is a listing of the individual's positive lifestyle behaviors. (40-item questionnaire re: physical activity, drug usage, driving habits, cholesterol level, medical history, and women's health issues. For IBM-PC)	National Wellness Institute
PERSONAL HEALTH APPRAISAL	There are two versions: The personal version is interactive, and the professional version can be used in either an interactive or batch-processing mode and can store and update profiles. The user's life expectancy is calculated at the end, and it includes an analysis of the user's "Cancer Early Warning Signs" and preventive health practices. (84-item questionnaire re: medical his-	MedMicro

(continued)

TABLE 7-4 Health Risk Assessment Instruments (continued)

Instrument	Description	Source
	MICROCOMPUTER-BASED HRAs	
	tory, occupational health information, lifestyle, and women's health. For IBM-PC)	
SPHERE	The 25-item questionnaire covers medical and lifestyle characteristics. Reports explain each user's risks and appraisal and achievable ages. Available in English and French. (For IBM-PC)	University of British Columbia
	SELF-SCORED QUESTIONNAIRES	
HOW DO YOU RATE AS A HEALTH RISK?	Booklet includes 40 questions on smoking, alcohol and other drugs, nutrition, weight control, exercise, stress, and safety. Provides suggestions to improve the individual's present condition.	Channing L. Bete Co., Inc.
HOPE HEALTH APPRAISAL	A complete health kit designed to help an individual manage his/her health risk and improve lifestyle.	International Health Awareness Center
HEALTHSTYLE: A SELF-TEST	2-page, 24-item questionnaire published by U.S. Public Health Service. Gives specific suggestions for reducing risks. Topics covered include nutrition, alcohol and drug use, smoking, fitness, stress, and safety.	ODPHP National Health Information Center
LIFESCORE-C	Designed for employee health programs. Results yield an individual score and can be batch-processed to yield a group profile. Questions cover lifestyle, environmental factors, family medical history, and utilization of health care. Scores are given for general health and life expectancy.	Center for Corporate Health Promotion (also available as LIFESCORE-M FOR IBM-PC)
	OTHER INSTRUMENTS	
INCREASED RISK ASSESSMENT	Check-off list related to carcinogenic exposure, genetic predisposition, personal history of cancer, and certain associated diseases. Next to each item is the associated cancer for which the person is at increased risk.	Costanza, Li, Green, and Patterson. Cancer prevention and detection: strategies for practice. In *Cancer Manual,* ed. 7. Boston: American Cancer Society, 1986.
C.A.R.E.S. (CANCER AWARENESS RISK EDUCATION SERVICE)	C.A.R.E.S. was designed to assist health educators in providing cancer risk reduction information to the general public. It is used on a Compaq 386 with 1024K of memory and an EGA board. User responds to questions about personal health history, family history, personal habits related to skin, lung, colorectal, breast, gynecologic, prostate, testicular, stomach, head and neck, and esophageal cancers. A comprehensive component on dietary habits, stress, and exercise is also included. The user receives a printed analysis of his/her personal risk for developing the cancers listed.	H. Lee Moffitt Cancer Center and Research Institute, Inc. P.O. Box 280179, Tampa, FL 33682-0179.

(continued)

TABLE 7-4 Health Risk Assessment Instruments (continued)

Instrument	Description	Source
	OTHER INSTRUMENTS	
CANCER RISK ASSESSMENT	Check-off questions for men and women related to cancer risks. Specific areas include skin, head and neck, lung, breast, colon-rectum, cervix, endometrium, vulva, vagina, prostate, testes.	White, L.N. Cancer risk assessment. *Semin Oncol Nurs* 2:184–190, 1986.
RISK APPRAISAL FORM	A Risk Appraisal Form that is practical and useful for office or clinic setting was developed. Questions are presented related to risk for cardiovascular disease, malignant diseases, auto accidents, suicide, diabetes. Scores are summarized to provide total number of risk factors for which the patient is in the highest risk level, and this is then converted to a percentage. Form indicates factors that provide low, medium, and high risk for patient.	Pender, N. Health promotion. In *Nursing Practice.* New York: Appleton-Century Crofts, 1982.

RESOURCES FOR HEALTH RISK ASSESSMENT INSTRUMENTS

Center for Corporate Health Promotion
1850 Centennial Park Dr.
Suite 520
Reston, VA 22091

Center for Research in Medical Education and Health Care
Jefferson Medical College
Philadelphia, PA 19107

Channing L. Bete Co., Inc.
200 State Rd.
South Deerfield, MA 01373

Compu Health Associates
13795 Rider Trail
Earth City, MO 63045

Control Data Corp.
StayWell/EAR Division
901 East 78th St.
Minneapolis, MN 55420

General Health, Inc.
3299 K. St., NW
Washington, DC 20007

Health Enhancement Systems
9 Mercer St.
Princeton, NJ 08540

Health Logics
111 Deerwood Pl
San Ramon, CA 94583

HMC Software Inc.
4200 North MacArthur Blvd.
Irving, TX 75038

International Health Awareness Center
157 South Kalamazoo Mall
Suite 482
Kalamazoo, MI 49007-4895

Lifestyle and Health Promotion
59 Monterrey Ave.
Kenner, LA 70065

Lifestyle Directions, Inc.
300 Ninth St.
Conway, PA 15027-1696

MedMicro
6701 Seybold Rd.
Suite 220A
Madison, WI 53719

National Wellness Institute
University of Wisconsin-Stevens Point
South Hall
Stevens Point, WI 54481

ODPHP National Health Information Center*
P.O. Box 1133
Washington, DC 20013

Prospective Medicine Center
Suite 219
3901 North Meridian
Indianapolis, IN 46208

Queue Inc.
562 Boston Ave.
Bridgeport, CT 06610

Regional Health Resource Center
Medical Information Laboratory
1408 West University Ave.
Urbana, IL 61801

St. Louis County Health Department
1001 East First St.
Duluth, MN 55805

University of British Columbia
Health Care and Epidemiology
5804 Fairview Crescent
Mather Building
Vancouver, BC V6T W5
Canada

University of California
Epidemiology and International Health
1699 HSW
San Francisco, CA 94143

University of Michigan
Fitness Research Center
401 Washtenaw Ave.
Ann Arbor, MI 48109-2214

University of Minnesota
Media Distribution
Box 734, Mayo Building
420 Delaware St., SE
Minneapolis, MN 55455

Well Aware About Health
P.O. Box 43338
Tucson, AZ 85733

Wellsource
15431 Southeast 82nd Dr.
Suite E
P.O. Box 569
Clackamas, OR 97015

Wisconsin Center for Health Risk Research
University of Wisconsin Center for Health Sciences
600 Highland Ave., Room J5/224
Madison, WI 53792

*Source for Health Risk Assessment Instruments (excluding "other instruments") and Resources: ODPHP National Health Information Center. *Healthfinder: Health Risk Appraisals.* Public Health Service, U.S. Department of Health and Human Services, Washington, DC: November, 1988. The *Healthfinder* includes other HRAs and can be ordered for $1.

to certain symptoms that can create problems in cancer prevention/detection. The history, therefore, is helpful not only in detecting early, vague symptoms but also in identifying signs and symptoms that the patient might deny if asked outright. In addition, the history helps to identify factors, such as a family history of genetic susceptibility, that may increase an individual's risk of specific cancers. In such situations, the physician may order special tests that are not included in the guidelines for the public in general.[123] A complete physical examination should follow the health history to provide objective data that can complement and verify the health history's subjective data.

For patients identified as having a high risk of cancer, advice should be given about avoiding additional exposure to carcinogens, and rigorous intervention may be indicated (e.g., excision of the colon in a patient with chronic ulcerative colitis before the appearance of cancer or removal of a dysplastic nevus to prevent progression to melanoma). In high-risk patients, screening might also be carried out more frequently and in greater detail than in low-risk patients. Women at high risk of breast cancer may need to have mammography and periodic physical examinations performed more frequently and started at an earlier age than women who are at low risk. The recommended schedule of prevention and detection procedures for the general population, as suggested by the American Cancer Society, are shown in Table 7-5.[28,29]

EDUCATION

Education of persons at high risk of cancer cannot be treated as something separate and distinct from general

TABLE 7-5 Summary of American Cancer Society Recommendations for the Early Detection of Cancer in Asymptomatic Persons at Average Risk

Examination	Sex	Age	Frequency
Sigmoidoscopy	M and F	50 and over	One exam every 3–5 years
Stool guaiac slide test	M and F	Over 50	Every year
Digital rectal examination	M and F	Over 40	Every year
Pap test and pelvic examination	F	All women who have been sexually active or have reached age 18	Every year. After 3 or more satisfactory consecutive, normal annual examinations, the Pap test may be performed less frequently, at the discretion of the physician.
Endometrial tissue sample	F	At menopause Women at high risk*	At menopause
Breast self-examination	F	20 and older	Every month
Clinical breast examination	F	20–39 40 and older	Every 3 years Every year
Mammography	F	35–39 40–49 50 and over	Baseline Every 1–2 years Every year
Health counseling†	M and F	Over 20	Every 3 years
Cancer checkup‡	M and F	Over 40	Every year

*History of infertility, obesity, failure to ovulate, abnormal uterine bleeding, or estrogen therapy.

†To include counseling about tobacco control, sun exposure, diet and nutrition, risk factors, sexual practices, and environmental and other occupational exposures.

‡To include examination for cancers of the thyroid, testicles, prostate, ovaries, lymph nodes, oral cavity, and skin.

Source: Fink[28]; Update January 1992.[29]

education of the public about cancer, although it has certain features. The aims of public education are

- to inform and educate about treatable forms of cancer and to reassure people that treatment is advantageous
- to persuade people, particularly those at special risk, to undertake preventive action, to undergo tests so that cancer can be detected at an earlier stage, or to seek medical advice quickly when recognizable signs of ill health occur.[124]

Consequently, organized cancer education attempts to maintain positive health behavior or to interrupt a behavior pattern that is linked to increased risks of cancer. The behavior usually is that of the persons whose health is in question, but often it includes the behavior of others who control resources or rewards for behavior, such as community leaders, parents, employers, peers, teachers, and health professionals. Whether it is at the primary, secondary, or tertiary stage of prevention, a cancer education program is an intervention to prevent disability, illness, or death or to enhance quality of life through voluntary change of cancer-related behavior.[125]

Areas that should be covered in educational programs include tobacco, alcohol, occupations and cancer, environmental pollutants, sexual activity, radiation, infective and genetic factors, and diet.[126] Each of these areas should be discussed in terms of the risks they impose for certain types of cancer, actions to reduce risks, signs and symptoms of specific cancers, screening and detection methods, and personal responsibility in prevention. To reduce fears that may prevent compliance, reassurance must be given that some forms of cancer respond well to treatment. These deep-seated fears influence behavior and often create situations in which the person knows what ought to be done but does not do it.

CONCLUSION

From experience to date, we know that more than 80% of the causes of cancer are theoretically avoidable. This tells us that cancer is not inevitable and that cancer prevention is feasible and practical. As LeMaistre[15] points out, "If we are willing to use the knowledge we now have about how to prevent cancer as effectively as we do the knowledge about how to cure cancer, then and only then will we be on the road to eliminating cancer." The concept of prevention is sound, but successful application will require that we move forward aggressively in two directions: (1) basic research in cancer prevention, and (2) understanding more about motivating human behavior change. A first step in refocusing our cancer prevention efforts occurred when a consensus was achieved that cancers are caused by specific risk factors in our environment and in our lifestyle. However, efforts at developing effective cancer prevention strategies have been hampered by the fact that the knowledge base and understanding of each risk factor varies. We must, therefore, acquire additional knowledge about each individual risk factor and determine how it affects the body. This information, combined with strong public education, will prove to be the cornerstone of cancer prevention.

REFERENCES

1. Robbins LC, Hall JH: *How to Practice Prospective Medicine.* Indianapolis, IN: Methodist Hospital of Indiana, 1970.
2. Schoenbach V: Appraising health risk appraisal. *Am J Pub Health* 77:409–411, 1987.
3. Higginson J: Existing risks for cancer. In Deisler P (ed.): *Reducing the Carcinogenic Risks in Industry.* New York: Marcel Dekker, 1984, pp. 1–19.
4. Bodnar B, Pedersen S: The nursing process. In Edelman C, Mandel C (eds.): *Health Promotion Throughout the Lifespan.* St. Louis: Mosby, 1986, pp. 44–71.
5. Rowe W: Identification of risk. In *Risk and Reasons: Risk Assessment in Relation to Environmental Mutagens and Carcinogens.* New York: Alan R. Liss, 1986, pp. 3–22.
6. Oleske D, Groenwald SL: Epidemiology of cancer. In Groenwald SL, Frogge MH, Goodman M, Yarbro CH (eds.): *Cancer Nursing: Principles and Practice* (ed. 2). Boston: Jones and Bartlett, 1990, pp. 3–27.
7. Newell G: Lifestyles and cancer prevention. In *Progress in Cancer Control IV: Research in the Cancer Center.* New York: Alan R. Liss, 1983, pp. 55–66.
8. Yarbro, JW: Carcinogenesis. In Groenwald SL, Frogge MH, Goodman M, Yarbro CH (eds.): *Cancer Nursing: Principles and Practices* (ed. 2). Boston: Jones and Bartlett, 1990, pp. 31–40.
9. Breslow L: Review and future perspectives of cancer screening programs. In Nieburgs H (ed.): *Prevention and Detection of Cancer. Part II. Detection.* New York: Marcel Dekker, 1978, pp. 1177–1212.
10. White L: Cancer risk assessment. *Semin Oncol Nurs* 2:184–190, 1986.
11. Boyd NF: The epidemiology of cancer: Principles and methods. In Tannock IF, Hill RP (eds.): *The Basic Science of Oncology.* New York: Pergamon Press, 1987.
12. Meili L: Epidemiology. In Otto SE (ed.): *Oncology Nursing.* St. Louis: Mosby Year Book, 1991, pp. 19–27.
13. Lin R, Kesseler I: A multifactorial model for pancreative cancer in man. *JAMA* 245:147–152, 1981.
14. Woods NH, Woods J: Epidemiology and the study of cancer. In Marino L (ed.): *Cancer Nursing.* St. Louis: Mosby, 1981, pp. 139–175.
15. LeMaistre C: Reflections on disease prevention. *Cancer* 62:1673–1675, 1988 (suppl).
16. Lovejoy N, Jenkins C, Wu T, et al: Developing a breast cancer screening program for Chinese-American women. *Oncol Nurs Forum* 16:181–187, 1989.
17. Million-Underwood S, Sanders E: Factors contributing to health promotion behaviors among African-American men. *Oncol Nurs Forum* 17:707–720, 1990.
18. Baquet CR, Ringen K: *Cancer Among Blacks and Other*

Minorities. Publication No. 86-2785. Washington, DC: U.S. Department of Health and Human Services, Public Health Service, National Institutes of Health, March 1986.
19. Roberson: Researcher questions high cancer rates for blacks. *Regional Cancer Report,* April 1986, 1–2.
20. Frank-Stromborg M, Olsen S (eds.): *Cancer Prevention in Minority Populations: Cultural Implications for Health Care Professionals.* St. Louis: Mosby, 1993.
21. Coreil J: Ethnicity and cancer prevention in a tri-ethnic urban community. *J Nat Med Assoc* 76:1013–1019, 1984.
22. Bassett M, Krieger N: Social class and black–white differences in breast cancer survival. *Am J Pub Health* 76:1400–1403, 1986.
23. Devesa S, Diamond E: Socioeconomic and racial differences in lung cancer incidence. *Am J Epid* 118:818–829, 1983.
24. Freeman H: Cancer in the socioeconomically disadvantaged. In *Cancer and the Socioeconomically Disadvantaged.* Atlanta: American Cancer Society, 1990.
25. Jenks S: War on cancer confronts poverty. *Med World News,* August 14, 1989, p. 31.
26. Satariano W, Swanson M: Racial differences in cancer incidence: The significance of age-specific patterns. *Cancer* 62:2640–2653, 1988.
27. Cardwell J, Collier W: Racial differences in cancer awareness. *Urban Health,* October 1981, pp. 29–31.
28. Fink D: *Guidelines for the Cancer-Related Checkup: Recommendations and Rationale.* Atlanta: American Cancer Society, 1991.
29. Update January 1992: The American Cancer Society Guidelines for the Cancer-Related Checkup. *CA* 42:44–45, 1992.
30. Gray N: Cancer risks and cancer prevention in the third world. In Vessey M, Gray M (eds.): *Cancer Risks and Prevention.* Oxford, Eng.: Oxford University Press, 1985, pp. 269–299.
31. Schulte P, Ringen K, Hemstreet G, et al: Risk assessment of a cohort exposed to aromatic amines. *J Occup Med* 27:115–121, 1985.
32. Schulte P, Ringen K, Hemstreet G, et al: Risk factors for bladder cancer in a cohort exposed to aromatic amines. *Cancer* 58:2156–2162, 1986.
33. Morrison A, Cole P: Urinary tract. In Schottenfeld D, Fraumeni J (eds.): *Cancer Epidemiology and Prevention.* Philadelphia: Saunders, 1982, pp. 925–937.
34. Wakefield J: Education of the public. In Fraumeni J (ed.): *Persons at High Risk of Cancer: An Approach to Cancer Etiology and Control.* New York: Academic Press, 1975, pp. 415–434.
35. Skegg D: Other drugs. In Vessey M, Gray M (eds.): *Cancer Risks and Prevention.* Oxford, Eng.: Oxford University Press, 1985, pp. 211–230.
36. Whitmore W: Bladder cancer: An overview. *CA* 38:213–221, 1988.
37. Scanlon, EF: Breast Cancer. In Holleb AI, Fink DJ, Murphy GP (eds.): *Clinical Oncology.* Atlanta: American Cancer Society, 1991, pp. 177–193.
38. Kelsey JL, Gammon MD: The epidemiology of breast cancer. *CA* 41:146–165, 1991.
39. Henderson D, Ross R, Bernstein L: Estrogens as a cause of human cancer: The Richard and Hinda Rosenthal Foundation Award Lecture. *Cancer Res* 48:246–253, 1988.
40. Hildreth NG, Shore RE, Dvoretsky PM: The risk of breast cancer after irradiation of the thymus in infancy. *N Engl J Med* 321:1281–1284, 1989.
41. Seidman H, Stellman S, Hushinski M: A different perspective on breast cancer risk factors: Some implications of the non-attributable risk. *CA* 32:301–313, 1982.
42. Berg J: Clinical implications of risk factors for breast cancer. *Cancer* 53:589–591, 1984.
43. Schatzkin A, Carter CL, Green SB, et al: Is alcohol consumption related to breast cancer? Results from Framingham Heart Study. *J Natl Cancer Inst* 81:31–35, 1989.
44. Harris RE, Wynder EL: Breast cancer and alcohol consumption. A study in weak associations. *JAMA* 259:2867–2871, 1988.
45. Schatzkin A, Jones Y, Hoover RN, et al: Alcohol consumption and breast cancer in the epidemiologic follow-up study of the first national health and nutrition survey. *N Engl J Med* 316:1169–1173, 1987.
46. Petrakis N, Ernster V, King M: Breast. In Schottenfeld D, Fraumeni J (eds.): *Cancer Epidemiology and Prevention.* Philadelphia: Saunders, 1982, pp. 855–870.
47. The Cancer and Steroid Hormone Study of the Centers for Disease Control and the National Institute of Child Health and Human Development: Oral-contraceptive use and the risk of breast cancer. *N Engl J Med* 315:405–411, 1986.
48. Schatzkin A, Greenwald P, Byar DP, Clifford CK: The dietary fat–breast cancer hypothesis is alive. *JAMA* 261:3284–3287, 1989.
49. Wynder E, Rose D, Cohen L: Diet and breast cancer in causation and therapy. *Cancer* 58:1804–1813, 1986.
50. Willett WC, Stampfer MJ, Colditz GA, et al: Dietary fat and the risk of breast cancer. *N Engl J Med* 316:22–28, 1987.
51. Stefanek ME: Counseling women at high risk for breast cancer. *Oncology* 4:27–38, 1990.
52. Herrero R, Brinton L, Reeves W, et al: Sexual behavior, venereal disease, hygiene practices, and invasive cervical cancer in a high-risk population. *Cancer* 65:380–386, 1990.
53. Villa L, Franco E: Ludwig Institute for Cancer Research Human Papillomavirus Study Group: Epidemiologic correlates of cervical neoplasia and risk of human papillomavirus infection in asymptomatic women in Brazil. *J Natl Cancer Inst* 81:332–340, 1989.
54. Lungu O, Sun XW, Felix J, et al: Relationship of human papillomavirus type to grade of cervical intraepithelial neoplasia. *JAMA* 267:2493–2496, 1992.
55. DeBuono B, Zinner S, Daamen M, et al: Sexual behavior of college women in 1975, 1986, and 1989. *N Engl J Med* 322:821–825, 1990.
56. Eddy DM: Screening for cervical cancer. *Ann Int Med* 113:214–226, 1990.
57. Hendershot GE: Coitus-related cervical cancer risk factors: Trends and differentials in racial and religious groups. *Am J Public Health* 73:299–301, 1983.
58. Brinton LA, Schairer C, Hasenszel W: Smoking and invasive cervical cancer. *JAMA* 255:3265–3269, 1986.
59. Carroll KK, Lipkin M, Weisburger JH: Diet's key role in preventing cancer. *Patient Care* 23:54–63, 1989.
60. National Research Council: *Diet and Health Report.* Washington, D.C.: National Academy of Sciences, 1990.
61. Council on Scientific Affairs: Dietary fiber and health. *JAMA* 262:542–546, 1989.
62. Willett WC, Stampfer MJ, Colditz GA, et al: Relation of meat, fat, and fiber intake to the risk of colon cancer in

a prospective study among women. *N Engl J Med* 323:1664–1672, 1990.
63. Kritchevsky D: Diet and cancer. *CA* 41:328–333, 1991.
64. Colon cancer gene offers new target for drug designers. *J NIH Res* 3:37, 1991.
65. Bufill JA: Colorectal cancer: Evidence for distinct genetic categories based on proximal or distal tumor location. *Ann Int Med* 113:779–788, 1990.
66. Fleischer DE, Goldberg SB, Browning TH, et al: Detection and surveillance of colorectal cancer. *JAMA* 261:580–585, 1989.
67. Ekbom A, Helmick C, Zack M, et al: Ulcerative colitis and colorectal cancer. *N Engl J Med* 323:1228–1233, 1990.
68. Di Bisceglie A: Hepatocellular carcinoma: Molecular biology of its growth and relationship to hepatitis B virus infection. *Med Clin North Am* 73:985–995, 1989.
69. Prevention of liver cancer. *WHO Tech Rep Ser* 691:1–30, 1983.
70. Kaklamai E, Trichopoulos D, Tzonou A, et al: Hepatitis B and C viruses and their interaction in the origin of hepatocellular carcinoma. *JAMA* 265:1974–1976, 1991.
71. Simonetti RG, Camma C, Fiorello F, et al: Hepatitis C virus infection as risk factor for hepatocellular carcinoma in patients with cirrhosis. *Ann Int Med* 116:97–102, 1992.
72. Falk H: Vinyl chloride–induced hepatic angiosarcoma. In Miller RW (ed.): *Unusual Occurrences as Clues to Cancer Etiology.* Tokyo: Japan Sci. Soc. Press, 1988, pp. 39–46.
73. Fleisher JM: Occupational and non-occupational risk factors in relation to an excess of primary liver cancer observed among residents of Brooklyn, New York. *Cancer* 65:180–185, 1990.
74. Rustigi VK: Epidemiology of hepatocellular carcinoma. *Gastroent Clin N Am* 16:545–551, 1987.
75. Regan LS: Screening for hepatocellular carcinoma in high-risk individuals. *Arch Intern Med* 149:1741–1744, 1989.
76. Kingsley LA, Rinaldo CR, Lyter D, et al: Sexual transmission efficiency of hepatitis B virus and human immunodeficiency virus among homosexual men. *JAMA* 264:230–234, 1990.
77. Beasley RP: Hepatitis B virus: The major etiology of hepatocellular carcinoma. *Cancer* 61:1942–1956, 1988.
78. Beasley RP, Hwang LY: Epidemiology of hepatocellular carcinoma. In Vyas GN, Dienstag JL, Hoofnagle JH (eds.): *Viral Hepatitis and Liver Disease.* Orlando, FL: Grune & Stratton, 1984, pp. 209–224.
79. Lisker-Melman M, Martin P, Hoofnagle JH: Conditions associated with hepatocellular carcinoma. *Med Clin N Am* 73:999–1009, 1989.
80. Fraumeni J, Blot W: Lung and pleura. In Schottenfeld D, Fraumeni J (eds.): *Cancer Epidemiology and Prevention.* Philadelphia: Saunders, 1982, pp. 564–582.
81. Hammond EC: Tobacco. In Fraumeni J (ed.): *Persons at High Risk of Cancer: An Approach to Cancer Etiology and Control.* New York: Academic Press, 1975, pp. 131–138.
82. Cigarette smoking among adults—United States, 1990. *JAMA* 267:3133, 1992.
83. Steenland K: Passive smoking and the risk of heart disease. *JAMA* 267:94–99, 1992.
84. Janerich D, Thompson WD, Varela LR, et al: Lung cancer and exposure to tobacco smoke in the household. *N Engl J Med* 323:632–636, 1990.
85. Harley NH, Harley JH: Potential lung cancer risk from indoor radon exposure. *CA* 40:265–275, 1990.
86. Mahboubi E, Sayed G: Oral cavity and pharynx. In Schottenfeld D, Fraumeni J (eds.): *Cancer Epidemiology and Prevention.* Philadelphia: Saunders, 1982, pp. 583–595.
87. Holmstrup P, Pindborg J: Oral mucosal lesions in smokeless tobacco users. *CA* 38:230–235, 1988.
88. Sankaranarayanan R, Duffy SW, Day NF, et al: A case-control investigation of cancer of the oral tongue and the floor of the mouth in southern India. *Int J Cancer* 44:617–621, 1989.
89. Mashberg A, Samit AM: Early detection, diagnosis, and management of oral and oropharyngeal cancer. *CA* 39:67–87, 1989.
90. Peto R: The preventability of cancer. In Vessey M, Gray M (eds.): *Cancer Risks and Prevention.* Oxford, Eng.: Oxford University Press, 1985, pp. 1–14.
91. Oreggia F, DeStefani E, Correa P, et al: Risk factors for cancer of the tongue in Uruguay. *Cancer* 67:180–183, 1991.
92. Weiss N: Ovary. In Schottenfeld D, Fraumeni J (eds.): *Cancer Epidemiology and Prevention.* Philadelphia: Saunders, 1982, pp. 871–880.
93. Ozols RF: The current status of the treatment of ovarian cancer. *Mediguide to Oncology* 11:1–5, 1991.
94. White L: The nurse's role in cancer prevention. In Newell G (ed.): *Cancer Prevention in Clinical Medicine.* New York: Raven Press, 1983, pp. 91–112.
95. Henderson B, Gerkins V, Pike M: Sexual factors and pregnancy. In Fraumeni J (ed.): *Persons at High Risk of Cancer: An Approach to Cancer Etiology and Control.* New York: Academic Press, 1975, pp. 267–284.
96. The Cancer and Steroid Hormone Study of the Centers for Disease Control and the National Institute of Child Health and Human Development: The reduction in risk of ovarian cancer associated with oral-contraceptive use. *N Engl J Med* 316:650–655, 1987.
97. Pritchard KI: Screening for endometrial cancer: Is it effective? *Ann Int Med* 110:177–179, 1989.
98. Gambrell RD: Estrogen-progesterone replacement and cancer risk. *Hospital Practice* 25:81–100, 1990.
99. Michell D: Contraception. *N Engl J Med* 320:777–787, 1989.
100. Persky V, Davis F, Barrett R, et al: Recent time trends in uterine cancer. *Am J Public Health* 80:935–939, 1990.
101. Crawford ED, Nabors WL: Diagnosing prostate cancer: Role of the primary care physician. *Primary Care & Cancer* 10:19–24, 1990.
102. Littrup PJ, Lee F, Mettlin C: Prostate cancer screening: Current trends and future implications. *CA* 42:198–211, 1992.
103. Greenwald P: Prostate. In Schottenfeld D, Fraumeni J (eds.): *Cancer Epidemiology and Prevention.* Philadelphia: Saunders, 1982, pp. 938–967.
104. Diagnosis and treatment of prostate cancer. *Senior Medical Review. AARP* 3:1–8, 1989.
105. Doll R, Peto R: *The Causes of Cancer: Quantitative Estimates of Avoidable Risks of Cancer in the United States Today.* New York: Oxford University Press, 1981.
106. Rose D, Boyar A, Wynder E: International comparisons of mortality rates for cancer of the breast, ovary, prostate, and colon, and per capita food consumption. *Cancer* 58:2363–2371, 1986.
107. Willson PC: Prostate cancer II: The nurse's role in screening and early diagnosis for primary disease and recurrence. *Nursing Interventions in Oncology.* (M.D. Anderson Cancer Center, Houston, TX) 4:4–5, 1992.

108. Council on Scientific Affairs: Harmful effects of ultraviolet radiation. *JAMA* 262:380–384, 1989.
109. Stewart DS: Indoor tanning: The nurse's role in preventing skin damage. In Reed-Ash C, Jenkins JF (eds.): *Enhancing the Role of Cancer Nursing*. New York: Raven Press, 1990, pp. 79–94.
110. Lawler PE, Schreiber S: Cutaneous malignant melanoma: Nursing's role in prevention and early detection. *Oncol Nurs Forum* 16:345–352, 1989.
111. Devereux DF: Diagnosis and management of dysplastic nevus syndrome and early melanoma. *Oncology* 4:73–83, 1990.
112. Koh HK, Lew RA, Prout MN: Screening for melanoma/skin cancer: Theoretic and practical considerations. *J Am Acad Dermatol* 20:159–172, 1989.
113. Lee JAH: The melanoma epidemic thus far. *Mayo Clin Proc* 65:1368–1371, 1990.
114. Campbell EM, Redman S, Sanson-Fisher WS: Screening for melanoma: A community survey of prevalence and predictors. *Med J Australia* 154:338–343, 1991.
115. Schottenfeld D, Warshauer M: Testis. In Schottenfeld D, Fraumeni J (eds.): *Cancer Epidemiology and Prevention.* Philadelphia: Saunders, 1982, pp. 947–957.
116. Shreyaskumar PR, Kvols LK, Richardson RL: Familial testicular cancer: Report of six cases and review of the literature. *Mayo Clin Proc* 65:804–808, 1990.
117. Karagas MR, Weiss NS, Strader CH, Daling JR: Elevated intrascrotal temperature and the incidence of testicular cancer in noncryptorchid men. *Am J Epidemiol* 129:1104–1109, 1989.
118. Koss L: Counseling persons who have family histories of cancer. In Fraumeni J (ed.): *Persons at High Risk of Cancer: An Approach to Cancer Etiology and Control.* New York: Academic Press, 1975, pp. 85–102.
119. Brinton LA, Nasca PC, Mallin K, et al: Case-control study of in situ and invasive carcinoma of the vagina. *Gynecol Oncol* 38:49–54, 1990.
120. Kelly P: Counseling persons who have family histories of cancer. In Newell G (ed.): *Cancer Prevention in Clinical Medicine.* New York: Raven Press, 1983, pp. 147–164.
121. Cohen J, Jaffe D: Holistic health—The future. In Edelman C, Mandle C (eds.): *Health Promotion Throughout the Life-Span.* St. Louis: Mosby, 1986, pp. 643–666.
122. Baeck M, Eisenberg M: Carcinogenic risk assessment: Concepts and issues. *Md Med J* 34:672–674, 1985.
123. Constanza M, Li F, Green H, et al: Cancer prevention and detection: Strategies for practice. In *American Cancer Society: Cancer Manual* (ed. 7). Boston: American Cancer Society, 1986, pp. 14–35.
124. Wakefield J: Education of the public. In Fraumeni J (ed.): *Persons at High Risk of Cancer: An Approach to Cancer Etiology and Control.* New York: Academic Press, 1975, pp. 415–434.
125. Green L, Rimer B, Elwood T: Public education. In Schottenfeld D, Fraumeni J (eds.): *Cancer Epidemiology and Prevention.* Philadelphia: Saunders, 1982, pp. 1100–1110.
126. Peto R: The preventability of cancer. In Vessey M, Gray M (eds.): *Cancer Risks and Prevention.* Oxford, Eng.: Oxford University Press, 1985, pp. 1–14.

Chapter 8

Assessment and Interventions for Cancer Prevention and Detection

Marilyn Frank-Stromborg, RN, EdD, NP, FAAN

Rebecca F. Cohen, RN, EdD, MPA, CPHQ

INTRODUCTION

Despite its long history, cancer became a relatively important health problem only during the twentieth century. It was among the first chronic diseases recognized as potentially "controllable," that is, amenable to public health strategies consistent with its magnitude and social impact. In 1937 the Congress of the United States took its first significant action on the problem of cancer by passing the National Cancer Institute Act. This law established the National Cancer Institute for purposes of conducting research relating to the cause, diagnosis, and treatment of cancer and the application of research results, with a view to the development and prompt widespread use of the most effective methods of prevention, diagnosis, and treatment of cancer.[1] Congressional intent toward the cancer problem was reaffirmed by the passage of the National Cancer Act of 1971. This act expanded activities

> to develop, through research and development efforts, the means to significantly reduce the morbidity and mortality from cancer by: preventing as many cancers as possible, curing patients who develop cancer, providing maximum palliation to patients not cured, rehabilitating treated patients to as nearly normal a state as possible.[2]

Although a clear expression of congressional intent existed regarding cancer control, results of the 1971 legislation tended to be in the direction of research. It had been hoped that the legislation would result in the following cancer control efforts: (1) to improve identification of techniques or methods with a potential for combating the disease, (2) to improve community testing of these technologic methods for safety and efficacy, (3) to provide for evaluation of the results of the testing, and (4) to enhance promotion of the appropriate general use of technologic techniques in the community through professional and public education. Obstacles existed, however, that made it much more difficult to initiate cancer control efforts than it had been to control other communicable diseases. One of the obstacles included the fact that physicians generally did not view cancer as epidemic in nature. It was believed that governmental action to establish public services for cancer diagnosis or treatment was an intrusion into physicians' freedom to practice. In addition, economic resistance to control measures, for example, by the tobacco industry, was assisted by the fact that the long latency period of cancer helped to make etiologic factors less identifiable. Finally, cancer's multiple etiology engendered an extensive research effort when an additional attack on the disease was mounted. Money for research and training of personnel was held onto tightly by special interest groups that resisted public expenditures from cancer control as a threat to their own existence.[3,4]

Thus organized cancer control in the United States has had three strong adversaries: the private medical world, the private industrial world, and the biomedical research establishment that emerged after the passage of the National Cancer Institute Act of 1937 and the subsequent creation of the National Institutes of Health in 1948. In some situations these forces, feeling threatened by cancer control, have developed strong lobbies against cancer control.

Can We Prevent Cancer?

The arguments that cancer can be prevented are familiar to almost everyone. Different populations throughout the world suffer from different kinds of cancer, but those who migrate tend to acquire the pattern of cancers characteristic of their new home. It is therefore concluded by scientists that the incidence of most kinds of cancers is determined by environment.[5,6] Research indicates that Americans could cut their incidence of cancer to little more than half the national average simply by adopting the lifestyle of the Seventh-Day Adventists and moving to the Rocky Mountain states or becoming Mormons and migrating to Utah.[7]

Evidence clearly illustrates that trying to change lifestyles may create some resistance.[8–12] Such attitudes as "there is not much a person can do to prevent cancer" and "scientists say everything causes cancer" create further resistance to the prevention of cancer.[13] Everyone knows about the link between cigarettes and lung cancer, and people expect to be exposed to lectures about the dangers of smoking. However, it has become customary to brush this aside and concentrate attention on modern industry as the supposed cause of most of our ills. It is attractive to distrust science and technology because they lay the blame on the imagined avarice of others rather than on one's own self-indulgence.[7]

In fact, some scientists[7,12] believe that there is really no evidence that any of the products of modern technology (except cigarettes) contribute to the common cancers. Thus most of the major cancers, except lung cancer, are not any more common today than they were 50 years ago.[7,12] It is suggested, however, that new industrial products be monitored for mutagenicity and carcinogenicity and that industries are deterred from adding hazardous ingredients or waste to our environment. However, cancer cannot be conquered simply by the surveillance and control of industry. To effectively conquer the common cancers, preventive measures must reach the individual and seek to modify personal habits and lifestyles.[7,12] For example, cancer of the lung is due to a highly addictive habit; cancer of the head and neck is associated with tobacco and excessive alcohol use; cancer of the large intestine and breast are most common in affluent countries and are thought to be related to diet; cancer of the skin is linked to ultraviolet rays and for some individuals is connected with increased leisure time.[10,12] The preventive strategies for these cancers may conflict with the immediate desires of some.[11] Apart from giving up smoking, sunbathing, and alcohol, the most recent change that we have been asked to make is in diet—the consumption of less fat, less cholesterol, and more fruits, vegetables, and cereals.[14–20]

Whether people will be willing to give up certain immediate desires for health and prolonged life remains to be seen. However, the National Cancer Institute has established as its "Year 2000 Cancer Control Objective" a 50% reduction in the cancer mortality rate.[10] It is the belief of the National Cancer Institute that through the application of current knowledge about cancer prevention, screening, and detection; access to the latest treatment; and continuing advances in cancer treatment, the 1980 mortality rate can be reduced by 20% to 50%. McGinnis et al.[10] have noted that in 1990 the target mortality rates for infants, children, and adults have been achieved whereas those for adolescents, young adults, and older adults have not.

LEVELS OF PREVENTION

How, then, can we approach the problem of cancer prevention? According to Edelman and Milio[21] we must begin by broadening our definition of prevention. Prevention, in a narrow sense, means averting the development of disease. In a broad sense, however, it consists of all measures, including definitive therapy, that limit the progression of disease at any point of its course. This concept is important because it implies that prevention can take place anywhere along the continuum of health. By adopting this definition, one could employ preventive strategies while healthy, during the phase of determining whether one has the disease, and during the phase of dealing with a disease already contracted. It has therefore been suggested that there are three levels of prevention: primary, secondary, and tertiary.[22,23] Each level of prevention occurs at a distinct point in the development of the disease process and requires specific interventions.

Primary Prevention

Primary cancer prevention involves activities undertaken to prevent the occurrence, or reduce the risk, of cancer in a population generally considered both physically and emotionally healthy.[24] Primary prevention is not therapeutic, does not use therapeutic treatments, and does not involve symptom identification. The purpose of primary prevention is decreasing the vulnerability of the individual or the population to illness or dysfunction through health-promoting strategies, as well as providing specific protection.[21,24–26]

Primary cancer prevention is true health promotion and includes activities such as[24]:

- identifying risk factors in individuals or groups
- counseling people for risk factor reduction
- identifying primary cancer prevention activities, such as stop-smoking programs
- planning and implementing new cancer prevention programs such as nutrition education programs; programs on the hazards of cigarette smoking, alcohol consumption, and poor diets; programs for the elderly and disadvantaged aimed at their health needs
- genetic screening
- periodic selective examinations
- conducting epidemiological research

Primary prevention must include teaching good health behaviors as well as delivering health care. The interpersonal and therapeutic nature of the doctor/nurse/patient relationship can create an ideal situation in which to instruct and encourage good health practices. Patients need to receive information during routine health maintenance exams, not after a diagnosis or illness is disclosed. Lay terms and simple sentences enhance understanding, and information should be organized, repeated, and have a personal impact on the individual. Also, it has been found that the greatest influence can be gained when the risk factor exposure is a matter of choice by the patient, such as with diet or smoking.[26,27]

Studies have indicated that when an individual perceives his or her susceptibility to cancer as high, views cancer as a serious disease, but perceives the benefits and barriers to action as low, the most favorable outcomes are obtained from behavioral approaches to prevention.[26,28] Motivation to take action is enhanced, and lifestyle changes are more easily achieved. However, in addition to possessing these important health beliefs, patients must know what forms of cancer are preventable, what modification techniques are possible, and how they can maintain the newly developed healthy lifestyle.[25,29,30]

One of the easiest ways to reach individuals in our society is through the work setting. The primary prevention role of the occupationally based nurse includes: (1) being actively involved in educating workers and supervisors in the proper use and handling of work materials; (2) educating employees about the importance of following recommended protective measures; and (3) instituting medical surveillance measures. Carrying out these activities in the workplace enables the nurse to provide programs that are convenient to the employees, makes follow-up and tracking of employees after a program easily accomplished, and allows programs to be targeted to identified high-risk employees.[31–34]

Nurses have also assumed innovative cancer prevention roles in ambulatory care and acute settings, within community health programs, and in basic nursing curriculums. Nationally the trend to include health promotion/"wellness" concepts in undergraduate and graduate nursing curriculums has helped to ensure that primary cancer prevention is addressed. In addition, there has been an increase in the number of nursing workshops and conferences devoted to primary and secondary prevention. Thus, within the last 10 years the role of the nurse in primary/secondary prevention has broadened, active involvement in a variety of settings has taken place, and nursing academic and continuing education programs have expanded their curriculums to prepare the nurse for an active and often nontraditional role in this area.[30,31,35–37]

In order to promote primary and secondary cancer prevention, nurses must possess knowledge and skills in such areas as risk factors associated with the development of cancer, factors affecting health behaviors, cancer screening and detection methods and recommendations for their utilization, teaching methods, and counseling techniques.[12,14,24,38–40]

Sirota et al.[25] state that it is important to help patients see why and how certain cancer risk-reduction strategies can fit into their lives. Various examples of motivational approaches that should be incorporated into primary prevention education have been identified:

- Begin preventive prescriptions at the onset of a patient relationship to set the tone for further preventive care.
- Promote the idea of "healthful lifestyle" rather than "disease prevention" to stress the positive and wide-ranging effects of lifestyle modification.
- Encourage participation by all family members who can serve as a support group for the patient, and promote the idea of prevention as necessary for everyone.
- Set realistic and achievable goals for major lifestyle modifications, and provide positive and constructive feedback to patients.
- Maintain the philosophy that patients are responsible for prevention—they can rely on the nurse for valuable health advice, but maintaining a healthful lifestyle is up to them.

Health promotion

Edelman and Milio[21] point out that health promotion efforts focus on maintaining or improving the general health of individuals, families, and communities. These activities are carried on at both the public level, such as government programs that promote adequate housing, and the personal level. There are two strategies of health promotion, passive and active. *Passive* strategies involve the individual as a passive participant or recipient. Examples include maintaining clean water and sanitary sewage systems and enforcing governmental regulations within industries to make sure that employees are protected from industrial agents/chemicals, lights, and injuries.[21] On the other hand, *active* strategies depend on the individual's adopting a proposed program of health promotion. Examples include changes in eating or exercise habits and enrollment in a stress management class.

Although health promotion is a desirable goal, the health care system in the United States responds to the most pressing matter at any moment. Health promotion lacks the demanding element of immediacy and thus tends to be regulated to lower levels of importance. Federal governmental policy advocates health promotion, as evidenced by the establishment of the Office of Health Information and Health Promotion and the publication of *Healthy People*.

Personal health promotion most commonly is provided by health education. However, because health education is concerned principally with creating changes in human behavior, it must involve more than the provision of health information and must be considered an important function of nurses, physicians, parents, and allied health professionals. The goal is to assist individuals to develop a sense of responsibility for their own health and a shared sense of responsibility for avoiding injury to the health of others. Health education encourages health-promoting habits, values, and attitudes that must be learned through practice. These, in turn, must be reinforced through systematic instruction in hygiene, bodily function, physical fitness, and use of leisure time. Another important goal of health education is to help the individual understand how to use health services appropriately.[21]

Specific protection

Specific protection focuses on protecting persons from disease by providing immunization and by reducing exposure to occupational hazards, carcinogens, and other environmental health risks. Primary prevention is considered health protection because it emphasizes shielding or defending the body from injury. Specific protection strategies include[21]:

- attention to personal hygiene
- use of environmental sanitation
- protection against occupational hazards
- protection from accidents
- use of specific nutrients
- protection from carcinogens
- avoidance of allergens

Finally, contrary to the popular belief that preventive medicine will decrease medical expenditures, it actually may *increase* the nation's steadily rising medical bills. However, preventive activities must be assessed in terms of health and not just cost, because there are certain preventive measures that will create enormous benefits in terms of health while increasing medical expenditures. Society must decide whether better health is worth the higher cost, and individuals must determine what best meets their own personal needs. The final choice depends on the value one places on health benefits, risks, and costs.[41,42]

Secondary Prevention

Secondary prevention activities include defining and identifying high-risk groups and groups with precursor stages of disease. It is important to acknowledge that there is no sharp break between primary and secondary prevention or between precursors and "early" stages of a disease.[23]

Secondary prevention ranges from early diagnosis/detection, screening, and treating early stages of disease to limiting disability by averting or delaying the consequences of advanced disease.

Early diagnosis and prompt treatment

Early detection is the identification of disease in an *individual*, when it is still localized, curable, or manageable, or the identification of a precancerous lesion. The individual may or may not be asymptomatic, and identification is made through tests, examinations, and observations. *Screening*, on the other hand, is an organized effort to find cancer in its early stages in a defined *population*. Screening for cancer is conducted at intermittent time intervals and is site-specific. Screening may be done through an organized program using one specific test, or it may use a battery of tests.[24,43] Examples of activities carried out to ensure early diagnosis and prompt treatment include[21,24,25,43]:

- case-finding measures, both on a individual basis and for the community as a whole
- screening procedures based on identified risk factors
- monthly breast self-examinations and mammography
- periodic Papanicoulaou (Pap) smears
- attending a cancer detection clinic
- seeking medical attention for one of cancer's seven warning signals
- prevention of complications and sequelae
- surgical removal of cancers
- digital rectal exams and sigmoidoscopy

There are three methods utilized in early detection: physical, cytologic, and biologic. Physical methods include: radiologic techniques, such as chest X ray and mammography; noninvasive techniques, such as nuclear magnetic resonance, CT scan, and ultra sound; and clinical examination. Examples of cytologic detection methods include: exfoliative cytology, such as Pap smears, sputum cytology, urine cytology, endometrial sampling, and gastric washings. Biological detection methods are laboratory tests that can detect tumor markers in body fluids.[24]

Early detection tends to focus on cancers that have a high incidence and in which early diagnosis contributes to increased survival. These cancers include: cervix, endometrium, breast, colon/rectum, oropharynx, testes, and skin. In addition, while lung cancer is not considered a cancer that is amenable to early detection, primary prevention is especially important because of the increase in lung cancer rates in women and its high correlation with cigarette smoking.[24]

Limiting disability

Providing adequate treatment to arrest a disease process and to prevent further complications and sequelae, as well as to provide facilities to limit disability and prevent death, are important functions in this category. Delayed recognition because of incomplete knowledge of some disease process in early secondary prevention results in the need to limit future disability in the late stage of secondary prevention. Certain economic environmental changes may aid in preventing sequelae, but the preventive measures primarily are therapeutic to arrest the disease and prevent further complications.[21]

Tertiary Prevention

Tertiary prevention takes place when a disability is permanent and irreversible. It involves minimizing the effect of disease and disability via surveillance and maintenance aimed at preventing complications and deterioration. Examples include chemotherapy, radiotherapy, pain control, and rehabilitation programs to help patients attain and retain an optimal level of functioning regardless of their disabling condition.[25]

ROLE OF THE NURSE IN PRIMARY AND SECONDARY CANCER PREVENTION

The National Cancer Institute (NCI) has proposed for the year 2000 that cancer mortality be reduced by 50%. This goal is partially based on the known link between cancer and smoking and will require active involvement by all health care professionals. Nursing professionals, comprising the largest health professional group in the United States, can play an important role in meeting this goal.

Frank-Stromborg and Rohan[30] have identified activities that should be undertaken by nurses as they carry out primary and secondary cancer prevention. These include: assessment, counseling, teaching, screening and detection, planning, acting as an advocate, and acting as a role model.

The nurse must begin any intervention by assessing the needs of the individual or target group. Intervention then can consist of one-on-one teaching or counseling; participating in planning, conducting, and evaluating new primary and secondary cancer prevention programs; serving as an information resource; or encouraging participation in existing cancer prevention and detection programs.[24,38,39]

Advocacy is an important aspect of cancer prevention. The nurse should act as an advocate to help promote and maintain healthier lives for people. Nurses must also encourage, or participate in, research that will investigate cancer prevention and learning methods on how to motivate changes in human behavior.[24,38,39]

A tremendous amount of effort has been put into early detection of breast cancer, but nurses must now be encouraged to investigate attitudes, behaviors, and knowledge related to cancers other than breast cancer.[30] The role of the nurse in primary and secondary cancer prevention must be broadened, and other health care professionals must recognize that this is a role in which nurses can and should actively participate.

CHEMOPREVENTION

Between 1950 and 1982 there was a steady increase in mortality rates despite marked improvements in both the diagnosis and treatment of cancer. In response to this the National Cancer Institute increased its emphasis on cancer prevention through the institution of chemoprevention clinical trials designed to test the roles of various nutrients in the reduction of cancer. *Chemoprevention* is the use of "defined chemicals or micronutrients to inhibit or reverse the process of carcinogenesis."[44, p.45] Chemoprevention agents are believed to have potential for both secondary and tertiary prevention of cancer.

The use of chemicals or micronutrients to try to prevent cancer has evolved from epidemiologic investigations and studies in vitro and in animals, as well as clinical studies.[45–49] In 1922 Mori first observed that diets low in fat-soluble vitamin A led to metaplastic changes of the epithelium and respiratory tract.[45] In 1926 Fujimaki detected that rats kept on a vitamin-A-deficient diet for a long period developed cancer of the liver. This finding gave evidence to a causality of nutritional factors or the lack of a certain defined substance for cancer incidence.[46] Scientists have also noted that vitamin A deficiency in the gastrointestinal system of rats resulted in loss of specific chemical epithelial functions that augmented neoplastic growth.[44,47] In 1941 Abels et al. linked vitamin A deficiency with human cancer by observing that when cancer patients were compared with a control group the cancer patients had lower serum values of vitamin A.[48] Numerous case-control studies have shown an inverse relation between the risk of cancer and the consumption of fruits and vegetables with a high content of beta-carotene.[49]

The agents being used today in clinical trials include vitamin A and its precursor beta-carotene, synthetic derivatives of vitamin A, vitamin C, vitamin D, vitamin E, folic acid, calcium, and the trace metal selenium. The Chemoprevention Program, one of the NCI's most recent cancer prevention programs, was initiated as a major research area after a number of working groups met between 1978 and 1981 to investigate the feasibility of a research effort in clinical and experimental chemoprevention. The major purpose of the program is to determine, in both animal models and human clinical trials, whether the introduction of synthetic or natural micronutrients or other low-molecular-weight substances into the diet can lower cancer incidence by preventing, halting, or reversing the carcinogenic process.[50]

Vitamin A

Retinoids

Retinoids are the natural derivatives and synthetic analog of vitamin A and are believed to be cytostatic agents in the prevention of epithelial carcinogenesis. It is known that retinoids can suppress carcinogenesis in a variety of epithelial tissues, including the skin, trachea, lungs, and oral mucosa in animals and humans.[51] Dietary sources of retinol include butter, whole milk, egg yolk, and liver.[44,52] The exact anticarcinogenic mechanism by which retinoids act is not understood, but recent research suggests that retinoids act primarily by regulating gene expression and may modulate the growth of premalignant cells or suppress the progression of premalignant cells to neoplastic lesions.[51]

Hong et al.[51] studied 103 patients who were disease-free after primary treatment for squamous cell cancers of the larynx, pharynx, or oral cavity. For a year these patients daily received either synthetic retinoid isotretinoin (13-*cis*-retinoic acid) or a placebo. The researchers concluded that daily treatment of high doses of isotretinoin was effective in preventing second primary tumors in patients who had been treated for squamous cell carcinoma of the head and neck. However, it did not prevent recurrences of the original tumor.

The chief obstacle to the long-term use of retinoids for prevention of cancer is their toxicity; most accumulate in the liver and can cause hepatic failure.[53] Fenretinide is a relatively nontoxic retinoid that has been recently synthesized. A long-term clinical trial investigating fenretinide's role in the prevention of second primary breast cancers is presently in progress.[54]

Beta-carotene

Beta-carotene is a plant-derived carotenoid with provitamin A (retinol) activity. It has been proposed as a possible preventive agent against cancer.[55] Beta-carotene, a precursor of vitamin A, is derived from leafy green and yellow vegetables and is converted to vitamin A in the gastrointestinal tract.[52] The mechanisms proposed to explain the anticarcinogenic effect of beta-carotene include the inactivation of reactive molecules and immunologic enhancement.[55] Beta-carotene acts as an antioxidant by deactivating carcinogenic free radicals and preventing them from transforming cells. It is known that carotenoids have a potent antioxidant effect that could reduce cancer risk by preventing tissue damage due to oxidation. This possibility is supported by data from a large number of observational epidemiologic studies, most of which have consistently found an inverse relation between the consumption of carotene-rich vegetables and cancer risk.[56] Greenberg et al.[55] conducted a clinical trial of beta-carotene in an effort to prevent basal cell and squamous cell cancer of the skin. Every day for over 5 years individuals who had recently had a nonmelanoma skin cancer received either 50 mg of beta-carotene or a placebo. The researchers reported that in persons with previous nonmelanoma skin cancer, treatment with beta-carotene did not reduce the occurrence of new skin cancers over the 5-year period of treatment and observation.

Vitamin C

Dietary sources of vitamin C are citrus fruits, fruit juices, and vegetables. Vitamin C appears to prevent the formation of nitrosamines, potential carcinogens resulting from metabolic reactions in the human digestive tract of nitrates, nitrites, and substances readily found in foods.[57]

It is known from epidemiologic studies that populations that have a high incidence of stomach cancer have a high intake of pickled, salt-cured, and smoked foods; types of foods that contain precursors of nitrosamines. It has been hypothesized that the addition of ascorbic acid to such a diet would inhibit the alteration of nitrates to nitriates and the formation of nitrosamines.[52] Nitrosamines are a potent carcinogenic agent. Olsen and Love point out that the data on the role of vitamin C ingestion and lowered risk for stomach, larynx, bladder, cervix, and esophagus cancer is controversial because several case-control studies have found no relationship between ascorbic acid and cancer risk.[52] Greenwald et al.[57] also note that current data from human studies do not support an association of vitamin C with several types of human cancer.[57]

Vitamin E

Vitamin E is similar to vitamin C in that it appears to prevent the formation of nitrosamines. This vitamin is present in a variety of foods, including vegetable oils, margarines, shortening, eggs, whole grains, and cereals. While there is presently no epidemiologic information on the association of vitamin E and cancer, there is limited evidence in laboratory models that vitamin E may inhibit tumorigenesis.[52,58,59]

Selenium

Selenium is an essential trace element found in seafood, meats, vegetables, whole grains, and milk. Numerous animal experiments have shown that selenium has a chemopreventive effect.[57] Laboratory animals fed selenium have shown a reduction in liver tumors, inhibition of carcinogenesis, reduced incidence of tumors following exposure to chemical carcinogens or ultraviolet light, a protective effect on the chemical induction of esophageal tumors, a decrease in the number of colon tumors, inhibition of the formation of papillomas, and inhibition of mammary carcinoma.[52,58,59]

Epidemiologic studies have demonstrated an inverse relationship between selenium intake and cancer. In some, but not all, case-control studies, selenium levels in the blood were significantly lower among cases with breast cancer than among controls, although an effect of disease on selenium levels cannot be excluded in these studies.[60] Death rates for cancers of the head and neck are lower in areas where the soil and crops contain higher levels of selenium.[58] High rates of colon and rectal cancer have been correlated with industrialization, high intake of fat, and low soil selenium.[57]

It is believed that selenium decreases the rate of proliferation of target cells and affects both initiation and promotion steps of carcinogenesis. It is theorized that the mechanism by which selenium offers a protective effect may be mediated through an increase in the activity of the selenium-dependent enzyme glutathione peroxidase. Selenium acts as an antioxidant when combined with glutathione peroxidase, and it functions in a manner similar to vitamins A, C, and E.[58]

In conclusion, only recently have chemoprevention trials focused on micronutrients. In 1992 a large-scale breast cancer prevention study began using the antiestrogen tamoxifen to prevent hormonally dependent breast cancer. The Breast Cancer Prevention Trial (BCPT) is designed for high-risk individuals. The BCPT is the first large chemoprevention study.[61] Since tamoxifen can inhibit the binding of estradiol to estrogen receptors in human breast tissue, it may produce a block in the developing breast cancer cells. Tamoxifen may be as effective in blocking the development of tumors as it is in the control of advanced disease.[62] The study will enroll 16,000 women aged 35 and older, who are at increased risk for breast cancer. Every day for at least 5 years in this randomized, double-blind study, half of the 16,000 women will take a 20-mg dose of tamoxifen and half will take a placebo.[62]

The next decade may well see profound changes in the area of cancer prevention if the results of the many ongoing NCI chemoprevention trials prove positive. If even a few provide positive results, the manner in which we view cancer management is likely to undergo a fundamental change.

DETECTION OF MAJOR CANCER SITES

In the last 10 years, physical assessment has become a vital part of the nursing role, regardless of the nurse's setting. The use of physical assessment techniques is not limited to nurses who have completed a nurse practitioner program. Rather, it is now routinely taught in all undergraduate nursing programs, and the expectations is that nursing students will incorporate the four cardinal techniques (inspection, palpation, percussion, and auscultation) into their daily clinical practice. Physical assessment techniques enable the nurse to assume an active role in the early detection of cancer.

Cancers of the lung, breast, cervix, colon/rectum, and prostate are among the cancers that result in the highest morbidity and mortality rates in the United States.[63] The nursing interventions for these five cancers and for skin, testicular, head and neck, and other gynecologic cancers will be discussed. Each of the following sections presents the nursing role in terms of obtaining the health history, conducting the physical examination, using screening tests for asymptomatic persons, and initiating patient education for primary and secondary prevention of the cancer.

Lung Cancer

It is estimated that 170,000 Americans in 1993 will be diagnosed with lung cancer.[64] It is the leading cause of death from cancer in men and women over 35 years old. Once considered a male disease, since the late 1980s it has replaced breast cancer as the chief cause of cancer deaths among women. Of all the known risk factors for lung cancer, the most important environmental carcinogen related to the increased incidence of lung cancer is cigarette smoking. Cigarette smoking is the largest single preventable cause of premature death and disability and the major single cause of cancer mortality.[65]

History assessment

When obtaining the history, the nurse should inquire into smoking habits, including marijuana use, occupational history, and the general respiratory environment in both the workplace and the home. Persons at high risk for lung cancer are those exposed to high levels of respiratory carcinogens in their workplace, in their general environment, and in their homes. Because of the risks of passive smoking, a detailed history should be taken of the number of smokers in the home and the length of time the individual has been exposed to the smoke environment.[66,67]

Although obtaining a detailed, lifetime occupational history is time-consuming, it is strongly recommended for anyone who has worked in shipyards or who is believed to have been exposed to asbestos; significant exposures may have been as brief as 1 month and may have occurred many years ago, even during World War II. Because the World War II work force was composed of women as well as men, the female patient should not be overlooked. The same type of detailed, lifetime occupational history should be obtained if exposure to other known carcinogenic respiratory agents, such as those found in the following occupations, is suspected: clothing and textile workers, laundry workers, meat wrappers and cutters, hairdressers, agricultural workers, chemical workers, electrical machinery manufacturers, and health care workers.[68] In the assessment of elderly persons, prior employment in settings unregulated by the National Institute of Occupational Safety and Health, the Occupational Safety and Health Act of 1970, or the Toxic Substances Control Act of 1976 must be considered because of possible exposure to toxic chemical or carcinogens that are no longer manufactured or permitted in unsupervised occupational settings.

An occupational history includes dates of employment, a list of current and longest-held jobs, average hours worked per week, exposure to potential hazards in the workplace, common illness in co-workers, and personal protective equipment worn on the job. Figure 8-1 presents a systematic approach to the occupational and environmental health history.[69]

Questions that should be included in the history and review of systems for lung cancer consist of the following items:

1. When was your last chest x-ray film?
2. When was your last tuberculin skin test? If positive, what was the treatment?
3. Do you presently smoke? How many packs a day and for how many years? (*Pack-years* equal packs per day times year of smoking.) What do you smoke? Are they filtered? What's your style of smoking? Have you ever tried to stop smoking? What happened? Do you have a "smoker's" cough? Who else in the home smokes, and how much do they tend to smoke a day?
4. Do you have bronchitis or asthma?
5. Have you ever had pneumonia?
6. Do you get short of breath with walking? climbing stairs? while resting? exercise?
7. Have you ever been told you have emphysema?
8. How many pillows do you sleep on? What happens if you don't?
9. Do you ever spit or cough up blood?
10. *Smokers:* What color is the sputum you cough up? Does it have a smell? How much is routinely coughed up in the morning?
11. What occupations have you had?
12. Chronic obstructive pulmonary disease: How often do you get flu shots? Have you been taught ways to drain the secretions from your lungs?
13. Have you ever had a pulmonary function test? What were the results?
14. Do you ever wheeze?
15. Do you cough a lot?

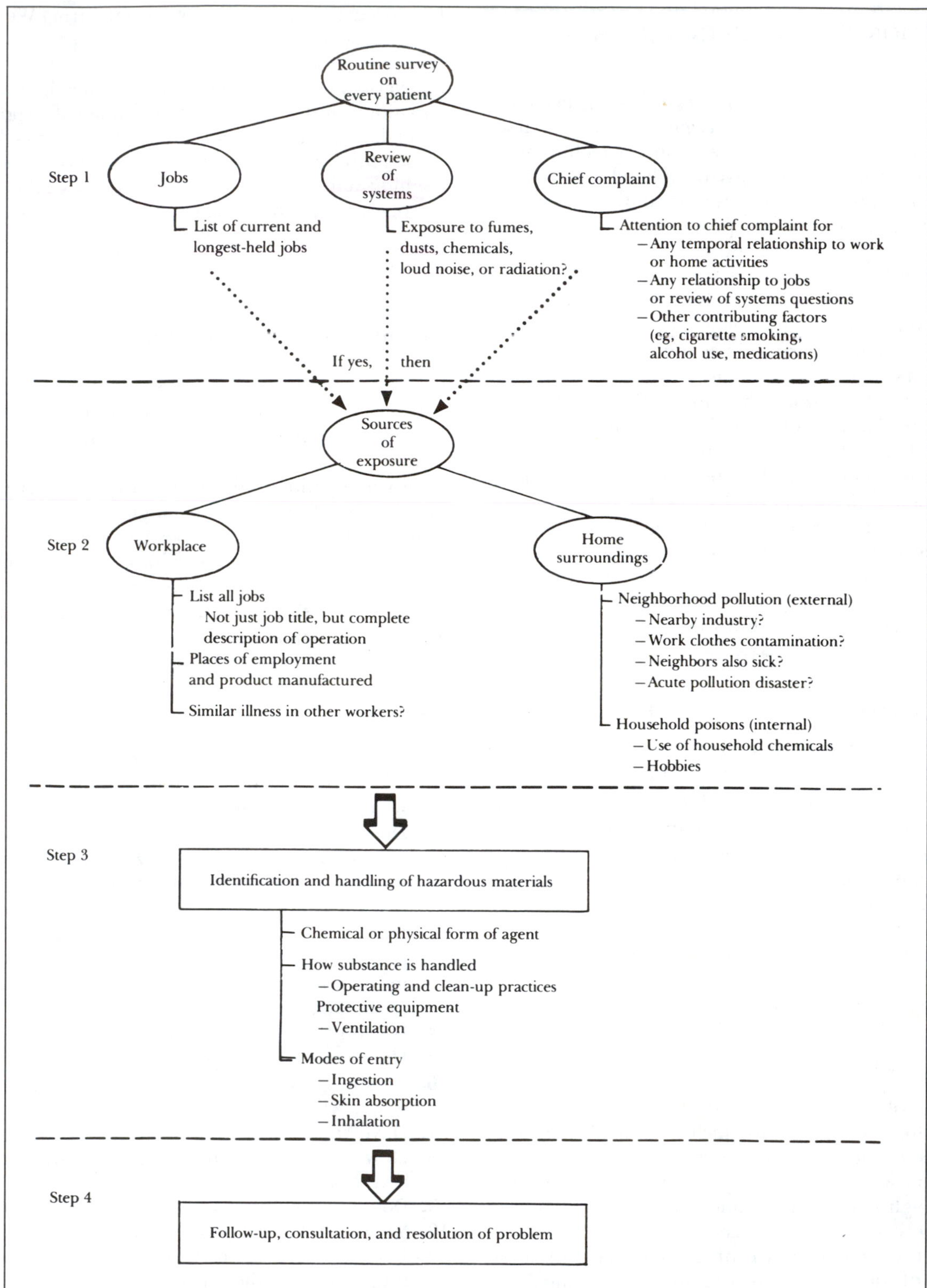

FIGURE 8-1 Systematic approach to the occupational and environmental health history. (Source: Goldman R, Peters J: The occupational and environmental health history. *JAMA* 246:2832–2836, 1981.)

16. Do you have any skeletal deformities? Or were you born with any skeletal conditions?
17. Have you had any broken ribs?
18. Do you have to purse your lips to breathe?
19. Are you aware of any sounds when you breathe?
20. Have you noticed any color changes of your lips or nails?
21. Are you now (or have you been at some time in the past) exposed to fumes, chemicals, dust, or radiation?

The majority of patients have no profound early symptoms, but most have some combination of cough, chest pain, weight loss, dyspnea, fever, fatigue, and transient hemoptysis. Because these symptoms are general in nature, they usually cause no alarm and delay diagnosis. The most frequently reported symptom of lung cancer is a cough that is productive and often associated with hemoptysis or chest pain. Cough may be the primary or only complaint in such varied diseases as congestive heart failure, asthma, upper respiratory infection, pneumonia, and bronchitis. The irritative cough may occur at night accompanied by mucoid expectoration. However, if the lung cancer is centrally located or if only the main carina is involved, the cough is nonproductive.

Later symptoms are increased frequency of early symptoms and some combination of wheezes, pleuritic pain, hoarseness, nerve disorders from local invasion, edema of head, neck, or arms, and dysphagia. There is a high index of suspicion in anyone with a history of smoking or exposure to carcinogenic agents who complains of pneumonitis that persists longer than 2 weeks despite antibiotic therapy. Unfortunately, the first symptoms of lung cancer are usually not alarming and therefore tend to be considered lightly by health professionals. Because elderly persons experience changes in respiratory structure and function, their initial vague respiratory complaints go unnoticed or are attributed to the aging process or chronic illnesses (e.g., congestive heart failure).

Physical examination

Inspection On inspection there may be many systemic, as well as localized, signs that will alert the practitioner to the possibility of lung cancer.

Finger clubbing This may be either an early or a late sign of thoracic disease, and it may be absent even in the presence of advanced disease. Clinically 5%–12% of the patients with carcinoma of the lung will have clubbing of the fingers. It also may be seen in other diseases such as industrial lung disease (e.g., asbestosis).[70] It is important to inspect the nails closely and to palpate them for sponginess. With clubbing, the nail bed becomes thickened and boggy, which is first observed by palpating the nail bed to elicit fluctuation. Clubbing usually occurs first in the thumb and the index finger and then spreads to the other fingers.

The changes associated with clubbing usually occur gradually over many weeks, months, and years. However, they have been noted to appear within a week of the onset of lung cancer. Clubbing is best assessed by viewing the finger from the side. A normal finger viewed from this direction has an angle of about 160° between the base of the nail and the skin next to the cuticle (Figure 8-2). In clubbing, this base angle is obliterated and becomes 180° or more.[71]

Barrel chest This is characterized by prominence of the sternum and a barrel-shaped configuration of the chest that appears to be held in a state of full inspiration.[72] This finding is associated with pulmonary emphysema or normal aging. Emphysema can be inherited, but the vast majority of persons with this disease have acquired it from a lifetime of smoking. Those with emphysema are at high risk for lung cancer. Typical physical findings of emphysema are pursed lips during breathing, retraction of the intercostal spaces during inspiration, use of accessory muscles during quiet respirations, and audible wheezes.

Abnormal breathing With obstructive types of pulmonary disease, expiration is prolonged and inspiration is gasping and may require the use of the accessory muscles of respiration in the neck and about the shoulder girdle.[73] Figure 8-3 shows the stance taken by individuals with pulmonary obstruction. This stance is called the "professorial attitude" because it resembles a professor lecturing.

Bulges on the thorax With the use of indirect lighting, the practitioner may observe a bulge on the chest. Neoplasm of the ribs may protrude and will be visible on inspection.

Breathlessness The patient's breathlessness during the history taking may indicate obstruction of the lungs.

Superior vena cava obstruction Obstruction of the superior vena cava is a common complication of lung cancer; approximately 80% of these cases are caused by undifferentiated neoplasms arising in proximal right bronchi.[74] The clinical picture is described by Buckingham:

> Edema of both eyelids, arms, and hands develops and will "pit" on pressure; . . . the face is a dusky blue color, the lips are deeply cyanotic; and the swollen, blue head sits on a thick "bull neck" which is distended by many large tense collateral views. The shoulders, chest, and upper abdomen are covered with a lacy collateral venous pattern.[73]

Palpation Palpation of the thorax includes testing for vocal fremitus, respiratory excursion, and compression and ascertaining the position and movability of the trachea. The following discussion presents physical signs of palpation that may indicate lung cancer.

Deviation and fixed trachea Normally the trachea is located in the midline and is freely movable. Localized disease may produce tracheal shift, or the trachea may be fixed by disease in the surrounding structures. Carcinoma of the lung rarely causes displacement except by producing atelectasis.[75]

Thoracic wall Palpation of the thoracic wall reveals masses.

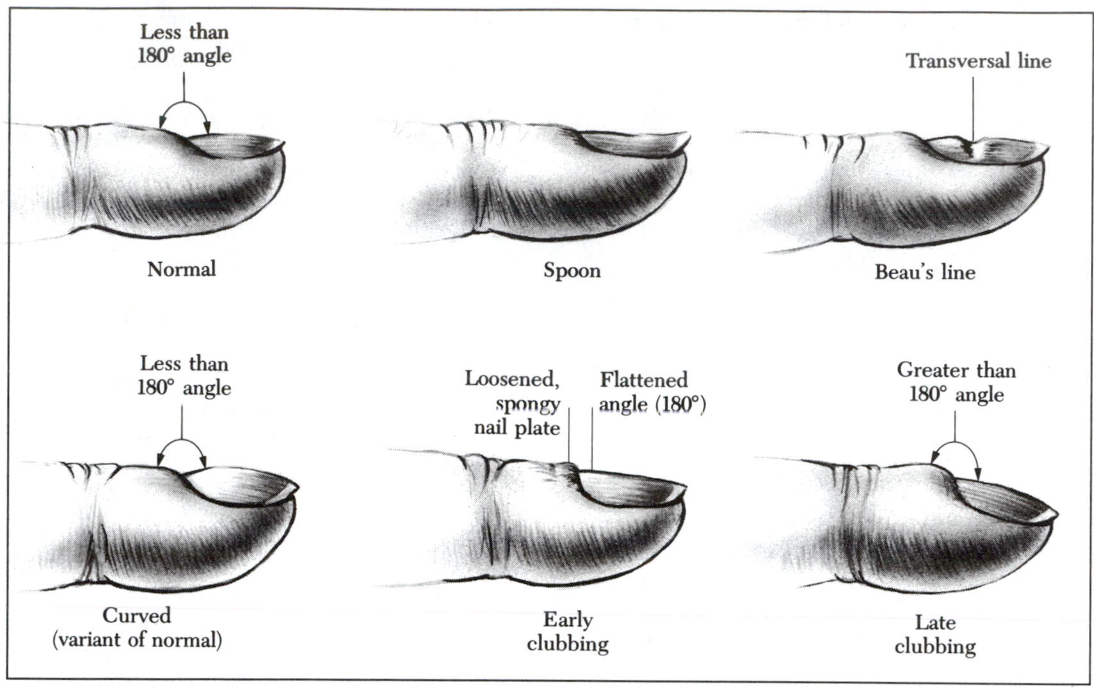

FIGURE 8-2 Normal and abnormal nails. (Source: Grimes J, Burns E (eds.): *Health Assessment in Nursing Practice* (ed. 2). Boston: Jones and Bartlett, 1987.)

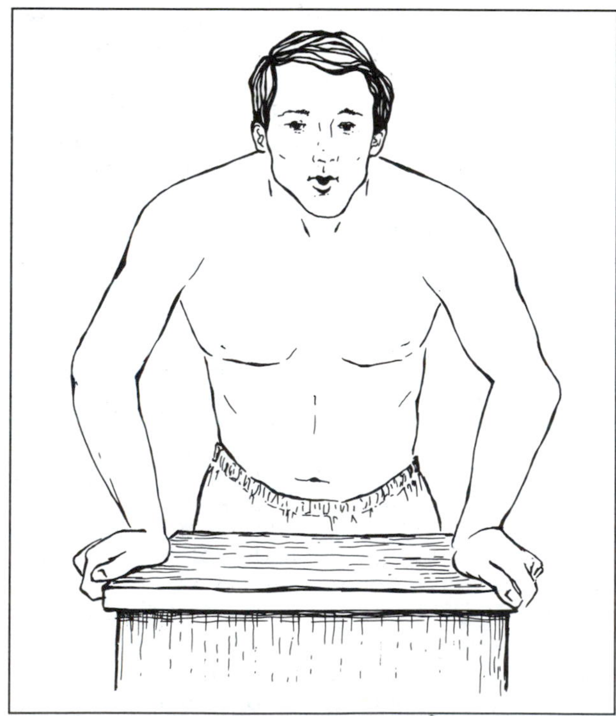

FIGURE 8-3 Patient fixes the arms and leans forward to use pectoral muscles as accessory inspiratory muscles for obstructed breathing. (Source: Buckingham W: *A Primer of Clinical Diagnosis* (ed. 2). New York: Harper & Row, 1979.)

Vocal fremitus Decreased or absent vocal fremitus indicates local bronchial obstruction from bronchial carcinomas, adenomas, or foreign bodies. Sound transmission through the bronchus is interrupted, causing the change in fremitus. Absent vocal fremitus also may indicate pleural effusions. Lung tumors immediately adjacent to the visceral pleura often cause early, insidious formation of pleural effusion that is responsible for the initial complaint of dyspnea.[74]

Percussion and auscultation These may provide the final clues to assessment of the individual who is at high risk for lung cancer. Auscultation is best done with the diaphragm of the stethoscope in a slow, methodical sequence of upper, middle, and lower zones and front, sides, and back. Physical signs that would require referral are discussed next.

Dullness Dullness on percussion indicates either pleural effusion or a consolidated lung. The normal sound percussed over the lung is resonance. Lung cancer is the most common cause of hemorrhagic pleural effusion in middle-aged and elderly male smokers. The early production of pleural fluid by most tumors produces the classic signs of pleural effusion: flatness, absence of fremitus, and breath sounds.[75] An excellent technique for assessing dullness in the thorax is the auscultatory-percussion technique. This technique is accomplished by having the examiner lightly percuss the patient's manubrium while listening with the diaphragm piece on the posterior chest wall (Figure 8-4[76]).

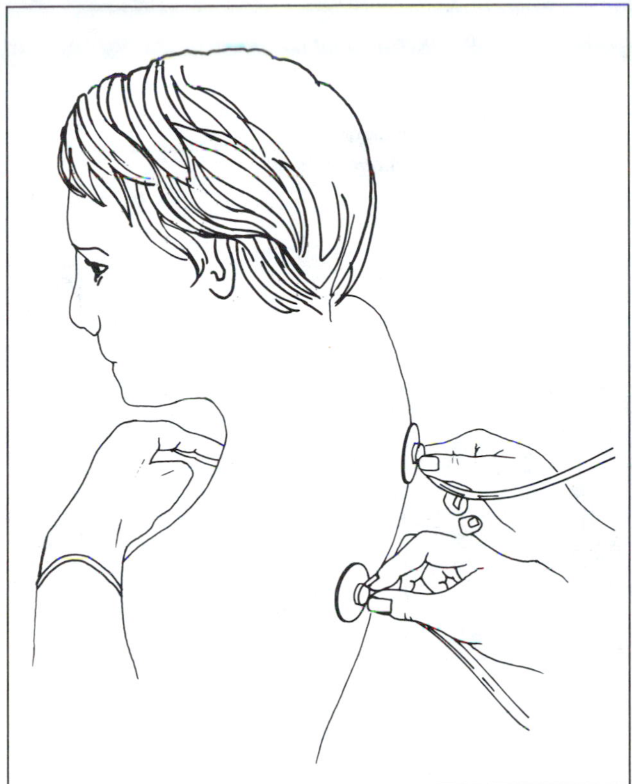

FIGURE 8-4 Auscultatory-percussion technique. (Source: Guarino J: Auscultatory-percussion, a technique for detecting unsuspected lung disease. *Diagnosis* January: 20–26, 1981.)

In the normal chest the sound on auscultatory percussion is resonant. If any pathologic condition exists between the sound source (manubrium) and the reception point (stethoscope), the sound produced is a duller tone than normal. This technique enables the examiner to detect small, deep areas of pathologic disease.

Decreased or absent breath sounds Breath sounds are decreased or absent when air flow is decreased or when fluid or tissue separates the air passages from the stethoscope.

Unilateral wheezing and the bagpipe sign Tumors in the main bronchus may cause a localized expiratory and/or inspiratory wheeze, or "honk," which sometimes is reproduced only when the individual lies on the affected side. When a continuous wheeze is heard at the end of expiration as air continues to whistle out past a partial obstruction, this is known as the *bagpipe sign*.[74]

Presence of whispered pectoriloquy, bronchophony, and egophony When the lungs are normal, whispered test words are faint and their syllables are not distinct when the examiner listens with a stethoscope over the lungs. When a lung is consolidated or compressed by a pleural effusion, transmission of voice sounds is altered. The sounds are louder, clearer than usual, and sometimes changed in quality. On the basis of these three criteria, the following changes are noted:

1. *Whispered pectoriloquy.* The patient whispers numerals (e.g., one, two, and three). Normally these sounds are muffled; in consolidation they are clearly transmitted.[77]

2. *Bronchophony.* When the patient says a number (e.g., 99), the sound normally is muffled. When the sound transmitted is a clear sound of the vocalized numerals, it is created by mucous- or fluid-filled alveoli or by cellular mass replacing alveolar tissue.[78]

3. *Egophony.* The patient says *e*, which normally results in a muffled, indistinct sound. In pleural effusion the *e* sound is heard as a nasal-sounding *a*.

In conclusion, there are no physical signs or symptoms in the early stage of lung cancer. The majority of physical signs the practitioner would discover during physical assessment are the result of late and far-advanced carcinoma of the lung. Figure 8-5 presents a synopsis of the physical findings commonly seen with tumors of different anatomic sites in the lungs. The majority of physical signs discussed previously are found in late or advanced lung cancer. The *only early* physical finding that most strongly suggests lung cancer is wheezing localized to a single lobe of the lung in an elderly person with a long history of smoking.

Screening tests for asymptomatic individuals

There are no recommended screening programs or tests for lung cancer because studies have not shown any evidence of a significant reduction in mortality from these programs. The American Cancer Society focuses on primary prevention: helping smokers to stop and keeping nonsmokers from starting.[79]

Smoking cessation

The greatest reduction in mortality can be achieved by cessation of smoking. Between 80% and 85% of deaths from lung cancer are directly attributable to smoking, thus making smoking the leading cause of cancer mortality in the United States.[80] Smoking in the United States is on the decline. Per capita cigarette consumption among adults fell from 4141 in 1974 to 3196 in 1987, and this is the lowest per capita consumption since 1944.[81] In general, smoking prevalence is decreasing across all race-gender groups, although at a slower rate for women than men.[82] However, there are distinct groups of Americans who start or who continue to smoke. In general, blue-collar workers, high school graduates, and men with lower incomes are more likely to smoke than men with college educations, white-collar occupations, and high-level incomes.[80] In contrast, women who work are more likely to smoke than housewives and women in households with low family incomes. The latest data collected by the National Health

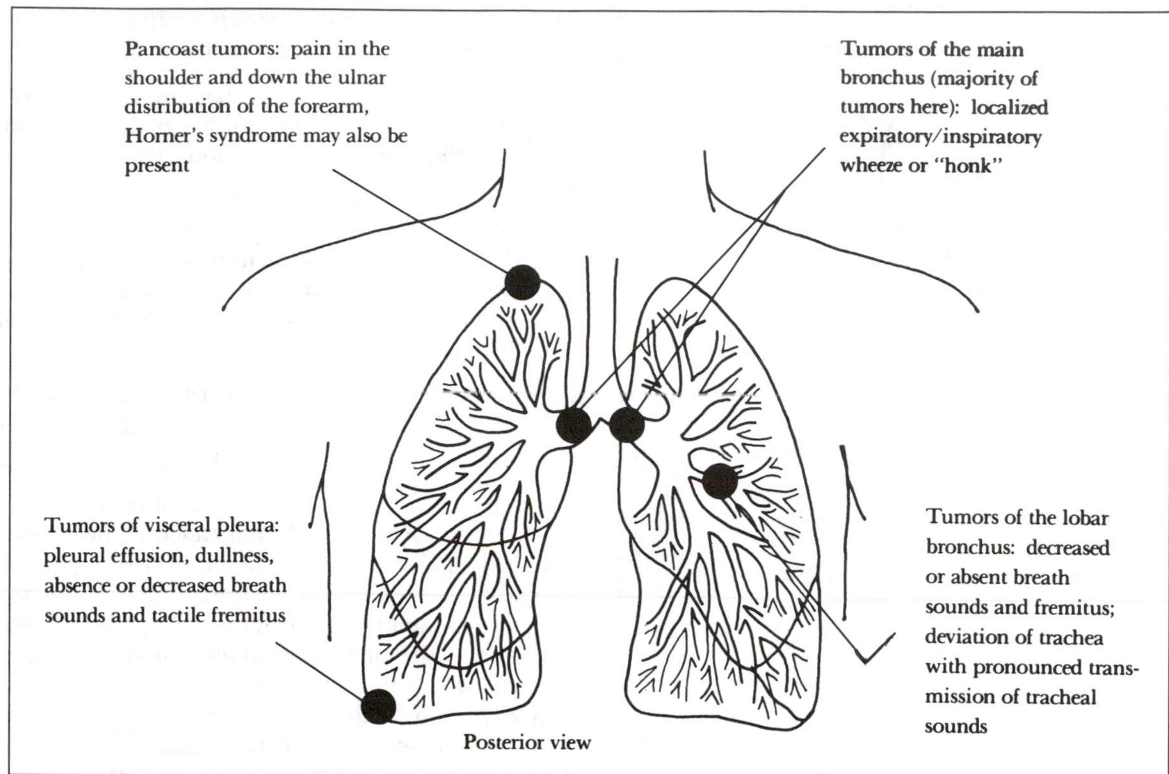

FIGURE 8-5 Synopsis of physical findings of lung cancer.

Interview Surveys indicate that educational level is the major demographic predictor of whether an individual will smoke cigarettes. Regardless of gender, a person who does not attend college is more than twice as likely to start smoking than the person who does. In addition, smoking cessation occurs more frequently in groups with higher levels of education than in groups with less education, and the gap is widening over time.[83]

Several cigarette advertising campaigns have been directed to groups that tend to smoke (women, minorities, and blue-collar workers) in order to recruit new smokers or to increase cigarette consumption among smokers.[84] Knowing the groups that tend to smoke and that are being targeted by the tobacco industry should assist health professionals in identifying and predicting patterns of cigarette use and in developing health promotion materials specifically designed for these high-risk groups.[85] The Yellow Pages at the back of this text list smoking cessation materials specifically written for blue-collar workers, minorities, and women.

Obviously, the nurse wants to monitor most aggressively those who smoke, who have had a history of heavy smoking, or who were employed in high-risk occupations. These individuals should have (1) a complete baseline respiratory assessment, (2) a thorough assessment of respiratory symptoms, and (3) physical assessment of their respiratory system at periodic intervals. Deviations from normal merit referral for chest x-ray studies and/or sputum cytologic findings. In this high-risk population a cold that lingers or "smoker's cough" that is accompanied by fatigue and weight loss should not be ignored.

One fallacy commonly heard about individuals who smoke is that because they have smoked for years, "what harm is there in letting them continue?" Nothing could be further from the truth or more detrimental to their health. Continual smoking damages not only their already compromised respiratory system but their cardiovascular system as well. Research clearly documents that smoking cessation results in improved sensory, respiratory, and cardiovascular status.[86] Fielding,[80] in a review on the health effects of smoking, noted that a British physician study reported that exsmokers who had not smoked for 5 years had a lung cancer mortality rate approximately 40% that of a current smoker. After 15 years without smoking the mortality rate of exsmokers was only slightly greater than that of nonsmokers. No one is ever too old nor has smoked too long to *stop* smoking.

The nurse should take a nonjudgmental approach with those who refuse or are unable to stop smoking. The 1988 surgeon general's report stated that "an extensive body of research has shown that nicotine is the drug in tobacco that causes addiction. However, the processes that determine tobacco addiction are similar to those that determine addiction to drugs such as heroin and cocaine."[87] Because of the addicting qualities of nicotine, many exsmokers are not able to give up the habit on the first attempt but must try three or more times before finally succeeding.[82] In the hope of reducing the adverse health consequences of smoking, health professionals frequently advise individuals who cannot quit to smoke fewer cigarettes, to smoke cigarettes with less than 10 mg of tar, to smoke filtered cigarettes, and to smoke only half of each cigarette. However, habitual smokers may compensate for the reduced number of cigarettes by taking in more smoke per cigarette ("oversmoking").[88]

The nurse needs to be aware and share with the smoking public that the introduction of smokeless cigarettes by tobacco companies (e.g., R.J. Reynolds) will expose smokers to the same levels of carbon monoxide and nicotine as conventional cigarettes.[89] Many authorities view the new smokeless cigarette as a novel device for nicotine delivery.

It is the nurse's responsibility to disseminate information actively and assertively on the disease potential of smoking whenever possible. Every assistance should be afforded to help those who want to stop smoking. Nurses who smoke are less likely to discuss health-promoting behaviors with patients, that is, the need to stop smoking or the various smoking cessation methods that can be employed to stop successfully.[90,91] It is essential that nurses act as role models by not smoking and by actively working at creating nonsmoking environments in both their employment and their home settings.

Nurses have frequent opportunities to advise smokers to quit either in health care settings or in the community. The importance of counseling smokers to quit is underscored by the research of Anda et al.[92] In their study of 5875 Michigan adults who smoked, of those who had seen a physician in the previous year, only 44% reported being told to quit smoking by a physician. In general, most smokers did not perceive physicians to be even minimally involved in their efforts to quit. In fairness to physicians, there may be a tendency for smokers to hear only what they want to hear.[93] For this reason, the U.S. Preventive Services Task Force recommends that smokers be exposed to a variety of intervention techniques on multiple occasions delivered by *both* physicians and nonphysicians to improve smoking cessation rates.[94] Kottke et al.[95] also found that the best results for helping smokers quit was to use a team of physicians and nonphysicians that employed multiple intervention modalities to deliver individualized advice on multiple occasions. The multiple smoking cessation interventions suggested by all authorities include the following:

1. direct, face-to-face advice and suggestions on smoking cessation
2. smoking cessation self-help materials that are culturally and educationally relevant to the individual person
3. referral to community smoking cessation programs
4. drug therapy when appropriate (e.g., nicotine gum, nicotine patch)
5. scheduled reinforcement with the smoker

Table 8-1 presents the process the nurse should follow to successfully assist the smoker in quitting, and

TABLE 8-1 Smoking Cessation Intervention Process

1. Initiate discussion of patient's smoking behavior
    - Review smoking history
    - Provide risk–benefit information, personalizing when possible
    - Assess health beliefs about smoking
2. Assess interest in smoking cessation
    - Determine patient's readiness to quit in terms of motivation, intention, and self-efficacy
3. Set the target quit-date
    - Pick a realistic calendar quit-date
    - Stop smoking "cold turkey"
4. Suggest smoking cessation strategies
    - Provide materials and referral sources
    - Describe preparatory techniques
        - List reasons for quitting
        - Become aware of smoking-related situations
        - Seek social support
        - Reduce number of cigarettes and/or amount of nicotine
        - Replace cigarettes with gum or food (preferably low-fat, low-calorie)
        - Eliminate environmental cues
        - Avoid, distract, delay
    - Discuss withdrawal symptoms
    - Review cognitive and behavioral strategies to use in high-risk situations—social, relaxation, work, and upsetting situations
5. Follow up
    - Encourage the maintenance of successful abstinence and discuss "slips"
    - Review relapse—motivate patient to resume cessation

Source: Gritz E: Cigarette smoking: The need for action by health professionals. Reprinted by permission from *Ca-A Cancer Journal for Clinicians* in (*CA* 38:194–212, 1988). Copyright 1988 American Cancer Society. Preparation of this article was supported by the National Cancer Institute of the National Institutes of Health (Grants CA36409 & CA43461).

Table 8-2 lists the factors associated with successful smoking cessation.[96] When individuals are referred to smoking cessation programs, it is advised that cost effectiveness be considered in the selection. Altman et al.[97] found that, although self-help programs had the lowest total cost and lowest time requirement for participants, their quit rate percentage was the lowest. In contrast, smoking cessation classes were expensive but had the most success in getting individuals to stop smoking.

A new development to assist smokers in quitting is the nicotine patch (e.g., Habitrol, Nicoderm, Prostep, Nicotrol, Nicolan, Nicotinell). These patches are available in three sizes that deliver 21 mg, 14 mg, or 7 mg of nicotine over 16–24 hours. The nicotine is either directly released through the skin or through a membrane system in contact with the skin. Side effects have been found to be minimal and include: mild-to-moderate sleep disturbances; skin reactions including transient itching, burning, and erythema; poorly defined body aches; and increased cough.

Significant changes in the social and work-related environments have occurred in this country that have resulted in less tolerance of smoking and that have made

TABLE 8-2 Factors Associated with Successful Smoking Cessation

Motivational Factors
Desire to overcome minor smoking-related symptoms (coughing, wheezing, shortness of breath)
Expectation of improved future health
Sense of personal vulnerability to risk
Desire to increase self-mastery and self-esteem
Expectation of many quitting benefits—health, freedom, social, and economic
Expectation of success
Expectation that benefits will outweigh difficulties
Support and encouragement from family (especially spouse), friends, work associates
Effective Quitting Skills
Quitting abruptly instead of tapering off
Using a variety of coping methods for withdrawal symptoms, such as deep breathing, positive thinking, and specific cigarette substitutes
Using a variety of methods to remain off cigarettes, such as avoiding temptations to smoke, finding alternative ways to relax and to cope with stress (such as hobbies or exercise), using substitute self-rewards to counteract sense of loss and prevent relapse
Taking a long-range, problem-solving approach
Social Supports/Psychosocial Assets
Personalized and medical quit-smoking advice and support
Encouragement, inspiration, and advice from exsmokers
Good psychosocial resources (such as education and income)
Smoking Habit Factors
Lower smoking rate and nicotine intake/dependence
Less reliance on cigarettes for regulation of negative effect
Past success in quitting for 6 months or more
Good stress management skills

Source: Orleans CT: Understanding and promoting smoking cessation: Overview of guidelines for physician intervention *Annu Rev Med* 36:51–61, 1985.

smokers more receptive to the antismoking messages of health professionals. The 1987 Bureau of National Affairs survey of 623 large corporations found that 54% had adopted some type of plan to restrict employee smoking. This was a 36% increase from a similar survey the previous year.[98] In the health care field more than 90% of hospitals have a smoking policy; 8% of those have banned smoking completely.[99] In addition, 43 states have passed laws that place limitations on smoking.[100] These antismoking policies appear to have a dramatic effect on the nation's smoking habits. Theoretically, they will encourage people to quit smoking by increasing the social pressure against it and by restricting the time available for it.

Gastrointestinal Cancer

Colorectal cancer incidence and mortality in the United States are second only to those of lung cancer. It is estimated that in 1993, 152,000 new colorectal cases will be diagnosed, and 57,000 people will die of this cancer. In both men and women 35 years of age and older, colorectal cancer is one of the leading causes of deaths from cancer.[64]

History assessment

Several conditions and health practices must be questioned to obtain a realistic picture of the patient's gastrointestinal system. For example, after the age of 50 years, approximately 25% of the population has demonstrable diverticulosis, and by age 80 years the proportion is 70%.[100] Slight rectal bleeding commonly is found with this disorder. Another condition that causes symptoms that mimic gastrointestinal cancer is depression. Depression is more common in the elderly than in the young because of increasing losses and limitations that accompany the aging process.[100] Some of the cardinal manifestations of depression are anorexia, constipation, and somatic pains. In addition, weight loss in the elderly may be due to nutritional disturbances rather than a malignancy. Loss of income, depression, decreased sensation of taste, loss of teeth, and difficulty swallowing all contribute to decreased food intake. Another important part of the nursing assessment is a thorough history of drug intake. The elderly tend to use aspirin frequently for the pain of arthritis and to abuse laxatives. Laxative abuse is the most common cause of diarrhea in this age-group, especially among women.[101] Considering these factors, the history and review of systems should include the following questions:

1. Do you have a history of cancer of the bowel or ulcerative colitis?
2. Have you ever been told you have polyps of the bowel? Gardner's syndrome? Have you had any polyps removed?
3. Do any of your relatives have (or have any had) bowel cancer?
4. Would you characterize your diet as consisting of more red meat than fish, veal, and poultry? Has your diet usually consisted of more starches and sweets than vegetables and fruits? Would you characterize your diet as being high in fats?
5. Do you take laxatives? If so, what kind, how often, what amount? How long have you taken laxatives?
6. Have you noticed a difference in your bowel habits? Do you have more constipation, more diarrhea? Do these two conditions seem to alternate?
7. What is your usual bowel habit? Has this changed in the last few years? Has the shape of your bowel movements changed recently?
8. Have you ever been told you have diverticulosis? ulcers? nervous stomach?

9. Have you had gastrointestinal x-ray studies within the last 2 to 3 years? Have you had a barium enema, proctoscope, or related procedure to examine your rectum and colon in the last 2 to 3 years? If you did, why was the test done and what were the results?
10. Do you take aspirin? How often and how much? What other medications (antacids, stool softeners, antispasmodics) are you now taking?
11. Are you familiar with at-home stool guaiac testing? Have you ever used this?
12. Do you have hemorrhoids or anal fissures?
13. Have you noticed any change in appetite? Are you experiencing nausea or vomiting?
14. Have you experienced any weight loss recently?
15. Do you have excessive gas? feelings of being bloated? abdominal pain?
16. Do you have the feeling after you have a bowel movement that you still have to go to the bathroom and expel more stool? Do you experience pain before, with, or after defecation?

The signs and symptoms of cancers of the colon and rectum often are related to the portion of intestine involved. Figure 8-6 identifies the most frequent presenting signs and symptoms of each area of the intestinal tract affected by cancer.

Physical examination

Inspection The assessment of the gastrointestinal system begins with inspection. The findings that may suggest cancer of the system include the following:

1. Nodular umbilicus. Abdominal carcinoma, especially gastric, may metastasize to the navel. This is called Sister Joseph's nodule.

2. Masses that distort the abdominal profile and indicate organomegaly.

3. Subcutaneous nodules under the skin that are visible with tangential lighting.

4. Distention. The abdominal profile should be inspected because neoplasms can distort the profile. The examiner may see distention of the lower half, lower third, or upper half of the abdomen.

5. Venous distention caused by blockage of the inferior vena cava, which can occur from spread of cancer. In this condition there is edema of the eyelids, a bluish face and lips, prominent neck veins, and pitting edema of the arms and large veins over the upper portions of the chest and shoulders.

6. Visible peristaltic waves, which may appear in normal persons with thin abdomens and may be accen-

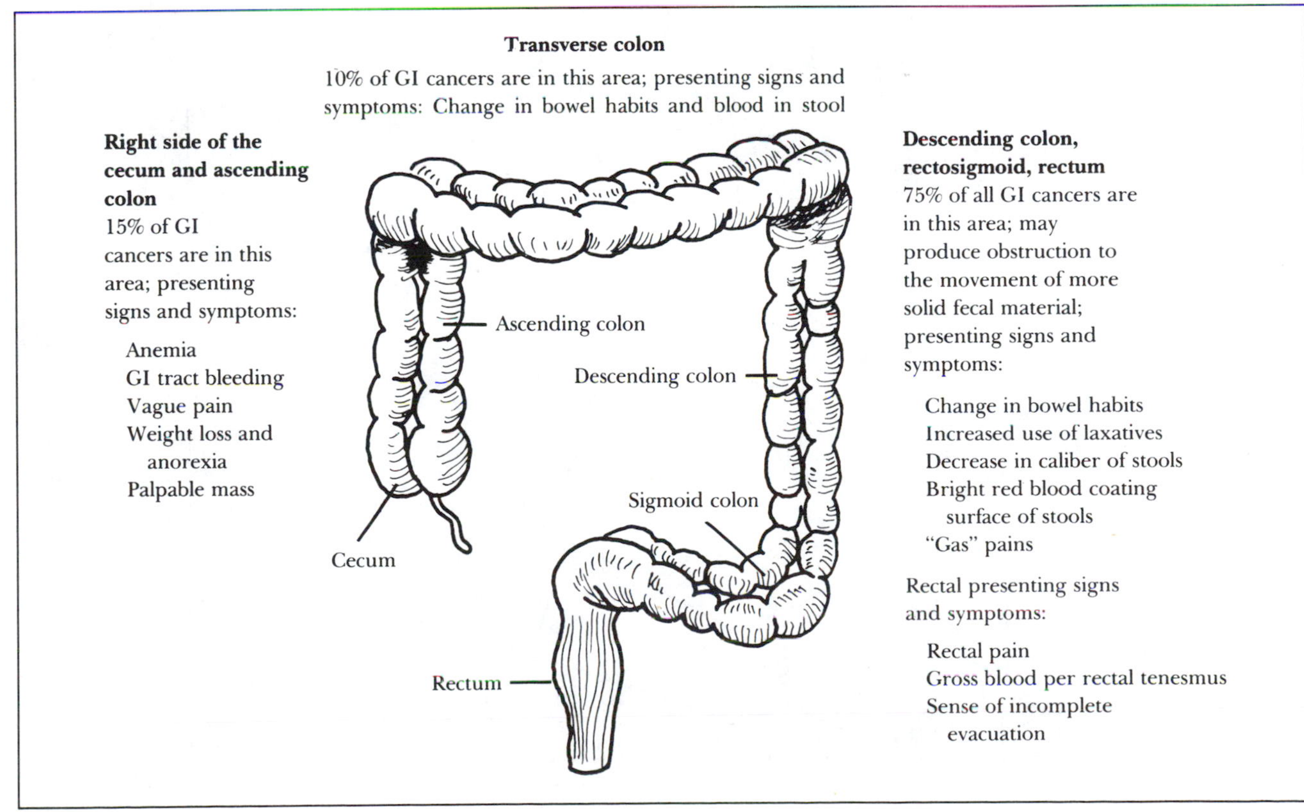

FIGURE 8-6 Presenting signs and symptoms of colorectal cancers based on location in the intestinal tract.

tuated in patients with obstruction to the forward passage of gastrointestinal contents. Small-bowel obstruction gives rise to a condition resembling a "bag of worms" or a "step ladder." Numerous segments of small bowel contract and relax in an irregular manner, and the peristalsis has no recognizable pattern.[72]

7. Bulging of the flanks may signal intraabdominal fluid.

Auscultation After a thorough inspection of the abdomen is performed with the use of tangential lighting, the abdomen should be auscultated. Bowel sounds that are heard without the use of a stethoscope are called *Borborygmi.* Bowel sounds heard with the stethoscope bell range from absent to frequent. The significance of the different types of bowel sounds includes the following:

- High-pitched, long, intense peristaltic rushes occur with any hypermotile state such as partial obstruction.
- High-pitched "tingling" sounds indicate a more complete mechanical intestinal obstruction.
- Extremely weak or infrequent sounds may also indicate bowel immobility.
- Absent bowel sounds, determined by listening to the bowel for at least *5 minutes,* may indicate advanced intestinal obstruction.

Another sound that may signal obstruction of the small intestines is a *succussion splash.* Succussion splash is produced by a combination of air and fluid in the gut when the examiner "tingles" the stomach or vigorously moves the abdomen. The sound resembles very loud splashes.

Some abdominal circulatory sounds also signal cancer (Figure 8-7). A bruit heard over the liver with the bell of the stethoscope when the patient takes a deep breath may indicate a hepatoma with arteriovenous shunting. In addition, a hepatic friction rub heard with the bell of the stethoscope may also indicate a hepatoma. A bruit heard over the pancreas may indicate pancreatic carcinoma. A murmur over the left hypochondrium is one of the rare physical signs that suggests an early carcinoma of the body of the pancreas. Thus auscultation of the abdomen may indicate a bowel obstruction, a hepatoma, or pancreatic carcinoma.

Palpation and percussion The information obtained from inspection and auscultation should alert the examiner to expected findings during palpation and percussion of the abdomen. It is important to remember

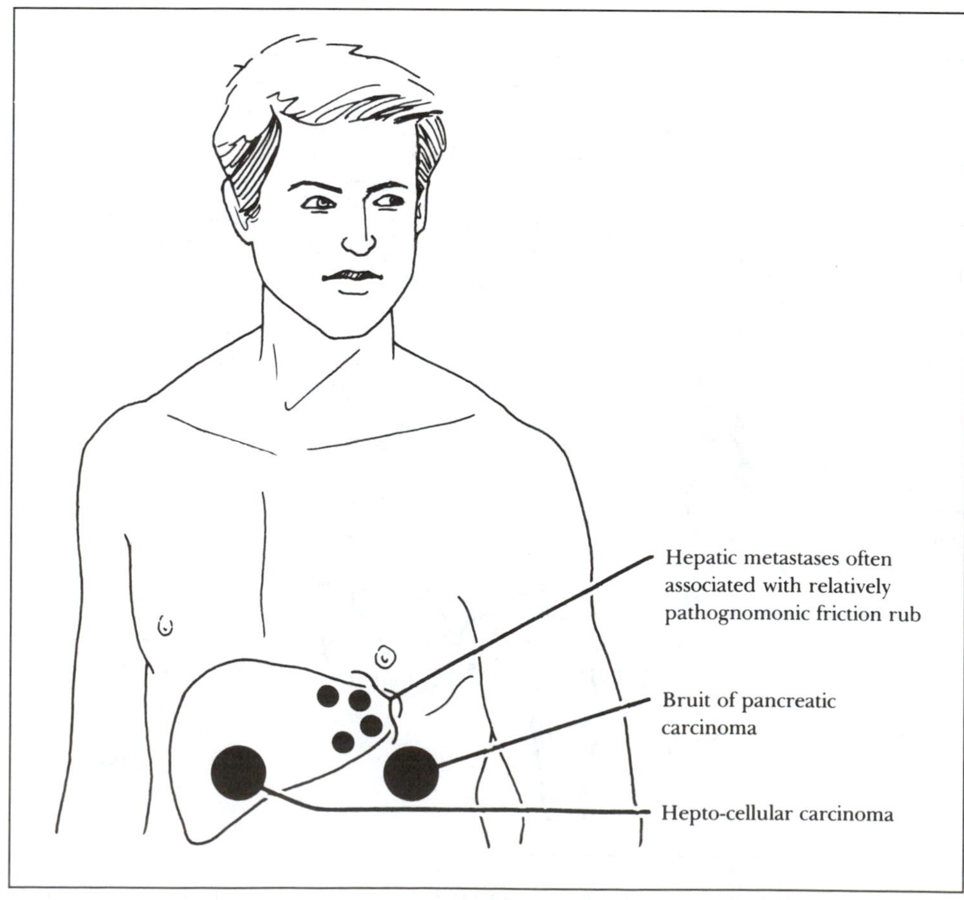

FIGURE 8-7 Abdominal sounds that indicate cancer.

that on palpation of the abdomen the organs that are normally palpated are the abdominal aorta, the edge of the liver, the lower pole of the right kidney, the descending colon and the sigmoid, and the ascending colon. The following findings on palpation and percussion merit further attention, and many signal colorectal cancer.

Hepatomegaly Total liver span is the best estimate of liver size because liver height cannot be determined by feeling only the edge. Palpation alone detects the inferior portion as it descends below the costal margin. A normal liver at the midclavicular line is 10–12 cm in span. Nodules on the liver or an irregular edge suggest malignancy.

Splenomegaly Because the normal spleen is rarely palpable, a spleen that descends below the left costal margin on deep inspiration is enlarged. Cancer conditions that enlarge the spleen are leukemias and lymphomas.

Enlargement of the colon Carcinoma of the colon may produce a palpable mass anywhere along the course of the colon.

Fluid Several tests can be used to determine if there is free fluid in the abdomen. The presence of intraperitoneal fluid is suspected when there is abdominal distention with bulging flanks and possibly an everted umbilicus. *Shifting dullness* and *fluid wave* are two tests frequently used to detect fluid in the abdomen. The *puddle sign* has the advantage of detecting small amounts of intraabdominal fluid. After the patient has been on hands and knees for several minutes, the examiner percusses the periumbilical area to detect a line between fluid and air, as in the determination of shifting dullness. As little as several hundred milliliters of ascitic fluid can be detected by this method.[75]

Rectal examination Half the cancers that occur in the rectum and colon are within reach of the examining finger. Lesions high in the rectum are sometimes felt more readily when the patient bears down as if having a bowel movement. On palpation the examiner may feel a *rectal shelf,* which, in men, is a stony hard mass above the prostate on the anterior rectal wall. In women it is felt as a stony hard mass in the cul-de-sac. The shelf indicates a carcinoma that has metastasized to the pelvic floor and therefore is a sign of advanced malignancy. Carcinoma of the rectum causes plateaulike, nodular, annular, and cauliflower masses in the rectum.[73]

• • •

Several physical findings in other parts of the body, which are not revealed in the abdominal examination, are typical in abdominal carcinoma. For instance, enlargement of a single node, usually in the left supraclavicular group, is the site of carcinomatous metastasis from a primary lesion in the upper portion of the abdomen. This node, called *Virchow's node,* is frequently behind the clavicular head of the left supraclavicular group. The Valsalva maneuver causes the node to rise, which enables the nurse to palpate Virchow's node.

Another physical finding that indicates abdominal carcinoma is *acanthosis nigricans,* a skin lesion. Acanthosis nigricans is probably the most well-known cutaneous marker of internal malignancy. It is a velvety, brownish skin eruption that strongly suggests an intestinal malignancy when it occurs in patients older than 40 years of age.[72,102]

Another systemic finding that is connected with pathologic findings of the gastrointestinal system is jaundice. Jaundice and accompanying steady pain may indicate hepatic or pancreatic lesions. Although painless obstructive jaundice is said to be a feature of carcinoma of the head of the pancreas, about 70% of patients with pancreatic cancer have some degree of anterior abdominal or back pain.[72] By means of daylight or fluorescent light the sclerae, the undersurface of the tongue, and the frenulum of the tongue should be examined for jaundice.

In conclusion, although there are many physical findings that suggest cancer of the gastrointestinal system, the findings that *most strongly* suggest cancer of the colorectal area are (1) a mass palpated in the rectum, (2) a palpable mass in the abdomen, and (3) evidence of blood in the feces. Nurses who work with the elderly or high-risk individuals in nursing homes, residential settings, acute-care institutions, and physician's offices are encouraged to take the time to thoroughly assess an individual's gastrointestinal complaints. Often the elderly will share their complaints with the nurse rather than the physician because they hesitate to bother the doctor with "trivial" problems.

Screening tests for asymptomatic individuals

Presently the two most important screening tests for asymptomatic persons are examination of the feces for occult blood and the digital rectal examination.[103] There is professional debate about the use of fecal occult blood tests as a mass screening tool. The results from the only true randomized controlled study in this country that assessed the effect of occult blood screening on colorectal cancer mortality has thus far failed to show any reduction in mortality.[104] The University of Minnesota School of Public Health has been amassing data on colorectal cancer detection since 1975. More than 46,000 people between the ages of 50 and 80 years have participated in the study. They were randomly assigned to three groups. One group was given an annual fecal occult blood test, another group was screened with the test every second year, and a control group was not offered the test. Only 2.3% of those with a positive slide result have been found to have colorectal cancer.[105] It is argued that although the test itself is inexpensive, the recommended follow-up diagnostic procedure is expensive. For instance, if 1 million people were screened, about 100,000 of them (10%) would show positive findings and the costs of the follow-up tests would be $50 million for the detection of 2300 colorectal cancers.[105]

Another problem with occult blood tests is the number of false-positive results that necessitate additional tests. It is recommended by the manufacturer that fecal occult test slides be rehydrated with a drop of water before development. This increases the sensitivity but decreases the specificity of the test.[106] The increased sensitivity after rehydration means that the number of false-positive test results increases as the specificity decreases. A Swedish study[106] documented that rehydration of Hemoccult II slides is necessary because significantly more carcinomas were found in the rehydrated group compared with the unrehydrated group of slides. Table 8-3 presents the causes of false-positive and false-negative test results in the use of Hemoccult slides.[107]

The American Gastroenterological Association and the American Society for Gastrointestinal Endoscopy recommend the following screening techniques for identification of colorectal adenomas and early detection of cancer. For the asymptomatic average-risk population, a digital rectal examination should be performed in persons 40 years of age and older, and fecal occult blood testing and flexible sigmoidoscopic examination in those 50 years of age and older.[108] In contrast, the U.S. Preventive Services Task Force states that there is

> insufficient evidence to make a recommendation either for or against fecal occult blood screening for individuals aged 45 years and older. Screening of individuals younger than age 45 years is not recommended. Based on the higher expected prevalence in individuals aged 45 years and older with a family history of colorectal cancer in a first-order relative, a stronger a priori argument can be made for screening in this group.[109]

TABLE 8-3 Causes of False-Positive and False-Negative Tests Using the Hemoccult Method

False-Positive Tests	False-Negative Tests
Meat in diet	Failure to employ high-residue diet
Medications; antibiotics, aspirin, anti-inflammatories, oral iron compounds	Vitamin C in diet
Diverticulosis	Time lag between specimen collection and specimen examination
Minor anorectal problems Hemorrhoids Fissures Proctitis	Failure to prepare slides properly or complete all six slides
Peroxidases in skins of vegetables and fruits (tomatoes and cherries)	Follow-up examinations that failed to detect lesion
Upper gastrointestinal pathology Gastritis from ASA ingestion Ulcer disease	Lesion not bleeding at the time of stool collection
Hiatus hernia	Outdated Hemoccult slides or reagent
Gastric malignancy	

Source: Sugarbaker P, Gunderson L, Wittes R: Colorectal cancer. In DeVita VT, Hellman S, Rosenberg SA (eds.): *Cancer: Principles and Practice of Oncology* (ed. 2). Philadelphia: Lippincott, 1986, pp. 795–884.

Although it is acknowledged that the role of fecal occult blood tests in the early detection of colorectal cancer is still being evaluated, the nurse should be aware of the following specific recommendations that will increase the accuracy of the test:

1. Duplicate samples should be taken from different parts of the feces each day for 3 consecutive days while the patient follows a meat-free diet.[110] It is important for the nurse to encourage the patient to collect stool for 3 consecutive days because not all bowel cancers bleed, and occult blood is not always uniformly distributed in feces. Increasing the numbers of tests may therefore address these two causes of false-negative tests.[111] Presently no scientific validation exists for a high-residue diet during the 3 days of stool specimen collection.[111]

2. During the 3 days of stool collection, patients should avoid:
- a. aspirin-containing compounds (cause false-positive reaction)
- b. antibiotics (cause false-positive reaction)
- c. anti-inflammatory drugs (cause false-positive reaction)
- d. ascorbic acid (cause false-negative reaction)
- e. foods high in peroxidase—broccoli, cabbage, potatoes, cantaloupe, turnips, apricots, apples, pears, horseradish (cause false-positive reaction)
- f. oral iron compounds (cause false-positive reactions)[112]

3. The stool specimens should be read within 6 days of collection because delay contributes to false-negative reactions.

Because of the false-positive and false-negative results frequently obtained with the present tests for occult stool by means of guaiac-impregnated cards, alternate methods to detect colorectal cancer are being sought. Several researchers have published preliminary data on immunochemical tests that do not rely on blood loss to detect gastrointestinal changes caused by cancer.[109,113,114] Clinical studies to validate the usefulness of these tests are being conducted. HemoQuant (SmithKline Diagnostics, Sunnyvale, Calif.) is a quantitative assay based on the conversion of heme to fluorescent porphyrins. It appears to be unaffected by dietary factors, specimen storage and hydration, and medication and seems to be as effective as the Hemoccult slide test. HemoQuant also distinguishes between heme that has been converted chemically during gut transmit and heme that has not, thus giving information about the level of bleeding in the gastrointestinal system. However, it costs several times as much as Hemoccult.[108,109]

In general, compliance with the collection of fecal occult blood tests tends to be poor, with rates of 22%–

30% reported.[111] Those who are most likely to be helped by screening (e.g., the elderly) are less likely to cooperate. Those studies that report good compliance usually deal with a highly motivated or selected group of volunteers.

The carcinoembryonic antigen (CEA) assay is not conclusive for the initial proven diagnosis of colorectal cancer.[103] A normal level does not rule out colon cancer, and elevated levels have been found in cancer of the pancreas as well as in nonmalignant diseases of the colon, lung, and liver. Because it is nonspecific, it is not considered a good screening test for colorectal cancer.

The American Cancer Society recommendations for screening asymptomatic patients for colorectal cancer are shown in Figure 8-8.

Additional nursing interventions

Nurses have a variety of roles in colorectal cancer detection. Not only are they practitioners, they also are educators, coordinators, counselors, and researchers. One of the most important roles the nurse assumes is that of educator. Two surveys conducted by the Gallup Organization for the American Cancer Society have

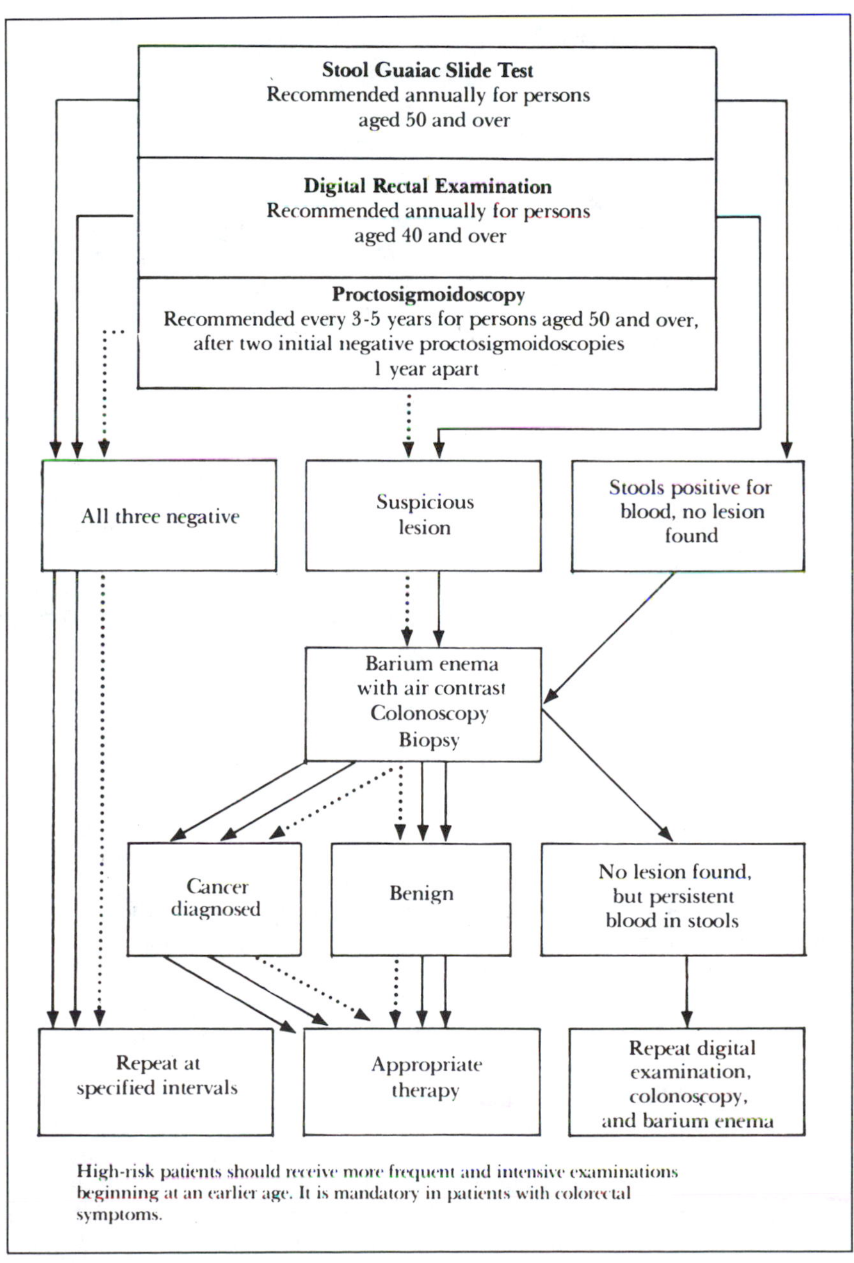

FIGURE 8-8 Diagnostic guide for asymptomatic patients. (Source: Leffall L: *Early Diagnosis of Colorectal Cancer.* New York: American Cancer Society [Professional Educational Publication 81-50M-No. 3311-PE], 1981.)

found that only a small percentage of the public has taken the necessary steps to detect colorectal cancer at its earliest stages.[115] The surveys also revealed that very few people were asking their physicians for the tests during regular physical examinations. There was also little knowledge about this type of cancer, and attitudes toward its early detection were pessimistic. A little more than one-third of Americans in the 40-plus age group knew that colorectal cancer was one of the most common forms of cancer. More than 40% believed that surgery for colorectal cancer would result in a permanent colostomy, and more than 50% had little faith that anything could be done to cure colorectal cancer. In addition, there were general misconceptions about the recommended early detection tests. Twenty-five percent believed that if no blood is found in a stool blood test, then the digital rectal and proctoscopic examinations would not be needed.

As educators, nurses can play an important role in colorectal cancer detection by (1) informing the general public about colon and rectum cancer, as well as by making a special effort to inform the elderly and other high-risk groups, and (2) encouraging the participation of the general public and high-risk groups in early detection of the disease through the use of a stool guaiac slide test, digital rectal examination, and, after 50 years of age, proctosigmoidoscopic examination. The most effective public education approach to general screening for colorectal cancer ("the cancer nobody talks about") is (1) to emphasize the effectiveness of the stool guaiac test, (2) to stress that it is painless and convenient (it can be administered in the privacy of one's home), and (3) to indicate the value of early detection of colorectal cancer (e.g., President Reagan's successful bout with a malignant tumor of the colon).[116]

Nurses who work in community organizations, clinics, nursing homes, retirement centers, geriatric day care centers, and hospitals are in ideal settings to provide education and plan and participate in colorectal screening programs. These screening programs could be conducted by community organizations such as the American Cancer Society, local service groups, and community religious groups, with the nurse coordinating the efforts.

Another role as educator relates to the following dietary recommendations of the American Cancer Society and the National Cancer Institutes to lower overall cancer risk including colorectal cancer.

1. Avoid obesity.

2. Decrease total fat intake. It is recommended that fat be only 30% of total calories. The year 2000 cancer control objective is to reduce average consumption of fat from 40% to 25% or less of total calories.[117] There are many simple methods to reduce dietary fat in the diet: (1) use low-fat cottage cheese instead of sour cream for dips, (2) use baked potatoes instead of French fries, (3) use nonstick pans or a cooking spray for grilling sandwiches instead of grilling them in oil, and (4) select bagels or whole wheat bread for breakfast instead of doughnuts, rolls, or croissants.

3. Consume more high-fiber goods, such as whole grain cereals, fruits, and vegetables. The year 2000 cancer control objectives are to increase the average consumption of fiber from 8–12 g/day to 20–30 g/day.

4. Include foods rich in vitamins A and C in the daily diet. Foods rich in carotene, a form in vitamin A, are carrots, tomatoes, spinach, apricots, peaches, cantaloupes. In general, dark green and deep yellow vegetables are rich in vitamin A.

5. Be moderate in the consumption of alcoholic beverages.

6. Be moderate in the consumption of salt-cured, smoked, and nitrite-cured foods.

7. Include cruciferous vegetables in the diet, such as cabbage, broccoli, brussels sprouts, kohlrabi, and cauliflower.[118–120]

Research supports the assumption that Americans will change their diet in an effort to be healthier. A survey in Illinois, conducted in 1982 and in 1986, found that 42% of the 46,830 subjects reported a major change in their diet since the first survey. Subjects reported eating less meat and pork and more fish and chicken, and there was a shift toward whole grains from refined grains and an increase in the number of times per week that subjects eat cruciferous vegetables.[121]

In the role of researcher, it is extremely important that nurses be knowledgeable about emerging information on the relationship between diet and colorectal cancer. Future research may establish definitive relationships, as well as additional relationships not presently known. Nurses also should be able to evaluate research findings. Those reports that are based on sound, ethical research principles may be judged appropriate for inclusion in patient education. Because of debate about the use of stool guaiac tests in screening programs in terms of lowering mortality from colorectal cancer, nurses need to remain alert to new research that either supports or refutes the use of this early detection test. Nurses also can plan or participate in the wide range of research projects related to colorectal cancer such as health behaviors, dietary habits, motives that facilitate early detection and dietary changes, and effective educational approaches for changing dietary patterns. Results certainly would benefit existing nursing practice as it relates to the prevention and early detection of colorectal cancer.

As practitioners, nurses are urged to use their physical assessment skills when they deal with individuals who have gastrointestinal complaints. Geriatric patients often share their symptoms first with a sympathetic nurse. Thus the nurse is in the ideal position to detect colorectal cancer in its *initial stages*. Physical assessment of the abdomen may reveal subtle clues of a pathologic condition that merits referral, one that otherwise might be overlooked by an elderly patient. Hospital-based nurses are cautioned not to assume that elderly patients must have had a thorough physical examination because they are in the hospital. If the complaints are not related to the gastrointestinal system, that system may not have been thoroughly assessed.

Prostate Cancer

Prostate cancer is currently the second most common cancer in American men. In men older than 75 years of age, it is estimated that the prevalence of prostate cancer is 500/100,000. The American Cancer Society estimates that in 1993 there will be 165,000 new prostate cases and 35,000 deaths caused by this cancer.[64] A large percentage of men have advanced disease at the time of diagnosis; approximately 35% have metastases to the bones or lymph nodes, and another 40% have extracapsular invasion.[122] Black American men have the highest incidence of prostate cancer in the world. Between 1937 and 1985 the incidence of prostate cancer increased 53.5% among white men and more than 100% in black men.[123] Prostate cancer increases in incidence with age more rapidly than any other cancer.

History assessment

There are *no* real symptoms of early, probably curable, disease. Most symptoms are related to late complications of stage C or D prostate cancer. Because many of the initial symptoms may be related to carcinomatous obstruction of the prostatic urethra, the inquiries made during the history should be about nonspecific urinary symptoms. The following questions are recommended:

1. Do you have to wait for your stream to begin?
2. Does your stream stop while you still have the urge to void?
3. Do you have to strain to urinate?
4. Does your stream seem very weak to you?
5. Do you have the urge to urinate but find you can't?
6. Have you noticed blood in your urine? Has your urine changed in color or smell at all?
7. Does the blood seem to come at the beginning or end of your stream?
8. Do you dribble after urinating?
9. Do you find you have to urinate more than you used to?
10. Do you have pain on urination?
11. Do you ever wet your pants?
12. How often do you urinate during the day? Do you get up at night to urinate? How often?
13. When was your last rectal examination? Why was this done? What was found?

Symptoms that suggest prostatic cancer are urinary difficulty manifested by a decrease in urinary stream and a frequency and urgency to urinate, often associated with pain. These symptoms also are found with prostatic enlargement (benign prostatic hypertrophy) that is extremely common in older men. The most frequent initial symptoms of prostate cancer are, in order of frequency, frequency of urination, difficult or painful urination, pain, complete urinary retention, and hematuria.[124]

Physical examination

An early diagnosis of prostate cancer can be done only by rectal palpation of the prostate (Figure 8-9). It is recommended that the examiner flex the distal finger joint 2–3 mm into the gland substance rather than keep the finger straight (Figure 8-10). The Valsalva maneuver during the rectal examination will bring the prostate gland closer to the examining finger. Early prostatic carcinoma is a nodule *within*, not *on*, the gland. Simply rubbing the gland is not effective for early detection of prostate cancer.[125]

The normal prostate on palpation is usually a rounded structure about 4 cm in diameter, feels firm rather than boggy, soft, or rock hard, and usually is not tender. Some examiners describe the consistency of the normal prostate as that of a pencil eraser. Cancer

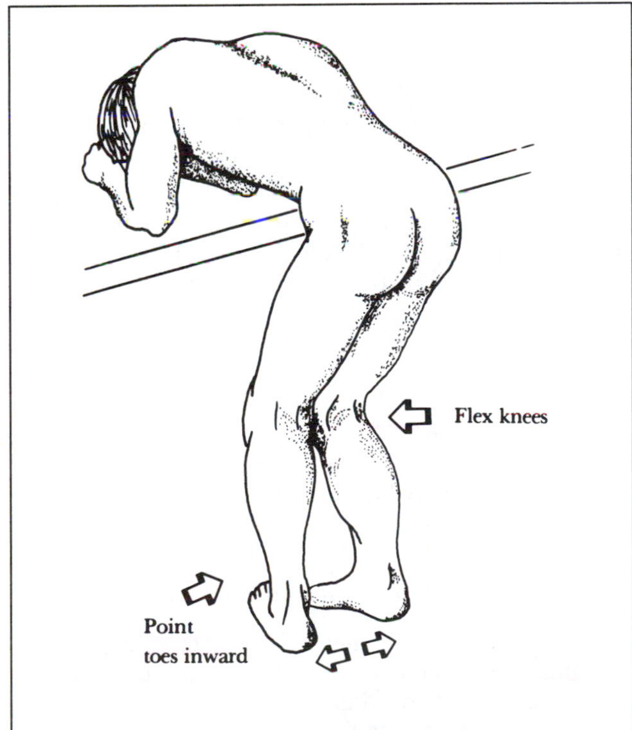

FIGURE 8-9 Recommended position for digital rectal examination. (Source: Adapted from Guinan P, Sharifi R, Bush I: Prostate cancer: Tips toward earlier detection. *Your Patient & Cancer* 4:37–42, 1984.)

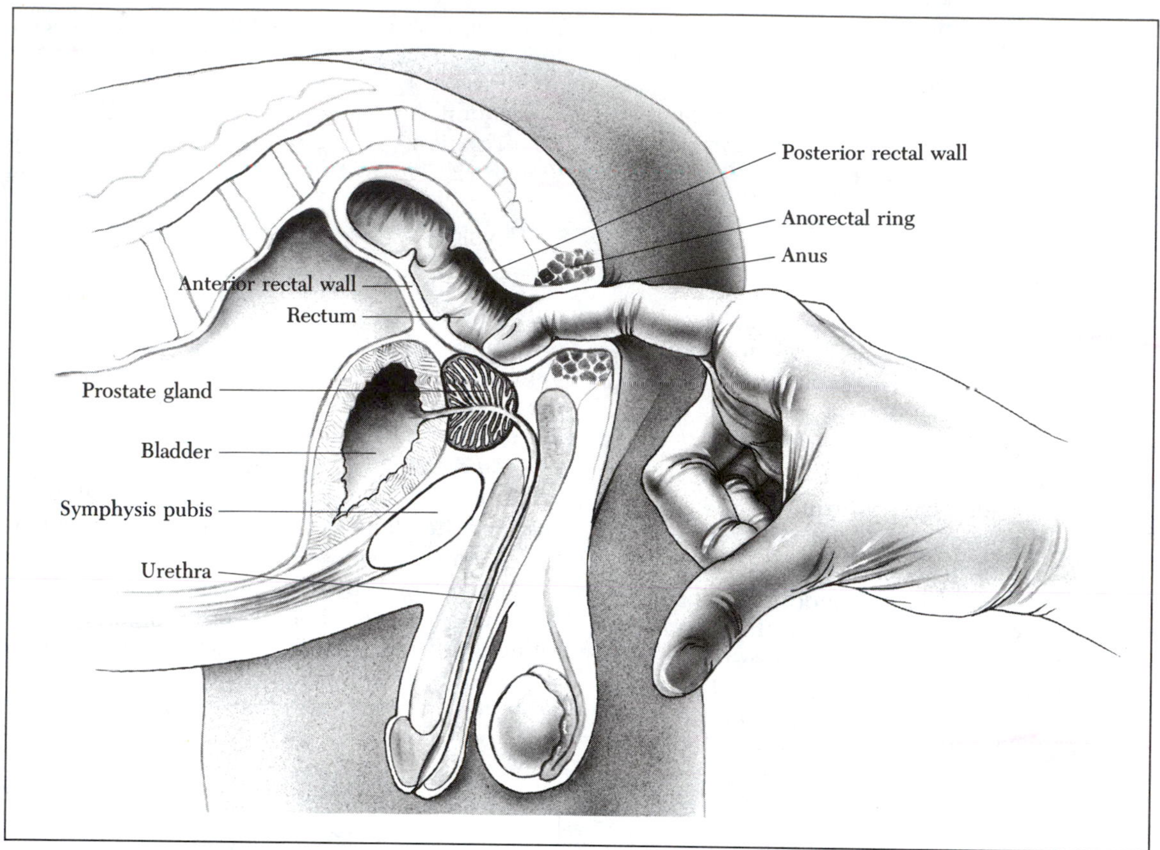

FIGURE 8-10 Technique for palpation of the prostate gland. (Source: Grimes J, Burns E (eds.): *Health Assessment in Nursing Practice* (ed. 2). Boston: Jones and Bartlett, 1987.)

of the prostate typically appears as a stony-hard nodule.[124] On the other hand, benign prostatic hypertrophy usually results in a diffuse enlargement of the prostate without masses.

It is extremely common to find in older men a diffusely enlarged prostate gland without masses (benign prostatic hypertrophy). Carcinoma of the prostate is manifested by a palpable hard nodule near the posterior surface of the prostate. As the carcinoma grows, the entire gland may become stony hard, or there may be several hard nodules.[75]

Screening tests for asymptomatic individuals

The most sensitive method of diagnosis of early prostate cancer is the digital rectal examination. Guinan et al.[126] compared the digital rectal examination with nine other laboratory tests designed to detect prostate cancer. Their data on 300 men suggest that the digital rectal examination is the most efficient test for the diagnosis of prostate cancer.

Research is being conducted to determine whether transrectal ultrasound has greater accuracy in the early detection of prostate cancer than the digital rectal examination.[127–129] The transrectal sonography, commonly used in Japan, involves a machine that is a large chair with a square hole through which an ultrasound probe protrudes. The probe is inserted into the rectum, and ultrasound images of the prostate are recorded on film. It is considered by most men to be less uncomfortable than a digital examination. Lee and colleagues[130–132] report that ultrasound is superior to the digital examination in a screening and detection program for prostate cancer in men older than 60 years of age. In their study of 784 men in this age group, findings of transrectal ultrasound examination alone resulted in biopsy recommendation for 83% of the biopsies performed, whereas digital examination resulted in biopsy recommendation for only 38%. A total of 22 cancers were found at biopsy, giving an overall detection rate of 2.8% and 1.3% for transrectal ultrasound and digital examination, respectively. Transrectal ultrasound demonstrated 100% (17/17) of tumors with the most favorable prognosis compared with 41% (7/17) for digital examination.[132]

A *tumor marker* is a biochemical indicator for the presence of a tumor. In clinical use the term refers to a molecule that can be detected in plasma or other body fluids.[133] Two tumor markers, prostate-specific antigen and prostatic acid phosphatase, are useful in monitoring therapy and disease progression of prostate cancer, but they have not as yet been shown to be specific or sensitive enough to use alone in the early detection of prostate cancer.

However, a new study has confirmed that the prostate-specific antigen (PSA) test *combined* with a digital rectal examination is the most effective screening technique for prostate cancer.[133] Researchers found that if rectal examination alone had been used, 32% of the early cancers would have been missed. Much controversy remains over how best to screen the general population, and some disagree over whether earlier detection will decrease mortality.[128] Klein[128] has developed a protocol for screening in all men over the age of 40 (see Figure 8-11).

One of the most important roles the nurse can assume in the detection of early prostate cancer is that of educator. All men older than 40 years of age, especially black American men, should be informed of the importance and rationale for yearly or biannual rectal examinations. Men with strong family histories of prostate cancer should be urged to *request and expect* rectal examinations at their annual physical inasmuch as early detection can result in cure and rectal examination is presently the most effective means of detecting early prostate cancer.

In some communities it may be necessary for the nurse to conduct the physical examination that includes the rectal examination for prostate as well as colorectal cancer. Female nurses who conduct physical examinations but omit the rectal assessment because of their embarrassment or the patient's discomfort must request a male physician or nurse practitioner to complete this portion of the examination rather than omitting it. In other settings it may be possible to develop a once-a-year volunteer transportation program that will enable infirm or geographically isolated elderly patients to have the recommended yearly examination. The development of a prostate screening program for each isolated, poor, or infirm elderly man is a problem all nurses should attempt to solve. At the very least the nurse should question all hospitalized elderly men about their last rectal examination and contact the physician about those men who have not had one within the last year (or who have "deferred" written on their chart next to "rectal examination").

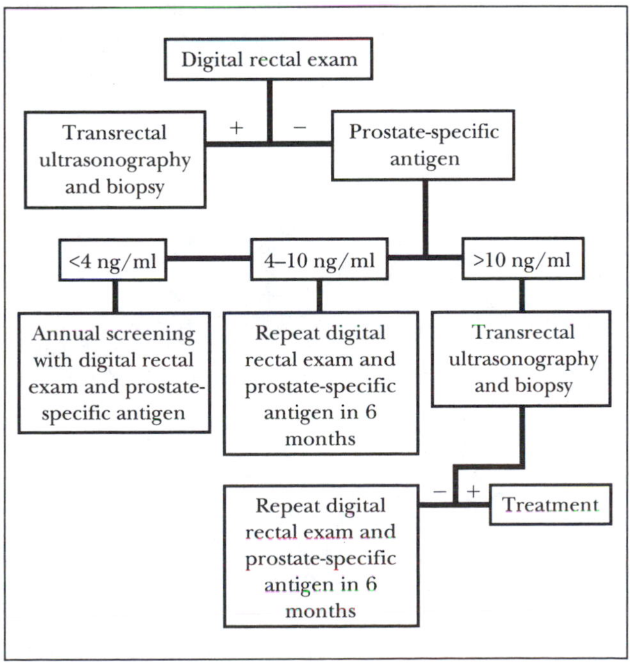

FIGURE 8-11 Practice guidelines for prostate cancer screening. (Source: Reprinted with permission from Klein EA: Prostate cancer: Current concepts in diagnosis and treatment. *Cleveland Clinic J Med* 59:383–389, 1992.)

Breast Cancer

Breast cancer is the most common cancer in women in the Western World.[134] It is the leading cause of cancer deaths in women 15 to 54 years of age and the second cause of cancer deaths in women older than 55 years of age.[64] It is estimated that in 1992, 181,000 women will be diagnosed with invasive breast cancer and 46,300 will die of the disease.[64] In women 40 years of age breast cancer develops each year in approximately 1/1000; by 60 years of age this rate rises to 2/1000 per year.[135] In the last 20 years the probability of breast cancer's developing in a woman's lifetime changed from 1/20 to 1/9.[134,136]

History assessment

Questions that may be asked during the history include the following:

1. Do you practice breast self-examination (BSE)?
   a. *"Yes" response:* How often do you do BSE? Where did you learn to do this? Do you feel comfortable doing BSE, or would you like me to go over it with you?
   b. *"No" response:* Have you ever been shown BSE? Would you be interested in learning BSE? Some women don't examine their breasts because they feel unsure, embarrassed, or frightened about doing it. Do you feel this way about BSE?
2. Have you ever been advised to have a mammogram? If you have had a mammogram, what were the results?
3. Do you experience sore breasts?
4. Have you ever been told you had "lumpy" or "cystic breasts"?
5. Have you noticed any color or temperature change on your breasts? Do you have trouble with scaly, itching nipples?
6. Have you ever had breast infections?
7. Have you ever had breast surgery or cosmetic surgery of your breasts? Tell me about the surgery that was done.
8. Do you have any sores or open wounds on your breasts?
9. Have you noticed any "dimpling" of your breasts?
10. Have you noticed any change in your nipples or discharge?

11. Have you ever been told that you had cancer of the breast?
12. Do you have or have you discovered any breast lumps?
13. Is there anyone in your family—grandparents, siblings, cousins, parents, aunts and uncles—who have or had cancer? Breast cancer? Can you remember how old your ________ was when she first was diagnosed as having breast cancer?
14. At what age (or grade in school) did you start menstruating? At what age did you stop menstruating?

The *most common* presenting complaint of women with breast cancer is a painless lump or mass in the breast. It is estimated that 90% of all palpable breast tumors are discovered by women themselves either accidentally or through planned self-examination.[136]

Physical examination

Inspection The physical examination begins with inspection of the breast with the woman sitting with her arms at her side, then sitting with her arms elevated, then sitting with pectoral contraction, and finally sitting bending forward (Figure 8-12). Visible signs of cancer of the breast include the following:

1. *Dimpling of the breast* results from a shortening of Cooper's ligaments as the tumor spreads in the breast.
2. *Unilateral flattening of the nipple* is caused by fibrosis and contraction of this fibrotic tissue, thus producing retraction signs, including flattening or deviation of the nipple.[77]
3. *Abnormal contours or flattening* becomes apparent as the woman changes positions. It is important to compare one breast with the other. An excellent position for observing this is when the woman leans forward.
4. *Peau d'orange,* orange peel skin, is caused by interference with the lymphatic drainage of the skin (Figure 8-13).
5. *Increased venous prominence* usually is unilateral. Carcinomas demand an increased blood flow; thus the dilated venous channels will be obvious on inspection.[137]
6. *Scaling or eczematoid lesions* of the nipple indicate Paget's disease, a slow-growing intraductal carcinoma.

It is essential that the woman be examined with good lighting (e.g., the use of a gooseneck lamp) so that subtle contours will be detected by the examiner. Also, the initial inspection *must* include all positions previously mentioned and shown in Figure 8-12; omitting a position may cause the nurse to miss important pathologic findings. The photographs in Figures 8-14 and 8-15 show the differences when the woman has her hands at her sides and when she raises her arms.

Palpation After inspection, the entire breast should be lightly palpated for thickening. This is accomplished by using the pads of your fingers. Palpation for thickening is done very lightly and slowly toward the nipple and enables the nurse to detect subtle differences in consistency in the breasts. This technique has evolved from 15 years of clinical practice as a nurse practitioner (MF-S). It should be viewed as a "scouting expedition" before palpation for masses is begun. If the woman complains of a lump, she should find it for the examiner. It is best to first palpate the normal breast. Cancer occurs as a hard, poorly circumscribed nodule, fixed to the skin or underlying tissue.

If cancer is suspected, the breast should be gently moved or compressed and observed for dimpling. A malignant lump that may be attached to the deep fascia

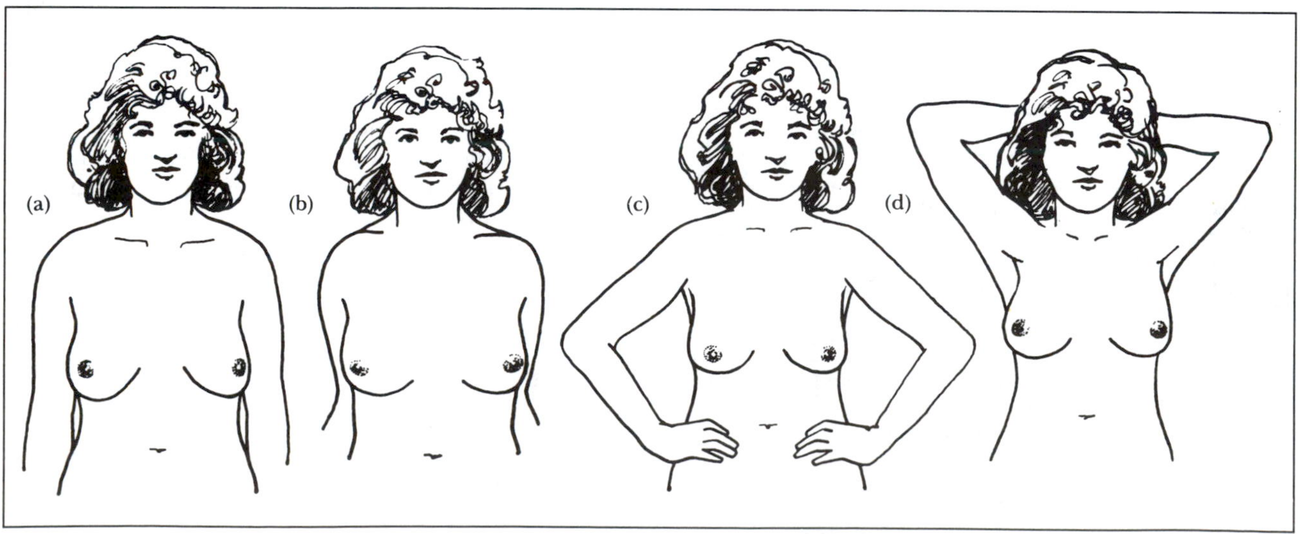

FIGURE 8-12 Positions for inspection of the breast. (a) Arms at side with woman relaxed; (b) arms at side pressed against body; (c) hands on waist pressed against body; (d) arms over head. (Source: Adapted from Olsen S: *Examinations for Detecting Breast Cancer.* Cancer Prevention Program, Wisconsin Clinical Cancer Center, 1300 University Ave-7C, Medical Science Center, Madison, WI 53706.)

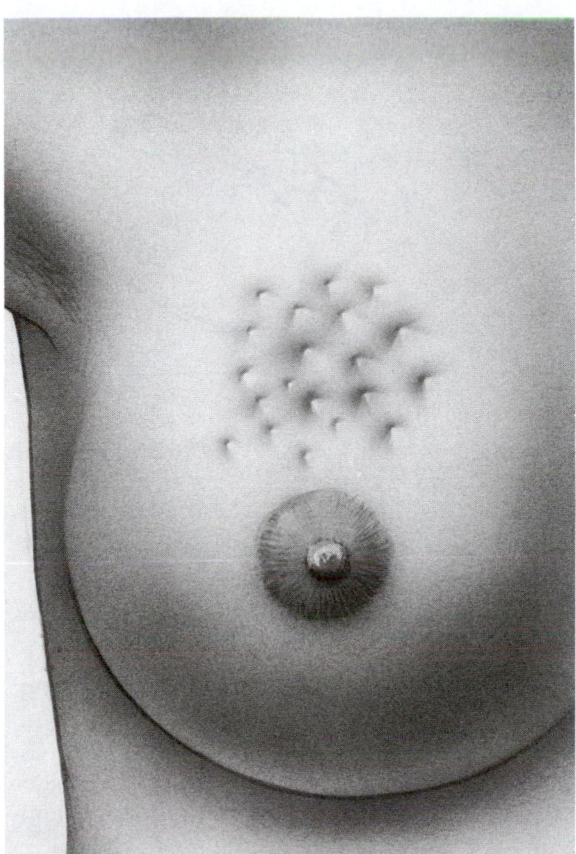

FIGURE 8-13 Peau d'orange. Note the rough, pitted appearance. (Source: Grimes J, Burns E (eds.): *Health Assessment in Nursing Practice* (ed. 2). Boston: Jones and Bartlett, 1987.)

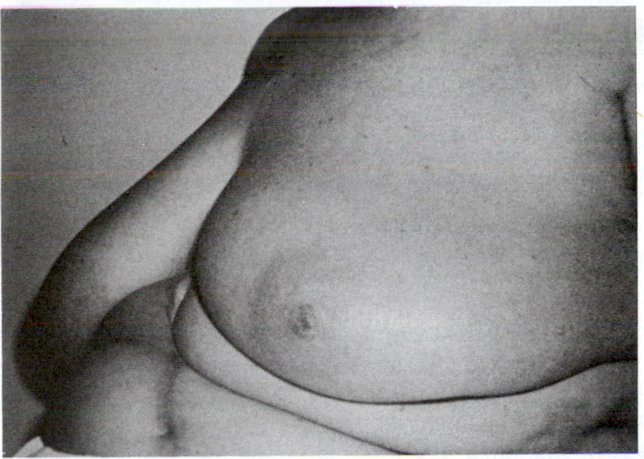

FIGURE 8-14 Woman sitting. Note that breasts appear normal. (Source: Rosemond G, Maier W: *Breast Cancer.* New York: Famous Teachings in Modern Medicine, Medcom, 1974.)

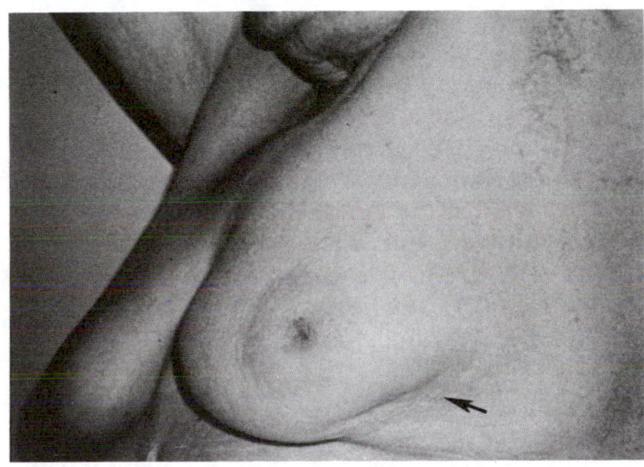

FIGURE 8-15 Woman raising her hands during breast inspection. Note dimpling, which becomes evident with this maneuver. (Source: Rosemond G, Maier W: *Breast Cancer.* New York: Famous Teachings in Modern Medicine, Medcom, 1974.)

will limit the mobility of the breast on the chest wall. The examiner checks for such a lump by having the patient place her hands on her hip; then the examiner moves the breast medially and laterally with the muscles relaxed and then with the muscles under tension by forced adduction.

The breasts need to be thoroughly palpated while the woman is supine with her arms above her head. One of us (MF-S) uses powder on the breasts to establish a frictionless surface. Palpation should be done with the flat part of the tips of three fingers. Using a spiral motion, rotate the fingers in small circles. It is recommended that the nurse start at the areolar margin and examine the breast by palpation in ever-widening concentric circles. Any mass that is felt should be charted as to its location, size, shape, consistency, discreteness, mobility, tenderness, erythema, and dimpling over the mass. Location of a nodule should be charted in terms of the quadrant, that is, right upper, left outer, and so forth. Special attention should be paid to the breast tissue along the inframammary crease. In its early stage cancer in this area may be hidden under the overlying breast tissue, and the normal induration of the inframammary crease can be confusing.[138]

Heymann[139] recommends that physical examination of a woman's breasts include right and left semilateral decubitus positions (Figure 8-16). The rationale for this is as follows: Lesions deep within the medial aspects, upper outer quadrants, or axillary tail, especially in large breasts, may be hidden within dense parenchyma or a thick layer of fat or may sink between ribs onto intercostal muscles when they are examined in the usual erect and supine positions (Figure 8-16a). By means of the right and left semilateral decubitus positions with both of the patient's arms elevated (Figure 8-16b), both breasts will fall dependently, thereby thinning the lateral aspects, upper outer quadrant, and axillary tail of the upper portion of the breasts and the medial aspect of the lower portion of the breast[139] (Figure 8-16c).

Next, the examiner needs to check for nipple discharge. Because the ducts are spoke wheellike, a dis-

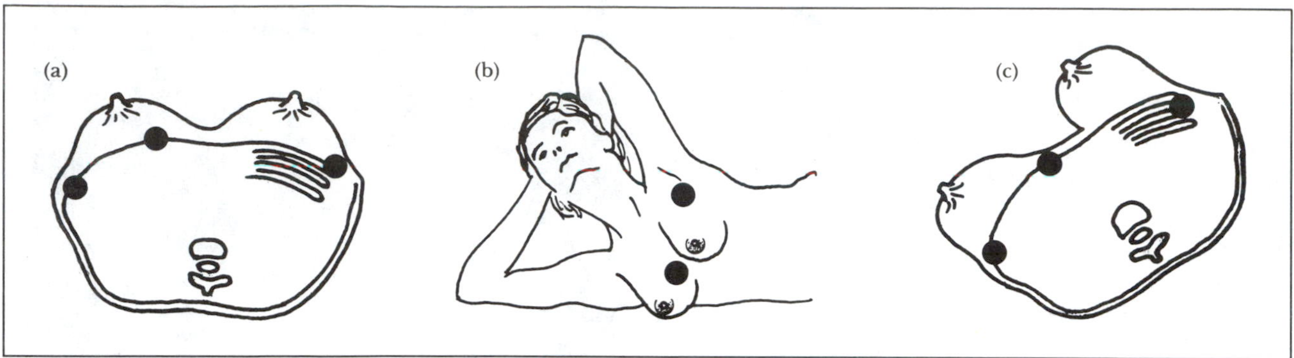

FIGURE 8-16 Semilateral decubitus breast examination. (a) Small masses obscured by breast parenchyma or ribs when breast is examined in upright or supine position; (b) semilateral decubitus position; (c) thinning of parenchyma with clarification of obscured masses when patient is in semilateral decubitus position. (Source: Adapted from Heymann A: Semilateral decubitus breast examination. *JAMA* 243:1713, 1980.)

charge from the 10 o'clock position indicates trouble in the upper inner quadrant, and so forth. The nipple should be gently compressed in *all* directions for the presence of discharge. Smears should be taken for cytologic examination of any suspicious discharge.

Because carcinoma of the breast may metastasize to regional lymph nodes, a careful palpation of the axillae and the supraclavicular regions is necessary. Most clinicians believe that the axilla is best palpated with the patient sitting erect and at a higher level than the examiner. Hard, fixed nodes palpated in the axillae or the supraclavicular region raise the suspicion of cancer. Normally, lymph nodes are felt as soft, movable structures.

When the clinician examines the breasts of the older woman, it should be kept in mind that the physiologic changes that normally occur with aging may simulate cancer of the breast. As a woman ages, there is atrophy of glandular elements that accentuates anatomic landmarks and reduces the amount of palpable tissue. Shrinkage and fibrotic changes of the breast may cause retraction of the nipple, and the terminal ducts are more visible. Both these changes may cause the examiner to suspect cancer. Because of the high incidence of breast cancer in elderly women, it is best to refer all suspicious findings rather than assume they are due to aging.

In conclusion, the physical signs that most *strongly* suggest cancer of the breast are dimpling, peau d' orange, abnormal contours of the breast, flattening of the nipple, palpable hard, poorly circumscribed nodules that are fixed to the skin or underlying tissue, and palpable hard, fixed nodes in the axillae or supraclavicular region.

Screening tests for asymptomatic individuals

Three methods used in screening for breast cancer are physical examination of the breast by the health professional, teaching the woman BSE, and mammography.

The American Cancer Society's revised recommendations for screening for breast cancer are as follows:

1. All women from age 20 years should perform BSE monthly.
2. Women 20–40 years of age should have a breast physical examination every 3 years, and women older than 40 years should have a breast physical examination every year.
3. Screening mammography should begin by age 40; women 40–49 years of age should have a mammogram every 1–2 years; and women older than 50 years of age should have a mammogram every year.[140,141]

The National Cancer Institute's cancer control objectives for the year 2000 are to increase the percentage of women from ages 50–70 years who have an annual breast examination and mammogram from 45% to 80%.[142] The mortality rate of carcinoma of the breast can be reduced by a combination of physical examination and mammography, as shown by a study conducted by the Health Insurance Plan of New York (HIP)[143]:

> About one-third of the cancers were detected on mammography alone, and were negative on initial clinical examination. At the same time, two fifths of the cancers were found on clinical examination alone, and were negative on mammography. About one fifth of the cancers were detected on both modalities. It was concluded that both modalities were needed for proper yield in screening.[134,p. 666]

The Breast Cancer Detection Demonstration Project (BCDDP) showed that mammography alone was responsible for the detection of 41.6% of 3557 cancers diagnosed in 280,000 women. In women 40–49 years of age, mammography alone detected 35.4% of 762 cancers. These percentages are better than the mass screening study of 160,000 women developed by HIP a decade earlier, which showed that mammography alone detected 33.3% of all cancers and 19.4% of the cancers in women 40–49 years of age. At 10 years, mortality is reduced 30% in women older than 50 years of age who are screened for breast cancer by mammography and physical examination. A study in Sweden duplicates the 30% mortality reduction found in the HIP study.[144] The BCDDP study also showed results consistent with the reduction in mortality from breast cancer found in the HIP and the Swedish study.[142] In all the studies, there is unequivocal benefit for those older than 50 years of age. However, the benefits for those 40–50 years of age have been widely debated in the literature.[143] In the HIP study women in the 40–49 age group exhibited only a 5% decrease in mortality.

A new analysis of the HIP data has found significant reductions in breast cancer mortality for women younger than 50 years of age, which may help settle the under-50 screening debate. The investigators attribute the new finding to longer follow-up and more efficient statistical methods. At the same time, recent analysis of the BCDDP data supports the new HIP findings that mammographic screening lowers mortality for the 40–49 age group. The National Cancer Institute, the American Cancer Society, and the American College of Radiology now recommend that women between 40 and 49 years of age have a mammogram every 1–2 years.[141,145,146]

Breast self-examination The importance of BSE is based on the fact that approximately 95% of breast cancers are self-discovered either accidentally or through planned examination. Because approximately 10% of cancers termed *interim cancers* will become apparent within a year of an examination with negative results, reliance has been placed on BSE to find these lesions. In the last few years there has been considerable debate about the value of BSE in reducing mortality and increasing survival rates.[147–150] The problem is that to date there have been no prospective randomized studies testing the benefits of BSE. The World Health Organization is sponsoring a prospective trial of BSE in Russia, and there is also a British randomized trial of breast cancer screening under way, but any data from these trials are several years away.[148] Because BSE has not been studied in a prospective, controlled trial with mortality as an outcome, the U.S. Preventive Services Task Force does not make a recommendation about the inclusion or exclusion of teaching BSE during the periodic health examination.[149] In addition, the World Health Organization does not recommend BSE screening programs as public health policy, although there is insufficient evidence to change them where they already exist.[149]

Although there probably is not sufficient evidence to justify BSE as a large-scale, community-based intervention, many authorities believe it should be encouraged as part of a woman's regular medical care.[142,151] A study by Huguley et al.[152] of 2093 women with breast cancer found that self-examiners tended to seek medical care more rapidly and to have earlier stages of disease at diagnosis than nonself-examiners. Five years after diagnosis the cumulative observed survival rates in breast cancer were 76.7% among self-examiners and 60.9% among nonexaminers ($p < 0.0001$). The researchers acknowledge that the observed survival advantage may be due to characteristics of the self-examiners other than BSE per se; however, they encourage BSE as an adjunctive technique for the early detection of breast cancer.[152]

In any discussion of BSE it must be remembered that the majority of American women do not practice monthly BSE. Although nearly all women (90%–99%) are aware of this early detection practice, only 15%–40% perform BSE monthly.[150] Bennett et al.[153] interviewed 616 women and found that women who were more likely to practice BSE on a frequent basis were living with their sexual partner, had a maternal history of breast disease, had been shown how to perform BSE, and were confident in their examination technique. They found no association between monthly BSE practice and formal education. Studies consistently have shown that lack of knowledge and low confidence are related to low rates of practice or no practice at all. In a review article on BSE, Kegeles[154] noted that knowledge of how it should be done and confidence in one's ability were the characteristics that consistently differentiated frequent from less frequent practitioners of BSE.[154] Table 8-4 provides several educational approaches to help women detect breast cancer early.

Many researchers, including those of the Gallup poll, found that personal instruction results in more frequent BSE than do films, pamphlets, or lectures. It also has been shown that individual contact is successful in bringing both low users of health services and women at high risk for cancer into cancer screening programs.[154] Self-instruction includes teaching a woman to do BSE by *using her own hand on her breast under the direct guidance of a professional.* Because women can be taught to detect lesions of 1 cm or less in their own breasts, those who practice regular BSE will detect tumors within a size range that will maximize chances for survival and minimize chances for axillary node involvement.[155] When teaching BSE, the nurse should also review the American Cancer Society guidelines, stressing the importance of a yearly physical examination by a health professional and mammographic examination at intervals determined by the woman's age.

Because a high percentage of cancerous lesions are potentially palpable, it is important for nurses to include one-on-one instruction in BSE techniques whenever possible. Research documents the effectiveness of personal instruction in self-examination techniques by registered nurses as part of a cancer education program through their place of employment.[136,156,157] In the BSE program reported by Styrd,[158] more than 60% of the eligible female employees participated in the program, and 1 year later 80% reported performing BSE some time during the 3 months before being surveyed. In addition, the proportion of employees who indicated they had performed BSE on a monthly basis increased significantly after the program ($p < 0.001$).

TABLE 8-4 Educational Efforts to Help Women Detect Breast Cancer Early

1. **Increase competence of women in doing BSE**
   a. Cognitive component—Educate women about importance of becoming familiar with their breasts in order to identify changes if they occur.
   b. Tactile-skill competence—Women are shown BSE and then *return* the demonstration. Women should be seen 6 months later to again demonstrate their technique and findings.
2. **Increase frequency and retain persistence of BSE**
   a. Habit component of BSE—Provide calendar or other stimulus memory aid noting date on which BSE should be performed.
   b. Memory component of BSE—Provide woman with a record form to be filled out each month; form should enable woman to chart findings.
   c. Reinforcement component of BSE—Offer praise whenever possible either verbally or through tangible rewards (ie, buttons, stickers).
3. **Reduce delay in reporting findings and increase access to physicians**
   a. Share the fact that BSE is not enough if something different is discovered. Need to have suspicious findings followed up by mammography and biopsy if necessary.
   b. Educate women about the favorable outcome of breast cancer that is found at stage I and the substantial risk in delay.
   c. Encourage woman to have physician who will welcome her if she finds differences in any monthly findings. Woman should change physicians if her present physician is not supportive of her early detection efforts.

Source: Kegeles S: Education for breast self-examination: Why, who, what, and how? *Prev Med* 14:702–720, 1985.

Primary nursing, as well as public health and occupational health nursing, afford the nurse excellent opportunities for BSE education. To date, there is some empirical evidence that supports nurses' ability to promote the practice of BSE in the acute care setting. Shamian and Edgar[159] studied the knowledge and the frequency pattern of 223 women taught BSE by nurse clinicians. They concluded that nurses influence positively the factual and proficiency knowledge base and the frequency of BSE practice. To reinforce personal instruction in BSE there could be posters, multimedia events such as slide-tape and films, and educational panels portraying the techniques of BSE. These methods, however, should reinforce, *not* replace, personal instruction.

Testicular Cancer

Although testicular cancer is relatively rare (1% of all cancers), it is the most common solid tumor in young men between 20 and 35 years of age.[160] A lesser peak occurs in early childhood. Testicular cancer, which is uncommon after 40 years of age, affects white men more than black. It is estimated that in 1993, 6600 men will be diagnosed with this cancer and 350 will die from testicular cancer.

History assessment

When obtaining the health history, the nurse should inquire about the following:

1. Do you have a history of undescended testicles? Was this surgically corrected? At what age?
2. Is there a history of mumps, orchitis, or testicular cancer in the family? History of inguinal hernia?
3. Did your mother take any type of hormones while she was pregnant with you?
4. Are you aware of any lumps in your scrotum?
5. Were there signs of early puberty as a child?
6. Have you noticed any changes in your genital organs or interest in sex?
7. Are you aware of any scrotal heaviness or heavy discomfort in the scrotum of lower portion of the abdomen and groin?
8. Are you aware of any breast swelling or nipple tenderness?
9. Do you practice testicular self-examination (TSE)? If not, have you ever been shown?
10. Are you aware of any recent trauma to the genital organs?

Although there is no direct proof that trauma causes testicular cancer, many men link swelling or a lump to a recent trauma. The most common presenting complaint is a painless enlargement of the testis, or "heaviness," which is noticed by about two-thirds of men.[161] Nodules in the testes are typically small, hard, and usually painless, and they are slightly more common in the right testis (52.3%) than in the left (47.7%).[162]

The major obstacle to early detection of testicular cancer is the delay that commonly occurs between initial detection of the lesion in the testis to the time of treatment. Approximately 6 months will elapse before treatment is either sought by the patient or begun by the physician.[161] The uninformed young man may ignore the unilateral enlargement for quite some time for the following reasons: (1) The man may hope that the testis will spontaneously revert to normal; (2) he may feel a certain pride in his enlarging sexual organ; (3) he may perceive the tumor as punishment for past sexual sins; (4) he may perceive the lack of pain as an indication that the lump is innocent; and (5) he may fear it is cancer.[161,163]

In 1978 Conklin and co-workers[164] explored the need for and the interest in a health education program about TSE at the University of Vermont. Although 58% of the 90 students interviewed had taken a health-related course in the previous 2 years, 75% had never heard of testicular cancer. None knew how to examine their testes correctly, and only one knew what to palpate for. In 1986 Blesch[165] surveyed a random sample of 233 professional men about their knowledge and perceptions of testicular cancer and TSE and found the same lack of knowledge about TSE as Conklin and colleagues. Of 129 responses, only 31.1% of the sample subjects were aware of TSE and only 9.5% practiced TSE. Although more than half the sample (61.2%) were aware of testicular cancer, 4 of 9 men with a personal history of undescended testis (a significant risk factor) had not heard of testicular cancer.[165] Because the effectiveness of TSE in lowering mortality has not been documented, there is debate about recommending this practice for men in screening programs.[142]

Physical examination

The examination begins with inspection of the scrotum. Cancer of the testes may be manifested by asymmetry of the scrotum. In most men the left side of the scrotal sac descends lower than the right because of the greater length of the left spermatic cord.[166] Another clue to the presence of a tumor in the scrotum is scrotal skin that appears stretched and thin over the tumor.

Palpation of the scrotal contents can be done with the man standing or in a recumbent position; however, the examination should be thorough and gentle because the testes are exquisitely tender to physical pressure.[167] The examiner must conduct the palpation as gently as possible to avoid eliciting the cremasteric reflex. Stimulation of the scrotum or inner thigh may elicit this reflex and cause the testes to be retracted into the inguinal canal (migratory testis). Several procedures are recommended for palpating the testes. Some authors advocate that the examiner palpate the scrotal contents with both hands to help differentiate the testicles from the other scrotal structures—epididymis, vas deferens, and spermatic cord. Palpating bimanually also improves the chances of detecting any weight differential between the testicles, an important clue to malignancy.[168] The bimanual procedure of using index and middle fingers to separate testes and scrotum so that the right testis and epididymis can be examined with left hand and vice versa is illustrated in Figure 8-17. DeGowin and DeGowin[75] recommend comparing both testes simultaneously by grasping one with each hand, using the thumb and forefinger. As is true with breast lesions, if the man has symptoms, the uninvolved testis should be examined first to provide a baseline comparison.[169]

A normal testicle has a somewhat rubbery, spongy consistency, and the consistency is uniform throughout with a surface free of lumps or indurations. Diffuse induration of the testis in the absence of discrete nodularity also may be the initial abnormality.[170] The most common sites for tumors are on the testicular anterior and lateral surfaces.[171] In the young male, the testis is apt to feel firm and smooth, whereas in the elderly male it may be very soft, almost mushy.[166] Even though the testes feel normal, each should be transilluminated. One may be atrophied and the normal size attained by a hydrocele.[75] Transillumination is helpful in distinguishing cystic from solid masses. Transillumination can be accomplished by aiming a small flashlight behind or on the side of the scrotum in a darkened room. It should be remembered that hydroceles may develop as a result of a tumor.[172] Typically, a testicular tumor occurs as a painless scrotal mass that does not transilluminate. The size may range from less than 1 cm to 10 cm in diameter.[160] The examiner needs to be aware that the scrotal skin overlying the tumor is rarely attached, although attachment may exist in lymphomatous involvement of the testis.[166]

Other areas should be checked to ascertain if there has been metastases; for example, a mass in the epigastrium or an enlarged left supraclavicular node (Virchow's node) may be palpable.[160] The examiner also should palpate the abdomen for retroperitoneal lymph node involvement. To feel any metastatic nodes the examiner will have to palpate the abdomen fairly deeply. Metastatic nodes usually lie at the level of, or slightly caudal to, the umbilicus. Ultrasonographic examination is often useful in further defining an abnormality of the testicular parenchyma.[170]

Education: testicular self-examination

There is a need for nurses to educate themselves, their colleagues, and their patients about testicular cancer and TSE. The major deterrent to early detection and treatment is young men's lack of knowledge of the great danger of testicular cancer and the lack of awareness of the need for regular self-examination.[165] Because the prognosis is good when the tumor is treated early, there is a vital need to educate the public about early detection and treatment. The majority of men discover the changes in the testes while bathing or showering, or it is found by their sexual partners. Only 4% of tumors are detected by clinicians doing a workup for infertility.[162]

Pediatric hospital and office-based nurses, pediatric nurse practitioners, and school nurses must instruct the parents of high-risk boys and adolescents, i.e., those who have or have had undescended testes, how to correctly palpate the scrotum and what physical findings are significant. These same children should be instructed in TSE as they mature. TSE techniques should be included in health education classes just as breast self-examinations are now routinely included in these classes. Education should emphasize the importance of reporting abnormal findings immediately because delay in reporting testicular lesions is common. Table 8-5 summarizes what should be taught during TSE.[173]

Nurses who work in the military, in occupational health settings, in physicians' offices, and in educational settings are in ideal clinical settings for teaching TSE and providing education that will dispel the myths that contribute to delay once a testicular lump is found.

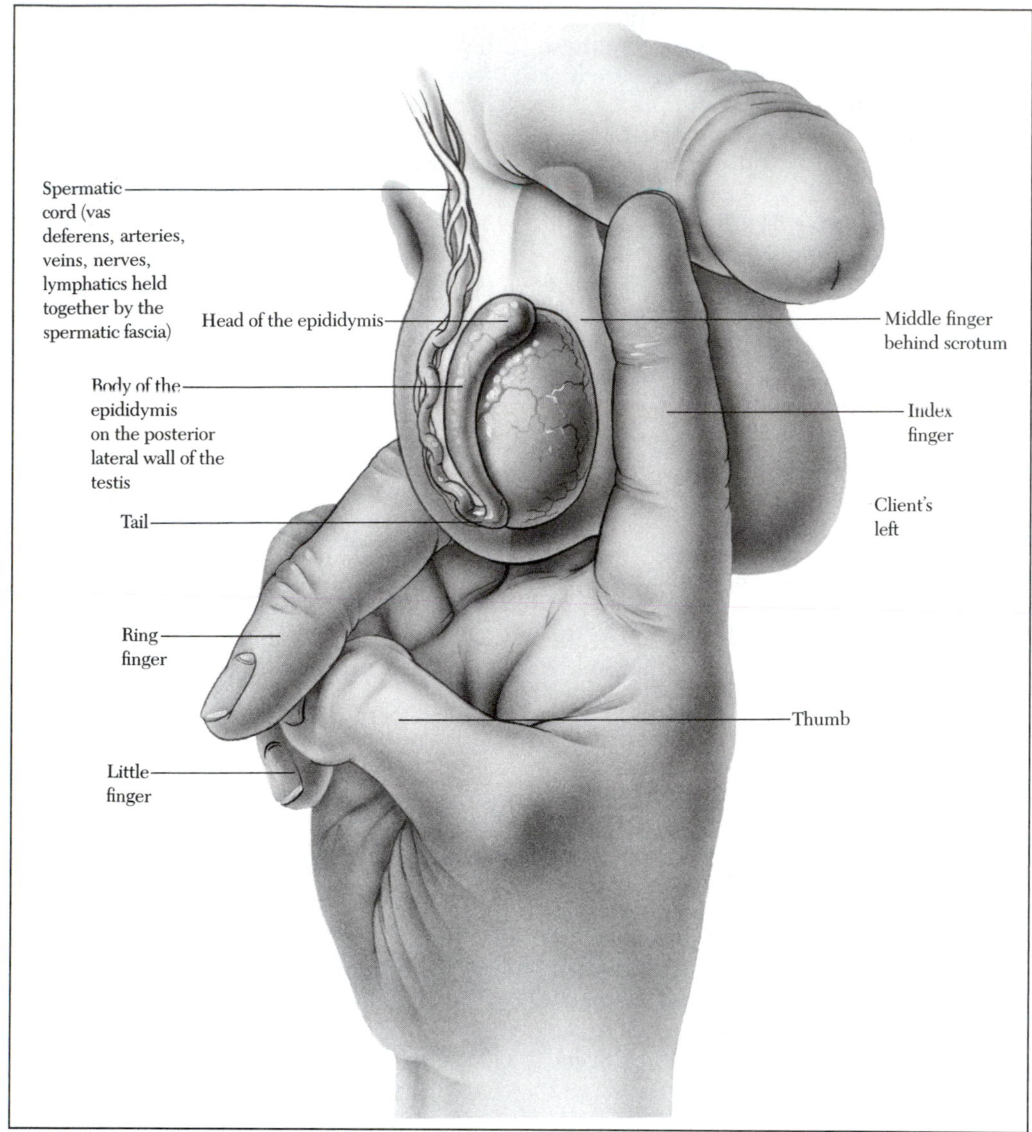

FIGURE 8-17 Palpation of the scrotum. (Source: Grimes J. Burns E (eds.): *Health Assessment in Nursing Practice* (ed. 2). Boston: Jones and Bartlett, 1987.)

Teaching TSE should be incorporated into routine physical examinations by the examining health professional. A nursing assessment of any male younger than 40 years of age should include a health history to elicit any subjective symptoms and established risk factors for testicular cancer. A man who complains of vague scrotal symptoms should be referred for a careful genital examination, and those men identified as being at high risk for testicular cancer should be instructed in TSE.

The following methods to disseminate information about testicular cancer and TSE have been proposed by Carlin[162]:

- Teach male clients in sexually transmitted disease clinics.
- Publish articles on TSE and early detection in local papers, radio, and television.
- Include discussions of TSE in all health education classes at the junior high and high school levels.
- Distribute TSE pamphlets to physicians' offices (especially offices of urologists), hospitals, pediatric clinics, clinics for women, infants, and children, immunization clinics, and other health care settings.
- Teach personnel in public health departments the importance of including discussions of testicular cancer and how to perform TSE when they work with parents of young boys and with men who attend the health clinic.
- Publish articles in college newspapers and offer health programs at the university infirmary on the early detection of testicular cancer.
- Discuss testicular cancer and TSE in all health-related programs for new military recruits.

TABLE 8-5 Summary Chart: Testicular Self-Examination (TSE)

- Perform monthly while bathing or showering. Lather hands with soap to increase the fingers' sensitivity.
- Hold the scrotum in the palm of the hands and compare each half of the sac for equal heaviness.
- Examine the side of the scrotal sac individually. Place index and middle fingers on the underside of the testis and the thumb on top. Palpate the ovoid-shaped testis for lumps. Locate the epididymis and palpate. It is a comma-shaped structure on top of and extending down behind the testicle. It is usually soft and slightly tender. Position the thumb and fingers into the deep groove between the anterior oval testis and the posterior epididymis. The testis is firmer than the epididymis.
- Identify the spermatic cord (vas deferens) that ascends from the epididymis. It is a smooth, firm, moveable, tubular structure.
- During TSE, apply gentle pressure. If there is pain, too much pressure is being applied.
- Examination of the testis should be done with a slow, gentle, rolling action. Check for any small lump, slight enlargement, or change in consistency.
- Repeat the same procedure for the opposite testicle.
- Report any changes found to a physician for immediate evaluation.

Source: White L: The nurse's role in cancer prevention. In Newell G (ed.): *Cancer Prevention in Clinical Medicine*. New York: Raven Press, 1983, pp. 91–112.

- Provide classes and written materials to male employees in occupational settings, particularly young men in the "high-tech" occupations.

In summary, the best defense against testicular cancer is a well-educated male population that practices TSE and understands the importance of seeking medical attention when a "lump" is discovered. Much progress has been made in the last 10 years in discussing and promoting breast self-examination among women. The time has come for nurses to address the issue of testicular cancer in the same forthright, open manner that breast cancer has been discussed so that men will incorporate this health practice into their lives.[174]

Skin Cancer

Cancers of the skin are the most common cancers in humans. In the United States it is estimated that in 1993, 32,000 people will be diagnosed with melanoma and 6800 will die of skin cancer.[64] Annually, new cancers of the skin will develop in more than 500,000 people in the United States.[175] Thus approximately one in three newly diagnosed cancers is a malignancy of the skin.

Malignant melanoma accounts for about 74% of all deaths that result from cutaneous cancers.[176] The mortality rate from malignant melanoma is increasing faster than that of any other cancer except lung cancer. Since 1930 the lifetime incidence of malignant melanoma has increased from 1/1500 people to 1/150—a tenfold increase.[177] Today the majority of persons with malignant melanoma are relatively young: The median age at diagnosis is 45 years.[178]

History assessment

When obtaining the health history, the nurse should inquire about the following:

1. Have you noticed any changes in any of your moles in terms of color, size, surface characteristics, sensation, areas around the mole, and elevation of the mole?
2. Are you aware of any skin lesions on your body that are new or don't seem to "go away"?
3. Are you aware of the development of any new moles?
4. Have you ever been told you should have a mole removed? Why were you told this?
5. Have you (or any members of your family) ever been told you have dysplastic nevi? Have you (or any members of your family) ever had skin cancer? melanoma? If yes, where was the cancer?
6. Do you feel you have a lot of moles? Where are the majority of these moles?
7. Do you sunbathe? How often? Do you use sunscreen?
8. Do you go to a tanning salon or use a tanning bed? How often?
9. Does your skin generally burn when in the sun or tan?
10. What is your occupation? Have you ever worked in a position in which you were outside for long periods of time? How long did you hold that job?
11. Have you ever worked in occupations in which you were exposed to tar and pitch, oils, paraffins, arsenic, X rays, or radium?
12. Were you ever burned, or do you have scarring from corrosive or thermal damage?
13. Do you have any outdoor recreational habits or hobbies that you consistently engage in?

When obtaining a health history, the nurse must inquire whether any of the aforementioned changes in moles have occurred. A history of change, often extending over a period of weeks or months, in a preexisting mole or the development of a new mole in an adult is of great importance and requires inspection. The nurse needs to be aware that almost half the melanomas arise in moles or pigmented areas; thus there should be a high index of suspicion in any mole that is changing or enlarging.[179]

Physical examination

It is essential that the entire integument be inspected during the examination of a patient. Skin assessment includes inspection of the inner lip mucosa, the axillae, the nail beds, the external genitalia, the webs between the toes, the soles of the feet, and the areas in skin folds.[180] This is best accomplished in a setting with good lighting (e.g., a gooseneck lamp) that enables the nurse to project the light obliquely across the body surface. A pen light can be used instead of a gooseneck lamp. A magnifying glass also allows closer inspection of minute details.[181]

All areas that are chronically exposed to the sun should be meticulously assessed, including the neck, ears, shoulders, face, scalp, arms, and hands. Areas that have been chronically exposed to sunlight are common sites for basal cell and squamous cell carcinomas. However, melanomas are found on head, neck, and trunk, which may or may not be exposed to sun, and on the legs in women; occurrence of maglignant melanoma is infrequent in rarely exposed or unexposed areas (breasts and bathing suit area of women and bathing trunk area of men).[182] The surface distribution of melanomas in black persons differs from that in white persons; the relatively depigmented palms, soles, nail beds, and mucous membranes are primary sites in almost all black patients.[183]

It is recommended that the entire posterior and anterior aspect of the body be viewed and the location of moles be mapped to serve as baseline data for future skin assessments. If a skin lesion is detected, the nurse has three responsibilities: accurate documentation (size, location, description of the lesion), referral of the patient to a physician for diagnosis, and follow-up for recurrent disease.[180]

There are three types of skin cancer: basal cell carcinoma, squamous cell carcinoma, and melanoma. The nurse should be aware of the following precancerous skin lesions: leukoplakia (found in the oral mucosa), senile and actinic keratoses, and dysplastic nevi. Table 8-6[176,184–186] lists the incidence, clinical characteristics, and common sites of actinic keratoses and basal cell and squamous cell skin cancer. Table 8-7 compares the clinical features of a normal mole, dysplastic mole, and malignant melanoma.

Education

Of all the known risk factors, ultraviolet radiation from the sun is the leading cause of skin cancer. Fortunately, the most carcinogenic of the ultraviolet wavelengths can be blocked by sunscreening agents. Sunscreens are rated according to *sun protection factor* (SPF), on a scale currently ranging from 2 to 35. An SPF of 2 in a sunscreen means that proper application allows users to stay in the sun twice as long as they could without any protection at all.[177] Sunbathing should be avoided during the 2-hour period around noon, because two-thirds of the day's ultraviolet light comes through during that time. Skin types are similarly rated from 1 to 6 according to intensity of sunburn in the first 30–45 minutes of unprotected exposure to the sun

TABLE 8-6 Incidence, Clinical Characteristics, and Common Sites of Premalignant Skin Cancers and Skin Cancer

Skin Carcinoma	Incidence	Clinical Characteristics	Common Sites
Actinic keratoses (senile keratoses, solar keratoses)	Most common premalignant keratoses; develop in persons with fair complexions as result of excessive exposure to light; located on sun-exposed areas	Appear as circumscribed dry patches with adherent scales on slightly red, inflamed skin	Most commonly found on the face and the backs of hands. 20% of cases lead to squamous cell carcinoma
Basal cell carcinoma	Most common form of skin cancer; occurs primarily in persons exposed to intense sunlight, especially fair-complexioned white persons with light eyes and hair	*Nodular basal cell carcinoma:* elevated papule to lesions with an ulcerated center, raised margin, and waxy or "pearly" border; firm	Commonly found on the nose, eyelids, cheeks, and neck
		Superficial basal cell carcinoma: plaque, usually with a crusted and erythematous center, flat, and defined margins	Commonly found on trunk and extremities
Squamous cell carcinoma	Less common than basal cell carcinoma: occurs primarily on areas exposed to actinic or ultraviolet (UV) radiation	Appearance varies from an elevated nodular mass to a punched-out ulcerated lesion or a large fungating mass. Unlike basal cell carcinoma, squamous cell tumors are opaque and aggressive	Commonly found on head and hands

Source: Adapted from Friedman et al,[176] Helm and Helm,[184] Epstein,[185] Gumport et al.[186]

TABLE 8-7 Comparison of Common Nevi, Dysplastic Nevi, and Malignant Melanoma

Characteristic	Common Nevi	Dysplastic Nevi	Malignant Melanoma
Color	Uniformly tan or brown	Variable mixtures of tan, brown, black, or red/pink within a single nevus; nevi may look very different from each other	Variegated colors ranging from various hues of tan and brown to black and sometimes intermingled with red and white
Shape	Round; sharp, clear-cut borders between the nevus and the surrounding skin; may be flat or elevated	Irregular borders; pigment may fade off into surrounding skin; always have a flat portion level with the skin, which often occurs at the edge of the nevus	Borders of early malignant melanomas usually irregular, notched or angular
Size	Usually <6 mm in diameter like this: ●	Usually >6 mm; may be >10 mm; occasionally <6 mm	Diameters of macular malignant melanomas often >5 mm (it is not unusual to see 1.0 to 1.5 cm); 98.5% had a diameter ≥5 mm
Number	In a typical adult: 10 to 40 are scattered over the body	Often very many (>100), but some people may not have an unusual number of nevi	
Location	Generally on the sun-exposed surfaces of the skin above the waist; the scalp, breasts, and buttocks rarely are involved	Sun-exposed areas: the back is the most common site, but also may be seen on the scalp, breasts, and buttocks	Relatively uncommon body areas that are always covered, especially the breast and pelvic area in women; sharp increase in incidence in the head, neck, trunk of men, and arms and lower legs of women

Source: Adapted from Friedman R, Rigel D, Kopf A: Early detection of malignant melanoma: The role of physician, examination and self-examination of the skin. *CA* 35:130–151, 1985.

after a period of no exposure. Skin type 1 burns easily and never tans, whereas skin types 5 and 6 rarely burn and tan well.

The following information about decreasing or eliminating skin cancer risks should be discussed with each patient:

1. Ultraviolet rays can penetrate thin clothing like cotton T-shirts; thus those who desire protective clothing should select hats, long-sleeved shirts, and beach robes rather than rely on T-shirts.
2. Persons with skin types 1 and 2 should avoid sunbathing.
3. Persons who live or vacation in areas of higher altitudes need to be aware that there is less atmosphere to filter out the ultraviolet rays so that the sun's effects are more intense.
4. Persons need to be informed that the sun's rays are reflected off snow, sand, and water and that significant sun exposure can result from activities on these surfaces.
5. As the ozone layer of the earth changes, persons need to be aware that this significantly changes the amount of ultraviolet radiation that reaches the earth.

Routine self-examination of the skin is the best defense against skin cancer, especially malignant melanoma. It is inexpensive, noninvasive, and totally free of danger. Periodic self-examination for melanoma and examination by others may result in improved survival.[187] It is recommended that persons older than 30 years of age who have fair skin and are subject to heavy sun exposures be taught skin self-assessment. Those with dysplastic nevus syndrome or a history of melanoma in a first-degree relative also should have regular medical examinations that include measurement and charting of location of unusual pigmented lesions.[176] It also is recommended that patients be given copies of blank body charts so that they can chart lesions found during self-skin assessment. Figure 8-18 illustrates the correct procedure for self-assessment of skin.

Along with self-assessment of the skin, patients should be instructed about the changes in moles that merit immediate medical attention: size, color, elevation, surface characteristics, and sensation. Melanoma is more likely to develop in individuals and families with a history of dysplastic nevus syndrome (DNS) than it is in most people. The initial diagnosis is based on a physical examination and confirmed by the removal and biopsy of several moles. Individuals with familial DNS should visit their clinician or dermatologist twice a year for assessment and follow-up. They also should conduct self-assessments of the skin on a monthly basis. Assistance usually is necessary because many of the nevi are present in areas such as the scalp or back that are difficult for the individual to inspect.

The elderly constitute the highest-risk group for skin cancer because of the number of years of exposure to the sun. It is estimated that 40%–50% of all those

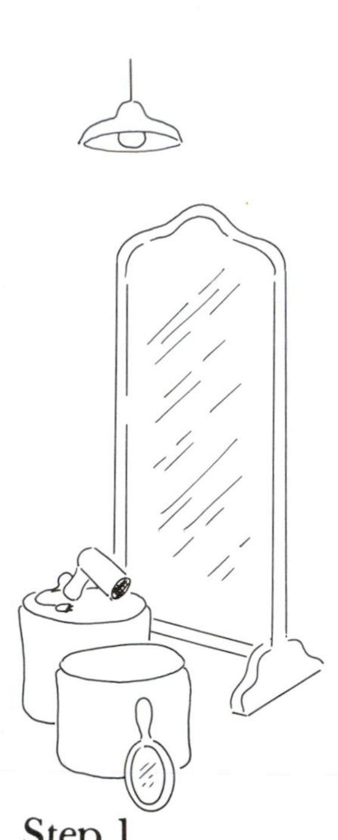

Step 1

Make sure the room is well-lighted and that you have nearby a full-length mirror, a hand-held dryer, and two chairs or stools. Undress completely.

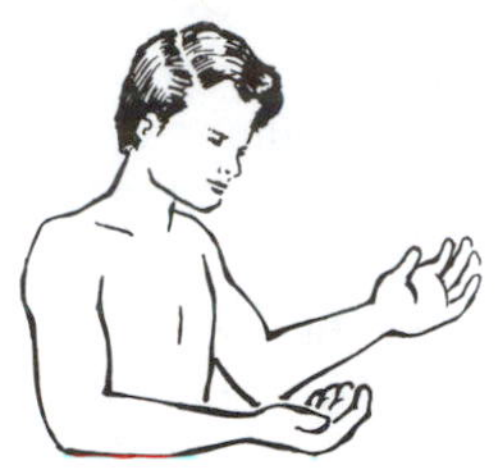

Step 2

Hold your hands with the palms face up, as shown in the drawing. Look at your palms, fingers, spaces between the fingers, and forearms. Then turn your hands over and examine the backs of your hands, fingers, spaces between the fingers, fingernails, and forearms.

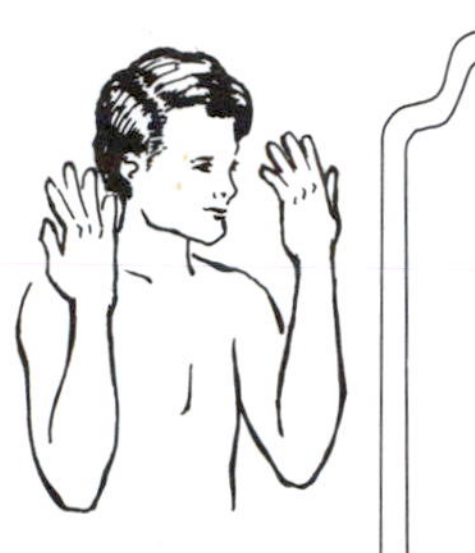

Step 3

Now position yourself in front of the full-length mirror. Hold up your arms, bent at the elbows, with your palms facing you. In the mirror, look at the backs of your forearms and elbows.

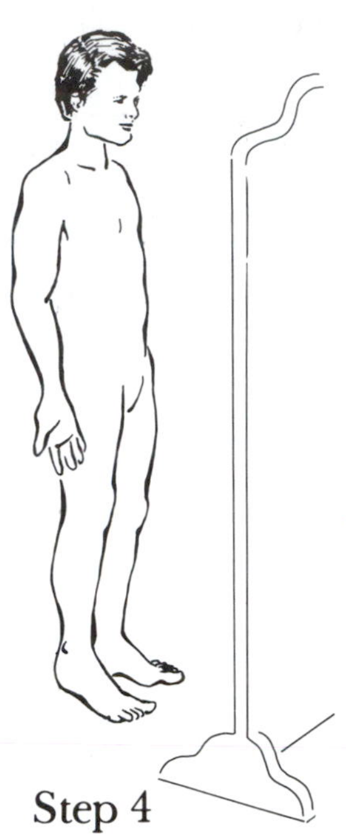

Step 4

Again using the full-length mirror, observe the entire front of your body. In turn, look at your face, neck, and arms. Turn your palms to face the mirror and look at your upper arms. Then look at your chest and abdomen, pubic area, thighs and lower legs.

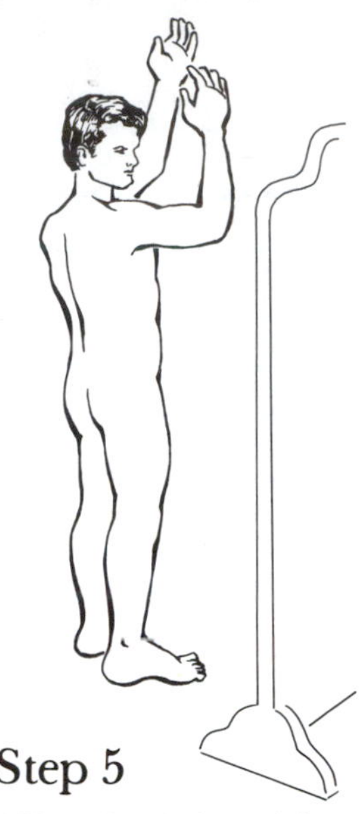

Step 5

Still standing in front of the mirror, lift your arms over your head with the palms facing each other. Turn so that your right side is facing the mirror and look at the entire side of your body—your hands and arms, underarms, sides of your trunk, thighs, and lower legs. Then turn, and repeat the process with your left side.

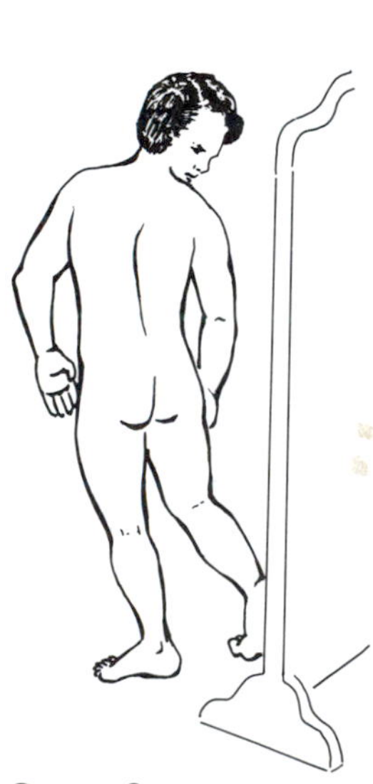

Step 6

With your back toward the full-length mirror, look at your buttocks and the backs of your thighs and lower legs.

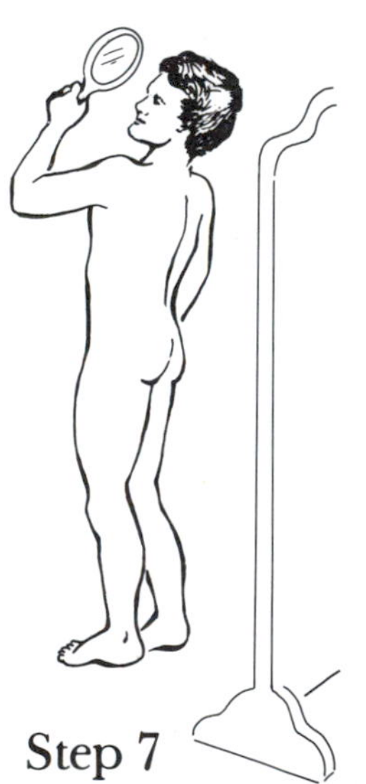

Step 7

Now pick up the hand-held mirror. With your back still to the full-length mirror, examine the back of your neck, and your back and buttocks. Also examine the backs of your arms in this way. Some areas are hard to see, and you may find it helpful to ask your spouse or a friend to assist you.

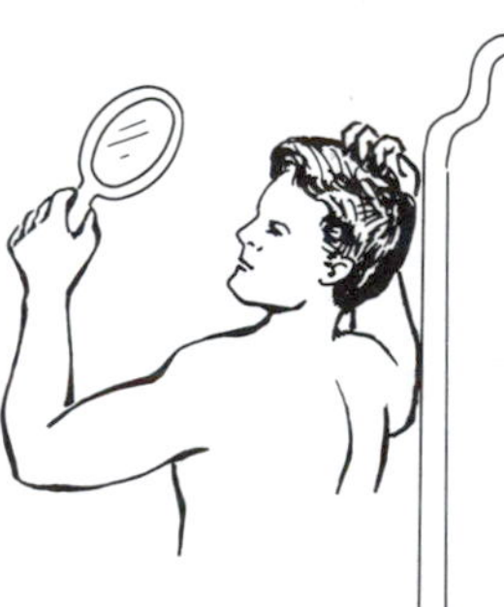

Step 8

Use the hand-held mirror and the full-length mirror to look at your scalp. Because the scalp is difficult to examine, we suggest you also use a hand-held blow dryer turned to a cool setting to lift the hair from the scalp. While some people find it easy to hold the mirror in one hand and the dryer in the other, while looking in the full-length mirror, many do not. For the scalp examination in particular, then, you might ask your spouse or a friend to assist you.

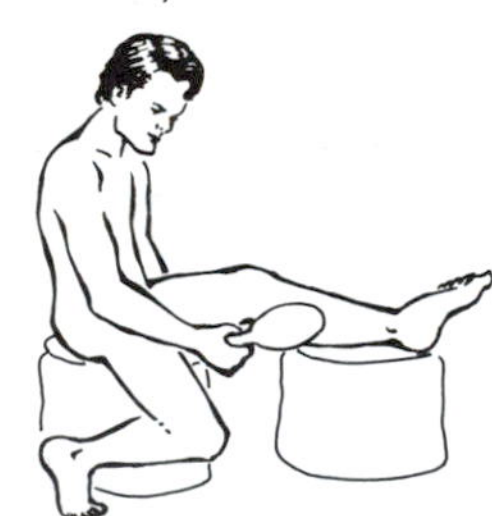

Step 9

Sit down and prop up one leg on a chair or stool in front of you as shown. Using the hand-held mirror, examine the inside of the propped-up leg, beginning at the groin area and moving the mirror down the leg to your foot. Repeat the procedure for your other leg.

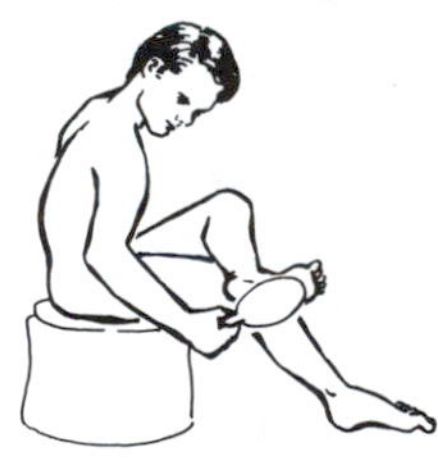

Step 10

Still sitting, cross one leg over the other. Use the hand-held mirror to examine the top of your foot, the toes, toenails, and spaces between the toes. Then look at the sole or bottom of your foot. Repeat the procedure for the other foot.

FIGURE 8-18 Self-examination of the skin. (Source: Friedman R, Rigel D, Kopf A: Early detection of malignant melanoma: The role of physician examination and self-examination of the skin. *CA* 35:130-151, 1985.)

who live to be 65 years of age will have at least one skin cancer during their lifetime.[188] Changes normally occur in the skin with age, which increase the risk of skin cancer. Keratoses, lentigines, and pigmented alterations develop with aging and in areas of chronic solar exposure. Elderly persons should be taught skin self-assessment and the importance of having a health professional examine any new lesions or changing lesions. Any setting where older adults congregate offers the nurse an excellent opportunity to provide an educational program on skin self-examination and early detection for skin cancer. Again, any areas that have been chronically exposed to the sun should be meticulously screened.

Oral Cancer

It is estimated that in 1993 there will be 29,800 new cases of oral cancer in the United States. The majority of these cancers (11,200) will be cancers of the mouth. There will be 7700 deaths from oral cancer.[64] These figures indicate that oral cancer incidence is not in decline nationally and that success in treatment has not made significant headway during the last decade.[189] Approximately 95% of all oral malignancies begin in the surface mucosa. Although the surface of the oral mucosa is easily inspected and palpated, by the time of diagnosis more than 60% of oral cancers have spread to the lymph nodes.[189]

History assessment

When the nurse obtains the health history, it is important to ask the following questions:

1. Do you smoke? How much do you smoke, and how many years have you smoked (pack-years)?
2. Do you chew tobacco or dip snuff? How long have you done this? How much tobacco do you use in a day? Can you describe where you place the tobacco in your mouth?
3. Do you smoke a pipe? How long have you smoked a pipe? Do you smoke a cigar?
4. Do you drink alcohol? Approximately how much alcohol do you drink in a day? What type of alcohol do you consume?
5. *For the patient from Southeast Asia or Central Asia:* Do you chew *betel quid?* Do you use betel quid with any form of tobacco (chewing or smoking)?[190]
6. Do you wear dentures? Do you have any sore spots in your mouth from your dentures? Do you inspect under your dentures at least weekly?
7. When was your last dental examination?
8. How often do you brush your teeth? floss your teeth?
9. Have you ever been in an occupation in which you spent a lot of time outside? Do you have any hobbies or sports interests that involve spending a great deal of time outdoors? Do you wear lip balm when outdoors to protect your lips?
10. Have you noticed any white or red sores in your mouth for longer than a month? any lumps, swelling, or rough spots?
11. Have you been aware of any limitation of tongue or jaw movement?
12. Have you noticed taste changes, dry mouth, speech changes, hoarseness, or chronic cough?
13. Are you aware of any sore or crusts on your lips?
14. Are you aware of any lumps or growing "bumps" in your neck or face?
15. Do you have problems with persistent halitosis that does not seem to respond to any home remedies?

Physical examination

The majority of oral cancers cause no symptoms in their early stages. most individuals who notice a white or bright red spot, "sore," or a swelling in their mouth attribute it to their teeth or dentures and thus seek the consultation of a dentist.

Physical examination of the mouth includes inspection, digital palpation, and olfaction of the oral cavity. The following maneuvers should be performed during the oral examination:

1. Have the patient extend the tongue and move it from side to side. The patient also should be asked to move the jaw from side to side and up and down. Limitation of normal movement could indicate that a tumor is interfering with muscle action.

2. Palpate the tongue with a gloved hand. Palpation may reveal a lesion not otherwise visible. Palpation of a hard lesion should be referred for biopsy to establish the diagnosis.[191]

3. Inspect the anterior two-thirds of the tongue by grasping the tip of the tongue with a piece of gauze and gently pulling the tongue forward and to each side. Lesions of the base of the tongue are most often overlooked and must be both inspected and palpated. The nurse should be aware that most tongue cancers appear on the lateral surfaces.

4. The floor of the mouth should be inspected by having the patient place the tongue on the hard palate. Squamous cell carcinomas frequently are found on the floor of the mouth. The floor of the mouth should be palpated bimanually, with the fingers of one hand in the floor of the mouth and the fingers on the other hand placed on the skin under the right side of the jaw.

5. Inspection of the mouth may reveal snuff keratosis from the use of snuff in one spot in the mouth and nicotine stomatitis from cigar or pipe smoking. Nicotine stomatitis is a diffuse white condition that contains numerous red dots. This lesion usually covers the entire hard palate and is almost always associated with pipe smoking and has minimal or no malignant potential. Complete resolution should occur with cessation of smoking.

Individuals who use smokeless tobacco may develop leukoplakias in the exact region where they hold the quid. The leukoplakia may vary from just a very mild whiteness, which may be difficult to see, to a very obvious white lesion.[192,193] When a white oral lesion is found, the area should be rubbed to see if it can be removed. White lesions that adhere to the surface are classified as keratotic and have a greater probability of malignancy, Leukoplakia occurs in men more commonly than in women, and the vast majority are seen in individuals older than 40 years of age.

In erythroplakia, also considered premalignant, a red plaque or well-defined red patches have a velvety consistency and often have tiny areas of ulceration. Erythroplakia (red) lesions usually have a more malignant histologic component than does leukoplakia.[191] Erythroplakia patches are characteristically painless and occur with about equal frequency in men and women who usually are older than 50 years of age.

6. While inspecting the lips, observe them for any skin changes, such as keratosis of the lips from excessive sun exposure and pipe smoking. Solar keratoses occur on sun-exposed surfaces and are flat, reddish-to-tan plaques that are usually scaly. In the earliest stages a cancerous lesion may appear as a small swelling or induration that may be difficult to see but that can be palpated. An area of roughness, induration, or granularity often is the best clue to the diagnosis of early carcinoma. The upper lip should be grasped between the index finger and the thumb and bidigitally palpated along its complete length to discover masses that may be located deep to the surface.[191]

7. Olfaction of the breath. An odor of sourness may indicate obstruction and fermentation, whereas fetid and foul odors may signal necrotic neoplasms indicative of advanced disease. All large, fungating oral cancers produce a marked halitosis; however, small oral cancers are not particularly associated with mouth odor.[192] Referral to a dentist may be necessary if the breath odors indicate advanced dental decay and poor oral hygiene.

8. Palpate the parotid, submandibular, and submental areas and the cervical lymph nodes.

Screening

Because alcoholics who smoke constitute the largest risk group for oral cancers, screening programs should be geared to this population. Any screening programs would have to be conducted in settings in which alcoholics could be approached as a group, such as in reform organizations, Salvation Army facilities for this population, shelters for the homeless, or alcoholic rehabilitation units. Although primary prevention by limiting alcohol intake and cessation of smoking is a more desirable goal, many alcoholics cannot be reached by these types of programs. Thus the more realistic approach with this group is to encourage periodic oral examinations so that cancer can be detected in the early stages.

It is important for the nurse to explain to individuals 40 years of age and older that it is necessary to have a complete oral and dental examination on a periodic basis to detect serious lesions. Individuals with complete dentures frequently believe they no longer require periodic oral examinations because of their loss of natural teeth.[194]

The use of smokeless tobacco (e.g., snuff and chewing tobacco) has risen dramatically in the last 10 years. The increase in the sales of smokeless tobacco, predominantly snuff, since the early 1970s has been estimated at 11% per year, representing an estimated 7–12 million users.[195] In the early 1970s a majority of users were men 50 years of age and older; now most are young men between 16 and 29 years of age. Nurses need to stress that smokeless tobacco is *not* a safe substitute for smoking. Long-term use of smokeless tobacco increases the risk of gingival and buccal carcinomas nearly 50-fold.[192] Many young people are not aware that smokeless tobacco is as addicting as cigarette smoking.[196] Information about the health hazards of smokeless tobacco should be shared with young people. Because so many users are very young children, it is advocated that education on the dangers of smokeless tobacco should begin with children as young as 6 and 7 years of age.[197] School nurses and nurses who work in settings with young people need to actively initiate educational programs on this subject or make sure that whenever smoking is discussed in health and science classes that the issue of smokeless tobacco also is addressed. In addition, parents, teachers, and athletic coaches should not neglect the powerful influence they can have as positive role models. Youngsters perceive the use of smokeless tobacco as "macho," and athletic coaches can have a tremendous influence in dispelling this myth. The Yellow Pages section at the back of this book lists sources for obtaining patient education materials on smokeless tobacco.

In summary, education first begins with the identification of persons at high risk for oral cancer. Depending on the risk factors identified, the individual could be referred to a physician or a dentist or taught oral self-examination for the early signs of cancer, or the nurse could conduct the oral examination at predetermined intervals. Grabau[198] found that about half those taught self-examinations for early signs of cancer continued these examinations at regular intervals. It is advocated that oral self-examination techniques need to be popularized in the same manner as breast self-examination techniques.

Gynecologic Cancer

It is estimated that in 1993 there will be 31,000 cases of endometrial cancers and 13,500 cases of cervical cancers. The anticipated mortality rates in this same period are expected to be 4400 deaths from cervical cancer and 5700 deaths from endometrial cancer.[64] The risk of endometrial cancer is age-related; the disease usually occurs in women 50–60 years old.

In stark contrast are the incidence and mortality rates for ovarian cancer. It is estimated that in 1993, 22,000 women would be diagnosed with this cancer and 13,300 would die of the disease. Ovarian cancer accounts for about 26% of all gynecologic cancer and about 52% of all genital cancer deaths. The greatest number of cases of ovarian cancer are found in the age group comprised of 55- to 59-year-old women.

History assessment

The health history should include questions that will elicit an accurate menstrual, obstetric, gynecologic, and sexual history. The majority of women at risk for cancer of the reproductive organs can be identified only after a thorough and complete gynecologic history has been obtained. The following questions will help identify high-risk women:

1. When was your last Pap smear? Do you remember the results? Was any follow-up done or recommended?
2. Have you ever been told that you have herpes? genital warts? Were the genital warts treated? What type of treatment was done for the genital warts? Have you been treated for pelvic inflammatory disease or any other sexually transmitted diseases?
3. Do you have any vaginal bleeding or discharge not connected with menses?
4. Do you have spotting between menstrual periods?
5. Do you have bleeding or spotting although you no longer have menstrual periods?
6. Do you have bleeding after intercourse or douching?
7. At what age did you start sexual activity?
8. Have you had a consistent sexual partner since beginning sexual activity, or have you had different partners?
9. What is the approximate number of sexual partners you have had?
10. What age did you start menstruation?
11. What age did you start menopause? When was your last period?
12. How many pregnancies have you had? How many live births? miscarriages? elective abortions?
13. Have you ever taken birth control pills? How long did you take birth control pills? Do you remember the name of the pill that you took?
14. Have you ever taken estrogens? How long did you take these? What was the dose that you were given? What follow-up tests were recommended for you while taking estrogens?
15. Have you ever had infertility problems? Have you ever had endometriosis? polycystic ovaries? Stein-Leventhal syndrome? uterine fibroids?
16. Are you aware of abdominal distention or vague abdominal discomfort?
17. Are you aware if your mother received diethylstilbestrol (DES) when she was pregnant with you?
18. Have you had any gynecologic surgery—hysterectomy, tubal pregnancy, sterilization, ovarian cysts, cancer?
19. Have you ever had office procedures for a gynecologic problem, such as cervical cautery and colposcopic examination?
20. Has your present sexual partner ever had a sexual partner who had cervical cancer?

Physical examination

The early signs and symptoms of gynecologic cancer are as follows. Ovarian cancer usually has no early manifestations. There may be vague abdominal discomfort, dyspepsia, indigestion, gas with constant distention, flatulence, eructation, a feeling of fullness after a light meal, or slight loss of appetite.[199] The majority of patients with endometrial cancer have unexplained bleeding. In postmenopausal women, abnormal bleeding takes the form of intermittent spotting or bleeding that the patient describes as a "very light period." A malodorous watery discharge may be noticed as an early sign. The symptoms of cervical cancer typically are abnormal vaginal discharge, irregular bleeding, elongation of menstrual period, or bleeding that may occur after douching or intercourse.[200]

The gynecologic examination includes *inspection* and *palpation*. The nurse should be aware of the following maneuvers performed during the gynecologic examination and related signs that indicate cancer.

Abdomen The abdomen must be thoroughly and slowly palpated to detect any masses, areas of tenderness, or inguinal adenopathy. A mass in the upper portion of the abdomen may suggest the presence of omental cake, the solid mass formed when the omentum is infiltrated with cancer, which is a sign of advanced ovarian disease. It may be palpated or detected by ballottement during the abdominal examination. Other signs of advanced ovarian cancer are abdominal distention and ascites.[199]

Vulva The vulva should be inspected and palpated for signs of cancer of the vulva: excoriation of skin because of pruritis, ulcers, lumps, leukoplakia, bleeding, atrophy of the labia, and narrowing of the introitus.[201]

Infection with human papillomavirus (HPV) may produce the typically raised exophytic tumors (warts) that can be seen with simple inspection of the vulva. There is, however, a variety of anogenital warts known as "flat" or "noncondylomatous" warts that may be invisible before the application of acetic acid. Several gauze pads (4-in. diameter) that are soaked in 3%–5% acetic acid should be compressed on the vulva and left in place for 10 minutes. After the compress is removed, the area should be inspected with a high-quality magnification lens for the *acetowhite reaction*. Acetic acid will cause the surface of both flat and exophytic warts to turn white.[202] Colposcopic examination also can be used to inspect lesions after acetic acid application. Further, carcinoma in situ also may appear as a hyperpigmented lesion. In addition, HPV can infect the entire lower female genital tract—the vagina and cervix. Patients with vulvar HPV lesions should have a thorough examination of the vagina, cervix, and perirectal epithelium with the use of an acetic acid compress application and a colposcopic examination.[202] In 1989 a minimum of 10% of the population, and probably much higher, was infected with HPV.[203] About half the individuals infected with HPV are carriers of the high-risk types of HPV virus.[16,18,64,66]

Vagina The vagina should be inspected and palpated for cancer—masses, vaginal bands, texture changes, ulcers, erosions, leukoplakia, pink blush, induration, telangiectasis, and erythematosus. Induration and nodulation may indicate submucosal vaginal lesions. Most squamous cell carcinomas are found in the posterior vaginal wall, but 25% involve the anterior wall and at least 15% arise from the lateral walls.[204] The majority of lesions occur in the upper third of the vagina.

The nurse may elect to do a Schiller's test on any suspicious area of the vagina or cervix. The mucosa is painted with an iodine solution (Lugol's solution), and the normal mucosa becomes brown whereas areas of abnormal epithelium remain uncolored. This test is merely an adjunctive aid to colposcopic examination or used when colposcopy is not available. It indicates a glycogen-free area and delineates biopsy sites.[201]

Cervix The cervix should be inspected and palpated, and a Pap smear should be taken for cytologic examination. To avoid contamination of the cell sample with foreign material, vaginal jelly should not be used before Pap smears are obtained. The cervical sample should contain cells from the squamous epithelium of the vaginal portion of the cervix, from the squamocolumnar junction (also known as the transformation zone), and from the endocervical epithelium.[203, 205] With aging the transformation zone becomes increasingly invisible as it moves into the endocervical canal. In women during and after menopause, a sample of the vaginal pool cells is obtained, in addition to the cervical smear, to identify cancer cells from the endometrium, tubes, and ovaries.

The nurse should inspect and palpate the cervix for position, shape, consistency, regularity, mobility, friability, and tenderness. The cervix is freely movable, firm, and smooth, and if it has been invaded by cancer, it becomes hard and immobile. In addition to rendering the cervix much harder than normal, malignancy produces a rough, granular surface and is likened to both the feel and appearance of a cauliflower.[166] However, the nurse needs to be cognizant of the fact that early carcinoma has an appearance that cannot be well differentiated visually from erosion. Cancer arising within the cervical canal may cause no abnormal appearance of the cervix.

Several physical changes may be apparent in the cervix that indicate possible patient exposure to DES in utero. Cervical ectropion, or cervical bumps or ridges ("cockscombs," "hoods," or "collars"), and other nonneoplastic changes are immediate clues to DES exposure. These physical signs merit referral to a physician.

The conventional Pap smear, taken in the usual manner for cervix cancer screening, is inaccurate for a diagnosis of endometrial lesions.[206] For this reason an annual suction curettage is recommended for menopausal women and women who have taken estrogen without progestational modification for a prolonged period after menopause. Suction curettage can provide an excellent sample and in most cases can be done in the office without need for anesthesia. Monitoring of women who have received long-term estrogen therapy will detect those whose endometrium is overstimulated (adenomatous hyperplasia), and appropriate referrals can be made.

Uterus and adnexa A bimanual examination of the uterus and adnexa should be done. The nurse should note the size, shape, mobility, position, tenderness, and consistency of the uterus. Uterine tenderness, immobility, or enlargement merits further investigation and appropriate referrals. An enlarged boggy uterus is an indication of advanced disease.

Ovaries Palpation of the ovaries in prepubertal girls or postmenopausal women also merits investigation because (1) normal ovary and tube are usually not palpable, (2) ovaries in these two groups of women are smaller than the usual ovarian size of 4 cm in its largest dimension, and (3) 3–5 years after menopause the ovaries usually have atrophied and are no longer palpable. In actively menstruating women, any ovarian enlargement that persists or increases more than 5 or 6 cm requires prompt referral.[199] In general the findings on the pelvic examination that can alert the nurse to a possible ovarian cancer are adnexal enlargement, fixation or immobility, bilateral irregularity or nodulation and masses, relative insensitivity of the mass, and bilaterality of the mass.

Rectovaginal palpation *Rectovaginal* palpation, as well as rectal palpation, should be done. It is extremely important that the anterior rectal wall in the region of the peritoneal rectovaginal pouch, or Douglas' cul-de-sac, be palpated. Thickening of this area occurs from spread of cervical carcinoma, whereas spread from ovarian cancer may be felt as a shelf, nodule, or handful-of-knuckles on rectal palpation.

Screening of asymptomatic individuals

The American Cancer Society recommends that all women who are, or who have been, sexually active or have reached 18 years of age have an annual Pap test and pelvic examination. After a woman has had three or more consecutive satisfactory normal annual examinations, the Pap test may be performed less frequently at the discretion of her physician.[207] Numerous other professional health organizations also have approved a similar or identical recommendation.

Cervical smears Because of the Pap test, the death rate from invasive cervical cancer has decreased by at least 70% over the last 40 years.[117] However, 15%–20% of American women do not have regular Pap testing.[207] The majority of women in whom cervical cancer develops have not had the test on a regular basis.

The importance of regular Pap smears was documented by Stenkvist and colleagues.[208] They studied 207,455 women for 10 years and found that when women were screened at least once, the incidence of cervical cancer dropped from 32/100,000 to 10/100,000 (a 75% decrease in invasive cervical cancer incidence among women who had smears taken at least once during the 10-year period). Among women with at least one normal smear, the incidence drops still lower, to 7/100,000. Because elderly women will constitute 17.3% of the adult population by the year 2020, screening programs for older, high-risk women will be needed.

Mandelblatt and Fahs[209] conducted a study of the cost effectiveness of a cervical cancer screening program for infrequently screened elderly women. The results of the Pap smears were abnormal in 11/816 women screened. This early detection of cervical neoplasia saved $5907 and 3.7 years of life per 100 Pap tests. The average medical costs per year of life extended by screening were included, and the program cost $2874 per year of life saved. The researchers concluded that the benefits from cervical cancer screening for elderly women can offset the costs of these programs.

Several factors contribute to false-negative results from Pap smears and other errors:

Patient error Patient error consists of women failing to have follow-up annual examinations, delay in seeing a physician while symptoms are present, and refusal to undergo diagnostic measures.

Physician error Physician error consists of failure to act on reports of abnormal cytologic findings, failure to perform a pelvic examination with a Pap smear, reading of Pap smears by untrained physicians, and diagnosis of "dysplasia," which is considered inconsequential by uninformed physicians.

Laboratory error Koss[203] reports in his excellent review article that studies have found a false-negative laboratory rate for invasive cancer of approximately 50%. The rate of screening errors for precancerous lesions was at least 28%.

Although nurses generally do not have control over laboratory errors, they can play a significant role in decreasing patient and physician error (1) by educating women about the early symptoms of gynecologic cancer and the necessity of seeking medical advice with these early symptoms; (2) by educating women about the recommended intervals for Pap smears; (3) by educating women, particularly older women, to the necessity of asking for a Pap smear when they have a physical examination; (4) by educating women to request information about the mechanism used by the health care setting to inform them about the results of their Pap smears: women with a history of abnormal or questionable Pap smear results should be encouraged to personally call about their results rather than rely on the health professional to alert them; (5) by educating women about the importance of receiving additional medical care with an abnormal or a questionable Pap smear finding; and (6) by performing Pap smears only after they are thoroughly versed in the proper procedures for obtaining a smear. Improperly done smears probably contribute to at least half of the 10%–35% false-negative rate generally reported for Pap smears.[210] Errors made by cytotechnologists may be minimized in the future by new experimental technologic techniques that measure the DNA content of standard Pap smears. Several groups of researchers are investigating the feasibility of automating the procedure of reading Pap smears on the basis of optical density of the specimens or DNA content of cell nuclei.[211,212] Studies are being conducted to determine the feasibility of these approaches.

Two classification methods are used to identify abnormal changes in the Pap smear. One method is the classification system accepted by the World Health Organization. This system identified two types of lesions, dysplasia and carcinoma in situ. The dysplasias are subdivided into very mild, mild, moderate, and severe grades, depending on the extent of involvement of the epithelium.[213] Another classification method is the cervical intraepithelial neoplasia (CIN) nomenclature. CIN is a contiuum of change and generally begins as a well-differentiated lesion (CIN 1, or mild dysplasia), passes through a less well-differentiated phase (CIN 2, or moderate dysplasia), and leads to an undifferentiated intraepithelial lesion (CIN 3).[205] CIN 3 is the severe dysplasia/carcinoma in situ in the World Health Organization system. Table 8-8 compares the commonly used Papanicolaou terminology and relationship to the

TABLE 8-8 Classification and Comparative Nomenclature of Cervical Smears

Class I
Normal smear
No abnormal cells
Class II
Atypical cells present below the level of cervical neoplasia
Class III
Smear contains abnormal cells consistent with dysplasia
Mild dysplasia = CIN 1
Moderate dysplasia = CIN 2
Class IV
Smear contains abnormal cells consistent with carcinoma in situ
Severe dysplasia and carcinoma in situ = CIN 3
Class V
Smear contains abnormal cells consistent with invasive carcinoma of squamous cell origin

CIN, cervical intraepithelial neoplasia.

Source: Nelson J, Averette H, Richart R: Dysplasia, carcinoma in situ, and early invasive cervical carcinoma. *CA* 34:307, 1984. Courtesy of James H. Nelson Jr.

CIN classification method, and Figure 8-19 is a schematic representation of precancerous cervical lesions.[214]

Colposcopic examination is an accurate and reliable method for evaluating the cervix and vagina of a woman with an abnormality revealed by Pap smear. This modality (a well-illuminated binocular microscope) not only provides visualization of the cervical transformation zone but also allows directed biopsy of specific areas of the epithelium, removing only small amounts of tissue.

Additional nursing interventions

Reaching those women who are at high risk for gynecologic cancer is one of the most challenging roles for nurses. Patient acceptance and increasing the availability of screening are areas that will require major effort on the part of nurses if the entire population at greatest risk is to be reached. Because cytologic screening is closely tied to obstetric care and contraceptive services, a higher proportion of women are screened among the groups that require such attention than among those that do not. This is effective for screening for cervical and vaginal cancer in the reproductive years but does not reach the postmenopausal women who are at risk for ovarian and endometrial malignancies. Nurses who work in retirement centers, extended care facilities, physicians' offices, factories, public health agencies, and ambulatory care settings are urged to provide health education programs that include the early signs and symptoms of ovarian, cervical, and endometrial cancer and to stress the need for gynecologic examinations after menopause as well as during the reproductive years. Female patients being followed routinely for chronic problems (such as hypertension, diabetes, heart condition, or chronic lung disease) should be asked when they had their last pelvic examination.

When appropriate, nurses should discuss the myths about menopause with women who are in their late 30s and early 40s. There are several significant barriers to early detection of gynecologic cancer in older women. Many women have the mistaken belief that once they are past childbearing years and/or are sexually inactive, they no longer need pelvic examinations. There are also physical changes that occur that make the gynecologic examination difficult for older women. There is decreased mobility of the femoropelvic structure, which leads to pain when they are put in the lithotomy position for a gynecologic examination. Nurses need to be aware of this physical barrier and suggest the use of the left lateral Sims' position instead of the traditional lithotomy position. Because the vaginal orifice may have narrowed with age, the insertion of the traditional speculum may cause discomfort or admit only the passage of one finger.

Nurses need to conduct educational programs in community settings that dispel these myths that surround menopause and aging and provide factual information on the early signs and symptoms of the common gynecologic cancers in older women, as well as discuss methods to make the gynecologic examination more comfortable for the woman. Women taking estrogens should be advised that they need to be routinely monitored by their physician in terms of an examination to detect endometrial cancer.[215,216]

Nurses need to be aware that older women are at high risk for endometrial, vulvar, vaginal, and ovarian cancer. Several premalignant conditions commonly found in elderly women predispose them to gynecologic cancers. These premalignant conditions are leukoplakic vulvitis, which precedes epidermoid carcinoma; lichen sclerosus et atrophicus, which precedes epidermoid carcinoma; and endometrial adenoma, which precedes hyperplastic lesions. Normal changes that occur with aging frequently obscure the early symptoms of cancer. The vaginal mucosa thins with aging, and there is a decrease in vaginal/cervical lubrication. Bleed-

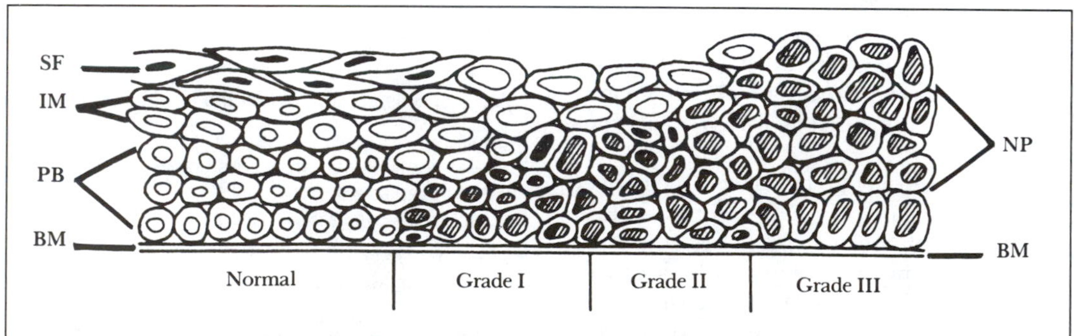

FIGURE 8-19 Cervical intraepithelial neoplasia *(CIN)*, showing infiltrating normal epithelium. CIN is dysplasia that occurs in the transformation zone. When CIN is suspected from abnormalities seen on a Pap smear of cervical secretions, a colposcopic examination should be done. (*SF* = superficial cells; *IM* = intermediate cells; *PB* = parabasal cells; *BM* = basement membrane; *NP* = neoplastic cells. *Grades* refer to degree of epithelium involved by dysplasia. *Grade I* = ¼ in thickness; *grade II* = ¼–¾ thickness; and *grade III* = ¾ to full thickness of epithelium. (Source: McCauley K, Oi R: Evaluating the Papanicolaou smear: Part I. *Consultant* 28(12):31-40, 1988.)

ing that results from endometrial or vaginal cancer is shrugged off as normal "postmenopausal bleeding" or attributed by health professionals to atrophic vaginitis and often is not followed up.[206]

Young women who have had venereal disease (syphilis, gonorrhea, genital herpes, or HPV infection) must be alert to the necessity of having regular Pap smears. Women with vulvar condyloma acuminatum should be referred for a thorough examination of the vagina, cervix, and perirectal epithelium with the use of acetic acid compress application, a colposcopic examination, and a Pap smear. It also is recommended that these women (and infected male partners) have frequent follow-up examinations to detect precancerous conditions caused by a latent virus in clinically and histologically normal tissue.[202] Infection of the genital tract by HPV is a common disease and often encountered in clinics for family planning, prenatal care, and sexually transmitted diseases. Women whose Pap smears indicate the presence of warty infections such as koilocytotic cells or who show cells consistent with squamous papilloma or warty atypia also should be referred to a physician for further evaluation.[217]

Nurses are urged to acquire physical assessment skills that will enable them to perform pelvic examinations. It has been documented that nurses who perform pelvic examinations can detect gynecologic malignancies, that patient acceptance and satisfaction are high, and that pelvic examinations done by nurses are cost effective.[206,218]

Nurses trained to conduct gynecologic examinations are in an ideal position to reach those women who are at highest risk for the development of various types of gynecologic cancers but who are least likely to use conventional screening programs or have routine health examinations, such as older women in residential settings or older poor women in the community. Nurses actively involved in conducting pelvic examinations also would increase the availability of screening programs and thus reach more women.[218]

REFERENCES

1. The National Cancer Institute Act, Aug 5, 1937. PL 244, 75th Congress, 1st Session. Chapter 565 (S. 2067).
2. The National Cancer Act of 1971. *JNCI* 48:577–584, 1972.
3. Schottenfeld D, Fraumeni JF: *Cancer Epidemiology and Prevention.* Philadelphia: Saunders, 1982.
4. Vessey MP, Gray M: *Cancer Risks and Prevention.* Oxford, Eng.: Oxford University Press, 1985.
5. Enstrom J, Austin D: Interpreting cancer survival rates. In Kruse L, Reese J, Hart L (eds.): *Cancer: Pathophysiology, Etiology and Management.* St. Louis: Mosby, 1979, pp. 28–37.
6. Bailar JC, Smith EM: Progress against cancer. *N Engl J Med* 314:1226–1232, 1986.
7. Hamburg D: Healthy people: The surgeon general's report on health promotion and disease prevention, background papers. Washington, DC: DHEW Publication No. (PHS) 79–55071A, 1979, p 162.
8. Schottenfeld D: *Cancer Epidemiology and Prevention: Current Concepts.* Springfield, IL: Thomas, 1975.
9. Pollner F: Debate over cancer survival rate is heating up. *Medical World News* 72:Apr 25, 1988.
10. McGinnis JM, Richmond JB, Brandt EN, et al: Health Progress in the United States: Results of the 1990 objectives for the nation. *JAMA* 268:2545–2552, 1992.
11. Fisher S: Cancer: Prevention, screening and early diagnosis. *Aust Fam Physician* 6:269–277, 1977.
12. Van Parifs LG, Eckhardt S: Public education in primary and secondary cancer prevention. *Hygiene* 111:16–28, 1984.
13. Slenker S, Spreitzer EA: Public perceptions and behaviors regarding cancer control. *J Cancer Educ* 3:171–180, 1988.
14. Kennedy BJ: Principles of cancer prevention. *Oncology Time* 6:2, 1984.
15. Blonston G: Cancer, the new synthesis: Prevention. *Science* 28:36–39, 1984.
16. Breslow L: A positive strategy for the nation's health. *JAMA* 242:2093–2095, 1979.
17. Whelan E: The politics of cancer. *Policy Review* 33:46, 1979.
18. Woods N, Woods J: Epidemiology and the study of cancer. In Marino L (ed.): *Cancer Nursing.* St. Louis: Mosby, 1981, pp. 139–175.
19. Becker CE, Coye MJ: *Cancer Prevention: Strategies in the Workplace.* Washington, DC: Hemisphere Publishing, 1986.
20. American Cancer Society: *Cancer Facts and Figures: 1988.* New York: American Cancer Society, 1988.
21. Edelman C, Milio N: Health defined: Promotion and specific protection. In Edelman C, Mandle CL (eds.): *Health Promotion Throughout the Lifespan.* St. Louis: Mosby, 1986, pp. 2–18.
22. Leavell H, Clark AE: *Preventive Medicine for Doctors in the Community.* New York: McGraw-Hill, 1965.
23. Fraumeni J: *Persons at High Risk of Cancer: An Approach to Cancer Etiology and Control.* New York: Academic Press, 1975.
24. Glasel M: Cancer prevention: The role of the nurse in primary and secondary cancer prevention. *Cancer Nurse* 8:5–8, 1985 (suppl 1).
25. Sirota H, Rubovits D, Cousins J, et al: Cancer control: Prevention. *Health Values* 12:33–36, 1988.
26. Valentine A: Behavioral dimensions in cancer prevention and detection. *Semin Oncol Nurs* 2:200–205, 1986.
27. Greenwald P: Prevention of cancer: Diet and nutrition. In DeVita VT, Hellman S, Rosenberg SA (eds.): *Cancer Principles and Practice of Oncology* (ed. 3). Philadelphia: Lippincott, 1989, pp. 167–180.
28. McGee R: The role of the nurse in cancer prevention. *Georgia Nurs* 1986.
29. Disease prevention: A link missing. *Arch Int Med* 149:1253, 1989.
30. Frank-Stromborg M, Rohan K: Nursing's involvement in the primary and secondary prevention of cancer: Nationally and internationally. *Cancer Nurs* 15:79–107, 1992.
31. Frank-Stromborg M: Nursing's role in cancer prevention and detection. *Cancer* 62:1833–1838, 1988 (suppl).
32. Cox A, Lovato C: Update: Collaborative efforts between AAOHN and the National Cancer Institute. *Occupational Health Nurs* 32:626–628, 1984.

33. McGuire R: Evaluation of cancer screening and education programs 1982. *Occupational Health Nurs* 30:25–29, 1982.
34. Ericksen M: The role of cancer prevention in workplace health promotion. *Health Values* 12:18–23, 1988.
35. White L: The nurse's role in cancer prevention. In Newell G (ed.): *Cancer Prevention in Clinical Medicine*. New York: Raven Press, 1983, pp. 91–112.
36. Lindberg S: Adult preventive health screening: 1987 update. *Nurse Pract* 12:19–41, 1987.
37. Heinrich J: Historical perspectives on public health nursing. *Nurs Outlook* 31:317–320, 1983.
38. Gianella A: Teaching cancer prevention and detection. *Cancer Nurs* 8:9–12, 1985 (suppl 1).
39. White L, Taylor D: *Cancer Prevention and Detection in Nursing Practice*. Houston: University of Texas System Cancer Center, MD. Anderson Hospital and Tumor Institute (no date), pp. 12–20.
40. LeMaistre C: Reflections on disease prevention. *Cancer* 62:1673–1675, 1988 (suppl).
41. Russel LB: Prevention often costs more. *Medical World News* (Jan 27):76, 1986.
42. Eddy DM: The economics of cancer prevention and detection: Getting more for less. *Cancer* 47:1200–1209, 1981.
43. McMillan S: Nurse's compliance with American Cancer Society Guidelines for Cancer Prevention and Detection. *Oncol Nurse Forum* 17:721–727, 1990.
44. Loescher LJ, Meyskens FL: Chemoprevention of human skin cancers. *Semin Oncol Nurs* 7:45–52, 1991.
45. Mori S: The changes in the paraocular glands which follow the administration of diets low in fat-soluble A with notes of the effects of the same diets on the salivary glands and the mucosa of the larynx and trachea. *Johns Hopkins Hospital Bulletin* 33:357–359, 1922.
46. Wrba H: Chemoprevention of cancer. In Eylenbosch WJ, Van Larebeke N, Depoorter AM (eds.): *Primary Prevention of Cancer*. New York: Raven Press, 1988, pp. 71–77.
47. Sporn MB: Retinoids and suppression of carcinogenesis. *Hospital Practice* 18:83–98, 1983.
48. Abels JC, Gorham AT, Pack GT, et al: Metabolic studies in patients with cancer of the gastrointestinal tract: I. Plasma vitamin A levels in patients with malignant neoplastic disease, particularly of the gastrointestinal tract. *J Clin Invest* 20:749–764, 1941.
49. Ziegler RG: A review of epidemiologic evidence that carotenoids reduce the risk of cancer. *J Nutr* 119:116–122, 1989.
50. Cullen JW: The National Cancer Institute's intervention trials. *Cancer* 62:1851–1864, 1988.
51. Hong, WK, Lippman SM, Itri LM, et al: Prevention of second primary tumors with isotretinoin in squamous-cell carcinoma of the head and neck. *N Engl J Med* 323:795–801, 1990.
52. Olsen SJ, Love RR: A new direction in preventive oncology: Chemoprevention. *Semin Oncol Nurs* 2:211–221, 1986.
53. Kelloff GJ, Malone WF, Boone CW, et al: Progress in applied chemoprevention research. *Semin Oncol* 17:438–455, 1990.
54. Formelli F, Clerici M, DePalo G, et al: Chronic oral administration of fenretinide, as a chemopreventive agent to breast cancer patients, does not affect plasma alpha-tocopherol concentration. *Ann Oncol* 2:446–447, 1991.
55. Greenberg ER, Baron JA, Stukel TA, et al: A clinical trial of beta carotene to prevent basal-cell and squamous-cell cancers of the skin. *N Engl J Med* 323:789–795, 1990.
56. Hennekens CH, Mayrent SL, Willett, W: Vitamin A, carotenoids, and retinoids. *Cancer* 58:1837–1841, 1986.
57. Greenwald P, Sondik E, Lynch B: Diet and chemoprevention in NCI's research strategy to achieve national cancer control objectives. *Ann Rev Public Health* 7:267–291, 1986.
58. *Cancer Prevention Research Summary—Nutrition*. U.S. Department of Health and Human Services, Public Health Service, National Institutes of Health. National Cancer Institute, Bethesda, MD. NIH Publication No. 85–2616, 1985.
59. Bakemeier A: The potential role of vitamins A, C, and E and selenium in cancer prevention. *Oncol Nurs Forum* 15:785–791, 1988.
60. Hunter DJ, Morris JS, Stampfer MJ, et al: A prospective study of selenium status and breast cancer risk. *JAMA* 264:1128–1131, 1990.
61. Harris JR, Lippman ME, Veronesi U, et al: Breast cancer (third of three parts). *N Eng J Med* 327:473–480, 1992.
62. *Breast Cancer Prevention Trial Will Recruit 16,000 Women:* National Cancer Institute, Office of Cancer Communications, National Institutes of Health, April 29, 1992.
63. Hospital discharge rates for four major cancers—United States, 1970-1986. *JAMA* 260:3412–3416, 1988.
64. Boring CC, Squires TS, Tong T: Cancer statistics, 1993. *CA* 43:7–26, 1993.
65. Garfinkel L, Silverberg E: Lung cancer and smoking trends in the United States over the past 25 years. *CA* 41:137–145, 1991.
66. Fielding J, Phenow J: Health effects of involuntary smoking. *N Engl J Med* 319:1452–1460, 1988.
67. Humble C, Samet J, Pathak D: Marriage to a smoker and lung cancer risk. *Am J Public Health* 77:598–560, 1987.
68. Stellman J, Stellman S: Occupational lung disease and cancer risk in women. *Occup Health Nurs* 31:40–46, 1983.
69. Goldman R, Peters J: The occupational and environmental health history. *JAMA* 246:2832–2836, 1981.
70. *Asbestos Exposure*. Washington, DC: National Cancer Institute, 1978; DHEW Publication No. 78–1622.
71. Grimes J, Burns E (eds.): *Health Assessment in Nursing Practice* (ed. 2). Boston: Jones and Bartlett, 1987.
72. Bouchier I, Morris J: *Clinical Skills. A System of Clinical Examination*. London: Saunders, 1976.
73. Buckingham W: *A Primer of Clinical Diagnosis* (ed. 2). New York: Harper & Row, 1979.
74. Rohwedder J: Neoplastic disease. In Guenter C, Welch M (eds.): *Pulmonary Medicine*. Philadelphia: Lippincott, 1977, pp. 300–320.
75. DeGowin E, DeGowin R: *Bedside Diagnostic Examination* (ed. 5). New York: Macmillan, 1987.
76. Guarino J: Auscultatory-percussion, a technique for detecting unsuspected lung disease. *Diagnosis*, January: 20-26, 1981.
77. Bates B: *A Guide to Physical Examination* (ed. 3). Philadelphia: Lippincott, 1983.
78. Burns K, Johnson P: *Health Assessment in Clinical Practice* (ed. 2). Englewood Cliffs, NJ: Prentice-Hall, 1980.
79. Ca screening: Auditing the payoff. *Medical World News* 26:42–55, 1985.
80. Fielding J: Smoking: Health effects and control. *N Engl J Med* 313:491–498, 1985.

81. Fiore M, Novotny T, Pierce J, et al: Trends in cigarette smoking in the United States. The changing influence of gender and race. *JAMA* 261:49–55, 1989.
82. Novello AC, Davis RM, Giovino GA: The slowing of the lung cancer epidemic and the need for continued vigilance. *CA* 41:133–136, 1991.
83. Pierce J, Fiore M, Novotny T, et al: Trends in cigarette smoking in the United States. Educational differences are increasing. *JAMA* 261:56–60, 1989.
84. Davis R: Current trends in cigarette advertising and marketing. *N Engl J Med* 316:725–732, 1987.
85. Ernster V: Trends in smoking, cancer risk, and cigarette promotion: Current priorities for reducing tobacco exposure. *Cancer* 62:1702–1712, 1988.
86. Hermanson B, Omenn G, Kronmal R, et al: Participants in the Coronary Artery Surgery Study: Beneficial six-year outcome of smoking cessation in older men and women with coronary artery disease. *N Engl J Med* 319:1365–1369, 1988.
87. Koop report equates nicotine with narcotic addiction. *Oncology & Biotechnology News* 2(6):3, 1988.
88. Benowitz N, Jacob P, Kozlowski L, et al: Influence of smoking fewer cigarettes on exposure to tar, nicotine, and carbon monoxide. *N Engl J Med* 315:1310–1313, 1986.
89. Cigarette chokes health experts. *Medical World News* 28:30, 1987.
90. Nurses' smoking habits and attitudes influence patients. *Cancer Lett* 1(12):4–5, 1987.
91. Johnson J: *Nurses: The Challenge to Action in Anti-Smoking Efforts.* New York: American Cancer Society [Professional Education Publication No. 80-50M-No 3340-PE], 1980.
92. Anda R, Remington P, Sienko D, et al: Are physicians advising smokers to quit? The patient's perspective. *JAMA* 257:1916–1919, 1987.
93. Smith J: Letter to the editor. *JAMA* 258:472, 1987.
94. U.S. Preventive Services Task Force: Recommendations for smoking cessation counseling. *JAMA* 259:2882, 1988.
95. Kottke T, Battista R, Defriese G, et al: Attributes of successful smoking cessation interventions in medical practice. A meta-analysis of 39 controlled trials. *JAMA* 259:2883–2889, 1988.
96. Orleans CT: Understanding and promoting smoking cessation: Overview and guidelines for physician intervention. *Annu Rev Med* 36:51–61, 1985.
97. Altman D, Flora J, Fortmann S, et al: The cost-effectiveness of three smoking cessation programs. *Am J Public Health* 77:162–165, 1987.
98. New rules extinguish "smoking lamp" in growing number of public places. *JAMA* 259:2809, 1988.
99. More "no smoking" signs seen in hospitals. *JAMA* 259:2814, 1988.
100. Schuster M: Disorders of the aging GI system. In Reichel W (ed.): *The Geriatric Patient.* New York: HP Publishers, 1978, pp. 73–81.
101. Evans J: Cancer of the colon and rectum. In Murphy G (ed.): *Cancer Signals and Safeguards.* Littleton, MA: PSG Publishing 1981, pp. 155–160.
102. Braverman I: *Skin Signs of Systemic Disease.* Philadelphia: Saunders, 1970.
103. Leffall L: *Early Diagnosis of Colorectal Cancer.* New York: American Cancer Society [Professional Education Publication 81-50M-No 3311-PE], 1981.
104. Collins J: Colon cancer screens unproven. *Medical World News* 29:77–78, 1988.
105. Minnesota study aimed at finding final answer on Hemoccult screening. *Cancer Lett* 13(30):4–6, 1987.
106. Kewenter J, Bjork S, Haglind E, et al: Screening and rescreening for colorectal cancer. *Cancer* 62:645–651, 1988.
107. Sugarbaker P, Gunderson L, Wittes R: Colorectal cancer. In DeVita VT, Hellman S, Rosenberg SA (eds.): *Cancer: Principles and Practice of Oncology* (ed. 2), Philadelphia: Lippincott, 1986, pp. 795–884.
108. Fleischer D, Goldberg S, Browning T, et al: Detection and surveillance of colorectal cancer. *JAMA* 261:580–585, 1989.
109. Knight K, Fielding J, Battista R: Occult blood screening for colorectal cancer. *JAMA* 261:587–593, 1989.
110. Rakel R: A clinician's guide: Tips on fecal occult blood testing. *Your Patient & Cancer* 3:33–38, 1983.
111. Simon J: Occult blood screening for colorectal carcinoma. A critical review. *Gastroenterology* 88:820–837, 1985.
112. Winawer S: Introduction to position papers from the Third International Symposium on Colorectal Cancer. *CA* 34:130–133, 1985.
113. Dorozynski A: Test for early detection of colorectal cancer under development. *Oncology & Biotechnology News* 1(2):3, 1987.
114. Colorectal ca found earlier with new quick office tests. *Oncology News/Update* 2(2):1–7, 1987.
115. Poll finds public misconceptions re colorectal cancer detection. *Oncology Times,* September 9, 1986, p. 25.
116. Callahan L: Colo-rectal cancer: Clinical trial/community outreach. Proceedings of the Fourth National Cancer Communications Conference. Washington, DC, National Institutes of Health, 1977, DHEW Publication No. (PHS) 78–1463.
117. Greenwald P, Sondik E, Lynch B: Diet and chemoprevention in NCI's research strategy to achieve national cancer control objectives. *Annu Rev Public Health* 7:267–291, 1986.
118. American Cancer Society Special Report: *Nutrition and Cancer: Cause and Prevention.* New York: American Cancer Society [Professional Education Publication 84-50M-No. 3389-PE], 1984.
119. Kritchevsky D: Diet and cancer. *CA* 41:328–333, 1991.
120. The Work Study Group on Diet, Nutrition, and Cancer: American Cancer Society Guidelines on diet, nutrition, and cancer. *CA* 41:334–338, 1991.
121. The changing diet: Illinois 1982–1986. *American Cancer Society Cancer Prevention Study II Newsletter* 5(2):3, Fall 1987.
122. Chodak G, Schoenberg H: Early detection of prostate cancer by routine screening. *JAMA* 252:3261–3264, 1984.
123. National Cancer Institute: *Cancer Among Blacks and Other Minorities: Statistical Profiles.* Washington, DC: NIH Publication No. 86–2785, March 1986.
124. Sagalowsky A, Wilson J: Carcinoma of the prostate. In Petersdorf R, Adams R, Braunwald E, et al (eds.): *Harrison's Principles of Internal Medicine* (ed. 10). New York: McGraw-Hill, 1983, pp. 795–798.
125. Guinan P, Sharifi R, Bush I: Prostate cancer: Tips toward earlier detection. *Your Patient & Cancer* 4:37–42, 1984.
126. Guinan P, Gilham N, Nagubadi S, et al: What is the best test to detect prostate cancer? *CA* 31:141–145, 1981.
127. Crawford ED, Nabors WL: Diagnosing prostate cancer:

Role of the primary care physician. *Primary Care & Cancer,* March:19-24, 1990.
128. Klein EA: Prostate cancer: Current concepts in diagnosis and treatment. *Cleveland Clinic J Med* 59:383–389, 1992.
129. Littrup PJ, Lee F, Mettlin C: Prostate cancer screening: Current trends and future implications. *CA* 42:198–209, 1992.
130. Lee F, Gray J, McLeary R, et al: Transrectal ultrasound in the diagnosis of prostate cancer: Location, echogenicity, histopathology and staging. *Prostate* 7:117–129, 1985.
131. Lee F, Gray J, McLeary R, et al: Prostatic evaluation by transrectal sonography: Criteria for diagnosis of early carcinoma. *Radiology* 158:91–95, 1986.
132. Lee F. Littrup P, Torp-Pedersen S, et al: Prostate cancer: Comparison of U.S. and digital rectal examination for screening. *Radiology* 168:389–394, 1988.
133. Catalona WJ, Smith DS, Ratliff TL et al: Measurement of prostate-specific antigen in serum as a screening test for prostate cancer. *N Engl J Med* 324:1156–1161, 1991.
134. Strax P: Mass screeing for control of breast cancer. *Cancer* 53:665–670, 1984.
135. Olsen S: *Examinations for Detecting Breast Cancer.* Cancer Prevention Program, Wisconsin Clinical Cancer Center, 1300 University Ave-7C, Medical Science Center, Madison, WI 53706.
136. Wilkes B: The development of a two-tier BSE educational program. In *Progress in Cancer Control III: A Regional Approach.* New York: Alan R. Liss, 1983, pp. 127–131.
137. Burnside J: *Adams' Physical Diagnosis* (ed. 15). Baltimore: Williams and Wilkins, 1977.
138. Scanlon E: A photo checklist for a better breast palpation. *Primary Care & Cancer* 7:13–20, 1987.
139. Heymann A: Semilateral decubitus breast examination. *JAMA* 243:1713, 1980.
140. Feig S: Mammography screening: Published guidelines and actual practice. *Recent Results Cancer Res* 105:78–88, 1987.
141. Update January 1992: The American Cancer Society guidelines for the cancer-related checkup. *CA* 42:44–45, 1992.
142. Greenwald P, Sondik E: *Cancer Control Objectives for the Nation: 1985–2000.* Washington, DC: National Institutes of Health, 1986. NIH Publication No. 86-2880, no. 8.
143. Dodd G: Screening for the early detection of breast cancer. *Cancer* 62:1781–1783, 1988.
144. Tabar L, Fagerberg C, Gad A, et al: Reduction in mortality from breast cancer after mass screening with mammography. *Lancet* 1:829–832, 1984.
145. New analysis of HIP study supports mammographic screening age 40–49. *Cancer Lett* 14(37):4–6, 1988.
146. Status of breast cancer research updated in overview compiled by NCI. *Cancer Lett* 14(32):3–5, 1988.
147. Frank J, Mai V: Breast self-examination in young women: More harm than good? *Lancet* 2:654–657, 1985.
148. Foster R, Costanza M, Worden J: The current status of research in breast self-examination. *NY State J Med* 85:480–482, 1985.
149. U.S. Preventive Services Task Force: Recommendations for breast cancer screening. *JAMA* 257:2196, 1987.
150. O'Malley M, Fletcher S: Screening for breast cancer with breast self-examination. A critical review. *JAMA* 257:2197–2203, 1987.
151. Feldman J; Breast self-examination—A practice whose time has come? *NY State J Med* 85:482–483, 1985.
152. Huguley C, Brown R, Greenberg R, et al: Breast self-examination and survival from breast cancer. *Cancer* 62:1389–1396, 1988.
153. Bennett S, Lawrence R, Fleischmann K, et al: Profile of women practicing breast self-examination. *JAMA* 249:488–491, 1983.
154. Kegeles S: Education for breast self-examination: Why, who, what, and how? *Prev Med* 14:702–720, 1985.
155. Study shows survival advantage for women who examine their breasts. *Medical World News* 25:31, 1984.
156. Boyle M, Michalek A, Bersani G, et al: Effectiveness of a community program to promote early breast cancer detection. *J Surg Oncol* 18:183 188, 1981.
157. Diem G, Rose D: Has breast self-examination had a fair trial? *NY State J Med* 85:479–480, 1985.
158. Styrd A: A breast self-examination program in an occupational health setting. *Occup Health Nurs* 30:33–35, 1982.
159. Shamian J, Edgar L: Nurses as agents for change in teaching breast self-examination. *Public Health Nurs* 4:29–34, 1987.
160. Garnick M, Scully R, Weber E, et al: Cancer of the testis. In Cady B (ed.): *Cancer Manual* (ed. 7): New York: American Cancer Society, Massachusetts Division, 1986, pp. 268–277.
161. Swanson D: Why you should conscientiously promote self-examination. *Consultant* 27(4):142–147, 1987.
162. Carlin P: Testicular self-examination: A public awareness program. *Public Health Rep* 101(1):98–102, 1986.
163. Borski A: Diagnosis, staging and natural history of testicular tumors. Proceedings of the National Conference on Urologic Cancer. New York, American Cancer Society, 1973 [Professional Education Publication No. 3080-PE].
164. Conklin M, Klint K, Morway A, et al: Should health teaching include self-examination of the testis? *Am J Nurs* 78:2073–2074, 1978.
165. Blesch K: Health beliefs about testicular cancer and self-examination among professional men. *Oncol Nurs Forum* 13(1):29–33, 1986.
166. Smith J, Hollenbeck Z: Genitalia. In Prior J, Silberstein J, Stang J (eds.), *Physical Diagnosis. The History and Examination of the Patient.* St Louis: Mosby, 1981, pp. 330–364.
167. Delp M, Manning R: *Major's Physical Diagnosis. An Introduction to the Clinical Process* (ed. 9). Philadelphia: Saunders, 1981, pp. 381–383.
168. Office urology: When your patient fears testicular cancer. *Patient Care* 9:102, 1975.
169. Frank-Stromborg M: The role of the nurse in cancer detection and screening. *Semin Oncol Nurs* 2:191–199, 1986.
170. Garnick M: Urologic cancer. In Rubenstein E, Federman D (eds.): *Oncology,* vol. 9. New York: Scientific American Medicine, 1988, pp. 1–17.
171. Murray B, Wilcox L: Testicular self-examination. *Am J Nurs* 78:2074–2075, 1978.
172. Malasanos L, Barkauskas V, Moss M, et al: *Health Assessment.* St Louis: Mosby, 1986, pp. 401–414.
173. White L: The nurse's role in cancer prevention. In Newell G (ed.): *Cancer Prevention in Clinical Medicine.* New York: Raven Press, 1983, pp. 91–112.
174. Frank-Stromborg M: Nursing's contribution to case finding and the early detection of cancer. In Marino L

(ed.): *Cancer Nursing*. St Louis: Mosby, 1981, pp. 176–233.

175. Kopf A: Prevention and early detection of skin cancer/melanoma. *Cancer* 62:1791–1795, 1988.
176. Friedman RJ, Rigel DS, Silverman MK, et al: Malignant melanoma in the 1990s: The continued importance of early detection and the role of physician examination and self-examination of the skin. *CA* 41:201–226, 1991.
177. Adler J, Gosnell M, Springen K, et al: The dark side of the sun. *Newseek,* June 9:60–64, 1986.
178. Legha S: Malignant melanoma. Pitfalls and controversies in diagnosis and treatment. *Consultant* 28(6):111–124, 1988.
179. Schleper J: Cancer prevention and detection: Skin cancer. *Cancer Nurs* 7:67–84, 1984.
180. White L, Patterson J, Cornelius J, et al: *Cancer Screening and Detection Manual for Nurses*. New York: McGraw-Hill, 1979, pp. 9–16.
181. Finley C: Malignant melanoma: A primary care perspective. *Nurse Practitioner* 11(4):18–38, 1986.
182. Fitzpatrick T, Rhodes A, Sober A: Prevention of melanoma by recognition of its precursors. *N Engl J Med* 312:115–116, 1985.
183. Smith T, Mihm M, Sober A: Malignant melanoma. In *Cancer Manual* (ed. 7). New York: American Cancer Society, Massachusetts Division, 1986, pp. 106–113.
184. Helm F, Helm J: On guard against skin cancer. In Murphy G (ed.): *Cancer. Signals and Safeguards*. Littleton, MA: PSG Publishing, 1981, pp. 67–80.
185. Epstein E: *Common Skin Disorders. A Manual for Physicians and Patients*. Oradell, NJ: Medical Economics, 1979.
186. Gumport S, Harris M, Kopf A: *Diagnosis and Management of Common Skin Cancers*. New York: American Cancer Society, 1974 [Professional Education Publication No. 3373-PE].
187. Rhodes A, Weinstock M, Fitzpatrick T, et al: Risk factors for cutaneous melanoma. A practical method of recognizing predisposed individuals. *JAMA* 258:3146–3154, 1987.
188. Diekmann J: Cancer in the elderly: Systems overview. *Semin Oncol Nurs* 4:169–177, 1988.
189. Wood N: Oral cancer: An overview. *Ill Dental J* 57:323, 1988.
190. Winn D: Smokeless tobacco and cancer: The epidemiologic evidence. *CA* 38:236–243, 1988.
191. Sawyer D, Wood N, Lehnert J: Examination, detection, diagnosis and referral. *Ill Dental J* 57:326–329, 1988.
192. Silverman S: Early Diagnosis of oral cancer. *Cancer* 62:1796–1799, 1988.
193. Holmstrup P, Pindborg J: Oral mucosal lesions in smokeless tobacco users. *CA* 38:230–235, 1988.
194. Kabot T, Heffez L, Bergschneider J: Prevention, detection and referral. Responsibility of the dental team: Prevention and patient education. *Ill Dental J* 57:324–325, 1988.
195. Squier C: The nature of smokeless tobacco and patterns of use. *CA* 38:226–229, 1988.
196. Benowitz N: Nicotine and smokeless tobacco. *CA* 38:244–247, 1988.
197. Schroeder K, Iaderosa G, Chen M, et al: Bimodal initiation of smokeless tobacco usage: Implications for cancer education. *Cancer Education* 2:15–21, 1987.
198. Grabau J: Oral/facial self-examination. In Nieburgs H (ed.): *Prevention and Detection of Cancer. Part I* (vol. 2), Prevention. New York: Marcel Dekker, 1978, pp. 2263–2274.
199. Williams T: Ovarian cancer. Fewest signs, greatest challenge. *Diagnosis* 3(5):53–60, 1981.
200. White L: Cancer prevention and detection: Cervical cancer. *Cancer Nurs* 7:335–345, 1984.
201. Beecham J, Helmkamp BF, Rubin P: Tumors of the female genital tract. In Rubin P (ed.): *Clinical Oncology for Medical Students and Physicians* (ed. 6). New York: American Cancer Society, 1983, pp. 428–481.
202. Mitchell MF, Sandella JA, White LN: Cervical cancer: The role of the human papillomavirus. In Hubbard SM, Greene PE, Knobf MT (eds.): *Current Issues in Cancer Nursing Practice Updates*. Philadelphia: Lippincott, 1992, pp. 1–9.
203. Koss L: The Papanicolaou test for cervical cancer detection. A triumph and a tragedy. *JAMA* 261:737–743, 1989.
204. Jones H: Vaginal cancer. Common signs, uncommon cause. *Diagnosis* 3(5):71–85, 1981.
205. Nelson J, Averette H, Richart R: Dysplasia, carcinoma in situ, and early invasive cervical carcinoma. *CA* 34:306–327, 1984.
206. Persky V, Davis F, Barrett R, et al: Recent time trends in uterine cancer. *Am J Pub Health* 80:935–939, 1990.
207. Fink D: Change in American Cancer Society checkup guidelines for detection of cervical cancer. *CA* 38:127–128, 1988.
208. Stenkvist B, Bergstrom R, Eklund G, et al: Papanicolaou smear screening and cervical cancer. What can you expect? *JAMA* 252:1423–1426, 1984.
209. Mandelblatt J, Fahs M: The cost-effectiveness of cervical cancer screening for low-income elderly women. *JAMA* 259:2409–2413, 1988.
210. Eddy DM: Screening for cervical cancer. *Ann Int Med* 113:214–226, 1990.
211. Diagnosing cervical cancer by measuring DNA content. *Primary Care & Cancer* 8:13, 1988.
212. Jones G: Densitometric screening found accurate for detecting cervical cancer. *Oncology & Biotechnology News* 2(2):3, 1988.
213. Lovejoy N: Precancerous lesions of the cervix. Personal risk factors. *Cancer Nurs* 10:2–14, 1987.
214. McCauley K, Oi R: Evaluating the Papanicolaou smear: Part I. *Consultant* 29(12):31–40, 1988.
215. Braunstein G: The benefits of estrogen to the menopausal woman outweigh the risks of developing endometrial cancer [Opinion: Pro]. *CA* 34:210–219, 1984.
216. Morrow C: The benefits of estrogen to the menopausal woman outweigh the risks of developing endometrial cancer [Opinion: Con]. *CA* 34:220–231, 1984.
217. Jones W, Saigo P: The "atypical" Papanicolaou smear. *CA* 36:237–242, 1986.
218. Stromborg M. Nord S: A cancer detection clinic: Patient motivation and satisfaction. *Nurse Pract* 4:10–14, 1979.

Chapter 9

Diagnostic Evaluation, Classification, and Staging

Sharon Saldin O'Mary, RN, MN

DIAGNOSTIC EVALUATION

Factors That Affect the Diagnostic Approach

The diagnosis and staging of cancer have been directly affected by rapidly changing technology in imaging modalities and biochemical analysis. Historically there has been a progression from the gross evaluation of a tumor mass at surgery to the assessment of genetic expression and structure of tumor cells to diagnose and predict the natural history of the disease.

Today the major goals of the diagnostic evaluation for a suspected cancer are to determine the tissue type of the malignancy, the primary site of the malignancy, the extent of disease within the body, and the tumor's potential to recur in the future. This information is the critical first step in planning the therapeutic management. The approach to the diagnostic evaluation depends on the following factors: the patient's presenting signs and symptoms, the patient's clinical status and ability to tolerate invasive procedures, the anticipated goal of treatment when the diagnosis is made, the biologic characteristics of the suspected malignancy, the diagnostic equipment available in the patient's community, and the third-party payer approval of diagnostic procedures.

Even with the sophisticated armamentarium presently available for cancer diagnosis, the key to survival continues to be early detection of disease. Early diagnosis of a precancerous lesion or a malignant neoplasm affords the very best opportunity for cure, extended survival, and less extensive treatment. For example, the nonpalpable breast mass found on a screening mammogram or the isolated tumor found incidentally on a chest film is more likely to be diagnosed as localized disease amenable to treatment and cure. More typically, the tumor goes undetected until specific signs or symptoms become apparent and the patient consults a health professional. Frequently, these symptoms include the complaints of weight loss, persistent pain, unexplained fever, fatigue, or one of the seven warning signals that have brought the early detection of cancer into public awareness.[1] Unfortunately, many of the people at greatest risk for developing cancer have an inadequate understanding of the importance of early detection of symptoms. A study of cancer knowledge among the elderly revealed an inability to recall more than one or two of the seven warning signals of cancer and a lack of awareness that elderly individuals have an increased cancer risk.[2] Table 9-1 identifies the most common warning signals of cancer, the significance of each signal or symptom, and the persons at greatest risk for developing an associated malignancy.[1,3]

The worst prognosis can be expected in those patients who delay seeking medical evaluation at the onset of their symptoms, in those cancers for which technologic methods are unavailable to make an early diagnosis, and in patients, with an unknown primary lesion. For the patient who presents with widespread extensive disease, the palliative goal of treatment may direct and abbreviate an otherwise exhaustive diagnostic work-up.

An effective clinical evaluation of the patient with a suspected malignancy includes a comprehensive history with the identification of known risk factors, a thorough physical examination, laboratory and imaging tests, and the histologic verification of the malignancy. Known biologic characteristics of the suspected malignancy and the typical routes of regional and distant metastases will direct the approach of further diagnostic and staging procedures. In some situations, extensive laboratory and imaging examinations precede tissue biopsy in the attempt to locate the primary tumor or an accessible tumor. In other patients, results of a biopsy specimen that confirm the presence of malignancy directs further testing that will be done to accurately stage the extent of disease. Those tests that are the least taxing to the patient and family, that are cost effective, and that yield the information necessary for treatment planning are considered. Obtaining tissue for histologic examination or cells for cytologic analysis is paramount in the diagnosis of malignancy and precedes any decision for treatment.

In the present era of cost containment in health care, the judicious selection and sequencing of diagnostic studies are stressed. The proper test is one that yields information on the suspicious site of malignancy and complements rather than merely confirms known information. The relative benefits of competing imaging technologies such as computed tomography and magnetic resonance imaging currently are being evaluated for several organ sites by the Radiology Diagnostic Oncology Group, a cooperative group funded by the National Cancer Institute.[4] The increased availability of sophisticated equipment, the fear of litigation, and pressure from patients and families are all factors that influence the physician to overinvestigate. At least one study has indicated that patients believed extensive test ordering correlated with physician quality.[5]

It is apparent that third-party payers, prospective payment systems, and managed care networks also play an important role as gatekeepers in the diagnostic evaluation. Unless patients are acutely ill, requiring hospitalization, it is likely that care will be delivered in the ambulatory setting. The 44% increase in hospital outpatient services in the last decade attests to this trend.[6]

Nursing Implications in Diagnostic Evaluation

Many opportunities exist for nurses to promote the early detection and diagnosis of cancer. As respected members of the health profession they are consulted formally and informally about perceived signs or symptoms of cancer. It is imperative not only that nurses be able to recognize and understand the meaning of a

TABLE 9-1 Seven Warning Signals of Cancer and Their Significance

Warning Signals	Significance of Warning Signal	Persons at Greatest Risk
Change in bowel or bladder habits	Changes in stool caliber and regular bowel function are frequent signs of colorectal cancer; dependent on the area of intestine involved. A change in bladder function, frequency, dysuria, retention, or hematuria may indicate prostate or bladder cancer.	*Colorectal cancer:* over age 40, personal or family history of polyps or colorectal cancer, family history of polyposis syndromes, inflammatory bowel disease *Prostate cancer:* over age 65, black males *Bladder cancer:* smokers, males, chemical exposure
Unusual bleeding or discharge	Any unusual bleeding or discharge can signify malignancy. Occult or bright red blood may be seen with colorectal cancer. Abnormal vaginal bleeding is the most frequent sign of endometrial or cervical cancer. A clear, milky, or bloody discharge from the nipple is the second-most common symptom of breast cancer. Hemoptysis is a sign of lung cancer. Hematuria is the most frequent sign of bladder cancer and is also seen in renal and prostate cancer.	*Endometrial cancer:* postmenopausal women over age 50, family history of endometrial cancer, obesity, diabetes, hypertension, prolonged estrogen administration *Cervix cancer:* first vaginal intercourse at early age, multiple sexual partners, genital human papillomavirus, smokers
A sore that does not heal	Delayed healing of a sore or a change in a skin lesion's size, color, or shape, particularly on a surface exposed to ultraviolet light, can represent basal cell or squamous cell cancer. Oral lesions and leukoplakia, particularly in tobacco or alcohol users, need careful follow-up. Persistent sores or itching of the vulva can indicate a preinvasive or malignant lesion.	*Skin cancer (nonmelanoma):* exposure to UV radiation, psoralens, and UV light, or chemical carcinogens; fair-skinned Caucasians *Oral cancer:* males, over age 40, tobacco users (chewed or smoked), pipe smokers, combined tobacco and alcohol use
Obvious change in wart or mole	A change in a mole's color and pigmentation pattern, irregularities in border or surface topography, or increasing size causes suspicion of malignancy. Occurs in areas protected from or exposed to the sun.	*Melanoma:* fair-skinned Caucasians with history of sun exposure, family or personal history of melanoma or dysplastic nevi, large congenital moles
Thickening or lump in breast or elsewhere	A painless lump or mass is most common presenting sign in cancer of the breast, testis, and soft-tissue sarcoma. Persistent enlarged lymph nodes can signify lymphoma or metastatic nodal disease.	*Breast cancer:* all women, particularly over age 50, personal or family history of breast cancer, nulliparity or first child after age 30 *Testis cancer:* males aged 20–35, undescended testes
Nagging cough or hoarseness	Persistent, productive cough is the most frequently reported symptom of lung cancer. Hoarseness may indicate lung, laryngeal, or thyroid cancer.	*Lung cancer:* all smokers, black males, history of asbestos exposure *Larynx cancer:* males over age 50, combined tobacco and alcohol use
Indigestion or difficulty in swallowing	Indigestion, gastroesophageal reflux, painful "spasms" after eating, or difficulty swallowing can be symptoms of cancer of the esophagus, stomach, or pharynx.	*Stomach cancer:* males over age 50, Japanese emigrants, history of pernicious anemia *Esophagus cancer:* males over age 60, history of Barrett's esophagus, achalasia, caustic injury to esophagus

clinical sign, but that they assess the individual's risk for cancer and then take responsibility for encouraging investigation and intervention.[7] Nurses can facilitate entry into the health care system by encouraging appropriate follow-up without delay, providing accurate information on cancer detection and diagnostic procedures, clarifying misconceptions, and referring to trusted health care providers or community programs. Frank-Stromborg and Rohan provide an extensive review of nursing involvement in cancer prevention and early detection and point out that efforts have been concentrated in the areas of breast, cervical, and lung cancer.[8]

Table 9-1's information on the significance of early warning signals of cancer can be used by nurses to design education programs for the community that target individuals who are at the highest risk for developing a malignancy and are most likely to delay seeking medical attention. The program content should stress the importance of recognizing symptoms early to improve survival. The rationale should be given for participating in screening or annual physical examinations that include rectal and pelvic examinations. Nurses proficient in physical assessment and screening techniques can perform early detection and diagnostic procedures, including digital rectal examinations, sigmoidoscopy, pelvic examinations and Papanicolaou tests, and testicular and breast examinations.[9,10,11] Integrating instruction on breast self-examination or testicular self-examination can be done by nurses in most practice settings. Displaying posters and pamphlets from the American Cancer Society that identify warning signals and recommendations for a cancer-related checkup is a free and effective way to reach many people. Educational programs will be most accessible if they are based in the community, church, work site, shopping center, health fair, senior center, or wherever participation can be maximized. Successful examples of this include a testicular and prostate cancer awareness program presented to 3000 men at their work site, a breast cancer screening and awareness program for Chinese American women at a Chinese YWCA, and a colorectal screening and education program in community black churches.[12,13,14]

Nurses are involved in providing support to patients facing the potential threat of cancer. The fear can motivate or totally immobilize an individual. The time between the attaching of meaning to a suspicious symptom, such as a breast lump, and the seeking of medical attention and the completion of diagnostic evaluation will vary in every situation, and for many reasons. However, the potential for stress, disruption, anxiety, and fear exists for every patient and family. Marino and Kooser separate the prediagnostic period from the diagnostic period to identify specific patient concerns and behaviors.[15] During the prediagnostic period, any patient delay in seeking attention depends on the perceived threat or importance attached to the symptom, the severity of the symptom, personal beliefs about cancer and treatment, and personal and financial resources. Once the individual acts on her or his concerns and seeks medical attention, the diagnostic period begins. Anxiety about the results of examinations and fear and curiosity regarding the technology of procedures are common.[16] The emotional impact of the cancer diagnosis, once confirmed, ranges from relief, disbelief, anger, depression, and hopelessness to intellectualization.[17,18] Guilt feelings from not seeking attention earlier or from lifestyles that may have contributed to the cancer are not uncommon.[15] Professional nurses in diverse settings are able to intervene by taking time to listen to concerns, respond to questions, and provide support.

Oncology nurses play a key role in providing information and support to reduce the stress of going through a diagnostic evaluation for a suspected malignancy. An accurate assessment of the patient's and family's desire to know, in addition to their ability to understand, is the first step in providing this much-needed support. Educational preparation for an examination should include an explanation of the procedure to be followed, as well as a description of any physical sensations that might be expected, such as pain, discomfort, and facial flushing. The purpose of the examination, what information can and cannot be gleaned from the examination, when the results can be expected, and from whom to expect them should be identified. Reinforcing verbal information with written materials targeted for the patient has proven to be helpful.[19,20]

Nurses also must be cognizant of any potential for complications during or after a procedure, including reactions to contrast agents, bleeding, vasovagal response, and the need for intravenous analgesia or conscious sedation. Nurses may be assisting with the procedure, performing the procedure, or providing postprocedure care.

Including the family members in all aspects of the diagnostic evaluation is helpful to the patient and family and to the health care team. Families are able to reinforce instructions and information, assist with examination preparation, observe for untoward effects from procedures as well as provide emotional support for the patient. An assessment of the entire family's adjustment to the cancer diagnosis may lead to referrals for more extensive support.

Other specific nursing interventions depend on identified nursing diagnoses. These include[21]:

1. knowledge deficits related to lack of exposure to or misconceptions about cancer
2. anticipatory grieving related to the stigma of cancer or probable prognosis
3. ineffective coping related to the meaning of the diagnosis, financial stress, inadequate support, and the demands of decision making
4. spiritual distress related to challenged belief because of diagnosis
5. fear of death, treatment, and body image changes related to inability to control events and knowledge deficit
6. self-care deficit related to effects of the malignancy

Laboratory Techniques

Laboratory studies are performed to help formulate or confirm a clinical diagnosis and to monitor the patient's response to or relapse from a specific therapy. The data provide information on the functioning of specific organs and metabolic processes that may be altered by disease or a malignant process.

Biochemical analysis of blood, serum, urine, and other body fluids identifies chemical and hematologic values outside the narrow, homeostatic range. Specific malignancies characteristically alter chemical composition of the blood, but no single value is diagnostic for a malignancy. For example, elevated serum levels of bilirubin, alkaline phosphatase, and glutamic-oxaloacetic transaminase are seen in approximately 50% of patients presenting with liver cancer, and the abnormalities are significant in their correlation with shorter survival. Nonspecific changes such as anemia, leukocytosis or leukopenia, and thrombocytosis or thrombocytopenia also may contribute to the diagnostic evaluation.

Tumor markers are proteins, antigens, genes, ectopically produced hormones, and enzymes that are expressed by the tumor (tumor derived) or produced by normal tissue in response to the tumor (tumor associated). Markers have been recognized in serum and body fluids, in tissue, and, with recent technologies like flow cytometry, at the cellular and genetic levels.

The value of a particular laboratory study or imaging technique often is reported in terms of sensitivity or specificity. *Sensitivity* establishes the percentage of patients with cancer who will have positive (abnormal) test results, known as *true-positive* results. Test results of patients with cancer that are negative (normal) are *false-negative* findings. *Specificity* establishes the percentage of patients without cancer who will have negative (normal) test results, known as *true-negative* results. Patients who are free of disease and show positive (abnormal) results are considered to have *false-positive* results. A clinically useful test will detect a malignant abnormality early in its development (sensitivity) and exclude nonmalignant sources for the abnormality (specificity). In reality, many tests are highly sensitive but not very specific.

Ideally, a tumor marker is produced exclusively by the tumor cell and not in other conditions (highly specific), is present and detectable in early, occult disease (highly sensitive), is detectable in levels directly reflecting tumor mass (proportional), predicts disease response and recurrence (predictive), and is cost effective and commercially available (feasible).[22] The only marker that approaches this ideal is human chorionic gonadotrophin in gestational trophoblastic tumors.[23] Several other markers are clinically useful in monitoring tumor activity during treatment and in detecting recurrent cancer but lack the specificity to be good screening tools. The assay for carcinoembryonic antigen is highly sensitive and correlates well with tumor burden and prognosis in gastrointestinal neoplasms.[24,25] It lacks specificity, however, because the antigen is expressed by benign as well as many different malignant cells.[26] Table 9-2 identifies several tumor markers and their clinical significance in the diagnosis and monitoring of cancer.[27–31]

Recent technological advances in monoclonal antibody production, radioimmunoassay, and flow cytometry have provided diagnostic and prognostic information in a variety of cancers. Techniques to produce monoclonal antibodies that detect specific tumor

TABLE 9-2 Selected Markers in the Diagnosis and Monitoring of Malignant Disease

Laboratory Test	Associated Malignancy	Comments
	ENZYMES	
Lactic dehydrogenase (LDH)	Lymphoma, seminoma, acute leukemia, metastatic carcinoma	Elevated in 50% of patients with advanced disease; also in hepatitis and myocardial infarction
Prostatic acid phosphatase (PAP)	Metastatic cancer of prostate, myeloma, lung cancer, osteogenic sarcoma	Elevated in 80% of patients with bone metastases from prostate cancer; also in prostatitis, nodular prostatic hypertrophy
Placental alkaline phosphatase (PLAP)	Seminoma, lung, ovary, uterus	Elevated in pregnancy
Neuron-specific enolase (NSE)	Small-cell lung cancer, neuroendocrine tumors, neuroblastoma, medullary thyroid cancer	
Creatine kinase-BB	Breast, colon, ovary, prostate cancers	Elevated in bowel infarction, renal failure, stroke
Terminal deoxynucleotidal transferase (TdT)	Lymphoblastic malignancy	
	HORMONES	
Parathyroid hormone	Ectopic hyperparathyroidism from cancer of the kidney, lung (squamous cell), pancreas, ovary, myeloma	Elevated in primary hyperparathyroidism
Calcitonin	Medullary thyroid, small-cell lung, breast cancer, and carcinoid	
Antidiuretic hormone (ADH)	Small-cell lung cancer, adenocarcinomas	Inappropriate secretion associated with pneumonia, porphyria
Adrenocorticotropic hormone (ACTH)	Lung, prostate, gastrointestinal cancers, neuroendocrine tumors	Elevated in Cushing's disease

(continued)

TABLE 9-2 Selected Markers in the Diagnosis and Monitoring of Malignant Disease (continued)

Laboratory Test	Associated Malignancy	Comments
	HORMONES	
Human chorionic gonadotrophin, beta subunit (B-HCG)	Choriocarcinoma, germ cell testicular cancer, ectopic production in cancer of stomach, pancreas, lung, colon, liver	Elevated in almost all choriocarcinoma, 60% of testicular cancer; also in pregnancy
	METABOLIC PRODUCTS	
5 Hydroxyindoleacetic acid (5 HIAA)	Carcinoid, lung	Drugs and diet interfere with test
Vanillylmandelic acid (VMA)	Neuroblastoma	Drugs and diet interfere with test
	PROTEINS	
Protein electrophoresis (urine—Bence Jones) (serum—immunoglobulins)	Myeloma, lymphoma	Elevated in connective tissue disease, benign monoclonal gammopathy, chronic renal failure
IgG	IgG myeloma	
IgA	IgA myeloma	
IgM	Waldenstroms macroglobulinemia	
IgD	IgD myeloma	
IgE	IgE myeloma	
	advanced neoplasms	
Beta-2 microglobulin	Myeloma, lymphoma	
	ANTIGENS	
Alpha fetoprotein (AFP)	Nonseminomatous germ cell testicular cancer, choriocarcinoma, gonadal teratoblastoma in children, cancer of the pancreas, colon, lung, stomach, biliary system, liver	Elevated in 80% of hepatocellular cancer, 60% of nonseminomatous germ cell cancer; also in cirrhosis, hepatitis, toxic liver injury
Carcinoembryonic antigen (CEA)	Cancer of the colon-rectum, stomach, pancreas, prostate, lungs, breast	Elevated in smokers, chronic obstructive pulmonary disease, pancreatitis, hepatitis, inflammatory bowel disease
Prostate-specific antigen (PSA)	Prostate cancer	Elevated in prostatitis, nodular prostatic hyperplasia
Tissue polypeptide antigen (TPA)	Breast, colon, lung, pancreas cancer	Marker for cell proliferation in benign or malignant disease
CA—125	Ovary (epithelial), pancreas, colon cancer	Elevated in >85% of ovarian cancer; also in endometriosis, pelvic inflammatory disease, peritonitis
CA—19-9	Pancreas, colon, gastric cancer	Differentiates benign from malignant pancreatobiliary disease
CA—15-3	Breast cancer	
CA—72-4	Gastric cancer	
	OTHER	
Lipid-associated sialic acid (LSA)	Leukemia, lymphoma, melanoma, most solid tumors	
Chromosome rearrangements (deletion, translocation, inversion)	Melanoma, small-cell lung, renal, testicular cancers, liposarcoma, neuroblastoma, lymphoma, leukemia, and others	
Amplified oncogenes		
myc	Neuroblastoma, small-cell lung cancer	
c-erbB	Glioblastoma, squamous cell carcinomas	
c-erbB$_2$	Breast, adenocarcinomas	

antigens have been important to the diagnosis, classification, localization, and treatment of several solid tumors, T- and B-cell lymphomas, and leukemia. Identified tumor antigens include surface immunoglobulins (cytoplasmic membranes), surface epitopes (antigen sites), antigens in various stages of cell differentiation, and enzymes.[32]

Radioimmunoassay, an important technique in the measurement of tumor markers, determines the amount of tumor antigen in a serum sample. A known amount of radio-labeled antigen combined with antibody is added to a serum sample. The patient's unlabeled antigen displaces the radio-labeled antigen, which permits quantification.

Flow cytometry rapidly measures and identifies DNA characteristics and cell surface markers that correlate with patient prognosis and are useful to diagnose a malignancy and monitor response to therapy. A cell sorter measures fluorescence and light scatter as cells flow past an excitation source. In hematologic and lymphoid malignancies, fluorescent-marked antibodies directed against specific cell surface antigens (T-cell antigens, common acute lymphocytic leukemia antigen) help to differentiate hematopoetic cell lines. The primary application of flow cytometry analysis in solid tumors has been to determine DNA content (ploidy) and the percentage of cells synthesizing DNA (the S-phase fraction). Normal DNA is characterized as diploid and contrasts with abnormal, disorganized DNA, which is aneuploid. The proliferative potential of a tumor is measured by the percentage of cells in the synthesis phase of the cell cycle. Both of these factors—aneuploidy and high S-phase fraction—correlate with the biologic aggressiveness of several tumors.[33,34] Breast cancer is a tumor in which DNA aneuploidy and high S-phase appear to be predictors of poor prognosis for women regardless of their node-negative or node-positive status. Although no standard for treatment has been established, some physicians and research protocols are incorporating this information into adjuvant treatment decisions.[35]

Tumor Imaging

Many diagnostic procedures are available to ascertain the presence of a tumor mass, localize the mass for biopsy, provide tissue characterization, and further assess or stage the anatomic extent of disease. Although diagnostic imaging has benefited from the technology that produced computerized tomography (CT) and magnetic resonance imaging (MRI), an important role remains for the conventional diagnostic procedures. Examinations are selected that are efficient in detecting suspicious lesions and that also result in the least risk, discomfort, and expense for the patient. Table 9-3 identifies preferred imaging procedures for tumor definition and staging in several organ sites.[36–50] Table 9-4 elaborates on the patient preparation and education for select examinations.[51,52] The following section discusses imaging techniques available for diagnosis and staging.

Radiographic techniques

Radiographic studies, or x-ray films, allow visualization of internal structures of the body. Distinction is made between normal and abnormal structure and function. X rays or gamma rays are passed through the body, are absorbed variably by tissues of differing densities, and react on specially sensitized film or fluoroscopic screens. Radiographs may be site specific, such as the standard chest film (Figure 9-1) or mammogram, or they may view the dynamic function of an entire organ system. For example, in a gastrointestinal series a continuous flow of X rays passes through the digestive tract to assess the action of peristalsis, to detect displacement of structures, and to visualize mucosal abnormalities.

Mammographic examination now is performed primarily in x-ray units dedicated solely to this procedure. These units are distinguished by the incorporation of a tissue compression device or cone that improves the quality of the image and reduces the amount of primary and scatter radiation. Imaging is done primarily by the film-screen mammography process. Assuring women that this examination offers a low dose of radiation and a high-quality mammographic image that is sensitive to abnormalities has been necessary to promote participation in screening efforts. Since 1987 the American College of Radiology (ACR) has provided accreditation

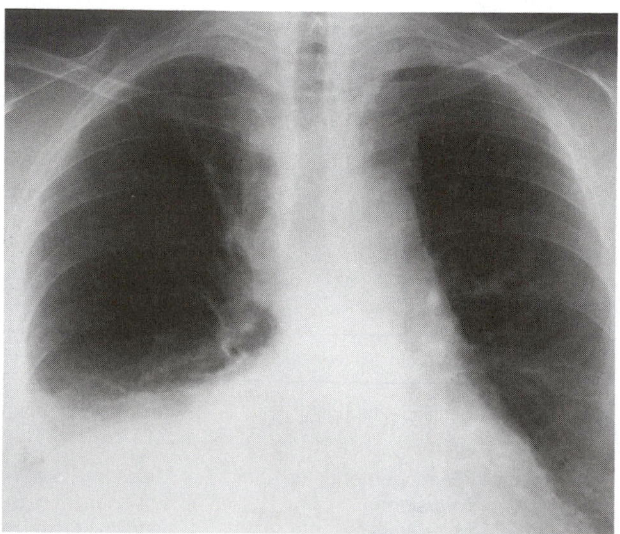

FIGURE 9-1 Initial chest x-ray film taken of a patient with small-cell lung cancer presenting with mediastinal adenopathy and right pleural effusion. (Source: Courtesy of Scripps Memorial Hospital, Department of Radiology, La Jolla, California.)

TABLE 9-3 Preferred Imaging Procedures for Tumor Definition and Staging

Site	Imaging Techniques	Comments
Central nervous system	MRI with contrast	MRI with contrast is superior to CT due to exquisite sensitivity of lesions <1 cm and lack of bone artifact in posterior fossa imaging
Head and neck	CT MRI	CT best for osseous change MRI superior for soft-tissue lesions, tumor–tissue interface, parapharyngeal spaces
Lung	CXR CT MRI	CXR good for detection of peripheral lesions CT preferred for parenchyma and mediastinal nodes MRI's advantage over CT is in chest wall, hilum, and mediastinal vascular invasion
Esophagus	Esophagram with contrast Endoscopic ultrasound (EUS) CT	Esophagram preferred for measuring lesion length, necessary for staging EUS superior to CT (except with severe stenosis) for depth of tumor invasion and lymph node assessment
Stomach	Barium studies with double contrast Endoscopic ultrasound	Barium studies good for detection EUS preferred over CT for staging due to better detection of small nodes
Colon	Barium enema with double contrast CT Endoscopic ultrasound	Most tumors originate in mucosa, where barium studies will detect 70%–90% of lesions CT assesses liver or distant node metastasis EUS is accurate in determining depth of tumor invasion and regional lymph nodes
Liver	Ultrasound (US) CT or MRI with contrast	US preferred for differentiating biliary obstruction from hepatic parenchymal disease CT has been preferred for imaging, but MRI with contrast may be equivalent
Bladder	Intravenous pyelogram (IVP) MRI or CT	IVP detects lesions >1.5–2 cm MRI preferred for bladder wall invasion, identifying large nodes and separating them from vessels
Kidney	Intravenous pyelogram CT	IVP preferred for detection CT with contrast provides 90% accuracy for staging
Musculoskeletal	X ray Bone scan CT or MRI	X ray for initial detection Bone scan more sensitive than X ray in identifying metastatic bone lesions (except multiple myeloma) CT preferred for intraosseous lesion; MRI preferred for extraosseous lesion or intraosseous lesion extending into bone
Breast	Mammogram	Mammography provides the standard for breast imaging; detects the 50% of breast lesions that are nonpalpable
Prostate	Transrectal ultrasound (TRUS) MRI or CT	TRUS is being evaluated as detection tool; detects extracapsular extension of lesion with 90% accuracy MRI preferred for staging seminal vesicle invasion
Endometrium	MRI	Primary staging is by surgery; MRI assists with staging of local and nodal disease
Ovary	Ultrasound or CT	Tumor mass >1 cm can be defined by US or CT; primary staging is by surgery
Lymphoma and Hodgkin's disease	CXR CT of chest and abdomen Lymphangiogram (LAG)	CRX required CT replacing need for LAG in non-Hodgkin's lymphoma; CT of abdomen images upper retroperitoneal and mesenteric nodes, liver, and spleen LAG has 95% sensitivity for imaging nodes in Hodgkin's disease and defines characteristic, abnormal, foamy lymph node architecture; doesn't visualize high celiac, splenic, hilar, or mesenteric nodes, requiring CT of abdomen

TABLE 9-4 Several Tumor Imaging Techniques with Instructions for Preparing the Patient

Tumor Imaging Examination	Patient Instructions	Comments
Barium studies	• Restriction of diet, smoking, and most medication before examination • Laxatives and enemas to cleanse bowel before colon examination • Will lie on tilting x-ray table, secured • Barium will taste chalky, milkshake consistency • Barium enema (BE) will feel cool, may cause cramping • Laxatives to clear barium after UGI • *Time:* 30–60 min	Bowel cleansing and procedure are exhausting for elderly patients. BE must precede UGI and small-bowel series. BE should follow other imaging examinations. Average cost for BE = $250.
Computerized tomography	• Diet restrictions before examination • Will lie still on adjustable table; x-ray tube rotates around patient to take many pictures • Machinery noisy • Test painless • May receive intravenous contrast dye; may feel burning sensation as injected • May report feelings of nausea, vomiting, flushing, itching, bitter taste • Drink fluids after examination to eliminate dye • *Time:* 30–90 min	Careful history required to determine prior adverse reaction to contrast. Average cost for CT of abdomen and pelvis = $1000.
Angiogram	• Diet restriction before examination • May receive sedative just before examination • Will lie still on x-ray table • Skin over selected artery site cleansed and anesthetized • Cannula passed into artery or vein • Contrast die rapidly injected, may feel burning sensation as injected • Several x-ray films taken • May report feelings of nausea, vomiting, flushing, itching, bitter or salty taste • Cannula removed after examination, pressure applied, limb immobilized • *Time:* 1–3 hr	Decreased use as diagnostic procedure. Being replaced by percutaneous procedures. Useful in preoperative planning and therapeutic embolization.
Lymphangiogram	• No diet restrictions • Blue dye injected into interdigital webs of feet; some discomfort • May discolor urine, stool, skin for 48 hr • Skin over lymphatic vessel on foot anesthetized • Small incision made on each foot, and cannula inserted • Contrast dye infused for 1–2 hr	Decreased use, but still has a role in staging Hodgkin's disease and lymphoma. Average cost = $700.

(continued)

TABLE 9-4 Several Tumor Imaging Techniques with Instructions for Preparing the Patient (continued)

Tumor Imaging Examination	Patient Instructions	Comments
	• May be uncomfortable during beginning of infusion, but must lie still • X-ray films taken after dye infused • *Time:* 2–3 hr • Must return following day for more x-ray films • *Time:* 30 min	
Magnetic resonance imaging	• No diet restriction • Remove anything affected by a magnet • Lie still on table, secured with Velcro straps • Table will move into narrow magnet opening • Knocking or beating sound in machinery is normal • Painless • May receive intravenous contrast dye • May report nausea, vomiting, itching if given contrast dye • *Time:* 45–60 min	Difficult to titrate medication for comfort and sedation during lengthy procedures. Average cost for MRI of abdomen = $600–$1200.
Ultrasonogram	• Diet restriction before examination • Full bladder for pelvic ultrasound • Will lie on exam table • Ultrasound gel applied over skin of area to be examined • Transducer passes over skin • May feel pressure; no pain • *Time:* 30 min	Increased use of probes introduced into the body (transrectal, transvaginal) for detection of cancer. Also has intraoperative use for intracranial and intraabdominal tumor localization. Average cost for abdominal ultrasound = $250.
Nuclear medicine imaging	• No diet restriction • Radioisotope injected before exam (15 min to 2 hr) • Will lie on scanner table, may have to vary positions • Scanner moves back and forth, taking several pictures • Procedure painless • Radioisotope harmless • *Time:* 30–60 min	Increased use of radioimmunoimaging using radio-labeled monoclonal antibodies. Average cost of liver and spleen scan = $500.
Endoscopy	• Diet restriction before examination • Mild sedation before procedure, but patient remains conscious • Intravenous infusion for medications and hydration *Oral:* • Local anesthetic sprayed in mouth • Flexible tube passed through mouth to level to be examined • Tongue and throat feel swollen; difficult to swallow	Screening sigmoidoscopy is recommended every 3–5 yr, beginning at age 50. Average cost = $100. Medicare does not pay for screening procedure. Colonoscopy requires more extensive preparation. Average cost = $350.

(continued)

TABLE 9-4 Several Tumor Imaging Techniques with Instructions for Preparing the Patient (continued)

Tumor Imaging Examination	Patient Instructions	Comments
	• May feel pressure and fullness if scope in stomach *Rectal:* • Prepared for exam with laxatives, enemas • Lubricated endoscope inserted anally • Feels cold, urge to defecate • May need to change positions during examination as scope is advanced • *Time:* 30–60 min	
Mammogram	• Breast is compressed between 2 plates on x-ray cassette • Compression may feel tight, but not painful • Radiation exposure is minimal and safe *Screening:* • Two views are taken of each breast: one view from head to foot (craniocaudal), the other lateral • *Time:* 15 min *Diagnostic:* • Three views taken of breast; craniocaudal, lateral, oblique • Spot compression and magnification films • *Time:* 30 min	Clinical breast exam and instruction on breast self-examination should be included. Average cost for screening mammogram = $100. Covered by Medicare.

of mammography facilities that has resulted in a standard of quality assurance. The accreditation process involves review of staff qualifications (radiologist, radiologic physicist, radiologic technologist, and the practitioner performing physical examination and providing instruction in breast self-examination), as well as testing the technical quality of the mammographic procedure (radiographic equipment, technique, image receptors, processing, image quality, and average dose of radiation to the breast).[53,54] The limiting dose for accreditation is a mean glandular dose of less than 400 mGy.[53] ACR accreditation is voluntary, and a list of qualified facilities can be obtained from a local American Cancer Society unit or the ACR.

Diagnostic mammography, indicated when symptoms or clinical findings exist, requires more views than the standard two-view mammogram used for screening, as well as spot compression and magnification views of suspicious spots. Frequently, mammographically guided needle localization of nonpalpable tumors is required for placement of a wire, needle, dye, or catheter near the suspicious lesion prior to biopsy and surgery (Figure 9-2).

Thermography, which images variations in radiant heat produced by bloodflow through the breast, now is considered to be an ineffective modality for breast cancer screening.[55]

Tomography provides a radiographic image of a selected layer or plane of the body that would otherwise be obscured by shadows of other structures. Tomograms are particularly helpful in evaluating small cal-

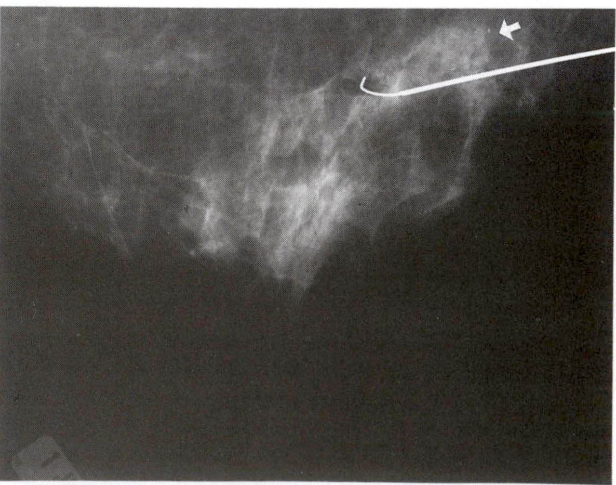

FIGURE 9-2 Mammographically guided needle localization of nonpalpable breast lesion with characteristic microcalcifications. (Source: Courtesy of Scripps Memorial Hospital, Department of Radiology, La Jolla, California.)

cified or cavitated lesions in the chest, hilar adenopathy, and mediastinal abnormalities.

Computerized axial tomography (CT or CAT) also provides sectional (axial, coronal, or sagittal) views of structures in the body. After serial x-ray exposures are taken through different angles of the body, a computer analyzes the information and provides a three-dimensional, reconstructed picture of the area studied. Computerized tomography is one of the most useful, informative, and available tests in the diagnosis and staging of malignancies. It is able to detect minor differences between tissue densities in any area of the body. Its major drawback is its production of artifact in areas of cortical bone content. Tissues surrounded by bone (such as the posterior fossa), the base of the skull, and the spine are most affected.[56] CT may be completed with or without contrast agents. Intravenous radioiodinated contrast enhances the projected image by highlighting the blood vessels. CT frequently is used to direct a needle to a tumor site for percutaneous biopsy. Figure 9-3 shows a large tumor of the liver imaged by CT with contrast.

Several radiographic examinations rely on contrast materials to enhance or outline the structures to be visualized. Angiography, venography, cholangiography, and urography, in addition to computerized tomography, all rely on the intravascular administration of iodinated contrast agents for optimal visualization of body structure and function. An example is the excretory radiograph, also known as the intravenous pyelogram (IVP), which is used in the initial diagnostic evaluation of renal masses.

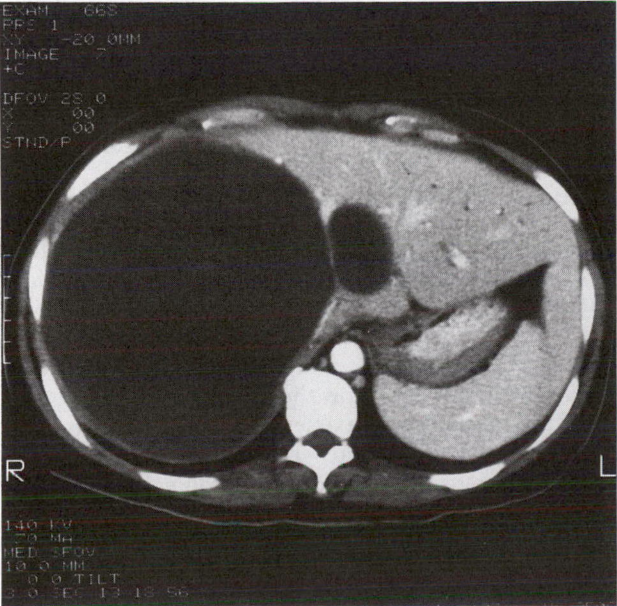

FIGURE 9-3 Contrast-enhanced CT of the abdomen revealing huge cystadenocarcinoma involving most of the liver. (Source: Courtesy of Scripps Memorial Hospital, Department of Radiology, La Jolla, California.)

Approximately 5% of the patients who undergo examinations with iodinated contrast material experience an adverse reaction to the contrast medium.[57] Most commonly this reaction includes nausea, localized pain at the injection site, a metallic or bitter taste, and a sensation of warmth and flushing, lasting from 1–3 minutes. Urticaria and facial edema may last 30–60 minutes.[58] These symptoms do not require treatment and will not progress to life-threatening reactions. The incidence of a severe reaction such as cardiopulmonary arrest is extremely uncommon, occurring in only 0.1% of patients.[57] There is not a good predictor for severe reactions; however, patients with any history of allergic response should be closely monitored. Patients considered at risk for reaction may receive a test dose of the contrast agent and be given premedication with diphenhydramine, adrenocorticotropic hormone, or epinephrine. At least one study refutes this practice, stating that even a test dose may be life-threatening and that premedication does not minimize or prevent adverse reactions.[58] Nonionic contrast agents are available at considerable expense for use with patients who have had serious reactions in the past.

An oily iodinated contrast material is employed in lymphangiography (LAG). The lymphatic vessels in each foot, or, less commonly, each hand, are injected to allow visualization of the lymphatic vessels and nodes. This is indicated in the diagnosis and staging of Hodgkin's and non-Hodgkin's lymphomas and in some pelvic cancers. In addition to the risk of a reaction to the iodine in the contrast medium, as described previously, there is a potential reaction of pulmonary microembolization. This is of greatest concern if the lymph channels of the upper portion of the body are imaged. The thoracic duct empties into the lungs, and a degree of embolization is likely to occur. Patients with compromised pulmonary reserve are at highest risk, since a significant decrease in lung diffusing capacity may occur. Symptoms to be observed for are shortness of breath, chest pain, hypotension, and cyanosis, which should last only a few hours. Nursing actions after lymphangiogram include instruction in deep breathing and coughing to keep the lungs expanded.

Intrathecal contrast agents are used in myelography and in computerized tomography. Radiographs of the subarachnoid space are taken after the injection of either an oily or a water-soluble contrast agent. The contrast agent will flow only to the point of obstruction, and more than one injection may be required. This is one reason why magnetic resonance imaging has become the superior examination for detection of spinal cord compression as well as for skeletal metastatic deposits. A water-soluble myelographic contrast agent often is used with computerized tomography if a single disease site within the spinal canal is suspected.[51]

Barium sulfate is a nonabsorbable, radiopaque agent used to enhance the contrast between the lumen of the gastrointestinal tract and adjacent soft tissues. Studies that use barium include esophagraphy, upper gastrointestinal (UGI) series, small-bowel series, barium enema, and hypotonic duodenography. Barium is ingested or introduced into the gastrointestial tract and allowed to coat the intraluminal surfaces. Radiographs are taken that can detect primary malignancies of the gastrointestinal organs or extrinsic compression from other tumor sites. Figure 9-4 presents a classic annular lesion of the colon imaged with radiopague contrast. By combining barium and air, a double-contrast study is performed that is more sensitive than barium alone in detecting primary gastrointestinal tumors.[59] There are seldom complications to this examination unless there is an obstruction or a perforation of the digestive tract. Retention of the barium may cause fecal impaction and discomfort in some patients. The administration of a laxative or an enema may be necessary to assist with bowel evacuation.

Meglumine diatrizoate (gastrografin), a contrast agent containing water-soluble iodine, can be used instead of barium.

Nuclear medicine techniques

Nuclear medicine imaging involves the intravenous injection or the ingestion of radioisotope compounds (technetium-99m methylene diphosphate, technetium-99m diethylenetriaminepentaacetic acid, technetium-99 sulfur colloid, iodine-123/131, or gallium-67 citrate), followed by the sensitive camera imaging of those organs or tissues that have concentrated the radioisotopes. Scans of the bones, liver and spleen, brain, thyroid, and kidneys are used in the detection of malignancy. Nuclear medicine studies are very sensitive and often will detect sites of abnormal metabolism or early malignancy several months before changes are seen on a radiograph. Gallium scans are particularly sensitive in detecting bronchogenic carcinomas and lymphomas. However, the increased use and the sensitivity of computerized tomography have replaced many radioisotope examinations.

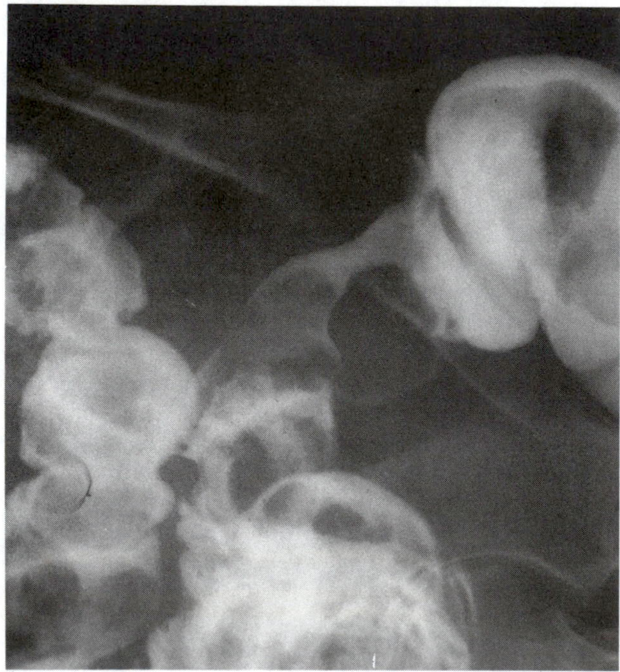

FIGURE 9-4 Barium enema visualizes annular, "apple core" lesion that is constricting the colon. (Source: Courtesy of Scripps Memorial Hospital, Department of Radiology, La Jolla, California.)

Positron emission tomography is an imaging modality that provides information based on the biochemical and metabolic activity of tissue. Infused biochemical compounds such as glucose are tagged with radioactive particles that emit positrons. The image is detected by gamma camera tomography. The best clinical application has been in brain imaging. It is particularly useful in differentiating low-grade tumors from high-grade tumors and in distinguishing treatment-induced tissue necrosis from recurrent tumor. Practical limitations of this modality are its expense and the need for a cyclotron to produce the isotopes.[60] Single-photon emission computed tomography uses commercially available radioisotopes and has much broader application.

Nuclear imaging with radio-labeled monoclonal antibodies is employed, thus far investigationally, to visualize microscopic sites of metastasis or suspected malignancy. This technique requires that a monoclonal antibody targeted against a specific tumor antigen be combined with tracer amounts of radioactivity, usually iodine-131 or iodine-123. After intravenous injection, the antibody binds to antigen on the tumor. These tumor sites then "light up" with imaging scanners. Sensitivity and specificity at levels of 90% have been achieved in some tumor types, occult lesions missed by other imaging modalities have been found, and the antibody has been administered without serious side effects.[61] In clinical trials, imaging has been successful in several disease sites, including the colon,[62] the breast[63] and the ovaries,[63] and in melanoma[64] and T-cell lymphomas.[65]

Ultrasonography

Ultrasonography (US) is a nonradiographic and noninvasive technique of imaging deep soft-tissue structures within the body. The reflecting echoes of high-frequency sound waves directed into specific tissues are recorded on an imaging screen. The echoes are variable, depending on the tissue density, and can be used to discriminate masses. A limitation of the examination is its inability to visualize through bone or air. Ultrasonography is most applicable in detecting tumors within the pelvis, the retroperitoneum, and the peritoneum of patients with cancer.[51] Masses greater than 2 cm in diameter can be detected and localized for possible percutaneous biopsy. Transrectal ultrasound is useful in guiding a needle biopsy of suspicious prostate lesions, but has not proven an effective screening tool. In the diagnosis of breast cancer, ultrasound is an important adjunct to mammography for distinguishing cysts from solid lesions with 98%–100% accuracy.

Magnetic resonance imaging

Magnetic resonance imaging (MRI) creates sectional images of the body, similar to computerized tomography, but does not expose the patient to ionizing radiation. Images are created by placing the patient within a powerful magnetic field that aligns the body's hydrogen nuclei in one direction. Radio-frequency pulses are used to excite the magnetized nuclei and change their alignment. Between radio-frequency pulses the nuclei return to a state of relaxation, and variable signals are transmitted on the basis of tissue characteristics. These signals are analyzed by the computer, and multiplaner (sagittal, coronal, and axial) images are produced with exquisite clarity. Magnetic resonance imaging can be enhanced with the intravenous paramagnetic contrast agents gadolinium diethylenetriaminepentaacetic acid (DTPA) and gadotetrate meglumine (DOTA).[66] These agents work by reducing tissue relaxation time, thus increasing signal intensity and image production. Adverse reactions to gadolinium DTPA, which are rare, include nausea, pain localized to the injection site, and headache occurring several hours after the examination. Anaphylactoid reactions to the contrast agent have been reported.[67]

Magnetic resonance imaging is most applicable in the detection, localization, and staging of malignant disease in the central nervous system, spine, head and neck, and musculoskeletal system. Contrast-enhanced MRI is the superior imaging modality in brain tumors (Figure 9-5).[68] MRI examination of the spinal cord essentially has eliminated the use of myelography in patients with cancer.[36]

Significant limitations do exist in the use of MRI. Patients with aneurysm or surgical clips, pacemakers, implanted pumps, tatooed eyeliner, or any ferromagnetic metallic implant cannot undergo MRI examination. The magnetic pull of the MRI is capable of dislodging the implant or interfering with its operation, or may actually remove the object from the patient's body. This excludes the MRI examination for acutely ill patients with life-support or monitoring devices. Nonferrous metallic implants may produce artifacts that distort the MRI image, but are generally safe for the patient. Implanted ports, frequently used in cancer patients to provide vascular, peritoneal, and epidural access, are made from many different materials. Shellock provides a list of ports that do not move or deflect during exposure to magnetic scanning.[69] Camp-Sorrell lists ports causing the least artifact, but concludes that attention must be paid to the manufacturer's recommendations as materials change and new ports are developed.[70] High-grade titanium and nonmetal ports produce the least or no artifact.

Claustrophobic patients may require sedation if they are to undergo an MRI scan, but they also benefit from explanations prior to the procedure, a support person nearby, verbal contact, MRI-compatible headphones, prisms or mirrors to allow a view outside of the tube, and relaxation techniques.[69] The cost (approximately 20% higher than an equivalent CT examination[71]), length of the examination (1–2 hours for a total scan of the spine), and somewhat limited availability of this diagnostic tool are additional disadvantages of the MRI.

(a)

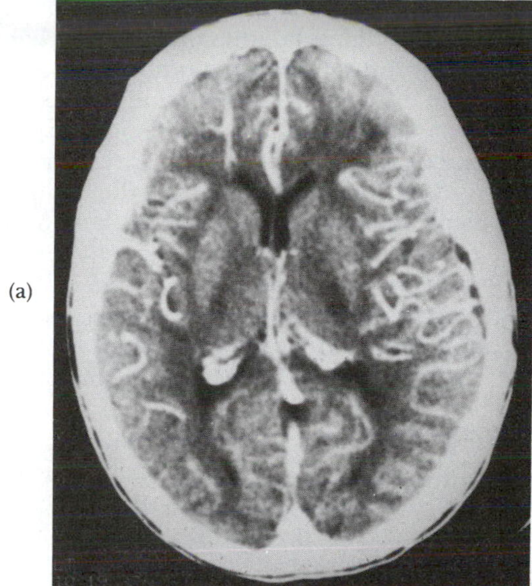

(b)

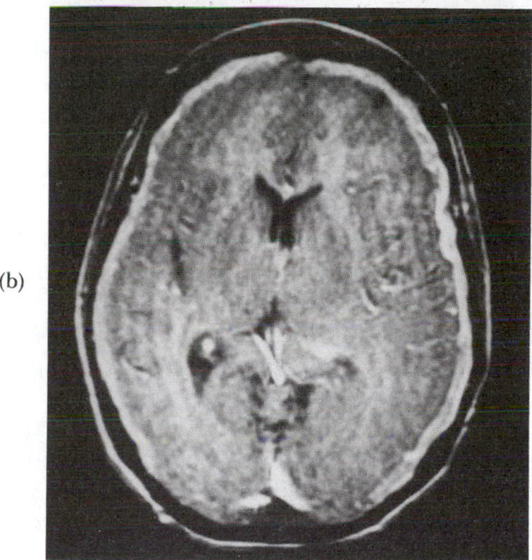

FIGURE 9-5 Contrast-enhanced CT (a) and contrast-enhanced MRI (b) of metastatic intracranial tumor. MRI shows "rind" of metastatic deposit around brain that was invisible on CT due to bone artifact. (Source: Courtesy of Scripps Memorial Hospital, Department of Radiology, La Jolla, California.)

Invasive Diagnostic Techniques

Endoscopy

Endoscopy is a method of directly visualizing the interior of a hollow viscus by the insertion of an endoscope into a body cavity or opening. The endoscope contains fiberoptic glass bundles that transmit light and then return an image to the optical head of the endoscope. The instrument may be rigid or flexible. Visual inspection, tissue biopsy, cytologic aspiration, staging the extent of disease, and the excision of pathologic processes are possible through the endoscope.

By passing a flexible scope through the mouth, endoscopic examinations can visualize directly the larynx, the upper airway passages and the bronchial tree, the esophagus, the stomach, and the upper duodenum. Visualization of the distal sigmoid colon, the rectum, and the anal canal is performed by means of a rigid scope. The entire large intestine can be viewed with a flexible colonoscope that is inserted anally.

Endoscopic retrograde cholangiopancreatography combines the diagnostic procedures of endoscopy and contrast-enhanced radiography to evaluate biliary tract obstruction and pancreatic masses.

The endoscopic ultrasound (EUS) may prove superior to other imaging modalities for assessing direct depth of tumor invasion and local lymph node status for esophageal, gastric, and colon malignancy. EUS, where available, is indicated to distinguish benign from malignant lesions, to stage neoplasms, to establish operability and surgical approach, and to determine response or recurrence.[72]

The cervix and vagina are visualized with the use of the magnification lens of the colposcope. Peritoneoscopy or laparoscopy permits assessment of surfaces within the peritoneal cavity by the insertion of a peritoneoscope through a small incision below the umbilicus. Thoracoscopy allows visualization of the visceral and parietal pleura, the mediastinum, and the diaphragm by means of a thoracoscope passed through an incision in the midaxillary line of the sixth to the eighth intercostal space.[73] The direct visualization of the tissues and organs of the mediastinum is performed under general anesthesia. The endoscope is introduced into the mediastinum through a small incision above the manubrium.

Biopsy

The importance of obtaining histologic or cytologic proof of malignancy cannot be overstated. Treatment decisions for cancers arising within the same organ differ on the basis of the histopathology report. An example is the very different treatment regimens for small-cell cancer of the lung and adenocarcinoma of the lung. Exactly what tissue is to be biopsied depends on several factors: the clinical status of the patient, the patient's willingness to undergo invasive procedures, the size and location of the identified tumor, and the amount of tissue needed by the pathologist for analysis.[74]

The cytologic examination of aspirated fluid, secretions, scrapings, or washings of body cavities may reveal malignant cells that have exfoliated from a primary or metastatic tumor. Tissue will not be obtained by this method, and the pathologist's ability to establish the primary site of the malignancy may be limited. Cancer of the cervix often is detected by the cytologic examination of cells acquired from a Papanicolaou smear.

The fine-needle aspiration biopsy, guided by palpation or an imaging technique, is extensively used and is available in the ambulatory setting. It provides not only cytologic information but also microhistologic information if adequate tissue fragments are obtained. Table 9-5 provides instructions for preparing the patient for an image-guided fine-needle aspiration biopsy.[75] Figure 9-6 shows a patient undergoing a CT-guided biopsy.

Stereotactic biopsy is another diagnostic procedure utilizing CT or MRI to establish the coordinates of a lesion before biopsy. The procedure is safe and relatively quick for lesions in certain areas of the brain. A stereotactic head frame is fixed to the skull under local anesthetic, the lesion is scanned for localizing landmarks, including the location of arteries and vessels, a small hole is made in the skull, and the biopsy is then directed by an instrument attached to the frame.

The biopsy provides tissue for histologic examination. The following are commonly recognized techniques for obtaining a biopsy: needle biopsy, incisional biopsy, excisional biopsy, punch biopsy, and bone marrow aspiration. These procedures and their nursing implications are discussed in Chapter 12. For a definitive diagnosis of malignancy it is imperative that the pathologist receive an adequate, representative, and well-preserved tissue specimen. A cytologic or histologic report that is negative for malignancy may only signify a specimen that is inadequate for diagnostic evaluation, thus necessitating repeat biopsy. Only a complete excisional biopsy can exclude malignancy with certainty. An equivocal biopsy specimen should be sent to an outside source for a second evaluation. The Armed Forces Institute of Pathology in Washington, D.C., is used by pathologists worldwide as a reference and for review.

Not infrequently, the biopsied tissue will confirm malignancy but the primary site or tissue of origin can-

TABLE 9-5 Instructions for Preparing the Patient for Image-Guided Fine-Needle Aspiration Biopsy

- Contrast agent may be required—intravenous or oral.
- Sedatives may be offered.
- Vital signs and oximetry will be monitored if intravenous sedation is used.
- Some pain may be experienced; local anesthetic is used.
- Skin at biopsy site is cleansed, and the needle inserted.
- Needle position is established by an imaging technique, eg, CT, ultrasound, or chest fluoroscopy.
- Syringe is attached to the needle, and the fluid and tissue are aspirated.
- Patient is observed for infection, bleeding, or increase in pain.

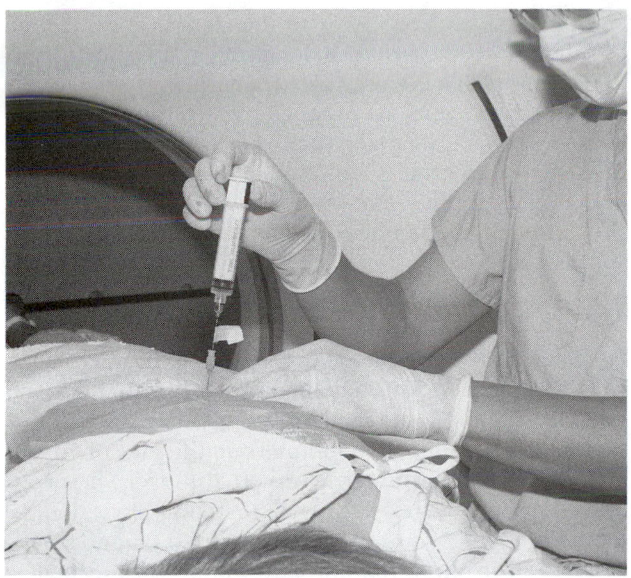

FIGURE 9-6 Patient undergoing CT-guided needle biopsy of retroperitoneal lymph node. (Source: Courtesy of Scripps Memorial Hospital, Department of Radiology, La Jolla, California.)

not be established by the pathologist or the clinician. An example is the patient who undergoes biopsy of a cervical node and is diagnosed with squamous cell carcinoma but for whom a thorough examination of the chest and head and neck area fails to yield the source of the malignancy. The goals for pursuing the primary site in this situation are discussed later in this chapter in the section on "Tumors of Unknown Origin."

CLASSIFICATION AND NOMENCLATURE

Basic Terminology

The terms *cancer* and *tumor* often are used interchangeably and inappropriately and can be misleading for patients, families, and professionals. A *tumor* is a swelling or mass of tissue that may be benign or malignant. *Cancer,* synonymous with *malignant neoplasm,* is an uncontrolled "new growth" capable of metastasis and invasion that threatens host survival.

The term *primary tumor* is used to describe the original histologic site of tumorigenesis. A *secondary,* or *metastatic, tumor* resembles the primary tumor histologically but sometimes may be so anaplastic as to obscure the cell of origin. A *second primary lesion* refers to an additional, histologically separate malignant neoplasm in the same patient. Although this is a relatively unusual occurrence, it must be excluded at the time of an apparent recurrence. Tables of probability for recurrence exist to guide the clinician in these determinations. A general rule is always to biopsy the first recurrence, because it may actually represent a new, curable or treatable malignancy. An example is the patient with a history of breast cancer who presents with suspicious lymph nodes and is found on biopsy to have lymphoma. However, some recurrences present in sites where the morbidity from biopsy is so significant that the lesion is treated without tissue confirmation. The patient with breast cancer presenting with a vertebral pedicle lesion is an example.

Benign and Malignant Tumor Characteristics

Certain biologic, histologic, and cytologic characteristics distinguish a benign tumor from a malignant tumor. However, with the exception of the properties of invasion and metastasis, which are found only in cancer, the differences between a benign process and a malignant process are relative. In some circumstances a definitive diagnosis of benign tumor versus malignant tumor cannot be made.[76] For example, a well-differentiated follicular carcinoma of the thyroid may be solitary and encapsulated and may mimic a benign adenoma of the thyroid. Occasionally a benign tumor will transform into a malignant tumor over time. An adenomatous polyp of the colon is an example of a relatively benign process that can transform into cancer of the colon if left untreated.

Most tumors will retain sufficient characteristics of the normal, differentiated cell to allow recognition of the type of tissue from which they were derived, which is the basis of distinguishing tumors in the histogenetic classification system (Table 9-6).[77,78] Specific nomenclature provides information on characteristics of the neoplasm. A suffix is added to the name of the tissue or cell type under pathologic study to designate its benign or malignant nature. Benign tumors usually end in the suffix *-oma,* the Greek root for "tumor." Most malignant tumors end in either the suffix *-sarcoma* or the suffix *-carcinoma,* depending on the tissues from which they arise. For example, lipoma is a benign tumor of fat tissue, and liposarcoma is a malignancy of fat tissue. *Sarcoma* specifies a malignant tumor of the connective tissues, that is, those tissues originating from the mesodermal embryonic layer. *Carcinoma* specifies a malignant tumor arising from epithelial tissues. Epithelium covers or lines surfaces in the body and arises from the ectodermal, mesodermal, or endodermal embryonic layers.

Tumor Classification System

The most relevant classification systems will universally communicate clinical and prognostic information. Tumors may be classified not only by their biologic behavior (benign versus malignant) but also by their tissue of origin.

To understand the nomenclature of tumors it is useful to review normal cell differentiation in the embryonic state. An early occurrence in the life of the embryo is the development of three primary germ layers: the ectoderm, the mesoderm, and the endoderm. The cells within these layers divide, specialize, and give rise to all cells, tissues, and organs within the body. The ectoderm differentiates into the skin and nervous system. The mesoderm differentiates into several organs and connective tissue: bones, blood, cartilage, fat, fibrous tissue, muscle, and blood and lymph vessels. The endoderm differentiates into the lining of the digestive and respiratory tracts, the bladder, and the urethra.

Virtually every cell type in the body is capable of transforming into a malignant cell. Chapter 3 provides a complete discussion of carcinogenic transformation. It is fairly well accepted that the malignant cell derives from a postembryonic cell that is arrested in the process of differentiation.

Most tumors will retain sufficient characteristics of the normal, differentiated cell to allow recognition of the type of tissue from which they were derived, which is the basis of distinguishing tumors in the histogenetic classification system (Table 9-6).[77,78] Specific nomenclature provides information on characteristics of the neoplasm. A suffix is added to the name of the tissue or cell type under pathologic study to designate its benign or malignant nature. Benign tumors usually end in the suffix *-oma,* the Greek root for "tumor." Most malignant tumors end in either the suffix *-sarcoma* or the suffix *-carcinoma,* depending on the tissues from which they arise. For example, lipoma is a benign tumor of fat tissue, and liposarcoma is a malignancy of fat tissue. *Sarcoma* specifies a malignant tumor of the connective tissues, that is, those tissues originating from the mesodermal embryonic layer. *Carcinoma* specifies a malignant tumor arising from epithelial tissues. Epithelium covers or lines surfaces in the body and arises from the ectodermal, mesodermal, or endodermal embryonic layers.

Carcinomas are further delineated by the prefixes *adeno-,* for tumors that arise from glandular epithelial tissue, and *squamous,* for tumors that originate from squamous epithelial tissues. Descriptive terms such as *cystic, follicular, papillary, medullary, exophytic,* and *polypoid* are added to further define histologic characteristics.

The suffix that refers to malignant tumors that resemble the primitive blastula phase in embryonic development is *-blastoma.* Examples are neuroblastoma and retinoblastoma.

Mixed tumors, such as adenosquamous carcinoma of the bronchi, represent tumors with mixed squamous and glandular elements but that arise from the same germ layer and tissue. Some tumors, although rare and highly malignant, have such primitive differentiation that characteristics of a carcinoma and sarcoma may be evident.[77,79]

Teratoma and its malignant counterpart, teratocarcinoma, arise from tissue of all three germ layers and have no relationship to the site of origin.[77]

Several exceptions exist to the classification system just described. For instance, lymphoma, melanoma, and hepatoma are malignant tumors with the *-oma* suffix. Additionally, some malignancies are named after the person who characterized them. Hodgkin's disease, Ewing's sarcoma, and Wilms' tumor are examples. The hematopoietic malignancies are classified separately by predominant cell type and their acute vs. chronic nature.

Tumors of Unknown Origin

As many as 9% of patients diagnosed with cancer each year are found to have a malignancy from an unknown primary site.[80] Most frequently the histologic classification will be adenocarcinoma, but the site of origin may never be determined, even on autopsy. The prognosis is poor, with an overall median survival of 5 months.[81] The goal of proceeding with a diagnostic investigation in this situation is to identify those malignancies, even if they are disseminated, that are potentially curable or palliated with known, effective treatment.[82] For example, lymphomas and germ cell tumors are potentially curable with systemic chemotherapy. Lesions in the nasopharynx may be cured with radiation. Local complications such as bowel obstruction, spinal cord compression, and pathologic fractures can be palliated with surgery or radiation treatment even when the primary site of malignancy is unknown. Hormonal therapy may be recommended if the presumptive diagnosis, based on tumor markers or hormone receptor analysis, is breast, prostate, or endometrial malignancy.

Patients and their families who are facing cancer from an unknown source present unique challenges for the nurse. Not only do they need information and preparation for extensive imaging and laboratory testing, but they also need support when these tests fail to yield a definitive diagnosis. It is often hoped, though not necessarily true, that a known primary source of malignancy will be more treatable or curable than an unknown primary. Coping with any cancer diagnosis is difficult. Coping with an "unknown" cancer accentuates the feelings of loss of control, anxiety, and frustration. The involved nurse can be most helpful by identifying psychosocial concerns and available support systems early in the diagnostic period, clarifying and reinforcing known information and the rationale for extensive testing, and providing hope and reassurance that treatment is offered for the most probable and most treatable source of malignancy.[83]

STAGING AND GRADING CLASSIFICATIONS

Staging the Extent of the Disease

The staging process is a method of classifying a malignancy by the extent of its spread within the body. It is

TABLE 9-6 Select Benign and Malignant Neoplasms Listed by Histogenetic Classification

Tissue of Origin	Benign Neoplasm	Malignant Neoplasm
Epithelial (Endodermal)		
Squamous	Squamous cell papilloma	Squamous cell or epidermoid carcinoma
Glandular	Adenoma	Adenocarcinoma
	Papilloma	Papillary carcinoma
	Cystadenoma	Cystadenocarcinoma
Respiratory tract		Bronchogenic carcinoma
Renal epithelium	Renal tubular adenoma	Renal cell carcinoma (hypernephroma)
Urinary tract	Transitional cell papilloma	Transitional cell carcinoma
Placental epithelium	Hydatidiform mole	Choriocarcinoma
Testicular epithelium		Seminoma
		Embryonal carcinoma
Liver	Liver cell adenoma	Hepatocellular carcinoma (hepatoma)
Biliary tree	Cholangioma	Cholangiocarcinoma
Stomach	Gastric polyp	Gastric carcinoma
Colon	Colonic polyp	Adenocarcinoma of the colon
Mesenchymal (Mesodermal)		
Connective		
Fibrous tissue	Fibroma	Fibrosarcoma
Adipose tissue	Lipoma	Liposarcoma
Cartilage	Chondroma	Chondrosarcoma
Bone	Osteoma	Osteosarcoma
Muscle		
Smooth muscle	Leiomyoma	Leiomyosarcoma
Striated muscle	Rhabdomyoma	Rhabdomyosarcoma
Endothelial		
Blood vessels	Hemangioma	Hemangiosarcoma
Lymphatic vessels	Lymphangioma	Lymphangiosarcoma
Hematopoietic and lymphoreticular		
Hematopoietic cells		Leukemias
Lymphoid tissue		Lymphomas
		Hodgkin's disease
Plasma cells		Plasmacytoma (multiple myeloma)
Neural (Ectodermal)		
Meninges	Meningioma	Meningeal sarcoma
Glia	Astrocytoma	Glioblastoma multiforme
Nerve cells	Ganglioneuroma	Neuroblastoma
		Medulloblastoma
Melanocytes	Nevus	Malignant melanoma
Mixed Tissues		
Kidney		Wilms' tumor
Salivary gland	Mixed tumor of salivary gland (pleomorphic adenoma)	Malignant mixed tumor of salivary gland

a clinical and histologic determination that depends on the natural course of each particular type of cancer. Staging is based on the premise that cancers of similar histologic features and site of origin will extend and metastasize in a predictable manner. Although most staging classifications are based on the anatomic extent of disease, other criteria are included for specific malignancies. For thyroid cancer, the age of the patient and the histologic diagnosis (papillary, follicular, medullary, or anaplastic) are included in the staging system. The histopathologic grade of the tumor is significant and included in staging of prostate cancer, soft-tissue sarcomas, primary malignant tumors of the bone, and brain tumors.

The objectives of solid-tumor staging are multiple: to aid in treatment planning, to give prognostic information, to assist in treatment evaluation, and to facilitate the exchange of information and comparative statistics among treatment centers.[84]

With the goal of developing an internationally consistent system of staging solid-tumor malignancy, the TNM committee of the International Union Against

Cancer (UICC) and the American Joint Committee on Cancer (AJCC) have agreed on the TNM staging system. The TNM staging system classifies solid tumors by the anatomic extent of disease, as determined clinically and histologically. Three categories are quantified, with gradations representing progressive tumor size or involvement. The extent of the primary tumor (T) is evaluated on the basis of depth of invasion, surface spread, and tumor size. The absence or presence and extent of regional lymph node (N) metastasis are considered, with attention to the size and location of the nodes. The absence or presence of distant metastasis (M) is assessed as the third category. A subscript may specify the site of metastasis. For example, M1PUL denotes pulmonary metastasis. The TNM system is further classified by whether the assessment is obtained clinically (cTNM or TNM), after pathologic review (pTNM), at the time of retreatment (rTNM), or on autopsy (aTNM). For reporting purposes, the TNM stage classification remains constant throughout the disease process. Progression of disease does not change the initial stage of disease. Table 9-7 presents the nomenclature of the TNM system for classification.[84]

It is important to distinguish the cTNM, based on a clinical exam, from the pTNM, which is determined after surgery when the true extent of the disease is known and treatment decisions can be made. This is particularly true in breast cancer, where the lymph node status (pN) is the most precise prognostic indicator and directs adjuvant therapy decisions. Surgical nurses are well aware of the support needed by the woman with breast cancer in the first 24–48 hours after lymphadenectomy while she is awaiting the pathologist's review of lymph nodes. Another example occurs in the treatment of prostate cancer when the discovery of tumor in the pelvic lymph nodes (pN) at the time of surgery precludes the anticipated radical prostatectomy.

After numerical values are assigned to the T, N, and M categories, they are clustered into one of four stages (I through IV), or stage O for carcinoma in situ. Stage IV consistently includes distant metastases (M1) and predicts the worst prognosis. All tumor sites are grouped differently on the basis of characteristics of the disease. A typical TNM grouping is depicted in Table 9-8.[85]

Several established and accepted staging classifications other than TNM exist for particular malignancies. Melanomas are staged histologically by the level of invasion of the primary lesion, since this is the major determinant of prognosis. The Clark levels of invasion are widely accepted. The TNM stages for melanoma incorporate Clark's classification into primary tumor (T) assessment. The Duke's staging system for colorectal cancer, with its many subsequent modifications, classifies colorectal tumors by their depth of invasion and presence of nodal metastasis. The International Federation of Gynecology and Obstetrics has an accepted staging system for cervical and endometrial cancers. Hodgkin's disease and non-Hodgkin's lymphoma are standardly described by the Ann Arbor classification,

TABLE 9-7 TNM Classification System for Describing the Anatomic Extent of Disease

TNM Definitions		
(T) Primary tumor		
	TX	Primary tumor cannot be assessed
	TO	No evidence of primary tumor
	Tis	Carcinoma in situ
	T1, T2, T3, T4	Increasing size and/or local extent of the primary tumor
(N) Regional lymph nodes		
	NX	Regional lymph nodes cannot be assessed
	NO	No regional lymph node metastasis
	N1, N2, N3	Increasing involvement of regional lymph nodes
(M) Distant metastasis		
	MX	Presence of distant metastasis cannot be assessed
	MO	No distant metastasis
	M1	Distant metastasis
TNM Classifications		
cTNM or TNM		*Clinical Classification:* Based on information obtained from the physical examination, laboratory and imaging studies, endoscopy, biopsy, and surgical exploration. Clinical staging uses all information available before the initiation of definitive treatment.
pTNM		*Pathologic Classification:* Based on information acquired before treatment, supplemented or modified by information from surgery and the pathologic examination of a resected specimen. This includes resected tumor (pT), lymph nodes (pN), and distant metastasis (pM).
rTNM		*Retreatment Classification:* Based on all information available after a disease-free interval or at the time of a second-look surgery. The extent or absence of disease recurrence is documented before retreatment planning is begun.
aTNM		*Autopsy Classification:* Based on all information available at the time of a postmortem examination. It is helpful in answering questions about the tumor's response to treatment, recurrence patterns, and the extent of disease at the time of death.

Source: Adapted from Beahrs OH, Henson DE, Hutter RVP, et al: *American Joint Committee on Cancer: Manual for Staging of Cancer* (ed. 4). Philadelphia: Lippincott, 1992, pp. 6–7.

which recognizes disease distribution and symptoms. Cancers of the brain are not entirely suited to the TNM system because there are no lymphatic structures to categorize nodal (N) involvement.

The nonsolid tumors do not conform to solid-tumor staging principles because of their disseminated nature. Leukemias are best classified according to their predominant cell types (i.e., lymphocytic or nonlymphocytic), cell maturation, and acute or chronic nature. Clinical and morphologic factors such as age, platelet and blast counts, and periodic acid-Schiff stain reaction are indicators of favorable or unfavorable prognostic

TABLE 9-8 A Typical Stage Grouping Based on TNM Classification

- *Stage I, T1, NO, MO:* Clinical examination reveals a mass limited to the organ of origin. The lesion is operable and resectable, with only local involvement, and there is no nodal and vascular spread. This stage affords the best chance for survival.
- *Stage II, T2, N1, MO:* Clinical examination shows evidence of local spread into surrounding tissue and first-station lymph nodes. The lesion is operable and resectable, but because of greater local extent there is uncertainty as to completeness of removal. The specimen shows evidence of microinvasion into capsule and lymphatics. This stage affords a good chance of survival.
- *Stage III, T3, N2, MO:* Clinical examination reveals an extensive primary tumor with fixation to a deeper structure, bone invasion, and lymph nodes of a similar nature. The lesion is operable but not resectable, and gross disease is left behind. This stage affords some chance of survival.
- *Stage IV, T4, N3, M+:* There is evidence of distant metastases beyond the site of origin. The lesion is inoperable. There is little to no chance of survival.

Source: Rubin P: Statement of the clinical oncologic problem. In Rubin P (ed.): *Clinical Oncology for Medical Students and Physicians: A Multidisciplinary Approach* (ed. 6). New York: American Cancer Society, 1983, p. 10.

categories in acute lymphoblastic leukemia. The French-American-British classification has some clinical significance in acute myeloblastic leukemia but is not a staging system. In chronic lymphocytic leukemia, two staging systems exist: the Rai classification, and a relatively new system prepared by the International Workshop on chronic lymphocytic leukemia.[86] For patients with myeloma there is a staging classification that correlates M proteins with myeloma cell mass to provide prognostic information.[87]

The AJCC, with the UICC, is currently developing staging systems for malignancies not yet classified by the TNM system. These include cancers of the small intestine, mesothelioma, spinal cord, carcinoid, and Kaposi's sarcoma. Additionally, they are likely to incorporate tumor markers into the present anatomic staging to produce a system with better prognostic indices.[88] This has important implications for patients with early-stage disease (based on anatomic staging) but who are actually at risk for recurrence based on other measurements of malignant potential and who will need further treatment. The 30% of women with node-negative breast cancer who eventually experience a recurrence are a good example. The staging system of the future will be an estimation of risk (of local extension and distant metastases) based on the sum of risks associated with anatomic stage, morphologic grade, biologic grade, and genetic potential.[89] In breast cancer this could include the TNM stage, degree of morphologic anaplasia, estrogen and progesterone receptor status, S-phase fraction and aneuploidy, epidermal growth factor receptors, and Her-2/neu, c-erB-2, or c-myc oncogene expression.[89]

Patient Performance Classification

A patient's physical performance status at the time of diagnosis and staging often will influence the type of treatment selected and provide prognostic information.[90] Bedridden patients are much less likely to respond to any treatment than those who are asymptomatic and able to maintain the activities of daily living. Performance scales that measure a patient's functional status are used frequently in the eligibility criteria for cooperative group clinical trials and also periodically to evaluate the effects of treatment and disease. It is important to evaluate whether aggressive, toxic treatment protocols actually will permit people to feel better and to maintain their optimum functional status. The most prevalent performance scales are the Karnofsky Performance Status scale, the Eastern Cooperative Oncology Group (ECOG) scale, and the World Health Organization (WHO) scale.[91, 92, 93] In an attempt to standardize this classification, the American Joint Committee on Cancer (AJCC) developed a simplified performance scale.[84] The four scales are compared in Table 9-9. Nurses need to be familiar with the scoring systems, for they may be able to contribute the most accurate information to a very subjective rating. Moderate interobserver reliability and weak correlation between the functional status score and the patient's self-assessment have been concerns with established scales.[94, 95]

Grading

Grading a malignant neoplasm is a method of classification based on histopathologic characteristics of the tissue. It assesses the aggressiveness or degree of malignancy of tumor cells by comparing the cellular anaplasia, differentiation, and mitotic activity with normal counterparts. Specific characteristics vary with each type of cancer.

In grading a tumor the pathologist's objective is to quantify information to assist with treatment planning and prognostic determinations. For selected tumors the grade of the tumor is considered more significant than anatomic staging in terms of prognostic value and treatment. In cancer of the prostate, a well-differentiated T1a tumor requires no specific therapy other than close observation; however, a poorly differentiated T1 tumor needs to be treated aggressively with radiation or radical prostatectomy if the lymph nodes are negative for disease.[96] In soft-tissue sarcomas the grade is the primary determinant of stage of disease and of prognosis. Cure rates for grade 1 sarcoma are 80%, whereas cure rates for grades 2 and 3 drop dramatically to 60% and 40%, respectively.[97] In other tumors, such as melanoma of the skin, testicular and thyroid cancer, and

TABLE 9-9 Comparison of Frequently Used Performance Status Scales

Karnofsky Scale		ECOG Scale		WHO Scale		AJCC Scale	
% Score	Status	Score	Status	Score	Status	Score	Status
100%	Normal; no complaints; no evidence of disease	0	Asymptomatic	0	Fully active, able to carry out all predisease activities without restriction	H0	Normal activity
90	Able to carry on normal activity; minor signs or symptoms of disease	1	Symptomatic; fully ambulatory	1	Restricted in strenuous activity but ambulatory and able to carry out light work or pursue sedentary occupation	H1	Symptomatic and ambulatory; cares for self
80	Normal activity with effort; some signs or symptoms of disease						
70	Cares for self; unable to carry on normal activity or to do active work	2	Symptomatic; in bed less than 50% of day	2	Ambulatory and capable of all self-care but unable to carry out any light work; up and about more than 50% of waking hours	H2	Ambulatory more than 50% of time; occasionally needs assistance
60	Requires occasional assistance, but able to care for most needs						
50	Requires considerable assistance and frequent medical care	3	Symptomatic; in bed more than 50% of day but not bedridden	3	Capable of only limited self-care; confined to bed or chair more than 50% of waking hours	H3	Ambulatory 50% or less of time; nursing care needed
40	Disabled; requires special care and assistance						
30	Severely disabled; hospitalization indicated, although death not imminent	4	Bedridden	4	Completely disabled; unable to carry out any self-care and confined totally to bed or chair	H4	Bedridden; may need hospitalization
20	Very sick; hospitalization necessary; active supportive treatment necessary						
10	Moribund; fatal processes progressing rapidly						
0	Dead						

neuroblastoma, histological grading has no application.

Two grading systems are commonly seen. One descriptively identifies the tumor as well differentiated (i.e., retaining most of the morphologic features and behavior of the normal cell of the tissue of origin), moderately well differentiated, poorly differentiated, or undifferentiated. The other system numerically grades from 1 to 3 or 4, with 1 being the most differentiated and 3 and 4 being the least well differentiated. Grade 4 applies to tumors with no specific differentiation. The AJCC recommends the following grading classification[84]:

- GX grade cannot be assessed
- G1 well differentiated
- G2 moderately well differentiated
- G3 poorly differentiated
- G4 undifferentiated

Certain problems exist with grading classifications:

A tumor's level of differentiation may vary with time. Several grades of malignancy may exist within one tumor, in which situation the tumor should be labeled as the least favorable level of differentiation. It is essential that an adequate and representative biopsy specimen has been obtained for a valid interpretation by the pathologist. Nurses aware of the significance of a malignant tumor's grade and stage, as well as new prognostic, molecular markers, will be able to respond realistically to the patient's questions about treatment and prognosis.

CONCLUSION

The diagnostic phase of a cancer illness is a time of adjustment, learning, anxiety, and uncertainty for the patient and the patient's family. With adequate knowledge of the symptoms of disease and of the diagnostic evaluation, nurses can help prepare patients, thereby easing the anxiety associated with the unknown. During this time nurses will interact with the patient in several health care settings—primary clinics, inpatient and outpatient units, and extended care units—as well as in the community. Oncology nurses have used their expertise to (1) facilitate early diagnosis of cancer by promoting awareness of "warning signals" of cancer and conducting screening programs, (2) educate and prepare patients for a diagnostic evaluation of suspicious signs or symptoms, (3) perform or assist with diagnostic procedures and interpret or clarify results, and (4) counsel and support the patient and family in a therapeutic relationship. Nurses are in pivotal positions to promote the detection of cancer at the earliest possible stage and to assist the patient and family to regain hope, control, and quality of life once the diagnosis of cancer has been determined.

REFERENCES

1. *Cancer Facts and Figures.* Atlanta: American Cancer Society, 1991.
2. Weinrich SP, Weinrich MC: Cancer knowledge among elderly individuals. In Ash CR, Jenkins JF (eds.): *Enhancing the Role of Cancer Nursing.* New York: Raven Press, 1990, pp. 217–233.
3. Fink DJ: Cancer detection: The cancer-related checkup guidelines. In Holleb AI, Fink DJ, Murphy GP (eds.): *American Cancer Society Textbook of Clinical Oncology.* Atlanta: American Cancer Society, 1991, pp. 153–176.
4. Gatsonis C, McNeil BJ: Collaborative evaluations of diagnostic tests: Experience of the RDOG. *Radiology* 175:571–575, 1990.
5. Marton KI, Sox HC, Alexander J, et al: Attitudes of patients toward diagnostic tests: The case of the upper gastrointestinal series roentgenogram. *Medical Decision Making* 2:439–448, 1982.
6. McNeil BJ: The changing financial picture in health: Impact on radiology and the use of new technologies. Radiological Society of North America '91:(PS), p. 21, 1991 (abstract).
7. Rovinski CA: Nurses and cancer's seven warning signals. *Cancer Nurs* 3:53–55, 1980.
8. Frank-Stromborg M, Rohan K: Nursing's involvement in the primary and secondary prevention of cancer. *Cancer Nurs* 15:79–108, 1992.
9. Melillo KD: Who needs health maintenance? *J Gerontol Nurs* 11:18–21, 1985.
10. Rosevelt J, Frankl H: Colorectal cancer screening by nurse practitioner using 60-cm flexible fiberoptic sigmoidoscope. *Dig Dis Sci* 29:161–163, 1984.
11. White L, Cornelius J, Judkins A, et al.: Screening of cancer by nurses. *Cancer Nurs* 1:15–20, 1978.
12. Martin J: Male cancer awareness: Impact of an employee education program. *Oncol Nurs Forum* 17(1):59–64, 1990.
13. Lovejoy NC, Jenkins C, Wu T, et al: Developing a breast cancer screening program for Chinese-American women. *Oncol Nurs Forum* 16(2):181–187, 1989.
14. Mitchell-Breen ME, Dodds ME, Choi KL, et al.: A colorectal cancer prevention, screening and evaluation program in community black churches. *CA* 39:115–118, 1989.
15. Marino LB, Kooser J: The psychosocial care of cancer clients and their families: Periods of high risk. In Marino LB (ed.): *Cancer Nursing.* St Louis: Mosby, 1981, pp. 53–66.
16. Peteet JR, Stomper PC, Ross DM, et al: Emotional support for patients with cancer who are undergoing CT: Semi-structured interviews of patients at a cancer institute. *Radiology* 182:99–102, 1992.
17. Frank-Stromborg M, Wright P, Segulla M, et al: Psychological impact of the cancer diagnosis. *Oncol Nurs Forum* 11(3):16–22, 1984.
18. Vettese T: Problems of the patient confronting a diagnosis of cancer. In Cullen JW, Fox BH, Isom RN (eds.): *Cancer: The Behavioral Dimensions.* New York: Raven Press, 1975, pp. 275–281.
19. Mahon, SM, Casperson D: Teaching women about mammography through use of a brochure. *Oncol Nurs Forum* 18(8):1375–1378, 1991.
20. Habegger D, Ellerhorst-Ryan JM: Needle localization for nonpalpable breast lesions. *Oncol Nurs Forum* 15(2):192–194, 1988.
21. Herberth L, Gosnell DJ: Nursing diagnosis for oncology nursing practice. *Cancer Nurs* 10:41–51, 1987.
22. Lovejoy NC, Thomas ML, Halliburton P, et al: Tumor markers: Relevance to clinical practice. *Oncol Nurs Forum* 14(5):75–82, 1987.
23. Braunstein GD, Vaitukaitis JL, Carbone PP, et al: Ectopic production of human chorionic gonadotropin by neoplasm. *Ann Intern Med* 78:39–45, 1973.
24. Wolmark N, Fisher B, Wieand HS, et al: The prognostic significance of preoperative carcinoembryonic antigen levels in colorectal cancer. Results from NSABP clinical trials. *Ann Surg* 199:375–381, 1984.
25. Zamcheck N: The present status of carcinoembryonic antigen (CEA) in diagnosis, detection of recurrence, prognosis and evaluation of therapy of colonic and pancreatic cancer. *Clin Gastroenterol* 5:625–638, 1976.
26. Bates SE, Longo DL: Use of serum markers in cancer diagnosis and management. *Semin Oncol* 14:102–138, 1987.
27. Tietz NW: *Clinical Guide to Laboratory Tests.* Philadelphia: Saunders, 1983.

28. Byrne CJ, Saxton DF, Pelikan PK: *Laboratory Tests: Implications for Nursing Care* (ed. 2). Menlo Park, CA: Addison-Wesley, 1986.
29. Rowley J: Principles of molecular cell biology of cancer: Chromosomal abnormalities. In DeVita VT, Hellman S, Rosenberg SA (eds.): *Cancer Principles and Practice of Oncology* (ed. 3). Philadelphia: Lippincott, 1989, pp. 81–97.
30. Park M, Woude GFV: Principles of molecular cell biology of cancer: Oncogenes. In DeVita VT, Hellman S, Rosenberg SA (eds.): *Cancer Principles and Practice of Oncology* (ed. 3). Philadelphia: Lippincott, 1989, pp. 45–66.
31. Ghosh BC, Ghosh L: *Tumor Markers and Tumor Associated Antigens*. New York: McGraw-Hill, 1987, pp. 1–10.
32. Ravel R: *Clinical Laboratory Medicine* (ed. 5). Chicago: Year Book Medical Publishers, 1989, pp. 69–89.
33. Madeya ML, Pfab-Tokarsky JM: Flow cytometry: An overview. *Oncol Nurs Forum* 19:459–463, 1992.
34. Williams NN, Daly JM: Flow cytometry and prognostic implications in patients with solid tumors. *Surg Gynecol Obstet* 171:257–266, 1990.
35. Collins-Hattery AM, Blumberg BD: S phase index and ploidy prognostic markers in node negative breast cancer: Information for nurses. *Oncol Nurs Forum* 18(1):59–62, 1991.
36. Bragg DG: State-of-the-art assessment: Diagnostic oncologic imaging. *Cancer* 64:261–265, 1989 (suppl).
37. Dillon WP, Harnsberger HR: The impact of radiologic imaging on staging of cancer of the head and neck. *Semin Oncol* 18(2):64–79, 1991.
38. Bragg DG: The application of imaging in lung cancer. *Cancer* 67:1150–1154, 1991 (suppl).
39. McClennan BL: Oncologic imaging, staging, and follow-up of renal and adrenal carcinoma. *Cancer* 67:1199–1208, 1991 (suppl).
40. Hricak H: Role of imaging in the evaluation of pelvic cancer. In DeVita VT, Hellman S, Rosenberg SA (eds.): *Important Advances in Oncology 1991*. Philadelphia: Lippincott, 1991, pp. 103–131.
41. Castellino RA: Diagnostic imaging evaluation of Hodgkin's disease and non-Hodgkin's lymphoma. *Cancer* 67:1177–1180, 1991 (suppl).
42. Tio TL, Cohen P, Coene PP, et al: Endosonography and computed tomography of esophageal carcinoma: Preoperative classification compared to new (1987) TNM system. *Gastroenterology* 96:1478–1486, 1989.
43. Norris CM, Cady B: Head, neck, and thyroid cancer. In Holleb AI, Fink DJ, Murphy GP (eds.): *American Cancer Society Textbook of Oncology*. Atlanta: American Cancer Society, 1991, pp. 306–328.
44. Sussman SK, Halvorsen RA, Illescas FF, et al.: Gastric adenocarcinoma: CT vs. surgical staging. *Radiology* 167:335–349, 1988.
45. Hatch TR, Barry JM: The value of excretory urography in staging bladder cancer. *J Urol* 135:49, 1986.
46. Johnson CD, Dunnick NR, Cohan RM, et al.: Renal adenocarcinoma: CT staging of 100 tumors. *Am J Radiology* 148:59–63, 1987.
47. Pettersson H, Gillespy T, Hamlin D, et al.: Primary musculoskeletal tumors: Examination with the MR imaging compared with conventional modality. *Radiology* 164:237–241, 1987.
48. Hendee WR, Manaster BJ, Harnsberger HR, et al.: Oncologic imaging. In Holleb AI, Fink DJ, Murphy GP (eds.): *American Cancer Society Textbook of Clinical Oncology*. Atlanta: American Cancer Society, 1991, pp. 643–677.
49. Salo JO, Kivisaari L, Rannikko S, et al.: Computerized tomography and transrectal ultrasound in the assessment of local extension of prostatic cancer before retropubic prostatectomy. *J Urol* 137:435–438, 1987.
50. Clouse ME, Harrison DA, Grassi CJ, et al.: Lymphangiography, ultrasonography, and computed tomography in Hodgkin's disease and non-Hodgkin's lymphomas. *J Comput Tomography* 9:1–8, 1985.
51. Borg SA, Rosenthal S: *Handbook of Cancer Diagnosis and Staging: A Clinical Atlas*. New York: Wiley, 1984.
52. *Diagnostics: The Nurse's Reference Library*. Nursing 81 Books. Springhouse, PA: Intermed Communications, 1981.
53. McLelland R, Hendrick RE, Zinninger MD, et al.: The American College of Radiology Mammography Accreditation Program. *Am J Radiology* 157:473–479, 1991.
54. Clark RA: Economic issues in screening mammography. *Am J Radiology* 158:527–534, 1992.
55. Paulus DD: Imaging in breast cancer. *CA* 37:133–150, 1987.
56. Bragg DG, Harnsberger HR, Thompson WM: Specialized techniques of cancer management: Radiologic techniques in cancer. In DeVita VT, Hellman S, Rosenberg SA (eds.): *Cancer Principles and Practice of Oncology* (ed. 3). Philadelphia: Lippincott, 1989, pp. 440–458.
57. Ehrlich RA, McCloskey ED: *Patient Care in Radiography*. St Louis: Mosby, 1989, pp. 139–167.
58. Shehadi WH: Contrast media reactions: Occurrence, recurrence, distribution patterns. *Radiology* 143:11–17, 1982.
59. Thompson WM: Imaging strategies for tumors of the gastrointestinal system. *CA* 37:165–185, 1987.
60. Treseler KM: *Clinical Laboratory and Diagnostic Tests: Significance and Nursing Implications* (ed. 2). Norwalk, CT: Appleton & Lange, 1988, pp. 556–559.
61. Goldenberg DM: Targeting of cancer with radiolabled antibodies. *Arch Pathol Lab Med* 112:580–587, 1988.
62. Goldenberg DM, Kim EE, Bennett S, et al: CEA radioimmunodetection in the evaluation of colorectal cancers and in the detection of occult neoplasms. *Gastroenterology* 84:524–532, 1983.
63. Epenetos A. Britton KE, Mather S, et al: Targeting of I-123 tumor-associated antibodies to ovarian, breast, and gastrointestinal tumors. *Lancet* 2:999–1005, 1982.
64. Siccardi AG, Buraggi GL, Callegaro L, et al: Multicenter study of immunoscintigraphy with radiolabeled monoclonal antibodies in patients with melanoma. *Cancer Res* 46:4817–4822, 1986.
65. Carrasquillo JA, Bunn PA, Keenan AM, et al: Radioimmunodetection of cutaneous T-cell lymphoma with 111In-labeled T101 monoclonal antibody. *N Engl J Med* 315:673–680, 1986.
66. Watson AD, Rocklage SM: Theory and mechanisms of contrast enhancing agents. In Higgins CB, Hricak H, Helms CA (eds.): *Magnetic Resonance Imaging of the Body*. New York: Raven Press, 1992, pp. 1257–1287.
67. Lufkin RB: Severe anaphylactoid reaction to GD-DTPA. *Radiology* 176:879, 1990.
68. Stack JP, Antoun NM, Jenkins JPR, et al: Gadolinium-DPTA as a contrast agent in magnetic resonance imaging of the brain. *Neuroradiology* 30:145–154, 1988.
69. Shellock FG: MRI biologic effects and safety considerations. In Higgins CB, Hricak H, Helms CA (eds.): *Magnetic Resonance Imaging of the Body*. New York: Raven Press, 1992, pp. 233–265.
70. Camp-Sorrell D: Magnetic resonance imaging and the implantable port. *Oncol Nurs Forum* 17(2):197–199, 1990.

71. Health Insurance Association of America: *Source Book of Health Insurance Data*. Washington, DC, 1990.
72. Nickl NJ, Cotton PB: Clinical application of endoscopic ultrasonagraphy. *Am J Gastroenterology* 85:675–682, 1990.
73. Sugarbaker PH, Roth JA: Specialized techniques of cancer management: Endoscopy. In DeVita VT, Hellman S, Rosenberg SA (eds.): *Cancer Principles and Practice of Oncology* (ed. 3). Philadelphia: Lippincott, 1989, pp. 423–439.
74. Neiman RS, Smith TJ: Biopsy principles, pathologic evaluation of specimens and staging. In *Cancer Manual* (ed. 8). Boston: American Cancer Society, Massachusetts Division, 1990, pp. 70–77.
75. Ell SR: Imaging techniques: Fine-needle aspiration of various organs and body sites. In Bibbo M (ed.): *Comprehensive Cytopathology*. Philadelphia: Saunders, 1991, pp. 615–620.
76. Bonfiglio TA, Terry R: The pathology of cancer. In Rubin P (ed.): *Clinical Oncology for Medical Students and Physicians: A Multidisciplinary Approach* (ed. 6). New York: American Cancer Society, 1983, pp. 20–29.
77. Pitot HC: *Fundamentals of Oncology* (ed. 3). New York: Marcel Dekker, 1986, pp. 21–33.
78. Robbins SL, Cotran RS: Neoplasia. In *Pathologic Basis of Disease* (ed. 2). Philadelphia: Saunders, 1979, pp. 141–187.
79. Sirica AE: Classification of neoplasms. In Sirica AE (ed.): *The Pathobiology of Neoplasia*. New York: Plenum Press, 1989, pp. 25–39.
80. Ultman JE, Phillips TL: Cancer of unknown primary site. In DeVita VT, Hellman S. Rosenberg SA (eds.): *Cancer Principles and Practice in Oncology* (ed. 3). Philadelphia: Lippincott, 1989, pp. 1941–1952.
81. Altman E, Cadman E: An analysis of 1,539 patients with cancer of unknown primary site. *Cancer* 57(1):120–124, 1986.
82. Robert NJ, Garnick MB, Frei E: Undifferentiated neoplasms and cancers of unknown primary: A clinicopathological perspective. In Fer MF, Greco FA, Oldham RK (eds.): *Poorly Differentiated Neoplasms and Tumors of Unknown Origin*. Orlando, FL: Grune & Stratton, 1986, pp. 541–555.
83. Yeomans AC, Washington JB: Occult primary malignancies. *Oncol Nurs Forum* 18(3):539–544, 1991.
84. Beahrs OH, Henson DE, Hutter RVP, et al: *American Joint Committee on Cancer: Manual for Staging of Cancer* (ed. 4). Philadelphia: Lippincott, 1992.
85. Rubin P: Statement of the clinical oncologic problem. In Rubin P (ed.): *Clinical Oncology for Medical Students and Physicians: A Multidisciplinary Approach* (ed. 6). New York: American Cancer Society, 1983, pp. 2–19.
86. Santoro A: Chronic leukemias. In Bonadonna G, Robustelli della Cuna G (eds.): *Handbook of Medical Oncology*. Milan, Italy: Masson, 1988, pp. 756–777.
87. Durie BGM, Salmon SE: A clinical staging system for multiple myeloma. *Cancer* 36:842–854, 1975.
88. Henson DE: Future directions for the American Joint Committee on Cancer. *Cancer* 69:1639–1644, 1992 (suppl).
89. Preisler HD, Raza A: The role of emerging technologies in the diagnosis and staging of neoplastic diseases. *Cancer* 69:1520–1526, 1992 (suppl).
90. Stanley KE: Prognostic factors for survival in patients with inoperable lung cancer. *J Nat Cancer Institute* 65:25–32, 1980.
91. Karnofsky DA, Abelmann WH, Craver LF, et al.: The use of the nitrogen mustards in the palliative treatment of carcinoma. *Cancer* 1:634–656, 1948.
92. Zubrod CG, Schneiderman M, Frei E, et al.: Appraisal of methods for the study of chemotherapy in man: Comparative therapeutic trial of nitrogen mustard and triethylene thiophosphoramide. *J Chron Dis* 11:7–33, 1960.
93. World Health Organization: *World Handbook for Reporting Results of Cancer Treatment*. Geneva: WHO, 1979.
94. Poelhuis EHK, Hart AAM, Burgers JMV, et al.: Assessment of quality of life: Scoring performance status in cancer patients. In Aaronson NK, Beckmann J (eds.): *The Quality of Life of Cancer Patients*. New York: Raven Press, 1987, pp. 93–99.
95. Hutchinson TA, Boyd NF, Feinstein AR: Scientific problems in clinical scales, as demonstrated in the Karnofsky index of performance status. *J Chron Dis* 32:661–666, 1979.
96. Shipley WU, Meares EM, Schwartz JH, et al.: Cancer of the prostate. In *Cancer Manual* (ed. 8). Boston: American Cancer Society, Massachusetts Division, 1990, pp. 284–294.
97. Suit HD, Mankin JH, Antman KH, et al.: Sarcomas of bone and soft tissue. In *Cancer Manual* (ed. 8). Boston: American Cancer Society, Massachusetts Division, 1990, pp. 315–326.

PART III

Treatment

Chapter 10

Quality of Life as an Outcome of Cancer Treatment

David F. Cella, PhD

INTRODUCTION

The term *quality of life,* or *health-related quality of life (HQL),* has emerged to organize and galvanize a collection of outcome evaluation activities in cancer treatment research over the past two decades. Prior to this, length of survival, regardless of its quality, was considered to be the only primary outcome in oncology treatment research. It is now widely accepted that in most circumstances *quality* of survival is as important as *quantity* of survival. This implies that a severely toxic treatment must be evaluated for its detrimental impact as well as its survival benefit. It also raises a less obvious point: that treatments can be considered efficacious if they improve the quality of life even in the absence of survival benefit. Thus, investigating the impact of cancer treatments on HQL is a two-tailed enterprise in which treatment toxicity is traded not only with survival time but also with posttreatment function and well-being.

HQL evaluation entails a multidimensional quantification of patient functional status, usually as perceived by the patient.[1-13] In the decades to come, treatment intensification strategies that increase toxicity are likely to continue, given the advent of hematopoietic growth factors and improved antiemetic regimens. This further increases the importance of evaluating toxicity, patient function, and patient preferences for treatment. HQL evaluation differs from classic toxicity ratings in two important ways: (1) It incorporates more aspects of function (e.g., mood, affect, social well-being) than those that typically have been attributed to treatment, and (2) it focuses on the patient's perspective.

THE ROLE OF NURSING

Nursing has always played a central role in the clinical appreciation and treatment of quality of life, as evidenced by interest in managing disease symptoms and treatment side effects. Symptoms and side effects represent a major component of HQL as it is understood today. Managing these problems has for centuries been the primary domain of nurses caring for people with cancer. Now, as HQL evaluation, which includes a detailed understanding of the relative impact of symptoms and side effects, figures prominently in the evaluation of cancer clinical trials, nurses find themselves well positioned to play a leadership role.

Since the early 1950s, most of the important large-scale oncology clinical trials have been conducted by one of the cooperative clinical trials organizations within the United States, Canada, Europe, and Australia. One cannot help noticing the rapid growth of interest shown by cooperative groups to include HQL evaluation in selected trials. For the first time since inception, *every* large cooperative clinical trials organization in Europe and North America is actively examining quality of life in some of its trials. In many groups (e.g., Southwest Oncology Group, Radiation Therapy Oncology Group, Eastern Cooperative Oncology Group) nursing has played a leadership role in these initiatives. This chapter presents background information to help the nurse-investigator understand and evaluate quality-of-life studies in oncology clinical trials, and a selected review of measures available to the investigator aspiring to participate in the broad-based evaluation of experimental cancer treatments.

EVALUATING METHODS OF ASSESSMENT

Along with the evolution of interest in HQL, many efforts to measure the construct have been created and promoted. A number of validated HQL measures have become accepted for use in oncology in particular[14-20] and chronic illness in general,[21-27] so it is increasingly unlikely that a single "gold standard" measure will ever emerge. The diversity of available measures is potentially valuable in that it provides the user with choices based on specific characteristics of a given disease site, clinical trial, or HQL domain of interest. This chapter provides the reader with some understanding of criteria to evaluate whether an HQL measure is likely to accomplish its stated purpose. Such an understanding can guide the reader who wishes to critically evaluate the development, initial testing, and field performance of a given measure.

Construct Definition as a Frame for Measurement

Any construct must be defined before it can be measured. HQL is no exception. There are many different definitions of HQL in the literature.[28-32] Disagreement about the definition of HQL or its dimensions does not mean that it cannot be measured. It does, however, suggest that all measures are not equivalent, so one must therefore be clear on the definition of HQL as put forth by the group that developed a particular measure. Definitions of HQL may differ across study groups and still be measured reliably and validly within the parameters of a definition. For example, most agree that important HQL domains include physical, mental, and social dimensions. Whereas virtually all currently accepted HQL measures provide some ability to separate physical and psychological dimensions, social functioning is much less evenly represented. Some measures cover social well-being and function more than others. For example, deHaes et al.[33] do not measure social functioning as a component, and yet their scale can be evaluated for reliability and validity within its range of item content. Regarding the social dimension of HQL, there may well be a distinction between social *well-being* (perceived social support, satisfaction with relationships, etc.) and social *functioning* (ability to see friends, leisure activity). Clearly, the most empirically substantiated distinction has been between the correlated, but distinct, dimensions of physical well-being and mental well-being.[33–35]

APPROACHES TO MEASURING HEALTH-RELATED QUALITY OF LIFE

Over time, two approaches to measuring HQL have evolved: psychometric and utility. These approaches have evolved as relatively independent of one another, largely because they were developed within different scientific disciplines. Psychometric approaches derive from psychology, whereas utility approaches derive from economics. Only recently have investigators considered integrating these two approaches. This remains a critical challenge in HQL measurement.

Psychometric Approach

The psychometric approach includes generic health profile measurement (e.g., Sickness Impact Profile[27]) and specific instruments intended to measure the multidimensional impact of a specific disease, treatment or condition (e.g., Functional Living Index—Cancer[17]). The psychometric approach places heavy emphasis on an individual's response and response variability across individuals. An important contribution of the psychometric approach is that it measures subjective or perceived well-being. Psychometric measures may or may not include a summary or total score. When available, only rarely have these summary scores been connected to patients' values for their current health status. This poses a problem, because without a rating of patient preference, one cannot appropriately make a decision about the value of a given treatment to a given patient. Very often, one of two patients with identical disease and treatment options declines therapy while the other accepts it enthusiastically. Because psychometric measures typically neither incorporate patient-specific weights for individual domains nor anchor states of health to a common standard, evaluating trade-offs between quality of life and length of life, or between one dimension of HQL and another, is difficult. This presents a challenge in a clinical trial where the primary purpose for integrating HQL measurement is to incorporate data on the impact of treatment on both length of life and quality of life into conclusions about treatment efficacy. The collection of patient preferences in clinical trials would allow evaluation of the effect of treatment on quality-adjusted survival as well as on conventional outcome measures. Further, the addition of patient preference assessments to clinical trial outcome evaluation can make it possible to distinguish patients who favor one treatment over another when both may have equivalent survival outcomes. A strategy for doing this has been described by Till and colleagues.[36]

Utility Approach

In contrast to the psychometric approach, the utility approach is explicitly concerned with treatment decision making, usually at a policy level. In this approach, treatments are typically evaluated as to their benefit compared in some way to their cost. The utility approach to health status measurement evolved from a tradition of cost-benefit analysis, into cost-effectiveness approaches and, most recently, cost-utility approaches.[37] The cost-utility approach extends the cost-effectiveness approach conceptually by evaluating the HQL benefit produced by the clinical effects of a treatment, thereby including the patient's (presumed) perspective. To be used this way, HQL must be measured as a utility since, by definition, utilities can be multiplied by time to yield a meaningful quantity. Two general cost-utility methods are the standard gamble approach and the time trade-off approach.[38] In the *standard gamble* approach, people are asked to choose between their current state of health and a "gamble" in which they have various probabilities for death or perfect health (cure). The *time trade-off* method is easier to perform and involves asking people how much time they would be willing to give up in order to live out their remaining life expectancy in perfect health. All utility approaches share in common the use of 0–1 scale in which 0 = death and 1 = perfect health. In practice, most cost-utility analyses employ expert estimates of utility weights, or, in some cases, weights provided by healthy members of the general public. It is often assumed that these weights are reasonable approximations of patient preferences. However, several studies have demonstrated that utilities obtained from patients are generally higher than those provided by physicians, which are, in turn, higher than utilities for the same health states obtained from healthy individuals.[39] There are practical impediments to collection of utilities directly from patients, including the complexity of the concepts involved and the requirement for an interviewer-administered questionnaire (often unfeasible in the cooperative group setting). In addition, utility assessments provide little information on important disease and treatment-specific problems and are probably less sensitive to changes in health status over time than psychometric data.[40,41] Finally, the few studies that have been done involving simultaneous measurement of utilities and health status have found them at best to be moderately correlated, with measures of mood and depression correlating more highly than other measures with utilities.[42]

A modified utility approach has been developed to evaluate the effectiveness of adjuvant chemotherapy for early-stage breast cancer.[43] This approach, the Quality-adjusted Time Without Symptoms and Toxicity (Q-TWiST), discounts survival time spent with toxicity or symptoms relative to disease-free survival off therapy. Like other decision analyses in cancer, no empirical data on patient preferences were obtained in these studies. Thresholds for decision making were determined by modeling actual survival data, and judgments were made by the investigators regarding where patient preferences were likely to fall relative to these threshold values. There is no theoretical reason that actual patient preference data could not have been used in the Q-TWiST analyses or other studies of quality-adjusted survival. If the relationship between psychometric data and utilities can be established, it will become possible to collect psychometric data and base utility estimates on the reports of patients rather than the best guesses of others.

In summary, the existing science of HQL measurement is organized around a presumed (but theoretically unsubstantiated) dichotomy between psychometric and utility approaches. Neither approach alone is sufficient to understand clinical trial outcome data. The psychometric approach provides the detailed perspective of the patient, but it does not generally tell us how important a given problem or set of problems is to a group of patients. The utility approach informs us about the relative value of various health states; however, because of its emphasis on a single summary score, it fails to reflect the specific problems that might emerge. To date, it has also usually relied on surrogates rather than on patients to provide the utility weights. A second reason to combine the two approaches is that an individual provider cannot be expected to work with either one alone. The psychometric approach can uncover specific areas of difficulty or dysfunction, yet patients may not consider these areas to be worthy of provider attention or a change in treatment. On the other hand, the utility approach does not generally reveal the nature of specific problems or dysfunctions, which clearly hampers the provider's efforts in planning interventions or treatment changes. In fact, identification of health dimensions uniquely important to an individual and quantifying patient status within those dimensions has been proposed.[44] These approaches can and must be integrated in order to continue to advance the field. Previous efforts to combine psychometric and utility approaches have been rare and, where present, poorly integrated.[45] An integrative approach could be applied in which a well-validated QL scale can be administered to a patient in a clinical trial (or in clinical practice, for that matter). This patient's total score can be converted to a standardized score that allows for both ease of communication and possible utility analysis.

EVALUATING PSYCHOMETRIC MEASURES

Asking a psychometric consultant if a given HQL measure is valid is like asking a bacteriologist if a given antibiotic is effective. Unless the measure is clearly invalid, the answer will always begin with a question such as: "Under what circumstances, and with which patients?" Just as there is no antibiotic for every infection, there is no HQL measure for every investigation. Similarly, when the question is: "Which HQL measure should I use for evaluating (*X*) treatment for (*Y*) disease," the answer has necessary contingencies: "At which phase of treatment?" "What differences do you expect?" In short, the investigator's task is to select the measure most likely to be effective for a given purpose. This is best accomplished by careful consideration of the purpose of the investigation, critical evaluation of the psychometric properties and known performance of available measures, and review of item content for relevance and appropriateness. This last activity is not trivial inasmuch as it can prevent selection of an otherwise-valid measure that will be insensitive for the application selected. For example, the short forms (e.g., SF-36) derived from the Medical Outcomes Study[22,23] have a long history of development and demonstrate good psychometric properties, but may be inappropriate at the high end of HQL (e.g., adjuvant chemotherapy) because they emphasize mobility and physical function over social well-being, sexuality, and body image. The issue of disease severity cuts across virtually all self-report measures of HQL, in that it becomes difficult if not impossible to obtain self-report HQL data from very weak, cognitively impaired, or emotionally upset patients. This is an unfortunate irony given that these patients are often the very ones for whom quality-of-life concerns take first priority in treatment decision making. Efforts to use surrogate ratings have been largely disappointing, showing that health providers and, to a lesser extent, family members cannot be considered as reliable surrogate raters.[46]

Reliability

Two synonyms for *reliability* are repeatability and consistency. *Repeatability* refers to the extent to which a measure, applied two different times (test-retest) or in two different ways (alternate form and interrater), produces the same score. Consistency refers to the homogeneity of the items of a scale. A measure's internal consistency is usually expressed in terms of Cronbach's coefficient α, because it is the most comprehensive strategy among those available, and can be easily done with most computer statistical packages.

A ruler is a perfectly reliable measure because it will always produce the same score when applied to the same object, whether done by the same person or two different people. No HQL measure can ever expect to achieve such perfection, expressed as a correlation coefficient of 1.0, but close approximations (e.g., correlations above .70) are important.[47] Other important things to keep in mind are discussed next.

Reliability is a matter of degree

Reliability is not a fixed property of a measure but rather a property of a measure used with certain people under certain conditions. Because of this, reported reliability cannot be assumed to be generalizable and therefore should be reevaluated in later applications. This may be unreasonable to expect of test-retest reliability, but certainly not of internal consistency or interrater reliability (when appropriate).

Reliability depends on the number of items

As the number of items goes up, so too does the reliability coefficient. It is this observation that led to the Spearman-Brown correction of the split-half reliability technique, which evaluates the internal consistency of a test by splitting it in half and correlating the two halves (Cronbach's α is the average of all split halves). In our effort to reduce the number of items in a scale so as to lower patient and staff burden, we cannot allow ourselves to go so far as to drop reliability below an acceptable level. Another important corollary to this basic principle is that subtests will usually have lower reliability than the total score, because they have fewer items. It would be acceptable, for example, to implement a measure that has Cronbach α coefficients ranging from, say, .65 to .80, for the subtests, and to .85 for the total score. One might be more cautious about interpreting data from the least internally consistent subtest, especially if it were the only one with significant results.

Reliability is increased by heterogeneous samples

This increase in reliability occurs because heterogeneous samples produce a greater spread of scores, which inflate the reliability coefficient. Therefore, a coefficient of .70 for a group of patients with advanced pancreatic cancer may reflect superior reliability compared to a coefficient of .80 obtained with a sample combining healthy and very ill people.

Validity

Validity refers to a scale's ability to measure what it purports to measure. A scale must be reliable in order to be valid, but it needn't be valid in order to be reliable. The ruler described earlier, for example, is certainly reliable; however, its validity must be clarified. As a measure of length, it can be demonstrated to be valid; in fact, it is a "gold standard" against which other measures of length could be compared. However, it has limited validity as a measure of weight. Length and weight are two different physical constructs, one of which is perfectly measured by a ruler, the other of which can be estimated by a ruler (assuming constant density). If we had no better measure of weight than a ruler, it could arguably be used as a reasonably valid approximation, but certainly not as a gold standard. In some sense, this is where we find ourselves today in HQL measurement: without a gold standard, trying to approximate a construct we agree is important and measurable. Data collected to substantiate this effort are validity data.

Validity has generally been subdivided into three types: content, criterion, and construct. *Content validity* is further divided into *face validity* (the degree to which the scale superficially appears to measure the construct in question), and *true content validity* (the degree to which the items accurately represent the range of attributes covered by the construct). Two things are important to understand about content validity. First, since content validity does not include statistical evidence to support inferences made from tests (the central feature of validity), some[48] do not consider content evidence to be a true measure of a scale's validity. Second, with a multidimensional construct such as HQL, content coverage should cut across at least three broad domains (i.e., physical, psychological, and social) in order to be considered valid from the perspective of item content. The scale reviewer can evaluate this by examination of the development strategy for the scale as well as the actual content of the items themselves, which may or may not be reflected by subtest scores.

Criterion validity is also subdivided into two types, *concurrent validity* and *predictive validity*. The distinction between the two is a function of when the criterion data are collected. Criterion data that are collected simultaneously with the scale data provide evidence of concurrent validity. Data that are collected some time after the scale data provide evidence for predictive validity. It is common to see scores on the self-report measure of HQL in question correlated to another "standard" that has been completed at the same time, provided as evidence of concurrent validity. Generally, when the method of completion is the same and the timing is concurrent, one would seek coefficients only slightly below the internal consistency coefficients for the reference and comparison scales. Similarly, test-retest reliability coefficients can be considered as upper bounds of predictive validity.

Construct validity extends criterion-related validity into a broader arena in which the scale in question is tested against a theoretical model and adjusted according to results that can, in turn, help refine theory. There are many different approaches to construct validation. One is to examine a matrix of correlations between the scale in question and the following: other measures of the same construct; measures of related constructs, measures of unrelated constructs; and different methods of data collection (e.g., self-report versus observer rating). This multitrait-multimethod matrix permits one to test for the presence of hypothesized high correlations (convergent validity) and hypothesized low correlations (discriminant validity).

Other contributions to construct validity can be derived from multidimensional scaling and factor analytic approaches that can confirm the presumed multidimensional nature of HQL. It might seem contradictory, but it may also help to conduct item analyses based on a unidimensional scaling model for the overall measure as well as the component subtests, given the fact that HQL dimensions are intercorrelated.

The ability of an instrument to differentiate groups of patients expected to differ in HQL is also an important validation of its sensitivity. A "known group technique"[49] can be employed in which patients with, for example, advanced disease are compared to those with limited disease to determine whether the HQL measure detects the differences known to exist between groups. The same could be done by comparing HQL scores of inpatients to those of outpatients, scores of patients receiving adjuvant therapy to those of a clinically comparable group receiving no therapy, scores of homebound patients to those of ambulatory patients, and so forth. Finally, the demonstration of an instrument's sensitivity or responsiveness to change over time, parallel to changes in clinical status[50] is an important example of its validity that can easily be neglected in early psychometric evaluations.

Some important things to keep in mind about validity are discussed next.

Validity is not absolute

Like reliability, validity should not be considered to be an absolutely achieved status of a measure. Validity data are cumulative, requiring ongoing updates and refinements. Related to this, validity is relative, in that a given measure might be valid (i.e., sensitive) in one setting and not in another. Consider a measure that emphasizes activities of daily living skills and physical sensations. Such a measure may be valid in the context of metastatic breast cancer, but insensitive in early-stage disease, where virtually all patients will score at the top of the scale. The potential for sample-dependent ceiling effects such as this (and for floor effects in the reverse case) warrants caution when selecting the best instrument for a given population.

An HQL measure should assess well-being in addition to impairment

A criterion of content validity is that a scale measure the full range of HQL. Given that the concept of HQL includes positive aspects of health status (well-being), it is important that a measure of HQL address well-being in addition to functional ability/limitations.

Statistical significance is not always clinically meaningful

Related to validity is the issue of meaningfulness of the data obtained. A comparison of treatment arms might indeed result in differences in HQL. But how much of a difference is clinically meaningful, as opposed to statistically significant? For a seven-point Likert scaling of symptoms, Jaeschke et al.[51] have suggested a difference of approximately 0.5 units as a minimal clinically important difference. For other types of scaling (e.g., linear analog), Jacobson and Truax[52] recommend a Reliable Change Index that estimates whether a change measured is real or just a consequence of imprecise measurement.

Acceptability of Measures

In addition to reliability and validity, the acceptability of an instrument to patients and staff is also very important. Intrusiveness or inappropriateness of items can damage the integrity of an HQL measure that might otherwise be quite sound. Also, while reliability and validity are certainly important, they are not static standards. Just as our understanding of HQL is evolving, so also should our measurement approaches.

QUALITY-OF-LIFE MEASURES FOR USE IN ONCOLOGY

The fact that there are now many available measures of HQL is both a blessing and a curse. It is a blessing in that it provides the user with choices based on specific characteristics of a given disease site or clinical trial. It is a curse in that it potentially fragments the field of HQL measurement, thereby impeding our ability to make comparisons across studies and measures. This section presents some of the more commonly used and adequately validated measures of HQL that have been designated as cancer-specific. The designation of cancer-specific is rather arbitrary in that some measures considered to be cancer-specific could be (and have been) applied to other diseases. Examination of item content of some of these measures reveals that indeed many of the concepts measured are generic rather than cancer-specific.

Psychometric Measures

Quality-of-Life Index (QLI)[21]

This scale is perhaps the best example of a "cancer-specific" scale that in reality measures generic health concepts. Although not the first cancer-specific quality-of-life measure to appear in the literature (e.g., see ref. 53), the QLI was certainly an early entry. Intended by its authors as conceptually equivalent to a neonatal Apgar score,[54] it was originally developed as a 10-point physician rating of five areas of functioning (activity, daily living, health, support, outlook). Since then, many have used this observer rating scale as a patient-rated scale, with reasonable success (e.g., see ref. 46). The

QLI was carefully constructed using expert advisory panels comprised of patients and professionals, and has been subjected to study in at least 28 empirical investigations. In their thorough review, Wood-Dauphinee and Williams[55] conclude that it is a well-validated global measure of HQL. Proxy ratings and reliability data for subscales of activity, daily living, and health are more robust than those for support and outlook. The QLI has demonstrated the ability to distinguish cancer patients with terminal disease from either patients with recent disease or ones who were engaged in active treatment.[64] The QLI has also been positively related to the Uniscale and Multiscale Measures of Quality of Life and self- and physician ratings of HQL in cancer patients,[55] although the relationship with the Karnofsky Performance Status (KPS) scale has been variable.

European Organization for Research and Treatment of Cancer Quality-of-Life Questionnaire—Core (EORTC-QLQ)[14,15]

This measure is a 36-item instrument consisting of both dichotomous responses (yes/no) and responses that utilize a 4-point rating scale ranging from "not at all" to "very much." The core instrument was developed from a conceptual model and measures physical, role, emotional, and social functioning, along with disease symptoms, financial impact, and global quality of life across different cultural contexts. Aaronson et al.[14] report α's for individual scales ranging from a low of .59 for a three-item subset of the physical functioning dimension to a high of .85 for the two-item global quality-of-life dimension. Multitrait scaling techniques using 156 tests of item discriminant validity yielded only one definite and three probable scaling errors and interscale correlations supported the notion of nonorthogonal dimensions ($p < .001$) in quality of life. Finally, Aaronson et al. demonstrated that the seven scales significantly predicted differences in patient clinical status.[14] The 36-item QLQ has been replaced with a 30-item version that reduces the number of physical- and emotional-functioning items and replaces the single concentration and memory item with two separate items.

Functional Living Index—Cancer (FLIC)[17]

This is a 22-item scale on which patients indicate the impact of cancer on "day-to-day living issues that represent the global construct of functional quality of life,"[17] using a 7-point Likert-type rating. The scale provides a total HQL score only. Although only a total score is available, factor analyses have consistently revealed two primary factors (physical and psychological) with other smaller factors also present. It might therefore be appropriate to create at least two subtest scores from this instrument. Convergent validity studies on the FLIC suggest that the emotional factor is more highly correlated with other well-validated measures assessing depression and anxiety than with measures of physical functioning. Conversely, the physical factor of the FLIC is more highly correlated with measures of physical functioning than with measures of emotional distress. The FLIC has been used extensively in oncology, with predominantly positive results.

Functional Assessment of Cancer Therapy (FACT) Scales[16,18]

This instrument is a 28–40-item compilation of a generic core (28 items) and six specific subscales, which reflect symptoms or problems associated with different diseases (e.g., breast, bladder, colorectal, head and neck, and lung cancers, and HIV infection).[18] The scale was developed from a model similar to that of the EORTC, using 135 patients with advanced cancer and 15 oncology specialists. It was then validated on a second sample of 630 patients with a variety of cancers at different stages. The measure yields a total HQL score and subtest scores for physical well-being, social/family well-being, relationship with doctor, emotional well-being, functional well-being, and disease-specific concerns. Six additional experimental items request information regarding how much each dimension affects HQL, using a rating scale that ranges from 0 ("not at all") to 10 ("very much so").

The 28-item FACT-G scale is able to distinguish metastatic ($M = 79.6$) from nonmetastatic disease ($M = 83.7$), $F(1,334) = 5.38, p < .05$. It also distinguishes between stage I, II, III, and IV disease, $F(3,308) = 2.94, p < .05$, and between inpatients and outpatients from different centers, $F(2,411) = 17.0, p < .001$. Concurrent validity is supported by Pearson correlations with the Functional Living Index—Cancer (.80) and a patient-completed version of the QL Index (.74). Initial evidence for construct validity is supported by: (1) moderate-to-high correlations with mood state as measured by the Taylor Manifest Anxiety Scale (.57) and a shortened version of the Profile of Mood States (.69); (2) moderate correlation with activity level as measured by the Eastern Cooperative Oncology Group five-point rating (−.56), and no correlation with social desirability as measured by a shortened version of the Marlowe-Crowne Social Desirability Scale (.03). Factor-analytic data from 545 patients with mixed cancer diagnoses yielded a six-factor solution (oblique rotation) accounting for 51% of the total variance.[18]

A unique feature of the FACT scales is that they provide supplemental valuative ratings that allow patients to provide domain-specific utility weights. These scales were developed primarily out of the psychometric tradition; however, there was an early eye toward movement into a utility approach as evidenced by two unique features. First, the 47 items (38 general; 9 site-specific) that were selected for version 1 of the FACT were drawn from a larger pool (over 200 possible items) according to patient ratings of item importance (utility weights) generated from the first-generation questionnaire. Second, each item on the second-generation questionnaire requires that the patient make two ratings: a rating of actual function or disability, and a rating of expectation that assesses whether a given symptom or rating was better or worse than expected. Thus it may provide an estimate of the acceptability of a given symptom or problem.

Cancer Rehabilitation Evaluation System—Short Form (CARES—SF)[19,20]

This is a 59-item self-administered rehabilitation and HQL instrument comprised of a list of statements reflecting problems encountered by cancer patients. Patients complete a minimum of 38 to a maximum of 57 items, depending on their treatments as well as on other medical and demographic factors. Statements are rated in terms of how applicable each is to them using a 5-point rating scale ranging from "not at all" to "very much." The measure yields a global score (summed ratings) reflecting overall HQL, five summary scores reflecting physical, psychosocial, medical interaction, marital, and sexual dimensions, and 31 subscales. Adequate test-retest reliability (10 days, $r = .92$ for global score, and ranges from .69 to .87 for subscales), internal consistency (α's for five subscales range from .67 to .83), and concurrent validity with other HQL measures (r's range from -0.50 to .74, $p < .0001$) are reported,[19] and the shortened form is correlated with the longer, 139-item version at $r = .98$. The global CARES score is sensitive to extent of disease in patients with colorectal, lung, and prostate cancer, and to improvement in HQL in patients with breast cancer over a 13-month period.[20] Summary scales, in part, have replicated global CARES scores, particularly in colorectal and lung disease.[20]

Linear Analogue Self-Assessment (LASA) Scales

LASA scales use a 100-mm line with descriptors at each extreme. Respondents are required to mark their current state somewhere along that line, which is then measured as a score in centimeters or millimeters from the 0 point. There are three noteworthy LASA scales for cancer patients. The original LASA scale of Priestman and Baum[53] was a 10-item scale for studying HQL in advanced breast cancer. This was later extended to 25 items in a study comparing chemotherapy and hormone therapy for advanced breast cancer.[56] These items included ten on symptoms and side effects, five on physical functioning, five on mood, and five on social relationships.

The other two LASA scales of note are the 31-item measure of Selby et al.,[57] which recently has been reduced to 29 items,[58] and the 14-item LASA of Padilla and colleagues.[59,60] Much of the Selby measure[57,58] was derived from the 12 Sickness Impact Profile (SIP) categories,[27] and supplemented with items to measure pain, mouth sores, concern with appearance, and other breast cancer-specific concerns. Test-retest reliability and internal consistency coefficients are above .70.[57,58] Concurrent validity coefficients with the appropriate SIP scales ranged from .28 to .98, with most above .60. Reliability coefficients on the Padilla et al. scale are acceptably high, with a factor analysis of 130 cancer patients revealing three factors (physical well-being, psychological well-being, symptom control) accounting for 73% of the total variance.[59] Padilla et al. have also developed a longer (23-item) measure for patients with colostomies.[60]

Linear analog scales are appealing because they are easy to administer and are usually presumed to have robust sensitivity due to interval scaling and a wide range of scores. They have also been criticized on the grounds that their sensitivity may be illusory and that it is difficult to know the minimal clinically significant difference. They also cannot be administered over the telephone, which can be limiting. However, they have performed rather well in studying individuals with metastatic breast cancer. For example, women receiving cytotoxic therapy were found to suffer more adverse physical reactions with a subsequent improvement in well-being on Priestman and Baum's scale, as long as there was an objective clinical response.[53] Later that decade, the much-quoted, counterintuitive results of Coates et al.[61] were reported in which women with metastatic cancer did better on continuous chemotherapy than those on intermittent chemotherapy. They used a very simple five-item linear analog scale along with the Spitzer QLI. Finally, Tannock et al.,[62] using the Selby LASA, demonstrated trends toward better HQL in women receiving higher dosages of cytotoxic chemotherapy as opposed to lower doses, presumably because of the increased tumor response and survival advantage gained from the increased dosage. All of these studies point to the same general conclusion about management of metastatic breast cancer: that the advantages of continuous cytotoxic chemotherapy outweigh the costs, assuming sufficient dosing and assuming the presence of measurable response to therapy. Taken together, these findings can provide valuable guidance in patient counseling and management with respect to the costs and benefits of cytotoxic chemotherapy in advanced breast cancer. In fact, Tannock has put forth a set of guidelines for managing metastatic breast cancer based on available treatment and HQL data.[63]

Medical Outcomes Study 36-Item Short-Form Status Health Survey (SF-36)[22,23]

The Medical Outcomes Study—Short-Form Health Status Survey (MOS SF-36) is a self-administered 36-item measure of eight health concepts: physical functioning, limitations in role functioning due to physical health problems, social functioning, bodily pain, general mental health, limitations in role functioning due to emotional problems, vitality, and general health perceptions.[22] It was developed to reproduce the previously well-validated, full-length scales, but in a shorter format. Responses vary as a function of the attribute measured, and range from dichotomous to a maximum of five possible choices. Its standardized scoring system yields a profile of eight health scores, which are summed scores of individual scale items (some of which have been reverse-scored), as well as summary indices. The SF-36 is reported to have satisfactory reliability (coefficients ranging from .73 to .94). Validity studies have demonstrated the ability to distinguish between patients with and without a chronic condition, discriminate levels of severity within a medical diagnosis, and reflect changes in health-related quality of life associated with changes in disease severity.[23]

Utility Measures

Quality of Well-Being (QWB) Scale[24–26]

The QWB is a utility measure of health-related QL. Kaplan and Anderson[24] focus on the qualitative dimension of functioning rather than exclusively on the psychological and social attributes of health outcomes, and use the term *health-related QL* to refer to the impact of health conditions on function. The Quality of Well-Being (QWB) scale is a 25-item list of symptom/problem complexes (CPX) covering the domains of mobility, physical activity, and social activity, each representing related but distinct aspects of daily functioning.[24] Community weights for each CPX control for its relative desirability, with higher weights reflecting more desirable states. The QWB is administered in a standardized interview and yields information about both specific states (CPX) and a total quality of well-being score (range = 0–1), expressed as the average of relative desirability scores. It is reported to demonstrate good test-retest reliability (*r*'s ranging from .78 to .99, with most correlation coefficients being above .90) over a 1-day period across different populations and health problems,[26] and adequate content, convergent, and discriminant validity.[25]

Quality-adjusted Time Without Symptoms and Toxicity (Q-TWiST)[43]

The only utility approach that was developed to be cancer-specific is the Quality-adjusted Time Without Symptoms and Toxicity (Q-TWiST) approach, which attempts to evaluate the effectiveness of adjuvant chemotherapy for early-stage breast cancer.[43] This approach was described earlier in the chapter, so it will only be commented on here. It discounts survival time by reducing it according to a predetermined utility weight (0–1 range), which accounts for the impact of disease symptoms and treatment side effects. The Q-TWiST approach does not clearly account for the effect of the time trade-off of most patients, who are usually quite willing to trade acute treatment toxicity for extended survival benefit. Like other utility methods, it does not, to date, generate the utility weights from patients themselves; rather, it depends on an assumed perspective. Given that it infers rather than measures patient preferences, the Q-TWiST approach may be regarded as related to but conceptually distinct from patient-rated HQL. It carries some advantages over approaches in that it is inexpensive to derive and allows for adjustment of survival time with the (presumed) HQL of that time. It may be possible to integrate the Q-TWiST approach with a psychometric scale or a patient preference scaling approach that increases sensitivity of measurement from the perspective of the patient.

CONCLUSION

This chapter provides a brief update of a sampling of cancer-specific health-related quality-of-life measures and approaches that have shown promise. Examination of sample measures is possible elsewhere.[4] Some of the measures described here have already contributed to an understanding of the diverse costs and benefits of cancer therapies. Most of the progress has been in the study of breast cancer and, to a lesser extent, lung, colorectal, and prostate cancers. It is certainly no coincidence that these are the most prevalent tumors. Further attention must be directed to less common (e.g., hematologic) malignancies as well as to intensive experimental therapies with severe toxicity and uncertain benefit (e.g., bone marrow transplantation with solid tumors). The "cancer-specific" issues in these areas may be sufficiently distinct to require new or appropriately adapted measurement. Because of their clinical experience and expertise, and because of their position at the forefront of cancer practice settings, nurses are in a unique position to assume leadership in evaluating the broad spectrum of costs and benefits associated with today's cancer therapies.

REFERENCES

1. Aaronson NK, Beckman J: *The Quality of Life of Cancer Patients.* Monograph Series of the European Organization for Research on Treatment of Cancer (EORTC), vol. 17. New York: Raven Press, 1987.
2. Barofsky I, Sugarbaker PH: Cancer. In Spilker B (ed.): *Quality of Life Assessments in Clinical Trials.* New York: Raven Press, 1990.
3. Osoba D (ed.): *Effect of Cancer on Quality of Life.* Boca Raton, FL: CRC Press, 1991.
4. Tchekmedyian NS, Cella DF (eds.): *Qualify of Life in Current Oncology Practice and Research.* Williston Park, NY: Dominus Publishing, 1991.
5. U.S. Department of Health and Human Services (DHHS), Public Health Service, National Institutes of Health: *Quality of Life Assessment in Cancer Clinical Trials: Report of the Workshop on Quality of Life Research in Cancer Clinical Trials.* Bethesda, MD: National Cancer Institute, 1990.
6. Moinpour CM, Feigl P, Metch B, et al: Quality of life end points in cancer clinical trials: Review and recommendations. *J Natl Cancer Inst* 81:485–495, 1989.

7. Cella DF, Tulsky DS: Measuring quality of life today: Methodological aspects. *Oncology* 4:29–38, 1990.
8. Gotay CC, Korn EL, McCabe MS, et al: Quality-of-life assessment in cancer treatment protocols: Research issues in protocol development. *J Natl Cancer Inst* 84:575–579, 1992.
9. Donovan K, Sanson-Fisher RW, Redman S: Measuring quality of life in cancer patients. *J Clin Oncology* 7:959–968, 1989.
10. Fayers PM, Jones DR: Measuring and analyzing quality of life in cancer clinical trials: A review. *Statistics in Medicine* 2:429–446, 1983.
11. Fetting JH: Evaluating quality and quantity of life in breast cancer adjuvant trials. *J Clin Oncology* 6:1795–1797.
12. Skeel RT: Quality of life assessment in cancer clinical trials—It's time to catch up. *J Natl Cancer Inst* 81:472–473, 1989.
13. Cella DF, Cherin EA: Quality of life during and after cancer treatment. *Comprehensive Therapy* 14:69–75, 1988.
14. Aaronson NK, Ahmedzai S, Bullinger M, et al: The EORTC Core Quality-of-Life Questionnaire: Interim results of an international field study. In Osoba D. (ed.) *Effect of Cancer on Quality of Life.* Boca Raton, FL: CRC Press, 1991.
15. Aaronson NK, Bullinger M, Ahmedzai S: A modular approach to quality-of-life assessment in cancer clinical trials. *Recent Results in Cancer Research* 111, 231–249, 1988.
16. Cella DF, Lee-Riordan D, Silberman M, et al: Quality of life in advanced cancer: Three new disease-specific measures. *Proc ASCO* 8:315 (#1225), 1989.
17. Schipper H, Clinch J, McMurray A, Levitt M: Measuring the quality of life of cancer patients: The Functional Living Index—Cancer: Development and validation. *J Clin Oncology* 2:472–483, 1984.
18. Cella DF, Tulsky DS, Gray G, et al: The Functional Assessment of Cancer Therapy (FACT) scale: Development and validation of the general version. *J Clin Oncology,* in press. To be published in March 1993.
19. Schag CAC, Ganz P, Heinrich RL: Cancer Rehabilitation Evaluation System—Short Form: A cancer-specific rehabilitation and quality of life instrument. *Cancer* 68:1406–1413, 1991.
20. Ganz PA, Schag CAC, Lee JJ, Sim MS: The CARES: A generic measure of health-related quality of life for patients with cancer. *Quality of Life Research* 1:19–29, 1992.
21. Spitzer WO, Dobson AJ, Hall J, et al: Measuring the quality of life of cancer patients: A concise QL index for use by physicians. *J Chron Dis* 34:585–597, 1981.
22. Ware JE, Sherbourne CD: The MOS 36-Item short-form health survey (SF-36): I. Conceptual framework and item selection. *Medical Care* (in press).
23. McHorney CA, Ware JE, Rogers W, et al: The validity and relative precision of MOS Short- and Long-Form Health Status Scales and Dartmouth COOP Charts: Results from the Medical Outcomes Study. *Medical Care* (In press).
24. Kaplan RM, Anderson JP: The general health policy model: An integrated approach. In Spilker B (ed.): *Quality of Life Assessments in Clinical Trials.* New York: Raven Press, 1990.
25. Kaplan RM, Bush JW, Berry CC: Health status: Types of validity and the Index of Well-Being: *Health Services Research* 11:478–507, 1976.
26. Anderson JP, Kaplan RM, Berry CC, et al: Interday reliability of function assessment for a health status measure: The Quality of Well-Being Scale. *Medical Care* 27:1076–1084, 1989.
27. Bergner J, Bobbitt RA, Carter WB, Gilson BS: The Sickness Impact Profile: Development and final revision of a health status measure. *Medical Care* 19:787–806, 1981.
28. Campbell A, Converse PE, Rodgers WL: *The Quality of American Life.* New York: Sage, 1976.
29. Till JE, McNeil BJ, Bush RS: Measurement of multiple components of quality of life. *Cancer Treatment Symposium* 1:177–181, 1984.
30. Calman KC: The quality of life in cancer patients—An hypothesis. *J Medical Ethics* 10:124–125, 1984.
31. Schipper H, Levitt M: Measuring quality of life: Risks and benefits. *Cancer Treatment Reports* 69:1115–1123, 1985.
32. George L, Bearon L: *Quality of Life in Older Persons: Meaning and Measurement.* New York: Human Sciences Press, 1980.
33. deHaes JCJM, vanKnippenberg FCE, Neijt JP: Measuring psychological and physical distress in cancer patients: Structure and application of the Rotterdam Symptom Checklist. *Brit J Cancer* 62:1034–1038, 1990.
34. Hays RD, Stewart AL: The structure of self-reported health in chronic disease patients. *Psychological Assessment* 2:22–30, 1990.
35. Ware J: Measuring functioning, well-being and other generic health concepts. In Osoba D (ed.): *Effect of Cancer on Quality of Life.* Boca Raton, FL: CRC Press, 1991, pp. 7–23.
36. Till JE, Sutherland HJ, Meslin EM: Is there a role for preference assessments in research on quality of life in oncology. *Quality of Life Research* 1:31–40, 1992.
37. Drummond MF, Stoddart GL, Torrance GW: *Methods for Economic Evaluation of Health Care Programmes.* Oxford, Eng.: Oxford University Press, 1987.
38. Torrance GW: Measurement of health state utilities for economic appraisal: A review article. *J Health Economics* 5:1–30, 1986.
39. Boyd NF, Sutherland HJ, Heasman KZ, et al: Whose utilities for decision analysis? *Med Decis Making* 10:58–67, 1990.
40. Tsevat J, Goldman L, Soukup JR, Lee TH. Stability of utilities in survivors of myocardial infarction. *Med Decis Making* 10:323, 1990.
41. Canadian Erythropoietin Study Group: Association between recombinant human erythropoietin and quality of life and exercise capacity of patients receiving hemodialysis. *Brit Medical J* 300:573–578, 1990.
42. Tsevat J, Cook EF, Soukop JR, et al: Utilities of the seriously ill (abstract). *Clin Res* 39:589A, 1991.
43. Gelber RD, Goldhirsch A, Cavalli F: Quality-of-life-adjusted evaluation of adjuvant therapies for operable breast cancer. *Ann Int Med* 114:621–628, 1991.
44. Llewellyn-Thomas HA, Sutherland HJ, Tritchler DL, et al: Benign and malignant breast disease: The relationship between women's health status and health values. *Med Decis Making* 11:180–188, 1991.
45. Feeny D, LaBelle R, Torrance GW: Integrating economic evaluations and assessments. In Spilker B (ed.): *Quality of Life Assessments in Clinical Trials.* New York: Raven Press, 1990, pp. 71–83.
46. Slevin ML, Plant H, Lynch D, et al: Who should measure quality of life, the doctor or the patient? *Brit J Cancer* 57:109, 1988.
47. Nunnally JC: *Psychometric Theory.* New York: McGraw-Hill, 1967.

48. Messick S: The once and future issues of validity: Assessing the meaning and consequences of measurement. In Wainer H, Braun HI (eds.): *Test Validity*. Hillside, NJ: Lawrence Erlbaum Associates, 1988.
49. Bohrnstedt GW: Measurement. In Rossi PH, Wright JD, Anderson AB (eds.): *Handbook of Survey Research*. New York: Academic Press, 1983.
50. Guyatt G, Walter S, Normal G: Measuring change over time: Assessing the usefulness of evaluative instruments. *J Chron Dis* 40:171, 1987.
51. Jaeschke R, Singer J, Guyatt GH: Measurement of health status: Ascertaining the minimal clinically important difference. *Controlled Clinical Trials* 10:407–415, 1989.
52. Jacobson NS, Truax P: Clinical significance: A statistical approach to defining meaningful change in psychotherapy research. *J Consul Clin Psychol* 59:12–19, 1991.
53. Priestman TJ, Baum M: Evaluation of quality of life in patients receiving treatment for advanced breast cancer. *Lancet* April 24:899–901, 1976.
54. Apgar V: Proposal for new methods of evaluation of newborn infants. *Anesth Analges* 32:260, 1953.
55. Wood-Dauphinee S, Williams JI: The Spitzer Quality-of-Life Index: Its performance as a measure. In Osoba D (ed.): *Effect of Cancer on Quality of Life*. Boca Raton, FL: CRC Press, 1991, pp. 169–184.
56. Baum M, Priestman T, West RR, Jones EM: A comparison of subjective responses in a trial comparing endocrine with cytotoxic treatment in advanced carcinoma of the breast. *European J Cancer* 16:223–226, 1980 (suppl 1).
57. Selby PJ, Chapman JAW, Etazadi-Amoli J, et al: The development of a method for assessing the quality of life of cancer patients. *Brit J Cancer* 50:13–22, 1984.
58. Boyd NF, Selby PJ, Sutherland HJ, Hogg S: Measurement of the clinical status of patients with breast cancer: Evidence for the validity of self assessment with linear analogue scales. *J Clin Epidem* 41:243–250, 1988.
59. Padilla GV, Presant C, Grant MM, et al: Quality of life index for patients with cancer. *Res Nurs Health* 6:117–126, 1983.
60. Padilla GV, Grant MM: Quality of life as a cancer nursing outcome variable. *Amer Nurs Sci* 8:45–60, 1985.
61. Coates A, Gebski V, Stat M (for the Australian-New Zealand Breast Cancer Trials Group): Improving the quality of life during chemotherapy for advanced breast cancer. *New Engl J Med* 317:1490, 1987.
62. Tannock IF, Boyd NF, DeBoer G, et al: A randomized trial of two dose levels of cyclophosphamide, methotrexate and fluorouracil chemotherapy for patients with metastatic breast cancer. *J Clin Oncology* 6:1377, 1988.
63. Tannock IF: Management of breast and prostate cancer: How does quality of life enter the equation? In Tchekmedyian NS, Cella DF (eds.): *Quality of Life in Oncology Practice and Research*. Williston Park, NY: Dominus (PRR), 1991.
64. Mor V: Cancer patients' quality of life over the disease course: Lessons from the real world. *J Chron Dis* 40:535, 1987.

Chapter 11

Principles of Treatment Planning

Mary B. Maxwell, RN, CS, PhD

INTRODUCTION

Because "cancer" includes more than 101 different disease entities involving virtually every organ system in the body, choosing among the therapeutic alternatives is a complex task. Fundamentally, treatment decisions in oncology are based on the location, cell type, and extent of the malignancy, with established modes of therapy (surgery, radiation, chemotherapy) directed toward the particular disease presentation. The aim of treatment is to cure if possible, causing minimal structural or functional impairment. If cure is not possible, then the aim is to control or palliate the disease. The sequence and intellectual considerations in cancer treatment planning are the same as in any problem-solving activity: gathering information, planning, executing the plan, and evaluating. In this chapter the factors involved in problem solving for cancer treatment are examined in detail. The material is organized temporally, following the usual sequence in planning treatment for a patient. An initial, brief historical look at treatment will set the stage for understanding the basis of contemporary therapy, from which projections can be made for the future.

The recipient of cancer treatment is a unique human being, and every aspect of the design and evaluation of therapeutic activities must take this into consideration. A therapeutic plan that seems indicated by abstract scientific analysis may have to be modified or changed by human events in the real world. Cancer treatment and care should be a humanistic application of established modes of therapy to a unique individual. Optimal treatment for both cure and palliation requires not only individualization of treatment but an approach that uses all therapeutic disciplines capable of improving results.

HISTORICAL PERSPECTIVES ON CANCER TREATMENT

In the haste to find more effective ways to treat cancer, new methods were and are continually being devised. Treatment assumptions that can seem so logical are often not borne out with time or by the application of rigorous scientific research methods. A hundred years from now, the treatments of today may seem as bizarre to clinicians as bloodletting and purging seem to us today. Understanding cancer involves unraveling the mysteries of the basis of life itself, and we are still far from this understanding. Until cancer can be prevented, therapeutic interventions will continue to evolve and change. Every year new discoveries are made and old methods modified or discarded. From the earliest times, the treatment of cancer has been based on the prevailing ideas about the etiology of the disease. In any era, such ideas stem from theories of the structure and functioning of the human body, the philosophic view of nature, and the available technology.[1]

Ancient Times

The Egyptians used arsenical ointment in 1500 B.C. to attack cancer's external manifestations, which were believed to be most important. Hippocrates cauterized cancer in the neck in the fourth century B.C. Celsus (30 B.C. to A.D. 38) excised breast cancer, leaving the pectoral muscles intact. Cato administered charcoal, and many therapists employed metallic salts, particularly copper and lead, treatments that persisted for centuries.

Dark Ages/Medieval Period

Galen (A.D. 131–203) classified tumors, and considered cancer a systemic disease caused by an excess of black bile humor, being thereby beyond the cure of operation. He advocated vegetable diets and purging, cautioning against eating walnuts. The theory of humors came from ancient Greek beliefs that universal elements (fire, air, wind, earth) and qualities (hot, cold, moist, dry) were assigned to four humors: blood, phlegm, yellow bile, and black bile.[1] Treatment for cancer in this era was mostly surgical, including lancing and bloodletting, aimed at releasing the offending collection of humor causing the cancer. The basic principle was first to purge the black humors and then to excise the affected area. These ideas predominated until the dawn of the eighteenth century.

The Enlightenment

As discoveries were made about anatomy and the lymphatic and circulatory systems, the humoral theories and the idea that cancer was a constitutional disease gave way to more scientific notions. In 1704 Valsalva advanced the theory that cancer was first a local lesion capable of cure by surgery, which then spread via the lymphatics to regional nodes, thus tending to recur as secondary lesions. The principles of modern cancer surgery are based on this theory.

The Nineteenth Century

John Hunter, father of scientific surgery, thought coagulated lymph was a cause of cancer and that tumors were nourished by lymph vessels. This led to a more chemical orientation in which corrosive acids or ferments of lymph were seen as culprits. Hunter removed local lymph nodes when possible and ligated vessels supplying the tumor. With the aid of the microscope and advances in chemistry and science in general, it later became accepted that the body was composed of fibers and tissues. The new tissue theories, coupled with findings from embryonic studies, led to a better understanding of cancer metastasis. This was followed by the cellular theory, which recognized cells as the basic structural units of tissues, including tumors. Toward the end of this era, the only available treatment, surgery, progressed in a dramatic manner due to the development of anesthesia and antiseptic techniques.

The Twentieth Century

An anatomic basis for cancer surgery arose about 100 years ago. *En bloc* resections (radical mastectomy, radical prostatectomy), in which the primary tumor as well as adjacent lymphatics and lymph nodes were removed in one continuous section, were deemed the proper cancer operation. Cancer surgery based on these considerations has persisted, with the goal being the surgical removal of every cancer cell. By the 1970s, however, the superradical procedures, such as hemicorporectomy and hindquarter operations, were seldom performed; patient survival had not been improved.

As a consequence of conceptual changes arising from new information about tumor biology, a biologic basis for cancer treatment emerged.[2] It became generally accepted that even the smallest solid tumor that could be diagnosed with contemporary methods was already systemic at the time of presentation. Since cancer is a systemic disease involving a complex spectrum of host–tumor interrelations, variations in local-regional therapy are unlikely to affect survival substantially. The primary aim of oncologic surgery became to reduce the tumor burden to a number of viable cells that could be destroyed by host immunologic factors, chemotherapy, or immunotherapy. If surgery was followed by one or more of these treatments, it was called *adjuvant* (aiding or assisting) *therapy*. More recently, *neoadjuvant therapy* (the use of drugs at the earliest possible time for induction) has been used for some tumors.[3,4] This involves giving a short course of chemotherapy prior to a surgical procedure, in an attempt to eliminate micrometastasis up front. These are examples of *multimodal therapy*, the integration of more than one antineoplastic therapy into a treatment program in order to improve therapeutic results, reduce toxicities (as compared to single modality treatment), or both.[5] The objective, to eradicate every malignant cell, remained the same, but the method for its accomplishment changed from exclusively surgical as other cancer treatment modalities became available.

Radiation Discovered

The discovery of X rays, radioactivity, and radium before the turn of the century was soon followed by the therapeutic application of the new agents. By 1899, a basal cell carcinoma had been cured by radiation.[6] It was thought that a miraculous new cure for cancer had been discovered because of the dramatic initial responses seen in the treatment of skin and superficial lesions. Then followed a period of disillusionment and pessimism as recurrence and serious injuries to normal tissues were realized. These first 25 years were the "dark ages" of radiotherapy. The physical nature and biologic effects of the new agents were not understood, and equipment was primitive. There was no reliable way to measure dose. Many scientists lost their lives through their work with radiation during this time. Because most of the earliest practitioners were surgeons, they used treatment methods involving single, massive exposures aimed at eradicating a tumor in a single treatment. As might be expected, those individuals who lived through the immediate postirradiation period, although they had impressive initial regressions of their lesions, usually developed serious complications as well as early recurrences. Starting in 1919, the technique of successive fractionated daily doses of radiotherapy evolved from clinical research. Impressive results became evident in the treatment of head and neck and cervical lesions. In the early 1950s, the emergence of megavoltage equipment greatly improved delivery. Recent technologic innovations such as beam-modifying devices, radiation sensitizers, and radioprotectors have enhanced the tumoricidal effect of radiation therapy. Where previously radiation was used only for palliation, it began to be used for cure in some situations.

Chemotherapy Introduced

Cancer chemotherapy had its origins in observations made of chemical warfare during World War I. Soldiers who breathed mustard gas suffered severe bone marrow suppression, aplasia, and death. It was hypothesized that these effects could be exploited in the treatment of cancer. Nitrogen mustard subsequently became the first chemotherapeutic agent to undergo clinical trials.

In the 1940s, the laborious task of ascertaining which of some 200,000 known chemicals possessed cancericidal properties was begun. Effective chemotherapeutic agents were produced by the synthesis of toxic radicals with chemical substances required by the malignant cell for division and multiplication. In the 1950s antibiotics (Adriamycin, Bleomycin) began to be used as antineoplastics. Thioguanine, mercaptopurine, and folic antagonists were introduced. The prospective, randomized clinical trial was introduced into clinical medicine as a mechanism for hypothesis testing, obtaining natural history information about the cancer, and for evaluating the worth of a particular treatment. The advent of clinical trials allowed cancer treatment to be based on rational choice rather than on anecdote and trial and error.[7]

Where at first single drugs were given continuously or daily over a period of time, the use of systemic chemotherapy has evolved to *pulse dosing* (high doses given intermittently), with multiple drugs being given concurrently (*combination chemotherapy*).[8] Because agents used in combinations are chosen for their overlapping toxicities as well as their sensitivity to a particular tumor, higher tumor cell kill can theoretically be achieved with each treatment, resulting in fewer side effects. *Biologic response modifiers,* agents meant to modulate biologic or immune responses that affect cancer, were introduced in the 1980s. These agents are described in Chapter 17. Biologic response modifiers may be considered a noncytotoxic type of chemotherapy. There are currently over 50 antineoplastic agents available (plus investigational drugs in testing stages) for treating cancers. Pharmacologic considerations, variables, and patient factors make for an infinite variety of combinations and sequences that have been, are, and will be tried for treatment.[9] *First-line drugs,* those used during initial treatment, are also those known to be most effective against the tumor and most likely to lead to remission, or "cure." If the tumor recurs, *second-line drugs* may be in order, because the patient failed on the drugs used initially (probably due to resistance). Second-line drugs are those with less activity against the tumor, but for which a response or a second remission may be possible if the tumor is sensitive to them. In some cases, such as hematologic malignancies, third- and fourth-line drugs may be possible.

The Cancer Team

Traditionally, surgeons had managed the treatment of most people with cancer. During the 1960s, medical oncology, an offshoot of internal medicine, became a specialty. Radiotherapy is a consultative discipline, and radiation oncologists see patients only on referral by other physicians. Whereas up to 30 years ago the primary qualifications for an oncology nurse were a kind heart and the ability to improvise,[10] the current variety and complexity of care opportunities has called forth a new breed of professional nurse. Advanced formal education, oncology nursing certification, and clinical sophistication are mandatory as nursing roles have expanded and nurses have assumed increased responsibility for all aspects of patient management. Modern cancer treatment and care has become a team effort involving the expertise of specialists from a variety of disciplines.

Treatment Centers

Because treatment approaches are not always clearly defined, the consultative assistance of qualified oncologic specialists is available to patients throughout the United States through tumor boards in hospitals with accredited cancer programs. Tumor boards allow a group of physicians specializing in cancer to meet, discuss particular cases, and give their opinions about the advantages and disadvantages of treatment alternatives. In many larger centers, there are even specialty tumor boards that review cases in one particular field (e.g., breast, urology, pediatrics).

Patients can now usually be treated in their own communities, avoiding the long periods away from home and family that used to be necessary. The care provided by the major cancer centers has become highly technological, palliative, or research oriented. Many community cancer centers have been established, as well as special oncology units in local hospitals, and hospices for the terminally ill. These cancer programs offer not only the latest treatment with state-of-the-art national protocols, but also rehabilitation and support programs for patients and families.

But the care of the person with cancer has not always been so enlightened. The first cancer hospital opened in Rheims in 1740 under the supervision of the Hotel Dieu (in Paris, the oldest hospital in Europe). In 1770, because of the superstition that cancer was contagious, the hospital was moved outside the city. The first cancer service in a general hospital was established in Middlesex Hospital in England. It consisted of 12 beds for patients who were permitted to remain until they either improved or succumbed. In the United States, the present Memorial Sloan-Kettering Cancer Center in New York City was established by J. Marion Sims, who was ridiculed and threatened for his efforts to treat cancer.

Because primary therapy has improved and combined methods offer a wide variety of interventions to manage the disease after recurrence, people with cancer are living longer. This often means additional therapeutic planning sessions and visits to the tumor board or cancer team as new problems arise. Figure 11-1 charts the usual sequence of events in planning cancer treatment.

FACTORS INVOLVED IN TREATMENT PLANNING

The Patient Presents

Any person with a health complaint who seeks health care may have cancer. Any complaints of weight loss, unexplained pain, unexplained loss of energy, or irregularities of the alimentary, respiratory, genital, urinary, or neurologic system, or concerns about lumps or bumps should alert the primary clinician to the possibility of cancer.

A Diagnostic Workup Is Begun

When neoplastic disease is suspected, a detailed history (including family and occupational information), physical examination, and hematologic, biochemical, and radiologic studies must be performed to establish the likelihood of cancer as the diagnosis and the necessity

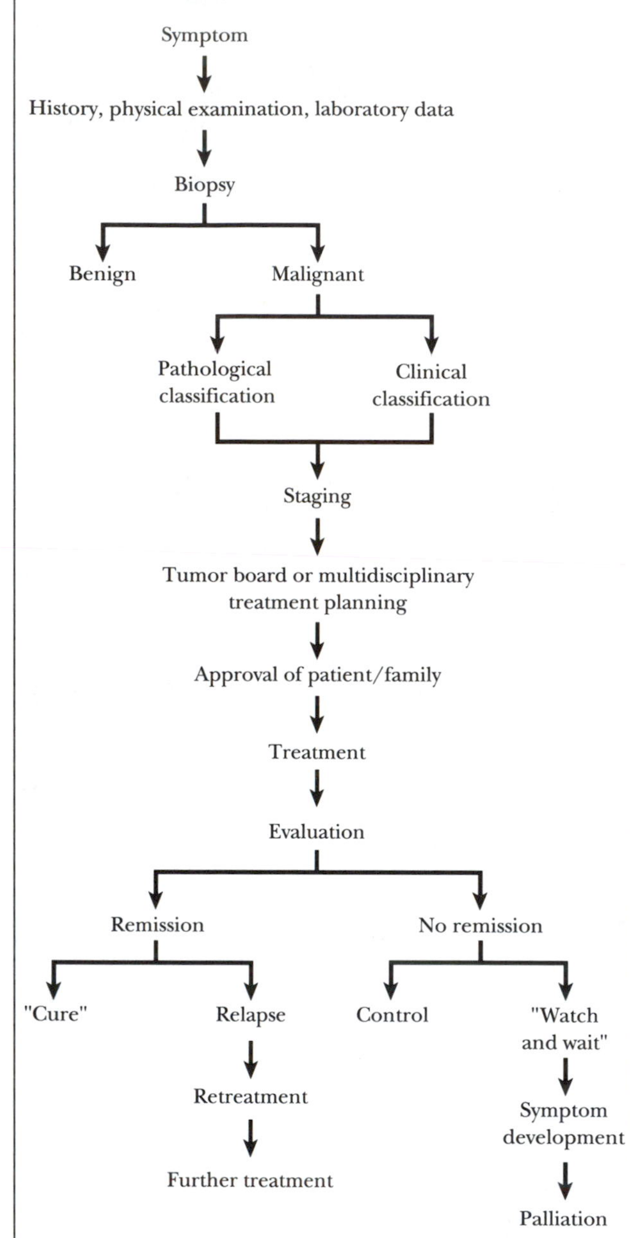

FIGURE 11-1 Usual sequence of events in planning cancer treatment.

for obtaining histologic proof. When the clinical evidence points to the presence of malignancy, the next step is to establish by biopsy the nature of the lesion.

A Biopsy Is Done

Histologic proof of malignancy is the cornerstone of diagnosis and treatment. It is crucial because neoplasms can masquerade as benign or inflammatory conditions, and vice versa. A biopsy is also a useful guide to prognosis, and a definitive diagnosis fosters the economical, orderly, and planned use of all available resources. It prevents hasty local treatment measures that might jeopardize later interventions. No matter how difficult it may be to obtain tissue (e.g., a suspected pancreatic tumor), proceeding to treat without a tissue diagnosis could lead to disaster if the lesion were later found to be benign. The site that is least risky to disrupt and most likely to provide the necessary information is biopsied. Chapter 12 describes methods for performing biopsies.

Any biopsy report that is equivocal or inconsistent with the clinical findings should be reviewed by an outside source (such as the Armed Forces Institute of Pathology) or a new biopsy should be obtained. Recurrent or metastatic disease requires the same critical diagnosis as the primary lesion.

The Biopsy Establishes the Diagnosis

The pathologist's report is crucial in oncology because it conveys the significance of a given neoplasm. The information is expressed in a kind of shorthand, condensing abundant information into a few terms. The language used must be understood by all involved and it must be simple enough to be practical for use in the clinical setting. It has been standardized so that cross-comparisons of different cancers in different persons in different geographic locations can be made.

The two major agencies involved in the standardization of the language of malignant disease are the International Union Against Cancer (UICC) and the American Joint Committee for Cancer Staging and End Results Reporting (AJCC). Not only does a common language assist the individual clinician in planning treatment and determining the patient's prognosis, but it assists oncology specialists around the world to share results of research and treatment outcomes.

Classifying the Tumor

Cancers are classified, or staged, via two main approaches: *pathological,* based on information about the tumor, and *clinical,* based upon information concerning the host. Table 11-1 compares these two systems, and Chapter 9 discusses classification in greater detail.

Pathological classification

The current and best pathological classification system is a combination of approaches: anticipated biologic behavior, histogenesis (tissue of origin), and grade.[11,12] In terms of *biologic behavior,* tumors can be divided into benign or malignant groups. A benign tumor is well circumscribed or encapsulated: microscopically, it appears orderly and is made up of cells similar to those of its parent tissue. A malignant tumor invades the organs from which it originated and eventually the surrounding tissues; it is made up of cells that vary greatly in size and shape and contain large,

TABLE 11-1 Tumor Classification Approaches: Pathological and Clinical

Approach	Describes	Based On	Performed By	When Performed	Information Provided	Useful For	Standardization
Pathological staging	Tumor	Microscopic examination of biopsy	Pathologist	Before first treatment		1. Diagnosis 2. Prognosis 3. Selection of treatment 4. Prevention of complications 5. Exchange of information 6. Research	Guidelines for reporting developed by College of American Pathologists and Joint Commission on Accreditation Health Care Organizations
a. Biologic behavior					a. Benign or malignant		
b. Histologic type					b. Cell tissue of origin		
c. Grade					c. Degree of malignancy		
d. Special studies, flow cytometry, cytogenetic, DNA probe analysis, electron microscopy, tumor markers					d. Differential diagnosis, quantification of cellular subpopulations		
e. Tumor size, margins, nodes, invasion		Microscopic examination of resected specimen		After surgical resection	e. Anatomic extent of disease		
Clinical staging a. Initial	Host	Physical exam, labs, x-rays, imaging, etc.	Clinician	a. Before first treatment	Extent of disease and organs involved	Same as for pathological staging	TNM staging system developed by International Union Against Cancer and American Joint Committee for Cancer Staging and End Results Reporting
b. Retreatment				b. After recurrence when further treatment needed			
c. Autopsy				c. At death			

hyperchromic nuclei and prominent nucleoli. Many mitotic figures are present in cancerous tissue, some of which are atypical, and lymph and blood vessels are often permeated with malignant cells.

Various suffixes are used to complete the nomenclature of tumors. The suffix *oma* implies, simply, tumor, and benign tumors are named by adding this suffix to the name of the cell type of tissue (such as fibroma or lipoma). Malignant tumors arising in epithelial tissues are known as *carcinoma. Sarcoma* refers to malignant tumors involving mesenchymal tissues. Because epithelial tissue contains three germ layers, neoplasms of the squamous epithelium are called *squamous cell carcinomas,* neoplasms of transitional epithelium are called *transitional cell carcinomas,* and those involving glandular epithelium are called *adenocarcinomas.*

Histopathologic type is a qualitative assessment whereby a neoplasm is categorized in terms of the tissue or cell type from which it has originated (e.g., lobular carcinoma, osteosarcoma, squamous cell carcinoma). Knowing the organ of origin does not provide much information, because tumors arising from different tissues in the same organ behave differently. Conversely, tumors of the same tissue from different organs behave in a similar fashion. For example, adenocarcinoma of the lung and adenocarcinoma of the rectum behave similarly, whereas adenocarcinoma of the lung and squamous cell carcinoma of the lung have different natural histories. The tissue of origin determines the behavior of a tumor, and the cell type can be relied on not to change. The general region of the tumor (e.g., lung, testicle) is primarily descriptive. A lesion with the same cell type but at a site other than the original site would indicate a *metastatic* tumor. A different cell type originating from another lesion anywhere in the body would indicate a *second primary* cancer. An important factor in cancer management is determining whether the tumor is in situ, microinvasive, or frankly invasive.

Histopathologic grade is a quantitative assessment of the extent to which the tumor resembles the tissue of origin. Grade is expressed in both numerical and descriptive terms. The language of grading refers to the appearance of the malignant cells and their degree of anaplasia or differentiation. Grading is done numerically from I to IV. Grade I indicates that the cells are so well differentiated that they closely resemble the normal parent cells. Grade IV tumor cells are so anaplastic that it is often difficult for the pathologist to determine their cell of origin. Grades II and III are intermediate designations. Grading can also be expressed by the terms "well differentiated" (Grade I), "moderately differentiated" (Grade II), poorly differentiated (Grade III), or undifferentiated (Grade IV).

Reports of the degree of cell differentiation are particularly important in deciding treatment approaches for tumors such as lymphomas. The prognostic value of grading varies with different types of tumors. For some, such as bladder cancers, the tumor grade is directly related to the ultimate prognosis of the patient, with the prognosis worsening as the cells become less differentiated. For other tumors, such as melanoma, grading has little or no prognostic value.

Sometimes the routinely assessed microscopic features of a cancer are not sufficiently conclusive for a firm diagnosis to be made. New technologies have provided the means for additional sophisticated studies to be performed on cells or tissues. For instance, electron microscopy, immunohistochemistry, in situ hybridization, and DNA probe analysis help distinguish between microscopic "look alikes." Flow cytometry permits rapid quantitative measurements of cellular characteristics.[13] Along with tumor markers and cytogenetics, all these special procedures are performed by the pathologist and may provide further information for critical diagnosis, prognosis, and treatment decisions. Before these procedures can have widespread application in clinical settings other than research institutions, however, certain problems must be solved. These include standardization and simplification of the technologies, selection of those that provide clinically meaningful information, and the conduct of large-scale clinical trials allowing multivariate statistical analysis to evaluate whether the new procedures actually improve on the present ability to diagnose and stage cancer patients.[14]

Quality assurance guidelines for information to be included in routine pathology reports for different types of primary cancers have been developed by the Cancer Committee of the College of American Pathologists (CAP) and the Joint Commission on Accreditation of Health Care Organizations (JCAH).[12]

Years of accumulated experience have shown that a tumor with a particular appearance of cells, with a certain level of differentiation, arranged in a certain way, and originating in a particular organ will behave in a predictable way. This knowledge permits the medical team to plan therapy based on collective information about what happened to numerous individuals with the same tumors in the past. For instance, a pathology report revealing a "seminoma" carcinoma of the testes means that metastasis to the nearby lymph nodes is likely. It also means that this type of tumor has a fairly good prognosis, because the primary lesion is usually resectable and lymph node metastasis is radiosensitive. High cure rates are expected, with only a 10% mortality rate. On the other hand, a report of an embryonal cell carcinoma of the testes is ominous. This type of tumor tends to metastasize early to the lung, liver, bone marrow, and brain. It is radioresistant, with a 50% mortality rate.

Clinical classification

Once the diagnosis is established, further testing is needed to assess the clinical extent of the disease. This process is called *staging*. There is no routine set of evaluations to be obtained on all patients. A knowledge of the natural history and patterns of spread of the particular neoplasm serve to focus and expedite the staging work-up. Whole-lung tomography, metastatic surveys, abdominal scans, bone marrow biopsies, or more routine procedures such as cystoscopy or chest x-ray film are meant to focus on areas of possible hidden metastasis. Staging procedures are expensive and should be ordered in a cost-effective manner.

When all the essential information is at hand, the patient's disease can be staged. This has been standardized by the TNM classification system.[15] By this system, the extent of disease is evaluated separately with respect to the primary tumor site (T), the regional lymph nodes (N), and the presence or absence of metastasis (M). The basic TNM model is expanded by using subcategories to describe how far the disease has progressed and the extent of metastasis if any. *Tis* indicates tumor in situ or tumor with all the histologic characteristics of malignancy except invasion. *T*, with the possible numbers 1, 2, 3, and 4, denotes increasing primary tumor extension. Increments of progressive lymph node involvement are indicated by N0, N1, N2, and N3. In like manner, M0, M1, M2, and M3 mean an advancing metastatic involvement and degree of organ impairment. On the basis of information about each of the TNM components, a stage designation can be assigned. Stage designations differ for each anatomic site, depending on the knowledge of spread and clinical behavior of the specific cancer. Stage designations have been developed for 40 primary tumor types. *Stage*

TABLE 11-2 Staging for Breast Cancer

PRIMARY TUMOR (T)	
TX	Primary tumor cannot be assessed
T0	No evidence of primary tumor
Tis	Carcinoma in situ: Intraductal carcinoma, lobular carcinoma in situ, or Paget's disease of the nipple with no tumor
T1	Tumor 2 cm or less in greatest dimension
T1a	0.5 cm or less in greatest dimension
T1b	More than 0.5 cm but not more than 1 cm in greatest dimension
T1c	More than 1 cm but not more than 2 cm in greatest dimension
T2	Tumor more than 2 cm but not more than 5 cm in greatest dimension
T3	Tumor more than 5 cm in greatest dimension
T4	Tumor of any size with direct extension to chest wall or skin
T4a	Extension to chest wall
T4b	Edema (including peau d'orange) or ulceration of the skin of breast or satellite skin nodules confined to same breast
T4c	Both T4a and T4b
T4d	Inflammatory carcinoma

LYMPH NODE (N)	
NX	Regional lymph nodes cannot be assessed (eg, previously removed)
N0	No regional lymph node metastasis
N1	Metastasis to movable ipsilateral axillary lymph node(s)
N2	Metastasis to ipsilateral axillary lymph node(s) fixed to one another or to other structures
N3	Metastasis to ipsilateral internal mammary lymph node(s)

PATHOLOGIC CLASSIFICATION (pN)	
pNX	Regional lymph nodes cannot be assessed (eg, previously removed, or not removed for pathologic study)
pN0	No regional lymph node metastasis
pN1	Metastasis to movable ipsilateral axillary lymph node(s)
pN1a	Only micrometastasis (none larger than 0.2 cm)
pN1b	Metastasis to lymph nodes, any larger than 0.2 cm
pN1bi	Metastasis in 1–3 lymph nodes, any more than 0.2 cm and all less than 2 cm in greatest dimension
pN1bii	Metastasis to 4 or more lymph nodes, any more than 0.2 cm and all less than 2 cm in greatest dimension
pN1biii	Extension of tumor beyond the capsule of a lymph node metastasis less than 2 cm in greatest dimension
pN1biv	Metastasis to a lymph node 2 cm or more in greatest dimension
pN2	Metastasis to ipsilateral axillary lymph nodes that are fixed to one another or to other structures
pN3	Metastasis to ipsilateral internal mammary lymph node(s)

DISTANT METASTASIS (M)	
MX	Presence of distant metastasis cannot be assessed
M0	No distant metastasis
M1	Distant metastasis (includes metastasis to ipsilateral supraclavicular lymph node(s))

STAGE GROUPING			
0	Tis	N0	M0
I	T1	N0	M0
IIA	T0	N1	M0
	T1	N1	M0
	T2	N0	M0
IIB	T2	N1	M0
	T3	N0	M0
IIIA	T0	N2	M0
	T1	N2	M0
	T2	N2	M0
	T3	N1	M0
	T3	N2	M0
IIIB	T4	Any N	M0
	Any T	N3	M0
IV	Any T	Any N	M1

Source: American Joint Committee on Staging: *Manual of Staging for Cancer* (ed. 4). Philadelphia: Lippincott, 1992. Reprinted with permission.

groupings involve combining the various classification elements of defined T, N, and M. Table 11-2 illustrates the staging of breast cancer.

Once a cancer is staged at a certain period of time, the stage of the tumor at that time is not subject to change. There are two main staging periods. The first, *pretreatment staging,* is based on tests and evidence gathered before the first treatment is begun. There are two aspects to pretreatment staging of a previously undiagnosed cancer: *clinical-diagnostic* staging, for patients who have had a biopsy but are otherwise in the preoperative phase of study, and *postsurgical resection-pathologic* staging, which includes a complete evaluation of the surgical specimen by a pathologist. Restaging, or reevaluation, may be done after a prescribed course of treatment to document remission. The second main staging period occurs if the patient has a recurrence following a disease-free interval and needs further treatment. This is termed *retreatment staging.* In addition, *autopsy staging* may occur to assess the extent of disease at death.

Previously, many other staging systems had been developed and modified, such as the Duke's classification for colorectal cancer and the Ann Arbor classification system for lymphomas. Consequently, data related to the management and prognosis of many cancers were not comparable. An attempt has been made to make the now-universally accepted TNM system consistent with several of these well-known classification systems already in use. The UICC published its pamphlet on the staging of cancer in 1987 and the fourth and latest edition of the AJCC's manual on cancer staging became available in 1992.[15,16] TNM information, data forms, and "pocket stagers" are readily available from any hospital's tumor registry. Since January 1991, TNM staging for all cancer patients is required for approval of cancer programs by the Commission on Cancer. To maintain approval status, implementation of this universal staging system for all tumor sites must be completed within two years. Future plans of the AJCC include improving uniformity in staging, expansion of the TNM system to include new prognostic markers (development of a prognostic index), the testing of prognostic indices using national and regional tumor registries, and development of staging systems for anatomic sites of types of cancer not yet classified by TNM (mesothelioma, carcinoid tumors). The goal of the AJCC is that all patients with cancer should be staged (universal staging).[17]

During the time of staging, additional factors that might influence the treatment plan must be considered. It is important to assess the patient's general clinical condition in terms of age, general debility, previous treatment for the same or other cancers, the presence of other major illness. Table 11-3 lists the many factors to evaluate and consider in the cancer treatment process.[18] Psychosocial status and family support can be evaluated in terms of discharge planning and home care needs during the course of treatment. The patient's educational background and medical sophistication have implications for the level and extent of patient education that will be needed.

TABLE 11-3 Factors Influencing Cancer Treatment Choices

Tumor Factors
Size
Anatomic location
Histology/aggressiveness
Sensitivity to chemotherapy or radiation
Natural history
Survival statistics
Treatment Factors
Availability of treatment modalities
Availability of research protocols/clinical trials
Experience of the treatment team
Potential morbidity/mortality
Prior cancer treatment
Patient Factors
Age
Sex
General health
Patient/family values and preferences
Physical performance status
Quality of life
Cardiac, renal, liver, bone marrow, and respiratory status
Immune system function
Psychological status
Life expectancy
Treatment Goals
Cure
Control
Palliation
Environmental Factors
Geographic distance from treatment center
Financial
Social network
Ethical Factors
Patient autonomy in decision making
Informed consent
Justice: individual rights to scarce and expensive resources vs. the public good

DETERMINING THE TREATMENT PLAN

A series of crucial decisions concerning management are now ready to be made. Careful integration of the extent of disease and the individual's condition with an extensive body of knowledge relating to treatment, anticipated complication rates, survival statistics, and other relevant clinical considerations will determine whether and when surgery, chemotherapy, radiation, chemotherapy, biotherapy, hormone therapy, bone marrow transplant, or "watch and wait" will be offered to the patient. The most effective, most definitive treatment aimed at cure for a given cancer is called *primary therapy.*

Should Treatment Be Aimed at Cure?

This is the vital question. In general, the oncologist tends to think of tumors with 5-year survival probabilities in the range of 1%–5% as having no or only minimal chance for cure. The oncologist will therefore ask whether any method can offer the person even such a small chance for cure. The risks involved must then be related to the person's age and condition. An intensive treatment program that offers a small chance for permanent cure may be justified for a young, vigorous adult but inappropriate for a frail, elderly person, even though their cancers may be of the same type and extent. A correct decision on whether to treat for cure is one of the most important decisions that the oncologist must make. Overly aggressive attempts can expose individuals who are incurable to needless morbidity, prolonged and expensive treatment, and distressing complications. On the other hand, therapeutic decisions that are too pessimistic may deprive the person who has a small but significant opportunity for cure of the chance to live out the rest of life. The patient's feelings and values are crucial to the decision. Some people, even knowing they have only a small chance for cure, will prefer an aggressive plan of action. Others will make it clear that they prefer to maximize quality of life.

Which Modality Should Be Used?

After it has been decided that treatment will be for cure, the next decision involves choosing the optimal modality or combination thereof. In the past, cancer was treated only by surgery *or* radiation *or* chemotherapy, depending on the stage of the disease. Two or three therapies may have been used, but they would have been used only one at a time in the above order. First, surgery if the tumor was localized, then radiation if there was actual or potential recurrence, and last, chemotherapy if the cancer involved vital organs or had spread to such an extent that more surgery and radiation were impossible. Today, this treatment strategy has been replaced by multimodality therapy. There is not universal agreement yet on what the optimal combination or best sequence of therapies is for many malignancies, but the following broad principles have evolved.

1. When tumors are large, locally aggressive, and contiguous to adjacent structures (e.g., head and neck tumors), radiotherapy might be given prior to surgery. This would cause tumor shrinkage and thus make the surgical resection easier. Intraoperative radiation also may be given during a surgical procedure,[19] such as in surgery for cancer of the pancreas.
2. Both radiation and chemotherapy may be given after surgery.
   - **a.** Radiation will usually be indicated if the tumor is found to be invading nearby tissues that cannot be surgically resected. Chemotherapy would be used to eliminate micrometastasis.
   - **b.** Radiation and chemotherapy have been combined in an attempt to produce a more powerful antitumor effect than either treatment can produce alone. Chemotherapy is sometimes used prior to radiotherapy to shrink a lesion, since radiation has a more effective tumoricidal action against smaller lesions.
3. The new biological therapies are being blended with standard radiotherapy and chemotherapy, but research on these combinations is still in the early stages. It is too early to know whether the addition of biologicals will be more effective than the standard treatment modalities.

A broad body of knowledge about all aspects of clinical oncology must be used by those planning cancer treatment, including an understanding of tumor growth and cell kinetics[20] as well as the anticipated results of surgery, chemotherapy, and radiotherapy, either alone or in combination with other procedures. Since cancer therapy is always evolving, cancer specialists must keep abreast of the most recent literature and attend professional meetings where research findings and other cancer information are presented. Each major modality has its advantages and its disadvantages, as illustrated in Table 11-4. Current treatment programs are designed to enable the greatest curative potential of each modality by using each to exploit the different biologic characteristics of a variety of cancers.

The best approach for treatment planning and evaluation is for an interdisciplinary group to share in the decision-making process. The surgeon specifies the therapeutic potential and resectability of the person's tumor. The radiation oncologist shares the expectation of curability by primary radiotherapy or the augmentation effect that radiotherapy might have prior to or following surgery and/or chemotherapy. The medical oncologist specifies the contribution that chemotherapy could make to cure the tumor and the potential for chemotherapeutic or hormonal palliation if surgical or radiotherapeutic cure are impossible. The pathologist explains the details of the biopsy and microscopic appearance of the tumor. The radiologist reviews the various radiographs and scans. Nurses may be involved in any number of ways: as enterostomal therapists, nurse practitioners providing case management, clinical trial coordinators, or discharge planners, to name a few. The nurse can participate in cancer treatment planning by providing a broad perspective on how a proposed treatment program will impact on the particular patient and family.

Because the basic principle of cancer therapy is to cure the person with the least functional and structural impairment, the interdisciplinary planning team considers how aggressive and radical a treatment should be based on the following factors: the aggressiveness

TABLE 11-4 Advantages and Disadvantages of Treatment Modalities

Treatment Modality	Advantages	Disadvantages
Surgery	• No biological resistance by tumors • No carcinogenic effects • May cure localized cancers • Gives the most accurate estimate of extent of disease and definition of histologic features of tumor	• No specificity for malignant tissues • Acute threat to life, possible morbidity • May result in deformity or loss of function • If cancer is disseminated, cannot cure: local/regional treatment only • May leave behind viable malignant cells
Radiation	• May be curative if disease is localized • Deliver large tumoricidal dose to a specific area • Minimal residual deformity or loss of function* • Palliative	• May develop side effects over a period of time • May leave behind viable malignant cells • Time-consuming • Has carcinogenic effect • If cancer is disseminated cannot cure: local/regional only • Some tumors not radiosensitive
Chemotherapy	• Systemic • Specificity for rapidly dividing (cancer) cells • Can cure some disseminated cancers • Potential for eliminating micrometastasis • Minimal residual deformity or loss of function • Potential to cure hematologic malignancies	• Biological resistance by tumor often develops • Affects rapidly dividing normal cells resulting in side effects over a period of time • Has carcinogenic effect • Less effective with large, bulky tumors • Some tumors not chemosensitive
Biologicals	• Not cytotoxic • Enhance immune system function	• Still primarily experimental • Often major side effects

*Exception: pediatrics, gonadal exposure

of the cancer, the predictability of spread, the morbidity and mortality that can be expected from the treatment, the cure rate, and the patient's desires. These are hard decisions, and the choice is often relative. What percentage of survival is acceptable for a debilitating surgical, radiotherapeutic, or chemotherapeutic maneuver? Is the tendency to be more radical justified as the chance for cure diminishes? Will a more conservative approach only lead to recurrence? The final decision must ultimately be personal judgment based on clinical experience and the experiences of others published in the literature. It is clearly in the patient's best interest to have the highly individualized prescription afforded by a multidisciplinary approach. The therapeutic aggressiveness of one member of the team is often tempered by the more conservative therapeutic bend of a colleague, and each member present brings a fresh approach. Although, in the majority of instances, the indications for one discipline or the other are clear-cut and noncompetitive, the decisions made by an interdisciplinary team are not easy. The construction of an overall treatment plan for the patient should provide for both immediate management and anticipated future developments.

The Benefit of Clinical Trials

Oncology clinicians, realizing the limitations of their own experience and of haphazard observations in general, turn for guidance to organized clinical trials. At present and for the future, these constitute the only sure foundation for therapeutic progress. Clinical trials involve objectivity, rigor, and the use of empirical data in a systematic manner. A randomized clinical trial can be defined as a carefully and ethically designed experiment that aims to answer a specifically framed question, such as determining which intervention is superior among alternatives. The study design is prospective in nature so the entire study group can be followed over time for the outcomes of interest. An absolute necessity is a valid protocol that covers all foreseeable eventualities and ambiguities. Clinical trials for chemotherapy drug testing proceed through several phases that are described in Chapter 14. The publication of the results of clinical trials allows clinicians around the world to evaluate outcomes and build on treatment successes. Replication of the experiments at other institutions ensures that treatment outcomes are not serendipitous.

Incidental advantages of clinical trials include the

freedom from having to make individual choices of treatment for each patient, and that the actual conduct of the trial can provide opportunities for a valuable exchange of ideas among the physicians involved. Clinical trials are not perfect. No trial can determine absolutely the best treatment for an individual. Also, it is hard to control the confounding variables that are possible with a human subject. Any type of therapy or combination thereof can be made the objective of a clinical trial. Most clinical trials are planned and organized under the auspices of a federally funded cooperative study group such as the Southwest Oncology Group (SWOG) or the Gynecology Oncology Group (GOG). Such cooperative groups achieve the goal of obtaining adequate numbers of study patients so that meaningful answers can be derived to improve therapeutic regimens for specific categories of malignant disease.

Selecting a Treatment Plan

Although in many instances the therapeutic decision is straightforward and clearly follows an established treatment pattern, there are often a variety of approaches that might be used. The optimal treatment plan from the physician's point of view would have the patient entered into an existing clinical trial (see Table 11-5). However, this is not always possible, for a number of reasons. The facility where treatment is to occur may not participate in a cooperative study group. There may not be a protocol available that fits the patient's stage of disease. If a protocol exists, the patient might be ineligible. The patient may refuse to be in a study for one reason or another.

An alternate approach is to use a conventional treatment program. Conventional or standard regimens are those that have been studied extensively, used for a long time, and widely accepted for common cancers. For instance, the MOPP regimen (nitrogen mustard, oncovin, procarbazine, prednisone) is a standard treatment choice for stage III or IV Hodgkin's disease, while CMF chemotherapy (cyclophosphamide, methotrexate, 5-fluorouracil) is a commonly used treatment for breast cancer. Conventional treatment programs involve drugs that are commercially available; clinical trials usually test recently developed investigational drugs that are available only to patients entered into a study. These newest drugs may provide a breakthrough not available with the older drugs, another reason why a clinical trial could offer the patient an advantage. On the other hand, the newest drugs may be less effective than those "tried and true."

If a patient is not eligible for a clinical trial and there is no conventional treatment program suitable for the case, the physician usually tries to find a study in the literature that documents a successful treatment program for the situation. Publications in journals usually involve larger numbers of patients and a longer post-treatment period for evaluating the effectiveness of the therapy. More details are provided in a journal article about side effects and dose modification than are provided in an abstract. If a journal article is unavailable, an abstracts publication could be used. Abstracts, that is, published synopses of oral presentations at professional meetings, offer few protocol details but often provide information about the latest drug combinations and doses being tried.

Finally, if no existing treatment programs are available, the physician puts together a protocol specific to the situation. Agents that are active against the tumor are specified for a regimen unique to that patient, the disease state, and the coexisting medical problems.

TABLE 11-5 Types of Treatment Plans (in order of preference by physician)

1. Clinical trial
2. Conventional treatment plan
3. Protocol published as journal article
4. Published abstract
5. Individualized treatment plan

ASSESSING RESPONSE TO TREATMENT

Responses to treatment may be classified as *objective* or *subjective* (Table 11-6). Objective parameters of the disease are measured before initiating therapy to give a baseline for evaluating treatment success or failure. Types of objective response parameters are listed in Table 11-7.[8] When the treatment course is completed, these indicators of response are measured again. This reevaluation, often called *restaging*, focuses particular attention on the disease parameters that were positive at diagnosis to signal a search for any remaining evidence that treatment should continue. Restaging does not imply that if a remission is obtained the patient reverts to a lesser disease stage. The stage ascribed at the time of diagnosis is the one that characterizes the illness throughout.

Survival Statistics

In oncology, it is difficult to evaluate the comparative efficacy of therapeutic interventions. If a person succumbs after being treated, therapy has clearly failed. On the other hand, normal recovery—with the return to health, weight gain, and the resumption of normal activity—is not conclusive evidence that a cure has been achieved. The nature of cancer is such that after a long time interval of apparent perfect health, the disease may reappear and the person die.

TABLE 11-6 Response Criteria for Assessing Treatment Outcomes

OBJECTIVE RESPONSE	
Complete response (CR)	Complete disappearance of signs and symptoms (for at least 1 month)
Partial response (PR)	50% or more reduction in sum of products of greater and lesser diameters of all measured lesions (for at least 1 month), with no new lesions appearing
Minimal response (MR)	Same as for PR but less than 50% reduction
Progression	25% or more increase in sum of products of greater and lesser diameters of all measured lesions, or appearance of new lesions
Stable disease	Measurable tumor does not meet criteria for CR, PR, MR, or progression
SUBJECTIVE REPSONSE	
• Patient feels better	
• Increased strength, decreased fatigue	
• Appetite improved, gains weight	
• Decrease in pain	

TABLE 11-7 Common Parameters for Assessing Objective Response to Treatment

Tumor size	Measured by palpation, x-ray films, radioisotope scans
Serum and urinary paraproteins, carcinoembryonic antigen	Decrease or increase
Peripheral white blood count	Decrease, increase, or blasts
Bone marrow biopsy	Types and condition of precursor cells
Gonadotropin titer	Decrease or increase
Pleural effusion status	Improves or worsens
Retroperitoneal nodes on abdominal CT scan	Larger, decreased in size,.or not enlarged
Organ function	Improved or worse

If at autopsy there is no evidence of tumor, a cancer can be said to have been cured. This is the only precise definition of "cure," but it is of little practical value. Freedom from clinical evidence of recurrent metastatic disease during the patient's lifetime is accepted by most clinicians as a reasonably reliable estimate of cure in a personal sense. In oncology, "cure" is a statistical term that applies to groups of cancer patients rather than to individuals.

The observation over time of individuals with cancer and the calculation of their probability of dying over several time periods is called *survival analysis.* A time interval is selected that must elapse without evidence of recurrence. The time at which survival can be called "cure" varies according to how soon after the primary treatment residual disease usually becomes evident. It is best understood as the time after treatment at which the annual death rate, given the age and sex of the treated person, is no longer greater than that of the normal population. Because this does not occur for 15–20 years after primary treatment in many tumors, 5-year survival rates, which have been customary to report the results of treatment, are important only in the more aggressive tumors (lung, pancreas). Since statistical cure is unlikely for the majority of cancer patients, it is apparent that despite our best treatment efforts, only palliation is usually achieved.

Patient Follow-up

Continued follow-up of patients is extremely important for the compilation of conclusive data. An integral part of a hospital's cancer program is a tumor registry or cancer data center. Information is compiled over time on each person diagnosed with cancer at that institution. These data not only aid in systematic follow-up of individuals with cancer but facilitate the hospital's evaluation of the effectiveness of different modes of therapy. Larger state, regional, and national cancer databases help in examining trends in cancer therapy and patient survival. The now widely used standardized methods of reporting the results of therapy are important to making such evaluation possible.

WHEN CURE IS NOT ACHIEVED

Should the disease recur, there may be a long period during which treatment is aimed at control. Cancer can thus be viewed as a chronic disease, similar to diabetes or heart disease, where cure is impossible and control is the objective. With some tumors, such as myeloma, cure is not yet an option, and therapy is aimed at control from the beginning. When relapse has occurred, survival can often be prolonged and improved with proper treatment.

Does the person have recurrent disease symptoms that require palliation? Radiation or even chemotherapy may be effective in relieving pain, bleeding, compression or obstruction of vital organs. A palliative surgical procedure may provide relief from a bulky tumor mass impinging on other organs. Palliative treatment should be used with discretion, based on sound clinical indications, and have a specific objective. It should minimize cost, inconvenience, discomfort, and risks, as well as be completed in the shortest possible time. Palliative measures may sometimes need to be used for people who are asymptomatic in whom the impending development of a catastrophic problem can be predicted, such as obstruction of the superior vena cava or a major bronchus, or a collapsing vertebral body. However, palliative treatment of most patients who are asymptomatic and incurable is usually deferred until the appearance of specific problems. Such persons should be followed closely to offer emotional support and for reassurance that appropriate palliative therapy will be initiated should the need arise.

FUTURE PROSPECTS

The evolution in cancer therapy over the years has been the result of technological advances and increasingly sophisticated knowledge about the structure and function of the human body and of cancer biology. As reviewed in this chapter, the current era of cancer treatment features rather crude interventions based on our best understanding of the disease: that cancer is usually systemic at presentation and that it involves a complex spectrum of host–tumor interrelations. Future efforts are being directed toward an increased understanding of these host–tumor interrelationships.[21] The rate of progress will depend on developments in molecular biology, immunology, and genetics as scientists delve deeper and deeper into the mysteries of both normal and abnormal microcellular function.

Postmodern strategies for cancer treatment may feature gene therapy, antineoplastic agents and delivery systems that exploit the difference between normal and malignant cells, the use of new and improved biologicals to prevent toxicity and extend the effectiveness of chemotherapy, and biological response modifiers to boost, direct, and restore the body's normal immune defenses.[22] As more is learned about the role of each biologic substance, more effective manipulation of the immune system will be possible. Chemoprevention, the use of agents to impede the carcinogenic process, will lower the rate of cancer incidence. Vaccines to prevent some cancers are in development. Ultimately, the only permanent solution to the cancer treatment problem is prevention.

REFERENCES

1. Gallucci BB: Selected concepts of cancer as a disease: From Greeks to 1900. *Oncol Nurs Forum* 12:67–71, 1985.
2. Fisher B: A biological perspective of breast cancer: Contributions of the national surgical adjuvant breast and bowel project clinical trials. *CA* 41:97–111, 1991.
3. Goldie JH: Scientific basis for adjuvant and primary (neoadjuvant) chemotherapy. *Semin Oncol* 14:1–7, 1987.
4. Harris DT, Mastrangelo MJ: Theory and application of early systemic therapy. *Semin Oncol* 18:493–503, 1991.
5. Scofield RP, Liebman MC, Popkin JD: Multimodality therapy. In Baird SB, McCorkle R, Grant M (eds.): *Cancer Nursing: A Comprehensive Text.* Philadelphia: Saunders, 1991, pp. 344–354.
6. Ahiya RK, Milligan AJ, Dobelbower RR: Radiation therapy in cancer management: Principles and complications. In Moossa AR, Martin C, Schimpff SC (eds.): *Comprehensive Textbook of Oncology.* Baltimore: Williams & Wilkins, 1986, pp. 257–268.
7. Kennedy BJ: Evolution of chemotherapy. *CA* 41:261–263, 1991.
8. Haskell CM: Principles of cancer chemotherapy. In Haskell CM (ed.): *Cancer Treatment* (ed. 3). Philadelphia: Saunders, 1990, pp. 21–39.
9. Krakoff IH: Cancer chemotherapy and biologic agents. *CA* 41:265–277, 1991.
10. Yarbro CH: The history of cancer nursing. In Baird SB, McCorkle R, Grant M (eds.): *Cancer Nursing: A Comprehensive Text.* Philadelphia: Saunders, 1991, pp. 10–20.
11. Pfeifer JD, Wick MR: The pathologic evaluation of neoplastic diseases. In Holleb AI, Fink DJ, Murphy GP (eds.): *Clinical Oncology.* Atlanta: American Cancer Society, 1991, pp. 7–24.
12. Hutter RV: The role of the pathologist in the management of breast cancer. *CA* 41:283–299, 1991.
13. Madeya ML, Pfab-Tokarsky JM: Flow cytometry. *Oncol Nurs Forum* 19:459–463, 1992.
14. Preisler HD, Raza A: The role of emerging technologies in the diagnosis and staging of neoplastic diseases. *Cancer* 69:1520–1526, 1992 (suppl).
15. Beahrs OH: Staging of cancer. *CA* 41:121–125, 1991.
16. American Joint Committee on Cancer: *Manual for Staging of Cancer* (ed. 4). Philadelphia: Lippincott, 1992.
17. Henson DE: Future directions for the American Joint Committee on Cancer. *Cancer* 69:1639–1644, 1992 (suppl).
18. Haskell CM: Introduction. In Haskell CM (ed.): *Cancer Treatment.* Philadelphia: Saunders, 1990, pp. 1–9.
19. Haibeck SV: Intraoperative radiation therapy. *Oncol Nurs Forum* 15:143–147, 1988.
20. Lind J: Tumor cell growth and cell kinetics. *Semin Oncol Nurs* 8:3–9, 199–217, 1992.
21. Yarbro JW: Future potential of adjuvant and neoadjuvant therapy. *Semin Oncol* 18:613–619, 1991.
22. Jenkins J: Biology of cancer: Current issues and future prospects. *Semin Oncol Nurs* 8:63–69, 1992.

Chapter 12

Surgical Therapy

Barbara Hansen Kalinowski, RN, MSN, OCN

INTRODUCTION

Greater understanding of the biology of cancer has dramatically altered the place surgery has in the treatment plan for individuals with cancer. The natural history of cancer is such that the initial treatment plan, whether single approach or multimodal therapy, is the critical opportunity to cure a person with cancer. Once disease recurs, cure is unlikely. Surgery is the treatment of choice for many tumors, but current understanding of tumor biology and advances in interdisciplinary cancer management have changed the reliance on surgery as the only form of curative therapy for cancer and has caused practitioners to reevaluate the magnitude of surgical resections. Approximately 55% of all individuals with cancer are treated with surgical intervention. Of the 40% that are treated by surgery alone, one-third are cured.[1] By using combinations of surgery, chemotherapy, radiotherapy, or biotherapy, disease-free intervals have been significantly lengthened and survival advantages have been realized.[2] Surgery can be used for prevention, diagnosis, definitive treatment, rehabilitation, or palliation.

Concepts and strategies used by oncology nurses in care settings other than the surgical arena are important to bring to the individual with cancer who is having surgery. This chapter will review the role surgery plays in the many aspects of cancer treatment. It will also highlight some areas of nursing care specific to caring for individuals with cancer who will be having surgery.

FACTORS INFLUENCING TREATMENT DECISIONS

Recent advances in tumor biology show the most promise for helping to determine the most appropriate surgical treatment for individuals with cancer.[3]

Tumor Cell Kinetics

An understanding of the biology and natural history of individual tumors is fundamental to the surgical treatment of cancer. Tumor cell characteristics such as growth rate, differentiation, metastatic potential, and metastatic pattern affect the treatment decision. It was once thought that cancer was essentially a mass of uncontrolled, rapidly proliferating cells that extended into surrounding tissues and lymph nodes and inevitably reached the circulatory system. With this in mind, surgeons felt that time was of the essence in curing cancer and that the lymph nodes had to be included in any resection because metastatic extensions would rest there. With these ideas guiding surgeons to extend the surgical margin and resect more tissue, extensive radical procedures such as hemicorporectomies and radical mastectomies were performed with better, but still disappointing, results. Such radical procedures have failed to significantly increase cure rates.[4–6]

In the past 20 years, an explosion of knowledge in the field of tumor biology has led clinicians to recognize that interdisciplinary collaboration and treatment planning are necessary to select the most effective treatment method for cancer.[3,7] Oncology practitioners must understand the potential of surgery, chemotherapy, radiation, and biotherapy to select the most effective course of therapy intelligently. The factors that affect the decision of whether an individual with cancer should be treated by surgery will be discussed in the following sections.

Growth rate

The rate of growth of a tumor is expressed in terms of volume-doubling time. The time it takes for a tumor mass to double in size depends on the cell cycle activity of proliferating cells comprising the tumor; the growth fraction, or number of cells that are proliferating in the tumor; and the rate of cell loss from the tumor. In general, tumors that are slow growing and consist of cells with prolonged cell cycles lend themselves best to surgical treatment because these types of tumors are more likely to be confined locally.[8]

Invasiveness

Any cancer cell remaining after treatment constitutes a potential risk for recurrence or metastasis if that cell is capable of proliferating. Therefore, a surgical procedure intended to be curative must involve resection of the entire tumor mass and normal tissue surrounding the tumor to ensure a margin of safety for removal of all cancer cells. Some cancers (e.g., melanomas) invade deeply into adjacent tissues, which either require extensive surgical procedures to remove the tumor mass or make surgery an impractical treatment option. Other tumors, such as basal cell carcinoma and chrondrosarcoma, are highly cohesive and are more amenable to complete surgical excision. Local, less radical procedures are performed for those particular tumors where research has demonstrated an equally effective result compared with radical surgery.[9–12]

Metastatic potential

The initial operation performed for removal of a cancer has a better chance for success than a subsequent operation performed for a recurrence; thus, knowledge of metastatic patterns of individual tumors is crucial for planning the most effective therapy.

Some tumors metastasize late or not at all, and, even if advanced, may be cured by aggressive therapy. Other tumors predictably metastasize to local or regional sites, and cure may be achieved by a procedure that involves removal of the primary tumor-bearing organ and the involved adjacent tumor sites or lymph nodes. Some tumors are known to metastasize early. In such cases surgery may not be warranted (e.g., lung cancer), or surgery may be used to remove all visible tumor in preparation for adjuvant system therapy or after a number of courses of chemotherapy to resect remaining disease (e.g., testicular cancer).[9–11]

Subclinical metastasis or occult disease is responsible for most recurrences when surgery has been the only treatment used. It is now believed that micrometastases are present in 50% of individuals by the time a tumor is large enough to be detected clinically.[13] Interdisciplinary planning and selection of the most appropriate treatment methods are important to improve survival and to lower an individual's risk of systemic metastasis.

Tumor Location

Once the location and extent of the tumor are determined through diagnostic and staging procedures, the clinician assesses the structural and functional changes that can be expected as a result of the surgical procedure. This assessment will assist the clinician and patient and family in weighing the benefits and risks involved in treatment. In some cases, the decision to treat an individual's cancer with surgery may rest solely on whether the tumor involves vital structures. Superficial and encapsulated tumors are more easily resected than those that are embedded in inaccessible or delicate tissues or those that have invaded tissues in multiple directions.

Physical Status

Careful preoperative assessment is critical for evaluating the significant factors that would potentially increase the risk of surgical morbidity and mortality. In-depth evaluation of respiratory, cardiovascular, nutritional, immunologic, renal, and central nervous (CNS) system status are important.[14] The severity of the underlying illness and comorbid conditions are considered in the decision regarding surgical therapy. The health care team assesses the patient's rehabilitation potential, particularly if the intended surgery will significantly alter normal physiologic function. In some cases the intended surgical procedure may produce physiologic alterations that are beyond that particular person's capabilities. The elderly often experience effects of aging that limit their dexterity and ability to manage difficult surgical deficits.[15] Since cancer incidence is much greater in elderly patients, age can be a factor to weigh in the treatment decision. In general, elderly patients have a higher surgical risk than younger patients. However, the elderly patient should also be treated as aggressively as possible but may require additional preoperative support (e.g., hyperalimentation, blood products). Elderly patients with cancer do not appear to have a higher risk or complication rate than their age-matched cohorts.[16]

Quality of Life

The goal of therapy for the person with cancer varies according to the stage of disease. Selection of the treatment approach includes consideration of the quality of the individual's life when treatment is complete. Research has shown that some radical surgical procedures are not warranted, either because they do not improve the end result or because they interfere unduly with the person's functional or psychological well-being. Multidisciplinary planning that includes the individual with cancer and significant others will facilitate the selection of a treatment plan tailored to that individual's unique needs and desires.

PREVENTING CANCER USING SURGICAL PROCEDURES

Certain conditions, diseases, and genetic or congenital traits are known to be associated with a higher risk of developing cancer. In some instances, surgical removal of nonvital benign tissue or an organ that is responsible for predisposing the individual to higher risk can lower incidence and possibly prevent occurrence of cancer. Polyposis is an excellent example of a condition that increases the individual's risk for developing colon cancer. Surgical excision of colon polyps is a relatively simple preventive procedure to reduce the person's risk for colon cancer.[17] Another, more complex situation is that of women who have a high risk for breast cancer. After careful review and thorough explanation, some women may elect to undergo prophylactic bilateral mastectomies to lower the risk of breast cancer.[18] The role of surgery in cancer prevention is somewhat limited at this time; however, future epidemiologic and etiologic findings may indicate a more extensive role for surgery.

DIAGNOSING CANCER USING SURGICAL TECHNIQUES

Each type of cancer responds differently to therapy; therefore, a histologic diagnosis is crucial to selecting effective treatment. Surgical techniques such as endoscopy, needle aspiration, incisional biopsy, excisional biopsy, and core needle biopsy are frequently used to obtain cells or tissue specimens for histologic examination.

An adequate biopsy requires careful planning by the physician. The biopsy specimen should contain both normal cells and tumor cells for comparison; it should be intact and not crushed or contaminated; and it should be labeled and preserved properly for complete evaluation. An important principle to note in the diagnosis of cancer is that only positive biopsy findings are definitive. A negative biopsy finding can mean no cancer, but it can also mean that the biopsy specimen was not representative of the tumor. If a high index of suspicion for cancer exists, another biopsy technique may be in order.

Before selecting the most appropriate biopsy technique, the surgeon will consider the possible treatment regimens that will be used if cancer is diagnosed. Because tumor cells can contaminate the biopsy site, tracts, or new tissue planes, either the biopsy site should be located so that it will be removed at surgery or the biopsy itself should contain the tumor in toto.[15] If multiple biopsies are to be taken, instruments that may have contacted the tumor should not be used for other sites. Aesthetic results are also considered during the biopsy so that incision lines and subsequent incisions will be located in cosmetically acceptable areas or folds if possible.

Use of incisional, excisional, aspiration, or core biopsy depends on tumor size, location, and growth characteristics. Figure 12-1 illustrates these four techniques when attempting to biopsy the breast.[19] Possible complications following any biopsy are pain, bleeding, hematoma, infection, dehiscence, and tumor cell seeding. Individuals should be instructed about biopsy site care and possible complications.

Individuals should know in advance when the biopsy results will be available and how the physician will give the results (e.g., phone call, in person). The individual should be informed as to whether the result will be known immediately (frozen section result) or whether the physician prefers to wait until the permanent sections have been prepared and interpreted, usually between 2 and 5 days later.

Needle biopsy

Needle biopsies are usually performed in an outpatient or office setting, since they do not require open surgical techniques. Cooperation and skill are required of the affiliated pathology or cytology lab when doing needle biopsy procedures to allow for an accurate diagnosis to be made. Local or topical anesthesia is commonly used. Table 12-1 lists specific details of each type of needle biopsy. An unfortunate limitation of either needle aspiration or core biopsy is the possibility that the tumor will be missed; therefore only a positive finding of malignancy is diagnostically significant.[20,21] Various types of biopsy needles are used. Some have carrier needles that shield and guide the actual biopsy needle, cup, or punch used to obtain the specimen. The carrier reduces the possibility of contaminating the needle tract with tumor cells from the specimen as the needle is withdrawn.

Surgical Biopsy

Surgical biopsies are careful and delicate procedures performed to secure a piece of tumor tissue larger than that possible with a needle (Table 12-1). *Excisional biopsy* is performed on small, accessible tumors to remove the entire mass and little or no margin of surrounding normal tissue. In some cases, such as tumors of the lip, nose, ear, or breast, excisional biopsy alone will be definitive therapy. The pathologist and the surgeon will determine whether the extent of the excisional biopsy is sufficient to eliminate the possibility of residual disease or whether more extensive surgery is indicated. Figure 12-2 illustrates a technique used to prepare tissue to allow visualization of the specimen margin.[19] The

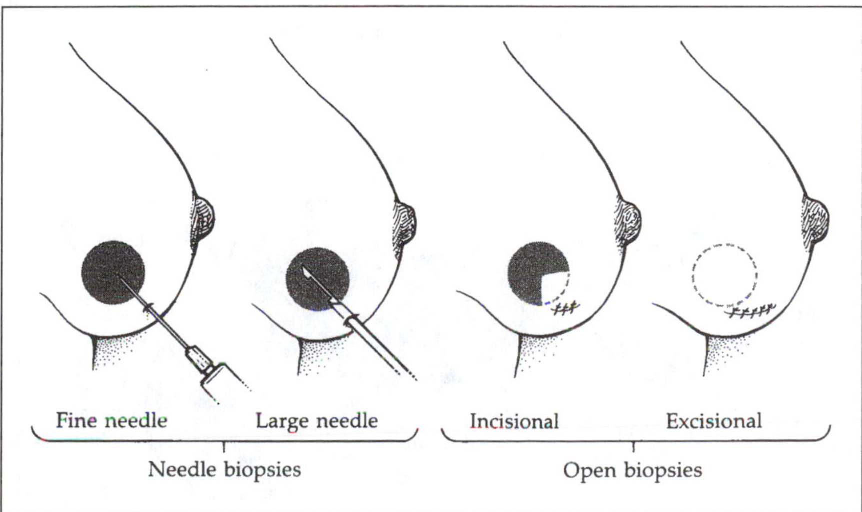

FIGURE 12-1 Possible approaches for breast biopsy. (Source: Love S: *Dr. Susan Love's Breast Book.* Reading, MA: Addison-Wesley, 1990. Reprinted with permission.)

TABLE 12-1 Approaches for Biopsy

Type	What Used For	Where Done	Rationale
Needle Biopsy			
Fine-Needle Aspiration: (21–22-g needle 5-cc syringe) local anesthesia	Solid, palpable lesion (ie, breast mass, thyroid nodule)	Outpatient setting Operating room	Involves only small amount of trauma to tissue, so if positive then surgical procedure is avoided. Used when there is a high level of suspicion of malignancy.
Steriotaxic Fine-Needle Aspiration: (21–22-g. needle, steriotaxic equipment) local anesthesia	Solid, nonpalpable lesion (ie, mammographic abnormality)	Outpatient setting Radiology center	Same as for fine-needle aspiration, but able to sample small, *nonpalpable* lesions.
Core-Needle Biopsy: (special cutting needle) local anesthesia; can use ultrasound to help guide	Solid, accessible tumor	Outpatient setting	Removes larger amount of tissue than fine-needle aspiration, may allow for more information (ie, hormone receptor tests).
Surgical Biopsy			
Excisional Biopsy: usually local anesthesia	Solid, palpable mass (ie, melanoma, breast mass)	Day surgery	Attempt is made to remove the whole mass only, without regard to clear margin. Result should be cosmetically acceptable.
Incisional Biopsy: usually local anesthesia	Solid, palpable large mass (ie, large, ulcerating or bleeding mass)	Day surgery	Biopsy is for diagnosis; mass is too large to remove without major surgery. May bleed profusely.
Endoscopy: (special endoscope) may use sedation	Solid mass in an accessible lumen (ie, colon, esophagus)	Outpatient setting Day surgery	May be for diagnosis or treatment. Avoids surgical trauma.

tissue is covered with ink, sliced, and then put on the slide for microscopic evaluation. *Incisional biopsies* are generally selected to diagnose large tumors that will require major surgery for complete removal. *Endoscopy* is a surgical technique used for diagnosis of tumors in accessible lumen.[22] Tumors of the gastrointestinal, genitourinary, or pulmonary system, and more recently the ductal system of the breast, can be diagnosed by inserting an optical instrument into the lumen to examine the area and secure a biopsy or secretions. Flexible instruments have made endoscopy more tolerable for the patient and more functional for the clinician.

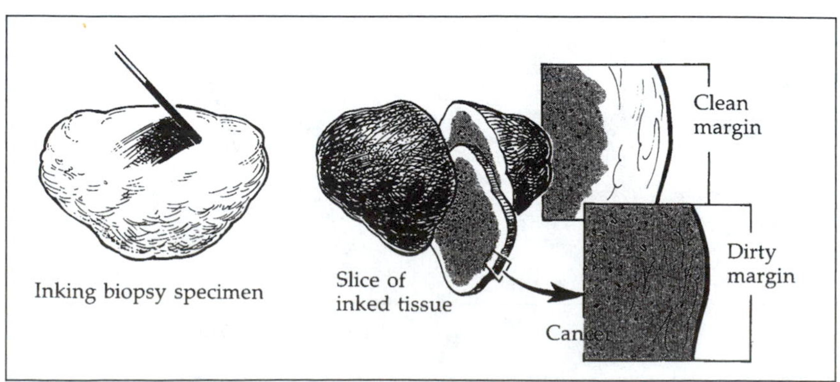

FIGURE 12-2 Technique for obtaining inked surgical margins. (Source: Love S: *Dr. Susan Love's Breast Book.* Reading, MA: Addison-Wesley, 1990. Reprinted with permission.)

STAGING CANCER USING SURGICAL PROCEDURES

Surgical procedures play a significant role in the diagnosis of cancer and in defining the extent of tumor involvement. For example, staging laparotomy is an important diagnostic measure for the pathologic staging of lymphomas. Exploratory surgical procedures can be done to diagnose most intracavitary tumors or to define the extent of tumor growth, size, nodal involvement, implants, or multiorgan involvement.

The American Joint Committee for Cancer Staging and End Results Reporting has developed a system for staging many cancers by site. The TNM classification defines the extent of solid tumors based on size and local extension (T), the presence or absence of nodal involvement (N), and the presence or absence of distant metastasis (M) and degree of organ dysfunction. (See Chapters 9 and 11 for more details on the TNM system.) Descriptions of staging and classification of each tumor are included throughout this text. Before recommending a surgical resection of the tumor for cure, the physician will undertake a search for evidence of distant metastasis. This metastatic work-up is important for accurate staging of disease. If distant metastases are present, radical or body-altering surgery is usually not indicated and the focus of treatment quickly shifts from local control to systemic treatment. Such a time can be difficult for the patient because the chance for cure is debated during this time.

During the diagnostic phase, including the biopsy and staging tests, the person with cancer will probably experience profound anxiety, which can be alleviated or reduced to some extent by astute nursing care. It is important to assess the factors that could possibly contribute to anxiety, such as previous hospitalizations, experience with other persons with cancer, influence of the mass media, formal and informal sources of information, and the person's developmental stage. The nurse should consider the person's understanding of the diagnostic procedures and the significance of the findings. Does the person generally understand the procedures, what to expect, and how he or she will feel afterward?[15]

Although seeking information is considered a healthy coping mechanism, only the patient can cue the nurse on how much information is adequate. Assessing the individual's learning needs will allow the nurse to teach the patient what he or she should know about the diagnostic procedures. Visual aids, pamphlets, slide tapes, and group sessions are all supplementary teaching techniques that have met with good results.

SURGERY FOR TREATMENT OF CANCER

After diagnosis, staging, and classification of the tumor, the interdisciplinary oncology team will propose the most appropriate plan and sequence of therapy. The goal of therapy is based on a collation of the patient's desires, general condition, and tumor stage and classification. The sequence and methods used will be guided by the most effective treatment protocols available for that particular tumor type. Surgical intervention may be the definitive treatment or may be part of a sequence of multimodal therapy. Preoperative chemotherapy or radiotherapy are used for some tumors, such as head and neck cancers.

Preoperative considerations include a thorough patient and family history and physical examination. Assessments are made of lifestyle habits, concomitant disease, general physical condition, nutritional status, hematologic status, and pulmonary status. Measures to improve the patient's overall status are initiated before surgery whenever possible.[14] In addition, an assessment of the patient's understanding of the surgery and rehabilitation should be completed. Involving the individual's significant others in preoperative teaching can often facilitate understanding and reduce anxiety (Table 12-2).

Surgery Aimed at Cure

Advances in our understanding of cancer biology have changed the surgical approach for cure from the "more is better" philosophy to an approach that considers tissue and functional preservation and relies more on effective use of radiotherapy, chemotherapy, or biotherapy. Tumors that are solid and accessible and have relatively well-defined margins can generally be surgically excised.

Excision of primary tumors

The type of surgical procedure selected for curative treatment of primary tumors depends on the specific tumor cell characteristics and site of involvement. In the preoperative period, the surgeon is challenged to identify those patients who will be treated best by limited or extensive surgery and to select the surgery and adjuvant therapies that will control local and distant disease.[15]

Local excision is used to resect small lesions when the entire tumor and a margin of safety can be encompassed. Tumors of the ear, skin, or lip are typical lesions where local excision can provide definitive therapy. Hemostasis and infection are the major postoperative concerns. Aseptic measures and prophylactic antibiotics provide control.

The magnitude of the surgical approach for many tumors has been greatly modified in recent years. A better understanding of the biology and natural history of specific cancers, combined with advances in adjuvant treatment modalities, has led to less radical surgery for some cancers. Breast cancer is probably the best example of a tumor that is approached much differently now because of our understanding of tumor biology.[6,23]

Major surgical resections are performed when the

TABLE 12-2 Preoperative Assessment/Teaching Guide

What to Assess	Teaching Strategies
Understanding of procedure	*Visual:* books, diagrams, models of equipment *Verbal:* Q & A session with patient and significant other, in person or on telephone; arrange network with patient who has had similar procedure
Understanding of process	Facility tour to include room and waiting area, explanation of expected sequence of events and the individual's anticipated participation
Preoperative physical condition • history and physical • special tests • hospital-specific requirements • previous therapy—especially chemotherapy or radiation • venous access devices	Discuss donating autologous blood Routine preoperative teaching (respiratory and circulatory exercises, wound care, catheter care, IVs, intensive care stay, etc)
Anxiety about procedure	Teach relaxation exercises Encourage use of techniques already helpful to patient (music, meditation) Discuss expectations of pain management Offer and discuss patient-controlled analgesia if available

tumor is surgically accessible, and there is hope that the tumor can be resected *en bloc* along with the necessary local or regional tissues and lymphatics. Surgical resections can greatly alter the person's body image as well as the structure and function of the person's body. Extensive surgery may be needed if the disease is to be eradicated and the person is to be given the chance to live a normal life span. There are obvious tradeoffs and concessions that the person with cancer must acknowledge. Striking a balance between length of life and quality of life is a major challenge in surgical oncology.

During the preoperative period, the nurse instructs the individual on what to expect in the postoperative period so that the person is aware of and can contribute to expected outcomes. It is important that the individual completely understand the outcomes of surgical therapy, as well as how surgery fits in the overall plan of therapy. Very often, the person and significant others have many questions and need information repeated and validated. Encouraging dialogue and allowing adequate time for instruction and verbalization of feelings and fears during the preoperative time period will enhance adjustment and acceptance of the surgical procedure during the postoperative period.

Discussion of nursing management and rehabilitation of the person following various surgical procedures is included in Part VI on the management of specific malignancies.

Surgery and adjuvant therapies

Surgery is a local therapy and thus is limited in what it can accomplish. Surgery was once the sole therapy for many solid tumors, such as carcinoma of the breast, colon, and head and neck. Survival rates for these cancers and others have not been satisfactory with surgery alone.[2] For this reason, combination or adjuvant therapies are being used to improve the rates of cure and disease-free survival. Adjuvant therapy can be given preoperatively, intraoperatively, or postoperatively. Surgery may be combined with radiotherapy for local tumor control. Chemotherapy is given to provide systemic control of micrometastases and distant metastases. In some situations, surgery is used to debulk or reduce the tumor mass to a size where radiation or chemotherapy can be most effective.[24] Ovarian cancer is often approached in this manner, since it is usually spread throughout the peritoneum by the time of diagnosis, and since debulking procedures improve therapeutic results. The individual may undergo definitive therapy for months or even years. This adjuvant approach to the treatment of the person with cancer requires a multidisciplinary team effort.

Excision of metastatic lesions

Surgery also may be done to resect a metastatic lesion if the primary tumor is believed to be eradicated, if the metastatic site is solitary, and if the patient can undergo surgery without major morbidity. Resection of the metastatic lesion is not indicated if there is evidence of additional metastatic disease or if the metastatic lesion is particularly aggressive or inaccessible. A solitary pulmonary lesion, a liver lesion, and a cerebral mass are examples of metastatic sites that may be amenable to resection with a curative intent.[15,25]

Surgery Aimed at Palliation

Many surgical procedures are performed for the palliation of the debilitating manifestations of cancer. These procedures are aimed at controlling the cancer and improving the quality of life for the person with cancer, even when all the cancer cannot be removed. If the quality of the person's life cannot be improved as a result of the surgery, then the surgery is not warranted. If the surgery carries an unnecessary risk of morbidity or mortality, it is also not indicated. Issues such as biologic pace of the disease, the person's life expectancy, and expected outcome of the palliative procedure all require careful consideration if the person is to benefit from the procedure. Open communication among the patient, the family, and the physician is of paramount importance. The patient must know the goals of the procedure and realistically understand the expected outcome. If the person's hope is unrealistic, the potential disappointment experienced postoperatively can be devastating. For instance, consider the person experiencing chronic pain who is offered a surgical procedure that can possibly alleviate suffering. It is more compassionate to ensure that the person understands and accepts that the pain may be relieved only temporarily rather than indefinitely. The person who lives with cancer knows well the meaning of palliation. Clinicians should always respect the courage and will of the individual with uncontrolled cancer and promote his or her active participation in the plan of care.

The goal of palliative surgery is to relieve suffering and minimize the symptoms of the disease. For example, palliative surgery may involve removal of a tumor that has become ulcerative and a likely source of infection or may involve the amputation of a nonfunctioning, painful limb with sarcoma. Some tumors are slow growing, and although metastatic sites are evident and the person is technically incurable, resection of the primary tumor is warranted to prevent future complications such as bleeding or obstruction. Several surgical techniques are used for palliation of cancer: fulgeration, electrocoagulation, lasers, photodynamic therapy, shunts, and bone stabilization procedures.[16,26,27]

Palliative procedures are not undertaken unless the clinician is reasonably confident that the wound will heal. For example, surgery is contraindicated for the person who has a local recurrence and lung metastasis following radiotherapy to an oropharyngeal lesion. In this case a surgical wound would probably not heal without extensive skin flap reconstruction, which would not be warranted in view of the distant metastasis.

Palliative surgery is particularly useful in relieving suffering caused by an obstructive process. Obstruction occurs in the respiratory, gastrointestinal, or urinary system. Surgical intervention such as a tracheostomy will restore airway patency, and a gastrostomy tube will facilitate adequate nutrition. Through palliative procedures, the individual can be supported while therapy is initiated to control the primary disease. Surgery may also be used to decompress vital structures (i.e., laminectomy) or to help in the control of pain (see Chapter 23).

Surgery for Rehabilitation

Although surgical procedures have long been used to treat cancer, their use in rehabilitation of individuals with cancer is fairly recent. Today, great emphasis is being placed on the quality of life for the person with cancer. With this emphasis has come an effort to develop techniques to restore an individual to as near a normal life as possible following surgery for cancer. Cosmetic or functional success has been achieved through breast reconstruction following mastectomy, facial reconstruction after head and neck surgery, and skin grafting following major resections for melanoma, to name a few.

Rehabilitation potential is considered before initiation of primary therapy. Careful interdisciplinary planning will assist the clinician to prepare the person emotionally and physically for both the primary treatment and subsequent rehabilitation. In preparing an individual for rehabilitation, the clinician strikes a fine balance between optimism and realism. Rehabilitative teaching and counseling generally are begun before primary surgical therapy is initiated. Some people fear that their desire for rehabilitative surgical procedures will be interpreted as valuing their physical appearance or function as more important than the length of their life. Nurses can assist the patient to see that rehabilitation is desirable and sometimes necessary for achieving the highest possible level of functioning.[28]

Rehabilitative success is measured not only by cosmetic improvement but also by improvements in function and self-esteem. As rehabilitative techniques improve, more people with cancer will select and enjoy the benefits of surgical rehabilitation.

CARING FOR THE INDIVIDUAL WITH CANCER WHO IS UNDERGOING SURGERY: SPECIAL CONSIDERATIONS FOR NURSING CARE

Nursing care of the person with cancer who is undergoing surgery follows many of the same principles as that for an individual undergoing noncancer-related major surgery, as well as concepts relative to caring for oncology patients in nonsurgical settings. Advances have been made in many areas of oncology care that can directly benefit the person with cancer who is having surgery. The nurse's role in coordination of care, education, and communication among the health care team is of utmost importance as surgical procedures become more complex, surgical stays become shorter, and patients undergo several forms of therapy in a short amount of time.

Surgical Setting

Traditionally, surgical procedures have been performed in a hospital setting, with preoperative testing done the night before surgery, preanesthetic agents routinely given, and a generous amount of time allowed for recuperation in the hospital before discharging a patient. In recent years, the health care delivery system has changed to accommodate many advances in surgical and anesthetic technique, as well as to respond to agencies urging cost-containment maneuvers.[29] In 1983, 20% of surgery was done on an ambulatory (same-day) basis. The American Hospital Association predicts that by 1995 about 60% of all hospital-based surgeries will be on an ambulatory basis.[30] This change in the method of delivery of care presents new challenges for nurses who are striving to interact fully with patients in various stages of crisis and aiming to ensure that adequate information is given, surgical procedures performed safely, and postoperative complications minimized.

Because of the change in length of stay, nurses must now rely more on communication via telephone and in writing rather than on face-to-face visits. Support systems must be identified well before the surgical procedure takes place. It is important to reinforce the importance of communication with health care professionals about any aspect of the surgical procedure.

Preoperative concerns/preventive strategies

Autologous blood donation

Depending on the type and length of the surgical procedure, the surgeon may suggest or patients may request donating one or more units of their own blood to bank prior to surgery. Some hospitals have their own autologous donation programs; others use the services of the American Red Cross Autologous Donor Program. It is important to schedule this donation well in advance of surgery. Blood can usually be donated from 42 days to 72 hours prior to surgery. Because of the small, but real, risk from homologous blood transfusions, most individuals are eager to donate their own blood.[31,32]

Anxiety/pain control

The issues of anxiety and pain as a result of surgical procedures should be addressed prior to the actual operation to allow patients to verbalize fears, to discuss previous experiences, and to be made aware of advances in pharmacologic methods of pain relief as well as to take advantage of behavioral methods of pain control and relaxation techniques. Carr et al.[33] recommend discussions in the preoperative period of expectations of pain and its relief to include dosing of analgesic medicine, availability of patient-controlled analgesia (PCA), units, use of rating scales to measure pain, and nonpharmacologic maneuvers to decrease pain and anxiety (Table 12-3). This level of awareness of concern about pain, more commonly found among clinicians who deal with chronic cancer pain, is now being welcomed in the acute care setting.[34] Relaxation and hypnosis have been used in the pediatric setting to help decrease the trauma of painful procedures.[35] These same techniques can be applied to the adult surgical population with effective results.[36,37] Relaxation, deep breathing, visualization, guided imagery, and self-hypnosis are all techniques available to help patients decrease anxiety and pain during painful procedures (i.e., bone marrow biopsy, needle localization, breast biopsy) as well as during the postoperative period. It is appropriate to bring these techniques into the surgical setting and to offer them to patients before painful procedures begin. Specially trained nurses may be available in the health care setting to provide training for hypnosis, meditation, or relaxation, but may also be able to coordinate referrals to other specialists in the institution or in the community for assistance in learning these techniques. As more individuals are incorporating these behavioral methods into their normal daily routine, it may be a matter of reminding patients to use skills already at their disposal (e.g., using Lamaze breathing during a painful procedure). As the patient care issue of pain control moves from a more chronic care setting to an acute care setting, nurses in positions to educate health care professionals should make it a priority to encourage and teach nonpharmacologic methods of pain relief while also reinforcing appropriate pharmacologic management. As with most aspects of caring for individuals with cancer, a team approach focused on communication is of the utmost importance and will benefit the person greatly.[37]

Nurses should be acutely aware of problems that can occur as a result of the cancer disease process itself, as well as possible postoperative complications. The person with cancer is cared for with a keen eye to complications in the following areas, which are common with this disease.

Nutrition

The nutritionally debilitated person with cancer is a poor surgical risk and often cannot undergo major surgery without preoperative correction of the underlying nutritional deficit. Because of the nutritional deficit, the individual might not be a candidate for adjuvant therapy either. When subjected to a major stress, such as surgical trauma or infection, the undernourished person is often unable to adapt with preservation of lean body mass, and will develop a negative nitrogen balance. As a result, the individual is at risk for poor wound healing, infection, pneumonia, and increased morbidity.[39,40]

An important first step in the management of the malnourished surgical cancer patient is to reverse protein calorie malnutrition and prevent weight loss. Once this is accomplished, the nutrition plan should be as aggressive as the anticancer plan. It is generally agreed that people who are nutritionally compromised should

TABLE 12-3 Nonpharmacologic Interventions for Pain Control[34]

Intervention*		Type of Evidence†	Comments
Simple relaxation (begin preoperatively)	• Jaw relaxation • Progressive muscle relaxation • Simple imagery	Ia, IIa, IIb, IV	Effective in reducing mild to moderate pain and as an adjunct to analgesic drugs for severe pain. Use when patients express an interest in relaxation. Requires 3–5 min of staff time for instructions.
	Music	Ib, IIa, IV	Both patient-preferred and "easy listening" music are effective in reducing mild to moderate pain.
Complex relaxation (begin preoperatively)	Biofeedback	Ib, IIa, IIb, IV	Effective in reducing mild to moderate pain and operative site muscle tension. Requires skilled personnel and special equipment.
	Imagery	Ib, IIa, IV	Effective for reduction of mild to moderate pain. Requires skilled personnel.
Education/instruction (begin preoperatively)		Ia, IIa, IIb, IV	Effective for reduction of pain. Should include sensory and procedural information and instruction aimed at reducing activity related pain. Requires 5–15 minutes of staff time.
TENS		Ia, IIa, III, IV	Effective in reducing pain and improving physical function. Requires skilled personnel and special equipment. May be useful as an adjunct to drug therapy.

*Selected references are included in this Clinical Practice Guideline. For more complete references, see: Acute Pain Management Guideline Panel: *Acute Pain Management: Operative or Medical Procedures and Trauma. Guideline Report.* AHCPR Pub. No. 92-0022. Rockville, MD: Agency for Health Care Policy and Research, Public Health Service, U.S. Department of Health and Human Services. In press.

†Insufficient scientific evidence is available to provide specific recommendations regarding the use of hypnosis, acupuncture, and other physical modalities for relief of postoperative pain.

Key to Type of Evidence

Ia Evidence obtained from meta-analysis of randomized controlled trails
b Evidence obtained from at least one randomized controlled trial
IIa Evidence obtained from at least one well-designed controlled study without randomization
b Evidence obtained from at least one other type of well-designed quasi-experimental study
III Evidence obtained from well-designed nonexperimental studies, such as comparative studies, correlational studies, and case studies
IV Evidence obtained from expert committee reports or opinions and/or clinical experiences of respected authorities

receive preoperative enteral or parenteral nutritional support, since studies have shown reductions in postoperative complications and surgical mortality from appropriate preoperative nutritional support.[41] Specific nursing measures to improve the nutritional status of patients are discussed in Chapter 27.

Hemostasis

Another common manifestation of cancer that can significantly increase the risk of postoperative complications is altered hemostasis, especially hypercoagulability and thrombosis.[42] Elevated clotting factors and shortened partial thrombopolastin and prothrombin times have been noted to occur in individuals with cancer. The person with cancer therefore is highly susceptible to minor changes in the hemostatic process. A person with cancer is more likely to develop postoperative thrombophlebitis than is a person without cancer.

The nursing management of the individual with cancer undergoing surgery is based on accurate assessment of hemodynamic parameters and an understanding of the implications of abnormalities in clotting factors that can result in bleeding tendencies and hemorrhage. The importance of early postoperative ambulation cannot be overemphasized. Because these individuals are at high risk for deep-vein thrombosis, the nurse observes the patient for signs and symptoms of this disorder. Bleeding abnormalities in individuals with cancer are discussed in more detail in Chapter 25.

Complications of Multimodal Therapy

The multimodal treatment of cancer has introduced a new set of challenges for health care providers in surgical oncology. Chemotherapy, radiation therapy, and biotherapy are now being given for certain tumors in various sequences: preoperative, intraoperative, and postoperative. The synergistic and augmented effect of these therapies can produce postoperative reactions and complications that may be difficult to manage.

Preoperative chemotherapy or radiotherapy, alone or in combination, is being used more frequently with particular tumors that have better response rates when multimodal therapy is sequenced in this manner. The timing and extent of surgery may require modification following radiation or chemotherapy, depending on the individual's response to therapy and the side effects experienced. Sometimes, surgical procedures become necessary during active radiation or chemotherapy treatment cycles, such as inserting vascular access devices, relieving obstructions, and repairing perforations.

Intraoperative radiotherapy and intraoperative chemotherapy are being researched for their potential to decrease recurrence and metastases. Radiotherapy or chemotherapy given intraoperatively involves the delivery of a single, high dose directly to the surgically exposed tumor or tumor bed. Intraoperative therapy requires extensive multidisciplinary collaboration. Patient and staff safety are carefully considered.[43] Potential side effects of intraoperative therapy are not yet fully known but appear to be similar to those of traditional delivery methods. Intraoperative treatments, used predominantly in major cancer centers, are administered for locally advanced abdominal and pelvic malignancies. Gastric, pancreatic, ovarian, bladder, and colorectal are a few of the tumor types being investigated.[43,44]

A major challenge in multimodal therapy is the problem of postoperative wound healing in the person who has previously received radiation to the surgical site. Radiation may cause long-term damage to the underlying tissues, such as fibrosis and obliteration of lymphatic and vascular channels.[45] Once the integrity of the tissue is damaged by radiation, additional traumas are not tolerated well. Postoperative wound dehiscence, infection, and tissue and bone necrosis are potential complications when surgery is performed on previously irradiated tissue.

TABLE 12-4 Possible Effects of Chemotherapy on Wound Healing[40,46]

Drug	When Delivered	Effects
Bleomycin	Intraoperatively	Decrease in fascial wound-bursting strength up to 7 days postsurgery
Doxorubicin	Early postoperative period, before wound has healed	Decrease in fascial wound-bursting strength
Corticosteroids	Perioperative period	Decreased granulation tissue and epithelialization

In some cases, it becomes necessary or highly desirable to initiate chemotherapy early in the immediate postoperative period. There are questions regarding the appropriate timing and effects of specific chemotherapeutic agents on wound healing. Table 12-4 outlines some of the potential postoperative complications as a result of intraoperative or early postoperative chemotherapy.[40,46] Given the trend toward more aggressive chemotherapy and radiotherapy, wound healing may become a significant problem in the future. These concerns point to the need for further research to determine the optimal doses and timing sequence for multimodal therapy.

The nurse should be aware of the overall plan for therapy, particularly the type and extent of treatment before and during surgery. This will allow the nurse to anticipate and to take measures to minimize the predictable postoperative complications that can occur with multimodal therapy.

Certain chemotherapeutic agents are toxic to specific organ systems, resulting in long-term side effects that can increase the individual's risk of surgical complications. Table 12-5 presents some of the agents that may have an effect on surgical outcome and wound healing.[47] The nurse needs to be aware of these effects

TABLE 12-5 Effects of Chemotherapy on Specific Organs[47]

Organ	Chemotherapeutic Agent	Effects
Respiratory system	Bleomycin	May predispose patient to postoperative acute adult respiratory distress syndrome
	Methotrexate Busulfan	May produce diffuse interstitial and alveolar pneumonitis
Renal system	Cis-platinum Streptozocin Methotrexate VP-16	Can result in persistant decrease in glomerular filtration rate (GFR)
Cardiac system	Doxorubicin Daunorubicin	With culumative dose of 500 mg/m² increased risk of intraoperative and postoperative congestive heart failure and pulmonary edema

and must focus assessments and nursing care toward minimizing complications and early detection of such. As new therapies become available and are used aggressively in an attempt to eradicate malignancies, the potential exists for different and more severe complications to occur. The nurse needs to seek knowledge about new therapies and apply that to the care of the individual undergoing surgery.

CONCLUSION

Surgery for cancer is the oldest form of cancer therapy still in use; however, there have been advances and changes in the scope of and reliance on surgical therapy. Almost all individuals with cancer will have some sort of surgical procedure, though not all will have surgery as part of their treatment plan. Current understanding of cancer biology and the natural history and progression of certain tumors has caused the role of surgery to be questioned and modified in many instances. Radical surgery is still a reasonable and valid approach for several tumor types, but not for others. Breast cancer is the most profound example of a less drastic surgical approach.[6]

Adjuvant therapy can lengthen survival and disease-free intervals and improve the quality of life. The potential side effects of adjuvant multimodal therapies present new challenges to health care practitioners.

Nurses who interact with individuals with cancer who are having surgery will find many useful practices and applicable concepts from other fields. Oncology clinical nurse specialists will find much satisfaction interacting with nurses in the operating room, the recovery room, and the surgical floors to learn what patients experience, as well as help with challenging assessments and postoperative complications.

Prospective clinical research, both physiologic and psychologic, that includes active participation of surgical practitioners is sorely needed.[48–50] Effective surgical cancer therapy depends on a solid integration of the biologic and clinical sciences of cancer. In addition to important strides in the understanding of the biology of cancer, clinicians have learned a great deal about the educational, psychologic, social, and rehabilitative needs of individuals who are undergoing surgical procedures for cancer therapy.[50,51]

REFERENCES

1. Morton DL, Economou JS, Haskell CM, Parker RG: Oncology. In Swartz SI, Shires GT, Spencer FC (eds.): *Principles of Surgery* (ed. 5). New York: McGraw-Hill, 1989, pp. 355–385.
2. Henderson IC: Adjuvant systemic therapy of breast cancer. In Harris JR, Hellman S, Henderson IC, Kinne D (eds.): *Breast Diseases*. Philadelphia: Lippincott, 1991, pp. 427–486.
3. Preisler HD, Taza A: The role of emerging technologies in the diagnosis and staging of neoplastic diseases. *Cancer* 9:1520–1525, 1992 (suppl.).
4. Herrera L, Luna P, Villarreal J: Perspectives in colorectal cancer. *J Surgical Oncol* 2:92–103, 1991 (suppl.).
5. Jeekel J: Can radical surgery improve survival in colorectal cancer? *World J Surg* 11:412–417, 1987.
6. NIH Consensus Conference: Treatment of early stage breast cancer. *JAMA* 265:391–394, 1991.
7. Steele G, Cady B: The surgical oncologist as the patient manager. In Steele G, Cady B (eds.): *General Surgical Oncology*. Philadelphia: Saunders, 1992, pp. 18–21.
8. Tannock IF: Principles of cell proliferation: Cell Kinetics. In DeVita VT, Hellman S, Rosenberg S (eds.): *Cancer: Principles and Practice of Oncology* (ed. 3). Philadelphia: Lippincott, 1989, pp. 3–13.
9. Douglass HO: Adjuvant treatment in colorectal cancer: An update. *World J Surg* 11:478–492, 1987.
10. Schuller DE, Laramore G, Al-Sarraf M, et al: Combined therapy for resectable head and neck cancer. *Arch Otolaryngol Head Neck Surg* 115:364–368, 1989.
11. Shepard FA, Ginsberg RJ, Patterson GA, et al: A prospective study of adjuvant surgical resection after chemotherapy for limited small cell lung cancer. *J Thorac Cardiovasc Surg* 97:177–186, 1989.
12. Siegel B, Mayzel K, Love S: Level I and II axillary dissection in the treatment of early-stage breast cancer. *Arch Surg* 25:1144–1147, 1990.
13. Liotta L: Overview of the biology of cancer invasion and metastasis. In Rosenberg S (ed.): *Surgical Treatment of Metastatic Cancer*. Philadelphia: Lippincott, 1987.
14. Ewer M, Ali MK: Surgical treatment of the cancer patient: Preoperative assessment and perioperative medical management. *J Surgical Oncol* 44:185–190, 1990.
15. Rosenberg SA: Principles of surgical oncology. In Devita VT, Hellman S, Rosenberg SA (eds.): *Cancer: Principles and Practice of Oncology* (ed 3). Philadelphia: Lippincott, 1989, p. 236–246.
16. Patterson WB: Surgical issues in geriatric oncology. *Semin Oncol* 16:57–65, 1989.
17. Ravikumar TS, Steele G: Colon cancer. In Steele G, Cady B (eds.): *General Surgical Oncology*. Philadelphia: Saunders, 1992, pp. 149–169.
18. Wapnir IL, Rabinowitz B: A reappraisal of prophylactic mastectomy. *Surg Gyn Obstet* 171:171–181, 1990.
19. Love S: *Dr. Susan Love's Breast Book*. Reading, MA: Addison-Wesley, 1990.
20. Bibbo M, Underhill S: Cytology of fine-needle aspiration. In Harris JR, Hellman S, Henderson IC, Kinne D (eds.): *Breast Diseases*. Philadelphia: Lippincott, 1991, pp. 297–300.
21. Flynn MB, Wolfson SE, Thomas S. et al: Fine needle aspiration biopsy in clinical management of head and neck tumors. *J Surg Oncol* 44:214–217, 1990.
22. Sugarbaker PH, Roth J: Specialized techniques of cancer management—Endoscopy. In DeVita VT, Hellman S, Rosenberg S (eds.): *Cancer: Principles and Practice of Oncology*. Philadelphia: Lippincott, 1989, pp. 423–440.
23. Kalinowski BH: Local therapy for breast cancer. Treatment choices and decision making. *Sem Oncol Nurs* 7:187–193, 1991.
24. Young RC, Fuks Z, Hoskins WJ: Cancer of the ovary. In

DeVita VT, Hellman S, Rosenberg S (eds.): *Cancer: Principles and Practice of Oncology*. Philadelphia: Lippincott, 1989, pp. 1162–1196.
25. Steele G, Ravikumar TS, Benotti PN: New surgical treatments for recurrent colorectal cancer. *Cancer* 65:723–730, 1990.
26. Russin DJ, Kaplan SR, Goldberg RI, et al: Neodymium-YAG laser. *Arch Surg* 121:1399–1403, 1986.
27. Dyck S: Surgical instrumentation as a palliative treatment for spinal cord compression. *Oncol Nurs Forum* 18:515–521,1991.
28. Schain WS, Wellisch DK, Pasnau RO, et al: The sooner the better. A study of psychological factors in women undergoing immediate versus delayed breast reconstruction. *Am J Psychiatry* 142:40–46, 1985.
29. Sangermano CA: Practice and principles of ambulatory surgery. In Meeker MH, Rothrock JC (eds.): *Alexander's Care of the Patient in Surgery* (ed. 9). St. Louis: Mosby Yearbook, 1991, pp. 964–979.
30. AHA predicts ambulatory surgery will be 60% of all operations. *Same-Day Surg* 13:71, 1989.
31. Tov P, Strauss RG, Stehling LC, et al: Predeposited autologous blood for elective surgery. *N Engl J Med* 316:517–20, 1987,
32. Lichtiger B, Huh YO, Armintor M, et al: Autologous transfusions for cancer patients undergoing elective ablative surgery. *J Surgical Oncol* 43:19–23, 1990.
33. Carr DB, Jacox A, Chapman CR, et al: *Pain Control After Surgery: A Patient's Guide*. Agency for Health Care Policy and Research pub. no. 92-0021. Rockville, MD: U.S. Department of Health and Human Services, 1992.
34. Carr DB, Jacox A, Chapman CR, et al: *Acute Pain Management: Operative or Medical Procedures and Trauma*. Agency for Health Care Policy and Research, Pub. no. 92-0032. Rockville, MD: U.S. Department of Health and Human Services, 1992.
35. Valante S: Using hypnosis with children for pain management. *Oncol Nurs* Forum 18:699–704, 1991.
36. Blankfield RP: Suggestion, relaxation, and hypnosis as adjuncts in the care of surgery patients: A review of the literature. *Am J Clin Hypnosis* 33:172–186, 1991.
37. Alberts MS, Lyons JS, Moretti RJ: Psychological interventions in the pre-surgical period. *Internat J Psychiatry Med* 19:91–106, 1989.
38. Paice JA, Mahon SM, Faut-Callahan M: Factors associated with adequate pain control in hospitalized postsurgical patients diagnosed with cancer. *Cancer Nurs* 14:298–305, 1991.
39. Falcone RE, Nappi JF: Chemotherapy and wound healing. *Surg Clin North Am* 64:779–794, 1984.
40. Ehrlichman RJ, Seckel BR, Bryan DJ, et al: Common complications of wound healing. *Surg Clin North Am* 71:1323–1351, 1991.
41. Daly JM, Redmond HP, Lieberman MD, et al: Nutritional support of patients with cancer of the gastrointestinal tract. *Surg Clin North Am* 71:523–536, 1991.
42. Kemplin S, Gould-Rossback P, Houland WS: Disorders of hemostasis in the critically ill cancer patient. In Howland WS, Carlon GC (eds.): *Critical Care of the Cancer Patient*. Chicago: Year Book, 1985.
43. Smith R: Intraoperative radiation therapy. In Dow KH, Hilderley L (eds.): *Nursing Care in Radiation Oncology*. Philadelphia: Saunders, 1992.
44. Haibeck SV: Intraoperative radiation therapy. *Oncol Nurs Forum* 15:143–147, 1988.
45. Chahbazian CM: The skin. In Moss WT, Cox JD (eds.): *Radiation Oncology: Rationale, Techniques, Results* (ed. 6). St. Louis: Mosby Year Book, 1989, pp. 83–111.
46. Smith RW, Sampson MK, Lucas CE: Effects of vinblastine, etoposide, cisplatin and bleomycin in rodent wound healing. *Surg Gynecol Obstet* 161:323–327, 1985.
47. Chabner BA, Myers CE: Clinical pharmacology of cancer chemotherapy. In DeVita VT, Hellman S, Rosenberg SA (eds.): *Cancer: Principles and Practice of Oncology*. Philadelphia: Lippincott, 1989, pp. 349–395.
48. Avis FP, Ellenberg S, Friedman MA: Surgical oncology research. *Ann Surg* 207:262–266, 1988.
49. Jacobs JR, Pajak TF, Snow JB, et al: Surgical quality control in head and neck cancer. *Arch Otolaryngol Head Neck Surg* 115:489–493, 1989.
50. Thorne SE: Helpful and unhelpful communication in cancer care: The patient perspective. *Oncol Nurs Forum* 15:167–172, 1988.
51. Morra ME: Choices: Who's going to tell the patients what they need to know? *Oncol Nurs Forum* 15:421–425, 1988.

Chapter 13

Radiotherapy

Laura J. Hilderley, RN, MS

THE CURRENT APPLICATION OF RADIOTHERAPY IN THE MANAGEMENT OF THE PERSON DIAGNOSED WITH CANCER

Radiotherapy often is combined with surgery or chemotherapy and immunotherapy, as well as being the sole treatment for cancer in some instances. For example, stage IIB adenocarcinoma of the endometrium is treated with preoperative radiation followed by hysterectomy, whereas Stage IIB squamous cell carcinoma of the cervix is treated with radiation alone.

The aim or intent of radiotherapy may be curative, as in skin cancer, carcinoma of the cervix, Hodgkin's disease, or seminoma. Treatment is vigorous and often lengthy, but the prognosis and probability of long-term survival make such an attempt worthwhile.

For certain other lesions, cure or eradication is not possible, and control of the cancer for periods ranging from months to years may be the aim. Recurrent breast cancer, some soft-tissue sarcomas, and lung cancer are examples of cancers controlled by radiotherapy in combination with surgery or chemotherapy.

Palliation may be another goal of radiotherapy. Relief of pain, prevention of pathologic fractures, and return of mobility can be achieved with radiation to metastatic bone lesions from breast, lung, and prostate tumors. Pain relief often is dramatic, and it is not uncommon for one individual to receive multiple palliative courses to different bony structures over the course of several years. Between such metastatic episodes the person can sometimes carry on a near-normal life. Palliative radiotherapy also is given for the relief of central nervous system (CNS) symptoms caused by brain metastasis or spinal cord compression. Hemorrhage, ulceration, and fungating lesions can be effectively reduced and in some instances eliminated by palliative radiotherapy.

"Anticipatory" palliation is a useful application of radiotherapy in treating potentially symptomatic lesions before they become a problem. Examples of anticipatory palliation include treatment of a mediastinal mass that threatens to produce a superior vena caval syndrome and treatment to a vertebral lesion when spinal cord compression is impending.

Although treatment techniques and equipment may vary, the fundamental principles of radiobiology and radiation physics form the basis on which a course of treatment is selected and designed for each patient. Understanding these principles will enable the oncology nurse to support and care for the person diagnosed with cancer receiving radiotherapy, meeting the emotional as well as the physical needs that result from the disease and the therapy.

APPLIED RADIATION PHYSICS

The use of ionizing radiation in the treatment of cancer is based on the ability of radiation to interact with the atoms and molecules of the tumor cells to produce specific harmful biologic effects. Ionization affects either the molecules of the cell or the cell environment.

An understanding of atomic structure is basic to understanding the ionizing effects of radiation. The atom, the basic unit of molecular structure, consists of two parts: the nucleus, containing positively charged protons and neutrons that have mass but no charge; and the shells (orbits), containing electrons (equivalent to the number of protons), each of which has a negative charge. Each shell can accommodate only a certain number of electrons; if this number is exceeded, a second or third shell is established more distant from the nucleus (Figure 13-1). The negatively charged electrons orbit the nucleus, held in place by the attractive

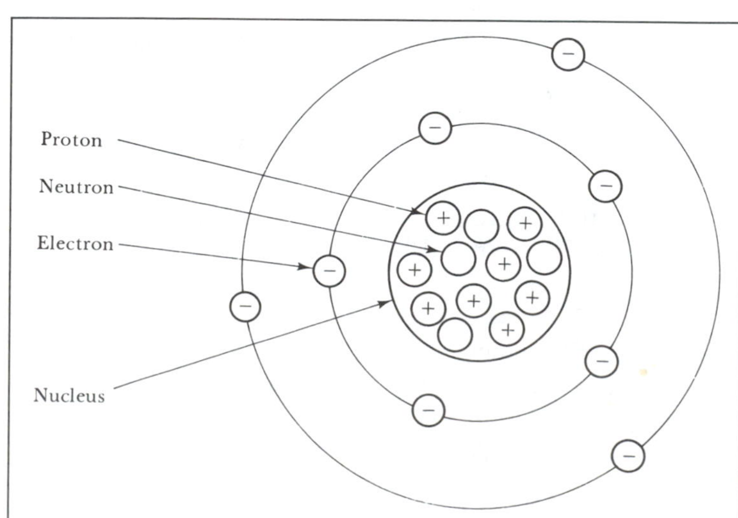

FIGURE 13-1 Basic structure of an atom. Protons, which are positively charged, and neutrons, which have no electrical charge, are the major components of the nucleus of an atom. The number of protons is equal to the number of negatively charged electrons orbiting the nucleus. Atoms of any given element may have different numbers of neutrons in the nucleus, thus giving atoms of the same element different atomic weights. An atom of a given element that differs only in its atomic weight is called an isotope.

force of the positive protons in the nucleus, thus maintaining a stable state. Certain atoms are known to be unstable, however, and it is in this process of decay or breakdown into a more stable state that alpha, beta, or gamma rays may be emitted. Radium, radon, and uranium are examples of unstable atoms that produce radiation.

Stable atoms also may be made to produce ionizing radiation through excitation, ionization, and nuclear disintegration. Radiation produced by these processes can be classified into two groups: *electromagnetic radiation* and *particulate radiation.* The electromagnetic spectrum can be further divided into five levels of decreasing wavelength:

1. radiowaves
2. infrared radiation
3. visible light
4. ultraviolet radiation
5. ionizing radiation

Ionizing radiation has the shortest wavelength and the greatest energy of the electromagnetic spectrum and is therefore the form of energy used in radiotherapy. A classification system for ionizing radiations is shown in Figure 13-2. As seen in the figure, the terms *X ray* and *gamma ray* both describe ionizing electromagnetic radiation and differ only in their means of production. That is, X rays are produced by specially designed equipment, and gamma rays are emitted by radioactive materials such as ^{60}Co undergoing nuclear transition. Both X and gamma rays have no mass, but rather are packets of available energy ready to be released on collision with a substance. Because they have no mass, X and gamma rays can penetrate much deeper into tissue before releasing their energy.

Particulate radiation, on the other hand, is composed of alpha and beta particles, as well as electrons and neutrons, which have a mass. The relatively large size of alpha particles allows them to penetrate only a short distance into tissue before collision and energy release take place; beta particles, which are smaller than alpha particles, will penetrate deeper but, because of their mass, do not have the ability to reach as deeply into tissues as do X and gamma rays. The significance of these variations in ability to penetrate tissue will be obvious when treatment beams and equipment are discussed.

X rays are produced when a stream of fast-moving electrons, accelerated by the application of high voltage (between the filament and the target), strikes the target, and the electrons give up their energy. This radiation loss occurs because the electron is attracted to and slowed down by the nucleus of the tungsten (target) atom. Figure 13-3 illustrates the basic structure of an x-ray tube.

In addition to X rays, some treatment machines (betatron, linear accelerators) are equipped to produce particle irradiation in the form of electrons. Electron energy is produced in an x-ray tube by bypassing one of the steps used to produce X rays (see Figure 13-3). Electrons from the heated tungsten filament are injected into the vacuum tube, are accelerated at a high velocity, and emerge from a window in the vacuum tube, thus bypassing the tungsten target and emerging as electron particles suitable for treating surface lesions and those located a few centimeters below the skin.

Electromagnetic and particulate radiations also are produced through the process of decay of radioactive elements and radioactive isotopes. This process, which produces radiation in the form of alpha, beta, or gamma rays, is illustrated as follows:

$$\text{atom } x \xrightarrow{\text{radioactive decay}} \text{atom } y + \text{radiation}$$

The time required for half the radioactive atoms present at any time to decay is known as the *half-life* of that radioactive element or isotope.

Because most radioisotopes are produced by neutron bombardment of stable elements (^{60}Co, ^{32}P, ^{182}Ta, ^{198}Au) or nuclear fission of uranium in a nuclear reactor (^{90}Sr, ^{137}Cs), they are referred to as *artificial isotopes* to distinguish them from naturally occurring radioisotopes such as ^{226}Ra and ^{222}Rn. Radioisotopes are listed in Table 13-1.

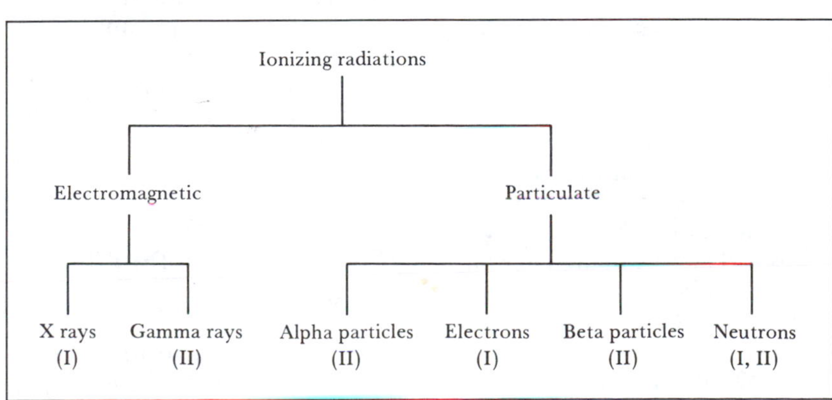

FIGURE 13-2 Classification system for ionizing radiations.

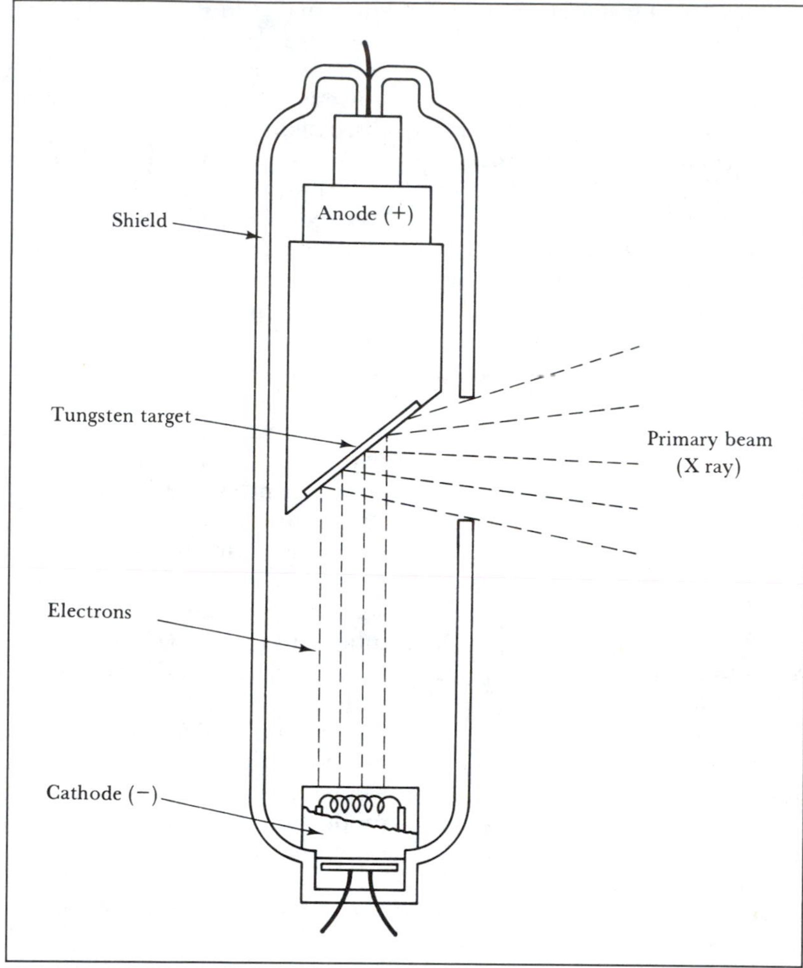

FIGURE 13-3 Basic structure of an x-ray tube. Electrons emitted from a heated tungsten filament are accelerated across a high-voltage source. These high-speed electrons then strike a positively charged tungsten target, producing X rays. The primary beam of radiation thus produced penetrates tissues. The greater the voltage, the greater the penetrating power of the beam.

EQUIPMENT AND BEAMS USED IN RADIOTHERAPY

The types of equipment and beams used in radiotherapy are numerous and vary considerably in their application to clinical practice. A large radiotherapy center will have available a selection suitable for the treatment of almost any malignancy in any part of the body. On the other hand, the equipment available in a private office or small general hospital may be limited to whatever is easiest to use and maintain.

Equipment can be classified according to use: external radiation, or *teletherapy* (radiation from a source at a distance from the body), or internal application, or *brachytherapy* (radiation from a source placed within the body or a body cavity).

A useful classification system of various beams, equipment, and radioactive materials is given in Figures 13-4 and 13-5. In addition to teletherapy and brachytherapy, radiotherapy can be administered systemically using radioisotopes. *Contact therapy* using ^{90}Sr isotopes for conjunctival lesions and *surface (mould) therapy* for superficial skin lesions are additional applications of brachytherapy.

Teletherapy Equipment

Conventional or orthovoltage equipment

Conventional or orthovoltage equipment produces X rays of varying energies, depending on the voltage used. The higher the voltage, the greater the depth of penetration of the x-ray beam. In selecting the proper

TABLE 13-1 Radioactive Isotopes Used in Radiotherapy

Isotope	Symbol	Half-Life	Emissions		
			Alpha	Beta	Gamma
Cesium	^{137}Cs	30 years			X
Cobalt	^{60}Co	5.3 years		X	X
Gold	^{198}Au	2.69 days		X	X
Iodine	^{131}I	8.0 days		X	X
Iridium	^{192}Ir	74.5 days		X	X
Phosphorus	^{32}P	14.3 days		X	
Radium	^{226}Ra	1622 years	X	X	X
Radon	^{222}Rn	3.83 days	X	X	X
Strontium	^{90}Sr	28 years		X	
Tantalum	^{182}Ta	118 days		X	X

beam for treatment of a particular lesion, the percentage depth dose of the beam must be known, as well as the depth within the body of the lesion. *Percentage depth dose* is defined as the percentage of the intensity of any given beam at a given depth in tissue compared with the presumed 100% dose level. The maximum, or 100%, level occurs at varying depths, depending mainly on the energy of the radiation being produced. Equipment in the range of 40–120 kV (1 kV = 1000 V) is suitable only for superficial skin lesions and those no deeper than 1 cm. Beams in the 250–400-kV range (orthovoltage) have greater penetration and have been in use for many years. There are, however, a number of disadvantages to orthovoltage beams in addition to the poor depth of penetration. Most important are the severe skin reactions, due to the fact that most of the dose is at skin level, and bone necrosis, which can result because bone absorbs more orthovoltage radiation than does soft tissue. As a result of bone absorption, tumor located distal to bone in the treatment field receives less than the desired dose of radiation.

Megavoltage equipment

Megavoltage equipment, operating at from 2–40 MeV (million electron volts) has distinct advantages over orthovoltage beams. The primary advantages of megavoltage therapy are (1) deeper beam penetration, (2) more homogeneous absorption of radiation (minimizing the excessive absorption by bone that occurs with

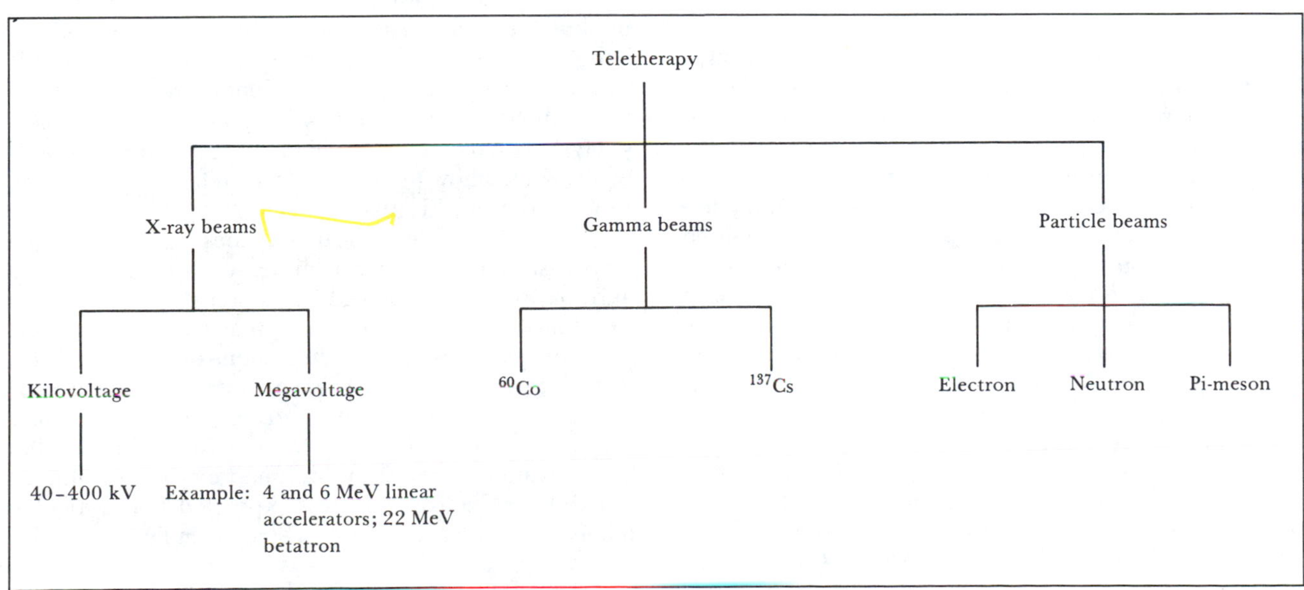

FIGURE 13-4 Classification system of teletherapy.

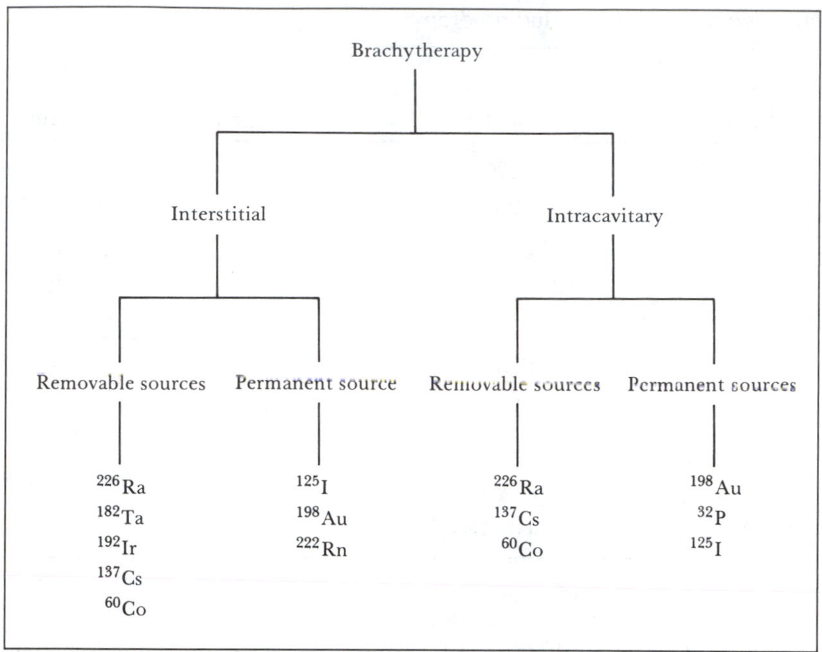

FIGURE 13-5 Radioactive sources used in brachytherapy.

orthovoltage treatment), and (3) greater skin sparing. Equipment used in megavoltage therapy includes the Van de Graaf generator, cobalt and cesium units, the betatron, and linear accelerators. Largely experimental units such as those producing heavy ions, neutron beams, and negative pi-meson particle beams will be briefly mentioned.

The Van de Graaf generator, operating at 2 million volts, was one of the forerunners in megavoltage equipment. Its use today is relegated primarily to the experimental laboratory, having been replaced in cancer therapy by more sophisticated equipment.

Cobalt-60 radiotherapy units were once the most common megavoltage equipment. The cobalt machine is easy to operate and maintain, having no complicated electronics, as do linear accelerators. Because the radiation source is a radioactive isotope of cobalt, it is undergoing constant decay, at the rate of about a 10% per year decrease in output. Cobalt sources are measured in curies (Ci), and 3000–9000 Ci typically are needed in a teletherapy unit. Gamma rays are emitted as the ^{60}Co atoms decay; with a half-life of 5.3 years, this means that the source would need to be replaced every 5–6 years to avoid lengthy treatment times. Cobalt units are also characterized by lower dose rates and a lower percentage depth dose compared with a linear accelerator of 10 MeV.

Cesium in the form of ^{137}Cs is also used in teletherapy units, primarily those outside the United States. Because of the low specific activity of a ^{137}Cs source, the source must be placed about 35 cm from the skin. This short source-to-skin distance (SSD) adds to surface skin dose by electron contamination, producing greater skin reactions. In comparison, ^{60}Co usually is placed at 80 cm SSD.

Linear accelerators, although more complex in terms of operation and maintenance than cobalt units, are widely used in most hospital-based radiotherapy departments as well as in the private practice setting. Linear accelerators have distinct treatment advantages, including the speed with which treatments can be given. Not only is this an advantage in terms of efficient use of time, but, more important, it means that the person being treated spends less time in awkward, sometimes uncomfortable positions. In addition, a sharply defined field of irradiation can be obtained, thus treating only the desired tissue volume.

Linear accelerators are so named because of the method of x-ray production, which involves accelerating electrons along a radiofrequency electromagnetic wave, achieving energies equivalent to those that could be obtained only in a conventional x-ray tube at excessively high voltage. Some linear accelerators are also equipped to allow use of the electron beam (particulate radiation) itself. Electron beam therapy is useful in relatively superficial lesions such as chest wall recurrence of breast cancer, skin cancers, and superficial nodes and may be used to provide a booster dose to a limited site following treatment with megavoltage therapy. Electron particles are the equivalent of beta particles, differing only in their origin (beta particles are produced by radioactive decay), and, because of their mass, they have limited penetration into tissue. This is a distinct advantage over X or gamma radiation in that almost all the electron energy is expended at a particular tissue depth, sparing whatever structures lie beyond the tumor site.

The betatron is a therapy machine that predates the development of the linear accelerator for electron therapy. Electrons produced from a heated tungsten filament are injected into a doughnut-shaped porcelain envelope and accelerated by a changing magnetic field. These high-velocity electrons range in energy from 10–30 MeV and are useful for deep-seated lesions. X rays (18–40 MeV) also may be produced by the betatron when the electron beam is directed at a tungsten target.

High-energy radiation

There are two basic forms of radiation used in radiotherapy, those classified as low LET (linear energy transfer) radiation, such as X rays, gamma rays, and electrons, and high LET radiation, such as neutron beams, heavy ions, and negative pi-mesons (pions). Basically, the difference between low and high LET radiation is in the deposition of energy in the tissue molecule. (See Figure 13-12 in the section entitled Radiobiology.) Low LET radiation could conceivably pass through a molecule without damaging it. In contrast, the number of ionizing events produced in molecules by high LET radiation is much greater.

High-energy radiation facilities are limited in distribution in the United States and elsewhere. Years of experimentation have shown that there are distinct advantages to this form of therapy, yet the cost of such facilities and the technologic sophistication needed to operate them have meant that they must remain as referral centers for very carefully selected individuals with cancer. According to Orton,[1] high LET radiation has several advantages over low LET radiation:

1. more biologically effective (greater relative biologic effectiveness [RBE])
2. reduced relative radioresistance of hypoxic cells in tumors (low oxygen enhancement ratio [OER])
3. less intertreatment recovery of tumor cells in fractionated dosage

Neutron beam therapy Fast neutrons are produced by a cyclotron, in which high-energy deuterons bombard targets of either beryllium or tritium. Neutron therapy is less expensive than other high LET energy producers; however, technologic problems and the low dose rate (5–6 cGy/min) are some of the disadvantages to this form of therapy.

Heavy-ion therapy Heavy ions, such as protons, helium, and nitrogen, are useful mainly for small tumors, because the dose distribution is best when treating a small volume. As the treatment volume increases, the OER will also increase.

Clinical trials with proton beam therapy are currently being conducted by the Proton Radiation Oncology Group, established in 1991. This cooperative group gathers data from the 13 centers around the world, three of which are located in the USA.[2]

Negative pi-meson therapy Negative pi-mesons (pions) are small, negatively charged particles found in the nuclei of atoms that "cement" protons and neutrons together. Pions are produced when protons are accelerated at approximately 131,000 miles/sec before striking a carbon target. The pions are then collected by a system of magnets, and the beam of high LET energy is directed at the target tissue. The first application of this form of treatment for human subjects took place at the Los Alamos Meson Physics Facility in Los Alamos, New Mexico, in 1974. The advantage of pion therapy, like other forms of high LET radiation, is that the beam can be shaped to fit the tumor precisely, thus minimizing the amount of radiation to surrounding normal structures. Pions can be aimed and stopped at a specific target site by adjusting the momentum of the particles.

Brachytherapy Equipment

Brachytherapy, the use of sealed sources of radioactive material placed within or near a tumor, is the treatment of choice for a variety of lesions. Brachytherapy frequently is combined with teletherapy and also may be used preoperatively and postoperatively.

Radioactive isotopes for brachytherapy application are contained in a variety of forms, such as wires (^{182}Ta), ribbons or tubes (^{192}Ir), needles (^{137}Cs, ^{226}Ra), grains or seeds (^{198}Au, ^{222}Rn), and capsules (^{137}Cs, ^{226}Ra). The source is selected by the radiotherapist according to the site to be treated, the size of the lesion, and whether the implant is to be temporary or permanent.[3]

Needles, wires, and ribbons (either preloaded or afterloaded) are particularly useful in treating head and neck lesions. Intraabdominal and intrathoracic lesions can be implanted with gold or iodine seeds introduced either through hollow needles or tubes or through a "seed gun" that injects the radioactive sources into the tumor bed. Isotopes implanted in this manner usually are permanent, and radiation precautions may be needed after the person is discharged.

Intracavitary radiotherapy most often is employed in the treatment of gynecologic lesions. A variety of techniques and types of equipment have been designed (Figure 13-6) to provide a desired dosage to the tissues around the radiation source.[4] Most gynecologic applicators are based on the "Manchester method."[5] According to this method, the radioactive source is contained in two vaginal ovoids separated by a spacer, and a central uterine tandem is added when both the corpus and cervix are to be treated. Many of these applicators are the afterloading type that can be positioned in the operating room and loaded with the radioactive source at a later time after the proper position has been checked by radiograph and the patient returned to her room. The afterloading method is most desirable because it prevents unnecessary radiation exposure to personnel.

Brachytherapy equipment and techniques have been a subject of intense interest and development in recent years. Standard applications and operative procedures as described earlier are still the most common method of treating with radioactive sources. However, the newer techniques involving high dose rate, remote afterloading procedures, and equipment are being utilized

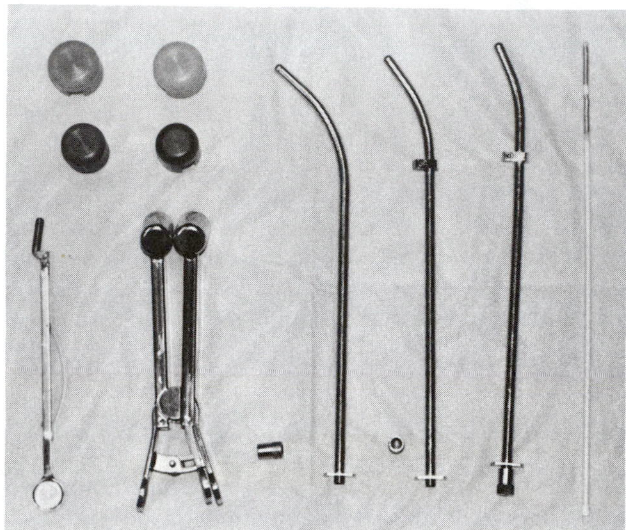

FIGURE 13-6 Examples of gynecologic applicators. Left to right: carrier for radioactive source to be inserted in colpostat; afterloading vaginal colpostats with plastic caps used to increase the size; afterloading uterine tandems; plastic tube containing radioactive sources to be inserted into tandem.

throughout the world and with increasing frequency in the United States.[6]

Use of high-dose-rate (HDR) sources for brachytherapy has distinct advantages over low-dose-rate (LDR) sources in that HDR produces the same radiobiologic effect in a shorter period of time. With standard brachytherapy techniques with LDR sources, the patient is hospitalized for up to 72 hours of continuous therapy. With HDR technique, 500–1000 cGy can be delivered in less than 10 minutes. Number of fractions and total dose must be chosen carefully for each body site and tumor type in order to produce the desired tumor effect while minimizing the effect on both early-responding (acute) and late-responding (chronic) normal tissues.

HDR brachytherapy can be used for intralumenal (lung, esophagus, bile duct), interstitial, intracavitary, and surface lesions. Under appropriate sedation, hollow catheters are placed within or adjacent to the lesion, the catheters are connected to the delivery system, and the appropriate dose is administered by propelling the radioactive source via catheter to the target site for the prescribed length of time. If the patient should require care (i.e., suctioning) before the treatment is completed, the radioactive sources simply are returned to the storage system via the catheter until care is completed.

Major advantages of the remote afterloading HDR technique include reduced exposure to personnel, flexible techniques, shorter treatment time, and outpatient options. In addition to the specialized equipment that must be acquired in order to utilize this method of brachytherapy, computer planning systems and physics programs must be added. A multidisciplinary team (including radiation oncologists, radiation therapists, physicists, nurses, and operating room personnel) usually is involved when remote afterloading brachytherapy is implemented. The nursing role in HDR brachytherapy is significant and must be incorporated into all phases of the procedure. Pretreatment teaching and patient assessment, treatment-phase support and monitoring of patient condition, and posttreatment education and follow-up are all nursing responsibilities. Nursing care during HDR for endobronchial lesions is detailed by Jordan and Mantravadi.[7] An excellent patient education booklet has also been published by Jordan and Buck.[8]

SIMULATION AND TREATMENT PLANNING

The decision to employ radiotherapy is made after consideration of a number of factors. Histologic confirmation of the diagnosis and staging of the disease by appropriate clinical, surgical, and laboratory procedures are necessary before a treatment decision can be made. In addition, such factors as the person's age and general condition, site of tumor, radioresponsiveness of the tumor, risk versus benefit, patient consent, and availability of treatment facilities must all be considered when selecting a plan of therapy.

When the decision has been made to treat a person with radiotherapy, the radiation oncologist devises the treatment plan, often utilizing an array of sophisticated equipment and involving a team of personnel.

One of the first steps in planning is localizing the tumor and defining the volume to be treated. Some lesions are visible and their dimensions can be determined clinically. However, often it is necessary to employ a simulator to determine treatment volume accurately. A simulator may have several component parts (Figure 13-7). It contains a diagnostic x-ray unit for visualizing the proposed treatment site. Fluoroscopic examination may also be done. From radiographs taken on the simulator, the physician can determine the field of treatment and draw in the proposed field outline on the radiograph. The radiation therapist (formerly called radiation technologist or radiographer) then duplicates these markings on the patient's skin using anatomic points and outlines projected onto the patient's skin by the simulator. Treatment portals can be identified by several small tattoos placed at the corners of the field. Tattooing is a simple process in which a drop of India ink is placed on the skin and a needle is used to introduce the ink into the skin, leaving a tiny permanent black dot. This procedure, which produces only momentary discomfort, can be distressing to the person if it is not explained carefully beforehand. For individuals receiving head and neck irradiation, where the field markings are particularly visible, tattoos may be substituted for lines once the reproducibility of the field has been ensured. In many

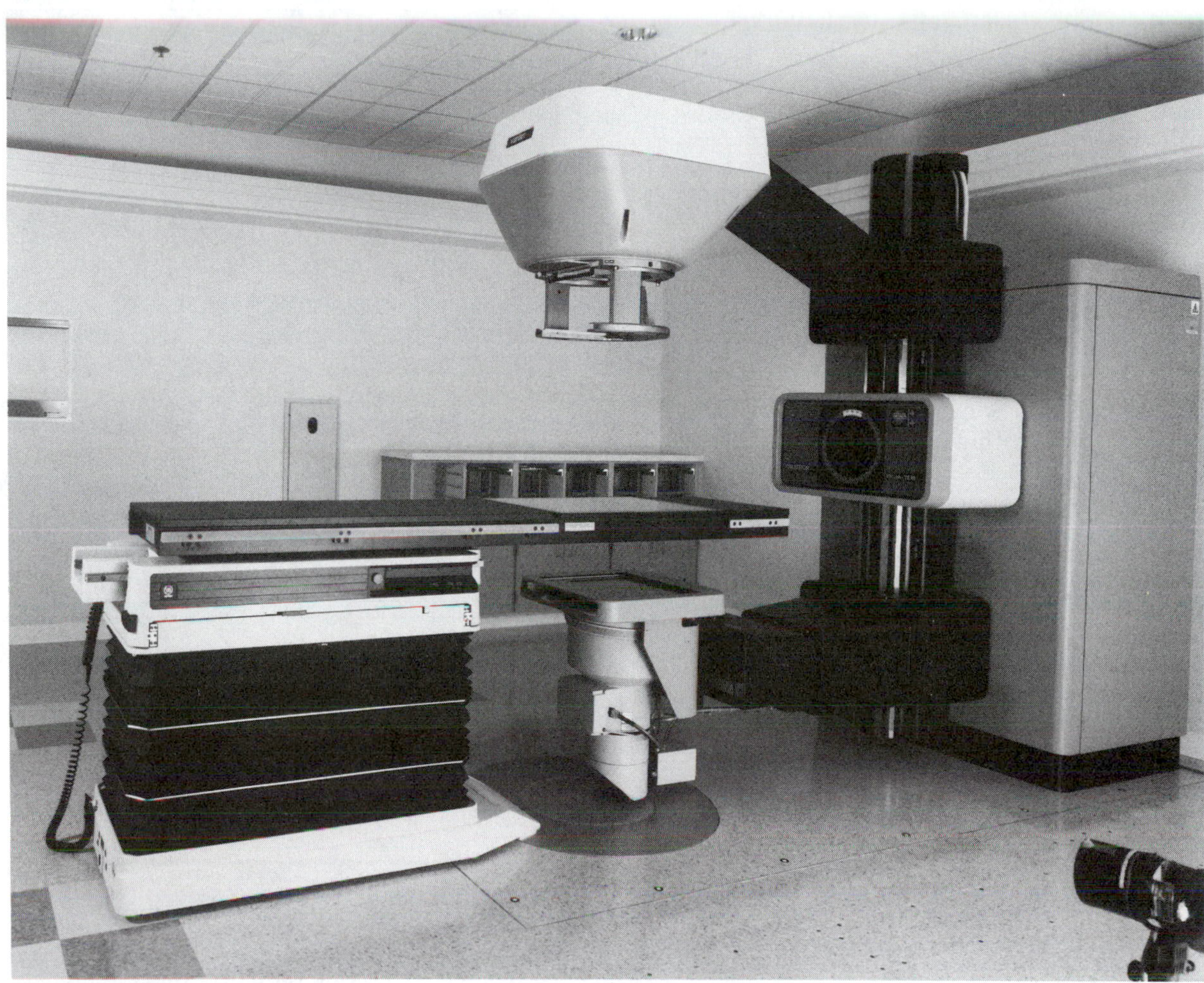

FIGURE 13-7 A Varian Ximatron™ C-Series radiation therapy simulator. (Photo courtesy of Varian Associates, Inc., Palo Alto, CA)

instances, however, tattoos are not placed until the end of the treatment course because a field may shrink or change as surface contours change and tumor volume shrinks. Tattoos are a useful means of identifying a previously treated area if a person returns for further therapy. Injection molding equipment has recently been employed to form masks or head holders of clear plastic. Field markings can be placed on these masks rather than on the skin, avoiding conspicuous facial marks.

Some simulators also are capable of transverse axial tomography. Tomography is a radiographic technique for showing detailed images of body structures at any given plane in the body. This technique obtains a three-dimensional view of the tumor and surrounding structures, allowing greater precision in planning and delivering treatment. Computerized tomography (CT scan) and magnetic resonance imaging (MRI) provide the radiation oncologist with even finer detail for treatment planning.

Some simulators are also equipped with an ultrasound device that produces an image of internal structures. This technique employs ultrasound (inaudible sound with frequencies ranging from 16,000 to 10 billion cycles per second [cps]) that is reflected back as an echo from the varying tissues it strikes. Differences in density and elasticity of tissues and organs produce differences in the echo, which are recorded as an image of the target structures. Ultrasound is another means of defining tumor volume and relationship to nearby vital structures.

Various restraining or positioning devices may be designed at the time of simulation to aid in immobilizing the person. Lying still in exactly the same position each day sometimes is difficult but is necessary to deliver the prescribed treatment to the prescribed volume. For children, especially, a custom-made body cast sometimes is used to ensure immobility. The adult also may be more accurately positioned by means of various headrests, armboards, handgrips, and the like.

An important part of simulation and treatment planning is shaping the field and determining what structures are to be blocked and protected from radiation. The therapy machine produces a rectangular field, which can, within limits, be made larger or smaller. However, that rectangular field must then be trimmed and shaped, with portions eliminated in varying patterns to meet individual requirements. Blocks to protect vital body organs and tissues are secured to a plastic tray that is then placed on the head of the treatment machine between the beam and the person being treated. *Portal films* (sometimes called *beam films*) are radiographs taken through the treatment machine to confirm the treatment field and the placement of blocks in the desired position.

During simulation, contours of the person's body may be obtained and then traced onto paper. Information from the tracings is fed into a computer, which then produces an isodose plot to guide the radiation oncologist and physicist in designing the best field arrangement possible. Some examples of various field arrangements for treating tumors in different locations are shown in Figures 13-8 and 13-9.

The physicist plays an important role in simulation and treatment planning. Working together, the physicist and radiation oncologist design the field arrangement, determine the dose calculations, monitor tumor response, and ensure accuracy of technical aspects. Physicists are also often involved in the maintenance and calibration of treatment machines.

For the person with cancer, simulation and treatment planning usually are the first introduction to the machinery of a radiotherapy department. Thorough and careful explanation about the purpose of this preliminary phase of treatment is important to allay anxiety about the procedures themselves and about the delay in getting treatment started. If the person can be helped to understand the importance of careful planning, the necessary steps will be accepted or at least tolerated better.

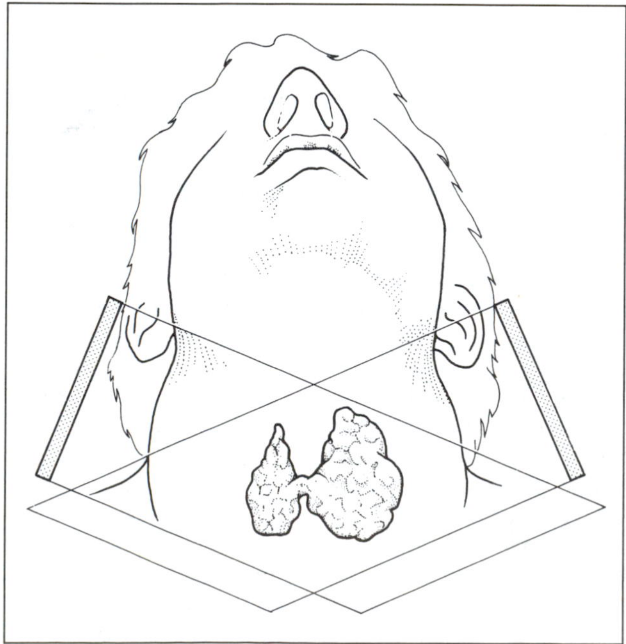

FIGURE 13-8 Two vertically wedged field arrangements for the treatment of thyroid carcinoma.

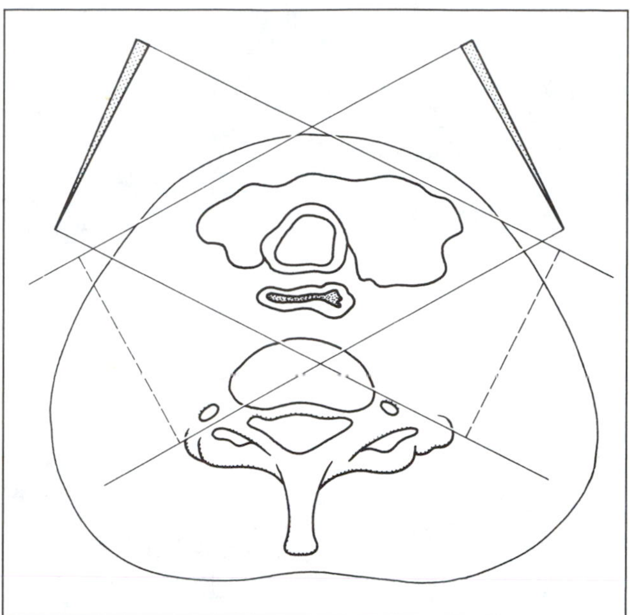

FIGURE 13-9 Cross section of the neck showing the zone of high-dose irradiation to a thyroid tumor; the dose to the spinal cord is low, although the skin dose is high.

RADIOBIOLOGY

The biologic effects of radiation on humans are the result of a sequence of events that follows the absorption of energy from ionizing radiation and the organism's attempts to compensate for this assault. Radiation effect takes place at the cellular level, with consequences in tissues, organs, and the entire body. Factors contributing to radiation response will be presented, and the reader is referred to Chapter 3 on cellular biology for background.

Cellular Response to Radiation

Radiation effect at the cellular level may be either direct or indirect. According to the target theory,[5,9] a *direct* hit occurs when any of the key molecules within the cell, such as DNA or RNA, are damaged. Among the types of damage observed after high-dose radiation of DNA molecules in vitro are (1) change or loss of a base (thymine, adenine, guanine, or cytosine), (2) breakage of the hydrogen bond between the two chains of the DNA molecule, (3) breaks in one or both chains of the DNA molecule, and (4) cross-linking of the chains after breakage. Such unrepaired breaks or alterations in the base lead to mutations, which bring about impaired cellular function or cell death.

An *indirect* hit, according to target theory, occurs when ionization takes place in the medium (mostly water) surrounding the molecular structures within the cell. Radiation absorbed by the water molecules results in a free radical when an electron is literally knocked out of orbit surrounding the ion. The resulting free radical is then available to join with the others, and this high degree of reactivity in itself can damage the macromolecules of the cell. Such free radicals may trigger a variety of chemical reactions, producing new compounds that are toxic to the cell. Figure 13-10 illustrates the ionizing effect of radiation on the water contained within a cell.

It generally is agreed that a direct hit (i.e., DNA damage and chromosomal aberrations) accounts for the most effective and lethal injury produced by ionizing radiation.[10] However, because of the relative proportion of water to DNA in a single cell, the probability of indirect damage through ionization of cellular water is much greater.

In addition to the damage produced by a direct or indirect hit, experimental evidence shows that radiation can cause damage to proteins, carbohydrates, and enzymes within the cell. Damage to these molecules, as well as alterations in the permeability of the cell membrane, also may be implicated in the ultimate effect of radiation at the cellular level.

The final products of the ionization of water molecules (HOH) by radiation are an ion pair (H^+, OH^-) and free radicals ($H^{\cdot}$, $OH^{\cdot}$), which are capable of damaging the cell. The ionization of water is shown in the following steps:

$$HOH \xrightarrow{\text{radiation}} HOH^+ + e^-$$

The free electron (e^-) is then captured by another available water molecule and, as shown in the next step, forms the second ion:

$$HOH + e^- \rightarrow HOH^-$$

Because the two ions (HOH^+, HOH^-) produced by these reactions are unstable, rapid breakdown occurs (in the presence of other, normal water molecules), forming yet another ion and a free radical as follows:

$$HOH^+ \rightarrow H^+ + OH^{\cdot}$$
$$HOH^- \rightarrow OH^- + H^{\cdot}$$

Although the resulting pair of ions (H^+, OH^-) have some potential for cellular damage through chemical reactions, they are more likely to recombine and form water (HOH). The free radicals ($H^{\cdot}$, $OH^{\cdot}$) are extremely reactive, and they too may simply recombine to form water. However, free radicals appear to be more likely to undergo chemical interactions with other free radicals, forming cytotoxic agents, as shown in this reactions:

$$OH^{\cdot} + OH^{\cdot} \rightarrow H_2O_2 \text{ (hydrogen peroxide)}$$

Free radicals that result from the interaction of radiation with water are capable of triggering a variety of chemical reactions within the cell and are therefore believed to be a major factor in the production of damage in the cell.

FIGURE 13-10 The effect of ionizing radiation on water molecules.

Cell cycle and radiosensitivity

According to Richter et al.,[11] radiosensitivity appears to be maximum during the M and G_2 phases of the cell cycle (Figure 13-11). Thus the maximum effect from radiation should occur just before and during actual cell division. Bergonie and Tribondeau[12] in early research formulated a law that says that the sensitivity of cells to irradiation is in direct proportion to their reproductive activity and inversely proportional to their degree of differentiation. A differentiated cell is one that is morphologically or functionally specialized (such as the erythrocyte) and does not undergo mitosis. An undifferentiated cell (such as the red blood cell stem cell or erythroblast) has few specialized morphologic or functional characteristics, and its primary purpose is to divide and provide new cells to maintain its own population. Because the effect of radiation is known to be greatest during mitosis, undifferentiated cell populations generally are most sensitive to radiation. In contrast, well-differentiated cells are relatively radioresistant.

Changes in mitotic activity due to radiation can be classified as *delayed onset* or *complete inhibition.* Delay in the onset of mitosis indicates that although damage occurred at some point during prophase, repair was accomplished and division takes place. *Complete inhibition* of mitosis, or cell sterilization, renders the cell incapable of division, although it may continue to live in a nonreproducing state.

Cell death

There are three types of cell death: mitotic (or genetic) death, interphase death, and instant death. *Mitotic death* occurs after one or more divisions and usually with much smaller radiation doses than those required to produce interphase death. *Interphase death* takes place many hours after irradiation and before the cell begins the mitotic process. *Instant death* occurs following extremely high doses of radiation and would take place only in the experimental laboratory or in the event of a nuclear accident.

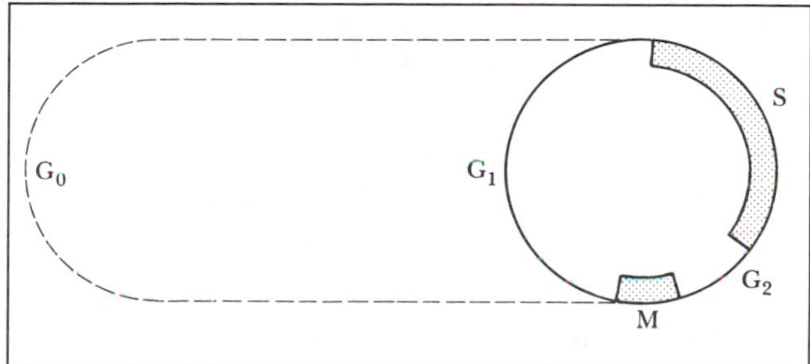

FIGURE 13-11 Stages in cell replication cycle: *S,* DNA synthesis; *G_2,* the gap between DNA synthesis and mitosis; *M,* mitosis; *G_1,* the gap between the end of mitosis and the start of DNA synthesis.

Other factors

A number of additional factors directly affect the biologic response to radiation and ultimately the treatment outcome. Among these are the oxygen effect, linear energy transfer, relative biologic effectiveness, dose rate, radiosensitivity, and fractionation.

Oxygen effect Well-oxygenated tumors show a much greater response to radiation, that is, are more radiosensitive, than poorly oxygenated tumors. Extensive laboratory and clinical research[10,13] has shown that the existence of oxygen tension between 20 and 40 mm Hg at radiation greatly enhances the radiosensitivity of the cells. Theoretically, the mechanism of the oxygen effect is related to the ability of oxygen to combine with the free radicals formed during ionization, producing new and toxic combinations. A second theory holds that the presence of oxygen at irradiation prevents the reversal (and thus the repair) of some of the chemical changes that occur as the result of ionization. The clinical significance of the oxygen effect is that oxygen modifies the dose of radiation needed to produce a given degree of biologic damage. The magnitude of the oxygen effect is expressed as the *oxygen enhancement ratio (OER)*. The OER is the ratio of radiation dose in the absence of oxygen (or hypoxia) to the radiation dose in the presence of oxygen required for the same biologic effect.

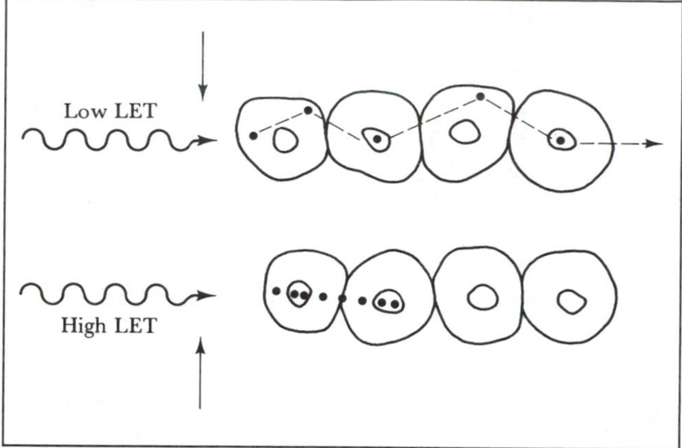

FIGURE 13-12 Comparison of the effects of low- and high-LET radiations on a population of cells. Notice the irregular path of the low-LET radiation, interacting with four cells, compared with the relatively straight path of the high-LET radiation, which is interacting with only two cells. However, the low-LET radiation produces only *one* hit in two nuclei, whereas the high-LET radiation produces *two* hits in two nuclei. (Source: Travis EL: *Primer of Medical Radiobiology*. Chicago: Year Book Medical Publishers, 1975, p 71. © 1975 Year Book Medical Publishers. Reproduced with permission.)

Linear energy transfer *Linear energy transfer (LET)* describes the rate at which energy is lost from different types of radiations while traveling through matter. Its usefulness is seen in designating the quality of radiation emitted from various radiations, such as X rays, neutrons, and alpha particles. Low-LET radiations (X and gamma rays) are sparsely ionizing, having a random pathway that results in few direct hits within the cell nucleus. Radiation of higher LET (alpha particles, neutrons, and negative pi-mesons) has a greater probability of interacting with matter and producing more direct hits (Figure 13-12).[9]

Relative biologic effectiveness Because different radiations have varying rates of energy loss, the biologic response will be different. Therefore, the term *relative biological effectiveness (RBE)* is used to compare a dose of test radiation with a dose of standard radiation that produces the same biologic response. The following formula is used to express RBE:

$$\text{RBE} = \frac{\text{Dose of reference radiation to produce a given biologic effect}}{\text{Dose of test radiation to produce the same biologic effect}}$$

Dose rate *Dose rate* refers to the rate at which a given dose is delivered by a treatment machine. Studies have shown low dose rates to be much less effective in producing lethal cell damage than high dose rates, primarily because low dose rates permit cell repair to occur before the lethal dose has been reached.

Radiosensitivity According to Bergonie and Tribondeau's law, ionizing radiation is most effective on cells that are undifferentiated and undergoing active mitosis.[12] Laboratory and clinical experience has shown this to be true in most tissues.

Fractionation *Fractionation,* or the dividing of a total dose of radiation into a number of equal fractions, is based on four important factors: repair, redistribution, repopulation, and reoxygenation,[9,10,14] commonly referred to as the four Rs of radiobiology.[15]

Repair Repair of intracellular sublethal damage by normal cells between daily dose fractions is one benefit of fractionation. The goal of fractionation is to deliver a dose sufficient to prevent tumor cells from being repaired while allowing normal cells to recover before the next dose is given. Although some tumor cells may be repaired between daily doses, they also may reoxygenate, rendering them more radiosensitive when the next dose is given. Thus although some degree of repair of tumor cells is possible between fractionated doses, repeated daily doses ultimately would lead to tumor control.

Redistribution Redistribution of cell age (within the cell cycle) as a result of daily radiation is advantageous because more tumor cells are made radiosensitive. Theoretically, with succeeding daily doses of radiation, more and more tumor cells would be delayed in cycle and reach the mitotic phase as the next dose is given, thus increasing the cell kill. Certain chemotherapeutic agents, such as methotrexate and hydroxyurea, are being used in combination with radiation to take advantage of this synchronization in the cell cycle.

Repopulation Repopulation of normal tissues takes place through cell division at some time during a multifraction treatment course. Fractionation of dose allows this repopulation in normal tissues, sparing them from some of the late consequences that might occur if repopulation (new growth) was inhibited. On the other hand, those tumor cells that do succeed in dividing while undergoing a fractionated course of radiotherapy usually are incapable of surviving because of the radiation effect. Thus fractionation favors normal tissue while still eradicating tumor.

Reoxygenation Reoxygenation is the fourth consideration favoring fractionation of the radiation dose. Whereas normal tissues usually are well oxygenated, tumors characteristically range from normal to hypoxic to anoxic. As discussed earlier, radiosensitivity is closely related to oxygen tension in the tumor cell; hypoxic or anoxic cells generally are radioresistant, whereas oxygenated cells are radiosensitive. Fractionating the dose allows time between treatments for the tumor to reoxygenate.

Tissue and organ response to radiation can now be understood on the basis of sensitivity of cellular components. It is important to note that tissues and organs are composed of more than one cell category, each cell category having different degrees of radiosensitivity. A second factor in determining tissue response is related to the parenchymal versus stromal substance found in that tissue. The parenchyma is composed of cells characteristic of the tissue or organ, and if those cells are radiosensitive (e.g., the testis), ionizing radiation has its greatest impact on the parenchyma. However, if parenchymal tissue is relatively radioresistant (e.g., the spinal cord), radiation response in that organ is due to the indirect effects on the stromal components (especially the vasculature) that support the parenchyma. Table 13-2 lists various organs according to their degree of radiosensitivity as measured by parenchymal hypoplasia.

TABLE 13-2 Degree of Radiosensitivity of Various Organs Based on Parenchymal Hypoplasia

Organ	Radiosensitivity
Lymphoid organs, bone marrow, blood, testes, ovaries, intestines	High
Skin, cornea, oral cavity, esophagus, rectum, bladder, vagina, cervix, ureters	Fairly high
Optic lens, stomach, growing cartilage, fine vasculature, growing bone	Medium
Mature cartilage or bone, salivary glands, respiratory organs, kidneys, liver, pancreas, thyroid, adrenals, pituitary gland	Fairly low
Muscle, brain, spinal cord	Low

CHEMICAL AND THERMAL MODIFIERS OF RADIATION

Radiosensitizers and Radioprotectors

The goal of radiotherapy is to achieve maximum tumor cell kill while minimizing injury to normal tissues (therapeutic ratio). Efforts to improve the therapeutic ratio have resulted in the development of certain compounds that act to increase the radiosensitivity of tumor cells or to protect normal cells from radiation effect. Combined modality therapy with both radiation and certain cytotoxic agents also takes advantage of enhanced tumor cell kill. Drugs such as doxorubicin, actinomycin-D, cyclophosphamide, bleomycin, and cisplatin often are used along with radiation to achieve greater cell kill than either therapy could achieve if used independently. When used alone, chemical modifiers of radiation therapy (radiosensitizers), however, generally are not cytotoxic like the chemotherapeutic agents.

Phillips[16] proposed several definitions useful in describing the various interactions of radiation with other agents. *Enhancement* or *potentiation* describes any radiation effect that is greater in the presence of the chemical than in its absence. If the effect is less than that caused by the most active agent in the combination, then this is known as *interference*. *Antagonism* is the term used to describe an outcome less than that of the least effective agent in a given combination. In clinical radiotherapy, enhancement by noncytotoxic sensitizers is called *radiosensitization*. Antagonism by protective compounds is called *radioprotection*.

Radiosensitizers are compounds that apparently promote fixation of the free radicals produced by radiation damage at the molecular level. The mechanism of this action is similar to the oxygen effect described earlier, in which biochemical reactions in the damaged molecules prevent repair of the cellular radiation damage. Free radicals (such as OH°) are captured by the electron-affinic radiosensitizers, rendering the molecules incapable of repair.

The two most biologically active radiosensitizing compounds first tested in phase II and III studies were metronidazole (Flagyl) and misonidazole (RO-07-0582). Major side effects are neurotoxicity, including peripheral neuropathies, and CNS symptoms of somnolence, confusion, and transient coma. Nausea and vomiting are also fairly frequent side effects that seem to be dose-related. Early clinical trials using misonidazole as a radiosensitizer indicated some degree of effectiveness in treatment of squamous carcinoma of the head and neck and of the uterine cervix. Overall results were disappointing, however, due to severe toxicity and only marginal improvement in tumor control. Brown[17] concludes that a new hypoxic cell radiosensitizer is needed. Misonidazole is the only such substance to have undergone extensive clinical trial evaluation, and most studies have failed to demonstrate a significant effect with the addition of misonidazole.

The compound SR-2508 (etanidazole) has been tested with promising results in phase I trials.[18] This member of the nitroimidazole group of compounds appears to be less toxic to the CNS tissue than misonidazole. It currently is being used in a number of phase II and III trials.

Early studies[19] with nitroimidazoles used in vitro showed that these radiosensitizers are also capable of cytotoxic activity in hypoxic cells after periods of long exposure. The high doses required to achieve actual cell kill in vitro have, however, prohibited their use in vivo for this purpose.

Misonidazole also has been shown to increase the cytotoxicity of alkylating agents, nitrosoureas, 5-fluorouracil (5-FU), cyclophosphamide, and melphalan.[20] However, the side effects commonly experienced with these agents are also apparently enhanced by the addition of misonidazole. This nonselective enhancement detracts from the potential benefits to be gained.

Radioprotectors are compounds that can protect aerated (nontumor) cells while having a limited effect on hypoxic (tumor) cells. This selective action thus serves to increase the therapeutic ratio by promoting the repair of irradiated normal tissues. Repair or return to a nondamaged state takes place through the chemical process of reduction. Free electrons are captured by the radioprotective substance and are thus unavailable to participate in further chemical reactions that lead to cellular damage. This process can be viewed as the opposite of what occurs when radiosensitizers are used.

The sulfhydryl groups contained in the nonprotein fraction of most cells aid in the reduction process following radiation damage. Thiophosphate compounds (such as cysteine and cysteamine), containing sulfhydryl and aminopropyl groups, were among the earliest radioprotectors synthesized. The compound that appears to be most useful at present is designated WR-2721.[21]

The study of radiosensitizers and radioprotectors has extended to phase II and III clinical trials in the continued effort to achieve better results in cancer treatment with radiotherapy. With combined therapy, toxicity can be increased and patient comfort may be compromised. Clinical trials are no longer confined to major cancer centers. Thus the nurse in a community hospital setting may be involved in caring for the person receiving radiosensitizers or radioprotectors.

Some nursing responsibilities in the use of radiosensitizers and radioprotectors would include:

1. providing patient and family education
2. participating in obtaining informed consent
3. administering investigational agents
4. timing and coordinating drug administration with radiotherapy treatment
5. observing and documenting expected and previously unreported effects and side effects
6. managing side effects, including developing interventions for those newly observed

A thorough discussion of the nursing implications for patients receiving chemical modifiers of radiation can be found in Noll.[22]

Combined Modality Therapy

Treatment of cancer with any single modality (surgery, chemotherapy, or radiation) does not always produce the desired effect of tumor eradication. Both chemotherapy and radiation therapy produce dose-limiting side effects that govern the extent of single modality treatment. In order to increase or improve the therapeutic index (ratio of tumor control vs. normal tissue damage), various combinations of chemotherapy and radiation have been studied for a number of years.

Ideally, a chemotherapeutic agent (or combination of agents) will shrink a tumor when given *prior to* local radiation (neoadjuvant chemotherapy); enhance or increase radiation cell kill when given *during* radiation (concomitant therapy); or control micrometastases and subclinical disease *after* a course of radiation (adjuvant therapy). Radiation and chemotherapy sometimes are given on a planned, alternating schedule using the so-called *sandwich technique*. This approach utilizes a split course of radiation in which the patient is treated with chemotherapy during a planned break in the total course of radiation therapy.[23]

Combined modality therapy is being used in the treatment of a variety of cancer types, including squamous cell cancer of the cervix, anus, head and neck, and lung. Cancers of the bladder, esophagus, pancreas, and stomach frequently are treated with both modalities in varying schedules. Vigorous combined modality therapy has allowed organ preservation for some individuals with carcinoma of the larynx, bladder, or anus.[23,24]

Some of the chemotherapeutic agents in common use for their radiosensitizing effect include cisplatin, methotrexate, doxorubicin, vinblastin, VP-16, mitomycin-C, 5-fluorouracil, actinomycin-D, and bleomycin. As would be expected, combined-modality therapy has the potential for enhanced side effects as well as enhanced tumor effect. Organ systems at greatest risk for toxicity are the gastrointestinal, integumentary, and myeloproliferative systems.

Nursing implications for care of the patient receiving combined-modality therapy are based on knowledge of any given individual's treatment plan and understanding of the principles of combined therapies. Coordination of treatment schedules sometimes is a nursing responsibility. More important, awareness of the drugs and radiation site and dose is an essential element in anticipating toxicities, monitoring acuity, and implementing appropriate care. Hirshfield-Bartek[25] and

Held and Volpe[23] present detailed nursing guidelines for assessment and management of the person receiving combined-modality therapy.

Hyperthermia

The use of hyperthermia to achieve a synergistic effect with radiotherapy has been studied and applied in clinical situations with considerable enthusiasm. Although it is technically arguable whether hyperthermia actually sensitizes tumor cells to radiation effect or simply combines to produce a greater effect than either modality can achieve on its own, researchers agree that this combined technique is warranted.[26–29]

The biologic basis for combining hyperthermia with radiation involves several factors. Heat is cytotoxic to cancer cells but is also destructive to healthy tissue if applied in excess of tolerable ranges. Controlled hyperthermia combined with radiation achieves tumor cell kill without excess toxicity.

Tumor cells are *least* radiosensitive during S-phase. Hyperthermia is *most* effective during S-phase; therefore, the combined effect on a tumor produces greater cell kill than either does alone. Similarly, hypoxic cells, which are generally radioresistant, have been found to be quite thermosensitive. Heat is also known to inhibit the repair of radiation damage, thus increasing the therapeutic ratio.

Valdagni et al.[30] reviewed the important parameters that may influence tumor response to combined hyperthermia and radiation therapy. Pretreatment parameters include tumor size, histologic findings, and disease site. Treatment parameters include total dose of radiation and dose per fraction, thermal dose, total and weekly number of hyperthermia sessions, and, finally, the sequencing of hyperthermia and radiation.

Hyperthermia is achieved in various ways, including immersion of the local area in a heated bath, ultrasound, microwaves, interstitial implants, and perfusion techniques. The choice of technique depends on whether local, regional, or whole-body hyperthermia is desired.[31–36]

Side effects of combined hyperthermia and radiation include local skin reaction, pain, fever, gastrointestinal effects, and cardiac arrhythmias. Late effects, such as necrosis and ulceration, can occur but do not seem to be significant enough to preclude continued use of this combined modality. Wojtas[37] details the nursing care of persons receiving hyperthermia treatments as well as the role nurses might take in administering the actual treatment. Table 13-3 provides an overview of the nursing care.

TABLE 13-3 Potential Nursing Responsibilities in Hyperthermia Treatment

Pretreatment evaluation phase
1. Assess suitability for treatment
2. Assess ability to tolerate treatment
3. Assess cardiac and neurologic status
4. Assess for presence of metal objects
5. Provide thorough patient and family education

Treatment phase
1. Vital signs, gastrointestinal preparation, sedation
2. Assist during surgical placement of thermometry probes
3. Position for comfort and access to applicator probes
4. Monitor patient throughout treatment
5. Provide physical and emotional support

Posttreatment phase
1. Clean and dress cannula sites
2. Observe and document thermal changes at treatment site
3. Provide discharge instructions
4. Manage subsequent local reactions

TISSUE AND ORGAN RESPONSE TO RADIATION

When discussing the effect of radiation on tissues, one must consider both the acute (or immediate) effects, seen within the first 6 months following treatment, and the late effects, seen after 6 months. In general, acute effects are due to cell damage in which mitotic activity is altered in some way. If early effects are not reversible, late or permanent tissue changes occur. These late effects can be attributed to the organism's attempt to heal or repair the damage inflicted by ionizing radiation.

The unit of radiation dose is called a *gray* (Gy). This term was officially adopted in 1985, replacing the term *rad* (an acronym for *r*adiation *a*bsorbed *d*ose). One Gy equals 100 rad. One cGy equals 1 rad.

In the following sections, radiation changes in normal tissues are presented according to body systems. It is important to remember that treatment volume, *dose rate* (number of cGy in a given unit of time), and *dose-time* factor (total number of cGy in a total number of days), as well as beam quality, may alter the tissue reaction. Except for those systemic effects described, radiation response is seen only in the tissues and organs that are within or immediately adjacent to the treatment field. Thus, an individual being treated to an abdominal field will not lose scalp hair from radiation, nor will the person being treated to the mediastinum develop radiation-induced diarrhea. Similarly, those persons undergoing brachytherapy will develop site-specific reactions to treatment, which vary with the site, dose, volume, and energy of the source. For example, cesium needle implants to the tongue will produce intraoral mucositis but usually no skin reaction. Application of a radioactive source intravaginally produces vaginal mucositis and often results in diarrhea due to the effect of radiation on the adjacent rectal mucosa. The important point to remember is that side effects from radiation are specific, and therefore preparation, teaching, and care must be planned for each individual.

Integumentary system

The outer layer of skin (epidermis) is composed of several layers of cells, with mature, nondividing cells at the surface and immature, dividing cells at the base. Normal mature cells constantly are being shed from the skin surface and replaced by new cells from the basal layer. This continual state of reproductive activity accounts for the high radiosensitivity of skin. Although the skin may be the primary site of radiation (as in skin cancer), it is also irradiated when any other site within the body is treated because radiation must pass through whatever tissues it encounters before reaching the target site. Depending on the equipment used and the beam quality, skin of the exit portal also may be affected. Erythema may be the only manifestation, or the skin reaction may progress to dry and then moist desquamation. Healing may be slow, but is usually complete and leaves minimal evidence of the acute damage except for changes in pigmentation. Fibrosis and atrophy may occur after high doses, as may ulceration, necrosis, and skin cancer. Such changes are uncommon with modern equipment and techniques. It is important to note that skin in certain areas, such as the groin, gluteal fold, axilla, and under the breasts, usually exhibits a greater and often earlier reaction to radiation due to the natural warmth and moistness in these areas and to friction caused by apposition of skin surfaces.

Use of the term *burn* or *radiation burn* to describe skin reactions is no longer appropriate. The severe skin reactions of the past are uncommon because of the skin-sparing effect of modern equipment. *Burn* implies accidental or unexpected damage, neither of which should take place in a controlled therapeutic setting. There are specific instances in which the person being treated will experience a severe reaction, especially when receiving electron beam therapy in the range of 5500–6000 cGy.

Skin reactions of this nature progress from a brisk erythema to a florid state, followed by a moist desquamation and loss of the epidermis. This, however, is an *expected* reaction because of the particular beam quality (see the earlier section entitled "Equipment and Beams Used in Radiotherapy"), and despite the severity of the acute reaction, the involved skin usually heals well.

Hair follicles and glands (sweat and sebaceous) are also radiosensitive. The radiosensitivity of the hair follicle is due to the relatively high rate of growth (mitotic activity) taking place; thus, these follicles are more susceptible to radiation damage. Under normal circumstances, hair grows and new hair is formed at a rate that keeps pace with the regular loss or shedding of the mature hair, with the net result being no obvious change in the amount of hair on the head. However, when the scalp is irradiated, the resulting inhibition of growth of new hair coupled with the accelerated hair loss due to damage to the follicle produces a net loss of hair, or *alopecia*. Epilation occurs in doses as low as a single dose of 500 cGy but is usually temporary. Regrowth may not begin for several months following the end of treatment, and the new hair may have a different quality or color. Higher doses (4500 cGy or greater) may produce permanent alopecia or delay regrowth for a year or more. Sebaceous and sweat glands usually will experience a decrease in activity during treatment and may cease functioning altogether at high doses (over 6000–7000 cGy). Return of function is proportional to the dose received.

Hematopoietic system

Red bone marrow is responsible for producing mature functional cells for the circulating blood. The stem cells are highly radiosensitive, and when large areas of red bone marrow (in the adult) are irradiated, including ilia, vertebrae, ribs, metaphyses of the long bones, skull, and sternum, the number of circulating mature cells decreases because production is suppressed. More erythroblasts (red blood cell precursors) are damaged by moderate doses than myeloblasts, but they recover rapidly, and thus anemia is not a prominent or early feature. Myeloblasts (white blood cell precursors) are suppressed at the same rate as erythroblasts, but the rate of recovery is much slower. Megakaryocytes (platelet precursors) are affected 1–2 weeks after exposure and take the longest time to recover (2–6 weeks).

Mature, nondividing blood cells in the circulating blood have a limited life span and are relatively insensitive to radiation. Peripheral blood does, however, reflect marrow activity. Thus, the person receiving radiotherapy may have depressed blood counts if sufficient radiation was given to active red bone marrow, especially if prior or concomitant chemotherapy has been given. The usual pattern seen in individuals whose marrow has been affected is a drop first in lymphocytes, then in neutrophils, and then in platelets and red blood cells. It sometimes is necessary to interrupt a course of radiotherapy for varying periods to allow the bone marrow to recover.

Radiation to the spleen alters its physiologic functions of hemolysis, red blood cell and iron storage, and antibody production, as well as causing shrinkage of the spleen itself.

Lymph nodes, like the spleen, are highly radiosensitive, whereas lymphatic vessels appear to be relatively radioresistant. Interference with lymphatic vessel function is thought to be caused by fibrotic changes and obstruction.

Gastrointestinal system

The gastrointestinal tract, from mouth to rectum, is lined with mucous membrane that contains layers of cells. A large proportion of these cells are undifferentiated and mitotic and are thus extremely radiosensitive. In addition, glandular tissue, ranging from large distinct bodies such as the parotids to multiple small mucous glands, is embedded in much of the mucous membrane. The effect of radiation on glandular tissue can be summarized as follows:

1. Initial swelling and edema of the epithelial lining of the ducts results in partial obstruction.
2. Secretion is inhibited by damage to the acini.
3. Atrophy and fibrosis occur as healing takes place, with permanent reduction in secretion, the amount depending on the dose received and the volume of mucous tissue irradiated.

Oral mucous membrane may develop a confluent mucositis, especially on the soft palate and the floor of the mouth, during the third and fourth weeks of therapy at the usual dose rate. Salivary function is altered as damage to the serous and mucous acini occurs, and saliva becomes viscous after moderate doses. Higher doses lead to atrophy of the salivary glands, with greatly diminished saliva and increased acidity. Such changes in saliva production and acidity often are permanent and are a factor in the development of radiation caries and infection. Alterations in the sense of taste occur early in treatment but are rarely permanent, depending on the dose of radiation received.

The esophagus and stomach also develop dose-dependent reactions. Changes in the glandular tissues of the stomach brought about by radiation are even more complex than those that occur in the glands of the oral mucous membranes. Gastric secretions, in addition to mucus, include pepsin and hydrochloric acid. When 1600 cGy are delivered in approximately 10 days to the stomach, all three secretions will be reduced; this may be accompanied by nausea, dyspepsia, and pyloric spasm. Inflammation of the mucosa (esophagitis and gastritis) occurs with moderate to high doses and produces dysphagia, anorexia, and sometimes nausea and vomiting. Late changes may include atrophy, ulcerations, and fibrosis.

The most sensitive area of the entire gastrointestinal tract is thought to be the small intestine. When one considers the length of the small intestine and also the fact that its loops overlap and fill a large portion of the abdomen, even a small radiation field of 5 × 8 cm on the abdomen will contain a large surface area of intestinal mucosa. Crypt cells (rapidly dividing, undifferentiated stem cells) arise from the base of the villi on a continuous basis to replace mature cells of the villi that are lost as part of the normal sloughing process. The high degree of radiosensitivity of these crypt cells and resultant changes in the intestinal villi account for the sometimes severe reactions that occur when abdominal or pelvic radiation is given.

Radiation reaction in the small intestine is characterized by shortening of the villi and loss of absorptive surface. Temporary reactions usually can be tolerated with minimal nutritional consequences. However, if reactions are prolonged and severe, as in some individuals receiving 5000–6000 cGy to the abdomen or pelvis, the nutritional consequences can be major. Shortening of the villi and denuding of the intestinal mucosa prevent adequate absorption of the end products of digestion, namely, amino acids (protein), simple sugars (carbohydrates), and glycerol and fatty acids (fats). Late changes following high doses of radiation include fibrosis, ulcerations, necrosis, and hemorrhage. Intestinal obstruction, although not common, can occur in a person receiving abdominal or pelvic irradiation. This is more likely to happen postoperatively, when the trauma of surgical manipulation combined with the previously discussed effects of radiation can result in paralytic ileus.

Such a reaction depends on many factors, including total dose, fractionation, volume, and site. Most individuals receiving pelvic irradiation experience only some degree of anorexia, nausea, diarrhea, or cramping, which can be managed readily with appropriate medication and diet.

The effect of radiation on the colon and rectum is similar to that seen in the small intestine, with the addition of the distressing symptom of tenesmus, which sometimes occurs when the anal sphincter is irradiated.

Liver

The liver is considered an accessory digestive organ and has been shown to be moderately radiosensitive. Although the parenchymal cells do have a regenerative capacity and are therefore vulnerable, the greatest damage produced by radiation to the liver is due to vascular injury. Early changes may be detectable only by liver function tests. However, radiation hepatitis is a possible consequence of doses over 2500 cGy, and the severity will depend on the volume irradiated.

Respiratory system

Mucous membrane lines the pharynx, trachea, and bronchi, and reactions that occur are due to the response of that sensitive tissue to irradiation. Hoarseness due to laryngeal mucous membrane congestion sometimes occurs. More significant in terms of radiation is the response of the bronchial tree and alveoli. Radiation pneumonitis, usually a transient response to moderate doses, is the result of changes in the alveolar wall plus the accumulation of exudate in the air sac, similar to pneumonia. Late changes are manifested by fibrosis in the lung tissue itself plus some thickening of the pleura. Such changes will compromise respiratory function in the area treated, but the degree of disability is related to the amount and condition of remaining untreated lung tissue.

Reproductive system

The cervix and uterine body are quite radioresistant and usually present no problem for the person being irradiated. However, vaginal mucous membrane responds to radiation much the same as the oral mucous membrane, with mucositis and inflammation. Following brachytherapy, vaginal stenosis due to permanent fibrotic changes is a potential problem. Radiation to the ovaries produces either temporary or permanent sterility, depending on the age of the person being treated and the dose of radiation. Permanent sterilization will occur at doses of 600–1200 cGy, and older women are sterilized at lower doses than younger women.

Maturation of graafian follicles and release of ova are essential for fertility. Radiation is most damaging to the intermediate follicle, thus preventing its development into a mature form. Small follicles are most radioresistant, and fertility may return if these small follicles are able to undergo repair and release ova. Mature graafian follicles are only moderately radiosensitive, and an ovum can be released, which accounts for the period of fertility that sometimes occurs after moderate doses of radiation.

In addition to sterility, hormonal changes (especially loss of estrogen production) and early menopause may occur. Perhaps most significant in terms of late or long-term consequences of radiation to the gonads in both the male and female is the potential for genetic damage. Chromosomal aberrations are a possibility that must be considered, especially at low doses. (For further reading on the genetic effects of radiation, the reader is referred to Travis,[9] BEIR III,[38] and Lushbaugh and Casarett.[39])

Radiation to the male testes damages and prevents maturation of the immature spermatogonia. Sterility can be permanent even after a dose of 500–600 cGy, and temporary sterility usually is seen following doses as low as 250 cGy.

Urinary system

Radiation-induced cystitis and urethritis are early and transient effects on the urinary tract that usually respond well to symptomatic treatment. Of major significance when considering the effect of radiation on the urinary system is damage to the kidneys in the form of nephritis. Early changes brought about by high doses of radiation lead to permanent fibrosis and atrophy, largely due to sclerosis of the vasculature. Renal failure and death can result. Protection of the kidneys is essential when the abdomen is irradiated.

Cardiovascular system

Damage to the vasculature of an organ or tissue (i.e., to stroma) can be the primary reason for the radioresponsiveness of that organ or tissue. Blood vessels (lined with epithelium) may become occluded when excessive cell production takes place during repair and regeneration in response to radiation injury. Thrombosis may be induced by the thickening that occurs during regenerative activity, thus further occluding the vessels. Late changes can be seen in the form of telangiectasia, petechiae, and sclerosis. The heart muscle itself is thought to be relatively radioresistant. However, at doses above 4000 cGy, pericarditis may occur in addition to the damage to the vasculature of the heart muscle.

Nervous system

The brain and spinal cord are considered to be relatively radioresistant, and peripheral nerves are even more so. However, therapeutic doses between 3000 and 6000 cGy have produced transient symptoms in the CNS, usually following a latent period in which no functional damage is seen. Especially noticeable is the response called *Lhermitte's syndrome,* which may occur following irradiation to the cervical cord. This syndrome is characterized by paresthesia in the form of shocklike sensations that radiate down the back and extremities when the neck is bent forward. Stretching of the cord in this manner compromises circulation, which may partially account for the sensations experienced. Myelopathy usually is transient, but at higher doses may lead to paralysis or paresis. When large volumes of the spinal cord (15 cm or more) are irradiated, doses of 4500–5000 cGy will produce transverse myelitis. The tissues of the nervous system are composed of a variety of cells, most sensitive of which are the neurons found in olfactory, gustatory, and retinal receptors. Radiation to these neurons can therefore alter or destroy the function of the particular sense organ. Because the nervous system is thought to be relatively radioresistant in itself, damage that does occur following radiation probably relates to vascular insufficiency. As described earlier, the vasculature of the body is radiosensitive. In addition, preexisting disorders such as diabetes, hypertension, and arteriosclerotic changes can enhance the effect of radiation on nervous tissue.

Skeletal system

Mature bone and cartilage are radioresistant and seldom present a problem in planning radiotherapy. However, late avascular necrosis can occur after high doses, causing pain and possible pathologic fracture. This is a relatively rare complication with supervoltage equipment.

Of much greater clinical significance is the effect of radiation on growing bone and cartilage. Children treated for spinal, thoracic, or abdominal tumors are susceptible to deformity as a result of radiation to the vertebrae. Failure to attain normal height due to spinal irradiation has occurred, as has shortening of a limb when the epiphyses are irradiated. Such orthopedic problems, although serious in themselves, may be considered a necessary compromise in terms of tumor eradication.

Systemic Effects of Radiation

Aside from or in addition to the specific local effects of radiation to tissues and organs already presented, the person receiving radiotherapy may experience certain subjective systemic effects, including nausea, anorexia, and malaise. Although the psychologic component of these symptoms cannot be overlooked, these systemic effects can theoretically be linked to the release of toxic waste products into the bloodstream resulting from tumor destruction. The presence of these toxins may account for the nausea and anorexia, whereas the increased metabolic rate required to dispose of the waste products might be partially responsible for the frequent complaint of fatigue. The physical effort needed to make a daily trip to the radiotherapy department for 4 or 5 weeks also may account for the malaise experienced by many individuals.

It is important to note that the response of the whole body (nausea, anorexia, malaise) to radiation of a limited site depends on the volume of the irradiated area, the anatomic site, and the dose. Consequently, not all individuals experience these systemic symptoms, and the degree of disability due to the symptoms will vary from mild to severe. Most individuals receiving radiotherapy tolerate treatment remarkably well and experience only mild systemic symptoms.

Whole-body and hemibody radiation

Whole-body and hemibody irradiation are relatively infrequent therapeutic applications of radiation. The effect on the person being treated varies with the dose, dose rate, and dose-time factor. For example, total-body irradiation of 150 cGy is being used in some centers in the treatment of chronic lymphocytic leukemia. This total dose is delivered at the rate of 5 cGy/day for 10 days, followed by a 2-week break, and then repeated for two more cycles to reach the total of 150-cGy. When total-body irradiation is delivered in this manner, which calls for small daily doses fractioned over a 10-week period, the side effects are negligible.

In contrast, radiotherapy given before bone marrow transplantation involves total body irradiation with 1000 cGy administered over 6–8 hours. Although the purpose of treatment in this instance is to suppress the bone marrow totally before transplantation with healthy marrow, this suppression presents a major problem in terms of patient management. With this high dose to the whole body, side effects are much greater and include nausea, vomiting, diarrhea, fever, erythema, alopecia, mucositis, parotitis, and pancreatitis, all of which occur in the immediate posttreatment phase. More severe skin reaction, cataracts, sterility, and major organ damage are delayed side effects.[40]

Hemibody radiation refers to treatment of the upper, middle or lower body in a single large fraction of approximately 500–800 cGy. This approach is used primarily for the person with widespread bone metastases to achieve rapid palliation of pain. Often, this individual has had one or several localized treatment courses, but no sooner achieves local pain relief than another site becomes problematic. Although individual sites can be treated sequentially, this is very time consuming as well as demoralizing for both patient and family. Treating a large volume in a single fraction is a viable alternative.[41]

Hemibody radiation, while generally effective in relieving pain, may produce significant side effects related to the site treated. Pretreatment medications such as antiemetics and steroids usually are administered for upper and mid-body treatment to alleviate nausea and possible radiation pneumonitis.

Lower hemibody radiation is better tolerated, although some patients experience brief periods of posttreatment nausea and occasional abdominal cramping or diarrhea. Bone marrow suppression is likely to occur because of the large volume treated. In addition, many patients who are candidates for hemibody treatment have had prior chemotherapy (and radiation) and are therefore already immunocompromised. Blood counts must be monitored pre- and posttreatment with hemibody radiation. If sequential hemibody treatment is required, there is usually a gap of several weeks between treatments to ensure marrow recovery.

Altered fractionation schedules

Standard treatment with radiation therapy calls for single daily fractions, given 5 days per week in daily doses in the range of 180 to 300 cGy. Patient tolerance, convenience, staff availability, and (most important) tissue tolerance are the factors governing today's standard fractionation schedules.

In the evolution of today's standard approach, numerous variations in time-dose relationships were tried, with results ranging from cure to severe radiation injury. Modern clinical experience with hyperfractionation began in the 1970s, progressing to randomized trials during the 1980s,[42] continuing into the 1990s. The development of flow cytometry allowed rapid measurement of tumor doubling time, increasing scientists' awareness of the danger of rapid tumor cell proliferation. These findings spurred further attempts to explore fractionation schemes in order to increase the therapeutic ratio of tumor cell kill versus normal tissue tolerance.

Two approaches to altered fractionation currently being explored are pure hyperfractionation and accelerated fractionation. Advanced, nonresectable, squamous cell carcinomas of various head and neck sites are the most frequent subject of these studies. *Hyperfractionation (HFX)* involves an increased number of fractions delivered over the same total treatment time as in standard fractionation. Typical doses are 115–125 cGy per dose, twice daily. *Accelerated fractionation (AFX)*, on the other hand, uses three fractions per day to achieve the same total dose as HFX while shortening overall treatment time by approximately 2 weeks.[43,44]

Horiot et al.[44] report that one study of HFX using two fractions per day has shown improved local-regional control without increasing incidence and severity of normal tissue damage, compared to a single fraction per day. Early results from an AFX study show that delivering three fractions per day is feasible; however, there is evidence of significant increase in acute morbidity and a trend indicating increased severe late effects.

One other alteration in standard fractionation schedule is the *dynamic* fractionation approach, in which doses are escalated over the length of the treatment course. One study calls for two fractions per day increasing from 150–200 cGy per fraction over 5 weeks.[43] Another study, cited by Fowler,[43] utilizes twice-daily fractions of 120–160 cGy plus two to four 200-cGy doses, achieving a total dose of 7200–7600 cGy in 5 weeks' time. As with any research, large prospective clinical trials are needed in order to determine efficacy as well as practicality of altered fractionation schedules in radiation oncology.

Chronic low-dose exposure

Chronic low-dose radiation exposure occurs to all persons, due to background radiation from naturally occurring radioactive substances and cosmic rays.[45,46] Such exposure is largely unavoidable and within the safe limits defined by federal regulations. Radiation workers are exposed to a somewhat higher level of ionizing radiation, but the allowable limit is well below that which is known to produce ill effects.

Total-body radiation syndrome

Total-body radiation syndrome refers to the effects of the acute exposure of the organism to doses of radiation received in a matter of minutes rather than hours or days. Acute exposure of human beings has been studied through data obtained from industrial and laboratory accidents, individuals exposed at Hiroshima and Nagasaki, Pacific Testing Grounds fallout exposure, and medical treatment procedures.[47] Doses of 150–2000 cGy delivered to the whole body in a short time produce life-shortening or lethal damage through effects on the hematopoietic, gastrointestinal, and central nervous systems. The April 1986 nuclear accident in Chernobyl, Ukraine, undoubtedly will produce additional significant information about the somatic and genetic effects of exposure to high levels of radioactivity. For greater detail and for information on the effects of radiation exposure to the embryo and fetus, the reader is referred to Travis.[9]

Radiation-induced malignancies in humans

The carcinogenic effects of radiation, often called "late effects," from both chronic low-dose exposure and acute exposure to the whole body are of particular interest and concern to the nurse, especially in providing support to the person who is hesitant about accepting treatment. The key to understanding lies in the fact that acute exposure and chronic low-dose exposure are the exceptions, occurring in radiation accidents, occupational exposure, and the early stages of the development of the science of radiotherapy. The usually prescribed therapeutic doses (in the range of 2500–6500 cGy) are believed to be less carcinogenic than lower doses given over a much longer time period. Theoretically, a cell that has survived in a damaged or altered state after low-dose irradiation may undergo carcinogenic mutation in the presence of other conditional factors. On the other hand, a cell that has been sterilized or destroyed by therapeutic doses of radiation should be incapable of malignant changes.

The most common malignancies associated with radiation exposure are skin carcinoma and leukemia, and evidence also implicates radiation in some sarcomas, thyroid carcinoma, and lung cancer.[48–51] Recent reports have suggested the possibility of inducing breast cancer in females by frequent radiographic exposure for screening for tuberculosis, other lung disease, and breast cancer itself.

Radiation carcinogenesis depends on a number of variables. These include a latent period of from 1 to 30 years, radiation dose, concomitant factors in the radiated organism's environment, and the actual fate of the cell as it responds to radiation injury. For a comprehensive review of radiation carcinogenesis, the reader is referred to Bucholtz.[52]

NURSING CARE OF THE PATIENT RECEIVING RADIOTHERAPY

Caring for the person receiving radiotherapy gives nurses an opportunity to put into practice all the theory and science acquired in their education and work experience. The person receiving radiotherapy is first and foremost a person with all the needs and problems generated by the diagnosis of cancer. Care cannot focus solely on the disease site (i.e., a "lung" patient, a "cervix" patient, a "Hodgkin's" patient, and so on). Nor can nursing care be based solely on meeting the immediate needs generated by treatment and its side effects without considering the individual's long-term needs. Nursing care must be individualized and holistic, intelligent and thoughtful, scientific and compassionate. All these qualities can be achieved in nursing care of the person receiving radiotherapy. By applying the scientific background material provided in earlier sections of this chapter and using specific nursing care measures detailed in the following pages, the nurse will be able to devise a comprehensive plan of care for each individual receiving radiotherapy.

Assessing the individual's situation is the first step in planning care. A number of questions must be asked and answered:

1. What is the diagnosis? The prognosis?
2. What is the goal of treatment?
3. Does the person know and understand the diagnosis?
4. Does the family (or significant others) know and understand the diagnosis?
5. What is the plan of treatment? Radiotherapy alone? Surgery? Chemotherapy? All three?

6. Will therapy be given on an inpatient or an outpatient basis?
7. What does the person know and understand about radiotherapy?
8. Where can the correct information about the individual's treatment plan be obtained?

When the person with cancer is an inpatient, the staff should begin this assessment on admission and build on the care plan as the diagnosis becomes available and treatment plans are formulated by the medical staff. Coping with the diagnosis may be the only crisis a particular person can handle at this early stage; elaborate plans and explanations about treatment may go largely unheard as the person struggles to resolve feelings about the diagnosis of cancer. In contrast, another individual moves quickly past the diagnosis and literally pleads to get treatment under way before a total care plan has been formulated. Each person must be assessed and managed on an individual basis.

In seeking answers to some of the assessment questions posed previously, the hospital nurse can turn to the patient's physician, the patient, and the family. After the person has been referred to a radiation oncologist and evaluated, the physician (and nursing staff from that department, if available) can provide further information that can be useful in devising the care plan.

What are some of the facts about radiotherapy the nurse must understand when caring for the person in the pretreatment phase? How can these facts be incorporated into the nursing care plan? Most individuals newly diagnosed with cancer have a number of misconceptions about treatment stemming from the experiences of other persons. The worst side effects are always the ones that are remembered and are often exaggerated in the retelling. Of course, side effects do occur, but their severity depends on such factors as treatment site, treatment volume, fractionation, total dose, and so on, and especially on the individual being treated. Knowing what side effects can be expected and, most important, knowing that measures are available to alleviate most symptoms can be reassuring to the person. In general, most individuals respond best to a reassuring pretreatment discussion in which side effects specific to their treatment are discussed, stressing that symptomatic relief is available. Knowing what to expect usually helps prevent the person from worrying that a treatment-related side effect represents a worsening or recurrence of disease. At this time the nurse can also mention briefly the reactions that will not occur. Some might argue that this only puts ideas into the anxious person's mind, but most people are reassured to know, for example, that they will not lose their hair or be nauseated if this is the case.

Thus nurses should know the facts about treatment site and potential side effects when they are caring for individuals before and during radiotherapy. Most people experience few or at least manageable side effects in today's modern and well-equipped radiotherapy departments and offices. Many individuals are able to continue working, perhaps with some changes in schedule, or manage a home and family just as they did before diagnosis and treatment. Others are debilitated by the disease or treatment, making it impossible to continue in their former roles.

In planning nursing care for the person receiving radiotherapy, another important consideration is the length of the treatment course. Specifically, it is important to determine the need for transportation following discharge and to help the individual and family obtain this transportation. Although some palliative treatment is given over a period of 7–10 days (often while the patient is hospitalized), most individuals receive radiotherapy for an average of 5 weeks, and some may be treated over 7 or 8 weeks. The person with stage III Hodgkins' disease receiving total nodal irradiation will be making trips to the radiotherapy department for approximately 3 months, with several 2-week breaks interspersed. Transportation must be arranged on a daily basis for these lengthy periods.

Some individuals are able and willing to drive themselves, and some have family and friends who can provide this service, but many, especially elderly persons, are without transportation on a steady basis and will need assistance. Sources of transportation vary, but some available services are as follows:

- senior citizens transportation (a federal or locally funded service in many parts of the United States)
- American Red Cross
- American Cancer Society
- religious groups (FISH)
- service and civic organizations

In addition to meeting transportation needs, explaining potential side effects, and dispelling misconceptions, the staff nurse or community nurse can provide a great service to the individual undergoing radiotherapy by describing the treatment facilities and equipment. People are sometimes frightened by the size and complexity of the equipment, the perceived impersonal attitude of the staff, and the fact that they must be alone in the room during treatments. Of course, no nurse can be familiar with every radiotherapy facility. However, nurses working in oncology settings or regularly caring for individuals with cancer should make it a part of their own education to visit and familiarize themselves with radiotherapy departments and facilities. Persons being treated and visitors sometimes are disturbed by the fact that a radiotherapy facility is in a basement or an underground location. Again, a factual explanation about the necessity for proper shielding will help allay some of these fears.

The well-informed nurse who is familiar with local radiotherapy facilities can provide the support and reassurance needed during the pretreatment phase of a person's illness. The confidence that familiarity brings can significantly increase the nurse's ability to meet some of the pretreatment needs of a person about to begin radiotherapy.

The personnel an individual comes in contact with during radiotherapy can play an important role in alleviating anxiety. The radiation oncologist, who prescribes, directs, and evaluates treatment, is primarily responsible for the person's care during treatment and for varying periods afterward. This often is done in conjunction with a family physician, oncologist, or surgeon. Nurses employed by a radiotherapy department can offer much of the supportive care needed to cope with the emotional and physical needs of the person being treated and the family. Symptomatic relief of side effects, nutritional support, and social and financial assistance are all nursing concerns. Coordination of complex treatment schedules and protocols also may be part of the nurse's role. Some departments employ one or more nurses to meet these patient needs, and in others an oncology nurse is shared by both medical and radiation oncology. The reality is that nurses are in short supply in radiotherapy departments, and nursing needs often go unmet. This is why the role of the staff nurse, office nurse, or community nurse is so important.

The person with whom the patient has the most frequent contact and establishes the closest relationship is very often the radiation therapist. The therapist is a highly skilled individual, certified by the American Society of Radiologic Technologists, and is responsible for giving the daily treatments under the direction of the radiation oncologist. Although the therapist's primary focus is the physics and mechanics of treatment, attention is also given to the person being treated as a human being with particular wants and needs. Nursing care sometimes is carried out by the therapist in departments where there are no nurses. However, it would be unfair to expect that a radiation therapist could or would be able to devote as much attention to nursing needs as to the technical responsibilities of the job. In recognition of this need for combined skills, some centers have employed, trained, and prepared nurses for certification as radiation therapists.

Regardless of who will be treating and caring for the person in a radiotherapy department, it is important and comforting for the individual and family to know that caring individuals are available who will try to make the total treatment experience as untraumatic as possible. Most individuals experience few or no treatment-related problems, and those who do can for the most part be managed effectively. The person being treated should be encouraged to ask questions, report symptoms, and regard radiotherapy as part of a total plan for managing the cancer.

Assessment of individual needs and implementation of nursing interventions are ongoing processes in oncology nursing. For individuals receiving radiotherapy, this is especially true because needs change as treatment progresses. Initial nursing concerns focus on diagnosis and the person's acceptance of treatment, preparation (both physical and psychologic) for treatment, transportation arrangements, and so on. As treatment progresses, many of the initial fears and misconceptions disappear, and the person settles into the somewhat routine process of coming for daily treatments. Expected side effects usually occur after 10–14 days, depending on dose, volume, and site. Individuals undergoing treatment frequently count the days and keep track of the number of treatments received. Although a plan has been made from the beginning prescribing the number of daily fractions, this plan is subject to change as the radiation oncologist deems appropriate. There are a number of reasons for adding to, subtracting from, or changing the plan, and if the person understands this from the beginning, changes will not be interpreted as signs of recurrence or disease progression. Although most individuals want to know how many treatments will be given so that they can adjust their activities accordingly, they should be helped to understand that this number is subject to change.

Apathy or a sense of futility may develop as treatment progresses and the person does not see any obvious changes in his or her disease. Visible lesions frequently can be observed to shrink or disappear with treatment, and this is encouraging. However, when a tumor is not visible or when treatment is an adjunctive measure in cases where no known lesion exists, the person being treated sometimes finds it difficult to continue in the absence of obvious and immediate benefits. This is especially true if side effects produce symptoms that are more troublesome than those created by the disease. Regardless of the setting, the nurse plays a vital role at this point in helping the person to accept and continue treatment for its long-term potential despite the immediate discomforts. A telephone call to the physician, nurse, or therapist in the department from the nurse caring for the person in another setting can be helpful in such situations.

SPECIFIC NURSING CARE MEASURES FOR PATIENTS RECEIVING RADIOTHERAPY

During a course of radiotherapy, certain treatment-related side effects can be expected to develop, most of which are site specific as well as dependent on volume, dose fractionation, total dose, and individual differences. Many symptoms do not develop until approximately 10–14 days into treatment, and some do not subside until 2 or more weeks after treatments have ended.

Nursing care measures and medical management described in the following sections reflect the policy and practices that have proved most effective in one particular practice. It should be noted that alternative means do exist for management and nursing care, any of which may be suitable to the particular setting in which they are practiced.

Fatigue

Fatigue or malaise is common among persons with cancer, and may be even more pronounced during and after a course of radiation treatment. Although a number of theories exist that attempt to explain radiation-induced fatigue, the mechanism is not well understood.[53,54]

Some of the potential contributors to the fatigue experienced with radiation treatment are relatively obvious and therefore may be amenable to interventions. Table 13-4 lists the more common factors contributing to fatigue.[55] Nursing assessment of the contributing factors is particularly important, for these factors can often be addressed. Pain management is especially important, since chronic, uncontrolled pain is one of the most wearisome challenges faced by some patients. Extra rest and a reduction in the normal activity level may be necessary during treatment. Individuals receiving radiation treatments should be encouraged to nap, go to bed early, or alter their daily schedule to allow for rest periods rather than to "fight it," as some are prone to do. Some individuals report that taking a nap immediately after returning home from their treatment gives them enough energy for the rest of the day. Others prefer to retire earlier than usual at night. The person who is bedridden at home or is hospitalized will need provisions for rest and quiet according to individual need.

Pretreatment patient education should include the potential for fatigue during treatment. With knowledge that treatment-induced fatigue usually is self-limiting, most patients are better able to tolerate this common side effect.

Anorexia

Anorexia occurs frequently among individuals receiving radiotherapy, regardless of the treatment site. Anorexia, like fatigue, is probably related to the presence in the person's system of the waste products of tissue destruction. Other possible causes for anorexia include anemia, inactivity, medications, alterations in the person's ability to ingest and digest foods, and psychologic factors. The cause often cannot be identified clearly, and therefore the symptom must be treated utilizing all the techniques known to encourage adequate intake. A self-perpetuating cycle of anorexia/weight loss/weakness/inactivity/anorexia can develop if the symptom is untreated. For detailed information on the management of anorexia and cachexia in the individual with cancer, see Chapter 27 in this text, and Iwamoto.[56]

TABLE 13-4 **Factors Contributing to Fatigue in the Patient Receiving Radiation Treatment**

- Recent surgery
- Prior or concurrent chemotherapy
- Pain
- Malnourishment
- Medications
- Frequency of treatment visits
- Maintaining usual lifestyle
- Tumor burden
- Anemia
- Respiratory compromise

Mucositis

The reaction produced by radiation to the mucous membranes in any part of the body (gastrointestinal, genitourinary, and respiratory systems) is called *mucositis.* Mucositis can be described as a patchy, white membrane that becomes confluent and may bleed if disturbed. This reaction is most visible when radiation is given to the mouth and oropharynx, and severe reactions cause considerable discomfort to the person. A number of measures can be employed in treating mucositis in the oral cavity, but it is first important to enlist the patient's cooperation in avoiding irritants such as alcohol, tobacco, spicy or acidic foods, very hot or very cold foods and drinks, and commercial mouthwash products (they are too astringent even when diluted). Although a 1:1 solution of hydrogen peroxide has been used for mouth care for many years, this solution can actually be very damaging to tissues if it is not diluted correctly. Normal saline is an acceptable solution, although it does little to refresh the mouth. One ounce of diphenhydramine hydrochloride (Benadryl) elixir diluted in 1 quart of water provides an ideal agent for mouth care in individuals with mucositis. The diphenhydramine hydrochloride solution provides a soothing, nontoxic, pleasant-tasting means for the person to rinse and gargle as needed. Mouth care should be done as often as every 3 or 4 hours and is especially important before mealtime. One technique is to use an air-powered spray apparatus to deliver a fine mist of the diphenhydramine hydrochloride solution, which can be directed at all surfaces of the mouth and oral cavity. This irrigation technique is effective in loosening retained food particles, breaking up the usually tenacious mucus, and soothing the mucosa. Care should be taken not to dislodge the plaquelike formations of mucositis, because dislodgement will cause bleeding and denude the mucosal surface. Outpatients can receive this irrigation treatment daily, as can inpatients when they are brought to the radiotherapy department for their radiation treatment. In addition, inpatients can be given mouth care by a modified technique at their bedside several times daily. A disposable irrigation bag is hung from an intravenous pole, using gravity to deliver a spray of solution to the mouth and oropharynx.

In addition to diphenhydramine hydrochloride mouth care solution, agents that coat and soothe the oral mucosa, such as Maalox, are sometimes used. Lidocaine hydrochloride 2% viscous solution may provide some relief from discomfort, but the anesthetic effect, especially on the tongue, is objectionable to some individuals. This active approach to mouth care for radiation-induced mucositis enables most individuals to tolerate the effects of radiation better. Occasionally, a break from treatment will have to be given when reactions are excessive, but constant, daily nursing support appears to be a factor in promoting tolerance of treatment.

Xerostomia

The dry mouth resulting from radiation to the salivary glands or portions of them is known as *xerostomia.* Alterations in taste frequently accompany xerostomia. Whether the condition is temporary or permanent depends on the dose received and the percentage of the total salivary tissues irradiated. During the course of radiation, little can be done to relieve this annoying symptom. The sensitivity of the mucous membranes precludes the use of saliva substitutes at this point, and frequent sips of water seem to be the best method of providing moisture. Saliva, though present, is thick and viscous, often causing the person to gag and to expectorate with difficulty. Frequent mouth care, especially before meals, will provide some relief. When a course of therapy has ended and any intraoral reaction has subsided, some individuals will benefit from the use of a saliva substitute to provide moisture and lubrication for 2- to 4-hour periods. During the night, xerostomia causes the person to awaken frequently with a dry, almost choking sensation that is relieved only by taking a drink of water. Some individuals find that using the saliva substitute allows them to sleep uninterrupted for several hours. A small container of this mixture can be carried easily in pocket or purse for use when the person is away from home. The formula for saliva substitute is as follows:

- Cologel 98.2 ml
- Glycerin 110.0 ml
- Saline 1000.0 ml

The solution should be mixed well and refrigerated. It is stable for 3 months. The person with xerostomia should use 1–2 teaspoons every 3 or 4 hours. The solution is swished in the mouth and swallowed. Several brands of saliva substitute are available for over-the-counter purchase.

Radiation Caries

Although it is a potential late effect of irradiation to the mouth and oropharynx, radiation caries can be greatly reduced or avoided by proper care before, during, and after a course of treatment. Absence or decrease in saliva and the altered pH produced by treatment promote decay. Before the start of therapy, a thorough dental examination and prophylaxis should be carried out. If extensive decay and generally poor dentition exist, full mouth extraction is usually the treatment of choice. However, if teeth are in good repair, a vigorous preventive program is begun to protect them from the late effects of radiation. This can include daily diphenhydramine hydrochloride mouth sprays for their cleansing effect, followed by a 5-minute application of fluoride gel. Brushing the teeth with a soft-bristled brush several times daily is also important. Such vigorous efforts to prevent decay in individuals receiving radiotherapy can be initiated by the nurse, and nursing support and encouragement are necessary in helping to ensure continuation of this preventive treatment when radiotherapy is completed.

A patient information sheet on oral and dental care is shown in Table 13-5.

Esophagitis and Dysphagia

When radiation is directed to the mediastinum, as, for example, in treating patients with cancer of the lung or breast or Hodgkin's disease, areas of the esophagus may receive a sufficient dose to produce symptoms of esophagitis.[56] This is a transient effect in which the esophageal mucous membrane becomes somewhat edematous, and mucositis can develop. The patient will first notice some difficulty in swallowing solids, which is often described as "a lump in my throat, only deeper." This may then progress to a definite esophagitis, which makes swallowing painful and can be responsible for a decrease in intake of foods and fluids. Newer treatment techniques are available that minimize this effect, and a treatment technique or schedule can be adjusted to allow the reaction to subside. The following mixture provides temporary relief from radiation esophagitis:

Radiotherapy mixture

Mylanta (Stuart)—450 ml (three 5-oz bottles)

Lidocaine hydrochloride viscous 2%—100 ml

Diphenhydramine hydrochloride elixir—60 ml

Shake well and refrigerate

Dosage: 1–2 tablespoons 15 min ac and hs

When esophagitis occurs, ensuring adequate nutrition becomes a major nursing concern. The person receiving treatment should be encouraged to substitute high-calorie, high-protein, high-carbohydrate liquids and soft, bland foods for their regular meals. Eggnogs, milk shakes, "instant" liquid meals, and commercially prepared liquid supplements all may be used between meals as well as substituted for solids. Blenderized foods from the person's regular diet are less expensive than commercial products, and the person with esophagitis should be encouraged to try this method.

The individual and family need continual encouragement and support through this difficult period. Weight loss caused by decreased intake can be inter-

TABLE 13-5 Dental Care for Patients Receiving Radiation to the Mouth Area

Before You Start Radiation Treatments:
Make an appointment with your dentist for dental prophylaxis. This includes inspection, polishing, scaling of teeth (if indicated), flossing, and repair or restoration of existing teeth. Daily fluoride treatments are necessary to help prevent future dental problems. Ask your dentist to recommend either a fluoride rinse or gel and applicator tray.

During a Course of Radiation Treatment:

Helpful Hints	Stay Away from These
• Use a soft toothbrush, brushing gently after meals and at bedtime.	• Do not use any commercial mouthwash.
• Use toothpaste if desired. Otherwise, just brush with lukewarm water.	• Avoid very hot foods and drinks.
• Use Benadryl mouthwash as a rinse and gargle 4–6 times daily or more often as needed. Directions for this mouthwash will be given to you.	• Do not drink alcoholic beverages.
• Eat a high-calorie, high-protein diet including plenty of liquids. Instant breakfast drinks and nutritional supplements such as Ensure and Meritene help add calories and protein.	• Do not smoke.
• Eat soft/bland foods if mouth is sore (eggs, custard, pudding, potato, cheese, milk and ice cream drinks).	• Avoid spicy, highly seasoned foods, and acidic foods such as oranges, grapefruit, and tomatoes.
• We will provide you with nutritional information and hints on food preparation.	

If You Wear Dentures:
Dentures or partial plates may be cleaned in your usual manner. If your mouth becomes irritated, we may ask you to stop wearing dentures except at mealtime.

Source: Courtesy of Philip G. Maddock, MD, and Laura J. Hilderley, RN, MS, Radiation Oncology, Warwick, RI.

preted by the person undergoing therapy as treatment failure and lead to a defeatist attitude. The temporary nature of the esophagitis and dysphagia should be emphasized.

Nausea and Vomiting

Of the potential side effects from radiotherapy, nausea or vomiting or both are probably the most distressing to the person being treated. Although nausea and vomiting are not common, the fear that they will occur causes great stress in many individuals. As with other side effects, treatment site and volume are the variables to be considered, along with preexisting conditions related to surgery, chemotherapy, and sites of disease. The patient's emotional state and apprehension about the disease and treatment are sometimes responsible for nausea when treatment is unlikely to be the cause.

Generally, the person receiving radiotherapy can be expected to experience some degree of nausea when treatment is directed to any of the following sites: whole abdomen or portions of it, large pelvic fields, hypochondrium, epigastrium, or para-aortic areas.

Some patients report nausea with whole-brain irradiation or wide mediastinal fields. However, the majority of patients experience little or no difficulty with this side effect. When nausea does occur, it usually can be controlled by antiemetics administered on a regular schedule and by adjusting the eating pattern so that treatment is given when the stomach is relatively empty. Delaying intake of a full meal until 3 or 4 hours after treatment is also helpful because nausea, if it occurs, will usually appear from 1 to 3 hours after treatment.

Diarrhea

Diarrhea, like nausea and vomiting, is not an expected side effect in most individuals receiving radiotherapy. However, it does occur if areas of the abdomen and pelvis are treated after about 2000 cGy have been given. Some individuals experience only an increase in their usual number of bowel movements, whereas others develop loose, watery stools and intestinal cramping. Occasionally, treatment must be interrupted to allow the bowel to recover from radiation effects, especially in elderly or debilitated individuals. When diarrhea and vomiting both occur, active intervention with intravenous fluids for short-term replacement may be needed, as well as a rest from treatment.

For most individuals with radiation-induced diarrhea, a low-residue diet and prescription of loperamide hydrochloride usually are sufficient. The low-residue diet may be all that is required in some instances. Many individuals are not sufficiently knowledgeable about foods and their composition to manage this on their own, and a low-residue diet sheet has been developed to supplement the teaching done by the nurse (Table 13-6). When reviewing the diet with the person being

TABLE 13-6 Low-Residue Diet for Control of Radiation-Induced Diarrhea

Foods Allowed	Foods to Avoid
BEVERAGES	
Skim or low-fat milk, tea, soda, Gatorade, ice milk, sherbet, low-fat yogurt (plain, vanilla, lemon), buttermilk	Coffee, beer, liquor, fruit juice, chocolate milk, cocoa, hot chocolate
BREADS AND CEREALS	
White bread and rolls, plain muffins, saltines, melba toast, cream of wheat or rice, farina, corn and rice cereals, well-cooked oatmeal	Dark, whole-grain breads, rolls and cereals (eg, whole wheat, cracked wheat, bran, pumpernickel, rye, granola, wheat germ, shredded wheat, bran flakes, cereals with dried fruits and nuts)
STARCHY FOODS	
White potatoes (no skin), plain spaghetti, macaroni, noodles, other pasta (no tomato sauce), white rice	Sweet potatoes, potato skins, brown or wild rice, pizza
VEGETABLES	
Well-cooked carrots, squash, green beans	All other vegetables (cooked or raw), especially cabbage, broccoli, brussels sprouts, baked beans, kidney beans, peas, radishes, cucumbers, corn
FRUITS	
Bananas, apples in any form (baked, raw, applesauce, apple juice)	All other fruits and juices
MEATS AND MEAT SUBSTITUTES	
Chicken (stewed, creamed, broiled, or baked, all without skin), turkey, lean beef, veal, pork, lamb, ham, fish, canned or well-washed clams, cottage cheese, hard cheese, eggs	All fried, tough, or spicy meats, hot dogs, sausage, poultry skins, gritty seafood, pork and beans, peanut butter
MISCELLANEOUS	
Broth, bouillon, consomme, creamed soups, salt, sugar, jelly, honey, plain jello, custard, tapioca pudding, other puddings (except chocolate), hard candies	All seasonings, jams, pickles, popcorn, olives, coconut, nuts, dried seeds, chocolate cake and chocolate cookies

Source: Courtesy of Philip G. Maddock, MD, and Laura J. Hilderley, RN, MS, Radiation Oncology, Warwick, RI.

treated (and with the individual preparing meals at home), it is especially important to emphasize the "Foods Allowed" and to point out that a daily multiple vitamin should be included. Vitamin C is notably lacking from the diet, as well as those vitamins found in leafy green vegetables. A favorite food from the "Foods to Avoid" list may be added now and then, if it does not increase symptoms. Diets such as this one should be individually designed to meet the particular geographic and ethnic food patterns of the population, hence the inclusion of well-washed clams and pasta without sauces on the sample.

Tenesmus, Cystitis, and Urethritis

Although infrequent, tenesmus, cystitis, and urethritis do occur in some individuals receiving pelvic irradiation. Tenesmus of the anal or urinary sphincter produces a persistent sensation of the need to evacuate the bowel or bladder. Relief sometimes can be obtained from gastrointestinal and urinary antispasmodics and anticholinergic preparations. The problem may persist, however, until after the course of treatment has ended.

Cystitis and urethritis resulting from radiation to the bladder area is distressing to the person being treated and usually is brought to the physician's or nurse's attention soon after it develops. A clean-voided urine specimen for culture and sensitivity testing should be obtained, and appropriate antibiotic therapy instituted if indicated. Usually, no infection is found, and treatment consists of urinary antiseptics and antispasmodics for symptomatic relief. High fluid intake is encouraged. Sitz baths, which are commonly prescribed for tenesmus, cystitis, and urethritis, are contraindicated if the perineal area is being irradiated. The added moisture will only enhance any potential or actual skin reaction.

Alopecia

The loss of hair is traumatic to most people, regardless of whether they are prepared for this change in body image. The needless fear of this loss is equally traumatic, and if patients are prepared for radiotherapy that does not include the scalp, they should be reassured that hair loss will not occur as a result of treatment.

During treatment of the whole brain, as in metastatic disease or for primary brain tumor, alopecia will occur and follows a typical pattern. At about 2500–3000 cGy fractionated over 2 or 3 weeks, the patient will notice excessive amounts of hair in the brush or comb and a gradual thinning of the hair. This continues for 2 or 3 weeks, and then quite suddenly most of the hair comes out, and the patient awakens to find the remainder of his or her hair on the pillow. The patient who is prepared for this with a wig or attractive scarves or caps will adjust to this change with less emotional trauma than one who is totally unprepared either emotionally or physically.

In some instances hair loss may occur regionally or in patches rather than over the entire scalp. Examples include the patient being treated for a pituitary lesion with a two- or three-field technique involving portals of approximately 6 × 6 cm or the person receiving mantle irradiation for Hodgkin's disease that includes the suboccipital lymph nodes. The latter patient will lose hair at the base of the scalp from the hairline to several centimeters above, with a strip remaining in the midline due to a block inserted to protect the spinal cord. Whenever possible, the person being treated with this or similar field arrangements in which patchy hair loss is expected should be advised to grow the hair longer. In some instances the long hair can be combed to cover areas of alopecia.

Care of the hair and scalp while receiving radiation to the scalp includes very gentle brushing or combing and infrequent shampooing. Permanent waves and hair coloring are contraindicated because of the potential harm to the irradiated skin of the scalp. Individuals being treated in the neck or facial areas should likewise avoid any procedures on the hair that involve the use of harsh chemicals, because such substances may run down onto treated skin. As in the case of irradiated skin in general, the scalp should be treated with care and caution for several months to a year or more after all healing has taken place. The top of the head, especially in males (who have less of a protective layer of hair), should be protected from sunburn with a cap. The forehead, ears, and neck also may exhibit more sensitivity to the sun than before radiation treatment was given.

Skin Reactions

The response of normal skin to radiation treatments varies from mild erythema to moist desquamation that leaves a raw surface similar to a second-degree burn. Because megavoltage and cobalt beams deliver the maximum dose beneath the skin, skin reactions have become less significant. Although an acute response may occur during the course of therapy in which brisk erythema progresses to dry and then moist desquamation, healing and cosmesis usually are satisfactory. Some individuals may exhibit a permanent tanning effect in the treatment area, with no change in the texture of the skin and subcutaneous tissues. Other individuals will have fibrosclerotic changes in the subcutaneous structures, and their skin will be smooth, taut, and shiny. Telangiectasia also may be evident.

Acute and chronic changes in irradiated skin depend on many factors that govern the severity and permanence of the radiation effect.[57,58] As in other treatment-related side effects, total dose, fractionation, and volume are important factors. Quality of the treatment beam and its percentage depth dose (see the section entitled "Applied Radiation Physics," earlier in the chapter) will determine the amount of skin sparing. Individuals treated with electron beams will exhibit considerable skin reactions when the electron beam is intended for lesions located on the skin or a few centimeters below the surface. Characteristics of the electron beam are such that maximum dose buildup occurs within 1 cm below the skin, especially at energies below 20 MeV. However, even more severe reactions that include area of moist desquamation and peeling will heal well, leaving some patchy depigmentation and telangiectasis.

Skin in some areas of the body, such as the groin, perineum, buttocks, inframammary folds, and axillae, has a relatively poor tolerance to radiation. This is due to the normal warmth and moisture found in these areas rather than any characteristic of the skin itself. Reactions to radiation in these sites are likely to be more severe than in adjacent areas receiving identical treatment.

Because moisture enhances skin reactions, the person being treated should be advised to keep the skin in the treated area as dry as possible. Bathing or showering is permissible, but long periods of soaking are inadvisable. Treated skin should be bathed gently with tepid water and mild soap. The area should be rinsed thoroughly and gently patted (not rubbed) dry. Lines or markings placed on the skin at simulation should not be removed until the radiation therapist advises the patient to do so. It may therefore be necessary for the patient to take sponge baths rather than tub baths or a shower for some time to avoid washing off the markings.

General guidelines to follow for care of the skin within the treatment site include the following:

1. Keep the skin dry.
2. Avoid using powders, lotions, creams, alcohol, and deodorants.
3. Wear loose-fitting garments.
4. Do not apply tape to the treatment site when dressings are applied.
5. Shave with an electric razor only. Do not use preshaves or aftershaves.

6. Protect the skin from exposure to direct sunlight, chlorinated swimming pools, and temperature extremes (hot water bottle, heating pad).

Such precautions are necessary throughout the course of treatment and until any skin reaction has disappeared afterward.

Specific measures useful in treating skin reactions include the use of a light dusting of cornstarch for pruritus from erythema and dry desquamation. If moist desquamation and denuded areas appear, a thin layer of A and D ointment may be applied, followed by a Telfa (nonstick) dressing to protect the clothing and the skin. The therapist or radiation oncology nurse should always be consulted regarding specific skin care measures appropriate to the individual.

When planning for skin care for the person receiving radiotherapy, it should be remembered that individuals often are treated by parallel opposing portals and only one of these portals may be marked to indicate the field. This means that in addition to the clearly marked portal on the person's abdomen or chest (for example), there may be a corresponding field on the posterior that needs the same careful attention. A telephone call to the nurse or therapist will provide the information needed to identify the treatment portal or portals. Tattoos that indicate the treatment site (as described in the earlier section entitled "Simulation and Treatment Planning") also may be present on the person's skin and may be helpful in determining which areas of skin require special care.

Skin care in radiotherapy varies considerably from one treatment center to another.[58] The radiotherapy nurse or physician should always be consulted about skin care if there is any question concerning institutional or office policy. Outpatients should be given explicit directions for managing at home, and written directions are very helpful in addition to the verbal instructions (see Table 13-7).

TABLE 13-7 Skin Care During Radiation

Skin over the area where you are receiving radiation therapy needs to be treated with gentle care. During your course of radiation treatment, please follow these guidelines:

Keep the treated area dry and free from irritation.

- Do not wash the treated area until the therapist tells you to. This may not be until 2 or 3 days after the start of treatments.
- Do not remove the lines or ink marks that have been placed on your skin until your therapist or doctor tells you to.
- When permitted, wash the treated skin gently, using a mild soap, and rinse well before patting dry. Always use warm or cool water, *not* hot water.
- Do not apply any lotions, creams, alcohol, aftershave, perfume, deodorants, etc. to the treated area.
- Heating pads and hot water bottles should not be used on treated skin.
- Avoid friction; that is, avoid clothing that is tight or may rub over the treated skin, such as shirt collars, ties, undergarments, belts.
- Men should use an electric razor if they are receiving treatment to the face and/or neck area. Do not use aftershave.
- If treated skin becomes reddened or tender, you may apply a thin layer of Vitamin A&D ointment. Be sure to tell us when this happens. If further irritation develops, we will give you special instructions or medications for skin care.
- Protect the treatment area from exposure to direct sunlight. While you are receiving a course of therapy, do not sunbathe or spend more than a few minutes in the bright sun if the treated area is exposed. We will give you special instructions about future sun exposure when you finish your course of treatment.

Source: Courtesy of Philip G. Maddock, MD, and Laura J. Hilderley, RN, MS, Radiation Oncology, Warwick, RI.

One area of skin care about which there usually is some question is the matter of exposure to the sun. Any restrictions on exposure apply only to the treated area or areas. No special precautions are needed for sites that normally are covered by clothing when outdoors. (One exception is skin that exhibits a moderate or severe reaction to radiation, which may become sunburned when protected only by a sheer or light fabric covering.) During treatment and for a month or more afterward, treated skin should not be exposed to direct sunlight. Individuals whose treatment site is exposed usually can go from home to car or elsewhere for brief periods without difficulty. However, during seasons when the sun is most intense or in locales where the exposure is more intense, even a brief trip outdoors without protective garments may enhance the reaction on treated skin, depending on the dose of radiation received. Caution and common sense should prevail.

When a course of radiotherapy has ended and after any reaction has subsided and healed, a cautious approach to sunbathing may be resumed. Previously treated areas may be exposed gradually (15 min/day), using a number 15 sunblock. Each person must determine his or her own tolerance to the sun and proceed accordingly.

Because of the skin-sparing effect of today's treatment machines, most individuals are able to enjoy outdoor activities without incident after their treatment course has ended. Again, it is important to emphasize caution and common sense. A patient information sheet for sense in the sun is shown in Table 13-8.

Bone Marrow Depression

When large volumes of active bone marrow are irradiated (especially the pelvis or spine in the adult), the effect on the marrow can be quite significant. Other areas of concern when large fields are treated include the sternum, ribs, metaphyses of the long bones, and

TABLE 13-8 Sense in the Sun After Radiation Treatment

Skin that has been treated with radiation will need special attention in the bright sunlight. When your course of radiation therapy is finished, you may have some dryness or raw areas in the treatment field. These will clear up in a few weeks with continuation of the special care instructions given to you during treatment.

Until the skin is completely healed, you should not expose the area to sunlight. When healing is complete, you may gradually begin to sunbathe, using a #15 sunscreen in the treated area, and increasing the exposure time very slowly and carefully. If the area becomes reddened or irritated—discontinue sun exposure. You may have to wait another season before trying again.

Wear a T-shirt, cover-up, broad-brimmed hat or some other means of protecting the treated skin. Remember that a thin, gauzelike layer of fabric does not block the harmful ultraviolet light.

Remember that the beach is not the only place where sunburns can occur. Use caution when riding in the car with your arm, neck, and face near a sunny window, when working in the yard or garden, at a ballgame or other summer outing, in a boat, and even when skiing on a bright sunny day.

While these instructions for special care refer primarily to skin that has been treated with radiation, we urge you to use care and common sense in general whenever the sun is bright.

Source: Courtesy of Philip G. Maddock, MD, and Laura J. Hilderley, RN, MS, Radiation Oncology, Warwick, RI.

skull. During simulation and treatment planning, provision is made for shielding as much of this active marrow as possible without compromising the treatment. Because of careful planning and trimming of fields to include only the necessary volume, the majority of people receiving radiotherapy are able to tolerate a course of treatment without experiencing bone marrow depression. Nonetheless, weekly blood counts should be done on all individuals receiving radiotherapy and two to three times weekly in some instances. The latter is necessary for individuals receiving concomitant chemotherapy or those who have had extensive chemotherapy before radiation. A notable example would be the person with Hodgkin's disease or non-Hodgkin's lymphoma who has received several cycles of combination chemotherapy. Individuals receiving total-body irradiation or splenic irradiation for chronic lymphocytic leukemia will require daily blood counts before treatment to avoid (or at least anticipate) a precipitous drop in the white blood cell or platelet counts.

For the person whose bone marrow is affected by treatment or a combination of factors, a number of support measures can be employed. Transfusions of whole blood, platelets, or other components may be necessary for the patient who has dangerously low counts, and treatment may have to be adjusted or interrupted. Nursing care should include observation of the person for signs and symptoms of bleeding, anemia, and infection. Patients and their families must be taught what to look for and to report to the physician, therapist, or nurse whenever symptoms occur.

Radiation Side Effects: Special Considerations

As previously stated, most people are less anxious if told ahead of time what specific side effects they may expect from their treatment. Knowing that diarrhea is quite likely to result from pelvic irradiation will help the person prepare for such an event, both in terms of dietary adjustments and in helping to avoid embarrassing accidents. There are, however, a number of side effects that do not occur with any predictability or regularity, and an individual being treated would not necessarily benefit from knowing about them ahead of time. The nurse, who is sometimes the first caregiver to whom a person may report symptoms, should be aware of these less common but possible side effects of radiotherapy to specific sites.

Transient myelitis

When lymph nodes in the cervical region are radiated, as in the mantle technique employed when treating patients with stage III Hodgkin's disease, the spinal cord is blocked to protect it from unnecessary radiation. However, a radiation effect on the spinal cord can still occur. Some individuals will experience paresthesia (a shocklike sensation radiating down the back and over the extremities) when flexing the neck. This is known as Lhermitte's syndrome and occurs after a latent period of 2–3 weeks after treatment to the site has ended. The symptoms usually improve gradually or spontaneously, leaving no permanent effect. The dose of radiation that can produce a transient myelopathy is well below the dose that results in a permanent injury to the spinal cord. A possible explanation for the symptoms found in Lhermitte's syndrome is the effect of radiation on the vasculature supplying the cervical cord. If the blood vessels are compromised by radiation injury, stretching or bending the neck can cause a temporary occlusion and decrease in blood supply to the cord, resulting in paresthesia. Paresthesias can be frightening to a person. However, the temporary nature of this effect can be stressed and the person reassured that this is a known side effect that sometimes occurs.

Parotitis

Parotitis is a painful swelling and inflammation of the parotid glands that sometimes occurs in individuals receiving radiation to the maxillomandibular area. It may occur with mantle irradiation for Hodgkin's disease, as well as with treatment to the area for other forms of cancer. The onset of symptoms is sudden and usually follows the first two or three treatments. Although uncomfortable, the symptoms subside almost as quickly as they arise, and no specific treatment is necessary.

Visual and olfactory disturbances

During radiation to the pituitary area, some individuals occasionally experience visual or olfactory disturbances, which can be distressing. Some have reported seeing lights or smelling something burning, among other things, after several treatments. The explanation for this phenomenon lies in the anatomic proximity of the optic and olfactory nerves to the hypophysis and the fact that ionization taking place in or near these structures can cause alterations in the sensations of sight and smell. A multiple-field technique is usually employed when treating patients with pituitary lesions to deliver a high dose to the tumor with a minimal dose to surrounding structures. However, the optic nerves, chiasma, and optic tract lie between the hypophysis and the bulk of the brain, and the olfactory bulb and tract lie superior and anterior to the hypophysis, which means that the olfactory and optic structures are likely to be included in the field arrangement. Again, reassurance and explanation tailored to the person's ability to understand are the best means of handling these disturbing but uncommon side effects.

Radiation recall

Although not technically a radiation reaction, *radiation recall* can occur in a previously irradiated site that exhibited mucositis or erythema. Radiation recall occurs in response to the systemic administration of certain chemotherapeutic agents (for example, actinomycin) several months to a year or more after radiation was received. Typically, the person develops intraoral mucositis or a skin reaction in the exact pattern corresponding to the previously treated radiation portal. Treatment is symptomatic, and the drug dosage or choice of agent may be modified if necessary.

NURSING CARE OF THE PATIENT WITH A RADIOACTIVE SOURCE

Nursing care of individuals being treated with implanted radioactive sources is a challenge that goes beyond basic medical-surgical theory and requires an understanding of radiation safety, biology, and physiologic manifestations. Rather than fear, the nurse should develop a healthy respect for all that is implicit in working with radioactive isotopes and proceed to plan and deliver optimum care under the special conditions encountered in each situation.

Radioactive materials for therapeutic usage are listed in Table 13-1 and specific sources for brachytherapy are outlined in Figure 13-5. In addition to being implanted in tissues or inserted into body cavities, some radioactive isotopes may be administered orally, intravenously, or by instillation. These materials are absorbed or metabolized by the body, and specific safety precautions are required, depending on the particular source and mode of administration. Adsorbed or metabolized isotopes used most commonly include ^{131}I, ^{32}P, and ^{198}Au, all of which are administered as colloids or solutions. Liquid souces such as these present a possibility of contamination of equipment, dressings, and linens, depending on the mode of administration and metabolism. In contrast, sealed sources such as ^{137}Cs and ^{226}Ra for implantation through a mechanical device are not metabolized and therefore are not excreted in body fluids.

The following information is necessary to provide safe and effective nursing care for individuals being treated with brachytherapy (sealed radioactive source placed within a body cavity or tissue) or with metabolized or adsorbed radiation:

1. What is the source being used?
2. What is the half-life of that source?
3. What is the type of emission (alpha, beta, gamma)?
4. How much radioisotope is being used (energy)?
5. What method of administration/application is being used?
6. Is the source metabolized? adsorbed? neither?

From this information, the nurse can plan and administer nursing care utilizing the appropriate precautions, including disposal of wastes and care of linens and equipment. This information will also help to determine whether radiation safety precautions are necessary after hospital discharge.

Radiation safety and radiation protection are the concern of every caregiver involved with brachytherapy patients. This includes the radiation oncologist, other physicians, nurses, therapists, physicists, and allied health workers who may come in contact with the person being treated. Leading this team is the radiation safety officer employed by the institution to implement radiation safety procedures and monitor all use of radioactive materials. Most institutions will also have a radiation safety committee composed of representatives from among the disciplines listed previously, whose responsibilities are the control and enforcement of the use of radioisotopes in the hospital as required by the Nuclear Regulatory Commission.

Three primary factors in radiation protection should be foremost in the minds of all personnel involved in care of the person being treated: *time, distance,* and *shielding.*

Time

The exposure to radiation that personnel receive is directly proportional to the time spent within a specific distance from the source. Nursing care must be planned and organized so that the nurse spends as little time as possible in close contact with the individual being treated while still providing for his or her needs.

Distance

As radiation is emitted from a point source, the amount of radiation reaching a given area decreases according to the law of inverse square. Figure 13-13 illustrates this principle.

Shielding

When a sheet of absorbing material is placed between a radiation source and a detector, the amount of radiation that reaches the detector decreases, depending on the energy of the radiation and the nature and thickness of the absorbing material (shield). The thickness of a shielding material that is required to reduce the radiation to half of its original quantity is referred to as the *half-value layer* (HVL). The HVL for ^{137}Cs (a commonly used radioactive source) is approximately 6 mm of lead or 10 cm of concrete. The practical implications of this should be evident.

When planning nursing care for the person with a radioactive source, time and distance are the two variables that can most readily be controlled. Because shielding from gamma radiation requires lead or concrete in the previously specified thicknesses, it is usually impractical to expect that much physical care can be given from behind such a shield. Portable radiation shields (similar in design to a moving blackboard on wheels) are available and do protect the caregiver who places it between himself or herself and the source. However, this is useful primarily in doing tasks within the person's room other than direct care. The so-called lead aprons used in diagnostic radiology are not of sufficient thickness to stop gamma rays and cannot protect the caregiver from exposure when caring for individuals with radium or cesium sources, for example.

Because shielding is not always possible or practical, time and distance are the two factors that nurses must incorporate into the care plan. Some of the ways in which exposure to personnel can be reduced are listed in Table 13-9.

Patient Education and Support

With all the emphasis on haste and elimination of nonessential care, it is sometimes easy to eliminate that most important consideration of emotional and social support of the person being treated. Individuals who are isolated for radiation precautions often feel "unclean" or "contaminated." The fact that visitors are allowed only at the doorway and that housekeeping personnel are barred from the room adds to this sense of isolation. Because the nurse also must limit the time spent in giving direct care, the person's sense of rejection often is heightened.

Planning and providing emotional support are major components of nursing care for all individuals, but

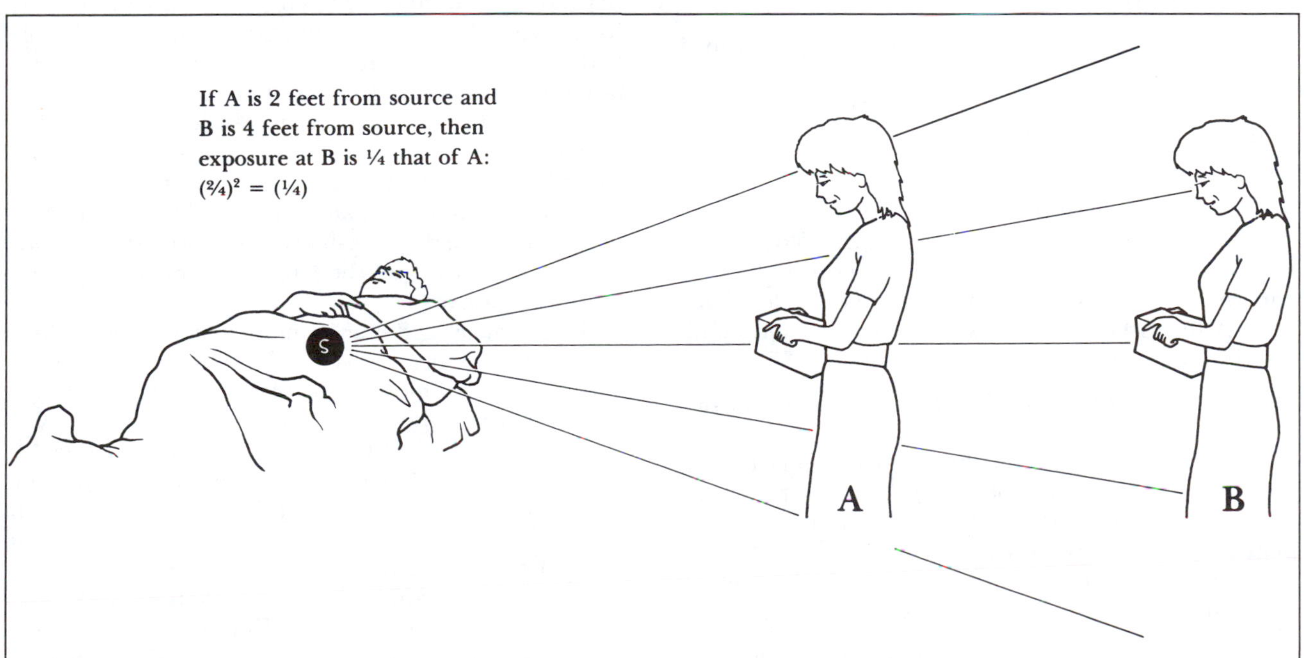

FIGURE 13-13 The inverse square law. As distance from a radiation source increases, exposure decreases by the square of that distance.

TABLE 13-9 Some Ways to Reduce Exposure to Personnel Providing Care for the Individual with a Radioactive Source

1. Use appropriate radiation precaution signs, wristbands, and tags.
2. Plan care to avoid delays at the person's bedside.
3. Eliminate the bedbath except for what the person can manage alone.
4. Change linens less frequently or only when soiled.
5. Prepare meal trays outside of the person's room instead of at the bedside (cut up meats, open containers, etc.).
6. Work quickly; concentrate on accomplishing the necessary tasks in as short a time as possible.
7. Position the bedside table, call bell, and television controls within easy reach of the person to avoid frequent return trips to the bedside.
8. Use appropriate monitoring devices and heed the information regarding total individual exposure.
9. Never care for more than two individuals at a time with radioactive sources.
10. Keep long-handled forceps and a shielded transport cart in the person's room at all times.
11. Use long-handled forceps to retrieve a radioactive source that has accidentally been dislodged.
12. Arrange the chair so that ambulatory individuals can be seated as far from the bed (and thus the caregiver) as possible while linens are being changed.

especially for those with an implant or other form of radioactive material. Preparation for these procedures should include all the following points of information:

1. *Description of the procedure.* For example, although performed in the operating room under anesthesia, insertion of vaginal tandem and ovoids will not involve a surgical incision.

2. *Possible change in appearance.* For example, individuals with needle implants in the facial region often request a mirror and should be prepared for their sometimes grotesque appearance while needles are in place.

3. *Anticipated pain or discomfort and measures available for relief.* For example, the presence of gynecologic applicators (such as in Figure 13-6) combined with bed rest and restricted movement often produces a low backache. Appropriate analgesics are prescribed and should be administered as needed.

4. *Potential short-term and long-term side effects and complications.* An example of a short-term side effect: Needle implants to the tongue usually produce edema, causing the tongue to be noticeably swollen during the procedure and for several days afterward. A long-term complication, such as occurs with vaginal brachytherapy, may result in scarring and the formation of adhesions that cause dyspareunia.

5. *Restrictions on activity while the radioactive sources are in place.* For example, individuals with gynecologic applicators in place are confined to bed for the duration of the treatment, which may be as long as 3–4 days.

6. *Visiting restrictions.* For example, policy varies depending on the availability of appropriate shielding devices and the energy of the sources being used. However, visitors usually are restricted from the person's room, and, when allowed, visits must be brief.

7. *Radiation precautions observed by hospital personnel.* For example, individuals should be reassured that their personal care needs will be met but that the nurses' time at the bedside and in the room will be restricted because of the presence of the radiactive sources.

The person also should be helped to prepare for such procedures by planning for suitable activities such as reading, handwork, television, and so on. Boredom and isolation sometimes are the most difficult part of treatment with a radioactive source. The nurse has a primary responsibility to meet those treatment-induced needs, as well as those of a physical nature.

With the proper application of the principles of radiation safety and careful attention to the special emotional needs of individuals being treated with brachytherapy, this challenge for nursing care can be met.

ADVANCES IN RADIOTHERAPY

Radiation oncology in the 1990s will be characterized by continual refinement of treatment techniques and expanded application of multimodal therapy. Numerous cooperative group studies employ radiation as primary or adjuvant therapy. Variations such as hyperfractionation (more than one treatment per day) for particularly resistant tumors are being tested. Whole-body or hemibody irradiation for widespread metastasis is providing rapid palliation for some individuals.[41]

Use of particle radiation such as fast neutrons, deuterons, helium ion beams, and negative pi-mesons will continue to be tested and refined for use in situations where conventional radiation is of little value. The expense and limited applicability of such treatment methods currently confine their use to a small proportion of cancer patients.

In February 1989, an announcement was made of the first proton beam accelerator built for hospital use. This device was moved out of the physics laboratory setting (Fermi Laboratory in Illinois, Harvard University, the University of California at Berkeley, as well as several sites abroad), where limited numbers of patients had been treated since the early 1970s. Loma Linda University Medical Center, Los Angeles, began using the $40 million treatment device in 1990.

Radio-labeled antibody therapy has been the subject of considerable interest and effort since the 1970s.[59] This treatment technique is based on the information acquired in recent years regarding immunobiology and the isolation of many tumor-specific monoclonal and polyclonal antibodies. Among the numerous radioactive isotopes that have been used therapeutically, ^{131}I and ^{90}Y, in particular, have been adopted for use in radio-labeled antibody therapy.

The underlying principle of radio-labeled antibody therapy involves attaching a radioactive isotope to the tumor-specific antibody to deliver therapeutic radiation directly to the target tumor. Theoretically, this avoids prolonged radiation exposure to healthy cells while delivering lethal or sublethal doses to the tumor. Among numerous phase I, II, and III clinical trials over the past two decades, some of the more significant results have been achieved in the treatment of hepatoma.[60] Studies involving treatment of intrahepatic biliary carcinoma, nonresectable, non-oat-cell carcinoma, and recurrent Hodgkin's disease are ongoing.[60]

Intraoperative radiotherapy (IOR) was developed in the United States during the late 1970s at Howard University and at Massachusetts General Hospital.[61] Unresectable tumors had been the primary target of IOR before the 1980s. By 1985, however, IOR was used increasingly in a prophylactic approach combined with resection of primary tumors, such as locally advanced colorectal carcinoma; pancreatic, gastric, and bladder cancers; and soft-tissue sarcomas.

Compared with external beam therapy, intraoperative radiotherapy has the advantage of increasing tumor dose in relation to normal tissue dose. After surgically exposing the target volume, a single, large fraction of radiation is delivered directly to the tumor site by a specially built cone attached to the therapy machine. The surgical procedure is then completed, and a further postoperative course of conventional radiotherapy is given. Some institutions give a preoperative rather than postoperative course of conventional radiotherapy, but rarely is IOR the definitive treatment.

There are a number of differences in the exact IOR procedures at the various institutions in the United States now using IOR.[62,63] Although some have installed radiotherapy equipment in an operating room or built a special room to perform the combined therapy, others have worked out a detailed procedure for transporting the fully anesthetized and surgically opened patient through the hospital corridors to the radiotherapy department. Despite the technical difficulties in performing IOR, it appears to have potential for further development and application in cancer management.

CONCLUSION

Radiotherapy in the treatment of cancer has indeed come a long way from its exciting beginning in the late 1800s. Much has been learned about the beneficial as well as the harmful effects of ionizing radiation. The 1990s continue to hold promise for advances in cancer treatment, with radiotherapy playing a major role in primary treatment as well as in combined modality approaches.

Along with advances in therapy there has been increased recognition of the important role of the nurse as educator and care provider for persons receiving radiation treatment and their families. As new radiation centers open and others are restructured, nurses are increasingly being added to the team of caregivers. Previously nurses had been involved somewhat peripherally in care of radiotherapy patients, but they are now taking a major role as collaborative caregivers with the radiation oncologist. Advances in nursing science and nursing care parallel advances in radiotherapy as a treatment modality.

REFERENCES

1. Berry RJ: Basic concepts in radiobiology: A review. In Mansfield CM (ed.): *Therapeutic Radiology: New Directions in Therapy*. New Hyde Park, NY: Medical Examination Publishing Co., 1983, pp. 1–15.
2. Suit H, Urie M: Proton beams in radiation therapy. *Natl Cancer Inst* 84:155–164, 1992.
3. Maddock PG: Brachytherapy sources and applicators. *Semin Oncol Nurs* 3:15–22, 1987.
4. Shell J, Carter J: The gynecological implant patient. *Semin Oncol Nurs* 3:54–66, 1987.
5. Hall EJ, Cox JD: Physical and biologic basis of radiation therapy. In Moss WT and Cox JD (eds.): *Radiation Oncology: Rationale, Technique, Results*. St. Louis: Mosby, 1989, pp. 1–57.
6. ———: *International Brachytherapy. Programme and Abstracts 7th International Brachytherapy Working Conference, Sept. 6–8, 1992, Baltimore/Washington*. Veenendaal, Netherlands: Nucletron International B.V., 1992.
7. Jordan L, Mantravadi RVP: Nursing care of the patient receiving high dose rate brachytherapy. *Oncol Nurs Forum* 18:1167–1171, 1991.
8. Jordan L, Buck S: A teaching booklet for patients receiving high dose rate brachytherapy. *Oncol Nurs Forum* 18:1235–1238, 1991.
9. Travis E: *Primer of Medical Radiobiology*. Chicago: Year Book Medical Publishers, 1975.
10. Hall EJ: *Radiobiology for the Radiologist* (ed. 2). Hagerstown, MD: Harper & Row, 1978.
11. Richter MP, Share FS, Goodman RL: Principles of radiation therapy. In Calabrese P, Schein PS, and Rosenberg SA (eds.): *Medical Oncology: Basic Principles and Clinical Management of Cancer*. New York: Macmillan, 1985, pp. 280–291.
12. Bergonie J, Tribondeau L: Interpretation of some results of radiotherapy and an attempt at determining a logical technique of treatment. *Radiation Res* II:587, 1959.
13. Gray LH: Radiobiologic basis of oxygen as a modifying factor in radiation therapy. *Am J Roentgenol* 85:805, 1961.
14. Withers HR, Peters LJ: Biologic aspects of radiotherapy. In Fletcher GH (ed.): *Textbook of Radiotherapy* (ed. 3). Philadelphia; Lea & Febiger, 1980, pp. 103–180.
15. Withers HR: Biologic basis of radiation therapy. In Perez CA and Brady LW (eds.): *Principles and Practice of Radiation Oncology*. Philadelphia: Lippincott, 1987, pp. 67–98.
16. Phillips TL: Chemical modification of radiation effects. *Cancer* 39:987–999, 1977.

17. Brown JM: Hypoxic cell radiosensitizers: Where next? *Int J Radiat Oncol Biol Physics* 16:987–993, 1989.
18. Coleman CN, Wasserman TH, Urtasun RC, et al: Phase I trial of the hypoxic cell radiosensitizer SR 2508: The results of the five to six week drug schedule. *Int J Radiat Oncol Biol Physics* 12:1105–1108, 1986.
19. Hall EJ, Miller R, Astor M, et al: The nitroimidazoles as radiosensitizers and cytotoxic agents. *Br J Cancer* 37 (suppl 3):120, 1978.
20. Phillips TL: Sensitizers and protectors. *Semin Oncol* 8:65–82, 1981.
21. Fowler JF: Chemical modifiers of radiosensitivity-theory and reality: A review. *Int J Radiat Oncol Biol Physics* 11:665–674, 1985.
22. Noll L: Chemical modifiers of radiation therapy. In Hassey-Dow K, Hilderley L (eds.): *Nursing Care in Radiation Oncology*. Philadelphia: Saunders, 1992, pp. 264–274.
23. Held J, Volpe H: Bladder preserving combined modality therapy for invasive bladder cancer. *Oncol Nurs Forum* 18:49–57, 1991.
24. Sischy B: The use of radiation therapy combined with chemotherapy in the management of squamous cell carcinoma of the anus and marginally resectable adenocarcinoma of the rectum. *Int J Radiat Oncol Biol Physics* II:1587–1593, 1985.
25. Hirshfield-Bartek J: Combined modality therapy. In Hassey-Dow K, Hilderley L (eds.): *Nursing Care in Radiation Oncology*. Philadelphia: Saunders, 1992, pp. 251–263.
26. Gonzalez D, van Dijk JDP, Blank LE, et al: Combined treatment with radiation and hyperthermia in metastatic malignant melanoma. *Radiother Oncol* 6:105–113, 1986.
27. Bicher HI, Wolfstein RS, Lewinsky BS, et al: Microwave hyperthermia as an adjunct to radiation therapy: Summary experience of 256 multifraction treatment cases. *Int J Radiat Oncol Biol Physics* 12:1667–1671, 1986.
28. Howard GCW, Sathiaseelan V, Freedman L, et al: Hyperthermia and radiation in the treatment of superficial malignancy: An analysis of treatment parameters, response and toxicity. *Int J Radiat Oncol Biol Physics* 3:1–8, 1987.
29. Valdagni R, Amichetti M, Pani G: Radical radiation alone versus radical radiation plus microwave hyperthermia for N3 (TNM-UICC) neck nodes: A prospective randomized clinical trial. *Int J Radiat Oncol Biol Physics* 15:13–24, 1988.
30. Valdagni R, Fei-Fei L, Kapp D: Important prognostic factors influencing outcome of combined radiation and hyperthermia. *Int J Radiat Oncol Biol Physics* 15:959–972, 1988.
31. Hand J, ter Haar G: Heating techniques in hyperthermia. *Br J Radiol* 56:969–970, 1983.
32. Guy A, Chou CK: Physical aspects of localized heating by radiowaves and microwaves. In Storm F (ed.): *Hyperthermia in Cancer Therapy*. Boston: GK Hall, 1983, pp. 279–304.
33. Scott R, Johnson R, Story K, et al: Local hyperthermia in combination with definitive radiotherapy: Increased tumor clearance, reduced recurrence rate in extended followup. *Int J Radiat Oncol Biol Physics* 10:2119–2123, 1984.
34. Bahman E, Perez C: Interstitial thermoradiotherapy: An overview. *Endocuriether/Hypertherm Oncol* 1:35–40, 1985.
35. Sapozink M, Gibbs F, Egger M, et al: Abdominal regional hyperthermia with an annular phased array. *J Clin Oncol* 4:775–783, 1986.
36. Shimm D, Cetas T, Oleson J, et al: Regional hyperthermia for deep-seated malignancies using the BSD annular array. *Int J Hypertherm* 4:159–170, 1988.
37. Wojtas F: Hyperthermia and radiation therapy. In Hassey-Dow K, Hilderley L, (eds.): *Nursing Care in Radiation Oncology*. Philadelphia: Saunders, 1992, pp. 307–319.
38. BEIR III: The effects on populations of exposure to low levels of ionizing radiation. Report of the Advisory Committee on the Effects of Ionizing Radiation (BEIR III). Washington, DC: National Academy of Sciences, National Research Council, 1980.
39. Lushbaugh CC, Casarett GW: The effects of gonadal irradiation in clinical radiation therapy: A review. *Cancer* 37:1111–1120, 1976.
40. Schryber S, LaCasse CR, Barton-Burke M: Autologous bone marrow transplantation. *Oncol Nurs Forum* 14:71–80, 1987.
41. Dudjak L: Alternatives in dose fractionation and treatment volume. In Hassey-Dow K, Hilderley L (eds.): *Nursing Care in Radiation Oncology*. Philadelphia: Saunders, 1992, pp. 285–294.
42. Thames HD: On the origin of dose fractionation regimens in radiotherapy. *Semin Radiation Oncology* 2:3–9, 1992.
43. Fowler JF: Intercomparisons of new and old schedules in fractionated radiotherapy. *Semin Radiation Oncology* 2:67–72, 1992.
44. Horiot JC, LeFur R, Schraub S, et al: Status of the experience of the EORTC Cooperative Group of radiotherapy with hyperfractionated and accelerated radiotherapy regimes. *Semin Radiat Oncol* 2:34–37, 1992.
45. Upton AC: The biological effects of low level ionizing radiation. *Sci Am* 246:41–49, 1982.
46. Harley N: Physics: Environmental sources of radioactivity levels and interaction with matter. In Upton AC, Albert RE, Burns FJ, et al (eds.): *Radiation Carcinogenesis*. New York: Elsevier Science, 1986.
47. Kato H, Schull WJ: Studies of the mortality of A-bomb survivors. Mortality, 1950–78. I. Cancer mortality. *Radiat Res* 90:395–432, 1982.
48. March HC: Leukemia in radiologists in a twenty-year period. *Am J Med Sci* 220:282, 1950.
49. Pack GT, Davis J: Radiation cancer of the skin. *Radiol* 84:436, 1965.
50. Conrad RA, Hicking A: Medical findings in Marshallese people exposed to fallout radiation: Results from a ten-year study. *JAMA* 214:316, 1970.
51. Stewart A: An epidemiologist takes a look at radiation risks. DHEW pub no. 73-8024. Washington DC: U.S. Government Printing Office, 1973.
52. Bucholtz J: Radiation carcinogenesis. In Hassey-Dow K, Hilderley L (eds.): *Nursing Care in Radiation Oncology*. Philadelphia: Saunders, 1992, pp. 342–357.
53. Piper BF, Lindsey AM, Dodd MJ: Fatigue mechanisms in cancer patients: Developing nursing theory. *Oncol Nurs Forum* 14:17–23, 1987.
54. Aistars J: Fatigue in the cancer patient: A conceptual approach to a clinical problem. *Oncol Nurs Forum* 14:25–30, 1987.
55. Hilderley L: Pain and fatigue. In Hassey-Dow K, Hilderley L (eds.): *Nursing Care in Radiation Oncology*. Philadelphia: Saunders, 1992, pp. 57–68.
56. Iwamoto R: Altered nutrition. In Hassey-Dow K, Hilderley L (eds.): *Nursing Care in Radiation Oncology*. Philadelphia: Saunders, 1992, pp. 69–95.
57. Sitton E: Early and late radiation-induced skin altera-

tions, Part I: Mechanisms of skin changes. *Oncol Nurs Forum* 19:801–807, 1992.

58. Sitton E: Early and late radiation-induced skin alterations, Part II: Nursing care of irradiated skin. *Oncol Nurs Forum* 19:907–912, 1992.
59. Bucholtz J: Radiolabeled antibody therapy. In Hassey-Dow K, Hilderley L (eds.): *Nursing Care in Radiation Oncology*. Philadelphia: Saunders, 1992, pp. 275–284.
60. Sitzman JV, Order SE, Klein JL, et al: Conversion by new treatment modalities of non-resectable hepatocellular cancer. *J Clin Oncol* 5:1566–1573, 1987.
61. Goldson A: Past, present, and prospects of intraoperative radiotherapy (IOR). *Semin Oncol* 8:59–64, 1981.
62. Kinsella TJ, Sindelar WF: Newer methods of cancer treatment: intraoperative radiotherapy. In DeVita VT, Hellman S, Rosenberg SA (eds.): *Principles and Practice of Oncology* (ed. 2). Philadelphia: Lippincott, 1986, pp. 2293–2304.
63. Smith R: Intraoperative radiation therapy. In Hassey-Dow K, Hilderley L. (eds.): *Nursing Care in Radiation Oncology*. Philadelphia: Saunders, 1992, pp. 295–306.

Chapter 14

Chemotherapy: Principles of Therapy

M. Tish Knobf, RN, MSN, FAAN

Henry J. Durivage, PharmD

INTRODUCTION

The past 50 years of cancer research have produced a wide variety of effective chemotherapeutic and hormonal agents (Figure 14-1).[1] Drug development and clinical drug trials during this period have been dramatically influenced by advances in basic science. The knowledge generated from these advances has increased our understanding about the behavior of tumors, the effect of tumor burden on therapy, metastatic processes and sensitivity, and resistance of tumor cells to chemotherapeutic drugs. This represents an outstanding example of the importance of the relationship of basic science and clinical practice. The generation of

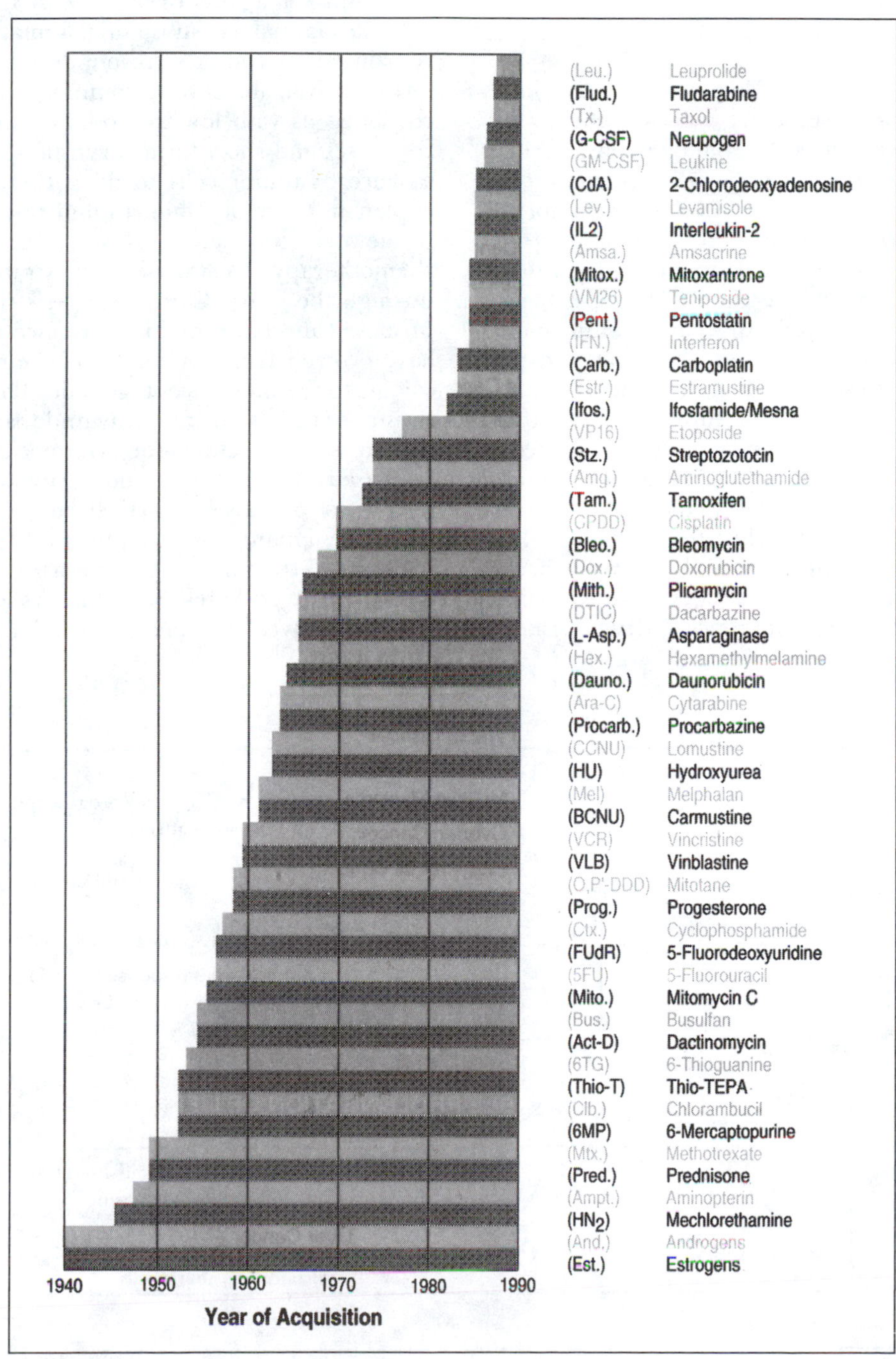

FIGURE 14-1 Acquisition of new anticancer drugs 1940–1990. (Source: Krakoff IH: Cancer chemotherapeutic and biologic agents. *CA* 41:264–278, 1991. Used with permission.)

new knowledge about cancer biology has, and continues to have, direct clinical application in medical oncology for study design, administration of therapy, selection of therapy, and development of strategies to overcome resistance to chemotherapeutic agents.

FACTORS INFLUENCING CHEMOTHERAPY EFFECTIVENESS

Responses to chemotherapy (Figure 14-2)[2] are influenced by the tumor, host factors, available chemotherapeutic drugs, and genetics. The biologic characteristics of tumors, such as growth rate, growth fraction, type, origin and proportion of tumor stem cells, tumor cell heterogeneity, and tumor burden, influence the approach and the outcome of treatment for both drug-sensitive and drug-resistance cancers.[3–5] Host factors influencing response include the patient's nutritional status, level of immune function, physical and psychologic tolerance to specific drugs/regimens, and the availability and effectiveness of supportive therapies. The response to a specific drug or drug regimen is related to the sensitivity of the specific tumor type and tumor cells, the dose, the toxicity, the route, and the schedule of administration. While tumor biology, host factors, and drugs are important influences on chemotherapeutic response, genetic changes in individual tumor cells that result in the emergence of drug resistance appear to be the most significant factors, explaining the limitations to cure with chemotherapy.[6]

HISTORICAL PERSPECTIVE ON CHEMOTHERAPY AND RESISTANCE

Advances in the treatment of many malignancies with antineoplastic agents over the past five decades have been substantial, yet substantial limitations to curability remain. Many complete responders fail to attain long-term survival, and several common tumors continue to challenge us with low to moderate initial therapeutic responses and short-term survival. The concept of resistance of tumor cells to drug therapy provides an explanation for our failures and our successes and a framework to review the history for the rationale of chemotherapy treatment and strategies employed through the years. Carter[7] suggests that views on the proposed mechanisms for resistance to drug therapy have evolved from kinetic to biochemical to pharmacologic to the most recent, genetic. The kinetic view of resistance represents the early understanding of tumor cells and the potential for cytotoxicity with drugs. It was based on the cell cycle and the hypothesis that drugs were most effective on actively dividing cells. Hematologic malignancies with highly proliferative cells were the focus of treatment, and clinical outcome supported the kinetic hypotheses. Solid tumors were observed as less responsive, explained by the kinetic factors of a

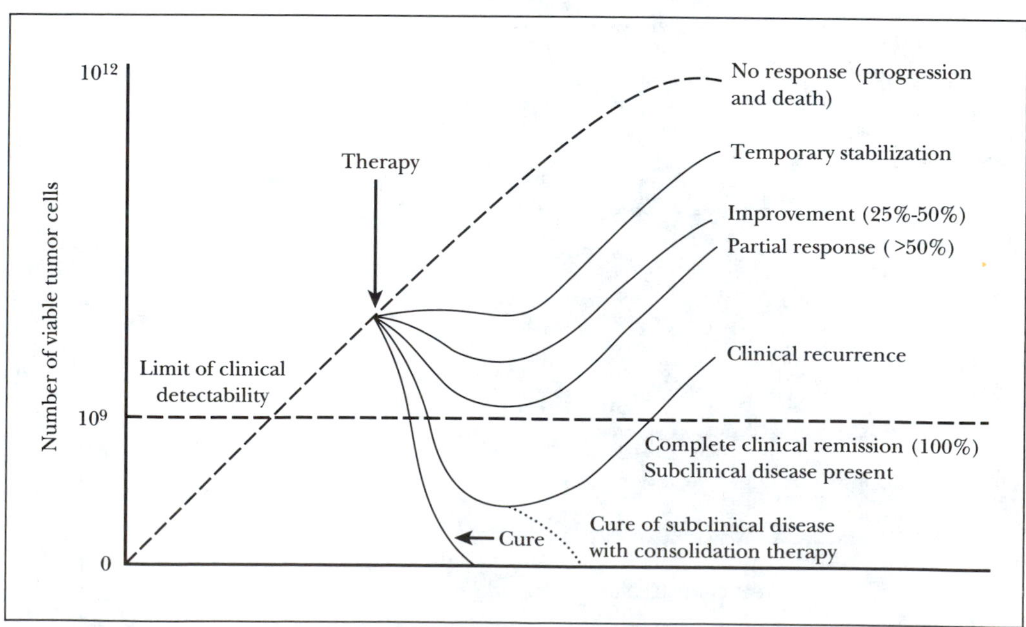

FIGURE 14-2 Possible responses to chemotherapy. (Source: Hubbard SM: Neoplastic processes. In Jones DA, Juronec MA, Dunbar CA (eds.): *Medical Surgical Nursing*. New York: McGraw-Hill, 1978, p. 145. Used with permission.)

long doubling time, low growth fraction, and a large percentage of cells in G_0, the resting phase.

Cell Cycle

While our knowledge of the mechanisms of cytotoxic therapy and resistance to drug treatment has broadened over the years, the cell cycle remains a critical component to understanding cell proliferation, tumor growth, and the rationale for chemotherapy. There are three potential cell populations: those that are actively dividing (cycling cells), those that leave the cell cycle after a certain point and differentiate (destined to die), and those that temporarily leave the cell cycle, remaining in a dormant state until reentry into the cycle.[8] This is true of all tissues, whether normal or abnormal. The cell cycle consists of five phases: G_1, G_2, S, M, and G_0 (Figure 14-3).[9] *Gap* is the term used for the time or phase between mitosis and S phase, represented by the capital letter *G*. The G_1 phase is primarily directed at RNA and protein synthesis and has the greatest variability in length, from 2–3 hours to several days.[10] Generally, a long G_1 phase reflects slow-growing cell populations, and a short or almost nonexistent G_1 phase reflects rapidly proliferating cell populations.[8] The G_2 phase is the time after cells complete DNA synthesis and are getting ready to enter mitosis, usually a brief period of time. The G_0 phase, often called a resting or dormant phase, represents cells that are out of the cycle but have the potential to reenter. They are active cells, however, and may continue to synthesize RNA and protein and carry out some differentiation functions.[10] The S phase is when DNA synthesis takes place; the time of the phase appears relatively constant, ranging from 8–30 hours.[11] It is important to note that the phase of DNA replication is short compared to the entire cell cycle. Thus, drugs such as the antimetabolites, which are active in the DNA replication phase, only affect a small fraction of cells for any given treatment. The M phase is mitosis, which results in cell division, producing two daughter cells; this is also a relatively short phase of the cycle, 30–90 minutes.[11]

The cell cycle time, growth fraction, rate of cell loss, and doubling time are important concepts related to tumor growth and treatment strategies. *Cell cycle time* is the interval between mitosis, for cycling cells. *Growth fraction* is the fraction or percentage of cycling cells within the overall population of cells. *Rate of cell loss* is the fraction or percentage of cells that die or go to other tissues. *Doubling time* is the time it takes a tumor to double its size. The critical factor is whether or not tumor cells are in the cell cycle; in fact, we know that proliferating tumor cells represent only a small percentage of the total tumor cell population. In summary, the cell cycle and cell cycle kinetics are essential factors in planning cancer treatment; alone, however, they do not provide a full understanding of tumor growth and explanation for observed therapeutic responses or failures.

Cell Kill Hypothesis

The kinetic concept that provided the early rationale for drug treatment and explanation for successes and failures was followed by biochemical and pharmacologic concepts. In the early to mid-1970s, the cell kill hypothesis and the Gompertzian model of tumor growth integrated the earlier concepts, producing major ad-

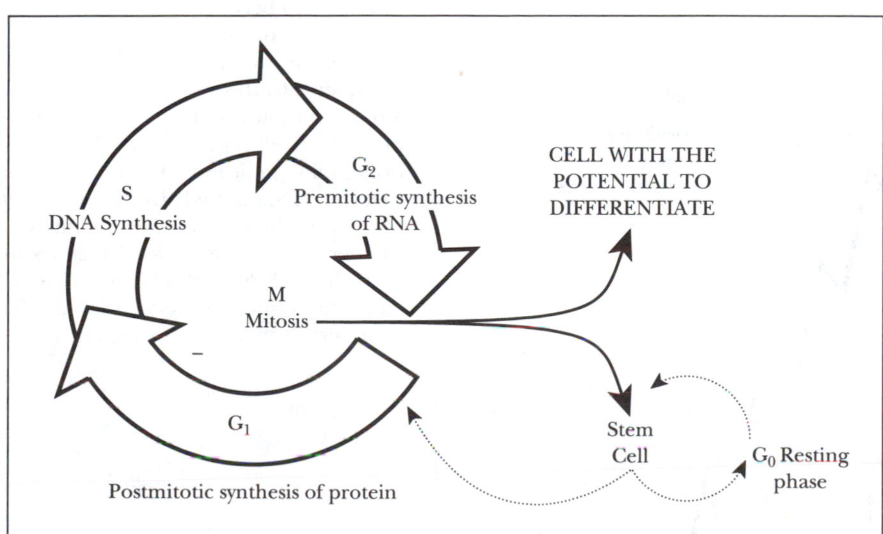

FIGURE 14-3 Cell cycle. (Source: Maxwell MB, Maher KE: Chemotherapy-induced myelosuppression. *Semin Oncol Nurs* 8:113–123, 1992. Used with permission.)

vances in our approach to treatment, toxicity, and supportive care.[7] The basis of the cell kill hypothesis is *log kill.* Chemotherapy drugs will kill a constant *proportion* of tumor cells, not a constant number; thus there is a relationship between cell number, treatment, and tumor cell survival.[12] If a chemotherapy treatment kills 99.9% of cells in a tumor with 10^{10} cells, it will reduce the tumor burden three logs, from 10^{10} to 10^7 (Figure 14-4).[10] The net tumor cell kill for a given treatment is the surviving tumor cells plus the cells that regrow before the next drug treatment. As illustrated in the example in Figure 14-4, a curative drug treatment program will produce a proportionate three-log kill, until all tumor cells are eliminated. It is critically important, however, to note that this model assumes that the tumor cells remain sensitive to the drug(s) throughout the entire course of treatment.

The Gompertzian model of tumor growth offered additional insight into our treatment successes and failures and our understanding of the relationship between treatment outcome and tumor cell burden. This model proposes an exponential growth curve for a tumor in the early stages followed by a decreasing growth rate and plateau as the tumor increases in size. Therefore, large tumors with low growth fractions would predictably fail to respond or have a poor response to the majority of antineoplastic drugs, which are directed at altering DNA metabolism. Alternatively, chemotherapy administered to patients with small tumors that have high growth fractions would result in a larger fraction of cells killed, since the population of proliferating cells would be greater.

These approaches, which evolved from the 1950s through the 1970s, directed the development of treatment strategies that continue to be the cornerstone of systemic drug treatment. Combination chemotherapy, adjuvant therapy, and prophylactic treatment of "sanctuary" sites represent major advances in medical oncology from this era. Yet clinical observations remind us that kinetic parameters alone fail to explain the variability of responsiveness, even in tumors that are initially drug sensitive, such as breast cancer, small-cell lung cancer, and other malignancies.

Drug Resistance

There are two major types of drug resistance, temporary and permanent. Temporary resistance is synonymous with the terms *relative resistance* and *biochemical resistance.* Factors related to this type of resistance include variations in drug bioavailability; metabolism or elimination; tumor present in sanctuary sites; limited drug diffusion; alteration in cell kinetics; host toxicity; and blood supply of the tumor.[3,13] While these factors pose barriers and challenges for successful treatment outcomes, strategies have been developed that can overcome some of these barriers; hence the terms *relative* and *temporary* resistance.

Permanent, or phenotypic, drug resistance is genetically based and is now thought to be the major factor for chemotherapy drug failure. In the early 1980s, Goldie and Coldman[5,14,15] proposed a genetic origin to explain cytotoxic drug resistance. The basis of their proposal came from early work done by Luria and Delbruck[16] with bacteria and resistance to antimicrobial

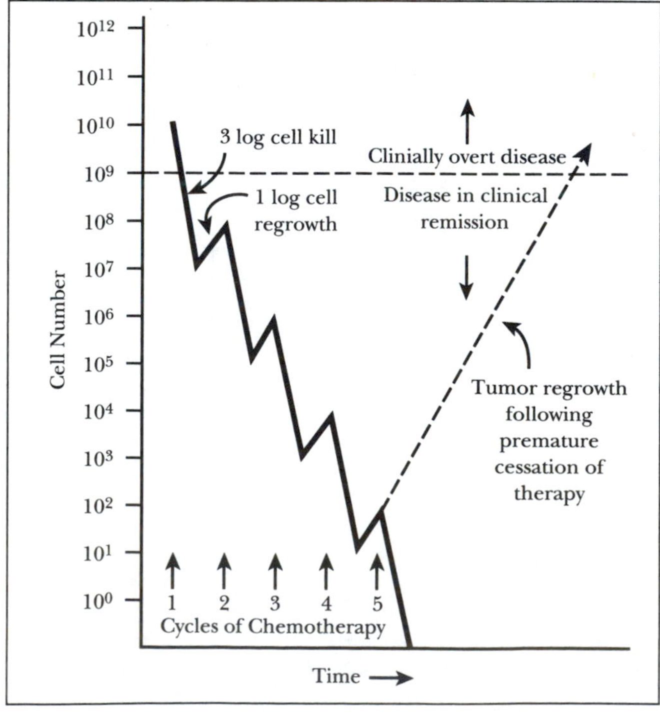

FIGURE 14-4 Relationship between tumor cell survival and chemotherapy administration. The exponential relationship between chemotherapy drug dose and tumor cell survival dictates that a constant proportion, not number, of tumor cells is killed with each cycle of treatment. In this example each cycle of drug administration results in 99.9% (three-log) cell kill, and one log of cell regrowth occurs between cycles. The broken line indicates what would occur if the last cycle of therapy were omitted: Despite complete clinical remission of disease, the tumor would ultimately recur. (Source: Cooper MR, Cooper MR: Principles of medical oncology. In Holleb AI, Fink D, Murphy G (eds.): *Clinical Oncology.* American Cancer Society, Atlanta: 1991, pp. 47–68. Used with permission.)

TABLE 14-1 Assumptions of the Goldie-Coldman Model of Drug Resistance

- Somatic mutation theory
- Genetic changes in cells
- Random nature to changes
- Genetic instability of neoplasms
- Cure means zero resistant cells
- Probability of resistant cells is a product of mutation rate and age of the tumor
- Tumor cells have stem cell capacity

TABLE 14-2 Genetic Changes in Cells

- Mutations
- Deletions
- Transposition of genetic elements
- Gene amplifications
- Chromosomal rearrangements
- Translocations

therapy. The work of Goldie and Coldman demonstrated that resistance to antibiotics occurred even if cells were not previously exposed to the drugs. Spontaneous genetic mutation provided the explanation for these observations. A fluctuation test was used to demonstrate that the number of resistant cells or clones varied (or fluctuated), dependent on when the spontaneous event happened, i.e., an early vs. a late mutation. This fluctuation analysis was later used to demonstrate a drug-resistant phenotype in tumor cells, resistant to a variety of chemotherapeutic drugs.[5]

The Goldie-Coldman model of drug resistance in cancer contains several assumptions (Table 14-1). The somatic mutation theory underlies the model, proposing that all biologic systems have an inherent probability of undergoing genetic variation as a consequence of random changes. The effect can be trivial or neutral or result in mutant cells with altered biological properties.[15] Tumor burden, tumor cell heterogeneity, and the known genetic instability of tumor cells increase the risk of genetic changes and the potential for development of mutant cells, i.e., drug-resistant cells or clones.[12,17,18] Genetic changes include mutations, deletions, transposition of genetic elements, gene amplifications, chromosome rearrangements, and translocations (Table 14-2). In addition to the actual genetic change, when the change occurred appears quite significant. The random nature of spontaneous mutation lends itself to a mathematical model that helps explain this phenomenon (Figure 14-5).[14] In the Goldie-Coldman model, the key to cure is zero resistant cells. The development of even one resistant phenotype will decrease the ability to attain cure since it will be resistant to the drug(s) even at maximum doses. The probability of at least one resistant cell is the product of the mutation rate and the size of the tumor.[14,15] The mutation rate is defined as the average frequency or probability of the appearance of a genetic variant with each cell division. The probability for cure will decrease with a higher mutation rate or a greater tumor burden. Figure 14-5 is a plot of probability of cure against an increasing tumor burden at two different mutation rates. Thus, increasing tumor size greatly diminishes the chance for cure because of the almost certain probability that at least one resistant mutation has occurred, if not more than one.

Phenotypic drug resistance is either intrinsic or acquired. *Intrinsic* resistance reflects tumor cell resistance to a specific drug without any prior drug exposure. *Acquired* drug resistance develops through a process of selection after treatment and represents some type of a permanent change in the nature of tumor cells themselves. Both of these forms of resistance provide an additional understanding about tumors that may fail to respond to initial therapy and those that respond but later relapse (Figure 14-2). The Goldie-Coldman

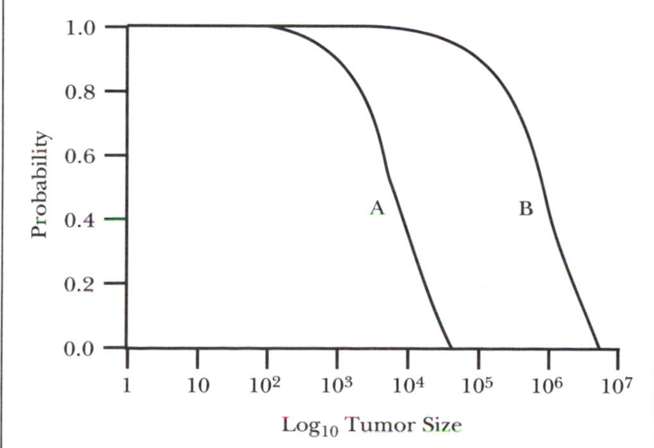

FIGURE 14-5 Plot of the mathematical relationships $P_0 = \exp(-\alpha(N-1))$, where P_0 = probability of zero resistant cells, α = mutation rate per cell generation, N = size of tumor, A: $\alpha = 10^{-4}$, B: $\alpha = 10^{-6}$. (Source: Goldie JH: Relevance of drug resistance in cancer treatment strategy. In Muggia FM (ed.): *Cancer Chemotherapy*. New York: Martinus Nijhoff, 1983, p. 9. Used with permission.)

model is basically a proliferative one, shifting the emphasis from cell kinetics to resistance; but like previous theories, it fails to incorporate tumor cell dormancy.[7] Yet the concept of resistance to explain chemotherapy successes and failures has been the driving force in laboratory research for the past decade. Several mechanisms of drug resistance have been discovered (Table 14-3). This research has expanded our knowledge and understanding of how drugs work, explains observed patient responses, and aids scientists in developing new strategies and approaches to treatment.[5,13,14,19,20]

Methotrexate has become a model to study acquired drug resistance at the molecular level.[20–22] The two most common mechanisms observed include overproduction of the target enzyme, dihydrofolate reductase (DHFR), due to amplification of the DHFR gene and impaired membrane transport. And at least three additional mechanisms have been identified in experimental studies: altered target protein (DHFR), defective metabolism, and availability of salvage pathways.[20] These mechanisms are not specific to methotrexate alone (Table 14-3); thus the research on methotrexate adds to our understanding of resistance to a variety of cytotoxic drugs.

Multidrug resistance (MDR) or pleiotropic drug resistance (PDR) is now a well-recognized phenomenon, in which exposure to a single drug is followed by cross-resistance to other drugs that are structurally unrelated and may have different mechanisms of action.[20,23–27] The initial drug involved appears to be a natural product, specifically, doxorubicin, daunorubicin, vincristine, vinblastine, etoposide, taxol, trimetrexate, mitomycin, or mitoxantrone.[24] While there is a wide variation in the structures of natural products, they are presumed to use a similar transport system, and drug transport appears to be the critical component in multidrug resistance. Alterations in how the drug gets in and out of the cell results in altered intracellular drug concentrations. Reduced drug accumulation within the cell and within the nucleus of the cell is inversely related to drug resistance. There are two proposed mechanisms for reduced drug accumulation: (1) drugs enter the cell at normal rates but are removed by an energy-dependent efflux pump, and (2) an energy-dependent barrier controls entry into the cell.[26] Available evidence suggests that the causative factor is P-glycoprotein, a 170,000-dalton glycoprotein (the P stands for permeability).[24] It is thought that drugs bind to P-glycoprotein and are actively pumped out of the cell (Figure 14-6).[24] This energy-dependent drug efflux appears more efficient in resistant cells and results in less intracellular drug.[20] The overexpression of P-glycoprotein is the predominant gene alteration responsible for multidrug resistance.[26] Expression of P-glycoprotein and the MDR phenotype have been documented in a substantial number of hematologic and solid tumors: acute lymphocytic leukemia, acute nonlymphocytic leukemia,

TABLE 14-3 Mechanisms of Resistance to Cytotoxic Drugs

- Defective transport
- Defective drug metabolism
- Altered nucleotide pools
- Increased drug activation
- Altered DNA repair
- Gene amplification
- Altered target protein
- Multidrug resistance

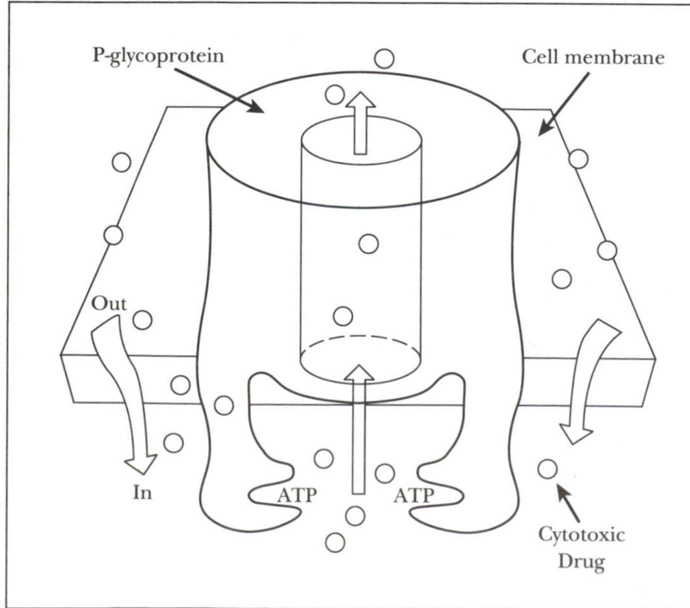

FIGURE 14-6 Model of P-glycoprotein demonstrating direct binding of the drug to the efflux protein. (Source: Dalton WS, Miller TP: Multidrug resistance. *PPO Updates,* 5:1–13, 1991.)

chronic leukemia, lymphoma, multiple myeloma, colon, renal cell, hepatoma, childhood sarcoma, adrenocortical, islet cell, carcinoid, and breast.[24]

THERAPEUTIC STRATEGIES

Cell kinetics, pharmacokinetics, mechanisms of actions of chemotherapy drugs, host toxicity, and clinical responses provided the basis for initial approaches to systemic cancer treatment. Dose, schedule, route of administration, drug synergy, and specific drug toxicity were major factors in the early development of combination chemotherapy.[28,29] Combination drug therapy remains a critically important strategy in oncology, but the basis for this approach has shifted to drug resistance.[23] The current understanding of mechanisms of resistance (intrinsic, acquired, and multidrug) provide the rationale for today's treatment strategies, specifically, combination drug regimens, scheduling, adjuvant therapy, sequencing, dose intensity, and agents to inhibit the function of P-glycoprotein in multidrug resistance.

Combination Chemotherapy

The major tenents in the initial research efforts to combine drugs include cycle specificity, different modes of action, varied toxicity, effectiveness of each single drug against a specific tumor type, drug synergy, maximum dose, and optimal schedule. The goal of maximum cell kill with tolerable toxicity remains unchanged, but the underlying principles of combination therapy today are tumor cell sensitivity to each of the drugs in a regimen, broad coverage of resistant cell lines in a heterogeneous tumor population, and minimizing or preventing the development of new resistant cell lines.[4,17] Intermittent high doses of drugs, alternating drugs, and minimizing the intervals between treatments are the major factors in planning treatment to prevent acquired drug resistance.[30]

The basic assumption of the Goldie-Coldman model of the development of a single resistant cell line has been extended to the probability of two resistant subpopulations.[31] Since all cells have stem cell capacity, it is possible that a doubly resistant phenotype may develop at the same time, or it may occur in sequence from a sensitive cell to a single resistant cell line to a doubly resistant cell line. Accepting this hypothesis, it is critical to develop combination drug strategies that would reduce both resistant cell lines in tandem, i.e., alternating noncross-resistant chemotherapy regimens. Underlying the potential success of this strategy are several factors: Each regimen must have an equivalent effect, and be completely noncross-resistant; maximum tolerated doses must be administered at minimal intervals; and all agents are to be given as concurrently as possible.[5] The goal is to maximize the kill of both sensitive and resistant cells with the least amount of regrowth between the treatment cycles (Figure 14-7). While this strategy appeared successful in the treatment of Hodgkin's disease,[32] it has been severely limited in the treatment of many solid tumors, virtually by the lack of a number of effective agents that can be combined to achieve equal effectiveness without cross-resistance. Recent data in the adjuvant treatment of node-positive patients with breast cancer, however, suggest a benefit to alternating doxorubicin with cyclophosphamide, methotrexate, and fluorouracil (CMF) over a sequence of eight courses of CMF followed by four cycles of doxorubicin[33] (Figure 14-7). The authors suggest that the prolonged administration of CMF in the sequential model may have allowed for the development of resistant cell lines, which were then refractory to the following cycles of doxorubicin.[34] While these results may provide some encouragement, the advantage of combining drugs and administering them by either a sequential or an alternating schedule has not been proven more beneficial than the administration of standard treatment. The outcome appears quite significantly influenced by tumor burden, heterogeneity of tumor cell populations, and resistant cells.

Dose

There is a definite relationship between drug dose and response for sensitive tumor cell populations. The therapeutic effect is compromised with inadequate drug dosing, which may commonly result from reductions in prescribed dose. This has regenerated a focus on dose as a significant outcome factor and created new ways to evaluate the impact of dose.[35] There are three parameters describing treatment as it relates to dose: size, total amount delivered, and rate.[36] The *dose size* is the amount delivered to the patient when corrected for pharmacologic variables, such as creatinine clearance and weight. The *total dose* is the sum of all doses of drug for an individual patient. *Dose rate* (or *dose intensity*) is the amount of drug delivered per unit of time. Hryniuk and Bush[37] developed a calculation of drug intensity that disregards the schedule of drug delivery (e.g., once a week, once every three weeks, daily times five). In this calculation, dose intensity is expressed as mg/m²/wk and represents the amount of drug delivered per unit of time. Regimens that are more dose intense have been retrospectively correlated with improved outcome in several tumors (e.g., breast, ovarian, colon), but there are potential limitations to the concept, such as the role of scheduling on outcome, growth fraction of the tumor, and degree of tumor burden.[38] Optimal dose intensity should be a composite of optimal drug dose and optimal duration of treatment, yet these are unknown for many of our current therapies.[38,39] The greatest potential effect of intense dosing is likely to be on sensitive cell populations, resulting in higher response rates and, hopefully, improved survival.[40] Continued efforts

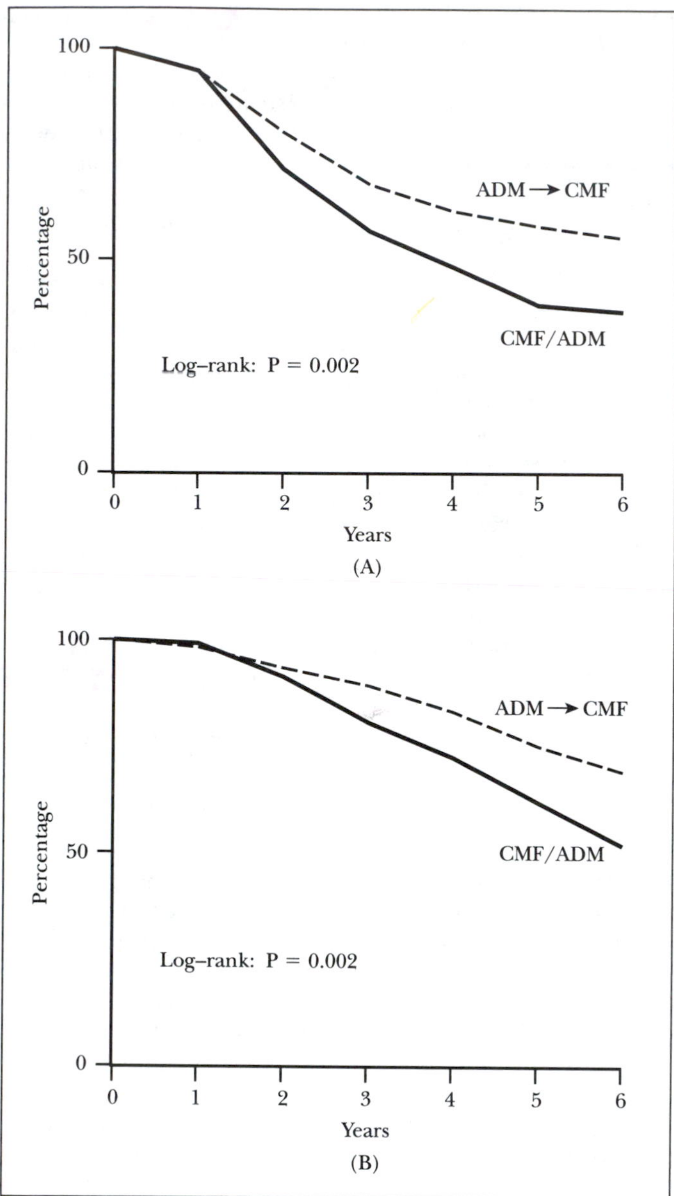

FIGURE 14-7 Six-year results in patients with three positive axillary nodes who received sequential (CMF/ADR) versus alternating ADR → CMF adjuvant chemotherapy. A = comparative relapse-free survival; B = comparative total survival. (Source: Bonadonna G: Evolving concepts in the systemic adjuvant treatment of breast cancer. *Cancer Res* 52: 2127–2137, 1992. Used with permission.)

in this area, such as the cumulative dose plot (planned dose intensity and total drug delivered), in prospective clinical trials may clarify and enhance our understanding of the dose–response relationship of current treatment regimens.[36]

Adjuvant Therapy

The rationale to treat small tumor burdens, that is, microscopic disease following primary (i.e., surgical) treatment, as a strategy to increase cure rates was soundly based on cellular kinetics, resistance theories, and animal data (Table 14-4).[33] The nearly two decades of adjuvant therapy in breast cancer provides a good tumor model to examine the effectiveness and limitations of systemic adjuvant treatment (multidrug chemotherapy, hormonal agents, or chemoendocrine combinations). Although adjuvant therapy reduces mortality in patients with Stage I and II breast cancer, the degree of benefit is much less than initially anticipated. There are several possible explanations for the clinical observations of continuing relapse.[5,14,33,39] The animal models tested represented tumors that are generally drug sensitive with high growth rates/fractions that do not likely reflect the average human breast tumor. Timing, tumor cell burden, heterogeneity, duration of therapy, specific drug(s), and resistant cells are important variables in evaluating the outcome of adjuvant treatment. Combination drug therapy is superior to single agents but dramatically less effective in patients with large tumor burdens (i.e., >10 positive nodes). Yet we also observe failures in women with supposed low tumor burdens (<3 positive nodes). Does this reflect devel-

TABLE 14-4 Clinical Observations, Laboratory Findings, and Biological Hypotheses Influencing the Beginning of Modern Adjuvant Chemotherapy for High-Risk Operable Breast Cancer

- By the time cancer becomes clinically detectable, it is advanced (near 30 doublings), and has had ample opportunity to establish distant micrometastases.
- Frequency of metastatic disease is directly related to tumor mass, and surgical cure rates drop as tumor volume at surgery increases.
- Tumor growth fraction is inversely related to population size.
- Effective drug kill follows first-order reaction kinetics.
- Combinations of drugs are superior to single agents and can eradicate 10–100 times as many cells.
- In transplantable tumors surgical adjuvant chemotherapy increases the long-term cure rates.
- The optimal kinetic conditions to achieve cure exist when microscopic foci of disease are present after curative surgery and/or radiotherapy.

Source: Bonadonna G: Evolving concepts in the systemic adjuvant treatment of breast cancer. *Cancer Res* 52:2127–2137, 1992. Used with permission.

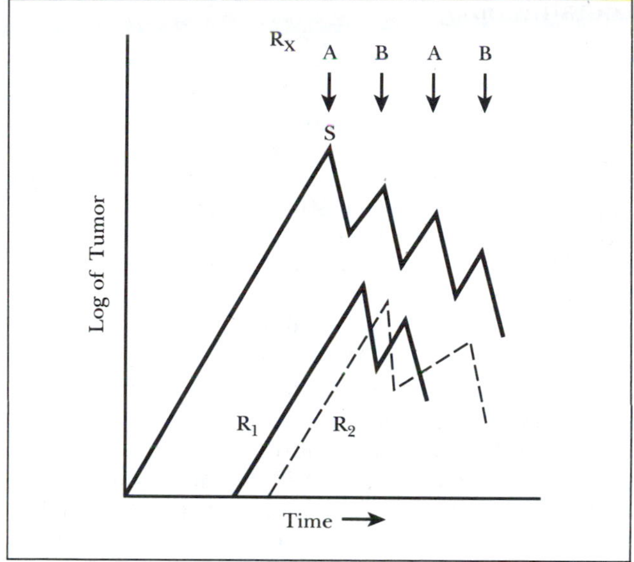

FIGURE 14-8 Schematic presentation of two noncross-resistant treatments (A and B) and potential effect on sensitive (S) and resistant cell populations (R1, R2). (Source: Goldie JH: Relevance of drug resistance in cancer treatment strategy. In Muggia FM (ed.): *Cancer Chemotherapy*. New York: Martinus Nijhoff, 1983, p. 18. Used with permission.)

opment of resistance, heterogeneous cell populations, inadequate dosing, or the timing of treatment? Answers remain unknown at this point, but it is clear that any or all of these factors may contribute to our inability to cure early-stage breast cancer with adjuvant therapy. Current strategies that consider these factors include alternating regimens (Figure 14-8),[14] neoadjuvant therapy, dose-intense regimens (with or without autologous bone marrow transplantation), and chemoendocrine combinations.

Modifying Agents

Other strategies for improving the effectiveness of antineoplastic drug treatment involve the use of modifying agents. Notable examples of drugs that have been used to enhance the efficacy of antineoplastic drugs are shown in Table 14-5.[41–53]

Reversing Multidrug Resistance

Major strategies to overcome multidrug resistance include: (1) increasing intracellular drug concentration using high doses of drugs; (2) alternating noncross-resistant chemotherapy regimens; (3) use of monoclonal antibodies or conjugates to target P-glycoprotein; and (4) use of drugs to inhibit the function of P-glycoprotein.[24] Attempts to inhibit P-glycoprotein function with drugs, which reverses resistance, represents a concentrated research effort. A variety of drugs, such as calcium channel blockers and calmodulin inhibitors, are capable of binding P-glycoprotein and, thus, of blocking the efflux of drugs in vitro.[13,24,54,55] This has been confirmed in vivo in clinical trials in patients who were drug resistant using verapamil, a calcium channel blocker. Unfortunately, cardiac toxicity is significant with the dose of verapamil that is required to reverse resistance. Such drugs are referred to as *chemosensitizers,* in that they increase intracellular drug concentration, resulting in greater cytotoxicity. The use of chemosensitizers appears to be a successful strategy in reversing drug resistance, but less toxic agents must be developed.

TABLE 14-5 Modifiers of Antineoplastic Drugs

Drug	Modifying Agent
Asparaginase	Methotrexate[41]
Cisplatin	Sodium thiosulfate[42] Amifostine (WR2721)[43]
Cytarabine	Cisplatin[44]
Floxuridine	Leucovorin[45,46]
Fluorouracil	Leucovorin[45–47] Interferon[48] PALA[49] Uridine[50] Methotrexate[51]
Methotrexate	Leucovorin[52]
Trimetrexate	Leucovorin[53]

Glutathione

Glutathione is the most abundant intracellular sulfhydryl-containing substance in most cells. Its formation is regulated by many cellular processes and is essential for the synthesis of DNA precursors. Glutathione enzymes, such as glutathione-S-transferase, are responsible for detoxifying harmful substances, scavenging free radicals, and repairing damage to DNA. Glutathione-S-transferase (GST) facilitates detoxification by attaching toxins with glutathione, resulting in the formation of a less toxic metabolite. Glutathione and glutathione-S-transferase have been implicated in the formation of cellular resistance to antineoplastic drugs of the alkylating class (e.g., nitrogen mustard, melphalan, cisplatin, and nitrosoureas).[56] Drugs that inhibit the activity of glutathione and/or glutathione-S-transferase, such as buthionine sulfoxime (BSO) and ethacrynic acid, are synergistic in animal models and have entered clinical trials in man.[57,58]

DRUG DEVELOPMENT

Preclinical Evaluation

In the United States all drugs and biological agents become commercially available only after careful preclinical testing followed by clinical trials in man.[59–64] The National Cancer Institute (NCI) and pharmaceutical firms have drug development programs. Drugs are screened from various sources, such as plant extracts or chemicals of a particular type. They are produced in sufficient amount to undergo testing in animal models of a particular disease. Thus, prospective anticancer compounds are tested against tumors implanted in mice and rats, as well as in a panel of tumor cell lines derived from human malignancies.[64,65] When a drug is found to have some level of activity against these tumor models, toxicology studies are done in at least two animal species. These studies are performed to examine toxic effects and to specifically determine the LD10 (i.e., dose of drug that is lethal to 10% of the animals) in mice. These studies are essential, because they allow for the prediction of a safe starting dose for human studies.[66]

Phase I Studies

In the United States all drugs undergo testing in phase I studies. Due to their obvious toxicities, phase I testing of antineoplastic drugs is done in patients with cancer who could potentially benefit from the drug (all other phase I studies are carried out in normal volunteers). The objectives of a phase I study are to evaluate acute toxicities, to establish the maximum tolerated dose (MTD) for a particular schedule of administration, and to analyze pharmacologic data so the drug can be delivered in the most effective manner during future studies.[67] The initial dose is customarily one-tenth of the LD10 in mice. Three patients are treated, and if no significant toxicity is seen, additional patients (in sets of three) receive higher doses of the drug. When significant toxicity is observed in an unacceptable number of patients (usually 50%) on a given dose level, the study is stopped. This dose is the MTD. The dose level one step below the MTD is used in subsequent, phase II studies.

Phase II Studies

Phase II trials seek to find anticancer activity. The chances of detecting an active drug are best when the phase II agent is administered before other treatments have been given. Patients who are eligible for phase II trials are, ideally, untreated patients. Most are patients with malignancies for which chemotherapy has shown little or no benefit, such as renal cell carcinoma, lung cancer, melanoma, and pancreatic cancer. At the end of a phase II trial, specific knowledge regarding tumor activity, administration techniques, precautions, modifications of dose, acute toxicity, and the necessary supportive care is more clearly delineated.

Phase III Studies

Phase III trials aim at defining the role of a drug in a cancer treatment regimen. For example, the effectiveness of a drug may be studied by comparing it with another treatment or by combining it with a standard treatment regimen. Evaluation of response, duration of response, toxicity, and quality of life are all elements used to determine the preferred treatment in a comparative study. When the study has been completed it should be known if the treatment is equal to or better than the standard therapy, whether it produces equivalent or less toxicity, whether it demonstrates the potential for combination with other agents, and finally, whether it has a significant positive effect on the quality of life and survival of patients treated.

Phase IV Studies

Phase IV trials are postmarketing studies. Their endpoints are usually aimed at defining new uses, dosing schedules, and additional information about risks and benefits of a commercially available drug.

CLINICAL TRIALS

A clinical trial is a scientific study designed to answer important clinical and biologic questions; it is carried out by *protocol,* a written guideline for the study. The protocol defines the essential elements of the study and how it will be conducted. From the discussion on drug development it should be clear that clinical trials provide the only mechanism to test the effectiveness of new therapies.[68] In the field of oncology almost all standard treatments arose from clinical trials.

The majority of patients and the public, when asked about clinical trials, have favorable views regarding the values of clinical research.[69] Patients participate in clinical trials to help other patients who will develop a similar medical condition in the future, to increase knowledge about their disease, to take advantage of increased monitoring as a part of a clinical study, and to obtain a second opinion about their disease.[69,70]

In the United States, only a few thousand patients each year are actually enrolled into clinical trials, despite the nearly one million patients diagnosed with cancer annually.[71,72] Although most oncologists believe they have an obligation to enroll patients into clinical studies, currently only around 2%–3% of the patients with cancer are so enrolled.[73,74]

The major reasons for poor patient accrual into clinical trials are due to issues about the individual physician–patient relationship, time, and money.[75–77] In a busy outpatient setting one may forget that a clinical trial is available. Protocols require time to read and to explain to the patient. Some studies are complex and may require extensive time by the physician and nurse for patient teaching. The treatment may or may not be totally reimbursed. Data collection procedures may seem onerous for the physician and the nurse who are also providing the direct care for the patients. There is no question that the reimbursement policies of insurance companies, health maintenance organizations (HMOs), and Medicare can adversely affect physician and patient participation in clinical trials.[78–81] Refusal to reimburse for the costs of a treatment that is offered as a part of a clinical study suppresses patient recruitment to clinical trials and slows the advancement of the field of oncology. A consensus conference sponsored by the NCI recommended that third-party payers reimburse for the costs associated with the *clinical care* but not the research costs of NCI-approved and other, selected clinical trials. Although these are all valid issues, it is to the advantage of everyone to be creative in the design and conduct of clinical trials and to provide the resources that will encourage patient recruitment and physician participation.

CLASSIFICATIONS OF ANTINEOPLASTIC AGENTS

Cytotoxic drugs are described by their chemical structure, cell cycle activity, and primary mode of action.[82] The classic categories include alkylating agents, antitumor antibiotics, plant alkaloids, and antimetabolites (Table 14-6). Alkylating agents are cell cycle nonspecific, and the primary mechanism of action is cross-linking strands of DNA, which prevents transcription of RNA and replication of DNA. Natural products represent a broad group of drugs and include the antitumor antibiotics, plant alkaloids, and enzymes. Antitumor antibiotics are cell cycle nonspecific and interfere with DNA function, although several other mechanisms may occur, such as alteration of the cell membrane or inhibition of certain enzymes. Plant alkaloids include topoisomerase inhibitors (etoposide, teniposide, CPT-11, topotecan) and mitotic inhibitors (vinblastine, vincristine). Topoisomerase inhibitors interfere with DNA replication by binding to DNA and the to-

TABLE 14-6 Classification of Cytotoxic Drugs

Alkylating Agents	Antimetabolites	Antitumor Antibiotics	Plant Alkaloids	Miscellaneous
Altretamine	Azacitidine	Bleomycin	Etoposide	Amsacrine
Busulfan	Chlorodeoxyadenosine	Dactinomycin	Taxol	Asparaginase
Carboplatin	Cytarabine	Daunorubicin	Taxotere	CPT-11
Carmustine	Edatrexate	Doxorubicin	Teniposide	Mitotane
Chlorambucil	Floxuridine	Epirubicin	Vinblastine	Piroxantrone
Cisplatin	Fludarabine	Idarubicin	Vincristine	Suramin
Cyclophosphamide	Fluorouracil	Mitomycin	Vindesine	Topotecan
Dacarbazine	Mercaptopurine	Mitoxantrone		
Ifosphamide	Methotrexate	PALA		
Lomustine	Mitoguazone	Plicamycin		
Mechlorethamine	Pentostatin			
Melphalan	Thioguanine			
Predismustine	Trimetrexate			
Procarbazine				
Streptozocin				
Thiotepa				
Uracil mustard				

poisomerase enzymes. Drugs from other classes (e.g., amsacrine, doxorubicin, mitoxantrone, daunorubicin) are thought to also inhibit topoisomerase activity in addition to their primary mechanism of action. The mitotic inhibitors, vinblastine and vincristine, are cell cycle specific, acting in the mitosis phase (Figure 14-3). They bind to microtubule proteins, blocking assembly, and cause metaphase arrest.[83] Taxol and taxotere, in contrast, promote assembly of the microtubule, which results in a very stable microtubule, though a nonfunctional one.

Antimetabolites are cell cycle specific, exerting their effect during the S phase (Figure 14-3). This class of drugs primarily interferes with DNA and RNA synthesis by blocking enzymes necessary for synthesis or by being incorporated into DNA or RNA. These drugs are most commonly subclassified as cytidine analogs, pyrimidines, purine analogs, ribonucleotide reductase inhibitors, adenosine deaminase inhibitors, and folic acid antagonists.[82]

While primary mechanisms of action may be similar for drugs within a class, the pharmacokinetics, secondary mechanisms of action, spectrum of activity, and host toxicity may vary widely. Information specific to the individual drug is critical for understanding treatment implications and expected outcomes.

PRACTICE CONSIDERATIONS

Understanding the rationale for treatment strategies is important to one's professional practice and for patient teaching and support. Facts related to drug preparation and potential drug interactions are also important and may influence the effectiveness and safety of the therapy. In Table 14-7, information on storage, reconstitution, stability, and compatibility has been synthesized to provide a practical and quick reference.[84–93]

Drug interactions result in an alteration in the pharmacokinetics or efficacy of a drug when administered in sequence or concurrently with another drug. The scope of the problem is not well defined in oncology, but the incidence of drug interactions increases the more drugs a patient is taking.[94] Many factors influence

TABLE 14-7 Injectable Cancer Chemotherapy Drugs: Reconstitution, Stability, Compatibility

Drug Name	Storage Prior to Use	Reconstitution/Dilution Sterile H_2O or NS May Be Used Unless Specified	Chemical Stability After Reconstitution/Dilution	Specific Compatibilities/ Incompatibilities
Amsacrine (AMSA)	Room	Add 1.5 ml (50 mg/ml) amascrine to diluent provided: yields 5 mg/ml	*Room:* 48 hrs Further diluted in 500 ml D5W + 1mEq $NAHCO_3$: 96 hr (room). Do **not** use sodium chloride solutions.	Should not be mixed with sodium-chloride-containing solutions
Asparaginase (Elspar)	Refrigerator	*IV:* 5 ml yields 2000 U/ml *IM:* 2 ml yields 5000 U/ml	*Room:* 8 hr *Refrigerator:* 14 days	Loss of potency occurs with use of 0.2-micron filter
Azacitidine (5-azacitidine)	Refrigerator	Add 20 ml to 100-mg vial to yield 5 mg/ml	*Room:* 30 min (5 mg/ml), 3 hr in D5W or LR (2 mg/ml), 2.4 hr in NS (2 mg/ml), 2 hr in NS or LR (0.2 mg/ml)	Electrolytes should not be added to solutions with azacitidine due to a destabilizing effect
Bleomycin (Blenoxane)	Refrigerator	Add 1 ml to yield 15 U/ml, 5 ml to yield 3 U/ml, or 3 ml to yield 5 U/ml	*Room:* 14 days *Refrigerator:* 28 days	Compatible with cyclophosphamide, doxorubicin, mesna, vinblastine, and vincristine; inactivated by ascorbic acid, hydrogen peroxide, methotrexate, and mitomycin
Carboplatin (CBDCA, Paraplatin)	Room	Add 5 ml to 50-mg vial, 15 ml to 150-mg vial, and 45 ml to 450-mg vial to yield 10 mg/ml	*Room:* 24 hr *Refrigerator:* 5 days Same stability as 1-mg/ml solution in D5-1/2 NS or D5-1/4 NS	Forms a precipitate when in contact with aluminum. Compatible with etoposide in NaCl or D5W for at least 24 hr at room temperature

(continued)

TABLE 14-7 Injectable Cancer Chemotherapy Drugs: Reconstitution, Stability, Compatibility (continued)

Drug Name	Storage Prior to Use	Reconstitution/Dilution Sterile H_2O or NS May Be Used Unless Specified	Chemical Stability After Reconstitution/Dilution	Specific Compatibilities/ Incompatibilities
Carmustine (BiCNU, BCNU)	Refrigerator	Add 3 ml ethanol provided to drug, further dilute with 27 ml to yield 3.3 mg/ml	*Room:* (0.2–3.3 mg/ml) 8 hr (14 hr if protected from light) *Refrigerator:* (0.2–3.3 mg/ml) 48 hr *Refrig:* 3 mo (in ETOH only, 2 mg/mL)	*Compatible* with cisplatin for 4 hr in glass container. *Incompatible* with polyvinyl chloride bags and sodium bicarbonate
Chlorodeoxyadenosine (2-CdA Leustatin)	Refrigerator	In solution, 1 mg/ml Allow to thaw at room temperature. Do **not** microwave	*Room:* 7 days *Refrigerator:* 14 days	None
Cisplatin (Platinol, CDDP)	Room	*10-mg vial:* 10 ml yields 1 mg/ml *50-mg vial:* 50 ml yields 1 mg/ml	*Room:* 72 hr *Refrigerator:* If <0.6 mg/ml, 96 hr Refrigeration may result in precipitation of solutions ≥0.6 mg/ml	Less stable in solutions without chloride ions; *incompatible* with fluorouracil, metoclopramide, mesna, sodium bicarbonate, and sodium thiosulfate
CPT-11 (Irinotecan)	Room	*In solution:* 20 mg/ml	*Room:* 24 hr	None
Cyclophosphamide (Cytoxan, Neosar, CTX)	Room	*100-mg vial:* 5 ml yields 20 mg/ml *200-mg vial:* 10 ml yields 20 mg/ml *500-mg vial:* 25 ml yields 20 mg/ml *1-g vial:* 50 ml yields 20 mg/ml *2-g vial:* 100 ml yields 20 mg/ml	*Room:* 7 days *Refrigerator:* 14 days (20 mg/ml); 28 days (4 mg/ml in NS) *Frozen:* 19 wk	*Compatible* with doxorubicin for 7 days at room temperature; also compatible with bleomycin, cisplatin, dacarbazine, and mesna
Cytarabine (Cytosar-U, Tarabine, Ara-C)	Room	Add 5 ml to 100-mg vial to yield 20 mg/ml; 10 ml to 500-mg vial to yield 50 mg/ml; 10 ml to 1-g vial or 20 ml to 2-g vial to yield 100 mg/ml	*Room:* 8 days, 15 days in plastic syringe (20–80 mg/ml), 28 days in Infusaid[R] pump *Refrigerator:* 15 days	*Incompatible* with carbenicillen, fluorouracil, heparin sodium, nafcillin, penicillin G sodium, and oxacillin *Compatible* with methotrexate, daunorubicin, vincristine, idarubicin, and etoposide
Dacarbazine (DTIC)	Refrigerator	Add 10 ml (100-mg vial), 20 ml (200-mg vial), or 50 ml (500-mg vial) to yield 10 mg/ml	*Room:* 24 hr *Refrigerator:* 96 hr	*Compatible* with cyclophosphamide, doxorubicin, dactinomycin, and methotrexate
Dactinomycin (Cosmegen, Actinomycin-D)	Room	Add 1.1 ml sterile H_2O to yield 500 mcg/ml Do **not** use preservative-containing solutions—a precipitate will form	*Room:* 2 mo	*Compatible* with dacarbazine *Incompatible* with solutions containing preservatives
Daunorubicin (Cerubidine)	Room	Add 4 ml to 20-mg vial to yield 5 mg/ml	*Room:* 48 hr *Refrigerator:* 72 hr	*Compatible* with cytarabine and etoposide *Incompatible* with fluorouracil, dexamethasone, and heparin

(continued)

TABLE 14-7 Injectable Cancer Chemotherapy Drugs: Reconstitution, Stability, Compatibility (continued)

Drug Name	Storage Prior to Use	Reconstitution/Dilution Sterile H_2O or NS May Be Used Unless Specified	Chemical Stability After Reconstitution/Dilution	Specific Compatibilities/ Incompatibilities
Doxorubicin (Adriamycin, Rubex)	Room	*In solution:* 2 mg/ml Dilute powder form with 5 ml (10-mg vial), 10 ml (20-mg vial), 25 ml (50-mg vial), or 75 ml (150-mg vial) to yield 2 mg/ml	*Room:* 35 days *Refrigerator:* 6 mo *Frozen:* 6 mo	*Compatible* with vincristine in NaCl for 5 days, room temperature; also compatible with cyclophosphamide, bleomycin, dacarbazine, and vinblastine *Incompatible* with aminophylline, cephalothin, dexamethasone sodium phosphate, diazepam, furosemide, fluorouracil, heparin, hydrocortisone, and methotrexate
Etoposide (Vepesid, VP-16)	Room	*In solution:* 20 mg/ml Further dilute to at least 0.4 mg/ml	*Room:* 0.4 mg/ml—72 hr 0.2 mg/ml—96 hr 20 mg/ml (in plastic syringe)—5 days	*Compatible* with cisplatin, carboplatin, cytarabine, daunorubicin, and mesna *Incompatible* with idarubicin
Floxuridine (FUDR)	Room	Add 5 ml to 500-mg vial to yield 100 mg/ml	*Room or refrigerator:* 14 days *Room* (0.5 mg/ml in NS or D5W): 7 days	*Compatible* in NaCl with heparin, calcium leucovorin, and dexamethasone
Fludarabine (Fludara, FAMP)	Refrigerator	Add 2 ml sterile H_2O to 50-mg vial to yield 25 mg/ml	25 mg/ml *(room):* 16 days 1–25 mg/ml (in D5W or NS at *room* temp): 16 days 0.04 mg/ml *(room or refrigerator):* 48 hr	None
Fluorouracil (Adrucil, 5FU)	Room	*In solution:* 50 mg/ml	*Room:* 14 days *Refrigerator:* (10 mg/ml in D5W) 16 wk	*Compatible* with leucovorin for 14 days at room temperature; also compatible with methotrexate, magnesium sulfate, potassium chloride, and vincristine *Incompatible* with cisplatin, cytarabine, daunorubicin, diazepam, doxorubicin, and idarubicin
Idarubicin (Idamycin)	Room	Add 5 ml NS to 5-mg vial, 10 ml to 10-mg vial to yield 1 mg/ml	*Room:* 3 days *Refrigerator:* 7 days	*Compatible* with cytarabine *Incompatible* with dexamethasone, etoposide, heparin, hydrocortisone, and fluorouracil
Ifosfamide (Ifex)	Room	Add 20 ml sterile or bacteriostatic H_2O to 1-g vial or 60 ml to 3-g vial to yield 50 mg/ml	*Room:* 7 days, 8 days in PVC portable infusion pump cassettes, 10–80 mg/ml in NS *Refrigerator:* 6 wk; same stability if further diluted to 0.6–20 mg/ml in D5W, NS, or LR	Chemically stable with mesna for 24 hr at room temperature in D5W or LR at equal concentrations
Mechlorethamine (Mustargen, nitrogen mustard)	Room	Add 10 ml to 10-mg vial to yield 1 mg/ml	*Room:* 1 hr *Refrigerator:* 6 hr	*Incompatible* with sodium thiosulfate

(continued)

TABLE 14-7 Injectable Cancer Chemotherapy Drugs: Reconstitution, Stability, Compatibility (continued)

Drug Name	Storage Prior to Use	Reconstitution/Dilution Sterile H_2O or NS May Be Used Unless Specified	Chemical Stability After Reconstitution/Dilution	Specific Compatibilities/ Incompatibilities
Melphalan (L-PAM)	Room	Add 10 ml diluent provided to 50-mg vial to yield 5 mg/ml Dilute with NS to 2 mg/ml with 0.45-μm filter prior to administration	*Room:* 0.1–5 mg/ml, 3 hr; 0.04 mg/ml (in 0.9% NS) 4.5 hr; administer within 1 hr of preparation	None
6-Mercaptopurine (6-MP)	Room	Add 50 ml sterile H_2O to 500-mg vial to yield 10 mg/ml; further dilute with D5W or NS (1–2 mg/ml final conc.) prior to administration	10 mg/ml at room or refrigerator temperature: 21 days 1–2 mg/ml in D5W or NS *(room or refrigerator):* 3 days	*Compatible* with methotrexate
Mesna (Mesnex)	Room	*In solution:* 100 mg/ml Dilute to 20 mg/ml with D5W, D5W + NS, or LR	*Room:* 20 mg/ml, 24 hr	*Incompatible* with cisplatin
Methotrexate (Mexate, Folex, MTX)	Room	*In solution:* 25 mg/ml Add 4 ml to 20-mg vial to yield 5 mg/ml Add 2 ml (50-mg vial), 4 ml (100-mg vial), 10 ml (250-mg vial) to yield 25 mg/ml Add 19.4 ml to 1-g vial to yield 50 mg/ml	*Room:* 4 wk *Refrigerator:* 3 mo (2–25 mg/ml *Frozen:* 30 days (50 mg/ 100 ml D5W), 12 wk (5 mg, 50 mg, or 1 g, in 50 ml NS)	*Compatible* with cephalothin, cytarabine, dacarbazine, furosemide, fluorouracil, hydrocortisone, leucovorin, mercaptopurine, sodium bicarbonate, vincristine, and amino acids *Incompatible* with bleomycin, doxorubicin, droperidol, idarubicin, prednisolone sodium, metoclopramide, and ranitidine in solution
Mitomycin C (Mutamycin)	Room	Add 10 ml (5-mg vial), 40 ml (20-mg vial), or 80 ml (40-mg vial) to yield 0.5 mg/ml	*Room:* 7 days *Refrigerator:* 14 days Diluted to 0.2–0.4 mg/ml: 3 hr in D5W, 12 hr in NS, 24 hr in LR	*Compatible* with heparin in NaCl
Mitoxantrone (Novantrone)	Room	*In solution:* 2 mg/ml Do **not** refrigerate	*Room:* 0.02–0.5 mg/ml in NS or D5W: 7 days	*Compatible* with hydrocortisone sodium succinate *Incompatible* with heparin and hydrocortisone sodium phosphate
PALA (Phosphonacetyl-L-aspartic acid)	Room	*In solution:* 100 mg/ml	*Room:* 1 mg/ml in D5W or NS: 14 days	None
Pentostatin (Deoxycoformycin, Nipent)	Refrigerator	Add 5 ml to 10-mg vial to yield 2 mg/ml	*Room:* 72 hr *Refrigerator:* 96 hr At 20 mcg/ml (*room* temp): 24 hr in D5W and 48 hr in NS or LR	None
Piroxantrone (Oxantrazole)	Refrigerator	Add 2.5 ml sterile H_2O to 50-mg vial to yield a 20-mg/ml solution	*Room and refrigerator:* 14 days Diluted to 0.1 mg/ml in D5W or NS, 72 hr at *room or refrigeration* temperatures	*Incompatible* with sodium bicarbonate
Plicamycin (Mithracin, Mithramycin)	Refrigerator	Add 4.9 ml sterile H_2O to 2.5-mg vial to yield 0.5 mg/ml Do **not** use D5W	*Room:* 24 hr *Refrigerator:* 48 hr Diluted to 24 mcg/ml in NS or D5W (*room* temp): 24 hr	*Incompatible* with cellulose esther filters, and iron and trace element solutions

(continued)

TABLE 14-7 Injectable Cancer Chemotherapy Drugs: Reconstitution, Stability, Compatibility (continued)

Drug Name	Storage Prior to Use	Reconstitution/Dilution Sterile H_2O or NS May Be Used Unless Specified	Chemical Stability After Reconstitution/Dilution	Specific Compatibilities/ Incompatibilities
Streptozocin (Zanosar)	Refrigerator	Add 9.3 ml NS or D5W to 1-g vial to yield 100 mg/ml	*Room:* 48 hr *Refrigerator:* 96 hr Diluted to 2 mg/ml in NS or D5W, same stability	None
Taxol	Refrigerator	Dilute to a final concentration of 0.3–1.2 mg/ml with NS or D5W in glass bottle	*Room:* 0.3–1.2 mg/ml in D5W or NS: 27 hr	*Incompatible* with PVC bags and infusion sets
Teniposide (Vumon, VM-26)	Refrigerator	*In solution:* 10 mg/ml Dilute to at least 1 mg/ml	*Room:* 0.1–0.4 mg/ml, D5W, or NS (glass container): 24 hr 0.1 mg/ml in NS (PVC container): 8 hr	None
6-Thioguanine (6-TG)	Refrigerator (3-yr stability at room temperature)	Add 5 ml of NS to 75-mg vial to yield a 15-mg/ml solution	15 mg/ml *(refrigerated):* 24 hr Further diluted in 500 ml NS or D5W *(room or refrigerated):* 24 hr	*Compatible* with thioguanine
Thiophosphoramide (Thio-TEPA)	Refrigerator	Add 1.5 ml sterile H_2O to 15-mg vial to yield 10 mg/ml isotonic solution	*Room:* 24 hr *Refrigerator:* 5 days *Room or refrigerator:* 15 days (0.5 mg/ml in LR)	None
Topotecan (Hycamptamine)	Refrigerator	Add 2 ml sterile H_2O to 5-mg vial to yield 2.5 mg/ml	*Room:* 0.02–0.1 mg/ml in NS or D5W: 48 hr	None
Trimetrexate (TMQ, TMTX)	Room	Add 1.9 ml sterile H_2O to 25-mg vial to yield 12.5 mg/ml	*Room:* 7 days (12.5 mg/ml), 24 hrs (4 mg/ml), 48 hr (0.1 mg/ml) Do **not** use chloride-containing solutions	*Incompatible* with chloride- or anion-containing solutions
Vinblastine (Velban, Velsar, VBL)	Refrigerator	*In solution:* 1 mg/ml Add 10 ml NS to 10-mg vial to yield 1 mg/ml	*Room:* 14 days *Refrigerator:* 30 days	*Compatible* with dacarbazine, doxorubicin, bleomycin, and metoclopramide *Incompatible* with furosemide, heparin, and Infusaid pumps
Vincristine (Oncovin, Vincasar, VCR)	Refrigerator	*In solution:* 1 mg/ml	*Room:* 30 days *Further diluted:* 96 hr *Frozen:* 4 weeks	*Compatible* with bleomycin, cytarabine, doxorubicin, fluorouracil, methotrexate, and metaclopramide *Incompatible* with furosemide, idarubicin, some in-line filters, and polysiloxan containers

Note: Certain drugs may only be compatible for a short time in solution (eg, at the Y-site of an IV during infusion). Other drugs may only be compatible at specific concentrations of each drug and in specific solutions. Please consult your pharmacist regarding the specific conditions under which these compatabilities apply.

the outcome of a drug reaction, including the specific drugs, dose, route, schedule, renal function, age, underlying disease, and hepatic function.[95] There are several proposed mechanisms of drug interactions (Table 14-8) that can result in additive toxicity, decreased effectiveness, or altered activity and outcome of nonchemotherapeutic agent(s). Multiple drug reactions with chemotherapeutic drugs have been reported (Tables 14-9, 14-10, 14-11). Pretreatment and ongoing assessment of the patient's current medications are essential to detect potential interactions and avert or minimize an adverse outcome.

TABLE 14-8 Mechanisms of Drug Interactions

Chemical or Physical Interactions
Acids and bases (protamine antagonizes the effects of heparin)
Adsorbent effects (charcoal and cholestryamine decrease absorption)
Incompatibilities of drugs in solution

Altered Gastrointestinal Absorption
Reduced absorbing surface area and circulation at the site of absorption (cancer chemotherapy and digoxin tablets)
Reduced GI flora (oral aminoglycosides can increase absorption of methotrexate)
Chelation complex

Protein-Binding Interactions
Displacement interactions (aspirin and other drugs displace warfarin, methotrexate, etc)
Significance depends on percentage of drug that is protein bound and drug affinities for plasma proteins

"Receptor" Interactions
Agonists and antagonists (opioid analgesics and naloxone)
Additive pharmacologic effects (anticholinergic effects)
Sensitization (general anesthetics sensitize the myocardium to the arrhythmogenic effects of catecholamines)
Masking (beta-blockers may mask hypoglycemia symptoms of insulin)
Synergy (leucovorin and 5-fluorouracil)
Reversal of cellular resistance (verapamil and doxorubicin)

Acceleration of Metabolism
Induction of hepatic microsomal enzymes (barbiturates, polycyclic hydrocarbons, rifampin may increase the metabolism of other drugs to inactive compounds (eg, quinidine, estrogens, methadone, propoxyphene) or may increase metabolism of other drugs (eg, cylophosphamide, meperidine) to active or toxic compounds

Inhibition of Metabolism
Decreased liver bloodflow (cimetidine and beta-blockers may decrease the metabolism of BCNU)
Inhibition of metabolic enzymes (allopurinol may inhibit xanthine oxidase and decrease the activation of 5-FU)
Inhibition of hepatic microsomal enzymes, thereby decreasing "first pass" metabolism (allopurinol slows the metabolism and enhances the pharmacologic effects of oral 6-mercaptopurine)

Alteration of Renal Excretion
Decreased renal bloodflow (nonsteroidal anti-inflammatory drugs may inhibit elimination of methotrexate)
Competition for tubular transport (probenecid and aspirin impede the elimination of penicillin and methotrexate)
Changes in urine pH may increase elimination of acidic drugs (eg, methotrexate, aspirin)
Additive nephrotoxicity

Diagnostic Interference
Chemical interference
Altered physiology (diuretics may cause hypokalemia and enhance the cardiotoxic potential of digoxin, amsacrine)

Source: Fischer DS, Knobf M, Durivage H: *The Cancer Chemotherapy Handbook* (ed. 4). St. Louis: Mosby-Yearbook (in press, 1993). Used with permission.

TABLE 14-9 Drug Interactions with Antineoplastic Drugs

Drug A	Drug B	Potential Outcome
Aminoglutethimide	Sedatives	Additive CNS depression
Asparaginase	Methotrexate	↓ effects of methotrexate
Bleomycin	Cisplatin	↓ elimination of bleomycin
Carmustine (BCNU)	Cimetidine	↓ metabolism of BCNU
Cisplatin	Bleomycin	↓ elimination of bleomycin
	Cytarabine	↑ ototoxicity
	Sodium thiosulfate	↓ cisplatin cytotoxicity
Cyclophosphamide	Mesna	↓ hemorrhagic cystitis
	Succinylcholine	↑ neuromuscular blockade
Cytarabine	Nephrotoxic drugs	↑ neurotoxicity of cytarabine
Doxorubicin	ADR-529 (dexrazoxane)	↓ doxorubicin cardiotoxicity
Floxuridine (FUDR)	Dexamethasone	↓ FUDR hepatotoxocity
5-Fluorouracil	Allopurinol	↓ 5-FU cytotoxicity
	Cimetidine	↑ 5-FU serum concentrations
	Interferon alfa	↑ 5-FU cytotoxicity
	Leucovorin	↑ 5-FU cytotoxicity
	Methotrexate	↑ 5-FU cytotoxicity
	PALA	↑ 5-FU cytotoxicity

(continued)

TABLE 14-9 Drug Interactions with Antineoplastic Drugs (continued)

Drug A	Drug B	Potential Outcome
Ifosfamide	Acetylcysteine	↓ hemorrhagic cystitis
	Mesna	↓ hemorrhagic cystitis
Interferon alfa	Theophylline	↓ theophylline clearance
6-Mercaptopurine (6-MP)	Allopurinol	↑ oral bioavailability of 6-MP
	Nondepolarizing muscle relaxants	↓ neuromuscular blockade
Methotrexate	Aspirin	↓ renal elimination of MTX, ↑ toxicity
	Leucovorin	↓ MTX cytotoxicity
	Nonsteroidal anti-inflammatory drugs	↑ MTX toxocity
	Probenecid	↓ renal elimination of MTX, ↑ toxicity
	Sulfonamides	↑ MTX protein displacement, ↑ toxicity
	Trimethoprim	Additive enzyme inhibition, ↑ toxicity
Mitomycin	Vinblastine	Acute pneumonitis
Mitotane	Spironolactone	↓ cytotoxicity of mitotane
Procarbazine	Ethanol	Disulfiram (Antabuse) reaction
	Sympathomimetics	Possible ↑ blood pressure
	Sedatives	Additive CNS depression
	Tyramine-containing food	? ↑ blood pressure
Thiotepa	Pancuronium (Pavulon)	↑ neuromuscular blockade

Source: Fischer DS, Knobf M, Durivage H: *The Cancer Chemotherapy Handbook* (ed. 4). St. Louis: Mosby-Yearbook (in press, 1993). Used with permission.

TABLE 14-10 Antineoplastic Drug Interactions with Digitalis Glycosides[96–98]

Digitalis Glycoside—Outcome	Antineoplastic Drugs (number of patients)
Digoxin: ↓ plasma levels (tablet formulation), no change (liquid formulation)	High-dose carmustine (3 patients) High-dose cyclophosphamide (1 patient) Carmustine and melphalan (1 patient) High-dose cytarabine (1 patient) High-dose cytarabine and cyclophosphamide (7 patients)
Digoxin: ↓ plasma levels	Cyclophosphamide, vincristine, prednisone ± procarbazine (17 patients) Doxorubicin, bleomycin, prednisone (3 patients) Cyclophosphamide, vincristine, cytarabine, prednisone (1 patient)
Digoxin and digitoxin: ↓ plasma levels of digoxin, no change in plasma levels of digitoxin	Cyclophosphamide, vincristine, prednisone ± procarbazine (11 patients) Cyclophosphamide, vincristine, cytarabine, prednisone (2 patients)

Source: Fischer DS, Knobf M, Durivage H: *The Cancer Chemotherapy Handbook* (ed. 4). St. Louis: Mosby-Yearbook (in press, 1993). Used with permission.

TABLE 14-11 Antineoplastic Drug Interactions with Warfarin[99–108]

Outcome of Drug Interaction	Antineoplastic Drugs (number of patients)
↓ prothrombin time and hematoma	Cyclophosphamide, methotrexate, 5-fluorouracil, vincristine, and prednisone (1 patient)
↓ prothrombin time, ↑ dose of warfarin required to maintain adequate anticoagulation	Aminogluthethimide (1 patient)
↑ prothrombin time and hematuria	Tamoxifen (1 patient)
↓ prothrombin time (3- to 5-fold increase in warfarin clearance)	Aminoglutethimide and cortisone acetate (2 patients)
↓ prothrombin time (dose-related increase in warfarin clearance)	Aminoglutethimide 125 mg q.i.d. (low dose) or 250 mg q.i.d. ("high" dose) (9 patients)
↑ prothrombin time, epistaxis, and hematuria	Cyclophosphamide, methotrexate, 5-fluorouracil (2 patients) ProMACE-MOPP (1 patient)
↓ prothrombin time, ↑ dose of warfarin required to maintain adequate anticoagulation	6-Mercaptopurine (positive rechallenge) (1 patient)
↑ prothrombin time	Levamisole and 5-fluorouracil
↑ prothrombin time	Etoposide and vindesine (1 patient)

Source: Fischer DS, Knobf M, and Durivage H: *The Cancer Chemotherapy Handbook* (ed. 4). St. Louis: Mosby-Yearbook (in press, 1993). Used with permission.

REFERENCES

1. Krakoff IH: Cancer chemotherapeutic and biologic agents. *CA-A J Clin* 41:264–278, 1991.
2. Hubbard SM: Neoplastic processes. In Jones DA, Juronec MA, Dunbar CA (eds.): *Medical Surgical Nursing.* New York: McGraw-Hill, 1978, p. 145.
3. DeVita, VT: The relationship between tumor mass and resistance to chemotherapy. *Cancer* 51:1209–1220, 1983.
4. DeVita VT: Principles of chemotherapy. In DeVita VT, Hellman S, Rosenberg SA (eds.): *Principles and Practice of Oncology.* Philadelphia: Lippincott, 1990, pp. 276–299.
5. Goldie JH, Coldman AJ: The genetic origin of drug resistance in neoplasms: Implications for systemic therapy. *Canc Res* 44:3643–3653, 1984.
6. Skipper HE, Simpson-Herren L: Relationship between tumor cell heterogeneity and responsiveness to chemotherapy. In DeVita VT, Hellman S, Rosenberg SA (eds.): *Important Advances in Oncology.* Philadelphia: Lippincott, 1985, pp. 63–77.
7. Carter SK: Some thoughts on resistance to cancer chemotherapy. *Canc Treat Rev* 11:3–7, 1984.
8. Baserga R: The cell cycle. *N Engl J Med* 304(8):453–459, 1981.
9. Maxwell MB, Maher KE: Chemotherapy-induced myelosuppression. *Semin Oncol Nurs* 8:113–123, 1992.
10. Cooper MR, Cooper MR: Principles of medical oncology. In Holleb AI, Fink D, Murphy G (eds.): *Clinical Oncology.* Atlanta: American Cancer Society, 1991, pp. 47–68.
11. DeVita VT: Cell kinetics and chemotherapy of cancer. *Canc Chemother Rep* 2:22–23, 1971.
12. Skipper HE, Schabel FM, Wilcox WS: Experimental evaluation of potential anticancer agents XII: On the criteria and kinetics associated with "curability" of experimental leukemia. *Cancer Chemother Rep* 35:1–111, 1964.
13. Ozols RF, Cowan K: New aspects of clinical drug resistance: The role of gene amplification and reversal of resistance in drug refractory cancer. In DeVita VT, Hellman S, Rosenberg SA (eds.): *Important Advances in Oncology.* Philadelphia: Lippincott, 1986, pp. 129–157.
14. Goldie JH: Relevance of drug resistance in cancer treatment strategy. In Muggia FM (ed.); *Cancer Chemotherapy.* New York: Martinus Nijhoff, 1983, pp. 1–30.
15. Goldie JH: Drug resistance and cancer chemotherapy strategy in breast cancer. *Breast Canc Res & Treat* 3:129–136, 1983.
16. Luria SE, Delbruck M: Mutations of bacteria from virus sensitivity to virus resistance. *Genetics* 28:491–511, 1943.
17. Dexter DL, Leith JT: Tumor heterogeneity and drug resistance. *J Clin Oncol* 4:244–257, 1986.
18. Spremulli EN, Dexter DL: Human tumor cell heterogeneity and metastasis. *J Clin Oncol* 1:496–509, 1983.
19. Chabner BA, et al: Cancer chemotherapy progress and expectations. *Cancer* 54:2599–2608, 1984.
20. Curt GA, Clendenimin NJ, Chabner BA: Drug resistance in cancer. *Canc Treat Rep* 68:87–99, 1984.
21. Bertino JR, Srimatkandada S, Carmen M, et al: Mechanisms of drug resistance in human leukemia. In Neth, Gallo, Greaves, Janka (eds.): *Modern Trends in Human Leukemia VI.* New York: Springer-Verlag, 1985, pp. 90–95.
22. Bertino JR, et al: Gene amplification and altered enzymes as mechanisms for the development of drug resistance. *Canc Treat Rep* 67:901–904, 1983.

23. Chabner BA: The oncologic end game. *J Clin Oncol* 4:625–638, 1986.
24. Dalton WS, Miller TP: Multidrug resistance. *PPO Updates* 5:1–13, 1991.
25. Ling V, Gerlach J, Kartner N: Multidrug resistance. *Breast Canc Res & Treat* 4:89–94, 1984.
26. Bradley G, Juranka PF, Ling V: Mechanism of multidrug resistance. *Biochimica et Biophysica Acta* 948:87–128, 1988.
27. Shoemaker RH, Curt GA, Carney DN: Evidence for multi-drug resistant cells in human tumor populations. *Canc Treat Rep* 67:883–888, 1983.
28. Reich SD: Rationale for anticancer drug dosing schedules. *Canc Nurs* 6:465–467, 1983.
29. Reich SD: The clinical application of drug dosing schedules in cancer therapy—Part II. *Canc Nurs* 7:59–61, 1984.
30. Bertino JR, O'Keefe P: Barriers and strategies for effective chemotherapy. *Semin Oncol Nurs* 8:77–82, 1992.
31. Goldie JH, Coldman AJ, Gudauskas GA: Rationale for the use of alternating non-cross resistant chemotherapy. *Canc Treat Rep* 66:439–449, 1982.
32. Santoro A, et al: Alternating drug combinations in the treatment of advanced Hodgkin's disease. *N Engl J Med* 306:770–775, 1982.
33. Bonadonna G: Evolving concepts in the systemic adjuvant treatment of breast cancer. *Canc Res* 52:2127–2137, 1992.
34. Moliterni A, Bonadonna G, Valagussa P, et al: Cyclophosphamide, methotrexate, and fluorouracil with and without doxorubicin in the adjuvant treatment of resectable cancer with one to three positive axillary nodes. *J Clin Oncol* 9:1124–1130, 1991.
35. DeVita VT: Dose-response is alive and well. *Clin Oncol* 4:1157–1159, 1986.
36. Coppin CM: The description of chemotherapy delivery: Options and pitfalls. *Semin Oncol* 14:34–42, 1987 (suppl).
37. Hryniuk W, Bush H: The importance of dose intensity in chemotherapy of metastatic breast cancer. *J Clin Oncol* 2:1281–1288, 1984.
38. Hryniuk WM, Peter JL: Implications of dose intensity for cancer chemotherapy. *Semin Oncol* 14:43–44, 1987.
39. Harris DT, Mastroangelo MJ: Therapy and application of early systemic therapy. *Semin Oncol* 18:493–503, 1991.
40. Coldman AJ, Goldie JH: Impact of dose-intense chemotherapy on the development of permanent drug resistance. *Semin Oncol* 14:29–33, 1987 (suppl).
41. Capizzi RL: Improvement in the therapeutic index of methotrexate by L-asparaginase. *Canc Chemother Rep* 6:37–41, 1975.
42. Howell, SB, Pfeifle CE, Wang WE, et al: Intraperitoneal cisplatin with systemic thiosulfate protection. *Ann Int Med* 97:845–851, 1982.
43. Glover DJ, Glick JH, Weile C, et al: Phase I/II trials of WR-2721 and cis-platinum. *Int J Rad Oncol Biol Phys* 12:1509–1512, 1986.
44. Atkins JN, Muss HB, Capizzi RL, et al: Phase I study of high-dose cytarabine and cisplatin in patients with advanced malignancy. *Canc Treat Rep* 69:897–898, 1985.
45. Erlichman C, Fine S, Wong A, et al: A randomized trial of fluorouracil and folic acid in patients with metastatic colorectal carcinoma. *J Clin Oncol* 6:469–475, 1988.
46. Grem JL: 5-Fluorouracil plus leucovorin in cancer therapy. *PPO Updates* 2:1–18, 1988.
47. Machover D, Goldschmidt E, Chollet P, et al: Treatment of advanced colorectal and gastric adenocarcinoma with 5-fluorouracil and high-dose folic acid. *J Clin Oncol* 4:685–689, 1986.
48. Wadler S, Lembersky B, Atkins M, et al: Phase II trial of fluorouracil and recombinant interferon alfa-2a in patients with advanced colorectal carcinoma. *J Clin Oncol* 9:1806–1810, 1991.
49. Kemeny N, Conti JA, Seiter K, et al: Biochemical modulation of bolus fluorouracil by PALA in patients with advanced colorectal cancer. *J Clin Oncol* 10:747–752, 1992.
50. Van Groeningen CJ, Peters GJ, Leyva A, et al: Reversal of 5-fluorouracil-induced myelosuppression by prolonged administration of uridine. *J Natl Cancer Inst* 81:157–162, 1989.
51. Bertino JR (ed.): Sequential methotrexate and 5-fluorouracil in the management of neoplastic disease. *Semin Oncol* 10:1–38, 1983 (suppl. 2).
52. Nirenberg A, Mosende C, Mehte B, et al: High-dose methotrexate with citrovorum factor rescue: Predictive value of serum methotrexate concentrations and corrective measures to avert toxicity. *Cancer Treat Rep* 61:779–783, 1979.
53. Lin JT, Bertino JR: Trimetrexate: A second-generation folate antagonist in clinical trial. *J Clin Oncol* 5:2032–2040, 1987.
54. Hait WN, Lazo JS: Calmodulin: A potential target for cancer hemotherapeutic agents. *J Clin Oncol* 4:994–1012, 1986.
55. Fine RL, Koizumi S, Curt GA, Chabner BA: Effect of calcium channel blockers on human CFU-GM with cytotoxic drugs. *J Clin Oncol* 5:489–495, 1987.
56. Ford JM, Hait WN: Pharmacology of drugs that alter multidrug resistance in cancer. *Pharmacol Rev* 42:155–199, 1990.
57. LaCreta F, Brennan J, Padavick K, et al: Phase I clinical, biochemical and pharmacokinetic study of buthionine sulfoxime (BSO) in combination with melphalan (L-PAM). *Proc Am Soc Clin Oncol* 10:104, 1991 (abstr.).
58. Freidman HS, Colvin OM, Griffith OW, et al: Increased melphalan activity in intracranial human medulloblastoma xenografts following buthionine sulfoxime-mediated glutathione depletion. *J Natl Cancer Inst* 81:524–527, 1989.
59. Johnson JR, Temple R: Food and Drug Administration requirements for approval of anticancer drugs. *Cancer Treat Rep* 69:1155–1159, 1985.
60. Buyse ME, Staquet MJ, Sylvester RJ (eds.): *Cancer Clinical Trials, Methods and Practice.* New York: Oxford University Press, 1984.
61. Piantadosi S: Principals of clinical trial design. *Semin Oncol* 15:423–433, 1988.
62. Spilker B: *Guide to Clinical Trials.* New York: Raven Press, 1991.
63. Simon RM: Design and conduct of clinical trials. In DeVita VT, Hellman S, Rosenberg SA (eds.): *Cancer Principles and Practices of Oncology* (ed. 3). Philadelphia: Lippincott, 1990.
64. Wittes RE: Current emphasis in the clinical drug development program of the National Cancer Institute. *PPO Updates* 1:1–15, 1987.
65. Boyd MR: Status of the NCI pre-clinical antitumor drug discovery screen. *PPO Updates* 3:1–12, 1989.

66. Grieshaber CK, Marsoni S: Relation of preclinical toxicology to findings in early clinical trials. *Cancer Treat Rep* 70:65–72, 1986.
67. VonHoff DD, Kuhn J, Clark GM: Design and conduct of phase I trials. In Buyse ME, Staquet MJ, Sylvester RJ (eds.): *Cancer Clinical Trials, Methods and Practice.* New York: Oxford University Press, 1984, pp. 210–220.
68. Wittes RE: How we know what we (think we) know. *J Clin Oncol* 4:827–829, 1986 (editorial).
69. Cassileth BR, Lusk EJ, Miller DS, et al: Attitudes toward clinical trials among patients and the public. *JAMA* 248:968–970, 1982.
70. Mattson ME, Curb DJ, McArdle R, et al: Participation in a clinical trial: The patient's point of view. *Controlled Clin Trials* 6:156–167, 1985.
71. Friedman, MA: Patient accrual to clinical trials. *Cancer Treat Rep* 71:557–558, 1987.
72. Hunter CP, Frelick RW, Feldman AR, et al: Selection factors in clinical trials: Results from the Community Clinical Oncology Program physician's log. *Cancer Treat Rep* 71:559–565, 1987.
73. Gelber RD, Goldhirsch A: Can a clinical trial be the treatment of choice for patients with cancer? *J Natl Cancer Inst* 80:886–887, 1988 (letter).
74. Wittes RE, Friedman MA: Accrual to clinical trials. *J Natl Cancer Inst* 80:884–885, 1988 (editorial).
75. Taylor KM, Morgolese RG, Soskoline CL: Physician's reasons for not entering eligible patients in a randomized clinical trial of surgery for breast cancer. *N Engl J Med* 310:1363–1367, 1984.
76. Levine AS: Clinical trials and the community physician. *Cancer* 51:2498–2502, 1983 (suppl. 12).
77. Brennan, MJ: Factors affecting patient's and doctor's decisions to participate in clinical trials in oncology. A thesis submitted to the Yale University School of Medicine in partial fulfillment of the requirements for the degree of Doctor of Medicine, 1989.
78. Wittes RE: Paying for patient care in treatment research—Who is responsible? *Cancer Treat Rep* 71:107–113, 1987.
79. Antman K, Schnipper LE, Frei E: The crisis in clinical cancer research. Third-party insurance and investigative therapy. *N Engl J Med* 319:46–48, 1988 (letter).
80. McCabe M, Friedman MA: Impact of third-party reimbursement on cancer clinical investigations: A consensus statement coordinated by the National Cancer Institute. *J Natl Cancer Inst* 81:1585–1586, 1989.
81. Friedman MA, McCabe MS: Assigning care costs associated with therapeutic oncology research: A modest proposal. *J Natl Cancer Instit* 84:760–763, 1992.
82. Fisher DS, Knobf MT, Durivage H: *The Cancer Chemotherapy Handbook* (ed. 4). St Louis: Mosby-Yearbook (in press, 1993).
83. Lobert S, Correia JJ: Antimitotics in cancer chemotherapy. *Canc Nurs* 15:22–33, 1992.
84. Trissel LA: *Handbook on Injectable Drugs* (ed. 6). Washington, DC: American Society of Hospital Pharmacists, 1990.
85. Koberda M, Zieske PA, Raghavan NV, Payton RJ: Stability of bleomycin sulfate reconstituted in 5% dextrose injection or 0.9% sodium chloride injection stored in glass vials or polyvinyl chloride containers. *Am J Hosp Pharm* 47:2528–2529, 1990.
86. Kirschenbaum BE, Latiolais, CJ: The stability of injectible medications after reconstitution and/or further dilution. *Parenterals* 4(5a):20–27, 44–48, 1986.
87. Stewart CF, Hampton EM: Stability of cisplatin and etoposide in intravenous admixtures. *Am J Hosp Pharm* 46:1400–1404, 1989.
88. Lokich JJ, Zipoli TE, Moore C, et al: Doxorubicin/vinblastine and doxorubicin/cyclophosphamide combination chemotherapy by continuous infusion. *Cancer* 58:1020–1023, 1986.
89. Seargeant LE, Kobrinsky NL, Sus CJ, et al: In vitro stability of daunorubicin, cytarabine, and etoposide. *Cancer Treat Rep* 71(12):1189–1192, 1987.
90. Hoffman DM, Grossano DD, Damin L, Woodcock TM: Stability of refrigerated and frozen solutions of doxorubicin hydrochloride. *Am J Hosp Pharm* 36:1536–1538, 1979.
91. Smith JA, Morris A, Duafala ME, et al: Stability of floxuridine and leucovorin calcium admixtures for intraperitoneal administration. *Am J Hosp Pharm* 46:985–989, 1989.
92. Waugh WN, Trissel LA, Stella VJ: Stability, compatibility, and plasticizer extraction of taxol injection diluted in infusion solutions stored in various containers. *Am J Hosp Pharm* 48:1520–1524, 1991.
93. Ratain MJ, Vogelzang NJ: Phase I and pharmacological study of vinblastine by prolonged continuous infusion. *Cancer Res* 46:4827–4830, 1986.
94. May FE, Stewart RB, Cluff LE: Drug interactions and multiple drug administration. *Clin Pharmacol Ther* 22:322–328, 1977.
95. Finley RSW: Drug interactions in the oncology patient. *Semin Oncol Nurs* 8:95–101, 1992.
96. Bjornsson TD, Huang AT, Roth P, et al: Effects of high-dose chemotherapy on the absorption of digoxin in two different formulations. *Clin Pharmacol Ther* 39:25–28, 1986.
97. Kuhlmann J, Wilke J, Rietbrock N: Cytostatic drugs are without significant effect on digitoxin plasma level and renal excretion. *Clin Pharmacol Ther* 32:646–651, 1982.
98. Kuhlmann J, Zilly W, Wilke J: Effects of cytostatic drugs on plasma level and renal excretion of beta-acetyldigoxin. *Clin Pharmacol Ther* 30:518–527, 1981.
99. Booth BW, Weiss RB: Venous thrombosis during adjuvant chemotherapy. *N Engl J Med* 305:170, 1981 (letter).
100. Bruning PF, Bonfrer JG: Aminoglutethimide and oral anticoagulant therapy. *Lancet* 2(8349):582, 1983 (letter).
101. Lodwick R, McConkey B, Brown AM: Life-threatening interaction between tamoxifen and warfarin. *Br Med J* 295:1141, 1987 (letter).
102. Lonning PE, Ueland PM, Kvinnsland S: The influence of a graded dose schedule of aminoglutethimide on the disposition of the optical enantiomers of warfarin in patients with breast cancer. *Cancer Chemother Pharmacol* 17:177–181, 1986.
103. Lonning PE, Kvinnsland S, Jahren G: Aminoglutethimide and warfarin. A new important drug interaction. *Cancer Chemother Pharmacol* 12:10–12, 1984.
104. Seifter EJ, Brooks BJ, Urba WJ: Possible interactions between warfarin and antineoplastic drugs. *Cancer Treat Rep* 69:244–245, 1985.
105. Spiers ASD, Mibashan RS: Increased warfarin requirements during mercaptopurine therapy. *Lancet* 2:221–222, 1974.

106. Spivack SD: Procarbazine. *Ann Intern Med* 81:795–800, 1974.
107. Stevenson HC: Potential adverse levamisole interactions with phenytoin and also with coumarin. *NCI Warning Letter,* July 10, 1991.
108. Ward K, Bitran JD: Warfarin, etoposide, and vindesine interactions. *Cancer Treat Rep* 68:817–818, 1984 (letter).

Chapter 15

Chemotherapy: Principles of Administration

Patricia E. Reymann, RN, MSN, OCN

CHEMOTHERAPY ADMINISTRATION

Oncology nurses today enjoy a vast and abundant array of educational and informational resources regarding chemotherapy administration. Standards or guidelines have been developed by the Oncology Nursing Society, American Society of Hospital Pharmacists, Occupational Safety and Health Administration, Intravenous Nurses Society, individual state boards of nursing, Environmental Protection Agency, and many other organizations.[1–8] Basic decision making in chemotherapy administration is now often guided by research and published clinical results that cover many situations encountered by oncology nurses in a variety of settings. The growing body of knowledge in this area allows nurses new to the area of oncology to become rapidly proficient and to experience the excitement of being on the cutting edge in oncology. It also entices the seasoned practitioner to forge ahead and sharpen that edge as changes in the health care system, altered patient expectations, and new technologies make advanced practice a constantly evolving challenge. This chapter deals with both basic and advanced principles in chemotherapy administration. It focuses on clinical practice, methods of drug delivery, and vascular access devices (VADs).

Professional Qualifications

Educational guidelines for nurses administering chemotherapy have been in existence since 1984 and are almost universally implemented in a variety of practice settings.[9] The *Oncology Nursing Society's Cancer Chemotherapy Guidelines* were expanded to five modules in 1988, with one specifically addressing "Recommendations for Cancer Chemotherapy Course Content and Clinical Practicum."[1] State boards of nursing have also recognized the need for specialized chemotherapy training and have enacted rules that require adherence to national standards.[10] Both the Intravenous Nurses Society and the Oncology Nursing Society have published position statements regarding the administration of antineoplastic agents and the preparation of the nurse.[11,12]

Basic qualifications for nurses administering antineoplastic agents include:

1. current licensure as a Registered Nurse
2. certification in CPR
3. intravenous therapy skills
4. educational preparation and demonstration of knowledge in all areas related to antineoplastic drugs (pharmacology, kinetics, handling, administration, side effect management, laboratory value monitoring, patient education, and resources)
5. demonstration of the skill of drug administration
6. ongoing acquisition of updated information and verification of continuing knowledge and skills
7. policies and procedures to govern specific actions (see Table 15-1)

Formal chemotherapy certification programs developed by and for oncology nurses are common and use a variety of teaching strategies. Program lengths vary from several days to several weeks. The most common approach involves organized lectures in a classroom setting, but some courses are designed independently, using videotapes, programmed instruction modules, and self-study materials. Programs should include a posttest to verify learning and some type of supervised clinical demonstration of the skill. Structured chemotherapy training has eliminated much of the fear and uncertainty for new oncology nurses and helps to ensure quality patient care and maintain high safety standards.[13,14] Chemotherapy certification also provides proof of formalized training and skill demonstration, which is extremely important from a professional liability perspective. Antineoplastic agents have potent or life-threatening side effects, and it is in the best interests of both the patient and the nurse that educational preparation be obtained and documented. Additionally, clinically oriented policies and procedures that are part of ongoing quality improvement help to provide a firm practical and legal foundation for this aspect of oncology nursing practice.

Handling Cytotoxic Drugs

Scientific articles regarding potential or actual hazards of cytotoxic drug exposure have been appearing in the medical, pharmaceutical, and nursing literature for over a decade.[2–4,15–21] Direct exposure to these cytotoxic agents can occur during admixture, administration, or handling and involve inhalation, ingestion, or absorption.[22–25] The drugs are known to be mutagenic, teratogenic, and carcinogenic. Additionally, exposure has been reported to result in rashes, skin discolora-

TABLE 15-1 Institutional Policies and Procedures That Should Be Established to Guide Oncology Nursing Practice in the Area of Chemotherapy Administration

- Staff education for chemotherapy and other specialty procedures (ie, VADs)
- Chemotherapy administration (all routes)
- Vesicant management
- Allergic reactions
- Safe drug handling and disposal
- Patient and family education
- Management of vascular access devices
- Documentation methods
- Outcome standards
- Oncology quality-improvement process

tions, scarring, blurred vision, and dizziness. Guidelines containing recommendations to prevent cytotoxic drug exposure to personnel and the environment have been established by the Occupational Safety and Health Administration (OSHA), Oncology Nursing Society, and American Society of Hospital Pharmacists.[2,4,25] Detailed drug handling guidelines are outlined in Table 15-2. Clearly, these guidelines and suggestions are to be used by those determining the actual policies and procedures of cytotoxic drug handling, since there are some differences of opinion, due primarily to lack of available research, regarding the extent to which measures must be taken to contain cytotoxic drugs.

TABLE 15-2 Cytotoxic Drug Handling Guidelines[2,4,25]

Preparation
- Don a disposable gown that is lint-free, low- or nonpermeable, long-sleeved, cuffed, and solid-fronted.
- Don a pair of powder-free, thick, surgical-quality latex gloves, ensuring that the cuffs of the gloves overlap the cuffs of the gown.
- Admix all cytotoxic drugs in a class II biologic safety cabinet (vertical air flow) that meets national standards and is inspected appropriately.
- Use a disposable, plastic-backed liner for the preparation area and appropriate equipment such as luer-lok syringes.
- Clean the cabinet daily with 70% alcohol, and decontaminate it weekly or if spills occur.
- Use aseptic technique.
- Take care to avoid drug dispersement by venting vials, handling ampules carefully, avoiding overfilling of containers, and adding diluents slowly.
- Attach and prime IV tubing before adding the cytotoxic drug to the IV solution.
- Wipe all syringes and containers, and label them appropriately, including a warning label indicating that the contents are cytotoxic.
- Do not clip or recap needles; discard all sharps in a convenient and appropriately labeled, puncture-proof container.
- Discard protective clothing and used materials in a separate trash bag labeled as cytotoxic.
- Wash hands.

Administration
- Receive appropriately labeled cytotoxic drugs in clean, dry syringes or bags of IV fluids. Syringes should be inside zip-close plastic bags. Inspect bags before opening to ensure no spillage within the bag.
- Wash hands and don protective clothing. If dripping or spashing can occur, this should include a disposable gown that is lint-free, low- or nonpermeable, long-sleeved, cuffed, and solid-fronted.
- Don a pair of powder-free, thick, surgical-quality latex gloves, ensuring that the cuffs of the gloves overlap the cuffs of the gown, if a gown is being worn.
- Place a plastic-backed absorbent pad over the work area to absorb any drips.

TABLE 15-2 Cytotoxic Drug Handling Guidelines[2,4,25] (continued)

- Use intravenous administration sets and syringes with luer-lok fittings.
- If the administration set is not attached to the intravenous fluids and primed by the pharmacist, it should be attached and primed with caution to prevent exposure of the drug to the environment. It may be primed into a gauze pad inside a zip-close bag, or it may be piggybacked to plain fluids and primed by retrograde flow ("back-primed").
- Secure all connections and Y-sites with tape.
- Keep a gauze pad at hand to wipe droplets off Y-sites or connecting points.
- Do not expel air from syringes. If air is in a syringe, hold it in such a way that the air is up near the plunger and simply stop pushing on the plunger when all of the drug is expelled and the air is reached.
- Do not use intravenous bottles with venting tubes.
- Monitor administration sets and connection sites for leakage.
- Do not clip or recap needles. Discard the needle-syringe unit into a convenient and appropriately labeled, puncture-proof container.
- Discard all gauze, tubing, bags, bottles, etc. in appropriately labeled bags, and seal. Remove gown and gloves and discard in a similar manner.
- Wash hands.

General Handling and Disposal
- Dispose of all sharps, containers, and cytotoxic waste according to appropriate state and federal guidelines (usually, incineration or burial in a hazardous waste landfill).
- Contain all grossly contaminated linen of treated patients within 48 hours in labeled double bags, and wash twice (same procedure as for infectious wastes).
- Obtain spill kits, and place them in the admixture and administration areas.
- Clean up spills using available kits and disposable towels or sponges. For large spills, double gloving is recommended.
- If direct exposure occurs, immediately rinse the area with running water. For eye exposure, rinse with an eye wash solution or sterile saline.
- Report all episodes of exposure to employee health or the equivalent resource.

Personnel
- Identify all personnel who handle cytotoxic drugs and their metabolites.
- Educate and train personnel in proper drug handling.
- Establish a mechanism to monitor cytotoxic drug handling practices, from receipt through disposal.
- Provide ready access to information regarding cytotoxic drugs.
- Address pregnancy and medical surveillance issues.
- Monitor all spills and occurrences of direct exposure through a quality-improvement program.
- Develop patient education materials as needed, particularly for use in the home.

A major area of controversy during drug administration is the need for protective clothing, which could be uniforms, lab coats, scrubs, or disposable gowns. Some institutions mandate specific garb; others leave it to the discretion of the individual to determine if spills or splashes are likely to occur. The OSHA standards regarding blood-borne pathogens require the *employer* to determine the risk of exposure for each task performed by an employee and to then specify the protective measure to be taken.[26] This approach probably will also be used when OSHA rewrites the cytotoxic drug handling guidelines.

It is well know that the drugs and their metabolites are excreted in the urine and stool beyond 48 hours after drug administration. The OSHA guidelines recommend gowning and gloving to handle excreta during this time frame; however, most nurses wear only regular exam gloves. Double gloving was a common practice at one time, but is now usually seen only when cleaning up large spills.

Personnel policies regarding pregnancy are quite varied, despite OSHA's suggestion that appropriate protective practices should reduce any potential reproductive hazards.[4] While OSHA recommends that employees be informed of potential risks and, if necessary, reassigned to other duties, it is not uncommon to find institutional policies that prohibit pregnant or lactating employees from working with cytotoxic drugs. Another personnel issue is medical surveillance, which usually includes a preemployment health assessment, a baseline CBC, and thorough documentation of any risk factors in the health history. It's becoming less common to require more extensive testing, for there are no data to support a cause-and-effect relationship between precautionary cytotoxic drug handling and abnormal physical or laboratory findings.

Patient education regarding cytotoxic drug handling is important so that patients and family members understand why gloves and/or gowns are being worn and not feel alienated by the practice. Education is a crucial element if chemotherapy is being provided in the home setting, since family members need to be instructed in drug containment practices. The health care professional should provide the patient with written instructions, such as those developed by Sansivero and Murray[27] or Blecke,[28] which specify that gloves be worn when working with the medications, used materials be placed in the provided containers, care be taken to avoid direct exposure, spills be cleaned up with the spill kit provided, and direct external exposure be managed with copious flushing and washing. They address a number of personal care areas, including hygiene (washing hands), personal contact (hugs are encouraged), and sexual intercourse (should be safe, but ask the physician or nurse if a condom should be worn).

Bingham very eloquently outlined the history of this occupational problem from the origin of chemicals designed to be cytotoxic through the epidemiologic proof of adverse effects.[29] Despite proof that exposure can be harmful, a large percentage of health professionals continue to disregard personal protective measures.[30] There appears to be a perception that low-level exposure is not harmful, since no absolute scientific quantification of exposure has been defined. It is not known if a little exposure is harmless or how much is too much or even if some drugs are more harmful than others. Given the fact that stiff financial penalties can be incurred if OSHA ascertains noncompliance with established guidelines, the minimum standards to be met include: (1) knowledge of the latest scientific information; (2) established policies and procedures; and (3) ongoing monitoring to ensure compliance and continuous quality improvement.

Patient and Family Education

Educating patients and their family members about cancer is usually started by the physician, who imparts the diagnosis of cancer, treatment options, risks and benefits, alternatives, and prognosis.[31,32] The nurse's role is defined by the *Oncology Nursing Society Standards of Oncology Education: Patient/Family,* and usually begins with clarifying information and disabusing misconceptions, especially the old wives tales that exist about cancer and cancer treatment.[33] Nurses are usually responsible for imparting specific information about treatment side effects and measures to recognize and minimize their consequences. Details regarding mouth care, skin care, wig shops, over-the-counter medications, food intake, and many other aspects of daily life are frequently addressed by the nurse. Identifying problems or side effects a patient might experience due to the chemotherapy as a whole rather than addressing each drug separately is usually easiest, due to the wide range of side effects encountered. Some basic steps to follow when planning and implementing patient education are included in Table 15-3.

It is very important in the preparation and planning stages to ensure adequate knowledge of the drugs, their side effects, and the treatment goal. Assessment of the patient should include the individual's response to the diagnosis, communication style, ability to read/comprehend information, family status, lifestyle, and treatment outcome expectations.

The patient and nurse should both be relaxed, with time to discuss the treatment and its side effects. Asking the patient if there are any questions helps to deal with concerns immediately and establishes an open exchange of information. Anxiety during the presentation is unavoidable, but the nurse should observe the patient's facial expression and body language to help measure the impact of the information on the patient, for it is sometimes necessary to probe for questions if the patient looks confused or to allow time for the facts to be assimilated. More complex instruction is required when a patient is entering a research protocol, since there is a written informed consent, usually several pages in length, that is read to the patient or reviewed in great detail. Participation in a research study is usually the

TABLE 15-3 Chemotherapy Patient Education Guidelines

Preparation

- Review policies, procedures, and documentation forms.
- Listen to experienced physicians and nurses when they are instructing patients, to gain ideas and hints.
- Read or review available educational materials, to become familiar with "patient" terminology.
- Identify learning needs and specific instructions for prevention and management of side effects (see Chapter 16).
- If using audiovisual equipment, know how it operates.

Planning

- Know the basics about the patient to be taught and the goal of the treatment plan. If necessary, read the chart or talk to others who have been involved in the care of the patient. It's especially important to know if the patient speaks and reads English, if that is the language being used.
- Have pertinent teaching materials available.
- If possible, separate the teaching session from the actual drug administration procedure.
- Advise the patient that information will be imparted, and determine if he or she desires the family members or a significant other to be present.
- Try to eliminate interruptions.

Presentation

- Introduce self and purpose.
- Determine if the patient has any specific questions or concerns to address before proceeding.
- Discuss the treatment process, ie, starting intravenous infusion, administering drugs, length of time, immediate events, expected follow-up, monitoring side effects, and home care. Describe any sensations the patient might have during the infusion/injection (eg, coolness, perirectal burning, lightheadedness, nasal stuffiness).
- Describe the potential side effects and interventions in order to minimize their consequences. Include specific information about what to look for, what's normal, how to take a temperature, where to buy a wig, which mouth care regimen to use, and other appropriate recommendations. Provide written information regarding when to call the physician or nurse.
- Avoid overloading the patient with information about rare or unusual risks of chemotherapy. Give written information regarding this aspect of his or her treatment and elaborate where appropriate.
- Ensure that informed consent has been obtained.
- Maintain a responsive atmosphere that is open to questioning.
- Give written instructions regarding activity, diet, hygiene, medications, and other self-care behaviors for the patient to follow for the next few days or weeks.

Follow-Up

- Document the encounter and the patient's response. (See Patient Teaching and Documentation Tool, Chapter 16.)
- Question the patient to assess his or her understanding of the information imparted.

TABLE 15-3 Chemotherapy Patient Education Guidelines (continued)

- When possible, observe the patient to determine if his or her actions indicate an understanding of the information (eg, hydration, mouth care, medications).
- It is optimal to contact the patient within 48 hours of drug administration to determine if there are any questions or problems to be resolved, especially if the patient and nurse are no longer together in the same setting (ie, hospital or home).

only circumstance under which the patient's signature on a written consent form is required by law. While some health care agencies require signed consent forms for all chemotherapy, many others consider that consent is granted when the patient allows the drug to be given.

Common questions asked by newly diagnosed patients reflect their fears and uncertainties and include: "Would you do this if you were me?" and "Am I going to die?" It's important for the nurse to remain nonjudgmental to realistically support the patient. Responses of "Sure, I'd do it" and "Everyone's going to die someday" do not address the underlying issues. More appropriate responses might include: "It sounds like you're wondering if you've made the right decision. Would you like to discuss how this treatment will affect you and your life?" or "Most people with a very serious illness such as cancer are concerned about dying. What makes you ask that question right now?" Other, more direct questions such as "Is my hair going to fall out?" are also sometimes difficult to answer because not all patients experience the same side effects. Frequently the best answer is a quantification of the issue (e.g., "probably," "most people do," or "most people don't") and reassurance on the positive possibility that if the problem occurs, there are frequently ways to minimize its consequences. Follow-up includes assessment of the patient's understanding of the information imparted and determination that the outcome has been achieved. Observation of the patient and questioning regarding actions and activities are usually sufficient to ensure comprehension. Documentation of the entire process is very important and can involve a detailed written note or a checklist-type form (see Chapter 16). Numerous forms are available in the literature for the nurse seeking a quick and easy way to document this very involved process.[34–39]

Cancer chemotherapy patient education is very detailed and involves interventions to meet changing and evolving needs of the patient and family. It must involve a series of encounters, both structured and unstructured, with a focus on defining and meeting the patient's goals. Barofsky describes a progression from compliance to adherence to therapeutic alliance.[40] In this model, the patient/family and the nurse move on a continuum from patient reporting of nurse-identified signs or symptoms, through patient questioning and considering options, to the eventual involvement of the patient in codecision making, self-care behaviors, and adoption of mutual goals. Progress toward therapeutic alliance takes time, but it promotes trust, compliance, and self-care, which are critical for patients on increasingly complex chemotherapeutic regimens in multiple care settings. A great deal of pertinent information on patient education is contained in Chapter 16.

Administration Principles

Chemotherapy administration is complex, due to the potency and purpose of the drugs, which have relatively low therapeutic indices, or a limited difference between a therapeutic dose and a lethal dose. It involves strong chemicals with radical side effects that can affect every system in the body. Overdosing can result in paraplegia, skin sloughing, renal failure, pulmonary dysfunction, or death. Underdosing can fail to control the cancer and result in disease progression or death. The nurse's role in drug calculation, delivery determination, administration, problem solving, symptom management, and follow-up with chemotherapy patients is increasing in sophistication and autonomy in most health care settings.[41]

Overlying these issues are the incredible advances made in chemotherapy administration and drug delivery systems as well as the health care industry itself during the last decade. There are more drugs than ever before, with new agents being marketed every year. Vascular access devices and ambulatory pumps are allowing innovations in drug combinations and scheduling. The setting is no longer the traditional hospital room. Most frequently it is an outpatient infusion center, a day hospital, a clinic, or a physician's office. More and more frequently, it is the patient's home. It's not unusual for patients to be diagnosed via outpatient procedures and to receive all treatments in the outpatient or home setting.[42,43] The medico-legal climate has intensified, and risk taking carries professional liability. Consumer awareness and right-to-know movements are at an all-time high. The use of investigational drugs is more common than ever, but still requires legal, signed informed consent, with specific information provided to the patient in written form. Reimbursement issues have also achieved prime consideration and frequently fall within the prerogative of the nurse to determine if the third-party payer will reimburse for the treatment and the setting. It's not unheard of for the setting and even to some extent the treatment itself to be altered to coincide with optimal reimbursement.[44,45] A 1991 report by the U.S. General Accounting Office revealed that 62% of the oncologists responding to a survey altered the setting while 8%–28% altered the cancer therapy because of reimbursement or other financial problems.[46]

Despite these changes and the complex choices they bring, the basic tenets of drug administration remain the same. These guidelines, listed in Table 15-4, are intended to highlight specific tasks involved in antineoplastic drug administration and are applicable in all practice settings. Issues specific to a particular route of administration (e.g., use of an Ommaya reservoir for intraventricular drug administration) are discussed later in this chapter. One patient preparation issue that is drug specific involves test dosing of bleomycin. While not a common practice, it is still ordered by some physicians because the first dose of bleomycin has been known to cause rare but severe allergic reactions, especially in patients with lymphoma.[47] When ordered, 0.5–1.0 unit of bleomycin is given IV, IM, or subcutaneously prior to the first dose of the drug. It is preferred to test dose 24 hours prior to administration, but it is commonly done 1 or 2 hours before the full dose, followed by very close observation. The anaphylactoid reactions include hypotension, rash, facial flushing, and bronchospasm, and can progress to anaphylaxis. The nurse should be prepared to handle these allergic manifestations if they occur; see Chapters 16 and 33 for specific information about drug hypersensitivity and allergic reactions.

Vesicant Extravasation Issues

One of the greatest challenges to nurses administering cancer chemotherapy is the realization that several of the most commonly administered drugs are vesicants, meaning that they cause tissue necrosis if they infiltrate or extravasate out of the blood vessel and into the soft tissue. While a few nonantineoplastic drugs are vesicants (e.g., Levophed and Dilantin), the number of antineoplastic vesicants is significant; they are listed in Table 15-5 along with the agents known to be irritating to the vein during drug administration.[48,49] It is critical that the nurse administering chemotherapy both be aware of those drugs that are vesicants and employ a number of safety measures to try and prevent extravasation.

When extravasation with a vesicant occurs, underlying tissue is damaged. The damage can be severe enough to result in physical deformity or a functional deficit, such as loss of joint mobility, loss of vascularity, or loss of tendon function. The following guidelines are suggested to minimize the risk of extravasation.

1. Be aware of certain patients at increased risk for extravasation:
   a. patients unable to communicate to the nurse about the pain of extravasation
   b. elderly, debilitated, or confused patients with general vascular disease
   c. any patient with very fragile veins
2. Generally, never infuse vesicants over joints, bony prominences, tendons, neurovascular bundles, or the antecubital fossa of the arms.

TABLE 15-4 Chemotherapy Administration Guidelines

Professional Preparation
- Have appropriate knowledge and skills.
- Review applicable policies and procedures.

Patient Preparation
- Verify patient identity (arm band, driver's license, verbalization of name).
- Ensure appropriate patient education.
- Ascertain adequate laboratory values.
- Measure and record baseline vital signs.
- Verify patient's allergy history.
- Assess venous access status (ie, need for VAD).
- Initiate pretreatment therapies, if ordered (eg, hydration, test dosing).

Drug Preparation
- Verify drug order (including body surface area and dosage calculations).
- Obtain prepared drug, and double check label for the correct drug, dose, route, and patient. If admixing, follow appropriate guidelines for cytotoxic drug admixture.
- Ensure rapid access to extravasation kit and medications necessary if allergic reaction occurs (parenteral diphenhydramine hydrochloride and hydrocortisone should be immediately available).
- Obtain necessary supplies and equipment for safe drug administration.
- Wash hands, and don gloves and appropriate protective clothing.

Venipuncture Guidelines
- Establish work area with plastic-backed pad.
- Organize materials, needle box, syringes, flush, IV start materials, and IV fluids.
- Select needle size and type according to setting, patient's veins, and treatment to be administered.
- Determine appropriate site for venous access, avoiding:
  - limbs with recent (ie, 30 min) venipunctures
  - limbs with axillary node dissections, extensive radiation therapy, or obstructive process
  - antecubital fossa (for peripheral sticks)
  - ecchymotic or sclerosed areas
  - bony prominences and joints
- Ensure adequate lighting and visualization of area to be accessed.
- Remove jewelry near access site.
- Select a large vein if administering drugs known to be irritating (mechlorethamine, BCNU, streptozotocin).
- Administer vesicants only at sites designated by established policies and procedures, specifically in areas with underlying subcutaneous tissue. Areas to be avoided when administering vesicants include veins over joints, bony prominences, neurovascular bundles, tendons, and areas of existing soft-tissue damage.
- For peripheral sites, begin at the most distal areas.
- Utilize an appropriate sterile technique for access.

TABLE 15-4 Chemotherapy Administration Guidelines (continued)

- Achieve a "clean" venipuncture and determine patency. The needle should not puncture through the back of the vein and then be resettled within the vein. There should be a brisk, immediate blood return and no swelling at the needle site.
- Secure needle with tape, but ensure visualization of the site.
- Flush needle with sterile NS, D5W, or other "plain" intravenous fluid to clear the line and establish patency. Observe the site at this time to ensure that swelling is not occurring at the needle site.

Drug Administration Guidelines
- Check patient's condition periodically during drug administration, and explain actions being taken, when appropriate.
- Monitor the status of the venous access site periodically during the process.
- Administer antiemetics (if not already given).
- Ensure drug containment at all times. Wipe any droplets at the connector or Y-site with a gauze pad.
- Administer chemotherapy drugs as ordered, using slow, steady pressure.
- Check for a blood return every few cc's and before and after each drug.
- Flush between each drug with sterile NS or D5W to avoid drug admixture and potential precipitation.
- When administering short-term drips or infusions, establish the infusion, taping all connections securely, and set the appropriate flow rate.
- Generally, place long-term infusions on an infusion pump.
- Flush after last drug with sterile NS or D5W.
- If appropriate, discontinue the IV needle. For peripheral sites, hold pressure manually over the site for a few minutes, then apply small, sterile dressing.

Postadministration Guidelines
- Discard all materials (needles, syringes, bags, tubing, gown, gloves, etc.) appropriately.
- Assess patient's status and provide for follow-up:
  - *Inpatient:* Call button within reach; fluids available, etc.
  - *Outpatient:* Transportation ready; return appointment and prescriptions obtained; telephone number of physician or nurse available
  - *Home care:* Caregiver available; telephone number of nurse-on-call available
- Document all actions (flow sheets or specialized forms are recommended). (See Chapter 16.)

3. Never give vesicants intramuscularly or subcutaneously.
4. Avoid giving vesicant drugs in areas where venous or lymphatic circulation is poor (e.g., operative side for a mastectomy patient, patient with superior vena cava syndrome) or that have been previously irradiated.
5. Make sure the peripheral IV site is fresh (less than

TABLE 15-5 Antineoplastic Vesicants and Irritants*

Commercially Available Vesicants[47,48]
Dactinomycin (Cosmegen)
Daunomycin (Cerubidine)
Doxorubicin (Adriamycin)
Estramustine (Estracyte)
Idarubicin (Idamycin)
Mitomycin-C (Mutamycin)
Nitrogen mustard (Mustargen)
Tenopiside (Vumon)
Vinblastine (Velban)
Vincristine (Oncovin)
Commercially Available Irritants
Carmustine (BCNU)
Dacarbazine (DTIC)
Etoposide (VP-16)
Mithramycin (Plicamycin)
Streptozotocin (Zanosar)

*There is some controversy regarding these lists, especially concerning mithramycin and streptozotocin. The practitioner is urged to remain up to date with current research and literature reports regarding these drugs as well as any new agents becoming commercially available

24 hours old). A brisk blood return and easy flow of fluids are to be determined before administering vesicants in any IV needle or catheter (peripheral or central).

6. Visualize the needle or catheter insertion site and observe the site continuously. (Never leave the patient unattended when administering a vesicant peripherally.)
7. When giving more than one chemotherapy agent, give the vesicant agent first.
8. Give vesicants in a steady, even flow, checking frequently for a blood return. When checking for a blood return, do so gently so as to avoid excessive pressure in the vein.
9. If a vesicant is ordered as an infusion, it is given through a central line and checked every 1–2 hours in health care facilities and every 2–4 hours when the patient is receiving vesicant infusions in the home.
10. Make immediately available in the setting an extravasation kit containing all materials necessary to manage an extravasation. Include in the kit a copy of the extravasation policy and procedure.

Despite these precautions, vesicant extravasation does occur, although the incidence is low among very experienced oncology nurses in cancer specialty settings (0.1%) and somewhat higher in general hospital settings (2%–5%).[50]

Detection of a vesicant extravasation in its earliest stage is most likely to result in the least possible soft-tissue damage. The nurse should be aware of the following symptoms that could indicate extravasation, although any or all of these symptoms may not occur:

- swelling (most common)
- stinging, burning, or pain at the injection site (not *always* present)
- redness (not often seen initially)
- lack of blood return (if this is *only* occurrence, the IV should be reevaluated; if still no blood return, consider other options); lack of a blood return *alone* is not always indicative of an extravasation

If an extravasation is suspected, the infusion is to be stopped immediately and the needle site inspected. The management of vesicant extravasation is discussed in Chapter 33.

ROUTES OF DRUG ADMINISTRATION

Chemotherapy was designed as a systemic treatment for cancer, having the ability to travel throughout the body via the bloodstream and damage or kill dividing cells. The first intravenous dose of chemotherapy was given to a lymphoma patient at Yale University in 1943, and since that time, major advances have continued to be made in available antineoplastic agents, dosing, scheduling, combinations, and routes.[7] It is now possible to direct drugs systemically as well as to almost every anatomic region in the body: to specific organs, inside body cavities, and to body spaces. Intravenous chemotherapy remains the most common route of drug delivery, but other systemic routes include oral, intramuscular, and subcutaneous. Regional drug delivery utilizes the following routes: topical, intraarterial, intraperitoneal, intrapleural, intravesical, intrathecal, and intraventricular. It is even possible to use these techniques to administer the drugs directly into the center of a tumor (intratumoral).

Topical

Cutaneous malignant lesions can be treated in a variety of ways, including the topical application of antineoplastic agents. This is most commonly done for cutaneous T-cell lymphoma, basal cell carcinoma, and squamous cell carcinoma. The agents used include nitrogen mustard for cutaneous T-cell lymphoma and fluorouracil for the two mentioned carcinomas.[51] The topical agent is usually applied once or twice daily until the lesions progress to the necrosis phase, which may take 1–3 weeks. The affected area is not washed vigorously during the treatment period. The expected result of topical antineoplastic administration is local sloughing of the affected area and eventual regranulization of normal tissue, so it is normal for the treated area to become red and tender, then to form a lesion that becomes necrotic, followed by superficial sloughing of the dead tissue and regrowth of healthy skin. It is unusual for the patient to experience any systemic side effects of the drugs unless the majority of the skin is being treated; but incidences of mild, delayed side effects such as nausea have been reported.

Special nursing considerations for these patients include:

1. patient education, with special consideration for body image issues
2. application of the drug using cotton swabs or non-metal applicators
3. close attention to application only in the prescribed (affected) area
4. careful avoidance of the eyes, nares, mouth, or other areas very close to mucous membranes
5. utilization of safe drug handling practices, e.g., gloves, and strict attention to drug containment
6. when using nitrogen mustard, having sodium thiosulfate available (to neutralize the nitrogen mustard) and applying it to areas of the skin that may be inadvertently treated (after removal of the drug)
7. application of dressings, if prescribed
8. observation for untoward sequelae, e.g., severe burning or rashes, which may result in discontinuation of therapy or subsequent dose reduction
9. monitoring disease response

Oral

A variety of antineoplastic agents are administered orally to treat numerous types of cancer (Table 15-6).[52] The oral route is convenient, economical, noninvasive, and oftentimes less toxic. Most oral drugs are well absorbed as long as the gastrointestinal tract is functioning normally.

The nursing responsibilities for oral drug administration include safe handling (gloves are considered acceptable if physical contact with the tablet or capsule is required) and monitoring for drug absorption and compliance with the prescribed therapy. If the patient experiences emesis immediately after drug ingestion and the pills or capsules cannot be visualized, the drug is usually not repeated. Several oral antineoplastic agents are also available in parenteral forms, providing an option for patients intolerant of or noncompliant with oral regimens. Other recommendations include:

1. Prescribe one "course" at a time, to avoid inadvertent overdosing, which could be life threatening or fatal.
2. Instruct the patient to take the medication on an empty stomach with water, to enhance absorption, unless the drug is tolerated better with food, as is the case with prednisone, cyclophosphamide, and tamoxifen.
3. Familiarize the patient with both generic and brand names of the drug, to avoid confusion or double dosing (many physicians prefer to prescribe brand name antineoplastic agents to avoid the possibility of the generics' not being bioequivalent).
4. Instruct the patient to maintain a record of drugs being taken.
5. Obtain a list of any drugs currently being taken by the patient to ensure compatibility.
6. Advise the patient to avoid any over-the-counter drugs unless first checking with the physician or nurse.
7. Question the patient at each visit regarding the medication, i.e., how much was taken, whether any doses were omitted, and why.

It is important that the patient comply with the treatment regimen to maximize the goal of therapy, i.e., remission or cure. Oral agents give the patient control over administration, and noncompliance is not common. However, tamoxifen can cause hot flashes and mood swings, cyclophosphamide and etoposide can cause emesis, and levamisole can cause neurotoxicity. A patient might decide to omit a dose in order to feel better temporarily. The patient needs to understand the importance of dosing and scheduling and how critical it is that the prescribed regimen be followed exactly. With therapy such as leucovorin following methotrexate, noncompliance could be fatal. It is common for patients receiving oral antineoplastic agents to be given a calendar with the doses indicated and space to record each dose. The nurse checks the previous treatment calendar and questions the patient about any omitted doses during each encounter. The regimen can often be modified to enhance the patient's tolerance of the side effects, e.g., administering an antiemetic to minimize nausea or changing the time of dose administration.

Intramuscular and Subcutaneous

Utilization of intramuscular (IM) or subcutaneous (SQ) antineoplastic drug delivery was uncommon in the past, since only a few drugs were indicated by this route. The development of the biologic agents (such as interferon, colony stimulating factors) has increased the number of drugs given IM or SQ. These convenient and quick routes are handled according to standard injection methods. Since some of the drugs can sting or burn, IM injections are usually given into large muscles, with the Z-track method being optional. Subcutaneous injections of small volumes (up to 3 ml) are in the usual sites and should be rotated if being given daily. Many drug manufacturers have distributed forms, charts, or posters that clearly outline the steps to follow for patients self-administering SQ medications (see Figure 15-1). One drug that is administered subcutaneously in a rather unique way is goserelin acetate (Zoladex®, ICI Pharma), a hormonal agent used in the treatment of breast cancer and prostate cancer. It is actually a dry drug pellet that is implanted in the soft tissue of the abdomen, where it gradually dissolves over a 28-day

TABLE 15-6 Oral Antineoplastic Agents[52]

Drug and Disease Indications	Dose and Schedule	Side Effects: Acute or Delayed	Pharmacokinetics	Comments
Cyclophosphamide (Cytoxan, Endoxan) Breast cancer Multiple myeloma Small-cell lung cancer Malignant lymphomas Leukemias	*Tab:* 25–50 mg *Dose:* 1–5 mg/kg/day 60–120 mg/m² Adjust dose in presence of renal dysfunction	*Nadir:* 7–14 days Bone marrow suppression (BMS) Anorexia, nausea, and vomiting Alopecia Hemorrhagic cystitis with gross or microscopic hematuria Amenorrhea Sterility	Activated in the liver Oral absorption in 1 hr 30% of drug excreted unchanged in urine	Vigorous hydration (3 liter/day). Encourage frequent voiding to prevent hemorrhagic cystitis (a sterile inflammation of the urinary bladder). If patient complains of burning on urination or bladder incontinence, urinalysis may reveal occult blood. Control by withdrawal of the drug and hydration. May take pills in divided doses early in the day and with meals or all at one time. Better tolerated with cold foods. Barbiturates and other inducers of hepatic microsomal enzymes may enhance toxicity, eg, cimetidine. Allopurinol may enhance BMS.
Chlorambucil (Leukeran) Leukemia Hodgkin's disease	*Tab:* 2 mg white *Dose:* 4–8 mg/m²day × 3–6 wk 16 mg/m²/wk every 4 wk	*Nadir:* 7–10 days Severe BMS Slight nausea and vomiting Occasional dermatitis Abnormal liver function Pulmonary fibrosis with prolonged use Second malignancy Sterility	Hepatic metabolism to active compound Renal excretion of 50% of unchanged drug	Good oral absorption. Concomitant barbiturate administration may enhance toxicity. Marrow suppression may be prolonged.
Busulfan (Myleran) Leukemia	*Tab:* 2 mg white *Dose:* 4–12 mg/day; for several weeks	*Nadir:* 10–30 days delayed marrow recovery Potentially teratogenic Pulmonary fibrosis with long-term use Dermatologic hyperpigmentation Gynecomastia Amenorrhea	Well absorbed Extensive hepatic metabolism to inactive compounds Renal excretion	Bone marrow recovery may be delayed; therefore caution is advised with long-term use. Hydration and allopurinol may be indicated to prevent hyperuricemia. Total cumulative dose: 600 mg. Long-term daily administration is not recommended owing to the risk of second malignancies with chronic alkylating agents.
6-Thioguanine Leukemia	*Tab:* 40 mg green/yellow *Dose:* 80–100 mg/m² Reduce dose if stomatitis occurs	*Nadir:* 7–28 days Stomatitis Diarrhea Hepatotoxicity	Variable, incomplete absorption Hepatic metabolism Renal excretion	Administer on an empty stomach. Does not require dose reduction when used in conjunction with allopurinol.
6-Mercaptopurine (6 MP) Leukemia	*Tab:* 50 mg off-white *Dose:* 80–100 mg/m²/day Titrate dose based on blood counts Reduce dose in presence of hepatic or renal dysfunction	*Nadir:* 10–14 days Nausea, vomiting Mucositis Diarrhea Drug fever Intrahepatic cholestasis Pulmonary toxicity with prolonged use	Incomplete oral absorption Hepatic inactivation Renal excretion 10% unchanged in 24 hr	Protect pills from light. Administer as single dose on an empty stomach. Increased toxicity with allopurinol (reduce dose by one-third to one-fourth of the original dose). Administer with caution to patients on sodium warfarin (Coumadin). Monitor liver function tests.
Hexamethylmelamine (Altretamine hexalene) Ovarian cancer	*Cap:* 50 mg clear *Dose:* 240–320 mg/m²/day	*Nadir:* 21–28 days Acute liver toxicity is dose-limiting; nausea and vomiting are dose-related Mild BMS Abdominal cramping Diarrhea Peripheral neuropathies Agitation, confusion	Variable absorption Rapid metabolism Urine excretion 90% in 72 hr	Pyridoxine 50 mg/day may decrease neuropathy. Take with food, prophylactic antiemetics. May worsen vincristine-related peripheral neuropathy.

(continued)

TABLE 15-6 Oral Antineoplastic Agents[52] (continued)

Drug and Disease Indications	Dose and Schedule	Side Effects: Acute or Delayed	Pharmacokinetics	Comments
L-phenylanine mustard (melphalan, alkeran) Multiple myeloma Ovarian cancer	*Tab:* 2 mg white *Dose:* 0.1–0.15 mg/kg/day × 2–3 wk Reduce dose with hepatic or renal impairment	*Nadir:* 10–18 days Nausea and vomiting usually mild Dermatitis Pulmonary fibrosis Long-term therapy can result in acute leukemia	Hepatic metabolism Renal excretion 20%–35% (10% unchanged) 20%–50% excreted in feces within 6 days	Protect pills from sunlight. Take on an empty stomach. BMS may be cumulative in older patients. Leukemogenic.
Lomustine (CCNU) Brain cancer Lymphomas	*Cap:* 100 mg green/green, 40 mg green/white, 10 mg white *Dose:* 100–130 mg/m² q 6–8 wk	*Nadir:* 28–42 days Severe cumulative BMS Nausea and vomiting 4–6 hr after dosing Anorexia Alopecia Stomatitis Hepatotoxicity	Absorbed rapidly (<60 min) Hepatic metabolism Renal excretion of 50% in 24 hr and 75% in 96 hr Crosses into CSF	Dispense one dose at a time to prevent accidental overdose. Take on an empty stomach just before bedtime. Pretreat with aggressive antiemetics. Protect pills from heat and humidity.
Hydroxyurea (Hydrea) Chronic myelocytic leukemia Melanoma Head and neck cancer	*Cap:* 500 mg *Dose:* 80 mg/kg/day every third day 750–1000 mg/m²/day × 5 Decrease dose in presence of renal dysfunction Store in tight container in a cool environment	*Nadir:* 13–17 days Acute nausea and vomiting Chronic and severe anemia Neurologic seizures and hallucinations Dermatitis Dysuria Azotemia	Well absorbed Hepatic metabolism Renal excretion of 80% of compound in 12 hr Crosses into CSF	Concomitant radiation and/or 5-FU may enhance neurotoxicity. Dysuria and renal impairment may occur. Consider pretreatment with allopurinol.
VP-16-213 (etoposide, VePesid) Lung cancer Testicular cancer	*Cap:*50 mg pink *Dose:* 2 × the intravenous dose or 100–200 mg/m²/day over 3–5 days every 3–4 wk	*Nadir:* 7–14 days (white blood cell count) Nausea and vomiting: 9–16 days (platelets) Alopecia Bone marrow suppression is dose limiting	Renal and hepatic metabolism Incomplete and variable absorption	Nausea is mild though can be more severe with oral route than with intravenous route.
Procarbazine (Matulane) Hodgkin's disease	*Cap:* 50 mg *Dose:* 100 mg/m²/day × 14 days every 4 wk; reduce dose in presence of hepatic or renal dysfunction	*Nadir:* 4 wk Bone marrow suppression, nausea, vomiting, and diarrhea gradually subside; flulike syndrome, paresthesias, neuropathies, dizziness, and ataxia	Well absorbed from the gastrointestinal tract Metabolized in the liver with a biologic half-life of about 1 hr 70% of the drug is eliminated by 24 hr in the urine, 5% appears as unchanged drug	Drug and food interactions can occur. Central nervous system (CNS) depression can occur with concomitant administration of procarbazine and CNS depressants. Hypertensive crisis can occur when procarbazine is administered with certain antidepressants (tricyclics and monoamine oxidase inhibitors) and tyramine-rich foods. Severe nausea and vomiting can occur if taken with ethanol, mixed drinks, and beer.
Methotrexate Squamous cell carcinoma Lung cancer	*Tab:* 2.5 mg yellow *Dose:* 2.5–10 mg/day PO or 15–30 mg/day PO × 5 days every 1–3 wk	*Nadir:* 7–10 days Nausea and anorexia can occur; stomatitis and ulcerations can occur and are dose-limiting.	Serum half-life is 2–4 hr Excreted by the kidneys	Dose is reduced with renal impairment; dosing on an empty stomach may enhance bioavailability. Excretion may be impaired in patients with simultaneous administration or weak acids such as salicylates or vitamin C; oral dosing is generally well tolerated. Avoid administration of methotrexate with ketoprotein or probenecid because toxicity of methotrexate may be enhanced.

Source: Adapted from Goodman M: Delivery of cancer chemotherapy. In Baird S, McCorkle R, Grant M (eds.): *Cancer Nursing: A Comprehensive Textbook*. Philadelphia: Saunders, 1991, p. 311. Used with permission.

1. Assemble and prepare supplies

- Select a clean, well-lit working surface
- Gather supplies:
  - A sterile syringe
  - Prepackaged alcohol wipes
  - A puncture-resistant container for disposal of needle and syringe
  - Medication and diluent vials
- Wash hands thoroughly

2. Reconstitute medication

- Flip tops of medication and diluent vials
- Wipe rubber stoppers with alcohol wipes
- Remove needle cap
- Pull the plunger back to the ______ mL mark on the syringe
- If the needle touches anything other than the injection site or the rubber stoppers, dispose of it and start again
- Inject air into the vial above diluent
  - Try not to inject air into the fluid

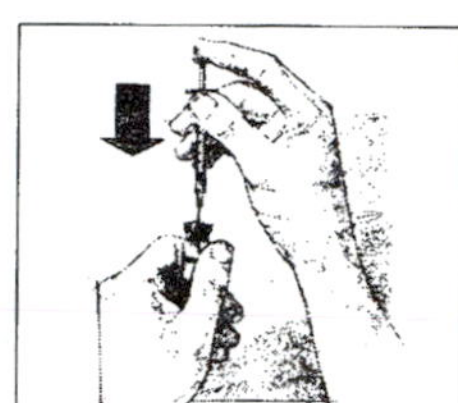

- Draw out diluent
  - Turn vial upside down, keeping the needle tip below the fluid level
  - Draw out diluent to the ______ mL mark on the syringe
  - Tap lightly and expel any air by pushing gently on the plunger
  - Insert the syringe with diluent into the rubber stopper of medication vial
  - Aim at the side of the vial; avoid air bubbles or foaming, push plunger to inject diluent
- Gently swirl until powder dissolves; do not shake

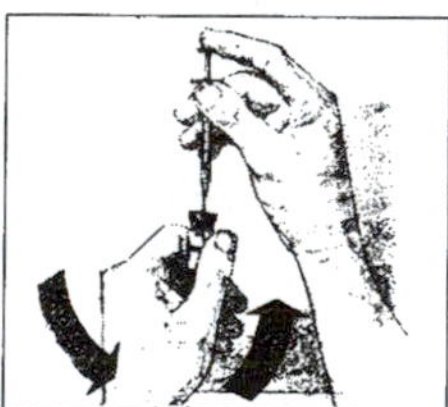

(If your doctor has prescribed a ready-to-use form, your medication will not need to be reconstituted. A half hour before you need it, take the vial out of the refrigerator and allow it to come to room temperature. Then proceed to step 3.)

Check the medication and be sure it is clear and colorless. If it is not, call your doctor, nurse, or pharmacist for further instructions

3. Prepare injection site

- Choose an injection site (see chart); rotate this site as you have been instructed

  With an alcohol wipe cleanse the site using a circular motion, and allow to dry for about 10 seconds

4. Withdraw prescribed medication from vial

- Turn the vial upside down, with the needle still in the rubber stopper

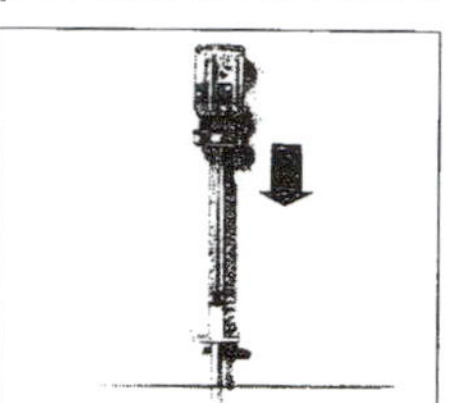

- Slowly withdraw medication to the ______ mL mark on the syringe
  - Again, tap the barrel of the syringe and expel any air by pushing gently on the plunger to remove any air bubbles; confirm you have the right amount of medication
- Remove the needle and syringe from the vial

5. Inject the medication

- Pinch the skin of the injection site between your thumb and forefinger
- Hold the syringe, just like a pencil, at a 45-90 degree angle to the skin, about 2 inches above the surface
- Use a quick, short motion to insert the needle as far as it will go
- Release grasp on the skin and gently pull back on the plunger a little

  If you see blood, don't inject the medication, remove the needle, dispose of the syringe and medication in the puncture-resistant container, and start over

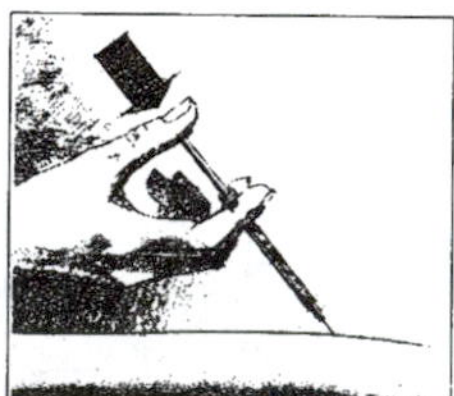

- Slowly inject all the medication
- Remove the needle at the same angle as it was inserted
- Press the site gently with an alcohol wipe until any bleeding has stopped

  If you make a mistake or forget an injection, call your doctor, nurse, or pharmacist

6. Dispose of supplies

- Dispose of syringes and needles in puncture-resistant container

  When it is two-thirds full, dispose of it the way you were instructed
- Throw away used vials immediately

Fill in specific information:

- Supplies to be used and where to obtain them ______________________________
- Name of drug ______________________________
- How often to inject ______________________________
- How to dispose of used supplies, if different from above ______________________________
- Name and telephone number of health care specialist ______________________________
- Specific side effects to watch for ______________________________
- Other special instructions ______________________________

FIGURE 15-1 Sample instruction sheet for patients injecting subcutaneous medication. (Courtesy of Immunex, Seattle, WA)

period. Figure 15-2 illustrates the injection process, which can include injection of a local anesthetic bleb (e.g., lidocaine) to minimize discomfort, since the needle is large (16-gauge).

Intravenous

Intravenous delivery, the most common of all antineoplastic drug administration routes, has been discussed extensively in several places in this chapter. Detailed nursing actions are included in Table 15-4. An excellent general source of comprehensive information about intravenous nursing practice is *Intravenous Nursing Standards of Practice,* developed by the Intravenous Nurses Society.[5]

There are some specific controversies regarding certain aspects of intravenous antineoplastic drug administration. Needle size preferences vary, with some nurses preferring large bore needles (18- or 19-gauge)

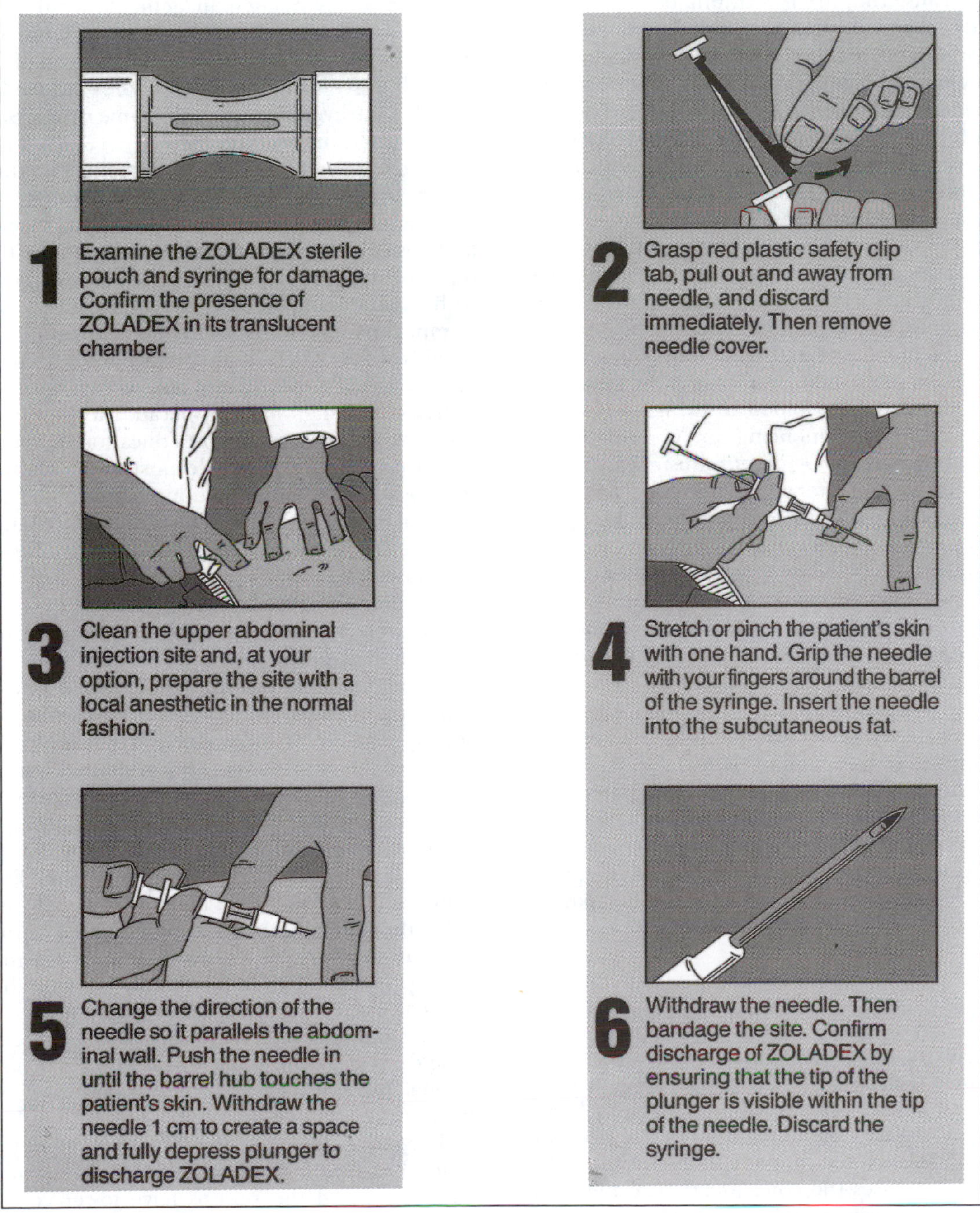

FIGURE 15-2 Zoladex administration guidelines (© 1991 ICI Americas, Inc. Courtesy of ICI Pharma, Wilmington, DE)

because they permit rapid administration of drug, thus decreasing the time an irritating drug is infusing, increasing the drug's dilution in large veins, and decreasing the time the patient is involved in this anxiety-producing procedure. Those preferring a smaller bore needle (21- or 22-gauge) do so because it is less likely to form scar tissue, can be inserted into a wider range of veins (i.e., smaller veins), is less painful on insertion, allows bloodflow around the needle to dilute the drug, and perhaps minimizes mechanical phlebitis.[1,49] Some practitioners prefer stainless steel, scalp vein needles (i.e., butterfly, 23- or 25-gauge) versus the over-the-needle catheters (i.e., Abbocath, Insyte). Needles are preferred because they are less traumatic to insert and have slightly lower infection and phlebitis rates. Catheters are preferred because they are less likely to infiltrate. In general, needles are preferred for one-time or short-term use (minutes to several hours), while catheters are preferred for longer use (hours to days) or when the patient is very active, e.g., during cisplatinum therapy involving large-volume hydration necessitating frequent trips to the bathroom.

While some nurses prefer the antecubital area because it contains large veins to facilitate rapid drug delivery, most nurses do not use it for antineoplastic drugs because it restricts patient mobility, increases the risk of dislodgement and extravasation, is a very vascular joint space that could be damaged by extravasation, and is preferred for blood drawing so it should not be overused. Drug sequencing can be controversial, depending on the drugs being administered. In general, antiemetics and pretreatments (i.e., anxiolytic agents) are given first, followed by the intravenous-push medications, short-term drip infusions (i.e., less than 2 hours), and finally any long-term or continuous infusions. The controversy arises with vesicants, which many nurses prefer to give first, while the vascular integrity is greatest and the vein is least likely to be irritated by other drugs. Some nurses prefer giving vesicants last or sandwiching them between the other drugs because the vesicants are irritating and patients have been known to complain of pain at the needle site due to venospasms occurring immediately after initiation of intravenous therapy. These and other controversial areas of antineoplastic drug administration are excellent opportunities for nursing research, to increase knowledge and enhance the quality of patient care.

Intraarterial

Intraarterial drug administration, a drug delivery practice that gained popularity in the early 1980s, involves cannulation of the artery providing a tumor's blood supply and subsequent administration of the drug directly through the arterial catheter to the tumor bed.[53] This practice increases the concentration of the drug to known areas of tumor and decreases the systemic drug concentration and thus the side effects. The primary utilization of this route is the hepatic artery for the management of potential or actual metastasis of colon cancer to the liver. It has also been used for hepatocellular carcinoma. The antineoplastic drugs used include fluorouracil, floxuridine, doxorubicin, and mitomycin C, among others.

The two methods of intraarterial drug delivery are external or internal. The external method involves radiographic placement of an arterial catheter (usually via the femoral artery) and attachment of the catheter to an external infusion pump for 3–7 days of drug delivery. The patient is required to lie flat during the infusion, with a pressure dressing over the catheter insertion site. Nursing management includes consistent patient care (e.g., fracture pans, log rolling) and monitoring of the site and infusion. Side effects of the drugs occur but are usually milder and/or delayed as compared to intravenous use of the same drugs. Since therapy is given intermittently for several courses, this approach is used initially to determine whether or not the treatment appears effective. For long-term use (6 months or longer) it is uncomfortable, inconvenient, and costly. A variation of this technique is the placement of an intraarterial port, which can be accessed with a noncoring needle attached to an ambulatory pump, thus increasing the patient's comfort and personal freedom. As with any situation of this nature, the patient must be willing and able to care for the device, to assess the site, and to operate the pump. Nursing care involves intense patient education in maintenance and use of the implantable port and monitoring for complications or malfunctions of both the port and external pump.[54,55] These activities are increasingly being managed by home care nurses and home infusion nurse specialists whose skills provide patients with a tremendous amount of freedom and security.

The internal, or implantable, method of intraarterial drug delivery involves the surgical placement of a totally implantable pump. The Infusaid pump (Infusaid, Inc., Norwood, MA) and the Synchromed Infusion System (Medtronics, Inc., Minneapolis, MN) are examples of subcutaneously implanted pumps, (see Figures 15-3 to 15-6). The catheter is inserted into the appropriate artery and then attached to the pump located in a surgically created subcutaneous pocket, usually in the lower abdomen or upper chest. The pump chamber is accessed via a noncoring needle and filled with either chemotherapy or heparinized sterile saline. The flow rates are dependent on pump design and are either preset prior to implantation or adjustable via an external electronic wand that communicates with the internal pump. Obviously, care and maintenance of these devices by the nurse requires a formalized educational program and ongoing monitoring of pump functioning.

The implantable pump offers the patient the greatest level of freedom when receiving intraarterial chemotherapy, and the pumps have lower complication rates than the external methods. One potential disadvantage is the cost; the pump plus the implantation can

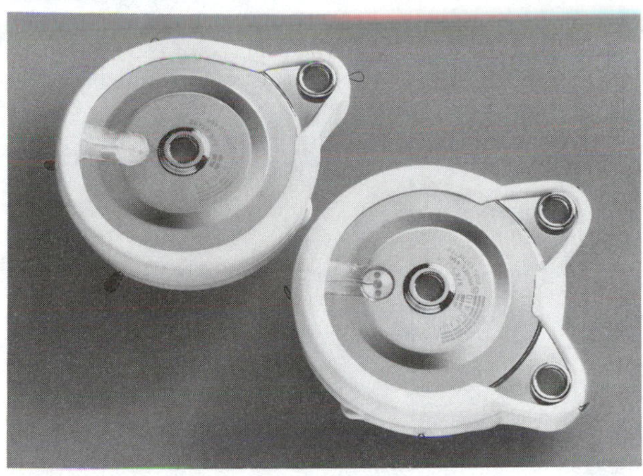

FIGURE 15-3 Infusaid pump, model 400, and model 400 dual-catheter pump. (Courtesy of Infusaid, Inc., Norwood, MA)

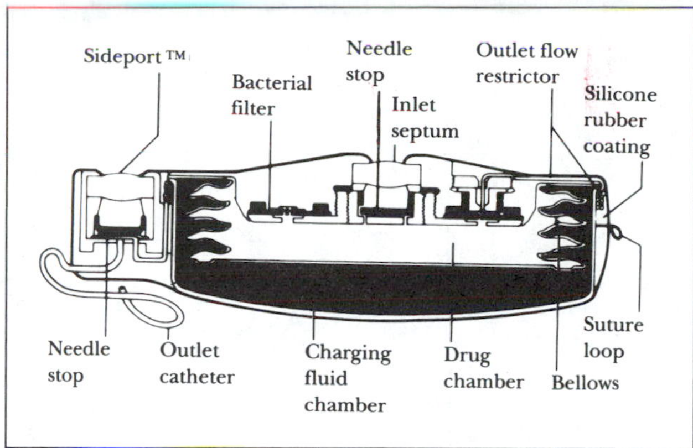

FIGURE 15-4 Schematic drawing of Infusaid pump, model 400. (Courtesy of Infusaid, Inc., Norwood, MA)

cost over $10,000.[56] When compared to intermittent hospitalization or an ambulatory pump, it is usually felt to be cost effective if therapy is anticipated for a minimum of 3–6 months or longer. In fact, long-term therapy with an external pump can eventually cost more due to the cost of disposable supplies.

Nursing considerations involve monitoring for drug side effects and potential pump complications, such as infection, occlusion, extravasation, and malfunction. Some very unique nursing actions are necessary when dealing with implantable pumps, such as not aspirating the center septum, monitoring or establishing pump flow rate, and detecting malfunctions. The oncology nurse is referred to the manufacturers' instructions and

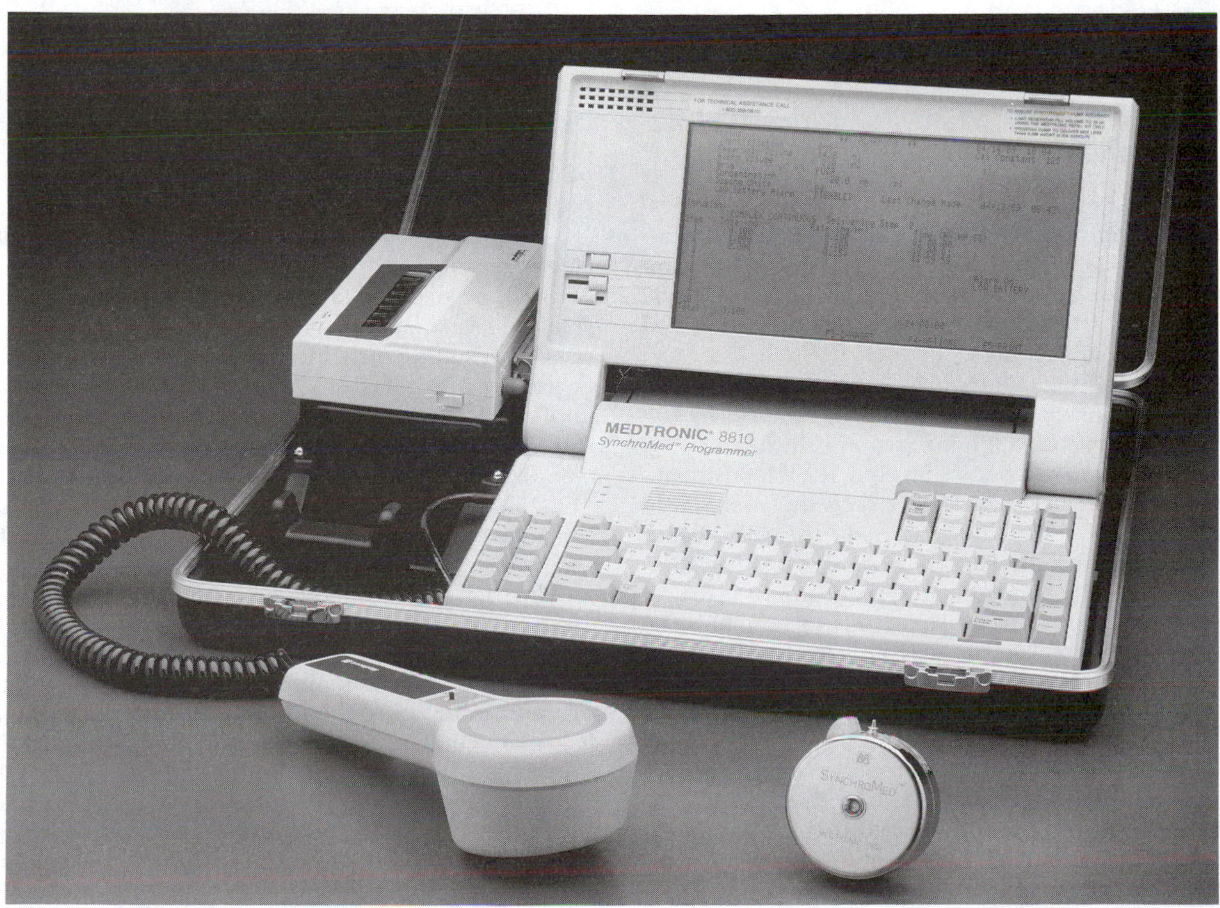

FIGURE 15-5 Synchromed infusion system. (Courtesy of Medtronic, Inc., Minneapolis, MN)

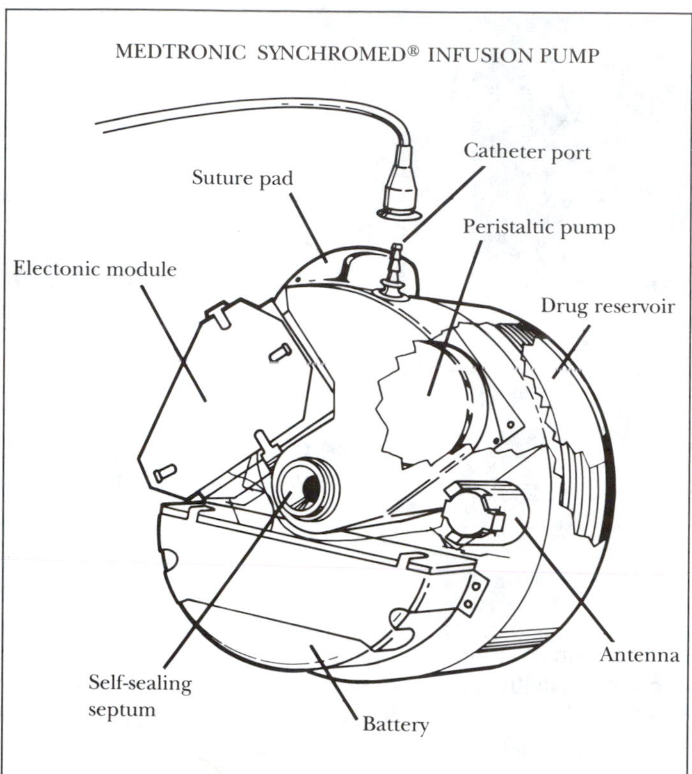

FIGURE 15-6 Schematic drawing of Synchromed infusion pump. (Courtesy of Medtronic, Inc., Minneapolis, MN)

guidelines regarding the management of these innovative and advanced nursing responsibilities.

Intraperitoneal

Regional delivery of chemotherapy into the peritoneal space has been found to be a safe and effective treatment for locally recurrent ovarian and colon cancers.[57,58] The antineoplastic agents used include cisplatinum, carboplatin, interferon, fluorouracil, and cytarabine, among others.

The semipermeable nature of the peritoneal space allows high concentrations of the drugs to be achieved at the tumor sites throughout the peritoneal space, but with lower concentrations entering the bloodstream. The procedure causes local side effects due to the large volume of fluid filling the space, and the drugs cause systemic side effects that are mild or delayed when compared to intravenous administration of the same drugs. It is possible with some of the drugs to minimize the systemic side effects by simultaneously infusing an agent intravenously to counteract drug side effects through the venous system. This is most commonly achieved during the intraperitoneal instillation of cisplatinum by infusing intravenous sodium thiosulfate, which appears to decrease the renal toxicities of the cisplatinum.[59]

There are three methods of accessing the peritoneal space: (1) intermittent placement of temporary indwelling catheters; (2) placement of a Tenckhoff external catheter; and (3) placement of an implantable peritoneal port.[60–64] Intermittent placement might be used if the therapy is planned for a short time, such as for symptom relief or palliation. Tenckhoff catheters or ports are placed when several months of therapy are planned, especially when the treatment goal is cure of minimal or microscopic residual disease. Tenckhoff catheters have the advantages of a very rapid flow rate (10–15 minutes for 2 liters) and the allowance of catheter manipulation to dislodge fibrin deposits, if necessary. The disadvantages are that it is external, thus requiring care and maintenance by the patient, and possibly resulting in an increased incidence of infection or leakage around the catheter. The advantages of the implanted port are that it is internal and requires no care when not accessed, and has a potentially lower rate of infection. Disadvantages include a slower flow rate (30–45 minutes for 2 liters), a needle stick is required for access, and a surgical procedure is necessary for removal.[60–64]

Nursing considerations include patient education, assessing the catheter or port patency, establishing access, administering systemic therapies as ordered, instilling the infusate, monitoring patient response to the procedure, draining the infusate (if ordered), side effect management, and documentation as outlined in Table 15-7.

Side effects of the drugs used for intraperitoneal chemotherapy are variable and depend on the agents being administered. Regardless of the drugs administered, complications specific to the intraperitoneal route include respiratory distress, abdominal pain, discom-

TABLE 15-7 Nursing Considerations in Intraperitoneal Drug Administration[63,65]

Patient Education

- Instruct the patient in the care of the catheter or port prior to its insertion.
- Immediately prior to initiating therapy, explain the drug administration process, side effects of the drugs, side effects of the route, and measures to manage/minimize the side effects.
- Teach the patient and/or family how to care for the catheter at home, if appropriate.

Pretreatment and Site Accession

- Verify the drug order and normal serum electrolyte levels.
- Insert a urinary catheter to straight drainage, if ordered, and initiate intake and output measurements.
- Ensure that intravenous therapy is proceeding as ordered. (IP cisplatinum infusions usually include prehydration for 12–24 hr with IV fluids containing potassium and magnesium supplements. A few moments before initiating the IP cisplatinum, IV sodium thiosulfate is begun, to neutralize the systemic cisplatinum and to prevent renal toxicities and severe nausea and vomiting.)
- Gather appropriate supplies and materials, and wash hands.
- Assess the area around the catheter or port for redness, edema, warmth, or tenderness.
- Organize materials, don gloves (and gown if desired).
- Access external catheter directly after a thorough povidone-iodine scrub of the external hub using aseptic technique, *or*
- Access implanted port using aseptic technique and a large-gauge, noncoring, 90° needle of appropriate length (usually 1–1.5 in.); anesthetize the skin surface prior to access, if desired, with 2% xylocaine or ice.
- Flush the catheter with 10–20 ml of nonbacteriostatic sterile saline; catheter should flush easily.
- Administer antiemetics, if ordered.

Drug Administration

- Initiate IV sodium thiosulfate, if ordered.
- Position patient comfortably in a semi-Fowler's position (elevate head of bed).
- Open the clamp on the tubing, and infuse the warmed IP chemotherapy at the prescribed rate (usually over 30 min to several hours)
- Stop infusion immediately if severe pain is experienced and check for catheter migration (usually with x-ray verification).
- Slow the rate of infusion if the patient experiences shortness of breath or discomfort.
- Administer analgesics as prescribed, if necessary.
- Apply blankets if patient feels chilled.
- Close the clamp on the tubing when the infusion is complete, and encourage repositioning from side to side every 15 min during the dwell time (usually 2–4 hr).
- Monitor patient's comfort levels, and observe for shortness of breath, abdominal discomfort, or diarrhea.

TABLE 15-7 Nursing Considerations in Intraperitoneal Drug Administration[63,65] (continued)

- After the prescribed dwell time, open the clamp to the drainage bag and allow the solution to drain. If flow is sluggish, check tubing for kinks, help patient roll from side to side, have patient use the Valsalva maneuver, apply manual pressure to the abdomen, or irrigate the catheter with normal saline.
- Recognize that the volume of drained fluid may be less than that infused, and reassure patient that the fluid will be reabsorbed and metabolized.
- Clamp tubing on drainage bag after fluid has drained (usually 30 min to 2 hr), and send specimen, properly labeled as cytotoxic, to cytology or dispose of in proper hazardous waste container.

Postadministration Care

- Flush catheter or port with nonbacteriostatic sterile saline; if using a port, follow with heparinized saline.
- Secure site using standard technique (ie, cap and secure catheter or remove needle from port, and cover site with a small dressing, if necessary).
- Establish IV fluids as prescribed, or discontinue IV needle.
- Assess patient's status; ensure ability to perform self-care, if appropriate.
- Document procedure in medical record.

fort, and diarrhea, which are due to increased intraabdominal pressure. Appropriate interventions to manage these problems include elevation of the head of the bed, instructing the patient to roll from side to side, and administering analgesics. Mechanical difficulties can occur, and include inflow or outflow occlusions caused by fibrin sheath formation over the catheter, other outflow occlusions, and catheter migration. Other complications include infection, chemical irritation of the peritoneal space, electrolytic imbalances, and (with an implantable port) drug extravasation.

In general, intraperitoneal chemotherapy is well tolerated by patients and provides a safe, effective treatment for the management of peritoneal disease, particularly ovarian carcinoma. Patients are frequently able to maintain a normal lifestyle, for this route is successfully utilized in inpatient, ambulatory, and home care settings, with fewer side effects than traditional intravenous therapy.

Intrapleural

Care of the patient with a pleural effusion traditionally involves insertion of chest tubes, drainage of the fluid, and sclerosis of the pleural space to prevent recurrence of the effusion. When the effusion is caused by malignant cells, the preferred treatment is sclerosis with an antineoplastic agent such as nitrogen mustard or bleomycin.[66] This is accomplished in the usual sterile manner by injecting the drug directly into the chest tube and clamping it for a specified time, e.g., 24 hours. The procedure can be repeated daily for several days if necessary. Nursing management of intrapleural chemotherapy includes patient education, safe drug handling, and side effect management. Nitrogen mustard is well known for its emetogenic properties, and treatment with adequate antiemetics is necessary. Also, severe pleural pain can accompany intrapleural nitrogen mustard, and a strong narcotic such as morphine sulfate is frequently ordered as a premedication and for 24–48 hours afterward. Use of a PCA pump is ideal for patient control of the analgesic agent to ensure adequate pain control. Bleomycin is not known to cause these symptoms but instead may cause mild nausea or fever and chills, similar to its intravenous side effect profile. In general, nursing care focuses on emesis control, pain control, respiratory status, chest tube security, and other comfort measures, depending on the drug utilized.

The process just described is a standard procedure that has been moderately successful for many years. The quest for newer and better forms of sclerosing therapy has led to a variety of alternatives that appear equally as good or better than traditional therapy. These include:

1. use of other agents, including methylprednisolone,[67] doxorubicin hydrochloride-containing poly (L-lactic acid) microspheres (ADR-MS),[68] and cisplatinum plus cytarabine[69] (all agents being used investigationally by some physicians)
2. insertion of small-bore percutaneously placed catheters or implantable ports with drainage and subsequent sclerosing instead of large-bore closed-tube thoracostomy[70,71] (see Chapter 30)
3. implantation of pleuroperitoneal shunts[72]

The most noteworthy of these advances is small-bore catheter placement, which is very easily accomplished with only mild discomfort and without the major trauma of regular chest tube insertion. Also, for recurrent pleural effusion, thoracentesis can be performed repeatedly via an implantable port, with the catheter portion in the pleural space and the portal on the lower rib cage. Acceptance and clinical utilization of these techniques is variable, and the oncology nurse is encouraged to be aware of the specific procedures used and the established policies describing the nurse's role in administering intrapleural chemotherapy.

Intravesical

Direct instillation of chemotherapy into the bladder has been proven to be a very effective and simple method of controlling superficial bladder cancer and carcinoma in situ. Agents such as thiotepa, doxorubicin, mitomycin C, and bacillus Calmette-Guerin (BCG) have all been shown to be effective, especially BCG. Instillation is usually weekly for 4–12 weeks and involves insertion of a urinary catheter, instillation of the drug (usually in 50–60 ml of sterile solution), and retention of the drug for 1 to 2 hours (with frequent movement to disperse the drug throughout the bladder) prior to unclamping the catheter or voiding. Some physicians prefer to have the urinary catheter remain clamped and in place for the dwell time. In this case, the fluid that drains from the catheter when it is unclamped should be contained and disposed of properly (i.e., sealed, then labeled as cytotoxic waste). If the physician prefers to withdraw the catheter after drug instillation and instructs the patient to void in 1–2 hours, the patient should flush the toilet twice after voiding. Local side effects such as bladder irritation or, with mitomycin C, dermatitis of the external genitalia can be experienced. A unique side effect of BCG is a "creepy-crawling" feeling sometimes referred to as "BCG-osis."[73,74] Patients report feeling as if their skin is creeping or little things are crawling on them. Administration of a mild sedative can be considered if this side effect occurs.

Nursing considerations for patients receiving intravesical chemotherapy include patient education (stressing hand washing and personal hygiene), drug administration, side effect monitoring, and safe drug handling. For most oncology nurses it is unusual to have experience with this method of drug delivery, since it is commonly performed in urologists' offices as a routine office treatment.

Intrathecal or Intraventricular

Cancer cells can cross the blood–brain barrier and appear in the cerebrospinal fluid (CSF), resulting in central nervous system involvement of the malignancy. This phenomenon is seen most commonly in leukemia (meningeal leukemia) and to a lesser extent in other malignancies, such as breast cancer, lymphoma, and rhabdomyosarcoma (meningeal carcinomatosis).[75,76] Unfortunately, available antineoplastic agents are unable to enter the CSF in sufficient concentrations to kill the cancer cells effectively, so chemotherapy is injected directly into the intrathecal or intraventricular space as prophylaxis or to manage existing disease. The antineoplastic drugs used include methotrexate, cytarabine, thiotepa, and interferon. When prepared for use by this route, the preservative-free drug is always admixed with a preservative-free diluent such as nonbacteriostatic sterile saline or Elliott's B solution.

The two primary methods of instillation are intrathecal and intraventricular. The intrathecal route is achieved by performing a standard lumbar puncture, using established techniques to ascertain placement, and injecting 10–12 ml of drug, followed by withdrawal of the needle. This procedure usually is performed by a physician or a nurse practitioner on a daily to weekly basis, depending on the protocol being followed. This method is quick and easy to perform but is disadvantageous because the drug may reach only epidural or subdural spaces. Even when it reaches the subarachnoid space, therapeutic levels of drug usually are not achieved in the ventricles. For this reason, many physicians prefer intraventricular drug administration.

Central instillation of drug into the ventricle can be achieved via an Ommaya reservoir (see Figure 15-7), which is placed by a neurosurgeon. A skin flap is created, and the Ommaya reservoir placed underneath the skin, with the catheter extending from the reservoir to the ventricle. Once the surgical site has healed, the only visible evidence of the device is a small bump on the head. Placement of this reservoir obviously involves greater risk than performance of a lumbar puncture, but it provides permanent intraventricular access for those patients in whom the intrathecal route is impractical or inaccessible. As with intrathecal therapy, preservative-free drug and diluent must be used, but the dose is usually slightly smaller, since its maximum effect is being realized. Ommaya reservoirs are usually accessed by specially trained nurses using sterile technique. The patient can be in a sitting, supine, or Trendelenburg position. The site is assessed for tenderness, redness, or warmth, and the reservoir is primed by depressing it lightly several times. It should refill rapidly. The area above the Ommaya reservoir is prepped with betadine in a standard circular motion, using three swabs (shaving a small area is desirable). Access is achieved using a small-gauge, noncoring needle, or a 25-gauge preprimed scalp vein needle, at an oblique angle. Cerebrospinal fluid is gentle aspirated, and if ordered can be sent for cytology or laboratory studies. The drug is administered slowly, and resistance should not be felt. The reservoir volume is approximately 1.5–2 ml, and the needle usually is flushed with a small volume of nonbacteriostatic saline to clear the drug from the needle prior to its removal. After needle withdrawal, it is common to gently palpate or "pump" the reservoir to aid in adequate drug dispersement. The patient frequently will hear a slight whooshing or squishing sound when the reservoir is depressed and then refills. No heparinization or intermittent flushing is necessary, as CSF flows freely through the device.[76–79]

Regardless of the specific delivery method, nursing considerations include patient education, assessment of the access site, administration (or assistance with administration) of the drug, safe drug handling, and side effect management. Even though intravenous drugs do not cross the blood–brain barrier in sufficient concentration to treat meningeal disease, the intraventricular drugs are quite capable of reversing the process and entering the systemic bloodstream. Side effects of the drugs, such as nausea, stomatitis, and mild myelosuppression, are to be anticipated. Special care should be taken with methotrexate, for doses are often high

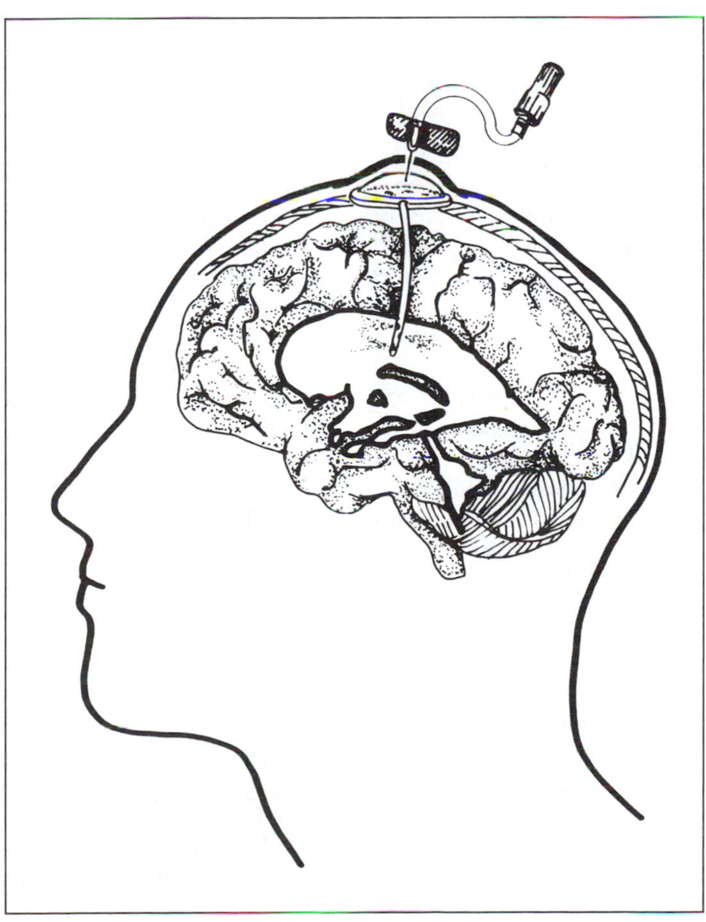

FIGURE 15-7 Ommaya reservoir placement.

enough to warrant administration of leucovorin to prevent unnecessarily severe toxicities. More information regarding side effect management of the drugs is contained in Chapter 16. The expected side effects related to the site of drug delivery can include headache, nausea, vomiting, ataxia, blurred vision, and, rarely, meningitis or paraplegia. The most serious complication (other than disease progression) for which to observe is infection, which is manifested by tenderness, redness, drainage, warmth or fever, stiff neck, and headache (with or without vomiting). Despite possible complications, the Ommaya reservoir is considered a safe and reliable aid to the intraventricular administration of antineoplastic agents.

VASCULAR ACCESS DEVICES

The development of central venous catheters (CVCs) and other types of long-term vascular access devices (VADs) has enhanced the lives of oncology patients but added a new series of concerns and challenges.[80–85] Device selection, patient selection, usage, maintenance, procedures, and complication management continue to be refined by practice and research.

There are many different kinds of catheters, needles, and implantable ports used for cancer chemotherapy delivery. Some of the major VAD types and features are outlined in Table 15-8. The nurse has a vital role in assessing the patient's vascular access needs and selecting or recommending placement of the proper device. Intermittent peripheral venous access is preferred for patients with good veins, on limited intermittent therapies not involving vesicant infusions. Even multiday infusional therapy can easily be administered through peripheral veins when vascular integrity is good. CVCs or ports should be considered in patients with poor veins, requiring multiinfusional therapy (e.g., the acute leukemia patient receiving chemotherapy, blood products, antibiotics, and TPN), long-term therapy, or continuous infusion of vesicants.

As with other aspects of chemotherapy administration, education of both the nurse and the patient and family are essential when dealing with vascular access devices. The oncology nurse should be well trained in all aspects of VAD care: selection, placement, postinsertion care, accessing, flushing, site care, troubleshooting, repairing, and removing. There is no universal standard of care for these devices, despite the fact that well over 500,000 VADs are placed annually.[87] The nurse is urged to be familiar with the particular brands of devices, the manufacturers' recommendations, existing clinical practice trends, and the established policies and procedures of the employing institution.[88,89] Patient and family education is vital, since many devices have self-care aspects that must be considered when selecting the VAD. Any patient having an external device (TCVC or PICC) must be able to flush, clean, and care for the device. Consideration should be given to the patient's ability to understand instructions, physical ability to manipulate the catheter, financial ability to purchase supplies, access to a clean area in the home, willingness to perform self-care activities, and compliance in reporting problems. Many excellent booklets and videotapes have been developed by VAD manufacturers and also by hospitals and health care agencies, but their usefulness depends on the nurse's assessment of the patient's ability to understand and comply with the actions described.[90]

General Management

The selection, care, and maintenance of the long-term devices is highly variable and will be addressed separately for nontunneled central venous catheters, tunneled central venous catheters (TCVCs), and implantable ports. Many of the major complications are handled in similar ways, so the management of complications will be addressed together for all the devices, immediately following this discussion of general management.

Nontunneled central venous catheters

Short-term use of a nontunneled central venous catheter, such as a standard subclavian line, is a common practice in urgent situations. When an immediate need for a central line arises, it commonly is placed by a physician at the bedside, in the intensive care unit, or in the emergency room. For oncology patients, it is primarily intended to provide immediate access until the emergency can be resolved. These devices are also used in oncology patients with the need for multiinfusional therapy beyond the capabilities of an existing tunneled CVC or implantable port. A multilumen subclavian catheter might be placed in an acute leukemia patient on chemotherapy, hydration, antibiotics, TPN, blood products, and other medications or a patient on a complex investigational drug protocol. The triple-lumen central catheter can augment the long-term device during the hospitalization and be removed prior to discharge.

For long-term use, the gap that exists between the trauma of subclavian lines and the investment in a long-term tunneled catheter or port has been closed with the use of peripherally inserted central catheters (PICCs).[91] From the patient's viewpoint, the PICC is the least expensive and most easily inserted long-term CVC, but it requires self-care capabilities and often even a caregiver, since it is located at the antecubital fossa and self-care has to be one-handed. These small-gauge, thin-walled catheters are inserted at the antecubital fossa into the basilic or cephalic vein (Figures 15-8 and 15-9). The procedure usually is performed by a physician or a specially trained nurse at the patient's bedside, and the catheter can be advanced into the superior vena

TABLE 15-8 Overview of Available Vascular Access Devices

Type	Description	Longevity	Comments
Peripheral needle Scalp vein Butterfly	• Stainless steel • Single lumen • 27–19-gauge	Minutes to days	• Excellent for short-term access, especially outpatient • Increased risk of infiltration with long-term use
Peripheral catheter Abbocath Insyte Streamline	• Catheter over needle • Teflon or polyurethane • Streamline is elastomeric hydrogel, which softens and expands one lumen size after insertion[86] • Single and double lumen • 26–14-gauge	Hours to days	• Excellent for multiday infusional therapy • Provides greater patient mobility since less likely to infiltrate • Streamline (Menlo Care, Inc.) has been known to remain patent and functioning for 1–2 weeks, due to its softer composition
Nontunneled central venous catheter Subclavian line Arrow (Arrow International Inc., Reading, PA)	• Polyurethane or silicone catheter • Single, double, and triple lumen	Hours to weeks	• Excellent for emergency need for CVC • Can augment existing VAD for acute care needs • Inserted at bedside by physician • High rate of trauma, infection compared to TCVC and port
Peripherally inserted central catheters (PICCs) C-PICS (Cook Critical Care, Bloomington, IN) Per-Q-Cath (Gesco International, San Antonio, TX) Groshong PICC (Davol Cath Tech Inc., Cranston, RI)	• Silicone elastomer or other polymers • Single and double lumen • 24–16-gauge	Weeks to months	• Excellent for continuous infusion over several weeks or months • Can be inserted at bedside by specially trained nurse • Quick, easy central access without surgical procedure • Requires external site care and routine flushing
Tunneled central venous catheter Hickman catheter (Davol Specialty Access Products Inc., Salt Lake City, UT) Raaf Cath (Quinton Instrument Co., Seattle, WA) Groshong catheter (Davol Specialty Access Products Inc., Salt Lake City, UT)	• Silicone catheter with Dacron cuff • Single, double, and triple lumen • 4.2–19.2 Fr; 40–90-cm length • Groshong has slit valve, requiring less flushing	Months to years	• Excellent for long-term, continuous, or intermittent therapy • Preferred for long-term TPN administration • Preferred by many for vesicant infusional therapy • Requires external site care and routine flushing
Implantable port Port-A-Cath (Pharmacia Deltec Inc., St. Paul, MN) Hickman Port (Davol Inc., Cranston, RI) Lifeport (Strato Medical Corp., Beverly, MA)	• Titanium, stainless steel, silastic, or plastic portal attached to catheter • Single and double lumen • Access with noncoring needle	Months to years	• Excellent for long-term, intermittent infusional therapy • No site care required, so excellent for patients unable to perform site care • Surgical procedure required for removal
Peripheral port PAS-Port (Pharmacia Deltec Inc., St. Paul, MN)	• Titanium portal attached to silastic catheter • Single lumen • Access with noncoring needle	Months to years	• Excellent for frequent, intermittent access, particularly for those patients with active lifestyles or body image concerns • No external site care

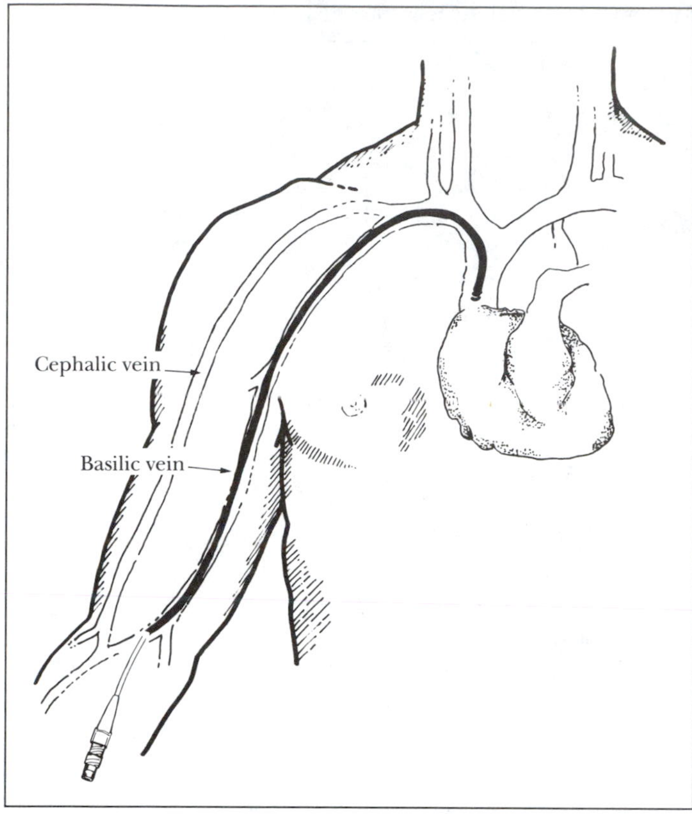

FIGURE 15-8 Peripherally inserted central catheter (PICC) placement.

cava, in which case x-ray verification of placement is required. A few state boards of nursing consider the placement of a central venous catheter to be outside the role of a professional nurse, so it is important for the nurse to verify that placement of a PICC is within the scope of nursing as defined by the state. Some states allow PICC insertion if it is considered a long-line catheter and is only advanced into the axillary or subclavian veins, in which case x-ray verification of placement is not necessarily required but is preferred, especially for vesicant administration. Formal training in the intricacies of PICC insertion is required, for the insertion techniques vary greatly among the specific devices and success is usually technique dependent and due to repeated practice.[91–95]

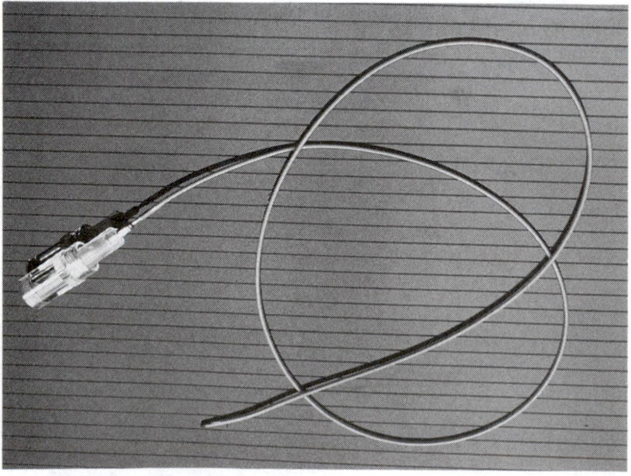

FIGURE 15-9 Groshong PICC—single lumen. (Photo courtesy of Bard Access Systems, Salt Lake City, UT)

PICCs are ideal for short-term access (one week to several months) in patients with adequate antecubital veins, self-care capabilities, and the need for a wide variety of intravenous therapies, including antibiotics, chemotherapy, TPN, and analgesics. The thin, flexible nature of the catheter does not lend itself well to blood withdrawal, but it is not contraindicated and may be successfully achieved with gentle application of pressure via the syringe used for blood withdrawal. The complication rate is similar to that for other VADs in terms of infection, clotting, and malfunction.[96–98] Some studies suggest a higher rate of phlebitis, which may be technique dependent or caused by powdered gloves. Meticulous attention to sterile technique during insertion and rinsing the powder off the gloves prior to handling the PICC seem to decrease these complications.[92] An overview of PICC features is given in Table 15-9.

Tunneled central venous catheters

The tunneled central venous catheter provides safe and reliable long-term access (months to years) with a

TABLE 15-9 PICC Overview

Catheter Features
• Multiple manufacturers and insertion techniques are involved.
• Composed of silicone elastomer or other polymers.
• Available in single- and dual-lumen styles.
• Sizes range from 16–24 gauge and 20–60 cm in length.
• Insertion kits with introducers are available from some manufacturers.
• Cost effective compared to all other VADs.
Placement
• Highly technique dependent; requires formal training.
• A sterile procedure; at bedside; performed by registered nurse or physician.
• Requires adequate antecubital veins and x-ray verification.
Usage
• Is excellent for central access for one week to several months.
• Blood withdrawal can be difficult.
• Requires regular flushing/heparinization (q 12–24 hr)
• Requires sterile dressing (changed q 5–7 days or prn).
• Easily removed by registered nurse at bedside.
• Over time, multiple insertions can cause venous scarring and decrease the ability to reuse the site.

low incidence of infection, suitable for almost all hematology/oncology patients and many others, as well. It continues to be well accepted and has been modified by the various manufacturers who now market similar devices. The unique features of the TCVC (see Figure 15-10) include a Dacron cuff around which granulation tissue forms, actually helping to hold the catheter in place. The 4–10-inch tunnel through which the catheter is channeled serves to prevent the easy passage of bacteria from the skin into the vein. Also, the cuff is thought to help stop bacteria traveling along the subcutaneous portion of the catheter. A second cuff (VitaCuff) impregnated with silver ions can be attached to any catheter to help decrease the infection rate[87] (see Figure 15-11). The catheter material is usually radiopaque silicone to aid insertion and subsequent placement verification. The external portion of the TCVC has a luer-lok hub (to allow direct access with an intravenous infusion set) or placement of a prn/heparin lock adapter (to allow access via a needle). Single-, double-, and triple-lumen TCVCs are available in various gauges and lengths.

One unique variation of a TCVC is the Groshong catheter (see Figure 15-12), which features a closed-end radiopaque tip. Flow through the catheter is achieved via a patented slit valve, which opens out into the bloodstream when fluid is infusing into the catheter, opens inward into the catheter lumen when blood is being withdrawn from the catheter, and remains

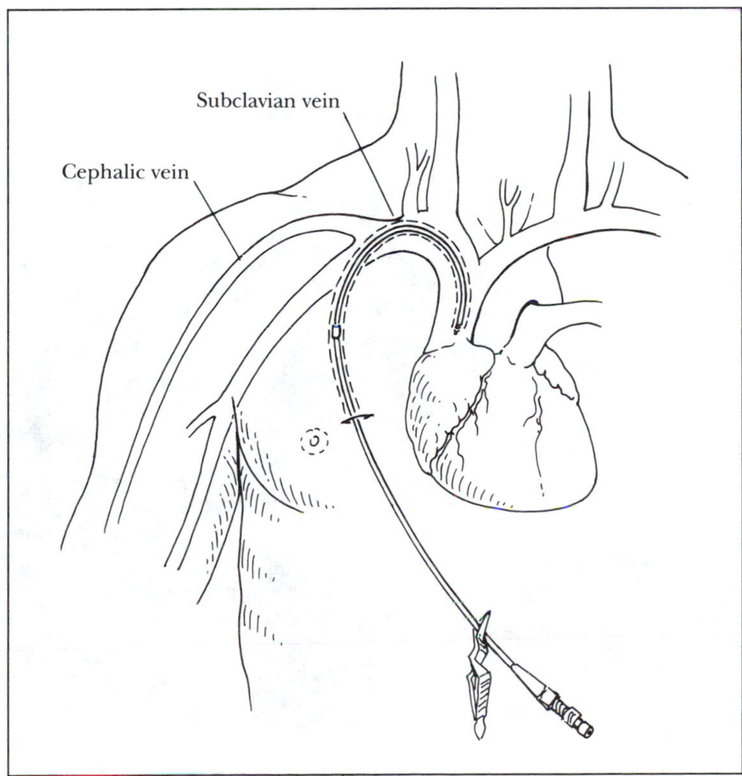

FIGURE 15-10 Tunneled central venous catheter placement.

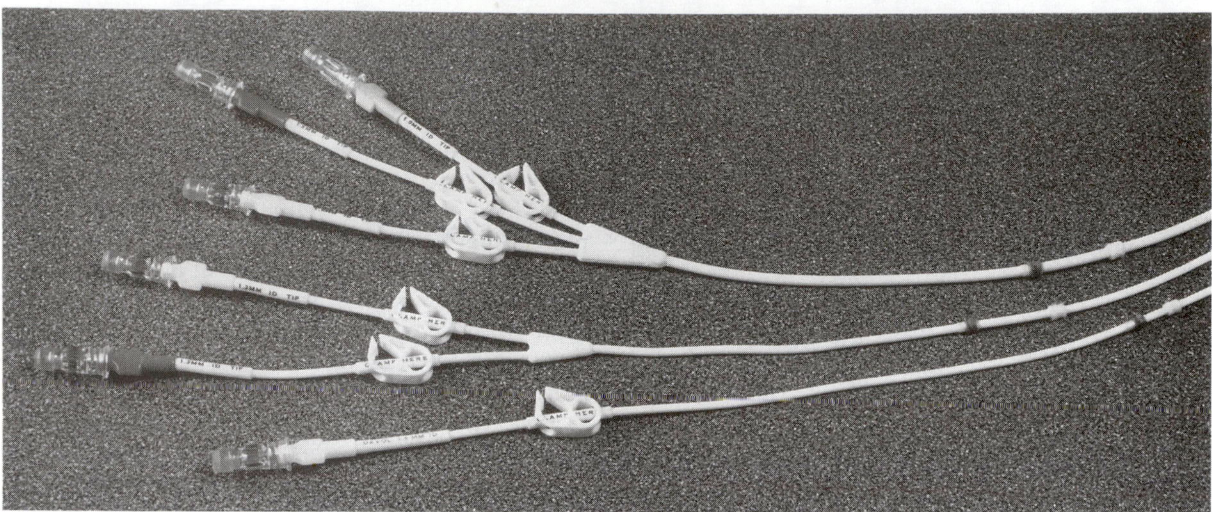

FIGURE 15-11 Hickman catheters—single, double, and triple lumen. (Courtesy of Bard Access Systems, Salt Lake City, UT)

closed when no pressure is being applied. Groshong catheter technology has been applied to the other VADs, and Groshong ports and PICCs are available, as well as the TCVC. This design prevents the need for regular heparinization of the catheter, which usually is flushed with sterile NS once a week when not in use, making it advantageous in those patients for whom heparin is contraindicated.

Patient selection is a key issue with the TCVC because it requires regular care and maintenance. The patient or significant other must be willing and physically able to clean the exit site, flush the catheter, change the cap, and assess and report complications. Lifestyle can be an issue, because of the catheter exit through the chest wall, which can be distressing or embarrassing to some patients, particularly adolescents. Also, whereas swimming in chlorinated pools is allowed by some practitioners, swimming in ponds, rivers, or the ocean usually is not recommended. The patient needs to be able to afford the equipment (needles, syringes, heparin or saline, and dressing materials) and have access to a clean area in the home in which to perform self-care.

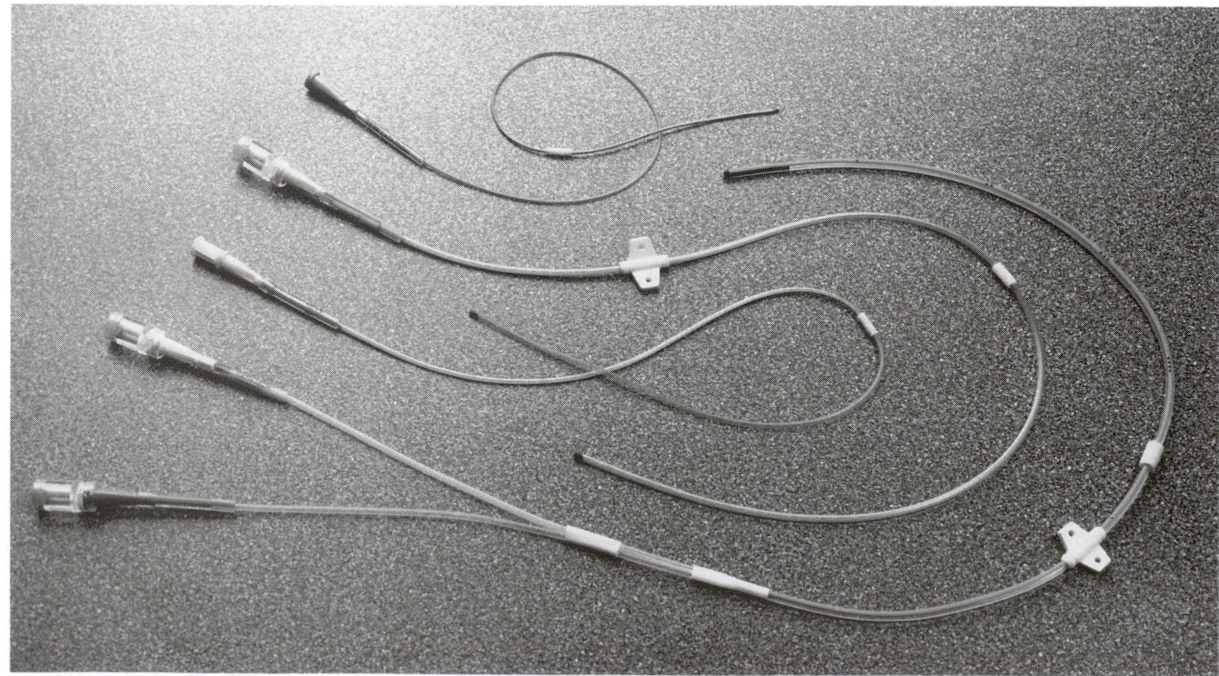

FIGURE 15-12 Various Groshong catheters (pediatric, CVC, TCVC, dual-lumen TCVC). (Courtesy of Bard Access Systems, Salt Lake City, UT)

There are several major advantages of the TCVC, including its elimination of needle sticks for those people who have a needle phobia (and do not want any needle sticks, even into implantable ports), and the ease with which it is removed when no longer needed for care. It also allows for a great deal of flexibility in terms of usage, being a preferred device for long-term TPN, vesicant therapy, and continuous infusions. It also is the only long-term device that offers a triple-access option. Finally, it is less expensive in terms of both the device and the insertion costs than an implantable port; however, there is some debate as to the long-term cost effectiveness, since supplies are needed for care and their cost depends on the regimen of care and frequency and type of flushing. An overview of TCVC features is given in Table 15-10.

Despite the common use of TCVCs for almost two decades, there is very little standardization of their insertion and care. Insertion is not without risks, and complications include pneumothorax and arterial puncture.[87,99] A variety of techniques is used for placement, and experienced oncology nurses are beginning to work with physicians and patients prior to insertion to help select a site that is convenient when considering clothing and body contours. Adequate instruction of the patient and family both before and after placement is critical to a successful experience with a TCVC.

Possible options for policies and procedures governing routine use of TCVCs include the following:

1. Requires sterile site care with dressings until the formation of granulation tissue and verification of normal absolute neutrophil counts, at which time site care involves bathing the chest wall and securing the catheter with tape to prevent dislodgement.
2. When not in use, requires daily, qod, or even weekly flushing with 5 ml of heparinized saline (10 u/ml).
3. Requires blood withdrawal for all laboratory tests (except coagulation studies), which can be achieved via vacutainer technique, if desired; vacutainer technique is preferred, since it minimizes the risk of accidental needle sticks.
4. Whenever blood has been aspirated into the catheter it is flushed with 20 cc of saline prior to hep-locking.
5. Must avoid intraluminal mixing of potentially incompatible drugs, which can be achieved by flushing with plain fluid between each drug.
6. Must avoid scissors, sharp objects, and needles longer than 1 inch.
7. Access is either direct or via prn/heparin lock adaptor cap; all connections must be taped.

Perhaps one reason there is so much variation in technique among states, settings, and facilities is because it does not really matter that much which type of dressing is used or how often and with what the catheter is flushed. Several small studies regarding dressings have suggested equivocal results. One study showed a slight increased risk of infection with transparent vs. gauze dressings, while the other showed no statistically significant difference between transparent, gauze, or no dressing.[100–102] In fact, the last study demonstrated the lowest infection rate in the no-dressing group. Similarly, Kelley et al.[103] analyzed existing data regarding flushing regimens, conducted a 3-year study, and concluded that weekly flushing with 100 u heparin/ml was safe and effective for 86.5% of study participants. Another group, routinely flushing with sterile saline weekly in pediatric patients, reported that the most striking finding of the study was the fact that the majority of infections occurred during the summer

TABLE 15-10 Tunneled Central Venous Catheter Overview

Catheter Features
- Multiple manufacturers.
- Composed of silicone or polyurethane with Dacron cuff.
- Available in single, double, and triple lumens.
- Sizes range from 4.2–19.2 Fr. and 40–90 cm in length.
- Inner diameter ranges from 0.7–1.6 mm, with a priming volume of 0.3–2.5 ml.
- Insertion kits with introducers are available from all manufacturers.
- Cost effective, especially with percutaneous insertion (eliminates operating room cost).

Placement
- Technique dependent; training or observation of the technique is strongly encouraged.
- A sterile procedure, performed by physician, usually in operating room, although some can be inserted percutaneously.
- Exit site on the nondominant side should be preselected by the nurse, with the patient erect and clothed to prevent placement at an inappropriate site, eg, under the breast.
- Groshong catheters require a reverse tunneling technique and cannot be trimmed at the proximal end.
- Can be placed through numerous veins, including the jugular, cephalic, and subclavian veins.
- Frequently placed under fluoroscopy; x-ray verification of placement is required.
- Suture should be placed at exit site to retain proper catheter placement until granulation occurs around the cuff (usually within 2 wk), and then the suture should be removed.

Usage
- Excellent for long-term access for several months to years.
- Preferred for TPN, vesicants, and continuous infusions.
- Requires regular flushing/heparinization (daily to weekly).
- Groshong requires weekly flushing with sterile NS when not in use.
- Requires exit site care.
- Blood withdrawal is easy; can use vacutainer technique.
- Usually removed by physician.

months, when children might be expected to be outside playing and swimming and are perhaps at high risk for infection.[104] Interpretation of these findings and resolution of some of these issues will continue to require continual assessment, documentation, and reporting of research study results.

One unique care issue related to TCVCs is breaking, puncturing, or cutting of the external portion of the catheter. This can be prevented by not using scissors or sharp objects near the catheter and limiting needles used for access to 1 inch in length or by using needleless systems. It is also advisable to avoid clamping the catheter continuously or, if clamping is desirous, padding and rotating the clamp site. As long as at least 2 inches of undamaged catheter exits the skin, it can be repaired using a repair kit available from the manufacturer. Most repair kits are generic, but others are designed only for a specific catheter, especially the double- and triple-lumen repair kits if the break is in the main portion of the catheter. Emergency repairs can be conducted via the following steps:[105,106]

1. Clamp catheter close to chest wall.
2. Clean catheter with alcohol at the most distal undamaged point.
3. Using sterile scissors, cut the catheter.
4. Remove the inner metal stylus from a 14-g or 16-g peripheral IV catheter, and insert the IV catheter into the TCVC until the cut edge touches the hub.
5. Secure with tape or suture.
6. Apply heparin lock adapter cap, unclamp, and gently flush catheter; heparinize or use in the normal manner.
7. Obtain a repair kit as soon as possible for permanent repair.

One major advantage of the TCVC is the ease with which it is removed by the physician when no longer needed or desired by the patient. Prior to withdrawal of the catheter, some catheter manufacturers suggest a very short surgical incision, under local anesthesia, to mechanically release the Dacron cuff from the subcutaneous tissues. Catheter removal is achieved by cleaning the exit site and then manually pulling on the catheter until it loosens in the tunnel. Pressure is then applied manually over the entrance site into the vein and maintained for several minutes after catheter removal. Steady, slow pressure is applied until the entire catheter is removed and inspected to ensure that it is intact, since breakage or splintering can occur. The exit site is dressed with a small dressing, if necessary. If the new cuff is not removed with the catheter, it may become infected at a later date.

Implantable ports

The implantable port has proven to be a unique development in vascular access devices because when it is not in use, it requires almost no care or maintenance (see Figures 15-13 and 15-14). A *port* is a hollow housing containing a compressed latex septum over a portal chamber that is connected via a small tube to a silicone or polyurethane catheter that is inserted into a blood vessel. It is placed subcutaneously and accessed percutaneously using a special noncoring needle. The needle has an offset bevel, which prevents coring the septum and allows 1000–3600 punctures per port, depending on manufacturer and needle size. These devices can be composed of stainless steel, titanium, silastic, or plastic (Figures 15-15 and 15-16). The plastic and titanium ports are advantageous because they cause little if any disturbance on x-ray film during imaging procedures. Ports are available with: (1) the catheter permanently attached to the portal housing, in which case the surgeon adjusts the length by trimming the distal portion of the catheter prior to insertion, or (2) the catheter separate from the portal housing, in which case the surgeon trims the proximal end prior to attaching and securing it to the portal during the implantation procedure. They are available in single and double designs, with the double port having two distinct portal chambers to prevent incompatible drug admixture. Most ports are accessed through the top. A portal design that provides access via the side, allowing the needle to be positioned parallel to the skin, has not been very well received and is not commonly used by practitioners today. An overview of port features is given in Table 15-11.[84,85,87]

Port routes There are five major routes for ports, each requiring entirely different nursing actions: venous port, arterial port, peritoneal port, intrapleural port, and epidural port. The unique portal design allows access to more than just the vascular system; and while

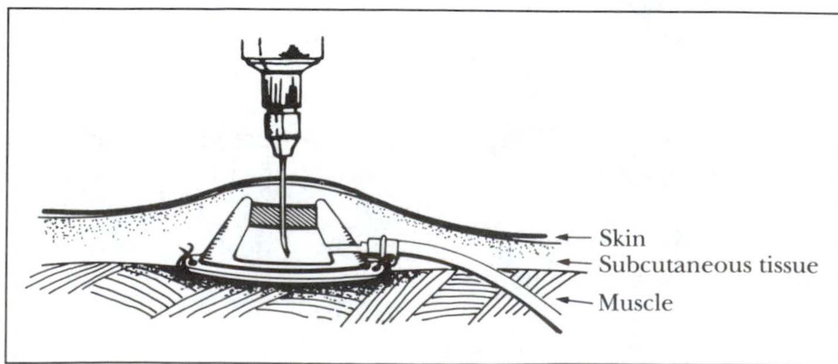

FIGURE 15-13 Schematic drawing of an implantable port.

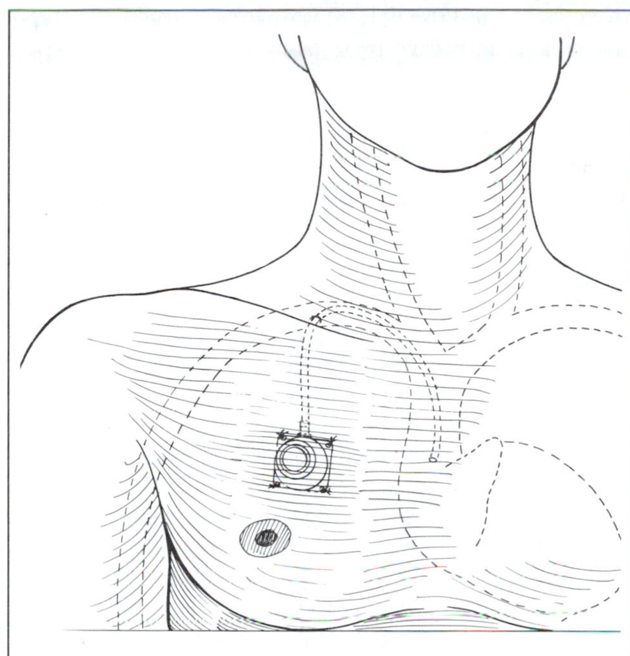

FIGURE 15-14 Venous port placement. (© 1990 Pharmacia Deltec, Inc. Courtesy of Pharmacia Deltec, Inc., St. Paul, MN)

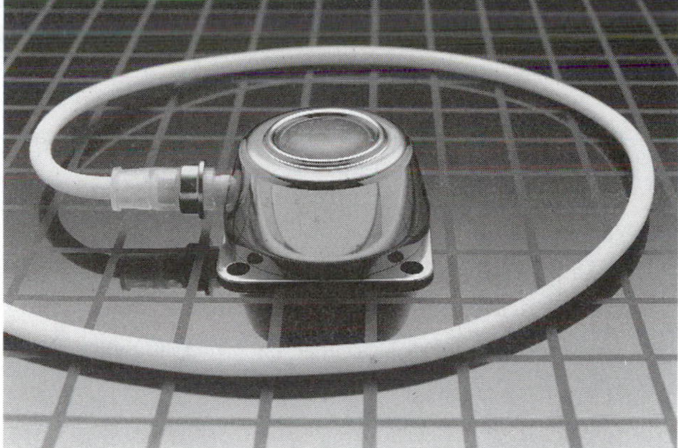

A

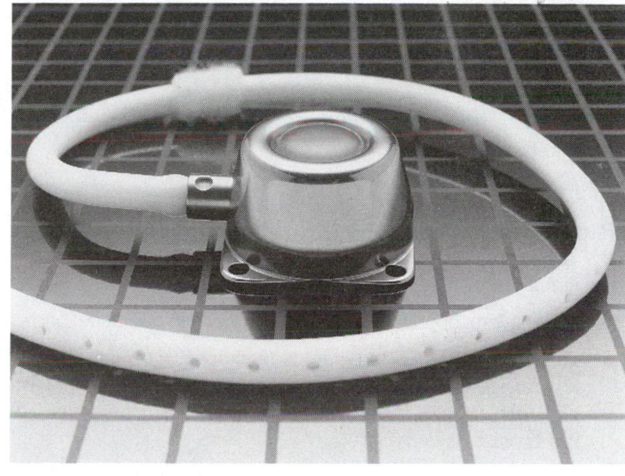

B

FIGURE 15-16 Port-a-Cath implantable ports. (a) Venous; (b) peritoneal. (© 1990 by Pharmacia Deltec, Inc. Courtesy of Pharmacia Deltec, Inc., St. Paul, MN)

the portal housings are all essentially the same, the catheters are designed and located differently. The arterial and epidural ports have specially designed catheters with very small lumens, since the flow rate through these devices is often as low as 2–3 ml per day. At the opposite end of the spectrum is the peritoneal catheter, which has a very large lumen and multiple exit sites to allow rapid infusion of fluids. The venous ports have varying-sized lumens and flow rates. Placement of these ports, illustrated in Figure 15-17, is usually over a bony structure in the left or right upper chest, lower chest, or lower abdomen. Usually, venous ports are placed in the upper chest area. Arterial ports can be placed in any of the sites. Peritoneal ports are consistently placed on the lower rib cage, but could be on the lower abdomen. Epidural ports could be at either of the lower positions. Unfortunately, there is no standardized placement of the different types of ports, which creates major problems for the nurse unfamiliar with a new patient. It is imperative that the type of device be determined prior to access of the port. It is not common, but it is important to remember that ports can be located in other areas of the body. For example, a port can be located over the lower rib cage and the attached catheter be inserted into the pleural space (see Chapter 30) or the peritoneum. It is important to know exactly where the catheter is and what it is to be used for. Most patients are given an identifying wallet card and information regarding their ports. If that information is

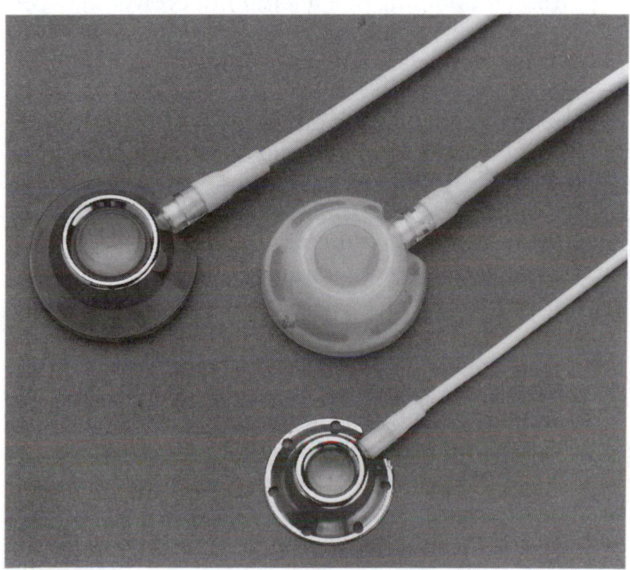

FIGURE 15-15 Various implantable port designs (Courtesy of Bard Access Systems, Salt Lake City, UT)

TABLE 15-11 Port Overview

Port Features
- Multiple manufacturers involved.
- Composed of stainless steel, titanium, or plastic, with catheter of silicone or polyurethane.
- Available with preattached or attachable catheters in single and double designs.
- Can be accessed with a noncoring needle, usually through the top; side-access models are available.
- Types include: venous, arterial, peritoneal, intrapleural and epidural.
- Venous variations include: central and peripheral insertion techniques.
- Available in pediatric and low-profile styles.
- Insertion kits with introducers are available from all manufacturers.
- Expensive, both in terms of port cost and implantation procedure.
- Possibly the least expensive of all VADs for routine care and maintenance.

Placement
- Technique dependent; training or observation of the technique is strongly encouraged.
- A sterile procedure, performed by surgeon in operating room.
- Exit site on the nondominant side should be preselected by the nurse, with the patient erect and clothed to prevent placement at an inappropriate site, eg, under the breast, in the breast, or under the arm.
- Groshong ports cannot be trimmed at the proximal end.
- Frequently placed with fluoroscopy; x-ray verification of placement required.
- Suture line should not be over the top of the port.
- Port should be accessed with an infusion set and a dressing applied prior to leaving the operating room if it is to be used immediately; some practitioners prefer to wait 5–7 days prior to use to allow swelling to go down.

Usage
- Can remain in place and functional for many years.
- Ideal for intermittent therapies.
- Can be accessed using noncoring needle, which should touch the bottom of the portal space and be held firmly by the latex septum.
- Ice or a local anesthetic can be used to decrease discomfort prior to accessing.
- When not in use, must be flushed monthly (usually with 3–5 ml of sterile 100 u/ml heparinized saline)
- For constant access, site care is provided and needle is changed per established policy (usually every 7 days or prn)
- Blood withdrawal is easy; can use vacutainer technique.
- Removal requires surgical procedure.

unavailable and the patient is unsure of the device type, then the health care professional must seek the operative note in the hospital chart to confirm device type and catheter route.

Nursing issues related to arterial, peritoneal, epidural, and intrapleural ports are summarized in Table 15-12 and have been discussed in some detail in the previous portion of this chapter dealing with routes of drug administration.

Port usage The major advantage of implantable ports over other vascular access devices is that they are implanted. The routine care of the venous port when not being used is to flush it once every 4 weeks with sterile heparinized saline (usually 5 ml of 100 u/ml solution).[107] It is an ideal choice for patients who are unable or unwilling to care properly for an external device, receiving intermittent therapies, concerned about body image, or physically active (especially if swimming in unchlorinated bodies of water). Its major disadvantage is that it requires a needle to pass through the skin and into the port for usage. The procedure of accessing the port could introduce infective organisms, cause a hematoma in a thrombocytopenic patient, cause anxiety in a patient with a needle phobia, or result in extravasation of fluid around the port if performed incorrectly or if the needle subsequently becomes dislodged. There is also a very remote chance that the device could extrude through the skin.[90]

Nursing management of ports involves assessing the site, accessing the device, infusing or withdrawing fluids, and flushing. The nurse should help select the portal site prior to implantation. With the patient erect and clothed, the nondominant side should be examined for a convenient location. Ideally, the port can be located over a rib in an area easy for the patient to visualize for care but not visible when clothed. Consideration should be given to clothing, brassiere straps, lifestyle (e.g., frequent holding of a telephone receiver between the head and chest) and physical activities (e.g., swimming). Thin patients may need low-profile ports; obese patients may need large ports. Also, in obese patients or large-breasted women, placement of the port near the sternum provides better needle stability and ease of access. Care should be taken to avoid placement of the port under the arm, under the breast, in the breast, or in the soft tissue of the abdomen (for nonvenous ports). The preferred site and an alternate should be marked on the skin as a reference for the surgeon. It is also helpful if the surgeon offsets the port pocket so that the suture line is 1–2 inches away from the top of the port.

Port access usually is achieved under sterile or aseptic technique after a betadine scrub using noncoring needles that can be either straight or bent at a 90° angle. The needle firmly penetrates the septum and is advanced until it touches the bottom of the portal chamber. The most popular access needles are actually infusion sets consisting of needle, tubing, and luer-

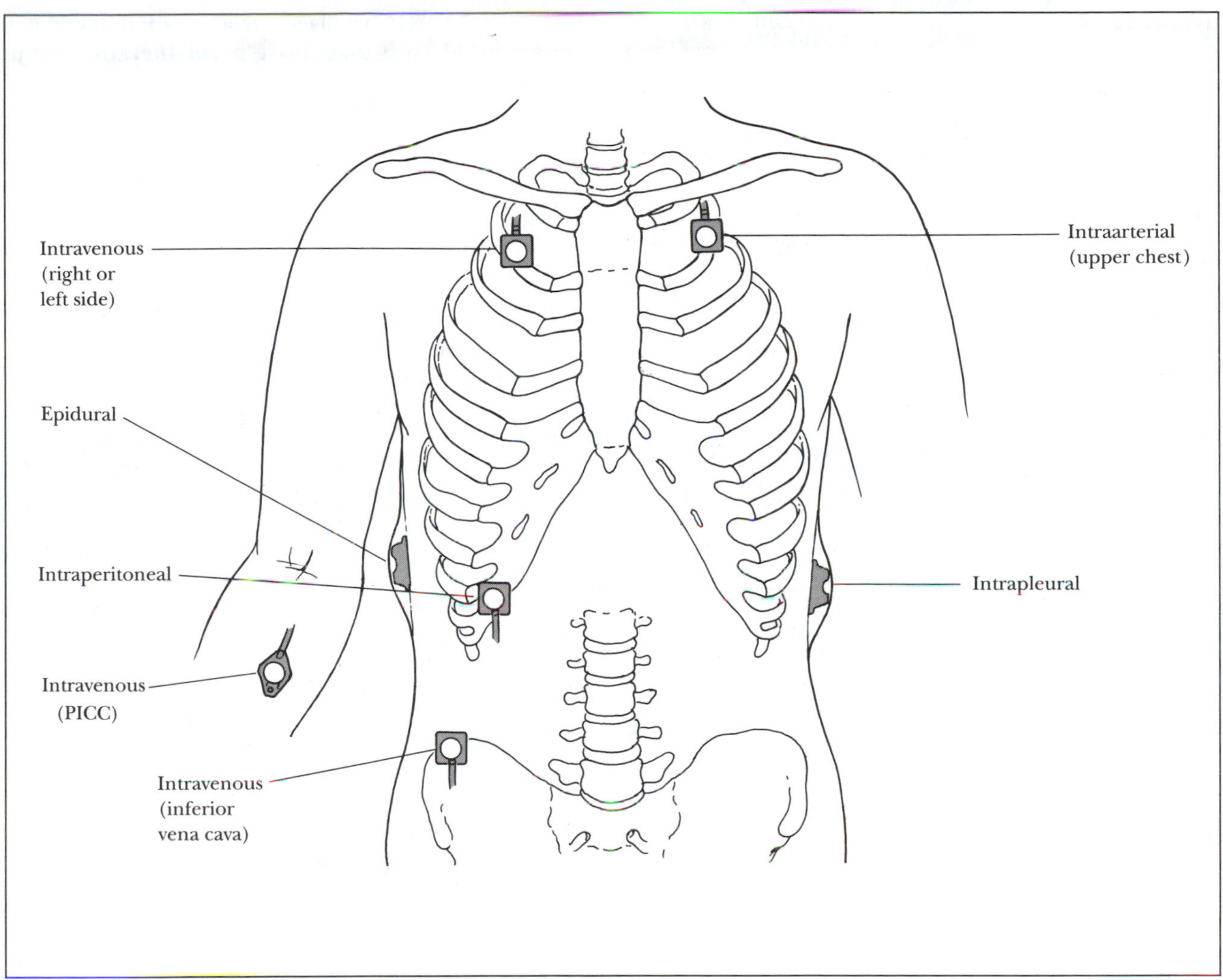

FIGURE 15-17 Implantable port placement sites.

lok hub and containing a Y-site and a clamp. These infusion sets allow great flexibility and multiple access and can be left in place for up to 7 days. For long-term access, a sterile dressing (usually transparent) is placed over the site and assessed on a daily basis. Redness, rash, or blistering of the skin around the port could be indicative of an allergic reaction to the tape or dressing, which is not uncommon and is resolved by using an alternative type of tape or dressing.

There are several other aspects of port accessing that are especially important to the patient. The area is tender and edematous for a week or so after implantation, causing manipulation of the device to be uncomfortable or even painful. Some practitioners prefer to wait until the site has healed and the edema is gone before using the port. When immediate use is desired, the port should be accessed and dressed securely in the operating room. For routine use once the site is healed, the needle stick usually is not a concern to most patients and causes little discomfort. An occasional patient will have a needle phobia or experience pain during insertion. Effective options to increase patient comfort include application of a small ice pack to the area for a few minutes or application of a topical anesthetic agent, to numb the area before accessing.

All types of medications and fluids can be administered through venous ports, but some problems have been noted with TPN, which can cause drug crystals or lipids to build up inside the portal housing and occlude the device. As with TCVCs, blood withdrawal can be accomplished for all laboratory studies except those involving coagulation, and the vacutainer technique can be utilized. There is a concern when administering continuous-infusion vesicants because the needle could become dislodged from the septum and remain under the skin, causing a port pocket extravasation. For this reason, vesicant infusions are monitored frequently (every 1–2 hours), and some practitioners prefer that

TABLE 15-12 Unique Types of Implantable Ports

Arterial

- Used to administer continuous or intermittent intraarterial chemotherapy.
- Catheter is placed into an artery, and portal is usually placed on the lower rib cage.
- Accessed and managed in the usual manner, except heparinization procedure may be different, with increased frequency (ie, weekly) or higher concentrations of heparin (100–1000 u/ml).
- Catheter has a small lumen and seems to form clots more easily than venous catheters; hence the need for at least weekly flushing.

Peritoneal

- Used to administer intermittent intraperitoneal chemotherapy for ovarian or colon cancer.
- Catheter is placed in the peritoneal space, and portal is usually placed on the lower rib cage but can be in the lower abdominal area.
- Accessed and managed in the usual sterile manner except 19-gauge noncoring needles are used to facilitate large-volume infusions; the portal is flushed after use with sterile saline, and heparinization usually is not required.
- Catheter has a very large lumen with several ridges or cuffs to secure placement and multiple exit holes in the distal portion for rapid fluid infusion.

Epidural

- Used to administer intrathecal or epidural medications, including chemotherapy and analgesics.
- Catheter is placed into the intrathecal or epidural space and tunneled through a long subcutaneous passage from the spinal area to the side of the abdomen, where the portal is placed on the lower rib cage or the abdominal area. The portal is designed with a 60-micron screen filter to remove particulate matter.
- Accessed using special 24-gauge noncoring needles, *always* with meticulous sterile technique, including sterile gloves, prep drape, and procedure tray.
- **Never to be flushed with heparin.**
- Preservative-free chemotherapy or morphine is instilled or infused into the port.
- After usage, 1–2 cc of sterile, preservative-free saline may be used to flush the line.
- Catheter has a small lumen (0.5-mm inner diameter), which is suitable for this type of drug delivery.

Intrapleural

- Used to drain pleural effusions periodically in patients who are unresponsive to sclerosing.
- Accessed with huber-point needle only.
- Patient's position is changed frequently during "tap."
- Flushed with 3 cc of saline. (See Chapter 30.)

PICCs or TCVCs be placed instead of ports if it is known in advance that this type of therapy may be necessary.

As with other VADs, the nurse is encouraged to know and assess for the signs and symptoms of complications prior to utilization of the device. The port should have a brisk blood return, easy flow of fluids, and no edema, redness, or pain. If any problems are noted, measures should be taken to resolve them; if necessary, verification of the patency of the port should be ascertained using x-ray film and/or venograms.

Peripheral implantable port A variation of the venous port that combines the properties of a PICC and a port is the peripherally inserted port.[108] The P.A.S.-Port (Peripheral Access System, Pharmacia Deltec, Inc., Minneapolis MN) allows the peripheral insertion of a port near the antecubital fossa (see Figures 15-18 and 15-19). Insertion and proper placement are achieved using an electronic device that enables insertion at the bedside or in the physician's office. The P.A.S.-Port is about half the size of a regular port and allows patients to experience the advantages of port placement (unobtrusive, long-term access, intermittent use) without having to expose the chest area to achieve access. It seems quite normal to a patient to simply extend his or her arm for "venipuncture" and treatment, so it has a high rate of patient acceptance. Access is achieved through a very short (0.5-inch) noncoring needle or infusion set. In all other aspects except placement, it is managed like a regular implantable venous port.

Complication Management

Occlusions, infections, and other complications can occur with all of the long-term vascular access devices. The incidence and type of complication depend on the device, insertion technique, care regimen, and to a great extent physiologic factors inherent in the introduction of a long-term catheter into the venous system.[109–111]

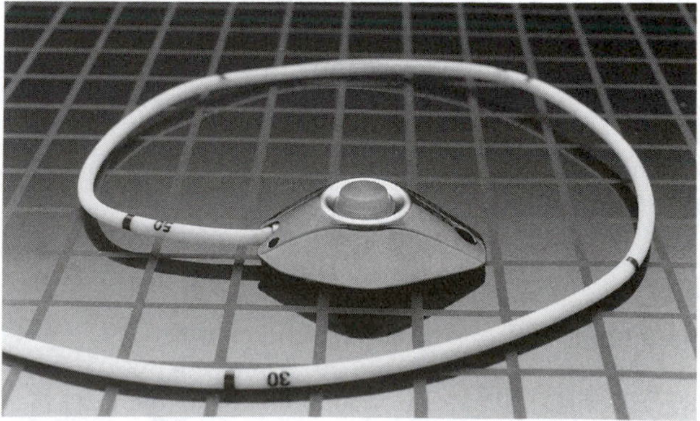

FIGURE 15-18 P.A.S.-Port (Peripheral Access System). (© 1990 Pharmacia Deltec, Inc. Courtesy of Pharmacia Deltec, Inc., St. Paul, MN)

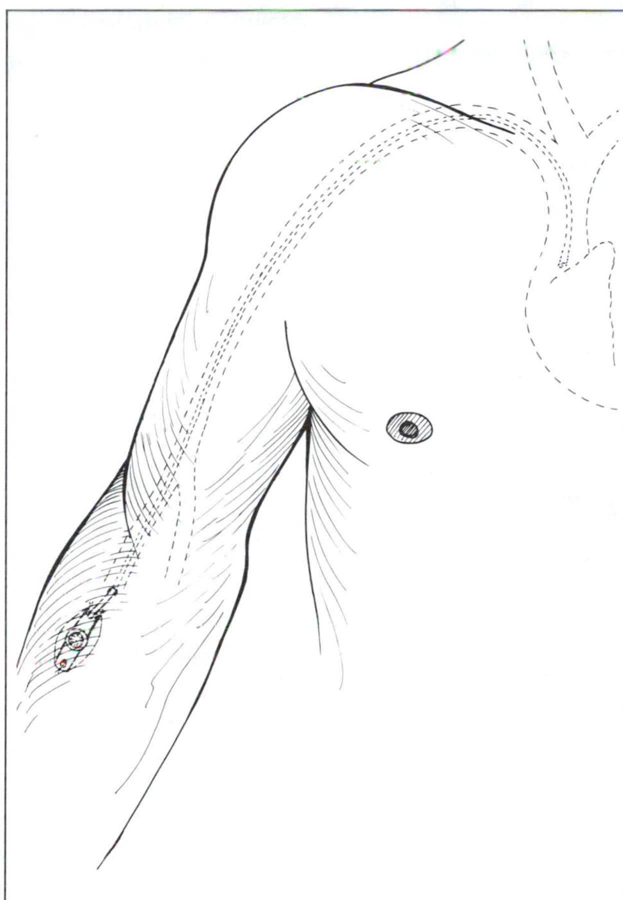

FIGURE 15-19 Schematic drawing of P.A.S.-Port placement (© 1990 Pharmacia Deltec, Inc. Courtesy of Pharmacia Deltec, Inc., St. Paul, MN)

Intraluminal catheter occlusion

The complete inability to withdraw blood or infuse fluid in a VAD is most commonly the result of a blood clot within the catheter. It can also be caused by incompatible drugs or lipids that have crystallized, precipitated, or obstructed the catheter. The nurse is instrumental in assessing the catheter and its most recent usage to determine which of these causes are most likely to have occurred. Blood clots can build up over time (i.e., sluggish catheter) but can also appear suddenly, for instance, in a port that is only accessed monthly. Drug precipitates tend to be more directly related to a recent infusion and are seen more often with TPN and lipids.[112] Measures to prevent either occurrence include the following.

1. Maintain positive pressure within the catheter when flushing.
2. Advise patient to avoid excessive manipulation (i.e., pinching or bending) of external catheters.
3. Vigorously flush with at least 20 cc of sterile NS after any blood has gotten into the catheter.
4. Document each patient's VAD experience, and adjust concentration, volume, and frequency of heparinized flush, as needed.
5. Question patient and family regarding actual catheter maintenance activities to assess compliance with recommended care and usage.
6. Flush between each drug with at least 10 cc of plain IV fluid to avoid incompatible drug admixture.
7. Vigorously flush catheter every 8–12 hours when administering TPN or lipids.
8. Avoid administering IV fluid or TPN containing visible precipitants (which is more likely to occur if the solution is more than 24 hours old).[113]

In the case of ports, the inability to infuse or aspirate usually is due to the needles being improperly placed in the septum rather than the portal. Advancing the needle into the portal usually will solve the problem.

Management of an occluded catheter when a blood clot is suspected involves the instillation of streptokinase or urokinase, which is almost universally successful.[114–116] Urokinase is less antigenic than streptokinase and is preferred by many practitioners. A dose of urokinase 5000 units in 1–3 ml is instilled using a 3-ml or larger syringe and a gentle to-and-fro motion. The catheter is then clamped for 30 minutes, after which an attempt is made to aspirate the catheter contents. If successful, the catheter is flushed and used; if unsuccessful the procedure is repeated.[117] If a second instillation of urokinase is unsuccessful, a variety of options exist. Some success has been obtained with a 24 "lock" of urokinase, while continuous infusions of urokinase for 4–24 hours have also been reported to clear occluded catheters successfully.[118,119] Tissue plasminogen activator (t-PA) has been reported to be successful in a small number of cases but remains investigational for this application.[120] Drug precipitants can be cleared using 0.1N hydrochloric acid for some crystals or ethanol 70% for lipid deposits.[113,121–124] The process is similar to that used for urokinase, with the gentle instillation of 0.2–1 ml of drug. After a dwell time of 30–60 minutes, an attempt is made to aspirate the catheter contents. If TPN is not involved and a specific drug is known or suspected, a pharmacist should be consulted about possible agents that might dissolve the precipitant and enable it to be aspirated from the catheter. Figure 15-20 describes a possible decision-making matrix to consider when dealing with a completely occluded catheter.

Extraluminal catheter occlusion

Catheter sluggishness or partial occlusion can be due to two extraluminal phenomena: fibrin sheath formation and thrombosis. The catheter position can also affect flow, so a partial occlusion, in the absence of pain or discomfort, should first be managed by instructing the patient to change positions, raise the arms, deep breathe, and/or cough (Figure 15-21). Each of these

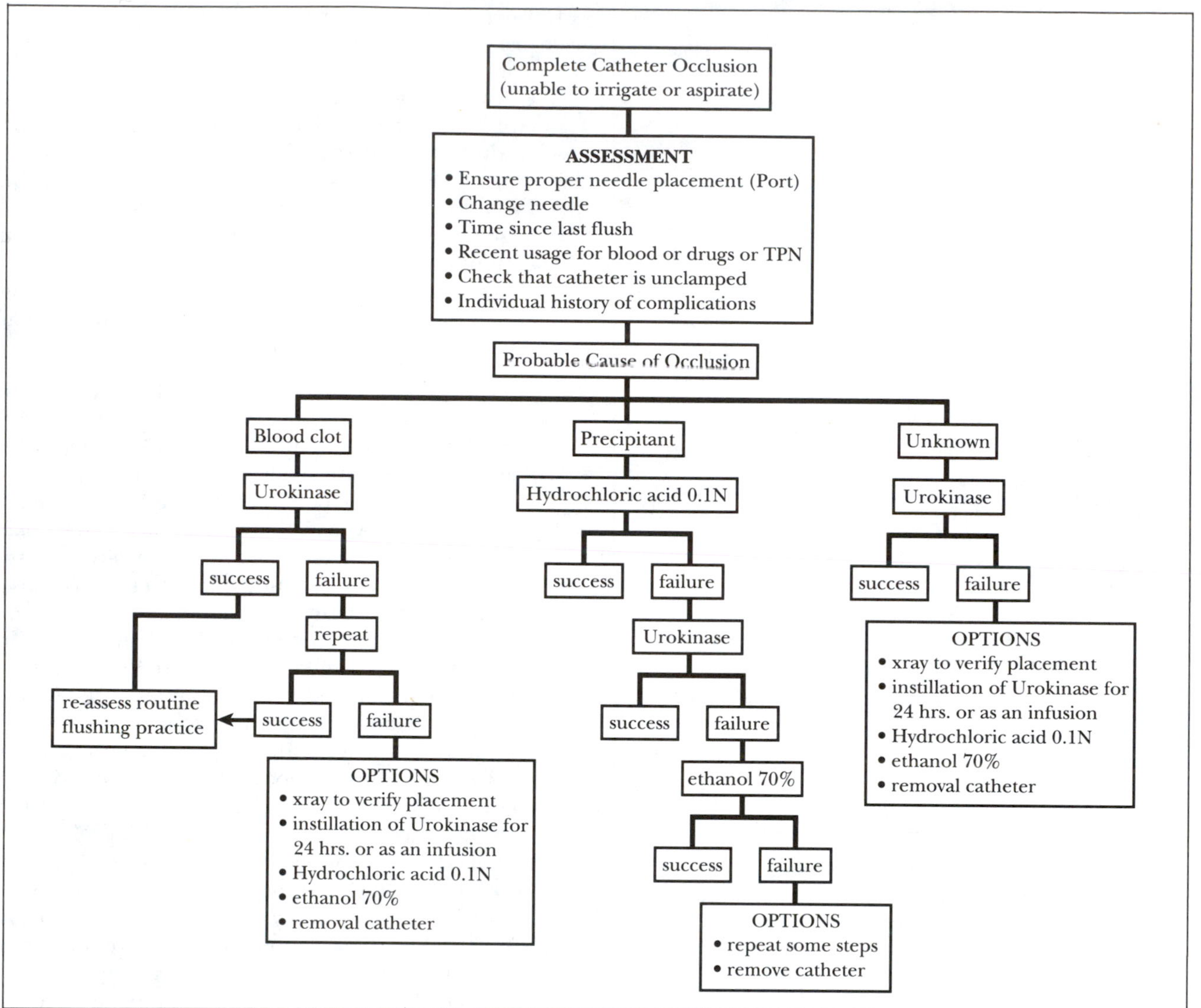

FIGURE 15-20 Managing complete catheter occlusion.

might release the open lumen of the catheter from the vein wall and allow easy flushing and blood withdrawal. If a withdrawal occlusion exists (flushes easily but backflow is very sluggish or nonexistent), fibrin sheath formation or thrombosis should be considered. Fibrin sheaths can form at the catheter insertion site and float, like a sleeve, around the outside of the catheter. If the sheath extends beyond the lumen, it can cause withdrawal occlusions. Lysis of the sheath usually is achieved by instilling urokinase 5000–10,000 units into the catheter with an extended dwell time of 1–24 hours.[111]

Venous thrombosis can be caused by a variety of factors, including endothelial injury, hypercoagulability, multiple catheters, catheter stiffness (i.e., polyvinyl chloride), catheter size (i.e., larger bore), and catheter placement (i.e., left side or in a smaller vein). The incidence of catheter thrombosis with clinical symptoms appears to be as high as 10%.[87,111] Actual incidence in the absence of clinical symptoms could be as high as 50%.[87,125,126] Signs and symptoms are related to impaired blood flow and include: edema of the neck, face, shoulder, or arm; prominent superficial veins; neck pain; tingling of the neck, shoulder, or arm; and skin color or temperature changes. A variety of radiographic studies can be used to diagnose and define the extent of the thrombosis accurately.

Management of venous thrombosis usually involves anticoagulants or thrombolytic agents. Several authors report success with the continuous infusion, centrally and/or peripherally, of urokinase for 4–24 hours.[118,119,127] It is recommended that all lumens of a multilumenal device be treated. The serum fibrinogen level should be maintained at 80–100 mg/dl by titration of the urokinase.[127] Prophylactic administration of low-dose warfarin (1 mg/day) appears to prevent or decrease the incidence of thrombus formation.[128,129]

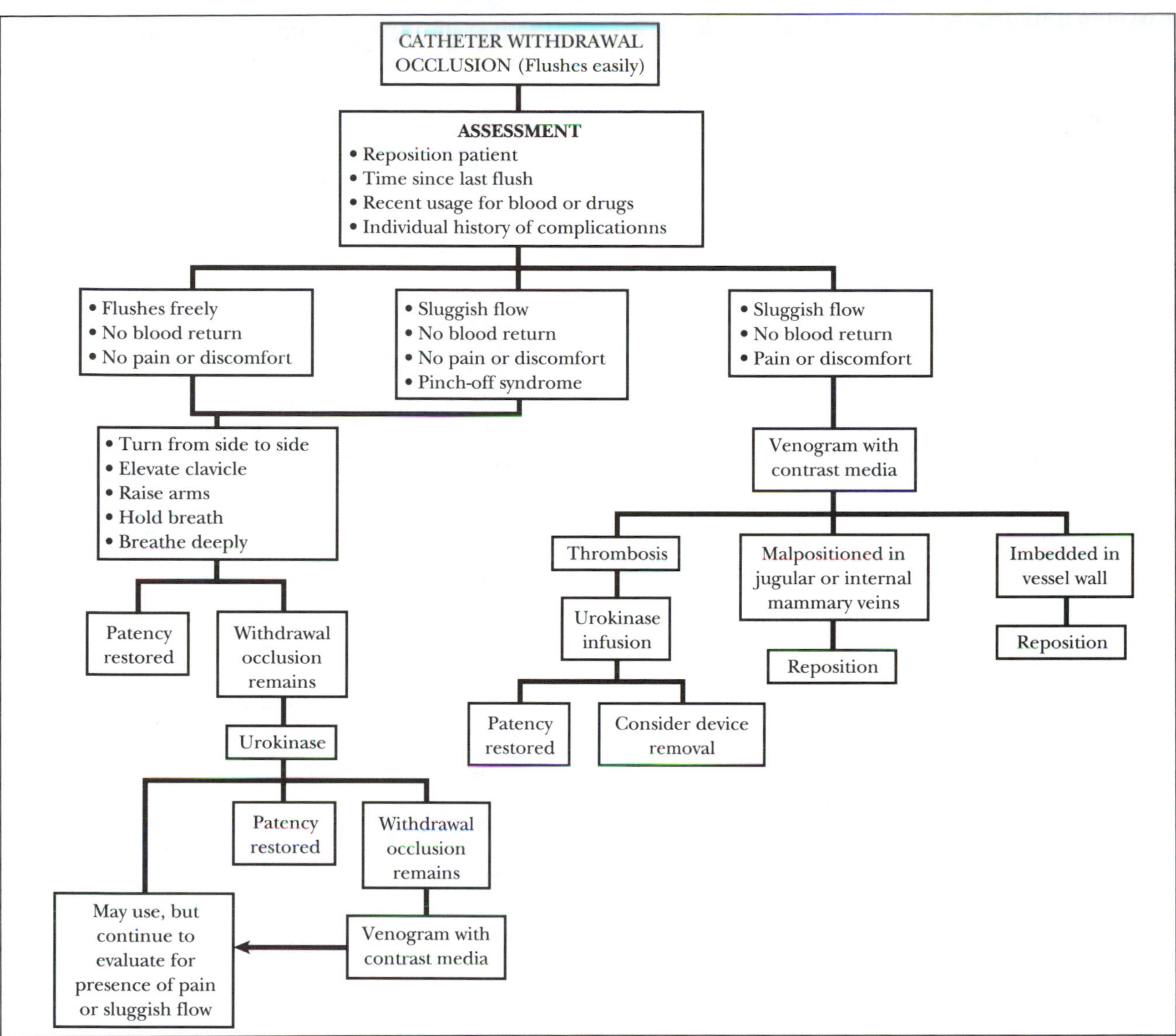

FIGURE 15-21 Managing catheter withdrawal occlusion.

Infection

Long-term central venous catheters are designed to minimize the risk of infection compared to regular venous catheters, but it still occurs in 2.7%–60% of devices.[87,109,110] This wide range is probably very dependent on the techniques used to insert and care for the VADs as well as the diagnoses and physical conditions of the patients involved. Infections can occur locally (on the skin), in the catheter tunnel/port pocket, or systemically. Infections are more common in patients with neutropenia (<500 granulocytes/mm³), those with multilumen catheters, and those receiving TPN or chemotherapy.

Local infections at the catheter exit site or over the skin around the port needle insertion site usually are due to organisms on the skin such as *S. aureus* and *S. epidermis*. Symptoms can include redness, warmth, discomfort, and exudate. Management includes culture of the area, increased frequency of dressing changes with meticulous site care, and administration of appropriate oral or IV antibiotics.[87,109,111] The needle should be removed from an implantable port if a skin infection occurs over the port, and it should not be reaccessed until the infection clears.

Infections in the catheter tunnel or port pocket usually involve a variety of different organisms and are manifested by redness, edema, tenderness or discomfort, exudate, skin warmth, and/or fever. After cultures have been taken, including aspiration of any port pocket exudate, appropriate IV antibiotic therapy is initiated.[87,109,111] If the causative organism is identified and appropriate antiinfective therapy fails to resolve the infection, consideration should be given to removal of the device.

Systemic infections can be thrombus-related or caused by intraluminal catheter colonization with a wide variety of infective organisms. Signs and symptoms include fever and chills. Blood cultures are taken through the device as well as peripherally and can be positive either in the device only or via both routes. Administration of appropriate antibacterial or antifungal therapy is initiated, and blood cultures are repeated. Failure to resolve the infection is cause to consider removal of the device.[87,109]

Preventing infection is a primary concern when caring for all types of VADs. Attention should be focused on the techniques used in routine maintenance, and care should be taken to employ measures to decrease the risk of infection. A new technologic development gaining popularity is the VitaCuff (Vitaphore, San Carlos, CA), which is impregnated with silver ions and can be attached to any catheter before insertion to provide an antimicrobial barrier within the catheter tunnel. It has been reported to decrease the incidence of catheter infections.[130] Another preventive measure successful in decreasing catheter infection rates is the "locking" of the device with a heparinized vancomycin solution (instead of only heparinized saline).[131] No toxicities or complications have been noted, and no patients have experienced bacteremia due to intraluminal colonization of vancomycin-susceptible organisms, although infection due to other organisms have occurred.[131]

Other complications

Occlusions and device malfunctions can occur for a variety of other reasons, and careful assessment of the device when occlusion occurs should always include consideration of malpositioning or breakage. Catheters can be kinked, compressed by tumor, compressed between the rib and clavicle ("pinch-off sign"), malpositioned due to patient manipulation ("twiddler's syndrome"), malpositioned for other reasons, severed, punctured, split, or separated.[132–134] The port access needle can be embedded in the septum; be inaccurately placed into the side of the port or catheter, instead of the portal housing; or become dislodged from the port and remain under the skin.

Thrombus formation can result in a retrograde flow of blood or fluid along the catheter tract, with subsequent extravasation into the subcutaneous tissues. Infusion of drugs into a severed, punctured, or separated catheter can also result in extravasation.[87] Prevention of vesicant extravasation is discussed elsewhere in this chapter, but it is prudent to reiterate that all vascular access devices should be patent and functioning appropriately before initiating vesicant therapy. Extravasation of vesicants into the chest wall or thorax can result in severe deformity, loss of function, or death.

All of the vascular access devices are popular, and manufacturers are developing new designs with innovative features every year. Oncology nurses frequently

TABLE 15-13 Vascular Access Devices: Product Selection Guidelines

VAD Selection Team Members

- Vascular or general surgeon
- Oncology nurse
- Purchasing representative
- Medical oncologist (optional or consultant to team)
- Others, as appropriate

Manufacturer Considerations

- Length of time in business
- Manufacturer vs. distributor
- Distribution system and supply turnaround
- Availability of representative (ie, locally or regionally)
- Reputation of reliability or quality
- Commitment to product (eg, R & D department)
- List of all customers using device
- Return policy
- Purchasing plan (eg, group discount)
- Price
- Training and in-service capabilities
- Availability of professional and patient education material

Device Selection

- Material (silastic vs. polyurethane; titanium vs. plastic)
- Ease of access; simplicity of use
- Design advantages (ie, preattached vs. attachable catheters)
- Lumen size and flow requirements
- Choice and size/type variations
- Supplies necessary for use, and their cost
- Standardization of design (to minimize errors)
- History of malfunctions and manufacturer's response
- Frequency of major design changes

VAD Selection Team Actions

- Examine VAD needs, ie, type, flow rate, infusion usage, patient population, and surgical preferences.
- Establish specifications, including points of view of all team members.
- Contact manufacturers for written material.
- Research subject matter, ie, infection rates, pros, cons, etc.
- Select 2–4 manufacturers to make individual presentations.
- Contact current users of devices from list provided by manufacturer.
- Use devices from 1–2 manufacturers on a trial basis, if necessary.
- Select most advantageous device(s).
- Implement educational plan and device usage.
- Evaluate device using preestablished expectations (specifications).
- Maintain records on usage, function, and complications.
- Publish process and utilization results.

review these new devices and are called on to evaluate their effectiveness. Table 15-13 contains product selection guidelines that might be useful in determining the product to be utilized by an individual health care institution. Cost containment is a growing concern, and the best price usually can be achieved if all of the devices selected come from a limited number of vendors, thus consolidating buying power. The oncology nurse contributes greatly to this interdisciplinary team by his or her clinical experience with the product and evaluation of specific outcome measures.

SUMMARY

Cancer chemotherapy administration is a rapidly evolving area of oncology nursing practice that offers exciting opportunities for both beginning and seasoned oncology nurses. The level of responsibility for monitoring patients receiving chemotherapy and managing many aspects of their care continues to increase. Expanded outpatient and home care settings, where the majority of chemotherapy is given, offer opportunities for triage assessment and nursing intervention at an increasingly autonomous level. The technical explosions in drug delivery systems are a constant informational challenge, as is maintaining the personal and rewarding relationships with patients for whom these advanced technologies are utilized.

Health care will continue to move toward more and more ambulatory and home care, with hospitals becoming virtually intensive care buildings. Reimbursement, lobbying, litigation, and legislation are predominant issues for the 1990s, and they will continue into the twenty-first century. The oncology nurse has a vital role in establishing effective policies and procedures, by serving on institutional practice or policy committees. An oncology clinical practice committee with responsibility for reviewing and recommending procedures can also serve to evaluate new technologies. Patient care evaluation and quality improvement is a key responsibility recognized by the Joint Commission on the Accreditation of Healthcare Organizations, which initiated clinical indicators for oncology to more closely monitor quality in the health care setting.[135]

REFERENCES

1. Oncology Nursing Society: *ONS Cancer Chemotherapy Guidelines, Modules I–V*. Pittsburgh, PA: Oncology Nursing Society, 1988.
2. American Society of Hospital Pharmacists: ASHP technical assistance bulletin on handling cytotoxic drugs in hospitals. *Am J Hosp Pharm* 42:131–137, 1985.
3. American Society of Hospital Pharmacists: *Safe Handling of Cytotoxic and Hazardous Drugs Study Guide*. Bethesda, MD: American Society of Hospital Pharmacists, 1990.
4. Occupational Safety and Health Administration: *Work Practice Guidelines for Personnel Dealing with Cytotoxic (Antineoplastic) Drugs*. Washington, DC: U.S. Department of Labor Publication 8–1.1, 1986.
5. Intravenous Nurses Society: *Intravenous Nursing Standards of Practice*. Belmont, CA: Intravenous Nurses Society, 1990.
6. AMA Council on Scientific Affairs: Guidelines for handling parenteral antineoplastics. *JAMA* 253:1590–1592, 1985.
7. Fischer DS, Knobf MT: *The Cancer Chemotherapy Handbook* (ed. 3). Chicago: Year Book Medical Publishers, 1989.
8. Tenenbaum L: *Cancer Chemotherapy: A Reference Guide*. Philadelphia: Saunders, 1989.
9. Oncology Nursing Society: *Cancer Chemotherapy Guidelines and Recommendations for Nursing Education and Practice*. Pittsburgh, PA: Oncology Nursing Society, 1984.
10. Alabama Board of Nursing: *Alabama Board of Nursing Administrative Code*. Montgomery, AL: Alabama Board of Nursing, 1990.
11. Rutherford C: Position paper—Administration of antineoplastic agents. *J Intraven Nurs* 15:8–9, 1992.
12. Oncology Nursing Society: *Position Statement—Preparations of the Professional Registered Nurse Who Administers and Cares for the Individual Receiving Chemotherapy*. Pittsburgh, PA: Oncology Nursing Society, 1991.
13. Krohner KM, Spitak AF: Cancer nursing education in the community hospital: Principles and practice. *Oncol Nurs Forum* 19:783–786, 1992.
14. Creaton EM, Leonard FE, Day AL: A hospital-based chemotherapy education and training program. *Cancer Nurs* 14:79–90, 1991.
15. Falck, K, Grohn P, Sorsa M, et al: Mutagencity of urine in nurses handling cytostatic drugs. *Lancet* 1:1250–1251, 1979 (letter).
16. Waksvik H, Klepp O, Brogger A: Chromosome analyses of nurses handling cytostatic agents. *Cancer Treat Rep* 65:607–610, 1981.
17. Anderson RW, Puckett W, Dana W, et al: Risk of handling injectable antineoplastic agents. *Am J Hosp Pharm* 39:1881–1887, 1982.
18. Rose W: The gray areas of antineoplastic therapy. *NITA* 10:202–208, 1987.
19. Barry LK, Booker RB: Promoting the responsible handling of antineoplastic agents in the community. *Oncol Nurs Forum* 12:41–46, 1985.
20. Valanis B, McNeil V, Driscoll K: Staff members' compliance with their facility's antineoplastic drug handling policy. *Oncol Nurs Forum* 18:571–576, 1991.
21. Caudell KA, Vredevoe DL, Dietrich MF, et al: Quantification of urinary mutagens in nurses during potential antineoplastic agent exposure. *Cancer Nurs* 11:41–50, 1988.
22. Dewerk-Neal A, Wadden RA, Chiou WL: Exposure of hospital workers to airborne antineoplastic agents. *Am J Hosp Pharm* 40:597–601, 1983.
23. Stellman JM, Aufiero BM, Taub RN: Assessment of potential exposure to antineoplastic agents in the health care setting. *Prev Med* 13:245–255, 1984.
24. Cloak MM, Connor TH, Stevens KR, et al: Occupational exposure of nursing personnel to antineoplastic agents. *Oncol Nurs Forum* 12:33–39, 1985.

25. Oncology Nursing Society: *Safe Handling of Cytotoxic Drugs.* Pittsburgh, PA: Oncology Nursing Society, 1989.
26. Department of Occupational Safety and Health Administration: Occupational exposure to bloodborne pathogens; final rule. *Federal Register* 46:64175–64182, 1991.
27. Sansivero GE, Murray SA: Safe management of chemotherapy at home. *Oncol Nurs Forum* 16:711–713, 1989.
28. Blecke C: Home chemotherapy safety procedures. *Oncol Nurs Forum* 16:719–721, 1989.
29. Bingham E: Hazards to health workers from antineoplastic drugs. *N Engl J Med* 313:1220–1221, 1985 (editorial).
30. Stajich GV, Barnett CW, Turner SV, et al: Protective measures used by oncologic office nurses handling parenteral antineoplastic agents. *Oncol Nurs Forum* 13:47–49, 1986.
31. U.S. Department of Health and Human Services: *Adult Patient Education in Cancer.* Bethesda, MD: U.S. Government Printing Office, 1982.
32. Chamarro T, Appelbaum J: Informed consent: Nursing issues and ethical dilemmas. *Oncol Nurs Forum* 15:803–807, 1988.
33. Oncology Nursing Society: *Standards of Oncology Education: Patient/Family and Public.* Pittsburgh, PA: Oncology Nursing Society, 1989.
34. Lynch M, Yanes L: Flowsheet documentation of chemotherapy administration and patient teaching. *Oncol Nurs Forum* 18:777–783, 1991.
35. Cushman KE: A tool for documenting chemotherapy administration quickly and completely. *Oncol Nurs Forum* 18:599–600, 1991.
36. Coker M, Lampert A: Teaching checklist for home infusion therapy. *Oncol Nurs Forum* 17:923–926, 1990.
37. Moore JM, Knobf MT: A nursing flow sheet for documentation of ambulatory oncology. *Oncol Nurs Forum* 18:933–939, 1991.
38. Pickett RR: Outpatient oncology chemotherapy documentation tool. *Oncol Nurs Forum* 19:515–517, 1992.
39. Hartman D, Knudson J: A nursing data base for initial patient assessment. *Oncol Nurs Forum* 18:125–432, 1991.
40. Barofsky I: Compliance, adherence, and therapeutic alliance: Steps in the development of self care. *Soc Sci Med* 12:369–376, 1978.
41. Akcasu N, Oswald D: A systemic approach to preparing for chemotherapy administration. *J Ped Oncol Nurs* 8:136–138, 1991.
42. Palmer P, Meyers FJ: An outpatient approach to the delivery of intensive consolidation chemotherapy to adults with acute lymphoblastic leukemia. *Oncol Nurs Forum* 17:553–558, 1990.
43. Sullivan DH, Gramm T, Hetzer P: Ambulatory care for patients with acute leukemia: An alternative to frequent hospitalization. *J Prof Nurs* 6:300–309, 1990.
44. Mannisto MM: Oncology practices in the 1990's. *Oncology Issues* 6:10–13, 1991.
45. Mortenson LE: Tight-money casualties in the war on cancer. *Wall Street Journal,* May 11, 1989.
46. U.S. General Accounting Office: *Off-Label Drugs—Reimbursement Policies Constrain Physicians in Their Choice of Cancer Therapies.* Washington, DC: U.S. General Accounting Office, PEMD-91-14, 1991.
47. Riggs CE: Antitumor antibiotics and related compounds. In Perry MC (ed.): *The Chemotherapy Source Book.* Baltimore, MD: Williams & Wilkins, 1992, pp. 318–358.
48. Recommendations for the management of extravasation and anaphylaxis. In *Oncology Nursing Society Cancer Chemotherapy Guidelines.* Pittsburgh, PA: Oncology Nursing Society, 1988.
49. Yarbro CH: Nursing implications in the administration of cancer chemotherapy. In Perry MC (ed.): *The Chemotherapy Source Book.* Baltimore, MD: Williams & Wilkins, 1992, pp. 873–883.
50. Rudolph R, Larson DL: Etiology and treatment of chemotherapeutic agent extravasation injuries: A review. *J Clin Oncol* 5:1116–1126, 1987.
51. Gilyon K, Kuzel T: Cutaneous T-cell lymphoma. *Oncol Nurs Forum* 18:901–908, 1991.
52. Goodman M: Delivery of cancer chemotherapy. In Baird S, McCorkle R, Grant M (eds.): *Cancer Nursing: A Comprehensive Textbook.* Philadelphia: Saunders, 1991, p. 311.
53. Neiderhuber JE, Ensminger W, Gyves J, et al: Regional chemotherapy of colorectal cancer metastatic to the liver. *Cancer* S3:1336–1343, 1984.
54. Cozzi E, Hagle M, McGregor ML, et al: Nursing management of patients receiving hepatic arterial chemotherapy through an implanted infusion pump. *Cancer Nurs* 7:229–234, 1984.
55. von Roemeling R, MacDonald M, Langevin T, et al: Chemotherapy via implanted infusion pump: New perspectives for delivery of long-term continuous treatment. *Oncol Nurs Forum* 13:17–24, 1986.
56. Lanning RM, Hrushesky WJM: Cost comparison of wearable and implantable drug delivery systems. *Proceedings of ASCO* 9:322, 1990 (abstr.).
57. Sugarbaker, PH, Gianola FJ, Speyer JL, et al: Prospective randomized trial of intravenous v. intraperitoneal 5FU in patients with advanced primary colon or rectal cancer. *Semin Oncol* 12:101–111, 1985 (suppl. 4).
58. Almadrones L, Yerys C: Problems associated with the administration of intraperitoneal therapy using the Port-a-Cath system. *Oncol Nurs Forum* 17:75–80, 1990.
59. Howell SB, Pfeifle CL, Wung WE, et al: Intraperitoneal cisplatin with systemic thiosulfate protection. *Ann Intern Med* 97:845–851, 1982.
60. Zook-Enck D: Intraperitoneal therapy via the Tenckhoff catheter. *J Intrav Nurs* 13:375–382, 1990.
61. Swenson KK, Eriksson JH: Nursing management of intraperitoneal chemotherapy. *Oncol Nurs Forum* 13:33–39, 1986.
62. Carney-Gersten P, Moore MD, Giuffre M: Intraperitoneal alpha interferon for ovarian cancer: A case report. *Oncol Nurs Forum* 17:403–407, 1990.
63. Malloy J: Administering intraperitoneal chemotherapy: A new approach. *Nursing* (January):58–62, 1991.
64. Hoff ST: Concepts in intraperitoneal chemotherapy. *Semin Oncol Nurs* 3:112—117, 1987.
65. Doane LS, Fisher LM, McDonald TW: How to give peritoneal chemotherapy. *Am J Nurs* 90:58–66, 1990.
66. Moores D: Malignant pleural effusions. *Semin Oncol* 18:59–61, 1991 (suppl. 2).
67. Bartal AH, Gazitt Y, Zidan G, et al: Clinical and flow cytometry characteristics of malignant pleural effusion in patients after intracavity administration of methylprednisolone acetate. *Cancer* 67:3136–3140, 1991.
68. Ike O, Shimizu Y, Hitomi S, et al: Treatment of malignant pleural effusions with doxorubicin hydrochloride-containing poly (L-lactic acid) microspheres. *Chest* 99:911–915, 1991.
69. Rusch VW, Figlin R, Godwin D, et al: Intrapleural cisplatin and cytarabine in the management of malignant

pleural effusions: A Lung Cancer Study Group trial. *J Clin Oncol* 9:313–319, 1991.
70. Parker LA, Charnock GC, Delany DJ: Small-bore catheter drainage and sclerotherapy for malignant pleural effusions. *Cancer* 64:1218–1221, 1989.
71. Walsh FW, Alberts WM, Soloman DA, et al: Malignant pleural effusions: Pleurodesis using a small-bore percutaneous catheter. *South Med J* 92:963–965, 1989.
72. Tsang V, Fernando HC, Goldstraw P: Pleuroperitoneal shunt for recurrent malignant pleural effusion. *Thorax* 45:369–372, 1990.
73. Herr HW, Badalament RA, Amato DA, et al: Superficial bladder cancer treated with bacillus Calmette-Guerin: A multivariate analysis of factors affecting tumor progression. *J Urol* 141:22–29, 1989.
74. Brosman SA, Lamm DL: The preparation, handling and use of intravesical bacillus Calmette-Guerin for the management of stage Ta, Ti, carcinoma-in-situ and transitional cell cancer. *J Urol* 144:313–315, 1990.
75. Obbens EA, Leavens ME, Beal JW, et al: Ommaya reservoirs in 387 cancer patients: A 15-year experience. *Neurology* 35:1274–1278, 1985.
76. Glover D, Glock JH: Oncologic emergencies. In Holleb AI, Fink DJ, Murphy GP (eds.): *American Cancer Society Textbook of Clinical Oncology*. Atlanta: American Cancer Society, 1991, pp. 513–533.
77. Wujcik D: Meningeal carcinomatosis: Diagnosis, treatment and nursing care. *Oncol Nurs Forum* 10(2):35–40, 1983.
78. Cornwell, CMcC: The Ommaya reservoir: Implications for pediatric oncology. *Pediatric Nurs* 16:249–251, 1990.
79. Esparza DM, Weyland B: Nursing care for the patient with an Ommaya reservoir. *Oncol Nurs Forum* 9:17–20, 1982.
80. Broviac JW, Cole JJ, Scribner BH: A silicone rubber atrial catheter for prolonged parenteral alimentation. *Surg Gynecol Obstet* 136:602–606, 1973.
81. Broviac JW, Cole JJ, Scribner BH: Prolonged parenteral nutrition in the home. *Surg Gynecol Obstet* 139:24–28, 1974.
82. Hickman RO, Buckner CD, Clift RA, et al: A modified right atrial catheter for access to the venous system in marrow transplant recipients. *Surg Gynecol Obstet* 148:871–875, 1979.
83. Raaf JH: Results from the use of 826 vascular access devices in cancer patients. *Cancer* 55:1312–1321, 1985.
84. Niederhuber JE, Ensminger W, Gyves JW, et al: Totally implanted venous and arterial access system to replace external catheters in cancer treatment. *Surgery* 92:706–712, 1982.
85. Welling RE, Hall JM, Meyer RL, et al: Implantable venous access devices: An alternative method of extended cancer care. *J Surg Oncol* 33:73–75, 1986.
86. Crocker KS, Devereaux GB, Ashmore DL, et al: Clinical evaluation of elastomeric hydrogel peripheral catheters during home infusion therapy. *J Intraven Nurs* 13:89–97, 1990.
87. Groeger JS, Lucas AB, Coit D: Venous access in the cancer patient. In DeVita VT, Hellman S, Rosenberg SA (eds.): *Principles and Practice of Oncology*. Philadelphia: Lippincott, 1991, pp. 1–14.
88. Oncology Nursing Society: *Access Device Guidelines: Recommendations for Nursing Education and Practice, Modules I–III*. Pittsburgh, PA: Oncology Nursing Society, 1989.
89. ACS Nursing Subcommittee: *Venous Access Devices Standards of Care*. Salt Lake City, UT: American Cancer Society, Utah Division, 1990.
90. Lucas AB: A critical review of venous access devices: The nursing perspective. In Hubbard SM, Greene PE, Knobf MT (eds.): *Current Issues in Cancer Nursing Practice*. Philadelphia: Lippincott, 1991, pp. 1–10.
91. Hadaway LC: An overview of vascular access devices inserted via the antecubital area. *J Intraven Nurs* 13:297–306, 1990.
92. Masoorli S, Angeles T: PICC lines: The latest home care challenge. *RN* (January):44–51, 1990.
93. Goodwin ML: The seldinger method for PICC insertion. *J Intraven Nurs* 12:238–243, 1989.
94. Kyle KS, Myers JS: Peripherally inserted central catheters: Development of a hospital-based program. *J Intraven Nurs* 13:287–290, 1990.
95. Lum PS, Soski M: Management of malpositioned central venous catheters. *J Intraven Nurs* 12:356–365, 1989.
96. May GS, Davis C: Percutaneous catheters and totally implantable access systems: A review of reported infection rates. *J Intraven Nurs* 11:97–103, 1988.
97. Graham DR, Keldermans MM, Klemm LW, et al: Infectious complications among patients receiving home intravenous therapy with peripheral, central or peripherally placed central venous catheters. *Am J Med* 91:95S–100S, 1991 (suppl. 3B).
98. Gullatte MM: Managing an implanted infusion device. *RN* (January):45–49, 1989.
99. Pessa ME, Howard RJ: Complications of Hickman-Broviac catheters. *Surg Gynecol Obstet* 161:257–260, 1985.
100. Hutchinson, SK, Waskerwitz M, Martin K, et al: Nonocclusive, clean permanent right atrial dressing change procedures compared with occlusive, sterile permanent right atrial catheter dressing change procedures in children with cancer. *J Pediatr Oncol Nurs* 7:71, 1990.
101. Conly JM, Grieves K, Peters B: A prospective, randomized study comparing transparent and dry gauze dressings for central venous catheters. *J Infect Dis* 159:310–319, 1989.
102. Petrosino B, Becker H, Christian B: Infection rates in central venous catheter dressings. *Oncol Nurs Forum* 15:709–717, 1988.
103. Kelly C, Dumenko L, McGregor, SE, et al: A change in flushing protocols of central venous catheters. *Oncol Nurs Forum* 19:599–605, 1992.
104. Wiernikowski JT, Elder-Thornley D, Dawson S, et al: Bacterial colonization of tunnelled right atrial catheters in pediatric oncology: A comparison of sterile saline and bacteriostatic saline flush solutions. *Am J Pediatr Hematol Oncol* 13:137–140, 1991.
105. Vial CD: Daily access of implanted venous ports, implications for patient education. *J Intraven Nurs* 13:294–296, 1990.
106. Welker DL: *Troubleshooting Vascular Access Devices*. Minneapolis, MN: Pharmacia Deltec, 1992.
107. Moore CL, Erikson KA, Yanes LB, et al: Nursing care and management of venous access ports. *Oncol Nurs Forum* 13:35–39, 1986.
108. Winters V, Peters B, Coila S, et al: A trial with a new peripheral implanted vascular access device. *Oncol Nurs Forum* 17:891–896, 1990.
109. Press OW, Ramsey PG, Larson EB, et al: Hickman catheter infections in patients with malignancies. *Medicine* 36:189–200, 1984.
110. Schuman ES, Winters V, Gross GF, et al: Management

of Hickman catheter sepsis. *Am J Surg* 149:627–628, 1985.
111. Wickham R, Purl S, Welker D: Long-term central venous catheters: Issues for care. *Semin Oncol Nurs* 8:133–147, 1992.
112. Breaux CW, Duke D, Georgeson KE, et al: Calcium phosphate crystal occlusion of central venous catheters used for total parenteral nutrition in infants and children: Prevention and treatment. *J Pediatr Surg* 22:829–832, 1987.
113. Duffy LF, Kerzner B, Gevus V, et al: Treatment of central venous catheter occlusions with hydrochloric acid. *J Pediatrics* 114:1002–1104, 1989.
114. Lawson M, Bottino JC, Hurtubise MR, et al: The use of urokinase to restore the patency of occluded central venous catheters. *A J Intraven Ther Clin Nutr* 9:29–31, 1982.
115. Hurtubise MR, Bottino GC, Lawson M, et al: Restoring the patency of occluded central venous catheters. *Arch Surg* 115:212–213, 1980.
116. Wachs T: Urokinase administration in pediatric patients with occluded central venous catheters. *J Intraven Nurs* 13:100–102, 1990.
117. Brown LH, Wantroba I, Simonson G: Reestablishing patency in an occluded central venous access device. *Critical Care Nurs* 9:114–121, 1989.
118. Bagnall HA, Gomperts E, Atkinson JB: Continuous infusion of low-dose urokinase in the treatment of central venous catheter thrombosis in infants and children. *Pediatrics* 83:963–966, 1989.
119. Curnow A, Idowu J, Behrens E, et al: Urokinase therapy for silastic catheter induced intravascular thrombi in infants and children. *Arch Surg* 120:1237–1240, 1985.
120. Atkinson JB, Bagnall HA, Gomperts E: Investigational use of tissue plasminogen activator (t-PA) for occluded central venous catheters. *J Paren Enter Nutrit* 14:310–311, 1990.
121. Holcombe BJ, Forloines-Lynn S, Garmhausen LW: Restoring patency of long-term central venous access devices. *J Intraven Nurs* 15:36–41, 1992.
122. Pennington CR, Pithie AD: Ethanol lock in the management of catheter occlusion. *J Paren Enter Nutrit* 11:507–508, 1987.
123. Thompson B, Veal D: Pharmacologic treatment of pediatric catheter occlusion. *Hospital Pharmacy* 27:137–141, 1992.
124. Shulman RJ, Reed T, Pitre D, et al: Use of hydrochloric acid to clear obstructed central venous catheters. *J Paren Enter Nutrit* 12:509–510, 1988.
125. Moss JF, Wagman LD, Riihimaki DU, et al: Central venous thrombosis related to the silastic Hickman-Broviac catheter in an oncologic population. *J Paren Enter Nutrit* 13:397–400, 1989.
126. Gray WJ, Bell WR: Fibrinolytic agents in the treatment of thrombotic disorders. *Semin Oncol* 17:228–237, 1990.
127. Fraschini G, Jadeja J, Lawson M, et al: Local infusion of urokinase for the lysis of thrombosis associated with permanent central venous catheters in cancer patients. *J Clin Oncol* 5:672–678, 1987.
128. Bern MM, Bothe A, Bistrian B, et al: Prophylaxis against central venous thrombosis with low-dose warfarin. *Surgery* 99:216–221, 1986.
129. Bern MM, Lokich JL, Wallach SR, et al: Very low doses of warfarin can prevent thrombosis in central venous catheters—A randomized prospective trial. *Ann Intern Med* 112:423–428, 1990.
130. Flowers RH, Schwenzer KJ, Kopel RF, et al: Efficacy of an attachable subcutaneous cuff for the prevention of intravascular catheter-related sepsis. *JAMA* 261:878–883, 1989.
131. Schwartz C, Hendrickson KJ, Roghmann K, et al: Prevention of bacteremia attributed to luminal colonization of tunnelled central venous catheters with vancomycin-susceptible organisms. *J Clin Oncol* 8:1591–1597, 1990.
132. Lum PS, Soski M: Management of malpositioned central venous catheters. *J Intraven Nurs* 12:356–365, 1989.
133. Gebarksi SS, Gebarski KS: Chemotherapy port "twiddler's syndrome": A need for preinjection radiography. *Cancer* 54:38–39, 1984.
134. Lafreniere R: Indwelling subclavian catheters and a visit with the "pinched-off sign." *J Surg Oncol* 47:261–264, 1991.
135. *AMH Accreditation Manual for Hospitals, 1992*. Oak Brook Terrace: Joint Commission on Accreditation of Healthcare Organizations, 1992.

Chapter 16

Chemotherapy: Toxicity Management

Dawn Camp-Sorrell, RN, MSN, OCN

INTRODUCTION

Chemotherapy is administered based on a dose–response relationship, i.e., the more drug administered, the more cancer cells killed. Characteristically, these agents have a narrow therapeutic index, with anticipated acute toxicities expressed in rapidly dividing normal tissues, such as the bone marrow, the gastrointestinal (GI) tract, the gonads, and the hair follicles. Acute and long-term toxicities from chemotherapy may also be a function of the drug's effect on specific cells of a given organ. The incidence and severity of toxicities are related to the drug's dosage, administration schedule, specific mechanism of action, concomitant illness, and specific measures employed to prevent or minimize toxicities. Chemotherapeutic agents cause side effects that can appear immediately, i.e., after a few days (acute), within a few weeks (intermediate), or months to years after chemotherapy administration (long term).[1]

Since virtually every organ is affected by chemotherapy, the toxicities of the drug will commonly determine the maximum amount of drug that can be administered safely. Side effects such as stomatitis, alopecia, myelosuppression, nausea, vomiting, anorexia, and diarrhea are common, depending on the agent administered.[2] These are expected side effects that can be managed effectively, and generally do not warrant reducing the dose or discontinuing the drug. *Toxic* effects refer to life-threatening, often dose-limiting effects characteristic of high dosages. Cumulative and irreversible damage to certain vital organs, such as the heart, limits the total dosage of chemotherapy.[3]

Providing nursing care to the patient receiving chemotherapy presents many challenges. Interventions focus on preventing or minimizing side effects caused by the chemotherapeutic agent. The key is to assess accurately the patient's status and to complete a health history to detect risk factors before initiating therapy that provides baseline data.[2] After the patient begins treatment, it is important to assess any changes from the baseline and to evaluate the effectiveness of interventions implemented.

PRETREATMENT EVALUATION: RISK ANALYSIS

Individuals with an overall weak physical condition and poor nutritional status are not likely to tolerate a vigorous treatment course.[3] Patients previously treated with multiple chemotherapy agents, radiation, or immunotherapy may lack marrow reserve, placing them at a higher risk for infection, bleeding, or anemia. The inability or unwillingness of an individual to perform self-care may increase the severity of a side effect and also delay the seeking of appropriate care from health care professionals.

Preexisting disorders such as hepatic or renal dysfunction can alter the absorption, distribution, metabolism, and excretion of chemotherapy, causing abnormal accumulations of the drug and its metabolites. Hypovolemia due to nausea/vomiting, diarrhea, inadequate dietary intake, third spacing, or hypoalbuminemia may increase the risk of acute renal failure.[4] Thus the patient could be placed at a higher risk for organ toxicities.

Since the incidence of cancer increases with age, nurses must be aware of possible additional risks for the elderly. Age-related changes in physical stature, body composition, kidneys, liver, and other organs influence the pharmacokinetic and pharmacodynamic properties of drug therapy, possibly prolonging the agent's half-life.[5] Many elderly people, especially those over age 85, are physically frail secondary to chronic and debilitating illness or poor nutrition or as a result of aging. Chronic illness such as arthritis, heart disease, diabetes, glaucoma, high blood pressure, cognitive deficits, and hearing and vision loss is common in the elderly. These conditions may interfere with the ability to perform basic activities of daily living and, consequently, elderly patients may be unable to perform preventive measures to minimize side effects.

Gradual but substantial changes occur in body composition with age. The percentage of body fat increases, with a corresponding decrease in muscle mass and percentage of body water. Decreases occur in cardiac output, kidney function, hepatic bloodflow, the ability to conjugate drugs, and the effectiveness of the immune system.[5,6] With advancing age the kidneys atrophy, bringing subsequent decrease in renal function. Vasoconstriction of the renal vasculature decreases renal bloodflow, glomerular filtration rate, and the ability to concentrate/dilute urine, resulting in a decreased creatinine clearance.[4]

Historically, elderly patients with cancer have not been treated as aggressively as their younger counterparts because it was speculated that the elderly would not be able to tolerate the stresses imposed by chemotherapy. This trend is changing, however, and many elderly patients now receive aggressive treatment for their cancer.[7–14] Numerous studies have looked at the consequences of treating older patients with chemotherapy. Although the study results are often variable and contradictory, the degree of tolerance to chemotherapy has depended on the type of malignancy and dose intensity.

In general, for many solid tumors, geriatric patients tolerate chemotherapy, used either for adjuvant or palliation therapy, as well as younger patients.[9] Geriatric patients with a systemic malignancy such as lymphoma or acute leukemia usually develop more treatment-related toxicity than younger patients. Leukemia in the elderly is frequently associated with poor prognostic features such as prior preleukemia, myelodysplastic syndrome, and chromosome abnormalities that may place them at an increased risk for toxicities such as infection.[8,10] However, geriatric patients can achieve complete response from chemotherapy if they survive the intensive initial therapy.[9]

A retrospective analysis was conducted on six Eastern Cooperative Oncology Group (ECOG) clinical trials for breast, lung, and colon cancers. Elderly patients were defined as 70 years or older in the lung and colon studies and 60–65 years of age in the breast studies. All patients had normal renal, hepatic, and cardiac function. When compared to nonelderly controls, the incidence of severe toxic reactions in the two groups was comparable.[11]

While it is critical to be knowledgeable regarding the potential problems the elderly may encounter as a consequence of physiologic aging, age alone has not been shown to be a significant factor in the incidence and severity of toxicity to chemotherapy.[12–14] The one exception has been hematologic toxicity, probably related to decreased marrow reserve and/or renal function. Health care professionals therefore should monitor hematologic values closely to minimize potential ill effects. Patients older than 70 years of age with normal renal and hepatic function and without serious medical conditions have been found to tolerate chemotherapy as well as individuals in younger populations.[9]

QUALITY OF LIFE AND CHEMOTHERAPY TOXICITY

Treatment considerations include the patient's quality of life, the impact chemotherapy will have on the patient's quality of life, and the patient's physical as well as mental well-being.[15] Complications or side effects of chemotherapy are weighed against its potential benefits. If tumor control or palliation is the goal, the side effects are weighed against such benefits of chemotherapy as pain control and prolonged survival time.

In the past, cancer treatment was evaluated by tumor response and survival rates rather than by functional ability or quality of life.[16] Currently, there is a movement to recognize and include quality of life as an acceptable end point in clinical trials, which has been influenced by viewing cancer as a chronic condition instead of as an acute event. Groups of cancer survivors have indicated to the health care community that quality of life is as important to the patient as is the overall therapeutic effect.[17]

Physical symptoms can result in significant distress that has a marked impact on the patient's quality of life.[18,19] It is important to realize that the patient's perception of cancer and chemotherapy treatment will influence how the patient reacts and ultimately adapts.[20] Side effects can impair a patient's abilities to function at work or at home, maintain sexual relationships, and engage in social activities. Feelings of helplessness are heightened, since patients are dependent on health care professionals to deliver their treatment. Anxiety can develop at key decision points, such as diagnosis, beginning of treatment, while awaiting test results, when the treatment plan is altered, or when the chemotherapy treatment plan has been successfully completed.[21] Chemotherapy-related changes in physical appearance are often described as a distressing aspect of cancer treatment. Weight changes and alopecia commonly occur and can be especially devastating because they can be viewed as public manifestations of having cancer.[20]

To help the patient cope with potential side effects, a trusting relationship between patient and nurse must be developed so that sufficient information can be provided for the patient to retain control over his or her care. An important aspect of establishing a partnership with the patient and family in the pretreatment phase is knowing what concerns about the treatment need to be explored and what information needs to be provided. Such information helps patients formulate questions about available options when making difficult decisions about their care. Feelings of control are enhanced, resulting in an improved functional status, sense of well-being, and performance of effective self-care.[22] Nurses must focus on developing practical interventions to reduce the psychological distress of treatment and to provide needed information, thereby increasing the patient's quality of life.

SELF-CARE

There is undeniable evidence that cost factors are dictating health care. Institutional, state, and federal regulatory bodies have assumed increasing jurisdiction over how and where patients will be treated. Diagnostic related groups (DRGs) and prospective payment, cost-control measures by other insurers, and increased out-of-pocket medical expenses by consumers have all combined to create a shift from hospital-based care to outpatient and home care settings.[23] The change from inpatient to outpatient administration of chemotherapy necessitates a shift in responsibility for managing treatment side effects from health care providers to patients and their families. To facilitate self-care, nurses must understand the nature, incidence, and relative severity of each side effect, as well as being aware of effective self-care activities for reducing the severity of side effects.

Dodd assessed self-care behaviors used for side effects from chemotherapy.[24] Via a self-care behavior questionnaire, 48 patients were asked to indicate how severe the side effects were and what actions were taken to alleviate those side effects. The side effects with the greatest frequency were nausea and vomiting (83%), loss of hair (75%), taste and smell changes (71%), and decreased appetite (69%). Patients initiated self-care most frequently for nausea and vomiting, constipation, and loss of hair.

In an attempt to test patients' self-care behavior, Dodd gave information on side effect management techniques to one of two groups of patients with cancer who were undergoing chemotherapy. Patients who received the information on side effect management reported initiating self-care behaviors with a higher degree of perceived effectiveness than those who did not receive this information. The informed patients also initiated self-care behaviors before side effects became persistent and severe.[25]

In another study, patients and family members were asked to describe self-care behaviors initiated by patients and their family members and to determine the relationship between patients and family members' affective states.[26] Data were collected over three cycles of chemotherapy from 42 patients and 40 family members. The independent variables were affective states (measured by the Profile of Mood Status), family functioning (measured by the Family Crises–Oriented Personal Scales), and self-care behavior (recorded in a Self-Care Behavior Log). Self-care behavior was defined as any activity initiated by patient, family, or friends to alleviate a side effect from chemotherapy.

Side effects reported most frequently were nausea (90%), fatigue (65%), vomiting (62%), mouth sores (31%), and weakness (31%). Patients did not delay in initiating self-care behaviors more than 24 hours, especially if a family member was present to help. However, with increasing severity of the side effect, patients became more immobilized, and delayed initiating self-care behaviors up to several days. The patients' mood disturbance was greater than the family members' during all three cycles, but the differences were more marked at the initiation of chemotherapy and decreased over time. These studies recommend that follow-up from the nurse be initiated at least 1–3 days postchemotherapy to assess the patients and to determine if side effects were being managed adequately. In addition, the studies concluded that patient education is essential to ensure that the patient and family understand what self-care measures need to be taken for side effects experienced.

Two other studies[27,28] evaluated the relationship between individual side effects and distress from chemotherapy using standard scales. Nausea, hair loss, and tiredness were reported by more than 80% of patients as the most distressing symptom. Vomiting was reported by 54%. The degree of distress reported by individuals correlated with the number of side effects experienced. Thus, a cumulative effect from experiencing several side effects had a greater impact on the patients' daily activities and quality of life.

Nail et al. studied the incidence of side effects from chemotherapy and the use of self-care activities, using a closed-ended approach provided by a self-care diary.[29] A total of 49 patients receiving chemotherapy on an outpatient basis were asked to complete the self-care diary on the second and fifth days after treatment. The self-care diary included a list of side effects that the patient might experience from chemotherapy and self-care activities that the patient might initiate to minimize individual side effects. Although there were 24 different drug combinations used, the most common regimens included 5-fluorouracil, cyclophosphamide, methotrexate, and doxorubicin.

Fatigue was the most frequently reported side effect (81%). Sleeping difficulty, nausea, and decreased appetite each were reported by approximately 50% of the subjects. The majority of side effects were rated as moderately severe, with the highest severity rating being for hair loss, followed closely by fatigue. Self-care activities used to gauge fatigue included obtaining extra sleep by napping, going to bed earlier, or sleeping later. The most effective activity for dealing with nausea was taking antinausea medication. The majority of patients' self-care activities were rated as slightly to moderately helpful. The authors recommend that nurses prepare patients for the occurrence of fatigue and review self-care activities directed to combating fatigue. Also, patients should be encouraged to use prescribed antiemetics.

This study also found that some patients believed that side effects from chemotherapy had to be endured. This was reinforced by health care professionals who did not tell patients what actions could be taken to alleviate the side effects. Several patients believed that if the interventions suggested did not alleviate the side effects, there were no other alternatives. These authors concluded that health care professionals either are not providing adequate information or are providing information in a form that the patient cannot absorb, retain, and recall when needed.[29]

Self-care activities are initiated pretreatment and are used throughout the treatment phase. Self-care activities are intended to manage or minimize chemotherapy side effects. In situations where patients are unable to participate or are unwilling, efforts must be made to include family members or visiting nurses to ensure compliance. Without compliance, the side effects could be severe and lead to further complications. Hospitalization and death may be the consequences of side effects that are not managed effectively.[26] From the studies just described it appears that the side effects that seem to be the most distressing to patients include fatigue, nausea, vomiting, alopecia, anorexia, and mouth sores. Nurses must continue to develop effective strategies to assist patients in minimizing these effects. Documenting effective strategies that have been successful, including those suggested by the patients, can serve as a useful resource for future teachings.

PATIENT EDUCATION AND FOLLOW-UP

Although teaching may be initiated while the patient is still hospitalized, most teaching regarding chemotherapy takes place in the outpatient setting and is provided by the nurse who will administer the drugs. The intent of teaching is more than to give information; it provides support and knowledge to empower the patient to manage self-care effectively.[30,31] For patient education to be most effective, it should begin early in the diagnostic phase and serve as a guide throughout treatments and follow-up care. Teaching patients about their treatment reduces fear, increases self-confidence, improves compliance, and enhances their participation in self-care.[30] The nurse is in a valuable position to identify what the patient needs to know about managing chemotherapy side effects and what resources are available to augment those teachings.

One approach to identifying the informational needs of the patients and family members is to focus on the various phases of cancer care: diagnosis, treatment, rehabilitation, survivorship, and recurrent disease. Goals of chemotherapy teaching include:

1. helping the patient adjust to the treatment
2. explaining how the treatment will affect the cancer
3. imparting the sequence of administration
4. recognizing and controlling side effects
5. encouraging self-care behaviors that minimize the side effects
6. listing side effects pertinent to report to the health care professional

All information offered to the patient must be documented in the patient's record (see Figure 16-1), for future reference as well as to comply with professional regulations.

An earlier study by Dodd indicated that despite the efforts of health care professionals, patients are not absorbing and retaining the information they need.[30] It was not uncommon for patients to attribute the majority of their symptoms to chemotherapy regardless of other medical conditions or medicines used. The symptoms most frequently attributed incorrectly to chemotherapy were nervousness, irritability, insomnia, and numbness/tingling of hands and feet. In conclusion the author stressed the importance of reinforcing teachings periodically, since retention without reinforcement is short-lived.

In the outpatient setting the nurse very frequently screens phone calls and triages the patient to assist in evaluating symptomatology and initiating the appropriate treatment measures. Most patient problems can be managed without the patient's needing to be seen on an emergency basis. It is important, however, for the nurse to be able to gather sufficient data to determine whether the patient needs medical intervention, and if so whether the patient will be cared for most appropriately in the outpatient setting or whether the patient needs emergency care. Figure 16-2 is a phone triage flow sheet listing basic steps that might be appropriate in managing patient problems over the phone. Obviously, the nurse needs to be highly knowledgeable about the patient's history, the last chemotherapy treatment, and whether this complaint is related to the treatment, and/or the disease, or is unrelated.

Objective and subjective data must be gathered methodically in order to formulate an opinion regarding the patient's deposition. Once consulting with the physician, the nurse once again speaks to the patient, either to gather more information or to relay instructions to the patient and/or family regarding care. Examples of specific phone triage flow sheets are included in the discussion of various chemotherapy side effects later in the chapter.

CHEMOTHERAPY TOXICITIES

Grading of Toxicities

Standardization of assessment and documentation of side effects is crucial in evaluating the therapeutic use of chemotherapy.[32] Specific therapies can be assessed by comparing their benefits with toxicity occurrence. To assess toxicity, the following information should be included in relation to chemotherapy administration[33]:

1. which toxicities occurred
2. toxicity severity
3. time of onset
4. duration of the effect
5. interventions incorporated to minimize the effect

It is important in the recognition and evaluation of toxicities to be able to discriminate between an expected versus a toxic reaction from chemotherapy and to distinguish these from the complications related to the cancer. For example, if a patient with lymphoma presents to the clinic with a complaint of paresthesias, numbness, and tingling, the patient must be evaluated for possible spinal cord compression from tumor progression versus peripheral toxicity from vincristine administration.

Using specific parameters and operational definitions to define the degree of a given toxicity ensures consistency in documenting observed reactions (see Table 16-1). Toxicity grading scales have been developed by the World Health Organization and various cooperative study groups to provide consistency in reporting. Adequate assessment and documentation of the side effect experienced, the patient's overall response to the regimen, and subsequent quality of life can be essential for evaluating the impact of treatment. Decisions regarding the need for appropriate adjustments in the treatment plan can be determined on the basis of sound, objective data documented by the nurse.[34]

Specific guidelines need to be taught and to be given in written form to the patient and caregiver to ensure they report any type of toxicity. Misinterpretation of the patient's report can make a significant difference in changes made in the treatment protocol. Nurses will continue to be challenged to design effective assessment and documentation systems that ensure accurate pa-

CHEMOTHERAPY TEACHING CHECK-LIST

Assessment Summary:

____

____

____

____

____

____

Patient
Name: ____________
Primary
Nurse: ____________

Drugs: ______________________________

____

____

LEARNING NEED	TEACHING INITIATED (DATE & INITIALS)	KNOWLEDGE CONFIRMED (DATE & INITIALS)	COMMENTS
1. Patient Education Booklets/Drug Cards			
2. Viewed Chemotherapy Video Other:			
3. Common Side Effects and Treatment			
a. Nausea and Vomiting – Antiemetics			
b. Stomatitis – Mouth Care			
c. Alopecia – Wigs/Scarves			
d. Decreased White Blood Cells – Infection Precaution			
e. Decreased Red Blood Cells – Fatigue			
f. Decreased Platelets – Bleeding Precaution			
g. Skin Changes – Hygienic Needs			
h. Loss of Appetite – Nutrition			
i. Diarrhea – Medication/Diet			
j. Constipation – Diet/Medication			
k. Flu-Like Symptoms			
l. Urine Discoloration			
m. Hemorrhagic Cystitis			
n. Other			
4. Specific Teaching			
a. Subcutaneous Injections			
b. Maintaining Adequate Nutrition			
c. Precautions to Report During Drug Administration:			
(1) Stinging, Burning Pain			
(2) Flushing of Face			
(3) Metallic Taste			
(4) Feeling of Numbness			
(5) Itching at Site (or generalized itching)			
(6) Allergic reactions			

FIGURE 16-1 Chemotherapy teaching checklist.

(continued)

LEARNING NEED	TEACHING INITIATED (DATE & INITIALS)	KNOWLEDGE CONFIRMED (DATE & INITIALS)	COMMENTS
d. Reproductive Changes * Dyspareunia * Menopausal Symptoms			
e. Activity			
f. Interaction with Other Drugs/Food			
g. Vascular access device			
h. Perineal Burning (Decadron)			
5. Symptoms to Report to Physician:			
a. Bleeding			
b. Prolonged Nausea or Vomiting			
c. Fever/Chills			
d. Stomatitis			
e. Diarrhea/Constipation			
f. Numbness or Tingling of Extremities			
g. Difficulty breathing or shortness of breath			
h. Other:			
6. Prescriptions given to patient with Instructions: ☐ Antiemetics ____________ ☐ Wig ☐ Blood Counts ☐ Other			
7. Schedule of Drug Treatment			
8. Instructions to obtain blood counts			
9. Follow-up or referral to community resources			

Comments: ____

____

____

____

Patient Signature: ____

RN Signature: ____

RN Signature: ____

FIGURE 16-1 Chemotherapy teaching checklist (continued).

tient observation and reporting of toxicities, especially in the home setting.

Systemic Toxicities

Bone marrow suppression

Myelosuppression is not only the most common dose-limiting side effect of chemotherapy but also potentially the most lethal.[35–38] All hematopoietic cells divide rapidly, regardless of their developmental stage, and are therefore vulnerable to chemotherapy. Proliferating progenitor cells that produce the mature granulocytes, erythrocytes, and thrombocytes in the peripheral circulation are commonly destroyed. As immature cells in the marrow and preexisting mature cells are destroyed, the nadir becomes apparent, usually 7–14 days after chemotherapy. At the same time, cells in the bone marrow are maturing and are ready to be released into the peripheral blood. Within a short period of time (3–4 weeks) the nadir will resolve.[38] However, when high doses are administered, the stem cell population may fail to repopulate quickly enough, resulting in a prolonged nadir period.

The majority of chemotherapy drugs cause some degree of myelosuppression.[36] Agents most active

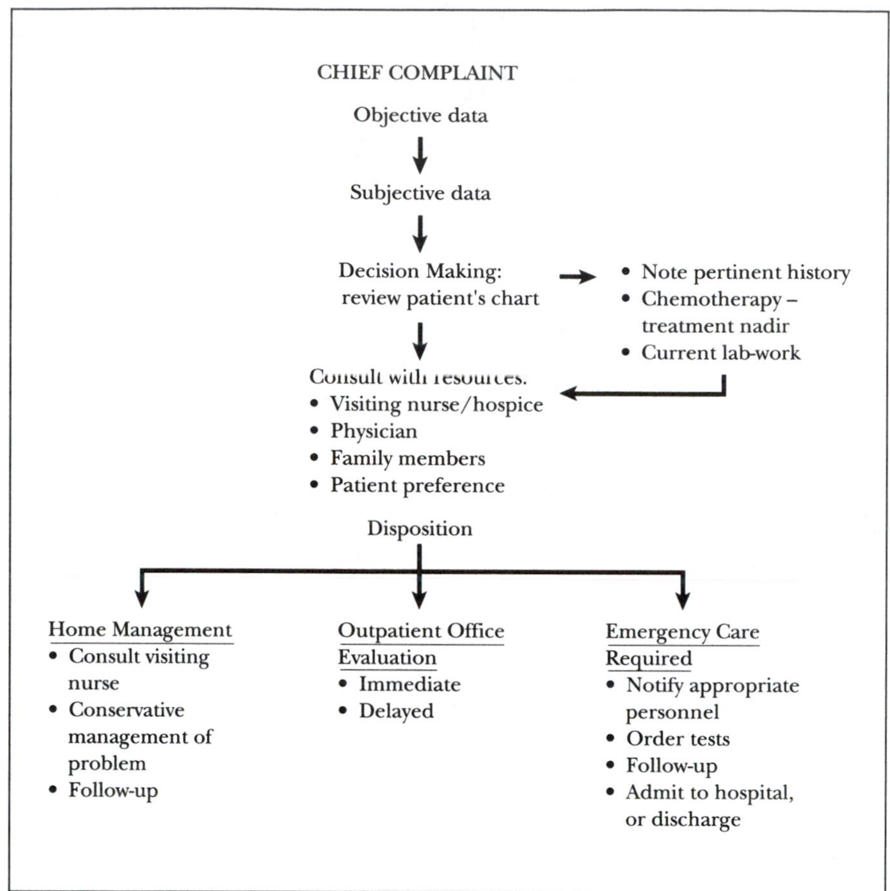

FIGURE 16-2 Phone triage flow sheet.

against cells that are cycling or those active during a specific phase of the cell cycle can produce rapid cytopenia. Because alkylating agents and nitrosoureas affect cycling cells as well as noncycling cells, these drugs are more likely to destroy the marrow stem cells. Antimetabolites, vinca alkaloids, and antitumor antibiotics are most damaging to cells that are in a specific phase of the cell cycle; thus, myelosuppression is less severe with these agents.[39] However, dose intensification and drug combinations can produce severe and prolonged neutropenia.

Younger patients are more tolerant of chemotherapy, due to their more cellular marrow and a decreased percentage of fat. Risk factors such as tumor cells in the bone marrow, prior treatment with chemotherapy or radiation, and a high negative nitrogen balance will compromise the marrow and increase the degree and duration of cytopenia.[39] It has been recognized that an increased risk of infection occurs among persons suffering from protein-calorie malnutrition, causing lymphopenia, diminished levels of the complement system, and a decrease of certain immunoglobulins.[40] In addition, myelotoxicity caused by chemotherapy and radiotherapy is enhanced by protein deprivation resulting from cancer cachexia.[41]

Differences in the lengths and kinetics of the life cycles of particular blood cells account for the frequency of neutropenia, thrombocytopenia, and anemia.[38] Maturation of cells in the bone marrow takes 8–10 days. The life span of platelets is 7–10 days. Thrombocytopenia usually occurs 8–14 days after chemotherapy and in most cases concomitantly with neutropenia. Chemotherapy may be held if the count drops below 100,000/mm^3. Manifestations of thrombocytopenia are easy bruising, bleeding from gums, nose, or other orifices, and petechiae on the upper and lower extremities, pressure points, elbows, and palate (see Figure 16-3).

Red blood cells (RBCs) have a life span of 120 days. Chemotherapy-induced anemia occurs rarely, because the bone marrow begins to recover before the number of circulating RBCs decreases significantly. Although low hemoglobin and hematocrit levels will not prevent administering chemotherapy, low levels affect how the patient feels and functions. Anemia is manifested by pallor, hypotension, headaches, irritability, and fatigue. Tachycardia and tachypnea may be present due to the hypoxic effects on the heart. Secondary problems include skin or mucous membrane breakdown arising from decreased tissue oxygenation, and cardiopulmonary stress. Anemia and thrombocytopenia can usually be corrected with blood component transfusions.[36]

TABLE 16-1 Grading Toxicities from Chemotherapeutic Agents

Toxicity	Grade 0	Grade 1	Grade 2	Grade 3	Grade 4
			HEMATOLOGIC		
WBC (1000/mm³)	>4.0	3.0–3.9	2.0–2.9	1.0–1.9	<1.0
Granulocytes (1000/mm³)	>2.0	1.5–1.9	1.0–1.4	0.5–0.9	<0.5
Platelets (1000/mm³)	>100	75–99	50–74	25–49	<25
Hemoglobin (g/100 ml)	>11	9.5–10.9	8.0–9.4	6.5–7.9	<6.5
Hemorrhage	None	Slight, no transfusion	Mild, 1–2 transfusions/ episode	Gross, 3–4 transfusions/ episode	Massive, >4 transfusions/ episode
Infection/fever	None	Temp; <38°C No antibiotics	Temp: 38°–40°C Broad-spectrum antibiotics	Temp: >40°C Antifungal coverage	Signs of sepsis: reevaluate medication
			GASTROINTESTINAL		
Nausea/vomiting	None	Slight nausea, 1 episode of vomiting Maintains intake	Occasional nausea, 2–5 episodes of vomiting Maintains intake	Frequent nausea, 6–10 episodes of vomiting Intake decreased	Constant nausea, >10 episodes of vomiting No intake
Diarrhea	None	2–3 stools	4–6 stools Moderate cramps	7–9 stools Severe cramps	>10 stools needs rehydration
Constipation	None	Dry, hard passage of painful stool Stool softner	No stool >2 days Laxatives	No stool >4 days Rule out obstruction or cause	—
Anorexia	None	Mild	Moderate, with weight loss	Severe Needs supplements	Life-threatening

The life span of the granulocyte is 6–8 hours after release from the marrow. Neutropenia typically develops 8–12 days after chemotherapy, with recovery in 3–4 weeks. Chemotherapy is usually withheld if the patient's white blood cell (WBC) count is between 1000 and 3000/mm³ or if the absolute neutrophil count (ANC) is below 1500/mm³. Neutropenia generally is defined as an ANC below 1500 cells/mm³. In normal individuals, neutrophils, including both the segmented and slightly less mature band forms, are found in concentrations ranging from 1830 to 7250 cells/mm³.[42] Profound neutropenia (grade 4) usually is defined as an ANC <500 cells/mm³.[43]

It is important to note that neutropenia can occur when total WBC count is within a normal range (4000–10,000/mm³). Consequently, quantitating the ANC is essential to achieving a correct assessment of neutrophil status. An ANC is calculated by multiplying the total WBC count by the differential proportion of combined band and segmented neutrophils in a blood sample.[43] Thus, in a patient with a WBC count of 4000 cells/mm³, a differential of 34% segmented neutrophils plus 3% band neutrophils yields an ANC of

$$4000 \text{ cells/mm}^3 \times 37\% = 1480 \text{ cells/mm}^3$$

Since the prime function of neutrophils is phagocytosis, neutropenia eliminates one of the body's prime defenses against bacterial infection.[44] Infections, due to invasion and overgrowth of pathogenic microbes, increase in frequency and severity as the ANC decreases. In addition, risk for severe infections increase when the nadir persists for more than 7–10 days.

Signs of an infection may not be apparent with the inhibition of phagocytic cells. The only response may be fever, and this at times may not be present. It is estimated that 80% of the infections that occur arise from endogenous microbial flora (GI or respiratory tract).[38] When the neutrophil count is less than 500, approximately 20% or more of febrile episodes will have an associated bacteriemia caused principally by aerobic gram-negative bacilli (*Escherichia coli, Klebsiella pneumoinis,* and *Pseudomonas aeruginosa*) and gram-positive cocci (coagulase-negative staphylocci, streptococci species, and *Staphylococcus aureus*).[45]

Chemotherapy-induced damage to the alimentary canal and respiratory tract mucosa facilitates the entry of infecting organisms; therefore pneumonia and sinusitis are commonly seen. The nurse must assess for inflammation at the sites most commonly infected, including the periodontium, pharynx, lower esophagus,

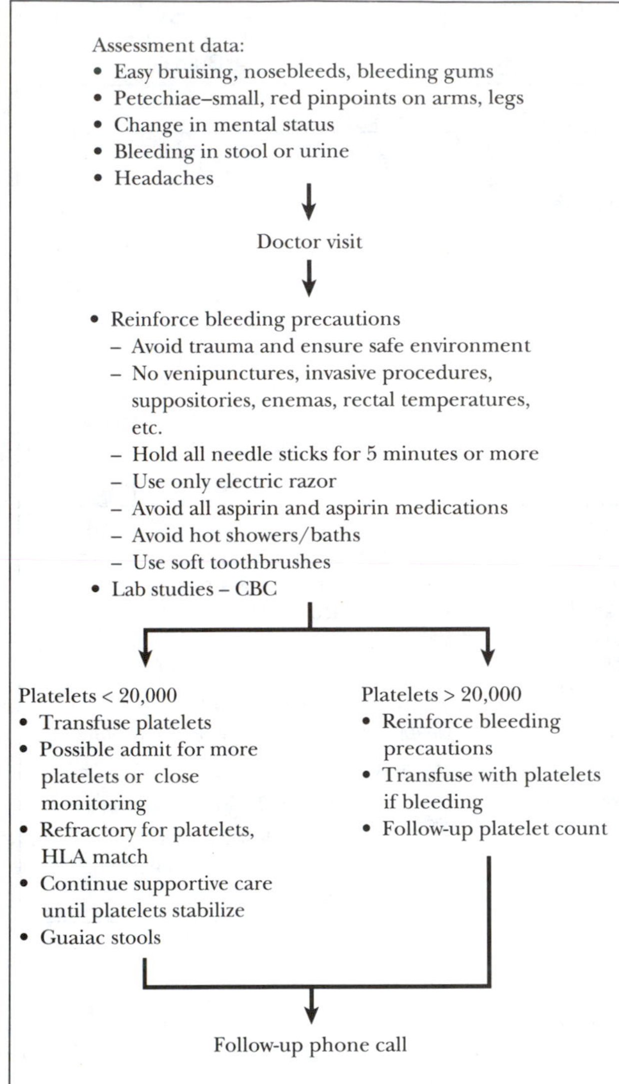

FIGURE 16-3 Thrombocytopenia phone triage flow sheet.

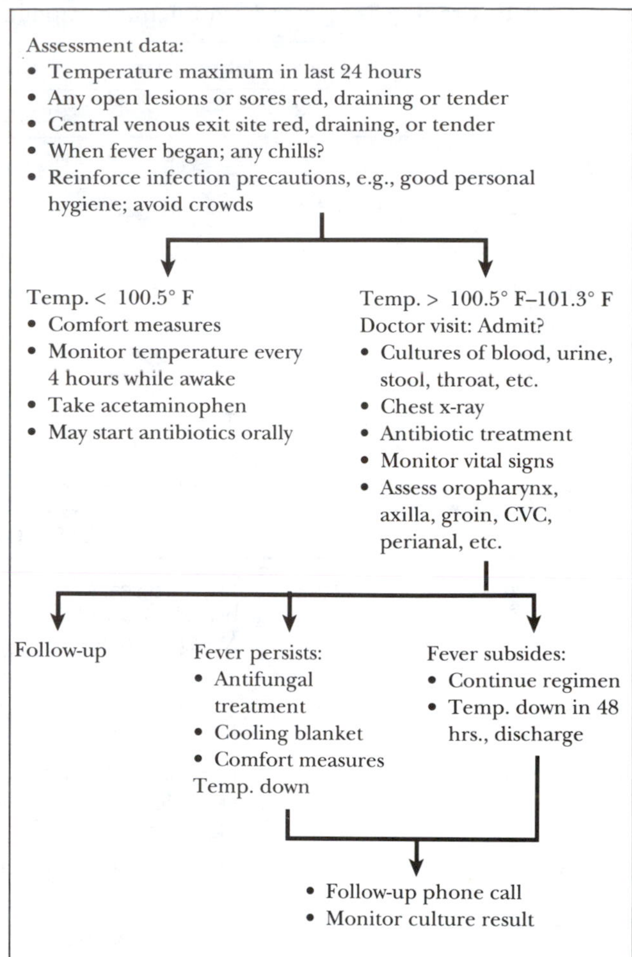

FIGURE 16-4 Fever phone triage flow sheet.

lung, perineum, anus, skin, and venous access exit sites. Prevention, early detection, good hand-washing technique, and prompt management of infections in patients with neutropenia are essential if sepsis and septic shock are to be avoided[36,42,44,46,47] (see Figure 16-4).

Once appropriate cultures are obtained, antibiotics are used to treat chemotherapy-induced infections: (1) until cultures indicate eradication of the causative organism, (2) for a minimum of 7 days, or (3) until the neutrophil count is greater than 500/mm^3.[45] To achieve a broad coverage, therapy with a broad-spectrum cephalosporin or penicillin in combination with an aminoglycoside has been the mainstay of empiric treatment in neutropenic patients for the past decade.[48] Fever persisting for over 3 days without identification of an infected site or organism suggests: (1) a nonbacterial cause, (2) resistance to the antibiotic, (3) emergence of a second bacterial infection, (4) inadequate antibiotic serum and tissue levels, (5) drug fever, or (6) infection at avascular sites (abscess).[49] At this point, antifungal therapy is started.[37,45,50] Antiviral drugs are usually counterrecommended unless mucosal lesions or viral disease is suspected.

Among all the problems identified with myelosuppression, infection is the most serious associated with significant morbidity and mortality.[45] For this reason, much attention has been focused on the therapeutic application of recombinant colony-stimulating factors (CSFs) to augment neutrophil counts. Hematopoietic growth factors are a family of glycoprotein hormones that act as natural regulators of hematopoiesis to promote the proliferation and differentiation of hematopoietic progenitor cells along multiple pathways.[51–53] While hematopoietic stimulants have not changed the decline rate of granulocytes, they have shortened the duration of neutropenia, thereby dramatically reducing the morbidity and mortality from infections. The discovery of CSFs offers hope that the myelosuppression associated with chemotherapy can be ameliorated and full dosages of chemotherapy can be used in cancer therapy.

Fatigue

Fatigue is a common adverse effect of cancer and its therapy; however, it is underdescribed in the literature as related to chemotherapy administration. When fatigue begins to have an adverse effect on the patient's well-being and interferes with activities of daily living, relationships, and compliance with medical therapy, interventions must be incorporated.[54]

Specific causative mechanisms underlying fatigue are unclear. Changes in skeletal muscle protein stores or metabolite concentration may be one physiologic mechanism.[55] Fatigue may result from the body's response to the accumulation of various metabolites and the metabolism of end products from cell destruction by chemotherapy. Other contributing factors could include other side effects, changes in energy usage, disease patterns, anemia, and psychological patterns.

Fatigue manifests as weariness, weakness, and lack of energy. The nurse must assess the onset, the duration, the intensity, the impact on lifestyle, and aggravating and alleviating factors.[56] Acute fatigue protects the individual from exhaustion, which usually dissipates with a good night's sleep. Chronic fatigue is described as a totally overwhelming experience. Chronic fatigue is not easily resolved, and a combination of approaches may be needed. Interventions to overcome fatigue include energy conservation, rest, setting priorities for activities, and delegating tasks.

Gastrointestinal

Anorexia Anorexia is a frequent complaint of patients with cancer and contributes to decreased caloric intake with subsequent weight loss. Weight loss often leads to cachexia and is indicative of a poor prognosis.[57] Anorexia or declining food intake implies alterations in food perception, taste, and smell that result from the effects of chemotherapy.[58] Abnormalities of carbohydrate, protein, and fat metabolism are central features of anorexia. Visceral and lean body mass depletion are common, along with muscle atrophy, visceral organ atrophy, and hypoalbuminemia.[59,60] Anorexia can lead to compromised immune status as manifested by decreased macrophage mobilization, depressed lymphocyte function, and impaired phagocytosis.[61]

Nutritional assessment is the first step in meeting the nutritional needs. This includes a physical assessment, a health history, and the obtaining of specific nutritional parameters (albumin, transferrin, nitrogen balance, and oxygen consumption). Other information to obtain during the initial interview include: financial resources for the purchase of food or supplements; persons responsible for purchasing, storing, and preparing food; and community resources available for food preparation and purchase. The interview and physical assessment can identify the usual nutritional patterns, the physiologic/psychological deficits affecting nutritional intake, and those individuals who are at high risk for the development of protein-caloric malnutrition.[62–64] A loss of more than 10% of body weight within the previous 6 months or an unintentional weight loss of more than 1 kilogram a week is considered a significant risk factor.

The success of maintaining nutritional status depends on a number of factors, including patient motivation, nutritional status at the time of diagnosis, site of the cancer, type of treatment, and severity of side effects. The patient must be taught that adequate nutrition is required for protein synthesis, cellular repair, and tissue growth. For patients receiving chemotherapy, an increase of 4.4 cal/kg and 2 g/kg of protein per body weight must be incorporated when developing a nutritional plan.[65] One strategy could be for the nurse to contract with the patient to increase the intake of calories and protein each day. Hyperalimentation, nutritional supplements, or enteral nutrition can be alternatives for sufficient nutritional intake. Short walks before meals and smaller more frequent meals may be helpful for the patient. Nutrition is an important aspect in providing care to the patient with cancer. Planning nutritional diets gives patients as well as families the ability to actively participate in their care.

Diarrhea Diarrhea is an increase in stool volume and liquidity resulting in three or more bowel movements per day. Diarrhea results from the destruction of the actively dividing epithelial cells of the GI tract. When these cells are destroyed, atrophy of the intestinal mucosa and shortening or denuding of the intestinal villa occur. The villi and microvilli become flattened, reducing the absorptive surface area and resulting in a "slick gut." Thus the intestinal contents move rapidly through the gut, reducing absorption of nutrients.[66]

The degree and duration of diarrhea depend on the agent, dose, nadir, and frequency of chemotherapy administration. Patients may experience abdominal cramps and rectal urgency with 5-fluorouracil-leucovorin therapy, which can evolve into nocturnal diarrhea or fecal incontinence leading to lethargy, weakness, orthostatic hypotension, and fluid/electrolyte imbalance. Without adequate management, prolonged diarrhea will cause dehydration, nutritional malabsorption, and circulatory collapse.[67]

Although 5-fluorouracil is the most common drug to cause diarrhea, other agents include methotrexate, actinomycin-D, doxorubicin, and daunorubicin. Recent manipulations of 5-fluorouracil metabolism with agents such as leucovorin and N-phosphonacetyl L-aspartic have potentiated its antitumor effect as well as increased diarrhea occurrence.[67]

Thorough evaluation to determine the cause of the diarrhea provides a firm foundation for planning interventions. Management may be limited to dietary measures, such as a low-residue high-caloric and protein diet, or pharmacologic measures. Stool cultures need to be obtained initially, to rule out an infectious process so appropriate therapy can be implemented. *Clostridium difficile* has been reported in patients receiving chemotherapy who have had prior antibiotic exposure. Antidiarrheal agents should never be given to counteract diarrhea resulting from an infection, since these agents slow the passage of stool through the intestines, prolonging the mucosa's exposure to the organism's toxins. Usually when the diarrhea is a result of an organism, it will resolve in a few days with the use of vancomycin or metronidazole.[68]

Pharmacologic intervention for diarrhea is varied. Anticholinergic drugs such as atropine sulfate and scopolamine reduce gastric secretions and decrease intestinal peristalsis. Opiate therapy binds to receptors on the smooth muscle of bowel, slowing down the intestinal motility and increasing fluid absorption. Loperamide is a long-acting opioid agonist, without central opioid activity.[67] Octreotide acetate, a synthetic analog of the hormone octapeptide, inhibits the release of gut hormones, including serotonin and gastrin from the GI tract. It effects the GI tract by prolonging intestinal transit time, increasing intestinal water and electrolyte transport, and decreasing GI bloodflow.[69,70] Octreotide acetate is indicated for patients who have excessive diarrhea as a result of GI resections or when other pharmacologic treatments have proven ineffective to manage chemotherapy-induced diarrhea.

Chemotherapy usually is administered despite the occurrence of diarrhea. However, diarrhea can be severe enough to be a dose-limiting toxicity of some chemotherapeutic agent combinations, specifically 5-fluorouracil and leucovorin. The nurse must carefully monitor the patient's status to provide appropriate therapy, such as antidiarrheal medications, fluid/electrolyte replacements, and perirectal care to prevent further complications (see Figure 16-5).

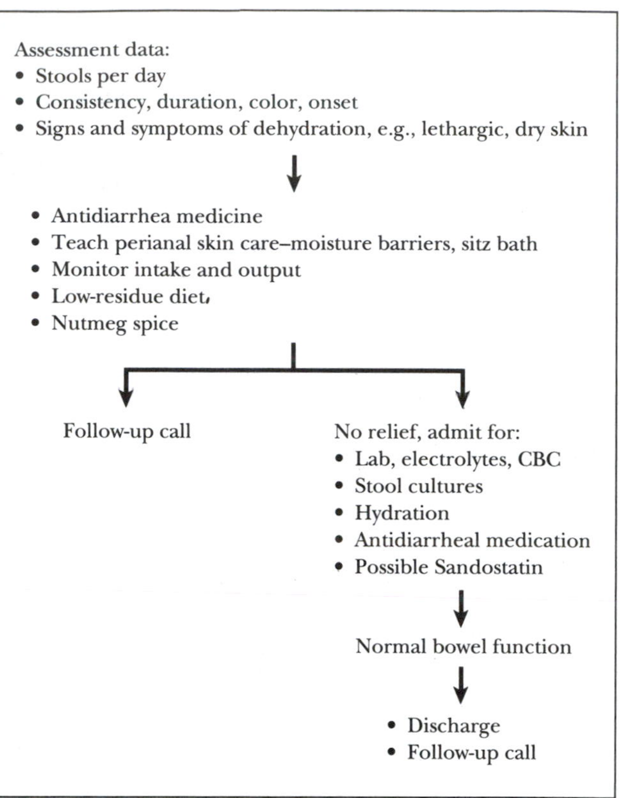

FIGURE 16-5 Diarrhea phone triage flow sheet.

Constipation Constipation is defined as infrequent, excessively hard and dry bowel movements resulting from a decrease in rectal filling or emptying.[37] Risk factors that contribute to constipation include narcotic/analgesics, a decrease in physical activity, a low-fiber diet, a decrease in fluid intake, and bed rest. Vincristine and vinblastine are the most common chemotherapy agents to cause constipation, as a result of autonomic nerve dysfunction manifested as colicky abdominal pain and ileus. Rectal emptying is specifically diminished because nonfunctional afferent and efferent pathways from the sacral cord are interrupted. Symptoms occur within 3–7 days of drug administration and may be accompanied by evidence of peripheral nerve dysfunction.[67,69]

Patients are instructed to be aware of bowel movements. If a bowel movement does not occur every other day, a laxative must be taken. If there are no results, the physician should be notified for further instructions. Laxative therapy or prophylactic stool softener is recommended prior to the use of vincristine or vinblastine, especially if the patient has a history of or is at risk for constipation. The patient should be encouraged to increase the amount of high-fiber foods in the daily diet as well as to increase fluid intake. The patient should be encouraged to increase physical activity, if that is tolerated. It should be stressed to the patient never to wait more than 3 days without a bowel movement to call the physician, since a complication such as impaction or ileus can arise (see Figure 16-6).

Nausea/vomiting During the past decade, the management of chemotherapy-related nausea and vomiting has vastly improved. Understanding the pathophysiology of the symptoms, the efficacy and limitations of pharmacologic interventions, and the use of nonpharmacologic techniques is essential in minimizing nausea and vomiting. Emesis is a complicated process that requires coordination by the vomiting center (VC) in the lateral reticular formation of the medulla (see Figure 16-7). The VC lies close to the respiratory center on the floor of the fourth ventricle and is directly activated by the visceral and vagal afferent pathways from the GI tract, chemoreceptor trigger zone (CTZ), vestibular apparatus, and the cerebral cortex. When the VC is stimulated, emesis is induced via impulses to the salivation and respiratory centers and to the pharyngeal, GI, and abdominal muscles.[71,72]

Vestibular-cerebellar afferent pathway areas transmit impulses to the cerebellum and then to the VC, which is experienced as motion sickness. When rapid motion change occurs, the receptors of the labyrinth in the inner ear are stimulated, which is associated with nausea.[73] Obstruction, irritation, inflammation, or delayed gastric emptying may stimulate the GI tract

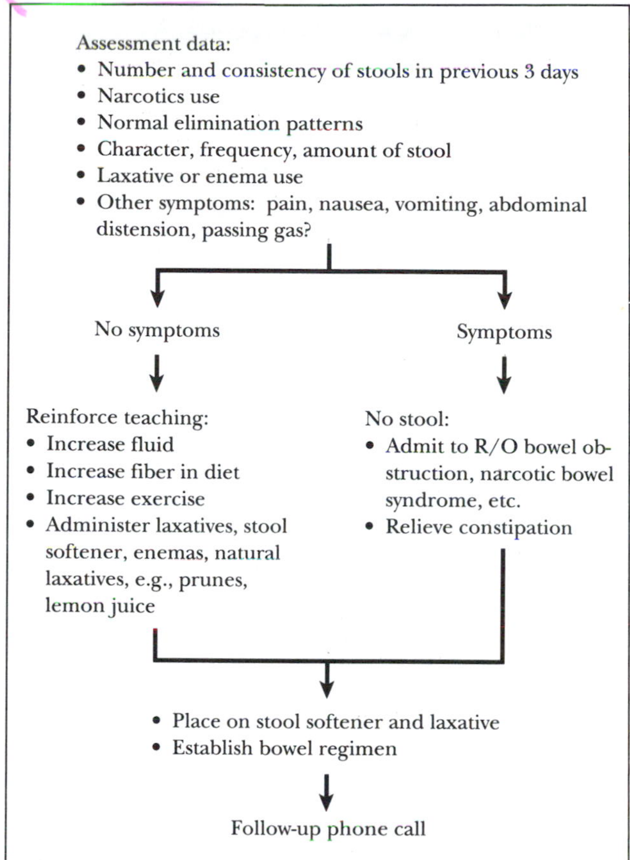

FIGURE 16-6 Constipation phone triage flow sheet.

through vagal visceral afferent pathways.[74] Conditioned and anticipatory response are controlled by the cerebral cortex and limbic system, which can be stimulated by sights, sounds, or odors that the patient associates with chemotherapy, thereby making the patient nauseated.[71]

The VC is rich in neurotransmitter receptors sensitive to chemical toxins in the blood and cerebrospinal fluid.[75] The major receptors are: dopamine, serotonin (5-HT3), and muscarinic cholinergic in the CTZ; muscarinic in the VC, vestibular apparatus, and the efferent vagal motor nuclei; and histamine in the VC and the vestibular apparatus.[72] A summary of the numerous factors involved in emesis, neurotransmitters, and pharmacologic management are summarized in Figure 16-8.

Although nausea, retching, and vomiting commonly occur together, they are considered separate conditions.[76,77] *Nausea* is described as a subjective conscious recognition of the desire to vomit and is manifested by an unpleasant wavelike sensation in the epigastric area, at the back of the throat, or throughout the abdomen. Nausea is mediated by the autonomic nervous system and accompanied by symptoms such as tachycardia, perspiration, lightheadedness, dizziness, pallor, excess salivation, and weakness.

Retching is a rhythmic and spasmodic movement involving the diaphragm and abdominal muscles controlled by the respiratory center in the brainstem near the VC. Negative intrathoracic pressure and positive abdominal pressure result in unproductive retching. When the negative pressure becomes positive, vomiting occurs. *Vomiting* is a somatic process performed by the respiratory muscles causing the forceful oral expulsion of gastric, duodenal, or jejunal contents through the mouth.[72,73]

Nausea and vomiting can be classified as acute, delayed, and anticipatory. *Acute* nausea and vomiting occur 1–2 hours after treatment, resolving within 24 hours. The pattern is determined by the emetogenicity of the chemotherapy and pretreatment with an antiemetic agent. *Delayed* nausea and vomiting persist or develop 24 hours after chemotherapy, perhaps due to the ongoing effect that the metabolites of chemotherapy continue to exhert on the CNS or GI tract. If nausea was controlled within the first 24 hours after therapy, delayed patterns are less likely to occur. However, despite effective antiemetic regimens, 93% of patients receiving a high dose of cisplatin experience delayed nausea and vomiting.[78,79] *Anticipatory* nausea and vomiting occur in 25% of patients as a result of classic operant conditioning from stimuli associated with chemotherapy. Such conditioned responses are experienced after a few sessions of chemotherapy and occur most commonly when efforts to control emesis are unsuccessful.[80–83]

It is possible to predict the degree and severity of nausea and vomiting as well as the onset and duration (see Table 16-2). Mechlorethamine, for example, induces emesis within 30 minutes of intravenous administration, whereas other highly emetic agents cause emesis at least 1 hour after infusion. With moderate to highly emetic drugs, emesis develops within 6 hours of administration. Drugs with low emetic potential usually cause emesis 12–48 hours after administration. Variability in occurrence and onset suggests that each drug may cause emesis via different mechanisms or by stimulating different pathways.[80,82] Rate and route of chemotherapy administration also affect emetic onset, intensity, and duration. For example, rapid infusion of cytarabine is more often associated with an earlier onset of severe emesis than is slower infusion.[75]

Management begins with obtaining an in-depth emetic history and developing a preventive action plan with antiemetics (see Table 16-3). Characteristics that affect the occurrence of nausea and vomiting include susceptibility to motion sickness, poor previous emetic control, and being young. Individuals with a heavy alcohol intake seem to have a decreased occurrence of nausea and vomiting.[83]

Successful antiemetic regimens interrupt the stimulation of the VC. Combination regimens must be individualized and developed according to the emetic potential of the chemotherapy regimen, expected duration of the nausea and vomiting, and current pattern of symptoms. Numerous combinations are being investigated extensively to eliminate the stimulation of

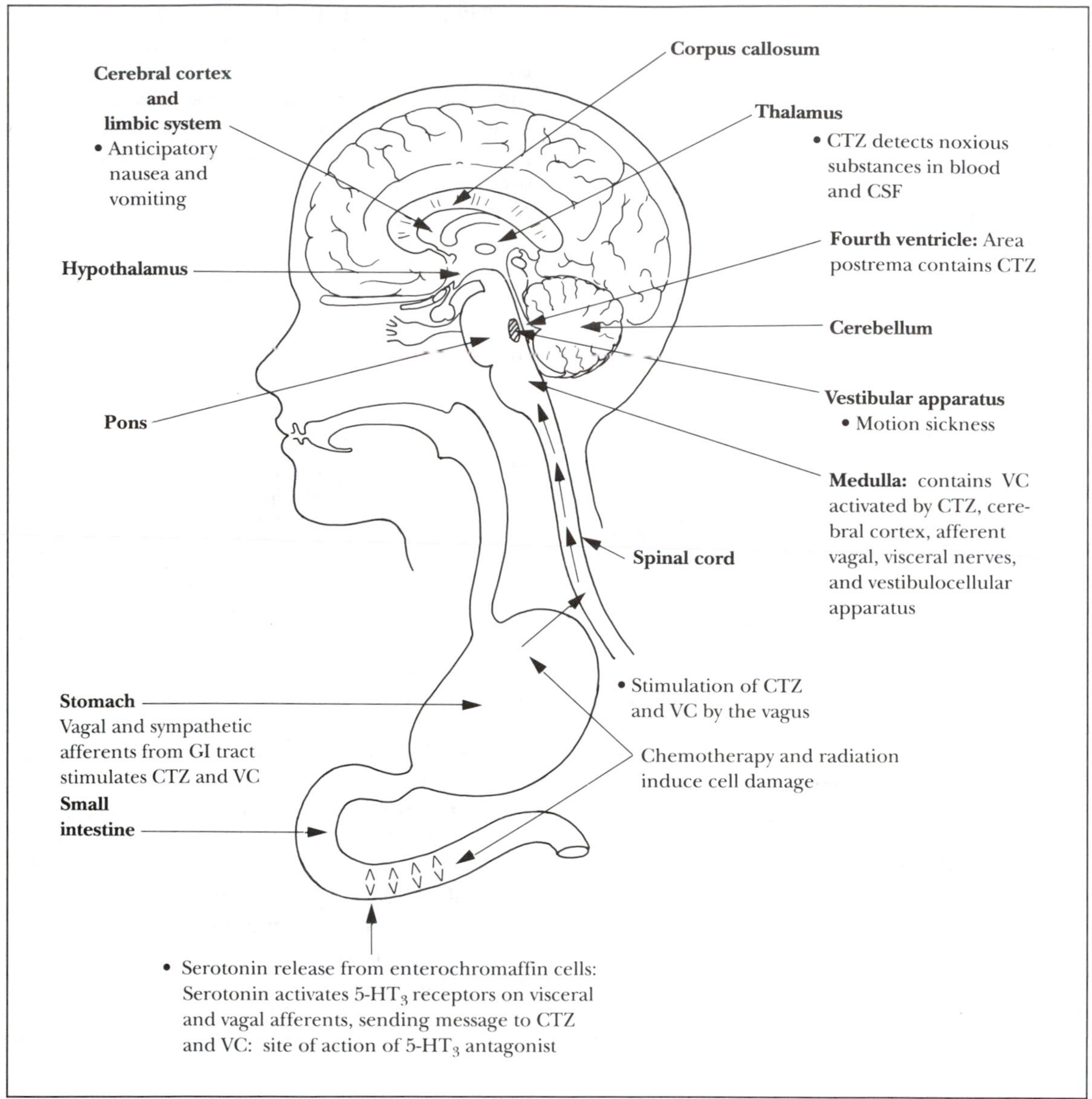

FIGURE 16-7 Pathways of nausea and vomiting.

the VC. These regimens use drugs with proven single-agent antiemetic activity, optimum doses, routes, and minimum overlapping toxicities (see Table 16-4).[82–87] For example, combinations of dopamine antagonists with steroids have been found to provide complete control of nausea and vomiting in up to 100% of patients undergoing high-dose cisplatin-base regimens. The combination of ondansetron and dexamethasone have been found more efficacious than ondansetron alone in controlling emesis.[88]

Behavioral interventions such as progressive muscle relaxation, hypnosis, and systematic desensitization can be taught to the patient to help interrupt the association of nausea and vomiting with chemotherapy. The nurse can try to minimize in the environment any aversive sounds or smells that could stimulate the VC. Distraction with audiotapes, radios, or television programs should be provided in the treatment area to help minimize nausea. Each of these techniques has been found effective in decreasing the frequency and duration of vomiting as well as in decreasing anxiety.[89,90]

It is important to teach the patient about the potential side effects of antiemetic therapy, such as drowsiness and diarrhea. If the patient is returning home after an emetogenic chemotherapy treatment, ensure that someone can provide transportation and care in the immediate hours following therapy. Phone follow-up 24–48 hours after treatment is essential to ensure that appropriate antiemetic management is being followed (see Figure 16-9).

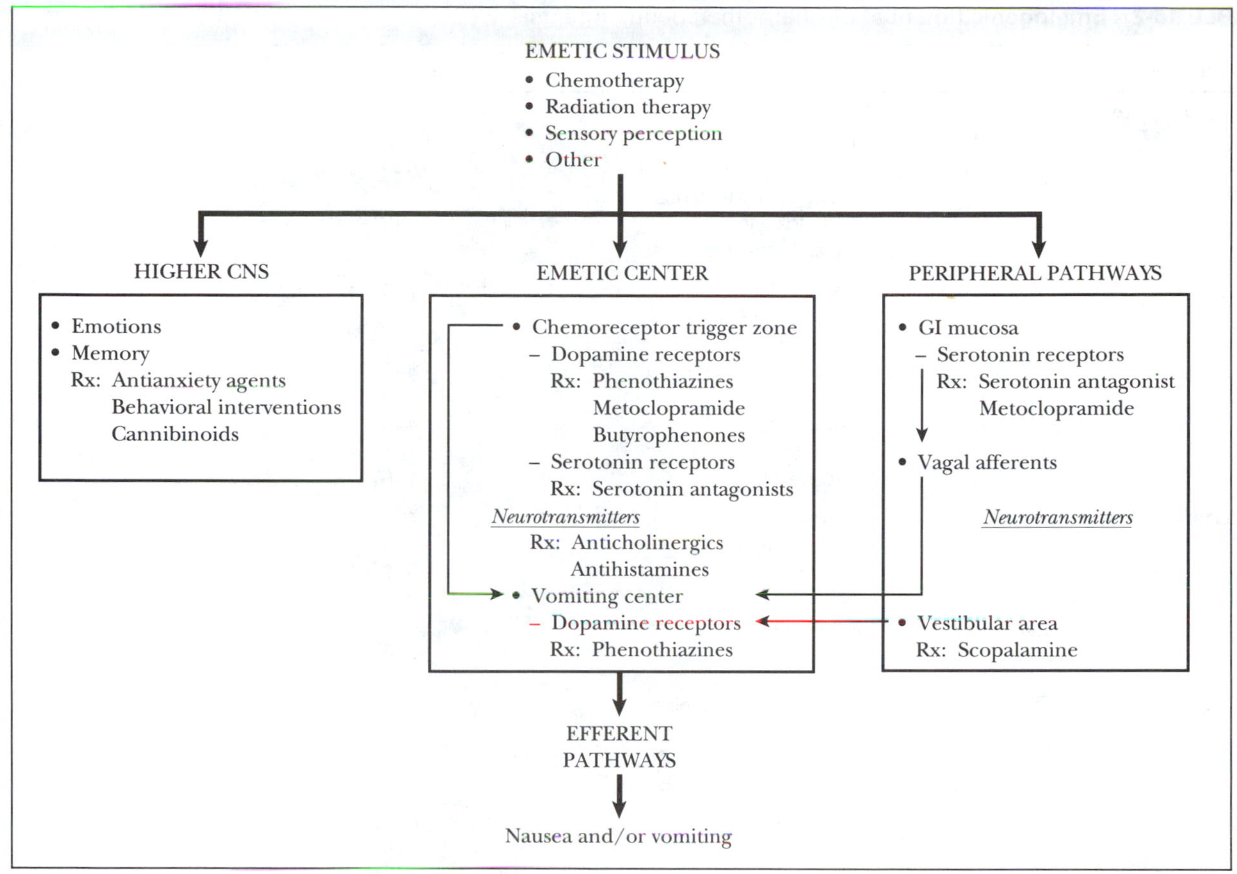

FIGURE 16-8 Physiology of chemotherapy-induced nausea/vomiting with proposed sites of action for interventions. (Published with permission of Wujcik, D: Current research in side-effects of high-dose chemotherapy. *Semin Oncol Nurs* 8:102–112, 1992.)

Organ Toxicities

Certain chemotherapy drugs may cause direct damage to specific cells of a given organ or cause indirect damage by the effects of cellular breakdown by-products. In general, organ toxicities are predictable based on the cumulative dose, the presence of concomitant organ dysfunction, the age of the patient, and the manner in which the drug is given. Of interest is the fact that the toxicity profile may be changing as a result of the more widespread use of dose-intensive regimens and CSFs. These approaches to managing the disease are likely to result in more organ toxicities as myelosuppression becomes less prominent. Each of the major organ toxicities will be discussed. Tables 16-5 through 16-10 provide a review of major toxicities in terms of risk factors, signs of toxicity, preventive measures, grading, and management.

Cardiotoxicity

Cardiotoxicity is described as an acute or chronic process. The acute form consists of transient electrocardiogram (ECG) changes, occurring in approximately 10% of patients receiving chemotherapy. Acute effects are immediate in onset and resolve quickly without serious complications. These effects are not dose related and are not an indication to stop the drug. Less than 5% of patients develop chronic cardiotoxicity from a cumulative drug effect requiring immediate discontinuation of the drug.[91,92] Chronic effects occur weeks or months after administration, involving nonreversible cardiomyopathy presenting as a classic biventricular congestive heart failure (CHF) with a characteristic low-voltage QRS complex. Signs and symptoms are classical for CHF, including complaints of a nonproductive cough, dyspnea, and pedal edema. Generally, it is poorly responsive to diuretics or digitalis, becoming progressively worse, with a 60% mortality.

Anthracyclines are known to cause cardiotoxicity by directly damaging the cardiac myocyte cells. The incidence of cardiotoxicity is 2%–3% after cumulative doses are administered.[92] Total cumulative dosages have been established at 550 mg/m² for doxorubicin and 600 mg/m² for daunomycin, with a decrease in dose to 450 mg/m² if mediastinal radiation has been administered.[93]

The mechanism of action occurs in the presence of

TABLE 16-2 Emetogenic Potential of Chemotherapeutic Agents

Incidence	Agent	Onset (hours)	Duration (hours)
Very High (>90%)	Cisplatin	1–6	24–48+
	Dacarbazine	1–3	1–12
	Mechlorethamine	0.5–2	8–24
	Melphalan—high dose	0.3–6	6–12
	Streptozocin	1–6	12–24
	Cytarabine—high dose	2–4	12–24
High (60%–90%)	Carmustine	2–4	4–24
	Cyclophosphamide	4–12	12–24
	Procarbazine	24–27	variable
	Etoposide—high dose	4–6	24+
	Semustine	1–5	12–24
	Lomustine	4–6	12–24
	Dactinomycin	2–5	24
	Pilcamycin	1–6	12–24
Moderate (30%–60%)	Doxorubicin	4–6	6+
	Mitoxantrone	4–6	6+
	5-Fluorouracil	3–6	24+
	Mitomycin C	1–4	48–72
	Carboplatin	4–6	12–24
	Daunorubicin	2–6	24
	L-Asparaginase	1–4	2–12
	Hexamethylmelamine	1–4	—
Low (10%–30%)	Bleomycin	3–6	—
	Cytarabine	6–12	3–12
	Etoposide	3–8	—
	Melphalan	6–12	—
	6-Mercaptopurine	4–8	—
	Methotrexate	4–12	3–12
	Vinblastine	4–8	—
	Hydroxyurea	—	—
	Teniposide	—	—
Very low <10%	Vincristine	4–8	—
	Chlorambucil	48–72	—
	Busulfan	—	—
	Thioguinine	—	—
	Hormones	—	—
	Steroids	—	—

oxygen, where the anthracyclines form a bond or union with iron or copper. These complexes inhibit lipid peroxidation, allowing a free oxygen radical to damage the myocytes directly. This results in a loss of myocardial fibrils, mitochrondrial changes, and cellular destruction.[93,94] As a result, the myocyte has limited contractility, leading to hypertrophy of the cardiac muscle, which increases the demand for oxygen.

In an attempt to decrease cardiotoxicity occurrence, altering the dose scheduling of doxorubicin to frequent lower doses has resulted in reduction of cardiotoxicity without compromise of antitumor effects.[94] Chemoprotectants are being evaluated to protect the cardiac tissue by blocking the anthracycline's damage to the myocytes.[95] Razoxane (ICRF-159), an investigational drug, has been shown to have chemoprotectant activity against daunomycin and doxorubicin in studies with mice. It appears that ICRF-159 competes with specific metals, such as iron, that are required for the anthracycline-induced cardiotoxicity. ICRF-187 is a similar compound currently being investigated that is more water soluble and easier to administer. This compound has permitted doses of doxorubicin up to 700 mg/m² to be administered without cardiotoxicity occurring.[96]

In an attempt to reduce further the cardiotoxicity from the anthracyclines, analogs that have greater antitumor activity and may have reduced cardiotoxicity have been developed. Epirubicin appears to be similar to doxorubicin, but the cardiotoxicity is significantly less. Patients can receive twice the cumulative dose of 1000 mg/m² before the risk of clinical cardiotoxicity begins to rise significantly.[97] Idarubicin, esorubicin, and aclarubicin also show less cardiotoxicity occurrence than doxorubicin. Although mitoxantrone has been associated with rare cardiac events, it is considered less cardiotoxic.[98,99]

TABLE 16-3 Antiemetic Therapy

Classification	Drugs	Availability/Dose	Schedule	Duration/ Half-Life	Comments
Benzodiazepines *Mechanism of action:* CNS depressant; interferes with afferent nerves from cerebral cortex; sedative *Common side effects:* Sedation, amnesia, confusion	Lorazepam (Ativan) Diazepam (Valium)	*Tablet:* 1–3 mg po or sublingual *IV:* 0.5–2.5 mg *Tablet:* 2–4 mg *IV:* 2–10 mg	q3–4 hr q4–6 hr	4–8 hr *Half-life:* 10–15 hr 4–8 hr *Half-life:* 30–40 hr	Reduces anticipatory nausea and vomiting. May aggrevate CNS effects of ifosfamide. Use with caution in patients with hepatic and renal dysfunction.
Butyrophenones *Mechanism of action:* Dopamine antagonist in the CTZ, esophagus, and stomach *Common side effects:* Sedation, hypotension, tachycardia, EPS	Droperidol (Inapsine) Haloperidol (Haldol)	*IM:* 2.5–10 mg *IV:* 0.5–2.5 mg *Tablet:* 3–5 mg *IM:* 1–2 mg *IV:* 1–3 mg	q3–4 hr q4 hr q2–6 hr	2–4 hr *Half-life:* 10 hr 2–6 hr *Half-life:* 12–18 hr	Diphenhydramine 25–50 mg po or IV will prevent EPS. EPS more common in young patients. May have additive effects. Use caution in patients with cardiac disorders.
Cannabinoids *Mechanism of action:* Suppresses pathways to VC (speculated) *Common side effects:* Sedation, dizziness, dysphoria, dry mouth, disorientation, impaired concentration, orthostatic hypotension, tachycardia	Dronabinol (Marinol)	*Tablet:* 5–10 mg	q4 hr	4–6 hr	May be difficult to obtain in outpatient setting. Elderly patients generally do not tolerate side effects. Generally used for second-line antiemetic therapy.
Phenothiazines *Mechanism of action:* Blocks dopamine receptor in the CTZ; inhibits VC by blocking autonomic afferent impulses via vagus nerve *Common side effects:* Sedation, orthostatic hypotension, EPS, dizziness, drowsiness	Prochlorperazine (Compazine) Promethazine (Phenergan) Thiethylperazine (Torecan) Chlorpromazine (Thorazine) Perphenazine (Trilafon)	*Tablet:* 5–25 mg *Sustained release:* 10–30 mg po *IM/IV:* 5–20 mg *Rectal:* 25 mg q4 hr *Tablet:* 12.5–25 mg *IM/IV:* 10–25 mg *Rectal:* 25 mg *Tablet:* 10 mg *IM:* 10 mg *Rectal:* 10 mg *Tablet:* 25–50 mg *IM/IV:* 25–50 mg *Rectal:* 25–100 mg *Tablet:* 4 mg *IM/IV:* 5 mg	q4–6 hr q10–12 hr q3–4 hr q4–6 hr q4–6 hr q4–6 hr q4–6 hr q4–6 hr	3–4 hr 10–12 hr 3–4 hr 3–4 hr 3–4 hr 3–4 hr 3–4 hr 3–4 hr	Administer IV dose over 15–30 min. EPS more common in person <30. Side effects can be cumulative in the elderly. Do not exceed 5 mg/min with IV dose Dystonia can occur with chlorpromazine, especially with IM. Chlorpromazine generally second-line antiemetic therapy. Diphenhydramine can prevent EPS and dystonia. Sustained-release form can prevent delayed nausea and vomiting.
Substituted Benzamide *Mechanism of action:* Dopamine antagonist; accelerates gastric emptiying and small-bowel transit; CTZ *Common side effects:* Sedation, diarrhea, anxiety EPS, fatigue, headache	Metoclopramide (Reglan)	*Tablet:* 5–10 mg *IV:* 1–3 mg/kg	q2–3 h × 3–5 doses	2–3 hr *Half-life:* 4–6 hr	EPS more common in young patients. Administer over 15 min to prevent intense anxiety. Use with caution in patients with renal dysfunction.

(continued)

TABLE 16-3 Antiemetic Therapy (continued)

Classification	Drugs	Availability/Dose	Schedule	Duration/ Half-Life	Comments
Steroids *Mechanism of action:* Antiprostaglandin synthesis activity? *Common side effects:* Insomnia, euphoria, anxiety, hypertension, edema	Dexamethasone (Decadron) Solu Medrol	*Tablet:* 10–40 mg *IV:* 4–20 mg *IV:* 125–250 mg	q3 hr q3 hr	*Half-life:* 2–3 hr	Rapid infusion causes perineal itching.
Antihistamines *Mechanism of action:* Histamine H-1; receptor antagonist *Common side effects:* Sedation, hypotension	Diphenhydramine (Benadryl)	*Tablet:* 25–50 mg *IM/IV:* 12.5–50 mg	q3–4 hr	*Half-life:* 5–8 hr	Prevents acute dystonic reactions. Use with caution in patients with hepatic dysfunction.
Serotonin Inhibitors *Mechanism of action:* Serotonin receptor; (5-HT3) antagonist *Common side effects:* Hypotension, headache, constipation, sedation minimal	Ondansetron (Zofran) Granisetron (BRL 43694A Investigational) Batanopride (BMY-25801 Investigational)	*IV:* 32 mg × 1 or 0.15 mg/kg × 3 *po:* 4-mg and 8-mg tablets IV and po *IV:* 1.2–8 mg/kg	q4 hr 30 min prior to chemo 2–3 hr × 3 doses	*Half-life:* 3–4 hr *Half-life:* 8–10 hr	Transient elevations of LFTs may occur with cisplatin and ondansetron administration. Single dose of BRL may be sufficient for a 24-hr time period. BMY has caused moderate to severe hypotension. ECG changes have been observed with BMY use. Ondanestron is not recommended for delayed or anticipatory nausea/vomiting.

VC, vomiting center; *CTZ,* chemoreceptor trigger zone; *EPS,* extrapyramidal symptoms; *LFTs,* liver function tests

Acute pericarditis has been reported with high-dose cyclophosphamide therapy (90–270 mg/kg) used in the bone marrow transplant (BMT) population with subsequent pericardial effusion and cardiac tamponade.[100] Cyclophosphamide damages the myocytes, similar to anthracyclines, where swelling and decreased contractility lead to less effective pumping of the heart. Hemorrhagic myocardial necrosis has been reported, with leakage of blood through capillaries. Toxicity ranges from minor, transient ECG changes and asymptomatic elevation of cardiac enzymes to fatal myopericarditis and myocardial necrosis.[101]

Myocardial ischemia has been reported with 5-fluorouracil infusion in patients with or without preexisting heart disease. Coronary vasospasm with resulting angina pectoris, myocardial infarction, S-T segment elevations, and ventricular ectopy has been described. The pathophysiology is unclear, although a direct cardiomyopathic effect from the release of vasoactive substances in the presence of 5-fluorouracil has been suggested.[102] It has been speculated that angina is a coronary artery spasm of the Prinzmetal's type, and it does respond to nitrates.[103] Cessation of therapy does not appear to be absolutely necessary, since patients who have such a syndrome can be pretreated with calcium antagonists known to prevent coronary artery spasm.

Asymptomatic bradycardia has been reported in about 30% of patients with ovarian cancer who have received taxol.[104] Other cardiac disturbances that have been reported in 5% of patients included atrioventricular conduction blocks, left bundle branch blocks, ventricular tachycardia, and symptoms of cardiac ischemia. In five patients who received both cisplatin and taxol, episodes of ventricular tachycardia occurred. The majority of taxol-related cardiac disturbances were not associated with clinical symptoms and were noted incidentally during continuous cardiac monitoring. The mechanism is unclear; however, it is speculated to be the result of the administration vehicle cremophor EL causing activation of selected cardiac-histamine receptors.[104]

Cardiac function should be evaluated throughout therapy for patients at high risk for cardiotoxicity or

TABLE 16-4 Combination Antiemetic Regimens

- When possible, antiemetics should be started 30 minutes prior to chemotherapy.
- When giving vesicant chemotherapeutic agents via a peripheral vein do not sedate patient until safe administration of the vesicant.
- All regimens designed for outpatient unless specified otherwise.

I. Low Emetic Potential
  A. Prochlorperazine 15 mg SR
     Lorazepam 1 mg po prn
  B. Thiethylperazine 10 mg po
     Dexamethasone 10 mg IV
  C. Droperidol 2–2.5 mg IV
     Dexamethasone 10 mg IV

II. Moderate–Severe Emetic Potential
  A. A • B • C • D (low dose)
     Lorazepam: 1 mg po or IV
     Diphenhydramine: 25–50 mg IV over 30 min
     Prochlorperazine: 15–20 mg IV over 30 min
     Dexamethasone: 10 mg IV

     At Hour of Sleep:
     Lorazepam: 1 mg po
     Diphenhydramine: 25 mg po
     Prochlorperazine: 15 mg SR po
  B. A • B • C • D (high dose)
     Lorazepam: 1–2 mg po q6 hr beginning 24 hr before morning of treatment
     Lorazepam: 1–2.5 mg IV
     Diphenhydramine: 50 mg IV
     Prochlorperazine: 20 mg IV infusion over 30 min q 3 hr × 2
     Dexamethasone: 20 mg IV

     At Hour of Sleep:
     Lorazepam: 2 mg po or SL
     Diphenhydramine: 50 mg po
     Prochlorperazine: 30 mg SR po and 15 mg SR in morning and q 12 hr prn
  C. Metoclopramide: 1–2 mg/kg 30 min prior and q2 hr for 2 additional doses
     Diphenhydramine: 50 mg IV
     Lorazepam: 1–2 mg po or IV
     Dexamethasone: 20 mg IV
  D. Metoclopramide: 1 mg/kg prior and q 2 hr for 2 additional doses
     Diphenhydramine: 50 mg IV
     Dexamethasone: 20 mg IV
     Diazepam: 5 mg IV
     Thiethylperazine: 10 mg supp q4–6 hr for 24 hr
  E. Metoclopramide: 1–2 mg IV 30 min prior and q2 hr for 2 additional doses
     Diphenhydramine: 50 mg IV
     Lorazepam: 1–2 mg po or IV
     Decadron: 20 mg IV
     continue
     Metoclopramide: 0.5 mg/kg po 4 × a day 1–4 days postchemotherapy
     Dexamethasone: 8 mg po bid days 1 & 2, 4 mg po bid days 3 & 4
  F. For inpatient receiving cisplatin daily for 5 days with 5FU or Vp_{16}:
     Prochlorperazine: 12 mg IV q8 hr with
     Diphenhydramine: 25 mg IV q8 hr

TABLE 16-4 Combination Antiemetic Regimens (continued)

     Lorazepam: 1–2 mg po q4–6 hr prn
     or
     Ondansetron: 0.15 mg/kg IV infusion over 15 min q8 hr × 5 days
     Lorazepam: 1 mg sublingually q4–6 hr
     Dexamethasone: 10 mg IV daily × 5, or 8 mg po bid days 1, 2, and 3 and 4 mg po bid days 4 and 5
  G. Ondansetron: 0.15 mg/kg IV infusion over 15 min, 30 min prior to chemotherapy and again in 2 hr
     Dexamethasone: 10–20 mg IV
     Lorazepam: 1–2 mg po

     At Hour of Sleep:
     Prochlorperazine: 15–30 mg SR
     Lorazepam: 1–2 mg po
     Diphenhydramine: 25–50 mg po

     This regimen works well for outpatient high-dose doxorubicin and cyclophosphamide or cisplatin and etoposide.
  H. Ondansetron: 32 mg IV infusion over 45 min, 30 min prior to chemotherapy (one dose only)
     Dexamethasone: 20 mg IV

     At Hour of Sleep:
     Prochlorperazine: 15–30 mg SR
     Lorazepam: 1–2 mg po
     Diphenhydramine: 25–50 mg po

those who will be receiving high dosages of an anthracycline. Methods to evaluate cardiac function include noninvasive monitoring with ECG, echocardiography, and radionuclide cardiography. An ejection fraction less than 55% of resting or a decrease of 5% or more from the resting value with exercise is considered abnormal. Further doses of chemotherapy are not recommended if the ejection fraction drops to 45% or less at rest or deteriorates to greater than 5% from baseline.[91] Although an endomyocardial biopsy can reveal damage to the myocytes prior to clinical detection, the procedure is costly and technically difficult and requires considerable expertise.

It has been recommended to obtain an ECG at 3 months and also at 1 year after the last anthracycline dose to determine cardiac status and risk for late abnormality. A radionuclide cardiac scan should be obtained with one of these tests to confirm cardiac status and to serve as a posttreatment baseline.[105,106] Low-risk patients have been defined as those receiving less than 200 mg/m² of an anthracycline and no mediastinal radiation or exhibiting no cardiac abnormality. Long-term follow-up has been recommended to include an ECG every 2–3 years, with a radionuclide cardiac scan with exercise stress every 5 years. High-risk patients are considered to have received more than 500 mg/m² of an anthracycline, to have received mediastinal radiation, or to have abnormal cardiac function. For long-term

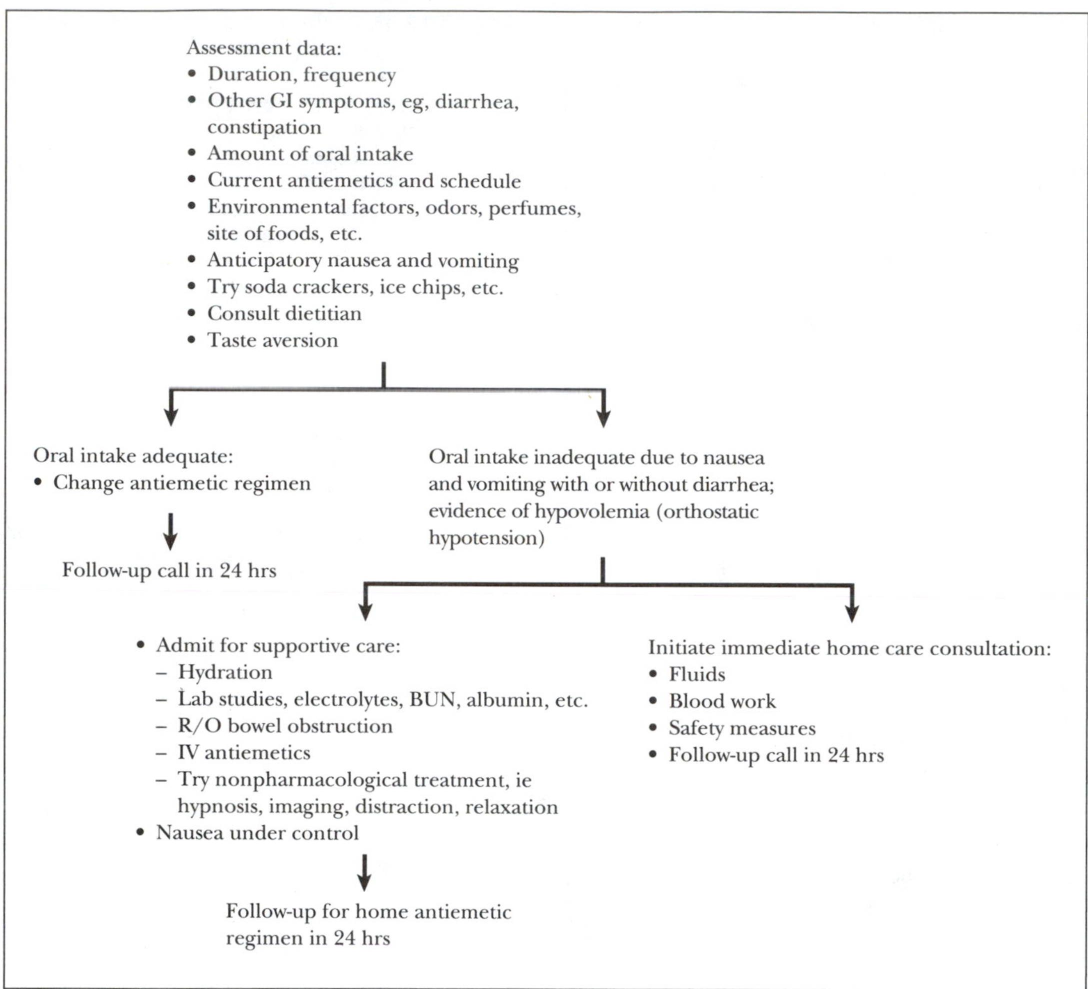

FIGURE 16-9 Nausea and vomiting phone triage flow sheet.

follow-up it has been recommended to include a minimum of an echocardiography yearly and a cardiac scan every 5 years if the patient remains asymptomatic.

Accurate documentation and monitoring of total cumulative dosages is essential. Cardiac assessment is imperative to evaluate for a third heart sound or gallop, which could indicate cardiac insufficiency. Cardiac monitoring may be necessary for administering high dosages of chemotherapy, such as with cyclophosphamide. Once the patient develops chronic cardiotoxicity, nursing interventions include teaching the patient about conservation of energy, managing fluid retention, and minimizing sodium in the diet. Supportive care with digitalis to enhance the cardiac output and with diuretics to manage fluid should also be instituted. Eventually the patient may need supplemental oxygen to relieve dyspnea. The degree of cardiac injury determines the limitations on activities of daily living the individual will experience. Few are prepared for this debilitating effect, and nurses must initiate interventions that will assist the patient and family in coping. Patients are also taught the importance of close cardiac follow-up, once the treatment is complete, to monitor for late cardiac effects (see Table 16-5).

Neurotoxicity

The clinical picture of chemotherapy-induced neurotoxicity can arise as a direct or an indirect damage to the central nervous system (CNS), peripheral nervous system, cranial nerves, or any combination of the three. The majority of patients experience temporary neurotoxicity; however, some will have permanent neurologic deficits. Significant neurotoxicity usually requires holding the treatment until the symptom resolves and reinstituting with a 50% dose reduction or discontinuing the drug.[107]

The central and peripheral nervous systems are protected against potentially neurotoxic effects by the blood–brain barrier and blood–nerve barriers. If intact, these barriers exclude most chemotherapeutic agents that are water soluble and also exclude relatively large molecules. Biopsies of damaged nerves from chemotherapy have demonstrated a mild decrease in

TABLE 16-5 Organ Toxicity of Chemotherapy Agents: Cardiotoxicity

Toxicity/ Symptoms	Grade	General Risk Factors	Chemotherapy Agent/Risk Factors	Mechanism of Damage	Protective/ Management Measures
• Tachycardia • Dyspnea • Nonproductive cough • Neck vein distention • Gallop rhythm • Rales • Pedal edema • Cardiomegaly • Dull or sharp precordial pain, may radiate to neck and shoulder • Friction rub (cardiac) • ST-T wave changes • Supraventricular • Tachyarrhythmias • T-wave flattening	*Cardiac Dysrhythmias:* 0 = None 1 = Asymptomatic, transient, requires no therapy 2 = Recurrent or persistent, no therapy required 3 = Requires treatment 4 = Requires monitoring. Hypotension, ventricular tachycardia, or fibrillation *Cardiac Function:* 0 = None 1 = Asymptomatic decline of resting ejection by less than 20% of baseline 2 = Asymptomatic, decline of resting ejection fraction by more than 20% of baseline 3 = Mild CHF, responsive to therapy 4 = Severe or refractory CHF	• Age • Cumulative dose • Schedule of drug administration • History of cardiac disease (ie, atherosclerosis, mitral valve prolapse, hypertension) • Use of combination drugs • Hepatic dysfunction • Prior mediastinum radiation • History of CHF • Prior anthracycline exposure	*Anthracyclines* • Doxorubicin (>550 mg/m^2) • Daunorubicin (>600 mg/m^2) • Dactinomycin • Doxorubicin-enhanced effect with: actinomycin, mitomycin, vincristine, melphalan, bleomycin cyclophosphamide *Mitoxantrone* (>160 mg/m^2) *Cyclophosphamide* • High dose (>144 mg/kg × 4 days) *5-Fluorouracil* *Taxol*	*Acute Changes:* • Hypereosinophilia of myocytes *Chronic Changes:* • Loss of contractile elements • Mitochondrial changes • Myocyte damage • Hemorrhagic myocardial necrosis • Fibrin deposition in interstitium • Coronary spasm of the Prinzmetal's type • Speculated to be related to Cremaphor EL, the administration vehicle that causes activation of selected cardiac histamine receptors	• Limit cumulative dose of doxorubicin to <550 mg/m^2 • Administer doxorubicin at lower doses more frequently • ECG before treatment • Radionuclide cardiac scan • Administer razoxane (ICRF-159) before anthracycline dose • Administer calcium channel blockers before anthracycline dose • Limit cumulative dose of daunorubicin to <600 mg/m^2 • Avoid alcohol, smoking, and cocaine use • Moderate exercise and low-fat, low-salt diet • Prevent thrombus with daily aspirin or Coumadin

the number of large-diameter myelinated nerve fibers, and ultrastructural studies have shown scattered degenerating nerve fibers both in the axon and in the myelin sheaths. Severity of neurotoxicity is usually dose related, with symptoms exhibited in a variable and unpredictable fashion.

The CNS is made up of collections of neurons and their connections organized into the brain and spinal cord areas. CNS damage primarily involves the cerebellum, which produces altered reflexes, unsteady gait, ataxia, and confusion. The peripheral nervous system is basically a set of communication channels located outside the CNS and consisting of the cranial and spinal nerves. Damage to the peripheral nervous system produces paralysis or loss of movement and sensation to those areas affected by the particular nerve. The autonomic nervous system (ANS) includes those peripheral nerves that regulate functions occurring automatically in the body, such as the cardiovascular, respiratory, and endocrine systems. Damage to the ANS causes ileus, impotence, or urinary retention.

Vincristine is well known for potential peripheral neuropathy characterized by myalgias, loss of the deep tendon reflex at the ankle, progressing to complete areflexia, distal symmetric sensory loss, motor weakness, foot drop, and muscle atrophy.[107] Autonomic neuropathy is characterized by ileus, constipation, impotence, urinary retention, or postural hypotension. The mechanism of damage is thought to involve disruption of the microtubules in the neural tissues, which thereby inhibits the mitotic spindle movements necessary for the mitosis phase of cellular reproduction.[108] Vincristine doses greater than 2 mg increase the risk of neurotoxicity.

Neuropathy related to cisplatin is reversible, although cases of persistent progression after the discontinuation of the drug have been reported.[109] Cisplatin affects the large-diameter fibers of the neural tissues, resulting in sensory changes. The earliest sign of peripheral neuropathy is decreased vibratory sense described as hand and feet paresthesias with the classic stocking glove distribution. Sensory loss occurs initially; and without dose modification, loss of the Achilles reflex, muscle weakness, and loss of the deep tendon reflex occurs. Symptoms of neuropathy are seen at cumulative doses of 300 mg/m^2 to 500 mg/m^2. As the neuropathy progresses, position sense is impaired, and a marked sensory ataxia develops.[110]

High tone loss is speculated to be related to the loss of hairs in the organ of Corti from cisplatin. Rapid drug delivery, simultaneous administration of aminoglycosides, and dehydration seem to increase the potential for ototoxicity. The loss can be reversed with discontinuation of the drug; however, permanent damage has been reported, resulting in the need for a hearing aid.[111] Carboplatin has minimal neurotoxicity at normal doses, exhibited as peripheral neuropathy and ototoxicity.[107]

Neurotoxicity characterized by metabolic encephalopathy manifested as blurred vision, subclinical electroencephalographic changes, urinary incontinence, motor system dysfunction, cranial nerve dysfunction, seizures, or irreversible coma has been reported in 5%–30% of patients treated with ifosfamide.[112] Signs have occurred within 2 hours of bolus administration and up to 28 days after therapy. Within 48–72 hours of cessation of ifosfamide, most abnormalities clear spontaneously.[113] Although the cause is not completely understood, the encephalopathy is thought to result from an accumulation of drug metabolites (chloracetaldehyde) causing direct CNS damage.

High-dose methotrexate (>1 g/m^2) occasionally causes encephalopathy after several courses, which usually is transient and reversible.[107] Intrathecal methotrexate may cause a chemical meningitis, with fever, headache, muscle rigidity, and cerebral spinal fluid leukocytosis. This is rare, but it occurs within hours of the intrathecal injection and resolves spontaneously.

5-FU may cause an acute cerebellar dysfunction, usually more common in the elderly. It is characterized by the rapid onset of gait ataxia, limb incoordination, dysarthria, nystagmus, and diplopia. Effects are reversible with drug withdrawal or dose reduction.

High-dose cytarabine can cause encephalopathy, leukoencephalopathy, and sometimes peripheral neuropathy with doses over 18 g/m^2. High doses increase the transport rate over the cell membranes, enhancing the intracellular drug concentrations and prolonging the cellular exposure to the drugs' metabolites. CNS toxicity usually occurs 5–7 days after the start of therapy.[114] Ocular toxicity (conjunctivitis, photophobia, burning, and decreased acuity), cerebellar, and cerebral dysfunction can also occur. Once the drug is stopped, the neurologic symptoms may resolve partially or completely.

Astute neurologic assessment is critical in patients receiving potentially neurotoxic agents. Sedatives, tranquilizers, and antiemetics, which are CNS depressants, must be used with caution since their usage may increase toxicity. In addition, other causes of these symptoms, such as electrolyte imbalances, metastasis, or other medical diseases, can cause similar effects. Neurotoxicity will affect patients by decreasing their mobility, ability for self-care, and ability to perform fine motor skills such as writing and buttoning a shirt. An occupational therapist may need to be consulted to help the patient adapt to loss of motor skills. Patients must be taught the importance of reporting any change in status, such as numbing and tingling of extremities. If neurologic deficits become severe, safety measures must be initiated to protect the patient from harm (see Table 16-6).

Pulmonary toxicity

Pulmonary toxicity usually is irreversible and progressive as a result of chemotherapy administration. The initial site of damage seems to be the endothelial cells, with an inflammatory-type reaction resulting in drug-induced pneumonitis. Another type of damage occurs as a result of an immunologic mechanism. Either the lung or the drug may act as the antigen in an allergic-type reaction.[115] Chronic exposure to chemotherapy causes an extensive alteration of the pulmonary parenchyma, with changes in the connective tissue, obliteration of alveoli, and dilatation of airspaces, known as "honey combing."[116] Continuous injury and repair result in restrictive lung disease, with a thickened, still interstitium, increased work of breathing, and a functionally reduced lung volume leading to impaired gas exchange. Hypoxemia results because oxygen does not diffuse in the damaged areas while perfusion continues.

Pulmonary toxicity usually presents clinically as dyspnea, unproductive cough, bilateral basilar rales, and tachypnea. The chest x-ray may be within normal limits, but can show a pattern of diffuse interstitial markings. Arterial blood gases reveal hypoxia with hypocapnia and respiratory alkalosis. The most sensitive pulmonary function test is the carbon monoxide diffusion capacity measurement that becomes abnormal before the onset of clinical symptoms. Other pulmonary function tests can show a restrictive pattern when pulmonary fibrosis has occurred. The best method to establish a histopathologic diagnosis is to obtain involved tissues by means of an open lung biopsy or a fiberoptic bronchoscopy. As a result, bacterial or fungal infections and metastasis can be ruled out.

Bleomycin is known to cause pulmonary toxicity. The incidence is 5% for a total cumulative dose of 450 units and 15% for higher dosages. Bleomycin is concentrated preferentially in the lung and is inactivated

TABLE 16-6 Organ Toxicity of Chemotherapy Agents: Neurotoxicity

Toxicity/ Symptoms	Grade	General Risk Factors	Chemotherapy Agent/Risk Factors	Mechanism of Damage	Protective/ Management Measures
Cerebellar: • Unsteady gait • Nystagmus • Ataxia • Dizziness • Seizures • Hemiparesis • Confusion • Coma *Autonomic:* • Ileus • Constipation • Impotence • Urinary retention • Postural hypotension *Peripheral/Cranial:* • Facial palsies • Diplopia • Paresthesia of hands and feet • Muscle atrophy • Foot drop • Loss of deep tendon reflexes • Areflexia • Sensory loss • Sensory perception loss • Hoarseness	*Neurocerebellar:* 0 = None 1 = Slight incoordination dysdiadokiness 2 = Intention tremor dysmetria, slurred speech 3 = Locomotor ataxia 4 = Cerebellar necrosis *Neurocortical:* 0 = None 1 = Mild somnolence or agitation 2 = Moderate somnolence or agitation 3 = Severe somnolence or agitation, confusion, disorientation, hallucination, aphasia 4 = Coma, seizures, psychosis *Neurosensory:* 0 = None 1 = Mild paresthesias, loss of deep tendon reflexes 2 = Mild or moderate objective sensory loss, moderate paresthesias 3 = Severe objective loss, or paresthesias that interfere with function *Neuromotor:* 0 = None 1 = Subjective weakness 2 = Mild objective weakness 3 = Objective weakness with impairment of function 4 = Paralysis	• Dosage • Cranial radiation • Intrathecal administration • Age • CNS depressants, ie, antiemetics, tranquilizers, and sedatives	*Ifosfamide:* • High doses • Cerebellar and cranial dysfunction	• Accumulation of drug metabolite (chloracetaldehyde) with direct CNS effect	
			Vincristine: • Dose related >2 mg/m² of unit dose • Hepatic dysfunction • Autonomic, peripheral dysfunction	• Disrupts microtubules in the neural tissues	• Place on bowel regimen • Oral diazepam 5 mg every 6 hr at the time of treatment, to manage muscle spasms
			Cisplatin: • Dose related • Renal dysfunction • Dehydration • Autonomic, peripheral dysfunction • Concurrent treatment with vincristine or etoposide	• Damages large fibers, resulting in sensory change • Damage/loss of inner hair cells in the organ of Corti	• Eliminate furosemide • Avoid concurrent administration of aminoglycosides • Audiometric testing for high risk • WR-2771 • Withhold therapy for severe toxicity, ie, muscle weakness or pain
			Methotrexate: • High dose (>1 g/m²) • Cerebellar dysfunction • Concurrent cranial radiotherapy • Intrathecal dose • Increases effect with cytarabine, daunorubicin, salicylates, sulfonamides, vinblastine, vincristine	• Demyelination of nerve fibers	• Neurologic recovery, start drug at 50% dose reduction • Monitor neurologic signs and symptoms • Monitor electrolytes • Institute safety measures
			Cytarabine: • High doses (>2 g/m²) • Cerebellar and peripheral effects		
			5-Fluorouracil: • Cerebellar dysfunction • Dose and schedule related		

by a hydrolase enzyme. This enzyme is relatively deficient in lung tissue as compared with other tissues, such as liver. These findings may explain the relative sensitivity of bleomycin to lung tissue causing: (1) early endothelial cell damage, (2) decrease in type I pneumocytes, with subsequent proliferation, and (3) migration of type II pneumocytes into alveolar spaces, inducing interstitial changes.[117] Following destruction of type I cells, repair is characterized by hyperplasia and dysplasia of the type II pneumocytes. Fibroblast proliferation, with subsequent pulmonary fibrosis, is probably the basis for irreversible changes induced by bleomycin.[117]

Cytarabine exerts a direct toxic effect on the pneumocytes and capillary endothelial cells to diminish the integrity of cell membranes and increase capillary permeability. A capillary leak syndrome, involving primarily the lung, occurs 2–21 days after the first dose, resulting in pulmonary edema and respiratory failure with features of adult respiratory disease (ARD). It appears to be related to high doses and continuous administration.[117]

Mitomycin C damage to the lung presents as diffuse alveolar damage with capillary leak and pulmonary edema. Incidence ranges from 3%–36%, occurring 6–12 months after therapy; however, occurrence may be after a brief exposure. If dyspnea occurs with a normal chest radiograph, it may be necessary to discontinue mitomycin from the treatment plan.[118]

Cyclophosphamide causes pulmonary toxicity in less than 1% of patients and is associated with high doses (120 mg/kg/day for 4 days). Histologic findings include endothelial swelling, pneumocyte dysplasia, edema, fibrosis, and fibroblast proliferation. The result of damage is alveolar hemorrhage and fibrin deposition.[115]

Carmustine inhibits lung glutathione disulfide reductase, which mediates the resultant cellular injury. Damage occurs after a long latency period, averaging 3 years, but may occur after only 6 weeks of therapy. High-dose carmustine has an incidence of 20%–30% when a cumulative dose of 1500 mg/m^2 is given. An insidious cough with dyspnea or sudden respiratory failure occurs. It has been suggested that this reaction may be more common when cyclophosphamide is given simultaneously.[115]

Methotrexate can also produce an acute or a chronic process related to endothelial injury.[119] Diffuse alveolar damage is characterized by the disappearance of type I pneumocytes, hyaline membrane formation, and the presence of inflammatory cells in the alveoli and interstitium. The incidence is less than 1%, with an acute onset of pulmonary edema producing ARDs or more gradual systemic toxicity, such as fever, chills, and malaise being present before the appearance of pulmonary symptoms. Radiographic features may be unique, with pleural effusion occurring alone or in conjunction with pulmonary infiltrates, peripheral consolidations, or chronic eosinophilic pneumonia. Discontinuation of the drug is not always required for recovery, and reinstitution of the drug may not result in recurring symptoms.[120]

Because lung damage usually is irreversible and progressive, it is imperative to detect evidence of pulmonary toxicity as early as possible. The causative agent may be discontinued or dose reduced to prevent further damage to lung tissue. High concentrations of inspired oxygen is toxic to the lungs, and the simultaneous administration of various chemotherapy drugs may induce lung damage. Nurses need to be aware of this phenomena and need to monitor the patient's oxygen saturation and breath sounds closely for early signs and symptoms of pulmonary toxicity.

When oxygen saturation is compromised due to restrictive lung damage, the patient experiences dyspnea on exertion or at rest. As a result, the patient will have an increased effort to perform simple activities of daily living. Nursing care is centered on teaching the patient to prioritize daily activities and to use breathing techniques such as pursed lips to lessen the effects of dyspnea. Supplemental oxygen therapy may be necessary to relieve the dyspnea. The family and patient must be taught how to administer the oxygen and what safety precautions to institute for oxygen therapy. Steroids are usually administered to lessen the pulmonary symptoms. To prevent further complications, the nurse must also teach the patient how to mobilize secretions by maintaining an adequate fluid intake and performing effective cough and deep breathing techniques (see Table 16-7).

Hepatotoxicity

Chemotherapy agents can cause a variety of hepatotoxic reactions. The initial site of damage seems to be the parenchymal cells. Obstruction to hepatic bloodflow results in fatty changes, hepatocellular necrosis, cholestasis, hepatitis, and venoocclusive disease (VOD). Hepatotoxicity usually is diagnosed initially by transient elevations of the hepatic enzymes during treatment that can progress to hepatomegaly, jaundice, and abdominal pain. Unless extensive fibrosis or necrosis has occurred, hepatotoxicity is reversible. For patients with hepatic dysfunction, the drug dose may need to be reduced or eliminated from the treatment plan.[121]

The incidence of VOD following high-dose chemotherapy in preparation for BMT is 20%, with a 50% mortality rate. Risk factors include increased age, hepatitis, and elevated SGOT before BMT. Clinical signs of VOD include insidious weight gain and jaundice that precede the development of abdominal pain, hepatomegaly, ascites, encephalopathy, and elevated bilirubin and SGOT laboratory values. VOD has also been documented after exposure to conventional or extremely high doses of a wide variety of chemotherapeutic agents, such as 6-mercaptopurine, cytarabine, thioguanine, dacarbazine, cyclophosphamide, carmustine, lomustine, busulfan, and mitomycin.[122]

TABLE 16-7 Organ Toxicity of Chemotherapy Agents: Pulmonary Toxicity

Toxicity/ Symptoms	Grade	General Risk Factors	Chemotherapy Agent/Risk Factors	Mechanism of Damage	Protective/ Management Measures
• Low-grade fever • Nonproductive cough • Dyspnea • Tachycardia • Diffuse basilar crackles • Wheezing • Pleural rub • Fatigue • Malaise • Chest pain • Night sweats • Tachypnea • Cyanosis	*Dyspnea:* 0 = None 1 = Asymptomatic with abnormal PFTs 2 = Dyspnea on exertion 3 = Dyspnea at normal activity 4 = Dyspnea at rest *Pulmonary Fibrosis:* 0 = Normal 1 = Radiographic changes, no symptoms 2 = N/A 3 = Changes with symptoms *Pulmonary Edema:* 0–2 = None 3 = Radiographic changes and diuretics required 4 = Requires intubation *Pneumonitis (Non-infectious):* 0 = Normal 1 = Radiographic change, symptoms do not require steroids 2 = Steroids required 3 = Oxygen required 4 = Requires assisted ventilation *Pleural Effusion:* 0 = None 1–4 = Present *ARDs:* 0 = None 1 = Mild 2 = Moderate 3 = Severe 4 = Life threatening	• Age • Preexisting lung disease, ie, COPD, TB • History of smoking • Cumulative dose • Long-term therapy • Mediastinal radiation • High inspired concentration of oxygen	*Bleomycin:* • Synergistic with vincristine • Cumulative dose >450 mg/m² • Oxygen exposure >50%	• Initial injury to capillary endothelium cells • Necrosis of type I epithelial cells • Hypertrophy of type II alveolar pneumocytes • Pulmonary fibrosis	• Assess for risk factors • Obtain baseline pulmonary function tests • Monitor cumulative dose • Limit cumulative dose • Limit oxygen to keep arterial PO_2 >60 mm Hg • Discontinue drug if dyspnea occurs • Assess for pulmonary symptoms • Administer steroids and oxygen • Monitor activities to minimize energy • Stop or reduce dose of drug • Fluid restriction • Administer diuretics • Follow-up with pulmonary function tests
			Mitomycin: • History of cyclophosphamide and/or methotrexate administration • Oxygen concentrations >50%	• Hypersensitivity reaction or immune complex related • Damage similar to bleomycin • Increased effect with VM-26, vincristine	
			Carmustine: • Dose related (>1500 mg/m²) • Concurrent administration with cyclophosphamide	• Inhibition of glutathione reductase in alveolar macrophages	
			Busulfan	• Hyperplasia and dysplasia of the type II pneumocytes	
			Cyclophosphamide: • High dose >120 mg/kg/day × 4 days	• Alveolar hemorrhage and fibrin deposition • Increased effect with cisplatin, VM-26, vincristine	
			Methotrexate	• Capillary leak syndrome, pulmonary edema • Interstitial pneumonitis	
			Cytarabine: • High doses (5 g/m²)	• Capillary leak syndrome	

VOD involves the partial or complete occlusion of the branches of the hepatic veins by endophlebitis and thrombosis. Normal hepatic circulation allows sinusoids to empty into the terminal hepatic venule through the small pores that penetrate the endothelial lining. When these pores are obstructed, the fluid and cellular debris become trapped, and eventually fibrosis of the venous walls occurs. Central hepatocellular necrosis occurs as well. Vascular engorgement results in hepatomegaly and ascites. As the hepatocytes degenerate and necrose, liver serum enzyme levels become elevated, which can lead to liver necrosis, fibrosis, and portal hypertension.[123,124]

In clinical studies pentoxifylline (PTX) has been shown to have a marked effect on cell mediators of inflammation and tissue injury. The therapeutic effect of PTX is to stimulate vascular endothelial production of noninflammatory prostaglandins (E and I series), enhancing regional bloodflow and promoting thrombolysis. These prostaglandins are responsible for the autoregulation of bloodflow in several organs, including the liver, promoting diuresis and maintenance of bloodflow. Studies suggest that PTX might preserve hepatic function and prevent VOD in the BMT population.[125]

Liver toxicity induced by high-dose methotrexate is transient and usually does not result in chronic liver disease. Elevation of hepatic enzyme levels is common, rising with successive courses and tending to be higher in patients treated on a daily schedule than those treated on intermittent schedules. All abnormalities usually resolve within 1 month following cessation of methotrexate therapy.[126]

High-dose cytarabine may induce intrahepatic cholestasis, possibly as a result of injury to the hepatocyte transport system. Changes are reversible; therefore they do not appear to limit cytarabine use.[127]

Fluorodeoxyuridine, usually administered as a continuous arterial dose, can cause chemical hepatitis, with rises in transaminases, alkaline phosphatase, and serum bilirubin levels. Stricture of intrahepatic or extrahepatic bile ducts can also occur. Toxicity appears to be both time and dose dependent. Liver function usually normalizes when the drug is discontinued. However, the development of biliary sclerosis is irreversible.[128]

Hepatocellular or cholestatic liver disease occurs with the administration of 6-mercaptopurine in daily doses exceeding 2 mg/kg. Histologic pattern includes features of intrahepatic cholestasis and parenchymal cell necrosis. Moderate elevations occur in transaminases, alkaline phosphatase, and serum bilirubin, with episodes of jaundice occurring 30 days after initiation of therapy.[121]

Amsacrine is concentrated in the liver, where it undergoes conjugation to glutathione and is excreted in the bile. Its half-life is prolonged in patients with hepatic dysfunction manifested as elevations in bilirubin and alkaline phosphatase values. A 40% dose reduction in patients with bilirubin greater than 2 mg/100 ml is recommended.[129]

Few guidelines exist for the use of drugs when hepatic dysfunction is present. Known hepatoxic drugs must be avoided when liver test results are abnormal. Impaired liver function delays excretion and results in increased accumulation in the plasma and tissues, especially for drugs such as doxorubicin, vincristine, and vinblastine, which are excreted primarily by the liver into the bile. It has been recommended not to administer or to reduce the dose of these agents if the serum bilirubin is between 1.5 and 3 mg/dl. If the SGOT is between 60 and 180 international units, the drug should be reduced by 50%.[121]

Hepatic toxicity is uncommon, but it can be a serious consequence of chemotherapy administration, ranging from transient enzyme elevations to permanent cirrhosis. Because there are many disease- and treatment-related factors that can be hepatotoxic, it is difficult to attribute hepatic toxicity definitely to specific agents. During chemotherapy administration, the nurse monitors liver function tests closely, since enzymatic changes may be the first clinical evidence of hepatotoxicity. Third spacing (the shift of fluid from the vascular space to the interstitial space) can occur as a result of hepatotoxicity. Signs of fluid shift are decreased blood pressure, increased pulse rate, low central venous pressure, decreased urine output, increased specific gravity, low levels of serum albumin, and hemoconcentration.[124] Albumin is administered to replace the plasma protein and hopefully assist with absorbtion of the fluid. Fluid restriction minimizes third spacing, which enhances renal bloodflow, decreases systemic congestion, and improves patient comfort. Other supportive care measures include diuretics, decreased protein intake, lactulose, and emotional support (see Table 16-8).

Hemorrhagic cystitis

Hemorrhagic cystitis is a bladder toxicity resulting from cyclophosphamide and ifosfamide therapy. Hemorrhagic cystitis ranges from microscopic hematuria to frank bleeding, necessitating invasive local intervention with instillation of scelerosing agents. Symptoms range from transient irritative urination, dysuria, suprapubic pain to life-threatening hemorrhage. Transient cystitis has an early onset and short duration due to the direct effect of the deposition of acrolein, a by-product of metabolism, on the urothelium.[130]

After oral or intravenous administration, cyclophosphamide is metabolized by hepatic microsomal enzymes to hydroxycyclophosphamide and later by target cells to phosphamide mustard (active) and acrolein (urinary metabolite). The binding of acrolein to the bladder mucosa results in inflammation and ulceration. Approximately 10% of people receiving cyclophosphamide experience microscopic hematuria.[122] Early diagnosis is accomplished by urine dipstick or visual observation of red-tinged urine. If necessary, a confirmed diagnosis can be accomplished by cystoscopy, which shows dis-

TABLE 16-8 Organ Toxicity of Chemotherapy Agents: Hepatotoxicity

Toxicity/ Symptoms	Grade	General Risk Factors	Chemotherapy Agent/Risk Factors	Mechanism of Damage	Protective/ Management Measures
• Elevated bilirubin, LDH, SGOT, alkaline, phosphatase, SGPT • Chemical hepatitis • Jaundice • Ascites • Decreased albumin • Cirrhosis • Hepatomegaly • Right upper quadrant pain • Fatigue • Anorexia • Nausea • Decreased clotting factor synthesis • Hyperpigmentation of skin	*Bilirubin:* 0–1 = Normal 2 = <1.5 3 = 1.5–3.0 4 = >3.0 *SGOT/SGPT:* 0 = Normal 1 = <2.5 2 = 2.6–5.0 3 = 5.1–20 4 = >20 *Alkaline Phosphatase:* 0 = Normal 1 = 2.5 2 = 2.6–5.0 3 = 5.1–20 4 = >20 *Liver Clinical:* 0–2 = No change 3 = Precoma 4 = Hepatic coma	• Prior liver damage, eg, hepatitis • Dose • Diabetes mellitus • Tumor involvement • Irradiation of liver • Alcoholism • Liver infections • Concurrent administration of hepatotoxic drugs, eg, phenothiazines • Age • Hepatic dysfunction • Total bilirubin >2 mg/100 ml	• Methotrexate • 6-Mercaptopurine • Cytarabine • Fluorodoxyuridine • Nitrosoureas • Eptoposide, high dose • Cisplatin, high dose • L-Asparaginase • Amsacrine • Cyclophosphamide, high dose • Doxorubicin • Vincristine • Vinblastine	*Direct Toxic Effects:* • Parenchymal cell damage • Intrahepatic cholestasis • Hepatic fibrosis • Fatty changes	• Pentoxycline • Reduce dose in presence of liver dysfunction for drugs metabolized in liver, eg, vincaalkaloids or doxorubicin • Avoid alcohol intake • Monitor liver function tests • If bilirubin >1.5 mg, reduce dose by 50% • If bilirubin >3.0 mg, reduce dose by 75%

crete bleeding capillaries or diffuse mucosal ulceration, hemorrhage, and necrosis.

When hemorrhagic cystitis develops, drug therapy probably should be discontinued. In many patients discontinuation will lead to amelioration of the symptoms without sequela; however, microhematuria can continue long after discontinuing cyclophosphamide.[130] When therapy is not stopped, up to 55% of patients have persistent symptoms. Extensive chronic bleeding and mucosal inflammation can produce long-term cystitis, irreversible bladder fibrosis, bladder contraction, and an increased risk for bladder cancer.[131]

In an attempt to prevent cyclophosphamide-induced hemorrhagic cystitis, several drugs have been investigated to decrease this toxicity by inactivating acrolein within the bladder. Intravesical instillation of N-acetylcysteine, a thiol compound, may produce sulfhydryl complexes and subsequent detoxification of acrolein. Prostaglandin E2 and sucralfate may have therapeutic roles as intravesical agents for acrolein inactivation. In high doses, mesna has been successful in protecting the bladder from the harmful effects of acrolein.[131]

Ifosfamide has a slower rate of metabolic activation into acrolein, allowing larger dosages to be administered as compared to cyclophosphamide. Mesna, a uroprotectant, contains a sulfhydryl group believed to bind acrolein within the urinary collecting system and detoxifies ifosfamide. Mesna is administered before ifosfamide administration and then intermittently up to 24 hours afterward to protect the bladder.[131]

Protection of the bladder from either drug focuses on hyperhydration, frequent voiding, and diuresis. If cystitis occurs, the treatment includes bladder irrigations through a three-way Foley catheter to clear developing clots. The various solutions that cause a protein precipitate to form over the bleeding surfaces include saline, potassium aluminum sulfate, silver nitrate, and formalin. Vasopressins such as amino caproic acid may be administered intravenously or orally to decrease clotting. Cystoscopy may be necessary to cauterize bleeders, if the bladder irrigations were ineffective in controlling the bleeding. As a last resort, a cystectomy may be necessary.

During administration of chemotherapy agents, the nurse should monitor the urine for blood, through dipsticking or observation. Strict intake and output measures are imperative to ensure minimal contact of arcolein with the bladder mucosa. The patient must be taught to maintain adequate hydration and to void frequently. If feasible, cyclophosphamide should be administered early in the day so the patient can drink fluids and void frequently without interruption of sleep. Insertion of a Foley catheter may be necessary when high doses of cyclophosphamide are administered, to ensure that the agent is being cleared from the bladder continuously (see Table 16-9).

Nephrotoxicity

Nephrotoxicity is a dose-limiting side effect of some chemotherapeutic agents. Serious fluid and electrolyte imbalances that can progress to renal failure are the result of the direct and indirect effects of these agents on the kidney. Prevention of nephrotoxicity primarily involves aggressive hydration, urinary alkalization, diuresis, and careful monitoring of laboratory values. The hospitalized patient receiving other potentially nephrotoxic drugs, such as aminoglycosides, should be assessed prior to administering the agent. For patients with preexisting renal disease or who exhibit early signs of renal toxicity, the dosage may need to be reduced or the agent eliminated from the treatment plan.

Many chemotherapy agents are both metabolized and excreted by the kidneys; others are merely excreted as metabolites or as unchanged drugs. The manner in which chemotherapy damages the kidney varies from direct renal cell damage to an obstructive nephropathy as a result of precipitate formation. Renal failure, acid/base disorders, or electrolyte abnormalities may also occur as a result of tumor lysis syndrome or uric acid nephropathy.[132]

Cisplatin can cause a mild to severe nephrotoxicity, with specific damage to the proximal and distal tubules. Platinum metal chelates in the renal tubules cause direct damage to the proximal tubular cells, damaging the tubular basement membranes, and can cause focal tubular necrosis.[133] Acute damage can occur within 3–21 hours after cisplatin administration, as evidenced by renal enzyme changes when precautions are not taken.[134,135] To avoid toxicity, patients should receive vigorous saline hydration of 1–2 liters as well as diuresis during therapy.

The use of mannitol in facilitating and inducing diuresis is a means of ensuring adequate urine flow. Mannitol possibly prevents immediate binding of cisplatin onto the renal tubules. Loop diuretics such as furosemide must be used with caution, since an increase in cisplatin toxicity has been reported.[136] Frequent determinations of renal function should be obtained, and if the creatinine clearance falls to less than 50 mg/ml, the drug should be withheld until renal function improves. Daily magnesium supplementation is indicated during cisplatin therapy, and electrolyte levels should be monitored frequently.[136]

The radioprotectant WR 2721 has been used in phase III trials with cisplatin. Data suggest that this compound provides protection against nephrotoxicity, ototoxicity, and neurotoxicity. WR 2721 is administered as a 15-minute infusion before cisplatin is administered. Reported side effects include flushing, nausea, vomiting, somnolence, and hypotension.[137] Another compound being used as a cisplatin chemoprotectant agent is diethyldithiocarbamate (DDTC). This compound reportedly removes tissue-bound platinum through chelation, without reversing cisplatin's antitumor activity. Protection is provided against nephrotoxicity, bone marrow suppression, and GI toxicity. DDTC is administered intravenously and can cause flushing, diaphoresis, chest discomfort, and uneasiness if given rapidly.[138]

TABLE 16-9 Organ Toxicity of Chemotherapy Agents: Hemorrhagic Cystitis

Toxicity/ Symptoms	Grade	General Risk Factors	Chemotherapy Agent/Risk Factors	Mechanism of Damage	Protective/ Management Measures
• Gross hematuria • Dysuria, urgency • Suprapubic pain	0 = None 1 = Micro only 2 = Gross, no clots 3 = Gross, with clots 4 = Requires transfusion	• Dose related • Pelvic radiation	*Cyclophosphamide:* • High dose (>2.5 g)	• Drug metabolite acrolein deposits and damages bladder mucosa *Synergistic Effect:* • Cisplatin • VM-26 • Vincristine	• Vigorous hydration • Frequent emptying of bladder, especially at night • Monitor urine for blood • 3-way Foley irrigation with saline, alum, or formaldehyde • Administer amino caproic acid IV or po
			Ifosfamide: • Single high dose vs multiple dose		• Mesna given in a dose of 20%–30% of ifosfamide q 4hr × 3

Standard doses of methotrexate are not associated with renal toxicity unless the patient has preexisting renal dysfunction. High doses (>1 g/m^2) can cause an obstructive nephropathy from precipitation of methotrexate or its metabolites (7-OH mtx) in the renal tubules. In general, urinary alkalization to maintain a urine pH greater than 7 with simultaneous administration of sodium bicarbonate or diamox prevents precipitate formation, permitting high-dose therapy.

Streptozocin in doses over 1.5 g/m^2 is associated with renal dysfunction in more than 65% of patients. Characteristically, streptozocin causes a tubulointerstitial nephritis and tubular atrophy due to direct damage of the tubules. This toxicity is manifested by hypokalemia, proteinuria, increased BUN, and increased creatinine levels.[134] Renal function tests and creatinine clearance test should be obtained before beginning streptozocin therapy. Patients who develop an elevation of serum creatinine, even if it subsequently returns to normal, are cautioned against receiving further streptozocin, since severe toxicity may occur.

Lomustine and carmustine can cause a delayed renal failure months or years following therapy. Azotemia and proteinuria are manifested, followed by progressive renal failure, often requiring dialysis. It appears that the incidence of renal failure increases dramatically after a total dose of 1500 mg/m^2.[139]

Mitomycin C has been associated with a syndrome of renal failure and microangiopathic hemolytic anemia. This toxicity occurs in approximately 20% of patients who have received a cumulative dose of 100 mg or more after approximately 6 months of therapy and is characterized by an abrupt onset of microangiopathic hemolytic anemia, thrombocytopenia, azotemia, proteinuria, and hematuria. It generally is reversible.[140]

Nurses play a vital role in preventing nephrotoxicity. Preventive management includes aggressive hydration, diuresis, urinary alkalinization, and careful monitoring of urine output. Renal function tests, especially creatinine clearance, should be monitored before administering nephrotoxic drugs. Patients that must receive other nephrotoxic drugs, such as aminoglycosides, should be monitored closely for early signs and symptoms of toxicity. Assessment of renal function should continue throughout treatment and periodically after the completion of therapy (see Table 16-10).

Gonadal toxicity

From the beginning of the use of chemotherapy in the treatment of cancer, gonadal failure, infertility, and premature menopause have been reported as consequences of chemotherapy. The likelihood that chemotherapy will affect a patient's fertility depends in part on the patient's gender, age, and the specific drugs. In contrast to males, the age of female patients is an important predictor of treatment-induced sterility. The aging ovary has progressively fewer germ cells, which are not replaced. Therefore, women over the age of 30 are less likely to regain ovarian function because they have fewer oocytes.[141–143] Treatment-induced gonadal function is quantified by elevation in the gonadotropins, follicle-stimulating hormone (FSH), and lutenizing hormone (LH), which reflects the efforts of the hypothalamic–pituitary axis to stimulate the injured gonads to function normally.[143,144]

Cycle-nonspecific drugs such as alkylating agents are the most detrimental to fertility.[143] Effects on fertility are presumably due to the constant mitotic cycles essential for spermatogenesis, compared with the relative inactivity of oocyte formation. Therefore the testes are more susceptible to injury from alkylating agents than the ovaries. Alkylating agents are most commonly associated with compromised fertility, and combination regimens have a greater effect than single agents. Busulfan causes amenorrhea, atrophic endometrium, and symptoms associated with menopause. Nitrogen mustard, chlorambucil, melphalan, and procarbazine cause ovarian atrophy. Cyclophosphamide elevates FSH levels, pointing to a direct toxic effect on the ovaries.[145]

It is difficult to define the effects of chemotherapy on gonadal function in children. Frequently, childhood cancers are treated with multimodality therapy combining chemotherapy and radiation therapy. In addition, children are in various stages of sexual and growth development. Presently, long-term follow-up is being conducted but has not been conclusive on long-term gonadal functions.

The testes of adult men are particularly vulnerable to chemotherapeutic agents. A progressive dose-related depletion of the germinal epithelial lining of the seminiferous tubule results in the disappearance of the spermatocytes and spermatogonia, leaving only Sertoli cells. Drug-induced testicular damage results in azospermia, oligospermia, and abnormalities of semen volume, motility, and sperm forms in postpubertal men. The incidence and length of time for recovery of spermatogenesis depend on the patient's age and the total drug dose. For example, cyclophosphamide produces azoospermia at a total dose of 9 grams, with a recovery of normal spermatogenesis in 100% within 31 months of treatment.[141,144] Male patients who desire to preserve childbearing ability may elect to utilize semen preservation, along with subsequent artificial insemination or in vitro fertilization.[146]

Chemotherapy affects fertility by injuring the germinal epithelium of the gonad. It is clear that prepubertal ovaries are profoundly affected histologically after chemotherapy. Ova become nonfunctional by direct injury or indirect injury resulting from loss of supporting follicular cells. These changes include focal stromal fibrosis, follicular maturation arrest, and reduction in numbers of ova despite exposure to lower total doses of drugs.[147–149] Women who develop amenorrhea after cytotoxic therapy often experience hot flashes, with menopausal blood levels of FSH, LH, and estradiol.

Over time, the more serious consequences of premature estrogen deprivation, such as osteoporosis and vaginal atrophy, can develop, but if not contraindicated can be effectively treated with hormonal replace-

TABLE 16-10 Organ Toxicity of Chemotherapy Agents: Nephrotoxicity

Toxicity/ Symptoms	Grade	General Risk Factors	Chemotherapy Agent/Risk Factors	Mechanism of Damage	Protective/ Preventive Measures	General Management
• Increased BUN, creatinine • Oliguria • Azotemia • Proteinuria • Decreased creatinine clearance • Hyperuricemia • Hypomagnesemia • Hypocalcemia	*Creatinine:* 0 = WNL 1 = <1.5 2 = 1.5–3.0 3 = 3.1–6.0 4 = >6.0 *Proteinuria:* 0 = No change 1 = 1+ or <3 g/liter 2 = 2–3+ or 3–10 g/liter 3 = 4+ or >10 g/liter 4 = Nephrotic syndrome *Hematuria:* 0 = None 1 = Micro 2 = Gross, no clots 3 = Gross, with clots 4 = Requires transfusion *BUN mg%:* 0 = WNL <20 1 = 21–30 2 = 31–50 3 = >50	• Age • Dose of agent • Preexisting disease of kidneys • Nutritional status • Duration of cancer therapy • Concurrent: Aminoglycoside therapy Amphotericin-B • Renal damage • Dehydration • Large tumor mass • Ileal conduits	*Nitrosoureas:* • Cumulative dose of 1200 mg/m^2 for carmustine and lomustine	• Direct cell damage in glomerulus • Chronic interstitial nephritis • Tubular atrophy	These following four measures apply to all drugs • Monitor renal function tests • Saline diuresis • Hydrate patient (3000 ml/day) • Decrease uric acid production with allopurinol	• Substitute analog drug • Reduce dose for creatinine clearance (normal 125 ml/min) *30–60 ml/min:* • Cisplatin—50% • Methotrexate—50% • Mitomycin—75% • Nitrosoureas—hold dose *10–30 ml/min:* • Cisplatin—hold dose • Mitomycin—75% *<10 ml/min:* • Cyclophosphamide—50% • Mitomycin—50%
			Mitomycin C: • Increased effect with vincristine and VM-26	• Direct cell damage in glomerulus • Microangiopathic hemolytic anemia • Tubular atrophy		
			Anthracyclines: • High dose (1.5 g/m^2/wk)	• Diffuse tubulointerstitial nephritis		
			Streptozotocin: • Dose (>1.5 g/m^2/wk)	• Tubulointerstitial nephritis • Tubular atrophy	• Stop drug if creatinine does not return to baseline	
			Cisplatin: • Multiple doses (>50 mg/m^2) • High dose • Increased effect with cyclophosphamide	• Direct cell damage in tubules • Necrosis of proximal and distal renal tubules	• Diuresis with mannitol • Administer WR-2721 15 min before administration • Administer DDTC	
			Methotrexate: • High dose (>1 g/m^2) • Enhanced effect with cisplatin	• Precipitation of metabolites in the acid environment of the urine • Obstructive nephropathy	• Maintain alkalinization of urine pH >7 • Administer leucovorin • Administer bicarbonate • Avoid vitamin C	

ment.[144] With failing ovary syndrome, there is a period of months or years of erratic ovarian function, with many months of amenorrhea interspersed with occasional normal menstrual periods.[143] Depending on the woman's age as well as the type and total dose of chemotherapy, ovarian function may resume after a period of time. Because the onset of chemotherapy-related ovarian failure is age related and progressive, a young woman might remain amenorrheic for several years and then begin to menstruate sporadically and even conceive during these cycles.[145,147] Attempts have been made to preserve ovarian function during chemotherapy through the use of oral estrogens, which produce negative feedback to the hypothalamic–pituitary axis, thereby decreasing gonadotropic stimulation of the ovaries.

For women who have conceived and must receive chemotherapy, few complications have been reported, provided the drugs are given in the second and third trimester.[148,149] The antimetabolites and alkylating agents administered during the first trimester cause teratogenesis. Even though chemotherapy agents are known to cross the placental barrier, second- or third-trimester chemotherapy exposure may result in low birth weight or prematurity.

In general, patients surviving cancer may be advised to wait at least 2 years after completion of therapy before attempting parenthood. This allows plenty of time for the elimination of chromosome breaks and damaged germ cells.[148–150] In women who conceive after receiving chemotherapy, the incidence of spontaneous abortion and fetal abnormality is not increased.[150]

Although many patients experience reproductive dysfunction during chemotherapy, information is still needed regarding the possibility of conception and the effects that could occur during chemotherapy administration. Birth control pills can be used if the patient does not have a cancer that is hormonally sensitive and the risk of cardiovascular side effects is not a concern. Intrauterine devices are not recommended when the patient is experiencing myelosuppression, since bleeding or infection could occur. Diaphragms, sponges, vaginal inserts, and condoms require careful attention to the insertion technique and personal hygiene after usage. A water-soluble lubricant may be needed if vaginal dryness is being experienced prior to intercourse.

Accurate information can make a significant difference in the patient's ability to deal with sexual concerns regarding chemotherapy. In general, most chemotherapy agents are excreted from the body in the first 72 hours following administration. Patients need to be instructed to use condoms and to avoid oral sex during this period in the event that the semen or vaginal secretions contain chemotherapy metabolites.

Female patients may need instruction on coping with ovarian dysfunction and guidance on managing hot flashes and vaginal dryness. Although high-dose chemotherapy may affect the male's ability to achieve or maintain an erection, usually this is not a problem. However, all patients may need to be counseled about decreased libido due to fatigue or the lack of sexual desire. Providing information that chemotherapy will not be transferred by kissing, hugging, or cuddling is reassuring and helps patients come to terms with feelings about cancer and sexuality.

SECONDARY/THERAPY-RELATED CANCERS

One of the most serious long-term consequences of cancer is that the treatment intended to cure the patient may contribute to the occurrence of a second malignancy.[151] *Second malignancy* refers to a new neoplasm that has developed after treatment of the initial or primary cancer.[152,153] It implies that the new neoplasm is related in some way to treatment that was not only cytotoxic but also carcinogenic. Although the risk for a secondary cancer is small, treatment for the primary cancer usually outweighs that risk.[151,154]

Therapy-related malignancies generally have a poor prognosis, and treatment is often unsuccessful. The mechanism of oncogenesis after treatment remains unclear but could relate to interactions between immunosuppressive factors, direct cellular damage produced by fibrotic tissue changes, or carcinogenic effects from other environmental carcinogens. Lethal damage to the neoplastic cell is the obvious intent of chemotherapy; yet if cellular damage is not repaired in the normal cell, malignant transformation and/or mutation can occur.[155] Long-term survivors of Hodgkin's disease who have received both chemotherapy and radiation have the highest incidence of secondary malignancies.[156] Other risk factors include the primary neoplasm, the natural history of the disease, the type of chemotherapy, the cumulative dose of the agent, the age of the patient during chemotherapy administration, the patient's immune status, and the patient's environment.[157,158]

The alkylating agents, nitrosoureas, and procarbazine are the agents most implicated in chemotherapy-related malignancies.[157–159] Although all alkylating agents have been implicated in producing a myelodysplastic disease or acute leukemia, melphalan is probably the most potent leukemogenic agent. Alkylating agents cause the two strands of DNA to become cross-linked so that DNA replication is inhibited. Due to a change in the structural configuration of guanine, miscoding of thymidine may occur, leading to abnormal base pairing.[151] Sister chromatid exchanges frequently occur after the use of alkylating agents and may be responsible for mutagenesis. Chromosomes 5 and 7 are involved in 90% of those with cytogenetic abnormalities. Observed deletions of all or part of those chromosomes strongly support the diagnosis of chemotherapy-associated acute leukemia. In addition, damage to the stem cells in the bone marrow by alkylating agents may result in the emergence of leukemic clones.[157]

After receiving alkylating agents, patients have a 1.6%–2.3% risk of developing acute nonlymphocytic leukemia (ANLL) within 10 years, peaking at 2–3 years.[159] Older patients have been found to have shorter intervals between treatment and preleukemic changes. This may be related in part to a declining immune status associated with age combined with long-term immunosuppressive effects of alkylating agents.[151]

The schedule of chemotherapy administration may have some bearing on the development of leukemia.[152] Patients with multiple myeloma who received intravenous doses of melphalan, carmustine, and cyclophosphamide had a rate of 0.7% in developing leukemia as compared to 2.6% of patients who received daily oral doses of melphalan. Multiple myeloma patients developed acute myelocytic or myelomonocytic leukemia at a risk of 2.5% at 5 years and 9.2% at 10 years.[157] Woman receiving melphalan for ovarian cancer are two or three times more likely to develop leukemic disorders than those receiving cyclophosphamide.[160] The interval between the onset of cyclophosphamide therapy and the occurrence of bladder, kidney, ureter, or urethra malignancy averaged more than 5 years, with a range of 1–12 years.[152]

Maintenance chemotherapy with chlorambucil and the use of mechlorethamine for induction seems to be a major contributor to the development of acute leukemia in Hodgkin's patients. The 10-year actual risk of ANLL was 10.9% in a series of 172 patients with Hodgkin's disease given radiation and chemotherapy.[155–157] This risk was 5.6% for patients under 40 years of age and 30.9% for those over 40. Risk also increased in direct proportion to the cumulative dose of alkylating agents as well as combination regimens.

Relative risks for developing leukemia after treatment for breast cancer with cyclophosphamide was 1.3%–2.7% and up to 30% with the use of melphalan and radiotherapy.[160,161] Increased risk was confined to women older than 50 years of age. It has been reported that etoposide may induce a leukemia with the morphologic and cytogenetic features of acute monoblastic leukemia rather than those seen with ANLL.[158] Patients with germ cell tumors treated with high-dose etoposide, cisplatin, and bleomycin are at an increased risk for developing myelodysplastic syndrome and acute myelocytic leukemia.[162]

Although the number of patients who develop a second malignancy is small, patients must be taught the importance of continual follow-up for the rest of their lives after treatment. The nurse may need to encourage patients to implement lifestyle changes to improve their health. The American Cancer Society warning signs of cancer should be taught to patients for their own follow-up. Patients who develop a second malignancy are a challenge to the nurse, especially when it involves a long-term survivor with whom there is a strong bonding relationship. It is imperative that the nurse assist the patient and family in coping with the diagnosis and impending treatment.

CONCLUSION

Advances in cancer therapy are made by continual investigations, evaluation of treatment results, and their incorporation into the practice of oncology. Because of the amount of time spent directly with the patient receiving chemotherapy, the nurse is often the health care provider best able to recognize subtle changes in the patient's status that could be indicative of pending complications from chemotherapy. Nursing responsibilities are multifaceted, and include patient education, ongoing physical assessments, identification of risk factors, and prompt therapeutic interventions with ongoing evaluation for modification.

Occurrence of side effects does not necessarily preclude withholding of chemotherapy but instead alerts nurses to the need for careful assessment, management, and evaluation. The nurse's assessment of a patient's response to treatment and assistance in preventing or managing side effects can make the difference in the patient's overall perceived quality of life. Once the treatment is complete, nurses can be instrumental in encouraging patients to have a yearly comprehensive physical examination to detect cancer recurrence, second malignancies, and other long-term effects of chemotherapy.

REFERENCES

1. Lilly LL: Side effects associated with pediatric chemotherapy: Management and patient education issues. *Ped Nurs* 16:252–255, 1990.
2. Camp-Sorrell D: Controlling adverse effects of chemotherapy. *Nurs 91* 4:34–42, 1991.
3. Goodman M: Managing the side effects of chemotherapy. *Semin Oncol Nurs* 5:29–52, 1989 (suppl. 1).
4. Lydon JL: Nephrotoxicity of cancer treatment. *Oncol Nurs Forum* 13:68–77, 1986.
5. Montamat SC, Cusack BJ, Vestal RE: Management of drug therapy in the elderly. *N Engl J Med* 321:303–309, 1989.
6. Annesley T: Pharmacokinetic changes in the elderly. *Clin Lab Sc* 3:100–102, 1990.
7. Blesch KS: The normal physiological changes of aging and their impact on the response to cancer treatment. *Semin Oncol Nurs* 4:178–188, 1988.
8. Leslie WT: Chemotherapy in older cancer patients. *Oncology* 6:74–80, 1992.
9. Walsh SJ, Begg CB, Carbone PP: Cancer chemotherapy in the elderly. *Semin Oncol* 16:66–75, 1989.
10. Yates J, Glidewell O, Wiernick P, et al: Cytosine arabinoside with daunorubicin or adriamycin for therapy of acute myelocytic leukemia. *Blood* 60:454–462, 1982.
11. Begg CB, et al: Are the elderly predisposed to toxicity from cancer chemotherapy? *Cancer Clin Trials* 3:369–374, 1980.
12. Begg CB, Carbone PP: Clinical trials and drug toxicity in the elderly: The experience of the Eastern Cooperative Oncology Group. *Cancer* 52:1986–1992, 1983.
13. Begg CB, Elson PG, Carbone PP: A study of excess hematologic toxicity in elderly patients treated on cancer chemotherapy protocols. In Yancik R (ed.): *Cancer in the Elderly: Approaches to Early Detection and Treatment.* New York: Springer-Verlag, 1989.
14. O'Reilly S, Klimo P, Conners J: Low-dose ACOP-B and VABE: Weekly chemotherapy for elderly patients with advanced stage diffuse large-cell lymphoma. *J Clin Oncol* 9:741–747, 1991.
15. Thomasma DC: Ethics and professional practice in oncology. *Semin Oncol Nurs* 5:89–94, 1989.
16. Schipper H, Levitt M: Measuring quality of life: Risks and benefits: *Cancer Treat Rep* 69:1115–1123, 1985.
17. Aaronson NK: Quality of life: What is it? How should it be measured? *Oncology* 2:69–74, 1988.
18. Holmes S, Eburn E: Patients' and nurses' perceptions of symptom distress in cancer. *J Adv Nurs* 14:840–846, 1989.
19. Ferrans CE: Quality of life: Conceptual Issues. *Semin Oncol Nurs* 6:248–254, 1990.
20. McCabe MS: Psychological support for the patient on chemotherapy. *Oncology* 5:91–107, 1991.
21. Cella DF, Cherin EA: Quality of life during and after cancer treatment. *Comprehensive Therapy* 14:69–75, 1988.
22. Morra ME: Choices: Who's going to tell the patients what they need to know? *Oncol Nurs Forum* 15:421–425, 1988.
23. Yasko JM, Verfurth M: Closing comment: Future trends. *Semin Oncol Nurs* 8:156–158, 1992.
24. Dodd M: Assessing patient self-care for side effects of cancer chemotherapy. Part 1. *Cancer Nurs* 5:447–451, 1982.
25. Dodd M: Self-care for side effects in cancer chemotherapy: An assessment of nursing interventions. Part II. *Cancer Nurs* 6:63–66, 1983.
26. Musci EC, Dodd MJ: Predicting self-care with patients' and family members' affective states and family functioning. *Oncol Nurs Forum* 17:394–400, 1990.
27. Holland JC, Lesko LM: Chemotherapy, endocrine ther-

apy and immunotherapy. In Holland JC, Rowland JH (eds.): *Handbook of Psychooncology.* New York: Oxford University Press, 1989, pp. 146–162.
28. Love RR, Leventhal H, Douglas V, et al: Side effects and emotional distress during cancer chemotherapy. *Cancer* 63:604–611, 1989.
29. Nail LM, Jones LS, Greene D, et al: Use and perceived efficacy of self-care activities in patients receiving chemotherapy. *Oncol Nurs Forum* 18:883–887, 1991.
30. Dodd M: Cancer patients' knowledge of chemotherapy: Assessment and informational interventions. *Oncol Nurs Forum* 9:39–44, 1982.
31. Fernsler JI, Cannon CA: The whys of patient education. *Semin Oncol Nurs* 7:79–86, 1991.
32. Miller AB, Hoogstraten B, Staquet M, et al: Reporting results of cancer treatment. *Cancer* 47:207–214, 1981.
33. Kisner DL: Reporting treatment toxicities. In Buyse ME, Staquet M, Sylvester RJ (eds.): *Cancer Clinical Trials: Methods and Practice.* New York: Oxford University Press, 1984, pp. 178–190.
34. Mili L: The community hospital perspective of clinical trials and the role of the nurse educator. *Semin Oncol Nurs* 7:280–287, 1991.
35. Link DL: Antibiotic therapy in the cancer patient: Focus on third generation cephalosporins. *Oncol Nurs Forum* 14:35–41, 1987.
36. Rostad ME: Current strategies for managing myelosuppression in patients with cancer. *Oncol Nurs Forum* 18:7–15, 1991 (suppl.).
37. Gootenberg JE, Pizzo PA: Optimal management of acute toxicities of therapy. *Pediatr Clin North Am* 38:269–297, 1991.
38. Maxwell MB, Maher KE: Chemotherapy-induced myelosuppression. *Semin Oncol Nurs* 8:113–123, 1992.
39. Hoagland HC: Hematologic complications of cancer chemotherapy. In Perry MC (ed.): *The Chemotherapy Source Book.* Baltimore: Williams & Wilkins, 1992, pp. 498–507.
40. Corman LC: The relationship between nutrition, infectin, and immunity. *Med Clin North Am* 69:519–531, 1985.
41. Balducci L, Hardy C: Cancer and malnutrition: A critical interaction. *Am J Hematology* 18:91–103, 1985.
42. Reheis CE: Neutropenia: Causes, complications, treatment, and resulting nursing care. *Nurs Clin North Am* 20:219–225, 1985.
43. Wujcik D: A case management approach to patients receiving G-CSF. *Oncol Nurs So Monograph* May:8–13, 1992.
44. Oniboni AC: Infection in the neutropenic patient. *Semin Oncol Nurs* 6:50–60, 1990.
45. Pizzo PA: Combating infections in neutropenic patients. *Hosp Pract* 22:93–110, 1989.
46. Nauseef WM, Maki DG: A study of the value of simple protective isolation in patients with granulocytopenia. *N Engl J Med* 304:448–453, 1981.
47. Gucalp R: Management of the febrile neutropenic patient with cancer. *Oncology* 5:137–148, 1991.
48. Koeppler H, Pflueger KH, Seitz R, et al: Three-step empiric treatment for severely neutropenic patients with fever: Ceftazidime, vancomycin, amphotericin B. *Infection* 17:142–145, 1989.
49. Hughes WT, Armstrong D, Bodey GP, et al: Guidelines for the use of antimicrobial agents in neutropenic patients with unexplained fever. *J Infect Dis* 161:381–396, 1991.
50. Sugar AM: Empiric treatment of fungal infections in the neutropenic host. *Arch Intern Med* 150:2258–2264, 1990.
the neutropenic host. *Arch Intern Med* 150:2258–2264, 1990.
51. Haeuber D: Future strategies in the control of myelosuppression: The use of colony-stimulating factors. *Oncol Nurs Forum* 18:16–21, 1991 (suppl.).
52. Vadhan-Raj S: Hematopoietic growth factors in chemotherapy-induced myelosuppression. *Cancer Bul* 43:208–214, 1991.
53. Sallerfors B, Olofsson T: Granulocyte-macrophage colony-stimulating factor (GM-CSF) and granulocyte colony-stimulating factor (G-CSF) in serum during induction treatment of acute leukaemia. *Br J Hematol* 78:343–351, 1991.
54. Aistars J: Fatigue in the cancer patient: A conceptual approach to a clinical problem. *Oncol Nurs Forum* 15:25–30, 1987.
55. St. Pierre BS, Kasper CE, Lindsey AM: Fatigue mechanisms in patients with cancer: Effects of tumor necrosis factor and exercise on skeletal muscle. *Oncol Nurs Forum* 19:419–425, 1992.
56. Piper BF, Lindsey AM, Dodd MJ: Fatigue mechanisms in cancer patients: Developing nursing theory. *Oncol Nurs Forum* 14:17–23, 1987.
57. Tchekmedyian NS, Hickman MN, Siau J, et al: Megestrol acetate in cancer anorexia and weight loss. *Cancer* 69:1268–1274, 1992.
58. Langstein HN, Norton JA: Mechanisms of cancer cachexia. *Hematol Oncol Clin North Am* 5:103–123, 1991.
59. Nelson K, Walsh D: Management of the anorexia cachexia syndrome. *Cancer Bul* 43:403–406, 1991.
60. Lindsey AM, Piper BF, Stotts NA: The phenomenon of cancer cachexia: A review. *Oncol Nurs Forum* 9:38–42, 1982.
61. Lin EM: Nutritional support: Making the difficult decisons. *Cancer Nurs* 14:261–269, 1991.
62. Eng-Hen N, Lowry SF: Nutritional support and cancer cachexia. *Hematol Oncol Clin North Am* 5:161–184, 1991.
63. Crosley MA: Watch out for nutritional complications of cancer. *RN* 48:22–27, 1985.
64. Nunnally C, Donoghue M, Yasko JM: Nutritional needs of cancer patients. *Nurs Clin North Am* 17:557–578, 1982.
65. Ramstack JL, Rosenbaum EH: *Nutrition for the Chemotherapy Patient.* Palo Alto, CA: Bull Publishing, 1990.
66. Wujcik D: Current research in side effects of high-dose chemotherapy. *Semin Oncol Nurs* 8:102–112, 1992.
67. Levy MH: Constipation and diarrhea in cancer patients. *Cancer Bul* 43:412–422, 1991.
68. Suppaiah L: Pseudomembranous colitis induced by *Clostridium difficile. Crit Care Nurs* 8:65–68, 1988.
69. Mitchell EP, Schein PS: Gastrointestinal toxicity of chemotherapeutic agents. In Perry MC (ed.): *The Chemotherapy Source Book.* Baltimore: Williams & Wilkins, 1992, pp. 620–634.
70. Katz MD, Erstan BL, Rose C: Treatment of severe diarrhea with octreotide in a patient with AIDS. *Drug Intell Clin Pharm* 22:134–136, 1988.
71. Borison HL: Anatomy and physiology of the chemoreceptor trigger zone and area postrema. In Davis CJ, Lake-Bakarr CV, Grahame-Smith DG (eds.): *Nausea and Vomiting Mechanisms and Treatment.* New York: Springer-Verlag, 1986, pp. 10–17.
72. Borison JL, McCarthy LE: Neuropharmacology of chemotherapy induced emesis. *Drugs* 25:8–17, 1983.
73. Morrow GR: The effects of susceptibility to motion sickness on the side effects of cancer chemotherapy. *Cancer* 55:2766–2670, 1985.

74. Akwar O: The gastrointestinal tract in chemotherapy-induced emesis. A final common pathway. *Drugs* 25:18–34, 1983.
75. Tortorice PV, O'Connell MB: Management of chemotherapy-induced nausea and vomiting. *Pharmacotherapy* 10:129–145, 1990.
76. Hogan CA: Advances in the management of nausea and vomiting. *Nurs Clin North Am* 25:475–497, 1991.
77. Wickham R: Managing chemotherapy-related nausea and vomiting: The state of the art. *Oncol Nurs Forum* 16:563–574, 1989.
78. Grunber SM: Advances in the management of nausea and vomiting induced by non-cisplatin containing chemotherapeutic regimens. *Blood Rev* 3:216 221, 1989.
79. Goodman M: Management of nausea and vomiting induced by outpatient cisplatin (Platinol) therapy. *Semin Oncol Nurs* 3:23–35, 1987.
80. Morrow GR: Chemotherapy-related nausea and vomiting: Etiology and management. *CA* 39:89–104, 1989.
81. Gralla RJ: The management of chemotherapy-induced nausea and vomiting. *Med Clin North Am* 71:289–299, 1987.
82. Gralla RJ: Progress in the development of antiemetics for chemotherapy-induced nausea and vomiting. *Cancer Bul* 43:407–411, 1991.
83. Aapro MS: Controlling emesis related to cancer therapy. *Euro J Cancer* 27:356–361, 1991.
84. Cubeddu LX, Hoffeman IS, Fuenmayor NT, et al: Efficacy of ondansetron and the role of serotonin in cisplatin induced nausea and vomiting. *N Engl J Med* 322:810–816, 1990.
85. Halperin JR, Murphy B: Extrapyramidal reaction to ondansetron. *Cancer* 69:1275, 1992.
86. Perez EA, Hesketh PJ, Gandara DR: Serotonin antagonists in the management of cisplatin-induced emesis. *Semin Oncol* 18:73–80, 1991 (suppl. 3).
87. Fraschini G, Ciociola A, Esparza L, et al: Evaluation of three oral dosages of ondansetron in the prevention of nausea and emesis associated with cyclophosphamide-doxorubicin chemotherapy. *J Clin Oncol* 9:1268–1274, 1991.
88. Roila F, et al: A double blind multicenter randomized crossover study comparing the antiemetic efficacy and tolerability of ondansetron versus ondansetron plus dexamethasone in cisplatinum-treated patients. *J Clin Oncol* 9:675–678, 1991.
89. Zeltzer LK, Dolgin MJ, LeBaron S, et al: A randomized, controlled study of behavioral intervention of chemotherapy distress in children with cancer. *Pediatrics* 88:34–42, 1991.
90. Cotanch PH, Strum S: Progressive muscle relaxation as antiemetic therapy for cancer patients. *Oncol Nurs Forum* 14:33–37, 1987.
91. Kantrowitz NE, Bristow MR: Cardiotoxicity of antitumor agents. *Prog Cardiovas Dis* 27:195–200, 1984.
92. Torti FM, Lum BL: Cardiac toxicity. In DeVita VT, Hellman S, Rosenberg SA (eds.): *Cancer: Principles and Practice of Oncology* (ed. 3). Philadelphia: Lippincott, 1989, pp. 2153–2169.
93. Bristow MR: Toxic cardiomyopathy due to doxorubicin. *Hosp Prac* 17:101–111, 1982.
94. Kaszyk LK: Cardiac toxicity associated with cancer therapy. *Oncol Nurs Forum* 13:81–88, 1986.
95. Dorr RT: Chemoprotectants for cancer chemotherapy. *Semin Oncol* 18:8–58, 1991 (suppl. 2).
96. Speyer JL, Green MD, Zeleniuch-Jacquotte A: ICRF-86 permits longer treatment with doxorubicin in women with breast cancer. *J Clin Oncol* 10:117–127, 1992.
97. Hurteloup P, Ganzina F: Clinical studies with new anthracyclines: Epirubicin, idarubicin, esorubicin. *Drugs Exp Clin Res* 12:233–246, 1986.
98. Crossley RJ: Clinical safety and tolerance of mitoxantrone. *Semin Oncol* 11:54–58, 1984 (suppl. 1).
99. Shenkenber TD, Von Hoff DD: Mitoxantrone: A new anticancer drug with significant clinical activity. *Ann Intern Med* 105:67–81, 1986.
100. Mill BA, Roberts RW: Cyclophosphamide-induced cardiomyopathy. A report of two cases and review of the English literature. *Cancer* 13:2223 2226, 1979.
101. Braverman AC, Antin JH, Plappert MT, et al: Cyclophosphamide cardiotoxicity in one marrow transplantation: A prospective evaluation of new dosing regimens. *J Clin Oncol* 9:1215–1223, 1991.
102. Oleksowicz L, Bruckner HW: Prophylaxis of 5 fluorouracil-induced coronary vasospasm with calcium channel blockers. *Am J Med* 85:750–751, 1988.
103. Kleiman NS, Lehane DE, Geyer CE, et al: Prinzmetal's angina during 5-fluorouracil chemotherapy. *Am J Med* 82:566–568, 1987.
104. Rowinsky EK, McGuire WP, Guarnieri T, et al: Cardiac disturbances during the administration of taxol. *J Clin Oncol* 9:1704–1712, 1991.
105. Steinherz LJ, Steinherz PG: Delayed anthracycline cardiac toxicity. *Prin & Prac Oncol* 5:1–15, 1991.
106. Steinherz LJ, Steinherz PG, Tan, CT, et al: Cardiac toxicity 4 to 20 years after completing anthracycline therapy. *JAMA* 266:1672–1677, 1991.
107. MacDonald DR: Neurotoxicity of chemotherapeutic agents. In Perry MC (ed.): *The Chemotherapy Source Book.* Baltimore: Williams & Wilkins, 1992, pp. 666–679.
108. Forman A: Peripheral neuropathy in cancer patients: Clinical types, etiology, and presentation. *Oncology* 4:85–89, 1990.
109. Holden S, Felde G: Nursing care of patients experiencing cisplatin-related peripheral neuropathy. *Oncol Nurs Forum* 14:13–19, 1987.
110. Mollman JE, Glover DJ, Hogan WM, et al: Cisplatin neuropathy: Risk factors, prognosis, and protection by WR-2721. *Cancer* 61:2192–2195, 1988.
111. Schaefer SD, Post JD, Close LG, et al: Ototoxicity of low and moderate dose cisplatin. *Cancer* 56:1934–1939, 1985.
112. Miller LJ: Ifosfamide induced neurotoxicity. *Cancer Bul* 43:456–457, 1991.
113. Anderson RN, Tandon DS: Ifosfamide extrapyramidal neurotoxicity. *Cancer* 69:72–75, 1991.
114. Conrad KJ: Cerebellar toxicities associated with cytosine arabinoside: A nursing perspective. *Oncol Nurs Forum* 13:57–59, 1986.
115. Cooper JA, White DA, Matthay RA: Drug-induced pulmonary disease. *Am Rev Respir Dis* 133:321–340. 1986.
116. Wickham R: Pulmonary toxicity secondary to cancer treatment. *Oncol Nurs Forum* 13:69–76, 1986.
117. Kreisman H, Wolkove N: Pulmonary toxicity of antineoplastic therapy. In Perry MC (ed.): *The Chemotherapy Source Book.* Baltimore: Williams & Wilkins, 1992, pp. 598–619.
118. Luedke D, Mclaughlin TT, Daughaday C, et al: Mitomycin C and vindesine associated pulmonary toxicity with variable clinical expression. *Cancer* 55:542–545, 1985.

119. White DA, Rankin JA, Stover DE, et al: Methotrexate pneumonitis. *Am Rev Respir Dis* 139:18–21, 1989.
120. Sostman HD, Matthay RA, Putman CE, et al: Methotrexate-induced pneumonitis. *Medicine* 55:371–388, 1976.
121. Perry MC (ed.): Hepatotoxicity of chemotherapeutic agents. In Perry MC: *The Chemotherapy Source Book*. Baltimore: Williams & Wilkins, 1992, pp. 635–647.
122. Wujcik D, Downs S: Bone marrow transplantation. *Crit Care Nurs Clin North Am* 4:149–166, 1992.
123. Rollins BJ: Hepatic veno-occlusive disease. *Am J Med* 81:297–306, 1986.
124. Keith JS: Hepatic failure: Etiologies, manifestations, and management. *Crit Care Nurs* 5:60–86, 1985.
125. Blanco JA, Appelbaum FR, Nemunaitis J, et al: Phase I-II trial of pentoxifylline for the prevention of transplant-related toxicities following bone marrow transplant. *Blood* 78:1205–1211, 1991.
126. Lewis JH, Schiff E: Methotrexate-induced chronic liver injury: Guidelines for detection and prevention. *Am J Gastroentrol* 88:1337–1345, 1988.
127. George CB, Mansour RP, Redmond J: Hepatic dysfunction and jaundice following high-dose cytosine arabinoside. *Cancer* 54:2360–2362, 1984.
128. Kemeny N, Daly J. Reichman B, et al: Intrahepatic or systemic infusion of fluorodeoxyruidine in patients with liver metastases from colorectal carcinoma. *Ann Intern Med* 107:459–475, 1987.
129. Applebaum FR, Shulman HM: Fatal hepatotoxicity associated with AMSA therapy. *Cancer Treat Rep* 66:1863–1865, 1982.
130. Stillwell TJ, Benson RC: Cyclophosphamide-induced hemorrhagic cystitis. *Cancer* 61:451–457, 1988.
131. Shepherd JD, Pringle LE, Barnett M, et al: Mesna versus hyperhydration for the prevention of cyclophosphamide-induced hemorrhagic cystitis in bone marrow transplantation. *J Clin Oncol* 9:2016–2020, 1991.
132. Patterson WP, Reams GP: Renal and electrolyte abnormalities due to chemotherapy. In Perry MC (ed.): *The Chemotherapy Source Book*. Philadelphia: Williams & Wilkins, 1992, pp. 648–665.
133. Safirstein R, Winston J, Goldstein, M, et al: Cisplatin nephrotoxicity. *Am J Kidney Dis* 8:356–357, 1986.
134. Vogelzang NJ: Nephrotoxicity from chemotherapy: Prevention and management. *Oncology* 5:97–112, 1991.
135. Daley-Yates PT, McBrien DC: A study of the protective effect of chloride salts on cisplatin nephrotoxicity. *Biochem Pharmacol* 34:2363–2369, 1985.
136. Corden BJ, Fine RL, Ozols RF, et al: Chemical pharmacology of high-dose cisplatin. *Cancer Chemother Pharmacol* 14:38–41, 1985.
137. Gandara DR, Perez EA, Wiebe V, et al: Cisplatin chemoprotection and rescue: Pharmacologic modulation of toxicity. *Semin Oncol* 18:49–55, 1991 (suppl. 3).
138. DeGregorio MW, Gandara DR, Hollerman WM, et al: High-dose cisplatin with diethyldithiocarbamate (DDTC) rescue therapy. Preliminary pharmacologic observations. *Cancer Chemother Pharmacol* 23:276–279, 1989.
139. Tuttle SE, Sharma HM, Bay WH, et al: Glomerular basement membrane splitting and microaneurysm formation associated with nitrosourea therapy. *Am J Nephrol* 5:388–394, 1985.
140. Hrozencik SP, Connaughton MJ: Cancer-associated hemolytic uremic syndrome. *Oncol Nurs Forum* 15:755–759, 1988.
141. Averette HE, Boike GM, Jarrell MA: Effects of cancer chemotherapy on gonadal function and reproductive capacity. *CA* 40:199–209, 1990.
142. Yarbro CH, Perry MC: The effect of cancer therapy on gonadal function. *Semin Oncol Nurs* 1:3–8, 1985.
143. Chapman RM: Gonadal toxicity and teratogenicity. In Perry MC (ed.): *The Chemotherapy Source Book*. Baltimore: Williams & Wilkins, 1992, pp. 710–753.
144. Chapman RM: Gonadal injury resulting from chemotherapy. *Am J Int Med* 4:149–161, 1983.
145. Shalet SM: Effects of cancer chemotherapy on gonadal function of patients. *Cancer Treat Rev* 7:141–152, 1980.
146. Sanger WG, Armitage JO, Schmidt MA: Feasibility of semen cryopreservation in patients with malignant disease. *JAMA* 244:789–790, 1980.
147. Nicosia SV, Matus-Ridley M, Meadows AT: Gonadal effects of cancer therapy in girls. *Cancer* 55:2364–2372, 1985.
148. Rustin GJS, Pektasides D, Bagshawe KD, et al: Fertility after chemotherapy for male and female germ cell tumors. *Intern J Androl* 10:389–392, 1987.
149. Gulati SC, Vega R, Gee T, Kozner B, et al: Growth and development of children born to patients after cancer therapy. *Cancer Inves* 4:197–205, 1986.
150. Mulvihill JJ, McKeen A, Rosner F, et al: Pregnancy outcome in cancer patients. *Cancer* 60:1143–1150, 1987.
151. Uhlenhopp MB: An overview of the relationship between alkylating agents and therapy-related acute nonlymphocytic leukemia. *Cancer Nurs* 15:9–17, 1992.
152. Hydzik CA: Late effects of chemotherapy: Implications for patient management and rehabilitation. *Nurs Clin North Am* 25:423–446, 1990.
153. Pape LH: Therapy-related acute leukemia: An overview. *Cancer Nurs* 11:295–302, 1988.
154. Fraser MC, Tucker MA: Second malignancies following cancer therapy. *Semin Oncol Nurs* 15:43–55, 1989.
155. Tucker MA, Coleman CN, Cox RS, et al: Risk of second cancers after treatment for Hodgkin's disease. *N Engl J Med* 318:76–81, 1988.
156. Koletsky AJ, Bertino JR, Farber LR, et al: Second neoplasms in patients with Hodgkin's disease following combined modality therapy. *J Clin Oncol* 4:311–317, 1986.
157. Kyle RS, Genta MA: Second malignancies after chemotherapy. In Perry MC (ed.): *The Chemotherapy Source Book*. Baltimore: Williams & Wilkins, 1992, pp. 689–702.
158. Ratain MJ, Kaminer LS, Bitran JD, et al: Acute nonlymphocytic leukemia following etoposide and cisplatin combination chemotherapy for advanced non-small cell carcinoma of the lung. *Blood* 70:1412–1417, 1987.
159. Tucker MA, Fraumeni JF: Treatment-related cancers after gynecologic malignancy. *Cancer* 60:2117–2122, 1987.
160. Valagussa P, Tancini G, Bonadonna G: Second malignancies after CMF for resectable breast cancer. *J Clin Oncol* 5:1138–1142, 1987.
161. Curtis RE, Boice JD, Stovall M, et al: Risk of leukemia after chemotherapy and radiation therapy for breast cancer. *N Engl J Med* 326:1745–1751, 1992.
162. Pedersen-Bjergaard J, Caugaard G, et al: Increased risk of myelodysplasia and leukemia after etoposide, cisplatin, and bleomycin for germ-cell tumors. *Lancet* 338:359–363, 1991.

Chapter 17

Biotherapy

Patricia F. Jassak, RN, MS, CS, OCN

INTRODUCTION

Biological therapies are becoming widely available for clinical use. Our knowledge of biologic agents and our ability to use them therapeutically continues to expand rapidly. Although the use of the combined therapeutic modalities of surgery, radiation therapy, and chemotherapy has resulted in increased survival for many persons with cancer, many types and stages of neoplastic disease remain unresponsive to our current treatment armamentarium.

In the search to control or cure cancer, the hypothesis that the immune system can be manipulated to restore, augment, or modulate its function has stimulated scientific inquiry since the beginning of this century. Evidence from both animal and human trials clearly indicates that under the proper circumstances, malignant tumors are susceptible to immunologic rejection. And so the search for effective biologic agents continues.

Fortunately, the future is brighter than the past, primarily as a result of four major technologic advances.[1–4] First, scientists continue to develop a broader understanding of the complex cellular structure of the immune system, which enables them to isolate new cellular components and to identify their function accurately. Second, advances in genetic engineering, also referred to as recombinant DNA technology, make it possible to clone genes and thereby produce large quantities of highly purified substances secreted by cells of the immune system for analysis and clinical use. Previously, isolation and purification were slow, cumbersome, and costly processes that produced small quantities and impure products. Third, advances in molecular biology continue to allow scientists to construct and alter molecules synthetically so that they can be investigated or their biologic activities changed. Fourth, technologic advances in laboratory equipment and computer systems aid researchers in their pursuit of the elusive substances of the immune system.

Scientists have pursued actively the use of immunologic approaches for cancer therapy for more than four decades. As a result of these technologic advances, *biotherapy,* the therapeutic use of biologic agents, also referred to as biologic response modifiers (BRMs), has emerged as the fourth modality of cancer therapy.

The reintroduction of biologic agents into the clinical setting has provided treatment strategies for diseases previously unresponsive to standard therapy. Durant[5] ponders the possibility that we have reached "the end of the beginning of the search for successful immunotherapy for cancer." He projects that the future of biotherapy will be limited only by how well we use our knowledge base and fit the puzzle pieces together.

Although the majority of agents classified as BRMs are, in fact, agents that modulate the immune system, biotherapy encompasses a broader range of approaches than previously considered under immunotherapy—in particular, those agents responsible for the growth and maturation of cells. A BRM is defined as any soluble substance capable of altering (modifying) the immune system with either a stimulatory or a suppressive effect.[6,p.178] Clark and Longo[7] classify BRMs into three major categories:

- agents that restore, augment, or modulate the host's immunologic mechanisms
- agents that have direct antitumor activity
- agents that have other biologic effects (agents interfering with tumor cells' ability to survive or metastasize; differentiating agents or agents affecting cell transformation)

A wide array of BRMs currently is approved for use in the clinical arena, including alpha- and gamma-interferon (IFN), interleukin-2 (IL-2), and colony stimulating growth factors (CSFs), including granulocyte colony stimulating factor (G-CSF) and granulocyte-macrophage colony stimulating factor (GM-CSF). Biologic agents such as monoclonal antibodies (MAbs), other interleukins, and tumor necrosis factor (TNF) remain investigational. The past decade has unveiled a tremendous amount of information about the activities and toxicities of biologic agents. Many of the clinical results are exciting, demonstrating responses in diseases previously unresponsive to our known arsenal of therapy. As we gain better insight into the individual's immune response to malignancy, we will learn techniques to manipulate successfully that response in a beneficial way.

HISTORICAL PERSPECTIVE

Two observations laid the early groundwork in immunology research: first, the observation of a spontaneous regression, in which the tumor becomes smaller and/or disappears without any apparent reason; second, the observation of prolonged survival, in which the patient lives longer than clinical experience or statistics would predict. Dr. William B. Coley, an early pioneer in the field of immunotherapy and a surgeon at New York's Memorial Hospital from 1891 until 1936, investigated why some patients with cancer appeared to be cured after surgical resection whereas others quickly relapsed. He identified that many of the patients who remained tumor-free had experienced after their surgery what we now call *septic episodes.* Clinically, Coley used live bacteria and, later, filtered toxins, referred to as *Coley's toxins,* to induce an infectious response in patients with cancer. These toxins were used clinically until approximately 1975, and provide the background for what is now called TNF.[8] These toxins may have aided the immune system to identify, detect, and destroy tumor cells.

The application of immunotherapy to cancer therapy has gained popularity only since the 1960s, when many clinical trials of bacterial agents were initiated—specifically, bacille Calmette-Guérin (BCG) and *Corynebacterium parvum.* These early experiments produced positive results in selective laboratory tumor models. In 1969, Mathe et al.[9] demonstrated positive therapeutic results in an initial clinical trial using BCG to treat children diagnosed with acute lymphoblastic leukemia. Subsequently, hundreds of clinical trials were undertaken with BCG for the treatment of leukemia and many types of solid tumors, with mixed results. Although survival as a result of BCG therapy was shown to increase among individuals with acute myelogenous leukemia, those with solid tumors were shown to derive no therapeutic benefit.[10]

Similarly, no substantial or significant improvement of response or survival rates was documented for individuals with leukemia, carcinoma of the head and the neck, colon, breast, cervix, and nonsmall-cell carcinoma of the lung and melanoma who received *C parvum.*[1,11] In addition, during this same period viruses were used to stimulate tumor cells to produce viral oncolysates, again in an attempt to manipulate the immune system to reject tumor cells. Although some of the early clinical trials showed positive results, the majority were discouraging and few if any could replicate the positive responses reported. Therefore, by the late 1970s most clinicians had a negative view of the promise of immunotherapy. Oldham and Smalley[1] attribute the early failure of immunotherapy as a treatment modality to the fact that initially most studies were conducted with the use of impure reagents, which resulted in variability of experimental procedure and lack of generalizable results. Oldham[2] believes that the future of biotherapy lies in the recent technologic advances that have allowed researchers to continue their quest. Major technological advances since 1970, as previously cited, have greatly expanded our ability to use BRMs therapeutically. Multiple recombinant products, including IFNs (r IFNs), IL-1, IL-2, IL-3, IL-4, IL-6, TNF, and CSFs, are now available for clinical use and investigation.

The 1980s saw cumulative positive clinical results in diseases previously deemed unresponsive. In 1986, α-IFN received approval from the Food and Drug Administration (FDA) for use in hairy-cell leukemia. Subsequently, in 1989, the FDA also approved α-IFN for use in AIDS-related Kaposi's sarcoma. History was made. In February and March 1991, two CSFs—G-CSF and GM-CSF, respectively—also were approved by the FDA. In May 1992, IL-2 joined the list of FDA-approved BRMs.

BRMs have established a therapeutic role in cancer therapy. It is important to emphasize that biologic agents must be evaluated slightly differently from other pharmacologic agents. Both the pharmacologic effect of the agent and the biologic response exerted by this approach must be measured and analyzed in order to understand clearly the overall effect of the BRM administered. A discussion of a variety of biologic agents under active clinical use and investigation follows.

ANTIBODY THERAPY (SEROTHERAPY)

The limiting factor in effective cancer therapy is its current lack of specificity. During the 1980s significant strides were made in the field of antibody therapy, which promotes specific targeting of cells through an antibody-antigen response. Antibody therapy is based on the knowledge that all cells (including tumor cells) typically have antigens present on their surface that are specific to that cell type. Although tumor-associated antigens are found mainly on tumor cells, they also may be present on normal cells in lesser quantities, thus allowing tumor cells to be targeted while sparing normal cells.

Hybridoma Techniques

In 1975, Kohler and Milstein[12] described a technique for the production of monoclonal antibodies. An animal (usually a mouse) is injected with the desired antigen (tumor cells). The mouse's lymphocytes recognize the antigen as foreign and produce antibodies. The immunized lymphocytes are removed from the mouse's spleen and fused with mouse malignant myeloma cells to form a "hybrid" (Figure 7-1).[13] This last step is done to form a "hybrid" (Figure 17-1).[13] This last step is done to make the lymphocytes immortal and therefore capable of unlimited cell division. The hybrid is then screened for antibody production and the antibody is concentrated and purified. The end result is a highly purified murine (mouse) monoclonal antibody directed against specific human tumor-associated antigens.
actly the same, hence the term *monoclonal antibodies* (MAbs). Thus, a hybridoma is the result of a fusion between two cell lines to form a hybrid that shares genetic information. The refinement of the hybridoma technique allowed scientists to obtain a pure antibody to a known antigen and facilitated the development of new therapeutic and diagnostic applications of antibodies in cancer therapy.[14]

Antibody Function

Monoclonal antibodies may be used alone (referred to as *unconjugated*) or in combination (*conjugated*) with radioisotopes, toxins, or chemotherapeutic drugs to stain, destroy, or identify cells with specific antigens on their cell surface. They also are used in vitro to remove tumor cells from bone marrow before autologous bone marrow transplantation and in conjunction with other biologic response modifiers, such as IFN and IL-2. An-

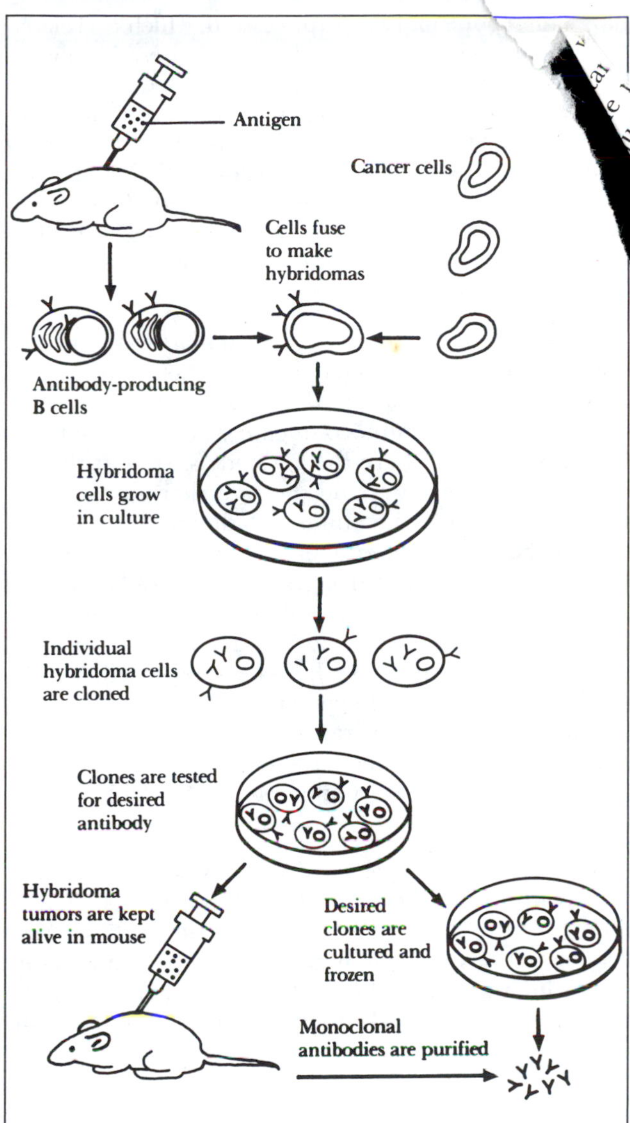

FIGURE 17-1 Use of hybridoma technique to make monoclonal antibodies. (Source: Schindler LW: *Understanding the Immune System.* NIH pub no. 88-529. Bethesda, MD: U.S. Department of Health and Human Services, July 1988, p. 28.)

tibodies can kill tumor cells through a variety of direct or indirect mechanisms.[15]

Direct tumor cell kill

Unconjugated monoclonal antibodies may kill tumor cells directly through several processes. The process of antibody-dependent cell-mediated cytotoxicity (ADCC) occurs when the antibody binding to the target cell acts as a signal to the effector cells to destroy the target cell (see Chapter 5). It is not yet known which cell type is the most important in vivo effector cell of ADCC; however, potential cells include lymphocytes, monocytes, and possibly neutrophils. Antibodies also may bind to the surface of the tumor cell, causing complement-dependent cytotoxicity to be initiated, which results in cell lysis. Opsonization is the process whereby tumor cells are coated by the antibody to facilitate clearance by the reticuloendothelial system.

Modulation of differentiation/growth

ıtibodies also are capable of blocking tumor cell e growth receptors for growth factors, providing t antiproliferative effect. This phenomenon has ye be demonstrated in vivo, because researchers mus st identify tumor-expressed growth factor receptors and then develop antibodies that are specifically capable of blocking the receptor but that are not active in promoting proliferation.

Regulation of immunity

Antibodies also may be used to regulate immunity. Attempts to develop an effective immunization program to prevent cancer or its recurrence have been impeded by the lack of a reliable supply of immunogenic vaccine of known reactivity.

Anti-idiotype as immunogen

Anti-idiotypic antibodies can be used as surrogate antigen, thus providing a possible solution to the supply and immunogenicity problems of a reliable cancer vaccine. An idiotype is the unique part of an antibody's variable region (Fab) that can in itself act as an antigen to trigger a complementary antibody. Antibodies complementary to idiotopes are termed *anti-idiotypic.* Anti-idiotypic antibodies can be used as a substitute for the original antigen in the preparation of vaccines against infectious microorganisms.

Unconjugated Monoclonal Antibodies

Murine MAbs have been used in clinical trials since the early 1980s to treat patients with acute lymphoblastic leukemia,[16] chronic lymphocytic leukemia,[17–19] B-cell lymphomas,[20–22] and T-cell leukemias and lymphomas.[17,23–26] Transient clinical responses have been reported.

In addition, the effect of murine MAbs has been studied in patients with gastrointestinal malignancies. Sears et al.[27] reported durable remissions, minimal toxicity, and a 17% response rate, which compares favorably with that achieved with 5-fluorouracil.

Most patients, however, did not benefit substantially despite known evidence of an antitumor effect. Attempts to improve response have included the use of in vitro incubation of peripheral blood mononuclear cells with antibody and γ-IFN before administration; however, limited response has been achieved.

Several clinical trials have evaluated murine MAbs in patients with metastatic melanoma.[28–35] For all studies combined, one complete response and seven partial responses are reported among a total of 54 patients. Although it is clear that MAbs directed against melanoma antigens are active, the development of human antimouse antibodies (HAMA) with repeated administration obliterates the clinical efficacy.

Immunoconjugates

The term *magic bullets* was coined at the turn of the century by Paul Ehrlich, who envisioned antibodies as carriers to deliver toxic agents directly to tumor cells. Immunoconjugates are formed when a variety of agents are linked to monoclonal antibodies. These agents include radioisotopes, plant and bacterial toxins, chemotherapeutic agents, and biologic agents.

Toxins

A variety of toxins are available for conjugation with antitumor antibodies, including ricin, diphtheria toxin, alpha-toxin, exotoxin, abrin, gelonin, saponin, and pokeweed antiviral protein.[36,37] Toxins are unique in their remarkable potency and are considered to be the most lethal substances known; a single molecule of toxin can kill a cell. Ricin-A chain has been conjugated with several antitumor murine antibodies to produce immunotoxins. Clinical trials with Ricin-A chain immunotoxins currently are under way in the treatment of melanoma, colorectal and breast cancer, and refractory leukemia. Spitler et al.[38] report that major toxicities include hypoalbuminemia, with secondary fluid shifts, dependent edema, and intravascular hypovolemia. To date, major tumor responses have yet to be achieved.

Chemotherapeutic agents

Chemotherapeutic agents conjugated to MAbs are called *chemoimmunoconjugates.* Agents used include chlorambucil, the anthracyclines, methotrexate, mitomycin C, and cisplatin. Theoretically, through conjugation, the antibody targets the chemotherapeutic agent to the tumor cells, alleviating the expected toxicity to normal cells. Thus, higher doses of chemotherapeutic agents potentially can be used with minimal systemic toxicity. Clinical trials remain in early phases, with therapeutic efficacy and toxicity still to be determined.

Isotopes

Diagnostic imaging Current diagnostic imaging also is limited by the lack of tumor specificity. Radio-labeled MAbs with the use of iodine (^{131}I), technetium, and indium (^{111}In) allow specific binding of these agents to tumor cells, thus enhancing the detection of tumor cells.[39–42] In diagnostic imaging these agents demonstrate sensitivity and specificity for tumor detection. Meredith et al.[43] report that the only side effect experienced in a phase I trial of I^{131} chimeric MAb was dose-dependent bone marrow suppression, which correlated with whole-body radiation dose estimates. In several instances imaging has been compromised because of the reticuloendothelial uptake of these immunoconjugates in the liver and spleen. These issues remain under study, and diagnostic use of radio-labeled immunoconjugates continues to be refined. It is anticipated that the use of radio-labeled MAbs will allow small tumors clinically undetectable by present technology to be identified.

Therapeutic radioisotopes Radio-labeled antibody therapy involves conjugation of an antibody active against a specific tumor antigen with a radioactive isotope. This radioimmunoconjugate is administered into the bloodstream, where the antibody seeks out the tumor and attaches to it, and the radioactive isotope internally irradiates the tumor. Radioimmunoglobulin therapy has been undertaken with the use of ^{131}I and ^{90}yttrium. Remissions through the use of radio-labeled polyclonal antiferritin antibodies have been reported in primary hepatomas (48%) and Hodgkin's disease (40%).[44] No acute toxicities have been reported.[45] Problems with nonspecific hepatic uptake, tumor vascularity, and choice and dose rate of the therapeutic isotope remain factors that need further refinement in the search for effective therapeutic radio-labeled immunoconjugates.

Immunobiologic agents MAbs may be linked to various lymphokines, cytokines, and hormones. These agents also may be used in conjunction with MAbs. Possible actions include increasing antigen expression, enhancing the action of cytotoxic cells, and altering the cellular membrane and vascular permeability of tumor cells.

Chimeric Antibodies

Murine MAbs have dominated the field of antitumor antibodies since the inception of hybridoma technology. In the 1980s, recombinant biologic techniques were utilized to develop a new type of antibody. The murine gene used to encode the portion of the antibody molecule that recognizes antigen was coupled with the human gene encoding the remainder of the immunoglobulin molecule. Thus, antigen specificity comes from the mouse genes, while the human Ig genes provide the other biologic functions. Recombinant technology is then used to produce the antibody in large, purified amounts.

The chimeric antibody (a mixture of human and murine antibodies) is capable of mediating immunologic functions similar to the original murine antibody. Initial reports indicated that chimeric antibodies have a longer circulating half-life and are less immunogenic than murine MAbs. However, these chimeric antibodies are still approximately one-sixth mouse origin and thus possess the ability to produce human antimouse immune responses.[46]

Human Antibodies

It is now possible to produce human antibodies, also referred to as combinatorial libraries or repertoire cloning.[46] Scientists identified that the genes coding for the antigen-binding fragments of human antibody could be expressed in bacteria. It was also found that the polymerase chain reaction (an enzymatic cloning technique) could be applied to produce millions of copies of a single DNA segment within a short time. This information can then be introduced into bacteriophage vectors (viruses that infect bacteria). Specificity is accomplished by using the antigen as a probe. The antigen recognizes only those phage vectors that express the specific antibody, code for it, and continue to replicate to produce that antibody. Human antibodies currently are under investigation in the clinical setting, most notably HA-1A, a human monoclonal antibody against endotoxin.[47] To date, clinical trials have not reported the development of human antihuman antibody (HAHA).

Problems with Antibody Therapy

Significant problems that have impeded the progress of antibody use for the treatment of cancer include the following.

Antigenic specificity. No true tumor-specific antigens have been isolated; only tumor-associated antigens or antigens that are proportionately overexpressed by tumors have been identified. Therefore it is critical that cross-reactivity with antigens on vital organs not occur, or at least that the antigen density be much lower on these organs than on tumor cells.

Antigenic modulation. Unlike the normal cell, the tumor cell surface antigen is shed or altered shortly after antibody administration. This effect may be overcome by the intermittent administration of the MAbs.

Antimouse antibodies. The human immune system recognizes mouse antibodies as foreign, triggers an immune response, and develops neutralizing antibodies to mouse immunoglobulin. Repeated treatments of MAb and chimeric antibodies have confirmed that significant toxicity and decreased efficacy can result from the development of indigenous human antimouse antibodies.

Monoclonal antibodies have yet to live up to their expected potential. Sands[48] identifies that improved immunologic reagents and better chelation chemistry in conjunction with a better understanding of tumor physiology should with time establish monoclonal antibodies as therapeutic options in the diagnosis and treatment of cancer.

Clinical Toxicities

Although anaphylaxis occurs infrequently, the nurse must be prepared to deal immediately with this acute toxicity. Its onset is predicted by the presence of a generalized flush and/or urticaria followed by pallor and/or cyanosis. Patients may complain of a tickle in their throat or impending doom; complaints of bronchospasm also are common. If any of these symptoms are present, stop the MAb infusion immediately, assess vital signs frequently, and alert the physician. Hypotension and unconsciousness may result.

Anaphylaxis is treated with 0.3-ml aqueous 1:1000 epinephrine injected subcutaneously if the patient is conscious and has a detectable blood pressure. Epinephrine 1:10,000 is administered by intravenous push for patients who cannot be aroused. Additional therapeutic measures may include the use of oxygen; the administration of antihistamines, corticosteroids, and aminophylline; and possibly cardiopulmonary resuscitation.

Common toxicities seen with the administration of MAbs include fever, chills, diaphoresis, rigors, malaise, pallor, weakness, generalized erythema, urticaria, pruritus, dyspnea, nausea, vomiting, diarrhea, and hypotension. Dillman[49] reports that the most common side effects of fever, rigors, chills, and diaphoresis occur within 2–8 hours following MAb administration.

CYTOKINES

The most exciting BRMs in the treatment of cancer are the cytokines. Cytokines are substances that are released from activated immune system cells that affect the behavior of other cells. Lymphokines are cellular products released by antigen-activated T-cells. Originally they were thought to be produced only by lymphocytes. It is now clear, however, that lymphokines are not restricted to lymphoid cells as previously identified, and thus the general term *cytokines* is now used to refer to them.[50] These cellular products activate a variety of biologic activities that may alter the growth and metastasis of cancer cells, including their ability to augment the responsiveness of T-cells to tumor-associated antigens, to enhance the effectiveness of B-cell activity, and to decrease suppressive functions of the immune system, thereby enhancing immune responsiveness. Cytokines may be administered directly to patients for control of cancer, or they may be used to manipulate the immune response in vitro to generate products that are used to treat individuals with cancer. Cytokines, currently FDA approved or under clinical investigation, are described in the next section.

Interferons

In the late 1940s virologists first noted that under certain conditions an infection of one virus protects for a time against infection by other viruses. In 1957, after much investigation, Isaacs and Lindemann[51] isolated a protein substance secreted by cells from a chicken embryo. Although this substance is not an antiviral agent itself, its presence appeared to interfere with virus activity in cells; hence it was called *interferon* (IFN). In the subsequent decade, researchers identified other properties of IFN, including its antiproliferative effects. Because isolation and preparation of interferon was at first difficult and costly, further information on its biologic activities was limited until the 1980s, when recombinant IFN became available in sufficient quantities for large-scale clinical trials (Figure 17-2). Although hopes were high that IFN's antitumor activity would constitute a major breakthrough in cancer treatment, initial results were modest and disappointing.[52,53]

Types of interferons

The IFNs are a family of naturally occurring complex proteins that belong to the cytokine family. Three major types of human IFN have been isolated: α-IFN, β-IFN, and γ-IFN. Each type originates from a different cell and has distinct biologic and chemical properties.[54–57] Table 17-1 identifies the types of IFNs, the

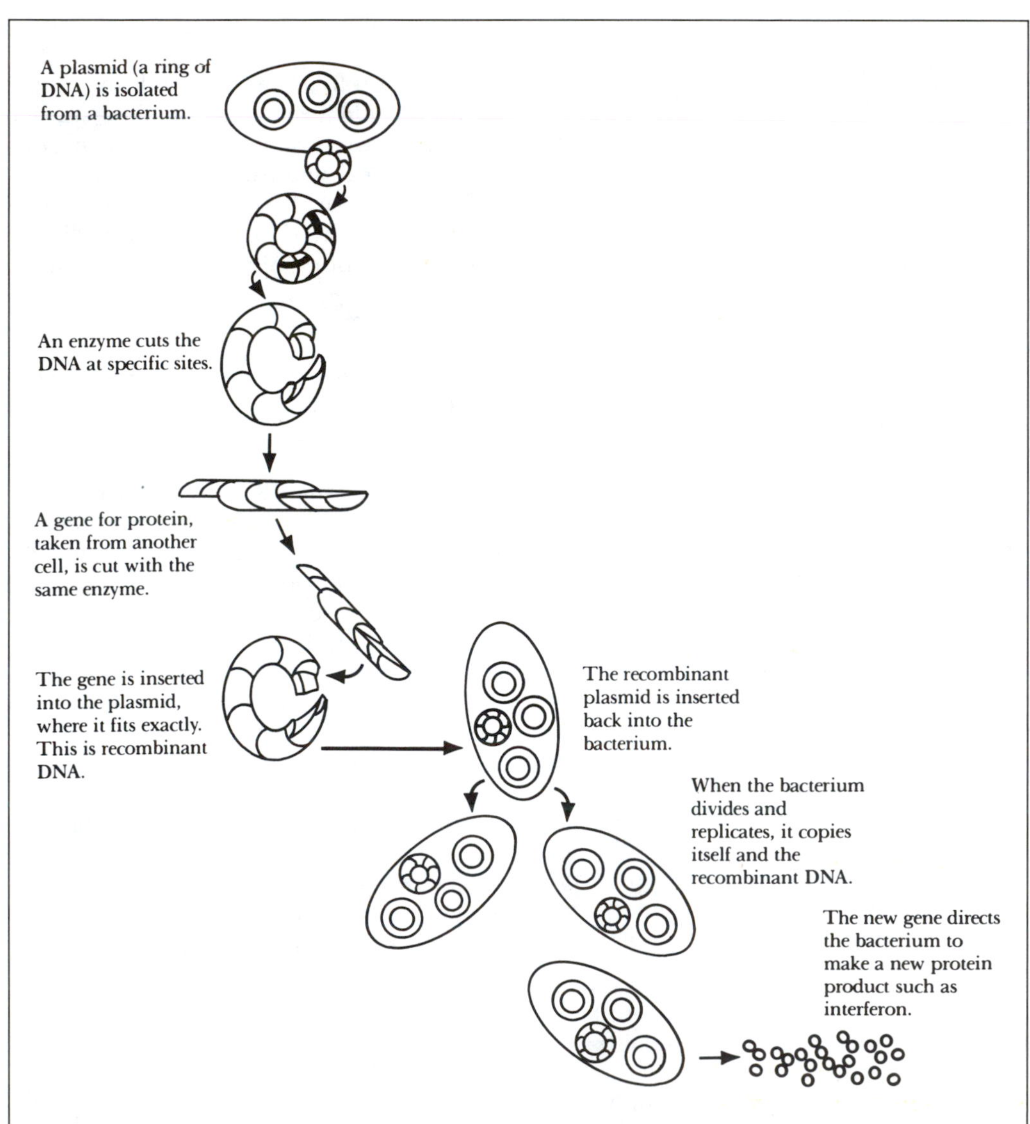

FIGURE 17-2 Recombinant DNA. Genetic engineering, known as recombinant DNA technology, allows scientists to pluck genes from one type of organism and combine them with genes of a second organism, inducing cells to make large quantities of human proteins, such as interferon and interleukins. Microorganisms also can be made to manufacture proteins from infectious agents, such as the hepatitis virus and the AIDS virus, for use in vaccines. (Source: Schindler LW: *Understanding the Immune System.* NIH pub. no. 88-529. Bethesda, MD: U.S. Department of Health and Human Services, July 1988, p. 29.)

TABLE 17-1 Interferons

Type	Agents That Stimulate Production	Interferon-Producing Cells	Cellular Effects
Alpha	B-cell mitogens, viruses, tumor cells	B-lymphocytes, T-lymphocytes; macrophages, and null cells	Antiviral,* antiproliferative,† immunomodulatory
Beta	Viruses	Fibroblasts	Antiviral, antiproliferative, immunomodulatory
Gamma	T-cell mitogens, specific antigens, interleukin-2	T-lymphocytes	Immunomodulatory,* antiproliferative,† antiviral

*Strongest activity.
†Moderate activity.

cells responsible for their natural production, and their major cellular effects. All three types are available in recombinant form. Alpha and gamma interferon are FDA approved; beta interferon remains investigational.

Cellular effects

The activity of the IFNs has been documented in three areas: antiviral, immunomodulatory, and antiproliferative.[58–62] All three types of IFN exhibit these cellular effects in various degrees. Clearly, the antiviral activity is the best defined, having played a significant role in IFN's original identification. IFNs protect a virally infected cell from attack by another virus and, in addition, inhibit intracellular replication of viral DNA as part of a primary defense response. All nucleated cells of vertebrates produce IFN when exposed to a virus. IFN then binds to specific receptors on the infected cell's surface and induces enzyme production that damages the viral DNA strands.

IFNs exert profound effects on the immune system. Immunomodulatory effects result from direct interaction with T-lymphocytes that stimulate the cellular immune response.[54,55,58,60,61] In vitro, the killing potential of natural killer (NK) cells is increased in the presence of IFN. The dose and route of IFN administration significantly affect NK cell activity.[58]

IFNs also exhibit an antiproliferative effect. Although the primary mechanism of the antiproliferative effect remains unclear, it is known that in tumor cells, IFN directly inhibits DNA and protein synthesis.[54,56,60,62] Furthermore, interferons increase tumor cell recognition by stimulating the expression of both human leukocyte antigens (HLAs) and tumor-associated antigens on tumor cell surfaces. IFNs also act to increase all cell phases, prolonging the overall generation time and thus inhibiting the rate of cell growth. Potentially, this action is in itself antiproliferative.

Therapeutic uses/clinical trials

Most research to date has involved the use of recombinant α-IFN (r α-IFN), which received FDA approval in 1986 for use in hairy-cell leukemia (HCL). Subsequently, its clinical indications were expanded to include Condyloma-acuminatum in 1988, AIDS-associated Kaposi's sarcoma in 1989, and chronic hepatitis C in 1991. Two recombinant forms of α-IFN are available: Roferon-A (Roche Laboratories, Nutley, NJ) and Intron A (Schering Corp., Kenilworth, NJ). Clearly, hematologic diseases have responded best to IFN therapy, with measurable responses occurring in the lymphoproliferative malignancies, such as hairy-cell leukemia, non-Hodgkin's lymphoma, and multiple myeloma and in chronic myelogenous leukemia and AIDS-associated Kaposi's sarcoma.[54,56,58–67]

Studies of solid tumors treated with IFN do not report as high objective response rates as those seen in the hematologic malignancies.[68] Tumors in which administration of systemic α-IFN has demonstrated good objective responses include renal cell carcinoma, malignant melanoma, and malignant carcinoid. A role for regional therapy with α-IFN has been identified, such as intravesical use in low-grade in situ bladder carcinoma (>50%),[69] intraperitoneal administration in minimal residual ovarian cancer (50%),[70] and intralesional therapy in cutaneous melanoma[71] and basal cell carcinoma.[72,73] Alpha-interferon is also under study in combination with fluorouracil (5-FU) in the treatment of colorectal cancer.[74] IFN has been shown to augment synergistically the cytotoxic effects of 5-FU and demonstrates greater therapeutic efficacy than 5-FU alone.[74–76]

The use of α-IFN in the treatment of chronic hepatitis C is now established.[77] Low-dose systemic α-IFN has demonstrated activity against the hepatitis B virus, with clinical evidence of the loss of the viral hepatitis B surface antigen.[78]

AIDS-associated Kaposi's sarcoma

Kaposi's sarcoma (KS) is the most common malignancy in patients with acquired immunodeficiency syndrome (AIDS). In the first clinical trial of α-IFN in AIDS-associated KS, Krown and colleagues reported that 5 of 12 patients demonstrated a partial or complete tumor response.[79] These data subsequently were confirmed in larger groups by other researchers who used various forms of r α-IFN. Response rates appear to be highest (range 13%–42%) when higher doses of α-IFN (20 million–30 million U/m²) are administered subcutaneously three times weekly.[79–81] No substantial evidence exists that supports the use of chemotherapeutic agents with α-IFN to improve KS tumor response.[82]

In vitro, α-IFN has been shown to suppress human immunodeficiency virus (HIV) replication.[83] Interestingly, studies have described an increased tumor response to α-IFN in a subset of patients with AIDS-associated KS.[80–82] These patients with AIDS-associated KS have a helper T4 cell count of more than 200/cu mm², lack "B" symptoms (fever, weight loss, night sweats), and have no prior history of opportunistic infections. This suggests that in AIDS-associated KS, α-IFN not only functions in an antiproliferative manner but also may be capable of modulating the patient's immune system. Thus, it is possible that interferon has a direct effect against HIV proliferation in individuals with AIDS.

On the basis of in vitro evidence of anti-HIV synergism, studies are exploring combinations of α-IFN with zidovudine (azidothymidine, AZT, Retrovir) and granulocyte-macrophage CSF.[84] These agents may be important in the treatment of AIDS and KS. Objective tumor responses were seen in 41% (7 of 17) patients. GM-CSF prevented the expected hematologic toxicity while producing no adverse effects on immune function or HIV activity. The flulike syndrome was responsible for the dose-limiting toxicity of this combined therapy.

Gamma-IFN (Actimmune) was approved by the FDA in 1991 to prevent infection in patients with chronic granulomatous disease. Prophylactic γ-IFN therapy led to a 70% reduction in the risk of infection for patients with both X-linked and autosomal traits compared to placebo.[85]

Ongoing phase I and II studies with the use of β- and γ-IFN continue. Antitumor responses of γ-IFN have been reported for renal cell carcinoma, melanoma, non-Hodgkin's lymphoma, Hodgkin's disease, and leukemia; however, data are limited and the role of this agent in the therapy of any of these diseases has yet to be established.[86–89]

The search to find the optimal immunomodulating and/or antiproliferative IFN dose and route continues. Studies that combine IFN with chemotherapeutic agents and with other cytokines to obtain optimal tumor response will be ongoing.

Administration

With the exception of the known FDA-approved indications and dosages, the optimal dose, route of administration, and frequency of IFN administration to treat other types of cancer must still be determined. IFN cannot be given orally because it is a protein substance and digestive enzymes would destroy it. Therefore, viable administration routes include subcutaneous, intramuscular, intravenous bolus, intravenous continuous infusion, intrathecal, intralesional, and intracavity. The route of administration of IFN has been shown to alter significantly the pharmacokinetics of this agent.[54–58] For example, the half-life of α-IFN administered intramuscularly or subcutaneously is approximately 2–4 hours, whereas the half-life of intravenous doses ranges from 6 to 8 hours.[59] Administration of IFN may cause local erythema and irritation at the injection site.

Clinical toxicities

Multiple systemic toxicities occur with the administration of the various types of IFN.[90] Most toxicities are dose-related; low doses of IFN are well tolerated, with minimal measurable toxicity, whereas high doses often require cessation of therapy. A summary of potential toxicities is found in Table 17-2.

Flulike syndrome A common reaction to any type of IFN is the occurrence of fever, chills, fatigue, and malaise. These symptoms are grouped together and referred to as a flulike syndrome. When patients continue to receive doses of IFN, tachyphylaxis or tolerance develops. If, however, the dose or schedule is altered, symptoms may recur. Less notable tachyphylaxis has been reported with γ-IFN.[91] This syndrome can be acute, appearing within hours after IFN administration; it can be subacute, consistently present with mild severity; or it can become chronic. Fevers, which range from 38°C to 40°C, occur 2–4 hours after injection. Fatigue can become so severe that further therapy may be limited.

TABLE 17-2 Interferon Toxicities

Flulike syndrome	**GI**
Fevers*	Nausea
Chills,* severe rigors	Vomiting
Malaise*	Diarrhea
Fatigue	Anorexia/weight loss
CNS	**Hematologic**
Headache	Leukopenia
Lethargy	Thrombocytopenia
Somnolence	Anemia
Seizures	
Confusion	**Cardiovascular**
Impaired concentration	Hypotension
Renal/hepatic	Tachycardia
Elevated transaminase	Arrhythmias
Proteinuria	Myocardial ischemia
	Integumentary
Reproductive	Alopecia
Impotence	Irritation at injection site
Decreased libido	

*Most common toxicities experienced

Source: Hahn MB, Jassak PF: Nursing management of patients receiving interferon. *Semin Oncol Nurs* 4:97,1988.

Musculoskeletal Patients commonly report the presence of myalgia, describing this as "aching" muscles. Low-back pain also has been reported.

Gastrointestinal Nausea and vomiting occur less frequently and usually can be managed with conventional antiemetics. Weight loss associated with IFN therapy has been reported to be significant, frequently resulting in more than 5% loss of total body weight within a 4-week period.[92]

Cardiovascular Although rare, hypotension has been documented with α- and γ-IFN administration and may be dose-related.[57,93] Those at risk for cardiac toxicities, the elderly and patients with a history of cardiac disease, should be thoroughly evaluated and consistently monitored if IFN therapy is undertaken. Other cardiac toxicities reported include arrhythmias, tachycardia, chest pain, and ischemia.

Renal/hepatic Increased hepatic enzymes, hyperbilirubinemia, proteinuria, and renal insufficiency have been documented. These toxicities appear to be dose-related and are monitored by laboratory studies.

Central nervous system (CNS) Symptoms that range from headache, mild confusion, somnolence, and seizure activity have been reported in patients receiving α-, β-,or γ-IFN. In most cases, patients return to baseline status within 96 hours after IFN is discontinued. At doses above 15 million U/day, acute CNS toxicity occurs more frequently, and further IFN therapy may be withheld.

Hematologic Neutropenia and thrombocytopenia have been reported in the use of all types of IFN. These reactions are thought to be both dose-related and dose-limiting. Frequently, neutropenia requires a dose reduction, temporary cessation of therapy, or discontinuation of the IFN. Coagulopathies, although rare, have been reported with γ-IFN.[91]

Miscellaneous Other toxicities reported include dry mouth and inflammation at the subcutaneous injection site. In addition to toxicity, another limiting factor in IFN therapy may be the development of neutralizing antibodies.[94] Because IFN is a recombinant molecule, it is potentially antigenic and can induce antibody formation as part of the immune response. Steis and colleagues[95] indicate that many factors influence the antibody response, including the underlying disease state, treatment schedule, cumulative dose, treatment duration, route of administration, blood sampling time, source of protein, and assay method. Renal cell carcinoma and KS have the highest incidence of reported antibody formation. What is not yet known is whether the presence of anti-IFN antibodies interferes with the biologic activity of IFN. Quesada et al.[96] report that when neutralizing antibodies developed in patients with renal cell carcinoma, tumor responses cease. Figlin, however, in summarizing the available data,[94] cites variances in tumor response concomitant with antibody formation. Clearly, the significance of neutralizing antibodies must be further evaluated.

Future use of IFN therapy

Future use of IFN therapy will expand its preliminary role in combination and adjuvant therapy. Potential combinations include IFN with other cytokine agents, such as IL-2, γ-IFN (due to different receptor sites and mechanisms of action), chemotherapeutic agents, with surgery or radiation therapy, and with hyperthermia.[78]

Interleukins

The ILs are among the most important regulatory substances produced by lymphocytes and monocytes. Multiple ILs have been isolated and identified; however, other than IL-1, IL-2, IL-3, IL-4, IL-6, IL-7, and IL-10, little is understood about their biologic effects. IL-2 is now FDA approved for use in metastatic renal cell carcinoma. Presently, IL-1, IL-4, and IL-6 are being studied actively in clinical trials, while IL-7 and IL-10 are in preclinical studies. Since IL-3 acts as a growth factor, it is discussed in the upcoming section on "Colony Stimulating Factors."

Interleukin-1

IL-1 is a family of at least two distinct glycoproteins produced by monocyte/macrophage fibroblasts and endothelial and smooth muscle cells. Two molecular forms of IL-1—IL-1α and IL-1β—were identified on purification of human IL-1.[97] IL-1 serves an important immunoregulatory role through a variety of biologic activities, which include (1) activation of T-cells to produce IL-2 and other cytokines, (2) induction of fibroblast proliferation, (3) induction of fever, promotion of bone resorption, and initiation of acute phase protein synthesis, (4) enhancement of antibody responsiveness through stimulation of helper T-cells and B-cells, (5) enhancement of cytotoxicity of lymphocytes, (6) induction of tumor-cell markers, and (7) provision of radioprotective properties.[97–100] Both IL-1α and IL-1β currently are under clinical study.

Scientists have found that IL-1 is identical to hematopoietin-1.[101] Hematopoietin-1 is a multilineage growth factor that allows macrophage (M), M-CSF, or IL-3 to stimulate proliferation and maturation of cells more primitive than those induced by either independently. Thus, hematopoiesis is regulated by IL-1's ability to induce proliferation of other CSFs and its synergistic action with the hormones or the primitive hematopoietic stem cells.[100]

IL-1α Recombinant human interleukin-1α (rhu IL-1α) is produced in *E. Coli* by Immunex Corporation and is just entering phase I clinical trials. The biologic activities of *E. Coli*-derived rh IL-1α suggest a variety of potential clinical applications, including prevention or reversal of iatrogenic neutropenia, reversal of thrombocytopenia, bone marrow transplantation, antiproliferative effects, infectious disease, dysmyelopoietic states, and combination therapy with other cytokines.

IL-1α is administered subcutaneously to rotating sites on the arms, abdomen, and thighs, with ice applied after injection to prevent bleeding. Most frequently reported clinical toxicities include fever, chills, headache, nausea/vomiting, tachycardia, asthenia, anorexia, hypotension, myalgia, and diarrhea. Hypotension has been the dose-limiting toxicity.[102,103]

IL-1β Recombinant human interleukin-1β (rhu IL-1β) was cloned, expressed and purified from *E. Coli* by Immunex Corporation and is undergoing clinical investigation and development by Syntax Research. IL-1β is synthesized in vivo by mononuclear phagocytes and a variety of other cells. It plays a key role in the immune system secondary to its ability to stimulate production of IL-2 and other cytokines.

Doses currently under study range from 1 to 1000 ng/kg given intravenously once daily for 2, 5, or 7 consecutive days as a 30- to 60-minute or continuous infusion. Toxicities experienced include fever (lasting between ½ and 3 hours), chills, and rigors; increased heart rate, respirations, and blood pressure; headaches; arthralgia; myalgia; and nausea/vomiting. Initial increases in blood pressure usually are followed by a return to baseline or mild-to-moderate hypotension requiring either no treatment or saline infusion alone. IL-1β produces a leukocytosis that peaks between 4 and 12 hours after administration and appears to be dose-related. Leukocyte counts return to 20% of baseline by 24 hours following administration. An increase in platelet counts also is seen, usually 5–6 days after initiation, and will remain elevated for between 20 and 24 days after cessation of treatment. Other changes in laboratory parameters include increased serum cortisol and glucose and decreased serum protein.

Further clinical investigation will determine the therapeutic effects of IL-1α and IL-1β.

Interleukin-2

IL-2, previously called T-cell growth factor, is a glycoprotein produced by helper T-cells after stimulation by mitogens or specific antigens and IL-1. Researchers have learned much about this lymphokine since Morgan et al. first described it in 1976.[104]

Cellular effects IL-2 binds to specific receptors on T-lymphocytes and on certain malignant lymphocytes, which may account for the specificity of IL-2 action in the immune response.[105] IL-2, which is an essential factor in the growth of T-cells, supports proliferation and augmentation of NK cells, is critical for the generation of lymphokine-activated killer (LAK) cells, and augments various other T-cell functions.[106–108] IL-2 also activates cytotoxic effector cells that produce a spectrum of secondary cytokines, such as TNF, IL-1, IL-6, and γ-IFN. It is hypothesized that these products play a significant role in the systemic toxicities of IL-2, although their antitumor effect is not yet fully understood.

Therapeutic uses/clinical trials IL-2 has been used as a single agent in a variety of doses and schedules, in conjunction with LAK cells or tumor-infiltrating lymphocytes (TILs), in combination with other biologic agents, and in combination with chemotherapeutic agents. IL-2 therapy produces objective tumor responses in 15%–45% of patients with renal cell carcinoma and malignant melanoma.

IL-2 alone or combined with LAK cells At the same time phase I studies of IL-2 were ongoing with recombinant IL-2, Rosenberg and colleagues[109] at the National Cancer Institute (NCI) were investigating the use and therapeutic value of IL-2 and LAK cells. On the basis of the positive results obtained in murine models in which LAK cells were generated in the laboratory from lymphocytes plus IL-2 and then systemically administered, this regimen was administered to 25 patients with advanced metastatic cancer in whom standard therapy had failed. This treatment is termed *adoptive immunotherapy;* it requires obtaining autologous lymphocytes by leukopheresis, incubating these cells with IL-2 to generate LAK cells, and then reinfusing the LAK cells in conjunction with additional doses of IL-2. Adoptive immunotherapy is an approach in which the tumor-bearing host passively receives cells that possess antitumor activity.

LAK cells are capable of selectively lysing tumor cells that are resistant to NK cells without affecting normal cells.[110] The adoptive transfer of these LAK cells plus recombinant IL-2 in individuals with advanced cancer resulted in regression of metastases from a wide variety of tumors, including melanoma, sarcoma, colon adenocarcinoma, and bladder cancer.[109] Objective responses, a reduction of more than 50% of disease volume, were seen in 11 of 25 patients. Complete tumor regression occurred in one individual with metastatic melanoma that was sustained for more than 10 months after therapy. Additional phase I and II studies of IL-2 substantiated the initially reported systemic toxicities and supported measurable clinical responses.[111–118] Numerous reports of IL-2 clinical trials are now found in the literature. IL-2 as a single agent appears as effective in achieving tumor response as IL-2 with LAK cells in patients with renal cell cancer.

Although far more knowledge of the therapeutic and immunologic activity of IL-2 must still be obtained, a few key points can now be summarized. Renal cell carcinoma and malignant melanoma are the solid tumors that have been studied extensively to date. Objective tumor responses have been reproduced, although many are partial responses and of limited duration. It is important to note, however, that these tumors previously did not respond to standard therapy; thus these responses must be viewed as noteworthy. Clearly, Rosenberg and colleagues[119] from the NCI surgical branch have the most extensive experience with IL-2. IL-2 alone is indicated for the treatment of metastatic renal cell cancer.

IL-2 and tumor-infiltrating lymphocytes A cell population obtained from tumor-bearing patients that appears to be more potent than LAK cells also was identified by Rosenberg and colleagues.[120,121] This subpopulation of lymphocytes, called tumor-infiltrating lymphocytes (TILs), infiltrate into tumors. By culturing single-cell suspension obtained from tumors with IL-2, TILs can be produced in large quantities and used to mediate the regression of metastatic tumors. TILs are functional without the administration of additional doses of IL-2, although low doses of IL-2 appear to enhance TIL's therapeutic efficacy.

A phase II study using high-dose IL-2 and TIL documented response rates of 36%–39% in patients with metastatic melanoma.[122] TIL cells are able to recognize unique tumor-associated antigens, making further delineation of the biologic characteristics of these antigens feasible.[123]

IL-2 in combination Numerous in vitro and preclinical animal studies have examined the use of various doses and schedules of IL-2 with other cytokines (including α-, β-, and γ-IFN, and TNF), MAbs, and chemotherapeutic agents.[124] Many of these combinations have entered clinical trials. Several studies are now investigating IL-2 in combination with α-IFN in an outpatient setting.[125,126]

Pharmacokinetics Aldesleukin's (Proleukin®) pharmacokinetic profile is characterized by high plasma concentrations following short IV infusion, with rapid distribution to the extravascular and extracellular space.[127] The drug is eliminated from the body via metabolism in the kidneys, with little or no bioactive protein excreted in the urine.

Initially 30% of the dose administered is delivered to the plasma, with 70% distributed to the liver, kidney, and lung. The primary route of clearance is the kidney, utilizing both glomerular filtration and peritubular extraction. This rapid clearance rate supports short, frequent dosage schedules.

Although higher doses of IL-2 can be administered through bolus intravenous infusion once or three times daily, at equal daily doses, continuous infusions of IL-2 produce greater toxicity and exert greater immunobiologic effects.[128a,128b] Differences in toxicities seen with different administration schedules are related to the agent's pharmacokinetics.

Clinical toxicities Administration of IL-2 results in multisystem toxicities that may be life-threatening.[128b–130] No organ system is spared. However, all side effects related to IL-2 administration are usually reversible; pretreatment laboratory values and physiologic states, with the exception of fatigue, generally return within 24–96 hours following cessation of therapy. These clinical toxicities are clearly related to dose, route, and schedule. Thus, at high dose (600,000 IU/kg) these systemic toxicities are a challenge to manage effectively, while at low doses of IL-2 (less than 18,000 IU/day) the severity and intensity of the toxicities lessen dramatically and are easily managed. Although neither the mechanism for the induction of these toxicities nor their pathophysiology is well known, considerable evidence suggests that the IL-2-induced production of other cytokines, IL-1, IL-6, γ-IFN and TNF, either contributes to or is totally responsible for these toxicities.[105,129–131]

Central nervous system Disorientation has been the major CNS toxicity observed.[132] Patients are carefully monitored for overt and subtle changes in mental status.[133] If signs and/or symptoms of disorientation—agitation, restlessness, increased anxiety—are present, subsequent IL-2 doses should be held or discontinued. Some patients may progress rapidly from confusion or agitation to somnolence, disorientation, or severe agitation, requiring the use of restraints. Although some studies have documented that neurotoxicity can progress even after therapy is stopped, generally these symptoms will resolve within 24–48 hours following the last dose of IL-2.

Cardiovascular/pulmonary Marked cardiovascular and pulmonary toxicities occur when IL-2 is administered at high dose. A capillary leak syndrome, characterized by marked extravascular fluid shifts, consistently occurs. IL-2 causes peripheral vasodilation, with a significant decrease in systemic vascular resistance and an increase in heart rate. Hypotension usually begins soon after the onset of treatment and is defined as a systolic BP less than 90 or a 20-mm Hg or greater decrease from baseline. Plasma protein fraction or albumin is administered initially. Fluid challenges are contraindicated and will increase the risk of fluid overload. Dopamine HC1 or phenylephrine HC1 (Neo-synephrine) is administered to keep the systolic BP greater than 90. Tachycardia occurs as a compensatory response to maintain cardiac output and vascular perfusion in the presence of hypotension. Cardiac dysrhythmias (sinus or supraventricular tachycardia) develop in approximately 10% of patients and respond to traditional medical management with digoxin or verapamil. Daily EKGs and increased vital sign monitoring for patients on vasopressors also are indicated. In addition, a decrease of 5% or greater in the left ventricular ejection fraction has been documented, which suggests either a direct or an indirect effect of IL-2 on the myocardium.[134, 135] These changes appear to be limited and reversible. Transient cardiac ischemia also has been reported. Myocardial infarctions, although rare, have occurred in four patients; one of them was fatal. Pulmonary congestion also is common. Oxygen saturation usually will be monitored by pulse oximetry, and patients may require oxygen therapy for dyspnea and diuretics for fluid management. The serum bicarbonate should be checked and replaced per physician order. If the serum bicarbonate is less than 15 mEq/l or the oxygen saturation is less than 90%–94%, the IL-2 dose may be held. An average weight gain of between 5% and 10% of total body weight also occurs, with 32%

of patients experiencing weight gains equal to or greater than 10% of their baseline weight. Appropriate prescreening should exclude patients with underlying cardiac or pulmonary risk factors. Thus, patients with histories of cardiac or pulmonary dysfunction are not eligible for treatment with IL-2.

Renal Oliguria, anuria, azotemia, and elevations of serum creatinine and blood urea nitrogen levels occur with IL-2 therapy. In addition, Kozeny et al.[136] noted a progressive respiratory alkalosis and hypophosphatemia, hypocalcemia, and hypomagnesemia. Serum BUN, creatinine, and electrolytes may reach ten times the patient's baseline value without the need for clinical intervention, if the increase is gradual and without other complications (e.g., marked fluid overload). Azotemia and elevated creatinine levels have occurred in all patients. However, a rapid rise in creatinine (daily doubling of value) may necessitate holding a dose of IL-2. Episodes of anuria, defined as the presence of less than 10 ml of urine per hour, lasting longer than 8 hours, occur in approximately 38% of patients. Patients may be started on low-dose dopamine to assist with renal perfusion. Normal renal function usually returns spontaneously after IL-2 therapy is stopped. Patients with prior nephrectomy appear at higher risk for nephrotoxicity and should be monitored closely.

Gastrointestinal Nausea and vomiting can be controlled effectively with the administration of antiemetics. Patients commonly experience diarrhea, which if severe may require administration of bicarbonate to correct deficiencies. Stomatitis occurs frequently but is not severe. Malaise and anorexia, although not treatment limiting, are most likely caused by the presence of γ-INF.

Hepatic Increased levels of serum bilirubin and liver enzymes occur with IL-2 therapy, as does a progressive hypoalbuminemia. Mild to moderate hepatomegaly without tenderness in the right upper quadrant of the abdomen is also commonly reported.

Hematologic Anemia, severe enough to warrant the transfusion of packed red blood cells, occurs in 77% of patients who receive IL-2. Criteria for transfusions include not only the hemoglobin and hematocrit values but also consideration of the patient's cardiopulmonary status and the need for hemodynamic support not achieved with crystalloid or colloid solutions. Thrombocytopenia ($<50,000/m^3$) is common; however, platelet administration rarely is clinically indicated. No evidence of disseminated intravascular coagulation or other severe coagulopathies has been reported, although an increase in prothrombin time can be measured in most patients.[137]

Integumentary A diffuse erythematous rash that is pruritic in nature and progresses to desquamation develops in all patients who receive IL-2. Skin desquamation can be severe, involving the soles of the feet, the palms of the hands, and moist intertriginous areas.

Flulike syndrome Fever, chills, rigors, and malaise are universal symptoms in all patients who receive IL-2. These symptoms can be managed to a degree by prophylactic administration of acetaminophen, diphenhydramine, and indomethacin. When chills or rigors are present, meperidine 25–50 mg intravenous push or lorazepam 1–2 mg intravenous push is effective. If hypotension is present, administering meperidine may further compound the clinical picture, whereas hypotension is a rare toxicity of lorazepam.

Endocrinologic Atkins et al.[138] noted the development of hypothyroidism in 20% of patients who received high doses of IL-2/LAK. Other reported endocrine effects of IL-2 include increases in blood levels of adrenocorticotropic hormone, cortisol, prolactin, growth hormone, and the acute-phase reactant C-reactive protein.

LAK cell reaction Mild to severe chills, followed by transient fever, have been reported within 0.5–1 hour following the first administration of LAK cells.[128b] These toxicities appear similar to those reported with granulocyte transfusions and therefore probably are directly related to LAK cell administration. Also noted is that patients generally report less severe reactions with subsequent LAK cell administration.

It remains unclear which of these toxicities are related to the immunomodulatory and antiproliferative effects of IL-2, and the subsequent production of other cytokines, or to purely toxic consequences of therapy that can and should be therapeutically altered.

Interleukin-4

Interleukin-4 is a natural product of activated T-lymphocytes, and it exerts multiple cellular effects on lymphocytes and monocytes, bone marrow progenitor cells, and endothelial cells of blood vessels. IL-4 is recombinantly produced in yeast and is currently undergoing phase I and II clinical trials. Preclinical studies suggest a role for rhu IL-4 in mediating antiproliferative effects. Lotze[131] reports objective tumor effects in patients with melanoma, renal cell carcinoma, and breast cancer when IL-4 is used in combination with IL-2. In addition, it is postulated that IL-4 might have a function as an anti-inflammatory agent since it suppresses the human monocyte production of TNF-α, IL-1, and prostaglandin E_2 (PGE_2).[131].

Clinical toxicities experienced with IL-4 appear to be dose-related. Potential toxicities include fever, chills, hypotension, nausea/vomiting, elevated liver enzymes, increased creatinine, weight gain, and marked nasal congestion. Chills typically occur within 30 minutes of the infusion and fever approximately 4–6 hours after initiation. These toxicities can be managed clinically using the interventions outlined earlier for IL-2.

Interleukin-6

Interleukin-6 is produced naturally primarily by monocytes, endothelial cells, and fibroblasts. It also is produced by B- and T-lymphocytes and some tumor cell lines.[139] Biologic properties of IL-6 identified include hematologic, antiproliferative, B-cell effects and inflammatory effects. Recombinant IL-6 is produced in *E. coli* and recently entered phase I clinical trials. Possible toxicities include elevated bilirubin and transaminases, chills, fever, nausea/vomiting, diarrhea, leukopenia, fatigue, somnolence, and anemia. The strategies used to manage the patient on IL-2 also can be effective for these patients.

Interleukin-7

Identification of the biologic properties of the IL-7 gene, just recently cloned and expressed, provided scientists with a more detailed understanding of its effects on lymphocyte growth and maturation.[140] IL-7 is produced by the bone marrow and thymic stromal cells. Several of the known biologic activities of IL-7 include: stimulation of the expansion of immature lymphoid cells,[140] induction of IL-2 production, and synergistic activity with IL-2 in thymic T-cell proliferation.[131] IL-7 is not yet in clinical trials, but it will be an interesting agent due to its activities on B- and T-lymphocytes.

Interleukin-10

Interleukin-10 also was recently cloned and expressed. Biologic activities of this agent include synergistic activity on both fetal and adult thymocytes with IL-7, IL-2, and IL-4, individually or in combination.[131] It is thought that IL-10, either alone or with IL-7, may function as a lymphopoietin, producing growth of both B- and T-cells.

It is clear from the foregoing description of additional interleukins that have been cloned, expressed, and in some cases recombinantly produced for further clinical investigation that multiple, intricate relationships exist between these cytokines. Lotze[131] suggests that the known and unknown complexities and relationships among the interleukins will provide the framework in our quest to understand the intricate balance and regulation of these cytokines. Once understood, these principles, regulating the immune system, can then be clinically applied to eradicate cancer effectively.

Tumor Necrosis Factor

In 1975, Carswell et al.[142] first identified TNF in the serum of mice injected with bacterial endotoxin (bacille Calmette-Guérin, or *C. parvum*) as the endogenous agent responsible for tumor necrosis. Further studies identified that TNF had cytotoxic or cytostatic in vitro effects on murine[142] and human[143,144] tumor cells, with no effect on normal cells. TNF, a naturally occurring agent, is produced by activated macrophages.[145–147] The gene that encodes human TNF was identified, cloned, and expressed in *E. coli*.[148] This highly purified recombinant human TNF demonstrated the same biologic activity spectrum as the isolated natural agent and thus became available for human investigation.

Concomitantly, research was under way to understand the pathophysiology of cachexia, often seen in patients with chronic diseases. Beutler and colleagues[149] isolated a molecule they called *cachetin,* believed to be an etiologic agent of cachexia, and structurally similar to TNF. Subsequently, molecular cloning studies confirmed that cachectin and TNF are identical substances.

Cellular effects

TNF is produced by endotoxin-activated macrophages; it travels through the bloodstream and binds to designated receptors located on cell membranes. Once bound to cell membranes, TNF initiates its cellular action. Early laboratory research with the use of murine models identified that the immediate effect of TNF on tumor cells is cytostasis, producing cell arrest in the G_2 phase of the cell cycle. Darzynkiewicz et al.[150] found this effect to prevail during the first 4 hours after exposure to TNF, with extensive cell lysis measurable after 7 hours and nearly complete cell lysis occurring after 24 hours. Research has identified that approximately one-third of human epithelial cancer cell culture lines are extremely sensitive to the cytolytic effects of TNF, whereas another one-third demonstrate cytostasis without lysis and another third are basically resistant to TNF.[143,151] Normal cell activity is affected only by a 100- to 10,000-fold increase in TNF concentration. Thus TNF selectively attacks tumor cells while sparing normal cells.[142,151]

TNF exhibits a broad range of biologic activity. In particular, TNF has been identified as a primary mediator of endotoxic shock.[152] Other biologic effects of TNF are summarized in Table 17-3.[153–161] The thera-

TABLE 17-3 Biologic Effects of Tumor Necrosis Factor

	Effect
Tumor cells	• Produces cytostasis
	• Induces cytolytic action
Normal cells	• Promotes production and activation of hematopoietic cells
	• Enhances function of effector cells
	• Stimulates activation of vascular/coagulation system
	• Induces secretion of other cytokines (GM-CSF, IL-1, IL-6)
	• Induces synthesis of collagenase and prostaglandin E_2
	• Increases expression of several cell-surface antigens
	• Induces secretion of small-molecule mediators of inflammation

GM-CSF, granulocyte-macrophage colony stimulating factor.
IL, interleukin.

peutic significance of the biologic activity of TNF is under phase I/II and phase III clinical investigation.

Pharmacokinetics

Chapman et al.[162] document that the serum half-life of intravenous bolus-administered recombinant TNF (rTNF) is approximately 20 minutes. Varying detectable serum TNF levels are reported for different routes of administration. With intravenous bolus TNF, serum levels were detectable at doses greater than 25 μg/m². Serum levels of rTNF were not detectable after subcutaneous administration except for one patient who received a dose of 250 μg/m². Jakubowski et al.[163] could not detect serum TNF levels in patients treated with intramuscular doses equal to or less than 100 μg/m². Much variability also exists in the time after injection that rTNF was detectable. This initial pharmacokinetic information suggests that the half-life of rTNF depends on the dose and route of administration.

Clinical trials

Since December 1985 more than 200 patients have participated in phase I studies of rTNF, receiving a fixed dose given repetitively by various routes and schedules. Phase I studies of 30-minute intravenous infusions administered for 5 days every other week have established the maximum tolerated dose of rTNF to be 150 μg/m²/day. This is similar to the work of Jakubowski et al.[163] in which rTNF was administered by intramuscular injection. Phase II clinical trials are under way to determine further tumor response, immune system modulation, dosage, route of administration, and toxicities.

Administration

In current clinical trials, rTNF is being administered by various routes, including intravenous bolus, continuous intravenous infusion, and subcutaneous and intramuscular injection. The optimal route and dosing schedule have yet to be established. Recombinant TNF is administered intravenously in a normal saline solution that contains human serum albumin at a concentration of 2 mg/ml. The intravenous tubing must be cleared with the admixture of normal saline and human serum albumin before the addition of rTNF to prevent the rTNF from adhering to the tubing. Because rTNF is an investigational agent, administration must conform to each institution's standards and policies for the use of investigational drugs.

Clinical toxicities

Experience with rTNF indicates that most patients experience side effects similar to those observed with the interferons and IL-2. As with IFN, tachyphylaxis will develop, in which the flulike syndrome will decrease with subsequent doses of rTNF. Most toxicities appear to be dose-dependent and are reversible, resolving within 48–96 hours after the drug is discontinued. Systemic toxicities of rTNF are summarized in Table 17-4. The most common toxicities are a flulike syndrome—which includes fever, chills, rigors, headaches, and fatigue—and a local reaction at the subcutaneous or intramuscular injection site.

Flulike syndrome Fever and chills generally occur within 1–6 hours following drug administration. Chapman et al.[162] note that different patterns for the onset of fever, chills, and rigors depend on the route of administration. Rigors may occur within 10 minutes following intravenous bolus administration of rTNF, and temperature rises within 20 minutes, with peak spikes recorded 1–2 hours after injection. After subcutaneous administration, rigors were reported to be milder and fevers peaked at 4–8 hours. Increases in dose did not alter fever increases. Fever, chills, and rigors are treated with acetaminophen and meperidine or lorazepam. Mild to severe fatigue, which lasts up to 3 days after subcutaneous administration but fewer than 24 hours after intravenous administration, has been reported, necessitating changes in the patient's daily activities. Headaches, described as dull and aching, occur frequently and respond to acetaminophen or narcotic analgesics.

Gastrointestinal Gastrointestinal toxicities associated with rTNF administration have been reported but do not appear to be dose-dependent.[162,163] Anorexia, nausea, vomiting, and diarrhea may occur. Antiemet-

TABLE 17-4 Recombinant Tumor Necrosis Factor Systemic Toxicities

Flulike syndrome Fever, chills* Rigors* Headaches*	**Hepatic** Increased bilirubin Increased ALT (SGOT) Increased alkaline phosphatase
Pulmonary Dyspnea	**Endocrine** Increased triglycerides Decreased cholesterol
Cardiovascular Hypotension Hypertension Supraventricular arrhythmias	**Gastrointestinal** Anorexia Nausea Vomiting Diarrhea
CNS Seizures Confusion Aphasia	**Integumentary** Inflammation at injection site (intramuscular, subcutaneous)
Hematologic Granulocytopenia Thrombocytopenia Increased circulating monocytes (monocytosis)	

*Most common.

ics, such as prochlorperazine, may be useful to control nausea. Significant weight loss has not been reported.

Cardiovascular Transient episodes of hypotension, in which the systolic blood pressure is 90 mm Hg or less, occur 1–11 hours after intravenous administration and 2–48 hours after subcutaneous administration at doses of 5 μg/m² or higher. This transient hypotension is treated effectively with intravenous saline infusions. Vasopressor agents have not been required. Hypertension also has been reported. It is believed that the hypertension episodes may be directly related to the presence of rigors that physiologically produce tachycardia and peripheral vasoconstriction. Supraventricular arrhythmias, although rare, also have been reported.

Hematologic Hematologic toxicities of rTNF include granulocytopenia, thrombocytopenia, and increased circulating monocytes. These toxicities appear to be dose-related, with larger decreases from baseline values observed at doses greater than 100μg/m²/day. No consistent changes in coagulation factors have been identified. Thus no evidence currently exists that patients who receive rTNF are at risk for the development of disseminated intravascular coagulation. These hematologic toxicities occur independent of administration route. Patients' hematologic values return to baseline on cessation of therapy.

Hepatic Moderate increases in liver enzymes and bilirubin have been reported.

Endocrine Increased serum triglyceride levels were detectable at doses greater than 50 μg/m²/day, whereas cholesterol levels decreased during most treatment courses.

Central nervous system Although rare, transient focal neurologic toxicities, such as seizures, confusion, and aphasia, have been reported. Sherman and colleagues[164] describe aphasic episodes that subsequently resolved without adverse clinical effects. The cause is unknown.

Pulmonary Dyspnea has been reported in patients who receive rTNF. Morice et al.[165] documented decreased gas exchange during treatment with rTNF, with return to near baseline values after therapy was discontinued. The cause of this toxicity is unknown but may be related to secondary alveolar endothelial damage.

Inflammation of injection site Subcutaneous and intramuscular injection of rTNF produces a local reaction at the injection site. Tenderness, erythema, induration, and vesiculation have been reported. This toxicity is dose-related, with increasing involvement and severity occurring at higher doses and with increased symptoms with continued drug administration. Local treatment measures of dry heat, cold packs, or warm soaks have been used with variable therapeutic response. Infiltration or phlebitis have not been reported with intravenous injection sites.

Colony Stimulating Factors

Blood cell growth is regulated by a complex structure of hematopoietic growth factors that mediate the proliferation, maturation, regulation, and activation of granulocytes, monocytes, macrophages, lymphocytes, erythrocytes, and platelets.[166] These critical elements that regulate hematopoiesis are called CSFs. All hematopoietic cell lines have their origin in a common source—the pluripotent stem cell. In November 1991 this pluripotent stem call was isolated in humans by SyStemix, Inc., a small biotechnology company in California. Haeuber and DiJulio[167] provide an excellent overview of the relationship of CSFs to normal hematopoiesis. CSFs acquired their name because, in agar cultures, they stimulate the growth of colonies of maturing blood cells from their hematopoietic precursors. Modern techniques of molecular biology, biochemistry, and recombinant technology have been used to isolate these elements and produce large quantities for clinical use.

CSFs are a group of naturally occurring glycoproteins also classified as cytokines. In general, CSFs are named for the major target cell lineage they affect. Thus granulocyte-macrophage CSF (GM-CSF) targets both the granulocyte and macrophage lineages; granulocyte CSF (G-CSF) targets only granulocytes; pleuripoietin IL-3 or multi-CSF targets the early cell lineage; and erythropoietin targets only the erythrocyte lineage. However, an overlap of the effects of one factor on other factors most probably occurs. Grosh and Quesenberry[168] in fact state that CSFs are not, as previously considered, lineage-specific. The actual role CSFs play in the regulation of hematopoiesis is unknown. Research suggests that G-CSF, GM-CSF, and IL-3 may serve as emergency signals to accelerate the production of leukocytes in the presence of inflammation or infection.[169] Thus it is hypothesized that the physiologic role of these particular CSFs may be to augment the production and function of mature granulocytes in pathologic disease states such as infection.

CSFs are used effectively in the treatment of disease states in which myelosuppression, anemia, and thrombocytopenia prevail and limit therapeutic treatment options.[170–177] CSFs allow increased and/or scheduled doses of chemotherapeutic agents to be given without the risk of long-term myelosuppression. They also are effective in other hematologic diseases in which abnormalities of blood cell components exist, such as congenital neutropenia and AIDS. CSFs that will be discussed include erythropoietin, G-CSF, GM-CSF, IL-3, and M-CSF. Other factors, such as thrombopoietin, although identified and isolated, have not yet been recombinantly produced, limiting their clinical investigation. The use of CSFs in clinical practice will be either prophylactic (i.e., to prevent expected complications) or therapeutic (i.e., administered to the patient once complications/need arises).

Erythropoietin

Erythropoietin (EPO) was the first CSF approved by the FDA (in June 1989). Erythropoietin has firmly established its role in the treatment of anemia caused by end-stage renal disease. When administered after dialysis treatments, erythropoietin is effective in stimulating erythropoiesis and either reducing or eliminating patient transfusion requirements.[178] Additional studies have identified that rHuEPO can ameliorate the anemia associated with AZT therapy in AIDS patients[179] and rheumatoid arthritis.[180] It is suggested that anemias that produce low endogenous serum Epo levels should be the most responsive to exogenous rHuEPO; however, this concept remains unclear.

Erythropoietin is produced by the liver and/or kidney in the presence of tissue hypoxia. The hormone then migrates to the hematopoietic tissue, where it activates the proliferation and differentiation of erythroid progenitor cells. Binding to specific receptors on the erythroid progenitor cells, EPO stimulates them to proliferate and to differentiate into mature erythrocytes. Grosh and Quesenberry[168] suggest that EPO also potentially modulates platelet production. Thus, the plasma concentration of EPO directly influences the rate of newer erythrocyte production. Anemia results when the system fails to increase the amount of circulating EPO in response to hypoxic episodes. The anemia related to cancer appears to be multifactorial in origin and has no clear-cut rationale.[181] Several studies have investigated the effect of EPO levels within the cancer population and found adequate hemoglobin rises (at least 2g/dl), subjective improvement in anemia-related symptoms, and statistically significant improvement in performance status.[182–187] It is anticipated that in 1993 EPO will be FDA approved to treat anemia in patients with cancer.

To treat anemia related to cancer, EPO is administered at a dose of 150 U/kg subcutaneously 3 times weekly. Hematocrit rises are detectable within 14–21 days following initiation of the drug treatment. Patients experience minimal side effects with this agent.

Granulocyte colony stimulating factor (G-CSF)

The regulatory function of G-CSF generally is known to be lineage-specific for the proliferation, maturation, and activation of granulocytes. G-CSF also has shown activity in early stem cells, stimulating erythroid and megakaryocyte production and inducing pre-B-cells.[168,188] G-CSF has demonstrated increased production of granulocytes, with corresponding bone marrow changes, in patients with solid tumors receiving standard doses and chemotherapy and following myeloablative treatment with bone marrow transplant and chronic neutropenic diseases.[168,188,189,192] G-CSF also has been used to stimulate stem cell mobilization prior to leukopheresis. In the transplant population, Sheridan[193] found that when G-CSF is administered in the postconditioning transplant regimen, platelet recovery occurs significantly earlier and neutrophil recovery also is accelerated.

Therapeutically, the leukocyte response is dose-dependent, and the schedule and route of administration are important. G-CSF (filgrastim, or Neupogen®) was FDA approved in February 1991 for chemotherapy-induced neutropenia, and is recombinantly produced in *E. coli.* The recommended dose is 5 μg/kg/day for up to 14 days. Administration usually is by subcutaneous injection; or if intravenous, a short (15-min to 1-hr) infusion is suggested. G-CSF is compatible only with dextrose.

Granulocyte-macrophage colony stimulating factor (GM-CSF)

GM-CSF has a broader spectrum of activity that affects all levels of granulocytes and stimulates the production of monocytes and macrophages. It also functions to induce these cells to produce a number of cytokines. Guttermann[171] reports that GM-CSF also produces a multilineage effect in some patients, which decreases the requirement for platelet and red cell transfusions, in addition to its effect on granulocytes. GM-CSF has been used to permit dose intensification and enhance myeloprotection by administering it both prior to the chemotherapeutic regimen and after the chemotherapy administration was completed.[194]

GM-CSF (sargramostim, or Leukine®) was FDA approved in March 1991 for neutropenia associated with autologous bone marrow transplantation and is recombinantly produced in yeast. Schering Corp. also manufactures a recombinant GM-CSF; however it is produced in *E. coli* and is still investigational. Thus, it is imperative to delineate which product is being used when reporting or interpreting the clinical information.

The recommended dose of GM-CSF is 250 μg/m²/day for up to 21 days. Administration can be either subcutaneous injection or intravenous infusion, ranging for a 2–6-hour duration. GM-CSF is compatible only in normal saline. Groopman et al.[172] reported that mild phlebitis occurred when GM-CSF was administered by continuous infusion through a peripheral vein. However, phlebitis did not occur when a central venous catheter was used. GM-CSF administered by subcutaneous injection may produce a local skin reaction at the injection site.[195] This reaction consists of an erythematous induration that persists for 3–5 days after each injection.

Clinical toxicities

One should never administer any CSF with an immediate effect on the progenitor cells (G-CSF, GM-CSF and IL-3) within the 24 hours preceding or following cytotoxic therapy. This time restriction is necessary because the cycling of the hematopoietic progenitor cells stimulated by the CSF will place more dividing cells at risk for destruction by the cytotoxic agents, producing an increase in cell kill instead of reducing the myelotoxicity of the regimen.[195]

Minimal toxicity has been associated with G-CSF therapy. Studies cite occasional reports of transient mild to moderate bone pain.[196] Glaspy and Golde[197] propose that the cause of this bone pain may be the rapid expansion of cells in the bone marrow.

GM-CSF therapy produces a wider array of systemic toxicities than does G-CSF.[188] Herrmann et al.[198] report facial flushing, mild myalgias, and bone pain with intravenous administration. Commonly reported toxicities that appear to be route- and dose-related include low-grade fever with chills that occur 4–6 hours after administration. Patients experienced reversible dyspnea during the initial 2–6 hours of continuous intravenous infusion. The cause of this toxicity is believed to be the rapid sequestration of neutrophils within the lung.[198] Generalized rashes and fluid retention also were described. It is quite possible that many of the side effects GM-CSF produces are related to its ability to stimulate multiple cytokines.[196,199] Bacterially derived *(E. coli)* GM-CSF has been reported to routinely cause a first-dose reaction characterized by transient flushing, tachycardia, hypotension, dyspnea, nausea/vomiting, musculoskeletal pain, and a decreased oxygen saturation.[199] The toxicities all have been reported to be reversible. Table 17-5 provides a summary of known toxicities for GM-CSF and G-CSF. Table 17-6 identifies salient points to review prior to administration of either G-CSF or GM-CSF.

TABLE 17-5 Colony-Stimulating Factor (CSF) Toxicities

Granulocyte-Macrophage CSF	Granulocyte CSF
Flulike syndrome	**Flulike syndrome**
Fever*	Fever
Chills, rigors	Myalgias*
Myalgias*	Headache
Headache	
Fatigue	**Integumentary**
	Generalized rash
Integumentary	
Facial flushing	**Miscellaneous**
Generalized rash	Bone pain*
Inflammation at injection site	
Hematopoietic	
Leukocytosis	
Eosinophilia	
Pulmonary	
Dyspnea	
Miscellaneous	
Bone pain*	
Fluid retention	

*Common toxicities reported.

Outpatients requiring treatment with G-CSF or GM-CSF need instruction in administration techniques, drug stability, and storage and may be asked to complete a daily symptom log to document toxicity trends. As of the end of 1992, Medicare did not cover reimbursement for outpatient use of G-CSF or GM-CSF, so arrangements for clinic/physician's office administration must be planned.

The effect of GM-CSF and/or G-CSF on leukemia remains unclear.[168,189,196] Laboratory and clinical research indicates that these CSFs are capable of inducing leukemic cell growth. It is possible that the use of CSFs in patients with acute myeloid leukemias stimulates the leukemic clone cell to proliferate (increased cell cycling), thus increasing its sensitivity to chemotherapeutic agents. However, the stimulation of the leukemic clone cell may also accelerate the malignant disease. Currently, phase II studies are investigating the efficacy and safety of this approach.

Interleukin-3 (multi-CSF)

IL-3 currently is under clinical investigation in phase I and II clinical trials. IL-3's primary function is that of a myeloid growth factor. In vitro IL-3 has been shown to stimulate the growth of and exert functional effects on neutrophil, monocytic, eosinophil, basophil, and thrombopoietic cell lines.[168,200] It is active on the primitive stem cell and also on the mature cells of multiple lineages. Biologic activities of IL-3 include activation of eosinophils, augmentation of the proliferation of blood monocytes and peritoneal macrophages, and production of basophil histamine release.[201]

IL-3 and GM-CSF share common binding sites, which provides a possible explanation for their similarity of biologic activities. A GM-CSF/IL-3 fusion protein (PIXY321) has been produced recombinantly in yeast, and may offer a substantial clinical benefit over either of the individual cytokines.[202] PIXY is being evaluated in phase I/II clinical trials.

Potential toxicities associated with IL-3 include fever, associated with headache, flushing, local erythema at the injection site, bone pain, lethargy, and nausea/vomiting.[203] Chills have been reported with IV bolus injection administration. The dose of IL-3 usually is 250 μg/m²/day. IL-3 is in phase II/III trials and is well tolerated.

Macrophage colony stimulating factor (M-CSF)

M-CSF, also referred to as CSF-1, demonstrates strong activity on differentiated macrophages and also affects neutrophil production.[168,204] M-CSF is under early clinical investigation and appears to produce a similar array of potential toxicities as previously described.

Clinical trials with CSFs have only begun to address the questions that will predict their future use. For example, can doses of chemotherapeutic agents be increased to obtain a better tumor response rate that

TABLE 17-6 Comparison of G-CSF and GM-CSF

	G-CSF	GM-CSF
Indications and Usage	• Chemotherapy-induced neutropenia • Peripheral stem cell mobilization	• Neutropenia associated with autologous BMT • Chemotherapy-induced neutropenia
Dosage	5-µg/kg/day up to 14 days	250 µg/m²/day up to 21 days
Administration	SC, IV infusion (15 min–1 hr)	SQ, IV infusion (2–6 hr)
Compatibility	D5	Saline
Contraindications	Known hypersensitivity to *E. Coli*	Known hypersensitivity to yeast-derived products
Drug Interactions	None	Lithium and corticosteroids may potentiate effects
Precautions	• Do not give 24 hr before or after chemotherapy • Because of the possibility of tumor growth, exercise precaution in use for myeloid malignancies • Leukocytosis (CBC 2×/wk) • Premature discontinuation of therapy—discontinue when absolute neutrophil count ≥ 10,000/mm³ or per study protocol	• Do not give 24 hr before or after chemotherapy • WBC count may increase rapidly; if absolute neutrophil count ≥ 20,000/mm³, reduce dose by one-half or discontinue • Because of possibility of tumor growth, exercise caution in use for myeloid malignancies
Warnings	None	• May cause fluid retention • Sequestration of granulocytes in pulmonary circulation—dyspnea • Serum creatinine, bilirubin, and hepatic enzymes may increase
Lab Monitoring	CBC 2×/wk	• CBC 2×/wk • Serum creatinine, liver enzymes for patients with history of renal/hepatic dysfunction

ultimately affects remission rates and overall survival? What long-term effect will CSFs have on the bone marrow? It can be clearly anticipated that CSFs will have a significant impact on the patient with cancer or hematopoietic dysfunction. Glaspy and Golde[205] point out that G-CSF and GM-CSF have entered second- and third-generation clinical trials investigating their use in a multitude of clinical areas, including allogenic BMT, in combination with other BRMs, peripheral stem cell harvest, dose intensification, compromised hosts, chemosensitization of myeloid leukemias, and in combination with each other to produce a wider array of biologic activities.

Gene Therapy

Biotherapy has successfully produced tumor responses in selected cancers. However, a large number of patients with cancer have no viable options to treat their disease effectively. Although attempts to modulate the immune system continue with new biologic agents, other avenues also are being actively pursued. Gene therapy is one such endeavor.[206] The first successful introduction of foreign genes into humans occurred in May 1989 at the NCI, by Rosenberg and colleagues, and continues today with the initiation of clinical trials utilizing gene therapy in patients with advanced cancer.[123,207] Rosenberg[207] defines gene therapy as "a technique in which a functioning gene is inserted into the cells of a patient either to correct a genetic error or to introduce a new function to the cell."

The prospect of gene therapy has produced significant scientific, legal, and ethical issues to consider. Multiple mechanisms have been established at various levels to promote the safe science of gene therapy. These include the NIH's Recombinant DNA Advisory Committee, the FDA, and the Institutional Internal Review Boards. All proposed gene transfer clinical studies must be evaluated by these groups, and only after stringent criteria are met can studies be implemented. Currently, gene therapy programs are limited in number due to the rigors and scientific support necessary to support the endeavor. Rosenberg[207] reports two patients have had positive results utilizing transduced [with a retroviral vector containing the neomycin phosphotransferase (Neo) gene] TIL cells.

Although gene therapy is in its infancy, possibilities

abound for its potential impact in treating patients with cancer. Clearly, early studies have demonstrated the ability and safety of gene therapy in humans. Future studies will seek to identify and clone genes responsible for human tumor-associated antigens. This will enable scientists to provide the specificity now lacking in our current arsenal of cancer therapy.

NURSING MANAGEMENT

General Nursing Implications

Many biologic agents will be investigated in humans during the 1990s for their immunomodulatory and/or antiproliferative effects. The nurse has a professional obligation to obtain specific information about these agents. Critical information the nurse must understand prior to the administration of any BRM includes the following.

1. What is the nature of this material? Does it contain tumor cells? Are they replicating? Does the material contain live organisms? Are they infectious? Does the material contain a foreign protein or other potentially allergenic substance? If so, what substance (for example, bacteria or yeast)?

2. Is this agent approved, or is it experimental? If experimental, is the agent exactly equivalent to the preceding agent? If not, how does it differ? Examples of differing agents might be interferons produced by different companies.

3. What equipment is needed, and what procedure should be followed to administer the agent? Does the agent require special admixture solutions? Does an antiseptic applied to the skin inactivate the bacteria in the vaccine? What handling and disposal precautions should be taken to protect the nurse and patient/family?

4. What are the potential toxicities? Will there be an immediate hypersensitivity reaction? What is the known pattern of expected toxicities?

5. What equipment and medication should be available to manage acute toxicities? What is an appropriate nurse-to-patient ratio to provide optimal observation and care?

6. Is an immune evaluation necessary?

7. How will this agent interact with other medication(s) the patient is receiving? Are certain medications contraindicated?

8. What additional information is needed before information can be provided to the patient/family? Does this agent cause potential danger to the family member who has intercurrent disease? An example of such danger is the administration of smallpox vaccine to the patient whose sibling has infantile eczema.

Nursing Interventions

Biotherapy is in the forefront of advancing medical science and merits continued personal study and consultation with medical investigators to maintain a current knowledge base. The nurse has an obligation to obtain accurate treatment information so that appropriate patient/family care and teaching are achieved.

Initially, the physician advises the patient and family of the purpose of therapy, the course of treatment and necessary procedures, and the precautions to be taken to prevent adverse reactions. Because many BRM agents remain investigational, it is a medical responsibility to obtain a signed statement of informed consent from the patient for all research protocols. It is critical that the nurse be involved directly and integrally in these discussions with the patient and family so that their needs for care specifically in the areas of education and emotional support can be determined and subsequently met.[208]

Because of the unique nature of BRMs, the patient must be encouraged to share information and observations concerning toxicities experienced. The nurse as an astute listener may gain a wealth of information that is vital to the ultimate evaluation of treatment efficacy and toxicities. This represents only one of many ways that nurses play an indispensable role in the research process.

Although each BRM agent has distinct biologic and chemical properties, nursing interventions focus on common areas that most BRMs share. These include the nature of the biologic agent as a medication, the diversity of organ-system toxicities, and the presence of an acute or a chronic flulike syndrome.[209]

The toxicities of each BRM agent depend on the dose, route of administration, and schedule. Nurses must be familiar with the particular agent in use, as well as the reported range of possible toxicities. This knowledge allows the nurse to predict the intensity, severity, and duration of potential toxicities. Effective measures to manage or prevent these toxicities then can be readily available. This knowledge base also aids in providing continued patient and family education and reassurance throughout therapy.

Administration of BRMs results in diverse organ-system toxicities. In particular, certain biologic agents are associated with unique side effects. IL-2 produces a capillary leak syndrome. The potential for anaphylactic or allergic reactions most commonly is associated with the administration of antibody therapy. Administration of TNF causes a local irritation at the injection site. Nursing assessment for organ toxicity involves establishing the patient's risk for development of such toxicity (in most cases, the eligibility criteria of research protocols will eliminate patients at increased risk for toxicities because of past or current medical history) and obtaining and documenting baseline values for future comparison.

Interferon has been viewed as the prototypic BRM agent because of its constellation of toxicities, its biologic nature, and the presence of an acute and a chronic flulike syndrome. An excellent review article of BRM-induced flulike syndrome is provided by Haeuber.[210] Management of this syndrome can be divided into three approaches: (1) treatment manipulation, i.e., changing dose or schedule; (2) administration of effective medications to block or minimize the effect, e.g., administration of meperidine or lorazapam at the onset of chills or rigors and premedication with acetaminophen and diphenhydramine; and (3) the practice of noninvasive nursing techniques, such as imagery and/or relaxation therapy. These measures, undertaken either alone or in combination, provide patient comfort and decreased toxicity without adverse effects.

Finally, the patient will, without doubt, look to the nurse for psychosocial support during this treatment endeavor. The nurse–patient relationship often is the critical factor in facilitating patient and family cooperation with the medical plan of care. Nursing research is beginning to examine the relationship between patients receiving BRMs and quality-of-life issues.[211,212] The element of patient responsibility and commitment to complete therapy, if at all feasible, should be emphasized.

The oncology nurse is at the forefront of new therapeutic modalities. The nurse's knowledge, capability, attitude, and expectations often are adopted by the patient undergoing BRM therapy. This awareness will assist the nurse to strive continually for excellence in planning and implementing each patient's care.

FUTURE PERSPECTIVES

The significant scientific and technologic breakthroughs represented by recombinant DNA and hybridoma techniques drastically have altered the nature of immunologic research. The ability to produce large quantities of purified biologic products and the ability to alter those products to generate more favorable cellular traits create unlimited therapeutic potential.

The ultimate success of biologic response modifiers as a fourth modality of cancer treatment lies in further understanding the unique complexities of the human immune system. Major research studies that involve BRM agents and components of the immune system are in progress; new paradigms are being proposed and constantly analyzed. These results stimulate hope that biotherapy will provide a means for the specific treatment of cancer without the problem of nonspecific toxicities. The future appears bright.

Oncology nurses with a major interest in biologic response modifiers share in the growing pains and opportunities of a new cancer modality. The clinical trials designed to define clearly more successful therapies for the treatment of patients with cancer will offer oncology nurses a multiplicity of new opportunities and challenges. In clinical practice the nurse will have the opportunity to make significant contributions. Sophisticated nursing care will be provided to individuals with complex organ toxicities.

Nurses will be active in developing and standardizing policies and procedures for monitoring patients receiving BRMs.[213] In addition, toxicities of BRMs may be subjective or subtle, making them difficult to observe, measure, and document accurately. Acute observation skills will be needed by nurses to enable them to detect and analyze the individual's response to the agent being studied. The nurse's attention to detail and observation of and communication with the patient will be crucial factors to the success of BRM clinical trials.

The possibilities for nursing research in the field of biotherapy are limitless.[214] Oncology nurses have an obligation to investigate current methods of caring for individuals receiving BRM agents and to make recommendations for improving that care. As new agents become available, nursing research studies should be designed to explore their implications for nursing practice and patient care. Nurse investigators and experienced oncology nurses also must assume their professional responsibility to disseminate new concepts in cancer management to other nurses in order to improve patient care through research, presentations, and publications. Nurses who care for persons with cancer need to understand this treatment modality and to participate actively in its further development. Progress will come. Oncology nurses must seek, earn, and nurture a role in the development of biotherapy.

REFERENCES

1. Oldham RK, Smalley RV: Immunotherapy: The old and the new. *J Biol Res Mod* 2:1–37, 1983.
2. Oldham RK: Biologicals and biological response modifiers: Fourth modality of cancer treatment. *Cancer Treat Rep* 68:221–232, 1984.
3. Mihich E: Future perspectives for biological response modifiers: A viewpoint. *Semin Oncol* 13:234–254, 1986.
4. Fauci AS, Rosenberg SA, Sherwin SA. et al: Immunomodulators in clinical medicine. *Ann Intern Med* 106:421–433, 1987.
5. Durant JR: Immunotherapy of cancer: The end or the beginning? *N Engl J Med* 316:939–941, 1987 (editorial).
6. Huffer TL, Kanapa DJ, Stevenson HC: *Basic Immunology for Paramedical Professionals.* Bethesda, MD: Clinical Investigations Sections, Biological Response Modifiers Program, National Cancer Institute, National Institutes of Health, 1985, p. 178.
7. Clark JW, Longo DL: Biological response modifiers. *Mediguide Oncol* 6:1–10, 1986.
8. Goodfield J: Dr. Coley's toxins. *Science* 84:68–73, 1984.
9. Mathé G. Amiel JL, Schwarzenberg L, et al: Active immunotherapy for acute lymphoblastic leukemia. *Lancet* 1:697–699, 1969.
10. Terry WD, Rosenberg SA (eds.): *Immunotherapy of Human Cancer.* New York: Excerpta Medica, 1982, pp. 55–60.

11. Smalley RV, et al: Biological response modifiers: Current status and prospects as anti-cancer agents. In Herberman RB (ed.): *Basic and Clinical Tumor Immunology.* Boston: Martinus Nijhoff, 1986.
12. Kohler G, Milstein C: Continuous cultures of fused cells secreting antibody of predefined specificity. *Nature* 256:495–497, 1975.
13. Schindler LW: *Understanding the Immune System.* NIH pub. no. 88-529. Bethesda, MD: Office of Research Reporting and Public Response, National Institute of Allergy and Infectious Diseases, and the National Cancer Institute, National Institutes of Health, 1988, pp. 28, 29.
14. Kohler G: Derivation and diversification of monoclonal antibodies. *Science* 233:1281–1286, 1986.
15. Harris OT, Mastrangelo MJ: Serotherapy of cancer. *Semin Oncol* 16:180–198, 1989.
16. Ritz J, Pesando JM, Sallan SE, et al: Serotherapy of acute lymphoblastic leukemia with monoclonal antibody. *Blood* 58:141–152, 1981.
17. Dillman RO, Shawler DL, Dillman JB, et al: Therapy of CLL and cutaneous T-cell lymphoma with T101 monoclonal antibody. *J Clin Oncol* 2:881–891, 1984.
18. Dillman RO, Shawler DL, Sobol RE, et al: Murine monoclonal antibody therapy in two patients with chronic lymphocytic leukemia. *Blood* 59:1036–1045, 1982.
19. Foon KA, Schroff RW, Bunn PA, et al: Effects of monoclonal antibody therapy in patients with chronic lymphocytic leukemia. *Blood* 64:1085–1093, 1984.
20. Meeher TC, Lowder J, Maloney DG, et al: A clinical trial of anti-idiotype therapy for B cell malignancy. *Blood* 65:1349–1363, 1985.
21. Meeher TC, Lowder J, Cleary ML, et al: Emergence of idiotype variants during treatment of B-cell lymphoma with anti-idiotype antibodies. *N Engl J Med* 312:1658–1665, 1985.
22. Rankin EM, Hekman A, Somers R, et al: Treatment of two patients with B cell lymphoma with monoclonal anti-idiotype antibodies. *Blood* 65:1373–1381, 1985.
23. Miller RA, Maloney DG, McKillop J, et al: In vivo effects of murine hybridoma monoclonal antibody in a patient with T-cell leukemia. *Blood* 58:78–86, 1981.
24. Miller RA, Levy R: Response of cutaneous T cell lymphoma to therapy with hybridoma monoclonal antibody. *Lancet* 2:226–230, 1981.
25. Miller RA, Oseroff AR, Stratte PT, et al: Monoclonal antibody therapeutic trials in seven patients with T cell lymphoma. *Blood* 62:988–995, 1983.
26. Bertram JH, Gill PS, Levine AS: Monoclonal antibody T101 in T cell malignancies: A clinical, pharmacokinetic and immunologic correlation. *Blood* 68:752–761, 1986.
27. Sears HF, Atkinson B, Herlyn D, et al: The use of monoclonal antibody in a phase I clinical trial of human gastrointestinal tumor. *Lancet* 1:762–765, 1982.
28. Sobol RE, Dillman RO, Smith JD. et al: Phase I evaluation of murine monoclonal anti-melanoma antibody in man: Preliminary observations. In Mitchell MS, Ottgen HF (eds.): *Hybridomas in Cancer Diagnosis and Treatment.* New York: Raven Press, 1982, pp. 199–206.
29. Goodman GE, Beaumier P, Helstrom I, et al: Pilot trial of murine monoclonal antibodies in patients with advanced melanoma. *J Clin Oncol* 3:340–352, 1985.
30. Oldham RK, Foon KA, Morgan AC, et al: Monoclonal antibody therapy of malignant melanoma: In vivo localization in cutaneous metastasis after intravenous administration. *J Clin Oncol* 2:1235–1244, 1984.
31. Vadhan-Raj S, Cordon-Cardo C, Carswell E, et al: Phase I trial of mouse monoclonal antibody against GD3 ganglioside in patients with melanoma: Induction of inflammatory responses at tumor sites. *J Clin Oncol* 6:1636–1648, 1988.
32. Dippold WI, Bernhard H, Dienes HP, et al: Treatment of patients with malignant melanoma by monoclonal ganglioside antibodies. *Eur J Cancer Clin Oncol* 24:S65–S67, 1988 (suppl. 2).
33. Coit D, Houghton A, Cordon-Cardo C, et al: Isolation limb perfusion with monoclonal antibody R24 in patients with malignant melanoma. *Proc Am Soc Clin Oncol* 7:248, 1988.
34. Lichtin A, Iliopoulos D, Guerry D, et al: Therapy of melanoma with an anti-melanoma ganglioside monoclonal antibody: A possible mechanism of complete response. *Proc Am Soc Clin Oncol* 7:247, 1988.
35. Cheung N-KV, Lazarus H, Miraldi FD, et al: Ganglioside GD2 specific monoclonal antibody 3F8: A phase I study in patients with neuroblastoma and malignant melanoma. *J Clin Oncol* 5:1430–1440, 1987.
36. Vitetta EX, Uhr JW: Immunotoxin. *Annu Rev Immunol* 3:197–212, 1985.
37. Pastan I, Willingham MC, Fitzgerald DJP: Immunotoxins. *Cell* 47:641–648, 1986.
38. Spitler L, delRio M, Khentigan A, et al: Therapy of patients with malignant melanoma using a monoclonal antimelanoma antibody ricin A chain immunotoxin. *Cancer Res* 47:1717–1723, 1987.
39. Halpern SE, Dillman RO: Problems associated with radioimmunodetection and possibilities for future solution. *J Biol Response Mod* 6:235–262, 1987.
40. Mach JA, Bucheggar F, Forni M, et al: Use of radiolabeled monoclonal anti-CEA antibodies for detection of human carcinomas by external photoscanning and tomoscintigraphy. *Immunol Today* 2:239–249, 1981.
41. Carrasquillo JA, Bunn PA Jr, Keenan AM, et al: Radioimmunodetection of cutaneous T-cell lymphoma with "inlabeled T101" monoclonal antibody. *N Engl J Med* 315:673–680, 1985.
42. Schlom J: Innovations in monoclonal antibody tumor targeting—Diagnostic and therapeutic implications. *JAMA* 261:744–746, 1989.
43. Meredith RF, Khazaeli MB, Plott WE, et al: Phase I trial of iodine-131-chimeric B72.3 (human IgG4) in metastatic colorectal cancer. *J Nucl Med* 33:23–29, 1992.
44. Order SE, Sleeper AM, Stillwagon GB, et al: Current status of radioimmunoglobulins in the treatment of human malignancy. *Oncology* 3:115–130, 1989.
45. Bucholtz, JD: Radiolabeled antibody therapy. *Semin Oncol Nurs* 3:67–73, 1987.
46. Burton DR: Human monoclonal antibodies: Achievement and potential. *Hosp Prac* 27:67–74, 1992.
47. Ziegler EJ, Fisher CS Jr, Sprung CL, et al: Treatment of gram-negative bacteremia against endotoxin, a randomized, double blind, placebo-controlled trial. *New Engl J Med* 324:429–436, 1991.
48. Sands H: Radiolabeled monoclonal antibodies for cancer therapy and diagnosis: Is it really a chimera? *J Nucl Med* 33:29–32, 1992.
49. Dillman JB: Toxicity of monoclonal antibodies in the treatment of cancer. *Semin Oncol Nurs* 4:107–111, 1988.
50. Dinarello CA, Mier JW: Current concepts, lymphokines. *N Engl J Med* 317:940–945, 1987.
51. Isaacs A, Lindemann JJ: Virus interference: The interferon. *Proc R Soc Lond* [Biol] 147:258–267, 1957.
52. Oldham RK, Smalley RV: The role of interferon in the

treatment of cancer. In Zoon KC, Noguchi PD, Lui TY (eds.): *Interferon Research: Clinical Application and Regulatory Consideration.* New York: Elsevier-North Holland, 1984.

53. Toufexis A, Jecius A: The big IF in cancer. *Time* March 31:60–66, 1980.
54. Oldham RK: Biologicals for cancer treatment: Interferons. *Hosp Pract* Dec. 15:71–91, 1985.
55. Borden EC: Interferons: Rationale for clinical trials in neoplastic disease. *Ann Intern Med* 91:472–479, 1979.
56. Kirkwood JM, Ernstoff MS: Interferons in the treatment of human cancer. *J Clin Oncol* 2:336–352, 1984.
57. Boonem EA, Oldham RK: Gamma-interferon: Physiology and speculation on its role in medicine. *J Biol Response Mod* 6:275–301, 1987.
58. Goldstein D, Laszlo J: Interferon therapy in cancer: From imaginon to interferon. *Cancer Res* 46:4315–4329, 1986.
59. Balmer CM: The new alpha interferons. *Drug Intell Pharm* 19:887–893, 1985.
60. Higgins PG: Interferons. *J Clin Pathol* 37:109–116, 1984.
61. Rinehart JJ, Young D, Laforge J, et al: Phase I/II trial of recombinant gamma-interferon in patients with renal cell carcinoma: Immunologic and biologic effects. *J Biol Response Mod* 6:302–312, 1987.
62. Harglum JE: Interferon: Mechanisms of action and clinical value. *Clin Pharm* 2:20–28, 1983.
63. Mitsuyasu RT: The role of alpha interferon in the biotherapy of hematologic malignancies and AIDS-related Kaposi's sarcoma. *Oncol Nurs Forum* 6:7–12, 1988 (suppl.).
64. Spiegel RJ: Clinical overview of alpha interferon. *Cancer* 59:626–631, 1987.
65. Groopman JE: Therapeutic options in hairy-cell leukemia. *Semin Oncol* 12:30–34, 1985.
66. Roth MS, Foon KA: Alpha interferon in the treatment of hematologic malignancies. *Am J Med* 81:871–882, 1986.
67. Quesda JR, Gutterman JU, Hersh EV: Treatment of hairy-cell leukemia with alpha interferons. *Cancer* 57:1678–1680, 1986.
68. Figlin RA: Biotherapy with interferon in solid tumors. *Oncol Nurs Forum* 6:23–26, 1987 (suppl.).
69. Torti FM, Shortliffe LD, Williams RD, et al: Alpha-interferon in superficial bladder cancer. A northern California oncology group study. *J Clin Oncol* 6:476–483, 1988.
70. Berek JS, Hacher NJ, Lichtenstein A, et al: Intraperitoneal recombinant α-interferon for "salvage" immunotherapy in stage III eipthelial ovarian cancer: A gynecologic oncology group study. *Cancer Res* 75:4447–4453, 1985.
71. Von Wussow P, Block B, Hartmann F, et al: Intralesional interferon-alpha therapy in advanced malignant melanoma. *Cancer* 61:1071–1074, 1988.
72. Greenway HT, Cornell RC, Tanner DJ, et al: Treatment of basal cell carcinoma with intralesional interferon. *J Am Acad Dermatol* 15:437–443, 1986.
73. Spiegel RJ: Additional indications for interferon therapy: Basal cell carcinoma, carcinoid and chronic active hepatitis. *Semin Oncol* 15:41–45, 1988 (suppl. 51).
74. Wadler S, Wiernil PH: Clinical update on the role of fluorouracil and recombinant interferon alfa-2a in the treatment of colorectal carcinoma. *Semin Oncol* 17(suppl 1):16–21, 1990.
75. Pazdur R: Fluorouracil and recombinant interferon alpha-2a in advanced gastrointestinal neoplasms. *Br J Haematol* 79:56–59, 1991 (suppl. 1).
76. Wadler S, Lembersky B, Atkins M, et al: Phase II trial of fluorouracil and recombinant interferon-2a in patients with advanced colorectal carcinoma: An eastern cooperative oncology group study. *J Clin Oncol* 9:1806–1810, 1991.
77. Kools AM: Hepatitis A,B,C,D, and E. Update on testing and treatment. *Postgrad Med* 91:109–114, 1992.
78. Baron S, Tyring SK, Fleischmann WR, et al: The interferons—Mechanisms of action and clinical applications. *JAMA* 266:1375–1383, 1991.
79. Krown SE, Real FX, Cunningham-Rundles S, et al: Preliminary observations on the effect of recombinant leukocyte α-interferon in homosexual men with Kaposi's sarcoma. *N Engl J Med* 308:1071–1076, 1983.
80. Groopman JE, Gottlieb MS, Goodman J, et al: Recombinant alpha-2 interferon therapy for Kaposi's sarcoma associated with the acquired immuno-deficiency syndrome. *Ann Intern Med* 100:671–676, 1984.
81. Abrams DI, Volberding PA: Alpha interferon therapy of AIDS-associated Kaposi's sarcoma. *Semin Oncol* 14 (suppl. 2): 43–47, 1987.
82. Krown SE: The role of interferon in the therapy of epidemic Kaposi's sarcoma. *Semin Oncol* 14:27–33, 1987 (suppl. 3).
83. Ho DD, Rota TR, Kaplan JC, et al: Recombinant human interferon alpha-A, suppresses HTLV-III replication in vitro. *Lancet* 1:602–604, 1985.
84. Krown SE, Paredes J, Bundow D, et al: Interferon-α, Zidovudine, and granulocyte-macrophage colony-stimulating factor: A phase I AIDS clinical trials group study in patients with Kaposi's sarcoma associated with AIDS. *J Clin Oncol* 10:1344–1351, 1992.
85. Gallin JI, Malech HL, Weening RS, and the International Chronic Granulomatous Disease Cooperative Study Group: A controlled trial of recombinant human interferon gamma to prevent infection in chronic granulomatous disease. *N Engl J Med* 324:509–516, 1991.
86. Van der Berg M, Edelstein M, Gerlis L, et al: Recombinant interferon (Immuneron): Results of a phase I trial in patients with cancer. *J Biol Response Mod* 4:264–272, 1985.
87. Vadhan-Raj S, Al-Katib A, Bhalla R, et al: Phase I trial of recombinant interferon gamma in cancer patients. *J Clin Oncol* 4:137–146, 1986.
88. Thompson JA, Cos WW, Lindgren CG, et al: Subcutaneous recombinant gamma interferon in cancer patients: Toxicity, pharmacokinetics and immunomodulatory effects. *Cancer Immunol Immunother* 25:47–53, 1987.
89. Ernstoff MS. Trautman T, Davis CA, et al: A randomized phase I/II study of continuous versus intermittent interferon gamma in patients with metastatic melanoma. *J Clin Oncol* 5:1804–1810, 1987.
90. Quesada JR, Talpaz M, Rios A, et al: Clinical toxicity of interferon in cancer patients: A review. *J Clin Oncol* 4:234–243, 1986.
91. Kirkwood JM, Ernstoff MS: A clinical update: The role of interferon in the biotherapy of solid tumors. *Oncol Nurs Forum* 6:3–6, 1988 (suppl.).
92. Mayer D, Hetrick K, Riggs C, et al: Weight loss in patients receiving recombinant leukocytes. A interferon (IFNrA): A brief report. *Cancer Nurs* 7:53–56, 1984.
93. Spiegel RJ: Intron A (interferon alpha-2b): Clinical overview and future directions. *Semin Oncol* 13:89–101, 1986 (suppl.).

94. Figlin RA: Biotherapy with interferon-1988. *Semin Oncol* 15:3–9, 1988 (suppl.).
95. Steis RG, Smith JW II, Urba WJ, et al: Resistance to recombinant interferon alpha-2a in hairy-cell leukemia associated with neutralizing anti-interferon antibodies. *N Engl J Med* 318:1409–1413, 1988.
96. Quesada JR, Rios A, Swanson D, et al: Antitumor activity of recombinant-derived interferon alpha in metastatic renal cell carcinoma. *J Clin Oncol* 3:1522–1528, 1985.
97. Oppenheim JJ, Kovacs EJ, Matsushima K, Durum SK: There is more than one interleukin 1. *Immunol Today* 7:45–56, 1986.
98. Dinarello CA: Interleukin-I and the pathogenesis of the acute-phase response. *N Engl J Med* 311:1413–1418, 1984.
99. Dinarello CA: Interleukin-1 and its biologically related cytokines. *Adv in Immun* 44:153–205, 1989.
100. Moore MA: Role of interleukin-1 in hematopoiesis. *Immunol Res* 8:165–175, 1989.
101. Zsebo KM, Wypch J, Yuschenkoff VN, et al: Effects of hematopoietin-1 and interleukin-1 activities on early hematopoietic cells of the bone marrow. *Blood* 71:962–968, 1988.
102. Dennis D, Chachoua A, Garrison L, et al: Biologic activity of interleukin-1 (IL-1) alpha in patients with refractory malignancies. *Pro ASCO* 11:255, 1992 (abstr. 230).
103. Vadhan-Raj S, Kudelka A, Garrison L, et al: Interleukin-1α (IL-1α) increases circulating platelet (plt) counts and reduces carboplatin (CBDCA)—Induced throbocytopenia. *Proc ASCO* 11:228, 1992 (abstr. 710).
104. Morgan DA, Ruscetti FW, Gallo R: Selective in vitro growth of T lymphocytes from normal human bone marrows. *Science* 193:1007–1008, 1976.
105. Ortaldo JR, Mason AT, Gerard JP, et al: Effects of natural and recombinant IL-2 on regulation of IFN production and natural killer activity: Lack of involvement of the TAC antigen for these immunoregulatory effects. *J Immunol* 133:779–783, 1984.
106. Ruscetti FW, Gallo RC: Human lymphocyte growth factor: Regulation of growth and function of T-lymphocytes. *Blood* 57:379–394, 1981.
107. Wanebo HS, Pace R, Hargett S, et al: Production of and response to interleukin-2 in peripheral blood lymphocytes of cancer patients. *Cancer* 57:656–662, 1986.
108. Ettinghausen SE, Lipford EII III, Mule JJ, et al: Systemic administration of recombinant interleukin-2 stimulates in vivo lymphoid cell proliferation in tissues. *J Immunol* 135:1488–1497, 1985.
109. Rosenberg SA, Lotze MT, Mueel LM, et al: Observations on the systemic administration of autologous lymphokine activated killer cells and recombinant interleukin-2 to patients with metastatic cancer. *N Engl J Med* 313:1485–1492, 1985.
110. Rosenberg SA: Immunotherapy of cancer by systemic administration of lymphoid cells plus interleukin-2. *J Biol Response Mod* 3:501–511, 1984.
111. Atkins MB, Gould JA, Allegretta M, et al: Phase I evaluation of recombinant interleukin-2 in patients with advanced malignant disease. *J Clin Oncol* 4:1380–1391, 1986.
112. Rosenberg SA, Lotz MT, Mueel LM, et al: A progress report on the treatment of 157 patients with advanced cancer using lymphokine-activated killer cells and interleukin-2 or high dose interleukin-2 alone. *N Engl J Med* 316:889–897, 1987.
113. West WH, Tauer KW, Yannelli JR, et al: Constant-infusion recombinant interleukin-2 in adoptive immunotherapy of advanced cancer. *N Engl J Med* 316:898–905, 1987.
114. Fisher RI, Coltman CA, Doroshow JH, et al: Metastatic renal cancer treated with interleukin-2 and lymphokine-activated killer cells. *Ann Intern Med* 108:518–523, 1988.
115. Dutcher JP, Gaynor ER, Boldt DH, et al: A phase II study of high dose continuous infusion interleukin-2 with lymphokine activated killer cells in patients with metastatic melanoma. *J Clin Oncol* 9:641–648, 1991.
116. Parkinson DR: Interleukin-2 therapy in patients with metastatic malignant melanoma: A phase II study. *J Clin Oncol* 8:1650–1656, 1990.
117. Dutcher JP, Creekmore SP, Weiss GR, et al: A phase II study of interleukin-2 and lymphokine-activated killer cells in patients with metastatic malignant melanoma. *J Clin Oncol* 7:477–485, 1989.
118. Weiss GR, Margolin KA, Aronson FR, et al: A randomized phase II trial of continuous infusion interleukin-2 or bolus injection interleukin-2 plus lymphokine-activated killer cells for advanced renal cell carcinoma. *J Clin Oncol* 10:275–281, 1992.
119. Rosenburg SA, Lotze MT, Yand JC, et al: Experience with the use of high dose interleukin-2 in the treatment of 652 patients with cancer. *Ann Surg* 210:474–485, 1989.
120. Yron I, Wood TA Jr, Spiess P, et al: In vitro growth of murine T cells. The isolation and growth of lymphoid cells infiltrating syngeneic solid tumors. *J Immunol* 125:238–245, 1980.
121. Rosenburg SA, Spiess P, Lafreniere R: A new approach to the adoptive immunotherapy of cancer with tumor-infiltrating lymphocytes. *Science* 233:1318–1321, 1986.
122. Rosenburg SA, Packard BS, Aebersold PM, et al: Use of tumor-infiltrating lymphocytes and interleukin-2 in the immunotherapy of patients with metastatic melanoma. *N Engl J Med* 319:1676–1680, 1988.
123. Rosenberg SA: The immunotherapy and gene therapy of cancer. *J Clin Oncol* 10:180–199, 1992.
124. Kriegel RL, Padavic-Shaller KA, Rudolph AR, et al: A-phase I study of recombinant interleukin-2 plus recombinant interferon. *Cancer Res* 48:3875–3881, 1988.
125. Figlin RA, Belldegrun A, Moldawer N, et al: Concomitant administration of recombinant human interleukin-2 and recombinant interferon alfa-2A: An active outpatient regimen in metastatic renal cell carcinoma. *J Clin Oncol* 10:414–421, 1992.
126. Atzpodien J, Korfer A, Franks CR, et al: Home therapy with recombinant interleukin-2 and interferon-α-2b in advanced human malignancies. *Lancet* 355:1509–1512, 1990.
127. Chiron Corporation—Cetus Oncology Corporation: Proleukin® Aldesleukin for injection. Package Insert, May, 1992.
128a. Thompson MS, Kempf RA, Harel W, et al: Influence of dose and duration of infusion of interleukin-2 on toxicity and immunomodulation. *J Clin Oncol* 4:669–678, 1988.
128b. Margolin KA, Rayner AA, Hawkins MJ, et al: Interleukin-2 and lymphokine-activated killer cell therapy of solid tumors: Analysis of toxicity and management guidelines. *J Clin Oncol* 7:486–498, 1989.

129. Siegel JP, Puri RK: Interleukin-2 toxicity. *J Clin Oncol* 9:694–704, 1991.
130. Herberman RB: Interleukin-2 therapy of human cancer: Potential benefits versus toxicity. *J Clin Oncol* 7:1–4, 1989.
131. Lotze MT: T-cell growth factor and the treatment of patients with cancer. *Clin Immunol Immunopathol* 62:547–554, 1992.
132. Denicoff KD, Rubinow DR, Papa MZ, et al: The neuropsychiatric effects of treatment with interleukin-2 and lymphokine-activated killer cells. *Ann Intern Med* 107:293–300, 1987,
133. Bernard JT, Ameriso S, Kempf RA, et al: Transient focal neurological deficits complicating interleukin-2 therapy. *Neurology* 40:154–155, 1990.
134. Lee RE, Lotze MT, Skibber JM, et al: Cardiorespiratory effects of immunotherapy with interleukin-2. *J Clin Oncol* 7:7–20, 1989.
135. Gaynor ER, Vitek L, Sticklin L, et al: The hemodynamic effects of treatment with interleukin-2 and lyphokine-activated killer cells. *Ann Intern Med* 109:953–958, 1988.
136. Kozeny GA, Nicolas JD, Creekmore S, et al: Effect of interleukin-2 immunotherapy on renal function. *J Clin Oncol* 6:1170–1176, 1988.
137. Parkinson DR: Interleukin-2 in cancer therapy. *Semin Oncol* 15:10–26, 1988.
138. Atkins MB, Mier JW, Parkinson DR, et al: Hypothyroidism after treatment with interleukin-2 and lymphokine-activated killer cells. *N Engl J Med* 318:1556–1563, 1988.
139. Kishimoto T: The biology of interleukin-6. *Blood* 74:1–10, 1989.
140. Namen AE, Lupton S, Hjerrild K, et al: Stimulation of B-cell progenitors by cloned murine interleukin-7. *Nature* 333:571–573, 1988.
141. Henney CS: Interleukin-7: Effects on early events in lymphopoiesis. *Immunol Today* 10:170–175, 1989.
142. Carswell EA, Old LJ, Kassel RC, et al: An endotoxin-induced serum factor that causes necrosis of tumors. *Proc Natl Acad Sci USA* 72:3666–3670, 1975.
143. Haranaka K, Satomi N: Cytotoxic activity of tumor necrosis factor (TNF) on the human cancer cells in vitro. *Jpn J Exp Med* 51:191–194, 1981.
144. Salmon SE, Young L, Scuderi P, et al: Antineoplastic effects on tumor necrosis factor alone and in combination with gamma-interferon on tumor biopsies in clonogenic assay. *J Clin Oncol* 5:1816–1821, 1987.
145. Old L: Tumor necrosis factor (rTNF). *Science* 230:630–632, 1985.
146. Currie GA, Basham C: Activated macrophages release a factor which lyses malignant cells but not normal cells. *J Exp Med* 142:1600–1605, 1975.
147. Mannel DN, Moore RN, Mergenhagen SE: Macrophages as a source of tumoricidal activity (tumor necrotizing factor). *Infect Immun* 30:523–530, 1980.
148. Aggarwal BB, Kohr WJ, Hass PE, et al: Human tumor necrosis factor: Production purification and characterization. *J Biol Chem* 260:2345–2354, 1985.
149. Beutler B, Milsark IW, Cerami A: Cachectin/tumor necrosis factor: Production, distribution, and metabolic fate in vivo. *J Immunol* 135:3972–3977, 1985.
150. Darzynkiewicz Z, Williamson B, Carswell EA, et al: Cell cycle-specific effects of tumor necrosis factor. *Cancer Res* 44:83–90, 1984.
151. Surgarman BJ, Aggarwal BB, Hass PE, et al: Recombinant tumor necrosis factor-alpha: Effects on proliferation of normal and transformed cells in vitro. *Science* 230:943–945, 1985.
152. Michie HR, Manogue KR, Spriggs DR, et al: Detection of circulating tumor necrosis factor after endotoxin administration. *N Eng J Med* 318:1481–1486, 1988.
153. Peetre C, Gullberg U, Nilsson E, et al: Effects of recombinant tumor necrosis factor on proliferation and differentiation of leukemic and normal hematopoietic cells in vitro. *J Clin Invest* 78:1694–1700, 1986.
154. Broxmayer HE, Williams De, Lu L, et al: The suppressive influences of human tumor necrosis factors on bone marrow hematopoietic progenitor cells from normal donors and patients with leukemia: Synergism of TNF and gamma interferon *J Immunol* 136:4487–4495, 1986.
155. Larrick JW, Graham D, Toy K, et al: Recombinant tumor necrosis factor causes activation of human granulocyte. *Blood* 69:640–644, 1987.
156. Nawroth PP, Stern DM: Modulation of endothelial cell hemostatic properties by tumor necrosis factor. *J Exp Med* 163:740–745, 1986.
157. Bevilacqua MP, Dober JS, Majeau GR, et al: Recombinant tumor necrosis factor induces procoagulant activity in cultured human vascular endothelium: Characterization and comparison with the actions of interleukin 1. *Proc Natl Acad Sci USA* 83:4533–4537, 1986.
158. Broudy VC, Kaushansky K, Segal GM, et al: Tumor necrosis factor type alpha stimulates endothelial cells to produce granulocyte/macrophage colony stimulating factor. *Proc Natl Acad Sci USA* 83:7467–7471, 1986.
159. Le J, Weinstein D, Gubler U, et al: Induction of membrane associated interleukin 1 by tumor necrosis factor in human fibroblast. *J Immunol* 138:2137–2142, 1987.
160. Michie HR, Spriggs DR, Manogue KR, et al: Tumor necrosis factor and endotoxin induced similar metabolic responses in human beings. *Surgery* 104:280–286, 1988.
161. Bachwich PR, Chensue SE, Larrick JW, et al: Tumor necrosis factor stimulates interleukin I and prostaglandin E_2 production in resting macrophages. *Biochem Biophys Res Common* 136:94–101, 1986.
162. Chapman PB, Lester TJ, Casper ES, et al: Clinical Pharmacology of recombinant human tumor necrosis factor in patients with advanced cancer. *J Clin Oncol* 5:1942–1951, 1987.
163. Jakubowski AA, Casper ES, Gabrilove JL, et al: Phase I trial of intramuscular administered tumor necrosis factor in patients with advanced cancer. *J Clin Oncol* 7:298–303, 1989.
164. Sherman ML, Spriggs DR, Arthur KA, et al: Recombinant human tumor necrosis factor administered as a five-day continuous infusion in cancer patients: Phase I toxicity and effects on lipid metabolism. *J Clin Oncol* 6:344–350, 1988.
165. Morice RC, Blick MB, Ali MK, et al: Pulmonary toxicity of recombinant tumor necrosis factor (rTNF). *Proc Am Soc Clin Oncol* 6:29, 1987.
166. Clark SC, Kamen R: The human hematopoietic colony-stimulating factors. *Science* 246:1229–1237, 1987.
167. Haeuber D, Dijulio JE: Hemopoietic colony stimulating factors: An overview. *Oncol Nurs Forum* 16:247–255, 1989.
168. Grosh WW, Quesenberry PJ: Recombinant human hematopoietic growth factors in the treatment of cytopenias. *Clin Immunology and Immunopath* 62:S25–S38, 1992.
169. Cannistra SA, Griffin JD: Regulation of the production and function of granulocytes and monocytes. *Semin Hematol* 25:173–188, 1988.

170. Gabrilove JL: Introduction and overview of hematopoietic growth factors. *Semin Hematol* 26:1–4, 1989.
171. Gutterman J: Clinical studies of granulocyte-macrophage colony stimulating factor. *Semin Oncol* 15:52–53, 1988.
172. Groopman JE, Mitsuyasu RT, Deleo MJ, et al: Effects of recombinant human granulocyte-macrophage colony-stimulating factor on myelopoiesis in the acquired immunodeficiency syndrome. *N Engl J Med* 317:593–598, 1987.
173. Vadhan-Raj S, Keating J, LeMaistre A, et al: Effects of recombinant human granulocyte-macrophage colony-stimulating factor in patients with myelodysplastic syndromes. *N Engl J Med* 317:1547–1552, 1987.
174. Gabrilove JL, Jakubowski A, Scher H, et al: Effect of granulocyte colony-stimulating factor on neutropenia and associated morbidity due to chemotherapy for transitional cell carcinoma of the urothelium. *N Engl J Med* 318:1414–1422, 1988.
175. Brandt BJ, Peters WP, Atwater SK, et al: Effect of recombinant human granulocyte-macrophage colony-stimulating factor on hematopoietic reconstruction after high-dose chemotherapy and autologous bone marrow transplantation. *N Engl J Med* 318:869–876, 1988.
176. Peters WP: The effect of recombinant human colony-stimulating factors on hematopoietic reconstitution following autologous bone marrow transplantation. *Semin Hematol* 26:18–23, 1989 (suppl. 2).
177. Antman KS, Griffin JD, Elias A, et al: Effect of recombinant human granulocyte-macrophage colony-stimulating factor on chemotherapy-induced myelosuppression. *N Engl J Med* 319:593–598, 1988.
178. Eschbach J, Egrie J, Downing M, et al: Correction of the anemia of end-stage renal disease with recombinant human erythropoietin: Results of a combined phase I and II clinical trial. *N Engl J Med* 316:73–78, 1987.
179. Fischl M, Galpin JE, Levin JD, et al: Recombinant human erythropoietin for patients with AIDS treated with zidovudine. *N Engl J Med* 322:1488–1493, 1990.
180. Pincus T, Olsen NJ, Russell IJ, et al: Multicenter study of recombinant erythropoietin in correction of anemia: III Rheumatoid arthritis. *Am J Med* 89:161–168, 1990.
181. Doweiko JP, Goldberg MA: Erythropoietin in cancer patients. *Oncology* 5:31–38, 43, 44, 1991.
182. Abels RI, Larholt KM, Krantz KD, Bryant EC: Recombinant human erythropoietin (r-HuEPO) for the treatment of the anemia of cancer. In MJ Murphy, Jr (ed.): *Blood Cell Growth Factors: Their Present and Future Use in Hematology and Oncology*. Dayton, OH: AlphaMed Press, 1991, pp. 121–141.
183. Henry D: Erythropoietin in the treatment of anemia associated with cisplatin chemotherapy. *Biotherapy and Cancer* 3:1–7, 1990.
184. Ludwig H, Fritz E, Kotzmann H, et al: Erythropoietin treatment of anemia of cancer. *Proc ASCO* 9:201, 1990.
185. Abels RI: Use of recombinant human erythropoietin in the treatment of anemia in patients who have cancer. *Sem in Oncol* 19:29–35, 1992 (suppl. 8).
186. Spivak JL: The application of recombinant erythropoietin in anemic patients with cancer. *Semin Oncol* 19:25–28, 1992 (suppl. 8).
187. Platanias LC, Miller CB, Mick R, et al: Treatment of chemotherapy-induced anemia with recombinant human erythropoietin in cancer patients. *J Clin Oncol* 9:2021–2026, 1991.
188. Lieschke GJ, Burgess AW: Granulocyte colony stimulating factor and granulocyte macrophage colony-stimulating factor (first of two parts). *N Engl J Med* 327:28–35, 1992.
189. Lieschke GJ, Burgess AW: Granulocyte colony-stimulating factor and granulocyte macrophage colony-stimulating factor (second of two parts). *N Engl J Med* 327:99–106, 1992.
190. Brochud MH, Scarffe JH, Thatcher N, et al: Phase I/II study of recombinant human granulocyte colony stimulating factor in patients receiving intensive chemotherapy of small-cell lung cancer. *Br J Cancer* 56:809–813, 1987.
191. Morstyn G, Lieschke GJ, Sheridan W, et al: Clinical experience with recombinant human granulocyte colony-stimulating factor. *Semin Hematol* 26:9–13, 1989 (suppl. 2).
192. Crawford J, Ozer H, Stroller R, et al: Reduction by granulocyte colony-stimulating factor of fever and neutropenia induced by chemotherapy in patients with small-cell lung cancer. *N Engl J Med* 325:164–170, 1992.
193. Sheridan WP, Begley CG, Juttner CA, et al: Effect of peripheral blood progenitor cells mobilized by filgrastim (G-CSF) on platelet recovery after high-dose chemotherapy. *Lancet* 339:640–644, 1992.
194. Vadhan-Raj S, Broxmeyer HE, Hittelman WN, et al: Abrogating chemotherapy-induced myelosuppression by recombinant granulocyte-macrophage colony-stimulating factor in patients with sarcoma: Protection at the progenitor cell level. *J Clin Oncol* 10:1266–1277, 1992.
195. Welte K, Bonilla MA, Gillio AP, et al: Recombinant human granulocyte colony-stimulating factor: Effects on hematopoiesis in normal and cyclophosphamide-treated primates. *J Exp Med* 165:941–948, 1987.
196. Moore MAS: The clinical use of colony stimulating factors. *Annu Rev Immunol* 9:159–191, 1991.
197. Glaspy JA, Golde DW: Clinical applications of the myeloid growth factors. *Semin Hematol* 26:14–17, 1989 (suppl. 2).
198. Herrmann F, Schulz G, Lindemann A, et al: Hematopoietic responses in patients with advanced malignancy treated with recombinant human granulocyte-macrophage colony-stimulating factor. *J Clin Oncol* 7:159–167, 1989.
199. Wing EJ, Magee M, Whiteside TL, et al: Recombinant human granulocyte/macrophage colony-stimulating factor enhances monocyte cytotoxicity and secretion of tumor necrosis factor α and interferon in cancer patients. *Blood* 73:643–646, 1989.
200. Oster W, Frisch J, Nicolay U, Schulz G: Interleukin-3. Biologic effects and clinical impact. *Cancer* 67:2712–2717, 1991.
201. Lindemann A, Ganser A, Herrmann F, et al: Biologic effects of recombinant human interleukin-3 in vivo. *J Clin Oncol* 9:2120–2127, 1991.
202. Williams DE, Park LS: Hematopoietic effects of a granulocyte macrophage colony stimulating factor/interleukin-3 fusion protein. *Cancer* 67:2705–2707, 1991.
203. Kurzrock R, Talpaz M, Estrov Z, et al: Phase I study of recombinant human interleukin-3 in patients with bone marrow failure. *J Clin Oncol* 9:1241–1250, 1991.
204. Munn DH, Cheung N-KV: Preclinical and clinical studies of macrophage colony stimulating factor. *Semin Oncol* 19:395–407, 1992.
205. Glaspy JA, Golde DW: The colony-stimulating factors: Biology and clinical use. *Oncology* 4:25–34, 1990.
206. Verma I: Gene therapy. *Sci Amer* Nov.:68–84, 1990.

207. Rosenberg SA: Gene therapy for cancer. *JAMA* 268:2416–2419, 1992.
208. Lynch MT: The nurse's role in the biotherapy of cancer: Clinical trials and informed consent. *Oncol Nurs Forum* 15:23–27, 1988 (suppl. 2).
209. Irwin MM: Patients receiving biological response modifiers: Overview of nursing care. *Oncol Nurs Forum* 14:32–37, 1987 (suppl.).
210. Haeuber D: Recent advances in the management of biotherapy-related side effects: Flu-like syndrome. *Oncol Nurs Forum* 16:35–41, 1989 (suppl.).
211. Rieker PP, Clark EJ, Fogelberg PR: Perceptions of quality of life and quality of care for patients with cancer receiving biological therapy. *Oncol Nurs Forum* 19:433–440, 1992.
212. Jackson BS, Strauman J, Frederickson K, Strauman TJ: Long-term biopsychosocial effects of interleukin-2 therapy. *Oncol Nurs Forum* 18:683–690, 1991.
213. Carter P, Engleking C, Rumsey K, et al: *Biological Response Modifier Guidelines. Recommendations for Nursing Education and Practice.* Pittsburgh, PA: Oncology Nursing Society, 1989.
214. Strauman JJ: The nurse's role in the biotherapy of cancer: Nursing research of side effects. *Oncol Nurs Forum* 15:35–39, 1988 (suppl.).

Chapter 18

Bone Marrow Transplantation

Patricia C. Buchsel, RN, MSN

INTRODUCTION

Bone marrow transplantation (BMT) has evolved during the past 30 years from an experimental procedure to an established and effective treatment for increasing numbers of selected patients. Between 1988 and 1990, 14,745 allogeneic or syngeneic BMTs were performed in 342 marrow transplantation centers worldwide[1] (Figure 18-1). Improvements in the management of graft-versus-host disease (GVHD) and cytomegalovirus pneumonia and the advancement of other supportive care measures are responsible for much of this growth.

The exact number of autologous bone marrow transplants performed to date is difficult to determine, and sources differ in their calculations. The International Bone Marrow Transplantation Registry (IBMTR) reports that centers that perform allogeneic BMTs do similar numbers of autologous BMTs, with a ratio of 1.08 (allografts) to 1.0 (autografts). The total number of autologous transplantations is expected shortly to surpass the number of allogeneic transplantations. With such an expanding population, oncology nurses working in the area will need to expand their skills to encompass hematology, pediatrics, ambulatory patients, home health care, critical care, research, and nursing administration.[2]

HISTORICAL PERSPECTIVES

The earliest marrow transplantation in humans was reported by Brown-Sequard in 1891. They described a procedure wherein an extract of marrow was given by mouth to patients with pernicious anemia and lymphadenoma.[3] In 1937, Schretzenmayr administered bone marrow intramuscularly. Although his studies were encouraging, they were not accepted by his peers.[4] These early attempts were soon followed by unsuccessful attempts to use marrow given by the intramedullary and intravenous routes.[4]

After World War II, studies of radiation-induced bone marrow failure led to treatments using infusions of bone marrow in aplastic anemia and radiation-in-

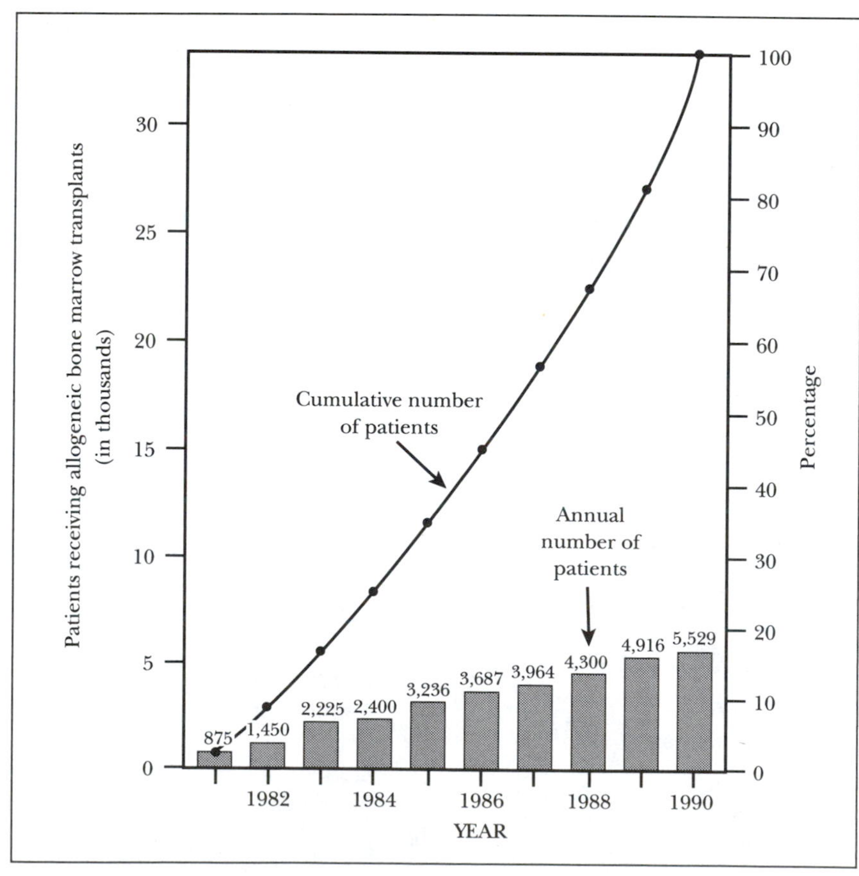

FIGURE 18-1 Annual and cumulative number of patients receiving allogenic bone marrow transplants worldwide, 1981–1990. (Source: Reproduced with permission from, Increasing utilization of allogeneic bone marrow transplantation: Results of the 1988–1990 survey. *Ann Intern Med* 116:509, 1992.)

duced bone marrow failure patients.[5] In 1949 and 1951, research in murine and canine models showed that animals given lethal doses of irradiation survived after parenteral infusion of bone marrow.[6]

The first modern human marrow transplants were conducted without success in patients with end-stage diseases. It was not until the mid-1960s that medical research focused on the importance of human tissue typing and applied these concepts to organ and marrow transplantation.[7] By the late 1960s, following the institution of histocompatible leukocyte antigen (HLA) typing to identify suitable sibling donors, successful human allogeneic transplants were carried out in increasing numbers. Simultaneously, the technology of platelet transfusions and methods of prophylaxis against infection were developed.[8,9]

In the 1980s, changes in pretransplant conditioning regimens, prophylaxis, and treatment of infectious diseases decreased transplant-related morbidity and mortality. Only a modest increase in leukemia-free survival rates occurred after identical-sibling BMT. This remains a major research priority today.

Autologous marrow transplantation, first reported more than 30 years ago, originally served as a salvage therapy for end-stage patients. During the last decade, autologous BMT has emerged as an increasingly important treatment for patients with hematologic and solid-organ malignancies. Thousands of patients without the matched donor necessary for allogeneic marrow transplantation can benefit from an autologous BMT. In addition, new dose-escalating chemotherapy regimens and supralethal doses of chemotherapy and irradiation can be administered as a treatment therapy, and the patient can be subsequently "rescued" from death with an infusion of his or her own previously harvested marrow.[10] Enhancing autologous marrow transplantation with the transfusion of peripheral blood stem cells in combination with the administration of hematopoietic growth factors is a phenomena of the 1990s, expected to increase exponentially the number of autologous BMTs.

Significant shifts in pretransplantation conditioning agents have occurred in recent years. Historically, total-body irradiation (TBI) plus cyclophosphamide (CY) has been the most common pretransplantation conditioning regimen. Currently, the use of fractionated (versus single dose) TBI and antileukemic drugs, such as high-dose etoposide and high-dose cytosine arabinoside, with TBI has increased markedly. The increased use of busulfan and CY without TBI for pretransplant conditioning is another important trend. This latter shift is an attempt to reduce the risk of leukemia relapse and to eliminate the late effects of irradiation, especially in the pediatric patient. Finally, the technique of T-cell marrow depletion to reduce the risk of graft-versus-host disease has been largely abandoned because of significantly high relapse rates in recipients of T-cell-depleted marrow infusions.[11]

Research to prevent and treat GVHD prompted significant changes in management techniques during the 1980s. Early in the decade most allogeneic marrow recipients received methotrexate alone or in combination therapy. Cyclosporine, a newly discovered immunosuppressive drug, emerged as an important treatment therapy and was used with corticosteroids to prevent GVHD.[12] By mid-decade, research demonstrated that cyclosporine with or without corticosteroids was a more effective treatment than other regimens. During the late 1980s, cyclosporine in combination with methotrexate was largely abandoned, and standard prophylaxis for GVHD currently is cyclosporine with corticosteroids.[1] Prophylaxis against viral infections, especially CMV infections, improved. Protective environments, including laminar airflow rooms and high-efficiency particulate air filters, were developed.

The number of older patients receiving BMT has increased, particularly in the treatment of chronic myelogenous leukemia, a disease affecting primarily older persons. Younger patients are undergoing transplantation for early acute leukemia, and transplantation for unrelated donors has increased by more than 8% in the last decade. Long-term survivorship has increased as a result of advances in medical technology, improved support of the immunosuppressed patient, and improved communication between long-term follow-up teams and referring physicians.[1] Currently, there are more than 2000 long-term survivors, defined as those patients who remain disease-free 1 year after BMT.[13]

CONCEPTS OF BONE MARROW TRANSPLANTATION

Replacing diseased marrow with healthy donor marrow is simple in concept. However, the toxicities of high-dose chemotherapy and irradiation used in preparative regimens make the treatment hard to implement successfully. Specialized medical and nursing care is required. The basic concepts of the BMT process are as follows.

- The dose of most chemotherapeutic agents administered to cure a patient's disease is limited by subsequent dose-related marrow toxicity.
- The availability of donor marrow for transplantation and engraftment make it possible to administer chemoradiotherapy in supralethal doses in an effort to kill malignant cells (preparative regimens for BMT).
- The patient is then rescued with donor marrow to prevent iatrogenic death (bone marrow transplantation).
- The infused marrow will reconstitute the patient's (host) hematopoietic and immunologic system, and the patient (host) will be rescued (engraftment).

TABLE 18-1 Process of Allogeneic Bone Marrow Transplantation: Sequence and Time of Events

Event	Time
1. Diagnosis of patient with disease treatable with BMT	Days (AA) to years (CML, CP)
2. Identification of histocompatible donor	2 wk
3. Evaluation of patient and donor for BMT	2 wk
4. Placement of multiple-lumen central catheter in patient	1 day
5. Admission to hospital for BMT	—
6. Initiation of pretransplantation conditioning regimen with high-dose chemoirradiation given either alone or in combination therapy	2–10 days
7. Admission of donor for marrow harvest	Day of BMT
8. Infusion of donor marrow into patient	Day of marrow harvest; several-hour infusion
9. Engraftment	2–4 wk
Acute complications	Day 0 to 100 days after BMT
10. Discharge to outpatient setting	30–40 days after BMT
11. Outpatient care	30–100 days after BMT
12. Late acute and early chronic complications	30–100 days after BMT
13. Return to referring health care team for continuing care	100 days after BMT
14. Chronic complications	100 days—4–5 yr after BMT

AA, Aplastic anemia; *CML,* chronic myelogenous leukemia; *CP,* chronic phase.

- Complications that follow BMT are the result of the high-dose chemotherapy and conditioning regimens used to prepare the patient to receive the donor marrow (acute and chronic complications).

Table 18-1 presents the sequence and time of events in the process of allogeneic BMT.

TYPES OF BONE MARROW TRANSPLANTATION

Originally, only patients with leukemia refractory to conventional therapy were considered for marrow transplantation. Successful marrow grafts are now performed in patients with a variety of hematologic and nonhematologic malignant disorders. The selection of marrow transplantation to treat any such disease is highly contingent on an available and appropriate donor source. Donor sources are allogeneic (related or unrelated), autologous (self), or syngeneic (twin). Alternative donor sources currently being investigated for possible use include fetal liver cells, umbilical cord blood, and cadaveric transplants.[14–16]

Syngeneic

A syngeneic marrow transplant is one in which the donor is an identical twin (who by definition is a perfect HLA match). Conditioning regimens are determined by the disease being treated.[7,12] A higher incidence of leukemic relapse has been reported in syngeneic than in allogeneic marrow recipients because of the demonstrated antileukemic effect of graft-versus-host disease.[9] This is known as graft-versus-leukemia effect, and will be discussed later in this chapter.

Allogeneic

Allogeneic marrow transplantation depends on the availability of an HLA-matched donor (Figure 18-2). GVHD, a complication unique to allogeneic marrow transplantation and a major impediment to successful transplantation, is discussed later in this chapter. Intensive supportive care with protective environments, gut decontaminants, prophylactic and therapeutic antibiotics, and red cell and platelet transfusions are required. Granulocyte transfusions are rarely used because of consistently poor results. Specialized nursing care is essential to manage these patients.[17]

Diseases treated with allogeneic BMT

Allogeneic transplantations are done most commonly for acute and chronic leukemia, lymphomas, multiple myeloma, severe aplastic anemia, genetic disease, immunologic deficiencies, and inborn errors of metabolism. Figure 18-3 identifies the diseases treated with allogeneic BMT and the frequency of these transplants.

Genetic disease Children with aplastic anemia, thalassemia, or Franconis anemia have received successful allografts. BMT for sickle cell anemia is under investigation; however, considerable controversy still exists in this area. The risks intrinsic to BMT for sickle cell anemia must be balanced against the expected morbidity and mortality of the disease. Weighing these risks is difficult, since the clinical course of sickle cell disease is quite variable. The cost effectiveness of using BMT for a disease with a 40-year life expectancy is also questionable.[18]

Immunologic deficiencies Cures have been reported in patients with congenital immunodeficiency diseases, including severe combined immunodeficiency disease syndrome (SCIDS), Wiskott-Aldrich syndrome, and some rare inherited disorders. Currently, marrow transplantation is a treatment choice only in the presence of an HLA-matched sibling.[19] The first human gene therapy experiment for the treatment of adenosine deaminase deficiency, a form of SCIDS, was recently described.[20] Considerable research is needed to understand the limitations and potential use of in vivo gene transfer therapy.

Inborn errors of metabolism Allogeneic BMT has been utilized successfully to treat diseases of inborn

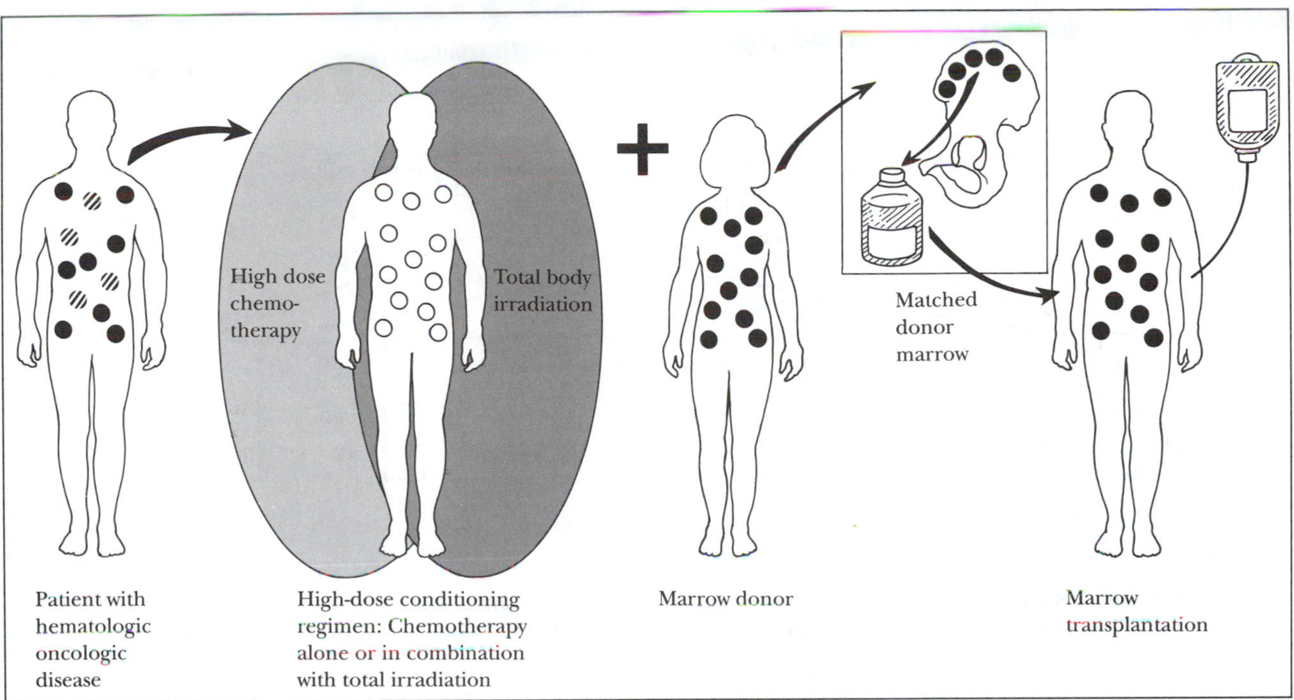

FIGURE 18-2 Schematic for allogeneic bone marrow transplantation.

errors of metabolism, such as Gaucher disease, chronic granulomatosis disease, osteoporosis, mucopolysaccharidosis (Hurler's syndrome), Sanfilipp B disease, and Maroteaux-Lamy syndrome. Lipidosis diseases include adrenoleukodystrophy (ADL) and metachromatic leukodystrophy (MLD). Treatment of these diseases has been limited to those patients with a histocompatible sibling. But as increasing numbers of volunteer donors become available, more unrelated donor searches may be initiated.[19]

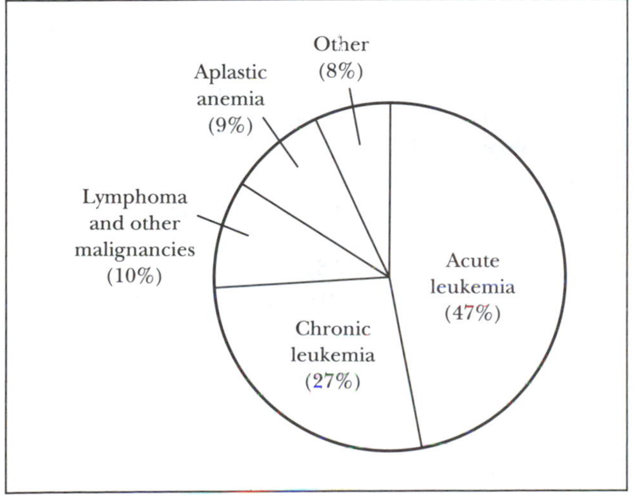

FIGURE 18-3 Diseases treated by allogeneic transplant, 1988–1990. (Source: International Bone Marrow Transplant Registry.)

Donors

Tissue typing

Human leukocyte antigen/mixed lymphocyte culture Selecting the most appropriate donor for a patient begins with an understanding of the major histocompatibility complex in humans, which is composed of a series of closely linked genetic loci on chromosome 6. The antigens located at HLA-A and HLA-B are defined serologically, and those of the HLA-A locus are detected by the mixed leukocyte culture (MLC) test. A locus identical with or closely related to HLA-D, called HLA-DR, can be serologically typed using B-lymphocytes.

A chromosomal region is known as a *haplotype*. Every person inherits one haplotype from each parent, and within any given family there can be only four haplotypes. There is approximately a 25% chance for a patient to be an HLA-match with a sibling[21] (Figure 18-4). Until recent years, most allogeneic transplantations were from HLA-identical siblings, but selected family members or unrelated phenotypically identical donors have been used successfully as marrow donors.

As the demand for marrow transplantation donors increases, faster and more accurate methods are needed to identify the most appropriate donor. One breakthrough in this area allows the identification of HLA allelic polymorphism directed at the DNA level by hybridization with sequence-specific ologonucleotide probes ("HLA ologotyping") after identification of DNA by polymerase chain reaction.[22]

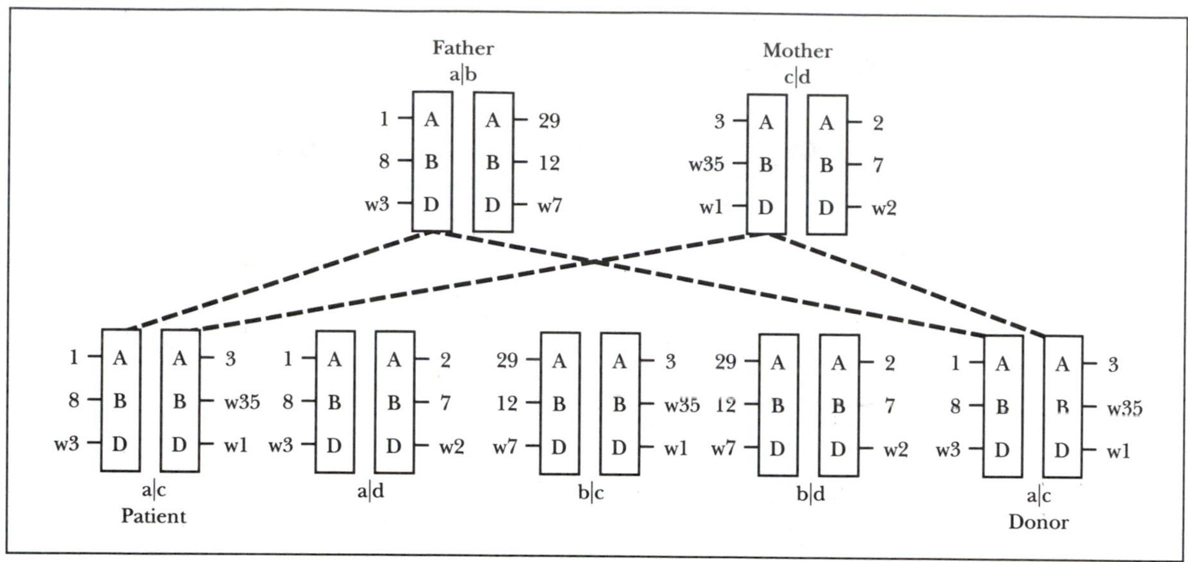

FIGURE 18-4 Diagram of possible combinations of human leukocyte antigen (HLA) region of chromosome 6 inherited from parents to sibling. The recipient and donor have inherited the same two haploytpes and are genotypically HLA identical.

ABO typing Major ABO-incompatible marrow grafting can be performed without significant hemolytic transfusion reactions. This is because effective techniques to remove red blood cells from donor marrow, and plasma exchange of patient marrow, have reduced the risk of such reactions.[23] Blood group typing, however, must be done on all patients and potential donors.[24] If unmanipulated incompatible ABO marrow is transfused, it, like any incompatible blood product transfusion, will cause a major hemolytic transfusion reaction, which can result in death. After transplantation, the patient's ABO type will become the same type as the marrow donor.

Marrow collection

Donor marrow is harvested in the operating room under sterile conditions, with the donor anesthetized under general or spinal anesthesia. The marrow is obtained from the posterior iliac crests in 2–5-ml aspirates, up to a total of 10 mg/kg to 15 mg/kg recipient body weight. If necessary, the anterior iliac crests and the sternum can be used. Although 150–200 aspirates are necessary to obtain sufficient marrow, only 6–10 skin punctures are made, with the aspiration needles redirected to different sites under the skin.[9] The heparinized marrow is screened through a series of progressively finer mesh screens to filter out bone particles and fat. Marrow is then placed in blood administration bags and infused into the patient within 2–4 hours.[5,9,17] The steps of marrow collection and harvest are outlined in Figure 18-5.

Unrelated donors The use of unrelated volunteer donors increased from 5% in 1988 to 8% in 1990. As of 1992, The National Marrow Donor Program (NMDP) has approved 53 BMT centers to perform allogeneic BMT for unrelated donors. There are 99 donor centers, and unrelated marrow harvests are performed at 80 approved collection centers. Since November 1991, the NMDP has facilitated 929 unrelated bone marrow transplantations.[25] Public education regarding the efficacy and benefits of unrelated donor marrow transplants, and the thrust to recruit black, Hispanic, Oriental, Jewish, and mixed European minority donors, makes possible marrow transplantation for thousands of patients without matched family donors.

Currently 650,000 unrelated donors are registered, and this number is expected to increase to more than 1 million by 1995 (personal communication, Claudio Anasetti, 1992). Improvements in genetic tissue typing with serologic and restrictive fragment-length polymorphism techniques hold promise for improving the reliability and speed of current screening methods. Scientific investigators working with unrelated donor transplants are striving to develop improved therapies to prevent the major complications of marrow rejection, GVHD, and infection.

Autologous

An autologous (self) marrow graft is a transplant in which a patient with a malignant disease receives his or her own marrow. This marrow is collected and cryopre-

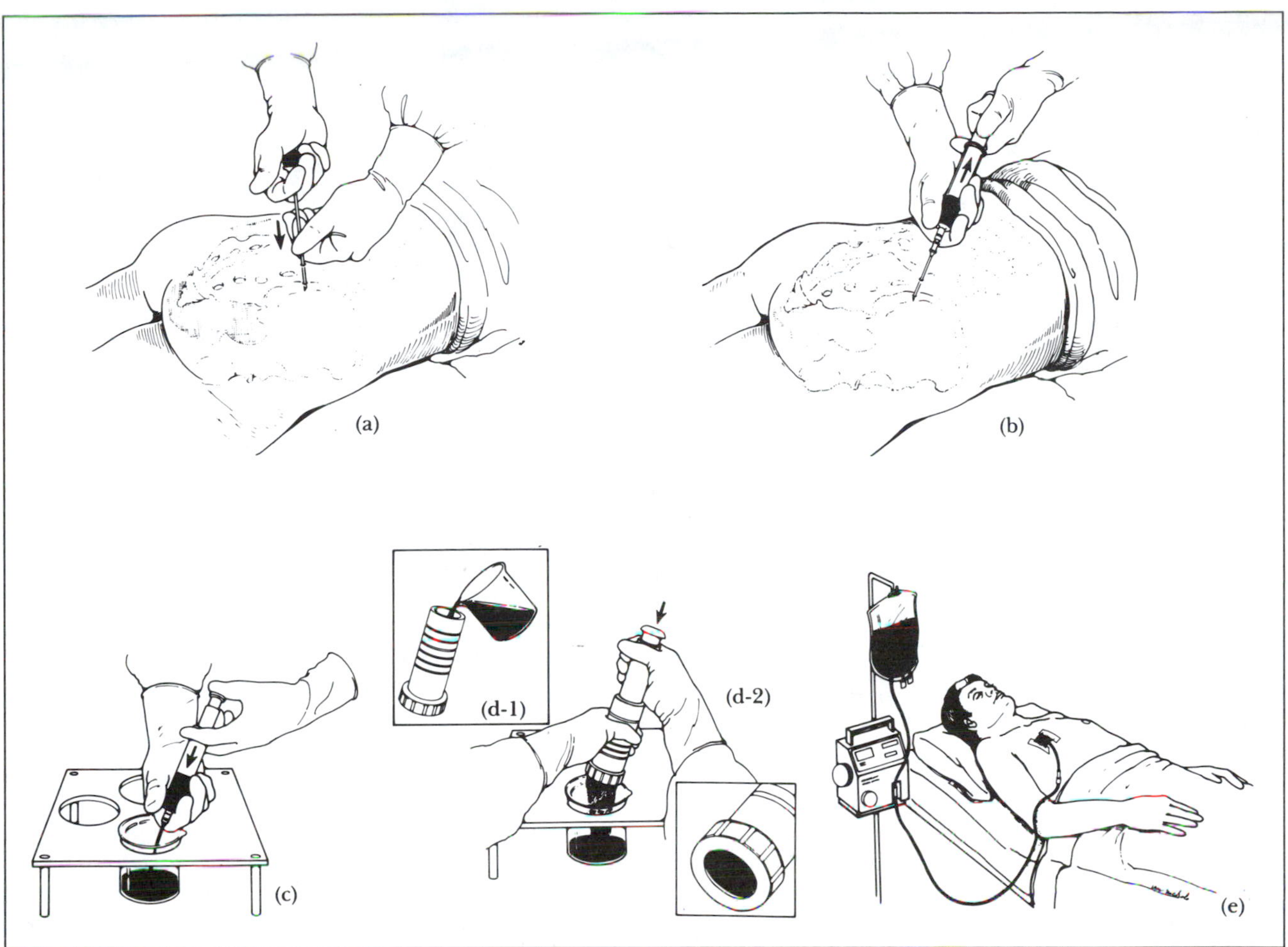

FIGURE 18-5 Figure series of steps in donor marrow aspiration and harvest. (a) Large-bore needle placed in the posterior iliac crest. (b) Multiple aspirations. (c) Marrow drawn up in large syringe. (d-1) Marrow placed in collection beaker; (d-2) strained through metal grid. (e) Marrow placed in a blood administration bag and administered through multilumen central catheter.

served during remission following high-dose preparative conditioning (Figure 18-6). One primary concern after autologous marrow transplantation is relapse of the malignancy. Relapse may be due to a failure of pretransplantation conditioning to eradicate residual host tumor cells successfully or to the contamination of the autologous donor marrow with malignant cells. For this reason, purging techniques are often used to "clean" the recipients marrow prior to reinfusion.[26] Purging techniques are discussed later in this chapter.

Diseases treated with autologous BMT

Autologous bone marrow transplantations (ABMTs) are being done with increasing frequency (Figure 18-7). Current clinical trials are studying the use of ABMT in breast, ovarian, colon, and small-cell lung cancers, melanoma, multiple myeloma, and malignant glioma. Advantages of autologous BMT are the absence of graft-versus-host disease and fewer BMT-related toxicities. Currently, experimental trials are focused on the treatment outcomes of ABMT versus outcomes for traditional treatment with chemotherapy and irradiation. The cost effectiveness of ABMT versus that of standard therapy is also being studied. Insurance coverage for the treatment of solid tumors with ABMT remains a major problem. ABMT is expensive and many third-party payers still classify it as an experimental therapy not covered under most policies.[26,27]

Marrow collection

Aspirations for an autologous transplant are obtained in a manner similar to that for allogeneic donor harvest; however, a larger total marrow volume may be needed if the marrow is to be purged or manipulated. Autologous marrow occasionally is infused immediately after the completion of the high-dose

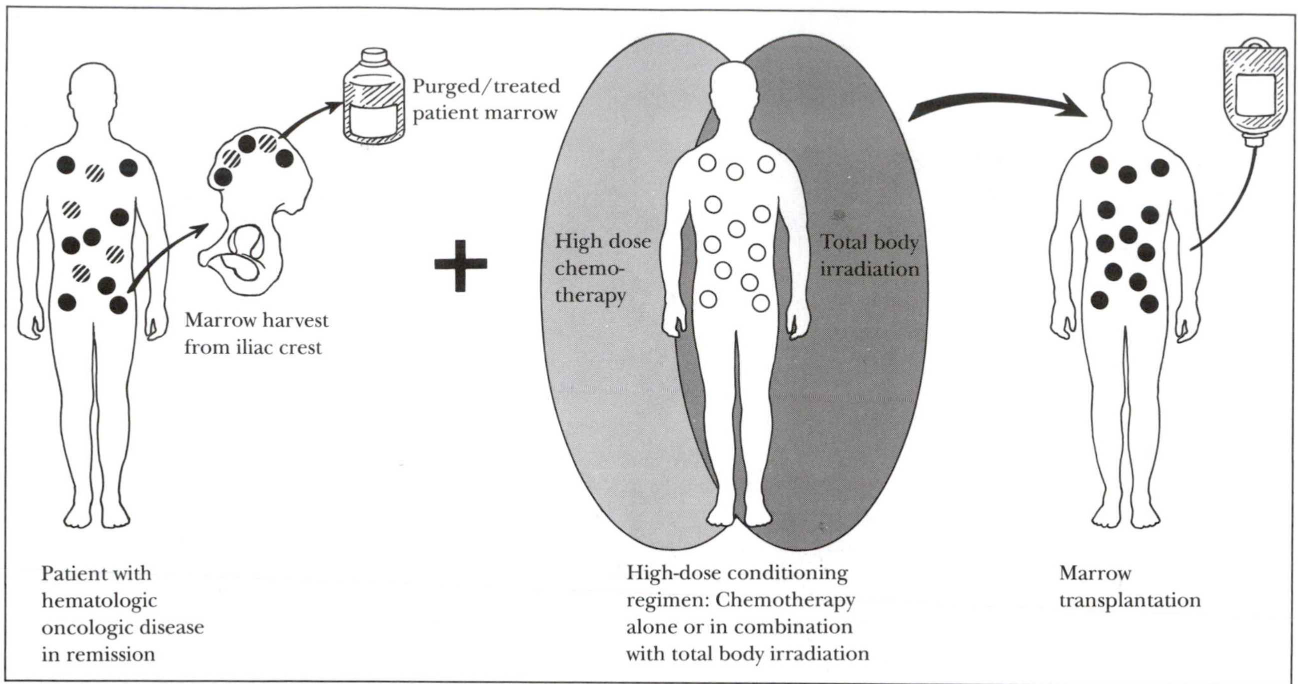

FIGURE 18-6 Schematic for autologous bone marrow transplantation.

preparative regimen. More often, the marrow is cryopreserved for use if the patient relapses. The length of time that marrow can be stored without compromising its viability is still unknown. Institutions vary in their policies on the stored marrow's "shelf life," and storage time ranges from 1 to 8 years.[21,26–28]

Purging techniques The purpose of purging autologous marrow is to remove malignant cells before the marrow is reinfused. There are three methods of purging marrow: physical, immunologic, and pharmacologic. Physical purging separates leukemic cells from marrow using lectin separation, centrifugation in density gradients, and counterflow evaluations. Immunologic purging uses immunotoxins and monoclonal antibodies alone or in combination with magnetic immunobeads.[29] Pharmacologic purging uses potent agents of mercocyanine 540, mafosfamide (ASTA-2-7557) 4-hydroperoxy-cyclophosphamide, or alkyl-lysophospholipids.[29]

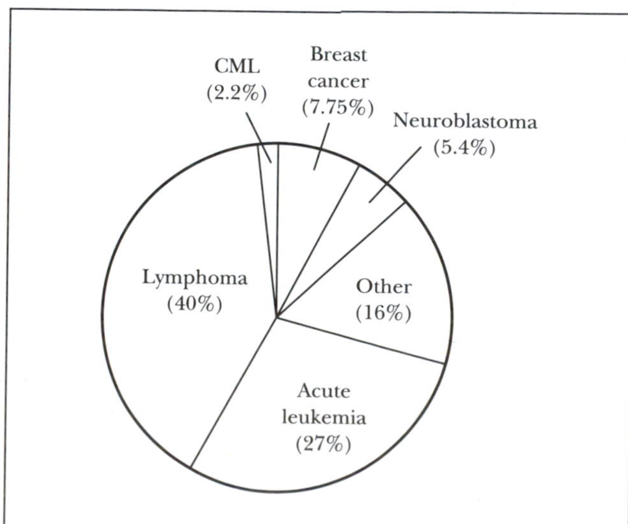

FIGURE 18-7 Diseases treated with autologous bone marrow transplantation.

Autologous peripheral stem cell transplant

Autologous peripheral stem cell transplantation (PSCT) holds promise as a curative therapy for selected patients with hematologic malignancies and solid tumors, including acute and chronic leukemias and lymphomas. Other oncologic diseases in current clinical trials with PSCT are breast, ovarian, sarcoma, small-cell lung, cervical, and brain cancers.[28–30]

The first successful PSCTs were performed in the 1970s in patients with chronic mylelogenous leukemia (CML).[27,30] Although initially encouraging, subsequent studies in 1979 and 1980 proved to be unsuccessful. Discouraged investigators shifted away from PSCT studies. In 1986, however, six international institutions simultaneously reported successful autologous PSCT for patients with diseases other than CML, and interest in PSCT was renewed.[31]

Likely candidates for PSCT are patients who are ineligible for autologous marrow transplantations because their marrow is hypoplastic from prior myeloablative therapies or those with metastatic marrow disease. Because PSCT is the subject of considerable investigation, several treatment protocols exist.

Collection and mobilization Collection and mobilization of peripheral stem cells via apheresis usually is done in the outpatient setting. Some centers use their own trained technicians or nurses; other contract with local blood banks or the American Red Cross to provide this service.

Mobilization is the term used to describe the process of either stimulating circulating hematopoietic stem cells with myelosuppressive chemotherapy or administering human recombinant growth factors during the collection period. A combination of these two techniques can produce more hematopoietic stem cells than when either technique is used alone.

In the actual procedure, peripheral stems are collected from the patient via venous access from a multilumen central catheter and are apheresed using a cell separation device programmed to collect either lymphocytes or low-density leukocytes. Generally, 6–10 stem cell collections are needed, and collections are done on separate days. The patient is connected to the cell separator for 2–4 hours per collection. Prior to each collection, a complete blood count is done to ensure that sufficient peripheral stem cells exist. To collect the cells, blood is withdrawn and separated and red blood cells, platelets, and plasma are returned to the patient. Multiple collections may be needed to obtain optimal cell count aliquots to perform the PSCT.[30,31] Optimal cell counts differ dramatically among research protocols and depend on the use of (1) recombinant human granulocyte–monocyte colony stimulating factor (rhGM-CSF) (2) mobilization techniques, (3) methods of cell culturing, and (4) collection equipment.[30,31]

Patients, like blood or platelet donors, may experience tingling or chilling sensations and lightheadedness during the procedure. Central catheter complications include hemothorax, venous thrombosis, line infection, and the inability to obtain adequate bloodflow secondary to catheter occlusion or malfunction.[32]

Once collected, cells undergo purification using a density gradient technique to reduce the number of contaminating red blood cells and granulocytes. Cells are then prepared for cryopreservation, similar to autologous marrow cryopreservation techniques, and stored in infusion bags. Two cryopreservation techniques currently exist, but the technique most often used is cryoprotectant dimethylsulfoxide (DMSO) at a concentraion of 10% by volume. Higher concentrations of DMSO are needed for peripheral stem cryopreservation (versus the previously mentioned autologous cryopreservation) because these cells contain 60% more mononuclear cells than do marrow cells. The cells are cooled and subsequently stored in liquid-phase (−196°C) or vapor-phase (−80°C) liquid nitrogen.

The second cryopreservation method uses dimethylsulfoxide at a concentration of 5% by volume combined with hydroxyethyl starch for cryopreservation. In this case, the peripheral cells are placed in a −80°C freezer for cooling and subsequently stored in the freezer. With each technique, the bags are flattened between two aluminum plates so that a thin monolayer preparation is obtained to allow uniform freezing.[33,34]

Transplantation of peripheral stem cells Immediately prior to peripheral stem cell transplantation, the cells are removed from storage and thawed or washed in a warm water bath. After thawing, they are infused as quickly as possible through a central or peripheral catheter over 2–4 hours. Some transplant center protocols allow for the infusion of PSCT in the outpatient center, followed by home care. Often, pretransplant conditioning with high-dose chemotherapy or total-body irradiation is done before PSCT. Centers may administer pretransplant conditioning in outpatient settings; others will admit the patient if complications cannot be managed on an outpatient basis.

Complications of infusion include nephrotoxicity as a result of red blood cell contamination, which may require hemodialysis. Cardiac toxicity may result from the infusion of DMSO. Dyspnea may occur and require oxygen administration. Once these crises pass, the care of the PSCT patient is similar to the care of autologous marrow transplantation recipients.[30–34]

The advantages and disadvantages of PSCT therapy, especially long-term effects, are the subject of considerable debate. Improved technologies are expected to decrease PSCT collections to one or two apheresis procedures, with hematopoietic growth factors rapidly restoring disease-free marrow function. Considerable research is still needed to determine the optimal use of PSCT to achieve long-term disease-free stem cell recovery with minimal toxicities.

PROCESS OF BONE MARROW TRANSPLANT

The oncology nurse in the referring physician's office or clinic can contribute significantly to the continuity of care for the BMT candidate, donor, and family. Anxiety associated with the decision to physically relocate to participate in an expensive life-threatening treatment has been well documented.[35,36] Community-based nurses can prepare and support BMT candidates, donors, and families by providing literature specific to BMT. The National Institutes of Health (NIH) provides material that explains the BMT process. Long-term survivors of BMT in the candidate's community may be an additional source of inspiration and information. Good communication between BMT coordinator nurses and community nursing care managers will enhance continuity of care between the community and the BMT center.

Pretransplant Evaluation and Preparation of the Patient

Marrow candidates require comprehensive evaluations to determine the patient's ability to sustain BMT. These evaluations, listed in Table 18-2, usually are done in outpatient facilities. A patient and family conference is

TABLE 18-2 Pretransplantation Preparation and Evaluation of Candidate and Donor for BMT

Evaluation	Candidate	Donor
Clinical evaluation		
• Histocompatible tissue typing (HLA, MLC, HLA-DR-RFLP)	X	X
• ECG, possible cardiac-ejection fraction, appropriate scans	X	X
• Complete history and physical examination	X	X
• Immunization history	X	X
• Diagnostic procedures (bone marrow aspiration, biopsies)	X	
• Oral examination	X	
• Pulmonary function test, arterial blood gases	X	
• Chest films	X	X
• Informed consent	X	X
• Nutritional evaluation	X	
• Psychologic evaluation, if recommended	X	X
• Gynecologic consultation for women of menstrual age	X	
• Appropriate consultations	X	X
• Sperm storage and ova storage if appropriate	X	
Laboratory evaluation		
• Complete blood count with differential and platelet count	X	X
• Chemistry profile	X	X
• Hepatitis screen		
non-A	X	X
non-B	X	X
A	X	X
B	X	X
C	X	X
• HIV antibody status	X	X
• Serologic test for syphilis	X	X
• ABO and RH groups	X	X
• CMV antibody status	X	X
• HCG	X	X
Preparation and intervention		
• Placement of right atrial catheter	X	
• Ferrous gluconate medication		X
• Preoperative and postoperative teaching regarding marrow harvest	X (autologous)	X
• Postoperative care and evaluation of marrow aspiration sites	X	X

RFLP, restriction fragment-length polymorphism; *HCG*, human chorionic gonadotropin.

held in the outpatient setting prior to the transplantation. The purposes of this conference are (1) to obtain informed consent, (2) to discuss expected risk and transplant-related morbidity and mortality, and (3) to discuss expected outcomes with the patient. A clear understanding of the BMT process is critical at this time. Often the patient discovers that actual survival statistics and other clinical data are very different from initial expectations. For example, a patient with acute myelogenous leukemia (AML) in second complete remission may have been told, prior to arrival at the center, that the statistical probability of a 5-year disease-free survival for the disease was 80%. In reality, the probability of disease-free survival is 50%.[37] Outpatient nurses can support the patient faced with the difficulties of accepting treatment realities and making critical treatment decisions.

Patient and family preparation for hospitalization can be conducted during the wait for hospital admission. Familiarizing the patient with laminar air flow rooms, protective isolation, and various complex treatment and research protocols can decrease the patient's anxiety concerning the procedures. Formalized instruction using videotapes and booklets is effective. Many BMT centers provide written information about their center, including maps, important telephone numbers, activities, and a glossary of BMT terms.

All patients have multilumen indwelling central catheters inserted before admission. Atrial catheters are essential to accommodate large volumes of parenteral fluids that will be required. Peripheral inserted catheters (PICs), placed by certified nurses, are gaining attention, especially for those patients receiving autologous bone marrow transplantation.

Gonadal failure caused by the high-dose chemotherapy and total-body irradiation used in preparative regimens is a concern for BMT patients. The option of sperm banking should be discussed prior to hospitalization in patients with adequate sperm counts.[2] Fertilized ova storage may be an option for women; however, ethical issues may arise if the woman should die during BMT.

Preparation of the Donor and Nursing Care

Selected allogeneic donors, in addition to being HLA matched, need to be relatively healthy, give informed consent, and be available for marrow harvest and platelet donation. Donors who are minors may present certain legal and ethical considerations. For example, the Illinois Supreme Court recently ruled that half-siblings cannot be required to undergo tissue-typing for a step-brother requiring a BMT.[38]

Although risks are minimal, donors need to be comprehensively evaluated prior to surgery, especially for the ability to tolerate general or spinal anesthesia. To minimize the risks of blood transfusion, donors weighing more than 50 kilograms donate a unit of autologous whole blood to be reinfused intraoperatively at the time of marrow harvest. Administration of erythropoietin to boost donor hematocrit levels before harvest is being studied (personal communication, Keith Sullivan, 1992).

Several factors influence the amount of counseling and education a donor needs prior to donation. These include the relationship between the donor, the patient, and the family, as well as the donor's own life responsibilities.[39,40] For example, donors often need to provide platelet support for the patient up to 3 months after marrow transfusion. This demand can create hardships for the donor. Donors can experience long-term psychological effects when the patient has died after the BMT. Long-term sequelae, including mood changes, lack of self-esteem, altered relationships, and guilt, can occur depending on the donor's perception of the success or failure of the BMT.[41,42] These studies, however, are dated and new research is needed. As with the patient, donors and their families can be effectively supported through eduction and written information to miminize anxiety and to promote realistic expectations.

Marrow donors usually are admitted to the hospital for marrow harvest the day of surgery and discharged 24 hours after surgery. Bolwell et al.[43] reported that outpatient marrow harvesting is feasible and that the need for red blood cell transfusions can be reduced by using red blood cells collected during the harvest. In Bolwell's study, researchers asked 211 marrow donors to describe the side effects of outpatient marrow donation. Of the 64% who responded, the most common side effects were pain at the donation site (90%), low-back pain (60%), nausea (43%), vomiting (31%), sore throat (43%), fever (18%), and bleeding at the donation site (6%). Similar complications are noted in marrow donors admitted for longer periods of time. Physical and psychologic follow-up care for the donor is essential.

Nursing care of the donor often is overshadowed by the attention given to the marrow recipient. Nurses can be instrumental in recognizing this phenomenon and making appropriate referrals to social workers or psychologists. Donors may be under stress due to separation from work and family, worries about lost income, and strained interpersonal relationships. Unrelated donors are typically harvested in a hospital away from the marrow recipient, for confidentially and convenience. Unrelated donors are not asked to remain available for future platelet transfusions to the marrow recipient. Nurses caring for unrelated donors should be sensitive to the ethical issues of confidentality, especially regarding the donor's motivations.[44]

THE BONE MARROW TRANSPLANT

Admission to the Hospital

Once patients have been thoroughly evaluated for BMT, they are admitted to the hospital and placed in a protective isolation room. Several isolation methods exist. The use of laminar air flow (LAF) rooms, to decrease infection-related morbidity and mortality, versus simple protective isolation is still under debate. Early studies showed that only patients with aplastic anemia admitted to LAF rooms survived longer when compared to patients not placed in LAF rooms.[45,46] There is no convincing evidence that patients cared for in LAF rooms have significantly higher survival rates than patients placed in conventional hospital rooms where reverse isolation, gloves, face masks, or filtered air are used.[47,48] Applicable research data on this topic in the past decade frequently have been confounded by an accompanying increase in oral nonabsorbable antibiotic administration.

Despite the uncertainty about the most effective protective isolation techniques, the use of LAF rooms and rooms with high-efficiency particulate air filters has increased during the past decade. Figure 18-8 depicts the basic laminar air flow room.

Patients transplanted in LAF rooms require specialized nursing care. These patients must undergo decontamination of their gastrointestinal tracts, skin, and body cavities. Decontamination techniques include ingestion of concentrated antibiotic solution, application of antibiotic powders or ointment in nostrils, ears, umbilicus, axillae, rectum, and groin areas, and bathing with sterile water and antibacterial soap. Nursing care of patients in LAF rooms includes supporting compliance with LAF medications as well as offering psychologic support. The loss of human touch can induce psychologic problems;[49] however, further nursing research is needed in this area.

Pretransplant Conditioning Regimens

Recipients of marrow transplant usually are admitted to the hospital 1 day prior to the start of their conditioning regimen. The methods used to prepare patients for grafting differ according to the underlying disease. Patients receive high-dose chemotherapy alone or with supralethal doses of irradiation. This serves to eradicate malignant cells and to prevent graft rejection by the patient's own immune system.[50]

Historically, cyclophosphamide (CY) in combination with total-body irradiation (TBI) has been the standard treatment used in BMT preparative regimens. CY is the most common chemotherapeutic agent because it provides tumor cell kill as well as immune ablation. Other agents sometimes used in combination with TBI include cytosine arabinoside and etoposide. The use of busulfan and cyclophosphamide without TBI has increased markedly during the late decade.[1]

Total-body irradiation is delivered in varying doses from cobalt or linear accelerator units. TBI offers optimal tumor cell kill because of its ability to penetrate the central nervous system and other privileged sites.[51] Lung shielding sometimes is used in efforts to reduce life-threatening pulmonary complications. TBI can be delivered in single or fractionated doses, but prevailing practice favors fractionated doses to reduce toxicities.[51] Pretransplant "booster" radiotherapy to previous tu-

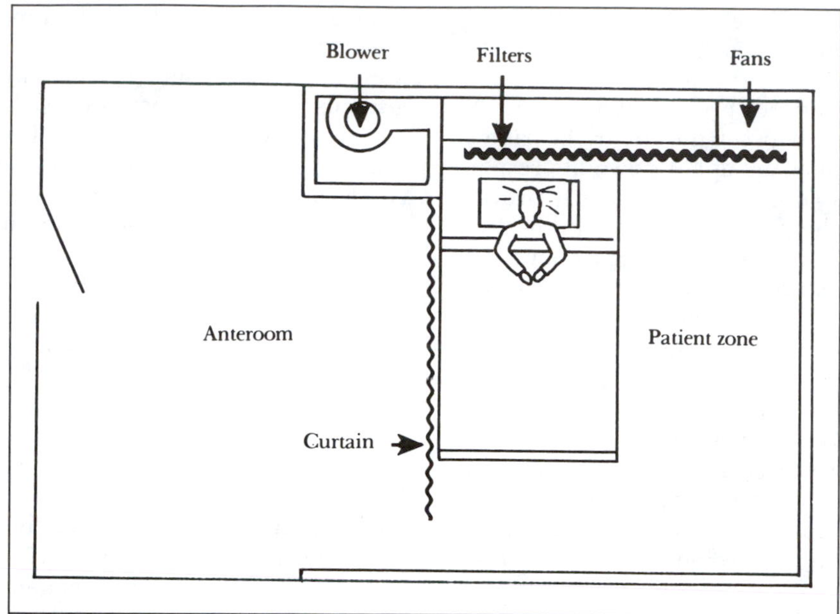

FIGURE 18-8 Diagram of a laminar air flow room. A plastic barrier separates the sterile patient zone from the outer zone. Patient decontamination may occur via drinking nonabsorbable antibiotics and application of antibiotic creams and powder to various body areas.

mor sites may be used in patients with bulky disease to reduce the chances of relapse.[52]

Marrow Infusion

The day of marrow infusion is "day 0," with subsequent days numbered from this time. The actual marrow infusion is a procedure similar to a blood transfusion. The marrow is infused through a central lumen catheter over the course of several hours. Marrow cells pass through the lung and home to the marrow cavity. Complications may include volume overload and pulmonary abnormalities from fat emboli. Symptoms similar to blood transfusion reactions can occur (i.e., chills, urticaria, and fever) and should be treated with antihistamines or antipyretics or by decreasing the rate of infusion.[53] Within 2–4 weeks, the marrow graft becomes functional, and peripheral platelets, leukocytes, and red cells increase in number. Intensive nursing care is required to prevent complications until the recipient's marrow recovers.

COMPLICATIONS OF BONE MARROW TRANSPLANTATION

Although BMT holds potential cure for a number of diseases, acute and chronic toxicities can complicate the posttransplantation course. Complications are the result of (1) high-dose chemotherapy and irradiation for conditioning regimens, (2) graft-vs-host disease (allogeneic), or (3) problems associated with the original disease.[54] The sequence of major complications following allogeneic BMT is presented in Figure 18-9. The major complications following autologous BMT are similar, except for GVHD.

Interrelationships of BMT Complications

The major symptoms of marrow transplant-related complications overlap (Figure 18-10) and are interrelated as follows.

- The chemoradiation therapy the patients receive would be fatal if the patients were not rescued with marrow infusion.
- Major complications after transplantation usually result from the chemoradiation used to prepare for transplantation or from the marrow transplantation, not from the original disease.
- Complications often occur simultaneously.
- Clinical manifestations of some complications may be sudden yet subtle.
- The clinical manifestations of different complications can be identical; one complication can cause or exacerbate another.

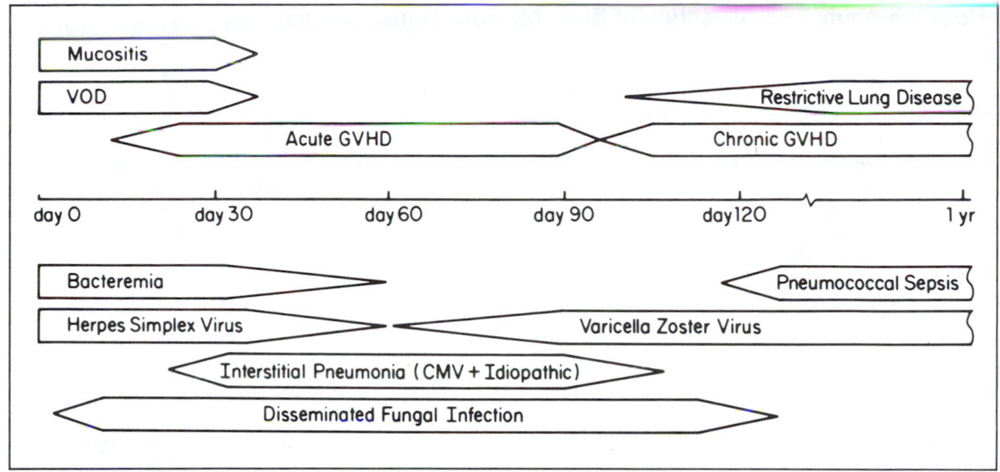

FIGURE 18-9 Temporal sequence of major complications after allogeneic bone marrow transplantation, from day 0 to 1 year after BMT. (Source: Press OW, Schaller RT, Thomas ED: *Complications of Organ Transplantation.* New York: Marcel Dekker, 1987, Fig. 1. Reprinted with permission of Marcel Dekker, Inc.)

- The treatment of one complication can cause or exacerbate another complication.
- The prophylaxis or treatment for one complication may have to be modified or terminated because of the development of another complication.

Nursing care of marrow recipients requires an ability to organize procedures and therapies aimed at prevention and treatment of transplant-related toxicities.[17]

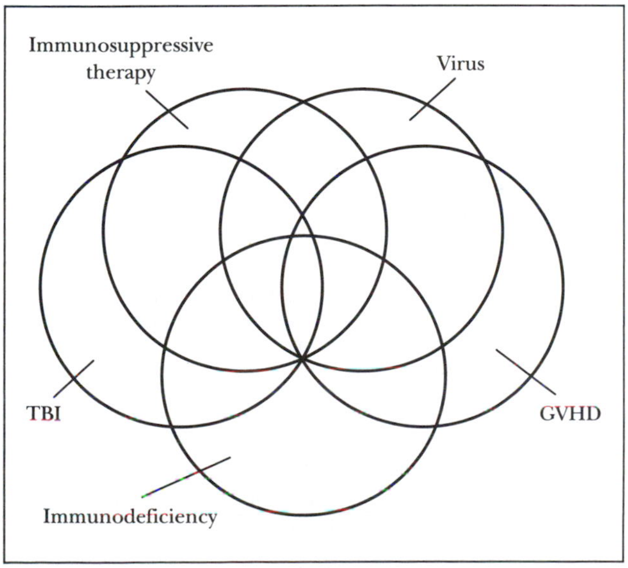

Immunosuppressive therapy
Virus
TBI
GVHD
Immunodeficiency

FIGURE 18-10 The multifactorial nature of acute and chronic complications following marrow transplantation. (Source: Degg JH: Delayed complications of marrow transplantation. *Marrow Transplant Reviews* 2:11, 1992. Reprinted with permission.)

Patients and families experience anxiety and stress associated with this treatment, and nurses require psychosocial nursing skills and the ability to interact with multidisciplinary teams to address patient needs. Table 18-3 lists times of increased anxiety for the marrow transplant recipient.

Acute Complications

Acute complications are seen several days after BMT and affect multiple organ systems. Because pretransplantation chemoradiotherapy ablates all cell lines, complications will be most severe until early engraftment. Table 18-4 presents a detailed summary of the cause, incidence, onset, manifestations, and interventions associated with acute complications of BMT.

Gastrointestinal toxicity

Mucositis The gastrointestinal tract is affected by TBI and chemotherapy preparative conditioning.

TABLE 18-3 Patterns of Psychosocial Response During Bone Marrow Transplantation

Phase	Identified Stressful Event
1	Making the decision to undertake a BMT
2	Preadmission
3	The conditioning regimen
4	Immunosuppression and germ-free isolation
5	Transplantation and waiting for engraftment
6	Hospital discharge and outpatient treatment

TABLE 18-4 Possible Acute Complications of Bone Marrow Transplantation

Complication	Cause	Incidence Rate (%)	Time of Onset after BMT (days)	Signs and Symptoms	Nursing Intervention	Medical Intervention
Gastrointestinal						
Oral mucositis	High-dose conditioning regimen of chemotherapy; TBI (immunosuppression) plus coexistent infection; HSV, methotrexate	100 Universal to chemotherapy and irradiation	0–28	Profuse, watery to thick ropy mucus, severe pain, bleeding ulceration, infection, potential airway obstruction, xerostomia	Assess nasal oral cavity for integrity of mucous membrane	Acyclovir for HSV infection; topical antibiotics: lidocaine, dyclonine, IV morphine
Esophageal mucositis	Same	100	Same	Esophageal dysphasia, bleeding, infection	Administer IV analgesic medication; provide frequent, vigorous oral care	IV morphine sulfate; daily chest film and CBC; viral cultures; parenteral support
Gastric mucositis	Same	100	Same	Anorexia, nausea, vomiting, bleeding, infection	Monitor with care I & O, fluids, and management of pain	Parenteral nutrition, biopsy, appropriate antibiotic therapy
Intestinal mucositis	Same	100	Same	Watery diarrhea, cramping pain, ulcerations, infections	Monitor vital signs q 4 hr; accurately measure I & O; manage pain	Surgical intervention; gut biopsy; antibiotic therapy
Gastrointestinal lower bowel toxicity	High-dose TBI and chemotherapy; GVHD	100	0–30	Nausea, vomiting, diarrhea	Monitor with care fluids and electrolytes, assessment of I & O; administer antiemetics, TPN	Antiemetics, fluid management, gut biopsy
Acute GVHD						
Skin	Reaction of immunocompetent donor T-lymphocytes against immunoincompetent host	40–50	10–70; median onset day 25 after BMT	Maculopapular rash on trunk, palms, soles, ears; generalized erythoderma with desquamation	Assess integumentary system; understand side effects of drugs used in treatment; provide psychologic support of patient	Immunosuppressive therapy with methotrexate, cyclosporine; treated T-cell–depleted donor marrow before BMT; antithymocyte globulin; corticosteroids; skin biopsy; analgesics
Liver	Same	40–50	Same	Elevated liver enzymes, alkaline phosphatase, right upper quadrant pain, heptatomegaly, jaundice	Monitor liver function tests	Liver biopsy
Gastrointestinal tract	Same	40–50	10–70	Green watery diarrhea, abdominal cramping, anorexia, nausea, vomiting	Monitor guaiac stool test, weight, accurate I & O, central venous pressure, CBC and electrolytes; administer antiemetics	Gut biopsy; differential diagnosis to rule out infection, VOD, gut rest, parenteral nutrition
Renal insufficiency	Nephrotoxins, amphotericin B, cyclosporine, methotrexate, aminoglycoside plus septic shock or cardiogenic	25	1–50	Decreased urine output, asymptomatic azotemia, proteinuria, hypertension, renal failure, thrombocytopenia pur-	Monitor vital signs, with postural BP; careful fluid management, accurate I & O; monitor serum creatinine,	Dialysis (5%–10% of BMT patients), removal or reduction of nephrotoxic drugs; correction of fluid electrolyte

(continued)

TABLE 18-4 Possible Acute Complications of Bone Marrow Transplantation (continued)

Complication	Cause	Incidence Rate (%)	Time of Onset after BMT (days)	Signs and Symptoms	Nursing Intervention	Medical Intervention
	shock or volume depletion because of diarrhea; hepatorenal syndrome of VOD			pura, thirst, dizziness; flat or distended neck veins, peripheral edema; doubling of baseline serum creatinine	BUN, electrolyte levels; monitor urine electrolyte collections, specific gravity q 4 hr; measure daily abdominal girth, weight; assess for peripheral edema; monitor patient during dialysis	and acid-base imbalance; treatment of infections
Hemorrhagic cystitis	High-dose cyclophosphamide	24	Immediately	Hematuria, dysuria, frequency, blood clots	Assess fluid intake; force fluids	Three-way catheters, continuous bladder irrigation
Venoocclusive disease	High-dose conditioning regimens; patients with previous liver disease; patients >15 yr old	21 (6% mortality rate) aplastic anemia (rare)	6–15	Weight gain >12%, ascites, hepatic metabolism, bilirubin >20 mg/dl, SGOT >40 mU/ml; right upper quadrant pain; encephalopathy, hepatomegaly	Carefully and frequently assess fluid balance; monitor weight BID, vital signs with postural BP, accurate I & O; measure abdominal girth daily, restrict fluid, sodium; monitor narcotics and, if indicated, hemodynamics; assess neurologic and mental changes	No known treatment; maintain intravascular volume and renal profusion; restrict sodium, maintain hematocrit >35%; albumin; low-dose dopamine; supportive care
Infection		100	0–30	Neutropenia, oral fever >38°C, sepsis, cough, lethargy	Provide LAF rooms; prevent infection; use good hand-washing techniques; wear mask in patient's room; provide surveillance, cultures, pan cultures; administer antibiotics; manage side effects of treatment drugs; regulate BP with pressor agents and hemodynamics monitoring; manage fluid and electrolyte acid-base balances; institute fever reduction measures	Prophylactic measures, protective isolation, LAF rooms, oral nonabsorbable antibiotics, low-bacteria diet, TMP-SMX for pneumocystis, acyclovir prophylaxis for HSV, passive immunization with CMV-Ig, IgG, CMV blood product screening, surveillance chest films, total-body skin cleaning, treatment with broad-spectrum prophylactic antibiotics; appropriate antibiotics for bacterial, viral, fungal, and protozoal infection
Bacterial		10				
Escherichia coli		5.5				
Staphylococcus epidermidis		35.9				
S. aureus		7.8				
Streptococcus spp.		6.3				
Viral						
Herpes simplex	Reactivation of latent virus	70–80	0–30	Pain, ulceration, bleeding, fever, infection	Provide vigorous mouth care; administer pain medication	Prophylaxis and treatment with IV acyclovir; analgesics

(continued)

TABLE 18-4 Possible Acute Complications of Bone Marrow Transplantation (continued)

Complication	Cause	Incidence Rate (%)	Time of Onset after BMT (days)	Signs and Symptoms	Nursing Intervention	Medical Intervention
CMV pneumonia	Reactivation of latent virus	70 in allogeneic 10 in autologous	60–70	Dyspnea, infiltrates on chest film; abnormal ABGs, PFTs; may be asymptomatic	Administer medication, chest auscultation	Diagnostic bronchoscopy, DGHP, CMV-Ig; bronchial washings
Fungal *Aspergillus* *(Candida)*	Immunosuppression caused by TBI and chemotherapy	10% unknown	0–30	Fever	Administer amphotericin B; monitor serum electrolytes, hydration status, side effects of amphotericin B; administer premedications to reduce drug reactions, eg, hydrocortisone, meperidine (Demerol), diphenhydramine (Benadryl)	Amphotericin B; endoscopic examination with biopsy
Alopecia	High-dose chemotherapy, TBI	100	7–10	Loss of body hair	Help patient cope with body image changes; acquaint patient with cosmetic head coverings	Psychologic support

ABG, arterial blood gas; *BID,* twice daily; *BP,* blood pressure; *BUN,* blood urea nitrogen; *CBC,* complete blood count; *CMV,* cytomegalovirus; *DHPG,* dihydroxyproproxymethylguanine; *HSV,* herpes simplex virus; *HZV,* herpes zoster varicella; *Ig,* immunoglobulin; *IgG,* immunoglobulin G; *I & O,* intake and output; *IV,* intravenous; *LAF,* laminar air flow; *PFT,* pulmonary function test; *SGOT,* serum glutamic oxaloacetic transaminase; *TBI,* total-body irradiation; *TMP-SMX,* trimethoprim-sulfamethoxazole (Bactrim); *TPN,* total parenteral nutrition.

Inflammation of the oral and pharyngeal tissues may occur 2–3 days after marrow infusion. Initially, oral tissues become hyperkeratotic; as mucositis continues, the cheeks, lips, and tongue become edematous. Patients often develop pharyngitis, complain of a sore throat, and have difficulty swallowing. Bleeding ulcerations may occur on the buccal mucosa or sides of the tongue. Concomitant herpes simplex lesions and other local or systemic secondary infections can further damage the oral mucosa.[55] The major symptom in all oral infections is protracted pain, which usually is treated with intravenous morphine.[56] Mucositis is further complicated by severe thrombocytopenia, and aspiration pneumonia can occur.[55] These problems resolve once engraftment occurs, and serious long-term problems are rare.

Nursing care includes supporting good oral hygiene measures with saline mouthwashes, use of toothettes, and flossing. Applications of ice bags or packs can control facial swelling and throat discomfort. Topical anesthetics may be useful for mild to moderate pain. Most patients, however, will require parenteral analgesics. Patient-controlled analgesia (PCA) delivery systems have been used successfully. Patients using PCA systems reported better pain control and reduced nausea and vomiting when compared to marrow recipients receiving continuous infusion analgesics.[56] Mucosal coating agents such as antacids, sucrafate, sodium alginate, and cellulose film may increase comfort and promote healing. Epstein et al.[57] demonstrated the effectiveness of benzydamine hydrochloride rinse in the reduction of oral mucositis. It is not clear if immunomodulators such as colony stimulating factors and cytokines reduce the incidence of mucositis.[58]

Nausea and vomiting Nausea and vomiting following chemotherapy and TBI is a consistent problem.[56] Protracted nausea and vomiting also may be caused by GVHD, CMV esophagitis, or gastrointestinal infections. In these cases, a differential diagnosis must be made and may include endoscopy with duodenal biopsy.[56] Nursing care of the patient with nausea and vomiting includes administration of antiemetics, careful recording of fluid intake and output, monitoring of acid and electrolyte balances, and psychologic support. The most frequently used antiemetic agents include high-dose metoclopramide, droperidol, metoclopramide, diphenhydramine, and lorazepam.[17,59] Most recently, the use of 5-HT_3 antagonists (ondansetron) has been found to be effective in pediatric marrow recipients.[60]

Diarrhea In the first weeks after BMT, diarrhea occurs as a result of chemoradiotherapy. This diarrhea seldom persists beyond day 15. Oral magnesium and nonabsorbable antibiotics (vancomycin, tobramycin, and nystatin) can cause mild diarrhea. Diarrhea associated with acute GVHD and infections is seen as early as day 7 in mismatched BMT patients;[56] this is discussed later in the chapter.

Hematologic complications

Transplant recipients are at high risk for hemorrhage and must be supported with red blood cells and platelets until the donor marrow becomes fully engrafted and functional. Marrow transplantation recipients who receive recombinant hematopoietic colony stimulating factors as an adjuvant therapy during marrow transplantation have demonstrated more rapid recovery of neutrophils compared to historical controls.[58] Blood products must be irradiated to destroy T-lymphocytes that can cause GVHD in the marrow recipient. Patients whose platelets become refractory to random platelet transfusions can receive HLA-matched platelets from family or community donors, and platelets that have undergone plasmapheresis from marrow donors yield optimal increments. Alloimmunization and platelet refractoriness contribute to a 1% case fatality rate from hemorrhagic complications.[61] Bleeding can occur from all body orifices and requires immediate intervention. Table 18-5 outlines clinical manifestations and interventions for management of hemorrhages.[17]

Hemorrhagic cystitis Twenty-four percent of marrow recipients develop hemorrhagic cystitis as a result of the urotoxic effect of acrolein metabolites in cyclophosphamide therapy used in conditioning regimens. Hemorrhagic cystitis can have a sudden onset, be delayed, or manifest itself months after BMT. Prevention of hemorrhagic cystitis involves continuous bladder irrigation and or aggressive intravenous (IV) therapy to flush cyclophosphamide metabolites from the bladder. Mesna (2-mercaptoethane sulfonate sodium) intravenous drug therapy has been shown to be of benefit in preventing hemorrhagic cystitis by combining with acrolein, but dosing must occur prior to manifestation of the problem.[61–64]

Acute graft-versus-host disease

GVHD is an immunologic disease that is a direct consequence of allogeneic marrow transplantation and occurs in an acute and chronic form. Despite prophylaxis with postgrafting in vivo immunosuppression, this disease remains a major impediment to successful marrow grafting and occurs in 30%–50% of HLA-identical recipients. GVHD is thought to be a graft–host response in which the grafted donor T-lymphocytes recognize disparate non-HLA host cell antigens and initiate cytotoxic injury directed against host (patient) tissue.[61,65] Acute GVHD targets the skin, liver, and gut.[65] Symptoms range from mild to severe, and the clinical states of acute graft-versus-host disease are outlined in Table 18-6. GVHD-related complications account for approximately 10% of all BMT deaths.[66]

Risk factors for the development of acute GVHD from HLA-matched transplantation are (1) patient and donor age greater than 18 years of age, (2) donor alloimmunization through transfusion or pregnancy, (3) mismatched-gender BMTs, (4) diagnosis of CML, and (5) CMV negativity in patient and donor.[66] Marrow recipients receiving unrelated donor transplants experience significantly worse GVHD than those receiving HLA-identical sibling transplants. However, there appears to be no significant difference in the occurrence of acute GVHD in unrelated BMTs than in mismatched related BMT.[67]

Clinical manifestations Clinical manifestations of acute GVHD typically begin with a maculopapular erythema that may be pruritic and may cover about 25% of the body. The disease can progress to a generalized erythroderma with frank desquamation and blistering similar to second-degree burns.[17,61,65]

Liver involvement may appear consistent with or subsequent to the onset of GVHD of the skin. On abdominal examination, patients may have pain in the right upper quadrant of the abdomen and hepatomegaly. In addition, increases in liver enzymes may be noted. Jaundice indicates progressive liver involvement.[17,61,65]

Gastrointestinal involvement of acute GVHD can result in nausea, vomiting, anorexia, abdominal cramping, and pain. A typical early symptom is green, watery diarrhea that may exceed 2 liters/day.[17,61,65]

Diagnosis The diagnosis of GVHD may be difficult to distinguish from symptoms secondary to infection or the high-dose conditioning regimens. Skin and liver biopsy and clinical, laboratory, and x-ray data help establish the differential diagnosis imperative to treatment.[65]

Prophylaxis and treatment One of the most important concepts in transplantation medicine is the prevention of GVHD and its related symptoms. Immunosuppressive medications are aimed at removing or inactivating T-lymphocytes that attack target organs.[61] Cyclosporine and methotrexate inhibit T-lymphocytes that are believed to be responsible for acute GVHD. Used in combination, they are more effective than either agent alone.[46] The use of T-cell depletion of donor marrow to decrease GVHD has been abandoned because of increased relapse rates and graft failure.[68] Other medications used to prevent and modify acute GVHD are antithymocyte globulin (ATG) and monoclonal antibodies. A new agent being studied is ZomaZyme-H65.[69] Another study reported success in the use of modified or "minidose" acute GVHD treatment protocols.[70]

TABLE 18-5 Prevention and Management of Hemorrhage in the Recipient of Bone Marrow Transplantation

Complication	Cause	Nursing Intervention	Medical Intervention
Nosebleed	High-dose chemotherapy and TBI (immuosuppression of megakaryocyte/erythrocyte lines)	Apply pressure and ice packs to nasal area; administer platelets; avoid invasive procedures	Daily CBC, blood product support, topical adrenalin and cocaine, ENT consult
Mouthbleed	Same as above	Assess airway for patency; provide vigorous mouth care, use toothettes, discourage toothbrushes; provide oral airway at bedside	Same; dental medicine consult
Cranial	Same as above	Frequent neurologic assessment for headache, seizure, confusion; lumbar puncture only with platelet count >50,000/mm³; avoid emesis and straining	Daily CBC; blood product support, neurologic consult; MRI, CT scans
Gastrointestinal	High-dose chemotherapy and TBI, mucosal irritation, infection, stress	Observe emesis and stools; avoid nasogastric tubes, enemas, rectal temperatures	Daily CBC; blood product support; endoscopy with platelets >50,000/mm³; coagulation studies
Invasive procedures	High-dose chemotherapy and TBI (immunosuppression of megakaryocyte/erythrocyte lines)	Place sandbags to surgical site after insertion of atrial catheters; avoid intramuscular injections	Platelet count >50,000/mm³; avoid cutdowns; use percutaneous procedures for Swan-Ganz catheters
Hemorrhagic cystitis	Same as above	Assess for blood in urine; irrigate bladder during administration of cyclophosphamide; use care in insertion of urinary catheters	Bladder irrigation; daily CBCs; IV hydration; blood product support
Menstrual bleeding	Same as above	Observe bleeding carefully (count number of sanitary pads); administer medroxyprogesterone acetate	Medroxyprogesterone acetate; daily CBCs; blood product support
Petachiae, bruising	Same as above	Turn patient frequently; avoid pressure sores; use eggshell mattress, sheepskin, alternating pressure mattress	

CBC, complete blood count; *CT,* computerized tomography; *ENT,* ear, nose, and throat; *IV,* intravenous; *MRI,* magnetic resonance imaging; *TBI,* total-body irradiation.

TABLE 18-6 Clinical Stages of Acute Graft-Versus-Host Disease

Stage	Skin	Liver	Gut
+ (mild)	Maculopapular rash <25% body surface	Bilirubin 2–3 mg/dl	Diarrhea 500–1000 ml/day
++ (moderate)	Maculopapular rash 25%–50% body surface	Bilirubin 3–6 mg/dl	Diarrhea 1000–1500 ml/day
+++ (severe)	Generalized erythroderma	Bilirubin 6–15 mg/dl	Diarrhea >1500 ml/day
++++ (life-threatening)	Desquamation and bullae	Bilirubin >15 mg/dl	Pain or ileus

Nursing implications Nursing care of patients with acute GVHD requires skillful assessment and management of its early complications. Drugs given to treat or prevent GVHD may have adverse side effects.[17] Nursing care includes management of burnlike wounds, abdominal pain, and voluminous diarrhea.[17] Frequent clinical reassessment is required to monitor fluid replacement, hyperalimentation, transfusion, and antibiotic therapy.[71] Large volumes of diarrhea mandate intensive nutritional assessment as well[17] (Table 18-4).

Renal complications

Renal complications after BMT occur in over 50% of marrow recipients and can be the result of one event or a combination of events.[63] Nephrotoxic drugs used for prevention and treatment of transplantation-related problems (e.g., amphotericin B, cyclosporine, methotrexate, aminoglycosides) are implicated in renal toxicities. These toxicities, superimposed on patients compromised with septic shock, volume depletion, or venoocclusive disease (VOD), act in concert to exacerbate renal hemodynamic complications further.[63,64]

Clinical manifestations/monitoring Clinical manifestations of renal complications include the abrupt onset of anuria,[62–64] which may be an early indication of acute tubular necrosis or acute renal failure. Anuria results from postrenal obstruction arising from cyclophosphamide-related hemorrhagic cystitis.[64] Renal failure, defined as a doubling of baseline creatinine, stems from tumor lysis resulting from high-dose chemotherapy. Early symptoms of renal failure include anuria, and acid–base imbalances from the lack of elimination of nitrogenous wastes, water, electrolytes, and acids.

Renal dysfunction in marrow transplant recipients usually is mild, and patients can be managed by dose adjustments of medications and careful fluid regulation. After allogenic transplantation, however, 5%–10% of patients will require renal dialysis; mortality is 85% in this group.[63]

Nursing implications Nursing assessment for acute tubular necrosis focuses on early recognition of symptoms of either prerenal or intrarenal failure. It includes the monitoring of routine vital signs, with postural blood pressures, determination of urine specific gravity, measurement of urine electrolytes, and determination of accurate intake and output of bodily fluids.[63] Complaints of thirst or dizziness or indications of mental confusion are also indicators of renal compromise. Distended neck veins or peripheral edema must be noted. Correct determination of abdominal girth and daily weight are important nursing assessments to distinguish between prerenal and intrarenal conditions. Knowledge of interactions and adverse effects of the pharmacologic agents given to the recipient is also imperative.[63]

Venoocclusive disease of the liver

Venoocclusive disease (VOD) is almost exclusive to BMT, and is the most common life-threatening complication of preparative-regimen-related toxicity for bone marrow transplantation.[72–74] Investigators currently disagree about known risk factors, morbidity and mortality outcomes, and the treatment for VOD. The diagnosis of VOD often is clouded by overlapping BMT-related symptoms. Risk factors for developing VOD include (1) patients with hepatitis before BMT, (2) those that receive high-dose irradiation in pretransplant conditioning regimens, (3) the use of antimicrobial therapy with acyclovir, amphotericin, or vancomycin, (4) and mismatched or unrelated allogeneic marrow grafts.[72]

Clinical manifestations Liver damage caused by chemoradiotherapy involves two histopathologic processes: (1) venule occlusion and/or venoocclusive process involving terminal hepatic venules and sublobular veins, and (2) hepatocyte necrosis. Clinical symptoms, which occur in the first weeks after transplantation, include fluid retention, sudden weight gain, abdominal distention, pain in the right upper quadrant of the abdomen, jaundice, hepatomegaly, icteric skin and sclerae, encephalopathy, possible bleeding, and elevated serum bilirubin levels.[63] These symptoms are the result of sinusoidal obstruction and intrasinusoidal hypertension, and morbidity ranges from 21% to 50%.[72–74]

Treatment Currently, there is no prevention or treatment for VOD, although researchers are exploring the use of heparin, prostaglandins, tumor necrosis factor, and ursodeoxcychoic acid. Symptom management and supportive measures to maintain the patient until the VOD has run its course are the mainstay of care. Treatment consists of fluid management, with diuresis and restriction of water. Hematocrit levels should be kept above 35% to maintain intravascular volume and renal perfusion.[17,74] An interesting note: Marrow recipients who require renal dialysis also have VOD because of liver–kidney hemodynamic interaction.[17,72–74]

Nursing implications Continuous and careful monitoring of the fluid status of the patient is a nursing responsibility. This includes weighing the patient twice a day, obtaining daily abdominal girth measurements, monitoring for signs of bleeding, and monitoring postural blood pressures.[63]

Pulmonary complications

Pulmonary complications are a major cause of morbidity and mortality, appearing as early and late sequelae of BMT. They occur as a result of chemoradiotherapy toxicity or bacterial, viral, or fungal infection in severely immunosuppressed patients.[75,76] Early complications, caused by severe mucositis, can occur days after marrow transplantation, and aspiration of secretions and blood can lead to upper airway obstruction that requires intubation.[75] Pulmonary edema caused by sodium excess and cardiomyopathy, myocarditis, and volume overload from VOD can occur immediately after transplant.[75] Interstitial pneumonia presents symptoms similar to those of adult respiratory distress syndrome (ARDS), and occurs early (before day 100) or late (after day 100) of transplantation.[75]

Clinical manifestations Manifestations of pneumonia may include nonproductive cough, dyspnea, hypoxemia, and fever. A chest x-ray may demonstrate evidence of interstitial infiltrates, and arterial blood gas levels may show hypoxia.[75,76] These symptoms have rapid onset in the compromised host, and the patient's condition deteriorates quickly.[17,75]

Differential diagnosis must be made rapidly to ensure appropriate treatment. Bronchoalveolar lavage and centrifugation culture, rather than an open lung biopsy, has improved the care of the marrow recipient with pneumonia by eliminating surgery and hastening identification of causative organisms and treatment.[67,76]

Interstitial pneumonia Interstitial pneumonia is a process that occurs in the interstitial spaces of the lungs. It occurs in approximately 35% of allogeneic marrow recipients and is the most frequent cause of death during the first 100 days after transplant.[78] The overall mortality rate from interstitial pneumonia is approximately 20% in allogeneic recipients transplanted for advanced hematologic malignancy.[77]

CMV pneumonia CMV pneumonia is the leading cause of infectious pneumonia after BMT. It occurs in 20% of patients who receive allogeneic marrow transplantation and has a fatality rate up to 85%.[77] The incidence of CMV pneumonia may be higher in the allograft versus autograph recipients because of prolonged periods of immunosuppression caused by medication.[77] Onset of early CMV is greatest between 5 and 13 weeks after transplantation. High-risk factors include (1) patients older than 30 years of age, (2) severe GVHD, (3) TBI conditioning regimen, (4) CMV seropositivity in patients, and (5) advanced hematologic malignancies.[77] The most effective prophylaxis against CMV pneumonia is the avoidance of viral infection by infusing only CMV-negative blood products in cases in which both donor and patient demonstrated CMV seronegativity prior to BMT.[77] Patients who receive screened blood products must continue to do so through day 100 after BMT. Patients who are seropositive and whose donors are seropositive may benefit from the use of antiviral agents such as acyclovir or from passive antibody prophylaxis with immunoglobulin.[78]

Historically, treatment of CMV pneumonia has been largely unsuccessful, despite the use of various antiviral drugs and immunotherapeutic agents used alone or in combination therapy.[78] However, treatment therapies that use combination ganciclovir and intravenous cytomegalovirus immunoglobulin have demonstrated a 40%–50% survival rate in marrow recipients whose diagnosis occurred during the initial episode of CMV pneumonia.[78]

Idiopathic pneumonia Idiopathic pneumonia accounts for 30% of all interstitial pneumonias in marrow recipients. It is believed to be a result of high-dose irradiation.[76,78] Idiopathic pneumonia is diagnosed when no specific organism is recovered in bronchial lavage washings or lung biopsy tissue.[78]

Other pneumonias Other pneumonias that occur may be caused by a virus (e.g., adenovirus, herpes simplex, or varicella zoster), bacteria, or fungus.[77] These account for 15% of pneumonia in marrow recipients, and may be successfully treated.[46,77] Most recently, respiratory syncytial virus (RSV) pneumonia has been identified in the BMT recipient.[79] Aerosolized ribavirin, successfully used in the neonate, has been used to manage BMT recipients with RSV, but research is needed to document treatment efficacy. *Pneumocystis carinii* pneumonia caused significant mortality in the early years of marrow transplantation, but has been successfully prevented by the use of prophylactic trimethoprim-sulfamethoxazole (TMP-SMX). Bacterial or fungal pneumonias are not a major cause of death in the marrow recipient.[80]

Nursing implications The median time of onset for interstitial pneumonias is 60–70 days following BMT. Typically, patients have been discharged from the acute-care setting and are being followed up in a clinic or a physician's office. Classic symptoms are related to the patient's inability to engage in daily activities and may manifest as fatigue, malaise, and/or dyspnea.[80] Patients must undergo routine chest x-rays and thorough physical examinations, including chest auscultation and determination of arterial blood gases in cases of suspected interstitial pneumonia. Readmission to the hospital is usually necessary, and patients may need respiratory support with mechanical ventilation.[80]

Neurologic complications

Neurologic and neuromuscular complications occur in 59%–70% of marrow recipients, with a resulting 6% fatality rate.[81] The underlying causes are pretransplant chemoradiotherapy, central nervous system infection, and immunosuppressive agents, such as cyclosporine, steroids, and intrathecal methotrexate. Neurologic complications from hemorrhage are rare because of the administration of prophylactic platelet transfusions to prevent bleeding. Recurrence of malignancy after BMT may occur in the CNS in up to 38% of the recipients who receive no posttransplant intrathecal prophylaxis.[13]

Leukoencephalopathy has been reported in the 7% of marrow transplant recipients who have had prior cranial irradiation and intrathecal methotrexate.[80] Symptoms include lethargy, somnolence, dementia, coma, and personality changes. Patients who receive cyclosporine for posttransplantation immunosuppression have documented hypomagnesemia, which can result in neurologic sequelae, such as seizure activity.[80–83] Magnesium dosing differs among institutions. Neurologic nursing assessments must be a part of the routine care of marrow recipients.[17]

Cardiac complications

Cardiac complications can develop within several days following administration of high-dose cyclophosphamide. Cardiomegaly, congestive heart failure, and fluid retention can develop, and can be managed with fluid balance to avoid iatrogenic pulmonary edema.[58] These symptoms usually resolve during the first 100 days after BMT and have a fatality rate of less than 1%.[58] Assessment of patients includes obtaining a history of previous therapy with cardiotoxic drugs (e.g., doxorubicin) and monitoring cardiac function with routine electrocardiograms, cardiac ejection fractions, and exercise tolerance tests during the first 100 days after BMT.[85]

Infection

Infections, as a result of profound immunosuppression caused by myeloablative therapy used in conditioning regimens and post-BMT immunosuppression, remain a major impediment to successful marrow grafting. The most common sites of infections are the gastrointestinal tract, oropharynx, lung, skin, and indwelling catheter sites.[78]

Dramatic improvements during the past decade have reduced marrow-transplantation-related infection through the development of antimicrobial therapy, immunomodulators, new diagnostic techniques, and changes in blood transfusion therapy.[78] The tempo and sequence of high-risk periods for bacterial, viral, fungal, and protozoal complications, which peak at predicted times after transplant, are well documented.[78]

The most common infections during the first month (preengraftment stage), are gram-negative and gram-positive bacterial infections, concomitant with fungal and herpes simplex virus. During the second and third months (early postengraftment stage), cytomegalovirus, fungi, gram-positive bacteria, and *Pneumocystis carinii* place marrow recipients at risk. After engraftment has been established, recipients are at risk for infection from encapsulated bacteria, varicella zoster, and *Pneumocystis carinii*.[78]

Preengraftment (days 0–30) The herpes simplex virus (HSV) types I and II, Epstein-Barr virus, cytomegalovirus, and varicella-zoster virus are the major viruses that occur in the first 30 days after BMT. Active HSV infection, caused almost exclusively by reactivation of HSV, is seen in 70%–80% of seropositive patients. Oral ulceration is the common clinical manifestation of HSV type I infection, and genital ulcerations are caused by HSV type II reactivation. The prophylactic therapy for HSV is acyclovir.

Neutropenia with concomitant damage to mucosal surfaces contributes to gram-negative bacteremia immediately after transplantation. Classic approaches to management have been semisynthetic penicillin, plus an aminoglycoside administered empirically at the first sign of fever during neutropenia. The advent of the fluoroquinolones (e.g., norfloxacin, ciprofloxacin) and development of effective regimens that do not include aminoglycosides have improved the control and treatment of gram-negative infections. Aminoglycoside, a known nephrotoxic agent, further compromises renal toxicity in many allogeneic marrow recipients who are receiving nephrotoxic immunosuppressive therapy with cyclosporine.[78,86] Monoclonal antibodies as adjunctive treatment against endotoxin (antilipopolysaccharide antibodies) are undergoing clinical trials, and, although early results are promising, these agents are expensive and limited to the treatment of gram-negative sepsis.[87]

Profound immunosuppression with resulting neutropenia concominant with denuding of the mucosa in the gastrointestinal tract places marrow recipients at risk for *Candida* infection. In addition, systemic *Candida* infections commonly occur during periods of neutropenia. The most common *Candida* species that cause infection are *C. tropicalis* and *C. albicans*. Amphotericin B is the agent of choice for the treatment of *Candida* infection.

Newer strategies being explored include prophylaxis with imidazole. Intravenous miconazole has been shown to be an effective prophylactic agent, but its use is limited by its cost. Fluconazole, now approved for clinical use, and iatraconazole, now in clinical trials, are currently being tested for prophylactic use. The advantages of fluconazole are that it can be administered either orally or intravenously and one daily dose may be sufficient.

Aspergillus is a major infectious problem during days 0–30. The portal of entry for *Aspergillus* infection is the respiratory tract, and the risk for *Aspergillus* infection increases with the duration and degree of neutropenia. Diagnosis from blood cultures is difficult, and percutaneous-needle, bronchoscopic, or open-lung biopsy may be used. Early diagnosis and aggressive treatment with high doses of amphotericin B in combination with flucytosine have improved survival outcomes in the marrow recipient.[78] Less common fungal pathogens that have emerged in recent years include *Trichosporon* spp., *C. lusitaniae, C. krusei*, and *Fusarium* spp. Aggressive therapy with high doses of amphotericin B and flucytosine is the recommended treatment.[78]

Early engraftment (days 30–90) Cytomegalovirus infection is the most significant infection during this phase and accounts for a 15%–20% mortality rate in marrow recipients. Risk factors are the presence of positive serologic titers, GVHD, and the degree of HLA tissue typing between patient and donor. The most severe CMV disease after BMT is interstitial pneumonitis, which is reviewed elsewhere in this chapter. CMV enteritis and retinitis occur less frequently in the marrow recipient.[88]

Bacterial infections are less frequent from day 30 to day 90 following marrow transplantation. Gram-positive infections associated with the central lumen catheter present a major risk for systemic infection. Gram-negative septicemia or infection related to flushing right atrial catheters has been documented in the outpatient setting.[89]

TABLE 18-7 Nursing and Medical Management of Infection in the Bone Marrow Transplant Recipient

Possible Infections	Incidence Rate	Cause	Nursing Management	Diagnostic Tools	Medical Management
			PHASE I: DAYS 0–30		
Bacterial					
Gram negative Gram positive	100%	High-dose chemotherapy and TBI; immunosuppressive drugs for TBI	Complete nursing assessments, with particular attention to mouth and central catheter site; vital signs q 2–4 hr;, administration of antibiotics; pan cultures in presence of fever or chilling; surveillance cultures; ice packs and cooling blankets	Blood and tissue cultures, chest x-rays, CAT scan	Prophylactic treatment with antibiotics, eg, fluoroquinolones (nafloxacin, ciprofloxacin), aminoglycosides, antilipopolysaccharide antibodies; LAF, HEPA filter rooms, masks, hand washing; colony stimulating factors
Viral					
Herpes simplex I and II, Epstein-Barr, CMV	70%–80%	CMV reactivation; high-dose chemotherapy and TBI	Complete nursing assessments, with particular attention to mouth, genital areas	Blood and tissue cultures, chest x-rays, acid-fast cultures	Prophylactic treatment with acyclovir
Adenovirus	5%	CMV reactivation; high-dose chemotherapy and TBI	Stool cultures	Stool cultures	Appropriate antibiotics
Fungal					
Candida tropicalis, albicans	100%	CMV reactivation; high-dose chemotherapy and TBI; broad-spectrum antibiotics	Complete nursing assessments, with particular attention to mouth and central catheter site; vital signs q 2–4 hr; administration of antibiotics; pan cultures in presence of fever or chilling; surveillance cultures	Blood and tissue cultures, chest x-rays, CAT scan, needle biopsy	Amphotericin B, imidazole, miconazole, fluconazole, iatraconazole
Aspergillus, Trichosporon spp., *C. lusitaniae, C. krusei, Fusarium* spp.	100%	High-dose chemotherapy and TBI	Complete nursing assessments, with particular attention to mouth and central catheter site; vital signs q 2–4 hr; administration of antibiotics; pan cultures in presence of fever or chilling; surveillance cultures	Percutaneous needle biopsy, bronchoscopy, open lung biopsy	Prophylactic treatment with antifungals, amphotericin B, flucytosine
			PHASE II: DAYS 30–90		
Bacterial	100%	High-dose chemotherapy and TBI; immunosuppres-	Complete nursing assessments, with particular attention	Blood and tissue cultures, chest x-rays, CAT scan	Prophylactic treatment with antibiotics eg, fluoro-

(continued)

TABLE 18-7 Nursing and Medical Management of Infection in the Bone Marrow Transplant Recipient (continued)

Possible Infections	Incidence Rate	Cause	Nursing Management	Diagnostic Tools	Medical Management
		sive drugs, with particular attention to central lumen catheter	to mouth and central catheter site; vital signs q 2–4 hr; administration of antibiotics; pan cultures in presence of fever or chilling; surveillance cultures		quinolones (nafloxacin, ciprofloxacin), aminoglycosides, antilipopolysaccharide antibodies; colony stimulating factors
Viral					
CMV pneumonia	20% allogeneic 2% autologous	CMV-positive recipient or donor; advanced hematologic malignancy; mismatched patients	Complete nursing assessment; assessment for cough, dyspnea, hypoxemia; vital signs q 2–4 hr; chest auscultation	Bronchial lavage and centrifugation culture, chest x-ray, arterial blood gases	Immunoglobulin, acyclovir, CMV-negative blood products; leukopoor; blood products
Respiratory syncytial virus (RSV)	Unknown	High-dose chemotherapy and TBI; RSV+	Complete nursing assessment; assessment for cough, dyspnea, hypoxemia	Bronchial washings	Ribavirin
Fungal					
Pneumocystis carinii pneumonia	80% or higher with GVHD	High-dose chemotherapy and TBI	Complete nursing assessment; determine patient compliance for TMP-SMX	Chest x-ray, CAT scans	Prophylactic treatment; aerosolized pentamidine treatments
		PHASE III: DAYS 100 TO 2 YEARS			
Bacterial					
Pneumonia, encapsulated bacteria, *Streptococcus pneumoniae, Neisseria* meningitidis, *Haemophilus influenzae,* septicemia, sinusitis	Unknown	High-dose chemotherapy and TBI; chronic GVHD	Complete nursing assessment; monitoring of chest x-rays; assessment for sinusitis, sepsis; assessment for patient compliance for medications	Chest x-ray, sputum culture	TMP-SMX prophylactically, appropriate antibiotic therapy; wearing mask, hand washing, avoiding crowds; immunizations after 1 yr without GVHD; immune testing with GVHD
Viral					
Varicella zoster virus	25%–40%	High-dose chemotherapy and TBI; reactivation of HZV	Complete nursing assessment, with attention to prodromal symptoms of pain, itching, burning		Acyclovir 500 mg/kg IV q 8 hr for 7–10 days; HZV immunoglobulin for sero-positive recipients exposed to HZV immunoglobulin

TBI, total-body irradiation; *CAT,* computerized axial tomography; *LAF,* laminar air flow room; *HEPA,* high-efficiency particulate air; *CMV,* cytomegalovirus; *RSV,* respiratory syncytial virus; *GVHD,* graft-versus-host disease; *TMP-SMX,* trimethoprim-sulfamethoxazole; *HZV,* herpes zoster varicella.

Fungal infections are problematic during this recovery phase, and marrow recipients with GVHD are at higher risk for infections than recipients without GVHD.[89] *Pneumocystis carinii* pneumonia accounts for 10% of interstitial pneumonitis in marrow recipients.[74,75,78] Open lung biopsy and bronchoscopic washings remain classic diagnostic measures, and trimethoprim-sulfamethoxazole (TMP-SMX) is effective as a preventive and therapeutic agent. Aerosolized pentamidine is an alternative therapy for those patients who report true allergies to TMP-SMX. Long-term effectiveness of aerosolized pentamidine has not been evaluated.

Clinical manifestations Fever is the cardinal symptom of infection.[17] The neutropenic condition of marrow recipients masks the classic infection-related symptoms of inflammation, pus formation, and elevated white blood cell counts. Consequently, cultures of blood, throat, urine, stool, and sputum are necessary to identify and treat pathogenic organisms.[17] Risk factors associated with life-threatening infections and measures to treat and prevent infections are outlined in Table 18-7.

Treatment Prevention and treatment of infection in the marrow recipient BMT patient is aimed at identifying the invasive organism and treating the accompanying infection with appropriate antibiotics. Antimicrobial therapy has proven to be successful, while granulocyte transfusions have been largely abandoned.[1] The role of immunoglobulin (IG) therapy in marrow transplantation is being studied; and potential uses of IG include (1) modifying or preventing CMV infections and CMV-related interstitial pneumonia, (2) decreasing GVHD, (3) preventing infections other than CMV, and (4) treating autoimmune complications of marrow grafting.[90] Results of studies indicate that IG given before and at 100 days posttransplant reduced the incidence of CMV pneumonia.[8,88,90]

Nursing implications Astute nursing assessments are important in determining the onset and course of infectious problems. Fever may be associated with GVHD and administration of blood and drug products. Steroid administration in immunosuppressed patients masks fever, and nurses need to be alert to the subtle signs of infection.[17] Current research is examining the effects of more palatable oral antibiotics for gastrointestinal decontamination. It is hoped that these drugs will provide optimal patient compliance while preventing bacterial and fungal infections.[17]

DISCHARGE FROM THE HOSPITAL

Hospital discharge after BMT averages 30–35 days.[91] The advent of peripheral stem cell transplantations with or without colony stimulating factors is shortening the length of hospital stays, reducing readmission rates, and allowing marrow recipients to return home sooner.

Guidelines to prepare the patient/family for discharge teaching are outlined in Table 18-8. Discharge

TABLE 18-8 Patient Guidelines upon Discharge from the Hospital

Report the following symptoms

- Fever >38.4°C (101.4°F)
- Difficulty flushing the central or peripheral catheter
- Bleeding of any kind
- Frequent urination or pain and burning on urination
- Redness, swelling, itching of skin
- Pain in any part of the body
- Cough, sneezing, runny nose, shortness of breath, or discomfort in the chest
- Light sensitivity to the eyes; blurring of vision, burning, itching, or sense of "grittiness" in the eyes
- Inability to sweat or perspire
- Redness, swelling, or drainage from the central catheter site
- Blisters around the mouth or in the genital area
- Any beeping or alarming of pump if receiving home infusion therapy

Further guidelines

- Report any problem or concern.
- Report all tests, examinations, and procedures.
- Take and record your medications. Renew all prescriptions immediately.
- Do not receive immunizations until advised by the physician.
- Avoid children or other persons who have had live-virus vaccines (such as the Sabin oral polio vaccine, measles, mumps, rubella, yellow fever, or small pox)

Personal health guidelines

- Avoid crowds for 6 months after bone marrow transplantation.
- Avoid swimming in public swimming areas until the central lumen or peripheral catheter is removed.
- Take a daily shower or bath using a mild soap. Use skin lotions without alcohol.
- Avoid sharing personal care items with family members, eg, towels, combs, washcloths.
- Daily, brush your teeth with a soft toothbrush and floss. Use saline rinses for a mouthwash, and avoid commercial mouthwashes.
- Practice safe sex; use condoms or dental dams.
- Keep your home environment clean. However, it is not necessary to sterilize personal items, such as dishes, and cooking areas
- Avoid cleaning cat litter boxes, fish bowls, and bird cages.
- Houseplants may remain in the home environment, but avoid cut flowers in water, which harbors bacteria.

teaching must involve the primary caregivers as well as the patient. Chielens and Herrick have described the discharge process and the role of the discharge planner.[92]

Discharge Criteria

Established discharge criteria for marrow recipients are becoming more liberal because of new trends in outpatient care. Antimicrobial and biotechnologic therapies have helped to diminish the effects of transplantation-related complications, and sophisticated infusion pump technology permits patients to receive numerous intravenous therapies in outpatient settings. In addition, economic pressures prompt earlier discharge for patients who, until recently, would have remained in the hospital for their care. Discharge criteria for marrow recipients differ among institutions and depend on the stability of the patient, the presence of skilled outpatient teams, and caregiver support at home.[92]

The following are representative discharge criteria common among marrow transplantation centers.

- availability of 24-hour outpatient medical care provided by a multidisciplinary outpatient BMT team
- oral intake 25%–50% of baseline nutrient requirements
- needing no more than 2500 ml of parenteral fluid every 24 hours
- nausea and vomiting controlled
- diarrhea controlled at <500 ml/day
- a platelet count supportable at 5000–15,000 mm^3
- granulocytes >500 mm^3 for 24 hours
- hematocrit >25%
- tolerating PO medications for 24 hours (i.e., narcotics, antihypertensives, cyclosporine, and prednisone)
- family support at home

Ideally, patients and a strong support person need to reside near the transplant center until 100 days after BMT, when the immune system has recovered sufficiently. Comprehensive outpatient care of the BMT recipient patient consists of daily-to-weekly clinic visits to assess the patient's stability. Blood products, parenteral nutrition, intravenous medications, research medications, and procedures can be delivered effectively in ambulatory care settings. Clear, consistent patient/family teaching aimed at prevention and early recognition of transplant-related problems must be emphasized. Patients and families are taught to prevent infections by avoiding crowds, school, and work for 1 year after BMT. Currently, the readmission rate is 50% for treatment of fever and neutropenia.[93]

CLINICAL MANAGEMENT OF THE BMT OUTPATIENT

The role of ambulatory care and home care for the marrow recipient is gaining importance in the face of earlier discharge of marrow recipients. Current research has been studying the efficacy and cost effectiveness of early discharge. Data concerning morbidity, mortality, nursing management, caregiver burden, and psychologic measures of care will be forthcoming. Larson[94] studied hospitalized patients' perception of needs during the first 4 weeks following BMT. By 30–34 days, BMT recipients were found to have an increase in positive thinking and physical activity, to want their families to be present, and to want physicians to be consistent and responsible in meeting their needs.

Outpatient Home Care

Outpatient care requires keen clinical management as well as nursing care delivered by oncology nurses highly knowledgeable of the BMT process, possible complications, and appropriate medications. Chronic complications of BMT may appear around 80 days after BMT. Clinical outpatient staff must be able to distinguish the tempo, duration, signs, and symptoms of acute and chronic GVHD, herpes, varicella zoster, cytomegalovirus, *Pneumocystis carinii* pneumonia, sexually transmitted diseases, and other transplantation-related problems.

Symptom management of the BMT outpatient is accomplished with a multidisciplinary team of physicians, nurses, dietitians, dentists, and social workers. Common marrow-transplant-related symptoms and their possible causes are shown in Table 18-9. The numerous tests and evaluations needed to assess, manage, and treat BMT recipients until they return home are presented in Table 18-10.

The goal of outpatient BMT nursing is to provide optimal care until individuals are stable enough to return home. Historically, marrow recipients remain under the care of the BMT team until approximately 100 days after BMT. Centers may differ slightly on this 100-day rule. For example, autologous BMT patients may be followed by the BMT team until 60 days after marrow transplant, whereas most allogeneic BMT recipients are asked to remain 100 days post-BMT. All patients experience at least 3 months of severe immune deficiency. Consequently, they are at considerable risk for bacterial, viral, and fungal infections. Evidence of improvement and return of immune function generally is seen between 6 and 9 months after BMT. Immune recovery is delayed in allogeneic patients with chronic GVHD.[77]

100-Day Evaluation

The 100-day workup evaluates the recipient's stability and risk factors for discharge home (Table 18-11). The

TABLE 18-9 Common Outpatient Marrow-Transplant-Related Symptoms and Their Possible Causes

Symptoms	Possible Causes
Fever	Bacterial (gram-negative, gram-positive sepsis), fungal infection *(Candida, Aspergillus)* Interstitial pneumonia (bacterial, viral, idiopathic) Herpes simplex virus, varicella zoster GVHD Hepatitis Granulocytopenia Blood product transfusions/drug toxicity Recurrent disease
Nausea, vomiting	GVHD Gastrointestinal infection (CMV, *Salmonella, Shigella, C. difficile*)
Diarrhea	Mucositis Leukoencephalopathy, encephalitis, subdural hematoma Septicemia Adrenal insufficiency Liver disease Cholecystitis, pancreatitis Hyperalimentation withdrawal Psychologic Drug toxicity
Bleeding	Thrombocytopenia GVHD, gut Hemorrhagic cystitis Drug-related (prednisone) Herpes simplex virus infection
Pruritus	Acute and chronic GVHD Herpes varicella zoster Drug toxicity Blood product transfusions
Rash	GVHD, HSV, drug toxicity
Fatigue	Drug-related (interferon) Altered sleep patterns Premature menopause Psychologic stress
Dyspnea	Sinopulmonary infection Restrictive, obstructive lung disease CMV pneumonia
Pain	Herpes zoster, relapse GVHD Peptic ulcer disease Mucositis Gastritis
Weight loss	Dehydration Mucositis GVHD Drug-related therapy Depression Malabsorption Body image
Vasomotor instability: nervousness, anxiety, irritability, depression	Leukoencephalopathy Premature menopause, drug toxicity Hypomagnesemia
Jaundice	GVHD Infection Drug toxicity Hepatitis
Body image changes	Alopecia Wearing a mask Drug-related (cyclosporine/prednisone) Hyperalimentation High-dose chemotherapy, TBI Presence of venous access catheter Early menopause/sterility Growth and development problems
Psychologic: role changes, adaptation/integration into community	Issues of survival Feelings of taking advantage of donor Rehabilitation needs Rebirth or Lazarus syndrome Survival syndrome Role changes within family

Source: Adapted with permission from Corcoran PC: Ambulatory care of the bone marrow transplant patient. *Puget Sound Quarterly, Oncology Nursing Society* 12:4–7, 1989.

patient's BMT course is reviewed, and a final discharge conference is scheduled with the physician, the patient, and the family. A nurse from the continuing care team attending this meeting can ensure continuity of care and bridge the gap between outpatient care and the outpatient's referring care physician.

GVHD is only one of the many potential long-term sequelae of BMT. Other potential transplantation-related problems are assessed before a marrow recipient's return to the care of the primary physician. Except for the GVHD evaluation, identical evaluations are performed on autologous recipients secondary to the effects of lethal conditioning regimens and other transplantation-related treatments. Marrow recipients view this "final" process with a mixture of anxiety and excitement. Relapse is a limiting factor in BMT, and it may be at this critical time that a patient is found to have relapsed. In this case, the patient and significant others are given the diagnosis, prognosis, and alternate plans of care. Options may include chemotherapy, irradiation, a second BMT, or hospice care. Outpatient nurses need to act as essential coordinators to orchestrate procedures and tests and to support the patient through this final phase of care.

Community-based physicians and nurses can expect to see a patient at least weekly for the first month alone. If no new medical problems develop and the patient is stable, these intervals can be lengthened to 2 weeks for

TABLE 18-10 Typical Assessments, Procedures, and Tests for Bone Marrow Transplantation Outpatients

- One to two clinic visits a week for full medical and nursing assessment to monitor for BMT-related problems
- Weekly assessments with the nutrition team for evaluation for parenteral support and nutritional counseling
- Once-a-month examination with the medical dental department to determine infection status of mouth for fungal, viral, and bacterial overgrowth
- Once-a-week consultations with social worker to assess ongoing psychological/social needs
- Consultation with gynecologists for all postpubertal women for evaluation of possible early menopause and sexual dysfunction
- Consultation visits with ophthalmologist, cardiologist, renal pulmonary physician, gynecologist, infectious disease physician as needed.
- Weekly evaluation of medication schedules and refills of medications

Procedures routinely required for BMT outpatient
- Daily to twice weekly blood draws to monitor blood chemistries, and engraftment and immune recovery status
- Once or twice weekly urine tests for infection surveillance
- Weekly throat cultures for infection surveillance
- Periodic bone marrow aspirations and biopsies for evaluation of engraftment and disease status
- Spinal taps of methotrexate for prophalaxis against central nervous system disease
- Skin biopsies for evaluation of graft-versus-host disease and diagnoses of other possible skin ailments
- Pulmonary function test and arterial blood gases for assessment of potential interstitial pneumonias
- Weekly surveillance chest x-rays for assessment of ongoing pulmonary complications

TABLE 18-11 Evaluation of Marrow Transplant Recipients Prior to Their Return Home

All marrow transplantation recipients
- Pulmonary function test and arterial blood gases for possible infection and obstructive/restrictive lung disease
- Bone marrow aspiration and biopsy to establish engraftment and disease state (remission or relapse)
- Complete blood counts and serum alkaline phosphatase, SGOT, bilirubin to evaluate hepatic function
- Follicle-stimulating hormone and testosterone levels to evaluate gonadal function
- Serologic indicators for return of immune function: ANA, AMA, ASMA, RA, IgA, IgM, IgE; C3, C4 (complement studies); immunoglobulin subclasses, immunoglobulin titer; direct Coombs test
- Repeated CAT scans and x-rays performed at pretransplant evaluation for comparison to determine possible underlying disease
- Medical-dental examination for dental caries, xerostomia
- Gynecologic examination for postpubertal woman for sexual counseling and prescribing of appropriate gonadal hormones

Allogeneic marrow transplantation recipients (chronic graft-host-disease)
- Physical assessment of the skin and skin biopsy to determine possible skin graft-versus-host disease
- Schirmer's tear test OS/OD to determine "dry" eye
- Physical assessment of the mouth to assess for chronic graft-versus-host disease

the next 2 months, and eventually to 3-week or monthly intervals depending on the patients' clinical status. Monitoring of liver function tests, chest x-rays, complete blood counts, food intake, and weekly weights (on the same scale) is considered routine care during this period. Nurses caring for BMT recipients spend a large part of their nursing time teaching and reassuring patients and families, assessing for infection and potential long-term complications, and interacting with long-term follow-up teams at the BMT center. Communication between community-based oncologists and long-term follow-up teams is essential to care for the growing number of long-term survivors of BMT. Nurses working in long-term follow-up settings triage and serve as liaison between BMT physicians and referring oncologists. Historically, all communication has been done by telephone. Facsimile (FAX) machines now facilitate the exchange of information and aid in early diagnoses of transplant-related problems.

As economic constraints in health care systems continue, more allogeneic marrow recipients will be sent home prior to the traditional 100th day after BMT. This will increase the demand for keen nursing assessment skills as well as for sophisticated long-term follow-up systems.

Copel and Smith[95] studied a select group of inpatient BMT nurses' knowledge of GVHD and found that nurses who participated in journal reading and who attended conferences relevant to GVHD scored higher than BMT nurses who did not. Like BMT nurses, community-based nurses will benefit from active participation in educational activities. Administrative managers are encouraged to budget time and money for nurses to pursue these opportunities.

Annual Assessments

Patients typically return to the BMT center for annual evaluations for up to 3 years following BMT, to test the marrow recipient for current or impending problems associated with the BMT. Outpatient nurses are extensively involved in annual assessments and procedures. Sensitive nursing support is needed because patients and families revisiting the facility will recall the emotional experiences associated with the BMT. The marrow recipient usually wants to visit with clinical staff. Patients may not understand when staff are too busy to stop and make hall visits. A solution to this dilemma may be a social event scheduled by clinic staff at which patients, family, and staff can renew acquaintances.

LATE COMPLICATIONS OF BMT

The number of marrow recipients living disease-free for years after BMT increases annually. It is estimated that there are approximately 2000 allogeneic marrow recipients alive 5 years after transplantation; some have survived more than 20 years.[96] Many recipients, however, will encounter late complications. Late complications caused by conditioning regimens are defined as those developing 100 days or more after transplant.[92] The incidence, time period, manifestations, and interventions of these late effects are outlined in Tables 18-12 and 18-13.

Chronic Graft-Versus-Host Disease (Allogeneic BMT)

Allogeneic marrow recipients are at considerable risk for chronic GVHD. Chronic GVHD typically develops more than 3 months after transplantation and differs from acute GVHD in both clinical presentation and target organs affected.[96–99]

TABLE 18-12 Nursing and Medical Management of Possible Late Effects of Bone Marrow Transplantation Caused by High-Dose Chemotherapy and/or Irradiation in Conditioning Regimens

Late Effect	Incidence Rate	Time Post-BMT	Signs and Symptoms	Nursing Management	Diagnostic Tools	Medical Management
Pulmonary complications						
Interstitial pneumonia Bronchiolitis obliterans	10%	3 mo to 2 yr	Cough, wheezing, dyspnea; decreased ability to perform daily living activities due to pulmonary insufficiency	Anticipatory teaching of pulmonary toilet; routine vital signs; chest A&P; monitor PFT and ABG	Bronchial lavage washings Decreased midexpiratory flow Open lung biopsy	Prophylactic—TMP-SMX Appropriate antibiotic therapy; ganciclovir; acyclovir; immunoglobulin Antimicrobial therapy; high-dose steroids; cyclosporine; prednisone; colony stimulating factors; corticosteroids; pentamidine, IV or aerozolized
Restrictive disease	20%		May be asymptomatic or cough		Total lung capacity, diffusion capacity	Respiratory therapy; bronchodilation
Obstructive disease	10%				Pulmonary function test; Ig, IgA levels	Immunosuppressive therapy
Neurologic complications						
Leukoencephalopathy	7%	1–5 mo	Lethargy, somnolence, dementia, seizures, spastic quadriplegia, coma, personality changes	Early intervention; multidisciplinary approach with special education program; routine neurologic assessments	Periodic head computer-assisted tomography (CAT) scans and psychometric evaluation	Symptomatic and supportive management
Impaired memory Learning disorders	Reported					

(continued)

TABLE 18-12 Nursing and Medical Management of Possible Late Effects of Bone Marrow Transplantation Caused by High-Dose Chemotherapy and/or Irradiation in Conditioning Regimens (continued)

Late Effect	Incidence Rate	Time Post-BMT	Signs and Symptoms	Nursing Management	Diagnostic Tools	Medical Management
Hypomagnesemia	Common occurrence		Tremors, seizures	Monitor magnesium serum levels		Magnesium replacement
Cataracts						
Total-body irradiation, fractionated	20%	1.5–3 yr	Poor vision	Anticipatory teaching of BMT risk factors; ophthalmologist recommendation	Examination with slit-lamp microscopy	Intraocular lens replacement
Total-body irradiation, single dose	50%	1.5–5 yr				
Psychological complications	5%–10%	Months to years	Depression, weight change; altered body image; survival syndrome; sibling rivalry; altered concentration; decreased IQ levels in children	Allow patient/family to verbalize feelings; identify coping mechanisms, personal strengths; refer to mental health resources	Psychological testing	Mental health evaluation and treatment from appropriate source
Impaired growth in children						
Irradiation only	100%	Months to years	Subnormal growth and development	Anticipatory teaching to patients/parents; annual evaluation of growth pattern; serial height/weight	Adrenocortical function; growth hormone; thyroid hormone	Possible appropriate hormone replacement; long-term follow-up
Late infectious complications						
Bacterial Encapsulated bacteria *Haemophilus influenzae* *Streptococcus pneumoniae* *Neisseria meningitidis*	>50%	3 mo to 1 yr	Fever, wheezing, rales, postnasal drip, signs of infection unexplained fever, otitis media, sinusitis, bronchopulmonary infection, septicemia	Preventive teaching; mask-wearing until 6 mo post-BMT; good handwashing techniques; avoid infectious persons (measles, chickenpox, mumps); avoid school/work, until 6 mo post-BMT; avoid hot tubs, public swimming pools until 6–9 mo post-BMT; limit number of sexual partners; avoid live-virus vaccines	Positive blood culture for bacteria, fungus, virus; abnormal chest x-ray studies, pulmonary function tests (PFT); pulmonary infiltrates; open lung biopsy; changes in CBC; decreased serum levels of IgG; impaired splenic reticulendothelia function	Appropriate antibiotic support
Cytomegalovirus *Pneumocystis carinii*	80%–100% 10%	3 mo to 1 yr	Fever, sepsis, hypotension, lethargy; cough dyspnea may be asymptomatic	Anticipatory preventive teaching; routine vital signs; chest auscultation and percussion (A&P); monitor PFT, arterial blood gases (ABG)	Chest x-ray studies, CBC, ABG, PFT; positive cultures for bacterial, fungal, and viral microorganisms; bronchoscopy; IgA, IgG levels	Prophylactic—TMP-SMX; appropriate antibiotic therapy; ganciclovir; acyclovir, immunoglobulin
Varicella zoster virus						
Without chronic GVHD	<50%	3 mo to 1 yr	Lesions, pain, malaise, tenderness, neurologic manifestation	Relieve pruritus, with calamine lotion; cool compresses; prevent secondary infection	Positive herpes zoster varicella (HZV) cultures	Strict isolation until lesions are crusting; IV acyclovir 500 mg/m² q 8hr × 7 days
With chronic GVHD	>75%					

(continued)

TABLE 18-12 Nursing and Medical Management of Possible Late Effects of Bone Marrow Transplantation Caused by High-Dose Chemotherapy and/or Irradiation in Conditioning Regimens (continued)

Late Effect	Incidence Rate	Time Post-BMT	Signs and Symptoms	Nursing Management	Diagnostic Tools	Medical Management
Dental						
Tooth decay	Known in children	3 mo to 1 yr	Oral sicca syndrome; abnormal tooth development	Oral assessments, preventative teaching	Panorex	Dental medicine consults
Aseptic necrosis of the bone	Reported	3 mo to 1 yr	Limited range of motion in legs/hips, joint contractures; pain, swelling in areas of head of femur	Assess for history of steroid therapy	Computer-assisted tomography	Antimicrobial therapy, femur head replacement
Genitourinary effects						
Bladder shrinkage Chronic urinary disorder Radiation nephritis Hemolytic uremic syndrome Delayed-onset nephrotic syndrome	Reported	4.5–26 mo	*Adenoviral,* CMV *Viral,* polyomaviruses, bladder infections, hematuria, dysuria, vague abdominal pain	Monitor urinary analyses, creatinine levels, assessment of urologic complaints, drug history for cyclosporine	Urinary analyses; culture and sensitivities; cystoscopy; increased serum creatinine levels	Appropriate antimicrobial therapy; urologic consultation
Graft failure—marrow dysfunction	HLA-matched marrow—rare HLA-mismatched—20% T-cell depleted—50% Autologous—20%		Profound immunosupression, infection, bleeding, hypoxemia, relapse	Assessment for pancytopenia	CBC, bone marrow aspiration and biopsy; determine engraftment with cytogenetic analysis, ABO blood type, red cell antigen, enzyme markers	Supportive therapy
Second malignancy	6%–22%	1–14 yr	Fever, fatigue, swollen glands, abnormal bleeding, pain, night sweats	Complete nursing assessments; knowledge of treatment prescription; promote routine cancer screening	CBC, diagnostic CAT scans, x-rays, needle biopsy	Traditional cancer therapy, chemotherapy, irradiation
Effects of high-dose chemotherapy (single agent)						
Females, prepubertal	Usually 0%		Usually no abnormalities; menarche onset 12–13 yr	Careful monitoring of development	Tanner sexual maturity scales	
Males, prepubertal	Usually 0%		Usually no abnormalities	Careful monitoring of development		
Females <26 yr	100%		Usually no abnormalities; return of menstrual period, median = 6 mo	Menstrual history; fertility counseling	Normal luteinizing hormone (LH); normal follicle-stimulating hormone (FSH)	
Females >26 yr	66%	Immediate	Premature menopause; sterility	Anticipatory teaching/counseling	LH levels; FSH levels	Cyclic hormone therapy
Males	33%	Immediate	Sterility	Anticipatory teaching/counseling; semen analysis; sperm storage prior to BMT	Testosterone levels	Testosterone therapy, if appropriate

(continued)

TABLE 18-12 Nursing and Medical Management of Possible Late Effects of Bone Marrow Transplantation Caused by High-Dose Chemotherapy and/or Irradiation in Conditioning Regimens (continued)

Late Effect	Incidence Rate	Time Post-BMT	Signs and Symptoms	Nursing Management	Diagnostic Tools	Medical Management
Effects of high-dose chemotherapy (high-dose cyclophosphamide and busulfan without TBI)						
Females	Unknown	Immediate	Sterility; premature menopause	Anticipatory teaching/counseling; menstrual history; fertility counseling	LH levels; FSH levels	Ova storage; cyclic hormone therapy
Males	Unknown	Immediate	Sterility	Anticipatory teaching; sexual counseling	Gonadotropin; low sperm counts	Sperm storage prior to BMT; testosterone therapy, if appropriate
Effects of high-dose irradiation						
Females, prepubertal	100%	Immediate	Delayed onset of puberty; failure to reach menarche	Anticipatory teaching/counseling	Tanner development scores; LH levels; FSH levels	Neuroendocrine evaluation; appropriate hormone therapy
Males, prepubertal	100%	Immediate	Delayed onset of puberty	Anticipatory teaching/counseling	Tanner development scores; testosterone levels	Neuroendocrine evaluation; testosterone therapy may be helpful
Males, adolescent	100%	Immediate	Sterility	Sperm storage prior to BMT	Tanner development scores; gonadotropin; sperm counts	Testosterone therapy
Females	95%–100%	Immediate	Premature menopause	Anticipatory teaching; sexual counseling	LH levels; FSH levels	Cyclic hormone therapy
Males	95%–100%	Immediate	Sterility	Sperm storage prior to BMT; anticipatory teaching/counseling	Gonadotropin; low sperm counts	Testosterone therapy

Source: Adapted from the *Oncology Nursing Forum* with permission from the Oncology Nursing Press, Inc. Corcoran-Buchsel P: Long-term complications of allogeneic bone marrow transplantation: Nursing Implications. *Oncol Nurs Forum* 13:61–70, 1986.

Chronic GVHD is a major cause of morbidity after allogeneic BMT and occurs in 33% of HLA-identical transplants, 49% of HLA-mismatched family members, and 64% of unrelated donor marrow transplantations.[96] In addition, the time to onset of chronic GVHD is shortened with greater allogeneic mismatch transplants. For example, onset for HLA-identical siblings is 201 days versus 159 days for mismatched family members versus 133 days for unrelated donors.[96] Chronic GVHD is a multisystem disorder of the skin, mouth, eyes, sinuses, liver, gut, vaginal mucosa, serosal surfaces, and pulmonary, nervous, urologic, hematopoietic, lymphoid, and endocrine systems.[97–99] Figure 18-11 depicts chronic GVHD of the skin. Clinical and pathologic findings resemble several naturally occurring autoimmune diseases, such as scleroderma, lupus erythematosus, lichen planus, rheumatoid arthritis, Sjögren's syndrome (sicca syndrome).[97–99]

Onset and classification

The onset of chronic GVHD may be progressive, quiescent, or de novo. *Progressive* onset, a direct extension of acute GVHD, has the poorest prognosis. *Quiescent* onset develops after clinical resolution of acute GVHD, and these patients have a fair prognosis. Patients with *de novo* onset have had no prior acute disease and have the best prognosis.

Chronic GVHD may be limited or extensive. Limited disease targets only the skin and liver and has a favorable course if untreated, whereas extensive disease affects numerous organ systems and can be fatal if not treated.

Clinical manifestations of chronic GVHD

Skin The skin is affected in more than 95% of patients diagnosed with chronic GVHD. Involvement

TABLE 18-13 Nursing and Medical Management of Late Effects of Bone Marrow Transplantation: Chronic Graft-Versus-Host Disease (GVHD)

Late Effect	Incidence Rate	Time Post-BMT (days)	Signs and Symptoms	Nursing Management	Diagnostic Tools	Medical Management
Skin	95%	100–400	Rough, scaly skin; malar erythema; generalized rash; hypo/hyperpigmentation; dyspigmentation; premature graying; alopecia, joint contractures; scleroderma; loss of sweating	Use of nonabrasive soaps, lotions, sunscreen; cosmetic support, makeup, wigs; range-of-motion activities; patient/family education; monitor compliance to treatment protocols	Skin biopsy positive for GVHD; Karnofsky score	Lanolin-based creams; possible systemic immunosuppressive therapy with cyclosporine, prednisone, Imuran
Liver	30%	100–400	Jaundice	Infection precautions until differential diagnosis is made; monitor LFTs; low-fat diet	Alkaline phosphatase; SGOT; bilirubin	Possible systemic immunosuppressive therapy with cyclosporine, prednisone, Imuran
Oral	80%	100–400	Pain, burning, dryness, irritation, soreness, loss of taste; lichenoid changes, atrophy, erythema in oral cavity; *Candida* infection; stomatitis; dental carries; xerostomia	Encourage soft, bland diet; dental hygiene education, soft toothbrush, flossing; saline rinses; dental medicine referral/recommendation; salivary gland stimulants, sugarless mints, artificial saliva	Labial mucosa biopsy positive for GVHD; secretory IgA levels; mouth culture positive for yeast organisms; mouth culture positive for bacterial and viral etiologies; radiographs	Possible systemic immunosuppressive therapy with cyclosporine, prednisone, Imuran; artificial saliva; clotrimazole troches or Nystatin; swish and swallow; appropriate topical medication; topical fluoride treatment; appropriate dental therapy
Ocular	80%	100–400	Grittiness, burning of eyes; dry eyes; sicca syndrome	Artificial tears; Schirmer's tear test; if <10 mm of wetting, refer to ophthalmologist	Keratoconjunctivitis; corneal ulceration; slit-lamp microscopy	Lacriset plugs; soft contact lens; punctal ligation for obliteration of tear duct outflow; keratoplasty; tarsorrhaphies
GI tract, esophagus	36%	100–400	Anorexia; difficulty eating; painful swallowing; retrosternal pain; weight loss; vomiting	Serial weights; high-calorie food supplements; recommend nutritional counseling	Barium swallow of esophagus and small bowel follow-through	Esophageal dilatation; possible systemic immunosuppressive therapy with cyclosporine, prednisone, Imuran; parenteral nutrition
Vagina	20%	100–400	Inflammation; stricture formation causing obstruction of menstrual flow; adhesions; dry vagina; painful intercourse; marital problems	Water-soluble lubricants; recommend sexual counseling and therapy	Papanicolaou smear	Vaginal stints; estrogen cream; surgical intervention

can include the entire integument and produce alopecia and nail ridging. Initially, patients will complain of itching and burning of the skin. Patchy hyperpigmentation, mottled-appearing skin, or dyspigmentation may occur. Fibrosis can result in joint contracture, skin ulcerations, and poor wound healing. Some patients have a sudden onset of erythema that can be activated by exposure to the sun.

Liver Liver disorders are observed in about 90% of patients with chronic GVHD. Pathologic findings are characterized by damaged or absent small bile ducts with concomitant severe cholestasis similar to that seen in primary biliary cirrhosis. Alkaline phosphatase, serum glutamic oxaloacetic transaminase (SGOT), and bilirubin levels are elevated. With treatment, bilirubin values return to normal within several weeks, but elevated

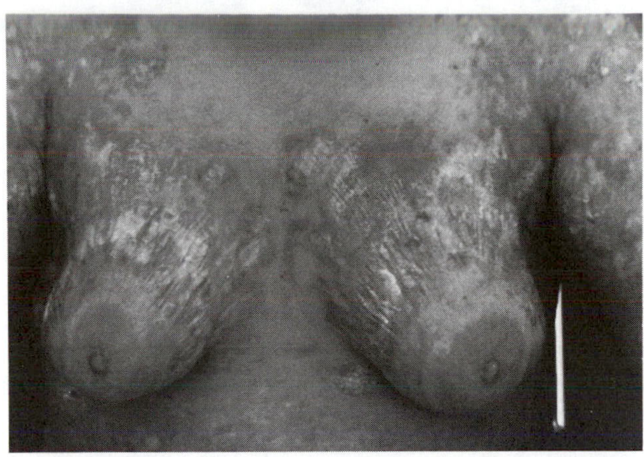

FIGURE 18-11 Chronic graft-versus-host disease of the skin.

alkaline phosphatase and SGOT may persist for months.[97–99] Nurses need to follow serial liver function laboratory values and be aware that jaundice in a patient 3–12 months after BMT may indicate liver involvement in chronic GVHD[96,97] (see Table 18-13).

Oral Oral mucosal involvement will develop in approximately 80% of patients with extensive chronic GVHD. Xerostomia and stomatitis are common symptoms. Lichenoid lesions can be confused with candidiasis.[99] Labial mucosa biopsy is a major diagnostic tool to screen for the presence of chronic GVHD. Salivary changes occur, and xerostomia may cause rampant tooth decay. Early subtle signs are complaints of changes in food tastes and burning after brushing of the teeth. The complete nursing assessment of the patient after transplantation must include examination of the oral cavity at each clinic visit.

Ocular Ocular involvement occurs in 80% of patients with extensive chronic GVHD. Major symptoms include burning, itching, and complaints of a "gritty" feeling in the eye. Unfortunately, these symptoms usually appear after corneal stippling has already occurred from lachrymal insufficiency. Schirmers's tear test may be employed four times a year to measure the tearing capacity of the eye. Supportive measures with artificial tear replacement and wearing glasses shielded to prevent entry of dust particles will prevent keratitis sicca, which can lead to corneal erosion, perforation, or scarring.[96–99]

Sinuses Sinusitis is common in patients with chronic GVHD and is caused by a combination of sicca syndrome involving the sinuses and the predisposition to gram-positive bacterial infections.[96–99]

Gastrointestinal tract Esophageal abnormalities, once a common complication in advanced cases of chronic GVHD, occur less frequently because of advances made in management of this disorder.[96–99] Symptoms include dysphagia, painful swallowing, and retrosternal pain caused by esophageal thinning. Patients may need to be readmitted to inpatient care for management of nutritional problems and pain. Upper and lower intestinal involvement can occur in chronic GVHD. Symptoms include diarrhea and abdominal pain. Malabsorption and submucosal fibrosis also have been documented in advanced cases.[96–99] Responsible nursing management requires early detection of nutritional deficiencies.

Vaginal Significant vaginal problems have been documented in women with chronic GVHD. Vaginal inflammation, stricture formation, and adhesions have occurred 1–3 years after transplantation. Stricture formation severe enough to require surgery to relieve menstrual obstruction with abdominal distention and pain is now rare. Vaginal atrophy may cause painful intercourse leading to sexual dysfunction. The use of a water-soluble, nonperfumed lubricating jelly during sexual intercourse helps women to overcome pain associated with the thinning of the vaginal mucosa and loss of natural lubrication. Treatment measures include vaginal dilation and use of topical estrogen cream in conjunction with immunosuppressive therapies for chronic GVHD. A routine gynecologic examination should be incorporated into the care of female recipients of BMT.

Other Problems in other organ systems will develop in 20% of patients with extensive chronic GVHD. The musculoskeletal system can be affected in a manner similar to rheumatoid arthritis and arthralgia, serosal effusions, joint contracture, and polymyositis. Dyspnea may be a manifestation of bronchiolitis obliterans.

Treatment

Most often, chronic GVHD does not manifest itself until after the patients return to their communities. A dangerous scenario could occur if chronic GVHD remained undetected by an oncology team unfamiliar with its clinical manifestations, diagnosis, and treatment. Consequently, allogeneic recipients have a battery of tests specific for diagnosing the presence of chronic GVHD; these were discussed earlier in the chapter (see Table 18-11). If chronic GVHD is present, appropriate treatment protocols are begun. Nurses involved in preparing allogeneic marrow recipients to return home may be coordinators of this "work-up," clinical assessments, and required tests. As more third-party payers mandate that marrow recipients return to their communities prior to 100 days post-BMT, referring physicians and the BMT center will need to cooperate in establishing the type and time of these evaluations.

Early detection and monitoring to detect subclinical chronic GVHD have proven key in preventing and treating chronic GVHD. Classic treatment of chronic GVHD is long-term administration of cyclosporine using a slow taper of 5%/week starting at week 7 following the transplant, followed by an abrupt taper. If acute GVHD flare-up occurs, the initial treatment is to reinstitute full-dose cyclosporine therapy. If resolution does not occur after several weeks, prednisone may be added and followed by a rapid taper.[99] Sullivan et al., in a prospective randomized study, found prednisone alone to be superior to prednisone with azathioprine in preventing GVHD.[102] The use of psoralen ultraviolet (PUVA) therapy has been effective for some cases of resistant chronic GVHD of the mouth and skin.[100]

Clinical trials using thalidomide for prevention and treatment of chronic GVHD are under way.[101] Other new treatment strategies under review are cytokine antagonists, oxpentifyline, and photopheresis monitoring.[96] Current and future studies will continue to control chronic GVHD while allowing a sufficient degree of chronic GVHD to preserve the graft-versus-leukemic effect (explained next). Nurses working within ambulatory settings will need to keep abreast of new treatment therapies for early detection, prevention, and treatment of chronic GVHD (see Tables 18-12 and Table 18-13).

Graft-versus-leukemic effect The graft-versus-leukemic (GVL) effect is a curious phenomenon that has been known in vitro since the early 1950s but is difficult to replicate artificially. The GVL effect was first observed in twins receiving syngeneic marrow transplantations. It was observed that syngeneic marrow transplant patients had a twofold higher relapse rate than allogeneic marrow patients who developed graft-versus-host disease. Studies ensued to identify techniques to remove T-cells, the cause of graft-versus-host disease, from donor marrow. T-cell depletion was successful in decreasing the incidence of graft-versus-host disease, but an increased incidence of graft failure and relapse was seen in patients receiving T-depleted allografts. As discussed earlier in this chapter, T-cell depletion has been largely abandoned, but research continues to seek the optimal balance of T-cell depletion to prevent graft failure yet preserve the antileukemic effect of GVHD. Recently, selected depletion of the T-cell, CD-8, from marrow transplant recipients reduced the incidence of acute GVHD from 50% to 20%, and graft failure to 10% without high relapse rates.[102,103]

Late Infectious Complications

As the immune system recovers, infectious complications generally decline. Marrow recipients with persistent acute GVHD or those who develop chronic GVHD, however, remain at considerable risk for infection due to immune dysfunction.[102] Long-term survivors without chronic GVHD are remarkably free of infections after 1 year. In contrast, patients in whom chronic GVHD develops remain at high risk for bacterial pneumonia, septicemia, and sinusitis, for their donor-derived immune systems have not yet matured and cannot adequately protect against invasive organisms[102,103] (Figure 18-12). The tempo and type of microbial infections follow a predicted path.

Varicella zoster virus (VZV)

Seropositive marrow recipients are at substantial risk for VZV infection. Median onset is 5 months after BMT and occurs in 25%–40% of patients. Reactivation occurs most often in marrow recipients with chronic GVHD; however, autologous BMT patients also are at risk. Aggressive antiviral therapy with intravenous acyclovir at 500 mg/kg every 8 hours for 7–10 days is the standard therapy.[78,102,103] Caution must be used in administering high-dose oral acyclovir (800 mg five times daily) because peak serum concentrations often are lower than the concentrations required to inhibit many VZV in vitro. For sero-negative marrow recipients exposed to VZV, early administration of VZV immunoglobulin may reduce the risk for infection.[77] Patients with nonspecific suppressor cells and chronic GVHD may be at greater risk for VZV as a result of prolonged immunosup-
pression.[102,103]

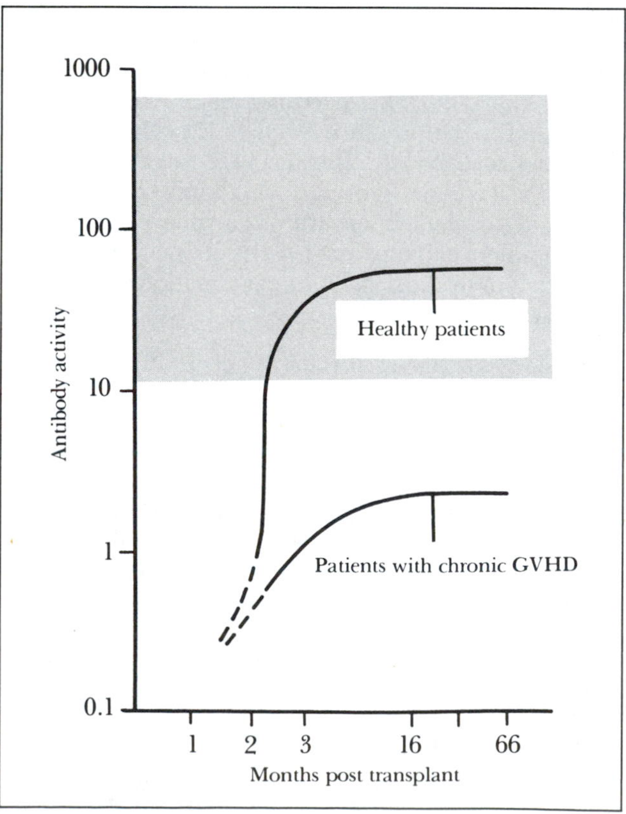

FIGURE 18-12 Effects of chronic graft-versus-host disease on the return of the immune system. (Source: Adapted from Witherspoon RP, Lum LG, Storb R: *Semin Hematol* 21:2–10, 1984. Reprinted with permission.)

Encapsulated bacteria

All marrow recipients with chronic GVHD are at risk for infection from encapsulated bacteria. The common cause is sinopulmonary infection caused by *Streptococcus pneumoniae, Neisseria meningitidis,* and *Hemophilus influenzae.* Resulting occult sinusitis and overwhelming sepsis can occur. All patients with chronic GVHD should receive antibiotic prophylaxis with penicillin or trimethoprim-sulfamethoxazole. Marrow recipients with IgG subclass 2 deficiency and recurrent sinopulmonary infection may benefit from intravenous immunoglobulin supplementation. Current research is focusing on the cost–benefit ratio of this therapy.[87]

A major concern after a BMT patient is discharged home is infection. Many transplantation teams, therefore, recommend that patients wear surgical masks for at least 6 months after transplant to reduce the risk of infections due to microorganisms, fungal spores, and pollen. Infection prophylaxis secondary to wearing a mask has not been studied; however, the mask does serve as a reminder to the patient and the community to take care when interacting with the patient. Immunizations are recommended after 1 year in patients without chronic GVHD and only after immune recovery testing for patients with chronic GVHD (see Table 18-12).

Pulmonary Complications

Restrictive pulmonary abnormalities are rarely observed in long-term survivors and are associated with chemoirradiation and recurrent pneumonia.[96] The incidence of restrictive disease peaks at 1 year. Obstructive pulmonary disease, which occurs in approximately 15% of long-term survivors with chronic GVHD, presents clinical and pathologic features of obliterative bronchiolitis. Late interstitial pneumonia occurs in 10%–20% of long-term survivors with chronic GVHD and carries a 50% mortality rate. Studies have identified specific pneumonias as idiopathic, CMV, varicella zoster, and *Pneumocystis carinii.* Twenty percent of patients with chronic GVHD will have restrictive lung disease, 10% will have obstructive lung disease, and 10% will be at risk for bronchiolitis obliterans.[102]

Complete nursing assessments of long-term survivors require careful histories and physical examinations. Specifically, inquire about changes in activities of daily living, perform chest auscultation and percussion, and monitor pulmonary capacities and volumes.[104]

Gonadal Dysfunction

Most transplant patients conditioned with TBI will demonstrate gonadal dysfunction. Patients prepared with chemotherapy alone recovery fertility and can successfully bear children. Table 18-12 describes possible gonadal dysfunction and related management in BMT recipients. The adverse effects of high-dose chemotherapy on gonadal function depends on the patient's age at the time of BMT. Girls and boys who are prepubertal at the time of BMT develop normally. Younger women (under 26 years of age) can expect return of menstrual periods, but only a few have borne children. Women over the age of 26 develop early menopause. Men usually return to normal gonadotropin levels and low to normal sperm counts, and can father children.[105]

TBI

Women Almost all female recipients conditioned with TBI have gonadal dysfunction, including sterility and early menopause. Cyclic oral or transdermal hormone replacement therapy commonly is used to reduce symptoms of premature menopause and to prevent long-term disorders, such as osteoporosis or vulvar and vaginal atropic changes. Vasomotor symptoms, such as hot flashes, sweating, palpitation, irritability, headache, sleep disturbances, and genitourinary tract symptoms, are common. Dysuria, vaginal dryness, dyspareunia, and vulva vaginitis are reported and are often the underlying cause of sexual dysfunction. In vitro fertilization plus artificial insemination currently is not advised; and until further research is done, this cannot routinely be recommended.[104,105]

The ideal time to prepare the patient and significant others is prior to BMT. Sensitive counseling by gynecologists, nurse practitioners, or staff nurses working in ambulatory and home care can support women with their intimate relationships. Sensitive lay information for understanding and managing sexual issues exists for the oncology patient and can be useful for the marrow transplant recipient.[104,105]

Men Most men conditioned with TBI preserve Leydig cell function and testosterone and luteinizing hormone production, but spermatogenesis usually is absent.[104,105]

Children Most prepubertal girls who receive TBI have primary ovarian failure, do not achieve menarche, and do not develop secondary sexual characteristics. A few prepubertal boys conditioned with TBI develop secondary sexual characteristics, but most have delayed onset of puberty. The children most profoundly affected are prepubertal boys who receive testicular irradiation prior to marrow conditioning. Testosterone therapy may be effective, but longer follow-up is needed.[104,105]

Sexual counseling prior to BMT is important for all marrow transplant candidates.[104,106] Pediatric long-term survivors require special consideration in assessing possible gonadal dysfunction. Children who fail to reach puberty require neuroendocrine evaluation, and young adolescents reaching puberty will need information about possible sterility. Oncology nurses who work with these families can be instrumental in assessing and teaching both parents and children.[103]

New pretransplantation conditioning regimens, aimed at decreasing toxicities, use high-dose busulfan and cyclophosphamide with TBI. Preliminary results[104] demonstrate that the combination of these two agents induces gonadal impairment, as measured by decreased levels of estradiol and elevated levels of luteinizing hormone and follicle-stimulating hormone. In males, testosterone and luteinizing hormone levels have remained normal while FSH is only slightly elevated.[105]

Growth in children Children who undergo conditioning with high-dose cyclophosphamide alone have normal growth and development.[105] TBI used in conditioning regimens causes abnormalities of growth and development in children. All children have decreased growth rates after TBI, and those who have chronic GVHD are the most significantly affected. Bone age does not seem to be as affected and often is consistent with chronological age, but adrenocortical function, growth hormone levels, and thyroid function have been subnormal in some children, especially those given prior prophylaxis with cranial irradiation.[104]

Establishing parental awareness of the potential late effects of irradiation is an important nursing function and should be addressed prior to and at regular intervals after transplant. Growth patterns should be evaluated annually, and those who demonstrate a decreased growth rate should be referred to a pediatric endocrinologist. Careful long-term follow-up through puberty will be necessary,[104] and growth hormone and appropriate sex hormone therapy may be indicated.

Thyroid Dysfunction

Thyroid dysfunction occurs in 30%–60% of patients prepared with a regimen including single-dose TBI.[105] Forty percent to 55% of children given high-dose TBI show a deficiency of growth hormone; in children with previous cranial irradiation, the incidence may be as high as 90%. As indicated earlier, sexual development may be severely impaired in both boys and girls receiving single-dose TBI.

Ophthalmologic Effects

Ophthalmologic effects include chronic GVHD and posterior capsular cataracts.[13,102] Cataract formation appears approximately 3.5 years post-BMT and is caused by TBI and long-term steroid therapy for GVHD. Lens shielding is not employed during TBI, because the eye is a potential site of leukemic relapse. Glucocorticoid therapy for treatment of GVHD increases the risk of cataract formation by 25% in patients who have had fractionated TBI or high-dose chemotherapy only. Patients may report poor vision and complain of grittiness, burning, or dryness of the eyes. Keratoconjunctivitis sicca or dry eye syndrome also is noted as an ocular complication. Sicca syndrome usually is associated with GVHD; however, it has been observed in patients without GVHD. Artificial tears can alleviate discomfort. The treatment of cataracts with surgical extraction is highly successful. An important nursing function is to educate and prepare patients for the possibility of cataract development and treatment, and to encourage annual eye examinations[13,102] (see Tables 18-12 and 18-13).

Graft Failure

Graft failure occurs rarely in an HLA-matched marrow transplantation. However, graft failure in patients who have had transplantation with HLA-mismatched or T-cell-depleted marrow typically occurs early, or months after transplantation.[13,102]

Graft failure differentiates into either primary graft failure or transient engraftment. *Primary graft failure* is the absence of hematologic recovery in patients surviving more than 21 days post-BMT. *Transient engraftment* is defined as complete or partial recovery of hematopoiesis, in the absence of moderate to severe GVHD, followed by recurrent pancytopenia. The causes for graft failure include immunologic rejection at the donor, minor histocompatible antigens, and inhibition of hematopoiesis by infection. Disease status at the time of transplantation, the degree of HLA compatibility, pretransplant treatment, preconditioning regimens, and immunosuppressive therapy for GVHD can also influence engraftment and outcome[13,102] (see Table 18-12).

Aseptic Necrosis

Aseptic necrosis of the bone, particularly of the humerus or femur head, has been observed in the long-term BMT survivor.[13,102] Aseptic necrosis usually develops in the head of the femur or humerus, and is a direct result of bone softening associated with steroid therapy. Patients can present with complaints of pain and limited range of motion. Nurses caring for marrow recipients need to examine closely the patient's medical history for prior or current steroid therapy.

Dental Effects

Dental effects related to pretransplant conditioning or to chronic GVHD can lead to oral hygiene effects and dental decay. Oral sicca, or dry mouth syndrome, is a common late effect causing oral caries, infection such as *Candida,* and other dental health problems. Radiation can directly affect dental and facial bone development, resulting in poor calcification and root blunting. Defects usually are more severe in the pediatric marrow recipient[107] (see Table 18-12).

Genitourinary Effects

Until recently, genitourinary toxicity has not been reported as a long-term sequela of BMT. Total-body irradiation, drug toxicity related to antimicrobial therapy, and cyclosporine are causative factors. The median time of onset is 9 months, with a range of 4.5–26 months. Renal insufficiency is characterized by increased serum creatinine, decreased glomerular filtration rate, anemia, hypertension, and proteinuria. Urinary effects caused by scarring from early onset of hemorrhagic cystitis can lead to bladder shrinkage and chronic urinary disorders.[108]

Radiation Nephritis

Radiation nephritis from radiation damage has recently been described and occurs approximately 5 months post-BMT. It is thought that multiagent preparative regimens are the underlying cause.[108]

Neurologic Complications

Central nervous system effects after irradiation and chemotherapy include subsequent impaired memory, shortened attention spans, and impaired verbal skills.[109] Pediatric BMT recipients, when tested against controls, performed less well.[13,105] Signs and symptoms of chronic leukoencephalopathy may not appear for months or even years after transplantation. Learning disabilities in children have been reported,[104] including abnormal motor, perceptual, behavioral, and language performance. Clinical signs and symptoms may be subtle and may require careful observation of the behavior of the pediatric patient. Neurologic and developmental assessments are a vital part of follow-up care.[13,104] (see Table 18-12).

Second Malignancy

Second malignancies have been observed in marrow transplant recipients and are considered to be a late sequela of this treatment modality.[109] Long-term immunosuppressive therapy used in recipients of solid organ grafts also have given rise to secondary neoplasms and infection from agents such as Epstein-Barr virus that might predispose patients to second malignancies after transplantation.[110]

The success rate of BMT has increased during the past 30 years, but relapse remains a major problem.[1] Most patients in whom relapse occurs have disease in host cells, which indicates that the conditioning regimen for transplantation was not sufficient to eradicate residual leukemic cells that found sanctuary in the marrow recipient. Late relapse in cells of donor origin has been detected by molecular analysis of donor and host DNA.[111] Marrow recipients receiving chemotherapy demonstrate a ratio of second malignancies similar to oncology patients receiving chemotherapy. Marrow recipients receiving TBI, however, have a 3.9-fold increase of second neoplasms compared to cancer patients receiving irradiation. Other risk factors are immunosuppression and viral infection[110,111] (see Table 18-12). Patients in whom relapse occurs after BMT need intensive supportive care, because families and patients feel they have exhausted not only their medical options but also their psychologic and economic strengths. Options for these patients may include a second transplant and hospice care. Nurses who work with the families of patients who ultimately will die of their original disease or of transplantation-related problems will be challenged to support patients and families on death and dying issues.[104]

Although marrow transplantation holds the promise of cure for many patients who would otherwise die of their disease, many problems exist and are the subject of ongoing research. Relapse of malignancy after marrow transplantation remains a significant impediment to successful transplantation. Conditioning protocols with new regimens of chemotherapeutic agents and hyperfractionated irradiation hold promise of obtaining optimal conditioning for BMT.[112]

Involved-field irradiation given in addition to TBI to patients with lymphoma may reduce relapse rates and irradiation toxicity. The extra irradiation may be given before or after BMT, and is being investigated in the hope of increasing tumor cell kill and lessening irradiation toxicities.[26] Monoclonal antibodies targeted to tumor or immunotoxins show encouraging early results.[113] Bone-seeking isotopes designed to ablate tumor cells in the marrow without creating additional toxicities to otherwise healthy organs show significant application to BMT.[26,113] Earlier transplantation for younger patients with CML and ALL are improving relapse rates.[1]

PSYCHOSOCIAL ISSUES

Patients

Research on the psychosocial issues unique to BMT is beginning to appear in the literature. Patients have consistently identified specific stresses associated with each phase of the BMT process[35] (see Table 18-3). Each phase is eclipsed by particular concerns and provides a framework for nurses who care for these patients to offer appropriate support through patient preparation and teaching.

Donors

Donors experience a variety of psychologic reactions before and after their marrow donation. Donor-related stresses have been identified; they were reviewed earlier in this chapter.

Family/Caregivers

Families may experience considerable psychologic, emotional, and social problems before and after marrow transplantation.[36,37] For example, transplant centers often are located far from familiar support systems, and relocation requires dramatic changes in every aspect of family dynamics. These changes include significant economic issues and medical consequences of marrow transplant. Families need to confront the long-term issues of caring for a recovering family member until the physical sequelae of treatment have vanished.[114] Strong social work teams are beneficial in transplant settings to prepare families for this experience and to identify community resources. This intervention lessens the likelihood of developing family-related dysfunctions. Studies examining the burden on the caregivers of BMT patients are currently under way.

Staff

Provision of psychologic support for staff members who care for patients undergoing marrow transplantation is essential to the quality of nursing care provided to marrow recipients and their families. Inherent to BMT nursing is chronic stress related to caring for patients whose condition may change rapidly. These nurses are challenged by family interactions as well as patient concerns, and they become part of a psychosocial team caring for acutely ill patients who may die. Excellence in patient care, staff retention, and emotionally healthy nurses can be the result of programs designed to support staff nurses. Implementation of successful programs has been described in the literature and requires a nursing administration committed to assist nurses in coping with the stresses of their environment.[115,116]

Quality of Life

Haberman and Bush[117] studied quality-of-life issues after BMT and found that BMT recipients surveyed 10 years after BMT report a quality of life similar to that of cancer patients 10 years after their oncologic treatment. Ferrell[118] reported the first quality-of-life instrument specifically for long-term follow-up of BMT recipients. This instrument measures physical symptoms (e.g., weight loss, frequent colds, skin changes, cataracts, sexual problems), psychologic symptoms (e.g., worry about recurrence of disease, adjustment to illness, social concerns, relationship adjustment, return to work), and spiritual well-being (e.g., sense of control, future goals).

Many sophisticated qualitative research studies in BMT are emerging. Studies of hope, meaning, and quality of life provide physical, psychologic, and social findings to help oncology nurses perform thorough and meaningful psychosocial assessments.[94,117–119]

Ethical Issues

Marrow transplantation can involve complex moral and ethical considerations. Informed consent for experimental procedures is standard, but the effectiveness of these explanations is poorly understood. The rights of children and their welfare continue to challenge medical and legal systems.[120] Broader social issues, such as allocation of resources, prolonged life support in the face of irreversible organ failure, and the competitive selection of marrow recipients, are being examined.[121,122] These and other complex questions provide opportunities for multidisciplinary studies of some of the major biopsychosocial issues of our time.

FUTURE APPLICATIONS

Stem Cell Technology

Research on techniques for separation of hematopoietic stem cells include studies of sedimentation techniques, monoclonal antibodies, and immunoabsorption columns. Application of these processes might enable infusion of leukemia-free marrow in autologous transplants.[113] These therapies may lessen the toxic effects of transplant therapy and allow patients to be discharged from the hospital more quickly. The use of peripheral stem cell or blood transplants, with or without colony stimulating factors, is increasing and will revolutionize methodologies, shorten recovery periods after marrow transplantation, and reduce the current costs of stem cell and marrow transplantation.[123] Clinical trials of radio-labeled antibody therapy and immunoconjugates followed by autologous BMT show promise for treatment in selected lymphomas.[124]

Alternate donor stresses are emerging. Fetal liver stem cell transplants have been reported in treatment of selected patients with severe combined immunodeficiency disease syndrome (SCIDS).[125] A small number of stem cell transplants using umbilical cord blood have been reported.[126] In utero transplantation of fetal hematopoietic stem cells has been documented.[127]

Gene Transfer

Gene transfer holds dramatic promise for future applications of BMT and other genetic diseases. This involves replacement of defective genetic material with healthy genes in marrow transplantation candidates with genetic diseases. Hematopoietic marrow stem cells probably would be used. Adenosine deaminase deficiency is the first disease to be treated with gene transfer therapy, and other genetic diseases, such as sickle cell anemia, will be treated with gene transfer therapy in clinical trials. The goal is to correct the sickle cell defect in the hematopoietic stem cell in concert with autologous transplantation of manipulated marrow for gene transfer.[16] Substantial preclinical improvements in transfer efficiency are required before wider clinical studies can be conducted.

CONCLUSION

The number of bone marrow transplantations will increase to unanticipated numbers, and a large majority of patient care will take place in outpatient settings. Expert training programs for physicians at large transplant centers will generate new transplantation teams to provide treatment to more patients.[1] Nurses on inpatient and outpatient units will interact more with third-party payers. BMT coordinators will assume more comprehensive roles in establishing safe and cost-effective care. The number of third-party-payer corporate case managers will increase and will influence the management of the patient. BMT education of these and other professionals will be crucial.

Growth of the unrelated donor pool could increase the allogeneic BMT population by 200% (personal communication, Claudia Anasetti, 1992). Existing transplantation resources, including physicians and nurses, hospital beds, blood banking and other supportive services, will require expansion. New models of care for stable BMT recipients will incorporate 24-hour clinics, day hospitals, infusion suites, and high-tech home health services.

Studies are under way to identify cost–benefit ratios and cost-effectiveness measures and to evaluate case management.[128–132] Centers of excellence are being identified by third-party payers who may limit reimbursement to BMTs received at an approved site.

The roles and responsibilities of oncology and bone marrow transplant nurses are rapidly changing. Nurses greatly influence the success of transplantation by the care given to marrow recipients before and after the procedure. BMT outpatients are more acutely ill than in the past and require new treatments and therapies. Nurses require in-depth, complex treatment protocols and the ability to continually assimilate new technologies. Unifying the goals of medical research and nursing care will continue to challenge multidisciplinary teams. Nursing management will be challenged to create an environment that promotes staff education and retention. As the number of patients undergoing marrow transplantation increases, the demand for BMT nurses of the highest professional caliber will continue to increase.

REFERENCES

1. Bortin MM, Horowitz MM, Rimm AA: Increasing utilization of allogeneic bone marrow transplantation. *Ann Intern Med* 116:505–512, 1992.
2. Corcoran-Buchsel PB, Ford RC: Introduction. *Semin Oncol Nurs* 4:1–2, 1988.
3. Quine WE: The remedial application of bone marrow. *JAMA* 26:1012–1013, 1896.
4. Santos GW: History of bone marrow transplantation. *Clin Haematol* 12:611–639, 1983.
5. Thomas ED, Storb R, Clift RA, et al: Bone-marrow transplantation. *N Engl J Med* 292:832–843, 895–902, 1975.
6. Barnes DWH, Corp MJ, Loutit JL, et al: Treatment of murine leukaemia with x-rays and homologous bone marrow. *Br Med J* ii:96–99, 1956.
7. Weiden PL, Flournoy N, Thomas ED, et al: Antileukemic effect of graft-versus-host disease in human recipients of allogeneic-marrow grafts. *N Engl J Med* 300:1068–1073, 1979.
8. Doney KC, Buckner CD: Bone marrow transplantation: An overview. *Plasma Ther Transfus Technol* 6:149–161, 1985.
9. Thomas ED, Sargur M: Bone marrow transplantation. In Cerilli J (ed.): *Organ Transplantation and Replacement.* Philadelphia: Lippincott, 1988, pp. 608–616.
10. Chao NH, Nademanee AP, Long GD, et al: Important bone marrow cytogenetic evaluation before autologous bone marrow transplantation for Hodgkin's disease. *J Clin Oncol* 9:1575–1579, 1991.
11. Goldman JM, Gale RP, Horowitz MM, et al: Bone marrow transplantation for chronic myelogenous leukemia in chronic phase: Increased risk of relapse associated with T-cell depletion. *Ann Intern Med* 108:806–814, 1988.
12. Storb R, Thomas ED: Allogeneic bone marrow transplantation. *Immunol Rev* 71:78–102, 1983.
13. Deeg JH: Delayed complications of marrow transplantation. *Marrow Transplant Reviews: Issues in Hematology, Oncology and Immunology* 2:10–16, 1992.
14. Zanjani EM, Harrison MR, Tavassoli M: In utero transplantation of fetal hematopoietic stem cells (HSC). *J Cellular Biochemistry* 16a:179, 1992 (abst. D 030) (suppl.).
15. Vilmer E, Broyart A, Lescoeur B, et al: HLA-mismatched cord blood transplantation in a patient with advanced leukemia. *J Cellular Biochemistry* 16a:214, 1992 (abst. 512) (suppl.).
16. Blazer BR, Lasky LC, Perentesis JP, et al: Successful donor cell engraftment in a recipient of bone marrow from a cadaveric donor. *Blood* 67:1655–1660, 1986.
17. Ford R, Ballard B: Acute complications after bone marrow transplantation. *Semin Oncol Nurs* 4:15–24, 1988.
18. Beutler E, Sullivan K: Marrow transplantation in sickle cell disease. In Forman SJ, Thomas ED, Blume K (eds.): *Bone Marrow Transplantation.* Cambridge, MA: Blackwell Scientific Publ, in press.
19. Parkman R: Bone marrow transplantation for genetic diseases. *Pediatr Ann* 20:677–681, 1991.
20. Blaese RM, Culver KW: Progress toward the application of gene therapy. In Nance SJ (ed.): *Clinical and Basic Science Aspects of Immunohematology.* Arlington, VA: American Association of Blood Banks, 1991, pp. 1–11.
21. Hansen RA, Clift ED, Thomas ED, et al: Marrow transplantation from donors other than HLA-identical siblings. *UCLA Symposium Bone Marrow Transplantation—Current Controversy,* 1988, 1989, pp. 616–624.
22. Tiercy JM, Morel C, Freidel AC, et al: Selection of unrelated donors for bone marrow transplantation is improved by HLA class II genotyping with oligonucleotide hybridization. *Pro Natl Acad Sci* 88:7121–7125, 1991.

23. Buckner CD, Clift RA, Sanders JE, et al: ABO-incompatible marrow transplants. *Transplant* 26:233–238, 1978.
24. Bensinger WI, Buckner CD, Thomas ED, et al: ABO-incompatible marrow transplants. *Transplant* 33:427–429, 1982.
25. Hanigan MJ: Unrelated bone marrow transplantation and the national marrow donor program: An update. Conference Proceed, University of Nebraska Medical Center, Omaha, 1992, pp. 71–75.
26. Appelbaum FR: Intensive chemotherapy or chemoradiotherapy with autologous marrow support as treatment for patients with solid tumors. *Hematol/Oncol Clin North Am* 2:345–351, 1988.
27. Spitzer G: The use of high-dose chemotherapy prior to marrow transplantation in the treatment of breast cancer. *Marrow Transplant Reviews: Issues in Hematology, Oncology and Immunology* 2:1–22, 1991.
28. Areman EM, Reed E, O'Shaunessey JA, et al: Cryopreservation and storage of human bone marrow: A survey of current practices. In Gross S (ed.): *Bone Marrow Purging and Processing.* New York: Alan R. Liss, 1990, pp. 523–529.
29. Schryber S, Lacasse CR, Barton-Burke M: Autologous bone marrow transplantation. *Oncol Nurs Forum* 14:74–80, 1987.
30. Antman KH: Marrow transplantation in patients with breast cancer. *Marrow Transplantation Reviews: Issues in Hematology, Oncology and Immunology* 1:23–25, 1992.
31. Kessinger A, Armitage JO, Smith DM, et al: High-dose therapy and autologous peripheral blood stem cell transplantation for patients with lymphoma. *Blood* 74:1260–1265, 1989.
32. Haire WD, Lieberman RP, Lund GB, et al: Thrombotic complications of silicone rubber catheters during autologous marrow and peripheral stem cell transplantation: Prospective comparison of Hickman and Groshong catheters. *Bone Marrow Transplant* 7:57–59, 1991.
33. Kessinger A, Achmit-Pokorny K, Smith DM, et al: Cryopreservation and infusion of autologous peripheral blood stem autografts. *Bone Marrow Transplant* 1:103–110, 1986.
34. Bell AJ, Hamblin TJ, Oscier G: Circulation stem cell autografts. *Bone Marrow Transplant* 1:103–110, 1986.
35. Haberman MR: Psychosocial aspects of bone marrow transplantation. *Semin Oncol Nurs* 4:55–59, 1988.
36. Durbin M: Bone marrow transplantation: Economic, ethical, and social issues. *Pediatrics* 82:774–778, 1988.
37. *Newsletter of the International Bone Marrow Transplant Registry.* Milwaukee, WI: International Bone Marrow Transplant Registry, 1992.
38. Curran WJ, Hyg SM: Beyond the best interests of a child: Bone marrow transplantation among half-siblings. *N Engl J Med* 324:1818–1819, 1992.
39. Dudjak LA: HLA typing: Implications for nurses. *Oncol Nurs Forum* 11:1130–1136, 1984.
40. Ruggiero MR: The donor in bone marrow transplantation. *Semin Oncol Nurs* 4:9–14, 1988.
41. Lesko LM, Hawkins DR: Psychological aspects of transplantation medicine. In Akhtat S (ed.): *New Psychiatric Syndromes: DSM-III and Beyond.* New York: Aronson, 1983, pp. 265–309.
42. Patenaude AF, Rappeport H: Psychological costs of bone marrow transplantation in children. *Am J Orthopsychiat* 49:409–422, 1979.
43. Bolwell B, Lichtin A, Sands K, et al: An analysis of complications of outpatient bone marrow harvesting. *Proc of Keystone Symposia on Molecular and Cellular Biology* p. 200, 1992 (abst.) (suppl.).
44. Weinberg P: The human leukocyte antigen (HLA) system, the search for a matching donor, national marrow donor program development, and marrow donor issues. In Whedon M (ed.): *Bone Marrow Transplantation: Principles, Practice, and Nursing Insights.* Boston: Jones and Bartlett, 1991, pp. 105–132.
45. Storb R, Prentice RL, Buckner CD, et al: Graft-versus-host disease and survival in patients with aplastic anemia treated with marrow graft from HLA-identical siblings: Beneficial effect of a protective environment. *N Engl J Med* 308:302–307, 1983.
46. Storb R, Deeg HJ, Whitehead J, et al: Methotrexate and cyclosporine compared with cyclosporine alone for prophylaxis of acute graft-versus-host disease after marrow transplantation for leukemia. *N Engl J Med* 314:729–735, 1986.
47. Russell JA, Poon MC, Jones AR, et al: Allogeneic bone-marrow transplantation without protective isolation in adults with malignant disease. *Lancet* 339:38–40, 1992.
48. Buckner CD, Clift RA, Sander JE, et al: Protective environment for marrow transplant patients: A prospective study. *Ann Intern Med* 89:893–901, 1978.
49. Whedon M (ed.): *Bone Marrow Transplantation: Principles, Practice, and Nursing Insights.* Boston: Jones and Bartlett, 1991.
50. Thomas ED: Bone marrow transplantation: A lifesaving applied art. *JAMA* 249:2528–2536, 1983.
51. Thomas ED, Fefer A: Bone marrow transplantation. In DeVita VT, Hellman S, Rosenberg SA (eds.): *Cancer Principles and Practice of Oncology* (ed. 2). Philadelphia: Lippincott, 1989, pp. 2320–2325.
52. Phillips G, Wolff S, Herzig G: Local radiotherapy followed by cyclophosphamide, fractionated total body irradiation and autologous marrow transplantation for refractory malignant lymphoma. *Blood* 62:228, 1983 (suppl. 1).
53. Freedman S, Hainsfield ME, McQuire DB, et al: Nursing considerations in the administration of blood component therapy. *Semin Oncol Nurs* 6:155–162, 1990.
54. Sullivan KM, Storb R: Allogeneic marrow transplantation. *Cancer Invest* 2:27–38, 1984.
55. Schubert MM, Sullivan KM, Truelove EL: Head and neck complications of bone marrow transplantation. In Peterson ED, Sonis ST, Elias EG (eds.): *Head and Neck Management of the Cancer Patient.* Boston: Martinus Nijhoff, 1986, pp. 401–427.
56. Hill HH, Chapman RC, Kornell JA, et al: Self-administration of morphine in bone marrow transplant patients reduces drug requirement. *Pain* 40:121–129, 1990.
57. Epstein JB, Stevenson-Moor P, Jackson S: Prevention of oral mucositis in radiation therapy: A controlled study with benzdamine hydrochloride rinse. *Internatl J Rad Oncol Biol Physics* 16:1571–1575, 1989.
58. Brandt SJ, Peters WP, Atwater SK, et al: Effect of recombinant human granulocyte-macrophage colony-stimulating factor on hematopoietic reconstitution after high-dose chemotherapy and autologous bone marrow transplantation. *N Engl J Med* 318:869–876, 1988.
59. Wolford JL, McDonald GB: A problem-oriented approach to intestinal and liver disease after marrow transplantation. *J Clin Gastroenterol* 10:419–433, 1988.
60. Hewitt M, Cornish D, Pamphilon D, et al: Effective emetic control during conditioning of children for bone mar-

row transplantation using ondansetron, a 5-HT 3 antagonist. *Bone Marrow Transplant* 7:431–433, 1991.

61. Press OW, Schaller RT, Thomas ED: Bone marrow transplant complications. In Toledo-Pereyra LH (ed.): *Complications of Organ Transplantation*. New York: Marcel Dekker, 1986, pp. 399–424.
62. Anderson RJ, Schrier RW: Acute renal failure. In Braunwald E, Isselbacher KJ, Petersdorf RG, et al (eds.): *Harrison's Principles of Internal Medicine*. New York: McGraw-Hill, 1987, pp. 1149–1155.
63. Ballard B: Renal and hepatic complications. In Whedon MB (ed.): *Bone Marrow Transplantation: Principles, Practice, and Nursing Insights*. Boston: Jones and Bartlett, 1991, pp. 240–261.
64. Klingemann H-G: Urinary tract. In Deeg HJ, Klingemann H-G, Phillips GL (eds.): *A Guide to Marrow Transplantation*. New York: Springer-Verlag, 1988, pp. 135–139.
65. Sullivan KM: Acute and chronic graft-versus-host disease in man. *Int J Cell Clon* 4:42–93, 1986 (suppl. 1).
66. Meyers JD: Infection in bone marrow transplant recipients. *Am J Med* 81:27–38, 1986 (suppl. 1A).
67. Weisdorf D, Hakke R, Blazar B, et al: Risk factors for acute graft-versus-host disease in histocompatible donor bone marrow transplantation. *Transplantation* 51:1197–1203, 1991.
68. Butturina A, Gale RP: T-cell depletion in bone marrow transplantation for leukemia: Current results and future directions. *Bone Marrow Transplant* 3:185–192, 1988.
69. Blume KG, Chao NJ: Surviving the cure. *Marrow Transplantation Reviews: Issues in Hematology, Oncology and Immunology* 2:7–14, 1992.
70. Yau JC, Dimopoulos MA, Huan SD: An effective acute graft-vs-host disease prophylaxis with minidose methotrexate, cyclosporine, and single-dose methoprednisolone. *Am J Hema* 38:288–292, 1991.
71. Ford R, Eisenberg S: Bone marrow transplant: Recent advances and nursing implications. *Nurs Clin N Am* 25:405–422, 1990.
72. McDonald GB, Sharma P, Matthews DE, et al: The clinical course of 53 patients with venoocclusive disease of the liver after marrow transplantation. *Transplant* 39:603–608, 1985.
73. Dulley FL, Kanfer EF, Appelbaum FR, et al: Venoocclusive disease of the liver after chemoradiotherapy and autologous bone marrow transplantation. *Transplant* 43:870–873, 1987.
74. Shulman HM, Hinterberger W: Hepatic veno-occulsive disease-liver toxicity syndrome after bone marrow transplantation. *Bone Marrow Transplant* 10:197–214, 1992.
75. Buckner CD, Meyers JD, Springmeyer SC, et al: Pulmonary complications of marrow transplantation: Review of the Seattle experience. *Exp Hematol* 12:1–5, 1984 (suppl. 15).
76. Sullivan KM, Meyers JD, Flournoy N, et al: Early and late interstitial pneumonia following human bone marrow transplantation. *Int J Cell Cloning* 4:107–121, 1986 (suppl. 1).
77. Crawford SW, Bowden RA, Hackman RC, et al: Rapid detection of cytomegalovirus pulmonary infection by bronchoalveolar lavage and centrifugation culture. *Ann Intern Med* 108:180–185, 1988.
78. Windgard JR: Management of infectious complications of bone marrow transplantations. *Oncology* 4:69–76, 1990.
79. Harrington RD, Hooten T, Hackman RC, et al: An outbreak of respiratory syncytical virus in a bone marrow transplant center. *J Infect Diseases* 165:987–993, 1992.
80. Gucalp R: Management of the febrile neutropenic patient with cancer. *Oncology* 5:137–144, 1991.
81. Davis D, Patchell RA: Neurologic complications of bone marrow transplantation. *Neurol Clin* 6:377–378, 1988.
82. Thompson CB, June CH, Sullivan KM, et al: Association between cyclosporine neurotoxicity and hypomagnesemia. *Lancet* 2:1116–1120, 1984.
83. Klingemann H-G: Central nervous system (CNS). In Deeg HJ, Klingemann H-G, Phillips GL (eds.): *A Guide to Marrow Transplantation*. New York: Springer-Verlag, 1988, pp. 135–139.
84. Meriney DK: Neurologic and neuromuscular complications of bone marrow transplantation. In Whedon MB (ed.): *Bone Marrow Transplantation: Principles, Practice, and Nursing Insights*. Boston: Jones and Bartlett, 1991, pp. 262–279.
85. Larsen RL, Barber G, Heise CT, et al: Exercise assessment of cardiac function in children and young adults before and after bone marrow transplantation. *Pediatr* 89:722–729, 1992.
86. Hughs WT: New drugs for infections in patients with cancer. *Cancer* 70:959–965, 1991.
87. Schulman KA, Glick HA, Rubine H, et al: Cost-effectiveness of HA-1A monoclonal antibody for gram-negative sepsis: Economic assessment of a new therapeutic agent. *JAMA* 266:3466–3471, 1992.
88. Sullivan KN, Kopecky K, Jocum J, et al: Antimicrobial and immunomodulatory effects of intravenous immunoglobulin in bone marrow transplantation. *Proc of the Twenty-Eighth Interscience Conference on Antomicrobial Agents and Chemotherapy*. Washington, DC: American Society for Microbiology, 1988, p. 216.
89. Buchsel P, Benson A, Counts G, et al: Etiology and prevention of gram negative septicemias (GNS) in bone marrow transplant (BMT) outpatients: Relation to nursing care of right atrial catheters (RAC). *Proc American Cancer Society First National Conference on Cancer Nursing Research*. Atlanta: American Cancer Society, 1989 (abst. 15).
90. Sullivan KM, Kopecky KJ, Jocom J, et al: Immunomodulatory and antimicrobial efficacy of intravenous immunoglobulin in bone marrow transplantation. *N Engl J Med* 323:705–712, 1990.
91. Chielens D, Herrick E: Recipients of bone marrow transplants: Making a smooth transition to an ambulatory care setting. *Oncol Nurs Forum* 17:857–862, 1990.
92. Buchsel PC: From hospital to home: Making the transition. In Whedon MB (ed.): *Bone Marrow Transplantation: Principles, Practice, and Nursing Insights*. Boston: Jones and Bartlett, 1991, pp. 240–261.
93. Buchsel P: Bone marrow transplants: Managing BMT patients in alternate site health care settings with infusion therapy. *Continuing Care* 11:27–36, 1992.
94. Larson PJ: Patients' perception of needs in the first four weeks after bone marrow transplant. *Oncol Nurs Forum* 19:313, 1992 (abst. 271).
95. Copel LC, Smith ME: Oncology nursing knowledge of graft vs host disease in bone marrow transplant patients. *Cancer Nurs* 10:243–249, 1989.
96. Sullivan KM, Mori M, Sander J: Late complications of allogeneic and autologous marrow transplantation. *Bone Marrow Transplant* 10:127–134, 1992.

97. Atkinson K, Horowitz MM, Gale RP, et al: Risk factors for chronic graft-versus-host disease after HLA identical sibling bone marrow transplantation. *Blood* 75:2459–2464, 1990.
98. Sullivan KM: Graft-versus-host disease. In Blume KG, Petz LD (eds.): *Clinical Bone Marrow Transplantation.* New York: Churchill-Livingston, 1983, pp. 91–129.
99. Atkinson K: Chronic graft-versus-host disease following marrow transplantation. *Marrow Transplantation Reviews: Issues in Hematology, Oncology and Immunology* 2:10–16, 1992.
100. Jampel RM, Farmer ER, Vogelsang GB, et al: PUVA therapy for chronic cutaneous graft-vs-host disease. *Arch Dermatol* 127:1673–1678, 1991.
101. Vogelsang GB, Hess AD, Santos GW: Thalidomide for treatment of graft-versus host disease. *Bone Marrow Transplant* 3:392–398, 1988.
102. Sullivan KM, Agura E, Anasett C, et al: Chronic graft-versus-host disease and other late complications of bone marrow transplantation. *Semin Hematol* 28:250–259, 1991.
103. Ferrara JLM, Deeg HJ: Graft-versus-host disease. *N Engl J Med* 324:667–674, 1991.
104. Corcoran-Buchsel P: Long-term complications of allogeneic bone marrow transplantation: Nursing implications: *Oncol Nurs Forum* 13:61–70, 1986.
105. Sanders JE, Seattle Marrow Transplant Team: Effect of bone marrow transplantation on reproductive function. In *Late Effects of Childhood Cancer.* New York: Wiley-Liss, 1992, pp. 95–101.
106. Schover, LR: *Sexuality and Cancer: For the Woman Who Has Cancer, and Her Partner.* Atlanta: American Cancer Society, 1988.
107. Dahllof G, Barr M, Bolme P, et al: Disturbances in dental development after total body irradiation in bone marrow transplant recipients. *Oral Surg Oral Med Oral Pathol* 65:41–44, 1988.
108. Jackett M, Perry EH, Daniels BS, et al: Hemolytic uremic syndrome following bone marrow transplantation. *Bone Marrow Transplant* 7:405–409, 1988.
109. Degg JH, Sanders J, Martin P, et al: Secondary malignancies after marrow transplantation. *Exp Hematol* 12:660–666, 1984.
110. Storb R, Prentice RL, Thomas ED, et al: Factors associated with graft rejection after HLA-identical marrow transplantation for aplastic anaemia. *Br J Haematol* 55:573–585, 1983.
111. Witherspoon RP, Fisher LD, Schoch G, et al: Secondary cancers after bone marrow transplantation for leukemia or aplastic anemia. *N Engl J Med* 321:784–789, 1989.
112. Thomas ED: The future of marrow transplantation. *Semin Oncol Nurs* 4:74–78, 1988.
113. Mullan F: Seasons of survival: Reflections of a physician with cancer. *N Engl J Med* 313:270–273, 1985.
114. Nims JW, Strom S: Late complications of bone marrow transplant recipients: Nursing care issues. *Semin Oncol Nurs* 4:47–54, 1988.
115. Sarantos S: Innovations in psychosocial staff support: A model program for the marrow transplant nurse. *Semin Oncol Nurs* 4:69–73, 1988.
116. Kelleher J, Jennings M: Nursing management of a marrow transplantation unit: A framework for practice. *Semin Oncol Nurs* 4:60–68, 1988.
117. Haberman M, Bush N: Quality of life after bone marrow transplantation. *Proc American Cancer Society Second National Conference on Cancer Nursing Research.* Atlanta: American Cancer Society, 1992, p. 28–B (abst.).
118. Ferrell B, Grant M, Schmidt G, et al: The meaning of quality of life for bone marrow transplant survivors: Part 2. Improving quality of life for bone marrow transplant survivors. *Cancer Nurs* 15:247–253, 1992.
119. Coxon VJ: Subjective perceptions of the demands of hospitalization and anxiety in bone marrow transplant patients. *Proc American Cancer Society Second National Conference on Cancer Nursing Research.* Atlanta: American Cancer Society, 1992, p. 27–B (abst.).
120. Serota FT, O'Shea AT, Woodward WT Jr, et al: Role of a child advocate in the selection of donors for pediatric bone marrow transplantation. *J Pediat* 98:847–850, 1981.
121. Crawford W: Decision making in critically ill patients with hematologic malignancy. *West J Med* 115:488–493, 1991.
122. Vaughan WP, Purtileo RB, Butler CD, et al: Ethical and financial issues in autologous marrow transplantation: A symposium sponsored by the University of Nebraska Medical Center. *Ann Intern Med* 105:134–135, 1986.
123. Bennett C, Greenberg P, Gulati SC, et al: GM-CSF decreases duration of cytopenia and hospitalization and in-hospital costs in patients with Hodgkin's disease treated with high-dose chemotherapy and autologous bone marrow transfusion. *Blood* 76:132a, 1990 (suppl. 1).
124. Press O, Eary J, Badger C, et al: Radiolabeled antibody therapy followed by autologous marrow transplantation for relapsed B cell lymphomas. *J Cellular Biochem* 16a:204, 1992 (suppl.).
125. Roncarolo MG, Bacchetta R, Touraine JL, et al: SCID patients reconstituted by fetal liver stem cells: Possible role of IL-10 in transplantation tolerance. *J Cellular Biochem* 16a:211, 1992 (abst. 613) (suppl.).
126. Takanori T, Ishii E, Harada M, et al: Autologous blood stem cell transplantation in advanced neuroblastoma. *J Cellular Biochem* 16a:22, 1992 (abst. 180) (suppl.).
127. Gale RP: Fetal liver transplants. *Bone Marrow Transplant* 9:11, 1992 (suppl. 1).
128. Chapman JR, Atkinson K, Lapsely H: Cost of bone marrow transplants using unrelated donors. *Blood Reviews* 5:112–116, 1991.
129. Hillner RE, Smith TJ, Christopher ED: Estimating the cost-effectiveness of autologous bone marrow transplantation for metastatic breast cancer. *Proc Am Soc Clin Oncol* 10:A60, 1991 (abstr.).
130. Boros L, Asbury RF, Chang AY, et al: Cost controls in autologous bone marrow transplantation. *Proc Am Soc Clin Oncol* 9:A388, 1990 (abst.).
131. Sullivan KM, Applebaum FR: Comparative trials of chemotherapy and bone marrow transplantation in acute nonlymphocytic leukemia. *Rinsko Ketsueki* 31:527–533, 1990.
132. Welch HG, Larson EB: Cost effectiveness of bone marrow transplantation in acute nonlymphoblastic leukemia. *N Engl J Med* 321:807–812, 1988.
133. Windgard JR: Health, functional status, and employment of long-term survivors after bone marrow transplantation. *Ann Intern Med* 114:114–113, 1991.

PART IV

Psychological and Social Dimensions of Cancer

Chapter 19

Overview: Psychosocial Aspects of Cancer

Rose F. McGee, PhD, RN

INTRODUCTION

The focus of the psychosocial dimension of cancer care is the unique needs of the individual at risk for or with cancer and the social groups affected by that individual. Each individual brings to the cancer experience unique personality traits and a personal socialization pattern different from all others. Understanding the uniqueness of the individual is achieved only through study of the commonalities of the "personality and social psychological"[1] aspects of illness.

To separate the dimensions of health care into physical and psychosocial is artificial, yet serves pragmatic purposes in narrowing the scope of the discussion. In fact, a whole body of literature exists on the study of psychosocial variables as a causative factor in carcinogenesis. Lickiss noted that reviews of cancer research in the nineteenth century indicated that "while tissue and cellular changes were the characteristic phenomena of cancer, both inherent susceptibility and extrinsic influences played a part in the genesis of these phenomena—by mechanisms unknown."[p.297] More recently, the study of psychosocial variables in the etiology of cancer has been focused on the immune and endocrine system mechanisms as probable causes of cancer.[3] Thus the study of psychosocial factors as causative is an evolving area of study in oncology that may provide future cues to prevention.

In the meantime, professional commitment to quality of care and to holistic care has resulted in a focus on psychosocial aspects of illness as outcome variables. Empirically, the prevalence of psychosocial distress in response to a diagnosis of cancer has been found to range from a rare occurrence to as high as 90% of all patients.[4] The burgeoning number of studies on variables that maximize self-actualization and minimize psychosocial distress offers new understandings with respect to the meaning of the cancer diagnosis and the response patterns of individuals and groups to the actual or perceived threat.

This chapter provides a conceptual foundation upon which the subsequent chapters in this part are based. It will discuss the ubiquitous threat of cancer and related factors, the psychosocial stressors, that intensify the fears of diagnosis, treatment, and outcome. For purposes of emphasis, individuals (in Chapter 20), and family, significant others, and professionals (in Chapter 21) will be discussed separately, but the interaction effect will be recognized as the essence of the process. Finally, psychosocial outcomes (in Chapter 22) of cancer experience will be explored. A basic assumption of the following discussion is that psychosocial responses to the cancer experience are determined by the characteristics of cancer, the person with or at risk for cancer, and the social system and environment of significance to the individual.

CHARACTERISTICS OF CANCER

One of the most indelible descriptions of cancer that I have heard was made by a patient following a routine follow-up visit that resulted in a diagnosis of recurrent disease. With a combination of anger, fear, and frustration, she said, "I hate this disease; it is so *sneaky*." The word *sneaky* may not appear in the literature, but is implied in the four characteristics of cancer selected for review in this chapter. The characteristics discussed include: the universal threat, social stigma, uncertainty, and chronicity.

Cancer Poses a Universal Threat

The only certainty in oncology is that cancer is an actual or potential threat to all humans. Statistically, one in three persons and three of every four families will experience cancer. But statistics apply to groups and serve a minimal purpose in assessing individual risks. A small percentage of the population can personalize risks because of a genetic predisposition to cancer. But for the majority, cancer risks are the product of unmeasurable, cumulative lifestyle and environmental events. Therefore, to live in the current physical and psychosocial environment is to be at risk for cancer. The particular risk varies with age, geographic location, and lifestyle choices, but no individual or social sector is exempt.

The prevailing Western view of cancer is that cancer is a treatable disease. The resulting societal expectation is that the individual will accept the diagnosis, seek care, and comply, with a fighting spirit.[5] Nevertheless, to the individual, cancer has been described as the "ultimate existential crisis."[6] For most persons, cancer is among the most feared of all diseases.[7] Reasons for fear of cancer include its occurrence without warning, uncontrollable spread of the disease, incurability beyond a certain point, association with pain and discomfort, social and professional attitudes of hopelessness, difficulty of diagnosis, mutilative treatment, unknown causation, and the fact that cooperation with treatment does not necessarily lead to successful outcomes.[8]

Furthermore, health in most cultures is valued and illness is experienced as a barrier to the achievement of valued goals; therefore, the perceived threat of cancer includes a subjective evaluation of the threat to health in general and the threat of cancer in particular. Smith[9] provided a multidimensional and hierarchical description of health that is useful in studying the impact of cancer on health in general. According to Smith, perceptions of health range from the most primitive level of absence of pathology, to maintenance of role functioning, to ability to adapt, to the highest level, which is self-actualization. Because of the problems of diagnosis and of determining spread or recurrence of disease, a perceived absence of pathology with respect to cancer is never certain among both the general population and persons previously diagnosed with cancer. Applying the hierarchy proposed by Smith, the constant threat of cancer is a general health threat that has the potential to alter achievement of societal roles and self-actualization.

The Stigma of Cancer Persists

The stigma of cancer has been traced historically by Cassileth[5] from the naming of the disease by Hippocrates as *karkinos,* meaning "crab," to the seventeenth and eighteenth century notion that cancer is contagious, which led to the use of "tumor" or other euphemisms to minimize isolation of persons with the diagnosis. During the nineteenth century, "tumors" were classified as benign or malignant, and further pathological delineation led to the contemporary understanding of cancer as a composite of many diseases.

Cassileth[5] described the last 50 years as an era in which cancer is no longer met with fearful retreat in Western cultures, but is met with more of a frontier spirit, as evidenced by the so-called "war on cancer." Nevertheless, the stigma of cancer continues with respect to social and individual perceptions. For individuals with cancer, insurance cancellations, job discrimination, and problems with reintegration into school and workplace are manifestations of the persistent social stigma of cancer.

Disease and Treatment Are Marked by Uncertainty

Delays in diagnosis, unpredictable prognoses, and short illness trajectories resulting in early death in apparently healthy individuals compound the uncertainties associated with cancer. Mishel defined uncertainty as the "inability to determine the meaning of illness-related events."[10,p.225] Uncertainty results from the inability to structure the meaning of illness-related stimuli into a cognitive schema for the illness events perceived.

Four stages of uncertainty in illness are proposed: the *antecedents* generating uncertainty; the *cognitive appraisal* of uncertainty, perceived as danger or opportunity; *coping efforts,* either to reduce uncertainty perceived as danger or to maintain uncertainty appraised as opportunity; and the state of *adaptation* resulting from effective coping (Figure 19-1).[10] Antecedents of uncertainty include stimuli frame and structure providers.[11]

Cancer is not a single disease. Therefore, the degree to which a specific malignancy serves as a stimulus for uncertainty is determined by the degree of: ambiguity concerning the state of the illness, complexity of treatment and the system of care, lack of information about the diagnosis and seriousness, and unpredictability of the disease course and prognosis. Accuracy of stimuli perception is influenced by altered perceptions, such as selected attention and altered cognitive processes caused by the disease or by emotional responses to the symptoms.[11] The more accurate the cognitive schema formed of the illness, the less uncertainty one experiences. Uncertainty may be perceived as either danger

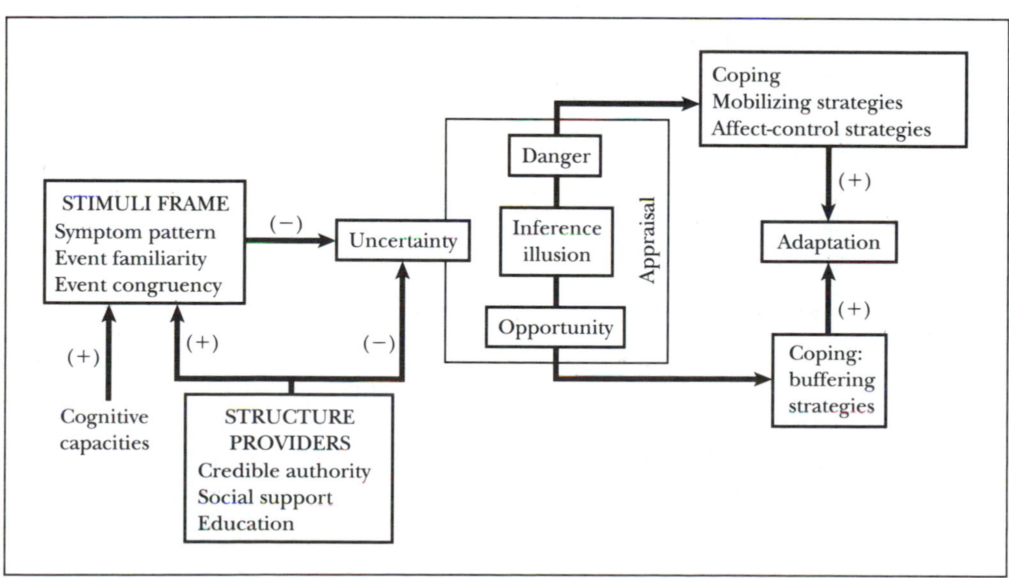

FIGURE 19-1 Model of perceived uncertainty in illness. (Source: Mishel MH: Uncertainty in illness. *Image* 20(4):266, 1988.)

or opportunity, depending on the individual's definition of the situation.

Structure providers, defined as "resources available to assist the person in interpretation of the stimuli frame,"[11,p.98] constitute the second component of the antecedents of uncertainty. Characteristics of the individual and social support systems influence interpretation of the stimuli. Education of the individual is one resource that enlarges the knowledge base and serves to enhance familiarity with illness events and thereby facilitate interpretation of information received from physicians, nurses, or other sources. Trust and confidence in health care professionals lessen uncertainty. Other social support systems serve a dual role in formulating and validating perceived meanings of the illness stimuli and providing feedback used for social comparisons.[11,12]

Social comparisons, by definition, include the process by which one determines "the desire to affiliate with others, the desire for information about others, and explicit self-evaluation against others."[13,p.569] Recent findings reflect a tendency for persons with cancer to make explicit self-evaluations against less fortunate individuals (downward evaluations) but to seek information and affiliation from more fortunate others (upward contacts). Downward evaluations in this case tend to foster self-esteem, upward contacts increase motivation and may lead to use of more credible sources among support systems.[13] Self-help and support groups are social comparison groups that patients may choose for affiliation; but the emergence of oncology as a specialty has resulted in forced affiliation with other individuals diagnosed with cancer by virtue of proximity in health care settings. The accuracy of cues perceived or information shared by similar patient populations will vary, making the effect on uncertainty unpredictable.

Other stages of the model of uncertainty (Figure 19-1) include appraisal of uncertainty as danger or opportunity, coping efforts either to reduce uncertainty perceived as danger or to maintain uncertainty appraised as opportunity, and the state of adaptation resulting from effective coping.[10] Mishel[10] proposed an ordering of coping strategies by resorting to affect-control strategies only if mobilizing strategies are not effective in reducing uncertainty. *Adaptation* is defined as "biopsychosocial behavior occurring within the range of behaviors of the individual."[10,p.231] Adaptation maintains activation, allowing achievement of goal-directed behaviors.

The Cancer Trajectory Is Manifest by Chronicity

Much has been written about the chronicity of cancer. Of significance with respect to management of psychosocial responses is the fact that simple crisis resolution models are not sufficient to address the scope of problems encountered with cancer. Mages and Mendelsohn[14] noted that people with cancer are confronted with a continuing series of stressors, rather than a single, time-limited crisis. The treatment is complex, often extended, and may cause irreparable damage to physical, mental, or social functioning. The lifelong fear of recurrence is one of the most disruptive aspects of the illness.

Corbin and Strauss[15] used the term *trajectory of illness* to refer to "management of the evolving course." *Trajectory* is defined as "the curve that a body describes in space from origin to first point of impact."[16,p.2425] The following quote further clarifies the concept.

> The management of chronic conditions is more than just a matter of controlling symptoms, or living with disability, or adapting to the psychological and social changes that long-term incurable illness brings to the lives of afflicted individuals and their families. It is all of these and more. Therefore, any approach to the nursing care of the chronically ill and their families must be comprehensive and reflect the diversity, multiplicity, and complexity of problems that chronic illness can bring.[15,p.155]

The trajectory framework originally evolved from in-depth study of the dying process and was designed to be applied to any chronic illness. The basic premise is that the illness trajectory can be shaped and managed over time and the nurse is the most likely person to coordinate these activities. An interactional effect is proposed, with disease and treatment influencing biographical fulfillment, identity, and performance of daily activities, and vice versa. Evans, for example, in describing a personal experience with cancer, related a vivid description of the interactional effect of internal and social variables on identity:

> There I was. I had cancer—the big "C." . . . The initial period of discovering my cancer caused the most trauma with both family and friends. . . . I could not cope with that look in their eyes. I did not want their sympathetic glances, their hushed tones. I had not changed inside. I was still the same person. Yet suddenly I seemed to have become different; I had become a cancer victim, losing my personal identity at home and in the hospital. I tried to retain a normal life. . . . It was then that I decided a personal survival plan would help and support me. [The doctors] were great. They just listened. I just hoped that I had enough strength to fight long enough for my life. Then the waiting period. Another form of purgatory—to regain normality while waiting to see if the cure will be effective. I was fortunate to receive the constant support of my family, friends, doctors, and nurses. My role was to find the inner strength and determination to fight back. I hope if I was ever put to the test again I would be able to fight back—I know now I would try. Life is far more precious to me now.[17,pp.17–18]

Trajectory phasing of changes in the course of the chronic illness[15] is exemplified by Evans as well. The eight phases of chronic illness are presented in Table 19-1.[15] Within or between phases, periods of reversal, plateau, or upward or downward movement may occur. Individuals, families, significant others, and professionals formulate trajectory projections based on

TABLE 19-1 Phases of Chronic Illness Trajectory

Phase	Definition
Pretrajectory	Before the illness course begins, the preventive phase, no signs or symptoms present
Trajectory onset	Signs and symptoms are present; includes diagnostic period
Crisis	Life-threatening situation requiring emergency or critical care
Acute	Active illness or complications that require hospitalization for management
Stable	Illness course and/or symptoms controlled by regimen
Unstable	Illness course and/or symptoms not controlled by regimen but not requiring hospitalization
Downward	Progressive deterioration in physical or mental status characterized by increasing disability and symptoms
Dying	Immediate weeks, day, hours preceding death

Source: Corbin JM, Strauss A: A nursing model for chronic illness management based upon the Trajectory Framework, *Scholarly Inquiry for Nursing Practice: An Internaional Journal* 5(3):155–174, 1991. Copyright Springer Publishing Company, Inc., New York, NY 10012. Used by permission.

knowledge, experience, hearsay, and beliefs.[18] Among these groups, projections can be similar or disparate, resulting in either facilitative or destructive effects on the management of the course of the disease. The plan to shape the trajectory is called the *trajectory scheme,* which functions to shape the overall illness course, to control symptoms, and to handle disability.

Available resources, past experiences, motivation, setting of care, lifestyles, beliefs, interactions among groups, type of illness, degree of physiological involvement, symptom distress, and the political and economic climate of health care influence trajectory management. The outcome goal is to maintain quality of life throughout all phases of the illness, and the nursing process is structured by the trajectory framework to achieve this goal. For example, nursing assessment includes determining strengths and weaknesses of the client and the family in managing the illness trajectory. Nursing care plans reflect mutual goal setting of the patient, family, significant others, and professional. Goals are phase-specific, such as "overcoming a plateau by enhancing self-care" or "dealing with an unstable phase by promoting symptom control." A third step involves identification of a target intervention, such as an inaccurate trajectory projection. Intervention, in this case, may focus on enhancing patient/family knowledge of the illness. Evaluation is focused on "progress toward change, rather than change itself."[15,p.170] Evaluation is dynamic, considering responses to changes in the illness, biography, and ability to perform activities of daily living over the illness trajectory. Further use of the model in practice is recommended to establish the usefulness and limitations of the model in various chronic illnesses.[15]

Defining chronic illness as "incurable" and identifying the last phase of the trajectory as "dying" are bothersome when applying this theory specifically to cancer during an era of longer survival and higher cure rates. Scott-Dorsett proposed instead a trajectory of cancer recovery.[19] The recovery model is oriented by survival versus dying, and emphasizes self-care over professional intervention. Recovery in this alternative model is composed of the processes of absorption (intake and integration of information), assimilation (synthesis and assignment of meaning), and accommodation (alterations, reconciliations, and transformations). Recovery is therefore "multidimensional, having physical, cognitive, and affective dimensions that are interrelated by structure, process, and outcome manifestations."[19,p.179] Self-care, social, and professional support can strengthen recovery and influence quality of life throughout the recovery process. The Integrated Cancer Recovery Model[20] is depicted in Figure 19-2.

Both trajectories stress the chronicity of cancer, the physical and psychosocial complexity of the course of the illness, and the awesome task of nursing in personalizing and coordinating the care of persons with cancer, especially in times of rapid change and escalating technology. The coexistence of both models may be mediated by changes in cancer and treatment. For example, the emergency of HIV-related cancers constitutes a group for which the dying trajectory is more applicable. Prior to the 1950s, children diagnosed with leukemia fit the dying course exclusively, but advances in treatment have made the recovery model increasingly more applicable.

In summary, the term, *trajectory*—used to describe the experiences of an individual moving through predictable and orderly responses to cancer—is simply not practical. In reality, patients describe the cancer experience as a roller coaster ride of real or probable cancer remissions and recurrences.

INDIVIDUAL RESPONSES TO CANCER

Help-Seeking Responses

The search for psychosocial resources to deal with the actual or potential threat of cancer generally is initiated in terms of self-appraisal, and can be conceptualized as expanding spheres to significant others and finally to members of the health care professions. Orem,[21] in emphasizing the self-care concept, heightened the awareness of the professional with respect to the fact that the initial help-seeking behaviors expand outward from the

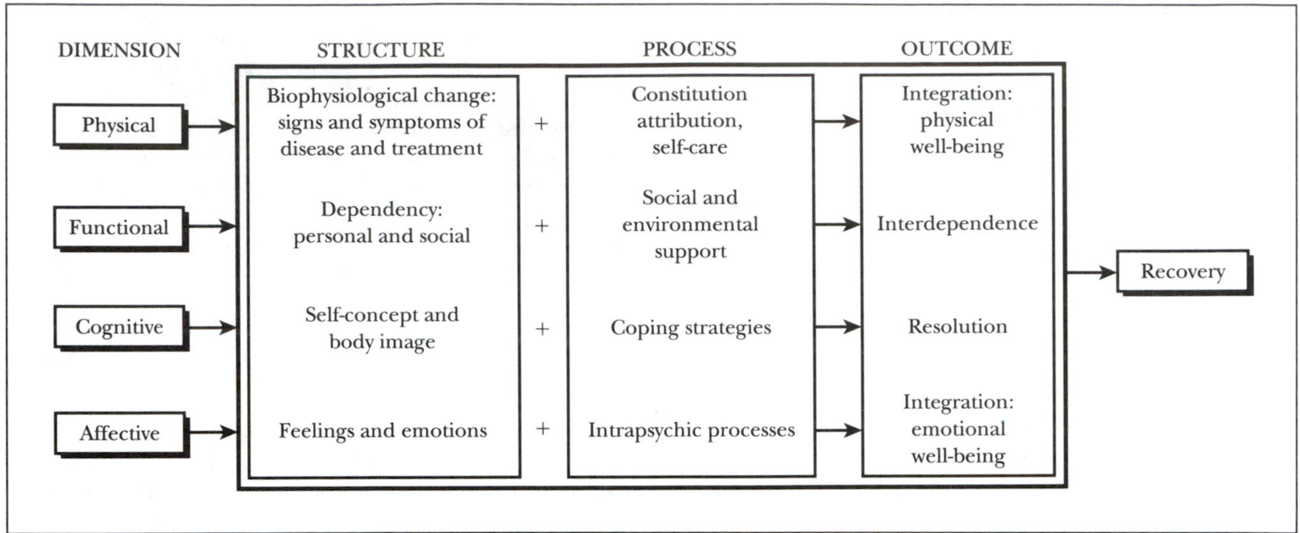

FIGURE 19-2 Integrated Cancer Recovery Model. (Source: Scott-Dorsett D: The trajectory of cancer recovery. *Scholarly Inquiry for Nursing Practice: An International Journal* 5(3):175–184, 1991. Copyright Springer Publishing Company, Inc., New York, NY 10012. Used by permission).

individual, to significant others, to the professional; likewise the return to health should be manifest by the professional's returning the responsibility for health care to the family and ultimately to the patient.

Culturally Determined Responses

The specific culture of the individual shapes the view of health in terms of the range of normal, cause-and-effect perceptions, and the language to describe deviations from normal. For example, in a culture in which life expectancy is short, cancer may be a less meaningful threat than in a culture in which the chronic diseases of aging are the leading causes of death.[22]

The repertoire of health and illness responses and behaviors of the individual are acquired primarily through lifelong socialization. For example, children of adults who resolve grief processes successfully have been found to adjust more constructively to losses later in life. However, cultural determinants of health behavior cannot be separated from socioenvironmental factors. Freeman,[23] in studying differences in help-seeking behaviors among African Americans with cancer found that socioeconomic factors were more strongly related than ethnicity to health behaviors that were related to lower survival. The socioeconomically disadvantaged must expend a preponderance of both material and psychosocial responses on daily survival; therefore, coping and health promotion responses are, of necessity, compromised. Nursing responses to delays in diagnosis, "noncompliant" behaviors, or self-neglect tend to be judgmental and accusatory when the sociocultural context of the individual is not explored sufficiently.

Furthermore, the culture, through socialization, shapes the more enduring aspects of the attitudes, beliefs, and values that constitute an individual's personality and that provide continuity in the reordering of the meaning of life and of a relationship to a higher being. Cancer can challenge lifelong values and beliefs and may result in changed cognitive, affective, and behavioral responses.[22] Affective responses identified as occurring most frequently among individuals with cancer are anxiety and depression. No one response, per se, is either adaptive or maladaptive. The appropriateness of the response to the psychosocially constructed reality of the situation and adaptability of the social network in acquiring new patterns of response, as indicated, determine the adaptive potential of the specific response.

Stress, Emotions, and Coping Responses

Psychological stress is defined by Lazarus and Folkman[24] as "a particular kind of relationship between person and environment . . . in which demands tax or exceed the person's resources."[25,p.3] Stress is further delineated as "a system of interdependent processes, including appraisal and coping, which mediate the frequency, intensity, duration, and type of psychological and somatic responses."[26,p.486]

Stress is not an inherent characteristic of the person or the environment, but is defined by the constantly changing individual appraisal of threat, harm, or challenge in the situation.[25] Appraisal of person–environment relationships is a cognitive process influenced by preexisting personality traits, developmental level, values, and perceived resources.[25]

Lazarus[25] described two forms of appraisal, primary and secondary. *Primary* appraisal includes perceptions of the meaning and potential outcomes of the situation

TABLE 19-2 Illustrative System Variables for the Stress and Emotion Process

Causal Antecedent →	Mediating Process →	Immediate Effect →	Long-term Effect
Person variables: values, commitments, goals		Encounter 1 . . . . 2 . . . 3 . . . *n* Within an encounter: Time 1 . . . . 2 . . . 3 . . . *n*	
General beliefs: self-esteem, mastery, sense of control, interpersonal trust, existential beliefs	Primary appraisal *(stakes)* Secondary appraisal *(coping options)*	Affect Physiological changes	Psychological well-being Somatic health/illness
Environmental variables: demands, resources, constraints, temporal aspects	Coping (including use of social support); problem-focused forms emotion-focused forms	Quality of encounter outcomes	Social functioning

Note: Although not shown here, the model is recursive. Also, note the parallelism between short-term and long-term effects.
Source: Lazarus RS: Theory-based stress measurement. *Psychological Inquiry* 1(1):3–13, 1990.

and thereby influences the type and intensity of emotional response. *Secondary* appraisal is more problem-focused and influences the coping strategies selected. Thus coping "consists of cognitive and behavioral efforts to manage specific external and/or internal demands that are appraised as taxing or exceeding the resources of the individual."[27,p.310] Empirical studies of stress indicate that both problem- and emotion-focused coping are used in stressful encounters. Both types of coping have multiple dimensions. Problem-focused coping includes confrontative and interpersonal strategies; emotion-focused strategies identified are distancing, escape-avoidance, accepting responsibility or blame, self-control over feelings, seeking self-support, and positive reappraisal.[28,29]

Application of stress management theory to the cancer experience makes the health professional attentive to the fact that the initial adaptive responses used by patients may be outmoded as the disease process and treatment change.[14] For example, denial may be adaptive in the early stages of the disease as a defense mechanism, allowing the adapting individuals to assimilate the impact of the illness in manageable increments of awareness. By the same token, persistent denial may block motivation or adaptive health behavior in later stages of the illness. Likewise, the preoccupation with self that is characteristic during diagnosis and recurrence may initiate problem-solving coping behaviors during these stressful events, but may alienate one's social and professional network if persistent.

A further implication of the usefulness of stress theory in understanding psychosocial responses is the consideration of the effect of cumulative stressors on the ability to adapt. Individuals come to the cancer experience with a history of stress responses. The individual who has been unsuccessful in resolving past stress situations, who is dealing with a number of stressors simultaneously, and who perceives minimal social support in the situation is at higher risk for psychosocial distress.

Recent theory by Lazarus and colleagues suggests the study of stress under the broader context of emotion.[27–29] *Emotion* is defined as "complex, organized psychophysiological reactions consisting of cognitive appraisals, action impulses, and somatic reactions."[27,p.310] The advantage of the emotion and stress model (Table 19-2)[25,p.4] is the provision of a theoretical base for measuring the multidimensionality of human responses to stress as opposed to many of the currently used unidimensional instruments. Furthermore, positive emotions, such as love or happiness, are included, as opposed to focusing exclusively on the more negative stress-induced reactions, such as anger, fear, and anxiety. The goal is to determine the effect of both positive and negative emotions on health.[25]

SOCIAL AND FAMILY RESPONSES TO THE STRESS OF CANCER

Cognitive appraisal of the stress of cancer includes perceptions of the existence and quality of social support systems. As noted earlier, social stigmas and prejudice against persons with cancer may impede coping, while supportive relationships at home and in the community may buffer individual responses. The return to work, for example, may influence the level of stress, depending on the perceived reactions of co-workers and the self-esteem of the individual. Postulated mechanisms of the buffering effect of perceived social support include diminishing the level of the perceived stress of the situation, facilitating coping effectiveness, and lessening the reactions of the individual to the stressors.[30] Recent efforts to facilitate reintegration into the school or workplace are based on the recognition of the role of social networks in facilitating coping with daily stress and the stress of illness.[31]

The family of origin or choice generally constitutes

the most important social support for the individual throughout the life span. When a person is diagnosed with cancer, the family becomes a source of information, nurturance, and validation.[32] In turn, the diagnosis of cancer becomes a stressor changing the family system[33] with respect to daily activities, expectations, roles, boundaries, patterns, and values.

The numerous theoretical frameworks in use for studying the family are derived primarily from these basic approaches: interactional, structural-functional, and developmental theories. The outline delineated in Table 19-3 provides an abbreviated overview of the theoretical components of each theory and general approaches to intervention.[35] These basic theoretical orientations have been expanded and restructured as the field of family therapy has grown. Numerous instruments to measure the concepts and test the major propositions have been developed and used for both clinical and empirical purposes. Further discussion of instruments will be found in Chapter 21.

Family forms have changed with changes in the social milieu. These trends include increased heterogeneity of lifestyles, influenced particularly by the expanding population of elderly, increased personal freedom of the individual, changes in philosophy and family values, and changing views of society.[35,p.92] The principal implication for the professional is that personal definitions of the family or family values may vary from those of patients. In essence, the family is defined by the patient, and values of the health care providers should not be imposed on others or interfere with interactional processes.

TABLE 19-3 Comparison of Family Theories

	Symbolic Interactionalism	Structual-Functional	Developmental
Defintion of Family	A dynamic, changing group of interacting personalities	A system organized by functional demands both at the internal level and as a subsystem of society	A unit of members advancing through various stages of the family life cycle
Basic Assumption	Human beings are actors as well as reactors, evoking meaning and values from the social milieu.	The family is a subsystem of society that must satisfy certain functional requirements if society is to survive at a given level.	Individuals and families must accomplish the tasks of each sequential stage of development to deal successfully with the successive stage.
Concepts	Interaction, social act, definition of the situation, significant other, communication, reference group, self, adaptation, role	Society, equilibrium, structure, function, role differentiation, instrumental behavior, expressive behavior, rules, boundaries	Development, role, position, norm, developmental tasks, family life cycle
Principal Proposition	Interactions and perceptions of relationships in the family are the basis for the development of self, self-esteem, and personality.	Clarity of boundaries is a measure of functional status; change in position of one family member changes the position of the others.	The family changes over time due to changes in age, composition, plurality patterns, school or job placement, and the function and status of the family within the context of the larger society.
Units of Analysis	Communication processes, patterns of interaction, individual definitions of the situation, rules of interaction, role taking, and social context or interaction	Transactional patterns, clarity of boundaries, role differentiation, subsystems, value systems, power structure, societal functions	Stages of the family life cycle, developmental tasks, critical periods, multiple generations, loss/addition of members, demoralization, crises of the life cycle
Assessment	Family interaction patterns, rules of communication, feedback mechanisms, perceptions, range of responses, power structure	Transaction patterns (conflict/coalitions, bonding, decision making, task allocation, role enactment, rules, communications), flexibility, sensitivity to member relationships, sources of support and stress, developmental stage	Family structure, sociocultural variables, stage-specific developmental tasks of individuals and family, tasks performance, current crisis, family attitudes toward crisis, tension reducing aspirations of family, loss/addition of members, demoralization, role or financial strains, threats to task or identity

(continued)

TABLE 19-3 Comparison of Family Theories (continued)

	Symbolic Interactionalism	Structual-Functional	Developmental
Diagnoses	Patterns of interaction (congruence, complementarity), dysfunctional communications (blaming, mixed messages, double binds, power struggles, failure to assume responsibilities)	Strains in relationships, lack of patterned relationships	Conformity, goals achievement, identity problems, resource problems
Intervention	Identify strengths and weaknesses of interaction patterns, determine degree of change possible, disturb family system, change communication patterns, evaluate goal attainment	Disrupt equilibrium, decrease stereotypic responses and increase alternate responses, change structure, change dysfunctional behavior, restructure alliances or interdependencies, evaluate effect of change in subsystem on total family system	Anticipatory guidance, crisis intervention, deal with grief and loss, enhance family resources
Therapeutic strategies	Role modeling, stress reduction, motivation, initiation	Care provider "joins" family, creates conditions that allow change, short-term therapy, evaluates outcomes.	Anticipatory guidance, crisis intervention, developmental task identification
Valued Outcomes	Happiness, adjustment, conformity, adaptation, mutual enjoyment, complementarity of needs	Creation and distribution of goods/roles, goal gratification, pattern maintenance.	Individual and family goal achievement, self-identity, resource availability, prevention of crises

PROFESSIONAL RESPONSES TO CANCER

Distancing

Distancing has been described as an unconscious versus a deliberate response of professionals, especially to persons who are dying.[36] Behaviors manifesting distancing include delays in answering call lights, infrequent visitations, failure to communicate, and maintaining "professionalism" in highly emotional situations. Maguire[37] found that "distancing tactics" are especially prevalent when the patient is not told the truth or when members of the health care team fail to communicate openly. Such behaviors enhance the loneliness and fear of the seriously ill.

Professionals who are well versed in the thanatology literature and have come to terms with death as a part of humanity appear to have less need to use distancing. Repeated losses are inevitable in the field of oncology. Professionals who feel comfortable in buffering these losses by allowing themselves to go through the grieving process are less likely to practice distancing as a self-serving behavior. Youll[36] suggests that personal qualities such as genuine concern, flexibility, and being a good listener further lessen professional distancing.

In contrast to distancing, nurses with high levels of interpersonal competence use communications strategically to effect behavioral changes, comfort, establish and maintain relationships, create a positive self-image for the patient, and relay information.[39] Strategic communication skills can be enhanced with study, evaluation, and the use of feedback. Use of communication experts to provide constructive feedback on videotape and audiotape monitoring are but two strategies for enhancing competence. Multidisciplinary conferences dealing with psychosocial needs of patients and families, led by a psychiatrist or a psychiatric nurse, have been found to facilitate communication skills by providing expert role models. Identification of objectives prior to the conference and follow-up evaluation of strategies that facilitated or blocked goal attainment provide the basis for self-evaluation and further skill development.

Caring

Historically, the importance of caring was assumed to be so universal to nursing that minimal attention was directed toward elucidating the theoretical and empirical aspects of the concept. Only recently has nursing followed the impetus originally set forth by theology and other disciplines to define and to study caring more systematically.[39]

Watson defined *caring* as a process that helps a person attain or maintain health or a peaceful death.[40,p.2] The professional aspects of care were further delineated by Leininger as cognitive and culturally learned action behaviors, techniques, processes, or patterns that help an individual, family, or community to maintain health. Emphasis is placed on care as a process, as action-oriented, and as helpful in intent. Curing is considered a subset of caring, or more specifically curing cannot occur without caring, but caring can occur without cure.[41]

Traditionally, medicine has been aligned with curing, which is based in science and technology, and nursing has been aligned with caring, which originated in the altruistic ideals of religious orders and is based on the psychosocial or so-called "soft" sciences. Valentine[39] traced the waxing and waning of the importance of the concept as the basis, focus, and status of the two professions were shaped by societal changes. Some argue that the caring dimension is waning in the present era of specialization and high technology, both of which foster fragmentation and depersonalization. Others argue that the emergence of the consumer demands for personalized services,[42] increasing emphasis on self-care, public misgivings regarding the motivations and healing potential of health care professionals, increasing incidence of chronic illnesses, decreasing rates of acute diseases, and economic constraints compel further attention to a collaborative relationship between health care providers, one that focuses on a team approach to caring rather than on a hierarchical or discipline-centered approach.

A recent content analysis of the nursing literature on the concept of caring revealed that caring has been defined as a human trait, moral imperative or ideal, affect, interpersonal relationship, and therapeutic intervention.[43,p.3] Caring among nurses generally refers to the quality of nurse–client (individual, family, or community) interactions and relationships.[44,p.74] The philosophy of caring is a moral commitment to protect human dignity. The caring commitment is grounded in human values such as kindness, helpfulness, concern, and love of self and others.[44]

Operationally, caring begins with interest in another, is expanded through knowledge, and becomes a commitment to assisting the person to exist and to grow. Empirical studies have shown that clients define caring behaviors among nurses as: both physical care that is humane (considerate, competent, gentle, timely, and accessible) and emotional care that includes concern, involvement, sharing, touching (when culturally condoned), voluntary presence, and humor. Nurses identified most of the same aspects as patients, with added concern for actions such as patient safety, planning for the future, and counseling. The primary consensus is that caring is the essence of nursing and that further study is imperative.[45]

A principal outcome of caring is to add meaning to the life of the caregiver and that of the recipient.[44] Mutual self-actualization is a recurrent theme of caring in the nursing literature. More specifically, the concept of *therapeutic reciprocity* has been operationally defined as "a mutual, collaborative, probabilistic, instructive, and empowering exchange of feelings, thoughts, and behaviors between nurse and client for the purpose of enhancing the human outcomes of the relationship for all parties concerned."[46,p.57] Two potentially negative outcomes of caring for the nurse are overinvolvement and burnout, both of which may be countered with supportive collegial relationships. Caring can be learned through strategies such as education, self-evaluation of clinical techniques, and role modeling.

Two recurrent client outcomes of caring identified by a literature review by Morse et al. include the subjective experience of the patient and the physical response of the patient.[43] Leininger[41] contends that caring should be culturally specific; otherwise, unintended, negative outcomes will result.

PSYCHOSOCIAL OUTCOMES

Self-Care

The goal of promoting self-care by clients has a long tradition in nursing, including the Nightingale model[47] and the Orem theory of nursing.[21] Broadly defined, self-care includes attempts of the individual to promote optimal health, prevent illness, detect symptoms, and manage chronic illness. Processes for achieving these goals include selecting healthy lifestyles, self-monitoring and assessing symptoms, perceiving and assigning meaning to symptoms, evaluating the severity of the situation, and determining treatment alternatives. Alternatives selected reflect sociocultural patterns, current stressors, and perceived resources; therefore, individuals can be expected to choose self-medications, denial, unproven methods, and spiritual cures, to name but a few alternatives, in addition to or instead of the traditional health care system.[48]

Self-care also is culturally specific;[49] therefore, the most successful selection of self-care strategies is based on knowledge of the cultural patterns of the recipient of care. Strategies include mutual goal setting, information giving, assisting with decision-making processes, assisting with problem-solving techniques, behavioral contracting, providing opportunities for expression of personal preferences, and professional support for patient decisions and preferences.

Outcomes of self-care behaviors include reduction in morbidity associated with the illness, increased use of health resources, lowered cost of health care, more effective coping strategies, enhanced role performance, increased independence in health-related and/or daily living activities, increased frequency of health promotion behaviors, and enhanced self-esteem and well-being.[50] Further research on self-care is ongoing, but the emerging tendency of special significance to nursing is that with aging, physical symptoms are more often attributed to aging than to pathology. The outcome is a delay in initiating self-care processes.[51] In oncology, delays in seeking treatment result in increased morbidity and mortality; therefore, the elderly should be a target group for empirical and clinical studies.

Survival

When psychosocial interventions are studied, the expected outcomes generally relate to improved mood, psychological adjustment, or decreased symptom distress. One of the rare studies of the prospective effect of psychosocial interventions on survival is worth noting,[52] primarily because one weakness of other studies may be the lack of longitudinal data or other methodological problems. The sample studied was 86 patients with metastatic breast cancer. A battery of psychological tests was administered to all subjects. Then subjects were randomly assigned to the intervention (1 year of weekly support groups and being taught self-hypnosis) or to the control group. Follow-up for the first year was every 4 months. At the end of 1 year the researchers found no evidence of improved survival within the treatment group. At the end of 10 years only three subjects survived, and a significantly longer survival time was found for the treatment group. Differences were attributed to the coping strategies learned in the support group, such as countering social isolation through developing strong relationships among group members, achieving more assertiveness in determining health care, finding meaning in the situation, and anticipatory grieving for losses.

Survival has been studied extensively in conjunction with clinical trials, but less systematically in terms of psychosocial intervention. Large, randomized, controlled, clinical trials may clarify the significance of survival as an outcome of psychosocial aspects of care.

Quality of Life

Schipper described *quality of life* as a relatively precise, operationally defined patient outcome variable.[52] The concept broadens the outcome measure from survival of the individual to the effects on the patient, family, and community. Quality of life, according to Cella[53] is a construct that has two aspects. First, survival is subjective, reflecting the concerns of the patient. Second, multiple dimensions are involved: physical, functional, emotional, and social.

The concept reflects the goals of alleviation of effects of illness and treatment, allaying negative emotional responses, promoting well-being, restoring the individual to societal roles, and achieving maximal physical, social, and psychological functioning. Further discussion of quality-of-life issues is found in Chapter 10.

SUMMARY

The importance of psychosocial nursing is reflected in the taxonomy of nursing diagnoses developed in a series of National Conferences for Classification of Nursing Diagnosis (NANDA). NANDA includes individual and family diagnoses that relate to physical, emotional, and social aspects of care. The diagnoses also reflect the fact that psychosocial responses include the potential both for distress and for growth. Nursing interventions to achieve the latter have been studied extensively, but methodological problems and the complexity of human behavior make the accumulation of definitive data a continuing challenge.

This chapter is intended to provide selected theoretical underpinnings of the subsequent chapters in this section. Implications for nursing practice are included, as appropriate, but will be discussed further in the following three chapters, which explore individual and family responses to cancer and survivorship.

REFERENCES

1. Cooper CL: The social psychological precursors to cancer. In Cooper CL (ed.): *Psychosocial Stress and Cancer.* New York: Wiley, pp. 21–33, 1984.
2. Lickiss JN: The growing edge: Psychosocial aspects of cancer. *Med J Austral* 1:297–302, 1980.
3. Greer S: Psychological enquiry: A contribution to cancer research. *Psycholog Med* 9:81–89, 1979.
4. Farber JM, Weinerman BH, Kuypers JA: Psychosocial distress in oncology outpatients. *J Psychosoc Oncol* 2:109–118, 1984.
5. Cassileth BR: The evolution of oncology as a sociomedical phenomenon. In Cassileth BR (ed): *The Cancer Patient: Social and Medical Aspects of Care.* Philadelphia: Lea & Febiger, 1979, pp. 3–15.
6. Weisman AD, Worden JW: The existential plight in cancer: Significance of the first 100 days. *Internatl J Psychiatry Med* 7:1–15, 1976/1977.
7. Cox T: Stress: A psychophysiological approach to cancer. In Cooper CL (ed.): *Psychosocial Stress and Cancer.* New York: Wiley, 1984, pp. 149–169.
8. Clark RL: Psychologic reactions of patients and health professionals to cancer. In Cullen JW, Fox BH, Isom RN (eds.): *Cancer: The Behavioral Dimensions.* New York: Raven Press, 1976, pp. 1–10.
9. Smith JA: The idea of health: A philosophical inquiry. *ANS* 3:43–50, 1981.
10. Mishel MH: Uncertainty in illness. *Image* 20:225–232, 1988.
11. Mishel MH, Braden CJ: Finding meaning: Antecedents of uncertainty in illness. *Nurs Res* 37:98–103,127, 1988.
12. Festinger L: A theory of social comparison processes. *Human Relations* 7:117–140, 1954.
13. Taylor SE, Lobel M: Social comparison activity under threat: Downward evaluation and upward contacts. *Psychological Rev* 96:569–575, 1989.

14. Mages NL, Mendelsohn GA: Effects of cancer on patients' lives: A personological approach. In GC Stone, F Cohen, NE Adler, (eds.): *Health Psychology: A Handbook.* San Francisco: Jossey-Bass, 1979, pp. 255–284.
15. Corbin JM, Strauss A. A nursing model for chronic illness management based upon the Trajectory Framework. *Scholar Inq Nurs Prac* 5:155–174, 1991.
16. Gove PB (ed.): *Webster's Third New International Dictionary of the English Language, Unabridged.* Springfield, MA: G&C Merriam, 1961, p. 2425.
17. Evans J: The cancer experience—A patient's view. In Pritchard AP (ed.): *Cancer Nursing: A Revolution in Care,* Proceedings of the Fifth International Conference on Cancer Nursing. London: Macmillan 1989, pp. 17–18.
18. Thorne SE, Robinson CA: Health care relationships: The chronic illness perspective. *Res Nurs Health* 11:293–300, 1988.
19. Dorsett DS: The trajectory of cancer recovery. *Scholar Inq Nurs Prac* 5:175–184, 1991.
20. Scott-Dorsett DW, Eisendrath SJ: Dynamics of the recovery process following diagnosis of breast cancer. *J Psychosoc Oncol* 3:53–65, 1986.
21. Orem DE: *Nursing: Concepts of Practice* (ed. 4). New York: McGraw-Hill, 1991.
22. Haney CA: Psychosocial factors in the management of patients with cancer. In Cooper CL (ed.): *Psychosocial Stress and Cancer.* New York: Wiley, 1984, pp. 201–227.
23. Freeman HP: Cancer in the socioeconomically disadvantaged. *CA:* 39:266–288, 1989.
24. Lazarus RS, Folkman S: *Stress, Appraisal, and Coping.* New York: Springer, 1984.
25. Lazarus RS: Theory-based stress measurement. *Psychological Inq* 1:3–13, 1990.
26. DeLongis A, Folkman S, Lazarus RS: The impact of daily stress on health and mood: Psychological and social resources as mediators. *J Personal Soc Psychol* 54:486–495, 1988.
27. Folkman S, Lazarus RS: The relationship between coping and emotion: Implications for theory and research. *Social Sci Med* 26:309–317, 1988.
28. Lazarus RS, Averill JR, Opton EM: Toward a cognitive theory of emotions. In Arnold MB (ed.): *Feelings and Emotions: The Loyola Symposium.* New York: Academic Press, 1970, pp. 207–232.
29. Lazarus RS, Kanner AD, Folkman S: Emotions: A cognitive-phenomenological analysis. In Plutchik R, Kellerman H (eds.): *Theories of Emotions.* New York: Academic Press, 1980, pp. 189–217.
30. House JS: *Work, Stress and Social Support.* Reading, MA: Addison-Wesley, 1981.
31. Clark JC, Landis LL: Reintegration and maintenance of employees with breast cancer in the workplace. *AAOHN Journal* 37:186–193, 1989.
32. Herndon A, Quinn WH: The family ecology of cancer. *J Psychosoc Oncol* 4:45–59, 1986.
33. McCubbin HI, Patterson JM: Family transitions: Adaptation to stress. In McCubbin HI, Figley CR (eds.): *Stress and the Family.* Vol I: Coping with Normative Transitions. New York: Brunner Mazel, 1983, pp. 5–25.
34. Nye FI, Berardo FM: *Emerging Conceptual Frameworks in Family Analysis.* New York: Macmillan, 1966.
35. Rubin RH: Epilogue: Families and alternative lifestyles in an age of technological revolution. In Macklin ED, Rubin RH (eds.): *Contemporary Families and Alternative Lifestyles.* Beverly Hills, CA: Sage, 1983, pp. 400–409.
36. Youll JW: The bridge beyond: Strengthening nursing practice in attitudes towards death, dying, and the terminally ill, and helping the spouses of critically ill patients. *Intens Care Nurs* 5:88–94, 1989.
37. Maguire P: Barriers to psychological care of the dying. *Brit Med J* 291:1711–1713. 1985.
38. Kasch CR, Lisnek PM: Role of strategic communication in nursing theory and research. *ANS* 7:56–71, 1984.
39. Valentine KL: History, analysis, and application of the carative tradition in health and nursing. *J NY State Nurses Assoc* 19:4–9, 1988.
40. Watson J: Nursing: The Philosophy and Science of Caring, Boston, MA: Little, Brown, 1979.
41. Leininger M: Some philosophical, historical, and taxonomic aspects of nursing and caring in the American culture. In Leninger MM (ed.): *Caring: An Essential Human Need.* Proceedings of Three National Caring Conferences. Thorofare, NJ: Charles B. Slack, 1981, pp. 133–143.
42. Curtin LL: Nursing in the year 2000: Learning from the future. *Nurs Manage* 17:7–8, 1986.
43. Morse JM, Solberg SM, Neander WL, et al: Concepts of caring and caring as a concept. *ANS* 13:1–14, 1990.
44. Nyberg J: Theoretic explorations of human care and economics: Foundations of nursing administration practice. *ANS*13:74–84, 1990.
45. Warren LD: Review and synthesis of nine nursing studies on care and caring. *J NY State Nurses Assoc* 19:10–16, 1988.
46. Marck P: Therapeutic reciprocity: A caring phenomenon. *ANS*13:49–59, 1990.
47. Nightengale F: *Notes on Nursing: What It Is and What It Is Not.* Philadelphia: Lippincott, 1859 (reprinted 1946).
48. Woods N: Conceptualizations of self-care: Toward health-oriented models. *ANS* 12:1–13, 1989.
49. Mechanic D: *Medical Sociology: A Selective View.* New York: Free Press, 1968.
50. Keller ML, Ward S, Baumann LJ: Processes of self-care: Monitoring sensations and symptoms. *ANS* 12:54–66, 1989.
51. Spiegel D, Bloom JR, Kraemer HC, Gottheil E: Effect of psychosocial treatment on survival of patients with metastatic breast cancer. *Lancet* 2:888–891, 1989.
52. Schipper H: Quality of life: Principles of the clinical paradigm. *J Psychosoc Oncol* 8:171–185, 1990.
53. Cella DF: Functional status and quality of life: Current views on measurement and intervention. In *Selected Papers from First National Conference on Cancer Nursing Research,* In *Functional Status and Quality of Life in Persons with Cancer.* Atlanta: American Cancer Society, 1989 (Publication #91-3332-02, pp. 1–12).

Chapter 20

Psychosocial Responses of the Patient

Jane Clark, RN, MN, OCN

INTRODUCTION

Psychosocial responses to cancer are influenced by factors that create the perceived reality of cancer for the individual. The reality of the cancer experience is complex and uncertain and results in psychosocial responses that are dynamic, nonlinear, and nonhierarchical and that vary in severity. The complex intrapersonal and interpersonal reactions to the cancer experience mandate that health care professionals share a common concern and maintain a high index of suspicion for the occurrence of dysfunctional psychosocial responses. Focusing on systematic and continuous assessment for signs and symptoms of psychosocial responses, identification of dysfunctional responses, development of interdisciplinary interventions to facilitate adaptive psychosocial responses, and evaluation of the effectiveness and efficiency of selected interventions to meet identified needs can improve both the quantity and quality of survival for people with cancer.

What is the basis of psychosocial care in oncology? Historically, clinical case studies of individuals and groups experiencing cancer were used to identify the unique psychosocial responses to cancer, to describe the types of coping patterns among persons with cancer, and to guide health care professionals in assisting the person with cancer to adapt to the diagnosis, the demands of treatment, and the demands of living with a cancer diagnosis. Yet just as significant variability exists in physiologic responses to cancer of different sites as well as within the same site, the variability of psychosocial responses is multiplied by the fact that each individual brings his or her values, beliefs, attitudes, personality, resources, and coping patterns to the cancer experience.

Efforts of health care professionals to understand the unique psychosocial responses of persons with cancer have been enhanced through qualitative studies of the relationship of selected psychosocial variables to:

1. Physiologic factors, such as site of cancer, histology, grade, stage of disease, or treatment modality
2. Care settings, including primary, secondary, and tertiary care hospitals, outpatient clinics, and the home
3. Temporal elements of the disease trajectory, ranging from screening to diagnosis, primary treatment, recurrence or relapse, death, or long-term survival
4. Developmental stage of the individual, with emphasis on the responses of children and older adults

Yet the findings from qualitative studies often yielded conflicting results. Thus, health care professionals began to examine conceptual and theoretical inconsistencies of both clinical and empirical data. Recently researchers have focused on developing clarity and specificity in describing the psychosocial responses of persons with cancer. The development of instruments with acceptable reliability and validity estimates among persons with cancer, expansion of research methodologies to include qualitative methods, and development of advanced statistical modeling procedures to study the interaction of psychosocial responses both as dependent and independent variables have contributed to understanding complex psychosocial relationships.

The focus of this chapter is the psychosocial responses that are of high incidence among persons with cancer. Responses selected include anxiety, depression, hopelessness, and altered sexual health. An operational definition of each response has been developed. Selected research and clinical instruments to measure the response are described and a review of representative research articles addressing the incidence and relationship of the response to the cancer experience is presented. Finally, areas for future nursing research are suggested.

ANXIETY

Anxiety has been described, with depression, as the most common psychosocial reaction experienced by persons with cancer. However, limited data exist on the occurrence and patterns of anxiety in persons with cancer. Often associated with transitions in the course of the disease or treatment, anxiety is described as a recurring response, varying in levels of intensity throughout the cancer experience.

Operational Definition

Operationally, anxiety can be defined as follows:

- An individual exists with the ability to respond affectively to changes in the environment.
- The individual perceives certain beliefs, values, and conditions essential to a secure existence.
- The individual experiences a nonspecific internal or external stimulus that is perceived as a threat to the secure existence.
- *The individual responds to the perceived threat affectively with an increased level of arousal associated with vague, unpleasant, and uneasy feelings defined as anxiety.*

Measurement Instrument: State-Trait Anxiety Inventory

The instrument used most commonly to measure anxiety among persons with cancer is the State-Trait Anxiety Inventory (STAI).[1] The STAI consists of two scales, the A-trait and A-state. Subjects are asked to respond to 20 items (A-state) on a 4-point scale (not at all, somewhat, moderately so, and very much so). Responses are summed to measure how the subject feels at a particular moment. Scores indicate the level of transitory anxiety characterized by feelings of apprehension, tension, and autonomic nervous system–induced symptoms: nervousness, worry, and apprehension.

The trait inventory is designed to measure general level of arousal and predict anxiety proneness. Subjects are asked to respond to 20 items (A-trait) on a 4-point scale (almost never, sometimes, often, and almost always). Again, responses are summed to measure disposition to respond to a stressful situation with varying levels of A-state intensity and the degree to which presenting stimuli are perceived as dangerous or threatening. Scores range from 20 to 80 for each scale, with a higher score representing higher levels of anxiety.

Reliability estimates for the STAI have been reported in the alpha coefficient range of .83 to .92. Construct validity has been reported as point biserial ranges of .60 to .73 and alpha ranges of .83 to .94. Concurrent validity has been established with the Taylor Manifest Anxiety Scale ($r = .79$ to .83) and the Affect Adjective Checklist ($r = .51$ to .52). In addition, construct validity with the known groups technique has been established.[1]

Patterns of Occurrence

The occurrence of anxiety as a response to the diagnosis and treatment of cancer was described in the literature by Lucente and Fleck,[2] who compared levels of anxiety between patients hospitalized with a diagnosis of cancer and with a nonmalignant condition. Findings indicated greater levels of anxiety in the group with a diagnosis of cancer. Similar findings have been reported by other researchers.[3,4]

Anxiety is increased at diagnosis and remains elevated in varying levels throughout the course of treatment regardless of treatment modality or setting. Surgery as a treatment modality in general elicits an anxiety response, yet when the surgery is for cancer, the response may be more severe. Morris and Royle[5] reported preoperative and postoperative levels of clinical anxiety among 20 patients with early breast cancer given a choice of surgery (simple mastectomy or wide excision and radiotherapy) and 10 patients not given a choice. Findings indicate that a significantly higher percentage of patients not offered a choice of surgery were clinically anxious preoperatively when compared with those patients given a choice ($p < .05$). For those patients offered a choice, no significant differences in clinical anxiety were found between those who had a simple mastectomy and those who had a wide excision and radiotherapy or between patients having surgery for benign breast disease ($n = 31$) and general surgical patients ($n = 20$).[5]

Oberst and Scott[6] reported no differences in anxiety scores among a group of patients with genitourinary cancer treated surgically with and without a resulting ostomy at five time periods from predischarge up to 180 days after discharge. Repeated measures ANOVA indicated that the pattern of anxiety scores were essentially linear with a significant time effect ($F(3,114) = 8.834$, $p < .0001$).[6]

To describe the emotional impact of surgical treatment for breast cancer within the first year after surgery, Gottschalk and Hoigaard-Martin[7] analyzed data collected from a collaborative study group supported by the National Cancer Institute. At 1 to 3 months after surgery, 118 women who had a unilateral mastectomy for stage I or II breast cancer had significantly higher mean death, mutilation, and total anxiety scores as measured by the Gottschalk-Gleser Content Analysis Scale than did 64 women who had a biopsy for benign breast disease, 69 women who had a cholecystectomy, and 78 women who had not had a major surgical intervention. However, significant reductions in mean mutilation, shame, and total anxiety scores ($p < .01$) were reported in the mastectomy group 10 to 12 months after surgery.[7]

Similar patterns of anxiety responses appear in the literature concerning radiation therapy as a treatment modality. In a study of 181 patients receiving external radiation therapy for cancer, Irwin et al.[8] found that all patients, male and female, exhibited higher anxiety scores than nonpatient norms before treatment. Yet higher anxiety scores were reported among female versus male patients before initiation of treatment, 1 week after treatment was completed, and 2 months after completion of therapy. Patients in general reported significantly higher anxiety during rather than after treatment.[8]

In another study, anxiety was examined among patients ($N = 45$) receiving external radiation therapy for cancer.[9] A pattern of anxiety responses emerged. Patients with lower anxiety scores (STAI) before treatment exhibited significantly higher A-state scores after treatment; patients with moderate anxiety scores exhibited little change in A-state scores; and patients with high anxiety scores exhibited a significant decrease in A-state scores after treatment. No such patterns of change were found for A-trait scores among any group, supporting the hypothesis that changes in scores were related to situational factors rather than personality factors.[9]

Andersen et al.[10] studied anxiety, as measured by the STAI, among 19 patients with gynecologic cancers receiving intracavitary radiation. A-state scores ranged in the 74th to 95th percentiles for all patients. As the time for treatment neared, anxiety increased for patients in both the low- and high-anxiety groups. When treatment was completed, high-anxiety patients had significantly lower A-state scores, while the low-anxiety patient group scores remained unchanged, indicating residual anxiety.

Anxiety related to chemotherapy and associated side effects has been implicated in the decision of patients either to reject treatment or to withdraw before completing the recommended therapy.[11] In a study of 78 stage II patients with breast cancer receiving adjuvant chemotherapy, anxiety was reported in 97% of the subjects, yet the levels of anxiety were represented by low scores, indicating mild distress.

Cassileth et al.[12] administered the STAI to 378 patients with cancer and 379 matched relatives. Mean anxiety scores among the patient group (37.2) were similar to scores among other physically ill patient groups yet were lower than scores among patients who were being treated for depression. Of note was the trend for state and trait anxiety scores to increase among patients under followup care, active treatment, and palliative care, respectively.

In a sample of 60 men cured of Hodgkin's disease, Cella et al.[13] studied the occurrence of persistent anticipatory nausea, vomiting, and anxiety after chemotherapy. Data generated from a semistructured interview revealed that 80% of the subjects who had completed chemotherapy at least 6 months before the study complained of anxiety when reminded of treatment.

In summary, increased levels of anxiety have been associated with a diagnosis of cancer. Patients treated with surgery, radiation therapy, and chemotherapy have also reported mild or moderate levels of anxiety. Yet anxiety at minimal or moderate levels may be motivating for the patient.

Impact of Anxiety on Patient Outcomes

Although increased levels of anxiety among persons with cancer have been documented, few researchers have studied the impact of increased anxiety on patient outcomes. Scott[4] studied the relationship of anxiety, critical thinking, and information processing during and after breast biopsy. Anxiety levels (STAI scores) among the 85 patients studied were extremely high and above group norms for acutely ill psychiatric patients. Women with high anxiety scores were found to have positively correlated critical thinking ability (Watson-Glaser Critical Thinking Appraisal) scores. In addition, critical thinking was substantially reduced at hospitalization when compared with 6 to 8 weeks after discharge.

Carey and Burish[14] studied the impact of anxiety as a predictor of behavioral therapy outcomes for 72 patients receiving chemotherapy. Findings indicated that pretreatment anxiety was associated with treatment outcome. Patients with low anxiety had significantly greater reduction in diastolic blood pressure, self-reported anxiety, and depression when compared with patients with moderate and high anxiety. However, pretreatment anxiety levels were not related to nausea levels.

Therefore, beginning empirical data indicate that anxiety is associated with selected patient outcomes. The strength and direction of the relationships between anxiety and selected psychosocial intervening and outcome variables remains to be defined.

Assessment Criteria

Anxiety has been recognized as an accepted nursing diagnosis category by the North American Nursing Diagnosis Association (NANDA).[15] As such, a preliminary definition, possible etiologies, and subjective and objective defining characteristics have been developed (Table 20-1).[15] Efforts have centered on developing specific criteria for deriving the diagnosis statement, yet the required clustering of signs and symptoms critical to the diagnosis are unclear. In addition, the criteria for fear and anxiety are remarkably similar except for the ability of the patient to identify the source of threat. Defining characteristics for anxiety include "fear"; defining characteristics of anticipatory anxiety include the designation of a "future/impending event perceived as a threat"; and contradiction exists over whether the consequences of the threat or the threat itself is the unspecified stimulus.

Consequently, the reliability and validity of the defining characteristics to predict the occurrence of anxiety are questioned. Thus, validation of the diagnosis with the perceptions of the patient is mandatory. Additional clinical research is needed to test the NANDA recommendations for definition and diagnostic criteria of anxiety. Critical characteristics to differentiate motivational versus dysfunctional anxiety also may be distinguished.

Nursing Interventions

Interventions are based on helping the patient to recognize the spectrum of manifestations of anxiety, to determine if the patient desires to do anything about the response, and to activate coping strategies to control anxiety levels.[16] Validation of observed manifestations of anxiety provides an opportunity for the patient to acknowledge or deny the presence of those manifestations and to prioritize the most disturbing responses. Although the manifestations may be classified by health care professionals as disturbing, the patient may perceive the level of anxiety experienced as positive and reject intervention.

However, if the patient expresses a desire to reduce the anxiety, the nurse has an opportunity to help the patient identify the threat, learn to modify responses to the stimuli, and channel the responses constructively. Based on the principles and assumptions of cognitive theory, the nurse may begin by exploring perceived patient concerns and helping the patient evaluate the concerns within the reality of the situation. Often the interventions of exploration and evaluation will result in the ability of the patient to focus on the threat or to appraise the stimuli in a different way, thus reducing anxiety.

Since the etiology of anxiety is defined as being nonspecific, interventions may focus on treating the symptoms by activating previously effective coping strategies or on teaching new strategies to control the anxiety.

TABLE 20-1 Nursing Diagnoses That Address Anxiety

Nursing Diagnosis	Definition	Defining Characteristics
Anxiety	Vague, uneasy feeling, the source of which is often nonspecific or unknown to the individual	Verbalizes apprehension, uncertainty, fear, distress, worry, verbalizes painful and persistent feelings of increased helplessness, inadequacy, regret, expresses concern (change in life events), fear of unspecified consequences, overexcited, rattled, jittery, scared, restlessness, focus on self, insomnia, increased perspiration, wariness, glancing about, poor eye contact, familial tension, voice quivering, increased tension, foot shuffling, hand and arm movements, trembling, hand tremor, shakiness
Mild Anxiety	Increased level of arousal associated with expectation of a threat (unfocused) to the self or significant relationships	Verbalizes feelings of increased arousal and concern, increased questioning, restlessness, increased awareness, attending, mild restlessness
Moderate Anxiety	Increased level of arousal associated with expectation of a threat (unfocused) to the self or significant relationships	Expressed feelings of unfocused apprehension, nervousness, or concern, verbalized expectation of danger, voice tremors, pitch changes, restlessness, increased rate of verbalization, pacing, hand tremor, increased muscle tension, narrowing focus of attention, diaphoresis, increased heart rate, respiratory rate, sleep or eating disturbances
Severe Anxiety (Panic)	Increased level of arousal associated with expectation of a threat to the self or significant relationships	Expressed feelings of unfocused, severe dread, apprehension, concern, or nervousness, inappropriate verbalization or absence of verbalizations, purposeless activity or immobilization, perceptual focus scattered, fixed, or inability to focus on reality, increased heart rate, hyperventilation, diaphoresis, increased muscle tension, dilated pupils, pallor
Anticipatory Anxiety	Increased level of arousal associated with a perceived future threat (unfocused) to the self or significant relationships	Indicators of anxiety (See Anxiety), future impending event perceived as a threat to physical or psychosocial self (unfocused)

Source: Gordon M: *Manual of Nursing Diagnosis.* New York: McGraw-Hill, 1987.

Each patient brings to the cancer experience a history of previous coping strategies that have been effective and ineffective in managing anxiety. The nurse has the opportunity to help the patient identify those strategies (Table 20-2)[17] used in the present milieu and evaluate the effectiveness of the strategies in reducing anxiety. For patients who desire to learn new strategies, the nurse may offer information through formal and informal education programs, assistance in problem solving through counseling, role modeling with anxiety-reducing techniques such as relaxation training or music therapy, or referral to support groups within the care institution and the community.

Few studies have been conducted among patients with cancer to determine the effectiveness of independent nursing interventions in reducing anxiety, yet available data indicate potential benefits for education programs, relaxation training, music therapy, and support groups. The following empirical studies are representative of the nursing literature with respect to the potential benefits of such interventions.

Johnson[18] reported on the effects of a patient education course on persons with a chronic illness. Fifty-two subjects were selected randomly from the patients with a first or recurrent diagnosis of cancer within a 12-month period. Preintervention measures of state anxiety (STAI), meaningfulness in life, and knowledge were obtained. Based on preintervention scores and demographic variables, subjects were paired. One subject from each pair was assigned randomly to the treatment group. Subjects in the treatment group attended eight educational sessions over a 4-week period. Con-

TABLE 20-2 Approach and Avoidance Coping Strategies

Approach Strategies	Avoidance Strategies
Information seeking	Denial of emotion
Participation in religious activities	Minimization of symptoms
Distraction	Social isolation
Expression of emotion and feeling	Passive acceptance
Positive thinking	Sleeping
Conservation of energy	Substance abuse
Maintenance of Independence	Avoidance of decision making
Maintenance of control	Blame others
Goal setting	Excessive dependency

Source: Adapted from Miller JF: *Coping with Chronic Illness: Overcoming Powerlessness.* Philadelphia: Davis, 1983.

tent for the sessions included learning about the disease, managing daily health problems, communication, feeling good about oneself, living within physical limitations, and community resources. The experimental group had statistically significant lower anxiety scores than the control group.

Cotanch and Strum[19] reported on the effects of progressive muscle relaxation (PMR) on anxiety, nausea, and vomiting associated with cancer chemotherapy. Sixty patients were randomized into an experimental group (PMR), a placebo control group (relaxing music), and a true control group (no intervention). A statistically significant difference was found for trait anxiety scores across courses of chemotherapy within the different treatment groups; however, no statistical difference was found for state anxiety scores. This finding is perplexing in view of the theoretical constructs of state and trait anxiety and other research findings presented previously.

Frank[20] studied the effect of music therapy and guided visual imagery on anxiety associated with chemotherapy-induced nausea and vomiting. In a single group ($N = 15$), pretest- and posttest-designed study, musical tapes and visual imagery aided by a scenic poster were used beginning 15 minutes before chemotherapy and continuing through chemotherapy administration (2 hours). All subjects received antiemetic drugs before chemotherapy administration. State anxiety scores as measured by the STAI were reduced significantly ($p < .001$). In addition, a significant negative correlation was found between the length of time the subject listened to the music and the postchemotherapy state anxiety score ($r = -.4984$, $p < .05$).[19]

In summary, a variety of behavioral interventions have been used successfully to alleviate anxiety associated with a cancer diagnosis and treatment. Each intervention represents an independent nursing action to modify the anxiety response exhibited among persons with cancer.

Future Directions for Nursing Research

Anxiety has been reported to be present subjectively and objectively among patients diagnosed with cancer across the disease trajectory. The vague, uneasy feelings defined as anxiety may serve a protective or disabling function for the patient with cancer. However, assessment criteria used in collaboration with the perceptions of the patient to determine the individual level of anxiety at which interventions to reduce anxiety should be instituted lack reliability and validity.

Although beginning research efforts have focused on the effectiveness of a variety of independent nursing interventions in reducing anxiety among persons with cancer, studies have been limited by sample size and heterogeneity, cross-sectional designs, single measures of anxiety, use of anxiety as both an independent and a dependent variable, and lack of randomized control groups. Intervention studies for anxiety reduction among persons with cancer have concentrated on applying the intervention across cancer populations at a variety of points in the cancer trajectory, yet definition of criteria by which to select a specific intervention for a specific person may be impossible or, at best, subjective. Finally, the effect of anxiety reduction on patient outcomes such as information processing, physiologic responses to cancer and cancer therapy, psychosocial adaptation, and sense of control have not been corroborated.

DEPRESSION

Depression is a ubiquitous response to actual or potential loss. Since cancer represents a potential loss of not only life, but also body parts and functions, roles, and relationships, depression has been identified as one of the most common responses to cancer. Yet the differential diagnosis of depression among persons with cancer is complicated by the coexistence of signs and symptoms of disease and treatment that are similar to those of depression.[21] In addition, depression resulting from a predisposition within the personality must be differentiated from a depressed mood associated with an adjustment disorder as a result of changes caused by cancer.[22]

In either case, depression can influence the quality of life of persons with cancer and their significant others. However, empirical and clinical reports indicate that depression is an underdiagnosed response among persons with cancer and, probably more critical, undertreated.[23] In the following section, depression is defined, research on depression among persons with cancer is described, assessment criteria are discussed, and nursing interventions are outlined.

Operational Definition

The following operational definition of depression is presented:

- An individual exists with the ability to respond cognitively, behaviorally, and affectively to stimuli in the environment.
- The individual perceives certain goals for the future and attributes the possibilities for success to the self.
- The attempts of the individual to attain goals are blocked.
- The individual attributes the failure to attain goals to personal inadequacies.
- *The perceived loss of self-esteem results in a cluster of affective (worthlessness, hopelessness, guilt, sadness), behavioral (change in appetite, sleep disturbances, lack of energy, withdrawal, dependency), and cognitive (decreased ability to concentrate, indecisiveness, or suicidal ideation) responses defined as depression.*

Measurement Instruments

A variety of instruments is available to assess depression. The majority of these instruments were developed to assess depression in psychiatrically ill patients. Items cluster about the characteristics associated with major depression as described in the *Diagnostic and Statistical Manual of Mental Disorders-Revised* (DSM-III-R). Limited reliability and validity data with respect to use in oncology populations have been reported.

Hamilton Rating Scale for Depression

The Hamilton Rating Scale for Depression (HRS-D)[24] is a 17-item, self-report scale used to assess cognitive, behavioral, and physiologic signs and symptoms typical of depression. Each item is rated for severity from 0 to 2 or from 0 to 4. Scores on each item are summed to produce a total depression score. A total score of greater than 25 indicates severe depression; 18 to 24, moderate depression; 7 to 17, mild depression; and less than 6, no depression. Reliability and validity estimates for the instrument for nononcology populations include interrater reliability ($r = .90$); construct validity by factor analysis resulting in four factors (retarded depression, somatic symptoms, anxiety reaction, and insomnia).[24]

Beck Depression Inventory

The Beck Depression Inventory (BDI)[25] is a 21-item self-report scale used to assess symptoms of depression. Each item is composed of a set of statements, graduating in severity of symptoms, measured on a scale of 0 to 3, with a higher score representing a more severe symptom. The subject chooses the statement in the set that most closely describes his or her current feeling. Total scores for the BDI are based on the number and severity of symptoms experienced. Subjects scoring in the 0 to 4 range are classified as not or minimally depressed; in the 4 to 7 range, as mildly depressed; in the 8 to 15 range, as moderately depressed; and in the 16 to 42 range, as severely depressed. Reliability estimates among psychiatric populations include internal consistency (KR_{20} alpha coefficients ranging from .88 to .94).

Other instruments

In addition to the instruments presented, other personality and mood inventories with depression subscales have been used to quantify the level of depression. The Minnesota Multiphasic Personality Inventory (MMPI),[26] Psychosocial Adjustment to Illness Scale (PAIS),[27] and Profile of Mood States (POMS)[28] have been used most frequently in studies of depression among persons with cancer. Reliability and validity estimates for the total instrument as well as subscales are reported in administration and scoring manuals for each instrument.

Patterns of Occurrence

The occurrence of depression among persons with cancer has been described in the literature. Petty and Noyes[29] reported that moderate to severe depression was found in 17% to 25% of hospitalized cancer patients. At least 20% of adult cancer patients will have a clinically significant syndrome of depression during the course of the disease.[30–32]

Factors that affect the occurrence of depression among persons with cancer have been described. Andersen and Hacker[33] reported on the psychosexual adjustment of 15 patients treated surgically for vulvar cancer. Data were collected through a semistructured interview and battery of psychosocial questionnaires: Katz Social Adjustment Scale, Symptom Checklist-90, and Dyadic Adjustment Scale. A mean score of 12.3 on the BDI was obtained for the sample, indicating a mild to moderate level of depression among these patients. Activity scores were correlated significantly and negatively with the measures of psychologic distress.

Goldberg et al.[34] reported on the relationship of the social environment and patient physical status to depression in 20 patients with lung cancer and their 18 spouses. Data were generated through a semistructured interview and a battery of psychological tests administered within 6 weeks of diagnosis and at 2-month intervals for 4 months. Physical status of the patient, as measured by the Karnofsky Scale, was related negatively to depressive symptoms as measured by POMS-D in patients.

The effects of age and marital status on emotional distress after mastectomy were studied by Metzger et al.[35] Data from interviews of 652 women who underwent a mastectomy 1 year before the study indicated that younger women were more likely to worry about disfigurement resulting from surgery but to have resources as buffers against depression. Married subjects were significantly less likely to worry about recurrence and experienced less depression.

Researchers have also attempted to differentiate depression associated with cancer from depression associated with a personality disorder. Robinson et al.[36] conducted a study to determine if the degree of self-reported anxiety and depression that is attributed to having cancer differs from current or past history of anxiety and depression attributed to other life events in 57 patients presently being treated for cancer. Findings indicated that patients who reported a history of anxiety or depression for reasons other than cancer had significantly higher anxiety and depression scores than those who did not report preexisting anxiety or depression. Patients who reported a history of depression or anxiety due to the diagnosis of cancer had self-rating scores on anxiety and depression that did not differ significantly from those of patients who reported no problems or "normal" symptoms.

Evaluations for depression among 62 patients with a diagnosis of cancer were reported by Bukberg et al.[37] DSM-III-R criteria for major depressive episodes were used to evaluate the presence of depression.[38] Twenty-six patients (42%) met the criteria for major depression, 14% had depressive symptoms that did not meet the criteria for major depression, and 44% had no depressive affect. The factor most clearly associated with depression was physical performance as measured by the Karnofsky Scale. Qualitative differences between depression in psychiatric and cancer patients were found. No subjects were found to have psychotic depressive symptoms, melancholia, feelings of worthlessness, or suicidal ideation.

In addition to describing the occurrence of depression among persons with cancer, researchers have studied the variations in occurrence and severity of depression across the disease trajectory. Layne et al.[39] reported significant differences in levels of depression as measured by the MMPI-D among patients with a diagnosis of cancer in the terminal phase, patients with a diagnosis of cancer who had been told that they would survive for at least 5 years, family members of patients in the cancer groups, and a normal group. Depression scores for the terminal group were significantly greater than those of the family member and normal groups ($p < .05$). The nonterminal patient group also had depression scores greater than those of the family member and normal groups, although the differences were not statistically significant.

Depression also has been explored as a predictor of adjustment to a diagnosis of cancer. Morris et al.[40] used standardized tests and structured interviews to identify factors that predicted psychological and social adjustment to mastectomy 2 years after surgery. High preoperative depression scores (HRS-D) were predictive of poor adjustment after mastectomy. Subjects who scored more than 10 on the HRS-D, with or without a history of depression, were significantly more likely to remain stressed by the mastectomy at 2 years ($p > .05$).

In summary, the focus of research related to depression among persons with cancer has been descriptive. The lack of assessment of preexisting depressive symptoms before the diagnosis of cancer, the presence of confounding physical and psychosocial responses related to the disease and treatment, and minimal reliability and validity estimates for instruments used among cancer populations result in significant limitations in previous research. Moreover, an emphasis on empirical studies that focus on independent nursing interventions to modify the depressive symptoms associated with the diagnosis of cancer is needed. With statistical modeling, knowledge of depressive responses within the context of other psychosocial variables inherent in the cancer experience may be enhanced.

Assessment Criteria

Reactive depression (situational) is defined as "an acute decrease in self-esteem or worth related to a threat to self competency."[15,p.210] Defining characteristics as established by NANDA are presented in Table 20-3.[15] Critical to establishing the diagnosis in physically ill persons is evaluation of selected defining characteristics commonly attributed to depression among the psychiatrically ill. Physiologic characteristics such as appetite disturbances, change in weight, sleep disturbance, and decreased energy are experienced frequently among persons with cancer as a result of disease or treatment. Furthermore, the psychosocial characteristics described for depression may occur in the person with cancer as a result of disease, treatment, or side effects (inability to concentrate, irritability, dependency, and anger). Therefore, the primary criteria for assessment of depression are that the characteristics are a change from previous functioning, are persistent, occur for most of the day, occur more days than not, and are present for at least 2 weeks.[38,p.219]

TABLE 20-3 Defining Characteristics of Situational Depression

Expressions of hopelessness, despair
Inability to concentrate on reading, writing, conversation
Change in physical activities, eating, sleeping, sexual activity
Continual questioning of self-worth (self-esteem)
Feelings of failure (real or imagined)
Withdrawal from others to avoid possible rejection (real or imagined)
Threats or attempts to commit suicide
Suspicion and sensitivity to words and actions of others related to general lack of trust of others
Misdirected anger toward self
General irritability
Guilt feelings
Extreme dependency on others with related feelings of helplessness and anger

Source: Gordon M: *Manual of Nursing Diagnosis.* New York: McGraw-Hill, 1987.

Nursing Interventions

The selection of nursing interventions for the treatment of patients with depression is based on identification of stimuli that have resulted in a loss of self-esteem as well as the defining characteristics present for the particular patient. If the patient presents with a long-standing history of depression, referral to another member of the health care team may be appropriate. Otherwise, concentration on the psychological and behavioral responses associated with depression offer beginning cues for selection of nursing interventions.

The nurse may begin by helping the patient to acknowledge feelings of hopelessness, despair, failure, anger, or guilt and by giving permission to discuss those feelings. Because the expression of the feelings is associated with a degree of risk-taking for the patient, the nurse must be open and accepting of the feelings.

Acceptance is demonstrated by attentive listening, acknowledgment of the feelings, and exploration of methods to deal positively with the feelings.

Sensitivity to potential increased vulnerability of the patient who shares feelings is a necessity. The nurse must assume the responsibility for emotional exposure of the patient and plan systematically for professional follow-up. Expression of depressive feelings may be both time-consuming and overwhelming for the patient and nurse; consultation with other health care personnel, namely, clinical nurse specialists in psychiatry, psychologists, and psychiatrists, may be indicated.

Besides giving permission for expression of feelings, the nurse has the opportunity to assist the patient to reappraise the situation cognitively with respect to aspects of the cancer experience and perceptions of self-esteem and self-competency. Accurate information about the plan of care and personal responses to treatment form the basis of cognitive reappraisal of the situation. Helping the patient focus on immediate goals of care often reduces the overwhelming feelings of powerlessness and helplessness associated with a chronic, life-threatening illness. Focusing on positive abilities of the patient, contracting short-term goals of care that the patient can achieve, and reinforcing patient attempts and successes to meet established goals provide the framework for effective nursing interventions in caring for the patient with depression.

In the milieu of the cancer experience, physical symptoms of the disease and treatment as well as lack of motivation accompanying depression may limit the ability of the patient to meet basic needs. Significant others as well as health care professionals may perceive the patient as generally helpless even in areas in which the patient is able to function independently. Enhancing self-competency and self-esteem may be accomplished by providing information about and role modeling self-care behaviors, negotiating goals for increasing independence in self-care as well as decision making, facilitating social interaction with others, and encouraging physical mobility.

Future Directions for Nursing Research

Although most persons with cancer are able to cope with the demands of illness and treatment with minimal psychosocial distress, criteria by which to predict those patients for whom the demands exceed interpersonal and intrapersonal resources are ambiguous. Furthermore, criteria to establish the diagnosis among medically versus psychiatrically ill patients are unclear.

Nursing interventions designed to effect positive outcomes for the patient diagnosed with depression are inherently time-consuming and may represent an unacceptable cost-benefit ratio in the acute care setting in light of the physical care demanded. However, if the goal of oncology care includes the quality as well as quantity of life, then intervention studies to compare both the effectiveness as well as costs of care in both inpatient and community settings for patients with depression are warranted.

HOPELESSNESS

Hopelessness is often described in the literature as a response of patients to the cancer experience; however, the response appears not to pervade the experience of the cancer patient but rather waxes and wanes with changes in perceived health, relationships, and spirituality. Described as both a unique response as well as one of a cluster of characteristics seen in other responses, hopelessness has been studied primarily within the framework of psychiatrically ill patients. Recently, however, health care professionals in general and nurses in particular have demonstrated increased interest in hopelessness and hope as both independent and dependent variables influencing the quantity and quality of the cancer experience.

Operational Definition

Operationally, hopelessness can be defined as follows:

- An individual exits within time and space.
- The individual has thoughts, feelings, and behaviors in response to stimuli in the environment.
- The responses an individual has to stimuli are based on the significance of the stimuli, potential responses identified, and calculated probabilities of success in creating a desired future.
- The individual, as an aspect of humanity, recognizes significant areas of life for which limited or no alternatives are identified or the probabilities of success in creating a desired future approach zero—the perceived reality for the individual.
- In an attempt to protect the individual against the despair generated by these areas of life, the individual seeks a personal or spiritual relationship, anticipating that interactions will lead to understandable, meaningful, or constructive outcomes in the future.
- *The interaction of thoughts, feelings, and behaviors resulting from the inability to mobilize internal and external resources sufficient to achieve a probability of success greater than zero or to create an understandable, meaningful, or constructive outcome in the future is defined as hopelessness.*

Measurement Instruments

Beck Hopelessness Scale

The Beck Hopelessness Scale (BHS)[41] is a 20-item, true-false scale designed to measure hopelessness in psychiatrically ill patients. Scores are calculated by sum-ming the scores on each statement. Scores range from 0 to 20, with a higher score representing a higher level of hopelessness. Scores of 0 to 3 represent no or minimal hopelessness; 4 to 8, mild hopelessness; 9 to 14, moderate hopelessness; and 15 to 20, severe hopelessness. Reliability estimates for the instrument include internal consistency as measured by the KR_{20} reliability coefficient = .93 among a sample of suicide attempters; concurrent validity between clinical ratings of hopelessness and instrument ratings ($r = .74, p < .001$); face validity established by a panel of psychiatric experts; and construct validity through factor analysis resulting in three factors (feelings about the future, loss of motivation, and future expectations)[41] with Eigenvalues > 1.000.

Nowotny Hope Scale

Conceptualized as a polar opposite to hopelessness, hopefulness has been measured by a number of instruments developed by nurse researchers. The Nowotny Hope Scale (NHS)[42] is a 29-item scale designed to measure hope on six dimensions: confidence in outcomes, relates to others, possibility of a future, spiritual beliefs, active involvement, and comes from within.[42] For each of the positively and negatively worded statements, the subject is asked to respond on a 4-point, Likert-type scale (1 = strongly agree to 4 = strongly disagree). Reliability and validity estimates for the instrument include internal consistency as calculated by Cronbach's coefficient alpha = 0.90; item-total correlations ranging from 0.3 to 0.7; item to subscale correlations ranging from 0.4 to 0.8; concurrent validity with the BHS ($r = .47, p = .001$); and construct validity through factor analysis resulting in six factors with Eigenvalues ranging from 9.8 to 1.4.[42]

Herth Hope Scale

The Herth Hope Scale (HHS)[43] is a 32-item self-report scale to which subjects respond either "applies to me" or "does not apply to me" to each item. Responses on each item are summed to produce a total hope score ranging from 0 to 32, with a higher score representing higher levels of hope. Reliability and validity estimates among persons with cancer include internal consistency as determined by Cronbach's coefficient alpha = 0.89; and construct validity through factor analysis resulting in three factors—positive expectancies, sense of personal competency and mutuality, and temporality with future orientation.[43]

Patterns of Occurrence

In recent years, the interest of health care professionals in the relationship of hope and hopelessness to the cancer experience has resulted in numerous anecdotal articles, a few descriptive studies, and a limited number of intervention studies. As early as 1966, Schmale and Iker[44] conducted a study of 40 women with abnormal cervical cytology suspicious of cancer. To test the hypothesis that the experience of specific feelings may facilitate or permit the clinical appearance of disease,[44] the researchers conducted an interview and administered a battery of psychological tests the day after a cone biopsy was done under general anesthesia. Content analysis of interviews was compared with preestablished criteria for hopelessness potential. A determination of "cancer" or "no cancer" was made for each subject. Thirty-one subjects (77.5%) were assigned to the correct grouping (x_c^2, 7.343; df, 1; $p = .007$).

Subsequent studies of hope among persons with cancer were focused on concept clarification, describing levels of hope across the disease trajectory, or instrument development for measuring hope. Using a grounded theory methodology, Hinds[45] developed an empirically derived definition of hopefulness through interviews with healthy adolescents, inpatient adolescents on a substance abuse unit, and a diagnostically heterogeneous adolescent group with cancer.

The induced definition of hopefulness had four dimensions that emerged from the data from the healthy and substance abuse adolescents (Table 20-4).[45] An additional attribute emerged from the adolescent cancer group, "the concern for and a focus on others in addition to self."[45,p.85] Thus, the resulting definition became "the degree to which an adolescent possesses a comforting or life-sustaining, reality-based belief that a positive future exists for self or others."[45] These data form the basis for additional study of the concept among adults.

In a similar study, the phenomena of hope and the hoping process were examined among 35 elderly patients with a diagnosis of cancer.[46] Hope was defined as a multidimensional dynamic life force characterized by confident yet uncertain anticipation of realistically possible and personally significant desirable future good

TABLE 20-4 Induced Dimensions of Hopefulness Among Adolescents

Dimension	Definition
Forced effort	The degree to which an adolescent tries to take on artificially a more positive view
Personal possibilities	The extent to which an adolescent believes that second chances for the self may exist
Expectations of a better tomorrow	The degree to which an adolescent has a positive although nonspecific future orientation
Anticipation of a personal future	The extent to which an adolescent identifies specific and positive future possibilities for self

Source: Hinds PS: Adolescent hopefulness in illness and health. *Adv Nurs Sci* 10:79–88, 1988.

having implications for action and for interpersonal relatedness.[46,p.380] Two spheres of hope, generalized and particularized, were identified, and six dimensions of hope were described—affective, cognitive, behavioral, affiliative, temporal, and contextual.

In a report on the development of an instrument to measure hope after a stressful event, Nowotny[42] described levels of hope among a sample of 150 patients with cancer. Scores on the NHS for the cancer patient group were not significantly different from scores of a sample of 156 well adults. Data were not collected on type of diagnosis, length of time since diagnosis, or type of treatment for the cancer patient sample.

Zook and Yasko[47] found hope levels decreased as time since diagnosis increased among a group of 26 patients with cancer receiving chemotherapy. In contrast, Greene et al.[48] reported no correlation between hope level and length of time since diagnosis.

The focus of more recent studies has been the description of the relationship of hope to other psychosocial variables in the cancer experience. Herth[43] reported a descriptive study to investigate the relationship between hope and coping in 120 adult patients with cancer undergoing chemotherapy in a variety of care settings. A significant relationship was found between level of hope and level of coping among subjects in hospital, outpatients, and home settings ($p < .05$). In addition, strength of religious convictions and performance of family role responsibilities, measured on one-item scales, were significantly related to the variables of hope and coping regardless of setting: subjects with a strong religious faith had significantly higher mean scores on the HHS than subjects with weak, unsure, or lost faith or who were without faith. Subjects who reported little or no interference in performing family role responsibilities had a significantly ($p < .05$) higher mean score on the HHS than did the group indicating severe interference.

Raleigh[49] studied 45 patients with cancer and 45 individuals with a nonthreatening chronic illness to describe the relationship between hope, locus of control, factors of illness, and personal factors. Raleigh reported no significant relationship between the level of hope and the identified personal and illness factors, yet these findings have been challenged.

To examine the relationship between hopelessness and locus of control, helpfulness of religious beliefs, and support from family and friends, Brandt[50] studied a sample of 31 women with breast cancer. Although all patients were receiving their first course of chemotherapy, variability existed in the time elapsed since initial diagnosis; that is, 42% of the sample had been diagnosed less than 6 months, while 26% of the sample had been diagnosed more than 24 months. Results indicate that the mean hopelessness score as measured by the BHS was 2.48, indicating minimal hopelessness. A statistically significant correlation ($r = .37$, $p < .05$) was found between hopelessness scores and locus of control scores (as measured by the Rotter I-E Locus of Control Scale). Patients who exhibited a more external locus of control expressed a greater level of hopelessness.[50] Perceived helpfulness of religious beliefs in coping with illness as measured by a one-item scale was found to be correlated significantly ($r = -.32$, $p < .05$) with lower levels of hopelessness. The author indicated minimal variability of scores on the religious beliefs question. Support from family and friends as measured by a one-item scale did not produce sufficient variability in scores to allow a Pearson correlation coefficient to be calculated.

Stoner[51] studied the relationship between personal and situational factors and hope in 58 white adults with cancer. Higher levels of hope ($p = .10$) were associated with being female, receipt of adequate information about disease and treatments, adherence by the subjects to their religious belief systems throughout illness, and lower socioeconomic status. Inability to carry out family role responsibilities, adverse effects of treatment, protracted illness, and greater severity of illness were not found to be associated with lower levels of hope.

In a subsequent study, Stoner and Keampfer[52] examined the effect of information with respect to life expectancy and phase of illness on levels of hope among a heterogeneous sample of 55 cancer patients. Although data indicated no significant differences in levels of hope between subjects according to the phase of illness (no evidence of disease, ongoing treatment, or terminal stage), a significant main effect for recalled life expectancy information on hope was shown ($F = 4.21$, $p < .05$). Subjects who did not remember receiving information about life expectancy had higher levels of hope than subjects who remembered receiving information.[52]

The relationship between hopefulness and participation styles with respect to treatment was studied among a sample of 256 patients with a diagnosis of cancer.[53] Selected findings of Stoner[52] were supported. The mean score on the BHS for the sample was 2.8, indicating minimal hopelessness. Levels of hope were found to correlate positively with medical status ($p < .05$); preference for active involvement in self-care ($p < .05$); and desire for as much information as possible ($p < .001$).

Hope as an intervening variable has been studied.[54] The relationship between locus of control, hope, and disease-free interval was examined among a convenience sample of 34 postmenopausal women with stage II breast cancer. Internal health locus of control was not found to be correlated significantly with disease-free interval; however, hope was found to be correlated positively and significantly ($p < .05$) with disease-free interval. Moreover, stressful life events were found to be intervening variables that had a significant negative correlation with disease-free interval.

Thus, hopefulness and hopelessness have been implicated in the development of cancer and in the quantity and quality of life after diagnosis of cancer. However, consistent conceptualization of hope and hopelessness remains elusive in the empirical studies reported. Ideally, future efforts in determining the relationship of hope and cancer will be targeted to demonstrate the biophysical-psychosocial connection between the variables.

Assessment Criteria

Hopelessness has been characterized by cognitive, affective, and behavioral responses (Table 20-5).[15] Few studies, however, have been conducted to establish the reliability and validity of the defining characteristics among clinical populations. Of even greater concern is the ability of the clinician to differentiate hopelessness from similar concepts such as depression and powerlessness using the accepted defining characteristics.

Nursing Interventions

Interventions for decreasing hopelessness and fostering hope among persons with cancer have been derived before development of conceptual and theoretical formulations. Based on conceptual models of the nature of hope and related variables, the following categories of interventions have been suggested: enhancing reality surveillance, fostering supportive relationships, enhancing personal power and abilities, and creating a future perspective.[55,56] Specific suggestions for implementation of each category are presented in Table 20-6.[55,56]

Future Directions for Nursing Research

Hope has been identified as a critical component of cancer care. As such, the necessity of conceptualizing hope and hopelessness within the context of the cancer experience, validating the defining characteristics of hope and hopelessness, describing the association of hope and hopelessness to other psychosocial variables, and evaluating the effectiveness of specific nursing interventions in fostering hope or protecting against hopelessness is apparent.

TABLE 20-5 Nursing Diagnosis: Hopelessness

Definition	A subjective state in which an individual sees limited or no alternative or personal choices available and is unable to mobilize energy on own behalf
Defining characteristics	Passivity Decreased verbalization Decreased affect Verbalization of despondent or hopeless content Lack of initiative Decreased response to stimuli Lack of involvement in care Turning away from speaker Closing eyes Shrugging in response to speaker Decreased appetite Increased sleep

Source: Gordon M: *Manual of Nursing Diagnosis*. New York: McGraw-Hill, 1987.

ALTERED SEXUAL HEALTH

The diagnosis of cancer poses potential threats to sexuality, how one perceives the self, how one perceives

TABLE 20-6 Interventions to Foster Hopefulness

Category	Interventions
Assist with reality surveillance	Review changes in and current health status Seek perceptions of patient with respect to health Confirm accurate perception Correct misconceptions of reality Encourage discussion of reality with others in same situation
Reinforce personal power and ability	Review perceived strengths of patient and family Include patient in planning care, goals, schedules Encourage review of past successes in stressful times Reward approximations of goals Encourage value of use of needed external resources
Encourage supportive relationships	Review number, types, and availability of supportive relationships Assist in helping patient ask for support needed Encourage continued contacts with supportive persons Respect relationship of patient to higher being Encourage expression of faith, if applicable
Create a future perspective	Review past occasions for hope Discuss meaning of hope from patient perspective Establish short-term goals with patient and family Evaluate progress in achieving goals on routine basis Encourage expressions of hopes for future

Sources: Clark JC: Hope as a critical factor in the cancer experience, in Pritchard AP (ed.); *Cancer Nursing: A Revolution in Care.* Proceeding of the Fifth International Conference on Cancer Nursing. London: Macmillan, 1989, pp. 117–119. Dufault K, Martocchio BC: Hope: Its spheres and dimensions, *Nurs Clin North Am* 20:379–391, 1985.

how others see the self, and how one behaves as a sexual being. As the nature of cancer has changed from an acute to a chronic illness, concerns of health care providers have expanded beyond survival to include factors that affect the quality of survival. Sexual health is one such factor.

Operational Definition

Operationally, sexuality can be defined as follows:

- An individual exists who has the ability to express himself or herself physically, psychologically, and socially with other human beings.
- The ability of the individual to distinguish self from and express self with others based on anatomic, physiologic, developmental, and psychosocial factors is defined as sexuality.
- The satisfactory, consistent, and rewarding expression of and distinction by one's sexuality results in a state of sexual health for the individual.
- The individual perceives a stimulus that impairs distinction or expression of sexuality.
- *The inability to express one's sexuality consistent with personal needs and preferences is defined as altered sexual health.*

Measurement Instruments

Derogatis Sexual Functioning Inventory

The Derogatis Sexual Functioning Inventory (DSFI)[57] is a 245-item, self-report instrument designed to measure the multidimensional concept of sexuality. Reported reliability and validity estimates include test-retest reliabilities for 10 subscales ranging from 0.42 to 0.96; internal consistency coefficients ranging from 0.56 to 0.97; and construct validity through factor analysis that revealed seven factors (body image, psychologic distress, heterosexual drive, autoeroticism, gender role, sexual satisfaction, and sexual precociousness).[57]

Sexual Adjustment Questionnaire

The Sexual Adjustment Questionnaire (SAQ)[58] is a 108-item instrument designed to measure sexual adjustment over time among patients with head and neck cancers. The questionnaire is completed by the subject at three separate points in time: Section A (37 items), 4 to 6 weeks after treatment; Section B (30 items), retrospective assessment before the diagnosis of cancer; and Section C (39 items), 16 to 20 weeks after treatment. Items include some questions evaluated on a 5-point Likert scale, several open-ended questions, and questions that require an explanation from the subject. Each section is composed of 7 subsections: desire, relationship, activity arousal, orgasm, techniques, and satisfaction. Scores on each item are summed to produce a total score for the subsection. High scores indicate more positive feelings of functioning, greater variety of sexual methods and activities, or a long-term relationship with a single partner. Reliability and validity estimates for the instrument include: test-retest reliability (2 to 4 weeks and 10 to 12 weeks apart) with Pearson correlation coefficients for the subsections ranging from .5389 to .9374; content validity evaluation by a panel of experts; and construct validity established by known-group technique (healthy subjects would be expected to score higher than cancer patients).

Patterns of Occurrence

The sequelae associated with radical surgery, radiation, chemotherapy, and biotherapy may threaten the sexual health of persons with cancer. Early studies on the effects of cancer on sexual health focused on barriers to return to previous levels of sexual function or, more specifically, intercourse. Anecdotal reports and descriptive studies provided the basis for identifying the potential risks to sexual health for site-specific and treatment-specific patient populations. Recently, however, researchers have expanded the concept of sexual health and sexuality to include the issues of self-concept and perceptions and behaviors of significant others.

Sexual behaviors

Abitbol and Davenport[59] published data related to the impact of treatment for cervical cancer on sexual function. Subjects (28 treated with radiation therapy only, 32 treated with surgery, and 15 treated with a combination of surgery and radiation) were interviewed about their sexual life before disease, sexual life 1 year after treatment, and other changes in sexual functioning. Approximately 40% of patients ($N = 75$) reported a decrease or abstinence in sexual activity after treatment. The radiotherapy group had the highest percentage of subjects reporting a decrease in sexual activity (25%). Other changes in sexual functioning identified primarily by the radiotherapy group were lack of libido (43%), pain or discomfort with intercourse (39%), shortened or narrowed vagina (54%), and fear of recurrence (15%). The authors recommended that clinicians assume a proactive posture in addressing the sexual concerns of cancer patients treated with radiation therapy regardless of age.

Subsequently, Jenkins[60] discussed the self-reported sexual changes in 27 women treated for endometrial and cervical cancer with surgery and radiation therapy. A statistically significant ($p < .05$) negative change in the frequency of intercourse, frequency of desire, frequency of orgasm, and enjoyment of intercourse was reported after treatment. Additional significant findings of the study included that 59% of the sample had received no preparation or information about sexual functioning, the majority of sexual information given was verbal versus written, and nurses had not provided any of the information about sexual functioning.

These findings were supported in a study of 60 women newly diagnosed with gynecologic cancers.[61] Twenty-nine of the subjects were sexually active before diagnosis. However, none of these subjects continued to have sexual intercourse after diagnosis either on recommendation of the physician or fear that intercourse would increase the risk for vaginal bleeding or discharge.

Surgery also has been implicated in changes in sexual health among women with vulvar cancer. Andersen and Hacker[62] reported on the psychosexual adjustment of 15 patients treated surgically for vulvar cancer. Data were collected through a semistructured interview and battery of psychosocial questionnaires. Measures of sexual functioning indicated that the sample reported limited capacity for sexual arousal, considerable sexual anxiety, inadequate sexual relationships, a discrepancy between actual and ideal frequency of intercourse, and lower body image scores than reported for healthy women.

The sexual function and psychosocial reactions among 25 women who had undergone vulvectomy and 15 of their partners indicated that more than two thirds of the patients reported a decrease in frequency of intercourse from pretreatment levels.[63] Ten women ceased sexual intercourse completely. Half the women reported being dissatisfied with sexual relationships and the occurrence of low spirits, lack of respect for their body, and not feeling like a "proper woman." These data are consistent with the findings of Jenkins[60] in that between 25% and 33% of patients perceived the information given to them before treatment as inadequate.

However, findings from related studies among women with breast cancer have not been consistent with the changes reported among women with gynecologic cancers. Woods and Earp[64] reported on 49 patients cured of stage I and II breast cancer. Four years after therapy, 81% of the sample reported no difference in sexual frequency and 63% reported being satisfied with sexual relationships. These findings were supported by the work of Jamison et al.[65] who interviewed 41 women with breast cancer. Seventy-six percent of the sample reported that the mastectomy had resulted in no difference or a positive effect on sexual satisfaction or orgasmic ability. Only 2.7% reported a decrease in sexual activity or interest.

In contrast, Taylor et al.[66] reported changes in the levels of affectionate behavior in the marriage ($r = .51$, $p < .001$) and patient perception of frequency of intercourse ($r = .32$, $p < .03$) that were associated with poor psychosocial adjustment among 78 women diagnosed and treated for breast cancer. Patients treated with modified radical mastectomy had significantly higher concern about body disfigurement and were affected significantly more negatively with respect to marital affection and sexual intercourse levels than were patients treated with lumpectomy.

Thus, data indicate that women with gynecologic cancers in general and those treated with radiation therapy are at risk for changes in sexual activity. In contrast, the diagnosis of breast cancer and treatment with surgery do not appear to place the patient at increased risk for changes in the frequency of sexual intercourse but, rather, for changes in self-concept.

Although empirical data are available for evaluating the potential risks of cancer and treatment among females, such data for males are limited. Blackmore[67] reported on the impact of orchidectomy on the sexuality of men with testicular cancer. Self-report questionnaires were distributed to three groups of subjects: group I, 20 men with stage I germ cell testicular tumors treated with unilateral orchidectomy within 2 years before the study; group II, 10 men who had undergone unilateral orchidectomy within 2 years before the study for reasons other than cancer; and group III, 15 men who had no history of cancer or testicular problems. Five sections of the DSFI (sexual drive, symptoms, affect, body image, and sexual satisfaction) were used as the basis for data collection. No statistically significant differences were found on any outcome sexuality variables among the three groups. In contrast, Schover et al.[68] found significant sexual morbidity among a sample of 84 men with a diagnosis of seminoma who were treated with radiation therapy. Problems reported included reduced semen volume (49%), reduced intensity of orgasm (33%), low rates of sexual activity (19%), low sexual desire (12%), erectile dysfunction (15%), difficulty reaching orgasm (10%), and premature ejaculation (14%).

Although treatment of prostatic cancer can affect sexual functioning (impotence and reduced frequency of intercourse and orgasm), limited empirical data are available to quantify the occurrence of sexual changes.[69] Banker[70] studied the preservation of potency among 100 men with prostate cancer treated with external radiation therapy. Subjects were interviewed before radiation therapy and again 1 year after treatment concerning frequency of intercourse, changes in sexual activity levels over the past 1 to 3 years, and ability to achieve and maintain a full erection. Forty-three percent of subjects ($n = 10$) who reported having intercourse with full erections less than three times per month before therapy maintained potency after treatment, compared with 73% of subjects ($n = 19$) who had intercourse with full erection more than three times per month.

In summary, researchers have identified the potential assaults to sexual health among males with genitourinary cancers, yet the data are limited with respect to threats to sexual health among persons with cancers of the head and neck, lung, and gastrointestinal tract. Also of interest is the lack of research related to the perceptions of significant others with respect to sexuality and perceptions of the patient with respect to self-concept.

Self-concept

Self-concept is defined as the total self-appraisal of appearance, background and origins, abilities, resources, attitudes, and feelings that culminate as a directing force in behavior.[71] Newman et al.[72] reported on the effect of Hickman catheters on the self-esteem of patients with leukemia. Self-esteem was measured on admission, on day 5, and on day 30.[73] Consecutive patients admitted with acute nonlymphocytic leukemia (ANLL) were assigned to two groups based on adequacy of venous access. Thirty patients were assigned to each group. Patients who received a Hickman catheter had initial self-esteem scores similar to and even slightly higher than those who did not. Self-esteem in both groups remained similar over the 30-day study period. However, one may question the appropriateness of the use of the Purpose in Life test to measure the self-esteem concept.

In contrast to the minimal surgical incision involved with a Hickman catheter placement, Weddington et al.[74] studied the psychological outcome of extremity sarcoma survivors undergoing amputation ($n = 14$) or limb salvage procedures ($n = 19$). No significant differences between group scores of cognitive capacity, symptoms, mood, body image changes, physical function, adjustment to illness and surgery, and lifetime prevalence of psychiatric disorders before or after surgery were noted.

Alopecia is one of the most common physiologic responses to chemotherapy. Baxley et al.[75] studied the effect of alopecia on the body image of 40 patients with cancer receiving chemotherapy. Subjects were divided into two groups based on the presence of alopecia. Each subject completed the Body-Cathexis-Self-Cathexis (BC-SC) Scale.[76] Significant differences on body cathexis scores ($t = 4.34$, $p < .001$) and self-cathexis scores ($t = 4.04$, $p < .0001$) were found between patients with and without alopecia. In addition, comparisons of scores for female and male patients in the alopecia group indicated a significant difference ($t = 2.91$, $p < .0009$) in that men with alopecia scored higher, indicating that they had a lower self-image than women with alopecia.

Evaluation of the impact of radical versus conservative surgery on disease-related and adjustment-related outcomes has been studied. Kemeny et al.[77] conducted a study of the differences in the psychosocial effects of mastectomy ($n = 27$) versus segmentectomy ($n = 25$) in women who were entered in a prospective randomized protocol for treatment of primary breast cancer. Questionnaires that were designed to evaluate psychosocial responses to treatment were sent to each subject who was at least 6 months past completion of treatment. Seven items were used to evaluate the emotional reaction to body image. Although responses to the items clustered around 3.0, "not sure," for the mastectomy patients, the segmentectomy patients had a significantly more positive assessment of themselves. Patients were asked to evaluate retrospectively changes in physical attractiveness before surgery, 6 months after surgery, and 6 months after completion of therapy. The mastectomy group rated themselves as significantly less physically attractive at 6 months after surgery ($p < .003$) and at the time of the questionnaire ($p < .04$). Mastectomy patients also had a significantly lower rating of femininity 6 months after surgery ($p < .01$) than patients in the segmentectomy group.[77]

In summary, the majority of empirical studies on the impact of cancer on sexual health have been descriptive in design and focused primarily on the effects of cancer and treatment on the frequency of sexual behaviors, particularly intercourse and orgasm, or on self-concept among females with gynecologic and breast cancer or on males with testicular and prostate cancer. However, the issues of perception of significant others' responses to the physical and psychological sequelae of cancer remain understudied. Additional empirical data are needed on the interaction of other variables, such as age, depression, and activity status, on the physical as well as psychosocial aspects of sexual health.

Assessment Criteria

Two nursing diagnoses related to sexual health have been approved by NANDA—sexual dysfunction and altered sexuality patterns.[15] Defining characteristics for each diagnosis are presented in Table 20-7.[15] Differential diagnosis of the two responses based on defining

TABLE 20-7 Nursing Diagnoses: Altered Sexual Health

Nursing Diagnosis	Definition	Defining Characteristics
Altered sexual patterns	The state in which an individual expresses concern regarding sexuality	Reported difficulties, limitations, or changes in sexual behaviors or activities
Sexual dysfunction	Perceived problem in achieving desired satisfaction of sexuality	Verbalizations of problem in sexuality Alterations in achieving perceived sex role Actual or perceived limitation imposed by disease or therapy Conflicts involving values Alteration in achieving sexual satisfaction Inability to achieve desired sexual satisfaction Frequent seeking of confirmation of desirability Alteration in relationship with significant other Change of interest in self and others

Source: Gordon M: *Manual of Nursing Diagnosis.* New York: McGraw-Hill, 1987.

characteristics is conceptually ambiguous in that the defining characteristic for altered sexuality patterns (reported difficulties, limitations, or changes in sexual behaviors or activities) provides the broad categories of the defining characteristics for sexual dysfunction.

Although conceptualization of the diagnoses related to sexual health requires clarification, the defining characteristics do emphasize subjective as well as objective criteria for evaluation of sexual health. Like other responses described in this chapter, the subjective responses and perceptions of the individual and, in this case, significant others must be considered when identifying a problem and planning care.

Nursing Interventions

Interventions for alterations in sexual health are based on assessment of the subjective perceptions and objective responses of the patient and significant others and careful delineation of the etiology of the problem. From the review of the literature, one is able to identify the most common etiologies of alterations to sexual health related to a diagnosis of cancer and the primary categories of nursing interventions.[78–80] However, the specific approach, suggestions, and resources used to treat the problem must be guided by the etiology of the problem and the perceptions and motivations of the patient or significant other.

Annon[78] has described a simple hierarchy of interventions for sexual problems known as the PLISSIT model (Table 20-8).[80] The system implies that for many problems, the simple acknowledgment and discussion of the perception of change in sexual health may be sufficient to help the patient or significant other resolve the problem. For other problems, especially those that existed before the diagnosis of cancer, referral to a professional for intensive individual or couple therapy may be indicated. For a detailed discussion on this intervention, see Chapter 32, Altered Body Image and Sexuality.

Approaches to treatment of changes in sexual health identified in the literature include education and counseling, yet few empirical studies have addressed the effectiveness of such interventions in ameliorating the symptoms associated with altered sexual health. Capone et al.[81] examined the effects of counseling on psychosocial rehabilitation in a study of 56 patients with gynecologic cancers and 41 patients who met the same criteria but served as controls. Forty-one (73%) of the experimental group and 25 (61%) of the control group were sexually active before initiation of treatment and not more than 6 weeks after diagnosis. Subjects in both groups were interviewed and completed a battery of psychological tests (Self-Rating Symptom Scale, Profile of Mood States, and Tennessee Self-Concept Scale). The experimental group received individual counseling based on crisis intervention principles. Counseling included helping the patient to shape reality-based expectations, facilitating adaptive changes in behaviors, enhancing reintegration of self, and teaching information-processing skills. Interviews and testing were repeated at 3, 6, and 12 months after treatment. Significant differences were found in comparative frequencies of intercourse between the counseling and control groups at 3 ($p < .04$), 6 ($p < .007$), and 12 ($p < .05$) months. Counseling was found to have a positive effect on the resumption of sexual intercourse during the first year after treatment.[81]

More recently, Cain et al.[82] described the psychosocial benefits of a cancer support group for women with a diagnosis of gynecologic cancer. After a psychosocial assessment within 1 month of diagnosis, subjects were assigned to one of three counseling groups: standard mode ($n = 31$), thematic individual mode ($n = 21$), and thematic group ($n = 28$). Each intervention was conducted for 8 weeks. Postcounseling data at 2 weeks and 6 months were obtained. Before the intervention, many of the subjects had significant disruption in sexual relationships. Women in the thematic individual and group counseling categories described significantly better sexual relationships at 6 months compared with baseline data ($F = 4.10$, $p < .02$).[82]

The two studies described are examples of innovative approaches to modify the threat of cancer to sexual health. However, the outcomes by which the effectiveness of the interventions were measured focus primarily on resumption of sexual intercourse. One might question that if sexual health is determined by how individuals perceive themselves, how they perceive that others see them, and how they behave in relationships with others, why were significant others not included in the intervention?

A second concern with respect to the interventions

TABLE 20-8 Levels of Sexual Counseling: The PLISSIT Model

P (Permission)	LI (Limited Information)	SS (Specific Suggestions)	IT (Intensive Therapy)
Legitimize sexual concerns Express sexual concerns with partner and health care team	Anticipatory guidance with respect to sexual concerns Provide information needed for rehabilitation	Cognitive reappraisal Coping skills for changes experienced in communication, roles, relationships Modify behaviors to accommodate limitations imposed by cancer or treatment	Referral to professional therapist

Source: Adapted from Shipes E, Lehr S: Sexuality and the male cancer patient. *Cancer Nurs* 5:375–381, 1982.

described is the lack of screening of patients for participation. Resource consumption of personnel, time, physical facilities, and materials required by such programs must be weighed against the benefits of the program. Therefore, selection of high risk patients for sexual dysfunction to participate in the program may increase the likelihood that sexual morbidity would be reduced. Screening would increase the probability of identifying those patients and partners with preexisting problems that may require more intensive therapy.

Future Directions for Nursing Research

Although sexual health is important, health care professionals have assigned limited value to and assumed a limited perspective of sexual health in relation to cancer care. Increasingly complex, multimodal, and lengthy treatment for cancer increases the risks of changes in sexual health among people diagnosed with cancer and their significant others.

Development of clinical and research instruments that have established reliability and validity for assessment of sexual health dimensions among people with cancer are needed. In addition, multimethods of assessing sexual health not only in the patient but also from the perspective of significant others are required if the interrelationships of the complex factors that contribute to sexual health are to be understood.

Definition, labeling, and validation of changes in sexual health among persons with cancer that require professional intervention are mandated by the level of concept clarification that currently exists. In addition, the effectiveness of educational, counseling, and anticipatory guidance interventions for selected patient and significant other populations should be evaluated.

CONCLUSION

Cancer threatens both the quantity and quality of life for the person who is faced with complex treatment plans, the uncertainty of recurrence, and integration of changed concepts of self, roles, and relationships resulting from the disease and treatment. The responses discussed in this chapter represent high-incidence phenomena described in the literature. One can see how little professionals know and understand about the incidence, contributing factors, variations of response, and long-term consequences of responses for the individual experiencing cancer. Thus, interventions designed to minimize the dysfunctional effects of the experience of cancer are, by the nature of our understanding of the phenomena, limited to "shot-gun," trial-and-error efforts. The specificity of interventions to particular patients based on a systematic appraisal of intrapersonal, interpersonal, social, and economic resources awaits the future.

REFERENCES

1. Spielberger C, Gorusch R, Lushene R: Manual for the state-trait anxiety inventory. Palo Alto, CA: Consulting Psychologists Press, 1970.
2. Lucente FE, Fleck S: A study of hospitalization anxiety in 408 medical and surgical patients. *Psychosom Med* 34:304–312, 1972.
3. Gottesman D, Lewis MS: Differences in crisis reactions among cancer and surgery patients. *J Consult Clin Psychol* 50:381–388, 1982.
4. Scott DW: Anxiety, critical thinking, and information processing during and after breast biopsy. *Nurs Res* 32:24–28, 1983.
5. Morris J, Royle GT: Choice of surgery for early breast cancer: Pre- and postoperative levels of clinical anxiety and depression in patients and their spouses. *Br J Surg* 74:1017–1019, 1987.
6. Oberst MT, Scott DW: Post discharge distress in surgically treated cancer patients and their spouses. *Res Nurs Health* 11:223–233, 1988.
7. Gottschalk LA, Hoigaard-Martin J: The emotional impact of mastectomy. *Psychiatr Res* 17:153–167, 1986.
8. Irwin PH, Kramer S, Diamond NH, et al: Sex differences in psychological distress during definitive radiation therapy for cancer. *J Psychosoc Oncol* 4:63–75, 1986.
9. Andersen BL, Tewfik HH: Psychological reactions to radiation therapy: Reconsideration of the adaptive aspects of anxiety. *J Personal Soc Psychol* 48:1024–1032, 1985.
10. Andersen BL, Karlsson JA, Anderson B, et al: Anxiety and cancer treatment: Response to stressful radiotherapy. *Health Psychol* 3:535–551, 1984.
11. Redd WH, Andrykowski MA: Behavioral intervention in cancer treatment: Controlling aversion reactions to chemotherapy. *J Consult Clin Psychol* 50:1018–1029, 1982.
12. Cassileth BR, Lusk EJ, Walsh WP: Anxiety levels in patients with malignant disease. *Hospice J* 2:57–69, 1986.
13. Cella DF, Pratt A, Holland JC: Persistent anticipatory nausea, vomiting, and anxiety in cured Hodgkin's disease patients after completion of chemotherapy. *Am J of Psychiatry* 143:641–643, 1986.
14. Carey MP, Burish TG: Anxiety as a predictor of behavioral therapy outcome for cancer chemotherapy patients. *J Consult Clin Psychol* 53:860–865, 1985.
15. Gordon M: Manual of Nursing Diagnosis. New York, McGraw-Hill, 1987.
16. Scandrett S: Cognitive reappraisal. In Bulechek GM, McCloskey J (eds.): *Nursing Interventions: Treatments for Nursing Diagnosis*. Philadelphia: Saunders, 1985, pp. 49–57.
17. Miller JF: *Coping with Chronic Illness: Overcoming Powerlessness*. Philadelphia: Davis, 1983.
18. Johnson J: The effects of a patient education course on persons with a chronic illness. *Cancer Nurs* 5:117–123, 1982.
19. Cotanch PH, Strum S: Progressive muscle relaxation as antiemetic therapy for cancer patients. *Oncol Nurs Forum* 14:33–37, 1987.
20. Frank JM: The effects of music therapy and guided visual imagery on chemotherapy induced nausea and vomiting. *Oncol Nurs Forum* 12:47–52, 1985.
21. Davis T, Jensen L: Identifying depression in medical patients. Image. *J Nurs Scholarship* 20:191–95, 1988.

22. Robinson JK, Boshier ML, Dansak DA, et al: Depression and anxiety in cancer patients: Evidence for different causes. *J Psychosom Res* 29:133–138, 1985.
23. Neilson AC, Williams TA: Depression in ambulatory medical patients. *Arch Gen Psychiatry* 37:999–1004, 1980.
24. Hamilton M: A rating scale for depression. *J Neurol Neurosurg Psychiatry* 23:56–62, 1960.
25. Beck AT, Beamesderfer A: Assessment of depression: The depression inventory. In Pichot P, Olivier-Martin R (eds.): *Psychological Measurements in Psychopharmacology: Modern Problems in Pharmopsychiatry* (Vol. 7). Basel: Karger, 1974, pp. 151–169.
26. Nelson LD: Measuring depression in a clinical population using the MMPI. *J Consult Clin Psychol* 55:788–790, 1987.
27. Derogatis LR, Melisaratos N: The DSFI: A multidimensional measure of sexual functioning. *J Sex Marital Therapy* 5:244–281, 1979.
28. McNair DM, Lorr M, Droppleman LF: Profile of mood states. San Diego: Educational and Industrial Testing Service, 1971.
29. Petty F, Noyes R: Depression secondary to cancer. *Biol Psychiatry* 16:1203–1220, 1981.
30. Derogatis LR, Morrow GR, Fetting J, et al: The prevalence of psychiatric disorders among cancer patients. *JAMA* 249:751–757, 1983.
31. Massie MJ, Holland JC: Diagnosis and treatment of depression in the cancer patient. *J Clin Psychiatry* 45:25–29, 1984.
32. Plumb M, Holland JC: Comparative studies of psychological function in patients with advanced cancer. II. Interviewer-rated current and past psychological symptoms. *Psychosom Med* 43:243–254, 1981.
33. Andersen BL, Hacker NF: Psychosexual adjustment after vulvar surgery. *Obstet Gynecol* 62:457–462, 1983.
34. Goldberg RJ, Wool MS, Glicksman A, et al: Relationship of the social environment and patients' physical status to depression in lung cancer patients and their spouses. *J Psychosoc Oncol* 2:73–80, 1984.
35. Metzger LF, Rogers TF, Bauman LJ: Effects of age and marital status on the emotional distress after a mastectomy. *J Psychosoc Oncol* 1:17–33, 1983.
36. Robinson JK, Boshier ML, Dansak DA, et al: Depression and anxiety in cancer patients: Evidence for different causes. *J Psychosom Res* 29:133–138, 1985.
37. Bukberg J, Penman D, Holland JC: Depression in hospitalized cancer patients. *Psychosom Med* 46:199–212, 1984.
38. Spitzer RL: *Diagnostic and Statistical Manual of Mental Disorders-Revised (DSM-III-R).* Washington, DC: American Psychiatric Association, 1987.
39. Layne C, Heitkemper T, Roehrig RA, Speer TK: Motivational deficit in depressed cancer patients. *J Clin Psychol* 41:139–144, 1985.
40. Morris T, Greer S, White P: Psychological and social adjustment to mastectomy: A two-year follow-up study. *Cancer* 40:2381–2387, 1977.
41. Beck AT, Lester D, Trexler L, et al: The measurement of pessimism: The hopelessness scale. *J Consult Clin Psychol* 42:861–865, 1974.
42. Nowotny ML: Assessment of hope in patients with cancer: Development of an instrument. *Oncol Nurs Forum* 16:57–61, 1989.
43. Herth KA: The relationship between level of hope and level of coping response and other variables in patients with cancer. *Oncol Nurs Forum* 16:67–72, 1989.
44. Schmale AH, Iker HP: The affect of hopelessness and the development of cancer. *Psychosom Med* 28:714–721, 1966.
45. Hinds PS: Adolescent hopefulness in illness and health. *Adv Nurs Sci* 10:79–88, 1988.
46. Dufault KJ: Hope of elderly persons with cancer (doctoral dissertation, Case Western Reserve University). *Diss Abstr Intl* 42:1820B, 1981.
47. Zook DJ, Yasko JM: Psychologic factors: Their effect on nausea and vomiting experiences by clients receiving chemotherapy. *Oncol Nurs Forum* 10:76–81, 1983.
48. Greene SM, O'Mahoney PD, Rungasamy P: Levels of measured hopelessness in physically-ill patients. *J Psychosom Res* 26:591–593, 1982.
49. Raleigh ED: An investigation of hope as manifested in the physically ill adult (doctoral dissertation, Wayne State University). *Diss Abstr Intl* 41:1313B, 1980.
50. Brandt B: The relationship between hopelessness and selected variables in women receiving chemotherapy for breast cancer. *Oncol Nurs Forum* 14:35–39, 1987.
51. Stoner M: Hope and cancer patients (doctoral dissertation, University of Colorado Health Sciences Center). *Diss Abstr Intl* 44:115-B, 1982.
52. Stoner M, Keampfer S: Recalled life expectancy information, phase of illness, and hope in cancer patients. *Res Nurs Health* 8:269–274, 1985.
53. Cassileth BR, Zupkis RV, Sutton-Smith K, et al: Information and participation preferences among cancer patients. *Ann Intern Med* 92:832–836, 1980.
54. Kerber A: Locus of control, hope, and disease-free interval (unpublished master's thesis), Emory University, Atlanta, GA, 1985.
55. Clark JC: Hope as a critical factor in the cancer experience. In Pritchard AP (ed.): *Cancer Nursing: A Revolution in Care.* Proceeding of the Fifth International Conference on Cancer Nursing. London: Macmillan, 1989, pp. 117–119.
56. Dufault K, Martocchio BC: Hope: Its spheres and dimensions. *Nurs Clin North Am* 20:379–391, 1985.
57. Derogatis LR: Psychological assessment of psychosexual function. *Psychiatr Clin North Am* 3:113–131, 1980.
58. Waterhouse J, Metcalfe MC: Development of the sexual adjustment questionnaire. *Oncol Nurs Forum* 13:53–59, 1986.
59. Abitbol MM, Davenport JH: Sexual dysfunction after therapy for cervical carcinoma. *Am J Obstet Gynecol* 119:181–189, 1974.
60. Jenkins B: Patients' reports of sexual changes after treatment for gynecological cancer. *Oncol Nurs Forum* 15:349–354, 1988.
61. Cain EN, Kohorn EI, Quinlan DM, et al: Psychosocial reactions to the diagnosis of gynecologic cancer. *Obstet Gynecol* 62:635–641, 1983.
62. Andersen BL, Hacker NF: Psychosexual adjustment after vulvar surgery. *Obstet Gynecol* 62:457–462, 1983.
63. Andreasson B, Moth I, Jensen SB, et al: Sexual function and somatopsychic reactions in vulvectomy-operated women and their partners. *Acta Obstet Gynecol Scand* 65:7–10, 1986.
64. Woods NF, Earp JA: Women with cured breast cancer. *Nurs Res* 27:279–285, 1978.
65. Jamison KR, Wellisch DK, Pasnau RO: Psychosocial aspects of mastectomy. I. The woman's perspective. *Am J Psychiatry* 135:432–436, 1978.
66. Taylor SE, Lichtman RR, Wood JV, et al: Illness-related and treatment-related factors in psychological adjustment to breast cancer. *Cancer* 55:2506–2513, 1985.

67. Blackmore C: The impact of orchidectomy upon the sexuality of the man with testicular cancer. *Cancer Nurs* 11:33–40, 1988.
68. Schover LR, Gonzales M, von Eschenbach AC: Sexual and marital relationships after radiotherapy for seminoma. *Urology* 27:117–123, 1986.
69. Heinrich-Rynning T: Prostatic cancer treatments and their effects on sexual functioning. *Oncol Nurs Forum* 14:37–41, 1987.
70. Banker FL: The preservation of potency after external beam irradiation for prostate cancer. *Int J Radiat Oncol Biol Phys* 15:219–220, 1988.
71. Labenne WD, Greene BI: *Educational Implications of the Self-Concept Theory*. Santa Monica, CA: Goodyear Publishing, 1969, p. 10.
72. Newman KA, Schnaper N, Reed WP, et al: Effect of Hickman catheters on the self-esteem of patients with leukemia. *South Med J* 77:682–685, 1984.
73. Crumbaugh JC: Cross validation of purpose-in-life test based on Frankl's concepts. *J Individual Psychol* 24:74–81, 1968.
74. Weddington WW, Segraves KB, Simon MA: Psychological outcome of extremity sarcoma survivors undergoing amputation or limb salvage. *J Clin Oncol* 3:1393–1399, 1985.
75. Baxley KO, Erdman LK, Henry EB, et al: Alopecia: Effect on cancer patients' body image. *Cancer Nurs* 7:499–503, 1984.
76. Jourard S, Secord PF: Body cathexis and personality. *Br J Psychol* 46:130–138, 1955.
77. Kemeny MM, Wellisch DK, Schain WS: Psychosocial outcome in a randomized surgical trial for treatment of primary breast cancer. *Cancer* 62:1231–1237, 1988.
78. Annon JS: *The Behavioral Treatment of Sexual Problems* (Vol. 1). Honolulu: Mercentile Printing, 1974.
79. Lamb MA, Woods NF: Sexuality and the cancer patient. *Cancer Nurs* 4:137–144, 1981.
80. Shipes E, Lehr S: Sexuality and the male cancer patient. *Cancer Nurs* 5:375–381, 1982.
81. Capone MA, Good RS, Westie KS, et al: Psychosocial rehabilitation of gynecologic oncology patients. *Arch Phys Med Rehabil* 61:128–132, 1980.
82. Cain EN, Kohorn EI, Quinlan DM, et al: Psychosocial reactions to the diagnosis of gynecologic cancer. *Obstet Gynecol* 62:635–641, 1983.

Chapter 21

Psychosocial Responses of the Family

Jane C. Clark, RN, MN, OCN

Robin R. Gwin, RN, MN, OCN

INTRODUCTION

The diagnosis of cancer, though assigned to the individual, has the potential to precipitate significant changes in the lives of the individual, members of the family unit, and community. Responses experienced vary among family members, across developmental stages of the family, with different illness demands, and with respect to economic and psychosocial resources. Anecdotal data and clinical observations have substantiated the theoretical assumption that a change in one element of the social system, in this case the patient diagnosed with cancer, will result in a ripple effect throughout the system.

Predictability with respect to family activities, roles, relationships, and communication patterns are threatened. Life for families facing cancer becomes more complex. Family members are challenged to learn new roles, self-care skills, and ways of relating to and communicating with each other, friends, and members of the health care team as they cope with the chronic nature of the cancer experience. Although the demands cancer places on the family members may be increased, few empirical studies have been conducted to identify the nature of these demands and to describe the psychosocial responses of the individual members or the family unit to the cancer experience.[1,2]

The majority of research on the family and cancer has focused on the responses of individual family members to the experience. Data are available to guide nursing assessment, intervention, and evaluation specifically for spouses and to a lesser extent for young, adolescent, and adult children of white, middle-class women with breast cancer. Databases are beginning to accumulate for family members of patients with lung cancer, of patients undergoing chemotherapy, and of terminally ill patients. However, few researchers have attempted to describe responses of nontraditional, multigenerational, or culturally diverse family units with respect to concepts discussed in theoretical models of the family, such as structure, function, interaction, and development. Thus, empirical contributions to guide nursing assessment and interventions for the family unit experiencing cancer are limited.

In this chapter, selected clinical and research instruments for evaluation of the family unit will be described. In addition, representative studies describing the demands that cancer places on family members and the identified needs of individual family members will be described. Factors that place the individual family member or family unit at risk for extreme responses will be identified. Concluding the chapter will be a review of selected interventions to modify responses of the family. Implications for further nursing research will be discussed.

INSTRUMENTS FOR EVALUATING THE FAMILY

Family APGAR The Family APGAR[3] is a screening questionnaire designed to assess family *A*daptability, *P*artnership, *G*rowth, *A*ffection, and *R*esolve from the perspective of the patient. The questionnaire consists of five questions to which patients respond on a 3-point scale indicating the frequency of satisfaction on the dimensions measured (almost always = 2; some of the time = 1; hardly ever = 0). Based on the definition of *family* as a "psychosocial group consisting of the patient and one or more persons, children or adults, in which there is a commitment for members to nurture each other,"[3,p.1232] the instrument does not assume the structural, institutional, or cultural boundaries of the traditional family. Reliability and validity data were not reported by the author.

Family Functioning Index The Family Functioning Index (FFI)[4] is a 15-item self-report instrument designed to assess the dynamics of family interaction in families that contain children. The instrument is intended for use as a predictive or intervening measure rather than as an outcome measure. Questions assess areas of marital satisfaction, frequency of disagreement, communication, problem solving, and feelings of happiness and closeness. Validity and reliability estimates for the instrument were determined by comparing scores on the FFI with clinical ratings by caseworkers, and by resulting high positive correlations of husband and wife scores. Five year test-retest reliability was reported as $r = .83, p < .001$.[5]

Feetham Family Functioning Survey The Feetham Family Functioning Survey (FFFS)[6] is a 21-item questionnaire designed to assess the family's ability to function as a unit within the community and within their own internal system. Items are intended to assess three constructs: family interactions with the community, the family relationship to various subsystems, and reciprocal relationships within the family structure. Respondents answer three questions on each item: "How much is there now?" "How much should there be?" and "How important is this to me?" on a 7-point, Likert-type scale ranging from *little* (1) to *much* (7). Scores for the three constructs are then determined. A discrepancy score is obtained by subtracting how much there should be from how much there is. Cronbach's alpha for the four measures range from .66 to 184. Test-retest reliability is reported to be .93 at a 2-week interval and .83 at a 5-year interval. Correlations between scores of husbands and wives were reported as .72.[6]

Family Inventory of Resources for Management The Family Inventory of Resources for Management

(FIRM)[7] is a 69-item self-report questionnaire designed to assess the ability of the family to deal with stressors. Each item is scored on a 4-point, Likert-type scale ranging from *not at all* (0) to *very well* (3). Four primary factors are evaluated: family strengths (esteem and communication), family strengths (mastery and health), extended family social support, and financial well-being. In addition, financial support and social desirability subscales have been measured. Scores are summed for each subscale. Cronbach's alpha for the FIRM is reported to be .89, with ranges for the alphas of the four primary subscales reported to be .62–.85. Total FIRM scores have been correlated with measures of family cohesion (.46), expressiveness (.27), conflict (−.30), and organization (.25).

Family Adaptability and Cohesion Evaluation Scales The Family Adaptability and Cohesion Evaluation Scales (FACES III)[8] is a 20-item self-report questionnaire designed to classify families into three general and 16 specific types on adaptability and cohesion dimensions. The instrument can be administered to individuals, couples, or families. Respondents give the frequency of a specific behavior on a 5-point scale ranging from *almost never* (1) to *almost always* (5). Cronbach's alpha for the instrument is estimated as .77 for cohesion, .62 for adaptability, and .68 for the total scale. Scores between family members vary considerably, with correlations ranging from .30 to .40. The authors recommend that the instrument be completed independently by multiple family members.

In summary, instruments with established reliability and validity estimates are available for the nurse to assess the family. The instruments vary in purpose, concepts measured, and length of time required for completion. The routine assessment of the family on entrance to the health care system and during the course of treatment, rehabilitation, survival, or death is recommended to improve the quality of care for members of the family and the patient.

NEEDS OF THE FAMILY

The family, like the person with cancer, has many needs as the cancer experience becomes a focus of daily living. Depending on the development stage of the individual and the family, organization of the family, roles within the family, and patterns of interaction, each family member may have different needs at different points in time across the cancer trajectory. A growing number of studies demonstrate that family members have perceived needs for information, communication skills, coping strategies, and support services.

Information

Families are in a unique position when faced with the task of getting information about cancer, cancer treatment, and prognosis. Increased use of home health care services, outpatient care, and hospice services has resulted in the family assuming a more active role in the care of the person with cancer across the disease trajectory. Yet few studies have addressed either the nature of the specific informational needs or the strategies used to obtain the needed information.

Northouse et al.,[9] in a review of communication literature, noted that obtaining information was one of the primary tasks facing family members of persons with cancer. Houts et al.[10] conducted a review of the information needs of families of cancer patients. Findings across 20 primary studies revealed that, in general, family members needed information, in understandable language, about the status of the patient, listing treatment plans, side effects, and prognosis. Furthermore, family members perceived that they needed anticipatory guidance about emotional responses of the patient across the cancer experience. When the family members were expected to provide home care, additional informational needs were identified related to caregiving skills and available support services for both the patient and the family member.[10]

Needs of family members change as the setting for care changes from acute care to outpatient/home arenas. Blank et al.[11] studied intrapersonal, interpersonal, and extrapersonal stressors identified by eight patients receiving cancer treatment on an outpatient basis and their eight caregivers. Caregiver needs based on intrapersonal stressors included treatment uncertainty, role responsibilities, fear of being alone, coping with the patient situation, and guilt. Caregiver needs based on interpersonal stressors included lack of support, relationship with the patient, the patient's activities of daily living, and lack of information. Needs based on extrapersonal stressors included finances and transportation.

Tringali[12a] studied cognitive, emotional, and physical family needs across three phases of illness: initial treatment, treatment at recurrence, and follow-up. For a convenience sample of 25 family members (blood relatives, spouses, or friends who accompanied the patient to the clinic), data indicated that family members ranked cognitive needs the highest across all phases of illness. Identified needs included having explanations in understandable terms and having honest answers about the disease, treatment, and prognosis. Participants also indicated the need for hope and to be able to trust the expertise and concern of care providers. For family members in the initial treatment sample, information about disease and treatment, patient responses, and how to manage the patient at home were considered most important. For the family members of patients with recurrent disease, the needs for honest information about the patient and for assurance that the best possible care was being provided by caring professionals were most critical. For family members in the follow-up sample, the need for honesty and hope remained significant.[11]

Informational needs for family members remained

consistent across spouses of patients with selected site-specific cancers. Northouse et al.[12b] studied the psychosocial adjustment of 50 newly diagnosed breast cancer patients who received surgical treatment and their spouses. Data were collected by interviews during hospitalization after mastectomy and again at 1 month after surgery. Survival was the primary concern of both spouses and patients during the hospitalization and 1 month after surgery. The spouses indicated that the most stressful phase of the breast cancer experience was the diagnostic phase (50%). Factors that contributed to the stressfulness of the diagnostic phase included the uncertainty of treatment decision and expectations as well as the frequent delays. Waiting for information about the patient following surgery contributed to the stress experienced during the hospitalization phase (44%), particularly on the day of surgery.

In 55 patient–spouse dyad interviews, Lewis et al.[13] noted that the major tasks of couples 1 year after initial diagnosis of breast cancer included finding, interpreting, choosing, and managing information related to the illness. Findings were corroborated in a study by Zahlis and Shands,[14] who interviewed 67 partners of women within 2.5 years of a breast cancer diagnosis. Data indicated that the majority of the partners identified the need to be educated about the disease and treatment, as well as the need to help make decisions. Demands that the illness had on the partners included reacting to the illness, adapting the lifestyle to meet the demands of the illness, being sensitive to the patient's needs, thinking about the future, and adapting to the impact on the relationship between the partner and the patient. Eleven respondents reported communication difficulties with partners.

Review of the literature indicates that information is critical. The type of information needed extends beyond the obvious details of the disease and treatment plan. Family members need information about resources available to address the added day-to-day demands of life in addition to cancer-related demands.

Nurses can address the informational needs of families facing cancer with a variety of strategies: individual instruction about specific concerns, group sessions on common concerns, audiovisual or written materials on disease and treatment concerns, and resources available to meet daily demands of family life.

All family members will not require the same types of information at the same time nor in the same format. Although some data exist about the informational needs of middle-class spouses, limited empirical data address the changing cancer information needs of the poor, culturally diverse and nontraditional families, children whose parents have cancer, and elderly parents whose adult children have cancer. The nurse evaluates the interpretation of information by the family. Information may need to be presented repetitively in different formats in order for learning and application of information to real-world problems to occur. The nurse is mandated by professional standards of practice to assume a role in providing information to patients and families facing cancer.

Communication

Communication patterns between the patient–spouse dyads[14] changed, in that the spouses became protective of the patient with respect to discussing distressful information and reported not sharing their feelings with patients. In spite of changed communication patterns, the majority of subjects reported increased closeness in patient–spouse and parent–child relationships.

Northouse et al.[9] reviewed 200 clinical papers and research studies printed over two decades to identify issues of communication among patients, health professionals, and family members. The authors argue that although the number of articles on communication issues among family members of persons with cancer is limited, the potential impact of communication issues on the care of the patient and the well-being of the family is far-reaching.

Communication becomes a primary issue among family members as caregiving demands increase. Data indicate that although the responsibilities of care are being shifted to the family, family members express concern over the difficulty in obtaining necessary information.[15–17] Second, as the demands of care increase, mood disturbances among family members, particularly anxiety and depression,[18,19] become more prominent. Yet family members have not communicated their concerns and responses to health professionals, and concern for care of family members by health care providers has been limited.

Just as data indicate that communication patterns have the potential to become strained between the patient and spouse facing cancer, indications are that communication patterns change between the parents and children within the family. Hymovich[20] conducted a semistructured, open-ended interview with parents with cancer and their spouses. Stressors identified included inadequate information and uncertainty regarding the illness. Parents disclosed that making decisions about what and how to communicate with the children about the illness were significant issues. Arranging child care and maintaining composure in front of the children were also constant concerns.

The importance of communication skills is never more critical than in a life-threatening situation. Communication is the way experiences are shared, perceptions are clarified, and new information is learned. The nurse can assume an important role in assessing communication styles in families living with cancer. Styles that are potential barriers to information gathering, decision making, and support development can be addressed with the individual family member or with the family unit. The nurse can intervene via one-on-one counseling, group sessions on communication, role modeling of facilitative communication, and role-playing communications with individual family members.

Coping Skills

Coping with the emotional responses of the patient as well as with their own responses were additional concerns expressed by family members, significant others, and caregivers. In Chapter 20, the individual responses of anxiety, depression, and hopelessness were discussed with respect to the diagnosis of cancer. Surprisingly, the responses of family members have been shown to be similar to those of the patient.

Germino[22] interviewed 50 newly diagnosed patients with cancer, their spouses, and adult children (N = 127) to study their perceptions of family functioning as determined by comparisons of family member concerns. Convergence of concerns centered on condition of the patient, diagnosis, and treatment. Concerns of spouses centered on managing their feelings and the feelings of others, relationships, and the demands imposed by cancer.

Oberst and James[18] conducted a study to determine the magnitude and pattern of crisis development among spouses of cancer patients (N = 40). Findings indicated that spouses experienced increased anxiety prior to discharge from the hospital, which was replaced by depression and anger at patients for egocentricity in the home-care period. Depression and anger were succeeded eventually by guilt. Moreover, spouses reported distress, anger, and frustration about the lack of support from professionals and all sources.[18,p.56] Spouses also had a higher incidence of emotional problems than did the patients at 10, 30, 60, 90, and 180 days postdischarge. In addition, spouses reported disruption in many lifestyle areas, including employment, home management, child care, social activities, and travel to and from the hospital. Thus, the acute hospitalization period precipitated significant psychological responses among spouses of patients with cancer that continued through the postdischarge, active treatment, home-care, and terminal phases of illness.

Findings of Oberst and James[18] were corroborated in a study of 43 patients with a variety of cancers treated with surgery and their spouses (N = 36).[22] Data were collected within 1 week presurgery and within 10–14 days postsurgery. Levels of distress reported by spouses remained constant over the study period, while distress levels for the patients decreased. Appraisal of the situation was identified as a significant factor in describing the spouse's response to the surgery.

A descriptive study of 28 caregivers of newly diagnosed patients with nonterminal, advanced cancer who were coping with the effects of surgery, radiation, and/or chemotherapy was reported by Perry and Roades de Meneses.[22] Caregivers were interviewed and completed the Jalowiec Coping Scale. Findings indicated that caregivers reported experiencing a variety of emotional responses, including increased stress (81%), fear (81%), anxiety (77%), inability to cope (77%), and emotional withdrawal (66%). Additional concerns expressed by the caregivers included fear of losing their loved one, uncertainty regarding the illness, and concern about keeping their own spirits up.

Depression has been noted as a primary response of family members experiencing cancer. The findings of Goldberg et al.[23] support the high incidence of depression among spouses (n = 18) of patients with lung cancer. Scores on the Profile of Mood States—Depression were measured within 6 weeks of diagnosis and at 2-month intervals for a total of 6 months. Spouses had elevated mean scores at the time of diagnosis (Time 1 = 14.7), and the mean scores remained elevated throughout the data collection period (Time 2 = 11.3, Time 3 = 10.6). In addition, scores of spouses on the Psychosocial Adjustment to Illness Scale, social environment subscale, were related significantly to the depression scores rather than to the physical status scores of the patient at all three time intervals.

Other psychosocial responses of spouses of patients with lung cancer were described by Cooper.[24] Fifteen patients with lung cancer and their spouses were interviewed to determine the effects of the diagnosis on the family. In content analysis of the interviews, the following effects were identified. Spouses experienced depression, shock, fear, and feelings of aloneness and helplessness at the time of diagnosis. Spouses also reported more symptoms of stress (nervousness, sleeplessness, loss of appetite, inability to concentrate, and irritability) than did patients.

Similar responses were reported by Kalayjian,[25] who analyzed the responses of 40 wives of patients with a diagnosis of cancer to an interview regarding coping difficulties resulting from the partner's diagnosis. The interviews were conducted 3–6 months after diagnosis. Depression, family changes, feelings of loneliness, and helplessness were described.

A comparison of psychological responses of patients with cancer and their next-of-kin family members (N = 210) was reported by Cassileth et al.[26] Patient and next-of-kin scores on three outcome measures, State-Trait Anxiety Inventory, Profile of Mood States, and Mental Health Index, were correlated significantly. Scores for both patients and next-of-kin indicated a decrease in psychological status related to the phase of the cancer experience; i.e., the psychological status was better for patients and next-of-kin during follow-up care versus active treatment versus palliative care.

Home care places additional demands on the physical, social, and emotional resources of the family. The response of spouses to home-care demands were described by Wellisch et al.[27] Records of home-bound, married cancer patients (N = 447) were reviewed to determine the types of psychosocial problems experienced by family members.[27,p.1] A standardized instrument to abstract the frequencies of psychosocial problem areas (Table 21-1)[27] was used for review. Findings indicated that families of male patients were more likely to feel overwhelmed by the demands of home care and were more likely to experience a severe mood disturbance than were families of female patients.

Age had a significant impact on the family variables studied. Families of patients 70 years or older were more likely to be overwhelmed by home care demands. Role disturbances were more likely to occur in families

TABLE 21-1 Psychosocial Problems Experienced by Family Members

- Impaired relationships with the family and/or significant others
- Impaired relationships with health care providers
- Somatic side effects of disease and treatment
- Difficulties in compliance with treatment
- Mood disturbances
- Difficulties in family roles
- Difficulties in self-management
- Financial difficulties
- Transportation difficulties
- Equipment difficulties
- Significant concerns about body image
- Denial
- Cognitive impairment

Source: Wellisch DK, Fawzy FI, Landsverk J, et al: Evaluation of psychosocial problems of the home-bound cancer patient: The relationship of disease and the sociodemographic variables of patients to family problems. *J Psychosoc Oncol* 1(3):4–5, 1983.

of patients age 50 years or younger, whereas mood disturbances were more likely to occur in families of patients 50 years or older.

Of note, the findings of the study indicated that the diagnosis of the patient, i.e., lung, breast, or cervical cancer, had a specific impact on the family outcome variables. The families of patients with lung cancer were more likely to exhibit significant mood disturbances and to be overwhelmed by the demands of home care. In contrast, families of patients with cervical cancer were more likely to experience disturbances in family relationships.[27]

Patterns of caregiver burden over time were described by McCorkle et al.[28] in a study of 17 patient–caregiver pairs. Caregivers consisted of 14 spouses, 2 parents, and 1 sibling. Findings indicated that for this sample, the number of patient problems was related to physical caregiving demands as well as financial impact on the caregiver at discharge from the hospital. Over a 6-month period, the condition of the patients improved, although reported caregiver burden levels remained unchanged. These findings support the emerging concern for the protracted course of caregiver burden and the implications for caregiver outcomes.

Gender differences have been demonstrated in several studies of caregiver burden. Siegel et al.[29] conducted a telephone interview with 295 cancer patient–spouse dyads to determine the prevalence and intensity of caregiver burdens. Data indicated that female caregivers were more likely than male caregivers to be the sole source of assistance and were less likely to use either formal or informal assistance. Both male and female caregivers reported social, time, and employment-related burdens, although female caregivers were more likely to experience time burdens. The presence of metastatic disease, increased number of reduced activity days for the patient, and increased number of patient symptoms resulted in increased incidence of physical, social, and time burdens for female caregivers.

Additional gender differences were described by Stetz[30] in semistructured interviews conducted in the home of 65 spouses of terminally ill adult cancer patients. Content analyses revealed nine categories of spouse caregiving demands (Table 21-2).[30] Gender differences were identified. Female caregivers had more difficulty with observing the physical deterioration of the spouse; male caregivers had more difficulty with home management.

Gustafson et al.[31] explored the association of needs and concerns with treatment effects and outcomes. Patients ($N = 376$) completed a set of standardized instruments. Qualitative interviews were conducted with 20 spouses. Female patients were more likely than male patients to report that their partners did not provide enough care and were more likely to have difficulty in asking their partners for assistance. Female patients found it more difficult to discuss emotional responses to cancer with their partners and reported that their partners were more distant.

How, then, do family members cope with the stressors and demands of living with the cancer experience? Spouses of 50 women with breast cancer reported relying on the emotional support of family, friends, and co-workers, information receiving, and maintaining a positive attitude. Religious faith and distraction were also identified as helpful coping strategies.[32]

Dibble[33] reported on a longitudinal, repeated-measures-design study of the coping strategies used by family members of cancer patients ($N = 100$) receiving chemotherapy to cope with their most important problem (patient's physical cancer-related health). The most frequently reported coping strategies involved talking with others, seeking information, and taking action. These strategies were categorized as direct-action strategies and were not different from those strategies used by the patients. When direct-action strategies to cope

TABLE 21-2 Perceived Spousal Caregiving Demands

- Management of physical care
- Management of household finances
- Standing by
- Alterations in caregiver's well-being and pattern of living
- Unmet expectations from the health care system
- Constant vigilance
- Cancer
- Anticipation of the future
- Alterations in relationship with ill spouse

Source: Stetz KM: Caregiving demands during advanced cancer: The spouse's needs. *Cancer Nurs* 10(5):260–268, 1987.

with the problem were rejected by the patient, family members shifted to more emotional-focused strategies.

A spectrum of confrontive, emotive, and palliative coping strategies were identified by 28 caregivers of newly diagnosed cancer patients under treatment.[22] Maintaining self-control (92%), trying and seeing what works (82%), and seeking information (82%) were the most common confrontive strategies used. Emotive strategies included worrying (78%) and preparing to expect the worst (61%). Palliative strategies included praying (85%), hoping that things would get better (75%), and using laughter (79%). Of note, 85% of the caregivers reported that they did not use any community resources or services.

Coping strategies used by families coping with chronic illness in the mother (diabetes, fibrocystic breast disease, and nonmetastatic breast cancer) were examined by Stetz et al.[34] Data supported the finding that coping strategies used by the families did not differ with the primary diagnosis of the mother. The most commonly used strategies involved the modification of roles and relationship rules within the family to meet the demands imposed by the illness. Other strategies included seeking help from sources outside the household family, and mobilizing action within the household family. Families were described as resourceful in developing coping strategies to meet their unique needs.

The type, amount, and usage of support systems and services needed by caregivers of differing age, sex, and socioeconomic status continues to be a concern for health care providers. However, minimal empirical data exist about these issues. The challenge of developing specific nursing interventions to address the coping needs of family members facing cancer depends on an accurate and thorough assessment of preexisting dysfunctional psychosocial responses and coping behaviors used by individual family members and the family unit in previous times of stress or crisis. For family members with preexisting problems, referral to a counselor, psychologist, or psychiatrist may be warranted early in the course of disease. For family units that have experienced other crises, the assessment provides the basis for supporting effective coping behaviors and for providing an opportunity to learn new coping skills. Group classes on stress reduction techniques, referrals to self-help groups, or individual counseling may be used to address coping needs. Again, the nurse assumes an active role in evaluating the effectiveness of coping skills and behaviors of the family throughout the cancer experience.

Support Services

Historically, clinicians and researchers have focused on support services designed to meet the physical care needs of the patient at home. While family members and caregivers have identified an assortment of needs, including home management, financial counseling, anticipatory guidance, transportation, and child care, a minimal number of programs to meet these needs are described in the literature. More significant are the findings related to the protracted patterns of needs and the perceived difficulties families and caregivers have in asking for support.

Ell et al.[35] conducted a longitudinal study of 143 cancer patient–significant other pairs. Subjects were interviewed at 3–6 months after the initial cancer diagnosis and then again in 6 months. Results indicated that contrary to expected results, significant others experienced a significant decrease in mental health scores, personal well-being scores, and an increase in distress levels between the time of diagnosis and 1 month after diagnosis. Few significant others reported having received assistance from a mental health worker (6%) or having attended a cancer support group (3%).

The difficulty that family members have in accessing support services was reported by Kalayjian.[25] Forty wives of patients diagnosed with cancer identified a range of coping difficulties, including family changes, depression, and changes in the behavior of children. Yet respondents experienced difficulty asking for additional support.

Weinert[36] conducted one of the few investigations of responses of special populations. In interviews with 420 cancer patients in rural areas who had caregivers in their homes, the researcher noted that satisfaction with the relationship for women was influenced positively by their perceived level of social support, the amount of care given by family members, and negatively influenced by care from informal sources.

Support patterns for spouse caregivers were described by Stommel and Kingry.[37] The researchers noted that when young children were in the home, support (13 hr/wk) was provided by family members outside the home. When adult children lived in the home, they contributed similar time to the care of the patient. However, support from family members outside the home dropped dramatically to less than 4 hr/wk.

Families and caregivers appear to "do the best they can" with the help of informal supports from nuclear and extended family members, friends, and community organizations, such as churches, and volunteer organizations, such as the American Cancer Society. However, data to describe and quantify the impact of the lack of perceived availability and use of support systems on outcomes of the cancer experience for the family and caregivers are still unavailable.

The nurse plays an important role in helping families to identify and access support that is available to meet the demands of cancer. Often, support systems will be activated early in the course of the disease, only to fade as the support needs become protracted. Helping family members recognize the importance of giving extended family and friends an opportunity to help, being specific about the type and amount of support needed, and acknowledging the benefits of support received is an important role for the nurse. Strategies such as role playing the asking for help may lessen the anxiety associated with the actual request. The nurse can help family members make a list of tasks that need to be done (grocery shopping, washing, cleaning the house, staying with the patient), the tasks that the family member wants to continue to do, the tasks that can be done by someone else, and those people or groups in the support system that may be contacted for assistance. Strategies requiring minimal time to let supporters know how meaningful their contributions have been to the family member and the patient can be suggested. Such strategies include notes in church bulletins; community newsletters or papers; written, duplicated updates on how things are going to all supporters; and development of a telephone tree.

EFFECT OF FAMILY AND CAREGIVER RESPONSES ON PATTERNS OF CARE AND ADAPTATION

The majority of studies in the area of family responses to a diagnosis of cancer have described the responses experienced in families of selected patient groups (site-specific or age-specific). However, empirical findings to quantify the impact of those responses on patterns of care or individual-member or family-level adaptation are limited.

Patterns of Care

Treatment choice

Minimal data exist to evaluate the effect of treatment choices on adjustment in spouses, specifically spouses from various cultures. Baider et al.[38] administered the Spielberger State-trait Anxiety Scale, the Beck Depression Rating Scale, and the Derogatis Psychosocial Adjustment to Physical Illness Scale to 64 Israeli women who had received treatment for breast cancer and 41 available spouses. Half of the women had had lumpectomy, the other half had had mastectomy. No significant differences in adjustment measures were found between the two groups of women or the two groups of spouses.

Use of hospice

Hays[39] conducted a retrospective-chart review of visits to 100 patients with cancer during the last 10 days of their lives to determine if the incidence of symptoms, family coping, and resources use were predictive of home and inpatient hospice use. The random sample of home care patients (Group I, home care only; Group II, home care/inpatient) were evaluated on physical symptoms of pain, nausea/vomiting, respiratory deficit, elimination, nutrition, and mental status; family coping patterns of anxiety and fatigue; and patterns of care, including length and frequency of home visits, discipliner visited, telephone contacts, home care episodes, and place of death. Patients who experienced more physical symptoms and more symptoms that were uncontrolled were more likely to require inpatient hospice services. An association of uncontrolled symptoms with increased anxiety and fatigue experienced by family members and demand for home care services also increased the use of inpatient hospice services.

Although data are limited, the responses of family members may play a role in the patterns of care for patients with cancer. Increasing concerns about the cost effectiveness of care across settings will mandate empirical data about the role and responsibilities of the family in health care.

Individual or Family-Level Adaptation

A longitudinal study of 143 cancer patient–significant other pairs was conducted to describe the psychological adaptation to the cancer experience.[35] Significant others experienced a significant decrease in mental health scores, personal well-being scores, and an increase in distress levels between the time of diagnosis and 1 month after diagnosis. Factors affecting the psychological adaptation included initial psychological status, educational level, and changes in the routine of the significant other. Significant others who functioned more poorly also had a lower sense of personal control, perceived inadequate emotional support, and greater stress from noncancer-related sources. Congruence between patient and significant other psychological functioning was not present in the study sample, suggesting differing adaptive trajectories or lack of a reciprocal cancer experience between the patient and the significant other.

Caregiver health

Certainly, the demands of cancer place an increased burden on caregivers in terms of physical, psychological, and social resources. Many times the health of the caregiver suffers as concern is focused on the health of the patient. Recent empirical studies have demonstrated the effects of cancer on caregiver health.

Factors associated with perceived level of health of 65 spouse caregivers of people with advanced cancer were explored by Stetz.[40] Cross-sectional data were obtained from interviews and supported the findings that older caregivers perceived health more negatively than younger caregivers. A stronger sense of purpose in life was positively associated with a positive perception of health, whereas higher levels of uncertainty were associated with a more negative perception of health.

Differences in individual outcomes between white and black caregivers were described by O'Hare et al.[41] Black caregivers described their health as poorer than did the white caregivers, felt that their health had declined as a result of caregiving demands, used more sick days during the previous 6 months, and reported less support from other family members. Lower income, minimal insurance coverage, and limited education among black caregivers contributed to the differences in the psychosocial responses noted.

The patient and family are described as the unit of care in oncology. The nurse should evaluate the effects of the physical and psychosocial demands on family members. Nurses can implement previously described strategies to provide critical information, to access resources, to develop and use effective coping strategies, and thereby decrease the negative effects of cancer on the family.

Marital relationships

Gritz et al.[42] studied the long-term effects of testicular cancer on marital relationships. The researchers interviewed 34 long-term survivors of testicular cancer and their wives 4 years after completion of treatment. Participants also completed the Profile of Mood States (POMS), CES-D, Sense of Coherence Score, and the Family Environment Scale. Findings indicate that the majority of couples experienced increased sense of cohesion, intimacy, communication, and sensitivity to feelings as outcomes of the testicular cancer experience.

Schover et al.[43] analyzed questionnaires on marital satisfaction from 84 men who had been treated with radiation therapy for seminoma. Nineteen percent ($N = 14$) reported being divorced subsequent to the cancer diagnosis, with 39% of those divorced indicating that cancer interfered with their marriage. Patients who divorced indicated that their relationships prior to the cancer diagnosis had been less happy than did those patients who remained married.

Relationships with and adaptation of children

Just as data indicate that relationships have the potential to become strained between the patient and the spouse facing cancer, indications are that relationships between parents and children within the family may also be at risk. Lichtman et al.[44] interviewed 78 patients with a diagnosis of breast cancer to describe changes in the relationships between patients and their children and to examine the factors that influence these changes. In addition to structured interviews, the subjects completed the Profile of Mood States, Self-Esteem Scale, Index of Well-being, and the Marital Adjustment Scale. Patients were also asked to provide the name of a significant other to be interviewed ($N = 63$).

Findings indicate 54% of patients ($n = 37$) reported that changes in the relationships with children occurred. The changes were characterized as improved (73%) and permanent (76%). Nineteen problem relationships were identified. Patients attributed the problems to changes in how the children were responding to the patient (28%) and how the patients were responding to the children (10%), changes in both response patterns (52%), and changes due to other reasons (10%). These findings were confirmed by interviews with identified significant others.

Deteriorated relationships were correlated significantly with a poor prognosis for the patient as well as with the severity of surgery. In addition, patient adjustment scores were predictive of perceived changes in relationships with children, in that patients with poor adjustment scores reported more changes and negative changes in relationships with children.

Changes in relationships with children differed significantly with respect to the gender of the child. Although patients reported similar problems with fears related to prognosis, rejection, and refusal to discuss cancer in both mother–son and mother–daughter relationships, the frequency and magnitude of the problems were greater in the mother–daughter relationships.

Birenbaum and Yancey[45] studied the adjustment of adolescent children to the parent's cancer experience. Comparisons were made between responses of adolescents and those of their parents. Perceptions of behavior problems in the adolescent child were consistent with normative ranges on the Child Behavior Checklist and with the perceptions of the spouse. However, behavioral problems in the child were perceived significantly higher by the patient than by either the spouse or the adolescent. Explanations for these differences among three family members were unclear.

Loss of a parent during adolescence has been documented as a critical event in the life of a child. Berman et al.[46] interviewed ten adolescents and the surviving parent within 6 months to 2 years following the death of a parent from cancer to describe responses experienced. The adolescents described open information sharing among the family unit during the illness; however, after the death, communication patterns changed. The adolescent reportedly assumed the protector role in shielding the remaining parent from discussing stressful feelings. The adolescents, as did the spouses in the previous studies, indicated that the protector role was extremely stressful and that they lacked sufficient support during this period. Discrepancies were reported between parents and adolescents in the changes in activities of daily living for the adolescents as well as in the sources of support for the adolescents. Adolescents perceived an increase in household responsibilities as well as more support from family and peers versus health professionals and clergy.

How do children cope with the cancer experience in the parent? Minimal data exist to describe the coping strategies of children of a parent with cancer. Based on content analysis of interviews of 81 children in white, middle-class families whose mothers were diagnosed with breast cancer in the past 2.5 years, children and families identified four primary coping strategies.[47] The children acted as if they were "in the mother's shoes" and focused on how they could help the mother rather than on how the mother and family could help them. The children and families tried to maintain "business as usual" to maintain family equilibrium and minimize the effects of the illness. Family time was used as a resource and a source of "group energy." Finally, the family and children made an effort to "put the illness on the table" or to understand the illness from the child's perspective. Children identified parents, other family members, young friends, and adult friends as sources of help in dealing with the illness. However, twice as many younger children than older children reported that no one helped them cope.

The impact of cancer on adult children has been the focus of study for several researchers. Germino[48] studied the responses of 38 adult children who had a parent with cancer. Demographic characteristics of the sample were different from most samples reported. Most of the subjects had only a high school education. Fifty percent of the subjects were unmarried and 27% were black. Adult children reported five major issues in dealing with the cancer experience: involvement in the parent's illness; disruption of current family relationships; unresolved relationship problems; fears, fantasies, and concern; and illness demands.

The relationships with adult children have the potential to become more complex when the adult child is a health care professional. In a cross-sectional study by Baird[49] of 27 nurse/daughters, the subjects were interviewed and asked to compare their perceptions of family relationships prior to and after the diagnosis of cancer. Nurse/daughter perceptions of roles changed with the diagnosis of cancer in the following ways: Roles expanded from that of information source to decision maker, intermediary, and caregiver. Even though the role changes were perceived as positive, nurse/daughters described role conflicts between daughter/nurse, sibling/nurse, and family member/nurse. Yet positive changes in communication patterns were identified by 59% of the sample. Parents and family members were perceived to be more open, closer, and more dependent after the diagnosis of cancer.

Recently, researchers have asked the question "Does cancer in the family effect the behaviors of adult children with respect to cancer surveillance and psychological functioning?" Wellisch et al.[50] examined the impact of a maternal history of breast cancer on knowledge, behaviors, and perceptions of 60 daughters and a comparison group matched for age, educational level, and race. Findings indicated no differences existed between the groups on frequency of breast self-examination (BSE) or mammography screening. However, daughters of breast cancer patients reported significantly less frequent intercourse, lower sexual satisfaction, and greater vulnerability to breast cancer. The authors indicate that these findings may reflect the perceptions of psychological vulnerability of the daughters, since they identified with the perceived responses of the mothers with breast cancer.

Findings of poor adherence to recommended breast cancer screening practices among high-risk women were supported in a study of 217 women with one or more first-degree relatives with a breast cancer diagnosis.[51] The impact of beliefs about breast cancer risks on surveillance behaviors was considered. Findings revealed that 94% of the women had regularly scheduled mammograms, but only 69% had regular clinical breast exams and only 40% performed BSE each month. Anxiety was a major determinant of adherence to recommended surveillance behaviors. Over 27% of the subjects reported psychological distress severe enough to warrant counseling. Women who reported more barriers to surveillance and fewer social supports had greater psychological distress.

In summary, children, regardless of age, are at risk for psychosocial consequences from parental cancer. The nurse should assess for the presence of children in the family and for the quality of communications and relationship that existed prior to the diagnosis of cancer. For families with relationships that were less than satisfactory prior to the diagnosis, referral for counseling or family therapy may be recommended. Open discussions with children about the illness, what will be done to treat the parent, and plans for caring for the child are encouraged. When possible, the child should be included in decision making. The child should be encouraged to talk with the parents about any concerns he or she has related to changes in family life required by the illness. The importance of continued contact with the ill parent even during lengthy hospitalizations is stressed. Telephone calls, videotapes, and visits to the hospital can decrease uncertainty and fear. Depending on the age of the child, referral to support groups for children of parents with cancer may be recommended.

Family-level adaptation

The relationships of family cohesion and adaptability, marital adjustment, and psychosocial adjustment to illness among 57 Caucasian women with breast cancer were explored by Friedman et al.[52] Based on the theoretical framework proposed by Olson et al.,[53] the researchers examined whether women who perceived that their families were balanced rather than extreme with respect to emotional connectedness and flexibility to change reported more positive levels of adjustment. Findings supported the notion that family cohesion is a desirable quality among women faced with a diagnosis of breast cancer. In fact, 34% of the respondents expressed a desire for more cohesiveness within the family, whereas no respondents indicated a desire for less cohesiveness. Data analyses revealed that women who reported the highest levels of family cohesion also reported more positive adjustment to breast cancer. No significant relationship was found between reported family adaptability and adjustment to breast cancer. Although the findings are not consistent with the propositions of the model offered by Olsen et al.,[53] the authors question if gender differences with respect to value of affection versus task-orientation could have contributed to the differences seen in the study sample.

Vess et al.[54] studied the effect of the pattern of reallocation of roles in the family on family functioning and the psychosocial environment. A total of 29 couples completed the Washington Family Role Inventory, the Marital Communication Inventory, the Family Environment Scale, and a structured interview at baseline Time 1 and again 5 months later at Time 2. Comparisons between the data sets indicated that families who experienced less disruption, role conflict, and role strain during the study period used achieved rather than ascribed role assignment, had older children who assumed additional role functions, and had higher levels of interspouse communication.

Lewis et al.[55] studied the spouse's perspective on family functioning of 48 fathers with school-age children and whose wife had breast cancer, diabetes, or fibrocystic breast disease. Data indicated that increased demands of illness were correlated with increased depression scores of the fathers. Spouses of women with breast cancer had higher levels of marital adjustment. Frequent demands of illness and increased levels of marital adjustment were correlated with coping behaviors that included family discussion, feedback, and reflecting. The fathers in this group reported more frequent interchange and strong father–child relationships as compared to the other fathers. Higher levels of marital adjustment and frequent interchange between father and child positively affected the function of the family.

Analysis of qualitative data by Hough et al.[56] described factors associated with well-adjusted or poorly adjusted families experiencing breast cancer. Well-adjusted families had the ability to find positive meaning in the experience: learning to value day-to-day living, creating a healthy balance of work and other activities in life, and feeling more empathetic with others. Perceived social support and fewer concurrent stressors also were factors that affected the positive adjustment in families.

ASSESSMENT CRITERIA FOR FAMILY PROBLEMS

The family is listed as a portion of four nursing diagnoses identified by the North American Nursing Diagnosis Association (NANDA): Alteration in family processes; Ineffective family coping: compromised; Ineffective family coping: disabling; and Family coping: potential for growth.[57] A comparison of each diagnosis is presented in Table 21-3.[57]

The complexities of assessment measures of the family are detailed by Lewis.[1] Yet the complexities of measures only reflect the complexities of the phenomenon of study, in this case the family coping with the cancer experience. Thus, the ideal assessment of families using multiple measures from multiple sources described by Lewis[1] offers the potential for collecting the most comprehensive and reliable database on which to base family-level services.

However, the personnel and time demanded by such an extensive assessment precludes application to all families in the clinical setting. Yet screening instruments described previously may serve to identify those families at high risk for dysfunctional responses to the cancer experience and to target families in need of a more comprehensive assessment and intervention.[58]

FAMILY-LEVEL NURSING INTERVENTIONS

Selection of nursing interventions for families facing cancer are based on the needs of the individual members of the family as well as on the needs expressed by the family unit. Family-level teaching with respect to the disease, treatment, rehabilitation, and/or prognosis; anticipatory guidance of family members throughout the cancer experience; single- and multiple-family group counseling; mobilization of health care and/or community resources; and referrals for intensive family therapy have been identified in the literature as strategies for family care.[59–66]

Although nursing interventions may be directed toward the individual members or the family unit, the majority of studies among families facing cancer have focused on the individual family members. Few empirical studies have been conducted to determine the effects of family-unit services. The effects of selected interventions on family outcomes will be discussed in the following section.

Cancer Information Service

Meissner et al.[61] described the use of a Cancer Information Service (CIS) to meet the information needs of the significant others (spouses, relatives, and friends) of people with cancer. A total of 750,000 calls to the CIS were received during a 4-year period. Twenty-five percent of the calls received were made by significant others of people with cancer. Significant others learned about the CIS primarily through health professionals, phone assistance, and publications. Callers most frequently requested information about site-specific cancers, treatment, and referral sources for second opinions. The CIS appears to offer the types of information identified as necessary by family members. However, CIS users were primarily female (70%), had greater than a twelfth-grade education (88%), and were white (89%). Thus, a large segment of the population is not using the service.

Formal Information Services

Derdiarian[62] studied the effects of an information intervention on informational needs, satisfaction, and coping. Sixty males who had recently been diagnosed with cancer and their spouses were randomly assigned to either an experimental group that received individualized formal information, counseling, referral, and cancer-related literature or a control group that re-

TABLE 21-3 Comparison of Family-Related Nursing Diagnoses

Nursing Diagnosis	Definition	Defining Characteristics
Alteration in Family Processes	Inability of family system (household members) to meet needs of members, carry out family functions, or maintain communications for mutual growth and maturation	Inability of family members to relate to each other for mutual growth and maturation, failure to send and receive clear messages, poorly communicated family rules, rituals, symbols, unexplained myths, unhealthy family decision-making processes, inability of family members to express and accept wide range of feelings, inability to accept and receive help, does not demonstrate respect for individuality and autonomy of members, rigidity in functions and roles, fails to accomplish current or past family developmental tasks, inappropriate boundary maintenance, inability to adapt to change, inability to deal with traumatic or crisis experience constructively, parents do not demonstrate respect for each other's views on childrearing practices, inappropriate level and direction of energy, inability to meet needs of members, family uninvolved in community activities (Gordon, 1987, p. 248).
Ineffective Family Coping: Compromised	Usually supportive primary person providing insufficient, ineffective, or compromised support, comfort, assistance, or encouragement that may be needed by client to manage or master adaptive tasks related to health challenge	Client expresses concern or complaint about significant other's response to health problem, significant person describes preoccupation with personal reactions to client's illness, disability, or other situational or developmental crisis, significant person describes or confirms inadequate understanding of knowledge base, which interferes with effective assistive or supportive behaviors, significant person attempts assistive or supportive behaviors with less than satisfactory results, significant person withdraws or enters into a limited or temporary personal communication with client at time of need, significant person displays protective behavior disproportionate to client's abilities or need for autonomy (Gordon, 1987, p. 296)
Ineffective Family Coping: Disabled	Behavior of significant person disables own capabilities and client's capacities to address effectively tasks essential to either person's adaptation to the health challenge	Neglectful care of client in regard to basic human needs and/or illness treatment, distortion of reality regarding client's health problem, including extreme denial, intolerance, rejection, abandonment, desertion, carrying on usual routines disregarding client needs, psychosomaticism, taking on illness signs of the client, decisions or actions by family that are detrimental to economic or social well-being, agitation, depression, aggression, hostility, impaired restructuring of a meaningful life for self, impaired individuation, prolonged overconcern for client, neglectful relationships with other family members, client's development of helpless, inactive dependence (Gordon, 1987, p. 300)
Family Coping: Potential for Growth	Family member has managed adaptive tasks involved with client's health challenge effectively and is exhibiting desire and readiness for enhanced health and growth in regard to self and in relation to the client	Family member attempts to describe growth impact of crisis on his/her own values, priorities, goals, or relationships, is moving in direction of health-promoting and enriching lifestyle that supports and monitors maturational processes, audits and negotiates treatment program and generally, chooses experiences that optimize wellness, expresses interest in making contact on a one-to-one basis or on a mutual-aid group basis with another person who has experienced a similar situation (Gordon, 1987, p. 294)

Source: Gordon M: *Manual of Nursing Diagnosis 1986–1987.* New York: McGraw-Hill, 1987.

ceived nondeliberate information. Findings indicated that the experimental group had a significant decrease in the scores on the information needs instrument and a significant increase in satisfaction scores over the 2-week study period. No significant changes were noted in the control group.

Spousal Support Groups

Sabo et al.[60] studied the responses of husbands of 24 patients who had undergone a mastectomy and the effects of a 10-week support group intervention in modifying those responses. All subjects were interviewed and completed a 37-item self-report instrument to evaluate gender expectations, self-esteem, depression, sexual compatibility, frequency of verbal communication about the mastectomy, and supportive attitude toward the wife prior to the intervention. Six husbands elected to attend the support group.

Interview findings indicated that the husbands had strong reactions of disbelief, alarm, isolation, and anxiety related to the role of support-giver for the wife. After the surgery, the husbands described assuming the role of protector to shield the wife from both his and her emotional reactions to the cancer experience, which resulted in strained communication patterns, distrust, and resentment. Comparison of pre–post scores on the instrument revealed that husbands who had attended the support group communicated significantly more with their wives about mastectomy issues than did husbands who had not attended the group sessions.

Risk Counseling

To address the need of family members for information about the cancer of the patient as well as personal risks for cancer, Kelly[63] described a program of risk counseling designed specifically for relatives of persons with cancer. Based on the expressed concerns of the relative, elements of the program may include biological and medical information about cancer risks, or a review of individual personality, lifestyle, and environmental risks. In addition, relatives may be counseled with respect to concerns about how to deal with tensions in the family, how to express concern for the family member with cancer, how to deal with personal physical and psychosocial responses to the cancer experience. Data related to the outcomes of the program were not reported by the author.

Psychotherapy

Goldberg and Wool[64] conducted a randomized prospective clinical trial to determine the effect of a program of social support counseling on newly diagnosed lung cancer patients ($n = 20$) and their significant others ($n = 23$). Patients and their significant others were divided into two groups. Group I served as the control group, and Group II significant others received scheduled counseling for 12 sessions following entry to the study. Counseling included five support functions: Maintain the integrity of the patient support system; promote a sense of autonomy of the patient; serve as an advocate for the patient in the health care system; encourage communication; and facilitate expression of feelings. Patients and significant others in both groups were interviewed and asked to complete the Psychosocial Adjustment to Illness Scale (PAIS) and the Profile of Moods Scale (POMS) within 6 weeks of diagnosis, and then 8 and 16 weeks later.

Findings indicated that patients and significant others in both groups had consistently low scores on the PAIS and POMS across the study period. The low scores were consistent with a positive adjustment to illness. In addition, no differences existed between the patients and significant others in Group I and II on the measures of emotional, social, and physical functioning. Although no differences were attributable to the intervention, the notion was raised that the majority of patients and significant others facing cancer are well adjusted without the need for intervention.

Formalized Support Services

Warren and Given[65] interviewed and collected self-administered questionnaires from 121 caregivers of persons with cancer to determine the effects of formalized cancer care services on the home caregiving situation. Thirty-nine percent ($n = 47$) of the caregivers identified themselves as users of formalized cancer care services. Surprisingly, the researchers found no significant differences in the caregiving situation, negative reactions, positive reactions, impact on schedule, impact on finances, impact on health, feelings of abandonment, and caregiver depression in the user versus the nonuser groups.

Social Support

Yancey[66] reported the findings from a longitudinal, correlational study of 37 adults (spouses and adult children) to determine the effect of social support on grief from death of a loved one related to cancer. Data indicated that perceived social support decreased significantly, and mood, as measured by the POMS, improved significantly from 1 to 6 months after the death. However, spouse subjects were significantly more distressed than child subjects throughout the study period. Scores on the Grief Resolution Index remained unchanged over the 5-month study period.

FUTURE DIRECTIONS FOR NURSING RESEARCH AND PRACTICE

The issues of family responses to a diagnosis of cancer go far beyond those discussed in this chapter. Even though selected psychosocial responses have been identified for spouses, patient–significant other dyads, caregivers, and children of adults with cancer, the effects of the interaction of those individual responses within the context of the family unit have not been studied systematically. The lack of data becomes even more critical when one considers the responses of nontraditional, multigenerational, and culturally diverse families. To date, research findings have been limited by methodology: consistent definition of the family, sample size, cross-sectional designs, and data collection from only one or two members of the family. Selection of family-level outcome variables, such as communication patterns, decision making, roles, patterns of interactions, responsibilities, and family development, is critical to future research on the family experience of cancer.

Gilliss and Davis[67] discussed research issues common to family research. Asking clinically relevant research questions, defining the unit of analysis, and differentiating statistically significant from theoretically or clinically significant findings were identified as areas that require attention in the design of future studies. In addition, the authors warned against limiting interventions for study to cognitive strategies. Use of affective and behavioral approaches and consideration of affective and behavioral outcomes are encouraged. Finally, the authors advocate justification for and acknowledgment of limitations associated with aggregation of data from multiple family members in evaluating family-unit-level responses.

Obviously, family-level services are neither needed nor available for every family faced with cancer. Yet screening instruments with established reliability and validity among families facing cancer and delineation of critical defining characteristics that predispose the family to dysfunctional responses are areas requiring additional study.

Finally, given the identification of high-risk or dysfunctional families, individual and family-level services to address expressed dysfunctional responses among cancer families are minimal. Multiple services and programs, primarily outside the realm of current services offered by tertiary and community hospitals, public health care and social agencies, and private and volunteer organizations, are needed to meet a spectrum of family needs. With the current climate of health care cost restraints, the issue of who should provide for and pay for the identified services becomes a crucial issue. Finally, the effectiveness of such services had programs in modifying the occurrence or resolution of dysfunctional responses in the family need to be evaluated.

REFERENCES

1. Lewis, FM: Family-level services for the cancer patient: Critical distinctions, fallacies, and assessment. *Cancer Nurs* 6:193–200, 1983.
2. Sales E: Psychosocial impact of the phase of cancer on the family: An updated review. *J Psychosoc Oncol* 9:1–18, 1991.
3. Smilkstein G: The family APGAR: A proposal for a family function test and its use by physicians. *J Fam Prac* 6:1231–1239, 1978.
4. Pless IB, Satterwhite BB: A measure of family functioning and its application. *Soc Sci Med* 7:613–620, 1973.
5. Satterwhite BB, Zweig SR, Iker HP, et al: The family functioning index—Five-year test-retest reliability and implications for use. *J Compar Fam Studies* 7:111–116, 1976.
6. Roberts CS, Feetham SL: Assessing family functioning across three areas of relationship. *Nurs Res* 3:231–235, 1982.
7. McCubbin HI, Comeau J: FIRM: Family Inventory of Resources for Management. In McCubbin HI, Thompson AI (eds.): *Family Assessment Inventories for Research and Practice*. Madison, WI: University of Wisconsin-Madison, Family Stress Coping and Health Project, 1987, pp. 145–160.
8. Olson DH, Portner J, Vell R: *Family Adaptability and Cohesion Evaluation Scales (FACES III)*. St. Paul, MN: University of Minnesota, Family Social Science, 1982.
9. Northouse PF, Northouse LL: Communication and cancer: Issues confronting patients, health professionals, and family members. *J Psychosoc Oncol* 5:17–46, 1987.
10. Houts PS, Rusenas I, Simmonds MN, Hufford DL: Information needs of families of cancer patients: A literature review and recommendations. *J Cancer Ed* 6:255–261, 1991.
11. Blank JJ, Longman AJ, Atwood JR: Perceived home care needs of cancer patients and their caregivers. *Cancer Nur* 12:78–84, 1989.

12a. Tringali C: The needs of family members of cancer patients. *Oncol Nurs Forum* 13:65–70, 1986.

12b. Northouse LL, Swain MA: Adjustment of patients and husbands to the initial impact of breast cancer. *Nurs Res* 35:221–225, 1987.

13. Lewis FM, Zahlis EH, Issel LM: The couple's experience with early stage breast cancer: A qualitative analysis. Presented at the Oncology Nursing Society Congress, San Francisco, CA, 1989.
14. Zahlis EH, Shands ME: Breast cancer: Demands of the illness on the patient's partner. *J Psychosoc Oncol* 9:75–93, 1991.
15. Krant MJ, Johnston L: Family members' perceptions of communication in late stage cancer. *Internat J Psychiatry Med* 8:203–216, 1977–1978.
16. Morrow GR, Hoagland AC, Mores IP: Sources of support perceived by parents of children with cancer: Implications for counseling. *Patient Counseling Health Ed* 4:36–40, 1982.
17. Wright K, Dyck S: Expressed concerns of adult cancer patient's family members. *Cancer Nurs* 7:371–374, 1984.
18. Oberst MT, James RH: Going home: Patient and spouse adjustment following cancer surgery. *Topics in Clinical Nurs* 7:46–57, 1985.
19. Keitel MA, Zevon MA, Rounds JB, et al: Spouse adjustment to cancer surgery distress and coping responses. *J Surg Oncol* 43:148–153, 1990.
20. Hymovitch DP: Parents with cancer: Parenting stressors and coping strategies. (Abstr.) Second National Conference on Cancer Nursing Research, January 30–February 1, 1992. Baltimore, MD: American Cancer Society. 47-C, 1992.
21. Germino BB: Family functioning as a measure of functional status. (Abstr.) First National Conference on Cancer Nursing Research, November 30–December 2, 1989, Atlanta, GA: American Cancer Society. 42, 1989.
22. Perry GR, Roades de Meneses M: Cancer patients at home: Needs and coping styles of primary caregivers. *Home Health Nurse* 7:27–30, 1989.
23. Goldberg RJ, Wool MS, Glicksman A, et al: Relationship of the social environment and patient's physical status to

depression in lung cancer patients and their spouses. *J Psychosoc Oncol* 2:73–80, 1984.

24. Cooper ET: A pilot study of the effects of the diagnosis of lung cancer on family relationships. *Cancer Nurs* 7:301–308, 1984.
25. Kalayjian AS: Coping with cancer: The spouse's perspective. *Arch Psychiat Nurs* 3:166–172, 1989.
26. Cassileth BR, Lusk RJ, Strouse TB, et al: A psychological analysis of cancer patients and their next-of-kin. *Cancer* 55:72–76, 1985.
27. Wellisch DK, Fawzy FI, Landsverk J, et al: Evaluation of psychosocial problems of the home-bound cancer patient: The relationship of disease and the sociodemographic variables of patients to family problems. *J Psychosoc Oncol* 1:1–15, 1983.
28. McCorkle R, Baird S, Luck E, et al: Relationship of patient psychosocial responses to caregiver burden over time. (Abstr.) Second National Conference on Cancer Nursing Research. Baltimore, MD: American Cancer Society. 66C, 1992.
29. Siegel K, Raveis VH, Mor V, Houts P: The relationship of spousal caregiver burden to patient disease and treatment-related conditions. *Ann Oncol* 2:511–516, 1991.
30. Stetz KM: Caregiving demands during advanced cancer: The spouse's needs. *Cancer Nurs* 10:260–268, 1987.
31. Gustafson L, Mood DW, Letzel E: Spousal and self-care concerns during radiation therapy. (Abstr.) Second National Conference on Cancer Nursing Research. Baltimore, MD: American Cancer Society. 19B, 1992.
32. Northouse LL: The impact of breast cancer on patients and husbands. *Cancer Nurs* 12:276–284, 1989.
33. Dibble SL: Patients' and families' coping strategies for their most important problem over time (OMEGA-COPE). (Abstr.) Second National Conference on Cancer Nursing Research. Baltimore, MD: American Cancer Society. 2B, 1992.
34. Stetz KM, Lewis FM, Primomo J: Family coping strategies and chronic illness in the mother. *Fam Relations* 38:515–522, 1986.
35. Ell K, Michimoto R, Mantel J, et al: Longitudinal analysis of psychosocial adaptation among family members of patients with cancer. *J Psychosom Res* 32:429–438, 1988.
36. Weinert C: Living with cancer: Support, assistance, and relationships. (Abstr.) Second National Conference on Cancer Nursing Research. Baltimore, MD: American Cancer Society. 23B, 1992.
37. Stommel M, Kingry M: Support patterns for spouse caregivers of cancer patients: The effect of the presence of minor children. *Cancer Nurs* 14:220–205, 1991.
38. Baider L, Rizel S, Denour AK: Comparison of couples' adjustment to lumpectomy and mastectomy. *General Hosp Psychiatry* 8:251–257, 1986.
39. Hays JC: Patient symptoms and family coping: Predictors of hospice utilization patterns. *Cancer Nurs* 9:317–325, 1986.
40. Stetz KM: The relationship among background characteristics, purpose in life, and caregiving demands on perceived health of spouse caregivers. *Scholarly Inquiry Nurs Prac* 3:133–153, 1980.
41. O'Hare PA, Malone BA, McCorkle R: Needs of black cancer patients and their caregivers post-hospitalization: A descriptive study. (Abstr.) Second National Conference on Cancer Nursing Research, January 30–February 1, 1992, Baltimore, MD: American Cancer Society. 80C, 1992.
42. Gritz ER, Wellish DK, Siau J, Wang HJ: Long-term effects of testicular cancer on marital relationships. *Psychosomatics* 31:301–312, 1990.
43. Schover LR, Gonzales M, von Essenbach AC: Sexual and marital relationships after radiotherapy for seminoma. *Urol* 27:117–123, 1986.
44. Lichtman RR, Taylor SE, Wood JV, et al: Relations with children after breast cancer: The mother-daughter relationship at risk. *J Psychosoc Oncol* 2:1–19, 1984.
45. Birenbaum LK, Yancey D: Children's response to parent's cancer. (Abstr.) Second National Conference on Cancer Nursing Research. Baltimore, MD: American Cancer Society. 10C, 1992.
46. Berman H, Cragg CE, Kuenzig L: Having a parent die of cancer: Adolescents' reactions. *Oncol Nurs Forum* 15:159–162, 1988.
47. Issel LM, Ersek M, Lewis FM: How children cope with mother's breast cancer. *Oncol Nurs Forum* 17:5–13, 1990 (suppl. 3).
48. Germino B: Impact of a parent's cancer on adult children: Role and relationship issues. Presentation at the Oncology Nursing Society Congress. May 13–16, 1992, San Diego, CA, 1992.
49. Baird SB: The effect of cancer in a parent on role relationships with the nurse/daughter. *Cancer Nurs* 11:9–17, 1988.
50. Wellisch DK, Gritz ER, Schain W, et al: Psychological functioning of daughters of breast cancer patients: Part I. Daughters and comparison subjects. *Psychosomatics* 32:324–336, 1991.
51. Kash KM, Holland JC, Halper MS, et al: Psychological distress and surveillance behaviors of women with a family history of breast cancer. *J Nat Cancer Inst* 81:24–30, 1992.
52. Friedman LC, Baer PE, Nelson DV, et al: Women with breast cancer: Perception of family functioning and adjustment to illness. *Psychosomatic Med* 50:529–540, 1988.
53. Olson DH, Sprenkle DH, Russell CS: Circumplex model of marital and family systems: I. Cohesion and adaptability dimensions, family types, and clinical applications. *Family Process* 18:3–28, 1979.
54. Vess JD, Moreland JR, Schwebel AI: A follow-up study of role functioning and the psychosocial environment of families of cancer patients. *J Psychosoc Oncol* 3:1–14, 1985.
55. Lewis FM, Woods NF, Hough EE, et al: The family's functioning with chronic illness in the mother: The spouse's perspective. *Soc Science Med* 29:1261–1269, 1989.
56. Hough EE, Lewis FM, Woods NF: Family response to mother's chronic illness: Case studies of well- and poorly adjusted families. *Western Nurs Res* 13:568–596, 1991.
57. Carpenito LJ: *Handbook of Nursing Diagnosis* (ed. 4). Philadelphia: Lippincott, 1991.
58. Zabora JR, Smith ED: Family dysfunction and the cancer patient: Early recognition and intervention. *Oncology* 5:31–41, 1991.
59. Heinricks RL, Coscarelli-Schag C: Stress and activity management: Group treatment for cancer patients and spouses. *J Consult Clin Psychol* 53:439–446, 1985.
60. Sabo D, Brown J, Smith C: The male role and mastectomy: Support groups and men's adjustment. *J Psychosoc Oncol* 4:19–31, 1986.
61. Meissner HI, Anderson DM, Odenkirchen JC: Meeting information needs of significant others: Use of the Cancer Information Service. *Patient Educ Counseling* 15:171–179, 1990.

62. Derdiarian AK: Effects of information of recently diagnosed cancer patients' and spouses' satisfaction with care. *Cancer Nurs* 12:285–292, 1989.
63. Kelly PT: Risk counseling for relatives of cancer patients: New information, new approaches. *J Psychosoc Oncol* 5:65–79, 1987.
64. Goldberg RJ, Wool MS: Psychotherapy for the spouses of lung cancer patients: Assessment of an intervention. *Psychother Psychosom* 43:141–150.
65. Warren B, Given B: Caregiver reactions to formal cancer services: Implications for care. (Abstr.) First National Conference on Cancer Nursing Research, November 30–December 2, 1989, Atlanta, GA: American Cancer Society. 108, 1989.
66. Yancey D: Effect of social support on grief from cancer death. (Abstr.) Second National Conference on Cancer Nursing Research. Baltimore, MD: American Cancer Society. 119C, 1992.
67. Gilliss CL, Davis LL: Family nursing research: Precepts from paragons and peccadilloes. *J Advanced Nurs* 17:28–33, 1992.

Chapter 22

Psychosocial Issues of Long-Term Survival from Adult Cancer

Susan Leigh, RN, BSN

Deborah McCaffrey Boyle, RN, MSN, OCN

Lois J. Loescher, RN, MS*

Barbara Hoffman, JD

INTRODUCTION

Early detection and effective multimodal therapies have increased significantly the numbers of cancer survivors to the extent that cancer is now considered a chronic, life-threatening illness rather than a terminal disease. In 1992, over 8 million Americans had histories of cancer, with 4 million surviving 5 years or more.[1] Cancers with a high and continually increasing 5-year relative survival rate are listed in Table 22-1.[1,2]

Traditionally, the health care community has been more interested in the aggressive medical treatment of cancers with high survival rates than with the quality of life and psychosocial aspects of long-term survival.[3] However, the burgeoning population of survivors makes evident the need to address quality of survival and the psychosocial consequences of cancer and its therapies. Long-term survivors have been found to experience problems ranging from minor, short-term difficulties to major psychosocial crises.[4–6] Determining which individuals are at greatest risk for psychosocial morbidity is critical for clinicians. But first the population being assessed must be defined.

DEFINITIONS OF SURVIVORSHIP

According to *Webster's College Dictionary: survivorship* is the state of being a survivor, a *survivor* is the person who survives, and *to survive* means to remain alive and continue to function and manage in spite of some adverse circumstance or hardship.[7] In the area of oncology, survivorship is a relatively new concept, and one with multiple meanings.

Cancer survivorship can be described as the experience of living through or beyond the illness; as such, it is a process, not a stage or a component of survival. Carter describes this process as a theme of "going through," and identifies a sense of movement through phases.[8] While this process encompasses all stages of survival, survivorship frequently is limited to a period of time more accurately defined as long-term survival.

TABLE 22-1 Cancers with High 5-Year Relative Survival Rates

Cancer	% White	% Black
Testicular cancer	92%	92%
Colon cancer	57	48
Cutaneous melanoma	81	65
Breast cancer	78	64
Hodgkin's disease	76	74
Prostate cancer	75	62
Cervical cancer	67	57

Sources: American Cancer Society: *Cancer Facts and Figures.* Atlanta: American Cancer Society, 1992. National Cancer Institute: Surveillance, Epidemiology, and End Results Program (SEER), Annual Cancer Statistics Review 1973–1987. NIH Publication No. 90-2789. Bethesda, MD: National Cancer Institute, 1990.

Another discrepancy arises when attempting to define *cancer survivor.* Medical definitions of a cancer survivor are specific and limited, and are not yet fully agreed on by the health care community. Historically, cancer survivors have been defined as individuals "cured" of their disease, with the "cured" state commencing 5 years after diagnosis.[1] The term *cure* traditionally applies to those individuals who have no evidence of disease with a minimal or nonexistent chance for recurrence.

Controversial aspects of associating long-term survival with cancer "cure" could be eliminated by basing the definition on the concept of control rather than "cure." Cancer itself constitutes many different diseases, each having distinct stages and behaviors and treated with a wide range of modalities. Some cancers, such as melanoma and early stages of breast cancer, are often "cured" once the cancer is physically removed. Other cancers, including stage I and stage II Hodgkin's disease, acute lymphocytic leukemias, and osteogenic sarcoma, may be considered cured following several courses of intensive multimodal therapy. Individuals with these types of cancers may, by definition, be considered "cured" at some time before the 5-year mark. Yet they are not classified as survivors by the medical community, since they are still not considered medically cured until the fifth year following diagnosis. Still other cancers, such as multiple myeloma and chronic leukemia, may not be "curable," but with continued treatment can be controlled, enabling patients to live for several years. Although these individuals are not "cured" in the medical sense, they are indeed survivors of a chronic disease. Finally, other cancers are initially labeled "incurable" or advanced at diagnosis, with expectations of inevitable death. The exceptional patient who unexpectedly survives this type of cancer diagnosis may be considered to have experienced either a "miracle cure" or a spontaneous remission.

Vought et al.[9] describe a survival paradigm or model that allows health care providers to rank the importance of the issues that a survivor might identify. The six components of the paradigm, listed here in descending order of importance, but not necessarily in order of occurrence, are:

1. basic survival (food, shelter, medical care)
2. physiologic self-concept (attractiveness, fitness, physical function)
3. psychologic self-concept (self-respect, integrity, autonomy)
4. proximal affiliation (intimate relationships)
5. distal affiliation (social relationships)
6. avocational component (recreation and play)

TABLE 22-2 Components of a Cancer Survival Paradigm

Focus	Critical Elements	Cancer-Related Barriers
Basic survival	Concern about resources for food, shelter, medical care	Limited finances, loss of job benefits, lack of adequate follow-up medical care
Physical self-concept	Physical attractiveness, fitness, maintenance of body function	Any body image alteration, energy reserve impairment, residual physical disability
Psychological self-concept	Self respect, integrity, autonomy	Use of self-blame, dependency, self-doubt; change from precancer lifestyle
Proximal affiliation	Relationships with family, lovers, and close friends	Fears about hereditary transmission, family stress related to illness, alterations in customary social support; sexual dysfunction; concern about disclosure
Distal affiliation	Relationships to co-workers and acquaintances	Shunning and isolationism; discriminatory practices; concern about disclosure
Avocational	Recreation, play, escape	Physical compromise; financial constraints; fear of distancing self from health care team

Source: Adapted with permission of the publisher from Vought CA, Dintruff DL, Fotopoulos SS: Adaptations to the constraints of cancer: Motivational issues. In Ahmed P (ed.): *Living and Dying with Cancer.* New York: Elsevier, 1981, pp. 205–219. Copyright 1981 by Elsevier Science Publishing Co., Inc.

Cancer-related barriers to this survival paradigm are listed in Table 22-2. Although Vought ranks physical self-concept as being highly important, psychosocial components make up the bulk of the model, indicating the overall importance of psychosocial issues.

SURVIVORSHIP AS A CONTINUUM

Utilizing the control definition enables cancer survivorship to be viewed as a continual, ongoing process rather than as an explicit event occurring at a predetermined time. Mullan[10] first proposed a continuum of survival stages, or "seasons," in lieu of the term *cure.* These "seasons" apply to everyone diagnosed with cancer, and consist of acute, extended, and permanent stages of survival.

The initial, *acute* stage of survival begins at diagnosis. Survivors are called *patients* in this stage and must deal with immediate effects of therapy in addition to their mortality. Life modifications that will become part of their present and their long-term future are begun, hopefully in consultation with a multidisciplinary rehabilitation team. Psychosocial support of the patient is critical in this stage, and usually is available to varying degrees in the hospital and clinic settings.

Following the acute stage, the survivor moves into the *extended* stage of survival. This stage begins when the disease is in remission or the survivor has finished the primary treatment course and starts consolidation or adjuvant therapies. Survivors at this stage often deal with issues such as altered body image and vocational disruptions, yet appropriate psychosocial intervention is more difficult to provide and may be unavailable.

Finally, from the extended stage, many move to the more *permanent* stage of survival that is most frequently associated with "cure." This stage evolves from the period of time when cancer activity or the chance of its return markedly decreases, and the disease is arrested permanently. Economic problems often surface in this stage along with concern for long-term and late effects of cancer treatment, and resources needed for continued support are essentially nonexistent.

Viewing cancer survivorship as an evolving process allows recognition of the fact that psychosocial issues of long-term survival can arise in any stage or phase of the survival continuum. Thus, in anticipation of long-term survival, psychosocial interventions begin at diagnosis rather than when the disease is considered medically "cured." This chapter will concentrate on psychosocial issues prevalent in the extended and permanent survival stages.

PSYCHOSOCIAL THEMES

Although many aspects of psychobiologic functioning encompass survivorship, studies confirm a relative lack of psychopathology in long-term survivors of cancer.[4,11–16] The major psychosocial themes to be anticipated in significant numbers of adults surviving cancer are:

1. psychosocial effects of long-term physiologic alterations
2. fears of relapse and death
3. dependence on health care providers
4. survivor guilt
5. uncertain future
6. social adaptation dilemmas
7. effects of survivorship on the family

Psychosocial Effects of Long-Term Physiologic Alterations

An individual's ability to cope within the trajectory of extended or permanent survival can be strongly influenced by physiologic compromise.[10,17] In an early study of 49 women 4 years postmastectomy, Woods and Earp[18] noted that subjects with more symptom distress associated with their surgery had greater degrees of depressive symptoms. Rieker, Edbril, and Garnick[19] later studied 74 men 2–10 years posttreatment for testicular cancer and found that those with resultant sexual impairment (i.e., infertility, ejaculatory dysfunction) reported more psychologic symptomatology and strained intimate relationships than men without long-term sexual impairment. Fobair et al.[5] then noted a relationship between persistent energy loss and depression in 403 Hodgkin's disease survivors evaluated approximately 9 years after completion of therapy. And more recently, in a small exploratory study by Loescher et al.,[20] long-term survivors who had completed therapy at least 2 years prior identified a heightened anxiety that prompted frequent self-monitoring of physical symptoms, no matter how vague these symptoms might appear. The survivors also requested continued access to information to help manage physical changes. Additional research that integrates the physical and psychosocial sequelae of surviving cancer will help identify those factors that enhance or detract from quality survival, and hopefully support additional health maintenance programs for the long-term cancer survivor.

Fears of Relapse and Death

Probably the most common concern of all cancer survivors is the fear of cancer recurrence.[15,20–24] Not knowing when and if cancer will reappear often negatively affects the survivor's sense of control over his or her life.[20,25,26] Commonly referred to as the "Damocles syndrome," death anxiety often fluctuates in intensity as the survivor deals with intermittent suspicious symptomatology.[16] Fear of relapse may present in a variety of forms, ranging from general uneasiness about the etiology of mild to moderate somatic complaints to pronounced anxiety or panic attacks that interfere with daily life. Exaggerated worry over somatic distress usually is most intense within 2 years following completion of therapy.[3,22] As time passes, a lessening of anxiety about relapse and recurrence may evolve. However, a heightened sense of vulnerability to illness frequently is a hallmark of the cancer survivor's long-term experience.[20,27] Thus, the health care community needs to be more receptive to survivors' needs for continued support, reassurance, and access to information.

Dependence on Health Care Providers

For many patients nearing the end of treatment, a significant ambivalence evolves. They are elated over the prospect of discontinuing therapy, yet fear distancing themselves from the health care team that helped them get to this extended survival stage.[24,28] Mullan[23] noted that as a fear of recurrence can lead to hypochondriacal behavior, so too can a fear of the physician's actually finding disease lead to physician avoidance.

Both the survivor's need to determine the nature of suspicious symptomatology and the physician's need to closely evaluate the patient following cessation of therapy necessitate an ongoing relationship between the patient and health care team.[20] Because routine check-ups and yearly comprehensive examinations can engender pronounced anxiety, the survivor needs access to ongoing education emphasizing the importance of continued health observation, promotion, prevention, and maintenance.[23,29–31]

Survivor Guilt

Waiting rooms may elicit reminders of the potential negative outcomes of cancer, causing survivors to question themselves: "Will I end up that way, too?" As comparisons are made to other patients, the phenomenon called "survivor guilt" may cause the survivor to ponder, "Why am I doing well and they aren't?"[12,31] As during the time of initial diagnosis, questions may arise as the survivor attempts to justify "why me?" or "why not me?" Hence, the survivor's period of follow-up care is characterized by mixed emotional reactions and multiple concerns.

Uncertain Future

Because of the prevailing perception that cancer results in a painful, lingering death, most people's immediate reaction to a diagnosis of cancer is the expectation of a shortened life span. Once successful completion of therapy is achieved, hope for continued survival often supercedes thoughts of death. Many survivors, however, change their lifestyle as a reaction to the possibility of dying younger than expected.

A critical evaluation of life's meaning and priorities seems to become of utmost importance. Survivors report greater appreciation of life and more satisfaction with life as a whole.[20,31] A significant value reassessment leads to heightened awareness of things taken for granted and lessened concern for the trivial. Mullan[10] characterized this phenomenon as "life rekindled." This enhanced appreciation of life and improved quality of life in the present represent important secondary benefits of having survived cancer.

Social Adaptation Dilemmas

Attempts to minimize memories of the treatment experience and to "get on with life" are not often easy tasks for the long-term survivor.[20] The transition from a sick role to a healthy role can be compromised by persistent physical debility (despite cessation of therapy), negative expectations from within the survivor's social support realm, personal concerns about the ability to readjust, and social stigma.

Similar to the survivor's ambivalent relationship with the health care team, confusion regarding available social support may deter social adaptation. On the one hand, the survivor may not want to be treated like a patient, yet may react negatively to the withdrawal of intense social support that was mobilized during the initial diagnosis phase.[24] Repeated explanations about one's health status to family, friends, acquaintances, employers, and insurers may drain the survivor's emotional resources, and the constant scrutiny from these individuals can be stressful. Also, dealing with relationships outside the immediate family unit can become more difficult if internal family needs are not met successfully.

In *Illness as Metaphor,* Susan Sontag[32] graphically describes the ability of cancer to elicit out-of-date feelings of dread, fear, and a sense of contagion. *Shunning,* a relatively subjective phenomenon of purposely avoiding the individual with cancer, may be a pervasive barrier to successful reorientation.[23,32] Even today the stigma of cancer pervades our society; Siegal and Christ[33] link "feelings of aversion" toward the person with cancer with the "physical mutilation and deterioration associated with the disease." Due to this continued social stigma and the increasing numbers of cancer survivors, it is no wonder that our society is now witnessing the development and expansion of cancer support and mutual aid networks.[34,35] To those survivors who fear or actually experience isolation from loved ones or peers, these groups offer opportunities for continued support, understanding, and friendship.

Family Effects

An abundance of information exists about the plight of the family coping with the active phases of cancer. However, there is little information about families coping with extended or permanent survival of a family member.[36] Premorbid family style is an important variable in assessing postillness coping.[16] Even the most supportive family member is not immune to experiencing psychologic stress within the long-term cancer continuum. The family's anxiety about the patient, i.e., worry over potential relapse and unfavorable social situations, may be exhibited by overprotectiveness and pervasive anxiety.[33] Marital discord and changes in sexual relationships can occur. Family members may not want to listen to or hear the survivor's concerns over potential relapse, since these can trigger their own sense of insecurity about continued long-term survival. Woods and Earp[18] identify "conversational isolationism" as a family's hesitance to discuss mutual concerns about the recurrence of cancer. As we acknowledge cancer as a family disease, we must be sensitive to the ramifications of survival for all members of the family unit.

EMPLOYMENT AND INSURANCE DISCRIMINATION

Many cancer survivors encounter ongoing socioeconomic impediments to full recovery. Concerns include regaining financial and work-related stability and maintaining medical insurance coverage. Access to insurance usually is through employment. But the issues of job discrimination and insurance-related problems are separate and complicated, and, therefore, will be addressed individually.

Employment Discrimination

Survivors' employment problems can be attributed to three predominant myths about cancer: (1) Cancer is a death sentence; (2) cancer is contagious; and (3) cancer survivors are an unproductive drain on the economy.[37–40] Meanwhile, current statistics indicate that more than half of all Americans diagnosed with cancer will survive their illness, that cancer is not contagious, and that cancer survivors have productivity rates similar to those of other workers.[1,41]

Categories of employment-related problems include: (1) dismissal, demotion, and reduction or elimination of work-related benefits; (2) situations arising from co-workers' attitudes about cancer; and (3) problems related to the survivors' attitudes about how they should be perceived by others in the workplace.[42] Discrimination can be as subtle as experiencing increased conflict with co-workers or as blatant as being fired or being rejected from promotion to a desired position.

The earlier work of both Wheatley et al.[43] and Stone[44] confirmed that the work performance of cancer survivors differed little, if any, from performance of others hired at the same age for similar assignments, and that up to 80% returned to work after being diagnosed. This employment-related information has been confirmed more recently by Crothers and Mellette for the American Cancer Society.[39,45] Yet an often-troublesome effect of a cancer history continues to be "job-lock," where one fears leaving an undesirable position because of the potential loss of medical insurance and other benefits.[46]

Certain federal and state laws prohibit employment discrimination against qualified individuals with a history of cancer. The Federal Rehabilitation Act of 1973 and the recent Americans with Disabilities Act prohibit employment discrimination against cancer survivors, that is, being treated differently because they are disabled or are regarded as being disabled. The Federal Rehabilitation Act applies only to employers who receive federal funding. The Americans with Disabilities Act prohibits discrimination against people with disabilities whether or not the employer receives any federal funding. As of July 26, 1990, this law applies to private employers with at least 25 employees. After July 26, 1994, the applicable law will target those businesses with 15 or more employees.[40] Most states prohibit discrimination against the disabled in general, while a few states explicitly protect those with histories of cancer. There can be a problem, though, when the legal system attempts to label all cancer survivors as handicapped or disabled when there often is no visible evidence of being either. This suggests the need for further clarification of terms through more explicit legislation.

Insurance Problems

With better access to treatment options, many cancer survivors are experiencing increased life spans after receiving more sophisticated medical care. The availability of adequate health insurance is rarely guaranteed, and the problems created when attempting to secure or obtain these benefits can be financially and emotionally devastating. The numerous barriers to insurability include refusal of new applications, policy cancellations or reductions, higher premiums, waived or excluded preexisting conditions, and extended waiting periods.[41,47] These barriers can also affect the spouse or family member who carries the insurance policy. Studies suggest that 25%–30% of cancer survivors experience some form of insurance discrimination.[41,47,48]

Because there is no state-mandated or federally mandated legal right to health insurance, individuals should examine carefully the specific terms of their policies and the applicable state law to determine a legal violation. An employer with more than 20 employees will be required under COBRA, a federal law passed in 1986, to offer a continuance of group medical coverage to those whose circumstances warrant reducing or changing work hours or leaving the job.[49] The affected employee is eligible for extended coverage up to 18 months, while spouse and dependents receive these benefits for 36 months.

Other sources of assistance for insurance problems are state insurance commissions that regulate insurance rates, policy conditions, and all aspects of coverage and benefits. These state agencies usually are available to individuals with questions and complaints concerning existing policies and insurability. In addition, a number of states have introduced high-risk pools for those considered medically uninsurable.[50] By requiring the major insurance companies to share in the risks and expenses, more people with preexisting conditions have the opportunity to purchase comprehensive insurance plans, albeit at higher premiums. Nurses should be familiar with the resources available to assist the survivor who has employment or insurance problems. These resources are available on local, state, and national levels, as described in Table 22-3.

TABLE 22-3 Local, State, and National Resources for Employment and Insurance Problems

Employment	Insurance
LOCAL	
• Disability and employment law attorneys • Local survivor organizations	• Insurance Department • Social Security, local office • Medicare • Medicaid • Group insurance plans • Open enrollment periods • Local survivor organizations
STATE	
• State Department of Labor, Civil Rights Division	• State Insurance Commission • High-risk pools (not applicable in all states)
NATIONAL	
• Federal Rehabilitation Act of 1973* • The Americans With Disabilities Act† • ERISA (Employee Retirement and Income Security Act)‡ • National survivor organizations	• COBRA (Consolidated Omnibus Budget Reconciliation Act)‡ • National survivor organizations

*Write to: Department of Justice, Civil Rights Division, Coordination and Review Section, Washington, DC 20530

†Write to: Equal Employment Opportunity Commission, Office of Communications and Legislative Affairs, 1801 L St. NW, Washington, DC 20507

‡Write to: Pension and Welfare Benefits Administration, U.S. Department of Labor, Room N-5658, 200 Constitution Ave. NW, Washington, DC 20210

REHABILITATION PARALLELS

In considering options for providing support for the long-term survivor of adult cancer, the concept of *rehabilitation* must be addressed. Early work by Mayer[51] noted that the concept of cancer rehabilitation encompasses the theme of quality survival—not how long a person lives, but how well that individual lives within the constraints of the disease. Veronesi and Martino[52] then stated that rehabilitation is the bridge that leads the patient from the condition of diversity to a condition of normality. When these two papers were authored in the 1970s, rehabilitation in the oncology setting essentially focused on hospitalized patients with physically disabling impairments, such as amputations and colostomies.[53] Little, if any, attention was given to the other areas of human functioning.

More recently, Watson[54] described *rehabilitation* as an appropriate umbrella concept applicable across the entire cancer continuum. Mellette[55] then expanded on this idea by suggesting that *prevention,* the avoidance of dysfunction in the first place, is the key word when discussing rehabilitation. If there is residual dysfunction, though, the nurse's role in cancer rehabilitation is to help the patient reduce the extent to which the cancer-related disability becomes a handicap or interferes with the ability to function in everyday life, however long that life may be. Because there is a paucity of information available on the long-term physiologic effects of cancer therapy for adults, the residual end products of therapy are unclear.[30] However, we know that as former patients cope with extended or permanent survival, many do not return to prior levels of functioning.[56] These survivors find they must develop strategies to cope with new situations and alterations in health status and functional abilities.

Rehabilitation in cancer care is particularly relevant as the numbers of cancer survivors increase. The growing acknowledgment of the physical, emotional, sexual, social, vocational, and economic implications of living with or beyond cancer suggests a more aggressive approach to both assessment and intervention planning for long-term survival (Table 22-4). Until recently, interest in this subset of people with a history of cancer has been negligible and certainly not comprehensive. The systematic follow-up of adult long-term survivors is virtually nonexistent in the United States. This nonpractice is incompatible with a model rehabilitative approach to cancer care that includes ongoing reassessment and redefinition of goals.[57]

Groenwald and Thaney[58] describe rehabilitation as a dynamic process, the antithesis of customary convalescence where a person is allowed passivity while nature takes its course. Preventive goal setting and restorative goal setting become critical parameters to the enhancement of a long-term survival trajectory characterized by minimal debilitation and a wellness orientation. Attention must also be directed to the potential ongoing and long-range financial burden imposed by cancer.[59–61]

TABLE 22-4 Foci and Objectives of a Comprehensive Assessment and Intervention Program for Adult Long-Term Cancer Survivors

Focus	Specific Considerations
Physical	• Follow up potential effects of cancer and multimodal therapies. • Recognize endurance, fatigue, energy reserve problems based on intensity of treatment. • Be aware of incidence of secondary malignancy from treatment, along with second or third primaries.
Emotional	• Acknowledge potential chronic anxiety associated with fear of recurrence. • Be alert to reactions to social stigma, changes in interpersonal relationships. • Be sensitive to family's adaptation to the cancer experience. • Acknowledge the potential existence of survivor guilt.
Sexual	• Consider interplay of fertility issues with coping strategies. • Consider intimacy needs as a subset of sexual satisfaction. • Discuss disclosure options relative to potential partners. • Anticipate concern about offspring health.
Social	• Discuss concerns about friends' and acquaintances' reactions to cancer history. • Recognize that life goals may be reprioritized. • Relate social adaptation to health status. • Encourage integration of family, friends, hobbies, and vacation into long-range plans.
Vocational	• Acknowledge potential job-related stress and co-workers' responses to cancer history. • Educate about possible discrimination at work. • Assist with vocational rehabilitation if necessary.
Economic	• Consider possible long-term financial burden. • Provide resources for insurance problems. • Encourage a balance between long-term and short-term goals.

Significant policy statements have been made by key groups that encourage future investigation into the development of rehabilitation models of cancer care. In

A new population lives among us today—a new minority of 5 million people with a history of cancer. Three million of these Americans have lived with their diagnoses for five years or more.

You see these modern survivors in offices and in factories, on bicycles and cruise ships, on tennis courts, beaches and bowling alleys. You see them in all ages, shapes, sizes and colors. Usually they are unremarkable in appearance; sometimes they are remarkable for the way they have learned to live with disabilities resulting from cancer or its treatment.

Modern medical advances have returned about half of the nation's cancer patients of all ages (and 59 percent for those under the age of 55) to a normal lifespan. But the larger society has not always kept pace in helping make this lifespan truly "normal": at least, it has felt awkward in dealing with this fledgling group; at most, it has failed fully to accept survivors as functioning members.

The American Cancer Society presents this Survivors' Bill of Rights to call public attention to survivor needs, to enhance cancer care, and to bring greater satisfaction to cancer survivors, as well as to their physicians, employers, families and friends:

1. Survivors have the right to assurance of lifelong medical care, as needed. The physicians and other professionals involved in their care should continue their constant efforts to be:
   - sensitive to the cancer survivors' lifestyle choices and their need for self-esteem and dignity;
   - careful, no matter how long their patients have survived, to take symptoms seriously, and not dismiss aches and pains, for fear of recurrence is a normal part of survivorship;
   - informative and open, providing survivors with as much or as little candid medical information as they wish, and encouraging their informed participation in their own care;
   - knowledgeable about counseling resources, and willing to refer survivors and their families as appropriate for emotional support and therapy which will improve the quality of individual lives.
2. In their personal lives, survivors, like other Americans, have the right to the pursuit of happiness. This means they have the right:
   - to talk with their families and friends about their cancer experience if they wish, but to refuse to discuss if that is their choice and not to be expected to be more upbeat or less blue than anyone else;
   - to be free of the stigma of cancer as a "dread disease" in all social relations;
   - to be free of blame for having gotten the disease and of guilt for having survived it.
3. In the work place, survivors have the right to equal job opportunities. This means they have the right:
   - to aspire to jobs worthy of their skills, and for which they are trained and experienced, and thus not to have to accept jobs they would not have considered before the cancer experience;
   - to be hired, promoted and accepted on return to work, according to their individual abilities and qualifications, and not according to "cancer" or "disability" stereotypes;
   - to privacy about their medical histories.
4. Since health insurance coverage is an overriding survivorship concern, every effort should be made to assure all survivors adequate health insurance, whether public or private. This means:
   - for employers, that survivors have the right to be included in group coverage, which is usually less expensive, provides better benefits, and covers the employee regardless of health history;
   - for physicians, counselors and other professionals concerned, that they keep themselves and their survivor clients informed and up to date on available group or individual health policy options, noting, for example, what major expenses like hospital costs and medical tests outside the hospital are covered and what amount must be paid before coverage (deductible);
   - for social policy makers, both in government and in the private sector, that they seek to broaden insurance programs like Medicare to include diagnostic procedures and treatment which help prevent recurrence and ease survivor anxiety and pain.

FIGURE 22-1 The cancer survivors' bill of rights. (Source: American Cancer Society.)

1988, Deborah Mayer and the Oncology Nursing Society (ONS) coordinated an invitational conference entitled "Addressing Barriers to Successful Cancer Rehabilitation."[62] Taking into account all of the definitions discussed in this chapter, the official ONS Position Statement on Rehabilitation states that cancer rehabilitation is "a process by which individuals, within their environments, are assisted to achieve optimal functioning within the limits imposed by cancer."[62] Three of the 15 proposed action items specifically address cancer survivors, and include recommendations to: (1) develop a system to identify cancer survivors; (2) develop a system for long-term follow-up and monitoring of cancer survivors; and (3) identify the needs of cancer survivors.[62] Also in 1988, the Cancer Survivor's Bill of Rights was published by the American Cancer Society "to call public attention to survivor needs" and "to enhance cancer care" (Figure 22-1). Finally, the Association of Community Cancer Centers has stated that the provision of rehabilitation services to cancer patients and their families should be a basic standard of care in the community.[63]

As increasing numbers of cancer patients survive, nurses can contribute to the quality and satisfaction of survivors' lives by developing a philosophy that is holistic in principle and rehabilitative in nature.[64] As Wells[65] noted in his address to the fifteenth Annual ONS Congress, nurses "must help others realize that rehabilitation is not a functional phenomenon; rather, it is a philosophy of care that must be relevant to all healthcare providers in the hospital." In discussing policy making in the health care arena, Mayer emphasized that "oncology nurses must become dissatisfied with the current way that they care for people surviving cancer.

They also must become more involved in translating this dissatisfaction into real programs and services."[66] Hassey-Dow[67] challenged oncology nurses in her 1990 Schering Clinical Lectureship to help map out survival trajectories, to develop and implement educational and supportive programs, and to make nursing referrals to appropriate local and national survivor groups and organizations. Finally, Loescher et al.[20,30,31] are strong proponents of adult long-term survivor clinics that address both physiologic and psychosocial needs while maintaining a focus on health maintenance and promotion. Rehabilitation as a component of the survivorship continuum must become an integral part of everyday oncology nursing practice.

RESOURCES AND INTERVENTIONS

Conflicting reactions to cancer survival can be a heavy burden for even the strongest of individuals. While grateful to be alive, the survivor may have difficulties adjusting to the trade-offs of survival, that is, the possible long-term and potentially unknown late effects of the disease and its treatment. As the health care industry succeeds in controlling and eradicating disease, so does its obligation to minimize the traumas of illness and medical intervention increase.

The availability of education, counseling, and supportive services becomes crucial in caring for those diagnosed with cancer. As more people live with cancer as a chronic illness, improvements in quality-of-life issues and survivor rights are a major concern. Even if support is available and adequate during the acute stage of care, an abrupt severance of this support can increase the trauma of readjusting to life as a nonhospitalized patient or cancer survivor.

From governmental agencies and medical institutions to grass-roots organizations, the collective cancer survivor population is being heard as it organizes, networks, and advocates for the rights to quality survival. Numerous model programs, encompassing both professional and peer support, are responding in a nationwide attempt to meet the changing needs of this expanding survivor population. However, before appropriate programs can be developed, in-depth interviews and studies must be undertaken to delineate the types of educational materials needed, the best methods for intervening, and the stages or timing to deliver information or intervention. Areas for consideration in planning interventions for long-term survivors of adult cancer include: undertaking individualized needs assessments, addressing educational needs, engaging in research, and developing model programs.

Assessing individual needs

As in acute phases of illness, it is imperative to continue assessing both the survivor's and the family's coping styles throughout the extended and permanent stages of survival. Included in this comprehensive and ongoing nursing assessment are strategies that help to resolve crisis intensity and enhance self-care. The survivor's age and developmental stage, socioeconomic background, type of cancer, prognosis, and treatment-related complications are important variables influencing individual needs. Examples of nursing diagnoses related to an individual needs assessment include: (1) ineffective patient or family coping related to ongoing surveillance for long-term effects from disease or treatment; (2) grieving related to loss of job after successful treatment for cancer; (3) alteration in sexuality related to difficulties in establishing intimate relationships; (4) knowledge deficit related to the recognition of cancer recurrence symptomatology.

Addressing educational needs related to survivorship

During the development of educational resources for survivors, nurses must continue to acknowledge the different needs and information preferences of individuals and families. Researchers at Stanford University found that patients want to be well informed about potential or expected problems.[68] Individuals who are avid information seekers may request specifics about cancer recurrence or anticipated problems relative to their diagnosis. Since fear of recurrence and worries about health are common among survivors, nurses can help reduce the stress associated with the unknown by anticipating crisis points and sharing this information with survivors. In the work by Loescher et al.,[20] continued access to information was a major need identified by survivors, and was deemed helpful in managing physical changes even though it did not necessarily diminish the sense of physical vulnerability. Examples of time-related crises that survivors may experience are anniversaries of diagnosis and treatment cessation, birthdays, holidays, yearly examinations, and the 5-year survival mark. Situation-specific crises include diagnosis disclosure to friends and co-workers, hearing stories about cancer, waiting for results of follow-up exams, symptomatology assessment, revealing past medical history, and establishing intimate relationships. If a crisis becomes unmanageable or persistent, nursing referrals can be made for an appropriate intervention.

Survivors and their families may want to know about potential secondary benefits of the cancer experience.[20,52] These benefits, frequently emphasized by survivors themselves, may include a new found zest for life, value reprioritization, and a greater sense of generalized well-being.

Promotion of a greater awareness of cancer survivorship issues should begin during basic nursing education. To sensitize student nurses to the continuing need for supportive care, interactions with long-term survivors are recommended.[51]

Engaging in research

While interest in studying the psychosocial aspects of the acute stage of survival has increased, there has been relatively little interest in gathering prospective, systematic, and longitudinal information about the latter stages of survival.[4] A comprehensive assessment format is needed to study the long-term needs of adult survivors, e.g., a format similar to those available for studying children.[69] Areas for potential research include: (1) the relationship of developmental stage to psychosocial sequelae; (2) description of survival trajectories; (3) family dilemmas during long-term survivorship; (4) the interrelationship of physical compromise and coping problems; (5) identification of the mediators of stress throughout survivorship; (6) association of the attitudes of the health care team with recurrence anxiety; and (7) how time influences fears of relapse.[27,31,64]

Developing model programs

Once survivor-specific assessments identify areas of individual need, a more general assessment of community resources already available for cancer survivors can then be performed. These two steps would logically precede the development of any formal survivor program. Including survivors themselves in the planning and implementation of these programs will enhance program development and reliability. A variety of support options, whether individual or group-related, allows interventions to be better tailored to the needs of the survivor.

The success of any cancer survivor program will depend on: (1) the commitment of the health care team to provide ongoing evaluation and planning for change as the patient lives with a history of cancer; (2) the identification of key individuals to coordinate activities within and among team members; (3) the involvement of the patient and family in the program from initial diagnosis; and (4) the effectiveness of communication among team members.[70] This approach encourages the early recognition of problems during therapy that is imperative for the possible prevention of long-term sequelae.

The majority of long-term survivor programs are nonhospital based and include national and local cancer hotlines, regional chapters of national organizations, and community networks that focus on peer support. The National Coalition for Cancer Survivorship (NCCS) (1010 Wayne Avenue, 5th floor, Silver Springs, MD 20910, 301/650-8868) serves as a resource to network individuals and groups concerned with cancer survivorship issues, and has increased access to information, referrals, resources, educational opportunities, and professional and peer support. Refer to the Yellow Pages at the back of this book for an extended list of resources.

Hospital- or community-based survivor programs can have multiple components. Comprehensive follow-up clinics provide surveillance for physical and psychosocial long-term effects. These clinics can be wellness oriented, emphasizing the importance of proper nutrition, the need for individualized exercise programs, and disease-prevention behaviors. Another component can help to clarify misconceptions about cancer and address survivor limitations by providing information about cancer survival to co-workers and employers. This information ultimately would be provided by the treatment team before the survivor returns to the workplace. Also, some programs offer survivor reunions within either individual hospitals or the community at large. Included in these reunions are those who continue to live with a history of cancer, their families and friends, and their health care providers.

All of these options and approaches for the development of long-term survivor programs become particularly important in light of the growing number of survivors. Programs need to deal with all developmental stages, ranging from the elderly[36] to the growing number of younger adult survivors.

CONCLUSION

Long-term survivorship of adult cancers has many psychosocial ramifications. The definitions of survivorship, the concept of survivorship as a continuum, major psychosocial themes, employment and insurance discrimination, rehabilitation parallels, and resources and interventions have been discussed.

Rosetta Poletti,[71] in her address to the Second European Conference on Clinical Oncology and Cancer Nursing, stated: "The goal of cancer nursing should be to assist the person to be a fully functioning person first and a cancer patient second." Within a framework of rehabilitation, support programs for cancer survivors can be developed in partnership with health care professionals and survivors, and focus on delivering optimal care during all stages of survival. Nursing, with its dynamic, holistic focus, is in an ideal position to promote the psychosocial rehabilitation of cancer survivors.

REFERENCES

1. American Cancer Society: *Cancer Facts and Figures*. Atlanta: American Cancer Society, 1992.
2. National Cancer Institute: Surveillance, Epidemiology, and End Results Program (SEER), Annual Cancer Statistics Review 1973–1987. NIH Publication No. 90–2789. Bethesda, MD: National Cancer Institute, 1990.
3. Fobair P, Mages NL: Psychosocial morbidity among cancer patient survivors. In Ahmed P (ed.): *Coping with Cancer*. New York: Elsevier, 1981, pp. 285–308.
4. Cella DF: Cancer survival: Psychosocial and public issues. *Cancer Invest* 5:59–67, 1987.
5. Fobair P, Hoppe RT, Bloom J, et al: Psychosocial problems among survivors of Hodgkin's disease. *J Clin Oncol* 4:805–814, 1986.

*Funded by Arizona Disease Control Research Commission 33640000000-1-1-AP-6621.

6. Goldberg RJ, Tull RM: *The Psychosocial Dimensions of Cancer.* New York: Free Press, 1983, pp. 40–80.
7. Costello RB (ed.): *Webster's College Dictionary.* New York: Random House, 1991.
8. Carter BJ: "Going through": A critical theme in surviving breast cancer. *Innovations Oncol Nurs* 5:2–4, 1989.
9. Vought CA, Dintruff DL, Fotopoulos SS: Adaptations to the constraints of cancer: Motivational issues. In Ahmed P (ed.): *Living and Dying with Cancer.* New York: Elsevier, 1981, pp. 205–219.
10. Mullan F: Seasons of survival: Reflections of a physician with cancer. *N Engl J Med* 313:270–273, 1985.
11. Weddington WW, Segraves KB, Simon MA: Current and lifetime incidence of psychiatric disorders among a group of extremity sarcoma survivors. *J Psychosom Res* 30:121–125, 1986.
12. Shanfield SB: On surviving cancer: Psychological considerations. *Compr Psychiatry* 21:128–134, 1980.
13. Chang PN, Nesbit ME, Youngren N, et al: Personality characteristics and psychosocial adjustment of long-term survivors of childhood cancer. *J Psychosoc Oncol* 5:43–58, 1987.
14. Tebbi CK, Mallon JC: Long-term psychosocial outcome among cancer amputees in adolescence and early adulthood. *J Psychosoc Oncol* 5:69–82, 1987.
15. Schmale AH, Morrow GR, Schmitt MH, et al: Well-being of cancer survivors. *Psychosom Med* 45:163–169, 1983.
16. Smith K, Lesko LM: Psychosocial problems in cancer survivors. *Oncol* 2:33–44, 1988.
17. Gotay CC: Quality of life among survivors of childhood cancer: A critical review and implications for intervention. *J Psychosoc Oncol* 5:5–23, 1987.
18. Woods NF, Earp JL: Women with cured breast cancer: A study of mastectomy patients in North Carolina. *Nurs Res* 27:279–285, 1978.
19. Rieker PP, Edbril SD, Garnick MB: Curative testis cancer therapy: Psychosocial sequelae. *J Clin Oncol* 3:1117–1126, 1985.
20. Loescher LJ, Clark L, Atwood JR, et al: The impact of the cancer experience on long-term survivors. *Oncol Nurs Forum* 17:223–229, 1990.
21. Cella DF, Lesko LM: Cancer survivors: Watch for signs of stress even years later. *Oncology Rounds (Primary Care and Cancer),* Burroughs Welcome Co., 1988, pp. 1–9.
22. Cella DF, Tross, S: Psychological adjustment to survival from Hodgkin's disease. *J Consult Clin Psychol* 54:616–622, 1986.
23. Mullan F: Re-entry: The educational needs of the cancer survivor. *Health Educ Q* 10:88–94, Spring 1984 (special suppl.).
24. Maher EL: Anomic aspects of recovery from cancer. *Soc Sci Med* 16:907–912, 1982.
25. Northouse LL: Mastectomy patients and the fear of cancer recurrence. *Cancer Nurs* 4:213–220, 1981.
26. Welch-McCaffrey D: Cancer anxiety and quality of life. *Cancer Nurs* 8:151–158, 1985.
27. Quigley KM: The adult cancer survivor: Psychosocial consequences of cure. *Semin Oncol Nurs* 5:63–69, 1989.
28. Gorsynski JG, Holland JC: Psychological aspects of testicular cancer. *Semin Oncol* 6:125–129, 1979.
29. Rose M: Health promotion and risk prevention: Application for cancer survivors. *Oncol Nurs Forum* 16:335–340, 1989.
30. Loescher LJ, Welch-McCaffrey D, Leigh SA, et al: Surviving adult cancer. Part 1: Physiologic effects. *Ann Intern Med* 3:411–432, 1989.
31. Welch-McCaffrey D, Hoffman B, Leigh SA, et al: Surviving adult cancer. Part 2. Psychosocial implications. *Ann Intern Med* 3:517–524, 1989.
32. Sontag S: *Illness as Metaphor.* New York: Vintage Books, 1979, pp. 5–6.
33. Siegel K, Christ GH: Hodgkin's disease survivorship: Psychosocial consequences. In Lacher MJ, Redman JR (eds.): *Hodgkin's Disease: The Consequences of Cure.* Philadelphia: Lea & Febiger, 1990, pp. 383–399.
34. Leigh S, Logan C: The cancer survivorship movement. *Cancer Invest* 9:571–579, 1991.
35. Rowland JH: Survivorship: Beyond just a movement. *Cancer Invest* 9:607–608, 1991.
36. Welch-McCaffrey D: Family issues in cancer care: Current dilemmas—future directions. *J Cancer Prog Mngmnt* 2:11–20, 1987.
37. Hoffman B: Employment discrimination based on cancer history: The need for federal legislation. *Temple Law Quarterly* 59:4–9, 1986.
38. Hoffman B: Cancer survivors at work: Job problems and illegal discrimination. *Oncol Nurs Forum* 16:39–43, 1989.
39. Crothers HM: Employment problems of cancer survivors: Local problems and local solutions. In *Proceedings of the Workshop on Employment, Insurance and the Patient with Cancer.* New Orleans: American Cancer Society, 1986, pp. 51–57.
40. Hoffman B: Employment discrimination: Another hurdle for cancer survivors. *Cancer Invest* 9:589–595, 1991.
41. Hoffman B: Taking care of business: Employment, insurance, and money matters. In Mullan F, Hoffman B (eds.): *Charting the Journey: An Almanac of Practical Resources for Cancer Survivors.* Mount Vernon, NY: Consumer Reports Books, 1990, pp. 97–142.
42. Feldman F: Female cancer patients and caregivers: Experiences in the workplace. In Stellman S (ed.): *Women and Cancer.* New York: Harrington Park Press, 1987, pp. 137–153.
43. Wheatley GM, Cunnick WR, Wright BP, et al: Employment of persons with a history of treatment for cancer. *Cancer* 33:441–445, 1974.
44. Stone RW: Employing the recovered cancer patient. *Cancer* 36:285–286, 1975.
45. Mellette SJ: The cancer patient at work. *American Cancer Society Professional Education Publication* 35:6–8, 1985.
46. Greenleigh Associates: Report on the social, economic and psychological needs of cancer patients in California. In *Proceedings of Western States Conference on Cancer Rehabilitation.* Palo Alto, CA: Bull, 1982.
47. Crothers H: Health insurance: Problems and solutions for people with cancer histories. *Proceedings of the 5th National Conference on Human Values and Cancer.* San Francisco: American Cancer Society, 1987, pp. 100–109.
48. Burton L, Zones J: The incidence of insurance barriers and employment discrimination among Californians with a cancer health history in 1983: A projection. American Cancer Society (Calif. division), 1982.
49. Consolidated Omnibus Budget Reconciliation Act (COBRA). 1986, 42 U.S.C. 300 bb *et seq.*
50. Trippler A: *Comprehensive Health Insurance for High-Risk Individuals: A State-by-State Analysis.* Fergus Falls, MN: Communicating for Agriculture, 1987.
51. Mayer NH: Concepts in cancer rehabilitation. *Semin Oncol* 2:393–398, 1975.
52. Veronesi U, Martino G: Can life be the same after cancer treatment? *Tumori* 64:345–351, 1978.

53. Ganz PA: Current issues in cancer rehabilitation. *Cancer* 65:742–751, 1990.
54. Watson PG: Rehabilitation philosophy: A means of fostering a positive attitude toward cancer. *J Enterostom Ther* 13:153–156, 1986.
55. Mellette SJ: Rehabilitation issues for cancer survivors: Psychosocial challenges. *J Psychosoc Oncol* 7:93–109, 1989.
56. Kudsk EG, Hoffman GS: Rehabilitation of the cancer patient. *Primary Care* 14:381–390, 1987.
57. Habeck RV, Romsaas EP, Olsen SJ: Cancer rehabilitation and continuing care: A case study. *Cancer Nurs* 7:315–320, 1984.
58. Groenwald SL, Thaney K: Rehabilitation. In Groenwald SL (ed.): *Cancer Nursing: Principles and Practice.* Boston: Jones and Bartlett, 1987, pp. 749–758.
59. Houts PS, Harvey HA, Simmonds MA, et al: Characteristics of patients at risk for financial burden because of cancer and its treatment. *J Psychosoc Oncol* 3:15–22, 1985.
60. McNaull FW: The costs of cancer: A challenge to health care providers. *Cancer Nurs* 4:207–212, 1981.
61. Baird SB: Economic realities in the treatment and care of the cancer patient. *Topics Clin Nurs* 2:67–80, 1981.
62. Mayer D: *An Invitational Conference Addressing Barriers to Successful Cancer Rehabilitation.* Proceedings of the 1988 Oncology Nursing Society President's Grant, Boston, August 1988.
63. Enck RE: ACCC standards: Past, present and future. *J Cancer Prog Mngmnt* 2:11–20, 1987.
64. Dudas S, Carlson CE: Cancer rehabilitation. *Oncol Nurs Forum* 15:183–188, 1988.
65. Wells RJ: Rehabilitation: Making the most of time. *Oncol Nurs Forum* 17:503–507, 1990.
66. Mayer DK: The healthcare implications of cancer rehabilitation in the twenty-first century. *Oncol Nurs Forum* 19:23–27, 1992.
67. Hassey-Dow K: The enduring seasons in survival. *Oncol Nurs Forum* 17:511–516, 1990.
68. Fobair P, Hoppe R, Bloom J, et al: Psychosocial problems among survivors of Hodgkin's disease. *J Clin Oncol* 4:805–814, 1986.
69. Fergusson J, Ruccione K, Wasderwitz M, et al: Time required to assess children for the late effects of treatment. *Cancer Nurs* 10:300–310, 1987.
70. Broadwell DC: Rehabilitation needs of the patient with cancer. *Cancer* 60:563–568, 1987.
71. Poletti R: *Living a Full Life with Cancer.* Proceedings of the Second European Conference on Clinical Oncology and Cancer Nursing. Amsterdam: ECCO, November 1983.

PART V

Manifestations of Cancer and Its Treatment

Chapter 23

Pain

Deborah B. McGuire, RN, PhD, FAAN

Vivian R. Sheidler, RN, MS

INTRODUCTION AND BACKGROUND

Definitions of Pain

Historically, pain has been a phenomenon not easy to define. During the seventeenth century, pain was viewed as a signal of bodily injury, with scant attention paid to its nonphysical aspects. This notion persisted until the twentieth century, when researchers began to formulate concepts of pain that recognized and included not only the physical "alarm" aspect but other neurologic activities, cultural factors, and individual personality and experiential variables as well. Despite these broader concepts, a precise definition of pain eluded workers in the field, for as Livingston wrote in 1943, "The chief difficulty encountered in a search for a satisfactory definition of pain is the fact that it can be considered from either a physiologic or psychologic approach. Any consideration of pain, by one approach alone, without due regard to the other, is incomplete."[1,p.62]

Reconciliation of these two disparate approaches proved very difficult, since a single definition seemed unable to satisfy everyone. Melzack and Wall highlighted this problem when they wrote in 1980 that "pain is such a common experience that we rarely pause to define it in ordinary conversation. Yet no one who has worked on the problem of pain has ever been able to give it a definition which is satisfactory to all of his colleagues."[2,p.9] In their view, pain was a "*category* of experiences, signifying a multitude of different, unique experiences having different causes, and characterized by different qualities varying along a number of sensory and affective dimensions."[2,p.71]

The need for a standard definition of pain, however, prompted the International Association for the Study of Pain (IASP) to form a subcommittee charged with developing a definition acceptable to both clinicians and researchers. The major result of their labors, published in 1979, was the following: "Pain is an unpleasant sensory and emotional experience associated with actual or potential tissue damage, or described in terms of such damage."[3] This definition accounted for both sensory and emotional aspects of pain as well as for pain of pathophysiological and psychological origin. It incorporated the essential elements of subjectivity and individual uniqueness in the pain experience.

In addition to this definition of pain, the IASP published a list of pain terms, with their definitions (e.g., *allodynia* and *causalgia*), which it viewed as a "minimum standard vocabulary for members of different disciplines who work in the field of pain."[3] Bouckoms wrote that the IASP definitions of pain and related terms provided a nontheoretical, relatively complete, valid taxonomy that was extremely useful to clinicians and researchers alike.[4] It is probably safe to say that in the 14 years since the IASP definition of pain was published, it has become commonly accepted and used by most pain specialists.

Since 1979, the IASP has continued its work on a taxonomy, or classification system, for pain. In 1986 it published additional pain terms with definitions, descriptions of chronic pain syndromes, and a classification and coding schema for these different syndromes.[5] Turk and Rudy [6] examined the reliability of two aspects of this schema—body location and presumed etiology. They found that physician raters demonstrated good interrater reliability when assessing location of pain in a heterogeneous chronic pain population, but only fair interrater reliability on etiology of pain. A more recent study[7] supports the clinical utility of the IASP coding schema as a means for deriving, coding, storing, and retrieving basic classification characteristics of pain.

Although the IASP publications just cited do not present a specific definition of acute pian, it is commonly accepted that chronic pain and acute pain are distinctly different phenomena. Bonica defined acute pain as "a complex constellation of unpleasant sensory, perceptual, and emotional experiences and certain associated autonomic, psychologic, emotional, and behavioral responses."[8,p.19] He emphasized that noxious stimulation from injury or disease to either cutaneous or deep tissues and the abnormal function of musculoskeletal or visceral tissues were the two major causes of acute pain. Furthermore, acute pain rarely has a strong psychopathologic or environmental component, as does chronic pain, and it may recur periodically when an individual has recurrent acute pathophysiologic processes, such as those commonly seen in persons with cancer.

Theories and Mechanisms of Pain

Closely related to definitions of pain are theories of what pain is and how it occurs. Various theories have been proposed over the years and, as with definitions of pain, began with one or two simple anatomical or clinical aspects of pain and then expanded to include a multitude of anatomical, neural, physiological, clinical, and psychological variables. Until the mid-twentieth century, several traditional but opposing theories of pain were prominent. Price[9] reviewed and discussed these "classical" theories. In addition to the classical theories that have been described, there are several current theories of pain.[9] Most notable of these is the *gate control theory of pain*, proposed by Melzack and Wall in 1965[10] and updated more recently.[11] Table 23-1 provides a brief overview of pain theories and their major tenets. Although the gate control theory is not perfect, it is the most comprehensive theory of pain yet proposed and serves an extremely useful purpose in explaining pain mechanisms for most health care givers. It is now abundantly clear that pain has a sensory component as well as a reactive (emotional) component. Much research is being conducted to elucidate the specific processes and phenomena responsible for producing the sensory and emotional puzzle called pain.

TABLE 23-1 Theories of Pain

Classical Theories	Major Tenets
Specificity Theory	• Pain one of four cutaneous stimuli: warmth, touch, cold, and pain • Pain results from specific pathways and receptors
Pattern Theory	• No specific nerve endings or fibers • Free nerve endings respond to stimuli, with different patterns of impulses
Summation Theory	• Specialized receptors • Chronic pain results from reverberating circuits in dorsal horn of spinal cord
Sensory Interaction Theory	• Rapidly conducting system inhibits transmission in a slowly conducting system • Interactions between input from large fibers and small fibers determine presence and severity of pain
Current Theories	**Major Tenets**
Gate Control Theory	• Nerve impulses are modulated in spinal cord by a gating mechanism • Gating mechanism is influenced by large and small fiber activity • Descending nerve impulses influence the gating mechanism • Central control trigger system activates cognitive processes • When output of transmission cells in spinal cord exceeds limits, action system is activated, causing complex patterns of experience and behavior
Parallel Processing Theory	• Spinothalamic projection systems consist of two tracts, responsible for sensory-discriminative and motivational-aversive reactions to pain • Higher central nervous system processes cause evaluative reactions • All three systems make up the "pain experience"
Sequential Processing Theory	• Affective-motivational state depends on sequential processes involving cognition

While it is not possible to describe these efforts in any detail in this chapter, a brief overview of general mechanisms of pain is provided next.

When considered strictly from the pathophysiologic and biochemical processes that cause it, pain experienced by patients with cancer is no different than pain experienced by other individuals. Etiological, clinical, and psychosocial characteristics of both tumor- and treatment-related cancer pain, however, distinguish it from other types of pain. These differences will be elaborated later in the chapter; in this section the basic mechanisms of pain in general are considered.

The perception of and response to pain are due to four distinct processes that operate simultaneously and are all required for pain to occur (Table 23-2).[12] The first of these processes, *transduction,* begins when a noxious (painful or tissue-damaging) stimulus affects a peripheral sensory nerve ending, depolarizing it and setting off electrical activity that initiates the whole phenomenon of pain perception. *Transmission,* the next process, consists of the series of subsequent neural events that carry the electrical impulses throughout the nervous system, from peripheral to central. *Modulation,* the third process, is a neural activity that controls pain transmission neurons, those originating in the periphery and/or the central nervous system. The fourth process, *perception,* is less an actual physiological/anatomical process than it is the vague subjective correlate of pain (how it feels) that encompasses complex behavioral, psychological, and emotional factors that are little understood. The reader interested in more detail is referred to Price,[9] Fields,[12] Bonica,[13] and Wall and Melzack.[14] Figure 23-1 shows schematically where transmission and modulation occur.

Cancer Pain as a Multidimensional Phenomenon

The notion of sensory and affective, or physiological and psychological, aspects of pain—developed and nurtured through the gate control theory of pain and its related model—has been used by researchers to develop a conceptual framework for cancer pain. Ahles and his colleagues[15] hypothesized five dimensions of the cancer pain experience: (1) *physiological* (organic etiology of pain), (2) *sensory* (intensity, location, quality), (3) *affective* (depression, anxiety), (4) *cognitive* (manner

TABLE 23-2 Mechanisms of Pain

Process	Anatomic and Physiologic Components	Description
Transduction	• Peripheral nerve fibers • Chemical substances	Noxious stimulus depolarizes peripheral nerve and sets off electrical activity
Transmission	• Afferent nerve fibers • Dorsal horn of spinal cord • Spinothalamic pathways • Thalamus and cortex	Neural events that occur subsequent to transduction and carry electrical impulses throughout nervous system, from peripheral to central
Modulation	• Periacqueductal gray • Descending neurons • Dorsal horn of spinal cord • Opiate receptors • Opioid peptides • Neurotransmitters	A central neural activity that controls transmission of pain impulses and contributes to variability of pain
Perception	• Transmission system • Modulation system • Cortical processes	Neural activities involved in transmission and modulation result in a subjective correlate of pain that encompasses complex behavioral, psychological, and emotional factors

Sources: Data from Price[9] and Fields.[12]

in which pain influences a person's thought processes, how the person views her- himself, or the meaning of pain), and (5) *behavioral* (pain-related behaviors such as medication intake and activity level). Since these investigators found little in the literature to support their multidimensional conceptualization, they conducted a systematic study in a group of 40 cancer patients with tumor-related pain to assess each of the five dimensions in their model. They used a variety of reliable and valid tools to assess the dimensions and found support for their conceptual model. When compared to cancer patients without pain, the subjects in the study had more depression, were more irritable, engaged in less physical activity, and took more medications. Those who believed that pain indicated progression of cancer had elevated depression and anxiety scores. Ahles et al.[15] suggested as a result of their findings that treatment for cancer pain consists of specific therapeutic modalities targeted to each of the five dimensions.

McGuire[16] adapted Ahles' conceptual framework to conduct a descriptive study of 40 cancer patients with pain and 40 without pain. In general, support was found for the five dimensions of the model. Patients with pain had more depression, poorer physical function, and more psychosocial and other problems than the pain-free patients. Another finding was that individuals with cancer pain practiced a number of cognitive and behavioral coping strategies that they reported as moderately effective at reducing and controlling their pain.[17]

In addition to these five dimensions of the multidimensional model of cancer-related pain, there is a sixth important area—the *sociocultural dimension.*[18] This involves various demographic, social, and cultural characteristics that are related to the experience of pain. The six dimensions contribute to the individual's perception of and response to pain. They are complex, interrelated, and as yet incompletely understood. A recent review of research literature indicates substantial support for this conceptualization of pain, for both cancer pain and other types of pain.[19] Further discussion of each dimension follows.

Physiologic dimension

Ahles et al.[15] originally described the physiologic dimension as consisting of the organic etiology of pain, specifying such causes as tumor that has metastasized to bone or infiltrated nerves or a hollow viscus. This definition was based on earlier work by researchers at Memorial Sloan-Kettering Cancer Center in New York. In 1979 Foley[20] described three types of pain observed in patients with cancer, each with a different etiology: (1) pain associated with direct tumor involvement, (2) pain associated with cancer therapy, and (3) pain unrelated to either the tumor or its treatment. From this initial schema, she and a number of colleagues developed a comprehensive listing of more specific causes of pain that fit within the first two categories.[21]

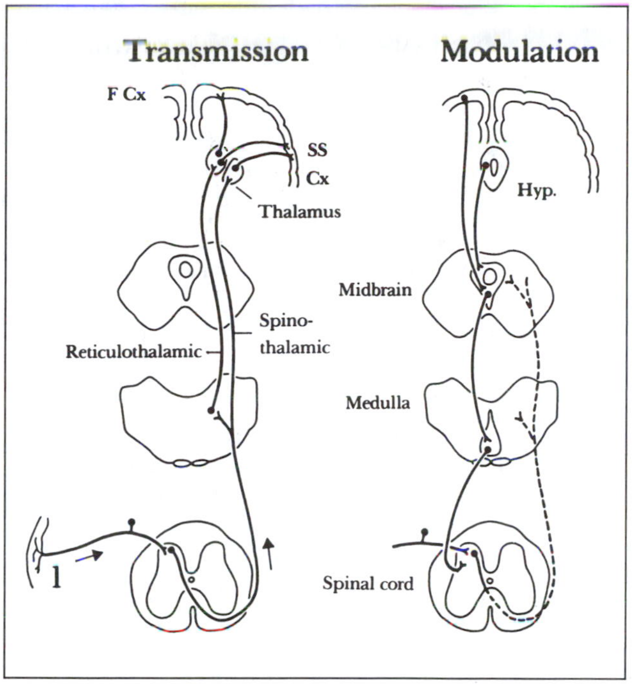

FIGURE 23-1 Pain transmission and modulation. **Left:** Transmission system for nociceptive messages. Noxious stimuli activate the sensitive peripheral ending of the primary afferent nociceptor by the process of transduction (*l*). The message is then transmitted over the peripheral nerve to the spinal cord, where it synapses with cells of origin of the two major ascending pain pathways, the spinothalamic and spinoreticulothalamic. The message is relayed in the thalamus to both the frontal (*F Cx*) and the somatosensory cortex (*SS Cx*). **Right:** Pain modulation network. Inputs from frontal cortex and hypothalamus (*Hyp.*) activate cells in the midbrain, which control spinal pain transmission cells via cells in the medulla. (Source: Reprinted with permission from Fields HL: *Pain*. New York: McGraw-Hill, 1987.)

TABLE 23-3 Types of Cancer-Related Pain

Tumor-Related	Treatment-Related
Infiltration of bone	**Diagnostic**
Base of skull	Mechanical injury
Vertebral bodies	Chemical irritation
Long bones	Inflammation
Infiltration of nerves	**Therapeutic (acute)**
Peripheral	Surgery
Plexus	Chemotherapy
Root	Radiotherapy
Epidural	
	Posttherapeutic (chronic)
Infiltration of hollow viscus	Surgery
Intestinal tract	Chemotherapy
Viscera	Radiotherapy
	Complications
	Tumor embolization
	Infections

Sources: Data from Coyle and Foley,[21] Chapman et al.,[22] Portenoy,[29] Payne,[30] and Kelly and Payne.[31]

Additional work on characterizing pain related to cancer therapy has been done.[22,23] The sources of pain associated with cancer treatment are many, ranging from initial diagnostic procedures causing acute, short-term pain, to standard therapeutic modalities (surgery, radiotherapy, chemotherapy) causing acute, short-term and/or chronic long-term pain. An example of acute, short-term pain is that associated with mucositis in patients receiving bone marrow transplantation.[24,25] Additional work is aimed at describing more fully treatment-related pain syndromes in specific populations, such as marrow transplant patients.[26] Additionally, recent literature from pediatric oncology strongly suggests that these pain etiologies and syndromes are also common in children with cancer pain.[27,28] Table 23-3 lists the major types of tumor- and treatment-related cancer pain.

The third type of pain described by Foley[20] was pain unrelated to either cancer or its treatment. She estimated that it accounted for 3%–10% of the pain seen in cancer patients. Individuals with cancer pain are just as likely as the average individual to have pain from migraine headache, osteoarthritis, or degenerative disk disease. The presence of such pain, however, is important, and should be carefully assessed to be sure that it is *not* cancer-related.

The work of Foley, Chapman, their colleagues, and others on etiology of cancer pain has led to a greater understanding of the epidemiology and pathophysiology of cancer pain, including three specific pain syndromes that occur in patients with cancer and are caused by tumor.[29] These syndromes of somatic, visceral, and neuropathic pain are characterized by pain of different qualities, located in different anatomical parts of the body, and caused by different mechanisms (Figure 23-2). All three syndromes are usually discussed in reference to tumor-related pain, but they may apply equally as well to treatment-related pain.[30,31] It is important to note that many cancer patients with pain will have one or more of these three syndromes simultaneously,[32] and that each syndrome responds differently to therapeutic modalities.[33]

Related to etiology of pain are two other characteristics. *Duration* of pain refers to whether pain is acute or chronic. Acute pain generally is due to tissue damage, is self-limited, and resolves when the tissue damage heals. There is a clear pattern of onset and resolution. When acute pain occurs, there may be hyperactivity of the autonomic nervous system, although this is not diagnostic of the presence of pain. Chronic pain is also usually due to tissue damage, but not always. It may

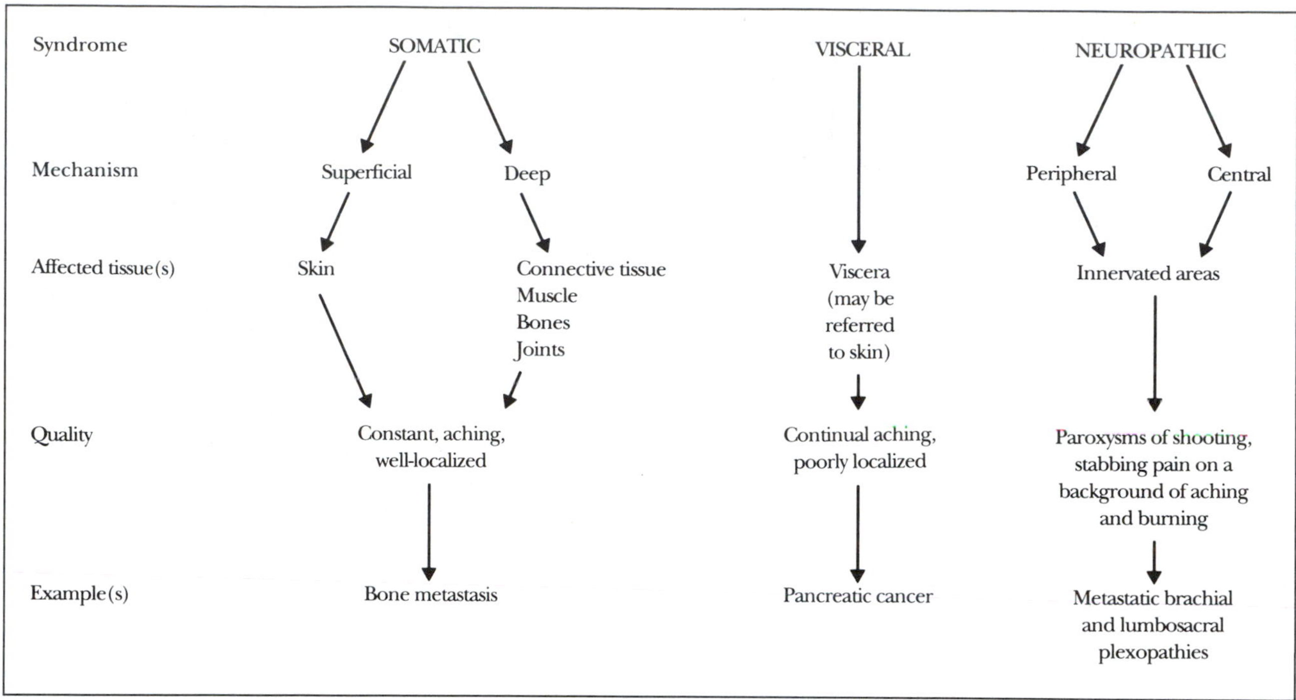

FIGURE 23-2 Pain syndromes in cancer.

last 3 months or more[5] and is usually accompanied by adaptation, rather than hyperactivity, of the autonomic nervous system. There is not always a clear pattern of onset and resolution. Cancer pain, whether caused by tumor or treatment, can be subdivided into acute and chronic pain; sometimes both types occur simultaneously.

The second characteristic related to etiology of pain is the *pattern* that pain displays. Melzack first described patterns of pain in a quantifiable way in his McGill Pain Questionnaire,[34] where he identified three separate patterns: (1) brief, momentary, or transient, (2) rhythmic, periodic, or intermittent, and (3) continuous, steady, or constant. The few researchers who have studied patterns of pain in cancer patients have found that about half of individuals experience pain that is constant, with just fewer than half experiencing intermittent pain and a very small number reporting brief or transient pain.[16,35–37] Arathuzik noted that in her sample of 80 breast cancer patients with pain, most had pain lasting for 1 to several hours at a time, and many had pain lasting all day.[38] Most cancer patients experience two or more patterns simultaneously.

In summary, the physiologic dimension of cancer pain includes organic etiology of the pain, which encompasses the specific anatomic sites affected. Additionally, duration and pattern of pain are inherent in this dimension. Together these factors constitute the physiologic portion of the multidimensional experience of cancer pain.

Sensory dimension

The sensory dimension of cancer-related pain is related to where the pain is located and what it feels like. Three specific components of this dimension are location, intensity, and quality.

The first component, *location* of pain, is an important component. Many cancer patients have been reported to have pain at two or more locations.[38–40] Given the patterns of metastasis or sites of involvement seen in many solid tumors and some hematologic malignancies, this finding is not surprising. The number of separate locations of pain has clear implications for the sensory dimension as well as for the entire pain experience.

Intensity of pain, or how strong it feels, is the second important component of the sensory dimension. Intensity is a perceived, and therefore a subjective, phenomenon, subject to individual pain threshold (the least stimulus intensity at which pain is perceived, according to Twycross and Lack[41]). Although intensity depends primarily on etiology of pain, individual threshold may be affected by a variety of factors, such as physical comfort, mood, medications, and social environment, thus causing perceived intensity of pain to increase or decrease. Intensity is the most commonly assessed aspect of pain, and is characterized by words such as *none, mild, moderate, severe, intolerable, excruciating, bad,* and *intense.*

The third component of the sensory dimension is the *quality* of pain, which refers to how it actually feels. Melzack and Torgerson[42] were among the first to systematically study words that people used to describe pain. They composed a list of 102 words from the clinical literature on pain, and organized them into classes that described sensory, affective, and evaluative properties of pain. Words placed in the sensory category referred to temporal, spatial, pressure, thermal, and other such aspects of pain. Examples of these sensory words are, respectively, *pulsing, radiating, penetrating, burning,* and *aching.* This initial work provided the foundation for the McGill Pain Questionnaire,[34] the first multidimensional measure of pain.

Some studies have revealed that patients with cancer pain use certain words more commonly than others to describe sensory aspects of their pain.[35–37,43–46] Words commonly used by patients in these studies included *sharp, tender, aching, throbbing, sore, stabbing, heavy, shooting,* and *gnawing.* Some authors distinguished between tumor- and treatment-related pain, but others did not, so it is not entirely clear which words describe which etiology. Nevertheless, the recurring word patterns found across time and in different groups of patients indicate that cancer pain is characterized by specific sensory qualities.

The sensory dimension of pain, as conceptualized by Ahles et al.,[15] consists of location, intensity, and quality. The nature of and relationships among these three components are unique to each individual and undoubtedly have a strong impact not only on the entire experience of pain but on the affective, cognitive, behavioral, and sociocultural dimensions as well.

Affective dimension

As defined by Ahles et al.,[15] the affective dimension consists of depression, anxiety, or other psychological factors or personality traits associated with pain. Of the five dimensions proposed by Ahles, this one had the most support in the literature. In 1987, ten studies were identified that examined relationships between pain in cancer patients and psychological factors or personality traits.[18] In 1988, Dalton and Feuerstein[47] reviewed literature relating to biobehavioral factors in pain as well as affective, behavioral, and cognitive responses to pain. Although their review included both anecdotal and research reports relevant to the affective dimension of pain, it was clear that little research existed. The chapter on pain in the previous edition of this text identified 21 studies related to the affective dimension of cancer pain[48] and, in tabular format, indicated what psychological parameters were measured and what their relationships were to pain. Recent research and review articles[24,38,46,49–51] also support the importance of the affective dimension in cancer pain.

It is evident that parameters relevant to the affective dimension of pain range from specific personality traits (e.g., neuroticism) to affective disorders (e.g., depression) to vague general concepts such as psychological well-being. Taking into account the strong and weak points of studies in this area, it is possible to conclude the following: (1) specific personality factors probably are not related to the experience of cancer pain, (2) there is little evidence that affective disorders such as depression and anxiety are *strongly* related to pain, and (3) much more research on the relationships among these many psychological parameters and the experience of cancer pain is needed.

Despite a limited body of research, it is quite clear from the clinical perspective that there is an affective component to the pain experience and that it influences the individual's response to pain. The critical issue here is that psychological variables important to a particular patient's pain experience must be identified and dealt with to effectively manage pain.

Cognitive dimension

The cognitive dimension of cancer pain, as conceived by Ahles et al.,[15] encompassed the manner in which the pain influences a person's thought processes or the manner in which the person views her- or himself. In their study, they found support for this dimension by assessing the meaning of each patient's pain. Almost two-thirds believed their pain was an indicator of progressive disease, and these individuals had significantly elevated anxiety and depression scores.

Spiegel and Bloom[52] found that in patients with metastatic breast cancer, the belief that pain indicated worsening disease was significantly correlated with reports of more pain, more anxiety, and more depression. Similarly, McGuire[16] found that 40% of patients considered pain an indicator of disease progression, and while they were more depressed than those without this view, the difference was not statistically significant. Barkwell[53] recently reported that cancer patients with pain ascribed meanings of challenge, punishment, and enemy to their pain. She found that patients who viewed pain as a challenge reported less pain and had lower depression and higher coping scores than those who viewed pain as punishment or an enemy. In a different vein, Jacox and Stewart[54] found that cancer patients with pain had a decreased health self-concept. These studies were all related to the way individuals view themselves. Less clear is the area of how pain influences an individual's thought processes; certainly more research is needed.

Several recent studies have examined the effects of opioid analgesics on cognitive function of patients with pain. They found that cognitive deficits occurred as opioids were first prescribed or when doses were adjusted upward but that the deficits were transient and that functioning returned to baseline when drug doses were stabilized for approximately 2 weeks.[55,56] Level and quality of cognition in relation to pharmacologic therapy appear to be part of the cognitive dimension of pain, since they may influence the ability of individuals to report pain.

Another aspect of the cognitive dimension is knowledge about pain and its management. Such knowledge can affect responses both to pain and to interventions. Rimer and colleagues[57] demonstrated that an educational intervention of nurse counseling and printed materials resulted in a higher likelihood of cancer patients with pain taking the proper dose of analgesic on the proper schedule.

Finally, several researchers have examined cognitive strategies used by cancer patients to cope with pain. Such strategies clearly fall within the cognitive dimension of pain since they result from cognitive processes. Specific strategies include various forms of distraction (e.g., reading, watching television), use of coping self-statements, reinterpretation of painful sensations, selective inattention, withdrawal, suppression of pain, and trying to accept pain.[17,53,58,59]

Behavioral dimension

The behavioral dimension of pain includes a variety of observable behaviors related to pain. Until recently, there was little research supporting this dimension of the cancer pain experience. Ahles et al.[15] focused on level of activity and intake of analgesics as manifestations of this dimension in their study. They found that cancer patients with pain spent significantly less time walking or standing than those who did not have pain. Furthermore, 77% of the patients with pain reported that people in their immediate environment could tell when they were in pain because of their facial expressions, changes in mood or activity, or verbal complaints.

Communication of pain to others was examined systematically by Bond and Pilowsky,[60] who studied the relationships among advanced cancer patients' subjective reports of pain, their communication of pain, and reactions of nurses caring for them. About one-quarter of their patients with pain did not communicate it to nursing staff, and their self-reported pain scores were lower than those of patients who had pain and reported it or who were offered analgesics by staff. In another study, these two researchers learned that patients who considered themselves "ill" reported considerable pain and tended to request analgesics frequently.[61]

Keefe and his colleagues[62] conducted a study of the behavioral manifestations of pain in patients with head and neck cancer who were undergoing treatment for their disease. Guarded movements and grimacing were found to be the major behavioral indicators of pain, with grimacing correlating significantly with patients' reports of pain intensity. In addition, the amount of time patients spent walking or standing tended to decrease over the treatment period and time spent reclining increased. Finally, as treatment progressed, the number of simple daily activities that caused pain increased significantly.

Another component of the behavioral dimension of pain consists of simple strategies or activities that patients engage in to control pain. Several studies have examined these activities. McGuire[35] noted that inpatients most frequently used analgesics, but one-third also reported lying still, restricting movement, or positioning and moving of affected body parts. In a survey of 351 hospitalized patients, some of whom had cancer, researchers noted that the most commonly cited (≥33%) pain reduction methods involved medications, rest or lying down, heat, and distraction.[63] Several studies found that cancer patients used an array of nonanalgesic, be-behaviorally-oriented pain control methods, including heat, distraction, position change, massage, nonnarcotic drugs, exercise, positioning, pressure/manipulation, immobilization, guarding, and use of analgesics.[49,58,59,64,65] McGuire[17] noted the use of a variety of behavioral and cognitive coping strategies by both inpatients and outpatients, who reported moderate effectiveness of these methods of relieving pain.

It is clear that the studies just described support the behavioral dimension of the cancer pain experience as conceptualized by Ahles et al.[15] The findings offer directions for therapeutic approaches as well, which will be examined in a subsequent section.

Sociocultural dimension

The sociocultural dimension of cancer pain consists of a variety of demographic, ethnic, cultural, spiritual, and related factors that influence a person's perception of and response to pain. There have been very few studies examining the relationships of any of these factors to cancer pain specifically, but the small body of research that has been conducted on sociocultural aspects of clinical pain is reviewed briefly next, since some of the findings may pertain to the individual with cancer pain.

A number of studies used experimentally induced laboratory pain to examine racial, age, religious, and ethnic differences in pain.[66] Although none of the studies reviewed in this paper allowed definitive conclusions about differences in pain response due to the factors studied, a strong role of culturally determined attitudinal factors in pain perception and response was clearly supported. In an updated review, Wolff[67] lamented that little progress had been made in studying and understanding the important role ethnocultural factors played in pain. He maintained, however, that cultural factors such as majority/minority group status seemed to be the most likely causes of differences in pain perception and response.

Lipton and Marbach[68] corroborated this idea in their study of interethnic differences and similarities in reported pain experiences of black, Irish, Italian, Jewish, and Puerto Rican patients with facial pain. All five groups were similar in their reported responses to pain; however, the factors that *influenced* their responses were quite different. For example, Italians were most influenced by duration of pain, while Jews and Puerto Ricans were most influenced by level of psychological distress. These researchers suggested viewing the relationship between ethnicity and the pain experience as a subtle continuum of behaviors, attitudes, and feelings.

A descriptive study of Arab Americans' perceptions of and responses to pain emphasized that cultural characteristics heavily influenced individual behaviors.[69] For example, vehement, persistent, and perhaps exaggerated verbal messages were the norm for this group, and reporting of pain was included. Endurance of pain was not a priority, since modern technology was available; endurance was easier if Arab Americans understood that the consequences of pain would be more positive. Pain generally was perceived as unpleasant, to be avoided, and to be controlled by all means. Individuals with pain often displayed more behavioral manifestations of pain and were more vocal about it to family members rather than to health care providers. Family members assumed a major role in trying to manage pain, primarily through usurping the decision making related to care.

Age, sex, and race have been examined in relation to expression of pain. Females and older individuals were found to have increased verbal expressions of pain.[70,71] One study revealed that blacks used more moderate words than whites in describing pain,[70] but another study demonstrated no significant differences.[72]

Only a few studies have focused on cancer patients with pain. The sociocultural variables studied have been mixed but have included sex, race, age, and cultural background. In a study of cancer inpatients, McGuire[35] noted that females and nonwhites had significantly lower scores on the McGill Pain Questionnaire than males or whites. In a subsequent study of inpatients and outpatients, she found that blacks and older patients had less pain (as measured by the McGill Pain Questionnaire) and depression.[16] A recent study by Greenwald[73] indicated that despite few differences between ethnic identity and pain report, the ways in which people described affective aspects of pain using the McGill Pain Questionnaire varied across ethnic groups. He concluded that specific ethnic identities still condition the individual expression of pain even though assimilation into the American population has occurred.

McMillan[74] found that cancer patients with pain who were older (over age 55) reported less pain intensity than those who were younger. On the other hand, another study[75] found that the pain intensity of patients who were over 65 years of age was similar to that of those under 65.

Cleeland and associates,[76] using the Brief Pain Inventory (BPI), compared American and Vietnamese patients with cancer pain. Only items related to pain severity and interference of pain in several life domains (e.g., activity, walking, sleep, work, relations with others, mood) were translated into Vietnamese. Their data suggested that these two groups of patients, from widely different cultural backgrounds, responded in a similar fashion to items rating the severity of their pain and its interference with daily living. The authors noted that Vietnamese patients, however, reported more severe pain despite fairly comparable cancers; it was hypothesized that this was due in part to the fact that 64% were receiving no analgesics at all whereas the remainder were taking nonopioids, specifically, a benzodiazepine-type of drug. Although the focus of this study was instrument development, it was clear that the two areas of concern—pain severity and interference—were important cross-culturally.

The research literature supporting the sociocultural dimension of cancer is just beginning to emerge. Only one recent review paper exploring relationships among culture, pain, and cancer could be found.[77] However, literature in noncancer populations and the slowly growing cancer literature make clear that ethnic and cultural factors are important in patients' perceptions of and responses to pain.

Implications of the multidimensional model

The multidimensional conceptualization of cancer pain, as initially defined by Ahles et al.,[15] expanded by McGuire,[18] and supported by the research of many investigators, provides the conceptual foundation for this chapter. The six dimensions are highly appropriate for assessment and management of cancer pain; each contributes in its own way to various aspects of these two critical processes. Additionally, the multidimensional framework allows the experience of cancer pain to be viewed as the complete, interrelated, interactive, and dynamic phenomenon that it is. Nursing assessment and management that are performed in a holistic, competent, and multidisciplinary manner will ensure that individuals with cancer pain achieve optimal quality of life regardless of the status of their disease.

SCOPE OF THE CANCER PAIN PROBLEM

Pain in the cancer patient has long been recognized as a challenging clinical problem. The Oncology Nursing Society's (ONS) position paper on cancer pain[78] emphasized the fact that cancer pain often is managed inadequately. Similarly, the National Institutes of Health (NIH) consensus statement on an integrated approach to the management of pain[79] highlighted the inadequacies of current approaches to pain. A comprehensive understanding of the scope of the cancer pain problem requires knowledge of its prevalence, significance, and professional issues involved in its management.

Prevalence

The American Cancer Society's 1992 statistics on cancer incidence and mortality[80] indicated that 1,130,000 would be diagnosed with cancer in 1992 and 520,000 would die of the disease. The incidence of cancer pain for all cancer diagnoses during all stages of the disease, however, has been difficult to quantify. Most studies report prevalence data rather than incidence data.

Coyle and Foley[21] identified several problems affecting the accuracy of prevalence data: (1) lack of systematic data collection and pain measurement techniques, (2) lack of documentation regarding the extent of patients' disease, (3) lack of identification of pain's etiology, and (4) inclusion of multiple cancer diagnoses as a single group. In spite of these problems, however, researchers have examined the prevalence of cancer pain, with the majority of reports appearing during the last 15 years.

The chapter on pain in the previous edition of this text[48] reviewed and discussed at length the literature on prevalence of cancer pain, presenting overviews in tabular format. In brief, prevalence of pain by clinical setting, regardless of cancer diagnosis, indicates that patients in hospice and specialty units report a higher prevalence of pain than patients in other settings. This observation can be understood by recognizing that patients with advanced, metastatic disease are often referred to these settings for terminal care. Patients with advanced disease report more severe pain than those who are in the early stages of their illness.

The severity of cancer pain, as opposed to the presence of pain, has been used as a means of reporting not only prevalence of pain but also its characteristics. Several studies cited in the chapter on pain in the previous edition of this text[48] revealed that patients with cancer-related pain described it as ranging from mild or moderate to severe or excruciating. Most patients, however, reported pain in the mild to moderate rather than the severe range.

Examination of pain prevalence data by cancer diagnosis shows the likelihood of pain becoming a significant problem with the progression of disease, particularly in common solid tumors such as lung and breast cancer. Several cancers, notably pancreatic and primary bone, exhibit relatively high prevalence rates of pain across all stages of disease.

Recent literature has addressed pain in children with cancer,[27,28] including prevalence and etiology. Very few studies of pain incidence or prevalence have been conducted in the pediatric oncology population, but the few data available suggest that between 25% and 78% of children may experience pain at some point during their cancer experience.

Taken together, the published studies on the prevalence of cancer pain indicate several important things. First, knowledge of cancer pain comes only from prevalence studies, since there are almost no published reports on the *incidence* of cancer pain. Second, pain clearly is more prevalent in those patients with advanced stages of disease and those being treated in hospice or specialty units. Third, certain common malignancies are more often associated with cancer pain, and it is these malignancies in which pain is better studied and understood. Finally, much of the available data are derived from patients with tumor- and/or treatment-related pain, rendering accurate rates for any specific type of pain difficult to ascertain.

Because of the complicated nature of cancer pain, with its different etiologies,[31] varied presentations,[32] multiple dimensions, and variety of treatments, and the previously mentioned problems with studying the incidence and prevalence of the problem, one can speculate that the true prevalence is much greater than existing reports indicate. Although cancer pain clearly is a multidimensional phenomenon, the impact on patients who have it, or their families and friends, is as yet little understood.

Significance

Aside from its high prevalence, cancer pain is a significant problem for a variety of reasons. It is already well known that individuals with cancer-related pain exhibit a variety of pain-related behaviors,[65] and experience many physical and psychosocial problems.[15,16,44,81–83] Additionally, the last 3–4 years have witnessed an explosion of clinical research, sociocultural, political, regulatory/legal, health policy and professional activities that have increased knowledge about pain and have influenced in both positive and negative ways how it is managed. These developments encompass quality of life, family and home care issues, suicide risk, ethical concerns related to use of advanced technologies, financial costs associated with cancer pain, regulatory influences on use of controlled substances, legal impediments to adequate management of pain, health policy initiatives in pain, increased emphasis on cancer pain by national and international agencies, and increased federal and private research funding opportunities. The brief discussion that follows provides a cursory overview of these developments and demonstrates the far-reaching significance of the cancer pain problem.

Quality of life is a construct that only recently has been examined in persons with cancer pain. Researchers have examined it as a domain of concern[46] as well as a potential outcome variable in treatment that included refining the psychometric properties of a quality-of-life assessment tool[50] and using a quality-of-life tool in the clinical arena to evaluate pharmacologic interventions with respect to impact on pain intensity as well as on the total person.[84] Additional research has documented the scope and extent of pain's influence on quality of life. For example, Strang and Qvarner[85] demonstrated in 84 patients with cancer-related pain that there was not only significant physical suffering but also negative influences on daily functional activities and concentration. Ferrell and colleagues[86] recently validated a conceptual model of quality of life in patients with cancer pain that included four domains: physical well-being and symptoms, social concerns, psychological well-being, and spiritual well-being. This research demonstrated quite clearly that quality of life was significantly affected by cancer pain, and that its assessment was important in evaluating both patients' responses to pain interventions and their overall status.

Quality of life also serves as a foundation for reexamining the current issue of suicidal ideation or actual suicide in persons with progressive cancer accompanied by severe pain. Foley[87] recently reviewed the issues surrounding patients' requests for physician-assisted suicide as an option in the face of uncontrolled pain and multiple other adverse symptoms. She emphasized that the past 15 years had produced a significant evolution in knowledge about cancer pain management, and that, in the experience of the Pain Research Program at Memorial Sloan-Kettering Cancer Center, suicidal ideation and requests for assistance "dissolve with adequate control of pain and other symptoms."[87,p.290] In essence, she called for the expansion of training and education of physicians and patients and families relative to pain management as the "first step in providing patients with access to care that will facilitate their choice of options."[87,p.290] In a discussion of barriers to adequate pain management, she emphasized the importance of quality of life, highlighting the psychological distress caused by pain. A study of 185 cancer patients with pain revealed suicidal ideation in 17% of the study population,[88] with most patients revealing no intent to act. Additional work demonstrated specific factors that may make patients more likely to engage in suicidal ideation: pain and suffering, advanced disease with poor prognosis, depression and hopelessness, delirium, loss of control, preexisting psychopathology, prior family or personal history of suicide, and exhaustion or fatigue.[89]

Coyle recently addressed the role of nursing in relation to current debates about euthanasia and physician-assisted suicide in patients with terminal cancer.[90] She emphasized the need for nurses to understand the issues surrounding these debates, including specific definitions, ethical principles underlying positions for or against euthanasia, and the positions of professional and global health organizations. She indicated that nurses also needed to understand the factors just cited that may make patients more vulnerable to considering suicide as an option, and to use all resources at their disposal to derive appropriate and individualized management plans for such individuals.

The impact of pain on family caregivers, particularly in the home environment, is an area that recently has been studied in some depth. A study of 85 family caregivers of patients with cancer pain[91] revealed that pain caused a significant burden for families. Their descriptions of pain centered on four themes: anatomic descriptions of pain, hidden pain (patient hides it), family fear and suffering, and overwhelming or unendurable pain. Families' experience of pain included three themes: helplessness, coping by denial of their own feelings (i.e., pretending to "be strong"), and a wish for the patient's death (a "welcome relief" from the suffering).

A second part of this same study[92] documented that family members played a major caregiving role in managing their loved one's pain. With respect to pharmacologic interventions, they decided what medications to give and when, monitored them around the clock, kept records, dealt with fears of addiction, and assumed total responsibility for pain medications. In the realm of nonpharmacologic interventions, they provided a number of physical interventions (e.g., positioning and/or mobility, massage, application of cold and heat) as well as cognitive interventions (e.g., being there, touch, talk). This research also revealed the questions and concerns family caregivers had about pain and its management, including their advice to professional caregivers (i.e., be there, offer hope, explain, be honest, listen, educate, give enough medicine) and their own personal perspectives (the future, understanding why, death, and fears about medications and handling pain at home).

Finally, data from this same study, conducted in a community hospital, a national cancer center, and a home-based community hospice, were examined in relation to caregiver burden and family factors influencing pain management.[93] Areas of burden included physical dimensions, psychological responses, and interference with normal activities. Families of patients cared for in all three sites rated patients' pain and distress as severe, but caregivers in the home hospice setting reported lower burden, better mood, less distress, and more feelings of being supported in their attempts to care for their loved one. This body of work illustrates quite nicely the significant impact pain has on the family system of cancer patients, and provides many directions for nursing practice.

Ethical concerns related to the use of high technology in medicine[94] are an emerging issue, particularly with respect to costs, access, social justice, informed consent, and autonomy. In the management of cancer pain, the potential for violations of accepted principles of biomedical ethics (autonomy, beneficence, nonmaleficence, and justice) has been clearly explicated.[95] Examples include decision making by health caregivers who as experts feel they can decide for patients, lack of respect for patients' values, inadequate concern for the vulnerability of people in pain, conflicts of interest when caregivers have ownership in companies manufacturing or distributing high-technology equipment, selection of therapies that may not provide the best benefits for patients, implementation of therapies that increase risk of harm, denial of access to needed therapy because of reimbursement issues, and use of inappropriate interventions to increase reimbursement. Whedon and Ferrell[96] provided an excellent discussion of considerations in using high-technology management in cancer patients with pain. They emphasized the *appropriate* use of such technology, delineating the need for specific guidelines in clinical practice and for use of pain management principles in deciding on, selecting, and implementing various advanced technologies.

The costs associated with caring for patients with cancer-related pain only recently have been explored empirically. Data from admissions records over a 12-month period in a national cancer center revealed that 26% of 5772 patients studied had at least one hospital admission for inadequately controlled pain, and that 54% of admissions for uncontrolled pain occurred within 2 weeks of the patient's most recent discharge.[97] The 255 readmissions for uncontrolled pain observed in this study were estimated to cost approximately $5 million over a 1-year period. The investigators suggested that predischarge education related to pain management and potential barriers to effective pain management in the home and/or community needs careful exploration. Because reimbursement for unplanned readmissions for pain control may be limited, tremendous costs to both patients and health care facilities may result.

A different twist on costs is provided by a landmark legal case that involved the inadequate management of pain in a terminally ill cancer patient admitted to a nursing home in North Carolina.[98] In this case, opioid analgesics were withheld from the patient by the nurse because of concerns about addiction, and other medications were substituted. The family of the patient proved that failure of the nurse and her employer to fulfill their obligations and responsibilities resulted in increased pain and suffering and in "emotional and mental anguish." This "inhuman treatment" resulted initially in a $15 million jury award for compensatory and punitive damages. Although the award was later set aside and a confidential settlement figure agreed on,[99] the case underscored the importance of ethical and professional obligations to relieve pain and suffering and of individualized plans of care for patients with pain.

Regulatory and legal developments also have come to the forefront in the cancer pain issue. Foley[100] discussed potential "criminal" factors associated with management of cancer pain, making the case that in today's drug-oriented society, these factors negatively affect how pain is managed. She cited the following specific factors: (1) drugs prescribed are lethal weapons; (2) drugs prescribed are controlled substances; (3) controlled substances are regulated by state and federal laws; (4) patients, physicians, pharmacists, and pharmaceutical companies must adhere to these laws or be indicted for a "crime." She called for a coordinated effort among regulatory agencies and health care professionals to "decriminalize" cancer pain, and discussed at length issues that contributed to poor pain management, for example, erroneous beliefs about addiction, substance abuse, and tolerance; and inadequate knowledge about pharmacologic therapy.

Other authors explicitly have addressed current international, national, and state regulations, laws, and policies agreeing that while they are not generally inappropriate, the way in which they often are interpreted and enforced is problematic[101–103] These authors also recommended against multiple-copy prescription programs at the state level, indicating that such programs, while resulting in rapid decreases in the number of prescriptions written for controlled substances, have had no effect on drug abuse. In contrast, data indicate that in states with triplicate prescription programs, cancer patients with pain are not receiving necessary drugs for pain relief. This problem is an international one as well. In Germany, Zenz and Sorge[104] demonstrated convincingly that strict governmental regulations and controls on opioid prescribing have resulted in significant undertreatment of pain, while drug abuse rates and related deaths have risen! They indicated that many physicians view morphine as "poison," and its prescription as "verging towards illegal practice." Such views and attitudes are culturally driven, according to Hill,[105] who posited that use and interpretation of laws reflected cultural influences, including barriers and pressures. He has, as have other authors across disciplines, called for increased efforts at educating both health care professionals and the lay public.

This brief review has highlighted several areas that demonstrate the far-reaching significance of the cancer pain problem. In addition, health policy initiatives and professional organizational efforts to reduce pain and improve its management are another recent and critically important development.[106,107] Such initiatives have occurred both within the United States and internationally. Increased funding opportunities for basic and applied research on pain are more available than in past years, with some agencies specifically targeting pain.[19,108]

Finally, another area of enormous significance to the cancer pain problem is the extensive evidence suggesting that cancer pain is poorly managed worldwide by health professionals from a number of disciplines. Nurses in particular suffer from a lack of research-based knowledge about the prevalence of pain, the impact it has on patients and others, and effective ways of managing it. The next section explores a number of professional issues that influence management of pain.

Professional Issues

Organizational efforts

Organizations and agencies involved with cancer treatment and pain management are directing their efforts toward improving pain management. Table 23-4 includes many of these groups. The ONS position paper[78] highlighted the fact that control of cancer pain is largely inadequate. Further, the paper pointed out that individuals with cancer pain have the right to have pain recognized as a problem and dealt with expedi-

TABLE 23-4 Major Agencies and Organizations Involved with Cancer Pain

Abbreviation	Name	Description	Resources
AHCPR	Agency for Health Care Policy and Research	Multidisciplinary federal agency, committee by invitation	Clinical guidelines for acute and postoperative pain;[168] guidelines for cancer pain[113]
APS	American Pain Society	Multidisciplinary organization	Quality assurance standards;[110] principles of analgesic use in the treatment of acute pain and cancer pain;[111] *APS Bulletin, APS Journal*
ASCO	American Society of Clinical Oncology	Predominantly medical and radiation oncologists	Cancer pain assessment and treatment curriculum guidelines;[112] *Journal of Clinical Oncology*
IASP	International Association for the Study of Pain	Multidisciplinary organization	Educational curriculum; taxonomy of pain syndromes;[5] *Pain*
NCI	National Cancer Institute	Multidisciplinary federal agency	Funding for pain research
NIH	National Institutes of Health	Multidisciplinary federal agency	Consensus statement for integrated management of pain;[79] funding for pain research
NCNR	National Center for Nursing Research	Federal agency	Priority expert panel state-of-the-science document;[19] funding for pain research
ONS	Oncology Nursing Society	Oncology nurses	Position paper on cancer pain;[78] Pain special interest group; *Oncology Nursing Forum*
	Various state initiatives	Multidisciplinary volunteer groups	Multiple publications, continuing professional education workshops
WHO	World Health Organization	International agency	Multiple publications, eg, *Cancer PainRelief*[109] and *Palliative Care*

ently. Similarly, the World Health Organization has designated the relief of cancer pain as one of the goals of its cancer control program.[109] Additionally, the NIH consensus statement[79] recommended using multiple treatment modalities to help control cancer pain. At a national level, the American Pain Society (APS) published quality assurance standards on pain management[110] and recently published the third edition of its principles for using analgesics to treat acute and cancer pain.[111] More recently, the American Society of Clinical Oncology (ASCO) issued a formal statement on the rights of patients to receive adequate pain management and published an educational curriculum for oncologists and oncologists in training.[112] The Agency for Health Care Policy and Research (AHCPR) is preparing clinical guidelines for the management of cancer-related pain.[113] The position papers, guidelines, and recommendations from these various groups have developed in part because of the compelling evidence documented over at least two decades that unrelieved cancer pain is a significant clinical problem.

Obstacles to successful management

There are a number of obstacles to successful pain management (Table 23-5). Inaccurate knowledge about pharmacologic principles represents a major problem area, as documented by many studies. Questionnaires administered to nurses, physicians, and students, as well as reviews of patients' records, indicate that in those with cancer pain, there are problems such as prolonged dosing intervals (i.e., not commensurate with the duration of action of the drug), lack of knowledge about equal analgesic doses, misconceptions about morphine's effectiveness as an oral analgesic, and use of doses too low to provide relief of pain.[114–120]

TABLE 23-5 Obstacles to Successful Pain Management

- Lack of understanding about pain
- Expectation that pain should be present
- Relief of pain not viewed as a goal of treatment
- Inadequate or nonexistent assessment
- Undertreatment with analgesics
- Inadequate knowledge of analgesics and other drugs
- Fears of addiction, sedation, and respiratory depression
- Inadequate knowledge of other interventions for pain
- Perceptual differences between patients and health care providers
- Legal impediments

A related pharmacologic problem stems from nurses' decision making in administering opioids. Cohen[121] found that patients received less opioid then the amount ordered, as demonstrated by the fact that 75.2% reported moderate to marked distress from pain. Furthermore, nurses' choices of amounts of opioid administered appeared to be irrational. Sheidler and colleagues[115] found that when nurses were given hypothetical patient vignettes in which changes were made in drug, dose, route, or interval, very few nurses were able to select the appropriate "new" order.

Issues surrounding addiction and potential toxicities of potent opioids also have been cited as reasons for suboptimal pain control.[122–127] Although some evidence strongly suggests that addiction is not a problem for individuals who require opioids,[128] nurses, physicians, and medical students fear iatrogenically induced addiction and certainly overestimate its risk when opioids are prescribed.[120,129–131]

Ferrell et al.[132] recently reviewed 14 pharmacology or medical-surgical nursing textbooks published since 1985 and found that only one out of 14 defined *opioid addiction* correctly and described accurately the likelihood of addiction developing with legitimate opioid use. This finding underscores the reason why there is so much confusion about addiction.

A more fundamental problem that nurses have demonstrated is a deficiency in the assessment of pain. A lack of basic assessment skills, failure to acknowledge and document the existence of pain, and inaccurate or nonexistent documentation when the problem is known to exist prohibit patients from receiving reasonable pain control.[39,116,133–135] Although there is strong evidence suggesting that systematic pain assessment and documentation can improve pain management,[136] these very basic nursing actions are not performed consistently.

Several other problems have been identified as obstacles to successful management of pain. The knowledge of the patient and family and the knowledge of physicians were identified by nurses as the most frequent barriers to pain relief.[137] Perceptual differences between patients and professionals about severity of existing pain have been documented by several investigators.[126,136,138] Complete relief of pain traditionally has not been viewed as a treatment objective.[117,121,139] And finally, the role of government agencies, such as the Drug Enforcement Agency, and existing legal statutes have contributed to inadequate prescribing by physicians because of fear of regulatory scrutiny.[102,140,141]

Improvements in management

Nurses and physicians have acknowledged their educational deficiencies related to cancer pain and its management.[116,125,142,143] The need for structured educational content in basic health professions educational programs has been encouraged.[78,79,144,145] In nursing, Spross and colleagues[78] delineated positions involving not only basic and graduate nursing school education but also continuing education. ASCO recommends education about cancer pain management for all fellowship training programs.[112]

There is evidence to suggest that changes in knowledge and attitudes can occur. Myers[125] found that after a 3-hour educational program about cancer pain, nurses' knowledge and attitude scores were significantly higher on an attitude inventory and an analgesia knowledge test than those of a group of nurses not receiving the program. Grossman and Sheidler[114] demonstrated that after a brief educational program, medical students and house officers were able to significantly improve their ability to correctly answer questions about changing patients' opioid prescriptions.

Formal educational programs, however, may not be sufficient to change practice. Max[146] proposed six possible ways of improving analgesic treatments for patients in pain: (1) make pain visible; (2) give practitioners useful tools; (3) make sure patients are part of the communication loop; (4) increase clinicians' accountability; (5) facilitate innovation and exchange of ideas; and (6) cooperate with authorities regulating opioids to help increase availability of opioids for cancer patients. In addition to these suggestions, there are other important components that should be in place. Developing a quality assurance program using the APS Quality Assurance Standards for Relief of Acute Pain and Cancer Pain[110] would be an important first step in sending a clear message on the value of pain management in an oncology clinical setting.[147]

Second, there must be opportunities to apply newly acquired knowledge in the clinical environment. Weissman et al.[148] described an educational format for disseminating pain information that involved a multidisciplinary team, patient consultations, and brief formal presentations about cancer pain. This approach allows for nurses, housestaff, attending physicians, and others to observe role models who place a high priority on cancer pain as an important clinical problem requiring resolution, and to gain experience in applying what they have observed and learned.

A third major factor necessary for changing practice is the support of administration. The ONS addressed this problem in its position paper, stating: "Effective cancer pain management, including the establishment of nurses' lines of accountability and responsibility of nurses, should be an organizational priority for nurse administrators."[78, p.944] Nursing and other administrators, by virtue of their control over budgets and allocation of resources, are in a position to make the assessment and management of cancer pain an important clinical priority for all staff.

A fourth factor important in improving the management of patients with cancer pain consists of major multidisciplinary programmatic initiatives, such as the World Health Organization Cancer Control Program and the Wisconsin Cancer Pain Initiative, that are designed and implemented solely to improve pain control. To achieve this objective, legislative and health policy activities aimed at overcoming sociopolitical obstacles to adequate management of pain must be undertaken.[78]

Delivery of pain management services

The delivery of pain management services is a controversial issue.[149] Individual practitioners who take care of oncology patients should possess basic skills in assessment and management. Recognizing the significant educational needs mentioned previously, some practitioners may feel more comfortable in referring a patient to a "specialist" for pain management, if one is available. A specialist may be an anesthesiologist, a medical or radiation oncologist, a neurologist, a neurosurgeon, a nurse, a pharmacist, a psychologist, a psychiatrist, or a social worker. Instead of an individual specialist, there may be a multidisciplinary pain team that can provide services.[150] When a referral is made to a specialist or to a pain team, several questions must be answered: (1) What is the level of responsibility of the consultant for the individual patient? (2) What role does the primary provider have after the consultation? (3) Does the patient incur significant additional costs by receiving care from a specialist or a multidisciplinary team? (4) If there are several options for a patient's pain management plan, how are decisions made, and who helps the patient and family with those decisions?

Gonzalez et al.[151] reported that in 64% of 276 patients referred for a pain consultation, the outcome of the evaluation (which usually required further diagnostic tests and analgesic changes) led to identifying the etiology of the pain problem. Metastatic disease was the most common cause of the pain. In addition, 22% of the patients received treatment for their pain problem with radiation, surgery, or chemotherapy. Walsh[152] described a palliative care service that saw approximately 400 patients per year. This consultant and management service was part of a hematology/medical oncology department, and was involved in research activities as well as providing full clinical services. Sheidler and Krumm[153] surveyed over 100 nurses involved in pain management activities, and found that of the 42 nurses who indicated they were from settings that had a formal pain team, 55% of the 38 physician-led "pain management teams" were under departments of anesthesiology. When clinical settings had a formal service, only 40% of the nurses associated with the group spent more than 50% of the day in pain-related activities, indicating that most were involved in activities other than pain management. Although the multidisciplinary approach to managing cancer patients' pain may be efficient, logical, and optimal, its true efficacy still needs to be established through careful evaluation.[154]

PRINCIPLES OF ASSESSMENT AND MANAGEMENT

Effective clinical assessment and management of cancer pain rests on recognition and use of a number of critical principles. Foley[155] delineated several of these for physicians: (1) complete assessment of the history of pain, (2) evaluation of the psychosocial status of the patient, (3) careful medical and neurologic exam, (4) use of appropriate diagnostic procedures to determine nature of pain, (5) early treatment with analgesics, (6) continual reassessment of patient's response to prescribed therapy, (7) reassessment of treatment approach or search for a new cause of pain, and (8) continuity of care from diagnosis to treatment. These principles were aimed at physicians practicing in acute care settings, but recent literature on the palliative care of cancer patients suggests that similar principles probably apply, although goals of care are different.[156,157] These activities clearly imply that establishing and treating the cause of pain is the physician's major goal in assessment, accompanied by the subsequent or concomitant treatment of the pain itself.[49,155]

The nursing role in assessment and management of pain, however, is different in many respects.[158] The ONS position paper[78] delineated the nurse's role as (1) describing pain, (2) identifying aggravating and relieving factors, (3) determining the meaning of pain, (4) determining its cause, (5) determining individuals' definitions of optimal pain relief, (6) deriving nursing diagnoses, (7) assisting in selecting interventions, and (8) evaluating efficacy of interventions. Although nurses certainly contribute to the goals of the physician and may perform some of these activities for physicians, their focus is on the individual as a whole person, and in his or her response to the pain. Their focus is on individual definitions of optimal pain relief, psychosocial and physical problems amenable to nursing interventions, and evaluation of the overall response to treatment. Additionally, nurses are interested in how pain affects an individual's significant others and support systems. The major emphasis is on decreasing pain and increasing comfort rather than on treating the cancer itself.

In addition, there are other principles of assessment and management that are implicit in successful nursing management of cancer pain. These principles consist of the use of a multidisciplinary approach in the delivery of pain management services, a well-conceived scope of practice for nurses, a thorough assessment and diagnosis, incorporation of guidelines and standards into clinical practice, and approaches to managing pain in special populations of individuals. Each of these areas is explored in the following sections.

Multidisciplinary Approach

The multidimensional conceptualization of cancer pain requires the involvement of multiple health care disciplines in assessment and management. Treatment approaches, delineated later in this chapter, consist of chemotherapy, radiotherapy, surgery, anesthetic techniques, pharmacologic agents, cognitive/behavioral methods, physical techniques, and many more. Clearly, there is no one best way to treat cancer pain, and no one best discipline or person prepared for managing cancer pain. Thus, input is required from specific health care professionals, including nurses, pharmacists, social workers, occupational therapists, physical therapists, psychologists, and physicians from many specialties and subspecialties (e.g., internal medicine, anesthesiology, surgery, radiation oncology, psychiatry).

Nursing's Scope of Practice and Responsibilities

Nurses are an integral part of the multidisciplinary team approach to managing cancer pain. The ONS position paper[78] delineated a number of positions related to the management of cancer pain and suggested strategies to achieve the positions. Important components of the paper included the nurse's scope of practice relevant to pain and specific nursing responsibilities. Both of these key areas will be briefly summarized next; the interested reader is encouraged to read the original source.

Oncology nurses, by virtue of their prolonged contact with cancer patients in a variety of settings, and by virtue of their relationships with these individuals and their families, are best prepared to assume a leadership role in the assessment and management of cancer pain. Assumption of such a role is consistent with the ONS's mission of improving the care of persons with cancer. The NIH consensus statement[79] described and endorsed a pivotal role for professional nurses in the management of pain.

The ONS position paper[78] delineated a scope of practice for nurses with different levels of expertise (e.g., nurses and oncology clinical nurse specialists). These levels of expertise were made operational with specific knowledge and skills associated with each level. For example, nurses should be capable of basic assessment of pain, development of a care plan, evaluation of the plan, recognition of ineffective interventions, and reporting of problems to appropriate health caregivers and/or supervisors. Clinical nurse specialists, on the other hand, should be able to perform sophisticated assessments, develop multidisciplinary treatment plans, coordinate contributions of the different disciplines, and evaluate and readjust the care plan as necessary.

Two positions set forth in the ONS position paper[78] dealt with the ethical and practice responsibilities of nurses in managing pain (Table 23-6). These positions, as well as all others, were based on several assumptions: (1) Patients have a right to relief of pain. (2) Unrelieved pain causes significant and unnecessary suffering for patients, families, friends, and health professionals. (3) Nurses and patients (i.e., society) have a social contract in which alleviation of pain and suffering is a tenet. (4) Nurses are often prevented from meeting this obligation because of inadequate education and a variety of sociocultural variables. (5) Nurses have sustained contact with patients and their significant others over the course of a cancer illness that make them key providers of care. (6) Cancer pain is an "orphan" problem with accountability for its relief unclear. (7) Cancer pain is a sociopolitical as well as a clinical problem.

It is clear that assumption of a leadership role in effective management of cancer patients' pain is a nursing responsibility. The scope of nursing practice delineated in the ONS paper provides the foundation for all positions relevant to nurses' roles and responsibilities in caring for persons with cancer-related pain.

Assessment and Diagnosis

Literature documenting nurses' problems with assessing cancer pain has been discussed previously. This section presents the rationale for and basic principles of assessment, assessment parameters, tools for assessing pain, nursing diagnoses resulting from pain assessments, and strategies for incorporating assessment into institutional practice.

Rationale and basic principles

Systematic nursing assessment of pain is important for several reasons.[159] First, it establishes a baseline from which to plan and begin interventions. Second, it assists in the selection of interventions. Third, it makes possible evaluation of the interventions. Assessment of pain is a critical process that aids in the clinical management of pain and, indeed, goes hand in hand with successful management. It is different from measurement of pain, which is used to quantify pain in a bias-free manner, and is generally carried out for research purposes.[158]

The timing of assessments is critical as well. Any cancer patient with pain who enters any health care setting should have an initial or baseline assessment. After the initiation of interventions, continuous or ongoing assessment is necessary for evaluation and revision of treatment plans. This approach to assessment is modeled on the nursing process. Collection of pain assessment data should be systematic and organized, just as the collection of general nursing data is.

The need for a complete nursing assessment of pain and documentation of the assessment was highlighted in several studies.[133,134] In addition, there are some "pitfalls" in assessment of pain. They include: (1) the belief that patients with pain will demonstrate changes in vital signs or display overt behavioral manifestations of pain, (2) the belief that all pain should have a documented organic cause, (3) the belief that pain in cancer patients may be of psychogenic origin ("all in the head"), (4) ascription of all pain in cancer patients to the tumor rather than to such "normal" problems as migraine headache or arthritis, and (5) feelings of being overwhelmed with clinical responsibilities and thus becoming insensitive to patients' pain and their related needs.

TABLE 23-6 Oncology Nursing Society Position Paper on Cancer Pain

POSITION STATEMENTS ON CANCER PAIN

Ethics
Individuals with cancer pain have a right to obtain optimal pain relief. Nurses caring for them have an ethical obligation to ensure exploration of everything possible within the scope of nursing practice to provide this relief.

Practice
Nurses caring for individuals with cancer pain must exercise leadership in identifying and assessing cancer pain and in planning, implementing, coordinating, and evaluating the interdisciplinary management of cancer pain.

- *Problem identification.* Nurses are responsible for identifying the problem of inadequate pain management in patients with cancer and for intervening responsibly to achieve optimal pain relief.
- *Assessment.* Nurses caring for individuals with cancer pain should perform initial and ongoing assessments of pain and communicate assessment data to colleagues.
- *Planning.* After assessing the individual experiencing cancer pain, the nurse develops a plan of care with the individual/significant other that includes: specific measurable goals and effective pain management interventions; incorporates specific pain management techniques based on mutual goal setting; specifies a schedule for the timing of interventions and of ongoing assessment of pain, pain relief, and side effects associated with pain therapy, as well as overall effectiveness of the regimen; and addresses nursing responsibilities as well as communication and other collaborative interventions with other health care providers involved in the individual's care.
- *Implementation and coordination.* Nurses are responsible and accountable for implementation and coordination of the plan for management of cancer pain.
- *Evaluation.* Nurses are responsible for evaluating patient responses to interventions for cancer pain control and for using evaluation data to revise the care plan. Nurses use all available clinical and administrative resources to ensure progress toward achieving relief or control of cancer pain.

Basic Nursing Education
Basic nursing education programs should have theoretical and clinical curriculum content related to cancer pain and its management.

Graduate Nursing Education
Graduate nursing education programs preparing advanced practitioners should provide advanced theoretical, research, and clinical curriculum content on cancer pain and management.

Responsibilities for Continuing Education
Nurses are responsible for regularly updating their knowledge of cancer pain assessment and management. Opportunities should exist to develop competence in areas of cancer pain assessment, management, and evaluation.

Patient and Public Education
Patient education is an essential element of cancer pain management and is a primary responsibility of nurses. Nurses have a responsibility to educate the public, patients, and significant others about the right to relief from cancer pain and the resources available for assessment and treatment of cancer pain.

Research
Cancer pain and pain management are research priorities for oncology nurses and the Oncology Nursing Society (ONS).

Research Utilization
Nurses have a responsibility to use research findings relevant to assessment and management of cancer pain in their practice and to facilitate the dissemination and use of these findings by others.

Nursing Administration
Effective cancer pain management should be an organizational priority for nurse administrators, including establishment of nurses' lines of accountability and responsibility.

Social Policy
ONS is committed to initiating legislative and health policy activities that will overcome sociopolitical obstacles to cancer pain management and to evaluating legislative and health policy actions that can influence cancer pain management.

Pediatric Cancer Pain
Children experiencing pain because of cancer have a right to optimal pain relief. The nursing process, as outlined in previous position statements in this paper, should include the use of developmentally appropriate assessments and interventions. Effective management of pediatric cancer pain should reflect an understanding of particular pediatric pain issues (e.g., the role of the parents, procedural pain).

Source: Reprinted from the *Oncology Nursing Forum* with permission from the Oncology Nursing Press, Inc. Spross JA, McGuire DB, Schmitt, RM: Oncology Nursing Society Position Paper on Cancer Pain Part I. *Oncol Nurs Forum* 17(4):595–603, 1990.

Awareness and avoidance of these "pitfalls" should help nurses perform good pain assessments.

Assessment parameters

The multidimensional conceptualization of pain described previously provides guidance in assessing pain. The range of assessment parameters is quite wide and represents each of the multiple dimensions of cancer pain. Key parameters that require assessment in each dimension are highlighted in Table 23-7. Basic techniques for assessing pain, including the very important pain history, are discussed in the previous edition of this chapter[48] and in other sources.[158–160]

Assessment tools

There is extensive literature on instruments to measure clinical pain, but a lengthy discussion is impossible here. The reader is referred to several recent publications in which this literature is reviewed and discussed, with a focus on practical application in both adult and pediatric populations.[27,28,161,162] There is also much literature on the assessment of cancer pain, with

TABLE 23-7 Assessment Parameters Using the Multidimensional Conceptualization of Cancer Pain

Physiologic	Sensory	Affective
• Location • Onset • Associated factors • Duration • Type of pain (acute or chronic) • Syndrome • Anatomy • Physiology	• Intensity • Quality • Pattern	• Distress • Anxiety • Depression • Mental state • Perception of suffering • Irritability/agitation • Pain Relief
Cognitive	**Behavioral**	**Sociocultural**
• Meaning of pain • Thought processes • Coping strategies • Knowledge • Attitudes/beliefs • Previous treatments • Influencing factors (positive and negative)	• Communication with others • Interpersonal relationships • Activities of daily living • Behaviors (pain-related, preventive, or controlling) • Use of medications • Sleep/rest patterns • Fatigue	• Ethnocultural/background • Family/social life • Work/home responsibilities • Environment • Familial attitudes/beliefs/behaviors • Personal attitudes/beliefs

some authors focusing on generic issues of assessment and/or reviewing available tools[163,164] and others reporting on the use of specific tools in selected cancer patients. Table 23-8 presents clinical, psychometric, and practical information about tools useful for assessing cancer pain in adult populations. Additionally, categories of tools for assessing pain in children with cancer are illustrated, and the interested reader is urged to consult the sources used in developing the pediatric tool section of Table 23-8. The general discussion presented next about types of tools, their appropriate uses, and considerations in selecting them should help readers select the best tool for a given situation.

Pain assessment tools can be classified by the number of dimensions of pain they assess.[161] Unidimensional tools focus on one dimension of the pain experience, such as the sensory dimension, and within that dimension may focus on a specific parameter, such as pain intensity (see Table 23-7). Ten-centimeter visual analogue scales (VAS) (anchors of *no pain* and *worst possible pain*) or verbal descriptor scales (VDS) (words such as *none, mild, moderate,* and *severe*) measuring pain intensity are examples of commonly used unidimensional tools. Although most VASs and VDSs are of the paper-and-pencil variety, a new format consisting of a 5 × 20-cm plastic device with a sliding marker moving within a groove that measures 10 cm recently was tested and found to be reliable and valid at assessing pain

TABLE 23-8 Tools for Assessing Pain

Tools	Dimension(s) Measured*	Patient Population(s)	Psychometric Properties	Advantages	Disadvantages
			ADULTS		
Brief Pain Inventory[76,171,172]	P, S, A, C, B, So	Cancer, rheumatoid arthritis, orthopedic	Test-retest reliability; construct, predictive validity	Brief, simple, self-administered, comprehensive	Provides fairly superficial information
McGill Pain Questionnaire (long form)[34–37,42,43,45,170]	P, S, A, C, B	Acute, chronic, cancer, experimental	Test-retest reliability; content, concurrent, construct, predictive validity	Comprehensive, versatile	Time-consuming (5–20 min), may be difficult for some individuals to understand or complete

(continued)

TABLE 23-8 Tools for Assessing Pain (continued)

Tools	Dimension(s) Measured*	Patient Population(s)	Psychometric Properties	Advantages	Disadvantages
McGill Pain Questionnaire (short form)[173]	S, A	Acute postoperative, obstetric, dental, musculoskeletal	Reliability not reported; concurrent validity	Brief, simple, self-administered	Reliability is unclear, needs further psychometric evaluation in other groups with acute and chronic pain
Memorial Pain Assessment Card[174]	S, A	Cancer	Reliability not reported; construct, concurrent validity	Brief, simple	Reliability is unclear, requires further psychometric evaluation and extension to additional acute and chronic pain populations
Numerical Rating Scale[161]	S	Acute, chronic (also used in children)	Reliability not reported; construct, concurrent validity	Brief, simple, more sensitive than verbal descriptor scale, less confusing than Visual Analogue Scale, can be administered in written or verbal form	Unidimensional, sensitivity to pain treatment is unknown
Pain Assessment Tool (PAT)/Pain Flowsheet (PFS)[136,175]	P, S, A, C, B, So	Cancer	Interrater reliability (PAT); content validity (PAT); construct validity (PFS)	Both PAT and PFS are comprehensive, PFS helpful in managing pain	PAT time-consuming to complete
Verbal Descriptor Scale[161,164,165]	S (pain intensity, relief)	Acute, cancer, chronic, experimental (also used in children)	Test-retest reliability; construct, concurrent validity	Brief, simple, easy to score	Lacks sensitivity, forces selection of only one word, even if no word satisfactorily describes pain intensity, can be difficult for persons with limited vocabulary
Visual Analogue Scale[27,161,164–166]	S (pain intensity, relief), A (depression, mood)	Acute, chronic, cancer (also used in children)	Test-retest reliability; construct, concurrent validity	Brief, provides a sensitive measure, scores can be analyzed as interval data	May be difficult for some individuals, scoring is awkward in the clinical setting and may be a source of error
			CHILDREN†		
Behavioral measures[178]	P, B	Postoperative, prolonged acute pain, during injections, cancer	Must read article(s) on specific tool(s) selected	Useful when self-report cannot be given or patient is preverbal	Does not allow for self-report
Self-report measures	S, A, C	Preschool, school-age, adolescent, injections, acute pain, chronic musculoskeletal pain, cancer	Must read article(s) on specific tool(s) selected	Allows self-report of various characteristics of pain, allows multidimensional assessment	May be difficult for preschoolers or for acutely ill youngsters

**P*, physiologic; *S*, sensory; *A*, affective; *C*, cognitive; *B*, behavioral; *So*, sociocultural.

†Sources: Ross DM, Ross SA: Assessment of pediatric pain: An overview. *ISS Compr Pediatr Nurs* 11:73–91, 1988; Beyer JE, Wells N: The assessment of pain in children. *Pediatr Clin North Am* 36:837–854, 1989.

intensity in cancer patients.[165] Pain relief can also be measured with VASs and VDSs simply by changing anchor and descriptor words. Although these scales have documented reliability and validity in measuring cancer-related pain,[161,164,166] they measure only one parameter of one dimension of pain and thus are limited in their representation of the total pain experience. However, because pain intensity is such a salient aspect of pain, these scales are an excellent means to evaluate the success of specific interventions for pain, most notably analgesics but also other interventions studied in randomized clinical trials.[167] Indeed, the APS quality assurance standards[110] recommended regular use of pain intensity and relief scales, as did the AHCPR guidelines for acute pain management.[168] Other unidimensional tools consist of body diagrams to assess location of pain[158] and rating scales to assess behavioral indicators of pain[169] (see Tables 23-7 and 23-8).

Multidimensional tools focus on two or more dimensions of the pain experience (see Tables 23-7 and 23-8). The McGill Pain Questionnaire (MPQ)[34] is perhaps the most well-known and best example, as it enables assessment of the sensory, affective, cognitive, and behavioral dimensions. The variety of available multidimensional tools is far more extensive than for unidimensional tools. The MPQ, although originally developed to measure multidimensional aspects of pain in many diseases, has been shown to be reliable and valid in a number of different cancer patient populations.[34–37,43,45,170] Another comprehensive multidimensional (sensory, affective, cognitive, behavioral, sociocultural) tool is the Brief Pain Inventory (BPI), developed initially for assessing pain in general but used fairly extensively for cancer pain.[76,171,172] The MPQ and BPI can be unwieldy in the clinical setting, so other researchers and clinicians have devised multidimensional tools that are short and easy to administer. For example, Melzack developed the short-form version of the MPQ[173] to assess sensory (including intensity and quality) and affective dimensions of pain. The Memorial Pain Assessment Card (MPAC) is another example.[174] It assesses pain intensity, pain relief, and mood (general psychologic distress) with VASs, and intensity with a series of verbal descriptors; thus it addresses sensory and affective dimensions of pain. Additional multidimensional methods for assessing pain have been developed to assist nurses in making both baseline and ongoing assessments, taking the form of comprehensive questionnaires, flow sheets, and time charts.[136,175,176]

Children with cancer pain represent a unique challenge to the nurse who wishes to assess pain. Because of their developmental characteristics, many of the assessment parameters already discussed are inappropriate. For example, infants and very young children lack verbal skills and therefore cannot tell others what their pain feels like, where it is located, and what makes it better or worse. Categories of measures include both behavioral and self-report.

Several instruments for measuring pain in children ages 3 years and older have been developed and tested[177] (see Table 23-8). These tools include the Oucher Scale[177] and the Children's Hospital of Eastern Ontario Pain Scale (CHEOPS), a behavioral scale for rating postoperative pain developed by McGrath and colleagues.[178] Additional tools recommended by McCaffery and Beebe[160] for assessing pain intensity in children include numerical scales (for ages 10 and older), the Wong/Baker Faces Rating Scale, the Eland Color Scale, and the Hester Poker Chip Scale. A discussion of each of these tools is beyond the scope of this chapter, but the reader who needs more information is referred to other sources.[27,28,179]

McCaffery and Beebe[160] urged nurses to use a multidimensional approach in assessing children's pain that included discussing pain with both child and family, obtaining the child's self-report if possible, identifying the presence of pathology with the potential to cause pain, observing behavioral manifestations of pain such as vocalizations or facial expressions, and considering a trial of analgesics with careful attention paid to the child's responses.

The choice of tools for assessing pain in both adults and children depends on several considerations.[158] Of foremost concern is the dimensions of pain that are most relevant in a given situation. For example, the behavioral dimension assumes primary importance in a preverbal child or in an adult cancer patient experiencing acute confusion or cognitive failure,[180,181] whereas the sensory and affective dimensions may predominate in an alert and oriented postoperative patient. The tool selected should be able to assess the relevant parameters of the dimension(s) of interest. The purpose of the assessment (i.e., baseline versus ongoing) is a second major consideration. In general, baseline assessments will require a more detailed and comprehensive tool, while ongoing assessments can use brief, simple tools.

A third consideration is related to the pain interventions being used. Effects of treatments aimed at the physiologic and sensory dimensions (e.g., analgesics) should be evaluated by assessing parameters such as location, intensity, and quality. Treatments aimed at the cognitive, affective, and behavioral dimensions (e.g., distraction and relaxation) should be evaluated using tools assessing parameters of those dimensions (see Tables 23-7 and 23-8). A fourth important area relates to specific patient and setting factors, such as age, cognitive abilities, type of pain, level of acuity, physical function, personal preference, and type of clinical setting (inpatient, outpatient, home, hospice). Some of these patient-related factors may influence whether the tools selected are subjective (patient self-report) or objective (observational) in nature.

Finally, issues related to time, feasibility, and relevance to the clinical setting are a major consideration. Important considerations include the amount of time required to complete tools, format and amount of writing, overlap with existing documentation, relevance of parameters to setting and to clinicians, personal comfort and preference, and lines of responsibility and accountability.

Nursing diagnoses and documentation

The outcome of a thorough baseline assessment of the cancer patient with pain should be nursing diagnoses that structure the design and implementation of the management plan. The North American Nursing Diagnosis Association (NANDA) included the diagnosis "Alteration in Comfort: Pain" in its 1988 taxonomy,[182] with two categories (pain and chronic pain). This diagnosis provided the framework for nursing management of patients with cancer pain in the ONS *Guidelines for Oncology Nursing Practice.*[183] Levin and colleagues[184] reported a validation study of selected nursing diagnoses, including "Alteration in Comfort: Pain." Although nurse respondents validated the diagnosis, they indicated that critical defining characteristics included the patient's verbalization of pain and a facial mask of pain.

A recent text on nursing diagnosis[185] placed pain and chronic pain under the general rubric of "Comfort, Altered." Defining characteristics included the major one (must be present) of the person reporting or demonstrating a discomfort, and a number of minor ones (may be present), for example, autonomic response in acute pain, guarded position, and facial mask of pain. This text also addressed factors related to pain such as pathophysiologic conditions (musculoskeletal disorders, visceral disorders, cancer, etc.); treatments (surgery, diagnostic tests); situational concerns such as immobility, stress, and overactivity; and maturational issues such as colic in infancy and recurrent abdominal pain in middle childhood.

McCaffery and Beebe[160] cited 18 other nursing diagnoses that the nurse should consider as part of the assessment process. These diagnoses include: anxiety, constipation, ineffective individual coping, diversional activity deficit, fatigue, fear, knowledge deficit (specify), impaired physical mobility, powerlessness, feeding self-care deficit, bathing/hygiene self-care deficit, dressing/grooming self-care deficit, toileting self-care deficit, sexual dysfunction, sleep pattern disturbance, social isolation, spiritual distress (distress of the human spirit), and altered thought processes. In Carpenito's text,[185] examples of NANDA-approved diagnoses that may be relevant are activity intolerance, anxiety, constipation, family coping, fatigue, and fear, among many others. Certainly the inclusion of *all* relevant nursing diagnoses will focus management efforts on the need for multiple disciplines to be involved in using multiple interventions for pain.

Of critical importance is the need for nurses to document their assessments and nursing diagnoses in a manner appropriate for their clinical settings. The APS quality assurance standards[110] recommended the documentation of pain intensity and pain relief on standard patient records, such as the vital sign sheet or patient flow sheet. Similarly, the AHCPR guidelines on acute pain management[168] suggested incorporation of assessment data into routine institutional records. Recent literature attests to the success of routine manual and computerized documentation systems for patient-controlled analgesia in the postoperative setting and for general care in a cancer pain management unit.[186,187] The use of standardized pain assessment and documentation appears to have a positive impact on pain intensity and to facilitate management of pain.[136]

Incorporation into Practice

Successful management of cancer pain will ultimately depend on the extent to which systematic processes, tools, documentation procedures, and lines of formal accountability and responsibility for pain management are incorporated into institutional settings. The ONS position paper,[78] as mentioned previously, places the *coordination* of pain management squarely on the oncology nurse. The issue for many nurses, then, is *how* to meet this responsibility. Although a detailed discussion is impossible within the context of this chapter, a few approaches deserve mention.

The position paper offered many strategies for clinicians, educators, and administrators, and should be consulted by those wishing to "institutionalize" pain assessment and management. Most important, the position paper urged the use of the APS quality assurance standards as a basis for incorporating pain into an institutional quality assurance system.[78] These standards very clearly spelled out how this goal could be accomplished and discussed the obvious advantages of such a strategy. Miaskowski and Donovan[147] recently described how the standards could be incorporated into an oncology nursing setting. Ferrell and colleagues[188] provided a helpful discussion of pain management as a quality-of-care outcome. The AHCPR guidelines for acute pain management should also be consulted and used.[168] They offered very specific ways to assess, document, and manage pain, including tools, procedures, and methods. Finally, the forthcoming AHCPR guidelines for cancer pain management[113] will certainly be useful in developing, implementing, and evaluating better ways of managing cancer pain in any clinical setting.

Special Populations

Because cancer is a group of diseases that affects individuals across the life span, the pain associated with it likewise occurs in groups of varying age, background, and clinical characteristics. Several populations—children, the elderly, individuals with substance abuse history, the critically ill, and persons with diverse sociocultural backgrounds, and the terminally ill—require special consideration in the areas of pain assessment and management. Specific issues relevant to pain in these groups generally have been neglected in the nursing literature on cancer pain.

Children

Assessment and management of pain in children with cancer have received little attention in the research arena.[189] The reasons for the paucity of published research are not entirely clear, but Stevens et al.[190] proposed that they included theories of pain that are inadequate to explain children's pain, methodologic and measurement difficulties, and clinical dilemmas brought about by differences in interpretation of children's behaviors coupled with nurses' and children's personal beliefs, values, fears, and pain experiences. The majority of existing research in children with cancer deals with the pain and distress of treatment-related procedures, such as bone marrow aspiration.[27,177,191]

Hester[192] recently reviewed research related to children's pain, covering the topics of prevalence of pain, children's perspectives on pain, assessment of pain, and management of pain. She concluded that although the volume of research in children's pain had increased dramatically over the past 20 years, much of it focused on measurement rather than on management of pain. She highlighted the need for studies of nonpharmacologic and pharmacologic interventions, and urged that the disparity between development of knowledge (i.e., research) and clinical practice be minimized, with the incorporation of research-based knowledge into practice as a major means for improving the care of children with pain.

The developmental level of children is directly related to how they perceive, interpret, and respond to pain, regardless of etiology.[193] Children's developmental stages have a number of implications for the assessment and management of their pain, and in fact can be used to help clarify a number of misconceptions that are held by health professionals and others about children with pain.

Generally speaking, the facts about children's pain can be represented by the following statements: There is significant evidence to indicate that neonates, including premature ones, do feel pain. Children who are verbally fluent may deny they have pain when in fact they *do* have it; this occurs when they have certain fears about pain or when they have adapted to it and do not realize it is worsening. Children's lack of willingness or ability to express pain or request treatment for it does *not* mean they do not have it. The child who sleeps, plays, or is otherwise distracted may still have a good deal of pain; such distractions are a common coping method used by children with pain. Children do *not* tolerate pain better than adults do. Opioids may be used safely in children provided there is an understanding of the pharmacokinetics and the children are properly observed; their use in all age groups, including teenagers, generally is safe. Pain is *not* a harmless entity in children, without side effects or life-threatening potential; it has been documented that presence of pain in neonates may be harmful, because of stressful reactions that can include prolonged crying leading to hypoxemia, and increased heart rate and blood pressure.[194] There is also the possibility of long-term psychological consequences from repeated episodes of acute pain or prolonged periods of unrelieved pain.[177]

The issue of undertreatment of children with pain is an important one. Although the evidence is not as massive as that documenting undertreatment of adults, there clearly is a problem in the pediatric arena. It was demonstrated that children who were hospitalized for surgery received very little of the analgesics ordered for them, and that, as compared to adults with the same diagnoses, they received 26 times *less* the amount.[195] Similarly, Schechter et al.[196] demonstrated that hospitalized children and adults with the same diagnoses were treated differently with respect to administration of opioids. Children were likely to have less opioids than adults. One of the reasons suggested for these findings included the possibility that beliefs and attitudes of nursing and medical staff affected administration of drugs.

In a follow-up study of the attitudes of physicians toward pain in children, Schechter and Allen[197] found that although 75% of the sample believed that children experienced adultlike pain by 2 years of age, 35% were somewhat or significantly concerned about the risks of addiction when using opioids. Pediatricians were significantly more likely than other specialists to view children as having adultlike pain and to prescribe opioids at earlier ages. While this study provided some explanation for differences in how adult versus pediatric patients with pain are treated, there probably are other, as-yet-unelucidated reasons as well.

A landmark document in the field of pediatric oncology was the report of the consensus conference on the management of pain in childhood cancer in 1990.[179] Key components of this report included assessment and methodologic issues in managing pain, disease-related pain, management of pain associated with procedures, and research priorities.

The subcommittee on assessment and methodologic issues recommended the development and use of a pain problem list for children with cancer. This list resulted from the assessment process, including pain history, and characterization and key features that may influence decisions regarding therapy, particularly with respect to the multiple dimensions of pain and the multiple disciplines involved in its management.

Interventions for pain in children with cancer should be tailored to the type of pain they are experiencing.[28,179,189] Pain that is acute in nature and related to operative procedures may be treated in the same manner as adult postoperative pain (i.e., with opioids, including patient-controlled analgesia if the patient is old enough). The AHCPR guidelines for acute pain management explicitly addressed the management of pain in children.[168] It is important to note that children metabolize opioids more quickly than adults do, so their doses may need to be scheduled more frequently.[189] Since needles and shots are uniformly hated by children, the intravenous route immediately postoperatively followed by the oral route when possible is the preferred strategy. Management of other types of treatment-related pain, such as that caused by esophagitis or oral mucositis, can be successfully implemented through the use of continuous intravenous and subcutaneous morphine infusions.[198]

The treatment of acute, procedure-related pain (e.g., bone marrow aspiration) is somewhat different. This type of pain usually is transient, though accompanied by a good deal of anxiety and fear. Interventions range from pharmacologic approaches (e.g., sedatives) to cognitive and behavioral techniques (e.g., distraction and imagery).[199] Sedatives, particularly the combination of meperidine, promethazine, and chlorpromazine ("DPT") should be used with caution, for they do not decrease pain and anxiety[189] and they may even bring on respiratory depression.[200] A number of authors[28,189] recommend the combined use of premedications and cognitive/behavioral techniques for procedures such as bone marrow aspiration. The efficacy of several techniques has been documented.[201,202] Recent research suggests that use of ethyl chloride as a topical anesthetic reduces the pain of procedures and is well received by both children and parents.[203]

The management of disease-related pain in children with cancer is a challenge. In the consensus conference report mentioned earlier,[179] the subcommittee on disease-related pain recommended the use of an algorithm for managing pediatric cancer pain. Guiding principles included: (1) tailoring the route of administration to patients' conditions, (2) using simpler rather than complex technological approaches, (3) providing a level of comfort the patients find satisfactory, (4) treating side effects aggressively, (5) titrating analgesic doses to clinical effect without adherence to "standard doses," and (6) trying the oral route of administration first. An analgesic ladder was described that began with nonopioids for mild pain and progressed to combinations of these drugs, with strong opioids for severe pain. The use of nonpharmacologic techniques was also recommended. Concurrent management of side effects and other symptoms, such as constipation, nausea, vomiting, urinary retention, and depression, was highlighted, with specific recommendations made regarding adjuvant analgesics. Finally, anesthetic and neurosurgical approaches were briefly discussed. This report offered a comprehensive and useful overview of managing pain in the pediatric cancer patient.

Finally, the management of pain due to terminal cancer is a challenging area, since the goal is pain relief without undue sedation. Oral analgesics administered around the clock often are very helpful. Since children metabolize narcotics more quickly than adults, drugs with a longer duration of action, such as methadone, are advisable and have been shown to provide adequate pain relief.[204,205] More recently, oral controlled-release morphine has been shown to be effective and safe when used in terminally ill children.[206] When pain is intractable, however, the parenteral route should be considered. A series of studies clearly demonstrated that continuous intravenous or subcutaneous infusions of morphine are safe and effective ways of relieving the pain of terminal cancer in children.[207,208]

In summary, assessment and management of cancer pain in children has been a significant clinical problem. Dispelling the misconceptions and misinformation that surround the assessment and management of pain in children is essential to achieving success. Although the research base of knowledge in this area is still limited, good assessment tools are continually being developed, and adequate interventions exist. The nurse caring for the pediatric cancer patient with pain plays a key role in managing this challenging problem, functioning within the scope of practice described by the ONS position paper.[78]

The elderly

The elderly population in the United States (individuals age 65 and older) more than doubled between 1950 and 1980 (from 12.3 million to 25.5 million), and one projection for the year 2030 is that the elderly population will increase to 64.3 million people.[209] As this population increases in number, one would expect to see a corresponding increase in the incidence of cancer and cancer-related deaths. Current American Cancer Society statistics indicate that for the five leading cancer sites, 51% of cancer deaths are in individuals between ages 55 and 74, and 36% are in individuals age 75 or older.[210]

The problem of cancer pain in elderly cancer patients has been grossly neglected,[211,212] and prevalence surveys of pain are lacking. Ferrell[213] recently reviewed 11 geriatric medicine textbooks and found only two with chapters on pain in the elderly, with negligible content about cancer-related pain. Research in this area has been limited, and much of what is known about pain in the elderly is based on empirical observations and anecdotal reports.

A misconception that lay individuals have about pain among the elderly is that pain is a normal sequela of aging.[160] As a result of this belief, elderly patients may not report pain as a problem since it is considered "normal." In one study of "younger" elderly versus "older" elderly, there was a trend for the older elderly to report pain less often.[214] Similarly, if health care professionals are told about pain from elderly patients, they may dismiss the complaint as insignificant since pain becomes a manifestation of the aging process. While it may be true that people develop more chronic diseases as they age,[215] the experience of pain does not need to be an expectation.

The normal process of aging creates unique problems in the management of cancer pain, especially as related to assessment. Ferrell et al.[216] found that 71% of patients in a long-term care facility had pain, with an average of five chronic medical conditions. With the prevalence of more chronic diseases, there potentially will exist multiple causes of the same complaint. The elderly experience greater alterations in the musculoskeletal system and are more vulnerable to acute and soft-tissue pain.[217] Chronic problems such as arthritis, degenerative disk disease, osteoporosis, and peripheral neuropathy may confuse the pain problem for individuals who also have cancer-related pain.

Another unique problem is that the elderly may experience significant sensory and cognitive impairment.[160,212,217,218] The symptoms associated with these potential impairments alert the health care professional to be especially astute in obtaining a careful, detailed pain history.[160,212,217] The risk of historical inadequacies through the underreporting of symptoms, memory deficits, and concomitant depression-related symptomatology may lead to an inaccurate pain diagnosis and inappropriate treatment. A very important piece of assessment data to obtain in the elderly is any change from baseline behaviors, usual routines, and social interactions. A gradual loss of physical health, changes in family structure, limited economic resources, and a loss of social status can greatly influence a patient's quality of life and, therefore, the problem of pain.[160,219,220] Newton stated: "elderly patients have a considerable morbidity due to inadequately treated pain, which includes confusion, withdrawal, agitation, anorexia, immobility, depression, and (perhaps) a predisposition to develop chronic pain."[217,p.244]

A third major unique problem is the issue of the sensitivity of elderly patients to both perception of pain and sensitivity to pharmacologic interventions. The literature about perceptual sensitivity reveals contradictions. Bayer et al.[221] reviewed symptoms of acute myocardial infarction in elderly patients and found that chest pain was reported less frequently than other symptoms, especially by patients over 85 years old. They proposed several explanations to account for this finding: higher pain threshold, autonomic dysfunction, or cortical failure from neurologic disease. Conversely, McMillan[74] found that younger cancer patients (under 55 years of age) reported significantly more intense pain than older patients (over 55). In a review of the relationship between age and experimentally induced pain, Harkins et al.[219] found no major age differences in pain sensitivity, but noted that interindividual changes in pain sensitivity may have accounted for some differences. Similarly, Bressler et al.[44] found no statistically significant differences in reports of pain intensity in cancer outpatients under versus over 60 years of age.

Issues related to sensitivity and response to pharmacologic interventions have been examined by several investigators. Physiological responses to medication in light of changes in absorption, distribution, metabolism, and excretion of drugs are a major concern in the elderly population.[160,209,218,222–224] The changes reflect the contribution of the gastrointestinal system, nutritional composites, and hepatic and renal function, and relate to studies demonstrating that with increasing age, the elderly reported an increase in pain relief when given the same opioid and dose as younger patients.[225] If increasing age is associated with a decrease in morphine clearance, then the toxicities from opioids and other drugs potentially are much greater.

An issue related to toxicity is whether the elderly are at greater risk for adverse drug reactions. Problems with study design and definitions of adverse reactions have contributed to the conflicting evidence in this area.[226] Since the elderly have more chronic diseases and take more medications for these illnesses, the risk of adverse drug reactions may be higher solely because of increased drug intake. Ferrell et al.[216] found that the average number of prescribed medications for the elderly in a long-term care facility was eight. Conn et al.[227] reported that the average number of prescribed medications for patients either recently discharged from a hospital or who were at home was five. The interactions of multiple drug therapies are also an important issue related to toxicities.

A fourth and final issue relevant to pain in the elderly follows naturally from the issues already discussed. If assessment of cancer pain in the elderly is complicated by the possibility of multiple causative factors, sensory and cognitive impairment, differences in sensitivity, and pain relief because of normal physiologic aging, does this population of patients receive adequate analgesic management? Several reports indicate that the elderly have fewer opioids prescribed for them than younger patients.[212,213,228, 229] Portenoy[211] raised a very important issue in this regard: If the elderly perceive pain less often, indicating a lower prevalence of pain, then less frequent prescribing of analgesics is appropriate. If, however, the elderly experience pain similar to the younger population of patients, and choose not to report the pain, *or* respond more slowly to painful stimuli, indicating a higher prevalence of pain, then underprescribing creates needless suffering. As in other areas related to cancer pain, more well-controlled, epidemiologic studies of the prevalence of pain in the elderly are needed to help delineate the scope of the problem in this vulnerable population and to assist in answering questions about appropriate management.

In summary, the problem of cancer pain in the elderly population is a very important one. As individuals enter the later stages of life, the risk of developing cancer increases, and thus the risk of cancer pain increases. Specific attention to the unique physiologic, pharmacologic, psychologic and sociologic issues for these individuals is crucial for appropriate, successful management of cancer pain. Here are some general recommendations for management of medications in the elderly:[223,230]

1. Evaluate carefully for treatable, underlying conditions.
2. Differentiate new acute pains from chronic pains.
3. Avoid interactions among drugs.
4. Begin with smallest doses of specific drugs; use one-half to two-thirds of "younger" dose.
5. Adjust dose to accommodate for hepatic and renal abnormalities.
6. Individualize and simplify regimens; use analgesics one at a time.
7. Consider visual and auditory abilities/disabilities when giving instructions and when labeling medications.
8. Address the adherence issue by ensuring that patients can afford prescribed medications, can obtain them from a pharmacy, and can open the containers.
9. Monitor for toxicity, efficacy, and compliance.
10. Use drugs with short half-lives.
11. Look for additive effects from multiple drugs, especially adjuvant analgesics.
12. Maximize drug dosages before changing to another drug prematurely.

Substance abuse history

The national problem of drug abuse creates unique and different management challenges for health care professionals when pain and substance abuse occur simultaneously. Coyle and Foley[231] identified three patient groups in this special population: (1) those currently in a methadone maintenance program, (2) those actively using illicit drugs, and (3) those who used illicit drugs previously, many years ago.

For the patient in a methadone maintenance program or with a long-standing prior history, health care providers need to be concerned about recidivism, especially during a time of stress associated with a cancer diagnosis and pain.[231] McCaffery and Beebe[160] suggested that the patient be asked whether using opioids will be detrimental to continued or sustained recovery from illicit drug use. Similarly, the patient should be asked to share any concerns about using opioids for pain relief. The use of aggressive nonopioid approaches should be maximized in this population.[160]

For the patient who is actively using illicit drugs, there may be a fear of being punished or treated unfairly by health care providers. In addition, fear of withdrawal symptoms and not having those symptoms treated properly are legitimate concerns.[232] The active substance abuser may be more of a concern to physicians and nurses. Twycross and Lack[41] discussed potential errors with this population: (1) pain is discounted so that no matter what the patient says, it is unlikely that adequate medication will be provided; or (2) the patient is treated as a nonaddict so higher doses are given than are actually needed.

With all patients having any previous or current substance abuse history, it is important that an adversarial relationship not begin or escalate between patient and staff. As with any other patient, the substance abuse patient's report of pain should not be questioned or doubted.[160] Appropriate medications should not be withheld as a form of punishment,[160] and pain relief should not become a bargaining tool.[232] Communication among all members of the health team, including the patient, about how pain will be managed should be instituted early in the course of contact with the patient. Sometimes a contract may be useful for establishing realistic goals between the health care provider and the patient. Regularly scheduled meetings to review the goals of care may avoid unnecessary conflict. In order to provide a consistent approach to management, several authors recommend having only one physician assume responsibility for writing all opioid orders and one nurse assume responsibility for coordinating nursing care.[231–233] The assistance of professionals experienced in substance abuse, analgesic management, and cognitive-behavioral approaches to pain may be helpful in developing a successful plan of care.

Individuals with a substance abuse history may require much higher doses of opioids for pain because of tolerance.[231] When a patient reports increasing pain that requires higher doses of opioids, the clinician should focus on the changing pain pattern as the reason for the need for more opioids and *not* on "drug seeking behavior." Twycross and Lack[41] recommended changing a patient from parenteral analgesics to oral or rectal routes so that the association between street drugs and pain relief is not present. Regardless of any history of substance abuse, the patient is entitled to receive reasonable, adequate care for a concomitant cancer pain problem. Obstacles to achieving this goal need to be discussed, examined, and resolved to ensure pain relief.

Critical care

Patients who receive aggressive treatment for their malignancy or patients who experience serious symptoms from their disease may require intensive critical care monitoring. Management of pain in the midst of problems such as sepsis, acute respiratory distress syndrome, cerebral edema and increasing intracranial pressure, and severe graft-versus-host disease is an enormous challenge. When patients are unable to speak because of endotracheal intubation or are unable to communicate because of central nervous system dysfunction, the health care provider must rely on other means of communication to assess and manage pain. A detailed review of this topic is beyond the scope of this chapter, but a recently edited book by Puntillo is an excellent source of information about pain assessment and management in the critically ill patient.[234]

Culturally diverse populations

Nurses' assessment and management of individuals with cancer pain can be influenced by a number of factors, ranging from attitudes, beliefs, and personal history of pain to stereotypical notions about how people of specific ethnocultural backgrounds respond to pain.[48] As the racial and cultural diversity of the United States increases, more and more nurses find themselves caring for patients of ethnocultural backgrounds different from their own. In this section, approaches for dealing with culturally diverse patient populations are discussed.

"The American health care system, its philosophies, and its practices have their roots in white, middle-class values and beliefs."[235] That is, in the American system of health care, provision frequently is not made for even acknowledging the individual's ethnocultural perspective, let alone understanding or using it in planning health care interventions. There is a tendency on the part of nurses and other health care providers to become ethnocentric—that is, to believe that their own health practices are superior to those of others.[236] Since nurses espouse the notion of holistic care, tailored to individuals' unique and specific needs, the idea of not only accepting but incorporating cultural diversity into plans for care is essential to achieving truly holistic care.

Different ethnic groups express pain and suffering differently.[237] Additionally, cultural background can influence choices of and responses to medical care and to the diagnosis of cancer itself.[77] The nurse's interpretation of individuals' behaviors and verbalizations related to pain should be based on knowledge of how the patient's culture views responses to pain.[236] Respect for cultures other than one's own, and for the fact that people have specific beliefs and behaviors that emanate from their cultural background, is known as cultural sensitivity.

Although providing nursing care for people who are culturally diverse can be extremely challenging, the nurse's commitment to delivering total care and supporting an individual's integrity and dignity can be exemplified by learning as much as possible about the individual's ethnocultural background and its influences on health and illness beliefs and behaviors.[238] In a review article on culture, pain, and cancer, Garro[77] noted that both patients' experiences and responses to pain *and* medical care itself are shaped by culture. She urged caregivers to focus on the cultural and personal meanings of illness and pain in order to better alleviate suffering.

Few studies have examined the relationship between cultural background and cancer pain. In one study of 78 Anglo and Hispanic children with cancer between the ages of 3 and 15, investigators sought to learn whether cultural heritage and acculturation affected perception and expression of pain and anxiety.[239] Although the children demonstrated similar behavioral responses to pain, the Hispanic parents were significantly more anxious than the Anglo parents. Little other literature exists in this area.

Several authors have made recommendations that should be useful to nurses caring for individuals of culturally diverse backgrounds. Fong[236] discussed the importance of developing rapport as the foundation of successful nursing interventions. She urged the use of good manners, maintaining a broad and open attitude, and maintaining flexibility. Kagawa-Singer[238] highlighted the importance of developing good communication with patients and their family, followed by facilitation of their integrating the disease process and its treatment into their lives. A key principle is the use of negotiation to achieve feasible treatment plans and to enlist the patient's and family's participation in reaching treatment goals. Similarly, Louie[240] made a number of recommendations to help avoid culture-related conflicts in the care of Chinese patients. These recommendations, however, are generically quite useful and include identification and achievement of mutual goals, compromise and integration of different health care practices into the care plan, identification and discussion of nursing interventions with patient and family, stressing the importance of health education, using vital teaching materials if language is a problem, and seeking additional information and assistance from cultural organizations and resources when necessary.

Although very little has been written specifically on dealing with cancer pain, or even with pain in general, in individuals of different cultural backgrounds, there is some literature on ethnocultural nursing practice that should prove helpful in dealing with specific cultural groups who experience cancer pain. Fong's[236] general discussion of ethnicity and nursing practice is extremely good, particularly with respect to cultural assessment. Kagawa-Singer[238] provided an excellent discussion of oncology nursing in people of Hispanic and Japanese American background. Reizian and Meleis[69] described the responses of Arab Americans to pain, and gave recommendations for nursing care, particularly in the critical care setting. Further information about individuals with Middle Eastern background is given in another article.[241] Louie[240] gave an excellent presentation on nursing the patient of Chinese background, and Capers[242] wrote about Afro-Americans and implications for care of these individuals.

Finally, in patients who are ethnoculturally different than their caregivers, as well as those who are similar, the area of spirituality is important. This construct is beginning to receive more attention, particularly as it relates to ethnocultural differences, the nursing process, chronic illness, and dying.[243] Of special note is Jacik's excellent chapter on the spiritual care of the dying adult.[244]

Palliative and terminal care

Twycross wrote in 1987 that "the aim of terminal care is to help the patient, despite the cancer and increasing physical limitations, to go on having a good quality of life until he dies."[245,p.173] Wanzer and colleagues described the physician's responsibility toward dying individuals, emphasizing the "art of deliberately creating a medical environment that allows a peaceful death."[246,p.846] The parallel for nursing is obvious—the nurse must practice the art of creating a nursing environment that allows a peaceful death.

In recent years, this approach has evolved into the new, multidisciplinary specialty of palliative care.[156,157] Weissman defined palliative care as "the active total care of patients at a time when their disease is not responsive to curative treatment."[157,p.67] Ventafridda noted that the aim of palliative care was "to give the patient . . . the highest quality of life possible."[156,p.394] and defined it as a global approach carried out by physicians, nurses, social workers, and volunteers. He described the following characteristics of palliative care:[156,pp.394–395]

1. It affirms life and regards dying as a normal process.
2. It neither hastens nor postpones death.
3. It provides relief from pain and other distressing symptoms.
4. It integrates the psychological and spiritual aspects of patient care.
5. It offers a support system to help the family cope during the patient's illness and in bereavement.
6. Investigations are kept to a minimum and treatment is directed to symptom control and psychosocial support and not to the underlying disease process.
7. Radiotherapy, chemotherapy, and surgery have a place in palliative care. They are used, however, in such a way to ensure that the symptomatic benefits of treatment clearly outweigh the disadvantages.

Philosophical, organizational, and practical aspects of providing palliative care to terminally ill individuals with cancer pain have been described for inpatient and home hospice settings,[244,247–250] the home care setting,[41,251,252] extended care facilities,[253] general inpatient and cancer settings,[152,254–256] and the special situation of children and adolescents.[257] Several key aspects of caring for these individuals exist, regardless of setting, and need to be considered by nurses who are involved in palliative care.

The focus of terminal care is on relief of pain and other symptoms and on psychologic support of both the patient and the family.[245] Teamwork is requisite to the success of these efforts. Death often is accompanied by great fear, a normal human response that is part of the survival instinct.[245] In the care of terminal illness, not only are the dying afraid of death, but the living are as well. Withdrawal from those who are dying is a common reaction, yet remaining with the individual is one of the most important aspects of terminal care. Jacik wrote: "Human presence is a priceless source of comfort to dying persons."[244,p.267] For those dying with pain, the knowledge that health care providers and others are not only present but continually focusing on relieving the pain serves as a great comfort.

Related to continual efforts at relieving pain are the issues of assessment and treatment, particularly when pain worsens or new pain appears. The goal of minimizing pain and increasing comfort in the terminally ill individual must not obstruct the normal response to complaints of pain or restrict the range of interventions that might be considered or attempted. There is no reason why terminally ill people with worsening or new symptoms of pain should be evaluated, diagnosed, and treated any differently than nonterminally ill persons with cancer pain. For example, the development of new and painful metastatic lesions of the bone in a home hospice patient should not preclude use of radiotherapy if appropriate, even if it means that the patient must be moved. The goal is increased comfort, and all possible means to achieve it should be considered.

A flexible and adjustable care plan to meet the patient's changing needs as the disease progresses is essential.[246] Recent research indicates that pain and other symptoms during the last 4 weeks of life assume tremendous variability.[258] Tailoring of palliative care to meet these diverse needs involves the use of multiple interventions, including pharmacologic therapies, and the expertise to use these interventions properly. Often there is inadequate knowledge of pharmacokinetics, neurology, and medical oncology.[259] Similarly, underutilization of opioids can erode patients' confidence in the medical system and bring their dying into sharper focus. Indeed, adjuvant drugs have not been used as often as they could be in the terminal or palliative care setting.[260] The World Health Organization guidelines for cancer pain relief have been applied successfully to terminal cancer patients with pain.[261] Although nonpharmacologic, noninvasive interventions for pain are appropriate in the terminal cancer patient, their use has not been addressed through systematic research. Since these interventions often are instituted by nurses, carefully planned studies of their effectiveness seem indicated.

In some clinical settings, such as hospice and home care, adjustments or modifications of interventions need to be made to accommodate the setting,[41,247] for example, the formulation of rectal diazepam, and systems such as reminder cards and special containers for home administration of opioids. Considerable creativity may go into devising methods for patients and their families to manage interventions on their own. Recent research has indicated the importance of addressing family factors that influence pain management, as well as the burdens home caregivers must deal with.[91–93] These activities, the ongoing need for assessment of pain, and coordination of pain management are well within the scope of practice for oncology nurses engaged in palliative care.

Summary

When caring for special populations with cancer pain, a number of basic principles and special considerations needs to be employed by nurses. Foremost is the need for a multidisciplinary approach. Exceedingly important as well, however, are a thorough understanding of the scope of nursing practice; accurate assessment and diagnosis; appropriate attention to developmental, clinical, and ethnocultural issues; and knowledge about palliative care. Awareness and use of the information just presented will help nurses to identify and assess cancer pain and to plan, implement, coordinate, and evaluate its interdisciplinary management.[78] Specific approaches to the management of cancer pain are presented next.

INTERVENTIONS

Methods for managing cancer pain can be categorized into three major approaches (Figure 23-3). In the first approach, treatment is aimed at the underlying pathology or organic etiology of the pain. In most cases, this approach consists of attempts to reduce or eradicate tumor. The second approach aims at changing the individual's perception or sensation of pain. A wide variety of techniques is available to help achieve this goal. The third approach consists of a number of interventions aimed at diminishing the emotional or reactive component of pain. Interventions from each of these three approaches may be, and commonly are, used simultaneously in a given individual.

With the wide variety of specific interventions available, a multidisciplinary treatment strategy clearly is the optimal approach to effective management of pain. In the following sections, specific interventions within each of the three major treatment approaches are discussed. Particular emphasis is put on the role of the nurse in relation to the intervention; some interventions will demand much more nursing knowledge and involvement than others.

Treatment of Underlying Pathology

Chemotherapy, radiotherapy, and surgery are the major modalities used to treat cancer when cure is the intent, but they can also be useful when palliation is the goal. Hormonal therapy, a fourth treatment modality used for palliative treatment of certain tumors, is discussed next, along with chemotherapy. Each of the three modalities has specific indications in the individual with cancer pain.

Chemotherapy and hormonal therapy

In 1979, Bonadonna and Molinari wrote: "The specific impact of medical treatment on pain produced by advanced cancer has not yet been the subject of a detailed report."[262,p.131] They proposed that the main reason was because responses to antineoplastic drugs generally were considered significant only if tumor regression was documented objectively. Improvement of subjective clinical phenomena such as pain was not regarded as meaningful. In 1983, Russell commented that "few reports on the results of chemotherapy give details of how pain relief is measured."[263,p.356] In 1989, MacDonald's[264] review of 24 phase II and III studies in patients with esophageal, stomach, pancreatic, and nonsmall-cell lung cancer published in the *Journal of Clinical Oncology* in 1986–1987 found that not one of them measured the impact of the chemotherapy on patients' pain. In only one study was pain even mentioned, and in that one it was viewed as a factor that could influence patients' responses to chemotherapy.

An argument was made for the importance of measuring pain relief as an outcome in cancer clinical trials, particularly those in individuals with poor-prognosis tumors, such as lung, pancreas, stomach, and esophagus.[264] Others[262] held the same view and stressed the importance of measuring pain relief when effective first-line chemotherapeutic regimens were used. The challenges of standardizing the measurement of pain in such endeavors may be partly addressed through the use of a clinical staging system for cancer pain, developed to include all the known prognostic factors for response to treatment.[265]

In the years since 1979, however, some evidence has accumulated to suggest that various chemotherapy drugs have some beneficial effects on cancer pain. Anecdotal data indicated that patients with breast and prostate cancer, and some leukemias and lymphomas, experienced very good to complete relief of pain from their chemotherapy.[262] In a very small sample of individuals with colorectal cancer, Estes et al.[266] reported that intraarterial 5-fluorouracil with or without whole-body hyperthermia was beneficial in helping to control pelvic pain. In a review of seven studies of single drugs, it was found that one study reported pain relief in women with breast cancer after treatment with doxorubicin.[263] In 11 studies using combination chemotherapy for bone metastases due to breast cancer, pain relief was reported as an outcome in all of them, ranging from 40% to 94%.[263]

Thus, it appears that some chemotherapeutic agents may provide some relief of pain in some types of tumors. It has been suggested that tumors where chemotherapy was unlikely to provide significant survival time but might palliate symptoms included gastrointestinal cancers, lung cancer, esophageal and prostate cancers, sarcomas, and melanoma. Further research is needed, however, to document the efficacy of chemotherapeutic regimens at relieving cancer pain.[267]

Hormonal therapy has been used for many years to treat breast and prostate cancers. It provides palliation with fewer side effects and may afford significant relief of pain, sometimes even for prolonged periods of time.[267] Investigators have reported good responses in painful bone metastases from breast and prostate cancers using a variety of therapies, including estrogen, androgen, progestin, aminoglutethimide, and corticosteroids.[268,269]

Radiotherapy

Radiation has long been used to treat painful bone metastases, most often in cancers of the breast, lung, and prostate.[262,267,270] In addition, it is standard treatment for relieving pain from epidural cord compression, and it may be helpful in relieving pain from headaches and increased intracranial pressure due to brain metastases.[271]

Radiotherapy also may be useful for pain resulting from nerve root infiltration, hepatic metastases, and advanced gynecologic, gastrointestinal, or upper aerodigestive cancers.[267] There appears to be no standardly prescribed doses of radiation for specific tumor problems, and there appears to be little correlation between dose of radiation and extent of relief or between dose required for relief and the histologic tumor type. Relief of pain can begin to occur within 24–48 hours of initiation of radiotherapy.[267]

The evidence of the efficacy of radiotherapy in relieving cancer pain caused by bone metastases is quite convincing. Ford and Yarnold[270] reviewed 11 studies and found that patients reported pain relief in 10 of them. Abrams and Hansen[267] cited several studies as well in which patients with prostate, lung, and breast cancers experienced significant relief of their pain following radiotherapy. A study by the Radiation Therapy Oncology Group (RTOG) indicated that 90% of individuals with bone metastases experienced some relief of their pain; 54% had complete relief, although initial pain intensity and site of the primary lesion affected responses to some degree.[272] A second RTOG study revealed that 73% of patients who had multiple symptomatic bone lesions experienced some relief of pain and 20% complete relief when treated with half-body radiation.[273] The advantages of this method of delivery included faster pain relief and less evidence of recurrence of pain in the treated area than conventional delivery methods.

Surgery

Surgery as a modality for treating cancer pain can take many forms, but the primary goal is palliative. Direct palliative surgery either helps resolve oncologic emergencies or other serious clinical situations such as bowel obstruction[274] or helps improve the therapeutic effects of the previous two modalities by reducing tumor burden. Indirect palliative surgery involves surgical ablation of endocrine glands in endocrine-related tumors, e.g., ovariectomy for advanced breast cancer. Three other forms of palliative surgery for individuals with pain consist of procedures to provide direct access to areas of tumor (e.g., implants of infusion pumps or radiation seeds), orthopedic procedures to prevent or repair fractures from metastatic disease,[275] and neurosurgical procedures performed on various areas of the CNS to interrupt the pain pathway (discussed separately later).

Although very few data are available to indicate the success of these various surgical approaches at relieving pain, many clinical situations show anecdotal relief of pain. Chalmers,[276] for example, described a number of orthopedic procedures useful in dealing with skeletal metastases. Table 23-9 shows clinical conditions and tumors that may benefit from various types of palliative surgery; relief of pain from these conditions is obviously an outcome of the surgical procedures.

The treatment modalities just described offer one approach to relieving cancer pain—treatment of the underlying pathology. Nursing responsibilities in relation to these methods are fairly standard, and quite similar to those when the same methods are used as first-line, curative therapies. In the second major approach to treating cancer pain, changing the perception and/or sensation of pain, the role and responsibilities of the nurse assume greater proportions.

Change in Perception/Sensation of Pain

As can be seen in Figure 23-3, the number of interventions in this approach is quite extensive. The most effective and commonly used techniques are discussed in some detail next. Techniques used less frequently, and with a lesser nursing role, are discussed only briefly. Pharmacologic therapy—consisting of nonopioids, opioids, and adjuvant drugs—is a major responsibility of nurses, and, as discussed previously, is an area about which much more knowledge and skill are needed.

Pharmacologic therapy

The pharmacologic management of cancer pain accounts for the major source of pain treatment. Regardless of *when* a patient presents with a pain problem as a result of cancer or its treatment, the use of various pharmacologic strategies must be incorporated into the plan of care.

During the past 14 years there have been a number of publications from physicians, nurses, pharmacists, and pharmacologists addressing the overall issue of pharmacologic management of cancer pain.[41,160, 277–283] This noninclusive, selected list of resources provides health care professionals with comprehensive information about pharmacologic management of cancer-related pain.

In order to understand pharmacologic management, one must be familiar with the terminology used to describe analgesics and their effects[160,284,285] (Table 23-10). These terms are especially important in understanding the actions of opioid drugs.

Nonopioids WHO's three-step analgesic ladder provides a framework for using analgesics. The use of nonopioids is included in all three steps of the ladder.[109] In the first step, these drugs are the primary therapy.

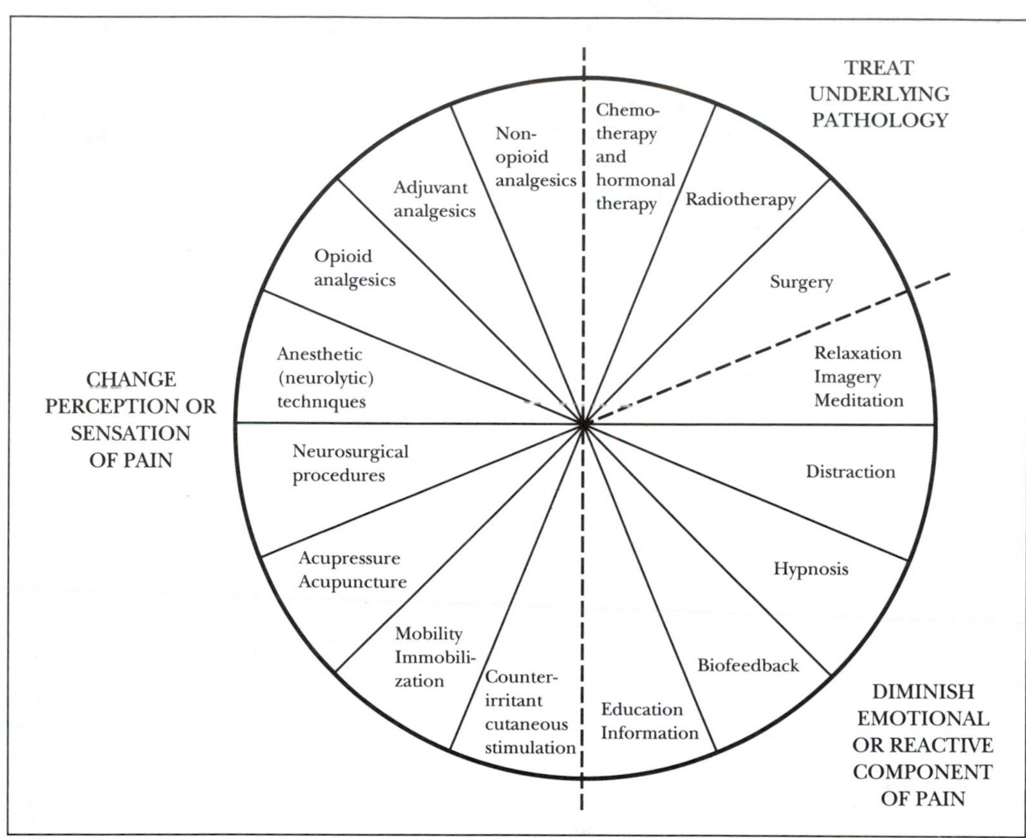

FIGURE 23-3 Three major approaches to treatment of cancer pain.

TABLE 23-9 Major Clinical Conditions Requiring Palliative Surgery for Pain

Clinical Condition	Tumor	Type of Palliative Surgery
Breast tumor	Ulcerating Fungating	Simple mastectomy
Abdominal cancer		
Intestinal occlusion	Colorectal carcinoma, ovarian, peritoneal carcinomatosis	Colostomy GI bypass
Intractable pelvic pain	Colorectal carcinomas	Intraarterial infusion (5-FU, nitrogen mustard)
Serious ascites	Breast, ovarian cancer	Peritoneovenous shunt
Acute urinary tract occlusion	*Upper tract:* flank and retroperitoneal tumor *Pelvic tract:* cancer of cervix, prostate, rectum	Nephrostomy Cutaneous ureterostomy, cystotomy
Rectovesical fistula		Colostomy
Rectovaginal fistula		Colostomy
Tumors of the extremities		
Large lesions	Sarcomas, epithelial tumors, metastatic visceral tumors	Reductive surgery (amputation) Disarticulation
Pathologic fracture	Metastases from lung, breast, prostate, renal, thyroid carcinomas Primary advanced bone and soft-tissue tumors	Amputation Prostheses Pins
Axial nervous system involvement		
Spinal cord compression	Metastases from lung, breast, prostate, renal, thyroid carcinomas Lymphomas, sarcomas	Decompressive laminectomy

Source: Azzarelli A, Crispino S: Palliative surgery in cancer pain treatment, in Swerdlow M, Ventafridda V (eds.): *Cancer Pain*. Lancaster, Eng.: MTP Press, 1987, pp. 97–103.

TABLE 23-10 Terminology in Analgesics

Efficacy	Degree of analgesia provided by a given dose of an analgesic administered under a particular set of conditions
Dose Response	Increase in dose accompanied by increase in effectiveness
Relative Analgesic Potency	Ratio of doses of two drugs
Relative Analgesic Potential	Relationship between efficacy and adverse effects
Half-Life	Time it takes a drug to fall to half its original concentration in the blood
Opiate Receptors	Specific recognition sites on which opioids produce their actions
Tolerance	A pharmacologic phenomenon that develops when a given dose of a drug produces a decreased effect or when larger doses must be given to obtain the effects observed from the original dose
Physical Dependence	An altered physiologic state produced by the repeated administration of a drug, and which necessitates the continued administration of the drug to prevent the appearance of withdrawal
Addiction	A behavioral pattern of drug use characterized by overwhelming involvement with its use; also known as *psychological dependence*

Sources: Data from McCaffery and Beebe,[160] Pasternak,[284] and Jaffe and Martin.[285]

In the second and third steps, they are used in conjunction with a weak opioid or a strong opioid.

Although nonopioid drugs differ in their chemical structure and classifications, they often are presented as two distinct categories—nonsteroidal anti-inflammatory drugs (NSAIDs) (which include aspirin), and acetaminophen. The similarities between categories are that they both have antipyretic and analgesic properties. Their site of action is primarily the peripheral nervous system, although a recent animal study indicates there may be a centrally acting component.[286] There have been reports of CNS toxicities with NSAIDs.[287] In addition, the nonopioids do not produce physical dependence, tolerance, or addiction, and they have a maximum ceiling effect for analgesic potential. Except for acetaminophen and choline magnesium trisalicylate, the NSAIDs have antiplatelet properties as well. This potential hematologic problem is caused by irreversible acetylation of platelet cyclooxygenase, which inhibits platelet aggregation.[12]

The mechanism of action for these drugs has been well described. The NSAIDs inhibit cyclooxygenase in peripheral tissues, which prevents arachidonic acid from converting to prostaglandin.[12,288] This action alters transduction in primary afferent nociceptors. Prostaglandins are associated with pain that results from injury or inflammation, and they can sensitize pain receptors to mechanical and chemical stimulation.

The indication for using nonopioids in patients with cancer pain is when pain is mild to moderate in intensity. Noncancer-related pain, such as that caused by arthritis, primary dysmenorrhea, muscle sprains, orthopedic injuries, and dental pain, commonly are treated with nonopioids. In cancer-related pain, NSAIDs are useful for: (1) metastatic bone pain, (2) pain from mechanical compression of tendons, muscles, pleura, and peritoneum, and (3) nonobstructive visceral pain.[289]

Studies using NSAIDs in individuals with cancer pain indicate that the drugs are efficacious in providing pain relief. Moertel[290] found aspirin (ASA) 650 mg to be superior to three other nonopioids (acetaminophen, phenacetin, mefenamic acid), three weak opioids (pentazocine, codeine, propoxyphene), and one phenothiazine (promazine). ASA and naproxen provided equal pain relief, with statistically significant improvement from baseline pain for both drugs.[291] In a study examining two different dosing schedules of naproxen, Levich et al.[292] reported that both schedules provided pain relief in approximately 80% of the patients after the same initial dose, but that the higher-dose group had greater pain relief without a significant increase in adverse side effects.

Diclofenac was compared to ASA/codeine combinations and nefopam (not available in the United States). Although patients in all three groups had improved pain relief, side effects were less frequent with diclofenac than with the other two analgesics.[293] In a single-dose, double-blind, placebo-controlled trial using three different dose levels of ketorolac (10, 30, and 90 mg) for cancer pain, all three ketorolac dosages were superior to the placebo. There was no difference in efficacy among the ketorolac dosages.[294] In a multidrug study of nine nonopioids, Ventafridda et al.[295] reported that the greatest pain relief was with naproxen, diclofenac, and indocin, and the least pain relief was with paracetamol (acetaminophen).

The combination of nonopioids and opioids administered simultaneously is designed to enhance analgesia.[296] One of the earliest studies with cancer patients demonstrated the beneficial effect of aspirin and morphine over morphine alone.[297] Another nonopioid, ibuprofen, was the drug of choice in two studies, the first involving two different doses of methadone[298] and the second involving a variety of scheduled opioids.[299] Both studies showed increased analgesic efficacy with the ibuprofen/opioid combination compared to the opioid alone.

The major potential toxicities from NSAIDs are gastrointestinal (GI) disorders (nausea, vomiting, epigastric pain, ulcers, bleeding, diarrhea, constipation).[288,300] The loss of the cytoprotective effect of prostaglandin on the GI epithelium contributes to these problems.[301] The elderly may have a significantly increased risk for developing peptic ulcer disease, especially with high doses.[302] Other potential toxicities include renal dysfunction, sodium and water retention, skin rashes, and headaches.[288,301,303]

The selection of a nonopioid for an individual patient often is based on individual preference and experience. Table 23-11 indicates many of the common drugs and doses. Portenoy[304] recommended a maximum ceiling of 1.5–2 times the recommended starting dose and continuing the drug for 2–3 weeks. Aspirin is considered by some to be a first-line nonopioid because it is relatively inexpensive and very efficacious.[41,109] Mannix and Rawlins[301] selected naproxen as their initial drug of choice because it is reasonably effective, comes in three formulations (tablet, suspension, and suppository), and can be given on a twice-a-day schedule so as to simplify drug administration. Table 23-12 list considerations in the use of nonopioids.

The benefits of nonopioids in patients who have pain of severe intensity and who require high doses of opioids has not been established. In designing analgesic

TABLE 23-11 Nonopioids Commonly Used in Analgesic Treatments of Cancer Pain

Name	Half-Life (hours)	Dosing Interval	Starting Dose (mg/day)	Maximum Dose (mg/day)
Acetaminophen	2–3	q 4 hr	2000	6000
Acetylsalicylic acid	2–3	q 4 hr	2000	6000
Choline magnesium trisalicylate	9–17	q 12 hr	2000	4000
Diclofenac	1–2	q 8–12 hr	75–100	200
Diflunisal	8–12	q 8–12 hr after loading dose	500–1000	1500
Ibuprofen	2	q 4–6 hr	1600	3200
Indomethacin	4–5	q 8–12 hr	50–75	150–200
Ketorolac	4–9	q 6 hr after loading dose	60–120	150
Naproxen	10–20	q 6–8 hr	750	1250

Sources: Insel PA: Analgesic-antipyretic and anti-inflammatory agents. Drugs employed in the treatment of rheumatoid arthritis and gout, in Gilman AG, Rall TW, Nies AS, et al (eds.): *Goodman and Gilman's The Pharmacological Basis of Therapeutics* (ed. 8). New York: Pergammon Press, 1990; *Physician's Desk Reference* (ed. 46). Montvale, NJ: Medical Economics Data, 1992; *Drug Evaluations Annual 1991.* Milwaukee: American Medical Association, 1990; *American Hospital Formulary Service Drug Information.* Bethesda, MD: American Society of Hospital Pharmacists, 1992.

TABLE 23-12 Considerations in the Use of Nonopioid Analgesics

Problem	Suggested Nonopiods
Need for strong anti-inflammatory activity	All drugs except acetaminophen
Need for parenteral route	Ketorolac
Risk of thrombocytopenia or other hematologic disorder	Acetaminophen, choline magnesium trisalicylate
Impaired renal function	Acetaminophen, diflunisal, sulindac
Altered gastrointestinal function	Acetaminophen, choline magnesium trisalicylate, salsalate
Compliance	Diflunisal, naproxen, piroxicam (longer half-lives)
Risk of significant adverse side effects	Avoid indomethacin, phenylbutazone, oxyphenbutazone
Need for chronic use	Avoid mefenamic acid, meclofenamate
Cost	Aspirin, acetaminophen

regimens for these individuals, however, nonopioids need to be considered either alone or in conjunction with an opioid.

Opioids Opioids, which interfere with pain perception in the CNS, are the most important category of drugs for use in the pharmacologic management of cancer pain. They are classified into three groups:

1. *Morphinelike opioid agonists.* These bind with mu and kappa receptors (mu receptors affect supraspinal analgesia, respiratory depression, euphoria, and physical dependence; kappa receptors affect spinal analgesia, miosis, and sedation); this group includes drugs such as codeine, fentanyl, hydromorphone, meperidine, morphine, and methadone.
2. *Opioid antagonists.* These have no agonist receptor activity (naloxone is a pure opioid antagonist).
3. *Opioid agonist-antagonists and partial agonists.* Agonist-antagonists, which include drugs such as pentazocine, butorphanol, and nalbuphine, act competitively at different receptor sites, and the partial agonists, which include buprenorphine, act at only one receptor site (mu).[285] It is generally accepted by cancer pain experts that opioid agonist-antagonist drugs have very limited usefulness in cancer pain management because of their propensity to induce opioid withdrawal. As a result, these drugs will not be discussed in this chapter.

There is certain information that is critical for physicians and nurses to know before prescribing and administering opioids. The specifics include: the mechanism of action, purpose and category, common starting doses, equivalences of other analgesics when needed, duration of effect, half-life, available routes, and unique side effects.[155] Table 23-13 contains information about the relative potencies of commonly used analgesics for mild to moderate pain and for severe pain.

TABLE 23-13 Relative Potencies of Commonly Used Analgesics

Mild to Moderate Pain	Oral Dose (mg)*
Codeine	30
Meperidine	50
Propoxyphene	65
Acetaminophen	650
Sodium salicylate	1000

Severe Pain	IM (mg)†	PO (mg)†	Plasma Half-Life (hr)	Average Duration of Action (hr)
Codeine	130	200	2.5–3	3–5
Meperidine	75	300	3–5	2–4
Oxycodone	15	30	2–3	3–5
Hydromorphone	1.5	7.5	2–3	3–6
Morphine	10	60§	2–3.5	4–5
Fentanyl‡	0.1	—	3–4	1–2
Levorphanol	2	4	11–16	4–5
Methadone	10	20	15–30	4–6
Oxymorphone	1	—	2–3	4–5

*Approximately equal to aspirin 650 mg.

†Approximately equivalent to morphine 10 mg IM. These values were determined from and based on clinical experience and single-dose studies of patients in acute pain.

‡Available as a transdermal patch.

§For chronic dosing, some pain experts believe that the oral morphine dose is approximately 20–30 mg, but this has not been demonstrated in any controlled trial.

Sources: Data from Foley,[155] Houde,[277] Inturrisi,[283] Jaffe and Martin,[285] Walsh,[329] and Houde.[334]

All opioid analgesics share common effects as a result of their action. Central nervous system, respiratory, cardiovascular, gastrointestinal, genitourinary, and dermatologic effects of these drugs are included in Table 23-14. The four most common side effects, however, are sedation, respiratory depression, nausea and vomiting, and constipation. The problem of sedation is addressed in the discussion about psychostimulants in a subsequent section.

If respiratory depression occurs, it can be treated easily and successfully with naloxone. The amount of naloxone a patient receives should be titrated to changes in respiratory rate. Rapid bolus injections of naloxone should be avoided in opioid-tolerant patients so as not to precipitate an abstinence syndrome response (nausea, vomiting, agitation, diaphoresis, intense pain). Respiratory depression is a concern when patients who have been maintained on opioid agonist drugs receive an anesthetic procedure that may totally eliminate their pain. The stimulus of pain on respiratory function is eliminated, which places the patient at risk for respiratory depression.

The chemoreceptor trigger zone (CTZ) in the brain is sensitive to chemical stimuli such as opioids. Similar to the effect of chemotherapy-related nausea and vomiting, the CTZ and the vomiting center can be stimulated to produce nausea and vomiting. In a retrospective review of 260 patients receiving opioids, Campora et al.[305] found that in patients who received morphine ($n = 71$), 18.3% had moderate/severe nausea and 28% had vomiting.

TABLE 23-14 Common Side Effects of Opioid Analgesics

System	Side Effect
Central nervous	Sedation, drowsiness, mental clouding, euphoria, analgesia, nausea, vomiting, ↓ physical activity, lethargy, mood changes
Respiratory	↓ Respiratory rate, ↓ ventilatory minute volume, ↓ tidal exchange, ↓ Po_2, ↑ Pco_2
Cardiovascular	Hypotension from peripheral vasodilation or histamine release
Gastrointestinal	*Stomach:* ↓ motility; *small intestine:* ↓ propulsive contractions, delayed digestion from ↓ biliary and pancreatic secretions; *large intestine:* ↓ or absent propulsive peristaltic waves, causing delay in passage of contents; *biliary tract:* ↑ pressure from morphinelike drugs, causing epigastric distress to biliary colic
Genitourinary	↑ Tone and amplitude of ureter contractions, ↑ tone of bladder muscles→urgency, ↑ tone of vesical sphincter
Dermatologic	Vasodilation of cutaneous blood vessels→ ↑ warmth and flushing of skin on face, neck, and upper thorax, sweating, pruritus

Source: Data from Jaffe and Martin.[285]

If a patient experiences opioid-related nausea and vomiting, there are many options available. Portenoy and Coyle[149] recommended the following: (1) Treat aggressively on initial presentation. (2) Use antiemetics that act at the CTZ, such as prochlorperazine and thiethylperazine. (3) Use metoclopramide if gastroparesis is a possible etiology of the nausea and vomiting. (4) Use an antivertigo drug such as cyclizine or scopalamine if symptoms worsen with movement. (5) Consider drug combinations. (6) Maximize dose response, especially if symptoms partially improve. (7) Prescribe antiemetics on an around-the-clock basis for 1–2 weeks.

Constipation can become a significant clinical problem for patients taking opioid analgesics if preventive measures are not instituted. The simplest dietary measures include encouraging patients to increase their fluid intake and dietary fiber consumption. The use of laxative preparations generally is necessary when patients must take opioids. Table 23-15 lists six categories of laxatives, their mechanisms of action, and commonly available preparations. Patients frequently require laxatives from more than one category, such as a stimulant laxative and a detergent laxative. More detailed guidelines regarding constipation management are available.[41,160,306,307]

There are inherent properties in opioids that can create potential problems for patients if health care professionals do not understand the distinctions among them. Table 23-10 includes definitions of *tolerance, physical dependence,* and *addiction.* Tolerance requires that doses of specific analgesics be adjusted to accommodate the pharmacologic phenomenon. Physical dependence is an issue when patients no longer require opioids for pain control and they must be tapered slowly off of them. It is also an issue if a patient inadvertently receives an agonist-antagonist drug causing acute withdrawal or if naloxone is required to reverse opioid-induced respiratory depression slowly. The problem of addiction was addressed earlier in this chapter, but to reiterate, addiction is not a problem for patients who require opioids for justifiable medical indications.

There has been considerable controversy over the last few years regarding the use of opioids for neuropathic pain.[149,308] Historically, neuropathic pain was thought not to be responsive to opioids. Portenoy et al.[308] suggested that patients may, in fact, just require higher doses of opioids to relieve neuropathic pain and that opioids should not be excluded as a viable option for patients who have neuropathic pain.

Specific drug selection A wide variety of opioids and combination opioids is available. Weak opioids such as codeine are used in step 2 of the WHO ladder, and strong opioids such as morphine are used in step 3.[109]

TABLE 23-15 Laxatives for Opiate-Induced Constipation

Category	Action	Common Preparations
Bulk	Increases size, weight, and frequency of stool; requires high fluid intake	Metamucil, Maltsupex
Saline	Draws water into intestinal lumen and distends bowel, changes stool consistency	Milk of magnesia, magnesium citrate
Stimulant	Increases motor activity by direct action on the bowel	Bisacodyl, senna, Ex-Lax, Cascara
Lubricant	Reduces friction and coats the stool	Mineral oil
Osmotic	Increases volume in colon; promotes water retention	Lactulose, sorbitol
Detergent	Reduces surface tension	Docusate; available in combination with stimulant laxatives

Sources: Data from Portenoy[306] and Levy.[308]

Various factors contribute to a specific opioid selection for an individual patient. One very important factor is the knowledge that has been gained through analgesic research. For example, meperidine is a drug that can produce significant CNS toxicities (agitation, tremors, myoclonus, seizures) as a result of normeperidine accumulation in plasma.[309] In addition, meperidine has poor oral efficacy[277] and should not be used for long-term analgesic management.

Another example for an opioid that has limited use in the United States is heroin. Supporters of the Compassionate Pain Relief Act (HR 5290) believed that heroin should be legalized for cancer pain management, as it is in England. The emotionalism associated with this issue supercedes the data that show that heroin is no better than morphine in providing pain control.[310,311] Heroin may be twice as potent as morphine and have a faster onset of analgesic effect, but in equal analgesic doses, morphine exhibits similar side effects.[312,313] In the sections that follow, the selected drugs discussed need special considerations when used to manage cancer pain.

Morphine Morphine probably is the most frequently used opioid analgesic for moderate to severe pain. It is used in the United States as well as in many foreign countries.[314–316] It is available as an oral, parenteral, rectal, and intraspinal preparation. The availability of long-acting morphine, which provides patients with 8–12-hour dosing schedules as opposed to 4-hour dosing, has contributed to improvements in patients' quality of life.[50] There can be considerable flexibility in dosing, since long-acting morphine comes in 15-, 30-, 60-, and 100-mg tablet sizes. Numerous studies, both controlled and uncontrolled, have demonstrated the efficacy and safety of long-acting morphine.[314,317–323] The design of these studies was similar: Patients were converted from their prestudy analgesic to short-acting morphine, the dose was titrated to achieve adequate pain relief for 24–48 hours, and then the short-acting morphine was converted to long-acting morphine.

Even though morphine is considered an effective oral analgesic,[41,324–326] its oral absorption rate is variable. Sawe et al.[327] demonstrated that oral morphine's bioavailability was 15%–64%. A related issue is the oral-to-parenteral ratio of morphine. The study that showed the oral:parenteral ratio of 6:1 (60 mg PO = 10 mg IM of morphine) was determined from a single-dose, postoperative study.[328] This number has been challenged by clinicians[41,329] who believe that based on clinical experience, the ratio is 2–3:1 (20–30 mg PO = 10 mg IM) in chronic dosing. This issue will be resolved best by a well-controlled clinical trial.[330]

One possible explanation for this analgesic effect of oral morphine in chronic dosing relates to a by-product of morphine metabolism, morphine-6-glucuronide. In patients with altered renal function, as well as in patients with normal renal function, morphine-6-glucuronide may be responsible not only for analgesia but also for the development of adverse side effects to morphine.[331–333]

Methadone and levorphanol Both of these opioid analgesics have prolonged plasma half-lives (see Table 23-13) that do not correspond to the average duration of action. When patients are initially placed on fixed schedules of these drugs, they are at risk of developing significant sedation and respiratory depression as the level in their plasma rises.[334,335] Houde[334] has continued to recommend that patients initially receive methadone on an as-needed basis to determine their optimal dose and schedule. Clinicians must be aware of the potential toxicities associated with analgesics that have long plasma half-lives.

Adjuvant analgesics Adjuvant analgesics are defined as those medications that enhance the action of pain-modulating systems.[12] In general, adjuvant analgesics are indicated primarily for uses other than pain management. The following categories of drugs are considered to be adjuvant analgesics: antidepressants, anticonvulsants, psychostimulants, corticosteroids, phenothiazines, and antihistamines. Each category is discussed briefly next.

Antidepressants The use of antidepressant medications for individuals with endogenous depression is considered standard treatment. These drugs act by inhibiting the uptake of neurotransmitters into nerve terminals.[336] They have been used in many chronic nonmalignant pain problems, such as postherpetic neuralgia, diabetic neuropathy, and migraine headaches.[337,338] In cancer pain, where their mechanism of action is not clear, their use has been for neuropathic pain often due to tumor infiltration of nerves.[339] This type of pain can be described as having a continuous, dysesthetic, burning quality.

Walsh[340] reviewed nine studies involving antidepressants and cancer pain. He found they often were prescribed in an attempt to decrease opioid use. Although these studies were beset with significant design and methodological problems, he concluded that the drugs were useful in an opioid-potentiating role in cancer pain.

Two additional studies using antidepressants in combination with other analgesics showed that patients' pain intensity decreased and analgesia improved, but the contribution of the antidepressants to decreased pain was unclear.[341] Amitriptyline doses (25–75 mg), methadone, and a nonopioid (aspirin, acetaminophen, or ibuprofen) were used in 14 patients for a duration of 14 days; patients reported a 74% decrease in pain intensity. Doxepin at a starting dose of 25 mg (titrated upward to a maximum of 225 mg) and piroxicam, a nonsteroidal anti-inflammatory drug, were used concomitantly. In this study patients reported analgesia within 48–72 hours.

In a randomized double-blind trial, Ventafridda et al.[342] compared trazadone and amitriptyline for patients with neuropathic pain. The analgesic efficacy of the drugs was similar. A partial list of antidepressants with starting and usual doses for cancer-related pain is given in Table 23-16. Dose changes at 1–2-day intervals in increments of 25 mg are recommended for these drugs.[343] The pain-relieving doses for antidepressants often are lower than those needed for treatment of depression. If patients do not achieve a therapeutic benefit within a few weeks of initiating the drug, then another drug should be considered.

The major side effects from antidepressants are anticholinergic. Sedation, dry mouth, constipation, postural hypotension, and urinary retention can be troublesome, especially if a patient is already receiving opioid analgesics and is experiencing similar problems.

Anticonvulsants The site and mechanism of the effectiveness of anticonvulsants for cancer-related pain are not well understood. They are a primary treatment for the pain caused by trigeminal neuralgia and have also been used for diabetic neuropathy and postherpetic neuralgia as well. Their effectiveness in chronic malignant pain has been supported by clinical observations and anecdotal experiences.

For patients who have neurogenic or neuropathic pain described as having a lancinating, stabbing quality, anticonvulsants may be beneficial.[344] Swerdlow and Cundill[345] studied 170 patients who had lancinating-type pain from a variety of etiologies. Each patient received four anticonvulsants (carbamazepine, clonazepam, phenytoin, valproate), proceeding from one to another after toxicity on each or lack of efficacy was demonstrated. Based on this study, the authors suggested that clinicians use carbamazepine or clonazepam as their first choice in treating lancinating-type pain.

Carbamazepine was used for 6 weeks in 13 patients for neurogenic pain caused by brachial plexus injury, peripheral nerve injury, and postherpetic neuralgia.[346] Toxicities from ataxia and rash caused six patients to withdraw from the study early, but five of seven reported pain relief at a maximum dose of 1200 mg/day. The patients in this study had pain for a duration of 6 months to 8 years.

Table 23-17 lists common doses and toxicities of four anticonvulsants.[12,347–349] The choice of one over another is based primarily on clinical judgment.

Psychostimulants Psychostimulants are useful in counteracting the sedation that accompanies opioid analgesics. If the sedation is present without any other CNS problems, such as delirium and confusion, and if pain occurs when the opioid dose is lowered, then psychostimulants may be indicated.

Two psychostimulants used for opioid-related sedation are amphetamines and methylphenidate. Amphetamines are a more powerful CNS stimulant than methylphenidate. They both decrease the central depression caused by other drugs. Their effects may be from cortical stimulation and/or reticular activating system stimulation.[350]

The more desirable side effects are increased alertness, increased ability to concentrate, mood elevation,

TABLE 23-16 Antidepressants for Cancer-Related Pain

Tricyclics	Usual Starting Dose (mg)	Usual Daily Dose (mg)
Amitriptyline	10–25	75–150
Nortriptyline	25–50	75–100
Imipramine	10–25	50–200
Desipramine	10–25	75–200
Doxepin	25–50	75–150
Second generation		
Trazadone	50 t.i.d.	150–250
Maprotiline	25	75–100

Sources: Data from Baldessarini[336] and Massie and Holland.[343]

TABLE 23-17 Anticonvulsants for Pain Management

Drug	Dose	Therapeutic Level	Toxicities
Phenytoin	150–200 mg b.i.d.	15–25 μg/ml	Drowsiness, dizziness, diplopia, ataxia
Carbamazepine	100–200 mg b.i.d. increase q.o.d. until pain-free or side effects, total daily dose 600–1200 mg/day	5–10 μg/ml	Drowsiness, dizziness, unsteadiness, gastric distress, anorexia, nausea
Clonazepam	0.5–1.5 mg/day, maximum 3–4 mg/day	20–80 ng/ml	Sedation, ataxia, behavioral disturbances
Valproic acid	15 mg/kg, maximum 3000 mg/day	50–100 μg/ml	Nausea, vomiting, indigestion, sedation

Sources: Data from Fields,[12] McEvoy,[348] and Rall and Schleifer.[349]

euphoria, and an increase in motor and speech activity. The more unpleasant side effects include confusion, agitation, dysphoria, apprehension, and fatigue.[350]

In an early study using morphine with or without dextroamphetamine, postoperative patients reported increased pain relief with the combination.[351] It has been only in the past few years that methylphenidate has been studied in cancer patients. In a controlled trial, Bruera et al.[352] demonstrated an increased analgesic effect and decreased sedation when methylphenidate (15 mg/day) was compared to a placebo. In a subsequent study, Bruera and his colleagues[353] found that 91% of patients reported improvement in somnolence 48 hours after treatment. They also found that patients became tolerant to the methylphenidate with an initial dose of 15 mg/day and a mean maximal daily dose of 42 mg ±6 after 39 ±20 days.

The limited trials with psychostimulants in patients with opioid-induced sedation indicate that sedation becomes less of a problem. As with other areas of pharmacologic management, more research is needed to clearly outline the benefits of these agents.

Phenothiazines/antihistamines According to Dundee and Moore, the origin of the myth for the potentiation of analgesics with promethazine came from "observations after its [promethazine's] use with large doses of pethidine [meperidine] or other analgesics, and erroneously attributing reductions in barbiturate dosage and side effects during anaesthesia to the promethazine."[354,p.96] Even though promethazine was reported to be antianalgesic to meperidine almost 30 years ago,[354] the potentiation myth is still widely believed today. Similarly, Keats et al.[355] found that promethazine did not increase analgesic efficacy or meperidine-induced respiratory depression or prevent meperidine-induced nausea and vomiting, but that it *did* increase the sedative effects of meperidine. Methotrimeprazine is the only phenothiazine with demonstrated analgesic properties.[356,357]

Hanks et al.[358] dispelled the myth about haloperidol potentiation from a retrospective review of 424 patients who received different doses of haloperidol and found no opioid-sparing effect.

Perhaps one of the best examples of erroneously applying research to clinical practice is with hydroxyzine. Beaver and Feise[359] compared 100 mg intramuscular hydroxyzine alone, morphine 8 mg IM alone, the combination of both drugs, and placebo in postoperative patients. In this *single-dose* study, the combination of morphine and hydroxyzine was superior to the other three groups. Hydroxyzine by itself was superior to placebo but less efficacious than morphine alone. Hydroxyzine seems to have analgesic properties, but it is not a potentiator of opioids, nor has it been shown to be less efficacious at a lower dose nor as an oral substitute (i.e., 25 mg PO QID).

Steroids Steroids are essential for managing the pain from epidural cord compressions, but their use as an adjuvant analgesic is based on limited data. Bruera et al.[360] compared methylprednisolone 32 mg/day to placebo in a 14-day randomized double-blind study to evaluate pain relief and other associated symptoms. Pain improved significantly with the methylprednisolone as opposed to with the placebo. The researchers found an improvement in appetite (77%) and in daily activity (68%) and a decrease in depression (71%) and in analgesic consumption (57%). Walsh[361] suggested that steroids could be used for problems such as bone metastases, lymphedema, mass effects from solid tumors, and brachial and lumbosacral plexopathies.

The known toxicities from steroids, particularly an increase in appetite and elevation of mood, may be desirable in some patients, especially those with advanced disease. The morbidity from other toxicities, such as proximal myopathy, steroid-induced hyperglycemia, and Cushingoid side effects, need to be considered seriously if steroids are used early in the treatment of a patient's pain problem.

Diphosphonates These powerful inhibitors of bone resorption are used for treating disorders such as Paget's disease and hypercalcemia of malignancy. Preliminary evidence indicates these drugs may be useful for treating bone pain from metastatic disease. Ernst et al.[362] found a statistically significant decrease in pain scores and an increase in activity level with clodronate 600 mg when compared to placebo in 24 patients with metastatic bone pain. In an open trial, Adami and Mian[363] gave clodronate 300 mg IV for 10 days to men with metastatic prostate cancer and reported notable improvement in bone pain. The use of diphosphonates for bone pain is still experimental. Future studies addressing efficacy, optimal dosing schedules, and toxicities are needed.

Routes of opioid administration The flexibility provided by many different routes of opioid administration allows the clinician to individualize a patient's analgesic regimen based on changing needs. There are five overall categories of routes of opioid administration: (1) oral, (2) parenteral (includes intramuscular, subcutaneous, and intravenous by intermittent bolus or infusion), (3) transdermal, (4) rectal, and (5) intraspinal (includes epidural, subarachnoid, and intraventricular by intermittent bolus, continuous infusion via external or implanted pumps). Each route is discussed briefly next.

Oral The oral route is an effective, comparatively inexpensive, and safe way for patients to receive opioids. Excluding oxymorphone and fentanyl, all of the opioid agonist drugs are available as oral preparations.

The oral route should be maximized for as long as possible. If a patient has an intact gastrointestinal system and can swallow the requisite number of pills or amount of liquid to achieve pain relief, then the oral route is the most appropriate route of administration.

Changing a patient to another route should be considered if high doses of oral opioids are ineffective or if toxicities occur that cannot be successfully treated. For example, if a patient has nausea with morphine, an aggressive trial of antiemetics should be tried before switching to another oral opioid or *any* parenteral route. Similarly, if a patient has received excellent pain relief with hydromorphone 12 mg PO every 4 hours and now reports increasing pain, the dose of hydromorphone should be increased as needed to achieve relief while efforts to determine the cause of the increased pain are under way. High doses of oral and parenteral opioids are common. The scheduling of oral medications should be on a fixed-interval basis[41,109] except in a few circumstances. These exceptions are: (1) initial dose titration for methadone and levorphanol,[328] (2) concomitant therapies, such as radiation and chemotherapy that may relieve pain, thus reducing the need for scheduled opioid analgesics, and (3) simultaneous scheduling with around-the-clock administration to provide for incident or breakthrough pain (this also applies to continuous infusions).

Parenteral Patients with acute pain, such as postoperative pain, often are the recipients of intermittent intramuscular or subcutaneous injections. For cancer-related pain, if a patient requires immediate pain relief and does not have peripheral or central venous access, then an occasional IM or subcutaneous injection might be indicated. Prolonged analgesic administration with multiple injections per day should be replaced with other routes that do not produce pain when drugs are administered.

Intravenous bolus is a common alternative to IM or subcutaneous injections. If scheduled bolus doses of intravenous opioids produce significant peak-and-trough effects, or if doses need to be given every 2 hours or less, then continuous parenteral infusion may be considered. Additional indications for infusional therapy are gastrointestinal problems such as uncontrollable vomiting or obstruction, inability to take the quantity of oral analgesic liquids or pills needed for pain relief, inadequate pain relief or unacceptable toxicities from intermittent bolus injections, and impracticality of frequent, repeated injections.[364]

The safety and efficacy of continuous intravenous infusions have been demonstrated.[198,364–367] Stuart et al.[366] reported in a retrospective review of 79 patients that all patients had baseline control of their pain, but 54% needed additional analgesics. The median duration of the infusion was 7 days (range 24–162 days), and the morphine dose range was 0.5–300 mg/hour. Fourteen patients experienced toxicities, which included hallucinations, sedation, respiratory depression, and diaphoresis. Ferris et al.[367] studied 135 patients receiving continuous infusions and found that 86% of the patients had good pain control without undue toxicity.

Continuous infusions provide the patient with steady blood levels of the opioid, and can avoid the potential side effects and the return of pain associated with intermittent dosing. Guidelines for initiating and managing continuous infusions have been based on clinical experience rather than on controlled studies.[364,368] These guidelines are very useful, especially since infusional parenteral therapy has become a common mode of drug delivery. A summary of these suggested guidelines is given in Table 23-18.

Continuous subcutaneous Continuous subcutaneous (SQ) infusions are alternatives to intermittent IM or subcutaneous injections and to continuous or bolus intravenous infusions if venous access is unavailable. With the availability of ambulatory, computerized infusion devices, continuous subcutaneous infusions have become a common analgesic delivery system.[369–376]

Morphine and hydromorphone have been the most commonly used opioids for subcutaneous administration. Small-gauge needles (25 or 27) are placed in the subcutaneous tissue, predominantly in the abdomen and anterior chest, but other sites can be used as well. Frequency of needle site changes has been quite variable. Reports have ranged from every 6 hours to every 21 days.[377] Brenneis et al.[375] studied 45 patients receiving subcutaneous infusions and found that the average duration of a needle remaining in place without toxicities was 7.3 days ± 5.2 (range 1–29).

For patients who are unable to use the oral route

TABLE 23-18 Suggestions for the Management of Continuous Intravenous Infusion of Opioid Drugs

1. All infusions should be administered with a flow-calibrated infusion pump.
2. Convert the patient's current opioid drugs to an equal-analgesic parenteral dose of the drug that will be used for the infusion.
3. If the drug to be used for the infusion is the same one the patient is currently receiving, divide the parenteral dose by 24 to determine the hourly infusion rate.
4. If the drug to be used for the infusion is a different drug, use only half of the parenteral dose, and then divide by 24 to determine the hourly infusion rate.
5. Administer a loading dose at the beginning of the infusion and with each increase in the infusion rate. The amount of the loading dose depends on the patient's current opioid requirements.
6. Titrate the infusion until the patient reports pain relief or unacceptable side effects. Titration may occur the following ways:
   a. Increase the infusion rate by 10%–20% every few hours if the patient is receiving close monitoring.
   b. Administer additional doses of a short-acting opioid (preferably the same drug as the infusion) every 1–2 hr as needed. Give 25%–50% of the hourly dose for PRN dosing. Increase the infusion rate every 12–24 hr by the amount equal to the total number of milligrams during the preceding period divided by the number of hours in that period. Use this method if the patient is not receiving close monitoring.

Source: Adapted from Portenoy RK: Continuous infusion of opioid drugs. *Med Clin North Am* 71:233–241, 1987.

as a result of vomiting or obstruction, lack of control with the oral route, and no venous access, this delivery system is a reasonable alternative. The system has been shown to be efficacious and safe. Toxicities have included local skin irritation, leakage, swelling, and discomfort at the needle site. Bruera et al.[374] reported that patients preferred this system for analgesic administration because they achieved better pain control and increased mobility and found it easy to administer. Moulin et al.[378] used a randomized, double-blind crossover design to compare SQ and IV hydromorhone infusions. They concluded that there were no significant differences between the two routes with regard to pain intensity, pain relief, mood, and sedation. In fact, they strongly recommended abandoning the IV route for management. In another prospective trial, Lang et al.[379] compared intermittent oral or SQ to continuous SQ and found statistically significant differences in pain relief and toxicities for the SQ route.

An important clinical issue for subcutaneous infusions is the volume and concentration of the drug infused. How do differences in volume and concentration contribute to pain relief and the occurrence of toxicities? Morphine and hydromorphone can be reconstituted to make concentrations as high as 60 mg/cc and 100 mg/cc, respectively.[380] The volume per 24 hours without the addition of substances like hyaluronidase has been reported at 24–48 cc/day.[369,374] Bruera et al.[372] reported on the successful use of hyaluronidase with a dextrose/saline solution to deliver subcutaneous hydration and opioid analgesics. The rate of infusion was 20–100 ml/hr.

Transdermal One of the newest opioid delivery systems is transdermal administration. Fentanyl, which is 75–100 times more potent than morphine, is the only opioid available via this route. It has been used in postoperative and cancer patients.[381–383] Calis et al.[384] have written an excellent review of the pharmacology, efficacy, and clinical issues related to transdermal fentanyl. Although randomized, well-controlled clinical trials using transdermal fentanyl are lacking, many open-labeled studies indicate that this delivery system provides effective pain relief.[385–388] The toxicities from transdermal fentanyl are similar to those from other opioid agonist analgesics.

There are several unique features of this delivery system that have important clinical implications. First, after removing a patch, it takes approximately 16 hours for the serum concentrations to fall 50%.[389] If patients experience significant sedation or respiratory depression, simply removing the patch does not eliminate the risk of further problems from drug toxicity. Second, variability in body temperature of 3°C can increase the serum concentrations by 25%.[390] Finally, variability in skin thickness can significantly affect serum concentrations. Thin skin can produce 1.5 times, broken skin 5 times, the normal serum value. Thus, an individual with thick skin may have less drug absorbed.[390] Payne[391] presented important clinical guidelines for using transdermal fentanyl, including the following: (1) follow similar principles for chronic opioid use; (2) use in patients with stable baseline pain and minimal incident pain; (3) provide liberal rescue analgesia, especially during the first 24 hours; (4) use rescue doses to calculate dose increases; (5) rotate skin sites; (6) clarify patient and family expectations; and (7) allow several weeks for therapeutic trial. Advantages and disadvantages of transdermal fentanyl are highlighted in Table 23-19.

Rectal With the advent of transdermal fentanyl and sophisticated pump technology, the use of the rectal route may not be as common an alternative to orally administered analgesics. There are rectal preparations available for nonopioids (e.g., acetaminophen, aspirin, indomethacin) and opioids (e.g., morphine, hydromorphone, oxymorphone).

Controlled trials using the rectal route of administration are lacking. Bioavailability of rectally administered morphine has been reported to be 31%–53.3%.[392–394] Exactly when the rectal route should be selected for patient use from all the available routes is unclear. Although there are three opioid agonist products commercially available, they do not allow flexibility in titration. For example, hydromorphone comes in 3-mg strengths, so patients who require high doses of hydromorphone would potentially need more suppos-

TABLE 23-19 Advantages and Disadvantages of Transdermal Fentanyl

Advantages	Disadvantages
FENTANYL TO ORAL	
• Convenient	• More expensive
• Continuous delivery	• Slower onset
• Long duration	• Slower titration
	• Difficult to reverse side effects immediately
FENTANYL TO IV/SQ	
• Less invasive	• Slower onset
• No needles or pumps	• Slower titration
• Less expensive	• Difficult to reverse side effects immediately
• Easy for caregiver	
• Requires less technical nursing time	• More experience with pump delivery systems

Sources: Data from Calis, Kohler, and Corso[384] and Payne.[391]

itories per dose. Similarly, even though morphine is available in 10-, 20-, and 30-mg strengths, the same problem for patients who require high doses occurs with morphine. Controlled-release morphine designed for rectal administration has been studied,[395] but it is not FDA-approved for rectal use. Cole and Hanning[396] described the advantages and disadvantages of the rectal route of opioid administration, which are summarized in Table 23-20.

Intraspinal The identification of opiate receptors in the brain and spinal cord[397] and the results of early animal work involving spinal opioids[398] provided the bases for the use of intraspinal opioid administration for cancer pain. One of the earliest studies demonstrated complete pain relief for a mean of 15 hours after a single 0.5-mg injection of morphine,[399] indicating that epidural opioids could provide analgesia without sensory, motor, or sympathetic involvement. Subsequent work revealed similar findings for low-dose administration and prolonged pain relief. Many later studies have demonstrated that patients require higher doses of opioid to achieve pain relief.[400–403] Plummer et al.[403] reported that in 284 cancer patients receiving intraspinal morphine, the minimum starting doses were 0.5–200 mg/day, the maximum doses were 1–3072 mg/day, not all patients responded to intraspinal administration.[400,404,405]

Max et al.[405] gave possible explanations for patients receiving pain relief of brief duration: (1) the patients had been on high doses of systemic analgesics prior to intraspinal administration; and (2) the patients also had neuropathic pain problems that did not respond well to opioids.

Arner and Arner[402] presented a hierarchy of response to intraspinal analgesic from different pain problems. From best response to least response these are: (1) somatic continuous pain, (2) visceral continuous pain, (3) somatic intermittent pain, (4) visceral intermittent pain, (5) neuropathic pain, either intermittent or continuous, and (6) cutaneous pain.

Morphine and fentanyl have been the most common agents used for intraspinal opioid administration. The combination of anesthetic agents such as bupivacaine and opioids has been used, especially in patients who have not been treated successfully with opioids alone.[406–408] Anesthetic agents, which act in part by reducing cell membrane permeability to sodium ions, act directly on the nerve roots.[409] Although there are added risks of motor, sensory, and sympathetic complications, the use of anesthetic agents can provide patients with effective pain relief.

TABLE 23-20 Advantages and Disadvantages of Rectal Opioid Administration

Advantages	Disadvantages
• Absorption is not delayed by alterations in GI tract, such as vomiting	• Wide variation in systemic availability
• Useful if patients have difficulty swallowing, are unconscious, or NPO	• Delayed or limited absorption due to small surface area
• Drug can be removed if an adverse drug reaction develops	• Defecation or constipation may impair absorption
• Digestive enzymes do not affect drug breakdown	• Rectal-wall enzymes or microorganisms may degrade drug
• No unpleasant taste	• Invasive
• Significant first-pass effect from the liver may be avoided	• Self-medication may be difficult or impossible
• Easier to learn than sophisticated pump technology	
• Low cost	

Source: Cole and Hanning.[396]

Criteria for determining the appropriateness of a patient for intraspinal opioids include:[409–413]

1. opioid-responsive pain, but unacceptable toxicities from systemic opioids
2. pain below the midcervical dermatome
3. neuroablative or anesthetic procedures unsuccessful or not indicated
4. life expectancy of more than 3 months
5. satisfactory home and family support
6. successful response to trial of opioids or anesthetic agent through temporary catheter

Penn and Paice[412] evaluated response to temporary catheter placement by assessing (1) decrease in systemic opioids, (2) degree of pain relief, and (3) improvement in activity level. Responses were categorized as excellent, good, poor, or failure.

Intraspinal opioids can be administered by an externally placed catheter, subcutaneous catheter with a reservoir or a port for injection (either as a bolus injection or continuous infusion), and a totally implantable pump as a continuous infusion. Factors that determine which type of system is used include life expectancy, clinician expertise, opioid and anesthetic needs, home care needs, and cost. For example, Bedder et al.[414] compared an external tunneled catheter to an implantable pump and found that the initial costs were approximately $6000 less for the external catheter; but at 6 months and 12 months, the implantable pump cost was approximately $4000 and $13,000 less, respectively.

Toxicities from these different techniques may include equipment-related problems, such as dislodgement, obstruction or occlusion, breakage, leakage from the catheter, and leakage of CSF. They may also include drug-related problems, such as urinary retention, pruritus, nausea, vomiting, and respiratory depression. The risk of infection is possible with all types of delivery systems. DuPen et al.[415] reported a 5.4% incidence of infection (1 per 1702 catheter days). The majority of the reported infections were exit-site or superficial epidural track infections. Catheters were removed only if a patient had a positive culture or an infection was present in the epidural space.

In addition to epidural and intrathecal opioid administration, the intraventricular route has been used. A catheter is placed in the frontal horn of the lateral ventricle, and an Ommaya reservoir is used for the injection site. Intraventricular opioids also have been given via an implanted pump.[416] Published reports indicated that patients obtain effective pain relief.[417–420] Toxicities have included somnolence, disorientation, hallucinations, pruritus, nausea, vomiting, respiratory depression, and dizziness. The intraventricular route for opioid administration is used infrequently and is considered experimental.

The basic knowledge nurses need to take care of patients receiving intraspinal opioids has been described.[421] This knowledge should include anatomy and physiology related to the neuroaxis, pharmacology of all agents, and potential complications related to type of procedure and agents used. Guidelines for patient monitoring, drug administration, and protocols involving potential complications and emergency situations need to be in place.

The nursing care of patients receiving intraspinal opioids can be divided into three major steps. The first step occurs before temporary catheter placement. The appropriateness of the therapy is determined, as discussed earlier. The patient and family have significant informational needs about the procedure, required diagnostic tests, costs, possible expected outcomes, alternatives, and home care requirements. Assessment, documentation, and evaluation of interventions at this time is important, since the patient is experiencing unrelieved pain or unacceptable toxicities or both.

The second step occurs after temporary catheter placement. During this time attempts to determine the effectiveness of the opioid or anesthetic agent occur. Olsson et al.[422] and Paice[423] have described care plans for patients receiving intraspinal opioids that include nursing diagnoses, patient outcomes, and nursing interventions. The nursing diagnoses include: (1) potential alteration in respiratory function; (2) potential alteration in comfort related to pruritus, nausea, vomiting, pain on injection, and inadequate pain relief; (3) potential alteration in elimination (urinary); (4) knowledge deficit regarding epidural analgesia; and (5) potential infection at the catheter site. At the end of this step a decision about inserting a permanent catheter or an implantable pump is made.

The final step occurs after a permanent device has been placed. In addition to the nursing care described in step 2, significant attention is given to optimizing the patient's dose in anticipation of discharge from the hospital. Plans for follow-up, outpatient management, and coordination of home care activities are critically important for the patient, who now has new equipment.

Patient-controlled analgesia Patient-controlled analgesia (PCA) has been used in patients who receive analgesics via the parenteral route and the epidural route. PCA has been used in postoperative patients since 1968,[424] but its use in cancer patients has been limited primarily to the last 10 years. PCA is designed to allow the patient to self-administer analgesics within preset programming parameters from special infusion pumps. Originally developed as a response to inadequate analgesic management in postoperative patients, PCA gives patients some independence in their care, allows individual response to analgesics to determine the amount of drug a patient will receive, and eliminates the usual lag time inherent in nurse-administered analgesics.

PCA is designed to avoid the peaks and troughs of conventional PRN parenteral administration.[425] PCA can be used in either of two ways: (1) bolus dosing only, or (2) bolus dosing with continuous infusion. Many pumps provide continuous infusion only as an option, which would be similar to standard infusion pumps.

The routes for PCA can be intravenous, subcutaneous, and epidural. Citron et al.[426] used intravenous PCA and subcutaneous PCA in 12 patients and found it to be safe and effective in both inpatients and outpatients. Bauman et al.[427] used PCA requirements to change patients to oral analgesic regimens. They also found PCA to be safe and efficacious. Even though patients used PCA more in the first 4 hours of administration than at any other time period, Citron et al.[426] reported no significant respiratory depression and sedation during the initial 4 hours.

PCA has also been successfully used in adolescents and adults to treat severe mucositis pain from the preparative regimen for a bone marrow transplantation.[428,429] Bruera et al.[430] reported similar efficacy and toxicity with subcutaneous PCA and subcutaneous continuous infusions in 22 patients. Each PCA bolus dose was equivalent to 4 hours of the infusion. Kerr et al.[431] reported that patients had improvement in pain control using PCA with subcutaneous and intravenous opioid infusions. Maximum hourly doses for the opioids in the study were hydromorphone 60 mg, morphine 80 mg, and meperidine 50 mg. Grochow et al.[432] used PCA to examine an unrelated research question concerning the duration of analgesia between intravenous methadone and morphine. The time between a patient's request and a nurse's administering the analgesic needed to be eliminated as a variable in the study. In a single-blind randomized study comparing PCA with and without continuous infusion in postoperative cancer patients, Hansen et al.[433] reported no significant differences between the two groups with regard to pain relief and sedation.

Sophisticated computer technology and demonstrated efficacy and safety have contributed to clinicians more commonly using PCA pumps in inpatient and outpatient settings. Ferrell et al.[434] identified some appropriate uses of PCA: (1) when the oral route is not available; (2) when the patient may benefit from increased self-control; and (3) as a useful modality for break-through pain. They also identified several inappropriate uses of PCA: (1) contraindicated in the sedated and confused patient; (2) when the oral route is inadequately tested; (3) potential conflict of interest if the owners of the equipment and the prescribers of the therapy are the same; (4) use only if it saves time; and (5) when there is inadequate training of staff.

The issues of appropriate use of PCA are only one aspect of a broader dilemma involving the use of technology in pain management. An ONS resolution addressing the appropriate use of technology in pain management included the use of intraspinal, intravenous, and subcutaneous infusions.[435] The resolution addressed the significant financial, physical, and psychologic burden that the use of high-tech therapies have on the patient and family. Although no one would argue that all patients are unequivocally entitled to receive pain relief, the process of selecting the methods to provide such relief is the issue. Ferrell and Rhiner[95] have used a biomedical ethical perspective in approaching this problem. The principles of autonomy, beneficence, nonmaleficence, and justice are relevant to the decisions whether to use high-tech therapies. Whedon and Ferrell[96] presented seven cases that involved the use of sophisticated therapies. These cases addressed the issues of patient selection, the need for a thorough assessment in determining the appropriateness of a treatment, informed consent, cost, family burden, conflict of interests, and morbidity. Indiscriminate use of therapies without clear indications and criteria is a major concern.

Nurses do not make the ultimate decision about whether a patient receives a specific high-tech therapy, but they are in a position to know what the benefits, risks, costs, and suitability are for an individual patient. Consider the following example. A patient is unable to take oral medications; the rectal route is not feasible; the patient does not have peripheral or central venous access; and the patient and family are worried about costs. Two potential alternatives to high-tech therapies can be considered. One option is the use of the subcutaneous route for doses every 4 hours of an opioid through the same administration set. For example, hydromorphone 10 mg (1 cc) SQ every 4 hours can be given through the same needle administration set, which is changed once or twice a week. Another option, if a continuous infusion is required to avoid fluctuating blood levels, is the use of the transdermal route with fentanyl and the subcutaneous route for intermittent PRN doses for break-through or incident pain.

Regardless of the analgesic a patient receives or the route through which it is administered, nurses have a pivotal role in assuring adequate management. The obstacles to successful cancer pain management are entrenched in issues related to analgesics. Nurses must have a solid foundation in the pharmacology of analgesics in order to assess the effectiveness of an individual regimen. This content includes knowing the commonly used analgesics and understanding duration of action, dosing schedules, equal analgesic doses and drugs, and side effects. Nurses need effective communication skills in conveying appropriate information about a patient's pain to physicians, other nurses, and other health care providers.

Anesthetic and neurosurgical modalities

Anesthetic, or nerve-block, procedures for cancer-related pain help modulate a patient's neural responses to noxious stimuli.[436] According to Swerdlow,[437] proper use of analgesic drugs should necessitate the use of nerve blocks in 20% of patients with cancer pain. Local anesthetic agents prevent generation and conduction of nerve impulses.[438] The use of these agents, in addition to agents used for neurolytic blocks, makes up the major focus of anesthetic interventions.

Nondestructive nerve blocks serve two functions: (1) they are used for treatment of intractable pain such as neuropathic pain caused by invasion or compression of intraspinal nerve roots; and (2) they are used for prognostic/diagnostic purposes in which they help differentiate between visceral and somatic pain, demonstrate neural pathways for individual problems, and help predict the efficacy of more permanent neuroablative procedures.[436]

Neurolytic (destructive) nerve blocks can lead to more prolonged pain relief than nondestructive nerve blocks. They are used in conjunction with other therapies, for they often do not provide complete pain relief.[437]

Three categorical criteria can be used for determining the appropriateness of a patient for a neurolytic block:[439]

- *Physiological*—evaluate the extent of disease, know the pathophysiology of the pain syndrome.
- *Cognitive*—explain risks, benefits to both the patient and the family.
- *Functional*—the benefit of loss of function in performing the procedure.

The choices of neuroablative procedures are based on anatomy and type of pain (nociceptive versus deafferentation). For example, patients with nociceptive or deafferentation pain arising from the abdominal viscera, as with pancreatic cancer, may benefit from a celiac plexus block.[439]

Destructive neurosurgical procedures most often are used when standard pharmacologic and nonpharmacologic strategies are no longer effective. Patients are carefully selected for these procedures due to the potential motor and sensory losses associated with their use. Common neurosurgical procedures are as follows:

- *Peripheral neurotomy*—destroys sensory modalities from peripheral nerve; not recommended for pain in extremities.
- *Rhizotomy*—eliminates all sensation entering dorsal spinal cord; preserves motor function; percutaneous procedure an option for debilitated patients.
- *Cordotomy*—involves interruption of ascending pain and temperature fibers in anterolateral spinal cord; preserves major sensory function; good for unilateral pain.
- *Myelotomy*—interrupts pain and temperature fibers as they cross before reaching opposite spinothalamic tract; used for bilateral pain.[440]

The nursing responsibilities for patients undergoing anesthetic and neurodestructive procedures include: (1) knowledge about the purpose of the procedure and how it is performed; (2) potential complications based on type of block, agent, and location; and (3) potential benefit of the procedure. An efficient way of obtaining some of this information is to participate in the explanation of the procedure to the patient and to talk with the anesthesiologist or neurosurgeon. Since this requisite information is based on the patient's individual pain problem, standard reference materials may provide incomplete information. The Core Curriculum for Neuroscience Nursing is a useful resource for patients undergoing neurodestructive procedures.[441]

Diminishing the Emotional and Reactive Components of Pain

Interventions included in this approach to management of cancer pain are those that do not affect the underlying pathology or alter the perception or sensation of pain but, rather, help in a variety of ways to decrease emotional reactions to pain. A recent review article discussed psychiatric complications in cancer patients with pain and their management; but since this content is beyond the scope of this chapter, the reader is referred to the article.[51] The nonpsychiatric, nonpharmacologic strategies encompassed in this major treatment approach are those that help individuals cope with their pain in a positive and proactive way.

It has long been known that both physicians and nurses have little information about nonpsychiatric, nonpharmacologic interventions; in fact, one survey[442] revealed that individuals with cancer had a greater awareness of them than did their health care providers. This same survey also indicated that respondents found the techniques helpful at reducing pain.

Aside from being little understood or used, the efficacy of these interventions has rarely been studied in a controlled way in the clinical environment.[443] The majority of evidence for their usefulness in treating cancer pain come from anecdotal reports. Although there are a number of methodologic and logistical difficulties inherent in conducting nonpharmacologic intervention studies with cancer patients,[444] there is still a need to describe and evaluate in a systematic way their usefulness in management of cancer pain. In particular, information is lacking about how they are best used in conjunction with pharmacologic approaches to therapy.

The role of these techniques is clearly that of an adjuvant to standard pharmacologic therapy.[445] Drugs are used to treat the somatic (physiologic and sensory) dimensions of pain, while nondrug methods are aimed at treating the affective, cognitive, behavioral, and sociocultural dimensions of pain. The benefits of many of the techniques are that they may increase sense of personal control, reduce feelings of helplessness, provide opportunities to become actively involved in care, reduce stress and anxiety, elevate mood, raise pain threshold, and thereby reduce pain.

Mayer[446] reviewed nonpharmacologic interventions, stressing that many of them were ideal components of nursing practice because they were within the average nurse's qualifications, did not require special equipment, were not subject to a physician's prescription or approval, did not interfere with standard medical therapies, and did not require informed consent. Indeed, these types of interventions are the major foci of clinical nursing texts dealing with pain management.[160,447]

Some of the treatment strategies aimed at diminishing the emotional and reactive components of pain are classified as cognitive, behavioral, or cognitive *and* behavioral techniques. *Cognitive* methods are those that attempt directly to modify thought processes in order to attenuate or relieve pain; they can be applied to thoughts, images, and attitudes. Examples include information, distraction, imagery, calming self-statements, identification of detrimental responses to pain, and informational or educational programs about pain and its management. *Behavioral* methods are those that modify physiologic reactions to pain or behavioral manifestations of pain. Examples include relaxation, meditation, music therapy, biofeedback, hypnosis, and various desensitization strategies. Sometimes both cognitive and behavioral techniques are used simultaneously. Relaxation with guided imagery is one example.

Another group of interventions that diminish the emotional and reactive components of pain are those that provide counterirritant cutaneous stimulation; examples include menthol ointments, heat, cold, and massage. Although these methods fall within the major treatment approach of changing perception or sensation of pain, they are included here because they are behavioral interventions that clearly are within the scope of nursing practice.

Another category of interventions that change perception or sensation of pain but also diminish affective reactions and are considered behavioral in nature uses mobility and/or immobilization as the basis of nursing actions. Most of these interventions are simple and can be initiated when ongoing assessment of pain suggests a need for them. In each of the following sections, selected interventions are briefly discussed, including the research evidence supporting their efficacy in cancer pain.

Counterirritant cutaneous stimulation

This group of methods is thought to help relieve pain by somehow physiologically altering the transmission of nociceptive stimuli; these methods are based on the gate control theory of pain. Mentholated ointments are rubbed onto the skin in a painful area; heat is applied with hot packs, a heating pad, a hot water bottle, or a shower or bath; cold is applied with cold packs, cold cloths, ice, gel packs, or cold water; massage is applied with fingers, hands, or various devices; transcutaneous electrical nerve stimulation is administered by placing electrodes on selected areas of the body, depending on location of pain. Some of these methods are home remedies used very frequently by many people with pain, and combinations are common (e.g., massage with mentholated ointment). The relief achieved may outlast the actual application of the counterirritant. Most of the research that used these methods is descriptive in nature,[58,63,64] although one fairly recent experimental study suggested that massage was an effective short-term intervention in male cancer patients with pain.[448]

The use of transcutaneous electrical nerve stimulation (TENS) in cancer pain has been studied infrequently. In one study,[449] beneficial effects from TENS were noted in two-thirds of the patients initially, but over time efficacy diminished. In another other study,[450] 37 patients were studied for a maximum of 30 days. There was a 96% marked reduction in pain intensity initially in those using TENS, but after 30 days there was only an 11% reduction. They reported that TENS was more effective in patients with head and neck pain and phantom limb pain.

Immobilization/mobilization

Even when good pharmacologic therapy has been instituted, some individuals may still experience pain on movement. Methods such as complete or partial immobilization of the body or parts of the body and positioning of specific body parts may be quite helpful. In other circumstances, mild exercise may help decrease pain, taking forms such as joint range of motion and stretching. And finally, rest or lying down may help in some instances, perhaps partly because of the relaxation that occurs. Again, the existing research is primarily descriptive[58,64] but does indicate benefit from these methods. One recent study examined the use of clinitron therapy and found it effective in promoting comfort in selected cancer patients.[451]

Distraction

Distraction is "directing one's attention away from the sensations or emotional reactions produced by a noxious stimulus; block[ing] awareness of the pain stimulus or its effects."[452] Distraction can be significantly helpful in reducing pain. A classic example is the focusing exercises (accompanied by relaxation techniques) taught in childbirth education classes. There are many individual distraction techniques and strategies; examples include conversation, verbalization to self or others, deep thinking, visualization and imagery, mind–body separation, routines/rituals, breathing exercises, counting, reading, and watching television. Caregivers do not always realize the broad scope and variety of distractive strategies; some may work for one individual and not for another.

The research that examines the methods just described falls into two categories—studies that asked patients to report what they used to help control cancer pain, and studies that used structured scales or questionnaires to collect this information. In the first group, several studies of both cancer inpatients and outpatients with pain[16,39,63–65,442] revealed that strategies such as heat, cold, distraction (including reading and television), relaxation, position change, exercise, inactivity, and massage helped to reduce pain to some degree. In one study that used a structured questionnaire to ascertain coping strategies,[17] patients with cancer pain employed a variety of cognitive and behavioral coping techniques (ignoring pain, reinterpreting the sensation, increasing physical activity, etc.) and rated them as moderately effective at reducing pain. Several other recent studies reported similar findings.[53,58,59]

Relaxation and guided imagery

Relaxation training helps produce physiologic and mental relaxation. The two most common methods are progressive muscle relaxation, which is the systematic tensing/relaxing of 16 muscle groups, and autogenic relaxation, which is the passive, quiet, and still use of autogenic phrases such as "my arms are warm and heavy." Training usually occurs in six to ten sessions with a therapist. Audiotapes can be used at home afterwards, and individuals are encouraged to practice and use their new skills. Guided imagery, in which an individual visualizes pleasant places or things, is frequently used in conjunction with relaxation.

The literature on these techniques in the cancer patient population is scanty. Bayuk[453] provided anecdotal evidence of the helpfulness of relaxation in a group of bone marrow transplant patients. Additionally, she emphasized the importance of establishing rapport prior to using the technique, educating patients, involving friends and family, and advising practice and use of skills. One study of relaxation as an intervention[83] found that patients who used relaxation or relaxation in combination with distraction reported mild to quite good or complete relief of pain. Another study[454] found that taped transcripts using guided imagery or progressive muscle relaxation were equally effective in reducing pain and distress. These two studies had small samples and methodologic problems, and little further research in this area has been published to date, so there is still a need to investigate the efficacy of these methods at reducing cancer pain, particularly when used with opioid analgesics.

Biofeedback

Biofeedback is "a process in which a person learns to reliably influence physiological responses of two kinds: either responses that are not ordinarily under voluntary control or responses that ordinarily are easy to regulate but regulation has broken down because of trauma or disease.[11,455] There are several biofeedback techniques, electromyography being the most common. It is taught in six to ten sessions and often combined with relaxation. The purpose of the technique is to decrease muscle tension and/or sympathetically mediated responses, such as vasoconstriction, that might produce or worsen pain. A decrease in variables that amplify pain (e.g., anxiety) may occur as well. Only a few studies have examined systematically the effects of biofeedback, one of them with relaxation as well.[456–458] Although biofeedback appeared helpful in the hospital setting, patients found it difficult to use at home, and the merits of its use are still unclear.

Hypnosis

Hypnosis is "a state of aroused, attentive focal concentration with a relative suspension of peripheral awareness."[459] It has been used for many years to relieve pain, relax muscles, and facilitate healing. When employed as a psychotherapeutic tool it can help alleviate symptoms, uncover forgotten memories, and facilitate behavioral changes. While an individual is under hypnosis, there are perceptual, motor, and cognitive alterations. With the help of a therapist or on one's own, several hypnotic strategies can be used for cancer pain: (1) block the pain from awareness; (2) substitute another sensation; (3) move pain to a smaller/less important area; (4) change the meaning of pain; (5) increase pain tolerance; or (6) dissociate part of the body from awareness.[460]

Although hypnosis has been in use for many years, the studies supporting its efficacy are fairly old, and are hindered by small sample sizes and nonexperimental designs. In a review of these studies, Twycross and Lack[41] concluded that most patients showed reduced pain using hypnosis. In an early prospective, controlled study of women with pain from metastatic breast cancer,[461] self-hypnosis training used in conjunction with a psychologic support group decreased pain and improved mood. This study was fraught with attrition problems and variable pain experiences (e.g., 41% of patients had no pain at the start of the study but developed it later), but it did provide beginning evidence for the helpfulness of hypnosis. A recent study using hypnosis and cognitive behavioral training in bone marrow transplantation patients suggested that hypnosis was effective in reducing reported oral pain due to mucositis.[462] More research on these techniques, however, is clearly needed.

Comprehensive cognitive/behavioral methods

Several individuals have proposed comprehensive cognitive and behavioral "treatment" packages for cancer pain. These proposals are based on cognitive and social learning models in which pain can be described in terms of objective qualities (e.g., location and intensity) and psychological significance. In Turk and Rennert's cognitive-social learning approach,[463] the goal is to help individuals modify thoughts, beliefs, or actions/behaviors that may exacerbate pain, depression, and anxiety, and to provide them with specific skills to cope with pain. There are unfortunately no data as yet on the efficacy of this treatment approach. In Fishman and Loscalzo's cognitive-behavior "specialized psychological approach,"[464] therapists provide short-term therapeutic interventions that are adaptable to the individual, with goals similar to those of Turk and Rennert.[463] Fishman and Loscalzo stated that their approach "can be very useful for both short-term and prolonged supportive care of cancer patients with pain" but provided only one case study as evidence. Another small body of work suggests that cognitive, educational treatment approaches are successful in helping patients better understand and adhere to pharmacologic treatment regimens.[57]

Miscellaneous methods

Other methods exist that diminish the emotional and reactive components of pain, and these include music therapy[465,466] and laughter therapy.[467] Almost no research exists to support their efficacy in relieving pain, although Beck's study[466] supported the use of music as an independent nursing intervention. Her sample, however, was very small, and the effects of analgesics were not controlled for. Clearly, additional research is needed in this area.

Summary and nursing implications

In summary, the evidence available from primarily descriptive research indicates that many of the nonpharmacologic, independent nursing techniques just described may be useful in alleviating cancer pain. The majority of these techniques are familiar to nurses or may be easily learned and are conducive to use in a variety of settings. References available to help nurses learn and understand these methods include heat, cold, and other cutaneous measures;[160,468,469] relaxation and imagery;[160,470–473] and distraction, including music therapy.[160,474,475] Many of these techniques require patient

TABLE 23-21 Use of Common Nursing Interventions for Pain

Intervention	Advantages/Disadvantages	Techniques
Cutaneous stimulation	*Adv:* Many methods available; eliminates or decreases pain sometimes after stimulation has stopped; produces relaxation and distraction. *Disadv:* May be viewed as curative; effects underestimated; tissue damage could occur; mild stimulation yields only mild pain relief	Superficial massage, pressure massage, vibration, superficial heat and cold, ice application and massage, menthol application to skin, transcutaneous electrical nerve stimulation (TENS)
Distraction	*Adv:* Increases pain tolerance; makes quality of pain more acceptable; improves mood and allows focusing on other things; gives sense of control *Disadv:* Effective use can cause others to doubt presence of pain; pain may recur or increase when distraction ceases, along with more fatigue and irritability; patient needs pain relief measure that allows rest (eg, analgesic) and that staff may be reluctant to give	Reading, watching TV, talking, singing/humming, rhyming, counting, word games, tactile/touch, rhythm, music, coping self-statements; try for auditory, visual, tactile, kinesthetic methods to stimulate all sensory modalities
Relaxation	*Adv:* Decreases oxygen consumption, respiratory rate, heart rate, and muscle tension; helps maintain normal blood pressure; increases alpha waves; aids sleep; helps decrease stress; improves problem solving; increases confidence and self-control; decreases fatigue; distracts from pain; increases effects of other pain treatments; elevates mood; decreases distress *Disadv:* People think they are relaxed when they are not; some have trouble accepting it or connect it with "psychologic" pain; it is *not* a substitute for drugs; it may not help with very severe pain; must be highly individualized for patient; and sometimes will not work at all	Deep-breathe/tense, exhale/relax; yawn; humor for relaxation; heartbeat breathing; jaw relaxation; slow, rhythmic breathing; peaceful past experiences; meditative relaxation script; progressive relaxation script; simple touch, massage, or warmth
Imagery	*Adv:* Forms and strengthens nurse–patient relationship; assists expressions about pain, exploration/understanding of pain and illness beliefs; increases confidence in ability to control pain; increases effects of other measures; decreases intensity of pain or changes sensation to more acceptable one *Disadv:* May connect it with "psychologic" pain; not a substitute for standard measures; not well accepted by all health care givers; unwanted side effects can occur; trial and error; does not work for all; time-consuming; emotionally exhausting	Subtle conversation; simple, brief symptom substitution; standardized imagery techniques; systematically individualized imagery techniques

Source: Adapted with permission from McCaffery M, Beebe A: *Pain: Clinical Manual for Nursing Practice.* St. Louis: Mosby, 1989.

and family education, and a willingness to try them as adjuncts to pharmacologic therapy. Finally, interventions such as hypnosis and biofeedback require specialized training and/or specific equipment and are best left to individuals who have or can obtain such training and equipment.

Table 23-21 presents the most commonly used nursing interventions for decreasing the emotional and reactive components of pain, along with advantages, disadvantages, and information on specific techniques. For more detail and clinical examples, the reader is referred to McCaffery and Beebe's excellent clinical manual on pain, especially Chapters 5–8.[160] In most cases, the use of these nonpharmacologic, distress-reducing interventions requires considerably more evaluation to determine efficacy in conjunction with analgesics.

CONCLUSIONS AND FUTURE DIRECTIONS

In this chapter the multidimensional phenomenon of cancer pain was presented, with special reference to the physiologic, sensory, affective, cognitive, behavioral, and sociocultural aspects of the experience. The importance of a multidisciplinary approach to management has been emphasized, with particular attention to the pivotal role of the nurse in this process. Various strategies for managing cancer pain have been presented, some of which call for more nursing involvement than others. Clearly, a great deal of information is readily available for nurses and other health professionals to use in achieving the best possible care for individuals with cancer pain. The challenge for the future is to utilize this knowledge to its fullest, to continue experimenting with new ways to treat pain, and to share the information gained with colleagues.

REFERENCES

1. Livingston WK: *Pain Mechanisms: A Physiologic Interpretation of Causalgia and Its Related States.* New York: Macmillan, 1943.
2. Melzack R, Wall PD: *The Challenge of Pain.* New York: Basic Books, 1982.
3. International Association for the Study of Pain Subcommittee on Taxonomy: Pain terms: A list with definitions and usage. *Pain* 6:249–252, 1979.
4. Bouckoms AJ: Recent developments in the classification of pain. *Psychosom* 26:637–642, 645, 1985.
5. International Association for the Study of Pain: Pain terms: A current list with definitions and notes on usage. *Pain* 3:S216–S221, 1986, (suppl.).
6. Turk DC, Rudy TE: IASP taxonomy of chronic pain syndromes: Preliminary assessment of reliability. *Pain* 30:177–189, 1987.
7. Brose WG, Cherry DA, Plummer J, et al: IASP taxonomy: Questions and controversies. In Bond MR, Charlton JE, Woolf CJ (eds.): *Proceedings of the VIth World Congress on Pain.* Amsterdam: Elsevier, 1991, pp. 503–507.
8. Bonica JJ: Definitions and taxonomy of pain. In Bonica JJ (ed.): *The Management of Pain,* Vol. 1, (ed. 2). Philadelphia: Lea & Febiger, 1990, pp. 18–27.
9. Price DD: *Psychological and Neural Mechanisms of Pain.* New York: Raven Press, 1988.
10. Melzack R, Wall PD: Pain mechanisms: A new theory. *Science* 150:971–979, 1965.
11. Melzack R, Wall, P: *The Challenge of Pain* (rev. ed.). London: Penguin, 1988.
12. Fields HL: *Pain.* New York: McGraw-Hill, 1987.
13. Bonica JJ (ed.): *The Management of Pain* (ed. 2). Philadelphia: Lea & Febiger, 1990.
14. Wall PD, Melzack R: *Textbook of Pain* (ed. 2). New York: Churchill Livingstone, 1989.
15. Ahles TA, Blanchard EB, Ruckdeschel JC: The multidimensional nature of cancer-related pain. *Pain* 17:277–288, 1983.
16. McGuire DB: Cancer-related pain: A multidimensional approach. *Dissert Abstr Internatl* 48(03), SecB:705, 1987.
17. McGuire DB: Coping strategies used by cancer patients with pain. *Oncol Nurs Forum* 14:123, 1987 (abstr.).
18. McGuire DB: The multidimensional phenomenon of cancer pain. In McGuire DB, Yarbro CH (eds.): *Cancer Pain Management.* Philadelphia: Saunders, 1987, pp. 1–20.
19. National Center for Nursing Research: *National Nursing Research Agenda: Volume 2. Symptom Management.* Bethesda, MD: NIH, U.S. Public Health Service, U.S. Department of Health and Human Services (in press).
20. Foley KN: Pain syndromes in patients with cancer. In Bonica JJ, Ventafridda V (eds.): *Advances in Pain Research and Therapy,* Vol. 2. New York: Raven Press, 1979, pp. 59–75.
21. Coyle N, Foley K: Prevalence and profile of pain syndromes in cancer patients. In McGuire DB, Yarbro CH (eds.): *Cancer Pain Management.* Philadelphia: Saunders, 1987, pp. 21–46.
22. Chapman CR, Kornell J, Syrjala K: Painful complications of cancer diagnosis and therapy. In McGuire DB, Yarbro CH (eds.): *Cancer Pain Management.* Philadelphia: Saunders, 1987, pp. 47–67.
23. Schreml W: Pain in the cancer patient as a consequence of therapy (surgery, radiotherapy, chemotherapy). *Rec Res Cancer Res* 89:85–99, 1984.
24. Gaston-Johansson F, Franco T, Zimmerman L: Pain and psychological distress in patients undergoing autologous bone marrow transplantation. *Oncol Nurs Forum* 19:41–48, 1992.
25. Altomonte V, McGuire DB, Peterson DE, et al: Patterns of mucositis and pain in patients receiving preparative chemotherapy and bone marrow transplantation. *Oncol Nurs Forum* 19:298, 1992, (abstr.).
26. Shivnan JC, Sheidler VR: Pain associated with bone marrow transplantation: Unique features and treatments. *Oncol Nurs Forum* 19:319, 1992 (abstr.).
27. Sutters KA, Miaskowski C: The problem of pain in children with cancer: A research review. *Oncol Nurs Forum* 19:465–471, 1992.
28. Patterson KL: Pain in the pediatric oncology patient. *J Ped Oncol Nurs* 9:119–130, 1992.

29. Portenoy RK: Cancer pain: Epidemiology and syndromes. *Cancer* 63:2298–2307, 1989.
30. Payne R: Cancer pain: Anatomy, physiology, and pharmacology. *Cancer* 63:2266–2274, 1989.
31. Kelly JB, Payne R: Pain syndromes in the cancer patient. *Neurol Clin* 9:937–953, 1991.
32. Banning A, Sjogren P, Henriksen H: Pain causes in 200 patients referred to a multidisciplinary cancer pain clinic. *Pain* 45:45–48, 1991.
33. Samuelsson H, Hedner T: Pain characterization in cancer patients and the analgetic response to epidural morphine. *Pain* 46:3–8, 1991.
34. Melzack R: The McGill Pain Questionnaire: Major properties and scoring methods. *Pain* 1:277–299, 1975.
35. McGuire DB: Assessment of pain in cancer inpatients using the McGill Pain Questionnaire. *Oncol Nurs Forum* 11:32–37, 1984.
36. Nicholson B, McGuire DB, Maurer VE: Assessment of pain in head and neck cancer patients using the McGill Pain Questionnaire. *The Journal* (official journal of the Society of Otorhinolaryngology and Head-Neck Nurses) 6:8–12, 1988.
37. Graham C, Bond SS, Gerkovich MM, et al: Use of the McGill Pain Questionnaire in the assessment of cancer pain: Replicability and consistency. *Pain* 8:377–387, 1980.
38. Arathuzik D: Pain experience for metastatic breast cancer patients. *Cancer Nurs* 14:41–48, 1991.
39. Donovan MI, Dillon P: Incidence and characteristics of pain in a sample of hospitalized cancer patients. *Cancer Nurs* 10:85–92, 1987.
40. Twycross RG, Fairfield S: Pain in far-advanced cancer. *Pain* 14:303–310, 1982.
41. Twycross RG, Lack SA: *Symptom Control in Far-Advanced Cancer: Pain Relief.* London: Pitman, 1983.
42. Melzack R, Torgerson WS: On the language of pain. *Anesthesiol* 34:50–59, 1971.
43. Dubuisson D, Melzack R: Classification of clinical pain descriptions by multiple group discriminant analysis. *Exp Neurol* 51:480–487, 1976.
44. Bressler LR, Hange PA, McGuire DB: Characterization of the pain experience in a sample of cancer outpatients. *Oncol Nurs Forum* 13:51–55, 1986.
45. Zimmerman L, Duncan K, Pozehl B, et al: Pain descriptors used by patients with cancer. *Oncol Nurs Forum* 14:67–71, 1987.
46. Padilla GV, Ferrell B, Grant MM, et al: Defining the content domain of quality of life for cancer patients with pain. *Cancer Nurs* 13:108–115, 1990.
47. Dalton JA, Feuerstein M: Biobehavioral factors in cancer pain. *Pain* 33:137–147, 1988.
48. McGuire DB, Sheidler VR: Pain. In Groenwald S, Frogge MH, Goodman M, Yarbro CH (eds.): *Cancer Nursing: Principles and Practice* (ed. 2). Boston: Jones and Bartlett, 1990, pp. 385–441.
49. Dorrepaal KL, Aaronsen NK, van Dam FSAM: Pain experience and pain management among hospitalized cancer patients: A clinical study. *Cancer* 63:593–598, 1989.
50. Ferrell BR, Wisdom C, Wenzl C: Quality of life as an outcome variable in the management of cancer pain. *Cancer* 63:2321–2327, 1989.
51. Massie MJ, Holland JC: The cancer patient with pain: Psychiatric complications and their management. *J Pain Sympt Manag* 7:99–109, 1992.
52. Spiegel D, Bloom J: Pain in metastatic breast cancer. *Cancer* 52:341–345, 1983.
53. Barkwell DP: Ascribed meaning: A critical factor in coping and pain attenuation in patients with cancer-related pain. *J Palliat Care* 7:5–14, 1991.
54. Jacox A, Stewart M: *Psychosocial Contingencies of the Pain Experience.* Iowa City: University of Iowa, 1973 (monograph).
55. Bruera E, Macmillan K, Hanson J, et al: The cognitive effects of the administration of narcotic analgesics in patients with cancer pain. *Pain* 39:13–16, 1989.
56. Sjogren P, Banning A: Pain, sedation and reaction time during long-term treatment of cancer patients with oral and epidural opioids. *Pain* 39:5–11, 1989.
57. Rimer B, Levy MH, Keintz MK, et al: Enhancing cancer pain control regimens through patient education. *Patient Educ Counsel* 10:267–277, 1987.
58. Wilkie DJ, Keefe FJ: Coping strategies of patients with lung cancer-related pain. *Clin J Pain* 7:292–299, 1991.
59. Arathuzik D: The appraisal of pain and coping in cancer patients. *West J Nurs Res* 13:714–731, 1991.
60. Bond MR, Pilowsky I: Subjective assessment of pain and its relationship to the administration of analgesics in patients with advanced cancer. *J Psychosom Res* 10:203–208, 1966.
61. Pilowsky I, Bond MR: Pain and its management in malignant disease: Elucidation of staff-patient transactions. *Psychosom Med* 31:400–404, 1969.
62. Keefe FJ, Brantley A, Manuel G, et al: Behavioral assessment of head and neck cancer pain. *Pain* 23:327–336, 1985.
63. Donovan MI: Nursing assessment of cancer pain. *Semin Oncol Nurs* 1:109–115, 1985.
64. Barbour LA, McGuire DB, Kirchhoff KT: Non-analgesic methods of pain control used by cancer outpatients. *Oncol Nurs Forum* 13:56–60, 1986.
65. Wilkie D, Lovejoy N, Dodd M, et al: Cancer pain control behaviors: Description and correlation with pain intensity. *Oncol Nurs Forum* 15:723–731, 1988.
66. Wolff BB, Langley L: Cultural factors and the response to pain: A review. In Weisenberg E (ed.): *Pain: Clinical and Experimental Perspectives.* St. Louis: Mosby, 1975, pp. 144–151.
67. Wolff BB: Ethnocultural factors influencing pain and illness behavior. *Clin J Pain* 1:23–30, 1985.
68. Lipton JA, Marbach JJ: Ethnicity and the pain experience. *Soc Sci Med* 19:1279–1298, 1984.
69. Reizien A, Meleis AI: Arab-Americans' perceptions of and responses to pain. *Crit Care Nurs* 6:30–37, 1986.
70. Miller JF, Shuter R: Age, sex, race affect pain expression. *Am J Nurs* 84:891, 1984.
71. Swanson DW, Maruta T: Patients complaining of extreme pain. *Mayo Clin Proc* 55:563–566, 1980.
72. Flannery RB, Sos J, McGovern P: Ethnicity as a factor in the expression of pain. *Psychosom* 22:39–40, 1981.
73. Greenwald HP: Interethnic differences in pain perception. *Pain* 44:157–163, 1991.
74. McMillan S: The relationship between age and intensity of cancer-related symptoms. *Oncol Nurs Forum* 16:237–241, 1989.
75. Ferrell BA, Ferrell BR: The experience of pain and quality of life in elderly patients. *Gerontol* 28:76A, 1988 (suppl.).
76. Cleeland CS, Ladinsky JL, Serlin RC, et al: Multidi-

mensional measurement of cancer pain: Comparisons of US and Vietnamese patients. *J Pain Sympt Manag* 3:23–27, 1988.
77. Garro LC: Culture, pain, and cancer. *J Palliat Care* 6:34–44, 1990.
78. Spross JA, McGuire DB, Schmitt R: Oncology Nursing Society position paper on cancer pain. *Oncol Nurs Forum* 17:595–614, 751–760, 825, 944–955, 1990.
79. National Institutes of Health: The integrated approach to the management of pain. *NIH Consensus Development Conference Statement* 6(3). Bethesda, MD: NIH, 1986.
80. American Cancer Society: *Cancer Facts and Figures 1992*. Atlanta: American Cancer Society, 1992.
81. Cleeland CS: The impact of pain on the patient with cancer. *Cancer* 54:2635–2641, 1984.
82. Ferrell BR, Schneider C: Experience and management of cancer pain at home. *Cancer Nurs* 11:84–90, 1988.
83. Norvell K, Zimmerman L: Psychological variables and cancer pain. *Oncol Nurs Forum* 16:160, 1989 (suppl.).
84. Ferrell B, Wisdom C, Wenzl C, et al: Effects of controlled release morphine on QOL for cancer pain. *Oncol Nurs Forum* 16:521–526, 1989.
85. Strang P, Qvarner H: Cancer-related pain and its influence on quality of life. *Anticancer Res* 10:109–112, 1990.
86. Ferrell BR, Grant M, Padilla G, et al: The experience of pain and perceptions of quality of life: Validation of a conceptual model. *Hosp J* 7:9–24, 1991.
87. Foley KM: The relationship of pain and symptom management to patient requests for physician-assisted suicide. *J Pain Sympt Manag* 6:289–297, 1991.
88. Saltzburg D, Breitbart W, Fishman B, et al: The relationship of pain and depression to suicidal ideation in cancer patients. *Proc Amer Soc Clin Oncol* 8:1215, 1989, (abstr.).
89. Breitbart W: Cancer pain and suicide. In Foley KM, Bonica JJ, Ventafridda V (eds.): *Advances in Pain Research and Therapy*. New York: Raven Press, 1990, pp. 399–412.
90. Coyle N: The euthanasia and physician-assisted suicide debate: Issues for nursing. *Oncol Nurs Forum* 19:41–46, 1992 (suppl.).
91. Ferrell BR, Rhiner M, Cohen MZ, et al: Pain as a metaphor for illness. Part I: Impact of cancer pain on family caregivers. *Oncol Nurs Forum* 18:1303–1309, 1991.
92. Ferrell BR, Cohen MZ, Rhiner M, et al: Pain as a metaphor for illness. Part II: Family caregivers' management of pain. *Oncol Nurs Forum* 18:1315–1321, 1991.
93. Ferrell BR, Ferrell BA, Rhiner M, et al: Family factors influencing cancer pain management. *Postgrad Med J* 67:S64–S69, 1991 (suppl.).
94. Ishay R: High technology in medicine—ethical aspects. *Israel J Med Sci* 25:274–278, 1989.
95. Ferrell BR, Rhiner M: High-tech comfort: Ethical issues in cancer pain management for the 1990s. *J Clin Ethics* 2:108–112, 1991.
96. Whedon M, Ferrell BR: Professional and ethical considerations in the use of high-tech pain management. *Oncol Nurs Forum* 18:1135–1143, 1991.
97. Ropchan R, Ferrell BR, Grant M, et al: Pain management as a nursing administration concern. *Oncol Nurs Forum* 19:317, 1992 (abstr.).
98. Angarola RT, Donato BJ: Inappropriate pain management results in high jury award. *J Pain Sympt Manag* 6:407, 1991.
99. Cushing M: The legal side: Pain management on trial. *Am J Nurs* 92:21, 22, 1992.
100. Foley KM: The "decriminalization" of cancer pain. In Hill SC, Fields WS (eds.): *Advances in Pain Research and Therapy*, Vol. 11. New York: Raven Press, 1989, pp. 5–18.
101. Joranson DE, Dahl JL: Achieving balance in drug policy: The Wisconsin model. In Hill CS, Fields WS (eds.): *Advances in Pain Research and Therapy*, Vol. 11. New York: Raven Press, 1989, pp. 197–204.
102. Angarola RT, Wray SD: Legal impediments to cancer pain treatment. In Hill CS, Fields WS (eds.); *Advances in Pain Research and Therapy*, Vol. 11. New York: Raven Press, 1989, pp. 213–231.
103. Portenoy RK: The effect of drug regulation on the management of cancer pain. *NY State Med J* 91:13s–18s, 1991.
104. Zenz M, Sorge J: Is the therapeutic use of opioids adversely affected by prejudice and law? *Rec Res Cancer Res* 121:43–50, 1991.
105. Hill CS: Relationship among cultural, educational, and regulatory agency influences on optimum cancer pain treatment. *J Pain Sympt Manag* 5:S37–S45, 1990 (suppl.).
106. Jacox A: Pain management: A health policy perspective. *Oncol Nurs Forum* 19:27–28, 1992 (suppl.).
107. Spross JA: Cancer pain relief: An international perspective. *Oncol Nurs Forum* 19:5–11, 1992 (suppl.).
108. National Institutes of Health: Exploratory Centers for Biobehavioral Symptom Management RFA: NR-92-02. *NIH Guide:* (2193), 1992.
109. World Health Organization: *Cancer Pain Relief*. Geneva: WHO, 1986.
110. American Pain Society Quality Assurance Standards for Relief of Acute Pain and Cancer Pain. In Bond MR, Charlton JE, Woolf CJ (eds.): *Proceedings of the VIth World Congress on Pain*. Amsterdam: Elsevier, 1990, pp. 186–189.
111. American Pain Society: *Principles of Analgesic Use in the Treatment of Acute Pain and Cancer Pain* (ed. 3). Skokie, IL: APS, 1992.
112. Ad Hoc Committee on Cancer Pain of the American Society of Clinical Oncology: Cancer pain assessment and treatment curriculum guidelines. *J Clin Oncol* 10:1976–1982, 1992.
113. Cancer Pain Management Guideline Panel: *Cancer Pain Management: Clinical Practice Guideline*. AHCPR (in press).
114. Grossman SA, Sheidler VR: Skills of medical students and house officers in prescribing narcotic medications. *J Med Educ* 60:552–557, 1985.
115. Sheidler VR, McGuire DB, Grossman SA, et al: Analgesic decision-making skills of nurses. *Oncol Nurs Forum* 19:1531–1534, 1992.
116. Fox LS: Pain management in the terminally ill cancer patient: An investigation of nurses' attitudes, knowledge, and clinical practice. *Mil Med* 147:455–460, 1982.
117. Watt-Watson JH: Nurses' knowledge of pain issues: A survey. *J Pain Sympt Manag* 2:207–211, 1987.
118. Charap AD: The knowledge, attitudes, and experience of medical personnel treating pain in the terminally ill. *Mt. Sinai Med J* 45:561–580, 1978.
119. Schauer PK, Wetterman TL, Schauer AR: Physicians' attitudes and knowledge about the management of cancer-related pain. *Conn Med* 52:705–707, 1988.
120. McCaffery M, Ferrell BR: Opioid analgesics. Nurses'

knowledge of doses and psychological dependence. *J Nurs Staff Dev* 8(2):77–84, 1992.
121. Cohen FL: Postsurgical pain relief: Patients' status and nurses' medication choices. *Pain* 9:265–274, 1980.
122. Morgan JP: American opiophobia: Customary underutilization of opioid analgesics. In Hill CS, Fields WS (eds.): *Advances in Pain Research and Therapy,* Vol. 11. New York: Raven Press, 1989, pp. 181–195.
123. Marks R, Sachar E: Undertreatment of medical inpatients with narcotic analgesics. *Ann Intern Med* 78:173–181, 1973.
124. Hauck SL: Pain: Problem for the person with cancer. *Cancer Nurs* 9:66–76, 1986.
125. Myers JS: Cancer pain: Assessment of nurses' knowledge and attitudes. *Oncol Nurs Forum* 12:62–66, 1985.
126. Weis OF, Sriwatanakul K, Alloza JL, et al: Attitudes of patients, housestaff, and nurses toward post-operative analgesic care. *Anesth Analg* 62:70–74, 1983.
127. Elliott TE, Elliott BA: Physician attitudes and beliefs about use of morphine for cancer pain. *J Pain Sympt Manag* 7:141–148, 1992.
128. Porter J, Jick H: Addiction rare in patients treated with narcotics. *N Engl J Med* 302:123, 1980.
129. Weissman DE, Dahl JL: Attitudes about cancer pain. A survey of Wisconsin's first-year medical students. *J Pain Sympt Manag* 5:345-349, 1990.
130. Edgar L, Hamilton J: A survey examining nurses' knowledge of pain control. *J Pain Sympt Manag* 7:18–26, 1992.
131. McCaffery M, Ferrell BR, O'Neil-Page E, et al: Nurses knowledge of opioid analgesic drugs and psychological dependence. *Cancer Nurs* 13:21–27, 1990.
132. Ferrell BR, McCaffery M, Rhiner M: Pain addiction: An urgent need for change in nursing education. *J Pain Sympt Manag* 7:117–124, 1992.
133. Camp LD: Comparison of medical, surgical and oncology patients' descriptions of pain and nurses' documentation of pain assessments. *J Adv Nurs* 12:593–598, 1987.
134. Dalton JA: Nurses' perceptions of their pain assessment skills, pain management practices, and attitudes toward pain. *Oncol Nurs Forum* 16:225–231, 1989.
135. Paice JA, Mahon SM, Faut-Callahan M: Factors associated with adequate pain control in hospitalized patients diagnosed with cancer. *Cancer Nurs* 14:298–305, 1991.
136. Faries JE, Mills DS, Goldsmith KW, et al: Systematic pain records and their impact on pain control. A pilot study. *Cancer Nurs* 14:306–313, 1991.
137. Ferrell BR, Eberts MT, McCaffery M, et al: Clinical decision making and pain. *Cancer Nurs* 14:289–297, 1991.
138. Grossman SA, Sheidler VR, Swedeen K, et al: Correlation of patient and caregiver ratings of cancer pain. *J Pain Sympt Manag* 6:53–57, 1991.
139. Rankin MA, Snider B: Nurses' perceptions of cancer patients' pain. *Cancer Nurs* 7:149–155, 1984.
140. Weissman DE, Joranson DE, Hopwood MB: Wisconsin physicians' knowledge and attitudes about opioid analgesic regulations. *Wisc Med J* 90:671–675, 1991.
141. Hill CS: Pain management in a drug-oriented society. *Cancer* 63:2382–2386, 1989.
142. Pritchard AP: Management of pain and nursing attitudes. *Cancer Nurs* 11:203–209, 1988.
143. Von Roenn JH, Cleeland CS, Gonin R, et al: Results of a physician's attitude toward cancer pain management survey by ECOG. *Proc Am Soc Clin Oncol* 10:326, 1991 (abstr.).
144. Pilowsky I: An outline curriculum on pain for medical school. *Pain* 33:1–2, 1988.
145. Ferrell BR, McGuire DB, Donovan MI: Knowledge and beliefs regarding pain in a sample of nursing faculty. *J Prof Nurs* 9:79–88, 1993.
146. Max MB: Improving outcomes of analgesic treatment: Is education enough? *Ann Int Med* 113:885–889, 1990.
147. Miaskowski C, Donovan M: Implementation of the American Pain Society Quality Assurance Standards for Relief of Acute Pain and Cancer Pain in oncology nursing practice. *Oncol Nurs Forum* 19:411–415, 1992.
148. Weissman DE, Abram SE, Haddox AD, et al: Educational role of cancer pain rounds. *J Cancer Educ* 4:113–116, 1989.
149. Portenoy RK, Coyle N: Controversies in the long-term management of analgesic therapy in patients with advanced cancer. *J Pain Sympt Manag* 5:307–319, 1991.
150. Williams A, Kedziera P, Osterlund H, et al: Models of healthcare delivery in cancer pain management. *Oncol Nurs Forum* 19:20–26, 1992 (suppl.).
151. Gonzales GR, Elliott KJ, Portenoy RK, et al: The impact of a comprehensive evaluation in the management of cancer pain. *Pain* 47:141–144, 1991.
152. Walsh TD: Continuing care in a medical center: The Cleveland Clinic Foundation Palliative Care Service. *J Pain Sympt Manag* 5:273–278, 1990.
153. Sheidler VR, Krumm SK: Pain management teams. Presentation at Oncology Nursing Society Congress, San Diego, May 1992.
154. Mohide EA, Royle JA, Montemuro M, et al: Assessing the quality of cancer pain management. *J Palliat Care* 4:9–15, 1988.
155. Foley KM: The treatment of cancer pain. *N Engl J Med* 313:84–95, 1985.
156. Ventafridda V: Palliative care: A new reality in medicine. *Rec Res Cancer Res* 121:393–398, 1991.
157. Weissman DE: Palliative medicine education: Bridging the gap between acute care and hospice. *J Cancer Educ* 6:67–68, 1991.
158. McGuire DB: Comprehensive and multidimensional assessment and measurement of pain. *J Pain Sympt Manag* 7:312–319, 1992.
159. Donovan MI: Clinical assessment of cancer pain. In McGuire DB, Yarbro CH (eds.): *Cancer Pain Management.* Philadelphia: Saunders, 1987, pp. 105–131.
160. McCaffery M, Beebe A: *Pain: Clinical Manual for Nursing Practice.* St. Louis: Mosby, 1989.
161. McGuire DB: Measuring pain. In Frank-Stromborg M (ed.): *Instruments for Clinical Nursing Research.* Norwalk, CT: Appleton & Lange, 1988, pp. 333–356.
162. Ross DM, Ross SA: Assessment of pediatric pain: An overview. *Iss Compr Pediatr Nurs* 11:73–91, 1988.
163. Syrjala KL: The measurement of pain. In McGuire DB, Yarbro CH (eds.): *Cancer Pain Management.* Philadelphia: Saunders, 1987, pp. 133–150.
164. Deschamps M, Band PR, Coldman AJ: Assessment of adult cancer pain: Shortcomings of current methods. *Pain* 32:133–139, 1988.
165. Grossman SA, Sheidler VR, McGuire DB, et al: A comparison of the Hopkins Pain Rating Instrument with standard visual analogue and verbal descriptor scales in patients with cancer pain. *J Pain Sympt Manag* 7:196–203, 1992.
166. Ahles TA, Ruckdeschel JC, Blanchard EB: Cancer-re-

lated pain—II. Assessment with visual analogue scales. *J Psychosom Med* 28:121–124, 1984.
167. Machin D, Lewith GT, Wylson S: Pain measurement in randomized clinical trials. *Clin J Pain* 4:161–168, 1988.
168. Acute Pain Management Guideline Panel: *Acute Pain Management: Operative or Medical Procedures and Trauma. Clinical Practice Guideline.* AHCPR Pub. No. 92-0032. Rockville, MD: Agency for Health Care Policy and Research, Public Health Service, U.S. Department of Health and Human Services, 1992.
169. Mateo OM, Krenzischek DA: A pilot study to assess the relationship between behavioral manifestations and self-report of pain in postanesthesia care unit patients. *J Post Anesth Nurs* 7:15–21, 1992.
170. Kremer EF, Atkinson JH, Ignelzi RJ: Pain measurement: The affective dimensional measure of the McGill Pain Questionnaire with a cancer pain population. *Pain* 12:153–163, 1982.
171. Daut RL, Cleeland CS, Flanery RC: Development of the Wisconsin brief pain questionnaire to assess pain in cancer and other diseases. *Pain* 17:197–210, 1983.
172. Cleeland CS: Measurement and prevalence of pain in cancer. *Semin Oncol Nurs* 1:87–92, 1985.
173. Melzack R: The short-form McGill Pain Questionnaire. *Pain* 30:191–197, 1987.
174. Fishman B, Pasternak S, Wallenstein SL, et al: The Memorial Pain Assessment Card: A valid instrument for the evaluation of cancer pain. *Cancer* 60:1151–1158, 1987.
175. McMillan SC, Williams FA, Chatfield R, et al: A validity and reliability study of two tools for assessing and managing cancer pain. *Oncol Nurs Forum* 15:735–741, 1988.
176. Walker VA, Dicks B, Webb P: Pain assessment charts in the management of chronic cancer pain. *Palliat Med* 1:111–116, 1987.
177. Beyer JE, Levin CR: Issues and advances in pain control in children. *Nurs Clin North Am* 22:661–676, 1987.
178. McGrath PJ, Johnson G, Goodman J, et al: The Children's Hospital of Eastern Ontario Pain Scale (CHEOPS): A behavioral scale for rating postoperative pain in children. In Fields HL, Dubner R, Cervero F (eds.): *Advances in Pain Research and Therapy,* Vol. 9. New York: Raven Press, 1985, pp. 395–402.
179. Schechter NL, Altman A, Weisman S (eds.): Report of the consensus conference on the management of pain in childhood cancer. *Pediatr* 86:5, 1990 (suppl.).
180. Stiefel F, Fainsinger R, Bruera E: Acute confusional states in patients with advanced cancer. *J Pain Sympt Manag* 7:94–98, 1992.
181. Bruera E, Fainsinger RL, Miller MJ, et al: The assessment of pain intensity in patients with cognitive failure: A preliminary report. *J Pain Sympt Manag* 7:267–270, 1992.
182. North American Nursing Diagnosis Association: *Proc 8th Natl Conf NANDA,* St. Louis, 1988.
183. McNally JC, Somerville ET, Miaskowski C, et al: *Guidelines for Oncology Nursing Practice* (ed. 2). Philadelphia: Saunders, 1991, pp. 125–142.
184. Levin RF, Krainovitch BC, Bahrenburg E, et al: Diagnostic content validity of nursing diagnoses. *Image: J Nurs Schol* 21:40–44, 1989.
185. Carpenito LJ: *Nursing Diagnosis: Application to Clinical Practice* (ed. 4). Philadelphia: Lippincott, 1992, pp. 211–248.
186. Bodnar B, Galligan A: An effective PCA documentation tool. *Nurs Manag* 23:48–50, 1992.
187. Schug SA, Zech D, Grond S: A computerized documentation system for cancer pain management units. *Comput Biol Med* 22:201–205, 1992.
188. Ferrell BR, Wisdom C, Rhiner M, et al: Pain management as a quality of care outcome. *J Nurs Qual Assur* 5:50–58, 1991.
189. Patterson KL, Klopovich PM: Pain in the pediatric oncology patient. In McGuire DB, Yarbro CH (eds.): *Cancer Pain Management.* Philadelphia: Saunders, 1987, pp. 259–272.
190. Stevens B, Hunsberger M, Browne G: Pain in children: Theoretical, research, and practice dilemmas. *J Pediatr Nurs* 2:154–166, 1987.
191. Broome ME, Lillis PP: A descriptive analysis of the pediatric pain management research. *Appl Nurs Res* 2:744–781, 1989.
192. Hester NO: Pain in children. *Annual Review of Nursing Research,* Vol. 10 (in press).
193. Katz ER, Kellerman J, Siegel SE: Behavioral distress in children with cancer undergoing medical procedures: Developmental considerations. *J Consult Clin Psychol* 48:356–365, 1980.
194. Beaver PK: Premature infants' response to touch and pain: Can nurses make a difference? *Neonatal Network* 6:13–17, 1987.
195. Eland JM, Anderson JE: The experience of pain in children. In Jacox AK (ed.): *Pain: A Sourcebook for Nurses and Other Health Professionals.* Boston: Little, Brown, 1977, pp. 453–476.
196. Schechter NL, Allen DA, Hanson K: Status of pediatric pain control: A comparison of hospital analgesic usage in children and adults. *Pediatr* 77:11–15, 1986.
197. Schechter NL, Allen D: Physicians' attitudes toward pain in children. *J Dev Behav Pediatr* 7:350–354, 1986.
198. Miser AW, Moore L, Greene R, et al: Prospective study of continuous intravenous and subcutaneous morphine infusions for therapy-related or cancer-related pain in children and young adults with cancer. *Clin J Pain* 2:101–106, 1986.
199. Broome ME, Lillis PP, McGahee TW, et al: The use of distraction and imagery with children during painful procedures. *Oncol Nurs Forum* 19:499–502, 1992.
200. Nahata MC, Clotz MA, Krogg EA: Adverse effects of meperidine, promethazine, and chlorpromazine for sedation in pediatric patients. *Clin Pediatr* 24:558–560, 1985.
201. Kuttner L: Favorite stories: A hypnotic pain-reduction technique for children in acute pain. *Am J Clin Hypn* 30:289–295, 1988.
202. Kuttner L, Bowman M, Teasdale M: Psychological treatment of distress, pain, and anxiety for young children with cancer. *J Dev Behav Pediatr* 9:374–381, 1988.
203. Zappa SC, Nabors SB: Use of ethyl chloride topical anesthetic to reduce procedural pain in pediatric oncology patients. *Cancer Nurs* 15:130–136, 1992.
204. Martinson IM, Nixon S, Geis D, et al: Nursing care in childhood cancer: Methadone. *Am J Nurs* 82:432–435, 1982.
205. Miser AW, Miser JS: The use of oral methadone to control moderate and severe pain in children and young adults with malignancy. *Clin J Pain* 1:243-248, 1986.
206. Goldman A: The role of oral controlled-release mor-

phine for pain relief in children with cancer. *Palliat Med* 4:279–285, 1990.

207. Miser AW, Miser JS, Clark BS: Continuous intravenous infusion of morphine sulfate for control of severe pain in children with terminal malignancy. *J Pediatr* 96:930–932, 1980.
208. Dothage JA, Arndt C, Miser AW: Use of a continuous intravenous morphine infusion for pain control in an infant with terminal malignancy. *J Assoc Pediatr Oncol Nurs* 3(4):22–24, 1986.
209. Gilford DM (ed.): *The Aging Population in the Twenty-First Century: Statistics for Health Policy.* Washington DC: National Academy Press, 1988.
210. Boring CC, Squires TS, Tong T: Cancer statistics 1992. *CA* 42:19–45, 1992.
211. Portenoy RK: Optimal pain control in elderly cancer patients. *Geriatr* 42:33–44, 1987.
212. Ferrell BA, Ferrell BR: Assessment of chronic pain in the elderly. *Geriatr Med Today* 8:123–134, 1989.
213. Ferrell BA: Pain in the elderly. In Watt-Watson JH, Donovan MI (eds.): *Pain Management: Nursing Perspective.* St. Louis: Mosby Year Book, 1992, pp. 349–369.
214. Thomas MR, Roy R: Age and pain: A comparative study of the "younger and older" elderly. *Pain Manag* 1:174–179, 1988.
215. Office of Technology Assessment: *Technology and Aging in America.* Publication No. OTA-BA-264. Washington DC: Office of Technology Assessment, 1985.
216. Ferrell BA, Ferrell BR, Osterweil D: Pain in the nursing home. *J Am Geriatr Soc* 38:409–414, 1990.
217. Newton PA: Chronic pain. In Cassel KY, Walsh JR (eds.): *Geriatric Medicine,* Vol. II, Fundamentals of Geriatric Care. New York: Springer-Verlag, 1984, pp. 236–274.
218. Lamy PP: Pain management, drugs, and the elderly. *J Am Health Care Assoc* 10:32–36, 1984.
219. Harkins SW, Kwentus J, Price DD: Pain in the elderly. In Bendetti C, Chapman CR, Morrica G (eds.): *Advances in Pain Research and Therapy,* Vol. 7. New York: Raven Press, 1984, pp. 103–121.
220. Ferrell BR, Grant MM, Riner M, et al: Home care: Maintaining quality of life for patient and family. *Oncology* 6:136–140, 1992 (suppl.).
221. Bayer AJ, Chadha JS, Farag RR, et al: Changing presentations of myocardial infarction with increasing old age. *J Am Geriatr Soc* 34:263–266, 1986.
222. Schmucker DL: Drug disposition in the elderly: A review of the critical factors. *J Am Geriatr Soc* 32:144–149, 1984.
223. Ouslander JG: Drug therapy in the elderly. *Ann Intern Med* 95:711–722, 1981.
224. Amadio P, Cummings DM, Amadio PB: Pain in the elderly: Management techniques. *Pain Manag* 1:33–41, 1987.
225. Kaiko RF, Wallenstein SL, Rogers AG, et al: Narcotics in the elderly. *Med Clin North Am* 66:1079–1089, 1982.
226. Nolan L, O'Malley K: Prescribing for the elderly. Part I: Sensitivity of the elderly to adverse drug reactions. *J Am Geriatr Soc* 36:142–149, 1988.
227. Conn VS, Taylor SG, Kelley S: Medication regimen complexity and adherence among older adults. *Image: J Nurs Schol* 23:231–235, 1991.
228. Faherty BS, Grier MR: Analgesic medication for elderly people post-surgery. *Nurs Res* 33:369–372, 1984.
229. Portenoy RK, Kanner RM: Patterns of analgesic prescription and consumption in a university-affiliated community hospital. *Arch Intern Med* 145:439–441, 1985.
230. Portenoy R: Pain management in the older cancer patient *Oncology* 6:86–98, 1992.
231. Coyle N, Foley KM: Alteration in comfort: Pain. In Baird SB, McCorkle R, Grant M (eds.): *Cancer Nursing: A Comprehensive Textbook.* Philadelphia: Saunders, 1991, pp. 782–805.
232. McCaffery M, Vourakis C: Assessment and relief of pain in chemically dependent patients. *Orthop Nurs* 11:13–27, 1992.
233. Hoffman M, Provatas A, Lyver A, et al: Pain management in the opioid-addicted patient with cancer. *Cancer* 68:121–122, 1991.
234. Puntillo KA (ed.): *Pain in the Critically Ill: Assessment and Management.* Gaithersburg, VA: Aspen, 1991.
235. Donnelly GF, Sutterley DC: From the editors (editorial). *Top Clin Nurs* 7:v, 1985 (entire issue on cultural diversity and nursing practice).
236. Fong CM: Ethnicity and nursing practice. *Top Clin Nurs* 7:1–10, 1985.
237. Douglas MK: Cultural diversity in the response to pain. In Puntillo KA (ed.): *Pain in the Critically Ill: Assessment and Management.* Gaithersburg, VA: Aspen, 1991, pp. 65–76.
238. Kagawa-Singer M: Ethnic perspectives of cancer nursing: Hispanics and Japanese-Americans. *Oncol Nurs Forum* 14:59–65, 1987.
239. Pfefferbaum B, Adams J, Aceves J: The influence of culture on pain in Anglo and Hispanic children with cancer. *J Am Acad Child Adolesc Psychiatry* 29:642–647, 1990.
240. Louie KB: Providing health care to Chinese clients. *Top Clin Nurs* 7:18–25, 1985.
241. Lipson JG, Meleis AI: Culturally appropriate care: The case of immigrants. *Top Clin Nurs* 7:48–56, 1985.
242. Capers CF: Nursing and the Afro-American client. *Top Clin Nurs* 7:11–17, 1985.
243. Carson VB (ed.): *Spiritual Dimensions of Nursing Practice.* Philadelphia: Saunders, 1989.
244. Jacik M: Spiritual care of the dying adult. In Carson VB (ed.): *Spiritual Dimensions of Nursing Practice.* Philadelphia: Saunders, 1989, pp. 254–288.
245. Twycross RD: Terminal care: Organization and technical aspects. In Swerdlow M, Ventafridda V (eds.): *Cancer Pain.* Lancaster, Eng.: MTP Press, 1987, pp. 173–184.
246. Wanzer SH, Federman DD, Adelstein SJ, et al: The physician's responsibility toward hopelessly ill patients. *N Engl J Med* 320:844–849, 1989.
247. Burchman SL: Hospice care of the cancer pain patient. In Abram SE (ed.): *Cancer Pain.* Boston: Kluwer, 1989, pp. 153–169.
248. Kane RL, Bernstein L, Wales J, et al: Hospice effectiveness in controlling pain. *JAMA* 253:2683–2686, 1985.
249. Austin C, Cody OP, Eyres PJ, et al: Hospice home care pain management: Four critical variables. *Cancer Nurs* 9:58–65, 1986.
250. Fainsinger R, Miller MJ, Bruera E: Symptom control during the last week of life on a palliative care unit. *J Palliat Care* 7:5–11, 1991.
251. Trotter JM, Scott R, MacBeth FR, et al: Problems of the oncology outpatient: Role of the liaison health visitor. *Br Med J* 282:122–124, 1981.

252. Ventafridda V, Ripamonti C, DeConno F, et al: Symptom prevalence and control during cancer patients' last days of life. *J Palliat Care* 6:7–11, 1990.
253. Degner LF, Fujii SH, Levitt M: Implementing a program to control chronic pain of malignant disease for patients in an extended care facility. *Cancer Nurs* 5:263–258, 1982.
254. Bruera E, MacMillan K, Hanson J, et al: Palliative care in a cancer center: Results in 1984 versus 1987. *J Pain Sympt Manag* 5:1–5, 1990.
255. Miller RD, Walsh TD: Psychosocial aspects of palliative care in advanced cancer. *J Pain Sympt Manag* 6:24–29, 1991.
256. Chan H, Woodruff RK: Palliative care in a general teaching hospital: Assessment of needs. *Med J Aust* 155:597–599, 1991.
257. Milch RA, Freeman A, Clark E: *Palliative Pain and Symptom Management for Children and Adolescents.* Alexandria, VA: Children's Hospice International, 1985.
258. Coyle N, Adelhardt J, Foley KM, et al: Character of terminal illness in the advanced cancer patient: Pain and other symptoms during the last four weeks of life. *J Pain Sympt Manag* 5:83–93, 1990.
259. Mount B: Challenges in palliative care (keynote address). *Amer J Hosp Care* 2:22–29, 1985.
260. Steitz AM: Analgesic utilization patterns in a hospice. *Oncology* 1:33–36, 1987 (suppl.).
261. Grond S, Zech D, Schug SA, et al: Validation of World Health Organization Guidelines for cancer pain relief during the last days and hours of life. *J Pain Sympt Manag* 6:411–422, 1991.
262. Bonadonna F, Molinari R: Role and limits of anticancer drugs in the treatment of advanced cancer pain. In Bonica JJ, Ventafridda V (eds.): *Advances in Pain Research and Therapy,* Vol. 2. New York: Raven Press, 1979, pp. 131–138.
263. Russell JA: Cytotoxic therapy—Pain relief and recalcification. In Stoll BA, Parbhoo S (eds.): *Bone Metastasis: Monitoring and Treatment.* New York: Raven Press, 1983, pp. 354–368.
264. MacDonald N: The role of medical oncology in cancer pain control. In Hill CS, Fields WS (eds.): *Advances in Pain Research and Therapy,* Vol. 11. New York: Raven Press, 1989, pp. 123–130.
265. Bruera E, MacMillan K, Hanson J, et al: The Edmonton staging system for cancer pain: Preliminary report. *Pain* 37:203–209, 1989.
266. Estes NC, Morphis JG, Hornback NB, et al: Intraarterial chemotherapy and hyperthermia for pain control in patients with recurrent rectal cancer. *Am J Surg* 152:597–601, 1986.
267. Abrams RA, Hansen RM: Radiotherapy, chemotherapy and hormonal therapy in the management of cancer pain: Putting patient, prognosis, and oncologic options in perspective. In Abram SE (ed.): *Cancer Pain.* Boston: Kluwer, 1989, pp. 49–66.
268. Pannuti F, Martoni A, Rossi AP, et al: The role of endocrine therapy for relief of pain due to advanced cancer. In Bonica JJ, Ventafridda V (eds.): *Advances in Pain Research and Therapy,* Vol. 2. New York: Raven Press, 1979, pp. 145–165.
269. Stoll BA: Hormonal therapy—Pain relief and recalcification. In Stoll BA, Parbhoo S (eds.): *Bone Metastasis: Monitoring and Treatment.* New York: Raven Press, 1983, pp. 321–342.
270. Ford HT, Yarnold JR: Radiation therapy—Pain relief and recalcification. In Stoll BA, Parbhoo S (eds.): *Bone Metastasis: Monitoring and Treatment.* New York: Raven Press, 1983, pp. 343–354.
271. Ashby M: The role of radiotherapy in palliative care. *J Pain Sympt Manag* 6:380–388, 1991.
272. Tong D, Gillick L, Hendrickson FR: The palliation of symptomatic osseous metastases: Final results of the study by the Radiation Therapy Oncology Group. *Cancer* 50:893–899, 1982.
273. Salazar OM, Ruben P, Hendrickson FR, et al: Single-dose half-body irradiation for palliation of multiple bone metastases from solid tumors: Final Radiation Therapy Oncology Group Report. *Cancer* 58:29–36, 1986.
274. Azzarelli A, Crispino S: Palliative surgery in cancer pain treatment. In Swerdlow M, Ventafridda V (eds.): *Cancer Pain.* Lancaster, Eng.: MTP Press, 1987, pp. 97–103.
275. MacDonald N: The role of medical and surgical oncology in the management of cancer pain. In Foley KM, Bonica JJ, Ventafridda V (eds.): *Advances in Pain Research and Therapy,* Vol. 16. New York: Raven Press, 1990, pp. 27–44.
276. Chalmers J: The management of bone metastases: Orthopaedic procedures. *Palliat Med* 1:121–127, 1987.
277. Houde RW: Systemic analgesics and related drugs: Narcotic analgesics. In Bonica JJ, Ventafridda V (eds.): *Advances in Pain Research and Therapy,* Vol. 2. New York: Raven Press, 1979, pp. 263–272.
278. Lipman AG: Drug therapy in cancer pain. *Cancer Nurs* 3:40–46, 1980.
279. Foley KM: The practical use of narcotic analgesics. *Med Clin North Am* 66:1091–1104, 1982.
280. McGivney WT, Crooks GM: The care of patients with severe chronic pain in terminal illness. *JAMA* 251:1181–1188, 1984.
281. Hanks GW: Opioid analgesics in the management of pain in patients with cancer: A review. *Palliat Med* 1:1–25, 1987.
282. Twycross RG: Opioid analgesics in cancer pain: Current practice and controversies. *Cancer Surv* 7:29–53, 1988.
283. Inturrisi CE: Management of cancer pain: Pharmacology and principles of management. *Cancer* 63:2308–2320, 1989.
284. Pasternak GW: Biochemistry and pharmacology of multiple mu opioid receptors. In Foley KM, Inturrisi CE (eds.): *Advances in Pain Research and Therapy,* Vol. 8. New York: Raven Press, 1986, pp. 337–344.
285. Jaffe JH, Martin WR: Opioid analgesics and antagonists. In Gilman AG, Rall TW, Nies AL, et al (eds.): *Goodman and Gilman's The Pharmacological Bases of Therapeutics* (ed. 8). New York: Pergamon Press, 1990, pp. 485–521.
286. Malmberg AB, Yaksh TA: Hyperalgesia mediated by spinal glutamate or substance P receptor blocked by spinal cyclooxygenase inhibitor. *Science* 257:1276–1279, 1992.
287. Goodwin JS, Regan M: Cognitive dysfunction associated with naprosyn and ibuprofen in the elderly. *Arthr Rheumatol* 25:1013–1015, 1982.
288. Insel PA: Analgesic-antipyretic and anti-inflammatory agents. Drugs employed in the treatment of rheumatoid arthritis and gout. In Gilman AG, Rall TW, Nies AL, et al (eds.): *Goodman and Gilman's The Pharmacological Basis of Therapeutics* (ed. 8). New York: Pergamon Press, 1990, pp. 638–681.
289. Ventafridda V, Fochi V, DeConno D, et al: Use of non-

steroidal anti-inflammatory drugs in the treatment of pain in cancer. *Br J Clin Pharmacol* 10:3435-3465, 1980.
290. Moertel CG: Treatment of cancer pain with orally administered medications. *JAMA* 244:2448–2450, 1980.
291. Turnbull R, Hills LJ: Naproxen versus aspirin as analgesics in advanced malignant disease. *J Palliat Care* 1:25–28, 1986.
292. Levich S, Jacobs C, Loukas DF: Naproxen sodium in treatment of bone pain due to metastatic cancer. *Pain* 35:253-258, 1988.
293. Minotti V, Patoria L, Roila F, et al: Double-blind evaluation of analgesic efficacy of orally administered diclofenac, nefopam, and acetylsalicylic acid (ASA) plus codeine in chronic cancer pain. *Pain* 36:177–183, 1989.
294. Staquet MJ: Double-blind study with placebo control of intramuscular ketorolac tromethamine in the treatment of cancer pain. *J Clin Pharmacol* 29:1031–1036, 1989.
295. Ventafridda V, De Conno F, Panerai AE, et al: Nonsteroidal anti-inflammatory drugs as the first step in cancer pain therapy: double blind, within-patient study comparing nine drugs. *J Int Med Res* 18:21-29, 1990.
296. Beaver WT: Aspirin and acetaminophen as constituents of analgesic combinations. *Arch Intern Med* 141:292–300, 1981.
297. Houde RW, Wallenstein SL, Rogers A: Clinical pharmacology of analgesics: A method of assaying analgesic effect. *Clin Pharmacol Ther* 1:163–174, 1960.
298. Ferrer-Brechner T, Ganz P: Combination therapy with ibuprofen and methadone for chronic cancer pain. *Am J Med* 77:78–83, 1984.
299. Weingart WA, Sorkness CA, Earhart RH: Analgesia with oral narcotics and added ibuprofen in cancer patients. *Clin Pharm* 4:53–58, 1985.
300. Allison MC, Howatson AG, Torrance CJ, et al: Gastrointestinal damage associated with the use of nonsteroidal anti-inflammatory drugs. *N Engl J Med* 327:749–754, 1992.
301. Mannix KA, Rawlins MD: The management of bone metastases: Nonsteroidal anti-inflammatory drugs. *Palliat Med* 1:128–131, 1987.
302. Griffin MR, Piper JM, Daughterty JR, et al: Nonsteroidal anti-inflammatory drug use and increased risk for peptic ulcer disease in elderly persons. *Ann Intern Med* 114:257–263, 1991.
303. Kantor TG: Control of pain by nonsteroidal anti-inflammatory drugs. *Med Clin North Am* 66:1053–1059, 1982.
304. Portenoy RK: Drug treatment of pain syndromes. *Semin Neurol* 7:139–149, 1987.
305. Campora E, Merlini L, Pace M, et al: The incidence of narcotic-induced emesis. *J Pain Sympt Manag* 6:428–430, 1991.
306. Portenoy RK: Constipation in the cancer patient: Causes and management. *Med Clin North Am* 71:303–311, 1987.
307. Levy MH: Constipation and diarrhea in cancer patients. *Cancer Bull* 43:312–422, 1991.
308. Portenoy RK, Foley KM, Inturrisi CE: The nature of opioid responsiveness and its implications for neuropathic pain: New hypotheses derived from studies of opioid infusions. *Pain* 43:273–286, 1991.
309. Kaiko RF, Foley KM, Grabinski PY, et al: Central nervous system excitatory effects of meperidine in cancer patients. *Ann Neurol* 13:180–185, 1983.
310. Kaiko RF, Wallenstein SL, Rogers AG, et al: Analgesic and mood effects of heroin and morphine in cancer patients with postoperative pain. *N Engl J Med* 304:1501–1505, 1981.
311. Twycross RG: Choice of strong analgesic in terminal cancer: Diamorphine or morphine? *Pain* 3:93–104, 1977.
312. Kaiko RF, Wallenstein SL, Rogers A, et al: Clinical analgesic studies of intramuscular heroin and morphine in postoperative and chronic pain. In Foley KM, Inturrisi CE (eds.): *Advances in Pain Research and Therapy*, Vol. 8. New York: Raven Press, 1986, pp. 107–116.
313. Inturrisi CE, Max MB, Foley KM: The pharmacokinetics of heroin in patients with chronic pain. *N Engl J Med* 310:1213–1217, 1984.
314. Ventafridda V, Saita L, Barletta L, et al: Clinical observations on controlled-release morphine in cancer pain. *J Pain Symptom Manag* 4:124–129, 1989.
315. Tsuneto S, Hayashi A, Miyazaki M, et al: Clinical survey of controlled release morphine for cancer pain relief in a Japanese hospice. *Postgrad Med J* 67:79–81, 1991 (suppl.).
316. Vijayaram S, Ramamani PV, Chandrashekhar NS, et al: Continuing care for cancer pain relief with oral morphine solution. One year experience in a regional cancer center. *Cancer* 66:1590–1595, 1990.
317. Homesley HD, Welander CE, Muss HB, et al: Dosage range study of morphine sulfate controlled release. *Am J Clin Oncol* 9:449–453, 1986.
318. Meed SD, Kleinman PM, Kantor TG, et al: Management of cancer pain with oral controlled-release morphine sulfate. *J Clin Pharmacol* 27:155–161, 1987.
319. Savarese JJ, Shepherd L, Krant MJ: Long-acting oral morphine in cancer pain analgesia. *Clin J Pain* 3:177–181, 1987.
320. Brescia FJ, Walsh M, Savarese JJ, et al: A study of controlled-release oral morphine (MS Contin) in an advanced cancer hospital. *J Pain Sympt Manag* 2:193–198, 1987.
321. Khojasteh A, Evans W, Reynolds RD, et al: Controlled-release oral morphine sulfate in the treatment of cancer pain with pharmacokinetic correlation. *J Clin Oncol* 5:956–961, 1987.
322. Thirwell MP, Sloan PA, Maroun JA, et al: Pharmacokinetics and clinical efficacy of oral morphine solution and controlled-release morphine tablets in cancer patients. *Cancer* 63:2275–2283, 1989.
323. Goughnour BR, Arkinstall WW, Stewart JH: Analgesic response to single and multiple doses of controlled-release morphine tablets and morphine oral solution in cancer patients. *Cancer* 63:2294–2297, 1989.
324. Walsh TD, Kadam BV: Morphine steady-state levels during repeated oral administration. *Br J Clin Pharmacol* 17:232, 1984.
325. Walsh TD, Grabinski PY, Kaiko RF: Clinical implications of morphine plasma levels in advanced cancer. In Foley RM, Inturrisi CE (eds): *Advances in Pain Research and Therapy*, Vol. 8. New York: Raven Press, 1986, pp. 31–35.
326. Ventafridda V, Oliveri E, Caraceni A, et al: A retrospective study on the use of oral morphine in cancer pain. *J Pain Sympt Manag* 2:77–81, 1987.
327. Sawe J, Dahlstrom B, Rase A: Morphine kinetics in cancer patients. *Clin Pharmacol Ther* 30:629–635, 1981.
328. Houde RW, Wallenstein SL, Beaver WT: Clinical measurement of pain. In de Stevens G (ed.): *Analgesics*. New York: Academic Press, 1965, pp. 75–122.

329. Walsh TD: Oral morphine in chronic cancer pain. *Pain* 18:1–11, 1984.
330. Kaiko R: Controversy in the management of chronic cancer pain: Therapeutic equivalents of im and po morphine. *J Pain Sympt Manag* 1:42–45, 1986.
331. Peterson GM, Randall CTC, Paterson J: Plasma levels of morphine glucuronide in the treatment of cancer pain: Relationship to renal function and route of administration. *Eur J Clin Pharmacol* 38:121–124, 1990.
332. Portenoy RK, Thaler HT, Inturrisi CE, et al: The metabolite morphine-6-glucuronide contributes to the analgesia produced by morphine infusion in patients with pain and normal renal function. *Clin Pharmacol Ther* 51:422–431, 1992.
333. Portenoy RK, Foley KM, Stulman, et al: Plasma morphine and morphine-6-glucuronide during chronic morphine therapy for cancer pain: Plasma profiles, steady state concentrations, and the consequences of renal failure. *Pain* 47:13–19, 1991.
334. Houde RW: Misinformation: Side effects and drug interactions. In Hill CS, Fields WS (eds.): *Advances in Pain Research and Therapy,* Vol. 11. New York: Raven Press, 1989, pp. 145–161.
335. Ettinger DS, Vitale PJ, Trump DC: Important clinical considerations in the use of methadone in cancer patients. *Cancer Treat Rep* 63:457–459, 1979.
336. Baldessarini RJ: Drugs and the treatment of psychiatric disorders. In Gilman AG, Rall TW, Nies AL, et al (eds.): *Goodman and Gilman's The Pharmacological Basis of Therapeutics* (ed. 8). New York: Pergamon Press, 1990, pp. 383–435.
337. Max MB, Lynch SA, Muir J, et al: Effects of desipramine, amitriptyline, and fluoxethine on pain in diabetic neuropathy. *N Engl J Med* 326:1250–1256, 1992.
338. Watson CPN, Chipman M, Reed K, et al: Amitriptyline versus maprotiline in postherpetic neuralgia: A randomized, double-blind crossover trial. *Pain* 48:29–36, 1992.
339. Portenoy RK: Practical aspects of pain control in the patient with cancer. *CA* 38:327–352, 1988.
340. Walsh TD: Antidepressants for chronic pain. *Clin Neuropharmacol* 6:271–295, 1983.
341. Richlin DM, Jamron LM, Novich NC: Cancer pain control with a combination of methadone amitriptyline and non-narcotic analgesic therapy: A case series analysis. *J Pain Sympt Manag* 2:89–94, 1987.
342. Ventafridda V, Caraceni A, Saita L, et al: Trazadone for deafferentation pain. Comparison with amitriptyline. *Psychopharm* 95:544–549, 1988.
343. Massie MJ, Holland J: The cancer patient with pain: Psychiatric complications and their management. *Med Clin North Am* 71:243–258, 1987.
344. McQuay HJ: Pharmacologic treatment of neuralgia and neuropathic pain. *Cancer Surv* 7:141–159, 1988.
345. Swerdlow M, Cundill JG: Anti-convulsant drugs used in the treatment of lancinating pain: A comparison. *Anaesthesiol* 36:1129–1132, 1981.
346. Rapoport WG, Rogers KM, McCubbin TD, et al: Treatment of intractable neurogenic pain with carbamazepine. *Scottish Med J* 29:162–165, 1984.
347. Fromm GF: Trigeminal neuralgia and related disorders. *Neurol Clin* 7:305–320, 1989.
348. McEvoy G (ed.): *American Hospital Formulary Service.* Bethesda, MD: Amer. Soc. Hosp. Pharm., 1992.
349. Rall TW, Schleifer LS: Drugs effective in the therapies of the epilepsies. In Gilman AG, Rall TW, Nies AL, et al (eds.): *Goodman and Gilman's The Pharmacologic Basis of Therapeutics* (ed. 8). New York: Pergamon Press, 1990, pp. 436–462.
350. Hoffman BB, Lefkowitz RJ: Catecholamines and sympathomimetic drugs. In Gilman AG, Rall TW, Nies AS, et al (eds.) *Goodman and Gilman's The Pharmacological Basis of Therapeutics* (ed. 8). New York: Pergamon Press, 1990, pp. 187–220.
351. Forrest WH, Brown BW, Brown CR, et al: Dextroamphetamine with morphine for treatment of post-operative pain. *N Engl J Med* 296:712–715, 1977.
352. Bruera E, Chadwick S. Brenneis C, et al: Methylphenidate associated with narcotics for the treatment of cancer pain. *Cancer Treat Rep* 71:67–70, 1987.
353. Bruera E, Brenneis C, Patterson AH, et al: Use of methylphenidate as an adjuvant to narcotic analgesics in patients with advanced cancer. *J Pain Sympt Manag* 4:3–6, 1989.
354. Dundee JW, Moore J: The myth of phenothiazine potentiation. *Anaesth* 16:95–96, 1961.
355. Keats AS, Telford J, Kurosu Y: "Potentiation" of meperidine by promethazine. *Anesthesiol* 22:34–41, 1961.
356. Beaver WT, Wallenstein SL, Houde RW, et al: A comparison of the analgesic effect of methotrimeprazine and morphine in patients with cancer. *Clin Pharmacol Ther* 7:436–446, 1966.
357. Bloomfield S, Simard-Savoie S, Bernier J, et al: Comparative analgesic activity of levomepromazine and morphine in patients with chronic pain. *Can Med Assoc J* 90:1156–1159, 1964.
358. Hanks GW, Thomas PJ, Trueman T, et al: The myth of haloperidol potentiation. *Lancet* 2:523–524, 1983.
359. Beaver WT, Feise G: Combination of analgesic effects of morphine sulfate, hydroxyzine and their combinations in patients with postoperative pain. In Bonica JJ, Albe-Fessard D. (eds.): *Advances in Pain Research and Therapy,* Vol. 1. New York: Raven Press, 1976, pp. 553–557.
360. Bruera E, Roca E, Cedaro L, et al: Action of oral methylprednisolone in terminal cancer patients: A prospective randomized double blind study. *Cancer Treat Rep* 69:751–754, 1985.
361. Walsh TD: Adjuvant analgesic therapy in cancer pain. In Foley KM, Bonica JJ, Ventafridda V (eds.). *Advances in Pain Research and Therapy,* Vol. 16. New York: Raven Press, 1990, pp. 155–169.
362. Ernst DS, MacDonald N, Paterson AHG, et al: A double-blind, crossover trial of intravenous clodronate in metastatic bone pain. *J Pain Sympt Manag* 7:4–11, 1992.
363. Adami S, Mian M: Clodronate therapy of metastatic bone disease in patients with prostatic carcinoma. *Rec Res Cancer Res* 116:67–72, 1989.
364. Portenoy RK, Moulin DE, Rogers A, et al: IV infusions of opioids for cancer pain: Clinical review and guidelines for use. *Cancer Treat Rep* 70:575–582, 1986.
365. Citron M, Johnston-Early A, Fossieck, B et al: Safety and efficacy of continuous intravenous morphine for severe cancer pain. *Am J Med* 77:199–204, 1984.
366. Stuart GJ, Davey EB, Wight SE: Continuous intravenous morphine infusions for terminal pain control: A retrospective review. *Drug Intell Clin Pharmacol* 20:968–972, 1986.
367. Ferris FD, Kerr IG, DeAngelis C, et al: Inpatient nar-

cotic infusions for patients with cancer pain. *J Palliat Care* 6:51–59, 1990.

368. Portenoy RK: Continuous infusion of opioid drugs. *Med Clin North Am* 71:233–241, 1987.
369. Coyle N, Mauskop A, Maggard J, et al: Continuous infusions of opiates in cancer patients with pain. *Oncol Nurs Forum* 13:53–57, 1986.
370. Dickson RJ, Howard B, Campbell J: The relief of pain by subcutaneous infusion of morphine. In Wilkes E (ed.): *Advances in Morphine Therapy, The 1983 International Symposium on Pain Control.* Royal Society of Medicine International Congress and Symposium Series #64. London: Royal Society of Medicine, 1983, pp. 107–110.
371. Miser AW, David DM, Hughes, CS et al: Continuous subcutaneous infusions of morphine in children with cancer. *Am J Dis Child* 137:383–385, 1983.
372. Bruera E. Legris MA, Kuehn N, et al: Hypodermoclysis for the administration of fluids and narcotic analgesics in patients with advanced cancer. *J Natl Cancer Inst* 81:1108–1109, 1989.
373. Drexel H, Dzien A, Spiegel RW: Treatment of severe cancer pain by low dose continuous subcutaneous morphine. *Pain* 36:169–176, 1989.
374. Bruera E, Brenneis C, Michaud M et al: Patient-controlled subcutaneous hydromorphone versus continuous subcutaneous infusion for the treatment of cancer pain. *J Natl Cancer Inst* 80:1152–1154, 1988.
375. Brenneis C, Michaud M, Bruera E et al: Local toxicity during subcutaneous infusion of narcotics: A prospective study. *Cancer Nurs* 10:172–176, 1987.
376. Bruera E, Brenneis C, Michaud M, et al: Continuous sc infusion of narcotics using a portable disposable device in patients with advanced cancer. *Cancer Treat Rep* 71:635–637, 1987.
377. Sheidler VR: New methods in analgesic delivery. In McGuire DB, Yarbro CH (eds.): *Cancer Pain Management.* Philadelphia: Saunders, 1987, pp. 203–222.
378. Moulin DE, Kreeft JH, Murray-Parsons N, et al: Comparison of continuous subcutaneous and intravenous hydromorphone for management of cancer pain. *Lancet* 337:465–468, 1991.
379. Lang AH, Abbrederis K, Dzien A, et al: Treatment of severe cancer pain by continuous infusion of subcutaneous opioids. *Rec Res Cancer Res* 121:51–57, 1991.
380. The United States Pharmacopeia, 21st rev., The United States Pharmacopeial Convention, Rockville, MD, 1984.
381. Caplan RA, Ready LB, Oden RV, et al: Transdermal fentanyl for postoperative pain management. *JAMA* 261:1036–1039, 1989.
382. Gourlay GK, Kowalski SR, Plummer JL, et al: The efficacy of transdermal fentanyl in the treatment of postoperative pain: A double-blind comparison of fentanyl and placebo systems. *Pain* 40:21–28, 1990.
383. Simmonds MA, Richenbacher J: Transdermal fentanyl: Long-term analgesic studies. *J Pain Sympt Manag* 7:S36–S39, 1992.
384. Calis KA, Kohler DR, Corso DM: Transdermally administered fentanyl for pain management. *Clin Pharm* 11:22–36, 1992.
385. Miser AW, Narang PK, Dothage JA, et al: Transdermal fentanyl for pain control in patients with cancer. *Pain* 37:15–21, 1989.
386. Herbst LH, Strause LG: Transdermal fentanyl use in hospice home-care patients with chronic cancer pain. *J Pain Sympt Manag* 7:S54–S57, 1992.
387. Levy MH, Rosen SM, Kedziera P: Transdermal fentanyl: Seeding trial in patients with chronic cancer pain. *J Pain Sympt Manag* 7:S48–S50, 1992.
388. Maves TJ, Barcellos WA: Management of cancer pain with transdermal fentanyl: Phase IV trial, University of Iowa. *J Pain Sympt Manag* 7:S58–S62, 1991.
389. Varvel JR, Shafer SL, Hwang SS, et al: Absorption characteristics of transdermally administered fentanyl. *Anesthesiol* 70:928–934, 1989.
390. Gupta SK, Southam M, Gale R, et al: System functionality and physiochemical model of fentanyl transdermal system. *J Pain Sympt Manag* 7:S17–S26, 1992.
391. Payne R: Transdermal fentanyl: Suggested recommendations for clinical use. *J Pain Sympt Manag* 7:S40–S44, 1992.
392. Westerling D, Lindahl S, Anderson KE, et al: Absorption and bioavailability of rectally administered morphine in women. *Eur J Clin Pharmacol* 23:59–64, 1982.
393. Johsson T, Christensen CB, Jordening H, et al: The bioavailability of rectally administered morphine. *Pharmacol Toxicol* 62:203–205, 1988.
394. Moolenaar F, Yska JP,Visser J, et al: Drastic improvement in the rectal absorbtion profile of morphine in man. *Eur J Clin Pharmacol* 29:119–121, 1985.
395. Hanning CD, Vickers AP, Smith G, et al: The morphine hydrogel suppository: A new sustained release rectal preparation. *Br J Anaesth* 61:221–227, 1988.
396. Cole L, Hanning CD: Review of the rectal use of opioids. *J Pain Sympt Manag* 5:118–126, 1990.
397. Pert CB, Snyder SH: Opiate receptor demonstration in nervous tissue. *Science* 179:1011, 1973.
398. Yaksh TL, Rudy TA: Analgesia mediated by a direct spinal action of narcotics. *Science* 192:1357–1358, 1976.
399. Wang JK, Nauss CA, Thomas JE: Pain relief by intrathecally applied morphine in man. *Anesthesiol* 50:149–151, 1979.
400. Zenz M, Schappler-Scheele B, Neuhaus R, et al: Long-term peridural morphine analgesia in cancer pain. *Lancet* 1:91, 1981.
401. Coombs DW, Maurer LH, Saunders RL, et al: Outcomes and complications for continuous intraspinal narcotic analgesia for cancer pain control. *J Clin Oncol* 2:1414–1420, 1984.
402. Arner S, Arner B: Differential effects of epidural morphine in the treatment of cancer-related pain. *Acta Anaesthesiol Scand* 29:32-36, 1985.
403. Plummer JL, Cherry DA, Cousins MJ, et al: Long-term spinal administration of morphine in cancer and non-cancer pain: A retrospective study. *Pain* 44:215–220, 1991.
404. Wang JK: Intrathecal morphine for intractable pain secondary to cancer of pelvic organs. *Pain* 21:99–102, 1985.
405. Max MB, Inturrisi CE, Kaiko RF, et al: Epidural and intrathecal opiates: Cerebrospinal fluid and plasma profiles in patients with chronic cancer pain. *Clin Pharmacol Ther* 38:631–641, 1985.
406. Sjoberg M, Appelgren L, Einarsson S, et al: Long-term intrathecal morphine and bupivacaine in "refractory" cancer patients. I. Results from the first series of 52 patients. *Acta Anaesthesiol Scand* 35:30–43, 1992.
407. DuPen SL, Kharasch ED, Williams A, et al: Chronic epidural bupivacaine-opioid infusion in intractable cancer pain. *Pain* 49:293–300, 1992.
408. Nitescu P, Appelgren L, Linder LE, et al: Epidural versus intrathecal morphine bupivacaine: Assessments of

consecutive treatments in advanced cancer patients. *J Pain Sympt Manag* 5:18–26, 1990.

409. Paice JA, Magolan JM: Intraspinal drug delivery. *Nurs Clin North Am* 26:477–498, 1991.
410. Krames ES, Gershow J, Glassberg A, et al: Continuous infusion of spinally administered narcotic for the relief of pain due to malignant disease. *Cancer* 56:696–702, 1985.
411. Penn RD, Paice JA, Gottschalk W, et al: Cancer pain relief using chronic morphine infusion: Early experience with a programmable implanted drug pump. *J Neurosurg* 61:302–306, 1984.
412. Penn RD, Paice JA: Chronic intrathecal morphine for intractable pain. *J Neurosurg* 67:182–186, 1987.
413. Onofrio BM, Yaksh TL: Long-term pain relief produced by intrathecal morphine infusion in 53 patients. *J Neurosurg* 72:200–209, 1990.
414. Bedder MD, Burchiel K, Larson A: Cost analysis of two implantable narcotic delivery systems. *J Pain Sympt Manag* 6:368–373, 1991.
415. DuPen SL, Peterson DG, Williams A, et al: Infection during chronic epidural catherization: Diagnosis and treatment. *Anesthesiol* 73:905–909, 1990.
416. Dennis GC, DeWitty RL: Long-term intraventricular infusion of morphine for intractable cancer of the head and neck. *J Neurosurg* 26:404–408, 1990.
417. Leavens ME, Hill CS, Cech DA, et al: Intrathecal and intraventricular morphine for pain in cancer patients: Initial study. *J Neurosurg* 56:241–245, 1982.
418. Lobato RD, Madrid JL, Fatela LV, et al: Intraventricular morphine for control of pain in terminal cancer patients. *J Neurosurg* 59:627–633, 1983.
419. Su CF, Liu MY, Lin MT: Intraventricular morphine produces pain relief, hypothermia, hyperglycemia and increased prolactin and growth hormone levels in patients with cancer pain. *J Neurol* 235:105–108, 1987.
420. Lazorthes Y, Verdi JC, Caute B, et al: Intracerebroventricular morphinotherapy for control of chronic cancer pain. *Prog Brain Res* 77:395–405, 1988.
421. American Association of Nurse Anesthetists Position Statement: Provision of pain relief by medication administered via continuous epidural, intrathecal, intrapleural, peripheral nerve catheters, or other pain relief devices, June 1990.
422. Olsson GL, Leddo CC, Wild L: Nursing management of patients receiving epidural narcotics. *Heart Lung* 18:130–138, 1989.
423. Paice JA: Intrathecal morphine infusion for intractable cancer pain: A new use for implanted pumps. *Oncol Nurs Forum* 13:33–39, 1986.
424. Sechzer PH: Objective measurement of pain. *Anesthesiol* 29:209–210, 1968.
425. Sheidler VR: Patient-controlled analgesia. *Curr Conc Nurs* 1:13–16, 1987.
426. Citron ML, Johnston-Early A, Boyer M, et al: Patient-controlled analgesia for severe cancer pain. *Arch Intern Med* 146:734–736, 1986.
427. Bauman TJ, Batenhorst RL, Graves DA, et al: Patient-controlled analgesia in the terminally ill cancer patient. *Drug Intell Clin Pharmacol* 20:297–301, 1986.
428. Hill HF, Saeger IC, Chapman CR: Patient-controlled analgesia after bone marrow transplantation for cancer. *Postgrad Med* 28:33–40, 1986.
429. Mackie AM, Coda BC, Hill HH: Adolescents use patient-controlled analgesia effectively for relief from prolonged oropharyngeal mucositis pain. *Pain* 16:265–269, 1991.
430. Bruera E, Brenneis C, Michaud M, et al: Patient-controlled subcutaneous hydromorphone versus continuous subcutaneous infusion for the treatment of cancer pain. *J Natl Cancer Inst* 80:1152–1154, 1988.
431. Kerr IG, Sone M, DeAngelis C, et al: Continuous narcotic infusion with patient controlled analgesia for chronic cancer pain in outpatients. *Ann Intern Med* 108:554–557, 1988.
432. Grochow LB, Sheidler VR, Grossman SA, et al: Does methadone provide longer-lasting analgesia than morphine? A randomized, double-blind study. *Pain* 38:151–157, 1989.
433. Hansen LA, Noyes MA, Lehman ME: Evaluation of patient-controlled analgesia (PCA) versus PCA plus continuous infusion in post-operative cancer patients. *J Pain Sympt Manag* 6:4–14, 1991.
434. Ferrell BR, Nash CC, Warfield C: The role of patient-controlled analgesia in the management of cancer pain. *J Pain Sympt Manag* 7:149–154, 1992.
435. Oncology Nursing Society: Resolution: Use of technology in pain management. 1991 Congress Oncology Nursing Society, San Antonio, TX, May 8–11, 1991.
436. Abram SE: The role of non-neurolytic blocks in the management of cancer pain. In Abram SE (ed.): *Cancer Pain.* Boston: Kluwer, 1989, pp. 67–76.
437. Swerdlow M: Role of chemical neurolysis and local anesthetic infiltration. In Swerdlow M, Ventafridda V (eds.): *Cancer Pain.* Lancaster, Eng.: MTP Press, 1987, pp. 105–128.
438. Ritchie JM, Greene NM: Local anesthetics. In Gilman AG, Rall TW, Nies AS, et al (eds.): *Goodman and Gilman's The Pharmacological Basis of Therapeutics* (ed. 8). New York: Pergamon Press, 1990, pp. 311–331.
439. Ferrer-Brechner T: Neurolytic blocks for cancer pain. In Abram SE (ed.): *Cancer Pain.* Boston: Kluwer, 1989, pp. 111–124.
440. Carson B: Neurologic and neurosurgical approaches to cancer pain. In McGuire DB, Yarbro CH (eds.): *Cancer Pain Management.* Philadelphia: Saunders, 1987, pp. 111–124.
441. Amidei CS: Pain and pain syndromes. In Cammermeyer M, Appeldorn C (eds.): *Core Curriculum for Neuroscience Nursing* (ed. 3). Chicago: American Association of Neuroscience Nurses, 1990.
442. Peteet J, Tay V, Cohen G, et al: Pain characteristics and treatment in an outpatient cancer population. *Cancer* 57:1259–1265, 1986.
443. Ahles TA: Psychological techniques for the management of cancer-related pain. In McGuire DB, Yarbro CH (eds.): *Cancer Pain Management.* Philadelphia: Saunders, 1987, pp. 245–258.
444. Ahles TA, Cohen RE, Blanchard ED: Difficulties inherent in conducting behavioral research with cancer patients. *Behav Ther* 7:69–70, 1984.
445. Breitbart W: Psychiatric management of cancer pain. *Cancer* 63:2336–2342, 1989.
446. Mayer DK: Non-pharmacologic management of pain in the person with cancer. *J Adv Nurs* 10:325–330, 1985.
447. Watt-Watson J, Donovan MI: *Pain Management: Nursing Perspective.* St. Louis: Mosby Year Book, 1992.
448. Weinrich SP, Weinrich MC: The effect of massage on pain in cancer patients. *Appl Nurs Res* 3:140–145, 1990.
449. Avellanosa AM, West CR: Experience with transcuta-

neous electrical nerve stimulation for relief of intractable pain in cancer patients. *J Med* 13:203–213, 1982.
450. Ventafridda V, Sganzerla EP, Fochi C, et al: Transcutaneous nerve stimulation in cancer pain. In Bonica JJ, Ventafridda V (eds.): *Advances in Pain Research and Therapy,* Vol. 2. New York: Raven Press, 1979, pp, 509–515.
451. Walsh Sr M, Brescia FJ: Clinitron therapy and pain management in advanced cancer patients. *J Pain Sympt Manag* 5:46–50, 1990.
452. McCaul KD, Malott JM: Distraction and coping with pain. *Psychol Bull* 95:516–533, 1984.
453. Bayuk L: Relaxation techniques: An adjunct therapy for cancer patients. *Semin Oncol Nurs* 1:147–150, 1985.
454. Graffam S, Johnson A: A comparison of two relaxation strategies for the relief of pain and its distress. *J Pain Sympt Manag* 2:229–231, 1987.
455. Blanchard EB, Epstein LH: *A Biofeedback Primer.* Reading, MA: Addison-Wesley, 1978.
456. Fotopoulos SS, Graham C, Cook MR: Psychophysiologic control of cancer pain. In Bonica JJ, Ventafridda V (eds.): *Advances in Pain Research and Therapy,* Vol. 2. New York: Raven Press, 1979, pp. 231–243.
457. Fleming U: Relaxation therapy for far-advanced cancer. *Practitioner* 229:471–475, 1985.
458. Fotopoulos SS, Cook MR, Graham C, et al: Cancer pain: Evaluation of electromyographic and electrodermal feedback. *Prog Clin Biol Res* 132D:33–53, 1983.
459. Spiegel D: The use of hypnosis in controlling cancer pain. *CA* 35:4–14, 1985.
460. Barber J, Gitelson J: Cancer pain: Psychological management using hypnosis. *CA* 30:130–136, 1980.
461. Spiegel D, Bloom J: Group therapy and hypnosis reduce metastatic breast carcinoma pain. *Psychosom Med* 45:333–339, 1983.
462. Syrjala KL, Cummings, C, Donaldson GW: Hypnosis or cognitive behavioral training for the reduction of pain and nausea during cancer treatment: A controlled clinical trial. *Pain* 48:137–146, 1992.
463. Turk DC, Rennert K: Pain and the terminally ill cancer patient: A cognitive-social learning perspective. In Sobel HJ (ed.): *Behavior Therapy in Terminal Care: A Humanistic Approach.* Cambridge, MA: Ballinger, 1981, pp. 95–123.
464. Fishman B, Loscalzo M: Cognitive behavioral interventions in management of cancer pain: Principles and applications. *Med Clin North Am* 71:271–287, 1987.
465. Bailey LM: Music therapy in pain management. *J Pain Symp Manag* 1:25–28, 1986.
466. Beck SL: The therapeutic use of music for cancer-related pain. *Oncol Nurs Forum* 18:1327–1337, 1991.
467. Erdman L: Laughter therapy for patients with cancer. *Oncol Nurs Forum* 18:1359–1363, 1991.
468. McAlary P: Relieving pain with heat or cold. *Nursing 88* July:64K–64N, 1988.
469. Spross JA: Cutaneous measures for pain. In Baird SB (ed.): *Decision Making in Oncology Nursing.* Toronto, Can.: Decker, 1988, pp. 74–75.
470. Mast D, Meyers J, Urbanski A: Relaxation techniques: A self-learning module for nurses: Unit I. *Cancer Nurs* 10:141–147, 1987.
471. Mast D, Meyers J, Urbanski A: Relaxation techniques: A self-learning module for nurses: Unit II. *Cancer Nurs* 10:217–225, 1987.
472. Cobb SC: Teaching relaxation techniques to cancer patients. *Cancer Nurs* 7:157–161, 1984.
473. Donovan MI: Relaxation with guided imagery: A useful technique. *Cancer Nurs* 3:27–32, 1980.
474. Munro S, Mount B: Music therapy in palliative care. *Can Med Assoc J* 4:1029–1034, 1978.
475. Spross JA: Behavioral intervention. In Baird SB (ed.): *Decision Making in Oncology Nursing.* Toronto, Can.: Decker, 1988, pp. 72–73.

Chapter 24

Infection

Jan M. Ellerhorst-Ryan, RN, MSN, CS

SCOPE OF THE PROBLEM

Incidence

Infection is the major cause of morbidity and mortality in individuals diagnosed with cancer. Infectious processes are implicated in at least 50% of deaths in persons with solid tumors and up to 80% of those with leukemia.[1,2] This may be due to the underlying disease, intensive treatment modalities, or prolonged hospitalization. To understand why individuals with cancer are susceptible to infection, it is necessary to understand normal host defenses and the mechanisms by which they are impaired by cancer and cancer therapy.

ANATOMY AND PHYSIOLOGY

Integumentary, Mucosal, and Chemical Barriers

Intact skin constitutes the most important physical barrier against invasion by both exogenous and endogenous organisms. The skin is made up of cornified layers of epithelial cells that cover the body and protect tissues against dehydration and invasion by harmful bacteria. When a break in the skin occurs, environmental microbes and those that normally inhabit hair follicles and sebaceous glands can enter the body and cause infection.

A second major defense against infection is the mucociliary activity found in the mucous membranes. The cilia of the epithelial cells that line the respiratory tract beat rhythmically to propel mucus and its entrapped foreign particles toward the nose and throat. In the gastrointestinal tract, the cilia propel bacteria and waste products to be removed in the feces. Microorganisms constitute up to 60% of the weight of the stool; therefore, an intact mucous membrane is essential to prevention of infection.

There are many other protective mechanisms in the body. Acid pH inhibits or prevents bacterial growth on the skin and in the stomach, the bladder, and the vagina. Microbicidal elements in prostatic fluid and tears also provide a protective effect.

Leukocytes

Leukocytes, particularly polymorphonuclear neutrophils (PMNs), represent a significant defense against infection. PMNs, which are also referred to as *polys* or *segs,* are short-lived white blood cells (WBCs) that respond quickly to bacterial invasion. They are the most numerous leukocyte, constituting 55%–70% of circulating WBCs. The primary function of PMNs is the destruction and elimination of microorganisms through *phagocytosis,* the process of engulfing and ingesting foreign matter. In addition, PMNs secrete *chemotactants,* chemical substances that alert the body to the presence of an invader. Chemotactants stimulate increased production of PMNs and macrophages and direct them to the site of invasion. Without sufficient numbers of PMNs, the body's ability to mount an inflammatory response is compromised.

Monocytes and Macrophages

Monocytes and macrophages constitute what was previously referred to as the reticuloendothelial system. *Monocytes* are released from the bone marrow before they complete the maturation process and are capable of only limited phagocytosis. After migrating into the tissues, full maturation occurs; the cells are then referred to as *macrophages.* Macrophages may survive from several months to several years.[3] They are highly phagocytic and play important roles in inflammation and in the cellular and immune responses. Following initial contact with a foreign protein, macrophages process and present antigens to lymphocytes, which stimulates the immune response and cytokine production. Monocytes also produce specific components required for the complement cascade.[4]

Lymphocytes

Lymphocytes, the cells responsible for cellular and humoral immunity, provide long-term protection against a variety of microorganisms. They usually constitute 25%–30% of the total WBC count. B-lymphocytes, responsible for humoral immunity, produce antibodies that neutralize, destroy, or facilitate phagocytosis of foreign proteins. T-lymphocytes provide cellular immunity and initiate a variety of activities that, directly or indirectly, result in elimination of microorganisms or other foreign substances. T-helper cells are the most numerous of T-lymphocyte subsets, normally making up over 75% of the total T-lymphocyte count. T-helper cells serve as the principal regulator of immune function through secretion of protein mediators (cytokines) that act on other cells involved in the immune and inflammatory responses.[5] Cytokines produced by T-helper cells include interleukins 2 through 6, gamma interferon, and granulocyte-macrophage colony stimulating factor. The immune response is discussed in greater detail in Chapter 5.

Cytokines

Cytokines are small protein hormones synthesized by a variety of leukocytes. Cytokines produced by mononuclear phagocytes (monocytes, macrophages, PMNs, and eosinophils) are referred to as monokines, whereas those secreted by T- and B-lymphocytes are called lymphokines.

Cytokines initiate and/or regulate a number of inflammatory and immune responses. They include interferons, interleukins, growth factors, and colony stimulating factors. Specific information about cytokines and cytokine activity is detailed in Chapter 5.

PATHOPHYSIOLOGY

Alterations in Nonspecific Defenses

Disruptions in protective barriers

Skin and mucous membrane integrity frequently is impaired by cancer and cancer therapy. Primary and metastatic tumor growth invades healthy tissue and disrupts normal circulation, resulting in ulceration and necrosis. Chemotherapy and radiation may further alter integrity of skin and mucosal surfaces, particularly in the gastrointestinal (GI) tract.

Diagnostic and treatment strategies typically include a variety of invasive procedures, including surgery, venipuncture, peripheral intravenous (IV) infusions, bone marrow biopsies and aspirations, central venous access catheters, "fingersticks," and bronchoscopy.

Host defenses are further compromised by neurologic impairments secondary to primary or metastatic disease involving the central nervous system (CNS). Examples include aspiration pneumonia due to loss of gag reflex and urinary tract infections associated with inability to empty the bladder.

Changes in normal flora

Undisturbed, endogenous microbial flora exist as a carefully balanced synergistic microenvironment within the host. Alterations in normal flora predispose persons with cancer to serious opportunistic or nosocomial infection.

Over 80% of infections developing in cancer patients arise from endogenous organisms, nearly half of which are acquired during hospitalization.[6,7] Institutional sources of potential infection include personnel, food, air, water, equipment, and procedures. The most significant factor contributing to transmission of infectious agents during hospitalization is poor hand washing by health care personnel.[6–10] The use of antibiotics commonly alters normal flora, allowing overgrowth of pathogenic organisms.

Obstruction

Obstruction, usually associated with solid tumors or lymphoma, may contribute to risk of infection by interfering with normal clearing and drainage mechanisms. Sites most often involved include the pulmonary system, the biliary tree, and the urinary tract.[11]

Granulocytopenia

There is a direct relationship between the number of circulating PMNs and the incidence of infection. Individuals whose granulocyte count is less than $1000/mm^3$ are considered to be granulocytopenic and at increased risk of infection (Figure 24-1). When the granulocyte count is less than $500/mm^3$, risk is significant.[11] As the length of therapy and duration of granulocytopenia increases, so does the incidence of sepsis.[12,13]

Because of the short life span of circulating PMNs, their number must be determined on a daily basis for granulocytopenic individuals. The absolute granulocyte count (AGC) is calculated using data from the total WBC and the differential, which specifies the percentage of WBCs by cell type. The differential also notes the presence of abnormal or premature WBCs. The AGC is determined by multiplying the percentage of PMNs and bands by the total number of WBCs. For example, a patient with a total WBC of 2200 $cells/mm^3$ has the following differential report:

33% PMNs
18% bands
42% lymphocytes
1% eosinophils
1% basophils
5% monocytes

To calculate the AGC, use the following formula:

$$\begin{aligned} AGC &= \text{Total WBC} \times (\%\ \text{PMNs} + \%\ \text{bands}) \\ &= 2200 \times (33\% + 18\%) = 1122 \end{aligned}$$

The individual in this example is not granulocytopenic, since the AGC is greater than 1000. Even when the

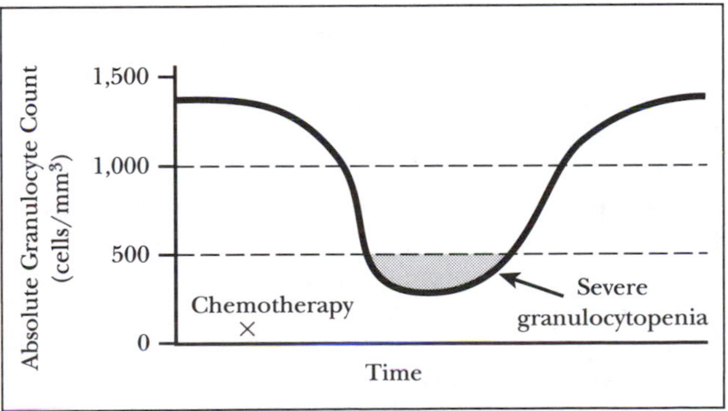

FIGURE 24-1 Chemotherapy cycle. Days of risk for infection vary according to type of chemotherapy agent administered and individual response to treatment. The fall in the granulocyte count may begin a few days after chemotherapy or may be delayed for more than a week. Severe granulocytopenia occurs when absolute granulocyte counts are less than 500, and may persist for several days, a week, or sometimes longer.

total WBC count is approximately the same from one day to the next, the percentage of PMNs and bands can still vary significantly. The WBC count alone does not always provide enough information to determine the presence of granulocytopenia.

Immunosuppression

Infection

Although infection commonly is viewed as a result of depressed immunity, certain infections actually contribute to impairment of immune function. Depression of lymphocyte function in vitro has been associated with a variety of viral infections, including cytomegalovirus (CMV), herpes simplex virus (HSV), and Epstein-Barr virus (EBV);[14] live vaccine (e.g., measles, mumps, and rubella); bacterial and mycobacterial infections, such as tuberculosis, leprosy, syphilis, and bacterial pneumonia; and fungal infections, such as candidiasis and coccidioidomycosis. It appears that both lymphocyte and macrophage functions may be abnormally depressed during and after acute infections, thereby extending susceptibility beyond the acute episode.[6]

Acquired immune deficiency syndrome (AIDS)

Acquired immune deficiency syndrome (AIDS) is characterized by loss of T-helper cells, resulting in progressive loss of immunocompetence, development of opportunistic infections and chronic wasting, impairment of the central nervous system, and emergence of unusual malignancies. The virus that causes AIDS, human immunodeficiency virus (HIV), has been isolated in blood, saliva, tears, urine, cerebrospinal fluid, semen, vaginal secretions, and breast milk. However, only blood, semen, and vaginal secretions have been proven to be vectors, with limited evidence to suggest that transmission via breast milk is possible.[15]

Common opportunistic infections associated with AIDS include CMV, HSV, herpes zoster, *Candida albicans, Cryptococcus, Pneumocystis carinii, Toxoplasma gondii, Cryptosporidium, Mycobacterium avium—intracellulare* (MAI), and tuberculosis.[16]

Infection with HIV is not synonymous with AIDS. AIDS is part of a continuum of illnesses related to infection with HIV. Many persons with primary HIV infection are asymptomatic even though they demonstrate seropositivity for antibodies to HIV. Others may have symptoms that can develop 2–6 weeks after infection, including fever, rigors, arthralgias, rash, abdominal cramping, and diarrhea. These symptoms may be accompanied by mild immunologic deficiencies, such as leukopenia, lymphopenia, and thrombocytopenia.[17]

AIDS-related complex or condition (ARC) is a vague term first applied to those persons with symptoms of immune deficiency but without opportunistic infection or AIDS-related malignancy. It generally is considered to be a prodromal phase, with manifestation of at least two clinical symptoms and at least two abnormal laboratory studies indicative of immune deficiency.[18] Immune thrombocytopenic purpura (ITP) is another AIDS-related diagnosis; it is evidenced by easy bruising, petechiae, mucosal bleeding, and varying degrees of lymphadenopathy.

Tumor-associated abnormalities

The types of infections that occur in persons diagnosed with cancer are somewhat predictable. Abnormal cell-mediated immunity in Hodgkin's disease and acute leukemia is associated with increased incidence of intracellular pathogens, including herpes zoster, *Cryptococcus neoformans, Brucella* species, *Myobacterium tuberculosis, Listeria monocytogenes, Salmonella* species, and *Toxoplasma gondii.* Other malignancies, such as advanced lung cancer and intracranial tumors, are associated with a decreased sensitivity to and decreased ability to respond to the challenging antigen.[7,19,20]

Individuals who are asplenic as a result of trauma, staging laparotomy for malignant lymphoma, hypersplenism, or sickle cell disease have impaired opsonization that can increase susceptibility to infection.[11,14,21] The risk of overwhelming sepsis and death in persons with asplenia, especially those with Hodgkin's disease, is at least 50 times greater than in the normal population. It has been noted, however, that individuals with Hodgkin's disease in complete remission had a 2.30% cumulative risk of overwhelming postsplenectomy infection, whereas the rate of infection increased to 15.25% for those in whom relapse had occurred.[22]

Febrile episodes occur frequently in individuals diagnosed with cancer. Although fever may be caused by the underlying cancer, 55%–70% of fevers result from infection, especially during periods of granulocytopenia.[4] Lymphomas, hypernephromas, and hepatomas can cause fever unrelated to infection.[8] In addition, tumor masses that cause local obstruction or compromise blood supply to normal tissue can predispose tissue to necrosis, local infection, and fever. Fever caused by an underlying cancer cannot be distinguished, on the basis of duration or degree of temperature elevation, from fever caused by infection. Excluding febrile episodes related to the administration of blood products and chemotherapeutic agents, which resolve spontaneously, fevers in the individual with cancer warrant thorough and prompt evaluation to rule out infection as the cause.

Nutrition

Cancer can affect an individual's nutritional status in several ways. The tumor can interfere with the functional capacity of gastrointestinal structures or organs and may cause inlet or outlet obstruction. Chronic obstruction can compromise the blood supply to surrounding tissue, especially if vascular impairment is severe or prolonged. The resulting necrosis and ulceration will predispose the affected areas to hemorrhage and infection.

Cachexia, a state of malnutrition and wasting, is often a debilitating manifestation of cancer. The exact mechanisms responsible for cachexia are not well understood. The rate of wasting does not appear to be related to the histologic findings of the tumor, the stage of the disease, or specific sites of involvement. Severity of cachexia may be unrelated to the quantity or quality of calories consumed, inasmuch as cachexia often develops without evidence of malabsorption.[23]

There is substantial evidence to support the existence of a relationship between malnutrition and a variety of immune deficiencies. Cell-mediated immunity is most often affected, with decreased numbers of lymphocytes and diminished response to antigen. Phagocytosis and the complement system are also impaired.[24,25] Immune defects related to nutritional deficiencies can be corrected by oral supplementation or parenteral nutritional support.

Cancer therapy

Surgery Surgery is commonly employed in diagnosis, staging, and treatment of individuals diagnosed with cancer. Various factors can increase the incidence of infectious complications in the individual undergoing surgery, including the duration of preoperative hospitalization, extent of surgery, length of the procedure, presence and degree of hemorrhage and tissue ischemia, nutritional status of the patient, prior chemotherapy or corticosteroid administration, and, most important, presence of infection or wound contamination during surgery. Preoperative prophylactic antibiotics may be given to provide protection during the operative risk period. The choice of antibiotic is based on the operative site, potential pathogens, presence of prior infection, or heavy colonization with particular microorganisms.[26]

The surgical wound is the most common site of infection during the postoperative period. Wound infections range in severity from minor inflammatory responses to major infections that can be life-threatening. Distinctive patterns of microorganisms usually are seen in different hospital environments. Each institution's infection control team monitors patterns, trends, and incidence of specific microorganisms resulting in infection. Special concern must be directed toward the detection of resistant organisms, which can develop with astonishing rapidity within the hospital environment, causing significant morbidity.

A greater risk of sepsis accompanies certain surgical procedures. Surgical instrumentation of the genitourinary (GU) and GI tracts are associated with higher incidence of morbidity and mortality.

Radiation therapy and chemotherapy Radiation therapy and chemotherapy interfere with essential metabolic functions of the cell and can cause inflammation and ulceration of normal tissues, predisposing to infection. Doses of chemotherapy and/or radiation that can be administered safely are determined by toxicity to normal tissues. Fractionation of radiation doses and administration of chemotherapy in intermittent cycles have been effective in enhancing therapeutic benefit while limiting toxicity. The major risks associated with therapeutic radiation and cytotoxic chemotherapy relate to the induction of granulocytopenia and immunosuppression.

Chemotherapy can induce immunologic defects that lead to bacterial, fungal, parasitic, or viral infection. Not all chemotherapeutic agents, however, produce immunologic compromise. The potential effects and side effects of each agent should be reviewed and incorporated into the patient's plan of care and assessment (see Chapter 16 for specific information concerning chemotherapy).

Hematologic competency can be adversely affected by radiation therapy. Leukocytes are the first to decrease, followed by platelets and erythrocytes. Blood counts should be monitored during radiation, especially if a large area is treated or if significant areas of bone marrow are included in the radiation field. Total body irradiation results in a substantial reduction in cellular immune function that persists for months to years.[11]

Depending on the total dose and type of radiation, skin and mucous membrane integrity may be impaired, thereby predisposing to infection.[27,28] Radiation reactions can include epilation, erythema, dry and moist desquamation, mucositis, and necrosis. Nursing care for the patient receiving radiation therapy is discussed in Chapter 13.

TYPES OF INFECTIONS

Bacteria

Changing patterns in bacterial infections are primarily the result of improvements in antibiotic therapy. During the 1950s and 1960s, *Staphylococcus aureus* was the most commonly identified organism in immunocompromised persons. Development of beta-lactamase–resistant penicillins provided highly effective therapy against *S. aureus* and led to the emergence of gram-negative organisms as the predominant pathogens. Empiric use of combination antibiotic therapy, incorporating third-generation cephalosporins, has greatly reduced the number of documented gram-negative infections. However, a recent resurgence of gram-positive infections is believed to be the result of increased use of central venous access catheters and the prevalence of methicillin-resistant strains of *Staphylococcus*.[6,12,29,30]

Gram-negative organisms

Despite current shifts in the patterns of infection, the primary cause of infection in granulocytopenic patients continues to be gram-negative organisms, especially *E. coli, K. pneumoniae, and P. aeruginosa.*[5] The most significant consequence of gram-negative infection is the potential for endotoxic or systemic shock. Endotoxins are lipopolysaccharide protein complexes found on the outer membrane of gram-negative organisms. The release of endotoxins initiates a cascade of events that, unless interrupted, will rapidly lead to death for the neutropenic patient. The actions of endotoxins include: release of endogenous pyrogens resulting in a febrile response; alteration of the vascular endothelium causing formation of microthrombi; activation of the complement, coagulation, and fibrinolytic systems; and release of bradykinin, histamine, and seratonin producing vasodilation and increased capillary permeability.[31] Without early detection and prompt initiation of treatment, endotoxic shock leads to hypotension, tissue ischemia, multisystem failure, and death.

Gram-positive organisms

S. aureus and *S. epidermidis* are responsible for most gram-positive infections occurring during periods of granulocytopenia; however, certain species of *Streptococcus* can also be encountered.[7] Although less common, infection with gram-positive organisms may result in shock through secretion of noxious proteins called exotoxins. The most well-known exotoxin, produced by *S. aureus,* is associated with toxic shock syndrome.

Treatment

Empiric antibiotic therapy is treatment initiated before the infecting organisms have been identified. To date, a standardized regimen for treatment of bacterial infections in granulocytopenic patients has not been defined. Selection of antibiotic agents must be individualized to consider the probable cause of infection and the likely site of origin, as well as institutional patterns of infection and antibiotic resistance. In general, the empiric antibiotic regimen selected should cover a broad spectrum of pathogens without significant risk for emergence of resistant organisms or drug-related toxicity.[11,32] Combination therapies commonly employed include an aminoglycoside plus either an antipseudomonal penicillin or third-generation cephalosporin.[32,33] Vancomycin often is added if gram-positive organisms are potentially involved.

Mycobacteria

Although mycobacterial infections are uncommon in persons with cancer, they tend to be associated with defects in cellular immunity. Latent infections with *M. tuberculosis* may be reactivated. *M. avium-intracellulare* (MAI) infection, common in persons with AIDS, has also been observed in persons with hairy cell leukemia.[11,34,35]

Treatment

While isoniazid is the treatment of choice for tuberculosis, it is not effective therapy for MAI. Combination therapy has been more successful in treating MAI, including amikacin, rifampin, ciprofloxacin, ethambutol, and clarithromycin.[36]

Fungi

In humans, fungi can exist in harmony with other endogenous flora in a carefully balanced synergistic microenvironment. Alterations in this environment, such as disrupted integumentary and mucosal barriers, treatment-induced granulocytopenia, immunosuppression, and alterations in normal flora can lead to invasive fungal infections. Fungal infections have become an increasingly important cause of morbidity and mortality in persons with cancer, particularly hematologic and lymphoreticular neoplasms.

Factors predisposing to fungal infection include severe, prolonged granulocytopenia, implanted vascular access catheters, administration of parenteral nutrition or corticosteroids, prolonged use of broad-spectrum antibiotics, and damage to oropharyngeal or GI mucosa due to disease or treatment.[30,33] Immunosuppressed persons who develop new or progressive pulmonary infiltrates while receiving broad-spectrum antibiotics present major problems for differential diagnosis. The possibility of fungal infection must be considered.

Candida

Candida is the most common cause of invasive fungal infection. The presence of *Candida* in the sputum, mouth, or throat cannot be definitively correlated with infection because *Candida* can reside harmlessly in the healthy host. However, the immunosuppressed person is at risk when granulocytopenia occurs and/or when cellular immunity is impaired. Broad-spectrum antibiotics alter the function of normal bacterial flora and, therefore, are associated with increased risk of fungal overgrowth and infection.

Dermatologic infections with *Candida* occur most frequently in skin folds, such as the groin, perineum, and perianal areas and under the breasts. Oral candidiasis (thrush) is a common yeast infection that can disseminate throughout the GI tract. Disseminated candidiasis often involves the lungs, kidneys, bones, joints, and central nervous system.

Aspergillus

Aspergillus is another common fungus that causes serious infections in persons with cancer, particularly in those who are granulocytopenic and/or are receiving immunosuppressive therapy. The fungus enters the host through the upper airway and typically causes pneumonia or sinus infection. Nosocomial transmission of *Aspergillus* has occurred in hospitals where spores contained in construction materials were disseminated through the ventilation system.

Aspergillosis is characterized by blood vessel invasion, which can lead to thrombosis and infarction of pulmonary arteries and veins. Blood cultures rarely are positive, even in disseminated aspergillosis. The infection is difficult to diagnose, often necessitating aggressive treatment before the diagnosis is confirmed. Without prompt and aggressive therapy with amphotericin, *Aspergillus* pneumonia is almost always fatal in granulocytopenic patients.[37,38]

Cryptococcus

Cryptococcus neoformans is a yeast found in soil and pigeon excreta and generally is acquired by inhalation. The infection appears most often in individuals with advanced Hodgkin's disease and other lymphomas. It commonly occurs as an insidious meningoencephalitis. Headache, vomiting, and diplopia without fever are typical symptoms. Cerebrospinal fluid examination reveals mononuclear pleocytosis and a low glucose level. Intrathecal administration of antifungal agents may be required for individuals whose cerebrospinal fluid does not clear with IV therapy. As with other fungi, cryptococcal infection can also occur in the lungs and disseminate to visceral organs.

Histoplasma

Histoplasmosis generally occurs as a pulmonary infection, usually in individuals with lymphoreticular neoplasms. The infection commonly disseminates, causing adenopathy and hepatosplenomegaly, which may be confused with the underlying neoplasm. Disseminated histoplasmosis can occur in persons whose cancer is in remission, as well as in those with active disease; therefore, histologic examination of biopsy material for *Histoplasma* is necessary if this organism is suspected as a cause of infection.

Phycomycetes

The Phycomycetes (*Mucor, Rhizopus,* and *Absidia*) are opportunistic fungi widespread in dust and air. The lungs, nasal sinuses, and GI tract are the three major sites of infection. After the fungi are inhaled into the lungs, the disease may disseminate to other body sites. Person-to-person transmission is rare.

Coccidioides

Coccidioides is found in the soil of the southwestern United States and typically enters the body by inhalation. The organism is rapidly phagocytized in persons who have a competent immune system and may cause no symptoms. Immunocompromised persons, however, are susceptible to the development of serious pulmonary infections.[26,39]

Treatment

Two major problems in treatment of fungal infections are the difficulty associated with culturing organisms from infected tissues and the limited number of effective agents available to manage severe fungal infections.

Amphotericin B is the drug of choice for treatment of systemic fungal infections. It is, however, associated with significant side effects and toxicities, including fever, chills, rigors, nausea, vomiting, hypotension, bronchospasm, and occasionally seizures. Premedication with acetaminophen and the addition of hydrocortisone sodium succinate to the IV solution generally reduce the reactions associated with the drug. IV meperidine (1 mg/kg) can be used to ameliorate fever and chills that frequently accompany the initial administration of amphotericin.[40]

The major toxicity of amphotericin is nephrotoxicity. With continued administration, elevated levels of creatinine and blood urea nitrogen can occur. Electrolyte imbalances, particularly hypokalemia, are common and warrant careful monitoring and treatment.

Flucytosine (5-FC) is another antifungal agent used for treatment of *Candida* and *Cryptococcus* infections. The major limitation to its use is the rapid onset of drug resistance. 5-FC is well-absorbed orally, with side effects including nausea, vomiting, diarrhea, myelosuppression, nephrotoxicity, and hepatotoxicity.[40] 5-FC commonly is used in combination with amphotericin.

Fluconazole is an oral antifungal agent that is well absorbed and is able to penetrate into cerebrospinal fluid, the eye, and peritoneal fluid. It is also available in parenteral form. Fluconazole most often is used to treat cryptococcal meningitis and oropharyngeal, esophageal, and systemic *Candida* infections. Side effects include exfoliative skin disorders (blistering, peeling, etc.), hepatotoxicity, and, less frequently, GI disturbances and headaches.

Ketoconazole, another oral antifungal agent, is used to treat disseminated and pulmonary coccidiodomycosis, candidiasis, and histoplasmosis. The most frequent side effects are nausea, vomiting, and diarrhea. Rare instances of hepatotoxicity have been reported. High-dose ketoconazole therapy has been shown to suppress adrenocorticoid secretion.[40]

Miconazole is a parenteral antifungal agent considered to be primarily a second-line therapy. It may be prescribed for treatment of candidiasis, coccidiodomycosis, and cryptococcus. For treatment of fungal meningitis, IV miconazole must be supplemented with intrathecal administration to achieve therapeutic drug levels. Side effects include hypersensitivity reactions, phlebitis, GI disturbances, and, less frequently, anemia and thrombocytopenia.[40]

Viruses

Viruses, the smallest-known infectious microorganisms, are visible only with the aid of an electron microscope. Viruses have no intrinsic energy system and consist of only a deoxyribonucleic acid (DNA) or ribonucleic acid (RNA) nucleus surrounded by a protein coat. Viruses are replicated by host cell mechanisms after invasion by a single virus. The primary virus invades the cell and initiates the formation of similar viruses by the host cell. Common viruses cause measles, mumps, rubella, respiratory infections, colds, and bronchitis. Most viral infections in granulocytopenic patients are caused by herpesviruses (HSV), varicella zoster (VZV), and CMV.

Herpes simplex

Herpes simplex virus (HSV) can cause serious infection in persons with cancer, either from primary exposure or from reactivation of a latent virus. Major sites of infection are the oropharynx, esophagus, eyes, skin, urogenital tract, and perianal area. In rare cases of HSV dissemination, pulmonary, CNS, and hepatic involvement may be seen.

Patients with impaired cell-mediated immunity are at increased risk for recurrent HSV infections resulting in extensive mucocutaneous ulceration. Progression of the ulcers occurs as the virus, unimpeded by T-cell response, spreads across the squamous epithelium.[41]

Varicella zoster

Infection with the varicella zoster virus (VZV; "chickenpox") can cause serious vesicular eruption in individuals with cancer, especially children, and results in a mortality rate of about 7%.[6] Following primary VZV infection, reactivation ("shingles") can occur, because the virus remains dormant in the spinal ganglia. Incidence of reactivation ranges from 5%–10% in patients with solid tumors to 35%–50% in those with Hodgkin's disease or following bone marrow transplant.[6] Radiotherapy can also increase the risk of VZV infection. Usually, the dermatomes that are involved with VZV lesions previously have been encompassed in a radiation field.

Diagnosis of VZV infection is based on a history of chickenpox, characteristic dermatomal distribution of vesicular lesions, and positive culture results. Since skin lesions (vesicles) can become confluent, meticulous skin care is required to prevent secondary bacterial infection.

The major complication of VZV infection is visceral dissemination, resulting in pneumonitis, hepatitis, and meningoencephalitis. However, even in the immunocompromised patient, disseminated VZV rarely is fatal.[42] The risk of visceral dissemination is increased in persons receiving chemotherapy during the time of infection, especially if lymphopenia occurs (<500 lymphocytes/mm^3). Disseminated VZV often is complicated by secondary bacterial infections.

Varicella is highly contagious, and the risk of spread to other seronegative immunocompromised persons is substantial, especially in adults with Hodgkin's disease and children with leukemia. Because of the severity of VZV infection in persons with cancer, infected patients have been treated with varicella zoster immune globulin (VZIG). When administered within 72 hours of exposure to VZV, VZIG generally modifies the infection to a subclinical or mild form. Management of persons with cancer who are seronegative and who have been exposed to VZV includes interruption of therapy and administration of VZIG. Whenever possible, cancer therapy should not be reinstituted until the end of the incubation period, approximately 21 days. When clinical evidence of VZV infection occurs in persons with cancer, immunosuppressive agents should be withheld until all skin lesions have dried and scabbed.

Cytomegalovirus

Cytomegalovirus (CMV) infection usually is a result of viral reactivation, particularly in association with immunosuppression. CMV is a common cause of interstitial pneumonitis in persons with impaired cellular immunity or following bone marrow transplant. CMV pneumonia characteristically occurs within 3 months of transplant and often is fatal.[43]

CMV retinitis is the most common opportunistic ocular infection noted in immunocompromised persons, especially those with AIDS. Direct viral invasion of retinal cells results in tissue damage, necrosis, and high risk of retinal detachment.[44] Less commonly, CMV will infect the GI tract, resulting in esophagitis, gastritis, or colitis.

Hepatitis virus

Hepatitis in persons with cancer can occur as a primary infection with one of the hepatitis viruses (A, B [HBV], or non-A non-B [NANBV]) or as a secondary infection with other viruses. HBV and NANBV are the major causative organisms in transfusion-related hepatitis.

Viral hepatitis occurs as an acute or a chronic infection. Asymptomatic carriers may exhibit mild hepatic dysfunction. Although transfusions of blood products constitute the primary route of transmission, nonparenteral transmission occurs through sexual intercourse and contact with contaminated saliva, urine, and feces. Risk of infection to hospital staff is high and warrants strict adherence to universal precautions outlined by the Centers for Disease Control and Prevention[45] (Table 24-1). The CDC guidelines have been incorporated into the rules pertaining to occupational exposure to blood-borne pathogens released by the Occupational Safety and Health Administration (OSHA).[46]

TABLE 24-1 Universal Precautions for Prevention of Transmission of Human Immunodeficiency Virus, Hepatitis B Virus, and Other Blood-Borne Pathogens

1. Never recap, bend, break, or clip needles.
2. Place needles and sharps promptly in an approved puncture-resistant container designated for needle disposal.
3. Use approved disposal containers in all areas.
4. Do not overfill containers.
5. Close container securely when three-quarters full.
6. Bag closed containers in red bags.
7. Protect open wounds from coming in contact with potentially infected materials.
8. Be sure to cover properly any broken skin surfaces.
9. Gloves are necessary when:
   a. drawing blood
   b. handling specimens that have obvious blood in them
   c. starting intravenous infusions (IVs)
   d. cleaning blood spills
   e. during cardiopulmonary resuscitation (CPR)
   f. suctioning (especially a new tracheostomy)
   g. changing dressings
10. Wear mask, gloves, and protective eyewear when:
    a. blood splattering may occur
    b. inserting or maintaining arterial lines
    c. doing oral care
    d. doing emergency procedures
    e. doing invasive procedures
    f. doing hemodialysis or hemapheresis
    g. doing peritoneal dialysis
11. Change gloves between patients.
12. Wash hands thoroughly before leaving the patient's room.

Source: Centers for Disease Control: Universal precautions for prevention of transmission of human immunodeficiency virus, hepatitis B virus, and other blood-borne pathogens. *MMWR* 37 (June 24):377–387, 1988.

Treatment

Acyclovir is an antiviral agent preferentially taken up by cells infected with HSV and VZV. Treatment with acyclovir decreases viral shedding from infected cells, accelerates healing of lesions, and decreases pain and itching. Acyclovir offers significant prophylaxis against recurrent infection for immunocompromised individuals, especially those who have had allogeneic bone marrow transplant. It is available in parenteral, oral, and topical forms; however, it is not well absorbed from the GI tract. Side effects are minimal, consisting primarily of nausea, vomiting, diarrhea, and anorexia. Phlebitis is common with IV administration.[40]

Vidarabine is an antiviral agent used primarily for VZV and HSV infections. Best used early in the course of infection, vidarabine is not particularly effective with disseminated infection. Toxicities include bone marrow suppression, GI disturbances, and neurologic effects such as tremor, confusion, and ataxia.[47]

Ganciclovir is used in treatment of CMV infection. It is a virostatic agent and, therefore, does not eliminate existing CMV but suppresses viral replication. Ganciclovir currently is available only as a parenteral agent, although clinical trials are under way to evaluate the efficacy of an oral form. The most significant toxicities of ganciclovir are neutropenia and thrombocytopenia. In patients with CMV retinitis for whom toxicity precludes continued systemic therapy, intravitreal administration may be attempted.[40]

Foscarnet is another virostatic agent that suppresses CMV replication. It may be prescribed for CMV infection that is resistant to ganciclovir. Oral absorption is poor; IV administration is required to achieve therapeutic serum levels. Primary side effects include anemia, nephrotoxicity, and hypocalcemia. Less common effects are mild CNS disturbances, including irritability, tremor, and headache.[48]

Protozoa and Parasites

Infections caused by protozoa and parasites are associated with defects in cell-mediated immunity. These organisms are ubiquitous, causing few problems, if any, in persons who are immunocompetent. However, in the immunocompromised host, these infections often are difficult to treat and, in some cases, can quickly become life-threatening.

Pneumocystis carinii

Pneumocystis carinii (P. carinii) is a protozoan that causes infection in malnourished infants, children with primary immunodeficiency disorders, persons with AIDS, and those with cancer undergoing immunosuppressive therapy. Clinical manifestations of infection include fever, nonproductive cough, tachypnea with intercostal retraction, and potentially life-threatening respiratory compromise. Rales are absent. Chest radiographs reveal hazy bilateral infiltrates, although some cases may present with unremarkable findings. Open lung biopsy is sometimes necessary to confirm the diagnosis.

Toxoplasma

Toxoplasma gondii (T. gondii) is an obligate intracellular parasite found in soil, cat excreta, and improperly cooked meats. It can remain encapsulated in host tissues, with reactivation of latent organisms causing infection. Persons at greatest risk include those with AIDS and those receiving immunosuppressive therapy for hematologic malignancies or prevention of organ transplant rejection. CNS involvement occurs in over 50% of infected individuals; however, the infection in immunocompromised persons often is disseminated at the time of diagnosis.[44]

Cryptosporidium

Although a common cause of enteritis in persons with AIDS, cryptosporidiosis has only occasionally been observed in other immunocompromised patients.[30] When severe deficiencies in cell-mediated immunity are present, cryptosporidiosis results in voluminous watery diarrhea and secondary malnutrition, dehydration, and electrolyte imbalance.

Treatment

Untreated *P. carinii* is fatal. Even with therapy, mortality is high. Treatment of choice for *P. carinii* is trimethoprim-sulfamethoxazole. Side effects include rash, nausea, vomiting, hepatotoxicity, and myelosuppression. In persons with known history of sulfonamide sensitivity, dapsone may be substituted in the antibiotic combination.[47]

Pentamidine is effective in treating *P. carinii* unresponsive to trimethoprim-sulfamethoxazole. Side effects, however, are troublesome and include azotemia, hypocalcemia, and hepatotoxicity. Rapid intravenous infusion can result in a precipitous fall in blood pressure. Severe, prolonged hypoglycemia has also been reported, usually associated with higher doses, longer duration of therapy, and retreatment within 3 months.[40]

Prophylactic treatment of high-risk patients most often is accomplished with trimethoprim-sulfamethoxazole. Alternative agents include aerosolized pentamidine, dapsone, and pyrimethamine plus sulfadoxine.

Treatment with pyrimethamine plus sulfadiazine has been effective against *T. gondii* in immunocompromised patients. Clindamycin can be substituted in patients with known allergies to sulfonamides.[47,49]

To date, there is no known treatment for cryptosporidiosis.

NURSING CARE OF THE PATIENT AT RISK FOR INFECTION

Prevention

Reducing environmental pathogens

Since most cancer care is delivered in the ambulatory setting, nursing care focuses on prevention of infection, measures to optimize the person's health, and aggressive interventions when needed. The patient and family need to be well informed about self-care measures, early detection, and expectations during therapy for infection. When an infection develops, prompt initiation of nursing measures is imperative to prevent life-threatening complications. (see Table 24-2).

TABLE 24-2 Nursing Care of Patient at Risk for Infection

Problem	Assessment	Nursing Intervention	Patient/Significant Other Teaching
Potential for systemic infection	a. *Patient history:* factors that compromise immune function (eg, cancer treatment, steroid use, nutritional status, chronic infections, HIV+) b. Absolute granulocyte count c. Vital signs d. Comprehensive physical assessment e. CSF Response to antimicrobial, colony stimulating factor therapy	a. Strict hand washing measures b. Appropriate protective measures (eg, private room, protective isolation, dietary restrictions) c. Adequate fluid/dietary intake d. Adequate periods of rest e. Aseptic technique for invasive procedures, dressing changes, etc.	a. Importance of hand washing b. Rationale for protective measures c. Importance of optimizing health status (eg, diet, rest, personal hygiene) d. Signs/symptoms of infection to report to health care team e. Ability to read thermometer
Potential/actual disruption of skin integrity	a. *Patient history:* recent trauma to skin or conditions that predispose to disrupted skin integrity b. *Physical assessment:* special attention to skin folds, wound sites; lesions suspicious for primary, recurrent malignancy c. Characteristics of open areas (eg, size, depth, discharge)	a. Meticulous personal hygiene, particularly to high-risk areas b. Electric razors, dressing supplies less likely to traumatize skin c. Moisturizing lotions, mild soaps to prevent drying, chapping, cracking of skin d. Adequate fluid, dietary intake e. Caution when moving bedfast patient f. Activity consistent with health status g. Special mattress to minimize pressure areas h. Cultures of suspicious areas i. Aseptic technique for dressing changes j. Referral to home care agency for postdischarge follow-up	a. Self-care information regarding maintenance of skin integrity (eg, avoidance of exposure to sun, use of skin care products) b. Rationale for precautions c. Signs/symptoms to report to health care team d. Proper techniques for wound care, dressing changes

(continued)

TABLE 24-2 Nursing Care of Patient at Risk for Infection (continued)

Problem	Assessment	Nursing Intervention	Patient/Significant Other Teaching
Potential/actual pulmonary infection	a. *Patient history:* dysphagia, diminished gag reflex, tobacco use, asbestos exposure, COPD, HIV+, radiation therapy to chest, pulmonary toxicity due to chemotherapy b. Respiratory rate, effort, use of accessory muscles c. Chest auscultation d. Recent changes in pulmonary status (cough, sputum, DOE, etc.)	a. Cough/deep breathing exercises b. Activity appropriate for health status c. Adequate hydration d. Staff/visitors with respiratory infection restricted e. TB testing f. Review of x-ray, lab test results g. Sputum specimen for culture h. Aseptic technique when suctioning i. Supplemental O_2	a. Proper performance of cough/deep breathing exercises b. Strategies for smoking cessation c. Signs/symptoms to be reported to health care team d. Home safety precautions when using O_2 e. Information about community resources
Potential/actual disruption of oral mucosa	a. *Patient history:* chemotherapy, radiation therapy to head/neck, HIV+, tobacco/alcohol use, periodontal disease, hydration/nutritional status b. *Physical assessment of oral cavity:* color, moisture, lesions, ulcerations, amount and character of saliva c. Patient's routine for oral hygiene, presence of oral pain	a. Oral hygiene plan—toothbrush, toothpaste, dental floss; cotton swab or Toothettes® if pain, bleeding preclude use of toothbrush b. Normal saline, ¼ str. hydrogen peroxide, or sodium bicarbonate mouth rinses. c. Bacterial, fungal, and viral cultures if oral pain present d. Adequate fluid intake e. Topical or systemic analgesia for oral or esophageal pain f. Water-soluble lubricant	a. Dietary modifications to reduce trauma to oral mucosa (avoidance of spicy foods, temperature extremes, high acid content) b. Consistent, thorough oral hygiene c. Avoidance of tobacco, alcohol d. Signs/symptoms to be reported to health care team e. Use of dentures for meals only if oral mucous membrane integrity disrupted
Potential/actual disruption of rectal mucosa	a. *Patient history:* diet, sexual practices, medications, chemotherapy, HIV+, change in bowel habits b. *Physical assessment of rectal area:* erythema, ulceration, hemorrhoids, bleeding c. Character, frequency of bowel movements	a. Dietary modifications to reduce rectal trauma (increase fiber for constipation; low residue for diarrhea) b. Avoid invasive procedures (eg, rectal temperatures, suppositories, enemas) c. Hygiene plan to prevent/minimize anorectal excoriation, promote comfort (eg, sitz baths, cotton balls or soft wipes instead of toilet tissue) d. Stool softeners or antidiarrheal agents	a. Factors that increase risk of infection and strategies to reduce risk; dietary modification, alternative sexual practices, etc. b. Signs/symptoms to be reported to health care team
Potential/actual genitourinary (GU) infection.	a. *Patient history:* benign prostatic hypertrophy, HIV+, bladder-toxic chemotherapy; symptoms of GU infection (dysuria, urinary, frequency, urgency, hematuria, pruritis, vaginal/penile discharge) b. *Physical assessment of genitilia:* lesions, ulcerations, discharge c. Characteristics of urine—color, turbidity, odor	a. Adequate hydration b. Urine specimen (straight catheter or clean catch) for culture and routine analysis c. Culture genital discharge, lesions d. Avoid in-dwelling urinary catheters e. Antispasmodic; analgesic agents as indicated	a. Rationale, importance of adequate hydration b. Signs/symptoms to be reported to health care team

Source: Adapted from Ellerhorst-Ryan JM: Nursing care plan for the immunocompromised patients. In Workman ML, Ellerhorst-Ryan JM, Koertga VH (ed.): *Nursing Care of the Immunocompromised Patient.* Philadelphia: Saunders, 1993.

The single most important intervention to prevent infection is meticulous hand washing by every person who enters the room or comes in contact with the individual at risk for infection. Neutropenic individuals are advised of their risk and are encouraged to remind family, visitors, and staff about hand-washing precautions.

When hospitalized, the patient is given a private room. Nursing assignments include consideration for whether a staff member has had a recent immunization or transmissible infection. Ideally, staff members caring for a patient with an active infection are not also assigned to a neutropenic patient. However, this precaution is probably unnecessary if thorough and meticulous hand washing is performed consistently. Visitors are also screened for recent immunization or transmissible infection.

When the AGC is less than 1000, live plants, cut flowers, and fresh fruit should not be brought into the patient's room. During times when granulocytes are adequate, bacterial content can be decreased by adding one teaspoon of chlorine bleach to each quart of water used in flower vases.[50] Water in pitchers, denture cups, and nebulizers is changed at least once a day.

During granulocytopenic episodes, invasive procedures are kept to a minimum, with adherence to strict aseptic technique when they are performed. In-dwelling urinary catheters are also avoided whenever possible. If catheter placement is necessary, the smallest lumen size available is selected and the duration of use kept as brief as possible. Communicating with laboratory staff to coordinate blood sampling can prevent unnecessary venipuncture.

Optimizing health status

Adequate nutritional intake during periods of increased risk requires a high-calorie, high-protein diet. If severe neutropenia is present, a low-bacteria diet may be prescribed, eliminating fresh fruit, raw vegetables, fresh eggs, cold cuts, and skim or chocolate milk.[50]

Fluid intake is monitored to ensure adequate hydration, especially during periods of nausea, vomiting, and diarrhea and when therapy includes agents with bladder and renal toxicity. IV fluid administration may be periodically needed.

Activities are organized to allow for periods of rest. Certain individuals may become frustrated or discouraged by their lack of stamina or endurance. Assisting them with realistic goal setting and planning may enable them to accomplish desired tasks without further compromising their health status.

Strategies to maintain skin and mucous membrane integrity are implemented. Meticulous personal hygiene is imperative, with strict attention to skin folds, including the axillae, perineum, groin, buttocks, and under the breasts. Mild soap and a water-soluble lubricant can help prevent drying of the skin. Shaving with an electric razor will reduce the occurrence of accidental cuts. Fingernails and toenails should be kept short; toenails that are difficult to trim should be brought to the attention of a podiatrist.

The optimal plan for oral hygiene includes use of a soft to medium toothbrush, toothpaste, and dental floss. However, periods of thrombocytopenia and oral stomatitis may require substitution of Toothettes® and normal saline. Oral care is performed after meals, at bedtime, and as needed while the patient is awake.

Enemas, rectal temperatures, and suppositories are likely to traumatize fragile rectal mucosa and are avoided as much as possible in the high-risk patient. Prophylactic stool softeners often are recommended, particularly if hemorrhoids are present.

Activity consistent with current health status is encouraged, to maintain optimal circulatory and pulmonary function. The patient is instructed and assisted in performance of coughing and deep breathing exercises.

Although impaired cellular immunity and neutropenia are the primary causes of immunosuppression in cancer patients, humoral immunity also can be affected by either disease or treatment. Impaired humoral immunity compromises the efficacy of immunization, especially if chemotherapy is administered at the same time. Persons with cancer, especially those with acute leukemia, should receive pneumococcal and other vaccines only while in remission, since antibody response is limited during chemotherapy.[10]

Education about infection risk begins at the time of diagnosis. The patient and family should be instructed about the impact of cancer and cancer treatment on the inflammatory and immune responses. They should also be taught about blood counts, anticipated time until the nadir is reached, and self-care activities to minimize risk of infection.

The patient and family are advised of signs and symptoms of infection that are to be promptly reported to the health care team. If the patient or caregiver is visually impaired or has difficulty reading a thermometer, a digital thermometer should be obtained.

Early Detection

Physical assessment

In spite of strict adherence to protective measures, prolonged or severe neutropenia will allow rapid progression of a localized infection to potentially life-threatening sepsis. When the inflammatory response is diminished or absent, classic signs and symptoms of infection—fever, erythema, edema, pain, and purulence—may not be present, making early identification difficult.

During neutropenic periods, patients need nurses with diligent physical assessment skills, including the ability to listen carefully to information provided by the patient and significant others and to identify subtle clues indicative of infection. The most reliable indicator of infection is a low-grade fever. A temperature elevation of 1° that persists for 24 hours may be the only evidence of infection.

Respiratory system The high incidence of pneumonia in immunocompromised patients mandates thorough assessment of the respiratory system. During hospitalization, chest auscultation is performed every 2–4 hours, depending on the extent of risk, and with each nursing visit when at home. Neutropenic patients may experience only slight temperature elevation and mild dyspnea when pneumonia is present. Assessment findings for upper respiratory infection range from pain, swelling, erythema, and discharge in nonneutropenic patients to vague discomfort and possibly mild erythema in neutropenic patients.

Oropharynx The oral mucosa is often traumatized by chemotherapeutic agents, especially the antimetabolites and antibiotics. Local infections can occur if inflamed or injured mucosal surfaces become colonized with bacteria, predisposing to systemic infection. Teeth and gums in poor condition can become a source of sepsis during periods of granulocytopenia. Stomatitis can compromise nutritional status and fluid intake and, when severe, necessitate interruption of chemotherapy.

The oral cavity is inspected regularly for white plaques, gingival edema, erythema, bleeding, and ulceration. Complaints of oral pain and dysphagia should be followed up with bacterial, fungal, and viral cultures.

Gastrointestinal system If a granulocytopenic patient receiving broad-spectrum antibiotics complains of dysphagia and/or retrosternal burning, *Candida* or HSV esophagitis must be considered. Disruption of intestinal mucosa by anticancer therapy facilitates bacterial invasion and increases the potential for sepsis. Gastritis, enteritis, and colitis typically present with nausea, vomiting, diarrhea, and abdominal pain or tenderness. Hepatitis results in fatigue, anorexia, early satiety, and clay-colored stools. The perirectal area should be inspected routinely for signs of inflammation, infection, hemorrhoids, and fissures. Complaints of perianal itching, tenderness, constipation, or pain with defecation can indicate early stages of perirectal cellulitis.

Central nervous system Subtle changes in neurologic function can signify either the onset of an infection or progression of malignancy. The development of any neurologic abnormality warrants immediate attention.

CNS infections present with a variety of symptoms, depending on the type and extent of infection. Typical complaints include headache, fever, meningismus, personality changes, focal neurologic signs, nuchal rigidity, altered mental status, and seizures.

Urinary tract Urinary tract infections (UTIs) are common in hospitalized persons, especially those with cancer who have fever and granulocytopenia. Classic symptoms of UTI are typically absent in neutropenic patients. Observation of urine characteristics—specifically, cloudy and foul-smelling—is usually more helpful. *Candida* infection can result in erythema and pruritis in the perineal area.

Skin Skin integrity should be assessed regularly, with special attention given to known areas of disruption or at increased risk of breakdown.

Cardiovascular system Symptoms of cardiovascular infection generally are nonspecific: fever, chills, malaise, night sweats. Indications of possible cardiac infection include new or changing murmurs, thromboemboli, unexplained heart failure, and arrhythmias.[44]

Nursing Care During Episodes of Infection

Infection in the neutropenic patient is always considered a potentially life-threatening emergency. Fatality rates during the first 48 hours range from 18% to 40%.[51]

Cultures are obtained from all potential sites of infection, including urine, sputum, wound, stool, and blood. If vascular access catheters are present, culture specimens are obtained both from peripheral veins and through the catheter.

After culture specimens have been obtained, empiric broad-spectrum antibiotic therapy is initiated promptly and the patient's response observed closely. Monitoring for efficacy of antimicrobial treatment includes assessing vital signs every 2–4 hours; reviewing reports of chest x-rays and laboratory data, including arterial blood gases, blood counts, chemistry profiles, culture results, and peak and trough antibiotic levels; and observing for signs of septic shock. If little or no improvement is apparent following 3–5 days of antibiotic treatment, cultures are repeated and the physician consulted about modifying the prescribed antimicrobial regimen.

Other supportive nursing care strategies include restoring circulatory fluid volume by administering IV fluids, blood or blood products, and vasopressors; maintaining adequate oxygenation through the use of supplemental oxygen and, when necessary, mechanical ventilation; and promoting optimal nutritional status by monitoring dietary intake, consulting with the dietitian, and conferring with the physician when enteral or parenteral nutrition is indicated.

Patients and family members should be informed of side effects of prescribed antibiotics, particularly those that are to be reported promptly to the health care team.

TREATMENT OF INFECTION

Approach to the Patient Without Granulocytopenia

Persons with cancer who are not immunocompromised or granulocytopenic can be treated with appropriate antibiotic therapy for the specific infectious agent identified. Cultures are performed before the initiation of therapy and if necessary, antibiotics are changed when the results of sensitivity testing are known. However, empiric treatment with a broad-spectrum antibiotic is initiated if a serious infection develops rapidly.

Approach to the Patient with Granulocytopenia and Fever

Persons with cancer who have fever during periods of granulocytopenia will have a thorough physical examination, chest radiograph, and appropriate laboratory studies. After cultures of all potential sources of infection have been obtained, empiric broad-spectrum antibiotic therapy will be initiated.

Granulocytopenic patients may not manifest clinical evidence of infection, because granulocytopenia prevents the mounting of an inflammatory response. Progression to systemic infection and septic shock usually is rapid. Therefore, individuals with granulocytopenia must be evaluated at frequent intervals for signs and symptoms of infection. Common sites of infection identified in patients with granulocytopenia and fever are listed in Table 24-3.

Empiric antibiotics

Empiric antibiotic therapy in the patient with fever and granulocytopenia reduces the number of infections that could become severe enough to be demonstrated by microbiologic culture or clinical documentation. The decreasing incidence of septic shock in this high-risk population suggests that prompt aggressive antibiotic therapy is effective in reducing the serious morbidity associated with gram-negative sepsis.[33] The particular empiric antibiotic regimen selected should meet the following criteria: provide broad-spectrum coverage for major pathogenic organisms; be synergistic and contain one bactericidal agent; and have minimal organ toxicity, satisfactory absorption by the route administered, consistent distribution to infected tissues, and adequate excretion.[32] Drug levels are monitored on a regular basis while the patient is receiving nephrotoxic antibiotics, and dosage adjustments are made when indicated to maintain safe therapeutic levels.

TABLE 24-3 Common Sites of Infections Identified in Febrile, Granulocytopenic Patients

Site	Percentage
Mouth and pharynx	25
Respiratory tract	25
Skin, soft tissue, and intravascular catheters	15
Perineal region	10
Urinary tract	5–10
Nose and sinuses	5
Gastrointestinal tract	5
Others	5–10

Source: Meunier F: Infections in patients with acute leukemia and lymphoma. In Mandell GL, Douglas RG, Bennett JE (eds.): *Principles and Practice of Infectious Disease* (ed. 3). New York: Churchill Livingstone, 1990, Table 2.

Isolation precautions and protected environments

Persons with cancer receiving intensive therapeutic regimens with total body irradiation, steroids, and chemotherapy are significantly more susceptible to infection than those receiving less intensive therapy. These severely immunocompromised persons often are placed on "protective" regimens intended to reduce the risk of infection. One such regimen, routine protective isolation, does not appear to reduce the risk of infection any more than does consistent frequent hand washing during patient care. Routine protective isolation fails to reduce the risk of infection from endogenous microorganisms or from colonization by contaminated hands of health care personnel.[52]

Efforts to exclude all microorganisms through use of patient isolator units (usually, laminar air flow rooms), nonabsorbable prophylactic antibiotics, and sterilization of the patient's food and water may prevent or delay the onset of some infection. Therefore, these procedures have been recommended by some investigators for immunocompromised patients who have a predictable period of significant risk.[53]

Laminar air flow rooms are protected environments developed to protect the compromised host from exogenous and endogenous sources of infection. In this sophisticated isolation system, air is circulated through high-efficiency particulate air filters capable of removing from the air particles larger than 0.3 μm with a greater than 99.7% efficiency. The unidirectional (laminar) air flow significantly reduces air turbulence, which decreases the potential for microbial contamination in the consistently clean, protected environment. Semiportable units with horizontal air flow can be installed in regular hospital rooms.

To create an environment as free of microorganisms as possible, patients undergo cutaneous and gastrointestinal decontamination with oral nonabsorbable antibiotics before entry into the room. All objects brought into the room are sterilized by steam or gas, and food is semisterile. Anyone who will be coming in physical contact with the patient wears gloves, mask, and gown.

The disadvantages of laminar air flow rooms are that the protective environment is elaborate, cumbersome, and expensive. In addition, the patient may experience depression due to social isolation and psychotic episodes because of sensory deprivation. Although laminar air flow rooms reduce incidence of infection and improve short-term survival, long-term survival has not been affected.

Granulocyte replacement

Initial attempts at granulocyte replacement were in the form of granulocyte transfusions. However, limited efficacy, cost, and serious complications, including development of lymphotoxic antibodies, made granulocyte transfusions impractical.[10]

Granulocyte colony stimulating factor (G-CSF) and granulocyte-macrophage colony stimulating factor (GM-CSF) are hormonelike glycoproteins that promote the proliferation and maturation of phagocytes. Studies have shown that the duration of granulocytopenia following chemotherapy administration is markedly decreased when G-CSF or GM-CSF are used. In addition, mean recovery time for neutrophils following BMT is significantly shorter with the addition of CSFs.[54] Nursing care of the patient receiving CSFs is discussed in greater detail in Chapter 17.

Approach to the Patient with Gram-Negative Sepsis

Shock develops in approximately 27%–46% of patients with gram-negative bacteremia,[9] resulting in inadequate tissue perfusion and circulatory collapse. Mortality rate approaches 80% unless vigorous treatment is begun promptly. The clinical syndrome is a result of a number of interrelated factors that include the direct effect of bacterial endotoxin on the cardiovascular system, activation of the protein cascade system, nutritional and hydration status of the patient, and the nature of the underlying disease. Signs and symptoms depend on the stage of shock, the causative organism, and the age of the patient. The first sign of impending shock in the immunocompromised host may be limited to a low-grade fever, shaking chills, and/or mild hypotension. Early recognition of sepsis and aggressive intervention are essential if irreversible damage to vital organs and subsequent death are to be averted (Table 24-4).

Early (warm) shock

Septic shock evolves through two phases that, although not always distinct, are characterized by different hemodynamic patterns. The early phase consists of vasodilation, decreased peripheral vascular resistance, normal to increased cardiac output, and mild hypotension. The signs of overt shock are not present in this phase. The patient may appear flushed, with warm extremities and adequate urinary output. Central venous pressures are low, as are left ventricular and diastolic pressures, and respiratory alkalosis is present. During the early phase, peripheral vasodilation results in loss of fluid to the interstitial spaces. If myocardial function and fluid replacement are adequate, the syndrome may not progress, provided immediate and appropriate antibiotic therapy is instituted. The duration of this early phase may vary from 30 minutes to 16 hours. However, if myocardial function is poor and volume replacement is inadequate, or if there is delay in initiating appropriate antibiotic therapy, severe life-threatening (late-phase) shock will develop.

Late (cold) shock

The late phase of septic shock is characterized by a profound reduction in cardiac output, increased peripheral vascular resistance, oliguria, and metabolic acidosis. These factors create a cycle of vasoconstriction, ischemia, and vasodilation, resulting in irreversible damage to the heart, vascular system, kidneys, liver, and vasomotor center of the brain.

Treatment of septic shock

The treatment of septic shock is based on two objectives: reversing the shock, and treating the underlying sepsis. Individuals in shock require adequate oxygenation, effective circulation and tissue perfusion, nutritional support, and immediate, appropriate broad-spectrum antibiotic therapy.

Persistent hypotension despite fluid replacement may be managed through administration of vasoactive

TABLE 24-4 Assessment of Patients with Septic Shock

Assessment Parameter	Early Shock	Late Shock
Temperature	Low-grade fever, possible shaking chill	Febrile
Cutaneous	Flushed, warm	Cold, clammy; acrocyanosis
Cardiovascular	Tachycardia, normal to slightly low blood pressure	Hypotension, moderate to severe; decreased cardiac output; peripheral edema
Renal	Transient decrease in urine output	Oliguria, anuria
Pulmonary	Hyperventilation	Pulmonary edema
Central nervous system	Alert, possible mild confusion, apprehension	Restlessness, anxiety, confusion, lethargy, coma
Gastrointestinal	Nausea, vomiting, diarrhea	Possible blood in stool or emesis

agents. In low to moderate doses, dopamine, the vasoactive agent of choice, increases arterial pressure without causing significant vasoconstriction and selectively increases renal, coronary, cerebral, and mesenteric flow.[40]

Any change in blood pressure, mental status, or urinary output in high-risk patients alerts the nurse to the probability of early shock. Once treatment has been initiated, nurses monitor closely for complications of shock, including disseminated intravascular coagulation (DIC), renal failure, gastrointestinal bleeding, and hepatic abnormalities (Table 24-5).

Finally, care is taken to meet the psychosocial needs of patients with septic shock and their significant others. The critical nature of septic shock, coupled with the intensive treatment regimen, can be overwhelming. Patients may face not only fear of death, but also loss of control and feelings of dependence. Nursing responsibilities include providing honest information, education, and assurance to both patients and family members.

Approach to the Patient with HIV Infection

Nursing care of persons with AIDS, with or without malignancy, presents a unique challenge. These individuals are at increased risk for opportunistic infection, not only because of HIV-related impairment of cellular immunity, but also because of granulocytopenia secondary to cancer treatment and/or antimicrobial therapy (e.g., ganciclovir). Most opportunistic infections are the consequence of T-helper cell depletion and are caused by mycobacterial, viral, fungal, or protozoal organisms. Antimicrobial therapy usually is continued indefinitely, since discontinuing treatment commonly results in recurrent symptoms of infection. Side effects of long-term antibiotic therapy and progression of AIDS typically result in anorexia, nausea, vomiting, diarrhea, and malabsorption, which further compromise the person's immune function.

TABLE 24-5 Complications of Septic Shock

Complication	Manifestation
Disseminated intravascular coagulation	Abnormal bleeding
Renal failure	Oliguria, increased specific gravity
Heart failure	Dyspnea, edema, tachycardia, distended neck veins
Gastrointestinal ulcers	Hematemesis, melena
Hepatic abnormality	Jaundice, hypoprothrombinemia, hypoalbuminemia

CONCLUSION

Persons with cancer are especially prone to develop infections as a result of impaired host defense mechanisms. Compromised immunity may be due to infection, nutritional deficiencies, tumor-associated factors, and/or cancer treatment. Most infections in this population are opportunistic in nature and involve gram-negative and gram-positive microorganisms, although viruses, fungi, and protozoa are also implicated.

Infection in the immunocompromised person with cancer can quickly progress to life-threatening sepsis. Diligent nursing care directed toward prevention, early detection, and aggressive treatment is of primary importance for patient survival during high-risk periods.

REFERENCES

1. Young LS: Treatment of established bacterial and fungal infections in patients with hematologic malignancies. In Wiernik PH, et al (eds.): *Neoplastic Diseases of the Blood.* New York: Churchill Livingstone, 1985, pp. 943–960.
2. Luna MA: Infection: The threat beyond cancer. *Diagn Med* 8:26–35, 1985.
3. Workman ML: Inflammatory responses. In Workman ML, Ellerhorst-Ryan JM, Koertge VH (eds.): *Nursing Care of the Immunocompromised Patient.* Philadelphia: Saunders, 1993, pp. 14–31.
4. Phair JP: Laboratory assessment of immunocompetence. In Shulman ST, Phair JP, Sommers HM (eds.): *Biologic and Clinical Basis of Infectious Diseases.* Philadelphia: Saunders, 1992, pp. 87–93.
5. Guyton AG: Resistance of the body to infection: II. Immunity and allergy. In Guyton AG (ed.): *Textbook of Medical Physiology.* Philadelphia: Saunders, 1991, pp. 374–384.
6. Pizzo PA, Meyers J: Infections in the cancer patient. In Devita VT, Hellman S, Rosenberg SA (eds.): *Cancer: Principles and Practice of Oncology* (ed. 3). Philadelphia: Lippincott, 1989, pp. 2088–2133.
7. Schimpff SC: Infections in patients with cancer: Overview and epidemiology. In Moosa AR, Schimpff SC, Robson MC (eds.): *Comprehensive Textbook of Oncology,* Vol. 2 (ed. 2). Baltimore, MD: Williams & Wilkins, 1991, pp. 1720–1732.
8. Masur H: Infections in critically ill immunosuppressed patients. In Parrillo JE, Masur H (eds.): *The Critically Ill Immunosuppressed Patient.* Rockville, MD: Aspen, 1987, pp. 215–242.
9. Martin MA: Epidemiology and clinical impact of gram-negative sepsis. *Infect Dis Clin North Am* 5:739–752, 1991.
10. Klatersky J: Infections in patients with cancer: Prevention. In Moosa AR, Schimpff SC, Robson MC (eds.): *Comprehensive Textbook of Oncology,* Vol. 2 (ed. 2). Baltimore, MD: Williams & Wilkins, 1991, pp. 1749–1753.
11. Schimpff SC: Infections in the immunocompromised host: An overview. In Mandell GL, Douglas RG, Bennett JE

(eds.): *Principles and Practice of Infectious Disease* (ed. 3). New York: Churchill Livingstone, 1990, pp. 2258–2265.

12. Lazarus HM, Creger RJ, Gerson SL: Infectious emergencies in oncology patients. *Semin Oncol* 16:543–560, 1989.
13. Oniboni AC: Infection in the neutropenic patient. *Semin Oncol Nurs* 6:50–60, 1990.
14. Robinson BE, Donowitz GR: Infections in patients with cancer: Host defenses and the immune-compromised state. In Moosa AR, Schimpff SC, Robson MC (eds.): *Comprehensive Textbook of Oncology*, Vol. 2 (ed. 2). Baltimore, MD: Williams & Wilkins, 1991, pp. 1733–1739.
15. Rutherford GW, Werdegar D: Epidemiology of acquired immunodeficiency syndrome. In Levy JA (ed.): *AIDS: Pathogenesis and Treatment*. New York: Marcel Dekker, 1989, pp. 1–36.
16. Koertge VH: Acquired immune deficiency syndrome. In Workman ML, Ellerhorst-Ryan JM, Koertge VH (eds.): *Nursing Care of the Immunocompromised Patient*. Philadelphia: Saunders, 1993, pp. 80–99.
17. Cohen FL: Clinical spectrum of HIV infection and its treatment. In Durham JD, Cohen FL (eds.): *The Person with AIDS: Nursing Perspectives*. New York: Springer, 1991, pp. 135–205.
18. Abrams DI: Persistent lymphadenopathy syndrome and immune thrombocytopenic purpura in HIV-infected individuals. In Levy JA (ed.): *AIDS: Pathogenesis and Treatment*. New York: Marcel Dekker, 1989, pp. 323–343.
19. Hellman S, Jaffe ES, Devita VT: Hodgkin's disease. In DeVita VT, Hellman S, Rosenberg SA (eds.): *Cancer: Principles and Practice of Oncology* (ed. 3). Philadelphia: Lippincott, 1989, pp. 1696–1740.
20. Gurevich I, Tafuro P: The compromised host: Deficit-specific infection and the spectrum of prevention. *Cancer Nurs* 9:263–275, 1986.
21. Armstrong D: Infection in the patient with neoplastic disease. In Wittes RE (ed.): *Manual of Oncologic Therapeutics*. Philadelphia: Lippincott, 1989/90, pp. 517–534.
22. Baccarani M, Fiacchini M, Galiene P: Meningitis and septicemia in adults splenectomized for Hodgkin's disease. *Scand J Haematol* 36:492–498, 1986.
23. Thom AK, Daly JM: Nutritional support of the cancer patient. In Wittes RE (ed.): *Manual of Oncologic Therapeutics*. Philadelphia: Lippincott, 1989/90, pp. 495–516.
24. Chandra RK: *Nutrition and Immunology*. New York: Alan R. Liss, 1988.
25. Dubey DP, Yunis EJ: Aging and nutritional effects on immune functions in humans. In Stites DP, Terr AI (eds.): *Basic and Clinical Immunology* (ed. 7). Norwalk CT: Appleton and Lange, 1991, pp. 190–193.
26. Hirschmann JV: Systemic prophylactic antibiotics in surgery. In Kass EH, Platt R (eds.) *Current Therapy in Infectious Disease—3*. Philadelphia: BC Decker, 1990, pp. 403–406.
27. Shank B: Radiotherapy: Implications for general patient care. In Wittes RE (ed.): *Manual of Oncologic Therapeutics*. Philadelphia: Lippincott, 1989/90, pp. 82–93.
28. Kinzie J: Radiation therapy. In Moosa AR, Schimpff SC, Robson MC (eds.): *Comprehensive Textbook of Oncology*, Vol. 2 (ed. 2). Baltimore, MD: Williams & Wilkins, 1991, pp. 1137–1143.
29. Kiehn TE, Armstrong D: Changes in the spectrum of organisms causing bacteremia and fungemia in immunocompromised patients due to venous access devices. *Eur J Clin Microbiol Infect Dis* 9:869–872, 1990.
30. Meunier F: Infections in patients with acute leukemia and lymphoma. In Mandell GL, Douglas RG, Bennett JE (eds.): *Principles and Practice of Infectious Disease* (ed. 3). New York: Churchill Livingstone, 1990, pp. 2265–2275.
31. Warren J: Sepsis. In Shulman ST, Phair JP, Sommers HM: *Biologic and Clinical Basis of Infectious Diseases*. Philadelphia: Saunders, 1992, pp. 475–490.
32. Wade JC: Infections in patients with cancer: Treatment. In Moosa AR, Schimpff SC, Robson MC (eds.): *Comprehensive Textbook of Oncology*, Vol. 2 (ed. 2). Baltimore, MD: Williams & Wilkins, 1991, pp. 1740–1748.
33. Karp JE, Merz WG, Dick JD, et al: Management of infectious complications of acute leukemia and antileukemia therapy. *Oncology* 4:45–54, 1990.
34. Maurice PDL, Bunker C, Giles F, et al: Mycobacterium avium-intracellulare infection associated with hairy-cell leukemia. *Arch Dermatol* 124:1545–1549, 1988.
35. Maziarz RT, Teepler I, Antin JH: Reversal of infection with Mycobacterium avium intracellulare by treatment with alpha-interferon in a patient with hairy-cell leukemia. *Ann Intern Med* 109:292–294, 1988.
36. Young LS, Inderlied CB: Mycobacterium avium complex infections. *AIDS Patient Care* 4:10–18, 1990.
37. Walsh TJ: Invasive pulmonary aspergillosis in patients with neoplastic disease. *Semin Respir Infect* 5:111–122, 1990.
38. Brown AE: Overview of fungal infections in cancer patients. *Semin Oncol* 17:2–5, 1990 (suppl. 6).
39. Phair JP: Fungal infections of the respiratory tract. In Shulman ST, Phair JP, Sommers HM (eds.): *Biologic and Clinical Basis of Infectious Diseases*. Philadelphia: Saunders, 1992, pp. 208–220.
40. United States Pharmacopeial Convention, Inc: *Drug Information for the Health Care Professional* (ed. 11). Rockville, MD: USPC Inc., 1991.
41. Yungbluth M: Infectious mononucleosis and viral infections of the upper respiratory tract. In Shulman ST, Phair JP, Sommers HM (eds.): *Biologic and Clinical Basis of Infectious Diseases*. Philadelphia: Saunders, 1992, pp. 120–137.
42. Whitley RJ: Varicella-zoster virus. In Mandell GL, Douglas RG, Bennett JE (eds.): *Principles and Practice of Infectious Disease* (ed. 3). New York: Churchill Livingstone, 1990, pp. 1153–1159.
43. Winston DJ, Ho WG, Champlin RE: Cytomegalovirus infection and interstitial pneumonia after bone marrow transplant. In Champlin R (ed.): *Bone Marrow Transplantation*. Boston: Kluwer Academic Publishers, 1990, pp. 113–128.
44. Ellerhorst-Ryan JM: Infections in the immunocompromised host. In Workman ML, Ellerhorst-Ryan JM, Koertge VH (eds.): *Nursing Care of the Immunocompromised Patient*. Philadelphia: Saunders, 1993, pp. 229–262.
45. Centers for Disease Control: Universal precautions for prevention of transmission of human immunodeficiency virus, hepatitis B virus and other blood-borne pathogens. *MMWR* 37 (June 24):377–387, 1988.
46. Occupational Safety and Health Administration, U.S. Department of Labor: Occupational exposure to bloodborne pathogens. *Federal Register* 56:64175–64182, 1992.
47. Bartlett JG: *Pocketbook of Infectious Disease Therapy*. Baltimore, MD: Williams & Wilkins, 1991.
48. Minor JR, Baltz JK: Foscarnet sodium. *DICP* 25:41–47, 1991.
49. Remington JJS, McLeod R: Toxoplasmosis. In Gorbach

SL, Bartlett JG, Blacklow NR (eds.): *Infectious Diseases.* Philadelphia: Saunders, 1992, pp. 1329–1343.

50. Yasko JM: *Guidelines for Cancer Care: Symptom Management.* Reston, VA: Reston Publishing, 1983.
51. Brandt B: Nursing protocol for the patient with neutropenia. *Oncol Nurs Forum* 17:9–15, 1990 (suppl. 1).
52. Lynch P, Jackson MM, Cummings JM, et al: Rethinking the role of isolation practices in the prevention of nosocomial infections. *Ann Intern Med* 107:243–245, 1987.
53. Wade JC, Schimpff SC: Epidemiology and prevention of infection in the compromised host. In Rubin RH, Young LS (eds.): *Clinical Approach to Infection in the Compromised Host* (ed. 2). New York: Plenum Medical Book, 1988, pp. 5–40.
54. Heauber D: Future strategies in the control of myelosuppression: The use of colony stimulating factors. *Oncol Nurs Forum* 18:16–21, 1991 (suppl. 2).

Chapter 25

Bleeding Disorders

Barbara Holmes Gobel, RN, MS

INTRODUCTION

Bleeding represents one of the most complex clinical challenges in the supportive care of the individual with cancer. The numerous and unique complications of each neoplasm, combined with the often toxic effects of various cancer treatments, create a difficult problem in the diagnosis and management of the individual with a bleeding disorder. Appropriate supportive measures are a vital aspect of the total care of these individuals. Supportive care may actually represent the difference between survival and death in an individual with a bleeding disorder. An exciting advancement in the supportive care of patients with cancer is the clinical availability of recombinant human growth factors. These factors are capable of stimulating the proliferation and maturation of bone marrow cells and promise to improve the results of chemotherapy. Growth factors may decrease the morbidity of current chemotherapy regimens, allowing drugs to be safely administered at higher doses or by a dose-intensity program.

Multiple hemostatic abnormalities may be involved in bleeding associated with cancer. Considerable differences exist in the presentation, proper management, and implications of these clinical problems. Minor bleeding may be the initial symptom that leads to the diagnosis of cancer. More severe bleeding may indicate the onset of a progressive or terminal disease. Because the morbidity and mortality of many bleeding problems are significant, prevention of the problem is clearly the best management plan. Rapid recognition, assessment, and knowledgeable treatment of the hemorrhagic complications of cancer will significantly improve quality of life, and, possibly, survival for the individual with cancer.

This chapter includes a review of normal platelet and erythrocyte physiology, hemostasis, and coagulation, the etiology of bleeding associated with cancer, and patient assessment. Care of the individual with cancer experiencing bleeding, including both nursing and medical support, is reviewed. Blood component therapy and its use in cancer therapy are covered, as is home transfusion therapy. Finally, future perspectives on the issue of bleeding associated with cancer are discussed.

NORMAL HEMATOPOIESIS

Normal hematopoiesis is the process by which blood cells are formed. During fetal development, the blood-forming organs include the spleen, the liver, and the bone marrow. The bone marrow is the primary site of hematopoiesis at the time of birth. During childhood this function takes place in the long bones, ribs, sternum, skull, pelvis, vertebrae, spleen, and liver. The major sites of blood cell development in adulthood include the vertebrae, ribs, sternum, skull, proximal epiphyses of long bones, pelvis, and spleen.[1] The proportion of fatty marrow increases with age, so that only half of the ribs and sternum are sites of hematopoiesis in the elderly.[2] The marrow provides a differentiating inducing environment, known as the *hematopoietic inductive microenvironment (HIM)*.[3]

All of the blood cell lines derive from a pluripotent *stem cell,* or common progenitor cell. These pluripotential stem cells are capable of extensive, possibly lifelong self-renewal and of differentiation to all cell lineages.[2] The stem cell normally is not in an active cell cycle.[4] When the cell is required to undergo division, as during injury or marrow depletion, a daughter cell leaves the stem cell pool and passes through a series of divisions and maturational changes. These changes culminate in the formation of the mature blood cells found in circulating blood. The processes of proliferation, differentiation, and maturation are mediated by various humoral factors. These factors are known to be predominantly an expanding set of hematopoietic growth factors, or *colony stimulating factors (CSFs).* Refer to Figure 25-1 for an outline of blood cell development and the factors that mediate this process.

Early on in blood cell development the progeny of the pluripotent stem cell forms a population of *multipotent progenitor cells.* These cells are uncommitted to any one cell line and have a limited self-renewing capacity. The CFU-GEMM (colony-forming unit) is an example of the multipotent stem cell for granulocytes, erythroid, monocyte, and megakaryocyte lines. This stem cell can develop into any one of these cell lines. The lymphoid cell line follows a separate course of differentiation and maturation.[3]

As cells continue to differentiate they become committed to specific cell lines. At this level, progenitor cells are called *unipotent* or *bipotent,* depicting their ability to follow, respectively, one or two cell lines. These cells include CFU-GM (neutrophil, monocyte, and macrophage), CFU-EO (eosinophil), BFU-E and CFU-E (erythroid), and CFU-MEG (megakaryocyte), and are considered committed stem cells.[1,3] Committed stem cells become increasingly differentiated and morphologically recognizable as belonging to a specific cell line. Ultimately the cell undergoes further division and becomes a mature component of the circulating blood.

Colony Stimulating Factors

Colony stimulating factors (CSFs) are a set of hormonelike glycoproteins or cytokines that mediate hematopoiesis for all of the blood cell lines.[5] These proteins govern the production of blood cells at every level of cell development, including the pluripotent stem cells.[6] CSFs appear to act on target cells via receptors on cell membranes. Different distribution of specific receptors may explain responsiveness to various CSFs.

Some of the CSFs appear to have their effect on more than one blood cell line. Interleukin-3 (IL-3), also called multi-CSF, is a growth factor for a variety of

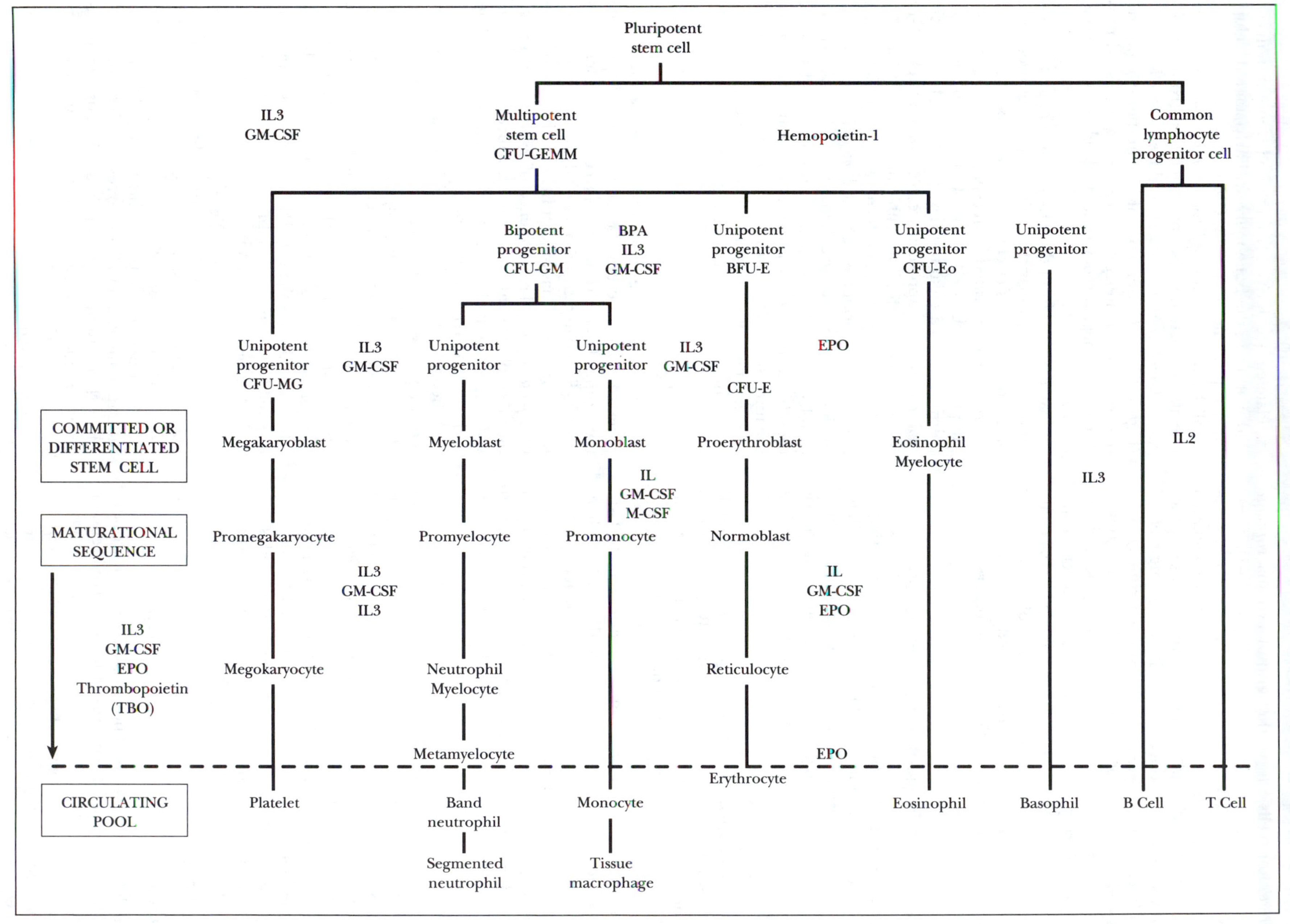

FIGURE 25-1 Hematopoiesis.

progenitor cells, as is the granulocyte-macrophage stimulating factor (GM-CSF) (see Figure 25-1). These CSFs stimulate the growth of multipotential hematopoietic progenitor cells and of cells already committed to myeloid, erythroid, or megakaryocytic lines.[7] Other CSFs stimulate production of cells along single blood cell lines. Granulocyte-CSF (G-CSF), macrophage-CSF (M-CSF), and erythropoietin (EPO) stimulate the growth of predominantly granulocytes, monocytes, and red blood cells, respectively.[8,9] CSFs appear to act on specific cells because of receptors that sit on the cell membrane. It is the different distribution of these specific receptors that may help explain why these cells are responsive to certain CSFs and not to others.

Erythrocyte Physiology and Function

The red blood cell (RBC) is a thin, biconcave disc-shaped cell with a thin membrane. The shape of the cell allows for oxygen transport and easy movement throughout the body. The normal RBC count in men is approximately 5.2 million cells/mm^3, and in women 4.7 million cells/mm^3.

RBCs are produced in the bone marrow from the pluripotent stem cell. Early stage of development is influenced by the following CSFs: BPA (burst-promoting activity), GM-CSF, and IL-3. The unipotent stem cell derived from the pluripotent stem cell is called the burst-forming unit (BFU-E [erythroid]), followed by a more differentiated progenitor cell called the CFU-E. Once the cell becomes committed to the erythroid line, its development is induced by erythropoietin (EPO). EPO is one of the earliest identified of the hematopoietic growth factors. EPO is produced primarily in the kidneys. A small percentage of EPO is produced in the liver. The kidneys produce EPO in response to hypoxia or hyperoxia.[7] Prostaglandin E and prostacyclin are also thought to induce renal EPO. The average life span of a red blood cell is 120 days. The cell becomes fragile as it ages, and it eventually ruptures, spilling its contents into the bloodstream. The contents of the cell, including the membrane, are completely recycled in the body.[1]

The major function of the RBC is the transport of hemoglobin, which carries oxygen to all tissues. The RBC also eliminates carbon dioxide, provides for hemoglobin synthesis and maintenance, and acts as a buffering agent in the blood.

Platelet Physiology and Function

Platelets, which are also known as *thrombocytes,* are anucleate, disc-shaped fragments of large marrow cells, or *megakaryocytes.* Platelets are formed when the mature, granular megakaryocyte sheds its cytoplasm. The cytoplasmic fragments are released in the marrow and subsequently into the bloodstream. The normal platelet count in men and women is approximately 150,000–400,000 cells/mm^3.

Platelets are derived from the pluripotent stem cell and mature in the bone marrow. Early-stage development is influenced by IL-3, GM-CSF, and EPO. Once a cell becomes committed to the megakaryocytic cell line, its production is also controlled by a growth factor called *thrombopoietin,* which is produced in the kidneys[10] (Figure 25-1). Under normal circumstances, any reduction in the platelet count causes an increased production of megakaryocytes and platelets in the bone marrow.

Platelets remain in the vascular system and are not found in extravascular fluid. Normally about two-thirds of the platelet mass circulates in the bloodstream, and the rest is concentrated in the spleen. The life span of the platelet is about 10 days. Most platelets die in repairing minor vascular injuries of daily life. Under normal conditions, approximately 30,000 platelets are formed each day for each cubic millimeter of blood.

Circulating platelets perform several functions. First and most important is that of *hemostasis,* or the formation of a mechanical hemostatic plug. A second platelet function is to furnish a phospholipid surface, thereby facilitating the action of the clotting factors of the intrinsic system, which is an important component of hemostasis. Finally, platelets are necessary for *fibrinolysis,* or lysis of the fibrin clot, and vessel repair.

Hemostasis

Hemostasis is the process by which the fluid component of blood becomes a solid clot, which prevents the escape of blood from the injured blood vessels. This process is initiated by vascular or tissue injury and culminates in the formation of a firm mechanical barrier, or a *platelet plug.* The sequence of events after injury includes: platelet adherence to structures in the vessel wall, aggregation of platelets to form a hemostatic plug, and local constriction and coagulation.

When blood vessel injury occurs, vasoconstriction initially provides a minimal degree of control of the bleeding. Within seconds, platelets are attracted to and adhere to the underlying layer of collagen of the exposed subendothelial tissue.[11] Platelets then release a number of components, including calcium, serotonin, proteolytic enzymes, cationic proteins, and nucleotide adenosine diphosphate (ADP). ADP causes platelets to swell and platelet membranes to become "sticky." This stickiness increases the adherence of platelets to one another. Increasing levels of ADP lead to clot contraction, degranulation, and ultimate fusion of the platelets. The end result of ADP-mediated platelet accumulation is the formation of a large platelet aggregate, or a hemostatic plug. This mass of platelets fills the gap in the vessel wall and arrests the bleeding, usually within 5 minutes. This primary hemostatic mechanism produces only a temporary cessation of bleeding.

Coagulation

Blood coagulation may be considered a mechanism for rapid replacement of an unstable platelet plug with

TABLE 25-1 Normal Coagulation Factors

Factor	Factor Name	Normal Range
I	Fibrinogen	142–366 mg/dl
II	Prothrombin	80%–120%
III	Tissue factor, tissue thromboplastin (extrinsic prothrombin activator)	80%–120%
IV	Calcium	8.5–10.5 mg/dl
V	Proaccelerin, accelerator globulin	50%–150%
VI	Not assigned	
VII	Proconvertin, serum prothrombin conversion accelerator (SPCA)	60%–140%
VIII	Antihemophilic globulin (AHG), antihemophilic factor (AHF)	60%–150%
IX	Plasma thromboplastin component (PTC), Christmas factor	60%–150%
X	Stuart-Prower factor	60%–150%
XI	Plasma thromboplastin antecedent (PTA)	60%–135%
XII	Hageman factor	50%–150%
XIII	Fibrin stabilizing factor (FSF)	Present

a stable fibrin clot. A series of interdependent, enzyme-mediated reactions ultimately act to activate fibrin. The fibrin clot is the final product of hemostasis.[11] When these enzymes or coagulation factors are stimulated, they become active in a sequential manner, not in numerical order (Table 25-1). This process often is referred to as the *coagulation cascade* (see Figure 25-2).

The formation of a fibrin clot is thought to occur through two separate pathways, the intrinsic pathway and the extrinsic pathway.[12,13] To generate a clot via the intrinsic pathway, components "intrinsic" to the whole blood are required. To generate a clot via the extrinsic pathway, components intrinsic to the whole blood are required in addition to an activating sub-

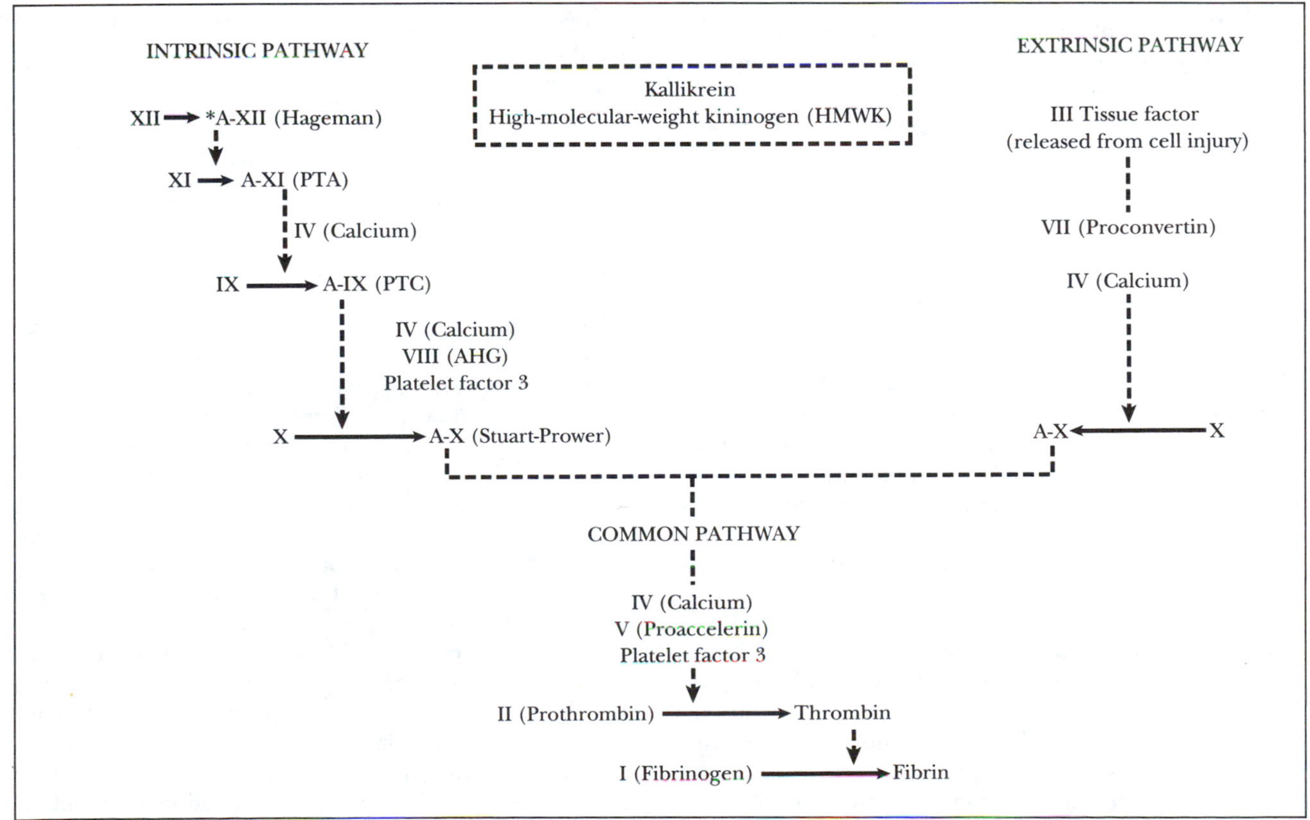

FIGURE 25-2 Blood coagulation.

stance, *tissue factor,* (or *tissue thromboplastin*), which is "extrinsic" to blood. The tissue factor is a cell surface protein that is expressed upon cellular injury.[11]

The intrinsic pathway of blood coagulation is initiated by activation of factor XII. Kallikrein and high-molecular-weight kininogen (HMWK) are proteins necessary for the intrinsic pathway sequence to proceed.[13] The specific factor or substance that stimulates the activation of coagulation factor XII, as well as its function, is unclear.[14] Factors VIII, IX, and XI all function as part of the intrinsic pathway until it converges with the common pathway. The presence of calcium ions is necessary for many of the enzyme conversions of the intrinsic pathway.

The extrinsic pathway begins with trauma to tissues that lie outside vessels. The pathway is initiated by a complex interaction between the tissue factor (released from cell injury) and factor VII. The reaction of tissue factor III with factor VII and calcium results in marked coagulant activity.[11] Factors III, VII, and IV function as part of the extrinsic system, then converge with the common pathway.

The interaction of the factors in both pathways leads to the stimulation of factor X. At this point, thromboplastin formation is complete. Thromboplastin is an essential factor for prothrombin-to-thrombin conversion. Subsequently, prothrombin is converted to thrombin by thromboplastin. Thrombin is the most powerful of the coagulation enzymes and acts on fibrinogen to form fibrin.[11] This fibrin network is an essential portion of a clot. The clot is soluble until it becomes polymerized by factor XIII (fibrin stabilizing factor), which converts it into a stable (insoluble) fibrin clot. Hemostasis is complete when the fibrin network alone is able to resist the hydrostatic pressure in the vessel.

Fibrin formation is an essential component of hemostasis, inflammation, and tissue repair. But it is a temporary reaction to an inciting stimulus. The fibrin clot must be remodeled and removed to restore normal tissue structure and function, as well as to restore normal bloodflow. This is done by the fibrinolytic system that controls the enzymatic degradation of fibrin.

Fibrinolysis

Fibrinolysis, or clot breakdown, is initiated by enzymes that are present in most body fluids and tissues (see Figure 25-3). These enzymes are known as *plasminogen activators.* They activate plasminogen (an inactive precursor of plasmin) to plasmin in the presence of thrombin. It is plasmin that is responsible for the lysis of fibrin clots. The breakdown of fibrinogen and fibrin results in polypeptides called *fibrin degradation products (FDPs).* FDPs are powerful anticoagulant substances. They have a destructive effect on fibrin in the platelet plug. They also are able to impair platelet aggregation, reduce prothrombin, and interfere with polymerization of fibrin. When these products are increased in the circulation there is a predisposition to bleeding.[15]

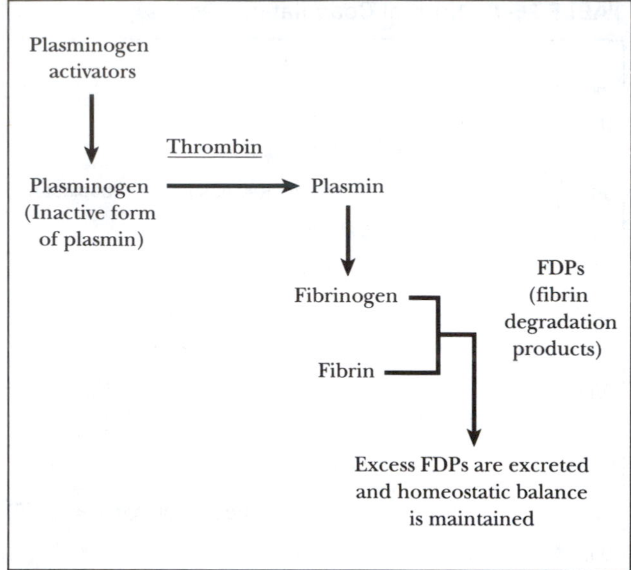

FIGURE 25-3 Fibrinolysis.

Under usual conditions of homeostasis the processes of coagulation and fibrinolysis are localized to the sites of injury. These processes constitute a threat to the organism if they extend beyond the site of injury to the general circulation. The blood carries natural anticoagulants that act to continually inhibit coagulation (i.e., heparin, antithrombin, and antithromboplastin).[16] A delicate balance between the processes of fibrin clot formation (coagulation) and clot breakdown (fibrinolysis) is necessary for effective hemostasis.

CAUSES OF BLEEDING IN CANCER

Tumor Effects

Bleeding is a common presenting symptom of cancer, generally occurring as a result of tumor extension and local tissue invasion. Blood loss and the resultant iron-deficiency anemia are frequently the initial signs of oropharyngeal, genitourinary, gynecologic, or enteric carcinomas.[17] Bleeding may present as excessive pinkish, viscous sputum, which is typical of bronchio-alveolar cell carcinoma, or as frank blood in the stool as a result of invasive left-sided colon cancer.

Frequently the most dramatic cause of bleeding in the individual with cancer is the invasion, erosion, and subsequent rupture of blood vessels. Any tumor involvement of vascular tissue or any tumor lying in close proximity to major vessels is seen as a threat of bleeding. Cancers of the large bronchi or lung may erode into the bronchial artery or branches of the pulmonary artery. Hemoptysis from tumor erosion into pulmonary blood vessels may appear as streaks of blood to gross blood loss. Head and neck tumors may also be associated with serious hemorrhage. Invasive neoplasms, particularly at the base of the tongue, can erode branches of the external carotid artery. Massive vaginal bleeding in individuals with pelvic tumor masses that invade major pelvic vessels is commonly seen in cervical carcinoma. Vaginal bleeding may also occasionally be seen with endometrial or ovarian carcinoma.

Other structural causes of bleeding that frequently occur in the individual with cancer include: cavitational and ulcerative effects of local infections at sites of vessels; destructive effects of radiotherapy on normal structures in the radiation field; and denuded remains of vessels at the site of radical cancer surgery. One example of a surgical cause of bleeding is the potential of a carotid artery rupture after a radical neck dissection. This can occur more frequently when the patient has received prior radiotherapy.

Minor incidents of vascular bleeding that are eventually expressed as chronic occult blood loss occur in individuals whose neoplasms produce abnormal proteins of very high viscosity. These paraproteins are common in individuals with myeloma and Waldenstrom's macroglobulinemia. Macroglobulinemia creates a circulating backflow in small vessels, thereby causing vascular rupture with resultant microscopic hemorrhage. A similar phenomenon is seen in individuals with acute leukemia with high white blood cell counts. Leukostasis, a potential complication of leukocytosis, results in aggregation and clotting of white blood cells in the microvasculature. This condition may mechanically stimulate obstruction, degeneration, and eventual disruption of small vessels, which results in bleeding.

Invasion and replacement of bone marrow by tumor may affect hematopoiesis. This process is called *myelophthisis,* and can result in anemia, thrombocytopenia, granulocytopenia, and impaired NK (natural killer) cell activity.[18] The decrease in production of normal marrow elements is thought to be a response to the physical "crowding out" of normal cells, competition for cellular nutrients, and the production by the invading cells' metabolic end products that are toxic to normal cells. Marrow infiltration may represent metastatic disease, or a primary disease process such as acute leukemia in which the leukemia cells "pack" the marrow.

Manifestations

Bleeding due to tumor effects may be manifested as symptoms ranging from minor incidents of vaginal bleeding to gross blood loss. Direct injury to major blood vessels can lead to acute bleeding and a true oncologic emergency. Specific symptoms depend on the site and extent of damage. Internal bleeding may present as massive hemoptysis, severe hematemesis, vaginal hemorrhage, loss of consciousness, or hypovolemic shock.

More gradual bleeding involving smaller circulatory structures is usually less obvious and therefore more difficult to diagnose. Melena due to colorectal carcinoma or the microscopic bleeding of macroglobulinemia can persist undetected until manifested by iron-deficiency anemia. A continual loss of 6–8 ml of blood per day eventually will precipitate classic iron deficiency, because the compensatory need for cell production exceeds the iron-producing capacity of the normal adult diet. A definitive diagnosis depends on demonstration of absent stainable iron stores in the individual's marrow. Other methods used to aid in the diagnosis of iron-deficiency anemia include the determination of the plasma iron levels, the unsaturated iron-binding capacity (UIBC), and the analysis of the serum ferritin level. The clinical picture of iron-deficiency anemia reflects a decreased plasma iron level, an increased UIBC, and a low serum ferritin level.[19] The homeostatic mechanisms in the body provide such remarkable compensatory adaptation that iron-deficiency anemia may be quite serious before the person actually develops significant symptoms. It is important to remember, therefore, that the onset of symptoms may reflect the rate of progression of the anemia better than does the severity. Fatigue, weakness, irritability, dyspnea, and tachycardia are typical clinical symptoms experienced by individuals with anemia.

Management

Tumors lying near or on major vessels generally are treated aggressively to avoid complications. Surgery, radiotherapy, and/or chemotherapy are treatment methods utilized to reduce or completely eliminate the neoplasm, if possible. If wound breakdown is in the neck area and carotid exposure occurs, wound debridement followed by a skin or skin-muscle flap carrying its own blood supply generally is done.[20] Prophylactic arterial ligation may be performed to minimize the risk of carotid hemorrhage. The patient who undergoes a bilateral ligation of the external carotid arteries runs the risk of a resultant stroke. Small transient bleeding usually occurs before vessel rupture. Careful observation can assist the caregiver in predicting and controlling such a complication (refer to Chapter 44). If vascular integrity is threatened by infection, antibiotic therapy is initiated. Preventing and treating infection is crucial in minimizing the potential for bleeding in the patient with cancer.

If acute bleeding occurs, direct methods to halt the hemorrhage are instituted immediately. Direct and steady pressure at the site of bleeding is applied. Mechanical pressure can be used if the site of bleeding is not directly exposed. Examples of mechanical pressure include insertion of an occlusion balloon catheter into the bronchus, and the use of nasal packing during epistaxis. Iced saline gastric lavages or enemas may help to control gastrointestinal bleeding. Hypovolemic shock is to be avoided in situations of acute hemorrhage. Whole blood is the blood component of choice to restore or maintain blood volume in acute life-threatening hemorrhage.[21] Whole blood restores circulatory volume and oxygen-carrying capacity simultaneously.

Minor vascular bleeding due to capillary destruction

is best controlled by treating the underlying malignancy. If iron-deficiency anemia has occurred, oral or parenteral iron supplements are indicated. Iron stores are replenished slowly, so iron therapy is continued for a prolonged period even after the malignancy has been treated.[19] If the hemoglobin level drops below 8–10 g/dl, blood replacement may be considered. Generally, blood replacement therapy is based on concurrent cardiac, pulmonary, or other conditions that can impair an individual's tolerance to anemia (see "Blood Component Therapy" later in this chapter). Clinical trials are under way to investigate the treatment of anemia of chronic disease, including cancer with recombinant human erythropoietin (rHuEPO).[22–24] rHuEPO is the first CSF approved by the U.S. Food and Drug Administration (June 1989) to be available for clinical use. The role of rHuEPO is firmly established in the treatment of the anemia of end-stage renal disease.[25–27] In this group of patients, erythropoietin has been found to be effective in stimulating erythropoiesis and reducing or eliminating transfusion requirements. One of the promising applications of rHuEPO is the treatment of anemia related to cancer chemotherapy, in particular, cisplatin-containing regimens, because of their nephrotoxic effects.[28] Clinical trials are being conducted to determine if the administration of rHuEPO, given at appropriate intervals, can maintain hemoglobin concentrations equal to 1 unit of packed red cells without significant side effects.[28,29] In the renal dialysis population, rHuEPO has been associated with hypertension, seizures, and arteriovenous shunt thromboses.[22]

Platelet Abnormalities

Abnormalities of platelet production, function, survival, and metabolism frequently occur in individuals with cancer. These abnormalities may be due to a variety of causes. Generally, they are due to mechanical or humoral effects of the tumor itself or to abnormalities in the host induced by the tumor.

Quantitative abnormalities

Thrombocytosis Thrombocytosis is a disorder in which there is an increased number of circulating platelets. Generally, the platelet count is only mildly elevated when thrombocytosis is due to cancer (400,000–600,000 cells/mm^3), but may on occasion be markedly elevated (>800,000 cells/mm^3).[30]

The mechanism by which thrombocytosis occurs is unknown, but the disorder commonly is associated with many types of neoplasms. Thrombocytosis is particularly common in the myeloproliferative disorders, such as chronic granulocytic anemia. It may also be seen in lung, ovarian, pancreatic, breast, kidney, and gastrointestinal carcinomas, Hodgkin's disease, splenectomized patients, and in individuals with widespread cancer.

The person with thrombocytosis usually is asymptomatic and does not require treatment. Thrombosis, usually venous, occurs in a small proportion of cases.[31] There are no data linking the likelihood of complications to the platelet count in thrombocytosis; however, counts greater than 1 million cells/mm^3 are considered hazardous due to the potential for thrombotic complications. The hazard is especially clear in individuals with concomitant symptomatic atherosclerosis.[30]

Thrombocytosis may disappear with effective therapy for the underlying disease. Individuals who experience complications related to thrombocytosis, such as venous thrombosis, can be treated by thrombocytopheresis. This treatment rapidly removes large numbers of circulating platelets. A platelet count can be reduced by 50% or more within a few hours. Concurrent with apheresis, the patient can be started on marrow suppressive therapy. Alkylating agents (busulfan, chlorambucil, cyclophosphamide, melphalan) and ionizing radiation (radioactive phosphorus) frequently are used to suppress the hyperproliferative marrow. These agents have a high leukemogenic potential.[32] Hydroxyurea can also be given to lower platelet counts, particularly to younger patients without symptoms. This agent, too, may have leukemogenic potential.[33,34] Anagrelide is an investigational agent currently being used to treat thrombocytosis in myeloproliferative diseases.[35] This drug has a powerful antiaggregating effect on platelets and has been found to lower the platelet count without altering the leukocyte count or the hemoglobin level. It is nonmutogenic and is not known to be leukemogenic. Drugs considered for the prevention of thrombotic complications in patients with thrombocytosis include aspirin and dipyridamole, due to their ability to interfere with platelet aggregation.[30]

Thrombocytopenia Thrombocytopenia, a reduction in the number of circulating platelets, is the most frequent platelet abnormality associated with cancer. This disorder may be due to a decrease in platelet production, a change in platelet distribution, platelet destruction, or vascular dilution.

Platelet production The most common cause of thrombocytopenia in patients with cancer is a disorder of production involving decreased megakaryocytopoiesis. This may be due to tumor invasion of the bone marrow or to an acute or delayed effect of chemotherapy or radiation therapy. When tumor invasion is the cause of the decrease in platelet production, the resulting thrombocytopenia is just part of the total picture of pancytopenia. A low platelet count is directly proportional to the degree of bone marrow infiltration by tumor cells.

Chemotherapy is the treatment most often associated with hematologic toxicity and bone marrow suppression. The effects of chemotherapy are due in large part to the particular drugs used, dosages, schedules, routes of administration, previous cancer treatments, concomitant therapy, and the person's age, nutritional status, and tumor type.[2] Acute chemotherapy-induced platelet toxicity usually is caused by the destruction of the proliferating cells of the platelet line,

CFU-MG. As these cells are destroyed, the circulatory platelets are cleared at the end of their life span, and the nadir of a person's blood cell count occurs. Considering that the average life span of a platelet is only 7 days, this accounts in part for the high incidence of thrombocytopenia related to chemotherapy.

The degree and duration of platelet toxicity related to various antineoplastic agents are the result of a number of factors, including the natural nadir of the drug, its potential for suppression, and cellular recovery time after the nadir. The major classification of these drugs also plays a part in how this toxicity is demonstrated. For example, cell-cycle-phase-nonspecific (CCNS) drugs, such as carmustine and lomustine, destroy cells in the resting phase of the cell cycle, damaging nonproliferating stem cells. These drugs can then have a delayed, prolonged, and cumulative suppressive effect.[2,36] The patient treated with carmustine will experience a platelet nadir approximately 3 weeks following treatment, and it may take as long as 8 weeks for platelet recovery to occur. Cell-cycle-phase-specific (CCS) drugs, such as bleomycin, cytarabine, and vincristine, have their impact on proliferating progenitor cells and do not destroy cells in the resting phase of the cell cycle. These agents have an earlier nadir and a shorter recovery time and tend to be less toxic. See Table 25-2 for a list of chemotherapeutic agents associated with moderate to severe thrombocytopenia.

The most significant factor that determines the risk of bone marrow depression related to radiation therapy is the volume of productive bone marrow in the radiation field. This risk factor is even more important than

TABLE 25-2 Chemotherapeutic Agents Associated with Significant Thrombocytopenia

Chemotherapeutic Agent	Degree of Suppression	Nadir (days)	Recovery (days)	Comments
Carmustine (BCNU)	Severe	28–42	35–42	Cell-cycle phase nonspecific (CCNS), cumulative toxicity
Lomustine (CCNU)	Severe	21–28	42	CCNS, cumulative
Streptozocin (Zanosar)				CCNS, cumulative
Mechlorethamine (nitrogen mustard)	Moderate	10–14	21–28	CCNS, cumulative
Busulfan (Myleran)	Moderate	21–28	42–56	CCNS, cumulative
Cyclophosphamide (Cytoxan)	Moderate (dose related—100 mg/m²)	7–14	21	CCNS, cumulative
L-phenylalanine (L-PAM, Melphalan)	Moderate	14–21	21–28	CCNS, cumulative
Triethylenethiphosphoramide (Thiotepa)	Moderate	14–21	40–50	CCNS
Chlorambucil (Leukeran)	Moderate	21–28	42–56	CCNS, cumulative
Dacarbazine (DTIC)	Severe (dose related—200 mg/m² IV daily × 5 days)	10–14	21–28	CCNS
Mitomycin-C	Severe	21–28	42–56	CCNS, cumulative
Doxorubicin (Adriamycin)	Moderate-severe (dose related)	10–14	21	CCNS
Plicamycin (Mithracin)	Moderate	14	21	CCNS
Dactinomycin (Actinomycin-D)	Severe	14	21–28	CCNS
Daunorubicin hydrochloride (Cerubidine)	Severe	10	21–28	CCNS
Epirubicin hydrochloride (Pharmorubicin)	Moderate	10–14	21	CCNS
5-Fluorouracil (5-FU)	Moderate (dose related—12–15 mg/kg)	9–21	21	Cell-cycle phase specific (CCS)
Cytarabine (Cytosar-U ARA-C)	Severe	10	21	CCS
Methotrexate (MTX)	Moderate (dose related—100 mg/m²)	10	14	CCS
Vinblastine	Moderate	10	21	CCS
Vindesine	Mild to moderate	3–6	7–10	CCS
Hydroxyurea (Hydrea)	Moderate	7	14	
Procarbazine (Matulane)	Moderate	14	21–28	

the therapeutic dose or the fractionation schedule.[2,37] Radiation-induced hematologic toxicity usually is caused by damage to the nonproliferating stem cells, or to the cells in the resting phase of the cell cycle. Radiation therapy is local treatment, except for total nodal or total body irradiation, and does not usually cause the nadirs in blood counts seen with chemotherapy. The localized nature of this treatment generally allows for the untreated marrow to compensate for the damage to the treated marrow.

Platelet distribution Thrombocytopenia due to an abnormal distribution of platelets can occur in cancer patients with hypersplenism. An enlarged spleen may sequester up to 90% of the platelet population, making them unavailable in the circulation. Tumor metastasis to the spleen, particularly due to lymphomas and lung, breast, prostate, colon, and stomach cancers are known to cause hypersplenism and subsequent platelet sequestration. The absence of a palpable spleen rules out this type of thrombocytopenic disorder. Sequestration of platelets with resultant bleeding may occur within the vascular channels of some tumors, such as giant hemangiomas. Surgical removal of the tumor or shrinkage of the tumor by low-dose radiation therapy is necessary for recovery of the platelet count.[38] Areas denuded from surgery, mucositis resulting from chemotherapy and/or microbial toxins, and necrotic tumor can also cause platelet aggregation and a decrease in circulating platelets.

If the primary cause of thrombocytopenia is platelet sequestration, the bone marrow will contain normal to increased numbers of megakaryocytes. This is due to the attempt of the bone marrow to compensate for the decreased number of circulating platelets. When splenomegaly is accompanied by marrow infiltration by tumor, the degree of thrombocytopenia is compounded, for the compensatory production of platelets will be inadequate.

Platelet destruction Thrombocytopenia can also be due to rapid platelet destruction, characterized by a dramatically shortened platelet life span and an abundance of megakaryocytes in the bone marrow. Although the platelet normally survives 8–10 days, it may live as little as a few hours.

This type of thrombocytopenia is seen in two situations. The first situation in which rapid platelet destruction occurs is immune thrombocytopenia, or idiopathic thrombocytopenic purpura (ITP). This disorder occurs most frequently in individuals with lymphoproliferative diseases, such as chronic lymphocytic leukemia, acute lymphocytic leukemia, and lymphoma.[39] ITP also has been found in association with extragonadal germ cell cancer. It is rarely associated with disseminated carcinomas.[40] The use of alpha-interferon therapy for cancer patients has also been identified with the development of immune thrombocytopenia.[41] The rapid destruction of platelets is due to an autoimmune process in which antibodies are formed against the individual's own platelets. This process results in normal or increased numbers of megakaryocytes in the absence of any other cause of peripheral platelet destruction, such as sepsis or disseminated intravascular coagulation.[39]

The second type of rapid platelet destruction is seen in conditions of increased platelet consumption. This can be observed in various clinical syndromes with intravascular coagulation. Disseminated intravascular coagulation (DIC) is discussed in depth later in this chapter in the section on "Hypercoagulability." In any condition involving increased platelet destruction, increased numbers of megakaryocytes will be present in the marrow as the body attempts to compensate for this abnormal state.

Platelet dilution Dilution is another cause of thrombocytopenia. It is thought that rapid reconstitution of the intravascular volume by the use of stored platelet-poor blood dilutes thrombocytes already present. Whole blood can be stored up to 21 days with minimal decrease in erythrocyte survival. The platelets in the whole blood, however, lose considerable effectiveness after 24 hours at usual storage temperatures of 4°C. This dilutional effect of platelets occurs in direct proportion to the amount of blood transfused.

Multiple-donor transfusions, possibly with incompatible platelet antigens, can stimulate an isoantibody response in the recipient. Studies of individuals with posttransfusion purpura have demonstrated the presence of platelet antibodies in the plasma, as well as microaggregation and lysis of platelets.[42]

Manifestations The platelet count is considered to be the single most significant factor for predicting bleeding in the individual with cancer. Gaydos, Freirich, and Mantel first reported an association between thrombocytopenia and an increased risk of bleeding in 1962.[43] The risk of spontaneous hemorrhage is considered to be greater than 50% when the platelet count is less than 20,000 cells/mm^3.

The platelet count is not the only determinant of a person's risk of bleeding. Concomitant infection, potential sources of bleeding, and a rapid decline in the platelet count commonly increase the risk of bleeding in an individual with cancer who is thrombocytopenic. Release of bacterial endotoxins from infection may stimulate a leukocyte response, which can enhance platelet consumption. Infection in the individual with thrombocytopenia increases the risk of bleeding. Potential sites of bleeding are numerous in the thrombocytopenic individual. They may be part of the disease process (e.g., necrotic tumor masses or intracranial bleeding) or treatment related (e.g., mucositis or sites of injections). Risk for bleeding is greater in an individual with a rapidly falling platelet count compared to one that is rising, even if the absolute platelet count is the same. When the count is returning to normal, the platelets in circulation tend to be younger and larger and are able to clot more effectively.[44]

Management Although thrombocytopenia may be the immediate cause of bleeding in individuals with platelet disorders, therapy must address the underlying cause of the decreased platelet level. When the decreased platelet production is due to tumor infiltration of marrow, the best therapy is treatment of the tumor itself. The hematologic complications will remain or worsen as long as the marrow involvement persists. Platelet transfusions are often given to maintain a safe level of circulating thrombocytes until tumor regression occurs and marrow function returns. If platelet production has been depressed by chemotherapy or radiotherapy, in addition to platelet support if necessary, the dosage or administration schedule can be altered to maintain safe levels of platelet production.[45]

The use of recombinant colony-stimulating growth factors in accelerating hematologic recovery following ablative chemoradiotherapy is an area of intensive investigation. Studies in both animals and humans have clearly shown that the administration of growth factors for granulocytes (rhG-CSF) and granulocytes-macrophages (rhGM-CSF) can reduce the hematopoietic toxicity that follows exposure to chemotherapy and radiation therapy.[46–51] GM-CSF possesses stimulating activities for granulocyte-macrophage, eosinophilic, and megakaryocytic progenitor cells in vitro.[52–54] Different effects of GM-CSF on platelet levels have been reported. Gianni et al.[55] reported that patients treated with continuous GM-CSF infusion (5.5 mg/kg/day) for 14 days after high-dose cyclophosphamide required fewer prophylactic platelet transfusions. Other studies have demonstrated earlier independence of platelet transfusions in some patients,[56] as well as a higher platelet nadir in patients treated with GM-CSF as compared to a control group.[47] A lack of platelet stimulation has been reported by other investigators.[57–60] According to Gianni et al., the lack of stimulation reported by these investigators might reflect differences in the myelotoxic damage underlying the conditions being treated with the growth factor.[55]

In addition to the intravenous route of administration, rhGM-CSF can effectively be administered by the subcutaneous (SC) route.[61–63] The ability to administer the drug SC allows patients to be discharged from the hospital and to be followed up in the outpatient setting. When the drug is administered SC, local reactions, ranging from redness to infiltrates, leading to cessation of rhGM-CSF have been reported.[57,64] DiVries et al.[64] reported that local reactions disappeared in most patients during the subsequent courses of treatment with GM-CSF. Reported side effects include a temporary generalized rash and pruritis, mild to moderate bone pain (sternum, ribs, shoulders, lower back and hip areas), and muscle pain.[64,65] Discontinuation of treatment, rest, and analgesics have been used effectively to relieve these reported symptoms. Other mild side effects include fever, chills, myalgia, headaches, decreased appetite, nausea, and flushing.[65–68] More serious reported toxicities include capillary leak syndrome and thrombosis.[47,69]

A second-generation blood cell growth factor currently is being investigated as a therapy for patients with chemotherapy-induced or radiation-therapy-induced thrombocytopenia and neutropenia. These phase 1 clinical trials are based on data from animal models that demonstrated that a combination of GM-CSF and IL-3 acts synergistically in stimulating hematopoiesis in primates.[70] This combination growth factor is manufactured by the Immunex® Corporation. The "Fact Sheet" published by the corporation describes this growth factor and the current clinical trials using the factor. PIXY321 is a fusion protein molecule that combines the biological effects of two immune system proteins: GM-CSF, which stimulates neutrophils, macrophages, and megakaryocytes, and IL-3, which is being investigated for its effect in promoting growth of megakaryocytes. Preclinical studies with PIXY321 have demonstrated rapid recovery of white blood cell and platelet levels in animals treated with cancer therapy. Phase 1 clinical trials are under way to study the effect of this growth factor in sarcoma patients undergoing chemotherapy for refractory solid tumors.

Platelet sequestration within a spleen enlarged due to malignancy is treated most effectively by aggressive tumor therapy. Chemotherapy and radiotherapy usually are most effective. Sequestration of platelets is at times reversible by the administration of epinephrine. Epinephrine causes a release of trapped platelets from an enlarged spleen.[71] Transient control of platelet sequestration has also been achieved with corticosteroid therapy. Steroids have a capillary stabilizing effect, which is important in minimizing the bleeding potential of thrombocytopenia. Splenectomy may be considered if other methods fail to control the sequestration of platelets.

High-dose intravenous immunoglobulin therapy has been advocated as a treatment choice for patients who are actively bleeding and who are alloimmunized to HLA-matched platelets.[72] Immunoglobulins provide a quick rise in the platelet count, with a radical decrease in bleeding. In the absence of active bleeding, the use of high-dose intravenous methylprednisone has been found as effective as high-dose intravenous immunoglobulins for the treatment of autoimmune thrombocytopenia.[73]

Platelet destruction by an autoimmune reaction rarely is treated by platelet transfusions. This therapy generally is ineffective and carries the risk of serious transfusion reactions. Should patients also require red cell therapy, it is recommended that they receive extensively washed red cells or frozen deglycerolized red cells. These preparations can provide less antigenic material.[74] The use of a leukocyte-poor blood filter when administering red cells may also minimize the chance of an antigenic reaction. Patients with severe chronic ITP (platelet counts lower than 30,000 cells/mm^3) usually are managed with corticosteroids or splenectomy. Resistant patients may require danazol or additional immunosuppressive therapy.[41]

Qualitative abnormalities

Platelet malfunction Patients with cancer may at times bleed despite normal platelet counts and/or coagulation factors. Alterations in platelet function may be responsible for the bleeding seen in these situations. The major abnormality noted in these patients is a decrease in the procoagulant activity of platelets, which is a measure of platelet factor III. This deficiency has been demonstrated in patients with chronic lymphocytic leukemia, acute leukemia, multiple myeloma, and macroglobulinemia.[75] Decreased platelet adhesiveness and decreased aggregation in response to ADP have been reported, especially in individuals with leukemia.[76] Abnormal platelet function also has been described in patients with thrombocytosis, associated with the myeloproliferative disorders. This may help to explain the increased incidence of hemorrhage in patients with an increased platelet concentration. These abnormalities may be due to the malignancy itself or to a partial release of the platelet contents after contact with malignant tissue.[75]

Numerous drugs are known to affect platelet function. At times some of these drugs are administered deliberately for their antithrombotic effect, with diminished platelet function being the therapeutic goal (e.g., heparin). For many of the other drugs, the decreased platelet function is an unwanted side effect. For all of the drugs known to affect platelet function, effect is measured by an abnormality of platelet function or bleeding time. Although all these drugs may be known to affect platelet aggregation or the bleeding time, only aspirin has been demonstrated to cause a significant increased risk of bleeding. (See Table 25-3 for a discussion of commonly used cancer care drugs that inhibit platelet function.) When aspirin is ingested, there is a predictable abnormality of impaired platelet aggregation with epinephrine, ADP, arachidonic acid, and low concentrations of collagen and thrombin.[77] This platelet aggregation abnormality associated with aspirin is so characteristic that abnormal platelet aggregation patterns of any etiology are often designated as "aspirinlike."[78] The decreased platelet aggregation can lead to bleeding. Aspirin also prolongs bleeding time, although this is less consistent than the platelet aggregation abnormality. Daily ingestion of 30 mg or more of aspirin can produce an increased bleeding time.[79] It has also been demonstrated that the bleeding time can be prolonged for up to 4 days after a single dose of aspirin, until normal platelet turnover results in a significant number of new platelets with normal function.[80]

The mechanism of action of nonsteroidal anti-inflammatory drugs appears to be similar to that for aspirin, that of inhibition of platelet aggregation. These drugs have only a temporary effect, causing inhibition only as long as the active drug is present in the circulation. Most of these drugs affect platelet function for only a few hours. One exception is piroxicam, which has a plasma half-life of more than 2 days.[81] The short half-life of these drugs suggests that they cause less risk of increased bleeding than does aspirin.[77]

Beta-lactam antibiotics, including the penicillins and cephalosporins, frequently are used in the cancer patient population. These antibiotics characteristically cause a prolonged bleeding time and abnormal platelet aggregation. These changes are seen after several days of high-dose parenteral therapy.[82] They may act by blocking ADP receptor activity on platelet membranes and, consequently, ADP-mediated platelet aggregation. The abnormalities can persist for several days after the antibiotics have been discontinued. The frequency of clinically significant hemorrhage due solely to the effect of antibiotics on platelet function is rare.[83] Moxalactam, however, is an antibiotic associated with a higher frequency of clinically significant hemorrhagic complications as compared to the other antibiotics.[83,84] Although its effect on bleeding time and platelet aggregation is no different than that of the other antibiotics, it has been implicated in the inhibition of synthesis of vitamin-K–dependent proteins. This process results in deficiencies of coagulation factors II, VII, IX, and X and impaired platelet function.[85]

Patients taking psychotropic drugs, such as tricyclic antidepressants and phenothiazines, may have impaired platelet aggregation and secretion responses to ADP, epinephrine, and collagen.[77] This effect has not been found to be associated with an increased risk of bleeding.

Administration of a few chemotherapeutic drugs has been found to be associated with abnormal platelet aggregation. Mithramycin, when administered to a total dose of 6–21 mg, has been associated with decreased platelet aggregation, increased bleeding time, and mucocutaneous bleeding.[86] BCNU and daunorubicin are both known to inhibit platelet aggregation and secretion, but are not linked to clinically significant bleeding caused by abnormal platelet function.

Management Management of hemorrhagic disorders due to platelet malfunction, such as when patients have a platelet factor III deficiency, frequently is aimed at the underlying cause. The patient will likely be treated with aggressive antineoplastic therapy. Drug-induced platelet abnormalities must be assessed carefully in respect to the patient's total clinical picture. Aspirin has been demonstrated to cause an increased risk of bleeding. Because of this risk, the patient with cancer should avoid taking this drug or any compounds containing aspirin. The clinical risk for bleeding associated with nonsteroidal anti-inflammatory drugs is much less than that for aspirin. However, they should be used cautiously in patients with already-low platelet counts. The potential for beta-lactam-induced bleeding in patients with cancer generally does not prohibit patients from being treated with appropriate antibiotic coverage. These patients need to be monitored closely for any signs or symptoms of bleeding. Bleeding studies, including the bleeding time, are monitored closely as well. Platelet transfusions can be used during periods of thrombocytopenia to avoid hemorrhage, as well as during periods of acute bleeding.

Hypocoagulation

Etiology and pathogenesis Malignancy or the metabolic alterations that frequently accompany it may pre-

TABLE 25-3 Commonly Used Cancer Care Drugs That Inhibit Platelet Function

Drug	Effects	Comments
	NONSTEROIDAL ANTI-INFLAMMATORY AGENTS	
Aspirin	• Impaired platelet aggregation • Prolonged bleeding time	Has been demonstrated to cause a significant increased risk for bleeding, especially when patients have conditions predisposing to hemorrhage.
Others Indomethacin (Indocin) Ibuprofen (Advil, Motrin, Nuprin, Rufen) Sulindac (Clinoril) Naproxen (Naprosyn) Phenylbutazone (Butazolidin) Mechlofenamic acid (Meclomen) Mefanamic acid (Ponstel) Diflunisal (Dolobid) Tolmetin (Tolectin) Piroxican (Feldene)	• Impaired platelet aggregation • Prolonged bleeding time, minimal and transient	Cause less risk of increased bleeding than aspirin; should be discontinued the day before surgery or an invasive procedure Has a half-life of more than 2 days; may increase slightly the risk of bleeding.
	β-LACTAM ANTIBIOTICS	
Penicillins Penicillin G Carbenicillin (Geopen) Ticarcillin (Ticar, Timentin) Methicillin (Staphcillin) Ampicillin (Polycillin, Omnipen) Nafcillin (Nafcil, Unipen) Piperacillin (Pipracil) Azocillin (Azlin) Mezlocillin (Mezlin) Temocillin Sulbenicillin Apalcillin **Cephalosporins** Cephalothin (Keflin, Seffin) Cefoxitin (Mefoxin) Cefotaxime (Claforan) Cefazolin (Ancef, Kefzol) Moxalactam (Moxam)	• Prolonged bleeding time • Impaired platelet aggregation	Effect on bleeding time occurs only in patients receiving large parenteral doses of antibiotics; effects may be greater in chronically ill patients with low serum albumin levels;[59] abnormalities do not subside for several days after drug discontinuance. Frequency of clinically significant hemorrhage due *only* to the effects of antibiotics on platelet function is rare.[58]
	PSYCHOTROPIC DRUGS	
Phenothiazines Chlorpromazine (Thorazine) Promethazine (Phenergan) Trifluoperazine (Stelazine) **Antidepressants** Amitriptyline Imiprimine (Tofranil) Nortryptaline (Pamelor)	• Impaired platelet aggregation and secretion response	Effect on platelets has not been associated with an increased risk of bleeding.
	CHEMOTHERAPY AGENTS	
Mithramycin	• Impaired platelet aggregation • Prolonged bleeding time • Mucocutaneous bleeding	Effects occur with total dose of 6–21 mg.
BCNU (carmustine) Daunorubicin (Daunomycin)	• Impaired platelet aggregation and secretion when added to platelet-rich plasma	Effect on platelets has not been found to cause clinically significant bleeding.

cipitate an imbalance in the coagulation factors, leading to an increased risk of bleeding. In 1974 Slichter and Harker[87] showed that these imbalances were related directly to tumor burden. Successful tumor therapy brought about a normalization of coagulation values. The most significant factor leading to a state of hypocoagulability is liver disease. Liver disease may be due to tumor invasion, chemotherapy, infection, or surgical resection. Liver disease interferes with the synthesis of plasma coagulation factors I, II, V, VII, IX, and X. In addition to decreasing the production of these factors, liver disease may also interfere with their functioning. Decreased liver function allows for diminished liver clearance of fibrin degradation products and activated clotting factors, which further inhibits the coagulation mechanism.

A deficiency of vitamin K may also cause a hypocoagulation syndrome. This may be seen in patients with neoplastic disease in which there is dietary lack of vitamin K, biliary obstruction, or malabsorptive states, or with intestinal sterilization due to antibiotic administration. A deficiency of vitamin K results in a greatly reduced chemical activation of vitamin-K–dependent proteins: factors II, VII, IX, and X. The result is a state of decreased hemostasis.

Individuals who undergo extensive surgical procedures and receive large amounts of frozen plasma may demonstrate a prolonged prothrombin time and a prolonged partial thromboplastin time. These individuals are prone to postsurgical bleeding. Frozen plasma has deficient levels of factors V and VIII, which can lead to an altered state of coagulation.[88]

A nonspecific plasma antagonist of several coagulation proteins has been described in various disease states, including neoplastic disease. These anticoagulants have been identified in the acute leukemias, lymphocytic lymphomas, and other disease states in which white cell turnover is rapid. These inhibitors have also been found to be highest at the onset of chemotherapy when there is lysis of white cells, and in disease relapse when there is a large tumor burden.[88]

Isolated factor deficiencies are also reported in neoplastic disease. Acquired von Willebrand's syndrome has been demonstrated to occur in solid tumors, hematologic malignancies, macroglobulinemia, and lymphoproliferative disorders. Patients with this syndrome demonstrate mucosal bleeding, bruising, and GI hemorrhage. Coagulation studies show a prolonged bleeding time and diminished or absent factor VIII procoagulant activity (factor VIII:C), von Willebrand factor antigen (VWF:Ag), and ristocetin cofactor activity. The factor VIII deficiency may be attributed to acquired inhibitors of coagulation proteins, which have been demonstrated in monoclonal IgG gammopathies, lymphoma, and macroglobulinemia.[39] The exact mechanism connecting the specific inhibitors and the underlying neoplastic disease is unclear. Factor XIII deficiency is also commonly affected by malignancy and liver disease.

Manifestations Conditions of decreased coagulability are less common than the other types of hemostatic alterations discussed in this chapter. Although any type of coagulation abnormality can lead to bleeding, they less frequently cause serious bleeding when they do occur. Hemorrhages tend to develop in the deeper areas of the body, such as the subcutaneous or intramuscular tissue. Bleeding into the joints, especially of the distal extremities, may be seen in the hypocoagulability states. A deficiency of any factor will lead to abnormal fibrin formation, which provides an ineffective matrix for normal fibroblastic proliferation and wound healing.

Management Effective tumor therapy generally is the best means of controlling hypocoagulability abnormalities. Plasma and plasma derivative therapy may be used discriminately in specific clinical situations. Specific replacement of diminished factors is difficult because of the complex nature of these abnormalities. Generally, the treatment of specific inhibitors of coagulation factors depends on the severity of the abnormality. Life-threatening bleeding requires therapy, but lesser symptoms may require observation only.[89]

Liver disease associated with hemorrhagic diathesis and a decrease in the production of the vitamin-K–dependent coagulation factors is at times treated by infusion of fresh-frozen plasma or prothrombin complex concentrates, when rapid correction of abnormalities is required. The therapeutic effectiveness of this therapy, however, is debated. Alternatively, albumin can be used as a volume expander when the patient is actively bleeding. Albumin is safer than plasma, since it carries no risk of hepatitis transmission. It may, however, precipitate congestive heart failure in patients with compromised cardiovascular function. The patient's cardiac and renal status must be monitored closely.[90] When there is an attempt to shorten a prolonged prothrombin time, as before a needle biopsy of the liver, prothrombin complex (containing prothrombin and factors VII, IX, and X) may be given. The usual initial dosage per kilogram of body weight of prothrombin complex is 40 U. Maintenance doses of 10–20 U are given daily until the patient's coagulation parameters normalize.[91] Plasma component therapy is always given intravenously.

Generally, parenteral vitamin K (Menaphthone, AquaMEPHYTON) is administered to correct the protein defects when this vitamin is deficient. Prothrombin complex concentrates can be used in rare situations of vitamin K deficiency with concomitant bleeding.[89] The patient is also instructed on the dietary sources of vitamin K (green leafy vegetables such as spinach, kale, and cabbage) if absorption of the vitamin is not a problem.

Isolated factor deficiencies are treated by specific plasma components. When factors V and VIII are deficient because the patient has received large amounts of frozen plasma, the infusion of several units of fresh plasma may correct the disorder. Patients who experience bleeding because of an acquired von Willebrand's syndrome, may be treated with infusions of fresh-frozen plasma and cryoprecipitate along with packed red cells and platelet concentrates to control the bleeding. The severity of the bleeding governs the amount and volume of plasma components given. Successful tumor therapy, including surgery, chemotherapy, or radiotherapy, may bring about the most significant response in the normalization of factor VIII-VWF complex parameters.[92,93] Factor XIII deficiency (or fibrin-stabilizing factor deficiency) is readily treated by replacement therapy with plasma or cryoprecipitate.

Hypercoagulability

Disseminated intravascular coagulation (DIC) is the most common serious hypercoagulable state occurring in individuals with cancer. It represents an inappropriate and exaggerated overstimulation of normal coagulation, in which both thrombosis and hemorrhage may occur simultaneously. This seemingly paradoxical situation results in hypercoagulation, in which multiple small clots are formed in the microcirculation of many organs, and fibrinolysis, in which there is consumption of clots and clotting factors. Ultimately the body becomes unable to respond to vascular or tissue injury through stable clot formation, and hemorrhage ensues. This syndrome is always secondary to an underlying disease process, such as malignancy, septicemia, obstetrical complications, or similar systemic stressors.

Although DIC is considered to be a common problem associated with malignancy, the incidence rate is difficult to estimate. The syndrome often remains undetected until severe hemorrhage occurs, and frequently is only discovered at the time of autopsy. Rickles and Edward[94] report that up to 92% of cancer patients have abnormal routine blood coagulation tests that are compatible with DIC. DIC contributes strongly to morbidity and mortality in patients with cancer, particularly when there is thrombosis or bleeding in the lung, central nervous system, or the gastrointestinal tract.[95] The mortality rate for DIC is in the range of 54%–68%, increasing with age, number of clinical manifestations, and severity of laboratory abnormalities.[96]

Etiology The most common cause of DIC is infection. It is believed that bacterial endotoxins, which are released from gram-negative bacteremia, activate the Hageman factor (XII). This factor initiates coagulation via the intrinsic pathway of hemostasis, as well as stimulating fibrinolysis.[96] DIC also is seen in the presence of gram-positive bacteremia, and with viremias. See Table 25-4 for a list of common causes of DIC in cancer.

Tumors themselves have been identified as stimulators of intravascular coagulation. The cancers most commonly associated with DIC include acute promyelocytic leukemia (APL) and the adenocarcinomas.[97] APL has a very high correlation with DIC (about 85%).[98] DIC associated with APL can occur before and in conjunction with chemotherapy administration.[99] It has been indicated that the tendency to bleed in persons with APL is associated with a white blood cell count of ⩾10,000 cells/mm³ at diagnosis.[100,101] A procoagulant substance has been identified on the promyelocytic blast cells that is similar to thromboplastin. This substance is believed to be released from granules on the promyelocytes, which subsequently initiate the clotting response.[102] The solid tumors most often associated with DIC are the mucin-producing adenocarcinomas, such as gastric, lung, pancreas, and prostate tumors. Solid tumors develop new vasculature, which have an abnormal endothelial lining thought to activate the procoagulant system.[97] Tumors may also release necrotic tissue into the circulation or tissue enzymes, which could activate the coagulation mechanism.

TABLE 25-4 Common Causes of Disseminated Intravascular Coagulation in Cancer

Neoplasms
- Solid tumors (lung, prostate, colon, stomach, breast, gallbladder, ovary, melanoma, pancreas, gastric)
- Leukemia (acute promyelocytic, acute myelogenous, chronic myelogenous, acute lymphoblastic)

Infections
- Gram-negative bacteria *(Pseudomonas, Meningococcus, Enterobacteriaciae, Salmonella, Hemophilus)*
- Gram-positive bacteria *(Pneumococcus, Staphlococcus),*
- Viremias (cytomegalovirus, hepatitis, varicella)
- Septic shock

Liver disease
- Obstructive jaundice
- Fulminant hepatic failure

Intravascular hemorrhage
- Multiple transfusions of whole blood
- Hemolytic transfusion reaction
- Minor hemolysis

Pathogenesis Disseminated intravascular coagulation is always secondary to an underlying disease process. The pathophysiology of DIC involves an extensive triggering of the coagulation system by the underlying disease, which results in abnormal activation of thrombin formation. This triggering mechanism may be direct, as with tissue thromboplastin associated with acute promyelocytic leukemia, or indirect due to endotoxins from gram-negative sepsis. Excess circulating thrombin may abnormally activate both coagulation and fibrinolysis, which upsets the balance of hemostasis.

Thrombin cleaves fibrinogen, which combines easily with circulating fibrin degradation products to form a soluble form of fibrin. At times this combination forms insoluble clots that deposit in the microvasculature of various organs. These fibrin thrombi are considered the hallmark of DIC. The lodged clots further trap circulating platelets, which results in the thrombocytopenia associated with DIC.[103] This entrapment of platelets impedes bloodflow, leading to tissue ischemia, hypoxia, and necrosis of multiple organs, along with consumption of clots and clotting factors.

The abnormal activation of thrombin also results in increased fibrinolysis. Thrombin not only acts to convert fibrinogen to fibrin, but also assists in the conversion of plasminogen to plasmin. Plasmin is responsible for the breakdown of fibrinogen and fibrin, which causes increased circulating fibrin degradation products that have strong anticoagulant properties. These then interfere with fibrin clot formation, as well as aiding in the consumption of clotting factors and platelets. The bleeding manifestations of DIC are caused by the combination of the consumption of platelets and certain clotting factors, plasmin's fibrinolytic properties, and the anticoagulant properties of the fibrin degradation products.

Manifestations DIC can present as a chronic coagulation disorder or an acute hemorrhagic diathesis, or it merely can be detected through various laboratory studies. Clinical symptoms may be similar to those of other thrombocytopenic conditions.

The patient generally is not critically ill from chronic DIC. It may produce minimal or no clinical manifestations. Easy and spontaneous bruisability may be present. Mild petechiae, ecchymosis, gingival bleeding, and minor gastrointestinal bleeding may be noted. Chronic DIC is more likely to cause thrombosis than bleeding. Laboratory tests may vary, but generally show minor coagulation abnormalities. Neurologic dysfunction occasionally can occur in chronic DIC as a result of small episodic cerebral bleeding. However, it is often mistaken for metabolic encephalopathy or metastasis.

Acute DIC (also called "uncompensated") occurs rapidly over hours to days. This condition rapidly depletes coagulation factors and inhibitors. Widespread thrombosis (purpura fulminans) and significant bleeding can occur. Overt hemorrhage involving multiple unrelated sites is not uncommon. The individual may display signs of shock and associated organ hypoxia.[104] Hemoptysis, intraperitoneal hemorrhage, and intracranial bleeding all may pose life-threatening situations for the patient with DIC.

There is no specific laboratory finding that is absolutely diagnostic of DIC. A battery of lab tests in conjunction with clinical evidence must be used to confirm the diagnosis, as well as to monitor response to treatment. A number of clinical conditions will affect these tests, which makes their interpretation difficult. For example, multiple blood product transfusions will dilute clotting factors or platelets, and liver disease with portal hypertension can lead to thrombocytopenia and the activation of the fibrinolytic system.

There is a classic triad of tests that is generally done to help support the diagnosis of DIC (see Table 25-5). They include the prothrombin time (PT), platelet count, and the plasma fibrinogen level. In DIC the PT is usually less than 15 seconds, which reflects decreased levels of clotting factors II and V and of fibrinogen. The platelet count drops below 150,000/mm^3. A low platelet count is considered a cardinal diagnostic finding in DIC. The count is below 50,000/mm^3 in about one-half of all cases of DIC.[100] In patients with acute leukemia and DIC, thrombocytopenia is more severe because of decreased thrombopoiesis. A low plasma fibrinogen level (150 mg/dl) results from the consumption of fibrinogen due to thrombin-induced clotting and from fibrinolysis in DIC. Other lab tests frequently used to detect DIC include FDP assays (increased in DIC), factor assays (decreased), partial thromboplastin time (PTT) (prolonged), antithrombin III assay (decreased), and protamine paracoagulant test (negative in DIC with severe hypofibrinogenemia). The diagnosis of chronic DIC is supported by the appearance of red cell fragments, called *schistocytes,* on peripheral blood smears. This is seen in all patients with chronic DIC, and in only 50% of patients with acute DIC. FDPs usually are elevated and induce platelet dysfunction.

TABLE 25-5 Clotting Studies of Disseminated Intravascular Coagulation

Test	Abnormality	Cause
Prothrombin time (PT)*	Prolonged	Elevated fibrin split products; decreased plasma clotting factor levels
Partial thromboplastin time (PTT)	Prolonged	Elevated fibrin split products; decreased plasma clotting factor levels
Platelet count*	Decreased	Platelet consumption
Plasma fibrinogen*	Low	Consumption of fibrinogen by the clotting cascade and by fibrinolysis
FDP assays	Increased	Fibrinogen destruction by plasmin
Factor assays	Decreased	Consumption of clotting factors
Antithrombin III assay	Decreased	Consumption of clotting factors
Protamine paracoagulant	Negative	Severe hypofibrinogenemia

*Classic triad of tests.

Management Treatment of the underlying malignancy is vital in treating the patient with a hypercoagulability abnormality, for the tumor is the ultimate stimulus. All other therapy, although effective on a short-term basis, will only provide an interval of symptomatic relief. Identification of and early treatment for other precipitating factors must also be done (e.g., sepsis, volume deficit, transfusion reactions).

Early detection of the signs and symptoms of DIC may allow for prompt diagnosis and treatment. Bleeding with resultant hemorrhage is the most common complication of DIC. It may be the first sign of underlying pathology.

Thrombus formation often occurs simultaneously with bleeding in DIC. Thrombi generally form in the superficial and smaller veins, and may be clinically undetectable. Subtle signs and symptoms of thrombi include red, indurated tender areas found in multiple organ sites. When thrombosis occurs, the signs and symptoms include: focal ischemia, acral cyanosis, superficial gangrene, altered sensorium, ulceration of the gastrointestinal tract, and dyspnea, which can lead to acute respiratory distress syndrome.

Heparin therapy for DIC associated with malignancy is controversial.[95,96,98,99,103,105] The controversy stems primarily from the lack of randomized trials of heparin therapy use in patients with DIC due to malignancy. There is also a controversy as to whether high-risk patients (e.g., a promyelocytic leukemia patient undergoing chemotherapy) should be treated prophylactically with heparin therapy.[98] The problem lies in the potential for unnecessarily exposing the patient to a risk of bleeding. Heparin therapy is used more frequently in the chronic DIC of malignancy associated with thrombotic, thromboembolic, or necrotizing complications.[95]

Heparin inhibits the formation of new clots by inhibiting factors IX and X, and may decrease the consumption of clotting factors. Heparin therapy for DIC generally is maintained until there is a disappearance of symptoms and a normalization of laboratory values. Large doses of heparin often are required to overcome intravascular clotting. A bolus of 10,000 U or more may be given, followed by a continuous IV infusion.[104] Heparin is given by continuous intravenous infusion to avoid peaks in drug effect caused by intermittent injections.

Another drug that may be used with DIC is epsilon-amino caproic acid (EACA, Amicar), a fibrinolytic inhibitor. The use of this drug in treatment of DIC is also controversial.[101] EACA can be used when the fibrinolysis of DIC has been resolved but uncontrolled bleeding persists. It is given to maintain platelet and fibrinogen levels, and only after intramuscular clotting has been brought under control, because it can lead to widespread fibrin deposition in the microcirculation and result in ischemic organ dysfunction.[106]

Once heparin therapy has begun, blood component therapy often is necessary, particularly in symptomatic, acute DIC. Platelets can be given if the platelet count drops below 30,000/mm^3. Packed red cells can be given if the patient is hemorrhaging. Fresh-frozen plasma also can be given for hemorrhage, since it contains all of the clotting factors, including antithrombin III. It can also be given for volume expansion. Albumin may be the component of choice for volume expansion for the reasons described previously. Specific coagulation factors may be given if laboratory data are able to identify the specific deficient factors. Antithrombin III is a coagulation factor that may be given to neutralize thrombin, plasmin, and activated forms of factors XII, XI, X, and VII. Cryoprecipitate (a concentrated source of fibrinogen and factor VIII) may be used to treat the hypofibrinogenemia that often occurs in DIC. Usually two to four bags per 10 kg are given initially, with each bag containing 10–12 ml of given factors. Depending on individual laboratory data, the patient may be given one or more bags per 15 kg of body weight per day.[91]

Prevention of further complications is another important goal in managing DIC. Any tight or restrictive clothing is removed if thrombophlebitis is suspected or apparent. If edema is present, it is measured daily. Elastic support stockings may help to minimize stasis and promote venous return. Other measures to decrease stasis and promote venous return include assisting the patient with leg lifts and/or elevating the legs to 15°–20° at intervals, and teaching the patient to wiggle his or her toes and perform ankle circles frequently while in bed. Compression to the knee vessels is minimized by avoiding placing anything under the knees while in bed (pillows, knee gatches), avoiding crossing of the knees or legs, and avoiding dangling the patient's legs over the side of the bed.

Patient education is a necessary component of care when a patient is at risk for DIC. Patients and families are taught to report any bleeding or unusual/abnormal symptoms. They are taught to save all excreta for the nurse to examine for blood. Finally, the patient and family will need excellent psychosocial support should the patient develop the paradoxical hemorrhage and thrombus formation of DIC.

PATIENT ASSESSMENT

Patient assessment begins with a thorough history and physical examination. Either component of the assessment may be comprehensive, when interviewing a patient suspected of having a malignancy, or cursory, when caring for an individual with acute blood loss due to the malignancy. The information gathered in the assessment is instrumental in preparing an appropriate plan of care for the patient.

Patient/Family History

The patient/family history is a vital component of the complete assessment. Because bleeding is a common problem in many malignancies, one must remain alert to findings that suggest hemostatic disorders. Patients may respond more openly and with greater ease if questions are focused toward activities of daily living, e.g., excessive bleeding while shaving, or prolonged bleeding after minor cuts and scrapes while cooking or cleaning. Key aspects of a comprehensive history for a patient at risk for bleeding include:

1. bleeding tendencies, including easy bruising, excessive nosebleeds, gingival bleeding, presence of petechiae, change in color of stools or urine, stomach discomfort, vision problems, and painful joints
2. family history of any bleeding abnormalities
3. drugs and chemicals taken that might interfere with the coagulation mechanism or that might uncover an important symptom for which the person is taking medication
4. general performance status that helps to identify the effects of the disease or the presence of complications
5. current blood component therapy, including reason for and response to therapy
6. nutritional status, to identify vitamin K or C deficiency or generalized malnutrition that will affect the person's hematologic system
7. presence of any signs/symptoms of anemia, which may signify undetected long-term bleeding.

Physical Examination

Observation is perhaps the most important measure in early detection of bleeding. Diagnostic signals can be subtle, including skin petechiae noticed while bathing the person, traces of blood as the person brushes her or his teeth, and oozing from venipuncture sites or sites of injections. These are examples of the types of information that can lead to early diagnosis of hemostatic problems, and might prevent an incident of spontaneous hemorrhage.

The major problem associated with active bleeding is hemorrhage. Although bleeding can occur from any part of the body, common sites of hemorrhage include the gums, nose, bladder, gastrointestinal tract, and brain. An examination of all body systems is done on a routine basis for any patient known to have a bleeding disorder (Table 25-6).

TABLE 25-6 Physical Examination of the Client with Actual or Potential Bleeding

Integumentary system (assess entire skin surface, including intertrigonous areas) Bruising, petechiae, purpura, ecchymoses, acrocyanosis (irregularly shaped cyanotic patches on the periphery of arms and legs associated with bleeding due to DIC); oozing from venipuncture sites or injections, biopsy sites, central lines, catheters, or nasogastric tubes
Eyes* and ears Visual disturbances, increased injection on the sclera, periorbital edema, subconjunctival hemorrhage (homogeneous red color that is sharply outlined on the sclera), headache, ear pain
Nose, mouth, and throat Petechiae on nasal/oral mucosa, epistaxis, tenderness or bleeding from gums or oral mucosa
Cardiopulmonary system Crackles, wheezes, stridor, dyspnea, tachypnea, cyanosis, and hemoptysis (all possible signs of bleeding in the lungs); vital sign changes, color and temperature of all extremities, peripheral pulses
Gastrointestinal system† Pain, bleeding, blood around rectum, tarry stools, frank or occult blood in stools, hemoptysis
Genitourinary system Bleeding, character and amount of menses, monitor intake and output (if urine drops below 30 ml/hr it may be due to acute tubular necrosis secondary to thrombi, bleeding, or hypovolemia)
Musculoskeletal system Check for complaint of painful joints while performing active or passive range of motion, which may indicate bleeding into the joints
Central nervous system Mental status changes, including restlessness, confusion, lethargy, dizziness, obtundation, seizures, or coma (may indicate intracranial hemorrhage or impaired tissue perfusion)

*Bleeding in the optic fundus could lead to permanent visual impairment.

†Guiac all excreta for blood.

Screening Tests

There are several screening tests that provide information regarding hemostatic function. These groups of tests give information about both phases of hemostasis and fibrinolysis. The hematologic alterations leading to bleeding are complex, and test results will vary depending on the degree of original coagulation dysfunction and the cascading effect of related hemostatic mechanisms. A brief discussion regarding some of the most common screening tests of hemostatic function follows. A more comprehensive list is given in Table 25-7.

Bleeding time

This test measures the time it takes for a small skin incision to stop bleeding. The results of the test depend on the platelet number and function and the ability of the capillary wall to constrict. The time varies from 1–9 minutes. The bleeding time is prolonged when there is a lack of platelets or in diseases affecting the blood vessel walls. Examples of disease states in which a prolonged bleeding time may be found include thrombocytopenia, von Willebrand's disease, infiltration of the marrow by tumor, and consumption of platelets in disseminated intravascular coagulation. Prolonged bleeding time is also found with drugs affecting platelet function, such as aspirin.

TABLE 25-7 Tests of Hemostasis

Test	Measures	Normal Value
	PLATELET FUNCTION	
Bleeding time	Platelet plug formation; response of small vessels	1–9 min
Platelet count	Number of circulating platelets	150,000–400,000/mm³
Clot retraction	Ability of platelets to support retraction of a clot	50% retraction within 1 hr; compare with normal value
Platelet aggregation	Ability of platelets to aggregate	Compare with normal control
Platelet phospholipid (factor 3) availability	Availability of platelet factor 3 for coagulation	Compare with normal control
	COAGULATION	
Partial thromboplastin time (PTT)	Intrinsic and common pathways	Varies; compare with normal control (usually 30–40 sec)
Prothrombin time (PT)	Extrinsic and common pathways	Varies; compare with normal control
Thrombin time	Fibrinogen concentration; structure of fibrinogen; presence of inhibitors	Varies; compare with normal value
Specific factor assays	Concentration of functional factor in plasma	50%–150% activity in pooled normal plasma
	FIBRINOLYSIS	
Assay of fibrinogen or fibrin degradation products (FDP)	Presence of FDP in serum	1:8; 10 mg/ml 1:4; 0–8 mg/ml 10 mg/ml

Platelet count

This test measures the actual number of circulating platelets per cubic millimeter of blood. Normal counts are considered to be 150,000–400,000/mm³. Counts below 100,000/mm³ are considered indicative of thrombocytopenia. Spontaneous hemorrhage generally is not a concern until the platelet count drops below 15,000/mm³. Thrombocytosis occurs when the count rises above 400,000/mm³.

Whole blood clot retraction test

This test measures the speed and extent of blood clot retraction in a test tube. The test is done to determine the degree of platelet adequacy. A normal clot shrinks to one-half its normal size in 1–2 hours and shrinks completely in 24 hours. Clot retraction is slower and will stay soft and watery with thrombocytopenia or with abnormally functioning platelets.

Prothrombin time (PT)

In this test tissue thromboplastin and ionized calcium are added to citrated plasma, and the time required for clotting is recorded. The test is measured against the time needed for a normal sample of blood to clot. PT is a measure of the factors involved in the extrinsic and common pathways in the clotting mechanism. Test results usually are given as the actual time, in seconds, and also are compared with a normal or control value. When the clotting factors exist in diminished quality, PT is prolonged. Prolonged PT values also are seen in liver disease (hepatitis and tumor involvement), in obstructive biliary disease (e.g., bile duct obstruction secondary to tumor), and with coumarin ingestion.[107]

Partial thromboplastin time (activated) (aPTT)

The aPTT is determined by adding phospholipid reagents to plasma in the presence of calcium chloride. The test is a sensitive measure of the intrinsic and common pathways of the clotting mechanism. Normal aPTT is 30–40 seconds. A prolonged aPTT is evidenced when any of the factors exist in inadequate quantities, as with consumptive coagulopathy, liver disease, and biliary obstruction, and as with circulating anticoagulants such as heparin.[108]

The PT and PTT taken together can give a fair indication of the nature of the clotting defect. If both the PT and PTT are normal, the vessels or platelets are probably defective. The defect is likely to be in the clotting mechanism if either the PT or PTT is prolonged. If both are prolonged, the defect is most likely in the common pathway.

Fibrin degradation products (FDP) test

This test is determined by adding peripheral venous blood to serum containing antifibrinogen degradation fragments. The measurement of FDPs provides an indication of the activity of the fibrinolytic system. Agglutination is demonstrated if the patient's blood contains the degradation fragments. FDP levels greater than 10 mg/ml indicate increased fibrinolysis, as seen in DIC and primary fibrinolytic disorders. No agglutination occurs if degradation products are absent in the patient's blood.

GENERAL NURSING CONSIDERATIONS FOR THE PERSON EXPERIENCING BLEEDING

The physical safety of the patient is always ensured to prevent trauma in individuals with diminished thrombocytic activity. Potential threats of injury in the environment are identified and then reduced or eliminated. Bumps or falls can be dangerous or even fatal in the individual with a low platelet count.

Diligent measures to maintain skin integrity are instituted. Electric razors are used to prevent cuts while shaving. The mouth and gums are easily damaged when the platelet count drops, and become an excellent potential source of infection. A systematic mouth care regimen should be used to minimize this problem. Soft-bristled toothbrushes help to avoid trauma to sensitive gums. When the platelet count drops below 20,000–30,000/mm^3, bristled toothbrushes are avoided and mouth swabs or toothettes are used. A nonirritating (alcohol-free) mouthwash is recommended. When the mouth and gums are irritated, dentures should not be replaced, particularly if they are ill-fitting. Patients requiring oxygen therapy via nasal cannula or endotracheal tube are assessed for irritation to the mucosa.

All unnecessary procedures are avoided, including intramuscular or subcutaneous injections, rectal temperatures or suppositories, and indwelling catheters. If the patient requires parenteral administration of medication, the intravenous route is used whenever possible. Intramuscular and subcutaneous injections place the patient at risk for the development of hematomas. Hematomas can become sites of infection when granulocytopenia is present. Injections, if unavoidable, are administered with the smallest possible gauge of needle. Pressure to the injection site is applied for several minutes, followed by the application of a pressure bandage to avoid hematomas. Similar care is taken at venipuncture sites.

Severe uterine hemorrhage can be a complication in thrombocytopenic women who are menstruating. Menses can be suppressed by pharmacologic agents, generally, progestational medications. In women whose menses are not suppressed, yet who have menstrual bleeding, careful napkin counts are done to help determine the volume of blood loss.

Forceful coughing, sneezing, or nose blowing can lead to bleeding. Epistaxis can be life-threatening in an individual with thrombocytopenia. The patient with epistaxis is placed in high Fowler's position. Ice packs, nasal packing, or topical adrenaline may also be used to decrease bleeding caused by small-vessel constriction within the nasal mucosa. Bowel strain caused by constipation can initiate rectal bleeding. Prescribed stool softeners may be necessary to avoid constipation. Instruction regarding proper diet and exercise to avoid constipation are also appropriate.

Hygiene is a problem in the patient who has active bleeding. The bleeding patient may require frequent baths and linen changes in order to feel and smell better. A room deodorizer may be needed, since blood exposed to air is malodorous.

Physical and emotional rest are essential when the patient is actively bleeding. Rest helps to decrease pulse rate and blood pressure, allowing for clot formation. A state of active bleeding is frightening and anxiety producing for the patient and family. A calm approach and reassurance are in order in managing a patient who is actively bleeding. Sedation can also be used to decrease anxiety and metabolic rate.

BLOOD COMPONENT THERAPY

Blood banking in the United States is a standardized industry heavily regulated by the federal government and some states. The blood banking industry is regulated by the federal government under Title 21 of the Code of Regulations. These regulations place stringent requirements on collection, testing, storage, and distribution of blood and blood components.[109]

The technological advances in blood transfusion therapy, which allows for aggressive transfusion support for patients with cancer who receive highly toxic treatment regimens, have led to a decrease in the morbidity and mortality of cancer and its treatment. Except in situations of extreme emergency, transfusion therapy is provided to correct deficiencies in a specific component of whole blood. Less than 10% of all necessary transfusions require whole blood.[110] Whole blood is removed from a donor and is then "fractionated" into the various components, i.e., red blood cells, platelets, plasma, and plasma proteins. This fractionation process is accomplished via refrigerated centrifugation or automated equipment using continuous-flow cell separations.

The entire collection system is sterile, disposable, and never reused. It is therefore impossible for a donor to contract a transfusion-transmitted disease. The collection system is considered a closed system, being open only at the tip of the needle.

Red Blood Cell Therapy

In any patient, the clinical concern for the adverse physiologic effects of anemia is usually the basis for considering red blood cell replacement. The decision to transfuse generally is based on an overall clinical picture, including any underlying cardiac or pulmonary condition or any concurrent conditions that might impair the patient's tolerance for anemia.[111] Among the causes of anemia frequently seen in cancer patients, the two most common include decreased red cell production secondary to myelosuppressive therapy and the primary disease process.

An attempt generally is made to keep a patient's hemoglobin level higher than 8 g/100 ml. It is customary in most centers to delay transfusions until the hemoglobin is lower than 8 g/100 ml or until the patient is symptomatic. A patient is transfused with a sufficient quantity of red cells to raise the hemoglobin level to at least 10 or 11 g/100 ml, and to even higher levels if the patient has a concomitant infection.[112] Physiologic signs of anemia (hyperventilation, rapid pulse, shortness of breath on exertion, rapid pulse, pallor, fatigue) should be relieved when the hemoglobin is raised to 10 or 11 g/100 ml.[72] If the patient is not actively bleeding, 1 unit of packed red cells should increase the peripheral hematocrit level by 3% and the hemoglobin by 1 g/dl.[113]

Packed erythrocytes usually are the therapy of choice. The advantage of packed red blood cells is that they provide more than 70% of the hematocrit of whole blood with only one-third of the plasma. This prevents unnecessary volume, electrolyte load, and anticoagulants that may otherwise be transfused. Leukocytes in red blood cell transfusions can cause reactions if the recipient has antileukocyte antibodies, which occurs in patients treated with multiple transfusions. Transfusion of packed red cells in these patients can cause fever and chills. The patient can become alloimmunized, or refractory to transfusions. This condition is demonstrated when a transfusion of a unit of red cells fails to achieve an expected increase in the hemoglobin level. The use of leukocyte-poor blood component therapy is indicated for these patients. Another major indication for leukocyte-poor blood products is with patients who have had prior febrile nonhemolytic transfusion reactions, or allergic reactions to packed erythrocytes.

Packed red blood cells are stored at 4°–6°C for a shelf life of 35 days. The shelf life can be extended to 42 days with the addition of certain solutions. The unit may also be frozen for storage for 7–10 years.[114]

Platelet Therapy

The use of platelet transfusions has proven to have tremendous therapeutic value in controlling and preventing hemorrhage in individuals with cancer. Generally the decision to transfuse is indicated when there is actual bleeding associated with thrombocytopenia, when the platelet count is greater than 20,000/mm^3 yet bleeding is present, and in patients with abnormally functioning platelets who are bleeding. Prophylactic platelet transfusions can be given in the absence of clinical hemorrhage but during periods of intense chemotherapy, to prevent spontaneous hemorrhage into the brain. Other factors that determine appropriateness of transfusion therapy are determined on an individual basis. The presence of infection and a rapid decrease in circulating platelets are factors that may suggest a decreased tolerance to thrombocytopenia.

Theoretically, one unit of platelets should increase the recipient's peripheral blood platelet level by 10,000–12,000 cells/mm^3. Traditionally, the attempt is made to maintain the patient's platelet count greater than 20,000/mm^3 to minimize the potential for spontaneous hemorrhage. More recent experience indicates that platelet counts in the range of 10,000–20,000/mm^3 can be monitored safely without the use of prophylactic transfusions.[115] Close observation of these patients to detect bleeding is essential.[116] In the absence of normal platelet production, platelet transfusions generally are required every 3 days. Concomitant infection, with fever, or active bleeding will increase platelet transfusion requirements.

Platelets can be given in fresh whole blood, platelet-rich plasma, or platelet concentrates (see Table 25-8). The concentrated method is the one most widely used today. As stated earlier, the use of fresh whole blood generally is used only in emergency situations in which there is severe and rapid hemorrhage. Platelet concentrates can be obtained from one donor and suspended in minimal plasma, by plateletpheresis techniques of closed-bag collection systems or by a blood cell separator. A donor can be pheresed frequently (up to every other day), if the donor's platelets provide the patient with good platelet count increases. One unit of platelets is routinely obtained from 500 ml of fresh whole blood.

Platelet survival

Several factors have been identified as important in determining posttransfusion platelet survival in an individual. Failure to achieve adequate increments in the circulating platelet count is often due to infection, fever, disseminated intravascular coagulation, or splenomegaly. Infection can enhance the consumption of platelets and increase the occurrence of hemorrhage. Patients with fever or sepsis require frequent transfusions to maintain an adequate platelet count. Patients with splenomegaly who are receiving platelet transfusions will have a reduced recovery of circulating platelets generally proportionate to the size of their spleen.[117] If platelets are being transfused while the person is actively bleeding, increased increments will not be detected by laboratory data. However, their effectiveness can be measured by clinical improvement and control of bleeding.

TABLE 25-8 Platelet Transfusion Therapy

Specific Component	Content and Volume	General Indications	Complications	Nursing Considerations
Random donor (RD) • Fresh—best • Frozen and cryopreserved (limited application because of poor recovery)	• Multiple donors (4+) approximately 200 ml • Plasma, WBCs, few RBCs	• Bleeding and bleeding prophylaxis • Platelet count <20,000/mm³	• Exposure of patients to multiple tissue antigens, which initiates antigen-antibody formation leading to refractoriness • Hepatitis (increased risk with pooled products) • Allergic reactions may be seen more often if leukocyte-poor-blood filter not used	• Gently agitate bag occasionally to prevent platelet clumping. • Rapid infusion (per patient tolerance). • Tubing should include a 170–220 micron in-line blood filter. Loukocyte-poor-blood filter may be required.
Single donor (SD) • Fresh (maximum effectiveness up to 6 hr)	• One donor • 1 unit—300 ml • Plasma, WBCs, RBCs	• Bleeding and bleeding prophylaxis • Severe febrile reactions • Often used once a patient is refractory to random donor platelets • Patients who require long-term platelet therapy	• Refractoriness to platelet may occur over time	• Rapid infusion (generally 30 min+). • Tubing as for RD. Leukocyte-poor-blood filter may be required.
Human-leukocyte-antigen (HLA) matched concentrate	• One donor compatible at the HLA complex • 1 unit—300 ml • Plasma, WBCs, RBCs	• When patients become refractory to RD and SD platelets	• Minimal	• HLA-matched platelets minimize patient exposure to multiple tissue antigens (HLA complex found on all blood cells—acts as a genetic monogram). • Rapid infusion (30 min+). • Tubing as for RD. Generally see more effective increases in the platelet count than with RD or SD.

Patients with fever due to infection can be premedicated with antipyretics prior to platelet transfusion, in an attempt to minimize platelet destruction. When a fever is caused by the platelet transfusion, i.e., febrile reaction to the transfusion, premedication can consist of antipyretics, corticosteroids, and/or antihistamines. Demerol may be given if the patient is having shaking chills. Certain antimicrobial drugs occasionally have also been found to cause platelet refractoriness, due to drug-induced antibodies. Drug-induced antibodies have been demonstrated against cotrimoxazole, amphotericin-B, and certain semisynthetic penicillins.[118]

Platelet survival is greatly decreased when alloimmunization to the platelet transfusion develops. Because of repeated exposure of patient/recipient platelets to the HLA antigens on the donor's platelets, patients eventually may become refractory to random donor platelets. The patient will require HLA-matched or leukocyte-poor transfusions to sustain an adequate platelet count and prevent bleeding (see Table 25-8).

Platelet increments may be negatively affected by leukoagglutinin reactions directed at non-HLA leukocyte antigens. In this situation donor platelets are contaminated with granulocytes.[72] Once transfused there is subsequent antibody formation, causing allergic symptoms. Symptoms include hives, skin flush, fever, and chills. These reactions can be avoided by leukocyte depletion from the platelet concentrate during preparation. The leukocyte-depletion process requires fresh platelets.[118] Patients can also be premedicated with antipyretics, coricosteroids, and antihistamines to minimize this reaction.

The preparation and storage of platelets are also important factors in determining the quality of the platelet transfusion. Platelets must be fresh and metabolically active to be most effective. Maximum effectiveness remains for up to 6 hours after being obtained. Storage longer than 24 hours at 22°C causes significant loss of platelet function due to release of ADP and alterations of platelet membrane permeability. Platelets can, however, be stored for up to 5 days. Platelets should be agitated gently during storage.

One therapy currently being investigated for the support of individuals refractory to all types of available transfusions is the use of intravenous gammaglobulin (IVIgG). Its use may inhibit the binding of alloantibodies to platelets, then delay their removal from the circulation.[119] Studies of this therapy report mixed results. Some studies report improvement of response to certain single-donor platelets and not to multiple-donor platelets.[119] Other studies report an improvement of response to multiple-donor platelets.[119–121] This therapy is expensive, but may be justified in the refractory patient with uncontrolled bleeding. The cost of administering an adequate dose of 2g/kg to a 70-kg adult is approximately $5000.[30]

Plasma Therapy

Plasma, like the other blood components, can be separated from whole blood via centrifugation. As blood is withdrawn from a donor, the red blood cells are packed by centrifugation, leaving about 70% of the platelets suspended in plasma. This platelet-rich plasma is then spun again to yield a platelet concentrate in approximately 50 ml of plasma. The remaining plasma is then removed and rapidly frozen at less than 18°C. The frozen plasma is called *fresh-frozen plasma* and contains all of the labile clotting factors and the plasma proteins. The plasma proteins can be isolated and removed from plasma, such as albumin and cryoprecipitate. Plasma and other blood components can also be obtained via apheresis.

The most common use of plasma and plasma components in cancer is with coagulation disorders associated with this disease. Plasma component therapy is also administered for severe bleeding, shock, and bleeding associated with infections.

A number of variables are used to determine the optimal dosage of plasma and plasma components as replacement therapy in coagulation disorders. The primary considerations include: severity of the deficiency, specific factor deficiency, severity of bleeding, possible danger of bleeding to the patient, and duration of therapy.[91] Replacement plasma usually is calculated in units, 1 unit of plasma equaling the activity present in 1 ml of normal human male plasma.

Another consideration in plasma therapy is the metabolic half-life of plasma and plasma derivatives. Replacement therapy is given in doses high enough to compensate for the decrease in the plasma level as it is metabolized.[89] The metabolic half-life varies for each of the factors. Plasma and plasma factors usually are infused rapidly, so the maximum plasma level is reached before metabolic changes or degradation occurs. Plasma component therapy is always given intravenously. (See Table 25-9 for further discussion of plasma therapy.)

Transfusion Complications

There are many hazards associated with the administration of blood component therapy. These hazards may cause immediate or delayed reactions. The major hazards include hemolytic and nonhemolytic transfusion reactions, transmission of diseases, and complications associated with intravenous therapy and transfusions. (See Table 25-10 for a complete list of transfusion reactions and Table 25-11 for the nursing management of transfusion reactions.)

Platelets generally can be transfused across incompatibilities of the major red blood cell antigens (ABO) unless there is gross red blood cell contamination into the transfusion pack. If significant spillage has occurred, the donor and recipient are matched by A,B,O antigens. If matching is not done when spillage occurs, hemolytic reactions are likely.[72]

Serious transfusion complications in patients who are significantly immunosuppressed (e.g., bone marrow transplant patients or leukemia patients undergoing induction chemotherapy) include the risk of developing graft-versus-host (GVH) disease and the rare transfusion-related acute lung injury (TRALI).[122] These complications can occur following the transfusion of blood products containing viable lymphocytes. The donor-competent T-lymphocyte immunologically attacks the immunocompromised host tissue after transfusion. This disease generally is manifested in the skin, liver, and gastrointestinal tract and can be fatal.[123]

It generally is recommended that all blood products given to the severely immunocompromised host be exposed to pretransfusion irradiation with 1500–3000 rads.[124] Irradiation of blood is done to inhibit proliferation of lymphocytes without impairment of platelets, red cells, or granulocytes.[98] Leukocyte-poor-blood filters, which are capable of removing nearly all leukocytes, can serve as an alternate approach to preventing GVH disease.[125]

TABLE 25-9 Commonly Used Plasma Components

Component	Content Volume and Route	Shelf Life	Indications	Complications	Nursing Considerations
Normal human plasma (fresh or frozen)	Plasma; all plasma proteins and clotting factors; 200 ml, IV route	1 yr frozen; 24 hr thawed	Blood loss; clotting factor deficiency; plasma volume expander without increasing the hematocrit	Volume overload; hepatitis and other infections; hypernatremia, hypocalcemia	Requires ABO compatibility; administer fresh-frozen plasma immediately after thawing to minimize deterioration of factors V and VIII; infusion should be slowed or stopped if patient demonstrates signs of citrate toxicity
Normal human serum albumin	Aqueous fraction of pooled plasma 5%: 250 ml and 500 ml; 25%: 25 ml and 50 ml, IV route	3–5 yr	Rapid volume expansion	No hepatitis risk	Monitor cardiac and renal function closely, for congestive heart failure may be precipitated by compromised function; each unit must be used immediately after opening since albumin contains no preservatives; rate of administration of 5% solution should not be >2–4 ml/min; rate of administration of 25% solution should not be >1 ml/min
Cryoprecipitate	Fibrinogen, factors VIII and XIII, von Willebrand factor, fibronectin; 10–20 ml, IV route	1 yr frozen; 6 hr thawed	Severe von Willebrand's disease; hypofibrinogenemia (DIC)	Hepatitis and other infections	Best to be ABO compatible; should be kept at room temperature until infused; administer within 3 min
Fibrinogen	Fibrinogen; 10 ml, IV route	1 yr frozen	Clotting disorders; hemophilia A or B		Monitor cardiac and renal function closely; administer rapidly; 1 U should raise level 10 U
Purified AHF concentrate	Factor VIII (lyophilized); IV route	Per pharmacy label	Severe von Willebrand's disease	High hepatitis risk (non-A, non-B)	Rate of administration is 2 ml/min, can be up to 10 ml/min; if patient's pulse increases significantly, rate of administration should be decreased
Heat-treated lyophilized prothrombin complex	Prothrombin factors VII, IX, X; IV route	Per pharmacy label	Bleeding disorders; hemophilia B; factor VIII inhibitor	High hepatitis risk (non-A, non-B); thrombosis	Monitor patient for signs/symptoms of thrombosis

Source: Gobel BH: Plasma and plasma derivative therapy for coagulation disorders. *Semin Oncol Nurs* 6:129–135, 1990. Reprinted with permission.

Leukocyte-Depleted Blood Products

Leukocytes remaining in donor blood collected for transfusion are responsible for many of the complications related to transfusion therapy, including immunologic effects and transmission of viral infections.[126–128] (see Table 25-12). The removal of leukocytes, more specifically the microaggregates of leukocytes that form in a spontaneous and progressive manner in stored blood products, is done extensively to prevent febrile nonhemolytic reactions as well as to prevent other complications.[125] It has been demonstrated that the likelihood of adverse reactions to blood component therapy is correlated with the absolute number of leukocytes transfused.[129]

The removal of leukocytes from stored blood products by conventional filtration methods generally can decrease the number of these cells to a point below the threshold for febrile reactions in a sensitized patient. (The pore size of a standard blood administration set in-line filter is 170 μm, and effectively removes gross fibrin clots.) The number of remaining leukocytes, however, may be sufficient to enhance or cause alloimmunization to blood products.[125] The remaining leukocytes are known to transmit viral infections as well. Some transfusion-induced infections are caused exclusively by white blood cells. Cytomegalovirus (CMV) can be eliminated by decreasing the number of white cells in the transfusion pack.[130] The need to decrease the number of transfused leukocytes to the lowest possible level continues to be investigated.

TABLE 25-10 Complications of Transfusions

Immediate
Febrile reactions, chills
Allergy—urticaria, anaphylaxis
Major hemolytic transfusion reaction
Bacterial contamination—shock, sepsis
Circulatory overload
Air embolism
Citrate toxicity
Hypocalcemia
Hyperkalemia
Hypothermia
Iron overload
Delayed
Delayed hemolytic transfusion reaction
Infection—hepatitis, retrovirus, cytomegalovirus, other
Graft-vs-host disease
Posttransfusion purpura
Alloimmunization

In addition to the traditional methods of leukocyte depletion of blood products (sedimentation, centrifugation, cell washing, and freeze-thaw deglycerolization), two methods of leukocyte depletion that currently are being extensively investigated include laboratory filtration and bedside filtration of blood components. The filters trap leukocytes by selective adsorption, with the most efficient medium being a nonwoven fiber mesh with a diameter less than 3 μm.[131] Most laboratory filters are capable of depleting 99% of the leukocytes present in a unit of blood, whereas the bedside filters deplete 99.9% (3 log) of the white blood cells.[132] Bedside filters require no special processing of the unit of blood and are not influenced by the age of the blood.[133] Currently, the leukocyte-depleting filters available for use in the United States are the Pall RC-100 (Glen Cover, NY) for red cells, the Pall PL for platelets, and the Sepacell (Asahi Medical Co., Ltd, Tokyo, Japan).

TABLE 25-11 Nursing Management of Transfusion Reactions

Type	Signs/Symptoms	Nursing Actions
Acute hemolytic	Fever, chills, decreased blood pressure, increased pulse rate, nausea/vomiting, flushing, back pain, decreased urine output, hematuria, dyspnea, anaphylaxis	1. Stop transfusion. 2. Maintain patent IV line. 3. Place in supine position. 4. Maintain open airway; provide CPR if necessary. 5. Obtain vital signs, and record. 6. Notify physician. 7. Monitor intake and output. 8. Administer fluids and medications per physician order. 9. Monitor vital signs. 10. Obtain blood and urine specimens. 11. Notify blood bank, and return remainder of blood to blood bank. 12. Document event. 13. Admit patient to hospital if outpatient.
Febrile nonhemolytic	Fever ± chills, headache, decreased blood pressure, increased pulse rate, dyspnea, chest pain, nausea/vomiting	1. Stop transfusion. 2. Maintain patent IV line. 3. Obtain and monitor vital signs, and record. 4. Assist in ruling out infection. 5. Notify physician. 6. Administer medications and fluids per physician order: acetominophen for fever, meperidine for chills, antihistamine for dyspnea. 7. Continue transfusion if symptoms not severe. 8. Notify blood bank. 9. Document event.
Allergic	Urticaria	1. Obtain and monitor vital signs, and record. 2. Slow transfusion rate. 3. Notify physician. 4. Administer medications per physician order: antihistamines. 5. Notify blood bank. 6. Document event.
Delayed hemolytic	Delayed (7–10 days to weeks) decreased hemoglobin, low-grade fever	Notify blood bank.

TABLE 25-12 Immunologic and Infectious Complications of Blood Transfusion Attributed to the Infusion of Donor Leukocytes

Immunologic consequences
Alloimmunization to human leukocyte antigens
Febrile transfusion reactions due to granulocytes
Transient immunosuppression/immune tolerance
Graft-versus-host reaction/disease
Transfusion-related acute lung injury (TRALI)
Transmission of blood-borne viruses (BBV)
Cytomegalovirus (CMV)
Human immunodeficiency viruses (HIV-1/2)
Human T-cell lymphotrophic viruses (HTLV-IIII)
Hepatitis B virus (HBV)
Human herpesvirus type 6 (HSV-6)
Epstein-Barr virus (EBV)

Source: Rawal BD, Davis E, Busch MP, et al: Dual reduction in the immunologic and infectious complications of transfusion by filtration/removal of leukocytes from donor blood soon after collection. *Trans Med Rev* 4:36–41, 1990. Reprinted with permission.

Home Transfusion Therapy for the Cancer Patient

There are a number of benefits to home transfusion therapy for the cancer patient. These include decreased cost (compared to receiving transfusions in the hospital), convenience for the patient and family of being able to stay home for needed blood components, psychological benefits, and the ability to be treated in a familiar environment with family available.[134,135] There are no legal constraints against transfusing patients at home, as long as the procedure is performed by licensed and qualified medical personnel.[136] However, regardless of precautions taken, the patient is at greater risk for complications than would be the case in a hospital setting (lack of sophisticated emergency equipment). Thus patients must be selected for home transfusion using appropriate criteria, and medical personnel administering the blood must be trained properly. The recommendations made follow those for out-of-hospital transfusion of the Transfusion Practices Committee of the American Association of Blood Banks.[137,138]

Selection criteria

The seven basic criteria for inclusion in a home transfusion therapy program include:[134]

1. physical limitations of the patient that make transportation difficult
2. stable cardiopulmonary status
3. absence of reactions to the most recent transfusion
4. a cooperative patient
5. presence of a responsible adult during and after transfusion
6. a telephone available for medical needs or need to call an ambulance
7. a diagnosis supporting the need for transfusion therapy

The person administering the transfusion should be a registered nurse with current venipuncture and intravenous therapy skills. The nurse should have completed a competency-based education program on transfusion therapy. Finally, the nurse should have supervision of her transfusion therapy skills prior to transfusing a patient in the home independently.

Preadministration considerations

Once the patient has been accepted as a candidate for home transfusion therapy, a number of appointments must be made and documents established. Appointments are made with the patient for pretransfusion blood samples and for the transfusions. Ideally, the pretransfusion blood sample collection is done the day before the scheduled transfusion, and by the nurse who will administer the blood. The samples are placed in an insulated container with appropriate request forms and are returned to the blood bank for processing. Once the informed consent has been signed by the patient, a means of identification is placed on the patient and must remain in place until after the transfusion. It is recommended that a commercial wrist band system that uses preprinted numbers be used, to increase patient safety.[139] Documentation records are established for each new patient, and include physician's written orders for the blood transfusion, a signed informed consent, laboratory results, nursing progress records, and a "Home Transfusion Flow Sheet." This form provides for complete documentation of the blood transfusion process (see Figure 25-4). Much of the information on the flow sheet can be filled out prior to the administration: patient's name and address, physician's name and phone number, and emergency information. All of this information needs to be verified on the day of the transfusion.

Administration considerations

Nurses who administer blood in the home setting take on a great deal of responsibility. Institutional policies and procedures must be adhered to closely in order to maximize patient safety. The home transfusion protocol outlined in Table 25-13 covers general administration considerations.

Posttransfusion considerations

Once the transfusion is complete, the nurse will discontinue the transfusion bag, yet maintain a patent IV line. The nurse remains with the patient for at least 30 minutes posttransfusion to observe the patient and to monitor vital signs. If the patient is stable at this time, the IV can be discontinued. All transfusion supplies are collected in a biohazard bag for disposal. If ordered, a

Date of transfusion: ______

Patient's name: ______ Patient's I. D. #: ______

Patient's address: ______

Patient's diagnosis: ______

Patient's blood type: ABO ______ Rh ______ CMV Neg. ______ CMV Pos. ______

Physcian's name: ______ Physician's phone #: ______

Order verified: ______ (Initials)

Name and location of emergency treatment facility: ______

Name and phone # of emergency/ambulance service: ______

Patient identity verified: Yes ______ No ______

Unique identifying number of the blood bag same as cross-matched unit recorded: Yes ______ No ______

Cross-matched units compatible: Yes ______ No ______

Parient's name and I.D. number on cross-match record verified with patient identification: Yes ______ No ______

Allergies: ______

Current Medications: ______

IV solution: ______

Time started: ______ By: ______ (Initials)
Amount infused: ______
Site of Infusion: ______
Device (type and gauge): ______

Premedications:

Acetaminophen ______ (dosage, route, time–initials)
Benadryl ______
Other ______

Filter type:

In-line ______ Leukocyte-poor ______

Restrictions:

Irradiation of products ______ Other ______

Blood component	Whole Blood #/ Pool #	Time Started	Time Complete	Volume Infused
Single-donor platelets ______	______	______	______	______
Random-donor platelets ______	______	______	______	______
HLA-matched platelets ______	______	______	______	______
Red blood cells ______	______	______	______	______
Whole blood ______	______	______	______	______

FIGURE 25-4 Home transfusion flow sheet. (Source: Adapted with the permission of The American Association of Blood Banks from Rutman et al.[137])

(continued)

Nurses notes:	Time	BP	T	P	R	Lung Sounds (when indicated)
Baseline	_____	_____	_____	_____	_____	__________
15 min	_____	_____	_____	_____	_____	__________
30 min	_____	_____	_____	_____	_____	__________
1 hr	_____	_____	_____	_____	_____	__________
1-1/2 hr	_____	_____	_____	_____	_____	__________
2 hr	_____	_____	_____	_____	_____	__________
2-1/2 hr	_____	_____	_____	_____	_____	__________
3 hr	_____	_____	_____	_____	_____	__________
3-1/2 hr	_____	_____	_____	_____	_____	__________
4 hr	_____	_____	_____	_____	_____	__________
Final	_____	_____	_____	_____	_____	__________

Suspected reaction: Yes _____ No _____

Symptoms: ______________________________

Amount infused: ______________________________

If yes, collect the following: Blood Sample __________ Urine Sample __________

Physician notified __________ (Initials)

* Return any blood bag to the blood bank when there is a suspicion of a blood transfusion reaction.

I have checked all information and find it to be correct. ______________________________
Signature

FIGURE 25-4 Home transfusion flow sheet (continued)

TABLE 25-13 Home Transfusion Protocol

Nursing Actions	Rationale
1. Gather supplies: • IV pole and pump (if required) • Blood filter (if required) • Saline • Appropriate blood tubing • Blood filters per institutional policies and procedures • Needles and syringes appropriate for type of vascular access device to be used • Transfusion flow sheet • Emergency drug kit (including epinephrine 1:10,000 and 1:1000 and diphenhydramine hydrochloride 50-mg, extra saline bag) • Transfusion reaction protocol • Emergency plan to transport patient (physician's phone #, hospital and ambulance phone #)	Most electromechanical pumps can safely administer red blood cell transfusions. See section on "Leukocyte-Depleted Blood Products." Combining other solutions (including glucose) with RBCs can cause agglutination or hemolysis of the RBCs. All blood components require an in-line blood filter of 170 micron, at minimum. Some centers require all blood component therapy to be transfused through leukocyte-depleting blood filters or similar device.
2. a. Check the physician's order to confirm the product type, dose, and rate of infusion. b. Review patient medical history/allergies, etc. c. Obtain blood component from blood bank, on departure to client's home.	All blood components must be administered with a physician's written order.

(continued)

TABLE 25-13 Home Transfusion Protocol (continued)

Nursing Actions	Rationale
• Check unit for patient's full name, patient's identification number, unique identifying numbers of the unit, the ABO and Rh type of the donor(s) and patient, expiration date. Cross-check with blood bank employee and sign off.	The major cause of acute fatal transfusion reactions is major ABO incompatibility related to clerical errors.
• Secure patient's record and interpretation of compatibility test to the blood container.	
• Examine unit for unusual color, clots, or excessive air.	Abnormalities can indicate contamination and/or improper collection or storage techniques.
3. Transport the blood at a temperature between 1°C and 10°C (cool but not frozen):	RBCs cannot be returned to storage if the temperature exceeds 10°C.
• Best achieved by transporting red blood cells in an insulated container with wet ice.	
• Transport platelets at room temperature (between 20° and 24°); **do not** transport with wet ice.	Platelets have best biologic activity if stored at room temperature.
4. Confirm patient identity:	As above.
• Verbally against the patient record.	
• Confirm patient identification using the medical bracelet or other identification means, and identify RBC compatibility on the tag attached to the unit and on all forms.	
5. Initiate blood component therapy:	May be required to alleviate allergic reactions.
• Explain procedure to patient/family.	
• Premedicate patient as ordered.	
• Establish baseline vital signs/record.	
• Start RBC transfusion slowly.	
• Observe for transfusion reaction.	Symptoms of a transfusion reaction (especially RBCs) are usually evident during infusion of first 50 ml of blood. Minimize the risk of bacterial contamination.
• Adjust flow rate per order.	
• Infuse RBCs within 4 hr.	
• Observe and monitor vital signs 30 min after completion.	
6. Documentation:	
• Patient identification procedure	All to be part of the legal record.
• General condition of patient and vital signs throughout procedure	
• Record medication on flow sheet, etc.	
• Record time of arrival/departure.	

posttransfusion blood sample can be obtained. Documentation of the entire blood transfusion process must be detailed and complete.

CONCLUSION

Patients with cancer are at risk for the development of bleeding due to multiple factors. Bleeding can occur as the result of the cancer itself or as a result of the treatment of the cancer. Bleeding associated with cancer may be occult and chronic, or acute and life-threatening as seen in the clotting and hemorrhage of DIC.

Treatment regimens for patients with cancer often are aggressive in nature and place the patient at risk for complications, including bleeding. The use of blood component therapy and the newer colony stimulating growth factors facilitates these aggressive treatment regimens. These sophisticated supportive care measures improve the prognosis of a number of malignancies. Care can be rendered in an acute care setting, an outpatient office or clinic, or in the patient's home. There is a greater need than ever with this increasing technology for nurses to be educationally prepared to meet the complex needs of these patients. Early detection of the signs and symptoms of bleeding can allow for prompt diagnosis and treatment of the disorder.

REFERENCES

1. Alkire K, Collingworth J: Physiology of blood and bone marrow. *Semin Oncol Nurs* 6:99–10, 1990.

2. Haeuber D, Spross JA: Alterations in protective mechanisms: Hematopoiesis and bone marrow depression. In Baird SB, McCorkle R, Grant M (eds.): *Cancer Nursing: A Comprehensive Textbook.* Philadelphia: Saunders, 1991, pp. 759–781.
3. Haeuber D, DiJulio JE: Hematopoietic colony stimulating factors: An overview. *Oncol Nurs Forum* 16:247–255, 1989.
4. Emerson SG: The stem cell model of hematopoiesis. In Hoffman R, Benz EJ, Shattil SJ, et al (eds.): *Hematology: Basic Principles and Practice.* New York: Churchill Livingstone, 1991, pp. 72–81.
5. Clark SC, Kamen R: The human hematopoietic colony-stimulating factors. *Science* 236:1229–1237, 1987.
6. Bagby GC, Segal GM: Growth factors and the control of hematopoiesis. In Hoffman R, Benz EJ, Shattil SJ, et al (eds.): *Hematology: Basic Principles and Practice.* New York: Churchill Livingstone, 1991, pp. 97–121.
7. Vadhan-Raj S: Clinical applications of colony-stimulating factors. *Oncol Nurs Forum* 16:21–27, 1989 (suppl.).
8. Broxmeyer HE, Williams DE: The production of myeloid blood cells and their regulation during health and disease. *CRC Crit Rev Oncol/Hematol* 8:173–226, 1988.
9. Broxmeyer HE, Vadhan-Raj S: Preclinical and clinical studies with hematopoietic colony stimulating factors and related interleukins. *Immunol Res* 8:185–201, 1989.
10. Sieff C: Hematopoietic growth factors. *J Clin Invest* 79:1549–1557, 1987.
11. Furie B, Furie BC: The molecular basis of blood coagulation. In Hoffman R, Benz EJ, Shattil SJ, et al (eds.): *Hematology: Basic Principles and Practice.* New York: Churchill Livingstone, 1991, pp. 1213–1231.
12. Ratnoff OD, Davie EW: Waterfall sequence for intrinsic blood clotting. *Science* 145:1310, 1964.
13. Nemerson Y: Sequence of coagulation reactions. In Williams WJ, Beutler E, Erslev AJ, Lichtman MA (eds.): *Hematology* (ed. 4). New York: McGraw-Hill, 1990, pp. 1295–1304.
14. Cool DE, MacGillivray RT: Characterization of human blood coagulation factor XII gene. Intron/exon gene organization and analysis of the 5'-flanking region. *J Biol Chem* 262:13662–13673, 1987.
15. Jennings BM: The hematologic system. In Alspach JG (ed.): *Core Curriculum for Critical Care Nursing.* Philadelphia: Saunders, 1991, pp. 675–747.
16. Bithell TC: Normal hemostasis and coagulation. In Leavell BS, Thorup OA (eds.): *Leavell and Thorup's Fundamentals of Clinical Hematology.* Philadelphia: Saunders, 1987, pp. 126–162.
17. Dutcher JP: Hematologic abnormalities in patients with nonhematologic malignancies. *Hematol Oncol Clin North Am* 1:281, 1987.
18. Sarzotti M, Baron S, Klingboll GR: El-4 metastases in spleen and bone marrow suppress the NK activity generated in the organs. *Int J Cancer* 39:118–125, 1978.
19. Beutler D: The common anemias. *JAMA* 259:2433–2437, 1988.
20. Swartz SS, Yuska CM: Common patient care issues following surgery for head and neck cancer. *Semin Oncol Nurs* 15:191–194, 1989.
21. Masouredis SP: Preservation and clinical use of erythrocytes and whole blood. In Williams WJ, Beutler E, Erslev AJ, Lichtman MA (eds.): *Hematology* (ed. 4). New York: McGraw-Hill, 1990, pp. 1628–1647.
22. Henry DH, Rudnick SA, Bryant E, et al: Preliminary reports of two double blind, placebo controlled studies using recombinant erythropoietin (rHuEPO) in the anemia associated with cancer. *Blood* 74:6a, 1989 (suppl. 1).
23. Ludwig H, Fritz E, Kotzman H, et al: Erythropoietin treatment for chronic anemia of malignancy. *Blood* 74:6a, 1989 (suppl. 1).
24. Oster W, Herrmann F, Gamm H, et al: Erythropoietin (EPO) for the treatment of anemia of malignancy due to neoplastic bone marrow infiltration. *Blood* 74:5a, 1989 (suppl. 1).
25. Eschbach J, Egrie J, Downing M, et al: Correction of the anemia of end-stage renal disease with recombinant human erythropoietin: Results of a combined phase I and II clinical trial. *N Engl J Med* 316:73–78, 1987.
26. Lim VS, DeGowin RL, Zavala D, et al: Recombinant human erythropoietin treatment in pre-dialysis patients. *Ann Intern Med* 3:108–114, 1989.
27. Erslev AJ: Erythropoietin coming of age. *N Engl J Med* 316:101, 1987.
28. Miller CB, Jones RJ, Piantadosi S, et al: Decreased erythropoietin response in patients with the anemia of cancer. *N Engl J Med* 322:1689, 1990.
29. Means RT, Olsen NJ, Krantz SB, et al: Treatment of the anemia of rheumatoid arthritis with recombinant human erythropoietin: Clinical and in vitro results. *Blood* 70:139a, 1987.
30. Williams WJ: Thrombocytosis. In Williams WJ, Beutler E, Erslev AJ, Lichtman MA (eds.): *Hematology* (ed. 4). New York:McGraw-Hill, 1990, pp. 1403–1406.
31. Buss DH, Stuart JJ, Lipscomb GE: The incidence of thrombotic and hemorrhagic disorders in association with extreme thrombocytosis: An analysis of 129 cases. *Am J Hematol* 20:365, 1985.
32. Adamson JW: Wither the platelet? *N Engl J Med* 318:1331–1332, 1988 (editorial).
33. Lofvenberg E, Nilsson T, Wahlin A, et al: Hydroxyurea treatment of myeloproliferative disorders. *Acta Med Scand* 222:169, 1987.
34. Schimke RT, Sherwood SW, Hill AB, et al: Over-replication and recombination of DNA in higher eukaryocytes: Potential consequences and biological implications. *Proc Natl Acad Sci, USA* 83:2157–2161, 1986.
35. Anagrelide Study Group: "Anagrelide," a therapy for thrombocythemic states: Experience in 577 patients. *Am J Med* 92:69–76, 1992.
36. Beaulieu LP, Tenenbaum L: Myelosuppression. In Tenenbaum L (ed.): *Cancer Chemotherapy: A Reference Guide.* Philadelphia: Saunders, 1989, pp. 135-163.
37. Hilderley L: Radiotherapy. In Groenwald SL, Frogge MH, Goodman M, Yarbro CH (eds.): *Cancer Nursing: Principles and Practice* (ed. 2). Boston: Jones and Bartlett, 1990, pp. 199–229.
38. Dachman AH, Ros PR, Shekitka KM, et al: Colorectal Hemangioma: Radiologic findings. *Radiology* 167:31–34, 1988.
39. Ey FS, Goodnight SH: Bleeding disorders in cancer. *Semin Oncol* 17:187–197, 1990.
40. Garnick MB, Griffin JD: Idiopathic thrombocytopenia in association with extragonadal germ cell cancer. *Ann Intern Med* 98:926–927, 1983.
41. McLaughlin P, Talpaz M, Quesada JR, et al: Immune thrombocytopenia following alpha-interferon therapy in patients with cancer. *JAMA* 254:1353–1354, 1985.

42. Kickler TS, Herman JS, Furihata TJ, et al: Identification of Bak[b], a new platelet-specific antigen associated with post-transfusion purpura. *Blood* 71:894–898, 1988.
43. Gaydos LA, Freirich EJ, Mantel N: The quantitative relation between platelet count and hemorrhage in patients with acute leukemia. *N Engl J Med* 266: 905–909, 1962.
44. Aderka D, Praff G, Santo M, et al: Bleeding due to thrombocytopenia in acute leukemias and reevaluation of the prophylactic platelet transfusion policy. *Am J Med Sci* 291:147–151, 1986.
45. Brown JK, Hogan CM: Chemotherapy. In Groenwald SL, Frogge MH, Goodman M, Yarbro CH (eds.): *Cancer Nursing: Principles and Practice* (ed. 2). Boston: Jones and Bartlett, 1990, pp. 230–273.
46. Bronchud MH, Scarff JH, Thatcher N, et al: Phase I/II study of recombinant human granulocyte colony-stimulating factor in patients receiving intensive chemotherapy for small cell lung cancer. *Br J Cancer* 56:809–813, 1987.
47. Antman KS, Griffin JD, Elias A, et al: Effect of recombinant human granulocyte-macrophage colony-stimulating factor on chemotherapy-induced myelosuppression. *N Engl J Med* 319:593–598, 1988.
48. Gabrilove JL, Jakubowski A, Scher H, et al: Effect of granulocyte colony-stimulating factor on neutropenia and associated morbidity due to chemotherapy for transitional-cell carcinoma of the urothelium. *N Engl J Med* 318:1414–1422, 1988.
49. Morstyn G, Campbell L, Souza ML, et al: Effect of granulocyte colony-stimulating factor on neutropenia induced by cytotoxic chemotherapy. *Lancet* 1:667–672, 1988.
50. Vadhan-Raj S, Buescher S, LeMaistre A, et al: Stimulation of hematopoiesis in patients with bone marrow failure and in patients with malignancy by recombinant human granulocyte-macrophage colony-stimulating factor. *Blood* 72:134–141, 1988.
51. Butturini A, De Souza PC, Gale RP, et al: Use of recombinant granulocyte-macrophage colony-stimulating factor in the Brazil radiation accident. *Lancet* II:471–475, 1988.
52. Robinson BE, McGrath HE, Quesenberry PJ: Recombinant murine granulocyte macrophage colony-stimulating activity and augments megakaryocyte colony stimulation by interleukin 3. *J Clin Invest* 79:1648–1652, 1987.
53. Bruno E, Miller ME, Hoffman R: Interacting cytokines regulate in vitro megakaryocytopoiesis. *Blood* 73:671–677, 1989.
54. Emerson SG, Yang YC, Clark SC, et al: Human recombinant granulocyte-macrophage colony-stimulating factor and interleukin 3 have overlapping, but distinct hematopoietic activities. *J Clin Invest* 82:1282–1287, 1988.
55. Gianni AM, Bregni M, Siena S, et al: Recombinant human granulocyte-macrophage colony-stimulating factor reduces hematologic toxicity and widens clinical applicability of high-dose cyclophasphamide treatment in breast cancer and non-Hodgkin's lymphoma. *J Clin Oncol* 8:768–778, 1990.
56. Nemunaitis J, Singer JW, Buckner CD, et al: Use of recombinant human granulocyte-macrophage colony-stimulating factor in autologous marrow transplantation for lymphoid malignancies. *Blood* 72:834–836, 1988.
57. Lieschke GJ, Maher D, Cebon J, et al: Effects of bacterially synthesized recombinant human granulocyte-macrophage colony-stimulating factor in patients with advanced malignancy. *Ann Intern Med* 110:357–364, 1989.
58. Phillips N, Jacobs S, Stoller R, et al: Effect of recombinant human granulocyte-macrophage colony-stimulating factor on myelopoiesis in patients with refractory metastatic carcinoma. *Blood* 74:26–34, 1989.
59. Herrmann F, Schulz G, Lindemann A, et al: Hematopoietic responses in patients with advanced malignancy treated with recombinant human granulocyte-macrophage colony-stimulating factor. *J Clin Oncol* 7:159–167, 1989.
60. Aglietta M, Piacibello W, Sanavio F, et al: Kinetics of human hemopoietic cells after in vivo administration of granulocyte-macrophage colony-stimulating factor. *J Clin Invest* 83:551–557, 1989.
61. Rifkin RM, Hersh EM, Hultquist SE, et al: Therapy of the myelodysplastic syndrome (MDS) with subcutaneously (SC) administered recombinant human granulocyte-macrophage colony-stimulating factor (GM-CSF). *Proc Am Soc Clin Oncol* 8:178, 1989 (abstr.).
62. Rifkin RM, Hersh EM, Hultquist SE, et al: Subcutaneous (SC) recombinant human granulocyte-macrophage colony-stimulating factor (GM-CSF) stimulates myelopoiesis in patients (pts) with bone marrow failure. *Proc Am Soc Clin Oncol* 8:178, 1989 (abstr.).
63. Champlin RE, Nimer SD, Oette D, et al: Granulocyte-macrophage colony-stimulating factor (GM-CSF) treatment for aplastic anemia (AA) or agranulocytosis. *Exp Hematol* 6:238a, 1988 (abstr.).
64. deVries EGE, Biesma B, Willemse PHB, et al: A double-blind placebo-controlled study with granulocyte-macrophage colony-stimulating factor for chemotherapy for ovarian carcinoma. *Cancer Res* 51:116–122, 1991.
65. Vadhan-Raj S, Keating M, LeMaistre A, et al: Effects of recombinant human granulocyte-macrophage colony-stimulating factor in patients with myelodysplastic syndromes. *N Engl J Med* 317:1545–1552, 1987.
66. Groopman J, Mitsyuasu R, DeLeo M: Effect of recombinant human granulocyte-macrophage colony-stimulating factor on myelopoiesis in the acquired immunodeficiency syndrome. *N Engl J Med* 317(10):593–598, 1987.
67. Antman K, Griffin J, Elias A, et al: Use of rhGM-CSF to ameliorate chemotherapy induced myelosuppression in sarcoma patients. Abstract No. 373. *Blood* 70:129a, 1987 (6, suppl. 1).
68. Brandt S, Peters W, Atwater S, et al: Effect of recombinant human granulocyte-macrophage colony-stimulating factor on neutropenia and associated morbidity due to chemotherapy for transitional cell carcinomas of the urethelium. *N Engl J Med* 318(22):1414–1422, 1988.
69. Mullins GM, Colvin M: Intensive cyclophosphamide (NCS-26271) therapy for solid tumors. *Cancer Chem Rep* 59:411–419, 1975.
70. Donahue RE, Seehra J, Metzger M, et al: S.C. Human IL-3 and GM-CSF act synergistically in stimulating hematopoiesis in primates. *Science* 241:1820–1923, 1988.
71. Silverstein MN: Diagnosis and treatment of polycythemia vera, agnogenic myeloid metaplasia, and primary thrombocytopenia. In Wierenik PH, Canellos GP,

Kyle RA, Schiffer CA (eds.): *Neoplastic Diseases of the Blood.* New York: Churchill Livingstone, 1984, p. 135.

72. Deisseroth A, Wallerstein R: Use of blood and blood products. In DeVita VT, Hellman S, Rosenberg SA (eds.): *Cancer: Principles and Practice of Oncology.* Philadelphia: Lippincott, 1989, pp. 2045–2059.
73. von dem Borne: High-dose IV methylprednisolone or high-dose IV gammaglobulin for autoimmune thrombocytopenia. *Br Med J* 296:249–250, 1988.
74. Vogelsang G, Kickler TS, Bell WR: Post-transfusion purpura: A report of five patients and a review of the pathogenesis and management. *Am J Hematol* 21:259–267, 1986.
75. Cook MB: Multiple myeloma. In Groenwald SL, Frogge MH, Goodman M, Yarbro CH (eds.): *Cancer Nursing: Principles and Practice* (ed. 2). Boston: Jones and Bartlett, 1990, pp. 990–998.
76. Shattil SJ, Bennett JS: Acquired qualitative platelet disorders. In Williams WJ, Beutler E, Erslev AJ, Lichtman (eds.): *Hematology* (ed. 4). New York: McGraw-Hill, 1990, pp. 1420–1433.
77. George JN, Shattil SJ: Acquired disorders of platelet function. In Hoffman R, Benz EJ, Shattil SJ, et al (eds.): *Hematology: Basic Principles and Practice.* New York: Churchill Livingstone, 1991, pp. 1528–1546.
78. Remaley AT, Kennedy JM, Laposata M: Evaluation of the clinical utility of platelet aggregation studies. *Am J Hematol* 31:188, 1989.
79. Kaullman R, Nieuwenhuis HK, de Groot PG, et al: Effects of low doses of aspirin, 10 mg and 30 mg daily, on bleeding time, thromboxane production, and 6-keto-PGF1a excretion in healthy subjects. *Thromb Res* 45:355, 1987.
80. Mielke CH Jr: Aspirin prolongation of the template bleeding time: Influence of venostasis and direction of incision. *Blood* 60:1139, 1982.
81. McQueen EG, Facoory B: Non-steroidal anti-inflammatory drugs and platelet function. *NZ Med* 99:358, 1986.
82. Sattler FR, Weitekamp MR, Ballard JO: Potential for bleeding with the new beta-lactam antibiotics. *Ann Intern Med* 105:924, 1986.
83. Brown RB, Klar J, Lemenshow S: Enhanced bleeding with cefoxitin or maxolactam: Statistical analysis within a defined population. *Arch Intern Med* 146:2159, 1986.
84. Sloand EM, Pierce P, Klein HG: Effect of albumin concentration on inhibition of platelet aggregation by beta-lactam antibiotics. *Blood* 74:405a, 1989 (abstr).
85. Lipsky JJ: Antibiotic associated hypoprothrombinanemia. *J. Antimicrob Chemother* 21:281, 1988.
86. Ahr DJ, Scialla SJ, Kimball DB Jr: Acquired platelet dysfunction following mithramycin therapy. *Cancer* 41:448, 1978.
87. Slichter SS, Harker LA: Hemostasis in malignancy. *Ann NY Acad Sci* 230:252–261, 1974.
88. Rao LV, Rapaport SI: Studies of a mechanism inhibiting the initiation of the extrinsic pathway of coagulation. *Blood* 69:645, 1987.
89. Gobel BH: Plasma and plasma derivative therapy for coagulation disorders. *Semin Oncol Nurs* 6:129–135, 1990.
90. Rice V: Understanding shock and how to treat it. II. Fluid resuscitation. *CINA J* 1:10–13, 16, 1989.
91. Menitove JE: Preparation and clinical use of plasma and plasma fractions. In Williams WJ, Beutler E, Erslev AJ, Lichtman MA (eds.): *Hematology* (ed. 4). New York: McGraw-Hill, 1990, pp. 1659–1673.
92. Rao KPP, Kizer J, Jones TJ, et al: Acquired von Willebrand's syndrome associated with an extranodal pulmonary lymphoma. *Arch Pathol Lab Med* 112:47–50, 1988.
93. Budde U, Dent JA, Berkowitz SD, et al: Subunit composition of plasma von Willebrand factor in patients with the myeloproliferative syndrome. *Blood* 68:1213, 1986.
94. Rickles FR, Edwards RL: Activation of blood coagulation in cancer: Trousseau's syndrome revisited. *Blood* 62:14–31, 1983.
95. Bunn PA, Ridgway EG: Paraneoplastic syndromes. In DeVita VT, Hellman S, Rosenberg SA (eds.): *Cancer: Principles and Practice of Oncology.* Philadelphia: Lippincott, 1989, pp. 1916–1923.
96. Siegrist CW, Jones JA: Disseminated intravascular coagulopathy and nursing implications. *Semin Oncol Nurs* 1:237–243, 1985.
97. Bick RL: Disseminated intravascular coagulation and related syndromes: A clinical review. *Semin Thromb Hemost* 14:299–338, 1988.
98. Goldberg MA, Girsburg D, Mayer RM, et al: Is heparin administration necessary during induction chemotherapy for patients with acute promyelocytic leukemia? *Blood* 69:187–191, 1987.
99. Cunningham I, Gee TS, Reich LM, et al: Acute promyelocytic leukemia: Treatment results during a decade at Memorial Hospital. *Blood* 73:1116–1122, 1989.
100. Kantarjian HM, Keating MJ, Walters RS, et al: Acute promyelocytic leukemia. *Am J Med* 80:789, 1986.
101. Dietz KA, Flaherty AM: Oncologic emergencies. In Groenwald SL, Frogge MH, Goodman M, Yarbro CH (eds.): *Cancer Nursing: Principles and Practice* (ed. 2). Boston: Jones and Bartlett, 1990, pp. 644–668.
102. Lisiewicz J: Disseminated intravascular coagulation in acute leukemia. *Semin Thromb Hemost* 14:339–348, 1988.
103. Young L: DIC: The insidious killer. *Crit Care Nurs* 10:26–33, 1990.
104. Griffin JP: Be prepared for the bleeding patient. *Nurs 86* 16:34–40, 1986.
105. Kingsley EC, Durie BG, Gareival HS: Acute promyelocytic leukemia. *West J Med* 146:322–327, 1987.
106. Feinstein DI: Treatment of disseminated intravascular coagulation. *Semin Thromb Hemost* 14:339–348, 1988.
107. Pagana KD, Pagana TJ: *Diagnostic Testing and Nursing Implications* (ed. 2). St. Louis: Mosby, 1986.
108. Beare PG, Rahr VA, Ronshausen CA: *Nursing Implications of Diagnostic Tests* (ed. 2). Philadelphia: Lippincott, 1985.
109. Food and Drug Administration: Title 21, Code of Federal Regulations. Washington, DC: U.S. Department of Health and Human Services, parts 600 and 601, 1989.
110. Masouredis SP: Preservation and clinical use of erythrocytes and whole blood. In Williams WJ, Beutler E, Erslev AJ, Lichtman MA (eds.): *Hematology* (ed. 4). New York: McGraw-Hill, 1990, pp. 1628–1647.
111. Pisciotto PT (ed.): *Blood Transfusion Therapy: A Physician's Handbook* (ed. 3). Arlington, VA: American Association of Blood Banks, 1989.
112. Pavel JN: Red blood cell transfusions for anemia. *Semin Oncol Nurs* 6:117–122, 1990.
113. Harmening D, Calhoun L, Polesky H: Blood preservation: Historical perspectives, review of metabolism, and current trends. In Harmening D (ed.): *Modern Blood*

Banking and Transfusion Practices (ed. 2). Philadelphia: Davis, 1980, pp. 2–7.

114. Jassak PF, Godwin J: Blood component therapy. In Baird SB, McCorkle R, Grant M (eds.): *Cancer Nursing: A Comprehensive Textbook*. Philadelphia: Saunders, 1991, pp. 370–384.
115. National Institutes of Health: *Transfusion Alert. Indications for Use of Red Blood Cells, Platelets, and Fresh Frozen Plasma*. Publication No. 89-2974a. Washington, DC: Author, 1989.
116. National Institutes of Health Consensus Conference: Platelet transfusion therapy. *Trans Med Rev* 1:195–200, 1987.
117. Fuller AK: Platelet transfusion therapy for thrombocytopenia. *Semin Oncol Nurs* 6:123–128, 1990.
118. Brand A, Claas FHJ, Falkenburg JHF, et al: Blood component therapy in bone marrow transplantation. *Semin Hematol* 21:141–153, 1984.
119. Ziegler ZR, Shadduck RK, Rosenfeld CS, et al: High-dose intravenous gammaglobulin improves responses to single donor platelets in patients refractory to platelet transfusions by intravenous gammaglobulin. *Am J Med* 76:199–203, 1984.
120. Kekomaki R, Elfenbein G, Gardner R, et al: Improved response of patient's refractory to random donor platelet transfusions by intravenous gammaglobulin. *Am J Med* 76:199–203, 1984.
121. Schiffer CA, Hagge DE, Aisner J, et al: High-dose intravenous gammaglobulin in alloimmunized platelet transfusion recipients. *Blood* 64:937–940, 1984.
122. VanBuren NL, Stroncek DF, Clay ME, et al: Transfusion related acute lung injury caused by an NB 2 granulocyte-specific antibody in a patient with thrombotic thrombocytopenic purpura. *Transfusion* 30:42–45, 1990.
123. Wedon MB: *Bone Marrow Transplantation: Principles, Practice and Nursing Insights*. Boston: Jones and Bartlett, 1991.
124. Leitman SF, Holland PV: Irradiation of blood products. Indications and guidelines. *Transfusion* 25:293–300, 1985.
125. Rawal BD, Davis E, Busch MP, et al: Dual reduction in the immunologic and infectious complications of transfusion by filtration/removal of leukocytes from donor blood soon after collection. *Trans Med Rev* 4:36–41, 1990.
126. Perkins HA: Transfusion-induced immunologic unresponsiveness. *Trans Med Rev* 2:196–203, 1988.
127. Holland PV: Prevention of transfusion associated graft vs-host disease. *Arch Pathol Lab Med* 113:285–291, 1989.
128. Adler SP: Cytomegalovirus and transfusions. *Trans Med Rev* 2:235–241, 1988.
129. Perkins HA, Payne R, Ferguson J, et al: Non-hemolytic febrile reactions. Quantitative effects of blood components with emphasis on isoantigenic incompatibility in leukocytes. *Vox Sang* II: 578–600, 1966.
130. Meyers DD: Infection in recipients of marrow transplants. In Remington JS, Swartz MN (eds.): *Current Clinical Topics in Infectious Disease*. New York: McGraw-Hill, 1985, pp. 261–292.
131. Nishimura T, Kuroda T, Mizoguchi H, et al: Advanced methods for leukocyte removal by blood filtration. In Brozovic B (ed.): *The Role of Leukocyte Depletion in Blood Transfusion Practice*. New York: Blackwell, 1988, pp. 35–40.
132. Sirchia G, Wenz B, Rebulla P, et al: Removal of leukocytes from red blood cells by transfusion through a new filter. *Transfusion* 30:30–33, 1990.
133. Wenz B: Clinical and laboratory precautions that reduce the adverse reactions, alloimmunization, infectivity, and possibly immunomodulation associated with homologous transfusions. *Trans Med Rev* 4:3–7, 1990.
134. Rutman R, Kakaiya P, Miller WV: Home transfusion for the cancer patient. *Semin Oncol Nurs* 6:163–167, 1990.
135. Whorton SS, McAbee B: The future role of home transfusion for the medical and surgical patient. In Snyder EL, Menitove E (eds.): *Home Transfusion Therapy*. Arlington, VA: American Association of Blood Banks, 1988, pp. 7–14.
136. Guilday TJ: Legal considerations of home blood transfusions. In Snyder EL, Menitove E (eds.): *Home Transfusion Therapy*. Arlington, VA: American Association of Blood Banks, 1988, pp. 41–52.
137. Rutman RC, Silberstein LE (eds.): *Out-of-Hospital Transfusions*. Arlington, VA: American Association of Blood Banks, 1989.
138. Rutman RC, Silberstein L, Mintz PD, et al: Blood transfusions outside the hospital. *Am J Nurs* 89:486–489, 1989.
139. Beck ML, Grindon AJ: Home transfusion therapy. *Transfusion* 26:296–298, 1986.

Chapter 26

Fatigue

Lillian M. Nail, RN, PhD

Maryl L. Winningham, RN, PhD, FACSM

INTRODUCTION

Everyone has experienced fatigue at some time. One popular view of the function of fatigue is that it serves to protect individuals from harm by keeping them from engaging in excessive amounts of physical or mental activity. Feelings of fatigue usually are attributed to physical exertion, psychological stress, and inadequate sleep and rest. People complain that fatigue changes their appearance, interferes with concentration, impairs physical performance, and makes them tense and irritable. Fatigue can interfere with all aspects of day-to-day life.

Acute fatigue is a relatively temporary state that is relieved by rest, although one night of undisturbed sleep may not provide complete relief. When fatigue persists over time, it is known as *chronic fatigue* or *chronic fatigue syndrome.*[1] Individuals with cancer may experience both acute and chronic fatigue as a result of the disease, as a side effect of treatment, and as a result of the psychological distress produced by the diagnosis of a potentially life-threatening condition.[2–6] The incidence of fatigue reported by cancer patients treated with surgery, radiation therapy, chemotherapy, or biologic response modifiers reached 90%.[7–13] Despite the prevalence of fatigue in cancer patients and the extent to which it can interfere with daily activities, there is limited research describing the time of onset, duration, pattern, and severity of fatigue; identifying factors that contribute to fatigue; or testing of interventions designed to prevent or ameliorate fatigue.

DEFINITION OF FATIGUE

Fatigue is a complex concept that has been associated with many other terms such as tiredness, exhaustion, weariness, drowsiness, malaise, weakness, asthenia, somnolence, lack of energy, and feeling "bushed" or "beat." Fatigue has been defined in terms of both objective performance and subjective experience. Early fatigue research focused on individuals' jobs or athletic performances. The aim of this research was to identify the causes of fatigue and find ways to improve performance. In this approach to understanding fatigue, an objective indicator of the point at which performance declines, such as exercise endurance or accuracy of completion of a mental task, is used to define fatigue.[14] Weakness is related to the objective view of fatigue, since it also represents a muscular performance deficit demonstrated on objective testing.

In the subjective experience approach, fatigue is conceptualized as involving both a feeling state and the impact of that state on the individual's perception of his or her ability to engage in usual activities.[4,6] In contrast to weakness, defined as the *inability* either to initiate or to maintain specific muscular activities, subjectively defined fatigue has a voluntary component, since individuals may push themselves to engage in a highly valued activity.

The subjective view of fatigue is most relevant to the concerns of nurses caring for individuals with cancer. The actions individuals take in response to fatigue will be based on their perceptions rather than on the results of a performance test or an evaluation of their level of fatigue made by another person. Some individuals will define their fatigue in terms of sensations, while others will define it in terms of their perceptions of their ability to engage in usual activities. Nursing care focuses on helping those who are at risk for fatigue or experiencing fatigue to plan for and deal with the experience.[1–4,6]

PATHOPHYSIOLOGY OF FATIGUE

Theories of Causation

Although causes of fatigue have been explored in numerous studies, no clear support for any of the major hypotheses has emerged. The majority of the research was conducted before 1970 using normal human subjects in performance test situations. Specific hypotheses about fatigue in cancer patients remain untested. The extent to which findings from research on fatigue in healthy normal subjects or trained athletes apply to individuals with cancer is not known.

Accumulation hypothesis

Early research on fatigue led to the accumulation hypothesis, which proposed that a build-up of waste products in the body produces fatigue. This hypothesis was supported when rapid accumulation of lactic acid, pyruvic acid, and other metabolic products was found during strenuous exercise, although subsequent research failed to relate the accumulation of waste products to the occurrence of fatigue.[15] Although it is common for fatigue in cancer patients receiving radiation treatment or chemotherapy to be attributed to the presence of by-products of cell death, to date no research has been conducted to test this hypothesis.

Depletion hypothesis

The depletion hypothesis was based on the idea that muscular activity is impaired when certain substances, such as carbohydrates, fats, proteins, adenosine triphosphate (ATP), and adrenal hormones are not readily available.[15] The relationship between nutrition and muscular activity is complex, involving both the supply and use of nutrients. When carbohydrates or fats are available for conversion into glycogen, protein is spared. With sustained muscle activity, glycogen is depleted, leading to fatigue.

The nutrition problems many cancer patients experience may lead to inadequate intake of nutrients; the way the body uses nutrients may change in the presence of cancer; and the tumor may successfully compete with normal tissues for available nutrients.[16] Therefore, indicators of changes in nutrition status, such as weight loss or changes in the nutrients available at the cellular level, should be associated with fatigue if the depletion hypothesis explains fatigue. However, the limited research in this area does not provide adequate support for this line of reasoning. For example, although weight loss was positively correlated with subjective postoperative fatigue in a group of general surgery patients, including some cancer patients, there was no association between fatigue and changes in specific muscle or plasma amino acids.[17] Tumor necrosis factor and cachectin are associated with muscle wasting that will contribute to fatigue.

The fatigue produced by anemia can also be thought of as an example of the depletion mechanism. Anemia decreases the blood's oxygen-carrying capacity, inhibiting the delivery of essential nutrients to the cells and decreasing the energy available to the organism. When anemic individuals who have experienced fatigue are treated with transfusions and subsequently demonstrate improvement in their hematocrit or hemoglobin values, they generally report a concurrent decrease in the severity of fatigue. Not all individuals with cancer who have anemia experience fatigue.[18a] There are many other variables that can affect fatigue in postsurgical patients. Despite the relationships between variables such as anemia, fluid volume deficit, nutritional status, and oxygenation, research examining these relationships is scanty. In addition, existing research is fraught with methodologic questions that must be addressed.

Biochemical and physiochemical phenomena

Changes in the production, distribution, use, balance, and movements of substances such as muscle proteins, glucose, electrolytes, and hormones may be important factors influencing the experience of fatigue.[15,19] Changes in the production and balance of hormones are central components of the Selye syndrome of stress response and may contribute to the fatigue experienced by individuals with cancer during physical or psychological stress.[20] Many of the drugs used to treat cancer or to manage side effects of treatment also can produce biochemical and physiochemical changes related to those believed to produce fatigue.[5]

Central nervous system control

In a 1970 review of the research on fatigue in animals and healthy human subjects, Grandjean concluded that central control of fatigue is vested in the reticular formation.[21] In Grandjean's neurophysiologic model of fatigue, the level of fatigue is determined by the balance between two opposing systems: the activating system and the inhibiting system. The *reticular activating system,* located in the reticular formation in the brain, controls alertness or wakefulness by stimulating the cerebral cortex and responding to both sensory stimulation and feedback from the cerebral cortex. The *inhibitory system,* believed to involve the cerebral cortex and the brain stem, depresses the activity of the reticular activating system. In Grandjean's model, both internal stimuli, such as thoughts and perceptions, as well as external stimuli (e.g., noise and light) stimulate the reticular activating system and promote wakefulness or alertness. The sustained arousal or wakefulness that occurs after environmental stimulation may be produced by release of adrenergic substances from the adrenal glands. Feelings of sleepiness or tiredness occur when the level of cortical stimulation of the reticular activating system is low, when there is little or no sensory input, or when the level of activity of the inhibitory system is high.

The neurophysiologic model of fatigue may explain the occurrence of fatigue in conditions of low stimulation, such as immobility produced by bed rest, even when there is little expenditure of energy. It also accounts for rapid decreases in feelings of fatigue when danger or excitement is perceived or a sudden increase in intensity or change in the nature of environmental stimuli occurs. The exploration of attentional fatigue in people with cancer has important implications for delivery of informational interventions.[22a]

Adaptation and energy reserves

Selye's approach to fatigue is that every individual has a certain amount of superficial energy available for adaptation and that fatigue occurs when that energy supply is depleted. Rest allows time for energy to be replenished from the individual's deep reserves so adaptation can continue.[20] As the reserves of adaptation energy are consumed, fatigue eventually leads to exhaustion and then to death. Selye's ideas incorporate accumulation, depletion, biochemical-physiochemical changes, and central nervous system (CNS) control, since all these may be involved in the individual's response to stressors. If rest was the antidote for fatigue, cancer patients who rested for prolonged periods of time would rate rest as completely effective in relieving fatigue. However, patients receiving chemotherapy rate rest as moderately rather than completely effective as a fatigue-relief measure.[22b]

The psychobiologic-entropy hypothesis

The psychobiologic-entropy hypothesis, which seeks to associate activity, fatigue, symptoms, and functional status, is based on the clinical observation that individuals who become less active as a result of disease and/or treatment-related symptoms lose energizing metabolic resources. According to Winningham, the initial cause of the decreased activity is less critical than the outcome of decreased activity and reduced functional status.[23] Decreased physical activity, regardless of the reason, leads to decreased energetic capacity (measured in terms of respiratory oxygen uptake or its correlate, calories consumed) for activity. This hypothesis is summarized in four propositions:[23]

1. Too much as well as too little rest contributes to feelings of fatigue.
2. Too little as well as too much activity contributes to feelings of fatigue.
3. A balance between activity and rest promotes restoration; an imbalance promotes fatigue and deterioration.
4. Any symptom that contributes to decreased activity will lead to increased fatigue and decreased functional status.

A fifth proposition suggests a conceptual basis for fatigue interventions: Any intervention that provides relief of a symptom that contributes to decreased activity may also serve to mitigate fatigue and promote functioning *providing that intervention does not have a sedating or catabolic effect.*[24] Thus, by enabling the patient to maintain normal activity levels, a psychosocial intervention, a biophysiologic intervention, or a combination of both may serve to alleviate fatigue, even if focused on a symptom not directly related to fatigue. Unfortunately, many pharmacologic agents used to relieve symptoms have sedative side effects or contribute to musculoskeletal breakdown.

The psychobiologic entropy hypothesis suggests that fatigue occupies a unique position among the constellation of distressing symptoms. Not only can it be a *primary* symptom (i.e., a direct consequence of preexisting conditions, disease or treatment), but it can be a *secondary* symptom (i.e., a *result* of the individual's *physiologic and/or psychosocial response* to other symptoms).[23] For example, if hair loss leads to feelings of social isolation and the individual becomes less active and more reclusive, the body's energy systems adjust to a lower level of activity, leading to increased feelings of fatigue in carrying on customary activities. Although anxiety may produce agitated behavior, often it is followed by exhaustion leading to increased feelings of fatigue. Healthy individuals maintain their energy basis for functional status by day-to-day, occupational, social, recreational, and leisure activities. During periods of disease- and treatment-imposed hypodynamia, these normal activities are decreased. Because the body's biochemical energy systems work on a 'use it or lose it' basis, the energy basis for functional status decreases, and normal activity demands become more fatiguing. Feelings of fatigue often are interpreted by patients as a signal to rest, resulting in accelerating fatigue and decreased functioning. Figure 26-1 shows the relationship between primary symptoms that may produce a decrease in activity and secondary fatigue that contributes to decreased functional status. There are three strategies for nursing interventions aimed at mitigating fatigue: (1) symptom alleviation, which may lead to maintenance of normal activities and energy maintenance, thereby minimizing the development of fatigue; (2) using an individualized activity/exercise program to prevent loss of energy efficiency; and (3) a combination of the two.

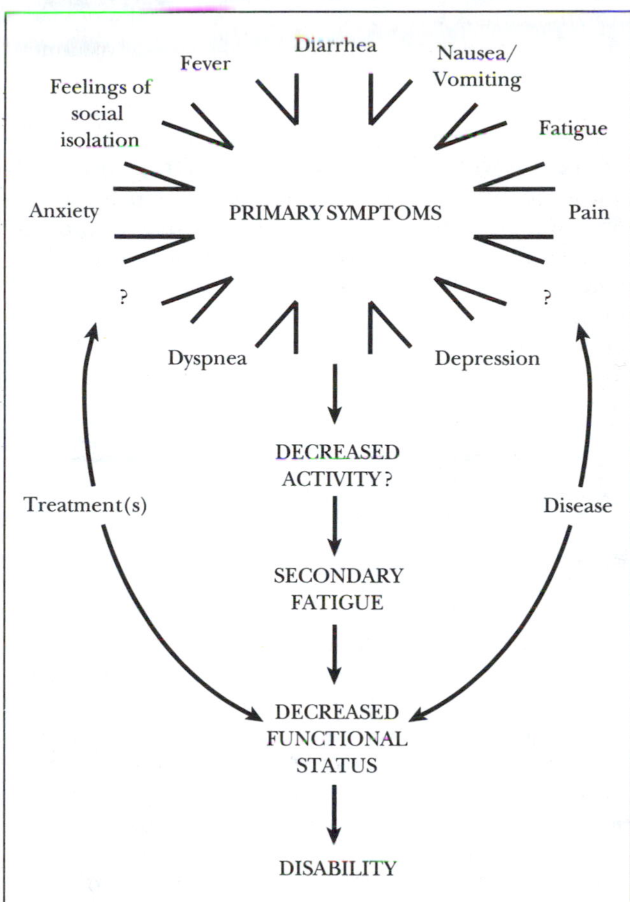

FIGURE 26-1 The psychobiologic-entropy model. (Source: © 1992 by Maryl L. Winningham, RN, PhD, FACSM. Used with express written consent of the author.)

Summary

Acute fatigue is an expected outcome of strenuous physical and mental activity and is believed to have the same sort of protective effect as acute pain. However, fatigue in individuals with cancer is more likely to resemble chronic fatigue than acute fatigue in that it may not respond to rest, persists over time, and often interferes with performance of usual daily activities.[25] Although there are many different hypotheses about the causal mechanisms of fatigue, none has been adequately tested in a population of cancer patients. However, all are potentially relevant to explaining at least some aspects of the fatigue experienced by individuals with cancer. Presently, the most reasonable approach to exploring the development of fatigue in individuals with cancer is to consider multiple factors.

Individuals with cancer experience biologic factors such as tumor burden, the physical stress of treatment, environmental changes during hospitalization, psychologic factors such as fear of death, changes in social relationships and roles, nutritional changes, and side effects of treatment or symptoms of the disease. In addition to the energy expenditure required to deal with symptoms or side effects, individuals with cancer may also experience disruption in their usual restorative activities when nausea, pain, or urinary frequency interferes with sleep and rest.

CANCER AND FATIGUE: PATHOPHYSIOLOGY AND PATHOPSYCHOLOGY

The phenomenon of fatigue recently has been recognized as important by researchers interested in the experiences of cancer patients. For example, 37% of patients treated for Hodgkin's disease were dissatisfied with the return of their energy many years posttreatment.[26] Weakness and fatigue were among the sources of greatest suffering reported by patients with lung cancer receiving various forms of treatment.[27] Somnolence syndrome, often viewed as synonymous with fatigue, was reported by all of the patients participating in a study of experiences following cranial radiation treatment.[28] Researchers and clinicians acknowledge the problems inherent in isolating causes of fatigue among patients with cancer diagnoses receiving multiple treatments, measuring a variable that does not have one widely accepted operational definition, and facing the reality that very few interventions have been identified to prevent or ameliorate fatigue.[29,30]

Treatment Effects

Surgery

Patients undergoing surgery experience direct tissue damage as well as the effects of anesthesia and analgesics. Fatigue is a consistent finding in patients who are recovering from surgery and is generally assumed to have multiple causes.[7,17,31,32] Fatigue may persist up to 6 months following surgery.[32] Since it is not unusual for patients to undergo several surgical procedures for diagnosis and initial treatment of cancer, the possible cumulative effects of multiple surgical procedures on fatigue are of concern to those who care for oncology patients. The effects of multiple surgical procedures on the severity and duration of postoperative fatigue have not been examined.

Radiation treatment

The majority of the side effects of radiation treatment are local and predictable based on the site of the treatment field. For example, individuals receiving radiation treatment to a pelvic field experience diarrhea, while those receiving treatment to the neck experience a sore throat. Fatigue is the only common *systemic* side effect of local radiation treatment and has been reported to be the most severe side effect of radiation during the last week of treatment.[11,12,33,34] In a sample of 30 patients who received radiation therapy and completed the Pearson Byars Fatigue Feeling Checklist daily throughout the course of their treatment, the mean level of fatigue increased over the course of treatment, with decreases in level of fatigue over the weekends (when patients were not treated).[11] A subgroup of the sample, consisting of patients with lung cancer, entered treatment with higher levels of fatigue than the other subjects and reported declines in fatigue before the end of treatment.

Weekly interviews of 96 patients undergoing radiation treatment revealed that fatigue was reported by 93% of the patients receiving treatment for lung cancer, 68% of the patients treated for head and neck cancer, 65% of the men treated for genitourinary cancer, and 72% of the women treated for gynecologic cancer. Among the patients with lung cancer, 60% reported fatigue at the first week of treatment compared with 5%–35% of the patients in the other three groups. In all four groups, fatigue declined gradually over the 3 months following treatment. Subjects reported that the fatigue was intermittent early in treatment but that it became continuous by the end of treatment, was worse in the afternoon or evening, and that resting or sleeping in the afternoon was helpful.[12]

The difference between the pattern of fatigue before and during radiation treatment reported by patients with lung cancer when compared with patients with other cancer diagnoses may be related to the characteristics of the disease. The high incidence of fatigue at the beginning of radiation treatment in patients with lung cancer may be explained by the increased energy expenditure required for breathing through partially obstructed airways. In research with healthy volunteers, decreases in airway diameter were associated with increased work of breathing.[35] If radiation treatment is successful in decreasing tumor size, individuals who enter treatment with some degree of airway obstruction are likely to experience some relief of fatigue as a result of the treatment.

The research on cancer patients' perceptions of fatigue as a side effect of radiation treatment is limited to patients receiving local radiation treatment. The experience of patients who receive total body irradiation in preparation for bone marrow transplantation has not been examined. Since patients who receive total body irradiation also receive a variety of drugs and undergo multiple medical procedures, their fatigue cannot be attributed to a single treatment modality and may be much different from that experienced by patients receiving local radiation treatment.

Chemotherapy

In general, the nature and severity of the side effects of cancer chemotherapy vary according to the type of drug(s) prescribed and the dose of the drug(s) (see Chapter 16). Despite variation among treatment regimens, fatigue is one of the most frequently reported side effects of chemotherapy.[8–10,36–46] In a prospective study of 66 patients with advanced colon or rectal cancer receiving either intravenous or intraperitoneal 5-fluorouracil (5-FU), 90% of the patients receiving intravenous 5-FU and 85% of the patients receiving intraperitoneal 5-FU reported on a questionnaire completed at home that they experienced fatigue following each cycle of chemotherapy.[8] For patients with lung cancer receiving combination treatment with radiation plus either of two drug regimens, fatigue increased compared with pretreatment levels in 68% of the patients in one group and 76% in the other at the completion of treatment.[39] Seventy-five percent of 61 patients with malignant lymphoma, 90% of whom were receiving treatment at the time of interview, reported fatigue as a side effect of chemotherapy.[10] In addition, fatigue was related positively to emotional distress.

Women receiving adjuvant chemotherapy for breast cancer have provided much information about side effects of treatment and quality of life during cancer chemotherapy. Forty-eight (96%) of 50 women receiving adjuvant chemotherapy for stage II breast cancer reported fatigue as a side effect of treatment, and many reported fluctuations in the level of fatigue depending on the phase of the treatment cycle.[43] Anecdotal data from these subjects characterize the fatigue as a lack of ambition, a feeling of slowness, and continuous feelings of tiredness.[42,43] Among 50 women receiving adjuvant chemotherapy for breast cancer and 28 women who had completed this treatment, fatigue received the highest physical distress rating among women currently receiving treatment and the second-highest rating among those who had completed treatment.[9] Although fatigue produced the most distress of any of the physical symptoms reported by the women under treatment, the mean level of distress fell between 2 and 3 on a scale of 1 (no distress) to 5 (great distress). The finding of a low level of physical distress among women with breast cancer was replicated in a sample of 107 subjects who completed a self-administered questionnaire, with the mean level of distress from fatigue, insomnia, nausea, and pain falling between 2 and 3 on the same 5-point scale.[44]

Among 128 women beginning a course of daily aminoglutethimide and medroxyprogesterone acetate for advanced metastatic breast cancer, fatigue appeared in 50% of the subjects and gradually disappeared during the first 6 weeks of treatment.[44] In a group of 56 patients with a variety of types of cancer beginning their first cycle of chemotherapy, 46 (82%) of the patients reported experiencing fatigue by the completion of the second treatment cycle.[40] Fatigue was the second-most distressing symptom, after pain, reported by 26 patients with a variety of solid tumors who participated in a phase I clinical trial, with the level of distress produced by fatigue similar to that reported by patients receiving adjuvant chemotherapy for breast cancer.[38]

These studies indicate that fatigue is the most prevalent side effect experienced by patients receiving chemotherapy for cancer. Fatigue is an important problem regardless of cancer diagnosis and type of drug treatment, although the time of onset, duration, pattern, and severity of the fatigue associated with chemotherapy and differences in the pattern of fatigue specific to individual drug regimens are not well documented.

Biologic response modifiers

Fatigue is described as the most important dose-limiting side effect of interferons.[30,47,48] In a small sample of patients with leukemia ($n = 11$) given two different types of interferon, 50% of the patients who received beta interferon and 60% of the patients who received gamma interferon experienced fatigue.[49] Findings of a phase I study of beta interferon demonstrated a positive relationship between dose and fatigue, with the incidence of fatigue reaching 100% at the highest dosage level administered in the protocol.[50] Findings of this study also suggest that patients may develop tolerance to some of the side effects of beta interferon, including fatigue. Interleukin-2 produces multiple systemic toxicities such as fatigue, chills, fever, and headaches that resemble those produced by the interferons.[51]

Based on the limited information available on the incidence and characteristics of fatigue associated with the use of biologic response modifiers, it appears that this cancer treatment modality is likely to produce fatigue that is more severe than that associated with surgery, radiation treatment, and the most commonly used chemotherapy regimens. The severity of the fatigue may exceed the individual's level of tolerance, either in terms of the sensation of fatigue or the impact of the fatigue on day-to-day activities, causing the person to terminate treatment. Since fatigue is a dose-limiting side effect of biologic response modifiers, a high priority for nursing care of individuals receiving this form of treatment is preventing and ameliorating fatigue.

Combined modality treatment

The majority of cancer patients who present for adjuvant chemotherapy or radiation treatment already have undergone a surgical procedure. Some patients receive concurrent radiation treatment and chemotherapy, while others receive radiation and biologic response modifiers. Research to determine whether the fatigue produced by sequential or combined modality treatment exceeds that produced by the most toxic treatment alone is needed to predict the responses of patients who receive multiple forms of cancer treatment.

Other Etiologic Factors

In addition to the direct effects of treatment, cancer patients experience a variety of problems that may produce fatigue.[2,4,6,52–54]

Physical factors

Physical problems such as pain, pruritus, urinary frequency, diarrhea, nausea, and vomiting may interfere with patients' ability to rest or sleep. Nutritional deficits, changes in nutrient metabolism, and alteration in fluid and electrolyte balance are produced by anorexia, taste changes, nausea, vomiting, stomatitis, esophagitis, mucositis, xerostomia, diarrhea, use of a restricted diet as part of an unproven method of cancer treatment, inappropriate use of a weight-reduction diet, hepatic and renal damage, side effects of medications, changes in absorption due to surgery, or diabetes. Bone marrow depression can produce anemia, bleeding, and increased susceptibility to infection, all of which are believed to produce fatigue. Some physical conditions increase energy expenditure, such as amputation of a limb or a neurologic deficit requiring the use of assistive devices for ambulation, weakness due to prolonged bed rest, a sensory deficit producing a need for increased vigilance, dyspnea, and decreased cardiac reserve. Alcohol and the use of prescription or nonprescription drugs also can contribute to feelings of fatigue, especially when the individual is using narcotics, sedatives, hypnotics, or antihistamines.

Psychosocial factors

Fatigue is often viewed as a symptom of anxiety and depression. Anxiety is associated with feelings of panic or tension and can produce agitation that may be followed by intense feelings of fatigue. Depression is a state of low energy and low levels of activity.[55] Receiving a diagnosis of cancer is certainly a frightening and stressful experience, and confronting a life-threatening disease can lead to depression. Conversely, feelings of anxiety and depression can result from the disruption in lifestyle produced by fatigue. When severe fatigue experienced as a side effect of cancer treatment forces the individual to decrease participation in social activities, transfer family responsibilities to others, and limit work activities, the person's response may include anxiety or depression as a result of the loss of usual social roles or inability to reach desired goals. The impact of the severity of fatigue and associated changes in activity depends on the individual's perception of what limitations are acceptable to the self and the family as well as expected duration of the limitations. These value judgments will differ substantially from person to person, with some individuals finding a week of fatigue following chemotherapy to be unacceptable and others regarding it as a perfectly acceptable experience.

For those who strive to maintain all their usual activities in addition to dealing with the demands of cancer treatment, fatigue may be the result of expending too much energy. For example, a person who maintains a full-time work commitment while commuting 1 or 2 hours a day for radiation treatment may experience fatigue as the daily commute is added to an already full schedule. Individuals who deny the effects of their illness and its treatment may find it difficult to set priorities for their activities and consequently may experience more fatigue than those who curtail some activities. The relationship between level of daily activities and fatigue in individuals undergoing cancer treatment has not been examined systematically.

NURSING CARE OF THE CANCER PATIENT WITH FATIGUE

The goal of nursing care for the patient with cancer who is experiencing fatigue is to assist the patient to maintain the highest quality of life. To reach this goal, the nurse must understand the possible causes of the person's fatigue and his or her values, coping resources, usual activities, and perception of fatigue.

Assessment

Level of fatigue

Since the patient's perception of fatigue will influence decisions about activities, participation in treatment, and overall quality of life, so-called objective ratings of fatigue made by health care professionals are less relevant to the patient's situation than assessments made by the patient. Fernsler found that when the problems reported by cancer patients receiving chemotherapy were compared with their nurses' reports of the problems they perceived the patients to be experiencing, patients reported three times the incidence of problems related to activity and rest than did their nurses.[56] In research on side effects of cancer treatment, various self-report measures have been used to obtain patients' ratings of the severity of fatigue or the distress produced by fatigue.[9,11,12,31,36] The measurement approaches used in these studies range from a single simple yes-no question to multiple adjective checklists. Although the multiple-item instruments are more likely than the single-item measures to be subjected to psychometric testing to assess their reliability and validity, the longer instruments are not readily incorporated in clinical interviews.[57,58] Clinicians often find it useful to ask if the person has experienced fatigue and then ask those responding affirmatively to rate the severity of their fatigue on a 5-point scale ranging from not at all to extremely severe.

The measures of fatigue based on health care providers' judgments or observations depend on observations of the individual's appearance, level of consciousness, activity level while in the hospital or during an outpatient visit, or patient reports of activity level. Using any measure of activity level as an indicator of fatigue is problematic in that it may represent a response to a variety of problems, such as nausea and pain, rather than a report of the sensation of fatigue. Measures of level of consciousness and appearance also are likely to represent multiple causes other than fatigue. In addition, this type of measure may not be very sensitive, since it is unlikely that the majority of patients experiencing fatigue will demonstrate marked changes in level of consciousness. The use of motor or mental task performance tests such as those used in research with healthy individuals has limited relevance to the clinical assessment of individuals with cancer.

Level of fatigue should be assessed at multiple points in time. Individuals who do not have fatigue when they begin treatment are likely to experience it at some point during treatment, and those whose fatigue does not gradually decrease once treatment is completed may require evaluation to determine if their fatigue is something other than an expected side effect of treatment. To assist patients in planning ways to deal with fatigue, the nurse must obtain information about both the daily pattern of fatigue and variations in fatigue in relation to the treatment cycle.

Usual activities

Information about the type and intensity of the individual's usual activities can be obtained by asking the patient to describe a typical day. The description should include the time the patient arises and retires, the number of times the patient awakens during the night, physical and mental activities performed during the day, the extent to which naps or rests are taken during the day, and a comparison of the current level of activity to the individual's level of activity before this episode of illness or the beginning of the present course of treatment. Individuals who report fatigue should be asked to describe what they do about it and to indicate the extent to which their self-care activities are effective in relieving their fatigue.

To assist the person to plan ways of modifying daily activities, the nurse determines who might be available to assume some of the individual's usual responsibilities and gains understanding of the meaning and value of each of the individual's activities. For example, a person who highly values maintaining his or her usual work role and places a lower value on recreation and entertainment will probably find it acceptable to suspend participation in sports and social events temporarily rather than take a leave of absence from work when experiencing fatigue as a side effect of cancer treatment. It is important to recognize that individuals experiencing fatigue over time may gradually downgrade their perception of the level of activity that is "usual." This process is analogous to changes in the body temperature set point in febrile conditions.

Additional assessment data

The assessment includes information about potential causes of fatigue. Chronic diseases such as diabetes, congestive heart failure, chronic obstructive pulmonary disease, Addison's disease, hyperthyroidism, hypopituitarism, renal or liver failure, anemia, and a variety of neurologic disorders as well as infection, pain, acute CNS changes, sleep disruption, overexertion, dehydration, electrolyte imbalances, malnutrition, anxiety, and depression may contribute to fatigue.[59-61] A careful review of the patient's medical and social history, including previous and current cancer treatment, laboratory data, and a thorough physical assessment, are essential in obtaining information about potential causes of fatigue.

Interventions

Despite the prevalence of fatigue as a side effect of cancer treatment, little attention has been given to determining the efficacy of the self-care activities patients use to deal with fatigue or to developing and testing new approaches to the problem. The types of interventions that are suggested for dealing with fatigue include providing preparatory information, decreasing activities, increasing sleep or rest, adjusting schedules to allow rest periods between activities, planning activities to coincide with the time the individual feels the most energetic, and encouraging exercise[3,4,45,62] (see Figure 26-2).

Preparatory information

Preparatory information is used to structure the person's expectations about receiving chemotherapy or radiation therapy. In one type of preparatory information, individuals are told about the pattern of fatigue expected as a side effect of treatment based on data collected from patients who have had the same treatment. Preparatory information, combined with suggestions about planning for rest periods, has had positive effects on patients' maintenance of usual activities when combined with similar information about various aspects of the experience of receiving radiation treatment for prostate cancer.[63] Although there are reports of research on the effects of providing other types of preparatory informational interventions in samples of patients receiving cancer treatment, none of them includes dependent variables relevant to level of performance of usual activities.

TEACHING GUIDE FOR FATIGUE

General Preparatory Information: All cancer patients beginning treatment should be prepared for the possibility that they may develop fatigue. For example, "Many patients receiving radiation treatment tell us that they experience fatigue during treatment. You may find this happening to you. If it does happen, please let us know so we can help you plan your activities around the tired feeling."

Assessment: Questions used to assess the cancer patient's level of fatigue and pattern of usual activities.

1. Have you felt fatigued over the past [*day, week, month*]? (if yes, ask questions 1a through 1c.)
   1a. How severe is the feeling of fatigue (on a scale of 1 = not at all severe to 5 = extremely severe)?
   1b. What time of day is the feeling of fatigue the lowest? What time of day is the feeling of fatigue most severe? How does the feeling of fatigue relate to your treatment? (How many days after chemotherapy, how many hours after radiation, etc.?)
   1c. What things have you tried to relieve the fatigue, and how well did each action work?
2. Please describe a typical day for you over the past week, beginning when you get up in the morning.
3. How does the day you just described differ from your usual day before this *illness* or before this *treatment?* (Probe: What additional things are you doing now that you did not do before? What things have you stopped doing or do less of?)
   3a. If activities have decreased, ask: Which of the changes you mentioned were made because of the fatigue?
4. For the things you are doing now, which ones are the most important for you to continue because they must be done? Which of these could be done by someone else?
5. What activities that you are now doing or stopped doing are things you really like to do?

Intervention Based on Assessment Data: First, determine if the patient has any signs or symptoms of other causes of fatigue such as infection, anemia, or poor control of diabetes. If the most likely explanation of the fatigue is as a side effect of cancer treatment:

1. Utilize data on the severity and pattern of fatigue to guide interventions. If the fatigue is severe, much more adjustment in activity is likely to be needed. If the fatigue is mild, the patient may decide to maintain activity at the present level but reorganize or restructure activities to take advantage of highest energy periods. For example, a manager in a local business is experiencing high levels of fatigue late in the afternoon but has no fatigue in the morning. She is concerned that her fatigue is interfering with her ability to conduct weekly staff meetings. A restructuring intervention would address rescheduling the staff meeting for morning when she does not feel fatigued and planning a different activity in the afternoon.
2. Build on what works for the patient. If the patient has identified activities that relieve the fatigue, such as going outside and walking in cold air, support the use of the intervention rather than trying to substitute something else. Discourage repeated use of interventions that are not working since they may be contributing to the fatigue.
3. When the patient cannot identify anything that works or helps, suggest decreasing activity and increasing rest. The patient may require assistance in identifying activities that can be eliminated. Focus on identifying the activities that are important to the patient and identifying which activities are essential and can be done by someone else. If the patient is interested in trying exercise, first screen for contraindications and follow the precautions listed in the references for this chapter.
4. For patients receiving treatment, provide reassurance that fatigue is an expected side effect of cancer treatment and that treatment-related fatigue gradually improves once treatment has ended. For patients experiencing fatigue as a symptom of advanced cancer, planning with the patient and caregivers to continue the most highly valued activities and monitoring activity to insure that the highly valued activities are given appropriate attention may be helpful.

FIGURE 26-2 Teaching guide for fatigue.

Rest and sleep

Rest is the most frequently recommended intervention for cancer patients who experience fatigue. Rest may take the form of a nap, a period of inactivity, a lower level of activity than usual, or a momentary respite from contact with others. Increasing the length of nighttime sleep may be considered a form of rest. However, increased sleep or rest may not improve fatigue for all individuals. Some have reported that sleep helps with fatigue only because they do not notice the fatigue while they are asleep, while others find sleep and rest to be extremely effective in relieving fatigue. Symptoms or treatment side effects that interfere with sleep and rest should be controlled to the extent possible. For example, when pain is not adequately controlled, the nurse can be an advocate for adequate pain control. Establishing a schedule for medication administration that does not interfere with the individual's desired rest time may also be helpful. The use of medication to induce sleep or relieve anxiety that interferes with sleep or rest may be appropriate for some individuals.

Rearranging activities

Rearranging activities to allow for rest periods or to shorten the time that high-energy output is required is another approach to dealing with limitations imposed by fatigue. Individuals may rearrange their weekly errands so they are spread throughout the week or schedule strenuous or high-priority activities at the time of day or week when they have the most energy. Some activities will be abandoned, performed in a different way, or shifted to another person. Rhodes et al.[45] provided a rich description of these changes in patients' lives as part of their research on self-care for the side effects of chemotherapy. Tiredness and weakness were the side effects that most interfered with self-care. The subjects limited energy expenditure through careful planning and scheduling, decreasing activities, and depending on others to complete some activities.

Exercise and activity

Some individuals have reported that exercise may play a role in relieving fatigue. In an exploratory study, breast cancer patients receiving chemotherapy who participated in a supervised, aerobic, interval training exercise program showed an improvement in mood that included perception of fatigue.[64] The same intervention program partially relieved nausea and improved functional capacity in women receiving adjuvant chemotherapy for breast cancer.[65,66] Further research is needed to determine the effects of different kinds of exercise on perceived fatigue in cancer patients. Although exercise has the potential to be a powerful intervention, it is not without risk. Considerations in recommending exercise should include adherence to published recommendations for safety.[18b,67–69] Individuals for whom exercise is not contraindicated can be encouraged to try short walks or their usual exercise to see if the activity relieves their fatigue.[70,71]

Manipulating the environment

Manipulating the environment to allow undisturbed time for sleep and rest as well as providing adequate stimulation to prevent boredom-related fatigue are nursing interventions used both in the hospital and the home. For the severely fatigued individual, it may be preferable for the nurse or a family member to perform activities of daily living for the person, even when the person can do them, so that he or she can conserve energy for other activities. The provision of care and opportunities for socialization should be scheduled individually to allow appropriate periods of rest and to take advantage of times of high energy for the activities the individual desires the most.

Posttreatment fatigue

When fatigue is experienced as a side effect of treatment, it does not disappear immediately once treatment ends. Individuals who have experienced fatigue during cancer treatment should be warned to expect a gradual lessening of fatigue over the months following treatment. The interventions that helped with fatigue during treatment may need to be continued, and activities should be resumed gradually. Individuals with advanced cancer may complete treatment and subsequently experience worsening of their fatigue. For these individuals, the side effects of pain medications and immobility may contribute to the fatigue. The use of assistive devices such as wheelchairs and grab rails, systematic planning of activities to include those most valued by the individual, and careful conservation of energy to ensure that adequate energy is available for highly valued activities are important in enabling the individual to maintain the best possible quality of life.[61]

Summary

Further research is needed to identify and test interventions designed to prevent or ameliorate fatigue. Eliminating problems or situations that produce fatigue or interfere with sleep and rest, rearranging or omitting some usual activities, providing information about fatigue so individuals view it as an expected side effect of treatment, increasing sleep and rest, and encouraging exercise are all possible interventions for cancer patients experiencing fatigue. Finding ways to deal with fatigue has the potential to improve the quality of life for cancer patients.

CONCLUSION

Although a number of hypotheses have been proposed to explain the causes of fatigue experienced as a symptom of cancer or as a side effect of cancer treatment, none has been adequately tested. Among the many side effects of cancer treatment, fatigue is the most prevalent but may be the most poorly understood.

The existing research on fatigue documents the incidence of fatigue among individuals receiving varying forms of cancer treatment. However, the measures of fatigue used in these studies represent a mix of patients' perceptions and those of physicians and nurses. Since the subjective view of fatigue is most relevant to patient care, both clinical assessment and further research should focus on obtaining the patient's assessment of the experience. To plan nursing care for the patient who is experiencing fatigue, the patient's pattern of usual activities and the relative importance or value of each activity must also be understood. In addition, data also should be obtained on a variety of physical and psychosocial factors that may produce fatigue.

The interventions routinely suggested to patients to lessen fatigue focus on increasing rest and decreasing the expenditure of energy. The specific activities suggested include naps, lengthening periods of sleep, rearranging schedules to spread strenuous activities over longer periods, and eliminating those activities that are unnecessary or are judged to be too taxing. Although some patients report using exercise to relieve fatigue, this intervention is not usually included in the clinical literature but is a subject of current research. Providing individuals with cancer with information about expected side effects of treatment, including fatigue, and assisting those who experience fatigue to plan alterations in their daily activities are important in helping individuals with cancer deal with their experience.

REFERENCES

1. Potempa K, Lopez M, Reid C, et al: Chronic fatigue. *Image* 18:165–169, 1986.

2. Alistars J: Fatigue in the cancer patient: A conceptual approach to a clinical problem. *Oncol Nurs Forum* 14:25–30, 1987.
3. Britton D: Fatigue. In Yasko JM (ed), *Guidelines for Cancer Care: Symptom Management.* Reston, VA: Reston, 1983, pp. 33–37.
4. Nail LM, King KB: Fatigue. *Semin Oncol Nurs* 3:257–262, 1987.
5. Piper BF: Fatigue. In Carrieri VK, Lindsey AM, West CM (eds), *Pathophysiological Phenomena in Nursing: Human Responses to Illness.* Philadelphia: Saunders, 1986, pp. 219–234.
6. Piper BF, Lindsey AM, Dodd MJ: Fatigue mechanisms in cancer patients: Developing nursing theory. *Oncol Nurs Forum* 14:17–23, 1987.
7. Christensen T, Hjortso NC, Mortensen E, et al: Fatigue and anxiety in surgical patients. *Acta Psychiatr Scand* 73:76–79, 1986.
8. Gianola FJ, Sugarbaker PH, Barofsky I, et al: Toxicity studies of adjuvant versus intraperitoneal 5-FU in patients with advanced primary colon or rectal cancer. *Am J Clin Oncol* 9:403–410, 1986.
9. Knopf MT: Physical and psychologic distress associated with adjuvant chemotherapy in women with breast cancer. *J Clin Oncol* 4:678–684, 1986.
10. Nerenz DR, Leventhal H, Love RR: Factors contributing to emotional distress during cancer chemotherapy. *Cancer* 50:1020–1027, 1982.
11. Haylock PJ, Hart LK: Fatigue in patients receiving localized radiation. *Cancer Nurs* 2:461–467, 1979.
12. King KB, Nail LM, Kreamer K, et al: Patients' descriptions of the experience of receiving radiation therapy. *Oncol Nurs Forum* 12:55–61, 1985.
13. Recombinant Human Interferon Gamma (S-6810) Research Group on Renal Cell Carcinoma: Phase II study of recombinant human interferon gamma (S-6810) on renal cell carcinoma: Summary of two collaborative studies. *Cancer* 60:929–933, 1987.
14. Grandjean EP: Fatigue: Its physiological and psychological significance. *Ergonomics* 11:427–436, 1968.
15. Simonson E: *Physiology of Work Capacity and Fatigue.* Springfield, IL: Thomas, 1971.
16. Lindsey AM: Cancer cachexia. In Carrieri VK, Lindsey AM, West CM (eds), *Pathophysiological Phenomena in Nursing: Human Responses to Illness.* Philadelphia: Saunders, 1986, pp. 122–136.
17. Christensen T, Kehlet H, Vesterberg V, et al: Fatigue and muscle amino acids during surgical convalescence. *Acta Chir Scand* 153:567–570, 1987.
18a. Maxwell MB: When the cancer patient becomes anemic. *Cancer Nurs* 7:321–326, 1984.
18b. St. Pierre B, Kasper CE, Lindsey M: Fatigue mechanisms in patients with cancer: Effects of tumor necrosis factor and exercise on skeletal muscle. *Oncol Nurs Forum* 19:419–425, 1992.
19. Taylor LA, Rachman SJ: The effects of blood sugar level changes on cognitive function, affective state, and somatic symptoms. *J Behav Med* 11:279–291, 1988.
20. Selye H: *Stress Without Distress.* Philadelphia: Lippincott, 1974.
21. Grandjean EP: Fatigue. *Am Ind Hyg Assoc J* 31:401–411, 1970.
22a. Cimprich B: Attentional fatigue following breast cancer surgery. *Res Nurs Health* 15:199–207, 1992.
22b. Nail LM, Jones LS, Greene D, et al: Use and perceived efficacy of self-care activities in patients receiving chemotherapy. *Oncol Nurs Forum* 18:883–887, 1991.
23. Winningham ML: How exercise mitigates fatigue: Implications for people receiving cancer therapy. In Johnson RM (ed), *The Biotherapy of Cancer V.* Pittsburgh: Oncology Nursing Press, 1992, pp. 16–21..
24. Winningham ML: The energetics of activity, fatigue, symptom management and functional status: A conceptual model. Presented at 1st International Symposium on Symptom Management, March 12, 1992, San Francisco.
25. Holmes GP, Kaplan JE, Gantz NM, et al: Chronic fatigue syndrome: A working case definition. *Ann Intern Med* 108:387–389, 1988.
26. Fobair P, Hoppe RT, Bloom J, et al: Psychosocial problems among survivors of Hodgkin's disease. *J Clin Oncol* 4:805–814, 1986.
27. Benedict S: The suffering associated with lung cancer. *Cancer Nurs* 12(1):34–40, 1989.
28. Faithfull S: Patients' experiences following cranial radiotherapy: A study of the somnolence syndrome. *J Adv Nurs* 16:939–946, 1991.
29. Irvine DM, Vincent L, Bubela N, et al: A critical appraisal of the research literature investigating fatigue in the individual with cancer. *Cancer Nurs* 14(4):188–199, 1991.
30. Piper BF, Rieger PT, Brophy L, et al: Recent advances in the management of biotherapy–related side effects: Fatigue. *Oncol Nurs Forum* 16(6):27–34, 1989, (suppl.).
31. Rhoten D: Fatigue and the postsurgical patient. In Norris CM (ed), *Concept Clarification in Nursing.* Rockville, MD: Aspen, 1982, pp. 277–300.
32. Rose EA, King TC: Understanding postoperative fatigue. *Surg Gynecol Obstet* 147:97–102, 1978.
33. Peck A, Boland J: Emotional reactions to radiation treatment. *Cancer* 40:180–184, 1977.
34. Andersen BL, Tewfik HH: Psychological reactions to radiation therapy: Reconsideration of the adaptive aspects of anxiety. *J Pers Soc Psychol* 48:1024–1032, 1985.
35. Shapiro M, Wilson K, Casar G, et al: Work of breathing through different sized endotracheal tubes. *Crit Care Med* 14:1028–1031, 1986.
36. McCorkle R, Young K: Development of a symptom distress scale. *Cancer Nurs* 1:373–378, 1978.
37. Meyerowitz BE, Watkins IK, Sparks FC: Psychosocial implications of adjuvant chemotherapy. *Cancer* 52:1541–1545, 1983.
38. Strauman JJ: Symptom distress in patients receiving phase I chemotherapy with Taxol. *Oncol Nurs Forum* 13(5):40–43, 1986.
39. Silberfarb PM, Holland JCB, Anbar D, et al: Psychological responses of patients receiving two drug regimens for lung carcinoma. *Am J Psychiatry* 140:110–111, 1983.
40. Cassileth BR, Farber JM, Lusk EJ, et al: Chemotherapeutic toxicity—the relationship between patients' pretreatment expectations and post-treatment results. *Am J Clin Oncol* 8:419–425, 1985.
41. Wander HE, Nagel GA, Blossey HC, et al: Aminoglutethimide and medroxyprogesterone acetate in the treatment of patients with advanced breast cancer. *Cancer* 58:1985–1989, 1986.
42. Meyerowitz BE, Watkins IK, Sparks FC: Quality of life for breast cancer patients receiving adjuvant chemotherapy. *Am J Nurs* 83:232–235, 1983.
43. Meyerowitz BE, Sparks FC, Spears IK: Adjuvant chem-

otherapy for breast carcinoma: Psychosocial implications. *Cancer* 43:1613–1618, 1979.
44. Ehlke G: Symptom distress in breast cancer patients receiving chemotherapy in the outpatient setting. *Oncol Nurs Forum* 15:343–346, 1988.
45. Rhodes VA, Watson PM, Hanson BM: Patients' descriptions of the influence of tiredness and weakness on self-care activities. *Cancer Nurs* 11:186–194, 1988.
46. Blesch KS, Paice JA, Wickham R, et al: Correlates of fatigue in people with breast or lung cancer. *Oncol Nurs Forum* 18:81–87, 1991.
47. Quesada JR, Talpaz M, Rios A, et al: Clinical toxicity of interferons in cancer patients: A review. *J Clin Oncol* 4:234–243, 1986.
48. Krown SE: Interferons and interferon inducers in cancer treatment. *Semin Oncol* 13:207–217, 1986.
49. Tamura K, Makino S, Araki Y, et al: Recombinant interferon beta and gamma in the treatment of adult T-cell leukemia. *Cancer* 59:1059–1062, 1987.
50. Grunberg SM, Kempf RA, Venturi CL, et al: Phase I study of recombinant beta interferon given by four-hour infusion. *Cancer Res* 47:1174–1178, 1987.
51. Jassak PF, Sticklin LA: Interleukin-2: An overview. *Oncol Nurs Forum* 13:17–22, 1986.
52. Chen MK: The epidemiology of self-perceived fatigue among adults. *Prev Med* 15:74–81, 1986.
53. Minden SL, Reich P: Nervousness and fatigue. In Blacklow RS (ed), *MacBryde's Signs and Symptoms* (6th ed). Philadelphia: Lippincott, 1983, pp. 591–621.
54. Silberfarb PM, Hauri PJ, Oxman TE, et al: Insomnia in cancer patients. *Soc Sci Med* 20:849–850, 1985.
55. Garber J, Miller SM, Abramson LY: On the distinction between anxiety and depression: Perceived control, certainty, and probability of goal attainment. In Garber J, Seligman MEP (eds), *Human Helplessness*. Orlando, FL: Academic Press, 1980, pp. 131–169.
56. Fernsler J: A comparison of patient and nurse perceptions of patients' self-care deficits associated with cancer chemotherapy. *Cancer Nurs* 9:50–57, 1986.
57. McNair DM, Lorr M, Droppleman LF: *Profile of Mood States Manual*. San Diego, CA: EdITS, 1971.
58. Lorr M, McNair D: *Profile of Mood States: Bi-Polar Form*. San Diego, CA: EdITS, 1982.
59. Minden SL, Reich P: Nervousness and fatigue. In Blacklow RS (ed), *MacBryde's Signs and Symptoms* (6th ed). Philadelphia: Lippincott, 1983, pp. 591–621.
60. Bruera E, MacDonald RN: Overwhelming fatigue in advanced cancer. *Am J Nurs* 88:99–100, 1988.
61. Billings JA: Weakness and fatigue. In Billings JA (ed), *Outpatient Management of Advanced Cancer*. Philadelphia: Lippincott, 1985, pp. 125–130.
62. Spross JA: Fatigue. In Baird SB (ed), *Decision Making in Oncology Nursing*. Philadelphia: Decker, 1988, pp. 76–77.
63. Johnson JE, Nail LM, Lauver D, et al: Reducing the negative impact of radiation therapy on functional status. *Cancer* 61:46–51, 1988.
64. MacVicar MG, Winningham ML: Promoting the functional capacity of cancer patients. *Cancer Bull* 38:235–239, 1986.
65. Winningham ML: Effects of a bicycle ergometry program on functional capacity and feelings of control in women with breast cancer. Diss., The Ohio State University, Columbus, OH, 1983.
66. Winningham ML, MacVicar MG: The effect of aerobic exercise on patient reports of nausea. *Oncol Nurs Forum* 15:447–450, 1988.
67. Winningham ML, MacVicar MG, Burke CA: Exercise for cancer patients: Guidelines and precautions. *Physician and Sportsmedicine* 14(10):125–134, 1986.
68. Winningham ML: The role of exercise in cancer therapy. In Watson RR, Eisinger M (eds), *Exercise and Disease*. Boca Raton, FL: CRC Press, 1992, pp. 63–70.
69. American College of Sports Medicine Preventive and Rehabilitative Exercise Committee: *Guidelines for Exercise Testing and Prescription* (4th ed). Philadelphia: Lea & Febiger, 1991:178–180.
70. Winningham ML, Glass EC, MacVicar MG: Rhythmic walking: Exercise for people living with cancer. Columbus, OH: The Ohio State University Cancer Center, 1990.
71. Winningham, ML: Walking program for people with cancer: Getting started. *Cancer Nurs* 14:270–276, 1991.

Chapter 27

Nutritional Disturbances

Annalynn Skipper, MS, RD, CNSD

Debra J. Szeluga, RD, PhD

Susan L. Groenwald, RN, MS

INTRODUCTION

Nutritional complications are a common consequence of cancer or its treatment. Malnourished individuals are more susceptible to infection and are less likely to tolerate or derive optimal benefits from therapy. In some studies malnutrition has been shown to be an important prognosticator of morbidity and survival.[1–4] Malnutrition also is an important issue in the quality of life of individuals with cancer.

In recognition of the serious consequences of malnutrition in cancer patients, scientists have examined a variety of problems related to nutrition to gain information for use in improving patient care. Among the most popular areas of inquiry are the role of nutrition in carcinogenesis; the effect of cancer on host metabolism; the use of parenteral infusates to improve the nutritional status of individuals with cancer; the identification of taste changes that alter eating habits; causes of anorexia in cancer; nutritional consequences of cancer therapy; and the impact of culture, values, and other societal factors on eating patterns of individuals. Much has been learned, but even more remains to be learned to establish nutritional therapy as a means of improving survival and the quality of life for individuals with cancer.

PATHOPHYSIOLOGY OF MALNUTRITION IN CANCER

Protein-calorie malnutrition occurs when the protein-calorie composition of the diet does not meet the individual's physiologic requirements. When dietary calories and protein are insufficient, adipose reserves and muscle are catabolized for energy. Thus, the first sign of malnutrition may be a reduction in fat stores and loss of muscle mass.

In cancer, local and systemic tumor effects result in a tremendous demand for nutrients. Dietary intake of protein and calories, regardless of quantity, may be insufficient to meet the demands of the tumor. Body stores of fat and protein are used. This parasitic process leads to loss of muscle protein, which results in weakness and debilitation; loss of subcutaneous fat, predisposing the individual to skin breakdown; impaired cellular and humoral immunity, increasing the individual's risk of infection; poor wound healing; apathy; and depression.

A variety of factors affect the development and severity of malnutrition related to cancer.[3]

Metabolic Effects of the Tumor

The most severe syndrome of malnutrition in cancer is cancer *cachexia,* which is characterized by profound and progressive loss of body weight, fat, and muscle. One-half to two-thirds of all individuals with cancer experience cachexia.[6] Progressive cachexia is one of the major causes of mortality in individuals with advanced cancer. Donaldson reports that in a series of autopsies of 500 individuals with cancer, cachexia was the only identifiable cause of death in 22% of cases.[7] Most frustrating about this devastating syndrome is the fact that little correlation has been made between cachexia and tumor extent, type, or location.

Research data suggest that cancer cachexia may be partially a result of paraneoplastic syndromes arising from the abnormal production of peptides by cancer cells.[6,10] In paraneoplastic syndromes, cells that do not normally produce certain peptides or hormones are altered by the cancer process. Genes responsible for hormone production that are usually repressed during the process of cell differentiation are depressed in cancer cells. Certain proteins, collectively termed *cytokines,* are released by the host in response to tumor, causing a number of metabolic alterations that result in profound nutritional consequences to the host.[11]

Altered carbohydrate metabolism

Carbohydrate metabolism in individuals with cancer is characterized by a number of aberrations.

Anaerobic glycolysis Normally, glucose is metabolized through the Embden-Meyerhof pathway to yield pyruvate; it proceeds either to glycolysis, of which lactic acid is the end product, or respiration, where the pyruvate is oxidized to carbon dioxide and water. Anaerobic glycolysis produces two adenosine triphosphate (ATP) molecules from each glucose molecule, whereas complete oxidation of glucose to carbon dioxide and water yields 36 ATP molecules. Thus, anaerobic glycolysis is far less efficient in energy production than is oxidative respiration.

Tumors predominantly use anaerobic glycolysis in glucose metabolism. The tumor uses glucose for its own growth, demanding increasing amounts as it enlarges.[12]

Increased rate of gluconeogenesis The lactic acid produced by anaerobic glycolysis is recruited back into glucose production (gluconeogenesis). This cycle of glucose to lactic acid and back to glucose is called the *Cori cycle* and is an energy-consuming process that occurs at an increased rate in individuals with cancer.[13] The energy required for gluconeogenesis cannot be supplied by lactic acid alone, so host reserves of amino acids and other sources make up the energy deficit. Young[14] estimates that the Cori cycle may account for a 10% increase in energy expenditure for an individual with cancer. As the tumor enlarges, a tremendous drain on body reserves to meet the excessive nutritive needs of the growing tumor results in vast depletion of body tissues.

Glucose intolerance A third aberration of carbohydrate metabolism present in individuals with cancer is glucose intolerance, which is evidenced by delayed clearing of intravenously or orally administered glucose. Glucose intolerance may be due to a defect of insulin response to hyperglycemia or a lack of tissue responsiveness to insulin.[13] However, because a number of clinical conditions are associated with glucose intolerance, such as bed rest, sepsis, and starvation, it is not possible to establish the tumor as the specific cause of the intolerance.[16]

Altered protein metabolism

Abnormalities of protein metabolism are common in individuals with cancer, especially those with cachexia. In the healthy adult, approximately 50 g of nitrogen is synthesized and broken down every day: only 10 g of nitrogen (approximately 62 g protein) is excreted per day.[17] Most of the amino acids that result from the breakdown of protein are reincorporated into protein synthesis.

Although an individual can lose 30% of body fat without serious consequences, loss of 30% of body protein content will result in death.[18] For this reason, cancer cachexia and the resulting loss of lean muscle mass present a serious hazard to the person with cancer. Serum albumin levels are frequently used as a measure of protein status. In individuals diagnosed with cancer, hypoalbuminemia is common. In a study of serum albumin levels of 222 individuals with cancer at various stages of disease, the mean concentration of serum albumin was 2.9 g/dl, compared with 4.0 g/dl in healthy adults.[19] Serum prealbumin, another hepatic protein, has been suggested as a predictor of survival in individuals with cancer.[20]

Increased uptake of amino acids by the tumor The apparent capacity of tumors to gain weight while the rest of the body wastes led some researchers to call the tumor a "nitrogen trap."[21] In its need for increasing amounts of glucose, the tumor draws on the host's protein reserves for gluconeogenesis.[22] The result is progressive muscle wasting. The amino acids taken up by the tumor are converted to lactic acid through the Cori cycle and are returned to glucose through gluconeogenesis.

Decreased protein synthesis Protein synthesis is decreased in individuals with cancer.[23] Although the decreased protein synthesis may be explained partially by poor intake and malnutrition, tumor factors also may play a role because protein synthesis is decreased even in individuals with normal food intake, possibly due to a decreased rate of synthesis of serum albumin.

Increased protein degradation Goodlad et al.[24] have demonstrated that muscle protein breakdown is accelerated in the tumor-bearing animal. Other researchers have demonstrated increased muscle protein degradation in humans with cancer.[25] Skeletal muscle is preferentially affected as opposed to cardiac muscle.

Protein loss Loss of protein through abnormal excretion or leakage can contribute significantly to depletion of protein stores and decreased muscle mass. In protein-losing enteropathies associated with some types of cancers such as gastric, colon, and esophageal carcinomas or carcinoid syndrome, release of an ectopic hormone causes ulceration of the mucosa of the gastrointestinal tract and loss of protein-rich exudate.[26] Fistulas, decubitus ulcers, or other exudative lesions also may be sources of protein loss.

Use of protein for energy needs In starvation in the healthy adult, adaptive processes cause the body to conserve protein and use body fat for energy needs. All stored energy in humans is in the form of adipose tissue. During fasting or starvation, fat depots are the first to be used to meet energy needs. In the case of cancer cachexia, however, such adaptation does not occur. Protein use by the tumor continues independent of the host's nutritional intake.

Altered lipid metabolism

There are conflicting laboratory observations regarding the degree to which lipid metabolism is altered in individuals with cancer. Theologides[9] hypothesizes that cancer cells synthesize and secrete a lipid-mobilizing factor that increases plasma fatty acids to meet the tumor's increased caloric requirements. Goodlad and Clark[27] provided evidence that mobilization of lipids from host tissues (hyperlipemia) occurs as a result of the tumor's excessive energy needs. The tumor exhausts its glucose supply and is forced to use fatty acids as an additional energy source.

Axelrod and Costa,[28] however, observed decreased mobilization of fat in individuals with cancer. They attribute the decreased fat mobilization to a normal homeostatic response to reduced caloric intake whereby the body conserves energy by decreasing its metabolism of fat. Waterhouse[29] corroborates Axelrod and Costa's observations through studies demonstrating that normal control mechanisms for inhibiting free fatty acid mobilization following ingestion of carbohydrates are intact in individuals with cancer.

Fluid and electrolyte disturbances

Tumors can affect renal function directly or indirectly through fluid and electrolyte abnormalities resulting from the action of ectopic hormones. The following are a few of the more common tumor-related fluid and electrolyte abnormalities that occur in individuals with cancer.

Hypercalcemia In some tumors, such as parathyroid, lung, kidney, ovary, or colon tumors, an ectopic parathyroidlike hormone causes deposition of calcium in renal tubules or other genitourinary structures and may result in a gradual or sudden onset of renal failure. Hypercalcemia also may cause a concentrating defect that leads to polyuria and water depletion (see Chapter 28).

Hyperuricemia In some leukemias and lymphomas, a rapid neoplastic cell growth phase is accompanied by increased catabolism of cellular nucleic acids. Hyperuricemia, hyperphosphatemia, and hyperkalemia occur as a result of the release of electrolytes from the resultant cellular breakdown. This situation also occurs in tumor lysis syndrome, in which cells are rapidly destroyed as a result of chemotherapy for lymphoproliferative diseases such as leukemia.

Hyperuricemia involves a sudden increase of uric acid in the plasma. Urate crystals may be deposited in the kidney, causing renal damage. The combined electrolyte disturbances may result in renal failure and cardiac arrest.

Hyponatremia A common presentation of some occult tumors, especially bronchogenic and oat cell carcinomas, is the syndrome of inappropriate antidiuretic hormone secretion (SIADH). SIADH secretion of ectopic antidiuretic hormone (ADH) by tumor cells is characterized by persistent urinary loss of sodium and excessive retention of water by the renal tubules. This produces a water excess characterized by reduced levels of serum sodium and serum osmolality but no edema.

Hypokalemia Renin-secreting tumors such as hypernephromas and renal juxtaglomerular cell tumors cause increased secretion of aldosterone, resulting in hypokalemic alkalosis. Aldosterone causes sodium and water retention in exchange for potassium and hydrogen ion excretion in the renal tubules. Prolonged hypokalemia damages the renal tubules, causing inability to concentrate urine. Polyuria and nocturia are clinical signs of hypokalemia.

Increased energy expenditure

Because of the excessive energy requirements of tumors, individuals with cancer cachexia have a greater energy expenditure then their normal counterparts.[30] Protein turnover and gluconeogenesis are energy-requiring metabolic processes that are increased in individuals with cancer, causing a tremendous drain on energy reserves.

Warnold et al.[31] assessed heart rate (as a function of oxygen consumption) to measure energy expenditure of individuals with cancer cachexia. They found that both the resting metabolic expenditure and daily energy expenditure were significantly greater in individuals with cancer cachexia than in individuals who had similar degrees of cachexia due to other disease processes.

In starvation in otherwise healthy adults, the body adapts by lowering its basal metabolic rate to conserve energy. In cancer, however, increased basal metabolic rate may be a frequent feature of advanced disease, even when food intake is significantly decreased.[32,33]

Altered taste

Taste changes occur frequently in individuals with cancer. In a study of 35 individuals with cancer, 25 complained of a general reduction in taste perception, or *hypogeusia*.[34] Twenty-two (88%) of the 25 respondents complained of aversion to meat. This perverted sense of taste, called *dysgeusia,* caused the individuals to refuse meat, fish, poultry, eggs, foods fried in oil or fat, and tomatoes. DeWys and Walter[35] reported that individuals with cancer have a decreased threshold for bitter, making bitter foods such as those high in protein less palatable, and an increased threshold for sweet, making sweet foods more difficult to taste.

Although the exact mechanisms responsible for taste changes in individuals with cancer remain unknown, nutritional deficiencies may play a role. Deficiencies of zinc, copper, nickel, niacin, and vitamin A have been implicated in decreased or altered taste sensations.

Recent research has focused on learned aversions as a major factor in the taste changes that occur in cancer. Learned food aversions develop when a food is associated with unpleasant symptoms such as nausea and vomiting, pain, and so forth.[36] Aversions seem to develop most rapidly to new and novel foods, but even the most familiar and favored foods may become aversive over time. Many substances including amphetamine, cyclophosphamide, ethanol, and lithium have been shown to produce profound food aversions.[37]

In children receiving chemotherapy, Broberg and Bernstein[38] have shown that the use of a scapegoat food item (a coconut or rootbeer candy) effectively reduced the impact of chemotherapy on the preference for normal menu items. Mattes et al.[39] and Andersen et al.[40] also demonstrated that the development of aversions to usual foods was reduced when adults consumed scapegoat foods just before their first course of therapy. Additional clinical research and application theories related to learned food aversions may produce other intervention possibilities.

Anorexia

It is well recognized that individuals with cancer experience metabolic abnormalities that induce or aggravate loss of appetite, or *anorexia,* which compounds the cachexia and weight loss associated with cancer. Anorexia is an initial symptom of cancer and is sometimes the first evidence of recurrence or progression. It is a nonspecific symptom of cancer that plagues almost all individuals with cancer at some point during their illness. Various factors contribute to loss of appetite and reduced food intake in individuals with cancer.

Central mechanisms The previously described metabolic alterations evoked by the tumor may cause appetite suppression by creating a false interpretation of satiety by the hypothalamus as a result of increased circulating lipids and peptides.[41] For example, the lactic acid produced by tumor metabolism or ketones resulting from lipolysis may be anorexigenic.

Neurotransmitters In recent years a variety of neurotransmitters have been investigated for their role in anorexia in cancer. Krause et al.[42] found that tumor-bearing animals have increased brain levels of the amino acid tryptophan and serotonin metabolites. Because decreased brain levels of tryptophan and serotonin seem to be associated with increased food intake in animals, these researchers hypothesized that the increased tryptophan levels and serotonin metabolism found in the brains of tumor-bearing animals may be responsible for the decreased food intake. Similar studies have been conducted on endorphins.[43] Although studies of the role of tryptophan and endorphins in cancer anorexia and cachexia offer exciting possibilities for clinical intervention through dietary and metabolite manipulation, definitive research is yet to be conducted.

Taste changes Taste changes lead to altered dietary habits and disinterest in food. Recent research has indicated that learned aversions to food may play a major role in the decreased food intake of individuals with cancer.[44] A positive taste experience is important in stimulating a variety of physiologic factors that contribute to the ingestion and digestion of food.[34] The volume and character of saliva and gastric secretions partially depend on the individual's taste experience. When food aversions or unpleasant taste changes occur, the taste stimulus may be insufficient to stimulate the physiologic responses necessary for effective ingestion and digestion of food, contributing to anorexia.

Physical discomfort Physical discomfort of any type may depress appetite and lead to reduced food intake. In addition, because eating is a motor activity that requires the expenditure of energy, a person who is immobile or fatigued may have loss of appetite or be unable to perform the motor functions necessary for eating.

Immunosuppression

The progressive growth of most neoplasms is accompanied by profound immunologic disturbances. Early in the disease process, the immune system is reasonably intact. As the disease advances and disseminates, alterations in humoral and cellular immunity occur.

Malnutrition has a number of deleterious effects on the immune system.[45]

Decrease in lymphoid tissues Lymphatic structures of the immune system, such as the spleen, lymph nodes, thymus, tonsils, and adenoids, are decreased in size, weight, and structure in malnourished individuals.[46] Because lymphatic structures participate directly in the immune response and also contribute to the number and function of immune cells, decrease in their size contributes to immunosuppression.

Decreased phagocytic activity Phagocytic activity and function are decreased in malnutrition. This decreased phagocytic activity apparently is due to deficiency of the protein necessary for synthesis of the neutrophils responsible for phagocytosis. The result is ineffective killing of bacteria.

Decreased T-lymphocyte function Malnutrition results in a decreased number of T lymphocytes in the peripheral circulation. T lymphocytes are responsible for the delayed hypersensitivity response to antigens, a response that is depressed in malnutrition. The greater the degree of malnutrition, the greater the deficiency of T lymphocytes and the lack of delayed hypersensitivity response. A total absence of delayed hypersensitivity response is called *anergy.*

Decreased B-lymphocyte function The percentage of B lymphocytes and the levels of immunoglobulins in the peripheral blood of malnourished individuals are frequently normal or elevated. Normal or elevated levels of B lymphocytes and immunoglobulins may be the result of repeated infections that occur as a result of the immune deficiency associated with malnutrition. As malnutrition progresses to severe, the percentage of B lymphocytes may decrease.

The complement system that participates with immunoglobulins in the destruction of bacteria is compromised in malnutrition, apparently as a result of a deficiency of protein necessary to synthesize the complement factors. Suppression of the complement system increases the individual's susceptibility to bacterial infection.

The degree of immunologic impairment is affected by the type of tumor, its extent, and the methods that are used to treat it. Cancer prognosis seems to be closely related to the degree of immunosuppression, and the degree of immunosuppression is related to the degree of malnutrition. The immune system works in concert with cancer treatment methods to destroy and eliminate tumor cells. Therefore, preservation of both nutritional status and immune system function is an important consideration in cancer therapy.

Mechanical Effects of the Tumor

The nutritional consequences of tumor destruction of local tissue depend on tumor location, type, and extent. A particularly invasive type of tumor may be more damaging to local tissue than an encapsulated tumor. However, if the encapsulated tumor is located within a constricted area, the pressure caused by tumor expansion will have more severe consequences. Table 27-1 shows some of the nutritional consequences of expanding tumors.

Nutritional Consequences of Cancer Treatment

Maintenance of adequate nutrition may become a problem if the person's ability to eat or absorb food is compromised by physiologic reactions to the treatment regimen. The following are the most common nutritional problems that result from cancer treatment.

TABLE 27-1 Nutritional Consequences of the Mechanical Effects of an Expanding Tumor

System	Local Tumor Effect	Nutritional Consequences	
Integument	Ulceration Decubiti Fistulas	Loss of fluid and electrolytes Loss of cellular components and nutrients Pain Infection—increased energy requirements Odor	Fluid, electrolyte, and protein disturbances; loss of appetite, loss of weight
Hematologic/immunologic	Inflammation; infection	Increased basal metabolic rate and energy requirements lead to weight loss	
	Bone marrow invasion	Infection increases energy requirements; anemia leads to fatigue and loss of appetite	
Cardiovascular	Hemorrhage	Loss of blood components and fluids; anemia causes fatigue and loss of appetite	
	Vascular obstruction	Ischemia; necrosis; inflammation; infection; edema; increased blood pressure; increased heart rate	
	Lymphatic obstruction	Edema; loss of protein; infection	
	Congestive heart failure	Edema; fatigue; shortness of breath	
Respiratory	Obstruction	Congestive heart failure; shortness of breath; edema; fatigue; effusions	
	Effusion	Shortness of breath; fatigue; loss of fluid and cellular components	
	Decreased lung capacity	Shortness of breath; increased energy requirements; loss of appetite; infection	
Genitourinary	Obstruction	Increased blood urea nitrogen; uremia; fluid and electrolyte disturbances	
	Ascites	Early satiety; hypoalbuminemia; fluid and electrolyte disturbances	
	Renal injury	Renal failure; fluid, electrolyte, and protein disturbances	
Gastrointestinal	Vomiting	Fluid and electrolyte disturbances	
	Mucositis	Pain; inability to swallow and eat	
	Obstruction	Impaired ingestion, digestion, and absorption; nausea, vomiting, and pain; nutritional deficiencies; jaundice	
	Constipation	Loss of appetite; nausea, vomiting, and pain	
	Diarrhea	Fluid and electrolyte disturbances	
	Fistulas	Loss of fluid and electrolytes, malabsorption	
	Liver dysfunction	Hypoalbuminemia; loss of fluid and electrolytes; malabsorption, ascites, and jaundice	
	Decreased digestive enzymes	Malabsorption; impaired digestion	
Central nervous	Pain	Loss of appetite	
	Confusion, somnolence	Missed meals	
	Increased intracranial pressure	Nausea and vomiting lead to fluid and electrolyte disturbances	
	Hypothalamic destruction	Hypernatremia; diabetes insipidus	
Endocrine			
Hyopthalamus	Lack of vasopressin	Diabetes insipidus leads to polyuria and dehydration	
	Somnolence	Missed meals	
	Increased body temperature	Increased basal metabolic rate; increased energy requirements	
Pituitary	Lack of ADH	Diabetes insipidus leads to polyuria and dehydration	
	Increased ACTH secretion	Cushing's syndrome—hyperglycemia, osteoporosis, hypertension, weight gain	
	Decreased ACTH secretion	Addison's disease—loss of appetite, decreased blood pressure, weight loss, hypoglycemia, hyperkalemia	
Adrenal	Adrenal hypersecretion	Cushing's syndrome	
	Adrenal insufficiency	Addison's disease	
Thyroid	Deficiency	Decreased metabolic rate; anemia	
	Hypersecretion	Increased basal metabolic rate; weakness	
Parathyroid	Deficiency	Hypocalcemia	
	Hypersecretion	Hypercalcemia	
Pancreas	Deficiency	Lack of pancreatic enzymes; malabsorption; hyperglycemia	
	Hypersecretion	Hypoglycemia	
Ovarian	Ascites	Hypoalbuminemia; early satiety; fluid and electrolyte disturbances	
Musculoskeletal	Pain, immobility, weakness, bone destruction	Loss of appetite; hypercalcemia; osteoporosis	

Anorexia

All the treatments for cancer may cause anorexia. The classic nausea and vomiting associated with many chemotherapeutic agents eliminate any interest in food for fear of the consequences. Constipation, immobility, dysphagia, odynophagia, fatigue, infection, and stomatitis—all consequences of cancer treatments—contribute to decreased interest in and sometimes aversion to food. Decreased food intake contributes to general weakness and weight loss.

Constipation

Constipation and adynamic ileus are major complications of the drug vincristine. Surgical procedures involving the alimentary tract may produce a transient constipation until bowel function is restored. Immobility and/or the administration of narcotics for pain contribute to constipation. Whatever the cause, constipation creates a full abdominal feeling and discomfort and contributes to anorexia.

Diarrhea

Diarrhea is most commonly the result of chemotherapy or abdominal radiation. The diarrhea associated with chemotherapy is part of general mucosal toxicity. The rapidly proliferating cells of the intestinal mucosa are highly susceptible to the effects of chemotherapy. Diarrhea is particularly severe after the administration of actinomycin D and 5-fluorouracil (5-FU) but also frequently occurs after the administration of thioguanine, methotrexate, floxuridine, hydroxyurea, the nitrosoureas, and 5-azacytidine. In severe cases the diarrhea may be accompanied by proctitis, ulceration, fistulas, and bleeding, which lead to dehydration, electrolyte imbalances, and malnutrition. In rare cases diarrhea may be so severe as to cause perforation of the bowel.

Abdominal irradiation also causes diarrhea as a result of mucosal toxicity. Altered function of the bowel and malabsorption occur during therapy but usually disappear when radiotherapy is stopped. In some cases symptoms of late radiation changes may occur within 1 year and up to 10 or more years following abdominal irradiation and include diarrhea, ulceration, fibrosis, fistula formation, and obstruction. Bowel resection may be required in severe cases.

Fistulas

In many cases surgery precedes the development of a fistula. The fistula may develop as a result of technical defects such as inadequate closure, unrecognized damage to internal structures, lack of blood supply to an anastomosis, or tension on an anastomosis. In cancer, fistulas may develop as a result of tissue necrosis adjacent to an expanding tumor or tissue destruction caused by chemotherapy or radiotherapy.

The complications of fistulas include loss of fluids and electrolytes, infection, and malnutrition due to loss of nutrients. The higher in the gastrointestinal tract the fistula is located, the more serious the complications and the higher the mortality rate.

Fluid and electrolyte imbalances

Fluid and electrolyte disturbances occur frequently as a result of cancer therapy. Vomiting, diarrhea, and fistulas may induce profound fluid and electrolyte imbalances through losses in excreta. Fluid volume is depleted, and sodium, chloride, and potassium are lost. Metabolic alkalosis may occur.

Surgical procedures may evoke fluid and electrolyte disturbances as a result of body fluid losses. In addition, surgical procedures may alter hormone secretion, indirectly affecting fluid and electrolyte homeostasis.

Treatment measures may indirectly alter fluid and electrolyte homeostasis as a result of kidney damage. In hyperuricemia resulting from a sudden increase in the release of uric acid after cytotoxic chemotherapy of lymphoproliferative diseases, urate crystals may be deposited in the kidney, resulting in renal shutdown and subsequent fluid and electrolyte disturbances.

Infection

All techniques used in cancer treatment predispose individuals to infection by suppressing the immune system. Chemotherapy and radiotherapy to sites of hematopoiesis damage hematopoietic tissue, impose neutropenia, and place the individual at risk for infection. Infection increases the metabolic demands on the host and may facilitate malnutrition.

Malabsorption

Intestinal malabsorption may occur as a result of several factors:

1. Interruption of the structure of the bowel. Surgical procedures such as intestinal resection reduce the absorptive surface of the gastrointestinal tract.

2. Damage to the absorptive surface of the bowel. Cytotoxic drugs and radiotherapy injure the epithelial cells that line the intestine. Damage to these epithelial cells flattens the intestinal villi and reduces the absorptive surface of the bowel, resulting in malabsorption of fat, protein, carbohydrate, vitamins, and minerals as well as loss of fluid.

3. Lack of the substance necessary for the absorption of nutrients. In liver dysfunction arising from surgical procedures, chemotherapy, or immunotherapy, lack of bile impairs the absorption of fats from the duodenum. Pancreatectomy eliminates the digestive enzymes that are important for the absorption of nutrients. Gastrectomy reduces or eliminates the gastric secretions that aid in the breakdown of foods to prepare for digestion and absorption. Bilateral vagotomy required in conjunction with esophagectomy induces significant malabsorption of fat and the clinical manifestation of steatorrhea.

Mucositis

The rapid turnover of epithelial cells of the mucous membranes makes them vulnerable to the toxicities of chemotherapy and radiotherapy. Because chemotherapy is a systemic treatment, all mucous membranes are at risk; however, the most common sites of mucositis are the oral cavity and the esophagus. Drugs that contribute to nutritional deterioration by rendering the person unable to eat because of painful oral mucosal toxicities include bleomycin, mitomycin, actinomycin D, methotrexate, mercaptopurine, thioguanine, vinblastine sulfate, daunorubicin, doxorubicin, and 5-FU.

Radiotherapy that includes mucosal tissue in the radiation field will lead to mucositis of the irradiated tissue. The development and severity of mucositis following radiation therapy depend on the dose of radiation and the method of administration. Mucositis usually disappears when therapy is discontinued; however, fibrosis with esophageal stricture may occur as a delayed effect of radiotherapy.

Nausea and vomiting

Nausea and vomiting are most commonly associated with the administration of antineoplastic drugs. The nausea and vomiting following chemotherapy are mediated by the chemoreceptor trigger zone located in the area postrema of the brain's fourth ventricle. Nausea and vomiting occur with many anticancer drugs and may be anticipatory.

As a result of the administration of some drugs, vomiting may be so severe as to require the dosage of the drug to be reduced or the chemotherapy to be interrupted. Drugs that may cause severe and prolonged nausea and vomiting include cisplatin, dacarbazine, cyclophosphamide, streptozotocin, actinomycin D, doxorubicin, and mechlorethamine. The nutritional consequences of prolonged vomiting are profound. The current practice of using combination antiemetic therapy involving a serotonin antagonist such as ondansetron (Zofran®) successfully minimizes nausea and vomiting with chemotherapy as well as radiation therapy. (Detailed discussion of the nausea and vomiting of chemotherapy and its treatment may be found in Chapter 16.)

Taste changes

Individuals receiving some antineoplastic drugs complain of experiencing a metallic taste during the intravenous administration of these agents. Drugs implicated include nitrogen mustard, cisplatin, and cyclophosphamide. Some individuals become so sensitized by this taste that they begin vomiting at the mere thought of the drug administration, even as they enter the waiting room of the outpatient clinic. Other taste changes have been documented in relation to the administration of specific drugs. 5-FU has been documented to cause decreased sensitivity to salty and sweet tastes.[47]

Radiotherapy to the head and neck region destroys taste buds and cells responsible for the secretion of saliva, resulting in a condition called *xerostomia*. The volume of saliva is decreased, and the saliva that is produced is viscid, acidic, and high in organic content. Individuals complain that food tastes like cardboard or cotton. Decreased taste perception and difficult mastication are the consequences, compounding the preexisting functional problems that result from extensive surgical procedures in the head and neck region.

Additionally, dental caries commonly result from the xerostomia and alteration in bacterial flora in the mouth.

NUTRITIONAL ASSESSMENT

Nutritional assessment is the critical first step in developing a comprehensive approach to nutritional management of the individual with cancer. For those with suspected nutritional problems, nutritional assessment serves as a foundation for the nutritional care plan and provides a baseline against which the effects of nutritional care can be measured. Nutritional reassessment is important for both hospitalized individuals and those receiving ambulatory care.

Nutritional Screening

Due to their disease and expected treatment, most individuals with cancer are candidates for nutritional screening. This procedure is usually performed shortly after hospital or clinic admission. It involves asking the patient a few questions about appetite, ability to eat, and recent weight change. The results of this brief interview as well as the individual's diagnosis and admission laboratory data are forwarded to a dietitian for evaluation. Nutritional screening programs for outpatients have also been developed.[48]

Physical Signs

Weight loss is the physical change that first leads many individuals with cancer to seek medical treatment. It is often the first gross sign of malnutrition as well. In advanced disease, weight loss is obvious with signs such as a protruding body skeleton and muscular wasting. The nurse conducting a general physical examination of the person with cancer should pay particular attention to the condition of the mucous membranes, skin, eyes, lips, oral cavity, nails, subcutaneous tissues, and muscles as indices of nutritional status. Manifestations of malnutrition include sparse, thin hair; pallor; dry, flaky skin; dull, sunken eyes; apathy; mouth lesions; muscle and tissue wasting; and edema. An evaluation of mental status, performance level, and the ability of an individual to feed himself or herself, prepare meals, or follow a nutritional care plan assists in formulating the nutritional plan.

Dietary History

A nutritional history informs the clinician about an individual's usual dietary intake. The nurse should obtain information about the type and quantity of food consumed, likes and dislikes, location and time of meals, the family living situation, difficulties with chewing or swallowing, nausea, vomiting, or diarrhea. Information about whether an individual has been prescribed a modified diet and about compliance with that diet is obtained.

Dietary recall

During a dietary recall, an individual is asked to record specific types and quantities of food consumed over a specific period of time (usually 24 hours). A checklist of common foods may be used to stimulate an individual's memory of food eaten. A food frequency list is another tool that may be used to quantify oral intake over a period of several days (usually a week).

The dietary recall is easy to use, but its accuracy depends on the skill of the person obtaining the history, the communication skills of the individual and the interviewer, and the individual's motivation.

Weighed inventory

A more accurate dietary history may be obtained by asking an individual to weigh food. In the hospital setting a nurse or dietitian may weigh the food. At home an individual may use standard household measures. Accuracy of this technique depends on the skill level and motivation of the individual performing the weighing. Also, individuals may alter intake to avoid weighing the food.

With both the dietary recall and weighed inventory methods of obtaining a dietary history, standard food tables are used to analyze nutrient intake. Nutrient deficits are noted and areas for potential improvement in nutrient intake are identified. The diet history also helps the clinician develop an individualized nutritional plan.

Anthropometric Measurements

Anthropometric measurements are physical measurements of the human body that are used to estimate body composition. Standard measurements for adults include weight, height, midarm circumference, and skinfold thickness.

Height

Height may be obtained by asking the patient or from the medical record. When self-reporting height, individuals tend to overestimate how tall they are.[49] Therefore, height is best measured using the ruler found with the standard hospital scale. For the recumbent patient, height can be measured by using a kneeheight caliper and comparing the results to tables.[50] An estimate of height can also be made by doubling the measurement taken from the sternal notch to the tip of the longest finger on the dominant hand.[51]

Weight

Body weight is one of the most important measures of the nutritional assessment. Several investigators have demonstrated that increased morbidity and mortality are associated with significant weight loss. Johnston et al.[52] found that dysgeusia, xerostomia, dysphagia, and mouth pain associated with head and neck radiation were greater and lasted longer in individuals with weight loss. DeWys[53] demonstrated that the median survival of cancer patients who experienced weight loss before receiving chemotherapy was half that of individuals who had not lost weight. Hickman et al.[54] found that individuals who weighed 20% less than their ideal weight had a complication rate of over 70% and a mortality rate of 42% after surgery for colorectal cancer. DeWys et al.[53] demonstrated that weight loss alone was a powerful independent prognosticator of survival in women with breast cancer. While weight is an important factor in assessing nutritional status and possibly in predicting the outcome of therapy, the benefits of weight repletion prior to therapy are unknown. Weight gain during cancer treatment is not often a practical goal; therefore, the focus of nutritional management is on weight maintenance.

An individual is weighed in light clothing and without shoes, using a lever or balance beam scale. Weight may be rounded to the nearest 0.5 kg. Current measured weight is then compared against usual and ideal weight.

Ideal weight can be obtained by several methods. The commonly used Hamwi equations[55] follow:

1. For women, ideal weight is estimated by adding 5 pounds for every inch the woman is over 5 feet tall to a figure of 100 pounds.
2. For men, ideal weight is estimated by adding 6 pounds for every inch the man is over 5 feet to a figure of 106 pounds.

A measured weight figure that falls within a range 10% above or below the ideal weight thus derived is interpreted as normal.

Several tables of ideal weight for height exist and may be in common clinical use. However, these tables represent normal weight for healthy individuals and should be used cautiously in interpreting the weight of individuals with cancer. The percentage of ideal weight is calculated as follows:

$$\text{Percentage of ideal body weight} = \frac{\text{Actual weight}}{\text{Ideal weight}} \times 100$$

Although the percentage of ideal body weight may be an indicator of weight loss, there are several limitations to using it as a standard. The index may not be an accurate measure of nutritional status. For example, the actual weight of a formerly obese individual may be close to the ideal weight; however, the person's weight is significantly lower than the pre-illness weight. The person may be malnourished, even though he or she is at ideal weight.

A more sensitive index of nutritional status is percent weight change. The formula for this calculation is in Table 27-2. The percent weight change indicates the extent of tissue loss as a result of inadequate nutrition. Questions that can be asked of an individual to accurately assess pre-illness weight include: How much did you weigh when you got married? How much did you weigh 10 years ago? 5 years ago? 1 year ago? The questions asked should provide a frame of reference and reveal whether weight loss occurred gradually over a long period or rapidly over a short period. Table 27-2 provides a means of evaluating weight loss over time. In evaluating weights obtained serially for the same patient, two factors deserve consideration:

1. *Calibration and accuracy of the scale.* It is best to use the same scale for each weighing. The zero point should be checked daily (or more often if the scale is moved), and the scale should be calibrated regularly (every few months) against the reference weight to maintain accuracy.

2. *Presence and degree of edema or dehydration.* Body fluid composition as well as intake and output can have a profound effect on daily weight fluctuations.

TABLE 27-2 Evaluation of Weight Change*

Time	Significant Weight Loss	Severe Weight Loss
1 wk	1%–2%	>2%
1 mo	5%	>5%
3 mo	7.5%	>7.5%
6 mo	10%	>10%

*Values charged are for percent weight change

$$\text{Percent weight change} = \frac{\text{Usual weight} - \text{actual weight}}{\text{Usual weight}} \times 100$$

Source: Blackburn GL, Bistrian BR, Maini BS, et al: Nutritional and metabolic assessment of the hospitalized patient. *J Parent Ent Nutr* 1:17, 1977.

Skinfold measurement

The skinfold thickness measurement is an indicator of subcutaneous body fat. Although the distribution of subcutaneous fat varies substantially from individual to individual, variations within an individual as a result of dietary alterations appear to occur proportionately throughout the body.[56] Therefore, a measurement of subcutaneous fat will reflect changes in total body fat. Skinfold thickness measurements can be taken from the subscapular or pectoral areas, abdomen, triceps, or biceps. The actual measurement obtained is the double thickness of the pinched skin plus the subcutaneous adipose tissue.

The skinfold thickness measurement is relatively reproducible provided that it is conducted by a trained clinician who does all the measurements on the same individual. However, variability of measurements obtained by different clinicians leads to criticism of skinfold measurements as indicators of nutritional status. While comparison to standards developed for healthy individuals may have limited use for individuals with cancer, serial measurements over time may have clinical utility.

Midarm muscle circumference

Arm muscle circumference has been shown to be a sensitive index of protein status that correlates significantly with serum albumin levels.[57] Once again, it is important that the same trained clinician perform all measurements, as measurements obtained by different clinicians can vary by as much as 5%. The methodology has been described elsewhere.[58] From measured arm circumference and triceps skinfold thickness, arm muscle circumference can be calculated.

$$\text{Arm muscle circumference (cm)} = \text{Arm circumference (cm)} - [0.314 \times \text{triceps skinfold (mm)}]$$

Triceps skinfold and midarm muscle circumference are measured during the initial examination and serially to determine changes in body composition.

Biochemical Measurements

Biochemical data provide important information about the actual deficiencies of specific substances in the body. Biochemical data are the most specific of the assessment parameters, detecting covert nutritional deficiencies and thus allowing early intervention.

The major biochemical parameters for assessing nutritional status can be divided into those that measure lean body mass and the transport proteins synthesized by the liver.

Transport proteins synthesized by the liver

Standard measurements of protein status include serum levels of albumin, transferrin, and prealbumin (transthyretin). Albumin has a half-life of 20 days, transferrin has a half-life of 8 days, and prealbumin has a half-life of 2 days. Therefore, serum albumin, transferrin, and prealbumin measurements assess the individual's long-term, intermediate, and short-term protein status, respectively.

Several investigators have found decreased plasma albumin levels to be associated with increased complication rates after cancer treatment.[54,59] Mullen et al.[60] observed that when the level of serum albumin was less than 3.0 g/dl, individuals had a postoperative complication rate that was 2.5 times greater than that of individuals with a higher serum albumin concentration. Thus, serum protein measurements can be used to identify an individual's risk of developing complications before therapy so that nutritional therapy can be instituted to prevent complications.

The plasma concentration of proteins measures the net result of protein synthesis versus protein degradation. However, plasma protein concentration is also affected by changes in the amount and distribution of body fluids, changes in capillary permeability, external losses, and ineffective lymphatic return. Therefore, hypoalbuminemia may be the result of a number of physiologic processes, including malnutrition.

Lean body mass

Urinary creatinine has long been considered an excellent index of lean body mass.[61] All muscle produces creatinine; therefore, the proportion of creatinine produced is directly proportional to the amount of muscle in the body. Creatinine excretion is fairly constant in an individual with normal renal function. In the individual with cancer or other malnourished individuals, creatinine excretion is decreased as muscle protein is degraded and used to meet energy requirements.

Twenty-four-hour urine collections are used to measure urinary creatinine for nutritional assessment. For reliable results, three collections are needed. Creatinine excretion is compared with ideal creatinine excretion for height to determine the *creatinine height index*, as follows.

$$\text{Creatinine height index} = \frac{\text{Actual urinary creatinine excretion}}{\text{Ideal urinary creatinine excretion}} \times 100$$

Ideal creatinine excretion is determined as 23 mg/kg of ideal body weight for males and 18 mg/kg of ideal body weight for females.[62]

Immunologic Measurements

Immune function is a critical measure of nutritional status. Cell-mediated immunity orchestrated by T lymphocytes is especially vulnerable to the effects of malnutrition. The degree of T-lymphocyte depresson correlates in an almost linear fashion with the degree of protein-calorie malnutrition.[63] Protein-calorie malnutrition places the individual at greater risk of infection and results in a poorer response to cancer therapy. Daly et al.[64] showed that individuals without an immune response averaged over 20 kg greater weight loss than individuals whose immune systems were functioning.

Two measurements are commonly used to evaluate immune function in relation to nutritional status: total lymphocyte count and skin sensitivity tests to recall antigens. The total lymphocyte count is derived from a complete blood count and calculated as follows:

$$\text{Total lymphocyte count} = \frac{\text{Percent lymphocytes}}{100} \times \text{WBC}$$

The total lymphocyte count is decreased in individuals with protein-calorie malnutrition.

The second major test of immune response is the skin sensitivity test. When cell-mediated immunity is impaired, there is a diminished response or lack of response to antigens to which the individual was previously exposed. This lack of response is called *anergy*.

An individual may be tested with a variety of antigens. The most common antigens are tetanus toxoid, diptheria toxoid, streptococcus, old tuberculin, candida, trichophyton, and proteus. The antigen is injected just under the skin. The induration is measured in millimeters at 24 hours and 48 hours.

Dionigi and colleagues[65] demonstrated that the skin test was an important prognosticator of postoperative complications in individuals with cancer undergoing surgery. Septic complications occurred in 37% of normoergic, 46% of hypoergic, and 83% of anergic individuals.

Several factors may limit the usefulness of the skin test in assessing nutritional status. Technical difficulties such as improper method of administration, reader variability, lack of previous exposure to the antigen, and so on may alter the individual's response to the antigen and provide false information. Concomitant diseases or therapies may be immunosuppressive and cause a lack of response. For example, because of general anesthesia, cell-mediated immunity can be depressed for as long as 2–3 weeks after surgery. In addition, immune components have high metabolic priority and thus are reduced only in severe malnutrition. Because of these limitations, several investigators do not recommend skin testing to measure immune status in a nutritional assessment.[66]

Summary

Table 27-3 summarizes the components of the nutritional assessment and provides a guide for collecting and evaluating both subjective and objective data. Once malnutrition is diagnosed, a therapeutic plan is established and implemented on the basis of the data obtained from the nutritional assessment. After the therapeutic plan is implemented, periodic reassessment should be done to evaluate the effects of therapy.

TABLE 27-3 Components of the Nutritional Assessment

Medical History	Physical Examination
Duration and type of malignancy Frequency, type, and severity of complications (infections, draining lesions, etc) Type and duration of therapy Specific chemotherapeutic agents used Radiation sites Antibiotics used Other drugs used Surgical procedures performed (site, type, date) Side effects of therapy (diarrhea, anorexia, nausea and vomiting) Concomitant medical conditions (diabetes, heart disease, liver failure, kidney failure, infection)	General appearance Condition of hair Condition of skin Condition of teeth Condition of mouth, gums, and throat Edema Performance status Identification of nutritionally related problems (fistula, pain, stomatitis, xerostomia, infection, constipation, diarrhea, nausea and vomiting, obstruction)
Dietary History	**Socioeconomic History**
24-hr recall of foods eaten, including snacks Composition of food taken in 24 hrs (calories and protein, caffeine, liquor) Time of day meals and snacks eaten Past or current diet modifications Self-feeding ability Special cancer diet Vitamins, minerals, or other supplements Modifications of diet or eating habits as a result of treatment or illness Foods withheld or given on the basis of personal or religious grounds (kosher, vegetarian, etc) Food preferences Food allergies or intolerances	Number of persons living in the home (ages and relationships) Kitchen facilities Income Food purchased by Food prepared by Amount spent on food per month Outside provision of meals
Anthropometric Data	**Biochemical Data**
Height Weight Actual weight as percentage of ideal Weight change as percentage of usual Triceps skinfold measurement Actual triceps skinfold as percentage of standard Midarm circumference Midarm muscle circumference Actual midarm muscle circumference as percentage of standard	Hematocrit Hemoglobin Serum albumin Serum transferrin Creatinine Creatinine height index Total lymphocyte count Delayed hypersensitivity response—skin testing Nitrogen balance Blood urea nitrogen Sodium, potassium, carbon dioxide, chloride Glucose

NUTRITIONAL MANAGEMENT

Malnutrition was once considered to be an inevitable consequence of advanced cancer. With the advent of relatively safe methods of delivering aggressive nutritional support and an increasing body of research demonstrating the positive effects of nutritional support on the quality and quantity of life for the person with cancer, clinicians now consider malnutrition an unnecessary and often preventable consequence of cancer. Aggressive nutritional therapy for individuals with cancer has been shown to decrease the morbidity and mortality of cancer and its therapy by preventing weight loss, maintaining or improving nutritional status, increasing responsiveness to therapy, minimizing side effects of therapy, improving the individual's sense of well-being, and improving the quality of life. The discussion of nutritional management in this section is concerned with the treatment of existing nutritional deficiencies as well as the prevention of deficiencies in the high-risk individual.

Controversies in Nutritional Support

Despite advances in the effectiveness of nutritional support therapies, controversy exists over whether nutritional therapy is contraindicated in some individuals with cancer. For example, there is concern that nourishing an individual with cancer may enhance tumor growth by improving the nutrient supply. As discussed earlier in this chapter, the energy requirements of a rapidly growing tumor take precedence over the individual's nutrient needs. Although tumor growth is stimulated in rats as a result of exogenously administered nutrients,[68] it is unclear whether the same phenomenon occurs in humans. Westin et al.[69] suggested that total parenteral nutrition (TPN) had no impact on human head and neck tumors, in contrast to findings in animals. Other studies[70,71] have shown that individuals with cancer who receive nutritional support have less chemotherapeutic toxicities, are able to tolerate larger doses of drugs, achieve positive nitrogen balance and weight gain, and live longer (for those who respond to treatment). In addition, improvement of the tumor's nutritional supply may stimulate the proliferation of malignant cells, inducing a more favorable response to chemotherapy or radiotherapy.[72]

Torosian et al.[72] demonstrated in an animal model that parenteral protein (with or without hypertonic dextrose) potentiates the tumor response to methotrexate without increasing host toxicity. One possible explanation for the enhanced tumor response to cycle-specific chemotherapy is increased induction of tumor cells into S-phase (synthesis), where the drug acts.[73]

Despite the initial enthusiasm for parenteral nutrition, several reviews suggest that routine provision of parenteral nutrition to individuals with cancer is not indicated.[74,75] One study concludes that with the exception of the bone marrow transplant patient, there are insufficient data to support routine aggressive nutrition support in the nonsurgical oncology patient.[76] For the malnourished individual with cancer who is undergoing surgery, there may be some benefit to preoperative nutritional support.[77] In a trial of perioperative nutritional support, no benefit to parenteral nutrition was realized except to the most severely malnourished patients.[78] However, in this trial, overfeeding may have resulted in an elevated infection rate. In view of the risks and expense of parenteral nutrition, the American Society for Parenteral and Enteral Nutrition (ASPEN)[79–81] and the American College of Physicians[82] have published guidelines for use of TPN. These guidelines suggest that routine use of parenteral nutrition is of limited benefit to individuals receiving chemotherapy. The ASPEN guidelines suggest that individuals with cancer be given aggressive nutritional support using the enteral or parenteral route only as an adjunct to aggressive treatment for tumor.

In addition, TPN is not indicated for the person whose life would be prolonged needlessly by its use. In fact, ethical decisions are reached by carefully considering factors including physiologic benefits and risks, patient preference, quality of life, cost, family concerns, and previous legal decisions.[83]

Establishing the Nutritional Therapy Plan

Identifying the goal of nutritional therapy

The first factor to be considered in selecting a nutritional therapy plan is the goal of the therapy. Is the goal of nutritional therapy weight gain? Weight maintenance? Restoration of immune function? Improvement of the person's sense of well-being? Prolongation of life? The therapeutic goal will determine the most effective method. The individual and family must participate in establishing the therapeutic goal.

Establishing the individual's caloric requirements

The average resting adult requires approximately 1200–1800 kcal/day (18–22 kcal/kg body weight) to maintain the basal metabolic rate (BMR). Any condition that increases energy expenditure, such as advanced cancer, sepsis, a healing wound, a draining fistula, or even simple exercise, increases the individual's caloric needs. Weight loss occurs when the energy expended is in excess of the calories consumed. The caloric intake necessary to maintain an individual's weight or cause the individual to gain weight must be determined on the basis of the nutritional assessment, and the results of nutritional therapy must be evaluated regularly so that adjustments can be made.

BMR is a measure of the amount of energy required to sustain life in a fasting, resting individual. BMR is determined primarily by an individual's body size; however, age, sex, and the stress of illness are also factors. Investigators found that energy requirements vary in individuals with cancer.[84,85] Not every individual is hypermetabolic. In fact, 25%–35% of patients are hypometabolic, 40%–50% are normometabolic, and only 25% are hypermetabolic. Therefore, because energy expenditure cannot be predicted accurately in cancer patients, measurement of energy expenditure by indirect calorimetry, when available, may be valuable for individualizing the caloric prescription.

When indirect calorimetry is not possible, Bell et al.[86] recommend the following formula based on the BMR calculated from the Harris-Benedict equations:

$$\begin{aligned}\text{Calories} &= 1.2 - 1.3 \times \text{BMR} \quad \text{where}\\ \text{BMR (men)} &= 66 + 13.8(\text{weight, kg})\\ &\quad + 5.0\,(\text{height, cm}) - 6.8\,(\text{age, yr})\\ \text{BMR (women)} &= 655 + 9.6(\text{weight, kg})\\ &\quad + 1.9\,(\text{height, cm}) - 4.7(\text{age, yr})\end{aligned}$$

These formulas do no apply to obese individuals because BMR is correlated with lean body mass. For obese individuals, ideal body weight is substituted for actual body weight in the formulas for BMR.

Activity level is the major variable in the energy requirements of individuals. A more active individual will require more calories per day to maintain or gain weight. Long et al.[87] estimated that the average hospitalized individual requires an addition of 20% to the BMR to adjust for minimal activities such as short walks, turning in bed, and walking from bed to chair. For the outpatient further increases in BMR may be based on activity levels.

Once caloric needs have been established, the composition of the diet and method of feeding may be determined.

Composition of the diet

Carefully planned dietary intake is important in providing the individual's energy requirements and the nutrients necessary to maintain important physiologic processes. Energy requirements are supplied primarily from carbohydrates and fat; lean tissue anabolism is supported by proteins, minerals, and vitamins. Energy requirements, present nutritional deficits, allergies, individual preferences, and conditions that affect digestion or absorption all must be considered.

Because there is no body protein reserve for energy as there is for fat in adipose tissue and carbohydrate in liver glycogen, the main aim of nutritional therapy is to protect or restore body protein. Nitrogen balance is an index of protein balance in the body. A positive nitrogen balance implies that body protein is intact: a negative nitrogen balance implies that body protein is being depleted.

An individual must take in both calories and protein to maintain a positive nitrogen balance. In the normal individual, at least 7%–8% of the total calories taken in must be provided by protein to maintain a positive nitrogen balance.[88] For the hypermetabolic individual, protein requirements will double and should be 15%–20% of the total calories or 1.5–2.0-g protein/kg body weight. In patients with liver and/or renal dysfunction, protein may need to be limited.

Enteral Nutrition

It has been demonstrated that the nutritional benefits of enteral and parenteral routes of feeding are comparable.[89,90] In addition, tube feeding is less expensive and more physiologic than TPN. The selection of one method of feeding over another is usually based on gastrointestinal function. The cost of enteral feeding is less than parenteral feeding, and with improved formulas, procedures, and equipment, the enteral route has become a popular approach to nutritional support. In addition, the benefits of enteral feeding in maintaining immune status are being illuminated.[91,92]

Oral feeding

If the individual is able to consume an adequate quantity of foods orally, a regular diet composed of the appropriate amount of protein and calories is preferred. The dietary plan is determined primarily by individual nutrient needs and food preferences. For those unable to eat adequate amounts, supplemental calories, protein, vitamins, and minerals may be indicated. Liquid nutritional formulas administered orally or by tube have been used for this purpose. In their study of head and neck cancer patients undergoing radiation therapy, Arnold and Richter[93] found that liquid nutritional supplements increased rather than supplanted usual food intake and resulted in improved serum albumin concentrations. However, they found no effect on weight loss or other adverse effects of radiation therapy between supplemented and nonsupplemented individuals with cancer.

Composition of the diet may be altered based on individual symptoms experienced as a result of the tumor or cancer treatments. Suggestions for alterations in diet to maximize oral intake are included in Table 27-4. Despite the well-known impact of cancer therapy on oral intake, there are limited data available to guide the clinician in providing dietary modifications to those with cancer. In a study of children receiving radiation, a gluten-free, lactose-free, low-residue diet resulted in prevention of acute and chronic radiation enteritis.[94] More recently, foods with neutral taste and odor have been used to increase the nutrient intake of those receiving chemotherapy.[95] It is generally the role of the nurse to observe and record the intake of and tolerance to diet. The nurse and dietitian will monitor and assess whether an individual is maintaining adequate nutritional status with the food ingested.

Enteral feeding

If oral intake alone cannot prevent weight loss, or if the person's physical condition prevents oral intake, tube (enteral) feeding may be indicated. Enteral feeding requires a functioning gastrointestinal tract with a minimum of 30 cm of functioning small bowel and an intact ileocecal valve. For those with tumors of the head and neck, lung, or upper gastrointestinal tract, feeding directly into the small intestine may be indicated.

Recent advances in enteral feeding have made this technique more practical to use. Small, soft nasoenteric feeding tubes are more comfortable than standard nasogastric tubes; percutaneous endoscopic feeding tube placement techniques enable long-term tube placement without general anesthesia. The "button" gastrostomy or jejunostomy, which leaves an individual with a small abdominal opening at the skin level rather than a tube protruding from the abdominal wall, is an important advance in maintaining body image.

Tube feedings may be administered by nasogastric or nasointestinal means. For a more permanent feeding, a surgically placed esophagostomy, gastrostomy, or jejunostomy tube may be indicated. A detailed discussion of tube feeding administration is available in Rombeau and Caldwell.[96]

Formula selection Liquid formulas for enteral feeding may be prepared from regular food, or commercial preparations may be purchased. Commercial

TABLE 27-4 Suggested Approaches to Problems That Interfere with Normal Nutrition

Problem	Intervention
Dysphagia	Eat soft or liquid foods Blenderize solid foods Moisten foods with cream, gravies, or oils Eat bland foods that are smooth in texture and tepid to minimize pain
Nausea/vomiting	Avoid acid foods such as citrus juice and tomatoes Eat salty foods, or add salt to foods Avoid overly sweet, greasy, or high-fat foods Drink clear, cool beverages Eat dry foods such as toast or crackers, especially after getting up in the morning Eat slowly and chew food thoroughly Eat small, frequent meals Frozen juice sticks or gelatin provide fluid Rest with the head elevated after eating Avoid rich, sweet foods Wear loose clothing Avoid favorite foods during chemotherapy to avoid developing an aversion to them Take antinausea, antiemetic, tranquilizing medications as prescribed
Early satiety	Eat five or six small meals per day Keep nutritious snacks available between meals Eat foods high in calories and low in fat Avoid greasy foods Chew foods slowly Avoid liquids with meals, take them ½ hour before or ½ hour after meals Drink nutritious liquids such as juice, milk, or milkshakes
Pancreatic insufficiency	Take digestive enzymes as prescribed Follow a diet low in fat and high in calories and protein Take commercial food supplements as prescribed
Anorexia	Eat small, frequent meals Make changes in diet or surroundings Try new recipes or foods, eat with friends, or go to a favorite restaurant Stimulate appetite with light exercise Time meals to coincide with the "best time" of the day Eat nutritious, high-protein snacks Avoid "empty calorie" foods such as coffee or diet soda Take medications with high-calorie foods or nutritional supplements Add powdered milk to foods during cooking to increase their protein content Drink a small glass of wine or fruit juice before meals to stimulate the appetite Avoid fatty foods Foods served cold (fruit, salads, sandwiches) may be easier to tolerate
Dumping syndrome	Eat foods low in concentrated carbohydrate, but high in protein Eat several small, dry meals during the day Avoid liquids with meals; take them ½ hour before or ½ hour after meals Avoid sugar, candy, jam, jelly, honey, desserts
Constipation	Drink at least 2 quarts of fluid daily Eat high-fiber foods such as fruits, vegetables, whole-grain breads and cereals, bran, dried fruits, and nuts Engage in light, regular exercise Utilize previously successful bowel stimulants
Diarrhea	Drink plenty of fluids to avoid dehydration Avoid milk or milk products, unless treated with lactase enzyme Electrolyte replacement fluids may be needed if diarrhea persists Avoid foods high in fiber Avoid high-fat, spicy, and gas-forming foods Eat foods rich in potassium (fruit and vegetable juices)
Dyspepsia	Avoid fatty foods Avoid spicy foods Elevate the upper trunk following meals Use antacids

(continued)

TABLE 27-4 Suggested Approaches to Problems That Interfere with Normal Nutrition (continued)

Problem	Intervention
Stomatitis	Eat soft or liquid foods Avoid irritating foods that are rough or acid Use warm saline irrigants to cleanse the mouth Cold or frozen foods may numb pain Avoid extremely hot beverages
Taste changes	Marinate red meat with sweet marinades or soy sauce Substitute poultry, fish, eggs, or cheese for red meat Serve meats chilled rather than hot (eg, chicken salad or cold sliced beef or chicken) Use high-protein liquid supplements if meat is not tolerated Rinse the mouth with carbonated water or suck on a lemon wedge before meals to clear the palate Mildly acid foods such as lemonade, tea with lemon, pickled foods, citrus fruits and juices may stimulate the taste buds Extra spices, onion, or garlic may improve the flavor of food Keep experimenting; foods previously avoided may now be acceptable due to taste changes
Xerostomia	Moisten foods with gravies or sauces Use artificial saliva as prescribed Use a blender or food processor to make foods easier to eat Soak foods in coffee, tea, milk, cocoa, or warm beverages Avoid dry foods such as crackers or toast Swallow liquid with each bite of food Use a humidifier or steam kettle in the room where food is eaten
General	Drink plenty of fluids Make mealtime pleasant with different surroundings and pleasant company Serve food attractively; use garnishes Experiment with recipes, flavorings, spices, types, and consistencies of food. Likes and dislikes may change from day to day Avoid empty calorie foods such as soda Eat high-calorie foods Take advantage of the best time of the day for eating Eat early in the day if energy levels are higher then Keep nutritious snacks handy to increase nutrient intake

formulas are convenient and ensure consistent nutritional composition and microbiological safety. Selection of the liquid formulas may depend on cost, the resources available for preparing liquid formulas at home, and individual preference for a formula made from regular food.

The most commonly used enteral formulas are those designed as complete diets. These are appropriate for the majority of enterally fed individuals with cancer. They provide 1 kcal/cc, are lactose-free, ready to feed, and isotonic. The macronutrient composition is approximately 12%–20% protein, 45%–60% carbohydrate, and 30%–40% fat. When fed at calorically adequate levels, these formulas provide adequate micronutrients (vitamins and trace minerals) for physiologically stressed individuals with cancer. For individuals who are volume-sensitive or who suffer early satiety, concentrated feedings providing 1.5–2.0 kcal/cc are available.[97] A number of formulas (e.g., high-branched chain amino acid, renal failure, and hepatic failure) are available for those with special needs. Cost and efficacy are considered in selecting these products. New enteral products are frequently introduced; therefore, it is advisable for the nurse to keep an updated product information file for clinical reference.

Complications of enteral feeding Gastrointestinal side effects, the most frequently noted complications of enteral feeding,[98] tend to lessen over time, making enteral feeding appropriate for long-term use.[99] Diarrhea is a common side effect of enteral feeding and has been attributed to formula-related factors including lactose content,[100] bacterial contamination,[101] and osmolality.[102] In addition, diarrhea in those receiving enteral feedings has been associated with hypoalbuminemia,[103] concurrent administration with hyperosmolar or sorbitol containing medications,[104,105] broad-spectrum antibiotics, or other mediations that produce diarrhea[106] (e.g., chemotherapy). Interestingly, when compared in prospective fashion, osmolality and lactose content of feedings have not been shown to affect the incidence of diarrhea.[107–109] At least one study has shown no benefit to elaborate progressions of enteral formula strength and rate.[110] Patterson et al. and Gottschlich et al. demonstrated that patients with hypoalbuminemia tolerated enteral feeding as well as those with normal serum albumin levels,[111,112] although others have found different results.[113]

If diarrhea does not resolve within 2–3 days, a medical work-up may be indicated. Antidiarrheal medication (synthetic or natural opiates) may be prescribed for those without *Clostridium difficile* or other contraindications. Pectin, a soluble fiber, has been shown to reverse liquid stool in normal subjects receiving enteral feedings.[114] However, commercial enteral formulas containing pectin are not yet available. Commercial fiber-containing formulas use an insoluble fiber source that has not been shown to have an effect on diarrhea in tube-fed patients when compared to patients fed with nonfiber-containing formulas.[115,116]

Fluid and electrolyte disturbances may be noted due to underlying disease. However, hypernatremia, hyperchloremia, azotemia, and dehydration may occur as a result of excessively high concentration of electrolytes and protein in the formula, inadequate fluid intakes, or renal insufficiency. Daily monitoring of fluid status including weights can help prevent fluid and electrolyte imbalance.

Hyperglycemia may be noted during the initial stages of feeding and may continue in individuals with diabetes. Regular monitoring of blood and urine glucose levels is recommended until test results are consistently negative. Those with diabetes may require adjustments in hypoglycemic agents if they receive continuous enteral feedings.

Parenteral Nutrition

Total parenteral nutrition is the intravenous infusion of a concentrated mixture of amino acids, glucose, fluid, vitamins, minerals, electrolytes, and trace elements into a central vein. Essential fatty acids, which are important in many metabolic processes, are often infused with the TPN solution in a lipid emulsion. Usually the superior vena cava is used because of its large diameter that allows concentrated solutions to be infused relatively safely without causing thrombophlebitis.

Indications

Total parenteral nutrition is indicated when it becomes impossible to use enteral feedings due to a nonfunctioning gastrointestinal tract. For example, individuals with cancer of the gastrointestinal tract often face partial or total obstruction as a result of expanding tumor, altered bowel function resulting from surgical manipulation, malabsorption syndromes because of irradiation of the bowel, dehydration, or cachexia as a result of fluid and electrolyte loss from fistulas. In the past, fistulas were a major cause of mortality for persons with gastrointestinal cancers. But technological advances in intravenous nutrition have made it possible to feed the individual while resting the gut and permitting the fistula to heal.

In addition, many persons were unable to complete a full course of cancer therapy because of malnutrition. TPN allows the bowel to rest, promoting healing of surgically disrupted tissue or allowing fistulas to close spontaneously.

Goal setting

Before TPN therapy is instituted, it is important for the nutritional support team to establish a measurable goal for the outcome of therapy. Examples of goals include continuation of TPN until the person gains a certain amount of weight, completes a regimen of chemotherapy or radiotherapy, or until a fistula heals. Establishment of a goal will enable the team to evaluate the effects of nutritional therapy and will allow the individual receiving TPN to participate in attaining the goal or assessing the progress made toward it.

The plan for TPN therapy should be discussed thoroughly with the individual and family. The goals of therapy should be discussed with the individual, as well as what to expect regarding catheter insertion, monitoring studies and their purposes, dressing changes, care of the infusion equipment, possible complications, and the expected duration of therapy.

Complications

Mullen suggests that the risks associated with TPN and their frequency, severity, and outcome depend on the following:[117]

1. patient population—nutritional status, histologic type of tumor, stage of disease, rate of progression, and and concomitant therapy
2. competence of the nutritional support team
3. competence of the institutional core staff—physicians, nurses, pharmacists, and house staff
4. rapidity with which innovations are used
5. organizational management of the nutritional support team

Three categories of complications are associated with TPN therapy: infectious, mechanical, and metabolic.

Infectious complications The incidence of infectious complications associated with TPN therapy has decreased substantially in the last decade as a result of attention to the importance of a regular program of catheter care involving strict aseptic technique. The incidence of infection decreases when there is an organized approach to TPN care such as through the services of a TPN team. Ryan et al.[118] studied 200 patients who had 355 catheters in 4492 hospital days. The sepsis rate of these individuals was only 3% when strict aseptic technique was maintained. When catheter care protocols were violated, the sepsis rate rose to 20%.

Individuals with cancer are frequently immunosuppressed as a result of malignancy. The added insult of immunosuppressive therapy such as chemotherapy or radiotherapy makes the individual vulnerable to overwhelming infection. The introduction of TPN through a central or peripheral line creates a real risk of infection. In addition, glucose and protein-rich TPN solutions provide an excellent medium for bacterial and fungal growth.

Infection results from contamination of the TPN solution, insertion site, or the equipment used or, more rarely, from seeding of the catheter tip by blood-borne infection. Skin microorganisms are the most frequent cause of sepsis. Offending organisms are either bacterial or fungal. Bacterial organisms include *Staphylococcus aureus, Staphylococcus epidermidis,* and gram-negative bacteria such as *Klebsiella. Corynebacterium* has been recognized as an organism causing infection in individuals receiving TPN. Its incidence is increasing, expecially in severely immunosuppressed individuals, such as those who have undergone bone marrow transplantation.

Also commonly implicated in TPN-related sepsis are the fungi *Candida albicans* and *Candida parapsilosis.*

Early detection of sepsis is an important nursing responsibility. The first sign of sepsis may be sudden glycosuria (or hyperglycemia) in the previously stable individual, which may precede any other clinical signs by as much as 24 hours.

Glycosuria is easily detected by the nurse who is conducting urine tests every 6 hours. Clinical signs of sepsis include fever, hypotension, tachycardia, and tachypnea.

In the presence of a temperature spike, peripheral blood and blood drawn from the catheter are cultured for bacteria and fungi. If both are positive, the catheter is the presumed source of the infection and may be removed if appropriate antibiotics fail to treat the infectious source. If the individual's condition deteriorates or the fever persists, the catheter must be removed. The proximal portion of the catheter is cultured for bacteria and fungi. If the catheter is found to be the source of the infection, symptoms of infection usually subside within 12–24 hours of catheter removal. If symptoms persist, other sources of infection are investigated. A new catheter cannot be inserted until all blood cultures are negative unless the lack of nutrients is deemed life-threatening[117] or intravenous access is essential but peripheral access is unavailable. If blood cultures and the catheter tip culture are negative and no other source of infection is identified, yet the patient becomes afebrile without antibiotics, the catheter is the presumed site of infection. Sepsis resulting from bacterial infection is treated with antibiotics; fungal infections are treated with a fungicidal agent such as amphotericin B.

Mechanical complications Mechanical problems can result from improper functioning of the central line due to blockage of the line from catheter crimping or thrombosis, malfunction of the infusion pump, or failure of the infusion set. Such mechanical problems can be minimized if the personnel caring for and using the equipment are knowledgeable and skilled and if there is a standardized protocol for care of the TPN equipment.

Thromboses are the most common mechanical problems associated with TPN therapy. Thrombosis of the catheter lumen is common, especially in individuals receiving intermittent feedings or when continuous infusions are interrupted. The incidence of thrombosis is reduced by the use of a heparin lock when the catheter is not in use.

If the lumen of the catheter becomes obliterated with a clot, patency may be restored by instilling streptokinase for clot lysis.

Thrombosis of the central vein is a rare but serious complication, requiring prompt removal of the catheter and administration of sodium heparin. Signs and symptoms of central vein thrombosis or thrombophlebitis include erythema; edema of the catheter insertion site; pain along the course of the vein; ipsilateral swelling of the arm, neck, or face; fever; tachycardia; tachypnea; and malaise.

Air embolism is a rare but potentially fatal complication of TPN therapy.[119] Air embolism can be prevented by clamping the tubing securely to prevent air from entering the system. The infusion system should be inspected regularly for leaks or cracks as part of the standard TPN protocol.

If the individual develops a significant air embolus, signs of sudden vascular collapse will be manifested by chest pain, apprehension, tachycardia, hypotension, and cyanosis progressing to seizures, loss of consiousness, and cardiac arrest. Even if the person must be resuscitated, the immediate emergency nursing action should be to position the person on the left side with the head down to allow the air to dissipate gradually through the pulmonary artery. This action may take several minutes, but it eliminates the vascular obstruction.

Precipitation of minerals, most commonly calcium phosphate, can occlude catheters when the concentration infused exceeds its solubility limit. Thus, the nurse should not coinfuse calcium and phosphate riders; riders should be hung consecutively, after flushing, and preferably into separate ports of the catheter.

Metabolic complications A variety of metabolic complications have been associated with TPN administration. Some of the most common complications are listed in Table 27-5. Most metabolic requirements are satisfied by the volume and content of the TPN solution. However, metabolic complications do occur. Weinsier et al.[120] reported that 67% of their 220 patients experienced at least one metabolic complication during TPN therapy.

The most common metabolic complication of TPN therapy is hyperglycemia, which occurs in approximately 15% of all individuals receiving TPN therapy.[117] Hyperglycemia results when the TPN infusion is too rapid, if insulin response is inadequate, or when there are increased insulin demands on the individual, such as occurs in sepsis.

Hyperglycemia is easily monitored by the nurse with the use of fractional urine tests or finger sticks for blood glucose every 6 hours. Clinical symptoms of hyperglycemia include dry mouth, flushed skin, thirst, malaise,

TABLE 27-5 Metabolic Complications of Total Parenteral Nutrition

Complications	Possible Causes
Glucose metabolism	
Hyperglycemia, glycosuria, osmotic diuresis, hyperosmolar, nonketotic dehydration and coma	Excessive total dose or rate of infusion of glucose; inadequate endogenous insulin; glucocorticoids; sepsis
Postinfusion (rebound) hypoglycemia	Persistence of endogenous insulin production secondary to prolonged stimulation of islet cells by high carbohydrate infusion
Amino acid metabolism	
Hyperchloremic metabolic acidosis	Excessive chloride content of crystalline amino acid solutions
Prerenal azotemia	Excessive amino acid infusion
Calcium and phosphorus metabolism	
Hypophosphatemia	Inadequate phosphorus administration; redistribution of serum phosphorus into cells and/or bone
Hypocalcemia	Inadequate calcium administration; hypoalbuminemia
Hypercalcemia	Excessive calcium administration; excessive vitamin D administration
Essential fatty acid metabolism	
Serum deficiencies of phospholipid linoleic and/or arachidonic acids	Inadequate essential fatty acid administration; inadequate vitamin E administration
Miscellaneous	
Hypokalemia	Inadequate potassium intake relative to increased requirements for protein anabolism; diuresis
Hyperkalemia	Excessive potassium administration; renal decompensation
Hypomagnesemia	Inadequate magnesium administration relative to increased requirements for protein anabolism and glucose metabolism
Hypermagnesemia	Excessive magnesium administration; renal decompensation
Anemia	Iron deficiency; folic acid deficiency; vitamin B_{12} deficiency; copper deficiency
Bleeding	Vitamin K deficiency
Elevations of SGOT, SGPT, and serum alkaline phosphatase	Enzyme induction secondary to accelerated glucose metabolism; possible hepatotoxicity secondary to amino acid imbalance; excessive glycogen and/or fat deposition
Zinc, copper, or chromium deficiency	Inadequate trace metal administration

Source: Adapted from Cupit GC: Total parenteral nutrition of the cancer patient. *Cancer Nurs* 2:66, 1979.

polyuria, nausea, or vomiting. If untreated, the hyperglycemia increases serum osmolality, causing fluid to shift from the intracellular to extracellular space. Osmotic diuresis occurs, with urine output as much as 800–900 ml in 1–2 hours, and results in dehydration. Hyperosmolar, hyperglycemic dehydration, if untreated, leads to convulsions, coma, and death.

Hyperglycemia is best treated by the addition of crystalline insulin to each TPN solution. Initial doses are 10 U.L. with gradual increases until the desired blood glucose level is achieved.

Occasionally, when hyperglycemia is significant (blood glucose 300–400 mg dl) and not well controlled with sliding-scale insulin, an insulin drip may be necessary to achieve "normoglycemia" (blood glucose 100–200 mg dl). To prevent life-threatening hypoglycemia, the insulin drip must be held when the TPN solution is not being infused.

Hypoglycemia occurs when too much insulin is administered or when the TPN infusion is interrupted or discontinued shortly after sliding-scale insulin is given. In the patient on a stable TPN regimen (even those with insulin as a component of the TPN mixture), the infusion usually can be stopped abruptly without significant hypoglycemia; however, the infusion should be tapered for an hour or two before discontinuation, if time permits. This is possible for patients receiving insulin as a component of the TPN mixture because intravenously administered insulin is only effective for a few minutes.

Symptoms of hypoglycemia include headache, drowsiness, dizziness, tachycardia, and tremor. Hypoglycemia is corrected when the TPN infusion is balanced against insulin administration.

Essential fatty acid deficiency occurs as a result of a prolonged reduction of fat intake. The symptoms of essential fatty acid deficiency include scaling of the skin over the lower calf and dorsum of the foot, alopecia, delayed wound healing, increased capillary fragility, and thrombocytopenia. Lipid emulsion should be administered regularly to individuals who receive TPN for longer than 14 days without dietary fat intake. DeWys and Kubota[121] recommend that a minimum of two to three bottles (250 or 500 ml per bottle) per week should be infused. Lipid emulsions prevent essential fatty acid deficiency, provide a concentrated energy source, are isotonic and therefore do not damage venous endothelium, and do not require insulin to promote nitrogen. Finally, provision of 25%–35% of the individual's calorie requirements as lipid may help reduce carbon dioxide production, which may be clinically significant in individuals with chronic obstructive pulmonary disease or those ventilator-dependent patients who retain carbon dioxide.[122]

The following is a list of guidelines for lipid emulsion infusion:

- Do not use the emulsion if the color or texture is inconsistent.
- Do not shake the container excessively.
- *Nothing* should be added to the lipid infusion—additives crack the emulsion.
- Infuse in the same line as the TPN solution using a Y-connector located near the infusion site.
- The lipid infusion should be hung higher than TPN or it will run up the TPN line.
- Do not use a filter.
- The initial maximum rate of infusion is 1 ml/min for the first 30 minutes. If no untoward reactions occur, increase the infusion rate to 500 ml over 4–12 hours.
- Observe the individual for untoward effects such as allergic reactions, dyspnea, cyanosis, nausea, vomiting, headache, flushing, fever, chills, pain in the chest or back, irritation at the infusion site, and diaphoresis.
- Discard any solution remaining in the container. Do not store it for later use.

If the individual experiences any of the untoward effects just mentioned, the lipid infusion should be discontinued. If the symptoms are a result of fat overload, the individual may receive sodium heparin intravenously to clear plasma lipids. Overall tolerance to the lipid infusion is monitored with routine serum triglyceride and cholesterol measurements.

Most of the other metabolic complications are deficiency states that can be avoided by appropriate replacement in the TPN solution. Trace metals have emerged as important factors in deficiency states resulting from long-term TPN therapy. However, most standard TPN solutions contain trace metals and vitamins.

Pharmacologic Treatment of Cachexia

Hormonal treatment of malignancy has recently received attention because of the potential for therapeutic efficacy with relatively little toxicity. Megestrol acetate is a synthetic derivative of progesterone that is used often in the hormonal treatment of patients with advanced breast cancer and prostrate cancer. Weight gain (10 or 20 pounds or more) and increased appetite are common side effects, even when the drug is administered at conventional doses (120–160 mg/day).[123–128] Regardless of the patient's pretreatment weight, type of cancer, extent of disease or response to therapy, weight gain is observed and is not due to edema. Although megestrol acetate is a potent inducer of lipocyte differentiation,[129] the mechanism by which megestrol acetate exerts its effects on appetite and anabolism has not been determined and is under investigation.

The use of megestrol acetate as a possible treatment for cachexia due to cancer or human immunodeficiency virus (HIV) has been proposed[130–133] because of initial anecdotal observations. The therapeutic efficacy and most effective dose of megestrol acetate are under investigation in several clinical trials of patients with cachexia due to cancer or HIV. Moreover, the appetite-stimulating effect of several other substances, including cyproheptadine, hydrazine sulfate, and cannabinoids, are being studied.[134]

Nutritional Therapy at Home

Many individuals are now able to carry out their own nutritional program at home. Home nutritional support is indicated especially for individuals who would otherwise not need to be hospitalized.

Tube feedings generally can be accomplished at home with little difficulty if the individual and family receive sufficient instruction. It is important that the regimen be as simple as possible. It should be written out for the individual and family, including goals for caloric intake and the desired weight gain. Instruction should include insertion of the tube (if applicable), preparation of the feeding, administration of the feeding, care and use of the equipment, documentation of intake, potential complications or side effects, and management of complications and equipment problems.

The individual and family have the opportunity to decide whether they would like to use blenderized home dietary formulas or commercially prepared formulas. The former are less expensive and give the individual and family more control in the food the individual receives and therefore more satisfaction. However, it is more difficult to ensure a nutritionally complete diet when a home formula is used. In addition, the risk of bacterial contamination is increased. Nonetheless, the individual's and family's ability to participate in decisions made about dietary intake plays an important role in their acceptance of the dietary regimen.

If the individual and family are intimidated by an electronic infusion pump, they should be encouraged to use continuous drip by gravity for the feedings. Feedings should be administered during family mealtimes to encourage the socialization that is associated closely with eating. If appropriate, feedings can be infused over night, allowing the individual freedom from the pump during the day. In addition, during the hiatus, the individual may develop an appetite and be able to enjoy small meals with the family.

Follow-up by a visiting nurse and regular visits to the outpatient department will reassure the individual and family that the therapy is being conducted properly. In addition, it allows the physician or nurse to evaluate the therapy and make necessary modifications.

Parenteral nutrition in the home is much more complicated and requires that the individual and family be capable of learning the technique, possess a high degree of motivation, and have adequate family support. Home TPN is indicated for individuals with fistulas, short bowel syndrome, severe radiation enteritis, or obstruction.

The individual who will be receiving long-term TPN at home will have a long-term central venous catheter (tunneled catheter or implanted port). The person must be instructed about catheter care and the infusion procedure in its entirety. If individuals are properly instructed and catheter care is meticulous, catheters may last up to 1 year or longer. The most frequent complication of home TPN is sepsis, requiring removal of the catheter.

For the person at home, the TPN fluid volume is 1000–2500 ml/24 hr. The total volume of TPN fluid often is administered overnight while the person is asleep to allow for mobility during waking hours. The solution is tapered during the last 2 hours of administration to prevent hypoglycemia on discontinuation.

The cost of home TPN is high but significantly lower than comparable therapy received in a hospital. Most major insurance companies and state medical aid programs reimburse individuals for home TPN. Close follow-up and evaluation by the TPN support team or visiting nurse are critical to the success of a home TPN program.

FUTURE TRENDS

Significant advances have been made in the last few decades regarding our knowledge about nutrition and cancer. Nutritional intervention has achieved the status of an important adjunct to cancer therapy through the premise that nutritional intervention supports and sustains the individual while the cancer therapy is destroying the tumor. Despite the tremendous gains in knowledge, however, much more remains to be learned.

The future of knowledge to be gained through nutritional research is promising. Health care professionals can look forward to the identification of factors that cause altered nutrition in individuals with cancer and new ways of applying this knowledge toward improving the quality of life for persons whose normal eating patterns are altered by cancer. For example, the brain peptides that are thought to cause anorexia in individuals with cancer are shown to play a role in cancer cachexia; antagonists to these peptides administered therapeutically may prevent the anorexia of cancer.

A major question yet to be answered in research about cancer and malnutrition is whether nutritional depletion on the individual with cancer is purely a manifestation of cancer that will resolve spontaneously after successful cancer therapy or whether nutritional intervention will actually improve treatment success. The challenge is for research to define areas where nutritional support will result in a measurable improved response to cancer therapy. More careful documentation of nutritional deficits at the beginning of nutritional and cancer therapy is needed so that changes can be measured. A concomitant need is for the identification of assessment parameters that can measure response to nutritional therapy. The goal is for nutritional assessment to be a prognosticator of outcome of cancer. Nurses must take a leadership role on behalf of individuals with cancer in this most important quest for improved patient care.

REFERENCES

1. Freeman M, Frankenman C, Beck J: Prognostic nutrition factors in lung cancer patients. *J Parent Ent Nutr* 6:122–127, 1982.
2. Richard KA, Detamore CM, Coates TD, et al: Effect of nutrition staging on treatment delays and outcome in stage IV neuroblastoma. *Cancer* 52:587–598, 1983.
3. Meguid MM, Meguid V: Preoperative identification of the surgical cancer patient in need of postoperative supportive total parenteral nutrition. *Cancer* 55:258–262, 1985.
4. Yamanaka H, Nishi M, Kanemakit, et al: Preoperative nutritional assessment to predict postoperative complications in gastric cancer patients. *J Parent Ent Nutr* 13:286–291, 1989.
5. Heber D, Beverly LO, Chi J, et al: Pathophysiology of malnutrition in the adult cancer patient. *Cancer* 58:1867–1873, 1986.
6. Kern KA, Norton JA: Cancer cachexia. *J Parent Ent Nutr* 12:286–298, 1988.
7. Donaldson SS: Nutritional consequences of radiotherapy. *Cancer Res* 37:2407–2413, 1977.
8. Costa G: Cachexia, the metabolic component of neoplastic disease. *Cancer Res* 37:2327–2335, 1977.
9. Theologides A: Cancer cachexia. *Cancer* 43:2004–2012, 1979.
10. Costa G, Donaldson S: The nutritional effects of cancer and its therapy. *Nutr Cancer* 2:22–29, 1980.
11. Beutler B: Cachexia: A fundamental mechanism. *Nutr Rev* 46:369–373, 1988.
12. Gold J: Cancer cachexia and gluconeogenesis. *Ann NY Acad Sci* 230:103–110, 1974.
13. Waterhouse C: How tumors effect host metabolism. *Ann NY Acad Sci* 230:86–93, 1974.
14. Young VR: Energy metabolism and requirements in the cancer patient. *Cancer Res* 37:2336–2347, 1977.
15. DeWys WM: Pathophysiology of cancer cachexia: Current understanding and areas for future research. *Cancer Res* 42:721s–726s, 1982(suppl).

16. Holroyde CP, Reichard GA: Carbohydrate metabolism in cancer cachexia. *Cancer Treat Rep* 65:55–59, 1981 (suppl 5).
17. Waterlow JC, Jackson AA: Nutrition and protein turnover in man. *Brit Med Bull* PS37PS:5–10, 1981.
18. Stein TP: Nutrition and protein turnover: A review. *J Parent Ent Nutr* 6:444–454, 1982.
19. Mider GB, Alling EL, Morton JJ: The effect of neoplastic and allied diseases and concentrations of the plasma protein. *Cancer* 3:56–65, 1950.
20. Bourry J, Milano G, Caldani C, et al: Assessment of nutritional proteins during the parenteral nutrition of cancer patients. *Ann Clin Lab Sci* 12:158–162, 1982.
21. Fenninger LD, Mider G: Energy and nitrogen metabolism in cancer. *Adv Cancer Res* 2:229–253, 1954.
22. Munro HN: Metabolic integration of organs in health and disease. *J Parent Ent Nutr* 6:271–279, 1982.
23. Lundholm K, Edstrom S, Ekman L, et al: Metabolism in peripheral tissues in cancer patients. *Cancer Treat Rep* 65:79–83, 1981(suppl 5).
24. Goodlad GAJ, Tee MK, Clark CM: Leucine oxidation and protein degradation in the extensor digitorum longus and soleus of the tumor-bearing host. *Biochem Med* 26:143–174, 1981.
25. Jeevanadam M, Tracey KJ, Schiller WR, et al: Effect of total parenteral nutrition on whole body protein kinetics in cachetic patients with benign or malignant disease. *J Parent Ent Nutr* 12:229–236, 1988.
26. Waldmann TA, Broder S, Strober W: Protein-losing enteropathies in malignancy. *Ann NY Acad Sci* 230:306–317, 1974.
27. Goodlad GAJ, Clark CM: Protein metabolism in the tumor-bearing host. *Acta Chir Scand* 498:137–140, 1980(suppl).
28. Axelrod L, Costa G: The contribution of fat loss to weight loss in cancer. *Nutr Cancer* 2:81–83, 1980.
29. Waterhouse C: Oxidation and metabolic interconversion in malignant cachexia. *Cancer Treat Rep* 65:61–66, 1981(suppl).
30. Knox LS, Crosby LO, Feurer ID, et al: Energy expenditure in malnourished cancer patients. *Ann Surg* 197:152–162, 1983.
31. Warnold I, Lundholm K, Shersten T: Energy balance and body composition in cancer patients. *Cancer Res* 38:1801–1807, 1978.
32. Arbeit JM, Lees DE, Corsey R, et al: Resting energy expenditure in controls and cancer patients with localized and diffuse disease. *Ann Surg* 199:292–298, 1984.
33. Lindmark L, Beenegard K, Eden E, et al: Resting energy expenditure in malnourished patients with and without cancer. *Gastroenterology* 87:402–408, 1984.
34. DeWys WD: Abnormalities of taste as a remote effect of neoplasm. *Ann NY Acad Sci* 230:427–434, 1974.
35. DeWys WD, Walters K: Abnormalities of taste sensation in cancer patients. *Cancer* 36:1888–1896, 1975.
36. Bernstein IL: Etiology of anorexia in cancer. *Cancer* 58:1881–1886, 1986.
37. Smith JC, Blumsack JT: Learned taste aversion as a factor in cancer therapy. *Cancer Treat Rep* 65:37–42, 1981(suppl 5).
38. Broberg DJ, Bernstein L: Candy as a scapegoat in the prevention of food aversions in children receiving chemotherapy. *Cancer* 60:2344–2347, 1987.
39. Mattes RD, Arnold C, Boraas M: Management of learned food aversions in cancer patients receiving chemotherapy. *Cancer Treat Rep* 71:1071–1078, 1987.
40. Andersen GV, Birch LL, Johnson PA: The scapegoat effect of food aversions after chemotherapy. *Cancer* 66:1649–1653, 1990.
41. Theologides A: Pathogenesis of cachexia in cancer. *Cancer* 29:484–488, 1972.
42. Krause R, Humphrey C, Von Meyenfeldt M, et al: A central mechanism for anorexia in cancer: A hypothesis. *Cancer Treat Rep* 65:15–21, 1981(suppl).
43. Lowy MT, Yim GKW: Similar feeding profiles in tumor-bearing and dexamethasone-treated rats suggest endorphin depletion in cancer cachexia. *Neurosci Abst* 6:518, 1980.
44. Bernstein IL: Physiological and psychological mechanisms of cancer anorexia. *Cancer Res* 42:715s–720s, 1982(suppl).
45. Dominioni L, Dionigi R: Immunological function and nutritional assessment. *J Parent Ent Nutr* 11:70s–72s, 1987(suppl).
46. Dionigi R, Campani M: Nutritional and immunological abnormalities in malignant disease. *Acta Chir Scand* 507:435–474, 1981(suppl).
47. Carson JS, Gormican A: Taste acuity and food attitudes of selected patients with cancer. *J Am Diet Assoc* 70:361–364, 1977.
48. White JV, Dwyer JT, Posner BM, et al: Nutrition screening initiative: Development and implementation of the public awareness checklist and screening tools. *J Am Diet Assoc* 92:163–167, 1992.
49. Pirie P, Jacobs D, Jeffrey R, et al: Distortion in self-reported weight and height data. *J Am Diet Assoc* 78:601–605, 1981.
50. Chumlea WC, Roche AF, Mukherjee D: *Nutritional Assessment of the Elderly Through Anthropometry.* Columbus, OH: Ross Laboratories, 1984.
51. Bernard MA, Jacobs DO, Rombeau JL: *Nutrition and Metabolic Support of Hospitalized Patients.* Philadelphia: Saunders, 1986, p. 27.
52. Johnston CA, Keane TJ, Prudo SM: Weight loss in patients receiving radical radiation therapy for head and neck cancer: A prospective study. *J Parent Ent Nutr* 6:399–402, 1982.
53. DeWys WD: Nutritional care of the cancer patient. *JAMA* 224:374–376, 1980.
54. Hickman DM, Miller RA, Rombeau JL, et al: Serum albumin and body weight as predictors of postoperative course in colorectal cancer. *J Parent Ent Nutr* 4:314–316, 1980.
55. Hopkins B: Assessment of nutritional status. In Shronts EP (ed), *Nutrition Support Dietetics Core Curriculum.* Silver Springs, MD: ASPEN, 1989, p. 24.
56. Heymsfeld SB, Casper K: Anthropometric assessment of the adult hospitalized patient. *J Parent Ent Nutr* 11:36s–41s, 1987(suppl).
57. Bistrian BR: Nutritional assessment and therapy of protein-calorie malnutrition in the hospital. *J Am Diet Assoc* 71:393–397, 1977.
58. Guenter PA, Smithgall JM, Rombeau JL: Skinfold measurements. In Rombeau JL, Caldwell MD, Forlaw L, et al (eds), *Atlas of Nutritional Support Techniques.* Boston: Little, Brown, 1991, pp. 24–33.
59. Kokal WA: The impact of antitumor therapy on nutrition. *Cancer* 55:273–278, 1985.
60. Mullen JL, Gertner MH, Buzley GP, et al: Implications of malnutrition in the surgical patient. *Arch Surg* 114:121–125, 1979.

61. Walser M: Creatinine excretion as a measure of protein nutrition in adults of varying age. *J Parent Ent Nutr* 11:73s–78s, 1987(suppl).
62. Blackburn GL, Bistrian BR, Maini BS, et al: Nutritional and metabolic assessment of the hospitalized patient. *J Parent Ent Nutr* 1:11–22, 1977.
63. Garre MA, Boles JM, Youinow PY: Current concepts in immune derangement due to under nutrition. *J Parent Ent Nutr* 11:309–313, 1987.
64. Daly JM, Dudrick SJ, Copeland EM III: Evaluation of nutritional indices as prognostic indicators in the cancer patient. *Cancer* 43:925–931, 1979.
65. Dionigi R, Gnes F, Bonea A, et al: Delayed hypersensitivity response (DHR) and infections in surgical cancer patients. *Brit J Surg* 66:900, 1979.
66. Miller CL: Immunological assays as measurements of nutritional status: A review. *J Parent Ent Nutr* 2:554–566, 1978.
67. Twomey P, Ziegler D, Rombeau J: Utility of skin testing in nutritional assessment: A critical review. *J Parent Ent Nutr* 6:50–58, 1982.
68. Edén E, Lindmark L, Karlberg I, et al: Role of whole-body lipids and nitrogen as limiting factors for survival in tumor bearing mice with anorexia and cachexia. *Cancer Res* 43:3707–3711, 1983.
69. Westin T, Stein H, Niedobitek G, et al: Tumor cytokinetic response to total parenteral nutrition in patients with head and neck cancers. *Am J Clin Nutr* 53:764–768, 1991.
70. Rossi MR, Uderzo C: Nutritional management of the childhood cancer patient. Recent results. *Cancer Res* 108:198–204, 1988.
71. Weisdorf SA, Lysne J, Wind D, et al: Positive effect of prophylactic total parenteral nutrition on long-term outcome of bone marrow transplantation. *Transplantation* 43:833–838, 1987.
72. Torosian MH, Mullen JL, Miller EE, et al: Enhanced tumor response to cycle specific chemotherapy by parenteral amino acid administration. *J Parent Ent Nutr* 7:337–345, 1983.
73. Torosian MH, Tsou KC, Daly JM, et al: Alteration of tumor cell kinetics by pulse total parenteral nutrition. *Cancer* 53:1409–1415, 1984.
74. Klein S, Simes J, Blackburn GL: Total parenteral nutrition and cancer clinical trials. *Cancer* 58:1378–1386, 1986.
75. Koertz RL: Parenteral nutrition: Is it oncologically logical? *J Clin Oncol* 2:534–538, 1984.
76. Lipman TO: Clinical trials of nutritional support in cancer: Parenteral and enteral therapy. *Heme/Oncol Clin North Am* 5:91–102, 1991.
77. Chen MK, Souba WW, Copeland EM: Nutritional support of the surgical oncology patient. *Heme/Oncol Clin North Am* 5:125–145, 1991.
78. Veterans Affairs Total Parenteral Nutrition Cooperative Study Group: Perioperative total parenteral nutrition in surgical patients. *N Engl J Med* 325:525–532, 1991.
79. ASPEN Board of Directors: Guidelines for use of home total parenteral nutrition. *J Parent Ent Nutr* 11:342–343, 1987.
80. ASPEN Board of Directors: Guidelines for use of total parenteral nutrition in the hospitalized adult patient. *J Parent Ent Nutr* 10:441–445, 1986.
81. ASPEN Board of Directors: Guidelines for use of enteral nutrition in the adult patient. *J Parent Ent Nutr* 11:435–439, 1987.
82. American College of Physicians: Parenteral nutrition in patients receiving cancer chemotherapy. *Ann Intern Med* 110:734–736, 1989.
83. Repka FR: Ethical considerations in nutritional support of cancer patients. *Top Clin Nutr* 1:50–55, 1986.
84. Dempsey DW, Mullen JL: Macronutrient requirements in the malnourished cancer patient. *Cancer* 55:290–294, 1985.
85. Merrick HW, Long CL, Gecor GP, et al: Energy requirements for cancer patients and the effect of total parenteral nutrition. *J Parent Ent Nutr* 12:8–14, 1988.
86. Bell SJ, Coffey LM, Blackburn GL: Use of total parenteral nutrition in cancer patients. *Top Clin Nutr* 1:37–49, 1986.
87. Long CL, Schaffel N, Geiger JW, et al: Metabolic response to injury and illness: Estimation of energy and protein needs from indirect calorimetry and nitrogen balance. *J Parent Ent Nutr* 3:452–456, 1979.
88. MacBurney MM: Determination of energy and protein needs in the hospitalized patient. *Am J Int Ther Clin Nutr* (Feb)10:18–27, 1983.
89. Fletcher JP, Little JM: A comparison of parenteral nutrition and early postoperative enteral feeding on the nitrogen balance after major surgery. *Surgery* 100:21–24, 1986.
90. Dempsy D, Mullen JL: Parenteral (glucose or glucose-lipid) vs enteral repletion in malnourished primates: A controlled crossover study. *Am J Clin Nutr* 45:1526–1532, 1987.
91. Alverdy JC, Chi HS, Sheldon GF: The effect of parenteral nutrition on gastrointestinal immunity. *Ann Surg* 202:681–684, 1985.
92. Alverdy JC, Aoys E, Moss GS: Total parenteral nutrition promotes bacterial translocation from the gut. *Surgery* 104:185–190, 1988.
93. Arnold C, Richter M: The effect of oral nutritional supplements on head and neck cancer. *Int J Rad Oncol* 16:1595–1599, 1989.
94. Donaldson SS, Lenon RA: Alterations of nutritional status. Impact of chemotherapy and radiation therapy. *Cancer* 43:2036–2052, 1979.
95. Menashian L, Flam M, Douglas-Paxton D, et al: Improved food intake and reduced nausea and vomiting in patients given a restricted diet while receiving cisplatin chemotherapy. *J Am Diet Assoc* 92:58–61, 1992.
96. Rombeau JL, Caldwell MD: *Enteral and Tube Feeding.* Philadelphia: Saunders, 1990.
97. Skipper A: Enteral formulas for specialized nutritional support. *J Am Diet Assoc* 86:654–658, 1986.
98. Cataldi-Betcher EL, Seltzer MH, Slocum BA, et al: Complications occuring during enteral nutrition support: A prospective study. *J Parent Ent Nutr* 7:546–552, 1983.
99. Zarling EJ, Parmar JR, Mobarhan S, et al: Effect of formula infusion rate, osmolality, and chemical composition upon clinical tolerance and carbohydrate absorption in normal subjects. *J Parent Ent Nutr* 10:585–590, 1986.
100. Walikie BC, Walikie JW: Relative lactose intolerance: A clinical study of tube fed patients. *JAMA* 238:948–951, 1977.
101. Kohn CL: The relationship between enteral formula contamination and length of enteral delivery set usage. *J Parent Ent Nutr* 15:567–571, 1991.

102. Heymsfield S, Bethel RA, Ansley JD, et al: Enteral hyperalimentation and alternative to central venous hyperalimentation. *Ann Intern Med* 90:63–71, 1979.
103. Brinson RR, Kolts BE: Hypoalbuminemia as an indicator of diarrheal incidence in critically ill patients. *Crit Care Med* 15:506–509, 1987.
104. Niemec PW, Vanderveen TW, Morrison JI, et al: Gastrointestinal disorders caused by medication and electrolyte solution osmolality during enteral nutrition. *J Parent Ent Nutr* 7:387–389, 1987.
105. Edes TE, Walk BE, Austin JL: Diarrhea in tube-fed patients: Feeding formula not necessarily the cause. *Am J Med* 88:91–93, 1990.
106. Kelly TWJ, Partick MR, Hillman KM: Study of diarrhea in critically ill patients. *Crit Care Med* 11:7–9, 1983.
107. Keohane PP, Attrill H, Jones BJM, et al: The roles of lactose and *Clostridium difficile* in the pathogenesis of enteral feeding associated diarrhea. *Clin Nutr* 1:259–264, 1983.
108. Pesola GR, Hogg JE, Eissa N, et al: Hypertonic nasogastric tube feedings: Do they cause diarrhea? *Crit Care Med* 18:1378–1382, 1990.
109. Keohane PP, Attrill HE, Love M, et al: Relation between osmolality of diet and gastrointestinal side effects in enteral nutrition. *Br Med J* 288:678–680, 1984.
110. Rees RG, Keohane PP, Grimble GK, et al: Tolerance of elemental diet administered without starter regimen. *Br Med J* 290:1868–1869, 1985.
111. Patterson ML, Domingues JM, Lyman B, et al: Enteral feeding in the hypoalbuminemic patient. *J Parent Ent Nutr* 14:362–365, 1990.
112. Gottschlich MM, Warden GD, Michel M, et al: Diarrhea in tube fed burn patients: Incidence, etiology, nutritional impact and prevention. *J Parent Ent Nutr* 12:338–345, 1988.
113. Ford EG, Jennings M, Andrassy RJ: Serum albumin (oncotic pressure) correlates with feeding tolerance in the pediatric surgical patient. *J Pediatr Surg* 22:597–599, 1987.
114. Zimmaro DM, Rolandeli RH, Koruda MJ, et al: Isotonic tube feeding formula induces liquid stool in normal subjects: Reversal by pectin. *J Parent Ent Nutr* 13:117–123, 1989.
115. Frankenfield DC, Beyer PL: Soy-polysaccharide fiber: Effect on diarrhea in tube-fed, head injured patients. *Am J Clin Nutr* 50:533–538, 1989.
116. Dobb GJ, Towler SC: Diarrhea during enteral feeding in the critically ill: A comparison of feeds with and without fibre. *Ins Care Med* 16:252–255, 1990.
117. Mullen JL: Complications of total parenteral nutrition in the cancer patient. *Cancer Treat Rep* 65:107–113, 1981(suppl 5).
118. Ryan JA Jr, Abel RM, Abbott WM, et al: Catheter complications in total parenteral nutrition: A prospective study of 200 consecutive patients. *N Engl J Med* 290:757–761, 1974.
119. Allen JR: Prevention of infection in patients receiving total parenteral nutrition. *Acta Chir Scand* 507:405–418, 1981(suppl).
120. Weinsier RL, Bacon J, Butterworth CE Jr: Central venous alimentation: A prospective study of the frequency of metabolic abnormalities among medical and surgical patients. *J Parent Ent Nutr* 6:421–425, 1982.
121. DeWys WD, Kubota TT: Enteral and parenteral nutrition in the care of the cancer patient. *J Med Assoc* 246:1725–1727, 1981.
122. MacFie J: Metabolic properties of intravenous fat emulsions during total parenteral nutrition (TPN). *Nutrition* 3:27–28, 1987(suppl).
123. Bonomi P, Pessis D, Nunting N, et al: Megestrol acetate used as primary hormonal therapy in stage D prostate cancer. *Semin Oncol* 12:36–39, 1985(suppl).
124. Morgan LR: Megestrol acetate v. tamoxifen in advanced breast cancer in postmenopausal patients. *Semin Oncol* 12:43–47, 1986(suppl).
125. Aisner J, Tchekmedyian NS, Moody M, et al: High-dose megestrol acetate for the treatment of advanced breast cancer: Dose and toxicities. *Semin Oncol* 14:48–55, 1987(suppl).
126. Tchekmedyian NS, Tait N, Abrams J, et al: High-dose megestrol acetate in the treatment of advanced breast cancer. *Semin Oncol* 15:44–49, 1988(suppl).
127. Sikic BI, Scudder SA, Ballon SC, et al: High-dose megestrol acetate therapy of ovarian carcinoma: A phase II study by the Northern California Oncology Group. *Semin Oncol* 13:26–32, 1986(suppl).
128. Creagan EG, Ingle JN, Schutt AJ, et al: A prospective randomized controlled trial of megestrol acetate among high-risk patients with resected malignant melanoma. *Semin Oncol* 12:152–155, 1989(suppl).
129. Hamurger AW, Parnes H, Gordon GB: Megestrol acetate induced differentiation of 3T3-L adipocytes in vitro. *Semin Oncol* 15:76–78, 1988(suppl).
130. Tchekmedyian NS, Tait N, Moody M, et al: Appetite stimulation with megestrol acetate in cachectic cancer patients. *Semin Oncol* 13:37–44, 1986(suppl).
131. Tchekmedyian NS, Tait N, Moody M, et al: High-dose megestrol acetate: A possible treatment for cachexia. *JAMA* 257:1195–1198, 1987.
132. Von Roenn JH, Murphy RL, Weber KM, et al: Megestrol acetate for treatment of cachexia associated with human immunity virus (HIV) infection. *Ann Intern Med* 109:840–841, 1988.
133. Aisner J, Parnes H, Hickman M, et al: Appetite stimulation and weight gain with megestrol acetate. *Semin Oncol* 17:2–7, 1990(suppl 9).
134. Bruera E: Current pharmacological management of anorexia in cancer patients. *Oncology* 6:125–130, 1992.

Chapter 28

Hypercalcemia

Jennifer M. Lang-Kummer, RN, MN

INTRODUCTION

Incidence

Primary hyperparathyroidism and malignancy are responsible for 90% of all cases of hypercalcemia (Table 28-1).[1] Overall, the incidence of primary hyperparathyroidism is twice that of malignancy-associated hypercalcemia and is most commonly described as a stable, asymptomatic disorder in an outpatient population of mostly elderly women.[2,3] In hospitalized populations, hypercalcemia due to malignancy is much more common because of the more severe symptomatology and the progressive nature of the syndrome when associated with cancer.[4] Since the hypercalcemia of malignancy is frequently associated with a high tumor burden and end-stage disease, hospitalizations for malignancy-associated hypercalcemia tend to be recurrent.

Hypercalcemia is a frequent complication of malignancy. About 10%–20% of cancer patients will develop hypercalcemia at some point during the course of their disease.[5] The incidence of hypercalcemia varies with the type of cancer, primarily due to the variability of the pathogenic mechanisms and circumstances responsible for the development of the condition.[3] Patients with lung cancer account for 25%–35% of reported cases, while 20%–40% of cases occur in patients with breast cancer. Hypercalcemia is also seen frequently in patients with multiple myeloma and with head and neck cancer, while it is rare in cancers of the stomach, duodenum, colon, rectum, biliary tract, and prostate.[1,3–7] The reported frequencies of malignancy-associated hypercalcemia by tumor type are summarized in Table 28-2.

Tumor histology is also a factor in the development of hypercalcemia in cancer patients. Although rare in patients with small-cell lung cancer, 23% of patients with squamous epidermoid cancer of the lung and 13% of those with large-cell anaplastic cancer of the lung will develop hypercalcemia.[8] Squamous histology also is the predominant feature for esophageal, head and neck, and many female reproductive system tumors, together making up 20% of cases.[9,10]

The high frequency of breast and lung cancer diagnoses among patients with hypercalcemia is related to the high overall incidence of these two types of cancers. Multiple myeloma, a relatively rare cancer, is the primary diagnosis in 10% of malignancy-associated cases. However, one-third of patients with multiple myeloma develop hypercalcemia, a high frequency rate for a disease with low prevalence.[10]

Hypercalcemia of malignancy is usually progressive, causes unpleasant symptoms, can cause the patient to deteriorate rapidly, and may be the cause of death in some patients refractory to treatment. In the early stages, symptoms may be vague and nonspecific and can be confused with symptoms resulting from treatments such as radiation therapy, chemotherapy or biologic response modifiers, brain metastases, or progressive disease. The pathophysiology of hypercalcemia is complex, varies with tumor characteristics, and usually involves at least two basic mechanisms: increased bone resorption and decreased renal calcium clearance. The recent addition of bisphosphonates to treatment regimens has expanded the options for management of hypercalcemic patients significantly. Nurses play an important role in recognition of patients at risk, patient and family teaching, early recognition and monitoring of response to symptoms and response to treatment, and, when all else fails, assisting the patient and family in the terminal phases of the illness.

TABLE 28-1 Causes of Hypercalcemia

Causes of Hypercalcemia
Hyperparathyroidism
Malignancy
Solid tumors without skeletal metastases (HHM)
Solid tumors with skeletal metastases
Hematologic malignancies
Granulomatous disorders
Sarcoidosis
Tuberculosis
Other granulomatous diseases
Immobilization
Spinal cord injury
Paget's disease
Fractures
Endocrine
Hyperthyroidism
Adrenal insufficiency
Pheochromocytoma
Drug-induced
Thiazides
Vitamin D intoxication
Vitamin A
Total parenteral nutrition
Lithium
Renal dialysis and transplantation

HHM = humoral hypercalcemia of malignancy

Definition

The normal range of serum calcium in adults is 8.5 to 10.5 mg/dl (2.13–2.63 mmol/l). Hypercalcemia is considered to exist when the serum calcium level exceeds 11.0 mg/dl (2.75 mmol/l).

PHYSIOLOGY OF CALCIUM HOMEOSTASIS

Calcium is essential for the maintenance of bones, teeth, clotting mechanisms, and intracellular metabolism. The majority of calcium (99%) is found in bone combined

TABLE 28-2 Frequency of Malignancy-Associated Hypercalcemia

Tumor Type	Fisken et al[4] (1980)	Fisken et al[1] (1981)	Mundy and Martin[3] (1982)	Blomqvist[6] (1986)	Combined Data No.	Combined Data %
Lung	54	24	25	24	127	27.3
Breast	44	20	18	33	115	25.7
Multiple myeloma	14	7	5	8	34	7.3
Lymphoma/leukemia	9	3	5	3	20	4.3
Head and neck	15	7	4	6	32	6.9
Renal	7	6	2	5	20	4.3
Prostate	3	1	2		6	1.3
Gastrointestinal	9	4	4	2	19	4.1
Esophagus	13	4		2	19	4.1
Ureters, bladder, urethra	15				15	3.2
Female genital	14	2			16	3.4
Others	12	4	2	2	20	4.3
Unknown primary	10	7	5	—	22	4.7
Total patients	219	89	72	85	465	

Source: Data have been combined from references 1, 3, 4, and 6 as follows: a 1-year prospective general hospital review,[1] a prospective general hospital review,[3] a 32-month retrospective general hospital review,[4] and a 1-year prospective oncology hospital review.[6]

with phosphate. The remaining 1% is divided evenly in the plasma between protein-bound (primarily albumin) and freely ionized forms. It is the freely ionized form that is biologically active. Maintenance of extracellular levels of ionized calcium within a narrow range is important for optimal function of numerous cellular and organ functions.[11] Because of the important role extracellular calcium plays in influencing cell membrane permeability, alterations in extracellular calcium levels will affect nerve excitability and muscle contractility.

Normal Calcium Homeostasis

Extracellular calcium levels are controlled tightly within a narrow range, primarily through the effects of three systemic hormones: parathyroid hormone (PTH), 1,25-dihydroxyvitamin D (the major biologically active metabolite of vitamin D), and calcitonin. Circulating levels of ionized calcium influence the secretion of each of these hormones through three negative-feedback loops.[12] PTH and 1,25-dihydroxyvitamin D influence extracellular calcium levels by controlling calcium transport across three organs: bone, kidney, and small intestine.

Although 99% of the body's calcium is stored in the skeleton, bone makes little contribution to calcium homeostasis in the healthy adult. The ability to control extracellular calcium levels is influenced primarily by the rate of calcium absorption from the intestine and the kidney's threshold for calcium resorption.[3] Renal regulation of calcium is controlled by PTH and 1,25-dihydroxyvitamin D. Only when pathologic states involving increased bone resorption (e.g., some malignancies, Paget's disease) occur do other homeostatic mechanisms come into play.

Calcitonin

Secreted by thyroid parafollicular cells, calcitonin inhibits bone resorption and thus acts as a counterregulator to PTH.[13] In healthy adults, calcitonin appears to play a minor role in calcium homeostasis, since abnormalities in calcium levels do not occur in the absence of the thyroid gland.[12] However, calcitonin can be an important inhibitor of bone resorption in pathologic states, although its effects are transient.[11]

Parathyroid hormone

Secreted by the parathyroid gland, PTH prevents serum calcium concentration from falling below the normal level directly by stimulating bone resorption and calcium liberation from the bony matrix and by calcium resorption in the renal tubules, and indirectly by influencing intestinal calcium absorption.

The direct effect of PTH on the kidney is to rapidly regulate and fine tune calcium balance.[3] Normally, the kidneys filter approximately 10 g of calcium each day,

98% of which is resorbed by the tubules, resulting in a net excretion of 150–200 mg/day. A fall in plasma calcium concentration stimulates the release of PTH and increased renal absorption of calcium. The primary role of PTH on the kidney appears to be maintenance of extracellular calcium levels between 7.5 and 11.5 mg/dl. Outside of that range, the ability of PTH to regulate extracellular fluid calcium levels is quite limited.[11]

Sixty-five percent of calcium filtered by the glomerulus is resorbed in the proximal tubules, 20%–25% in the ascending limb of Henle's loop, and 10% in the distal convoluted tubules. In the proximal tubule, calcium resorption is closely linked with sodium and water resorption and is not influenced by PTH. Since phosphate resorption is inversely related to calcium resorption, PTH's actions in the proximal tubule are directed at inhibition of water, sodium, calcium, bicarbonate, and phosphate resorption.[14] When patients are dehydrated, renal blood flow is decreased and sodium resorption is enhanced. Calcium resorption accompanies sodium resorption, so dehydration can potentiate hypercalcemia by this mechanism.[11] PTH-mediated resorption of calcium occurs in the ascending limb of the loop of Henle and in the distal tubule. In the distal convoluted tubule, about 1000 mg are resorbed daily and is under the effect of PTH enhanced by 1,25-dihydroxyvitamin D.[11,12,14] In normal individuals the fractional excretion of calcium increases as the serum calcium increases to the point at which renal capability for calcium excretion is exceeded, usually 600 mg/day.[11,12]

In the skeleton, PTH plays a mediating role in bone resorption by stimulating the number and activity of bone osteoclasts, leading to the release of calcium and phosphate into the circulation.[14] The exact mechanisms through which this occurs have not yet been identified.

1,25-dihydroxyvitamin D

Vitamin D is hydroxylated from 25-hydroxyvitamin D by enzymes found in the liver, gut, and kidney. 25-hydroxyvitamin D is the major circulating and storage form of vitamin D. In the proximal tubules of the kidney, 25-hydroxyvitamin D is hydroxylated by 1-alpha hydroxylase to 1,25-dihydroxyvitamin D, primarily under the influence of PTH.

In the gastrointestinal tract, 1,25-dihydroxyvitamin D stimulates the absorption of dietary calcium in response to low circulating levels of calcium. The net absorption of calcium from the gut is roughly equal to renal calcium excretion, about 150–200 mg/day. Calcium is absorbed from the gut through an active transport process and a passive diffusion process. While both of these processes are complex and imperfectly understood, the active transport process appears to occur through calcium binding with a protein regulated by 1,25-dihydroxyvitamin D. The passive diffusion process also appears to be mediated by 1,25-dihydroxyvitamin D.[11] Dietary intake of calcium influences the efficiency of calcium absorption from the gut. 1,25-dihydroxyvitamin D acts to increase efficiency of calcium absorption when dietary calcium intake decreases. While the effect of PTH on renal resorption of calcium occurs on a minute-to-minute basis, 1,25-dihydroxyvitamin D's effect on intestinal calcium absorption is less responsive to immediate changes in serum calcium levels and thus is responsible primarily for chronic calcium homeostasis.

A number of disease states influence circulating levels of 1,25-dihydroxyvitamin D and thus intestinal calcium absorption. In some types of hypercalcemia, 1,25-dihydroxyvitamin D levels may be increased, probably through extrarenal synthesis of 1,25-dihydroxyvitamin D, and include primary hyperparathyroidism, sarcoidosis, and T-cell or B-cell lymphomas.[11]

In addition to its effect on calcium absorption in the gut, 1,25-dihydroxyvitamin D works in concert with PTH by acting directly on bone calcium mobilization by stimulating osteoclastic bone resorption and enhancing osteoblastic bone mineralization. In the bone marrow, 1,25-dihydroxyvitamin D plays an important role in the differentiation of cells of the monocyte-macrophage lineage and in enhancing the production of interleukin-1 by monocyte-macrophage cells.

In the kidney, 1,25-dihydroxyvitamin D works in concert with PTH to enhance calcium resorption and against PTH to enhance phosphate resorption.[11]

Homeostatic responses to increased calcium loads

With an increased extracellular fluid calcium load, the secretion of PTH is suppressed; this decreases physiologic calcium release from bone and inhibits intestinal calcium resorption. This inhibitory effect occurs as a result of decreased renal synthesis of 1,25-dihydroxyvitamin D. In addition, decreased PTH results in increased urinary calcium excretion. The kidney is the principal route by which a calcium load can be cleared.[10] To protect against an increased extracellular calcium level of hypercalcemic proportions, the kidney can increase calcium excretion approximately fivefold to a maximum of approximately 600 mg/day.[11] Mild hypercalcemia impairs glomerular filtration and urinary concentrating ability, creating a polyuric state. This predisposes a patient to dehydration and prerenal azotemia. Once the renal compensatory mechanisms are exceeded, further renal insufficiency enhances calcium resorption and phosphate wasting in the proximal tubule, further exacerbating the development of hypercalcemia and renal failure.[10]

The role of bone in calcium homeostasis

Skeletal bone serves as the body's calcium reservoir. In the healthy adult before middle life, bone resorption and formation are in balance and occur as a renewal process in response to the need for repair and to local mechanical factors such as weight bearing and fluid pressure.[11,15] Only small amounts of skeletal calcium are exchanged daily with the extracellular fluid, and under most circumstances the exchange of calcium with extracellular fluid by the process of bone resorption and bone formation is in balance.[11] However, in disease states the contribution of skeletal calcium to extracellular calcium levels assume a larger role. There are two mechanisms through which skeletal calcium can enter extracellular fluid: bone remodeling and calcium exchange between the bone surface and extracellular fluid. This second mechanism is not well understood.

Bone remodeling

The bone cells primarily concerned with the process of bone formation and resorption, known as *bone remodeling,* are the osteoclasts, osteocytes, and osteoblasts (Table 28-3). Incitement of bone remodeling is thought to be directed at the osteocyte, which prepares the bone surface for osteoclastic activity and liberates chemical messengers that not only attract osteoclasts but also initiate osteoblast precursor proliferation.[15] Thus, normal bone remodeling activity can be said to be "coupled" both geographically and chronologically; bone resorption is coupled with bone formation. "Uncoupling" refers to the failure of bone formation to follow the resorption process.[16]

The process of bone remodeling occurs in discrete units throughout the skeleton, and the location and frequency of bone remodeling activity appear to be influenced primarily by mechanical factors such as weight bearing; by the activity of the osteotropic hormones PTH, 1,25-dihydroxyvitamin D, and calcitonin; and by the presence of local factors such as prostaglandins, regulatory proteins, and constituents of the organic matrix.[11,15]

Local events lead to an increase in osteoclast activity that involves the formation of a mature multinucleated osteoclast from its precursor, differentiation of the committed progenitors, and then activation of the preformed cell. Bone is resorbed by the osteoclast through a process of extracellular degradation and proteolysis. The resorption phase of the remodeling process lasts for approximately 10 days and is followed by a reversal process. In the reversal process, osteoclastic resorption ceases and the resorption bay is occupied by mononuclear cells. Thereafter a team of osteoblasts aggregates at the resorption site, and repair of the defect and bone formation follows.[11] The repair and bone formation process is estimated to take 3 to 5 months. The action of PTH promotes the cellular differentiation of osteocytes, osteoblasts, and their precursors, while 1,25-dihydroxyvitamin D promotes the differentiation and fusion of osteoclasts (Table 28-4). At physiologic levels of these hormones, bone remodeling takes place in an orderly and coupled manner (Figure 28-1). High levels of PTH and 1,25-dihydroxyvitamin D, on the other hand, stimulate large volumes of osteocytic and osteoclastic breakdown and resorption of calcified matrix.[14] Hormones that act as growth factors for osteoclast progenitors include the bone-resorbing cytokines interleukin-1, tumor necrosis factor, and transforming growth factor alpha.[11] An elevated serum acid phosphatase can indicate the presence of osteoclastic bone catabolism, as seen in metastatic skeletal involvement as well as other disease states. An elevated serum alkaline phosphatase indicates osteoblastic activity, which can be seen in states of high bone turnover: Paget's disease, prostate cancer with blastic skeletal involvement, or healing of a bone fracture.

Since normal bone remodeling is a coupled process, skeletal calcium generally plays an insignificant role in calcium homeostasis. Although not important to the understanding of calcium homeostasis in the healthy adult, local and humoral factors that influence the liberation of calcium from bone in pathologic states assume more significance.

Pathophysiology

In the 1960s, malignancy-associated hypercalcemia was thought to be a simple paraneoplastic syndrome caused

TABLE 28-3 Cells Responsible for Bone Remodeling

Cell	Origin	Function
Osteoblasts	Undifferentiated mesenchymatous cells	Bone-forming cells that secrete collagen; differentiation is promoted by PTH
Osteocytes	Osteoblasts buried within osteocytic lacunae in bone matrix	Responsive to PTH; liberates collagenase, which prepares bone surface for osteoclast resorption; communicates with osteoclasts through liberation of prostaglandin E
Osteoclasts	Mononuclear* bone marrow cells	Multinuclear bone cells that erode and resorb previously formed bone; chemotactic factors attract to osteocyte prepared bone; differentiation and fusion promoted by IL-1, 1,25-dihydroxyvitamin D; function inhibited by calcitonin

*Osteoclast precursors are mononuclear cells that fuse to form large multinuclear units.

PTH, parathyroid hormone.

Source: Adapted from Taylor BM, Weller LA: Hypercalcemia, in Groenwald SL (ed), *Cancer Nursing: Principles and Practice* (1st ed), 1987, p. 292.

TABLE 28-4 Hormonal Mediators of Calcium Homeostasis and Bone Remodeling

Organ	Parathyroid Hormone	1,25-dihydroxyvitamin D	Calcitonin
	Secreted by parathyroid gland in response to ↓ Ca^{++}	Synthesized in liver, kidney, and gut	Secreted by thyroid parafollicular cells in response to ↑ Ca^{++}
Bone	Promotes coupled bone remodeling through stimulation of osteocyte activity, number and activity of osteoclasts, differentiation of osteoblasts	Promotes differentiation and fusion of osteoclasts, differentiation of cells of monocyte lineage, stimulation of osteoclasts and osteoblast bone mineralization	Inhibits osteoclast bone resorption
Kidney	Maintains serum Ca^{++} levels between 7.5–11.5 mg/dl; mediates calcium resorption in Henle's loop and distal tubule; influences renal hydroxylation of 25-hydroxyvitamin D to 1,25-dihydroxyvitamin D	Enhances Ca^{++} resorption in concert with PTH in distal tubule; enhances PO_4 resorption	
Small intestine		Stimulates absorption of dietary Ca^{++} through active transport and passive diffusion	

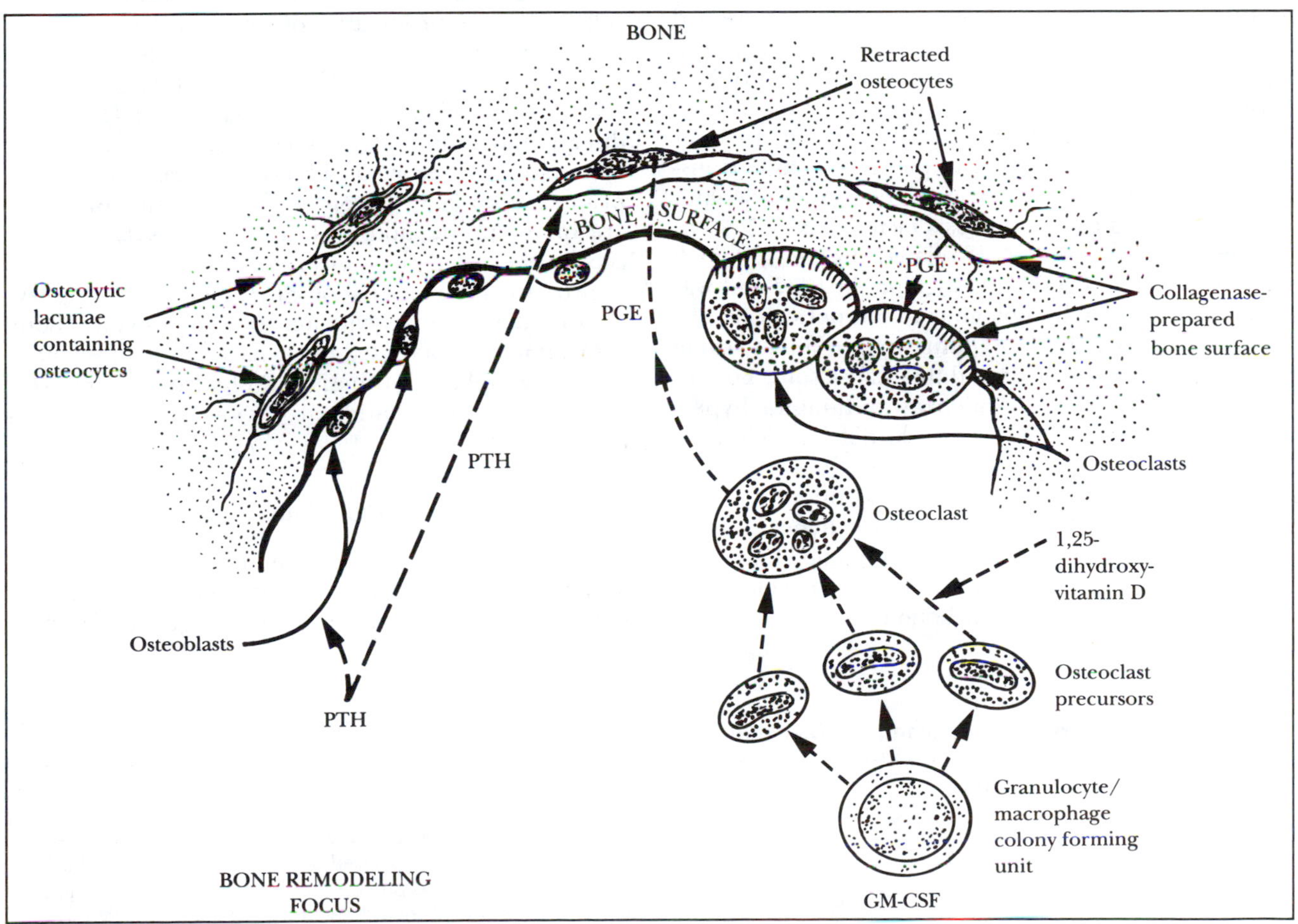

FIGURE 28-1 Coupled bone remodeling. *Bone Resorption:* Osteocytes retract within lacunae under the influence of PTH, liberating collagenase and messengers such as PGE. Collagenase prepares the bone surface for osteoclast resorption. The presence of PGE attracts osteoclasts to the bone surface. Osteoclast precursors, derived from granulocyte-macrophage colony-forming units, differentiate and fuse to form multinuclear osteoclasts under the influence of 1,25-dihydroxy-vitamin D. *Bone Formation:* Osteoblasts differentiate under the influence of PTH, secreting collagen and mineralizing bone. Some osteoblasts become buried within osteocytic lacunae during the bone-forming process to become osteocytes. Osteoblasts recycle Ca^{++} liberated during the bone resorption process to mineralize new bone. (PTH, parathyroid hormone; PGE, prostaglandin E; GM-CSF, granulocyte-macrophage colony-stimulating factor.)

either by an excess of circulating PTH or by bone resorption mediated by primary or metastatic tumor cells in direct contact with bone.[2,12,17] We now know that malignancy-associated hypercalcemia is not related to either of the two mechanisms noted above but is a complex metabolic complication in which the primary defect is an increase in bone resorption that exceeds both bone formation and the kidney's ability to excrete extracellular calcium.[12] No single mechanism can explain the abnormalities in calcium transport in bone, kidney, and intestine in various cancers. Based on our current understanding of the factors mediating bone resorption in different kinds of cancer, there are three general categories of hypercalcemia: solid tumors without associated metastases (also known as humoral hypercalcemia), solid tumors with associated metastases, and hematologic malignancies.[13]

Humoral hypercalcemia of malignancy

Hypercalcemia that develops in patients with solid tumors without bone metastases is thought to be due to tumor-produced systemic mediators of increased bone resorption (Table 28-5). Most humoral hypercalcemia of malignancy tumors are thought to produce parathyroid hormone-related proteins or transforming growth factor alpha (TGF-alpha).[13,20] Other cytokines and factors that have been implicated include transforming growth factor beta (TGF-beta),[20] interleukin-1 (IL-1),[21,22] and tumor necrosis factor (TNF).[23]

The existence of a PTH-related protein (PTHrP) was reported by several investigators in 1987 and was found to be highly homologous to but not exactly like PTH.[24–26] The PTHrP is hypothesized to bind to some but not all PTH receptors and thus cause some but not all possible PTH effects. Patients with humoral hypercalcemia of malignancy (HHM) do not have elevated levels of 1,25-dihydroxyvitamin D and do not have increased levels of intestinal calcium absorption, as is seen with elevated PTH levels in primary hyperparathyroidism. Additionally, HHM is accompanied by an uncoupling of osteoblastic and osteoclastic activities such that bone resorption exceeds bone formation, and hypercalcemia and hypercalciuria occur to a greater degree than that which occurs with primary hyperparathyroidism.[27] The hypercalcemic effect of PTHrP is related to increased bone resorption, increased renal tubular calcium resorption, and phosphate wasting.[28,29]

Several authors have suggested that perhaps PTHrP is responsible for the hypercalcemic/hypophosphatemic renal effects of HHM, while another agent such as TGF-alpha works in concert with PTHrP to enhance bone-resorbing activity.[10,12,13,18,26,30,31] While the roles of IL-1, TNF, and G-CSF have not been clearly defined, there is evidence that these factors produced by normal host immune cells act synergistically with PTHrP and TGF-alpha to increase bone resorption through osteoclast activation (Table 28-6).[13,32]

1,25-dihydroxyvitamin D

Hypercalcemia in patients with Hodgkin's and non-Hodgkin's lymphomas historically has been attributed either to the direct action of skeletal metastases on bone cells or to the production of an osteoclast-activating factor.[2] Several investigators have reported the presence of elevated levels of circulating 1,25-dihydroxyvitamin D in hypercalcemic patients with Hodgkin's disease and non-Hodgkin's lymphoma without bony metastases that resolved with effective treatment of the primary disease.[33–37] Proposed mechanisms of action are tumor production of 1-alpha-hydroxylase, which acts on the circulating substrate 25-hydroxyvitamin D to produce, independent of PTH, high circulating levels of 1,25-dihydroxyvitamin D that enhance bone resorption and increased intestinal transport;[36,38] monocyte-macrophage synthesis of 25-hydroxyvitamin D;[39] and synthesis of 1,25-dihydroxyvitamin D by disease-activated macrophages.[40]

Tumors with skeletal metastases

The cause of hypercalcemia in cancer patients with skeletal metastases such as breast cancer, multiple myeloma, and lymphoma is more heterogenous, particu-

TABLE 28-5 Humoral Hypercalcemia of Malignancy

Factor	Source	Action
PTHrP	Tumor cells	↑ osteocyte and osteoclast activity; ↓ osteoblast activity (uncoupled bone resorption); ↑ renal calcium resorption and phosphate wasting; no stimulation of renal 1,25-dihydroxyvitamin D synthesis ⩾ no ↑ intestinal Ca^{++} transport
1,25-dihydroxyvitamin D	Tumor-produced hydroxylase, which converts circulating substrates to 1,25-dihydroxyvitamin D; (?) synthesis by disease-activated macrophages	Enhanced intestinal Ca^{++} transport; ↑ differentiation and fusion of osteoclast precursors; ↑ bone resorption.
TGF-alpha	Most solid tumors	↑ production of osteoclast progenitors, osteoclast activation; (?) stimulation of PGE

TABLE 28-6 Local Cytokines (Osteoclast-Activating Factors) and Growth Factors Influencing Bone Resorption

Factor	Source	Action
IL-1	Monocytes/macrophages	Stimulates production and fusion of osteoclast precursors (inhibited by calcitonin but not PGE)
PGE	Tumor cells Monocytes Osteocytes	Stimulates osteoclast bone resorption, shape change, collagenase release; stimulates lymphokines and OAF
TNF-alpha (cachectin)	Monocytes	Stimulates osteoclast activation
TNF-beta (lymphotoxin)	Lymphocytes	Stimulates osteoclast activity
IFN-gamma	Lymphocytes	Inhibits cytokine-mediated bone resorption
CSF-GM	Lymphocytes	Increases proliferation of osteoclast precursors and monocyte-macrophage precursors
CSF-1, CSF-M	Monocytes	Increase proliferation of osteoclast precursors and monocyte-macrophage precursors

larly in breast cancer.[42,43] Many cancers invoke their hypercalcemic effect through a combination of humoral and local cell-mediated mechanisms. Among the implicated factors are prostaglandins of the E series (PGE), TGF-alpha, and the cytokines known as osteoclast-activating factor (OAF).[10–12,17]

PGE_2 is a potent osteoclast stimulator that has been demonstrated to mediate hypercalcemia by stimulating bone resorption in several animal models.[12] A prostaglandin synthesis inhibitor, indomethacin, was shown to alleviate hypercalcemia in animals, but similar results have not been found in humans; fewer than 10% of patients with hypercalcemia have been found to be responsive to optimal doses of indomethacin.[10,12,43]

Breast cancer Hypercalcemia occurs in up to 40% of women with breast cancer.[42] Although the majority of patients with hypercalcemia have widespread metastases, not all patients with metastases develop hypercalcemia.[41,42] Hypercalcemia and bone lesions are more common in estrogen-receptor positive tumors, and in those patients in whom hypercalcemia occurs, extensive bone metastases are almost always present.[11]

Cultured breast cancer cells have been shown to resorb bone directly in vitro through tumor secretion of lysosomal enzymes and collagenase.[44] New evidence indicates that direct bone resorption by tumor cells is a minor component of the bone destruction that occurs with metastatic cancer.[18] The fact that hypercalcemia of breast cancer is generally responsive to osteoclast inhibitors indicates that osteoclast activation is the major mechanism associated with hypercalcemia.[11] TGF-alpha, TGF-beta, and prostaglandins have also been implicated (Table 28-7). Prostaglandins released by breast cancer cells have been reported to stimulate osteoclast bone resorption. Hypercalcemia in breast cancer patients is generally unresponsive to prostaglandin inhibitors, making understanding of the precise role of PGE in the pathogenesis of hypercalcemia difficult. It is known that hormonally manipulated breast cancer cells do release prostaglandins.[11]

Factors not produced by tumor cells also may be responsible for increased bone resorption at the metastatic site. The presence of breast cancer cells at the bone surface may be sufficient to stimulate a cell-mediated immune response and production of TNF-beta, TNF-alpha, or IL-1, all of which are potent bone-resorbing factors.

Some patients with estrogen-receptor-positive metastatic breast cancer treated with estrogens or antiestrogens suddenly develop hypercalcemia that may be associated with bone pain within 1 month of starting estrogens, androgens, or tamoxifen. Known as *tumor flare,* it is associated with a temporary period of accelerated tumor growth shortly after beginning additive hormonal therapy. Tamoxifen-induced hypercalcemia occurs 4 to 10 days after the initiation of hormonal therapy and has a rapid onset.[45] Tumor flare is generally self-limiting and is thought to indicate a hormonally responsive tumor. The hypercalcemia is probably due to tumor release of PGE, which accelerates bone resorption. A decision to withdraw the hormone temporarily or to treat the patient with a prostaglandin inhibitor such as indomethacin or glucocorticoids without terminating the hormonal agent is usually influenced by the degree of hypercalcemia and its responsiveness to therapy.[9,12,45]

PTHrP appears to play a greater role in the pathogenesis of hypercalcemia in breast cancer patients with and without skeletal metastases than was previously appreciated. Several investigators have reported that a PTHrP-mediated mechanism of hypercalcemia may be involved in as many as 65% of breast cancer patients regardless of the presence or extent of bone metastases.[42,46,47]

Hematologic malignancies Multiple myeloma is one of the malignancies most frequently associated with

TABLE 28-7 Hypercalcemia in Tumors with Skeletal Metastases*

Tumor Type	Implicated Factors	Features
Breast carcinomas with skeletal involvement	TGF-alpha; TGF-beta; PGE; Cell-mediated immune response with production of TNF-alpha, TNF-beta, or IL-1; preceding with PTHrP	↑ osteoclastic bone resorption without bone formation; ↓ intestinal Ca^{++} absorption; normal renal Ca^{++} resorption
Some estrogen-receptor–positive breast cancers with skeletal involvement	PGE release mediated by tamoxifen, androgens, or estrogens	Self-limiting hypercalcemia within 1 month of starting therapy—"tumor flare"
Multiple myeloma	OAFs: IL-1, TNF-alpha, TNF-beta, CSF-GM, CSF-1; preceding in combination with PTHrP	↑ osteoclast bone resorption with ↓ osteoblast activity; ↓ GFR; ↓ intestinal Ca^{++} absorption; normal renal Ca^{++} resorption except as influenced by ↓ GFR
T-cell lymphomas/leukemias and some B-cell lymphomas with and without bone metastases	1,25-dihydroxyvitamin D; OAFs, IL-1, TNF-alpha and beta; PTHrP	↑ osteoclastic bone resorption; ↕ intestinal Ca^{++} absorption depending on presence of 1,25-dihydroxyvitamin D or PTHrP

hypercalcemia, which occurs in 20%–40% of all myeloma patients at some time during the disease.[48] Hypercalcemia is more common in myeloma than in any other hematologic malignancy and can be either a presenting symptom or an indicator of terminal disease.[11] Intractable bone pain is a prominent presenting symptom in 80% of patients.[49] Hypercalcemia in myeloma can be expected whenever patients become bedridden and may be caused by or contribute to renal failure.[50]

The pathophysiology of hypercalcemia in myeloma is different from that in most solid tumors. In most solid tumors, increased bone resorption and decreased urine calcium excretion are the cause. However, in myeloma the cause is increased bone resorption and decreased glomerular filtration.[51] Hypercalcemia in patients with myeloma is almost always accompanied by renal insufficiency due to impaired glomerular filtration caused by Bence Jones protein; uric acid nephropathy; pyelonephritis; or occasionally amyloidosis, which results in an inability to clear ultrafilterable calcium through the glomerulus.[12,48,51]

Hypercalcemia in myeloma always occurs in the presence of extensive bone destruction occurring adjacent to collections of myeloma cells.[11] The possible causative factors for hypercalcemia in myeloma include osteoclast-activating factors IL-1 and tumor necrosis factors alpha and beta, as well as the bone-resorbing cytokines CSF-GM and CSF-1 (CSF-M). Whether these factors are tumor produced or are produced by normal immune cells in response to the presence of myeloma cells is not yet clear. In addition to the increased osteoclastic activity that takes place in myeloma, there is also evidence to support the presence of decreased osteoblastic activity as part of the pathologic process.[49]

Hypercalcemia in patients with B-cell lymphomas is uncommon, occurring in up to 4% of patients.[50] However, HTLV-I– and HTLV-II–associated adult T-cell lymphoma/leukemias (ATCL) are frequently associated with hypercalcemia, occurring in as many as 50% of patients.[11,52] In lymphomas, hypercalcemia is usually seen in patients with bone involvement, but humoral factors have also been found to play a part.[10] As previously discussed, elevated levels of 1,25-dihydroxyvitamin D have been found in lymphoma patients without bone metastases. The presence of PTHrP has been demonstrated in more than half of patients with myeloma and adult T-cell lymphoma/leukemia, indicating that HHM is involved in some cases.[27,53,54] The osteoclast-activating factors IL-1 and tumor necrosis factors alpha and beta have also been implicated as causes of hypercalcemia in these patients. Most likely the cause of hypercalcemia will be found to be a combination of tumor-produced humoral and local osteoclast-activating factors. What differentiates the hypercalcemia found in myeloma from that found in lymphomas is the presence of renal insufficiency associated with myeloma.

Other factors Immobilization, dehydration, poor nutrition, inappropriate use of diuretics, and generalized wasting all play important roles in the pathogenesis of malignancy-associated hypercalcemia.

Local mechanical forces such as weight bearing are important to stimulate bone formation. Individuals with a preexisting state of high bone turnover are more likely to experience increased hypercalciuria and bone resorption when immobilized.[10] Passive range-of-motion exercises may be useful in maintaining muscle and joint mobility but are not helpful in preventing hypercalcemia due to immobilization. Weight bearing is more important.

Dehydration occurs as a result of diminished fluid intake (due to nausea, vomiting, or anorexia) as well as polyuria and inability to concentrate urine due to hypercalcemic interference with the effects of antidiuretic hormone (ADH) on the tubules.

Thiazide and potassium-sparing diuretics act on the

distal tubule to enhance calcium but not sodium reabsorption. Thus, administration of such diuretics produces not only volume depletion but also a hypercalcemic effect.

CLINICAL MANIFESTATIONS

The clinical presentation of hypercalcemia is variable, influenced not only by the degree of hypercalcemia, the rapidity of onset, and the patient's general physical and mental condition, but also by the kidney's ability to maintain calcium homeostasis. Hypercalcemia that develops slowly and gradually is associated with few if any symptoms. Conversely, a rapidly expanding tumor burden associated with a progressively increasing rate of bone resorption may suddenly overwhelm renal compensatory mechanisms, producing a rapid and symptomatic rise in serum calcium levels. This is particularly true in HHM.

Signs and Symptoms

Because of calcium's role in maintaining cell membrane permeability, hypercalcemia produces symptoms in almost all organ systems. Symptoms are numerous, vague, and nonspecific. Since many cancer patients with hypercalcemia have large tumor burdens and will die in less than 6 months (particularly those with HHM), symptoms of hypercalcemia may be confused with those of end-stage disease.[3,55] Recognition of symptoms is important for early identification and treatment of the syndrome to reduce the risk of coma, irreversible renal failure, or a terminal cardiac event (Table 28-8). The symptomatology of hypercalcemia is potentially reversible with treatment, and active treatment correlates with a better outlook.[5] However, it is most important to remember that the development of malignant hypercalcemia is usually associated with a poor prognosis.[5,55] Common symptoms of hypercalcemia in order of reported frequency are fatigue, anorexia, weight loss, bone pain, constipation, polydipsia, muscle weakness, nausea and vomiting, mental changes, and polyuria[1] (Table 28-8).

Gastrointestinal

Elevated extracellular calcium levels depress smooth muscle contractility, leading to delayed gastric emptying and decreased gastrointestinal motility. Anorexia, nausea, vomiting, abdominal pain, and constipation are early and common symptoms in hypercalcemia patients.[56,57] These symptoms may be exacerbated by the disease itself or by cytotoxic therapy.[3] The development of obstipation and ileus are late findings associated with high serum calcium levels and are probably exacerbated by dehydration.

TABLE 28-8 Symptoms of Hypercalcemia

System	Mechanism	Signs and Symptoms
Gastrointestinal	Depressed smooth muscle contractility causes delayed gastric emptying and decreased intestinal motility	Early: Nausea, vomiting, anorexia, constipation Late: Obstipation and ileus; weight loss
Neuromuscular	Depressed excitability of neurons	Early: lethargy, drowsiness; restlessness, mood changes Mid: mental status changes, poor calculation, decreased attention span, somnolence Late: psychotic behavior, marked confusion, slurred speech, stupor, coma
	Impaired electrical conduction and cell membrane permeability in skeletal muscles	Early: muscle weakness, fatigue Late: profound muscle weakness, hypotonia
	? PGE-mediated bone resorption	Bone pain
Renal	Interference with action of ADH on renal collecting tubules → inability to concentrate urine and then volume contraction followed by ↓ GFR	Early: polyuria Mid: polydipsia Late: prerenal azotemia
Cardiovascular	Impaired electrical conduction and cell membrane permeability; altered intracellular metabolism; arterial vasoconstriction	Early: hypertension Mid: sinus bradycardia, prolonged PR interval, shortened QT interval, dysrhythmias especially in digitalized patients Late: Prolonged QT interval due to widened T wave, coving of ST segment, AV block, asystole

ADH, Antidiuretic hormone; *Early,* mild hypercalcemia (<12 mg/dl); *GFR,* glomerular filtration rate; *Late,* severe hypercalcemia (>15 mg/dl); *Mid,* moderate hypercalcemia (12–15 mg/dl); *PGE,* prostaglandin E.

Neuromuscular

Elevated extracellular calcium levels affect both the central nervous system (CNS) and neuromuscular function.[56,57] Initial CNS dysfunction can present as personality changes, impaired concentration, mild confusion, drowsiness, and lethargy.[56,57] Patients with rapidly advancing hypercalcemia may lapse into stupor or coma, usually at serum calcium levels greater than 15 mg/dl. Neurological manifestations are usually much more prominent in the elderly and may persist for several days after normalization of serum calcium levels.

Personality changes occur subtly and are often unnoticed by the family or individual. Extreme restlessness, irritability, overt confusion, and progressive deterioration in cognitive function may develop. In a study of hospitalized patients with hypercalcemia, Mahon[56] reported increasing problems with memory span and attention span, inability to calculate, inappropriate conversation, slow mentation, and inappropriate behavior in patients with corrected serum calcium levels greater than 12.1 mg/dl.

Neuromuscular involvement is primarily neuropathic, involving decreased muscle strength and a decrease in respiratory muscular capacity. Impairment of skeletal muscle electrical conduction and cell membrane permeability leads to profound muscle weakness and hypotonia, usually with severe hypercalcemia.[57]

Renal

Hypercalcemia interferes with the action of ADH on the kidney's collecting tubules, causing an inability to concentrate urine and polyuria (a syndrome similar to nephrogenic diabetes insipidus). Subsequent volume contraction, which is exacerbated by nausea and vomiting, decreases the glomerular filtration rate (GFR). Decreased GFR stimulates sodium and water reabsorption in the proximal tubule. Since sodium and calcium are absorbed in parallel, hypercalcemia is exacerbated. In addition, evidence indicates that TGF-alpha also acts on the kidney's proximal tubule to enhance the resorption of calcium, while distal tubular calcium resorption is influenced by PTH and PTHrP.[12] The downward spiral continues with the development of nitrogen retention, acidosis, and eventual renal failure. Renal failure is most common in patients with multiple myeloma.[12]

Cardiovascular

Calcium ions affect not only smooth, skeletal, and cardiac muscle contractility and cell membrane permeability but also influence conduction of electrical impulses within the heart. Hypertension may occur due to the direct effect of hypercalcemia on arterial smooth muscle.[58] Hypercalcemia results in bradycardia, shortened QT intervals in moderate hypercalcemia, and prolonged QT intervals with calcium levels above 16 mg/dl. Prolonged QT intervals are due to widening of the T wave, with coving of the ST segment.[58,59] Prolonged PR intervals and significant dysrhythmias may also occur, particularly in patients taking digitalis.[60] Since the effects of digitalis are mediated partly by membrane-bound calcium, digitalis toxicity may be potentiated.[58] Atrioventricular block and asystole may occur when the serum calcium level reaches 18 mg/dl.[56,57]

Laboratory Assessment

An elevated serum calcium (corrected for abnormal protein values) is diagnostic. Calcium is found in the serum in three forms: 45% protein bound (primarily to albumin); 45% freely ionized; and 10% complexed to ions such as sulfate, phosphate, or citrate. It is the freely ionized form that is biologically active. Normally, freely ionized calcium is in equilibrium with protein-bound calcium. When there is an abnormality in serum protein levels, serum calcium determinations may not represent true ionized calcium levels. Rarely, in multiple myeloma, a monoclonal protein may have an affinity for calcium and be associated with elevated protein-bound but normal ionized calcium levels, thus creating an illusion of an elevated serum calcium level.[3]

The more common finding in cancer patients is hypoalbuminemia, in which more calcium may be ionized due to low levels of serum albumin available for binding. Ionized serum calcium levels provide a more accurate means of measuring calcium when serum proteins are abnormal. A normal serum calcium is 8.5–10.5 mg/dl (2.13–2.63 mmol/l), while a normal serum ionized calcium level is 4.2–5.2 mg/dl (1.05–1.3 mmol/l). When ionized calcium levels are not available, total serum calcium levels can be corrected to reflect ionized serum calcium more accurately. A frequently used formula is:

$$\text{Corrected calcium (mg/dl)} = \text{Measured calcium} + [4 - \text{albumin (g/dl)}] \times 0.8$$

or

$$\text{Corrected calcium (mmol/L)} = \text{Measured calcium} + [40 - \text{albumin (g/dl)}] \times 0.02$$

In the first example, 0.8 mg/dl of calcium is added (to the laboratory determination of serum calcium) for every 1 g/dl the serum albumin is less than 4.0, which is used as the mid-range normal value for serum albumin.[57]

TREATMENT

Hypercalcemia results from a combination of excessive bone resorption and impaired renal calcium excretion. Treatment must therefore be directed at both causes. Most important initially is improving renal calcium excretion by correcting those factors impairing renal function, usually dehydration and diminished GFR. Second, bone resorption must be eliminated either by eliminating the primary cause (treating the primary tumor) or by inhibiting osteoclast function to prevent recurrence of hypercalcemia. Unless the primary tumor or skeletal metastases can be controlled, all antihypercalcemia interventions tend to be palliative. In a retrospective study of 126 hospitalized hypercalcemia cancer patients, Ralston[55] reported that median survival in these patients was 30 days but that antihypercalcemic therapy produced improvement of symptoms and facilitated patient discharge from the hospital during the terminal stages of their illness.

There are several pharmacologic approaches to the treatment of patients with hypercalcemia, but specific therapy regimens for different hypercalcemic etiologies have not yet been developed (Table 28-9). The degree of urgency with which the hypercalcemia is treated depends on the serum calcium level and the patient's symptomatology. Patients with corrected serum calcium levels above 13.0 mg/dl or symptomatic patients with a calcium level less than 13.0 mg/dl should be treated aggressively, whereas asymptomatic patients with lower calcium levels require more specific but less urgent treatment.[3,12]

In patients with recurrent humoral hypercalcemia and end-stage disease where all cancer treatment options have been exhausted, physicians may, after discussion with the patient and family, elect not to treat further episodes of hypercalcemia, allowing the patient to lapse into a coma and, shortly thereafter, die. Since hypercalcemia can be associated with such unpleasant but manageable symptoms as mental status changes, nausea and vomiting, and abdominal pain, early dialogues among the physician, patient, and family are essential in order to determine what constitutes a "quality death" for the patient.[61] Ralston reported that only 28% of patients treated for hypercalcemia in his study actually died of uncontrolled hypercalcemia. The remainder died of other tumor-related complications after the hypercalcemic event.[55] The recent advent of the bisphosphonates for the treatment of hypercalcemia

TABLE 28-9 Available Therapy for Malignant Hypercalcemia

Therapy	Dosage	Comments
Tumor ablation	Tumor-specific	Only definitive approach to long-term resolution of hypercalcemia
Saline	5–8 liter IV in first 24 hr, then 3 l/day	Restores plasma volume, ↑ renal Ca^{++} excretion; continue until Ca^{++} is <12.0 mg/dl; may require cardiac and CVP monitoring with compromised cardiovascular or renal function.
Furosemide	Diuretic dose 20 mg q 4–6 hr; calciuretic dose 80–100 mg q 1–2 hr	Diuretic dose to control overhydration; calciuretic doses require ICU monitoring to replace electrolyte and fluid losses.
Bisphosphonates		
Etidronate (Didronil)	7.5 mg/kg/d IV over 2–3 hr × 3–7 days, then 5–10 mg/kg/dl PO for up to 3 mo	Prevent osteoclast bone resorption; when effective, calcium level will normalize in 3–5 days; contraindicated in renal failure; given with saline hydration; adverse effects include taste perversions, nausea and vomiting, fever; osteomalacia with long-term use.
Pamidronate (Aredia)	60–90 mg in 1000 ml IV fluid as single dose over 3–24 hr	Inhibits bone resorption without impairing bone mineralization. Higher doses for more severe hypercalcemia; onset of action within 24 hr, longer duration of action; adverse effects same as above but dose-related, intravenous infusion site reactions in 7% of patients.
Calcitonin plus a glucocorticoid	200 MRC units q 12hr IM/SQ Hydrocortisone 100 mg PO q 6hr	Rapid onset of action; ↑ renal calcium excretion; safe in patients with cardiac or renal failure; most effective in hematologic malignancies.
Plicamycin	15–25 μg/kg (max 1500 μg) as single dose IV over 4 hr; can be repeated in 48 hr	Onset of action within 24–48 hr; variable duration of action; adverse effects increase with cumulative dosage and include thrombocytopenia, hepatic and renal toxicity, nausea and vomiting. Extravasation causes cellulitis at injection site.
Phosphate	1–3 g/dl in divided doses	Prevents intestinal Ca^{++} absorption and inhibits mineral and bone matrix resorption; dose-limiting diarrhea usually occurs at 2 g/dl. Chronic administration accompanied by loss of effectiveness. Contraindicated in patients with renal failure and serum phosphorus levels >3.8 mg/dl.
Gallium nitrate	200 mg/m²/dl continuous IV infusion over 5–7 days	Inhibits osteoclast bone resorption. Median duration of response is 6 days. More effective than calcitonin or etidronate in achieving normocalcemia. Adverse effects include asymptomatic hypophosphatemia and nephrotoxicity. Five-day continuous treatment limits outpatient use.

has changed physician approaches to decision making in this area. Bisphosphonates are effective when administered as a single 4-hour infusion and in some cases when administered orally, making them quite useful in outpatient treatment.

General Measures

Initial measures should involve correcting volume contraction and removing factors that may exacerbate hypercalcemia, such as thiazide diuretics, vitamins A and D, and, in some breast cancer patients, hormonal agents. Discontinuation of tamoxifen is not always indicated. Medications whose actions are potentiated by hypercalcemia, such as digoxin, should be adjusted.

Mobilization in an effort to promote weight bearing should be encouraged whenever possible. Except in some patients with lymphoma in whom elevated levels of 1,25-dihydroxyvitamin D enhance intestinal calcium absorption, restriction of dietary calcium is without scientific basis. However, calcium supplementation in intravenous hyperalimentation formulas should be discontinued because of the intravenous route of administration.

Hydration and Saline Diuresis

The cornerstone of all hypercalcemic therapy is to expand volume, correct dehydration and renal insufficiency, and promote calciuresis. In patients with mild hypercalcemia and normal renal function, oral hydration may be all that is required.[62] In symptomatic patients, intravenous hydration is indicated. Since sodium and calcium are excreted in parallel, calciuresis can be promoted by administering high volumes of normal saline, usually at 250–300 ml/hr, until corrected serum calcium levels are less than 12.0 mg/dl. Measurement of fluid intake and output and body weight, and frequent assessment for signs of fluid overload are important. Patients with compromised cardiovascular function or renal failure may need central venous pressure and cardiac monitoring during therapy. Hypokalemia, hypomagnesemia, and hypophosphatemia commonly occur.[3,63] Hyperosmolar states due to some patients' inability to excrete high sodium loads have been observed.[3]

Loop Diuretics

Once rehydration has been established, loop diuretics such as furosemide may be used to enhance calcium excretion. Use of such diuretics, which block calcium and sodium reabsorption across the ascending limb of Henle's loop, is controversial. Mild to moderate hypercalcemia can usually be managed by saline diuresis alone, and the benefit of adding furosemide to saline diuresis has not been documented.[3,12,63]

There is a difference between the diuretic and calciuretic doses of furosemide.[3] Doses of 20 mg every 4–6 hours are usually sufficient to manage overhydration in patients with compromised cardiovascular or renal function.[62] To achieve a calciuretic effect, the recommended dose of furosemide is 80–100 mg every 1–2 hours.[58] Patients treated with high doses of furosemide should be monitored in an intensive care setting to ensure that fluid and electrolyte losses are carefully replaced and that extracellular fluid volume is not depleted. Depletion of extracellular fluid volume in the hypercalcemic patient ensures reabsorption of calcium from the proximal tubule and further exacerbation of the hypercalcemia. Side effects of high-dose furosemide are severe potassium and magnesium loss, but some authors have reported that calcium levels can be decreased 2–4 mg/dl in 24–48 hours with this approach.[58]

Clinical improvement in mental status and relief of nausea often occur in younger patients within 24 hours of rehydration, but serum calcium levels may not normalize except in cases of mild hypercalcemia.[63] Once rehydration and improvement in renal function have been achieved, inhibition of osteoclastic bone resorption must be attained in order to achieve and maintain a normocalcemic state. Although antitumor therapy is the treatment of choice when available, pharmacologic inhibition of bone resorption is usually indicated in order to prevent the movement of calcium from bone into extracellular fluid. Several treatment regimens are available, and all are nonspecific, but choices are made based on the agent's side effects and the severity of the hypercalcemia.

Calcitonin

Calcitonin, a 32 amino acid polypeptide normally produced by the parafollicular cells of the thyroid gland, produces transient (24–72 hours) inhibition of bone resorption through its direct effects on osteoclast formation. Calcitonin also acts directly on the kidney to promote urinary calcium excretion and can be used safely in patients with dehydration or renal failure. Onset of action is rapid, with declines in serum calcium within 4–6 hours of the first dose. Best responses are seen in patients with multiple myeloma and other hematologic neoplasms.[3] Unfortunately, inhibition of bone resorption is short and tachyphylaxis or "escape" from therapeutic effect limits its usefulness, but use of calcitonin in severe hypercalcemia can buy time while antineoplastic or other antihypercalcemic therapy is started. Administration in combination with glucocorticoids appears to be more effective because corticosteroids overcome the effect of renal tubular resistance to calcitonin, possibly through inhibition of PTHrP production.[62,64,65]

Synthetic calcitonin can be administered subcutaneously at a starting dose of 4–12 units/kg body weight every 8–12 hours or as rectal suppositories at a dose of 300 mg three times daily for 7 days. Side effects are mild and include nausea and vomiting, flushing, skin rashes, and occasionally allergic reactions. It has been recommended that skin testing be performed before initiation of treatment.[11]

Rectal administration of calcitonin suppositories for 3 days in combination with a single dose of the bisphosphonate pamidronate has been reported to be more effective, with earlier reductions in serum calcium and a higher efficacy, than with administration of pamidronate alone.[66] Intranasal administration of calcitonin is currently under investigation.

Glucocorticoids

Glucocorticoids (prednisone and hydrocortisone) are most effective in hypercalcemia associated with multiple myeloma, other hematologic diseases, and sometimes breast carcinoma. Hypercalcemia associated with other solid tumors is responsive only 30% of the time.[62] Glucocorticoids may be effective in hypercalcemia due to myeloma because they inhibit bone resorption mediated by osteoclast-activating factors or because they cause a decrease in calcium either by a direct tumor cytolytic effect or by inhibiting tumor-produced prostaglandin.[58] Glucocorticoids also increase urinary calcium excretion and decrease intestinal calcium absorption. This latter effect may be important in those lymphomas that can hydroxylate 25-hydroxyvitamin D to produce high circulating 1,25-dihydroxyvitamin D levels, which stimulate intestinal calcium absorption. The benefits of long-term use of glucocorticoids outweigh potential side effects (Cushing's syndrome, osteomalacia), since most patients do not survive for more than 3–6 months. Side effects of glucocorticoids usually do not occur until after 3 months of administration.[11]

Glucocorticoids used alone are not as effective as when used with calcitonin.[62] Both can be used in patients with renal or cardiac failure who are dehydrated, and they therefore are useful for treatment of hypercalcemia when saline diuresis is contraindicated. The advantages to combined use are a more rapid response and prevention of the escape phenomenon encountered with use of calcitonin alone.[3,58] The usual dosage is prednisone 40–100 mg/dl in divided doses.[63]

Plicamycin

Plicamycin (mithramycin) is a cytotoxic drug with antihypercalcemic effects, probably through its toxic effects on osteoclasts[63] and irreversible impairment of osteoclast bone resorption.[11] Plicamycin has been associated with thrombocytopenia and with renal and hepatic toxicity. Nausea, vomiting, and toxic effects are related to cumulative dosage and rarely occur with the first or second dose. Since the drug is excreted through the kidneys, toxicity is more likely in patients with impaired renal function. Hypocalcemia and tetany also have been reported. Although some authors recommend use of this agent only when other less toxic regimens have failed,[12,58,62] its ease of administration in the ambulatory setting as well as cost constraints encourage its use as a first-line approach to moderate hypercalcemia. Plicamycin's major disadvantages are cumulative myelotoxicity with thrombocytopenia, which may interfere with administration of myelotoxic anticancer therapy, and renal toxicity, which may further impair renal function in patients who already have renal insufficiency due to hypercalcemia.[11,63]

Plicamycin is administered intravenously at a dose of 25 micrograms/kg (maximum dose 1500 mg) either as a slow bolus injection or as a 4-hour infusion. Bolus injections are associated with a higher incidence of nausea and vomiting. Reduction in serum calcium occurs within 48 hours and normocalcemia usually occurs after a single dose.[11,63] The dose may be repeated if no detectable lowering of serum calcium occurs within 48 hours. Once the serum calcium is lowered, the duration of action is variable and unpredictable, lasting from 3 days to a week or more. Treatment is not repeated until hypercalcemia returns.[58,62] Extravasation is associated with local irritation and cellulitis at the injection site. A change in the injection site and application of warm compresses are recommended by the manufacturer should extravasation occur (Miles Laboratories package insert).

Phosphates

Intravenous administration of inorganic phosphates rapidly decreases extracellular fluid calcium concentration by promoting skeletal calcification. Unfortunately, extraskeletal calcification also occurs and is associated with, among other things, impairment of renal function due to nephrocalcinosis. Intravenous phosphates should not be employed except as a last resort.[62]

Oral phosphates are less toxic in patients with normal renal function and serum phosphorus levels less than 4.0 mg/dl and are useful for chronic treatment of hypercalcemia once serum calcium levels have been reduced with other drugs. Phosphates prevent intestinal calcium absorption by forming poorly soluble Ca-PO_4 salts in the intestinal lumen, which makes less calcium available for absorption, and also by impairing conversion of 25-hydroxyvitamin D to 1,25-dihydroxyvitamin D (a major stimulator of intestinal calcium transport). In addition, phosphates inhibit mineral and bone matrix resorption. Soft tissue and skeletal calcification also occurs to a lesser extent than with intravenous phosphates, but lung and renal calcification has been documented with chronic administration.[3] The most common and also most limiting side effect is diarrhea, since phosphates are administered in the form of sodium or potassium salts, Fleets Phospho Soda being one of the preparations most commonly prescribed. The usual starting dosage is 1 g/dl in divided doses with titration of the dose upwards to a maximum of 3 g/dl. Dose-limiting diarrhea usually occurs at 2 g/dl.[63] Despite an initial response, chronic administration is often accompanied by loss of effectiveness.[3] No randomized prospective studies have evaluated the efficacy of oral phosphates. Phosphates are contraindicated in patients with renal failure and serum phosphorus levels greater than 3.8 mg/dl.

Prostaglandin Inhibitors

Aspirin, indomethacin, and nonsteroidal anti-inflammatory drugs have been tried, but only on occasion is there an antihypercalcemic response.

Bisphosphonates

The bisphosphonates (synonymous with diphosphonates or biphosphonates) are analogs of pyrophosphate, a naturally occurring substance that has an affinity for bone. They are effective inhibitors of osteoclast bone resorption apparently by binding tightly to calcified bone matrix and preventing osteoclast bone resorption.[67,68] Two bisphosphonates are currently FDA-approved for treatment of hypercalcemia: etidronate and pamidronate. A third bisphosphonate, clodronate, is widely used in Europe but is not available in the United States.

Etidronate

Etidronate (Didronel,® MGI Pharma) is available in both intravenous and oral formulations. Etidronate has been shown to be more effective than either saline hydration alone[69] or calcitonin after saline hydration.[67] It has been demonstrated to be safe with few side effects and is most effective when administered intravenously to the hydrated patient at a dose of 7.5 mg/kg daily administered over at least 2 hours for 3–7 days followed by oral maintenance therapy at a dose of 5–10 mg/kg/day.[11] Side effects reported in fewer than 10% of patients included altered taste during etidronate infusion, nausea and vomiting,[69] and fever postinfusion.[70] Renal toxicity (elevated serum creatinine) was reported to have occurred in 12% of patients receiving etidronate in one study.[69] Toxicities associated with long-term use (more than 3 months) of etidronate include impaired mineralization of bone and increases in serum phosphate.[67] Serum calcium levels usually normalize within 4–5 days, and median duration of effect for intravenous etidronate in one study was reported to be 29 days.[69]

Pamidronate

Pamidronate (Aredia,® Ciba), a second-generation bisphosphonate approved for treatment of moderate to severe malignant hypercalcemia in 1992, has been demonstrated to be more effective than etidronate.[70] It inhibits bone resorption without preventing bone mineralization. Pamidronate has a rapid onset of action, with serum calcium levels responding within 24 hours and reaching nadir by 7 days and a longer duration of action than that seen with other therapies.[70–72] There appears to be a significant dose-response relationship, with more severe hypercalcemias requiring higher doses in order to achieve normocalcemia.[71] Serum calcium responses are faster in patients receiving 4-hour infusions rather than the recommended 24-hour infusion.[73] A combination of intravenous pamidronate and calcitonin suppositories has been demonstrated to have a more rapid onset and better efficacy than intravenous pamidronate alone in a small study of 34 patients.[66] The recommended dose of pamidronate for moderate to severe hypercalcemia is 60–90 mg in 1000 ml of fluid (0.45% or 0.9% saline or 5% dextrose) administered as a single infusion over 24 hours in well-hydrated patients. The dose may be repeated after 7 days if needed. Side effects are dose related and include postinfusion temperature elevations (approximately 1°C 24–48 hr postinfusion), nausea, anorexia, taste perversions, asymptomatic hypophosphatemia, hypokalemia, hypocalcemia, and hypomagnesemia. Seven percent of patients receiving pamidronate in one study were reported to experience infusion site reactions consisting of redness, swelling, induration, or pain at the intravenous catheter insertion site.[70]

Clodronate

Clodronate is a highly effective bisphosphonate that has been studied extensively in Europe. Trials were halted in the United States when it was reported that several patients had developed leukemia after being treated with this agent, although it continues to be used in Europe.[11]

Gallium Nitrate

Gallium nitrate is a cytotoxic drug that has been found to inhibit bone resorption and restore normocalcemia with few side effects in 75%–85% of patients.[74] In a randomized double-blind trial, 50 patients received either a 5-day infusion of gallium nitrate or intramuscular injections of salmon calcitonin every 6 hours for 5 days. Eighteen of 24 patients receiving gallium nitrate achieved normocalcemia, compared with 8 of the 26 patients receiving calcitonin. Median duration of normocalcemia before other cytotoxic or hypocalcemic therapy was 6 days with gallium nitrate and 1 day with calcitonin.[75] Gallium nitrate has also been compared to etidronate. Gallium nitrate was administered by continuous infusion at a dose of 200 mg/m^2/dl for 5 days, while etidronate was administered as a 4-hour infusion at a dose of 7.5 mg/kg/day for 5 consecutive days. Normocalcemia was achieved by 82% of patients in the gallium group compared to 43% of patients treated with etidronate.[76]

Potential side effects in gallium-treated patients include asymptomatic hypophosphatemia and nephrotoxicity. A major disadvantage to the use of gallium nitrate is the 5-day continuous treatment regimen, which makes outpatient treatment inconvenient.

CONCLUSION

Hypercalcemia is a common metabolic complication of malignancy with vague symptoms that can often be confused with those of other paraneoplastic syndromes as well as those of end-stage disease. Nurses caring for cancer patients must be cognizant both of patients at risk and of their associated risk factors. In an exploratory study of hospitalized and ambulatory hypercalcemic patients, 88% of the patients were not aware that hypercalcemia might occur, and 80%–95% were not aware of the various symptoms of hypercalcemia.[77] Counseling of patients and families regarding prevention and recognition of early symptoms enables therapy to commence before extreme debilitation develops (Table 28-10). Patient and family education regarding the purposes and goals of therapy promotes coping with yet another complication of cancer. Meticulous monitoring of fluid and electrolyte balance is essential for effective medical treatment. If hypercalcemia becomes refractory to treatment, nursing measures that facilitate coping with issues related to death and dying are essential.

Although theoretical knowledge regarding humoral and local factors associated with hypercalcemia is advancing, current therapies are nonspecific, aimed at osteoclast inhibition rather than at the mediating bone-resorbing factor itself. The development of specific antagonists to local and humoral hypercalcemic factors would theoretically improve treatment of malignant hypercalcemia.

TABLE 28-10 What You Should Know About Hypercalcemia—A Patient Guide

Calcium is normally stored in the bones and a small amount is found circulating in the bloodstream. Proper levels of calcium in the bloodstream are needed to maintain body functions. Normally, the kidneys regulate the amount of calcium circulating in the bloodstream. When this balance is offset by kidney disease, cancer in the bone, or another cause, hypercalcemia occurs.

Hypercalcemia occurs when the amount of calcium circulating in the bloodstream is too high. Some types of cancer are more likely than others to be associated with hypercalcemia. Treatment of the disease process (cancer) is the best way to manage hypercalcemia.

WHAT YOU CAN DO TO REDUCE YOUR RISK OF DEVELOPING HYPERCALCEMIA

Hypercalcemia cannot always be prevented. However, you may be able to reduce your risk of developing hypercalcemia by following these guidelines:

- Remain as active as possible. Walking, standing, or sitting is good because such activity stimulates new bone formation and keeps excess calcium in the bones, not in the bloodstream.
- Drink at least 3 quarts of fluid per day. Dehydration prevents the kidneys from excreting excess calcium. If nausea or vomiting prevent you from maintaining an adequate fluid intake, notify your doctor or nurse.
- If possible, avoid taking thiazide diuretics (fluid pills) such as hydrochlorthiazide (Diuril™), which can impair the kidney's ability to excrete calcium.

TABLE 28-10 What You Should Know About Hypercalcemia—A Patient Guide (continued)

- Avoid taking vitamins A and D unless prescribed by your doctor.
- Unless your health care provider suggests otherwise, maintain a normal diet. The calcium in your diet will *not* increase your risk of hypercalcemia.

SYMPTOMS OF HYPERCALCEMIA

The symptoms of hypercalcemia are due to the effects of excess calcium on the function of muscles and the nervous system. Early symptoms of hypercalcemia may be difficult for you or your family to identify because they are similar to the symptoms that you may already be experiencing due to your illness or your treatment. It is important that both you and your family report any change or worsening in the symptoms you experience. If you are developing hypercalcemia, the earlier that you get treatment, the less likely you are to experience severe symptoms. Treatment for high levels of calcium in the bloodstream usually requires hospitalization, while lower levels may be treated on an outpatient basis. Common early symptoms of hypercalcemia include the following:

- nausea, vomiting, or loss of appetite
- constipation and/or abdominal pain
- extreme fatigue or muscle weakness
- bone pain
- increased thirst or excessive urination
- sleepiness, difficulty thinking or concentrating
- inappropriate behavior or conversation

Physician's name and number ______________________
Nurse's name and number ______________________

REFERENCES

1. Fisken RA, Heath DA, Sommers S, et al: Hypercalcemia in hospital patients: Clinical and diagnostic aspects. *Lancet* 1:202–207, 1981.

2. Mundy GR, Ibbotsen KJ, D'Souza SM, et al: The hypercalcemia of cancer: Clinical implications and pathogenic mechanisms. *N Engl J Med* 310:1718–1727, 1984.
3. Mundy GR, Martin TJ: The hypercalcemia of malignancy: Pathogenesis and management. *Metabolism* 31:1247–1277, 1982.
4. Fisken RA, Heath DA, Bold AM: Hypercalcemia—a hospital survey. *Q J Med* 49:405–418, 1980.
5. Myers WP: Hypercalcemia associated with malignant disease. In *Endocrine and Nonendocrine Producing Tumors.* Sixteenth Annual Clinical Conference on Cancer, MD Anderson Hospital and Tumor Institute. Chicago: Year Book Medical Publishers, 1973, pp. 147–171.
6. Blomqvist CP: Malignant hypercalcemia—a hospital survey. *Acta Med Scand* 220:455–463, 1986.
7. Monno S, Nagata A, Furuta S: Hypercalcemia of cancer in the digestive tract. *J Clin Gastroenterol* 9:78–82, 1987.
8. Bender RA, Hansen H: Hypercalcemia in bronchogenic carcinoma: A prospective study of 200 patients. *Ann Intern Med* 80:205–208, 1974.
9. Stewart AF, Romero R, Schwart PE, et al. Hypercalcemia associated with gynecologic malignancies: Biochemical characterization. *Cancer* 49:2389–2394, 1982.
10. Strewler GJ, Nissenson RA: Nonparathyroid hypercalcemia. *Adv Intern Med* 32:235–258, 1987.
11. Mundy GR: *Calcium Homeostasis: Hypercalcemia and Hypocalcemia.* London: Martin Dunitz, 1989, pp. 1–126.
12. Mundy GR: The hypercalcemia of malignancy. *Kidney Int* 31:142–155, 1987.
13. Mundy GR: Pathophysiology of cancer-associated hypercalcemia. *Semin Oncol* 17:10–15, 1990.
14. Habener JF, Rosenblatt M, Potts JT: Parathyroid hormone: Biochemical aspects of biosynthesis, secretion, action and metabolism. *Physiol Rev* 64:985–1040, 1984.
15. Peck WA, Rifas L, Cheng SL, et al: The local regulation of bone remodeling. *Adv Exp Med Biol* 108:255–259, 1986.
16. Meunier PJ: Cellular mechanisms of bone remodeling evaluated at the intermediary level of organization of bone. *Adv Exp Med Biol* 208:247–254, 1986.
17. Broadus AE, Mangin M, Ikeda K, et al: Humoral hypercalcemia of cancer: Identification of a novel parathyroid hormone-like peptide. *N Engl J Med* 319:556–563, 1988.
18. Mundy GR, Ibbotsen KJ, D'Souza SM: Tumor products and the hypercalcemia of malignancy. *J Clin Invest* 76:391–394, 1985.
19. Gowen M, MacDonald BR, Hughes DE, et al: Immune cells and bone resorption. *Adv Exp Med Biol* 208:261–273, 1986.
20. Linkart TA, Mohan S, Jennings JC: Copurification of osteolytic and transforming growth factor beta activities produced by human lung tumor cells associated with humoral hypercalcemia of malignancy. *Cancer Res* 49:271–278, 1989.
21. Fried RM, Voelkel EF, Rice RH, et al: Two squamous cell carcinomas not associated with humoral hypercalcemia produce a potent bone resorption-stimulating factor which is interleukin-alpha. *Endocrinology* 125:742–751, 1989.
22. Sato K, Fujii Y, Kasono K, et al: Production of interleukin alpha and a parathyroid hormone-like factor by a squamous cell carcinoma of the esophagus (EC-GI) derived from a patient with hypercalcemia. *J Clin Endocrinol Metab* 67:592–601, 1988.
23. Sabatini M, Yates AJ, Garrett IR, et al: Increased production of tumor necrosis factor by normal immune cells in a model of the humoral hypercalcemia of malignancy. *Lab Investig* 63:676–682, 1990.
24. Burtis WJ, Wu T, Bunch C, et al: Identification of a novel 17,000-dalton parathyroid hormone-like adenylate cyclase-stimulating protein from a tumor associated with humoral hypercalcemia of malignancy. *J Biol Chem* 262:7151–7156, 1987.
25. Mangin M, Webb AC, Dreyer BE, et al: Identification of a cDNA encoding a parathyroid hormone-like peptide in messenger RNAs from a human tumor associated with humoral hypercalcemia of malignancy. *Proc Natl Acad Sci* 85:597–601, 1988.
26. Ikeda K, Mangin M, Dreyer BE, et al: Identification of transcripts encoding a parathyroid hormone-like peptide in messenger RNAs from a variety of human and animal tumors associated with humoral hypercalcemia of malignancy. *J Clin Invest* 81:2010–2014, 1988.
27. Stewart AF, Horst R, Deftos LJ, et al: Biochemical evaluation of patients with cancer-associated hypercalcemia: Evidence for humoral and non-humoral groups. *N Engl J Med* 303:1377–1383, 1980.
28. Bonjour JP, Rizzoli R, Pizurki L: Action of tumoral PTH-related peptide on phosphate and calcium transport. *Progress Clin Biological Res* 332:39–49, 1990.
29. Insogna KL: Humoral hypercalcemia of malignancy. The role of parathyroid hormone-related protein. *Endocrinol & Metab Clin NA* 18:779–794, 1989.
30. Jacobs JW, Simpson E: Hypercalcemia of malignancy. *Adv Exp Med Biol* 208:357–366, 1986.
31. Nagata N, Yasutomo Y, Kugai N, et al: Parathyroid hormone-related protein and transforming growth factor activities in an extract from a breast cancer associated with humoral hypercalcemia of malignancy. *Jap J Clin Oncol* 19:353–359, 1989.
32. Sato K, Fujii Y, Kasono K, et al: Paraneoplastic syndrome of hypercalcemia and leukocytosis caused by squamous carcinoma cells (T3M-1) producing parathyroid hormone-related protein, interleukin 1 alpha, and granulocyte colony stimulating factor. *Cancer Res* 49:4740–4746, 1989.
33. Mercier RJ, Thompson JM, Harman GS, et al: Recurrent hypercalcemia and elevated 1,25-dihydroxyvitamin D levels in Hodgkin's disease. *Am J Med* 84:165–168, 1988.
34. Breslau NA, McGuire JL, Zerwekh JE, et al: Hypercalcemia associated with increased serum calcitriol levels in three patients with lymphoma. *Ann Intern Med* 100:1–7, 1984.
35. Rosenthal N, Insogna KL, Godsall JW, et al: Elevations in circulating 1,25-dihydroxyvitamin D in three patients with lymphoma associated hypercalcemia. *J Clin Endocrinol Metab* 60:29–33, 1985.
36. Mudde AH, van den Berg H, Boshuis PG, et al: Ectopic production of 1,25-dihydroxyvitamin D by B-cell lymphoma as a cause of hypercalcemia. *Cancer* 59:1543–1546, 1987.
37. Devogelaer JP, Lambert M, Boland B, et al: 1,25-dihydroxyvitamin D in lymphoma: Two case reports. *Clin Rheumatol* 9:404–410, 1990.
38. Fetchik DA, Bertolini DR, Sarin PS, et al: Production of 1,25-dihydroxyvitamin D_3 by human T-cell lymphotrophic virus-1-transformed lymphocytes. *J Clin Invest* 78:592–596, 1986.
39. Hayes ME, Bayley D, Drayson M, et al: Metabolism of 25-hydroxyvitamin D3 by blood derived macrophages from a patient with alveolar rhabdomyosarcoma during short-term culture and 1 alpha, 25-dihydroxyvitamin D3 after long term culture. *J Steroid Biochem & Molec Biol* 38:301–306, 1991.

40. Adams JS: Vitamin D metabolite-mediated hypercalcemia. *Endocrinol & Metab Clin NA* 18:765–778, 1989.
41. Percival RC, Yates AJ, Gray RE, et al: Mechanism of malignant hypercalcemia in carcinoma of the breast. *Br Med J (Clin Res)* 291:776–779, 1985.
42. Isales C, Carcangiu ML, Stewart AF: Hypercalcemia in breast cancer: Reassessment of the mechanism. *Am J Med* 82:1143–1147, 1987.
43. Ralston SH: The pathogenesis of humoral hypercalcemia of malignancy. *Lancet* 2:1443–1446, 1987.
44. Eilon G, Mundy GR: Effects of inhibition of microtubule assembly on bone mineral release and enzyme release by human breast cancer cells. *J Clin Invest* 67:69–76, 1981.
45. Legha S, Powell K, Budzan A, et al: Tamoxifen-induced hypercalcemia in breast cancer. *Cancer* 47:2803–2806, 1986.
46. Gallacher SJ, Fraser WD, Patel U, et al: Breast cancer-associated hypercalcemia: A reassessment of renal calcium and phosphate handling. *Ann Clin Biochem* 27:551–556, 1990.
47. Grill V, Ho P, Body JJ, et al: Parathyroid hormone-related protein: Elevated levels in both humoral hypercalcemia of malignancy and hypercalcemia complicating metastatic breast cancer. *J Clin Endocrinol Metab* 73:1309–1315, 1991.
48. Mundy GR: Pathogenesis of hypercalcemia of malignancy. *Clin Endocrinol* 23:705–714, 1985.
49. Mundy GR, Bertolini DR: Bone destruction and hypercalcemia in plasma cell myeloma. *Semin Oncol* 13:291–299, 1986.
50. Muggia FM: Overview of cancer-related hypercalcemia: Epidemiology and etiology. *Semin Oncol* 17:3–9, 1990.
51. Mundy GR: Hypercalcemic factors other than parathyroid hormone-related protein. *Endocrinol Metab Clin NA* 18:795–806, 1989.
52. Kiyokawa T, Yamaguchi K, Takeya M, et al: Hypercalcemia and osteoclast proliferation in adult T-cell leukemia. *Cancer* 59:1187–1191, 1987.
53. Fukumoto S, Matsumoto T, Watanabe T, et al: Secretion of parathyroid hormone-like activity from human T-cell lymphotropic virus type *T*-infected lymphocytes. *Cancer Res* 49:3849–3852, 1989.
54. Moseley JM, Danks JA, Grill V, et al: Immunocytochemical demonstration of PTHrP in neoplastic tissue of HTLV-1 positive human adult T-cell leukemia/lymphoma: Implications for the mechanisms of hypercalcemia. *Br J Cancer* 64:745–748, 1991.
55. Ralston SH, Gallacher SJ, Patel U, et al: Cancer-associated hypercalcemia: Morbidity and mortality. Clinical experience in 126 treated patients. *Ann Intern Med* 112:499–504, 1990.
56. Mahon SM: Signs and symptoms associated with malignancy induced hypercalcemia. *Cancer Nurs* 12:153–160, 1989.
57. Bajorunas DR: Clinical manifestations of cancer-related hypercalcemia. *Semin Oncol* 17:16–25, 1990 (suppl. 5).
58. Fields ALA, Josse RG, Bergsagel DE: Metabolic emergencies: Hypercalcemia. In DeVita VT, Hellman S, Rosenberg SA (eds), *Cancer Principles and Practice of Oncology*. Philadelphia: Lippincott, 1985, pp. 1866–1872.
59. Poe CM, Radford AI: The challenge of hypercalcemia in cancer. *Oncol Nurs Forum* 12:29–34, 1985.
60. Coward DD: Cancer-induced hypercalcemia. *Cancer Nurs* 9:125–132, 1986.
61. Boisaubin EV, Lynch GR: Hypercalcemia of advanced malignancy: Decision making and the quality of death. *Amer J Med Sci* 301:314–318, 1991.
62. Fetchik DA, Mundy GR: Hypercalcemia of malignancy: Diagnosis and therapy. *Comprehen Ther* 12:27–32, 1986.
63. Ritch PS: Treatment of cancer-related hypercalcemia. *Semin Oncol* 17:26–33, 1990.
64. Hosking DJ, Stone MD, Foote JW: Potentiation of calcitonin during the treatment of hypercalcemia of malignancy. *Eur J Clin Pharmacol* 38:37–41, 1990.
65. Kasono K, Isozaki O, Sato K, et al: Effects of glucocorticoids and calcitonin on parathyroid hormone-related protein (PTHrP) gene expression and PTHrP release in human cancer cells causing humoral hypercalcemia. *Jap J Cancer Res* 82:1008–1014, 1991.
66. Thiebaud D, Jacquet AF, Burckhardt P: Fast and effective treatment of malignant hypercalcemia. Combination of suppositories of calcitonin and a single infusion of 3-amino 1-hydroxypropylidene-1-bisphosphonate. *Arch Intern Med* 150:2125–2128, 1990.
67. Singer FR: Role of the bisphosphonate etidronate in the therapy of cancer-related hypercalcemia. *Semin Oncol* 17:34–39, 1990.
68. Coleman RE: Bisphosphonate treatment of bone metastases and hypercalcemia of malignancy. *Oncology* 5:55–60, 1991.
69. Singer FR, Ritch PS, Ringenberg QS, et al: Treatment of hypercalcemia of malignancy with intravenous etidronate. A controlled, multicenter study. The Hypercalcemia Study Group. *Arch Intern Med* 151:471–476, 1991.
70. Gucalp R, Ritch P, Wiernik PH, et al: Comparative study of pamidronate and etidronate disodium in the treatment of cancer related hypercalcemia. *J Clin Oncol* 10:134–142, 1992.
71. Thiebaud D, Jaeger AF, Jacquet AF, et al: Dose-response in the treatment of hypercalcemia of malignancy by a single infusion of the bisphosphonate AHPrBP. *J Clin Oncol* 6:762–768, 1988.
72. Coleman RE, Rubens RD: 3(amino-1, 1-hydroxypropylidene) bisphosphonate (APD) for hypercalcemia of breast cancer. *Br J Cancer* 56:465–469, 1987.
73. Sawyer N, Newstead C, Drummond A, et al: Fast (4-h) or slow (24-h) infusions of pamidronate disodium (aminohydroxypropylidene diphosphonate (APD)) as single shot treatment of hypercalcemia. *Bone & Mineral* 9:121–128, 1990.
74. Todd PA, Fitton A: Gallium nitrate. A review of its pharmacological properties and therapeutic potential in cancer-related hypercalcemia. *Drugs* 42:261–273, 1991.
75. Warell RP Jr, Israel R, Frisone M, et al: Gallium nitrate for acute treatment of cancer-related hypercalcemia: A randomized, double-blind comparison to calcitonin. *Ann Intern Med* 108:669–674, 1988.
76. Warrell RP Jr, Murphy WK, Shulman P, et al: A randomized double-blind study of gallium nitrate compared with etidronate for acute control of cancer-related hypercalcemia. *J Clin Oncol* 9:1467–1475, 1991.
77. Coward D: Hypercalcemia knowledge assessment in patients at risk of developing cancer induced hypercalcemia. *Oncol Nurs Forum* 15:471–476, 1988.

Chapter 29

Hormonal Disturbances

Ada M. Lindsey, RN, PhD

INTRODUCTION

Abnormal hormone secretion can occur as a consequence of malignant neoplastic growth.[1-11] This abnormal secretion was labeled *ectopic hormone production* because the hormone synthesis occurred in nonendocrine tissues. The continued development of localization and measurement techniques has shown that what was originally believed to be ectopic hormone production was in many cases a somewhat erroneous conception. It is now known that hormones are secreted from many normal cells not normally classified as being endocrine; that is, nonendocrine tissues secrete a variety of hormones in small quantities. These molecules are all polypeptide or glycoprotein hormones, or *hormone precursors*. To date, such steroid hormone production has not been observed.[2,3] With more sensitive immunochemical, biochemical, and molecular biologic technologies, some hormone precursor molecules, hormones, and encoding mRNAs have been found in cells not originally thought to make those products.[2-4] However, it is in tumors that these products are synthesized in amounts that produce clinical syndromes, and they are produced without the normal regulatory feedback.

Regardless of whether the label *ectopic* remains descriptive, there are a variety of paraneoplastic hormonal syndromes that are associated with some malignancies. For example, "ectopic" secretion of adrenocorticotropic hormone (ACTH) from lung tumors is one of the more commonly observed hormonal abnormalities. In normal circumstances, ACTH is secreted from the anterior pituitary gland in response to stimulation from corticotropin-releasing hormone released from the hypothalamus and in response to circulating levels of glucocorticoids (e.g., cortisol) released from the adrenal cortex. However, in some cases of lung cancer, as well as in other cancers, with the alterations that occur with cell transformation into malignant cell growth, these nonendocrine cells synthesize and secrete specific hormones. Normally, these cells are from organs and tissues, such as lung tissue, that are not endocrine glands, per se, but when they become transformed, some will synthesize hormone(s) or other peptides. In some cases the hormone molecules produced by the malignant nonendocrine cells are exactly like the biologically active hormone that is normally produced by the respective endocrine gland. In some cases only fragments of a hormone or the larger precursor hormone molecule may be produced. In that circumstance, if the fragments or precursor are not capable of producing a biologic response in the target organs, there would be no clinical evidence of the ectopic hormone secretion. However, if the hormone produced by the malignant cells is biologically active, the target organ for the specific hormone will respond. If the hormone is produced in sufficient quantity, the abnormal secretion will become clinically evident as an endocrine syndrome. For example, there have been cases of lung cancer where the initial or presenting symptoms reflected a Cushing's syndrome resulting from excess glucocorticoid/cortisol production by the adrenal glands in response to the ectopic production of ACTH from the lung tumor. These syndromes also may occur some time after the cancer has been diagnosed.

In normal circumstances, hormone secretion is very finely controlled and regulated; what is unusual in the ectopic secretion of hormones is that the malignant nonendocrine cells that produce these hormones are not sensitive to the control or regulatory feedback systems that exist for the endocrine glands. The ectopic production of the hormone goes unchallenged by the usual regulatory mechanisms, resulting in excess secretion of the hormone. Depending on the hormone produced, some of the resulting endocrine abnormalities may be more immediately life-threatening than the cancer itself. Thus, it is imperative to recognize the variety and the significance of hormonal disturbances that may result from the production of hormones by malignant tumors of nonendocrine origin.

Many tumors synthesize protein or polypeptide molecules. Some of these are hormones or hormone fragments; others have become known as *tumor markers*, such as alpha feto-protein and carcinoembryonic antigen (CEA); and investigations on others are still in progress. The systemic effects of these tumor products are referred to as *paraneoplastic phenomena*. In addition to the endocrine paraneoplastic syndromes, other paraneoplastic syndromes have been described. These include neurologic, hematologic, renal, and cutaneous syndromes, and even cachexia is classified as a paraneoplastic phenomenon.[1] As tumor products are identified and assays are developed or improved for increased sensitivity and specificity, measurement of these tumor products can be used for cancer detection and as indicators of disease recurrence and tumor response to treatment.

Tumors also can arise in endocrine glands and may result in hormonal abnormalities. In contrast to ectopic secretion, the release of hormone from endocrine cells is labeled *entopic*. The hormonal disturbances that occur with endocrine gland malignancies are presented in Chapter 40.

Incidence

Originally thought to be rare, the occurrence of abnormal hormone production by malignant cells is now considered to be more common.[3] Many cancers are not associated with any clinically apparent paraneoplastic syndrome. However, the incidence varies by type of cancer. For example, lung cancer, particularly small-cell lung cancer, is more often associated with paraneoplastic endocrine syndromes. In one report of 84 small-cell lung cancer patients, 14% had a demonstrated endocrine syndrome.[12] Earlier reports show a much lower incidence, and later reports show a higher incidence.[1,3] One author purports that 50% of lung carcinomas produce biologically active ACTH.[3] The real incidence of paraneoplastic endocrine syndromes remains somewhat speculative. Secretory abnormalities may exist, but if the secretory products are not biologically active, a clinical syndrome does not result. Specific syndromes are described in the "Clinical Manifestations" section of this chapter, and the tumor types associated with each syndrome are identified.

Definitions

Entopic refers to the production of hormones by endocrine cells. *Ectopic* hormone production has been the term used to describe the production of hormones by malignant cells that are of nonendocrine origin. Because it is now known that some normal nonendocrine tissues synthesize some hormones in very small quantities, the term *ectopic* is not so accurate a description, but it is still used. *Paraneoplastic endocrine syndrome* is the term used when a tumor produces biologically active substances and these tumor by-products enter the circulation and cause remote effects, resulting in some physiologic alteration. The focus of this chapter is on examples of ectopic (nonendocrine tissue) hormone production observed in association with cancer.

ANATOMY, PHYSIOLOGY, AND SCIENTIFIC PRINCIPLES

Understanding the normal anatomical structures and physiological regulation and functions of the neuroendocrine system provides the basis for elucidating and interpreting the hormonal alterations that can occur with ectopic secretion from nonendocrine malignant tissue. Significant scientific advances in delineating the mechanisms of action and regulation as well as in the measurement of hormones have been made. These advances, in addition to those made in the field of genetics, have contributed to the development of knowledge about the endocrine syndromes observed in association with cancer.

Neuroendocrine Structures

The major central neuroendocrine structures include the hypothalamus, the pituitary, and the connecting hypothalamic-pituitary stalk. The hypothalamus and the pituitary are in very close proximity; the vascular connections (i.e., the hypophyseal-portal system between the two structures) are located in the stalk. The hormones released via these structures directly enter the bloodstream and circulate to the peripherally located target endocrine glands. The hormones from the hypothalamus are produced and released via neurons, while those from the pituitary are produced and released by endocrine cells. The majority of the hypothalamic hormones have a stimulatory or an inhibitory action on the anterior pituitary gland cells. Two hypothalamic hormones, antidiuretic hormone and oxytocin, are released via hypothalamic neurons in the posterior pituitary, where they enter the circulatory system. The secretion rates of hormones are not constant. The hypothalamus is influenced by circadian rhythms and as a result some of the hormones have a characteristic diurnal secretory pattern. Some hormones are secreted in a pulsatile rhythm and others, such as those involved in ovulation and menstruation, have a complicated secretory pattern. All the hypothalamic and pituitary hormones are derived from amino acids and are thus classified as polypeptide/protein hormones.

The target organs, the peripherally located endocrine glands, respond to the centrally released hormones by producing and releasing another hormone or by some other biologic response. The release of glucocorticoids (e.g., cortisol) by the adrenal cortex in response to the pituitary release of ACTH is one example, while the conservation of water by the renal tubules illustrates the example of a biologic response, in this case, to the release of the hypothalamic antidiuretic hormone (ADH) or arginine vasopressin (AVP).

Most peripheral endocrine glands are regulated primarily through the hypothalamic pituitary neuroendocrine axis. However, some peripheral endocrine glands have other regulatory mechanisms; these include the parathyroid glands, the insulin-producing islets of the pancreas, the thymus gland, and the gastrointestinal endocrine cells. For example, the circulating levels of calcium influence the secretion of parahormone, and the circulatory levels of glucose influence the secretion of insulin.

Some of the hormones produced by these target organs are polypeptides (e.g., insulin); some, such as cortisol, estrogen, testosterone, and aldosterone, are steroids; the thyroid hormones are classified as iodothyronines; and epinephrine and norepinephrine are catecholamines.

The neuroendocrine structures of major importance include the hypothalamus, the connecting hypophyseal-portal system, the pituitary gland, and the target endocrine glands and tissues. The hormones produced by the endocrine cells and some hypothalamic neurons are chemical signals that are transported by the circulatory system to their specific sites of action.

This description presents the classical endocrine system. However, in recent years many more substances have been identified and characterized. These substances have been labeled hormones because they are released, circulate, and have effects distant to the cells producing them. Examples include CNS and gastrointestinal peptides such as neurophysin and bombesin, and even the growth factors and immune response mediators.

Neuroendocrine Regulation and Function

The regulation of neuroendocrine function is based on a very responsive feedback system that involves stimulation and inhibition. The hormones secreted from the hypothalamus are used as a beginning point. Some of these, such as thyrotrophin-releasing hormone (TRH), stimulate production of anterior pituitary hormones; others, such as somatostatin, are inhibitory. Stimulatory hormones from the hypothalamus cause a specific anterior pituitary hormone to be released, and it in turn stimulates the release of hormone from its peripherally located target endocrine gland. Thus, TRH stimulates thyroid-stimulatory hormone (TSH) from the anterior pituitary gland, which in turn stimulates release of thyroxine and triiodothyronine from the thyroid gland. In many cases the end product, such as cortisol (resulting from CRF stimulation of ACTH and subsequent production of cortisol from the adrenal cortex) acts in an inhibitory way on the hypothalamus and on the anterior pituitary, resulting in decreased release of CRF. Refer to Figure 29-1 for a diagrammatic representation of this feedback system of regulation.

There are other models of regulation. For example, ADH secretion by the hypothalamic neurons is sensitive to osmotic pressure, blood volume, and blood pressure. Pain, stress, and emotional states also influence ADH secretion. ADH plays a role in the conservation of water and in the maintenance of plasma osmolality, blood pressure, and volume. The renin-angiotensin-aldosterone system is involved in the control of the internal fluid and electrolyte environment. The regulation of this system also is a different model from that shown in Figure 29-1, but in each case feedback mechanisms are involved in regulation. The biologic effects resulting from the initial hormone stimulation serve as the inhibitory mechanisms resulting in a decrease in hormone release. For example, when sufficient quantities of water have been conserved by the renal tubule cells in response to ADH, the change in osmotic pressure, blood volume, and/or blood pressure results in a decrease in the release of ADH from the hypothalamic neurons.

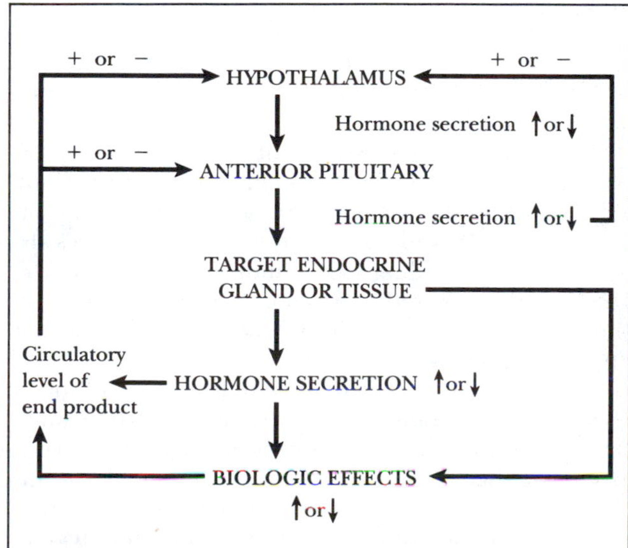

FIGURE 29-1 Diagrammatic representation of neuroendocrine feedback regulation mechanisms. (Key: + stimulatory; − inhibitory; ↑ increase; ↓ decrease.)

The regulation of the gonadotrophin-releasing hormone (GnRH or LHRH), follicle-stimulating hormone (FSH), luteinizing hormone (LH), and the estrogen and progesterone system is even more complex and not completely elucidated. Secretions occur in cyclical patterns and change over the life span.

Trophic hormones have several general functions. Many stimulate the synthesis of their specific cell receptors, some induce differentiation of cells, some stimulate cell mitosis, and some stimulate other cell functions. Thus, the stimulation of target tissue may result in an increase of the cells' sensitivity to the hormone, an increase in the number of functional cells, and an increase in other specific cell activities.

From this brief overview it is apparent that many factors are involved in the normal regulation of neuroendocrine function. The factors vary depending on the system. However, the regulation includes the capacity to sense minute environmental changes in the internal milieu and in some cases in the external world. The regulation includes the ability of the system, in response to changes, to increase or decrease synthesis and release of hormones or other biologic effects; a chain of events results in modulation of the system.

In the case of hormone production by nonendocrine malignant cells, the regulatory system is not effective. The production of the hormone is not a result a trophic hormone stimulation, but occurs as the result of gene expression in the undifferentiated, transformed malignant cells, and these cells are not responsive to a decrease in the trophic (stimulating) hormone or other regulatory feedback mechanisms to which normal endocrine cells respond. Thus, these nonendocrine tissue hormones are produced in excess and are not subject to usual control mechanisms. There have been some cases reported where there is evidence that the releasing hormone and the stimulatory or trophic hormone have both been synthesized by the same malignant tumors.[13,14]

Glands

The hypothalamus, although not considered a gland, does synthesize and secrete hormones that stimulate the synthesis and secretion of the pituitary gland trophic hormones. The target glands for these trophic hormones include the pineal gland, the thyroid gland, the adrenal gland, the ovary, and the testis. Other hormone-secreting tissues include the pancreatic A and B cells, the parathyroid, the adrenal medulla, C cells of the thyroid, gastrointestinal hormone-secreting cells, and the placenta. In addition to the endocrine cells, these glands or tissues comprise other structural and functional components. One common feature is that the hormones are released directly into the circulatory system.

Hormones

Hormones known to be produced by neurons originating in the hypothalamus include corticotrophin-releasing hormone (CRH), thyrotrophin-releasing hormone (TRH), gonadotrophin-releasing hormone (GnRH or LHRH), somatostatin (SRIF), antidiuretic hormone (ADH), and oxytocin. These latter two are released directly into the circulation at the posterior pituitary; the former are released into the hypophyseal-portal system, which goes to the anterior pituitary.

Hormones produced by the pituitary include growth hormone (GH or somatotrophin), adrenocorticotrophin hormone (ACTH), thyrotrophin hormone (TSH), luteinizing hormone (LH in females and interstitial cell-stimulating hormone, ICSH, in males), prolactin (PRL), and melanocyte-stimulating hormone (MSH). ACTH is synthesized in the form of a large precursor molecule containing MSH, B lipotrophin, beta-endorphin, and met-enkephalin; these latter peptides have morphine-like properties.[1]

Some of the peptide hormones generally characterized as originating from gastrointestinal-secretory cells have been found to occur in extrahypothalamic areas of the brain. These hormones include gastrin, substance P, and cholecystokinin (CKK). Some of the hypothalamic and pituitary hormones have also been found in other discrete locations within the central nervous system. These include TRH, SRIF, ACTH, and GnRH.

Other hormones are released from the peripheral target glands and tissues—for example, epinephrine from the adrenal medulla, aldosterone and glucocorticoids from the adrenal cortex, thyroxine from the thyroid, calcitonin from the C cells of the thyroid, insulin from the pancreatic B cells, glucagon from pancreatic A cells, estrogens from the ovary, and testosterone from the testis. Hormones are released from the placenta and also from the gastrointestinal tract secretory cells; the liver and kidney are the major source for the cholecalciferol metabolites (vitamin D).

Hormones are classified by their primary chemical composition. The four major classifications are: (1) the amine group, including the catecholamines, norepinephrine, and epinephrine; (2) the iodothyronines, (i.e., thyronine and triiodothyronine); (3) the peptide, protein, and glycoprotein group, which includes a large number of hormones; and (4) the steroids. Examples of the peptide hormones are ADH or vasopressin, oxytocin, TRH, GnRH, SRIF, and the angiotensins. Insulin, glucagon, prolactin, calcitonin, and ACTH are protein hormones, and examples of glycoprotein hormones are FSH, luteinizing hormone, and TSH. Peptides are small chains of amino acids, while proteins are larger chains of amino acids; i.e., polypeptide chains are linked to create larger structures. Glycoproteins are created intracellularly by the addition of sugars to various specific locations on the protein structure. The peptide/protein class of hormones are synthesized by intracellular DNA-RNA actions. The synthesis of estrogens, progesterone, testosterone, glucocorticoids (e.g., cortisol), and aldosterone also occurs intracellularly, but through a complicated orderly sequence of enzymatic steps. Iodothyronines are also synthesized through a series of enzymatic steps.

It is significant that of the nonendocrine tissue production of hormones observed to occur with malignant tumors, all the hormones have been of the peptide/protein class, where the synthesis occurs via DNA-RNA direction. Because a number of specific enzymatic steps are involved sequentially in the synthesis of other classes of hormones, this synthetic process is much more difficult and thus unlikely to occur as a paraneoplastic phenomenon. However, the end result in some circumstances of ectopic hormone production is the excess secretion of some nonprotein hormones such as cortisol. For example, the Cushing's syndrome that occurs with excess unregulated cortisol secretion is the result of the ectopic production of the protein hormone adrenocorticotrophin, by nonendocrine malignant cells. The excess ACTH stimulates the cortisol production by the adrenal cortex.

Some hormones are produced as larger molecules and are called *precursors* or *prohormones.* These larger molecules must be cleaved or separated to yield the biologically active hormone. Such is the case for ACTH, which is part of the larger pro-opiomelanocortin molecule. Similarly, insulin is initially part of a larger molecule. Separation is required for biologic activity. The glycoprotein hormones have sugars added to their protein structure to confer their biologic activity.

Most hormones are transported in the circulatory system attached to carrier proteins specific for the hormone, such as the sex hormone–binding globulin that carries estrogen and testosterone. Many hormones also are carried by binding to albumin. However, it is only the free, or unbound, hormone that is available as the biologically active molecule and can interact with its cell-specific receptors.

Hormones are very effective in low concentrations; they have a physiologic range of 10^{-7} to 10^{-12} mol/l. The action time frame of hormones is generally comparable to their chemical classification. Epinephrine and norepinephrine are effective in milliseconds, the peptides (e.g., angiotensin and ADH) within minutes, the proteins and glycoproteins (e.g., insulin, calcitonin, and TSH) within minutes to hours, the steroids (e.g., estrogen, cortisol, and aldosterone) within hours, and the iodothyronines (e.g., thyroxine) are effective over days.

Target Tissues/Receptors

Since hormones circulate in the bloodstream they would be accessible to virtually all tissues. What accounts for the specificity of hormone "recognition" is the presence of receptors in the target tissues. These receptors recognize the hormone specific for the particular target tissue. Some hormones have receptors in many types of tissues, while some have specific receptors in only one or a few types of tissue. For example, receptors specific for growth hormone are found in almost all cells, while receptors for ADH are localized in renal tubule cells. Some hormone-specific receptors are located on the cell surface; others are located intracellularly. In the case of the peptide/protein hormones, the hormone-specific receptors are located on the cell surface. When the hormone is bound to the receptor, a series of actions evolve; depending on the target organ, the result could be the synthesis and release of a hormone, as is true for ACTH action on the adrenal cortex that stimulates release of the glucocorticoids. Alternatively, some protein hormones when binding with their specific target cell receptors result in other types of biologic activity, such as occurs with insulin interacting with peripheral tissues effecting entry of glucose and decrease of lipolysis. The specific receptors of steroid hormones are located intracellularly. Lipid hormones cross cell membranes and interact with a cytosol receptor; this hormone-receptor complex moves into the cell nucleus, where the cascade of hormone action begins.

The receptors for all hormones, whether on the cell surface or intracellular, are protein structures. The receptors are specific for their respective hormone. The number of receptors and the amount of hormone binding to the receptors influence the magnitude of the hormone response. There is evidence that the number of receptors is regulated as well as the binding capacity. Thus, the receptors have a major role in specific hormone action in addition to the amount of circulating biologically active free hormone.

PATHOPHYSIOLOGY

All cells in an individual have the same genetic material, the entire genome. Through the processes of cellular differentiation and specialization, depending on the tissue, specific genes will be expressed while others are not expressed, creating the differences in cells and ultimately cell function. It is thought that in the malignant transformation of cells some of the genes that are not ordinarily expressed in the normal differentiated cell of a particular tissue are expressed or become activated in the malignant cells.[5–7,11] This may account for the expression of genes that code for the synthesis of the peptide/protein hormones in nonendocrine malignant cells. The only hormones produced ectopically are the peptide class. No steroid hormones or catecholamines have been found in ectopic production.[5] However, all the polypeptide hormones have occurred in ectopic production from tumors of nonendocrine origin. Some of the peptides synthesized by the malignant cells are exactly like the normally secreted hormone from endocrine cells, and some are only fragments or deviate in other ways. It is only in those cases where the tumor product has sufficient biologic activity that a clinical syndrome will become evident.

In addition to hormones, tumor cells may synthesize other biologically recognized entities, such as antigens. Responses to these abnormally produced substances can result in remote or systemic effects. Cases in which these effects result in some recognized physiological alteration are also classified as paraneoplastic syndromes. In some cases, based on associated clinical evidence, the biologically active substance is presumed to exist, but the specific substances have not been identified. Conversely, a biologic function has not been identified for all the substances that have been elaborated by tumor cells. In addition, the host immune response to the tumor may result in paraneoplastic phenomena, now thought to be one explanation for the presence of tumor necrosis factor (TNF) and other cytokines in association with cachexia. It is estimated that at some time during the course of cancer at least half of the patients will be affected by some paraneoplastic phenomenon.[5] The systemic effects may be a greater problem than that resulting from the local tumor growth. As is true of ectopic hormone secretion, some paraneoplastic syndromes may precede the diagnosis of the malignancy, or they may occur at any time following the diagnosis. In both situations the syndromes will be reversed only when tumor treatment is effective. Some therapies are effective in reducing the effects of the syndromes, but complete eradication depends on effectiveness of treatment of the tumor. Symptom management also may be possible for some of these syndromes when treatment of the malignancy fails.

Expression of the oncofetal proteins, carcinoembryonic antigen (CEA) and alpha-fetoprotein, has occurred with different malignancies. While these abnormally produced proteins do not result in a syndrome, measurement of the tumor-produced proteins has been used to monitor response to anticancer therapies.

Originally it was thought that the malignant cells that produced ectopic hormones had a common embryonic origin, such as the neural crest. Cells originating from the neural crest are characterized by their capacity for amine precursor uptake and decarboxylation (APUD), processes involved in peptide hormone synthesis.[15] These cells are widely distributed and were believed to result in the ectopic hormone production. However, this concept no longer explains all the ectopic hormone production that has been observed to occur in many other morphologic cell types.[5,7,11,16,17] Also, there is evidence to suggest that all the neuroendocrine cells may not have a common embryologic origin. Thus, the concept of activation of some genetic expression in malignant cells ordinarily not expressed in normally differentiated cells, as previously described, is the more widely accepted explanation for the occurrence of paraneoplastic syndromes including ectopic hormone production. Recent evidence that some hormones are found and/or produced in small quantities by nonendocrine cells may lead to other explanations for the production of hormones by nonendocrine malignant cells.[3,9]

CLINICAL MANIFESTATIONS

The clinical manifestations of the paraneoplastic syndromes vary depending on the type of substances produced by the malignant tumor. A tumor may produce more than one hormone or product. It is known that many peptides are produced by malignant cells. In many cases, no clinical syndrome will occur because the tumor product is not biologically active. These may be hormone fragments or prohormones (larger precursor molecules) where cleavage of the larger molecule did not occur (because enzymes responsible for the specific cleavage were not present), or the hormone structure may be altered. Only those products that are biologically active and that are secreted in sufficient excess will result in a clinical syndrome. Paraneoplastic syndromes have been reviewed in detail.[1–11] The syndromes resulting from the more commonly occurring "ectopically" produced hormones are described next.

Glands

Malignancies arising in endocrine glands may or may not result in hormonal disturbances. If this occurs, the hormonal secretions may be increased or decreased; however, the secretion is entopic. The affected gland may remain responsive to the regulatory feedback mechanisms, or this control may be compromised. When the malignancy arises in an endocrine gland, the hormonal changes observed may vary from patient to patient. Multiple endocrine neoplasias (MEN) have been reported.[11] Several endocrine glands are involved, and the result is alteration in secretion of hormones from the multiple affected glands. The more common malignancies arising in endocrine glands are described in Chapter 40.

Endocrine glands also are affected when the malignancy arises in nonendocrine tissue and the malignant cells produce hormones. The ectopic hormone, if biologically active, will affect its specific target tissue. Some nonendocrine tissue tumors secrete more than one hormone; in those cases more than one endocrine gland or endocrine responsive tissue will be affected.

Hormones and Target Tissues

The hormones that are produced "ectopically" by malignant tumors are in the peptide/protein class. However, these hormones may be trophic to an endocrine gland that secretes a steroid hormone, and thus the clinical syndrome results from increased entopic steroid hormone production from the endocrine gland that was stimulated by the tumor-produced peptide hormone. An example is Cushing's syndrome, where the entopic production of cortisol results from stimulation of the adrenal cortex by the ectopically produced peptide hormone ACTH.

Hormones and hormone precursors that have been observed to be secreted in association with tumors include ACTH, corticotrophin-releasing hormone, ADH, growth hormone–releasing hormone, prolactin, chorionic gonadotrophin, calcitonin, glucagon, somatostatin, and many others.[1–3,5,9] Hormone disturbances from ectopic production and the resulting clinical syndromes observed more commonly in association with malignant tumors are described in the following subsections.

Ectopic ACTH production

Ectopic production of ACTH occurs most often in association with small-cell lung cancer.[1–3,9,18,19] It also has been observed to occur with other lung cancer types and in a variety of other tumors such as carcinomas of the pancreas or thymus; medullary carcinoma of the thyroid; carcinoma of the breast, ovary, testis, stomach, colon, and prostate; and from other sites, especially those neoplasms originating from neural crest tissue such as pheochromocytoma and neuroblastoma.

The ACTH molecule is part of a larger structure, pro-opiomelanocortin, which also contains melanocyte-stimulating hormone and beta-endorphin.[1,9,18] Thus, clinical evidence of ectopic secretion may include increased pigmentation. Clinical evidence of biologically active ectopic ACTH results from the ACTH stimulatory effect on the adrenal cortex and the subsequent increased glucocorticoid production. Symptoms include muscle weakness and atrophy, edema, hypertension, and psychosis. High serum ACTH and plasma cortisol levels, hyperglycemia, abnormal glucose tolerance, elevated urinary cortisol, urinary 17-hydroxycorticoids, and hypokalemia are diagnostic of ectopic ACTH production.[1,2,6] Other classical features of Cushing's disease (such as centripetal obesity, moon facies, "buffalo hump," and cutaneous striae) are seen infrequently in those with ectopic secretion except when the tumor grows slowly.[2,5,11] If the tumor is growing very rapidly the Cushing syndrome characteristics may not appear; in cases where tumor growth is less rapid the symptoms that appear may range from a few abnormalities to the entire classical features of the syndrome.

In ectopic ACTH production, use of dexamethasone (8 mg/day) most often will not suppress ACTH or plasma cortisol.[1,5,11,14] This dexamethasone suppression test is used to distinguish between an endocrine pathology, where suppression of secretion occurs, and ectopic production, where suppression usually does not occur, although cases have been reported where suppression has occurred with ectopic production.[1,9,20] In some there is evidence that the tumor is producing the corticotropin-releasing hormone.[7,13,14,21] Responses to the administration of metyrapone and ovine corticotropin-releasing factor also are used in making the differential diagnosis of ectopic ACTH production.[20–23] Measurement of ACTH levels in specimens aspirated from intrathoracic tumors has been used to identify the ectopic production of ACTH.[24] If tumor therapy is not effective, levels of cortisol can be decreased with the administration of agents that inhibit cortisol production, such as aminoglutethimide, metyrapone, and ketoconazole.[1,5,11,25]

Ectopic ADH production

Arginine vasopressin (AVP)/ADH is produced ectopically most often in carcinomas of the lung (small-cell) and colon.[1,2,5,11,26,27] It has also occurred with other lung cancer types; in carcinoma of the adrenal cortex, pancreas, colon, and prostate; and in Hodgkin's disease. Clinically these patients may have hyponatremia (sodium <130 mEq/l) and inappropriate high urine osmolality (>500 mOsm/kg) resulting from renal sodium loss (>20 mEq/l) and water retention. There may be no symptoms if the individual does not take in excess fluids. However, with water intoxication, symptoms of inappropriate antidiuretic hormone syndrome (SIADH) will occur. Neurologic and behavioral symptoms include lethargy, agitation, altered mental status including confusion, and psychotic behavior. Seizures and coma may also occur; in some cases death may result.[1,26,28] The treatment is directed at the tumor; however, initially it may be necessary to direct treatment at the clinical problems of SIADH.[1,27]

Arginine vasopressin (AVP) is normally secreted from the hypothalamic neurons with a carrier protein, neurophysin. Neurophysin also has been found in ectopic secretion.[1,9,27,29] As yet there is no known demonstrable clinical syndrome associated with excess production of neurophysin. Researchers who have used the measurement of neurophysin to determine tumor response to therapy suggest it may be a good tumor marker, particularly in patients with small-cell lung cancer.[29]

Several studies have reported elevated plasma levels of atrial natriuretic peptide (ANP) as a plausible explanation for the inappropriate natriuresis that occurs with SIADH.[27,30,31] It is suggested that ANP may be secreted in response to the increased volume load resulting from the elevated plasma levels of AVP. In addition, ANP may account for the increased glomerular filtration rate and decreased aldosterone secretion observed with SIADH.[31] ANP also may contribute to the escape from arterial hypertension because of its effects on vascular smooth muscle. There has been a case report of ectopic presence of ANP and AVP with small-cell lung cancer.[32] Clinical and biochemical evidence suggests that some tumors, especially small-cell lung carcinomas, may produce more than one hormone ectopically.[32,33] One example is AVP and ACTH.[33] The simultaneous presence of two syndromes presents a very challenging clinical situation.

Ectopic gonadotropin production

The three hormones classified as gonadotropins are follicle-stimulating hormone (FSH), luteinizing hormone (LH), and human chorionic gonadotropin (HCG). These hormones all have common alpha subunits but distinct beta subunits, and in each case, biologic activity requires the presence of combined alpha and beta subunits.[1,3,9] Levels of FSH and LH vary normally over time and age, and ectopic production has not yet been well documented. HCG is normally produced by the placenta; thus, in cases where an ectopic gonadotropin hormone production is suspected, the measurement of HCG is common. It also has been used to monitor therapy. Although HCG is normally produced by the placenta, using radioimmunoassay (RIA) and radioreceptor assays, an HCG-like material has been found in extracts from all tissues.[1–3,9,11] The HCG-like material differs from that produced by the placenta and by tumors in that it has no or few carbohydrates attached to the protein structure, while the placental HCG is a glycoprotein. The HCG that does not have the sugars attached is much less biologically active and is rapidly cleared from the bloodstream. The biologically active HCG that has been produced ectopically by tumors has resulted in gynecomastia in men, oligomenorrhea in premenopausal women, and precocious puberty in children.[1,11,34] Tumors in addition to those in the pituitary gland found to secrete HCG include germ cell tumors of the ovary and testis and those arising from extragonadal sites, and gestational trophoblastic tumors such as hydatidiform mole and choriocarcinoma. HCG secretion also has been reported for other tumors such as lung, breast, pancreas, GI, and prostatic cancer.[1–3] The types of cancer with which ectopic HCG occurs are relatively uncommon, and thus the expression of the clinical syndromes resulting from HCG production also is less common. Treatment is directed to the tumor.

Ectopic calcitonin production

Increased calcitonin levels have occurred in patients with lung (especially small-cell) cancer, breast, gastric, and colon cancer and in carcinoid tumors. Normally, calcitonin is produced by the C cells of the thyroid. Production is frequently increased in individuals with medullary carcinoma of the thyroid. Calcitonin action results in the release of calcium from the bone and an increase in the urinary excretion of calcium and phosphate. Although calcitonin participates in the regulation of serum calcium, there is to date no recognized clinical syndrome resulting from its ectopic production.[1,9]

Ectopic PTHrP production/hypercalcemia

Hypercalcemia (serum calcium >11.0 mg/dl) that occurs with malignancy results from several mechanisms. In addition to bone metastases, one of the mechanisms is the ectopic production of parahormone (PTH) by malignant tumors.[11] Ectopic production of growth hormone or vitamin D also could influence serum calcium levels because absorption of calcium from renal tubules and the gastrointestinal tract is stimulated by GH, vitamin D, and PTH. There is controversy about whether PTH production results in hypercalcemia.[1,9,35]

Current evidence suggests that hypercalcemia is rarely the result of ectopic PTH; however, other tumor-produced factors that have parathyroidlike hormone activity have been reported.[1,9,35–37] A parathyroid hormone-related protein (PTHrP), a bone-resorbing factor, and prostaglandins (PGE, 1 and 2) have been produced by tumors and can result in hypercalcemia.[1,5,7] Parathyroid hormone-related protein (PTHrP) is produced by many tumor cells, especially squamous cell carcinomas, but it also is expressed by breast, ovarian, pancreatic, and renal carcinomas.[37] As a result of its effects on increasing bone resorption and decreasing calcium excretion, PTHrP is a major factor involved in the humoral (i.e., without bone metastases) hypercalcemia of solid tumors.[38] PTHrP also produces phosphaturia and hypophosphatemia, which is consistent with humoral hypercalcemia. There is some evidence that the ectopic secretion of PTHrP by breast cancers may contribute to the growth of bone metastases.[39] Investigators have found significantly more PTHrP localization in breast cancer skeletal metastases than in nonskeletal metastases.[39] If this holds true, PTHrP may become a useful marker to identify those breast cancer patients at greater risk for developing bone metastases and for targeting more effective earlier treatment. There is potential for development of drugs that are antagonists to the receptors and thus would block the adverse biologic effects.

Tumors that produce PTHrP also commonly produce transforming growth factor-alpha. Much remains unknown about this factor, but it is thought to have a role as a regulatory factor in osteoclast formation and thus may be involved in the hypercalcemia of malignancy.[37] It is plausible that cytokines, such as interleukin-1 and TNF, may be the mediators of humoral hypercalcemia seen with hematogenous malignancies and with some solid tumors.[37,38]

While tumor necrosis factor has been shown to affect bone resorption, TNF is not produced by tumor cells but by macrophages. While TNF may contribute to the hypercalcemia of malignancy, it is produced as a host immune response, not as an ectopic product from the tumor.[37] Tumor cells stimulate normal host immune cells to produce TNF.

Hypercalcemia not resulting from metastasis to bony structures is associated more frequently with carcinoma of the lung, head and neck, ovary, and kidney. It also occurs with lymphomas and leukemias that have been shown to produce bone-resorbing factors.[5,35] Symptoms associated with hypercalcemia include anorexia, nausea, vomiting, lethargy, weakness, and mental confusion.[36]

Ectopic GHRH production

A number of tumors have produced growth hormone–releasing hormone (GHRH). These include carcinoid tumors, pancreatic islet cells, small-cell lung cancer, thyroid medullary carcinoma, and endometrial cancer.[1,2,9,11] In some cases there is no evidence of clinical abnormality,but there are cases where GHRH has stimulated the secretion of growth hormone and the classic features of acromegaly have resulted.[7,41–45] This is particularly true for slow growing bronchial carcinoid tumors. Acromegaly induced by ectopic GHRH production is rare, but it does occur. The treatment is directed at the tumor; signs of acromegaly will regress with tumor regression.

Other paraneoplastic syndromes

Syndromes other than those resulting from ectopic hormone production have been associated with a variety of malignancies; cachexia, fever, neurologic, and dermatologic syndromes are examples.[5] These paraneoplastic syndromes are thought to result from tumor-produced factors or from host responses to the tumor-produced factors. In general, these are not described as resulting from abnormal hormonal secretions. An example is the remote nervous system effects that are demonstrated in a variety of neurologic dysfunction syndromes.[46–48]

Subacute sensory neuropathy and encephalomyelitis are illustrative of these paraneoplastic syndromes. Cases examples and descriptions of these syndromes have been reviewed in detail.[47–50] The central and/or the peripheral nervous system may be involved; pathologically inflammatory infiltrates occur, and there is loss of neurons. These syndromes, similar to the ectopic hormone syndrome, are most frequently associated with lung cancer, more particularly small-cell lung cancer.[49,52–54] They also have been reported in patients with breast, ovarian, and other cancers.[50] In some cases the neuropathy precedes the cancer diagnosis. Evidence now suggests that these syndromes are the result of the effects of autoantibodies, implicating autoimmunity as the pathogenic mechanism. Tumor cells, particularly from small-cell carcinomas, may have antigens similar to neuronal tissue, and if antibodies are made against the tumor antigens they also may recognize similar neuronal tissue antigens.[53]

There is some evidence that some nonneuronal tumors express neuronal antigens, and this abnormal expression is thought to be the antigenic stimulus that results in the autoimmune or antionconeural immune response leading to destruction of neurons.[51] The tumor antigens trigger the antibody production, and these antibodies cross-react with the neuronal antigens. Although not considered to be hormonal disturbances, these nervous system paraneoplastic phenomena are briefly summarized here because there is similarity in the underlying mechanisms for the ectopic hormone production and the abnormal production of neuronal antigens by some tumors—that is, the expression of proteins by some tumors that are not ordinarily expressed by the cell types involved. In both of these cases of abnormal protein expression by the tumor, small-cell lung carcinomas are more frequently involved than are other tumor types. Additional research may elucidate other explanations or mechanisms. These and other less frequently occurring paraneoplastic phenomena such as dermatomyositis and paraneoplastic skin lesions are reviewed elsewhere in more detail.[1,5,9]

Ectopic production

The evidence that some polypeptide hormones are found normally in small amounts in nonendocrine tissue changes somewhat the meaning of *ectopic production.* As more information is obtained, it is possible that the term *ectopic* may not be used to describe these hormonal syndromes. One general characteristic, however, is that the ectopic, nonendocrine-tissue hormone production by tumor cells appears to be autonomous. The hormone synthesis by malignant nonendocrine tissue does not respond to the regulatory feedback mechanisms as occurs for hormones produced entopically.

ASSESSMENT

The paraneoplastic syndrome may be the presenting symptoms for which some individuals seek medical attention.[1,6,23] The syndrome can occur at any time during the course of the cancer illness. Thus, the nurse needs to be alert to signs and symptoms associated with the specific ectopic hormone production.[5,55] It is also important to be knowledgeable about the tumors that are more frequently associated with ectopic hormone production and the more commonly observed syndromes. For example, many paraneoplastic syndromes have occurred in association with small-cell lung cancer. When the cancer is treated effectively, the syndrome also will diminish.

History

If the paraneoplastic syndrome occurs after the cancer is diagnosed, usually the history will have been recorded previously. If the diagnosis of cancer has not been made, a careful history must be taken. In taking the individual's history, the usual procedure is followed. Questions about the specific symptoms focus on onset, duration, and severity; for example, when the symptoms were first apparent, under what circumstances they occur, and whether there have been changes in severity. It also is important to identify any other known diseases. If the individual presents with symptoms characteristic of an endocrine syndrome and also has symptoms frequently associated with cancer, the history needs to focus on questions that may help to identify or rule out a possible malignancy. The history should elicit any evidence of weight loss, changes in diet, fatigue, weakness, and other changes in usual patterns. For the person with a known malignancy, the history should include information about the type, stage, treatment used, and evidence of any paraneoplastic syndromes. The history provides information that can guide the physical examination and the diagnostic studies.

Physical Examination

The primary focus of the physical exam is derived from the history and presenting symptoms. Hypertrophy or other structural changes in the endocrine gland, such as a nodule, may be found during the physical examination. Hyperplasia or hypertrophy may result from excess trophic hormone stimulation of the endocrine gland. Tumor growth within the gland can change the structure. Recognition of these changes during the exam will depend on the location of the affected tissue. For example, testicular and thyroid gland changes are more easily determined due to their accessibility for palpation. The location of the gland also influences whether the individual will notice sensations associated with glandular hypertrophy. In cases of thyroid enlargement, the individual may feel a tightness in the neck or a pressure sensation on the trachea. If the pituitary gland is enlarged, the symptoms may include a bilateral loss of the temporal visual field and headache. Because the pituitary is almost surrounded by bone and dura, enlargement causes pressure on the optic nerve chiasm, resulting in visual loss.

The physical examination also should identify changes that may be associated with ectopic hormone syndromes, such as hyperpigmentation or gynecomastia. Results of the exam provide direction for selecting appropriate diagnostic tests.

Diagnostic Studies

First it is necessary to determine if there are alterations in secretion of the suspected hormone(s). Radioimmunoassay techniques have been developed to measure hormone precursor molecules, hormone fragments, and subunits, as well as the biologically active hormone.

Because hormones circulate in very low concentrations, the assays need to be sensitive to minute amounts of specific hormone. A number of hormones or their metabolites are excreted in the urine. Thus, in addition to determination of blood levels of specific hormones, urine may be collected for measurement of selected hormones or their metabolic products.

When excess hormone production is identified, it is important to determine if the alteration is a paraneoplastic syndrome, or due to a malignancy of an endocrine gland, or the result of a benign change in endocrine tissue.[7,10,56] Serial monitoring of hormone levels over time may be included in the diagnostic evaluation, as the typical secretory pattern for specific hormones may not be apparent with ectopic production.

Determination of an abnormally high level of the suspected hormone by radioimmunoassay is necessary for the diagnosis of ectopic production. Measurement of the hormones involved in the feedback control mechanisms of the specific hormone in question also is necessary. Responses to the administration of stimulatory and/or inhibitory hormones are useful in determining if the hormone production is ectopic.[1,20,21] Because ectopic hormones are produced autonomously, it is unusual for changes in hormone level to occur in response to stimulation or inhibition of the hormones involved in the feedback regulatory system. Other evidence that the secretion is ectopically produced is that the hormone level decreases with tumor removal or other successful tumor therapy. High concentrations of the hormone in the tumor or a difference in hormone concentration across the arteriovenous gradient of the tumor tissue are evidence of hormone production by the tumor.[1,7,23,24]

In all cases, it is important to use diagnostic procedures that allow differentiation between an ectopic paraneoplastic syndrome and some other plausible diagnosis. For example, diuretics and some chemotherapeutic agents such as cyclophosamide and vincristine can result in hyponatremia; it is important to determine whether the hyponatremia is associated with these agents or reflects SIADH.[1,26,28] When patients with small-cell lung cancer experiencing SIADH are treated with high doses of cyclophosamide and are hydrated, the symptoms of SIADH may be exaggerated.

Monitoring levels of the specifically identified hormone(s) as well as other tumor products such as CEA is useful in determining tumor response to therapy. The presence of a known tumor marker suggests malignancy.

When the excess hormone secretion is thought to be paraneoplastic and the cancer has not been diagnosed, other diagnostic procedures, such as radiographic imaging techniques, computed tomography scans, and magnetic resonance imaging techniques are used.

The nurse's role includes explanations to the patient and family about the specific diagnostic procedures, ensuring accurate collection of specimens such as urine, and assisting the patient and family to cope with all the attendant circumstances associated with the diagnostic procedures.[6,55] The nurse may be involved in the administration of the stimulatory or suppressive test agents. Recording the specific times of administration is imperative for correct interpretation.

INTERVENTIONS

If the paraneoplastic syndrome is life-threatening, treatment must be directed at correcting or altering the hormonal disturbance. However, the most effective therapy for paraneoplastic syndromes is the eradication of the tumor and metastases. When tumor therapy is effective, the excess ectopic hormone secretion is alleviated and usually there is regression of the syndrome.

If antitumor therapy is not effective, other symptom-reducing strategies may be used. For example, fluid restriction may be necessary for ameliorating symptoms associated with SIADH. Fluid restriction to 500 ml/day or less may be necessary to control hyponatremia. Chemotherapy that requires hydration may need to be postponed for several days to allow plasma osmolality to increase by using fluid restriction; this will occur over a week or more.[1] Infusion of 3% hypertonic saline and furosemide (1 mg/kg) may be used if the patient has severe symptoms or is comatose as a result of SIADH.[5,26] The goal is to increase serum sodium and to decrease retention of water to raise plasma osmolality to 270 mOsm/kg. If cancer treatment fails, and there is recurrence of SIADH, demeclocycline can be used to block the action of ADH on the renal tubule cells. Urea administered orally also has been used to create obligatory diuresis.[1]

Use of drugs that block hormone receptors or block hormone synthesis may be necessary. An analogue of somatostatin can be used to control acromegaly caused by ectopic GHRH production. It decreases circulating levels of GH and somatomedin C. Treatment to decrease symptoms of tumor-related hypercalcemia is directed at decreasing serum calcium levels; the initial approach is the administration of 2–3 liters of saline per day and furosemide. Drugs that block or inhibit bone resorption may be used; these include calcitonin, mithramycin, and etidronate.[35,40] Hypercalcemia is discussed in detail in Chapter 28.

The aims of therapy would be to prevent the synthesis of excess hormone or to prevent hormone-receptor interaction. The best resolution of paraneoplastic syndrome occurs with tumor regression.

FUTURE TRENDS

There is need for more specific and sensitive assays for known hormones and tumor markers, as well as increased understanding of malignant cell aberrations that result in the abnormal (or abnormally expressed) synthesis of peptides. There is also a need to develop agents that are selectively effective in blocking the actions of these factors or in preventing their synthesis. The greatest need is for effective anticancer therapies.

All of these areas require laboratory research and clinical trials. Nurses will continue to make their contributions to these efforts. One current challenge for nurses is to continue to test the effectiveness of various nursing therapies in assisting the patient and family to alleviate or diminish the distressing consequences of these syndromes and of the cancer experience.

REFERENCES

1. Bunn PA Jr, Ridgway EC: Paraneoplastic syndromes. In DeVita VT, Hellman S, Rosenberg SA (eds), *Cancer Principles and Practice of Oncology*. Philadelphia: Lippincott, 1989, pp. 1896–1940.
2. Rose DP: Ectopic hormone production and neoplasia. In Sirica AE (ed), *The Pathobiology of Neoplasia*. New York: Plenum Press, 1989, pp. 461–475.
3. Odell WD: Paraendocrine syndromes of cancer. *Adv Intern Med* 34:325–352, 1989.
4. De Lellis RA: Tumor markers in endocrine malignancies. *Clin Lab Med* 10:39–57, 1990.
5. Griffin TW, Rosenthal PE, Costanza ME: Paraneoplastic and endocrine syndromes. In Cody B (ed), *Cancer Manual*. Boston: American Cancer Society Massachusetts Division, 1986, pp. 373–390.
6. Lindsey AM, Piper BF, Carrieri V: Malignant cells and ectopic hormone production. *Oncol Nurs Forum* 8:13–15, 1981.
7. Melmed S, Rushakoff RJ: Ectopic pituitary and hypothalamic hormone syndromes. *Endocrinol and Metab Clin* 16(3):805–821, 1987.
8. Mundy GR: Ectopic hormonal syndromes in neoplastic disease. *Hosp Prac* April 15:179–194, 1987.
9. Odell WD: Humoral manifestations of cancer. In Wilson JD, Foster DW (eds), *Williams Textbook of Endocrinology*. Philadelphia: Saunders, 1985, pp. 1327–1344.
10. Root AW, Diamond FB, Duncan JA: Ectopic and entopic peptide hormone secreting neoplasms of childhood. *Adv Pediatr* 32:369–415, 1985.
11. Stolinsky DC: Paraneoplastic syndromes: *West J Med* 132:189–208, 1980.
12. Lokich JJ: The frequency and clinical biology of the ectopic hormone syndromes of small cell carcinoma. *Cancer* 50:2111–2114, 1982.
13. Suda T, Kondo M, Totani R, et al: Ectopic adrenocorticotropin syndrome caused by lung cancer that responded to corticotropin-releasing hormone. *J Clin Endocrinol Metab* 63:1047–1051, 1986.
14. Schteingart DE, Lloyd RV, Akil H, et al: Cushing's syndrome secondary to ectopic corticotropin-releasing hormone-adrenocorticotropin secretion. *J Clin Endocrinol Metab* 63:770–775, 1986.
15. Pearse AGE: Endocrine tumors of neural crest origin: Neurolophomas, apudomas and the APUD concept. *Med Biol* 52:3, 1974.
16. Odell WD, Wolfsen AR: Hormones from tumors: Are they ubiquitous? *Am J Med* 68:317–318, 1980.
17. Stevens R, Moore G: Inadequacy of APUD concept in explaining production of peptide hormones by tumors. *Lancet* 1:118–119, 1983.
18. Carbone DP, Minna JD: Molecular biology of lung cancer. In Broder S (ed): *Molecular Foundations of Oncology*. Baltimore, MD: Williams & Wilkins, 1991, pp. 339–366.
19. Richardson GE, Johnson BE: Paraneoplastic syndromes in lung cancer. *Cur Opinion Oncol* 4:323–333, 1992.
20. Nieman LK, Chrousos GP, Oldfield EH, et al: The ovine corticotropin-releasing hormone stimulation test and the dexamethasone suppression test in the differential diagnosis of Cushing's syndrome. *Ann Int Med* 105:862–867, 1986.
21. Malchoff CD, Orth DN, Abboud C, et al: Ectopic ACTH syndrome caused by a bronchial carcinoid tumor responsive to dexamethasone, metyrapone and corticotropin-releasing factor. *Am J Med* 84:760–764, 1988.
22. Cagliero E, Lorenzi M: The corticotropin-releasing factor test in the diagnosis of ectopic ACTH secretion. *West J Med* 146:614–615, 1987.
23. Finding JW, Tyrrell JB: Occult ectopic secretion of corticotropin. *Arch Intern Med* 146:929–933, 1986.
24. Doppman JL, Loughlin T, Miller DL, et al: Identification of ACTH-producing intrathoracic tumors by measuring ACTH levels in aspirated specimens. *Radiology* 163:501–503, 1987.
25. Farwell AP, Devlin JT, Stewart JA: Total suppression of cortisol excretion by ketoconazole in the therapy of the ectopic adrenocorticotropic hormone syndrome. *Am J Med* 84:1063–1066, 1988.
26. List AF, Hainsworth JD, Davis BW, et al: The syndrome of inappropriate secretion of antidiuretic hormone (SIADH) in small-cell lung cancer. *J Clin Oncol* 4:1191–1198, 1986.
27. Moses AM, Scheinman SJ: Ectopic secretion of neurohypophyseal peptides in patients with malignancy. *Endocrinol Metab Clin North Am* 20:489–506, 1991.
28. Poe CM, Taylor LM: Syndrome of inappropriate antidiuretic hormone: Assessment and nursing implications. *Oncol Nurs Forum* 16:373–381, 1989.
29. North WG, Ware J, Maurer LH, et al: Neurophysins as tumor markers for small cell carcinoma of the lung. *Cancer* 62:1343–1347, 1988.
30. Cogan E, Debieve M-F, Philipart I, et al: High plasma levels of atrial natriuretic factor in SIADH. *N Engl J Med* 314:1258–1259, 1986.
31. Manoogian C, Pandian M, Ehrlich L, et al: Plasma atrial natriuretic hormone levels in patients with the syndrome of inappropriate antidiuretic hormone secretion. *J Clin Endocrinol Metab* 67:571–575, 1988.
32. Shimizu K, Nakano S, Nakano Y, et al: Ectopic atrial natriuretic peptide production in small cell lung cancer with the syndrome of inappropriate antidiuretic hormone secretion. *Cancer* 68:2284–2288, 1991.
33. Pierce ST, Metcalfe M, Banks ER, et al: Small cell carcinoma with two paraendocrine syndromes. *Cancer* 69:2258–2261, 1992.
34. Wurzel RS, Yamase HT, Nieh PT: Ectopic production of human chorionic gonadotropin by poorly differentiated transitional cell tumors of the urinary tract. *J Urology* 137:502–504, 1987.
35. Canfield RE: Rationale for diphosphonate therapy in hy-

percalcemia of malignancy. *Am J Med* 82:1–5, 1987 (suppl. 2A).
36. Chevinsky AH, Berelowitz M, Hoover HC: Adenosquamoasmous carcinoma of the colon presenting with hypercalcemia. *Cancer* 60:1111–1116, 1987.
37. Mundy GR: Ectopic production of calciotropic peptides. *Endocrinol Metab Clin N Am* 20:473–487, 1991.
38. Strewler GJ, Nissenson RA: Peptide mediators of hypercalcemia in malignancy. *Ann Rev Med* 41:35–44, 1990.
39. Powell GJ, Southby J, Danks JA, et al: Localization of parathyroid hormone-related protein in breast cancer metastases: Increased incidence in bone compared with other sites. *Cancer Res* 51:3059–3061, 1991.
40. Singer FR, Fernandez M: Therapy of hypercalcemia of malignancy. *Am J Med* 82:34–41, 1987 (suppl. 2A).
41. Barkan AL, Shenker Y, Grekin RJ, et al: Acromegaly due to ectopic growth hormone (GH)-releasing hormone (GHRH) production: Dynamic studies of GH and ectopic GHRH secretion. *J Clin Endocrinol Metab* 63:1057–1064, 1986.
42. Roth KA, Wilson DM, Eberwine J, et al: Acromegaly and pheochromocytoma: A multiple endocrine syndrome caused by a plurihormonal adrenal medullary tumor. *J Clin Endocrinol Metab* 63:1421–1426, 1986.
43. Sano T, Saito H, Yamasaki R, et al: Production and secretion of immunoreactive growth hormone–releasing factor by pheochromocytomas. *Cancer* 57:1788–1793, 1986.
44. Boizel R, Halimi S, Labat F, et al: Acromegaly due to a growth hormone–releasing hormone–secreting bronchial carcinoid tumor: Further information on the abnormal responsiveness of the somatotroph cells and their recovery after successful treatment. *J Clin Endocrinol Metab* 64:304–308, 1987.
45. Garcia-Luna PP, Leal-Cerro A, Montero S, et al: A rare cause of acromegaly: Ectopic production of growth hormone–releasing factor by a bronchial carcinoid tumor. *Surg Neurol* 27:563–568, 1987.
46. Dropcho EJ: The remote effects of cancer on the nervous system. *Neurol Clin* 7:579–603, 1989.
47. Chad DA, Recht LD: Neuromuscular complications of systemic cancer. *Neurol Clin* 9:901–918, 1991.
48. Posner JB: Paraneoplastic syndromes. *Neurol Clin* 9:919–936, 1991.
49. Moll JWB, Henzen-Logmans SC, Vecht CJ: Anti-neuronal antibodies in paraneoplastic neurological disorders with small cell lung carcinoma. *Clin Neurol Neurosurg* 92-3:223–228, 1990.
50. Waterhouse DM, Natale RB, Cody RL: Breast cancer and paraneoplastic cerebellar degeneration. *Cancer* 68:1835–1841, 1991.
51. Furneaux HM, Rosenblum MK, Dalmaw J, et al: Selective expression of Purkinje-cell antigens in tumor tissue from patients with paraneoplastic cerebellar degeneration. *N Engl J Med* 322:1844–1851, 1990.
52. Kimmel DW, O'Neill BP, Lennon VA: Subacute sensory neuronopathy associated with small cell lung carcinoma: Diagnosis aided by autoimmune serology. *Mayo Clin Proc* 63:29–32, 1988.
53. Budde-Steffen C, Anderson NE, Rosenblum MK, et al: Expression of an antigen in small cell lung carcinoma lines detected by antibodies from patients with paraneoplastic dorsal root ganglionopathy. *Cancer Res* 48:430–434, 1988.
54. Dalman J, Furneaux HM, Gralla RJ, et al: Detection of the anti-Hu antibody in the serum of patients with small cell lung cancer—a quantitative Western Blot analysis. *Ann Neurol* 27:544–552, 1990.
55. Lind JM: Ectopic hormonal production: Nursing implications. *Semin Oncol Nurs* 1:251–258, 1985.
56. Freeman DA: Steroid hormone-producing tumors in man. *Endocrine Rev* 7:204–220, 1986.

Chapter 30

Malignant Effusions and Edemas

Mary B. Maxwell, RN, CS, PhD

INTRODUCTION

Fluid derangements are common in patients with cancer. Abnormal leakage from the blood and lymph vessels into tissues (edema) or cavities (effusions) occurs with many kinds of malignancy. Usually associated with advanced disease but sometimes occurring as the presenting symptom, effusions and edemas interfere with normal body function at the site where they develop and add new problems to those manifestations already present as a result of the underlying cancer and its treatment.

Although all cancers can metastasize to any of the body's serous cavities, *malignant effusions* occur most commonly in the pleural space of the lung (pleural effusion), the peritoneal cavity in the abdomen (ascites), or the space surrounding the heart (pericardial effusion). The brain and the extremities are frequent sites for *malignant edemas.* This chapter discusses normal fluid regulation in relation to fluid derangements seen in cancer patients and compares and contrasts the various edematous states. The pathophysiology, clinical manifestations, assessment, and interventions for the six most common malignant fluid retention sites are presented.

NORMAL FLUID REGULATION

The distribution pattern of body water is termed *fluid spacing. First spacing* describes a normal distribution of fluid in both the extracellular and intracellular compartments. *Second spacing* refers to an excess accumulation of interstitial fluid (edema), while *third spacing* is fluid retention in areas that usually have no fluid or a minimum of fluid (effusion). Edema or effusion represent a disturbance in the normal distribution of extracellular fluid.

Extracellular fluids are separated into interstitial and intravascular compartments by the semipermeable membranes surrounding capillaries and cells. These membranes serve as the points where exchange takes place between each cell and its respective fluid environment (the interstitial fluid) and between the interstitial fluid and the plasma within the circulatory system. Various pressures as described by Starling's Law influence fluid movement across the capillary membranes (Figure 30-1). More fluid moves out of the intravascular into the interstitial compartment than returns via the capillary membrane. The lymphatic capillaries take up the excess interstitial fluid and return it to the bloodstream

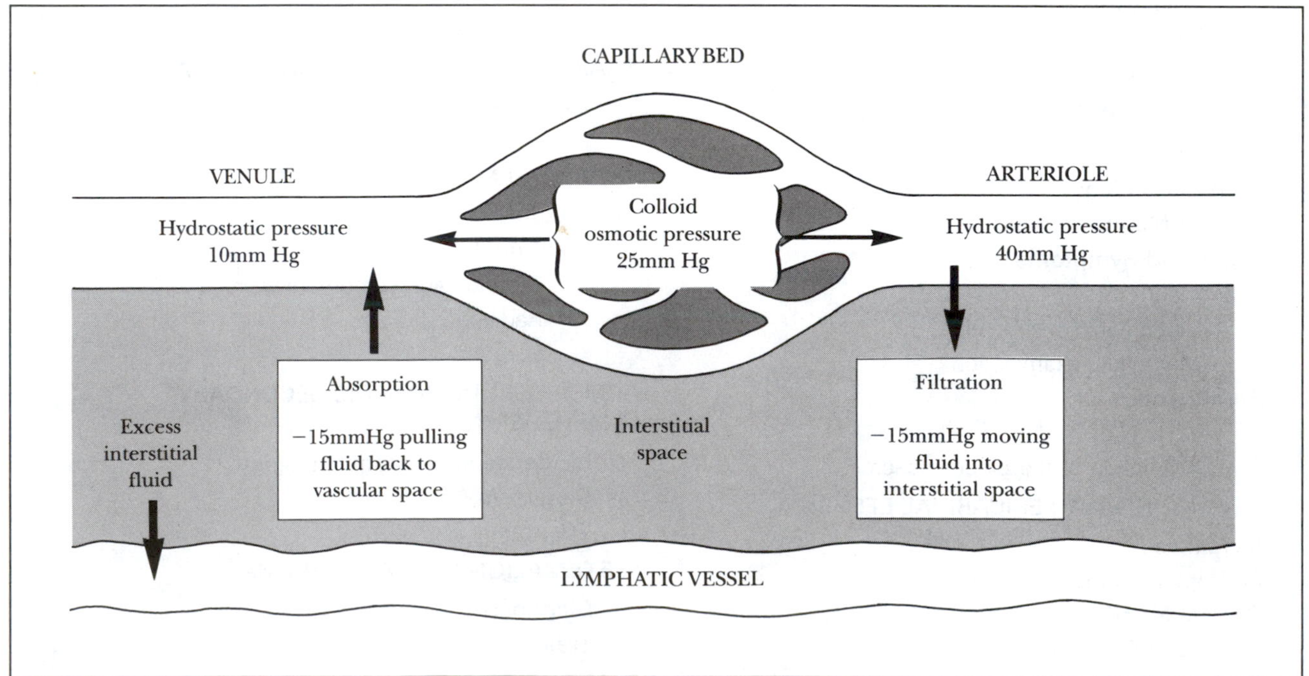

FIGURE 30-1 As described by Starling's Law, the colloid osmotic pressure, hydrostatic pressure, capillary permeability, diffusion, and filtration pressure are all factors influencing fluid movement across the capillary membrane from the blood to the interstitial space.

via the lymphatic and thoracic ducts. Lymphatic drainage is particularly important for the removal of proteins that leak into the interstitial spaces, thereby keeping the interstitial osmotic pressure low. Edema results from any augmentation of the forces influencing movement of fluids from the intravascular compartment into the interstitial compartment.

FLUID DISTURBANCES IN CANCER

Effects of Cancer and Cancer Treatment

Cancer, either a primary tumor or metastatic lesion, can affect fluid pressure dynamics in several negative ways: by direct extension of tumor, seeding of body cavities with malignant cells, lymphatic or venous obstruction, and/or causing severe hypoproteinemia (Table 30-1). Also, cancer treatments can affect or be altered by effusions/edemas. For instance, methotrexate given at routine doses can cause excessive myelosuppression in a patient who is experiencing third spacing. Edema can be a toxic side effect of growth factors given to a patient with a chronic inflammatory disease or an acute infection.[1] As a result of the syndrome of inappropriate antidiuretic hormone (SIADH), the severe fluid imbalance termed "water intoxication" can occur. It usually develops in patients with lung cancer or one receiving antineoplastic agents or analgesics (cytoxan, vincristine, morphine).

TABLE 30-1 Causes of Malignant Edema (According to Underlying Physiologic Mechanism)

HYDROSTATIC PRESSURE ABNORMALITIES
Increased Capillary Fluid Pressure
Increased venous pressure
Vein obstruction
Tumor
Thrombophlebitis
Increased total volume with decreased cardiac output
Fluid overload
Sodium and water retention, increased aldosterone from:
Decreased renal blood flow
Renal failure
Increased aldosterone
Corticosteroid therapy
Inability to metabolize aldosterone
Liver metastasis
ONCOTIC PRESSURE ABNORMALITIES
Decreased Capillary Oncotic Pressure
Loss of serum protein
Anemia
Bleeding
Decreased protein intake
Malnutrition
Decreased albumin production
Liver metastasis
Increased Interstitial Oncotic Pressure
Increased capillary permeability to protein
Inflammatory reactions
Seeding of cavity surfaces with tumor cells
Infection
Obstructed lymphatics: decreased removal of tissue fluid and protein
Malignant disease
Surgical removal of lymph nodes

General Considerations: Similarities and Differences

Benign versus malignant

Of the six fluid retention states discussed in this chapter, all except lymphedema are directly due to cancer. Lymphedema is a benign iatrogenic problem secondary to radical cancer surgery. Nonmalignant edema, always a possibility for a patient with cancer, should be considered in the differential diagnosis for any fluid accumulation.

Incidence

Much of the data on incidence of effusion and edema are from autopsy reports in earlier years, when postmortems were routinely carried out. Since autopsies are currently performed for only 10% of cancer deaths,[2] the actual incidence of metastases and malignant fluid retention is less clear today. It is surmised that the incidence of these later complications is on the rise because longer survival after diagnosis is occurring as a result of improved treatments for primary disease.[3] The only fluid retention state decreasing in incidence is lymphedema. While pericardial effusion is seen only in end-stage disease, in contrast, pleural effusion, ascites, and cerebral edema may be the first indication of cancer.

Rapid versus slow accumulation

Cavities and tissues can accommodate surprisingly large volumes of fluids if the abnormal liquid accumulates slowly over time. However, a rapid increase in volume, even a small amount, tends to overwhelm compensatory mechanisms, and life-threatening symptoms can occur. Malignant effusions and edemas usually begin slowly but then increase and expand exponentially.

Assessment

Many more malignant pleural effusions than pericardial effusions are symptomatic. Thus, pericardial effusions are more difficult to diagnose. Often the patient's history and physical exam point to the likely etiology of the effusion/edema. The most helpful diagnostic tools for pleural effusion are the chest x-ray and examination of the pleural fluid, while the echocardiogram is the most important diagnostic tool in pericardial effusions. The physical examination helps determine the diagnosis with ascites, lymphedema, and pedal edema. Brain lesions causing cerebral edema are usually diagnosed with computerized tomography (CT).

Transudates versus exudates

Fluid accumulation at an effusion site can be classified as either a transudate or an exudate. Classification has diagnostic implications and can be a distinguishing characteristic between a malignant or a nonmalignant cause. A *transudate* is a low protein fluid that has leaked from blood vessels due to mechanical factors, as in cirrhosis, congestive heart failure, or nephrotic syndrome. In contrast, an *exudate* is protein-rich fluid that has leaked from blood vessels with increased permeability. Most malignant effusions are exudates, caused by irritation of the serous membrane by sloughed cancer cells or solid tumor implants. The malignant exudate contains cells or cellular debris released by the resulting inflammation. Transudates and exudates can be distinguished by fluid protein to serum protein ratios and fluid LDH to serum LDH ratios.[3]

Treatment

For effusions, systemic treatment is usually employed first if the underlying cancer is responsive to chemotherapy. Otherwise, local therapy for malignant effusions is similar: Drain the fluid, attempt to obliterate the third space, and prevent reaccumulation. No single clearly superior approach for local control of any of the effusions has been demonstrated by randomized clinical trial. A variety of treatment techniques have been advocated. Treatment for lymphedema and pedal edema involves application of local measures to the affected limb and possible administration of diuretics. Cerebral edema is treated quite differently, with steroids and radiation therapy. The main goals of treatment for malignant effusions and edemas are similar (see Table 30-2). Specific therapy depends upon the site where the fluid has accumulated and the individual patient and tumor-related factors (Table 30-3).

TABLE 30-2 Goals of Treatment for Malignant Effusions or Edemas

Goals
Short-term Goals
Determine underlying cause
Relieve discomfort
Prevent fluid reaccumulation
Long-term Goals
Prevent complications
Prolong survival
Enhance quality of life

TABLE 30-3 Factors Influencing Treatment Choices for Malignant Effusions/Edemas

PATIENT-RELATED FACTORS
Presence and degree of symptoms
Age
Performance status
Concomitant medical problems
Estimated life expectancy
Motivation
Quality of life
TUMOR-RELATED FACTORS
Primary or metastatic cancer
Responsiveness to chemotherapy or radiation
Natural history of tumor type: histology, aggressiveness
Location and extent of tumor
Availability of therapies
Prior therapies
Concurrent therapies

Source: Reprinted (adapted) from the *Oncology Nursing Forum* with permission from the Oncology Nursing Press. Gobel BH, Lawler, PE: Malignant pleural effusions, *Oncol Nurs Forum,* 12(4):49–59, 1985.

Nursing care

Although most patients will develop edemas or effusions when their cancer is advanced, ongoing *assessment* of each cancer patient for signs or symptoms of fluid retention is crucial so interventions can be instituted early. When fluid accumulation occurs, the patient and family will need *emotional support* to counteract the stress and fears associated with advancing disease, cosmetic appearance changes, and the necessity for further medical intervention. With the treatment of effusions, the nurse will probably *assist* with potentially painful diagnostic and/or sclerosing procedures. Important nursing interventions include minimizing discomfort, providing reassurance, and *monitoring* the patient during and after these procedures for untoward reactions. *Patient education* will prepare the patient and family for tests and procedures as well as teaching them to recognize and report side effects or complications. *Prevention* is important, particularly with lymphedema. Keeping records of fluid intake and output, evaluating the rate of fluid reaccumulation after cavity drainage, monitoring electrolytes and proteins, and helping the patient with a sodium restricted diet may be important in some edemas. *Skin care* of the affected area is necessary with ascites, pedal edema, and lymphedema. *Pain evaluation and control* are often in order since the abnormal fluid accumulation can put pressure on nerve endings in surrounding structures. *Medications* (steroids, diuretics) may need to be administered and assessment for iatrogenic complications

TABLE 30-4 Nursing Care Plans for Patients with Malignant Effusions or Edemas

Effusion or Edema Type	Plans	Reference
Pleural effusion	Nursing management during chest tube insertion and pleural sclerosing	Rossetti[9,pp.106–197]
	Thoracostomy management in the home (patient education)	Hewitt[14,p.20]
Pericardial effusion	Nursing plan of care for patients experiencing cardiac tamponade	Joiner et al[19,p.57]
	Nursing care plan for patients with pericardial window surgery for cardiac tamponade	Wojciechowicz[23,pp.31–33]
	Nursing interventions for common complications of medical treatment for pericardial effusion	Mangan[21,p.1220]
Peritoneal effusion	Patient care standards for patients with peritonevenous shunt	Kehoe[30,pp.525–527]
Lymphedema	Nursing interventions for patients with lymphedema	Getz[40,pp.180–182]
	Guidelines for the care of the patient with altered tissue perfusion (lymphedema)	Kennelly and Yurkovic[45,pp.387–391]

completed. If life-threatening cardiac tamponade or brain herniation occurs, *emergency care* is needed. Using the elements emphasized here, a complete plan of care for actual and potential problems specific to the fluid retention state should be developed for each patient. Additional detailed nursing care plans are available for selected aspects of fluid retention management (Table 30-4).

LUNG: MALIGNANT PLEURAL EFFUSION

Incidence

Although it is usually stated that approximately half of all newly diagnosed pleural effusions in adults are malignant,[4] there have been no recent reports on the incidence of pleural effusion. Table 30-5 shows the tumor types associated with malignant pleural effusion and the incidence for each type.

Fifty percent of all cancer patients will develop pleural effusion at some time during their disease.[5] It may be the first sign of malignancy. In one series, 46% of patients with carcinoma of the pleura had pleural effusion as a presenting finding.[6] Pleural effusion later in the disease progression is an ominous sign, but it does not necessarily mean the beginning of the terminal stage. A median survival time of 14 months for breast cancer patients with effusions has been reported, compared to 6 months for patients with lung and other tumors and 16 months for patients with mesothelioma.[7] Most patients (90%) will have effusions of more than 500 ml, and approximately one-third will present with bilateral pleural effusions.[8]

Pathophysiology

Normally, fluid is constantly being filtered across the pleural space from the parietal pleural surface and reabsorbed through the visceral pleura. Five to ten liters of fluid moves through the pleural space each 24 hours.[8] The space between these two pleura contains a small amount of fluid (5–15 ml) that acts as a lubricant allowing the two surfaces to move without friction. The parietal pleura contains nerve endings for pain, but the visceral pleura does not. In the presence of a massive effusion process, the interpleural space may contain as much as 1500 ml of fluid (Figure 30-2).

There are five ways that fluid equilibrium in the pleural space can be disturbed by cancer, either directly

TABLE 30-5 Incidence of Pleural Effusion Related to Tumor Type

Tumor Type	Incidence (%)
Lung cancer	35
Breast cancer	23
Adenocarcinoma, unknown primary	12
Leukemia/Lymphoma	10
Reproductive tract	6
Gastrointestinal tract	5
Genitourinary tract	3
Primary unknown	3
Others	5

Source: Adapted with permission from *CA—A Cancer Journal for Clinicians* 41:165–179, 1991.

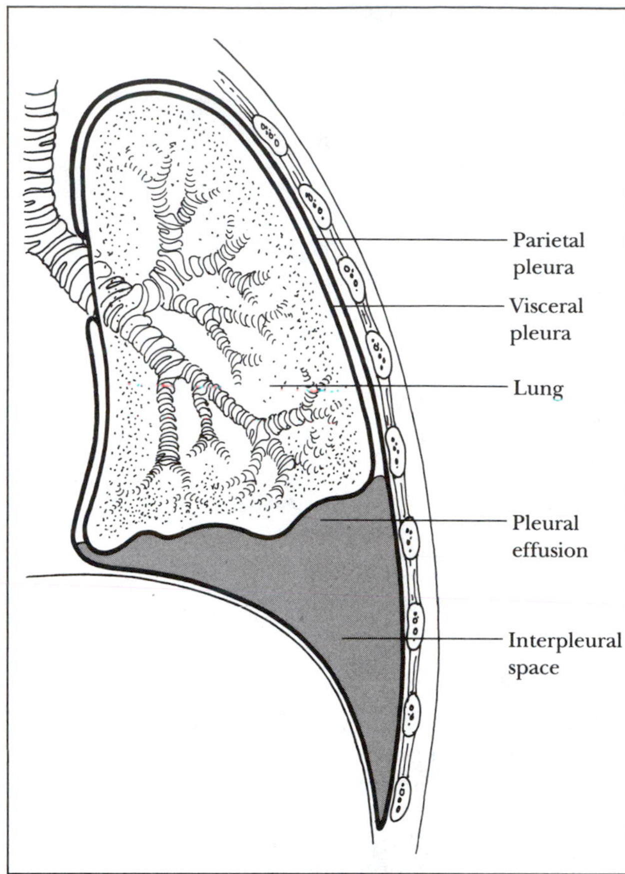

FIGURE 30-2 In the lung, fluid is constantly being filtered across the intrapleural space from the parietal pleural surface and reabsorbed through the visceral pleura. When obstruction by malignant processes prevents reabsorption, fluid accumulates in the intrapleural space and pleural effusion results.

by origination in the pleura or indirectly via metastatic spread.

1. Most commonly, implantation with cancer cells on the pleural surface leads to increased capillary permeability and leakage from the intravascular to the interstitial compartment. This occurs with pleural effusions in patients with solid tumors such as lung cancer.

2. Obstruction of pleural or pulmonary lymphatic channels by malignant processes can prevent reabsorption of fluid. This is seen in pleural effusions related to lymphomas or breast cancer.

3. The pulmonary veins can be obstructed by tumor, leading to increased capillary hydrostatic pressure in the visceral pleura. This is another mechanism seen in lung cancer.

4. The pleural space colloid osmotic pressure may be increased by necrotic malignant cells being shed into the pleural space. This leads to a reduced absorption of fluid by the visceral pleural capillaries. It may be seen with lung and breast cancers.

5. The thoracic duct may be perforated, producing a chylous pleural effusion. This sometimes occurs with lymphoma.[3]

In addition, tumor-related pathologies that can cause pleural effusion include superior vena cava syndrome (SVCS) (about 30% of patients with SVCS develop pleural effusions[9]), endobronchial obstruction with atelectasis, postobstructive pneumonitis, and pericardial constriction.

Clinical Manifestations

The extent of alteration of respiratory function depends on the amount and rate of pleural fluid accumulation as well as the patient's underlying pulmonary status. The fluid accumulation restricts lung expansion, reduces lung volume, alters the ventilation and perfusion capacity, and results in abnormal gas exchange and hypoxia. Malignant pleural effusion may develop slowly over a period of several months. Pleural effusions due to noncancer causes usually have a more abrupt onset.

When pleural effusion develops in the patient with advanced cancer, it is often difficult to sort out the respiratory effects of the pleural fluid accumulation as opposed to shortness of breath due to thoracic muscle weakness and general debilitation. Breathing difficulties may also be aggravated by the side effects of chemotherapeutic agents (bleomycin and methotrexate) or prior lung irradiation.

Signs and Symptoms

Common presenting symptoms and signs are distressing to most patients (Table 30-6). Dyspnea is related to pulmonary compression. Cough is caused by compression of bronchial walls by fluid.[8] Dull, aching, continuous chest pain is the most common symptom and points to parietal pleural metastasis. Pleuritic chest wall pain is usually more intense and associated with parietal pleural inflammation.[8] The degree of subjective symptoms produced by a pleural effusion is not as dependent on the amount of fluid involved as on the rapidity with which it has accumulated. If the effusion has developed over a short period of time, the patient may be in extreme respiratory distress.[10] Although the majority of cancer patients with pleural effusions are symptomatic, 23% are not, with the effusion being found incidentally.[6]

Diagnosis

Radiographic examination

Chest x-rays are important in visualizing free fluid in the pleural cavity and relating the accumulation to

TABLE 30-6 Assessment of the Patient with Suspected Pleural Effusion

SUBJECTIVE INDICATORS
Dyspnea Orthopnea Dry, nonproductive cough Chest pain, chest heaviness
OBJECTIVE INDICATORS
Labored breathing Tachypnea Dullness to percussion Restricted chest wall expansion Impaired transmission of breath sounds
LABORATORY INDICATORS
Fluid visualized on chest X ray Positive pleural fluid cytology

other structures. Most pleural effusions begin in the subpulmonic area between the lung and the diaphragm and appear as an elevated diaphragm on the affected side. The fluid casts an opaque shadow that has the same density as the heart. The larger the effusion, the more opaque it will appear. A pleural effusion will not be detected on a posterior-anterior chest film unless it contains at least 200–300 ml of fluid. A small effusion shows haziness at the base of the lung and obliterates the costophrenic angle. A lateral decubitus x-ray film is the best way to identify a small effusion, because gravity will cause the fluid to shift to a position along the dependent lateral rib cage where it is easier to visualize.[10]

Clues to the type of cancer causing the pleural effusion may be seen on X ray. Mediastinal shift away from the effusion points to a disseminated nonthoracic tumor, such as breast or ovary. If the mediastinum is shifted toward the effusion, carcinoma of the lung, with some degree of bronchial obstruction, is probably involved. Mesothelioma or fixed central nodal metastasis is indicated if no mediastinal shift is seen.[4] If there is suspicion of pleural mesothelioma, CT can be useful.[3]

Pleural fluid examination

Any new pleural effusion must be aspirated to confirm the presence of malignant cells and to rule out nonmalignant causes. Pleural fluid cytologic analysis yields a definitive diagnosis in approximately 70% of patients with malignant pleural effusion.[7] Thoracoscopy with direct pleural biopsy leads to a diagnosis 100% of the time. If possible, the pleural fluid should be removed at the same time as the diagnostic thoracentesis. This measure provides immediate relief for the distressing symptoms of large (1000–1500 ml) effusions.[3] Fluid should be removed slowly to avoid reexpansion pulmonary edema.

It is important to determine whether the fluid is an exudate or a transudate. Since malignant effusion is almost always an exudate, a transudative fluid would indicate a nonmalignant cause. The aspirated fluid is sent for cultures, gram and acid-fast stains, cell counts, and chemistry studies. Characteristics of the fluid that are helpful diagnostically are appearance (straw-colored, bloody, turbid, or milky) and levels of glucose, amylase, protein, LDH, and lymphocytes.[3] A bloody effusion is the single strongest indicator of malignancy.[8]

Treatment

How the malignant pleural effusion is treated depends on the type of tumor and previous therapy (Figure 30-3). Small, asymptomatic effusions caused by lymphomas, leukemias, breast cancer, small-cell lung cancer, and ovarian cancer are first treated with systemic chemotherapy or hormonal therapy. Unless the patient has been aggressively treated in the past and the tumor has become resistant to certain drugs, these types of tumors will usually respond and the effusion will disappear. Patients with chemotherapy-resistant tumors (melanoma, non–small-cell lung cancer) will require alternative treatment approaches. If the underlying disease is unresponsive to therapy and the patient is symptomatic, palliative measures should be implemented.

Removal of fluid

Relief of symptoms is a short-term treatment goal that is usually achieved when the pleural fluid is mechanically drained. However, the fluid tends to reaccumulate when it is not possible to control the underlying cancer. Long-range treatment goals are directed toward the obliteration of the pleural space so that pleural fluid cannot reaccumulate.

Thoracentesis In thoracentesis, pleural fluid is removed by needle aspiration through the chest wall. The patient is placed in an upright sitting position with arms and shoulders raised. This elevates and separates the ribs to make the needle insertion easier. After the thoracentesis is completed and the pleural fluid has been drained, the patient is assessed for complications such as pneumothorax, pain, hypotension, or pulmonary edema. Patient education and support as well as medication and local anesthesia are important measures to prevent anxiety and discomfort during any of these therapeutic procedures.[12,13]

Although thoracentesis alone is effective for diagnosis, palliation, or relief of acute respiratory distress, it is of little value for treating recurrent malignant effusions because the fluid usually reaccumulates quickly. In one study of 94 patients, the average reaccumulation time was four days and there was a 97% chance of recurrence within a month of the thoracentesis.[3] The

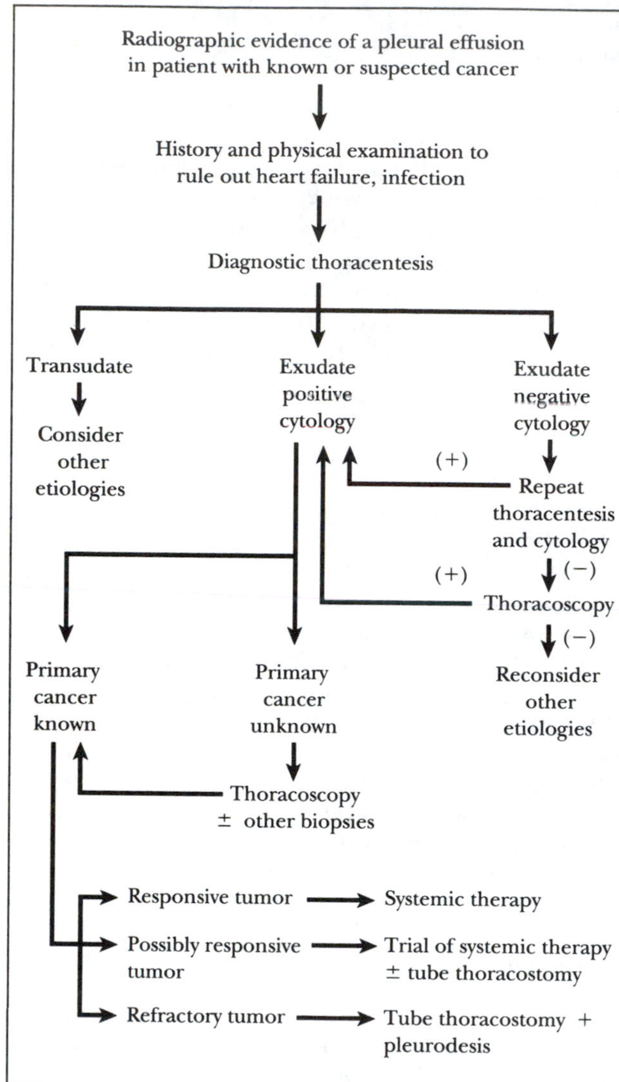

FIGURE 30-3 Algorithm for diagnosis and management of malignant pleural effusion. (Source: Reprinted with permission of Ruckdeschel.[16])

risks of repeated thoracentesis include hypoalbuminemia, electrolyte imbalance, pneumothorax, fluid loculation, and infection.

Thoracentesis via an implanted port and intrapleural catheter is an alternative approach that can be advantageous for the patient whose cancer is refractory to treatment and thus will likely experience repeated pleural fluid reaccumulation.[51] Pleural fluid removal via an implanted port and intrapleural catheter can be completed by the nurse in the ambulatory or home setting. (See Figure 30-4.) Using the implanted port reduces the risk of pneumothorax and infection that can occur with repeated traditional percutaneous aspiration approaches. In addition, there can be significant reduction of health care resources consumed since nurses can evacuate the fluid accumulation before the symptoms of effusion become disabling. There is also a reduced need for repeat radiologic examinations. Since a Huber point needle is used to access the implanted port, the patient experiences less pain than occurs with the large-gauge thoracentesis needle or a thoracostomy tube. Ease of performing the thoracentesis procedure, along with reduced pain and anxiety, significantly improves the patient's experience.

Thoracostomy tube A thoracostomy tube may be inserted to facilitate fluid drainage and then left in place to assess the degree of fluid reaccumulation. However, chest tube drainage alone is only partially effective. Measures to prevent fluid reaccumulation are also needed. Nursing assessments while a thoracostomy tube is in place include observing for pneumothorax, pain, hypotension, and pulmonary edema as well as care of the closed-chest drainage system.[14] Care is taken to ensure that the chest tube remains patent since exudate fluid tends to clot. Thoracostomy tubes can also be used to instill sclerosing agents into the pleural space.

Obliteration of the pleural space

If the pleural space can be obliterated, then the reaccumulation of pleural fluid may be prevented. Obliteration is achieved by instilling a chemical agent that causes the visceral and parietal pleura to become permanently adhered together. The chemical agent causes mesothelial fibrosis and the obliteration of small pleural blood vessels.[3]

Chemical agents Many chemicals have been used over the years as sclerosing agents to prevent pleural effusion recurrence. Chemical sclerosing does not prolong the patient's life but may enhance quality of life by relieving symptoms and reducing the time a patient spends in the hospital. Agents used for pleural instillation in the past (nitrogen mustard, atabrine, 5FU, talc) have had side effects, such as nausea and vomiting, hypotension, pain, and bone marrow depression.[10] Bleomycin[15] and tetracycline are the two most commonly used chemical agents currently.[3] Both agents control malignant pleural effusion in 70% or more of patients.[16] Tetracycline has been popular due to its overall efficacy, convenience, low cost, and minimal morbidity. Patients may be successfully retreated with tetracycline sclerosis if the effusion recurs.[8] A recent 13-center randomized trial compared tetracycline 1 g and bleomycin 60 u. With bleomycin there was a longer median time to recurrence or progression of the effusion, and the recurrence rate was lower.[4] An advantage of bleomycin is that it can be used without thoracostomy tube drainage for patients with smaller effusions.

The selected sclerosing agent is instilled into the pleural space via the thoracentesis needle or the thoracostomy tube. Since the overall objective is to expose as much of the pleura as possible to the chemical, most of the pleural fluid will have been removed and the lung reexpanded before the agent is instilled. The pa-

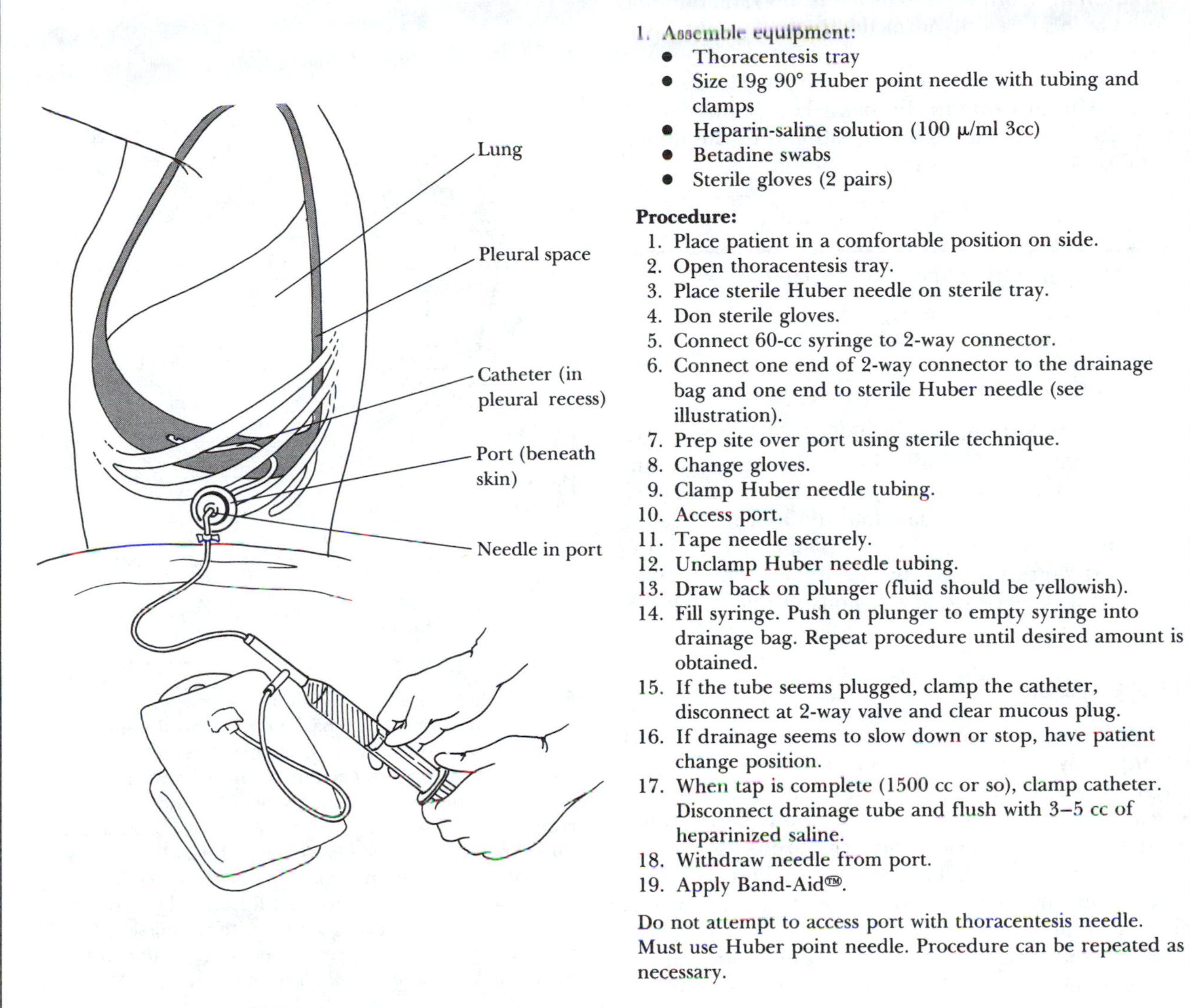

1. Assemble equipment:
   - Thoracentesis tray
   - Size 19g 90° Huber point needle with tubing and clamps
   - Heparin-saline solution (100 μ/ml 3cc)
   - Betadine swabs
   - Sterile gloves (2 pairs)

Procedure:

1. Place patient in a comfortable position on side.
2. Open thoracentesis tray.
3. Place sterile Huber needle on sterile tray.
4. Don sterile gloves.
5. Connect 60-cc syringe to 2-way connector.
6. Connect one end of 2-way connector to the drainage bag and one end to sterile Huber needle (see illustration).
7. Prep site over port using sterile technique.
8. Change gloves.
9. Clamp Huber needle tubing.
10. Access port.
11. Tape needle securely.
12. Unclamp Huber needle tubing.
13. Draw back on plunger (fluid should be yellowish).
14. Fill syringe. Push on plunger to empty syringe into drainage bag. Repeat procedure until desired amount is obtained.
15. If the tube seems plugged, clamp the catheter, disconnect at 2-way valve and clear mucous plug.
16. If drainage seems to slow down or stop, have patient change position.
17. When tap is complete (1500 cc or so), clamp catheter. Disconnect drainage tube and flush with 3–5 cc of heparinized saline.
18. Withdraw needle from port.
19. Apply Band-Aid™.

Do not attempt to access port with thoracentesis needle. Must use Huber point needle. Procedure can be repeated as necessary.

FIGURE 30-4 Thoracentesis via an Implanted Port. (Source: Procedure compliments of Michelle Goodman, RN, MS, Rush-Presbyterian-St. Luke's Medical Center.)

tient will be asked to move around and change position frequently to help distribute the agent. Nursing management during chest tube insertion and pleural sclerosing includes patient education and reassurance, pain control, positioning, and the management of the chest tube drainage as well as maintaining the drainage system.[9] Chest tube insertion and pleural sclerosing can be difficult and painful procedures for patients, who may already be debilitated due to their underlying disease.

Newer investigational methods for controlling malignant pleural effusion by pleural space obliteration include antibody-guided radiation using tumor-associated monoclonal antibodies radiolabeled with ^{131}I. *C. parvum* is being used as a sclerosing agent to elicit a potent inflammatory and antitumor effect.[3] Other biological agents are being studied in current trials.

Surgical methods If a pleural effusion remains uncontrolled after other approaches have been tried, surgery is another option. If a patient has a good life expectancy and a good performance status, pleural stripping is advocated. Success rates approach 90%, but there can be serious complications, such as persistent air leak, bleeding, pneumonia, and empyema.[3] Talc poudrage and pleurectomy have been reported to be effective in some cases. Also, a pleuroperitoneal shunt has been developed for control of malignant effusions. The shunt is inserted into the subcutaneous tissue and pleural fluid is diverted to the peritoneal cavity via manual compression of the shunt's valve pump. The patient must be motivated, because he is required to conscientiously pump the valve intermittently (100 times five times a day) to prevent clogging. Failure of the shunt has plagued this procedure.[8]

Radiation Although external beam radiation may be used as local treatment for mediastinal tumors (lymphoma and lung), hemithoracic radiation is not recommended as a first-line management of malignant pleural effusions due to the hazard of pulmonary fibrosis. Radiation is limited to treatment of the underlying disease, not the resultant effusion.

HEART: MALIGNANT PERICARDIAL EFFUSION

Incidence

Autopsy series indicate metastasis to the heart and pericardium occurs in 8%–20% of cases.[3,17] However, only 30% of affected patients are symptomatic.[18] Since pericardial effusion is not easily detected by routine tests, it is often not discovered while the patient is alive. Lung and breast cancer are the most common tumor types associated with pericardial effusions (Table 30-7).

Pathophysiology

The pericardial sac, or cavity, that surrounds the heart is completely closed. Two layers make up the sac: a tough outer fibrous pericardium called the parietal pericardium and an inner layer of serous pericardium called the visceral pericardium (Figure 30-5). Malignant pericardial effusion collects within this cavity. The cavity ordinarily contains less than 50 ml of fluid, which serves as a lubricant.

Pericardial metastasis results from lymphatic or hematogenous spread or from direct invasion by an adjacent primary tumor. Tumor implants may stud the pericardial surface or completely encase the pericardium. Pericarditis secondary to prior radiation therapy can cause severe pericardial thickening. The majority of pericardial effusions result from obstruction of lymphatic and venous drainage of the heart. This obstruction disturbs the intrapericardial pressure and results in fluid build-up. The effects of pericardial fluid accumulation are largely dependent on the rate of exudation, the physical compliance capacity of the pericardial cavity, ventricular function, myocardial size, and blood volume. If the fluid accumulation is gradual, usually the case with metastatic spread, the pericardium can stretch to accomodate up to four liters of fluid. Rapid build-up of even 150–200 ml can trigger a cardiac-oncologic emergency.[8,19]

TABLE 30-7 Incidence of Pericardial Effusion Related to Tumor Type

Tumor	Incidence (%)
Lung cancer	37
Breast cancer	22
Leukemia and lymphoma	17
Sarcoma	4
Melanoma	3
Others	19

Source: Adapted with permission from *CA—A Cancer Journal for Clinicians* 41:165–179, 1991.

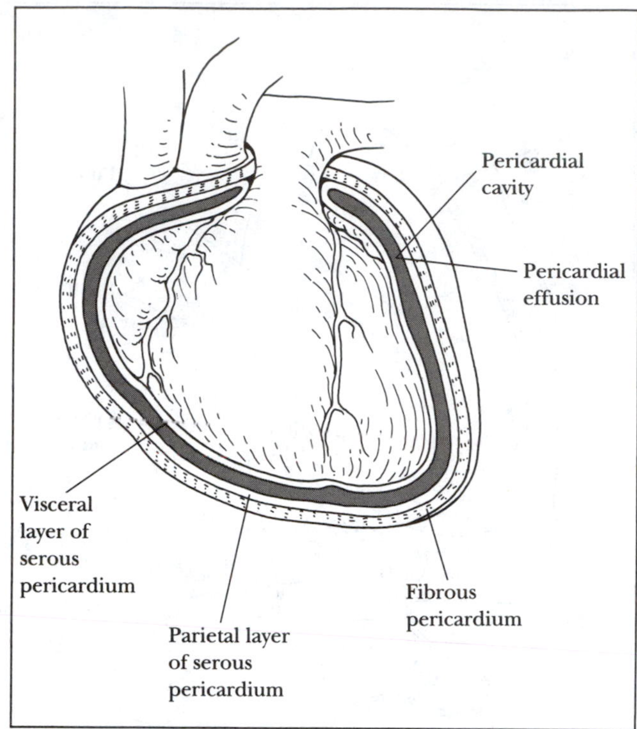

FIGURE 30-5 The pericardium is composed of two main compartments, the parietal pericardium and the visceral pericardium. Where the great vessels attach to the heart, these layers become continuous with each other to form the pericardial space. If venous or lymphatic drainage of the heart becomes obstructed by tumor-related processes, seepage of fluid through the visceral pericardium into the pericardial space leads to pericardial effusion. (Source: Reprinted [adapted] from the *Oncology Nursing Forum* with permission from the Oncology Nursing Press. Mangan C: Malignant pericardial effusion, *Oncol Nurs Forum* 19(8):1216, 1992.

Clinical Manifestations

Pericardial effusion interferes with cardiac function as the fluid burden occupies space and reduces the volume of the heart in diastole. Systemic circulatory effects of decreased cardiac output and impaired venous return lead to generalized congestion. The body tries to compensate in several ways, such as: (1) a tachycardia is created by adrenergic stimulation to offset decreased stroke volume; (2) systemic and pulmonary venous pressure increase in an attempt to improve ventricular filling; (3) the adrenergic stimulation increases the ejection fraction, leading to increased peripheral resistance that will support arterial blood pressure.[19]

Signs and Symptoms

Most patients with pericardial effusions are asymptomatic, so cardiac involvement may be overlooked. The patient may have only nonspecific symptoms at first: dyspnea, cough, and chest pain. Often the patient is treated for right heart failure or complaints related to the underlying tumor. The clinician should have a high index of suspicion for pericardial involvement whenever cancer patients exhibit cardiovascular symptoms.[20] If not diagnosed early, pericardial effusion can lead to a life-threatening emergency.

Signs and symptoms of a developing pericardial effusion are often insidious (Table 30-8). These findings can be subdivided into three clinical stages, from mild effusion to tamponade.[21] Cardiac tamponade is characterized by impaired hemodynamic function due to increased intrapericardial pressure that overcomes normal compensatory mechanisms. Cardiac tamponade is the most severe symptom complex and is an oncologic emergency.[19,21] In addition to the symptoms in Table 30-8, the patient with cardiac tamponade will position himself in an upright, forward-leaning stance for maximum relief, have anxiety, an ashen face with facial plethora, and vague gastrointestinal complaints due to visceral congestion.[8] When cardiovascular collapse is imminent, severe symptoms, profuse perspiration, and altered mental status can also occur. Cardiac tamponade is seen in 16% of patients symptomatic for pericardial effusion[18] and is more common in breast cancer than lung cancer patients.

Nursing management of patients in tamponade includes measures to minimize activity and promote adequate respiration, elevation of the head of the bed, and administration of oxygen and medications to relieve anxiety and pain. Intravascular volume maintenance with intravenous fluids, vasopressors, and other cardiac medications may be in order while preparation is made for pericardiocentesis or surgical intervention. Ongoing assessment for complications is imperative to prevent a fatality from occurring.[19]

TABLE 30-8 Assessment of the Patient with Suspected Pericardial Effusion (in Order of Frequency Encountered)

Signs and Symptoms	Frequency (%)
SUBJECTIVE INDICATORS	
Dyspnea	79
Cough	47
Chest pain	27
Orthopnea	26
Weakness	20
Dysphagia	18
Syncope	4
Palpitations	3
OBJECTIVE INDICATORS	
Pleural effusion	51
Tachycardia	50
Jugular venous distention	45
Hepatomegaly	37
Peripheral edema	35
Pulsus paradoxus	31
Hypotension	31
Distant heart sounds	17
Rales	15
Pericardial rub	12
LABORATORY INDICATORS	
Echocardiographic fluid	100
Abnormal ECG	91
Abnormal chest x-ray	87
Positive pericardial fluid cytology	79
Positive pericardial biopsy	55

Source: Adapted with permission from Press AW, Livingston R: Management of malignant pericardial effusion and tamponade, *JAMA* 257:1088–1092. Copyright 1987, American Medical Association.

Diagnosis

Radiography

Echocardiography (ECHO) is the fastest, least invasive, and most precise method for visualization and quantification of malignant pericardial effusion. It also allows for evaluation of ventricular function. However, it may take too much time to perform in a cardiac tamponade emergency. An upright AP x-ray view of the chest reveals cardiomegaly ("water bottle heart"), but is not diagnostic. Bilateral pleural effusion, mediastinal widening, and hilar adenopathy can be observed. A small pericardial effusion may not be apparent on X ray. Difficult-to-detect lesions may be better visualized by CT.

Electrocardiography

ECG changes with neoplastic pericarditis or effusions include tachycardia, premature contractions, low

QRS voltage, and nonspecific ST and T wave changes. Electrical alterans can occur with large effusions or with tamponade.[8,19]

Pericardial fluid examination

Fluid withdrawn from the pericardial cavity by pericardiocentesis (needle aspiration using a subxyphoid approach) that has a bloody appearance is indicative of malignancy, especially with lung cancer. Such fluid is always exudative. Cytologic examination can reveal tumor cells, but false-negatives are possible. The ability to make the diagnosis based on cytology can be difficult, particularly with effusions due to lymphoma or leukemia.[8]

Treatment

Medical and surgical treatment options for pericardial effusions have significant advantages and disadvantages.[17] Choice of treatment depends on the physiologic impairment caused by the effusion and the degree of tamponade. If the patient is asymptomatic, it is usually expedient to simply watch and wait (Figure 30-6).

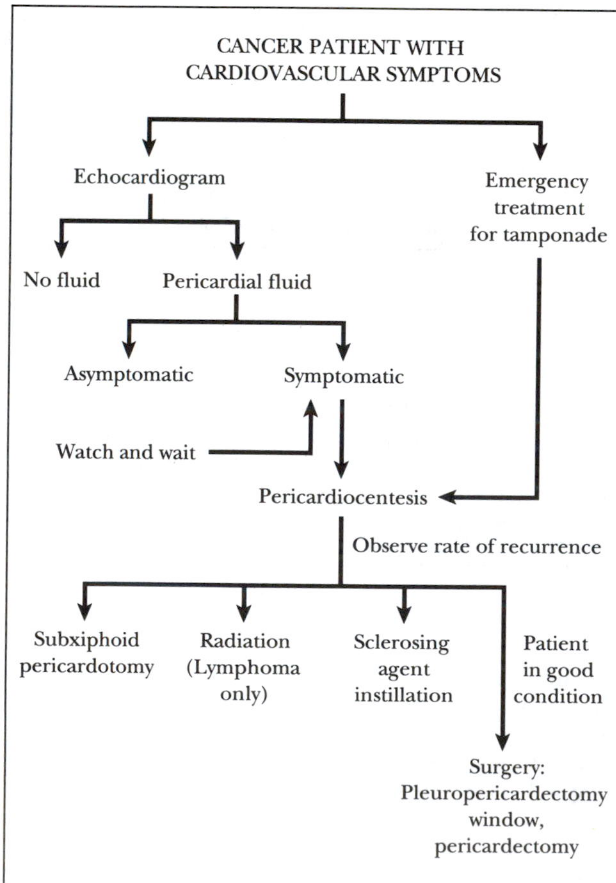

FIGURE 30-6 Algorithm for diagnosis and management of malignant pericardial effusion.

Removal of fluid

Pericardiocentesis alone Percutaneous pericardiocentesis (performed since 1840) guided by echocardiography (ECHO), is an important diagnostic tool and is useful for initial drainage of fluid from the pericardium. This leads to dramatic relief of patient symptoms with minimal risk.[8] Using ECHO to guide the procedure decreases the risk of puncturing the heart. Pericardial drainage alone as treatment for effusion has been equivocal, with most patients relapsing a short time after the tap. The complication rate ranges from 10%–25%.[17] Pericardiocentesis is crucial with cardiac tamponade. Nursing care during the pericardiocentesis includes explaining the procedure to the patient and attempting to reduce anxiety and discomfort; positioning the patient in a semi-Fowler's position; maintaining asepsis; and having available a good light source, defibrillator, and emergency medications. The nurse must continuously monitor the patient and the EKG during the pericardiocentesis, and afterwards monitor for complications such as pneumothorax, myocardial laceration, and coronary artery laceration.[22] Other emergency support measures may be needed first, such as IV fluids, oxygen, and drugs to increase cardiac output and blood pressure.[19,21,22]

Subxiphoid pericardiotomy Under local anesthesia using a subxiphoid approach, subxiphoid pericardiotomy allows for a longer period of drainage and permits examination of the pericardial space as well as obtaining a pericardial biopsy. Complications are rare, and effusion usually does not recur.[23] Nursing care is the same as for pericardiocentesis.

Obliteration of the pericardial space

Pericardiocentesis with sclerosing agent instillation Sclerosing agents are instilled into the pericardial cavity via pericardiocentesis, but they are associated with significant toxicity. Sclerosing agents used in pericardial effusions include tetracycline, 5-fluorouracil, radioactive gold or phosphorus, quinacrine, and thiotepa.[24] The degree of response varies with each agent.[24] Effusions recur in approximately 50% of the patients thus treated.

Surgery Surgical intervention, including pleuropericardial window via thoracotomy and pericardiectomy, is generally reserved for medically appropriate patients whose malignant effusion is unresponsive to other therapies or who have required repeated pericardiocentesis. General anesthesia and thoracotomy are required. Cardiac tamponade symptoms are usually present.

A nursing care plan for patients with tamponade undergoing pericardial window surgery includes preoperative measures to maintain blood pressure and heart rate, maintain urine output and mental status, provide sufficient oxygen, and decrease pain and anxiety. Nursing measures postoperatively include prevention of infection, atelectasis, pleural effusion, and pneumothorax, as well as ongoing assessment for cardiac arrhythmias due to surgical irritation or the presence of the pericardial catheter. Prevention of anxiety and pain and bleeding due to the catheter and maintaining free-flowing pericardial drainage are important.[23]

Recurrence following surgical intervention is rare. A reported experience with subxiphoid partial pericardiectomy, with or without a sclerosing agent concluded that this procedure is a safe and effective treatment for malignant pericardial effusions.[25] It was suggested that patients with symptomatic malignant pericardial effusions be treated first with subxiphoid partial pericardiectomy, thus reserving sclerosant instillation for those patients who have persistent drainage after surgery.[25]

Radiation The use of external beam radiation is primarily reserved for pericardial effusions due to lymphomas, which are highly radiosensitive.[8] Approximately 50% of cases will respond. Carcinoma of the lung and breast are also sufficiently radiosensitive for radiation to be considered in the treatment plan.

ABDOMEN: MALIGNANT PERITONEAL EFFUSION

Incidence

Malignant peritoneal effusion (ascites) is most common in patients with ovarian cancer (Table 30-9). Ascites will be found at presentation in 33% of these patients, and over 60% will develop ascites at some time before death.[26] Ascites also develops in patients with gastrointestinal malignancies, though it typically develops later in the course of the disease. The appearance of ascites in patients with advanced disease is prognostically grim, and palliation is usually all that can be offered. Life expectancy is a few months.

TABLE 30-9 Tumors Associated with Malignant Peritoneal Effusion

Ovary	Gastric
Endometrial	Pancreatic
Breast	Lymphoma
Colon	Mesothelioma

Pathophysiology

The peritoneal cavity is covered by a serous lining composed of the visceral peritoneum that lines and supports the abdominal organs, and the parietal peritoneum. The parietal peritoneum covers the abdominal and pelvic walls and the undersurface of the diaphragm (Figure 30-7). As with the other third spaces, a small amount of fluid lubricates the cavity. Normally, the volume of peritoneal fluid is regulated by the pressure gradient balances described previously, with lymphatic channels draining 80% of all lymphatic peritoneal fluid.[12] When the production of peritoneal fluid exceeds the ability of the lymphatic channels to drain the cavity (the thoracic duct may be dilated five to ten times normal size), ascites develops.

The most common cause of ascitic fluid build-up is tumor seeding the peritoneum, resulting in obstruction of the diaphragmatic and/or abdominal lymphatics. This occurs primarily with gynecologic cancers. Excess in-

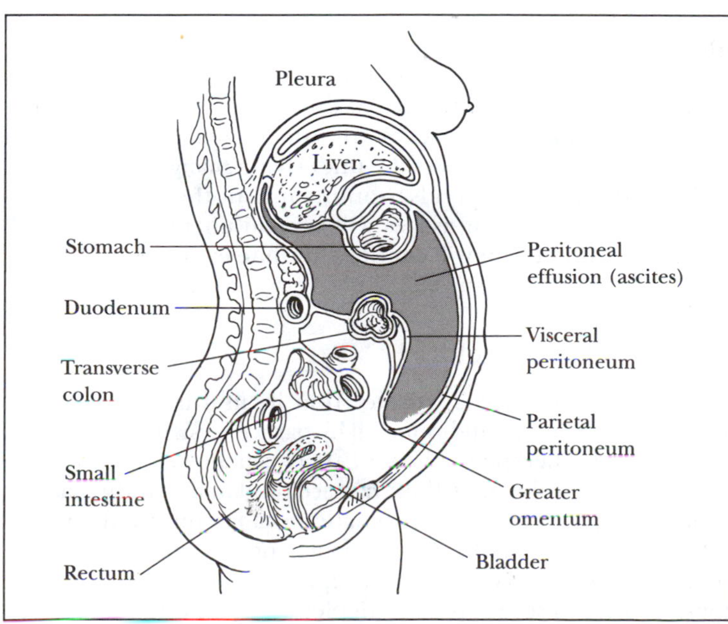

FIGURE 30-7 The peritoneal cavity is covered by the visceral peritoneum that lines and supports the abdominal organs, and the parietal peritoneum that covers the abdominal and pelvic walls and the undersurface of the diaphragm. If, due to malignant processes, the volume of fluid accumulating in the peritoneal space exceeds the capacity of lymphatic channels to drain the cavity, ascites develops. (Source: Adapted from Pick TP, Howden R [eds]: *Gray's Anatomy* [rev. Am. ed from 15th Eng. ed], New York: Bounty Books, 1977, p. 900.)

traperitoneal fluid production may also be a factor contributing to ascites. The tumor itself may elaborate humoral factors that cause increased capillary leakage of proteins and fluids into the peritoneum. In patients with diffuse liver metastasis and venous obstruction, hypoalbuminemia and low serum protein may play a part in the development of a transudative ascites.

Clinical Manifestations

The pressure of the ascitic fluid volume on nearby organs is uncomfortable and restrictive for patients. Several liters of ascitic fluid can be accommodated in the abdomen. Some people report gaining 50–60 pounds of body weight as a result of the excess fluid. This massive accumulation of fluid leads to negative body image changes, anorexia, early satiety, and difficulty breathing and walking. Subjective, objective, and laboratory findings illustrate the typical profile of a person with ascites (Table 30-10). Most physical signs appear after one liter or more of fluid is present.

Diagnosis

Peritoneal effusion is diagnosed primarily by physical exam, with malignant characteristics confirmed by paracentesis. An abdomen filled with more than 500 cc of fluid appears as a single curve from the xiphoid process to the pubis, with the umbilicus frequently everted. The following signs are characteristic of free fluid: bulging flanks, typanny at the top of the abdominal curve, elicitation of a fluid wave, and shifting dullness. A small effusion is hard to detect. The "puddle sign" is said to detect as little as 120 cc of free fluid in the abdominal cavity. To elicit the puddle sign, the patient lies prone for 5 minutes, then rises on elbows and knees. A stethoscope is applied to the most dependent part of the abdomen, and the clinician flicks the near flank with a finger repeatedly. As the stethoscope is moved across the abdomen away from the examiner, the sound becomes louder. Small volumes of fluid in the abdomen can also be detected by ultrasonic examination. Detecting ascites in obese patients is difficult, even when it is marked.

Treatment

Many treatment approaches have been tried, but optimal intervention has yet to be found.[26] No controlled trials comparing alternative therapies have been reported. It is difficult to carry out research in patients whose longevity is limited to only a few months. An algorithm for the management of the patient with ascites includes the multiple factors influencing selection of treatment (Figure 30-8). Nursing care measures focus on maintaining fluid and electrolyte balance, comfort measures, and early recognition of complications.

TABLE 30-10 Assessment of the Patient with a Peritoneal Effusion

SUBJECTIVE INDICATORS
Increasing abdominal girth—"clothes don't fit"
Indigestion and early satiety
Swollen ankles
Easy fatigability
Shortness of breath
Constipation
Reduced bladder capacity
OBJECTIVE INDICATORS
Weight gain
Distended abdomen
Fluid wave
Shifting dullness
Bulging flanks
Everted umbilicus
Stretched skin
LABORATORY INDICATORS
Abdominal flat plate: generalized ground-glass appearance, air-filled small-bowel loops occupy central position and are separated by fluid between loops
Ultrasound
Abdominal CT
Paracentesis
Gross character on inspection: bloody, serous, milky, turbid
Cell count and differential
Chemistries: total protein, LDH, CEA, amylase levels
Cytology
Microbiology: Gram stain and culture

Source: Adapted with permission from Baker AR, in DeVita VT, Hellman S, Rosenberg SA (eds): *Cancer: Principles and Practice of Oncology* (3d ed). Philadelphia: Lippincott, 1989.

Diet and diuresis

Although diet and diuresis are important as therapy for patients with ascites due to cirrhosis, sodium restriction and diuretics are usually ineffective in malignant ascites. Unless the underlying malignancy causing the ascites responds to antineoplastic therapy, the pathophysiology of ascites will remain unaltered and fluid accumulation will continue despite exogenous fluid restriction measures.

Removal of fluid

Paracentesis Aside from its usefulness as a diagnostic tool, fluid removal by paracentesis alone achieves little therapeutic benefit. It is usually reserved until a large volume of fluid has accumulated and the patient is profoundly symptomatic because the fluid reaccumulates rapidly. Of particular note, removal of two to three liters of fluid and repeated paracentesis taps can lead to severe protein depletion and electrolyte abnor-

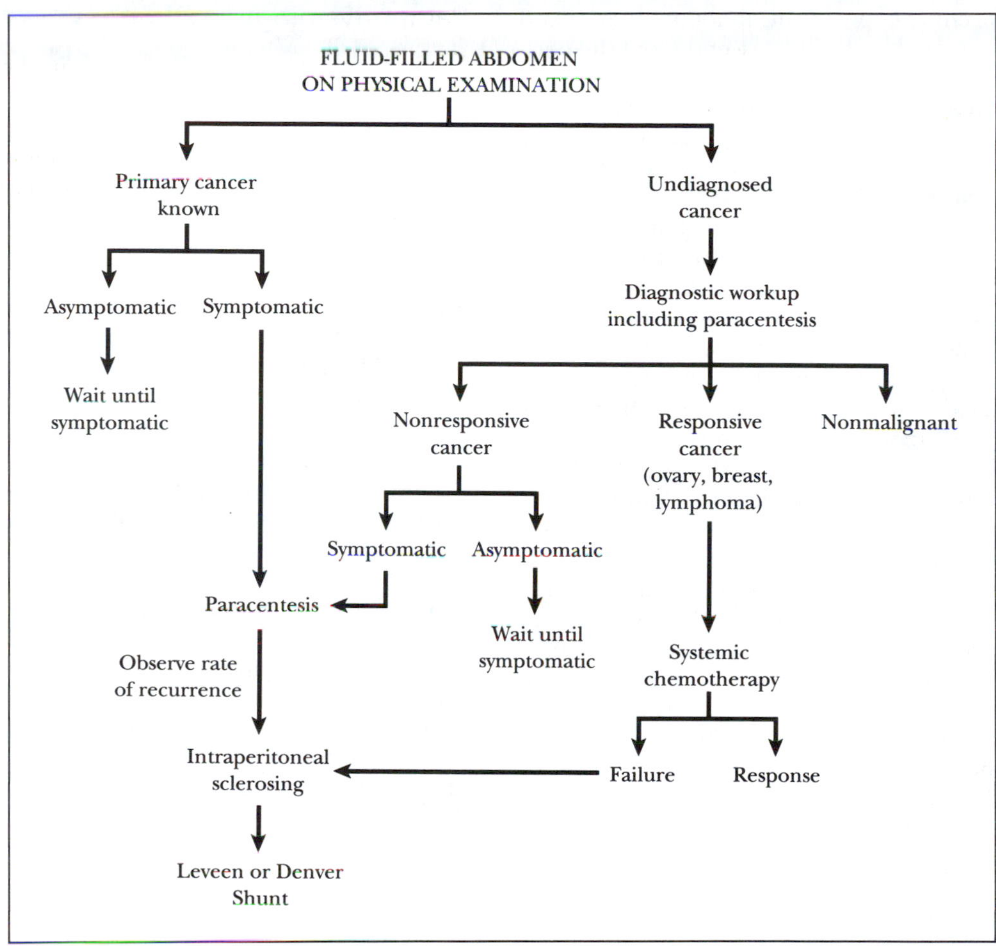

FIGURE 30-8 Algorithm for diagnosis and management of malignant peritoneal effusion.

malities. Injury to the viscera and the introduction of infection can occur. Although caution is urged regarding removing large volumes of ascitic fluid rapidly, there has been recent anecdotal evidence that rapid decompression via paracentesis is not harmful with malignant ascites, probably because the mechanism of its production differs from that of cirrhotic ascites.[27]

Obliteration of the intraperitoneal space In the past, intracavity therapy has consisted of instillation of a radioactive colloid suspension (no longer in favor today) or a chemotherapeutic agent. The chemotherapy instillation is designed to provoke an inflammatory response leading to sclerosis of the peritoneal space linings. Although sclerosing therapy is effective in treating malignant pleural effusions, it is less successful with ascites.[26] Modest responses to bleomycin instillation for palliation have been reported with no significant side effects. Adriamycin, nitrogen mustard, and tetracycline instillations have been tried with small groups of patients. Cisplatin has been administered intraperitoneally.

Access to the peritoneal cavity for drug administration is an important technical problem. The peritoneum can be entered on a temporary basis with various catheters, but repeated puncture of the abdominal wall and peritoneum is risky. Adhesions can occur, which increases the risk of bowel perforation and peritonitis. The Tenchoff catheter is often used to provide repeated access to the peritoneum. It can remain in place indefinitely and allows peritoneal fluid sampling in addition to drug instillation. Problems with the Tenckoff catheter have been poor return following drug and fluid instillation and abdominal pain or discomfort necessitating catheter removal.[12] Positive experience using a Groshong catheter for draining malignant ascites has recently been described as an alternate to conventional paracentesis.[28] Use of the Groshong catheter prevents needle access and does not require surgical removal upon completion of chemotherapy. Complex dressing changes like those required by the Tenchoff catheter are unnecessary.

Peritoneovenous shunting Shunt devices (Leveen ® and Denver ®) can be used to recirculate ascitic fluid continuously to the intravascular space. One end of a catheter is implanted in the peritoneal cavity and a tube is channeled through subcutaneous tissue to the superior vena cava where the other end is implanted. A pressure differential between the abdominal cavity and the thoracic vein enables fluid to ascend from the peritoneal cavity into the superior vena cava. Since neoplastic ascites tends to contain more particulate matter than other fluid types (usually an exudate), a Denver shunt may be preferred because it has a subcutaneous pump that can be manually compressed to prevent clogging of the tubing.[29] Despite this potential advantage, a functional superiority of one over the other of these devices has not been documented in the literature,[26] leaving the choice to the clinician's personal preference.

Peritoneovenous shunting is no panacea. It is usually reserved for patients when all other treatment options have failed. Median survival time after shunt placement is 2–4 months, so it is difficult to obtain objective evaluation criteria. When the shunt is functioning well, it provides good palliation. Complications can occur, with clotting occurring most frequently, but sometimes disseminated intravascular coagulation and pulmonary embolism develop. In some instances, postoperative complications might be predicted by a preoperative procedure designed to assess patient tolerance to the proposed permanent shunt. Termed *peritoneovenous autotransfusion,* this preoperative evaluation can be accomplished by using an external shunting system trial over 48 hours.[30]

Nursing care of the patient with a peritoneovenous shunt includes teaching the patient and family the purpose and care of the shunt, signs and symptoms of problems with the shunt, recognition and prevention of infection, and alleviating anxiety. In addition, nursing care includes measures related to the peritoneal effusion and advanced cancer.

BRAIN: MALIGNANT CEREBRAL EDEMA

Incidence

Cerebral edema results from an increase in brain volume caused by an increase in the fluid content of the brain.[31] There are three major types of cerebral edema: *vasogenic* edema (extracellular, the most common type); *cytotoxic* edema (intracellular, due to metabolic abnormalities); and *interstitial* edema (due to cerebrospinal fluid blockage). Malignant cerebral edema is the vasogenic type caused by increased permeability of the cerebral capillary endothelial cells. Although the edema can be iatrogenic, caused by radiotherapy or chemotherapy, most cerebral edema accompanies primary or metastatic brain tumors or carcinomatous meningitis. Any cancer can metastasize to the brain; brain metastasis occurs in 25%–35% of all cancer patients. Lung cancer accounts for most of the metastatic lesions in the brain (40%–50%), followed by breast cancer (13%), melanoma, renal carcinoma, and others.[32]

Pathophysiology

Mechanisms thought to play a role in the formation of malignant cerebral edema are (1) direct injury to the vascular endothelium by the expanding tumor, (2) dysplastic vascular structures within tumor lesions, (3) biochemically mediated alterations of capillary permeability (including the excretion of a permeability factor by tumor cells),[33] and (4) a less stable blood-brain barrier integrity. Capillary permeability varies depending on histology and tumor size. Within an individual brain tumor there are significant variations in capillary permeability among regions of tumor necrosis and those of active tumor growth.[34] Edema develops as water and ions passively diffuse into the brain extracellular space to maintain isotonicity. The white matter of the brain is primarily affected (Figure 30-9). The progression of edema through brain tissue occurs as bulk fluid flow regulated by cerebral perfusion pressure. It is possible for edema fluid to travel along the longitudinal tracts of the white matter and thus increase local extracellular water content at a distance from the focal tumor.[35]

The tumor continuously produces edema fluid. There can be great differences in the volume of edema, depending on the level of productivity of that particular tumor.[36] How cerebral edema leads to neurologic dysfunction is not clear, but it is probably related to ischemic effects of the mass itself and/or toxic inhibition of local neuron activity induced by metabolic abnor-

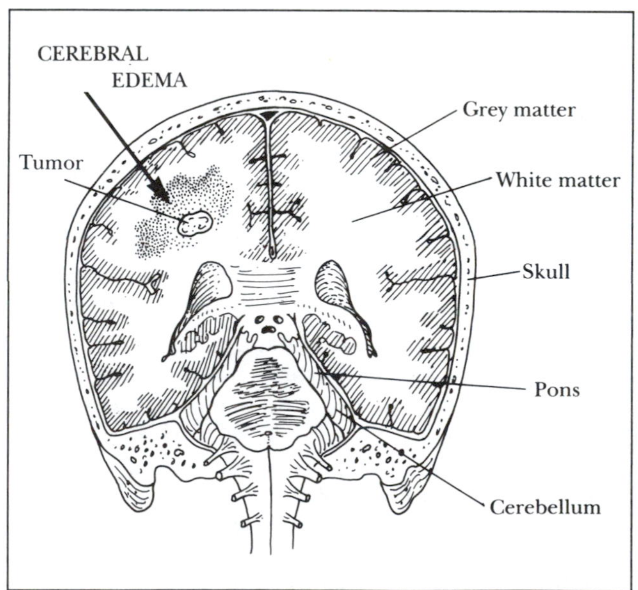

FIGURE 30-9 Vasogenic edema of the brain due to a primary tumor or metastatic lesion is characterized by increased permeability of brain capillary endothelial cells. The white matter of the brain is primarily affected. The progression of edema through the white matter of brain tissue occurs as bulk flow regulated by cerebral perfusion pressure.

malities in the surrounding extravascular fluid. When the edema exceeds the limits of compensatory mechanisms, brain herniation can occur.

Clinical Manifestations

Malignant cerebral edema produces diffuse signs and symptoms reflecting its more global effects on brain functioning, as opposed to the focal signs and symptoms caused by direct destruction of tissue by tumor.[35] Most patients with metastatic brain tumors have regional swelling of tissue, mostly in the cerebrum. In such patients the clinical deficits manifested are more often caused by peritumoral edema than by the tumor mass itself.[31] Subtle early changes in the patient's status are vague and usually only observed by someone who knows the patient well. Family members may notice the patient's lack of persistence in tasks, undue irritability, emotional lability, inertia, faulty insight, forgetfulness, reduced range of mental activity, indifference to common social practices, and lack of initiative and spontaneity. These early symptoms are often incorrectly attributed to worry, anxiety, or depression. Patients themselves often complain only of being weak, tired, or dizzy. As time progresses, the symptoms become more pronounced (Table 30-11).

Seizure is the most common acute onset symptom. Headache, another common early symptom, is due to distortion and traction of pain-sensitive structures by the edema. Intermittent at first, headache usually is present in the morning and gradually increases in duration and frequency. Other indications of brain edema can be generalized or focal. Clinical signs may be observed that relate to specific parts of the brain, and these can be localized to the affected area by neurological assessment.[38]

TABLE 30-11 Assessment of the Patient with Cerebral Edema

Signs and Symptoms	Frequency (%)
SUBJECTIVE INDICATORS	
Headache	53
Weakness, focal	40
Mental disturbance	31
Seizures	15
Gait disorder	20
Visual disturbance	12
Language disturbance	10
OBJECTIVE INDICATORS	
Hemiparesis	66
Impaired cognition	77
Sensory loss, unilateral	27
Papilledema	26
Ataxia	24
Aphasia	19
LABORATORY INDICATORS	
Computerized tomography (CT) brain	
Magnetic resonance imaging (MRI)	

Source: Adapted with permission from Wright DC, Delaney TF, in DeVita VT, Hellman S, Rosenberg SA (eds): *Cancer: Principles and Practice of Oncology* (3d ed). Philadelphia: Lippincott, 1989.

Diagnosis

Neurologic examination, CT scanning, and magnetic resonance imaging (MRI) are the primary studies used for diagnosing a brain tumor mass. MRI is best for visualizing cerebral edema.[38] Surgery, such as stereotactic biopsy, is required for a definitive tissue diagnosis if a primary site is not in evidence elsewhere in the body.

Treatment

Aggressive therapy is warranted to sustain or restore neurologic function. The principal treatment regimen is radiation therapy. In addition, patients receive supportive care and steroids to reduce edema. Patients with edema due to carcinomatous meningitis are aggressively treated with intrathecal chemotherapy. In most patients, neurologic symptoms resolve or improve with treatment. Improvement is often maintained until the patient succumbs to systemic disease.[37]

Nursing management of patients with cerebral edema focuses on assessment, medication administration, management of side effects associated with these medications, the institution of safety and seizure precautions, and prevention of complications of immobility. Interventions may be targeted to the patient's specific neurologic deficits. The nurse must be sensitive to changes in vital signs and be able to intervene rapidly. With advanced cerebral edema and the resultant intercranial hypertension, changes in vital signs such as bounding radial pulse, elevated temperature, and respiratory impairment may be seen. Early detection of brain herniation is essential to preserve brain function. Decreased level of consciousness, change in pupil size and reaction to light, and altered motor response, in addition to other vital signs changes, should alert the nurse to impending brain herniation, an oncologic emergency.[38]

Steroids and osmotherapy

The single most important adjunctive treatment to combat the effects of vasogenic cerebral edema is the use of glucocorticoids (dexamethasone, prednisone). These drugs rapidly reduce the rate of edema fluid formation by the tumor (by 30%) by inhibiting the capillary permeability factor produced by tumor cells.[36] The aim of steroid therapy is to reduce intracranial pressure and increase cerebral blood flow. The usual starting dose of dexamethasone is 16 mg/day in four divided doses. Dexamethasone is the preferred agent because of its minimal salt-retaining properties and relative potency. Mannitol is an osmotherapy agent that can be used to reduce profound cerebral edema on a temporary basis.[35]

Once radiotherapy has relieved the neurologic symptoms caused by the edema, steroids are slowly tapered to prevent Addison's crisis. Steroid withdrawal can result in headache, lethargy, postural dizziness, or nausea, even if there is no laboratory evidence of adrenal insufficiency. These symptoms can confuse the clinician, since they mirror symptoms associated with either adrenal suppression or progressive edema.[34]

Dexamethasone dose as high as 100 mg/day have been used for patients who are refractory at lower doses. Patients failing to improve after a 7-day trial at 100 mg/day are rapidly tapered to the lowest dose that will maintain stable neurologic functioning. The continued long-term use of steroids can lead to serious toxic effects such as cataracts, hyperglycemia, peptic ulcer, and osteoporosis. The effects of long-term therapy should be considered in the nursing plan of care.[39]

Radiation therapy

Ionizing radiation to the underlying tumor is the most effective way to decrease malignant edema as well as tumor bulk. Since it is assumed microscopic tumor is present with metastatic disease, the radiation port usually encompasses the whole brain. Treatment typically lasts 2–3 weeks. Interstitial brachytherapy (the implantation of seeds containing iodine 120 or iridium 192) can sometimes be used to achieve a high-dose "local" boost to the tumor while minimizing radiation exposure for normal brain tissue. Despite initial response rates of 80%, radiation accomplishes little in terms of survival. Medial survival after treatment is 3–6 months.[35]

Surgery

Surgical decompression may be in order in selected cases of resistant or relapsing cerebral metastasis. Surgical decompression or debulking can rapidly reduce the effect of the mass and remove the source of edema production. Neurosurgical procedures have significant associated risk, such as infection, hemorrhage, and operative mortality. Appropriate patient selection is a critical factor for successful surgical outcome.

ARMS/LEGS: IATROGENIC SECONDARY LYMPHEDEMA

Incidence and Pathophysiology

Unlike the other effusions and edemas, postsurgical lymphedema of the arm or leg is a benign condition. Arm lymphedema was the frequent postoperative sequelae of the most common treatment for all types of breast cancer in the past: radical mastectomy with axillary node dissection followed by radiation. With the less invasive breast cancer treatments in use today, arm lymphedema occurs much less frequently. Even so, lymphedema continues to affect 5%–10% of women who have a modified radical mastectomy.[40]

Mechanical interruption (surgical technique) and radiation often produce lymphatic obstruction, the most common cause of lymphedema. Usually the more radical the surgery or radiation, the more severe the edema. Other factors contributing to the development of lymphedema are obesity,[41] insufficient muscle contraction, inflammation, trauma, formation of fibrosclerotic tissue within the lymph vessel, and scarring secondary to radiation therapy or infection. Narrower and fewer lymph channels remain, fluid transport is insufficient, and swelling occurs. Chronic lymphedema is a late postoperative complication that can occur anywhere from 6 weeks to 20 years after surgery. For most women, the affected arm becomes enlarged within the first year after mastectomy.[42] The unpredictable and often delayed nature of lymphedema is postulated to be due to smoldering infection associated with subclinical lymphangitis.[43]

Lymphedema of the leg may develop after groin dissection. Groin dissection is performed for the treatment of metastatic disease from primary tumors (melanoma, squamous cell carcinoma, or soft tissue sarcomas) located in the anatomic area drained by the inguinal lymph nodes. The incidence of leg lymphedema after this type of surgery increases gradually over time, and by the fifth postoperative year is estimated to occur in 80% of patients.[44] However, a more recent study has shown that improved surgical technique and a preventive regimen of leg elevation and elastic stockings reduced the overall incidence of mild to moderate lymphedema to 20%, with no severe cases occurring.[44]

The pathogenesis of lymphedema of the lower extremities (eventually including the genitalia) after groin dissection or radiation therapy is similar to that of the arm. Progressive interstitial fibrosis follows the mechanical interruption of lymph flow caused by the surgery and scarring ensues. If the edema is severe, the result is the classic brawny, nonpitting, firm form of soft tissue swelling. The edematous extremity is painful, can become contracted, and compromises the patient's ability to walk.

Rarely, a malignant lymphedema of the extremities occurs in a patient with an advanced, untreated lymphoma who has ignored earlier symptoms. Cancer cells obstruct lymph vessels or lymph nodes through intraluminal propagation or by external compression. This patient will usually respond to systemic treatment and the edema will subside.

Diagnosis

Assessment for extremity lymphedema includes monitoring the circumference of the limb, condition of the skin, mobility of the extremity, signs of infection, nutritional status, impairment of circulation, and constriction caused by clothing or other objects.

Measurements of the arm circumference are taken prior to surgery and at each postoperative visit. The arm is measured 5.0 and 10.0 cm above and below the olecranon process. Measurement sites are documented and consistent for each patient. Leg measurements are done similarly at the level of the calf. Lymphedema is defined as present if there is a difference in measurement of 1.0 cm to 1.5 cm compared to the unaffected extremity. It can be classified as mild (less than 3 cm), moderate (3.0–5.0 cm) or severe (more than 5 cm).[42]

Treatment

The goals of therapy are primarily aimed at prevention, to increase the flow of lymph away from the limb and minimize formation of new lymph fluid. Elevation, progressive mild exercise, and massage help mobilize fluid out of the limb. Use of an elastic sleeve is important to reduce the potential of stagnation of lymph fluid. Compliance and proper use are critical factors.[42] Prophylactic measures to prevent new fluid from forming include elastic support sleeves or stockings; sodium restriction; and avoidance of infection, excessive use of the limb, local heat, and trauma to the limb. Nursing care is usually divided into primary, secondary, and tertiary interventions.[40,42,45] The primary nursing interventions for lymphedema involve measures to prevent the complication. These begin preoperatively, with assessment of the patient's educational needs, nutritional status, and arm measurements. Instruction on postoperative hand and arm care and postoperative exercises should also occur at this time.

The secondary phase of nursing management is directed towards the early detection and initial treatment of lymphedema. The patient should be alerted to the signs and symptoms of lymphedema, the arms/legs should be measured at regular intervals, the affected limb should be elevated, massage therapy may be instituted, an elastic wrap or sleeve to the affected extremity may be needed, discomfort should be managed, and hand and arm care measures and exercises should be continued. The patient should be taught to recognize and prevent infection.

Tertiary care is associated with the long-term care of the patient with lymphedema and includes elevation of the arm, continued hand and arm care measures and exercises, massage therapy, elastic wrap or sleeve to the extremity, pain control, and assessment of the patient for general functioning and ability to perform activities of daily living. The National Lymphedema Network publishes a quarterly newsletter that focuses on the care of people living with lymphedema (221 Post Street, Suite 404, San Francisco, CA 94115).

Diuretics are usually not helpful. Long-term use of diuretics is reserved for cases of generalized low protein edemas in which the total body sodium content is elevated. In contrast, lymphedema is caused by the stagnation of proteins in the interstitium (a high-protein edema) and not by retention of sodium.

FEET: MALIGNANT PEDAL EDEMA

Peripheral, or dependent, edema is common in patients with far advanced cancer. Among the multiple causes are the lack of normal muscular activity, which would ordinarily return fluids from the periphery to the central circulation; hypoalbuminemia; venous or lymphatic obstruction; compromised circulation; malnutrition; and hyperaldosteronism. As much as 10 lb of liquid can accumulate in the lower extremities before it is recognizable as pitting edema.[46] Many patients will tolerate this fluid accumulation with no discomfort and require no special therapy other than elevation of the legs several times a day. However, patients and families are often disturbed by the cosmetic unsightliness of the swollen feet and ankles, especially when shoes no longer fit, and they may request more definitive intervention.

Diagnosis

Measurement of the ankle is useful to record changes in circumference and note the effectiveness of treatment measures. Pitting can be assessed by pressing the thumb into the patient's skin over a bony surface.[46] The edema of advanced cancer is bilateral; a unilateral edema would lead to a search for a treatable cause such as thrombophlebitis. Serum albumin or serum total protein levels will indicate whether hypoalbuminemia is present, as will serum total proteins. The prealbumin level is a quick and accurate test that indicates malnutrition.[47]

Treatment

Three approaches can be taken in an attempt to relieve ankle edema.[46] First, the patient's nutritional status may be improved with concentrated dietary supplements. Particularly important is protein.[48] Overt sodium can be eliminated from the diet; however, most patients are eating little food at this point and have stopped eating salty foods at earlier stages of the illness. Water should be restricted if the patient is hyponatremic. Second, there is an effort to improve venous blood return by elevation of the legs while sitting, wearing of support stockings, eliminating clothing that constricts the lower legs, and gentle exercise. Third, diuretics may be helpful and can be tried on a short-term basis.[49] A typical diuretic regimen starts with low-dose hydrochlorothiazide and cautiously proceeds through progressively larger doses of spironolactone to furosemide until a diuretic response is achieved.[50] Serum electrolytes, BUN, and creatinine are monitored during such a trial.

CONCLUSION

When fluid accumulates abnormally in the cancer patient, the consequences can range from life-threatening to merely irksome. A variety of interventions can be employed, mostly for palliation, depending on the amount of fluid present and the site where it is retained. Aggressive medical and nursing care can alleviate discomfort and may prolong life, or at least maintain its quality. The best hope for eliminating malignant effusions and edemas would be to discover a cure for cancer, or at least more effective therapies.

REFERENCES

1. Maxwell MB, Maher KE: Chemotherapy-induced myelosuppression. *Semin Oncol Nurs* 8(2):113–123, 1992.
2. Hill RB, Anderson RE: The autopsy in oncology. *CA* 42:47–56, 1992.
3. Olopade OI, Ultmann JE: Malignant effusions. *CA* 41:166–179, 1991.
4. Moores DW: Malignant pleural effusion. *Semin Oncol* 18:59–61, 1991(suppl).
5. Leff A, Hopewell PC, Costello J: Pleural effusion from malignancy. *Ann Intern Med* 88:532–537, 1978.
6. Chernow B, Sahn SA: Carcinomatous involvement of the pleura. *Am J Med* 63:695–702, 1977.
7. Martini N, Bains MS, Beattie EF: Indications for pleurectomy in malignant effusions. *Cancer* 35:734–738, 1975.
8. Pass HI: Treatment of malignant pleural and pericardial effusions. In DeVita VT, Hellman S, Rosenberg SA (eds), *Cancer: Principles and Practices of Oncology* (3d ed). Philadelphia: Lippincott, 1989, pp. 2317–2327.
9. Rossetti AC: Nursing care of patients treated with intrapleural tetracycline for control of malignant pleural effusion. *Cancer Nurs* 8:103–109, 1985.
10. Wegmann JA, Forshee, T: Malignant pleural effusions: Pertinent issues. *Heart and Lung* 12:533–543, 1983.
11. Hausheer FH, Yarbro JW: Diagnosis and treatment of malignant pleural effusion. *Semin Oncol* 12:54–75, 1985.
12. Zehner LC, Hoogstraten B: Malignant effusions and their management. *Semin Oncol Nurs* 1:259–268, 1985.
13. Gobel BH, Lawler PE: Malignant pleural effusions. *Oncol Nurs Forum* 12(4):49–54, 1985.
14. Hewitt JB, Janssen WR: A management strategy for malignancy-induced pleural effusion: Long-term thoracostomy drainage. *Oncol Nurs Forum* 14(5):17–22, 1987.
15. Ostrowski MJ: An assessment of the long-term results of controlling the reaccumulation of malignant effusions using intracavity bleomycin. *Cancer* 57:721–727, 1986.
16. Ruckdeschel JC: Management of malignant pleural effusion: An overview. *Semin Oncol* 15(3):24–28, 1988(suppl).
17. Hawkins JW, Vacek JL: What constitutes definitive therapy of malignant pericardial effusion? Medical vs. surgical treatment. *Am Heart J* 118:428–432, 1989.
18. Thurber DL, Edwards JE, Archor RW: Secondary malignant tumors of the pericardium. *Circulation* 26:228–241, 1962.
19. Joiner GA, Kolodychuk GR: Neoplastic cardiac tamponade. *Crit Care Nurs* 11:50–58, 1991.
20. Press OW, Livingston R: Management of malignant pericardial effusion and tamponade. *JAMA* 257:1088–1092, 1987.
21. Mangan CM: Malignant pericardial effusions: Pathophysiology and clinical correlates. *Oncol Nurs Forum* 19(8):1215–1221, 1992.
22. Estes ME: Management of the cardiac tamponade patient: A nursing framework. *Crit Care Nurs* 5(5):17–26, 1985.
23. Wojciechowicz V: Peripheral window surgery for cardiac tamponade. *Crit Care Nurs* 5(5):28–33, 1985.
24. Missri J, Schechter D: When pericardial effusion complicates cancer. *Hosp Prac* 23:277–286, 1988.
25. Chan A, Rischin D, Clarke CP, et al: Subxiphoid partial pericardiectomy with or without sclerosant instillation in the treatment of symptomatic pericardial effusions in patients with malignancy. *Cancer* 68:1021–1025, 1991.
26. Baker AR: Treatment of malignant ascites. In DeVita VT, Hellman S, Rosenberg SA (eds), *Cancer: Principles and Practice of Oncology* (3d ed). Philadelphia: Lippincott, 1989, pp. 2328–2332.
27. Ratliff CR, Hutchinson M, Conner C: Rapid paracentesis of large volumes of ascitic fluid. *Oncol Nurs Forum* 18:1461, 1991.
28. Hrozencik SP, Ness EA: Intraperitoneal chemotherapy via the Groshong catheter in the patient with gynecologic cancer. *Oncol Nurs Forum* 18:1245, 1991.
29. Klopp A: Shunting malignant ascites. *Am J Nurs* 84:212–213, 1984.
30. Kehoe C: Malignant ascites: Etiology, diagnosis, and treatment. *Oncol Nurs Forum* 18:523–530, 1991.
31. Fishman RA: Brain edema. *N Engl J Med* 293:706–711, 1975.
32. Ryan LS: Nursing assessment of the ambulatory patient with brain metastasis. *Cancer Nurs* 4:281–291, 1981.
33. Ito U, Reulen HJ, Tomita H, et al: A computed tomography study on formation, propagation, and resolution of edema fluid in metastatic brain tumors. In Long D et al (eds), *Advances in Neurology* (vol 52). New York: Raven Press, 1990.
34. Weissman DE: Glucocorticoid treatment for brain metastases and epidural spinal cord compression: A review. *J Clin Oncol* 6:543–551, 1988.
35. Wright DC, Delaney TF: Treatment of metastatic cancer to the brain. In DeVita VT, Hellman S, Rosenberg SA (eds), *Cancer: Principles and Practice of Oncology* (3d ed). Philadelphia: Lippincott, 1989, pp. 2245–2261.

36. Reulen HJ, Huber P, Ito U, et al: Peritumoral brain edema. In Long D, et al (eds), *Advances in Neurology* (vol 52). New York: Raven Press, 1990.
37. Cairncross JG, Posner JB: Neurological complications of systemic cancer. In Yarbro JW, Bornstein RS (eds), *Oncologic Emergencies*. New York: Grune & Stratton, 1981.
38. Saba MT, Magolan JM: Understanding cerebral edema: Implications for oncology nurses. *Oncol Nurs Forum* 18:499–505, 1991.
39. Harper J: Use of steroids in cerebral edema: Therapeutic implications. *Heart and Lung,* 17:70–73, 1988.
40. Getz DH: The primary, secondary, and tertiary nursing interventions of lymphedema. *Cancer Nurs* 8:177–184, 1985.
41. Werner RS, McCormick B, Petrek J, et al: Arm edema in conservatively managed breast cancer: Obesity is a major predictive factor. *Radiology* 180:177–184, 1991.
42. Knobf MK: Primary breast cancer. Physical consequences and rehabilitation. *Semin Oncol Nurs* 1:214–224, 1985.
43. Witte CL, Witte MH, Dumont AE: Pathophysiology of chronic edema, lymphedema, and fibrosis. In Staub NC, Taylor AE (eds), *Edema*. New York: Raven Press, 1984, pp. 521–542.
44. Karakousis CP, Heiser MA, Moore RH: Lymphedema after groin dissection. *Am J Surg* 145:205–208, 1983.
45. Kennelly LF, Yurkovic CA: Altered tissue perfusion, peripheral, related to lymphedema. In McNally JC, Somerville ET, Miasknowski C (eds), *Guidelines for Oncology Nursing Practice*. Philadelphia: Saunders, 1991, pp. 387–391.
46. Maxwell MB: Pedal edema in the cancer patient. *Am J Nurs* 82:‘1225–1228, 1982.
47. Maxwell MB: Cancer, hypoalbuminemia, and nutrition. *Cancer Nurs* 4:451–458, 1981.
48. Chlebowski RT: Nutritional support of the medical oncology patient. *Hematol/Oncol Clin North Am* 5:147–159, 1991.
49. Flombaum C, Isaacs M, Scheiner E, et al: Management of fluid retention in patients with advanced cancer. *JAMA* 245:611–614, 1981.
50. Billings JA: Fluid accumulation—edema and effusions. In Billings JA (ed), *Outpatient Management of Advanced Cancer*. Philadelphia: Lippincott, 1985, pp. 106–110.
51. Leff RS, Eisenberg B, Braisden CE, et al: Drainage of recurrent pleural effusion via an implanted port and intrapleural catheter. *Ann Intern Med* 104(2):308–309, 1986.

Chapter 31

Sexual and Reproductive Dysfunction

Linda U. Krebs, RN, MS, OCN

INTRODUCTION

Although increasingly recognized as consequences of cancer or cancer therapy, sexual and reproduction dysfunctions often have been dismissed as normal side effects about which the caregiver can do little or nothing. Indeed, these dysfunctions often have gone underdiagnosed or underrated, or both, because of lack of concern, information, or knowledge on the part of the caregiver or because of fear, lack of knowledge, or embarrassment on the part of the patient or family. Often problems related to sexuality and reproduction are not addressed unless the patient is extremely assertive or presents to the health care provider in a crisis situation.[1]

Unfortunately, of all the complications associated with cancer, difficulties in the ability to be sexually intimate or to bear children have remained major problems that affect all aspects of the patient's and family's lives, sometimes influencing choices for therapy.[2,3] For some patients, sexual or reproductive dysfunctions may be temporary, with full recovery expected when therapy is completed. For many others, however, alterations in sexual or reproductive function are permanent, requiring adaptations in management of intimate relationships and lifelong plans to bear and raise children. Even short-term, temporary alterations can have long-term effects on the patient and family, affecting lifestyles and life choices.

Sexuality and reproductive ability are integral components of life, involving all aspects of our being.[4] Various factors may affect the cancer patient's sexuality and reproductive capacity, including the biologic process of cancer, the effects of treatment, the alterations caused by cancer and treatment, and the psychologic issues surrounding the patient and family.[5] Physiologic problems of infertility and sterility, changes in body appearance, and the inability to have intercourse are enhanced by the psychologic and psychosexual issues of alteration in body image, fear of abandonment, loss of self-esteem, alterations in sexual identity, and concerns about self. Without appropriate education, counseling, and support, it may be difficult for the patient and family to adapt to the alterations that cancer can produce.

PHYSIOLOGY OF GONADAL FUNCTION

Gonadal function is regulated by the pituitary and the hypothalamus. The pituitary is divided into two distinct parts, the anterior and posterior portions. The pituitary is attached to the hypothalamus by the pituitary or hypophysial stalk, through which runs a minute blood vessel system, the hypothalamic-hypophysial portal vessels.[6,7]

The secretion of hormones by the anterior pituitary is controlled by hormones called *hypothalamic-releasing* or *-inhibiting hormones*. These are secreted within the hypothalamus and then spread via the portal vessel system to the anterior pituitary, where they act to influence glandular secretion. When produced in appropriate amounts, these hormones institute a feedback mechanism that shuts off hormonal secretion at the hypothalamus and/or pituitary level.[2,6–9]

In gonadal function, luteinizing hormone-releasing hormone (LHRH) or gonadotropin-releasing hormone (GnRH), is secreted by the hypothalamus and stimulates the anterior pituitary to produce luteinizing hormone (LH) and follicle-stimulating hormone (FSH). LH and FSH stimulate the testis or ovary to produce the appropriate hormones. When blood levels of these hormones are adequate, the hormones will exert a negative feedback on the pituitary, thus decreasing secretion.[2,6–9]

FSH and LH play major roles in the control of male sexual function. LH acts on the interstitial Leydig cells to produce testosterone; FSH, in conjunction with testosterone, is responsible for the conversion of spermatogonia into spermatocytes. A reciprocal inhibition of hypothalamic/anterior pituitary secretion of gonadotropic hormones by testicular hormones keeps the level of hormones stable. In this system the hypothalamus secretes GnRH, which causes the anterior pituitary to secrete LH. LH stimulates the Leydig cells to produce testosterone. The testosterone then negatively feeds back to the hypothalamus, inhibiting production of GnRH. Spermatogenesis is controlled in much the same manner, with FSH stimulating the Sertoli cells to convert spermatides into sperm. The Sertoli cells then secrete a hormone called inhibin that, through negative feedback, causes a decrease in FSH production, thus keeping spermatogenesis at a constant rate[2,6–9] (Figure 31-1).

The female hormonal system, like the male, consists of three levels of hormones: GnRH from the hypothalamus, LH and FSH from the anterior pituitary, and estrogen and progesterone from the ovary. In the nonpregnant female, monthly rhythmic changes in the rates of secretion of female hormones and responding change in the sexual organs result in the female sexual (menstrual) cycle. As a result a single mature ovum is released from an ovary and the endometrium of the uterus is prepared for implantation. FSH is responsible for growth of the ovarian follicle, which eventually will become the mature ovum. At the beginning of menstruation, FSH and LH increase, causing rapid cellular growth in about 20 follicles. Eventually one follicle begins to outgrow the others, causing atresia of the remaining follicles. During follicle growth, estrogen is secreted, probably causing a positive feedback that results in a surge of LH. This surge of LH, which occurs 2 days before ovulation, is necessary for follicular growth and ovulation. Around the time of ovulation the ruptured follicle, under the stimulation of LH, becomes the corpus luteum that secretes both estrogen and progesterone. After several days the estrogen and progesterone

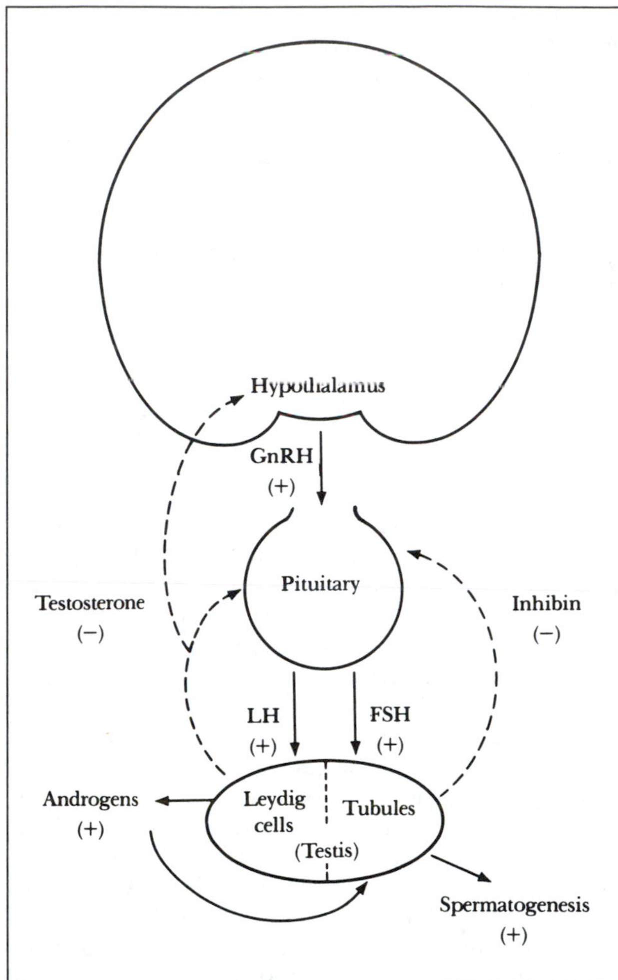

FIGURE 31-1 Normal testicular function. FSH, follicle-stimulating hormone; GnRH, gonadotropin-releasing hormone; LH, luteinizing hormone. (Source: Adapted from Yarbro and Perry,[2] Guyton,[6] and Gill.[7])

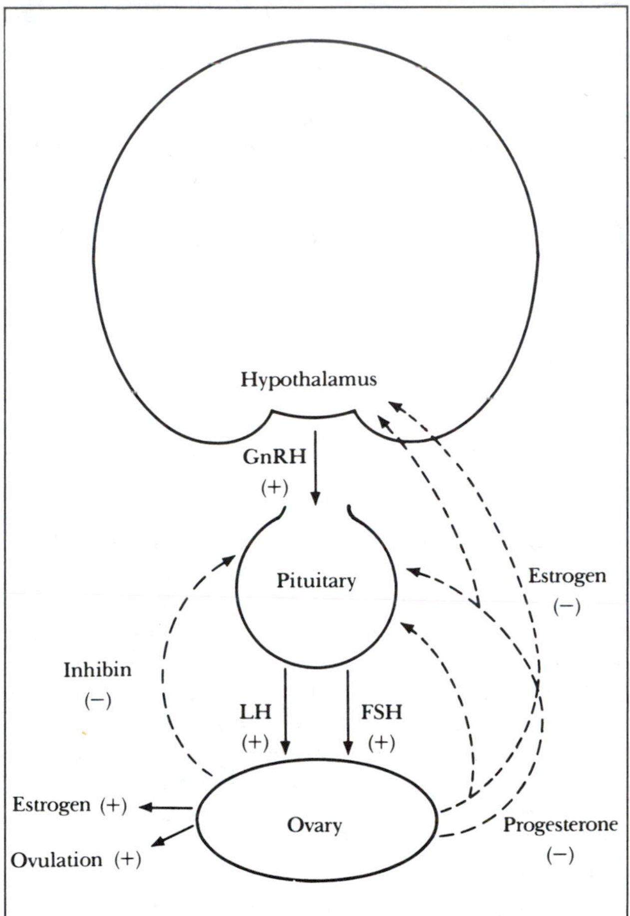

FIGURE 31-2 Normal ovarian function. FSH, follicle-stimulating hormone; GnRH, gonadotropin-releasing hormone; LH, luteinizing hormone. (Source: Adapted from Yarbro and Perry,[2] Guyton,[6] and Gill.[7])

create a negative feedback to decrease secretion of FSH and LH. The corpus luteum, which also secretes inhibin, slowly degenerates, creating a loss of the feedback mechanism and an associated rise in secretion of FSH and LH, beginning a new ovarian cycle and leading to menstruation[2,6–9] (Figure 31-2).

Ovarian failure and germinal aplasia can occur as a result of disease, therapy, nutritional status, psychologic factors, or any combination of these. Ovarian failure also is related to age; as women near menopause, ovarian failure is more likely. In failure, damage to ovarian follicles causes decreased levels of estrogens and progesterones. This results in increased levels of LH and FSH with no compensating feedback mechanism. In addition, inhibin may be produced and react further to alter FSH production. Ovulation ceases, menstruation becomes erratic or ceases, and early menopause often results[2,6–9] (Figure 31-3). In the male, damage to the Leydig cells results in decreased testosterone production; LH and FSH will be elevated. Initially, Leydig cell activity may be compensated enough to produce adequate amounts of testosterone, but continued damage results in temporary, but more often permanent, sterility[2,6–10] (Figure 31-4).

EFFECT OF CANCER THERAPY ON GONADAL FUNCTION

Surgery

Some surgical procedures for cancer of the gastrointestinal and genitourinary tracts cause sexual dysfunction through the removal of sexual organs, through damage to nerves that enervate sexual organs, or through alteration in normal function. In addition, surgery on head and neck areas and the breast or amputations may alter body image and affect sexual identity. Organ dysfunction, either through loss of or alteration in normal function, is most common in can-

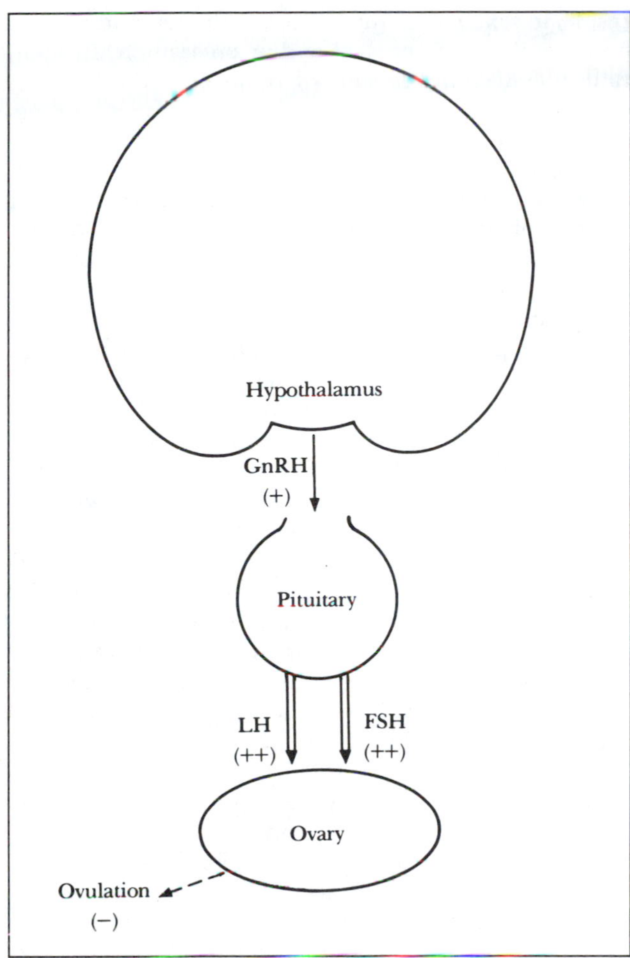

FIGURE 31-3 Ovarian failure. FSH, follicle-stimulating hormone; GnRH, gonadotropin-releasing hormone; LH, luteinizing hormone. (Source: Adapted from Yarbro and Perry,[2] Guyton,[6] and Gill.[7])

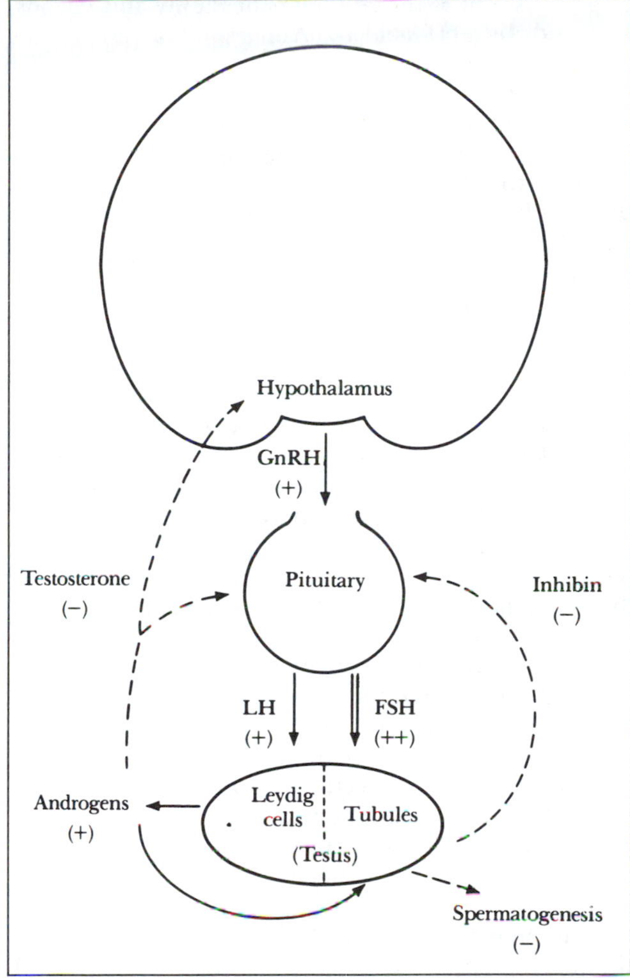

FIGURE 31-4 Germinal aplasia. FSH, follicle-stimulating hormone; GnRH, gonadotropin-releasing hormone; LH, luteinizing hormone. (Source: Adapted from Yarbro and Perry,[2] Guyton,[6] and Gill.[7])

cers of the colon, rectum, bladder and associated urinary structures, and male and female genital tracts. Even when organs are not removed, normal function may be disrupted through the removal of tumor tissue surrounding an organ, through lymph node dissection, or through associated physiologic and psychologic abnormalities related to the type of surgery.

Cancer of the colon and rectum

Surgery for cancer of the colon or rectum may cause sexual dysfunction in both men and women. In general, sexual dysfunctions in women are more commonly related to psychosocial issues, whereas in men dysfunctions may be both organically or psychosocially caused. The most common surgery for colon cancer is some degree of colectomy with or without a colostomy. Whenever possible, primary anastomosis is performed. Cancer of the rectum and anus, however, may require anterior or abdominoperineal resection (APR). If possible, sphincter-preserving surgery without need for an ostomy may be done. Although such surgery is usually performed only for mid-rectal or high-rectal lesions, local excision of lesions in the distal third of the rectum may be possible if the lesion meets the criteria denoting minimal likelihood of metastases.[11] Excision is followed by radiotherapy and chemotherapy. In addition, the use of the end-to-end anastomosis stapling device has allowed for more secure anastomoses at lower levels, minimizing the need for colostomy.[12] The use of multimodality therapy has also minimized the size of surgical resections.[13] In general, the type of surgery will be associated with tumor location and available surgical techniques.[11,12]

For the patient who requires an APR, sexual dysfunction may be related to the placement of a colostomy, to removal of or interference with sexual organ function, or some combination of the two. A colostomy can be associated with sexual dysfunction because of patients' negative changes in body image and self-esteem, as well as the responses of family and friends. In a study by McDonald and Anderson[14] of 420 patients with rectal cancer, 265 had a permanent colostomy. Of these individuals, 16% felt severely stigmatized because of the colostomy. Of those who were married or widowed since surgery, 48% of men and 27% of women younger than 65 years old (n = 116) felt that their married life had suffered as a result of the colostomy.

For the woman with an APR, the ovaries or uterus may be removed at the time of surgery in addition to colostomy, thus causing dysfunction from primary inability to bear children or from alterations in normal hormonal patterns. In addition, women may have part of the vagina removed, or healing of the perineal wound may result in vaginal scarring that causes painful or incomplete vaginal intercourse. A decreased incidence of orgasm and vaginal lubrication, reduced libido, and dyspareunia have also been noted.[12,15–18]

For the man who has an APR, sexual dysfunction is more severe, with a suggestion that permanent sexual dysfunction may be as high as 80%.[19] Although men may lose the ability to obtain or maintain an erection, 30%–35% maintain the ability to have an orgasm, and 25%–50% maintain the ability to ejaculate.[20,21] In a study by Andersen[18] it was reported that 30%–60% of men who have an APR will experience decreased desire, 30%–75% will have erectile dysfunctions, and 65%–85% will have ejaculatory dysfunctions. Age appears to be a factor, with the older patient more likely to suffer complete or incomplete erectile impotence.[22,23] This is most likely due to damage to parasympathetic and sympathetic nerves that control both erection and ejaculation. In addition to erectile dysfunction, decreased amount and/or force of ejaculation or retrograde ejaculation may occur. This occurrence may be temporary or permanent and adds to the trauma of this surgery because of its unpredictable outcome. For all patients the removal of rectal tissue appears to be the most common denominator to organic sexual dysfunction. If the rectum remains intact, there rarely is an associated sexual dysfunction without direct tumor invasion.[24–26] Koukouras et al.[27] reported sexual dysfunction, as denoted by cessation of sexual relationship, absence of erection, absence of ejaculation, or inability to penetrate, to be 15% in men who had a high anterior resection, whereas 54% of men with an APR experienced some type of dysfunction.

Cancers of the genitourinary tract

Bladder cancer The treatment of bladder cancer may alter sexual function in men and women. Repeated cystoscopy for local treatment of transitional cell cancer has been noted to cause pain with coitus for women, transient pain during erection and ejaculation in men, and temporary decrease in desire for both.[28] Transurethral resection or partial cystectomy may result in mild pain or dyspareunia; however, normal sexual function should not be altered.[29] Radical cystectomy results in sexual dysfunction for both men and women because of organ removal and/or enervation. In men, radical cystectomy consists of removal of the bladder, prostate, seminal vesicles, pelvic lymph nodes, and occasionally the urethra.[29] It has been noted that about 15% of men who undergo radical cystectomy will recover full erection potential and that men older than 60 years of age are more likely to be negatively affected. Retrograde or no ejaculation may also result.[21] Orgasm may be experienced but is usually less intense and without ejaculate.[18] For these men the increasing availability and use of penile prostheses and the ability to perform revascularization of the penis have made erectile dysfunction a more manageable problem.[16,28] Boyd and Schiff[30] reported on 19 men who had inflatable penile prostheses implanted following surgery for transitional cell cancer. All were satisfied with appearance and function. For the woman who has radical cystectomy, the surgery usually includes removal of the bladder and urethra, the uterus, ovaries, fallopian tubes, and the anterior portion of the vagina. Although vaginal reconstruction usually is performed, the resulting vagina may be more narrow and shallow and provide less lubrication than before surgery, leading to difficulty with penetration. In addition, the removal of the ovaries with associated estrogen loss leads to dryness, inelasticity of the vagina, dyspareunia, and menopausal symptoms. Vaginal dilation and the liberal use of lubrication may provide relief.[18,23,31,32] For both sexes, urinary diversion is a necessity with radical cystectomy, resulting in alterations in self-esteem and body image.[33] In the past the ileal conduit, which necessitated the continuous use of an ostomy appliance, was the most common method for urinary diversions. Today the surgical development of a Kock pouch, or continent reservoir, has become more widely employed, resulting in overall improved sexual adjustment due to decreased odor and leakage.[29,34] Combined modality therapies are being investigated that will allow for tumor reduction while maintaining the bladder. Success of these interventions should have direct effects on subsequent sexual function.[35]

Penile cancer/cancer of the male urethra Cancer of the penis and male urethra are rare, with fewer than 500 cases reported in the United States in 1991.[36] Treatment includes total or partial penectomy, radiation therapy, or topical chemotherapy, with radiation therapy or chemotherapy used for small, early lesions. Partial penectomy does not result in loss of erectile, ejaculative, or orgasmic abilities, whereas erectile ability obviously is absent with total penectomy.[18,28,29] Desire remains, and stimulation of the remaining genital tissue can produce orgasm.[37,38] Ejaculation, through the perineal urethrostomy, should continue. New techniques to create a penis have been used after a total penectomy. A semirigid or inflatable prosthesis restores the ability to have intercourse.[28,29,37–39] A Mayo Clinic study reported a successful placement rate of 90%–95% and an 8% mechanical failure rate in the 3-year study period of patients with penile implants. Eighty-nine percent of subjects and mates felt satisfied with function and appearance.[40]

Testicular cancer Testicular cancer, which represents about 1% of all cancers in men, is the leading cause of cancer in young men.[21] The treatment of testicular cancer includes an orchiectomy and possibly retroperitoneal lymph node dissection and/or removal of a pelvic mass. Unilateral orchiectomy will not result in infertility or sexual dysfunction providing that the contralateral testis is normal and the individual is fertile at diagnosis. Infertility before any definitive therapy is well documented and may be related to hormonal imbalance or the result of subacute chronic illness.[41–43] If bilateral orchiectomy is performed, sterility and decreased libido, related to loss of testosterone, will result. Retroperitoneal lymph node dissection done for staging or as treatment for stage II disease may result in temporary or permanent loss of ejaculation, whereas potency and the ability to have an orgasm remain.[28,29,41,43,44] Narayan et al.[43] reported that 100% of 55 patients who underwent peritoneal lymphadenectomy reported loss of ejaculation, with 45% regaining function within 3 years following surgery. Nerve-sparing procedures with careful adherence to surgical boundaries and identification of sympathetic fibers has resulted in an almost 80% preservation or return of ejaculation following lymphadenectomy.[41] Retrograde ejaculation has been noted in 25% of patients, whereas decreased libido, decreased pleasure at orgasm, and erectile dysfunction have occurred in 10%–38% of these men.[16,28,29,39,45] Gritz et al.[46] reported on the psychosexual status of 34 men and their partners a median of 4 years following treatment for testicular cancer. All men had a unilateral orchiectomy followed by additional surgery, chemotherapy, or radiation therapy. At the time of follow-up, 23% reported alterations in body image, 29% reported a decrease in sexual satisfaction, 20% an occasional problem with erection, and 38% a decrease in frequency of intercourse. Of those who underwent retroperitoneal lymphadenectomy, 50% reported the inability to ejaculate and 54% experienced a decrease in the quality of orgasms. Forty-one percent of the couples desired children and expected to conceive, or adopt if necessary, in the future. For those individuals desiring to maintain fertility, sperm banking should be discussed and arranged prior to therapy.

Prostate cancer Prostate cancer, because it generally occurs in men older than 50 years of age, often is not considered in terms of its potential to cause sexual dysfunctions. However, because sexual concerns are not necessarily related to age and because therapy for prostate cancer frequently causes sexual dysfunction, counseling and management of potential problems need to be addressed. Therapy for prostate cancer consists of various combinations of surgery, chemotherapy, radiation therapy, and hormonal manipulation, all of which have a potential to alter sexual function. Surgical treatment of prostate cancer includes prostatectomy (accomplished through transurethral, perineal, or transabdominal approaches) or bilateral orchiectomy. Transurethral resection of the prostate generally does not cause impotence or erectile dysfunction; however, retrograde ejaculation occurs in approximately 90% of all patients. Transabdominal resection of the prostate results in retrograde ejaculation in 75%–80% of patients and may cause erectile dysfunction. The perineal approach, or radical prostatectomy, includes removal of the prostate, seminal vesicles, and vas deferens and may result in permanent damage to erectile function with concomitant loss of emission and ejaculation.[24,29,47] Nerve-sparing or potency-sparing surgery was developed by Walsh in the 1980s and, according to Church,[48] probably has been the most significant surgical development in the treatment of prostate cancer. Prior to the development of this procedure, 2%–15% experienced urinary incontinence and 80%–90% experienced impotence. Eggleston and Walsh[49] evaluated 100 patients who had radical prostatectomies that incorporated nerve-sparing surgical techniques and reported that potency was maintained in approximately 86% of patients. Walsh and Schlegel[50] evaluated 320 men 1 to 5 years following surgery. Of the 259 who were potent prior to surgery and who had sexual partners, 192 (74%) were currently potent. Potency appeared to return gradually over a period of months to years. Bilateral orchiectomy causes sexual dysfunction through gradual diminution of libido, impotence, gynecomastia, and penile atrophy.[16,29] Various methods, including the use of penile prostheses, suction or vacuum devices, intracorporeal injections of papaverine hydrochloride or prostaglandin E-1, or medications such as yohimbine hydrochloride, have been used to restore erectile potential. Fear of failure may also play a role. Since return of full erection potential may take as long as 2 years, it is suggested that the patient wait a minimum of 6 months after surgery to see if function will be restored.[28,29,51–53] With new techniques, sterility in individuals with retrograde ejaculation is not as frequent. Because of the ability to separate sperm from urine, artificial insemination of the mate may be possible.[54]

Gynecologic malignancies

Surgical management of gynecologic malignancies includes surgery of the vulva, vagina, uterus and uterine cervix, ovary and fallopian tube, and pelvic exenteration. Although the majority of gynecologic surgeries are invisible assaults to femininity, sexual identity and sexual functioning are often permanently affected. It is imperative that sexual and reproductive counseling be provided to the patient and family before surgical intervention because most surgeries permanently alter fertility and may alter sexuality.

Vulvar cancer Vulvar cancer represents 1% of all cancers found in women, with approximately 85% occurring in postmenopausal women.[55] Treatment will not alter fertility but may affect sexuality, with 21%–90% of women reporting cessation of all sexual activities following radical vulvectomy.[56,57] Therapy for carcinoma in situ or preinvasive disease may include simple vulvectomy, wide local excision, skinning vulvectomy, topical 5-fluorouracil cream, or laser therapy. In general, good cosmetic results occur with treatment of early disease except for the simple vulvectomy, which removes the labia and subcutaneous tissue, with retention of the clitoris. Introital stenosis may result but may be easily managed through the use of lubrication and vaginal dilators. DiSaia[58] recommends conservative treatment with wide local excision and skin graft for the woman with early disease in order to maintain body image and minimally affect sexuality. Radical vulvectomy, which removes the labia minora and majora and the clitoris and usually includes a groin node dissection, frequently results in delayed wound healing, altered body image, abnormalities in sensory perception of the genital area, leg edema, decreased range of motion in lower extremities, altered orgasmic potential, and introital stenosis.[16,41,55,59] New methods for evaluation of lymph nodes prior to radical surgery may allow for more limited surgeries with less compromise to sexuality.[60] All women need education on the effects of removal of tissue and on body image prior to surgery to promote self-esteem, function, and compliance with care.

Vaginal cancer Vaginal cancer is rare. Surgery for the majority of gynecologic cancers results in some abnormality and/or need for reconstruction of the vagina. A shortened vagina can cause considerable sexual dysfunction because of vaginal length and width, lack of lubrication, or pain on intercourse. Total vaginectomy without reconstruction precludes vaginal intercourse; however, there are multiple techniques for vaginal reconstruction.[39] Reconstruction can be accomplished using the large or small bowel. Because of its thicker wall, the large bowel is usually preferred.[61] It has been noted that in 30%–70% of patients who do have reconstruction there is a return of orgasmic sensations if they existed before surgery.[62] Despite this finding, reconstruction should not be considered a panacea for sexual dysfunction, with women complaining that the new vagina is too large, too small, or has a persistent, annoying discharge.[63]

Cervical cancer and endometrial cancer Invasive cancer of the uterine corpus and cervix are the first and second most common gynecologic malignancies, representing 10% of all cancers in women.[36] Treatment for cervical intraepithelial neoplasia and carcinoma in situ includes conization, laser therapy, cryosurgery, or simple hysterectomy.[60,61,63] All but the last usually do not affect fertility (conization may result in cervical stenosis or incompetence), nor should they cause any physiologic sexual dysfunction. Simple hysterectomy precludes further child bearing but should not affect sexual functioning, although numerous authors have noted that altered sexual identity and/or body image may result in sexual dysfunction.[24,64–66] Treatment for invasive disease is usually radical hysterectomy, consisting of removal of the uterus and cervix, supporting structures, and upper third of the vagina and pelvic lymph nodes. For cancer of the endometrium, the ovaries and fallopian tubes also may be removed. If oophorectomy is included, menopausal symptoms with hot flashes and decrease in vaginal lubrication and elasticity may severely alter sexual functioning. Zussman et al.[66] noted that 33%–46% of women who had a radical hysterectomy, including oophorectomy, reported decreased sexual desire, whereas Jenkins[67] and Schover et al.[68] noted alterations in frequency of desire, orgasm, and frequency and enjoyment of intercourse in women who had abdominal hysterectomy and bilateral salpingo-oophorectomy and had received pelvic radiation for cervical or endometrial cancer. Schover et al.[68] reported that 15% of these women became celibate within 1 year of treatment. Although sexual feeling should not be altered after a radical hysterectomy, delayed bowel and bladder function may occur and necessitate discharge from the hospital with a urinary catheter. Long-term catheter placement may alter body image and affect sexuality. Intercourse can be accomplished through securing the catheter to the abdomen and making changes in coital position.[59,69] It also should be remembered that many women measure femininity by the ability to bear children. If this ability is removed, sexual dysfunctions may occur even in the absence of organic cause.[24]

Ovarian cancer Ovarian cancer represents approximately 25% of gynecologic cancers and frequently is seen in the premenopausal female. Initial treatment is surgery, usually consisting of a radical hysterectomy with bilateral salpingo-oophorectomy and omentectomy. Fertility is lost and the associated menopausal symptoms occur. In the young woman with ovarian teratoma or borderline malignant epithelial neoplasia, it is possible to maintain fertility if disease is confined to one ovary and is of low grade; however, it is most common for radical surgery to be performed.[70–72] Treatment usually continues with combination chemotherapy, thus further compounding sexual and reproductive dysfunctions.

Pelvic exenteration

Although pelvic exenteration may be performed in the man or woman with advanced colorectal or bladder cancer, the most common indication for pelvic exenteration is a locally advanced gynecologic malignancy. A pelvic exenteration that is anterior preserves the rectum, whereas a posterior exenteration preserves the bladder. A total pelvic exenteration involves removing the vagina, uterus, ovaries, fallopian tubes, bladder, and rectum (in the man, the prostate, seminal vesicles, and vas deferens are removed).[60,63,73,74] In patients with total pelvic exenteration a urinary conduit and colostomy also are created; a neovagina may be constructed.[60,61,73] In the woman, reproductive and sexual dysfunction are profound. Andersen and Hacker[75] reported that 80%–90% of women surveyed ceased all sexual activity except kissing. Dysfunction related to removal of all pelvic organs with resulting ostomies is obvious. In addition, body image, sexual identity, and self-esteem are disturbed, and appropriate interventions and education need to be provided. In the woman with vaginal reconstruction, intercourse will be possible; however, the physiologic and psychologic ramifications of this surgery may result in inability and/or lack of desire to participate in sexual activities.[76]

Breast cancer

Although some surgeries may not be strictly related to sexual functioning, they may cause dysfunction as a result of the psychologic issues related to the particular body part. Probably the most likely assault to body image and sexual identity with resultant sexual dysfunction is surgical removal of all or part of the breast. Although fertility is not altered by mastectomy or lumpectomy, the inability or difficulty in breast-feeding should pregnancy be accomplished may be a major assault to the woman's femininity. In addition, removal or partial removal of a breast may result in sexual dysfunction because of fear of rejection, physical discomfort, anxiety about initiating sexual activities, feelings of being defective or different, or any combination of these factors.[77,78] Rutherford[79] noted that loss of even part of the breast can be seen as an alteration of self, with resultant alterations in body image and sexuality.

Although it has been previously reported that the use of breast-preserving surgery (lumpectomy) has been shown to cause significantly less alteration in body image, sexual desire, and frequency of intercourse,[63,77,78] recent studies[80–83] showed no difference between women receiving lumpectomy and radiotherapy and women undergoing mastectomy. What appears to be of significance is the opportunity or perceived opportunity to select the surgical technique employed. Thus, choices should be offered whenever possible. If breast-preserving surgery is not an option, breast reconstruction can be considered. The ability to have breast reconstruction has been shown to bolster sexual self-esteem and decrease reactions to body image alterations.[84] If such options are limited, sexual dysfunction, which should be temporary, may become permanent. Education and ongoing counseling should be available and may provide positive functional outcomes.

Head and neck cancer

Although not generally considered an area responsible for sexual dysfunction, surgical treatment for cancers of the head and neck region are responsible for varying degrees of alteration in body image leading to changes in sexuality and intimacy. Results of disease and treatment are readily apparent. Even with reconstructive surgery or the use of prostheses to ameliorate deformities, sexuality may be affected by the alterations in sensation, breathing, voice, the ability to use the mouth and tongue, or similar abnormalities. Presurgical counseling and long-term follow-up may be necessary for sexual rehabilitation.[69,85,86]

Radiation Therapy

Radiation therapy can cause sexual and reproductive dysfunction through primary organ failure (e.g., ovarian failure and testicular aplasia), through alterations in organ function (e.g., decreased lubrication and impotence), and through the temporary or permanent effects of therapy not associated with reproduction (e.g., diarrhea and fatigue). Permanent effects most commonly are related to total dose, location, length of treatment, age, and prior fertility status.[54,87–89] In the woman, fertility depends on follicular maturation and ovum release. Radiation therapy to the ovaries has its most direct effect on the intermediate follicles. If these follicles are damaged by radiation and insufficient small follicles remain, permanent sterility results.[90] In the man, although the Leydig cell and mature sperm are relatively radioresistant, immature sperm and spermatogonia are extremely radiosensitive. Small doses of radiation will begin the process of infertility, which, depending on total dose, may be permanent.[7]

In women, temporary or permanent sterility is related to the dose of radiation, the volume of tissues radiated, the time period the ovaries are exposed to radiation, and the woman's age.[88–92] Because a woman has fewer oocytes as she nears menopause, radiation injury at that point in the life span is more likely to be permanent. Balducci et al.[54] and Hilderly[90] noted that a radiation dose of 600–1200 cGy is capable of inducing menopause; however, younger women appear to be more resistant to this effect. In addition, although age is an important factor, doses <400 cGy may result in temporary sterility whereas doses >400 cGy often result in permanent sterility. The number of oocytes is one of the most important factors in permanent sterility, with 95% of young women becoming sterile with a radiation dose >2000 cGy. In women older than 40 years of age, 600 cGy often is associated with subsequent menopause and the associated menopausal symptoms of hot flashes, amenorrhea, dyspareunia, loss of libido, and vaginal atrophy.[88,93] For some women the use of exogenous estrogens may alleviate these side effects.[68]

For women, movement of the ovaries out of the radiation field (oophoropexy), with appropriate shielding, has helped maintain fertility even when relatively high doses of radiation have been given. Ovaries can be moved to the midline of the uterus or to the iliac crests. In young women or those desiring to maintain both reproductive capacity and hormonal function, ovarian transposition, with the ovaries moved to the upper abdomen, can be undertaken.[88] In a study by Horning et al.,[94] 8 of 19 patients treated with total lymphoid irradiation for Hodgkin's disease had reversible amenorrhea and 7 eventually became pregnant. Even with oophoropexy and appropriate shielding, 30%–50% of all patients who receive more than 600–1000 cGy will have permanent menstrual cessation.[95,96]

In addition to sterility or transient infertility, radiation therapy can produce other sexual dysfunctions, which may be temporary or permanent. Decreases in sexual enjoyment, ability to attain orgasm, libido, and frequency of intercourse and sexual dreams, as well as vaginal stenosis or shortening and decreased lubrication and sensation have been reported in women treated with radiation therapy. Painful intercourse and menstrual changes have also been reported.[92,97–101]

In men, temporary or permanent azoospermia also is a function of age, dose, tissue volume, and exposure time. When the testis is exposed to radiation, a reduction in sperm count begins within 6 to 8 weeks and continues for up to 1 year after completion of therapy. Doses of <500 cGy usually are associated with temporary sterility, whereas doses of >500 cGy usually result in permanent sterility.[90] The return of normal spermatogenesis is related to total testicular dose, with a dose of <100 cGy taking 9 to 12 months for recovery, whereas 200 to 300 cGy may take 2 to 3 years and 400 to 600 cGy more than 5 years to infinity.[102] Kinsella et al.[103] reported on 27 male adults with soft tissue sarcoma who were treated with high-dose radiation therapy. The testes were not in the primary field and were shielded; however, significant scatter radiation still was received. In 11 of 27 patients who received <50 cGy, no abnormalities resulted, whereas in 6 patients with exposures of 50–150 cGy exposures, FSH was elevated 200% and testosterone was decreased. In the 10 patients who received >150 cGy, FSH was increased, whereas LH and testosterone were decreased; thus, testicular function was inadequate to support spermatogenesis. Fossa et al.[104] evaluated the long-term morbidity of infradiaphragmatic radiotherapy in men with testicular cancer and noted that 23% of those previously thought to be fertile were found to be infertile following doses ranging from 36Gy to 50Gy. Gonadal dysfunction has been reported in survivors of childhood acute lymphoblastic leukemia who received at least 12 Gy testicular irradiation.[105,106] In a follow-up of 60 long-term survivors, Sklar et al.[106] found that 50% of men exposed to craniospinal and extended abdominal field radiation experienced decreased testicular volume, abnormal germ cell function, and elevated FSH levels. Due to the morbidity of even low-level testicular radiation, Kinsella et al.[107] suggest that those not requiring primary testicular irradiation receive additional testicular shielding to alleviate infertility sequelae.

The majority of men treated by external beam for prostate cancer have temporary or permanent impotence. Impotence is thought to be caused by fibrosis of pelvic vasculature or radiation damage of pelvic nerves. Van Heeringen et al.[108] reported that 25% of men were impotent, 67% experienced decreased frequency, and more than 50% experienced decreased libido following radiation for localized cancer of the prostate. Herr[109] reported that 40 of 41 patients treated by lymphadenectomy remained potent if interstitial therapy was used, whereas Carlton et al.[110] noted that only 25% of patients treated with internal and external therapy plus lymphadenectomy became impotent. This suggests that interstitial therapy may be less likely to cause impotence. In patients treated for testicular cancer, Schover and von Eschenbach[111] noted that 10% of 121 patients reported erectile dysfunction, and 38% experienced a decrease in pleasure of orgasm. The inability to gain and maintain an erection may begin as early as 2 weeks into treatment and may last several weeks after treatment.[111] Occasionally impotence does not occur until after radiation therapy is completed. In these patients the effects usually are not reversible.[112] In addition to difficulty in gaining or maintaining erection, a decreased libido, inability to ejaculate, inability to lubricate, inability to achieve orgasm, and decreased sexual pleasure are common findings in men who receive radiation to the pelvis.

Along with direct assaults to sexual and reproductive function by radiation therapy, the general side effects and accompanying psychologic effects frequently can alter sexual function. Severe fatigue can limit all activity. Nausea, vomiting, and diarrhea can decrease energy, sexual desire, and feelings of desirability and can interfere with a sense of general well-being. Inflammation, pain, and limited range of motion may make sexual activities difficult or impossible. In addition to physical limitations, fear, depression, anxiety, stress, body image alterations, and lowered self-esteem may be additional burdens.[113] The appropriate use of energy-conserving strategies, medications, lubricants, prostheses, time, and counseling may alleviate side effects, promote a sense of well-being, and improve sexual function.

Chemotherapy

Chemotherapy-induced reproductive and sexual dysfunction is related to the type of drug, dose, length of treatment, age and sex of the individual receiving treatment, and length of time after therapy. In addition, the use of combination therapy with multiple agents and drugs given to combat side effects of chemotherapy also plays a role in infertility or sexual dysfunction.

Infertility and sterility after chemotherapy have been noted since the early 1970s, with reports of amenorrhea and azoospermia after single-agent or combination therapy.[114] Adult men are more likely to experience long-term side effects regardless of age, whereas women are more apt to have permanent cessation of menses as they near the age of 40 years.[115,116] The primary agents that induce infertility are the alkylating agents, but other drugs have been implicated, in particular cytosine arabinoside, 5-fluorouracil, vinblastine, vincristine, cisplatin,[117] and procarbazine. Combinations of these drugs appear to prolong infertility[115,118–122] (Table 31-1).

Men

Infertility occurs in men primarily through depletion of the germinal epithelium that lines the seminiferous tubules. On testicular biopsy the interstitial Leydig cells appear normal, whereas the tubules are abnormal, contain Sertoli cells, and have depleted or absent germinal epithelium. Clinically, testicular volume decreases, oligospermia or azoospermia occurs, and infertility results.[123]

Single-agent and combination chemotherapy have been reported to cause germinal aplasia, with alkylating agents the most extensively studied. Richter et al.[124] reported that doses of chlorambucil <400 mg cause progressive oligospermia, whereas doses >400 mg have caused azoospermia and permanent germinal aplasia. They also studied cyclophosphamide and noted that doses as low as 50–100 mg/day for 2 months resulted in azoospermia. Recovery time related to total dose and length of time since the completion of treatment. Nijman et al.[45] studied the gonadal function of 54 patients with testicular cancer who received chemotherapy with cisplatin, vinblastine, and bleomycin (PVB) after surgery. They noted, as have others,[125,126] that 72% of these men were infertile before treatment. Two years following therapy, 48% remained infertile, with increased levels of LH and FSH. Stoter et al.[127] evaluated 48 men with testicular cancer who had been treated with PVB plus maintenance chemotherapy. With a minimum follow-up of 7 years, 40% reported a negative alteration in sexual life, with 21% experiencing decreased sexual desire, 8% experiencing erectile dysfunction, and 15% experiencing ejaculatory dysfunction. Drasga et al.[126] reviewed 69 patients with disseminated testicular cancer treated with PVB ± doxorubicin; 41 patients were part of a prospective study and 28 part of a retrospective study. In the prospective group only 6.6% of patients were able to meet sperm-banking requirements; the others had severe oligospermia or azoospermia. With a median of 17 months' follow-up, 100% of these men continue to be infertile. In the retrospective group, 46% had a normal sperm count at the time of evaluation. Thirty-two percent have successfully impregnated their wives. Male patients treated with cisplatin, doxorubicin, and dacarbazine (PADIC) for osteosarcoma were noted to be infertile during active treatment. However, within 2 years after completion of treatment, 70% had attained normal sperm counts. Those receiving more than 600 mg/m² cisplatin were more likely to remain infertile.[128] It appears that in some instances fertility may improve with time.

The most widely studied combination chemotherapy has been mechlorethamine, vincristine, procarbazine, and prednisone (MOPP) used in the treatment of Hodgkin's disease. Chapman[116] reported frequent sexual dysfunction and decreased fertility in men treated with MOPP. This is corroborated by Cunningham et al.,[129] who noted that only 1 in 10 men receiving MOPP and 1 in 13 receiving MOPP plus pelvic radiation were able to impregnate. Viviani et al.[130] reported that azoospermia developed in only 54% of patients treated with doxorubicin, bleomycin, vinblastine, and dacarbazine (ABVD), whereas azoospermia occurred in 97% of patients treated with MOPP. In addition, 100% of those treated with ABVD had complete restoration of spermatogenesis, whereas only 14% of those treated with MOPP had return of spermatogenesis.

Hormonal manipulation and treatment with estrogens are well known as a cause of sexual dysfunction. The majority of patients who receive antiandrogen therapy experience a major reduction in interest in sexual intercourse and are unable to attain or maintain an erection.[131] Gynecomastia and decreases in libido, sexual excitement, and the ability to achieve sexual fulfillment are significant problems.[92,121,132]

TABLE 31-1 Chemotherapeutic Agents Affecting Sexual or Reproductive Function

Agent	Complication
Alkylating	
Busulfan	Amenorrhea, oligospermia, azoospermia, decreased libido, ovarian dysfunction, erectile dysfunction
Chlorambucil	
Cyclophosphamide	
Melphalan	
Nitrogen mustard	
Antimetabolites	
Cytosine arabinoside	As for alkylating agents
5-Fluorouracil	
Methotrexate	
Antitumor Antibiotics	
Doxorubicin	As for alkylating agents
Plicamycin	
Dactinomycin	
Plant Products	
Vincristine	Retrograde ejaculation, erectile dysfunction
Vinblastine	Decreased libido, ovarian dysfunction, erectile dysfunction
Miscellaneous Agents	
Procarbazine	As for alkylating agents
Androgens	Masculinization (women)
Antiandrogens	Gynecomastia, impotence
Estrogens	Gynecomastia, acne
Antiestrogens	Irregular menses
Progestins	Menstrual abnormalities, change in libido
Aminoglutethamide	Masculinization (women)
Corticosteroids	Irregular menses, acne
Interferons	Transient impotence

Source: Data from Yasko,[92] Dodd,[101] Schilsky and Erlichman,[115] Burke,[118] Otto,[119] Gasel,[120] Guy,[121] and Goodman.[122]

Women

Women experience sexual and reproductive dysfunction from chemotherapy as a result of hormonal alterations or direct effects that cause ovarian fibrosis and follicle destruction. Previous sexual health may also play a role. FSH and LH levels are elevated and estradiol is decreased, leading to amenorrhea, menopausal symptoms, dyspareunia, and vaginal atrophy and dryness.[118,123]

Like men, women experience reproductive dysfunction from both single-agent and combination chemotherapy; however, age appears to play a more significant role in infertility in women than in men, with women younger than 35 years old able to tolerate much higher doses of chemotherapy without resultant infertility. Amenorrhea has been noted in women with breast cancer who receive 40–120 mg/day of cyclophosphamide.[133] Busulfan, which may be used to treat chronic myelogenous leukemia, also induces amenorrhea.[134] Chapman et al.[135] reported that amenorrhea developed in 49% of patients treated with MOPP, 34% experienced irregular menses, and 17% maintained normal menses. Of those with irregular or normal menses, 30% later experienced irreversible amenorrhea. Other investigators[129,136,137] have reported that permanent amenorrhea occurred in 26%–50% of women treated with MOPP combination chemotherapy and that permanent amenorrhea and early menopause were more common with advancing age. Indeed, in women less than 25 years of age, 80% continued with normal menses. In women over 25 years of age, amenorrhea appeared to occur gradually after cessation of treatment. It was noted in a study of ABVD plus radiation therapy versus MOPP plus radiation therapy that 50% of women over 30 treated with MOPP plus radiation therapy had prolonged amenorrhea.[138] In contrast, none of the women younger than 30 years and none of the women receiving ABVD plus radiation therapy noted this side effect. Other combination therapy also has been reviewed with similar results.[139]

It appears that any combination of drugs that contains an alkylating agent is apt to cause infertility, and as women near menopause, permanent cessation of menses is more likely. When hormonal manipulation includes androgens, not only are sexual and reproductive function affected but also body image and feelings of sexual identity. Appropriate support and counseling should be provided.

Children

The effect of chemotherapy on gonadal function in children has been extensively studied.[140–142] Primary effects include delayed sexual maturation and alterations in reproductive potential. Levy and Stillman[142] note that although the effects of chemotherapy are different in girls and boys, the primary effects appear to be age-related. Prepubescent boys seem to be minimally affected by chemotherapy and progress into and through puberty without major difficulty. Young men treated during puberty, however, appear to be more likely to have gonadal dysfunction with profound effects on both germ cell production and Leydig cell function, with a resultant increase in FSH and LH and a decrease in testosterone levels.[143,144] The majority of girls treated with combination therapy appear to have normal ovarian function.[2,145]

Other issues

No discussion of gonadal dysfunction from chemotherapy is complete without acknowledgment that drugs used to manage chemotherapy side effects can alter sexual function. Impotence, decreased sexual desire, decreased sense of sexual fulfillment, and decreased ability to achieve orgasm all have been associated with these agents[92,114,120,132,146–148] (Table 31-2).

Biologic Response Modifiers

Little information is available on the sexual and reproductive dysfunctions associated with the biologic response modifiers (BRMs). In part, this lack of information is due to the continued experimental nature of the agents and their use primarily in advanced cancer patients. As use of these agents becomes more frequent in individuals who are less ill, the effects on gonadal function will become more apparent.

TABLE 31-2 Cancer-Associated Drugs That Affect Sexual and Reproductive Function

Agent	Complication
Antiemetics/Sedatives/ Tranquilizers	
Prochlorperazine Chlorpromazine Diazepam Lorazepam Metoclopramide Scopolamine	Sedation, orgasm without ejaculation, impotence, decreased sexual interest, decreased intensity of orgasm
Antihistamines	
Diphenhydramine	Sedation, decreased sexual interest
Antidepressants	
Amitriptyline Imipramine	Impotence, altered libido
Narcotics	
Morphine Hydromorphone Codeine	Decreased libido, sedation, impaired potency
Miscellaneous	
Ketoconazole	Decreased libido
Cimetadine	Impotence
Steroids (See Table 31-1)	

Source: Data from Yasko,[92] Schilsky and Erlichman,[115] Glasel,[120] Kaempfer,[132,147] and Brager and Yasko.[148]

Some information is available on the use of the interferons, in particular alpha-interferon, alone or in combination with other agents. A decrease in libido has been reported with alpha-interferon, and animals exposed to interferon have demonstrated an increased rate of spontaneous abortions.[149] Mangold and Robinson (personal communication, 1988) stated that patients have reported decreased sexual desire and pleasure and difficulty in attaining and maintaining an erection. In addition to drug-induced dysfunction, the usual side effects of fatigue and flulike symptoms affect interest in and comfort with sexual activities. Nursing research on the subject of gonadal dysfunction related to BRMs is extremely important.

Bone Marrow Transplantation

Until recently, few reports were available concerning the sexual and reproductive dysfunctions associated with bone marrow transplantation (BMT). Ostroff and Lesko[150] present a comprehensive review and note that late effects of BMT include chronic fatigue, body image alterations, gonadal dysfunction, and infertility. Women experienced decreased sexual desire and satisfaction, vaginal atrophy and decreased vaginal lubrication, and painful intercourse. Men frequently experienced premature ejaculation due to prolonged abstinence. They report that the standard germ-free environment and long hospitalization affect sexuality and intimacy. They note that sexual interest and activity increase as health improves. Belec[151] evaluated 24 patients following BMT and noted that 50% experienced lack of energy and fatigue severe enough to impede normal activities. Cust et al.[152] reported on 36 women who were treated for leukemia with BMT and total-body irradiation (TBI). Twenty experienced vaginal dryness and 18 women reported dyspareunia. Forty percent complained of feelings of loss of femininity.

Sanders et al.[153] evaluated patients following BMT ± TBI. They noted that in those receiving BMT with TBI that all had primary gonadal dysfunction. Recovery of ovarian function occurred in less than 10% of the women, and 94% of men remained azoospermic. Milliken et al.[154] reported three successful pregnancies in two women following BMT for acute leukemia. TBI was not used. They felt that the ability to conceive or father a child after BMT appeared to be related to age (older patients were less likely to reverse gonadal dysfunction) and treatment with TBI. Sexual and reproductive implications of treatment should be discussed and counseling provided prior to, throughout, and following treatment.

Sexual Counseling

All patients should receive information concerning the possible side effects of disease and treatment on sexuality and reproduction. Patients deserve the opportunity to have their sexual problems thoughtfully identified, and good communication among all parties is essential.[155] Potential side effects and possible methods for management should be discussed with the patient (and partner if available) at diagnosis, throughout treatment, and during follow-up visits.

Loescher et al.[156] evaluated the impact of the cancer experience on 17 long-term survivors. Patients repeatedly listed problems and concerns related to sexuality and reproductive function, including concerns about alterations in physical function and libido, problems with erection and ejaculation, and infertility.

Auchincloss[157] suggests that in order to effectively assess a patient for alterations in sexuality, the nurse must understand the patient's medical, psychiatric, and psychosexual status, evaluate present relationships, and provide recommendations and encouragement. Nurses should include sexuality in their assessment of all patients and should provide hope, reassurance, and basic information.[23] Anderson and Schmuch[63] developed the ALARM model for assessment of sexual dysfunction. The model provides a structure for assessing information similar to that suggested by Auchincloss. (See Table 31-3.)

Once sexual functioning has been assessed, interventions are necessary to maintain optimal sexual functioning and to promote adaptation to the sexual and reproductive side effects of disease and treatment. Interventions should include the patient's partner whenever possible. The PLISSIT model is another method of intervention (see Table 31-4). This model can help the majority of patients without the need for intensive therapy.[158] In order to maintain integrity and to improve quality of life, it is essential that all patients are counseled about sexual dysfunction, that open communication is encouraged, and that interventions are individualized and of value.

TABLE 31-3 Evaluation of Sexual Dysfunction

ALARM Model[63]	Auchincloss Model[23,157]
A—Activity (sexual)	Evaluate sexual status:
L—Libido/Desire	Present sexual function
A—Arousal and Orgasm	Past experiences
R—Resolution/Release	Relationships
M—Medical Data	Evaluate medical, psychological, and cancer status

Source: Data from Andersen and Schmuch[63] and Auchincloss.[23,157]

TABLE 31-4 PLISSIT Model for Evaluation of Sexual Dysfunction

P —Permission
LI —Limited Information
SS—Specific Suggestions
IT —Intensive Therapy

Source: Annon.[158]

FERTILITY CONSIDERATIONS AND PROCREATIVE ALTERNATIVES

Mutagenicity

Mutagenicity is the ability to cause an abnormality in the genetic content of cells, resulting in cell death, alteration(s) in growth and replication, or no noticeable alteration in cell function. Mutagenicity following radiation therapy in mice has been documented; however, the mutagenic effects following radiation or chemotherapy in humans are less clear.[159] Possible germ cell mutations may not be evident for generations of offspring.[160–162]

Numerous researchers have investigated pregnancy outcomes of children and adolescents exposed to chemotherapy or radiotherapy as a method to adequately assess mutagenicity following therapy.[163–167] Mulvihill et al.[163] reviewed 12 retrospective case series of pregnancies in cancer survivors. There were 1573 pregnancies and 1240 live-born infants with 46 (4%) birth defects (which is comparable to the rate among the general population). The researchers noted only two instances of possible mutants. Hawkins[165] evaluated 2286 survivors of childhood cancer who were exposed to chemotherapy, radiotherapy, or both. In women who had received radiotherapy to the abdomen or gonads there was an increased rate of miscarriage (19%) for first pregnancies. No statistical difference for congenital anomalies was seen. Senturia and Peckham[166] evaluated children fathered by men treated with chemotherapy for metastatic testicular cancer and reported no statistical difference in congenital anomalies, although they did note a higher than expected rate of cardiac abnormalities. Green et al.[167] examined the records of 306 men and women treated with chemotherapy for pediatric malignancies. No difference was noted in the rate of congenital anomalies; however, they did note that 10% of babies born to mothers who were given dactinomycin had structural congenital cardiac defects. In all studies it has been difficult to specifically implicate germ cell mutations as the cause of adverse outcomes to pregnancies. Follow-up over several generations of patients and their offspring will be needed before definitive answers are obtained.

Teratogenicity

Teratogenicity is the ability of a toxic compound to produce alterations in an exposed fetus. Both chemotherapy and radiotherapy are known to have teratogenetic effects on the fetus, causing spontaneous abortion, fetal malformation, or fetal death especially during the first trimester. Low-dose radiation has also been implicated in fetal malignancy.[160,161,168,169] Mulvihill et al.,[163] in their study of fetal exposure to radiotherapy or chemotherapy during gestation, noted a 28% abnormal outcome (spontaneous abortion or birth defects). Of five conceptions exposed only to radiotherapy, two were electively aborted, one was stillborn, and two were carried to term. All had some form of congenital malformation.

Fetal damage probably does not occur at doses <10 cGy and is only rarely reported at doses <50 cGy.[54] Radiation exposure during the first trimester represents the greatest risk to the fetus, with exposure ≥100 cGy resulting in fetal death, microcephaly, eye anomalies, and intrauterine growth retardation. In the second or third trimester, fetal death is unlikely, but growth retardation, sterility, and cataracts are common findings.[169]

Chemotherapy, particularly when received during the first trimester, has been related to congenital abnormalities, with approximately 10% of fetuses experiencing some type of anomaly. In general, the alkylating agents and antimetabolites have been most often associated with fetal malformations. Chemotherapy during the second or third trimesters may cause premature birth or low birth weights, but congenital abnormalities are not increased over the normal pregnancy incidence.[168,170,171] Doll et al.[170] noted that the timing of chemotherapy is critical, with the period of teratogenicity limited to the time of embryonic organogenesis. They state that effects also are related to drug dose, length of exposure, frequency of administration, and type and number of drugs administered (Table 31-5).

Reproductive Counseling

Discussions concerning fertility and reproduction issues need to be held prior to the onset of therapy and should continue well into posttreatment and follow-

TABLE 31-5 Teratogenetic Effects of Chemotherapy

Agent	Complication
Alkylating	
Busulfan	Spontaneous abortions
Chlorambucil	Skeletal malformations
Cyclophosphamide	
Nitrogen mustard	
Antimetabolites	
Cytosine arabinoside	Spontaneous abortion
6-Mercaptopurine	Skeletal malformations
5-Fluorouracil	
Methotrexate	
Miscellaneous	
Procarbazine	Atrial/septal defects
Glucocorticoids	Spontaneous abortions
Daunorubicin	Spontaneous abortions
Vinblastine	Spontaneous abortions

Source: Data from Balducci et al.,[54] Glasel,[120] Kaempfer,[160] Robinson and Krebs,[168] and Accola and Summerfield.[171]

up.[172] Current fertility status, desire for future child bearing, and contraception practices should be investigated during initial assessment.[173] Potential alterations should be openly discussed and referrals made as appropriate. Counseling for possible risks of mutagenicity, increased cancer risk, and unknown sequelae of treatment for progeny should be included.[174] Birth control methods need to be implemented to minimize the possibility of an unplanned pregnancy during therapy. In addition, methods to maintain fertility during therapy should be investigated.

For those receiving radiotherapy, appropriate shielding of the testes or ovaries or oophoropexy to position the ovaries outside the radiation field may be of benefit. Birth control pills in women and gonadotropin-releasing hormone analogues in men may protect the germ cells from damage by chemotherapeutic agents.[175,176] Studies in these areas continue, with results unclear.

Because it is often difficult to predict when an individual receiving chemotherapy is infertile, it is extremely important that methods to prevent pregnancy are discussed and appropriate drugs or devices provided. It has also been suggested that following cancer therapy an individual should wait a minimum of 2 years before attempting conception. This suggestion is made both to prevent pregnancy during the time recurrence is most likely and to allow for the recovery of spermatogenesis or ovarian function if it has been temporarily altered by therapy.[168,173,177]

Sperm Banking

Semen storage for use in artificial insemination has been available for many years. Although initially used to establish pregnancy in infertile couples, sperm banking has more recently also been used to preserve procreation abilities in men undergoing cancer therapy. The option to bank sperm unfortunately will not be available to every man undergoing cancer therapy. As previously noted, many men will be subfertile or infertile at the time of diagnosis. In addition, since sperm banking needs to be completed prior to initiation of therapy, anyone with rapidly progressing disease frequently cannot delay the start of therapy to complete the cryopreservation process. Redman et al.[178] investigated 79 men treated for Hodgkin's disease who had pretreatment semen analysis. Of these individuals, 28% were considered to be infertile at diagnosis. Of these men, 44 were followed posttherapy, and only 20% had normal sperm counts at a median of 27 months' follow-up. Eleven couples attempted pregnancy using the cryopreserved semen; thus far only three inseminations have been successful. Milligan et al.[179] reported on semen cryopreservation in 2219 men treated for cancer. Only 133 attempted conception, resulting in 27 pregnancies in 23 couples. Of the 27 pregnancies there were 21 live births and 6 miscarriages. Averette et al.[137] reported on 157 patients. Of these there were 22 inseminations resulting in 6 pregnancies. Of importance were sperm counts >20 × 10^6/ml and postthaw counts >30%. Fossa et al.[180] question the use of cryopreservation in metastatic testicular cancer. Of 91 patients, only 53 (58%) were able to cryopreserve sperm, resulting in four attempts to conceive but only one pregnancy.

Even if artificial insemination is never completed, the knowledge that semen has been banked and is available when needed can provide a significant psychological boost for the male undergoing cancer therapy.[181] All aspects of the sperm banking process, from initial visit through the completion of the insemination, should be fully discussed with the patient so that informed decisions can be made.

In Vitro Fertilization/Embryo Transfer

In vitro fertilization, used for male infertility due to low sperm counts or for female infertility due to severe endometriosis, immunologic infertility, or absent or damaged fallopian tubes, has undergone remarkable technological advances, with more than 30,000 fertilization cycles undertaken each year.[182,183] In vitro fertilization requires ovarian stimulation followed by ova retrieval via ultrasound-guided needle aspiration of the preovulatory follicles. Laparoscopy also may be used. The retrieved oocytes are then incubated with sperm for 5–26 hours. Following incubation, these embryos are transferred to the uterus and released. The woman remains hospitalized and on bed rest for about 6 hours. Following discharge, she is encouraged to rest for 48–72 additional hours. Initial results of a single oocyte-retrieval procedure have resulted in a pregnancy rate of 10%–16%. It has been shown, however, that after 4 to 6 attempts, the rate of successful pregnancies may approach 50%–60%.[182,184] Fedele et al.[185] reported on a woman with a tubal adenocarcinoma treated with salpingectomy. Following in vitro fertilization and embryo transfer, she delivered a normal male child. The patient remains alive and well. Other methods to attain fertility include the use of cryopreserved oocytes and zygotes, with pregnancy rates about 40%.[186,187]

PREGNANCY AND CANCER

Although pregnancy complicated by a diagnosis of cancer is a rare event, it creates multiple problems for all concerned. Uncertainty about the prognosis of mother and fetus, the rigors of treatment, and the long-term sequelae of cancer for patient, infant, and family compound events that normally are surrounded by a myriad of conflicting emotions. Only with comprehensive care by many health care and ancillary individuals can a positive outcome for mother, fetus, and family be anticipated.

Cancer is the second leading cause of death in the reproductive years. It is estimated that cancer complicates about 1 in 1000 pregnancies, and approximately 1 in 118 women with cancer also have a concomitant pregnancy. The most commonly associated cancers are those of the breast, cervix, ovary, and colorectum and lymphoma, leukemia, and malignant melanoma, the cancers most commonly seen during the reproductive years.[71]

In general, most cancers do not adversely affect a pregnancy, nor does the pregnancy adversely affect the cancer outcome, although it is possible that the treatment necessary to manage the cancer may have an adverse affect on the pregnancy. Therapeutic abortion has not been shown to be of benefit in altering disease progression and should not be considered unless continued pregnancy will compromise treatment and thus prognosis. The wishes of the patient and family must be considered, with therapeutic options, including prognosis for mother and fetus, fully explained.

It was previously believed that cancer associated with pregnancy was more aggressive and the outcome for all patients dismal. It is now recognized that delay in diagnoses may be a more likely cause of advanced disease at the time of diagnosis. Diagnosing cancer during a pregnancy is difficult, and signs and symptoms of the disease may be misconstrued or underestimated. Treatment options should be evaluated as though the patient were not pregnant, and therapy instituted when appropriate.[71,168,177,188]

Medical Management of Commonly Associated Cancers

Breast cancer

Breast cancer is the cancer most commonly associated with pregnancy, representing 1 cancer for every 3000 pregnancies.[71,168,177] Parente et al.[189] noted that collected series show a range from 1 to 7 breast cancers per 10,000 pregnancies. In terms of all women with breast cancer who are still in their child-bearing years, 1 in 3 will be pregnant at the time of diagnosis.[71,168]

Breast examination should be part of the initial prenatal visit. Although breast enlargement during pregnancy makes examination difficult, it is essential that all women have a thorough examination. If the woman does not practice breast self-examination (BSE), BSE education should be included. If a mass is felt, prompt evaluation is necessary. Although a mammogram is difficult to interpret because of density of the breast, it may be safely undertaken if appropriate fetal shielding is used. Even if a mammogram shows negative results, a breast mass must be investigated until a definitive diagnosis is made.[71,168]

Treatment of breast cancer should be as in the nonpregnant patient. Biopsy with the patient under local anesthesia has not been shown to cause fetal harm and should be performed without delay.[190] Once a definitive diagnosis is made, further therapy can be tailored to time of gestation, physician recommendations, and patient wishes. In general, modified mastectomy with lymph node sampling is the standard treatment for early disease. Depending on gestational age, adjuvant chemotherapy can often be delayed until after delivery. For the woman desiring breast-conserving surgery, lumpectomy with lymph node sampling may be done if she is close to term, but radiation therapy and chemotherapy will be delayed until delivery. For advanced disease, surgery and chemotherapy should be undertaken without delay. Therapeutic abortion may be suggested during the first trimester in order to prevent chemotherapy exposure to the fetus.[71,170,190–192]

Chances for survival has been considered poor, with reports of 30%–57% survival rates.[193,194] Most authors note that when patients are matched stage for stage with nonpregnant control subjects, there appear to be no differences in survival rates.[193–195]

Further pregnancies following a breast cancer diagnosis have been considered controversial. Some authors[177,189]suggest that all women refrain from any pregnancies, whereas others[193,196] suggest that a further pregnancy may actually protect against recurrence. Most authors now suggest a wait of 1–3 years after treatment for stages I and II and up to 5 years for stages III and IV.[61,195,196]

Breast-feeding after breast cancer diagnosis also has been highly debated. On the basis of breast cancer in mice, it has been suggested that breast-feeding is contradicted;[60] however, no information on human beings is available. Hassey[197] stated that breast-feeding should no longer be discouraged and, in fact, should be recommended if the woman desires. For the woman who has received primary breast radiation, it has been suggested that breast-feeding occur only on the nonirradiated side, primarily because of the possible increase in mastitis associated with breast-feeding in the irradiated breast.

Cancer of the cervix

The cancer second most commonly associated with pregnancy is cancer of the cervix, which occurs in 1 in 400 pregnancies. Approximately 1 in every 100 women diagnosed with cervical cancer will be pregnant at the time of diagnosis. Carcinoma in situ is most commonly found, with invasive disease seen in only 2%–5% of all cases. Signs and symptoms are similar to those found in the nonpregnant patient, with the majority of pregnant patients experiencing vaginal bleeding or discharge.[198] Diagnosis is most commonly made by Papanicolaou smear. If the smear is abnormal, colposcopy with appropriate biopsies should be undertaken. Cone biopsy is rarely indicated but may be undertaken to confirm a diagnosis of microinvasion. However, it is not without risks and is associated with a 30% complication rate, including hemorrhage, premature delivery, and infection.[60,72,168]

For carcinoma in situ the pregnancy may be allowed to continue. Biopsy should be repeated every 6 to 8 weeks and, unless there is progression, definitive therapy delayed until after delivery. If frank invasion is found, treatment consistent with standard practice for nonpregnant women should not be delayed. During the first two trimesters, surgery or radiation therapy without therapeutic abortion usually is undertaken. Early stage disease (IA and IB) may be treated with radical hysterectomy and pelvic lymph node dissection, while in advanced disease, radiation therapy is the most common treatment. During the third trimester, fetal viability usually can be awaited and the baby can be delivered by cesarean section, after which the appropriate cancer therapy is given.[60,71,168,198–200]

Controversy exists over the safety of vaginal delivery. It has been suggested[60] that vaginal delivery may disseminate the cancer or cause hemorrhage or infection; thus, cesarean section is recommended. Others have suggested that vaginal delivery actually may be associated with an improved overall survival and should be allowed if possible.[201] Gordon et al.[202] reported the fourth case of recurrence in an episiotomy after vaginal delivery. They suggest that careful follow-up for recurrence is essential. To date, no definitive answer is available.

Ovarian cancer

Ovarian masses are common during pregnancy, occurring once in every 81 pregnancies. In general, only 2%–5% of these are malignant, for an estimated 1 in 9000 to 1 in 25,000 case ratio. Most patients are asymptomatic, with an adnexal mass noted at the first prenatal visit.[168,184] There are a variety of ways to approach a pelvic mass during pregnancy. Orr and Shingleton[203] suggest that a mass >5 cm that lasts into the second trimester should be explored. Roberts[198] suggests that any mass >6 cm or symptomatic be immediately evaluated, whereas Barber[61] states that a unilateral, encapsulated, movable mass <10 cm can wait until the second trimester for evaluation.

If malignancy is diagnosed, treatment should proceed as in the nonpregnant patient. Early disease (stage IA) of low-grade histologic findings can be managed by unilateral oophorectomy and biopsy of the other ovary. The pregnancy may be allowed to continue. For all other stages, standard therapy of radical hysterectomy, omentectomy, node biopsy, and peritoneal washings should be carried out. If the patient is near term, a cesarean section, followed by the appropriate therapy, may be performed. Unfortunately, 30%–50% of all patients will be diagnosed with stage III or IV disease. Although recent management of stage III disease has resulted in improved survival, in general, the prognosis for long-term survival is poor.[60,61,198,204] As in the treatment of all cancers, the wishes of the patient must be considered. It is not uncommon for a pregnant woman with advanced disease to delay treatment until the fetus is viable. Palliative treatment should be instituted at the earliest possible time.

Malignant melanoma

Malignant melanoma is one of the most rapidly increasing cancers, with a predicted incidence of 1 in 100 Caucasians by the year 2000. It occurs most often in a preexisting mole in fair-haired individuals with blue or green eyes and an inability to tan when exposed to the sun, and the peak incidence is during the third and fourth decades.[203,205]

It has been suggested[206] that melanoma arising during pregnancy is associated with poor prognosis because it is hormonally influenced and thus exacerbated by pregnancy. At present this has yet to be definitely proven. What is known is that melanoma that occurs during pregnancy more often is found on the trunk, a melanoma site associated with a poor prognosis. In addition, all pigmented areas darken during pregnancy, making diagnosis of early changes more difficult. Biopsy and removal of questionable lesions are indicated. There appears to be no difference in survival between the pregnant and nonpregnant woman with melanoma.[206–210]

Treatment consists of wide excision with skin graft if necessary. Lymph node dissection remains controversial. Adjuvant therapy is being investigated, but no definite answers are available. The benefits of chemotherapy and biologic response modifiers remain unclear. For patients with advanced disease, therapeutic abortion followed by palliative chemotherapy is advised. For the patient with brain metastasis, surgery or radiation therapy with appropriate fetal shielding may be undertaken.[203,208]

Malignant melanoma is known to metastasize to the placenta and fetus. The placenta should be carefully evaluated at delivery and the baby monitored for development of melanoma.[71,168,208,211–213] Further pregnancies should not be undertaken until at least 2 years after diagnosis and treatment.[214]

Lymphomas

Both non-Hodgkin's lymphoma (NHL) and Hodgkin's disease (HD) occur with pregnancy, although the incidence is rare, with Hodgkin's disease occurring in 1 in 6000 pregnancies and NHL rarely associated.[60] Hodgkin's disease usually occurs as asymptomatic lymphadenopathy of the cervical, supraclavicular, or mediastinal regions. Disease confined to the neck or axilla usually can be treated with radiation therapy used with fetal shielding. Because more extensive disease requires combination chemotherapy, a therapeutic abortion is suggested during the first half of pregnancy. During the last half of pregnancy, therapy will be defined by the stage of the pregnancy. If viability is imminent, therapy may be delayed or single-drug treatment instituted and delivery awaited. For rapidly progressing disease, combination chemotherapy should be instituted immediately.[60,71,168]

Fewer than 50 cases of NHL and pregnancy have been reported in the literature. Steiner-Salz et al.[215]

reported on 6 cases of NHL that complicated pregnancy, and they reviewed an additional 22 cases. Therapy consisted of chemotherapy or radiation therapy, or both. Seventeen patients died within 9 months of delivery, six infants died shortly after birth, and the remaining patients and offspring are believed to be alive and well. Although NHL is known to metastasize to the placenta and fetus and thus requires careful observations at delivery, NHL has not developed in these infants.[211,212]

Leukemia

Leukemia occurs in 1 in 75,000 pregnancies. Diagnosis is often made on routine complete blood count. Treatment should be instituted immediately unless the fetus is viable or near viability. If the fetus is viable, delivery should not be delayed. If the fetus is near viability, leukaphereses may be utilized until delivery is possible. Therapeutic abortion is suggested in the first trimester to avoid fetal exposure to chemotherapy.[216] In a study of 20 children born of 18 women with acute leukemia, one infant was stillborn and two others died within 90 days of birth. Five of the 18 women remain alive; the other 13 died of recurrent leukemia. The 17 remaining children developed normally without apparent psychologic or physiologic abnormalities.[217] In another report,[218] perinatal mortality was as high as 50%, with 75% of mothers dying within 7 months of delivery. Leukemia also may spread to the placenta and fetus; thus, placental and fetal monitoring are important aspects of delivery and postpartum care.[211,212]

Effects of Treatment and Malignancy on the Fetus

Surgery

Maternal surgery can be safely accomplished with minimal risk to the fetus.[60,203] Pelvic surgery is more easily accomplished during the second trimester. There is little risk to the fetus from short exposure to anesthetic agents after the first trimester. Adequate ventilation and prevention of hypotension are of prime importance.[203] As long as competent surgeons and anesthesiologists with appropriate fetal monitoring equipment are available, no harm to the fetus should occur.[177]

Radiation

Radiation doses of >250 cGy during pregnancy have been associated with fetal damage—for example, mental retardation, skin changes, and spontaneous abortions (depending on stage of gestation). Low doses of radiation associated with diagnostic x-ray studies (<0.5 cGy) are probably not harmful if adequate fetal shielding is provided. Radiation to the pelvis should be avoided.[219,220] Long-term effects of low-dose radiation remain unknown, but the concerns of chromosomal aberrations and an increase in childhood cancer in children exposed in utero remain. Follow-up over many generations may be necessary to determine the exact effects.[60,220]

Chemotherapy

Chemotherapy has been administered prior to and concurrent with pregnancy.[221] As previously noted, chemotherapy during the first trimester has been associated with fetal wastage, malformations, and low birth weights. Many studies indicate that the incidence of fetal malformations is low (<10%) and may be minimized or avoided with careful selection of agents. Latent effects are still unknown, and offspring need continuous evaluation.

Maternal–fetal spread

Only a few cancers spread from the mother to the fetus, with melanoma, NHL, and leukemia the most common. Because few series have been compiled, the exact incidence is unknown. Rothman et al.[211] reviewed 11 cases and Potter and Schoeneman[212] 24 cases of maternal cancer that metastasized to the infant. Seventeen of the 35 women had metastatic melanoma. Fifteen infants died of cancer; an additional 6 died of events unrelated to cancer. Dildy et al.[222] reviewed cases of maternal malignancy metastatic to products of conception and reported on 53 cases. The most common cancer was malignant melanoma. Metastasis to the placenta occurred in 12 cases and spread to the fetus in 7 cases. The second most common were the hematologic malignancies (leukemia and lymphoma), involving 8 instances of placental spread and 4 cases of fetal spread. Breast and lung cancer were next; however, no cases of spread to the fetus have been reported. Because of the rare incidence of metastatic involvement to the infant, evaluation of the placenta and fetus is essential in women with disseminated cancers.

Nursing Management of the Pregnant Patient

Nursing management of the pregnant patient with a concomitant diagnosis of cancer can be extremely complicated. Interventions including psychosocial, educational, and ethical considerations must be developed and implemented. It has been suggested that pregnancy and cancer be treated as a high-risk event with all the associated needs.[71] Careful explanations of all aspects of care, with special emphasis on support of the patient and her family, need to be included. Normal activities of pregnancy may be delayed or prevented by disease or treatment, and fears of fetal demise, cancer therapy, and death may prevent resolution of ambivalence toward pregnancy and establishment of emotional affiliation to the growing child. Ethical considerations become apparent as plans for pregnancy are contrasted with needs for therapy. In some instances, therapeutic abortion may be necessary for optimal treatment; in other instances, therapy delays may be requested to provide for the safety of the fetus. Nonjudgmental care by health care personnel is essential during these difficult times.

Nursing care of the woman with cancer and her baby is extremely complex and of utmost importance. With a focus on educational interventions, psychological support, and coordination of care, the nurse has an important role in the final outcome. Treatment plans; coordination of follow-up; education about cancer, pregnancy, and treatment; and emotional support of the patient and significant others are integral components of the comprehensive care needed by the pregnant woman with cancer. Without these essential elements, it may not be possible to provide the necessary care for a positive or improved maternal and fetal outcome.

CONCLUSION

Sexual and reproductive dysfunction in cancer patients occurs much more frequently than previously recognized. Almost every patient exposed to cancer or cancer treatment has the possibility of experiencing some form of sexual dysfunction at some point during the illness. With cancer survival rates improving and with the understanding that sexual and reproductive function are important to all individuals, it is essential that sexuality and sexual function be assessed and evaluated prior to therapy and that appropriate interventions be implemented throughout treatment and the follow-up period.

REFERENCES

1. Ganz PA: Current issues in cancer rehabilitation. *Cancer* 65:742–751, 1990.
2. Yarbro CH, Perry MC: The effect of cancer therapy on gonadal function. *Semin Oncol Nurs* 1:3–8, 1985.
3. Yasko JM, Green P: Coping with problems related to cancer treatment. *CA* 37:107–125, 1987.
4. Smith DB: Sexual rehabilitation of the cancer patient. *Cancer Nurs* 12:10–15, 1989.
5. Fisher SG: The psychosexual effects of cancer and cancer treatment. *Oncol Nurs Forum* 10:63–68, 1983.
6. Guyton AC (ed): Endocrinology and reproduction. In *Human Physiology and Mechanism of Disease* (4th ed). Philadelphia: Saunders, 1987, pp. 563–654.
7. Gill GN: Endocrine. In West JB (ed), *Best and Taylor's Physiological Basis of Medical Practice* (11th ed). Baltimore: Williams & Wilkins, 1985, pp. 844–933.
8. Emslie-Smith D, Paterson CR, Schratcherd T, et al (eds): Reproduction. In *Textbook of Physiology*. Edinburgh: Churchill Livingstone, 1988, pp. 323–335.
9. Marieb EN (ed): Reproductive system. In *Essentials of Human Anatomy and Physiology*. Menlo Park, CA: Addison-Wesley, 1987, pp. 311–333.
10. Hobbie WL, Schwartz CL: Endocrine late effects among survivors of cancer. *Semin Oncol Nurs* 5:14–21, 1989.
11. Jessup JM, Steele G: Rectal and anal carcinoma. In Steele G, Cady B (eds); *General Surgical Oncology*. Philadelphia: Saunders, 1992, pp. 171–183.
12. Wicks LJ: Treatment modalities for colorectal cancer. *Semin Oncol Nurs* 2:242–248, 1986.
13. Cantril ST, Schoeppel P: Carcinoma of the anus: A review. *Semin Oncol Nurs* 4:203–299, 1988.
14. MacDonald LD, Anderson HR: Stigma in patients with rectal cancer: A community study. *J Epidemiol Community Health* 38:284–290, 1984.
15. Dobkin KA, Broadwell DC: Nursing considerations for the patient undergoing colostomy surgery. *Semin Oncol Nurs* 2:249–255, 1986.
16. Lamb MA, Woods NF: Sexuality and the cancer patient. *Cancer Nurs* 4:137–144, 1981.
17. Donovan MI (ed): Teaching the patient about sexuality. In *Cancer Care: A Guide for Patient Education*. New York: Appleton-Century-Crofts, 1981, pp. 257–289.
18. Andersen BL: How cancer affects sexual functioning. *Oncology* 4:81–88, 1990.
19. De Bernardinis G, Tuscano D, Negro P, et al: Sexual dysfunction in males following extensive colorectal surgery. *Int Surg* 66:133–135, 1981.
20. Hurney C, Holland J: Psychosocial sequelae of ostomies in cancer patients. *Cancer* 35:170–183, 1985.
21. Shipes E, Lehr S: Sexuality and the male cancer patient. *Cancer Nurs* 5:375–381, 1982.
22. Danzi M, Ferulano GP, Abate S, et al: Male sexual function after abdominoperineal resection for rectal cancer. *Dis Colon Rectum* 26:665–668, 1983.
23. Auchincloss SS: Sexual dysfunction. In Holland JC, Rowland JH (eds), *Handbook of Psychooncology*. New York: Oxford University Press, 1989, pp. 383–413.
24. Glasgow M, Halfin V, Althausen AF: Sexual response and cancer. *CA* 37:322–333, 1987.
25. Williams JJ, Slack WW: A prospective study of sexual function after major colorectal surgery. *Br J Surg* 67:772–774, 1980.
26. Burnham WR, Leonard-Jones JE, Brooke BN: Sexual problems among married ileostomists. *Gut* 18:673–677, 1977.
27. Koukouras D, Spiliotis J, Scopa CD, et al: Radical consequence in the sexuality of male patients operated for colorectal carcinoma. *Eur J Surg Oncol* 17, 285–288, 1991.
28. Schover LR, von Eschenbach AC, Smith DB, et al: Sexual rehabilitation of urologic cancer patients: A practical approach. *CA* 34:66–74, 1984.
29. Bachers ES: Sexual dysfunction after treatment for genitourinary cancer. *Semin Oncol Nurs* 1:18–24, 1985.
30. Boyd SD, Schiff WM: Inflatable penile prostheses in patients undergoing cystoprostatectomy with urethrectomy. *J Urol* 141:60–62, 1989.
31. Watt RC: Nursing management of a patient with a urinary diversion. *Semin Oncol Nurs* 2:265–269, 1986.
32. Schover LR, Fife M: Sexual counseling of patients undergoing radical surgery for pelvic or genital cancer. *J Psychol Oncol* 3:21–41, 1986.
33. Shipes E: Sexual functioning following ostomy surgery. *Nurs Clin North Am* 22:303–310, 1987.
34. Mansson A, Johnson G, Mansson W: Quality of life after

cystectomy: Comparison between patients conduit and those with caeca reservoir diversion. *Br J Urol* 62:240–245, 1988.
35. Held J, Volpe H: Bladder preserving combined modality therapy for invasive bladder cancer. *Oncol Nurs Forum* 18:49–57, 1991.
36. American Cancer Society. *Cancer Facts and Figures—1992.* Atlanta, GA: American Cancer Society, 1992.
37. Dobkin PL, Bradley I: Assessment of sexual dysfunction in oncology patients: Review, critique, and suggestions. *J Psychosocial Oncol* 9:43–74, 1991.
38. Witkin MH, Kaplan HS: Sex therapy and penectomy. *J Sex Marital Ther* 8:209–221, 1982.
39. Donovan MI, Girton SE (eds): Self concept. In *Cancer Care Nursing* (2d ed). Norwalk, CT: Appleton-Century-Crofts, 1984, pp. 506–556.
40. Furlow WL: Sexual consequences of male genitourinary cancer: The role of sex prosthetics. In Vaeth JN (ed), *Frontiers of Radiation Therapy and Oncology.* Basel, Switzerland: Karger, 1980, pp. 104–107.
41. Lange PH, Chang WY, Fraley EE: Fertility issues in the therapy of nonseminomatous testicular tumors. *Urol Clin North Am* 14:731–747, 1987.
42. Blackmore C: The impact of orchiectomy upon the sexuality of the man with testicular cancer. *Cancer Nurs* 11:33–40, 1988.
43. Narayan P, Lange PH, Fraley EE: Ejaculation and fertility after extended retroperitoneal lymph node dissection for testicular cancer. *J Urol* 127:685–688, 1982.
44. Lamb MA: Alterations in sexuality and sexual functioning. In Baird SB, McCorkle R, Grant M (eds), *Cancer Nursing—A Comprehensive Textbook.* Philadelphia: Saunders, 1991, pp. 831–849.
45. Nijman JM, Koops HS, Kremer J, et al: Gonadal function after surgery and chemotherapy in men with stage II and III nonseminomatous testicular tumors. *J Clin Oncol* 5:651–656, 1987.
46. Gritz ER, Wellisch DK, Wang H, et al: Long-term effects of testicular cancer on sexual functioning in married couples. *Cancer* 64:1560–1567, 1989.
47. Heinrich-Rynning T: Prostatic cancer treatments and their effects on sexual functioning. *Oncol Nurs Forum* 14:37–41, 1987.
48. Church PA: Prostate cancer. In Steele G, Cady B (eds), *General Surgical Oncology.* Philadelphia: Saunders, 1992, pp. 275–285.
49. Eggleston JC, Walsh PC: Radical prostatectomy with preservation of sexual function: Pathological findings in the first 100 cases. *J Urol* 134:1146–1148, 1985.
50. Walsh PC, Schlegel PN: Radical pelvic surgery with preservation of sexual function. *Ann Surg* 208:391–400, 1988.
51. Einhorn C: Helping the prostate surgery patient face sexual dysfunction. *Innovations Urol Nurs* 3:1, 9, 1992.
52. Meredith CE: Treatment options for men with erectile dysfunction. *Innovations Urol Nurs* 3:2–4, 8, 11, 1992.
53. Morales A, Condra MS, Owen JE, et al: Oral and transcutaneous pharmacologic agents in the treatment of impotence. *Urol Clin North Am* 15:87–93, 1988.
54. Balducci L, Phillips DM, Gearhart JG, et al: Sexual complications of cancer treatment. *Am Fam Physician* 37:159–172, 1988.
55. Lamb M: Vulvar cancer. Patient information booklet. *Oncol Nurs Forum* 13:79–82, 1986.
56. Andersen BL, Turnquist D, LaPolla J, et al: Sexual function after treatment of in situ vulvar cancer: Preliminary report. *Obstet Gynecol* 71:15–19, 1988.
57. Weijmar Schultz WCM, Van de Weil HBM, Bouma J, et al: Psychosexuality after cancer of the vulva. *Cancer* 66:402–407, 1990.
58. DiSaia PJ: Conservative management of the patient with early gynecologic cancer. *CA* 39:135–154, 1989.
59. Lamb MA: Psychosexual issues: The woman with gynecologic cancer. *Semin Oncol Nurs* 6:237–243, 1990.
60. DiSaia PJ, Creasman WT: *Clinical Gynecologic Oncology* (3d ed). St Louis, MO: Mosby, 1989.
61. Barber HRK: *Manual of Gynecologic Oncology* (2d ed). Philadelphia: Lippincott, 1989.
62. Hubbard JL, Shingleton HM. Sexual function of patients after cancer of the cervix treatment. *Clin Obstet Gynecol* 12:247–264, 1985.
63. Andersen BL, Schmuch G: Sexuality and cancer. In Holleb AL, Fink DJ, Murphy GP (eds); *American Cancer Society Textbook of Clinical Oncology.* Atlanta, GA: American Cancer Society, 1991, pp. 606–616.
64. Morgan S: Sexuality after hysterectomy and castration. *Women Health* 3:5–10, 1978.
65. Masters WF, Johnson VE (eds): *Human Sexual Response.* Boston: Little, Brown, 1966.
66. Zussman L, Zussman S, Sunley R, et al: Sexual response after hysterectomy-oophorectomy: Recent studies and reconsideration of psycho-genesis. *Am J Obstet Gynecol* 140:725–729, 1981.
67. Jenkins B: Patients' reports of sexual changes after treatment for gynecologic cancer. *Oncol Nurs Forum* 15:349–354, 1988.
68. Schover LR, Fife M, Gershenson DM: Sexual dysfunction and treatment for early stage cervical cancer. *Cancer* 63:204–212, 1989.
69. Shell JA: Impact of cancer on sexuality. In Otto S (ed), *Oncology Nursing.* St. Louis, MO: Mosby Year Book, 1991, pp. 430–451.
70. Lamb MA, Bargman C, Brozovich K: Ovarian cancer. Patient information booklet. *Oncol Nurs Forum* 12:83–88, 1985.
71. Krebs LU: Pregnancy and cancer. *Semin Oncol Nurs* 1:35–41, 1985.
72. Martin LK, Braly PS: Gynecologic cancers. In Baird SB, McCorkle R, Grant M (eds), *Cancer Nursing—A Comprehensive Textbook.* Philadelphia: Saunders, 1991, pp. 502–535.
73. Hampton BG: Nursing management of a patient following pelvic exenteration. *Semin Oncol Nurs* 2:281–286, 1986.
74. Hubbard SM, Jenkins J: An overview of current concepts in the management of patients with testicular tumors of germ cell origin. II. Treatment and strategies by histology and stage. *Cancer Nurs* 6:125–139, 1983.
75. Andersen BL, Hacker NF: Psychosexual adjustment following pelvic exenteration. *Obstet Gynecol* 61:331–338, 1983.
76. McKenzie F: Sexuality after total pelvic exenteration. *Nurs Times* 84:27–29, 1988.
77. Schain WS: The sexual and intimate consequences of breast cancer treatment. *CA* 38:154–161, 1988.
78. Schain WS: Breast cancer surgeries and psychosexual sequelae: Implications for remediation. *Semin Oncol Nurs* 1:200–205, 1985.
79. Rutherford DE: Assessing psychosocial needs of women experiencing lumpectomy. *Cancer Nurs* 11:244–249, 1988.
80. Fallowfield LJ, Hall A: Psychosocial and sexual impact

of diagnosis and treatment of breast cancer. *Br Med Bull* 47:388–399, 1991.
81. Fallowfield LJ, Hall A, Maguire GP, et al: Psychological outcomes of different treatment policies in women with early breast cancer outside a clinical trial. *Br Med J* 301:575–580, 1990.
82. Schover LR: The impact of breast cancer on sexuality, body image and intimate relationships. *CA* 41:112–120, 1991.
83. Holmberg L, Omne-Ponten M, Burns T, et al: Psychosocial adjustment after mastectomy and breast-conserving treatment. *Cancer* 64:969–974, 1989.
84. Andersen BL: Sexual functioning morbidity among cancer survivors: current status and future research directories. *Cancer* 55:1835–1842, 1985.
85. Metcalf MC, Fishman SH: Factors affecting the sexuality of patients with head and neck cancer. *Oncol Nurs Forum* 12:21–25, 1985.
86. Dropkin MJ: Coping with disfigurement and dysfunction after head and neck cancer surgery: A conceptual framework. *Semin Oncol Nurs* 5:213–219, 1989.
87. Witt ME, McDonald-Lynch A, Grimmer D: Adjuvant radiotherapy to the colorectum: Nursing implications. *Oncol Nurs Forum* 4:17–21, 1987.
88. Granai CO, Amado PM, Goldstein AS, et al: The effects of cancer therapy on fertility. *Clin Adv Oncol Nurs* 3:1,3,7–9, 1991.
89. Feldman JE: Ovarian failure and cancer treatment: Incidence and interventions for the premenopausal woman. *Oncol Nurs Forum* 16:651–657, 1989.
90. Hilderley LJ: Radiotherapy. In Groenwald S, Frogge MH, Goodman M, Yarbro CH (eds), *Cancer Nursing: Principles and Practice* (2d ed). Boston: Jones and Bartlett, 1990, pp. 199–229.
91. Yasko JM (ed): Sexual dysfunction. In *Care of the Client Receiving External Radiation Therapy*. Reston, VA: Reston, 1982, pp. 192–231.
92. Yasko JM (ed): Sexual and reproductive dysfunction. In *Guidelines for Cancer Care: Symptom Management*. Reston, VA: Reston, 1983, pp. 269–287.
93. Stair J: Sexual dysfunction: Infertility. In McNally JC, Sommerville ET, Miaskowski C, Rostad M (eds), *Guidelines for Oncology Nursing Practice* (2d ed). Philadelphia: Saunders, 1991, pp. 345–349.
94. Horning SJ, Hoppe RT, Kaplan HS, et al: Female reproductive potential after treatment for Hodgkin's disease. *N Engl J Med* 304:1377–1382, 1981.
95. Ray GR, Trueblood HW, Enright L, et al: Oophoropexy: A means of preserving ovarian function following pelvic megavoltage radiotherapy for Hodgkin's disease. *Radiology* 96:175–180, 1970.
96. Baker JW, Peckham MJ, Morgan RL, et al: Preservation of ovarian function in patients requiring radiotherapy for paraaortic and pelvic Hodgkin's disease. *Lancet* 1:1307–1308, 1972.
97. Seibel MM, Freeman MG, Graves WL: Carcinoma of the cervix and sexual function. *Obstet Gynecol* 55:484–487, 1980.
98. Fisher SG: Sexuality. In Johnson BL, Gross J (eds), *Handbook of Oncology Nursing*. New York: Wiley, 1985, pp. 363–379.
99. Jenkins B: Sexual healing after pelvic irradiation. *Am J Nurs* 86:920–922, 1986.
100. Shell JA, Carter J: The gynecological implant patient. *Semin Oncol Nurs* 3:54–66, 1987.
101. Dodd MJ: *Managing Side Effects of Chemotherapy and Radiation Therapy: A Guide for Nurses and Patients*. Norwalk, CT: Appleton and Lange, 1987.
102. Rowly MJ, Leach DR, Warner GA, et al: Effects of graded doses of ionizing radiation on human testes. *Radiat Res* 59:665–678, 1974.
103. Kinsella TJ, Shapiro E, Fraass BA et al: Testicular injury following high dose conventionally fractionated irradiation. *Int J Radiat Oncol Biol Phys* 9S:136–137, 1983.
104. Fossa SD, Aass N, Kaalhus O: Long-term morbidity after infradiaphragmatic radiotherapy in young men with testicular cancer. *Cancer* 64:404–408, 1989.
105. Costillo LA, Craft AW, Kernahan J, et al: Gonadal function after 12-Gy testicular irradiation in childhood acute lymphoblastic leukaemia. *Med Pediatr Oncol* 18:185–189, 1990.
106. Sklar CA, Robison LL, Nesbit ME, et al: Effects of radiation on testicular function in long-term survivors of childhood acute lymphoblastic leukemia: A report from the Children's Cancer Study Group. *J Clin Oncol* 8:1981–1987, 1990.
107. Kinsella TJ, Trivette G, Rowland J, et al: Long-term follow-up of testicular function following radiation therapy for early-stage Hodgkin's disease. *J Clin Oncol* 7:718–724, 1989.
108. van Heeringen C, DeSchryver A, Verbeek E: Sexual function disorders after local radiotherapy for carcinoma of the prostate. *Rad Oncol* 13:47–52, 1988.
109. Herr HW: Preservation of sexual potency in prostatic cancer patients after iodine implantation. *J Am Geriatr Soc* 27:17–19, 1979.
110. Carlton CE, Hudgins PT, Guerriero WG, et al: Radiotherapy in the management of stage C carcinoma of the prostate. *J Urol* 116:206–210, 1976.
111. Schover LR, von Eschenbach AC: Sexual and marital counseling with men treated for testicular cancer. *J Sex Marital Ther* 10:29–40, 1984.
112. Goldstein I, Feldman M, Deckers P, et al: Radiation-associated impotence. *JAMA* 251:903–910, 1984.
113. Shell JA: Knowledge deficit related to radiation therapy. In McNally JC, Sommerville ET, Miaskowski C, Rostad M (eds), *Guidelines for Oncology Nursing Practice* (2d ed). Philadelphia: Saunders, 1991, pp. 62–69.
114. Longo DL, Fisher RI: Medical problems in long-term survivors of Hodgkin's disease. *Internal Med Spec* 4:165–171, 1983.
115. Schilsky RL, Erlichman C: Late complications of chemotherapy: Infertility and carcinogenesis. In Chabner B (ed), *Pharmacologic Principles of Cancer Treatment*. Philadelphia: Saunders, 1982, pp. 109–128.
116. Chapman RM: Effect of cytotoxic therapy on sexuality and gonadal function. *Semin Oncol* 9:84–94, 1982.
117. Wallace WHB, Shalet SM, Crowne EC, et al: Gonadal dysfunction due to cis-platinum. *Med Pediatr Oncol* 17:409–413, 1989.
118. Burke MB, Wilkes GM, Berg D, et al: *Cancer Chemotherapy: A Nursing Process Approach*. Boston: Jones & Bartlett, 1991.
119. Otto SE. Chemotherapy. In Otto S (ed), *Oncology Nursing*. St. Louis, MO: Mosby Year Book, 1991, pp. 292–316.
120. Glasel M: Effects on sexuality. In Tenenbaum L (ed), *Cancer Chemotherapy—A Reference Guide*. Philadelphia: Saunders, 1989, pp. 195–204.
121. Guy JL: Medical oncology—the agents. In Baird SB, McCorkle R, Grant M (eds), *Cancer Nursing–A Compre-*

hensive Textbook. Philadelphia: Saunders, 1991, pp. 266–290.
122. Goodman M: Delivery of cancer chemotherapy. In Baird SB, McCorkle R, Grant M (eds), *Cancer Nursing—A Comprehensive Textbook.* Philadelphia: Saunders, 1991, pp. 291–319.
123. Schilsky RL, Lewis BJ, Sherins RJ, et al: Gonadal dysfunction in patients receiving chemotherapy for cancer. *Ann Intern Med* 93:109–114, 1980.
124. Richter P, Calamera JC, Morgenfeld MC, et al: Effect of chlorambucil on spermatogenesis in the human with malignant lymphoma. *Cancer* 25:1026–1030, 1970.
125. Viviani S, Ragni G, Santoro A, et al: Testicular dysfunction in Hodgkin's disease before and after treatment. *Eur J Cancer* 27:1389–1392, 1991.
126. Drasga RE, Einhorn LH, Williams SD, et al: Fertility after chemotherapy for testicular cancer. *J Clin Oncol* 1:179–183, 1983.
127. Stoter G, Koopman A, Vendrik CP, et al: Ten-year survival and late sequelae in testicular cancer patients treated with cisplatin, vinblastine and bleomycin. *J Clin Oncol* 7:1099–1104, 1989.
128. Meistrich ML, Chawla SP, DaCunha MF, et al: Recovery of sperm after chemotherapy for osteosarcoma. *Cancer* 63:2115–2123, 1989.
129. Cunningham J, Mauch P, Rosenthal DS, et al: Long-term complications of MOPP chemotherapy in patients with Hodgkin's disease. *Cancer Treat Rep* 66:1015–1022, 1982.
130. Viviani S, Santoro A, Bon Pante V, et al: Gonadal toxicity after combination chemotherapy for Hodgkin's disease: Comparative results of MOPP vs ABVD. *Eur J Cancer Clin Oncol* 21:601–605, 1985.
131. Rousseau L, Dupont A, Labrie F, et al: Sexuality changes in prostate cancer patients receiving antihormonal therapy combining the antiandrogen flutamide with medical (LHRH agonist) or surgical castration. *Arch Sex Behav* 17:87–98, 1988.
132. Kaempfer SH: Male sexual dysfunction. In Baird SB (ed), *Decision Making in Oncology Nursing.* Toronto: Decker, 1988, pp. 164–165.
133. Warne GL, Fairley KF, Hobbs, JB, et al: Cyclophosphamide-induced ovarian failure. *N Engl J Med* 289:1159–1162, 1973.
134. Belohorsky B, Siracky YJ, Sandor L, et al: Comments on the development of amenorrhea caused by myleran in cases of chronic myelosis. *Neoplasia* 4:397–402, 1960.
135. Chapman RM, Sutcliffe SB, Malpas JS: Cytotoxic-induced ovarian failure in women with Hodgkin's disease. II. Effects on sexual function. *JAMA* 242:1171–1181, 1979.
136. Andrieu JM, Ochoa-Molina ME: Menstrual cycle, pregnancies and offspring before and after MOPP therapy for Hodgkin's disease. *Cancer* 52:435–438, 1983.
137. Averette HE, Boike GM, Jarrell MA: Effects of chemotherapy on gonadal function and reproductive capacity. *CA* 40:199–209, 1990.
138. Santoro A, Bonadonna G, Valagussa P, et al: Long-term results of combined chemotherapy-radiotherapy approach in Hodgkin's disease: Superiority of ABVD plus radiotherapy versus MOPP plus radiotherapy. *J Clin Oncol* 5:27–37, 1987.
139. Gershenson DM: Menstrual and reproductive function after treatment with combination chemotherapy for malignant ovarian germ cell tumors. *J Clin Oncol* 6:270–275, 1988.
140. Meadows AT: Follow-up and care of childhood cancer survivors. *Hosp Prac* 15:99–108, 1991.
141. Heiney SP: Adolescents with cancer—Sexual and reproductive issues. *Cancer Nurs* 12:95–101, 1989.
142. Levy MJ, Stillman RJ: Reproductive potential in survivors of childhood malignancy. *Pediatrician* 18:61–70, 1991.
143. Rivkees SA, Crawford JD: The relationship of gonadal activity and chemotherapy-induced gonadal damage. *JAMA* 259:2123–2125, 1988.
144. Blatt J, Poplack DG, Sherins RJ: Testicular function in boys after chemotherapy for acute lymphoblastic leukemia. *JAMA* 304:1121–1124, 1981.
145. Byrne J, Mulvihill JJ, Myers MH, et al: Effects of treatment on fertility in long-term survivors of childhood or adolescent cancer. *N Engl J Med* 317:1315–1321, 1987.
146. Wilson B: The effects of drugs on male sexual function and fertility. *Nurs Pract* 16:12–24, 1991.
147. Kaempfer SH: Female sexual dysfunction. In Baird SB (ed), *Decision Making in Oncology Nursing.* Toronto: Decker, 1988, pp. 162–163.
148. Brager BL, Yasko J (eds): Sexual and reproductive dysfunction. In *Care of the Client Receiving Chemotherapy.* Reston, VA: Reston 1984, pp. 287–297.
149. Roferon A (package insert). Nutley, NJ: Roche Laboratories, 1987.
150. Ostroff JS, Lesko LM: Psychosexual adjustment and fertility issues. In Whedon MB (ed), *Bone Marrow Transplantation—Principles, Practice and Nursing Insights.* Boston: Jones and Bartlett, 1991, pp. 312–333.
151. Belec RH: Quality of life: Perceptions of long-term survivors of bone marrow transplantation. *Oncol Nurs Forum* 19:31–37, 1992.
152. Cust MP, Whitehead MI, Powles R, et al: Consequences and treatment of ovarian failure after total body irradiation for leukaemia. *Br Med J* 299:1494–1497, 1989.
153. Sanders JE, Buckner CD, Amos D, et al: Ovarian function following marrow transplantation for aplastic anemia or leukemia. *J Clin Oncol* 6:813–818, 1988.
154. Milliken S, Powles R, Parikh P: Successful pregnancy following bone marrow transplantation for leukaemia. *Bone Marrow Transp* 5:135–137, 1990.
155. Granai CO, Amado PM, Goldstein AS, et al: Female sexuality and cancer. *Clin Advances Oncol Nurs* 3(2):1–3, 7–9, 1990.
156. Loescher LJ, Clark L, Atwood JR, et al: The impact of the cancer experience on long-term survivors. *Oncol Nurs Forum* 17:223–229, 1990.
157. Auchincloss S: Sexual dysfunction after cancer treatment. *J Psychosocial Oncol* 9:23–42, 1991.
158. Annon JS: *The Behavioral Treatment of Sexual Problems.* Honolulu, HI: Mercantile Printing, 1974.
159. Mulvihill JJ, Byrne J: Genetic counseling of the cancer survivor. *Semin Oncol Nurs* 5:29–35, 1989.
160. Kaempfer SH: The effects of cancer chemotherapy on reproduction: A review of the literature. *Oncol Nurs Forum* 8:11–18, 1981.
161. Kaempfer SH, Wiley FM, Hoffman DJ, et al: Fertility considerations and procreative alternatives in cancer care. *Semin Oncol Nurs* 1:25–34, 1985.
162. Byrne J: Fertility and pregnancy after malignancy. *Semin Perinatol* 14:423–429, 1990.
163. Mulvihill JJ, McKeen EA, Rosner F, et al: Pregnancy outcome in cancer patients—experience in a large cooperative group. *Cancer* 60:1143–1150, 1987.
164. Mulvihill JJ, Myers MH, Connelly RR, et al: Cancer in

offspring of long-time survivors of childhood and adolescent cancer. *Lancet* 2:813–817, 1987.

165. Hawkins MM: Is there evidence of therapy-related increases in germ cell mutation among childhood cancer survivors? *J Natl Cancer Inst* 83:1643–1650, 1991.
166. Senturia YD, Peckham CS: Children fathered by men treated with chemotherapy for testicular cancer. *Eur J Cancer* 26:429–432, 1990.
167. Green DM, Zevon MA, Lowrie G, et al: Congenital anomalies in children of patients who received chemotherapy for cancer in childhood and adolescence. *N Engl J Med* 325:141–146, 1991.
168. Robinson WA, Krebs LU: Oncologic disease. In Abrams R, Wexler P (eds), *Medical Care of the Pregnant Patient: Concepts and Management.* Boston: Little, Brown, 1983, pp. 307–319.
169. Brent RL: The effect of embryonic and fetal exposure to x-ray, microwaves and ultrasound: Counseling the pregnant and nonpregnant patient about these risks. *Semin Oncol* 16:347–368, 1989.
170. Doll DC, Ringenberg QS, Yarbro JW: Antineoplastic agents and pregnancy. *Semin Oncol* 16:337–346, 1989.
171. Garber JE: Long-term follow-up of children exposed in utero to antineoplastic agents. *Semin Oncol* 16:437–444, 1989.
172. Accola KM, Sommerfeld DP: Helping people with cancer consider parenthood. *Am J Nurs* 79, 1580–1583, 1979.
173. Kaempfer SH: Reproductive planning. In Baird SB (ed), *Decision Making in Oncology Nursing.* Toronto: Decker, 1988, pp. 166–167.
174. Hoskins IA: Genetic counseling for cancer patients and their families. *Oncology* 3:84–92, 1981.
175. Chapman RM, Sutcliffe SB: Protection of ovarian function by oral contraceptives in women receiving chemotherapy for Hodgkin's disease. *Blood* 58:849–851, 1981.
176. Glode LM, Robinson W, Gould SF. Protection from cyclophosphamide-induced testicular damage with an analog of gonadotropin releasing hormone. *Lancet* 1:1132–1134, 1981.
177. Lowitz BB: Pregnancy and sexual function. In Casciato DA, Lowitz BB (eds), *Manual of Clinical Oncology* (2d ed). Boston: Little, Brown, 1988, pp. 403–410.
178. Redman JR, Bajoruna DR, Goldstein MC, et al: Semen cryopreservation and artificial insemination for Hodgkin's disease. *J Clin Oncol* 5:233–238, 1987.
179. Milligan DW, Hughes R, Lindsay KS: Semen cryopreservation in men undergoing cancer chemotherapy—a UK survey. *Br J Cancer* 60:966–967, 1989.
180. Fossa SD, Aass N, Molne K: Is routine pretreatment cryopreservation of semen worthwhile in the management of patients with testicular cancer? *Br J Urol* 64:524–529, 1989.
181. Kaempfer SH, Hoffman DJ, Wiley FM: Sperm banking: A reproductive option in cancer therapy. *Cancer Nurs* 6:31–38, 1983.
182. Speirs AL: The changing face of infertility. *Am J Obstet Gynecol* 158:1390–1394, 1988.
183. Meacham RB, Lipshultz LI: Assisted reproductive technologies for male factor infertility. *Curr Opinion Obstet Gynecol* 3:656–661, 1991.
184. Seibel MM: A new era in reproductive technology: In vitro fertilization, gamete intrafallopian transfer, and donated gametes and embryos. *N Engl J Med* 318:828–834, 1988.
185. Fedele L, Cittadini E, Bortolozzi, et al: Successful in vitro fertilization and embryo transfer after limited surgery for tubal adenocarcinoma. *Cancer* 64:1546–1547, 1989.
186. Levran D, Dor J, Rudak E, et al: Pregnancy potential of human oocytes—the effect of cryopreservation. *N Engl J Med* 323:1153–1156.
187. Abdalla HI, Barber RJ, Kirkland A, et al: Pregnancy in women with premature ovarian failure using tubal and intrauterine transfer of cryopreserved zygotes. *Br J Obstet Gynaecol* 96:1071–1075, 1989.
188. Zemlickis D, Lishner M, Degendorfer P, et al: Maternal and fetal outcome after invasive cervical cancer in pregnancy. *J Clin Oncol* 9:1956–1961, 1991.
189. Parente JT, Amsel M, Lerner R, et al: Breast cancer associated with pregnancy. *Obstet Gynecol* 71:861–864, 1988.
190. Hoover HC: Breast cancer during pregnancy and lactation. *Surg Clin North Am* 70:1151–1163, 1990.
191. Barnavon Y, Wallack K: Management of the pregnant patient with carcinoma of the breast. *Surg, Gynecol, Obstet* 171:347–352, 1990.
192. Van der Vange N, van Dongen JA: Breast cancer and pregnancy. *Eur J Surg Oncol* 17:1–8, 1991.
193. Peters MV: The effect of pregnancy in breast cancer. In Forrest APM, Kunkler PB (eds), *Prognostic Factors in Breast Cancer.* Edinburgh: Livingston, 1968, pp. 65–89.
194. Nugent P, O'Connell TX: Breast cancer and pregnancy. *Arch Surg* 120:1221–1224, 1985.
195. Petrek JA, Dukoff R, Rogato A: Prognosis of pregnancy-associated breast cancer. *Cancer* 67:869–872, 1990.
196. Danforth DN: How subsequent pregnancy affects outcome in women with a prior breast cancer. *Oncology* 5:23–35, 1991.
197. Hassey KM: Pregnancy and parenthood after treatment for breast cancer. *Oncol Nurs Forum* 15:439–444, 1988.
198. Roberts JA: Management of gynecologic tumors during pregnancy. *Clin Perinatol* 10:369–382, 1983.
199. McGee JE: Management of cervical dysplasia in pregnancy. *Nurs Pract* vol. xii, no. 3:34, 37, 41–42, 1987.
200. Hannigan EV: Cervical cancer in pregnancy. *Clin Obstet Gynecol* 33:837–845, 1990.
201. Lee RB, Neglia W, Park RC: Cervical carcinoma in pregnancy. *Obstet Gynecol* 58:584–589, 1981.
202. Gordon AN, Jensen R, Jones HW: Squamous carcinoma of the cervix complicating pregnancy: Recurrence in episiotomy after vaginal delivery. *Obstet Gynecol* 73:850–852, 1989.
203. Orr JW, Shingleton HM: Cancer in pregnancy. *Curr Probl Cancer* 8:1–50, 1983.
204. King LA, Nevin PC, Williams PP, et al: Treatment of advanced epithelial ovarian cancer in pregnancy with cisplatin-based chemotherapy. *Gynecol Oncol* 41:78–80, 1991.
205. Rifkin RN, Thomas MR, Mughal TI, et al: Malignant melanoma—profile of an epidemic. *West J Med* 149: 43–46, 1988.
206. Riberti C, Marola G, Bertani A: Malignant melanoma: The adverse effect of pregnancy. *Br J Plast Surg* 34:338–339, 1981.
207. Shiu MH, Schohenfeld D, Maclean B, et al: Adverse effect of pregnancy on melanoma: A reappraisal. *Cancer* 37:181–187, 1976.
208. Houghton AN, Flannery J, Viola MV: Malignant melanoma of the skin occuring during pregnancy. *Cancer* 48:407–410, 1981.
209. Slingluff CL, Reintgen DS, Vollmer RT, et al: Malignant

melanoma arising during pregnancy: A study of 100 patients. *Ann Surg* 211:552–559, 1990.

210. Wong JH, Sterns EE, Kopald KH, et al: Prognostic significance of pregnancy in stage I melanoma. *Arch Surg* 124:1227–1231, 1989.
211. Rothman LA, Cohen CJ, Astarloa J: Placental and fetal involvement by maternal malignancy: A report of rectal carcinoma and a review of the literature. *Am J Obstet Gynecol* 116:1023–1024, 1973.
212. Potter JF, Schoeneman M: Metastasis of maternal cancer to the placenta and fetus. *Cancer* 25: 380–388, 1970.
213. Anderson JF, Kent S, Machin GA: Maternal malignant melanoma with placental metastasis: A case report with literature review. *Pediatr Pathol* 9:35–42, 1989.
214. Mackie RM, Bufalino R, Morabito A, et al: Lack of effect of pregnancy on outcome of melanoma. *Lancet* 337:653–655, 1991.
215. Steiner-Salz D, Yahalom J, Samuelov A, et al: Non-Hodgkin's lymphoma associated with pregnancy: A report of six cases, with a review of the literature. *Cancer* 56:2087–2091, 1985.
216. Henderson ES: A selected overview. In Gunz FW, Henderson ES (eds), *Leukemia* (4th ed). Orlando, FLA, Grune & Stratton, 1983, pp. 785–798.
217. Aviles A, Niz J: Long-term follow-up of children born to mothers with acute leukemia during pregnancy. *Med Pediatr Oncol* 16:3–6, 1988.
218. Lilleyman JS, Hill AS, Anderkon KJ: Consequences of acute myelogenous leukemia in early pregnancy. *Cancer* 40:1300–1303, 1977.
219. Dekaban AS: Abnormalities in children exposed to x-radiation during various stages of gestation: Tentative timetable of radiation injury to the human fetus. Part I. *J Nucl Med* 9:471–477, 1968.
220. Jankowski CB: Radiation and pregnancy: Putting the risks in proportion. *Am J Nurs* 86:260–265, 1986.
221. Schapira DV, Chudley AE: Successful pregnancy following continuous treatment with combination chemotherapy before conception and throughout pregnancy. *Cancer* 54:800–803, 1984.
222. Dildy GA, Moise KJ, Carpenter RJ, et al: Maternal malignancy metastatic to the products of conception: A review. *Obstet Gynecol Survey* 44:535–540, 1989.

Chapter 32

Altered Body Image and Sexuality

Susan Dudas, RN, MSN

INTRODUCTION

Self-concept is a significant factor in the recovery and rehabilitation of the person with cancer. Body image and sexuality are integral parts of a person and must be given as much attention in a nursing care plan as other physical, emotional, and spiritual needs. How changes in body image should be managed depends primarily on the patient's perception of these changes and the reactions of people who are important to the patient. The nurse needs to accurately assess the impact of an altered body image and the significance of sexuality to ensure that the patient is given the information and attention necessary to cope with these concerns.

This chapter is concerned with the assessment of changes in body image and sexuality in the person diagnosed with cancer. Interventions to help the patient cope with body image changes and sexuality issues will also be discussed.

CONCEPT OF BODY IMAGE

Carlson[1] has defined self-concept as "all unconscious and conscious perceptions, cognitions, information, feelings, goals, and evaluations that refer to the self." Self-esteem includes all evaluative aspects of the self-concept: perceptions of self, self-acceptance, self-approval, and self-expectations. Basic to self-esteem and self-concept is the concept of *body image;* body image includes those elements that refer to the physical self. Concepts of body image and self-concept are, according to Klopp,[2] "dynamic constructs which are developed and changed both by private perceptions and social feedback." The attitudes and beliefs one has about self are influenced by significant others and significant events in one's life. Norris[3] cites body image as the interpersonal experience of feelings and attitudes towards one's body but also acknowledges body image as a "social creation." This view is reflected in how cultural and societal attitudes, as well as those of significant others, influence body image. Schilder[4] also extended the body image concept to include a sociologic meaning for both the individual and society as well as the individual's personal or psychologic investment in his or her body and body parts. Body image and self-concept are important concepts in understanding behavior, because if a change in body image is unacceptable to the individual, the way that individual views and values self may also be altered.[5]

The most commonly used definition of body image is that of Schilder,[4] who referred to body image as the "picture of our body, formed in the mind's eye." He also recognized body image as a part of normal psychology and noted the impact of sensory input on body image. Feelings about intelligence, mobility, and physical capacity to endure pain and stress, as well as how our bodies look and how they function, also are components of body image.

Thus, body image is affected by physical factors and sensations as well as by emotional and social reactions; body image relates to one's actual appearance and body function as well as to how one perceives the self and what one perceives as an "ideal" body or image. In current American society, an ideal body, for example, often emphasizes youth, beauty, and slimness. The ideal image of oneself and the real image must coincide or be compatible; if there is a discrepancy between what is idealized and what is real, a conflict in body image may develop and may affect health and personality.[5] The internalized view of one's appearance affects behavior, as well as one's emotional outlook. The concept that an internal body image mechanism exists has been supported by Altabe,[6] but research is needed on how to more readily obtain patients' views of their body image in order to identify those who will need more assistance in their adaptation to changes in body image.

Researchers use several different instruments in their studies on body image aspects. Secord and Jourard[7] described "body cathexis" as the degree of satisfaction or dissatisfaction with the various parts or processes of the body. They developed the Body Cathexis-Self Concept (BC-SC) scale to appraise body cathexis and found a strong relationship between body cathexis with various parts or processes of the body and one's self concept. Body image inventories are often derived from this classic scale. However, body image is a multidimensional construct that requires a multimethods approach for study.[8] Brown and colleagues[9] have analyzed the Body-Self Relations Questionnaire (BSRQ), an attitudinal body-image instrument used by several researchers. This instrument does not restrict the body image construct to attitudes about physical appearance. The BSRQ takes into account cognitive and behavioral components as well as affective components and is used to determine subjects' attitudes toward physical appearance, physical fitness, and health. Another tool related to body image issues is the Body Esteem Scale (BES), which also has a multidimensional focus on self-esteem.[10] These instruments are some resources for researchers to use as they investigate the impact of changes in body image on the adaptation and rehabilitation of patients with cancer.

Because cancer and its treatment may cause alterations in body appearance and function, oncology nurses should consider potential or actual body image disturbance as a nursing diagnosis. It is important for nurses to increase their awareness of those persons with cancer who are at greatest risk for body image disturbances.

CANCER AND BODY IMAGE

Cancer, its treatment, and resulting changes in appearance, abilities, and function often cause a change in body image and can negatively affect a person's self-esteem. Emphasis on physical attractiveness places an additional burden on individuals who sustain disfigurement or dysfunction from illness. Changes in body image that are not realistically integrated into the patient's self-concept hinder adaptation and adjustment. Such body image changes are viewed as threats or major losses. Any alteration to the body is a threat to the body image as perceived by the individual patient and can result in the patient's feeling worthless as a person, physically unattractive or even repulsive, and unable to be valued or loved.[11] As patients go through a process of mourning for these losses, they may express these feelings as anger, depression, pessimism, or withdrawal.[11]

Problems in coping with changes in body image caused by cancer affect the patient's ability to learn, to be motivated for self-care, and to resume the role in the family that he or she held before the cancer diagnosis. Nurses should be concerned with body image factors in order to help cancer patients be comfortable and realistic about their physical selves. They cannot make assumptions about a patient's reactions to cancer and its sequelae without verifying these perceptions with the patient.[12] Nursing assessment of the state of the patient's self-esteem and perspective of his or her body image is important; awareness of these aspects is necessary to foster the cancer patient's potential for rehabilitation and improved quality of life. More than half of the 323 ambulatory cancer patients in one study[13] perceived the diagnosis and treatment of cancer as changing their physical appearance and said that these changes made them feel worse; in addition, the majority felt moderately or strongly negative about these changes. These patients primarily referred to changes in their body image or changes in their emotional outlook as factors affecting their changed feelings about themselves.

Damage or an alteration to the body usually causes conflict between the image that has been established over time and current reality.[14] If the patient does not change the image of his or her physical self, self-esteem may decrease because the patient may have some expectations that can no longer be met. Changing self-assessments in ways that are congruent with reality is a necessary part of the adjustment process.[1] Norris[3] has identified factors that contribute to the ability of persons to adapt to changes in the appearance, structure, or function of the body:

1. the nature of the threat
2. the meaning that the change has for the person
3. the person's own coping ability
4. the responses from significant others
5. the help available to the patient and his or her family

Additional factors are the time available to prepare for and absorb the meaning of the change and to experience and accept the changes in the body.

Certain types of cancer are more likely to affect body image. The major cancers associated with altered body image and altered functions that may result in body image disturbances include: breast cancer that results in a mastectomy or changes related to radiation therapy, head and neck cancer that results in residual defects, colorectal or bladder cancer that requires an ostomy, gynecologic cancer that affects the woman's genitalia or reproductive organs, and prostate or testicular cancers. Patients receiving chemotherapy for cancer may also have physical changes that affect body image. Changes in reproductive functioning, such as fertility problems associated with cancer chemotherapy or radiation therapy, effects of chemotherapeutic agents on gonadal function and pregnancy, parenting issues, and alternative options such as sperm banking are discussed elsewhere in this book.

Breast Cancer

In much of today's society the breast is valued in terms of fertility and femininity and is symbolic of sexuality. Women who undergo mastectomy for the treatment of breast cancer may suffer manifestations of psychologic maladjustment that cause them to feel rejected, sexually mutilated, and depressed.[15] These feelings may contribute to a poor self-image, a sense of worthlessness, difficulties in interpersonal relationships, a decline in sexual activity and, in some cases, deterioration of marriage.[15] Many patients with breast cancer become socially isolated and withdraw from social contacts.[16] One cannot assume that age is a factor, making the younger woman more vulnerable to body image disturbances than the older woman; other factors are more likely to be the issue. For example, mastectomy for a woman who has a strong marital relationship that has lasted over many years is not likely to be as threatening as for a young divorcee who depends on her physical appearance to initiate new relationships with men.[17] Loveys and Klaich[18] caution nurses that a diagnosis of breast cancer does not impose one standard set of problems for every woman. In their interviews with 79 women newly diagnosed with breast cancer, all of whom were of child-bearing age, they identified 14 domains of illness demands that included physical changes, reconstructing the self, uncertainty, loss (referring to both the breast and to hair loss), acceptance of the illness, and social interaction or support, as well as other domains.

Changes in treatment methods for breast cancer, such as the use of lumpectomy in lieu of modified mastectomy in selected patients and the use of radiation therapy, have been oriented to improving cosmetic outcome of therapy. However, nurses should not assume that body image changes are not as significant with these techniques as with mastectomy. Although women undergoing radiation therapy generally have fewer negative feelings regarding body image changes,[19,20] it is necessary to consider individual perspectives of the situation. Although the breast is retained in these techniques, radiation therapy, for example, can cause changes in the texture of the breast tissue and the contour of the breast, thickening of the skin, discoloration of the skin, and, in the case of simultaneous chemotherapy, it may cause severe skin reactions, which can affect the patient's body image.[19,20] In addition to the physical alterations associated with surgical procedures and radiation therapy, side effects, such as alopecia, weight gain, and early menopause, are commonly encountered in women with breast cancer who are receiving adjuvant chemotherapy. These side effects often result in a lowered body image.[15]

Fallowfield and co-workers[21] studied 101 women who were treated for early breast cancer and found that slightly more of the patients who underwent a lumpectomy followed by radiotherapy had affective disorders and anxiety states as compared to women who underwent mastectomy. They also found that patients in the lumpectomy group often expressed deep concern that they had received the "wrong operation" and that the surgeon might not have removed all the cancer, and they feared recurrence. The researchers caution health care providers that counseling services should be provided for all women treated for breast cancer, not just for those who undergo mastectomy. Even though the nurse may view a lumpectomy and axillary resection as less traumatic for the woman with breast cancer, it is important to remember that "any visual or perceived change in the breast affects the woman's perception of her 'self' as well as her physical being."[19] Wainstock[22] also notes that breast-conservation procedures do not protect women from problems with psychosocial adjustment, though there is a degree of protection from difficulties in body image in those women who undergo breast-conservation procedures. Foltz[23] concluded from her review of studies related to body image and cancer that, although generally lesser surgery or immediate cosmesis does reduce distress related to altered body image in the immediate posttreatment period, the concerns and distress of all patients are similar at 1 year, regardless of the procedure.

Confrontation with an altered body image occurs at different times with different people and also may occur unexpectedly even when someone perceives that he or she has handled a situation well. A female patient, for example, on being informed that she had breast cancer decided definitely that a modified mastectomy was appropriate for her. She was very confident before and after the operation and verbalized her reasons for this decision, handling the loss of her breast matter-of-factly. However, when she went to purchase a breast prosthesis, she faced herself in a full-length mirror and felt particularly vulnerable. She expressed how surprised she felt by her sad and anxious feelings on being measured for the prosthesis and viewing herself in the mirror; she had thought that she had accepted her mastectomy in a very realistic and positive way with no display of regret or sadness prior to this time.

Because of advances in plastic and reconstructive surgery, breast reconstruction is an option for women with mastectomy. The goal is to provide symmetry and preserve body image.[19] This procedure can be done at the time of mastectomy or later. Schain and co-workers[24] found in their study of 63 patients who had breast reconstruction that wanting to wear a wider range of clothing and eliminating the need for an external prosthesis were the common reasons for choosing reconstructive surgery; less common was the desire to improve sexual relations or to improve marital state. Winder and Winder[25] reviewed multiple studies to determine the basis for decisions to have breast reconstruction. In addition to eliminating the need for a prosthesis and to be able to wear more attractive clothing, other reasons for selecting breast reconstruction were to increase self-esteem and to improve their appearance. Some of the barriers to women's considering reconstruction as an option include the cost of the procedure, the fear of another surgical experience (if not done at time of mastectomy), and the concern about others' reactions to their having the cosmetic procedure.[25] In her review of studies on self-concept, Foltz[23] noted, for example, that reconstruction may not always be seen by marital partners as a positive action. Nurses also need to be careful that their own views about breast reconstruction do not bias them in working with patients undergoing mastectomy. For example, if nurses do not provide information about breast reconstruction because they do not believe it is important or necessary, the patient is denied knowledge on which to base a decision.

The choice for or against reconstruction, however, cannot be made until the patient both cognitively and emotionally recognizes that the breast is gone.[25] The time required for this acknowledgment to occur varies considerably among individual patients, although Schain and co-workers[24] found that patients who had reconstructive breast surgery at the time of mastectomy or within 1 year had significantly less recalled distress about their mastectomy than those who had it more than 2 years later.

Ironically, as reconstruction procedures have become more appealing to many mastectomy patients, the safety of silicone used for implants has come under scrutiny, bringing new concerns for these patients. Implants have been viewed as emotional lifesavers by some women, but now women may be fearful of breast reconstruction because of the publicized problems associated with implant materials. Knobf and Stahl[26] have summarized the options regarding breast reconstruction, and the topic is discussed in Chapter 38.

Ongoing acceptance of the woman's concern with body image over time must be a part of nursing care. An accepting and nonjudgmental attitude about how patients react to breast cancer and its treatment is essential because the reactions can be so varied. Some women react to what they view as coercion by persons to have them select breast reconstruction even though they may feel no need for the procedure. A unique reaction to mastectomy, for example, is that of a well-known author and poet who had a tree branch tattooed on her right chest, where her breast was removed for cancer. A picture of her in the nude with her hands outstretched is on the front cover of her book and also is available in a poster format.[27] On the poster these words declare her perceptions about her mastectomy and experience with cancer:

> I am no longer afraid of mirrors where I see the sign of the amazon, the one who shoots arrows. There was a fine red line across my chest where a knife entered, but now a branch winds about that scar and travels from arm to heart. Green leaves cover the branch, grapes hang there and a bird appears. What grows in me now is vital and does not cause me harm. I think the bird is singing. I have relinquished some of the scars.
>
> I have designed my chest with the care given to an illuminated manuscript. I am no longer ashamed to make love. Love is a battle I can win. I have the body of a warrior who does not kill or wound. On the book of my body, I have permanently inscribed a tree.[27]

Head and Neck Cancer

Facial appearance is an important component of body image. Aversion to visible deformities, especially in the face, is well documented.[28,29] Aggressive treatment of head and neck cancer that removes large portions of bony and soft tissue from the head and neck results in extensive defects, often causing professionals as well as the patient to wonder if the result is worth it. These visible defects, which affect both appearance and functions (i.e., speech, eating, swallowing, salivary control, and chewing) result in alterations in body image that require sensitive nursing care to assure patients that they need not expect rejection, loss of sexual appeal, or even repulsion as a result of the defects.[30] Unless patients adjust to an altered body image, they will not be successfully rehabilitated in spite of the restoration of cosmetic appearance and function.

Dropkin and colleagues[28] developed a Disfigurement/Dysfunction Scale to quantitatively measure the perception of visible disfigurement and dysfunction after head and neck surgery for the treatment of cancer. The scale technique measures others' perceptions of the relative severity of 11 common disfigurements and 8 commonly associated dysfunctions. Their study documented that procedures viewed as "most severe were associated with major structural alteration in the center of the face or that region that provides the greatest audiovisual stimuli in interaction with others"[28, p. 569] (i.e., orbital exenteration and radical maxillectomy). The scale has been used as a way to determine patients' ability to cope with disfigurement and dysfunction by measuring the impact of specific alterations in body image through observation of self-care and "social affiliation behaviors."[31]

Cancers Resulting in Ostomies

Patients with surgically constructed stomas, either colostomies or urostomies, frequently have disturbances of body image. Klopp[2] examined the relationship between body image and self-concept at varying lengths of time after ostomy surgery and reported that, because control of elimination is learned as a private, controlled function, the necessity of an ostomy and loss of sphincter control result in a changed body image. Others[12,32] have noted that persons with stomas often have poor psychosocial outcomes, including failure to return to occupations, withdrawal from social and intimate contacts, depression, and anxiety. These patients are concerned with the visibility of urine or stool on their bodies and on the potential visibility (or detectability) to others during social or intimate contact. Behaviors often associated with the construction of a stoma include social isolation, sexual dysfunction, anxiety, and dependency.[2,12,32] In contrast to these reports, however, Tomaselli and co-workers found that body image after ostomy surgery improves over time; the majority of subjects in their study returned "back to normal" about 6 months after surgery.[33]

Oberst and Scott[34] in their study of surgically treated cancer patients found that patients with ostomies were slower to return to pre-illness functional levels and had greater psychologic distress than nonostomy patients. This finding gives impetus to the practice of nurses' intervening early to help ostomy patients adjust to body image changes, but also acknowledging the need for adequate time for rehabilitation.

Side Effects of Chemotherapy

Even if no anatomical alterations occur, side effects of cancer treatments may cause distressing symptoms that interfere with the patient's body image. These symptoms include alopecia, pain, nausea, vomiting, diarrhea, weakness, fatigue, muscle atrophy, and neurologic changes. Women may feel unattractive when loss of hair from the head, axilla, and pubic area results from therapy. One study[35] of 44 cancer patients found that, regardless of sex, alopecia negatively affected a person's body image. Appropriate wigs in styles worn previously, hats, turbans, or attractive scarves can be used effectively, but some patients may find this intervention inadequate and withdraw from social interactions.

It is important for the nurse working with the cancer patient to realize that the impact of changes in body image may fluctuate during the cancer experience. Priorities vary at different times for different individuals. Nurses cannot assume that body image changes mean the same to each person.

A female patient who had ovarian cancer and was to receive chemotherapy that would result in alopecia sobbed uncontrollably when she was informed that she would lose her stunning black hair. She had been stoic and courageous in having four major surgeries in the treatment of her cancer, but she was devastated by the threat of alopecia, which she viewed as cruel and unjust. However, after several months when her cancer progressed in spite of chemotherapy, she inadvertently went out to her garden without her wig and talked with her neighbors without realizing that she was not wearing it. When she came into the house and looked in the mirror and saw her bald head, she simply laughed. Her priority at this time was to have a day without pain; her hair loss had decreased in importance. This is also an illustration of the time factor that Norris[3] has identified as being important in experiencing and accepting changes in the body.

Even when body changes are not visible, the patient may experience a disturbance in body image. For example, when premature menopause results from chemotherapy, as in some young women who have had Hodgkin's disease, body image disturbances may occur; nursing interventions to support the sense of self-worth are necessary for these women.[36]

The self-esteem of some patients is dependent on physical strength, endurance, and productivity; such patients may have increased difficulty when side effects of fatigue and weakness occur. Because productivity is so important to them, they may exceed their capacity for work and become ill due to exhaustion. Sometimes nurses may actually foster this by their emphasis on all the patients are able to do in spite of therapy, putting even higher expectations on the patient. Nurses may believe that the patient has no problem in this area, because he or she is able to keep up with considerable activity; from the patient's perspective, however, productivity and activities may have changed so drastically from the premorbid style that the patient actually feels like a worthless failure. The nurse does not have a complete picture of the person's premorbid lifestyle, but the patient compares the current situation with the pre-illness pattern of activity and productivity. If the patient's pattern of activity and attitude about the changes occurring as a result of the cancer are not determined, opportunities for identifying body image disturbances may be missed. The nurse is increasingly likely to see more of these types of patients because of the increased numbers of women who manage work, family, and self-care achieving a view of themselves as "superwomen." Such women may feel like failures when they cannot keep up with their usual responsibilities because of the effects of fatigue and other symptoms caused by chemotherapy. Emphasizing the individual patient's remaining abilities rather than the disabilities is an important focus of the nurse in promoting acceptance of an altered body image related to altered functioning.

PROMOTING ADJUSTMENT TO AN ALTERED BODY IMAGE

The goal of promoting a healthy and realistic attitude toward a positive body image requires support for the patient to accept a new or changed body image. To reach this goal, the nurse helps prevent disturbances in body image by providing emotional support as patients grieve for the loss of a body part or body function. Patients need assurance that such grieving is appropriate and normal, and they need time to prepare for and absorb the meaning of the change and to experience and accept the changes in the body. Following Norris's framework for interventions,[3] the nurse will need to discuss changes in body image with the patient to assess how the patient perceives the threat. Attentive listening is a major intervention in this process.

Touching, spending calm and unrushed time with patients, and conveying sincere interest are ways to convey acceptance and caring. The nurse should be cautious, however, in using touching as a means of support; some patients of certain cultures may find this intrusive and inappropriate. It is wise for the nurse to update her or his knowledge about cultural beliefs and attitudes in order to be supportive to the many patients of various cultures who become cancer patients. Providing information and teaching patients to appropriately manage procedures involved with body changes will help patients gain control; this also will enhance body image and self-concept. Enabling patients to manage necessary procedures or care efficiently may also be helpful in ensuring that the body change does not become the focus of their lives. This principle is a major aspect of rehabilitation protocols after head and neck surgery. Dropkin et al.[28] emphasize how the patient's taking over irrigation and self-care techniques after head and neck surgery helps improve body image perceptions. Support for their self-esteem may help patients accept and adapt to changes. It is important for nurses to avoid pushing or forcing patients to accept change. Readiness is an important factor to assess. Acceptance of change takes time; just as adjusting to grief and loss varies widely in terms of time and manner, so does adjustment to changes in body image vary.

The nurse can play an influential role in helping patients express anger and grief during the mourning process and cope with these feelings. Assisting patients to deal with the change in their bodies and not make the changes the focus of their lives reinforces their self-esteem. Patients need to understand the full situation to avoid placing undue restrictions on themselves because of cancer or its treatment. Some may also need help to not use cancer as an excuse for unsuccessful relationships but instead to resume social relationships satisfactorily.[12]

Watson[37,38] studied the effects of short-term counseling on ostomy patients' self-concept. Participants cited the following feelings about their experiences: (1) anger at having the ostomy and the change in physical condition, (2) grief and revulsion at losing bowel or bladder control, (3) fears regarding their sexuality, (4) feelings of ugliness because of the presence of the ostomy, and (5) feelings of worthlessness caused by the need for the ostomy. She demonstrated that patients who were counseled with empathetic understanding, positive regard, genuineness, and concreteness (based on the Carkhuff Helping Model) achieved independence and competence in ostomy care, an improved self-concept, and social involvement outside of the home more readily than did a control group. In addition, problem-solving skills were developed to facilitate a positive adaptive response. Thus, attention paid to self-concept (and potential or actual body image disturbances) with provision of counseling and teaching was beneficial for these patients.

The role of the family cannot be overemphasized in terms of sustaining the person with cancer, but this support can be more freely given and be more realistic if the spouse, partner, or significant others are prepared for the patient's changes. It is important to remember that there has to be an ongoing assessment of the family's response to the patient's illness, treatment, and changes. Northouse,[39,40] for example, has documented the need for an ongoing assessment of patients with breast cancer and their husbands. She found that difficulties in psychosocial adjustment are not confined to the early phase of illness but persist over time for both patients and husbands. Spouses need to be involved and informed about ways to support cancer patients' self-esteem. The family must be prepared for any physical changes resulting from cancer or its treatment; it is necessary to help the family avoid displaying fear or revulsion to physical changes that may have occurred. Children can be particularly helpful in this situation if they have a secure and special relationship with the patient. This author has seen grandchildren unconcerned with their grandfather's facial disfigurement after head and neck surgery, responding to the grandparent as the same person they had always known. These positive reactions helped the grandfather more readily adjust to body image changes. Admittedly, some children may be fearful of these changes and avoid the person; such children need guidance and reassurance from the person who has had the radical surgery and body changes. Enlisting members of patients' support systems to validate and reinforce their value and importance is another intervention that may help enhance self-esteem and promote adjustment to changes in body image.[36]

Orienting patients and their families to mutual self-help groups, such as the United Ostomy Association, Reach to Recovery, CanSurMount, and I Can Cope, can be helpful to patients who are adjusting to changes in body image. Sharing their concerns with others who have had similar experiences and have resolved some of their negative reactions to body changes may help patients make their own adjustments. Nurses need to be cautious, however, that they do not force patients to participate in these groups. Not everyone benefits from such activities. Some patients have adequate opportunities to express their concerns with family members and significant friends and do not desire to make their altered body and cancer the focus of their lives by socializing only with others who have similar illnesses.

One of the areas in which psychologic factors such as body image changes and altered self-concept can adversely affect relationships in the family and with significant others is in the area of sexual relationships. A person's perception of his or her body image affects self-esteem and is closely linked to sexuality. Body image changes, therefore, may contribute to feelings of sexual inadequacy.[41]

ALTERATION IN SEXUAL FUNCTIONING

Closely tied to the concepts of self-esteem, self-concept, and body image is the aspect of sexuality. Sexuality, or sexual health is defined by the World Health Organization[42] as the integration of somatic, emotional, intellectual, and social aspects of sexual being in ways that are positively enriching and that enhance personality, communication, and love. Sexuality is concerned with the biologic, psychologic, sociologic, spiritual, and cultural aspects of life. Sexuality has been recognized as a significant part of nursing care of patients with cancer, as documented by the fact that sexuality is the ninth standard developed by the Oncology Nursing Society.[43] Because sexuality is an integral part of living and an essential part of a person's personality and behavior, it should be a significant part of any nursing care plan.[12,44]

Because cancer may threaten a person's biopsychosocial status, oncology nurses often work with patients who have concerns about their sexuality. Cancer and cancer therapy may temporarily or permanently affect behavior used to express sexual identity. Cancer of the bladder, prostate, testes, and penis, for example, may affect libido, erection, orgasm, and ejaculation in the male patient.[32] Sexuality, however, involves more than the single act of intercourse.[44] Changes in appearance and physiologic changes that affect function may cause patients to doubt their masculinity or femininity.[41] Side effects of treatments for cancer may result in anxiety, depression, dependency, and anger, which may interfere with sexual desire and the maintenance of satisfactory relationships. Thus, adverse effects on sexual functioning may occur as a result of the stress associated with the cancer experience itself. Foltz,[23] in her review of studies related to effects of cancer and cancer treatment on sexual aspects of self-concept, concluded that the incidence, magnitude, and duration of sexual dysfunction are mediated by the site of disease, treatment-associated injury determined by disease site, treatment modality, marital status, and age. She further suggests that sexual disability may be determined less by body image alteration (defined as perceived sexual attractiveness) than by other psychosexual and treatment-related physiologic change.

BARRIERS TO INTERVENTIONS FOR SEXUALITY

There are varieties of sexual expression, as well as sexual preferences, so patients must receive the right kind of information for their situation. Concerns about body acceptability, sexual ability, libido, partners' enjoyment, and rejections are not unusual, especially in new relationships. However, persons experiencing cancer and body changes that threaten their sexuality are even more vulnerable to these fears and stresses related to sexual functioning.

Nurses may be reluctant to discuss sexuality with their patients or even to include sexuality as part of assessment. They often do not see sex as a priority topic for discussion with cancer patients compared to information on treatments or medications. They often think patients are too concerned with other health problems to be concerned with sexual issues. Nurses may be uncomfortable discussing sexual matters because they feel inadequately informed or because their beliefs regarding sex may be rigid and they do not think such a discussion is appropriate. They may think that other health professionals can handle this aspect. It may be difficult for nurses to avoid basing their actions on their own values regarding sexuality. They may believe that they do not wish to invade the patient's privacy, since sexuality is very personal and the patient may be offended. Yet, these same nurses may not hesitate to ask patients about other personal factors such as bowel and bladder function or hygiene values and beliefs. Avoiding inquiries into sexuality may give patients the impression that sex is no longer appropriate for them. Nurses need to listen carefully to what their patients say, because they may give subtle cues that indicate a desire to discuss these sexual concerns.

Williams and co-workers[45] studied nurses' attitudes toward sexuality in cancer patients. They found in their sample of 211 registered nurses that only 3% responded "always" and 27% responded "never" to a question concerning how often they had offered to discuss sexual concerns with patients in the past month. "Seldom" or "sometimes" was a common response to this question. Only 19% responded "frequently" or "very frequently." The majority of the nurses in this study did not feel sexual counseling was part of their role or that addressing the sexual needs of cancer patients was a major component of nursing care. These findings draw attention to the need for greater emphasis on sexual aspects in the assessment and care of cancer patients and to the need for educating nurses about sexual issues in the provision of nursing care. Fisher and Levin[46] also investigated the sexual knowledge and attitudes of 120 professional nurses caring for oncology patients. They found that the nurses had significantly lower knowledge scores and more conservative attitudinal scores related to heterosexual relations, masturbation, and abortion than medical students and graduate nurses who had been tested a decade before. This is a surprising finding in an era of increased sexual education and openness about sexuality and reinforces the need to assess nurses for their knowledge and practice regarding sexuality issues.

NURSING CARE ISSUES REGARDING SEXUALITY

Nurses need to be aware of and comfortable with their own sexuality and they need to examine their own values regarding sex and sexuality in order to provide assistance to the patient who is experiencing problems in this area. Nurses should recognize their own biases regarding sexuality to be assured that they are not forcing their own attitudes and biases on the patient or that they are not failing to inform the patient of other options because the options do not fit into their own value systems. Determining whether their values are in conflict with the values of their patients is a necessary process for nurses. If there is a conflict of values, they need to refer these patients to other persons who may be more helpful, rather than omit opportunities for assistance. They cannot deny patients the information they need to function in satisfying sexual relationships. They need to consider the sociocultural factors on which the person's sexual value system is based.[47] Age, religious and ethnic background, education, and specific illness ramifications are factors that should be taken into consideration. Issues on sexual morality are taught differently among different religions, yet members of a specific religious denomination may also have different beliefs and practices.[47] Thus, when nurses identify the religion of their patients, they cannot assume that these patients abide by traditional teachings. Again, it is important to obtain the patient's specific views on these matters and not to act on assumptions.

One of the first ways a nurse can affirm the view that the patient is still a sexual being is to discuss sexual issues with that patient, who may be reluctant to bring up the topic. Bringing up the topic in a matter-of-fact manner acknowledges the patient as a sexual person. The nurse's behavior should communicate to patients that their sexual concerns are respected and justified; nurses must reflect open-mindedness and tolerance, regardless of their personal sexual beliefs and practices.

It is important for nurses to recognize their own preconceived notions about age, gender, and expectations about sexual behavior. Nurses cannot assume that all patients follow their sexual behavior or practices. Nor can they assume that all persons are interested in sex; for example, some persons may not have valued sex previously and may use cancer as an excuse for reducing sexual activity in their relations with their partners. Interviews can be conducted to discover the patient's feelings about sexual aspects of life after experiencing cancer, its treatment, and its effect on him- or herself and his or her families.

It is also important not to make assumptions about sexual preference or behavior, and not to press for information if it is not readily given. Stevens and Hall[48] reviewed studies on the interactions of lesbians with health care providers, finding that lesbians said health care workers were judgmental, nonsupportive, and negatively responsive when their identity as lesbians became known. In fact, these persons often did not identify themselves as lesbians because they feared it would hinder the quality of their health care. They described being responded to with ostracism, invasive personal questioning, shock, embarrassment, and fear, and they also felt that their partners had been mistreated and their confidentiality breached. The respondents also noted that questions asked by health care providers assumed that their female clients were heterosexual, that their partners were male, and that their sexual activity involved intercourse. They often felt "forced to make an announcement" of their lesbian identity. These researchers concluded that lesbians often do not feel comfortable about seeking health care because of experiences with nonempathetic responses when they do and that they even feel at risk of harm in some health care situations. The need for improved understanding of this group is further evident in another study that found lesbian phobia common among female nursing students and that a significant number of the 120 students sampled believed that lesbians were a high-risk group for AIDS.[49]

Sexual concerns are probably most often discussed after ostomy surgery because there is evidence that sexual problems frequently occur after this surgical procedure. Impotence, for example, is a frequent occurrence in patients undergoing abdominoperineal resection for rectal cancer or radical cystectomy. Erectile impotence, the persistent inability to achieve or maintain a penile erection to permit coitus, is of deep concern to male patients after such surgery. Impairment of sexual function also may occur after orchidectomy for treatment of testicular cancer and can have profound effects on self-image, masculinity, and sexual identity.[50] This is particularly significant since cancer of the testicle is the most common malignancy in men between 25 and 34 years of age. Fear of venereal spread of cancer or cancer as a punishment for past sexual conduct and concern about future sexual dysfunction may come to the forefront when patients are allowed to explore sexual concerns.[51]

Gloeckner[52] studied the impact of sexuality and body image disturbances on patients with ostomies and found that 60% of the participants reported that they felt a decrease in sexual attractiveness. It is difficult to separate sexuality from feelings of attractiveness and desirability. The loss of body functions is a source of anxiety about sexual functioning as well as about interpersonal relationships. Fear of sexual or social rejection may be a factor that leads some cancer patients to isolate themselves and avoid taking risks necessary to develop intimate relationships. It should be obvious that to ignore discussions about sexuality with patients who have ostomies is to omit a significant aspect of the nursing care plan.

Less often, more subtle situations can bring about concern for sexuality issues. For example, peripheral neuropathy can result from antineoplastic agents such as vincristine or cisplatin. These drugs can affect sexual functioning because sensations of touch, loss of muscle control and proprioception, and discomfort, as well as loss of strength and endurance, can interfere with sexual activity.[53] For these patients there is a need to identify and use appropriate alternative means of expressing sexuality and receiving sexual pleasure.

Patients who have undergone radical surgery may feel threatened in their self-worth if they sense that caregivers are withdrawing or are uncomfortable about coping with their changes. Patients who have undergone head and neck surgery have described the negative impact of facial appearances on their sexual relationships, citing deficits caused by tongue changes, misshapen mouths, interference by nasogastric tubes, and facial disfigurement.[30] Sexual counseling should focus on helping patients understand their own abilities and disabilities so they can make knowledgeable choices and decisions regarding sexual aspects of their illness. It is important to keep patients from placing undue restrictions on themselves because of having cancer or using cancer as an excuse for insecure relationships.[54]

INTERVENTIONS TO ENHANCE SEXUAL FUNCTIONING

Nurses can educate themselves in the area of sexuality by reviewing films, attending sexuality conferences and workshops, and reading books and journals such as *Medical Aspects of Human Sexuality,* to broaden their knowledge base and views on sexuality. They also need to review or obtain a sound knowledge base in anatomy and physiology of normal sexual responses to be able to understand alterations resulting from cancer and its treatment. Oncology units may benefit their nursing staffs by obtaining the services of a qualified consultant to help nurses cope with the sexual needs of their patients and also to discuss specific issues involving selected patients.

As stated previously, assessment is the first step in determining the need for interventions related to sexuality. This requires interviewing the patient regarding sexual issues. Open-ended and direct questions may be used, along with active listening, reflection techniques, and avoidance of judgmental comments that can close discussions quickly. Table 32-1 provides examples of questions that can be integrated into an overall nursing assessment interview to obtain information on sexuality and sexual concerns. These interviews should begin

TABLE 32-1 Nursing Assessment of Sexuality Issues in the Cancer Patient—Options for Questions*

Goals	Options for Questions
To determine the patient's self-concept and feelings of body image and To determine the extent of stress imposed by symptoms (eg, alopecia, fatigue, etc)	What currently makes you feel good about yourself?[60] How do you see yourself since your surgery or treatment?[41,60] How do you think others see you?[60] Has there been any change in the way you feel about your personal appearance?[58] Do you think there has been any change in you personally since you had your surgery (or were diagnosed with cancer)?[58] Do you see yourself differently as a result of your surgery or cancer treatment?
To provide opportunity for initial discussion regarding effect of cancer on sexuality and To facilitate exploration of sexual concerns	Please describe changes you have made in your life as a result of your cancer. What changes do you anticipate making as a result of having cancer (or cancer surgery)?[58,59] Has treatment affected the way you feel about yourself as a woman? man? Has the cancer (or treatment) interfered with you being a mother, father, or spouse? How has the diagnosis of cancer altered how you feel about being a young man or young woman?[56] Some other single women who have had a mastectomy (or other surgery) often have concerns about how they will handle telling significant men in their lives about the mastectomy (or other surgery). They have been reluctant to start new relationships. How do you think you would handle this if it should happen to you? Has treatment affected your roles as a wife, mother, or worker? (husband, father, worker?)[55] How has your cancer, surgery, treatment, affected your relationships (eg, with spouse, significant other, family, children)?
To obtain specific information on patient's sexual interest, practices, and concerns	Have you had any difficulties in sexual relationships prior to getting this diagnosis? Has this changed any since your diagnosis/treatment? Other patients often wonder if there will be changes in their sexual relationships with their spouse after this type of surgery/treatment. Tell me a little about the place that sexuality has in your relationship with your spouse or significant other.[51] Some couples have intercourse every day, some a couple of times a week, and still others not at all. About how often do you have intercourse?[57] Frequently, men are concerned about sexual activity after a prostatectomy (or other surgery). How has the cancer diagnosis affected your sex life so far?[51] Are you currently active with a partner? How often do the two of you have some sexual activity together?[51] Have you had changes in your breast tissue or breast sensation since radiation therapy that may have had an effect on satisfaction with foreplay or intercourse?[59] Has your sexual activity changed during treatment?[55] Have you experienced a change in sexual desire, excitement, or orgasm?[55] Do you have difficulty obtaining or maintaining an erection?

*These are options for questions or comments to facilitate discussion with the patient. The nurse varies the order or choice of question, depending on the comfort level of the nurse and the patient with each other as well as with the type of question. The nurse needs to observe the patient's appearance, body language (including posture and tone of voice), and any change in affect such as withdrawal, crying, or inappropriate responses or unwillingness to discuss questions. The nurse should note the language the patient uses in sexual discussion. If a specific problem is identified, then questions explore the onset, history of the problem, and perceptions about the cause and treatment events.

with the least sensitive sexual matters, usually starting with general questions.[51] The interview and the specific questions asked should be based on the patient's specific diagnosis and treatment issues likely to affect sexuality, on the type of relationship the nurse has with the patient, and on how comfortable the nurse is in seeking information on sexuality. For example, when an atmosphere of trust and comfort has been created, discussions of the more intimate aspects of sexuality can begin.[17] Determining the patient's views on sexuality can clear the air for further discussions or for referral to other experts who may be able to handle the specific problem or issue more effectively. Assessment also includes an awareness of the appropriate time for counseling; a sexual issue may arise earlier than when the nurse planned to discuss the issue. During assessment of knowledge and attitudes, teaching strategies can be used to clarify information, provide facts, and dispel myths. Such misconceptions may include, for example, the belief that cancer is transmitted sexually or that sex causes cancer.[55]

A sexual-adjustment questionnaire (SAQ), originally designed for use with head and neck patients, has been modified for use with other postsurgical patients.[61] The information gained from use of the SAQ may help clarify the kinds and frequency of sexual problems experienced by cancer patients and identify patients at higher risk of postoperative sexual problems. Another assessment tool, titled by its acronym BASIC ID, has been used by Fontaine[62] to assess behavior, affect, sensation, imagery, cognition, interpersonal relationships, and drugs in assessment for sexual concerns or problems.

When it is expected that the cancer and its treatment are likely to affect sexual functioning, a thorough assessment requires the nurse to determine the patient's level of understanding about sexual functions in general and to learn how important sexual functioning is in the person's life. The nurse should take into consideration the patient's previous level of sexual activity and ascertain previous methods of sexual expression.[54] Nurses may erroneously assume that older patients do not consider sexuality an important element in their lives; they may learn later that, in reality, sexuality was a major concern and actually required attention that was not provided. It is important to listen to the patient's real concerns.[54] For example, in older patients, sexuality may mean close companionship, opportunities to touch and be touched, body image, or sexual intercourse and making love.[63] Just as it is inappropriate to avoid sexual discussions, it is also inappropriate to make assumptions about the person's sexual status and to emphasize sexual activities to a patient who has placed minimal significance on sexual activity in the past.[12] Some patients may not wish to discuss their sexual views or behavior, and they should not be forced to do so.

Mobility limitations, positioning, changes in body image, and increased dependence on others for hygiene and personal care are all factors that affect the patient's confidence in sexual relationships.[54] Patients who are undergoing chemotherapy may not have the energy to engage in even limited sexual activities. Fatigue and other symptoms may interfere with sexual relationships when, for example, the patient is too fatigued and weak and unable to be a partner in the sexual act. Couples can be advised that intimacy can be expressed by close body contact, lying together, showing caring feelings, and touching; sexual intercourse is not the only expression of sexual experience. Leiber and co-workers[64] studied 38 patients receiving chemotherapy for advanced cancer and found that patients and spouses of both sexes experienced simultaneously an increase in desire for physical closeness (e.g., simple proximity, holding hands, embracing, and kissing) and a decrease in the desire for sexual intercourse.

Alterations in sexual patterns can result from the cancer or its symptomology, or from its treatment (e.g., chemotherapy or radiation), or they may occur when there is a change in appearance after surgery that affects the person's body image and self-concept. Feminization resulting from hormonal therapy, for example, may have a negative effect on body image of the male patient and result in a decreased desire for sexual activities.

Assessment requires investigation into a patient's perspectives on how illness will affect or has affected sexuality and how the patient and significant others have responded to these changes. To determine any other possible causes of alterations in sexual function, questions should be raised regarding medications that the patient is taking. For example, large amounts or chronic use of cocaine, narcotics, or marijuana inhibit sexual performance, and alcohol in large amounts inhibits performance and desire. In addition, antihypertensive agents, tranquilizers, sedatives, antidepressants, some antihistamines, and some antispasmotics are known to affect sexual functioning.[65] Awareness of the effects of specific drugs and specific illnesses on sexuality is essential if the nurse is to ask appropriate questions in any sexual assessment.

Timing of counseling on sexuality varies; for some persons it may be an immediate concern, while for others the diagnosis, the prognosis, and the surgical procedure have to be assimilated before the patient is ready to discuss sexual concerns.[66] This author recalls a female, middle-aged patient whose first question of the nurse after an emergency transverse colostomy was "Will this affect my having sex?" The depth of discussions should be guided by the patient's needs at the specific time. Another patient with familial polyposis refused to have surgery, in spite of the fact that his father had died of colon cancer and he had been informed of the definite likelihood of his having cancer if surgery and an ileostomy were not performed, when he learned that his sexual functioning might be altered by the surgical procedure.

Sexual Counseling

The PLISSIT model, a commonly used model for sexual counseling, consists of four levels of interventions.

Permission, limited information, specific suggestions, and intensive therapy are the levels that form the acronym, P-LI-SS-IT.[67] As implied in their names, the first three tend to require brief therapy, whereas the last requires longer and more intensive therapy. Nurses usually can assist patients with the first three levels of interventions, but the last level requires more expertise unless they have had additional education and experience. Zalar[68] believes that the graduate professional nurse should be able to competently assist patients with needs involving permission and limited information because the interventions are viewed as preventive. Nurses may be better able than other health professionals to establish the trusting relationships necessary for brief sexual counseling, because of their frequent and lengthy contacts with patients and their families in hospitals and communities.[68]

It is appropriate to refer patients to other nurses or other personnel at any of the levels if the nurse is not comfortable with dealing with the needs of patients or believes that someone else may be able to respond to the patient more effectively. Nurses need to recognize their abilities, limitations, biases, and knowledge bases in working with patients and to determine which level of sexual counseling is needed for specific patients.

Permission

At the first level of counseling the nurse creates a permissive atmosphere or introduces the topic of sexual concerns in such a way as to suggest that it is one that can be discussed. Permission is first promoted when the nurse asks a patient about sexual concerns or suggests that it is an appropriate topic for discussion. This level indicates to the patient that sexual concerns are normal and expected. Providing time to discuss sexual concerns is an appropriate activity at this level. In the case of the cancer patient, it is characterized by discussion of the impact of cancer and treatment on sexuality. An attitude is conveyed that sexual concerns, needs, and feelings related to sexual function are appropriate for discussion and that the nurse is willing to discuss these aspects with the patient, spouse, or significant other. Active listening on the part of the nurse helps the patient explore the problem.

Limited information

The second level of counseling continues to convey the willingness to discuss sexuality, but, in addition, the nurse provides information to help clarify concerns the patient may have as well as to eliminate myths and misconceptions. Anticipated changes related to the surgery or other treatments are aspects to be discussed, with provision of specific suggestions for actions. For example, fear of hurting the patient or making the cancer worse (especially when the genitalia are involved in the cancer) is often an area of concern that needs clarification. Information about results of surgery (for example, the loss of vaginal lubrication associated with menopause that results from bilateral oophorectomy) is warranted. If surgery or other therapy causes loss of sensation in essential areas, the couple may require more information on how to continue to enjoy physical intimacy. In cases in which sexual intercourse is no longer possible, patients and partners can be helped to recognize the importance and effectiveness of touching and caressing. It is important to encourage open communication and honest sharing of feelings and concerns between partners so that patients can let partners know their desires and fears and to allow enough time for both partners to become accustomed to the loss of a body part or change in appearance.[12,54]

Specific suggestions

The third level of sexual counseling is appropriate when support and limited information are not adequate for the particular patient. Specific suggestions are given and followed up to monitor their effectiveness. For example, a patient who is paraplegic as a result of a spinal tumor needs specific information about management of the urinary catheter and preparation for sexual intercourse, depending on the level of injury and whether the patient is a female or male. The use of sexual foreplay, erotic literature, alternatives to vaginal intercourse, and masturbation and the finding of other effective erogenous zones on the body may be discussed as a means for a couple to achieve sexual gratification. Any interventions that are recommended, however, should be within the framework of the patient's religious and spiritual beliefs and cultural practices to avoid inciting distrust and distress in the patient and partner.[47] This requires nurses to intervene with sensitivity, compassion, and respect for beliefs and values that may be different from their own. Suggestions about changing positions to increase comfort or decrease fatigue are another aspect to discuss. It is important to be sensitive in discussing alternate methods, because some couples will not wish to have this information and may think it is inappropriate.

There are several strategies for enhancing sexual expression after the patient and partner express their goals for sexual activity. For some, increasing their willingness to communicate their feelings about sexual activity with the partner may be sufficient to help the couple work together to resolve the issues. Other partners may need encouragement to experiment with various methods, such as fantasy, activation of erogenous zones, changing positions, and finding alternative methods to achieve sexual satisfaction. For some patients, teaching ways to stimulate and maintain erections or referral for penile implants may be an appropriate intervention. Others may benefit from planned schedules to capitalize on times of peak energy for sexual pleasure. Patients can be advised to use alternate positions so that they can choose the position that requires the least expenditure of energy. Advising the use of water-based lubrication for the woman who has had surgery, chemotherapy, or radiation therapy that interferes with vaginal lubrication is helpful. For the patient with an ostomy, guidance on managing ostomy appliances to prevent leakage during sexual activity and ways to avoid odor and noise from the stoma may be the appropriate intervention.

Intensive therapy

The fourth level requires referral when adequate progress is not being made at the other levels and when more depth in counseling is needed for complex problems. Nurses should recognize when there is a need for more competent and expert sexual therapists to obtain adequate and appropriate support for the patient and partner. Referral to a qualified therapist can be one of the nurse's most important actions.[66] Intensive therapy may be necessary to deal with sexual problems that existed prior to the cancer experience. Extensive psychologic counseling may be necessary, for example, when reconstructive surgery of genitalia is needed or when the use of prosthetic devices, such as penile implants, may be necessary.

The level of the nurse's participation in the PLISSIT model is based on the nurse's knowledge, experience, and own comfort level with sexual discussions. Shipes and Lehr[32] propose that approximately 70% of all sexual concerns can be dealt with in all types of settings by nurses using the first three levels (P-LI-SS) of the model and that the remaining 30% require referral to a qualified therapist for intensive therapy (IT). However, the nurse should be careful not to delve into alternate methods of sexual experiences without gaining permission from the patient. A full assessment of the couple's attitudes is necessary to determine their values and comfort level. Some expectations regarding alternate methods may be threatening to some couples; in some cases the discussion is inappropriate and can actually increase the sexual concerns of the couple. Keen sensitivity to the needs of individual patients is extremely important. A knowledgeable, nonjudgmental nurse with good communication skills can play an important role, through effective sexual counseling, in enhancing a patient's quality of life.[50,60]

CONCLUSION

In this time of shorter hospital stays, increased demand on nurses, increased acuity of hospitalized patients, and the intensity of the clinical setting, there needs to be an increased awareness of psychosocial needs of patients in the area of body image and sexuality if quality care is to be achieved. For continuity of care, nurses must relay areas of concern to those providing follow-up care. If these issues are not adequately addressed in the hospital situation, they should at least not be lost to future health care givers. Since cancer patients are surviving for longer periods, it is important for nurses to include more interventions regarding the aspects of adjustment to body image and altered sexual functioning related to cancer in order to improve the quality of their lives.

Research is needed to determine the relationship between cancer and its treatment and the impact on body image and sexuality. Research is also needed to develop effective techniques for assessing those persons at high risk of body image disturbances and sexual difficulties. These techniques will be helpful in identifying those persons who are most vulnerable and in need of specific interventions. Research into the most helpful approaches and interventions for working with patients with body image disturbances and sexual dysfunction will be valuable in improving the quality of life of our patients with cancer.

REFERENCES

1. Carlson CE: Psychosocial aspects of neurological disability. *Nurs Clin North Am* 15:309–320, 1980.
2. Klopp AR: Body image and self-concept among individuals with stomas. *J Enterostom Ther* 17(3):98–105, 1990.
3. Norris CM: Body image: Its relevance to professional nursing. In Carlson CE, Blackwell B (eds), *Behavioral Concepts and Nursing Interventions* (2d ed). Philadelphia: Lippincott, 1978, pp. 5–36.
4. Schilder P: *The Image and Appearance of the Human Body.* London: Kagan, Paul, Trench, Trubner, 1935.
5. Bramble K: Body image. In Lubkin IM, *Chronic Illness Impact and Interventions* (2d ed). Boston: Jones and Bartlett, 1990, pp. 218–231.
6. Altabe MN: The social cognition of body image: Validity of the body image construct (self perception) (doct. diss.). University of South Florida, 1991.
7. Secord PF, Jourard SM: The appraisal of body cathexis: Body cathexis and the self. *J Consult Psychol* 17:343–347, 1953.
8. Fawcett J, Frye S: An exploratory study of body image dimensionality. *Nurs Res* 29:324–327, 1980.
9. Brown TA, Cash TF, Mikulka PJ: Attitudinal body image assessment: Factor analysis of the Body-Self Relations Questionnaire. *J Pers Assessment* 55:135–144, 1990.
10. Franzoi SL, Shields, SA: The Body Esteem Scale: Multidimensional structure and sex differences in a college population. *J Pers Assessment* 48:173–178, 1984.
11. Shipes E: Psychosocial issues: The person with an ostomy. *Nurs Clin North Am* 22:291–302, 1987.
12. Dudas S: Psychosocial aspects of patient care. In Smith D, Johnson DE (eds), *Ostomy Care and the Cancer Patient,* Orlando, FL: Grune & Stratton, 1986, pp. 93–102.
13. Frank-Stromborg M, Wright P: Ambulatory cancer patients' perception of the physical and psychosocial changes in their lives since the diagnosis of cancer. *Cancer Nurs* 7:117–130, 1984.
14. Dudas S, Carlson CE: Cancer rehabilitation: Implications for nursing. *Oncol Nurs Forum* 15:183–188, 1988.
15. Kriss R: Self image and sexuality after mastectomy. In Bullard DG, Knight SE (eds), *Sexuality and Physical Disability: Personal Perspectives.* St. Louis, MO: Mosby, 1981, pp. 185–192.

16. Wellisch DK: The psychologic impact of breast cancer on relationships. *Semin Oncol Nurs* 1:196–199, 1985.
17. Schover LR: The impact of breast cancer on sexuality, body image and intimate relationships. *CA* 41:112–120, 1991.
18. Loveys BJ, Klaich K: Breast cancer: Demands of illness. *Oncol Nurs Forum* 18:75–80, 1991.
19. Knobf MKT: Primary breast cancer. Physical consequences and rehabilitation. *Semin Oncol Nurs* 1:214–224, 1985.
20. Rutherford DR: Assessing psychosexual needs of women experiencing lumpectomy: A challenge for research. *Cancer Nurs* 11:244–249, 1988.
21. Fallowfield LJ, Baum M, Maguire GP: Effects of breast conservation on psychological morbidity associated with diagnosis and treatment of early breast cancer. *Brit Med J* 293:1331–1334, 1986.
22. Wainstock JM: Breast cancer: Psychosocial consequences for the patient. *Semin Oncol Nurs* 7:207–215, 1991.
23. Foltz AT: The influence of cancer on self-concept and life quality. *Semin Oncol Nurs* 3:303–312, 1987.
24. Schain WS, Wellisch DK, Pasnau RO, et al: The sooner the better: A study of psychological factors in women undergoing immediate versus delayed breast reconstruction. *Am J Psychiatry* 142:40–46, 1985.
25. Winder AE, Winder BD: Clarifying a woman's choice for breast reconstruction. *Patient Educ Counsel* 7:65–75, 1985.
26. Knobf MT, Stahl R: Reconstructive surgery in primary breast cancer treatment. *Semin Oncol Nurs* 7:200–206, 1991.
27. Metzger D: TREE. Oakland, CA: Wingbow Press, 1983.
28. Dropkin MJ, Malgady RG, Scott DW, et al: Scaling of disfigurement and dysfunction in postoperative head and neck patients. *Head Neck Surg* 6:559–570, 1983.
29. Dropkin MJ: Coping with disfigurement and dysfunction after head and neck cancer surgery: A conceptual framework. *Semin Oncol Nurs* 5:213–219, 1989.
30. Metcalfe MC, Fischman SH: Factors affecting the sexuality of patients with head and neck cancer. *Oncol Nurs Forum* 12:21–25, 1985.
31. Dropkin MJ: Rehabilitation after disfigurative facial surgery. *Plast Surg Nurs* Winter:130–134, 1985.
32. Shipes E, Lehr S: Sexuality and the male cancer patient. *Cancer Nurs* 5:375–381, 1982.
33. Tomaselli N, Jenks J, Morin KH: A longitudinal study of body image changes in ostomy patients. Poster presented at International Association Enterostomal Therapists 24th Annual Conference, Las Vegas, 1992.
34. Oberst MT, Scott DW: Post discharge distress in surgically treated cancer patients and their spouses. *Res Nurs Health* 11:223–233, 1988.
35. Baxley KO, Erdman LK, Henry EB, et al: Alopecia: Effect on cancer patients' body image. *Cancer Nurs* 7:499–503, 1984.
36. Feldman JE: Ovarian failure and cancer treatment: Incidence and interventions for the premenopausal woman. *Oncol Nurs Forum* 16:651–657, 1989.
37. Watson PG: The effects of short-term post-operative counseling on cancer/ostomy patients. *Cancer Nurs* 6:21–29, 1983.
38. Watson PG: Postoperative counseling for cancer ostomy patients. *J Enterost Ther* 10:84–91, 1983.
39. Northouse L: A longitudinal study of the adjustment of patients and husbands to breast cancer. *Oncol Nurs Forum* 16:511–515, 1989.
40. Northouse LL, Cracchiolo-Caraway A, Appel CP: Psychologic consequences of breast cancer on partner and family. *Semin Oncol Nurs* 7:216–223, 1991.
41. Cooley ME, Cobb SC: Sexual and reproductive issues: Hodgkin's disease Part I. *Cancer Nurs* 9:189–193, 1986.
42. World Health Organization Technical Report Series (No. 572): *Education and Treatment in Human Sexuality: The Training of Health Professionals.* Geneva: World Health Organization, 1975.
43. Oncology Nursing Society and American Nurses' Association, Division on Medical-Surgical Nursing Practice: *Outcome Standards for Cancer Nursing Practice,* Washington, DC: American Nurses' Association, 1979.
44. Smith D: Sexual rehabilitation of the cancer patient. *Cancer Nurs* 12:10–15, 1989.
45. Williams HA, Wilson ME, Hongladarom G, et al: Nurses' attitudes toward sexuality in cancer patients. *Oncol Nurs Forum* 13:39–43, 1986.
46. Fisher SG, Levin DL: The sexual knowledge and attitudes of professional nurses caring for oncology patients. *Cancer Nurs* 6:55–58, 1983.
47. Hogan RM: Influences of culture on sexuality. *Nurs Clin North Am* 17:365–375, 1982.
48. Stevens PE, Hall JM: Stigma, health beliefs and experiences with health care in lesbian women. *IMAGE* 20:69–73, 1988.
49. Eliason MJ, Randall CE: Lesbian phobia in nursing students. *West J Nurs Res* 13:363–374, 1991.
50. Blakemore C: The impact of orchidectomy upon the sexuality of the man with testicular cancer. *Cancer Nurs* 11:33–40, 1988.
51. Schover LR: Sexual rehabilitation of the ostomy patient. In Smith D, Johnson DE (eds), *Ostomy Care and the Cancer Patient.* Orlando, FL: Grune & Stratton, 1986, pp. 103–119.
52. Gloeckner MR: Perceptions of sexual attractiveness following ostomy surgery. *Res Nurs Health* 7:87–92, 1984.
53. Holden S, Felde G: Nursing care of patients experiencing cisplatin-related peripheral neuropathy. *Oncol Nurs Forum* 14:13–19, 1987.
54. Dudas S: Rehabilitation concepts of nursing. *J Enterost Ther* 11:6–15, 1984.
55. Cooley ME, Yeomans AC, Cobb S: Sexual and reproductive issues for women with Hodgkin's disease II. Application of PLISSIT model. *Cancer Nurs* 9:248–255, 1986.
56. Klopovich PM, Clancy BJ: Sexuality and the adolescent with cancer. *Oncol Nurs Forum* 1:42–48, 1985.
57. MacElveen-Hoehn P: Sexual assessment and counseling. *Semin Oncol Nurs* 1:69–75, 1985.
58. Morris CA: Self-concept as altered by the diagnosis of cancer. *Nurs Clin North Am* 20:611–630, 1985.
59. Schwarz-Appelbaum SI, Dedrick I, Jusenius K, et al: Nursing care plans: Sexuality and treatment of breast cancer. *Oncol Nurs Forum* 11:16–24, 1984.
60. Swanson B, Cronin-Stubbs D, Sheldon JA: The impact of psychosocial factors on adapting to physical disability: A review of the research literature. *Rehabil Nurs* 14:64–68, 1989.
61. Waterhouse J, Metcalfe MC: Development of the Sexual Adjustment Questionnaire. *Oncol Nurs Forum* 13:53–59, 1986.
62. Fontaine KL: Unlocking sexual issues. Counseling strategies for nurses. *Nurs Clin North Am* 26:737–743, 1991.
63. Allen ME: A holistic view of sexuality and the aged. *Holistic Nurs Pract* 1:76–83, 1987.
64. Leiber L, Plumb MM, Gerstenzang ML, et al: The com-

munication of affection between cancer patients and their spouses. *Psychosom Med* 38:379–388, 1976.

65. Woods NF: Toward a holistic perspective of human sexuality: Alterations in sexual health and nursing diagnoses. *Holistic Nurs Pract* 1:1–11, 1987.
66. Shipes E: Sexual function following ostomy surgery. *Nurs Clin North Am* 22:303–310, 1987.
67. Annon JS: The PLISSIT Model: A proposed conceptual scheme for the behavioral treatment of sexual problems. *J Sex Educ Ther* 2:1–15, 1976.
68. Zalar MK: Role preparation for nurses in human sexual functioning. *Nurs Clin North Am* 17:351–363, 1982.

Chapter 33

Integumentary and Mucous Membrane Alterations

Michelle Goodman, RN, MS, OCN

Lori A. Ladd, RN, MSN

Sandra Purl, RN, MS, OCN

INTRODUCTION

The effects of radiation therapy and chemotherapy on the skin and mucous membranes can be profound. The oncology nurse is commonly faced with the challenge of deciding how to minimize and manage these complications of treatment. This chapter focuses on how and why these complications occur and common management strategies. In addition, because this chapter deals primarily with the skin and measures to promote healing, chemotherapy drug extravasation and the management of malignant ulcerating wounds will be discussed.

ANATOMY AND PHYSIOLOGY

Integument

Skin

The skin is the largest organ of the body, receiving approximately one-third of the heart's oxygenated blood. The skin is composed of three layers: the impermeable multilayered epidermis; a tough, durable but porous layer called the dermis; and a lipid, rich, deep layer called the subcutaneous tissue (Figure 33-1).

The epidermis is a stratified (multilayer) squamous epithelium that arises from the outer germ layer, the ectoderm. The epidermis forms a resistant surface cover and permeability barrier of varying thickness in different parts of the body. For example, the epidermis on the palms of the hands and the soles of the feet is usually thicker than the epidermis in other parts of the body. The epidermis renews itself continuously through cell division in its deepest layer (basal layer) and undergoes keratinization to produce scales that are shed from the outer layer (stratum corneum). It is avascular, receiving its nutrient support from the underlying dermis.

The epidermis is separated from the dermis by an anatomic dermal-epidermal junction that welds the two layers together. This interface, consisting primarily of dermal papilla, gives support to the basal cells of the epidermis and acts as a barrier to the movement of inflammatory and neoplastic cells between the dermis and epidermis.

The dermis lies between the epidermis and subcutaneous adipose tissue. It gives the skin its strength, elasticity, and softness. The dermis protects deeper structures from injury and contains blood vessels that regulate body temperature and provide nourishment to the epidermis. The dermis also interacts with the epidermis during wound repair.

The subcutaneous tissue lies beneath the dermis and is composed primarily of adipose tissue that serves as a cushion to physical trauma, an insulator to temperature change, and an energy reservoir. Nerves, blood vessels, and lymphatics that serve the skin course through this tissue.

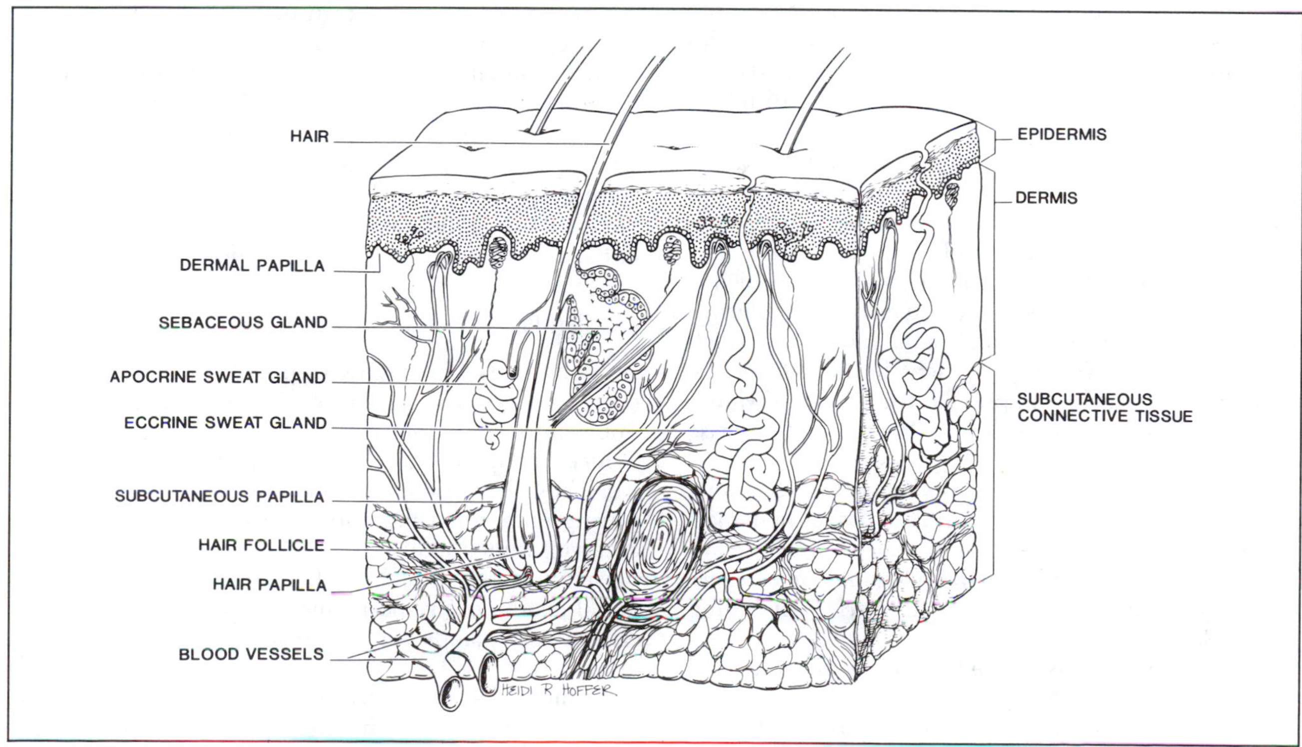

FIGURE 33-1 The structures of the skin.

The functions of the skin are many and include protection, regulation of body temperature, sensory perception, and vitamin D production, which is necessary for bone and teeth formation. In addition, the skin contains an interactive system of immunologic elements including dermal lymphocytes, mast cells, mononuclear phagocytes, and Langerhans cells, which provide an active system of immunologic defense.[1]

Intact skin is the first line of defense against bacteria and foreign substances, physical trauma, heat, or rays. If this barrier is weakened for any reason, permeability to bacteria, drugs, rays, and so on is increased. Protection against the environment is accomplished by (1) eccrine gland sweating, (2) insulation by the skin and the subcutaneous tissue, (3) regulation of cutaneous blood flow (vasoconstriction and vasodilation), and (4) muscle activity (e.g., shivering). Receptors for heat, cold, pain, and touch are present in the skin, making it possible for the skin to receive sensory stimuli. Another function of the skin is excretion. For example, loss of water and salt through excessive sweating is important for maintaining water balance in the body. Finally, because the skin is the part of the body visible to others, it is a way of communicating feelings and is involved in an individual's body image. The appendages of the skin are the hair, nails, apocrine and eccrine sweat glands, and sebaceous glands. The anatomy and physiology of each appendage will be discussed briefly.

Hair

Hair, a product of the epidermis, is composed of tightly fused keratinized cells. Hairs are distributed widely over all body surfaces, being absent only on the lips, palms of the hands, soles of the feet, and nipples of the breast. Hair varies in thickness, length, and color in different parts of the body and among different people.

Each body hair develops from a hair follicle (a follicular involution of the epidermis). The full portion of the hair projecting from the surface of the skin is the hair shaft; the portion under the skin is the hair root. At the base of the root is the hair bulb, which is lodged in the hair follicle. At the hair bulb the dermis pushes up to form the dermal papilla, through which the blood and nerve supply reach the hair. Over the surfaces of the dermal papilla lie the rapidly dividing stem cells (regeneration time of 24 hours) that give rise to the hair.

Hair growth and loss in humans occurs randomly so that hair loss is continuous, unlike in other mammals in which hair growth and loss are seasonal. There are three phases in the hair growth cycle: anagen, catagen, and telogen. Duration of each phase varies depending on body location of hair.

The *anagen phase* is the metabolically active period involving the growth of a hair from a follicle. The average hair root produces 0.35 mm of hair shaft daily, or 1 cm in 28 days. An average of 85%–90% of scalp hairs are in this anagen growth phase at any one time, but this may vary from 35%–100%. Scalp hair remains in anagen for 2–6 years, or an average of 3 years.[2] Approximately 3% of scalp hairs enter the *catagen,* or transitional, *phase* at any one time. Hair growth is slow or intermittent during this 2- to 3-week period in which involution of the hair root occurs. During the *telogen,* or resting, *phase,* all activity ceases. About 12% of scalp hairs are in this phase, which lasts approximately 3 months. It is normal to lose 25–100 telogen hairs each day and even more when the hair is washed.

In contrast to scalp hair, hairs located elsewhere on the body (legs, eyelashes, pubic area) have a shorter anagen phase and longer catagen and telogen phases, which explains why these hairs remain short. For example, the eyebrows actively grow for up to 30–60 days and then rest for approximately 105 days.

The function of hair is both physical and psychosocial in humans. Physically, hair plays a less important role in humans than in most mammals by protecting the surface of the skin and offering temperature regulation by conserving body heat. Specifically, scalp hair decreases exposure of the scalp to ultraviolet rays and minimizes loss of body heat from the head. Eyelashes and hairs lining the nose and ears act as filters to dust and other air-borne contaminants.

Psychologically, hair contributes greatly to body image and is closely associated with secondary sexual characteristics.

Nails

The nail is a specialized epidermal structure made of keratinized cells cemented together. Specifically, nails are modifications of the stratum corneum and lucidum of the epidermis. Nails are found on the dorsal surfaces of the terminal phalanges of the fingers and toes. They rest on the nail bed, composed of the germinal layer of the epidermis and underlying dermis. The visible part of the nail, called the *body,* is highly vascular, resulting in the pink color seen through the semitransparent structure. The nail shapes the fingers and greatly enhances the coordinated fine motion of the finger.

Glands

In humans there are two types of sweat glands: apocrine and eccrine. Apocrine glands have a duct that opens into a hair follicle, whereas eccrine glands have a duct that opens onto the skin surface independent of a hair follicle. Most of the apocrine sweat glands regress during embryonal life and are found only in limited areas in adults: axillae, nipples, periumbilical region, perineum, and genitalia. These glands become functional just before puberty and atrophy with age. Apocrine sweat glands are odiferous and increase evaporative heat loss.[3]

Some 1.6–4 million eccrine sweat glands are present over the entire body. These glands are especially plentiful in the palms, soles, and axillae and least abundant on the back. The main function of these glands is to cool the body through secretion and evaporation of water. Eccrine sweat glands secrete a thin watery solution, primarily composed of sodium chloride and some sulfates, phosphates, and urea, known as perspiration.

The sebaceous glands are small, sacculated granular organs located in the dermis. Although not grossly visible, sebaceous glands are found in most parts of the skin, particularly on the face, scalp, upper chest, and back. They are not found on the palms or soles. The size and number of sebaceous glands vary from area to area. Each gland opens directly into a hair follicle and is lined by a cuboidal epithelium. Sebaceous glands continually secrete a mixture of fat, fatty acids, and cell remnants called *sebum* that is emptied into the hair shaft. Sebum keeps the skin and hair lubricated, pliable, and waterproof.

Mucous Membranes

Epithelial membranes are formed in the body by epithelia combined with connective tissue. The major epithelial membranes are the serous membranes, mucous membranes, and the cutaneous membrane or skin. Serous membranes line the body cavities that do not open to the exterior, such as organs of the respiratory, digestive, excretory, and reproductive tracts. The skin is continuous with the mucous membranes. The function of the mucous membranes depends on their location in the body but may include absorption, transport, or secretion of mucus for lubrication of tissue surfaces. The rapidly proliferating cells of the epithelial layer of the mucous membranes make these membranes sensitive to the effects of both radiation and chemotherapy.

The oral mucosa is the body organ that forms a continuous lining of the oral cavity from the mucocutaneous junction of the lips to the oropharynx. The oral mucosa separates the interior of the oral cavity from the complex underlying organs. Because the oral mucosa is exposed to an aggressive environment in which injury and cell death are everyday occurrences, the epithelial lining of the mucosa constantly renews itself, with cell production meeting cell replacement needs. Maintenance of the integrity of the oral mucosa depends on continuous stem cell replication at the basement membrane. Epithelial cells produced at the basement membrane migrate upward to the mucosal surfaces to replace cells lost as a result of normal sloughing. Complete replacement of the epithelial layer occurs approximately every 7 days.

The mucous membranes of the oral mucosa play a vital role in maintaining homeostasis. The primary function of the oral mucosa is to provide a first line of defense against infection. This is accomplished primarily by the epithelial lining of the mucosa. If, however, the integrity of the mucosa is altered and does not succeed in barring unwanted substances, the lamina propria of the connective tissue provides a second line of defense. Similar to the skin, the oral mucosa can both receive and transmit stimuli from the environment (e.g., heat, cold, pain, touch, and pressure). Sensory innervation of the oral mucosa is provided largely by the connective tissue component.

ALTERATIONS TO THE INTEGUMENT

Radiation Effects

The skin-sparing capabilities of newer megavoltage, high-energy equipment, and sophisticated treatment planning methods have reduced the incidence of severe tissue complications once associated with radiation therapy. However, certain acute and late side effects of radiation occur due to the effects of radiation on normal tissue and are, for the most part, expected and unavoidable.

The major effect of radiation on dividing cells is reproductive death, which leaves the cell unable to produce viable progeny capable of reproduction. The radiosensitivity of cells determines the degree to which they will be susceptible to injury from radiation as well as when that injury will manifest itself. Cells in a renewal system with rapid turnover and having little or no differentiation (e.g., skin cells, mucous membranes, hematopoietic stem cells) are radiosensitive. Cells that do not divide regularly or at all and are highly differentiated (e.g., muscle cells, nerve cells) are radioresistant. Damage from radiation is apparent early, within weeks to months of first exposure, in radiosensitive cells and is classified as an acute effect of radiation. In contrast, radioresistant cells may not manifest damage for months to years after exposure to radiation. These effects are classified as late effects of radiation.[4–6]

Acute effects of radiation are usually considered temporary, as the normal cells affected are often capable of repair. Late radiation effects are usually permanent and often become more severe as time goes on. The severity of acute and late effects are dependent upon dose-time-volume factors.[7] Higher doses given over shorter periods of time to larger volumes of tissue will result in more severe acute reactions. Acute damage results from the depletion of actively proliferating parenchymal or stromal cells and is characterized by vascular dilation, local edema, and inflammation. The severity of late effects is more dependent upon the total dose delivered and the volume of tissue irradiated.[8] It appears that damage to endothelial or connective tissue results in late effects that occur as a result of narrowing or occlusion of small vasculature and fibrosis.[4,5]

It is important to note that the presence or severity of acute effects cannot be used to predict late effects of radiation. Late reactions such as tissue necrosis or dense tissue fibrosis can occur independently of acute reactions.

Side effects from radiation therapy, both acute and late, are local. That is, only those tissues within the irradiated area will be affected. The following discussion will focus on specific tissues of the integument and mucous membranes, their response to radiation, and symptom management.

Acute radiation skin effects

Rarely can radiation treatments be delivered to a target without first penetrating the skin and its supporting connective tissue. The cells of the skin are highly radiosensitive due to their rapidly proliferating cell population. Maintenance of the skin's integrity depends on the consistent rate of mitotic reproduction in the basal cell layers. Radiation disrupts this balance, resulting in alterations in the skin's integrity.

The acute skin reactions associated with radiation therapy include erythema, dry desquamation, pruritis, hyperpigmentation, and moist desquamation (Table 33-1).[5,6,9–13] Not all patients will experience all degrees of skin reaction, and many will have several occur simultaneously. For example, brisk erythema may surround patches of moist desquamation or moist and dry desquamation may exist in adjacent areas being treated with photon and electron beams (see Figures 33-2 to 33-4—Plates 1–3, respectively).

Several factors determine the degree, onset, and duration of radiation-induced skin reactions.[4,6,8,10–12]

1. *Dose-time-volume factors:* Higher doses given over shorter periods of time to larger volumes will result in more severe acute skin reactions.

2. *Equipment:* The energy or particular beam quality of a machine will influence the surface or skin dose. Electrons will produce greater skin reactions than photons. Electron therapy is often used to deliver high doses to superficial structures such as skin lesions, chest wall recurrence of breast cancer, and dermal lymphatics.

3. *Bolus material:* Placing tissue-equivalent material on the skin reduces the skin-sparing effect of radiation therapy, allowing for maximum dose at the level of the skin. This approach is used to treat chest wall recurrence.

4. *Tangential fields:* This approach is used to deliver a more homogeneous dose to the treatment area, but it simultaneously increases the skin dose. This approach is used in the treatment of breast cancer.

5. *Concomitant chemotherapy:* The use of radiosensitizing chemotherapeutic agents such as doxorubicin, 5-fluorouracil, and actinomycin-D often result in increased severity of skin reactions.

6. *Anatomic location:* Treatment of areas of skin apposition (e.g., axilla, groin, skin folds) is prone to increased reactions secondary to warmth, moisture, and lack of aeration. Patients with ostomies, draining wounds, or tracheostomies in the treatment field are prone to more severe reactions as secretions may create a bolus effect. Treatment delivered over a bony prominence or surgical site may result in increased skin reactions due to alterations in vasculature and circulation.

7. *Patient-related considerations:* Normal age-related changes including thinning of the epidermis and dermis, diminished elasticity, and decreased dermal turgor result in delayed healing. Nutritional status must also be considered as appropriate nutrients are needed for cellular repair and wound healing.

Late radiation skin effects

The late skin reactions associated with radiation therapy include photosensitivity, pigmentation changes, atrophy, fibrosis, telangiectasia, and, rarely, ulceration and necrosis (Table 33-2).[4–6,10,11,13]

Not all patients will have noticeable late effects, and those who do will experience them in varying degrees. Factors that may increase the risk and severity of late effects include dose and volume of irradiated tissue (higher total doses delivered to larger volumes) and altered physiological integrity of the tissue. For example, tissues with surgical changes such as fibrosis and those with severely depleted sweat and sebaceous gland functioning are more prone to late radiation skin effects. The potential for late effects limits the total dose that can be delivered to a particular target, which in turn may affect cure.

Nursing considerations

Nurses play an important role in minimizing and managing the effects of radiation on skin. Nursing responsibilities include skin assessment, patient education, and management of skin reactions.

Initial assessment of the skin in the irradiated field including the exit site is necessary in order to determine the condition of the skin prior to treatment. Documentation should include the patient's present skin condition including surgical changes (edema, scars, unhealed wounds), preexisting skin disorders (skin cancers, psoriasis, maceration), medical conditions (especially those that may affect healing), medications (including past and present chemotherapeutic agents), age-related factors, and nutritional status. Knowledge of the individual's overall plan of treatment is necessary to identify treatment-related factors that may enhance skin reactions.

Skin assessment should be performed prior to initiation of treatment, at least weekly during treatment, 1–2 weeks following completion of treatment, and at each follow-up appointment thereafter. Consistency in assessment and documentation is imperative. Careful use of terminology related to radiation skin reactions will help prevent inconsistencies in reporting of toxicity. Grading scales are available and provide an objective system of categorizing impaired skin integrity. A commonly used system for grading acute radiation toxicity is one devised by the Radiation Therapy Oncology Group (RTOG) (Table 33-3).[14]

Patient education precedes initiation of radiation therapy and promotes self-care behaviors and optimal

TABLE 33-1 Acute Effects of Radiation on Skin

Tissue Response	Onset/Duration	Clinical Presentation	Physiological Rationale
Erythema			
Phase I (transient)	Within hours to days of first treatment Resolves after several days but will recur if treatment continues	Faint, often unnoticed redness	Thought to be a vascular response to extracapillary cell injury
Phase 2 (erythema proper)	Following 2–3 wk of standard fractionated radiation therapy Resolves 20–30 days following last treatment	Redness that outlines treatment field Intensifies as treatment continues	Intensity greater with higher radiation doses and larger treatment fields (greater amount of vasculature)
		Increased skin temperature	Increased blood flow through dermis from vasodilation
		Edema	Capillary vasodilation with endothelial swelling and increased capillary permeability. Histamine and serotonin are released and microcirculation increases tissue perfusion allowing infiltration of the area by leukocytes.
Dry desquamation	Following 3–4 wk of standard fractionated radiation therapy Resolves 1–2 wk after completion of treatment	Dryness, flaking, and peeling often accompanied by itching	Each dose of radiation destroys a fixed percentage of basal cells. Surviving basal cells become cornified and are shed at an increased rate. Noncycling basal cells are stimulated and cell cycle time is shortened.
Pruritis	Occurs most commonly when exposure exceeds 20–28 Gy	Itching	Thinning of the epidermis with decreased sebaceous and sweat gland function results in dehydration of the stratum corneum, the water-retaining skin layer.
Hyperpigmentation	Following 2–3 wk of standard fractionated radiation therapy Usually resolves 3 mo to 1 yr following completion of treatment, but may be chronic	Tanned appearance	Cornified basal cells carry more melanin into superficial layers of the epidermis and radiation stimulates tyrosinase to convert tyrosine to melanin. Increased melanocyte activity causes cells to become darker. Darker-skinned people may have more hyperpigmentation because they traditionally have more melanin.
Perifollicular hyperpigmentation		Brown dots at hair follicles	Hyperpigmentation of the epithelial cells surrounding hair follicles
Moist desquamation	Following 40 Gy or with trauma/ excess friction Recovery usually 2–4 wk after completion of treatment	Brilliant erythema Sloughing skin Exposed dermis Serous exudate oozing from surface	Destruction of epithelium. All basal cells have been destroyed and no new cells are yet formed.
		Pain	Nerve endings in the dermis are exposed.
Skin regrowth following moist desquamation	Dependent upon severity Usually complete 2–3 mo following completion of treatment	Small areas of epithelium develop New skin is smooth, pink, thin, and dryer	Epithelial cells migrate via proliferation from outside the treatment field and through peripheral migration.
		Gradual thickening of skin over time, but skin does not regain former thickness	Migration occurs best over moist healthy tissue. Fewer sweat and sebaceous glands result in chronic dryness.

Source: Data from Strohl RA;[5] Perez CA, Brady LW;[6] Dangel RB;[9] Lewis F, Levita M;[10] Dow KH, Hilderly LJ;[11] Margolin SG et al.;[12] Hassey KM, Rose CM.[13]

TABLE 33-2 Late Effects of Radiation on Skin and Connective Tissue

Tissue Response	Onset/Duration	Clinical Presentation	Physiological Rationale
Photosensitivity	Begins during treatment and is lifelong	Enhanced erythema over skin exposed to UV radiation from sun and tanning beds/booths	Destruction of melanocytes in the irradiated dermis and slower melanin production following irradiation reduce the skin's ability to protect itself from UV rays.
Pigmentation changes			
Hyperpigmentation	Refer to Table 33-1		
Hypopigmentation	May begin anytime following resolution of hyperpigmentation Permanent	Lack of skin color	Radiation doses necessary to eradicate cancer may permanently destroy melanocytes, which results in the skin's inability to form pigment.
Atrophy	Following epidermal regrowth Permanent	Thin and fragile epidermis	Newly formed epidermis is thinner. The epidermis thickens over time, but never attains its preirradiation thickness.
Fibrosis	Usually begins 4–6 mo following completion of treatment May worsen over time	Dense, hard, uneven skin texture If extensive, may cause considerable induration	Fibroblasts, responsible for producing collagen, demonstrate uneven cellular division resulting in faulty collagen remodeling. Fibrotic tissue results, giving the skin an uneven texture.
Telangiectasia	Occurs up to 8 yr following radiation therapy Permanent	Purple-red, spiderlike appearance of blood vessels in skin	Dose and fraction size–dependent. Basement membrane thickening results in a decreased permeability of material through capillary walls. With capillary occlusion, there are fewer functioning small vessels and a decreased capacity for capillary regeneration. This results in increased pressure of blood flow through remaining undamaged superficial structures.
Ulceration and necrosis	Infrequent May occur up to 20 yr following treatment Usually occurs as a result of inflammation and trauma to previously irradiated tissue	Painful ulcers with red, raised edges and a shaggy, necrotic base Usually shows little or no tendency to epithelialize or contract Despite local treatment, ulcers tend to deepen and become more painful	Although the mechanism is not clear, late ulceration and necrosis occur as a result of connective tissue damage. Electron microscopic studies suggest that permanent damage to fibroblasts and their precursor cells prevents stem cell replication, angiogenesis, and wound contraction. Occasionally, sustained vascular occlusion and tissue ischemia may be responsible for ulceration and necrosis.

Source: Data from Rubin P;[4] Strohl RA;[5] Perez CA, Brady LW;[6] Lewis F, Levita M;[10] Dow KH, Hilderly LJ;[11] Hassey KM, Rose CM.[13]

TABLE 33-3 Acute Radiation Toxicities—Radiation Therapy Oncology Group Scale

	0	I	II	III	IV
Skin	No change	Follicular erythema Dull redness Epilation Dry desquamation	Moderate edema Moist Bright erythema	Moist pitting edema	Necrotic Ulceration Hemorrhage
Mucous membranes	No change	Erythema	Patchy mucositis	Fibrinous mucositis Severe pain	Necrotic Ulceration Hemorrhage
Salivary glands	No change	Mild mouth dryness Thickened saliva Slightly altered taste	Moderate dryness Thickened saliva Markedly altered taste	Compete dryness	Acute salivary gland necrosis
Pharynx and esophagus	No change	Mild dysphagia or painful swallowing—may require anesthetic, nonnarcotic analgesia, soft diet	Moderate dysphagia or painful swallowing—may require narcotic analgesia, puree, or liquid diet	Severe dysphagia or painful swallowing Dehydration or weight loss requiring feeding tube, hyperalimentation, or IV fluids	Complete obstruction, ulceration, perforation, fistula
Upper gastrointestinal	No change	Anorexia with ≤5% weight loss from baseline Abdominal discomfort and nausea and/or vomiting not requiring medications	Anorexia with ≤15% weight loss Abdominal pain and nausea and/or vomiting requiring antiemetics and/or analgesics	Anorexia with ≥15% weight loss requiring nutritional support Severe abdominal pain despite medication Nausea and/or vomiting requiring NG or parenteral support	Ileus, subacute or acute obstruction, perforation, GI bleeding requiring transfusion, abdominal pain requiring tube decompression or bowel diversion
Lower gastrointestinal	No change	Increased frequency Change in quality Rectal discomfort No medications needed	Diarrhea requiring parasympatholytic drugs Minimal mucus discharge Rectal or abdominal pain requiring analgesics	Diarrhea requiring parenteral support Severe mucus or blood discharge requiring sanitary pads Abdominal distention	Acute or subacute obstruction, fistula, or perforation, GI bleeding requiring transfusion, pain requiring tube decompression or bowel diversion

Source: Winchester D, Cox JD.[14]

outcomes. Patients and their significant others require information regarding the anticipated skin reactions (both acute and late), probable time frame for each reaction including onset and duration, and skin care guidelines to be followed during and after radiation. Table 33-4 offers frequently recommended skin care guidelines. Written instructions are provided as an aid to patient learning and as a reference for future use. Patients should be informed that side effects usually do not occur for 2-3 weeks after beginning treatment, that they are usually gradual and become more severe as treatment progresses, and that most resolve 2-3 weeks after treatment is completed. It is also important to reassure patients that management of side effects and maintaining comfort is a priority. The importance of compliance with recommended skin care guidelines is reinforced frequently during the treatment course.

Management of basic skin care needs during and after radiation therapy is fairly standard, as are the approaches to management of reactions. Management of reactions such as severe dry desquamation with pruritis and moist desquamation is not well documented in the literature. Interventions are based on management goals and what is known about ideal wound-healing environments. Goals include promoting comfort and healing as well as prevention of infection and fluid loss. A clean, moist wound bed permits epithelial cells to migrate from healthy areas to areas of desquamation.[15] Table 33-5 reviews some of the commonly used interventions for severe acute skin reactions.[9–11,16,17] A

TABLE 33-4 Skin Care Guidelines During and After Radiation Therapy

While receiving radiation therapy, the skin in the treatment area may become dry, reddened, tanned, and sensitive. Skin changes are usually gradual and become noticeable after 2 or 3 weeks of treatment, becoming more obvious as treatment continues. Care must be taken to protect the skin and prevent trauma. *The following guidelines pertain only to the skin within the radiation treatment field.*

Guidelines	Rationale
DURING TREATMENT	
Shower or bathe using lukewarm water. Gently wash the area using fingertips. Rinse well and pat dry with soft cloth.	Extreme temperatures may further compromise vasculature. Mechanical irritation such as vigorous rubbing may cause trauma and an increased rate of superficial cell loss.
Avoid harsh soap. If it is necessary to use a cleaning solution, use baking soda and water (½ box to one tub of water) or a creamy mild soap made for sensitive skin (Basis, Neutrogena, Ivory).	Perfumed soaps contain chemicals and heavy metal ions that irritate sensitive skin and may enhance skin reactions from radiation therapy. Mild soaps help to decrease the incidence of folliculitis and local skin infections.
Do not apply any ointment, cream, lotion, deodorant, perfume, cologne, powder, cosmetics, or home remedy to the skin unless specifically instructed to do so. Pure, unscented, kitchen cornstarch may be used in place of deodorant or to decrease itching. Apply lightly to *dry* skin using a powder puff or cotton ball.	Many products contain heavy metal ions and chemicals as described above. Cornstarch helps to reduce pruritis as well as moisture build-up, especially in the axilla, under the breast, and in skin folds. It must only be used on dry areas as its use on moist areas can promote fungal growth (by forming a glucose-rich environment), thereby increasing the risk of infection.
If instructed, apply a recommended mild, water-soluble lubricant to reduce itching and discomfort. Apply 2–3 times/day. Do not apply for at least 3 hr before treatment.	Use of water-soluble, mild aloe-based lubricant containing no heavy metal ions or perfumes is frequently recommended during radiation to prevent trauma from itching, promote comfort, and stimulate fibroblast formation. Examples include Natural Care Gel® (Bard) and Skin Balm® (Carrington Laboratories).
Avoid shaving if possible. If it is necessary to shave, use an electric razor.	Shaving increases the rate of superficial cell loss resulting in earlier dry desquamation and can lacerate the skin thereby increasing the risk of infection.
Avoid extreme temperatures. Do not use water bottles, heating pads, sun lamps, ice bags, etc.	Irradiated skin has a decreased sensitivity to temperature, which can place the area at a higher risk for injury. Extreme temperatures may further compromise vascular reactions in the capillaries within the treatment area.
Avoid tight fitting clothing made of irritating fabric. Clothes made of cotton or cotton blends are preferred over wool and polyester. If skin becomes irritated from clothing, change to a mild detergent such as Ivory Snow® or Dreft®.	Mechanical irritation caused by tight fitting clothes results in discomfort and trauma to fragile skin. Cotton clothing promotes air exchange and decreases moisture build-up.
Avoid exposing skin to sun. Use wide-brimmed hats, long sleeves, and gloves to prevent exposure. Always apply a sunscreen with an SPF of 15 or higher before sun exposure, even under lightweight clothing.	Destruction of melanocytes in the irradiated epidermis and a slower rate of melanin production in new epidermal cells render the skin at higher risk for sunburns.
Do not apply tape or adhesive bandages to skin in the radiation treatment field.	Removal can result in mechanical trauma to the already compromised epidermis.
Drink at least 3 qt of fluid each day.	Radiation to the skin and sweat and sebaceous glands causes dryness and itching. This is characterized by dehydration of the stratum corneum, the water-retaining layer of skin.
AFTER TREATMENT	
Continue following the above guidelines for 2–3 wk after the completion of treatment.	The acute effects of radiation are cumulative and may be at their peak 5–7 days after the last treatment. Great care must be taken to protect and preserve the fragile irradiated skin.
Apply an unscented hydrophilic emollient (lotion or cream) 2–3 times each day for 1–2 mo after treatment and then daily. Examples of moisturizers include Lubriderm®, Alpha Keri®, Nivea®, and Eucerin®. Application to damp (not wet) skin such as after bathing will help to seal in moisturizers.	Obliteration of sweat and sebaceous glands will cause permanent dryness to some degree. Lifetime use of a moisturizer should be encouraged to keep the skin lubricated and prevent fissuring.
Always avoid exposing previously irradiated skin to the sun. When this is not possible, use a sunscreen with an SPF of 15 or greater.	Melanocytes in the epidermis have been destroyed by radiation, and production of new cells and regeneration is slow and often not complete. Lifetime care must be taken to protect skin from injury.

Source: Data from Strohl RA;[5] Dangel RB;[9] Lewis F, Levita M;[10] Dow KH, Hilderley LJ;[11] Hassey KM, Rose CM;[13] Ratliff C.[16]

team approach to managing side effects is most efficient and beneficial. Together, radiation oncologists, nurses, technologists, and patients can often devise a plan that will meet the needs of the patient while ensuring optimal treatment outcomes.

Tissue fibrosis, ulceration, and necrosis are late radiation skin effects and tend to be chronic in nature; therefore, they can significantly impact a patient's quality of life. Tissue fibrosis occurs in varying degrees from unnoticeable to severe. Moderate to severe fibrosis is occasionally seen in patients who have received surgery and radiation to the head and neck region and to the breast. Significant mobility restriction, pain, and lymphedema can result. Scar tissue integration therapy administered by registered physical or massage therapists is often extremely helpful in regaining mobility and pain reduction. Scar tissue integration therapy "breaks up" or loosens and redistributes scar tissue to increase mobility, decrease pain, and enhance lymphatic drainage. Qualified professionals are able to assess a patient's condition to determine appropriateness of this intervention. Following initiation of therapy, patients are usually instructed on exercises and techniques that can be done at home, which can make this therapy extremely cost-effective.[18,19]

In patients with fibrosis, ulcerations, and necrosis, pain may be a significant problem. A pain management program should be developed to ensure optimal relief of pain. Nonsteroidal anti-inflammatory agents are often effective in managing chronic pain of this nature; however, narcotic analgesia may become necessary. For basic principles of pain assessment and management in the oncology population, see Chapter 23.

Management goals include promoting comfort and healing as well as prevention of infection and fluid loss. Theses wounds are often chronic and worsen over time; therefore, assessment of patient compliance and economic status should accompany wound assessment in order to develop an appropriate plan of care. A thorough nutritional assessment must also be performed. Successful wound healing requires adequate stores of protein, carbohydrates, fat, vitamins, and minerals.[12,15]

Wound care is individualized, based on the assessment and what is known about the optimal environment for wound healing. Wound beds should be moist, clean, free of debris and eschar, and without evidence of infection. Chronic radiation ulcers are heavily colonized with bacteria, which is responsible for the foul odor often associated with these wounds. Keeping the

TABLE 33-5 Management of Severe Acute Radiation Skin Reactions

Agent	Application	Rationale	Comments
	DRY DESQUAMATION WITH PRURITIS		
1. Lubricants—water-soluble, aloe-based such as Natural Care Gel® (Bard Pharmaceuticals) and Skin Balm® (Carrington Laboratories)	Increase frequency to PRN Avoid application 3 hr prior to treatment	Decreases itching to increase comfort, stimulates epithelialization, and reduces the risk of skin cracking and fissure formation	Discontinue use if moist desquamation occurs
2. Mild astringent soaks such as Domeboro® solution (Miles Laboratories)	Dissolve one tablet or packet in one quart of water (not one pint as suggested on package). Soak clean cloth in solution, lightly wring out, and apply to irritated area for 15 min 3–4 times a day May be used in sitz bath for irritation from pelvic irradiation	Causes contraction of tissue and reduces inflammation by forming a protective film over the area, which aids in reducing or preventing fluid loss and infection Anti-inflammatory response and cooling effect promote comfort Provides gentle debridement of dead cells and exudate	Solution may be kept for 1 wk if refrigerated in a sealed glass container May be used for dry and moist desquamation
3. Topical steroids—mild	Apply as directed—usually 0.25% b.i.d. or t.i.d. Avoid application 3 hours prior to treatment May be used in rectal preparations such as Anusol HC® (Parke-Davis), Preparation H® (Whitehall Laboratories), and Proctofoam® (Reed and Carnrick)	Anti-inflammatory and antipruritic actions Often used when there is a risk for mechanical trauma from scratching or when sleep disruption occurs from pruritis	Use is controversial as topical steroids may result in further thinning of the epidermis causing the skin to be more susceptible to injury

(continued)

TABLE 33-5 Management of Severe Acute Radiation Skin Reactions (continued)

Agent	Application	Rationale	Comments
		MOIST DESQUAMATION	
1. Mild astringent soaks (see above)			
2. Hydrogel primary wound dressings such as Vigilon (Bard Pharmaceuticals) and Spenco Second Skin (Spenco Medical)	Remove film from one side and place hydrogel portion on the wound or skin. Cover with nonadherent dressing such as Telfa and secure with paper tape placed outside of the radiation treatment field. May be used following mild astringent soaks	Composed of 98% water and 2% cellulose fiber Maintains moist environment, protects newly formed epithelial cells from trauma, and increases comfort by covering exposed nerve endings Mildly absorbent	Expensive Difficult to secure Must not be allowed to dry Dressing can be removed and reapplied for routine soaks and cleaning Must be removed during radiation treatment
3. Wound cleansers such as Biolex Wound Cleanser (BARD) and Caraklenz (Carrington Laboratories), and epithelial stimulants such as Biolex Wound Gel (Bard) and Wound Dressing (Carrington Laboratories)	Cleanse wound with gentle spray b.i.d. or t.i.d. Apply liberal amount of gel to denuded area and cover with nonadherent dressing such as Telfa. Secure with paper tape placed outside of the radiation treatment field, or flexible netting.	Cleanser aids in debridement and maintenance of wound bed pH. Does not harm proliferating fibroblasts Wound gel maintains moist environment and stimulates epithelialization Promotes comfort by covering exposed nerve endings	Expensive Difficult to secure Gel must be applied liberally to avoid drying between dressing changes Must be removed during radiation treatment
4. Occlusive hydrocolloid dressings such as DuoDerm® (Convatec), Restore® (Hollister), Cutinova hydro® (Beiersdorf, Inc.)	Cleanse wound Choose dressing size that provides 1¼-in. margin around wound. Apply as directed on package. Dressing can remain in placed for up to 7 days Removal—use great care to prevent harm to new skin. If necessary, small amounts of sterile saline may be used to aid in removal.	Maintains moist environment Promotes rapid epithelialization and aids in debridement. Isolates wound against bacterial contamination Promotes comfort by covering exposed nerve endings and preventing friction Absorbent	Cost-effective Do not use if infection is present May produce a malodorous yellow-brown fluid that may be mistaken as an infection. If this occurs, remove dressing, cleanse wound, and apply new dressing if needed. Should not be used during treatment as daily removal disturbs wound bed

Source: Data from Dangel, RB;[9] Lewis F, Levita M;[10] Dow KH, Hilderley LJ;[11] Ratliff C;[16] Hutchinson JJ, McGuckin M.[17]

wound clean and managing infection helps to minimize odor while maintaining the integrity of the skin surrounding the wound. Table 33-6 lists various products used in managing wounds of this nature.

If conservative treatment is unsuccessful in providing wound closure, definitive debridement of the ulcer and underlying fibrotic bed with surgical closure of the wound may be attempted. Surgical wound closure is often unsuccessful for the following reasons: (1) irradiated tissue is fibrotic and unyielding, making it prone to dehiscence; (2) healthy tissue often cannot be reached surgically because the ulcers are so deep; and (3) radiation injury extends beyond the ulcer to surrounding tissues.[15,19] Myocutaneous flaps are the preferred method for surgical closure of radiation ulcers due to the rich vascular supply they provide to ischemic tissue and the greater resistance to infection.

Chemotherapy Effects

Hyperpigmentation

Numerous chemotherapeutic agents are associated with altered pigmentation of the skin. While the etiology of this purely cosmetic reaction is poorly understood, it is possible that the drug or a metabolic byproduct of the drug stimulates melanocytes to produce increased quantities of melanin. It is unclear why some drugs are associated with widespread hyperpigmentation and others cause darkening confined to specific areas such as the nails, mucous membranes, or tongue.

Hyperpigmentation occurs more commonly in dark-skinned individuals and in persons receiving alkylating agents or antitumor antibiotics. Patients receiving busulfan often experience hyperpigmentation involving the neck, upper trunk, nipples, and abdomen. This

TABLE 33-6 Agents Used in Wound Management

Classification	Indication/Rationale	Product Examples
Absorption	Draining, noninfected wounds Absorbs exudate, maintains moist environment Some facilitate debridement	Wound filler products Debrisan Beads and Paste® (Johnson & Johnson) Bard Absorption Dressing® (Bard) Comfeel Ulcus Powder and Paste® (Coloplast-Kendall) Duoderm Granules and Paste® (Convatec) Calcium Alginate Dressing-Kaltostat® (Calgon Vestal Labs) Sorbsan® (N.I. Medical)
	See above Reduces pain Prevents mechanical trauma	Occlusive hydrocolloid dressings Comfeel Ulcus® (Coloplast-Kendall) DuoDerm CGF and Extra Thin® (Convatec) Restore® (Hollister) Cutinova hydro® (Beiersdorf, Inc.)
	Absorbs exudate Decreases frequency and number of dressing changes	Nonadherent dressings Lyo Foam® (Acme United Corp.) ExuDry® (Frastec Wound Care Products) Sanitary pads and disposable diapers with nonadherent lining
Antibiotics	Use in presence of known infection Positive wound cultures of $>10^5$ bacteria	Topical or systemic Agent dependent upon organism
Antiseptics	May be irritating to healthy skin surrounding wound	Hibiclens® (Stuart Pharmaceuticals) Acetic acid 0.25%–5%
	Often caustic to wound	Hydrogen peroxide 1%
	Use with caution	Povidine iodine 1% Sodium hypochlorite 0.5% (Dakins)
Cleansers	Aid in debridement Soften eschar Nontoxic to proliferating fibroblasts pH-adjusted	Biolex Wound Cleanser® (Bard) Granulux® (Dow B. Hickman, Inc.) Caraklenz® (Carrington Laboratories)
Debriding agents	Topical debridement of eschar and necrotic tissue	Granulex® (Dow B. Hickman, Inc.) Elase® (Parke-Davis)
	May cause local irritation and disrupt granulation	Travase® (Sutilains) Santyl® (Kaal) Dakins solution
Deodorizers		
Sprays	Applied on dressing, act as odor antagonist—not to be applied directly to wound	Dignity® (Convatec) Medi-Aire® (Bard)
Solutions and Ointments	Applied directly to wound, act as odor antagonist and antibacterial agent to reduce odor and promote healing	Chloresium Ointment and Solution® (Rystan)
Dressings	Applied over wound—charcoal absorbs odor	Lyofoam-C® (Acme United Corp.) Carbonet® (Smith & Nephew, Inc.)
Epithelial stimulants	Create and maintain moist environment pH-adjusted	Biolex Wound Gel® (Bard) Carrington Wound Gel® and Carrington Hydrogel Wound Dressing®—(Carrington Laboratories)
Hemolytic agents	Arrest small vessel bleeds to provide hemostasis	Silver nitrate cauterizing stick Surgical topical thrombin—Thrombogen® (Johnson & Johnson) Absorbables—Gelfoam® and Xeroform® (Sherwood Medical)
Hydrogel dressings	Maintain moist environment Reduce pain Minimal absorption	Elasto Gel® (Southwest Technologies) Spenco Second Skin® (Spenco Medical) Vigilon® (Bard)
Skin barriers	Protect healthy intact skin surrounding wound Should not be applied directly to wound	Sween-A Peel® (Sween) Bard Protective Spray® (Bard) Tincture of benzoin zinc oxide ointment Moisture Barrier Ointment (Bard) Stomahesive

complication occurs with increasing frequency in individuals also experiencing busulfan-induced pulmonary fibrosis.[20]

Hyperpigmentation associated with cyclophosphamide may be diffuse or confined to the palms, soles, nails, or gums. Skin contact with carmustine or nitrogen mustard can result in a contact dermatitis followed by postinflammatory hyperpigmentation.[21]

Hyperpigmentation has been noted following 5-fluorouracil therapy, especially in those patients who receive high-dose weekly infusions with or without citrovorum factor (leucovorin). Hyperpigmentation occurs most readily in sun-exposed areas. Serpiginous hyperpigmented streaks overlying veins used repeatedly for infusions of 5-fluorouracil occur without any clinical evidence of cutaneous inflammation, phlebitis, or sclerosis (Figure 33-5).

Bleomycin also may cause a change in pigmentation over the veins into which the drug is given. However, bleomycin is more commonly associated with hyperpigmentation over pressure points (elbows) or with linear streaks occurring in areas of intense scratching, presumably due to a localized vasodilation that results in an increased concentration of the bleomycin in the skin (Figure 33-6).[22,23]

Doxorubicin, busulfan, cyclophosphamide, 5-fluorouracil (5-FU), and etoposide have been associated with hyperpigmentation of the oral mucosa and tongue, especially in African Americans (Figure 33-7). Doxorubicin and 5-FU also may cause skin darkening over the interphalangeal and metacarpophalangeal joints (Figure 33-8). The mechanism of this effect is not known, but the phalangeal darkening decreases once therapy is terminated.

Hypersensitivity

Cutaneous hypersensitivity reactions (HSRs) to chemotherapy occur infrequently and tend not to be dose-related. Cutaneous manifestations of immediate HSRs (type I reactions) generally present as urticaria and angioedema. L-asparaginase, for example, is a polypeptide of bacterial origin that causes HSR in 10%–20% of patients receiving the drug.[24] Acute urticaria is the most frequent manifestation of L-asparaginase HSR, with 10% of these patients progressing to life-threatening anaphylaxis.[20]

Taxol has been observed to cause hypotension, rash,

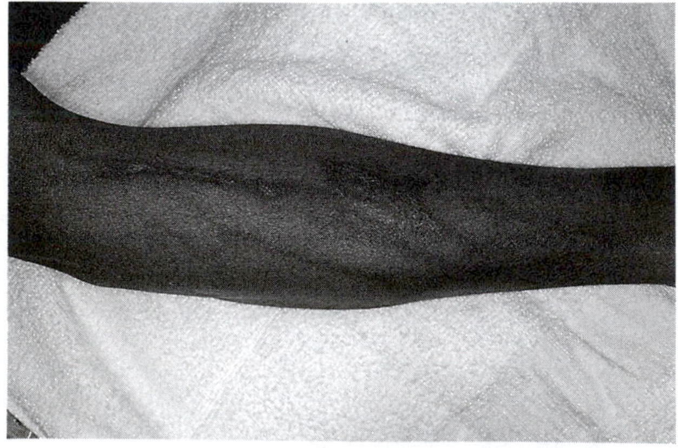

FIGURE 33-5 Serpiginous hyperpigmentation following 5-fluorouracil infusion.

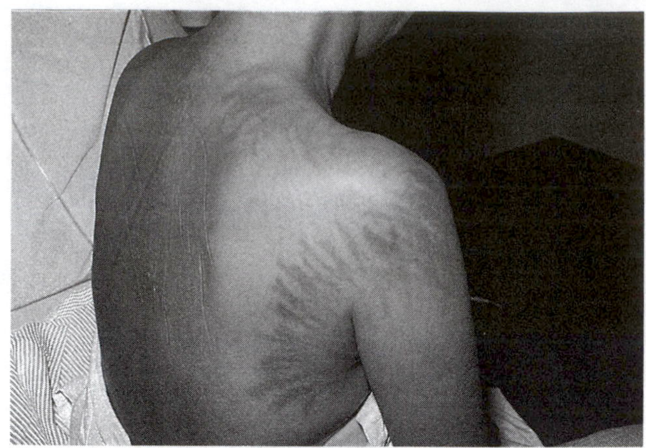

FIGURE 33-6 Flagellate streaks of hyperpigmentation in an Asian woman occurring in areas of intense scratching following intracavitary (intrapleural) bleomycin.

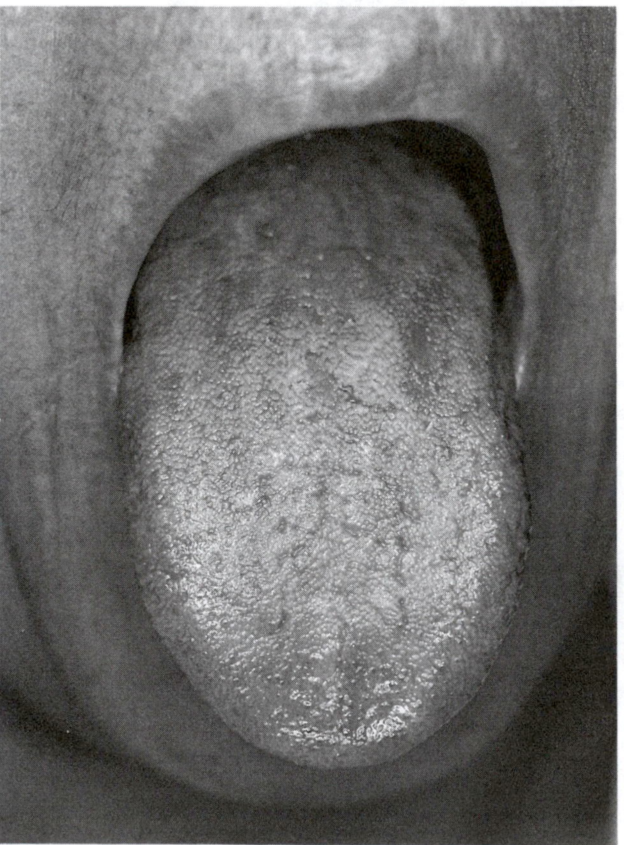

FIGURE 33-7 Black tongue following doxorubicin.

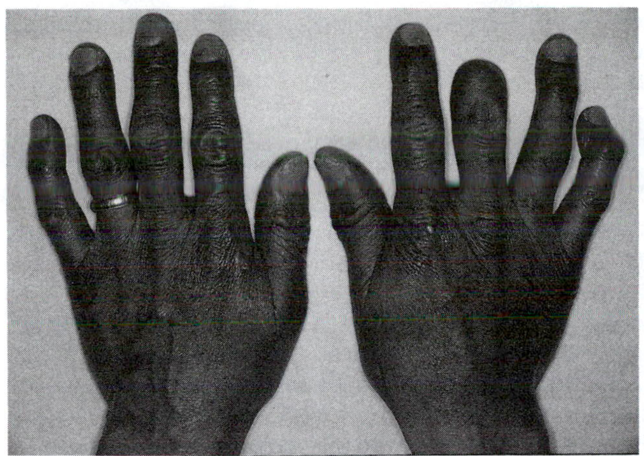

FIGURE 33-8 Skin darkening over the interphalangeal and metacarpophalangeal joints.

dyspnea, and bronchospasm within 10 minutes of initiating the drug, suggesting a nonimmunologic anaphylactoid reaction.[25] The cause of this HSR is felt to be due to the drug vehicle, Cremophor EL. Measures to minimize HSR with taxol include prolonging drug infusion time (6–24 hours) and using a three-drug prophylactic regimen consisting of an antihistamine, a corticosteroid, and an H-2 receptor antagonist. Despite these precautions, approximately 10% of patients will experience HSRs.

Parenteral cisplatin, carboplatin, and iproplatin (CHIP) can cause a type I HSR in approximately 5% of patients. The manifestations of this reaction include anxiety, pruritis, cough, dyspnea, angioedema, bronchospasm, rash, urticaria, and hypotension. These symptoms are generally relieved by prompt administration of antihistamines.[25]

Teniposide and parenteral etoposide can cause HSR with the initial dosing, manifesting as dyspnea, wheezing, hypotension, urticaria, pruritis, angioedema, facial flushing, and rash.[26] The incidence is higher with teniposide as it is formulated with Cremophor EL. Decreasing the infusion rate and premedicating with an antihistamine and a steroid generally permits further drug administration.

Other drugs producing rash, urticaria, or angioedema include procarbazine, cytarabine, levamisole, alpha interferon, interleukin, anthracycline antibiotics, melphalan, and methotrexate.

A common side effect of aminoglutethimide is a morbeliform, maculopapular skin rash sometimes associated with fever. The rash usually disappears and does not necessitate cessation of therapy. Rarely it can progress and cause desquamation. Hydrocortisone may be given in higher than usual doses for the first 2 weeks of therapy in an attempt to decrease severity of the skin rash.

Dactinomycin folliculitis presents as diffuse erythematous papules over the face and trunk resembling acne, appearing approximately 5 days after therapy. The rash resolves in 3–5 days. Folliculitis has also been reported following administration of high-dose methotrexate.

Erythema multiforme has been infrequently associated with chemotherapeutic agents. Patients receiving high-dose combination chemotherapy are more at risk for erythema multiforme. This reaction is characterized by target lesions over the extremities, often involving the mucous membranes. Busulfan, etoposide, procarbazine, hydroxyurea, bleomycin, methotrexate, and cytarabine have been associated with such lesions, which occasionally develop into generalized blistering (toxic epidermal necrolysis).[20]

Acral erythema

An intensely painful erythema, scaling, and epidermal sloughing from the palms and soles followed by desquamation and reepithelialization of the skin has been reported with continuous infusions of 5-FU,[27] doxorubicin, high-dose cytarabine,[28] and floxuridine (FUDR) (see Figure 33-9—Plate 4). This condition, also called *palmar-plantar erythrodysesthesia syndrome,* may represent a direct toxic effect on the epidermis and dermal vasculature or an accumulation of the chemotherapeutic agent in eccrine structures and sweat, causing erythema of the palms and soles, where there is a high concentration of eccrine glands.[23] Chemotherapy is usually suspended until symptoms subside and is then resumed at a lower dose. However, the symptoms usually recur and may necessitate cessation of therapy.

Pruritis

Etiology Pruritis or itching may be localized or generalized and is associated with many medical conditions. Pruritis may occur in conjunction with thyroid disease, diabetes, anemia, polycythemia, leukemia, multiple myeloma, adenocarcinoma, Hodgkin's disease, and non-Hodgkin's lymphoma. It may also occur as a consequence of obstructive biliary disease or a treatment side effect such as dry desquamation following radiation therapy, as a reaction to opiate analgesics, or an allergic dermatitis following chemotherapy. For example, aminoglutethimide has been associated with a pruritic rash that usually resolves spontaneously. Interleukin can cause a macular erythema most prominent on the head and neck region, with burning and pruritis.

Pruritis may also be a symptom of infection or a reaction to antibiotics. Whatever the cause, the urge to scratch can be overwhelming and distressing to the individual, as it commonly interferes with rest and sleep and can result in skin breakdown and infection.

Assessment Assessment requires a thorough evaluation of the possible cause of the itching and any factors that might aggravate the condition. If the itching is due to a drug reaction, the condition is generally short-lived and subsides when the drug is stopped or gradually dissipates following antihistamine therapy despite continued administration of the offending agent. When the pruritis is due to Hodgkin's disease, the itching goes away with successful therapy; if relapse should occur, the pruritis is often the presenting symptom.

The characteristics of the pruritis and the patient's history will further assist in management and include the following: (1) localization, onset, duration, and intensity of the itching; (2) prior history of pruritis; (3) past or present cancer, cancer treatment, noncancer systemic disease, or use of analgesics or antibiotics; and (4) presence of infection. The nurse carefully examines all areas of the skin for any obvious signs of infection or drug reaction, as well as environmental conditions and level of hydration that may contribute to pruritis.

Management Nursing care focuses on three areas: skin care, environmental control, and administration of therapeutics.[29,30]

Dry skin, whether caused by cancer therapy, dehydration, or aging, is subjectively uncomfortable and may lead to itching, skin cracking, and fissure formation. Adequate hydration promotes healthy skin. Drinking 3000 cc of fluid per day and eating a diet rich in iron, zinc, and protein promotes skin integrity. Medicated baths (AVEENO Colloidal Oatmeal Bath®) can be soothing, especially if antipruritic. Local anesthetic creams (e.g., Lanacaine®), emollient lotions (e.g., Lubriderm®, AlphaKeri®, Nivea®) may be useful. Soaps made especially for sensitive skin such as AVEENO Oatmeal Bar®, Neutrogena®, or Basis® should be used when skin cleansing is required. The patient is encouraged to employ alternate cutaneous stimulation methods to relieve the urge to scratch. These include massage, pressure, or rubbing the area with a soft cloth.

Environmental factors include keeping the room humidity at 30%–40% and the room temperature cool. Cotton clothing and sheets should be washed in hypoallergenic soaps. Distractions such as music, imagery, or relaxation may ease the itch sensation.

Medications may be recommended based on the etiology of the pruritis. If the itch is related to a drug reaction, an antihistamine and corticosteroid may be useful. If it is due to biliary obstruction, cholestyramine is often indicated. When itching is related to an infection, antibiotics or antifungal agents are indicated. Other pharmacologic measures include Periactin, aspirin, and Atarax. Dosages may be increased at the hour of sleep since pruritis generally worsens in the night.

Photosensitivity

There are three main types of ultraviolet radiation: ultraviolet A (UVA), ultraviolet B (UVB), and ultraviolet C (UVC). UVA is far more damaging to the skin than once believed. It penetrates deeply into the skin, destroying collagen and elastic fibers of connective tissue. UVA is commonly used in tanning salons. UVB penetrates only as far as the epidermis, causing erythema of a sunburn and is responsible for skin cancer. UVC is generally absorbed by the upper atmosphere, but because of the thinning of the ozone layer, UVC will likely contribute to skin damage in the future.

Photosensitivity is an enhanced skin response to ultraviolet radiation. This enhanced response may present like a sunburn with erythema, edema, blisters, hyperpigmentation, and desquamation or peeling. Rarely, photoallergy similar to a contact dermatitis with immediate wheal and flare reactions or delayed reactions may occur.

Photosensitivity is caused by a variety of topical or oral medications such as analgesics, antidepressants, antimicrobials, diuretics, antihistamines, nonsteroidal anti-inflammatory agents, and cytotoxic drugs. Photosensitivity has been reported following skin exposure to UV light following administration of 5-FU, dacarbazine, vinblastine, and high-dose methotrexate. In general, the exposed area becomes erythematous within a few hours and gradually subsides. Dacarbazine, however, has been associated with pruritis and erythematous edematous eruptions on the face, neck, and dorsal surfaces of both hands when sun exposure occurred within 1–2 hours following drug administration.[31]

Patients with cancer often are taking several different prescription and nonprescription medications, many of which can cause photosensitivity reactions. This fact highlights the importance of the oncology nurse obtaining a complete list of all medications that the patient has taken recently or is currently taking. In addition, patients are commonly receiving both radiation and chemotherapy, which further enhances the potential for photosensitivity.

Melanin commonly protects the skin by absorbing UV radiation from the sun. However, following radiation therapy the skin's ability to protect itself from UV rays is decreased as a result of destruction of melanocytes in the irradiated epidermis and the slower rate of melanin production in new epidermal cells in the radiation field. The newer and thinner epidermis after radiation is more easily damaged and is susceptible to all types of injuries: infectious, chemical, and physical.[32]

Nurses are responsible for educating patients on the dangers of exposure to UV radiation following treatment with radiation or certain chemotherapeutic agents. Verbal and written instructions concerning ways to reduce the risk of developing a photosensitivity reaction are given to the patient. Patients are instructed to avoid tanning booths and to limit their exposure to the sun, particularly between the hours of 10 a.m. and 3 p.m. when the harmful rays are most intense.

Because clouds allow 80% of the sun's UV light to reach the earth's surface, patients are still vulnerable to UV light on cloudy days. Therefore, protective clothing or a hat must be worn to protect areas of irradiated skin.

Most important, nurses provide instructions regarding the proper use of sunscreen based on the individual's skin type. Sunscreens contain a sun protection factor (SPF), which defines the ratio of the time it takes to develop erythema with the sunscreen applied compared with the time it takes to develop erythema without the sunscreen. For example, an individual who can only be in direct sunlight for 30 minutes without erythema may, by applying a sunscreen with an SPF of 8, remain outside for 240 minutes (30 × 8) without burning. The higher the SPF number, the more complete the sun protection. Products with an SPF higher than 15 are generally recommended for use in a tropical climate or for protection following chemotherapy or radiation therapy. Physical sun blocks with an SPF of 25 or more are available and recommended for children and fair-skinned individuals. In general, the greater the SPF, the greater the chance of skin irritation. Some sunscreens and blocks are water-resistant, but in general they should be applied frequently and directly to the skin. To maximize its effectiveness, sunscreen should be applied at least 15–30 minutes before sun exposure and as often as indicated by activities in which the individual is engaged. While some companies are developing products that are long-lasting and stay on until washed off with soap, most water-resistant products will provide protection for up to 40 minutes of continuous water exposure, while waterproof products will protect for up to 80 minutes of continuous water exposure.

TABLE 33-7 Irritant Chemotherapeutic Agents

ANTINEOPLASTICS
Carmustine (BCNU)
Dacarbazine (DTIC)
Streptozotocin (Zanosar)
Fluorouracil (5-FU)
Cisplatin (Platinol)
Mitoxantrone (Novantrone)
Plicamycin (Mithracin)
Teniposide (Vumon)
Etoposide (Vepesid)
Taxol
BIOLOGICALS
Tumor necrosis factor
Interleukin-2
GMCSF (Sargramostim)

Vesicant Chemotherapy Extravasation

Chemotherapy drug extravasation is a known complication of cancer treatment. The occurrence of extravasation of vesicant chemotherapeutic agents is probably underreported, but according to the literature the incidence ranges from 0.5% to 5% of patients receiving peripheral intravenous chemotherapeutic agents[33,34] and 6.4% of patients (n = 300) receiving vesicant chemotherapy via implanted vascular access ports.[35]

The most benign, inconsequential local reaction to chemotherapy is venous flare (see Figure 33-10—Plate 5). This reaction occurs most commonly in patients receiving doxorubicin and is characterized by a localized erythema, venous streaking, and pruritis along the injected vein. Vogelzang[36] reported a 3% incidence of venous flare in patients receiving doxorubicin. This localized allergic reaction is distinguishable from an extravasation by the absence of pain or swelling and the presence of a blood return. Once this important distinction is made, it is safe to continue injecting the agent. Flushing the vein with saline and slowing the injection rate appear to ease the symptoms, which dissipate without treatment within 20–30 minutes of the injection.

Another local tissue reaction characterized by pain, venous irritation, and chemical phlebitis can occur with certain nonvesicant chemotherapy agents. These agents are called *irritants* and are listed in Table 33-7. While any drug given in concentrated form in sufficient amount can cause tissue damage if infiltrated, these agents are not associated with ulceration if infiltrated. Irritants cause intravascular irritation often accompanied by pain (described as achiness or as tightness) during the infusion only and may, as is the case with carmustine, be a function of the diluent. With some irritants like dacarbazine or streptozotocin, increasing the dilution or slowing the drip rate will ease the pain associated with the infusion.

The most devastating skin reactions caused by chemotherapy occur when a vesicant agent is infiltrated causing an extravasation injury. The degree of injury to local tissues is related to the vesicant properties of the drug infiltrated, the concentration of the drug, and the amount of the drug infiltrated. For example, in the animal model 0.2 ml of doxorubicin at a concentration of 2 mg/ml produces a 1cm-diameter lesion taking 7 or 8 weeks to heal.[37]

By definition, an *extravasation* is the infiltration of a vesicant chemotherapeutic agent. A *vesicant* is a drug that, if infiltrated, is capable of causing pain, ulceration, necrosis, and sloughing of damaged tissue. While all vesicants are capable of causing significant ulceration and morbidity due to pain, tissue necrosis, and potential loss of function of the affected area, this rarely occurs when these drugs are given by professional nurses who are trained in the proper techniques of chemotherapy drug administration. Although infiltration of vesicant agents can occur even when these drugs are given by properly trained individuals, the sequelae are usually inconsequential and the wound usually heals spontaneously over time.

To infiltrate a vesicant agent is traumatic for patient and nurse, but it is not an act of negligence. In many situations the patient is elderly with small frail veins, or obese with deep and difficult-to-access veins. In such cases the occurrence of an extravasation is more a function of venous integrity than the administration technique. Patients should be thoroughly informed regarding the vesicant potential of the drugs they are receiving and the importance of reporting any pain, burning, or stinging during the injection.

To ensure the best outcome possible in the event of an extravasation, the nurse must be able to recognize that an infiltration has occurred and act appropriately. When vesicant agents are administered by nurses and physicians who are not trained in the skills of chemotherapy administration, the subtle early signs and symptoms of an extravasation may go unnoticed, resulting in extensive tissue damage and possible loss of function, even amputation (see Figures 33-11 and 33-12—Plates 6 and 7, respectively). Table 33-8 lists vesicant chemotherapy agents as identified by the Oncology Nursing Society Cancer Chemotherapy Guidelines and Recommendations for Management of Chemotherapy Drug Extravasation Module V (1992).

Prevention and assessment

Because there are no universally effective, optimal means of treating vesicant extravasation, the best approach is prevention. The Cancer Chemotherapy Guidelines and Recommendations for the Management of Vesicant Extravasation (Module V, 1992) is an excellent resource for nurses and physicians to implement preventive care and for the design of appropriate policies and procedures in individual practice settings. The official position of the Oncology Nursing Society is that all personnel who administer chemotherapy should receive training in chemotherapy drug administration and management of toxicities including drug extravasation.

TABLE 33-8 Vesicant Chemotherapeutic Agents

Agent
Dactinomycin (Actinomycin D)
Daunomycin (Cerubidine)
Doxorubicin (Adriamycin)
Mitomycin-C (Mutamycin)
Mechlorethamine (nitrogen mustard, mustargen)
Vinblastine (Velban)
Vincristine (Oncovin)
Vindesine (Eldisine)
Amsacrine (M-AMSA)
Epirubicin
Idarubicin (Idamycin)
Esorubicin
Pyrazofurin (Pyrazomycin)
Menogril (Tomasar)
Maytansine
Vinorelbine (Navelbine)

Institutionally approved guidelines for extravasation management should be readily available, reviewed, and revised regularly as appropriate. The physician's guidelines or institutional protocol for the management of a presumed or proven extravasation should be readily available wherever vesicant drugs are administered and instituted immediately in the event of an extravasation. The procedure for documenting and reporting an actual or suspected extravasation should be clearly defined. Table 33-9 depicts a sample chemotherapy drug extravasation record.[38]

The signs and symptoms of an extravasation may be very obvious or extremely subtle. The one obvious sign of drug infiltration is a bleb formation at the injection site that is readily apparent in a superficial vein, or swelling that occurs in more deeply accessed veins. In the absence of pain, swelling, or diffuse induration, an extravasation may go unnoticed, especially when the vein lies deeply in an obese limb. In this situation a large amount of drug can infiltrate, especially if the drug is injected very slowly.

Pain can be an early or late symptom depending upon the patient's ability to report this sensation. If a patient is elderly and confused or heavily sedated, symptoms may go unreported. Any antiemetics, sedatives, or analgesics that may affect the patient's ability to readily report any change in sensation at the injection site should be withheld until after the vesicant has been safely administered. The report of any change in sensation such as pain, stinging, or burning at the injection site warrants further investigation to ensure an intact vein. The vesicant injection is stopped immediately and the vein is aspirated to ensure a blood return. In the absence of any swelling, pain, or evidence of infiltration, the injection of the vesicant may continue following a copious (30–40 cc) saline flush. If the patient again complains of discomfort despite the presence of a blood return and absence of swelling, the site should be flushed with saline once more and the intravenous discontinued. Drug administration is resumed at another appropriate site despite the absence of any evidence of extravasation. Mitomycin has been associated with subtle extravasation; therefore, in the presence of any discomfort, the nurse is cautioned to immediately stop the injection, flush copiously with saline, and restart the IV despite the absence of any objective signs of extravasation.

A blood return should be assessed every 1–2 cc of drug administration. The presence of a blood return is valuable to determine venous access but does not always ensure an intact vein. A blood return can be obtained in the presence of an extravasation as the needle may extend partially through the vein, allowing for a subtle leakage of the vesicant into the subcutaneous tissues. In this situation the blood return will be weak instead of full and brisk. On the other hand, the absence of a blood return in no way confirms an extravasation. The needle bevel or cannula tip may upon aspiration become positioned against the vein wall, preventing appropriate and obvious blood return. In this

TABLE 33-9 Chemotherapy Drug Extravasation Record

Date ______
Time ______

Patient ______ Risk Factors ______

Drug ______ Dilution mg/ml ______

Method of Administration: Two-syringe technique IV push ______
Side-arm ______
VAD: Port ______ External catheter ______
Type of needle ______
Other: ______

Amount infiltrated ______ Amount aspirated ______
Size of infiltration (note size in cm) ______

Location of Extravasation

Hand: Dorsal Surface			*Arm:* Ventral Surface		
hand ______	rt ______	lt ______	forearm ______	rt ______	lt ______
forearm ______	rt ______	lt ______	wrist ______	rt ______	lt ______
wrist ______	rt ______	lt ______	ac fossa ______	rt ______	lt ______

VAD: Describe ______
other ______ Photograph yes ______ no ______

Process Documentation:

S: (Patient's Symptoms) ______

O: (Clinical Signs) ______

A: (Assessment) suspected extravasation ______ definite extravasation ______

P: (Plan of care) ______ Physician notified: Date ______ Time ______ Initials ______

Follow-up (document with serial photographs): ______

Source: Goodman M: Delivery of cancer chemotherapy, in Baird SB, McCorkle R, Grant M (eds): *Cancer Nursing: A Comprehensive Textbook.* Philadelphia: Saunders, 1991, pp. 291–319.

situation the clinician may choose to restart the intravenous or rely on other measures of assessing venous integrity. Often the patient does not have numerous venous access sites from which to choose. While one would always want to spare the patient another needle stick, it is often better to restart the intravenous elsewhere, especially when, after flushing with saline, there remains any doubt of an intact vein.

Rarely, if ever, is the administration of chemotherapy an emergency situation, meaning that if the nurse determines that the patient has no optimal means of safely receiving the vesicant agent, then the nurse should confer with the physician regarding placement of a vascular access device, after which the drug may be administered. In the current milieu of cancer treatment and variety of short- and long-term vascular access devices available, the nurse should not feel compelled to administer vesicant agents in less than optimally safe circumstances. These devices (see Chapter 15) have become a common method of drug delivery and, depending on the patient's individual treatment plan, may be recommended prior to beginning chemotherapy.

While generally considered a reliable and safe means of drug delivery, implanted ports and, less commonly, tunneled catheters do sometimes result in extravasations of vesicant agents. In the case of implanted ports, the cause of drug extravasation is usually a misplaced or displaced needle. In this situation the drug extravasates into the port pocket or area surrounding the port. Another mechanism for drug extravasation from ports involves retrograde subcutaneous leakage from percutaneously inserted catheters obstructed by a fibrin sheath.[39] Extravasation may also occur into the subcutaneous tunnel either from thrombosis and back tracking or from a damaged or fractured central venous catheter. Extravasation may also occur into the intrathoracic cavity as a complication of catheter placement.

Prior to injecting or infusing a vesicant into a tunneled central venous catheter (e.g., Hickman, Raaf, or Groshong) or a nontunneled centrally or peripherally placed central venous catheter (e.g., PICC), examine the exit site for leaks and the insertion site for evidence of swelling or venous thrombosis. Catheter displacement may be evidenced by the appearance of the cuff extruding from the exit site or an obviously more white segment of catheter at the exit site indicating that the catheter has been pulled or slipped out of place. Observe the insertion site (usually the ipsilateral supraclavicular area) for evidence of swelling during fluid bolus. Any evidence of swelling or subjective complaints by the patient of pain or discomfort during fluid bolus warrants investigation.

The presence of a blood return from an implanted port or a tunneled catheter usually confirms catheter tip placement. However, it is not uncommon for a catheter to be properly placed, without evidence of catheter damage, and still have an absent or intermittent blood return. The catheter or port is still safe to use provided it flushes easily without subjective complaints. If, however, the patient complains of discomfort with fluid injection or flow demonstrates resistance, becomes sluggish, or does not flow freely with gravity, it is possible that the catheter tip is somehow intermittently obstructed, the catheter has drifted or migrated into a smaller ancillary vein, or it has otherwise become bent or coiled preventing back flow of blood (Figure 33-13 and Figure 33-14). It is important in these situations to determine catheter placement by radiologic means. The injection of fluid or chemotherapy should be withheld pending physician examination.

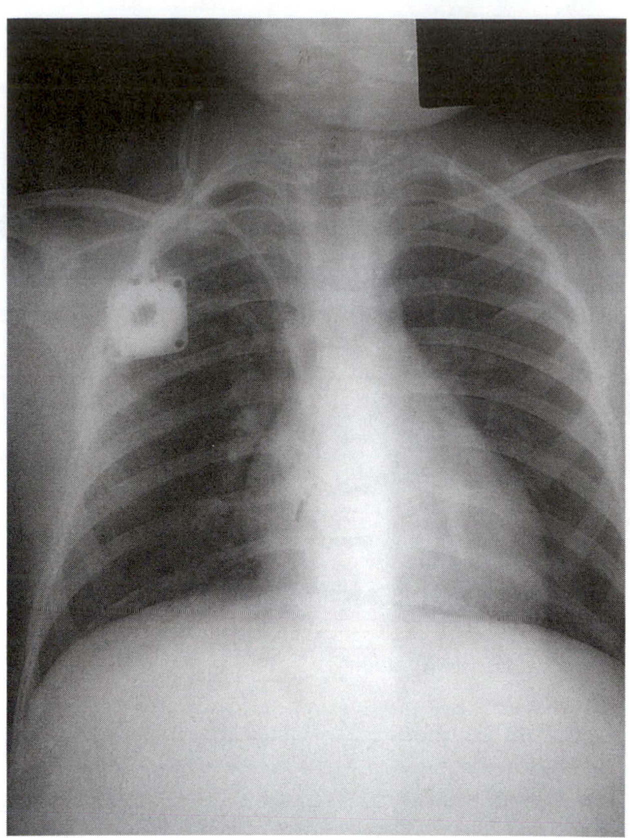

FIGURE 33-13 Catheter bent causing resistance during infusion and lack of blood return.

When giving vesicant agents through a port, whether by simple injection or long-term infusion, it is important to use a 90-degree bent huber point needle rather than a straight needle. Straight needles can easily become dislodged because there is no way to stabilize them regardless of how brief the injection time. Patients are instructed to report any pain, burning, tightness, stinging, or discomfort over the chest area during the injection or infusion. When injecting a vesicant, the blood return is assessed before the injection and at the conclusion of the injection. During the short-term or long-term infusion of a vesicant, assessment of blood return is variable depending upon the status of the patient. In some situations where the patient is confused or uncooperative, it is reasonable to question whether it is safe to use a port for long-term vesicant infusions because these needles can become dislodged even under the best of conditions.

It is difficult to determine how frequently a catheter should be aspirated during the infusion of a vesicant in the hospitalized individual to determine the presence or absence of a blood return. If the catheter or port never had a blood return prior to instituting the vesicant infusion, then assessment of the site every hour as one would any intravenous infusion seems appropriate. If a blood return is known to exist, then assessment of blood return will vary from institution to institution, but the beginning of each shift seems appropriate, with hourly visual examination of the infusion/insertion site. More frequent catheter aspiration such as the beginning and end of each shift or every 4 hours would appear excessive and could significantly increase risk for infection.

The ideal catheter for infusion of vesicant agents in the outpatient/home environment is the tunneled externally based catheter or PICC line. In some situations

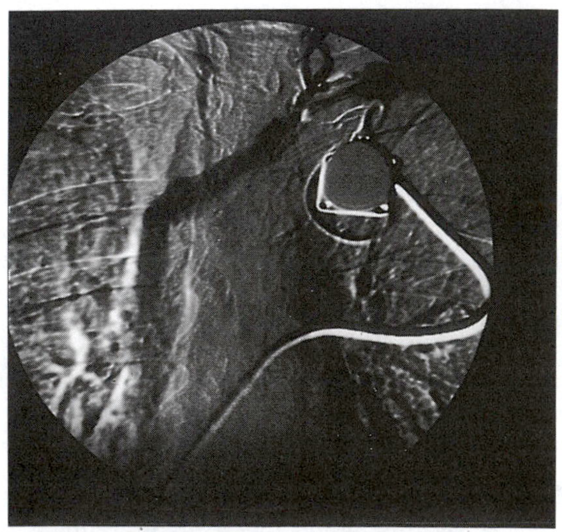

FIGURE 33-14 Catheter coiled around port as demonstrated by digital subtraction venogram.

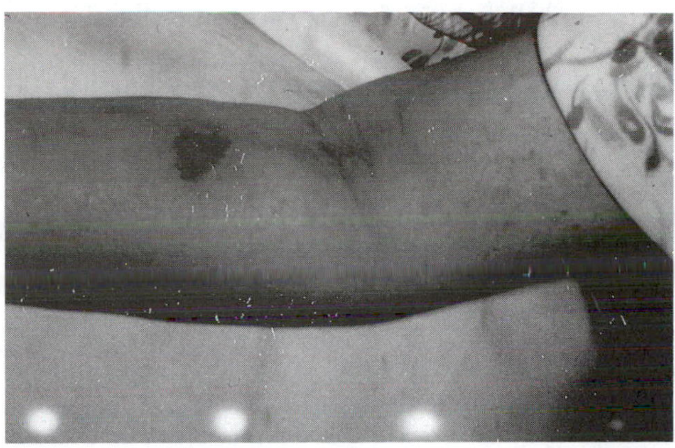

FIGURE 33-19 Mitomycin C extravasation 10 days after injection.

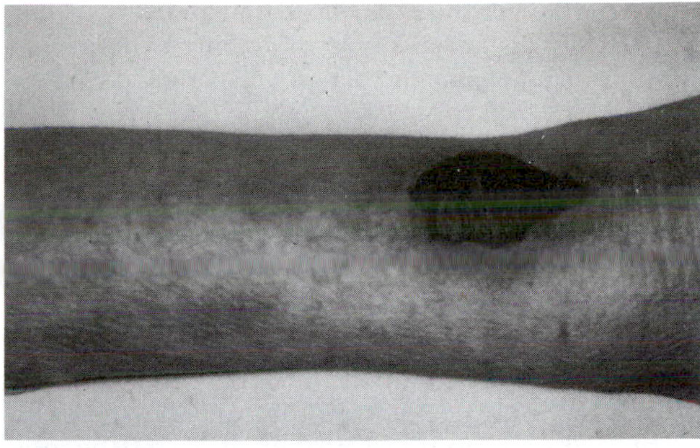

FIGURE 33-20 On day 28, satellite extravasation ulcer appeared on the dorsum of the wrist.

where a port is already in place, this device can safely be employed for vesicant infusions provided the patient is capable of regularly assessing the site for proper needle placement.

Management

If a frank extravasation has occurred, it will usually be obvious to patient and nurse at the time it occurs. In some situations, however, the actual symptoms are delayed for 24–48 hours. The patient may report a redness over the injection site that is warm to touch. Most often these delayed symptoms indicate that only a small amount of drug actually infiltrated. Figure 33-15 (Plate 8) depicts a doxorubicin extravasation 12 days after drug administration. There was no pain with movement of the area, which healed spontaneously without local treatment. Figure 33-16 (Plate 9) demonstrates erythema and edema at the injection site 1 week after doxorubicin administration. At the time of administration, blood return was lost and the patient complained of slight pain at the site. The drug was stopped. After flushing with saline, slight swelling was noted over the area. Ice was applied. This area progressed to blister formation in 3 weeks with clear demarcation of the damaged area (see Figure 33-17—Plate 10), which was surgically excised (see Figure 33-18—Plate 11).

In the case of mitomycin C, satellite lesions, while uncommon, may appear at sites distant from where the drug was actually given. On day 10 following mitomycin injection, an ulcer was reported at the injection site (Figure 33-19). There was no complaint of pain or evidence of extravasation at the time the drug was given. On day 28, a new ulcer formed on the dorsum of the wrist (Figure 33-20). On day 37, another new lesion was noted behind the left ear (Figure 33-21). All lesions eventually healed without surgical intervention.

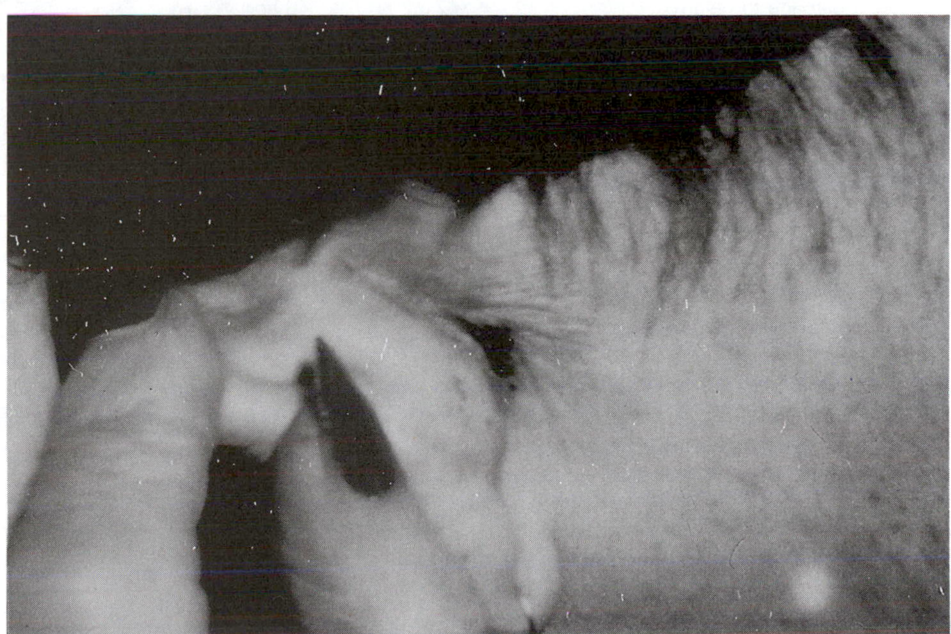

FIGURE 33-21 New satellite lesion on day 37 noted behind the ear.

When there is cause to believe that an extravasation of a vesicant agent has occurred during drug administration, prompt nursing action will, in general, minimize tissue damage (see ONS Guidelines and Recommendations for Management of Extravasation Module V, 1992). The nurse is responsible for ensuring that all antidotes and diluents are readily available and accessible. The following outlines appropriate steps to be taken if an extravasation is suspected.

1. Stop the administration of the chemotherapeutic agent. If injecting through the side arm of a free flowing intravenous, stop the fluid flow immediately. Failure to do so further disperses the infiltrated drug into the tissues.
2. Disconnect the intravenous tubing or syringe and attach an empty 10-cc syringe. Attempt to aspirate any residual drug in the tubing and at the site. Stabilize the extremity and tape the syringe in place.
3. If unable to aspirate any blood or residual drug from the tubing, remove the needle. Gentle apply a sterile 2 × 2 gauze pad over the needle entrance site.
4. Prepare the antidote according to institutional policy and procedure (see Table 33-10).
5. Replace syringe with antidote-filled syringe and inject the antidote.
6. If the needle has been removed, inject the antidote subcutaneously into the extravasation site using a single injection of a 25-g needle.
7. Remove the needle.
8. Avoid applying direct manual pressure to the site.
9. Photograph the extravasation site prior to applying a loose sterile dressing.
10. Apply a warm compress in the event of a plant alkyloid extravasation 15 minutes or more QID for 24 hours.
11. Apply ice for 15 minutes or more every 3–4 hours for 24–48 hours as tolerated in the event of an anthracycline extravasation.
12. Notify the attending physician that an extravasation has occurred or is suspected.

TABLE 33-10 Management of Selected Vesicant Extravasations

Chemotherapeutic Agent	Mechanism of Tissue Damage and Clinical Course	Pharmacologic Antidote	Local Management	Comments
Doxorubicin (Adriamycin)	Binds to nucleic acids leading to prolonged tissue damage Drug is steadily released from dead or dying cells, thereby causing damage to neighboring cells	None	Apply ice for 15 min every 3–4 hr as tolerated for 24–48 hr[41] Elevate the extremity for 48 hr Resume normal activities after 48 hr Physical therapy may be appropriate to prevent stiffness and neuralgia Topical dimethylsulfoxide (DMSO) 99% applied six times daily to the site for 2 wk may minimize ulceration.[42] Further study is needed to establish use. <50 mg hydrocortisone subcutaneous injection has been recommended,[43,44] but there is no scientific rationale for its use[41]	Less extensive (1–2 cc/2 mg/ml) extravasations tend to heal spontaneously More extensive (>3 cc) extravasations follow an indolent course, usually causing ulceration, eschar formation, and pain Surgical intervention with skin grafting may be required If surgical debridement is not performed once painful necrosis is apparent,[40] the tissue damage can be progressive[41]

(continued)

TABLE 33-10 Management of Selected Vesicant Extravasations (continued)

Chemotherapeutic Agent	Mechanism of Tissue Damage and Clinical Course	Pharmacologic Antidote	Local Management	Comments
Daunorubicin (Cerubidine)	Binds to nucleic acids leading to prolonged tissue damage. (See doxorubicin) Severe pain may be noted during infusion of the drug Cellulitis may occur without extravasation	None	Ice or local cooling has not been beneficial, but may be used to increase comfort Heat increases ulceration Surgical excision is usually needed to remove necrotic tissue and locally entrapped drug[40] Little information is currently available. Extravasations may be managed like doxorubicin extravasation	The role of topical DMSO has not been determined in situations involving daunomycin extravasation[45]
Epirubicin Idarubicin (Idamycin)	Both drugs have vesicant properties similar to doxorubicin	None	Little information is currently available. Extravasations may be managed like doxorubicin extravasation	
Mechlorethamine (nitrogen mustard, mustargen)	Drug rapidly fixes to tissues, causing immediate tissue damage Drug is probably not recycled locally Immediate, often intense pain is noted if extravasated Thrombophlebitis of the injected vein is common Perivenous hyperpigmentation may occur following a single injection	Isotonic sodium thiosulfate Mix 4 ml 10% sodium thiosulfate with 6 ml sterile H_2O or 1.6 ml 25% sodium thiosulfate with 8.4 ml sterile H_2O Yield 10 cc 1/6 molar solution sodium thiosulfate	Inject 1–4 ml 1/6 molar solution of sodium thiosulfate through existing IV line or subcutaneously if IV has been removed Inject 1 ml for each mg extravasated Topical cooling may promote comfort but does not appear to minimize ulceration[41]	Sodium thiosulfate neutralizes nitrogen mustard[46] Initiate local treatment immediately Ensure availability of sodium thiosulfate and sterile water for injection in extravasation kit prior to initiating injection of nitrogen mustard
Vincristine (Oncovin) Vinblastine (Velban) Teniposide (Vumon)	These agents do not bind to DNA, but inhibit mitosis. Tissue damage tends to follow a more indolent course	Hyaluronidase (Wydase) (refrigerate) Mix 150 u/ml hyaluronidase with 1 ml of sodium chloride	Inject 1.4 ml through existing IV line or subcutaneously if IV has been removed Administer 1 ml for each ml extravasated	Both hyaluronidase and heat act to enhance the systemic absorption from subcutaneous spaces[47]

(continued)

TABLE 33-10 Management of Selected Vesicant Extravasations (continued)

Chemotherapeutic Agent	Mechanism of Tissue Damage and Clinical Course	Pharmacologic Antidote	Local Management	Comments
Vindeside (Eldisine) Vinorelbine (Navelbine) Etoposide (Vepesid)	Pain, localized swelling, and erythema typically occur if these drugs are extravasated Blister formation may occur within a week of extravasation and gradually resolve without frank ulceration If ulceration does occur, healing is often prolonged, taking 5–6 mo Symptoms of vindesine extravasation may be delayed. Ulceration and delayed healing (6 mo) have been noted		Apply warm compress 15 min four times a day for 48 hr	Local cooling, vitamin A cream, and hydrocortisone injection significantly increase vinca alkaloid skin ulcers[41] Vinblastine may be associated with an intense aching along the injected vein 12–24 hr after the injection, persisting for 3–4 days. Systemic analgesics may be necessary.
Mitomycin C (Mutamycin)	Frank and obvious mitomycin C extravasation is associated with intense pain gradually resulting in painful ulceration, necrosis, and eschar formation Surgical debridement is usually necessary where significant extravasation has occurred Delayed skin ulceration may appear at a previous injection site following injection in the opposite arm Extravasation may occur without any evidence of pain or swelling at the site with delay of ulceration occurring weeks to months later[50]	None	DMSO may provide some benefit in the treatment of mitomycin C extravasation, but further research is needed The role of sodium thiosulfate in the management of mitomycin extravasation is yet to be determined and warrants further research	Mitomycin C may cause dermal ulceration at sites distant from injection site[48] Glucocorticoids appear to offer no therapeutic benefit in the treatment of immediate or delayed mitomycin C extravasations,[49] and may even worsen ulceration[51] Neither heating nor cooling has proven therapeutic

(continued)

TABLE 33-10 Management of Selected Vesicant Extravasations (continued)

Chemotherapeutic Agent	Mechanism of Tissue Damage and Clinical Course	Pharmacologic Antidote	Local Management	Comments
Dactinomycin (Actinomycin D)	Dactinomycin is a potent intercalating agent that causes intense pain and ulceration if extravasated	None	Ice may be applied to the site to increase comfort Elevate area for 48 hr Resume normal activities after 48 hr Consult plastic surgeon if pain persists for >7–10 days	Neither topical cooling nor DMSO is effective local treatment for extravasation of dactinomycin[45] Heat may significantly enhance tissue damage

13. Instruct the patient on local care, systemic analgesics, and plan for follow-up.
    a. Elevate the extremity for 48 hours.
    b. After the first 48 hours the patient should be encouraged to use the extremity normally. Failure to do so may result in stiffness, neuropathy, and causalgia.[40]
    c. Arrange for a return appointment once or twice weekly depending on the amount of drug suspected to have extravasated and the patient's individual concerns.
    d. Photograph the site weekly as appropriate. Document degree of erythema, induration, pain, and whether there is evidence of ulceration or necrosis.
    e. If pain persists beyond 7–10 days, confer with physician regarding a plastic surgery consultation, especially if there is evidence of ulcer demarcation.[40]
    f. Consider physical therapy consultation to encourage normal use of the extremity during healing.
14. Complete extravasation documentation record (Table 33-9), paying special attention to subjective complaints and objective observations of the details immediately surrounding the extravasation event.

Extravasation from a central venous catheter (tunneled, nontunneled, implanted port, or PICC line) may be substantial before detected since infusions are not monitored constantly and the vesicant may be more diluted than when given by intravenous injection. Therefore, pain at the site may not be noted early. Dressings over the port site may mask swelling. Because infusions tend to be given very slowly, a considerable amount of drug can extravasate without obvious evidence of leakage. In the case of an implanted port, the cause is usually needle dislodgement from the port septum, where the needle is found lying in the subcutaneous tissue. The degree of tissue damage will depend on the concentration of the drug and amount infiltrated. In some cases there may be no tissue breakdown; in others, wide excision including mastectomy may be required for the wound to heal.

If an extravasation is suspected from a central venous catheter, the infusion is immediately stopped and the physician is notified. An attempt should be made to estimate the amount of drug extravasated. It may be possible to aspirate residual drug from the site. An antidote can be administered if available. Otherwise, the needle should be removed. Efforts to manually express fluid from the site should be avoided. Instead, a sterile dressing should be applied over the needle entrance site and changed frequently. Ice or warm packs should be applied per institutional policy and procedure. Appropriate documentation (extravasation documentation record) is completed, and plans for careful follow-up and additional consultation with a surgeon may be appropriate.

HAIR

Radiation Effects

Hair follicles in the active growing phase (anagen) represent the most rapidly proliferating cell population in the human body. This rapid mitosis of epithelial cells in the hair root renders it quite radiosensitive, making alopecia a common local effect of radiation therapy. While scalp hair is the most radiosensitive, other terminal hairs are also susceptible to the effects of radiation. In order of radiosensitivity are scalp, beard, eyebrow, eyelash, axillary, pubic, and fine hair of the body.

In the normal adult scalp, 85%–90% of hairs are in the anagen phase, with only 10% in the telogen or resting phase. Radiation causes premature conversion of hair follicle cells from the anagen to the telogen phase, which results in new hairs being shed at an increased rate. Radiation also affects hair growth and weakens the hair shaft, making it more susceptible to breakage.[16]

A number of factors determine the extent and duration of radiation-induced alopecia, including the individual's normal hair growth rate, the area being treated, the dose per fraction, and the total dose delivered to an area. Hair loss is either complete or partial depending on the treatment field. Complete scalp hair loss is usually seen in patients receiving whole-brain irradiation as treatment for primary or metastatic brain cancer; whereas patients who receive radiation to a portion of the brain will experience hair loss limited to the area treated.

Although hair loss patterns vary slightly, radiation-induced alopecia follows a somewhat predictable pattern. Hair thinning usually begins to occur after 2–3 weeks of treatment at a dose of 25–30 Gy and continues for an additional 2–3 weeks. Significant or complete hair loss occurs after a dose of 45–55 Gy has been delivered. While hair loss resulting from radiation to the scalp cannot be prevented, measures should be taken to reduce trauma to the remaining hair and the skin of the exposed scalp. General care of the hair and scalp is reviewed in Table 33-11. If hair regrowth occurs, it usually begins 8–9 weeks following completion of treatment. New hair usually has a slower growth rate, a finer

TABLE 33-11 Nursing Diagnoses Related to Alopecia

Diagnosis	Expected Outcome—Patient Will:	Nursing Interventions
I. Knowledge deficit regarding alopecia related to chemotherapy and/or radiation therapy	I. A. Verbalize understanding of the cause and expected sequelae of treatment-induced alopecia B. Identify available resources related to alopecia	I. A. Assess patient's risk for hair loss related to treatment. B. Inform patient of precise time of hair loss and how it will occur (complete, partial) if possible. C. Explain rationale for alopecia specific to chemotherapy and/or radiation therapy. Discuss: 1. Why hair falls out with specific therapy 2. Variability of hair loss depending on therapy 3. Possibility of hair regrowth—stress regrowth when appropriate 4. Potential change in color and texture of new hair when regrowth occurs D. Encourage verbalization of misconceptions regarding alopecia related to treatment. E. Provide literature and resources related to alopecia.
II. Potential disturbance in body image and/or self-concept related to thinning or complete loss of hair	II. A. Verbalize feelings regarding hair loss and identify coping measures B. Describe appropriate interventions to minimize degree and impact of alopecia	II. A. Assess the impact of hair loss on patient and significant other(s). Encourage verbalization of fears and concerns. B. Identify ways to support patient's feelings in such areas as self-worth, masculinity and femininity, social contacts, and work activities. C. Encourage patient to speak with others who have experienced and adjusted to hair loss. D. Offer tips to minimize degree of alopecia: 1. Shampoo gently one to two times/week with a mild protein-based shampoo. Check with radiation therapist before washing hair if marks have been placed on scalp. 2. Rinse well with lukewarm water and gently pat dry with soft towel. 3. Use a soft-bristled hairbrush or wide-toothed comb to reduce stress on the hair shaft. 4. Use a satin pillowcase to minimize rubbing friction on scalp hair while lying down. 5. Avoid use of hot rollers, hair dryers, curling irons, permanents, and hair dyes—all can dry the scalp and damage sensitive hair follicles.

(continued)

TABLE 33-11 Nursing Diagnoses Related to Alopecia (continued)

Diagnosis	Expected Outcome—Patient Will:	Nursing Interventions
		6. Avoid rollers in the hair while sleeping, braids, pony tails, or corn rows. 7. Consider a short haircut—may reduce the weight on the hair shaft and make it easier to manage loose hairs. 8. Utilize hair-preserving measures when appropriate and ordered by physician. E. Provide information regarding wigs or hairpieces prior to hair loss. Include information on: 1. Types of wigs (synthetic vs. human; machine-made vs. hand) 2. Cost, fit, and style 3. Area retailers or available wig banks such as a cancer society 4. Reimbursement—prosthetic coverage a. Health insurance companies (provide physician prescription; need invoice from retailer providing service) b. Tax deduction as medical expense F. Identify wig alternatives. 1. Scarves, turbans, bandannas, sports caps, hats 2. Use of wardrobe, makeup, and jewelry to highlight other features and help to "feel good about oneself" G. Encourage use of eyebrow pencil, false eyelashes, wide-brimmed eyeglasses to minimize loss. H. Inform patient of "Look Good . . . Feel Better Program." Call 1-800-395-LOOK for information.
III. Alteration in protective mechanisms of hair: A. Potential for impaired skin integrity related to scalp hair loss B. Potential for eye injury related to loss of eyebrows and eyelashes	III. A. Verbalize knowledge of scalp care when hair loss is evident B. Identify measures to minimize eye injury related to loss of eyebrows and eyelashes	III. A. Inform patient of the protective mechanisms of hair (scalp, eyebrows, eyelashes). B. Instruct patient on scalp care: 1. Wash scalp gently with mild shampoo one to two times/week. 2. Use a head covering to protect scalp from wind, cold, and sun. 3. Always apply a sunscreen with a sun protection factor of 15 or more when sun exposure is expected. 4. While receiving radiation therapy, apply a water-soluble, mild lubricant such as Natural Care Gel® (Catalin Corp), or Skin Balm® (Carrington Laboratories) two to three times daily. Do not apply 3 hours before receiving treatment. 5. With chemotherapy cycles or after radiation treatments are completed, apply a hydrophilic lubricant containing no perfume two to three times daily. Examples include Lubriderm®, Eucerin®, and Special Care Cream®. Continue applying until hair regrowth begins. 6. Ensure wig lining is comfortable and nonirritating. C. Instruct patient on measures to protect eyes from injury (eg, use of sunglasses, wide-brimmed hats, false eyelashes).

texture, and may have a different color. Regrowth is unlikely if alopecia persists for greater than 6 months. The likelihood of hair regrowth also diminishes with age and higher doses of radiation.[13,16]

Hair loss is often a devastating side effect of irradiation to the scalp. Clinicians need to recognize the potential impact of alopecia on a patient's quality of life and take measures to enhance coping. The probability of hair loss, its extent, and duration are addressed at the onset of treatment. Patients should be encouraged to discuss their feelings regarding hair loss, whether it is to be temporary or permanent, and great care must be taken not to minimize the potential impact on self-image. It is often helpful for patients to prepare for probable alopecia by procuring a wig before it becomes necessary. This often reduces the anxiety associated with the uncertain timing of hair loss and makes it easier for a stylist to match color and style. Encourage patients to question their insurance companies regarding coverage for a "scalp prosthesis for treatment-induced alopecia." Some companies will reimburse with a physician's prescription and/or letter. Table 33-12 reviews suggestions for wig procurement and insurance reimbursement.

To minimize or delay hair loss and scalp irritation, basic hair and scalp care guidelines should be instituted at the onset of treatment. The duration and extent of hair loss are dependent upon self-care, individual hair growth patterns, and total radiation dose delivered to an area. Although purely speculative, some clinicians theorize that the drug Minoxidil (Upjohn) may decrease the time needed for hair regrowth following radiation-induced alopecia. Even more uncertain is whether or not the drug would have any impact on what is considered to be permanent radiation-induced alopecia. This is clearly an area worthy of research.

Although controversial, hair transplantation by a punch or graft technique is the only reported treatment for permanent radiation-induced alopecia. Limited success for this procedure is thought to be a result of the compromised vascularity of irradiated skin. While it is reported that grafts take, the number of hairs that result per graft is poor. In cases where success has been reported, good technical cosmetic results have improved the patient's quality of life.[52]

TABLE 33-12 Tips for Wig Selection

1. Select and purchase a wig prior to hair loss so hair color and style can be matched. If hair has thinned or complete loss has occurred, bring photographs to match.
2. Bring someone along whose opinion you trust.
3. If you need or want privacy, phone for an appointment or consultation.
4. Where to purchase: department stores, hair salons, and full-service wig stores. Ask your nurse or physician for area resources or contact your local cancer society.
5. Types of wigs: Wigs vary—human hair wigs are more costly and need more servicing; synthetic wigs are less expensive, easier to style, washable, and need less care. *Both look natural.*
6. Price: Ask what is included in the cost. Consider charges for fitting, altering, styling, accessories such as wigstand, shampoo, etc.
7. How to look natural: Consider *fit* (close on your head and feeling comfortable), *color* (choose one close to your own), *style* (hand-made vs. machine-made). For men, hand-tied is best choice because of the need for close styling.
8. How many wigs: Life expectancy of a wig worn on a daily basis given proper care is 6 months; therefore, two wigs are preferred if hair loss is expected to be greater than 6 months.
9. Care of wig:

   synthetic—wash with cold water using a capful of wig shampoo, do not brush when wet, and keep away from excess heat
   human hair—as you care for normal hair
10. How to obtain insurance coverage for wig:
    - Get prescription from physician—"cranial therapeutic prosthesis for medical indication."
    - Obtain receipt from person servicing the wig.
    - Know your rights as the insured party and process claim.
    - If claim denied—appeal and ask for review by medical review board.
11. Alternative options to wigs: cap and hairpiece combinations
    - HEADLINER (Designs for Comfort, Inc., 1-800-443-9226)
    - SWEETIE CAP (Lan Care, Inc., 1-309-762-4800)

Chemotherapy Effects

Alopecia

Alopecia is the most common cutaneous side effect of chemotherapy and often one of the most distressing.[53,54] Extent of hair loss may range from thinning of the scalp to total body hair loss. Although certainly not a life-threatening event, loss of hair has a profound psychological impact on the patient and the patient's acceptance of treatment. Some patients may even refuse potentially curative therapy for fear of this side effect.

Hair follicles are vulnerable to the effects of chemotherapy because of their high mitotic and metabolic activity. At any given time an average 85% of scalp hair follicles are in the anagen (proliferative) phase, while the majority of other body hair follicles (e.g., eyebrows, pubic, axilla) are in the telogen (resting) phase. This explains why scalp hair loss is a more common and severe occurrence than the loss of other body hair. However, with long-term therapy, pubic, axillary, and facial hair may also be lost.

Chemotherapy-induced alopecia occurs by two mechanisms affecting either the hair root or the hair shaft. Higher doses of chemotherapy or more potent epilators destroy enough cells to cause complete atrophy of the root and loss of the hair root bulb. Hair falls out spontaneously or is lost easily when combed or washed. Drugs of less intensity slow the cellular mitotic rate, causing partial atrophy of the bulb and narrowing of the hair shaft. Narrow, weakened hair shafts break off easily at the point of constriction. However, the root remains intact and active in the scalp, leaving a thinning pattern of hair.

Unlike natural hair loss, chemotherapy-induced alopecia occurs rapidly and becomes apparent over a 2- to 3-week period following a dose of chemotherapy. Assuming the human scalp is composed of an average of 100,000 hairs, alopecia is clinically evident when 25% of hair is lost. Hair loss is diffuse and asymptomatic, although some patients have described intense scalp discomfort 1–2 days prior to hair shedding.

Fortunately, the cytotoxic injury to hair follicles is essentially temporary. After discontinuation of the epilating drugs, regrowth is visible in 4–6 weeks. Regrowth may even occur during active treatment because of developed drug resistance by cells of the hair matrix. As hair grows back, changes in hair pigmentation (lighter or darker), hair texture (finer or coarser), and hair type (straight or curly) may be evident. This change is usually temporary, with hair returning to its original type within 1 year. While extremely rare, prolonged and possibly irreversible alopecia has been reported in patients undergoing busulfan/cyclophosphamide conditioning regime for allogeneic bone marrow transplantation.[55] The possibility of this occurrence and impact on quality of life for long-term survivors must be considered.

The severity and duration of chemotherapy-induced hair loss is related to several drug factors including the type of drug or combination of drugs, dose of drug (acute and cumulative), method of administration and pharmacokinetics, as well as patient-related factors. Contrary to patient perceptions, the majority of cytotoxic drugs do not cause hair loss. Rather, hair loss is a common side effect of a number of drugs that are used frequently in cancer treatment. Cytotoxic agents with the potential to cause alopecia when given alone or in combination include: bleomycin, cyclophosphamide, dactinomycin, daunorubicin, doxorubicin, etoposide, 5-FU, hydroxyurea, ifosfamide, methotrexate, mitomycin, mitoxantrone, melphalan, taxol, and vinblastine. Doxorubicin (doses greater than 50 mg/m^2) and cyclophosphamide (doses greater than 500 mg/m^2) particularly are known to induce epilation after two cycles.[56] Combination therapy with both drugs almost always produces severe alopecia.

Bolus intravenous administration of chemotherapy results in immediate peak serum levels with subsequent exposure and damage of sensitive growing hairs resulting in hair loss. Infusions over several hours or longer are associated with a greater likelihood of alopecia. The risk of alopecia appears to be decreased with low-dose continuous infusion. This may be related to the fact that high peak serum levels are necessary to cause hair loss.

Since the liver is the organ of metabolism for most drugs, hepatic dysfunction can result in prolonged serum levels of drug. Abnormal hepatic function has been associated with severe hair loss in patients treated with doxorubicin even when preventive measures were used.[57,58]

A patient-related factor that may influence the degree of scalp hair loss includes the variability of scalp hair growth among individual patients. The percentage of scalp hairs in the anagen phase at any given time is variable; therefore, individuals who have relatively few hairs in this proliferative phase will be less sensitive to the epilatory effects of chemotherapy. Additionally, the condition of the patient's hair before treatment is a factor that must be considered—damaged hair may potentiate the risk for alopecia.

Other factors such as noncytotoxic drugs (e.g., heparin, propranolol, ibuprofen) and medical conditions (e.g., malnutrition, chronic stress, hypothyroidism) may also contribute to or cause alopecia in the cancer patient.[59]

Prevention of alopecia

Since the 1960s, considerable efforts have been directed to reducing the incidence and severity of alopecia using empirical methods like scalp tourniquet[60–62] and scalp hypothermia.[65] Neither method has proven particularly useful and they are not widely employed, especially in cases of dose-intensive chemotherapy.

Scalp hypothermia may be more advantageous than scalp tourniquet in hair preservation because it not only causes scalp vasoconstriction but also reduces cellular uptake of drug by hair follicles that are temperature-dependent. Additionally, scalp hypothermia may lower the metabolic rate of cells, making hair follicles less susceptible to the epilatory effects of chemotherapy.[66]

Research on scalp hypothermia has focused on doxorubicin-induced alopecia for several reasons. There is a high incidence of reported hair loss with doxorubicin, which has widespread and routine clinical efficacy in a number of cancers. Furthermore, its pharmacokinetics makes it an ideal choice: a short initial distribution phase with a rapid fall in plasma concentration during the first 15–30 minutes following injection making it possible to minimize the amount of hair loss.

The earliest study on scalp hypothermia was reported by Luce et al.,[62] in which a plastic helmet was attached to a room air conditioner to cool patients' scalps. The control group lost 80% of hair compared to 30% hair loss in the experimental group. Subsequent studies demonstrated that cooling the scalp to 25°C or less[63,67] and wetting the hair before applying the cooling device (to minimize trapped air) can reduce and sometimes prevent alopecia. Scalp hypothermia is less effective with high doses of doxorubicin, especially when used in combination with cyclophosphamide.[65]

The use of hair preservation techniques has not been recommended for all patients; in particular, it is contraindicated for those with hematologic malignancies, solid tumors that originate in the scalp, or those who have a high incidence of scalp metastases. Opponents caution that methods used to decrease blood flow to the scalp during chemotherapy administration could create a drug sanctuary, thereby protecting tumor stem cells from cytotoxic therapy. However, others report that the risk of cutaneous metastases as the first site of recurrence is negligible and they routinely recommend scalp hypothermia for a number of solid tumors including breast, ovarian, and osteosarcoma.[68]

Several cases of scalp metastases following the use of hypothermia have been reported.[69,70] Therefore, risk of scalp micrometastases must be considered when treating patients with curative intent. Currently, hypothermia is only recommended where the goal of therapy is control or palliation or in situations where the patient would otherwise refuse potentially curative adjuvant therapy.

In the early 1970s, when the FDA first approved the use of commercially available hypothermia devices, few questions were raised regarding their safety and efficacy in chemotherapy-induced alopecia. They were determined to be "substantially equivalent" to cold packs that were marketed to decrease hemorrhaging and swelling. In 1990 the FDA requested manufacturers of these devices to provide clinical data documenting their safety and effectiveness in prevention of chemotherapy-induced alopecia. When no documentation was submitted, the FDA halted the manufacturing and distribution of commercially available cooling devices.

Even though commercial devices are unavailable for purchase, some institutions still provide scalp hypothermia for selected patients. For patients considering hair preservation techniques, discussion must include weighing the benefits (hair preservation) versus the risks (developing scalp metastases at a later date). Some institutions require the patient to sign an informed consent that becomes part of the patient's medical record.[71]

The stigma associated with hair loss has promoted research with products that have shown efficacy in male pattern baldness such as Minoxidil. Although known to induce hair regrowth and prevent hair loss in male pattern baldness, Minoxidil 2% topical solution has shown no benefit in prevention of chemotherapy-induced alopecia.[75] Further research may be beneficial to evaluate Minoxidil's role in accelerating regrowth of hair following treatment-related alopecia.

Nursing Care

Hair contributes greatly to body image and is associated closely with one's sexuality. Consequently, the potential or actual loss of one's hair can have a devastating emotional impact on a patient.

In light of the uncertainty of hair-preserving techniques, more emphasis needs to be placed on the psychological support of the patient experiencing hair loss from cancer treatment and on helping the patient find appropriate ways to adapt to alopecia (Table 33-11).

It is essential that the nurse give the patient and family an adequate appraisal of the potential and degree of hair loss and approximately when it will occur. While this is not always known, many times it is; for instance, when high-dose doxorubicin and cyclophosphamide are used, hair loss is nearly complete by 3 weeks. As previously discussed, it is often helpful for patients to prepare for probable alopecia by procuring a scalp prosthesis (wig or hairpiece) before it becomes necessary.

Although alopecia is not preventable, certain measures may minimize or delay hair loss and scalp irritation. For example, some clinicians advise patients to cut long hair short in anticipation of hair loss. Short hair may make hair loss less noticeable, make remaining hair appear thicker, and possibly decrease the weight on the hair shaft. On the other hand, if hair is thinning or radiation therapy is given to a portion of the scalp causing a balding area, longer hair may be a better style to camouflage thinning or lost hairs. Patients should begin using basic hair and scalp care guidelines at the onset of treatment.

Once hair loss is significant, necessitating a wig or head covering, the patient may be advised to shave the remaining scalp hairs. This practice allows the hair to grow in at the same length, often permitting the patient to go without a wig sooner. In addition, shaving the head rids the patient of the problem of continuous shedding of hair.

The use or nonuse of hair care practices such as blow drying, perming, or coloring hair is controversial and an area for further nursing research. Some claim these practices cause the hair to become brittle and fall out faster during chemotherapy, while others have not found these practices to be related to postchemotherapy hair loss.

The nurse is often the preferred person to assist patients in coping with personal images needs.[76] Ehmann et al.[76] describe an independent oncology nursing consultative service developed to intervene with patients at risk for alopecia. Other enterprising nurses have provided patients with an "Alopecia Packet" that includes a booklet describing hair loss and a cotton turban head covering.[77] Patient information materials are widely available and may facilitate nursing interventions for patients adapting to hair loss.

Finally, guidelines are available for enhancing the appearance of patients undergoing chemotherapy and/or radiation therapy. The "Look Good . . . Feel Better" program is a national program developed by the American Cancer Society, the Cosmetic, Toiletry and Fragrance Association (CTFA) Foundation, and the National Cosmetology Association. Appearance mirrors positive attitude, and positive feelings enhance one's ability to cope.

Hirsutism

Androgens are efficacious in the treatment of women with breast cancer, especially postmenopausal women with bone metastases. Troublesome side effects include loss of hair in the frontotemporal portion of the scalp (male pattern baldness) and hirsutism. *Hirsutism* is characterized by an excessive growth of hair in androgen-dependent areas of the body including the upper lip, chin, chest, abdomen, and anterior aspects of the thighs. The intensity of this side effect depends on the amount of drug taken, with distribution of hair returning to normal after the androgen is discontinued. Clinicians need to be aware that this excess hair growth may cause a great deal of distress and lead to refusal of treatment and noncompliance.

Nursing interventions are aimed at providing emotional support for altered body changes. Excess hair can be removed by tweezing or shaving; however, electrolysis is not recommended because of the increased possibility of skin irritation and infection. If the hair is fine, bleaching may mask the condition.

NAILS

While similar to that of a hair follicle by virtue of its rapidly proliferating cell population, the radiosensitivity of a finger or toenail is not usually of consequence in patients receiving radiation therapy. Rarely are these structures included in the radiation treatment field; however, there are exceptions. Patients receiving low-dose total body irradiation (12–15 Gy) prior to bone marrow transplantation usually have minimal nail effects, while those patients whose nails receive higher doses (25–30 Gy), as seen in treatment for mycosis fungoides, may lose the nail(s). Radiation to the nail can result in decreased growth rates and the development of ridges when the nail attempts to grow. While nothing can be done to prevent nail changes when these structures are irradiated, patients need to be aware of the potential effects.[6,11]

Changes in the fingernails and toenails are commonly seen during chemotherapy. Pigmentation is seen most commonly and occurs with more regularity and intensity in African Americans than in whites. The pigment generally is deposited at the base of the nail, causing transverse dark bands that correlate with the times the drug was administered. This reaction occurs most commonly with doxorubicin and cyclophosphamide but has been reported with melphalan, 5-FU, daunomycin, and bleomycin. If continuous infusion therapy of these drugs is given, the nails darken evenly.

Beau's lines (transverse white lines or grooves in the nail) indicate a reduction or cessation of nail growth in response to cytotoxic therapy. A partial separation of the nail plate (onycholysis) can be seen with 5-FU, doxorubicin, and bleomycin therapy.[20]

GLANDS

Sebaceous glands are composed of cells that are destroyed and used in the production of sebum, which keeps the skin and hair lubricated and pliable. These cells undergo replacement through continuous cellular proliferation and, as a result, are radiosensitive. The loss of oil in the skin secondary to impairment or destruction of sebaceous glands is in large part responsible for the acute and late skin effects associated with irradiated skin such as pruritis and inelasticity.[6,13,16]

Irradiation of sweat glands can also contribute to the dryness of treated skin. The cells of sweat glands have long lives with a slower renewal system, making them only moderately radiosensitive. Complete and permanent destruction of sweat gland function occurs with a skin dose greater than 30 Gy delivered in 3 weeks, leaving the skin dry and itchy.

Great care must be taken to protect dry, irradiated skin as it is more susceptible to fissuring, subsequent infection, and late necrosis. Table 33-4 reviews basic postirradiation skin care.

ALTERATIONS OF THE MUCOUS MEMBRANES

Mucositis is a general term that describes the inflammatory response of mucosal epithelial cells to the cytotoxic effects of chemotherapy as well as localized radiation therapy. Painful ulceration, hemorrhage, and secondary infection may develop when mucositis is not detected early or continues untreated. Since all mucous membrane–covered surfaces exhibit similar patterns of growth, replacement, and function, any mucous membrane–bearing site in the gastrointestinal (GI) tract from mouth to rectum or the vagina can be adversely affected by cancer treatment.

Gastrointestinal Mucositis

The epithelial cells lining the gastrointestinal mucosa renew rapidly, which enables them to replace cells lost from general "wear and tear" that occurs when food is chewed, swallowed, digested, and eliminated from the body. Toxicity (mucositis) results when these mucosal cells damaged by cancer treatment are unable to adequately repair and replace normal cell loss. Manifestations of GI toxicity that will be discussed include: mucositis in the oral cavity (stomatitis), in the esophagus (esophagitis), and in the intestines as diarrhea (enteritis).

Stomatitis

The oral mucosa is a major site for complications secondary to cancer treatment, affecting approximately 400,000 patients annually.[78] It has been reported that 40% of non–head and neck cancer patients treated with conventional therapy develop oral complications.[79] However, the incidence is greater for patients in high-risk categories such as those with leukemia, those receiving radiation therapy to the head and neck region, and those receiving more complex and intense treatment modalities such as bone marrow transplantation (BMT). Woo et al.[80] reported the development of significant mucositis in 75% of BMT patients.

Oral complications resulting from treatment may be acute and/or chronic. Acute reactions include mucosal inflammation and ulceration, infection, and mucosal bleeding. Chronic complications occur as a result of changes in healthy tissue and include xerostomia, taste alterations, trismus, and soft tissue and bone necrosis. In BMT patients, acute and chronic oral graft-versus-host disease (GVHD) is also observed.

The many factors contributing to the occurrence and severity of these complications are listed in Table 33-13. Recognition of these stressors and development of pretreatment and treatment strategies to minimize or prevent oral problems may result in decreased frequency, decreased morbidity, and an increase in patient well-being.

Chemotherapy-induced stomatitis

Chemotherapy affects the oral mucosa either directly at the cellular level where the drug is destroying proliferating cells (direct stomatotoxicity) or indirectly as a result of the drug's myelosuppressive action (indirect stomatotoxicity).[81] (See Figure 33-22.)

Risk factors The risk of developing chemotherapy-induced stomatitis is not the same for all patients nor is it equal in similar drug regimens. Both patient-related and drug-related factors influence the incidence and severity (Table 33-14).

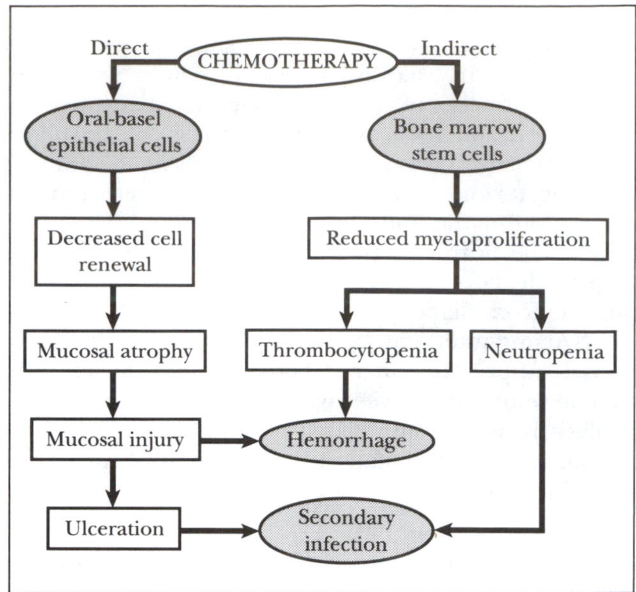

FIGURE 33-22 Stomatotoxic effects of chemotherapy. (Source: Adapted with permission from Lockhart PB, Sonis ST: Relationship of oral complications to peripheral blood leukocyte and platelet counts in patients receiving cancer chemotherapy. *Oral Surg* 48:21–28, 1979.)

TABLE 33-13 Factors Contributing to Stomatitis in the Cancer Patient

Poor oral hygiene
Preexisting dental problems
Dental caries
Periodontal disease
Partially erupted third molars
Exposure to irritants
Chemical (citrus fruits, spicy foods)
Physical (coarse food, ill-fitting dental prosthesis)
Thermal (extremes in food temperatures)
Tobacco and alcohol
Dehydration
Malnutrition
Drug therapy
Antibiotics
Chemotherapy
Steroids
Radiation therapy
Head and neck area
Surgical manipulation
Immunosuppression and myelosuppression
Cancer
Cancer therapy

The frequency of oral problems is two to three times higher in patients with hematologic malignancies than with solid tumors. Patients undergoing BMT experience severe and prolonged mucositis due to the direct stomatotoxic effects of immunosuppressive drugs, total body irradiation, and the indirect effect of the pancytopenia and aplasia.[82] Stomatitis occurs more commonly in younger and older patients. The higher mitotic index of the oral mucosa and higher incidence of hematologic malignancies in the younger patient population may explain the age-related risk factor.

Preexisting oral disease (e.g., dental caries, periodontal disease, partially erupted third molars) as well as poor oral hygiene and local irritants (e.g., ill-fitting dental prostheses, tobacco, alcohol) will predispose chemotherapy patients to an increased risk of oral complications. Furthermore, research has substantiated that oral complications can be reduced or eliminated by meticulous oral assessment with interventions before, during, and between courses of chemotherapy.[82]

One of the most important variables influencing stomatotoxicity is the choice of cytotoxic agent. Stomatitis may be seen in association with numerous chemotherapeutic agents, but it occurs most commonly with the antimetabolites and antitumor antibiotics (Table 33-15 and Figure 33-23—Plate 12).

Although stomatotoxicity generally is dose-related and is more common with higher doses, patients differ in their ability to tolerate a given dose or combination. There is no way to predict which new patient will manifest oral mucositis and which will not, given the same dose of the same drug. However, those who develop stomatitis with one cycle of therapy will almost assuredly develop recurrence in subsequent courses unless the drugs or doses are changed.[83] This is especially the case when the body is unable to adequately eliminate a stomatotoxic drug. For example, in the presence of renal dysfunction or liver dysfunction, excretion of methotrexate and doxorubicin may be compromised respectively. Stomatotoxic drugs used in combination or combined with head and neck irradiation may also increase the degree of stomatitis. Mucositis is observed more often with 5-FU when combined with other mucositis-producing drugs such as methotrexate and doxorubicin and when 5-FU is given concurrently with leucovorin to augment its cytotoxicity.[84]

Direct stomatotoxicity Direct stomatotoxicity results from the cytotoxic action of drugs on the cells of the oral basal epithelium causing a decrease in the rate of cell renewal. The sequelae are a thinned atrophic mucosa and initiation of an inflammatory response (stomatitis). Most often affected are the nonkeratinized mucosal areas including the buccal and labial mucosa, tongue, soft palate, and floor of the mouth. Rarely is the gingiva, or hard palate, involved.[85]

Histologic changes can occur within 5–7 days of initial drug exposure. A dry mucosa, tongue or lips; burning sensation in the oral cavity; and increased salivation result. Visible signs of inflammation and oral ulceration can be observed 7–14 days following therapy, just prior to the granulocyte nadir. Without complications and further insult from repeated drug administration, stomatitis is self-limiting and gradually reverses itself within 2–3 weeks. However, if a break in mucosal integrity occurs, secondary infection leading to sepsis can occur.

Oral pain is the major clinical problem associated with stomatitis. Pain results due to sloughing of the superficial epithelium, inflammation of the oral mucosa, and ulceration, making it difficult for patients to practice adequate oral hygiene, eat properly, and communicate. Treatment of drug-induced stomatitis is essentially palliative, involving topical anesthetics, analgesics, coating agents, and cleansing mouthwashes.

Xerostomia Another potential direct effect on the oral mucosa following chemotherapy is *xerostomia,* a decrease in the quality and quantity of saliva. Patients complain of dry mouth and accumulation of thick, ropy saliva that can interfere with nutrition, taste, and speech. Xerostomia is transient, with treatment aimed at lubricating the oral mucosa and alleviating pain. However, if prolonged, xerostomia may precipitate oral caries as well as candidal infections. Saliva substitutes or frequent rinses with ice water usually provide sufficient relief.

Taste alterations Patients receiving chemotherapy may be susceptible to taste alterations in which there is actual or perceived changes in taste sensations. The drugs cause direct injury to taste cells composing the

TABLE 33-14 Factors Affecting Chemotherapy-Induced Stomatotoxicity

PATIENT-RELATED
Type of disease (incidence higher in hematologic vs. solid tumor)
Age of patient (frequency greater in younger vs. older)
Condition of oral cavity pretreatment (poor oral hygiene practices and preexisting oral disease increase risk)
Level of oral care (risk decreases with oral assessment and interventions prior to, during, and between treatment)
DRUG-RELATED
Drug (most frequently associated with antimetabolites and antitumor antibiotics)
Dose (more common with higher cumulative doses)
Administration schedule (eg, incidence increased with continuous infusion 5-FU vs. intravenous bolus 5-FU)
Drug metabolism (risk increases with impaired renal and hepatic function)
Concomitant therapy (increased risk with stomatotoxic drugs used concurrently with head and neck irradiation)

TABLE 33-15 Chemotherapeutic Drugs with Potential to Cause Stomatotoxicity

- Antimetabolites
  - Cytosine arabinoside
  - Floxuridine
  - 5-Fluorouracil*
  - 6-Mercaptopurine
  - Methotrexate*
  - 6-Thioguanine
- Antibiotics
  - Bleomycin*
  - Dactinomycin*
  - Daunomycin
  - Doxorubicin*
  - Mitomycin
- Alkylating agents
  - Cyclophosphamide
  - Nitrogen mustard
- Plant alkaloids
  - Vinblastine
  - Vincristine
- Miscellaneous
  - Hydroxyurea
  - Procarbazine

*Frequently associated

taste buds, resulting in taste changes that vary widely and are highly individualized. Commonly induced changes include lowered threshold for bitter taste, increase threshold for sweet taste, and complaints that a metallic taste is present. Chemotherapy drugs frequently associated with taste alterations are cyclophosphamide, dacarbazine, doxorubicin, 5-FU, methotrexate, nitrogen mustard, and vincristine.

Some agents like doxorubicin and methotrexate may alter taste acuity, while others like cyclophosphamide and vincristine can be tasted while injected. Chemotherapy-induced taste alterations can further be influenced by poor oral hygiene, infection of the oral cavity, dentures (causing decreased taste sensations), and unpleasant odors. Nursing interventions are aimed at maintaining optimal nutrition. Eating hints should be customized in accordance with each patient's change in taste appreciation.

Indirect stomatotoxicity Chemotherapeutic drugs can affect not only the cells of the oral mucosa but also other cell pools, especially those in the bone marrow. Reduced myeloproliferation is manifested by neutropenia and thrombocytopenia; infection and hemorrhage secondary to myelosuppression can then occur.

Since leukocytes and oral mucosal cells have similar cell renewal rates, changes in the oral status correlate with the timing of myelosuppression. Stomatitis is frequently observed near the nadir of leukocytes, with subsequent resolution often preceding bone marrow recovery by 2–3 days.[81] Improvement in the status of the oral mucosa can therefore be predictive of a recovering white blood cell count.

The oral cavity is susceptible indirectly to infection because of chemotherapy-induced neutropenia. Patients with a granulocyte count less than 1000/mm^3 have a greater than 50% chance of developing an opportunistic infection—bacterial, viral, or fungal.[86] Infections of the oral cavity will be discussed elsewhere in this chapter. It is important to remember than when a patient's granulocyte count is significantly reduced, classic signs of inflammation may be absent.

Oral bleeding and hemorrhage are indirect stomatotoxic sequelae from chemotherapy-induced thrombocytopenia. Bleeding results when the oral mucosa is traumatized or because of underlying periodontal disease and may occur anywhere in the mouth. The gingiva is the most common source. The lower the platelet count, the greater the possibility of bleeding. As a general guideline, gingival bleeding may occur whenever the platelet count is less than 20,000/mm^3 and generally is more severe in patients with preexisting periodontal disease or poor oral hygiene. For patients at risk, oral hygiene regimens should be modified to the less vigorous traumatic measures. Bleeding precautions should be exercised with oral hygiene measures for patients at risk. Management of bleeding with topical coagulants (thrombin-soaked gauze) and pressure is often helpful.

Oral graft-versus-host disease

Acute and chronic graft-versus-host disease (GVHD) is a significant complication of patients who undergo allogeneic BMT. Oral involvement has been reported in 33%–75% of patients with acute GVHD and nearly 80% of those with chronic GVHD.[87] Cultures are necessary to distinguish candidiasis and herpetic stomatitis from oral GVHD. Oral ulceration and pain are complications of acute GVHD and a sclerodermalike picture in chronic GVHD. Treatment strategies include systemic immunosuppressive therapy; topical steroids, which may or may not be beneficial; and fluoride therapy for patients at risk for caries secondary to xerostomia.

Radiation-induced stomatitis and oral complications

Dental evaluation and prophylactic care Oral mucosal side effects of radiation therapy can begin early in the treatment course and progressively worsen. Treatment to the oral cavity may result in stomatitis, hypogeusia (loss of taste), and xerostomia. If the esophagus is included in the treatment field, patients may experience esophagitis and/or dysphagia. While stomatitis, esophagitis, and dysphagia are usually temporary, taste alterations and xerostomia may be permanent in varying degrees. Other effects of radiation are less common and usually do not manifest for months to years after the completion of treatment. These effects include trismus, dental caries, tissue fibrosis, and tissue necrosis.

Regardless of dentition status, patients should have a thorough oral examination by the dentist at least 2–3 weeks before any therapy is initiated if possible. This will ensure adequate time for treatment of infections if present and for healing if invasive procedures are required. The pretreatment dental evaluation is comprehensive and serves to establish a baseline, identify risk factors for developing complications, and allow development of a realistic preventative program designed to meet the needs and abilities of the individual. Any preexisting oral problems including decay, infection, and source of irritation should be assessed. A thorough cleaning to reduce bacteria that can result in local and systemic infection may include root planing, scaling, and curettage. Dentures and prosthetic devices are evaluated and adjusted to ensure fit and prevent friction. Teeth with caries and/or periodontal disease should be repaired or extracted if necessary.

Daily fluoride treatments and good oral hygiene can significantly reduce the incidence of radiation-induced oral complications. A custom-made fluoride carrier or tray is designed by the dentist to deliver topical fluoride. Patients should be instructed on proper brushing and flossing if not contraindicated. Fluoride gel, 0.4% stannous fluoride and 1% sodium fluoride, is then placed in the carrier, which is inserted over the teeth and left in place for 5–10 minutes daily. Bedtime is a preferred time of day as eating or drinking should be avoided for 30 minutes to 1 hour after use.

Oral care and status must be assessed frequently during and after the completion of treatment. Although recommendations vary, it is suggested that patients at risk for developing oral complications be followed by a dentist before treatment, during treatment if complications arise, and 2 months following completion of treatment as acute effects have resolved. Routine dental evaluation is then every 6 months for 2 years and then annually.

Consideration of these factors is important in educating patients as well as in developing a plan of care based on actual and potential problems. Table 33-16 reviews potential radiation-induced gastrointestinal toxicities.

TABLE 33-16 Radiation-Induced Gastrointestinal Toxicities—Direct and Indirect

Tissue Response	Risk Factors: Onset/Duration	Clinical Presentation	Physiological Rationale
Stomatitis	10 Gy	Mucosa appears white. Tenderness and increased sensitivity to extreme temperatures, acidic foods and fluids, and spicy or rough textured foods	Radiation results in a decrease in mitotic activity and subsequent retention of superficial cells, allowing cells to proceed to a higher degree of keratinization. Aggravated by alcohol and smoking.
	20–25 Gy Progressively worsens Usually resolves 2–3 wk after treatment completion	Pain and burning first associated with eating and progressing to a continuous sensation Erythema	Increased sensitivity of nerve endings. Microvascular changes result in vascular congestion and increased capillary permeability.
		Mucosal thinning and sloughing	As cells are lost, they are not sufficiently replaced by epithelial stem cells.
		Edema Mucosal surface red	Mucosa becomes swollen as a result of vascular congestion and hyperemia.
		White or tan, glistening membrane	Fibrinous exudate composed of serum and dead cells covers some areas. Mucosa is very thin and easily ulcerated.
	Trauma	Painful ulceration leaving bright red mucosa	Membrane is friable, fragile, and easily traumatized.
Esophagitis		Refer to Stomatitis	Refer to Stomatitis.
	20 Gy	Difficulty swallowing solids Mild to moderate dysphagia	Microvascular changes result in vascular congestion and increased capillary permeability.
	20–30 Gy Usually resolves 2–3 wk after treatment completion	Substernal burning sensation Pain with swallowing May become progressively worse	Epithelial cells are destroyed without sufficient replacement cells being produced.
Taste alterations	10 Gy exponential to 30 Gy	Diminished taste acuity Increased sensitivity to bitter and salty—appears first and lasts longest Decreased sensitivity to sweets	Indirectly, a function of changes in the oral mucosa and salivary glands (xerostomia). Directly, a result of damage of the microvilli of taste cells.
	>30 Gy Resolution: Partial: 20–60 days after treatment completion Complete: 60–120 days after treatment completion	May be unable to distinguish tastes	

(continued)

TABLE 33-16 Radiation-Induced Gastrointestinal Toxicities—Direct and Indirect (continued)

Tissue Response	Risk Factors: Onset/Duration	Clinical Presentation	Physiological Rationale
Taste alterations, continued	May have permanent alterations	Food may continue to taste bland, papery, or salty	Diminished salivary flow alters the electrolyte balance in the remaining saliva, creating altered taste perceptions.
Xerostomia	Dependent upon salivary glands within treatment field		
	10–20 Gy 50% decrease in saliva	Dry, smooth, shiny mucosa	Damage to salivary glands (major and/or minor) reduces amount of saliva produced.
	>30 Gy 75% decrease in saliva	Thick, ropy saliva	Serous secretions are diminished first, leaving only mucin-type saliva.
	May be permanent	Difficulty chewing and swallowing	Progressive inflammation and degeneration of acinar and ductal cells result in replacement by fibrinous connective tissue infiltrated with lymphocyte and plasma cells.
Oral flora changes	Onset with xerostomia and stomatitis	Fungal and bacterial infection Erythema and burning sensation May have scattered irregular areas of white plaque that may or may not be easily removed—often difficult to distinguish from fibrinous exudate of stomatitis Prime sites: tongue, buccal mucosa, and mucosal surfaces under dentures	An indirect function of radiation. Xerostomia results in a decrease in the volume of saliva and in the antimicrobial compounds responsible for chemical and mechanical debridement. Plaque and microorganisms accumulate. Increase in cariogenic and decrease in noncariogenic bacteria.
Dental caries	Onset—variable Permanent risk	Decay—all teeth at risk Begins as diffuse demineralization of teeth and can progress to rampant decay	An indirect function of radiation. Xerostomia impairs the mechanical and chemical defenses against dental decay (refer to Oral flora changes). Decreased pH prevents saliva from acting as a buffer.
Mucosal atrophy	Following repair of acute mucosal injury Permanent	Thinned, shiny epithelium	Permanent decrease in keratinization and changes in microvasculature.
Fibrosis of subepithelial tissues	Several months following treatment completion Progressive and permanent	Severity/degree ranges from small induration to hard, stony fibrosis Contraction and shrinkage of tissue over time	Faulty collagen remodeling results in fibrotic tissue replacing submucosa. Perivascular and periglandular fibrosis. Increased susceptibility to chemical and mechanical trauma.
Soft tissue necrosis	Following repair of acute mucosal injury Permanent risk Induced by chemical or mechanical trauma	Pain and ulceration of epithelium and underlying tissue	Extracapillary fibrosis, inhibition of vascular remodeling, and vascular occlusion impairs the ability of tissue to respond to injury.
Bone necrosis (osteoradionecrosis)	Uncommon Progressive and irreversible	Constant throbbing pain—most severe at night and during mastication	Bone exposed by soft tissue damage is susceptible to infection by oral cavity bacteria.

(continued)

TABLE 33-16 Radiation-Induced Gastrointestinal Toxicities—Direct and Indirect (continued)

Tissue Response	Risk Factors: Onset/Duration	Clinical Presentation	Physiological Rationale
Bone necrosis (osteoradionecrosis)	Trauma-induced or spontaneous (rare)	Fistula formation Pathological fracture	Radiation causes cellular and vascular injury within bone. Regional blood vessels thicken and result in bone hypoxia and disorganization of remodeling abilities. Destruction of osteocytes, absence of osteoblasts, and lack of new osteoid cells.
Trismus	May develop during treatment—usually 3–6 mo after treatment completion Permanent if untreated	Tonic muscle spasms Restriction in mouth opening Pain with swallowing	Fibrosis of the muscles of mastication and/or fibrotic changes in the capsule of the temporomandibular joint.
Nausea and vomiting	Dependent upon treatment field	Complaint of nausea with or without emesis	Direct response to mucosal irritation by radiation.
	May occur within hours of receiving first treatment	Often accompanied by weight loss and dehydration	Indirect response to presence of toxic waste products of cellular destruction.
	Usually resolves within 2–3 days following treatment completion		Stimulation of the vomiting center resulting from radiation-induced release of serotonin from enterochromaffin cells of the gastrointestinal tract.
Enteritis			
Acute	20–30 Gy Progressively worsens as total dose increases Resolution usually begins 3 wk after treatment and is complete after 3 mo	Increased frequency Change in fecal consistency to loose or watery Intestinal cramping (tenesmus)	Transient mucosal atrophy and infiltration of the lamina propria with leukocytes and plasma cells. Mucosal epithelial damage results in malabsorption of lactose, fat, bile acids, and vitamin B_{12}. Fat malabsorption results in decreased bile salt reabsorption, which then acts as a cathartic in the colon by inhibiting water reabsorption and stimulating peristalsis. Carbohydrate malabsorption results in unabsorbed sugars producing an osmotic effect that causes dilation and peristalsis.
Chronic	6 mo–5 yr after treatment completion Progressive	Diarrhea, steatorrhea, abdominal cramping and pain, nausea and vomiting, malabsorption, and obstruction	Refer to malabsorption syndromes above. Progressive ischemia results in diffuse collagen deposition, mucosal atrophy, and tissue fibrosis.
		Luminal narrowing, perforation, fistula formation	Mucosal ulceration and necrosis.
		Partial or complete obstruction	Adhesions occur between the loops of the bowel.

Source: Data from Perez CA, Brady LW;[6] Dudjak LA;[88] Bashiri H, Suen JY;[89] Ingall JF et al;[91] Iwamoto R;[92] Gilpin JL;[93] Kuten A et al;[94] Witt ME et al;[95] Dreizen S et al.[98]

Stomatitis The toxicities experienced as a result of radiation are directly related to the total dose delivered to a specific anatomical structure. Higher doses of radiation given to larger volumes over shorter time periods increase severity of oral complications, as does hyperfractionation. The type of radiation used (external beam and/or interstitial brachytherapy) will influence incidence of stomatitis, as will multimodality therapy. Agents such as cyclophosphamide, 5-FU, and doxorubicin can have radiosensitizing effects and enhance oral complications. Lastly, individual patient factors including pretreatment condition of the oral cavity, nutritional status, and continued use of alcohol and tobacco will impact oral tolerance.[88–90]

Stomatitis resulting from radiation damage ranges in severity from tenderness to severe pain and ulceration. It is self-limiting and usually resolves 2–3 weeks after completion of treatment if infection and further trauma are avoided. If severe, a break in treatment may be necessary in order to promote comfort, facilitate healing, and ensure willingness to complete treatment.

Poor nutritional status, use of irritants such as tobacco and alcohol, and large dental fillings and permanent prosthetic appliances have been found to significantly influence the onset, degree, and duration of stomatitis.[91] Dentures and appliances should be removed during treatment if possible. Nutritional deficiencies and smoking have both been shown to cause considerable delays in healing. Smoking cessation should be encouraged and facilitated if possible and nutritional deficiencies corrected.

As stomatitis and subsequent pain develop, patients are often unable to maintain an adequate intake of food and fluid. Early intervention and education can prevent or reduce the malnourishment that often accompanies stomatitis. Patients and their significant others need to understand the importance of nutrition and hydration and their impact on comfort, infection prevention, healing, and overall tolerance of treatment. Weight and hydration status are closely monitored.

Patients may be reluctant to report pain and an inability to eat and should therefore be assessed frequently. Patients should be assured that measures can be taken to reduce the discomfort should it occur. Use of systemic analgesia and topical anesthetic should be encouraged and their efficacy evaluated. Narcotic analgesia may be necessary. Appropriate management of pain will help to ensure that patients perform the oral care necessary to promote comfort and healing and prevent infection.

Taste changes (hypogeusia) Alteration in taste sensation is a result of direct and indirect radiation changes in the oral mucosa, salivary function, and taste cells. Taste changes usually occur early in a course of therapy and worsen as the accumulated dose increases. Complete taste loss may occur. Although usually not permanent, alterations in or loss of taste may take several months to resolve.

Hypogeusia can significantly impact nutritional status and quality of life as patients no longer find pleasure in eating. A positive correlation has been found between taste changes and weight loss in patients receiving radiation therapy.[96,97] Therefore, early intervention is necessary in order to reduce the potential for problems resulting from weight loss and malnourishment (see Chapter 27).

Xerostomia Xerostomia is one of the most common and can be one of the most devastating sequelae of radiation to the head and neck. It is a direct result of radiation damage and subsequent change in salivary function. Salivary glands are highly radiosensitive with a drastic decrease in secretion evident after just 10 Gy that is usually permanent after 40 Gy.[98] Although some patients may report subjective improvement, this is more likely a result of adaptation than actual improvement in function. Unfortunately, doses used in an attempt to cure cancers of the head and neck exceed 40 Gy, making xerostomia a chronic problem with serious implications. Younger patients, such as those treated for Hodgkin's disease, may show some improvement in salivary function over time.[92]

Adequate salivary gland function is essential for maintaining the integrity of the oral cavity. Saliva contains organic and inorganic compounds that provide significant protective capacity. Its buffering ability protects teeth, it serves to chemically and mechanically remove cellular and bacterial debris, and it acts as a barrier to irritants. In addition, saliva contains antibacterial agents, lysosomes, and immunoglobulin A, all of which influence the defense against bacterial and viral invasion.[88,91,93] Inadequate saliva creates difficulty in speaking, chewing, and swallowing, as well as altering the environment of the oral cavity making it more prone to dental caries, mucosal lesions, pain, and infection.

Strategies to prevent xerostomia include studies aimed at using radioprotective agents and drugs such as pilocarpine that are currently in progress and may be promising for the future.[90] Until that time when this condition can be prevented or minimized, treatment is palliative, directed at promoting comfort and maintaining the integrity of the oral cavity.

Nursing assessment should include a review of medications that may contribute to xerostomia, including antihistamines, decongestants, anticholinergics, diuretics, tricyclic antidepressants, opioids, and phenothiazines. Avoiding these agents or using acceptable alternatives when possible will prevent a synergistic effect.[99]

Nutrition is often a problem for patients with xerostomia. Thick, ropy saliva makes eating and swallowing difficult and unpleasurable. Oral care before meals will help to freshen the mouth and stimulate appetite. Increasing fluid intake during meals and snacks will help to lubricate food and ease swallowing. Patients should be instructed to avoid dry, bulky, spicy, and acidic foods as they are more difficult to chew and swallow and can potentially damage friable mucosa. Softening or moistening food with milk or gravy may be helpful. Intake of adequate fluid, at least eight glasses per day unless contraindicated, and maintaining adequate air humidification may help to prevent drying and cracking of the mucous membranes. The use of humidified air is often beneficial, especially at night when frequent waking occurs from dryness. Many patients find it necessary to carry containers of water or other liquids for use throughout the day.

Irritants such as tobacco, alcohol, carbonated beverages, and caffeine should be avoided as they can dry and irritate the mucous membranes. Commercial mouthwashes contain astringent and antiseptic agents that may be drying and irritating and should be avoided. Commonly used in the past, lemon glycerin is also contraindicated as it dries and irritates the mucosa and can decalcify teeth.

Lubricating agents such as saliva substitutes are frequently used; however, they are expensive and have variable success. In the United States these products are primarily composed of carboxymethylcellulose solutions with a viscosity and electrolyte composition aimed at approximating normal saliva. They may help to temporarily decrease discomfort and buffer the hyperacidity associated with xerostomia. Lubricating agents may assist in protecting tissues under dental appliances and dentures by increasing the bond and reducing irritation. Vegetable or corn oil swished in the mouth may be a cost-effective alternative for artificial lubrication. Research aimed at identifying an effective lubricating agent should be a priority as this malady can greatly impact a patient's quality of life.

Use of proteolytic enzymes, papain and amylase, is known to effectively dissolve and break up thick saliva in some patients. Papain is found naturally in papayas and papaya juice, is used in commercial meat tenderizers, and can be purchased over the counter. Eating or drinking papaya or swabbing the oral cavity with meat tenderizer before meals has been recommended.[92] Pineapple contains amylase, an enzyme also helpful in cleansing the tongue and mouth. To avoid potential stinging in the mouth, eating frozen pineapple slices has been suggested.[99]

Stimulating residual parenchyma to produce more saliva is often possible and useful. *Sialogogues* are agents that stimulate the secretion of endogenous saliva and include gustatory stimulants such as sugar-free lemon candy, masticatory stimulants such as sugar-free gum, and systemic stimulants. Recently, systemic treatment with parasympathomimetic agents such as pilocarpine has shown promise in stimulating remaining salivary gland function. Systemic agents are not yet widely used and should be used with caution due to their side effects of bradycardia, hypertension, and gastrointestinal upset.[100]

Less commonly used to manage xerostomia are salivary reservoirs and reconstructive surgery. Saliva reservoirs contain artificial saliva and are constructed within a maxillary or mandibular denture. They may not be appropriate for patients with only minimal resorption of the mandibular alveolar process or a shallow palatal vault. Surgical restoration of a secretory mucosa may be possible with reconstruction using gastric mucosa; however, long-term efficacy of the technique is yet to be determined.

Not only is xerostomia extremely uncomfortable, but its sequelae can have serious consequences. Infection, rampant dental caries, and tissue necrosis are all indirect effects of radiation damage to salivary glands. These effects can be rapid, pronounced, persistent, and often irreversible.

Xerostomia creates an alteration in the normal oral flora as well as a decrease in antibacterial capabilities. As a result of xerostomia, an increase is seen in oral fungal populations, a lowered pH results in an increase in oral yeast flora, and there is an increase of cariogenic bacteria with a decrease in noncariogenic bacteria.[89,94] These alterations render a patient extremely susceptible to infection, especially if accompanied by immunosuppression, stomatitis, poor oral hygiene, malnourishment, tumor involvement, or altered protein synthesis.

Prevention and early detection of infection are essential. Teaching and reinforcing the need for meticulous oral and dental care coupled with frequent assessment of the oral cavity are necessary. Cleansing agents such as those used in managing stomatitis may be effective in mechanical and chemical debridement of accumulated plaque and microorganisms, a function no longer performed by saliva. Maintaining a clean and moist oral cavity will help to prevent trauma and ulceration, which becomes a breeding ground for microorganisms.

Prompt and appropriate medical treatment becomes necessary should an infection develop. Pathogenic organisms allowed to spread systemically will greatly compromise the patient. If an infection develops during radiation treatments, a suspension of treatment may be necessary until the complication resolves. This can potentially compromise the outcome of treatment.

Depending upon the organism identified, treatment may include local and/or systemic therapy. Fungal infections are frequently treated with topical antifungal agents such as nystatin or clotrimazole troches. These agents should be used in a clean mouth and allowed to remain in place for 15 minutes; therefore, a patient should not eat or drink anything for this period of time. Long-term use of oral troches should be avoided as they contain large quantities of sugar that may result in dental caries. It is important to note that ketoconazole requires acidity for dissolution and can therefore be ineffective or less effective in patients taking antacids or stomatitis cocktail solutions containing antacids. Prophylactic use of antifungal agents may be used successfully in patients at risk.

Bacterial infections are usually the result of gram-negative bacteria and are treated with aggressive oral care and broad-spectrum antibiotics when necessary. Preventing ulceration of the epithelium can greatly reduce the risk of bacterial infection.

Radiation-induced soft tissue and bone necrosis Although less common, necrosis of soft tissue and bone following radiation to the head and neck is possible, and measures must be taken to prevent its occurrence. Necrosis can occur at any time after tissue has been irradiated and is usually precipitated by trauma.

Soft tissue necrosis is a result of chemical, mechanical, or microbial insult. It is very painful, slow to heal, and enlarges rapidly unless treated. Prevention is best; however, if necrosis does occur, early irrigation with saline and baking soda rinses is usually employed. Antibiotics are given when necessary. The cause of trauma should be determined and corrected if possible.

Failure to effectively manage soft tissue necrosis can result in exposure of underlying bone. This tends to occur most frequently in patients with chronic and advanced periodontal disease. Poor oral hygiene and exposure to irritants also contribute to exposure of bone.

Osteoradionecrosis is uncommon and can be a direct or indirect effect of radiation injury. It is usually precipitated by soft tissue necrosis; however, pathological fractures can occur. Osteoradionecrosis results in severe pain, usually at night and during mastication, and can be accompanied by fistula formation.

Treatment, if early, begins with gentle debridement using saline irrigation. More aggressive debridement of dead or nonviable bone may become necessary. Antibiotic packs and systemic antibiotic therapy are used when infection is present. If osteoradionecrosis is severe and persistent, hyperbaric oxygen may be used either alone or in combination with surgery.[101] If bone is viable and noninfected, a full thickness tissue graft may be used to cover the exposed bone.[89]

Radiation-induced trismus *Trismus* is the result of fibrosis of the muscles of mastication and/or fibrotic changes in the capsule of the temporomandibular joint. Restriction in mouth opening, tonic muscle spasms, and pain can limit access to the oral cavity and impair chewing. Treatment is best accomplished when initiated early. Repetition of jaw exercises should be used prophylactically in patients at high risk and should be initiated in others immediately after a problem develops. Patients are instructed to open their mouth as wide as possible 25 times. This is to be repeated three to four times each day. If severe, various appliances such as wedges, screws, springs, and elastics may be necessary. Surgical intervention to release fibrotic tissue is used only as a last resort.[89,92]

Nursing care

Assessment Identification and treatment of oral complications secondary to chemotherapy and/or radiation therapy must be based on a comprehensive oral and dental assessment that includes examination of the physical condition of the oral mucosa, patient's perception of any changes in oral sensations and function, and a dental evaluation with radiographic films as necessary. Assessment requires adequate knowledge of the anatomy and physiology of the oral cavity and the effects of radiation and chemotherapy on the structure and function of the oral mucosa.

Assessing the oral cavity requires adequate lighting, removal of all dental prostheses, and inspection and palpation of all mucosal surfaces. Use of a glove, tongue blade, and dental mirror facilitates a thorough exam.

Critical to assessment is the availability of an oral assessment tool that can describe and quantify the physical and functional condition of the oral cavity. A reliable and valid tool will ensure consistency in reporting, thereby facilitating initial and ongoing assessment. Additionally, a clinically useful tool enables stomatotoxic protocols to be identified and the efficacy of varied oral care regimens and interventions to be evaluated.

Eilers and associates[102] developed an oral assessment guide (OAG) based on clinical experience and nursing and dental literature (Table 33-17). The OAG utilizes three levels of descriptors to define oral health and function. Research validates the clinical usefulness of the OAG in BMT and hematologic patients receiving chemotherapy and/or radiation therapy.[102,103] Applicability in the clinical setting is strengthened because the OAG is understandable and requires only 3–4 minutes to complete.

Ideally, a baseline assessment of the oral cavity should be done prior to the initiation of treatment. When possible, time should be allowed for completion of any necessary dental care to ensure that the oral cavity is free from preexisting sources of irritation and infection. This is especially important in the patients receiving radiation to the oral cavity. Pretreatment oral care documentation decreases not only the development of stomatitis but also the incidence of oral infection. Once treatment is initiated, an oral assessment should be repeated at regular intervals; outpatients should be instructed on self-assessment.

Nursing management of stomatitis will depend on its severity, which is often described as mild, moderate, or severe. A grading system depicting degree of severity of mucosal damage includes the following:

Grade 1— erythema of oral mucosa

Grade 2—isolated small ulcerations (white patches)

Grade 3—confluent ulcerations (white patches) covering more than 25% of oral mucosa

Grade 4—hemorrhagic ulceration

Management Table 33-18 describes a protocol for oral care based on assessment and grade of stomatitis.[104] Table 33-19 depicts various oral cleansing agents and devices, different means of lubricating and coating the oral cavity, and basic solutions and measures to manage oral discomfort.

Since it is apparent that systematic performance of oral care may be of greater significance in reducing the destructive effects of radiation and chemotherapy rather than the actual agents used,[88] developing a plan of care that the patient finds acceptable may be of greater im-

TABLE 33-17 Oral Assessment Guide (OAG)

Category	Tools for Assessment	Methods of Measurement	Numerical and Descriptive Ratings		
			1	2	3
Voice	Auditory	Converse with patient	Normal	Deeper or raspy	Difficulty talking or painful
Swallow	Observation	Ask patient to swallow To test gag reflex, gently place blade on back of tongue and depress	Normal swallow	Some pain on swallow	Unable to swallow
Lips	Visual/palpatory	Observe and feel tissue	Smooth and pink and moist	Dry or cracked	Ulcerated or bleeding
Tongue	Visual/palpatory	Feel and observe appearance of tissue	Pink and moist and papillae present	Coated or loss of papillae with a shiny appearance with or without redness	Blistered or cracked
Saliva	Tongue blade	Insert blade into mouth, touching the center of the tongue and the floor of the mouth	Watery	Thick or ropy	Absent
Mucous membranes	Visual	Observe appearance of tissue	Pink and moist	Reddened or coated (increased whiteness) without ulcerations	Ulcerations with or without bleeding
Gingiva	Tongue blade and visual	Gently press with tip of blade	Pink and stippled and firm	Edematous with or without redness	Spontaneous bleeding
Teeth or dentures (or denture-bearing area)	Visual	Observe appearance of teeth or denture-bearing area	Clean and no debris	Plaque or debris in localized areas (between teeth if present)	Plaque or debris generalized along gum line or denture-bearing area

Source: From Eilers J, Berger AM, Petersen MC: Development, testing and application of the oral assessment guide, *Oncol Nurs Forum* 15:325–330, 1988. Reprinted with permission of June Eilers, University of Nebraska Medical Center, Omaha, NE.

portance than the employment of complicated regimens. Because reinforcement promotes compliance, nurses should continually review with the patients the individual plan of care and assess its continued acceptability.

Generally, the recommendation is that routine oral care be performed at least after meals and at bedtime and that the frequency be increased as the severity of stomatitis increases.

Mouth rinses enhance the removal of loosened debris and should be nonirritating and nondehydrating. Several solutions for rinsing have been studied and include normal saline, sodium bicarbonate, and hydrogen peroxide, as well as various combinations of these. As yet, the optimal mouthwash for stomatitis has not been determined. Normal saline may be the least damaging; sodium bicarbonate is effective as a cleansing agent, but some patients complain of an unpleasant taste; hydrogen peroxide breaks down new tissues and should be avoided when fresh granulation surfaces are visible in the mouth.

The lips should be lubricated as often as necessary to keep them moist and comfortable. Moisture within the oral cavity is maintained with lubricating agents such as saliva substitutes. Although saliva substitutes have the physical characteristics of saliva, they lack antibacterial factors, a function of normal saliva. A thin layer of water-soluble lubricant may be applied to the lips as well as the oral mucosa for lubrication.

Various topical formulations available to relieve the pain and inflammation of stomatitis are categorized as mucosal coating agents, anesthetic agents, and systemic analgesics. Nursing management of oral pain follows the same principles as management of other cancer-related pain: subjective and objective assessment of the pain, treatment aimed at the cause of the pain, and evaluation of the effectiveness of interventions. A limitation to the use of topical agents is their generally

TABLE 33-18 Stomatitis: Oral Care Protocol[104]

I. Potential Stomatitis (Grade 0)
  A. Assess oral cavity daily
  B. Encourage routine oral hygiene regimen pc and hs
    1. Brush with soft toothbrush (eg, Oral-B® 35 or 40) and nonastringent fluoride toothpaste using Bass technique
    2. Floss with unwaxed dental floss
    3. Rinse with mouthwash of patient preference—avoid mouthwashes with high alcohol content
    4. Remove, cleanse, and replace dental prostheses after oral care; store nightly in denture antiseptic solution (eg, Efferdent®) (*Note:* Change solution daily to prevent growth of pathogens)
    5. Apply lip lubricant (eg, Blistex, lipstick)
  C. Use oxidizing agent prn for mucolytic area
    1. 3% hydrogen peroxide and water (1:4 mixture)—swish, gargle, and expectorate (*Note:* Mix just prior to use to maintain oxidizing effect)
    2. Sodium bicarbonate solution (eg, 1 tsp in 8 oz water)—swish, gargle, and expectorate
    3. Rinse with warm water or saline
    4. Remove thick, tenacious mucus with a swab as needed
  D. Provide daily fluoride treatment for patients with xerostomia and prophylactic use for patients receiving head and neck irradiation
  E. Use prophylactic chlorhexidine mouth rinse 15 ml—swish, gargle, and expectorate every 8 hours for high-risk patients
  F. Consult dentist

II. Mild or Moderate Stomatitis (Grade 1 or Grade 2)
  A. Assess oral cavity twice daily
  B. Follow oral hygiene regimen (see IB above) every 2 hr while awake and every 6 hr during the night
    1. Use normal saline mouthwash if no crusts are present
    2. Alternate oxidizing agent with warm saline mouthwash if crusts are present
    3. Omit flossing if pain results or bleeding occurs with a low platelet count
    4. Remove, cleanse, and do not replace dental prostheses except for meals; store nightly in denture antiseptic solution (eg, Efferdent®) (*Note:* Change solution daily to prevent growth of pathogens)
  C. Culture any suspicious oral lesions
    1. Culture for: viral, fungal, aerobic and anaerobic; send for Gram stain
    2. Use prophylactic oral antifungal, antiviral, and antibacterial agents per physician order as needed
  D. Apply topical anesthetics ac and prn for local pain control
    1. Lidocaine HCL viscous 2% or 5%
      a. apply directly on lesion(s) with cotton swab
      b. dilute 1 tablespoon with saline—"swish and spit" 10 min ac and hs; "swish and swallow" if throat is sore (*Note:* may cause decreased or absent gag reflex)
    2. Cetacaine or Hurricane® spray—1 to 2 sprays to mouth as needed
    3. "Stomatitis cocktail": mixture of equal parts lidocaine viscous, diphenhydramine HCl elixir (12.5 mg/5 ml) and Maalox®—"swish and spit" 15–30 ml every 4 hr prn; "swish and swallow" if throat is sore (*Note:* May cause decreased or absent gag reflex)
    4. If xerostomia is not present: mixture of 50% Kaopectate® and 50% diphenhydramine HCl elixir (12.5 mg/5 ml)—"swish and spit" 15–30 ml every 4 hr prn
    5. Zilactin-hydroxypropyl cellulose or Oratect Gel® topical application—apply directly on lesion(s) with cotton swab prn
  E. Use oral analgesics for systemic pain control
    1. Take 1.5 hr ac and prn
    2. Schedule dose at regular intervals (eg, every 3–4 hr) if pain is constant
    3. Titrate to pain control; may need alternate route of administration
  F. Provide oral lubricants (eg, Moi-stir® swabs) or "artificial salivas" (eg, Xero-Lube®) for patients with xerostomia
  G. Adapt diet to ensure maximum nutrition and fluid intake
    1. Encourage frequent small feedings with soft, bland foods; increase fluids to three liters/day
    2. Recommend diet high in protein and calories; add nutritional supplements (eg, Ensure®, Sustacal®) as needed
    3. Avoid irritants
      a. chemical (citrus fruits, spicy foods)
      b. thermal (extremes in food temperatures)
      c. physical (coarse foods)
      d. tobacco and alcohol
    4. Consult dietician prn

III. Severe Stomatitis (Grade 3 or Grade 4)
  A. Assess oral cavity every 8 hr
  B. Assess for evidence of infection; culture any suspicious lesion(s) as in IIC
  C. Institute aggressive and timely antimicrobial therapy as ordered by physician
  D. Cleanse mouth every 2 hr while awake and every 4 hr at night
    1. Alternate warm saline mouthwash with antifungal or antibacterial oral suspension
    2. Use oxidizing agent (see IB) for mucolytic area every 4 hr followed by saline rinse
  E. Gently brush teeth every 4 hr avoiding trauma to gums; substitute soft foam toothettes if bleeding occurs or brushing is too painful
  F. Apply lip lubricant every 2 hr; if lips are bleeding or ulcerated, apply warm saline soaks every 4 hr for 20 min
  G. Remove, cleanse dental prostheses—do not replace; store in denture antiseptic solution (eg, Efferdent® (*Note:* Change solution daily to prevent growth of pathogens)
  H. Institute local pain control measures as in IID above
  I. Use systemic analgesics as needed, especially ac
  J. Provide adequate nutritional and fluid intake
    1. Liquid or pureed diet
    2. Intravenous fluids to prevent dehydration
    3. Enteral or total parenteral nutrition may be needed until healing occurs

Abbreviations: ac = before meals; pc = after meals; hs = at bedtime; prn = as required

Source: From Goodman M, Stoner C.[104]

TABLE 33-19 Prevention and Management of Peri-Oral Complications of Cancer Treatment

BASIC ORAL CLEANSING

Recommend routine oral cleansing after meals and at bedtime; increase frequency as stomatitis worsens; lip lubricant as needed

Avoid commercial mouthwashes and lemon glycerin swabs because they are drying and irritating to mucosal epithelia

Plan	Action	Active Ingredient	Schedule	Comments
Cleansing Mouthrinses				
Normal saline	Mechanical plaque control—removes and washes away loose debris Physical—moistens and soothes oral mucosa	Isotonic sodium chloride	Routine: four times daily (after meals and at bedtime)	Nonirritating No unpleasant taste Mixture preparation: 1 teaspoon salt in one quart warm water; use sterile saline if granulocytopenic or mouth ulcers present
Sodium bicarbonate solution	Mechanical plaque control—loosens hardened crusts and debris Mucosolvent Reduces acidity	Sodium bicarbonate	Routine: four times daily (after meals and at bedtime)	Decreases odor Unpleasant taste reported Mixture preparation: 1 tsp baking soda in 8 oz water for thick paste of sodium bicarbonate; water applied to gingival sulcus for use in mechanical plaque debridement
Hydrogen peroxide (3% solution)	Mechanical plaque control—loosens hardened crusts and debris Mucosolvent Germicidal		Routine: four times daily (after meals and at bedtime)	Unpleasant taste Use with caution on ulcers or fresh granulation surfaces—may break down tissue Chronic use may alter normal oral flora and predispose to Candidal infections Mixture preparation: dilute 3% hydrogen peroxide to ¼ strength. *Note:* Mix just prior to usage to maintain oxidizing effect Refrigerated solution may also provide local anesthetic effect
Antimicrobial Mouthrinse				
Peridex	Broad-spectrum antimicrobial agent used to suppress oral microflora and prevent dental plaque formation Decreases bacterial cloud in mouth Prevents oral candidal infections	Chlorhexidine digluconate	15 ml rinse for 30 sec three times daily Do not swallow Avoid eating or drinking 1 hr following use	Prophylaxis for therapy-induced mucositis (high-risk patients) Most common local side effect from long-term use is staining of teeth and tongue. No systemic toxicity has been reported

(continued)

TABLE 33-19 Prevention and Management of Peri-Oral Complications of Cancer Treatment (continued)

BASIC ORAL CLEANSING

Plan	Action	Active Ingredient	Schedule	Comments
Cleansing Devices				
Toothbrush	Mechanical cleansing and removal of debris		Toothbrushing four times daily (after meals and at bedtime)	Cleansing instrument of choice Bass technique of brushing recommended
Toothette	Stimulate circulation to oral mucosa Removes debris more gently than toothbrush		Every 4 hr and as needed	Recommended for cleansing when platelet count falls below 20,000 Use unflavored if stomatitis is present

MAINTENANCE OF MOISTURE

Cleanse cracked or ulcerated lips with gauze soaked in normal saline; encrusted lips with gauze soaked in sodium bicarbonate or H_2O_2 solution

A dry mouth (xerostomia) contributes to taste disturbances, which may affect appetite and nutritional status; radiation to the oral cavity is associated with xerostomia

Fluoride treatment recommended to prevent dental caries secondary to xerostomia

Plan	Action	Active Ingredient	Schedule	Comments
Lipcare				
K-Y Jelly®	Lubricates lips Prevents cracking and bleeding	Sodium carboxymethylcellulose Sodium alginate Glycerin	Apply as needed for moisture	Nonirritating Water-soluble Can be applied on oral mucosa also Safe for use in patients receiving oxygen
Petrolatum (eg, Vaseline®, petroleum jelly)	Lubricates lips Prevents evaporation of moisture	Petrolatum	Apply as needed for moisture	Unpleasant taste Forms occlusive film on lips Harmful if aspirated
Oral Cavity Care				
Orabalance®	Relief of dry mouth		Use after rinsing mouth and after every brushing	A nondrying moisturizing gel May be applied around the teeth and along gum line
Saliva substitutes (eg, Moi-Stir®)	Mouth-moistening salivary supplement	Sorbitol, sodium carboxymethylcellulose and electrolytes present in saliva	Apply as needed for xerostomia	Available in oral swabsticks and spray
(eg, Xerolube®)	Mouth moisturizer Caries inhibition	Carboxymethylcellulose	5 ml orally as needed for xerostomia	Includes fluoride as an added benefit
Sialogogues				
Pilocarpine	Stimulates salivary tissue by its muscarinecholinergic agonist properties	Pilocarpine	Adult dosage: 2.5–7.5 mg two to four times daily	Investigational use for patients with postradiation xerostomia Not recommended for use in patients with cardiovascular problems, unstable hypertension, or gastrointestinal ulcers

(continued)

TABLE 33-19 Prevention and Management of Peri-Oral Complications of Cancer Treatment (continued)

RELIEF OF PAIN AND INFLAMMATION

Pain from isolated areas of mucositis or ulceration is best managed with localized topical anesthetics and coating agents; topical rinses may be helpful for confluent, generalized ulcerations

Systemic analgesics may be necessary to alleviate moderate to severe oral pain and enhance oral intake

Plan	Action	Active Ingredient	Schedule	Comments
Coating Agents				
Orabase®	Topical anesthetic for localized areas of pain	Benzocaine 20%	Dry lesion(s) and apply as needed for pain	Quick onset of action—30 sec, but short duration of action—5–15 min Does not change consistency after application
Hurricane®	Topical anesthetic	Benzocaine 20%	Apply as needed to lesion(s) for pain	Available as spray, liquid, or gel Onset of action—30 sec, duration 15 min No systemic absorption
Oratect-gel®	Topical anesthetic	Benzocaine 20%	Dry lesion(s) and apply as needed up to four times daily	Gel dries in about 30–60 sec to form a protective film Maximum protection lasts about 2 hr Film dissipates gradually over 6 hr Do not try to mechanically remove Mild, transient stinging when applied
Zilactin®	Provides a protective coating and leads to pain relief	Tannic acid 7%	Dry lesion(s) and apply four times daily	Forms protective film over oral ulcers that can last 5 hr Gel forms an opaque white film inside the mouth and a transparent film extraorally when dried Mild, transient burning sensation with application of gel
Topical Anesthetic Rinses				
Xylocaine viscous 2% solution	Topical anesthetic for generalized areas of pain	Lidocaine HCl	15 ml swish and spit every 3 hr as needed for pain (not to exceed 120 ml in 24 hr)	Onset of action is 5 min Duration of action is approximately 20 min Systemically absorbed Watch for CNS and cardiac toxicity Swish and swallow for brief pain relief (eg, before meals)
Dyclonine Hydrochloride 0.5% or 1% solution	Topical anesthetic for generalized areas of pain	Dyclone	15 ml swish and spit as needed for pain	Minimally absorbed Decreasing potential for CNS and cardiac toxicity

(continued)

TABLE 33-19 Prevention and Management of Peri-Oral Complications of Cancer Treatment (continued)

RELIEF OF PAIN AND INFLAMMATION				
Plan	Action	Active Ingredient	Schedule	Comments
Combination "mixtures" (eg, viscous xylocaine 2%, Benadryl® elixir 12.5 mg/ml, Maalox®)	Topical anesthetics for general areas of pain	Lidocaine Diphenhydramine Magnesium hydroxide	15 ml swish for 1 min, then spit or swallow four times daily	Benadryl may exacerbate xerostomia
Ulcerease®	Anesthetic mouthrinse	Buffered solution of glycerin and liquified phenol (0.6%)	15 ml swish for 15 sec, then spit every 2 hr as needed	Contains no alcohol Use full strength May apply directly to ulcers with cotton swab after rinsing
Sucralfate suspension	Binds to ulcerated tissue protecting it from further insult and may promote healing	Sucralfate (Sulfated sucrose and aluminum hydroxide)	1 g/15 ml swish (pc and hs) 15 ml four times daily—swish for 1–2 min, then spit	No anesthetic action Suspension may aggravate nausea
Vitamin E	Promotes healing of mouth ulcers and controls pain	Tocopherol	1 ml (400 mg/ml) of vitamin E oil applied topically to oral lesions twice daily	Anecdotal and research-based studies conclude vitamin E may help speed healing of chemotherapy-induced stomatitis
Systemic Analgesics				
Nonsteroidal anti-inflammatory agents (eg, Trilisate®)	Mild to moderate pain	Choline magnesium trisalicylate	1500–3000 mg	Longer duration of action than aspirin No effect on platelets Minimal GI side effects
Narcotic agents (eg, morphine)	Moderate to severe pain	Morphine sulfate		

short duration of action (20 minutes to 1 hour). This duration may only provide adequate relief for eating. Extensive oral pain is an indication for systemic analgesics used in increasing levels of potency to obtain adequate pain relief. Analgesics should be given around the clock and alternate routes considered if the oral pain prevents swallowing of pills.

Two factors must be kept in mind when using topical agents. First, because they work on contact, the mouth should be cleansed before application of the agent to permit contact with the oral mucosal surface. Secondly, when applying topical agents directly to painful areas, gloves are advised to prevent the possible spread of infection. Whether topical anesthetics are used as rinses to "swish and spit" or to "swish and swallow," side effects such as diminished gag reflex need to be monitored.

Maintenance of nutrition during this period is also essential. A diet high in calories and protein is needed to promote healing. Nutritional supplements may be indicated. Cold, soft foods such as yogurt or ice cream are soothing and well tolerated. Dehydration can occur when severe stomatitis develops, and total enteral or parenteral nutritional support may be necessary until stomatitis resolves.

Stomatitis can have a great impact on a patient's quality of life and compliance with therapy. A standard of nursing care to assess, plan, interview, and evaluate is necessary to prevent or minimize this distressing side effect, to decrease the incidence of infection, and to prevent nutritional deficits.

Although the treatment of stomatitis remains palliative and symptom-oriented, studies are ongoing evaluating prophylactic measures to alleviate this side effect. It is only recently that researchers have identified an animal model for chemotherapy-induced mucositis—the Golden Syrian hamster.[105] With this animal model, new agents and optimal use of existing treatments may perhaps be studied.

Oral mucositis is a major toxic effect related to 5-FU, a frequently used cytotoxic drug. Several clinical trials have focused on appropriate measures to prevent this side effect. A pilot study by Clark and Slevin[106] found allopurinol rinses beneficial in decreasing the severity of stomatitis in six out of six patients receiving 5-FU alone. In a subsequent study, 77 patients treated with 5-FU ± leucovorin were randomly assigned to use either a placebo or allopurinol mouthwash. Results were convincingly negative and demonstrated no protective effect of allopurinol; furthermore, a nonsignificant trend toward more mucositis was observed with those patients rinsing with allopurinol.[107] Further investigation is warranted before incorporating this procedure into routine clinical practice.

The use of oral cryotherapy has proven beneficial in minimizing oral stomatitis due to doxorubicin as well as 5-FU and leucovorin. In a study by Mahood et al.,[108] 95 patients receiving 5-FU and leucovorin on 5 consecutive days were randomized to no treatment or ice chips for 30 minutes beginning 5 minutes prior to chemotherapy. Those in the treatment group experienced less stomatitis. It would appear that ice effectively causes vasoconstriction, thereby minimizing blood flow to the oral cavity preventing uptake of 5-FU by oral mucosal cells. Both doxorubicin and 5-FU have a short half-life, which makes cryotherapy a logical approach to prevention of stomatitis.

The efficacy of topical sucralfate suspension for prophylaxis of chemotherapy-induced mucositis has also been studied.[109,110] Sucralfate is thought to work by binding to the inflamed areas of the mucosa, thereby forming a protective barrier against further mucosal damage. A placebo controlled study evaluated treatment with sucralfate in patients receiving cisplatin and continuous 5-FU for 5 days. A significant reduction ($p = 0.04$) in objective measurements of mucositis was seen among 23 evaluable patients as well as a trend in patient preference for the sucralfate rinse.[109]

Of interest is the role that growth factors may play in stomatitis prevention. Research trials with colony stimulating factors (e.g., G-CSF) administered to patients undergoing chemotherapy have incidentally reported a decrease in the occurrence and severity of stomatitis along with restoration of neutrophil counts and function.[111]

Other preventive measures reported in the literature include supplemental beta carotene and prostaglandin E compounds. Prophylactic use of antimicrobial rinses will be discussed in the next section.

Infections of the Oral Cavity

Infection is the most clinically significant oral problem secondary to treatment with chemotherapy and/or localized radiation therapy. The mouth, inhabited by both normal and opportunistic pathogens, provides ideal conditions for microbial growth, particularly in the granulocytopenic patient. The risk of serious infection is directly related to the degree and duration of granulocytopenia.

Integral to the pathogenesis of infection in the cancer patient is impairment of normal host-defense mechanisms. Cytotoxic therapy weakens host defenses by layering the oral flora and salivary quantity and composition. An overgrowth of normal oral microorganisms results in invasion of both endogenous and exogenous pathologic organisms capable of producing oral infections. Mucosal disruption becomes an important portal of entry and compromises the integrity of the oral mucosa as the first line of defense. Pathogenic organisms can further contaminate the lungs and the GI tract, disseminating infection systemically.

Pathogenicity of normal oral flora increases with poor oral hygiene and in the presence of oral disease. It has been shown that as oral hygiene measures are decreased, the presence of microbial populations increases. Periodontitis, a common oral disease in the general population, causes a tenfold increase in bacterial and fungal organisms in the mouth.[112] The discomfort and pain associated with stomatitis from either chemotherapy or radiotherapy often result in decreased intake of nutrients and fluids, which can lead to malnutrition and dehydration. Depletion of protein stores and malnutrition increases the risk of infection by altering the integrity of the epithelial barrier and depressing the immune system. Research suggests that adequate nutritional status as evidenced by normal serum albumin levels and optimal pretherapy weight may decrease the rate of oral infection.

Immunosuppression due to the treatment of cancer or the cancer itself further increases a patient's susceptibility to oral infection. Specifically, immunosuppression depresses phagocytic activity, interferes with the inflammatory response, abolishes antibody production, and inhibits the development of delayed hypersensitivity.

Bacterial, fungal, and viral infections are all common; *Streptococcus* species, *Candida* species, and herpes simplex virus are the major oral infectious pathogens.[113] Each infection has certain clinical features, such as the white or "cottage-cheese" appearance of *Candida albicans* or the painful vesicular lesions of herpes simplex, that assist in identification of the pathogen. However, the task is difficult at times, particularly when one is trying to differentiate between noninfectious therapy-induced lesions and those caused by pathogenic organisms. Ultimately, proper identification of the responsible pathogen requires culture. Management will vary depending on the pathogenic organism. The most frequent cause of oral infection is fungal. *C. albicans* is the predominating organism and pseudomembranous candidiasis (oral thrush) the most common clinical manifestation. Due to discoloration by tobacco and food stains, oral thrush occasionally appears as a thick brown coating on the tongue surface.

Oral *Candida* infections are traditionally treated with topical antifungal agents such as nystatin (Mycostatin), oral rinses, or clotrimazole (Mycelex) troches. The nystatin liquid must be swished in the mouth for 5 minutes and then spit or swallowed, four times daily. The troche, given five times a day, must be sucked in the mouth until dissolved (approximately 30 minutes). If xerostomia secondary to radiation is present, it will take a longer time to dissolve. Patients should be instructed to cleanse the mouth before administrating the agent and not to eat or drink for at least 30 minutes after application. This will permit drug contact with the mucosal surfaces to exert an antifungal effect.

Alternatives for oropharyngeal candidiasis refractory to topical treatment are the systemic oral antifungal agents: ketoconazole (Nizoral) 200 mg daily or fluconazole (Diflucan) 100 mg daily.[114] Fluconazole is also available for intravenous use. Increased compliance due to once-a-day dosing is an advantage; however, fluconazole is potentially liver-toxic. Absorption of ketoconazole is dependent on gastric acidity; therefore, patients are instructed to avoid the use of antacids and other medications that alter gastric pH within 2 hours of taking ketoconazole. A course of low-dose intravenous amphotericin B (Fungizone) is indicated for nonresponsive infection and in severe esophageal and disseminated candidal infections.

The value of prophylactic antifungal agents to prevent systemic infection is controversial. Chlorhexidine mouthrinses have also been studied as an adjunct in managing patients at high risk for developing mucositis and infection. Although no consistent findings are available, several studies have reported the effectiveness of chlorhexidene in modifying candidiasis.[115,116]

Herpes simplex virus (HSV) is the most common viral pathogen affecting the oral cavity. Since the appearance of HSV resembles other infectious lesions or therapy-induced stomatitis, culturing of suspicious lesions is mandatory. Optimally, vesicle fluid should be obtained for culture. When no vesicles are present, the base of the lesion should be swabbed using a viral culture swab. Swabs used for nasopharyngeal cultures (calcium alginate swabs) inactivate the virus and should not be used. Furthermore, gloves should always be worn when swabbing suspicious lesions as HSV is highly infective.

Reactivation of latent HSV is the cause of the majority of HSV infections. Immunocompromised patients who are seropositive are at risk. The more intense the immunosuppression, the greater the risk (e.g., BMT patients are at high risk). For patients with limited tissue involvement, acyclovir (Zovirax) ointment can be applied topically every 3–6 hours while awake. Patients should be instructed to use gloves or cotton swabs when applying ointment, since autoinoculation with the virus can occur. Extensive tissue involvement or disseminated herpes requires systemic acyclovir therapy either orally or parenterally. Acyclovir prophylaxis may be used to prevent infection in selected high-risk patient populations (e.g., seropositive BMT or leukemic patients).[117] Optimum dose and schedule for prophylaxis have not been determined.

The vast majority of bacterial infections may affect three sites in the mouth: the gingiva, the mucosa, or the teeth. A bacterial culture isolate and positive blood culture confirms the diagnosis; however, clinical features (e.g., pain, fever, oral lesions) may be present without a positive blood culture. Parenteral antibiotic therapy based on causative organism is the treatment of choice. The effectiveness of chlorhexidine (Peridex) rinses in the prevention of local and systemic infections in immunocompromised patients has been reported differently in the literature. Results are inconclusive because of variances in the study design including differences in the concentration of chlorhexidine used, duration of use, and concomitant use of broad-spectrum antibiotics. Table 33-20 outlines the clinical features, diagnosis, and management of oral infections.

Esophagitis

The mucosal lining of the esophagus histologically is the same as the oral cavity and is lined with stratified squamous epithelial cells. Destruction and inadequate

TABLE 33-20 Infections of the Oral Cavity

Infection	Clinical Features	Diagnosis	Management	Comment
Bacterial				
Gingival	White, necrotic pseudomembrane Pain Fever Lymphadenopathy	+ bacterial culture ± blood culture	Parenteral antibiotics (gram-negative coverage plus beta-lactam antibiotics) Local debridement of bacterial plaques Aggressive oral hygiene Prophylactic chlorhexidine mouthrinse for high-risk patients	Resembles acute necrotizing ulcerative gingivitis (ANUG). More common in patients with preexisting periodontal disease Calculus and plaque removal recommended prior to therapy
Odontogenic	Tooth pain Fever	Dental examination including radiographs ± blood culture	Extraction of infected tooth Fluoride treatment	Third molars are most often involved Pretreatment dental examination and extraction are recommended

(continued)

TABLE 33-20 Infections of the Oral Cavity (continued)

Infection	Clinical Features	Diagnosis	Management	Comment
Mucosal	Painful ulceration Fever	+ bacterial culture + blood culture	Broad-spectrum parenteral antibiotics Aggressive oral hygiene Prophylactic chlorhexidine mouthrinse for high-risk patients	Normal signs of inflammation and infection may be absent in neutropenic patients
Gram-negative bacilli (eg, *Pseudomonas* spp.)	Raised dry, yellowish lesion encircled by a reddened halo; center turns purple to black with necrosis			
Gram-positive cocci (eg, *Streptococcus* spp.)	Yellowish-white exudate enclosed by an erythematous halo			
Fungal				
Candida albicans	Pseudomembranous: white, raised cottage cheese-like plaques Painless when undisturbed Raw, bleeding, painful surface results when scraped off Atrophic: localized to confluent erythema of oral mucosa Patchy depapillation of dorsum of tongue Painful Fever rare with only oral involvement	+ fungal culture for *Candida* spp. + smears: Gram-stained Potassium hydroxide Wet preparation	Antifungal agents Topical: Nystatin oral rinse/troche Clotrimazole troche Systemic Oral ketoconazole Oral fluconazole Nonresponsive: Parenteral amphotericin B Value of prophylactic antifungal agent is controversial Chlorhexidine mouthrinse has been effective in modifying candidal infections	Patients with oral *Candida* are at significant risk for spread to esophagus and systemically Radiation-induced xerostomia predisposes oral mucosa to fungal infection
Viral				
Herpes simplex (HSV)	Prodromal symptoms of tingling, itching pain followed by eruption of small vesicles that ulcerate and become encrusted Common areas of occurrence: lips and circumoral region Fever, malaise, and lymphadenopathy may be present	+ viral culture ↑ HSV serum titer	Antiviral agent: Acyclovir Topical: Acyclovir ointment (eg, lip lesions or herpes labialis) Systemic: Acyclovir Prophylactic: Acyclovir for high-risk seropositive patients	Reactivation of HSV is the most common cause of viral infection in the neutropenic cancer patient Seropositive patients for HSV are at greater risk
Varicella zoster	Unilateral vesicular lesions along trigeminal nerve			

replacement of these epithelial cells by radiotherapy or chemotherapeutic agents result in an inflammatory response called *esophagitis*. Similar to stomatitis, esophagitis can progress to include ulceration, hemorrhage, and secondary infection and can cause sufficient pain to make eating very difficult. Treatment may be discontinued temporarily to allow recovery of these cells, which parallels recovery of the white blood cell count.

Most common early symptoms of esophagitis include dysphagia (difficulty in swallowing), odynophagia (painful swallowing), and epigastric pain. Esophageal pain that worsens and becomes continuous and substernal indicates progressing esophagitis.[118]

Radiation-induced esophagitis Radiation used to treat esophageal cancer; Hodgkin's disease; and head and neck, breast, and lung cancer often requires that the esophagus receives a radiation dose high enough to induce esophagitis. Esophagitis is a common and expected transient side effect. It occurs as a result of vascular changes and an inability for cell renewal to keep up with epithelial cell loss. This results in erythema and mucosal irritation.

Onset of esophagitis is dose-related and may be enhanced or hastened by concomitant chemotherapy or dietary indiscretions, especially alcohol. Symptoms often begin with a report of difficulty in swallowing liquids and a feeling as though there is a "lump in the throat." After 2–3 weeks of therapy, symptoms may progress to pain, often caused by swallowing; a burning sensation; and dysphagia. If the reaction becomes severe, the pain and burning sensation may be continuous and debilitating. A treatment break may be necessary to prevent or correct dehydration and malnutrition.

Treating esophageal cancer requires higher doses delivered directly to the esophagus. This places these patients at a higher risk for developing an esophageal ulceration, perforation, and/or fistula during or after treatment completion. Careful treatment planning, often utilizing an esophagram, is therefore employed in an attempt to predict and prevent this complication.

While resolution of the acute effects of radiation usually begins 2–3 weeks following treatment completion, late effects may be seen 1–5 years later. Late complications include epithelial thickening, microvascular changes, and fibrosis of muscle and connective tissue. Ulceration is seen less frequently, with the incidence increasing when doses greater than 70 Gy have been delivered. If fibrosis and luminal stenosis become severe, repeated esophageal dilation may become necessary. If this procedure is unsuccessful, a gastrostomy may be necessary for nutritional intake and adequate hydration.

Nursing considerations Risk factors for developing esophagitis include alcohol consumption, tobacco use, ulcer disease, and esophageal exposure to radiation.

Ongoing assessments should be performed at least weekly and should include weight, dietary and hydration status, and blood chemistry if indicated. This along with the patient's report of pain or difficulty swallowing should be carefully documented. Use of a grading scale such as that in Table 33-3 will help to ensure consistency in assessment and documentation.

Patients and their significant others must be educated regarding the possible acute and late side effects of therapy, probable time frame for their onset and duration, and self-care measures to help alleviate the side effects. Table 33-21 offers self-care guidelines to assist patients experiencing esophagitis and dysphagia. Compliance with recommended guidelines should be assessed and the importance frequently reinforced during a patient's treatment course.

Although management of esophagitis varies greatly, all management is directed at symptom relief and supportive care. Interventions are initiated to minimize irritation and promote comfort. This is best accomplished through diet manipulation, anesthesia, and systemic analgesia when needed.

If nutritional status becomes compromised, patients may benefit from commercially prepared supplements. A nutritionist may be helpful in determining which

TABLE 33-21 Self-Care Guidelines for Esophagitis (Sore Throat) and Dysphagia (Difficulty Swallowing)

While receiving chemotherapy or radiation to the neck or chest, you may begin to develop a sore throat or a feeling like food is getting stuck when you swallow. This usually begins gradually after about 2 weeks of treatment and may become more severe as treatment continues. It is temporary and will begin to gradually get better about 2 weeks after treatment is finished.

The following guidelines were designed to help you to be more comfortable during treatment and to make sure that you are eating and drinking enough liquids.

1. Tell your nurse or doctor if you have a sore throat or are having trouble swallowing.
2. Change your diet to include foods that are soft and moist. Using sauces and gravies is helpful.
3. Avoid foods that are spicy, salty, dry, or rough in texture.
4. Drink at least eight glasses of liquid each day. Fruit nectar is often very soothing. Avoid alcoholic beverages, citrus juices, and carbonated beverages—they will irritate your throat.
5. Avoid very hot foods.
6. Eat or drink cold foods such as ice cream, frozen juice bars, and Jell-O. This may help to soothe the throat, especially before eating a meal.
7. Take small bites and chew foods well.
8. Use a straw to make swallowing easier.
9. Avoid using commercial mouthwashes because they often contain alcohol, which can irritate your throat.
10. Try not to smoke. It can be difficult to stop smoking during a stressful time, but your nurse or doctor can provide you with some helpful suggestions.
11. Placing a cool air humidifier with tap water in the room where you spend most of your time during the day and where you sleep at night may help to keep your mouth and throat from getting dry.
12. If your doctor prescribes medicine to help with the pain and discomfort, do not be afraid to take it. Taking this medicine will make you more comfortable and help you to eat and drink.
13. Notify your nurse or doctor if taking pills becomes difficult. Some, but not all, pills can be crushed and taken in ice cream or applesauce.
14. Keep your mouth fresh and clean. Baking soda (1 tsp mixed in 1 qt of water) works well to rinse your mouth and gargle. This can be done every 2 hr.
15. If it becomes more difficult to eat, change your foods to include very soft, blended, and/or liquid foods. Your nurse or doctor may suggest liquid food supplements.
16. Tell your nurse or doctor if you notice any of the following:
    - being unable to drink fluids
    - dizziness, extreme tiredness, or weakness
    - chills or fever of 100.8°F or higher
    - urinating small amounts of dark urine

products would best meet the individual needs of the patient. Some patients may require a feeding tube, usually gastrostomy, if esophagitis becomes severe. Occasionally, a tube will be placed prior to initiating treatment if nutritional problems are anticipated.

Local anesthetics are often used to help alleviate the pain associated with esophagitis. Temporary relief may occur after using over-the-counter preparations such as liquid antacids, Aspergum® (Plough, Inc.), and children's acetaminophen elixir. For moderate to severe esophagitis, numerous "cocktail" recipes exist. Most contain common ingredients including viscous Xylocaine 2% to anesthetize and liquid antacids to coat and soothe. Many contain diphenhydramine elixir to reduce inflammation; however, this may burn and cause an increase in the dryness of already compromised mucous membranes. As an alternative, nonsteroidal anti-inflammatory agents may be used, if not contraindicated by existing gastric ulcers or thrombocytopenia. Patients using viscous Xylocaine should be aware that their gag reflex may be diminished. Local anesthetics are usually prescribed every 3–4 hours as needed and/or 15–30 minutes before meals.

Sucralfate suspension is also used to treat radiation- and chemotherapy-induced esophagitis. It is suggested that it promotes comfort and possibly healing by binding to proteinaceous exudate in exposed mucosa. The ingredients of sucralfate suspension are: sucralfate 12 g dissolved in 60 ml water, Benylin syrup 60 ml, and Maalox suspension to a total of 180 ml. Patients are instructed to use 15 ml after meals and at bedtime—swish in clean mouth for 2 minutes and then swallow.[119]

If pain and discomfort are not relieved with topical anesthetic preparations, it may be necessary to add narcotic analgesics. Acetaminophen with codeine or morphine elixirs are often utilized as tablets and may be difficult to swallow. The alcohol content of elixirs may further irritate mucosa.

Superimposed *Candida* infections may also present significant problems for cancer patients. *Candida* esophagitis may or may not be symptomatic. Symptoms, when they exist, are often difficult to distinguish from treatment-induced esophagitis and may include dysphagia and pain. Prompt and appropriate medical treatment is necessary in order to prevent a systemic spread. Esophageal candidiasis is most commonly treated using ketoconazole, fluconazole, or nystatin oral suspension.[120]

Chemotherapy-induced esophagitis Any patient who develops oral mucositis postchemotherapy is at risk for spread to the esophageal mucosal tissue. Prior or concurrent radiation may augment the severity and extent of mucosal injury. Some drugs such as dactinomycin and doxorubicin potentiate radiation injury to the esophagus, while others including 5-FU, hydroxyurea, procarbazine, and vinblastine produce an additive toxic effect with irradiation. It is not uncommon for a stomatotoxic agent to be discontinued during treatment with radiation and restarted once radiation is completed.

Both infectious and noninfectious causes may result in clinically significant esophagitis. In immunocompromised patients who are granulocytopenic and receiving antibiotics, an infectious esophagitis is most common. Fungal, viral, and bacterial organisms can all be responsible. Candida is the most likely cause and can be fatal if disseminated systemically. Herpes simplex should also be considered in the differential diagnosis. Patients who have received extensive chest wall or mediastinal radiation can present with symptoms clinically identical to an infectious esophagitis.[121]

It is essential to determine the cause of esophagitis so that appropriate therapy can be given. Flexible endoscopy with brushings is more accurate than radiographic examination of the esophagus to identify the correct cause in immunocompromised patients. Biopsy, culture, and histologic examination are necessary for definitive diagnosis. If a biopsy is not possible, a trial course of empiric therapy can be given.

Nursing management is discussed in the preceding section on radiation-induced esophagitis.

Enteritis

Radiation-induced enteritis Treatment of pelvic and abdominal malignancies usually necessitates inclusion of a portion of the bowel within the radiation treatment field. Although improvements in equipment, tumor and normal tissue localization techniques, and treatment planning have significantly reduced the severity of acute and chronic radiation enteritis, its occurrence remains a common effect of treatment.

Cells of the epithelial lining of the intestinal mucosa have a short life cycle. Rapid mitosis is necessary in order to maintain a balance between cell renewal and cell death that occurs as a result of the frequent, normal trauma from passage of feces. This renders the intestinal mucosa quite radiosensitive and vulnerable to treatment-induced enteritis. Radiation doses necessary for tumor control range from 47–75 Gy or more, which exceeds the normal tissue tolerance.[95,122] Table 33-22 reviews patients at risk and dosages required for developing severe radiation enteritis.

Radiation enteritis can be classified as acute, occurring during treatment; and chronic or persistent, with symptoms at greater than 6 months. A lack of acute enteritis does not preclude the development of chronic radiation enteritis; however, there is a positive correlation between the occurrence of severe acute enteritis and the development of chronic radiation enteritis.[123]

Several factors influence the degree, onset, and duration of radiation-induced acute and chronic enteritis.[6,122,124,125]

1. *Dose per fraction:* Higher doses given over shorter time periods result in greater toxicity.
2. *Volume of tissue (field size):* Treatment delivered to larger volumes will cause more side effects. Boost techniques or coning down reduces the volume of

TABLE 33-22 Gastrointestinal Radiation Tissue Tolerance

Cancer Site	Expected Total Dose for Severe Enteritis
Cervix	40 Gy + implant
Uterus	40–50 Gy + implant
Ovary	30–40 Gy
Testes	24–40 Gy
Hodgkin's disease	40–50 Gy
Prostate	50–65 Gy
Colon and rectum	30–50 Gy
Bladder	40–50 Gy
Renal	40–50 Gy
Abdominal lymph nodes	30–50 Gy

Source: Adapted from O'Brien PH, Jenrette JM, Garvin AJ: Radiation enteritis, *Am Surg* 53:501–504, 1987.

tissue included in the treatment field after a predetermined dose has been delivered.

3. *Treatment technique/plan:* The use of a four-field technique (anterior, posterior, right, and left laterals) helps to spare a portion of the bowel. Use of pretreatment contrast studies and computer-assisted planning to provide more individualized dosimetry decreases the incidence of chronic radiation enteritis.
4. *Bowel displacement techniques:* Attempts to move part of the small bowel out of the radiation field may include:
   a. treatment with a full bladder to elevate the small bowel
   b. patients lying in a prone position on a Styrofoam platform or "belly board" that has a cut-out area designed to allow abdominal contents to fall forward
   c. surgical placement of an omental sling or pedicle flap to support the small bowel in the upper abdomen (this technique is less commonly used due to the surgical procedure required).
5. *Previous abdominal surgery and/or radiation therapy:* These predispose patients to developing adhesions.
6. *Concomitant chemotherapy:* Significant enhancement of intestinal injury has been reported with actinomycin-D, doxorubicin, 5-FU, and cisplatin.
7. *Patient-related considerations:* Factors including compromised nutritional status, preexisting bowel disorders, diabetes, and hypertension may enhance enteritis.

Consideration of these factors is important in anticipating toxicities and educating patients. Table 33-16 reviews gastrointestinal toxicities.

Acute radiation enteritis Although variable, it is estimated that 85% of patients receiving radiation therapy to the abdomen or pelvis will develop some degree of enteritis due to the highly radiosensitive nature of the epithelium.[5,95] The severity ranges from a mild change in frequency and consistency to excessive diarrhea and cramping. Most patients report an increase in frequency to three to five bowel movements daily and a loose or watery consistency. Diarrhea accompanied by tenesmus may occur during or soon after abdominal or pelvic irradiation.

Radiation enteritis is the result of cellular and vascular changes, alterations in absorption, and a decrease in enzyme activity. Morphological changes seen with increasing doses include an increased rate of cell loss from intestinal villi that exceeds the capability of reproduction by crypt cells and a shortening of the villi resulting in a reduction in the total epithelial surface.[95]

Although temporary, acute radiation enteritis can cause significant problems. A frequent need and sense of urgency can prevent patients from participating in work and social activities. If severe, a reduction in daily fraction size or an interruption in treatment may be necessary, and fluid and electrolyte imbalances may require intravenous support. Attempts should be made to prevent the potentially serious complications associated with acute radiation enteritis.

Nursing considerations The role of the nurse in managing a patient at risk for developing acute radiation enteritis includes assessment, symptom management, and patient education. An initial assessment should include normal patterns of elimination as well as recent changes including frequency, amount, color and consistency, history of bowel disorders, use of laxatives and antidiarrheals, and food intolerances. Nutritional and hydration status must also be determined. Careful and complete documentation of the initial assessment will serve as a baseline for future comparison.

Ongoing assessment should be at least weekly and includes any changes in elimination, abdominal tenderness, bowel sounds, weight, and hydration status. A complete blood count and chemistry panel may be indicated. In addition, assessment of the skin and mucous membranes of the perianal areas should be performed as diarrhea may further compromise these tissues. Documentation of toxicities can be accomplished by using a standard scale such as that found in Table 33-3.

Patients and their significant others should be educated as to the potential side effects of treatment including diarrhea, cramping, and mucosal irritation as well as the usual time of onset and resolution. Patients must understand the need to report changes and should also be reassured that appropriate interventions will be employed when the side effects occur. The importance of maintaining adequate food and fluid intake must be stressed.

Treatment of acute radiation enteritis begins when symptoms begin and is dependent upon the severity. Dietary changes, specifically a low-fat, low-fiber diet, is usually initiated at the first sign of radiation enteritis and is often the only treatment necessary. Table 33-23 includes dietary guidelines for managing enteritis. Many

TABLE 33-23 Dietary Guidelines for Enteritis

This diet is planned to help reduce the chance that you will develop diarrhea during radiation therapy or to lessen its effects should it develop. Please start this diet as soon as you are instructed.

This diet restricts the intake of foods that are (1) *high in roughage* (the indigestible parts of plants); (2) *fatty foods* such as fats, oils, fatty meats, fried foods, or rich desserts that may be poorly absorbed; and (3) foods that might cause increased intestinal activity, such as hot peppers, regular coffee, and alcohol.

Follow this diet for at least 2 weeks after your course of treatment is completed. Slowly and cautiously resume your normal eating pattern. By adding one new food at a time, you will know if a certain food causes diarrhea. Simply leave that food out of your diet for another month and then try it again.

FOOD GROUPS	
Vegetables	
Include:	Cooked young vegetables such as beets, carrots, green pepper; strained tomatoes; peeled squash; tomato paste, sauce, and puree; potato without skins
Avoid:	Raw vegetables; cooked broccoli; cabbage; green beans; cauliflower; brussels sprouts; celery; peas and dried beans (of all kinds); spinach; onions; corn; any vegetables cooked in butter, margarine, or cream sauces
Fruits and Juices	
Include:	Cooked or canned fruit without seeds or skins and fresh ripe bananas; fruit nectars; apple, grape, or cranberry juices with added vitamin C
Avoid:	Raw fruits (except bananas); dried fruits such as currants, raisins, and prunes; orange and grapefruit juice
Bread, Muffins, Crackers, Cereals, Other Grains	
Include:	Enriched bread without seeds; melba toast; muffins (plain, corn, and English); plain crackers; refined cereals (Cream of Wheat, rice, cornflakes, etc); converted white rice; pasta; plain pancakes or waffles
Avoid:	Whole-grain breads such as whole wheat, sprouted wheat, or bran; breads with seeds, nuts, fruit skins; whole grains such as bran or whole wheat; crackers with seeds such as sesame, etc
Fats	
All foods should be baked, broiled, or boiled without added fats. Meat should be well trimmed. Use butter, margarine, or mayonnaise *sparingly* on bread, vegetables, and starches.	
Meats, Fish, Poultry, Eggs, and Other Protein Foods	
Include:	All chicken, turkey, fish, lean beef, lamb, and veal; liver; tofu (broil, bake, *do not fry*); eggs; cheese such as low-fat cottage cheese; processed skim milk cheeses; part-skim mozzarella and ricotta; Velveeta; American string cheese; Parmesan
Avoid:	Fried foods; sour cream; cream cheese; poultry skin; fatty meats; nuts; gravies

TABLE 33-23 Dietary Guidelines for Enteritis (continued)

Desserts	
Include:	Frozen juice bars; sherbet; pudding made with nonfat milk; Jell-O; angel food cake; arrowroot cookies; ginger snaps; vanilla wafers; frozen yogurt; hard candies; jelly beans
Avoid:	Frostings made with milk or fats; pies; puddings; custards made with whole milk; whipped toppings; chocolate cake
Beverages	
Include:	Water; weak or decaffeinated tea; ginger ale or 7-Up–type soft drinks; decaffeinated colas and Gatorade®. All should be iced and stirred to reduce the fizz.
Avoid:	Regular coffee; Dr. Pepper; Mountain Dew; alcohol
Milk	
Include:	Skim milk; low-fat milk; powdered skim milk; buttermilk; evaporated skim milk; low-fat yogurt; chocolate milk; vanilla ice milk; frozen yogurt
Avoid:	Whole milk; evaporated milk; cream; ice cream

patients develop a lactose intolerance during treatment. If this occurs, reducing or eliminating lactose in the diet is necessary. Products such as lactaid or lactose-free milk may be recommended to ensure adequate intake of calcium and riboflavin. Elemental diets have been recommended by some to decrease the prevalence and severity of radiation enteritis; however, others have found no significant benefit.[126]

If dietary changes do not sufficiently control acute radiation enteritis, pharmacologic management is implemented (see Table 33-24). Conservative treatment with mild antidiarrheals such as Pepto Bismol® or Kaopectate® may be helpful initially. Diphenoxylate (Lomotil®) or loperamide (Imodium®) may also be prescribed. Anticholinergics, antispasmodics, and/or bile salt sequestrating agents may also be prescribed when appropriate.

Management of severe diarrhea may include the use of opiates such as opium tincture, paregoric elixir, and codeine to decrease peristalsis. Sandostatin® given subcutaneously may also be used to control diarrhea by suppressing the secretion of serotonin and gastroenteropancreatic peptides possibly contributing to diarrhea. Based on the presumption that radiation increases prostaglandin secretion and evidence that certain prostaglandins may be responsible for diarrhea in some patients, antiprostaglandin compounds such as salicylates and choline magnesium trisalicylate (Trilisate®) are now under study. Clinical trials are under way to determine if these agents may be useful in preventing or managing acute and chronic radiation enteritis.

Nursing care must also focus on skin care in the perianal area. Table 33-4 offers skin care guidelines for use during and after completion of radiation therapy.

TABLE 33-24 Suggested Pharmacologic Management of Diarrhea

Drug	Active Ingredient	Adult Dosage	Comments
		NONPRESCRIPTION DRUGS	
Kaopectate® Caplet—750 mg Liquid—600 mg/ml	Attapulgite	Initial: 2 caplets or 30 ml Repeat as needed after each loose stool (maximum: 12 caplets in 24 hr)	Attapulgite is a clay-containing material Acts as an absorbent Does not decrease gastric motility
Donnagel® Tablet—600 mg Liquid—600 mg/15 ml	Attapulgite plus three anticholinergics (atropine, scopolamine, lyoscyamine)	Initial: 2 tablets or 30 ml, then 1 tablet or 15 ml every 3 hr as needed	Absorbent plus anticholinergic activity Useful in diarrhea associated with abdominal cramping
Pepto-Bismol® Tablet Liquid (one tablet = 15 ml liquid)	Bismuth subsalicylate	Initial: 2 tablets or 30 ml Repeat every ½–1 hour as needed (maximum: 8 doses in 24 hr)	Antisecretory May temporarily turn stool black or darken tongue Contains salicylates Also relieves associated abdominal cramping
Metamucil® Flavored powder Wafers	Psyllium Hydrophilic mucilloid	One to three doses daily prepared per product label instructions	Absorbent Bulk-forming natural fiber Encourage additional fluids for optimal benefit
Imodium A-D® Caplet—2 mg Liquid—1 mg/5 ml	Loperamide HCl	Initial: 2 caplets or 20 ml, then 1 caplet or 10 ml after each loose stool (maximum: four caplets or 4.0 ml/24 hr, unless otherwise directed by physician)	Antiperistaltic activity No central opioid activity found at normal therapeutic doses Also available as prescription drug
Amphojel® Suspension 320 mg/5 ml	Aluminum hydroxide gel	20–40 ml four times daily	Absorbent Popular use as an antacid—alternate with magnesium-containing antacids to avoid swings from diarrhea to constipation
Imodium® Capsule—2 mg	Loperamide HCl	Initial: 2 capsules, then 1 capsule after each unformed stool (maximum: 8 capsules in 24 hr)	Nonnarcotic Antiperistaltic activity Unlike Lomotil® and codeine, no central opioid activity found at normal therapeutic doses Also available as nonprescription drug (Imodium A-D)
Lomotil® Tablet Liquid One tablet = 5 ml	Diphenoxylate HCl (2.5 mg) plus atropine sulfate (0.025 mg)	1–2 tablets (5–10 ml) three to four times daily (maximum: 8 tablets/40 ml in 24 hr)	Opiate Schedule V controlled drug Atropine added to discourage drug abuse High doses (40–60 ml) may cause opioid activity including euphoria
Codeine Tablet—15 mg, 30 mg, 60 mg	Codeine sulfate	PO: 30–60 mg every 4–6 hr as needed	Opiate Schedule II controlled drug More constipating than morphine

(continued)

TABLE 33-24 Suggested Pharmacologic Management of Diarrhea (continued)

Drug	Active Ingredient	Adult Dosage	Comments
NONPRESCRIPTION DRUGS			
Codeine, continued			30 mg equivalent to 5 mg Lomotil or 2 mg Imodium
Tincture of opium Liquid: 10% opium, 19% alcohol base	Opium	PO: 0.6 ml every 4–6 hr as needed	Opiate Schedule II controlled drug 6 mg morphine equivalent per 0.6 ml dose Anise flavor Dilute with water prior to taking
Paregoric Liquid: camphorated tincture of opium 0.4%, 45% alcohol base	Opium	PO: 5–10 ml taken one to four times daily	Opiate Schedule III controlled drug 2 mg morphine equivalent per 5 ml dose Brown liquid appears milky when water is added
Sandostatin 1 ml ampul for subcutaneous use only .05 mg/ml 0.1 mg/ml 0.5 mg/ml	Octreotide acetate	SQ: 50–200 mcg given two to three times daily	Antisecretory Side effects: pain at injection site nausea headache

Absorbents—decrease fluidity of stool by absorbing water.

Adsorbents—hold noxious substances (toxins, bacteria) on drug surface preventing their absorption.

Opiates—decrease intestinal motility, thereby reducing stool frequency.

Antisecretory—inhibit GI endocrine secretion and/or inhibit secretion of fluids and electrolytes.

Should dry or moist desquamation occur, methods should be employed to promote healing and comfort (Table 33-5).

Chronic radiation enteritis While the diagnosis of acute radiation enteritis is easily made based on clinical findings, the diagnosis of chronic enteritis is not. It can occur months to years following treatment, and its clinical features are often attributed to a recurrence of a malignancy. In any patient who received previous abdominal pelvic irradiation, chronic radiation enteritis should be suspected and attempts made to diagnosis. Unfortunately, there are no specific noninvasive screening tests available to make this diagnosis, and those utilized are often inconclusive for various reasons. Diagnostic tests utilized include small bowel follow-through, single-contrast barium infusion, and biochemical and hematologic testing. Correlation of diagnostic findings with the clinical history and presentation is necessary for a correct diagnosis.

Chronic radiation enteritis most frequently occurs 6 months to 5 years following completion of treatment, although it may occur earlier or much later in some patients. It is estimated that 5%–15% of patients who received a dose greater than 55 Gy to the abdomen or pelvis may develop chronic enteritis.[127,128] It is suggested that this may be a conservative estimate due to the retrospective nature of the data and the number of patients lost to follow-up.[129]

Progressive endarteritis is thought to be responsible for chronic changes in the alimentary tract. Mucosal ulceration and infarction necrosis may occur and partial or complete obstruction may develop as a result of adhesions.

Conservative treatment of chronic radiation enteritis is preferred unless a patient presents with an acute problem requiring surgical intervention, such as complete obstruction or perforation. Diets low in fat and residue and free of gluten and lactose are frequently used to manage diarrhea and malabsorption problems. Antidiarrheal agents, antispasmodics, bile sequestrating agents, and broad-spectrum antibiotics may be used to treat obstructive and malabsorption symptoms.

Although resolution is usually temporary, a conservative approach is often used in treating patients with a partial bowel obstruction. Surgical intervention may become necessary as symptoms tend to recur without treatment of the underlying problem. Conservative treatment includes decompression with a nasogastric tube and support with parenteral fluids. This is followed by maintenance on a soft-liquid diet.[130]

Repeated episodes of partial bowel obstruction often occur, necessitating surgical intervention. Intractable diarrhea and abdominal pain are also indications for surgery. It is important to note that there is often an increased risk of surgical complications including poor vascularity and impaired wound healing in irradiated tissue. When possible, patients should be free of infection and nutritionally stable at the time of surgery. Hyperalimentation provided prior to surgery has been shown to greatly reduce morbidity and mortality.[131]

Controversy exists over the choice of surgical procedure to employ when attempting to repair chronic radiation enteritis. The choice of procedure is often dependent upon the presenting symptoms as well as clinical findings at the time of surgery. If extensive disease is found, a bypass procedure is usually recommended. However, if only a single discrete area of disease is found, resection and primary anastomosis is the preferred treatment.[132]

Nursing considerations The role of the nurse in managing a patient with chronic radiation enteritis includes assessment, symptom management, education, and emotional support.

Patient assessment should focus on abdomen and bowel status. Any changes or complaints indicative of progressing enteritis require prompt attention. This would include abdominal pain, hypo- or hyperactive bowel sounds, nausea and/or vomiting, a change in bowel movements, rectal bleeding, and impaired nutrition/hydration status.

Patients and their significant others should be educated as to the signs and symptoms of chronic enteritis and the importance of seeking medical attention should enteritis become worse. Dietary changes should be reviewed with special attention placed on those items that can be included, as opposed to just those that must be avoided. If medications are prescribed, written instructions on use and potential side effects should be provided.

Chemotherapy-induced enteritis Destruction of rapidly proliferating cells of the intestinal mucosa by chemotherapeutic agents may also lead to enteritis and diarrhea. Epithelial cells in the small intestine (villi and microvilli) are more vulnerable to destruction than cells in the sigmoid colon, which have a longer cell cycle time. Slavin et al.[133] observed that the epithelial damage occurs histologically in three stages:

1. initial injury (cellular atypia and maturation arrest)
2. progressive injury (cellular necrosis and epithelial denuding)
3. regeneration (resumption of mitotic activity and mucosal repair)

A rapid transit of intestinal contents is stimulated by these alterations and diarrhea results; adequate absorption of nutrients, fluids, and electrolytes is prevented. Without complications and supervening infections, normalization of the mucosa occurs 7–10 days after initial injury.

Diarrhea, the passage of loose watery stools rather than the usual pattern of bowel elimination, is often accompanied by abdominal cramping and rectal urgency. With excessive passing of stools, initiation and breakdown of anal tissue can occur and become a source of infection. Severity is documented through the use of a grading scale and can range from minimal symptoms (two to three stools over baseline) to bloody diarrhea.

Chemotherapy-induced diarrhea most often results from the cytotoxic effects of the antimetabolites (cytosine arabinoside, 5-FU, and methotrexate) and the antitumor antibiotics (dactinomycin and doxorubicin). The degree and duration of diarrhea depend on the drug, dose, scheduling, and duration of the therapy. The drug 5-FU is probably the most toxic of these. Bloody diarrhea has been associated with mucositis caused by high-dose 5-FU and is considered a grave complication.[134] Weekly administration of 5-FU causes less toxicity than 5-FU given over 5 consecutive days. Attempts to augment the cytotoxicity of 5-FU with modulating compounds such as leucovorin and PALA have potentiated this toxic effect.[135,136]

In the cancer patient, diarrhea can be caused by the cancer itself (e.g., GI tumors) or can be a preexisting condition that is exacerbated by its treatment. Other contributing factors in the patient receiving chemotherapy include: radiation therapy to the abdominal-pelvic region, acute graft versus host disease, antibiotics, fecal impaction, alterations in diet, anxiety, and increased stress.

Diarrhea can also be related to GI mucosal changes due to infection or antibiotic-associated colitis. If suspected, based on patient history, examination of stool should include smears for pus, blood, fat, ova, or parasites; *Clostridium difficile* toxin; and stool culture and sensitivity. Antidiarrheal drugs that inhibit gut motility should be used cautiously or avoided until infectious causes are ruled out because they could slow elimination of pathogens from the GI system. Since many cancer patients require antibiotic therapy at some point in their course of therapy, they are at risk for antibiotic-associated colitis (pseudomembranous colitis). The cause is overgrowth of *C. difficile* in the colon; almost all antibiotics can be responsible.

Neutropenia may be responsible for the increased incidence of *C. difficile* in leukemia patients. Neutropenic enterocolitis is a rare condition that can occur during treatment of hematologic malignancies, mainly lymphomas and leukemias; however, it may occur in any patient who is neutropenic and receiving chemotherapy.[137] Clinical symptoms are nonspecific and include fever, diarrhea, bloody stools, and abdominal pain in the lower quadrant.

Intestinal candidiasis is rarely documented antemortem. A high index of suspicion is warranted in patients receiving any combination of chemotherapy, radiotherapy, corticosteroids, and antibiotics. Diagnosis requires elimination of other causes of diarrhea. A negative fungal culture of the oropharynx should not rule out involvement distally in the GI tract. A stool culture positive for mycelia correlates well with candidal infection.[134] The best diagnostic tool when possible is endoscopy with brushings and biopsy. Clinically stable, nonneutropenic patients may be treated initially with oral fluconazole (Diflucan); neutropenic or unstable patients require systemic amphotericin B.[138]

Viral infections, herpes simplex, and varicella zoster are common after BMT, although acute GVHD is the most common cause of diarrhea. Treatment choice is acyclovir.[139]

Nursing management is as discussed in the section on acute radiation enteritis.

ALTERATIONS OF THE GENITOURINARY MUCOUS MEMBRANES

Radiation-Induced Cystitis and Urethritis

Radiation therapy employed to treat cancers of the genitourinary system, such as prostate, cervix, and bladder cancers, often results in a temporary irritation of the bladder and/or urethra. This irritation can be annoying and can cause considerable discomfort. Acute reactions tend to subside within 2–3 weeks after treatment completion (see Table 33-25). Due to the similarity of symptoms to a urinary tract infection, a clean catch urine specimen is sent for culture and sensitivity, and antibiotics are prescribed as needed. A positive culture is unusual.[128]

Treatment is directed at reducing irritation. Patients should be instructed to increase fluid intake as dilute urine will cause less irritation. Urinary anesthetics (Pyridium®) and antispasmodics (Urispas®, Ditropan®) are frequently used for symptom management.[126,128]

Chronic cystitis is much less common, with an occurrence of about 15% in patients who have received high-dose irradiation (65–70 Gy). These patients will have considerable bladder contraction and submucosal hemorrhage. While there is no preventive treatment available, the risk decreases when physical irritation is minimized. Trauma from infection and mechanical instrumentation and catheterization should be avoided. If hemorrhage becomes severe, hyperbaric oxygen may be used to reverse hematuria.[128]

Radiation-Induced Vaginitis

Risk Factors

Radiation therapy used in the treatment of gynecologic and colorectal malignancies frequently results in significant acute and chronic alterations in the vaginal mucosa. The rapidly proliferating cells of the mucosa as well as its secretory glands are quite radiosen-

TABLE 33-25 Radiation-Induced Genitourinary Toxicities

Tissue Response	Onset/Duration	Clinical Presentation	Physiological Rationale
Cystitis			
Acute	30–40 Gy Resolution—2 wk after treatment completion	Bladder irritation, dysuria, frequency and urgency	Mucosal and submucosal inflammation. Capillary engorgement.
Chronic	6 mo after high-dose radiation (65–70 Gy)	Frequency	Bladder volume diminished due to chronic replacement of detrusor muscle with fibrous deposits.
		Hemorrhagic cystitis	Decreased capillary permeability results in increased pressure of blood flow.
Urethritis	30–40 Gy Resolution—2 wk after treatment completion	Pain and burning with urination	Mucosal and submucosal inflammation. Epithelial cells are destroyed without sufficient replacement cells being produced.
Vaginitis	May begin during treatment and is chronic	Vaginal discharge, spontaneous and contact bleeding, dyspareunia, pruritis, dysuria, or pain	Epithelial cell loss results in thinning of the vaginal lining and loss of elasticity.
		Fibrosis and stenosis	Diminished estrogen production is a direct result of radiation change. Adhesion formation.

Source: Data from Yeoh EK, Horowitz M;[129] Smith DH, Decrosse JJ;[131] Martin PL et al.[143]

sitive, similar to those of the oral mucosa. This coupled with the high doses needed to control these malignancies places the vagina at high risk for radiation-induced complications.

The effects of radiation on the vaginal mucosa include erythema, inflammation, atrophy, fibrosis, hypopigmentation, telangiectasia, inelasticity, and ulceration. Clinical manifestations are reviewed in Table 33-24. The physiological rationale for these changes is quite similar to that of the skin and gastrointestinal mucous membranes. If preventive measures are not taken following pelvic irradiation, partial or complete vaginal occlusion can occur as a result of stenosis and adhesion formation. This combined with vaginal dryness can have serious implications in that sexual intercourse and pelvic examination become difficult, painful, and occasionally not feasible. Surgical intervention may become necessary to restore patency.[141]

Fibrosis and vaginal stenosis may develop as a result of adhesions and can manifest as early as during the immediate postirradiation period when acute reactions are beginning to resolve. Women who are able to continue having intercourse during treatment have considerably less adhesion formation.[126] Adhesions develop most frequently at the areas receiving the highest doses of radiation. This includes the area between the ectocervix and vaginal mucosa, and the anterior and posterior surfaces of the upper third of the vagina. If adhesions are left unmanaged, they can result in occlusion, stenosis, and vaginal shortening. Stenosis is generally limited to the upper third of the vagina. It has been estimated that 80% of all women will develop some degree of stenosis and occlusion following treatment with radiation to the pelvis.[128]

Patients at greatest risk for developing radiation vaginitis are those who have received treatment for cervical cancer. These patients often receive doses in excess of 100 Gy with a combination of external beam and brachytherapy. Direct effects of high-dose radiation on the vaginal mucosa and estrogen production combined with mechanical trauma induced by brachytherapy applicators and packing can result in severe trauma to the vaginal mucosa and underlying tissue.[142]

Less commonly seen, but nonetheless the most serious complication of high-dose radiation, is tissue necrosis. A result of trauma and severe vascular damage, necrosis can result in vesicovaginal and/or rectovaginal fistula formation and hemorrhage. Conservative management is usually attempted for necrosis. This includes estrogen cream, antibiotic therapy, debridement, and antiseptic douches.[141] Tissue necrosis can cause severe pain that is often unresponsive to systemic therapy. Use of nonpharmacologic pain interventions may be beneficial when combined with systemic therapy.

Fistula formation and hemorrhage often require surgical management; however, outcomes are often poor due to the severely damaged vasculature of irradiated tissue. Urinary or bowel diversion or total pelvic exenteration is occasionally necessary.

Nursing considerations

Postirradiation vaginitis can have significant consequences if not managed appropriately. Nursing interventions begin early, prior to treatment, to prevent or minimize its debilitating effects. The goals of intervention are to promote comfort and sexual expression and to ensure that complications do not impede medical follow-up.

Nurses also need to be cognizant of the increased risk of vaginal infections in patients who have received radiation to the pelvic area and should assess for signs and symptoms of an infection. Patients should be instructed to always report fever, changes in vaginal drainage, and pain. Early identification of an infection and prompt medical intervention will help to alleviate discomfort and prevent serious complications.

Discussing sexuality and the sexual organs can be very difficult for many people and so it is often avoided. The implications of this can be fear and anxiety when patients complete treatment; anger because they were not aware of potential long-term consequences; and poor compliance with interventions. Patients and their significant others must be educated prior to radiation therapy as to the acute and late effects of radiation, as well as to the planned treatment for postirradiation vaginitis.

Treatment for radiation vaginitis usually begins 2 weeks after the completion of radiation when the acute reactions have begun to subside. Management is by vaginal dilatation and use of vaginal estrogen preparations. Dilatation can be accomplished through sexual intercourse and/or use of a vaginal dilator designed to minimize fibrosis and stenosis. Vaginal dilatation should take place at least three times per week.

Vaginal estrogen preparations such as Premarin® and Estrace® may be in the form of a cream or vaginal suppository. They are relatively easy to use and appear safe in the treatment of radiation vaginitis. Vaginal preparations are absorbed systemically and result in high sustained levels of estrogen in the systemic circulation; therefore, their use should be avoided in patients with medical or oncologic conditions in which systemic estrogen therapy is contraindicated. Patients need to know that the use of estrogen preparations will need to be permanent as high-dose radiation results in chronic estrogen deprivation. Patients treated prophylactically with estrogen preparations after radiation have been found to have less bleeding, dyspareunia, and narrowing of the vaginal caliber. Its use promotes epithelial regeneration and helps to prevent mucosal atrophy.[143]

Patients are instructed to begin vaginal dilatation approximately 2 weeks after completing treatment. Dryness and some fibrosis may have already begun to occur, and they should be instructed to always use a water-soluble lubricant during vaginal intercourse to reduce discomfort and prevent irritation and trauma. The purpose of dilatation must be reinforced. Not only is it important for sexual intercourse, but a patent vagina is necessary in order to perform pelvic exams that are needed to monitor disease status.

The use of a dilator may be quite distressing for some women. Fear of pain as well as a connotation of masturbation can reduce compliance. Nurses need to assess patients' feelings regarding its use and correct any misconceptions. Sensitivity and compassion are of utmost importance when reviewing the procedure with patients. Patients should be given verbal and written instructions on proper use of the dilator and should be encouraged to express any fears or concerns regarding its use. If possible, a dilator should be provided by the radiation oncology department. This will prevent embarrassment often experienced when purchasing one. Table 33-26 includes patient instructions for using a vaginal dilator.

If patients are sexually active and have intercourse at least three times per week, use of a dilator is not necessary. If they are sexually active but have intercourse less than three times per week, use of a dilator is necessary.

Patients are encouraged to continue having intercourse; however, body image changes and fear of pain often interfere. Speaking with a patient's significant other, with the patient's permission, may be beneficial.

TABLE 33-26 Use of a Vaginal Dilator

Vaginal dilatation is recommended for all women who have received radiation to the pelvis. This is to reduce the scar tissue that may form after treatment, which can cause the vagina to narrow. Dilatation can be accomplished through sexual intercourse and/or use of a vaginal dilator. Dilators are designed to keep the vagina open so that pelvic examination and/or sexual intercourse is not uncomfortable.

Vaginal dilators come in different sizes. Your nurse or doctor will decide which size you should use and if or when you need to change to a different size. Use the dilator three times each week.

1. Insert the dilator either lying in bed with knees bent or by standing with one foot up on a step or the toilet. Both positions will allow for relatively easy insertion.
2. Before you insert the dilator, apply a *water-soluble lubricant* on the dilator. Recommended lubricants include, but are not limited to: Astroglid®, K-Y Jelly®, Lubrin®, and Replens®.
3. Gently insert the rounded tip of the dilator into the vagina. Insert it as far as possible and hold the dilator in place.
4. Leave the dilator in place for 10–15 minutes. You should not feel pain or discomfort when the dilator is in.
5. Remove the dilator and rinse it with soap and water. Do not be alarmed if you notice a small amount of blood when you use the dilator the first few times.
6. Use the dilator three times a week unless you have sexual intercourse more than three times a week.

Please let your nurse or doctor know if you do not think you will be able to insert the dilator, if you have difficulty using the dilator, or if you have any increased bleeding or pain.

Occasionally, the fragile vaginal mucosa is irritated by semen. Use of a nonlubricated condom and water-soluble lubricant may help prevent irritation. Water-soluble lubricants must always be used. Reinforcement of the need to continue vaginal dilatation should be provided at each follow-up visit. Review of proper technique is often necessary.

Chemotherapy-Induced Vaginitis

Potentially any drug known to cause oral mucositis may also be associated with painful irritation and inflammation of the vagina. Because the vagina is near the vulva, women may experience both vulvar and vaginal irritation (vulvovaginitis). Other factors contributing to vaginitis besides cytotoxic therapy include exposure to pelvic irradiation, antibiotic therapy, immunosuppressive therapy, and change in pH of the vagina.

Symptoms may occur 3–5 days after chemotherapy is given and resolve 7–10 days later. The nurse should inquire as to whether the patient is experiencing any discomfort because such information may not be easily volunteered. Signs and symptoms to report include vaginal discharge, itching, odor, pain, soreness, bleeding, or dyspareunia. The vulvar and vaginal membranes should be inspected for signs of impaired integrity such as erythema, swelling, or ulceration.

Nursing interventions are directed toward measures to decrease inflammation of mucous membranes, to increase comfort, and to minimize complications.[147] Comfort can be provided with cold compresses or cool sitz baths for relief of pruritus and warm compresses for severe inflammation. Patients are instructed to wear cotton-lined underpants and to avoid pantyhose and tight fitting clothes. Analgesics may be needed for severe discomfort or pain. Exposure to physical and chemical irritants (e.g., tampons, genital deodorant sprays, deodorant-containing vaginal pads or liners) should be avoided to decrease inflammation of the mucous membranes.

The importance of recognizing specific treatable causes such as *Candida* vaginitis must be emphasized. Laboratory tests and cultures are valuable to determine causative organisms (e.g., potassium hydroxide-prepared slide identifies *Candida*). Medical treatment is based on etiology and includes topical and systemic medications.

The treatment of choice for *Candida* vaginitis is miconazole nitrate (nystatin) or clotrimazole (Gyne-Lotrimin®) cream or suppositories. When vaginal creams are prescribed, patients should be taught not to use tampons, which will absorb the medication. If a suppository is ordered, the patient should be instructed where it is to be placed (i.e., vaginally, not rectally). The importance of completing the course of therapy should be stressed since recurrence is common if therapy is stopped early. Trichomonas vaginitis is treated systemically with metronidazole (Flagyl); it is further recommended that the partner also receive therapy.

Prevention of chemotherapy-induced vaginitis includes educating the patient regarding good personal hygiene measures. The nurse's goal is to help the patient maintain a healthy vagina, thereby reducing the potential for secondary vaginal infections. The perineum should be cleansed following each urination and bowel movement with mild soap and water and then pat- or air-dried. Soap and water remove most odors from noninfectious causes; persistent genital odor should be investigated. An unresearched but popular hygiene practice recommends front to back wiping to prevent vaginal and urethral contamination with fecal organisms. Routine douching is not recommended.

Patient and family education should also include sexual activity guidelines. The patient is instructed to use a water-based lubricant during vaginal intercourse to avoid mucosal irritation. Condoms should be used to prevent transmission of organisms through nonintact mucosa. Vaginal intercourse should be avoided in the presence of mucosal ulcerations and while neutrophil and platelet counts are low. Alternative methods of sexual activity should be suggested.

MALIGNANT WOUNDS

Description

Malignant wounds can be one of the most debilitating and frustrating sequelae of cancerous infiltration of the epithelium. In addition to the detrimental effect on quality of life, if unmanaged these wounds can be the source of anemia, electrolyte imbalances, and a portal for infection.

Fortunately, these wounds are uncommon; however, when they do occur they are challenging and difficult to manage. Malignant wounds are most often seen in patients with cancers of the breast, stomach, lung, uterus, kidney, ovary, colon, and bladder; melanoma; sarcoma; and lymphoma. Mucosis fungoides is a T-cell lymphoma involving the skin that can develop into fungating lesions.

Malignant wounds are characterized by excessive purulent drainage, odor, and infection. They develop from local extension or tumor embolization into the epithelium and its supporting structures. Vascular permeability is altered in malignant wounds, persisting to provide a constant source of nutrients and oxygen to cells, thereby enhancing unregulated growth. Malignant cells continually secrete growth factors and have platelet-type functions that continually add new vasculature and collagen to support malignant growth. As the lesion increases in size, it "outgrows" and loses its vasculature, resulting in fragile capillaries. Poor vascular perfusion and altered collagen synthesis result in tissue ischemia and necrosis.[145–147]

Malignant wounds may develop at the primary cancer site or at a distant site due to metastasis. The latter, coupled with variability in appearance, often results in misdiagnosis until a lesion has become large and fungating.

A variety of treatments used alone or in combination have been reported. Choice of treatment is often based upon whether the disease is local or disseminated and whether the goal is to cure or simply palliate.

When definitive treatment is planned, local control is usually attempted with surgery, radiation, and/or hyperthermia. Surgical extirpation with or without radiotherapeutic sterilization is often successful in providing pain relief and eliminating infection, drainage, and odor. This procedure is contraindicated in patients with extensive disseminated disease.

Hyperthermia used alone or in conjunction with radiation therapy and cytotoxic drugs has shown impressive response. Hyperthermia has direct cytotoxic effects on heat-sensitive hypoxic cells, sensitizes cells to radiation, and enhances the cytotoxic effect of some radiosensitizing agents.

Microwaves or ultrasound are used to deliver local heat. The goal is to maintain a temperature of 42°C–44°C for 30–60 minutes. Hyperthermia should be delivered 30 minutes before or 30 minutes after radiation. The procedure is repeated two to three times per week. More frequent application has been shown to cause thermotolerance of some cells. Technical problems and an inability of some patients to tolerate heat often limit the use of hyperthermia.[6,145]

Management of disseminated disease is most often attempted with hormonal manipulation, immunotherapy, and/or chemotherapy. Unfortunately, malignant wounds accompanied by disseminated disease carry a very poor prognosis.[146–148]

The goal in palliative management of malignant wounds is not to heal the wound, but to improve quality of life by alleviating the distressing symptoms of the wound. Radiation is often the first choice of therapy and may be combined with hyperthermia and/or chemotherapy.[6,146,148]

Nursing Considerations

The nurse's role in caring for a patient with a malignant wound is profound. Care requires flexibility, creativity, knowledge of normal wound healing and the pathophysiology of malignant wounds, and often unending patience. Unfortunately, little has been published regarding malignant wounds and their management. These wounds have a very poor prognosis for healing. Malignant wounds do not undergo normal healing due to the inability of epithelial cells to migrate over active tumors and their altered vascularity. Nonetheless, principles of normal wound healing and management should be the basis for planning care.

The goals of management should include minimizing the negative impact on quality of life, promoting comfort, maintaining an environment conducive to healing, maintaining and promoting the integrity of the skin surrounding the wound, and preventing fluid and electrolyte imbalance from excessive drainage.

Nursing responsibilities in managing this patient population include assessment, planning, evaluation, and patient education. Initial assessment and documentation should include wound characteristics—amount of drainage, presence of odor and infection, and measurement.

Based on assessment and principles of wound healing, a wound management program should be planned. Patients and their significant others should be encouraged to participate in the planning, implementation, and evaluation of care. They need to understand the difficulty in managing these wounds, have a realistic expectation for intervention, and realize that many changes in treatment strategy may be necessary. An acceptable and realistic plan of care will improve patient compliance and improve quality of life.

Considerations in developing a wound care regimen include goal of therapy (e.g., odor control, infection control, minimizing drainage), financial resources, product availability, ease of treatment, patient's ability to perform intervention, and availability of caregivers. Poor compliance will occur if patients cannot afford or obtain supplies; therefore, creative management is necessary. Table 33-6 includes many classifications of agents used in wound management, the rationale for their use, and product examples. The information is by no means exhaustive. A decision to use any product or combination of products is acceptable if based on principles of wound healing. Unless otherwise indicated, products should be used according to the package insert.

In order to maintain an optimal environment with control of infection, odor, and drainage, certain interventions are required. The following discussion will include debridement, infection control, hemostasis, wound care, and odor control.

Debridement

Malignant wounds often contain large amounts of necrotic tissue and eschar that contribute to infection and odor and therefore should be removed. Debridement may be chemical or mechanical. Chemical debridement may be appropriate in the presence of a moderate amount of necrotic tissue or eschar. Great care must be used in ensuring that caustic agents do not disrupt normal tissue.

Gentle mechanical debridement is usually preferred and may be accomplished with vigorous wound irrigation using a large syringe. Wet to dry dressings are contraindicated as they are counterproductive and may induce trauma and bleeding when removed. If eschar is dense, it may act as a splint to prevent wound contraction. This may require surgical removal. Maintaining a debrided state will help to prevent infection, control odor, and reduce drainage.

Infection control

Malignant wounds frequently become infected from bacterial infiltration. Escherichia coli; pseudomonas aerugenosa; and strains of staphylococcus, proteus, and klebsiella are common in these wounds, especially those with incomplete debridement. It is important to differentiate between normal wound inflammation with the presence of colonizing microorganisms and the presence of invading microorganisms. Organisms found in wound fluid are not necessarily invading. A positive wound culture of $>10^5$ bacteria is indicative of infection. In this case, antibiotics are appropriate and may be ordered based upon the specific organism. Topical antibiotics are often more successful due to the diminished vasculature and presence of necrotic tissue that may impede systemic therapy.[15] Proper wound care and cleaning will help to prevent infection.

Hemostasis

Malignant wounds frequently bleed due to fragile vasculature and capillary oozing. If not managed, this can result in acute or chronic anemia. Bleeding is most often a result of trauma and can usually be prevented by proper wound care. Trauma can be greatly reduced by keeping wounds moist and using nonadherent dressings. If a wound and its dressing do become dry, soaking the dressing in normal saline before removal will help to prevent trauma.

Hemolytic agents may be necessary to arrest small vessel bleeds. If unable to arrest bleeding with these agents or if bleeding is severe, radiation delivered in doses of 2–4 Gy per day may be given until bleeding stops.

Cleansing

Wounds must be kept clean and free of debris if infection, drainage, and odor are to be controlled. Cleansing with a mild soap and water or nontoxic cleanser will help to remove necrotic tissue with minimal trauma.

Antiseptic agents commonly used in the past are not considered appropriate for most patients due to the caustic effect on cells and the rapid inactivation by many body fluids. If used, great care must be employed to protect healthy tissue. Agents should be rinsed thoroughly from the wound with water or normal saline.[15,146]

Wound dressing

Maintaining a moist wound environment is necessary in order to prevent trauma from drying and fissuring, stimulate epithelial cell migration over any normal tissue, and facilitate resurfacing. Angiogenesis of tumors can be enhanced by fibrinolysis, which is stimulated by a moist environment. This tumor vascularization can in turn enhance the effectiveness of radiation and chemotherapy.

Moist wound environments can be attained using any number of wound care products. Wound fillers are very absorbent and can be used on noninfected wounds. Epithelial-stimulating wound gels, if applied liberally and not allowed to dry, also maintain a moist, pH-adjusted environment. Occlusive hydrocolloid dressings have limited use in this type of wound due to their uneven texture, which makes application and occlusion difficult. Petroleum-impregnated dressings should be avoided as they inhibit aeration and increase anaerobic bacterial growth.

Dressings should be chosen that conceal and collect drainage and minimize odor and unnecessary expense. Nonadherent dressings should be used to prevent trauma to the wound bed during dressing changes. Cost-effective alternatives include sanitary pads and disposable diapers with nonadherent linings. These items are inexpensive, easy to obtain, and very absorbent. Care should be taken to avoid plastic placed next to the skin.

Maintaining the normal tissue surrounding the wound is important. Irritation by caustic agents, wound drainage, and tape used to secure dressings should be avoided.

Skin barriers and creative alternatives to tape can be used to prevent irritation. Montgomery Straps and flexible netting are alternatives. If it is necessary to use tape, hydrocolloid dressings can be applied to healthy skin and used as a base for securing tape.

Odor management

Odor can be the most debilitating consequence of malignant wounds as it greatly impacts quality of life and normalcy. Patients often withdraw and avoid social situations because of the offensive odor.

The odor of these wounds is a result of bacterial invasion and the presence of debris and necrotic tissue. Attempts should be made to eliminate the cause of odor or, when this is not possible, to disguise the odor.

Frequent cleansing will help to eliminate bacteria and excessive drainage. Chlorophyll-containing ointment and solution (Chloresium®) applied directly to the wound may significantly decrease or eliminate odor. If used, patients, caregivers, and health care team members should be aware of its green color. It has also been suggested that chlorophyll tablets taken orally may help to control odor. No detrimental effects have been reported from use of these agents.

If the cause of odor cannot be eliminated, various deodorizing sprays and solutions and charcoal-containing dressings are available that may help to reduce offensive odors. Charcoal dressings tend to be quite expensive, which may limit their acceptability for long-term use. Suggesting that patients reserve use of these dressings for times when frequent dressing changes are not possible or when fear of odor is especially profound (as in social situations) may be financially feasible and help to promote socialization.

Although unconventional, odor control using yogurt or buttermilk, either applied topically or taken orally, has been found to be useful. Although the mechanism is not clear, it is postulated that the low pH of lactobacilli directly affects wound odor by inhibiting the growth of odor-producing organisms that require an alkaline medium for growth.

Regardless of the treatment regime planned, ongoing and frequent assessment is necessary. Patients need to feel as though alternatives are available should an intervention fail. Case studies are presented to demonstrate the care and course healing malignant wounds. See Tables 33-27 and 33-28 and Figures 33-24 and 33-25.

The psychosocial implications of malignant wounds cannot be understated. Patients often are unable to separate wound from self and may feel as though their body is rotting. Isolation may result from embarrassment, shame, and guilt. Health care providers must treat patients with respect and compassion in order to improve self-concept.

In order to provide optimal care for patients with malignant wounds, nurses need to report successful interventions. Only through study and dissemination of information will health care providers be successful in managing malignant wounds and their subsequent consequences and in ensuring patients' optimal quality of life.

REFERENCES

1. Stenn KS, Bhawan J: The normal histology of the skin. In Farmer ER, Hood AF (eds), *Pathology of the Skin*. Norwalk, CT: Appleton and Lange, 1990, pp. 3–36.
2. Parker F: Structure and function of the skin. In Orkin M, Maibach HI, Dahl MV (eds), *Dermatology*. Norwalk, CT: Appleton and Lange, 1991, pp. 1–14.
3. Holbrook KA: Structure and development of the skin. In Soter NA, Baden HP (eds), *Pathophysiology of Dermatologic Diseases* (2d ed). New York: McGraw-Hill, 1991, pp. 3–44.
4. Rubin P: Late effects of chemotherapy and radiation therapy: A new hypothesis. *Int J Radiat Biol Phys* 10:5–34, 1984.
5. Strohl RA: The nursing role in radiation oncology: Symptom management of acute and chronic reactions. *Oncol Nurs Forum* 15:429–434, 1988.
6. Perez CA, Brady LW: *Principles and Practice of Radiation Oncology* (2d ed). Philadelphia: Lippincott, 1992.
7. Bloomer W, Hellman S: Normal tissue responses to radiation therapy. *N Engl J Med* 293:8–83, 1975.
8. Chahbazian CM: The skin. In Moss WWT, Cox JD (eds), *Radiation Oncology, Rationale, Techniques, Results* (6th ed). St. Louis, MO: Mosby, 1989, pp. 83–111.
9. Dangel RB: Pruritis and cancer. *Oncol Nurs Forum* 13:17–21, 1986.
10. Lewis F, Levita M: Understanding radiotherapy. *Cancer Nurs* 11:174–185, 1988.

TABLE 33-27 Case Study #1

Case:	85-year-old white female with no previous medical history presented with stage IV unresectable, locally advanced breast cancer. A large exophytic, foul-smelling, fungating lesion replaced the entire right anterior chest wall. She received 3 months of Halotestin and Tamoxifen with no improvement in the mass and experienced increasing weakness and a 25-lb weight loss during this period.
Plan:	Palliative Treatment
Medical:	External beam radiation therapy delivered to a total dose of 60 Gy over 6 weeks to the entire right chest wall. Hyperthermia was given twice weekly in 1-hour sessions. Concomitant radiosensitizing mitomycin and continuous 5-fluorouracil were given during weeks 1 and 6.
Nursing:	Chest wall care four times daily 1. Half-strength Domeboro solution applied as a soak for 15 minutes for gentle debridement of necrotic tissue. 2. Cara-Klenz wound cleanser sprayed on entire area to aid in debridement and maintain low pH for bacterial control. 3. Plain yogurt was applied liberally to entire area for odor control and maintenance of moist environment. 4. Lesion was covered with nonadherent dressings and held in place with flex-net. (NOTE: After discharge from hospital, a disposable diaper with nonadherent lining was used as a dressing and held in place with flex-net. This proved to be very absorbent and cost-effective. All plastic edges were kept away from skin.) 5. Daily shower.
Outcome:	Immediately after initiating vigilant nursing care, drainage decreased and odor improved, with a significant reduction in necrotic tissue. An impressive decrease in the size of the lesion was noted during the course of combined therapy. Treatment was tolerated well with no associated pain and minimal toxicities (neutropenia at nadir and fatigue).
Follow-up:	In the 2 weeks following completion of therapy, the lesion continued to decrease in size, with a subsequent reduction in odor and drainage. Areas of moist desquamation replaced tumor superiorly, medially, and inferiorly. Wound care was decreased to three times daily.

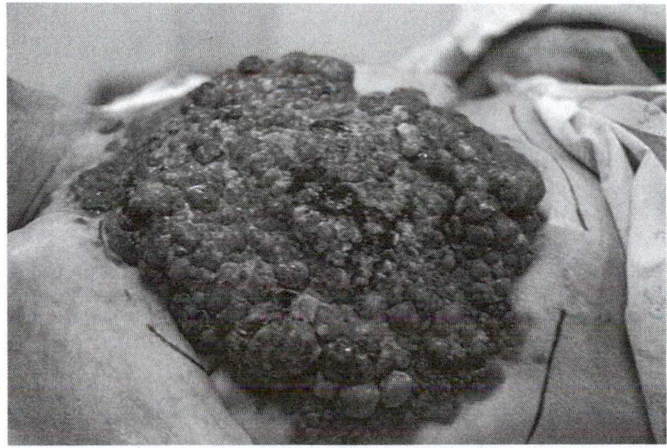

(a) Fungating lesion at onset of treatment.

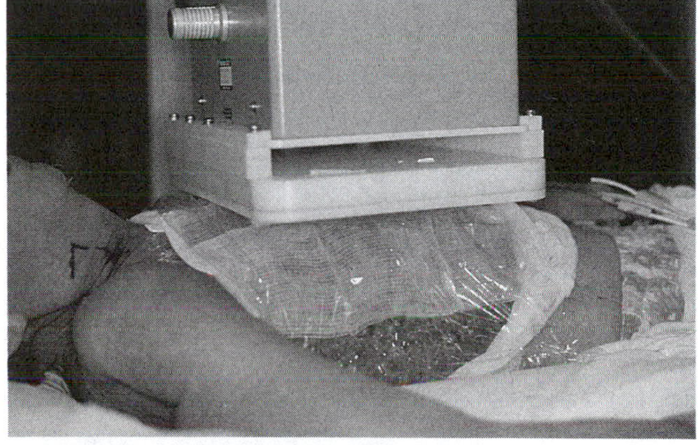

(b) Patient receiving hyperthermia.

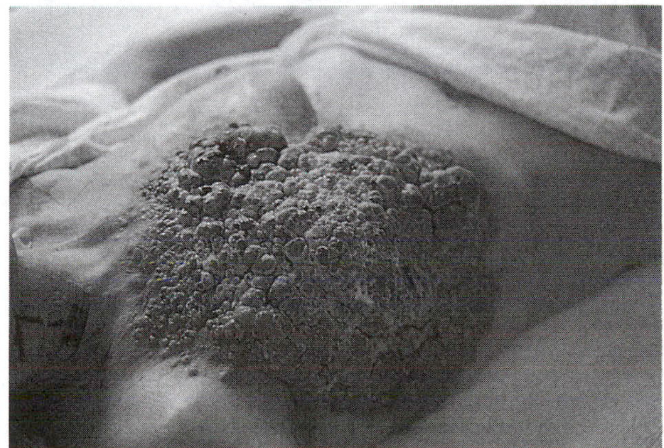

(c) Lesion after initiating wound care and 4 weeks of combined therapy.

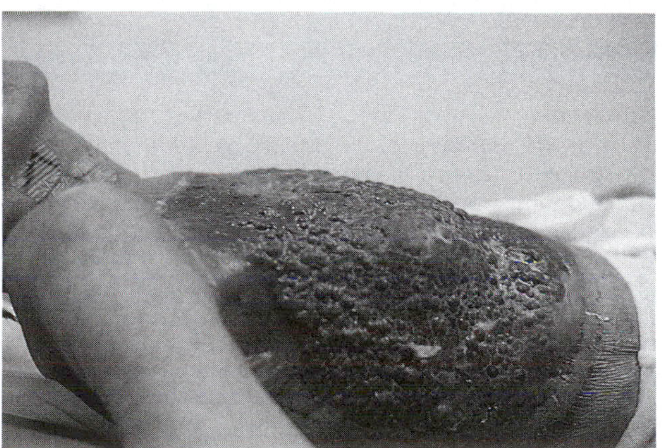

(d) Lesion 2 weeks after completion of therapy with continuing wound care.

FIGURE 33-24 Case Study #1

TABLE 33-28 Case Study #2

Case:	51-year-old white male who presented with a massive ulcerating right neck mass. Biopsy revealed squamous cell carcinoma. Primary site of disease was thought to be pyriform sinus.
Plan:	
Medical:	External beam radiation therapy delivered to a total dose of 70 Gy to right posterior neck using 9 mev electrons. Concomitant cisplatin and 5-fluorouracil. Treatment was delivered every other week for six cycles.
Nursing:	Wound care three times daily 1. Half-strength Domeboro solution applied as a soak for 15 minutes for gentle debridement. 2. Biolex Wound Cleanser® sprayed on the mass to aid in further debridement and maintenance of wound pH. 3. Biolex Wound Gel® liberally applied to maintain a moist wound bed, promote comfort, and stimulate re-epithelization. 4. Lesion was covered with a nonadherent dressing (Telfa®) and secured with paper tape placed outside of the radiation treatment field.
Outcome:	Rapid and dramatic decrease in size of mass. Tolerated treatment with minimal toxicities. Nutritional and hydration status well maintained via gastric tube placed prior to initiation of treatment. Moderate amount of tissue fibrosis.
Follow-up:	Local control of right neck disease. Died 6 months after treatment as a result of distant metastases.

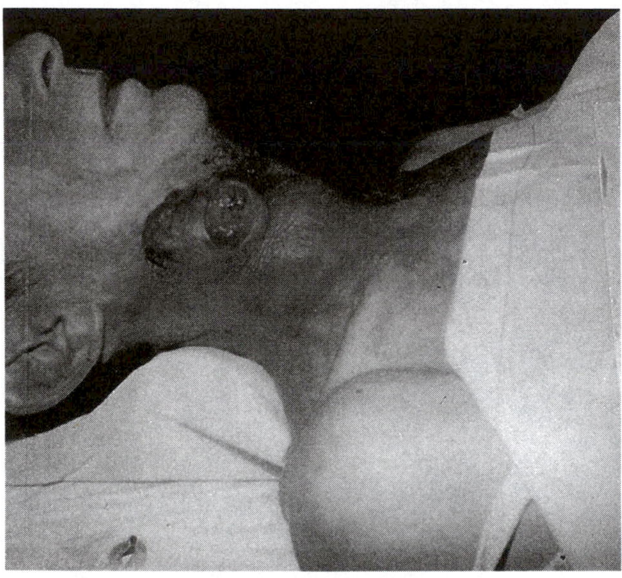

(a) Onset of treatment.

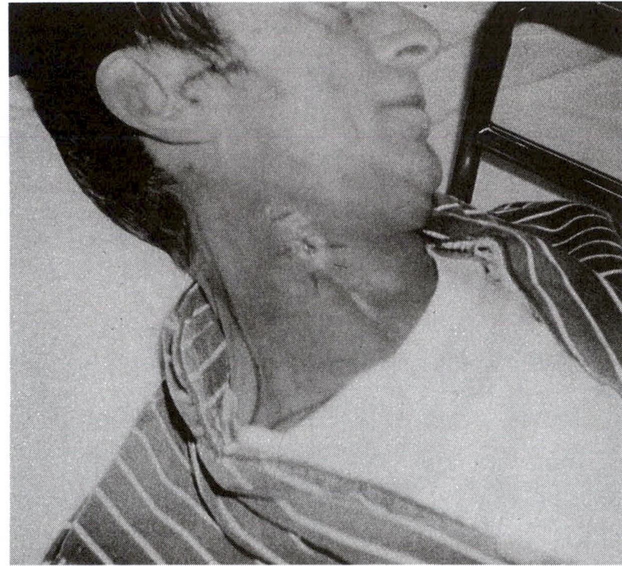

(b) After second cycle of combined therapy.

FIGURE 33-25 Case Study #2

11. Dow KH, Hilderley LJ: *Nursing Care in Radiation Oncology*. Philadelphia: Saunders, 1992.
12. Margolin SG, Breneman JC, Denman DL, et al: Management of radiation-induced moist skin desquamation using hydrocolloid dressings. *Cancer Nurs* 13:71–80, 1990.
13. Hassey KM, Rose CM: Altered skin integrity in patients receiving radiation therapy. *Oncol Nurs Forum* 9:44–50, 1982.
14. Winchester D, Cox JD: Standards for breast conservation. *CA* 42:134–162, 1992.
15. Eaglstein W, Rudolph R, Shannon ML: New directions in wound healing. *Wound Care Manual* 1:1–99, 1990.
16. Ratliff C: Impaired skin integrity related to radiation therapy. *J Entero Ther* 17:193–198, 1990.
17. Hutchinson JJ, McGuckin M: Occlusive dressings: A microbiologic and clinical review. *Am J Infect Cont* 18:257–268, 1990.
18. Hardy MA: The biology of scar formation. *Phys Ther* 69:1014–1024, 1989.
19. Millon R, Parsons J, Mendenhall W: Scar tissue. In Vaeth J, Meyer J (eds), *Radiation Tolerance of Normal Tissue*. New York: Karger, 1989, pp. 83–100.
20. DeSpain JD: Dermatologic toxicity. In Perry MC (ed), *The Chemotherapy Source Book*. Baltimore, MD: Williams & Wilkins, 1992, pp. 531–547.
21. Vonderheid EC: Topical mechlorethamine chemotherapy. *Int J Dermatol* 23:180–186, 1984.
22. Siegel RD, Schiffman FJ: Systemic toxicity following intra-cavitary administration of bleomycin. *Chest* 98(2):509, 1990.

23. Kerker BJ, Hood AF: Chemotherapy induced cutaneous reactions. *Sem Dermatol* 8(3):173–181, 1989.
24. Clavell LA, Gelber RA, Cohen HJ, et al: Four agent induction and intensive asparaginase therapy for treatment of childhood acute lymphocytic leukemia. *N Engl J Med* 315:657–663, 1986.
25. Weiss RB: Hypersensitivity reactions. In Perry MC (ed), *The Chemotherapy Source Book.* Baltimore, MD: Williams & Wilkins, 1992, pp. 553–569.
26. Canal P, Bugot R, Chatelut E, et al: Phase I pharmacokinetic study of intraperitoneal teniposide (VM26). *Eur J Cancer Clin Oncol* 25:815–820, 1989.
27. Lokich JJ, Moore C: Chemotherapy associated palmar plantar erythrodysesthesia syndrome. *Ann Intern Med* 101:798–800, 1984.
28. Burgdorf WHC, Gilmore WA, Garick RG: Peculiar acral erythema secondary to high dose chemotherapy for acute myelogenous leukemia. *Ann Intern Med* 97:61–62, 1982.
29. Bord MA, McCray ND, Shaffer S: Alteration in comfort: Pruritis. In McNally JC, Somerville ET (eds), *Guidelines for Oncology Nursing Practice* (2d ed). Philadelphia: Saunders, 1991, pp. 143–147.
30. Dangel R: Pruritis and cancer. *Oncol Nurs Forum* 13(1):17–21, 1986.
31. Serrano G, Aliaga A, Febrer I: Dacarbazine-induced photosensitivity. *Photoderm* 6:140–141, 1989.
32. Chahbazian CM: The skin. In Moss WT, Cox JD (eds), *Radiation Oncology, Rationale, Techniques, Results* (6th ed). St. Louis, MO: Mosby, 1989, pp. 83–111.
33. Laughlin RA, Landeen JM, Habal MB: The management of inadvertent subcutaneous adriamycin infiltration. *Am J Surg* 137:408–412, 1979.
34. Ignoffo RJ, Friedman MA: Therapy of local toxicities caused by extravasation of cancer chemotherapeutic drugs. *Cancer Treat Rev* 7:17–27, 1980.
35. Brothers TE, Niederhuber JE, Roberts JA, Ensminger WD: Experience with subcutaneous infusion ports in three hundred patients. *Surg Gynecol Obstet* 66:295–301, 1988.
36. Vogelzang NJ: Adriamycin flare: A skin reaction resembling extravasation. *Cancer Treat Rep* 63:2067–2069, 1979.
37. Desai MH, Teres D: Prevention of doxorubicin-induced skin ulcers in the rat and pig with dimethylsulfoxide (DMSO). *Cancer Treat Rep* 66:1371–1374, 1982.
38. Goodman M: Delivery of cancer chemotherapy. In Baird SB, McCorkle R, Grant M (eds), *Cancer Nursing: A Comprehensive Textbook.* Philadelphia: Saunders, 1991, pp. 291–319.
39. Gemlo BT, Rayner AA, Swanson RJ, et al: Extravasation: A serious complication of the split-sheath introducer technique for venous access. *Arch Surg* 123:490–492, 1988.
40. Rudolph R, Larson DL: Etiology and treatment of chemotherapeutic agent extravasation injuries: A review. *J Clin Oncol* 5:1116–1126, 1987.
41. Dorr RT: Antidotes to vesicant chemotherapy extravasations. *Blood Rev* 4:41–60, 1990.
42. Olver IN, Aisner J, Hament A, et al: A prospective study of topical dimethylsulfoxide for treating anthracycline extravasation. *J Clin Oncol* 6:1732–1735, 1988.
43. Rudolph R, Stein RS, Pattillo RA: Skin ulcers due to adriamycin. *Cancer* 38:1087–1094, 1976.
44. Reilly JJ, Neifeld JP, Rosenberg SA: Clinical course and management of accidental adriamycin extravasation. *Cancer* 40:2053–2056, 1977.
45. Soble MJ, Dorr RT, Plezia P, et al: Dose-dependent skin ulcers in mice treated with DNA binding antitumor antibiotics. *Cancer Chemother Pharmacol* 20:33–36, 1987.
46. Merck Sharp & Dohme Company: *Mustargen Official Prescribing Information Physician Desk Reference* (39th ed). Oradell, NJ: Medical Economics Co, 1985, pp. 1337–1339.
47. Laurie SWS, Wilson KL, Kernahan DA, et al: Intravenous extravasation injuries: The effectiveness of hyaluronidase in their treatment. *Ann Plast Surg* 13:191–194, 1984.
48. Argenta LC, Manders EK: Mitomycin C extravasation injuries. *Cancer* 50:1080–1082, 1983.
49. Johnston-Early A, Cohen M: Mitomycin C induced skin ulceration remote from infusion site. *Cancer Treat Rep* 65:5–6, 1981.
50. Wood HA, Ellerhorst-Ryan JM: Delayed adverse skin reactions associated with mitomycin C administration. *Oncol Nurs Forum* 11:14–18, 1984.
51. Dorr RT, Soble M, Liddil JD, et al: Mitomycin C skin toxicity studies in mice: Reduced ulceration and altered pharmacokinetics with topical dimethylsulfoxide. *J Clin Oncol* 4:1399–1404, 1986.
52. Ayres S: Hair transplantation. In Epstein ED (ed), *Skin Surgery* (6th ed). Philadelphia; Saunders, 1987, pp. 198–279.
53. Coates A, Abraham S, Kaye S, et al: On the receiving end—patient perception of the side effects of cancer chemotherapy. *Eur J Cancer Clin Oncol* 19:203–208, 1983.
54. Baxley KO, Erdman LK, Henry EB, et al: Effect on cancer patients' body image. *Cancer Nurs* 7:499–503, 1984.
55. Baker BW, Wilson CL, Davis AL, et al: Busulfan/cyclophosphamide conditioning for bone marrow transplantation may lead to failure of hair regrowth. *Bone Marrow Transplant* 7:43–47, 1991.
56. Seipp CA: Adverse effects of treatment: Hair loss. In DeVita VT Jr, Hellman S, Rosenberg SA (eds), *Cancer: Principles and Practice of Oncology* (3d ed). Philadelphia; Lippincott, 1989, pp. 2135–2136.
57. David J, Speechley V: Scalp cooling to prevent alopecia. *Nurs Times* 83:36–37, 1987.
58. Symonds RP, McCormick CV, Maxled KJ: Adriamycin alopecia prevented by cold air scalp cooling. *Am J Clin Oncol* 9:454–457, 1986.
59. Keller JR, Blausey LA: Nursing issues and management in chemotherapy-induced alopecia. *Oncol Nurs Forum* 15:603–607, 1988.
60. Hennessey JD: Alopecia and cytotoxic drugs. *Br Med J* 2:1138, 1966 (letter).
61. Lovejoy NC: Preventing hair loss during adriamycin therapy. *Cancer Nurs* 2:117–121, 1979.
62. Luce JK, Raffetto TJ, Crisp IM, et al: Prevention of alopecia by scalp cooling of patients receiving adriamycin. *Cancer Chemo Rep* 57:108–109, 1973(abstr).
63. Dean JC, Griffith KS, Cetas TC, et al: Scalp hypothermia: A comparison of ice packs and the Kold Kap in the prevention of doxorubicin-induced alopecia. *J Clin Oncol* 1:33–37, 1983.
64. Satterwhite B, Zimm S: The use of scalp hypothermia in the prevention of doxorubicin-induced hair loss. *Cancer* 54:34–37, 1984.
65. Parker R: The effectiveness of scalp hypothermia in preventing cyclophosphamide-induced alopecia. *Oncol Nurs Forum* 14:49–53, 1987.

66. Kennedy M, Packard R, Grant M, et al: The effects of using Chemocap on occurrence of chemotherapy-induced alopecia. *Oncol Nurs Forum* 10:19–24, 1982.
67. Guy R, Parker H, Shah S, et al: Scalp cooling by thermocirculator. *Lancet* 1:937–938, 1982.
68. Dean JC, Solomon SE, Griffith KS: Prevention of doxorubicin-induced hair loss with scalp hypothermia. *N Engl J Med* 301:1427–1429, 1979.
69. Wittman G, Cadman E, Chen M: Misuse of scalp hypothermia. *Cancer Treat Rep* 65:507–508, 1981.
70. Middleton J, Franks D, Buchanan RB, et al: Failure of scalp hypothermia to prevent hair loss when cyclophosphamide is added to doxorubicin and vincristine. *Cancer Treat Rep* 69:373–375, 1985.
71. Sorrell DC: Scalp hypothermia devices: Current status. *ONS News* 6(8): 1,5, 1991.
72. Wood LA: Possible prevention of adriamycin-induced alopecia by tocopherol. *N Engl J Med* 312:1060, 1985.
73. Perez JE, Macchiavelli M, Leone BA, et al: High-dose alpha-tocopherol as a preventative of doxorubin-induced alopecia. *Cancer Treat Rep* 70:1213–1214, 1986.
74. Ingle R, Johnson DH: Failure of high dose Vitamin E to prevent doxorubicin-induced alopecia. *Oncol Nurs Forum* 15:163, 1988(suppl).
75. Granai CO, Frederickson H, Gajewski W, et al: The use of Minoxidil to attempt to prevent alopecia during chemotherapy for gynecologic malignancies. *Eur J Gynaecol Oncol* 12(2):129–132, 1991.
76. Ehmann JL, Sheehan A, Decker GM: Intervening with alopecia: Exploring an entrepreneurial role for oncology nurses. *Oncol Nurs Forum* 18:769–773, 1991.
77. Eilers J: Alopecia article well received. *Oncol Nurs Forum* 16:155, 1989, (letter).
78. National Institute of Health Consensus Development Panel: Consensus statement: Oral complications of cancer therapies. *NCI Monographs* 9:3–8, 1990.
79. Sonis ST, Sonis AL, Lieberman A: Oral complications in patients receiving treatment for malignancies other than of the head and neck. *J Am Dent Assoc* 97:460–472, 1978.
80. Woo SB, Sonis ST, Sonis AL: The role of herpes simplex virus in the development of oral mucositis in bone marrow transplant recipients. *Cancer* 66:2375–2379, 1990.
81. Lockhart PB, Sonis ST: Relationship of oral complications to peripheral blood leukocyte and platelet counts in patients receiving cancer chemotherapy. *Oral Surg* 48:21–28, 1979.
82. Beck SL: Prevention and management of oral complications in the cancer patient. In Hubbard SM, Greene PE, Knofb MT (eds), *Current Issues in Cancer Nursing Practice Updates.* Philadelphia: Lippincott, 1992, pp. 1–11.
83. Peterson DE, Schubert MM: Oral toxicity. In Perry MC (ed), *The Chemotherapy Source Book.* Baltimore, MD: Williams & Wilkins, 1992, pp. 508–528.
84. Poon MA, O'Connell MJ, Moertel CG, et al: Biochemical modulation of fluorouracil: Evidence of significant improvement on survival and quality of life in patients with advanced colorectal carcinoma. *J Clin Oncol* 7:1407–1418, 1989.
85. Sonis ST: Epidemiology, frequency, distribution, mechanisms, and histopathology. In Peterson DE, Sonis ST (eds), *Oral Complications of Cancer Chemotherapy.* The Hague, Netherlands; Martinus Nijhoff, 1983, pp. 1–12.
86. Carl W: Oral manifestations of systemic chemotherapy and their management. *Semin Surg Oncol* 2:187–199, 1986.
87. Schubert MM, Sullivan KM: Recognition, incidence, and management of oral graft-versus-host disease. *NCI Monographs* 9:135–141, 1990.
88. Dudjak LA: Mouth care for mucositis due to radiation therapy. *Cancer Nurs* 10:131–140, 1987.
89. Bashiri H, Suen JY: Dental considerations. In Suen J, Myers E (eds), *Cancer of the Head and Neck.* New York: Churchill Livingstone, 1989, pp. 179–196.
90. Oral complications of cancer therapies: Diagnosis, prevention, and treatment. *National Institutes of Health Consensus Development Conference Statement* 7:1–32, 1989.
91. Ingall JF, Saper JR, Kish J, et al: Rehabilitation of head and neck cancer patients. *Head and Neck* Jan/Feb:1–13, 1992.
92. Iwamoto R: Alterations in oral status. In Baird SB, McCorkle R, Grant M (eds), *Cancer Nursing: A Comprehensive Textbook.* Philadelphia: Saunders, 1991, pp. 742–758.
93. Gilpin JL: Xerostomia: A review for dental hygienists. *J Dent Hyg* 2:111–114, 1989.
94. Kuten A, Ben-Aryeh H, Berdicevsky I, et al: Oral side effects of head and neck irradiation: Correlation between clinical manifestations and laboratory data. *Int J Radiat Oncol Biol Phys* 12:401–405, 1986.
95. Witt ME, McDonald-Lynch A, Grimmer D: Adjuvant radiotherapy to the colorectum: Nursing implications. *Oncol Nurs Forum* 14:17–21, 1987.
96. DeWys WD: Abnormalities of taste as a remote effect of a neoplasm. *Ann NY Acad Sci* 230:427–434, 1974.
97. Bolze M, Fosmire GJ, Stryker JA, et al: Taste acuity, plasma zinc levels, and weight loss during radiotherapy: A study of relationships. *Radiology* 144:163–169, 1982.
98. Dreizen S, Daly TE, Drane JB, et al: Oral complications of cancer radiotherapy. *Postgrad Med* 61:85–92, 1977.
99. Shepard KV: Xerostomia in cancer patients. *Palliative Care Letter 2:* insert 1, 1992.
100. Schuller DE, Stevens P, Clausen KP, et al: Treatment of radiation side effects with oral pilocarpine. *J Surg Oncol* 42:272–276, 1989.
101. Mansfield MJ, Sanders DW, Heimbach RD, et al: Hyperbaric oxygen as an adjunct in the treatment of osteoradionecrosis of the mandible. *J Oral Surg* 39:585–589, 1981.
102. Eilers J, Berger AM, Petersen MC: Development, testing, and application of the oral assessment guide. *Oncol Nurs Forum* 15:325–330, 1988.
103. Kenny SA: Effect of two oral care protocols on the incidence of stomatitis in hematology patients. *Cancer Nurs* 13:345–353, 1990.
104. Goodman M, Stoner C: Mucous membrane integrity, impairment of, related to stomatitis. In McNally J, et al (eds), *Guidelines for Oncology Nursing Practice* (2d ed). Philadelphia : Saunders, 1991, pp. 241–246.
105. Sonis ST, Tracey C, Shklar G, et al: An animal model for mucositis induced by cancer chemotherapy. *Oral Surg Oral Med Oral Pathol* 69:437–443, 1990.
106. Clark PI, Slevin ML: Allopurinol mouthwash and 5-fluorouracil induced oral toxicity. *Eur J Surg Oncol* 11:267–268, 1985.
107. Loprinzi CL, Cianflore SG, Dose AM, et al: A controlled evaluation of an allopurinol mouthwash as prophylaxis against 5-FU–induced stomatitis. *Cancer* 65:1879–1882, 1990.
108. Mahood D, Dose AM, Loprinzi C, et al: Inhibition of fluorouracil-induced stomatitis by oral cryotherapy. *J Clin Oncol* 9:449–452, 1991.

109. Pfeiffer P, Madsen EL, Hansen O, et al: Effect of prophylactic sucralfate suspension on stomatitis induced by cancer chemotherapy. *Acta Oncol* 29:171–173, 1990.
110. Solomon MA: Oral sucralfate suspension for mucositis. *N Engl J Med* 315:459–460, 1986.
111. Gabrilove JL, Jakubowski A, Scher H, et al: Effect of granulocyte colony-stimulating factor on neutropenia and associated morbidity due to chemotherapy for transitional-cell carcinoma of the urothelium. *N Engl J Med* 318:1414–1422, 1988.
112. McElroy TH: Infection in the patient receiving chemotherapy for cancer: Oral considerations. *JAMA* 109:454–456, 1984.
113. Wingard JR: Infectious and noninfectious systemic consequences. *NCI Monographs* 9:21–26, 1990.
114. Meunier F, Aoun M, Gerald M: Therapy for oropharyngeal candidiasis in the immunocompromised host: A randomized double-blind study of fluconazole vs. ketoconazole. *Rev Infect Dis* 12:364–367, 1990(suppl 3).
115. Ferretti GA, Ash RC, Braun AT, et al: Control of oral mucositis and candidiasis in marrow transplantation: A prospective double-blind trial of chlorhexidine digluconate oral rinse. *Bone Marrow Transplant* 3:483–493, 1988.
116. Weisdorf DJ, Bostrom B, Rather D, et al: Oropharyngeal mucositis complicating bone marrow transplantation: Prognostic factors and the effect of chlorhexidine mouth rinse. *Bone Marrow Transplant* 4:89–95, 1989.
117. Saral R: Management of acute viral infections. *NCI Monographs* 9:107–110, 1990.
118. Nunnally C, Donoghue M: Esophagitis. In Yasko JM (ed), *Nursing Management of Symptoms Associated with Chemotherapy*. Colombus, OH: Adria Laboratories, 1986, pp. 50–53.
119. Wilkes GM: Sucralfate suspension for mucositis. *Oncol Nurs Forum* 13:71–72, 1986.
120. Francis P, Walsh T: Current approaches to the management of fungal infections in cancer patients. *Oncology* 6:81–90, 1992.
121. Pizzo PA, Meyers J: Infections in the cancer patient. In DeVita VT Jr, Hellman S, Rosenberg SA (eds); *Cancer: Principles and Practice of Oncology* (3d ed). Philadelphia; Lippincott, 1989, pp. 2088–2133.
122. Phillips TL, Fu KK: Quantification of combined radiation therapy and chemotherapy effects on critical normal tissues. *Cancer* 37:1186–1200, 1976.
123. Bourne RG, Kearsley JH, Grove WD, et al: The relationship between early and late gastrointestinal complications of radiation therapy for carcinoma of the cervix. *Int J Radiat Oncol Biol Phys* 9:1445–1450, 1983.
124. Whitehouse GH: Complications of hysterectomy and radiotherapy. In Whitehouse GH (ed), *Gynaecological Radiology*. Boston: Blackwell Scientific Publications, 1981, pp. 160–179.
125. Snijders-Keilholz A, Trimbos JB: A preliminary report on new efforts to decrease radiotherapy related small bowel toxicity. *Radiol Oncol* 22:206–208, 1991.
126. Shell JA, Carte J: The gynecological implant patient. *Semin Oncol Nurs* 3:54–66, 1987.
127. Schofield FF, Holden D, Carr HD: Bowel disease after radiotherapy. *J Soc Med* 76:463–466, 1983.
128. Coia LR, Moylan DJ: *Therapeutic Radiology for the House Officer*. Baltimore, MD: Williams & Wilkins, 1984.
129. Yeoh EK, Horowitz M: Radiation enteritis. *Surg Gynecol Obstet* 165:373–379, 1987.
130. Rubin P: The Granz Buschke lecture: Late effects of chemotherapy and radiation therapy: A new hypothesis. *Int J Radiat Oncol Biol Phys* 10:5–34, 1984.
131. Haddad GK, Grodinsky C, Allen H: The spectrum of radiation enteritis: Surgical considerations. *Dis Colon Rectum* 26:590–594, 1983.
132. Smith DH, Decosse JJ: Radiation damage to the small intestine. *World J Surg* 10:189–194, 1986.
133. Slavin RE, Dias MA, Saral R: Cytosine arabinoside induced gastrointestinal toxic alterations in sequential chemotherapeutic protocols. *Cancer* 42:1747–1759, 1978.
134. Mitchell EP, Schein PS: Gastrointestinal toxicity of chemotherapeutic agents. *Semin Oncol* 9:52–57, 1982.
135. O'Dwyer PJ, Paul AR, Walczaka J, et al: Phase II study of biochemical modulation of fluorouracil by low-dose PALA in patients with colorectal cancer. *J Clin Oncol* 8:1497–1503, 1990.
136. Arbuck SG: Overview of clinical trials using 5-fluorouracil and leucovorin for the treatment of colorectal cancer. *Cancer* 63:1036–1044, 1989.
137. Mower WJ, Hawkins JA, Nelson EW: Neutropenic enterocolitis in adults with acute leukemia. *Arch Surg* 121:571–573, 1987.
138. Francis P, Walsh TJ: Current approaches to the management of fungal infections in cancer patients. *Oncology* 6:81–92, 1992.
139. Lightdale CJ, Sloyer AE, Sherr C: Bowel dysfunction. In Wittes RE (ed), *Oncologic Therapeutics 1989/1990*. Philadelphia: Lippincott, 1990, pp. 557–561.
140. DeVries CR, Freiha FS: Hemorrhagic cystitis: A review. *J Urol* 143:1–8, 1990.
141. Chamorro T: Cancer and sexuality. In Baird SB, Donehower MG, Stalsbroten VL, et al (eds), *A Cancer Source Book for Nurses* (6th ed). Atlanta, GA: American Cancer Society, 1991, pp. 141–149.
142. Gusberg SB, Runowicz CD: Gynecologic cancers. In Holleb AI, Fink DJ, Murphy GP (eds), *Textbook of Clinical Oncology*. Atlanta, GA: American Cancer Society, 1991, pp. 481–497.
143. Martin PL, Yen SSC, Burnier AM, et al: Systemic absorption and sustained effects of vaginal estrogen creams. *JAMA* 242:2699–2700, 1979.
144. Clark JC: Mucous membrane integrity, impairment of, related to vaginal changes. In McNally J, et al (eds), *Guidelines for Cancer Nursing Practice* (2d ed). Philadelphia: Saunders, 1991, pp. 248–251.
145. Foltz AT: Nursing care of ulcerating metastatic lesions. *Oncol Nurs Forum* 7:8–13, 1980.
146. Ivetic O, Lyne PA: Fungating and ulcerating malignant lesions: A review of the literature. *J Adv Nurs* 15:83–88, 1990.
147. Bunn PA, Fuks Z: Cutaneous lymphomas. In DeVita VT Jr, Hellman S, Rosenberg S (eds), *Cancer: Principles and Practice of Oncology* (3d ed). Philadelphia: Lippincott, 1989, pp. 1799–1807.
148. Wood DK: The draining malignant ulceration: Palliative management in advanced cancer. *JAMA* 244:82–821, 1991.

Chapter 34

Oncologic Emergencies

Kathleen A. Dietz, RN, MA, MS

Anne Marie Flaherty, RN, MS

INTRODUCTION

Individuals with cancer often experience medical emergencies as a result of the disease process or the treatments. As more effective and aggressive treatments are discovered, patients with cancer live longer and therefore have a greater likelihood of complications from either the treatment or the disease. Some oncologic emergencies, however, can be the presenting symptoms of the malignancy. Prompt diagnosis and treatment of an oncologic emergency can enable further treatment of the primary cancer and thus prolong life. This chapter highlights the most frequent oncologic emergencies that confront the nurses who care for these patients. Clinical pathways have been included to provide the nurse with an overview to guide the care of persons experiencing the various oncologic emergencies.

SEPTIC SHOCK

Scope of the Problem

Definition

Septicemia, a systemic invasion of the blood by microorganisms, can lead to the life-threatening syndrome known as *septic shock*. Septic shock is a profound syndrome characterized by hemodynamic instability, coagulopathies, and alterations in metabolism.

Incidence

The incidence of sepsis and septic shock has increased since the 1930s due to the widespread use of invasive medical devices, corticosteroids and chemotherapy, and enhanced longevity of persons who are susceptible to sepsis (e.g., diabetics).[1,2] Usual sites of bloodstream invasion include skin, pulmonary, gastrointestinal, and genitourinary systems.[3] It is estimated that 400,000 cases of septicemia occur annually in the United States. Of these, 200,000 persons will develop septic shock, and for 100,000 people the outcome will be fatal.[4,5]

Mortality rates are high (>75%) for cancer patients in whom septic shock develops. Rapid and aggressive therapy is needed.[6]

Anatomy, physiology, and scientific principles

Microorganisms, bacterial or fungal, responsible for septic shock can enter the blood either by local invasion of a blood vessel or by entering the venous system via the lymphatic vessels. Endotoxins are produced by gram-negative bacteria, whereas gram-positive organisms produce exotoxins; both cause the release of chemical mediators and hormones and initiate the inflammatory response. Antigen-antibody complexes are formed, activating the complement protein system. The complement proteins directly destroy organisms, enhance phagocytosis, promote chemotaxis, release histamine, activate the kinin system, promote vasodilation, and increase capillary permeability.[7] Plasma leaks into interstitial tissues and causes depletion of intravascular volume, which leads to hypotension.[8] Tissue perfusion is compromised secondary to fluid in the lungs, decreased circulating oxygen-carrying blood, and microemboli caused by the activation of factor XII and the clotting process.[9]

Septic shock is classified into two patterns: early hyperdynamic shock and late hypodynamic shock. In the early or hyperdynamic phase of shock, cardiac output increases and systemic vascular resistance decreases in an attempt to maintain adequate tissue perfusion. The blood pressure may be normal initially, but it soon falls as vasodilation persists and the respiratory rate increases in an attempt to provide oxygen. As hypoxemia develops, cells shift from aerobic to anaerobic metabolism, leading to metabolic acidosis. Pulmonary edema and adult respiratory distress syndrome can develop in the early phase of septic shock.[6] In the advanced or hypodynamic phase of shock, there is vasoconstriction of the splanchnic, pulmonary, and renal circulation, which produces ischemia of the abdominal organs, impaired alveolar gas exchange, and decreased urine output. This compensatory vasoconstriction actually decreases cardiac output, venous return, and blood pressure by trapping blood in vascular beds.[10] Progressive lactic acidosis results from the prolonged anaerobic metabolism. Increasing blood lactose levels indicate critical systemic tissue hypoperfusion and thus can predict a poor outcome.[8] As septic shock progresses, multiple organ failure syndrome develops, in which respiratory and renal failure occur, poor cerebral perfusion leads to coma, and inadequate perfusion of heart muscle leads to ischemia, arrhythmias, and death.

Pathophysiology

Sepsis is the most common cause of shock in the cancer patient.[6] Cancer patients are at risk of infections that may lead to septic shock because of the local effects of tumor growth, immunologic effects of neoplastic disease or treatment, iatrogenic factors, and nosocomial sources.[11] Local tumor growth (e.g., cancer of the skin, head and neck, and gastrointestinal tract) can disrupt normal mucocutaneous barriers, thus enabling invasion by endogenous or acquired pathogens.[11] Likewise, such tumors as head and neck or lung cancers may obstruct natural passages, causing retention or aspiration of secretions that result in pneumonia. Cellular immunity is impaired in Hodgkin's disease and also in persons receiving radiotherapy and chemotherapy. Cancers that involve B lymphocytes, such as multiple myeloma, chronic lymphocytic leukemia, and Waldenström's macroglobulinemia, may impair humoral immunity. Splenectomy for staging or treatment purposes (e.g., in lymphoma and leukemia) can increase the risk of infection. Neutropenia may be caused by the cancer itself but is also a potential side effect of radiation and chemotherapy.

Autologous and allogenic bone marrow transplant, and more recently peripheral stem cell rescue, allow more aggressive anticancer therapy to be given in an attempt to treat both hematologic and solid malignancies. Invasive procedures, such as placement of vascular access devices, chest tubes, stents, and urinary catheters, can alter the patient's barriers against infection. Hospital-acquired organisms may be transmitted by humidifiers, respirators, flowers, and most especially by hospital personnel. In patients who receive long-term antibiotic therapy, resistant organisms often develop, or there may be overgrowth of normal endogenous bacteria or fungi.

Clinical Manifestations

When caring for individuals with cancer, a high index of suspicion and close monitoring are essential to recognizing persons at high risk of septic shock.[12,13] The clinical picture varies from patient to patient.

The sepsis syndrome includes tachycardia, fever or hypothermia, tachypnea, and evidence of inadequate tissue perfusion.[14] The clinical picture of a person with sepsis reflects derangements in cardiac function, vascular resistance, capillary permeability, cellular metabolism and volume homeostasis.[5] See Table 34-1.

Fever or shaking chills in the granulocytopenic and/or immunosuppressed patient may herald a life-threatening infection that can lead to septic shock if left untreated. Vital signs and level of consciousness are monitored closely. In hyperdynamic or "warm" shock, cardiac output increases, causing a rise in blood pressure, an increased heart rate, and a widened pulse pressure[3] (Figure 34-1). The skin is warm as a result of vasodilation and respiratory rate increases because

TABLE 34-1 Early and Late Signs of Impending Septic Shock

Early
Fever or hypothermia
Rigors
Tachycardia
Hypertension
Late
Bilateral rales
Oliguria
Mental status change
Cyanosis
Hypotension
Adult respiratory distress syndrome

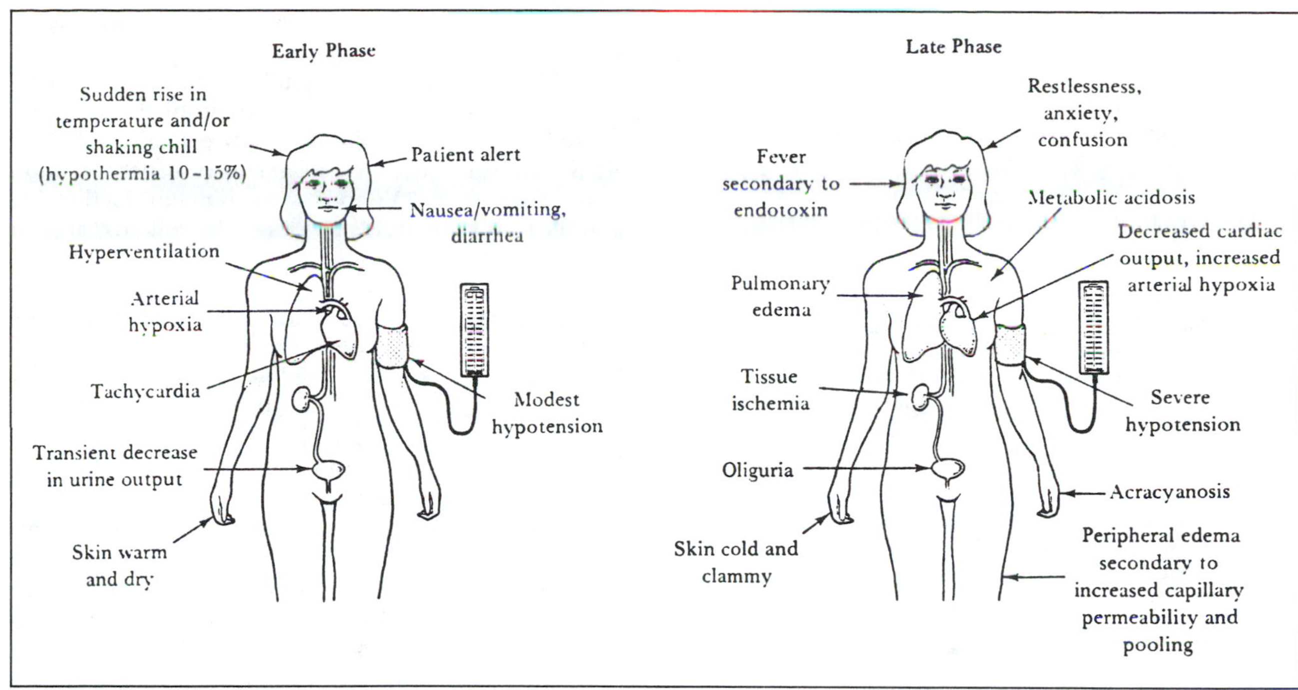

FIGURE 34-1 Sepsis and septic shock.

of capillary leakage in the lungs, causing hypoxia. Since there is a high incidence of associated adult respiratory distress syndrome, bilateral rales will be auscultated if pulmonary edema develops.[15,16] Mental status often deteriorates early, as evidenced by lethargy and confusion. Urine output may be normal to increased initially, but as blood flow to vital organs is reduced, oliguria develops. In the hypodynamic or "cold" shock phase, the patient is cool, clammy, and cyanotic, the pulse is rapid and thready, and the blood pressure begins to fall with a narrowing pulse pressure.[3,17] Arterial blood gases will initially show respiratory alkalosis, but as anaerobic metabolism persists, a combination of metabolic and respiratory acidosis occurs. Decreased venous return leads to pulmonary edema, adult respiratory distress syndrome, coma, and death.

Assessment

Cancer patients at greatest risk of septic shock have granulocyte counts of less than 100/mm^3.[6] During early sepsis a low $PaCO_2$ indicates respiratory alkalosis, which in the later stage progresses to a metabolic acidosis and elevation of lactic acid levels to more than 1–2 mmol/l above normal.[6] In cancer patients, rapid muscle wasting, negative nitrogen balance, decreased intravascular volume, and renal dysfunction contribute to elevated blood urea nitrogen levels.[6] When disseminated intravascular coagulation occurs in association with sepsis, thrombocytopenia and coagulation abnormalities (e.g., prolonged prothrombin and activated partial thromboplastin time and decreased fibrinogen) may be noted.

Interventions

Knowledge of the pathophysiology of the various cancers, treatment protocols, patient history, physical assessment, and results of laboratory tests provides the data base necessary to predict which individuals are at risk of septic shock. Early identification may prevent an episode of fever from becoming a critical event. Because death from septic shock can occur rapidly among cancer patients, immediate therapy is necessary. The primary therapeutic intervention is directed toward controlling sepsis. See Figure 34-2. Administration of empiric broad-spectrum antibiotics is instituted immediately after appropriate microbiology cultures are obtained.[18]

Blood cultures should be taken peripherally and from vascular access devices. The choice of antibiotics is based on the likely sources of infection, the host immune status and the known patterns of resistance and sensitivity developed at a given institution.[5]

A recommended initial approach for neutropenic patients includes administration of an aminoglycoside, an extended-spectrum penicillin active against anaerobes and *Pseudomonas aeruginosa*, and a cephalosporin for staphylococcal and *Klebsiella* coverage. If *Staphylococcus epidermidis* is suspected or if *Corynebacterium* is identified, an agent such as vancomycin should be added to the regimen.[6,18]

In women with sepsis following gynecologic surgery, infection with *Bacteroides* species, particularly *B. fragilis,* should be suspected. If shock develops in the presence of prolonged antibiotic therapy and persistent neutropenia, a fungal source is suspected and treatment with

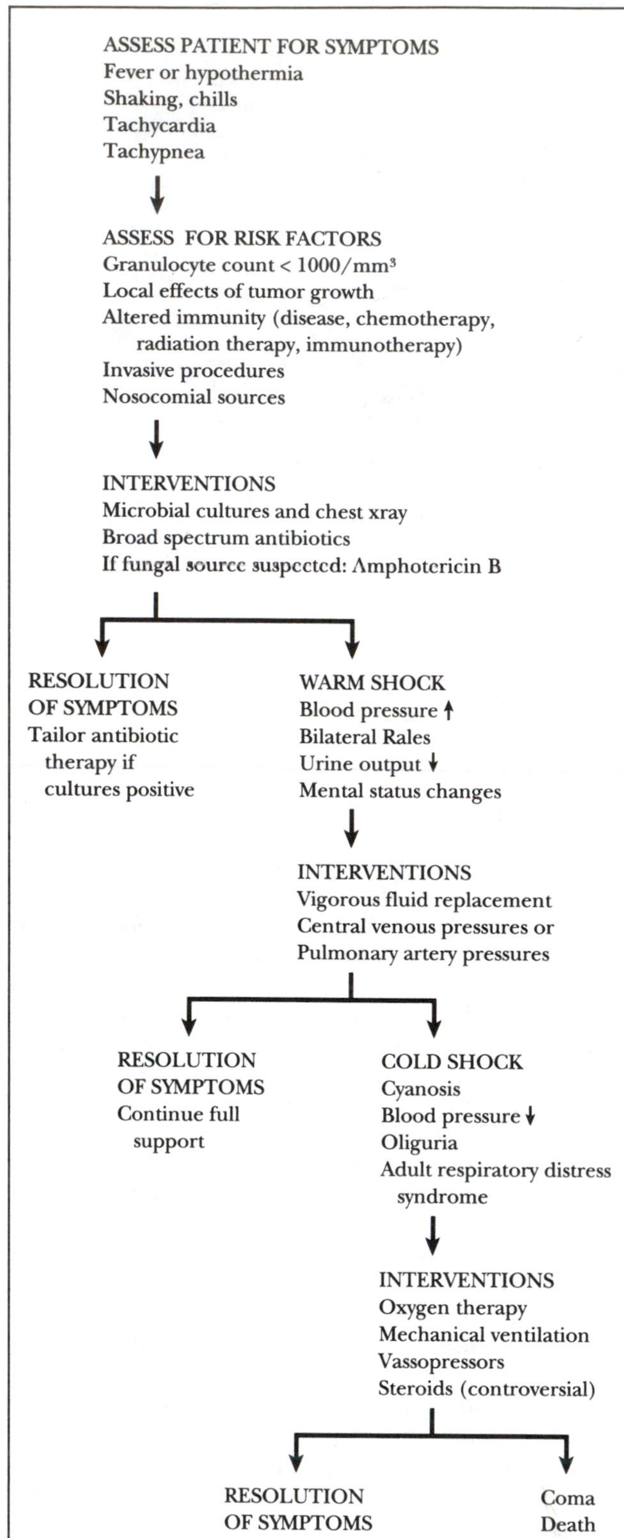

FIGURE 34-2 Clinical pathway for septic shock.

amphotericin B is initiated. An infectious agent may not be identified in 30% of cancer patients with sepsis.[6] Antibiotic therapy must not be delayed, even in the absence of a positive blood culture. Prompt institution of an appropriate antibiotic regimen is associated with improved survival and a decrease in the frequency of septic shock.[4]

Additional measures are taken in an effort to stabilize the patient and to gain time until the source of sepsis is controlled or eliminated. See Table 34-2. Vital signs, urine output, and level of consciousness are monitored frequently.[19] Venous access is maintained for the administration of fluids, crystalloids, colloids, and vasopressors. Fluid status is closely monitored. Vigorous fluid replacement is given to expand plasma volume that is depleted because of diffuse capillary leakage. Unless the patient exhibits signs of fluid overload, a fluid challenge of 500 ml within 20–30 minutes is infused.[20] Crystalloid solutions, such as normal saline or Ringer's lactate, or colloids, such as albumin, are administered to increase intravascular volume.[5,21,22] Fresh frozen plasma can be given in an infusion of 250 ml every 10–20 minutes until a mean arterial pressure of 80 mm Hg is reached.[6] Controversy exists over the use of crystalloids versus colloids for volume replacement.[6,18,19] Blood and colloid solutions expand the intravascular volume more rapidly and with less fluid. When crystalloids are given, peripheral edema often develops and may be mistaken for fluid overload.[5] Central venous pressure or pulmonary artery pressures must be monitored to ensure proper replacement of fluid and intravascular volume without complications of fluid overload.

When vital signs do not improve in response to fluids, vasopressors such as dopamine or levarterenol are given in an attempt to maintain cerebral, coronary, and renal perfusion. Administering norepinephrine to patients refractory to dopamine has been considered controversial; however, recent data support its usefulness.[4]

High-dose corticosteroids may be administered early in the course of shock to produce anti-inflammatory activity and enhance survival. However, if steroids are given later in the course, they may delay death without effecting survival.[9] One commonly used approach is to give methylprednisolone, 30 mg/kg intravenously every 6 hours, during the initial 24 hours after septic shock is diagnosed.[6] Typically, steroids are given only when adrenal insufficiency is suspected since steroids may cause superinfection and have failed to demonstrate improved survival.[1,8]

Airway patency is maintained and nasopharyngeal suctioning is instituted as necessary. Oxygen therapy is administered, and if respiratory status continues to decompensate, intubation and mechanical ventilatory assistance are indicated.[16] Arterial blood gases and

TABLE 34-2 Nursing Diagnoses for Septic Shock

Potential for infection due to inadequate secondary defenses and immunosuppression
Altered protection due to deficient immunity
Hyperthermia due to infection
Altered tissue perfusion due to sepsis syndrome

electrolytes are monitored, and the physician is immediately notified of results. Since metabolic acidosis occurs as anaerobic metabolism develops, intravenous injections of sodium bicarbonate are given to maintain the blood pH within the normal range. An indwelling urinary catheter is used to assist in monitoring of renal perfusion. Hypotensive patients are placed in the Trendelenberg position to promote venous return, and skin is assessed for color, temperature, and moisture.

The effectiveness of the therapies administered is assessed by continuous monitoring of blood pressure, central venous or pulmonary artery pressure, apical rate, frequency and character of respirations, skin color and temperature, level of consciousness, and urinary output.[12,19] Multiple organ failure syndrome encompassing pulmonary, hepatic, gastrointestinal, and renal failure may be recognized as early as 12 hours or as late as 7–10 days after the initiation of sepsis and septic shock.[5]

When therapy is effective, the vital signs should stabilize, pressure should reflect proper intravascular volume, and urine output should be adequate. Maintaining this high level of care is paramount to the resolution of septic shock.

The mortality rate associated with septic shock is estimated at between 50% and 90%. The higher rates are observed among persons with hematologic malignancies.[9] The frequency of shock and the mortality rate increase if the patient does not mount an initial febrile response, as may occur in patients who are taking steroids or who are severely debilitated.[6]

Future Trends

Currently, new avenues for the treatment of sepsis are being explored. Gram-negative sepsis accounts for approximately 30% of overall episodes of sepsis.[23] Patients with gram-negative sepsis without the symptoms of shock have a much better prognosis.[21] Endotoxin activates monocytes; stimulates the release of tumor necrosis factor (TNF), interleukin-1 (IL-1), interleukin-6 (IL-6), and platelet activating factor; and has direct effects on the coagulation cascade and the complement system.[2,24] In experimental studies, administration of large doses of TNF duplicates many of the signs and symptoms of septic shock, including hypotension, neutropenia, edema, and pulmonary permeability.[2] Recently a human monoclonal antibody, HA-IA, was found to block the toxic effects of endotoxin and decreased mortality by 39%.[23] Anti-TNF and IL-1 receptor antagonists are also being investigated.[23]

Wolff[21] has suggested that future treatments for gram-negative sepsis may include:

1. antibiotics directed at the bacteria
2. monoclonal antibodies against bacterial endotoxins
3. agents that block or interfere with the mediators (cytokines) responsible for many of the adverse effects that result in hypotension and the associated high mortality rate.

DISSEMINATED INTRAVASCULAR COAGULATION

Scope of the Problem

Definition

Disseminated intravascular coagulation (DIC), an abnormality of the coagulation system, is characterized by widespread clotting within arterioles and capillaries and simultaneous hemorrhage. DIC can be acute or chronic. Acute DIC must be treated as a medical emergency, whereas chronic DIC produces coagulation abnormalities, with or without clinical manifestations, that can be medically managed.[25,26]

Incidence

DIC is not a primary disorder; it is always a reflection of another event that is occurring in the body (Table 34-3). The DIC syndrome is seen in fewer than 15% of persons with cancer and can be related to either the disease process or the treatment protocol.[26] In malignancy, tissue injury occurs, expressing procoagulant material, usually tissue factor, on the surface of the circulating tumor cells or on the vasculature surface.[25] Solid tumors develop new vasculature, which has an abnormal endothelial lining that may activate the procoagulant system. It is also thought that tumors may release into the circulation necrotic tissue or tumor enzymes that could activate the coagulation system.[26] Solid tumors associated with DIC include mucin-producing adenocarcinomas, such as gastric, lung, pancreas, and prostate tumors (Table 34-4).[27]

TABLE 34-3 Conditions Associated with Acute DIC

Conditions
Intravascular hemolysis
Bacteremia (gm−, gm+)
Viremia (CMV, hepatitis, varicella)
Mucin-producing adenocarcinoma (gastric, lung, pancreas, prostate)
Hematologic malignancy (leukemia, lymphoma)
Prosthetic devices (LeVeen shunt)
Liver disease (↑ FSP)

TABLE 34-4 Disseminated Intravascular Coagulation and Common Malignancies

Gastrointestinal	Ovary
Pancreas	Melanoma
Prostate	Acute leukemia
Lung	Myeloma
Breast	Myeloproliferative syndromes

Source: Bick RL: Disseminated intravascular coagulation and related syndromes: A clinical review in *Seminars in Thrombosis and Hemostasis* (vol 14, no 4) (New York: Thieme Medical Publishers, 1988).

Anatomy, physiology, and scientific principles

Normally, the body has a steady state between clot formation (thrombosis) and clot dissolution (fibrinolysis).[28] When a vessel is severed or ruptured, the wall of the vessel contracts to reduce blood flow. The endothelium loses its normal smoothness and becomes wet and sticky, allowing the endothelial surfaces to become glued together. On coming into contact with this sticky endothelial surface, platelets which are usually round or oval disks, assume bizarre, irregular forms with irradiating processes that adhere to the endothelial surface and to other platelets forming a plug. Since the platelet plug is relatively unstable, procoagulants from both the traumatized vascular wall and the adhering platelets act to form a stable clot.

For clotting to be effective, both platelets and the 13 different clotting factors are required. These clotting factors are proteins involved in a series of enzymatic reactions that have a cascading or domino effect. The clotting cascade is initiated either by the intrinsic mechanism (via factor XII) when the blood itself is traumatized or by the extrinsic mechanism (via factor VII) when there is tissue injury (Figure 34-3). Factor X is the common pathway for the intrinsic and extrinsic systems and converts prothrombin to thrombin in the presence of factor V, platelets, and calcium. Both calcium and lipid are essential for clotting; calcium is normally present in the body, and lipid is provided by platelet membranes. Prothrombin is an unstable plasma protein that is continually produced by the liver. Vitamin K, produced by the intestinal flora, is required by the liver for the normal function of prothrombin. Thrombin is the enzyme responsible for converting fibrinogen to a fibrin clot, which is stabilized by factor XIII. Once healing has occurred, the anticlotting system is activated and plasmin dissolves the clot, resulting in the release of fibrin split products (FSPs). These degradation products are normally cleared by the liver. The normal homeostatic balance between the procoagulant and anticoagulant systems prevents thrombosis and hemorrhage.

In DIC, both microvascular thrombosis and bleeding from numerous sites occur simultaneously. Fibrinogen is consumed by thrombin-induced clotting and plasmin-induced fibrinolysis. Persons with DIC have decreased macrophage clearing function, thereby aggravating the process by limiting the removal of activated clotting factors.[25] Likewise, coagulation takes place so rapidly that the liver is unable to clear the FSPs. When a large quantity of FSPs are circulating, they produce a feedback inhibition of clotting and have an anticoagulant effect. At the same time, the consumable factors I, II, V, and VIII and platelets are depleted by the extensive microvascular clotting.

Pathophysiology

Patients with solid tumors may have laboratory evidence of a low-grade, chronic DIC that does not produce clinical manifestations. Thrombosis, manifested by deep venous thrombosis, phlebitis, or pulmonary embolism, is seen in 25% of persons with disseminated cancer.[25,29] Thrombosis occurs more frequently in the postoperative period, in association with bacterial sepsis

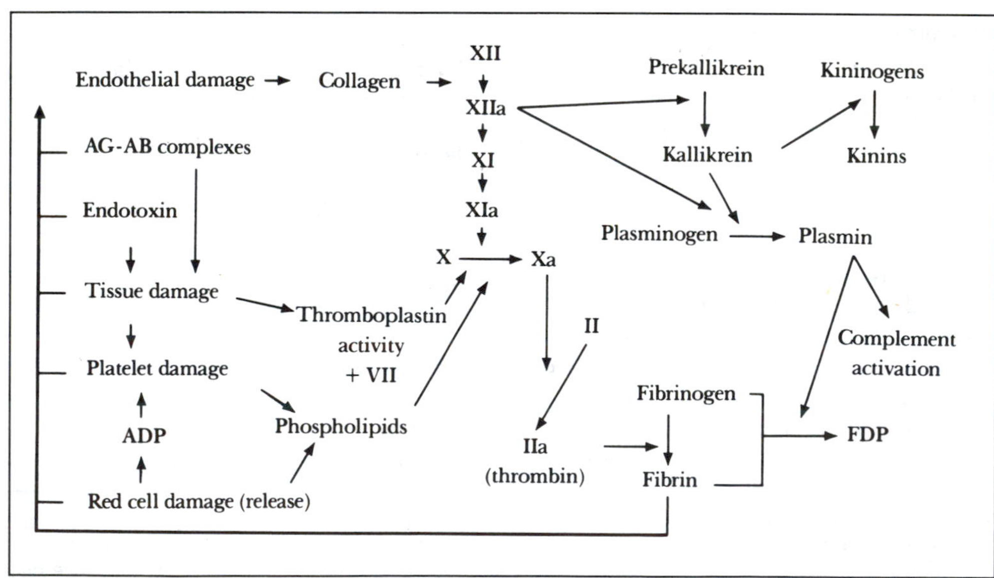

FIGURE 34-3 A schema of the triggering mechanisms in disseminated intravascular coagulation. (AG-AB, antigen-antibody.) (Source: RL Bick: Dissemated intravascular coagulation and related syndromes: A clinical Review, in *Seminars in Thrombosis and Hemostasis* [vol 14, no 4]. New York: Thieme Medical Publishers, 1988. Reprinted by permission.)

and in conjunction with hormonal therapy and chemotherapy.[27] In cancer-related chronic DIC, hemorrhage occurs less frequently than thrombosis.[25] Patients with cancer of the pancreas or prostate, however, will usually have overt signs of DIC. A study at the Mayo Clinic showed that a coagulation screening should be performed before prostate surgery, since there appears to be a direct correlation between preoperative laboratory findings of DIC and postprostatectomy blood loss.[6]

It is presumed that clot promoting agents from the tumor gain access to the circulation.[27] Patients with cancer of the body or tail of the pancreas may experience "migratory thrombophlebitis" as a result of ductal obstruction with subsequent release of trypsin into the systemic circulation. Trypsin acts like thrombin and activates the coagulation cascade, causing thrombosis.[26]

Persons with acute promyelocytic leukemia (APL) have a high incidence of DIC (about 85%),[30] which can occur both before and in conjunction with chemotherapy.[31–33] During conventional therapy for APL, DIC almost uniformly worsens and may be associated with increased mortality related to hemorrhage, renal failure, and adult respiratory distress syndrome (ARDS).[25] Studies indicate that in persons with APL the tendency to bleed is associated with a white blood cell count of ≥10,000/mm^3 at diagnosis.[31,34] This bleeding diathesis is thought to be due to the release of procoagulant material from granules on the promyelocytes. Autopsy studies of individuals with APL have revealed diffuse thrombosis with fibrin deposition in 15%–25% of cases.[35] Likewise, in patients with large tumor burdens, as occurs with some other leukemias and lymphomas, DIC may develop during treatment when cells are rapidly lysed.[36]

Complications of cancer therapy are also associated with DIC. *Meningococcus* and other gram-negative organisms causing sepsis may provide the triggering event that initiates the clotting cascade.[37] Endotoxins can activate factor XII, induce a platelet-release reaction, cause endothelial sloughing, and initiate a release of granulocytic procoagulant materials—all mechanisms capable of initiating the clotting cascade.[26] Gram-positive bacterial sepsis and acidosis associated with DIC occur in a similar fashion. Viremias, most commonly involving varicella, hepatitis, and cytomegalovirus, are also associated with DIC, possibly because of an antigen-antibody activation of factor XII.

Intravascular hemolysis (e.g., hemolytic transfusion reaction) can cause DIC by the release of red cell adenosine diphosphate or red cell phospholipoproteins, which may activate the procoagulant system.[26] Foreign surfaces in the circulatory system may cause the generation of microthrombi and subsequent fibrinolysis leading to DIC. This may be an obstacle to the use of prosthetic devices. The LeVeen shunt and other peritoneovenous shunts placed to alleviate intractable malignant ascites are also associated with both acute and chronic DIC. The DIC may be a result of both placement of a foreign device and the fact that ascitic fluid precipitates procoagulant activity.[26,38]

Clinical Manifestations

DIC has been defined as the presence of two or more of the following coagulation abnormalities[30] (see Table 34-5):

1. prothrombin (PT), 3 or more seconds greater than control
2. activated partial thromboplastin time (APTT), 5 or more seconds greater than the upper limit of the normal range
3. thrombin time (TT) prolonged by 3 or more seconds more than control
4. fibrinogen (Fib) less than 150 mg/dl
5. fibrin split products (FSP) equal to or greater than 40 μg/ml

No single coagulation abnormality will definitely diagnose DIC. In acute DIC, the PT is prolonged in 75% of patients, and the APTT is prolonged in only 50%–60%. Thrombin time is often normal in persons with DIC. Fibrin split products are elevated in 85%–100% of patients with acute DIC.[26] Fibrinogen levels have been reported as normal in up to 57% of patients with acute DIC.[36] The mean fibrinogen in patients with metastatic disease and normal hemostasis is approximately 450–500 mg/dl. Therefore, in the absence of liver involvement, a finding of a fibrinogen level of 200–250 mg/dl or less should be considered abnormal.[25] Fibrinogen is an acute-phase reactant in infection, causing the fibrinogen level to be normal in DIC associated with infection. Serial fibrinogen levels should be determined to ascertain whether there is a downward trend. In acute DIC, fibrinogen levels should be monitored at 12-hour intervals.[25]

Protamine sulfate or ethanol gelation tests will be positive in persons with acute DIC, and the platelet count will be decreased as a result of consumption. The degree of thrombocytopenia in DIC averages about 60,000 mm^3.[26] In patients with leukemia and DIC, thrombocytopenia is more severe because of decreased thrombopoiesis. The likelihood of bleeding is increased when the fibrinogen level is less than 100 mg/dl with concomitant thrombocytopenia.[27]

Red cell fragments called *schistocytes* can be seen on peripheral blood smears in all patients with chronic DIC but in only 50% of patients with acute DIC. Fibrin split products are usually elevated in chronic DIC and induce platelet dysfunction.[26]

TABLE 34-5 Disseminated Intravascular Coagulation

Two or More Coagulation Abnormalities	
Prothrombin	≥3 sec more than control
PTT	≥5 sec more than control
Thrombin	≥3 sec more than control
Fibrinogen	<150 mg/dl
FSP	≥40 mcg/ml
Decreased platelet count	

Assessment

Persons with cancer who are considered at risk of DIC should be monitored closely.[39] Observation and reporting of early signs of bleeding will aid in the diagnosis of DIC.[39] (See Table 34-6.) Patients with acute DIC will usually have clinical evidence of bleeding from at least three unrelated sites.[26] The organ systems most often compromised by bleeding include the skin, heart, lungs, gastrointestinal tract, and central nervous system.[39] Current evidence indicates that DIC can result in pulmonary changes associated with ARDS.[25] Signs of internal bleeding include anxiety, restlessness, confusion, tachycardia, tachypnea, abdominal tenderness, and increased abdominal girth. The person may have headaches, change in mentation, epistaxis, conjunctival hemorrhage, periorbital petechiae, bleeding gums, hemoptysis, diffuse ecchymoses, joint pain, and oozing of blood from wounds, previous injection sites, or bone marrow aspiration sites.[20,39] Women should be asked whether menses has been unusually prolonged or heavy and whether there is midcycle spotting. Emesis, urine, and stool are tested for the presence of occult blood if frank bleeding is not apparent.[40]

Patients with chronic DIC commonly have gingival bleeding; spontaneous, large cutaneous ecchymoses; and mild to moderate genitourinary or gastrointestinal bleeding. Pulmonary hemorrhage is an early and prominent sign of chronic DIC in the patient with cancer.[26] Patients at risk for thrombosis-related DIC should have all extremities assessed for symmetry, temperature, color, and pain. Dyspnea, chest pain, tachycardia, and cough may be indicative of pulmonary embolism.

Interventions

The major and only effective treatment for DIC is treatment of the underlying cause of the syndrome.[37] Aggressive management of the underlying cause (tumor- or therapy-related) must be undertaken immediately in cases of acute DIC. Concomitant interventions to control DIC include administration of platelets and fresh frozen plasma to replace consumable factors as well as cryoprecipitate to replace fibrinogen.[36,37] Fresh frozen plasma or antithrombin III concentrates neutralize excess thrombin and slow the DIC process. (See Figure 34-4.)

Heparin, although controversial, may be given to inhibit factors IX and X, thereby halting the clotting cascade.[30,31,33,34,41,42] Also, heparin may prolong the effects of transfusions of platelets or fresh frozen plasma.[25] Heparin is given in a continuous intravenous infusion to avoid peaks in the effect that result from intermittent subcutaneous injections. The usual administration of heparin is a controlled infusion of 7.5 U/kg per hour with incremental increases of 2.5 U until the fibrinogen level reflects an upward trend.[31] Heparin therapy is contraindicated in patients in whom excessive bleeding occurs in a closed space so that it compromises vital function (e.g., intracranial, intraspinal, pericardial, or paratracheal bleeding).[36] The heparin infusion should be stopped immediately if the person complains of headache, displays signs of intracranial bleeding, or has observable frank bleeding (e.g., gastrointestinal bleeding). Epsilon-aminocaproic acid (EACA), 1 g/hr intravenously, has been given in conjunction with heparin therapy to maintain platelet and fibrinogen levels, but its use is controversial.[32,36,41,43] EACA should not be used in the great majority of patients with DIC because inhibition of the fibrinolytic system may lead to widespread fibrin deposition in the microcirculation and result in ischemic organ dysfunction or failure.[32,36]

In patients with DIC caused by septicemia, anticoagulant therapy is usually not indicated since the DIC most often resolves after the initiation of antibiotic therapy and no difference in survival has been shown when heparin was given.[36] Anticoagulant therapy is initiated only if the patient with septicemia has evidence of fibrin deposition, acral or dermal ischemia, venous or arterial thromboembolism, or bleeding associated with thrombocytopenia and decreased fibrinogen level after a trial of antibiotic therapy.[26,36]

During acute DIC, the patient is assessed for signs of bleeding or increased bleeding. (See Table 34-7.) A quiet environment is maintained, and vital signs with neurologic checks are recorded every 2–4 hours. Medications are given to suppress symptoms that will increase intracranial pressure (e.g., coughing or vomiting). Patients are assisted during ambulation after receiving medications that cause drowsiness or orthostatic changes. Medications that interfere with platelet function, such as aspirin-containing products or nonsteroidal anti-inflammatory drugs, should be avoided.[37,44] Bleeding should be prevented and minimized by institution of bleeding precautions.[45] Caution should be exercised so as not to disturb an established clot. When airway suction is indicated, suction pressure is lowered to prevent damage to the tracheal mucosa.[40]

An accurate record of blood loss should be kept by counting of wound dressings or vaginal pads and meas-

TABLE 34-6 Early and Late Signs of Impending Disseminated Intravascular Coagulation

Early
Anxiety, restlessness
Tachycardia, tachypnea
Headache
Conjunctival hemorrhage
Periorbital petechiae
Oozing blood
Bleeding gums
Late
Change in mentation
Joint pain
Tarry stool, melena, BRBPR
Frank hematuria
Hemoptysis

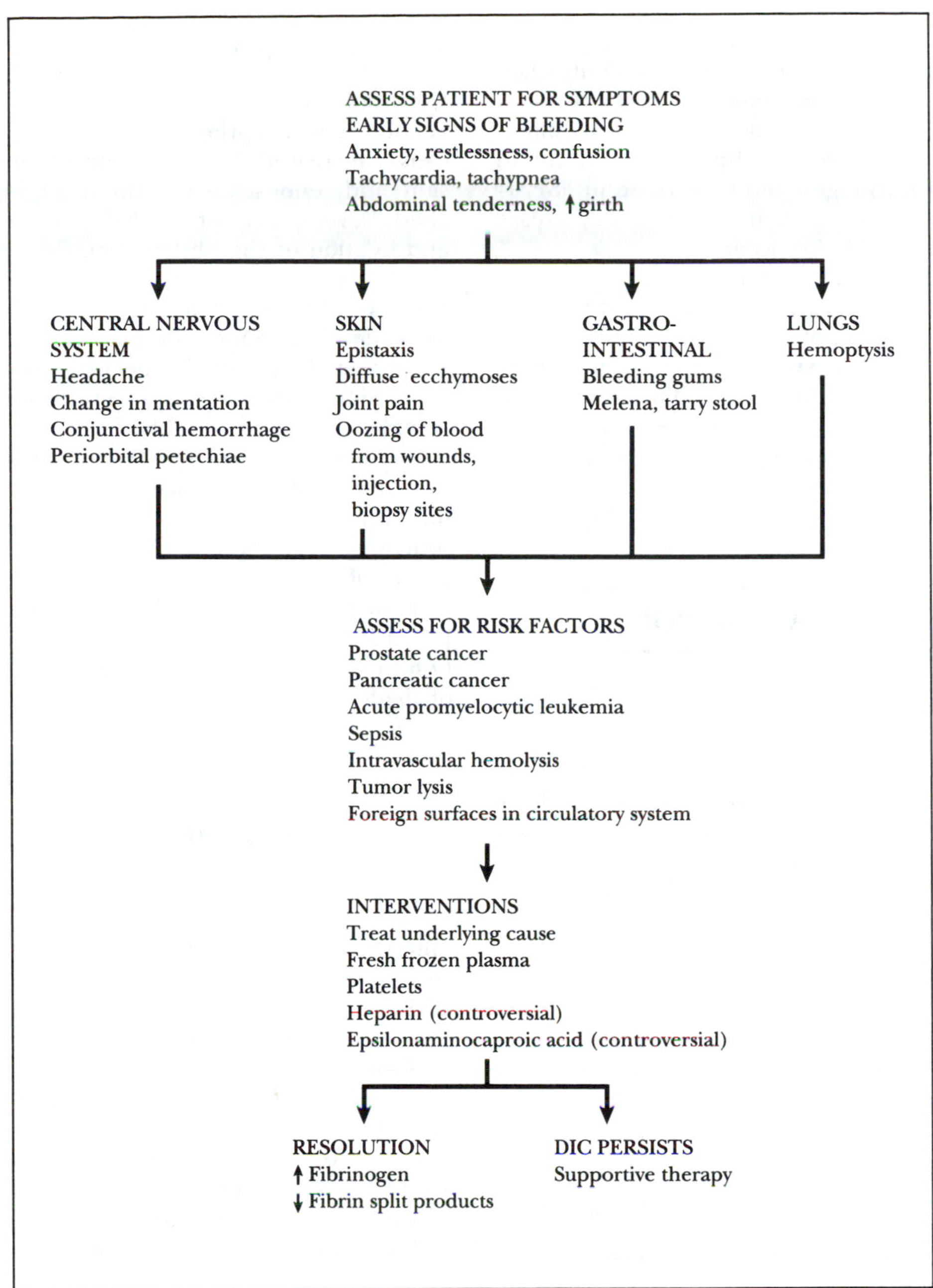

FIGURE 34-4 Clinical pathway for disseminated intravascular coagulation.

urement of emesis, urine, or stool containing frank blood.[46,47] Venipunctures should be kept to a minimum. The patient should be monitored for signs of cardiogenic shock, including hypovolemia, hypoxia, hypotension, and oliguria.[48]

TABLE 34-7 Nursing Diagnoses for Disseminated Intravascular Coagulation

Potential for injury due to abnormal blood profile
Altered tissue perfusion due to bleeding and abnormal clotting

Clinically manifest chronic DIC associated with solid tumors can be effectively treated with subcutaneous injections of heparin or antiplatelet agents, such as aspirin or dipyridamole.[26] It should be noted that oral warfarin has been shown to be ineffective.[36] Persons with superficial or deep vein thrombosis need elevation of the extremity and frequent applications of warm compresses. Superior vena cava syndrome can occur when there is thrombus formation around a permanent central venous access device.

Prognosis

Resolution of acute DIC will be accomplished only when the underlying cause of this medical emergency is successfully treated. Evaluation is accomplished by monitoring the coagulation screen and platelet count for an upward trend in fibrinogen and a decrease in FSP. If the patient is not receiving chemotherapy, an increase in platelet count should also occur.

When the process that triggers an acute episode of DIC is removed, the intravascular clotting process is stopped, and blood component therapy is given as indicated, there is a 75% survival rate and low morbidity in patients with classic acute DIC.[26] The lowest incidences of hemorrhagic deaths in patients with APL and acute DIC, with or without heparin therapy, are 14% and 15%, respectively.[30,31]

SUPERIOR VENA CAVA SYNDROME

Scope of the Problem

Definition

Superior vena cava syndrome (SVCS) is the result of compression of the superior vena cava by tumor that leads to a characteristic pattern of upper body manifestations. If untreated, SVCS can lead to airway obstruction.

Incidence

SVCS is rarely an emergency but may be the presenting sign of a malignancy. SVCS occurs in approximately 3%–4% of the oncology population; yet 97% of all cases of SVCS are due to cancer.[49,50]

Anatomy, physiology, and scientific principles

The superior vena cava is the major vessel that returns blood from the head, upper chest, and arms to the right atrium of the heart. It is a thin-walled vessel with relatively low intravascular pressure. The superior vena cava is surrounded by rigid structures, including the right mainstem bronchus, vertebral bodies, sternum, lymph nodes, and the aorta, which has high intravascular pressure.[51] The presence of an expanding mass or lymphadenopathy in the mediastinum will compress the superior vena cava due to lack of room for expansion within the chest.

Pathophysiology

Three pathophysiologic states can cause an obstruction of the superior vena cava:

1. external compression of the vessel by tumor or lymph nodes
2. direct invasion of the vessel wall by tumor
3. thrombosis of the vessel

Occlusion of the superior vena cava causes reduced venous return to the right atrium, and this in turn causes increased venous pressure, venous hypertension, and venous stasis in the head, arms, and upper chest. Development of SVCS depends upon the degree and location of the obstruction, the aggressiveness of the tumor, and the competency and efficiency of collateral circulation.[52] The azygos venous system is critical to the development of adequate collateral circulation.[53] If untreated, the syndrome progresses from venous congestion to thrombosis, cerebral edema, pulmonary complications, and possibly death.[52]

Two malignancies, lung cancer and lymphoma, are most frequently the cause of SVCS. Small-cell is the most common histologic type of lung cancer.[53] A benign source of SVCS observed in the oncology population is thrombus formation around a central venous catheter, such as those placed for long-term therapy, and pacemaker wires. SVCS can also be induced by radiation fibrosis, which can cause a stricture or narrowing of the SVCS.[52]

Clinical Manifestations

Superior vena cava obstruction causes elevated venous pressure and congestion, resulting in an array of signs and symptoms that are hallmarks of this syndrome. The severity of symptoms is related to the rapidity of onset and the adequacy of collateral circulation to help reduce venous congestion.[51] (See Table 34-8.)

Clinical characteristics include shortness of breath, facial edema, trunk and upper extremity edema, neck and chest vein distention, cough, hoarseness, and stridor. The conjunctiva may also be engorged. Neurologic symptoms are related to increased intracranial pressure and include headache, dizziness, visual disturbances, and occasionally alterations in mental status. A rapidly

TABLE 34-8 Early and Late Signs of Impending SVCS

Signs
Early
Facial, trunk and upper extremity edema
Pronounced venous pattern on trunk
Neck vein distention
Cough
Late
Hoarseness
Stridor
Engorged conjunctiva
Headache
Dizziness
Visual disturbances
Change in mental status
Respiratory distress

developing SVCS may be fatal, whereas gradual onset of SVCS allows the collateral circulation to shunt enough blood to minimize complications.[50] Airway obstruction can occur with rapidly developing SVCS, leading to respiratory failure.

Assessment

In addition to clinical evidence, a radiograph of the chest will usually reveal a mediastinal mass or adenopathy. Extensive diagnostic tests to establish SVCS are unnecessary. In the past, prompt treatment of SVCS with mediastinal irradiation was initiated, regardless of the type of underlying malignancy. Recently, however, oncologists believe that most cases of SVCS do not represent a life-threatening emergency and that invasive tests to establish the histopathologic diagnosis of the underlying malignancy are well tolerated.[54,55] Type of treatment, future therapy, and prognosis are dependent on a definitive tissue diagnosis. Therefore, a tissue specimen should be obtained if the patient's clinical condition permits. Respiratory and neurological status usually determine if this is feasible. Biopsy is easily performed if abnormal tissue, such as an enlarged supraclavicular lymph node, is readily accessible.[56] If the patient already has a diagnosis, then treatment for that particular malignancy should commence immediately to reverse SVCS.

Interventions

Patients with severe SVCS who are experiencing acute respiratory distress, massive edema, acute neurological changes, and markedly elevated venous pressure require immediate intervention to avoid respiratory arrest.[54] In a life-threatening crisis with no tissue diagnosis, fractionated irradiation of the mediastinum is the treatment of choice. High doses of fractionation, 300–400 cGy per day, are given initially, followed by 200 cGy doses to complete a cumulative 3000–3500 cGy dose to the obstructing tumor site.[57] It should be noted that this scenario is the rare exception with SVCS, and every effort should be made to obtain a tissue diagnosis before initiating therapy.

In the usual course of SVCS, tissue diagnosis is obtained and proper treatment for the underlying disease is initiated. For example, small-cell lung cancer is very responsive to combination chemotherapy. When SVCS occurs in patients with small-cell lung cancer, chemotherapy is initiated immediately. If there is a lack of tumor response or if SVCS continues to progress, mediastinal irradiation can be added to the treatment regimen. In non–small-cell lung cancer, radiation therapy is the treatment of choice.

Lymphomas are extremely radiosensitive. Therefore, fractionated radiation for SVCS is reasonable. Combination chemotherapy is usually preferred to reverse the SVCS and control systemic disease, followed by local consolidation with radiation to large mediastinal masses.[53] Chemotherapy is also the preferred treatment if the patient has already undergone previous mediastinal radiation therapy.

The timing of systemic chemotherapy and/or mediastinal irradiation is crucial so that optimal therapy is administered with the least amount of normal tissue damage and maximal tumor destruction. Steroids and anticoagulant therapy are sometimes used in the treatment of SVCS, but this is controversial and the benefits have not been clearly established. Although an inflammatory reaction is usually not associated with SVCS, steroids are probably indicated when respiratory distress is present.[58]

Anticoagulants can prevent thrombosis in the presence of decreased circulatory time and decreased blood flow through the obstructed vessel, and fibrinolytic agents may reduce intramural thrombi.[59] A new approach to the treatment of SVCS due to thrombosis is the use of tissue type plasminogen activator (rTPA) rather than traditional fibrinolytic agents. Initial results are very favorable.[60] Catheter-induced SVCS, most often the result of thrombosis, is treated with fibrinolytic therapy such as streptokinase or urokinase and possibly catheter removal. Urokinase is probably superior because it has fewer complications such as hemorrhage, pyrexia, and allergic reaction.[60]

Surgical intervention is rarely used for the treatment of malignant SVCS. One of two approaches, superior vena cava bypass graft and stent placement, may be performed for the patient with a good prognosis who has chronic or recurrent SVCS and has exhausted other treatment options. The graft creates a new vessel that circumvents the obstruction; the stent is inserted into the superior vena cava to dilate and expand the narrowed lumen of the vessel.[61]

Figure 34-5 describes the clinical pathway for SVCS and highlights critical decisions and interventions for this syndrome. Nursing care of patients experiencing SVCS is directed toward maintaining adequate cardiopulmonary status, monitoring the progression of SVCS, assisting with medical intervention, and reducing the patient's anxiety.

Invasive or constrictive procedures are avoided in the upper extremities because of impaired venous return and the potential for hemorrhage. Blood pressure measurements are taken on the thigh, using the popliteal pulse, and venipuncture is performed on the lower extremities. The administration of chemotherapeutic agents that are irritants or vesicants is of considerable concern. There is some controversy about the safety of administering these substances via the peripheral veins of the lower extremities. Upper extremity administration is avoided since SVCS causes pooling of the irritant or vesicant in the upper thorax, with inadequate drug distribution and possible phlebitis or thrombosis.[52] Probably the safest route for administration of chemotherapy during the acute phase of SVCS is surgical cannulation of the femoral vein, either temporarily or with placement of a Silastic cuffed catheter, such as a Hickman or a Broviac catheter.

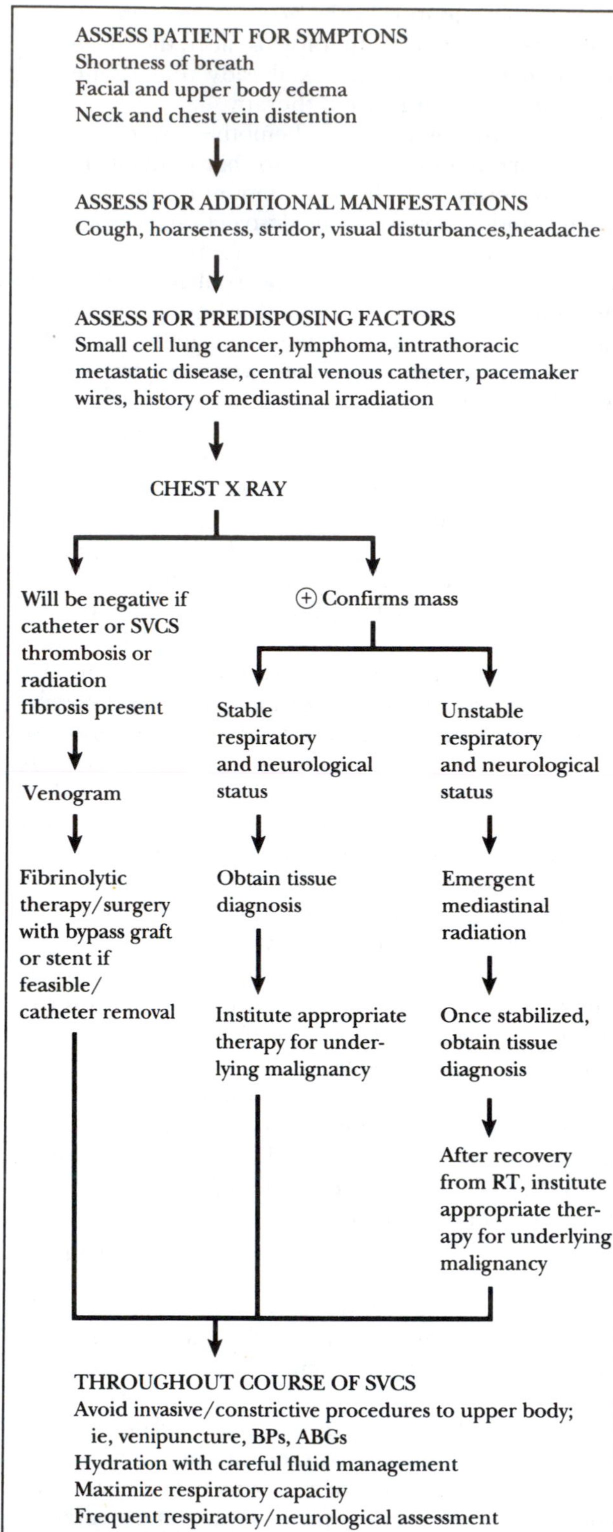

FIGURE 34-5 Clinical pathway for superior vena cava syndrome.

Fluid management during and after administration of chemotherapy is also a challenge. Although kidney function needs to be preserved, care is taken to avoid overhydration and subsequent exacerbation of SVCS. The use of diuretic agents may be necessary to maintain an adequate fluid balance.

Patients require careful monitoring of respiratory, neurologic, and hemodynamic status during the acute phase of SVCS. Coagulation profiles are monitored routinely if anticoagulants are administered. Positioning the patient comfortably with the head elevated will help maximize breathing and allay anxiety. A calm environment with visible support will significantly reassure the patient who is experiencing this crisis. It is important to stress that the physical appearance is temporary and will subside once the SVCS is resolved. Table 34-9 lists the most common nursing diagnoses when treating a patient with SVCS.

Resolution of the clinical manifestations is adequate evidence of effective treatment. This may occur within 24 to 72 hours after the initiation of therapy. Thrombus is usually suspected if the syndrome does not respond rapidly. Fibrinolytic therapy and surgery may then have to be pursued. If diagnostic evaluation of the underlying malignancy is incomplete, it can begin or proceed, once the clinical condition of SVCS improves.

The prognosis for the resolution of SVCS is favorable, but overall survival depends on the prognosis of the underlying malignancy. More than 50% of patients with SVCS have either a complete (38%) or a partial (23%) response to treatment of the syndrome.[62a] Recurrence of SVCS is infrequent in the lymphoma population, but may be seen in patients with small-cell lung cancer. After resolution of SVCS, rehabilitation is rather rapid, with disappearance of the physical effects. Thereafter, routine follow-up care provided for the oncology patient is sufficient.

Future Trends

Superior vena cava syndrome is a relatively rare entity; it is most often caused by an intrathoracic malignancy. The major trends in the management of SVCS are toward determining the underlying cause prior to treatment and evaluating new fibrinolytic therapies. SVCS is fairly well tolerated in most patients and is a true medical emergency only in rare cases of airway obstruction. New and evolving therapies for the most prevalent underlying malignancies, lung cancer and lymphomas, will have the greatest impact on the resolution of SVCS.

TABLE 34-9 Nursing Diagnoses for SVCS

Ineffective breathing pattern due to venous congestion
Potential for decreased cardiac output due to decreased venous return
Knowledge deficit of treatment for SVCS
Potential for altered cerebral tissue perfusion due to increased intracranial pressure

CARDIAC TAMPONADE

Scope of Problem

Definition

Cardiac tamponade is a life-threatening emergency in which excessive fluid accumulation in the pericardial space creates pressure of such magnitude that the heart's ability to fill and pump is severely compromised. Decreased cardiac output and impaired systemic perfusion result. The prognosis is dependent on the rapidity of this fluid accumulation, degree of pressure, and prompt diagnosis and treatment.

Incidence

Neoplastic involvement of the heart most often is not evident except postmortem. Approximately 20% of oncology patients have cardiac or pericardial disease on autopsy, yet less than one-third of these patients had clinically evident pericardial effusion and only 16% had cardiac tamponade.[62b,63] Of these symptomatic patients, many die from their pericardial disease, but only a small proportion are diagnosed prior to their demise.

Anatomy, physiology, and scientific principles

The pericardial space, a double-layered serous membrane between the visceral and parietal layers of the serous pericardium, normally holds 25–35 ml of pericardial fluid, which originates in lymphatic channels and acts as both lubricant and cushion.[64,65] Intrapericardial pressure results from the amount of fluid in this space and the elasticity or flexibility of the pericardium. Normally, intrapericardial pressure is close to that of intrapleural pressure, and both pressures are several millimeters of mercury lower than ventricular diastolic pressure.[66] This gradient assists in ventricular filling.

Pathophysiology

Increased fluid or fibrosis and thickening of the pericardium can raise the intrapericardial pressure to the point where the pressure interferes with the heart's function. Development of cardiac tamponade results from three pathophysiological changes: disruption in pressure gradients, decreased diastolic filling, and decreased stroke volume and cardiac output.[67]

Intraventricular diastolic pressure rises as a result of higher intrapericardial pressure. This prevents adequate filling of the ventricle during diastole, causes venous congestion, and thereby decreases cardiac output. Multiple physiological changes occur as other pressures are subsequently affected, including an elevated central venous pressure and a lowered left atrial pressure (Figure 34-6). The compensatory mechanisms that attempt to counteract these pressures and maintain cardiac output are an increase in heart rate (tachycardia) and peripheral vasoconstriction, which in turn help maintain arterial pressure and venous return. Peripheral vasoconstriction decreases renal blood flow, and this leads to water and sodium retention and an increase in blood volume.[67]

If these compensatory mechanisms fail and intervention does not reverse the syndrome of progressive pericardial effusion, then cardiac output falls and impedes coronary artery flow, leading to severe myocardial ischemia, further cardiac decline, and eventual circulatory collapse.[68]

Cardiac tamponade is caused by either an abnormal accumulation of fluid in the pericardial space or, less commonly, constrictive fibrosis of the pericardium. Both cancer and cancer therapy can initiate these changes. Pericardial effusion and constrictive pericarditis can be caused by metastatic tumors involving the pericardium through direct extension or by hematogenous or lymphatic spread. Tumors that most commonly metastasize to the pericardium include lung cancer, breast cancer, leukemia, Hodgkin's disease, lymphoma, melanoma, gastrointestinal tumors, and sarcomas. Although rare, primary tumors of the heart, including mesothelioma and sarcoma, can also involve the pericardium.[64] Hemopericardium can occur in patients with thrombocytopenia or other coagulopathies.[69]

Radiation therapy, especially when it involves high doses to the mediastinum, can damage the pericardium, causing a constrictive pericarditis and/or pericardial effusion.[68] Doses ranging from 4000–6000 cGy, delivered to a large portion of the heart, may induce either acute or chronic pericarditis, which can progress to cardiac tamponade with or without an effusion.[70] About 5% of patients who receive significant doses of radiation develop constrictive pericarditis, often within the first year following radiotherapy.[71]

The rate of onset and severity of pericardial effusion and cardiac tamponade are determined by the rate of fluid accumulation, compliance of the pericardium, myocardial size, and intravascular volume.[72,73] Patients with a compliant pericardium, thick myocardial wall, and large intravascular volume are less symptomatic and tolerate larger effusions.[72] Regardless of other factors, a rapidly occurring effusion will present very dramatically due to the lack of time for compensatory mechanisms to impact on cardiac function. Primary tumors of the heart tend to develop effusions more quickly than metastatic tumors.[74]

Clinical Manifestations

The patient with impending cardiac tamponade may complain of retrosternal chest pain, shortness of breath, and weakness. (See Table 34-10.) The chest pain is relieved somewhat by leaning forward but is more severe when the patient is in the supine position.[68] The

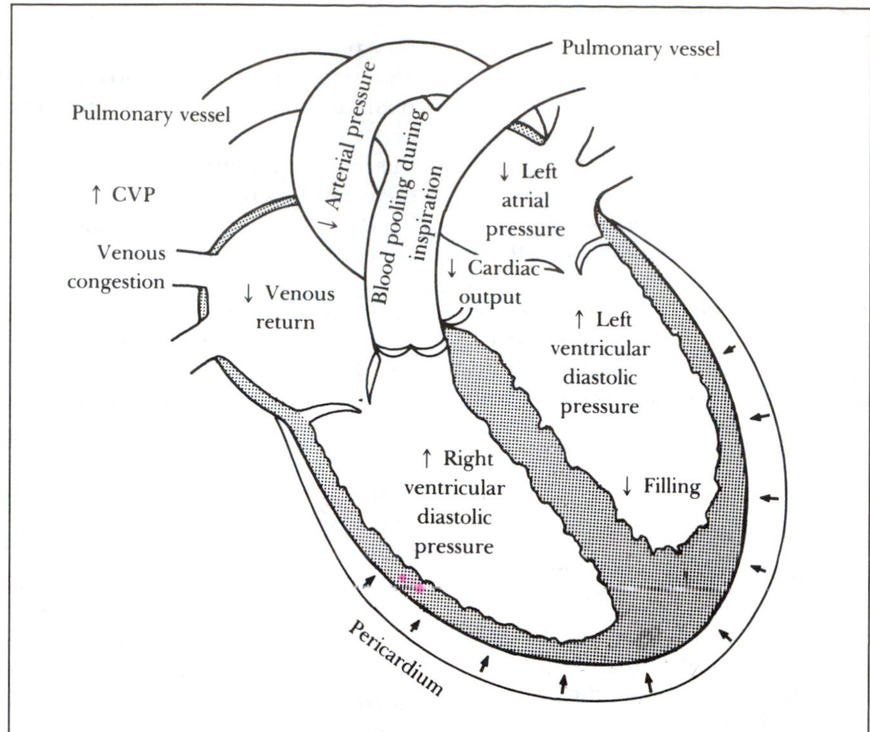

FIGURE 34-6 Cardiovascular effects of increased intrapericardial pressure. Intraventricular diastolic pressure rises as a result of higher intrapericardial pressure. This prevents adequate filling of the ventricle, causing venous congestion, decreased cardiac output, lowered left atrial pressure, and elevated central venous pressure. (↑, Increased; ↓, decreased.)

primary clinical signs of cardiac tamponade are venous distention, distant heart sounds, and paradoxical pulse.[75] Venous distention can mimic heart failure, with jugular neck vein distention, orthopnea, hepatic congestion, and possible bilateral pleural effusions.[65] Neck vein distention will usually increase during inspiration if the tamponade is significant. Hepatojugular reflux may be present and is determined by pressing on the right upper quadrant for 60 seconds while the patient is supine with head elevated so that jugular pulsations are seen. If there is a rise in jugular pressure, then reflux is present.[67]

TABLE 34-10 Early and Late Symptoms of Impending Cardiac Tamponade

Early
Weakness
Retrosternal chest pain
Shortness of breath
Venous distention
Distant heart sounds
Paradoxical pulse
Late
Hypotension
Tachycardia
Diminished arterial pulse palpated during inspiration
Cough
Peripheral edema
Diaphoresis
Abdominal distention, nausea, vomiting
Confusion
Cyanosis

Hypotension and tachycardia are usually present and reflect a decreased cardiac output. Distant heart sounds and dullness over the precordium occur when tamponade is caused by pericardial effusion. Conversely, heart sounds will be easily heard and a friction rub and atrial arrhythmia may be present if tamponade is caused by tumor encroachment and/or constrictive pericarditis.[76]

A paradoxical pulse is defined as a pulse that is significantly weaker during inspiration than during expiration.[77] Systolic blood pressure is normally 8–10 mm Hg lower during inspiration and is attributed to increased blood volume in the lungs, decreased venous return, and decreased stroke volume, thereby causing a difference of more than 10 mm Hg in systolic blood pressure at inspiration and expiration.[69] If cardiac tamponade is severe, a palpated arterial pulse may also diminish during inspiration.

Additional findings include dyspnea, cough, narrowed pulse pressure, cyanosis, diaphoresis, confusion, and peripheral edema. Abdominal tenderness, nausea, and vomiting may occur secondary to hepatomegaly and intestinal edema.[72]

Assessment

Assessment of the patient begins with a thorough history and physical exam and identification of risk factors and signs and symptoms associated with cardiac tamponade. On exam, two key signs, pulsus paradoxus and hepatojugular reflux, are determined.

If the clinical signs suggest cardiac tamponade, the echocardiogram is the easiest, most sensitive, and accurate tool with which to determine the presence of pericardial effusion. Large or small (15 ml or less) accumulations of fluid can be observed easily. With posterior effusions, two echos rather than one are seen with a single heart beat; the space between the echos indicates the size of the effusion or the thickness of the pericardium.[78]

A computerized tomography scan can also be helpful in estimating the volume of the effusion and visualizing the thickness of the pericardium. A radiograph of the chest will usually reveal a cardiac silhouette that is enlarged and globular in shape, like a bottle. An electrocardiogram is not a sensitive diagnostic tool for cardiac tamponade, but it can show low-voltage, nonspecific ST and T changes and electrical alternans, where P waves and QRS complexes vary in size.

Interventions

Management of the patient with cardiac tamponade begins with early recognition and prompt diagnosis. Populations at risk—patients with cardiothoracic malignancies and widely disseminated disease—should be skillfully assessed, particularly if shortness of breath, fatigue, tachycardia, or hypotension is present.

Once cardiac tamponade is suspected, supportive therapy is instituted to stabilize the patient while preparations are made for an emergency pericardiocentesis.[75] Supportive therapy includes volume expanders such as saline solution, 5% Plasmanate, or fresh frozen plasma given to improve cardiac filling pressures and to compensate for a decreased cardiac output.[69,70] Cardiac output can be further maximized by infusions of vasoactive agents such as isoproterenol, epinephrine, or dopamine.[69,75,79] Oxygen should be given as needed, but intubation with positive pressure breathing should be avoided since this would further decrease venous return and increase intrapleural and intrapericardial pressures.[75] Table 34-11 lists the major nursing diagnoses that apply to patients with cardiac tamponade.

The decision to perform a pericardiocentesis is based on the "rule of 20": central venous pressure greater than 20 mm Hg, pulsus paradoxus greater than 20 mm Hg, and pulse pressure less than 20 mm Hg.[65,80] Pericardiocentesis involves placement of a 16-gauge needle into the pericardial sac from a left subxiphoid approach while the patient is supine and the head of the bed is elevated 30 degrees. Under echocardiogram guidance and with a V lead attached to the needle, a syringe is used to withdraw pericardial fluid. This fluid may be sent for cytologic study and culture, but false-negative cytologic findings in the face of a malignant effusion are quite common.

TABLE 34-11 Nursing Diagnoses for Cardiac Tamponade

Decreased cardiac output due to elevated intrapericardial pressure
Impaired gas exchange due to decreased cardiopulmonary perfusion

During pericardiocentesis the patient's hemodynamic status and electrocardiogram are closely monitored. The nurse observes the patient for possible complications, which include: puncture of the right atrium or ventricle, arrhythmia, infection, injury to the lungs, laceration of the coronary artery, and inadvertent injection of air into the heart.[78] These complications are rare, however, when echocardiogram and ECG guidance are used.

Although pericardiocentesis will immediately reverse cardiac tamponade, more permanent resolution is sought through systemic therapy or local treatment to prevent reaccumulation of fluid. If effective systemic therapy is an option, as it is in some hematologic malignancies, it should be instituted as soon as the emergent tamponade is resolved. Following pericardiocentesis, further palliation may be obtained through surgical intervention. Three types of surgery are available: subxiphoid pericardotomy/pericardial window, pleuropericardial window, and total pericardectomy.

Currently, subxiphoid pericardial window is the most frequent surgical intervention since it can be performed under local anesthesia within one hour. This may also be performed instead of pericardiocentesis if tamponade has not occurred and the patient is stable enough to undergo the window. A small incision is made under the xiphoid, the pericardium is exposed, a small square of tissue is removed, and a catheter to chest tube drainage may be placed to completely drain the fluid.

Postoperatively, observe the patient for the following potential complications: infection due to invasive procedures and catheters, arrhythmias due to irritation from pericardial catheter, bleeding from the incision or pericardial catheter, and atelectasis, pleural effusion, pneumothorax, or costochondritis related to surgery.[80] Although subxiphoid pericardial window is heralded as a safe, effective treatment for cardiac tamponade, recurrence of the effusion can occur. Creation of a pericardial window is a fairly successful surgical procedure with a greater than 90% response rate and about 10% rate of recurrence.[64]

For recurrent pericardial effusions, prolonged palliation, or major pericardial involvement, pleuropericardial window and total pericardectomy are surgical options that require anterior thoracotomies and general anesthesia. The subxiphoid pericardial window is probably as effective as the pleuropericardial window and involves less risk.[64] For patients with a favorable prognosis who are considered free of malignant disease who have constrictive pericarditis, total pericardectomy by thoracotomy may be the treatment of choice if a large resection of pericardium is required to control the effusion. Total pericardectomy carries a high morbidity and should be chosen for a very limited population.[64]

Some oncologists prefer drainage and sclerosing therapy by means of a catheter insertion similar to the approach for pleural effusions. Common sclerosing agents are tetracycline, quinacrine, thiotepa, nitrogen mustard, and 5-fluorouricil. Sclerosing is successful in about 50% of the attempts and causes transient chest pain, arrhythmias, nausea, and fever.[64]

Recent advances in intracavitary therapy, the instillation of cytotoxic agents into a body cavity to destroy cancer cells rather than sclerosing the cavity, have been applied to the treatment of malignant pericardial effusions. Markman and Howell [81] have effectively treated recurrent pericardial effusions with intrapericardial instillation of cisplatin, 10 mg in 50 ml normal saline solution administered daily for 5 days.

Corticosteroids can help alleviate the inflammation of constrictive pericarditis as a short-term measure. Radiation therapy has also been used to prevent recurrent pericardial effusions in radiosensitive tumors but carries the risk of damage to the pericardium and myocardium. Long-term resolution is a challenge since there is a significant rate of recurrence of pericardial effusions. Figure 34-7 illustrates a clinical pathway for cardiac tamponade and highlights the critical decisions and interventions for the emergency.

Development of a pericardial effusion is a significant prognostic indicator. It usually occurs in the face of widely metastatic cancer or a rapidly progressing cardiothoracic malignancy. No studies have compared the prognosis of patients with or without pericardial effusion in various types of cancer.[75] In small trials of different treatment options available for pericardial effusions caused by a variety of cancers, overall average survival ranges from 3–17 months.[82–84] Death is most often attributed to the disseminated cancer and not to cardiac complications.

For patients who have an acute episode, tamponade is usually reversible and recovery is rapid once effective treatment is initiated. Rehabilitation requirements are short term. The patient's status, however, is monitored through frequent office visits. Resolution of the effusion and/or cardiac tamponade is ultimately achieved by treatment of the underlying cancer.

Chronic pericardial effusion, constrictive pericarditis, and unsuccessful treatment can severely debilitate the cancer patient, who already has a limited outlook for survival. Home care needs may include assistance with activities of daily living, assistive devices, oxygen therapy, and possible admission to an extended care facility or hospice. Supportive care is critical during the terminal phase of the disease.

Future Trends

Since effective treatments for cancer have prolonged overall survival, the incidence of metastasis to the pericardium and cardiac complications of cancer treatment is increasing. When recognized and treated early, pericardial effusion and cardiac tamponade are reversible emergency conditions. Tumor encroachment and invasion of the heart will most often cause fatal cardiac tamponade.

Further research is needed to evaluate the use of intracavitary instillation therapy as compared to and in combination with subxiphoid pericardial window. The goal would be to combine a safe, effective, and immediate intervention with one that prevents recurrence of the effusion.

HYPERCALCEMIA

Scope of the Problem

Definition

Hypercalcemia is a metabolic disorder that can occur in persons with cancer as a result of increased bone resorption caused by either bone destruction by tumor invasion or increased levels of parathyroid hormone (PTH), osteoclast-activating factor (OAF), or prostaglandin produced by the cancer.[85,86] If adequate renal clearance of calcium is not preserved, hypercalcemia can develop. Untreated or uncontrolled hypercalcemia can lead to life-threatening alterations in cardiac, neurologic, and renal function.

Incidence

The two most common causes of hypercalcemia are primary hyperparathyroidism and cancer. Hypercalcemia is the most common life-threatening metabolic abnormality in patients with cancer and will occur in 10%–20% of patients during the course of the illness.[85,87,88] The occurrence of hypercalcemia often heralds a lack of control of the malignant disease process.[89] See Table 34-12.

Anatomy, physiology, and scientific principles

Normal serum calcium levels are maintained by absorption of calcium from the gastrointestinal tract, secretion of PTH and calcitonin, effects of vitamin D,

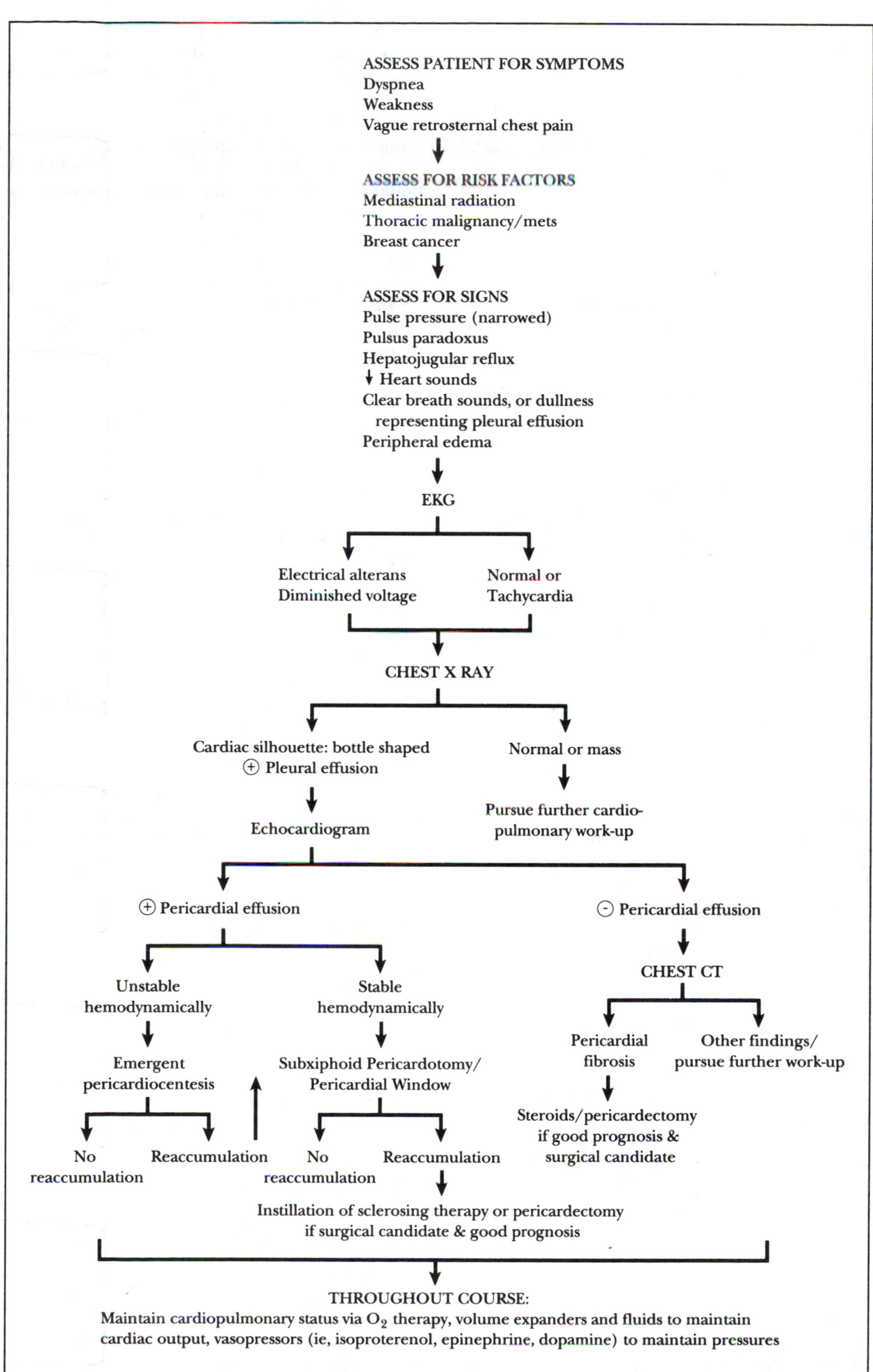

FIGURE 34-7 Clinical pathway for cardiac tamponade.

TABLE 34-12 Incidence of Cancer-Associated Hypercalcemia

Breast cancer	30%–40%
Multiple myeloma	20%–40%
Head and neck cancer	2.9%–25%
Renal cell cancer	3%–17%
Lymphoma	0.3%–4%

Source: Data from Muggia FM,[89] Silverman P.[94]

deposition or resorption of calcium from bone, renal clearance of calcium, and binding of calcium to serum proteins, usually albumin.[90]

PTH, produced by the parathyroid gland, promotes the release of calcium from bone when the calcium level in the extracellular fluid surrounding the parathyroid is low. PTH stimulates osteoclasts to break down bone structure, thus liberating calcium phosphate crystals. PTH increases gastrointestinal absorption of calcium by stimulating the active-transport system to move calcium from the intestinal lumen to the blood. In addition, vitamin D stimulates calcium absorption from the intestine. PTH also stimulates increased renal tubular absorption of calcium while reducing reabsorption of phosphate to lower extracellular phosphate concentration.[91] Calcitonin, secreted by the thyroid, is part of a feedback mechanism to lower serum calcium by inhibiting bone resorption and opposing the effects of PTH. Ninety-nine percent of body calcium is bound in bone and teeth. The other 1% is present in the plasma as ionized (0.5%) and protein-bound (0.5%) calcium.[85] When serum albumin levels are reduced, there is a disproportionate increase of ionized (free) calcium in the blood. Ionized (free) calcium is the critical component in clinical hypercalcemia.

Prolonged immobilization is associated with increased resorption of calcium from the bones.[92] Dehydration results in a decreased glomerular filtration rate (GFR) and an increased sodium resorption to conserve water, which then increases calcium reabsorption and decreases calcium excretion, respectively. An elevated serum calcium level causes a decrease in smooth muscle tone of the gastrointestinal tract, resulting in anorexia, nausea, vomiting, and constipation. Likewise, a renal tubular defect can cause an inability to conserve water as evidenced by polyuria and polydipsia, with worsening dehydration, and the vicious cycle of hypercalcemia persists. Decreased GFR may be a side effect of some chemotherapeutic or antibiotic medications and could contribute to hypercalcemia.

Pathophysiology

Persons at greatest risk of hypercalcemia include those with bone metastases from primary tumors of the breast, lung, and kidney because of extensive bone destruction and release of calcium into the extracellular fluid.[93] Hypercalcemia also occurs in persons with osteolytic bone lesions and with hematologic malignancies such as multiple myeloma and lymphomas, particularly HTLV-1 associated T-cell lymphoma or leukemia. Squamous cell lung cancer and carcinoma of the head and neck are thought to produce PTH, OAF, and prostaglandin, which stimulate bone resorption.[93]

Other factors that contribute to the occurrence of hypercalcemia in cancer patients include hyperparathyroidism, immobilization, anorexia, nausea, vomiting, dehydration, and renal failure. Cancer patients have an increased incidence of primary hyperparathyroidism, which should be considered in the differential diagnosis.[85,86]

Several humoral mediators of cancer-related hypercalcemia have recently been identified, including a PTH-related protein and transforming growth factor alpha, both of which are frequently produced by tumor in conjunction with the cytokines interleukin 1 (IL-1) and tumor necrosis factor (TNF).[85,94,95] IL-1 and TNF may be produced by normal host immune cells that have been stimulated by the tumor. It is hypothesized that humoral-mediated hypercalcemia of malignancy may be due to the concerted action of tumor products and the products of normal host cells on both bone and kidney.[85]

Prostaglandin has been associated with increased bone resorption following hormonal therapy. It should be noted that as treatment with estrogen or anti-estrogen is initiated in patients with breast cancer, there is a potential for an acute increase in serum calcium.[94,95]

Hypercalcemia with hematologic malignancy is due to the release of OAF by the malignant cells. In vitro, several cytokines including IL-1, lymphotoxin, and TNF, (all members of the OAF family) have each been found to be potent stimulators of osteoclastic bone resorption.[94]

Clinical Manifestations

Mundy and Martin[96] outlined three categories of patients with hypercalcemia and indications for treatment:

1. Patients with serum calcium levels of 10.5–12.0 mg/dl (2.62–3.0 mm/l) who are asymptomatic should be observed carefully and may be given chronic therapy as outpatients.
2. Patients with serum calcium levels of 12–13 mg/dl (3.0–3.25 mm/l) who are asymptomatic require specific but nonurgent therapy.
3. Patients with serum calcium levels of 13 mg/dl (3.25 mm/l) or higher and any patients with symptoms require emergency treatment of hypercalcemia.

In patients with malignancy, the clinical manifestations of hypercalcemia are often related to the rapidity of onset. Therefore, some patients may develop symptomatic hypercalcemia when the serum calcium level is only marginally increased but the rise occurs rapidly.[97]

It is important to note that since calcium is bound to protein, the serum calcium level must be "corrected" for albumin less than 4 to obtain an accurate measure of the calcium level. The formula for this calculation is:[96]

$$\text{"Corrected" total serum calcium (TSC)} = \text{Measured TSC} + (4.0 - \text{serum albumin}) \times 0.8$$

Serum phosphorus level is variable in patients with malignant hypercalcemia, reflecting the influence of diet, glucose intake, antacid use and renal function.[85] Hypokalemia occurs in 52% of patients with normal renal function who are not taking potassium-depleting medications.[85,90] It appears that there is an inverse relationship between serum calcium and serum potassium. Also, people with malignant disease tend to have decreased oral intake and increased potassium loss from the gastrointestinal tract caused by the disease and/or its treatment.[90]

Assessment

Knowledge of the specific cancers and factors that contribute to hypercalcemia is necessary for determination of who is at risk for this metabolic emergency.[98] Clinical characteristics are usually related to the effects of increased calcium on smooth, skeletal, and cardiac muscle. (See Table 34-13.) The main systems affected include gastrointestinal, neuromuscular, cardiac, and renal. The effects of hypercalcemia on the gastrointestinal tract can be manifested as anorexia, nausea, vomiting, constipation, abdominal pain, and dehydration.[85,94,98,99] Neuromuscular manifestations are lethargy, confusion, stupor, convulsions, and hyporeflexia.[85,94,99,100] Abnormalities in cardiac function may be bradycardia or tachycardia and electrocardiographic abnormalities reflecting an increased PR interval and a decreased QT interval. Polyuria, polydypsia, and decreased renal concentrating ability invariably occur and accelerate the development of dehydration, contraction alkalosis, and progressive renal insufficiency.[85,94] Dry mucous membranes, poor skin turgor, rapid thready pulse, and orthostatic hypotension may signify dehydration. Cancer patients who have hypercalcemia usually experience a progressive course with recurrent episodes.

The nursing diagnoses useful when caring for patients with hypercalcemia are listed in Table 34-14.

TABLE 34-13 Early and Late Symptoms of Impending Hypercalcemia

Early
Anorexia, nausea, vomiting
Abdominal pain, constipation
Lethargy
Polyuria, polydypsia
Poor skin turgor
Dry mucous membranes
Late
Dehydration
Confusion, stupor
Hyporeflexia, convulsions
Bradycardia, tachycardia
Orthostatic hypotension

Interventions

Tumor control or reduction of tumor burden is the only long-term measure that is effective for reversing hypercalcemia (Figure 34-8).[88,93,101] Cancer therapy and emergency medical intervention must be instituted for patients who have symptoms or who have a serum calcium level of 13 mg/dl or more. For cancer patients, severe hypercalcemia is a medical emergency that requires vigorous hydration to restore the normal volume of extracellular compartment fluid, increase glomerular filtration, and promote urinary calcium excretion. Infusion of 4–6 liters of normal saline solution (0.9%) each day for 48 hours will raise the glomerular filtration rate and interfere with calcium reabsorption in the proximal tubule.[88,93,94,102] Serum calcium will likely decrease by 2–3 mg/dl over 1–2 days.[101] Parenteral furosemide, 40–80 mg every 4–6 hours, can produce sodium diuresis, which in turn causes calcium diuresis. Many experts agree that diuretics should only be given when there are signs of fluid overload.[88,93,101]

When hypercalcemia is emergent, fluid and electrolyte balance is monitored closely. Fluid balance is assessed by monitoring intake, output, and weight and observing for edema of lower extremities or sacrum, noting distended neck veins and shortness of breath, and auscultating the lungs for rales. Serum electrolytes are monitored closely since vigorous hydration can lead to hypokalemia, hyponatremia, hypocalcemia, and hypomagnesemia.[94,103] Likewise, blood urea nitrogen and creatinine are monitored to evaluate the adequacy of renal function.

Intravenous mithramycin, 15–25 μg/kg body weight, is given in a single dose to inhibit bone resorption of calcium; it usually decreases serum calcium within 12 hours, with a peak effect at 48–96 hours.[88,93,94,101] Intravenous mithramycin, initially developed as a cytotoxic agent, may cause nausea and vomiting, bone marrow suppression, clotting abnormalities, and hepatic and renal changes. Mithramycin is administered

TABLE 34-14 Nursing Diagnoses for Hypercalcemia

Potential fluid volume deficit due to hypermetabolic state
Constipation due to hypercalcemia
Potential for injury due to altered mental status
Potential fluid volume excess due to IV fluid administration

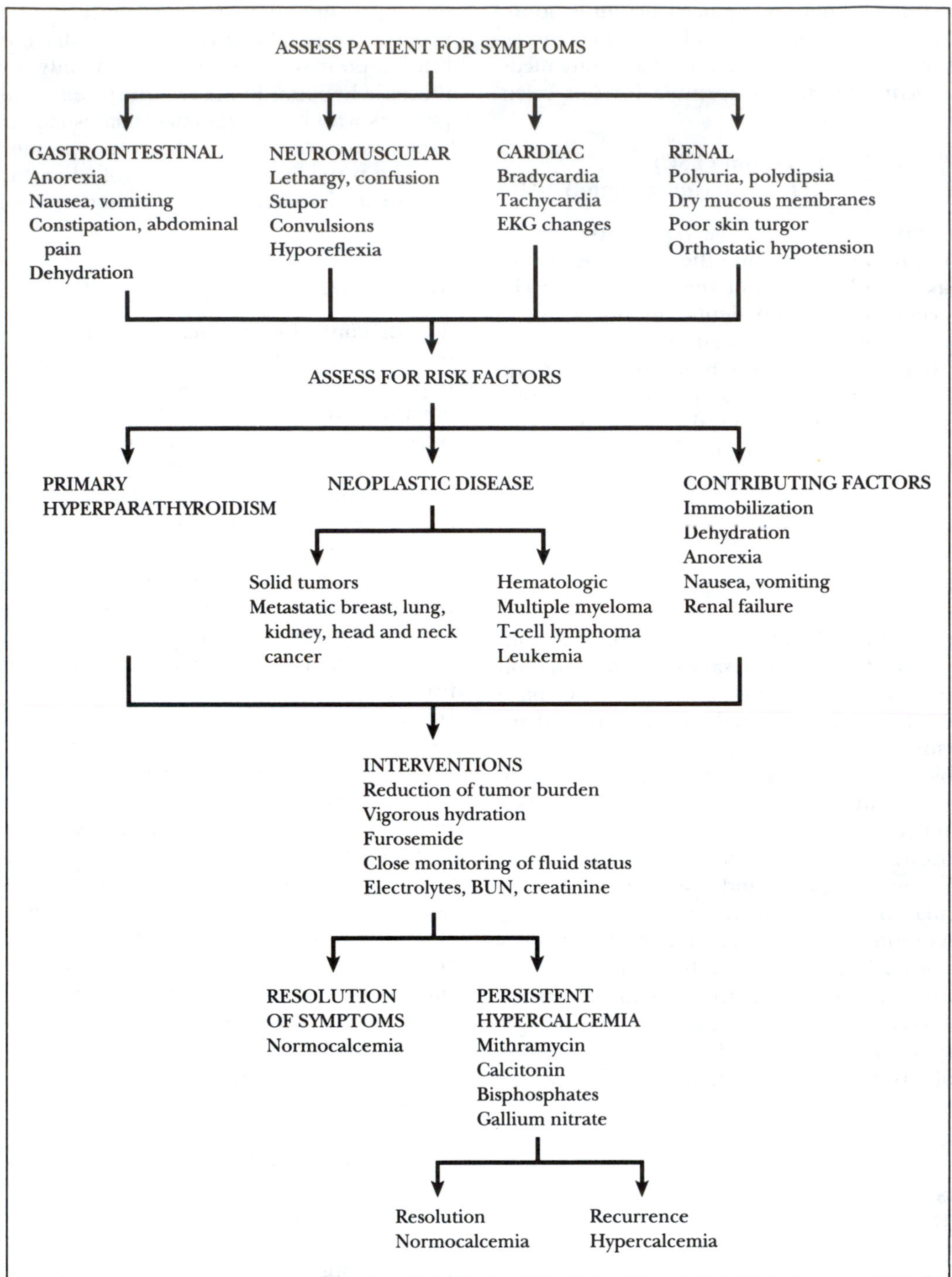

FIGURE 34-8 Clinical pathway for hypercalcemia.

cautiously through an intravenous line since infiltration can cause tissue necrosis at the site. Antiemetic agents are administered, but they may cause increased lethargy, particularly if liver function is compromised. The limiting toxic effects associated with mithramycin are thrombocytopenia and bleeding diathesis despite a normal platelet count.[85,104] Prothrombin and partial thromboplastin levels are monitored and precautions are instituted to prevent bleeding, especially when other antineoplastic agents are given concomitantly. Mithramycin is nephrotoxic, eliminated by the kidneys, and cannot be used when renal function is impaired. Many cancer patients have impaired renal function as a result of previous antibiotic or cytotoxic therapy. Patients with multiple myeloma may have impaired renal function from Bence-Jones proteinuria.[96]

Calcitonin, 4 Medical Research Council units per kilogram of body weight subcutaneously every 12 hours, also can inhibit bone resorption, with a rapid effect, but the duration of the response is limited.[88,101] Serum calcium level is reduced by 2–3 mg/dl.[101] However, the effect is transient and limited to 24–72 hours, despite repeated administration. This phenomenon "may be due to down-regulation of calcitonin receptors on bone cells which occurs in the continued presence of calcitonin."[96] Glucocorticosteroids (e.g., hydrocortisone, 100 mg intravenously every 6 hours) are often administered concomitantly to prevent this phenomenon.[88] Since there is a risk of anaphylaxis with calcitonin injections, skin testing is done before administration. Epinephrine, antihistamines, and oxygen should be available for emergency use.

Phosphate, 75 mmol intravenously, although extremely toxic, may be administered as a single injection if other measures fail to promote the precipitation of inorganic calcium phosphate.[96] Intravenous phosphates act within minutes of administration; however, there is danger of hypotension, hypocalcemia, renal failure, and visceral calcification.[86]

Bisphosphonates are potent inhibitors of osteoclastic bone resorption. Currently there are three bisphosphonates in clinical trials to determine their usefulness as antihypercalcemic agents. Etidronate 7.5 mg/kg/day IV, clodronate 300–600 mg IV, and pamidronate 30 mg IV have each proven to be effective in producing normocalcemia within 5–9 days.[102] As with other interventions, however, these will not prevent recurrence of hypercalcemia within 2 to 4 weeks unless there has been successful treatment of the underlying tumor. Oral clodronate 1600 mg po every day may be given after the initial intravenous dose to prolong the effect.[102] At this time, the bisphosphonates are only available in IV form.

The bisphosphonates are well tolerated and are relatively free of side effects, although Pamidronate can produce transient temperature elevation.[85] Repeated long-term use of etidronate, however, can cause osteomalacia. Clinical trials of clodronate have been suspended in the United States because of its potential leukemogenicity.[85,88]

Gallium nitrate, 200 mg/m² in continuous intravenous infusion for 5 days, has been shown to be an effective agent in decreasing serum calcium salts in the bone.[86,87,105,106] Warrel et al.[87] conducted a multicenter clinical trial comparing gallium nitrate and etidronate and found that normocalcemia was produced in 82% of patients receiving gallium nitrate and 43% of patients receiving etidronate.

Oral phosphate, 1–3 g three times daily, may be given to control chronic, mild hypercalcemia when the serum phosphorus level is less than 3.7 mg/dl: however, diarrhea may be a dose-limiting side effect.[88,94,96,102] When oral phosphates are prescribed, the patient is taught that perianal care after defecation is necessary to prevent skin breakdown caused by the caustic effect of excreted phosphate. If perianal pain or excoriation develops, sitz baths are encouraged and anesthetic ointment is applied. Indomethacin and oral steroids may be prescribed for patients with hypercalcemia, but the effectiveness of these agents is controversial.[85,94,96,102] Patients who are taking steroids or indomethacin are taught that immunosuppressive agents may mask fever as an early sign of infection, and precautionary measures are reviewed.

Recognition of the early signs of hypercalcemia is an important nursing intervention to prevent further complications of hypercalcemia.[107] Patients and family members are taught to observe for these symptoms, and the importance of frequent ambulation or mobilization of extremities is stressed.[88,93,94,98,106,108] Analgesic agents are administered before mobility exercises if chronic pain is a problem. However, any new bone pain must be reported, since patients at risk of hypercalcemia may develop pathologic fractures.[108] Patients at risk of hypercalcemia are encouraged to drink 2–3 liters of fluid each day to prevent dehydration and promote urinary excretion of calcium.

Thiazide diuretics inhibit calcium excretion; therefore they are contraindicated in persons who are at risk of hypercalcemia. Likewise, the dosage of digitalis preparations may need to be lowered and digitalis toxicity carefully assessed, since the action of digitalis is potentiated in a hypercalcemic state.[109]

Prognosis

Emergent hypercalcemia can be reversed in 80% of episodes with aggressive, immediate intervention. However, the duration of normocalcemia may last only a few days to 3 weeks unless there is control of the underlying tumor that is causing the hypercalcemia.

TUMOR LYSIS SYNDROME

Scope of the Problem

Definition

Acute tumor lysis syndrome (ATLS) is a complication of cancer therapy that occurs when a large number of rapidly proliferating tumor cells are lysed. It is characterized by the development of acute hyperuricemia, hyperkalemia, hyperphosphatemia, and hypocalcemia with or without acute renal failure.[110]

Incidence

ATLS is most commonly seen in cancer patients with high-grade lymphoma or acute lymphoblastic leukemia, since these cancer cells are particularly sensitive to treatment and will rapidly lyse.[111-113] In addition, immature lymphoblasts contain an abnormally high level of phosphorus, which is released when the cells are lysed.[114] In untreated persons with cancer, ATLS can also develop when there is a rapidly growing large tumor mass that undergoes profound cell destruction.[115,116] The syndrome has also been described in patients with acute myelogenous leukemia, chronic myelogenous leukemia in blastic transformation, and non-Hodgkins lymphoma.[111,115] Although rare, ATLS has been reported to occur in patients with small-cell lung cancer, metastatic breast cancer, and metastatic medulloblastoma.[115,117] In patients with solid tumors, the syndrome is usually milder since there is a slower responsiveness to chemotherapy.

Anatomy, physiology, and scientific principles

Within the cell are the minerals potassium and phosphorus and nucleic acids that form DNA and RNA. When the cell membrane is ruptured, released nucleic acids are converted by the liver into uric acid while potassium and phosphorus are released into the bloodstream, causing abnormally high levels of these minerals and a decrease in calcium (Figure 34-9). An inverse relationship exists between phosphorus and calcium; increased serum phosphorus results in decreased serum calcium because serum phosphorus binds with circulating calcium.

Pathophysiology

Many chemotherapeutic agents destroy tumor cells while the cells are dividing; likewise, cells that are undergoing division are more sensitive to radiation therapy. Therefore, cancer patients with massive tumor burdens that are rapidly dividing are at risk of ATLS, particularly as treatment is instituted.

When a large number of cells are lysed within a short period of time, the result is ATLS characterized by acute hyperuricemia, hyperkalemia, hyperphosphatemia and hypocalcemia, and/or acute renal failure.[115,118-120] The degree of metabolic abnormality depends on the adequacy of renal function, since uric acid, potassium, and phosphorus are excreted in the urine.[118,121] These metabolic abnormalities can develop alone or in combination. Acute renal failure results from intratubular precipitation of uric acid or calcium phosphate crystallization.[110,111,121]

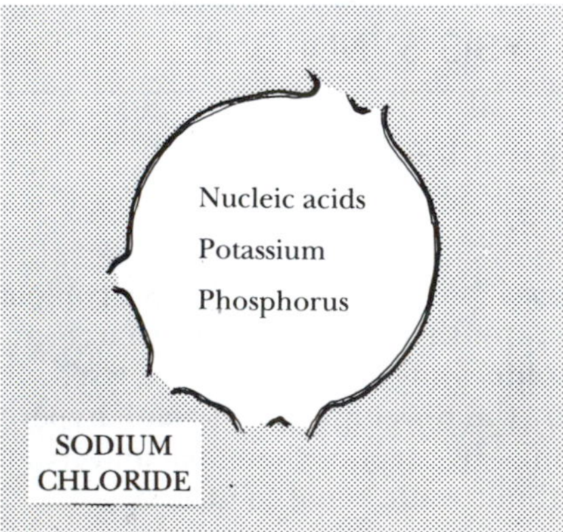

FIGURE 34-9 Intracellular contents are released into the circulation when cell lysis occurs such as following chemotherapy. When massive numbers of cells lyse, the potential for acute tumor lysis syndrome increases.

Clinical Manifestations

Pretreatment serum potassium levels may be elevated because of dehydration; compromised renal function; acidosis resulting from sepsis; adrenal insufficiency as steroids are tapered; and medications such as indomethacin, potassium supplements, and potassium-sparing diuretics.[116] Signs of hyperkalemia include weakness, paresthesia, muscle cramps, ascending flaccid paralysis, bradycardia, ECG changes, diarrhea, and nausea.

Clinical indicators of hyperphosphatemia include oliguria, anuria, and renal insufficiency. Patients with hypocalcemia may exhibit muscle twitching, carpopedal spasm, tetany, laryngospasm, paresthesia, convulsions, hypotension, and ECG changes. Hypomagnesemia, acute pancreatitis, vitamin D deficiency, diarrhea, multiple blood transfusions, and anorexia are predisposing factors for hypocalcemia.[116] Alkalemia resulting from sodium bicarbonate infusion may lower ionized calcium and aggravate symptomatic hypocalcemia.[117] Medications that may potentiate hyperphosphatemia and hypocalcemia include phosphates, furosemide, mithramycin, gallium nitrate, and anticonvulsants.[116]

Signs of hyperuricemia and compromised renal function include nausea, vomiting, diarrhea, lethargy, edema, flank pain, hematuria, crystalluria, azotemia, oliguria, and anuria.[111] Thiazide diuretics potentiate hyperuricemia.

Assessment

When cancer patients with rapidly proliferating tumors are receiving cytotoxic therapy, ATLS should be anticipated. (See Table 34-15.) Patients with large tumor burdens in combination with high white blood cell count, lymphadenopathy, splenomegaly, and elevated lactate dehydrogenase are at particularly high risk. They will require close monitoring of metabolic parameters, including potassium, phosphorus, calcium, uric acid, blood urea nitrogen, and creatinine levels. For high-risk pa-

TABLE 34-15 Early and Late Symptoms of Impending Tumor Lysis Syndrome

Early
Weakness, paresthesia
Muscle cramps
Nausea, vomiting, diarrhea
Lethargy
Late
Ascending flacid paralysis
Bradycardia, hypotension
Oliguria, anuria, edema
Hematuria, crystalluria
Azotemia, flank pain
Carpopedal spasm, laryngospasm
Tetany, convulsion

tients, baseline renal function is assessed before the initiation of aggressive antineoplastic therapy.

Interventions

Knowledge of cancer patients who are at risk of acute tumor lysis syndrome and close monitoring for hyperuricemia, hyperkalemia, hyperphosphatemia, hypocalcemia, and impaired renal function are essential.[114,122] Electrolytes should be measured every 6–8 hours and serum phosphorus, calcium, magnesium, uric acid, creatinine, and blood urea nitrogen levels measured at least daily.[110] Adequate renal function must be preserved during treatment for cancers associated with ATLS. (See Table 34-16.) Uric acid crystallization in the renal tubules causing obstruction, decreased glomerular filtration, and/or acute renal failure is a major complication that can be prevented by prophylactic alkalinization of urine, thus increasing the solubility of uric acid. This is accomplished by maintaining the urine pH at a level greater than 7, with the use of sodium bicarbonate and vigorous intravenous hydration to decrease the uric acid concentration in the urine.[110,115,120,123] A recommended fluid regimen is D5W/0.45NS with sodium bicarbonate, 60 mEq/l, at 150 ml/hr. Sodium bicarbonate administration should be discontinued once serum uric acid has normalized since overly vigorous alkalinization may accelerate phosphate precipitation in the renal tubules.[110] Also, alkalosis may predispose the patient to neuromuscular irritability by further lowering the calcium level.[110]

Potassium and magnesium may need to be replaced if deficits in these electrolytes appear.[121] Simultaneous hydration and diuresis promote the excretion of phosphorus and potassium. Urine output should be maintained at a minimum of 100 ml/hr. Diuretics may be administered as adjunctive therapy, particularly when the person has a coexisting condition (e.g., impaired cardiac function) that could potentiate the risk of fluid overload. If adequate urine output is not achieved, furosemide 40–80 mg intravenously, or mannitol 12.5 g intravenously, may be given to promote diuresis.[110,121] Fluid balance is assessed by monitoring of intake, output, and weight and observation for edema of lower extremities or sacrum. Distended neck veins or shortness of breath should be noted and the lungs should be auscultated for adventitious sounds (rales). Decreased urine output, hematuria, and urine pH <7 are reported immediately. Meticulous records of intake and output are necessary to monitor effectiveness of therapy.

If ATLS is a potential complication of the cytotoxic therapy, allopurinol is generally given as a prophylactic measure.[120] Allopurinol decreases uric acid levels by interfering with purine metabolism. If tumor lysis syndrome develops, allopurinol 600–900 mg/day is given and then reduced to 300–450 mg/day after 3–4 days.[110] It may cause a skin rash within 7 days of initial dosage, requiring palliative relief measures with lotion or diphenhydramine hydrochloride.

Persons with cancer that infiltrates the kidney (e.g.,

TABLE 34-16 Prevention and Management of the Metabolic Complications of Acute Tumor Lysis

Control of hyperuricemia
Begin allopurinol administration at a dose of 600–900 mg/day and reduce to half after 3–4 days.
Urinary alkalinization
Maintain urine pH ≥7 by addition of 50–100 mEq of $NaHCO_3$ to each liter of IV fluid
Acetazolamide 250–500 mg IV daily if above measure is ineffective or serum HCO_3 >27 mEq/l
Discontinue urinary alkalinization once hyperuricemia is corrected (serum uric acid <10 mg/dl)
Forced diuresis
Maintain urine flow at >150–200 ml/hr with infusion of 5% dextrose 0.5NS at 200 ml/hr
Initiate low-dose dopamine and diuretics in patients with preexisting evidence of fluid retention (marked edema or ascites) or oliguria
Do not insert Foley catheter unless patient has altered mental status or evidence of urinary retention
Maintain fluid balance
Avoid fluid overload: administer IV furosemide (20–100 mg q 4–8hr) if urine output falls below fluid intake
Obtain daily weights
Maintain scrupulous records of intake and output
Monitoring of blood chemistries
Serum electrolytes, BUN, creatinine, uric acid, calcium, phosphorous, magnesium q 6–8hr during the first 72 hr following chemotherapy
Acute hyperkalemia
Initiate hypertonic glucose and insulin infusion, Kayexalate and furosemide
Hyperphosphatemia
Initiate hypertonic glucose and insulin infusion, and oral antacids

lymphoma or leukemia) may require radiation therapy to the kidney area before they receive chemotherapy, which should reduce the overall tumor burden.[110,121] Also, leukapheresis may be employed when the white blood cell count is extraordinarily elevated (e.g., 100,000/mm³) to reduce both the tumor burden and the risk of tumor lysis syndrome. If the aforementioned interventions fail to promote adequate renal function, dialysis may be necessary.

If hyperkalemia develops, an intravenous solution of 50% glucose (25 g) is administered to raise plasma insulin levels, thereby causing an intracellular shift of potassium. It is recommended that 1 unit of regular insulin be given with each 4 g of glucose administered.[121] An ion exchange resin, such as Kayexalate (Winthrop-Breon) may be given orally or rectally in conjunction with sorbitol to promote excretion of potassium in feces.[115] Oral Kayexalate is given in a dose of 15–30 g with 50 ml of 20% sorbitol two to four times daily. If the patient is unable to tolerate oral medications, then a retention enema of 50 g in 200 ml of 20% sorbitol, held for 30–60 minutes, is recommended.[121] If cardiac or neuromuscular toxicity is exhibited, calcium gluconate is given to decrease these symptoms.

Hypocalcemia and hyperphosphatemia are treated by administration of calcium supplements and phosphate-binding antacids, such as Amphogel (Wyeth) or Basaljel (Wyeth). Pulse rate, rhythm, and ECG should be monitored frequently and changes should be reported. Serum potassium, phosphorus, calcium, uric acid, blood urea nitrogen, and creatinine levels should be monitored every 6 hours, or as ordered.

Prognosis

The occurrence and resolution of ATLS are dependent on the tumor's responsiveness to the radiation and/or chemotherapy administered. Since cytolysis occurs within 7 days following treatment, ATLS usually resolves during that time frame if adequate renal function has been maintained and metabolic parameters have been corrected. (See Figure 34-10.) If a person who has a hematologic malignancy and a rapidly rising white blood cell count has a relapse, there is usually a recurrence of ATLS when therapy is instituted again.

SYNDROME OF INAPPROPRIATE ANTIDIURETIC HORMONE

Scope of the Problem

Definition

Syndrome of inappropriate antidiuretic hormone (SIADH) is a paraneoplastic disease that develops when excessive amounts of antidiuretic hormone (ADH) are present, exerting an effect on the kidney and causing water intoxication.

Incidence

SIADH occurs in approximately 1%–2% of patients with cancer.[124] It is most frequently associated with small-cell lung cancer and may even be the presenting symptom of the disease.

Anatomy, physiology, and scientific principles

Antidiuretic hormone (ADH), also referred to as arginine vasopressin, is produced by the hypothalamus and stored in the posterior lobe of the pituitary. In response to either an increase in plasma concentration (serum osmolality) or a decrease in plasma volume, ADH is secreted. ADH increases the permeability of the distal tubules of the kidney, which then conserve water. As a result, plasma osmolality is lowered by the dilutional effect of additional water and plasma volume increases.[125] A feedback loop of osmoreceptors in the hypothalamus and pressoreceptors in the left atrium and carotid sinus monitor plasma osmolality and circulation volume to adjust ADH secretion appropriately. When a person becomes dehydrated, plasma osmolality is increased and plasma volume is depleted. As a result, ADH is secreted, causing water retention and return of normal plasma concentration and volume.

Pathophysiology

SIADH is usually associated with an excess of ADH resulting from ectopic production, abnormal stimulation of the hypothalamus-pituitary network, or if ADH effects of the kidney are mimicked or enhanced. The resulting pathophysiologic state is *water intoxication.* When excessive amounts of water are retained, plasma osmolality drops and dilutional hyponatremia occurs. In addition, urinary excretion of sodium increases, causing further hyponatremia, and urinary osmolality becomes inappropriately higher than plasma osmolality.[126] Hyponatremia occurs from both water retention and increased urinary excretion. Table 34-17 lists many of the etiological factors in SIADH according to pathological mechanism.

The tumors most frequently associated with ectopic ADH production are small-cell tumors of the lung. ADH levels are elevated in approximately 50% of the cases of small-cell lung cancer, while only about 10% have clinically evident SIADH.[127–129] Other malignancies that produce inappropriate levels of ADH are gastrointestinal cancers, thymoma, lymphoma, Hodgkin's disease, bladder and prostate cancer, and some sarcomas.[126,130]

Certain antineoplastic agents, drugs, and chemicals (e.g., cyclophosphamide, vincristine, chlorpropamide, morphine, nicotine, and ethanol) can induce SIADH.[126]

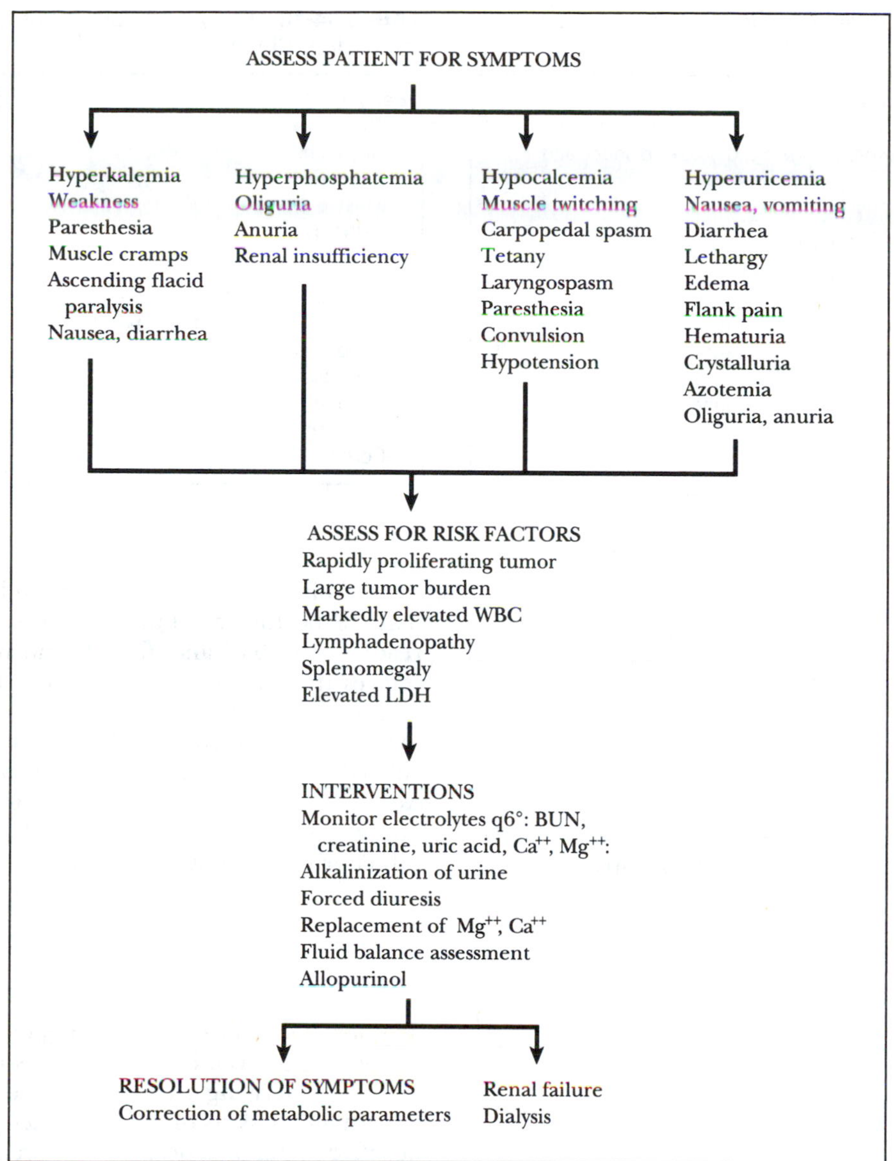

FIGURE 34-10 Clinical pathway for tumor lysis syndrome.

Some agents directly stimulate ADH secretion; others affect the renal tubules. Cisplatin administration has been associated with the development of SIADH, but whether it increases ADH secretion or affects the renal tubules has not been established.[131] Other medical conditions, such as pulmonary and central nervous system infections, neurologic trauma, anesthesia, prolonged intubation with positive pressure breathing, and primary or metastatic brain tumors, can also cause SIADH. While SIADH is most frequently associated with ectopic hormone production in small-cell lung cancer, patients with these other conditions also receive the above mentioned chemotherapy with vigorous hydration and are at risk to develop brain metastasis.[132]

Hyponatremia in the patient with small-cell lung cancer can also be caused by a mechanism unrelated to ADH. Recent reports indicate that a circulating hormone, atrial natriuretic peptide (ANP), has been elevated in these patients, while ADH levels were normal. The ANP was not secreted by tumor but by atrial tissue via an unknown mechanism. ANP causes sodium uresis by inhibiting renin, aldosterone, and vasopressin.[133]

Clinical Manifestations

The primary clinical characteristics of SIADH are those manifestations of water intoxication. The severity depends on the degree of abnormality of the serum sodium and plasma osmolality as well as the rapidity with which the syndrome develops. Neurological symptoms

TABLE 34-17 Potential Etiologic Factors Contributing to the Development of SIADH

Ectopic production of ADH
Malignancies: Small-cell lung cancer, pancreatic cancer, lymphoma, thymoma, Hodgkin's disease, bladder and prostate cancers
Pulmonary infections
Abnormal stimulation of ADH production
CNS trauma: hemorrhage, stroke
CNS infection: meningitis, abscess
CNS tumors: primary and metastatic
Stress, shock, positive pressure breathing, pain, dehydration
Chemotherapy: vincristine, vinblastine
Nicotine
Induced ADH effects on renal tubule
Narcotics: morphine, tranquilizers, barbiturates
General medications: thiazide diuretics, potassium supplements, chlorpropamide, acetominophen, isoproterenol
Anesthetics
Chemotherapy: cyclophosphamide, cisplatin

Source: Data from Schaefer SL,[136] Poe CM.[134]

TABLE 34-18 Early and Late Symptoms of Impending SIADH

Early
Thirst
Headache
Anorexia
Muscle cramps
Lethargy
Late
Nausea, vomiting
Weight gain without edema
Hyporeflexia
Confusion
Oliguria
Seizures
Coma

are attributed to the effects of cerebral edema. (See Table 34-18.) In persons with mild hyponatremia (serum sodium less than or equal to 130 mEq/l), thirst, headache, anorexia, muscle cramps, and lethargy may be seen. As the serum sodium levels fall below 125 mEq/l, nausea, vomiting, weight gain, hyporeflexia, and confusion may ensue. Severe hyponatremia (serum sodium <115 mEq/l) can cause seizures, coma, and death.[134]

Other clinical characteristics may include decreased urine output (less than 400 ml/24 hr) and unexplained weight gain without evidence of edema.[135]

Assessment

Identification of patients at risk of SIADH and of its manifestations aids in recognition and treatment of this emergency. Initially, symptoms are vague and easily attributed to side effects of therapy or tumor. Assessment of blood and urine chemistries and physical manifestations will help confirm the diagnosis of SIADH.

Hyponatremia (or serum sodium less than 130 mEq/l) is not solely diagnostic of SIADH. It may be due to rigorous hydration or recent diuretic administration. Hyponatremia associated with a low serum osmolality, high urine sodium level, and high urine osmolality is indicative of SIADH. Table 34-19 lists the laboratory parameters used to diagnose SIADH. Adrenal, renal, and thyroid function are normal in SIADH. Blood urea nitrogen and serum uric acid levels may be low as a result of the expanded intravascular volume.

Radioimmunoassay of plasma and urine ADH levels may be performed, but these are costly, not always readily available, and may be normal in certain instances that are not due to ectopic production or pituitary stimulation.[126] A water load test can be performed to definitively diagnose SIADH by administering a calculated amount of water and measuring urine output, osmolality, and specific gravity.[134,136] This test should not be performed if the serum sodium is less than 125 mEq/l or the patient is symptomatic.[126]

Interventions

The management of SIADH depends on the severity of the hyponatremia, the patient's clinical condition, and the underlying cause of the syndrome. Initial therapy usually consists of water restriction to induce a net negative water balance. In the oncology population, most often the underlying malignancy and its ectopic hormone production are causing SIADH. If the patient's condition permits, systemic chemotherapy should be instituted immediately, since no other medical intervention will effectively suppress tumor production of ADH. Most chemotherapy regimens require adequate hydration, so this situation demands critical assessment and monitoring skills to manage the patient's fluid and electrolyte status.

In mild hyponatremia the minimal amount of hydration during chemotherapy administration with nor-

TABLE 34-19 Laboratory Values in SIADH

Serum sodium	<130 mEq/l
Plasma osmolality	<280 mOsm/kg
Urine osmolality	>330 mOsm/kg
Urine sodium	>20 mEq/l

mal saline solution and subsequent fluid restriction of 500 ml/24 hr will control the syndrome until the tumor regresses. Moderate SIADH, when the serum sodium level is less than 125 mEq/l and the patient has symptoms, may require infusion of normal saline solution and electrolytes and diuresis with furosemide before initiation of systemic chemotherapy to treat the underlying tumor.

Patients who are severely hyponatremic (serum sodium level less than 120 mEq/l) and experiencing profound neurologic changes may require 3% hypertonic saline infusions and furosemide diuresis.[137] Systemic chemotherapy may have to be delayed for several days until the patient's fluid and electrolyte balance and neurologic status are improved. When neurologic status is impaired, patient safety is a priority and a protective environment is provided.

Some of the systemic chemotherapy agents currently used to treat small-cell lung cancer are vincristine, cyclophosphamide, and cisplatin. When managing patients with SIADH who are receiving these chemotherapeutic agents, one should consider the ADH effects and toxicities associated with each particular agent. Vincristine, cisplatin, and cyclophosphamide may exacerbate SIADH. Fluid restriction may promote hemorrhagic cystitis with cyclophosphamide, nephrotoxicity with cisplatin, and uric acid nephrolithiasis from tumor lysis. If hydration is critical to the administration of chemotherapy, normal saline solution is used with or without furosemide diuresis. Weight, neurologic status, intake and output, plasma and urine osmolality, and urine and serum sodium levels are carefully monitored and used as critical parameters for management. Any other medications that can induce SIADH must be withheld and substitutions made if possible.

SIADH that is chronic or recurs despite systemic chemotherapy may require therapy with demeclocycline (900–1200 mg/24 hr). Demeclocycline can partially inhibit the action of ADH, but it induces a reversible diabetes insipidus.[138] The absorption of demeclocycline, as with tetracycline, is affected by foods high in calcium. It is best absorbed on an empty stomach. Side effects include azotemia, photosensitivity, hematologic toxicity, and suprainfections.[139]

SIADH commonly occurs as a presenting symptom of small-cell lung cancer. Nursing interventions are directed toward reversing SIADH; administering chemotherapy and managing its side effects; educating the patient and family about the disease, treatment, side effects and self-care measures; and also providing support to the patient and family during this crisis. Since most therapy for lung cancer is administered on an outpatient basis, education and home care instructions are essential. Patients are taught about fluid restrictions, measurement of intake and output, signs and symptoms of hyponatremia, and when a condition indicates the need to contact the physician. Table 34-20 lists the nursing diagnoses that apply to patients with SIADH.

TABLE 34-20 Nursing Diagnoses for SIADH

Fluid volume excess due to ↑ ADH secretion and/or other contributing factors
Knowledge deficit of self-care measures to monitor and alleviate SIADH
Potential for injury due to risk of seizures and/or cerebral edema

Reversal of SIADH is evident when the serum sodium level approaches normal. When the permeability of the renal tubules to water normalizes, not only the serum sodium level but the plasma and urine osmolality and the urine sodium value also return to normal. Mental status improves and other symptoms resolve as fluid and electrolyte balance is restored. This balance must be restored slowly since rapid changes in serum sodium and water levels can cause shrinkage of neurons, leading to cerebral edema and seizures.[134]

Untreated, SIADH can progress to seizure, coma, and death. The insidious onset of SIADH can delay early diagnosis; therefore, the nurse must be aware of the population at risk and of the predisposing factors. Involvement of the patient and family is crucial in effective management, since compliance with fluid restriction, monitoring of symptoms, and reporting of changes is necessary to reverse SIADH. Figure 34-11 provides a clinical pathway for SIADH and highlights the critical decisions and intervention for this syndrome.

The overall prognosis for the cancer patient with SIADH depends on the underlying cause. SIADH usually resolves as the tumor regresses, but it can persist despite tumor control. It may recur and suggest tumor progression, but recurrence is sometimes seen with stable disease during the maintenance phase of chemotherapy.[126] Neurologic impairment from water intoxication is usually reversible and does not require long-term rehabilitation. Frequent assessment of the patient and monitoring of the serum sodium level is needed in the initial period following SIADH.

Future Trends

Because of the increased incidence of small-cell lung cancer and other tumors associated with ectopic production of ADH, the incidence of SIADH is increasing. Future research is geared toward better control of small-cell lung cancer and other cancers, prevention of lung cancer through smoking cessation and clean air acts, and medications that reduce circulating ADH or its release from tumors. While no drugs can stop ectopic production of ADH, some narcotic antagonists have been studied in animals for their effectiveness in inhibiting ADH release from the pituitary.[130]

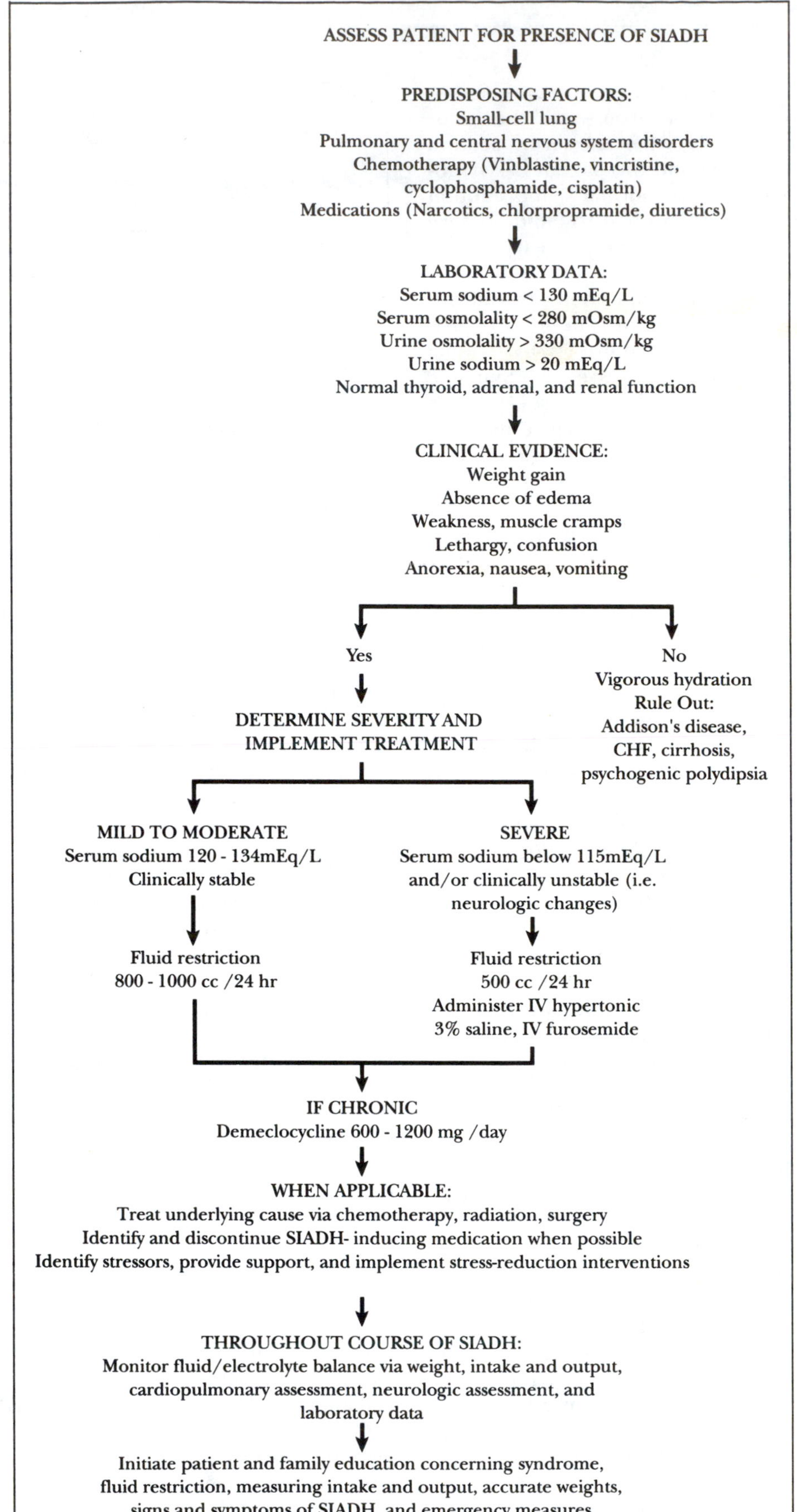

FIGURE 34-11 Clinical pathway for SIADH. (Source: Adapted from Poe CM, and Tayen LM.[134])

SPINAL CORD COMPRESSION

Scope of the Problem

Definition

Spinal cord compression (SCC) refers to a malignant process in which tumor encroaches upon the spinal cord or cauda equina. The same complex of symptoms, disease process and treatment applies to compression of either the cord or the cauda equina.[140]

Incidence

For the oncology patient, spinal cord compression is a neurologic emergency that requires prompt diagnosis and intervention so that neurologic function can be preserved and maintained. It is estimated that spinal cord compression develops in about 5% of patients with systemic cancer and that approximately 95% of these cases are due to metastasis to the vertebral column.[141–143] As a result of prolonged survival and increased incidence of those particular cancers prone to bone metastasis, the incidence of spinal cord compression may actually be rising. Spinal cord compression can cause partial or complete paralysis, requiring extensive nursing care and even assisted ventilation. Early recognition and treatment can maintain quality of life for the oncology patient.

Anatomy, physiology, and scientific principles

The spinal cord is surrounded by three connective tissue membranes, known as the leptomeninges, and bony structures or vertebrae. The leptomeninges include: the innermost layer closest to the cord, the pia mater; the arachnoid mater; and the dura mater, or the outermost layer. Between the pia and the arachnoid maters is the subarachnoid space through which cerebrospinal fluid circulates. The subdural space is located between the arachnoid and dura maters; the epidural space is found between the dura mater and osseous membrane of the vertebrae (See Figure 34-12.)

The spinal cord spans the length of the vertebral column, ending at the space between the first two lumbar vertebrae. The *cauda equina* refers to the group of lumbar and sacral nerve roots emerging from the end of the cord.[140] The vertebral column supports the body and provides flexibility and mobility. Each vertebra consists of a vertebral body, two laminae, two pedicles, and a spinous process. The vertebral column protects the spinal cord and enlarges in the cervical and lumbar

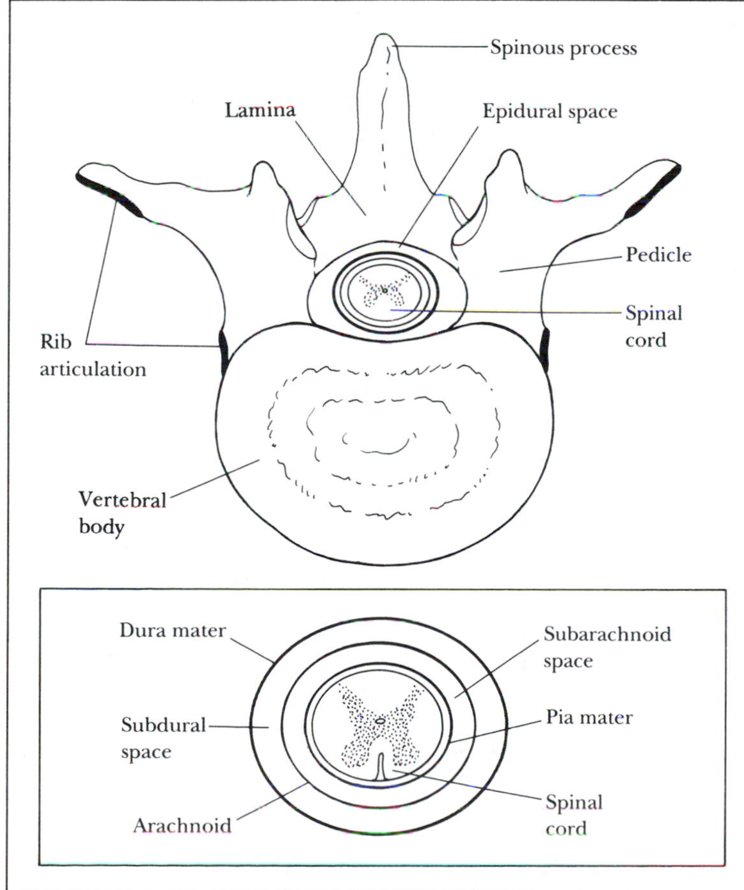

FIGURE 34-12 Cross-section of vertebra and spinal cord. The vertebra consists of the vertebral body, pedicles, laminae, and spinous process. The spinal cord spans the length of the vertebral column in the canal formed by the vertebrae. The cross-section of the spinal cord in the inset illustrates the leptomeninges or membranes surrounding the spinal cord and spaces between the membranes.

areas to accommodate expansions of the spinal cord.[140] The spinal cord consists of ascending and descending nerve tracts that send impulses to the brain and the peripheral nerves. This conduit transmits sensory and motor signals.[144]

Pathophysiology

Spinal cord compression can be classified according to the location of the tumor causing compression as intramedullary, intradural, extravertebral, or extradural.[145,146] Intramedullary and intradural tumors are usually primary malignancies such as ependymona, astrocytoma, glioma, neurilemmona, and meningioma.[144] Metastasis to the interior cord and dura mater are rare.[142] Intramedullary and intradural metastasis occur through hematogenous spread from the paravertebral and extradural venous plexus, growth along nerve roots from paravertebral tumors, or seeding from leptomeningeal metastasis.

Extravertebral lesions that extend through the intervertebral foramina are usually tumors of contiguous structures, such as mediastinal and retroperitoneal lymph nodes from lymphomas, germ cell tumors, and neuroblastomas.[140]

Extradural or epidural lesions are most frequently associated with spinal cord compression. These lesions are usually caused by bone metastasis to the vertebrae. Compression of the spinal cord occurs either by direct extraosseous extension of the tumor into the epidural space or, less often, by vertebral collapse and displacement of bony elements into the epidural space.[147,148] Usually the cord is compressed anteriorly by tumors that develop between the dura and the periosteum and cause destruction of the vertebral bodies, laminae, pedicles, and epidural tissues.[145]

Extradural compression of the spinal cord under any circumstance leads to ischemia and edema of the spinal cord and also mechanically distorts and damages neural tissue. Intramedullary involvement can destroy actual cord tissue.[149,150] The rate and degree of compression and resulting cord damage are responsible for the array of clinical manifestations. The spinal cord has sensory, motor, and autonomic functions, and the amount of damage can range from minor neurologic changes to complete paralysis (paraplegia).

Epidural metastasis is most frequently associated with cancers that metastasize to bone, such as cancers of the breast, lung, prostate, and kidney; multiple myeloma; and melanoma. Lymphomas have a high correlation with spinal cord compression because of direct extension through the intervertebral foramina. In the past decade the incidence of lymphoma-induced spinal cord compression has declined as a result of the use of aggressive radiation early in the treatment of lymphoma.[142,151] Other cancers that can cause spinal cord compression include unknown primary, sarcoma, neuroblastoma, gastrointestinal cancers, and thyroid cancer.[141]

The site of epidural metastasis and cord compression is related to the type of the primary cancer. In their classic study of cord compression, Gilbert and colleagues[151] concluded that lung and breast cancers most often cause thoracic spinal cord compression, whereas gastrointestinal cancers most frequently metastasize to the lumbosacral spine. Breast cancer is also related to vertebral subluxation or dislocation of the cervical spine. The relationship between primary tumors and epidural metastases is due to anatomic location, vascular supply, and venous drainage. Figure 34-13 illustrates the incidence of epidural metastasis by location on the spinal cord and primary cancer.[151]

Clinical Manifestations

Over 95% of patients with spinal cord compression have pain as the presenting symptom.[152] Thirty-three percent of patients who present with back pain and a normal neurological exam have a greater than 75% block of the spinal cord.[151] The pain is either radicular or localized. Radicular pain follows the distribution of the segmental dermatome of the involved nerve roots; lumbosacral and cervical radicular pain tends to be unilateral, while thoracic is usually bilateral.[140] Thoracic radicular pain is most often described as a constrictive band around the chest or waist. This is a significant symptom since approximately 53% of patients with radiculopathy have greater than 75% blocks in their spinal column.[151] See Table 34-21.

Central back pain is caused by vertebral collapse or stretching of the periosteum of the involved bony structure. The pain is usually located within one or two vertebrae of the actual compression.[140,151] Regardless of

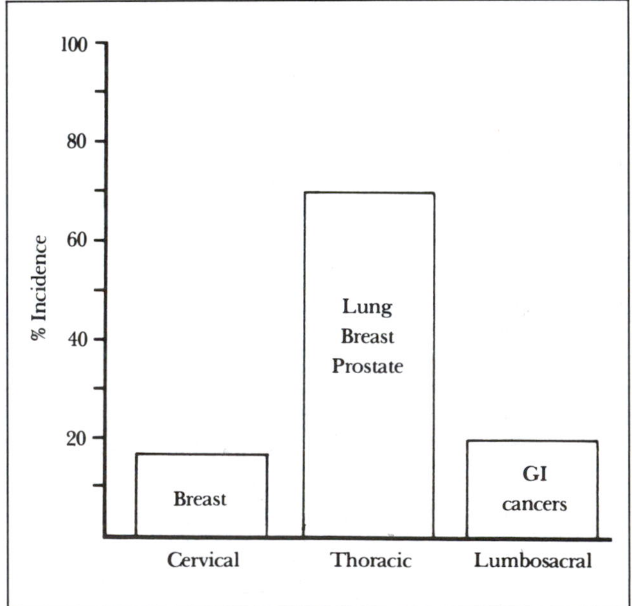

FIGURE 34-13 Primary cancers responsible for most cord compressions specific to location on spinal cord.

TABLE 34-21 Relationship between Symptoms/Neurologic Findings and Significant Spinal Cord Compression

Symptom/Neurologic Finding	Percent of Patients with >75% Blockage
Back pain alone	33%
Radiculopathy	53%
Motor weakness	95%

Source: Data from Schaeffer SL,[140] Gilbert RW, Kim JH, Posner JB.[151]

the nature of the pain, it can be elicited by percussion of vertebra near the level of the compression and, depending on the location of the compression, by either straight leg raising or neck flexion. The pain can be aggravated by coughing, sneezing, or Valsalva maneuver. The pain is different from that of a herniated disc in that it is not relieved by lying down.[140]

Sometimes it may be difficult to distinguish pain due to preexisting bone metastasis from pain related to spinal cord compression. The hallmark indicator to early detection of spinal cord compression is the pain changing location, intensity, or nature. Prompt diagnostic evaluation needs to be performed.

Motor weakness is usually the next symptom to evolve in this emergency, but it is rarely the presenting symptom. About three-fourths of patients are obviously paraparetic at the time of diagnosis and even more are discovered by neurologic exam. The weakness is usually described as heaviness or stiffness. Approximately 95% of patients with motor weakness were found to have a greater than 75% block in the spinal cord.[151]

Sensory loss occurs next usually in the form of numbness and paresthesia but can progress to loss of light touch, pain, then thermal sensation. Sensory loss of proprioception, deep pressure, vibration, or position represents a more severe cord compression. Sensory loss can progress to motor loss or paralysis, which holds a poor prognosis.[140] The type and degree of sensory and motor loss will relate to the level and degree of spinal cord compression.

Autonomic dysfunction caused by spinal cord compression includes various bladder and bowel disturbances. Urinary symptoms include difficulty initiating void, retention, overflow, and incontinence. A neurogenic bladder can be diagnosed by first having the patient void, then performing a urinary catheterization. If the postvoid residual amount is greater than 150 ml, urinary retention is present.[147] Bowel problems may begin as difficulty expelling stool and loss of feeling and progress to constipation or incontinence. Poor sphincter tone is a late sign of autonomic dysfunction.[140] Sensory loss, autonomic dysfunction, and poor sphincter control are present in about half of the patients when the compression is diagnosed and usually indicate progressive disease.[151]

Assessment

The importance of early recognition and diagnosis of spinal cord compression cannot be overemphasized. The single critical prognostic factor in spinal cord compression is the neurologic status before the initiation of therapy. The less extensive the injury to the cord before treatment, the greater the likelihood of full ambulation, sensation, and bowel and bladder control after treatment.[141,151] The converse is also true: Compromised neurologic status before treatment would indicate that posttreatment recovery will probably be limited. See Table 34-22.

Even if back pain is the only symptom, spinal cord compression should be suspected in cancer patients. Radiographs of the spine will demonstrate vertebral body collapse, pedicle erosion, osteolytic lesions, or paraspinal masses in more than 85% of cases of epidural metastasis.[142,153] These films are an inexpensive and readily available diagnostic tool. A bone scan can also be helpful in the identification of vertebral body metastasis, but often this has already been established and does not differentiate cord compression. Also, benign processes are evident on bone scan.

In the past, myelography was the definitive diagnostic tool for spinal cord compression. Oil-based iodinated contrasts were used to visualize the spinal cord, until metrizomide, a water-soluble nonirritative agent, was developed. Oil-based dyes had the advantage of remaining in the cerebrospinal fluid (CSF) to allow future films, but metrizomide has the advantages of providing better visualization on myelography, enhanced visualization on CT scan, and fewer side effects. The contrast is injected via a lumbar puncture into the subarachnoid space, and flow is observed to identify any defects. These defects are measured in approximate percentages to describe the degree of tumor involvement in the epidural space. A complete block is present when no contrast flows above the level of the tumor. A cervical puncture is performed to identify the upper level of the block. CSF is withdrawn before the instillation of the contrast and sent for cytologic study, cell count, and determination of glucose and protein levels. Examination of CSF will diagnose leptomeningeal metastasis.[154]

Magnetic resonance imaging (MRI) has emerged as

TABLE 34-22 Early and Late Signs of Impending Spinal Cord Compression

Early
Back pain, radicular or localized
Motor weakness
Sensory loss
Late
Motor loss
Urinary retention, overflow, incontinence
Difficulty expelling stool, constipation, incontinence
Poor sphincter control

the safest and most definitive diagnostic tool for spinal cord compression.[147,154,155] MRI is noninvasive and provides better visualization of neural tissue and distinguishes extradural, intradural, and intramedullary and extravertebral masses. MRI also visualizes neural tissue above and below the mass. Myelography with contrast does not provide such detailed visualization and requires two punctures, one above and one below the blockage in order to accurately define a complete spinal cord compression. In addition, when performing myelography on patients with a complete blockage, approximately 14% will develop rapid neurologic deterioration as a complication of the procedure.[156]

The disadvantages of MRI are primarily patient convenience and machine availability. Complete MRI visualization of the spinal column takes approximately 2 hours while the patient lies flat in a noisy, claustrophobic atmosphere. Since this technology is fairly new, machine availability may be limited in smaller facilities or rural areas. Also, as this state-of-the-art tool becomes more widely used, appointment availability may become less limited.

Interventions

Timely treatment of spinal cord compression is as important as rapid diagnosis. Neurologic deficits can quickly progress and render the patient paraplegic if intervention is not initiated immediately. Controversy exists concerning the initial treatment of choice: radiation therapy, surgical decompression, or a combined approach of surgery followed by irradiation.

Radiation therapy is the treatment most often used for patients with epidural metastasis and spinal cord compression.[142] The radiation port extends one to two vertebral bodies above and below the compression. A total dose of 3000–4000 cGy is delivered in fractionated doses over a few weeks. The side effects of radiation to the involved area are minimal and relate to location on the spinal column. Over all, the radiation treatments are well tolerated. Patients with preexisting bone metastasis and less than optimal bone marrow function may incur further suppression of marrow function due to radiation effects.

Surgical decompression with laminectomy or vertebral body resection can promptly relieve spinal cord compression. In the past, a posterior approach removing the lamina and spinous processes was used; complete tumor resection was impossible since most epidural metastases are anterior to the spine.[154] The primary goal was decompression by providing alternate space for the tumor and spine stabilization. The alternative is the anterior approach, which involves vertebral body resection via a thoracotomy. It was performed infrequently in the past due to inability to adequately stabilize the spine. However, new acrylic materials and advances in surgical technique have been developed to overcome this barrier and enable the successful use of the anterior approach for decompression.[157]

With the traditional posterior laminectomy approach, surgery followed by radiation offered the same results as radiation alone.[143] Now, with the availability of the anterior surgical approach, surgery is offered to patients when one of the following conditions is present: pathological fracture with spinal instability or compression by bone, radiation-resistant tumor with neurological deficit, unknown tissue diagnosis, relapse at a previous site of radiation, or failure to respond to radiation with rapid neurological deterioration.[154] Clearly, the morbidity associated with surgery for patients with advanced cancer makes the surgical approach appropriate for only a highly select group. In most instances, surgery is followed by radiation, except for those patients who failed or relapsed after previous radiation. Chemotherapy may be used with extremely chemosensitive cancers, such as lymphoma and Hodgkin's disease, or as an adjuvant to either surgery or radiation.

Regardless of the type of treatment, steroids are included as part of the management of spinal cord compression. Steroids are initiated as soon as there is a high degree of suspicion, even before a definitive diagnosis is made. Low-dose steroid (e.g., dexamethasone 4 mg orally twice or four times daily) is initiated and continued until a definitive diagnosis is made. If a high degree of block is diagnosed, high-dose steroids are administered, usually a 100mg bolus of dexamethasone given intravenously, followed by 24 mg orally every 6 hours for 2 days then rapidly tapered.[142,158] The purpose of steroid therapy is to reduce spinal cord edema and pain. With certain tumors, steroids have an oncolytic effect.[159] Frequently, severe and sometimes fatal complications are associated with prolonged steroid use. These include gastric ulceration and bleeding, hyperglycemia, immunosuppression, hypertension, psychosis, and osteoporosis.[160] Greenberg and his colleagues compared high-dose steroids to more traditional dosages and found that higher doses relieved pain more effectively and had a low incidence of complications.[161] See Figure 34-14 to review the clinical pathway for spinal cord compression.[162]

Patients with spinal cord compression develop clinical problems that are determined by the rapidity of onset, level and degree of compression, presenting symptoms, type of treatment, and response to treatment. Patient assessment is crucial throughout this emergency for evaluation of neurologic status and preservation of maximal function. Assessment includes monitoring of sensory and motor function as well as urinary and bowel function. Intensive care may be needed if acute decompensation occurs, resulting in respiratory arrest, increased intracranial pressure, seizures, or autonomic dysreflexia.

Since more than 95% of patients with spinal cord compression have pain, knowledge of the principles of analgesia in the oncology population is essential. Effective analgesia is established early and adjusted as steroids and treatment reduce pain. The variety of analgesic agents and the types of administration tech-

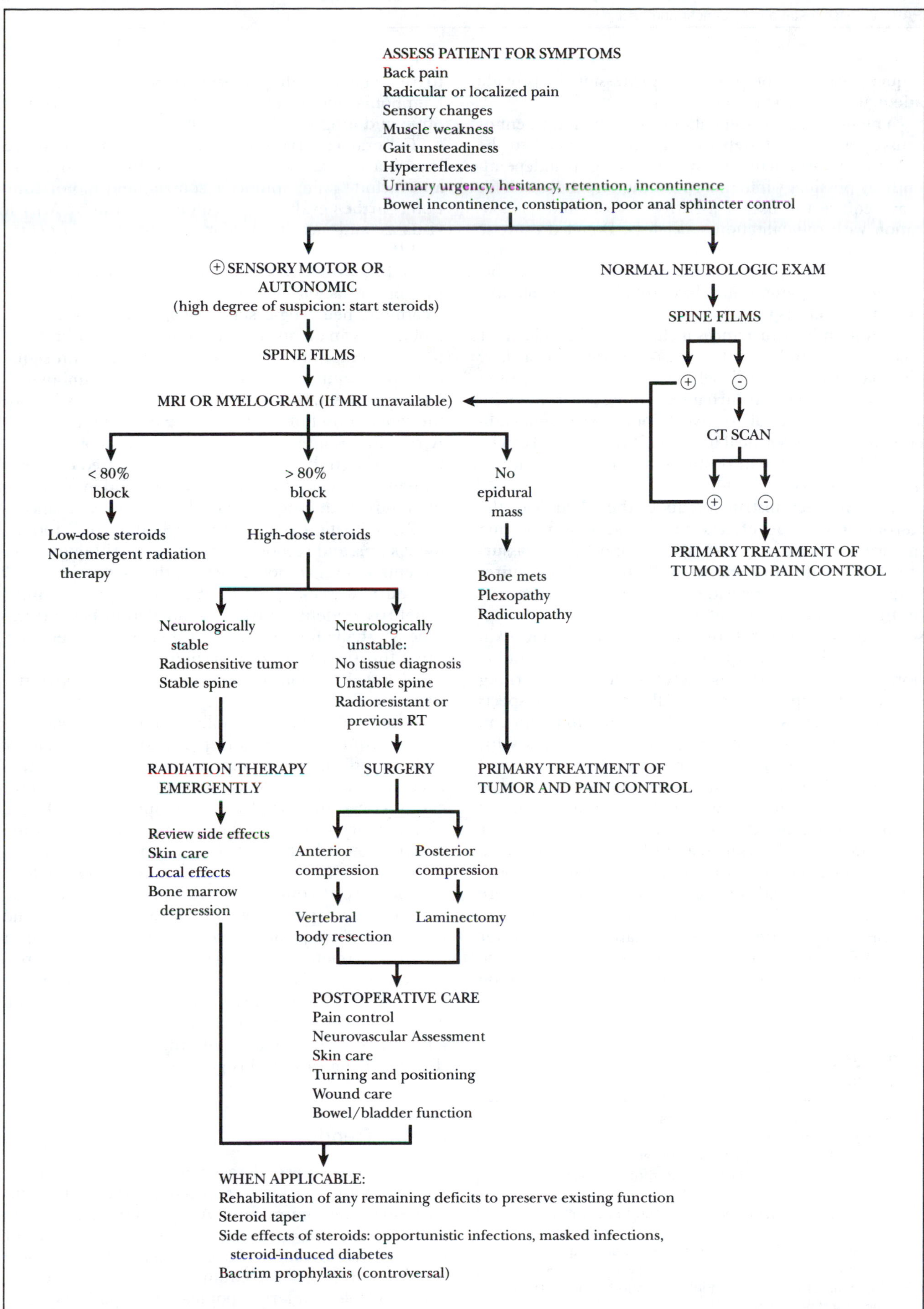

FIGURE 34-14 Clinical pathway for spinal cord compression. (Source: Data from Portnoy RK, Lipton RB, Foley KM.[163])

niques available help health professionals provide adequate relief for patients.

The nurse assists the patient in the management of sensory and motor deficits. The patient needs to be able to perform activities of daily living as independently as possible while incorporating any deficits. This may require the use of assistive devices and collaboration with rehabilitation specialists. Detailed exercise regimens should be reinforced and facilitated by the nurse. Preserving and maximizing function are a priority since many patients may have rehabilitative potential after treatment is initiated.

Autonomic disturbances include bowel and bladder incontinence and retention. Establishment of a daily elimination regimen will help manage incontinence and retention. Urinary disturbances can be reversed by institution of a schedule of hydration, intermittent catheterization, and perineal hygiene. Bowel control can be established with the appropriate use of diet, laxatives, and suppositories.

Patients need instruction about the schedule of the steroid taper, side effects, and conditions requiring medical care. Patients also need support and reassurance during this stressful time. If the patient requires surgery, the nurse provides routine postlaminectomy or thoracotomy care that includes neurovascular assessment, pain control, turning and positioning, skin care, wound care, and rehabilitation.[163] During radiation therapy the nurse instructs the patient concerning side effects and measures to alleviate them, inspects skin, and assesses toxicities and response to treatment. Table 34-23 lists the potential nursing diagnoses for patients with spinal cord compression.

Comparison of response rates shows that the type of tumor determines the response rate and that the various treatments currently yield similar results for each tumor type. Bruckman and Bloomer[141] pooled data from several studies to analyze satisfactory response rates of patients with various types of tumor who were treated for spinal cord compression. Satisfactory response rates were defined as ambulation and sphincter control for more than 3 months after treatment. The percentages of patients who had a satisfactory response to treatment according to primary cancer are as follows: lymphoma and myeloma, 50%; breast and prostate, 30%; and lung and kidney, 10%.[141]

TABLE 34-23 Nursing Diagnoses for Spinal Cord Compression

1. Pain due to spinal cord compression
2. Sensory alteration due to disruption in sensory function
3. Potential for injury due to sensory and motor deficits
4. Impaired physical mobility due to motor weakness/paralysis
5. Constipation/bowel incontinence due to neurologic impairment
6. Urinary retention/incontinence due to neurologic impairment
7. Potential for impaired skin integrity due to immobility and decreased sensation
8. Self-care deficits due to neurologic deficits

General criteria for evaluation of treatment response are measured through neurologic examination and include pain, sphincter control, and motor function. Further evaluation includes CT scan or MRI to visualize and measure tumor response to treatment.

Effective treatment of spinal cord compression is related to prolonged survival.[158] The most important prognostic factor in spinal cord compression is pretreatment neurologic status. Approximately 80% of ambulatory patients remain ambulatory after treatment, whereas only 30%–40% of patients with significant pretreatment motor dysfunction are ambulatory after treatment.[142,160] Other prognostic factors include the rate of onset of symptoms and type of malignancy. A rapidly progressing syndrome has a poor recovery rate. In the study of response rates discussed earlier,[141] patients with lymphoma and myeloma did much better than those with lung, prostate, breast, or renal cancers.

Rehabilitation potential is dependent on pretreatment status and response to treatment. Although some patients will regain lost function, the vast majority will not. Several weeks after radiation therapy, maximum benefit is evident. Further rehabilitation beyond this time is usually not possible; the goal is to preserve existing function. If surgical decompression is successful, rapid rehabilitation is expected after postoperative recovery.

After treatment is completed, intensive follow-up care is required to assess response to treatment, assist with the adjustment to any motor or autonomic dysfunction, and monitor existing neurologic status. Home care services, such as physical therapy or home health aid, may need to be obtained and coordinated. Additional follow-up care related to the primary disease and its systemic treatment and monitoring is also needed.

Spinal cord compression can produce devastating sequelae for a patient who is already physically and emotionally compromised by the diagnosis of cancer and its treatment. Nurses play a vital role in early recognition of spinal cord compression. Prompt diagnosis and treatment help ensure neurologic preservation and a higher quality of life for the patient. Symptom management and rehabilitation are the primary goals that direct nursing care in this population.

Future Trends

Investigation is needed regarding the best treatment modality for the various tumor types, level, degree, and location of the compression. A prospective study using specific criteria to determine the most effective type of treatment is warranted. Surgical technique and spine stabilization materials continue to evolve to make surgery available to a larger population of patients.

Further study is also indicated with regard to appropriate dosage and schedule of steroids. Controversy exists as to high-dose versus low-dose steroids. There is a lack of specific criteria to determine high or low dose, timing of taper, and length of treatment. The development of MRI has begun to positively impact on the speed and safety of diagnosing spinal cord compression. This diagnostic tool is becoming more clinically useful and available to more patients.

CONCLUSION

Radiation therapy, chemotherapeutic agents that affect bone marrow function, and primary malignancies of the bone marrow (i.e., leukemia) predispose the patient to prolonged periods of neutropenia. Sepsis is the most common cause of septic shock in patients with cancer. Appropriate nursing diagnoses and interventions may prevent an episode of neutropenic fever from progressing to septic shock. New avenues of treatment, including human monoclonal antibody, anti-TNF, and IL-1 receptor antagonists are being investigated in an attempt to reverse the sepsis syndrome.

Septic shock is one process that can initiate disseminated intravascular coagulation (DIC), an abnormality of the clotting process that results in massive clotting and simultaneous hemorrhage. Patients with gastric, prostate, and pancreatic cancers as well as those with acute promyelocytic leukemia (APL) are also prone to DIC. Successful treatment of DIC is dependent on treatment of the underlying cause.

Intrathoracic malignancies are most often associated with superior vena cava syndrome (SVCS) and cardiac tamponade secondary to pericardial effusion. SVCS is a rare emergency resulting from compression of the superior vena cava and is associated with upper body edema, venous congestion, and possible respiratory distress. In the past, treatment of SVCS often precluded diagnosis of the underlying malignancy. Current practitioners prefer definitive diagnosis before initiation of treatment. The prognosis of SVCS is dependent on treating the underlying malignancy.

Pericardial effusion, with or without cardiac tamponade, is easily reversible, provided it is recognized early. Unfortunately, early symptoms of fatigue, shortness of breath, and chest discomfort can be attributed to the effects of disease or treatment. Cardiac tamponade is usually caused by fluid accumulation and increased intrapericardial pressure but can also be caused by inflammation and inelasticity of the pericardium. The outcomes of SVCS and cardiac tamponade depend on the speed with which the emergency develops and on prompt diagnosis and treatment.

Various metabolic abnormalities are associated with cancer, its treatment, and necessary supportive therapy. Three of the most common metabolic emergencies in the oncology population are hypercalcemia, tumor lysis syndrome, and syndrome of inappropriate antidiuretic hormone (SIADH). When cancer infiltrates bony structures, life-threatening problems associated with the release of calcium into the blood arise. Hypercalcemia can also result from inappropriate production of PTH, OAF, and prostaglandin by tumors. Successful long-term treatment of hypercalcemia is dependent on tumor control and regression, but vigorous hydration and calcium-inhibiting agents can reverse an emergent episode of hypercalcemia. Clinical trials are being conducted to determine the most effective bisphosphonate and route of administration for the treatment of hypercalcemia.

Individuals with massive tumor burden, such as Burkitt's lymphoma, lymphoblastic leukemia, or any rapidly growing cancer, are at risk of tumor lysis syndrome. This syndrome is characterized by hyperkalemia, hyperphosphatemia, hyperuricemia, and hypocalcemia, and if not recognized early may cause renal failure as large numbers of sensitive tumor cells are destroyed. Tumor lysis syndrome is most successfully treated when it is anticipated and adequate renal function is maintained.

Syndrome of inappropriate antidiuretic hormone is a paraneoplastic syndrome characterized by ectopic tumor production of this hormone. It is most frequently associated with small-cell lung cancer but can also be initiated by various medications, including those used to treat small-cell lung cancer. Again, this syndrome is most successfully reversed by removal of the underlying cause, but anticipation and planning can greatly reduce the degree of morbidity.

Spinal cord compression is one of the most common neurologic emergencies facing the patient with cancer. Prompt recognition and treatment preserve neurologic function and prevent permanent deficits, such as paraplegia and bowel and bladder incontinence or retention. Magnetic resonance imaging has emerged as the safest and most clinically useful diagnostic tool in spinal cord compression. Although radiation therapy has been the primary treatment modality, new techniques are making surgical treatment a more feasible option for a select group of patients.

Since cancer is not one disease with one treatment, the oncology nurse must be familiar with the various cancers, treatment protocols, and associated medical emergencies. This knowledge, along with the patient's history, physical assessment, and results of laboratory tests, provides the nurse with the database necessary to predict which individuals are at risk and allow for the planning and nursing interventions required to prevent a critical event.

REFERENCES

1. Parrillo, JE: Management of septic shock: Present and future. *Ann Intern Med* 115:491–493, 1991.
2. Bone RC: The pathogenesis of sepsis. *Ann Intern Med* 115:457–469, 1991.

3. Houston MC: Pathophysiology of shock. *Crit Care Nurs Clin North Am* 2:143–149, 1990.
4. Parrillo JE, Parker MM, Natanson C, et al: Septic shock in humans. Advances in the understanding of pathogenesis, cardiovascular dysfunction, and therapy. *Ann Intern Med* 113:227–242, 1990.
5. Gileski WJ: Sepsis. What it is and how to recognize it. *Surg Clin North Am* 71:749–764, 1991.
6. Groeger JS: Shock states and cancer. In Howland WS, Carlon GC (eds), *Critical Care of the Cancer Patient.* Chicago: Yearbook Medical Publishers, 1985, pp. 296–317.
7. Vander AJ, Sherman JH, Luciano DS (eds): *Human Physiology—The Mechanisms of Body Function* (2d ed). New York: McGraw-Hill, 1975.
8. Rackow EC, Astiz ME: Pathophysiology and treatment of septic shock. *JAMA* 266:548–554, 1991.
9. Cunnion RE, Parrillo JE: Cardiovascular disease. In Parrillo JE, Masur H, *The Critically Ill Immunosuppressed Patient.* Rockville, MD: Aspen, 1987, pp. 3–38.
10. Clowes GH: Stresses, mediators and responses of survival. In Clowes GH (ed), *Trauma, Sepsis and Shock: The Physiological Basis of Therapy.* New York: Dekker, 1988, pp. 11–54.
11. Gucalp R, Dutcher JP: Fever and infection. In Dutcher JP, Wiernik PH (eds), *Handbook of Hematologic and Oncologic Emergencies.* New York: Plenum, 1987, pp. 153–184.
12. Fromme L, Mesa D, Outlaw E: Septic shock. In Brown MH, Kiss ME, Outlaw EM, et al (eds), *Standards of Oncology Nursing Practice.* New York: Wiley, 1986, pp. 469–472.
13. Mason CA: Septic shock. *J Assoc Pediatr Oncol Nurses* 4(3–4):25–31, 1988.
14. Bone RC, Fisher CJ, Clemmer TP, et al: Sepsis syndrome: A valid clinical entity. Methylprednisolone severe sepsis study group. *Crit Care Med* 17:389–393, 1989.
15. Perry AG: Shock complications: Recognition and management. *Crit Care Nurs Q* 11:1–8, 1988.
16. Littleton MT: Pathophysiology and assessment of sepsis and septic shock. *Crit Care Nurs Q* 11:30–47, 1988.
17. Truett L: The septic syndrome: An oncologic treatment challenge. *Cancer Nurs* 14:175–180, 1991.
18. Karakusis PH: Considerations in the therapy of septic shock. *Med Clin North Am* 70:933–944, 1986.
19. Barry SA: Septic shock: Special needs of patients with cancer. *Oncol Nurs Forum* 16:31–35, 1989.
20. Peters JI, Utset OM: Shock in the ICU: When to suspect, how to determine its cause. *J Crit Illness* 4(7):77–93, 1989.
21. Wolff SM: Monoclonal antibodies and the treatment of gram-negative bacteremia and shock. *N Engl J Med* 324:486–488, 1991.
22. Roach AC: Antibiotic therapy in septic shock. *Crit Care Nurs Clin North Am* 2:179–186, 1990.
23. Ziegler EJ, Fisher CJ, Sprung CL, et al: Treatment of gram-negative bacteremia and septic shock with HA-1A human monoclonal antibody against endotoxin. A randomized, double-blind, placebo-controlled trial. The HA-1A Sepsis Study Group. *N Engl J Med* 324:429–436, 1991.
24. Bone RC: A critical evaluation of new agents for the treatment of sepsis. *JAMA* 266:1686–1691, 1991.
25. Colman RW, Rubin RN: Disseminated intravascular coagulation due to malignancy. *Semin Oncol* 17:172–186, 1990.
26. Bick RL: Disseminated intravascular coagulation and related syndromes: A clinical review. *Semin Thromb Hemost* 14:229–338, 1988.
27. Ratnoff OD: Hemostatic emergencies in malignancy. *Semin Oncol* 16:561–571, 1989.
28. O'Brian BS, Woods S: The paradox of DIC. *Am J Nurs* 78(11):1878–1880, 1978.
29. Tallman MS, Kwaan HC: Reassessing the hemostatic disorder associated with acute promyelocytic leukemia. *Blood* 79:543–553, 1992.
30. Goldberg MA, Girsburg D, Mayer RM, et al: Is heparin administration necessary during induction chemotherapy for patients with acute promyelocytic leukemia? *Blood* 69(1):187–191, 1987.
31. Cunningham I, Gee TS, Reich LM, et al: Acute promyelocytic leukemia: Treatment results during a decade at Memorial Hospital. *Blood* 73:1116–1122, 1989.
32. Happ M: Life threatening hemorrhage in children with cancer. *J Assoc Pediatr Oncol Nurses* 4(3–4):36–40, 1988.
33. Drapkin RL, Gee TS, Dowling MD, et al: Prophylactic heparin therapy in acute promyelocytic leukemia. *Cancer* 41:2484–2490. 1978.
34. Kantarjian HM, Keating MJ, Walters RS, et al: Acute promyelocytic leukemia. *Am J Med* 80:789, 1986.
35. Lisiewicz J: Disseminated intravascular coagulation in acute leukemia. *Semin Thromb Hemost* 14:339–348, 1988.
36. Feinstein DI: Treatment of disseminated intravascular coagulation. *Sem Thromb Hemost* 14:351–362, 1988.
37. Fruchtman S, Aledort LM: Disseminated intravascular coagulation. *J Am Coll Cardiol* 8:159B–167B, 1986.
38. Tempero MA, Davis RB, Reed E, et al: Thrombocytopenia and laboratory evidence of disseminated intravascular coagulation after shunts for ascites in malignant disease. *Cancer* 55:2718–2721, 1985.
39. Rooney A, Haviley C: Nursing management of disseminated intravascular coagulation. *Oncol Nurs Forum* 12:15–22, 1985.
40. Bell TN: Disseminated intravascular coagulation and shock. *Crit Care Nurs Clin North Am* 2:255–268, 1990.
41. Rosen N, Kaufman D, Young RC: Medical emergencies in patients with solid tumors. In Parrillo JE, Masur H (eds), *The Critically Ill Immunosuppressed Patient.* Rockville, MD: Aspen, 1987, pp. 481–498.
42. Kingsley EC, Durie BG, Gareival HS: Acute promyelocytic leukemia. *West J Med* 146:322–327, 1987.
43. Schwartz BS, Williams EC, Conlon MG, et al: Epsilon-aminocaproic acid in the treatment of promyelocytic leukemia and acquired alpha$_2$-plasma inhibitor deficiency. *Ann Intern Med* 105:873–877, 1986.
44. Pilapil F: Disseminated intravascular coagulation (DIC). In Brown MH, Kiss ME, Outlaw EM, et al (eds), *Standards of Oncology Nursing Practice.* New York: Wiley, 1986, pp. 459–463.
45. Division of Nursing, Memorial Sloan-Kettering Cancer Center, New York, 1984.
46. Young LM: DIC: The insidious killer. *Crit Care Nurs* 10:26–33, 1990.
47. Siegrist CW, Jones JA: Disseminated intravascular coagulopathy and nursing implications. *Semin Oncol Nurs* 1:237–243, 1985.
48. Bavier AR: Alterations in hemostasis. In Johnson BL, Gross J (eds), *Handbook of Oncology Nursing.* Bethany, CT: Flescher, 1985, pp. 506–516.
49. Donoghue M: Superior vena cava syndrome. In Yasko JM (ed), *Guidelines for Cancer Care: Symptom Management.* Reston: Reston Publishing, 1983, pp. 145–162.

50. Helms SR, Carlson MD: Cardiovascular emergencies. *Semin Oncol* 16(6):463–470, 1989.
51. Simpson JR, Perez CA, Presant CA, et al: Superior vena cava syndrome. In Yarbro JW, Bornstein RS (eds), *Oncologic Emergencies.* New York: Grune & Stratton, 1981, pp. 43–72.
52. Schaefer SL: Oncologic complications: Superior vena cava syndrome. In Otto SE (ed), *Oncology Nursing.* St. Louis, MO: Mosby Year Book, 1991, pp. 468–526.
53. Yahalom J: Oncologic emergencies: Superior vena cava syndrome. In DeVita VT, Hellman S, Rosenberg SA (eds), *Cancer Principles and Practice of Oncology* (3d ed). Philadelphia: Lippincott, 1989, pp. 1971–1977.
54. Lopez MJ, Vincent RG: Malignant superior vena cava syndrome. In Kapoor AS (ed), *Cancer and the Heart.* New York: Springer-Verlag, 1986, pp. 206–212.
55. Little AG, Golomb HM, Ferguson MK, et al: Malignant superior vena cava obstruction reconsidered: The role of diagnostic surgical intervention. *Ann Thorac Surg* 40:285–288, 1985.
56. Lokich JJ, Goodman RL: Superior vena cava syndrome. *JAMA* 231:58–61, 1975.
57. Perez CA, Presant CA, Amburg AL: Management of superior vena cava syndrome. *Semin Oncol* 5:123–134, 1978.
58. Varricchio C: Clinical management of superior vena cava syndrome. *Heart Lung* 14:411–416, 1985.
59. Adelstein DJ, Hines JD, Carter SG, et al: Thromboembolic events in patients with malignant superior vena cava syndrome and the role of anticoagulation. *Cancer* 62:2258–2262, 1988.
60. Greenberg S, Kosinski R, Daniels J: Treatment of SVC thrombosis with rTPA. *Chest* 99(5):1298–1301, 1991.
61. Spross J, Stern R: Nursing management of oncology patients with a superior vena cava obstruction syndrome. *Oncol Nurs Forum* 6(3):3–9, 1979.
62a. Lopez MJ, Sala JM: Malignant superior vena cava syndrome: A 15 year experience. *Mo Med* 79:810–815, 1982.
62b. Theologides A: Neoplastic cardiac tamponade. *Semin Oncol* 5:181–192, 1978.
63. Thurber DL, Edwards JE, Achoe RW: Secondary malignant tumors of the pericardium. *Circulation* 26:228–241, 1962.
64. Pass HI: Treatment of malignant pleural and pericardial effusions. In DeVita VT, Hellman S, Rosenberg SA (eds), *Cancer: Principles and Practice of Oncology* (3d ed). Philadelphia: Lippincott, 1989, pp. 2317–2327.
65. Schafer SL: Oncologic complications. In Otto SE (ed), *Oncology Nursing.* St. Louis, MO: Mosby Yearbook, 1991, pp. 468–526.
66. Helms SR, Carlson MD: Cardiovascular emergencies. *Semin Oncol* 16(6):463–470, 1989.
67. Estes ME: Management of the cardiac tamponade patient: A nursing framework. *Crit Care Nurs* 5(5):17–26, 1985.
68. Shabetai R: Diseases of the pericardium. In Wyngarden JB, Smith LH (eds), *Cecil's Textbook of Medicine.* Philadelphia: Saunders, 1988, pp. 362–367.
69. Groeger J: Shock states and cancer. In Carlon G, Howland W (eds), *Critical Care of the Cancer Patient.* Chicago: Yearbook Publishers, 1985, pp. 296–317.
70. Appelfeld MM, Cole JF, Pollock SH, et al: The late appearance of chronic pericardial disease in patients treated by radiotherapy for Hodgkin's disease. *Ann Intern Med* 94:338–341, 1981.
71. Zehner LC, Hoogstraten B: Malignant effusions and their management. *Semin Oncol Nurs* 1(4):259–264, 1985.
72. Joiner GA: Neoplastic cardiac tamponade. *Crit Care Nurs* 11(2):50–58, 1991.
73. Press OW, Livingston R: Management of malignant pericardial effusion and tamponade. *JAMA* 257:1088–1092, 1987.
74. Gilbert I, Henning RJ: Adenocarcinoma of the lung presenting with pericardial tamponade: Report of a case and review of the literature. *Heart Lung* 14:83–87, 1985.
75. Kapoor AS: Malignant pericardial effusion and cardiac tamponade. In Kapoor AS (ed), *Cancer and the Heart.* New York: Springer-Verlag, 1986, pp. 216–231.
76. Hancock EW: Constrictive pericarditis: Clinical cues to diagnosis. *JAMA* 232:176, 1975.
77. Basmajian JV, Burke MD, Burnett GW, et al: *Illustrated Stedman's Medical Dictionary* (24th ed). Baltimore, MD: Williams & Wilkins, 1982, p. 1171.
78. Glover D, Glick JH: Oncologic emergencies. In Holleb AI, Fink DJ, Murphy GP: *American Cancer Society Textbook of Clinical Oncology.* Atlanta, GA: American Cancer Society Inc., 1991, pp. 513–533.
79. Concilus E, Bohachick P: Cancer: Pericardial effusion and tamponade. *Cancer Nurs* 7:391–398, 1984.
80. Wojciechowicz V: Pericardial window surgery for cardiac tamponade. *Crit Care Nurs* 5(5):28–33, 1985.
81. Markman M, Howell SB: Intrapericardial instillation of cisplatin in a patient with a large malignant pericardial effusion. *Cancer Drug Delivery* 2:49–52, 1985.
82. Osuch JR, Khandikar JD, Fry WA: Emergency subxiphoid pericardial decompression for malignant pericardial effusion. *Am Surg* 51:298–300, 1985.
83. Shepherd FA, Morgan C, Evans WK, et al: Medical management of malignant pericardial effusion by tetracycline sclerosis. *Am J Cardiol* 60:1161–1166, 1987.
84. Woll PJ, Knight RK, Rubens RD: Pericardial effusion complicating breast cancer. *J R Soc Med* 80:490–491, 1987.
85. Bajorunas DR: Disorders of endocrine function. In Groeger JS (ed), *Critical Care of the Cancer Patient* (2d ed). St. Louis, MO: Mosby Year Book, 1991, pp. 192–225.
86. Borenstein M: Metabolic emergencies in cancer. *Top Emerg Med* 8(2):75–81, 1986.
87. Warrel RP, Murphy WK, Schulman P, et al: A randomized double-blind study of gallium nitrate compared with etidronate for acute control of cancer-related hypercalcemia. *J Clin Oncol* 9:1467–1475, 1991.
88. Ritch PS: Treatment of cancer-related hypercalcemia. *Semin Oncol* 17:26–33, 1990(2 suppl 5).
89. Muggia FM: Overview of cancer-related hypercalcemia: Epidemiology and etiology. *Semin Oncol* 17:3–9, 1990(2 suppl 5).
90. Deconti RC: Management of hypercalcemia of neoplastic disease. *Curr Concepts Oncol* (Spring):7–13, 1985.
91. Vander AJ, Sherman JH, Luciano DS: *Human Physiology: The Mechanisms of Body Functions* (2d ed). New York: McGraw-Hill, 1975.
92. Coward DD: Cancer-induced hypercalcemia. *Cancer Nurs* 9(3):125–132, 1986.
93. Mundy GR, Yates AJ: Recent advances in pathophysiology and treatment of hypercalcemia of malignancy. *Am J Kidney Dis* 14:2–12, 1989.
94. Silverman P, Distelhorst CW: Metabolic emergencies in clinical oncology. *Semin Oncol* 16:504–515, 1989.

95. Mundy GR: Pathophysiology of cancer-associated hypercalcemia. *Semin Oncol* 17:10–15, 1990(2 suppl 5).
96. Mundy GR, Martin TJ: The hypercalcemia of malignancy: Pathogenesis and management. *Metabolism* 31: 1247–1277, 1982.
97. Bajorunas DR: Clinical manifestations of cancer-related hypercalcemia. *Semin Oncol* 17:16–25, 1990(2 suppl 5).
98. Mahon SM: Signs and symptoms associated with malignancy-induced hypercalcemia. *Cancer Nurs* 12:153–160, 1989.
99. Ralston SH, Gallacher SJ, Patel U, et al: Cancer associated hypercalcemia: Morbidity and mortality. Clinical experience in 126 treated patients. *Ann Intern Med* 112:499–504, 1990.
100. Einzig AI: Hypercalcemia in malignancy. In Dutcher JP, Wiernik PH (eds), *Handbook of Hematologic and Oncologic Emergencies.* New York: Plenum, 1987, pp. 17–27.
101. Stewart AF: Therapy of malignancy-associated hypercalcemia: 1983, *Am J Med* 74:475–480, 1983.
102. Heath D: The treatment of hypercalcemia of malignancy. *Clin Endocrinol* 34:155–157, 1991.
103. Poe CM, Radford AI: The challenge of hypercalcemia in cancer. *Oncol Nurs Forum* 12(6):29–34, 1985.
104. Hasling C, Charles P, Mosekilde L: Etidronate disodium in the management of malignancy-related hypercalcemia. *Am J Med* 82:51–54, 1987(suppl 2A).
105a. Singer FR, Fernandez M: Therapy of hypercalcemia of malignancy. *Am J Med* 82:34–41, 1987(suppl 2A).
105b. Mundy GR, Ibbottson KJ, D'Souza SM, et al: The hypercalcemia of cancer. *N Engl J Med* 310:1718–1728, 1984.
106. Warrel RP, Israel R, Frisone M: Gallium nitrate for acute treatment of cancer-related hypercalcemia. *Ann Intern Med* 108:669–674, 1988.
107. Moore JM: Metabolic emergencies. In Johnson BL, Gross J (eds), *Handbook of Oncology Nursing.* Bethany, CT: Fleschner, 1985, pp. 459–470.
108. Waters HF, Stuckey PA: Oncology alert for the home care nurse: Hypercalcemia. *Home Health Care Nurse* 6:32–36, 1988.
109. Henry P, Seery R, Outlaw E: Hypercalcemia. In Brown MH, Kiss ME (eds), *Standards of Oncology Nursing Practice.* New York: Wiley, 1986, pp. 488–493.
110. Flombaum CD: Electrolyte and renal abnormalities. In Groeger JS (ed), *Critical Care of the Cancer Patient* (2d ed). St. Louis, MO: Mosby Year Book, 1991, pp. 140–164.
111. List AF, Kummet TD, Adams JD, et al: Tumor lysis syndrome complicating treatment of chronic lymphocytic leukemia with fludarabine phosphate. *Am J Med* 89:388–390, 1990.
112. Simmons ED, Somberg KH: Acute tumor lysis syndrome after intrathecal methotrexate administration. *Cancer* 67:2062–2065, 1991.
113. Cohen LF, Balow JE, McGrath IT, et al: Acute tumor lysis syndrome: A review of 37 patients with Burkitt's lymphoma. *Am J Med* 68:486–491, 1980.
114. Moore JM: Tumor lysis syndrome. In Johnson BL, Gross J (eds), *Handbook of Oncology Nursing.* Bethany, CN: Fleschner, 1985, pp. 470–476.
115. Silverman P, Distelhorst CW: Metabolic emergencies in clinical oncology. *Semin Oncol* 16:504–515, 1989.
116. Henry P, Seery R: Tumor lysis syndrome. In Brown MH, Kiss ME, et al (eds), *Standards of Oncology Nursing Practice.* New York: Wiley, 1986, pp. 473–479.
117. Hussein-Am, Feun LG: Tumor lysis syndrome after induction chemotherapy in small-cell lung carcinoma. *Am J Clin Oncol* 13:10–13, 1990.
118. Loosveld OJ, Schouten HC, Gaillard CA, et al: Acute tumor lysis syndrome in a patient with acute lymphoblastic leukemia after a single dose of prednisone. *Brit J Haematol* 77:122–123, 1991.
119. Sparano J, Ramirez M, Wiernik PH: Increasing recognition of corticosteroid-induced tumor lysis syndrome in non-Hodgkin's lymphoma. *Cancer* 65:1072–1073, 1990.
120. Marcus SL, Einzig AI: Acute tumor lysis syndrome, prevention and management. In Dutcher JP, Wiernik PH (eds), *Handbook of Hematologic and Oncologic Emergencies.* New York: Plenum, 1987, pp. 9–16.
121. Flombaum C: Electrolyte and renal abnormalities in the cancer patient. In Howland WS, Carlon GC (eds), *Critical Care of the Cancer Patient.* Chicago: Yearbook Medical Publishers, 1985, pp. 114–142.
122. Patterson KL, Klopovich P: Metabolic emergencies in pediatric oncology: The acute tumor lysis syndrome. *J Assoc Pediatr Oncol Nurses* 4(3–4):19–24, 1988.
123. Nace CS, Nace GS: Acute tumor lysis syndrome: Pathophysiology and nursing management. *Crit Care Nurs* 5(3):26–34, 1985.
124. Silverman P, Distelhorst CW: Metabolic emergencies in clinical oncology. *Semin Oncol* 16(6):504–515, 1989.
125. Burry M, Martens L: ADH: Antidiuretic hormone and its inappropriate secretion. *Cancer Nurs* 76(2):41–43, 1980.
126. Bunn PA, Riggway EC: Paraneoplastic syndromes. In DeVita VT, Hellman S, Rosenberg SA (eds), *Cancer Principles and Practice of Oncology* (3d ed). Philadelphia: Lippincott, 1989, pp. 1902–1905.
127. Lokich JJ: The frequency and clinical biology of the ectopic hormone syndromes of small cell carcinoma. *Cancer* 50:2111–2114, 1982.
128. Hansen M, Hansen HH, Hirsch FR, et al: Hormonal polypeptides and amine metabolites in small cell carcinoma of the lung with special reference to stage and subtypes. *Cancer* 45:1432–1437, 1980.
129. Hainsworth D, Workman R, Greco FA: Management of the syndrome of inappropriate antidiuretic hormone secretion in small cell lung cancer. *Cancer* 51:161–165, 1983.
130. Moses AM, Blumenthal SA, Streeten DH, et al: Acid base and electrolyte disorders associated with endocrine disease, pituitary and thyroid. In Arieff AI, Defronzo RA (eds), *Fluid, Electrolyte, and Acid Base Disorders* (Vol 2). New York: Churchill-Livingston, 1985, pp. 872–877.
131. Ritch PS: Cis-dichlorodiamineplatinum II induced syndrome of inappropriate antidiuretic hormone. *Cancer* 61:448–450, 1988.
132. Minna JD, Pass H, Glastein EJ, et al: Cancer of the lung. In DeVita VT, Hellman S, Rosenberg SA (eds), *Cancer Principles and Practice of Oncology* (3d ed). Philadelphia: Lippincott, 1989, pp. 591–705.
133. Kamoi K, Ebe T, Hasegawa A, et al: Hyponatremia in small cell lung cancer: Mechanisms not involving inappropriate ADH secretion. *Cancer* 6(5):1089–1093, 1987.
134. Poe CM, Taylor LM: Syndrome of inappropriate antidiuretic hormone: Assessment and nursing implications. *Oncol Nurs Forum* 16(3):373–382, 1989.
135. Coleman P: Antidiuretic hormone: Physiology and pathophysiology—A review. *J Neurosurg Nurs* 199–204, Dec 11, 1979.

136. Schaefer SL: Oncologic complications: SIADH. In Otto S (ed), *Oncology Nursing*. St. Louis, MO: Mosby Year Book, 1991, pp. 468–523.
137. Hantman D, Rossier B, Zohlman R, et al: Rapid secretion correction of hyponatremia in the syndrome of inappropriate secretion of antidiuretic hormone: An alternative treatment to hypertonic saline. *Ann Intern Med* 78:870–875, 1973.
138. Kleger A, Lovett D: Electrolyte abnormalities in cancer patients. In Yarbro W, Bornstein R (eds), *Oncologic Emergencies*. New York: Grune & Stratton, 1981, pp. 215–246.
139. McEvoy G: American Hospital Formulatory Service. AHFS: Drug Information, Bethesda, MD: AHFS, 1991, pp. 323–324.
140. Schaefer SL: Oncologic complications: Spinal cord compression. In Otto SE (ed), *Oncology Nursing*. St. Louis, MO: Mosby Year Book, 1991, pp. 468–526.
141. Bruckman JE, Bloomer WD: Management of spinal cord compression. *Semin Oncol* 5:135–140, 1978.
142. Cairncross JG, Posner JB: Neurological complications of systemic cancer. In Yarbro JW, Bornstein RS (eds), *Oncology Emergencies*. New York: Grune & Stratton, 1981, pp. 73–96.
143. Black P: Spinal metastasis: Current status and recommended guidelines for management. *Neurosurgery* 5:726–746, 1979.
144. Pallet PS, O'Brien MT: Anatomy and physiology of the spinal cord. *Textbook of Neurological Nursing*. Boston: Little, Brown, 1985, pp. 110–132.
145. Chernecky CC, Ramsey PW: *Critical Nursing Care of the Client with Cancer*. Norwalk CT: Appleton-Century-Crofts, 1984, pp. 195–201.
146. Hickey JV: *The Clinical Practice of Neurological and Neurosurgical Nursing*. Philadelphia: Lippincott, 1986, pp. 483–492.
147. Flynn DF, Shipley WU: Management of spinal cord compression secondary to metastatic prostatic carcinoma. *Urol Clin North Am* 18(1):145–152, 1991.
148. Black P. Metastatic tumors of the central nervous system: Spinal metastases. In Abeloff MD (ed), *Complications of Cancer*. Baltimore, MD: Johns Hopkins University Press, 1979, pp. 313–356.
149. Findley JP: Nursing management of common oncologic emergencies. In Ziegfeld CR, Cossman JT, McMillan SC, Strohl, RA (eds), *Core Curriculum for Oncology Nursing*. Philadelphia: Saunders, 1987, pp. 321–332.
150. Klein PW: Neurologic emergencies in oncology. *Semin Oncol Nurs* 1:278–284, 1985.
151. Gilbert RW, Kim JH, Posner JB: Epidural spinal cord compression from metastatic tumor: Diagnosis and treatment. *Ann Neurol* 3:40–51, 1978.
152. Siegal TA, Siegal TZ: Current considerations in the management of neoplastic spinal cord compression. *Spine* 14(2):223–228, 1989.
153. Posner JB: Neurological complications of systemic cancer. *Med Clin North Am* 55:625–646, 1971.
154. Delaney TF, Oldfield EH: Spinal cord compression: Oncologic emergencies. In DeVita VT, Hellman S, Rosenberg SA (eds), *Cancer Principles and Practice of Oncology* (3d ed). Philadelphia: Lippincott, 1989, pp. 1978–1986.
155. Glover D, Glick JH: Oncologic emergencies: Spinal cord compression. In Holleb AI, Fink DJ, Murphy GP (eds), *American Cancer Society Textbook of Clinical Oncology*. Atlanta, GA: American Cancer Society, 1991, pp. 513–533.
156. Hollis PH, Malis LI, Zappullo RA: Neurological deterioration after lumbar puncture below complete spinal subarachnoid block. *J Neurosurg* 64:253, 1986.
157. Sundaresan N, Galicich JH, Lane JM, et al: Treatment of neoplastic epidural cord compression by vertebral body resection and stabilization. *J Neurosurg* 63:676–684, 1985.
158. Marlenson JA, Evans RG, Lie MR, et al: Treatment outcome and complications in patients treated for malignant epidural spinal cord compression. *J Neuro-Oncol* 3:77–84, 1985.
159. Posner JB, Howieson J, Cvitkovic E: Disappearing spinal cord compression: Oncolytic effects of glucocorticoids and other chemotherapeutic agents on epidural metastases. *Ann Neurol* 2:409–413, 1977.
160. Greenberg HS, Kim JH, Posner JB: Epidural spinal cord compression from metastatic tumor: Results with a new treatment protocol. *Ann Neurol* 8:361–366, 1980.
161. McEvoy GK: American Hospital Formulary Service Drug Information '91. Bethesda, MD: American Hospital Formulary Service, 1991.
162. Portnoy RK, Lipton RB, Foley KM: Back pain in the cancer patient: An algorithm for evaluation and management. *Neurology* 37:134–137, 1987.
163. Dyck S: Surgical instrumentation as a palliative treatment for spinal cord compression. *Oncol Nurs Forum* 18(3):515–521, 1991.

Chapter 35

Late Effects of Cancer Treatment

Ida Marie (Ki) Moore, RN, DNSc

Kathleen S. Ruccione, RN, MPH

INTRODUCTION

More than 5 million Americans with a history of cancer are alive today; 3 million of these cases were diagnosed 5 or more years ago. At least half these individuals can be considered biologically cured.[1] For children, in particular, 63% survive 5 years or more from the time of diagnosis, an improvement of 40% since the early 1970s. In fact, the current estimate is that by the year 2000, one in every 1000 young adults from 20 to 29 years of age will be a survivor of childhood cancer.[2]

Biologic cure refers to a patient who has no evidence of disease, has the same life expectancy as a person who never had cancer, and ultimately dies of unrelated causes.[3] Given the state of the art in cancer treatment, this cure is not without consequences. These consequences, or *late effects,* result from physiologic changes related to particular treatments or to the interactions among the treatment, the individual, and the disease. In contrast to the acute side effects of chemotherapy and radiation that are due to the death of proliferative cells in tissues with relatively rapid renewal, late biologic toxicity is believed to progress over time and by different mechanisms.

Late effects can appear months to years after treatment and can be mild to severe to life-threatening. They can be clinically obvious, clinically subtle, or subclinical. Their impact depends on the age and developmental state of the patient. Young people may rebound from the acute toxicities of treatment better than adults, but the growing child may be more vulnerable to the effects of delayed toxicities. A great unknown is what will happen to individuals who received intensive treatment in their youth as they age. Although we may not be able to detect any obvious side effects soon after the completion of treatment, the effect of even subtle tissue damage on the process of aging is unknown. For adults the cumulative effects of mild but permanent treatment toxicity in hearts, lungs, and kidneys when combined with hereditary predisposition to particular health problems and environmental exposure to pollutants are unknown. This chapter summarizes what is currently known about the long-term consequences of treatment on organ systems and on the development of second malignancies. The treatments associated with specific late effects and individual risk factors are discussed. For many late toxicities the specific mechanisms of pathogenesis are not well understood. This content is included whenever possible.

CENTRAL NERVOUS SYSTEM

Neuropsychologic, neuroanatomic, and neurophysiologic changes can occur as a result of central nervous system (CNS) treatment. These late effects have been observed in children with acute lymphoblastic leukemia (ALL) and brain tumors and in adult small-cell carcinoma of the lung (SCCL) patients, all of whom received CNS treatment for the primary tumor or as prophylaxis against meningeal disease.

Neuropsychologic Effects

The most frequently described neuropsychologic late effects of CNS treatment include significant decrements (10–20 points on the *WIS-R*) in general intellectual potential and academic achievement scores,[4–10] as well as specific deficits in visual-motor integration, attention, memory, and visual-motor skills.[6,11–20] Nonverbal, or performance, skills seem to be particularly vulnerable to the deleterious effects of CNS treatment,[15–17] and deficits in these areas may be among the first to appear.

An important hallmark of neuropsychologic late effects is that they do not become apparent until 24–36 months following treatment.[4,7,8] For example, Obetz et al.[21] found that 48% of children with ALL who had received treatment that involved the CNS more than 2 years prior to the time of evaluation had neuropsychologic or neuroanatomic abnormalities. This latency between CNS treatment and the manifestation of neuropsychologic late effects also has been observed in other patient populations.[10,18,19]

To overcome the problem of obtaining reliable pretreatment measures of intellectual functioning, several studies of children treated with cranial radiation have used healthy siblings' scores as a baseline estimate because the intelligence scores of siblings show high correlation. The findings from these studies demonstrated that children whose treatment involved the CNS were functioning at a significantly lower level than their healthy brothers and sisters[22–26] and that the differences became more marked over time.[22]

The type of CNS treatment that has been most closely associated with neuropsychologic deficits is cranial radiation in combination with intrathecal (IT) chemotherapy. Numerous studies have compared children with ALL who received 2400 cGy of whole-brain radiation in combination with IT methotrexate with those who received only IT methotrexate for CNS prophylaxis. The findings provide strong evidence that radiation is closely linked to long-term functional problems.[3,7,11,18,21,24,26–28] Although less is known about the effects of intrathecal chemotherapy, several studies suggest that there are no deficits, or that the deficits are less severe.[27,29]

There may be a synergistic effect between cranial radiation and chemotherapy that increases the magnitude of the toxicity. Robinson et al.[5] found that longer duration of chemotherapy was closely associated with lower intelligence quotient (IQ) scores in children with ALL who were treated with 2400 cGy, and Duffner et al.[10] reported that adjuvant chemotherapy was a significant risk factor associated with declines in IQ in patients with brain tumors who received radiation. The schedule of administration of intrathecal methotrexate when used in combination with whole-brain radiation may influence intellectual function. Balsom and associates[30] found that full, performance, and verbal scale IQ scores were consistently higher in girls who received IT methotrexate prior to and during cranial radiation than in the corresponding control group who received (IT) methotrexate concurrent with whole-brain radiation.

It is difficult to systematically determine if a radiation-dose response relationship exists for neuropsychologic sequelae. There is modest evidence that young children who received whole-brain radiation doses of less than 1000 cGy in preparation for bone marrow transplantation are neurologically and intellectually normal.[31–33] Tameroff et al.[34] reported that children who received either 1800 or 2400 cGy of whole-brain radiation and IT methotrexate had significantly lower full and performance IQ and visual motor integration test scores than those who received only IT methotrexate; however, there were no significant differences between the scores of children in the two radiation groups. In contrast, higher doses of radiation (e.g., 2400–4800 cGy), which frequently are used in the treatment of brain tumors or micrometastasis in SCCL, tend to result in more severe impairments.[26,35–38]

Age at the time of CNS treatment is an important risk factor for neurologic sequelae.[4,7,8,11,25] Children who receive at least 2400 cGy of cranial radiation before the age of 3,[10,25] 4,[38] or 5[6,18] years are at greatest risk for neuropsychologic late effects. This age-at-time-of-treatment effect has been attributed to the deleterious effects of radiation and chemotherapy on the processes of brain development that occur during early childhood.[40,41] There are no reported studies of the significance of age at the time of CNS treatment with lower doses of radiation. In addition to age, recent evidence suggests that girls are more severely affected than boys in terms of general cognitive performance such as IQ scores.[42] Balsom et al.[30] found that the protective effect of pre-irradiation IT methotrexate was most significant in girls less than 5 years of age at the time of CNS treatment.

Neuroanatomic Effects

Computed tomography (CT) and magnetic resonance imaging (MRI) have been used to evaluate structural changes after CNS treatment. Brouwers et al.[43] found that the CT scans of 13 of 23 (57%) long-term survivors of ALL who received 2400 cGy of whole-brain radiation showed abnormalities. Similarly, there are reports that 73% of children with brain tumors[44] and from 70%–100% of those with SCCL[12,21] treated with higher radiation doses have neuroanatomic changes that are unrelated to the tumor itself.

Atrophy and decreased subcortical white matter are the most frequently reported abnormalities. Atrophy usually is manifested as ventricular dilatation and widening of the subarachnoid spaces; it has been reported in 25%–51% of patients treated with cranial radiation.[44–47] Periventricular hypodensity, believed to represent decreased white matter, has been documented in 26% of patients with brain tumors[44] and 45% of those with SCCL;[21] however, it has occurred less frequently in patients with ALL who received 1800–2400 cGy of radiation.[41,45,48]

Other less common neuroanatomic abnormalities include calcification[26,34,45,47] and leukoencephalopathy.[12,35] As with neuropsychologic effects, these neuroanatomic changes are associated most closely with cranial radiation, although mild indications of atrophy and white matter degeneration have been reported in up to 20% of children who received only IT methotrexate.[46,47]

These studies of neuroanatomic pathologic conditions suggest that higher radiation doses result in a greater incidence and severity of abnormalities. Age at the time of CNS treatment also may be important. Davis et al.[44] reported that children with brain tumors who receive irradiation before the age of 3 years are at greatest risk for abnormalities, and Tsurada et al.[49] found that the highest incidence of white matter degeneration in adult patients with brain tumors occurred in those older than 60 years of age. This finding is of interest because it suggests that the aging, as well as the developing, brain may be more vulnerable to the deleterious effects of cancer treatment involving the CNS.

Mechanisms of Pathogenesis

The pathogenesis of delayed injury to normal tissue after treatment of the CNS is not well understood. Sheline et al.[50] suggest that demyelination may be important in the early stages of delayed injury, with ischemia becoming progressively significant over time. Oligodendroglia, the myelin-producing cells in the CNS, are proliferative during early childhood and therefore radiosensitive. Damage to or a reproductive loss of glial cells from radiation can disrupt the myelin membrane that insulates axons. Antigens released from the damaged glial cells initiate an autoimmune response that can also contribute to the pathogenesis of delayed tissue damage.[51]

A synergistic relationship between radiation and methotrexate may account for progressive demyelination.[52,53] The reduction of dihydrofolate to tetrahydrofolate, which is necessary for 1-carbon transfers in phospholipid synthesis, is inhibited by methotrexate. Procarbazine, which frequently is used in combination with methotrexate in the treatment of SCCL, can further this neurotoxicity by potentiating the methotrexate-induced depletion of the 1-carbon pool.[21] The result is disruption and loss of integrity in phospholipid membranes, such as the myelin sheath. An interference with phospholipid synthesis has been hypothesized as the underlying mechanism of demyelination[53] and a contributing factor to the pathogenesis of delayed tissue damage.[54,56] Degenerative changes of glial cells, disruption of myelin sheaths, thickened capillary walls, and necrotizing and sclerotic microangiopathy have been documented in children who died of leukoencephalopathy (progressive white matter destruction) and had been treated with a cumulative dose of 2000 cGy of cranial radiation and intravenous methotrexate.[56]

Myelin basic protein (MBP) has been used as a marker for the disruption in synthesis or increased breakdown of myelin following CNS treatment. Elevated MBP has been measured in the cerebral spinal fluid of patients with ALL who have clinical and neuroradiologic evidence of leukoencephalopathy.[57,58] In one study the persistent release of MBP correlated with the progression of neurotoxicity.[58] Patients with elevations in MBP had received CNS treatment involving either 2400 cGy of whole-brain radiation in combination with IT methotrexate or triple IT therapy with methotrexate, hydrocortisone, and cytosine arabinoside. Children without evidence of leukoencephalopathy, however, did not have elevations in MBP in the cerebral spinal fluid with neuropsychologic and/or neuroanatomic sequelae.

Damage to the endothelial cells of the microvasculature is believed to play an important role in the pathogenesis of delayed injury following CNS treatment.[52,53,59,60] These cells may be particularly vulnerable to the damaging effects of radiation because of their replicating capacity.[59] The consequences of endothelial cell damage include increased synthesis and density of collagenous tissue and loss of the tight intracellular junctions that form the blood-brain barrier. These pathologic changes result in decreased perfusion, increased blood-brain barrier permeability, and disruption of active transport mechanisms. The net effect is inflammation, ischemia, and loss of parenchymal tissue function. Vascular changes have been documented in animals treated with low to moderate doses of radiation[61] and in human beings who received 1500–6000 cGy.[56,62]

Vision and Hearing

In addition to the long-term effects of CNS treatment involving neuropsychologic function and neuroanatomy, visual deficits and hearing loss also can occur. Enucleation, which may be necessary in the treatment of ocular tumors such as retinoblastoma, is the most disabling visual deficit. Cataracts have been associated with cranial irradiation and long-term corticosteroid therapy.[63] They may be detected on a visual examination or require a slit-lamp examination.

Hearing loss in the high-tone range is most closely associated with cisplatin.[64] Recent evidence from a limited study of children with brain tumors suggests that treatment with high doses of cranial irradiation within 10 months of cisplatin administration increases the sensitivity to the ototoxic effects of this drug in young children. Profound hearing loss occurred in all frequency ranges.[65] The investigators postulated that postirradiation hyperemia may have increased the sensitivity of the cochlea to cisplatin damage. Recurrent otitis media, a common problem in children receiving chemotherapy, as well as the use of antibiotics that are ototoxic, also can contribute to hearing loss.

ENDOCRINE SYSTEM

Cancer treatment can adversely affect a number of endocrine functions, including metabolism, growth, secondary sexual development, and reproduction. These late effects result from damage to the target organ (i.e., thyroid, ovary, and testis), and/or the hypothalamic pituitary axis. Table 35-1 summarizes the major endocrine sequelae, related risk factors, and recommendations for evaluation and treatment.

Thyroid

Direct damage to the thyroid gland causes primary hypothyroidism with a decreased production of thyroxine (T_4) and triiodothyronine (T_3). These hormones have biologic effects on oxygen consumption, the central and peripheral nervous systems, skeletal and cardiac muscle, carbohydrate and cholesterol metabolism, and growth and development.[66] Primary hypothyroidism can be compensated when there is only partial organ damage and some function is preserved. The compensated state is maintained by an increased production of thyrotropin-releasing factor (TRF) and thyroid-stimulating hormone (TSH) from the hypothalamus and pituitary. This chronic overstimulation is of concern because it is believed to increase the risk of malignant transformation in previously damaged cells.

Overt or compensated primary hypothyroidism has been documented in 4%–80% of patients who received radiation to the neck for Hodgkin's disease, other lymphomas, and carcinomas.[67–76] Damage to the thyroid gland usually occurs after radiation doses of more than 2000 cGy in multiple fractions. Sklar et al.,[76] however, documented hypothyroidism in 47% of children who received a single dose of 750 cGy of whole-body radiation in preparation for bone marrow transplantation. In general, the incidence and severity of thyroid dysfunction appear to increase with higher radiation doses and may be due to damage to thyroid follicular cells, thyroid vasculature, or connective tissue. There are no chemotherapeutic agents that have been associated with long-term thyroid damage.

The importance of age at time of irradiation has been difficult to assess. Although hypothyroidism usually develops 3–4 years after treatment, it can occur as late as 7–14 years afterward.[73,77] Glatstein et al.[67] reported a higher incidence of dysfunction in patients

TABLE 35-1 Endocrine Late Effects and Associated Risk Factors

Ovaries	Chemotherapy	Radiation	High Risk	Evaluation	Treatment
Ovaries	Procarbazine Cyclophosphamide Nitrogen mustard Busulfan (age-dependent)	400–800 cGy Age-dependent	Older > younger age Abdominal and pelvic tumors Hodgkin's disease Spinal radiation (ALL, brain tumors)	LH FSH Estradiol	Oophoropexy before treatment Replacement hormones
Testes	Procarbazine Cyclophosphamide Nitrogen mustard Busulfan	≤400 cGy: Azospermia with recovery possible ≥600 cGy: Permanent azoospermia ≥2400 cGy: Leydig cell damage (↓ testosterone)	Pelvic tumors Testicular tumors Testicular leukemia Hodgkin's disease	LH FSH Testosterone	Sperm banking before treatment Transposition of testicles before treatment Replacement hormones
Thyroid	None currently identified	>2000 cGy overt or compensatory hypothyroidism: Graves' disease ≥750 cGy TBI for BMT: hypothyroidism	Younger > older age Hodgkin's disease Head and neck tumors Brain tumors Leukemia (cranial rad) Bone marrow transplantation	Free triiodothyronine Thyroxine Antithyroid and antichromosomal autoantibodies (follow-up to 15 yr)	Replacement hormones
Hypothalamic: pituitary axis	None currently identified	≥2400 cGy: Hypothalamic dysfunction ≥4000 cGy: Pituitary dysfunction	CNS tumors Head and neck tumors Leukemia with CNS irradiation	Growth chart Growth hormone Pulsatile test Stimulation test Somatomedian-C LH, FSH Prolactin	Replacement hormones Bromocriptine

ALL = acute lymphocytic leukemia; *BMT* = bone marrow transplantation; *FSH* = follicle-stimulating hormone; *LH* = luteinizing hormone; *TBI* = total body irratiation; *CNS* = central nervous system.

Source: Hobbie WL, Schwartz CL: Endocrine late effects among survivors of cancer, *Semin Oncol Nurs* 5:15, 1989. Reprinted with permission.

treated before the age of 20 years, which was attributed to an increased sensitivity of the thyroid in younger individuals or to an induced sensitivity from prolonged iodine release in the contrast used in lymphangiograms.[74] Others have found that age at time of irradiation is not a significant risk factor.[78,79]

When the hypothalamic pituitary axis is in the field of radiation to the nasopharynx of the CNS, secondary hypothyroidism can occur. Decreased levels of TRF, TSH, T_3, and T_4 have been reported in patients who received at least 5500 cGy of external beam radiation for nasopharyngeal, paranasal sinus, or brain tumors that did not involve the hypothalamus or pituitary.[80,81] These studies found no difference in the development of secondary hypothyroidism between children and adults; however, the majority of subjects were adults. As with primary thyroid dysfunction, secondary hypothyroidism may not develop until years after the completion of therapy.

Growth

Growth hormone deficiency with short stature is one of the most common long-term endocrine consequences of radiation to the CNS in children. Growth impairment with deficient growth hormone release and decreased linear growth rate has been found in 50%–100% of children with brain tumors who received 2400 cGy or more of cranial or craniospinal radiation.[36,82–88] Children with ALL who received radiation for CNS prophylaxis have demonstrated a similar pattern of growth disturbances.[89–94] Pituitary dysfunction requires radiation doses of at least 4000 cGy, but damage to the hypothalamus occurs with lower doses.[95] Although the belief has been that growth disturbances as a result of hypothalamic damage require doses of at least 2400 cGy,[95,96] Starceski et al.[97] observed a 25% decline in height percentile in children treated with 2400 cGy and 14% in children treated with 1800 cGy. In both groups, growth velocity decreased significantly over 3 years following treatment and did not recover. Sanders et al.[98] observed partial growth hormone deficiency in 6 of 18 children who received total body irradiation in preparation for bone marrow transplantation. A dose-response relationship has been demonstrated, with higher doses resulting in more significant growth abnormalities.[95] Clayton and Shalet[99] found that dose of whole-brain radiation (from 27–47.5 Gy) and time from irradiation were significant predictors of growth hormone (GH) deficiency. The overall incidence of GH deficiency (74%) 5 years after treatment was comparable across radiation doses; however, children who received 30 Gy or more of radiation developed growth hormone deficiency earlier. The fewer the number of fractionations for a given radiation dose, the greater the risk of long-term sequelae.[89] Children treated with cranial radiation before the age of 5 years are believed to be more susceptible to growth deficits,[91] which may become most apparent during periods of rapid growth.[100] Growth retardation may be more pronounced in children who receive cranial and spinal irradiation because of spinal shortening.[85]

Secondary Sexual Development and Reproduction

Chemotherapy, specifically alkylating agents (e.g., cyclophosphamide, mechlorethamine, busulfan, and procarbazine) can cause permanent damage to the gonads. Primary ovarian failure, with amenorrhea, decreased estradiol, and elevated gonadotropins (luteinizing hormone and follicle-stimulating hormone), has been reported in women who received these agents for Hodgkin's disease,[101–103] breast cancer,[104,105] and ovarian germ cell tumors.[106] In younger patients, ovarian damage is manifested as failure to develop secondary sexual characteristics or as arrested pubertal development.[107] Shalet[108] observed ovarian dysfunction in 4 of 12 girls with ALL who received cyclophosphamide. In 3 patients, normal pubertal development subsequently occurred, which suggests that both transient and permanent damage can occur.

Damage to the germinal epithelium of the testis with decreased or absent spermatogonia can occur in males treated with alkylating agents.[109] Leydig cell damage is unusual; thus, testosterone production and pubertal development are not affected.[109] Testicular damage with azoospermia is most frequent in males with Hodgkin's disease who received MOPP (mechlorethamine, vincristine, procarbazine, and prednisone)[110–113] but also has been observed in males with ALL treated with cyclophosphamide and cytosine arabinoside.[114]

Age at time of treatment, sex, total drug dose, and the use of combinations of alkylating agents are important risk factors for gonadal failure. The quiescence of the prepubertal gonad provides some protection, whereas the incidence of gonadal damage increases with age and stage in pubertal development. The testis appears to be more sensitive than the ovary to the damaging effects of therapy. Rivkees and Crawford[112] reported that the incidence of gonadal dysfunction increased from 0% in prepubertal girls and 14% in prepubertal boys to 71% in sexually mature women and 95% in mature men. Byrne et al.[115] found that the fertility of men treated with alkylating agents was half that of the fertility of control subjects, whereas the fertility of women was unimpaired.

The risk of gonadal failure also increases with greater total doses of alkylating agents and the use of more than one drug, such as in MOPP therapy. For example, Koyama et al.[104] found that the dose of cyclophosphamide that resulted in amenorrhea was 5.2 g in women older than 40 years and 20.4 g in those 20–29 years of age. Similarly, 64% of men treated with less than three cycles of MOPP had recovery of spermatogenesis, whereas those treated with more than five cycles had persistent azoospermia.[116]

Radiation is another cause of gonadal dysfunction. Pathologic changes in women who receive radiation to the ovaries include reduced numbers of oocytes, inhibited follicle development, atrophic ovaries, and strong fibrohyalinization.[117,118] Older women are at greater risk for ovarian failure following radiation. The ovaries may be preserved in women who receive 800 cGy; however, ovarian failure has been reported in 100% of women older than 40 years of age treated with 400 cGy.[119,120]

The testis is extremely sensitive to the damaging effects of radiation. The threshold dose required to damage the germinal epithelium is as low as 300–900 cGy,[121] whereas the Leydig cells are more resistant, with permanent damage occurring following doses at 2000 cGy.[122] Scatter to the ovaries and testes as a result of abdominal or craniospinal irradiation also can result in long-term damage.[123,124] In a large retrospective cohort study of 2283 survivors of childhood cancer, Byrne et al.[115] found that radiation therapy directed below the diaphragm depressed fertility in men and women by approximately 25%, and combined therapy involving infradiaphragmatic radiation and alkylating agents reduced fertility to almost 50% of that in the control subjects. However, testicular damage and ovarian failure occur infrequently after treatment for leukemia with regimens that do not include alkylating agents or cytosine arabinoside, and there does not appear to be an increased frequency of adverse pregnancy outcome (i.e., spontaneous abortions and stillbirths) compared to the general population.[125]

Radiation to the cranium or nasopharynx can damage the hypothalamic pituitary axis, causing secondary gonadal failure. Subnormal levels of luteinizing hormone (LH), follicle-stimulating hormone (FSH), and prolactin-inhibiting factor (PIF) have been found in both sexes treated for head and neck tumors with 400–7800 cGy of radiation.[80,126] In addition to the effects of low LH and FSH levels on ovarian and testicular function, the decrease in PIF and resultant increase in prolactin caused irregular menses, anovulatory periods, low testosterone, reduced libido, and impotence.[80,127]

IMMUNE SYSTEM

Immunosuppression has long been recognized as one of the most serious acute toxic effects of chemotherapy and radiation. A more recent discovery is that certain aspects of immune function can be adversely affected for years after the completion of treatment. These immunologic late effects have been studied most thoroughly in patients treated for leukemia, Hodgkin's disease, and breast cancer.

The early studies of children who received combination chemotherapy for ALL measured immune system recovery by absolute lymphocyte, T-cell, and B-cell counts and by immunoglobulin production.[128,129] A rebound of these parameters within the first 12 months was observed and may have contributed to the assumption that immunocompetence is restored during this time period.

More recent studies provide compelling evidence for persistent immunologic impairments following radiation and chemotherapy. The lymphopenia that occurs immediately after radiation usually involves both cellular (T-cell) and humoral (B-cell) immunity.[130] The time required for recovery of these cell populations, however, is very different.[131–134] The B-lymphocytes gradually repopulate within 12 months,[133,135] whereas T-lymphocyte depletion is much more prolonged. Of particular significance is the finding that suppressor T-cells recover more rapidly than T-helper cells, which seem to be particularly radiosensitive. The result is an inversion of the helper-to-suppressor ratio that can persist for as long as 10 years following local radiation for breast cancer,[133,134] nodal radiation for Hodgkin's disease,[135,136] and total body irradiation prior to bone marrow transplantation.[137] Decreased lymphocyte proliferative capacity, natural killer cells, and immunoglobulin production associated with defective suppressor-cell immunoregulation and an abnormal helper-to-suppressor cell ratio also have been observed in patients treated with multiagent chemotherapy for Hodgkin's disease[138] and leukemia.[139–141] In addition, a pronounced long-term effect on plasma cell and immunoglobulin production, with a possible effect on T-cell function, also has been observed in children with ALL.[139,140]

The immunosuppressive effects of specific chemotherapeutic agents are not well known. The use of radiation in conjunction with multiagent chemotherapy can result in more frequent and more severe immune system impairment.[142] Larger volumes of irradiated bone marrow and greater total radiation doses result in more severe hematopoietic depression and more prolonged recovery. In a study of 32 patients with lymphoma who received either mantle or mantle with inverted Y radiation, bone marrow recovery was observed following doses of 2000 cGy, but recovery was markedly limited after 4000 cGy.[143] Compensation by hyperactivity of the nonradiated marrow persisted for up to 10 years after radiation. Bone marrow regeneration also has been found to be slower and less extensive in older patients (20 years of age or older).[144]

The clinical significance of these long-term alterations in immune function is not well understood. There is no evidence that patients with persistent immunologic abnormalities are at greater risk for infections. One group of patients who is at increased risk of infections are those who have undergone splenectomy. Overwhelming bacterial infections, primarily pneumococcal, are a major concern to these individuals because of the protective role of the spleen against encapsulated organisms. Persistent immune defects have not been linked to the occurrence of second malignancies. This may change, however, as survival time increases for larger numbers of patients.

CARDIOVASCULAR SYSTEM

The use of anthracyclines, such as daunorubicin and doxorubicin, has improved survival in patients with acute leukemias, lymphomas, pediatric solid tumors, and other cancers. One of the most serious late effects of these drugs is cardiac toxicity, which typically presents as cardiomyopathy, with clinical signs of congestive heart failure. Recent evidence, however, indicates that structural damage to the heart can occur in the absence of clinical signs. Steinherz et al.[145,146] detected abnormalities of contractility and rhythm, apparently related to myocardial fibrosis, on echocardiograms obtained 4 to 20 years after anthracycline therapy. These investigators also have documented cardiac failure, dysrhythmias, and sudden deaths many years following completion of therapy. Some of the patients with these late complications had no early symptoms. Myocardial fibrosis was present on autopsy in all cases of sudden death.[145,146]

The risk of cardiotoxicity is related to cumulative dose,[145–147] schedule of administration (continuous versus intermittent), and presence of other factors such as mediastinal irradiation.[148] Cumulative doses of 550 mg/m^2 have been associated with cardiac toxicity;[149,150] similar abnormalities can occur after lower doses in adults and children.[151] Lipshultz and colleagues[147] found that 57% of children with acute leukemia treated with doxorubicin developed abnormalities of left ventricular afterload or contractility. The cumulative dose of doxorubicin was the most significant predictor of abnormal cardiac function. Table 35-2 includes a summary of cardiotoxicity, methods of assessment, and suggestions for intervention.

Individuals who received radiation therapy to a field that includes the heart, such as mediastinal radiation for Hodgkin's disease or other lymphomas, also are at risk for cardiotoxicity. Radiation-induced cardiotoxic-

TABLE 35-2 Biologic Late Effects on Selected Organ Systems

Body System	Health Problem	Associated Treatment Modality	Method of Assessment	Management and Nursing Considerations
Cardiovascular	Cardiomyopathy	Anthracycline chemotherapy Risk increased with lifetime cumulative dose >550 mg/m², mediastinal irradiation	Detection is difficult: ECG, echocardiogram, scans may be inadequate Monitor with clinical observation for shortness of breath, weight gain, edema	Careful monitoring of anthracycline dosage to limit lifetime dose If congestive heart failure develops, support care with digitalis, diuretics, sodium restriction, provision of adequate rest periods
	Pericardial damage	Mediastinal irradiation (eg: 4000–6000 cGY)	Clinical observation for chest pain, dyspnea, fever, paradoxic pulse, venous distention, friction rub, Kussmaul's sign Abnormalities visible on chest film	May be self-limiting If pericardial effusion occurs; treatment may include anti-inflammatory agents, pericardiectomy
	Peripheral vascular disease	Vinblastine	History of digital cold sensitivity	Avoidance of cold
Respiratory	Pulmonary fibrosis	Lung irradiation Some chemotherapeutic agents Risk increased with larger lung volume in radiation field, dose: 4000 cGy, radiation sensitizing chemotherapeutic agents	Clinical observation for dyspnea, rales, cough, decreased exercise tolerance, pulmonary insufficiency Monitor with physical examination, chest film, pulmonary function tests	Health education for smoking prevention/cessation Supportive care with provision of adequate rest periods Vigilance re: development of pulmonary infection
Musculoskeletal	Scoliosis, kyphosis	Radiation therapy for intra-abdominal tumor in which vertebrae absorb radiation unevenly	Regular physical examination May not become apparent until adolescent growth spurt	Referral to orthopedist for rehabilitative measures, instruction regarding normal weight Maintenance to make problem less noticeable
	Spinal shortening (decrease in sitting height)	Spinal irradiation (eg, for medulloblastoma); direct effect of radiation on growth centers of vertebral bodies	Serial measurements of sitting height (crown to rump)	Referral to orthopedist Anticipatory teaching regarding disproportion between shorter-than-usual trunk and normal leg length as full growth is attained; reassurance that disproportion probably will not be obvious to others but may be a problem in fitting clothing
	Increased susceptibility to fractures, poor healing, deformities, or shortening of extremities	Irradiation to lesions in long bones (eg, Ewing's sarcoma)	Regular physical examination	Referral to orthopedist Teaching about protective measures such as avoiding rough contact sports
	Facial asymmetry	Surgery plus irradiation to head and neck area (eg, for rhabdomyosarcoma) causing altered growth in facial bones	Physical examination Early evaluation by reconstructive surgeon	Anticipatory guidance regarding possible adjustment problems with visible deformity Referral to family counseling to manage or prevent adjustment and behavior problems

(continued)

TABLE 35-2 Biologic Late Effects on Selected Organ Systems (continued)

Body System	Health Problem	Associated Treatment Modlity	Method of Assessment	Management and Nursing Considerations
	Dental problems: gingival irritation and bleeding; tooth loosening, migration (can lead to peridontal disease); delayed/arrested tooth development	Radiation therapy to maxilla mandible areas; chemotherapy	Clinical observation with dental examination	Many dental problems can be minimized or prevented with good oral hygiene with flossing/brushing, gingival massage, use of plaque-disclosing tablets/solutions; preradiation therapy flouride prophylaxis; dental evaluation 2 wk postradiation; orthodontic treatment for malocclusion; extraction of damaged, nonfunctional teeth
Gastrointestinal	Chronic enteritis	Radiation therapy Risk increased with doses >5000 cGy, previous abdominal surgery, radiation-sensitizing chemotherapeutic agents	Clinical observation for pain, dysphagia, recurrent vomiting, obstipation/constipation, bloody or mucus-containing diarrhea, malabsorption syndrome	Nutritional consultation for diet plan to diminish symptoms while providing adequate nutrition for growth and development to fit family routine, ethnic or cultural customs; dietary modifications may include low-fat, low-residue, gluten-free, free of milk and milk products If enterostomy is performed, coordination with enterstomal therapist for patient family teaching about stoma care
	Hepatic fibrosis, cirrhosis	Radiation therapy Some chemotherapeutic agents	Clinical observation for pain, hepatomegaly, jaundice Monitoring with liver function tests and liver scans may be inconclusive, thus, periodic liver biopsy may be necessary	Supportive care with nutritional consultation
Kidney and urinary tract	Chronic nephritis (may lead to renal failure, cardiovascular damage)	Radiation to renal structures Risk increased with concomitant chemotherapy	Clinical observation and monitoring with blood pressure readings, urinalysis, CBC, BUN	If progressive renal failure develops, supportive care (possibly dialysis and/or transplantation)
	Chronic hemorrhagic cystitis	Chemotherapy (cyclophosphamide) Risk increased with pelvic radiation, inadequate hydration before, during, and after chemotherapy	Clinical observation for dysuria, urinary frequency, hematuria Monitoring with urinalysis	Ensure adequate hydration before, during, and after chemotherapy (3000 ml/m²/24 hr) Bladder hemorrhage may be treated with formalin instillation and/or fulguration of bleeding sites
	Unilateral kidney	Nephrectomy for Wilms' tumor	Clinical observation for dysuria, urinary frequency, flank pain, hematuria Monitoring with urinalysis	Health education to avoid injury to remaining kidney (eg, contact sports) If urinary tract infection develops; identification of causative organism, antibiotic treatment, repeat urinalysis Medic-Alert identification bracelet/tag

Source: Adapted from Ruccione K, Weinberg K: Late effects in multiple body systems, *Semin Oncol Nurs* 5:6–8, 1989. Reprinted with permission.

ity is manifested primarily as congestive heart failure. An acceleration of coronary artery disease that results in angina and myocardial infarction may occur in some patients.[148] Pericardial damage secondary to mediastinal irradiation is another cardiovascular complication.[152] Patients may have overt symptoms and/or abnormalities that are visible on x-ray examination. Pericardial damage may be self-limiting, but life-threatening pericardial effusions also can occur.[153] In general, peripheral vascular disease is a rare cardiovascular late effect. However, approximately 50% of patients with germ cell tumors of the testes treated with cisplatin, vinblastine, and bleomycin report having Raynaud's phenomenon.[154] Vinblastine is the suspected cause, but there is no evidence of a dose effect.

PULMONARY SYSTEM

Pneumonitis and pulmonary fibrosis are the major biologic late effects of treatment to the pulmonary system (see Table 35-2). These problems can be caused by chemotherapy, radiation therapy, and recurrent respiratory infections in immunosuppressed patients.[155,156] Pulmonary fibrosis occurs in 1%–5% of patients who receive bleomycin for treatment of Hodgkin's disease, non-Hodgkin's lymphoma, testicular cancer, and head and neck tumors.[157] The effect is dose-related, and the incidence of fibrosis increases to at least 10% if the cumulative dose exceeds 450 U.[158] Other factors that contribute to the toxic effects of bleomycin on the pulmonary system are advanced age and concurrent radiation therapy to the lungs.

Alkylating agents, primarily busulfan, and the nitrosourea agents (e.g., lomustine and carmustine) also have been associated with the development of pulmonary fibrosis. Busulfan currently is used as part of the preparative regimen for bone marrow transplantation in patients with leukemia. Although acute pulmonary toxicity appears to be less than that following total body irradiation, long-term follow-up is needed to determine the actual incidence and severity of late toxic effects of busulfan. Pulmonary fibrosis also has been observed in some patients treated with nitrosourea agents for brain tumors, lymphomas, and a variety of solid tumors. The risk is related to total cumulative dose, the patient's age, number of cycles of chemotherapy, and underlying disease.[159]

Pulmonary fibrosis is the most common type of chronic lung damage following radiation therapy. Obstructive lung disease also can occur. Pulmonary damage is more likely when higher radiation doses are used and when larger lung volumes are irradiated. Radiation therapy also can potentiate the long-term toxicity induced by other agents such as bleomycin and nitrosoureas.

GASTROINTESTINAL SYSTEM

Radiation and radiation-enhancing chemotherapeutic agents can have long-term effects on the gastrointestinal tract and the liver.[160] Although rare, vascular abnormalities and altered digestive system activity can result in malabsorption.[161] Late effects in the liver are more common and include hepatic fibrosis, cirrhosis, and portal hypertension. Radiation therapy in combination with radiation-enhancing agents, such as actinomycin D and possibly vincristine, can result in hepatic fibrosis. Portal hypertension can occur if the fibrosis is severe.[162] Methotrexate also has been linked to hepatic fibrosis and cirrhosis (although the use of citrovorum factor may minimize or prevent these effects), and methotrexate in combination with 6-mercaptopurine can result in cirrhosis with portal hypertension.[163] Finally, the administration of blood products as part of the supportive care of myelosuppressed patients can cause chronic hepatitis. Table 35-2 includes a summary of late biologic toxic effects in the gastrointestinal tract.

RENAL SYSTEM

Nephritis and cystitis are the major long-term renal toxicities that result from cancer treatment (see Table 35-2). Damage to the nephrons and bladder has been documented in patients treated with cyclophosphamide, ifosfamide, and cisplatin. The hemorrhagic cystitis that can occur following cyclophosphamide therapy may persist, and the risk is increased by concurrent pelvic radiation.[164,165] Radiation also can damage the kidneys. Radiation doses of 2000 cGy or less may minimize the risk of renal toxicity, whereas concurrent administration of radiation-enhancing drugs increases the risk.[166,167] Clinical manifestations of nephritis include proteinuria, hypertension, anemia, and progressive renal failure, although early detection and intervention may prevent irreversible damage. The compensatory hypertrophy of the remaining kidney following nephrecotomy for renal tumors such as Wilms' tumor has not been associated with any biologic consequences. However, urinary tract infections or trauma to the remaining kidney obviously can be a serious problem.

MUSCULOSKELETAL SYSTEM

The treatment most frequently associated with late effects in the musculoskeletal system is radiation. Stature already achieved at the time of radiotherapy, radiation dose, and volume of tissue irradiated are all risk factors.[168] Children treated at an early age (younger than 6 years) and those undergoing puberty are at high risk because of rapid growth and development. Uneven irradiation to the vertebrae, soft tissue, and muscles (e.g., radiation to one side of the body) for the treatment of intra-abdominal tumors frequently results in scoliosis or kyphosis, or both. Silber and colleagues[168] have developed a mathematical model for predicting adult stature in children successfully treated for cancer outside the CNS. The model is based on radiation dose adjusted for radiation site and attained height at the time of irradiation. Although more recent therapies have been modified to minimize these problems, skeletal abnormalities may occur in some children and tend to become more apparent during periods of rapid growth such as the adolescent growth spurt.[169] In a recent study of 31 children successfully treated for Wilms' tumor with surgery, chemotherapy, and radiation (orthovoltage or megavoltage), 10 children developed an orthopedic abnormality requiring intervention or a scoliotic curve greater than 20.[170] There were no orthopedic defects among children treated with megavoltage radiation. Other factors associated with the occurrence of significant late orthopedic problems were higher radiation dose (mean dose of 2890 cGy) and larger irradiated field (150 cm^2).

Spinal shortening, another radiation-related effect, is caused by damage to the growth centers in the vertebral bodies.[171] Children who receive spinal radiation frequently do not achieve their full height potential; those who receive craniospinal irradiation are at great risk for growth retardation because of central (hypothalamic-pituitary), as well as direct (skeletal), effects.

The late effects on long bones include functional limitations, shortening of the extremity, osteonecrosis, increased susceptibility to fractures, and poor healing.[148] Radiation is the treatment most commonly associated with these problems; however, prolonged use of corticosteroids also can have degenerative effects. Finally, surgical procedures such as amputation or limb disarticulation have obvious immediate and lasting cosmetic, as well as physical, consequences.

Altered growth of facial bones following maxillofacial or orbital irradiation or surgery causes facial asymmetry. This is a difficult problem that frequently occurs in children treated for tumors such as rhabdomyosarcoma. Maxillofacial irradiation also can cause a number of dental problems such as foreshortening and blunting of the roots, incomplete calcification, delayed or arrested tooth development, caries, and loosening.[172,173] Recently, dental problems in patients who were treated with chemotherapy have been reported and include abnormal occlusion, hypoplasia, enamel opacities, and radiologic abnormalities.[174]

SECOND MALIGNANT NEOPLASMS

It has been clearly established that adults and children who have received chemotherapy or radiation therapy, or both, for a primary malignancy are at increased risk for the development of a second malignant neoplasm. For example, in patients with Hodgkin's disease there is a 77-fold increased risk of the development of leukemia within 4 years of initial treatment.[175] For children the overall risk is estimated to be at least 10 times greater than the cancer incidence among age-matched children,[176] with a 20-year cumulative probability of 12%.[177] Malignant transformation of normal cells is due to nonlethal damage to the DNA that is not repaired. Alkylating agents and ionizing radiation are the treatments most closely linked to a second malignant neoplasm. In addition to the type and dose of treatment received, the risk of the development of a second cancer depends on several predisposing factors. Some tumors have a common underlying etiologic factor. For example, patients with bladder cancer are at greater risk for the development of lung cancer because both tumors are associated with smoking.[178] Genetic susceptibility is a second factor.[176] Children with the genetic form of retinoblastoma (which is usually bilateral) have a much higher incidence of sarcomas (as a second malignant neoplasm) than those with the nongenetic form of the disease.[179–181]

Second Malignancies Following Chemotherapy

Acute nonlymphocytic leukemia (ANL) following treatment with alkylating agents is the most common chemotherapy-related second malignant neoplasm. The disease usually is preceded by a period of prolonged pancytopenia and can occur as early as 1.3 years following the initiation of chemotherapy for the primary malignancy. The incidence of treatment-related ANL peaks at 5 years and plateaus at 10 years following treatment.[182]

ANL following Hodgkin's disease has been studied intensively in large cohorts of patients.[182–189] The overall cumulative risk has been reported to be 3.3% at 15 years postdiagnosis but varies from 0.6% in patients who received only radiation therapy to 17% in those treated with combination chemotherapy.[182,190,191] Coleman[185] reported that the average length of survival after the diagnosis of ANL was 6 months. The treatment regimen with the greatest leukemogenic potential is MOPP, presumably due to the mechlorethamine and procarbazine.[182,184–191] A dose-response relationship between alkylating agents and the occurrence of a second malignant neoplasm has been reported;[190,191] Aisenberg[184] has suggested that leukemia is most likely to develop in patients who received more than six cycles of MOPP or similar drug regimens that contain alkylating agents. The addition of radiation to the MOPP regimen does not appear to significantly increase the risk of ANL,[179] whereas the recent use of ABVD (doxorubicin, bleomycin, vinblastine, and dacarbazine) and a regimen involving procarbazine, melphalan, and vinblastine have not been found to carry an increased risk of acute leukemia, which is attributed to lower total dose of alkylating agents.[182,190–192] The risk of ANL in children previously treated for Hodgkin's disease has been associated with disease relapse, treatment with alkylating agents and radiation, and splenectomy.[193,194]

In patients with multiple myeloma the risk is unusually high, more than 200 times that of the incidence in the general population, for the development of ANL. In a study of 364 patients the cumulative risk of ANL reached 17.5% at 50 months of follow-up.[195] The drug most closely associated with ANL was melphalan, although multiple myeloma may also be associated with an increased risk of ANL that is unrelated to treatment.[189]

Although the incidence is not as great as with Hodgkin's disease or multiple myeloma, treatment-related acute leukemia has occurred in patients with non-Hodgkin's lymphoma,[196–198] breast cancer,[199,200] gastrointestinal cancer,[201,202] lung cancer,[203,204] germ cell tumors in men,[205] and ovarian cancer[206,207] and in survivors of childhood cancer.[208,209] Alkylating agents, primarily cyclophosphamide and melphalan, have been linked to the occurrence of ANL. ANL was two to three times more likely to develop in women who received melphalan for the treatment of ovarian cancer than in those who received cyclophosphamide, which suggests that, of the two drugs, melphalan has the greater leukemogenic potential.[210] There is also concern among some cancer researchers that etoposide may increase the risk for ANL.[204]

Second Malignancies Following Radiation

Sarcomas of the bone and soft tissue are the most common second malignant neoplasm after radiation therapy. Although the latency period can be as short as 5 months,[211] it ranges from 10 to 20 years following radiation.[212] The incidence has been found to peak at 15 to 20 years after the initial diagnosis.[212,213] Malignant transformation can occur in doses ranging from 1000–8000 cGy. The relative risk increases from 8 following doses of 1000–2000 cGy to 40 following doses of 6000 cGy.[212,213] It has been postulated that the decreased risk

TABLE 35-3 Selected Studies of Risk of Acute Nonlymphocytic Leukemia in Patients Treated for Several Types of Cancer

Series	Total Number of Patients	Number of Leukemias Observed	Relative Risk	Cumulative Risk (no. yr follow-up)
Hodgkin's disease				
Tucker et al[182]	1507	28	66	3.3% ± 0.6% (15)
Valagussa et al[183]	1329	27		3.6% ± 0.9% (12)
Tucker et al[191]	1036	12	89	4.2% ± 1.9% (20)
Coleman et al[187]	730	8	86	
Blayney et al[188]	193	12*	96	10% ± 3% (15)
Multiple myeloma				
Bergsagel et al[195]	364	14	214	17% ± 4% (4)
Ovarian cancer				
Greene et al[206]	1399	12	67	4.7% ± 1.6% (7)
Greene et al[210]	3363	28	23.5	8.4% ± 1.6% (10)†
Non-Hodgkin's lymphoma				
Gomez et al[197]	117	4	341	NA
Greene et al[198]	517	9	105	7.9% ± 3.2% (10)
Child cancer				
Tucker et al[191]	9170	22	14	0.8% ± 0.2% (20)
Breast cancer				
Fisher et al[199]	8483	43*	NA	<2% (10)
Gastrointestinal cancer				
Boice et al[201]	1402	6	1.6‡	NA
Boice et al[202]	3633	17*		3.2% (7)
Lung cancer				
Chak et al[203]	158	3	316	25% ± 13% (3.1)
Ratain et al[204]	119	4	NA	44% ± 24% (2.5)

*Includes myelodysplastic disorders.
†Cumulative risk among women treated with chemotherapy only.
‡Risk not statistically significant.
NA, data not available.
Source: Adapted from Fraser MC, Tucker MA: Second malignancies following cancer therapy, *Semin Oncol Nurs* 5:43–55, 1989. Reprinted with permission.

following doses of 8000 cGy is due to the phenomenon of cell killing rather than nonlethal cell damage.

In a large study of 9170 survivors of childhood cancer, 48 cases of bone cancer occurred as opposed to the 0.4 expected (relative risk 133).[212] The risk was highest among children treated for retinoblastoma (relative risk 999) and Ewing's sarcoma (relative risk 649) but also was increased significantly in patients treated for rhabdomyosarcoma, Wilms' tumor, and Hodgkin's disease. Of the patients with sarcoma, 84% had received radiation, and 83% of the subsequent tumors occurred within the field of radiation.

ANL following radiation therapy is uncommon but has been reported in childhood cancer[190,213] and non-Hodgkin's lymphoma.[187] Women with breast cancer treated with postoperative radiation also have a slightly increased risk of ANL.[199] In addition to sarcomas and leukemia, a variety of other solid tumors have been linked to treatment with radiation. Carcinomas of the breast can occur in girls treated with pulmonary irradiation,[190] and a slightly excessive number of tumors of the bladder, rectum, uterus, bone, and connective tissue has been reported in women who received radiation for gynecologic cancer.[214,215] Brain tumors can occur after cranial irradiation for CNS prophylaxis in childhood ALL.[216,217] Finally, lung cancer following mantle radiation for Hodgkin's disease has been reported.[219] The average latency period was 7 years, and smoking was a contributing factor in only 53% of patients. Table 35-3 summarizes the findings from selected studies on the risk of ANL in patients treated for various types of cancer.

Twenty-four second malignant neoplasms of the CNS were found in a cohort study of 9720 children treated for ALL.[218] This represented a 22-fold excess of CNS tumors. All CNS tumors developed in children treated with cranial radiation; the risk was greatest in children who were 5 years of age or younger at the time of diagnosis.[218]

CONCLUSION

This chapter has provided a comprehensive review of the biologic late effects that can be caused by curative cancer therapy. Long-term surveillance for these toxic effects is a recent and challenging area for oncology nurses and physicians. A long-range perspective is essential because the latency period for some late toxicities is many years after completion of treatment and the consequences of permanent tissue damage across the life span are unknown.

General recommendations for long-term follow-up include an annual physical examination with a complete blood cell count and urinalysis. Evaluation of specific toxicity to organ systems and second malignancies depends on the initial diagnosis, type and amount of treatment received, and host risk factors. For some late toxicities, surveillance guidelines have been standardized. The Cardiology Committee of the Children's Cancer Study Group recently published guidelines for cardiac monitoring of children during and after anthracycline therapy.[220] Recommendations for late cardiac follow-up include: (1) an ECG and echocardiogram every 2–3 years and (2) a radionuclide angiocardiogram and 24-hour continuous taped ECG every 5 years posttherapy.[220] These recommendations may serve as a model for establishing long-term evaluation guidelines for all late toxicities. However, for all biologic late effects a careful balance must be struck between monitoring and the creation of needless anxiety that could hinder the patient's overall rehabilitation and emotional adjustment.

REFERENCES

1. *Cancer Facts and Figures: 1992.* Atlanta, GA: American Cancer Society, 1992, pp. 3–30.
2. Meadows AT, Hobbie WL: The medical consequences of cure. *Cancer* 58:524–528, 1986.
3. van Eys J: Living beyond cure: Transcending survival. *Am J Pediatr Hematol Oncol* 9:114–118, 1987.
4. Meadows AT, Massari DJ, Fergusson J, et al: Declines in IQ scores and cognitive dysfunctions in children with acute lymphoblastic leukemia treated with cranial irradiation. *Lancet* 2:1015–1018, 1981.
5. Robison LL, Nesbit ME, Sather HN, et al: Factors associated with IQ scores in long-term survivors of childhood acute lymphoblastic leukemia. *Am J Pediatr Hematol Oncol* 6:115–121, 1984.
6. Moore IM, Kramer JH, Ablin AR: Late effects of central nervous system prophylactic leukemia therapy on cognitive functioning. *Oncol Nurs Forum* 13:45–51, 1986.
7. Lansky SB, Cairns NU, Lansky LL, et al: Central nervous system prophylaxis. *Am J Pediatr Hematol Oncol* 6:183–190, 1984.
8. Stebhens JA, Kisker CT: Intelligence and achievement testing in childhood cancer: Three years postdiagnosis. *J Dev Behav Pediatr* 5:184–188, 1984.
9. Moehle KA, Berg RA, Ch'ien LT, et al: Language-related skills in children with acute lymphocytic leukemia. *J Dev Behav Pediatr* 4:257–261, 1983.
10. Duffner PK, Cohen ME, Parker MS: Prospective intellectual testing in children with brain tumors. *Ann Neurol* 23:575–579, 1988.
11. Chak LK, Zatz IM, Wasserstein P, et al: Neurologic dysfunction in patients treated for small cell carcinoma of the lung: A clinical and radiological study. *Int J Radiat Oncol Bio Phys* 12:385–389, 1986.
12. Frytak S, Earnest F, O'Neill B, et al: Magnetic resonance imaging for neurotoxicity on long-term survivors of carcinoma. *Mayo Clin Proc* 60:803–813, 1985.
13. Pfefferbaum-Levine B, Copeland DR, Fletcher JM, et al: Neuropsychological assessment of long-term survivors of childhood leukemia. *Am J Pediatr Hematol Oncol* 6:123–128, 1984.
14. Fletcher JM: Neurobehavioral effects of central nervous systems prophylatic treatment of cancer in children. *J Clin Exp Neuropsychol* 10:495–538, 1988.

15. Goff JR, Anderson HR, Cooper PF: Distractability and memory deficits in long-term survivors of acute lymphoblastic leukemia. *J Dev Behav Pediatr* 1:158–163, 1980.
16. Kramer JH, Moore IM: Verbal learning deficits in long-term survivors of acute lymphoblastic leukemia. *Proc Am Psychol Assoc* 97:401, 1985(abstr).
17. Kramer JH, Moore IM: Age at time of treatment effect on mnemestic functioning following CNS irradiation and intrathecal methotrexate. *J Clin Exp Neuropsychol* 7:627, 1985(abstr).
18. Copeland DR, Fletcher JM, Pfefferbaum-Levine B, et al: Neuropsychological sequelae of childhood cancer in long-term survivors. *Pediatrics* 75:745–753, 1985.
19. Ellison N, Bernath A, Kane R, et al: Disturbing problems of success: Clinical status of long-term survivors of small cell lung cancer. *Proc Am Soc Clin Oncol* 1:149, 1982(abstr).
20. Rodgers J, Britton PG, Morris RG, et al: Memory after treatment for acute lymphoblastic leukemia. *Arch Dis Child* 67:266–268, 1992.
21. Obetz SW, Smithson WA, Groover RV, et al: Neuropsychological follow-up of children with acute lymphoblastic leukemia. *Am J Pediatr Hematol Oncol* 1:207–213, 1979.
22. Twaddle V, Britton PG, Craft AC, et al: Intellectual function after treatment for leukaemia or solid tumors. *Arch Dis Child* 58:949–952, 1985.
23. Taylor HG: Postirradiation treatment outcomes for children with acute lymphoblastic leukemia: Clarification of risks. *J Pediatr Psychol* 12:395–411, 1987.
24. Moss HA, Nannis ED, Poplack DG: The effects of prophylactic treatment of the central nervous system on the intellectual functioning of children with acute lymphocytic leukemia. *Am J Med* 71:47–52, 1981.
25. Jannoun L: Are cognitive and educational development affected by age at which prophylactic therapy is given in acute lymphoblastic leukemia? *Arch Dis Child* 58:953–958, 1983.
26. Silverman CL, Palkes H, Talent B, et al: Late effects of radiotherapy on patients with cerebellar medulloblastoma. *Cancer* 54:825–829, 1984.
27. Rowland JH, Glidewell OJ, Sibley RF, et al: Effects of different forms of central nervous system prophylaxis on neuropsychological function in childhood leukemia. *J Clin Oncol* 2:1327–1335, 1984.
28. Pavlovsky S, Castano J, Leigurda R, et al: Neuropsychological study in patients with ALL. *Am J Pediatr Hematol Oncol* 5:79–128, 1983.
29. Tamaroff M, Miller DR, Murphy ML: Immediate and long-term post-therapy neuropsychologic performance in children with acute lymphoblastic leukemia treated without central nervous system radiation. *J Pediatr* 101:524–529, 1982.
30. Balsam WR, Bleyer WA, Robison LL, et al: Intellectual function in long-term survivors of childhood acute lymphoblastic leukemia: Protective effect of pre-irradiation methotrexate. A Children's Cancer Study Group study. *Med Pediatr Oncol* 19:486–492, 1991.
31. Kaleita T, Tesler A, Feig SA: Prospective neurodevelopmental studies: Two children treated with total body irradiation and bone marrow transplantation for acute leukemia in infancy. *Prog Bone Marrow Transplant* 1:157–164, 1987.
32. Smedler AC, Bergman H, Bolme P, et al: Neuropsychological functioning in children treated with bone marrow transplantation. *J Clin Exp Neuropsychol* 10:325–326, 1988.
33. Halberg F, Wara W, Kramer JH, et al: Total body irradiation in infancy: Effect on growth and development after bone marrow transplant for SIDS. *Int J Radiat Oncol Biol Phys* 15:154, 1988(abstr).
34. Tamaroff M, Salwen R, Miller D, et al: Neuropsychological sequelae in irradiated (1800 rads [r] and 2400 r) and non-irradiated children with acute lymphoblastic leukemia (ALL). *Proc Amer Soc Clin Oncol* 4:C-644, 1985(abstr).
35. Duffner PK, Cohne ME, Thomas PR, et al: The long-term effects of cranial irradiation on the central nervous system. *Cancer* 56:1841–1846, 1985.
36. Berry MP, Jenkins DT, Green GW, et al: Radiation treatment for medulloblastoma. *J Neurosurg* 55:43–51, 1981.
37. Mulhern RK, Crisco JJ, Kim LE: Neuropsychological sequelae of childhood brain tumors: A review. *J Child Clin Psychol* 12:66–73, 1983.
38. Packer RJ, Zimmerman RA, Bilaniuk LT: Magnetic resonance imaging in the evaluation of treatment-related central nervous system damage. *Cancer* 58:635–640, 1986.
39. Chin HW, Maruyama Y: Age at treatment and long-term performance results in medulloblastoma. *Cancer* 53:1952–1958, 1984.
40. Dobbing J, Sands J: Quantitative growth and development of the human brain. *Arch Dis Child* 48:757–767, 1973.
41. Davison AN, Dobbing J: Myelination as a vulnerable period in brain development. *Br Med J* 22:40–44, 1966.
42. Waber DP, Tarbell NJ, Kahn CM, et al: The relationship of sex and treatment modality to neuropsychologic outcome in childhood acute lymphoblastic leukemia. *J Clin Oncol* 10:810–817, 1992.
43. Brouwers P, Riccardi R, Fedio P, et al: Long-term neuropsychological sequelae of childhood leukemia: Correlation with CT brain scan abnormalities. *J Pediatr* 106:723–728, 1985.
44. Davis PC, Hoffman JC, Pearl GS, et al: CT evaluation of effects of cranial radiation therapy in children. *Am J Neuroradiol* 7:639–644, 1986.
45. Peylan Ramu N, Poplack D, Pizzo D, et al: Abnormal CT scans of the brain in asymptomatic children with acute lymphoblastic leukemia after prophylactic treatment of the central nervous system with radiation and intrathecal chemotherapy. *N Engl J Med* 298:815, 1978.
46. Ochs JJ, Berger P, Brecher ML, et al: Computed tomography brain scans in children with acute lymphoblastic leukemia receiving methotrexate alone as central nervous system prophylaxis. *Cancer* 45:2274–2278, 1980.
47. Ochs JJ, Parvey LS, Whitaker JN, et al: Serial cranial computed tomography scans in children with leukemia given two different forms of central nervous system therapy. *J Clin Oncol* 1:793–798, 1983.
48. Kramer JH, Norman D, Brant-Zawadski M, et al: Absence of white matter changes on magnetic resonance imaging in children treated with CNS prophylaxis therapy for leukemia. *Cancer* 61:928–930, 1988.
49. Tsurada JS, Kortman KE, Bradley WG, et al: Radiation effects on cerebral white matter: MR evaluation. *Am J Radiat* 149:165–171, 1987.
50. Sheline GE, Wara WM, Smith V: Therapeutic irradiation and brain injury. *Int J Radiat Oncol Biol Phys* 6:1215–1228, 1980.
51. Caveness WF: Experimental observations: Delayed necrosis in the monkey brain. In Gilbert MA, Kagan AR (eds), *Radiation Damage to the Nervous System*. New York: Raven Press, 1980, pp. 1–38.

52. Cassarett G: Basic mechanisms of permanent and delayed radiation pathology. *Cancer* 37:1002–1010, 1976.
53. Committee for Radiation Oncology Studies: Normal tissue tolerance and damage. *Cancer* 37:2046–2055, 1976.
54. Allen JC: The effects of cancer therapy on the nervous system. *J Pediatr* 93:903–909, 1978.
55. Greasey W: Basic mechanisms of tissue injury by chemotherapy. *Cancer* 37:999–1002, 1976.
56. Price RA, Jamieson PA: The central nervous system in childhood leukemia. II. Subacute leukoencephalopathy. *Cancer* 35:306–318, 1975.
57. Mahoney DH, Fernbach DJ, Glaze DG, et al: Elevated myelin basic protein level in the cerebral spinal fluid of children with acute lymphoblastic leukemia. *J Clin Oncol* 2:58–61, 1984.
58. Gangji D, Reaman GH, Cohen SR, et al: Leukoencephalopathy and elevated levels of myelin basic protein in the cerebral spinal fluid of patients with acute lymphoblastic leukemia. *Medical Intelligence* 303:19–21, 1980.
59. Packer R, Meadows AT, Rorke L, et al: Long-term sequela of cancer treatment on the central nervous system in childhood. *Med Pediatr Oncol* 15:241–253, 1987.
60. Hopewell JW: Late radiation damage to the central nervous system: A radiobiological interpretation. *Neuropathol Ap Neurobiol* 5:329–343, 1979.
61. Tiller-Boricich JK, Fike JR, Phillips TL, et al: Pathology delayed radiation brain damage: An experimental canine model. *Radiat Res* 110:161–172, 1987.
62. Deck MD: Imaging techniques in the diagnosis of radiation damage to the central nervous system. In Gilbert HA, Kag AR (eds), *Radiation Damage to the Nervous System.* New York: Raven Press, 1980, pp. 107–127.
63. Wharam MD: Radiation therapy. In Altman AJ, Schwartz AD (eds), *Malignant Diseases of Infancy, Childhood and Adolescence.* Philadelphia: Saunders, 1983, p. 103.
64. Piehl IJ, Meyer D, Perlia CP, et al: Effects of cisdiammine dichloroplatinum (NSC-119875) on hearing function in man. *Cancer Chemother Rep* 58:871–875, 1974.
65. Walkwe DA, Pillov J, Waters KD, et al: Enhanced cisplatin ototoxicity in children with brain tumors who have received simultaneous or prior cranial irradiation. *Med Pediatr Oncol* 17:48–52, 1989.
66. Ganong WF: The thyroid gland. In Ganong WF (ed), *Review of Medical Physiology.* Palo Alto, CA: Appleton & Lange, 1987, pp. 262–275.
67. Glatstein E, McHardy-Young S, Brast N, et al: Alterations in serum thyrotropin (TSH) and thyroid function following radiotherapy in patients with malignant lymphoma. *J Clin Endocrinol Metab* 32:838–841, 1971.
68. Shalet SM, Rosenstock JD, Beardwell CT, et al: Thyroid dysfunction following external irradiation to the neck for Hodgkin's disease in childhood. *Radiology* 28:511–515, 1977.
69. Smith RE, Adler RA, Clark P, et al: Thyroid function after mantle radiation in Hodgkin's disease. *JAMA* 245:46–49, 1981.
70. Donaldson SS, Glatstein E, Rosenberg SA, et al: Pediatric Hodgkin's disease. II. Results of therapy. *Cancer* 37:2436–2447, 1976.
71. Ramsay N, Kim T, Coccia P, et al: Thyroid dysfunction in pediatric patients after mantle held radiation therapy for Hodgkin's disease. *Proc Am Soc Clin Oncol* 19:331, 1978(abstr).
72. Mortimer RH, Hill GE, Galligan JP, et al: Hypothyroidism and Graves' disease after mantle irradiation: A follow-up study. *Aust NZ J Med* 16:347–351, 1986.
73. Josensuu H, Viikari J: Thyroid function after postoperative radiation therapy in patients with breast cancer. *Acta Radiol Oncol* 25:167–170, 1986.
74. Fuks Z, Glatstein E, Marsa G, et al: Long-term effects of external radiation on the pituitary and thyroid glands. *Cancer* 37:1157–1161, 1979(suppl).
75. Mauch PM, Weinstein H, Botnick L, et al: An evaluation of long-term survival and treatment complications in children with Hodgkin's disease. *Cancer* 51:925–932, 1983.
76. Sklar C, Kim T, Ramsay N: Thyroid dysfunction among long-term survivors of bone marrow transplantation. *Am J Med* 73:688–694, 1982.
77. Constine LS, Rubin P, Woolf PD: Hyperprolactinemia and hypothyroidism following cytotoxic therapy for central nervous system malignancies. *J Clin Oncol* 5:1841–1851, 1987.
78. Samaan N, Scholtz P, Yang KP: Endocrine complications after radiotherapy for tumors of the head and neck. *J Lab Clin Med* 109:361–362, 1987.
79. Nelson DF, Reddy KV, O'Mara RE, et al: Thyroid abnormalities following neck irradiation for Hodgkin's disease. *Cancer* 42:2553–2562, 1978.
80. Schimpff SC, Diggs CH, Wiswell JG, et al: Radiation-related thyroid dysfunction: Implications for the treatment of Hodgkin's disease. *Ann Intern Med* 92:91–98, 1980.
81. Samaan NA, Vieto R, Scholtz PN, et al: Hypothalamic, pituitary and thyroid dysfunction after radiotherapy to the head and neck. *Int J Radiat Oncol Biol Phys* 8:1857–1867, 1982.
82. Richards GE, Wara WM, Grunbach MM, et al: Delayed onset of hypopituitarism: Sequelae of therapeutic irradiation of central nervous system, ear, and middle ear tumors. *J Pediatr* 89:553–559, 1976.
83. Shalet SM, Beardwell CT, Aarous BM, et al: Growth impairment of children treated for brain tumors. *Arch Dis Child* 53:491–494, 1978.
84. Bamford FN, Morris Jones PH, Pearson D, et al: Residual disabilities in children treated for intracranial space-occupying lesions. *Cancer* 37:1149–1151, 1976.
85. Braumer R, Rappaport R, Prevot C, et al: A prospective study of growth hormone deficiency in children given cranial irradiation, and its relation to statural growth. *J Clin Endocrinol Metab* 68:346–351, 1989.
86. Pasqualini T, Diez B, Domene H, et al: Long-term endocrine sequelae after surgery, radiation therapy and chemotherapy in younger children with medulloblastoma. *Cancer* 59:801–806, 1987.
87. Oberfield SE, Allen JC, Pollack J, et al: Long-term endocrine sequelae after treatment of medulloblastoma: Perspective study of growth and thyroid function. *J Pediatr* 108:219–223, 1986.
88. Ahmed SR, Shalet SM, Beardwell CG: The effects of cranial irradiation on growth hormone secretion. *Acta Paediatr Scand* 75:255–260, 1986.
89. Shalet SM, Beardwell CG, Morris Jones PH, et al: Growth hormone deficiency after treatment of acute leukemia in children. *Arch Dis Child* 51:489–493, 1971.
90. Wells RJ, Foster MB, D'Ercole JD, et al: The impact of cranial irradiation on growth of children with acute lymphoblastic leukemia. *Am J Dis Child* 137:37–39, 1983.
91. Blatt J, Bercu BB, Gillin C, et al: Reduced pulsatile growth hormone secretion in children after therapy for acute lymphoblastic leukemia. *J Pediatr* 104:182–186, 1984.
92. Berry DH, Elders MJ, Crist WM, et al: Growth in chil-

dren with acute lymphoblastic leukemia: A Pediatric Oncology Group study. *Med Pediatr Oncol* 11:39–45, 1983.
93. Hakami N, Mohammad A, Meyer J: Growth and growth hormone of children with acute lymphoblastic leukemia following central nervous system prophylaxis with and without cranial irradiation. *Am J Pediatr Hematol Oncol* 2:311–316, 1985.
94. Robison LL, Nesbit ME, Sather HN, et al: Height of children successfully treated for acute lymphoblastic leukemia: A report from the late effects study committee of Children's Cancer Study Group. *Med Pediatr Oncol* 13:13–21, 1985.
95. Shalet SM, Bearwell CG, Pearson E, et al: The effect of varying doses of cerebral irradiation on growth hormone production in childhood. *Clin Endocrinol* 5:287–290, 1976.
96. Cicognani A, Cacciari E, Veechi V, et al: Differential effects of 18- and 24-Gy cranial irradiation on growth rate and growth hormone release in children with prolonged survival after acute lymphoblastic leukemia. *Am J Dis Child* 141:550–552, 1986.
97. Starceski PJ, Lee PA, Blatt J, et al: Comparable effects of 1800- and 2400-rad cranial irradiation on height and weight in children treated for acute lymphoblastic leukemia. *Am J Dis Child* 141:550–552, 1987.
98. Sanders JE, Pritchard S, Mahoney P, et al: Growth and development following marrow transplantation for leukemia. *Blood* 68:1129–1135, 1986.
99. Clayton PE, Shalet SM. Dose dependency of time of onset of radiation-induced growth hormone deficiency. *J Pediatr* 118:226–227, 1991.
100. Brauner R, Czernichow P, Rappaport R: Greater susceptibility to hypothalamopituitary irradiation in younger children with acute lymphoblastic leukemia. *J Pediatr* 108:3332, 1986.
101. Chapman R, Sutcliffe S, Malpas J: Cytotoxic-induced ovarian failure in Hodgkin's disease. II. Effects on sexual function. *JAMA* 242:1882–1884, 1979.
102. Chapman R, Sutcliffe S, Malpas J: Cytotoxic-induced ovarian failure in women with Hodgkin's disease. I. Hormone function. *JAMA* 242:1877–1881, 1979.
103. Andrieu J, Ochoa-Molina ME: Menstrual cycle, pregnancies and offspring before and after MOPP therapy for Hodgkin's disease. *Cancer* 52:435–438, 1983.
104. Koyama H, Wada T, Nishizawa Y, et al: Cyclophosphamide-induced ovarian failure and its therapeutic significance in patients with breast cancer. *Cancer* 39:1403–1409, 1977.
105. Jordan VC, Fritz NF, Tormey DC: Endocrine effects of adjuvant chemotherapy and long-term tamoxifen administration on node-positive patients with breast cancer. *Cancer Res* 47:624–630, 1987.
106. Gershenson DM: Menstrual and reproductive function after treatment with combination chemotherapy for malignant ovarian germ cell tumors. *J Clin Oncol* 6:270–275, 1988.
107. Hobbie WL, Schwartz CL: Endocrine late effects among survivors of cancer. *Semin Oncol Nurs* 5:14–21, 1989.
108. Shalet SM: The effects of cancer treatment on growth and sexual development. *Clin Oncol* 4:223–238, 1985.
109. Hensle T, Burbige K, Shepard B, et al: Chemotherapy and its effect on testicular morphology in children. *J Urol* 131:1142–1144, 1982.
110. Sherins RJ, Olweny CLM, Ziegler JL: Gynecomastia and gonadal dysfunction in adolescent boys treated with combination chemotherapy for Hodgkin's disease. *N Engl J Med* 299:12–16, 1978.
111. Whilthead E, Shalet SM, Morris Jones PH, et al: Gonadal function after combination chemotherapy for Hodgkin's disease in childhood. *Arch Dis Child* 57:287–291, 1982.
112. Rivkees SA, Crawford JD: The relationship of gonadal activity and chemotherapy-induced gonadal damage. *JAMA* 259:2123–2125, 1988.
113. Green DM, Brecher BL, Lindsay AN, et al: Gonadal function in pediatric patients following treatment for Hodgkin's disease. *Pediatr Oncol* 9:235–244, 1981.
114. Shalet SM, Hann IM, Lendon M, et al: Testicular function after combination chemotherapy in childhood for acute lymphoblastic leukemia. *J Pediatr* 94:719–722, 1981.
115. Byrne J, Mulvihill JJ, Myers MH, et al: Effects of treatment on fertility in long-term survivors of childhood or adolescent cancer. *N Engl J Med* 317:1315–1321, 1987.
116. de Cunhna MF, Meistrich ML, Fuller IM, et al: Recovery of spermatogenesis after treatment for Hodgkin's disease: Limiting dose of MOPP chemotherapy. *J Clin Oncol* 2:571–577, 1984.
117. Nicosia S, Matus-Ridley M, Meadows AT: Gonadal effects of cancer therapy in girls. *Cancer* 55:2364–2372, 1985.
118. Himelstein-Braw R, Peters H, Faber M: Morphological study of the ovaries of leukemic children. *Br J Cancer* 38:82–87, 1978.
119. Ash P: The influence of radiation on fertility in man. *Br J Radiol* 53:271–278, 1980.
120. Fischer B, Bheung A: Delayed effect of radiation therapy with or without chemotherapy on ovarian function in women with Hodgkin's disease. *Acta Radiol Oncol* 23:43–48, 1984.
121. Shalet SM, Beardwell CG, Jacobs JG, et al: Testicular function following irradiation of the human prepubertal testis. *Clin Endocrinol* 9:483–490, 1978.
122. Shalet SM, Horner A, Ahmed SR, et al: Leydig cell damage and testicular function combination chemotherapy in childhood for acute lymphoblastic leukemia. *Med Pediatr Oncol* 13:65–68, 1985.
123. Hamre MR, Robison LL, Nesbit ME, et al: Effects of radiation on ovarian function in long-term survivors of childhood acute lymphoblastic leukemia: A report from the Children's Cancer Study Group. *J Clin Oncol* 5:1759–1765, 1987.
124. Shalet SM, Beardwell CG, Morris Jones PH, et al: Ovarian failure following abdominal irradiation in childhood. *Br J Cancer* 33:655–658, 1976.
125. Green DM, Hall B, Zevon M. Pregnancy outcome after treatment for acute lymphoblastic leukemia during childhood or adolescence. *Cancer* 64:2335–2339, 1989.
126. Saman N, Vieto R, Schultz B, et al: Hypothalamic, pituitary and thyroid dysfunction after radiotherapy to the head and neck. *Int J Radiat Oncol Biol Phys* 8:1857–1867, 1982.
127. Buvat J, LeMarie A, Burat-Herbaut M, et al: Hyperprolactinemia and sexual function in men. *Horm Res* 22:196–203, 1984.
128. Hitzig WH, Pluss HJ, Joller P, et al: Studies on the immune status of children with acute lymphocytic leukemia. II. In remission with and without cytostatic treatment. *Clin Exp Immunol* 26:414–418, 1976.
129. Borella L, Green AA, Webster RG: Immunologic rebound after cessation of long-term chemotherapy in acute leukemia. *Blood* 40:42–51, 1972.

130. Hancock BW, Bruce L, Whitman MD, et al: The effects of radiotherapy on immunity in patients with cured localized carcinoma of the cervix uteri. *Cancer* 53:884–887, 1984.
131. Job G, Pfreundschuh M, Baner M, et al: The influence of radiation therapy on T lymphocyte subpopulations defined by monoclonal antibodies. *Int J Radiat Oncol Biol Phys* 10:2077–2081, 1984.
132. Rotstein S, Blomgren H, Petrini B, et al: Long-term effects of the immune system following local radiation therapy for breast cancer. I. Cellular composition of peripheral blood lymphocyte population. *Int J Radiat Oncol Biol Phys* 11:921–925, 1985.
133. Rotstein S, Blomgren H, Petrini B, et al: Long-term effects on the immune system following local radiation therapy for breast cancer. IV. Proliferative responses and induction of suppressor activity of the blood lymphocyte population. *Radiother Oncol* 6:223–230, 1986.
134. Waserman J, Blomgren H, Petrini B, et al: Effect of radiation therapy and vitro x-ray exposure on lymphocyte subpopulations and their functions. *Am J Clin Oncol* 5:195–208, 1982.
135. Haas GS, Halperin E, Poseret D, et al: Differential recovery of circulating T cell subsets after nodal irradiation for Hodgkin's disease. *J Immunol* 132:1026–1030, 1981.
136. Fuks Z, Strober S, Bobrove AM, et al: Long-term effects of radiation on peripheral blood of patients with Hodgkin's disease. *J Clin Invest* 58:803–814, 1976.
137. Ueda M, Harada N, Shiobara S, et al: T lymphocyte reconstitution in long-term survivors after allogeneic and autologous transplantation. *Transplantation* 3:552–556, 1981.
138. Van Rijswijk RF, Sybesma JPH, Kater L: A prospective study of the changes in the immune status before, during and after multiple agent chemotherapy for Hodgkin's disease. *Cancer* 51:637–644, 1983.
139. Layward L, Ledvinsky RJ, Butler M: Long-term abnormalities in T and B lymphoblastic leukemia. *J Haematol* 49:251–258, 1981.
140. Paolucci P, Layward L, Hayward AR, et al: Increase and inhibition of pre-B cell proliferation in culture by T cells. *Clin Exp Immunol* 43:336–341, 1979.
141. Katz J, Walter BN, Bennetts GA, et al: Abnormal cellular and humoral immunity in childhood acute lymphoblastic leukemia in long-term remission. *West J Med* 146:179–187, 1988.
142. Workman ML: Immunologic late effects in children and adults. *Semin Oncol Nurs* 5:36–42, 1989.
143. Parmentier L, Morardet N, Tubina M: Late effects on human bone marrow after extended field radiotherapy. *Int J Radiat Oncol Biol Phy* 9:1303–1311, 1983.
144. Sacks EL, Goris ML, Glatstein E: Bone marrow regeneration following large field radiation. *Cancer* 42:1057–1065, 1978.
145. Steinherz LJ, Steinherz P, Tan C, et al: Cardiac toxicity 4–20 years after completing anthracycline therapy. *Proc Am Soc Clin Oncol* 8:296, 1989(abstr).
146. Steinherz LJ, Steinherz P, Tan C: Cardiac failure more than six years post anthracyclines. *Proc Int Soc Paediatric Oncol:* 19:136, 1987(abstr).
147. Lipshultz SE, Colan SD, Gelber RD, et al: Late cardiac effects of doxorubicin therapy for acute lymphoblastic leukemia in childhood. *N Engl J Med* 324:808–815, 1991.
148. Ruccione K, Weinbert K: Late effects in multiple body systems. *Semin Oncol Nurs* 5:4–13, 1989.
149. Von Hoff DD, Layward MW, Basa P, et al: Risk factors for doxorubicin induced congestive heart failure. *Ann Intern Med* 91:710–717, 1979.
150. Von Hoff DD, Rozencweig M, Piccart M: The cardiotoxicity of anticancer agents. *Semin Oncol* 9:23–33, 1982.
151. Pratt CT, Ransom JL, Evans WE: Age-related adriamycin cardiotoxicity in children. *Cancer Treat Rep* 62:1381–1384, 1978.
152. Muggia FM, Cassileth PA: Constructive pericarditis following radiation therapy. *Am J Med* 11:116–123, 1968.
153. Martin RG, Ruckdeschel JC, Chang P, et al: Radiation related pericarditis. *Am J Cardiol* 35:216–220, 1975.
154. Roth BJ, Greist A, Kubilis PS, et al: Cisplatin-based combination chemotherapy for disseminated germ cell tumors: Long-term follow-up. *J Clin Oncol* 6:1239–1247, 1988.
155. Libshitz JI, Southard ME: Complications of radiation therapy: The thorax. *Semin Roentgenol* 9:41–49, 1971.
156. Ginsberg AJ, Cormis RI: The pulmonary toxicity of antineoplastic agents. *Semin Oncol* 9:35–51, 1982.
157. DeLena M, Guzzon A, Monfardini S, et al: Clinical, radiologic and histopathologic studies on pulmonary toxicity induced by treatment with bleomycin (NSC-125066). *Cancer Chemother Rep* 56:343–356, 1972.
158. Blum RH, Carter SK, Agre K: A clinical review of bleomycin: A new antineoplastic agent. *Cancer* 31:903–913, 1973.
159. Aronin PA, Mahaley MS, Rudnick SA, et al: Prediction of BCNU pulmonary toxicity in patients with malignant gliomas. *N Engl J Med* 303:183–188, 1980.
160. Donaldson SS, Jundt S, Ricour C, et al: Radiation enteritis in children: A retrospective review, clinicopathologic correlation, and dietary management. *Cancer* 35:1167–1178, 1975.
161. Jaffe N: Biological consequences of cancer and its treatment and their relationship to current treatment planning. *Am J Pediatr Hemat Oncol* 9:62–67, 1987.
162. D'Angio GJ, Pearson D: Radiation therapy. In Bloom HGJ, et al (eds), *Cancer in Children.* Berlin: Springer-Verlag, 1975, pp. 217–241.
163. Jaffee N: Late sequelae of cancer therapy. In Sutow SS, Fernbach DJ, Vietti TJ (eds), *Clinical Pediatric Oncology*, St Louis, MO: Mosby, 1984, pp. 810–832.
164. Aron BS, Schlesinger A: Complications of radiation therapy: The genitourinary tract. *Semin Roentgenol* 9:132–145, 1974.
165. Bennett AH: Cyclophosphamide and hemorrhagic cystitis. *Urology* 111:603–606, 1974.
166. D'Angio GJ, Farber S, Maddock CL: Potentiation of x-ray effects by actinomycin-D. *Radiology* 73:175–177, 1959.
167. Tefft M, Lattin PB, Jerab B, et al: Acute and late effects of normal tissues following combined chemo- and radiotherapy of childhood rhabdomyosarcoma and Ewing's sarcoma. *Cancer* 37:1202–1213, 1976.
168. Silber JH, Littman PS, Meadows AT: Stature loss following skeletal irradiation for childhood cancer. *J Clin Oncol* 8:304–312, 1990.
169. Probert JC, Parker BR: The effects of radiation therapy on bone growth. *Radiology* 114:155–162, 1975.
170. Rate WR, Bulter MS, Robertson WW, et al: Late orthopedic effects in children with Wilms' tumor treated with abdominal irradiation. *Med Pediatr Oncol* 19:265–268, 1991.
171. Shalet SM, Gibson B, Swindell R, et al: Effect of spinal irradiation on growth. *Arch Dis Child* 62:461–464, 1987.
172. Jaffe N, Toth BB, Hoar RE, et al: Dental and maxillo-

facial abnormalities in long-term survivors of childhood cancer. Effects of treatment with chemotherapy and radiation to the head and neck. *Pediatrics* 73:816–823, 1984.

173. Hazra TA, Shipman B: Dental problems in pediatric patients with head and neck tumors undergoing multiple modality therapy. *Med Pediatr Oncol* 10:91–95, 1981.
174. Maguire A, Craft AW, Evans RGB, et al: The long-term effects of treatment on the dental conditions of children surviving malignant disease. *Cancer* 60:2570–2575, 1987.
175. Roller AC, Pembrook L, Plese L, et al: One-in-five Hodgkin's patients still at risk after 15 years. *Oncol Nurs Update* 2:13, 1987.
176. Meadows AT: Second malignant neoplasms in childhood cancer survivors. *J Assoc Pediatr Oncol Nurs* 6:7–11, 1989.
177. Li FP, Cassady R, Jaffee N: Risk of second tumors in survivors of childhood cancer. *Cancer* 35:1230–1235, 1975.
178. Fraser MC, Tucker MA: Second malignancies following cancer therapy. *Semin Oncol Nurs* 5:43–55, 1989.
179. Meadows AT: Second malignant neoplasms in children: An update from the Late Effects Study Group. *J Clin Oncol* 3:532–538, 1985.
180. Meadows AT, Strong LC, Li FP, et al: Bone sarcoma as a second malignant neoplasm in children: Influence of radiation and genetic predisposition. *Cancer* 16:2603–2606, 1980.
181. Tucker MA, D'Angio GI, Boice JD, et al: Bone sarcomas linked to radiotherapy and chemotherapy in children. *N Engl J Med* 317:588–593, 1987.
182. Tucker MH, Coleman CN, Cox RS, et al: Risk of second cancers after treatment for Hodgkin's disease. *N Engl J Med* 318:76–81, 1988.
183. Valagussa P, Santoro A, Fossati-Bellani F, et al: Second acute leukemia and other malignancies following treatment for Hodgkin's disease. *J Clin Oncol* 4:830–837, 1986.
184. Aisenberg AC: Acute nonlymphocytic leukemia after treatment for Hodgkin's disease. *Am J Med* 75:449–454, 1983.
185. Coleman CN: Secondary neoplasms in patients treated for cancer: Etiology and perspective. *Radiat Res* 92:188–200, 1982.
186. Coleman CN, Kaplan HS, Cox R, et al: Leukemia, non-Hodgkin's lymphoma and solid tumors in patients treated for Hodgkin's disease. *Cancer Surv* 1:733–744, 1982.
187. Coleman M, Easton DF, Horwich A, et al: Second malignancies and Hodgkin's disease—The Royal Marsden Hospital experience. *Radiother Oncol* 11:229–238, 1988.
188. Blayney DW, Longo DL, Yound RC, et al: Decreasing risk of leukemia with prolonged follow-up after chemotherapy and radiation for Hodgkin's disease. *N Engl J Med* 316:710–714, 1987.
189. Green MH: Epidemiologic studies of chemotherapy related acute leukemia. In Castellani A (ed), *Epidemiology and Quantitation of Environmental Risk in Humans from Radiation and Other Agents.* New York: Plenum, 1985, pp. 499–514.
190. Meadows AT: Second malignant neoplasms. *Clin Oncol* 4:217–261, 1985.
191. Tucker MA, Meadows AT, Boice JD, et al: Cancer risk following treatment of childhood cancer. In Boice JD Jr, Franmem JF Jr (eds), *Radiation Carcinogenesis: Epidemiology and Biological Significance.* New York: Raven, 1981, pp. 211–224.
192. Valagussa P, Santoro S, Kenda R, et al: Second malignancies in Hodgkin's disease: A complication of certain forms of treatment. *Br Med J* 280:216–219, 1980.
193. Pui CH, Hancock ML, Raimondi SC, et al: Myeloid neoplasia in children treated for solid tumors. *Lancet* 336:417–421, 1990.
194. Meadows AT, Obringer AC, Marrero O, et al: Second malignant neoplasms following childhood Hodgkin's disease: Treatment and splenectomy as risk factors. *Med Pediatr Oncol* 17:477–484, 1989.
195. Bergsagel DE, Bailey AJ, Langley GR, et al: The chemotherapy of plasma cell myeloma and the incidence of acute leukemia. *N Engl J Med* 301:743–748, 1979.
196. Pedersen-Bjergaard J, Ersboll J, Sorensen HM, et al: Risk of acute nonlymphocytic leukemia and preleukemia in patients treated with cyclophosphamide for non-Hodgkin's lymphomas. *Ann Intern Med* 103:195–200, 1985.
197. Gomez GA, Aggarwal KK, Han R: Post-therapeutic acute malignant myeloproliferative syndrome and acute nonlymphocytic leukemia in non-Hodgkin's lymphoma: Correlation with intensity of treatment. *Cancer* 50:2285–2288, 1982.
198. Greene MH, Yound RC, Merrill JM, et al: Evidence of a treatment dose response in acute nonlymphocytic leukemias which occur after therapy of non-Hodgkin's lymphoma. *Cancer Res* 43:1891–1898, 1983.
199. Fisher B, Rockete H, Fisher ER, et al: Leukemia in breast cancer patients following adjuvant chemotherapy or postoperative radiation: The NSABP experience. *J Clin Oncol* 3:1640–1658, 1985.
200. Lerner HJ: Acute myelogenous leukemia in patients receiving chorambucil as long-term adjuvant chemotherapy for stage II breast cancer. *Cancer Treat Rep* 62:1135–1138, 1979.
201. Boice JD, Greene MH, Killen JY, et al: Late effects of low dose adjuvant chemotherapy in colorectal cancer. *J Natl Cancer Inst* 64:501–511, 1980.
202. Boice JD, Greene MH, Killen JY, et al: Leukemia and preleukemia after adjuvant chemotherapy of gastrointestinal cancer with semustine (methyl-CCNU). *N Engl J Med* 309:1079–1084, 1983.
203. Chak LY, Sikie BL, Tucker MA, et al: Increased incidence of acute nonlymphocytic leukemia following therapy in patients with small cell carcinoma of the lung. *J Clin Oncol* 2:385–390, 1984.
204. Ratain MJ, Kaminer LS, Bitran JD, et al: Acute nonlymphocytic leukemia following etoposide and cisplatin combination chemotherapy for advanced non-small cell carcinoma of the lung. *Blood* 70:1412–1417, 1987.
205. Redman JR, Vugrin D, Arlin ZA, et al: Leukemia following treatment of germ cell tumors in men. *J Clin Oncol* 2:1080–1087, 1984.
206. Greene MH, Boice JD Jr, Greer GE, et al: Acute nonlymphocytic leukemia after therapy with alkylating agents for ovarian cancer. *N Engl J Med* 307:1416–1421, 1982.
207. Kaldor JM, Day NE, Pettersson F, et al: Leukemia following chemotherapy for ovarian cancer. *N Engl J Med* 322:1–6, 1990.
208. Tucker MA, Meadows AT, Boice JD Jr, et al: Leukemia after therapy with alkylating agents for childhood cancer. *J Natl Cancer Inst* 78:459–464, 1987.
209. Moss TS, Stauss LC, Das L, et al: Secondary leukemia following successful treatment of Wilms' tumor. *Am J Pediatr Hemat/Oncol* 11:158–161, 1989.
210. Greene MH, Harris EL, Gershenson DM, et al: Me-

phalan may be a more potent leukemogen than cyclophosphamide. *Ann Intern Med* 105:360–367, 1986.

211. Meadows AT, D'Angio GJ, Mike V, et al: Patterns of second malignant neoplasms in children. *Cancer* 40:1903–1911, 1977.
212. Tucker MA, D'Angio GJ, Boice JD, et al: Bone sarcomas linked to radiotherapy and chemotherapy in children. *N Engl J Med* 317:588–593, 1987.
213. Schwartz AD, Lee H, Baum ES: Leukemia in children with Wilms' tumor. *J Pediatr* 87:374–376, 1975.
214. Boice JD Jr, Blettner M, Kleinerman RA, et al: Radiation dose and second cancer risk in patients treated for cancer of the cervix. *Radiat Res* 116:3–55, 1988.
215. Storm HH: Secondary primary cancer after treatment for cervical cancer: Late effects of radiotherapy. *Cancer* 61:679–688, 1988.
216. Rimm IJ, Li FC, Tabell NJ: Brain tumors after cranial irradiation for childhood acute lymphoblastic leukemia. A 13 year experience from the Dana Farber Cancer Institute and The Children's Hospital. *Cancer* 59:1506–1508, 1987.
217. Gilmann PA, Miller RW: Cancer after acute lymphocytic leukemia. *Am J Dis Child* 135:311–312, 1981.
218. Neglia JP, Meadows AT, Robison LL, et al: Second neoplasms after acute lymphoblastic leukemia in childhood. *N Engl J Med* 325:1330–1336, 1991.
219. List AF, Doll DC, Greco A: Lung cancer in Hodgkin's disease: Association with previous radiotherapy. *J Clin Oncol* 3:215–221, 1985.
220. Steinherz LS, Graham T, Hurwitz R, et al: Guidelines for cardiac monitoring of children during and after anthracycline therapy: Reports of the Cardiology Committee of the Children's Cancer Study Group. *Pediatrics* 89:942–949, 1992.

PART VI

The Care of Individuals with Cancer

Chapter 36

AIDS-Related Malignancies

Theresa A. Moran, RN, MS

INTRODUCTION

For decades, scientists and medical researchers have attempted to prove or disprove the hypothesis of immune surveillance and the evolution of cancer. As research in this area continues, it appears that human immunodeficiency virus (HIV) infection contributes yet another piece of evidence that supports the hypothesized link. The devastation wreaked by HIV on the immune system, particularly the cell-mediated arm, results in the diagnosis of a malignancy at some point during the illness in approximately 70% of those with acquired immunodeficiency syndrome (AIDS).[1] Neoplasms of all organs and body systems also have been reported in patients whose serum is positive for HIV antibody. The three most common malignancies in AIDS are Kaposi's sarcoma (KS), non-Hodgkin's lymphoma (NHL), and primary central nervous system (CNS) lymphoma. These diseases have been referred to as *opportunistic* malignancies because they occur in patients with preexisting immunodeficiency; for example, in persons with primary immunodeficiency, in those who undergo therapeutic immunosuppression, and now in persons with HIV infection. Because these individuals are immunosuppressed, the aforementioned cancers proliferate rapidly.

KAPOSI'S SARCOMA

In 1872 Dr. Moritz Kaposi first described the lesions of Kaposi's sarcoma in seven men of Mediterranean or Jewish ancestry. In 1947 the literature indicated that only 500 cases had been reported, and by 1960 only 1200 total cases had been documented in the 100 years since the disease was first described. The incidence in the general population was estimated to be two to six cases per 100 million people; thus, dermatologists and oncologists were not likely to diagnose this rare malignancy in the course of their professional careers. Beginning in the 1970s, however, the incidence of KS increased dramatically. As more sophisticated technologic advances brought on the era of organ transplantation, an increasing number of reports documented the occurrence of this malignancy in patients who were chemically immunosuppressed to prevent organ rejection.[1,2] With the development of new drugs, oncologists began seeing KS in patients treated with antineoplastic agents. Reports from Africa in the late 1970s revealed that KS was endemic in certain areas of the continent. In 1981 KS was reported in yet another population, that of previously healthy, young, homosexual men who were neither receiving chemotherapy nor undergoing organ transplantations.[3,4] This outbreak of what was once believed to be a rare skin cancer initially was considered an isolated anomaly, but as other cities in the United States began noting the increasing numbers of young men with KS, it became obvious that a new phenomenon was occurring. Controversy exists over whether KS is a malignancy at all or simply a highly dysplastic phenomenon.[5,6] In addition to KS, other opportunistic infections, primarily *Pneumocystis carinii* pneumonia, were diagnosed in this same population.[3,4]

In an effort to determine the cause of this KS outbreak, researchers began examining the immune systems of these young homosexual men. All were found to have some degree of immunosuppression.[4] In 1982 these findings led to the clinical definition of a new disease, acquired immunodeficiency syndrome (AIDS), in which the underlying immunodeficiency resulted in the appearance of indicator diseases.[7] One of the indicator diseases was the diagnosis of KS in a person younger than 60 years of age. In 1987 the diagnosis of AIDS was expanded to include the advent of KS in a person of any age who is seropositive for HIV antibody.[8]

Epidemiology

Before the occurrence of HIV infection, KS was divided into the following categories: classic KS (non-African), African KS (endemic), and KS that occurred in transplant recipients. Cases of classic KS are found in the United States and Europe. Predominantly a disease that occurs in men, it has a male/female ratio of 10–15:1 and primarily affects men of Mediterranean or Jewish ancestry in the fifth to eighth decades of life.[2] This malignancy is characterized as an indolent, slow-growing cutaneous nodule or plaquelike lesion. In 88% of those diagnosed, lesions will be confined to the lower extremities, distal to the knee, without invasive or disseminated disease. Treatment generally is not indicated because of its indolent nature. It is predictably a chronic, fairly benign malignancy that is rarely fatal.[2]

In contrast, African KS (endemic) is a malignant disease that affects persons of all ages, including children, and is found almost exclusively in black Africans. Cases of KS appear to cluster near the equator in the eastern half of the continent. African KS affects men twice as often as women, with a male/female ratio of 2.5:1.[9] Clinical presentations range from one similar to that observed in classic KS (nodular and indolent skin lesion) to a florid, infiltrative, and highly aggressive lymphadenopathic form that progresses rapidly and is frequently fatal.[9]

Transplant recipients experience an increased incidence of KS as high as 150 to 200 times the number of cases found in the general population.[10] Transplant KS also affects men at a higher incidence than women (2–3:1), and presentations can range from localized skin lesions to disseminated visceral and mucocutaneous disease. A correlation seems to exist between the degree of immunosuppression and the incidence of KS. The more depressed the immune system, the greater the incidence of KS. Spontaneous remissions have been documented in transplantation patients whose immunosuppression has been reversed.[10]

The fourth category, AIDS-associated KS, was first described in 1981 and is distinctly different from the other categories of KS (Table 36-1).[11] It is 20,000 times more likely to occur in an HIV-infected individual than in the general population and 300 times more likely than in other immunosuppressed groups.[12] Additionally, within the HIV-infected population it seems that those patients who acquire HIV through sexual transmission are more likely to develop KS than those whose source is injection drug use. Twenty-one percent of homosexual/bisexual men have an index diagnosis of KS, compared to only 1% of hemophiliacs affected with HIV. Interestingly, women are four times more likely to develop KS if their partners are bisexual. This suggests that, in addition to HIV infection, another sexually transmitted organism may play an important role in the development of KS.[12]

Clinical presentation ranges from localized skin lesions to disseminated disease that involves multiple body organs. KS that occurs with AIDS tends to be a highly aggressive disease. Interestingly, it appears that patients diagnosed with KS later than July 1984 may have a more severe form of the disease. Patients with KS diagnosed before then had a mean survival duration of 122.9 weeks, while those diagnosed after July 1984 had a mean survival duration of 71.9 weeks.[13] The reasons for this difference are unclear. Northfelt et al.[13] did not elaborate on demographic data of the population or on any concomitant infection. The authors hypothesized that patients diagnosed earlier in the epidemic had a more intact immune system than those diagnosed later. Despite the aggressiveness of AIDS-related KS, patients rarely die as a direct result of KS. Overall, the mortality rate in this group is approximately 41%, with more than 60% of all patients alive at 1 year and more than 50% alive at 22 months. This rate contrasts with the average survival rate of 18 months for all persons diagnosed with AIDS.[1] Patients with only KS and no opportunistic infections tend to live longer, and there are a number of anecdotal reports of persons with AIDS-related KS who have survived from 3–7 years.[10] The cause of death in patients with AIDS-related KS is usually from concomitant opportunistic infections or the pathologic effects of HIV itself.

Etiology

Earlier in the epidemic, there appeared to be a strong link between immunosuppression and KS, even though the degree of immunosuppression provided no predictive ability. Recently, there has been a report of the appearance of KS in six HIV-negative gay men.[14] This recent report lends support to the hypothesis that a sexually transmitted agent may in fact be responsible for the development of KS and may be more readily expressed in the presence of HIV. There may also exist a large population infected with this KS-causing agent that remains symptom-free unless they become immunosuppressed.[14]

When KS was first reported, it was the initial indicator disease in 30%–35% of all diagnosed cases. A steady decline has been noted, however, in the proportion of AIDS-KS cases among total AIDS cases.[15] It appears that in the gay population a decline of 20% per year has been noted; in other populations with AIDS-KS, a 10% decline per year has been reported.

TABLE 36-1 Clinical Features of Kaposi's Sarcoma

Groups	Clinical Features	Response to Therapy
Classic: elderly men, especially of Jewish, Mediterranean ancestry	Indolent; cutaneous lesions of legs, feet; immunologic attrition of aging	Local radiation: good control; rarely fatal.
Endemic: black Africans	Variable; children: aggressive, lymphadenopathic; adults: usually indolent, affects extremities; no underlying immunodeficiency	Systemic chemotherapy; poor response in lymphadenopathic form; excellent response in indolent, adult form.
Renal transplant recipients	Aggressive, localized to visceral involvement; chemotherapy-induced immunosuppression	Controlled by stopping immunosuppressive medications
AIDS-related	Aggressive, disseminated disease with cutaneous, visceral, and lymphadenopathic involvement; virally induced immunodeficiency	Systemic chemotherapy: response rates of 25%–50% Radiation therapy: good response but recurrence common: palliative not curative Treatment selection is complex; need to control tumor without exacerbating immunodeficiency.

Source: Adapted from Volberding PA: Kaposi's sarcoma in AIDS, in Levy JA (ed), *AIDS, Pathogenesis and Treatment*. New York, Dekker, 1989, p. 349.

It has been suggested that this decline reflects behavior change, as correlated with a decreased risk of developing sexually transmitted diseases.[13] Other possible explanations for this reduction in incidence of initial diagnosis include medical advancements that enable opportunistic infections to be diagnosed earlier than KS and the elimination of a co-factor that promotes the development of KS. Some researchers link the decreased incidence of KS to the decreased use of "poppers," or amyl nitrate, believed to be a co-factor in the development of AIDS-related KS.[16] This connection was suggested in several studies; however, large enough cohorts have not been collected and studied to document a causal relationship. Another group of researchers believes that hereditary or genetic predisposition plays an important role in the development of KS in both immunocompetent and immunodeficient populations. These researchers postulate that men infected with HIV who carry the human leukocyte antigen (HLA)-DR5 allele may be at an increased risk for KS development. Again, a causal relationship has not been established, and the postulate remains controversial.[17]

KS seems to be a disease found predominantly in homosexual and bisexual men with AIDS. Other groups diagnosed with AIDS (women, children, or men who are heterosexual or intravenous drug users, or both) do not have as high an incidence of KS as homosexual men with AIDS.[18,19] One study found the DNA of cytomegalovirus (CMV) in the nucleus of cells of KS lesions, which suggests a viral cause of KS.[20] Serologic testing demonstrates that as many as 94% of all homosexual men may have been infected by CMV, as evidenced by antibodies to CMV.[21] CMV also has been isolated from the blood, semen, gastrointestinal tract, central nervous system (CNS), and lungs of patients with AIDS, which suggests the possible role of latent CMV infection in AIDS-related KS. In fact, a decline in CMV seroconversion has also been noted in recent years. Together with high CMV antibody seroprevalence, this viral link may offer an explanation for the predominance of KS in homosexual men.

It is also important to remember that statistics for KS are kept only on initial diagnosis of AIDS. There are few reports that examine the development of KS at any point during the AIDS illness. Northfelt et al.,[13] however, reported the San Francisco experience and indeed did note a decline in the report of KS at any time during the illness. This may reflect, however, the expanded definition of AIDS and the increased number of AIDS cases being reported under that expanded definition.

Detection

Detection of KS is typically by self-observation of cutaneous lesions. This makes patient education in lesion identification an important method of detection. Additionally, all health care providers should routinely perform a careful visual examination of cutaneous surfaces of all persons who are seropositive for HIV or who are in a high-risk group for AIDS. Visual inspection includes the skin of the head (including the sclera), neck, torso, extremities, perirectal area, palms of the hands, soles of the feet, and the oral cavity. Biopsy specimens of suspicious lesions are examined. KS also may be a differential diagnosis in patients with enlarged lymph nodes or with pulmonary symptoms and a chest film with abnormal findings.

Pathophysiology

After histologic examination the pathologist has the responsibility of diagnosis. All types of KS (endemic, classic, transplantation-induced, and epidemic) are microscopically similar. Descriptions of lesions include interlacing bands of spindle cells, with vascular structures in a network of reticular and collagen fibers. As the integrity of this network is lost, clefts usually occur among the vascular structures, which allows the extravasation of red blood cells. Lymphatic and blood vessels are present throughout the lesion and on its periphery. The nuclei of the spindle cells are frequently pleomorphic. Hemosiderin, extravasated red cells, and red cells that phagocytose the hemosiderin may be found between spindle cells. An inflammatory response involving histiocytes, lymphocytes, and plasma cells also may be seen.

Diagnosis can be difficult, especially in early or immature lesions. This stage has been referred to as the *macular stage*. Changes in this stage may be subtle, and the pathologist may observe only abnormally dilated vessels surrounding normal superficial vasculature. There may be little or no inflammatory response at this stage. Nuclear pleomorphism may be seen in mitosis, with nuclear atypia. As the lesion matures and becomes a plaque, it demonstrates more extensive neoplastic involvement, with proliferation through many layers, including the dermis and occasionally the adipose layers. A marked inflammatory response occurs at this stage, with a corresponding increase in numbers of spindle cells and extravasation of red cells. The prominence of hemosiderin deposits also is noted at this time. As the lesion advances toward nodular formation, these effects become more exaggerated. Spindle cells are dense, with considerable reticulum deposition.[17,22–24]

Clinical Manifestations

The clinical presentation of AIDS-related KS resembles that of KS in transplant recipients. Multicentric skin lesions may be observed on any part of the body—the disseminated mucocutaneous and visceral disease frequently affects the lymphatic, pulmonary, gastrointestinal, cardiac, renal, biliary, and adrenal systems. There is no characteristic site of initial involvement as there is in the classic form of the disease. Lesions can be found on almost any skin surface, including the palms of the hands, soles of the feet, genitals, and head and neck. These lesions generally do not metastasize; instead, they are multicentric (i.e., each lesion is a primary lesion unto itself). The lesions range in pigmentation from brown, brown-red, purple, dark red, to violet; in rare cases they may appear to be deep blue-purple, resembling ecchymosis. They may be raised bullous nodules or flat plaquelike lesions. In either presentation they do not blanch when pressure is applied and are not painful unless they are responsible for structural damage or impinge on vital organs or nerves. Black patients commonly have nodular lesions, and white patients tend to have either nodular or plaquelike lesions. As with HIV infection, the average age range for AIDS-related KS is from 20–40 years.

This tumor can involve not only the skin but also the mucocutaneous surface of the buccal mucosa, the hard and soft palate, and the gums, as well as the sclera of the eyes. In fact, at the time of initial diagnosis of KS, approximately 72% of patients will already have involvement of one or more organ systems.[1] Internal organs most frequently affected include lymph nodes (81%), gastrointestinal tract (33%), and the lungs (11%).[1,25] KS in these organ systems can cause severe morbidity. Lesions also have been found in the liver, pancreas, adrenal glands, spleen, testes, and heart. Symptoms caused by these lesions usually are minimal.[1,20]

As HIV infection progresses, the immune system becomes increasingly suppressed; with it the occurrence and severity of KS also increase. Increasing numbers of skin lesions may be found all over the body surface. The multicentric skin lesions continue to enlarge, frequently coalescing with each other to form one large confluent lesion, often encompassing as large an area as the thigh, shin, or forearm. Malignant cells may involve the lymph nodes, thus compromising lymphatic drainage and blood circulation, resulting in severe edema distal to the affected area and stasis ulcers from edematous tissue. The lymph node involvement may be so severe as to cause major shifts in body fluids, limiting the flow of vital protein from lymph to plasma. The patient may succumb to anasarca, which is due to internal coalesced lesions and a decreased total serum protein/albumin resulting from the shift of fluid.

Additionally, when the gastrointestinal tract is involved, the patient may have a protein-losing enteropathy.[26] In this instance, protein is not absorbed from the gastrointestinal tract, which results in a decreased total serum protein/albumin level. In cases where progression of KS involves the lung, symptoms include dyspnea and shortness of breath, eventually culminating in fatal respiratory distress.[25,27,28]

Staging

The ability to classify patients with similar stages of the disease would enable researchers to compare data and patient outcome, and to this end Laubenstein,[29] Krigel et al.,[30] and later Mitsuyasu[15] proposed staging systems for AIDS-related KS (Table 36-2).[17,30] These researchers recognized that there are some patients with KS whose prognosis is better than others. The reasons are not clear, nor have all the variables been examined. Some studies have correlated the relationship between the absolute CD4 lymphocyte count and prognosis. For example, the lower the CD4 value in a patient with KS, the poorer the prognosis. A person with a helper/suppressor (H:S) ratio of greater than 0.5 (>1:2) and a CD4 lymphocyte count of greater than 300/mm³ has a relatively good prognosis. A helper/suppressor ratio of less than 0.2 (<1:5) and a CD4 lymphocyte count of less than 100/mm³ indicates a very poor prognosis. The area in between these values is of unclear prognostic value.[31–33] Other data also indicate that patients with head and neck involvement,[34] patients with prior or concomitant opportunistic infections, and patients exhibiting "B" symptoms (weight loss, fevers, chills, night

TABLE 36-2 Staging of Epidemic Kaposi's Sarcoma

Stage	NYU Staging System*	Mitsuyasu Staging System†
I	Cutaneous, locally indolent	Limited cutaneous (<10 lesions or one anatomical area)
II	Cutaneous, locally aggressive with or without regional lymph nodes	Disseminated cutaneous (>10 lesions or more than one anatomical area)
III	Generalized mucocutaneous and/or lymph node involvement‡	Visceral only (GI, lymph node)
IV	Visceral	Cutaneous and viscera, or pulmonary KS
Subtype		
A	No systemic signs or symptoms	No systemic signs or symptoms
B	Systemic signs; weight loss (10%) or fever (>100°F orally, unrelated to an identifiable source of infection lasting >2 wk)	Fevers >37.8°C unrelated to identifiable infection lasting >2 wk, or weight loss >10% of body weight

* Kringel RL et al: Kaposi's sarcoma: A new staging classification, *Cancer Treat Rep* 67:531, 1983.
† Mitsuyasu RT, Groopman JE: Biology and therapy of Kaposi's sarcoma, *Semin Oncol* 11:53, 1984.
‡ Generalized-more than upper or lower extremities alone; includes minimal GI disease defined as <5 lesions and <2 cm in combined diameters.
Source: Groopman J, Broder S: Cancer in AIDS and other immunodeficiency states, in DeVita VT, Hellman S, Rosenberg SA (eds); *Cancer Principles and Practice of Oncology.* (3d ed). Philadelphia, Lippincott, 1989, p. 1962.

sweats, diarrhea) all have a shorter life expectancy than those without these factors. With the exception of the lung, organ involvement does not seem to influence prognosis, nor does tumor burden correlate with prognosis.[35]

In 1989 the Oncology Committee of the National Institute of Allergy and Infectious Diseases (NIAID)–sponsored AIDS Clinical Trials Group (ACTG) developed a proposal for uniform evaluation, response, and staging criteria for KS. This system, similar to the tumor-node-metastasis (TNM) system, utilized the extent of tumor, the immune status, and other systemic illnesses (TIS) that were AIDS-related, to determine the stage of disease (Table 36-3).[36] Patients are assigned to either a good risk or poor risk category depending on the extent of the tumor, immune system status, and other systemic illnesses. In addition to the staging system developed by the NIAID-ACTG, this group also developed criteria for a standardized format of documenting the extent of KS on both initial and subsequent evaluation, as well as response definitions that include assessments of lesion nodularity and tumor-associated edema, supplementing the more traditional method for evaluating tumor response. This new system should allow for more accurate assessment of patients with KS and more meaningful outcomes from research studies.

TABLE 36-3 Recommended Staging Classification

	Good Risk (0) (All of the Following)	Poor Risk (1) (Any of the Following)
Tumor (T)	Confined to skin and/ or lymph nodes and/ or minimal oral disease*	Tumor-associated edema or ulceration; extensive oral KS; gastrointestinal KS; KS in other nonnodal viscera.
Immune system (I)	CD4 cells ≥200/mm³	CD4 cells ≤200/mm³
Systemic illness (S)	No history of opportunistic infection or thrush; no "B" symptoms†; performance status ≥70 (Karnofsky)	History of opportunistic infection and/or thrush; "B" symptoms; performance status <70 (Karnofsky); other HIV-related illness (eg, neurologic disease; lymphoma)

* Minimal oral disease is nonnodular KS confined to the palate.
† "B" symptoms: unexplained fever, night sweats, >10% involuntary weight loss, or diarrhea persisting more than 2 weeks.
Source: Krown S, Metroka C, Wernz J: Kaposi's sarcoma in the acquired immune deficiency syndrome: A proposal for uniform evaluation, response, and staging criteria, *J Clin Oncol* 7:1206, 1989. (Reprinted with permission.)

Assessment

A complete history and physical examination is indicated, including the patient's past history of drug use, sexual practice, and ethnic ancestry, along with close examination of the sclera, oral cavity, and integumentary system. Suspicious lesions must be biopsied before a diagnosis can be established. Visual inspection of lesions alone is insufficient to establish a diagnosis. Experienced physicians who care for patients with AIDS reflect anecdotally on lesions that appeared to be symptomatic of KS but were not histologically confirmed; conversely, examination of tissue from lesions that did not resemble those of KS proved to be diagnostic of KS. A lesion that visually suggested KS may be an immature lesion and thus does not show the distinctive pathologic changes that are diagnostic of KS. Repeat biopsies of other suspicious lesions at a later date (e.g., in 2 weeks) may in fact yield a diagnosis of KS.

Examination of preparations from a 3-, 4-, or 6-mm punch biopsy of skin lesions is the most common method of diagnosis. Patients with KS involvement of the oral cavity should be referred to an oral surgeon for a diagnostic biopsy. Suspicious lymph nodes are best evaluated by means of an open (excisional) biopsy. Suspected KS involvement of other organs requires more invasive diagnostic procedures. For example, documentation of lung involvement requires a bronchoscopic examination. Similarly, documentation of gastrointestinal lesions requires endoscopic examination of the upper or lower tract. Lesions visualized by means of bronchoscopy or endoscopy may be examined by biopsy, but because of the submucosal and highly vascular nature of the tumor, removal of tissue from these sites may cause bleeding and increased morbidity. For this reason, visual inspection and identification may be adequate for diagnosing lung or gastrointestinal involvement.

Documenting organ involvement by other means can be difficult. KS that involves the lung cannot be diagnosed or distinguished from other causes of respiratory distress by means of chest films. An upper gastrointestinal series may demonstrate lesions in the gut, but the cause remains unknown without visual inspection by endoscopy or tissue biopsy. Because it appears that the presence or absence of organ involvement, with the exception of the lung, does not affect survival, documentation of extent of disease is not useful in treatment decisions. If treatment of a specific site is to be initiated (e.g., radiation therapy to treat enlarged lymph nodes), then tissue diagnosis must be determined.[33,34] There are several reports in the literature of patients having both KS and another malignancy in the same lymph node.

Patients with AIDS-related KS also may show laboratory abnormalities that probably are more related to HIV infection than to KS. These include elevated erythrocyte sedimentation rate (ESR), mild anemia, and leukopenia. Depressed test results with cosyntropin stimulation, elevated serum transaminase levels, and depressed platelet count may result from KS involvement of the adrenal glands, liver, or spleen respectively.

Treatment

Medical

Before the epidemic of AIDS and HIV infection, the KS seen in the United States was primarily classic KS (i.e., indolent, slow growing, and chronic), which required little or no treatment. In the transplant recipient the reversal of immunosuppression by withdrawing immunosuppressive drugs generally resolved the problem. In AIDS-related KS, treatment of the malignancy provides only temporary remission or stabilization of disease and does not improve survival rate. The main goal of treatment is to lessen morbidity.

As with other malignancies, three treatment options exist: surgery, radiation therapy, and chemotherapy. Other than enabling the provider to establish a diagnosis, surgery has almost no role in the treatment of KS. Radiation therapy is highly effective and plays a role in local control of lesions and in cosmetic effect. This treatment, however, is not free of side effects and affects patients with KS in the same manner as it does others who receive radiation therapy. Irradiation of tonsillar or oral lesions, for example, may cause severe stomatitis because of a preexisting *Candida* infection. Chemotherapeutic agents are useful in the treatment of AIDS-related KS when a systemic effect is necessary and the benefits of treatment outweigh the risks to the patient. Guidelines for treatment of AIDS-related KS are outlined in Table 36-4.[11,15,37]

Patients with aggressive or extensive disease who have an absolute neutrophil count greater than 1000/mm^3 may receive weekly single-agent chemotherapy. Those single agents include doxorubicin, 10–15 mg/m^2; vinblastine, 0.1 mg/kg; vincristine, 2 mg; or etoposide 150 mg/m^2. A patient with rapidly progressing disease, with disease unresponsive to single-agent therapy, or with lung involvement may be offered combination chemotherapy consisting of doxorubicin, bleomycin, and vincristine, administered every other week on the basis of the patient's complete blood cell count (CBC) or single-agent etoposide either orally or intravenously.[38] Overall, lung involvement is a poor prognostic sign. Patients who are unable to tolerate aggressive chemotherapy because of a low CBC receive a weekly course of either bleomycin or vincristine, alternating with vinblastine every other week.[11,16,37,39]

Interferon also has shown efficacy in the treatment of AIDS-related KS. Trials of recombinant alpha-interferon began in 1981, and since that time a select group of patients has been identified as favorable responders to alpha-interferon.[40] Their characteristics include CD4 counts greater than 200/mm^3, no prior AIDS-defining diagnosis, and no "B" symptoms. Objective responses in this group of patients ranged from 42%–79%.[41,42] Recommended dosages range from 18–30 million units subcutaneously injected every day, 5 days a week. Due to both subjective (fevers, chills, myalgias) and objective side effects (neutropenia, thrombocytopenia, transient elevated transaminases), the usual dose tolerated is approximately one-quarter to one-half the recommended dose.

To minimize systemic side effects, investigators also have explored the use of intralesional recombinant tumor necrosis factor and intralesional vinblastine for local control. Results from using intralesional recombinant tumor necrosis factor (rTNF) were disappointing. While 15 of the 16 patients treated with intralesional rTNF evidenced objective responses, the intense local inflammatory response was thought to be the cause of tumoricidal activity rather than the rTNF.[43]

The response of KS lesions to chemotherapy can be dramatic. The lesions frequently will decrease in size, flatten, and lose their pigmentation; however, they do not completely go away. The area remains pigmented, both after treatment with chemotherapy or radiation therapy or both.

Nursing

Nursing care includes assessment of the patient in terms of the health–illness continuum. Consideration is given to the psychosocial aspects of the disease, as well as to the physical status of the patient. A determination of the patient's risk group and whether KS is the patient's first diagnosis or one in a long line of indicator diseases will help the nurse establish a plan of care.

Although great strides have been made to reduce phobia concerning AIDS and homosexual men, it is important to remember that the patient may be explaining his sexual preference to his family for the first time and informing them that he has a fatal disease. Emotional support is crucial. If the patient is an intravenous drug user, philosophic dilemmas may arise concerning the patient entering drug rehabilitation programs. Realistic goals are necessary in this patient population because of both drug-seeking and manipulative behavior.

The complications associated with the use of chemotherapeutic agents in patients with KS are similar to the complications experienced by other patient populations receiving the same agents. Nausea, vomiting, anorexia, stomatitis, and alopecia all occur with the same frequency as in other populations. What appears to differ in the AIDS population is the severity of the complications. For this reason, nurses should be aggressive in the assessment of potential complications, alert the physician promptly, and implement appropriate nursing interventions. It also should be remembered that these patients have an underlying illness that predisposes them to other opportunistic infections and malignancies.

Patients with KS, on receiving the first dose of vinca alkaloids, may experience severe jaw pain. Although

TABLE 36-4 Guidelines for Therapy in AIDS-Related Kaposi's Sarcoma

Group	Recommendations	Regimen
Minimal KS; <25 cutaneous lesions, stable disease, no history of opportunistic infections and/or "B" symptoms	No treatment with expectant observation for disease progression	No treatment
	or	
	Experimental immunomodulators and/or antiviral drugs	Alpha-interferon, 20–50 million units qd; SQ, IM or IV
	or	or
		Azidothymidine, 200 mg q 4hr, PO
	Vinblastine or other single-agent therapy	Vinblastine, 4–8 mg/wk, IV or Vincristine, 2 mg/wk or qowk, IV Doxorubicin, 15–20 mg/m²/wk, IV Vinblastine/Vincristine, doses as above; each drug used individually on an alternating weekly basis
Minimal KS; <25 cutaneous lesions, stable disease, prior history of opportunistic infections and/or "B" symptoms	Vinblastine or other single-agent therapy	Vinblastine; doses as above, or Vincristine; doses as above, or Doxorubicin; doses as above, or Vinblastine; vincristine; doses as above
	and	
	Experimental immunomodulators and/or antiviral drugs if used in conjunction with cytotoxic agents	Alpha-interferon or azidothymidine; doses as above
Advanced KS; extensive disease, prior to history of opportunistic infection and/or "B" symptoms	Etoposide or doxorubicin as single-agent therapy	Etoposide, 150 mg/m² qd × 3 days, then 28 days, IV doxorubicin; doses as above
	or	
	Multiple-agent chemotherapy with doxorubicin, bleomycin, and vinblastine	Doxorubicin, 40 mg/m² q wk–28 days, IV; bleomycin, 15 units/m² q 15 days, IV; vinblastine, 6 mg/m² q 21 days, IV
KS with severe neutropenia or thrombocytopenia	Vincristine with or without bleomycin	Vincristine; doses as above with or without bleomycin; doses as above
Pulmonary KS	Etoposide or doxorubicin with or without radiation therapy	Etoposide; doses as above
Localized, bulky KS lesion of oral cavity, face, legs, or lymph nodes	Radiation therapy	Local therapy, 800–3000 cGy; fractionation or slow dose administration to oral cavity or oropharynx

Source: Volberding PA: Kaposi's sarcoma in AIDS, in Levy JA (ed), *AIDS, Pathogenesis, and Treatment* (New York, Dekker, 1989), pp. 352–354; Mitsuyasu RT: Kaposi's sarcoma in the acquired immunodeficiency syndrome, in Sande MA, Volberding PA (eds), *The Medical Management of AIDS*. Philadelphia: Saunders, 1988, pp. 296–302.

this reaction is a reported side effect of treatment with the vinca alkaloids, patients with AIDS and KS seem to have an increased incidence. Treatment with vinca alkaloids should be discontinued in patients with this reaction because they may cause irreversible nerve damage.[44]

NON-HODGKIN'S LYMPHOMA

Epidemiology

Beginning in 1982, physicians in San Francisco, Los Angeles, and New York noted an increased incidence of NHL in homosexual patients. Because they believed that this incidence of NHL was somehow linked to the same immunodeficiency seen in AIDS, they began to prospectively collect blood for evaluation of the immune system. In fact, the immune deficiencies found in these patients with NHL were similar to those found in other patients with AIDS. Because cancer in and of itself is immunosuppressive, this finding alone did not establish a diagnosis of AIDS. It did, however, initiate further investigation. When the HIV antibody test became available, these patients with NHL were found to be seropositive. Thus, the link to HIV disease was demonstrated, and a new category of malignancy was added to the case definition of AIDS. NHL in a person who also is seropositive for HIV antibody or has positive culture results is considered to affirm a diagnosis of AIDS.[8,45–47]

It is difficult to determine the impact of HIV-related NHL on cancer statistics. Approximately 41,000 cases of NHL will be diagnosed in 1992;[48] however, the percentage of those cases that are HIV-related cannot be determined because statistics concerning tumors do not account for HIV status. Because the reporting of AIDS cases to the Centers for Disease Control (CDC) now is required by law, the incidence of HIV-related NHL eventually may become known. It has been estimated that NHL has been diagnosed in 4%–10% of patients with AIDS. It is important to remember, however, that the CDC requires reporting of index diagnosis only and that HIV-testing of all NHL has not become part of the standard work-up. In one review by the French Registry of HIV-associated tumors, 33% of NHL occurred in patients already diagnosed with AIDS (56/168).[49] If U.S. statistics parallel the French data, one can assume that there has been a fair amount of underreporting. Of interest in the French review is the histology of the tumors. They reported three distinct categories of AIDS-related NHL: large-cell lymphoma (LCL), immunoblastic lymphoma (IL), and Burkitt's-like lymphoma (BL). They also associated the first two lymphoma histologies with severe immune suppression, defined as a median CD4+ of 99 cells/μL and compared with BL, with a median CD4+ of 270 cells/μl. This finding has significance in the pathogenesis of NHL. It is known that LCL and IL are associated with immune suppression, while BL is not, suggesting perhaps another reason for the development of BL in HIV-positive persons.[49]

A brief mention should be made of the controversy that exists around antiretroviral agents, specifically azidothymidine (AZT) and the development of NHL. The question continues to be asked whether the use of AZT increases the likelihood of developing NHL. While AZT has been shown to cause malignancies in laboratory animals, the dosages administered were 3 to 24 times higher than the recommended human dose. It is now generally recognized that the increased survival attributed to AZT increases the likelihood of developing NHL. Data exist showing that the incidence of developing NHL in long-term survivors of HIV is comparable whether the patient takes AZT or not.[50]

Etiology

The connection between cancers and viruses has not been fully established; however, there are some malignancies in which a causative viral agent has been isolated. One such association exists between the malignancy known as African lymphoma, or Burkitt's lymphoma, which is a type of high-grade NHL, and Epstein-Barr virus (EBV). In 1962 Dr. Dennis Burkitt described a malignant lymphoma in African children that was typically extranodal in origin, with an affinity for facial bones. There appeared to be an increased incidence of this malignancy in regions of high temperature and rainfall. This suggested to Burkitt some type of insect vector as a method of infection (or transmission). Since then, serologic studies and tissue cultures have established a constant association with the DNA-containing herpes virus known as EBV and the development of Burkitt's lymphoma.[47] Although the significance of the geographic distribution remains unclear, it has been hypothesized that malaria or some other insect-borne infection results in a reticuloendothelial hyperplasia that may be a necessary co-factor for the oncogenic virus in the development of the malignancy. EBV also has been implicated as the causative agent in nasopharyngeal carcinoma and in the development of NHL in transplant recipients; it also has been suggested as an important etiologic agent in AIDS-NHL.[47]

Of interest is that similar research involving patients with AIDS could not causally link EBV to HIV-related NHL. Although the EBV genome has been isolated in 30%–50% of the DNA of HIV-positive patients with NHL, a direct relationship is not apparent.[51,52] The role of EBV in the development of NHL remains unclear; however, even though the viral link cannot be causally established, it is strongly suspected. Ziegler[53] hypothesized that once infection with HIV occurs, EBV may trigger lymphocyte proliferation that remains unchecked as a result of immune dysfunction caused by HIV. This proliferation, in turn, may allow the expression of two oncogenes, resulting in a polyclonal or monoclonal NHL.[53] Confusingly, Kaplan et al.[54] report on EBV-positive serum in a small series of AIDS-NHL patients. In the 14 patients whose tissue was tested, four specimens were EBV-positive, and in a fifth patient EBV was recovered from one tumor site but not the second tumor site, leading Kaplan et al. to hypothesize that EBV may be a "passenger" virus and not responsible for malignant transformation. There also seem to be distinct differences in EBV positivity between tumor histology and site of involvement. MacMahon et al.[52] reported that large-cell lymphomas were more frequently EBV-positive (65%), whereas the small, non-cleaved cell (Burkitt's-like) lymphomas are less likely to be EBV-positive (20%) in the HIV-infected individuals. They also reported a consistent association of EBV to primary CNS lymphoma in the HIV-infected individual. Twenty-one specimens of brain tissue from HIV-positive CNS lymphoma patients were examined for EBV, and all 21 tested positive, suggesting a different pathogenesis from the systemic form of the disease.

It is now known that therapeutic immunosuppression increases the risk of lymphoma development. For example, the risk for transplant recipients has been estimated to be between 35 and 200 times greater than that for the general population.[55]

Pathophysiology

AIDS-associated NHLs are predominantly B-cell malignancies, typically intermediate to high grade. However, there have been a few isolated reports of lymphomas that are T-cell in origin in men who show HIV seropositivity. The significance of these few cases is unclear; the numbers are small and may simply represent the normal distribution of T-cell lymphoma in the general population. Only through an increase in the frequency of this type of lymphoma can significance be determined. In the meantime it remains an interesting phenomenon.[56,57]

Most cases of AIDS-NHL also have been associated with a previous history of persistent generalized lymphadenopathy. Benign follicular hyperplasia is a typical histologic finding upon biopsy, which suggests that this lymphoma may arise from a polyclonal B-cell activation. This polyclonal B-cell lymphoproliferation may be a complex result of EBV and HIV infection.[51,58–61] Current research is underway on the role of human T-lymphotropic virus type I as a co-infecting retrovirus in the development of lymphomas in AIDS.[62] Few patients have been identified as being co-infected, and it appears that their course of disease is determined more by their HIV infection.[63]

If the process of AIDS-associated NHL begins in a lymph node, the growing tumor causes structural damage, including effacement of the normal node architecture, replacement of normal cellularity by uniform and/or grossly abnormal cells, and the random extension of cellular proliferations beyond the original structural confines of the node. Development of lymphoma, however, is not limited to lymph nodes or the spleen; all organs have lymphocytes within their boundaries that are capable of transforming and forming tumors.

Clinical Manifestations

In the general population the earliest sign of NHL unrelated to AIDS is usually a painless, enlarged, discrete lymph node located in the neck. Although most patients have no symptoms, approximately 20% may experience "B" symptoms, including fever, night sweats, and weight loss.[51] Patients who do not have AIDS frequently have a history of intermittent lymphadenopathy that has been present for several months. Although axillary or inguinal lymph nodes may be the first to enlarge, this enlargement is not common. Frequently, there is involvement of Waldeyer's ring, epitrochlear nodes, the testes, and the gastrointestinal tract. The liver and bone marrow may be involved. There is a higher incidence of CNS involvement in patients with NHL unrelated to AIDS who have bone marrow involvement. The disease will be localized in fewer than 10% of patients who do not have AIDS.[64] Because of the diffuse presentation of lymphoma, non-AIDS NHL should be included in the differential diagnosis of patients with superior vena cava syndrome, acute spinal cord compression, solitary thyroid nodules, isolated tumor nodules of the skin, bone tumors, unexplained anemias, testicular masses, or solitary brain lesions.

In contrast to the presentation just described, patients with HIV-related NHL have very advanced disease, which frequently involves extranodal sites. In one of the first studies[64] of 90 cases of AIDS-NHL, 19% were classified as intermediate-grade diffuse large cell; 28% as high-grade, large-cell immunoblastic; and 36% as high-grade, small, noncleaved lymphomas. This presentation remains unchanged, with greater than 50% of patients presenting as high grade.[49,54] Extranodal sites most commonly involved include the CNS, bone marrow, bowel, and the anorectum; less commonly involved is the myocardium. In addition, these extranodal sites may be the only site of disease; that is, peripheral lymphadenopathy may be absent. If nodal sites are involved, there does not appear to be any predisposition to specific nodes.[60–64] In addition, these patients also may have underlying signs and symptoms of HIV infection, AIDS-related complex, or AIDS, including wasting, anorexia, nausea, vomiting, and fever, which confounds the work-up and makes diagnosis difficult.

Assessment

The diagnosis and classification of lymphoma can be made only by means of a biopsy specimen that is examined by a pathologist. Fine-needle aspirations may be helpful in differentiating a benign versus a malignant process, but, because of insufficient tissue yield, they are not useful in classifying the lymphoma. To fully assess HIV-related NHL, the patient's status must be staged and graded. Staging—that is, determining the extent of disease involvement—is accomplished by means of the Ann Arbor staging classification system (see Chapter 47). The staging work-up includes a careful history, which notes the presence or absence of "B" symptoms, and a complete physical examination with special attention to Waldeyer's ring, the liver, and the spleen. Laboratory tests include CBC, differential cell and platelet count, sedimentation rate, serum chemistries, and liver function tests. The laboratory tests are not specific to lymphoma; they can indicate the overall wellness of the patient and are helpful in screening for hypercalcemia, hyperphosphatemia, and hyperuricemia. A chest film and computed tomography (CT) scans of the chest, abdomen, and pelvis also are indicated. These usually are not indicated for patients with NHL in the general population, but because of the extensive extranodal involvement characteristic of HIV-related NHL they are extremely important. A bilateral bone marrow biopsy and aspiration, as well as a lumbar puncture, should be performed. Once all the tests are complete, the patient is assigned a staging number that can help predict responsiveness to treatment.

If AIDS has not been previously diagnosed, an HIV

antibody test is indicated. It is important to note that not all swollen lymph nodes are malignant; benign reactive lymphadenopathy is a common finding in this HIV-seropositive population and is postulated to be an adaptive physiologic response to HIV insult. Abdominal masses or lymph nodes in a person who is HIV seropositive could be related to *Mycobacterium avium-intracellulare* infection; thus, it is essential to obtain a biopsy specimen and compare it with normal tissue before a diagnosis is made. It is unusual for patients with HIV-related NHL to present at a stage lower than stage III.[54,65,66]

Treatment

Medical

Once the disease is staged and graded, treatment for NHL may begin. Treatment options can be determined on the basis of method (surgery, radiation therapy, and chemotherapy), as well as by grade of tumor. Low-grade tumors are uncommon in the population infected with HIV; in the general population the tumors are indolent and slow growing, requiring no treatment until they impinge on a vital structure or cause symptoms. At that time, radiation therapy to the affected site usually is sufficient to treat the tumor, although chemotherapy may be used as well. Intermediate-grade tumors are more common in the population infected with HIV and may account for as much as 50% of HIV-related NHL. This grade of tumor in the general population can be treated with either chemotherapy or radiation therapy, depending on the stage at presentation.

The remaining HIV-related NHL occurs as high-grade, advanced stage disease. DiCarlo et al.[65] found that 41% of patients with HIV-related NHL had high-grade disease. Ahmed et al.[66] found that all patients with HIV-related NHL in their review had either intermediate or high-grade disease.

The treatment of choice for advanced intermediate/high-grade lymphoma is combination chemotherapy. The most active and effective single agent used in the treatment of NHL is cyclophosphamide. Other drugs that are effective include methotrexate, doxorubicin, vincristine, vinblastine, prednisone, and cytosine arabinoside. Generally, these agents are used in some combination. The most common regimens include M-BACOD (methotrexate, doxorubicin, cyclophosphamide, vincristine, dexamethasone), MACOP-B (methotrexate, doxorubicin, cyclophosphamide, vincristine, prednisone, bleomycin), and CHOP (cyclophosphamide, doxorubicin, vincristine, prednisone) (see Chapter 47 for a description of these regimens). Initial responses to chemotherapy usually are dramatic, with shrinkage of the tumor noted within 24 hours. But the response is not usually long-lived. Typically, patients remain disease-free while receiving chemotherapy; relapse occurs within 4–6 weeks after the discontinuation of chemotherapy. Once chemotherapy is reinstituted, response rates are somewhat diminished. The neutropenia that results from treatment may be severe (attributed to poor bone marrow reserve as a result of either HIV or *M. avium intracellulare*) and sometimes precipitates an opportunistic infection. Research trials being conducted by the ACTG are examining the use of growth factors to support the bone marrow in AIDS-related NHL patients being treated with chemotherapy. It is important to remember that these patients have an underlying immune disorder and that, whatever the outcome, they still have HIV infection and AIDS.

Radiation therapy may be useful for patients with limited bulky disease, for those who are unable to tolerate chemotherapy either because of poor health or low blood counts, for local control, or in some instances, for CNS prophylaxis. Surgery plays no role in the treatment of NHL other than to obtain a biopsy specimen.

Results and prognosis

As with other types of cancer, a group of patients can be identified who will respond better to treatment and demonstrate a better prognosis. Kaplan, et al.[54] identified a "good" prognosis category that included indicators such as prior AIDS diagnosis, Karnofsky performance status, site of disease, and CD4 count (Table 36-5). In addition, they identified a treatment-related indicator, the dose of cyclophosphamide received by the patient; however, they caution that these indicators were not the result of a randomized trial, and that many confounding variables exist.

Nursing

Nursing care of patients with AIDS-related NHL is no different from the care of those patients in the gen-

TABLE 36-5 Prognosis and Survival Trends in Treated Patients with AIDS-Associated NHL

Good Prognosis	Median Survival (months)	Poor Prognosis	Median Survival (months)
No prior AIDS diagnosis	8.3 ± 1.5	Prior AIDS diagnosis	2.2 ± 7.7
KPS >70%	6.8 ± 1.7	KPS <70%	3.8 ± 1.1
No extranodal sites	12.2 ± 3.0	Extranodal nodal	3.4 ± 1.0 4.2 ± 1.3
CD4 + >100	24 ± 3	CD4 + <100	4.1 ± 1.0
Treatment			
Cyclophosphamide (CTX) <1 g	12.2 ± 1.7	CTX >1 g	4.6 ± 1.3

Source: Adapted from Kaplan L, Abrams D, Feigal E, et al: AIDS-associated non-Hodgkin's lymphoma in San Francisco, *JAMA* 261:719–724, 1989.

eral population with non-AIDS-related NHL, with the exception of the emotional (psychosocial) aspect.

It should be noted that patients with large, bulky, high-grade disease are at high risk for tumor lysis syndrome. The exact numbers of patients with tumor lysis syndrome are unknown; some clinicians estimate that it may occur in as many as 10% of patients, whether or not their NHL is related to HIV. Anecdotally, it appears that patients with HIV-related NHL have a high incidence of this phenomenon. Tumor lysis syndrome generally occurs when the patient is initially treated. It is the result of the lysing of rapidly growing tumor cells that spill their contents into the general circulation, causing a metabolic imbalance. This results in hypocalcemia, hyperkalemia, hyperphosphatemia, and hyperuricemia. If left uncorrected, this condition may result in renal failure and death. The treatment of choice is prevention. Therefore, any patient suspected of being at high risk for tumor lysis should receive vigorous hydration (300–500 ml/hr) and may receive sodium bicarbonate to alkalinize the urine and prevent hyperuricemia nephropathy. However, sodium bicarbonate interferes with phosphate excretion and should be stopped prior to the administration of chemotherapy. In addition, allopurinol, a drug that blocks the conversion of metabolic wastes to uric acid, should be administered either intravenously or orally. The patient's urine output needs to be monitored every hour, and the physician should be alerted to any sign of urinary insufficiency. Serum chemistry levels are monitored every 6 hours in patients who are at high risk for tumor lysis, and in some cases the patient may need to be transferred to the intensive care unit. Dialysis may be necessary if the patient's electrolyte levels continue to rise and renal function deteriorates. Generally, there is less morbidity if the patient receives dialysis before renal failure occurs.

Although tumor lysis occurs in most patients 48–72 hours after the initiation of chemotherapy, some patients with HIV-related NHL may have this phenomenon sooner, usually within 24 hours.[67] However, all patients with HIV-related NHL should be observed for a full 72-hour period for any sign of tumor lysis syndrome. These signs and symptoms include decreased urine output and increased lethargy. If the patient is being monitored by telemetry, arrhythmias may be noted.

It also should be noted that some patients with HIV-related NHL have some form of tumor lysis before they receive treatment. This may be due to the tumor cells replicating and dying at an extraordinary rate, spilling their cellular contents into the general circulation.[68] These patients also may have tumors that produce lactic acid, causing metabolic acidosis before treatment.[68]

The complications of this group are the same as those experienced by all patients with NHL: neutropenia-related sepsis, thrombocytopenia, and untreated tumor lysis syndrome.

PRIMARY CENTRAL NERVOUS SYSTEM LYMPHOMA

Epidemiology

Primary CNS lymphoma is a rare malignancy, accounting for 0.3%–2% of all newly diagnosed lymphomas.[69] Although it can affect immunocompetent hosts, most of those diagnosed with primary CNS lymphoma are immunocompromised. Therefore, those with primary immunodeficiency, acquired immunodeficiency, and iatrogenic immunologic abnormalities (organ transplant recipients) are at increased risk for the development of primary CNS lymphoma.[70–72] In the case of organ transplant recipients, primary lymphoma involving the brain accounts for 50% of lymphomas in this population; it is common enough to predict its occurrence 28 months after transplantation.[73] It is not surprising then that primary CNS lymphoma develops in those infected with HIV who have subsequent severe immune dysfunction, defined as CD4 counts less than $75/mm^3$. Before the AIDS epidemic, primary CNS lymphomas were noted in the 50–70-year-old age range.[74] In the general population the average time from onset of symptoms to disease is 1–2 months. Unfortunately, patients with AIDS are also at risk for the development of infectious CNS disease. Cryptococcosis and toxoplasmosis are AIDS-related opportunistic infections of the CNS. The differential evaluation of these diseases can prolong and complicate the diagnostic process; yet, in the setting of HIV infection, a complete evaluation of all possible pathologic causes is required.

The early medical literature reflects the confusion encountered in attempting to identify the cell of origin for primary CNS lymphoma. Perithelial sarcoma, reticulum cell sarcoma, and microglioma were a few of the names used to classify primary lymphoma involving the brain. It is now accepted that the cell of origin is the same as that causing NHL elsewhere in the body. The transformed cell, which multiplies in an area that does not allow expansion, is the cause of most presenting symptoms. In approximately 30% of all cases, this neoplasm will be multicentric, arising in several different areas of the brain at the same time.[71] This presentation is similar to that described in either spontaneously occurring tumors or in tumors arising in immunodeficient states.

Clinical Manifestations

Two retrospective reviews[74,75] of a total of 26 patients revealed that the most frequently observed symptoms of HIV-associated CNS lymphomas included confusion, lethargy, and memory loss (12/26) and alterations in personality and behavior (5/26). Of the 26 patients, hemiparesis or aphasia was seen in seven, three patients had seizures, two had cranial nerve palsy, one had headache as the only symptom, one had headache associated with a lack of coordination, and one had no symptoms. Further review by So et al.[74] revealed that although only three patients had seizures initially, seizures later developed in four additional patients. More than half the patients also reported more specific symptoms that consisted of focal seizures and progression of focal neurologic symptoms over days or weeks. In a review by Gill et al.,[75] all six patients studied had disease within the cranium; four had disease in the frontoparietal region, and two had involvement of the pons cerebellum.

These clinical manifestations are typical of spontaneous primary CNS lymphoma. They also are typical symptoms caused by other mass lesions in the CNS. This similarity in symptomatology often makes it difficult to distinguish between CNS lymphoma and vascular and infectious disorders. The most common explanation for a mass lesion in the CNS is toxoplasmosis, which occurs in 10% of patients with AIDS.[76] Because of the morbidity associated with brain biopsy, primary CNS lymphoma is usually a diagnosis of exclusion. That is, the patient with CNS symptoms and a demonstrated brain mass will generally be treated empirically for toxoplasmosis for approximately 2 weeks. If the lesion fails to respond to treatment, the diagnosis of primary CNS lymphoma will then be considered. At this point a brain biopsy could yield a definitive diagnosis; however, due to the invasiveness of the procedure for the patient in obtaining a biopsy and to the dismal response of primary CNS lymphoma to treatment, a presumptive diagnosis may be established.

In most patients the radiographic findings from the CT and magnetic resonance imaging (MRI) examinations will reveal single or multiple discrete lesions. Prior to the use of a contrast medium on CT scanning, low-density lesions will appear, and a shift of midline structures also may be apparent. After the administration of contrast material, the lesion will characteristically appear enhanced. Reports differ on the type of enhancement; both uniform and patchy nodular enhancement with varying degrees of surrounding edema have been reported.[74,75] Primary CNS lymphoma usually appears as single or multiple discrete lesions and exhibits a characteristic pre- and postcontrast appearance. Some primary CNS lymphoma patients, however, have demonstrated ring-enhancing lesions on CT scan that are frequently indistinguishable from lesions seen in patients with cerebral toxoplasmosis. It is important to remember that a diagnosis of lymphoma cannot be determined by scans alone. In addition, MRI does not contribute to the differential diagnosis, although MRI may be useful in revealing lesions undetectable by the CT scan and may provide alternate biopsy sites.[74,75]

Examination of cerebral spinal fluid (CSF) may reveal some abnormalities; however, the results are nonspecific and useful only in that they indicate some abnormality in the CNS. Tests ordered on CSF include toxoplasmosis titers, the Venereal Disease Research Laboratory (VDRL) test, and cytologic examination. Cytologic findings will be positive in approximately 50% of patients who have CNS lymphoma.[77] This result, however, tends to depend on the volume of CSF obtained. Toxoplasmosis titers and VDRL results can help rule out toxoplasmosis and syphilis as causes for behavioral changes and altered mental status.

Treatment

Medical

It appears that whether or not patients with AIDS-associated CNS lymphoma are treated, the outcome remains the same. In a review by So et al.[74] they noted that in one study six patients experienced a highly aggressive course and died within 2 weeks. In another, 7 of 20 patients underwent treatment with radiation therapy.[75] Doses ranged from 3000–6000 cGy. Of the four patients who had CT scans after radiation therapy, three showed dramatic improvement. However, only 2 of 7 patients were alive at 2 months. Most patients die of the concomitant opportunistic infections frequently experienced in AIDS. In a review by Gill et al.,[75] 4 patients were treated with subtotal resection of the tumor, followed by whole brain radiation and systemic chemotherapy. One patient remained alive at 28 months after diagnosis. It should be noted that the diagnosis of this particular patient was based on a pathologic finding of low-grade lymphoma. The other patients survived less than 2 months. An average survival time of 1.7–2.7 months has been reported.[75]

In a third retrospective review, 55 patients with primary CNS lymphoma who were treated with whole-brain radiation were evaluated. Complete radiological responses were reported in 17%, with 52% of patients achieving a partial response. Clinical improvement was evidenced in 76%. Although responses were good, they were short-lived. In one group of 29 patients, the median survival was 119 days. Cause of death in the majority of patients was an opportunistic infection. There were no deaths attributable to unchecked primary CNS lymphoma.[78] Short survival was also reported by Formenti et al.[79] In this review, 6 of 10 patients with primary CNS lymphoma had a prior history of opportunistic infection and, treated with whole-brain irradiation, demonstrated complete responses. Again, the responses were not durable. Median survival in this group was 5.5 months.[79]

Nursing

Nursing responsibility in the care of these patients includes a thorough assessment, paying particular attention to any focal findings, motor incoordination, and cognitive deficits. Safety in the environment must be considered in both the acute care setting and the home. Provisions for activities of daily living also must be anticipated and a long-term plan developed. For example, if the patient cannot be maintained at home, plans should be made for transfer to a skilled nursing care facility. Providing emotional support to the patient and family is essential, whether this be through referrals to counselors or by the nurse. Ethical issues may be encountered when treatment is discussed. A determination should be made as to whether the patient is mentally competent to make decisions; if not, it should be determined who is the next of kin or whether someone has been authorized power of attorney. If the patient is deemed incompetent, has no next of kin, or has not transferred power of attorney, then a legal guardian will need to be appointed by a court of law to make decisions for the patient.

Complications

The most frequent complication in the treatment of AIDS-associated CNS lymphoma is the patient's mental deterioration to the point of becoming moribund and comatose. The reason for this downhill course associated with treatment is unclear. Unfortunately, there appears to be no preventive intervention. It may be a function of general debilitation caused by HIV, by HIV involvement of the brain, by the treatment itself, by a combination of these, or by another factor that has yet to be explored. Current research is not encouraging. Combining chemotherapy and radiation therapy in an attempt to control or eliminate the primary CNS lymphoma is currently being explored, but the research is confounded by the low numbers of enrollable patients and their rapid deterioration. As a result, the hope is for an effective antiviral agent that will control the HIV infection and for regeneration of the immune system through the use of immunomodulators.

OTHER MALIGNANCIES AND HUMAN IMMUNODEFICIENCY VIRUS

Kaposi's sarcoma, non-Hodgkin's lymphoma, and primary CNS lymphoma account for approximately 95% of all cancers diagnosed in patients with AIDS, but they are not the only malignancies seen in persons who are seropositive for HIV antibody.[80] Nor are they the only malignancies that develop in the presence of immune dysfunction. It is reported in the transplant population that there is a 100-fold increase in the development of vulvar and anal cancers and a 14-fold increase in cervical cancer.[81] Hodgkin's disease, squamous cell cancers of the rectum, nasopharyngeal cancers, malignant melanomas, and multiple myelomas have all been reported in patients infected with HIV. The difference between the indicator malignancies (KS, NHL, and primary CNS lymphoma) and other malignancies in individuals with HIV is the frequency with which they occur. There is a significantly greater incidence of the indicator malignancies in those who are seropositive for HIV. The same is not true for the other malignancies described in AIDS patients. Although these cancers may be seen in AIDS patients, no epidemiologic link or direct causal relationship has been established. HIV positivity does not prevent the development of any other cancer at the same rate seen in those who are seronegative. It is useful to know, however, the HIV status of a patient with a malignancy because response to therapy is typically poor in the person with HIV infection. It is reasonable to expect an increasing incidence of virally linked malignancies (e.g., hepatomas and cervical cancer) as the incidence of AIDS and HIV infection continues to rise.[82] Of great concern are women infected with human papilloma virus (HPV). Early reports show an increased HPV positivity in HIV-infected women (49%) compared with 25% of the general population. In addition, women who are both HIV/HPV infected are 42 times more likely to have cytologic changes.[83] Men who are HIV/HPV positive are also more likely to have cytologic changes. Thirty-nine percent of men examined had abnormal anal cytologies, and in 54% of these patients the DNA of HPV was identified in the cytology.[84]

CONCLUSION

The care of patients with a malignant disease who also are infected with HIV presents a demanding challenge for nurses. In addition to the already difficult task of managing the care of a patient receiving chemotherapy, infection with an immunosuppressive virus must be taken into account. The patient also may be receiving antiviral agents or immunomodulators, or both. Sorting out the side effects, as well as providing a comprehensive plan of care for these patients, presents an opportunity to participate in the nursing challenge of the 1990s.

REFERENCES

1. Longo DL, Seis RG, Lane HC, et al: Malignancies in the AIDS patient: Natural history, treatment strategies, and preliminary results. *Ann NY Acad Sci* 437:421–430, 1984.
2. Steis R, Broder S: A general overview. In DeVita VT, Hellman S, Rosenberg SA (eds), *AIDS Etiology, Diagnosis, Treatment and Prevention.* Philadelphia: Lippincott, 1985, pp. 299–338.
3. Centers for Disease Control: Kaposi's sarcoma and *Pneumocystis* pneumonia among homosexual men—New York City and California. *MMWR* 30:305–308, 1981.
4. Centers for Disease Control: Follow-up on Kaposi's sarcoma and *Pneumocystis* pneumonia. *MMWR* 30:409–410, 1981.

5. Brooks JJ: Kaposi's sarcoma: A reversible hyperplasia. *Lancet* 2:1309–1311, 1986.
6. Costa J, Rabson AS: Generalized Kaposi's sarcoma is not a neoplasm. *Lancet* 1:58, 1983.
7. Centers for Disease Control: Update on acquired immune deficiency syndrome (AIDS)—United States. *MMWR* 31:507–514, 1982.
8. Centers for Disease Control: Revision of the CDC surveillance case definition for acquired immunodeficiency syndrome. *MMWR* 35:3S–15S, 1987.
9. Rosenberg SA, Suit H, Baker L, et al: Sarcomas of the soft tissue and bone. In DeVita VT, Hellman S, Rosenberg SA (eds), *Cancer Principles and Practice of Oncology*. Philadelphia: Lippincott, 1982, pp. 1036–1093.
10. Krigel R, Friedman-Kien A: Kaposi's sarcoma in AIDS. In DeVita VT, Hellman S, Rosenberg SA (eds), *AIDS Etiology, Diagnosis, Treatment, and Prevention*. Philadelphia: Lippincott, 1985, pp. 185–212.
11. Volberding P: Kaposi's sarcoma in AIDS. In Levy J (ed), *AIDS, Pathogenesis and Treatment*. New York: Dekker, 1989, pp. 349–358.
12. Beral V, Peterman T, Berkleman R, et al: Kaposi's sarcoma among persons with AIDS: A sexually transmitted infection. *Lancet* 335:123–127, 1990.
13. Northfelt D, Kahn J, Volberding P: Treatment of AIDS-related Kaposi's sarcoma. *Hematol/Oncol Clin North Am* 5:297–310, 1991.
14. Friedman-Kien A, Saltzman B, Cao Y, et al: Kaposi's sarcoma in HIV-negative homosexual men. *Lancet* 335:168–169, 1990.
15. Mitsuyasu RT: Kaposi's sarcoma in the acquired immunodeficiency syndrome. *Infec Dis Clin North Am* 2:511–523, 1988.
16. Haverdos HW, Pinsky PF, Drotman DP, et al: Disease manifestation and homosexual men with acquired immunodeficiency syndrome: A possible role of nitrites in Kaposi's sarcoma, *Sex Transm Dis* 23:203–208, 1985.
17. Groopman J, Broder S: Cancer in AIDS and other immunodeficiency states. In DeVita VT, Hellman S, Rosenberg SA (eds), *Cancer Principles and Practice of Oncology* (3d ed). Philadelphia: Lippincott, 1989, pp. 1953–1970.
18. Garrett T, Lange M, Ashford A, et al: Kaposi's sarcoma in heterosexual intravenous drug users. *Cancer* 55:1146–1158, 1985.
19. Nissenblatt M: Cancers and AIDS. In Gong V (ed), *Understanding AIDS*. New Brunswick, NJ: Rutgers University Press, 1985, pp. 65–74.
20. Urmacher C, Myskowski P, Ochoa M, et al: Outbreak of KS with CMV infection in young homosexual men. *Am J Med* 74:569–575, 1982.
21. Drew L, Mintz L, Miner R: Prevalence of cytomegalovirus in homosexual men. *J Infect Dis* 143:188–192, 1981.
22. McNutt N: Kaposi's sarcoma. In Theirs B, Dobson R (eds), *Pathogenesis of Skin Disease*. New York: Churchill Livingstone, 1986, pp. 459–474.
23. Caro W, Bronstein B: Tumors of the skin. In Moschella S, Hurley H (eds), *Dermatology* (vol 2) (2d ed). Philadelphia: Saunders, 1985, pp. 1639–1671.
24. MacKie R: Tumors of the skin. In Rook A, Ebling F, Wilkinson E, et al (eds), *Textbook of Dermatology* (vol 3). London: Blackwell Scientific Publications, 1986, pp. 2375–2478.
25. Meduri G, Stover D, Lee M, et al: Pulmonary Kaposi's sarcoma in the acquired immune deficiency syndrome: Clinical, radiographic and pathologic manifestations. *Am J Med* 81:11–18, 186.
26. Laine L, Plitoske E, Pardash G: Protein-losing enteropathy in acquired immunodeficiency syndrome due to intestinal Kaposi's sarcoma. *Arch Intern Med* 147:1174–1175, 1988.
27. Kaplan L, Hopewell P, Jaffe H, et al: Kaposi's sarcoma involving the lung in patients with acquired immunodeficiency syndrome. *J AIDS* 1:25–31, 1988.
28. Brown R, Huberman R, Vanley G: Pulmonary features of KS. *Am J Radiol* 139:659–660, 1986.
29. Laubenstein L: Staging and treatment of Kaposi's sarcoma in patients with AIDS. In Friedman-Kien A, Laubenstein L (eds), *AIDS: The Epidemic of Kaposi's Sarcoma and Opportunistic Infections*. New York: Masson, 1984, pp. 51–56.
30. Krigel R, Laubenstein L, Muggia F: Kaposi's sarcoma: A new staging classification. *Cancer Treat Rep* 67:531–534, 1983.
31. Krigel R: Prognostic factors in Kaposi's sarcoma. In Friedman-Kien A, Laubenstein L (eds), *AIDS: The Epidemic of Kaposi's Sarcoma and Opportunistic Infections*. New York: Masson, 1984, pp. 69–72.
32. Taylor J, Afrasia R, Fahey J, et al: Prognostically significant classification of immune changes in AIDS with Kaposi's sarcoma. *Blood* 76:666–671, 1986.
33. Afrasiabi A, Mitsuyasu R, Nishanian R, et al: Characteristics of a distinct subgroup of high-risk persons with KS and good prognosis who present with normal T4 cell number and T4:T8 ratio and negative HTLV/LAV serologic test results. *Am J Med* 81:969–973, 1986.
34. Gnepp D, Chandler W, Hyams V: Primary Kaposi's sarcoma of the head and neck. *Ann Intern Med* 100:107–114, 1984.
35. Safai B, Sarngadharan M, Koziner B, et al: Spectrum of KS in the epidemic of AIDS. *Cancer Res* 45:6465–6485, 1985(suppl 9).
36. Krown A, Metroka C, Wernz J: Kaposi's sarcoma in the acquired immunodeficiency syndrome: A proposal for uniform evaluation, response, and staging criteria. *J Clin Oncol* 7:1201–1207, 1989.
37. Mitsuyasu R: Kaposi's sarcoma in the acquired immunodeficiency syndrome. In Sande M, Volberding P (eds), *The Medical Management of AIDS*. Philadelphia: Saunders, 1988, pp. 296–302.
38. Laubenstein L, Krigel R, Odajnk C, et al: Treatment of epidemic Kaposi's sarcoma with etoposide or a combination of doxorubicin, bleomycin, and vinblastine. *J Clin Oncol* 2:1115–1120, 1984.
39. Safai B: Kaposi's sarcoma and other neoplasms in acquired immunodeficiency syndrome. In Gallin J, Fauci A (eds), *Advances in Host Defense Mechanism*, (vol 5), *Acquired Immunodeficiency Syndrome (AIDS)*. New York: Raven Press, 1985, pp. 59–73.
40. Krown A: The role of interferon in the therapy of epidemic Kaposi's sarcoma. *Semin Oncol* 14:24–33, 1987(suppl 3).
41. Volberding P, Gotlieb M, Rothman J, et al: Therapy of Kaposi's sarcoma in acquired immunodeficiency syndrome (AIDS) with alpha-2 recombinant IFN. *Proc Am Soc Clin Oncol* 2:53, 1983(abstr).
42. Volberding P: Therapy of Kaposi's sarcoma in AIDS. *Semin Oncol* 11:60–67, 1984.
43. Kahn J, Kaplan L, Volberding P, et al: Intralesional re-

combinant tumor necrosis factor-α for AIDS-associated Kaposi's sarcoma: A randomized double blind trial. *J AIDS* 2:217–221, 1989.

44. Luce J: Personal communication, Aug 3, 1989.
45. Kaplan L, Wofsy C, Volberding PA: Treatment of patients with acquired immunodeficiency syndrome and associated manifestations. *JAMA* 257:1367–1372, 1987.
46. Diffuse, undifferentiated non-Hodgkin's lymphoma among homosexual males—United States. *MMWR* 31:277–279, 1982.
47. Aisenberg A: Malignant lymphoma. *N Engl J Med* 288:883–890, 1973.
48. *Cancer Facts and Figures: 1992.* Atlanta, GA: American Cancer Society, 1992.
49. Roithmann S, Tourani J, Andrieu J: AIDS-associated non-Hodgkin's lymphoma. *Lancet* 338:884–885, 1991.
50. Chapman M, Minor J: Lymphoma in AIDS patients receiving long-term antiretroviral therapy. *Am J Hosp Pharmocol* 49:174–175, 1992.
51. DeVita VT, Jaffe E, Mauch P, et al: Lymphocytic lymphomas. In DeVita VT, Hellman S, Rosenberg SA (eds), *Cancer Principles and Practice of Oncology* (3d ed). Philadelphia: Lippincott, 1989, pp. 1953–1970.
52. MacMahon E, Glass J, Hayward S, et al: Epstein-Barr virus in AIDS-related primary central nervous system lymphoma. *Lancet* 338:969–973, 1991.
53. Ziegler J: AIDS and cancer. *Ann Inst Pasteur Immunol* 138:253–260, 1987.
54. Kaplan L, Abrams D, Feigal E, et al: AIDS-associated non-Hodgkin's lymphoma in San Francisco. *JAMA* 261:719–724, 1989.
55. Kaplan L: AIDS-associated lymphomas. In Sande M, Volberding P (eds), *The Medical Management of AIDS.* Philadelphia: Saunders, 1988, pp. 307–315.
56. Nasr S, Brynes R, Garrison C, et al: Peripheral T-cell lymphoma in a patient with acquired immune deficiency disease. *Cancer* 61:947–951, 1988.
57. Presant C, Gala K, Wiseman C, et al: Human immunodeficiency virus associated with T-cell lymphoblastic lymphoma in AIDS. *Cancer* 60:1459–1461, 1987.
58. Yarchoan R, Redfield R, Broder S: Mechanisms of B-cell activation in patients with acquired immunodeficiency syndrome. *J Clin Invest* 78:439–447, 1986.
59. Ziegler J: Lymphomas and other neoplasms associated with AIDS. In Levy J (ed), *AIDS, Pathogenesis and Treatment.* New York: Dekker, 1989, pp. 359–370.
60. Knowles D, Chamulak G, Subar M, et al: Lymphoid neoplasia associated with the acquired immunodeficiency syndrome (AIDS). The New York University Medical Center experience with 105 patients (1981–1986). *Ann Intern Med* 108:744–753, 1988.
61. Italian Cooperative Group for AIDS-Related Tumors, 1988: Malignant lymphomas in patients with or at risk for AIDS in Italy. *J Natl Cancer Inst* 80:855–860, 1988.
62. McGrath M: Personal communication, Aug 3, 1989.
63. Pieri KL, Murphy E: The clinical significance of HTLV-I and HTLV-II infection with the AIDS epidemic. In Volberding P, Jacobson M (eds), *AIDS Clinical Review 1991.* New York: Dekker, 1991, pp. 39–57.
64. Ziegler J, Beckstead J, Volberding P, et al: Non-Hodgkin's lymphoma in 90 homosexual men—relation to generalized lymphadenopathy and the acquired immunodeficiency syndrome. *N Engl J Med* 311:565–570, 1984.
65. DiCarlo E, Amberson J, Metroka C, et al: Malignant lymphomas and the acquired immunodeficiency syndrome. *Arch Pathol Lab Med* 110:1012–1016, 1986.
66. Ahmed S, Wormser G, Stahl R, et al: Malignant lymphomas in a population at risk for acquired immune deficiency syndrome. *Cancer* 60:719–723, 1987.
67. Kaplan L: Personal Communication, June 29, 1992.
68. Warrell R Jr, Bockman R: Oncologic emergencies. In DeVita VT, Hellman S, Rosenberg SA (eds), *Cancer Principles and Practice of Oncology* (3d ed). Philadelphia: Lippincott, 1989, pp. 1996–1997.
69. Henry J, Heffner R, Dillard S, et al: Primary malignant lymphomas of the central nervous system. *Cancer* 34:1293–1302, 1987.
70. Frizzera G, Rosai J, Dehner L, et al: Lymphoreticular disorders in primary immunodeficiency: New findings based on an up to date histologic classification of 35 cases. *Cancer* 46:692–699, 1980.
71. Good A, Russo R, Schnitzer B, et al: Intercranial histiocytic lymphoma in rheumatoid arthritis. *J Rheumatol* 5:75–78, 1978.
72. Frizzera G, Hanto D, Gaji-Peczalska K, et al: Polymorphic diffuse B-cell hyperplasia and lymphomas in renal transplant recipients. *Cancer Res* 41:4262–4279, 1981.
73. Levin V, Sheline G, Gutin P: Neoplasms of the central nervous system. In DeVita VT, Hellman S, Rosenberg SA (eds), *Cancer Practice and Principles of Oncology* (3d ed). Philadelphia: Lippincott, 1989, pp. 1557–1611.
74. So Y, Beckstead J, Davis R: Primary central nervous system lymphoma in acquired immunodeficiency syndrome. A clinical and pathological study. *Ann Neurol* 20:566–572, 1986.
75. Gill P, Levine A, Meyer P, et al: Primary central nervous system lymphoma in homosexual men. *Am J Med* 78:742–748, 1985.
76. Mills J: *Pneumocystis carinii* and *Toxoplasmosis gondii* infections in patients with AIDS. *Rev Infect Dis* 8:1001–1011, 1986.
77. Casciato D, Lowitz B: Neuromuscular complication. In Casciato D, Lowitz B (eds), *Manual of Clinical Oncology.* Boston: Little, Brown, 1988, pp. 468–483.
78. Baumgartner J, Rachlin J, Beckstead J, et al: Primary central nervous system lymphomas: Natural history and response to radiation therapy in 55 patients with acquired immunodeficiency syndrome. *J Neurosurg* 73:206–211, 1990.
79. Formenti S, Gill P, Lean E, et al: Primary central nervous system lymphoma in AIDS: Results of radiation therapy. *Cancer* 63:1101–1107, 1989.
80. Levine A: Non-Hodgkin's lymphomas and other malignancies in the acquired immune deficiency syndrome. *Semin Oncol* 14:34–39, 1987(suppl 3).
81. Penn I: Secondary neoplasms as a consequence of transplantation and cancer therapy. *Cancer Detect Prevent* 12:39–57, 1988.
82. Friedman S: Gastrointestinal and hepatobiliary neoplasms in AIDS. *Gastroenterol Clin North Am* 17:465–486, 1988.
83. Maiman M, Fruchter R, Serur E, et al: Human immunodeficiency virus infection and cervical neoplasia. *Gynecol Oncol* 38:377–382, 1990.
84. Palefsky J, Gonzales J, Greenblatt R, et al: Anal intraepithelial neoplasia and anal papilloma-virus infection among homosexual males with group IV HIV disease. *JAMA* 263:2911–2916, 1990.

Chapter 37

Bone and Soft Tissue Sarcoma

Patricia A. Piasecki, RN, MS

INTRODUCTION

Bone and soft tissue malignancies are so uncommon that they are not listed among the five leading cancer sites. They occur in all age groups. Diagnosis and treatment of these lesions are complex. Teamwork is essential. Key members of the health care team include the patient and family, the orthopedic surgeon, medical oncologist, roentgenologist, pathologist, radiation oncologist, thoracic surgeon, physical therapist, nurse, prosthetist, and social worker. Increased knowledge about bone and soft tissue sarcomas and a multidisciplinary approach to treatment have improved the results of bone and soft tissue tumor treatment in recent years.

EPIDEMIOLOGY

The incidence of primary malignant bone and soft tissue tumors is remarkably low. These tumors account for a small percent of malignant tumors diagnosed in the United States.[1] The American Cancer Society estimated in 1991 that 2000 new cases of bone cancer were discovered annually. Incidence is slightly higher for men. The estimated number of deaths that occurred in 1991 from bone cancer is 1050, which represents a decrease over prior years. In 1991, 5800 new cases of soft tissue cancer were discovered. The estimated death toll from soft tissue tumors was 3300.[1]

ETIOLOGY

At present, relatively little is known regarding the cause of primary bone and soft tissue tumors. Consequently, prevention and detection of bone and soft tissue sarcoma remain difficult because few risk factors have been identified. Prior cancer therapy in the form of high-dose irradiation has been linked to the development of bone and soft tissue sarcoma. Chemicals such as vinyl chloride gas, arsenic, and dioxin or agent orange have been associated with the formation of soft tissue sarcomas. Exposure to alkylating agents such as melphalan, procarbazine, nitrosoureas, and chlorambucil predisposes patients to sarcomas.[2] Immunosuppressed patients such as renal transplant recipients and persons with AIDS have a higher risk for soft tissue sarcomas. Neurofibromatosis patients have a 10% chance of one of their tumors transforming to a neurofibrosarcoma.[3] Prolonged lymphedema following a mastectomy can lead to a lymphangiosarcoma.[4]

Evidence of a familial tendency in bone cancer has been demonstrated by reports of siblings with osteosarcoma, Ewing's sarcoma, and chondrosarcoma. Bone and soft tissue sarcomas may be only part of a complex of different tumors that cluster in families.[5] These findings suggest that common susceptibility may be the critical factor in predisposition to diverse forms of cancer.

Malignant bone neoplasms have been associated with a number of preexisting bone conditions. Paget's disease primarily predisposes individuals to osteosarcoma but occasionally to fibrosarcoma, chondrosarcoma, and giant cell tumor. The incidence of sarcomas in patients with symptoms of Paget's disease is 0.8%.[6] It has been proposed that the mechanisms responsible for the relationship are prolonged growth, an overstimulated metabolism, or both. These mechanisms are also implicated in the occurrence of bone tumors associated with hyperparathyroidism, chronic osteomyelitis, old bone infarct, and fracture callus.

Other factors such as syndromes of skeletal maldevelopment and skeletal growth patterns have been implicated in the etiology of bone cancer. These factors are discussed here in conjunction with the specific bone tumor type to which they apply.

Molecular genetics are being studied in musculoskeletal tumors, and genetic therapy may be a trend in the next decade. Osteosarcomas are noted to occur if both alleles at the RB1 and P53 are altered. These genes are tumor-suppressor genes.[7,8] Similar studies in chondrosarcoma cell lines are being performed. Neurofibrosarcoma patients have a loss of tumor suppressor gene on chromosome 17P.[9] Ongoing research in this area is occurring.

PATHOPHYSIOLOGY

Primary malignant bone and soft tissue tumors are derived from the cells that have a common ancestry, namely the mesoderm or ectoderm. One group of bone and soft tissue tumors is produced by cells characterized by their ability to produce collagen. This group includes the osteogenic tumors arising from osteoblasts, the chondrogenic tumors arising from chondroblasts, and the fibrogenic tumors arising from fibroblasts. Another group originates in the bone marrow reticulum and includes round cell tumors such as Ewing's sarcoma and reticulum cell sarcoma. The third group arises in blood vessels of the bone and includes the angiosarcomas. Soft tissue sarcomas such as alveolar soft part sarcomas and epithelioid sarcomas have no known cellular origins.

Little can be said regarding the pathophysiology of bone and soft tissue tumors in general because of the individualized behavior demonstrated by the different types of tumors. Nearly every bone and soft tissue in the skeleton may be affected; however, individual tumors have a predilection for certain locations. Most often, soft tissue sarcomas arise in the extremities but can involve head and neck and retroperitoneum areas. In addition, there are differences in cellular characteristics and in the progression of disease. In general, bone and soft tissue tumors tend to involve contiguous tissue and muscle aggressively and metastasize early to the lungs via the hematogenous route. Occasionally, soft tissue sarcomas can spread to regional lymph nodes.

ASSESSMENT

Patient History

The evaluation of pain is a major focus in the patient interview. Obtaining information regarding the location, onset, duration, and quality of the pain assists in the differential diagnosis. It is important to rule out a traumatic injury to the area, which could result in a condition such as hematoma or myositis ossificans that can resemble tumors. More commonly, an injury merely brings a preexisting neoplasm to the attention of the individual. Bone tumor pain often has a gradual onset and may be present for a few months before the person seeks medical advice. An abrupt onset of pain does not necessarily rule out the presence of bone tumor because a pathologic fracture may be the presenting symptom. Pain can be radicular. For example, a tumor of the hip can radiate pain via the obturator nerve and present with knee pain. Musculoskeletal tumor pain often is constant and worse at night. The severity of pain steadily increases as the tumor enlarges. Over-the-counter medications may not relieve the pain.

Soft tissue sarcomas present as painless masses, unless they are impinging on nerves, blood vessels, or viscera. Other presenting symptoms such as a history of swelling need to be assessed during the patient interview. Attention is given to symptoms suggestive of pulmonary metastasis. A history of hemoptysis, chest pain, cough, fever, chills, weight loss, malaise, exposure to toxic substances, radiation, or travel out of the country is noted.

To determine potential problems and needs, a psychosocial assessment should be incorporated into the initial interview. The individual may have a life-threatening tumor that may require mutilating surgery. The nature of family, peer, love relationships, and other support systems is explored. It often is helpful to identify the person in whom the patient most frequently confides and the patient's usual coping strategies when confronting stress. To further delineate possible resources, the significance of relation, work, and leisure activities is assessed.

Physical Examination

The physical examination of the individual with a suspected bone or soft tissue lesion involves inspection and palpation of the affected area. Inspection may reveal a visible mass or swelling. Dilated surface veins may be evident. A firm, nontender, warm enlargement may be palpated over the affected portions, although malignant bone tumors are not always visible or palpable. Dimensions of the soft tissue mass should be noted. Evaluation for adenopathy and hepatomegaly also is performed. Limitations in motion of proximal joints are noted. Muscle atrophy can occur in a chronic setting and can be documented by measuring the affected and nonaffected limb. An analysis of the gait will most likely reveal an antalgic gait for a lower extremity tumor, as the patient will shorten the time spent on the affected limb. An assessment of neurovascular function of the affected limb is done.

Diagnostic Studies

Evaluation of the individual with symptoms suggestive of bone or soft tissue sarcoma necessitates the collaboration of the radiologist, orthopedic surgeon, and pathologist. Before any diagnostic conclusions are made, the person's clinical history is reviewed, as well as the radiologic and histologic features of the lesion.

Radiographs, although they frequently do not yield a specific diagnosis, provide the opportunity to view the location and the anatomy of the bony lesion, as well as the status of surrounding tissue (Figure 37-1). In general, radiographic changes can be appreciated only when the tumor is far advanced. Three basic patterns of tumor destruction that may be viewed radiographically are described as geographic, moth-eaten, or permeative. These patterns (Figure 37-2) may be correlated with the pathologic aggressiveness or quiescence of the tumor and may occur alone or in combination with one or both of the other patterns.[10] The geographic pattern indicates that the tumor has a slow rate of growth. It is characterized by a large, well-defined hole in which the edge of completely destroyed bone interfaces with the edge of bone that is completely intact. The moth-eaten pattern indicates a moderately aggressive tumor. It is characterized by multiple holes that tend to coalesce. This pattern implies severe cortical destruction. Finally, the permeative pattern indicates an aggressive tumor with a strong capacity for infiltration. It is characterized by multiple tiny holes in cortical bone. These holes diminish in size and number in the peripheral areas of the lesion. The moth-eaten pattern indicates that the tumor has breached the cortex and has extended longitudinally within the bone. Soft tissue sarcomas may have negative radiographs, as radiographs best image bony tissue and poorly image the soft tissues.

Several other radiologic methods can be used in the evaluation of primary malignant bone and soft tissue cancer. These include bone scans, arteriography, computed tomography (CT), fluoroscopy, and magnetic resonance imaging (MRI). A bone scan is not helpful in distinguishing one bone condition from another but

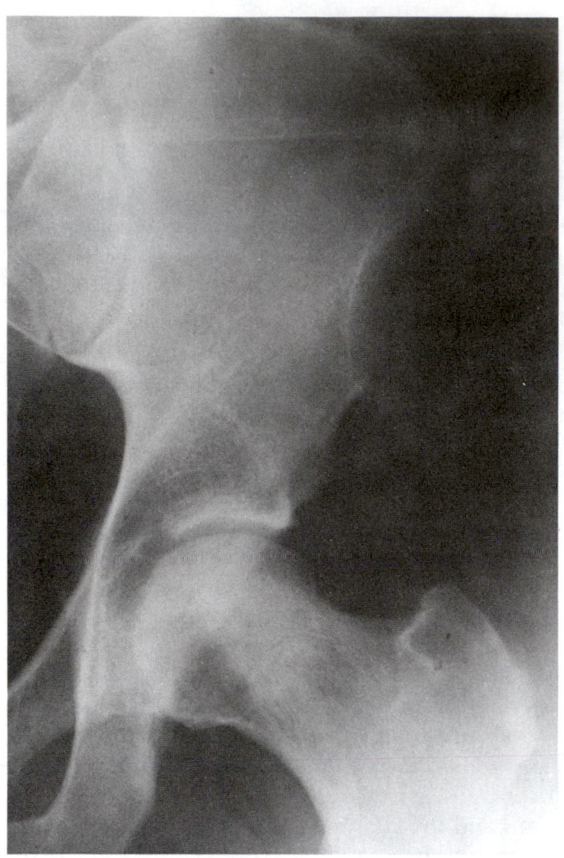

FIGURE 37-1 Radiograph of 67-year-old man with primary osteosarcoma of the femur.

is useful in verifying the presence of abnormal bone when plain radiographs show normal findings. A bone scan helps to detect or exclude the presence of additional lesions in the skeleton. Likewise, arteriography is not diagnostic but aids in the planning of surgical, radiation, and perfusion chemotherapy treatments by outlining tumor margins and mapping arterial blood supply to the tumor. CT provides an evaluation of the true extent of the disease. Fluoroscopy is used in the operating room to document the location in the bony lesion from which the biopsy specimen is taken.

MRI uses a magnetic field to produce an image. The MRI is superior to a CT scan in demonstrating the tumor extent in marrow and soft tissue and in detecting recurrence in the presence of surgical clips and metallic prostheses.[11] Ultrasonography is useful in determining size and density of the soft tissue mass. It measures the reflection of continuous high-frequency sound waves.

Biopsy is crucial for diagnosis. The biopsy should include the most representative section of the lesion as determined by the imaging. Biopsy tissue can be obtained by use of an incisional or needle technique.

Incisional biopsy is the most common type of biopsy used for bone and soft tissue lesions. With the patient under general anesthesia, an incision is made over the tumor mass and through to the soft tissue. Bone biopsies are more painful, weaken the bone, and need to be processed in the pathology department for a few days before diagnosis is made. Incisional biopsy yields a larger volume of tissue for examination.

The location and size of the incision are equally important to the surgeon and radiation oncologist. If

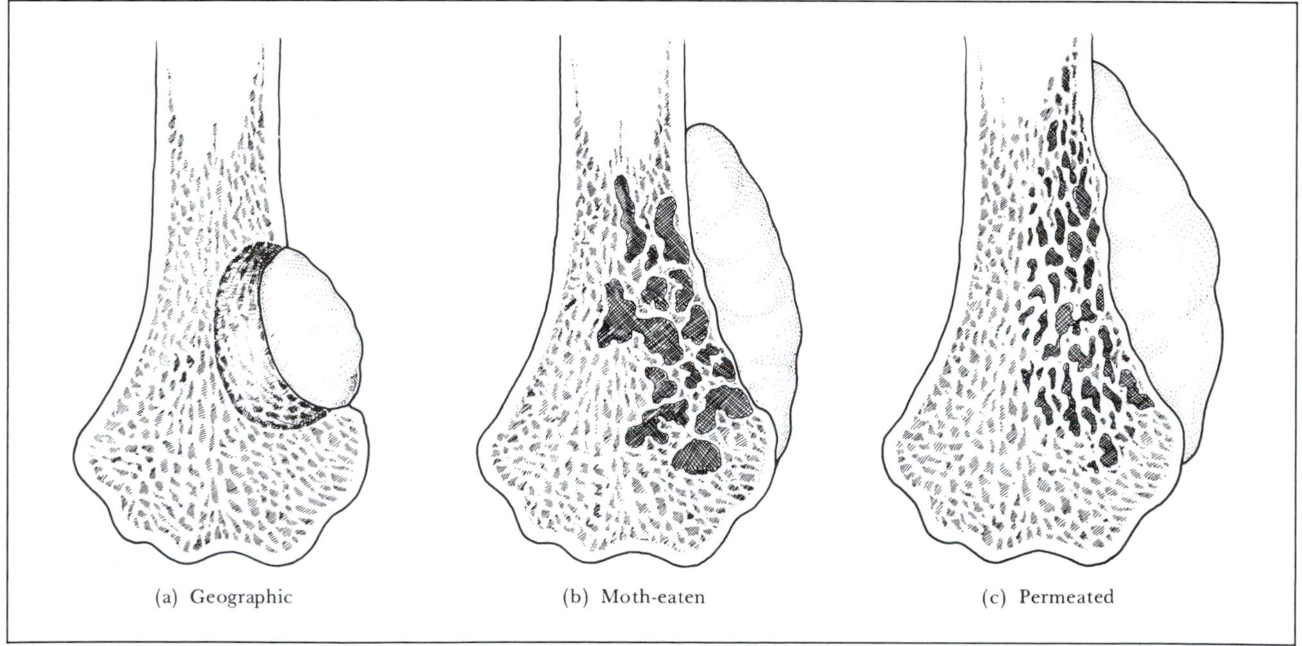

FIGURE 37-2 Radiographic patterns of tumor destruction. (a) Geographic pattern, indicating a slow rate of tumor growth. (b) Moth-eaten pattern, indicating moderately aggressive tumor growth. (c) Permeated pattern, indicating aggressive tumor growth. (Source: Lodwick GS: Solitary malignant tumors of the bone. *Semin Roentgenol,* 1:293–313, 1966.)

hindquarter or forequarter amputation eventually is indicated, the biopsy scar must not compromise the skin flap. Therefore, it is advisable for the orthopedic oncologist rather than the referring surgeon to perform the biopsy. If resection of the tumor is performed, the site of the biopsy incision is removed *en bloc* with the tumor. The radiation oncologist includes the incision site in the field of treatment. The patient has less tissue injury with a smaller field of radiation.

Frozen sections are done during incision biopsy to ensure that representative material has been obtained. In circumstances in which clinical and radiologic findings are high, suggestive of a particular lesion, frozen sections are obtained with the intention of performing surgery while the patient is still anesthetized. For many bone tumors, however, it is advisable to await permanent paraffin sections.

Needle biopsy is utilized on the basis that it is technically simple, involves minimal patient risk, is cost- and time-effective, may be repeated without any ill effects, and makes it possible to extract material from different depths of the tumor. This biopsy can be done by the surgeon under anesthetic; in some centers, radiologists perform CT-guided needle biopsies using sedation. In addition, it is always possible to do incisional biopsy if the diagnosis remains unclear. Although positive results of biopsy nearly always are accurate, biopsy yields a 25% false-negative rate. For this reason, needle biopsy generally is not the preferred method except in individuals with known metastatic disease.

In general, laboratory studies are not helpful in the diagnosis of musculoskeletal tumors. There are a few exceptions, which will be addressed in conjunction with the specific tumor type to which they apply.

Metastatic disease is screened for with a CT of the chest and regional lymph nodes. Node exam is done only if palpable on physical examination.

CLASSIFICATION AND STAGING

The classification of bone and soft tissue tumors currently is based on histologic patterns. These patterns correlate in general with the gross appearance, radiologic features, and biologic behavior of the tumor. Uncertainty with regard to the definition of terms used in pathologic nomenclature and classification not only complicates the treatment of bone tumors but also impedes research efforts aimed at the development of staging classification for musculoskeletal tumors. Consequently, the American Joint Committee on Cancer has recommended that *International Histological Classification of Tumors*, published by the World Health Organization, be used for specific definitions of histologic typing.[12]

The World Health Organization scheme of classification (Table 37-1) is based on the type of differentiation shown by the tumor cells and the type of intracellular material they produce.[13] The main types of primary bone and soft tissue tumors are listed according to whether they are bone-forming, cartilage-forming, marrow-forming, vascular-forming, nerve-forming, or other connective tissue type.

The surgical staging system for musculoskeletal sarcomas includes surgical grade, surgical site, and presence of metastases (Table 37-2). Stage I includes low-grade lesions with low incidence of metastases, such as periosteal osteosarcoma and giant cell tumors. Stage II includes high-grade lesions with high incidence of metastases, such as classic osteosarcoma and angiosarcoma. The site is noted to be "A," which indicates an intracompartmental lesion, or "B," which indicates an extracompartmental lesion. Anatomic compartments have barriers to tumor extension. In bone, these barriers are cortical bone and articular cartilage; in joints, articular cartilage and joint capsule; and in soft tissue, the major fascial septa and the tendinous origins and insertions of muscle. Lesions that involve the neurovascular bundle are extracompartmental. Stage III includes any site or grade lesion with metastases. Another system developed by the American Joint Committee of Cancer includes surgical grade, site, presence of metastases, and nodal involvement (Table 37-3).

TREATMENT/NURSING CARE

The goals of treatment of primary malignant bone and soft tissue cancer include eradication of the tumor, avoidance of amputation when possible, and preservation of maximum function. The primary lesion is managed by surgery, radiotherapy, or chemotherapy, or a combination of these therapies. To a limited extent, immunotherapy is being evaluated for its usefulness as an adjuvant treatment. Treatment is highly individualized because an optimal treatment program has not been identified.

Surgery

Surgical management of primary neoplasia of the bone is strongly influenced by the histopathologic features of the lesion, the anatomic site of the lesion, and the physical size of the lesion. Clinical and radiographic data also are considered because they provide further information about the biologic behavior of a given lesion.

In the past 20 years, research indicated that no procedure short of ablation would control or eradicate aggressive forms of osteosarcoma, fibrosarcoma, and chondrosarcoma.[15] Historically, the amputation included the joint above the tumor. Tumors in inaccessible areas such as the pelvis, spine, or skull pose unique and difficult problems, with treatment frequently aimed at palliation.

TABLE 37-1 Histologic Typing of Primary Bone Tumors and Tumorlike Lesions

- Bone-forming tumors
  - Benign
    - Osteoma
    - Osteoid osteoma and osteoblastoma (benign osteoblastoma)
  - Malignant
    - Osteosarcoma (osteogenic sarcoma)
    - Juxtacortical osteosarcoma (parosteal osteosarcoma)
- Cartilage-forming tumors
  - Benign
    - Chondroma
    - Osteochondroma (osteocartilaginous exostosis)
    - Chondroblastoma (benign chondroblastoma; epiphyseal chondroblastoma)
    - Chondromyxoid fibroma
  - Malignant
    - Chondrosarcoma
    - Juxtacortical chondrosarcoma
    - Mesenchymal chondrosarcoma
- Giant cell tumor (osteoclastoma)
- Marrow tumors
  - Ewing's sarcoma
  - Reticulosarcoma of bone
  - Lymphosarcoma of bone
  - Myeloma
- Vascular tumors
  - Benign
    - Hemangioma
    - Lymphangioma
    - Glomus tumor (glomangioma)
  - Intermediate or indeterminate
    - Hemangioendothelioma
    - Hemangiopericytoma
  - Malignant
    - Angiosarcoma
- Other connective tissue tumors
  - Benign
    - Desmoplastic fibroma
    - Lipoma
  - Malignant
    - Fibrosarcoma
    - Liposarcoma
    - Malignant mesenchymoma
    - Undifferentiated sarcoma
- Other tumors
  - Chordoma
  - Ameloblastoma of long bones
  - Neurilemmoma (schwannoma, neurinoma)
  - Neurofibroma
- Unclassified tumors
- Tumorlike lesions
  - Solitary bone cyst (simple or unicameral bone cyst)
  - Aneurysmal bone cyst
  - Juxtaarticular bone cyst (intraosseous ganglion)
  - Metaphyseal fibrous defect (nonossifying fibroma)
  - Eosinophilic granuloma
  - Fibrous dysplasia
  - "Myositis ossificans"
  - "Brown tumor" of hyperparathyroidism

Source: Schajowicz F, Ackerman LV, Sissons HA: *International Histological Classifications of Tumours,* Monograph no 6. Geneva: World Health Organization, 1972.

TABLE 37-2 Surgical Stages of Musculoskeletal Sarcomas

Stage	Grade	Site
IA	Low (G_1)	Intracompartmental (T_1)
IB	Low (G_1)	Extracompartmental (T_2)
IIA	High (G_1)	Intracompartmental (T_1)
IIB	High (G_1)	Extracompartmental (T_2)
III	Any (G) Regional or distant metastasis	Any (T)

Source: Enneking WF, Spanier S, Goodman M: A system for surgical staging of musculoskeletal sarcomas, *Clin Orthop,* 153:105–119, 1980.

In 1984, the National Institutes of Health held a conference to evaluate the efficacy of limb-sparing surgery. Experts reported their experiences with 2000 individuals diagnosed with sarcoma. The same disease-free survival rate was reported for individuals who underwent limb-sparing surgery as for those who underwent amputation.[16]

The traditional contraindications for limb salvage are as follows: (1) inability to attain adequate surgical margin; (2) neurovascular bundle involved by tumor; and (3) age group—that is, children younger than 10 years old, because of resultant limb length discrepancy.

An expandable prosthesis was developed in the early 1980s. The implantation of this prosthesis into the resected bone allows retention of the skeletally immature child's limb. Every 6–12 months, surgery is performed to expand the prosthesis. The long-term outcome of these implants is unknown.[17]

Another option for skeletally immature patients with malignant neoplasm is the Van Nes rotationplasty. The procedure is utilized for distal femur lesions that otherwise would require an above-knee amputation. First, the bone and soft tissue of the thigh are resected while preserving the sciatic nerve. The proximal tibia is internally fixed to the proximal femur after rotating it 180°. The foot is backwards. The foot is then used to fit a below-knee prosthesis on.[18] The bone takes approximately 3 months to heal. The prosthetic fitting ensues. Due to the unusual anatomy, prosthetic fitting and rehabilitation can be prolonged. The advantage of this surgery is that the limb is retained and, therefore,

TABLE 37-3 Anatomic Staging

RULES FOR CLASSIFICATION

Clinical Staging. Clinical staging includes physical examination, clinical laboratory tests, and biopsy of the sarcoma for microscopic diagnosis and grading.

Pathologic Staging. Pathologic staging consists of the removal of the primary tumor, nodes, or suspected metastases.

PRIMARY TUMORS (T)

TX	Primary tumor cannot be assessed
T0	No evidence of primary tumor
T1	Tumor 5 cm or less in greatest dimension
T2	Tumor more than 5 cm in greatest dimension

REGIONAL LYMPH NODES (N)

NX	Regional lymph nodes cannot be assessed
N0	No regional lymph node metastasis
N1	Regional lymph node metastasis

DISTANT METASTASIS (M)

MX	Presence of distant metastasis cannot be assessed
M0	No distant metastasis
M1	Distant metastasis

TUMOR GRADE (G)

GX	Grade cannot be assessed
G1	Well differentiated
G2	Moderately well differentiated
G3–4	Poorly differentiated; undifferentiated

STAGE GROUPING

Stage IA	G1	T1	N0	M0
Stage IB	G1	T2	N0	M0
Stage IIA	G2	T1	N0	M0
Stage IIB	G2	T2	N0	M0
Stage IIIA	G3–4	T1	N0	M0
Stage IIIB	G3–4	T2	N0	M0
Stage IVA	Any G	Any T	N1	M0
Stage IVB	Any G	Any T	Any N	M1

Source: American Joint Committee on Cancer: *Manual for Staging of Cancer.* Philadelphia: Lippincott, 1988.

function is improved both in terms of energy and rigorous physical endeavors. The disadvantage of the surgery is the unusual limb appearance when the prosthesis is off. Complications include nonunion and infection.[19] It is another surgical option for young sarcoma patients.

Limb salvage is indicated for lesions that tend to metastasize late, such as periosteal osteosarcoma and locally aggressive chondrosarcomas that have not invaded soft tissue.[20] Wide resection is necessary in limb surgery to ensure adequate tumor excision.

If the tumor extends to the incision surface at any point or cannot be removed entirely, amputation at a more proximal level may be indicated. Amputation also is indicated if a nonfunctional limb would result from a salvage procedure.

Radical resection with reconstruction

In the preoperative period, it is necessary to discuss with the patient and family the postoperative management and rehabilitation of the patient with radical resection and reconstruction. The patient, especially a younger one, needs to be aware that implant failure may occur and that further surgery, including amputation, may be necessary.

Postoperative management in terms of levels of activity, mobilization, joint motion, weight bearing, the use of bracing devices, or external immobilization will vary according to the amount of bone and soft tissue resected, location, and stability of the implant or graft. When more extensive surgery is done, the actual function cannot be predicted as readily as when an amputation is planned. It is important to clarify this postoperatively.

Prevention of postoperative complications begins with preoperative teaching in conjunction with follow-up after surgery. The extensive nature of most resections requires longer exposure to anesthesia, necessitating attention to pulmonary hygiene. In the preoperative period the individual is familiarized with the pulmonary regimen. The patient is instructed in isometric exercises and ankle pumps to prevent venous stasis. Malignancies, along with immobilization, increase the risk of deep vein thrombosis and pulmonary embolism.

The nurse conducts a baseline assessment of neurovascular function distal to the surgical site. Because nerve injury may occur during the surgical procedure, the assessment provides the opportunity to observe for changes in sensation and motor function that occur. A splint may be ordered until the nerve recovers.

Blood loss and anemia can result from extensive tumor resection and reconstruction. These patients may be somewhat anemic preoperatively due to adjuvant treatments. Patients with malignancies cannot donate autologous blood but may elect to have their families and friends donate the 4–6 units of blood that may be necessary. Banked blood from the hospital is also available. A drainage tube is placed in the wound for 24–48 hours to prevent hematomas or seromas. Iron supplementation may be prescribed. The nurse monitors the patient's vital signs and laboratory values.

Position restrictions are determined by the surgeon based on operative findings and personal management philosophies. Limb elevation, length of bed rest, and other restrictions are noted in the chart. Patients who undergo hip arthroplasty return from surgery with an abductor pillow or balanced suspension traction. The traction is kept on for a few days and then converted to an abductor pillow. For approximately 6 weeks postoperatively, patients are restricted from flexing the hip over 90°, leg crossing, or side lying without a pillow between the legs. If these positions are not followed, a dislocation of the hip may occur, which is very painful, and often the leg shortens. The patient will need to have the hip relocated under sedation or general anesthesia. Occasionally an open reduction is required. Following a dislocation, a hip spica cast or hip orthosis is applied for 6 weeks to allow the soft tissue to heal.

Postoperative pain occurs after these extensive procedures. Initially, pain is managed with epidural catheter continuous infusions of narcotics or a patient-controlled analgesic pump. As pain decreases, milder narcotic tablets such as hydrocodone and nonsteroidal anti-inflammatory tablets are prescribed. Patients are frequently discharged on these oral medications.

Wound necrosis can occur if large flaps are used to close the wound, especially if the surgical site was previously irradiated. Conservative treatments such as debridement and frequent dressing changes may also be utilized. Plastic surgeons may be required to employ a muscle flap or split thickness skin grafts to close the wound that does not heal primarily.

Postoperative infection remains a significant concern because adjuvant therapies such as chemotherapy may adversely affect patient immunity. Patients are given broad-spectrum antibiotics for 48 hours or longer after surgery. Prophylactic oral antibiotics may be used for weeks or months. Patients are advised in lifelong prevention of implant infection, which could result from a hematogenous source. For example, an abscessed tooth could spill bacteria into the bloodstream and infect the implant. Written instructions are given to the patient (Figure 37-3). Considerable bone damage can occur before detection of infection. Once infection is identified, treatment involves removal of the graft or implant, insertion of drains, immobilization, intravenous antibiotic therapy for 6 weeks, and/or antibiotic therapy for 6–12 months. Amputation of the limb is a possibility if complications occur. Consequently, the nurse must be vigilant in observing for signs of infection and in teaching patients about signs and symptoms to report.

Assessment for pneumonia, pulmonary embolism, and deep vein thrombosis is done during the postoperative period. Prophylactic anticoagulation with coumarin, sequential compressive embolic devices, and antiembolic stockings are often utilized.

Functional independence and a gradual adaptation to the changes in body image are the goals of rehabilitation. Resection often involves muscle tissue; therefore, physical therapy regimens often are used to improve and develop muscle tone. Assistive walking and brace devices may be needed if motor function is limited temporarily or permanently. For lower extremity resections, leg length discrepancies may necessitate gait retraining or may be managed simply through the use of shoe lifts. Finally, the importance of safety within the home environment cannot be overemphasized. The length of hospital stay ranges from 7–14 days. Most patients who are discharged to their previous home environment are able to negotiate stairs. Lifelong activity restrictions, such as no jogging, heavy lifting, or racquet sports, may be imposed and thereafter may alter the individual's career and recreation.

IMPLANT INFECTION PRECAUTIONS

Your allograft and/or metallic prosthetic implant does not have your body's natural protection against infection. Bacteria can enter your bloodstream and infect your implant. Here is a list of possible sources of infection and countermeasures.

Source of Infection	What to Do
Invasive Procedures: Surgery Proctoscope Cystoscope Endoscope	Notify your doctor so antibiotics can be given to protect your implant.
Dental Procedures: Cleaning Extraction Root canal Drilling	Notify your doctor or dentist prior to your appointment so antibiotics can be started before your procedure.
Wound or abrasion that is red or pus-filled; drainage; fever, chills	Immediately see your doctor to determine if antibiotics are needed.
Infection in urinary tract, ears, throat, etc.	Immediately see your doctor to determine if antibiotics are needed.

FIGURE 37-3 Implant infection precautions list

After wide resection, reconstruction to provide stability can be accomplished through the use of metal and synthetic materials; the use of bone *autografts*, which are those transplanted from one area to another in the same individual; or the use of bone *allografts*, which are those transferred between two genetically different members of the same species. The three most common methods of reconstruction after sarcoma resection are arthrodesis, arthroplasty with metallic or allograft implant, and intercalary allograft reconstruction. Careful consideration should be given to type of reconstruction, particularly in view of the patient's functional needs.[21]

Arthrodesis, or fusion, results in a stiff joint, which is a handicap for the individual. This form of reconstruction, however, is sturdy and permits activities such as running and jumping. Revision surgery is less likely with this procedure. There are a variety of surgical techniques for arthrodesis that use metallic implants, allograft implants, or autograft bone (Figure 37-4). Complications include infection and nonunion. In 1985 Otis and colleagues[22] found that patients who underwent segmental replacement have lower energy cost during gait than those with above-the-knee amputation, which could be a consideration in elderly patients, who frequently have compromised cardiac status.

Arthroplasty with metallic or bone allograft implant

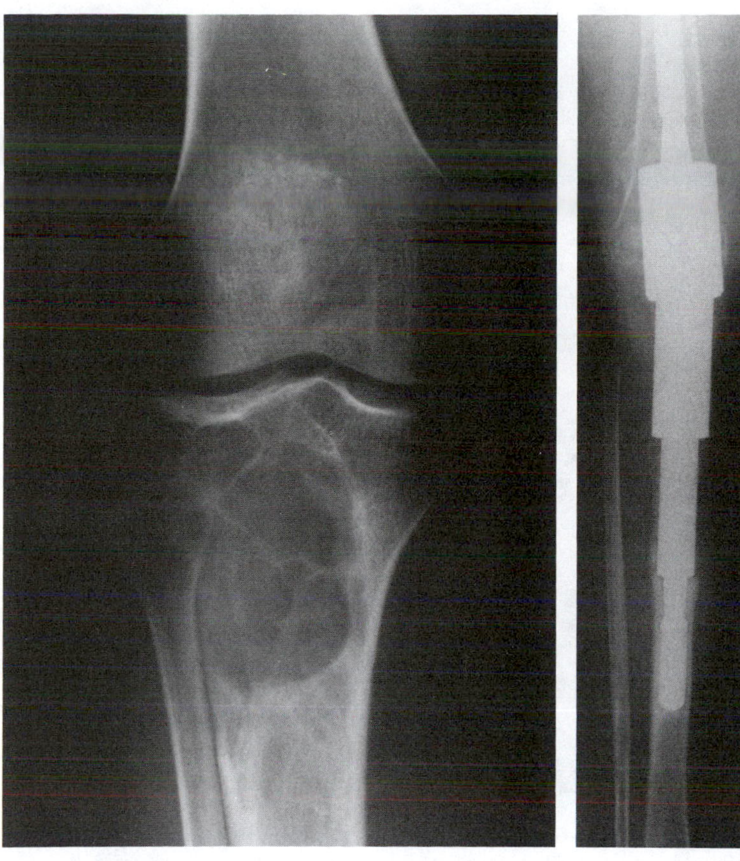

FIGURE 37-4 Radiograph of 30-year-old woman with fibrosarcoma of the proximal tibia who underwent a wide excision of the tumor and received a segmental arthrodesis. She is disease-free after 6 years.

or a combination of metal and allograft allows maintenance of joint function (Figure 37-5). The implant, however, is an artificial joint and will not tolerate percussive activities such as jogging and racquet sports or heavy lifting. Complications include infection, implant fracture, loosening of implant, and nonunion. In any limb salvage surgeries, muscle flaps, and skin grafting may be necessary to assist in wound closure.

Allografts

The use of allograft bone in tumor reconstruction has gained acceptance since the 1960s. In 1990, according to the American Association of Tissue Banks, an estimated 450,000 patients received transplants of bone, tendon, ligaments, and connective tissue. Allograft tissue can be custom sized in the surgical suite. There is no donor site morbidity or size limitation. There is improved joint stability and function by suturing allograft soft tissue attachments to host tissue. This is not possible with metallic implants. Allograft or cadaveric bone is procured in an operating room after consent is obtained from the next of kin. Often the donors have been involved in a motor vehicle accident or other fatal event. They may also donate heart, heart valves, lungs, liver, kidneys, corneas, and blood vessels. The donors were healthy and under 60 years of age. Thorough history and serological tests are performed to screen for viral or bacterial contamination. The chance of transplanting a human immune deficiency virus (HIV) allograft is calculated to be one in over a million.[23]

The bone is frozen, which diminishes its immune response. Bone allograft recipients do not require immunosuppressive agents, which are often given to organ recipients.[24] Freezing does inhibit cartilage viability, even when cryopreservation agents such as glycerol are applied to the articular surfaces. In a recent study by Enneking and Mindell,[25] 16 retrieved cadaveric allografts were found to have no chondrocytes. When a bone is needed by a surgeon, the medical director of the tissue bank selects an appropriate sized allograft utilizing recipient and allograft radiographs. Tissue typing is not performed. The tissue serves as a scaffold for the new host bone to grow into. The term *osteoconduction* describes this growth of capillaries and osteoprogenitor cells of the host into the allograft.

Osseous and osteochondral intercalary allografts provide a theoretically superior alternative to metallic implants because they provide joint mobility and are biologic materials.

In an intercalary allograft the allograft is placed between two segments of the host bone (Figure 37-6). The allograft actually heals to the host bone after being secured by metallic plates and screws. Research indicates successful results in the replacement of long bone tumors with fresh-frozen allografts.[26–28] Degenerative

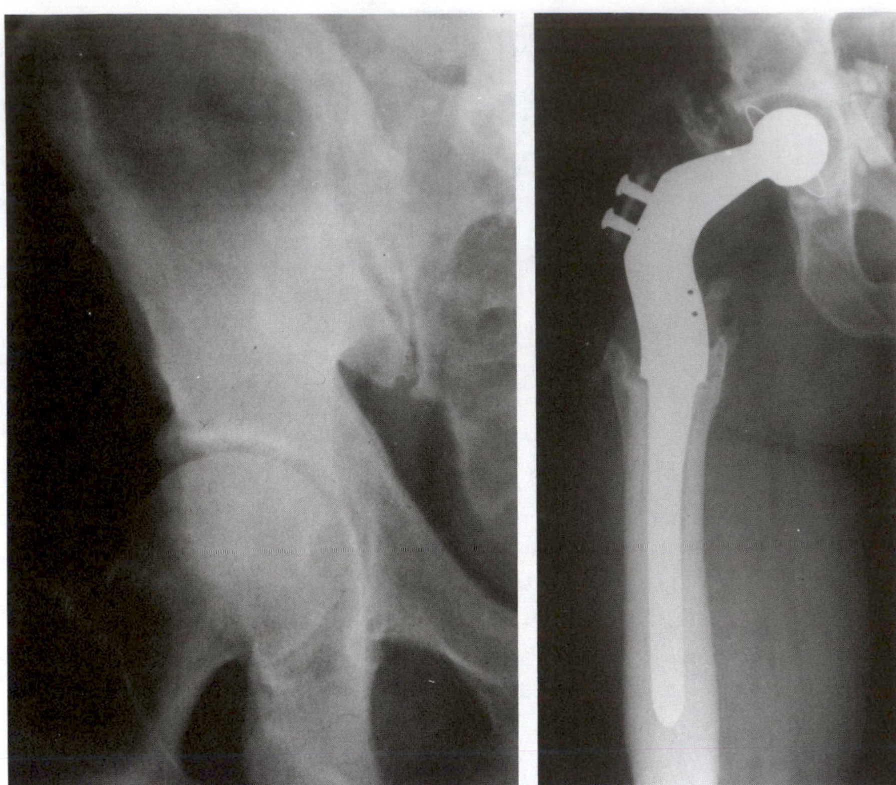

FIGURE 37-5 Radiograph of 25-year-old man with osteosarcoma of the proximal femur who underwent a wide excision of the tumor with proximal one-third femur replacement with a metallic implant. He is disease-free after 10 years.

arthritis can occur in osteoarticular allografts but can be managed by nonsteroidal anti-inflammatory medications, another osteoarticular allograft, or composite implant.[29,30]

Long-term activity restrictions for individuals undergoing allografts are the same as for those receiving metallic implants. However, the individual needs to limit weight bearing and often must wear a cast or brace, sometimes for up to 6–12 months, until the allograft is healed to the host bone. Complications of this procedure include infection, allograft fracture, and nonunion. The incidence of infection is reported to be 5%.[31] Nonunions may require an autogenous iliac bone graft for 1 year following surgery. Chemotherapy retards allograft healing; postoperative chemotherapy increased complications from 44%–51% in three series of studies.[32–34] The future of allograft reconstruction appears promising for individuals whose bone is destroyed by malignant tumors.

Metastatic sarcoma

The role of surgery in the management of disseminated disease has gained support in recent years. Sarcomas frequently metastasize to the lung before involving other sites. If untreated, most patients with pulmonary metastases will die within 18 months. Individuals in whom lung metastases develop are good candidates for resection, provided the primary tumor is controlled, there is no indication of other visceral metastatic disease, and the pulmonary nodules are resectable. CT of the chest and chest roentgenogram are performed at the time of diagnosis and every 3 months thereafter to assess for extent of disease. Wedge excision is the preferred procedure for lung lesions. The nodule is adequately resected without compromising lung function. The only factor predictive of survival after relapse is if the patient can be rendered surgically disease-free. Patients generally recover rapidly after a thoracotomy. The 5-year actuarial survival cure is 50%.[36]

Radical resection without reconstruction

In soft tissue sarcomas and in bone sarcomas in expendable bones such as a fibula, clavicle, and sections of the pelvis, the resection is performed without any need for reconstruction. The nursing care is similar to those with reconstruction. No lifelong infection concerns exist as no implants are placed.

Amputation preparation

The psychologic needs of the individual who undergoes amputation should be considered during preoperative preparation. It is reasonable to assume that the person facing an amputation has fears regarding death,

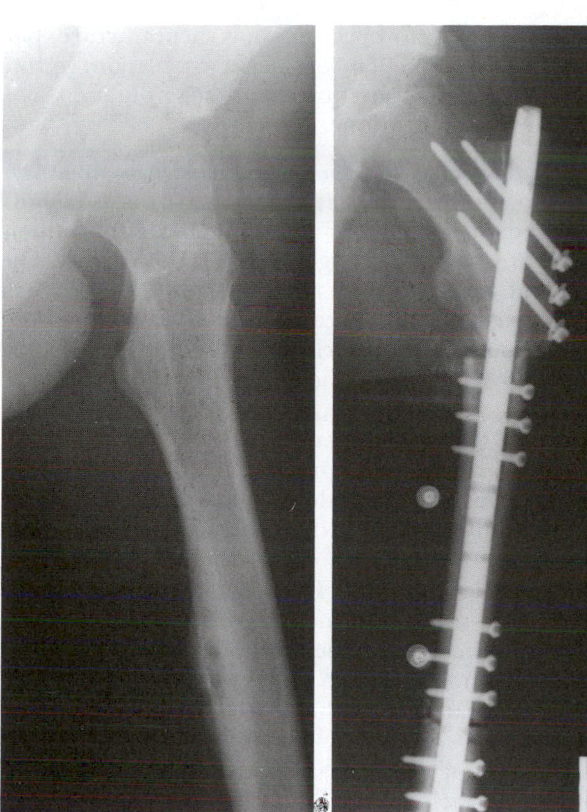

FIGURE 37-6 Radiograph of 18-year-old man with periosteal osteosarcoma of the diaphysis of the femur. He underwent a wide excision of the tumor with an intercalary allograft reconstruction. In the postoperative radiograph, it is difficult to detect the junction between the allograft and host bone. The individual is disease-free after 5 years.

disability, and deformity. In addition, the person may be concerned about the potential loss of social and economic self-sufficiency. These fears and concerns may lead to changes in self-esteem, which can be manifested by anxiety and depression. All these factors will affect the individual's readiness to learn and ability to participate in rehabilitation. Consequently, the plan of care includes interventions aimed at minimizing fear, decreasing anxiety, and promoting realistic optimism. The individual and family may wish to express their fears and doubts. Efforts are made to integrate their expectations with reality by providing accurate information from nursing and medical staff regarding the postoperative recovery period and future rehabilitation.

The individual having a hemipelvectomy may harbor fears concerning sexual adequacy. If appropriate, a woman needs to be reassured that pregnancy and normal delivery are possible after surgery. A decision concerning future pregnancies, however, may be influenced by the fact that the prosthesis cannot be worn during pregnancy. Impotence in a man often is related to age. Loss of erectile power is due primarily to a decrease in blood supply; however, pelvic nerve function may be compromised. Most men recover potency over time. The younger the individual, the more rapid the recovery of potency.

To reduce anxiety it sometimes is helpful for the person undergoing surgery to meet preoperatively those individuals who will be involved in his or her postoperative care. Depending on the institution's program, this may include physical and occupational therapists, the prosthetist, the social worker, and the psychologist. Likewise, in some instances it may be helpful to arrange a preoperative visit from a person with an amputated limb who has mastered his or her prosthesis and achieved independence. Information regarding local organizations that train such volunteers can be obtained from the American Cancer Society. Care is taken in assessing which individuals could benefit by interaction with these resources. An overload of information may serve only to increase the person's anxiety and fear.

The nurse consults social service personnel to inform the patient and family about financial resources and rehabilitation programs available in the state. There is generally underutilization of available resources for individuals with cancer. Other support is available through groups such as the American Cancer Society and American Handicapped Association.

It is important for the nurse to help establish realistic expectations regarding the patient's postamputation function. Many individuals who have lower extremity amputation can expect a return to full function and a relatively normal active life through the use of a lower limb prosthesis and occasional walking aids. Amputees resume activities such as downhill skiing, swimming, basketball, and cycling with or without recreational prostheses. It is estimated that 20,000 amputees participate in sporting activities, with more than 5000 participating in organized competition.[37] The person who has a hemicorporectomy is wheelchair-bound. Hemipelvectomy prostheses will approximate only soft tissue, and the use of a walker or crutches will be necessary for additional stability. Because of the significantly increased energy expenditure required, it may be necessary for the person with a more proximal amputation to spend more time in a wheelchair. Elderly patients or those with cardiac conditions may find prosthetic use tiring and may need to use at least a cane.

Ideally, the goal for the individual is independent function with the use of prostheses. In evaluating rehabilitation potential, the nurse considers other factors such as age, effects of adjuvant therapy, the existence of unrelated disease, and the person's attitude. Prosthetic rehabilitation requires cooperation, coordination, tremendous physical energy, and a comfortable prosthesis.[38] Lane and colleagues[39] have found that amputees who have received doxorubicin and bleomycin have greater resting heart rates, decreased walking velocity, and increased oxygen requirements. The longer the stump, the lower the energy cost. With this information, they have found that patients with lightweight prosthetic devices and supervised cardiovascular training three times a week increased their gait velocity and reduced net energy cost.[39]

The nurse learns from the physician whether the patient will have an immediate postsurgical prosthetic fitting or a conventional delayed prosthetic fitting. This decision is made before surgery, which permits adequate preparation of the individual for the postoperative care regimen.

Phantom limb phenomenon Preoperative teaching includes a frank discussion of phantom limb sensation and pain. It is a frightening experience for an individual with a recent amputation to feel sensation or pain, or both, in a limb that no longer exists. Consequently, the person who is not adequately prepared may neglect to report the occurrence of the phantom limb phenomenon and may harbor doubts about his or her sanity.

All individuals who have had an amputation can expect to feel some phantom limb sensation, whereas only 35% of those experience phantom limb pain.[40] Phantom limb sensation is described as an awareness of the position or existence of the limb. Itching, pressure, or tingling sensations may be described. Phantom limb pain is described as severe cramping, throbbing, or burning pain in various areas of the amputated limb. Phantom limb sensations usually are experienced shortly after surgery. Phantom limb pain usually occurs for 1–4 weeks after surgery and may be triggered by fatigue, excitement, sickness, weather change, stress, and other stimuli. The incidence and severity of phantom limb pain are greater when the amputation site is more proximal. For many individuals, phantom limb pain resolves gradually in a few months. However, the pain becomes worse over the years for 5%–10% of those who have amputations of limbs. It is suggested that increased severity of phantom limb pain after a few months may be a symptom of locally recurrent cancer in a stump or it may be a sign of a neuroma.

Phantom limb pain is poorly understood but seems to depend on a combination of physical and emotional factors. The physical component relates to the surgical interruption of neural reflex pathways, with resultant transmission of abnormal patterns of nerve impulses. Melzack[40] noted a correlation between the length of time a person experiences limb pain before surgery and the incidence and duration of phantom limb pain. Other factors that contribute to phantom pain include the maladaptive use of pain for secondary gain, the availability of support systems, and the ability to cope with loss.[41]

A variety of measures are used to alleviate phantom limb pain. Relief may be obtained simply by applying heat to the stump or by pressure, such as with elastic bandages. Distraction and diversion techniques may decrease the person's awareness of the pain. Tranquilizers, muscle relaxants, or local anesthesia are occasionally effective in managing the pain. Psychotherapy and behavioral therapy also may be useful. Procedures that are available for intractable pain include hypnosis, nerve blocks, sympathectomy, cordotomy, acupuncture, biofeedback, and transcutaneous nerve stimulation. In rare cases, revision of the stump with reamputation at a higher level may be done.

Amputation of the lower extremity Preoperative preparation of the individual having a lower extremity amputation incorporates all considerations routinely given to any person undergoing general anesthesia. The individual who is to have a hemipelvectomy will need to know that a urethral catheter will be inserted and that preoperative bowel cleansing and antibiotics will be given to decrease the bacterial count of the intestinal tract.

General strengthening measures and mobility training should be initiated preoperatively by a physical therapist. Pull-ups provide effective preparation for walking with crutches. Active and active-resistive exercises of the unaffected extremity maintain and increase muscle strength. The person also should be instructed in transfer maneuvers from bed to chair to commode. Finally, the person should be instructed to ambulate with the use of a walker or crutches. Control of weight bearing on the affected side should be emphasized.

The goals of postoperative care are to use modern prostheses, to achieve the highest level of function possible, and to minimize the negative psychosocial consequences of amputation. The actual postoperative care varies according to whether the individual has had an immediate prosthetic fitting or a conventional delayed prosthetic fitting.

Immediate postsurgical prosthetic fittings consist of a rigid dressing and cast that is applied to the stump at the time of surgery. A socket on the distal end of the cast is designed so that a pylon prosthetic unit can be attached to the cast (Figure 37-7). Restraining straps that go over the shoulder or attach to the waistband contribute to controlled pressure, improved stump shaping, and tissue support provided by the cast.

If a conventional delayed prosthesis fitting is planned, the patient will return from surgery with the stump covered with a dressing and an elastic bandage. To shrink and shape the stump, elastic bandages or elastic stump shrinkers are used until the first fitting (Figure 37-8). The individual is fitted with a temporary or intermediate prosthesis at approximately 3–6 weeks, when acute swelling has decreased. An intermediate prosthesis, however, lacks a cosmetic covering. Ambulation with weight bearing is encouraged as tolerated. Approximately 3 months after surgery, the individual is fitted with a permanent prosthesis, with or without immediate postsurgical fitting.

The relative advantages and disadvantages for immediate and delayed prosthesis fitting are summarized in Table 37-4.

With the conventional delayed fitting, drains frequently are inserted during surgery to remove blood and serous drainage. The nurse observes for signs of

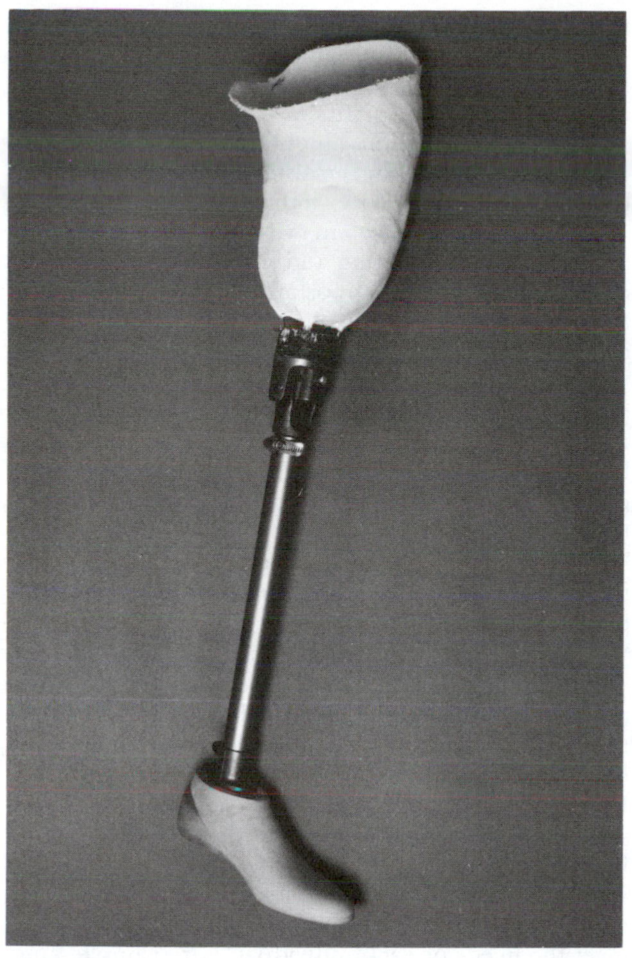

FIGURE 37-7 Immediate postsurgical prosthetic fitting with a pylon prosthetic unit attached to the cast.

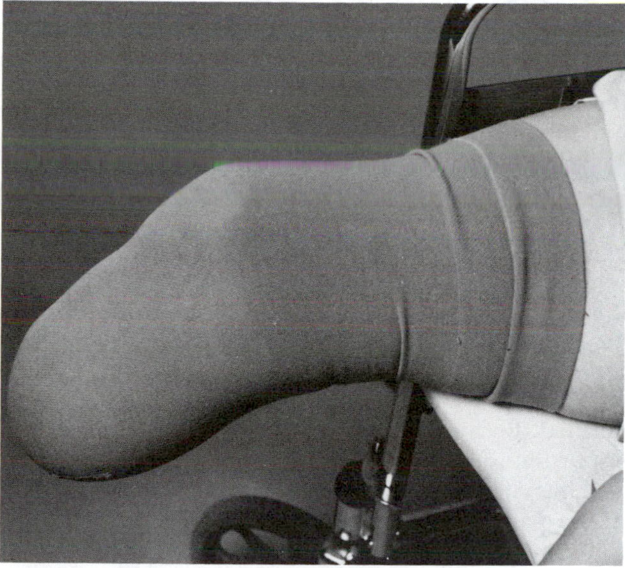

FIGURE 37-8 Elastic stump shrinker applied to shape stump.

hemorrhage such as excessive bleeding through the dressing or an increase in pain, tenderness, or swelling of the stump.

The stump usually is elevated for 24 hours after surgery to prevent edema and promote venous return. To prevent hip contractures, the individual is assisted into the prone position three to four times a day for a minimum of 15 minutes and encouraged to assume that position for sleep. Exercises to maintain muscle tone and prevent edema, joint contractures, and muscle atrophy are initiated on the first postoperative day. Exercises include active range of motion, strengthening exercises for the upper extremities, and hyperextension of the stump.

Stump care involves frequent wrapping with elastic bandages or stump shrinkers to facilitate stump shrinking. Dangling and transfer to a chair are encouraged on the first postoperative day. Crutch walking is started as soon as the person is strong enough. Sutures or staples are removed approximately 2 weeks after surgery. Temporary prosthetic fitting will occur at 3–6 weeks. For the individual having a hemipelvectomy, mobilization also is possible on the second or third postoperative day. The permanent prosthesis may be fitted

TABLE 37-4 Relative Advantages and Disadvantages of Delayed Versus Immediate Prosthetic Fitting

	Delayed Fitting	Immediate Fitting
Advantages	Wound can be inspected for healing. Skin can be conditioned by Ace wraps and stump shrinkers	Better emotional adjustment with immediate substitute limb. Motivation increased with early ambulation. Decreased stump edema, pain, phantom limb pain, and contractures (caused by pressure of device).
Disadvantages	Edema delays shrinking and shaping of stump. Continuous rewrapping with elastic bandages is required. Ambulation is delayed. Attention must be given to prevention of contractures and other complications of immobility.	Wound cannot be visualized. Temporary prosthesis is heavy. Poor gait pattern can develop because of heavy prosthesis and discomfort in early ambulation period. Prosthetist must go to operating room to apply.

within 12 weeks. A sitting or bucket prosthesis also is needed for an individual with a hemipelvectomy because of the absence of an ischium on which to sit. Until the bucket prosthesis is fabricated, a pillow is placed under the surgical site for balance.

With immediate prosthetic fitting, hemorrhage is less likely because of the compression effects of the cast. However, evidence of blood staining on the cast should be noted. The rigid cast also minimizes acute swelling; however, the stump is routinely elevated for 24 hours. Care must be taken to prevent the cast from slipping off the stump, which would rapidly lead to edema and wound disruption. Should this occur, the stump should be wrapped with an elastic bandage and the surgeon notified. Because the wound cannot be visualized, it is important to monitor for signs of infection such as fever, increased white blood cell count, and significant stump pain. Such symptoms would necessitate immediate removal of the cast for wound inspection.

Nursing management includes cast care. The skin near the edges of the cast should be inspected for friction ribs, swelling, or discoloration. In addition, the cast should be inspected routinely for cracks. The rigid cast assists in the prevention of hip and joint contractures.

Ambulation with the pylon and crutches or walker is initiated on the first or second postoperative day. The length of time permitted for ambulation increases gradually. The individual advances to the use of parallel bars and to crutches while bearing touch-down weight on the pylon. The sutures and cast are removed. A stump shrinker is applied 2 weeks after surgery. After the swelling is diminished, fitting for a permanent prosthesis is undertaken at 12 weeks after surgery. Chemotherapy may increase stump swelling and delay fitting of the permanent prosthesis.

The primary nurse assumes the responsibility for coordinating the efforts of the health professionals involved in the care during hospitalization of a person undergoing amputation, as well as for making the appropriate referrals to those professionals in the community who will become involved in the person's total rehabilitation. This may include a referral to a community nurse, community physical therapist, and local rehabilitation programs involved with vocational rehabilitation. Most individuals with amputated limbs are capable of returning to work with restrictions.

The primary nurse also contributes to improved health and the prevention of complications through patient and family education. Teaching the individual how to care for the stump is an essential element of the rehabilitation program. The person needs to be responsible for daily stump hygiene with the use of a mild soap and water. The person also should be instructed to avoid the use of skin creams, oils, and rubbing alcohol. Daily inspection for redness, blisters, or abrasions should be incorporated into the person's routine. The stump socks or elastic wraps should fit properly and be changed daily. When the wound has healed, the individual can prevent edema by putting on the prosthesis immediately after arising and keeping it on all day. The person with an immediate postsurgical prosthetic fitting also should be instructed regarding cast care and inspection for fit.

The individual also is taught how to put on and care for the prosthesis. The prosthesis socket is wiped out daily with a damp, soapy cloth. Care is taken to thoroughly remove the soap and to dry the socket to prevent a source of skin irritation and prosthesis rust. The individual is taught the importance of never attempting to make mechanical adjustments to the prosthesis. Discomfort or difficulties in the use necessitate an immediate visit to the prosthetist.

The primary nurse and physical therapist review the exercises that contribute to achievement of the highest level of functioning with grace and coordination. Exercises that contribute to balance and movement patterns include standing, weight shifting, heel and toe balance, rocking, hip hiking, and stair climbing. The individual is advised to practice these exercises after discharge from the hospital.

The physician and prosthetist collaborate in the planning of the prosthetic device to be constructed. The prosthetist ultimately is accountable for the construction and fit of the prosthesis and should be certified by the American Board for Certification of Prosthetists. Lower limb prostheses generally consist of a socket, suspension such as a waistband or suction or latex sleeve, knee joint, ankle joint, and foot (Figure 37-9). Many varieties of these components are available; consequently, numerous combinations can be developed to meet the needs of each individual. For example, knee joints are available that provide either mechanical or hydraulic assistance in controlling the swing phase of walking and that provide increased stability during standing. Energy-storage prosthetic feet such as the Seattle foot are made with a flexible heel that releases the energy of foot fall at terminal stage to help initiate swing phase. These features, however, increase weight, cost, and maintenance. An above-knee prosthesis weighs approximately 3 kg and a below-knee prosthesis 1 kg. In designing the prosthesis, consideration is given to the person's age, ability, endurance, financial status, occupation goals, and motivation as well as comfort, fit, alignment, safety, ease of application, and appearance. The primary nurse can assess these factors and communicate them to the prosthetist. Figure 37-10 shows an endoprosthesis for the individual with a hemipelvectomy before application of the cosmetic urethane foam cover pictured in Figure 37-11.

After discharge, the individual with an amputation should be seen by the prosthetist every 4–6 weeks for the first postoperative year. It is the responsibility of the community health nurse to observe for problems related to fit, comfort, physical stress, or psychologic maladjustment. These problems then should be explored with the individual and/or the prosthetist or physician. The rehabilitation process is complete when the individual has attained an optimal level of inde-

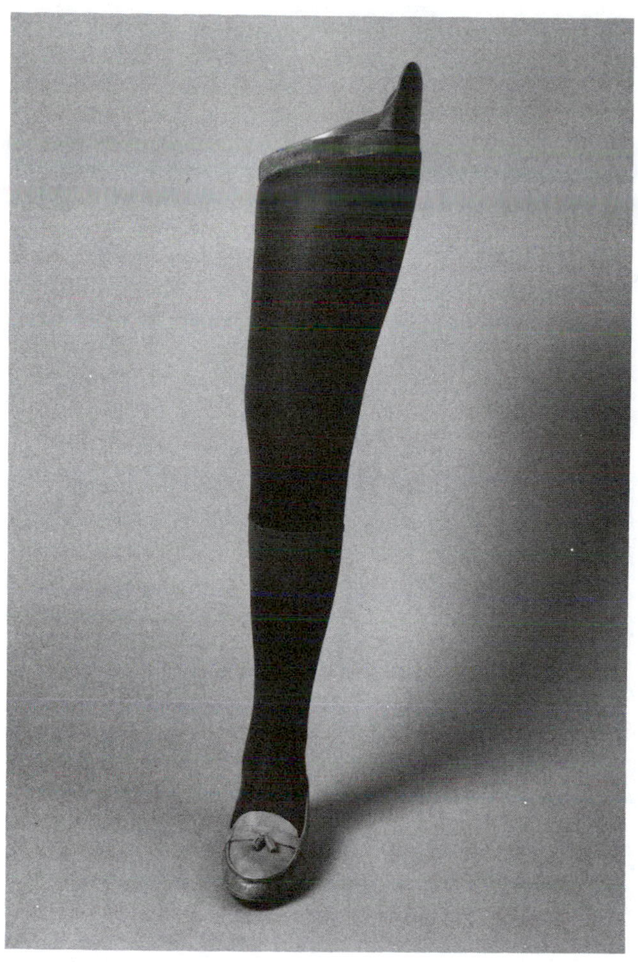

FIGURE 37-9 Lower limb prosthesis for an above-knee amputation showing the socket, suction suspension, joints, and foot.

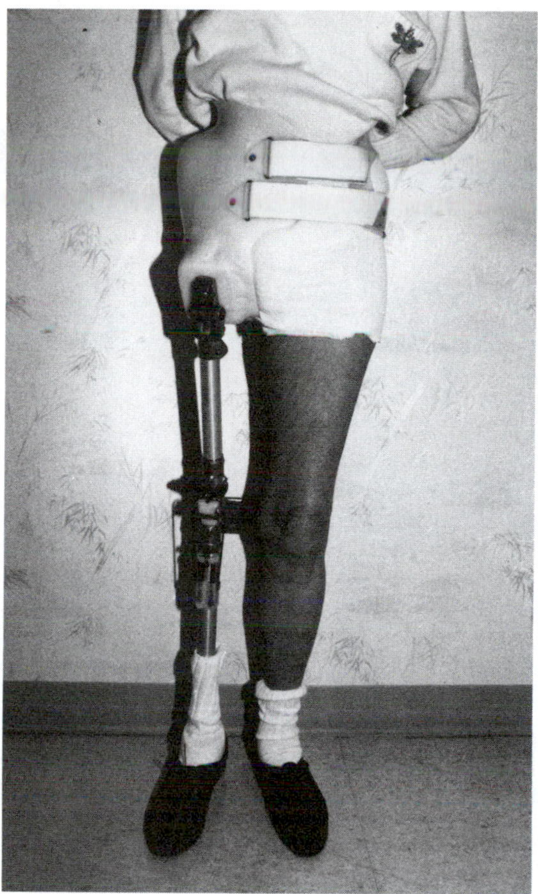

FIGURE 37-10 Hemipelvectomy endoprosthesis.

pendence and successfully incorporated the prosthesis into the body image.

Amputation of the upper extremity Many of the considerations concerning preoperative, postoperative, and rehabilitative care that were discussed in the preceding section apply to individuals having an upper extremity amputation. There are, however, some significant differences.

Upper limb prostheses are far less satisfactory than those created for lower extremities in both appearance and function. The functional capabilities of the prosthesis for upper extremity amputation decrease as the level of amputation becomes more proximal. Power and motion are supplied in only a comparatively gross fashion. The most functional terminal (hand) device is a hook. The development of a substitute for the complex actions of the intricate muscles of the hand has thus far been impossible. Adequate cosmetic appearance can be obtained at the expense of function. Polyvinyl cosmetic gloves with realistic skin creases, veins, and hair are available. Skin tones are matched; shade changes that occur in the normal hand as a result of position and season cannot be reproduced. In addition, the glove must be replaced frequently because ink, newsprint, and other stains are impossible to remove.

Conventional prostheses for the upper extremities consist of a hand terminal device, a harness to supply force from the proximal muscles, appropriate segments between them, including a socket for the stump, and cable system that provides motion at the terminal device and/or the elbow (Figure 37-12). Abduction of the scapula or flexion of the shoulder on the side of the prosthesis initiates movement. Flexion and extension of the wrist usually are omitted, although wrist units in flexed or extended positions are available. Pronation and supination are achieved by rotating the terminal device with the opposite hand. Likewise, opening and closing of the terminal device are accomplished through the use of the opposite hand.

Prostheses for interscapulothoracic amputations are fitted over the upper portion of the chest. Motion is severely limited because sources of power are unavailable. Some force can be initiated from the opposite shoulder and chest expansion. The primary function of the prosthesis, however, is cosmetic. Rejection of the upper extremity prosthetic devices occurs more often

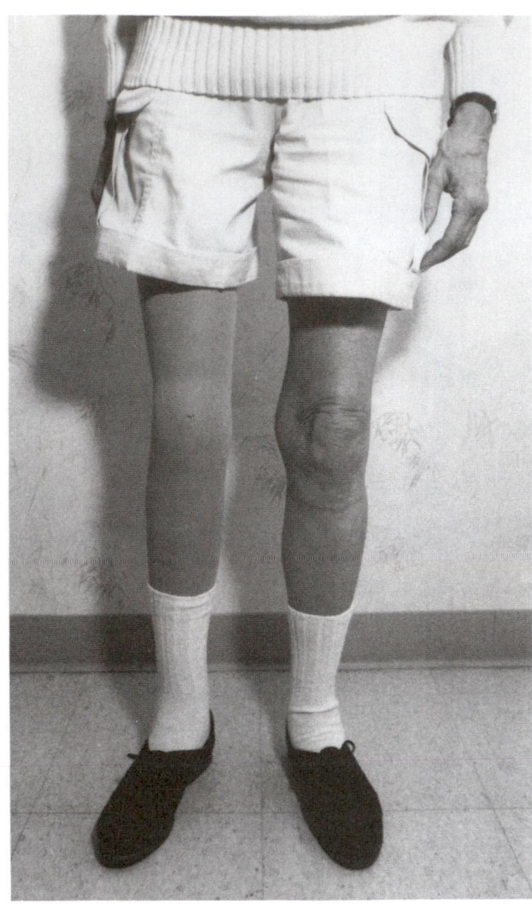

FIGURE 37-11 Hemipelvectomy endoprosthesis with cosmetic urethane foam cover.

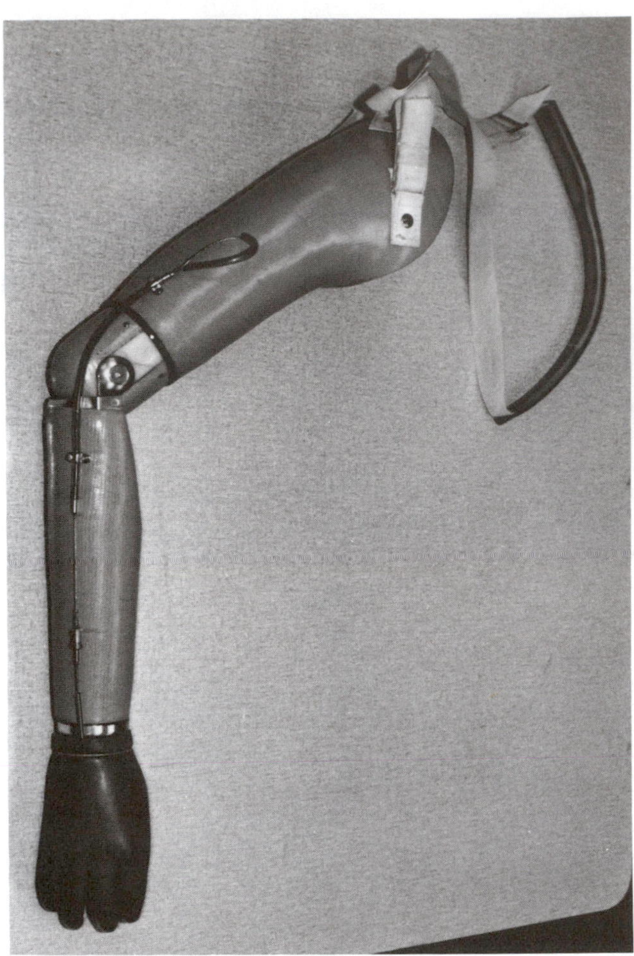

FIGURE 37-12 Upper extremity prosthetic device showing a cable system, elbow joint, and hand terminal device.

than with prostheses of the lower extremity because of a combination of poor function, low cosmetic value, and lack of motivation.

Upper extremity prosthetic research has been directed at the development of myoelectric limb substitution. In this system, electrical impulses from the contraction of extensor and flexor muscle in the stump are picked up by electrodes in the socket and are in turn amplified, switching on and off electrical motors in the prosthesis. An external battery pack may be worn to provide an additional electrical supply. Opening and closing of the terminal device, pronation and supination, and elbow flexion can be provided. The individual must be assessed first for the ability to elicit and control myoelectric signals. The advantages include an increase in control with less energy expenditure and improved physical appearance. The disadvantages include electrical interference or inadvertent contraction of the muscles with user coughs or stretches and the cost of the device.

The reality is that the inadequacy of available upper limb prostheses can be disappointing for the person with an upper limb amputation. The nurse, in conjunction with the physician, provides realistic information regarding the functional and cosmetic features of the upper extremity prostheses. It is important to discuss with the individual the negative social stigma attached to the hook, as well as its functional capabilities. Equal emphasis should be placed on the functional limitations and cosmetic value of the glove. Some individuals are willing to sacrifice function to obtain the best cosmetic replacement.

As with lower extremity amputations, immediate or delayed postsurgical prosthesis fitting is possible. When delayed fitting is planned, the individual will return from surgery with a soft dressing and elastic bandages covering the stump. Compression of the surgical area is to be avoided until healing takes place.

As with the lower extremity amputation, independence and an adapted body image can be facilitated through the provision of psychologic support, patient and family education, and appropriate referral to community resources. Rehabilitation goals emphasize use of the remaining arm for activities of daily living. The patient should be evaluated preoperatively by an occupational therapist for information on one-handedness. Vocational rehabilitation assumes particular importance for the individual with an upper extremity amputation because the ensuing disability could prevent the resumption of previous employment.

Radiotherapy

The use of radiotherapy in the management of primary or metastatic malignant bone or soft tissue sarcoma depends on the radiosensitivity of the particular tumor type. Most bone tumors are relatively unresponsive to radiation. Consequently, radiation is reserved for palliation and may be used in conjunction with chemotherapy for inoperable tumors or in conjunction with surgery to reduce the tumor load of partially resectable tumors. Conventional radiation doses for palliative treatment of primary bone tumors often results in fibrosis and contractures that lead to amputation even if the tumor is controlled. Neutron beam therapy, however, which is produced by heavy particle accelerators, can deliver higher doses with fewer complications. At the Fermilab Neutron Therapy Facility in Batavia, Illinois, 25 individuals were treated with neutron beam therapy for bone sarcoma in the axial skeleton or when surgery was refused for cosmetic or emotional reasons. The local control rate was 44% and the crude survival rate was 39%.[42] Neutron beam irradiation may be an effective option for nonresectable sarcoma.

In contrast, radiotherapy plays an integral role in the management of Ewing's sarcoma and soft tissue sarcomas. Complications of treatment include tendon contractures, edema of the involved extremity distal to the site of irradiation, cessation of growth of the extremity, and nonhealing fractures.

Regional hyperthermia is a technique of raising the temperature in a tumor to 42°C for approximately 1 hour. In a study of 40 patients with advanced sarcoma, regional hyperthemia along with ifosfamide plus etoposide was employed. There were 38 assessable patients and only 6 had a complete response.[43] It can be a painful procedure for patients, with high systematic temperature and tachycardia occurring during the procedure. Complications include local infection, thrombosis, burns, and hematoma. It is a treatment option not utilized commonly in the United States for sarcoma.

Chemotherapy and Immunotherapy

Since the addition of postoperative chemotherapy to the treatment of bone sarcomas in the early 1970s, survival rates have increased from 20% to more than 50%.[44] Currently, chemotherapy is given preoperatively as well as postoperatively. The rationale for preoperative chemotherapy is to treat the micrometastasis; to decrease the primary tumor size, thereby increasing the likelihood of limb salvage surgery; and to assess the effectiveness of the chemotherapeutic agents for 2–3 months.[45] The route of chemotherapy is either intravenous or intraarterial. The duration of treatment ranges from 6–12 months. Adjuvant chemotherapy for soft tissue sarcomas is considered experimental, as will be discussed later.

Toxic effects are decreased by administering agents to counter the effects. Ifosfamide can cause hemorrhagic cystitis, but mesna can inactivate metabolites in urine and prevent this complication.[46] High-dose methotrexate can cause renal toxicities, but calcium leucovorin or citrovorium factor can ameliorate this toxicity. The systemic effects of chemotherapy such as neutropenia and thrombocytopenia may create wound complications.[47] Neutropenia may increase incidence of infection but not necessarily impede wound healing. Chemotherapy is tremendously important in the treatment of sarcoma, and any complications are accepted and treated appropriately.

SARCOMAS

Osteosarcoma

Epidemiology and etiology

Osteosarcoma is the most common osseous malignant bone tumor, accounting for an estimated 20% of such lesions.[15] Its incidence is greatest in individuals between 10 and 25 years of age, and it affects males twice as often as females. The incidence of osteosarcoma peaks again in older adults with Paget's disease.

The increased incidence of osteosarcoma during adolescence has been correlated with skeletal growth patterns, which in turn may account for the greater overall occurrence in males.

Pathophysiology

Osteosarcoma appears to arise from primitive bone-forming mesenchyma in the medullary cavity. Proliferating connective tissue generally gives rise to tumor osteoid and bone directly. The proliferating connective tissue also may form some tumor cartilage that undergoes rapid osseous transformation.

Periosteal osteosarcoma, a variant of osteosarcoma, was originally described by Unni et al.[48] It occurs as a hard mass on the bone surface, especially tibia and knee. The tumor is confined to the periosteum and cortex without a medullary component. Tumors are low to intermediate grade.

Parosteal or juxtacortical osteosarcomas occur also on bony surfaces, especially posterior femur and humerus. They are often low grade. Raymond[49] recommends that both subvariants be called *surface osteosarcoma*.

The histologic pattern of osteosarcoma is so variable that no two specimens are exactly alike. Specimens have varying mixtures of malignant bone, malignant cartilage, and malignant stroma. Consequently, the tumor may be described as osteoblastic, chondroblastic, or fibroblastic, depending on which component is dominant. Whatever the pattern, the essential criteria for the diagnosis of osteosarcoma are the presence of frankly sarcomatous stroma and the formation of tumor osteoid and bone by malignant connective tissue.

The most frequent sites of osteosarcoma include the distal end of the femur, the proximal end of the tibia, and the proximal end of the humerus. Osteosarcomas may be discovered in the iliac bone, vertebral column, mandible, and in rare cases the scapula, clavicle, or bones in the hands and feet. Humeral and tibial lesions have a better prognosis.[50]

Metastatic spread occurs primarily to the lungs by the hematogenous route. Radiologic evidence of pulmonary or bony metastases usually appears within 24 months of the definitive surgery. Late metastasis in one or more of the other bones occurs occasionally, often in the presence of pulmonary metastases.

Assessment

The individual with osteosarcoma typically has pain and a mass. The pain becomes more severe at night.

If the tumor is allowed to follow its natural course, the affected limb becomes swollen and its superficial veins significantly dilated. In individuals with rapidly growing tumors, weight loss and anemia may be seen. In addition, pathologic fractures are not uncommon. The duration of symptoms varies from weeks to 6 months or more before medical advice and treatment are sought.

Half the individuals with osteosarcoma have an elevation in the serum alkaline phosphatase level. This level, which represents osteoblastic activity, tends to decline after removal of the tumor and to return to the initially high level in the presence of pulmonary metastasis. In the normal growing child the levels are elevated. Other laboratory data do not appear to be significant in the diagnosis of osteosarcoma.

The classic radiologic features of osteosarcoma include cortical bone destruction, extension of the tumor into soft tissue, and periosteal new bone formation that may appear in a perpendicular striated, or "sunburst," pattern. These findings can be diagnostic on plain radiographs.

Treatment

The 5-year survival rate for individuals treated with surgery alone or irradiation and surgery has been approximately 10%–20%.[51] The high mortality rate is due principally to pulmonary metastasis, which is assumed to be present microscopically at time of presentation. Reports evaluating adjuvant chemotherapy after surgery for osteosarcoma indicate a significant prolongation of the disease-free interval. Reports from the 1970s show that the 5-year survival rate increased from 40%–60% with the use of adjuvant chemotherapy using single agents.[52] Current chemotherapy protocols have used doxorubicin, high-dose cyclophosphamide, ifosfamide, cisplatin, or high-dose methotrexate with leucovorin rescue. Most agents, with the exception of methotrexate or ifosfamide, are given on an outpatient basis. The drugs are given via an intravenous or intraarterial route. Bacci and colleagues[53] and Glasser and colleagues[50] demonstrated an 87% disease-free state at 2 years to 77% at 5 years. When preoperative or primary chemotherapy is used, effectiveness is assessed at the time of tumor resection. This regimen allows in vivo study of the tumor cells. During the 8–20 weeks of preoperative chemotherapy, physical examination of the tumor site is performed to assess for effectiveness of treatment by indices such as decreased pain and swelling. If there is 90% tumor necrosis, the high-dose methotrexate regimen is continued postoperatively for 6 months. The greater the necrosis, the greater the survival. If tumor necrosis is less, the chemotherapy is changed to another effective, non–cross-resistant agent. The course is extended to 8–12 months.

The improved results of chemotherapy have sparked interest in limb salvage resections. The chemotherapy can result in a decrease in soft tissue component and ossification of bony component. There is concern that if preoperative chemotherapy is not effective, the delay in surgery could allow tumor growth. The limb salvage criteria apply to these patients. Amputations are indicated for patients with large and invasive tumors. The occurrence of occult medullary extension or skip metastasis within a single bone or across joints is uncommon, which allows cross bone amputation with wide margins of normal tissue. Disarticulation, which results in greater disability and no greater overall survival, is performed as a last resort.[54] It is advisable to obtain a second opinion if an amputation is recommended. Local recurrence is as frequent in amputation surgery as in limb salvage surgeries (under 5%).[55] Resumption of chemotherapy after definitive surgery is delayed for 1–3 weeks.

Significant improvement of patient survival with metastatic disease has been demonstrated in the 1980s. Of patients with osteosarcoma who had thoracotomies for metastases, 41% were free of disease more than 4 years after surgery.[44] No patients survived the development of pulmonary metastases unless they had surgical resection of gross disease. In these situations, chemotherapy is given after thoracotomy to eradicate microscopic disease.

Radiation currently is reserved for palliation or inoperable cases. Significant morbidity and mortality were reported when irradiation alone was used for treatment of the primary tumor.

Chondrosarcoma

Epidemiology and etiology

Chondrosarcoma accounts for approximately 13% of malignant bone tumors. The incidence is greatest in individuals between 30 and 60 years of age and among males.

The occurrence of chondrosarcomas has been associated with syndromes of skeletal maldevelopment. Transformation of cartilaginous exostosis, enchondromas, or chondroplasia to chondrosarcoma has occurred. Chondrosarcoma also occurs in individuals with Ollier's disease, a syndrome of polyosteotic benign cartilage tumors.

Pathophysiology

Chondrosarcoma arises from the cartilage and never has osteoid tissue.

There are both primary and secondary chondrosarcomas. The former include central chondrosarcomas, which arise in the medullary cavity. The latter include those chondrosarcomas that arise from benign tumors.[56]

The diagnosis of chondrosarcoma is based on cytologic changes of the cartilage cells. A cartilage tumor is considered malignant in the presence of many cells with plump nuclei, that is, more than a few cells with two such nuclei or clumps of chromatin.

The most frequent sites of chondrosarcoma include the pelvic bone, long bones, scapula, and ribs. Less frequent sites include bones of the hand and foot, the nose, the maxilla, and the base of the skull.

Most chondrosarcomas do not tend to metastasize early but rather remain slow growing and locally invasive. When advanced chondrosarcoma does become aggressive, it tends to metastasize via venous channels to the lungs and heart. Regional lymph nodes occasionally may be involved.

Assessment

Individuals with chondrosarcoma usually have a relatively long but unremarkable history. Medical advice often is sought for a slow-growing mass with intermittent dull, aching pain at the tumor site. Physical examination can reveal a firm enlargement over the affected area. Joints may be swollen and exhibit restricted motion if they are near the affected area.

Radiographs of chondrosarcoma show a lobular pattern with or without calcification. If calcification is present, it usually is seen in a circular or semicircular pattern. Central chondrosarcomas in the long bones may show thickening of the cortex because of swelling of the shaft. The peripheral chondrosarcoma may demonstrate a vast, dense, blotchy appearance. Ragged, irregular, radiopaque streaks extending away from the central part of the lesion may be seen.

Treatment

When the diagnosis of chondrosarcoma has been established, surgery is indicated. If the tumor is of central origin and has not extended through the cortex, wide resection and reconstruction are considered. Limb salvage surgery or amputation are options.

At present, chondrosarcoma remains nearly totally refractory to chemotherapeutic efforts because chondrosarcomas usually have a poor blood supply. Consequently, drugs given intravenously do not reach the tumor in concentrations that are high enough to be effective. The benefit of chemotherapy as an adjuvant to surgery has not been established.

Radiotherapy has limited effectiveness and is reserved for palliation of advanced or inoperable chondrosarcomas.

Individuals with a diagnosis of chondrosarcoma have a considerably better prognosis than those with osteosarcoma. The overall survival rate of individuals treated with wide resection or amputation has been reported to be 67% at 5 years and 50% at 10 years.[57] In this series, survival correlated well with the designated histologic grade of the lesion. The estimated 10-year survival rate of individuals with grade 1 tumors is 87% and that of individuals with grade 2 tumors is 41%. For those with grade 3 lesions, the 5-year survival rate is 44%, and the 10-year survival rate is 27%.

Fibrosarcoma

Epidemiology and etiology

Fibrosarcoma is rare, accounting for fewer than 4% of primary malignant bone tumors.[56] This type of neoplasm may occur at any age but is rare in children. There is no evident sex predominance.

Paget's disease may be a predisposing factor in the development of fibrosarcoma. In addition, the tumor may develop as a sequel to therapeutic irradiation or may develop at the site of an old bone infarct. Chronic osteomyelitis or fibrous dysplasia also may be a predisposing factor in the development of fibrosarcoma.

Pathophysiology

Fibrosarcoma is a malignant fibroblastic tumor that fails to develop tumor osteoid or bone in its local invasive growth site or in its metastatic foci. Periosteal new bone may be laid down as a direct extension of the tumor.

Like osteosarcoma, fibrosarcoma usually originates within the medullary cavity. It eventually penetrates the overlying cortex and extends into the periosteum and muscle. Occasionally a fibrosarcoma may arise periosteally and extend into the interior of contiguous bone.

Histologic findings show that fibrosarcomas range from well differentiated to poorly differentiated. Rapidly growing tumors reflect cytologic changes such as moderate anaplasia, cell irregularity, and many mitotic figures, and they tend to metastasize early. Less aggressive fibrosarcomas develop more slowly, taking longer to penetrate the cortex of the bone. Some fibrosarcomas are surprisingly indolent in their growth patterns and may show very little change over a period of years.

The femur and the tibia are the most common sites of occurrence and account for 50% of all fibrosarcomas.[54] The neoplasm also may be observed in the humerus, radius, ulna, skull, and facial and pelvic bones. Metastasis occurs primarily to the lungs.

Assessment

People with fibrosarcoma, like those with other primary bone tumors, usually have initial pain and swelling of the affected area.

The diagnosis of fibrosarcoma is based on histologic study. The degree of differentiation of the malignant fibroblasts, the cellular pattern, and the amount of collagen produced vary. The poorly differentiated tumors are more aggressive.

Treatment

When the diagnosis of fibrosarcoma has been established, radical surgery is indicated. A radical resection may be considered for a well-differentiated tumor or low-grade tumor that is still confined to the cortex. Amputation is an option. Fibrosarcoma is considered to be radioresistant; consequently, the use of radiotherapy is reserved for inoperable tumors. Adjuvant chemotherapy programs after surgical treatment are being evaluated for reducing the incidence of microscopic residual metastatic disease.[54]

The prognosis for fibrosarcoma is guarded. The 5- and 10-year survival rates after radical surgery have been reported at 21.8% and 28% respectively.[54] Individuals with poorly differentiated lesions have a poor prognosis.

Ewing's Sarcoma

Epidemiology and etiology

Ewing's sarcoma accounts for 5% of all malignant bone tumors.[54] Eighty percent of such tumors are diagnosed in individuals younger than 30 years of age, and 66% more males are affected than females. These patients are younger than any other patient affected by primary malignant bone tumors. The development of Ewing's sarcoma has not been strongly linked to any specific etiologic factor.

Pathophysiology

Ewing's sarcoma is a primitive, multicentric tumor that appears to be derived from the mesenchymal connective tissue framework of bone marrow. The tumor usually arises in the marrow spaces in the shaft of long bones and rarely involves the epiphysis.

On microscopic examination, Ewing's sarcoma is characterized by the presence of uniform cells with indistinct borders. These cells are packed closely together and contain prominent round or ovoid nuclei and have finely divided chromatin.

No one site seems to predominate in the development of Ewing's sarcoma. The tumor commonly is situated in the pelvis and the diaphyseal or metadiaphyseal regions of long bones. Ewing's sarcomas metastasize early and most frequently involve the lungs. The lymph nodes and the skull are other frequent sites of metastasis. On autopsy, a considerable portion of skeleton is affected. It is unclear whether these bone lesions represent metastatic spread or independent development of disease in multiple sites. Metastasis may be present in nearly 20% of individuals at the time of diagnosis.

The individual with Ewing's sarcoma frequently has a history of pain that has become increasingly severe and persistent. In addition to local pain, the person may complain of disability or stiffness in a corresponding joint. The physical examination usually reveals a palpable and tender mass. The temperature of the overlying skin is increased, and small superficial blood vessels may be seen.

Assessment

Many individuals have fever, anemia, high erythrocyte sedimentation rates, and sometimes leukocytosis at presentation. These symptoms can lead to an incorrect diagnosis of osteomyelitis. It has been observed that such findings result in a fulminating disease course that ends in death within a few months. Individuals who did not initially have such findings tended to survive longer. Glaubiger and colleagues[58] noted that normal lactic dehydrogenase, small distal primary lesion (8 cm), and absence of metastasis were better prognostic factors for the patient with Ewing's sarcoma.

Radiographs of Ewing's sarcoma show bone destruction that involves the shaft. Varying amounts of periosteal thickening may be present, with "onion" layers of laminated subperiosteal new bone. A large soft tissue mass frequently will be visualized as well.

Treatment

Initially, treatment consisted of radiation with chemotherapy. Local recurrence rates of 21%–30% were theorized to be caused by small foci of persistent tumor retained in each lesion.[59,60] Integrated therapy with radiation and/or surgery in combination with chemotherapy is the treatment of choice for Ewing's sarcoma.

Surgery or radiation alone will not prevent the appearance of tumor foci elsewhere in the skeleton nor pulmonary metastasis. Consequently, primary chemotherapy, as prophylactic therapy for micrometastases and to decrease tumor bulk in order to lessen need for local therapy, is used as part of the initial treatment for all patients. Using actinomycin, doxorubicin, vincristine, and cyclophosphamide, Bacci et al.[55] reported an actuarial 5-year disease-free survival rate of 40%–50%. Ifosfamide is an agent with a response rate approaching 50%.[62] Two randomized studies (Intergroup Ewing's Sarcoma studies IESS-I and IESS-II) confirmed that multiagent chemotherapy along with local treatments improve overall survival and control of local disease.[63] The rates of 5-year disease-free state and survival were 50%–64% and 57%–70%, respectively. The agents in these two studies include vincristine, actinomycin D, doxorubicin, and cyclophosphamide. Treatment duration is usually 6 to 12 months and is often administered in an outpatient setting. Local treatment (surgery and/or radiation) begins approximately 3 months after chemotherapy starts.

The tumor is extremely radiosensitive and capable of being cured locally with 50 Gy by means of shrinking fields. Improved techniques and the use of supervoltage radiation contribute to effective irradiation of the tumor without unacceptable damage to normal bone, skin, and subcutaneous tissue. The radiation oncologist may modify dosage when doxorubicin and actinomycin are given as they are radiation potentiators. The National Cancer Institute reports a 3% incidence of radiation-induced sarcoma after combined chemotherapy and radiation in Ewing's patients.[61] Physical therapy for gentle range of motion exercises during radiotherapy and for 6–12 months after therapy improves leg function.

Surgery combined with radiotherapy improves the local control rate. Surgery can decrease the need for extremely high radiation doses.[62] Limb salvage and amputation are both options to be considered. The goal is to eradicate the tumor and maintain function. This goal is considered by both surgeon and patient during the planning of treatment.

Patients with metastases at the time of presentation are similarly treated, with a 5-year survival rate of 30%. Ifosfamide is often utilized as a single agent for patients who have relapsed. There is ongoing research to evaluate its effectiveness as part of standard therapy for relapsed Ewing's patients.

Soft Tissue Sarcomas

Epidemiology and etiology

The histological subtypes of soft tissue sarcomas include malignant fibrous histiocytoma, liposarcoma, fibrosarcoma, synovial sarcoma, rhabdomyosarcoma, and leiomyosarcoma. They occur over 50% of the time in extremities and the remainder in the head and neck and retroperitoneum. The etiology of these tumors includes exposure to herbicides and other chemical exposure. Prior radiotherapy for oncological diseases and neurofibromatosis can lead to increased risk of soft tissue sarcomas.

Pathophysiology

Soft tissue sarcomas invade surrounding tissue along the anatomic planes. They compress surrounding tissue and form a pseudocapsule, which contains tentacles of tumor. A marginal excision will never cure a soft tissue sarcoma. The local recurrence rate of this procedure is close to 100%.

Nodal metastases are common with specific subtypes: synovial sarcomas (17%), epithelioid sarcomas (20%), and rhabdomyosarcomas (12%).[64] Lymph node involvement is a poor prognostic sign.

The more proximal lesions are usually larger since, in the retroperitoneum, buttock, or thigh, they can be disregarded until they are massive. A tumor smaller than 5 cm in size and superficial is felt to have a better prognosis.

Some histological subtypes such as rhabdomyosarcomas, synovial sarcomas, and malignant histiocytomas are considered poor prognosticators due to their high grade. However, any high-grade soft tissue sarcoma is ominous. Detectable pulmonary metastasis is more common in the high-grade soft tissue sarcomas. Typically, the first 2 years will reveal metastases and local recurrences. Rhabdomyosarcomas in children are very sensitive to chemotherapy.

The 5-year survival percentages of soft tissue sarcomas range from 30% to 95% based on subtype and grade.[9] The range for extremity sarcomas is 90%–95%, for trunk sarcomas 50%–75%, and for retroperitoneal lesions 30%–50%. In each of the three locations, higher grade sarcomas have a poorer survival rate.

Treatment/Nursing care

Surgery It is not uncommon for the surgeon to surgically remove a mass and, after routine pathologic examination, learn it is a malignant sarcoma. In this situation, microscopic tumor is usually found at the surgical site. A local recurrence is almost guaranteed. It is recommended that a reexcision of the tumor bed be performed immediately following the definitive diagnosis of sarcomas. Patients need to understand the need for the two excisions. Occasionally, the second surgical excision will reveal no evidence of microscopic tumor cells. The explanation needs to be reinforced that it is vital to ensure that no cells are left behind in order to avoid a local recurrence.

In the optimal situation, imaging (Figure 37-13) is performed prior to biopsy of the tumor. If the tumor is small and superficial, a primary myectomy (*en bloc* resection of tumor) may be recommended. The patient is informed that no biopsy will be done prior to the resection. The advantage behind this surgical decision is to avoid leaking cells during biopsy and also to avoid a second surgery. The disadvantage of this approach is that occasionally the final histology will reveal a be-

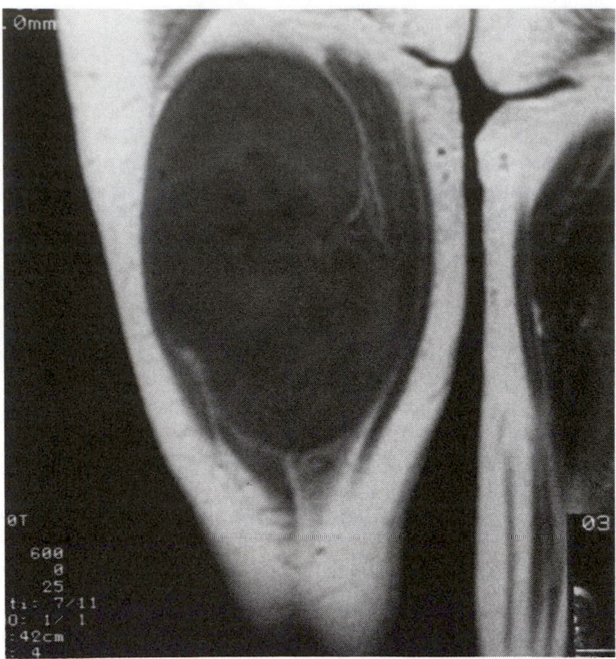

A

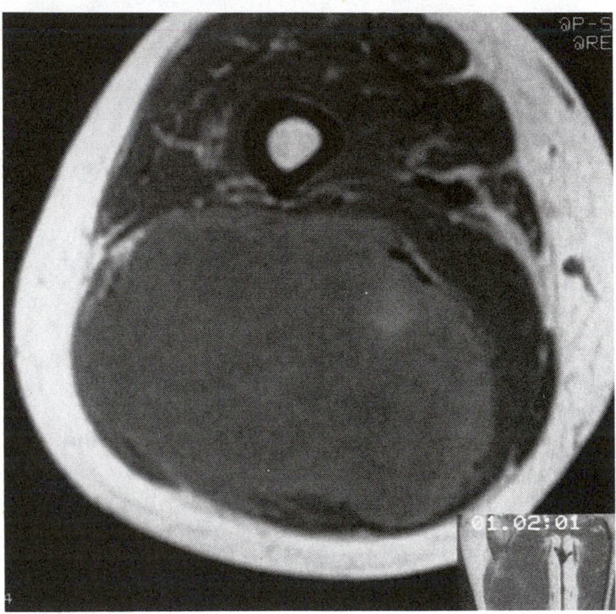

B

FIGURE 37-13 MRI imaging of a 62-year-old female with an enlarging posterior thigh mass. Biopsy revealed a liposarcoma. Both axial (a) and coronal (b) reveal the large mass, which was treated with preoperative irradiation and limb salvage surgery.

nign diagnosis, which could have been removed in a less radical manner. In most cases an incisional biopsy is performed.

The surgery timing is based on the decision for whether radiation is necessary. If radiation is deemed unnecessary, as in either a subcutaneous or intramuscular tumor with no impingement on neurovascular structure, a limb salvage surgery is performed.

In a study of 56 patients with soft tissue sarcomas treated with limb salvage surgery with no radiation, four local recurrences were observed. Forty-seven of these patients had high-grade tumor. A recurrence rate of less than 10% is acceptable.

A wide excision is defined as more than 3 cm of normal tissue. If the pathologist notes a lesser margin, radiation is given. The nursing care following limb salvage surgery of this type is covered under the section "Radical Resection Without Reconstruction."

Amputation was the surgical treatment prior to advances in both radiation oncology and limb salvage surgery. Luckily, amputation is reserved today for tumors that involve neurovascular structures and would require surgical removal of these structures, leaving a dysfunctional limb. Patients with fungating tumors or tumors that are radio- and chemo-insensitive are other amputee candidates. Amputation may be advisable in tumors involving the foot, as a wide margin is impossible to attain. Nursing care is covered under the section on amputation.

Radiation—external beam The advantage of postoperative radiation is that it allows for thorough histological grading and diagnosis. There is no delay in surgery. Wound healing is uncomplicated. At the time of surgery the tumor margin can be outlined with radiopaque clips. The radiation can be more accurately administered. Currently, this radiation timing is utilized for sarcomas that are widely resected with or without a close margin. The dosage is 60–65 Gy to the tumor bed with 45–50 Gy to all tissues disrupted during the procedure.

Preoperative radiation has the advantage of a small treatment area with fewer complications. It does require more preplanning with the surgeon and radiation oncologist. The patient may be rendered a candidate for limb salvage surgery with preoperative irradiation if the tumor has regressed. A radiation series administered preoperatively has a 10% complication rate, which is higher than postoperative radiation programs.[66] This may reflect patient selection with larger tumors. Wound healing was the primary problem. Surgery is delayed for 4–6 weeks following the cessation of radiation. If margins are close, additional radiation may be ordered.

Another theoretical advantage of preoperative radiation is that the pseudocapsule surrounding the tumor becomes thicker in an experimental swarm rat.[67] A tumor with a thicker rind or encapsulation is easier and safer to remove.

Eilber et al.[68] developed a regimen of doxorubicin and irradiation preoperatively. The chemotherapy was given intraarterially followed by 35 Gy of radiation. Local tumor control approached 90%, but the complication rate was very high at 35% and consisted of wound sloughs and fractures. Lowering the radiation dose only reduced the complication rate to 25%. Nevertheless, some centers continue to use this method.

Brachytherapy is a technique where catheters are placed in the tumor bed during surgery and 1–2 days later loaded with radioactive sources such as iridium 192. This method is utilized with a large, deep tumor that is close to a neurovascular bundle. It is a technically tedious procedure. A randomized prospective study of 117 patients who received brachytherapy were found to have decreased local recurrence as compared to patients receiving external beam.[69] The wound complication rate was 22%, which is significantly higher than with the external beam group.

Chemotherapy Patients with soft tissue sarcomas often achieve improved local control but frequently develop distant metastases. Initially, studies using chemotherapy, specifically doxorubicin, were solely for patients with metastatic soft tissue sarcoma. These patients had prolonged survival.

Based on these results, clinical trials were designed to examine the role of adjuvant chemotherapy in the management of soft tissue sarcoma. Single-agent studies utilizing doxorubicin showed no improvement in disease-free survival or survival.[70–73] In the search to find better chemotherapy agents, multiagent trials for soft tissue sarcoma were initiated. One study showed improved disease-free survival but no improvement in overall survival utilizing doxorubicin and cyclophosphamide.[72] Recently, ifosfamide is another drug that has been effective. The role of chemotherapy in the adjuvant setting for soft tissue sarcoma is still in its infancy. Further trials are needed to determine its utility in this disease.

METASTATIC BONE TUMORS

The incidence of metastatic bone tumors has decreased because of the advent of multimodal treatment approaches to controlling local disease and distant metastases. When metastatic bone tumors do occur, they significantly affect musculoskeletal function and decrease life expectancy. Pain, functional limitation, and coping with the knowledge of recurrent disease place the individual under considerable stress. Metastasis to bone occurs by means of one of three mechanisms: direct extension of the tumor to adjacent bone, arterial embolization after passage through the right cardiopulmonary circulation, and direct venous spread through the pelvic and vertebral veins (Batson's plexus). A number of tumors have a predilection for metastasizing to bone. These include primary tumors of the lung, breast, prostate, kidney, and thyroid. Gastric, colonic, pancreatic, and testicular tumors also have been shown to metastasize to bone. Ten percent to 15% of patients with metastatic disease present with an unknown primary.[74] The earliest sites of metastases include spine, ribs, and pelvis. More than 90% occur in the axial skeleton. These lesions are most often seen in patients over 40 years of age and in multiple sites. Solitary bony lesions should be worked up like a primary lesion, with local imaging such as MRI and biopsy.[75]

The individual with a metastatic bone lesion typically has initial dull, aching bone pain. Bone pain will increase steadily as the day progresses, peaking in the night hours and interfering with usual sleep patterns. The tumor invades the bone and can weaken it, resulting in pathological fractures. Pain, both local or leg pain, is most often seen in spine metastases. Neurological dysfunction can precede pain in lesions of the thoracic spine (e.g., heavy limb sensation, leg buckling). Tenderness and/or warmth over the lesion may be found on physical examination. In addition, loss of range of motion of involved joints and an antalgic gait may be noted.

Diagnostic evaluation includes conventional radiography and bone scanning techniques that frequently reveal multiple lytic lesions. Biopsy is not necessary if the appearance of the lesion is consistent with the known primary tumor. Biopsy, often needle, is indicated in the absence of a known or suspected primary tumor that will facilitate treatment of primary carcinoma. Abnormal laboratory studies may reveal clues as to the location and nature of the cancer. For example, hypercalcemia in the presence of a normal alkaline phosphatase level is associated with breast carcinoma, and elevations of serum acid phosphatase occur with prostatic cancer.

Once the diagnosis of a metastatic bone lesion has been established, treatment may include surgery, chemotherapy, or radiotherapy. The goals of surgical interventions are augmenting the material strength of the bone, increasing resistance to fracture, improving functional use of the part, and resuming ambulatory status. Even a bedridden patient with metastatic carcinoma with a femur fracture would benefit from surgery, if only for comfort. This may be accomplished through prosthetic arthroplasty, including allograft arthroplasty or the use of an intramedullary stabilizing device.[76] Bone cement or methyl methacrylate is used to fill the cavity created by the tumor and to stabilize the implant.

Individuals treated prophylactically for an impending pathological hip fracture have fewer complications, a lower incidence of stabilization failure, and a high level of postoperative ambulation.[77] Fifty percent of cortex should be destroyed in a weight-bearing bone to be considered an impending fracture.[74] Radiographs can reveal the amount of cortex loss. Nursing should encourage the patient to protect the involved bone and should include carefully transferring patients. However, a pathological fracture can occur with a turn in bed.

Spine lesions may need additional imaging with MRI, CT scan, or myelogram. Spinal lesions are most often treated nonoperatively with steroids, radiation, and bracing. The indications for surgical intervention of metastatic spinal disease include intractable pain unresponsive to nonoperative management, progressive neurological changes during or after radiotherapy, presence of radioresistant tumor, decompression of neural element, or spinal instability.[78] The surgery can include Harrington rods or prosthetic body replacements.

Amputation is indicated for tumors of the lower extremity that cannot be stabilized or that continue to fracture despite surgical intervention. Amputation also is an option for nonhealing lesions that do not respond to local care or radiotherapy.

Radiotherapy may be used to shrink the tumor to facilitate surgical intervention or for palliation of pain. Doses range from 20–30 Gy. In addition, radiation may be used postoperatively as adjuvant therapy or alone in cases in which surgical intervention would not provide any benefits. After internal fixation of involved bone, radiation is given to kill tumor cells and allow the surgical implant to maintain anatomic alignment. If the patient survives 6 months, near normal bone structure may be restored.[79]

Chemotherapy also is used to reduce the tumor cell mass. Chemotherapy and its effect on normal cell function, however, interfere adversely with wound healing. If chemotherapy has been used before surgery, it is necessary to delay surgery until the leukocyte count is near normal. Similarly, institution of chemotherapy in the postoperative phase should be delayed until adequate collagen synthesis has occurred, usually 1–2 weeks.

CONCLUSION

The treatment of bone and soft tissue sarcomas is complex. The overall survival rates have improved since the late 1970s. Progress can be attributed to factors such as improved staging, adjuvant chemotherapy, and pulmonary resections. With the advent of limb salvage surgery, fewer patients are having amputations without altering their survival rates. It is hoped that ongoing studies on chemotherapy, surgery, radiation, and molecular genes will continue to show improved survival rates for bone and soft tissue sarcoma.

REFERENCES

1. American Cancer Society: *Cancer Facts and Figures, 1991.* New York: American Cancer Society, 1991.
2. Tucker M, D'Angio G, Boice J, et al: Bone sarcomas linked to radiotherapy and chemotherapy in children. *N Engl J Med,* 317:588–593, 1987.
3. Sorenson SA, Mulvihill J, Nielsen A: Long-term follow-up of Von Recklinghausen neurofibromatosis survival and malignant neoplasms. *N Engl J Med,* 314:1010–1015, 1986.
4. Hajdu SI, Rosen G: Sarcomas. In Calabresy P (ed), *Medical Oncology: Basic Principles and Clinical Management.* New York: Macmillan, 1985, pp. 1193–1225.
5. Miller RW: Deaths from childhood leukemia and solid tumors among twins and other sibs in the United States, 1960–67. *Natl Cancer Inst Monogr,* 46:203–209, 1971.
6. Uhthoff H: *Current Concept of Diagnosis and Treatment of Bone and Soft Tissue Tumor.* Berlin: Springer-Verlag, 1984.
7. Hansen M: Molecular genetic consideration in osteosarcoma. *Clin Orthop Rel Res,* 270:237–246, 1991.
8. Araki N, Uchida A, Kimura T, et al: Involvement of the retinoblastoma gene in primary osteosarcomas and other bone and soft tissue tumors. *Clin Orthop Rel Res,* 270:271–277, 1991.
9. Mazanet R, Antman K: Sarcomas of soft tissue and bone. *Cancer,* 68:463–473, 1991.
10. Lodwick G: Solitary malignant tumors of bone. *Semin Roentgenol,* 1:293–313, 1966.
11. Zimmer W, Berquist T, McLeod R, et al: Bone tumor magnetic resonance imaging versus computed tomography. *Radiology,* 155:709–718, 1985.
12. American Joint Committee on Cancer: *Manual for Staging of Cancer* (3d ed). Philadelphia: Lippincott, 1988.
13. Schajowicz I, Ackerman V, Sissons HA: International histological classification of tumours. Monograph no. 6. Geneva: World Health Organization, 1972.
14. Enneking WF, Spanier S, Goodman M: A system for surgical staging of musculoskeletal sarcomas. *Clin Orthop,* 153:106–119, 1980.
15. Dahlin DC, Unni K: *Bone Tumors.* Springfield, IL: Thomas, 1986.
16. Consensus Conference: Limb-sparing treatment of adult soft tissue sarcoma and osteosarcomas. *JAMA,* 254:1791–1794, 1985.
17. Lewis M: The use of an expandable and adjustable prosthesis in the treatment of childhood malignant bone tumors of the extremity. *Cancer,* 57:499–502, 1986.
18. Krajbich J: Modified Van Nes rotationplasty in the treatment of malignant neoplasms in the lower extremities of children. *Clin Orthop Rel Res,* 262:74–77, 1991.
19. Cammisa F, Glasser D, Phil M, et al: The Van Nes tibial rotationplasty. *J Bone Joint Surg,* 72A(10):1541–1547, 1990.
20. Simon M, Aschliman M, Thomas N, et al: Limb-salvage treatment versus amputation for osteosarcoma of the distal end of femur. *J Bone Joint Surg* [AM], 68:1331–1337, 1986.
21. Sim FH, et al: Reconstruction of musculo-skeletal defects about the knee for tumor. *Clin Orthop,* 221:188–201, 1987.
22. Otis J, et al: Energy cost during gait in osteosarcoma patients after resection and knee replacement and after above-the-knee amputation. *J Bone Joint Surg* [AM], 67:606–610, 1985.
23. Buck B, Malinin T, Brown M: Bone transplantation and human immunodeficiency virus. *Clin Orthop Rel Res,* 249:129–136, 1989.
24. Piasecki P, Rodts M: Bone banking: Its role in skeletal tumor reconstruction. *Orthop Nurs,* 4(5):56–60, 1985.
25. Enneking WF, Mindell ER: Observations on massive retrieved human allografts. *J Bone Joint Surg,* 73A(8):1123–1142, 1991.
26. Parrish FF: Allograft replacement of all or part of the end of a long bone following excision of a tumor: Report of twenty-one cases. *J Bone Joint Surg* [AM], 55:1–22, 1973.
27. Mankin HJ, Fogelson FS, Thrasber AZ: Massive resection and allograft transplantation in the treatment of malignant bone tumors. *N Engl J Med,* 294:1247–1255, 1976.
28. Gitelis S, Heligman D, Quill G, et al: The use of large allograft for tumor reconstruction and salvage of the failed total hip arthroplasty. *Clin Orthop,* 231:62–70, 1988.
29. Piasecki P: The nursing role in limb salvage surgery. *Nurs Clin North Am,* 26(1):33–41, 1991.

30. Power R, Wood D, Tomford W, et al: Revision osteoarticular allograft transplantation in weight-bearing joints. *J Bone Joint Surg,* 73B(4):595–599, 1991.
31. Tomford W, Thongphasuk J, Mankin H, et al: Frozen musculoskeletal allografts. *J Bone Joint Surg,* 72A(8):1137–1150, 1990.
32. Eilber FR, Morton DL, Eckardt J, et al: Limb salvage for skeletal and soft tissue sarcomas. *Cancer,* 54:2579–2589, 1984.
33. Dick H, Malinin T, Mnaymneh W, et al: Massive allograft implantation following radical resection of high-grade tumor requiring adjuvant chemotherapy treatment. *Clin Orthop,* 197:88–95, 1985.
34. Gebhardt M, Flugstad D, Springfield D, et al: The use of bone allografts for limb salvage in high-grade extremity osteosarcoma. *Clin Orthop Rel Res,* 270:181–196, 1991.
35. Goorin A, Shuster J, Baker A, et al: Changing pattern of pulmonary metastases with adjuvant chemotherapy in patients with osteosarcoma: Results from the multiinstitutional osteosarcoma study. *J Clin Oncol,* 9(4):600–605, 1991.
36. Snyder C, Saltzman D, Ferrell K, et al: A new approach to the resection of pulmonary osteosarcoma metastases. *Clin Orthop Rel Res,* 270:247–253, 1991.
37. Michael J, Gailey R, Bowker J: New developments in recreational prostheses and adaptive devices for the amputee. *Clin Orthop Rel Res,* 256:64–75, 1990.
38. Williamson V: Amputation of the lower extremity: An overview. *Orthop Nurs,* 11(2):55–65, 1992.
39. Lane J, Kroll M, Rossbach P: New advances and concepts in amputee management after treatment for bone and soft tissue sarcoma. *Clin Orthop Rel Res,* 256:22–28, 1990.
40. Melzack R: *The Challenge of Pain.* New York: Basic Books, 1983.
41. Sherman R, Ernst J, Barja R, et al: Phantom pain: A lesson in the necessity for careful clinical research on chronic pain problems. *J Rehabil Res Dev,* 25(2):7–10, 1988.
42. Cohen L, Hendrickson J, Mansell J, et al: Response of sarcomas of bone and of soft tissue to neutron beam therapy. *Int J Radiat Oncol Biol Phys,* 10:821–824, 1984.
43. Issels R, Prenninger S, Nagele A, et al: Ifosfamide plus etoposide combined with regional hyperthermia in patients with locally advanced sarcomas. *J Clin Oncol,* 8(11):1818–1829, 1990.
44. Schaller R, Haas J, Schaller J, et al: Improved survival in children following resection of pulmonary metastases. *J Pediatr Surg,* 17:546–555, 1987.
45. Malawer M: Impact of short course of neoadjuvant chemotherapy and the choice of surgical procedure for high grade sarcoma of extremities. *Proc Am Soc Clin Oncol,* 8:320, 1989.
46. Elias A, Ryan L, Aisner J, et al: Mesna, doxorubicin, dacarbazine regime for adults with advanced sarcoma. *Semin Oncol,* 17(2):41–49, 1990.
47. Silane M, Oot-Giromini B: Systemic factors that affect wound healing. In Eaglstein W, Baxter C, Mertz P (eds), *New Directions in Wound Healing.* Princeton, NJ: Squibb, 1990.
48. Unni KK, Dahlin DC, Baebout JW: Periosteal osteogenic sarcoma. *Cancer,* 3:2476–2485, 1976.
49. Raymond K: Surface osteosarcoma. *Clin Orthop Rel Res,* 270:140–148, 1991.
50. Glasser D, Lane J: Stage IIB osteogenic sarcoma. *Clin Orthop Rel Res,* 270:29–39, 1991.
51. Campanacci M, Bacci G, Gaetano S, et al: The treatment of osteosarcoma of the extremities. *Cancer,* 48:1569–1581, 1981.
52. Sutow WW, Gehan E, Dyment P, et al: Multidrug adjuvant chemotherapy of osteosarcoma: Interim report of Southwest Oncology Group studies. *Cancer Treat Rep,* 62:265–270, 1978.
53. Bacci G, Picci P, Pignatti G, et al: Neoadjuvant chemotherapy for non-metastatic osteosarcoma of the extremities. *Clin Orthop Rel Res,* 270:87–98, 1991.
54. Sim FH: Diagnosis and treatment of bone tumors: *A Team Approach.* Thorofare, NJ: Slack, 1983.
55. Bacci G, Springfield D, Capanna R, et al: Neoadjuvant chemotherapy for osteosarcoma of the extremity. *Clin Orthop,* 224:268–276, 1987.
56. Schajowicz F: *Tumors and Tumor-like Lesions of Bone and Joints.* New York: Springer-Verlag, 1981.
57. Gitelis S, Bertoni S, Picci P, et al: Chondrosarcoma of bone. *J Bone Joint Surg* [AM], 63:1248–1257, 1981.
58. Glaubiger D, Makoch R, Schwarz J, et al: Determination of prognostic factors and their influence on therapeutic results of Ewing's sarcoma. *Cancer,* 45:2213–2219, 1980.
59. Bacci G, Picci P, Gherlinzoni I, et al: Localized Ewing's sarcoma of bone: Ten years' experience at the Instituto Ortopedico Rizzoli in 124 cases treated with multimodality therapy. *Eur J Cancer Clin Oncol,* 21:163–173, 1985.
60. Rosen G, Caparros B, Nirenberg A, et al: Ewing's sarcoma: Ten year experience with adjuvant chemotherapy. *Cancer,* 47:2204–2213, 1981.
61. Donaldson S: The value of adjuvant chemotherapy in the management of sarcomas in children. *Cancer,* 55:2184–2197, 1985.
62. Magrath I, Sandlund J, Raynor A, et al: A phase II study of ifosfamide in treatment of recurrent sarcomas in young people. *Cancer Chemother Pharmacol,* 18(2):25–28, 1986 (suppl).
63. Jaffee N: Chemotherapy for malignant bone tumors. *Orthop Clin North Am,* 20(3):487–503, 1989.
64. Rosenberg S: Combined treatment approaches to soft tissue sarcomas. *Hosp Prac,* 151–166, 1987.
65. Rydholm A, Gustafson P, Rooser B, et al: Limb-sparing surgery without radiotherapy based on anatomic location of soft tissue sarcoma. *J Clin Oncol,* 9(10):1757–1765, 1991.
66. Suit H, Mankin H, Wood S, et al: Preoperative, intraoperative and postoperative radiation in the treatment of primary soft tissue sarcoma. *Cancer,* 55:2659–2667, 1985.
67. Gitelis S, Thomas R, Templeton A, Schajowicz F: Characterization of the pseudocapsule of soft tissue sarcomas. *Clin Orthop Rel Res,* 246:285–292, 1989.
68. Eilber F, Morton D, Eckardt J, et al: Limb salvage for skeletal and soft tissue sarcomas, multidisciplinary preoperative therapy. *Cancer,* 53:2579–2590, 1984.
69. Brennan M, Hilaris B, Shiru M, et al: Local recurrence in adult soft tissue sarcoma, a randomized trial of brachytherapy. *Arch Surg,* 122:1289–1293, 1987.
70. Eilber I, Giuliano A, Huth J, et al: A randomized prospective trial using post-operative adjuvant chemotherapy in high grade extremity sarcoma. *Am J Clin Oncol,* 11:39–45, 1988.
71. Antman K, Amato D, Pirrpich M, et al: A preliminary analysis of a randomized intergroup trial of adjuvant doxorubicin for soft-tissue sarcomas. In Salomon (ed), *Therapy of Cancer V.* New York: Grune & Stratton, 1987, pp. 725–734.
72. Chang A, Kinsella T, Glastein E, et al: Adjuvant chemotherapy for patients with high grade soft tissue sarcomas of the extremity. *J Clin Oncol,* 6:1491–1500, 1988.

73. Bramwell V, Mouridsen H, Santora A, et al: Cyclophosphamide vs. ifosfamide: Final report of a randomized phase II trial in adult soft tissue sarcoma. *Eur J Cancer Clin Oncol,* 23(2):321–322, 1987.
74. Nielsen O, Munro A, Tannock I: Bone metastases. Pathophysiology and management policy. *J Clin Oncol,* 9(3):509–524, 1991.
75. Frassica F, Gitelis S, Sim F: Metastatic bone disease: General principles, pathophysiology, evaluation and biopsy. In Elbert RE (ed), *Instructional Course Lectures.* Park Ridge, IL: American Academy of Orthopaedic Surgeons, 1992, pp. 293–300.
76. Jaffe M, Goorin A, Link M, et al: Reconstruction for defects of the proximal part of the femur using allograft arthroplasty. *J Bone Joint Surg* [AM], 70:507–516, 1988.
77. Gitelis S, Hammerberg K, Sheinkop S, et al: Surgery in the management of metastatic hip disease. *Orthopedics,* 5:1004–1011, 1982.
78. Asdourian P: Metastatic disease of the spine. In Bridwell K, Dewald R (eds), *Textbook of Spinal Surgery.* Philadelphia: Lippincott, 1991, pp. 1187–1241.
79. Shocker J, Brady L: Radiation therapy for bone metastasis. *Clin Orthop,* 169:38–43, 1982.

Chapter 38

Breast Cancer

Michelle Goodman, RN, MS, OCN

Diane D. Chapman, RN, MS

INTRODUCTION

Breast cancer is the most common cancer in women and the leading cause of death for women 40–44 years of age. It is second to lung cancer as the leading cause of cancer death in all women. The incidence of breast cancer increases rapidly with age until menopause, after which time it increases more slowly with advancing years.[1] Over 70% of all breast cancer occurs in women who are 50 years of age or older. The National Institutes of Health consensus development conference statement emphasized that in the next decade, more than 1.5 million women (186,000 in 1992) in the United States will be newly diagnosed with invasive breast cancer and, of that number, 30% will die of their disease.[2] Screening methods, particularly mammography, have become more precise, permitting earlier diagnosis, which in part accounts for the dramatic increase in incidence in breast cancer between 1982 and 1987.[1] However, more research in the area of chemoprevention, systemic therapies, and access to preventive health care and early detection for the socioeconomically disadvantaged are needed to change the current mortality rates from this disease.[3]

In 1963, the lifetime risk of breast cancer was about 5.5%, or 1 in every 18 women, with an estimated life span of 72 years.[4] Current statistics indicate that the average woman in her early 60s has a projected lifetime risk of almost 10% of developing breast cancer. In general, breast cancer incidence varies across the country, but is about 1 in every 9 women.[5] This increasing incidence is predominantly in women under 55 years of age and in black women. Possible reasons for this increased incidence are that there are more women who are living longer into the cancer-prone years, there is better statistical reporting, and there are better screening methods. In addition, changes in dietary and socioeconomic habits, hormonal milieu, increasing exposure to carcinogens, and decreasing immunocompetence may contribute to this increased incidence of breast cancer.[6,7]

While the incidence of breast cancer has increased over the past 30 years, the mortality rate has remained stable, reflecting better cure rates for earlier staged lesions. This apparent progress may in part be related to a better understanding of the natural history of breast cancer.

Historically, breast cancer has been considered a disease that remains localized until some time in which metastasis occurs via the lymph nodes and later spreads beyond regional nodes to distant sites. The possibility that hematogenous spread would occur early, prior to lymph node involvement, was proposed nearly two decades ago and supports the concept that breast cancer is a systemic disease at the time of clinical diagnosis.[8]

It is now widely accepted that breast cancer is not one disease but rather protean, differing in histologic, biologic, and immunologic characteristics. Phenotypic heterogeneity exists within individual breast neoplasms such that drug resistance, both intrinsic and acquired, occurs, rendering unresponsive cell lines unopposed and capable of establishing metastatic sites. Whether or not the individual with breast cancer survives the disease is determined by numerous factors, but the outcome primarily depends upon the intrinsic growth rate of the tumor, which varies dramatically; the age of the woman at diagnosis; and numerous biologic parameters that ultimately define the natural history of the disease.

The interdisciplinary team utilizes various clinical, histologic, and pathologic findings to define, as precisely as possible, the particular characteristics of a breast cancer that will determine the most appropriate treatment plan for a given patient. As a member of this team, the nurse must be aware of the factors affecting the selection of the treatment plan as well as the various treatment strategies to prevent and manage the complications of the disease and its treatment.

ETIOLOGY

Risk Assessment

Experimental and clinical data indicate that the development of breast cancer is not a chance event. The genesis of breast cancer seems to be a multiphasic process involving many factors that are influential in the ongoing duel between tumor growth potential and host resistance.

Attempts are being made to reveal the etiology of breast cancer through an intense study of its epidemiology. As populations are identified in whom the incidence of the disease is increased, a genetic, hormonal, or biochemical factor may be identified that is considered significant in etiology. Epidemiologic features, when statistically correlated with incidence of disease, designate a particular factor as a "risk factor." Each risk factor merely serves as one piece of the puzzle because there are so many different factors that either increase or decrease a woman's risk of developing breast cancer. Table 38-1 separates current risk factors for breast cancer according to their degree of importance in our understanding of the etiology of breast cancer.

TABLE 38-1 Risk Factors

PRIMARY	
Female	
Age >50	
Country of origin:	North America Northern Europe
Family history:	Personal history of breast cancer
	Two or more first-degree relatives with breast cancer
	Bilateral/premenopausal breast cancer in first-degree relative
Biopsy histology:	Atypical hyperplasia
	Carcinoma in situ (DCIS and LCIS)
SECONDARY	
Postmenopausal obesity	
Early menarche (<12) coupled with late menopause (>55); onset of regular cycles within 1 year of menarche	
First full-term pregnancy >35 years of age	
Use of oral contraceptives prior to age 20 and persisting for 6 or more years	
Ionizing radiation to chest with exposure occurring prior to age 35	
Benign breast disease	
OTHER	
Nulliparous	
Estrogen replacement therapy	
Alcohol	
Diet	

Hormonal Factors

The hormone environment has long been recognized as a major factor in the development of breast cancer. This is well demonstrated in that gender is the most significant risk factor for the development of the disease. Women are 100 times more likely to develop breast cancer than men. Additionally, after a diagnosis of breast cancer has been made, the relationship of the tumor estrogen receptor with the response to hormonal manipulation strongly suggests a hormonal connection. The significance of early menarche (before 12), nulliparity or parity after 35, and late menopause (after 55) are well-known events that are considered risk factors for development of breast cancer. All of these events are linked to the type and duration of exposure to endogenous hormones that may impact on the development of breast cancer.

The relevance of breast cancer risk to early menarche and/or late menopause is correlated with the length of ovarian function. Additionally, women who experience early menarche with onset of regular cycles within a year are proposed to be at three times the normal risk. A woman with 40 or more years of ovarian function has twice the risk compared with those who have ovarian function for 30 or fewer years. Conversely, those with natural or surgical menopause before the age of 45 without replacement therapy are believed to have two times a reduction in risk.[9] Women who have their first full-term pregnancy after the age of 35 have a greater risk than nulliparous women.

Hormones play a significant role in the development of breast cancer, though the extent to which this role affects the genesis and outcome of the disease is relatively unknown at this time. While hormones themselves are not inherently mutagenic, it is surmised that they may act as initiators or promoters in that they alter cell proliferation, differentiation, and atrophy.[10,11]

The endocrine system circulates three estrogens in a woman's body; estriol, estrone, and estradiol. Estriol is not considered to be a factor in cancer genesis. In fact, it is thought to have an oppositional effect to the carcinogenic action of estrone and estradiol. Estrone may be used in the treatment of hormone deficiencies. It is considered to be less active than estradiol. Estradiol is a potent estrogen that is the primary ingredient in exogenous hormone therapy. Estradiol is the dominant hormone present during the premenopausal years, and estrone may play a significant role during the postmenopausal years.

Several studies have considered the relationship between the excretion of estrogens and breast cancer. The results have been more consistent with postmenopausal than with premenopausal women. These studies examined the levels of urinary hormone excretion, plasma hormone concentrations, and estradiol distribution and binding protein concentrations. A comparison of results indicated the postmenopausal patients with breast cancer were exposed to more estrogens than the controls. No difference was reported in the premenopausal group.[11]

More recent speculation involves the effect of progesterone on the risk of breast cancer. Breast epithelial mitosis, which varies significantly within the menstrual cycle, peaks during the luteal phase.[12] This finding has suggested that progesterone and estrogen may contribute to the risk of breast cancer. However, studies that have measured progesterone in premenopausal women found that progesterone levels were decreased rather than increased in patients with breast cancer.[11]

Pregnancy (full term) has been reported to exert a deterrent effect on the development of breast cancer. This is generally thought to be based on the change in the hormonal milieu. The exact mechanism is unknown, but speculation includes the effects of the alteration of prolactin and/or estriol. Prolactin has been recognized as having a direct effect on the growth of human breast epithelial tissue and is associated with the generation of mammary tumors in the rat. The decrease in prolactin levels during pregnancy may account for this protective effect.[13] Furthermore, there is a significant increase in estriol compared with estrone and estradiol during pregnancy.

This preventive effect may be more pronounced with pregnancies at a young age (<20) and is enhanced by subsequent pregnancies.[13] Additionally, the benefit conferred on these women continues to be a positive factor during the extent of their lifetime. Breast feeding may not impart the protective element once thought. The rationale is that, although nursing may delay ovulation, the safeguard may only be related to parity, and there is inconsistent evidence supporting the benefit of lactation.[14]

The role that endogenous estrogens may play in the development of breast cancer suggests that exogenous therapy may be instrumental in the development of breast cancer. Animal studies have shown that exogenous estrogens, some progesterones, and some estrogen/progesterone combinations cause mammary tumors in rats and mice.[15] The information on the use of hormone therapy is limited in its consistency, owing to the disparity of dosages and duration as well as the current inability to assess cohort lifetime effects as well as multigenerational effects.

Oral contraceptives have been marketed since the 1960s. The question of a connection between oral contraceptives (OC) and breast cancer has resulted in inconsistent and controversial reports.[16] Pike and associates[17] reported an increase in risk for those who use the oral contraceptive pill before a first full-term pregnancy. The second study confirmed an additional risk related to age and duration of use. Those who used the pill before age 25 for 4–6 years showed a relative risk of 2.0, and a risk of 4.9 was attributed to those who used the pill for more than 6 years. Another study was conducted that showed increased risk before the first pregnancy, but no difference was noted with use after the first pregnancy. A study published in 1989 showed a relative risk correlation with duration of use (1.43 for 49–96 months and 1.74 for 97 or more months' use). However, this study also looked at the relative risk of use before and after the first pregnancy and found no significant difference.[18] A review of the literature suggests the use of OC during the middle reproductive years seems to pose no additional risk. Another increase in risk has been associated with the use of OC during the perimenopausal years.[19] The risk may possibly be due to delaying menopause by creating and maintaining a hormonal environment that mimics that of a menstruating woman.[12]

The question of risk in relation to estrogen replacement therapy (ERT) is equally murky, with little replicated evidence of increased risk. Recent studies associate risks that vary in relation to duration and type of replacement. One study, which did not address dosage, reported a slight increase in risk with long-term use of estrogens, which may be increased by the additional use of progestins.[11] A large study looked at postmenopausal use of ERT and found the risk was decreased in those women who took ERT compared with those who did not (0.98 vs. 1.8), and risk seemed to be dose-related. The women who took ERT before 1958 had 2.3 times the risk compared with other users of ERT.[20] Long-term therapy did not confer increased risk, and there was no comment on combination (estrogen and progestin) replacement therapy. Mills[21] showed a slight increase in risk in women using ERT with an additional risk if these women had also used OC, suggesting that the duration of exposure increases the risk.[21]

Current evidence suggests either no effect on breast cancer risk from ERT or an elevation in risk of less than twofold with very long-term use or relatively high doses. Any potential effect of ERT on breast cancer risk must be considered with the therapy's established protective effect against osteoporotic fractures and increased risk of endometrial cancer and probable decreased risk for coronary artery disease.[7]

Family History

Along with age and gender, family history of breast cancer is a primary indicator of the potential risk of developing the disease. Many people, including physicians, erroneously estimate risk factors. This is due to the wide range of risk associated with a family history of breast cancer dependent upon the age and known risk factors of the patient, the ages and number of first- and second-degree relatives with breast cancer, and whether the cancer is unilateral or bilateral. A woman who has a first-degree relative with unilateral breast cancer has 2.3 times the normal risk, which corresponds to approximately a 20% lifetime risk. There are conflicting reports on whether a higher risk is associated with unilateral premenopausal breast cancer. A woman with two first-degree relatives who have breast cancer has a 13.6 relative risk of developing the disease.[22] The greatest risk is associated with a first-degree premenopausal relative with bilateral breast cancer. A lifetime risk for a 30-year-old sister of this patient is estimated at 50%.[9]

The issue of lifetime risk is inferred in virtually all of these studies and is assumed to be true. The question of lifetime risk was addressed by examining data from 9000 women to determine if risk associated with family history remained stable or varied with age. Although the mechanism is unknown, the findings suggest that family history may only be a determinant for women below the age of 60.[23]

Most women (approximately 70%) who develop breast cancer have no known risk factors. Familial and hereditary breast cancer account for a very small proportion of the diagnosed cases (20% and 9% respectively). The majority of breast cancers are considered to be *sporadic,* which is defined as no history of breast cancer through two generations. *Familial or polygenic* breast cancer is described as a family history of one or more first-degree relatives with breast cancer. *Hereditary or genetic* breast cancer is defined as a positive family history, often with related cancers (e.g., ovarian), consistent with an autosomal dominant factor that includes onset at an early age (less than 40), an excess of bilaterality, and other multiple cancers. Hall and colleagues[24] have tested women simultaneously for genetic linkage and heterogeneity of breast cancer in families. Their findings suggest both the presence of a gene for early-onset breast cancer on chromosome 17q21 and linkage heterogeneity of the disease. The ultimate goal of gene mapping is to be able to identify a crucial gene, characterize it, and thereby gain an understanding of the molecular predisposition of breast cancer in families. This information could conceivably lead to new methods of breast cancer therapy.[25]

For the woman who has breast cancer, there is a 2%–14% risk of developing a second primary breast cancer.[20] Over time, risk increases .05% per year. Therefore, a woman diagnosed at age 35 would carry a 40% risk of developing a second primary breast cancer by age 75.

An increased risk of breast cancer also may be associated with primary ovarian or endometrial cancer, but this risk is low, estimated at less than two times the normal.[9]

Diet

The wide range of variance in breast cancer rates worldwide and dramatic increases in migrant populations may reflect one or several factors that influence the risk of breast cancer. The risk of breast cancer is greatest in developed countries, especially those of North America and northern Europe. The risk is lowest in developing third-world countries. Apart from a genetic influence, diet has been investigated as the most plausible variant.

Japan is known to have a low incidence of breast cancer. However, when Japanese women migrate from Japan to Hawaii where the incidence of breast cancer is high, they experience a significant increase in breast cancer incidence. By the second generation, the incidence rate parallels that of daughters of Japanese women born in Hawaii, suggesting a dietary influence. Diet, however, may not be the only factor in cancer genesis of migrants. The new culture may provide accessibility to risk factors that may not have been an issue in the country of origin. Changes in exercise habits, alcohol and drug use, hormone therapy, and smoking may be experienced, which could confound the diet correlation.

Diets high in fats have been implicated in countries that have shown a sudden increase in incidence rates, as well as high-risk countries. Reports of positive correlations with meat and dairy products have been issued, but additional case studies have largely failed to support the data.[26,27]

There is still controversy regarding at which time of life dietary habits may be most influential in the development of breast cancer. Looking at current diet regimes in relation to breast cancer would not be helpful if perimenarchal diet were the determining factor. The possible significance of diet at this time of a woman's life corresponds to a physical environment of accelerated growth and development of the breasts. These mammary tissues may potentially be altered by or sensitized to hormones produced by an excess of dietary fat.

The relationship of dietary fats and breast cancer is largely based on consistent findings in animal studies. Rats ingesting a high-fat diet demonstrated an increase in breast malignancies over those on a low-fat diet.[28] It has been speculated that this connection may be linked to the amount and ratios of hormones produced by the endocrine system. The proliferation of breast tissue may be altered by changes in estrogen, pituitary, and thyroid function, which are sensitive to dietary changes.[26]

Obesity

Obesity confers a slight increased risk overall, but demonstrates more of a risk for those women who are postmenopausal than any other age group.[29] Although one study shows a correlation between obesity and premenopausal breast cancer,[30] thin women are considered to be more at risk than obese women. However, thin women are more likely to have small, nonmetastatic tumors.[26] Obese women, in general, may be more at risk for recurrence, but this may be explained by detection bias owing to the large amount of body fat that could obscure clinical findings.

A possible explanation of the discrepancy between pre- and postmenopausal risk may be linked to hormonal influences. Obesity during childbearing years has been associated with a decrease in the level of progesterone, which reduces cell proliferation in the breast. Obese postmenopausal women have no ovarian function and have both higher rates of conversion of androstenedione to estrogen in adipose tissue and lower levels of sex hormone–binding globulin than do thinner women.[6] Additionally, the enzyme responsible for converting estrone to estradiol is present in adipose breast tissue, and the rate of conversion has been positively correlated to body weight.[29]

Alcohol

According to a meta-analysis,[31] the literature favors a positive association between alcohol and breast cancer risk. The biological mechanisms of the association are not known. Whether the increased risk involves exposure to circulating cytotoxic by-products of alcohol, its effect on hepatic function, or a possible alteration in the cell membrane permeability in breast tissue or other mechanisms is yet to be determined. The most compelling evidence suggests that the relationship between alcohol and breast cancer risk is greatest for women who consume more than two drinks per day.[32,33] However, this connection is not strong enough at this point to conclude a causality exists between the use of alcohol and breast cancer.

Radiation

The carcinogenic effect from both low- and high-dose ionizing radiation has been well documented. Survivors of the atomic bombs exhibited an increase in breast as well as other cancers. A risk of breast cancer has been associated with radiation therapy for a broad spectrum of health problems including chronic mastitis, tuberculosis, tinea capitis, thymus disorders, and adult and childhood cancers.[9,34–37] The risk increases with dosage, especially if a woman is exposed in the period of young adulthood.

The concern about the effects of radiation has generated some apprehension regarding the potential harm of repeated mammograms and chest radiographs. The doses for these procedures are extremely small, and the potential benefit far outweighs the risk. A mammogram emits a dose of .15 cGy, and a chest film generates approximately .002 cGy to each breast.[38] The radiation exposure from a mammogram is similar to the radiation exposure incurred from flying 400 miles in an airplane.

Proliferative Disease

The presence of proliferation on a pathology slide indicates a presence of increased cell growth. According to Page and DuPont, the term *proliferative breast disease* "indicates that proliferative alterations are noted by histology and that they indicate a disease by their demonstrated link to an increased risk of subsequent carcinoma."[39,p.119] These risks have been categorized as *slight,* which is associated with one and one-half to two times the normal risk; *moderate,* which is associated with four to five times the normal risk; and *marked,* which is associated with eight to ten times the normal risk.

Proliferative disease without atypia falls into the slightly increased risk category. This classification includes examples of common types of epithelial hyperplasia, which may be subcategorized as mild, moderate, or florid. The degree refers to the number of cells present relative to the basement membrane of a lobular unit or duct. Since two cells are usually present above the basement membrane, the presence of three or more cells is described as mild hyperplasia. The presence of five or more cells constitutes moderate hyperplasia, and an increased progression of these changes characterizes florid hyperplasia. Twenty percent of breast biopsies contain moderate or florid hyperplasia. The presence of papilloma and sclerosing adenosis also falls in the slight risk category.[39–41]

The moderate risk category includes atypical ductal hyperplasia and atypical lobular hyperplasia. These risk statistics are not lifetime estimates, but are limited to 10–15 years after biopsy, which is the limit of most benign breast disease follow-up. Atypical hyperplasia has some, but not all, of the characteristics of carcinoma in situ.[39]

Ductal carcinoma in situ (DCIS) and lobular carcinoma in situ (LCIS) are characterized by an eight- to tenfold increased risk of developing invasive cancer. DCIS lesions are often singular, and conservative treatment with local excision is an accepted treatment. Lobular carcinoma in situ may be associated with increased risk within both breasts. Mastectomy with close follow-up of the other breast is often the treatment of choice, although some clinicians feel LCIS may be treated with local excision and close follow-up that employs mammograms twice a year and clinical exam every 3–4 months. Improvements in mammography sensitivity have made this approach more feasible.[39]

Carcinoma in situ has been referred to as a "precancerous condition." This definition reflects the potential capabilities of the cells, rather than the histopathologic characteristics. The nomenclature of *carcinoma in situ* refers to a localized process confined to a duct or a lobule that is incapable of spreading. A carcinoma in situ that remains in the breast is capable of transforming to an invasive cancer but does not necessarily do so.

Nonproliferative Disease

Approximately 70% of biopsies reflect cellular changes that impart no risk or a very small risk to the patient. These include usual, moderate, or florid hyperplasia; sclerosing adenosis; and papilloma, which have been addressed previously. In addition, some nonproliferative changes are recognized to bestow no increased risk to the patient. These are adenosis, apocrine change, duct ectasis, and usual mild epithelial hyperplasia.[39]

Apocrine change is often accompanied with the diagnosis of a cyst. These cells may form tufted or papillary clusters instead of the characteristic single cell layer. *Adenosis* and *duct ectasia* refer to an increase in the number of cells in a gland and a dilation of a duct. Epitheliosis or mild epithelial hyperplasia is associated with common configurations seen with slightly increased number of cells at the basement membrane.[40]

PREVENTION OF BREAST CANCER

While it is conceivable to determine the possibility of developing breast cancer based on risk factors, it is virtually impossible to predict with certainty who will or will not develop breast cancer in a lifetime. The unknown etiology of breast cancer coupled with conflicting data regarding the identification of risk factors as well as how these risk factors influence the genesis of breast cancer makes preventive action difficult. To prevent an event from occurring, one must know the cause. Unfortunately, there is a paucity of information regarding the origin of breast cancer. As mentioned earlier in this chapter, some elements have been recognized to be primary risk factors in the development of breast cancer and others may be secondary or possible risk factors. Even this information is limited at best, because 70% of the women with breast cancer have no identifiable risk factors.

Research concerning prevention and early detection of breast cancer is critically important in the reduction of mortality from breast cancer. Of the more than 150,000 women diagnosed yearly, only 50% will be diagnosed with stage I disease, and approximately 30% of these women will subsequently die of their disease. Assuming a tumor doubling time to be approximately 100 days, or 30 doublings before a tumor reaches a size that is clinically detectable (1×10^9 cells), means a woman has the disease 8 years before its presence is known. Newer, even more sophisticated methods of detecting breast cancer or preventing further proliferation of these undetectable pathological breast cancers must be on the forefront of clinical research efforts. As nurses, our role in educating the public, promoting research, and recruiting of women into these research studies cannot be overemphasized.

Chemoprevention

Chemoprevention for breast cancer has been proposed to possibly alter the course of disease for those with known risk factors. Several dietary micronutrients have been touted for their presumed protective capabilities in animal studies, but they remain controversial for human use. Vitamin A and its retinoid derivatives offer some promise for chemoprevention. Vitamin A can affect the growth and differentiation of epithelial tissue. Breast cancer is considered a disease of the breast epithelial cells, and the retinoids may have the capacity to alter the oncogenic course.[42] Studies examining the effects of the synthetic retinoid 4-HPR in preventing breast cancer in high-risk women and preventing a second primary cancer in the contralateral breast are being conducted. Vitamins A, E, and C in foods act as antioxidants, which defend against free radicals and aid in stimulating the immune response. However, it is difficult to attribute these qualities to specific micronutrients because of the multiple components of vegetables and fruits.[42]

The most promising breast cancer prevention intervention to date is NSABP P-1, the randomized study using tamoxifen to determine if the breast cancer can be prevented in women with known high risk.

The influence of hormones in breast cancer is uniformly recognized. Because of this known association, physicians and scientists have long entertained the possibility of an anti-estrogen that may prevent breast cancer. Tamoxifen was introduced in the 1960s and is the most widely used drug for breast cancer in the United States. It was first introduced as a treatment for advanced breast cancer in postmenopausal women.[43] Since then, tamoxifen has been found to be effective in the treatment of premenopausal women with advanced disease.[44] It has also been found to increase disease-free survival in node-negative, ER-positive disease,[45] as well as node-positive disease.[46] The fact that women taking tamoxifen for primary breast cancer have also experienced a reduction in the expected incidence of contralateral breast cancer strengthens the possibility of a chemoprotective effect.

The enrollment into this study will be based on the amount of risk factors and the relative weight each factor is assigned.[47] Because of the increased risk with advancing age, any woman over 60 is eligible. No one below the age of 35 is eligible. Women over 35 with diagnoses of LCIS that have been treated with local excision are eligible. A woman between the ages of 35 and 59 must have a risk of developing breast cancer equal to a 60-year-old woman.

The study will last for a minimum of 5 years. The participants will be expected to comply with the schedule for daily medication, clinical examinations, and mammography.

Side effects are an important consideration when any drug is taken electively. The common toxicities reported are similar to menopausal symptoms; hot flashes, vaginal discharge, and irregular menses. Rare events include ocular changes, thromboembolic disease, and second primary cancers of the liver and endometrium.

Although tamoxifen is considered an anti-estrogen and, therefore, an antagonist, it may also act as an agonist. As an antagonist, tamoxifen competes with estradiol for the receptor sites in the nucleus. This mechanism causes an estrogen blockade and impedes growth of malignant cells. Although the exact action of the drug is unknown, several explanations have been postulated. Tamoxifen may alter the growth factors that regulate breast cell proliferation,[48] bind to cytoplasmic antiestrogenic binding sites thereby increasing intracellular drug levels,[49] inhibit the amount of free estrogen available to the cell,[50] stimulate natural killer cells,[51] or affect the endocrine regulation of breast cancer cells.[52]

Tamoxifen also exhibits agonist activity, which was recognized in the early trials. This agonist mechanism suggests beneficial action regarding osteoporosis and cardiovascular disease, both of which are significant factors of morbidity and mortality in postmenopausal women.[53]

Nurses across the country are instrumental in the identification of women who are eligible for the Breast Cancer Prevention Trial, the education of the public, recruitment of women to the study, and compliance with the treatment, as well as assessment of toxicity and data collection. Clinicians and families are enthusiastic about the potential outcome of this study, which may provide information on the possible feasibility of chemoprevention and innovative insights into the cause and evolution of breast cancer.

Exercise

The role of exercise in the prevention of breast cancer has not been widely studied. The endorsement of exercise is presented in the context of reducing or counteracting known risk factors. Women who exercise tend to have less body fat, which impacts their hormone milieu. Ovarian function is altered by strenuous exercising, which may delay menarche or create irregular menses or an amenorrheic state. Exercising may reduce the risk of breast cancer for postmenopausal obese women by reducing the amount of free estrogen stored in body fat.

Prophylactic Mastectomy

A *prophylactic mastectomy,* that is, the removal of the majority of breast tissue, may be warranted in certain high-risk women; however, controversy exists over how much risk is enough to justify performing this procedure. Women for whom a prophylactic mastectomy may be indicated have been identified as those with some or all of the following conditions:[25,54]

1. A family history of documented hereditary breast cancer consistent with an autosomal dominant factor. Women who are presumed to be gene carriers may have a breast cancer risk ranging from 50%–100% depending on family history.
2. A personal risk of at least 50% for developing breast cancer.
3. A proven history of breast cancer in one breast and nodularity of cystic disease in the opposite breast. The incidence of a second breast cancer in the opposite breast is estimated to be 15%–20%.
4. Chronic cystic mastitis or a diagnosis of atypical hyperplasia with repeated surgical biopsies.
5. An overwhelming fear of breast cancer such that the possibility of developing breast cancer interferes with her daily life.

The patient must be presented with a clear, in-depth evaluation of her current and potential risk, stressing that a 50% risk also carries a 50% possibility of *not* developing the disease. It is important for the woman to take adequate time in weighing the risk versus benefit of this procedure. The complications are similar to those for a mastectomy. However, if reconstruction is added to this procedure, capsular contracture is a relatively frequent occurrence.[55]

Optimally, women at high risk for breast cancer should be followed by close surveillance utilizing mammograms and frequent clinical examinations, preferably through a comprehensive breast center. Provided such surveillance is feasible, this alternative is an important, even reassuring, alternative for the woman considering prophylactic mastectomy.

SCREENING AND DETECTION

Chemoprevention only applies to high-risk women at this time. Consideration needs to be directed to the 70% of women without significant risk factors who will develop breast cancer. In addition to research into more sophisticated methods to detect subclinical disease, efforts need to be directed toward educating the public to use the health promotions available to provide for early detection. The standard of breast care should include monthly breast self-examination (BSE), regular clinical exams by trained professionals, and periodic mammography.

Early detection reduces the mortality of breast cancer and provides a 90% survival rate for 5 years. The survival rate decreases significantly with regional and distant metastatic disease. The early detection efficacy of breast self-examination, clinical exam, and mammography has been documented.[56] Unfortunately, the literature reveals that BSE and mammography are generally grossly underutilized; strides need to be made in these areas before dramatic reductions in mortality will be seen.

BSE

It is estimated that monthly BSE is performed by approximately one-third of adult women. Lack of proficiency is one of the most consistent barriers to BSE practice. This can be alleviated through an education process that provides verbal and written information as well as demonstration and return demonstration. Many women find the use of demonstration models helpful in increasing confidence and proficiency.

Women should be instructed by a trained professional to begin monthly BSE at age 20. Since 90% of breast lumps are found by the woman or her partner, BSE has the capability to be the primary screening tool for many women. Proficient self-examiners have the potential of finding cancers at an earlier stage, thereby improving prognosis and increasing survival.

The nurse can play a major role in the educational process by promoting and initiating instruction of BSE in the community as well as the health care environment and reinforcing the skill by asking for a return demonstration immediately and each time the patient presents to the office or clinic. The American Cancer Society endorses three methods of self-examination; circular, vertical, and wedge. Regardless of style preference, it is important to note that BSE training should have three basic components: (1) a visual exam using a mirror; (2) a palpation exam in the shower and in the supine position on the bed; and (3) proper technique emphasized during the instructional and return demonstration session, i.e., area, motion, number and position of fingers, and pressure type (Figure 38-1).

The monthly exam should be done 5–7 days after menses stops in premenopausal women or on an appointed day of the month for postmenopausal women. It may be helpful to instruct these women to do BSE on the day that corresponds to their date of birth or the day retirement or Social Security checks arrive. This method is easier to remember than the first or last day of the month. Emphasizing one exam a month cannot be stressed enough. Women who examine themselves more than once (some may examine daily, thinking this offers them better protection) confuse the issue because breast tissue changes can vary from slight to dramatic during the month and they may be unable to determine the normal architecture of their breasts when a problem does arise.

The exam should begin with a visual inspection before a mirror. The woman stands before a mirror with arms relaxed, looking for any changes in breast symmetry, size, and shape, including changes in the skin or nipple/areolar complex (e.g., puckering, dimpling, color of skin). The woman should turn to the side to inspect the lateral aspect of each breast as well. The visual inspection is repeated with arms overhead and with arms pressing on the hips. The reason for these position changes is that the pressure on the underlying muscle alters the appearance of the breast tissue, which may enhance the detection of an abnormality. The visual exam is concluded with the woman leaning forward to inspect the breasts while they are suspended.

The next step is the exam in the shower. Soaping the hand and skin allows the fingers to glide easily over the skin. Raising the arm adjacent to the breast to be examined, the opposite hand is used for BSE. The flat pads of the first three fingers should be used to apply enough pressure to penetrate the dense breast tissue.

The self-examination begins at the axilla, applying gentle, moderate, and deep pressure with the first three fingers in small dime-sized concentric circles, being careful to glide the fingers across the area without lifting the hand away. After the axilla is completed, the exam continues to include the entire breast along with the infraclavicular nodes. After the palpation exam is completed, the woman gives her nipple a slight squeeze to elicit any discharge that may be present, looking for pink or bloody drainage. The other breast is examined in a similar manner. Areas of concern may be new skin thickening, a lump, or mass in the breast or nodal areas.

The final part of the monthly exam includes palpation in the supine position, again with the arm raised on the side of the breast to be examined. If the woman is large breasted, a towel placed under the shoulder will help spread out the breast tissue to enhance examination.

Mammography

Eleven groups, including the AMA, NCI, and ACS, have agreed to recommend guidelines for breast cancer screening. Their recommendations note that mammography and clinical breast exams provide the best protection for early detection and both must be incorporated for maximum benefit[57] (see Table 38-2). Asymptomatic women should begin screening mammography by the age of 40 and continue with screening

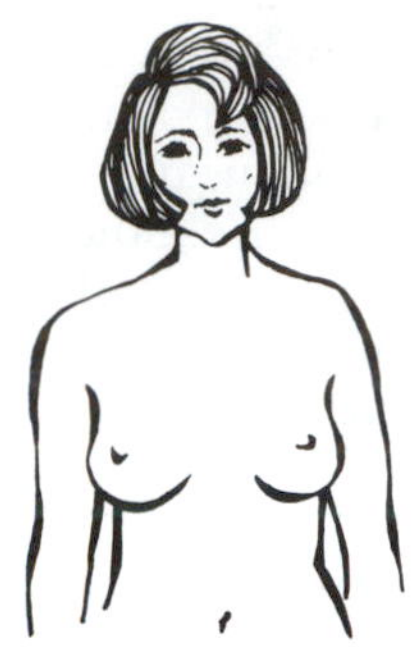

1. Stand before a mirror. Inspect both breasts for anything unusual such as any discharge from the nipples or puckering, dimpling, or scaling of the skin.

The next two steps are designed to emphasize any change in the shape or contour of your breasts. As you do them, you should be able to feel your chest muscles tighten.

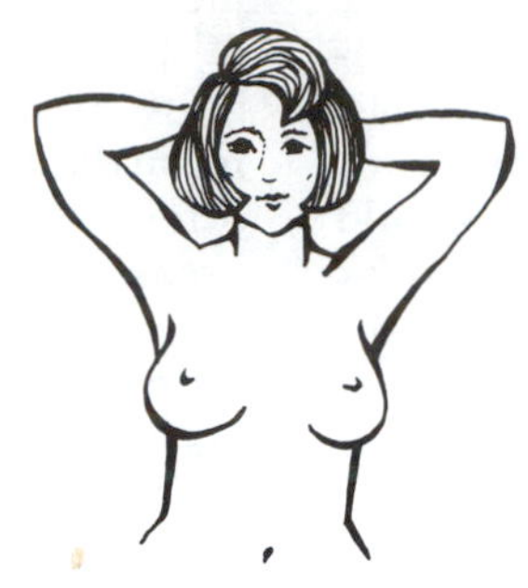

2. Watching closely in the mirror, clasp your hands behind your head and press your hands forward.

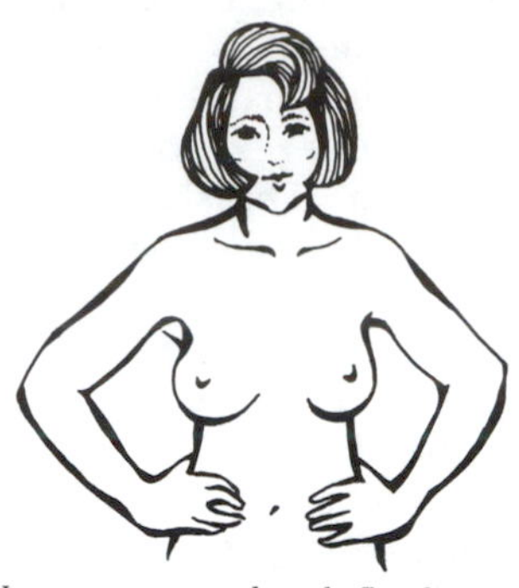

3. Next, press your hands firmly on your hips and bow slightly toward your mirror as you pull your shoulders and elbows forward.

Some women do the next part of the exam in the shower because fingers glide over soapy skin, making it easy to concentrate on the texture underneath.

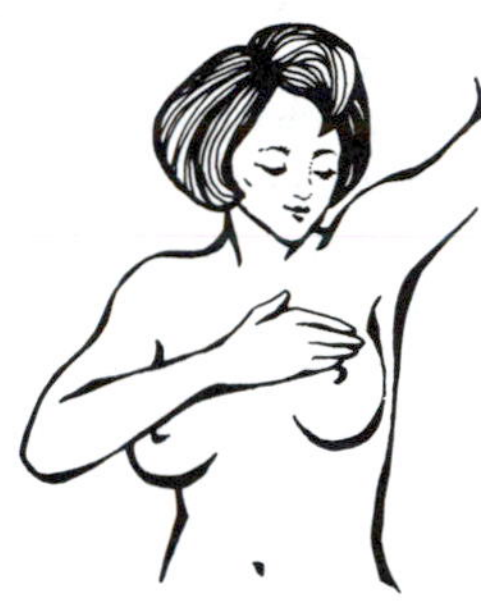

4. Raise your left arm. Use three or four fingers of your right hand to explore your left breast firmly, carefully, and thoroughly. Beginning at the outer edge, press the flat part of your fingers in small circles, moving the circles slowly around the breast. Gradually work toward the nipple. Be sure to cover the entire breast. Pay special attention to the area between the breast and the underarm, including the underarm itself. Feel for any unusual lump or mass under the skin.

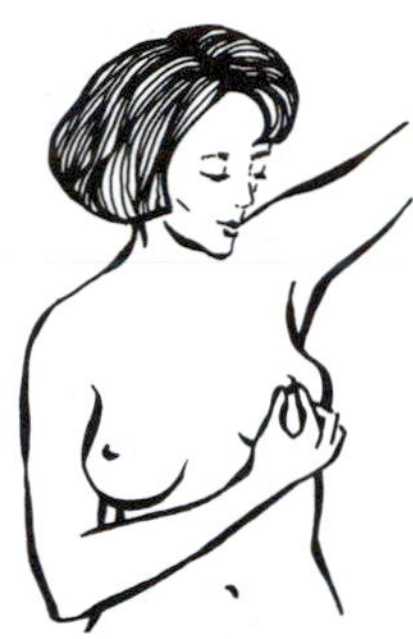

5. Gently squeeze the nipple and look for a discharge. (If you have any discharge during the month—whether or not it is during BSE—see your doctor.) Repeat steps 4 and 5 on your right breast.

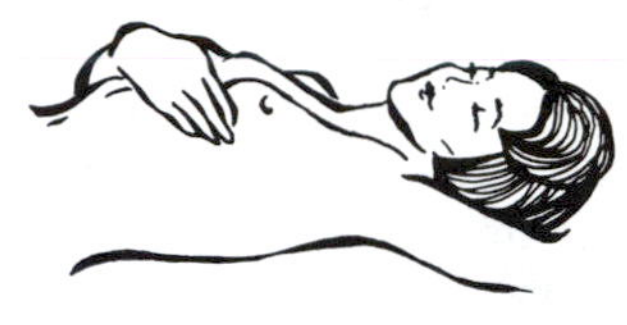

6. Steps 4 and 5 should be repeated lying down. Lie flat on your back with your left arm over your head and a pillow or folded towel under your left shoulder. This position flattens the breast and makes it easier to examine. Use the same circular motion described earlier. Repeat the exam on your right breast.

FIGURE 38-1 Breast self-examination instructions.

mammography and clinical exams every 1–2 years as recommended by their physician. These organizations believe these guidelines will have a significant effect on the early detection rate for the 40–49 age group. Women 50 and older are encouraged to have yearly screening mammography and clinical exams.

Mammograms are generally not recommended for women under age 35 because younger breasts tend to be dense, which causes the mammogram to appear white and contains very little contrast. After the age of 35, a woman's breast begins to be replaced by fat, which can be easily imaged.

Although it is accepted that young women's breasts are difficult to image, there has been an increase in the number of mammograms ordered for woman under 30. A retrospective study was conducted that evaluated the clinical influence of mammograms of 76 patients aged 18–29.[58] The patients were referred for evaluation of a palpable mass or a primary complaint other than a dominant mass (e.g., lumpy breasts, family his-

TABLE 38-2 Breast Screening Guidelines

Screening Method*	Age	Frequency†
BSE	>20	Monthly
Professional clinical exam	20–40	Every 3 years
	>40	Every 1–2 years
	>50	Every year
Mammogram	>40	Every 1–2 years
	>50	Every year

*All three components must be present to ensure early detection.

†The clinician may recommend mammography at an earlier age and/or more frequent clinical examinations for women with increased risk factors.

tory of breast cancer, discharge, enlarged lymph nodes). The study indicated that the radiographic findings did not influence clinical management and recommended alternative diagnostic tools be used including sonography and fine-needle aspiration.

Screening mammography has been proven to be beneficial in studies conducted in the United States and Europe. These studies confirmed reductions in mortality as well as technical improvements in the detection of malignancies. Because mammography is considered to be such an integral part of the screening and detection process, the NCI has set a goal for an 80% utilization rate for screening mammography by the year 2000.[60] This goal seems lofty given that it has been recently estimated that only 15%–20% of women over 50 have ever had a mammogram.

Several possible explanations for this phenomenon have been elicited from patient and physicians. There seems to be a general lack of awareness on the part of physicians and patients regarding the benefits and recommended guidelines for screening. Physicians expressed concern about radiation risk, noncompliance of patients, and overtreatment (i.e., unnecessary biopsies). Patients relate fear of discovering a malignancy, concern about discomfort during mammography, and cost of the examination.

Many of these issues may be addressed by educating patients and members of the health care field about the demonstrated value of mammography. The confusion about disparate guidelines has been addressed to form a consensus (see preceding discussion). Part of the educational process must address fears of mastectomy and the advantages of early detection, which often results in saving the breast through breast conservation surgery.[61]

Equipment and technical issues are easily addressed. The risk of harmful radiation from a mammogram is negligible, and the benefit far outweighs the perceived risk to the patient. Discomfort from breast compression has been generally considered to be a barrier to mammography. Two surveys looked at discomfort as a possible deterrent to mammography. One study reported that patients who understood the procedure usually found the compression acceptable.[62] Another study indicated that the expected compression complaints were minimal and the discomfort issue may be overestimated.[63]

Cost is an issue that is difficult to address. The cost may vary from approximately $50.00 to $200.00. The high end reflects diagnostic mammograms, which are recommended when a clinical or prior mammographic abnormality is known to exist. Screening mammograms are less expensive and appropriate for the asymptomatic woman. Medicare now will cover screening mammograms for women every other year. Some city and county facilities offer free screening mammograms. Businesses interested in health promotion have begun providing on-site mobile mammography units free of charge or at a nominal fee. Facilities and centers may offer a reduced price to coincide with Breast Cancer Awareness Month in October.

Women who "shop" for their yearly mammogram may be doing themselves a disservice if the mammogram is taken at a different facility each time. Facilities may differ with respect to the expertise of the radiologist and the technique employed. Potentially, an abnormality could be overlooked or a stable abnormality will be recommended for biopsy because comparison films are not available. This problem can be avoided by always bringing old films for comparison or having yearly mammograms at the same institution.

DIAGNOSTIC EVALUATION

Routine mammography may reveal a large spectrum of breast pathology ranging from equivocal benign conditions, to those that may mimic suspicious or malignant processes, to those that are considered malignant until proven otherwise. The appearance of these lesions is often a coincidental finding on a screening mammogram of an asymptomatic woman. However, if there is a palpable abnormality, additional diagnostic tools will be utilized to isolate the abnormality and provide more specific information for the clinician.

The diagnostic evaluation of breast lesions may be a simple one-step procedure or it may progress to a multilevel process. There are several noninvasive and low-invasive diagnostic tools that aid the clinician in identifying lesions within the breast. There are a series of steps that may be taken before determining which lesions actually need open (excisional) biopsy. Figure 38-2 and Figure 38-3 describe the steps involved in the diagnostic evaluation of a nonpalpable and a palpable breast mass.

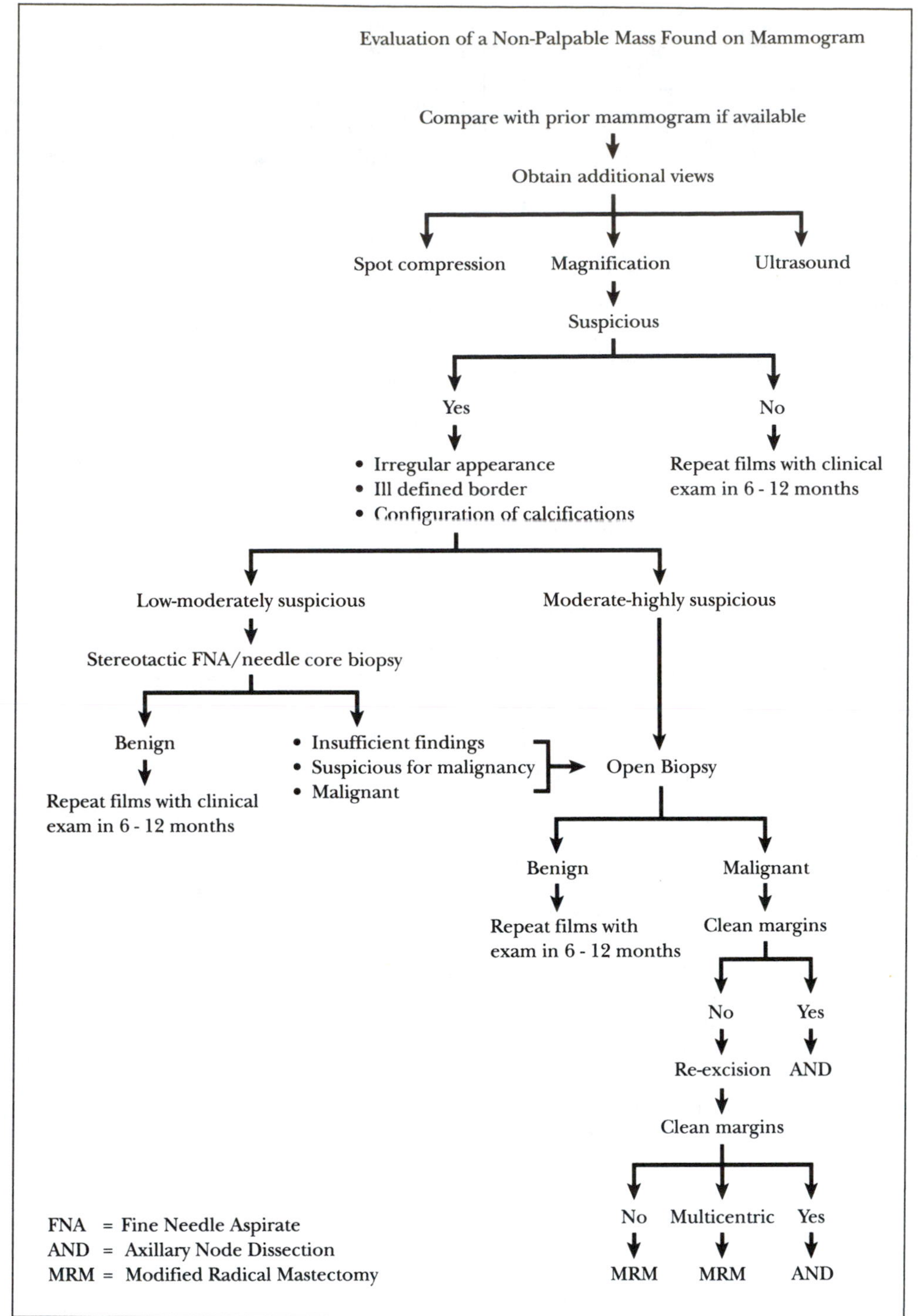

FIGURE 38-2 Evaluation of a non-palpable mass found on mammogram.

Characteristics of Benign versus Malignant Breast Disease

Nearly eight of ten lumps that are biopsied are found to be benign. The clinical differences between benign and malignant disease are clear. An obvious mobile mass that is encapsulated or circumscribed with a distinct barrier from adjacent tissues is most likely to be a fibroadenoma or cyst, particularly in a premenopausal woman. Malignant disease, on the other hand, usually has less distinct boundaries and lack of mobility because of tumor infiltration into adjacent tissues. A benign lesion is often soft and smooth with regular borders, whereas a malignant lesion is a firm, three-dimensional area with irregular borders.

Benign disease is frequently associated with bilat-

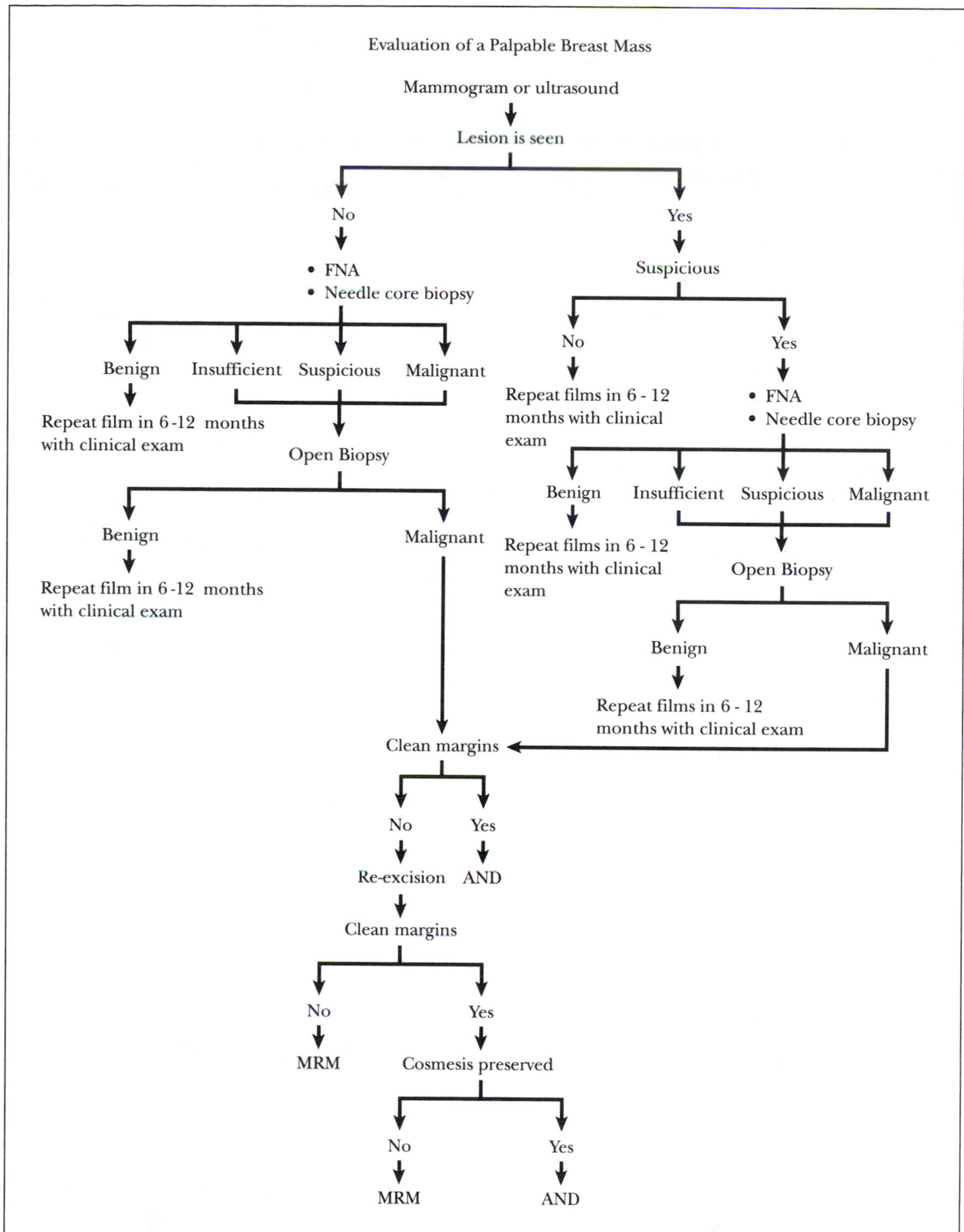

FIGURE 38-3 Evaluation of a palpable breast mass.

eral, diffuse breast pain and tenderness that is more prominent at the time of the menstrual period. Often this pain radiates to the axilla. Pain is not a common symptom of breast carcinomas, but it may be present with more advanced local disease. Pain in this situation is characterized as focal, constant, and nonradiating and is not related to the menstrual period.

Benign disease is usually clear on transillumination, whereas malignant disease is opaque. Malignant disease is usually a solitary, unilateral lesion; benign disease may be multiple bilateral lesions. Nipple discharge is most often a sign of benign disease but can indicate breast cancer if it is pink or bloody, spontaneous and unilateral. Nipple ulceration or scaly skin at the nipple is suspicious of Paget's disease, an early form of breast carcinoma.

Clinical manifestations that are more suspicious of malignant disease are nipple retraction or elevation, which may be due to tumor fixation or infiltration into the underlying tissues. Skin dimpling or retraction also may be present and is possibly due to invasion of the suspensory ligaments and fixation to the chest wall. Heat and erythema of the breast skin may be related to inflammation, but they are also signs of inflammatory breast carcinoma. Skin edema, or *peau d' orange* (Figure 38-4), is characteristic of malignant disease. The edema is thought to be due to the invasion and obstruction of dermal lymphatics by tumor. Ulceration of the skin with secondary infection may be present. The presence of isolated skin nodules indicates invasion of blood vessels and lymphatics. This often results in implantation of tumor emboli in adjacent tissues and indicates that distant metastases are likely. Clinical presentation may also include, or be limited to, signs of local or distant metastatic disease.

Mammograms

Screening mammograms

Screening mammograms are used for routine breast surveillance for the asymptomatic patient. The goal of screening mammography is to detect a malignancy before it becomes clinically apparent. It is important to have an appreciation for what mammography can accomplish. A 10-mm tumor containing 10^9 or 1 billion cells is palpable by clinical examination. Mammography can improve this by about six or seven doublings, or approximately 20% of the life of the tumor. Detection at 10^7 by mammography or 10^9 by palpation (usually by a trained professional) occurs still earlier than the discovery of a tumor of the size ordinarily encountered in clinical practice (BSE).

Clinical detection through the use of BSE generally occurs when a tumor is 33 mm, or 10^{10} cells, and is by no means early in the biologic history of the cancer. Therefore, mammography is an important consideration in the triad of early detection of breast cancer.

The routine screening mammogram provides a high-sensitivity study at the lowest possible cost. A highly sensitive study enables the radiologist to detect any discrete abnormality, thereby reducing the false-negative reports. The technology employed can be either xeroradiography or film-screen. The current trend is toward film-screen mammography.

A woman should consider the institution where the mammogram is performed. There are several important guidelines to follow to ensure that the mammogram and report reflect state-of-the-art technology and interpretation. A facility should be accredited by the American College of Radiologists, which has developed a voluntary mammography accreditation program that offers the opportunity for peer review and evaluation of equipment, image quality, radiation dosage, and staff qualifications. To qualify for accreditation, the facility must be directed by a Board-certified radiologist and the technologists must be certified or have an equivalent license.[63] One can call 1-800-ACR-LINE for current information on accredited hospital and clinics.

The screening mammogram usually consists of four views, two per breast (Figures 38-5 and 38-6). A

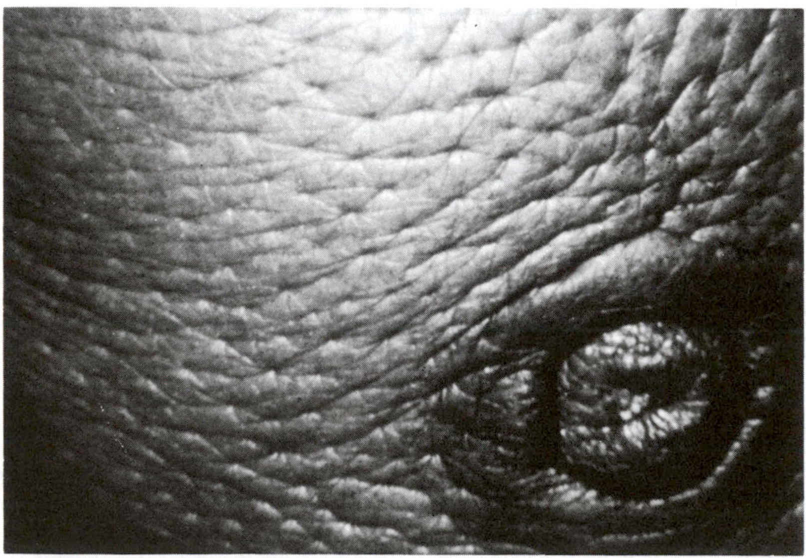

FIGURE 38-4 *Peau d'orange;* characteristic of lymphatic and dermal invasion by adenocarcinoma (inflammatory carcinoma).

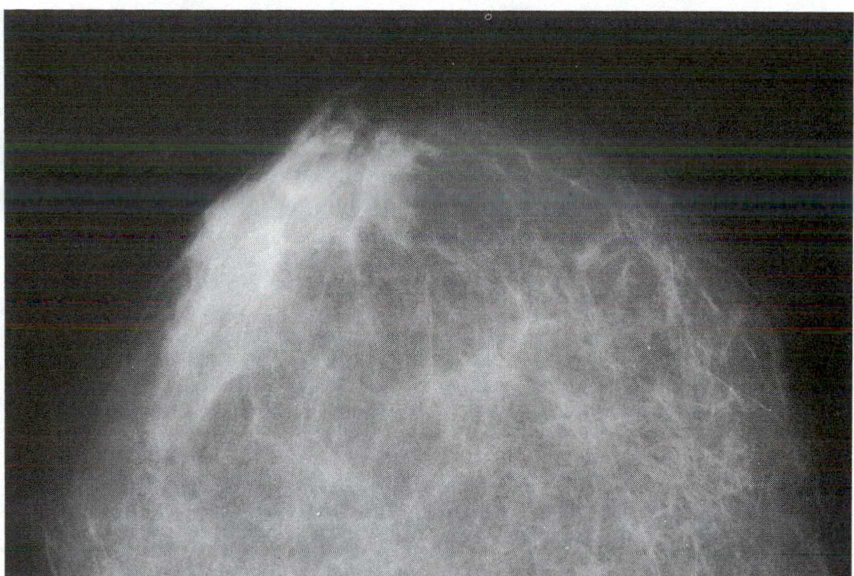

FIGURE 38-5 Screening mammography of an asymptomatic breast from above (craniocaudal view).

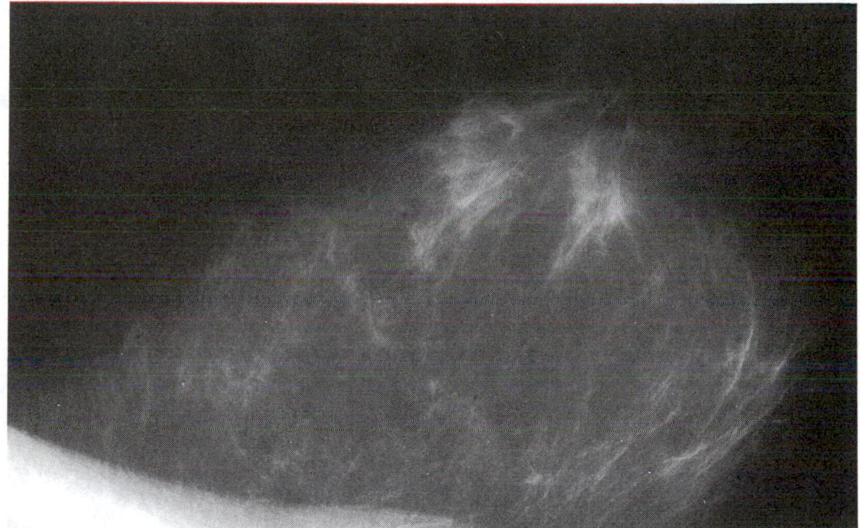

FIGURE 38-6 Screening mammography of an asymptomatic breast from the side (mediolateral view). Note the inclusion of the axilla and the pectoralis muscle, which ensures that the entire breast is imaged.

mediolateral oblique and a crainocaudal view of each breast enables the technologist to image as much breast as possible (i.e., the axillary tail and pectoralis muscle).

A screening mammogram allows the radiologist to detect characteristic benign and malignant masses. Benign masses include cysts, fibroadenomas, and inframammary lymph nodes, all of which have defined borders. Malignant lesions may present as spiculated or ill-defined masses, architectural distortion, asymmetric densities, and microcalcifications (Figures 38-7 and 38-8). Additionally, subtle abnormalities may be noted by the radiologist that require further studies to determine if pathology exists.[64]

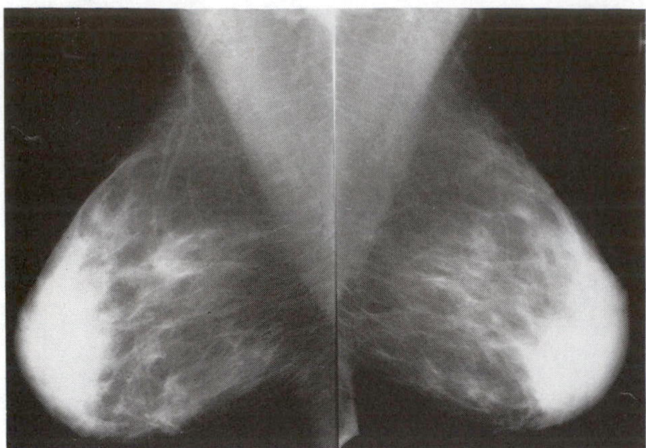

FIGURE 38-7 The mediolateral views show the appearance of an asymmetric density.

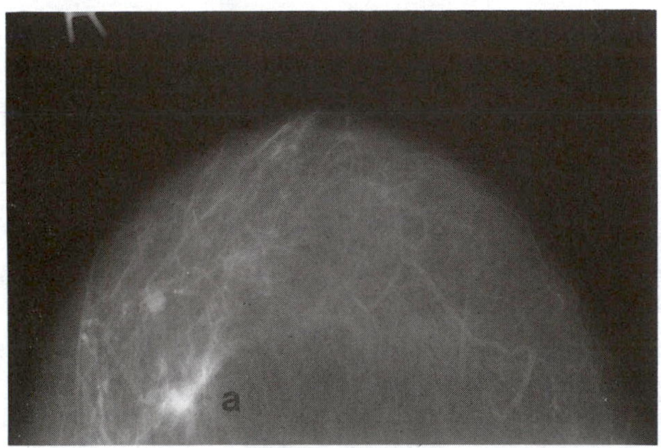

FIGURE 38-8 A craniocaudal view demonstrates the presence of spiculated nodule.

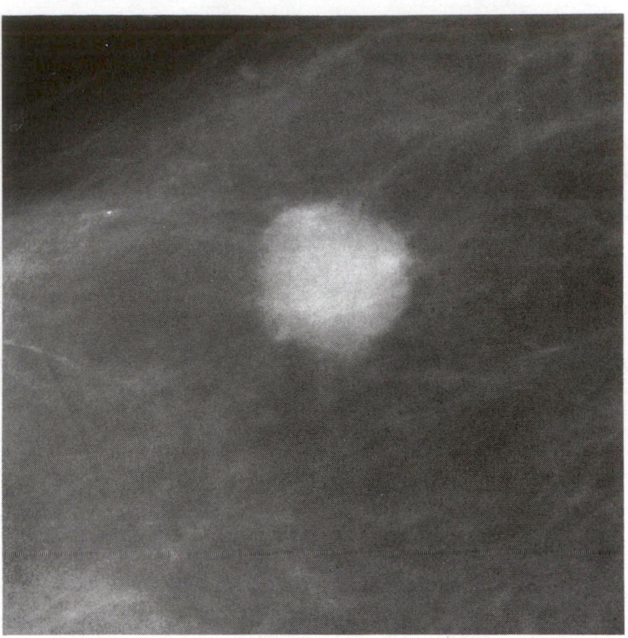

FIGURE 38-9 Magnification of the nodule provides a more accurate picture of the irregular border noted on screening mammogram. Note that the border is not clearly defined, but appears fuzzy or hazy, which is especially demonstrated on the left side. The irregular appearance makes this nodule suspicious for cancer.

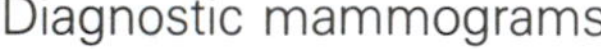

Diagnostic mammograms

A diagnostic mammogram is performed when the patient reports specific symptoms, suspicious clinical findings exist, or an abnormality has been found on a screening mammogram. A diagnostic film uses additional views of the affected breast as well as the possibility of localized compression and magnification views to increase the specificity of identifying the abnormality.[60] The area in question is locally compressed and/or magnified, which enables the radiologist to comment more accurately on the lesion (Figures 38-9 and 38-10).

Diagnostic mammography provides the radiologist with additional detail to render a more specific diagnosis, which may preclude the need for an open biopsy. However, if the diagnosis is nonspecific and the lesion has a low-suspicion threshold and is felt to be benign, the radiologist may recommend repeat films in six months to ensure the area in question has not changed. This information must be discussed with the patient, as some people are uncomfortable waiting to be reexamined mammographically and may prefer to have the abnormality sampled or excised.

Sonogram

A sonogram or ultrasound is used to determine whether a known lesion is solid or cystic. Ultrasounds are appropriate to investigate palpable lesions in young women whose breasts have the dense fibroglandular tissue that may obscure a lesion in the breast. Ultrasounds are also useful in pregnant women, who need to be spared radiation when an abscess or galactocele is suspected, or in recently lactating women whose breasts are extremely dense.

While sonograms are useful in determining if a lesion is solid or cystic, the sensitivity and specificity are not the same caliber as mammograms. They should not be used for screening purposes (Figure 38-11).[64]

FIGURE 38-10 New microcalcifications were seen on a routine mammogram. The radiologist requested magnified views, which revealed a small area of clustered microcalcifications (top) as well as microcalcifications that tend to branch (below). Both are suspicious for cancer.

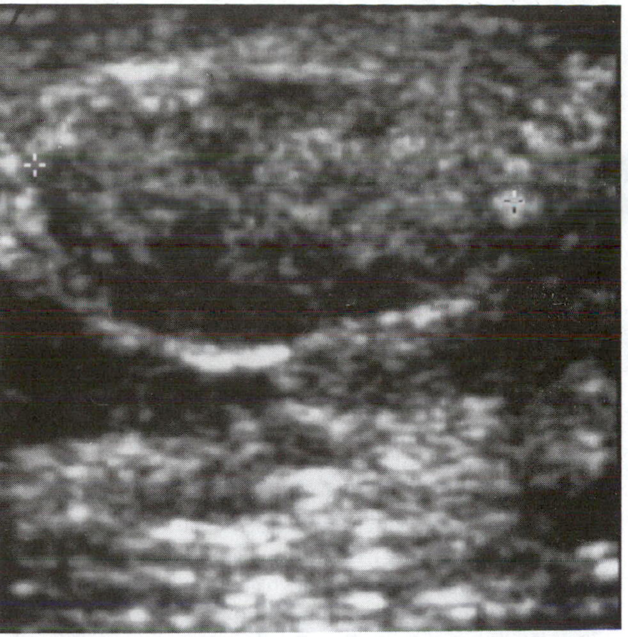

FIGURE 38-11 An ultrasound of a palpable mass reveals the characteristics of a fibroadenoma (between the crosses), which is a benign nodule.

MRI

MRI (or MRM, magnetic resonance mammography) of the breast is a relatively new procedure that may allow for earlier detection based on the ability of this test to determine smaller lesions and finer detail. It is superior to ultrasound in imaging the parenchyma, axilla, or chest wall. MRI evaluates the rate at which the contrast initially enters the breast tissue. Malignant lesions tend to exhibit an increased enhancement within the first 2 minutes. It is limited in the detection of calcifications, which excludes its use for many nonpalpable lesions. MRI may be best viewed as a complement to mammography and clinical exam to distinguish between a benign or malignant lesion in the hope of preventing benign biopsies.

Fine-Needle Aspiration

Fine-needle aspiration (FNA) is employed when an abnormality is known to be solid or to determine if the lump is a cyst. FNA may also be used to confirm a clinically apparent positive diagnosis. FNA is a simple office procedure that can be performed with or without local anesthetic using a small 20- or 22-gauge needle.

If the lump in question is a cyst, the area should resolve after the aspiration is completed. Cysts may return in the same area or in other areas of the breast and the patient may require repeated aspirations over time. If a lump is solid, it is still possible to obtain a cytology sample by making several passes into the lesion using the same entry point. This method will retrieve small cell samples from several sites within the lesion and reduce the false-negative result.

It should be mentioned, however, that a lesion that does not demonstrate a malignant histology may still remain clinically suspicious to the physician. In cases such as these, a biopsy will often be recommended.

Stereotactic Needle-Guided Biopsy

The stereotactic biopsy is relatively new in the United States. This procedure was developed in Sweden and tested there at the Karolinska Institute and the University of Kiel in Germany before being introduced to the United States. This method of biopsy is mainly used to target and identify mammographically detected, nonpalpable lesions in the breast.[65]

While mammography offers the best detection of early breast cancer, mammography often cannot distinguish between benign or malignant tumors.

Approximately 60%–80% of recommended biopsies are for benign abnormalities. The stereotactic biopsy permits diagnosis of benign disease without the trauma or scarring of an open biopsy. The basic principle of stereotactic biopsy is to immobilize the breast from fixed horizontal and vertical coordinates to calculate the exact position of the lesion within a three-dimensional field.[66]

The procedure takes place in a specially equipped operating room. The room contains breast-imaging equipment and an examination table that has an opening at the front end through which the breast is suspended as the patient lies in a prone position. This positioning is necessary to examine and target the precise area to be sampled. (See Figure 38-12.)

After proper placement is confirmed by stereoradiographs, the breast is locally anesthetized and a double-lumen coaxial needle is inserted under sterile conditions. The outer needle serves as the localizer and remains in place during the cytology and histology sampling. A syringe is then attached to the inner needle and an aspirate is taken. During this procedure the physician will often reinsert the needle within a 1-cm area to obtain additional samples.[67]

Following the aspirate, a 16–20-gauge needle is inserted several times, which allows two or three core biopsy samples to be taken. The cytology and histology samples are then sent to the pathology department. The cytology results are available within the hour, and the histology results are reported in approximately 2 days.

Stereoradiographs are taken again to identify the exact area from which the samples are taken. The area is then marked with methylene blue and a small hook wire is inserted in the event an excisional biopsy is warranted. If the immediate result is benign, the wire is removed and the patient is discharged.

Wire Localization Biopsy

The preparation for the wire-localized biopsy is somewhat similar to the stereotactic method. The difference lies in the goal of the procedure. The aim of this biopsy procedure is to assist the surgeon in locating the nonpalpable lesion for the purpose of excisional biopsy. The character of the abnormality is identified after biopsy.

The needle-localized biopsy targets the area via mammography using the craniocaudad and mediolateral views. Once the area is anesthetized, a double-lumen needle is inserted into the area that has been calculated by the planes of the mammograms. A set of

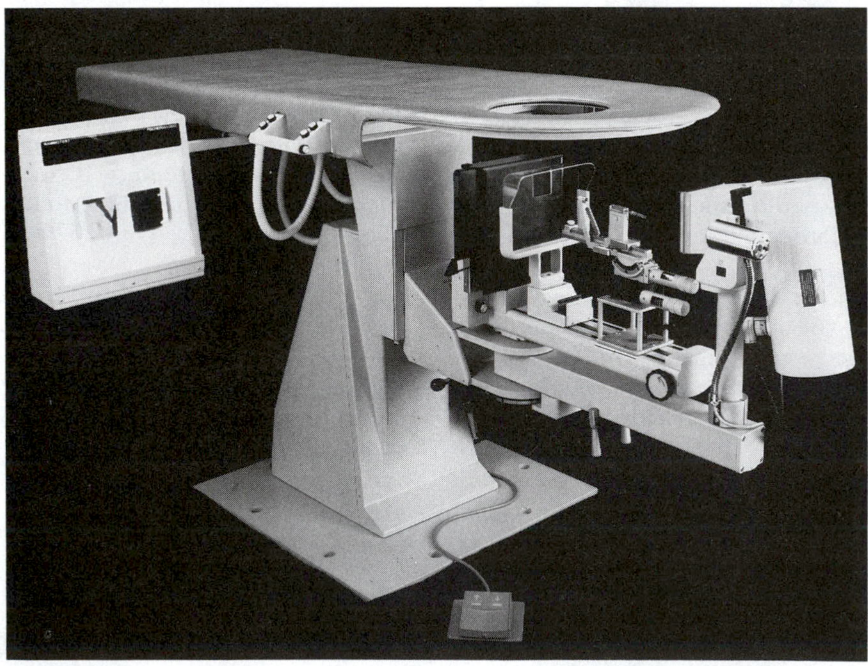

FIGURE 38-12 The stereotactic table allows for localization of the nonpalpable lesion between the Plexiglas plates below the opening from which the breast hangs down. Some machines allow for the procedure to be done in a sitting position, which is less favorable due to the possibility of syncope. (Photo courtesy of Fisher Imaging, Denver, CO.)

repeat mammograms is then taken to ensure proper placement.

Once proper placement has been determined, the area may or may not be marked with a combination of blue dye and radiopaque contrast. The outer needle is removed, leaving a thin hook wire marking the area of concern, and this wire is then taped to the skin of the breast to prevent dislodgement. The patient is sent to the operating room with the mammograms that note the area to be excised.[68] After the biopsy a specimen mammogram of the tissue is taken to ensure the abnormality has been removed.

Open Biopsy

The excisional biopsy is the most invasive diagnostic procedure. There are several reasons for recommending an excisional biopsy; (1) Sonogram findings show the lesion to be solid, (2) the cytology and/or histology results are insufficient, (3) the clinical or mammographic findings are suspicious, or (4) the patient with a probable low-risk lesion requests a biopsy to allay her anxiety.

The objective of this biopsy is to remove the lump or area identified, along with a small amount of surrounding normal tissue. This is done by using curvilinear or circumareolar incision over the lesion after the area has been anesthetized. The use of circumareolar incisions for distant lesions is not recommended, and radial incisions should not be used because of poor cosmetic results. After the tumor is removed, the skin is closed without approximating breast tissue or fat. This method results in less deformity at the biopsy site. The excised tissue is identified and sent to pathology for histopathological diagnosis.

An incisional biopsy that removes only part of the lesion is rarely performed. If the tumor is very large and a diagnosis is needed, FNA or needle-core biopsy is usually sufficient and an incisional biopsy is not necessary.

MULTIDISCIPLINARY BREAST CENTERS

The increasing public awareness of breast cancer treatment options and the recognized controversies in breast cancer detection and management, together with oncologists' and institutions' commitment to provide optimum care, have spearheaded the concept of the multidisciplinary breast center. The design of these centers is, in essence, a response to the fact that treatment of breast cancer has become a complicated process necessitating specialized, collaborative management that is often beyond the scope of an individual practitioner. The purpose and goals of a multidisciplinary breast center include, but are not limited to, the following:

1. to provide a comprehensive interdisciplinary evaluation and planning in the management of all aspects of breast disease
2. to provide prompt and timely evaluation and diagnosis of potential breast disease implementing current methodology and state-of-the-art diagnostic tools
3. to participate in and support national protocol studies that investigate new surgical and adjuvant treatment modalities
4. to provide careful surveillance of women at high risk for breast cancer, thereby minimizing the anxiety associated with the knowledge that one has an increased risk for developing the disease as well as reducing the risk of patients being lost to follow-up
5. to provide educational materials and the opportunity to learn about early detection measures (e.g., BSE) and the possibility of participating in breast cancer prevention studies as well as research studies aimed at early detection and management of malignant breast cancer
6. to provide educational opportunities for medical students, Fellows, general practitioners, nurses, and others involved in the care of the woman with breast disease as well as providing a mechanism for peer review of the oncologist in practice
7. to provide highly specialized assessment and diagnostic procedures that enable prompt decision making in the evaluation of a breast mass, which conceivably minimizes unnecessary surgical biopsies
8. to provide the woman and family with the necessary information to allow her to make an informed decision regarding her choices for treatment in a prompt and timely manner
9. to offer educational programs to the community that include instruction in BSE and information on risk factors and the importance of utilizing the current methods available to promote early detection

Ideally, the comprehensive breast center should have a full complement of disciplines available to provide an expert opinion regarding assessment of diagnostic and histopathological data; prognostic indicators; and surgical diagnostic and treatment options including systemic chemo/endocrine therapy, radiation treatment, and surgical reconstructive techniques when warranted. A psycho-oncologist and social worker provide counseling regarding body image issues, sexual concerns, and anticipated changes in lifestyle for those patients dealing with a potentially life-threatening disease.

The oncology clinical nurse specialist is often viewed as the coordinator of the comprehensive breast center. It is imperative that this professional possesses specialized knowledge in all aspects of breast cancer and its treatment as well as a compassionate, yet controlled, approach to the evaluation of a suspected breast cancer. It is not uncommon for women to telephone the breast center, frantic with fear and apprehension, expressing a need to be seen as soon as possible. Regardless of the schedule, this is exactly what needs to occur if possible. Such understanding and prompt attention to the woman's needs and concerns will help to establish a trusting and caring relationship, which is vital considering the possible diagnostic outcome. This approach to patient management is critical to the success of a comprehensive breast center.

The nurse coordinator ensures that all materials (slides, x-rays) necessary for a comprehensive evaluation are present at the time of the consultation. The nurse informs the patient and family of the sequence of events once the appointment is established. This includes which doctor(s) the patient will see and when, how materials will be reviewed, and the critical role the patient plays in the decision-making process. Emphasis is placed on the fact that often there is more than one approach to management of the problem and that once informed of her options, the patient is the ultimate decision maker. The nurse can be instrumental in ensuring that information is delivered in a manner that will enhance the patient's understanding and ability to make an informed decision.[69]

In addition to facilitating the process of informed consent and decision making, the nurse is also instrumental in providing BSE instruction to all patients.[70] The nurse also will be called on to answer questions regarding diagnostic tests, therapy regimens, clinical trials, postoperative events, and potential complications of treatment. The nurse may see patients postoperatively in the hospital to provide continuity of care as well as instruction concerning general postoperative care including infection precautions. Ideally, the nurse coordinator will be able to provide exercise instruction prior to surgery and evaluate understanding and potential for compliance during the period following hospitalization. Additionally, the nurse utilizes every opportunity to lecture to professionals and the public concerning breast cancer as a health issue and methods available for early detection. In addition, time should be set aside specifically to accept or return phone calls concerning questions related to breast cancer risk specifically as well as other pertinent issues.

The design of a comprehensive breast center should reflect the goals of providing a complete, efficient, yet personal evaluation of the patient. The exam rooms should be large enough to accommodate the patient, family/significant other, as well as the team of physicians. The clinical area should have additional smaller consult rooms where the patient may be seen by individual consultants based on her individual concerns and needs.

A physician conference room should be available to provide an area for viewing films, pathology slides, and reports. Diagnostic tests and outpatient surgery suites positioned on site facilitate a quick and efficient diagnostic process.

These centers are successful because they meet a growing need for a multidisciplinary and comprehensive approach to the care of the woman with breast disease and because they are philosophically based on the premise that women are entitled to all the information available to make an informed decision regarding their choice of treatment.[70]

PATHOPHYSIOLOGY—CELLULAR CHARACTERISTICS

The majority of primary breast cancers are adenocarcinomas located in the upper outer quadrant of the breast (Figure 38-13). The most common types of breast tumors are summarized in Table 38-3. Infiltrating ductal carcinoma may take various histologic forms; either well differentiated and slow growing, poorly differentiated and infiltrating, or highly malignant and undifferentiated with many mitoses.[71] This variant of adenocarcinoma primarily affects women in their early 50s. The overall 10-year survival rate is 50%–60%.

Invasive lobular carcinoma occurs in the same age range as ductal carcinoma, accounts for 5%–10% of all

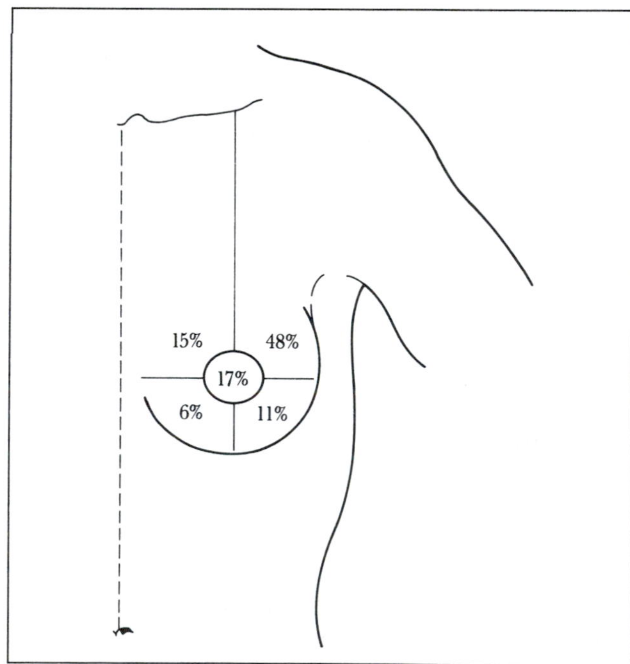

FIGURE 38-13 Incidence of breast cancer according to location.

breast cancers, and is frequently bilateral. The prognosis is similar to ductal carcinoma.

Tubular carcinoma is fairly uncommon and represents a well-differentiated adenocarcinoma of the breast. These cancers typically occur in women aged 55 and older. The presence of microcalcification is characteristic and facilitates early mammographic discovery. Axillary metastasis is uncommon.

Medullary carcinomas account for 5%–7% of malignant breast tumors, occurring most commonly in younger women (<50 years of age). These tumors may be quite large and circumscribed and may be bilateral.

Mucinous or colloid carcinoma is uncommon, occurring in women 60–70 years of age. This tumor type is characterized by the presence of large pools of mucin interspersed with small islands of tumor cells. Metastasis to axillary lymph nodes occurs in about one-third of patients and distant metastasis occurs late.

Other malignant tumors of the breast include sarcomas, papillary carcinoma, apocrine, invasive cribriform, and Paget's disease.

PROGNOSTIC INDICATORS

Pathologist and clinicians continue to attempt to identify morphologic and phenotypic characteristics of tumors that will reflect the innate biologic aggressiveness of the individual breast cancer. The identification of various prognostic indicators is valuable because such efforts help define the natural history of breast cancer, identify various subsets of high-risk women who might benefit most from more aggressive therapies, as well as establish prognosis with increasing accuracy. For example, the presence of vascular, lymphatic, or blood vessel invasion portends probable dissemination of cancer and a lower survival rate and short-term failure, usually within 18 months. Inflammatory carcinoma characterized by clinical and microscopic involvement of the dermal lymphatics by adenocarcinoma has long heralded a poor prognosis.[71]

Valuable parameters for determining the prognosis for patients with breast cancer include the status of the axillary lymph nodes, size of the tumor, the invasive nature of the neoplasm, multicentricity, nuclear grade, estrogen-progesterone receptor levels, cell proliferative indices, DNA ploidy, and measures of immune competence.

Axillary Lymph Node Status

The presence or absence of axillary node status has long been recognized as a key feature in determining prognosis in breast cancer (Figure 38-14). Clinical assessment of the axillary nodes carries a 30% false-positive and false-negative rate. Pathological staging of the lymph nodes is mandatory.[71] However, in one study, 17% of stage I breast cancer patients initially diagnosed with no evidence of metastatic disease in lymph nodes had occult axillary metastatic disease when reexamined pathologically.[72] Once involvement is determined, important issues are whether the metastases are micro-

TABLE 38-3 Histologic Types of Breast Cancers

Histological Type	Percentage of Occurrence	Clinical Features	Metastatic Pattern	Prognosis
Infiltrating ductal carcinoma	75%	Stony hardness to palpation Prominent lump	Axillary lymph nodes (common) Bone Lung Liver Brain	Poor
Infiltrating lobular carcinoma	5%–10%	Diffuse, ill-defined thickness Multicentric Bilaterality (30%)	Axillary lymph nodes (common) Occult lymph node micrometastasis may occur Meningeal surfaces	Poor
Tubular	2%	May be quite large	Axillary lymph nodes (uncommon) Distant metastases uncommon	Moderate
Medullary	5%–7%	Well circumscribed Rapid growth rate Bilaterality	Approximately 40% of cases demonstrate lymph node involvement at diagnosis	Moderate
Mucinous (Colloid)	3%	Slow growing, bulky	Axillary lymph node involvement in less than ⅓ of cases at diagnosis	Favorable

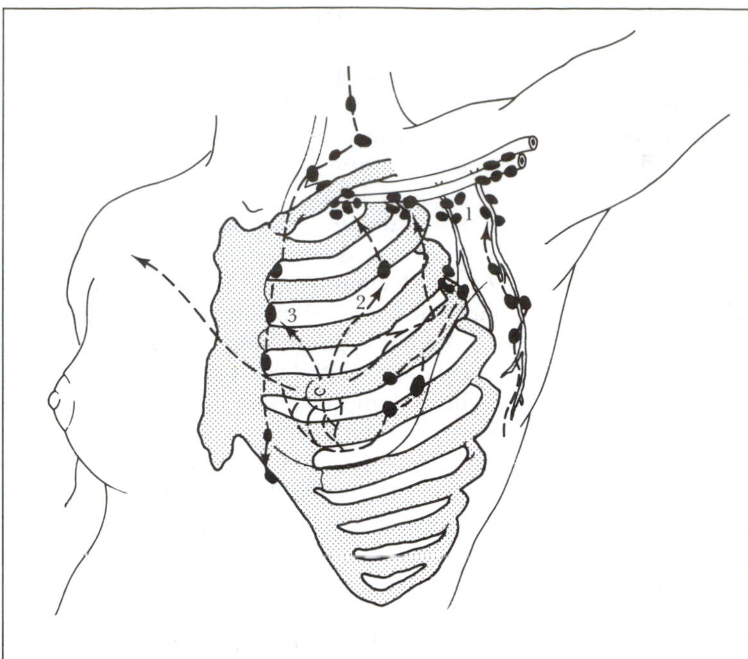

FIGURE 38-14 Lymphatics of the breast leading to (1) axillary nodes, which are distributed over a large area from the lateral aspects of the breast proper to the axillary vessels; (2) interpectoral chain leading to interpectoral node (circle detail) and to high nodes in the axilla; (3) chain of the internal mammary leading frequently to node in second interspace and to supraclavicular and cervical nodes. The lymphatics of the breast may empty into the opposite axillary nodes.

scopic or macroscopic, the number of nodes involved, the levels of involvement, and whether the lymph node capsule has been invaded.[73] Extranodal extension is significant prognostically only when the metastases are confined to one to three nodes.[74] Staging of axillary nodes requires pathologic view of at least four axillary nodes.[75]

Seventy percent of patients with negative nodes survive 10 years. Prognosis worsens as the number of positive lymph nodes increases. Recurrence of disease is seen in approximately 75% of women with axillary metastases. Metastases to the internal mammary nodes have the same significance as those to the axillary nodes. Internal mammary node metastases occur more readily in patients who have medial or lateral lesions. Internal mammary nodes are not commonly sampled but are invaded in 10% of patients when axillary nodes are negative. This may help to explain the recurrence patterns in some axillary node–negative women.[76,77]

The correlation between survival and number of involved nodes has been expanded from that originally used (i.e., 0, 1–3, 4+) to include additional fractions of 4–6, 7–9, and 10 or more involved nodes (Table 38-4).[78]

TABLE 38-4 Recurrence Rates in 20,547 Women with Breast Cancer According to the Number of Histologically Involved Axillary Nodes

Number of Positive Nodes	Recurrence at 5 Years
0	25%
1–3	40%
4–6	49%
7–9	58%
10+	78%

Source: Adapted from Nemoto T, et al.[78]

Tumor Size

Prior to the more widespread use of mammography, less than 8% of women with node-negative breast cancer had tumors that were less than 1 cm in diameter with a relative overall 5-year survival of nearly 99%. Patients with tumors measuring 1–3 cm have a relative 5-year survival of approximately 91%, while those with tumors measuring more than 3 cm have a 5-year survival of 85%.[79] Recurrence rates for patients with tumors greater than 3 cm is more than 50%, however. Therefore, consideration toward other prognostic indicators is necessary to determine the appropriate approach to systemic therapies.

Cell Proliferative Indices and DNA Ploidy

Research indicates that assessment of cell proliferative potential has important prognostic significance, especially in node-negative breast cancer. Using flow cytometry it is possible to measure DNA content and proliferative activity (S-phase fraction) of a tumor. Patients whose tumors have an abnormal amount of DNA (aneuploid tumors) have a worse prognosis compared to those who have a normal amount of DNA (diploid tumors).[80–83]

Tumors with positive estrogen receptor protein tend to demonstrate a low proliferative activity (low S-phase fraction) and tend to be more diploid than aneuploid. Comparatively, tumors that are estrogen receptor negative tend to have a high S-phase fraction reflecting a more aggressive metastatic potential.

Tumor proliferative activity in invasive breast cancer has also been measured by an immunoperoxidase procedure using the monoclonal antibody Ki-67, which reacts with a nuclear antigen throughout the cell cycle (G_1, S, G_2, and M) of proliferating cells.[84] Patients with tumors containing a high mitotic rate, high nuclear grade, negative estrogen receptors, as well as premenopausal disease tend to have high numbers of Ki-67 positive cells (>15%). In a study of node negative breast cancer, long-term follow-up showed a significant correlation of 5-year disease-free survival and Ki-67 staining, with higher staining correlating with lower survival.[84]

Histological Grade

The more differentiated the tumor cells, the better the prognosis. Tumors are generally classified as well differentiated, moderately well differentiated, or poorly differentiated according to their degree of anaplasia. Such factors as nuclear size and shape, mitotic figures, and degree of tubule formation determine differentiation and likewise predict aggressiveness and metastatic potential of tumor cells. Approximately 10% of patients have grade 1 (well differentiated) tumors and, of these patients, greater than 90% have estrogen receptor positive tumors; the majority are diploid and have a 5-year disease-free survival rate of over 90%.[85] Therefore, in node-negative disease, grade may be a reliable tool for assessing the need for adjuvant therapy.

Epidermal Growth Factor Receptor

The idea that estrogen plays a significant role in the pathogenesis and initial proliferation of breast cancer is an accepted one. The fact that some cells develop estrogen independence during proliferation in part accounts for variance in clinical behavior and response to treatment in estrogen dependent (ER+) and estrogen independent (ER−) breast cancer. Mori et al.[86] found that patients' breast cancer tissue that stained positive for epidermal growth factor tended to be estrogen receptor negative, suggesting that estrogen may exert inhibitory action on epidermal growth factor receptor (EGFR) production through binding to the estrogen receptor. In the absence of this inhibition, the EGFR may actually increase proliferation of breast cancer cells. Research in this area may lead to new approaches to controlling the growth and development of breast cancer cells.

c-erb B-2 Oncogene

A frequently studied proto-oncogene in breast cancer is c-erb B-2. Overexpression or amplification of this oncogene occurs in 10%–35% of human breast cancers and correlates positively with a poor prognosis in node-positive disease. This gene, which is also known as *neu* or HER-2 or HER-2/*neu*, is similar structurally and functionally to EGFR.[87] Studies concerning the relative prognostic importance of the c-erb B-2 oncogene are conflicting. Gullick et al.[88] demonstrate that the prognostic effect of this oncogene is equivalent in node-positive and node-negative patients, but they point out that, in order to reliably demonstrate prognostic effect of c-erb B-2 expression, large numbers of patients are required. This is because node-negative patients have a better prognosis than node-positive patients. They relapse and die less frequently. In addition, c-erb B-2 is expressed relatively infrequently.[87]

While studies concerning the significance of c-erb B-2 oncogene overexpression vary, there is substantial evidence that it is a useful prognosticator in breast cancer. Overexpression occurs more frequently in more advanced tumors that are more poorly differentiated.[89,90] Findings of Allred et al.[91] indicate that overexpression of c-erb B-2 oncogene is associated with poor clinical outcome (40% disease-free survival at 5 years compared to 80% in patients with c-erb B-2 negative tumors) in a subset of node-negative patients with small, ER-positive, invasive tumors. The possibility that c-erb B-2 could function as a growth factor receptor in ER-positive tumors supports the idea that this oncogene also plays a role in drug resistance.

Cathepsin D

Cathepsin D is a lysosomal enzyme that is synthesized in normal tissues but that may be overexpressed and secreted in certain breast cancers and appears to have a direct role in invasion and metastasis.[92] High cathepsin D levels increase the probability of recurrence (60% at 5 years) and poor survival in aneuploid node-negative breast cancer.[92,93] Table 38-5 summarizes information concerning possible prognostic indicators in breast cancer.

CLASSIFICATION AND STAGING

Once a breast cancer has been diagnosed, a complete evaluation of the disease is initiated to establish stage of disease and the most appropriate approach to treatment. Such planning and evaluation are optimally orchestrated by a comprehensive breast center where all

TABLE 38-5 Prognostic Indicators in Breast Cancer

Clinical/Pathologic Parameter	Method of Analysis	Value		Ref.	Significance/Additional Comments
		No. of Nodes	% 10-Year Survival		
Axillary lymph node status	Surgical pathologic examination	0 1–3 4+	70 40 15	72–80	Axillary lymph node status is the most important predictor of disease recurrence and survival. Approximately 30% of women with surgical/pathologic negative nodes will experience recurrence of their breast cancer following local therapy.
Occult micrometastatic lymph node involvement	Immunohistochemical methods and serial sectioning			94	Detection of occult micrometastatic disease in axillary nodes of node-negative disease correlates with a poorer prognosis.
Tumor size		≤1 cm 1–2 cm >2 cm		83 95,96	In tumors less than 1 cm (node negative), local therapy is usually adequate (5-year relapse-free survival 96%). In node-negative disease, tumors 1–2 cm in diameter with a high S-phase fraction have a 5-year relapse-free survival of 52%. In tumors greater than 2 cm, there is substantial relapse rate and aggressive therapy is generally indicated.
DNA analysis (content) Diploid Aneuploid	Flow cytometric analysis or Static cytophotometry	Diploid—DNA index of 1 (normal) Aneuploid—DNA index of >1.2 (abnormal)		82 81	S-phase fraction alone or in combination with ploidy may be more important prognostically than ploidy alone.
Proliferative indicators (measure growth fraction) S-phase fraction (SPF)	Titrated thymidine labeling Flow cytometry Immunohistochemistry	Low % of cells in S-phase (variable: generally <10%) High % of cells in S-phase (variable: >10%)		 98 97	A high-S-phase fraction is associated with a rapidly proliferating tumor and a worse prognosis. Diploid tumors have a lower risk for recurrence than aneuploid tumors. SPF provides useful prognostic information for predicting disease free survival for node-negative breast cancer patients with small ER positive tumors.
K-67 monoclonal antibody		High level of staining (>20% of tumor cells) is predictive of recurrence		84	Indicates cycling cell fractions that include parts of G^1 and G^2 phases of the cell cycle as well as S-phase.

(continued)

TABLE 38-5 Prognostic Indicators in Breast Cancer (continued)

Clinical/Pathologic Parameter	Method of Analysis	Value	Ref.	Significance/Additional Comments
Histologic grade (differentiation)	Histopathologic examination	Grade 1—well differentiated	96	The presence of glands is a strong indicator of good prognosis.
A combined histologic grading system takes into account mitotic activity, nuclear pleomorphism, and tubule formation		Grade 2—moderately well differentiated Grade 3—poorly differentiated	85	The presence of mitoses is a strong indicator of poor prognosis. High histologic grade is strongly associated with a high SPF.
Growth rate (tumor doubling time [dt])	Serial mammography	Tumor doubling time (dt) <75 to >130 days		The tumor growth rate correlates with the incidence of metastases 3 years following local treatment. Tumors with a dt of >130 days tend to be ER+, grade 1, whereas tumors with a dt between 75–100 days tend to be ER−, grade 3.
Epidermal growth factor receptor (EGFR)	Immunocytochemical assay	EGFR <20 fm/mg protein (favorable) >25 fm/mg protein (unfavorable)	86	May potentially facilitate proliferation of breast cancer cells in estrogen receptor negative breast cancer.
c-erb B-2 protein (HER 2 *neu* oncogene)	Immunohistochemical staining of cell surface membranes of tumor cells Immunoblotting	<2000 fm/mg protein Overexpression is reported as present or absent	87 88	Overexpression of c-erb B-2 protein may directly contribute to the malignant conversion of cells and have a direct impact on cellular growth control.
			90	Overexpression of c-erb B-2 is more common among tumors with poor nuclear grade and advanced stage.
			91	Overexpression of c-erb B-2 is associated with an increased mortality and may be an independent prognostic variable for survival in node positive patients. Controversy exists whether this oncogene is a reliable predictor of prognosis in node-negative women.
Cathepsin-D autocrine growth factor	Western blot analysis Immunohistochemical assay	Negative: <30 fm/mg protein (favorable) Positive: >60 fm/mg protein (unfavorable)		May be an important indicator of metastatic potential; may facilitate spread of cancer cells.
			85	High levels of cathepsin-D correlate with early relapse.
			91–93	Node-negative patients with high Cathepsin-D aneuploid tumors have a higher rate of relapse compared to cathepsin-D negative tumors.

(continued)

TABLE 38-5 Prognostic Indicators in Breast Cancer (continued)

Clinical/Pathologic Parameter	Method of Analysis	Value	Ref.	Significance/Additional Comments
Cytoplasmic P24 protein P24 is an estrogen-regulated secretory protein that is generally not detectable in normal breast tissue	Immunocytochemical analysis using a monoclonal antibody to P24 protein	Positive: >10% of cells show cytoplasmic staining for P24 protein Negative: <10% of cells show cytoplasmic staining for P24 protein	99	Patients with P24-positive tumors have significantly higher response to treatment, more prolonged duration of response, and duration of survival from diagnosis of metastatic disease compared to P24-negative disease. ER-positive tumors commonly stain positive for P24 protein compared to ER-negative tumors. P24 positivity occurs more commonly in histologic grade 1 and 2 tumors.
ER and PR receptors	Immunocytochemical staining (ER-ICA) Tumors that are positive for both ER and PR have a 75% response rate. ER+/PR− tumors have a response rate of only 30%	ER− <10 fm/mg protein ER+ >10 fm/mg protein PR− <10 fm/mg protein PR+ >10 fm/mg protein	77	About 60%–70% of primary breast cancers contain ER and 40%–50% have PR. Receptor content may change over time.
			100	Patients with receptor (+) tumors have a lower rate of recurrence and longer survival than those with receptor (−) tumors.

disciplines consult with the patient concerning her decisions regarding therapy.

In the initial evaluation, the diagnostic mammogram is utilized to look for evidence of tumor multicentricity or for evidence of bilaterality. The history and physical exam; routine blood work including complete blood counts, liver function tests, serum calcium; and a chest film are complete prior to the initial planning session. A bone scan and/or bone films are only indicated if there is a suspicious area suggesting tumor involvement. Likewise, a liver scan would only be indicated if liver function tests were abnormal.

Following the pretreatment evaluation, the patient is clinically staged on the basis of the characteristics of the primary tumor, the physical examination of the axillary nodes, and the presence of distant metastases. As previously mentioned, the clinical evaluation is inaccurate and, because of the prognostic significance of axillary node involvement, a pathologic stage is necessary to determine stage of disease.[100]

The pathologic staging recommended by the American Joint Committee on Cancer (AJCC)[101] is described in Table 38-6. This system is relatively complicated and can be simplified in terms of the most critical components, that is, whether or not nodes are involved and whether distant metastases are known to be present.

TABLE 38-6 Pathologic Staging System

PRIMARY TUMOR (T)	
Tx	Primary tumor cannot be assessed
T0	No evidence of primary tumor
Tis*	Carcinoma in situ: intraductal carcinoma, lobular carcinoma in situ, or Paget's disease of the nipple with no tumor
T1	Tumor 2 cm or less in greatest dimension
	T1a—0.5 cm or less in greatest dimension
T	T1b—more than 0.5 cm, but not more than 1 cm in greatest dimension
1	T1c—More than 1 cm, but not more than 2 cm in greatest dimension
T2	Tumor more than 2 cm, but not more than 5 cm in greatest dimension
T3	Tumor more than 5 cm in greatest dimension
T4†	Tumor of any size with direct extension to chest wall or skin
	T4a—Extension to chest wall
	T4b—Edema (including *peau d'orange*) or ulceration of the skin of the breast or satellite skin nodules confined to the same breast
	T4c—Both (T4a and T4b)
	T4d—Inflammatory carcinoma

(continued)

TABLE 38-6 Pathologic Staging System (continued)

REGIONAL LYMPH NODES (N)	
NX	Regional lymph nodes cannot be assessed (eg, previously removed)
N0	No regional lymph node metastasis
N1	Metastasis to movable ipsilateral axillary lymph node(s)
N2	Metastasis to ipsilateral axillary lymph node(s) fixed to one another or to other structures
N3	Metastasis to ipsilateral internal mammary lymph node(s)

DISTANT METASTASIS (M)	
MX	Presence of distant metastasis cannot be assessed
M0	No distant metastasis
M1	Distant metastasis (includes metastasis to ipsilateral supraclavicular lymph node(s)

STAGE GROUPING			
Stage 0	Tis	N0	M0
Stage I	T1	N0	M0
Stage IIA	T0	N1	M0
	T1	N1	M0
	T2	NO	M0
Stage IIB	T2	N1	M0
	T3	N0	M0
Stage IIIA	T0	N2	M0
	T1	N2	M0
	T2	N2	M0
	T3	N1,N2	M0
Stage IIIB	T4	Any N	M0
	Any T	N3	M0
Stage IV	Any T	Any N	M1

*Paget's disease associated with a tumor is classified according to the size of the tumor.

†Chest wall includes ribs, intercostal muscles, and serratus anterior muscle, but not the pectoral muscle.

Source: From the American Joint Committee on Cancer: *Staging for Breast Carcinoma* (3 ed), Atlanta, GA: American Cancer Society, 1989.

Stage I—localized disease only

Stage II—axillary nodal involvement pathologically

Stage III—more advanced locoregional disease without distant metastasis

Stage IV—distant metastases are present

TREATMENT ALTERNATIVES

Local-Regional Management

The current hypothesis governing the design of treatment alternatives for the woman with breast cancer contends that invasive breast cancer is a systemic disease involving complex host–tumor interactions and that variations in local regional therapy are unlikely to affect survival outcomes.[102,103] This hypothesis has been tested, and studies confirm that the vast majority of women, including those with stage I and II breast cancer with positive or negative nodes, can be treated by breast conservation procedures (lumpectomy, partial mastectomy, segmental resection, or quadrantectomy) and breast irradiation.[104,105] Patients who die from breast cancer have distant occult metastases at the time of local therapy or metastases from inadequately treated local or regional disease.[106] To this end, the possibility of multicentric tumors and the presence of nodal involvement become critical.

Multicentricity occurs frequently in breast cancer (9%–75%).[107] In patients with clinically occult, nonpalpable breast cancers detected by mammography, Schwartz and colleagues[108] reported a 44% incidence of multicentricity.

In NSABP, B-06 patients with stage I or stage II breast cancer (tumor size ≤4 cm) were randomized to total mastectomy or to segmental mastectomy alone, provided that margins of resection were free of tumor. All patients had axillary dissection. Results indicate that disease-free and overall survival were similar in all groups; however, those having breast radiation had significantly fewer breast recurrences compared to those having segmental mastectomy alone (10% vs. 39%).[109] These findings confirm the now standard approach to breast preservation, employing adjuvant radiation therapy to control multicentric disease. Most surgeons will advocate a wide local excision or partial mastectomy with a 1–2-cm margin of normal tissue as breast preservation surgery. The principal objective of this procedure is a cosmetic one, and if clean margins are not obtained, the mammogram reveals extensive macrocalcifications, the tumor is multicentric, there is a subareolar mass, or cosmesis is unacceptable, then a total mastectomy or modified radical mastectomy is appropriate.

The extent of axillary dissection is generally determined by the size of the primary tumor and the presence of palpable nodes. A low-level dissection is appropriate for in situ carcinoma where microinvasion is noted on pathologic examination of the primary lesion. Patients with invasive breast cancer require a level I and II dissection or a full dissection, depending upon whether axillary nodes are found to be positive for tumor. More extensive dissections are associated with breast and arm edema, especially when radiation is also used.

A modified radical mastectomy involves the removal of all breast tissue and nipple areola complex, and level I and II axillary node dissection. The pectoralis muscle is preserved. A horizontal incision is made because it is cosmetically more acceptable. Modified radical mastectomy is indicated for larger, multicentric disease or where cosmesis is otherwise not achievable. Modified radical mastectomy may also be employed as definitive treatment following local recurrence in patients who fail conservative surgery and radiation. In general, patients with noninvasive or focally invasive tumors have excellent prognoses following salvage mastectomy. However, patients with predominately invasive recurrent tumors are at significant risk for further relapse.[110]

Carcinoma in situ is becoming more of an issue in local control of breast cancer, owing to the success of mammography in detecting these small cancers. Lobular carcinoma is distinctive in that it does not present in any discernible clinical or mammographic manner, but is usually discovered by the pathologist during the removal of a benign condition. In 20%–30% of cases, lobular carcinoma tends to be bilateral, and the majority are multicentric.[106] Untreated lobular carcinoma carries an equal risk of development of invasive cancer in each breast. Treatment options range from observation including annual mammography with frequent physical examination, ipsilateral mastectomy with contralateral biopsy, or bilateral mastectomy with immediate or delayed reconstruction.

Intraductal carcinoma generally presents as clustered microcalcifications on mammography and rarely carries risk of axillary node involvement. Options for treatment include total mastectomy with low axillary dissection, wide excision followed by radiation, or wide excision alone. Because ductal carcinoma in situ frequently extends beyond the area of microcalcifications, a wide excision should include tumor-free margins around this area. Invasive carcinoma develops in about 30%–50% of patients within 10 years when excisional biopsy alone is selected as definitive treatment.[111] This accounts for the more widespread use of total mastectomy and low axillary dissection as definitive treatment, especially where poor prognostic parameters, such as ploidy and high nuclear grade, are present.[112] Research comparing the benefits of excision combined with radiation or excision alone for intraductal carcinoma demonstrates a recurrence rate of 10% after radiation, suggesting a benefit from radiation while conserving cosmesis.[113] In 1986, the NSABP initiated a prospective randomized trial to examine the natural history of ductal carcinoma in situ and the worth of segmental mastectomy (lumpectomy) alone versus segmental mastectomy plus ipsilateral radiation therapy. Until the findings of this study are definitive, breast-conserving surgeries are indicated only where it is possible to remove all mammographic evidence of disease and tumor-free margins.[103]

The role of radiation in the treatment of localized breast cancer has evolved over the years and is now standard treatment, making breast preservation a realistic possibility. In selected patients, irradiation of the regional lymph node areas may reduce regional recurrence and distant dissemination.[114] With an equivalent survival rate and preservation of the breast, conservative surgery plus radiation is now considered preferable to mastectomy for the majority of women. The major criteria for selecting patients for breast-conserving surgery and radiation therapy are, first, the feasibility of resecting the primary tumor without causing major cosmetic deformity and, second, the likelihood of tumor recurrence in the breast.[115] Mammography will usually reveal the extent of microcalcifications and whether or not multiple tumors in the breast can be removed without sacrificing cosmesis.

When residual tumor cells extend away from the primary tumor site, larger doses of radiation are required to control disease, and consideration needs to be given to the fact that the radiation dose that can be tolerated by the entire breast is smaller than the dose directed to the primary site.[115]

Likewise, radiation is more successful when complete resection of all gross disease has been accomplished. A reexcision of the primary site may be necessary to ensure an adequate tumor bed prior to radiation. In patients with close or involved margins, a boost to the primary site of at least 60 Gy may be needed to achieve sterilization of the bed.

Radiation doses to the breast are delivered using supervoltage equipment and tangential fields to minimize lung and heart exposure. The whole-breast dose ranges from 45–50 Gy delivered in about 5 weeks. Whether or not a boost is given depends upon the type of local excision and risk for local recurrence. The morbidity of a boost of moderate size and dose delivered either by electron beam or interstitial implantation is small.[115] However, in patients with a history of diminished lung capacity, radiation may be contraindicated.

The cosmetic result following partial mastectomy and radiation therapy is generally considered to be good. Breast edema, telangiectasia, and arm edema initially occur with radiation, and the cosmetic result may decline somewhat over the 3 years following therapy.

Radiation following modified radical mastectomy is reserved for patients with a high risk of local recurrence. Risk factors include tumors greater than 5 cm in diameter, positive axillary nodes, tumor involvement at the surgical resection, tumor invasion of muscle, or extranodal extension into the axillary fat. When chemotherapy is also employed, radiation is generally given concurrently to minimize local recurrence.[116]

Adjuvant Systemic Therapy

Early stage I and II breast cancer

Approximately 20 years of clinical research concerning the natural history of breast cancer supports the biological hypothesis concerning the presence of micrometastatic disease at diagnosis. Table 38-7 describes the factors influencing the design of adjuvant chemotherapy trials in curable breast cancer.[117] Scientific efforts have concentrated on finding optimal regimens of systemic therapy that can potentially destroy circulating tumor cells. The need for such research is paramount considering that nearly 90% of women newly diagnosed with breast cancer are potentially curable. Of that number, nearly 50%, or 70,000 women diag-

TABLE 38-7 Factors Influencing the Beginning of Modern Adjuvant Chemotherapy for High-Risk Operable Breast Cancer

By the time cancer becomes clinically detectable, it is advanced (near 30 doublings), and has made ample opportunity to establish distant micrometastasis.
Frequency of metastatic disease is directly related to tumor mass, and surgical cure rates drop as tumor volume at surgery increases.
Tumor growth fraction is inversely related to population size.
Effective drug kill follows first-order reaction kinetics.
Combination of drugs is superior to single agents and can eradicate 10–100 times as many cells.
In transplantable tumors, surgical adjuvant chemotherapy increases the long-term cure rates.
The optimal kinetic conditions to achieve cure exist when microscopic foci of disease are present after curative surgery and/or radiotherapy.

Source: With permission from Bonadonna G: Evolving concepts in the systemic adjuvant treatment of breast cancer, *Cancer Res* 52:2127–2138, 1992.

TABLE 38-8 Early Breast Cancer Trialists' Collaborative Group (Meta-Analysis)

14% overall reduction in the odds of death for those who received chemotherapy
CMF reduced the odds of death 23% (37% reduction in women younger than 50 years of age and a 9% reduction for older women)
16% overall reduction in the odds of death for women who took tamoxifen (20% reduction among women 50 years of age or older)
A longer duration of chemotherapy (12 months) was no better than 6 months of chemotherapy
At the 10-year analysis, polychemotherapy increased survival over that seen at 5 years
In women <50, ovarian ablation was associated with significant improvement in overall survival (25%)
Adjuvant immunotherapy (BCG) had no influence on recurrence-free or overall survival

Source: Data from Early Breast Cancer Trialists' Collaborative Group.[124]

nosed each year will have node-negative disease.[118] The results of prospective clinical trials suggest that the rate of disease recurrence in patients with node-negative breast cancer can be reduced 20%–50% by adjuvant therapy.[110,120–122] This led to the conclusion at the NIH Consensus Development Conference on Early Stage Breast Cancer held in 1990 that, although "the majority of patients with node-negative breast cancer are cured by breast conserving treatment or total mastectomy and axillary node dissection, the rate of local and distant relapse following local therapy for node-negative breast cancer is decreased by both combination cytotoxic chemotherapy and by tamoxifen."[123,p.4]

The Early Breast Cancer Trialists' Collaborative Group involved a worldwide meta-analysis of the results of randomized trials involving 75,000 women with early (stage I and II) breast cancer.[124] This large statistical analysis demonstrated that overall optimal use of adjuvant therapy can significantly improve long-term survival in women with stage I and II breast cancer. In addition, tamoxifen as well as ovarian ablation was shown to significantly reduce the incidence of contralateral breast cancer. Table 38-8 summarizes pertinent findings of the meta-analysis.

The ability of adjuvant chemotherapy to increase disease-free intervals has been observed in clinical trials, but its effect on overall survival has not been demonstrated until recently. The meta-analysis demonstrates a clinically relevant reduction in tumor mortality due to adjuvant chemotherapy.

Stage I (node-negative) breast cancer In certain subsets of women with node-negative breast cancer, the incidence of metastatic disease approaches 50%.[125] Combination chemotherapy can effectively reduce the annual odds of recurrence by at least 30% in this population. To accomplish this, the majority of patients will receive therapy unnecessarily because they have been cured by surgery alone or by virtue of the natural history of their disease were destined to fail, regardless of systemic therapy.

Currently, there are important prognostic indicators that help to determine a woman's risk of recurrence, such as ploidy, proliferative indices, and tumor grade, but no one parameter is indicative of recurrence (Table 38-5). Most clinicians agree that all women with node-negative breast cancer should receive adjuvant chemotherapy, especially those with larger tumors,[103] although not all agree with this approach.[117] Women with the lowest risk of recurrence are those with tumors less than 2 cm, a grade I malignancy, positive estrogen/progesterone receptors, and a low proliferative rate. In contrast, those with tumors larger than 3 cm, grade III malignancy, negative estrogen/progesterone receptors, and a high rate of proliferation are most at risk for recurrence. Table 38-9 summarizes selected clinical trials involving therapy of women with node-negative breast cancer.

Clinically, node-negative and node-positive patients are eligible for the NSABP B18 trial, which evaluates preoperative versus postoperative chemotherapy. Because the chemotherapy is given prior to surgery, it is possible to evaluate the response of the tumor and lymph nodes and to correlate this to disease-free survival and overall survival. It is also possible that the chemotherapy will permit more conservative surgery and decrease the incidence of ipsilateral tumor recurrence.

The NSABP protocol B-19 compared two differ-

TABLE 38-9 Cooperative Studies of Adjuvant Systemic Therapy in Node-Negative Disease

Study and Patient Eligibility Criteria	Design	Primary Research Question
NSABP B-18: ER/PR status unknown, node-negative or node-positive patients with palpable operable breast cancer whose diagnosis is established by FNA or core biopsy (all patients who have lumpectomy receive radiation)	Total mastectomy or lumpectomy + axillary dissection + AC × 4 vs AC × 4 followed by total mastectomy or lumpectomy plus axillary dissection	Will preoperative chemotherapy effectively prolong disease-free survival and overall survival compared to the same regimen given postoperatively? Will preoperative chemotherapy permit more conservative surgery and decrease the incidence of ipsilateral breast cancer recurrence? Will response of the primary tumor to preoperative chemotherapy correlate in any way to disease-free survival and survival?
NSABP Protocol B19: ER-negative, lumpectomy or total mastectomy and axillary dissection	M–F + L vs CMF	Is there a universally standard chemotherapy regimen for node-negative, ER-negative breast cancer? Recent findings indicate that CMF is superior to M–F + L.
NSABP Protocol B20: ER-positive, lumpectomy or total mastectomy and axillary dissection	TAM alone vs TAM + M–F + L vs TAM + CMF	Does the addition of tamoxifen to chemotherapy increase disease-free survival and overall survival significantly more than tamoxifen alone in ER-positive breast cancer?
NSABP Protocol B21: Occult invasive disease <1 cm, ER/PR status unknown, lumpectomy	TAM alone vs TAM + RT vs RT alone	What is appropriate therapy for clinically occult invasive breast cancer?
Intergroup Study 0102: ER-positive, high SPF, <2 cm tumor or ER-positive, ≥2 cm tumor or ER-negative tumors regardless of size	CAF ± TAM vs CMF ± TAM	Is cyclophosphamide, doxorubicin, and 5-fluorouracil superior to standard CMF in high-risk, node-negative breast cancer patients with or without tamoxifen?

Abbreviations: *TAM* = tamoxifen; *RT* = radiation, *CMF* = cyclophosphamide, methotrexate, 5-flurouracil; *AC* = adriamycin, cyclophosphamide; *CAF* = cyclophosphamide, adriamycin, 5-flurouracil; *M–F + L* = methotrexate, 5-flurouracil plus leucovorin.

ent chemotherapy regimens known to be effective in node-negative breast cancer. One regimen involves methotrexate followed in 1 hour by 5-fluorouracil (M-F). Leukovorin calcium (L) is begun 24 hours after the methotrexate. This regimen is compared to the standard cyclophosphamide, methotrexate, and 5-fluorouracil (CMF) therapy. Information gained in this study may help to identify a potentially universal, standard treatment for node-negative women. Recent analysis of this study indicates that both regimens offer at least a 30% risk reduction for recurrence, but CMF was superior to M-F + L overall. In the case of a woman with a small (<1-cm) tumor, either regimen is considered adequate therapy. The M-F + L appears to be less toxic in terms of myelosuppression and hair loss and does not have the leukemogenic potential of an alkylating agent–containing regimen. Furthermore, in premenopausal women, M-F + L does not affect gonadal function.

In a previous study, tamoxifen was found to be useful in premenopausal and postmenopausal, estrogen-positive, node-negative patients, representing a 30% reduction in risk of recurrence.[126] NSABP protocol B-20 asks whether chemotherapy (CMF or M-F + L) added to tamoxifen is superior to tamoxifen alone in node-negative women.

NSABP protocol B-21 considers whether or not long-term treatment with tamoxifen (with or without breast irradiation) is effective in prolonging disease-free survival in patients with occult invasive cancer less than 1 cm in clinical or mammographic size. Previous studies have demonstrated that tamoxifen reduces the incidence of local recurrence after lumpectomy and radiation and significantly decreases the incidence of contralateral breast cancer.[124,126] Consequently, the results of this study will help to determine whether or not radiation is necessary after lumpectomy, the impact of tamoxifen on recurrence, and whether the premise that tamoxifen prevents contralateral breast cancer will be upheld.

Intergroup study 0102 asks whether a doxorubicin-based regimen (cyclophosphamide, doxorubicin, 5-fluorouracil) (CAF) is superior to CMF in node-negative women deemed to be at high risk on the basis of tumor size (2 cm or larger) and proliferative activity (SPF). It is hoped that the benefits of doxorubicin in advanced breast cancer may prove of even greater benefit in patients with early, but high-risk disease.

Stage II (node-positive) breast cancer Women with tumor involving the lymph nodes are recognized as having a greater likelihood for distant recurrence and death. Postoperative chemotherapy, especially for premenopausal women age 50 and younger, is widely accepted.

Early clinical trials involving CMF confirmed the importance of nodal extent and established an inverse relationship between number of nodes and treatment outcomes.[127,128] These studies also demonstrate the efficacy of 6 months versus 12 months of CMF. CMF for 6 months has been the standard approach to node-positive breast cancer against which other regimens have been and are being compared. One such clinical trial was NSABP B-15. In this study, patients who received adriamycin and cyclophosphamide (AC) every 3 weeks for four courses did as well as those who received CMF for 6 months. While patients receiving AC experienced more immediate and profound hair loss, they experienced less nausea over time, visited health professionals one-third as often, and completed their therapy in much less time compared to those receiving CMF.

The efficacy of chemotherapy in postmenopausal women has not been sufficiently demonstrated. Tamoxifen has proven efficacy and, in a study involving almost 1200 patients, tamoxifen plus chemotherapy (AC) has shown greater benefit than tamoxifen alone.[129] In addition, this study failed to demonstrate an unfavorable interaction between chemotherapy and tamoxifen when administered simultaneously.[130]

In a summary study, Intergroup study 0100 compares CAF and concurrent or delayed tamoxifen with tamoxifen alone in post-menopausal, ER-positive, node-positive patients. This study will help to confirm or deny the worth of tamoxifen as standard therapy for this subset as well as further delineate the role of tamoxifen in the prevention of contralateral breast cancer.

Intergroup study 0101 is designed for premenopausal women with ER-positive tumors. All women entered on the study will receive 6 months of chemotherapy. The luteinizing hormone-releasing hormone (LHRH) antagonist, goserelin acetate (Zoladex: ICI Pharma, Wilmington, DE) with or without tamoxifen will be given following chemotherapy. Because tamoxifen does not totally block the effects of circulating estrogen, the addition of Zoladex may help to create a total estrogen blockade in these ER-positive patients.

In the absence of new chemotherapeutic agents, efforts to improve outcome in node-positive patients have focused on giving available drugs more effectively. Dose intensification may effectively increase intracellular drug concentration. With the addition of colony simulating factors, it may be possible to ameliorate the dose-limiting toxicity of myelosuppression, possibly preventing the need for dose reductions or treatment delays. Giving optimal doses at regular frequent intervals is also an important strategy in preventing resistance and ultimate recurrence of disease.

The specific objectives of Intergroup study 0108 are to compare the efficacy and toxicity in node-positive, receptor-negative breast cancer patients receiving either CAF or a 16-week multidrug regimen. The CAF regimen is given on days 1 and 8 every 28 days for six cycles in standard doses using oral cyclophosphamide. Patients on the 16-week multidrug regimen receive cyclophosphamide by mouth, doxorubicin, vincristine, and methotrexate by intravenous push, and 5-fluorouracil as a 2-hour infusion, 20 hours after the methotrexate. This regimen alternates with a 48-hour infusion of 5-FU every other week. This 4-month course of intensive therapy delivers the maximum amount of drug over a relatively brief time period. Because women with receptor-negative, node-positive disease represent a poor prognostic group, the use of a more intensified aggressive treatment is justified.

The use of this protocol emphasizes the potential benefit of drug scheduling. In this 16-week protocol, patients receive sequential methotrexate and 5-fluorouracil alternating with 5-fluorouracil infusion. Both measures attempt to enhance tumor cell kill by increasing exposure of 5-fluorouracil to tumor cells that cycle relatively slowly.

In 1989, the NSABP began Protocol B-22, the goal of which was to evaluate the effect of dose intensification and increased cumulative dose of postoperative adriamycin and cyclophosphamide (AC). The study involved all node-positive women regardless of ER status. This study closed mid-1991, and while it is too early to determine its worth, the conduct of the study is known, and this helped to establish optimal dose intensity for NSABP B-25.

The NSABP B-25 is a sequel to B-22 that looks at the value of not only dose intensification but also cumulative dose. All patients receive standard dose adriamycin. The cyclophosphamide dose is doubled and given for two courses in one group and for four courses in another group. The third group receives standard-dose cyclophosphamide for four courses. All patients receive colony stimulating factors. Tamoxifen is begun on day 1, continuing for 5 years (50 years and over age group).

This is an important study because it will help to delineate the role of dose-intensive chemotherapy in high-risk women. In addition, because colony stimulating factors are given, it is hoped there will be fewer dose reductions and less myelosuppression. Further, the findings of this study will help to define the role of dose intensity as it relates to autologous marrow transplant in high-risk breast cancer. (Table 38-10 summarizes selected studies in node-positive breast cancer.)

Locally advanced breast cancer (stage III)

Locally advanced breast cancer is associated with high risk of developing distant metastases. The larger the size of the primary tumor and the greater the number of histologically positive lymph nodes, the greater

TABLE 38-10 Cooperative Studies of Adjuvant Systemic Therapy in Node-Positive Breast Cancer

Study and Patient Eligibility Criteria	Design	Primary Research Questions
ECOG 4188 (Intergroup 0100): Postmenopausal, ER-positive, mastectomy ± radiation	TAM vs CAF × six cycles + TAM for 5 years vs CAF × six cycles followed by TAM for 5 years	How does TAM alone compare with chemoendocrine therapy in postmenopausal ER-positive patients? Is there a difference in response rate between patients who receive TAM concurrent with chemotherapy compared with those who receive TAM after the last course of chemotherapy?
ECOG 5188 (Intergroup 0101): Premenopausal, ER-positive, lumpectomy + axillary dissection ± radiation, mastectomy ± radiation	CAF × six cycles vs CAF followed by goserelin acetate × 5 years vs CAF followed by goserelin acetate ± TAM for 5 years	Is the addition of goserelin acetate to CAF with or without TAM superior to CAF alone?
ECOG 3189 (Intergroup 0108): ER-/PR- negative tumor ≥5 cm, mastectomy with or without radiation	CAF × six cycles vs 16-week multidrug regimen	Is a 16-week multidrug regimen superior to standard CAF in the treatment of ER-negative, node-positive breast cancer? Are the toxicities of the two regimens comparable?
NSABP protocol B-25: All age groups, node positive (1 or more) ER positive or negative, lumpectomy + axillary dissection + RT or mastectomy ± RT	AC: comparison of three dose schedules every three weeks I: A—60 mg/m² × 4 C—1200 mg/m² × 4 vs II: A—60 mg/m² × 4 C—2400 mg/m² × 2 vs III: A—60 mg/m² × 4 C—2400 mg/m² × 4 plus TAM × 5 years (all patients >50)	Will giving larger but fewer doses of cyclophosphamide (dose intensification) in combination with adriamycin and colony stimulating factors effectively prolong disease-free survival and survival more than the same cumulative dose of cyclophosphamide given over a prolonged period of time? Will increasing dose intensity as well as cumulative dose of cyclophosphamide more effectively prolong disease-free survival and survival than the same dose intensity but for a shorter period of time?

the risk of metastasis and death.[132,133] These tumors by virtue of their size (>5 cm) are not amenable to treatment by breast-conserving surgery, and modified radical mastectomy is generally the treatment of choice if surgery is possible. Clinical characteristics of locally advanced disease include large or unresectable primary tumors, fixed axillary nodes, involvement of internal mammary nodes, and the classic inflammatory carcinoma. While distant metastasis are presumed to be present, it is not clinically apparent at staging.

If the tumor is fixed to the chest wall, inflammatory carcinoma is present, significant ulceration exists, or the axillary nodes are fixed to one another or other structures, the situation is generally considered to be inoperable due to the almost certain risk of recurrence.[134,135] The presence of supraclavicular lymph nodes is considered distant metastasis rather than locally advanced breast cancer; however, in the absence of more distinct distant metastasis, these patients are often grouped with locally advanced breast cancer.

The prognosis of these patients is rarely improved by local therapy alone, and while many physicians approach these patients with a purely palliative intent, the role of systemic therapy is becoming more widely accepted. Results are superior when chemotherapy is combined with radiation.[136–138] The use of primary (neoadjuvant) chemotherapy has resulted in significant tumor regression in 60%–90% of women.[136] The advantages of this approach include in vivo assessment of response. Significant tumor shrinkage may permit resection in a previously unresectable disease and even less extensive surgical procedures. Primary chemotherapy also provides immediate treatment to presumed metastasis that would otherwise be delayed by local therapy. Primary chemotherapy also prevents/avoids the theoretical postsurgery growth spurt of metastatic disease. Combined modality therapy employing primary chemotherapy results in complete disappearance of disease in many patients including those with inflammatory cancer.[135] Some studies report significant improvement in disease-free intervals and survival 5–14 years after treatment.[138,139] Not all studies report such findings. Rubens and colleagues[140] utilized chemotherapy (CMF) and tamoxifen together with radiation therapy. There was a significant improvement in disease-free survival, but no significant overall survival.

High-dose chemotherapy with autologous bone marrow rescue and hematopoietic growth factor support is currently an option for treatment for women with high-risk advanced disease. The toxicities of this treatment are significant, with a mortality rate of up to 20%. The principal causes of death include infection, hemorrhage, and organ damage. The therapeutic benefit of ABMT has yet to be definitively established in breast cancer.

Other areas of research include the use of alternating non–cross-resistant regimens in an attempt to treat potentially resistant heterogenous cell lines.[141,142] Table 38-11 describes chemotherapy regimens commonly used to manage advanced local disease.[100]

Nursing Considerations in the Care of the Woman with Localized Breast Cancer

The majority of women who suspect a breast cancer or are told they have a suspicious lump will seek information from friends or others who have experience with the disease. Women today are active health consumers who commonly seek information regarding their options. It is not uncommon for the nurse to be called upon for advice concerning where a woman might go for a consultation concerning how a suspicious mass should be investigated. If a comprehensive breast center is available in the area, the woman should be referred to the center for an opinion. In any case, the woman should not delay in seeking medical attention; indeed, most women view the need for a definitive diagnosis as a psychological emergency.[143,144] Fortunately, nurses and physicians who specialize in breast cancer realize this and generally mobilize resources to provide a swift and accurate assessment of the breast problem. While a breast cancer diagnosis causes significant emotional, social, economic/vocational upheaval, such distress eases over time as therapy is planned and carried out. Most women actively participate in the decision-making process and are able to clearly articulate their need for information throughout treatment planning and months of therapy. To be a supportive advocate for the woman and her family, the nurse must be knowledgeable concerning the options for therapy, the goals of therapy, measures to minimize complications of treatment, and the various resources that may need to be mobilized throughout the treatment period and beyond.

For rehabilitation to be optimal, the nurse pays careful attention to the woman's expressed need for information at each juncture of treatment. Seeking

TABLE 38-11 Adjuvant Chemotherapy Regimens in Advanced Localized Breast Cancer

Acronym	Drugs	Dose (mg/m^2)	Cycle Frequency	Duration
CMF ± P	Cyclophosphamide Methotrexate 5-fluorouracil Prednisone	100, PO days 1 to 14 40, IV days 1 and 18 600, IV days 1 and 18 40, PO days 1 to 14	Every 28 days	6 cycles
CMF	Cyclophosphamide Methotrexate 5-fluorouracil	600, IV day 1 40, IV day 1 600, IV day 1	Every 21 days	12 cycles
CMVP	Cyclophosphamide Methotrexate 5-fluorouracil Vincristine Prednisone	60, PO daily 15, IV weekly 400, IV weekly 0.625, IV weekly for 10 weeks 30, PO daily for 14 days 20, PO daily for 14 days 10, PO daily for 14 days	NA	1 year
FAC	5-fluorouracil Adriamycin Cyclophosphamide	500, IV days 1 and 8 50, IV day 1 500, IV day 1	Every 21 days	6 cycles
CAF	Cyclophosphamide Adriamycin 5-fluorouracil	100, PO days 1 and 14 30, IV days 1 and 8 500, IV days 1 and 8	Every 28 days	6 cycles
AC	Cyclophosphamide Adriamycin	600, IV day 1 60, IV day 1	Every 21 days	4 cycles

Source: Modified from Osborne CK: Breast cancer, in Wittes RE (ed), *Manual of Oncologic Therapeutics,* Philadelphia: Lippincott, 1992, pp. 146–153.

information is a valuable coping device and yet rarely useful unless the woman recognizes the need for it. The right amount of accurate information will help the woman formulate questions and will facilitate decision making, decrease anxiety, and enhance overall adjustment to the illness and treatment.[145]

How well a woman adjusts psychologically and socially to the diagnosis and treatment will depend upon her previous coping strategies and emotional stability. In addition, social support has consistently been found to influence a woman's adjustment through treatment.[146] The threat to emotional, social, sexual, and physical well-being is multifaceted, and the relative impact of these factors on adjustment varies from patient to patient and assumes varying degrees of importance at different stages of treatment.

A strong source of social support will be extremely valuable throughout all phases of treatment. While the most important sources of social support are the woman's spouse, her family, and friends,[147] other sources of support may also be needed to maintain a strong social network. The roles of the psycho-oncologist, the social worker, and various support groups are important adjuncts to the care of these women and their families.

The patient's need for information will vary considerably throughout each phase of treatment. It is not uncommon for the treatment plan to include surgery, radiation, and chemotherapy. For many women the time of active treatment lasts at least 6 months, and most do not feel rehabilitated for up to a year following their diagnosis. If reconstruction is planned, this rehabilitation phase will be extended.

Surgical considerations

The current options for surgical management of stage I and II breast cancer include breast-preserving surgery and radiation or modified radical mastectomy.

The cosmetic result of breast-preserving surgery is generally considered to be acceptable, as body image is maintained. Prior to surgery, it is important to emphasize that the breast will appear different from the other breast depending on the size of the breasts and amount of tissue removed. Scar tissue may form causing some contracture over time, but most women find the cosmetic result acceptable, especially when wearing a bra.

Complications following breast-preserving surgery include arm edema, seroma formation and wound infection, shoulder dysfunction, upper extremity weakness, fatigue, and limitations in mobility.[148,149] Complications more specific to axillary node dissection include nerve injury and axillary vein thrombosis.

Postoperative complications following mastectomy include wound infection, flap necrosis, and seroma formation. A transverse incision is associated with less skin flap necrosis compared to the less cosmetically acceptable vertical incision. Seromas occur in about 10% of patients and generally resolve following aspiration. Antibiotics may be indicated to manage infection.

Lymphedema following mastectomy may be transient or permanent and may occur in the early postoperative period or much later. Lymphedema is more likely to occur in women who have postoperative radiation to the axilla, infection, seroma formation, or flap necrosis or who are obese.

Nursing care of the postmastectomy patient centers on wound care, with special attention to maintaining functioning wound drains. If drains become blocked, the wound is more likely to develop a seroma/hematoma leading to infection and possibly flap necrosis. Drains may be irrigated if necessary to maintain suction and an adherent flap. Drains are usually removed within 2–4 days following surgery.

Postmastectomy exercises to maintain shoulder and arm mobility may begin as early as 24 hours after surgery. The woman is instructed to maintain the affected arm in the adducted position but to perform limited exercises involving the wrist and elbow. Flexing fingers and touching the hand to the shoulder are encouraged. Squeezing a ball is discouraged, as it increases blood flow and, if done too vigorously, leads to swelling in the early postoperative period (see Table 38-12—"Postmastectomy Exercises" and Table 38-13—"Hand and Arm Precautions").

Prior to discharge, the patient should have clear instructions regarding wound care. Initial care of the wound involves maintaining a clean incision with dressing changes daily if indicated. A return appointment is usually made to remove stitches. At that time the patient should receive specific instructions regarding postmastectomy exercises. A mild analgesic may be indicated to promote arm mobility during exercises and prevention of shoulder dysfunction.

Care of the axilla involves avoiding the use of depilatory creams, strong deodorants, and shaving under the arm for approximately 2 weeks following surgery.

Instructions regarding breast self-exam and follow-up are best given during the first outpatient visit after surgery. Introducing the patient to various prosthesis and mastectomy bras can occur in the hospital, but women are generally more ready to receive this information once the surgery is behind them. Most are not advised to wear a prosthesis until the wound has healed completely (6–10 weeks). In this time period, the woman may want to meet with a Reach to Recovery or Y-ME volunteer who will assist her in learning about resources in her area for purchasing a prosthesis. There are many different kinds of prostheses; some are foam filled, liquid silicone filled, or are the more permanent self-adhering variety. It is important that the prosthesis fits properly and that the weight is similar to the remaining breast. Insurance pays for most prostheses provided a prescription or letter demonstrating medical necessity is submitted.

The woman alone or together with her husband

TABLE 38-12 Postmastectomy Exercises

When to Begin	Purpose	Exercises: Perform Exercises 5–10 Times Each, Three Times a Day
Postoperatively days 1–5	Prevent and/or reduce swelling	• Position arm against your side in a relaxed position. Elbow should be level with your heart, and the wrist is just above the elbow when resting. • Rotate wrist in a circular fashion. • Touch fingers to shoulder and extend arm fully.
After drains are removed	Promote muscle movement without stretching	• While standing, brace yourself with your other arm and bend over slightly, allowing your affected arm to hang freely. Swing the arm in small circles and gradually increase in size. Make 10 circles—rest—repeat in the opposite direction. • Swing arm forward and back as far as you can without pulling on the incision. • While standing, bend over slightly and swing arms across the chest in each direction. • While sitting in a chair, rest both arms at your side. Shrug both shoulders, then relax. • While sitting or standing, pull shoulders back, bring the shoulder blades together.
After sutures are removed	To stretch and regain full range of motion. To gain mobility of your shoulder, you must move it in *all* directions, several times a day	• While lying in bed with arm extended, raise arm over your head and extend backwards. • While lying in bed, grasp a cane or short pole with both hands across your lap. Extend arms straight up and over your head and return. • Repeat, rotating the cane clockwise and then counterclockwise while over your head. • While standing, extend arm straight over your head and down. • Extend your elbow out from your side at a 90° angle—hold it for 10 seconds—relax. • Extend your arm straight out from your side even with your shoulder—extend arm straight up toward the ceiling. • Stand at arms' length facing a wall. Extend arms so your fingertips touch the wall. Creep fingers up the side of the wall, stepping forward as necessary. Repeat the procedure going down the wall—keep arms extended. • Stand sideways to the wall. Extend arm out so fingers touch the wall. Creep up the wall a little more each day. • Use hand and arm normally (see hand and arm precautions).
After 6 weeks	To strengthen arm and shoulder and to regain total use of arm and shoulder	• Begin water aerobics. • Begin overall fitness program. • Begin aerobics, Jazzercise, or other resistive exercises.

(spousal designate) should have the opportunity to discuss any physical or emotional concerns regarding sexual relations. Evidence is mounting to support the contention that, while the diagnosis of breast cancer and the loss of a breast are certainly emotionally distressing for all concerned, they do not result in an increased prevalence of psychiatric disorders or sexual dysfunction.[150–152] The woman's overall psychological health, relationship satisfaction, and prior sexual relations are far stronger predictors of sexual health than the extent of breast surgery. As a group, however, younger women have consistently been found to experience more episodes of depression, anger, resentment, sexual problems, and fears of recurrence compared to older women.[153,154]

Chemotherapy

Perhaps a more important consideration in the occurrence of sexual dysfunction throughout the months following surgery is the effects of chemotherapy and hormone therapy.[150,153,155,156] Many premenopausal women who receive chemotherapy will experience ovarian failure and early menopause, especially if an alkylating agent is included in the treatment regimen. The probability of premature menopause occurring and being permanent increases for women over age 35.[157] In a study by Knopf,[158] 56% of premenopausal and 41% of postmenopausal women receiving CMF or CMFVP reported decreased frequency and quality of sexual relations. Seventy-two percent of the premenopausal

TABLE 38-13 Patient Information—Hand and Arm Precautions

Do not permit injections, blood samples, or vaccinations to be done on your affected arm unless specifically recommended by a physician who is aware of your surgery.
When trimming cuticles, take extra care not to tear hangnails.
Wear heavy gloves when gardening and digging or handling thorny plants.
Always use a thimble when sewing to avoid pinpricks, and wear rubber gloves while washing dishes.
Protect your arm from burns, especially from small appliances such as irons or frying pans, and from the sun.
Be sure your hand and arm are well protected with an elbow-length mitt when reaching into a hot oven.
Always have blood pressure measurements taken on the opposite arm.
Avoid arm constriction from tight elastic, sleeves, or jewelry.
Do not carry heavy objects—especially grocery bags or luggage—or push heavy furniture.
Apply a good lanolin cream several times daily if your skin appears dry.
Treat cuts and scratches by washing the area well and applying an antiseptic. Contact your physician if signs of infection, redness, warmth, or swelling occur.

Source: With permission from Cooley ME, Erikson B: Rehabilitation, in Fowble B, Goodman RL, Glock JH, Rosato EF (eds), *Breast Cancer Treatment: A Comprehensive Guide to Management*, St. Louis, MO: Mosby Year Book, 1991, pp. 511–583.

women had menopausal symptoms, and more of these women reported changes in sexual relations compared with those who did not experience menopausal symptoms.

Premenopausal women who receive chemotherapy should be clearly informed of their risk for temporary or permanent ovarian failure. Women experiencing ovarian failure generally experience less subjective desire and arousability, vaginal dryness, vulvar/vaginal soreness, a burning pain, and light spotting after intercourse. Women should be encouraged to use a water-soluble lubricant during vaginal intercourse to minimize discomfort.

Other menopausal symptoms that commonly occur in women receiving chemo/hormonal therapy include hot flashes, sweats, and irregular menses. Hot flashes and profuse perspiration may be most troublesome at night and may interfere with sleep. Some women may benefit from lowering the thermostat in the home, especially where they sleep. Avoiding highly seasoned foods, caffeine, and alcohol may minimize the frequency of hot flashes. Dressing in loose-fitting cotton clothing and in layers, so a sweater or jacket can be removed during a hot flash, is advised. Women can try vitamin E, 800 IUs per day or, if this is ineffective, Bellargel-S®, one tablet twice daily[159] may be prescribed. A low-dose clonidine patch (Catapress Transderm®) may effectively control hotflashes. Side effects of clonidine include a dry mouth, headache, irritability, and dizziness.[160] Although no significant changes in blood pressure or pulse have been noted with low-dose clonidine, the patient's blood pressure should be checked once or twice a week during the first few weeks on clonidine therapy.

Weight gain is a troublesome side effect of therapy and is commonly felt by patients to occur because of water retention. In fact, it is due to increased caloric intake.[161] Significant correlations exist between weight gain and subjective feelings of unhappiness, worry, and increased distress regarding appearance when these women were compared to women who lost or maintained their weight.[158] Factors contributing to weight gain include prednisone, oral cyclophosphamide, taste changes, increased appetite, depression, mild nausea that is relieved by eating, and psychological distress.[145,162–165]

Women need to receive nutritional counseling regarding the avoidance of weight gain at the outset of therapy. Some gain as much as 15 pounds and find it very difficult to lose once therapy is over. This adds to their increased distress and is avoidable with counseling.

Fatigue is a common subjective complaint associated with adjuvant therapy, and symptoms such as total body tiredness, forgetfulness, and wanting to rest increase over time throughout therapy.[166,167] Women should be encouraged to interject rest periods into their normal schedule and, if possible, to begin a regular exercise program such as walking or water aerobics. In addition to combating fatigue, exercise helps to minimize nausea associated with treatment. Nausea and vomiting with chemotherapy is predictable based on the type of chemotherapy or hormone therapy treatment. Patients on methotrexate and 5-FU experience less nausea and vomiting than women receiving CMF. Oral cyclophosphamide is associated with more prolonged nausea compared to intravenous cyclophosphamide. Women on higher doses of adriamycin and cyclophosphamide experience intense nausea and vomiting for 48–72 hours following therapy if appropriate antiemetics are not employed. Most women will usually not experience nausea and vomiting on the first day of their therapy especially when given 32 mg of ondansetron (Zofran®) plus 20 mg of dexamethasone over 45 minutes as a single dose. However, the nausea and vomiting are worse on the second and third day posttreatment. Therefore, patients need a clear plan for managing these unpleasant symptoms for at least 72 hours posttreatment. Ondansetron, 8 mg orally every 6–8 hours, prochlorperazine, 15-mg spansules, and lorazepam, 1 mg every 12 hours for 2 days following therapy, are effective in minimizing these symptoms.

Adriamycin and cyclophosphamide (AC) are commonly used in curable breast cancer, which means many women experience total alopecia within 2½–3 weeks of beginning therapy. This is highly distressing and contributes greatly to feelings of loss and body image changes. Women need to be aware of when and how hair loss will occur and have a plan to manage hair loss. Some women prefer shaving their heads or cutting the hair very short to minimize the constant and annoying shedding of their hair. The American Cancer Society's "Look Good, Feel Better" program is an excellent support and resource for women experiencing not only hair loss but body image changes in general.

Women on methotrexate-5-fluorouracil therapy do not lose significant amounts of hair and rarely require a wig. Women receiving CMF experience gradual thinning over the 6–8 months of therapy and may require a wig only towards the end of treatment. Hair begins to grow back within a month of ending therapy at a rate of ¼ inch per month with some variation. Women, especially younger ones, often are able to go without a wig or head covering within 4 months of therapy. Large earrings, a little more makeup, and hair mousse enable a woman to feel attractive and stylish in the early recovery period (see Chapter 33 for a more complete discussion of alopecia).

Radiation

Radiation generally begins within 3–4 weeks following chemotherapy. Women commonly experience fatigue, some nausea, but primarily skin changes and arm and breast swelling. Breast edema is unique to patients undergoing breast-preserving surgery and radiation and usually appears during the treatment or within 1–6 months of treatment. Breast edema is more common in women who have had an axillary dissection where more than 11 nodes are removed and in those also receiving adjuvant chemotherapy. Skin reactions occur in all patients and generally present as itching, dryness, scaling, redness, and tenderness. The breast may feel sore and warm to touch. Patients are instructed not to use soap to wash the area and to pat dry. Dry desquamation can progress to a moist desquamation with infection. (For a complete discussion on skin care changes during radiation, see Chapter 33.)

Arm edema occurs in about 10% of patients who have axillary dissection in addition to radiation.[168] Symptomatic pneumonitis characterized by a dry cough and low-grade fever is infrequent, but can appear within 2–3 months of therapy and is more common in women receiving methotrexate-5-FU concurrently. Brachial plexopathy manifesting as paresthesias, with or without arm and hand weakness, may be transient or permanent, but is an infrequent complication. Rib fractures and cardiac complications are also rare and relate to dose and whether concurrent chemotherapy is also given.

Pregnancy and the Woman with Curable Breast Cancer

The fact that women are delaying parenting into their mid-30s, the increasing incidence of cancer in premenopausal women, early detection measures, and successful treatment outcome make the issue of pregnancy a particularly important topic. Having a diagnosis of breast cancer is frightening and makes one poignantly aware of mortality and the experiences one truly wants in life before dying. Parenting is something some women have an intense desire to experience. Approximately 25% of all breast cancer patients will develop their disease during their childbearing years.[169] Approximately 7% of premenopausal women have one or more pregnancies after treatment for breast cancer, with 70% of these occurring within the first 5 years after treatment.[170,171]

The most important considerations in the potential effect of pregnancy in a woman with a history of breast cancer are whether or not the hormonal changes from pregnancy might stimulate growth of occult disease, the risk for genetic alterations in offspring, and the woman's overall risk for recurrent breast cancer.

While it is true that hormone changes of pregnancy may potentially influence the behavior of a breast cancer, there are no data to suggest that pregnancy subsequent to successful breast cancer treatment worsens a woman's prognosis.[171,172] In women who have node-negative disease, it is unreasonable and scientifically unfounded to encourage a delay of 2 years before attempting pregnancy. These women may gain nothing but lost time by waiting. Even early-stage patients who experience a local recurrence following breast conservation therapy remain curable by mastectomy. On the other hand, for patients at high risk for recurrence, there is no time span beyond which their risk lessens.

Counseling the woman who wishes to become pregnant following successful breast therapy involves, above all else, attention to what is known concerning prognosis as it relates to pregnancy and the individual woman's prognosis. The decision must be reinforced as hers alone. The best service the professional can offer is to help the patient and her family understand the uncertainties and risks involved.

BREAST RECONSTRUCTION

Breast reconstruction has come to be regarded as a viable and acceptable component in the treatment of breast cancer. In the past decade, improved procedure techniques and advances in the manufacture of implants have enabled many women to retain their self-confidence and body image, thereby enhancing their quality of life. Prior to the advent of plastic surgery for the treatment of breast cancer, many women found the external prostheses cumbersome and consequently felt it necessary to alter their activity and/or selection of clothing due to fear of displacement or discomfort of the prosthesis.

Despite the recent findings equating the two surgical procedures (mastectomy vs. lumpectomy plus radiation), in terms of survival, many women either choose or are advised to have a mastectomy. This decision may be based on a variety of circumstances including histologic findings, emotional or body image issues, financial considerations, or accessibility of medical resources.

A woman who presents with diffuse microcalcifications or multicentric disease throughout the breast is not considered a suitable candidate for breast preservation.[173] Some patients are troubled by the fact that, although the cancer appears to have been removed, an occult lesion may remain, and consequently they will choose to remove the breast. Additionally, cosmesis may be compromised because too great a proportion of breast tissue needs to be removed to ensure clear margins. Patients who are responsible for a substantial portion of their medical bills may forego the cost of radiation treatments and choose mastectomy. Other women find that suitable medical facilities for radiation treatments may require extensive travel time or are geographically unavailable.

Implants are considered to be safe and effective treatment despite recent media attention to the contrary. Citing the potential harmful effects of silicone implants revealed in an ongoing investigation, the FDA imposed a moratorium on the use of silicone implants for augmentation and issued guidelines to limit the use of silicone implants for reconstruction.

To qualify for placement of silicone implants, certain criteria must be met. The surgeon informs the patient of the possible side effects as well as documents that the patient fulfills an "Urgent Need" that has been predetermined by the FDA. Additionally, the patient is enrolled in a registry to aid in the long-term tracking of these patients.

Initially, the criteria were very stringent, but the revised guidelines issued in August 1992 expanded the eligibility regulations. The patient must be 18 years of age or older. Women who have experienced cancer, other disease, or trauma may have immediate or delayed reconstruction. Implants may be placed in any woman who currently has silicone implants and needs replacement or revision for medical or health reasons resulting from augmentation or mastectomy surgery. Women with congenital defects or severe asymmetry are considered candidates for silicone implants. Additionally, women who require augmentation of the unaffected breast for any of the preceding reasons may have an implanted silicone prosthesis. Additional information on current guidelines issued by the FDA is available from the American Society for Aesthetic and Plastic Surgery or the American Society of Plastic and Reconstructive Surgeons at 1-800-635-0635.

The patient exclusion criteria includes pregnancy or lactation, tissue abnormalities, and increased risk due to other treatment or psychological issues. Women who demonstrate active infection, lupus, or scleroderma or uncontrolled diabetes are not candidates for the procedure. Patients experiencing radiation damage, problems with vascularization, or who have inadequate tissue available are considered to be ineligible. The surgeon may declare any patient unsuitable who possesses any other physical or psychological condition that will compromise compliance and/or success of the surgical procedure.

Although implants are considered a viable and acceptable choice, other avenues continue to be explored. Autologous transplants have provided a suitable alternative to the inert prosthesis in certain circumstances. These procedures include latissimus dorsi flap, TRAM (transverse rectus abdominis muscle) flap, and free transfer of abdominal or gluteal tissue.[174]

The silicone implant was introduced in the 1960s, and the basic design remains relatively unchanged today. The saline tissue expander is used as a temporary device or may function as a more permanent implant to remain in place until more is known regarding the potential risk of the silicone implants.

The timing of the consultation is very important because of the myriad of considerations to be addressed prior to surgery. In the past the general rule of thumb was to delay reconstruction, sometimes waiting months to years. Currently, surgeons who recognize that the psychological trauma associated with the loss of a breast may be lessened by more timely reconstruction will, after careful assessment, offer the patient immediate reconstruction. However, the woman's general health and/or treatment plan may indicate that a delay in reconstruction be considered.

The ideal candidate is one who has early-stage disease without nodal involvement and low risk factors for recurrence. Heavy smokers may be advised to quit smoking or significantly reduce daily use to ensure an adequate blood supply. The surgeon will also attempt to identify those who may be subject to additional problems such as hypotension or hypoxia, which may compromise circulation and impact on the success of the surgical procedure.[173] Patients who present with extensive local or metastatic disease may need further evaluation regarding chemotherapy and/or radiation therapy, which may necessitate a minor or significant delay in reconstruction due to immunosuppression and/or skin changes.

During the initial consultation the surgeon additionally evaluates and addresses the patient's and family's expectations of surgery. This may be done through the use of before and after pictures as well as the surgeon's frank explanation of the expected outcome. A patient with realistic expectations is more likely to accept the expected imperfections when these aspects are known prior to surgery. The goals of reconstructive surgery are to achieve "acceptable" symmetry and softness, correct any deformity caused by prior treatment, and construct an adequate nipple areolar complex.

Silicone Implants

Silicone implants are used for reconstruction when the surgeon has ascertained that adequate skin is or will be available postmastectomy. The surgery is usually done in stages (i.e., the implant is placed during one procedure, the nipple areolar complex is constructed during another procedure, and some additional surgery may be needed subsequently to attain the desired cosmetic result).

An ideal candidate for a silicone implant is a woman who is small breasted with a minimum of ptosis on the contralateral breast. If the patient's opposite breast needs revision to achieve symmetry, an implant placement and/or mastopexy will be performed at the same time.

The procedure entails incising part of the mastectomy scar or using the mastectomy incision to form a pocket beneath the chest wall muscles and inserting the silicone prothesis. Placing the implant beneath the chest wall muscles helps counteract the expected firmness due to capsular contraction and supports the implant.[174]

The complications that may arise are progressive contracture, hematoma, infection, and flap necrosis. Contracture is an expected sequela of silicone implants and is the result of scar tissue enveloping the prothesis. However, some patients will experience increasing contracture that alters and deforms the breast. New implants are being designed with an attempt to reduce the incidence of contracture, which has been calculated at 35%–55%.[175,176] Hematomas occur infrequently and are most often surgically drained. Infections happen rarely and are most often successfully treated with antibiotics or removal of the implant in extreme cases. Flap necrosis can be serious and, if extensive, may necessitate the removal of the prosthesis. Usually, the necrosis involves a small amount of tissue that is excised.[173]

Saline Tissue Expanders

Saline expanders are used when an inadequate supply of skin is available at the mastectomy site or when a large and/or ptotic breast is required. Tissue expansion is the most frequently used reconstructive procedure.[177] The expander is placed behind the chest wall muscles using the lines of the mastectomy incision.

The expanders have a filling port that is either located remotely or on the anterior of the implant. After allowing sufficient time for wound healing, a series of injections is performed as an office procedure. The saline expanders, which are partially filled at the time of insertion, usually require 60–120-cc injections on a weekly or biweekly basis. The expansion continues until the device is overinflated by approximately 50%, usually in 6–8 weeks.[174] The overfilled expander is left in place for several months to allow for accommodation of the stretched tissue. This overfilling helps to promote a more natural, supple contour of the reconstructed breast (Figure 38-15). The expander is then removed and a permanent prosthesis of lesser fluid volume is placed.

Contracture is a complication that may hinder or prevent further expansion. Deflation can occur spontaneously or as a result of needle puncture. Expanders with remote ports are less likely to be accidentally deflated.

Latissimus Dorsi Flap

The latissimus dorsi flap is used when inadequate skin is available at the mastectomy site and/or if additional tissue is needed to fill the supraclavicular hollow and create an anterior axillary fold following a radical mastectomy (Figure 38-16). An ellipse of skin along with the latissimus dorsi muscle is rotated onto the mastectomy site. The viability of the tissue is maintained through the thoracodorsal vessels (Figure 38-17).

Flap necrosis is rare due to the abundant vascularization of the area. This surgery takes 3–4 hours, approximately double the time needed for an implant procedure.

TRAM Flap

The transverse rectus abdominis muscle flap has been commonly referred to as the "tummy tuck." During

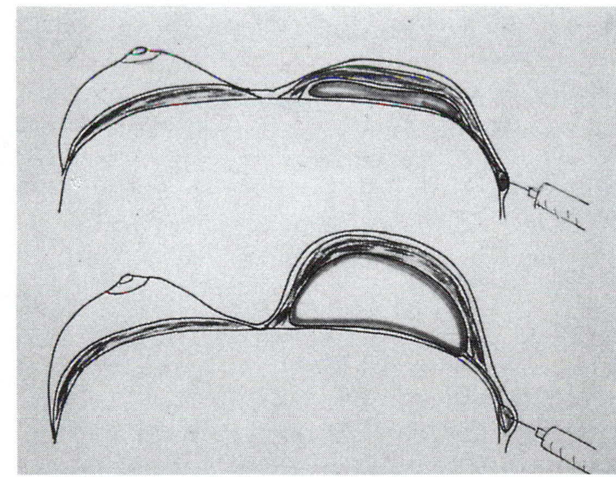

FIGURE 38-15 The horizontal view illustrates the overexpansion that is needed to allow for a more natural suppleness when the permanent prosthesis is implanted. (Courtesy of Dr. Craig Bradley, MD, Senior Attending Plastic and Reconstructive Surgery RPSLMC, Chicago.)

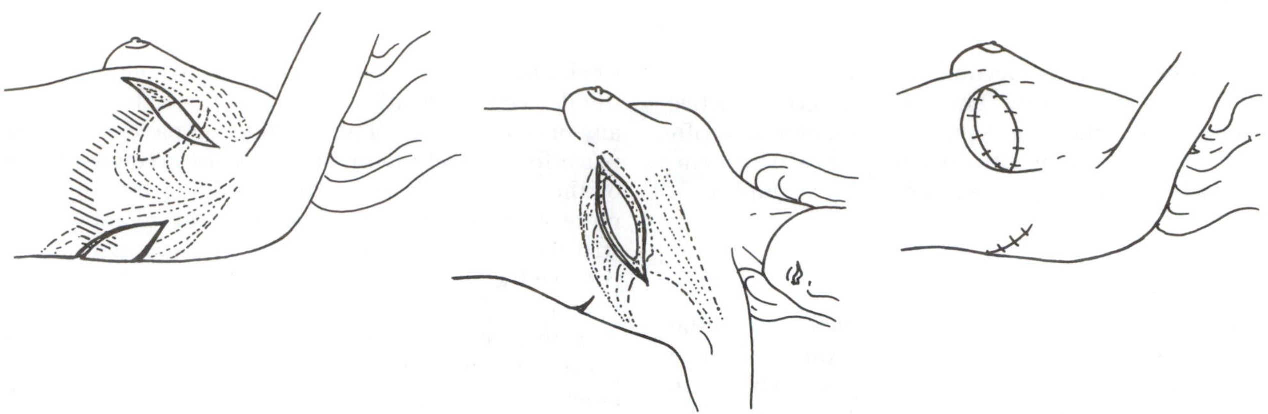

FIGURE 38-16 A diagram of the latissimus dorsi procedure. (Courtesy of Dr. Craig Bradley, MD, Senior Attending Plastic and Reconstructive Surgery RPSLMC, Chicago.)

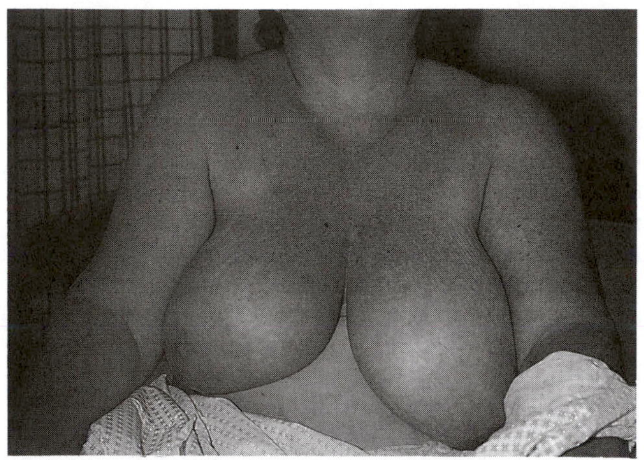

A

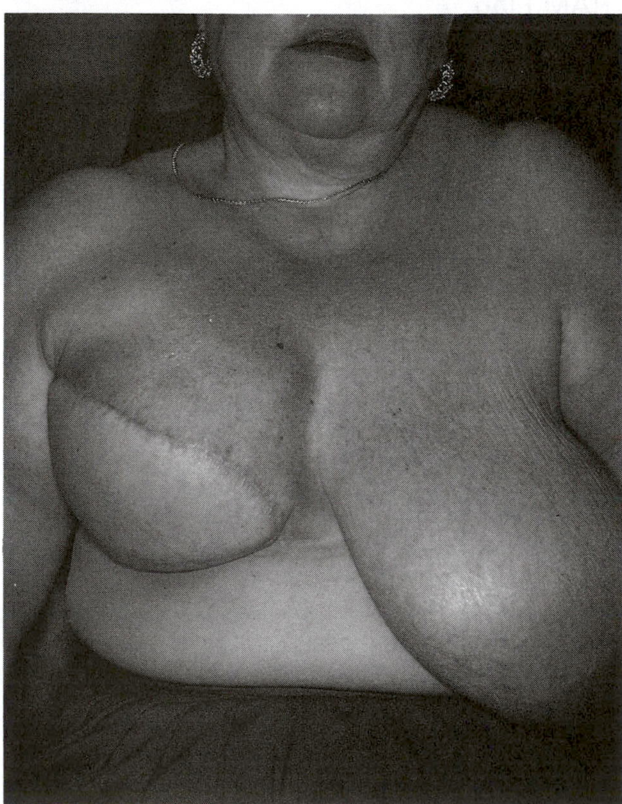

B

this procedure a low transverse ellipse incision is made and abdominal muscle and fat are tunneled under the abdominal skin to the mastectomy site. Tissue viability and perfusion are retained by the abdominal rectus muscle (Figure 38-18 and Figure 38-19).

Possible complications are hernia at the donor site, which can be remedied by the placement of synthetic mesh, and flap necrosis, which may be largely avoided by careful selection of the candidates. Obese patients (>20% overweight), those with circulatory problems, smokers, and those over 65 are not considered eligible for this procedure.[173]

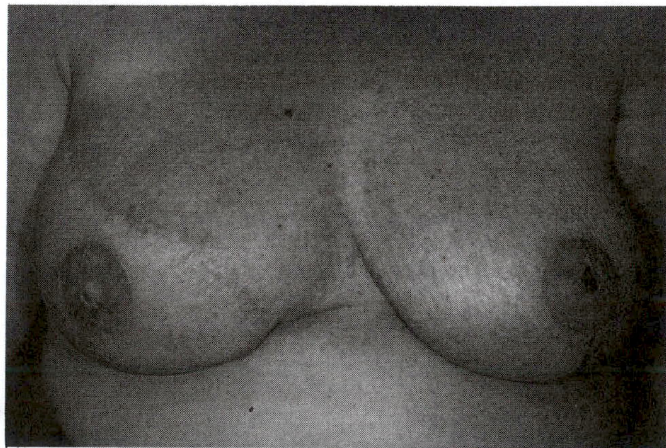

C

FIGURE 38-17 Three pictures illustrate a large woman (a) before the procedure, (b) after the mastectomy and latissimus dorsi flap and, (c) after mastopexy was performed to reduce the size of the other breast. Note the appearance of the tattooed nipple, which closely resembles the reduced breast. (Courtesy of Dr. Craig Bradley, MD, Senior Attending Plastic and Reconstructive Surgery RPSLMC, Chicago.)

Free Flap

The free flap represents the newest technique in reconstructive surgery. This procedure entails removing a portion of the skin and fat from the buttocks or lower abdomen and grafting it to the mastectomy site with microvascular anastomoses. This is a complicated procedure that demands microsurgical technique from two teams of surgeons; one to remove the flap and one to prepare the recipient vessels. The success of this operation depends on the reliability of the anastomoses of the vessels to ensure adequate nourishment of the tissues. The main complication is failure to maintain sufficient perfusion in the postop period. Tissue death will ensue within 6 hours if flow is interrupted and cannot be sustained.[177]

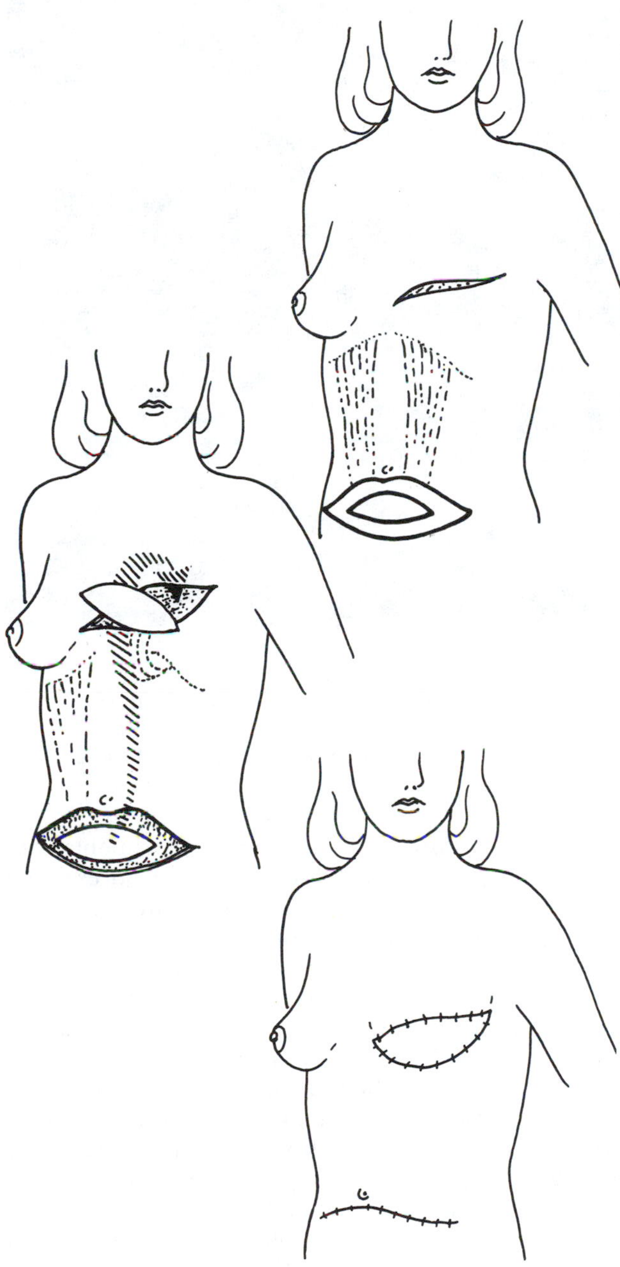

FIGURE 38-18 A diagram of the TRAM flap procedure. (Courtesy of Dr. Craig Bradley, MD, Senior Attending Plastic and Reconstructive Surgery RPSLMC, Chicago.)

Nipple Areolar Construction

The nipple-areolar complex is the final phase of the reconstruction process. The symmetry and cosmetic result of the breast mound should be satisfactory before this procedure is performed. The nipple should closely match the opposite side in size and pigment.

Tissue may be taken from the opposite breast if there is an adequate supply or if mastopexy has been performed. Previously, the nipple was often "banked" to the patient's thigh or groin to be used later. This method has fallen out of favor due to the risk of introducing potentially malignant tissue to the disease-free breast.

If the areola in the opposite breast is too small to permit adequate tissue transfer, other pigmented areas may provide suitable substitute tissue. Areas commonly used are the inner thigh, supraclavicular, and postauricular. Some of these grafts fade with time, and tattooing may be needed to darken the area at a later date. Local tissue is often used, followed with tattooing (Figure 38-20).

Maintaining projection is a challenge that has been met by construction of pedicle flaps. These techniques employ folding the skin to achieve a slightly protuberant nipple. The most popular method is the skate flap technique, in which the skin is raised and folded to achieve a natural nipple profile.

Complications are rare with this reconstruction, but those that may occur are failure to maintain suitable projection of the nipple, graft failure, and fading of the pigmented areas.[178]

METASTATIC BREAST CANCER

Approximately 10% of women diagnosed with breast cancer have metastatic disease at clinical presentation, and 30%–40% of women diagnosed with and treated for potentially curable breast cancer will have metastatic disease and eventually die. The majority of patients who relapse (80%) do so within 2 years of the diagnosis. The median survival time for stage IV disease is 2–3 years; however, reports of 5-year survival range from 12%–35% and 10-year survival from 5%–22%.[179]

The most common mode of metastasis is via the lymphatics, whereby the cells may be transported to

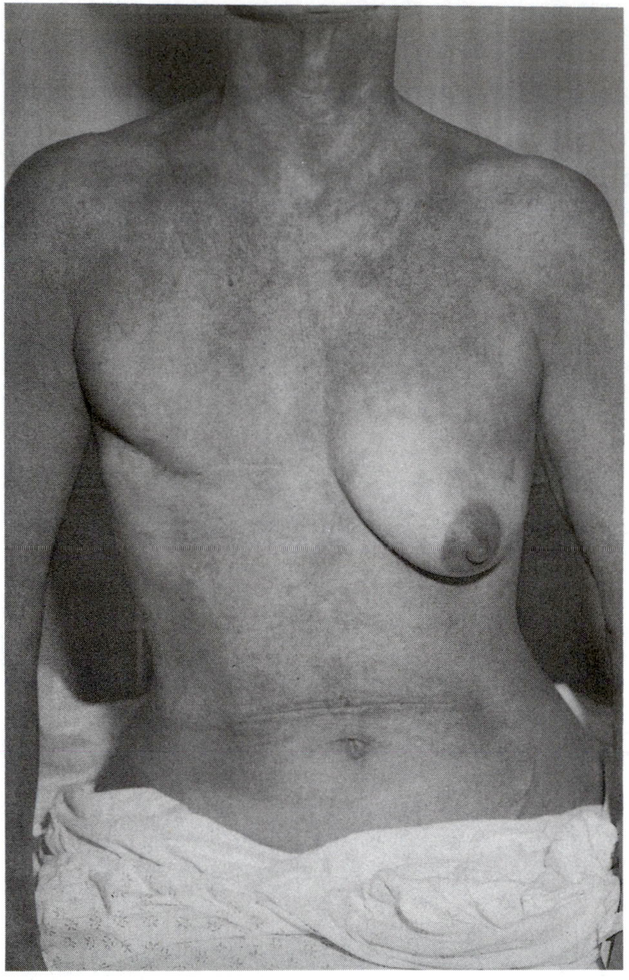

A

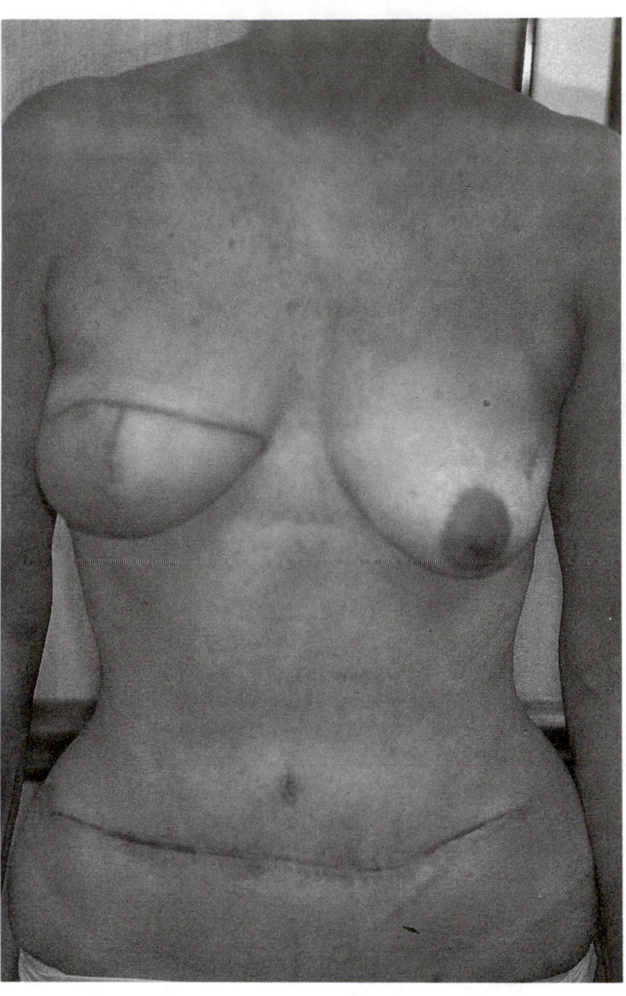

B

FIGURE 38-19 First picture shows a patient (a) after mastectomy and before the TRAM flap. The second and third pictures show the (b) anterior and (c) lateral view of the same patient shortly after the procedure. The scars will fade with time. (Courtesy of Dr. Craig Bradley, MD, Senior Attending Plastic and Reconstructive Surgery RPSLMC, Chicago.)

local and more distant regional nodes. Conversely, breast cancer cells may enter the lymphatics by direct penetration. More virulent cancer cells can directly enter the blood vessels and spread to distant sites without evidence of lymph involvement. Once blood borne, malignant cells adhere to the vascular endothelium, stimulating endothelial retraction and exposing the underlying basement membrane, whereby a metastatic deposit and invasion of the structure occurs.

Breast cancer most commonly metastasizes to bone (>50% of patients), specifically the spine, ribs, and proximal long bones. Patients will commonly complain of localized, deep-seated, unrelenting pain. Pathologic fracture of the proximal femur may occur spontaneously despite efforts to protect the weakened bone. Likewise, persistent back pain may herald a compression fracture and possible neurologic impairment. Hypercalcemia may reflect bone resorption due to tumor growth and resultant osteoclastic stimulation. Bone marrow metastasis occurs frequently in patients with extensive multifocal bone disease, generally presenting as bone marrow failure or as fleeting nocturnal pain.[180]

Loss of appetite and abnormal liver function tests are early symptoms of liver involvement. Late symptoms include pain, abdominal distention, nausea, emesis, periodic fever, jaundice, and generalized weakness. Pulmonary involvement may begin as a subtle, nonproductive cough or shortness of breath. Lymphangitic pulmonary spread is an ominous sign of rapidly progressive disease. Pleural effusions can progress slowly over time and respond temporarily to drainage and sclerosing. Renal involvement generally presents as oliguria and/or uremia in a woman with deteriorating mental status. Brain metastasis usually occurs in the supratentorial region, multiple sites, or as carcinomatous meningitis presenting as cranial nerve palsies, altered mentation, seizures, and/or focal paresis. Local cancer spread to the chest wall usually presents as a

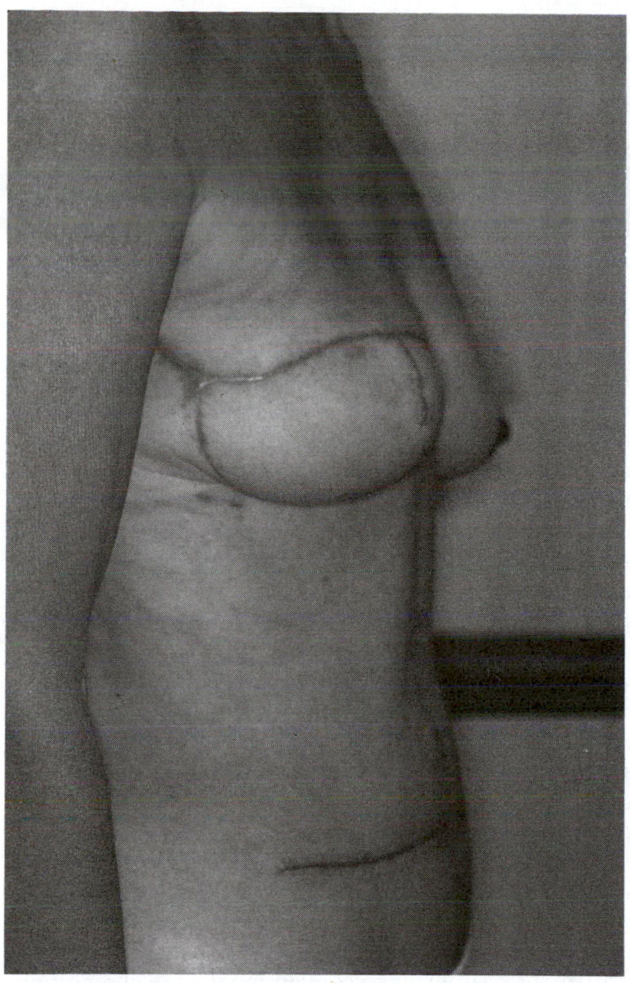

C

FIGURE 38-19 (continued)

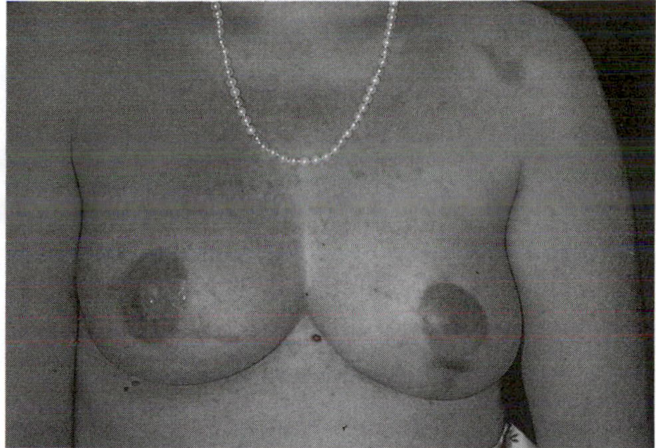

FIGURE 38-20 Right breast reconstruction following a modified radical mastectomy. Unilateral nipple tattoo on the right is compared to the patient's own unaffected nipple on the left following mastoplexy. (Courtesy of Dr. Craig Bradley, MD, Senior Attending Plastic and Reconstructive Surgery RPSLMC, Chicago.)

painless subcutaneous nodule along the mastectomy scar and adjacent chest wall areas. These lesions may respond well to local therapy, but distant disease is presumed to be present.

The management of patients with metastatic breast cancer is aimed at judicious use of local and systemic measures that palliate symptoms and improve quality of life. The initial choice of therapy is generally the one that is the least toxic and carries with it the highest response rate.[181] The basic strategy is to achieve optimal control of the disease and temporize for as long as possible. Local and systemic therapies are added periodically as needed until they have outworn their usefulness. For many women, especially those with hormone receptor positive disease, this can mean many years of quality of life.

It may be difficult for a woman with metastatic disease to understand why her doctor is not recommending more aggressive treatment. The idea that a new or different treatment is introduced only with evidence of disease or troublesome symptoms causes some women to ask why the treatment was not given to prevent the problem before it occurred. The answer is based on the desire not to make the woman more ill than her disease is making her and the knowledge that these therapies, including chemotherapy, have only a small effect on the median survival of women with metastatic disease. The goal is to get as much mileage out of each therapy as possible without compromising quality of life unless temporarily and absolutely necessary. However, an exception involves the patient who is asymptomatic or minimally symptomatic, is desirous of therapy, and is not likely to require significant palliation for 3–6 months. In this situation it is entirely appropriate and optimal that the woman be introduced to innovative and experimental treatment protocols ongoing in cancer centers and cooperative cancer study groups. Their participation in these studies is critically important to women who desire more than what is currently available as well as to the overall research effort in breast cancer.

Defining Extent of Disease

An assessment of the extent of disease is made to determine the most appropriate therapeutic approach and to determine response to therapy. Such clinical studies as chest film, liver scan, bone scan, MRI, and cytologic analysis of the cerebral spinal fluid may be indicated based on the woman's symptoms. Tumor measurements are taken periodically to determine response to therapy. Serum carcinoembryonic antigen (CEA) and Ca153 are important markers that indicate tumor activity often before clinical symptoms appear.

Chemotherapy

Women who have a disease-free interval of less than 2 years, have hormone receptor negative disease, are refractory to hormone therapy, or have aggressive disease in the liver or pulmonary system are candidates for chemotherapy[100] (Table 38-14).

Combination chemotherapy results in higher response rates compared to single agents. Response rates vary from 50%–70% and can last for 9–12 months. The rate of complete response (percentage of individuals in whom all evidence of disease disappears) consistently has been only 10%–20% of cases.[182]

Currently, methotrexate-5-fluorouracil plus leucovorin, cytoxan-methotrexate-5-fluorouracil, mitoxantrone-thiotepa, or cytoxan-adriamycin-5-fluorouracil are among the more commonly used regimens. Doxorubicin-containing regimens have shown a 10%–20% better response rate, but currently offer no significant survival advantage over combinations not containing doxorubicin. For women who are elderly and prefer a regimen that does not cause hair loss or significant nausea, mitoxantrone and thiotepa or methotrexate-5-fluorouracil + leucovorin are available. For women who fail on first line therapy, 5-FU may be given as a continuous infusion with or without leucovorin with good results, even in those who previously failed on 5-FU.[183,184]

The majority of combination regimens are administered either monthly or in divided doses twice a month. Once a response is documented and ensured, lengthening the interval between treatments is useful to decrease cost and inconvenience to the patient and does not ordinarily sacrifice therapeutic benefit.

Individuals with slow growing disease and those with rapidly progressing disease will benefit from chemotherapy. The response of women to cytotoxic agents is not significantly related to the predominant site of disease. Women with visceral metastases as well as those with bony involvement will respond. Although radiologic evidence of bone healing may take as long as 6 months, subjective improvement occurs within a shorter time.

Newer approaches to treatment of metastatic breast cancer are currently ongoing. Verapamil, tamoxifen, and high dose phenothiazines may be effective in blocking drug resistance, thereby facilitating increased cellular uptake of drugs like doxorubicin and vincristine.[185] The use of chemohormonal therapy, specifically tamoxifen and doxorubucin, may afford a degree of synergism. Alternating non–cross-resistant combinations of agents may also prove useful in attempting to increase survival in metastatic disease. Phase II and III clinical trials involving taxol, a plant-derived anticancer drug, are ongoing and appear promising, with 50% response rate in metastatic breast cancer. Monoclonal antibodies directed against tumor cells can, when coupled with chemotherapy, possibly increase specificity of chemotherapy while sparing normal tissues.[186]

Most studies involving autologous bone marrow rescue in breast cancer are appropriate only for very good-risk metastatic disease. The treatment usually involves standard or high-dose induction chemotherapy to induce a good tumor response followed by dose-intensive chemotherapy and reinfusion of the bone marrow.[187] If the patient experiences a good response to the first ABMT, the procedure may be repeated a second time.

Current evidence does not demonstrate that high-dose chemotherapy with autologous bone marrow transplant is superior to conventional-dose chemotherapy for treatment of metastatic breast cancer.[188] Furthermore, the risk of transplantation is high in terms of mortality, organ failure, toxicities, and quality-of-life measures.

TABLE 38-14 Commonly Used Regimens for Advanced Breast Cancer

Acronym	Drugs	Dose (mg/m²)	Response Rate (%)	Median Duration of Response (months)
CMF ± P	Cyclophosphamide	100, PO days 1 to 14	49%–59%	5–8
	Methotrexate	40, IV days 1 and 8		
	5-fluorouracil	600, IV days 1 and 8		
	Prednisone	40, PO days 1 to 14; repeat every 28 days		
FAC	5-fluorouracil	500, IV days 1 and 8	50%–75%	6–10
	Doxorubicin	50, IV day 1		
	Cyclophosphamide	500, IV day 1; repeat every 21 days		
AC	Doxorubicin	40, IV day 1	40%–80%	6–12
	Cyclophosphamide	200, PO days 3 to 6; repeat every 21 days		
CAF	Cyclophosphamide	100, PO days 1 to 14	60%–80%	10–12
	Doxorubicin	30, IV days 1 and 8		
	5-fluorouracil	500, IV days 1 and 8		

Source: With permission from Osborne CK: Breast cancer, in Wittes RE (ed), *Manual of Oncologic Therapeutics,* Philadelphia: Lippincott, 1992.

A goal of research in this area is to identify and treat patients with very low tumor burden or those who have sensitive responding tumors but are clearly incurable by conventional methods. The Eastern Cooperative Oncology Group trial (EST2190) will examine bone marrow transplant as adjuvant intensive therapy in breast cancer patients at risk for early relapse (stage II or III with at least ten involved axillary nodes). The results of this study and others will help to define the role of transplant therapy in breast cancer.

Endocrine Therapy

Women who have estrogen receptor positive breast cancer demonstrate a consistently superior survival after recurrence compared to women who are estrogen receptor negative.[189,190] Endocrine therapy is one of the major forms of treatment of the woman with metastatic breast disease. It is well known that the growth of normal mammary tissue is influenced by a variety of steroid hormones. Normal mammary cells contain cytoplasmic receptor sites for each of the hormones known to influence the growth and function of the mammary gland, specifically, estrogen, progesterone, and prolactin.

Steroid hormones can promote the growth of a breast cancer if the cells are hormonally dependent. In a woman who has a hormonally dependent tumor, estrogen enters the cell and binds to a specific cytoplasmic receptor protein called *estrophillin* or estrogen-receptor protein. The estrogen-receptor hormone complex is then believed to undergo transformation and enter the cell nucleus to promote tumor growth. It is thought that if the source of estrogens is removed by surgical ablation or medication manipulation, or if the hormone's access to the estrogen-receptor protein is blocked by anti-estrogens, the chain of action is broken and the tumor regresses. Tumor cells that lack the cytoplasmic estrogen-receptor protein should not be expected to regress with hormonal or anti-estrogen therapy.

The amount of estrogen-receptor protein present in a tumor remains relatively constant throughout the course of a woman's disease, and its measurement provides information about the degree of hormone dependency of a tumor.

Premenopausal women have a lower incidence of receptor-positive tumors (30%) than postmenopausal women (60%), and perimenopausal women have the lowest rate (10%).

Receptor-negative disease is usually associated with a short disease-free interval and more aggressive disease. Receptor-positive tumors are generally associated with a long disease-free interval between initial treatment and recurrence. These women often have slow growing disease, usually in soft tissue or bone.

In summary, treatment with hormonal therapy, either additive or ablative, is indicated when there are metastases, the metastases are not amenable to treatment by surgery or radiotherapy, the disease is not life-threatening, and the tumor is estrogen-receptor positive. Because endocrine therapies generally have the same efficacy, the least toxic is used first. In postmenopausal women, tamoxifen is used first. In premenopausal women, it is arguable whether oophorectomy or tamoxifen is less toxic (Table 38-15).[191]

Estrogens

In women who are 5 or more years past menopause, the administration of pharmacologic doses of estrogens (diethylstilbestrol [DES], 5 mg orally two or three times per day) can result in an objective remission in about 35% of the cases, lasting several months to many years. The average duration of response is 1 year. DES has been found to be comparable to tamoxifen in efficacy.[192] Administration of high doses of exogenous estrogens suppresses pituitary follicle-stimulating hormone (FSH) and luteinizing hormone (LH) and therefore the production of endogenous estrogens.

At the initiation of therapy, nausea and occasional vomiting may occur for a few days. Nausea and vomiting accompanied by progressive lethargy or polyuria are symptoms of hypercalcemia, which may occur with the initiation of therapy but is not necessarily an indication for discontinuing therapy. The woman taking estrogens should be instructed to limit sodium intake and be aware that she is likely to retain fluid and have decreased bladder tone as a result of estrogen administration. Diuretics are frequently needed to control fluid retention. Increased pigmentation of the nipples and areolas and enlargement of the breasts are other side effects.

Objective evidence of tumor regression is seen most often in women with soft tissue disease. When the disease is reactivated, estrogen therapy is terminated. Estrogen withdrawal occasionally will result in a reinduction of a brief partial remission. Individuals may experience uterine bleeding with estrogen withdrawal. Women who respond to estrogen therapy and then experience a relapse may benefit from other forms of endocrine therapy.

Androgens

Androgens are most effective in women who are 5 or more years postmenopause. The overall response rate is 20%. Androgens exert their therapeutic effect by opposing endogenous estrogens. Androgen therapy may be added to oophorectomy in women under 35 years of age, but response rates are low. In the postmenopausal woman, androgens are indicated for the treatment of soft tissue or bone metastases. For visceral or pulmonary lesions, the response rate is less than that achieved with estrogens.[193]

Several androgens are available. The most widely accepted is fluoxymesterone (Halotestin), 20 mg per day orally. About 3 months of therapy with fluoxymesterone is needed before the maximum benefit is

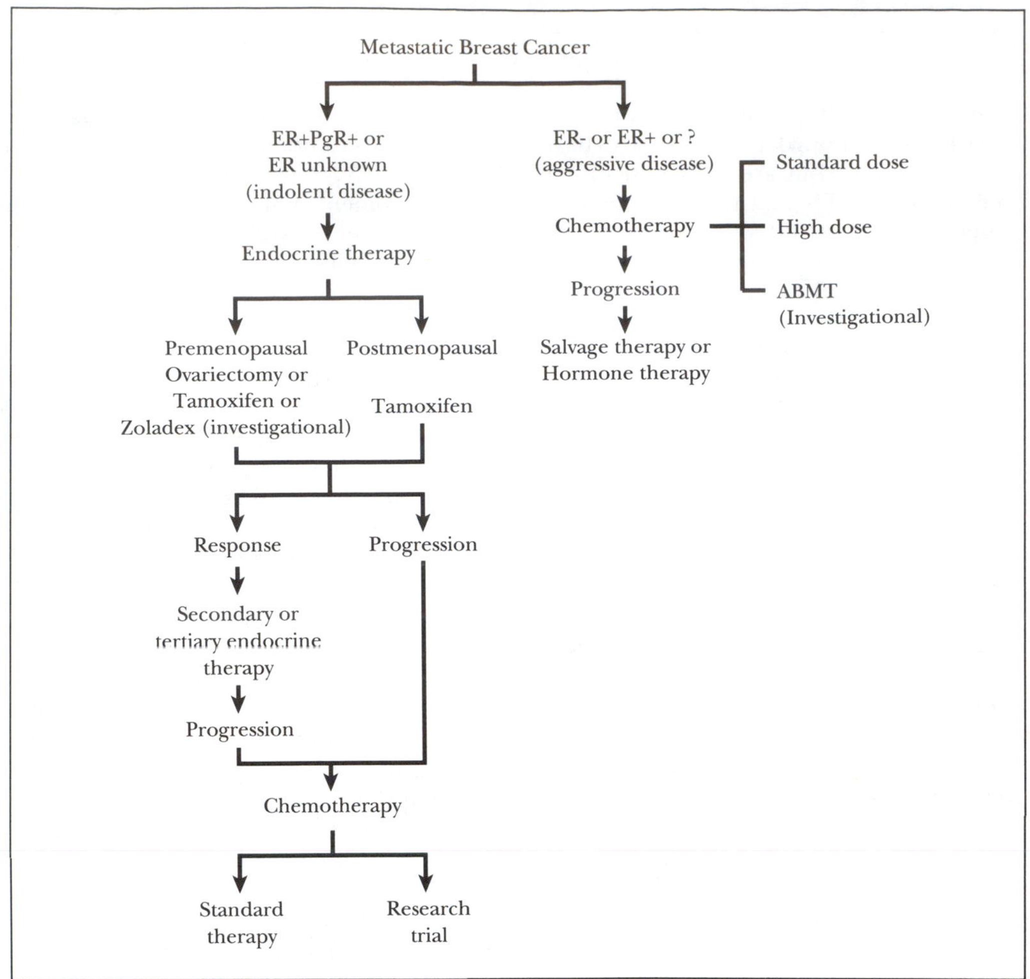

FIGURE 38-21 Therapeutic Options in Metastatic Breast Cancer (Source: Henderson IC, et al.[191])

achieved. The systemic effects of fluoxymesterone include fluid retention, erythrocytosis, and masculinization. The woman may experience an increased libido, hair loss, amenorrhea, and occasionally anorexia and nausea. In the woman who is premenopausal or early menopausal, there is the danger of precipitating hypercalcemia in the first few weeks of androgen therapy, and serum calcium levels should be monitored.

Progestins

Megestrol acetate is a progestational agent with a response rate of 26%–30%, with a median duration of up to 22 months.[194] The standard dose of megestrol acetate is 160 mg once a day. This drug is generally tolerated as well as tamoxifen and is comparable in efficacy. The most important side effect is weight gain, which occurs in up to 50% of patients. This weight gain is related primarily to increased food intake and increases with higher doses.[195] Other side effects include hot flashes, vaginal bleeding, hypercalcemia, tumor flare, and thrombophlebitis.

Corticosteroids

Pharmacologic doses of corticosteroids (prednisone, 30 mg orally every 8 hours, or dexamethasone, 6 mg orally every 8 hours) can result in an objective response in approximately 30% of women with metastatic breast disease. Corticosteroids suppress pituitary adrenocorticotropic hormone (ACTH) secretion, thereby opposing estrogen-progesterone secretion from the adrenals. The response generally lasts only 3 months. Corticosteroids are often used as adjuncts to radiotherapy of cerebral metastasis, in chemotherapy of advanced liver and lung metastasis, and in the management of hypercalcemia. The rate of response with steroids is not as great as with ablative procedures, nor is the duration of response as long. Because of their anti-inflammatory action, steroids can reduce peritumor edema, thereby relieving symptoms of cerebral and pulmonary metastasis. Steroids also increase the individual's appetite and feeling of well-being and can reduce pain from bone or visceral metastasis. The side effects and complications may be serious and include bleeding peptic ulcer, muscle weakness, hypertension, infection, edema, glucose intolerance, moon facies, and osteoporosis.

Anti-estrogens

Tamoxifen is a potent anti-estrogen and is indicated for the treatment of both primary and metastatic disease. Although the process is not clear, anti-estrogens effectively compete with estrogen-receptor sites, thereby blocking the effect of estrogens on target tissues. Tamoxifen can increase response rates when it is added to conventional adjuvant chemotherapy in metastatic breast disease. The standard practice is to use hormones alone in patients who are likely to respond and then proceed with chemotherapy sequentially in an effort to spare the patient from the side effects of long-term chemotherapy. Tamoxifen can produce remissions similar to those obtained with other forms of endocrine therapy that last more than 10 months. Tamoxifen, 20 mg daily, has been shown to induce remission in women who have previously responded or failed to respond to oophorectomy. Currently, tamoxifen is the first-line hormone therapy in metastatic breast cancer in postmenopausal women with estrogen receptor positive tumors.[196]

Tamoxifen has some important advantages over estrogens. It does not produce side effects such as nausea, urinary incontinence, breast tenderness, or fluid retention, which occur commonly with estrogen therapy. Furthermore, tamoxifen may be useful in some premenopausal and perimenopausal women, but this has yet to be definitely proven. The best response from tamoxifen has been seen in postmenopausal women with soft tissue and lung metastasis rather than bone metastasis. The most common side effects of anti-estrogens are hot flashes, mild nausea, fluid retention with ankle swelling, vaginal cornification, and postmenopausal bleeding.[196] Tumor flare of bone pain and hypercalcemia in patients with bone disease may occur transiently at the onset of therapy and are usually interpreted as a favorable antitumor response, although this is not well substantiated in the literature.

Oophorectomy

Surgical oophorectomy, tamoxifen,[197] and ovarian radiation are equally effective in removing endogenous sources of estrogens in premenopausal and some perimenopasual women and may be indicated in women with estrogen receptor positive tumors. Oophorectomy is not indicated in women with estrogen receptor negative tumors. The controversy over prophylactic versus therapeutic oophorectomy has, for the most part, been settled. Researchers have found that there is no therapeutic benefit to prophylactic oophorectomy in premenopausal women.[198] Oophorectomy is therefore reserved for women with recurrent or metastatic disease, provided their disease at time of recurrence is not life-threatening. Delaying oophorectomy is important to evaluate response and predict response to subsequent hormonal therapy.

About 32% of women who undergo oophorectomy obtain remission of disease, which may last for approximately 1 year. Women who experience an objective response to oophorectomy are candidates for additional endocrine therapy.

Secondary ablative procedures

In the past, adrenalectomy or hypophysectomy resulted in objective remission in about 32% of women who responded to previous endocrine therapy. These procedures are no longer performed to treat women with disseminated breast cancer. The results of medical adrenalectomy with aminoglutethimide (Cytadren) therapy are equivalent to those of surgical ablation without the risks of surgery and permanent adrenal suppression. Aminoglutethimide effectively blocks the conversion of androstenedione to estrone in peripheral tissue and inhibits the conversion of cholesterol to pregnenolone, thus blocking all adrenal steroid synthesis. It also inhibits the peripheral conversion of androgens to estrogens. Hydrocortisone replacement is needed because of adrenal suppression. The side effects of aminoglutethimide administration include lethargy and skin rash occurring 7–10 days after initiation of therapy. If these reactions should occur, the aminoglutethimide is not discontinued, nor should the dose be decreased. The administration of increased doses of hydrocortisone for a week or more is effective in alleviating the rash. Figure 38-21 reviews treatment options for women with metastatic breast cancer.

Research in hormone therapy for metastatic breast cancer

There are a few new anti-estrogens showing promise in breast cancer. Toremifen demonstrates some responses in women with metastatic breast cancer, but the toxicity profile is not insignificant, especially when compared to the toxicity profile of tamoxifen. In women who failed to respond to tamoxifen or whose disease progressed on tamoxifen, few experience objective responses to toremifen.[199] Toxicities included nausea and vomiting, hot flashes, fatigue, inability to think clearly, and vaginal bleeding.

RU486 (Mifepristone), an antiprogestin and anti-gluco-corticoid, has shown promise in women with estrogen and progesterone-positive tumors who have failed conventional hormone manipulation.[200,201] RU486 has been extensively studied as an abortifacient in Europe and is currently not available in this country despite its obvious therapeutic benefit in breast cancer.

4HPR (Fenretinide) is a derivative of vitamin A that has shown substantial cancer chemopreventive and therapeutic benefit against breast cancer in animals. There is evidence to suggest that synergy exists between 4HPR and tamoxifen, but its efficacy in breast cancer is unknown.[202] A phase I study being conducted by the Illinois Cancer Council (Protocol 88B3) will help to determine the efficacy of this drug in women with metastatic breast cancer.[203] Prospective randomized studies employing 4HPR and tamoxifen will further delineate the role of this drug in the prevention and management of this disease.

Fadrozole, a new aromatase inhibitor, has shown good therapeutic effect as second-line treatment in postmenopausal women with metastatic breast cancer.[204] Toxicity is comparable to conventional hormone therapy and includes hot flashes, nausea and vomiting, fatigue, and loss of appetite.

MALE BREAST CANCER

Male breast cancer accounts for less than 1% of all breast cancers.[5] The anatomic structures of the male breast are the same as those of the female breast. It is the hormonal stimulation present in the female breast and absent in the male breast that accounts for the development and physiologic differences between the male and female breast. This lack of hormonal stimulation also may explain the comparatively low incidence of male breast cancer. However, the disease in both sexes is similar in terms of epidemiology, natural history, and response to therapy.[205]

The incidence of breast cancer is increased in men who have undergone sex-change procedures. The administration of estrogens results in lobular development and enlargement of the male breast. Hormonal imbalance and gynecomastia are characteristic of Klinefelter's syndrome, and the incidence of breast cancer is increased in men 20 to 66 times that of an average male, with a risk of breast cancer of 3%.[206]

The administration of DES to men with carcinoma of the prostate has been associated with male breast cancer but is a rare occurrence. While it is true that large numbers of men receiving DES for prostatic carcinoma do not exhibit an increased incidence of breast cancer, it is important to note that the life expectancy of these men is relatively short, and breast cancers may indeed be present but not yet manifested.

Breast cancer occurs most frequently in men 50–70 years old. It appears that after 40 years of age, the Sertoli cells (elongated cells in the seminiferous tubules) secrete increasing amounts of estrogens. The majority of male breast cancers (75%) are known to be estrogen receptor positive. They typically arise from ductal elements and present as infiltrating ductal carcinoma, which is commonly fixed to underlying fascia and skin. Nipple retraction and a bloody discharge may be present.

A painless, centrally located subareolar mass is usually the first symptom that brings the man to seek medical attention. Pectoral fixation, involvement of skin, nipple changes, and discharge are commonly present because of limited breast disease and delay in seeking medical attention. These factors may account for the increased frequency of widespread disease and early invasion of local and regional lymphatics. Ulceration may occur early in the course of the disease and carries a relatively poor prognosis. A bloody discharge from the nipple and nipple inversion may be present. Because of its relatively central location, male breast cancer can be expected to metastasize to the internal mammary nodes. The lungs and bony skeleton are the most common metastatic sites.

Because of the low incidence and relatively small number of patients, it is difficult to conduct controlled clinical trials to aid in establishing appropriate therapy. The treatment of male breast cancer is based in principle on the treatment of female breast cancer. The modified radical mastectomy has been the mainstay of therapy. The skin and underlying fascia are frequently involved, requiring skin grafting. Adjuvant radiotherapy, hormonal manipulation, and chemotherapy are the main methods of treatment.

With evidence of extensive disease, hormonal manipulation (orchiectomy, aminoglutethimide, or tamoxifen) is indicated unless the disease is life-threatening or aggressive, in which case chemotherapy would be indicated. The response rate to chemotherapy is about 44%, and it remains an option but is second-line therapy.[207]

Orchiectomy appears to remove the source of estrogen and androgen in recurrent male breast cancer and can result in a prompt remission. With recurrent disease, further hormonal manipulation, including tamoxifen, aminoglutethimide, progestin, and DES, may be beneficial. Aminoglutethimide, tamoxifen, and other forms of hormone manipulation are relatively ineffective without orchiectomy. However, Buserelin, or goserelin acetate, effectively reduces testosterone to castration levels and may be an important alternative to men who refuse orchiectomy.

COMPLICATIONS OF METASTATIC DISEASE

Bone Metastasis

Many individuals with breast cancer will, throughout the course of their illness, experience pain due to bony destruction by tumor. The individual may complain of pain over the rib cage, which is aggravated by a cough, or pain in the leg when rising from a sitting position. The person may also report feeling as if his or her back was strained while bending to pick something off the floor. In general, the pain is constant and grows progressively more severe. A radiograph of the area may demonstrate bony destruction and may be the first sign of metastasis or progression of disease. Bone pain may precede the development of skeletal radiographic changes by several weeks. Destructive bone lesions must be 1.0–1.5 cm in diameter and associated with a 30%–50% loss of bone mineral content before they can be detected with conventional radiography. A bone scan is therefore indicated to determine the extent of disease. A more sensitive method than radiography for detecting metastatic disease, a bone scan should be obtained in all individuals with symptoms suggesting skeletal involvement.

In addition to radiography, examination of peripheral blood or serum chemistries may indicate metastatic disease. Anemia, thrombocytopenia, leukocytosis, and immature forms of circulating nucleated red blood cells may indicate metastasis to the bone marrow. Elevation of the serum alkaline phosphatase level may be observed with either bone or liver involvement. The serum calcium level also may be increased and indicates significant bone destruction. Individuals who complain of back pain should have a thorough neurologic examination as well as radiographic evaluation of the spine. An MRI may be necessary to determine whether spinal cord compression is present or imminent.

For the individual who has had a long disease-free interval, a bone biopsy may be needed to document metastatic disease in bone. This is particularly true for the person who has no evidence of other metastatic deposits.

In addition to being painful, destructive lesions involving the femur or the humerus are highly susceptible to fracture. If fracture of the diseased bone should occur, severe vascular or neurologic damage may ensue, as well as immobility and severe pain. Irradiation in doses of 30–40 Gy to symptomatic areas often results in effective pain relief and recalcification of bone. If a fracture is pending or has occurred, surgery to stabilize the bone by internal fixation or replacement of the femoral head may be necessary. This is followed by 25–30 Gy of irradiation. This palliative surgery should allow the individual to remain ambulatory, thus decreasing the hazards of immobility such as hypercalcemia, deep vein thrombosis, and pneumonia. Physical therapy is instituted in the postoperative period and after discharge to ensure optimal rehabilitation.

In individuals with widespread bone involvement, radiation is given to areas that are painful and disabling. In cases where one or more fractures are pending, surgery is indicated and offers the least morbidity. The nurse should be particularly aware of the vulnerability of a person with metastatic bone lesions. Simply turning the person in bed can result in fracture of the affected area. The customary ways of repositioning patients in bed are contraindicated for the individual with disease in the clavicle. Lifting beneath the person's arms puts pressure on the clavicle and may cause a fracture. A pull sheet should be used to reposition the person with known disease in the hip, ribs, or vertebrae. At least two persons are needed to reposition the patient properly so that correct body alignment is ensured. The nurse also should be aware of the intense pain often associated with a fracture and institute an aggressive pain management protocol.

Spinal Cord Compression

Spinal cord compression constitutes an emergency because of the potential for developing paraplegia. Compression may be secondary to epidural tumor or altered bone alignment due to pathologic fracture. The initial signs and symptoms may be extremely subtle. Pain is usually present for several weeks before the development of additional neurologic symptoms. Imminent compression should be suspected in individuals who have known bone metastases, progressive back pain associated with weakness, paresthesias, bowel or bladder dysfunction, or gait disturbances. An MRI is performed as soon as the diagnosis is suspected to determine the exact level of the compression and identify other occult extradural lesions.

If the individual is found to have compression with an isolated extradural mass, radiotherapy combined with corticosteroids may produce optimal results and return of ambulation. The person is usually fitted with a brace or maintained on bed rest throughout the course of radiotherapy. Decompression laminectomy may be indicated for individuals who develop spinal cord compression and in whom the diagnosis of epidural metastasis is in doubt, or whose neurologic deficits continue to worsen while they receive radiotherapy. Fewer than 50% of these individuals can be expected to regain ambulatory function. The degree of recovery of function correlates directly with the length of time the patient experiences symptoms prior to therapeutic interventions.

Brain Metastasis and Leptomeningeal Carcinomatosis

Brain metastasis occurs in about 30% of individuals diagnosed with breast cancer and is often associated with devastating physical and emotional problems. The most frequent signs and symptoms of intracranial metastasis are headaches, seizures, visual defects, motor weakness, and mental changes. Symptoms generally subside with total brain irradiation and chronic steroids.

Most chemotherapeutic agents do not achieve a therapeutic concentration in the brain or cerebral spinal fluid (CSF). This is why the central nervous system may be considered a potential sanctuary for tumor cells. Leptomeningeal metastases occur most likely by hematogenous spread through the capillary structure of the choroid plexus or by rupture of cerebral metastases that subsequently involve the subarachnoid space. The diagnosis of leptomeningeal metastases is made by lumbar puncture and analysis of the CSF. Headache and changes in mental status are the most common symptoms of meningeal carcinomatosis. Cranial nerve dysfunction also may be present. Ocular muscle paresis is common, as are facial weakness, hearing loss, and vision loss.

Treatment generally involves total brain irradiation (24–30 Gy in eight to ten fractions). This is commonly followed by intraventricular-intrathecal chemotherapy given through an ommaya reservoir. Methotrexate, cytosine arabinoside, steroids, and thiotepa may safely be given intrathecally. Treatment usually includes methotrexate and thiotepa given twice weekly initially, then once a week until there is no evidence of metastatic cells in the CSF.

Chronic Lymphedema

The overall prevalence of lymphedema in breast cancer is 8%. It is most common in women who have had axillary dissection followed by radiation in excess of 46 Gy.[208] With the recent trend toward more conservative surgical resection with minimal axillary dissection for the individual undergoing mastectomy, the problem of massive lymphedema is less common. When axillary dissection is done, there may be transient edema initially; however, it is unusual for edema to persist beyond 3 months after surgery.

The most common causes of chronic lymphedema are infection and tumor recurrence, or tumor enlargement in the axilla. When this occurs, there is an increased resistance to venous flow and a disturbance in oncotic pressure that develops in the affected arm. The longer the edema persists, the more difficult it is to manage. Lymph is an excellent culture medium, and infections such as cellulitis and lymphangitis can flourish. The individual is instructed to elevate the hand above the elbow and the forearm higher than or level with the heart whenever possible. If edema persists or worsens, the individual is instructed in the use of an elastic stockinette to aid in venous flow. The stockinette is measured precisely to ensure that it fits properly and does not constrict venous flow. The individual wears the stockinette when out of bed. While the individual is sleeping, the arm is positioned to aid venous flow. Therapeutic retrograde massage is also a useful form of conservative treatment.[209] The individual is instructed to care for the skin and fingernails very carefully to avoid infection. Infection enhances lymphedema and slow regeneration of lymphatics. Individuals with chronic lymphedema are also instructed to control their weight and, in some situations, to lose weight.

For the individual who has massive edema without evidence of infection, a program of intermittent compression with an extremity pump may be necessary. The arm usually is treated daily as tolerated for 3–4 hours in the morning and 3 to 4 hours in the afternoon. When the arm reaches 1+ pitting edema, the treatment is discontinued and the arm is measured for a compression support. A compression pump is strictly contraindicated when there is evidence of acute phlebitis, perivascular lymphangitis, or cellulitis.

The lymphedematous arm is cosmetically unattractive and can be functionally useless. The arm can cause tremendous strain on the neck and shoulder muscles, which can result in pain. The woman may have difficulty adjusting her wardrobe to provide for the increasing size of her arm. Furthermore, the edematous arm can rarely be concealed adequately and can renew feelings of disfigurement and depression associated with the mastectomy that the woman may have resolved before the lymphedema occurred. When function of the arm is affected, the woman may not be able to work or perform activities of daily living. These limitations may not have been imposed on the woman following her mastectomy. Efforts should be made to discuss the goals and rationale of management with the woman, thereby enlisting her cooperation and participation in the planned treatment regimen.

PREGNANCY AND BREAST CANCER AS A SIMULTANEOUS EVENT

The current literature reports the incidence of concurrent pregnancy or lactation and breast cancer to be 0.2%–3.8%.[211] The diagnosis of breast cancer during pregnancy occurs in about 10% of eligible patients. The average patient is in her fourth or early fifth decade of life, has had multiple pregnancies but relatively few deliveries, and has a long interval since a previous pregnancy or childbirth.

The prognosis of women diagnosed with breast cancer during pregnancy has generally been poor, but today there is new optimism. It is now realized that the poor prognosis is more likely due to the increased incidence of delay in diagnosis in this population of women and subsequent discovery and treatment of advanced disease than it is due to the pregnancy itself. When compared with nonpregnant breast cancer patients of the same age, disease stage, and histologic grade, the prognosis for these patients is actually no worse.

Although the techniques of early detection and diagnosis in a pregnant patient can be difficult to perform because of the physiological changes in the breast, they are no less essential. Breast examinations should be performed as a regular part of prenatal care, and all women should be encouraged to practice BSE throughout the duration of the pregnancy. Any suspicious lump should receive a prompt work-up as previously outlined. The effectiveness of mammography may be compromised by the increased density of the breast and, if it is performed, the fetus should be shielded. The risk to the fetus in the event a breast biopsy is needed is minimal.

The treatment of breast cancer in this population of women is determined by the extent of the disease present and the term of pregnancy or lactation. In general, the same treatment principles apply. Early-stage disease should be surgically treated with little risk to the fetus. Radiation therapy is not recommended due to potential hazards to the fetus. Chemotherapy, if indicated, should not be administered during the first trimester, but can be more safely used in the second and third. Antimetabolites, specifically folic acid antagonists, when given during the first trimester, have consistently been shown to be teratogenic. As exposure to a drug increases over time, the frequency and severity of the teratogenic effects also increase.[211] There is also a threshold effect, meaning that below a certain dose the incidence of death, malformation, growth retardation, or functional deficit is not greater than controls.[212] Research concerning the use of antiemetics in pregnancy are understandably limited. Metaclopramide has been compared with prochlorperazine or a placebo to treat hyperemesis of pregnancy. Metoclopramide was somewhat superior to prochlorperazine and placebo.[213] Ondansetron is associated with minimal toxicities, and while there are no human data, reproductive studies have been done in rats with no evidence of harm to the fetus. Overall, it appears that antiemetics cause minimal toxicity.[214]

A therapeutic abortion during the first trimester is not necessary, nor has it been found to be therapeutically beneficial. A more advanced disease stage needs effective, urgent palliation and may indicate the need for termination of an early pregnancy to promptly begin treatment for the breast cancer. If the diagnosis is made in the third trimester, local therapy is carried out and adjuvant therapy is instituted once the child is born. When chemotherapy is deemed crucial because of more aggressive disease. cesarean section at the earliest opportunity may be recommended. There is no evidence that chemotherapy given in the latter months of pregnancy will harm the fetus. However, while infants may be described as phenotypically normal, subtle impairments in growth and development may go unnoticed, increasing the need for these children to be followed over time.[215,216]

REFERENCES

1. Miller BA, Feuer EJ, Hankey BF: Recent incidence trends for breast cancer in women and relevance of early detection: An update. *CA* 43:27–41, 1993.
2. National Institutes of Health Consensus Development Conference Statement: *Treatment of Early Stage Breast Cancer.* Bethesda, MD: National Institutes of Health, 1990.
3. Kirkman-Liff B, Kronenfeld J: Access to cancer screening devices for women. *Am J Public Health* 82(5):733–735, 1992.
4. Shimkin MB: Cancer of the breast. *JAMA* 183:358, 1963.
5. American Cancer Society: *Cancer Facts and Figures—1992.* Atlanta, GA: American Cancer Society, 1992, pp. 1–22.
6. Leis HP: Prognostic parameters for breast cancer. In Bland KI, Copeland EM (eds): *The Breast: Comprehensive Management of Benign and Malignant Disease.* Philadelphia: Saunders, 1991, pp. 331–346.
7. Kelsey JL, Gammon MD: The epidemiology of breast cancer. *CA* 41(3):146–165, 1991.
8. Fisher B: Biology and clinical considerations regarding the use of surgery and chemotherapy in treatment of primary breast cancer. *Cancer* 40:574–587, 1977.
9. Mant D, Vessey MP: Epidemiology and primary prevention of breast cancer. In Bland KI, Copeland EM (eds): *The Breast: Comprehensive Management of Benign and Malignant Disease.* Philadelphia: Saunders, 1991, pp. 235–246.
10. Key TJ, Pike MC: The role of oestrogens and progestagens in the epidemiology and prevention of breast cancer. *Eur J Cancer* 24:29–43, 1988.
11. Bergkvist L, Adami HO, Persson I, et al: The risk of breast cancer after estrogen and estrogen-progestin replacement. *N Engl J Med* 321:293–297, 1989.
12. Potten CS, Watson RJ, Williams GT: The effect of age and menstrual cycle upon proliferative activity of the normal human breast. *Br J Cancer* 58:163–170, 1988.
13. Bruzzi P, Negri E, LaVecchia C, et al: Short term increase in risk of breast cancer after full term pregnancy. *Br J Med* 297:1096–1098, 1988.
14. Lippman M: Epidemiology of breast cancer. In Lippman M, Lichter AS, Danforth DN (eds): *Diagnosis and Management of Breast Cancer.* Philadelphia: Saunders, 1988, pp. 1–8.
15. Petitti DB: Animal models of sex steroid hormones and mammary cancer: Lessons for understanding studies in humans. In Institute of Medicine, Division of Health Promotion and Disease Prevention: *Oral Contraceptives and Breast Cancer.* Washington, DC: National Academy Press, 1991, pp. 152–164.
16. Pike MC, Henderson BE, Casagrande JT, et al: Oral contraceptive use and early abortion as risk factor for breast cancer in young women. *Br J Cancer* 43:72–76, 1981.
17. Pike MC, Krailo MD, Henderson BE, et al: Breast cancer in young women and use of oral contraceptives: Possible modifying effects of formulation and age at use. *Lancet* 926–930, 1983.
18. UK National Case-Control Study Group: Oral contraceptive use and breast cancer risk in young women. *Lancet* 973–982, 1989.
19. Lipnick RJ, Buring JE, Hennekens CH, et al: Oral contraceptives and breast cancer. *JAMA* 255(1):58–61, 1986.
20. Dupont WD, Page DL, Rogers LW: Influence of exogenous estrogens, proliferative breast disease and other variables on breast cancer risk. *Cancer* 63:948–957, 1989.
21. Mills PK, Beeson L, Phillips RL, et al: Prospective study of exogenous hormone use and breast cancer in Seventh Day Adventists. *Cancer* 64:591–597, 1989.
22. Sattin RW, Rubin GL, Webster L, et al: Family history and the risk of breast cancer. *JAMA* 253(13):1908–1913, 1985.
23. Roseman DL, Strauss AK, Shorey W: A positive family history of breast cancer: Does its effect diminish with age? *Arch Intern Med* 150:191–194, 1990.
24. Hall JM, Lee MK, Newman B: Linkage of early-onset familial breast cancer to chromosome 17q21. *Science* 250:1684–1689, 1990.
25. Skolnick MH, Cannon-Albright LA: Genetic predisposition to breast cancer. *Cancer* 70:1747–1754, 1992.
26. London S, Willett W: Diet and the risk of breast cancer. *Hematol/Oncol Clin North Am* 3(4):559–575, 1989.
27. Winick M: Calories and cancer. *Hematol/Oncol Clin North Am* 5(1):1–5, 1991.
28. Rose D: Introduction to the proceedings of a workshop on new developments on dietary fat and fiber in carcinogenesis. *Prev Med* 16:449–450, 1987.
29. Morabia A, Wynder EL: Epidemiology and natural his-

tory of breast cancer. *Surg Clin North Am* 70(4):739–752, 1990.
30. Ingram D, Nottage E, Ng S, et al: Obesity and breast disease: The role of the female sex hormone. *Cancer* 64:1049–1053, 1989.
31. Longnecker MP, Berlin JA, Orza MJ, et al: A meta–analysis of alcohol consumption in relation to risk of breast cancer. *JAMA* 260:652–656, 1988.
32. Hiatt RA, Klatsky AI, Armstrong MA: Alcohol consumption and the risk of breast cancer in a prepaid health plan. *Cancer Res* 48:2284–2287, 1988.
33. Richardson S, Vincenzi I, Pujol H, et al: Alcohol consumption in a case–control study of breast cancer in southern France. *Int J Cancer* 44:84–89, 1989.
34. Modan B, Chetrit A, Alfandary E, et al: Increased risk of breast cancer after low-dose radiation. *Lancet* 629–630, 1989.
35. Parker RG, Grimm P, Enstrom JE: Contralateral breast cancers following treatment for initial breast cancers in women. *Am J Clin Oncol* 12(3):213–216, 1989.
36. Hildreth NG, Shore RE, Dvoretsky PM: The risk of breast cancer after irradiation of the thymus in infancy. *N Engl J Med* 321:1281–1284, 1989.
37. Miller AB, Howe GR, Sherman GJ, et al: Mortality from breast cancer after irradiation during fluoroscopic examinations in patients being treated for tuberculosis. *N Engl J Med* 321:1285–1289, 1989.
38. Page DL, Dupont WD: Anatomic markers of human malignancy and risk of breast cancer. *Cancer* 66:1326–1335, 1990.
39. Page DL, Simpson JF: Benign high risk and premalignant lesions of the MAMMA. In Bland KI, Copeland EM (eds): *The Breast: Comprehensive Management of Benign and Malignant Disease*. Philadelphia: Saunders, 1991, pp. 113–134.
40. Page DL, Dupont WD: Premalignant conditions and markers of elevated risk in the breast and their management. *Surg Clin North Am* 70(4):831–850, 1990.
41. Osborne MP, Telang NT: Primary prevention of breast cancer. In Bland KI, Copeland EM (eds): *The Breast: Comprehensive Management of Benign and Malignant Disease.* Philadelphia: Saunders, 1991, pp. 246–261.
42. Dorgan JF, Schatzkin A: Antioxidant micronutrients in cancer prevention. *Hematol/Oncol Clin North Am* 5(1):43–63, 1991.
43. Cole MP, Jones CT, Todd ID: The new anti-estrogenic agent in late breast cancer: An early clinical approach of ICI 46474. *Br J Cancer* 25:27–275, 1971.
44. Sawka CA, Pritchard KI, Paterson HG, et al: Role and mechanism of action of tamoxifen in premenopausal women with metastatic breast carcinoma. *Cancer Res* 46:3152–3156, 1986.
45. Fisher B, Constantino J, Redmond C, et al: A randomized clinical trial evaluating tamoxifen in the treatment of patients with node negative breast cancer who have estrogen receptor positive tumors. *N Engl J Med* 320:479–484, 1989.
46. Cummings FJ, Gray R, Tormey DC, et al: Adjuvant tamoxifen versus placebo in elderly women with node-positive breast cancer: Long term follow-up and causes of death. *J Clin Oncol* 11:29–35, 1993.
47. NSABP Protocol P-1: A clinical trial to determine the worth of tamoxifen for preventing breast cancer. Pittsburgh, PA: National Surgical Adjuvant Breast and Bowel Project, 1992.
48. Knabbe C, Lippman ME, Wakefield LM: Evidence that transforming growth factor–B is a hormonally regulated negative growth factor in human breast cancer cells. *Cell* 48:417–428, 1987.
49. Murphy LC, Sutherland RL: Antitumor activity of clomiphene analogs *in vitro*: Relationship to affinity for the estrogen receptor and another high affinity anti-estrogen-binding site. *J Clin Endocrinol Metab* 57:373–379, 1983.
50. Jordan VC, Fritz NF, Tormey DC: Long term adjuvant therapy with tamoxifen: Effects on sex hormone binding globulin and antithrombin III. *Cancer Res* 47:4517–4519, 1987.
51. Berry J, Green BJ, Matheson DS: Modulation of natural killer cell activity by tamoxifen in stage I post–menopausal breast cancer. *Eur J Cancer Clin Oncol* 23:517–520, 1987.
52. Pollak M, Constantino J, Polychronakos C, et al: Effect of tamoxifen on serum insulin–like growth factor I levels in stage I breast cancer. *JNCI* 82(21):1693–1697, 1990.
53. Vogel VG: High risk populations as targets for breast cancer prevention trials. *Prev Med* 20:86–100, 1991.
54. Pennisi VR: The prevention of breast cancer by subcutaneous mastectomy. *Surg Clin North Am* 57:1023–1027, 1987.
55. Bostwick J: Breast reconstruction after mastectomy. *Cancer* 15:1402–1411, supplement, 1990.
56. McLellan GL: Screening and early diagnosis of breast cancer. *J Fam Pract* 25(5):561–568, 1988.
57. Breast cancer screening guidelines agreed on by AMA, other medically related organizations. *JAMA* 262(9):115, 1989.
58. Williams SM, Kaplan PA, Petersen JC, et al: Mammography in women under age 30: Is there clinical benefit? *Radiology* 161:49–51, 1986.
59. Bassett LW, Gambhir S: Breast imaging for the 1990s. *Semin Oncol* 18(2):80–86, 1991.
60. Bassett LW, Manjikian V, Gold RH: Mammography and breast cancer screening. *Surg Clin North Am* 70(4):775–800, 1990.
61. Jackson VP, Lex AM, Smith DJ: Patient discomfort during screen–film mammography. *Radiology* 168:421–423, 1988.
62. Stomper PC, Kopans DB, Sadowsky NL, et al: Is mammography painful? *Arch Intern Med* 148:521–524, 1988.
63. Vyborny CJ, Schmidt RA: Mammography as a radiographic examination: An overview. *Radiograph* 9(4):723–763, 1989.
64. Winchester DP: Evaluation and management of breast abnormalities. *Cancer* 66:1345–1347, 1990.
65. Dowlatshahi K, Jokich PM, Schmidt R, et al: Cytologic diagnosis of occult breast lesions using stereotaxic needle aspiration. *Arch Surg* 122:1343–1346, 1987.
66. Dowlatshahi K, Yaremko LM, Kluskens L, et al: Nonpalpable breast lesions: Findings of stereotaxic needle-core biopsy and fine-needle aspiration cytology. *Radiology* 181:745–750, 1991.
67. Schwartz GF, Feig SA: Management of patients with nonpalpable breast lesions. *Oncology* 5(10):39–48, 1991.
68. Fisher B: Experiences in the evolution, technique, and results of breast conservation for the treatment of mammary cancer. In Bohmert HH, Leis HP, Jackson IT (eds): *Breast Cancer: Conservative and Reconstructive Surgery*. New York: Thieme Medical Publishers, 1989, pp. 40–57.

69. Frank-Stromberg M, Rohan K: Nursing's involvement in the primary and secondary prevention of cancer: Nationally and internationally. *Cancer Nurs* 15(2):79–108, 1992.
70. Durant JR: How to organize a multidisciplinary clinic for the management of breast cancer. *Surg Clin North Am* 70(4):977–983, 1990.
71. Hutter RV: The role of the pathologist in breast cancer management. *Cancer* 66:1363–1372, 1990.
72. Wilkinson EJ, Hauss LL, Hoffman RG, et al: Occult axillary lymph node metastases in invasive breast cancer: Characteristics of the primary tumor and significance of the metastases. *Pathol Annu* (PTZ) 17:67–91, 1982.
73. Leis HP: Prognostic parameters for breast carcinoma. In Bland KI, Copeland EM (eds): *The Breast: Comprehensive Management of Benign and Malignant Disease*. Philadelphia: Saunders, 1991, pp. 331–346.
74. Mambo NC, Gallagher HS: Carcinoma of the breast: The prognostic significance of extranodal extension of axillary disease. *Cancer* 39:2280–2285, 1977.
75. Kinne DW: Staging and follow-up of breast cancer patients. *Cancer* 67:1196–1197, 1991.
76. Donegan WL: Prognostic factors: Stage and receptor status in breast cancer. *Cancer* 70:1755–1764, 1992.
77. Jones SE, Moon TE, Bonadonna G, et al: Comparison of different trials of adjuvant chemotherapy in stage II breast cancer using a natural history data base. *Am J Clin Oncol* 10:387–395, 1987.
78. Nemoto T, Vana J, Bedwani RN, et al: Management and survival of female breast cancer: Results of a national survey by the American College of Surgeons. *Cancer* 45:2917–2924, 1980.
79. Carter CL, Allen C, Henson DE: Relation of tumor size, lymph node status, and survival in 24,740 breast cancer cases. *Cancer* 63:181–187, 1989.
80. Joensuu H, Tolkkanen S, Klemi PJ: DNA index and S-phase fraction and their combination as prognostic factors in operable ductal breast carcinoma. *Cancer* 66:331–340, 1990.
81. Rosen PP, Groshen S, Saugo PE, et al: A long term follow-up study of survival in stage I and stage II breast carcinomas. *J Clin Oncol* 7:355–366, 1989.
82. O'Reilly SM, Camplejohn RS, Barnes DM, et al: DNA index, S-phase fraction histological grade and prognosis in breast cancer. *Br J Cancer* 61:671–674, 1990.
83. Sigurdsson H, Baletorp B, Bord A, et al: Indicators of prognosis in node-negative breast cancer. *N Engl J Med* 322:1045–1053, 1990.
84. Sahin AA, Ro J, Ro JY, et al: Ki-67 immunostaining in node-negative stage I/II breast carcinoma. *Cancer* 68:549–557, 1991.
85. McGuire WL, Clark GM: Prognostic factors and treatment decisions in axillary node-negative breast cancer. *N Engl J Med* 326(26):1756–1760, 1992.
86. Mori T, Morimoto T, Komaki K, et al: Comparison of estrogen receptor and epidermal growth factor receptor content on primary and involved nodes in human breast cancer. *Cancer* 68:532–537, 1991.
87. Perren TJ: c-erb B-2 oncogene as a prognostic marker in breast cancer. *Br Med J* 63:422–426, 1991.
88. Gullick WJ, Love SB, Wright C, et al: c-erb B-2 protein overexpression in breast cancer is a risk factor in patients with involved and uninvolved lymph nodes. *Br J Cancer* 63:434–437, 1991.
89. Lovekin C, Ellis IO, Locker A, et al: c-erb B-2 oncoprotein expression in primary and advanced breast cancer. *Br J Cancer* 63:439, 1991.
90. Park S, Hazan R, Fisher ER, et al: Pathological findings from the National Surgical Adjuvant Breast and Bowel Project: Prognostic significance of erb B-2 protein overexpressed in primary breast cancer. *J Clin Oncol* 8:103–112, 1990.
91. Allred DC, Clark GM, Tandon AK: HER-2/*neu* in node-negative breast cancer: Prognostic significance of overexpressing influenced by the presence of *in situ* carcinoma. *J Clin Oncol* 10:599–605, 1992.
92. Rochefort H, Capony F, Garcia M: Cathepsin D in breast cancer: From molecular and cellular biology to clinical application. *Cancer Cells* 2:383–388, 1990.
93. Isola J, Weitz S, Visakorpi T, et al: Cathepsin D expression detected by immunohistochemistry has independent prognostic value in axillary node-negative breast cancer. *J Clin Oncol* 11:36–43, 1993.
94. International Breast Cancer Study Group: Prognostic importance of occult axillary lymph node micrometastases from breast cancer. *Lancet* 335:1565–1568, 1990.
95. O'Reilly SM, Camplejohn RS, Barnes DM, et al: Node negative breast cancer: Prognostic subgroups defined by tumor size and flow cytometry. *J Clin Oncol* 8:2040–2046, 1990.
96. Page DL: Prognosis and breast cancer: Recognition of lethal and favorable prognostic type. *Am J Surg Pathol* 15(4):334–349, 1991.
97. Clark GM, Matheiu MC, Owens MA: Prognostic significance of S-phase fraction in good risk node negative breast cancer patients. *J Clin Oncol* 10:428–432, 1992.
98. Frierson HF: Ploidy analysis and S-phase fraction determination by flow cytometry of invasive adenocarcinomas of the breast. *Am J Surg Pathol* 15(4):358–367, 1991.
99. Seymour L, Bezwoda WR, Meyer K: Tumor factors predicting for prognosis in metastatic breast cancer. *Cancer* 66:2390–2394, 1990.
100. Osborne CK: Breast cancer. In Wittes RE (ed): *Manual of Oncologic Therapeutics*. Philadelphia: Lippincott, 1992, pp. 146–153.
101. American Joint Commission on Cancer: Staging for Breast Carcinoma (3d ed). Atlanta, GA: American Cancer Society, 1989.
102. Fisher B: Laboratory and clinical research in breast cancer: A personal adventure: The David A. Karnofsky Memorial Lecture. *Cancer Res* 40:3863–3874, 1980.
103. Fisher B: A biological perspective of breast cancer: Contributions of the National Surgical Adjuvant Breast and Bowel Project Clinical Trials. *CA* 41(2):97–111, 1991.
104. Fisher B, Redmond C, Fisher ER, et al: Ten year results of a randomized clinical trial comparing radical mastectomy and total mastectomy with or without radiation. *N Engl J Med* 312:674–681, 1985.
105. Fisher B, Redmond C: Lumpectomy for the treatment of breast cancer: An update of the NSABP experience. *J Natl Cancer Inst,* in press.
106. Kinne DW: The surgical management of primary breast cancer. *CA* 41(2):71–84, 1991.
107. Liagos MD, Westdahl PR, Rose MP: The concept and implications of multicentricity in breast carcinoma. *Pathol Annu* 16:83–102, 1981.
108. Schwartz GH, Patchesky AS, Feig SA, et al: Multicentricity of non-palpable breast cancer. *Cancer* 45:2913–2916, 1980.

109. Fisher B, Redmond C, Poisson R, et al: Eight year results of a randomized clinical trial comparing total mastectomy and lumpectomy with or without irradiation in the treatment of breast cancer. *N Engl J Med* 320:822–828, 1989.
110. Abner AL, Recht A, Eberlein T, et al: Prognosis following salvage mastectomy for recurrence in the breast after conservative surgery and radiation therapy for early stage breast cancer. *J Clin Oncol* 11:44–48, 1993.
111. Betsill WL, Rosen PP, Lieberman PH, et al: Intraductal carcinoma: Long term follow-up after treatment by biopsy alone. *JAMA* 239:1863, 1978.
112. Rosato EF, Curcillo PG: Surgical considerations in the management of breast cancer. In Fowble B, Goodman R, Glick JH, Rosato EF (eds): *Breast Cancer Treatment: A Comprehensive Guide to Management.* Chicago: Mosby Year Book, 1991, pp. 89–104.
113. Fisher E, Sass R, Fisher B, et al: Pathologic findings from the National Surgical Adjuvant Breast Project (B-06) Intraductal Carcinoma (DCIS). *Cancer* 57:197–202, 1986.
114. Marcial VA: Primary therapy for limited breast cancer. *Cancer* 65:2159–2164, 1990.
115. Dewar JA, Benhamou S, Benhamou E, et al: Cosmetic results following lumpectomy, axillary dissection, and radiotherapy for small breast cancers. *Radiother Oncol* 12:273–280, 1988.
116. Recht A, Come SE, Gelman RS, et al: Integration of conservative surgery, radiotherapy, and chemotherapy for the treatment of early-stage, node-positive breast cancer: Sequencing, timing, and outcome. *J Clin Oncol* 9:1662–1667, 1991.
117. Bonadonna G: Evolving concepts in the systemic adjuvant treatment of breast cancer. *Cancer Res* 52:2127–2137, 1992.
118. Andersson I, Aspegren K, Jamzon L, et al: Mammographic screening and mortality from breast cancer: Malmo-mammographic screening trial. *Br Med J* 297:943–948, 1988.
119. Fisher B, Constantino J, Redmond C, et al: A randomized clinical trial evaluating tamoxifen in the treatment of patients with node-negative breast cancer who have estrogen-receptor-positive tumors. *N Engl J Med* 320: 479–484, 1989.
120. Fisher B, Redmond C, Nikolay V, et al: A randomized clinical trial evaluating sequential methotrexate and fluorouracil in the treatment of patients with node-negative breast cancer who have estrogen-receptor-negative tumors. *N Engl J Med* 320:473–478, 1989.
121. Mansour EG, Gray R, Shatila AH, et al: Efficacy of adjuvant chemotherapy in high-risk node-negative breast cancer. *N Engl J Med* 320:485–490, 1989.
122. Lippman ME: Proceedings of the NIH Consensus Development Conference on adjuvant chemotherapy and endocrine therapy for breast cancer. *Natl Cancer Inst Monogr* 1:1, 1986.
123. Dorr FA (ed): Proceedings of the NIH Consensus Development Conference on Early Stage Breast Cancer. *Natl Cancer Inst Monogr:*1–19, 1990.
124. Early Breast Cancer Trialists' Collaborative Group: Systemic Treatment of Early Breast Cancer by Hormonal Cytotoxic or Immune Therapy: Part I and II. *N Engl J Med* 339:1–15, 71–85, 1992.
125. Winchester DP: Adjuvant therapy for node negative breast cancer. *Cancer* 67:1741–1743, 1991.
126. Fisher B, Constantino J, Redmond C, et al: A randomized clinical trial evaluating tamoxifen in the treatment of patients with node negative breast cancer who have estrogen receptor positive tumors. *N Engl J Med* 320:479–484, 1989.
127. Bonadonna G: Conceptual and practice advances in the management of breast cancer: Karnofsky Memorial Lecture. *J Clin Oncol* 7:1380–1397, 1989.
128. Bonadonna G, Valagussa P, Rossi A, et al: Ten year results with CMF based adjuvant chemotherapy in resectable breast cancer. *Cancer Res Treat* 5:95–115, 1985.
129. Fisher B, Redmond C, Legault-Poisson S, et al: Postoperative chemotherapy and tamoxifen compared with tamoxifen alone in the treatment of positive-node breast cancer patients aged 50 years and older with tumors responsive to tamoxifen: Results from the National Surgical Adjuvant Breast and Bowel Project B-16. *J Clin Oncol* 8:1005–1018, 1990.
130. Fornander T, Rutqvist LE, Cedermark B, et al: Adjuvant tamoxifen in early breast cancer: Occurrence of new primary tumors. *Lancet* 1:117–120, 1989.
131. Healey B, Tormey DC, Gray R, et al: Arterial and venous thrombotic events in ECOG adjuvant breast cancer trials. *Proc ASCO* 6:208, 1987(abstr).
132. Duggan D: Local therapy of locally advanced breast cancer. *Oncology* 5(12):67–72, 1991.
133. Carter CL, Allen C, Henson DE: Relation of tumor size, lymph node status and survival in 24,470 breast cancer cases. *Cancer* 63:181–187, 1989.
134. Wallgren A: Clinical trials of locally advanced breast cancer. *Acta Oncol* 29:357–360, 1990.
135. Hortobagi GN: Comprehensive management of locally advanced breast cancer. *Cancer* 66:1387–1391, 1990.
136. Swain S, Lippman M: Systemic therapy of locally advanced breast cancer: Review and guidelines. *Oncology* 3:21–28, 1989.
137. Rubens R, Bartelink H, Engelsman E, et al: Locally advanced breast cancer: The contribution of cytotoxic and endocrine treatment to radiotherapy. An EORTC Breast Cancer Cooperative Group Trial. *Eur J Cancer Clin Oncol* 25:667–678, 1989.
138. Hortobagi GN, Buzdar AN: Locally advanced breast cancer: A review including the M.D. Anderson experience. In Ragaz T, Ariel T (eds): *High Risk Breast Cancer.* Berlin-Heidelberg: Springer Verlag, 1991, pp. 382–413.
139. Hortobagi GN, Ames FC, Buzdar NA, et al: Management of stage III primary breast cancer with primary chemotherapy, surgery, and radiation therapy. *Cancer* 62:2501–2516, 1988.
140. Rubens RD, Bartelink H, Engelsman E, et al: Locally advanced breast cancer: The contribution of cytotoxic and endocrine treatment to radiotherapy. An EORTC Breast Cancer Cooperative Group Trial. *Eur J Cancer Clin Oncol* 25:667–678, 1989.
141. Spittle MF, Hill BF, Ostrowski MJ, et al: A randomized, prospective, comparative multicenter trial of a single combination versus alternating combinations of antitumor drugs in advanced breast cancer. *Eur J Cancer Clin Oncol* 23:1155–1162, 1987.
142. Tormey D, Gelman R, Falkson G: Prospective evaluation of rotating chemotherapy in advanced breast cancer. *Am J Clin Oncol* 3:1–18, 1983.
143. Romsaas EP, Malec JF, Javenkoski BR, et al: Psychological distress among women with breast problems. *Cancer* 57:890–895, 1985.

144. Hughes J: Emotional reactions to the diagnosis and treatment of early breast cancer. *J Psychosom Res* 26:277–283, 1982.
145. Knobf MK: Symptoms and rehabilitation needs of patients with early stage breast cancer during primary therapy. *Cancer* 66:1392–1401, 1990.
146. Bloom JR: Social support, accommodation to stress and adjustment to breast cancer. *Soc Sci Med* 16:1329, 1982.
147. Sinsheimer L, Holland JC: Psychosocial issues in breast cancer. *Semin Oncol* 14(1):75, 1987.
148. Fowble B: Local-regional treatment options for early invasive breast cancer. In Fowble B, Goodman RL, Glick JH, Rosato EF (eds): *Breast Cancer Treatment: A Comprehensive Guide to Management*. St. Louis, MO: Mosby Year Book, 1991, pp. 25–88.
149. Cooley ME, Erikson B: Rehabilitation. In Fowble B, Goodman RL, Glick JH, Rosato EF (eds): *Breast Cancer Treatment: A Comprehensive Guide to Management*. St. Louis, MO: Mosby Year Book, 1991, pp. 511–583.
150. Schover LR: The impact of breast cancer on sexuality, body image and intimate relationships. *CA* 4(2):112–119, 1991.
151. Psychological Aspects of Breast Cancer Study Group: Psychological response to mastectomy: A prospective comparison study. *Cancer* 69:189–196, 1987.
152. Vinokur AD, Threatt BA, Caplan RD, Zimmerman BL: Physical and psychosocial functioning and adjustment to breast cancer: Long-term follow-up of a screening population. *Cancer* 63:394–405, 1989.
153. Vinokur AD, Threatt BA, Vinokur-Kaplann D, et al: The process of recovery from breast cancer for younger and older patients: Changes during the first year. *Cancer* 65:1242–1254, 1990.
154. Stevens LA, McGrath MH, Druss RG, et al: The psychological impact of immediate breast reconstruction for women with early breast cancer. *Plast Reconstr Surg* 73:619–628, 1984.
155. Feather BL, Kaiser SB, Rucker M: Mastectomy and related treatments: Impact of appearance satisfaction on self-esteem. *Home Econ Res J* 17:127–139, 1988.
156. Anderson BL, Jochimsen PR: Sexual functioning among breast cancer, gynecologic cancer, and healthy women. *J Consult Clin Psychol* 53:25–32, 1985.
157. Sherins RJ, Mulvihill JJ: Gonadal dysfunction. In DeVita VT Jr, Hellman S, Rosenberg SA (eds): *Cancer: Principles and Practice of Oncology* (3d ed). Philadelphia: Lippincott, 1989, pp. 2170–2180.
158. Knobf MT: Physical and psychological distress associated with adjuvant chemotherapy in women with breast cancer. *J Clin Oncol* 4:678–684, 1986.
159. Bergmans M, Merkos J, Corbey R, et al: Effect of bellargel regard on climacteric complaints: A double blind placebo controlled study. *Maturitas* 9:227–234, 1987.
160. Magamani M, Kelver M, Smith E: Treatment of menopausal hot flashes with transdermal administration of Clonidine. *Am J Obstet Gynecol* 156(3):561–565, 1987.
161. Grindel CG, Cahill CA, Walker A: Food intake of women with breast cancer during the first 6 months of chemotherapy. *Oncol Nurs Forum* 16:401–407, 1989.
162. Knobf M, Mullen J, Xistris D, et al: Weight gain in women with breast cancer receiving adjuvant chemotherapy. *Oncol Nurs Forum* 10:28–33, 1983.
163. Foltz AT: Weight gain among stage II breast cancer patients: A study of five factors. *Oncol Nurs Forum* 12:21–26, 1985.
164. Huntington MO: Weight gain in patients receiving adjuvant chemotherapy for carcinoma of the breast. *Cancer* 56:472–474, 1985.
165. Goodwin PJ, Panzarella T, Boyd NF: Weight gain in women with localized breast cancer: A descriptive study. *Br Cancer Res Treat* 11:59–66, 1988.
166. Piper B, Freidman L, Hartigan K, et al: Fatigue patterns over time in women receiving CMF chemotherapy for breast cancer. *Proc Oncol Nurs Soc* 16:217, 1989(abstr).
167. Love RR, Leventhal H, Easterling DV, et al: Side effects and emotional distress during cancer chemotherapy. *Cancer* 63:604–612, 1989.
168. Beadle GF, Harris JR, Silver B, et al: Cosmetic results following primary radiation for early breast cancer. *Cancer* 54:2911, 1984.
169. Danforth DN: How subsequent pregnancy affects outcome in women with prior breast cancer. *Oncology* 5(11):23–29, 1992.
170. Hassey KM: Pregnancy and parenthood after treatment for breast cancer. *Oncol Nurs Forum* 15:439–444, 1988.
171. Donegan WL: Breast cancer and pregnancy. *Am J Obstet Gynecol Oncol* 244–252, 1977.
172. Mignot L, Morvan F, Sarrazin D, et al: Breast carcinoma and subsequent pregnancy. *Proc Am Soc Clin Oncol* 5:57, 1986.
173. Bostwick J: Breast reconstruction after mastectomy. *Cancer* 66:1402–1411, 1989.
174. Handel N: Current status of breast reconstruction after mastectomy. *Oncology* 5(11):73–83, 1991.
175. Burkhardt BR: Capsular contracture: Hard breasts, soft data. *Plast Reconstr Breast Surg* 15(4):521–532, 1988.
176. Gybert L, Asplund O, Jurell G: Capsular contracture after breast reconstruction with silicone-gel saline filled implants: A 6 year follow-up. *Plast Reconstr Surg* 85(3):372–377, 1990.
177. McGraw JB, Cramer AR, Horton CE: Breast reconstruction following mastectomy. In Bland KI, Copeland EM (eds): *The Breast: Comprehensive Management of Benign and Malignant Disease*. Philadelphia: Saunders, 1991, pp. 656–692.
178. Bostwick J (ed): Skate flap. In *Plastic and Reconstructive Breast Surgery*. St Louis, MO: Quality Med Publishing, 1990, pp. 1156–1160.
179. Smith IA: Recurrent disease. In Harris JR, Hellman S, Henderson IC, et al (eds): *Breast Diseases*. Philadelphia: Lippincott, 1987, pp. 369–384.
180. Nicolson GL, Hug V: Breast cancer growth and metastases. *MD Anderson Oncol Case Rep Rev* 5(4):1–11, 1990.
181. Henderson IC, Garber JE, Breitmeyer JB, et al: Comprehensive management of disseminated breast cancer. *Cancer* 66:1439–1448, 1990.
182. Canellos GB: Systemic therapy of breast cancer. *Med J Aust* 148:88–91, 1988.
183. Jabboury K, Holmes FA, Hortobagyi G: 5-fluorouracil rechallenge by protracted infusion in refractory breast cancer. *Cancer* 64:793–797, 1989.
184. Loprinzi CL: 5-fluorouracil with leukovorin in breast cancer. *Cancer* 63:1045–1047, 1989.
185. Vogel CL: Treatment of metastatic breast cancer. *Semin Oncol Nurs* 7(3):194–199, 1991.
186. Scheinberg DA, Houghton AN: Current status of an-

titumor therapy with monoclonal antibodies. *Oncology* 1:31–40, 1987.

187. Ayash LJ, Antman K, Cheson BD: A perspective on dose intensive therapy with autologous bone marrow transplantation for solid tumors. *Oncology* 5(3):25–41, 1991.
188. Eddy DM: High dose chemotherapy with autologous bone marrow transplantation for the treatment of metastatic breast cancer. *J Clin Oncol* 10(4):657–670, 1992.
189. Donegan WL: Prognostic factors, stage and receptor status in breast cancer. *Cancer* 70:1755–1764, 1992.
190. Ruder AM, Lubin F, Wax Y, et al: Estrogen and progesterone receptors in breast cancer patients. *Cancer* 64:196–202, 1989.
191. Henderson IC, Garber JE, Breitmeyer JB: Comprehensive management of disseminated breast cancer. *Cancer* 66:1439–1448, 1990.
192. Ingle JN, Ahmann DL, Green SJ, et al: Randomized clinical trial of diethylstilbestrol versus tamoxifen in postmenopausal women with advanced breast cancer. *N Engl J Med* 304:16–21, 1981.
193. Ingle J: Additive hormone therapy in women with advanced breast cancer. *Cancer* 53:766–777, 1984.
194. Schacter LP, Rozencweig M, Cannetta R, et al: Overview of hormonal therapy in advanced breast cancer. *Semin Oncol* 17(6):38–46, 1990.
195. Cruz JM, Muss HB, Brockschmidt JK, et al: Weight changes in women with metastatic breast cancer treated with megestrol acetate: A comparison of standard versus high dose therapy. *Semin Oncol* 17(6):63–67, 1990.
196. Wolter J: Tamoxifen: A review. *Female Patient* 16:71–80, 1991.
197. Sunderland MC, Osborne CK: Tamoxifen in premenopausal patients with metastatic breast cancer: A review. *J Clin Oncol* 9:1283–1297, 1991.
198. Sheh SP, Allegra JC: Endocrine therapy of breast cancer. In Bland KI, Copeland EM (eds): *The Breast: Comprehensive Management of Benign and Malignant Disease.* Philadelphia: Saunders, 1991, pp. 937–947.
199. Vogel CL, Shemano I, Schoenfelder J, et al: Multicenter phase II efficacy of toremifine refractory patients with advanced breast cancer. *J Clin Oncol* 11:345–350, 1993.
200. Barden S, Vignon F, Chalbos D, et al: RU486: A progestin and glucocorticoid antagonist inhibits the growth of breast cancer cells via the progesterone receptor. *J Clin Endocrinol Metab* 60:692–697, 1985.
201. Romieu G, Maudelonde T, Elmann A, et al: The antiprogestin RU486 in advanced breast cancer: Preliminary clinical trial. *Bull Cancer* 74:455–461, 1987.
202. Bakker GH, Setyono HB, Portengen H, et al: Treatment of breast cancer with different antiprogestins: Preclinical and clinical studies. *J Steroid Biochem Mol Biol* 37(6):789–794, 1990.
203. Illinois Cancer Council Protocol #88B3: Pilot study (Phase I) of tamoxifen and a vitamin A analogue (4-HPR) in patients with metastatic adenocarcinoma of the breast. Chicago: Illinois Cancer Council, 1991, pp. 1–40.
204. Raats JI, Falkson HC: A study of fadrozole, a new aromatase inhibitor in post-menopausal women with advanced metastatic cancer. *J Clin Oncol* 10:111–116, 1992.
205. Donegan WL: Cancer of the breast in men. *CA* 41(6):339–351, 1991.
206. Evans DB, Crichlow RW: Carcinoma of the male breast and Klinefelter's syndrome: Is there an association? *CA* 37:246–251, 1987.
207. Bezwoda WR, Hesdorffer C, Dansey R, et al: Breast cancer in men: Clinical features, hormone receptor status, and response to therapy. *Cancer* 60:1337–1340, 1987.
208. Larsen D, Weinstein M, Goldberg I, et al: Edema of the arm as a function of the extent of axillary surgery in patients treated with stage I-II carcinoma of the breast treated with primary radiotherapy. *Int J Radiat Oncol Biol Phys* 16:1575–1582, 1986.
209. Brennan MJ: Lymph edema following surgical treatment of breast cancer: A review of pathophysiology and treatment. *J Pain Symp Manag* 7:110–116, 1992.
210. Fowble B: Special considerations. In Fowble B, Goodman RL, Glick JH, Rosato EF (eds): *Breast Cancer Treatment: A Comprehensive Guide to Management.* St. Louis, MO: Mosby Year Book, 1991, pp. 528–549.
211: Doll DC, Ringenberg QS, Yarbro JW: Antineoplastic agents and pregnancy. *Semin Oncol* 16:337–346, 1989.
212. Barnicle M: Chemotherapy and pregnancy. *Semin Oncol Nurs* 8(2): 124–132, 1992.
213. Harrington RA, Hamilton DW, Brogden RN, et al: Metoclopramide: An updated review of its pharmacological properties and clinical use. *Drugs* 25:451–494, 1983.
214. Leathem AM: Safety and efficacy of antiemetics used to treat nausea and vomiting in pregnancy. *Clin Pharmacol* 5:660–668, 1986.
215. Garber JE: Long term follow-up of children exposed *in vitro* to antineoplastic agents. *Semin Oncol* 16:337–444, 1989.
216. Zemlickis D, Lishner M, Degendorfer P, et al: Fetal outcome after in utero exposure to cancer chemotherapy. *Arch Inter Med* 152(3):573–576, 1992.

Chapter 39

Central Nervous System Cancers

Jo Ann Wegmann, RN, PhD

INTRODUCTION

The brain and spinal cord represent a closed system of intricately functioning structures. Tumor involvement within the central nervous system (CNS) is associated with a high degree of morbidity and mortality. The CNS also is a common site for metastatic lesions and often reflects advanced systemic disease. The incidence of brain metastases is increasing, probably due to increased disease-free intervals, better local control of cancer, and longer survival of patients with cancer. Recognition of this increasing incidence has implications for nursing in terms of treatment, quality of life, and rehabilitation potential. Treatment and long-term management of the patient at home are also assuming greater importance.

ANATOMY AND PHYSIOLOGY

The intracranial cavity contains the cerebral hemispheres, the cerebellum, and the brain stem. Each of the cerebral hemispheres has four lobes: frontal, temporal, parietal, and occipital (Figure 39-1). Below the cerebral hemisphere is the diencephalon, which contains the thalamus, basal ganglia, hypothalamus, and pineal gland. The midbrain, pons, and medulla make up the brain stem. The cerebellum is attached to the brain stem by three pairs of peduncles. The cerebellum has two hemispheres and a midline region called the vermis.

The cranial nerves have fiber pathways entering and exiting the brain and cranial cavity. The olfactory and optic nerves (I and II) are associated with the cerebral hemispheres. The third and fourth cranial nerves, the occulomotor and trochlear, receive their fibers from the midbrain. The trigeminal nerve (V) is located between the midbrain and the pons; it has fibers running through the medulla, pons, and midbrain. The abducens and facial nerves (VI and VII) are located in the pons, with the abducens lying at the pontomedullary junction. The vestibulocochlear nerve (VIII) has fibers in the pons and in the medulla. The remaining cranial nerves—IX through XII (glossopharyngeal, vagus, spinal accessory, and hypoglossal)—are associated with the medulla (Figure 39-2). Symptoms of cranial nerve dysfunction provide valuable information for localizing an intracranial tumor.

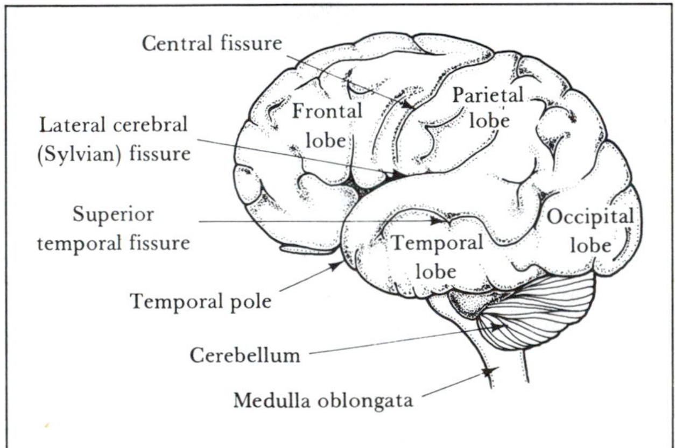

FIGURE 39-1 The four lobes of the cerebral hemispheres.

The brain is supported and protected by the skull, meninges, and cerebrospinal fluid (CSF). The meninges consist of the tough dura mater below the skull, the arachnoid lining the dura, and the pia mater, which adheres directly to the surface of the brain. Cerebrospinal fluid circulates through the subarachnoid space, supporting and cushioning the brain and spinal cord (Figure 39-3).

The dura mater is a dense, tough layer of connective tissue. It is attached to the periosteum, from which it receives small blood vessels. Two large partitions, or dural reflections, provide support for parts of the brain. These are the falx cerebri surrounding the cerebral hemispheres and the tentorium cerebelli, which wraps between the occipital lobes and the cerebellum. The edge of the tentorium runs along the midbrain. The space between the tentorial notch, or incisura, and the midbrain is small. This narrow space is the only passageway between the supratentorial and subtentorial regions (Figure 39-4).

Cerebrospinal fluid is formed in ventricles and circulates through the brain and spinal pathways. The choroid plexuses of the lateral, third, and fourth ventricles are responsible for the majority of CSF production. The flow of CSF is from the lateral ventricles through the intraventricular foramen, into the third ventricle, through the aqueduct of Sylvius, and into the fourth ventricle. Cerebrospinal fluid exits from the ventricular system via the foramen of Magendie and the foramina of Luschka. Fluid circulates around the brain and the spinal cord. It is absorbed into the dural venous sinuses. The sagittal sinus is an important site of reabsorption.

Blood flow to the brain is supplied by the two internal carotid arteries and the two vertebral arteries. The internal carotid arteries supply approximately 80% of this blood flow. The internal carotid bifurcates to form the anterior and middle cerebral arteries. These arteries supply blood to the frontal, temporal, and parietal lobes. The vertebral arteries enter the base of the skull and join to form the basilar artery. The cerebellum and the brain stem receive blood from the posterior cerebral artery. This artery supplies the occipital lobes and inferior and medial aspects of the temporal lobes.

Collateral circulation to the brain is provided by an intact circle of Willis (Figure 39-5). The posterior communicating arteries provide a connection between the

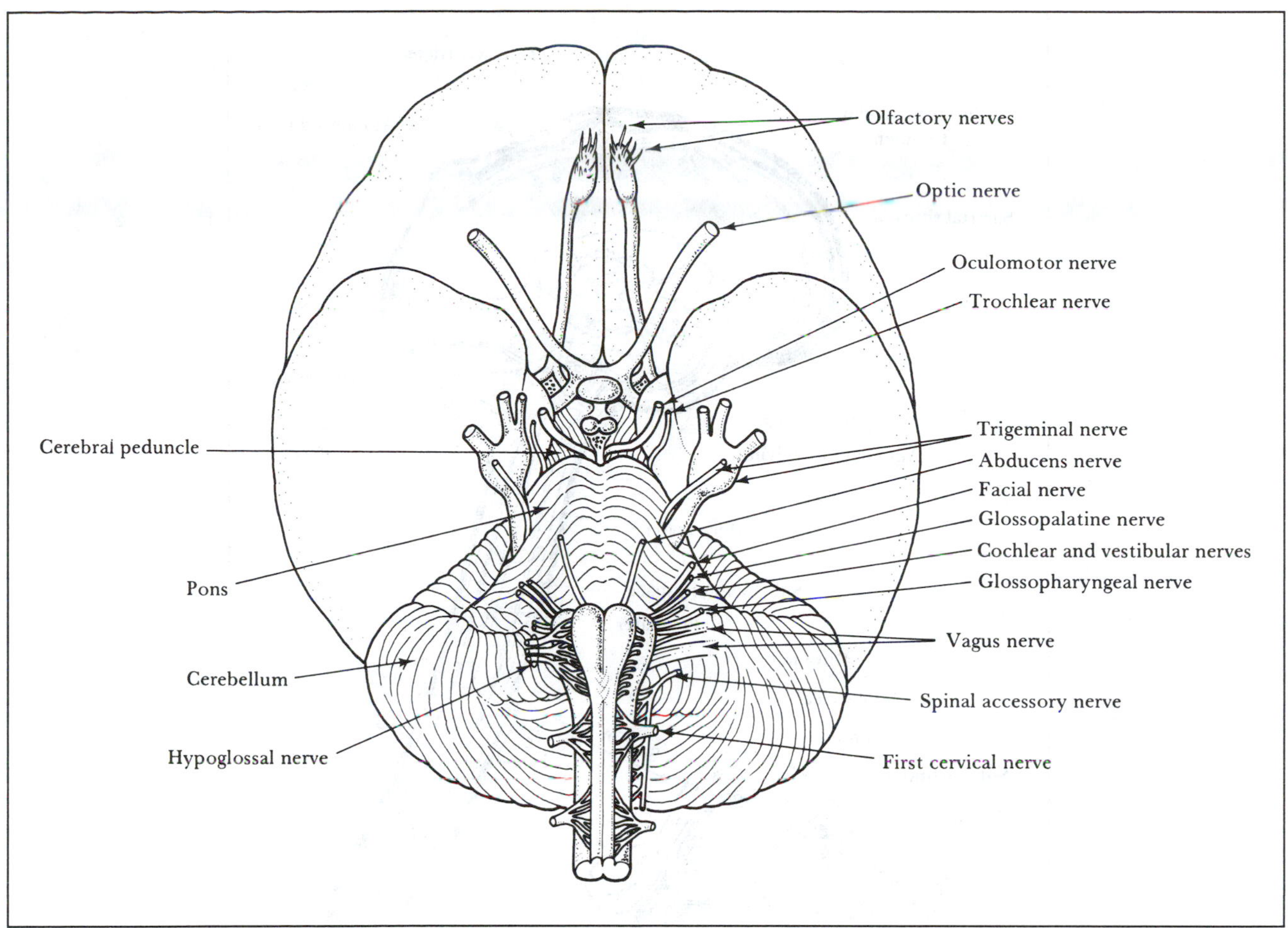

FIGURE 39-2 Sagittal representation of the brain.

internal carotid and posterior cerebral arteries. The two anterior cerebral arteries are connected by the anterior communicating artery. Blood can be shunted from one area of the brain to another in the event of sudden occlusion. This is possible only when the communicating arteries are present; these arteries are not present in all individuals.

Blood flow to the brain remains constant between systemic arterial pressures of 60 and 145 mm Hg. This regulatory mechanism is called *autoregulation.* Cerebral blood flow and blood volume in the brain are controlled through adjustments in the size of blood vessels. The cerebrovascular resistance (vasoconstriction or vasodilation) regulates blood flow in accordance with metabolic needs. It also maintains a normal intracranial pressure despite fluctuations in arterial pressure and venous drainage.

Cerebral blood vessels dilate in response to decreased pH and increased $PaCO_2$. Decreased $PaCO_2$ also will increase cerebral blood flow through vasodilatation. Declining $PaCO_2$ causes a constriction of cerebral blood vessels and a decrease in blood flow. A decline in $PaCO_2$ can occur as a result of decreased metabolic demand or hyperventilation.

Intracranial pressure (ICP) is maintained within the normal range by the autoregulatory mechanism. The two major determinants of ICP in normal and abnormal conditions are the arterial blood pressure and the intracranial venous pressure.[1] Arterial blood pressure increases with certain activities: sneezing, coughing, isometric muscle contraction, and performance of a Valsalva maneuver. Venous pressure is increased by obstruction of blood outflow. This is accomplished by jugular compression, flexion-extension of the neck, and rotation of the neck.[2] Because intracranial veins do not have valves, pressure in the venous system can be transmitted to the cranium. Increased intrathoracic or intraabdominal pressure can obstruct venous outflow. Activities that increase thoracic and abdominal cavity pressures include positive end-expiratory pressure (PEEP) treatments, hip flexion, Valsalva maneuvers, and lying on the abdomen. Elevating the head of the bed promotes venous drainage.

In the autoregulating brain, ICP remains constant despite changes in systemic arterial blood pressure and intracranial venous drainage. Loss of autoregulation means that cerebral blood flow and volume will fluctuate passively with systemic blood pressure. Activities

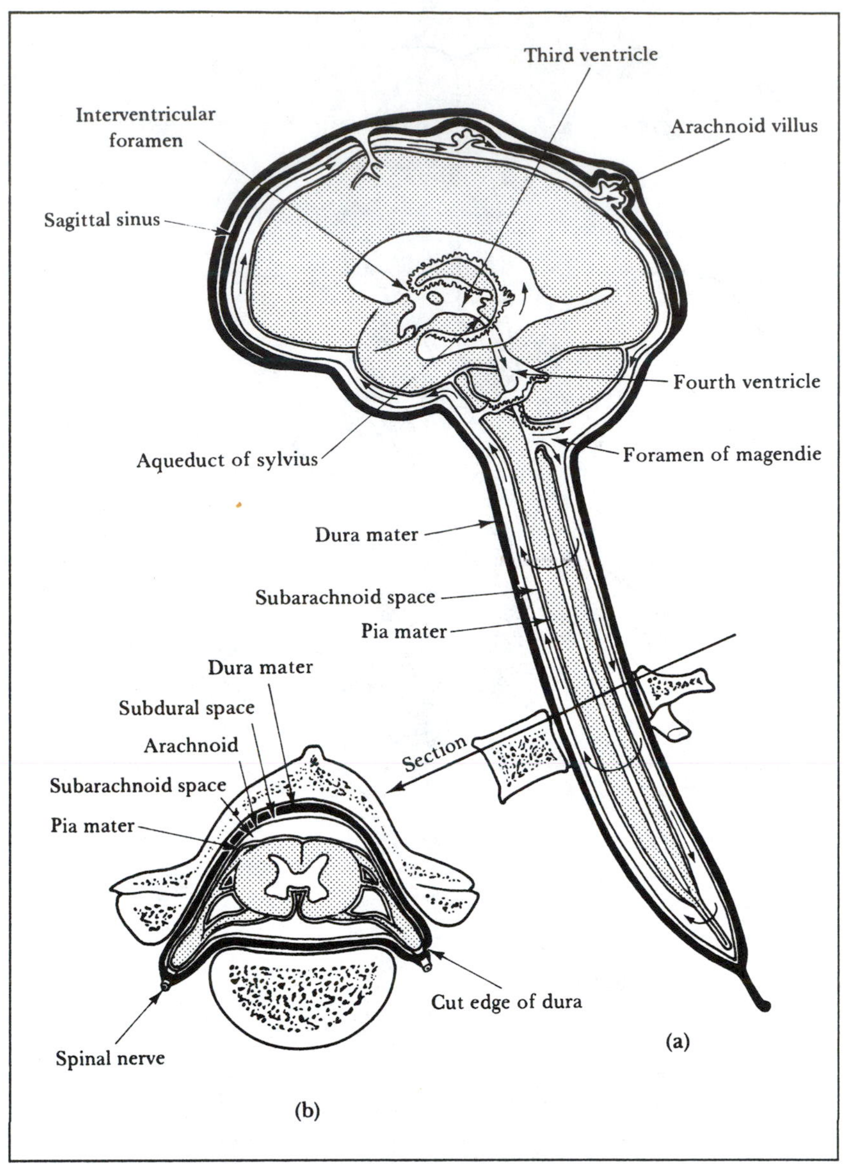

FIGURE 39-3 Circulation of cerebrospinal fluid.

that affect blood pressure and intracranial venous pressure will have significant effects on ICP.

EPIDEMIOLOGY

The most prevalent malignant CNS tumor is the tumor within the intracranial system, or the brain tumor. More than 50% of primary brain tumors are malignant and infiltrate the brain substance. Metastatic intracranial tumors occur predominantly in middle-aged individuals because the rate of metastasis increases with each decade of life, reaching a peak during the seventh decade in men and the sixth decade in women.

There are approximately 16,700 new cases of primary brain and CNS tumors and 11,500 deaths from CNS tumors each year in the United States.[3] Malignant brain tumors account for 1.5% of all cancer in the United States.[3] The death rate from brain and nervous system involvement is slightly higher for males than for females. Five-year survival rates for brain and nervous system cancer have been slowly increasing, with a 24% survival rate for white and a 32% survival rate for blacks.[3]

Most malignant CNS tumors are metastatic from a distant site. The most common primary sites include lung, breast, and colon. Metastatic brain tumors occur with equal frequency in all races, and incidence rates are slightly higher for males.[4] The lung is considered the primary tumor site with greatest propensity for brain metastases; of the 28% of the total cancer deaths in the Unites States that were due to lung cancer, a significant number involve metastatic brain lesions.[3]

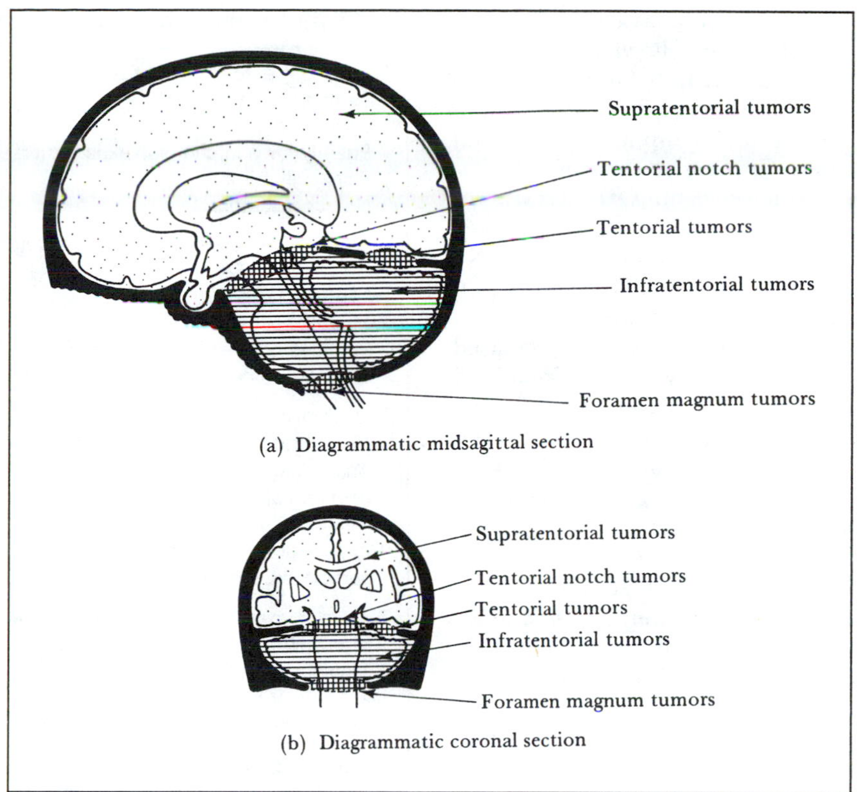

FIGURE 39-4 Localization of intracranial tumors.

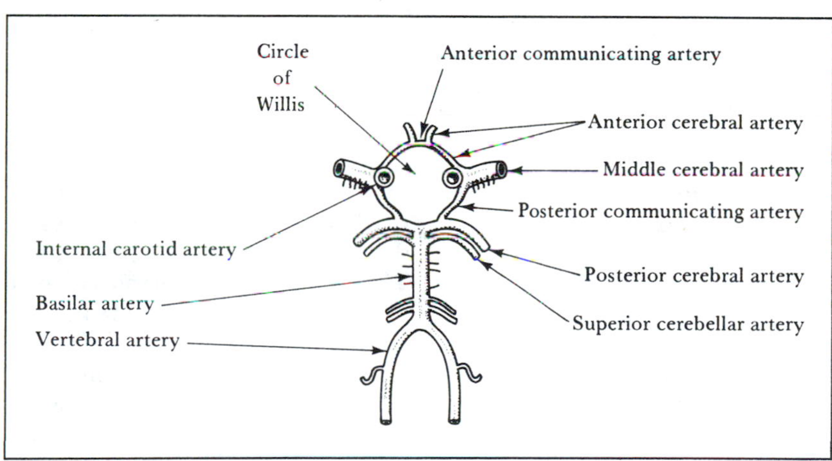

FIGURE 39-5 Circle of Willis.

Incidence of primary malignant brain tumors is smaller, estimated at 5 per 100,000 individuals. At least 10% of nontraumatic neurologic disease results from primary brain tumors.[5] A somewhat higher incidence of CNS cancer also has been found in persons with poor response to immunosuppressive agents, and a familial tendency is implicated for some brain tumors, particularly glioblastoma[6] and retinoblastoma.[7]

ETIOLOGY

Specific causes of the various CNS tumors remain speculative. Prophylactic radiation therapy of the brain in children with other malignancies (e.g., leukemia) has been linked with the subsequent appearance of malignant brain tumors.[8,9] Radiation gliomas are uncommon, but are believed to possibly occur following therapy for acute lymphocytic leukemia (ALL).[10] Similarly, an increased incidence of both primary and metastatic brain tumors, including intracranial lymphoma, has been found following immunosuppressive therapy.[11]

Evidence as yet is inconclusive, but several researchers suggest that certain occupational exposures may predispose an individual to the development of CNS tumors. These include exposure to vinyl chloride, plutonium, and petroleum.[12,14] Another area of occupational concern is that of electronics, where increased risk of astrocytic brain tumors may exist.[13] Combined exposures of occupational and environmental factors have been explained, with suggested formulas to determine interactions among such factors as smoking and exposure to asbestos.[15] It is recognized that there is a need for more systematic efforts to investigate interaction phenomena.

Further epidemiological evidence suggests an association between exposure to extremely low-frequency electromagnetic fields and increased incidence of cancer.[16] Occupational concern exists about the lack of data regarding cancer-causing elements of magnetic fields. To date, few studies have been performed regarding incidence of either childhood leukemia or CNS malignancy and exposure to magnetic fields.[17]

PATHOPHYSIOLOGY

Classification of primary CNS tumors is based on the presumed cell type of the tumor. The distinction between benign and malignant tumors is seldom made in epidemiologic studies of CNS tumors because of the variety of symptoms. Yet, several models for classification exist, based on embryogenetics, grading systems, and other histological classifications. A decade ago, collaboration of various groups resulted in the universal histological classification of CNS tumors.[18] This classification provided a uniform international nomenclature that considered both histological type and degree of malignancy.[19] This classification is shown in Table 39-1.

This classification represents the universally accepted histological classifications of CNS tumors. Diagnostic classification and staging are discussed later in this chapter.

Primary brain tumors arise from neuroepithelial cells (glial cells), and are called gliomas. Glial cells are among the few neural cells that are capable of division. Gliomas include astrocytic tumors, oligodendroglial tumors, ependymal and choroidplexus tumors, pineal cell tumors, neuronal tumors, and poorly differentiated embryonal tumors. Those of astrocytic origin are the most common.[20]

TABLE 39-1 Histologic Classification of CNS Tumors

Tumors of neuroepithelial tissue
Astrocytic tumors
Oligodendroglial tumors
Ependymal and choroidplexus tumors
Pineal cell tumors
Neuronal tumors
Poorly differentiated and embryonal tumors
Glioblastoma
Medulloblastoma
Medulloepithelioma
Primitive polar spongioblastoma
Gliomatosis cerebri
Tumors of nerve sheath cells
Neurilemmoma (schwannoma, neurinoma)
Anaplastic (malignant) neurilemmoma (schwannoma, neurinoma)
Neurofibroma
Anaplastic (malignant) neurofibroma (neurofibrosarcoma, neurogenic sarcoma)
Tumors of meningeal and related tissues
Meningioma
Meningeal sarcomas
Xanthomatous tumors
Primary melanotic tumors
Tumors of the blood vessel origin
Hemangioblastoma (capillary hemangioblastoma)
Monstrocellular sarcoma
Germ cell tumors
Germinoma
Embryonal carcinoma
Choriocarcinoma
Teratoma

Neuroepithelial tumor cells are often found diffusely in the perivascular spaces and subpial region of the cortex. Such a tumor may appear to be multicentric. These tumors may spread via the CSF to distant parts of the nervous system. Metastases of primary neuroepithelial tumors outside the CNS are rare.[21] The most common primary CNS tumors of the adult are discussed in the following sections.

Astrocytoma

Astrocytomas are the largest group of primary brain tumors of one cell type. In adults, astrocytomas are ranked third in frequency (10%) after glioblastomas and meningiomas.[6] Their incidence is greatest in individuals in the fifth and sixth decades of life, with the incidence being somewhat higher in males than in females.[22]

Astrocytomas generally arise in the cerebral hemispheres of adults and develop in the central and subcortical white matter. Infrequently they may arise in the corpus striatum.[22] These tumors are generally solid but may present as cystic lesions such as cerebellar and spinal cord astrocytomas.[4] The histologic patterns of astrocytomas are varied. Grade I astrocytomas consist of well-differentiated astrocytes, whereas grade IV tumors demonstrate significant pleomorphism, cellularity, numerous mitoses, necrosis, and sometimes giant cells. Grades II and III are considered to be intermediate stages.

Astrocytoma grades III and IV (glioblastoma multiforme) may have multiple foci of origin. They are considered highly malignant because of their infiltrative character and lack of capsulation. Areas of necrosis and hemorrhage with frequent mitoses occur. Sloughing of tumor cells around necrotic foci is characteristic of these tumors. Vascular changes such as endothelial proliferation, thrombosis, and fibroblastic proliferation are features of these tumors.[4]

Oligodendroglioma

Fewer than 5% of primary brain tumors are oligodendrogliomas. These tumors present as typically circumscribed, spongy, and vascular masses, usually located in the frontal lobes. Calcification is a usual finding within the tumor and adjacent brain tissue.[4,6]

Cellular pleomorphism in the form of multinucleated giant cells of the Langhan type is a feature of this tumor. Other anaplastic features include abundant necrotic zones and proliferation of blood vessels. Oligodendrogliomas are slow-growing tumors, most commonly presenting as a seizure disorder. Of interest, these tumors have shown a unique chemosensitivity to procarbazine, CCNU, and vincristine, enhancing research interest in this rare tumor.[23]

Glioblastoma

Glioblastoma is the most common (60%) of the primary adult brain tumors.[6] Glioblastomas arise in the cerebral hemisphere of adults, with a somewhat higher incidence in men than in women. They typically occur during the fifth and sixth decades of life. Glioblastomas have a predilection for the frontal lobe.

Glioblastoma presents with necrosis, pseudopalisading, fistulous vessels, vascular endothelium proliferation, and areas of old and fresh hemorrhages.[18] This is typically a grade IV tumor. Thrombosis and fibroblastic proliferation are also present.

Primary Malignant Lymphomas

Primary central nervous system lymphoma is a rare form of neoplasm, formerly representing less than 1% of primary brain tumors. However, in the last 10 years the number of cases has tripled. There is an increasing incidence of these tumors in the immunosuppressed patient (either inherited or acquired immunosuppression). Those populations at greatest risk include transplant recipients, AIDS patients, and those with congenital immunodeficiencies. There is also a slightly higher incidence in men than women. Approximately 3% of AIDS patients will develop CNS lymphoma.[24]

These non-Hodgkin's lymphomas are mainly of B-cell origin. Studies suggest that the Epstein-Barr virus plays a role in its development. This tumor may arise primarily in any part of the cerebrum, cerebellum, or brain stem and may be either monofocal or multifocal. Perivascular and meningeal spread results in shedding of cells into the CSF.[25]

CNS lymphoma presents in various ways. One may see localized neurological dysfunction, apathy, confusion, or personality changes. Most of the AIDS-related primary brain lymphomas are reported to be of high or intermediate grade.[26]

Spinal Cord Tumors

CNS tumors include intraspinal tumors, which occur with considerably less frequency than intracranial tumors. Intraspinal tumors may be primary (approximately 15% of primary CNS tumors)[25] or metastatic (Figure 39-6). Regardless of pathophysiology, intraspinal tumors may result in spinal cord compression.

Cord compression is considered an oncologic emergency, as discussed elsewhere in this text. Compression rapidly results in irreversible neurologic changes; therefore, rapid surgical removal of the tumor is of utmost importance to relieve edema and related pressure.

Typically spinal cord tumors become clinically manifested in one of three ways.[25] Sensorimotor spinal tract syndromes compress the cord and cause destruction of cord tracts; initial asymmetric motor disturbance results. Radicular-spinal cord syndrome results in pain in the distribution of a sensory nerve root; the pain is intensified by straining and radiates in a distal direction, away from the spine. A syringomyelic syndrome results from an intramedullary tumor and produces a mixed sensorimotor tract syndrome.

Diagnosis of cord compression is established by spinal radiographs, CSF examination, and MRI. Of particular importance to nursing are the ongoing assessment of neurologic status, prompt determination of a potential problem with compression, and immediate intervention to prevent irreversible neurologic damage and loss.

Metastatic Tumors

The incidence of metastatic brain tumors is estimated at 24% of individuals who die from cancer.[27] Brain

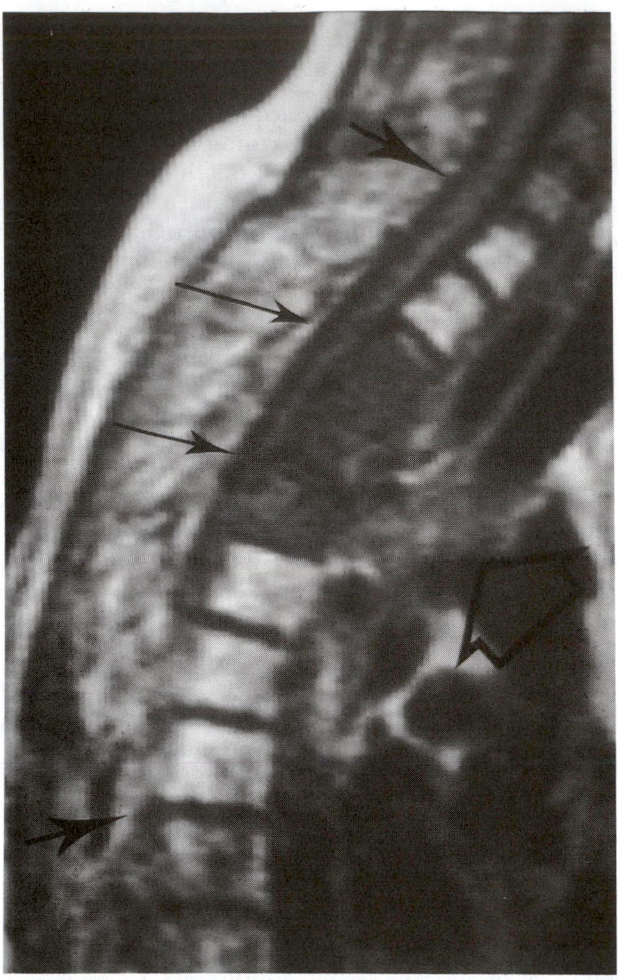

FIGURE 39-6 MRI showing invasion and destruction of thoracic vertebrae. (Courtesy Radiology Department Rush-Presbyterian-St. Luke's Medical Center, Chicago.)

metastases are present at autopsy in 10%–20% of individuals with systemic cancer.[5]

Intracranial metastases occur at three main sites: the skull and dura, the brain itself, and meninges. The skull and dura are infiltrated by tumors that metastasize to the bone, particularly metastatic tumors of the breast and prostate. These metastases are believed to reach the skull via Batson's vertebral venous plexus, a valveless system of veins that runs the length of the vertebral column from the pelvic veins to the large venous sinuses of the skull, bypassing the systemic circulation.[25]

Metasases to the brain occur by hemotogenous spread, with a third originating in the lung.[25] The example of metastases from the lung is described here. From the lungs, cancer cells may enter the pulmonary veins and reach the left atrium and ventricle. Tumor cells transported in this manner are widely dispersed and are ultimately deposited in the capillaries. Once within the arterial circulation, tumor cells readily travel to the brain and liver. Tumor cells may return to the heart, enter the arterial circulation, and become generalized. Metastasis to the brain then occurs.

The most common site of metastasis in the brain is the cortex. Within the cortex is the terminal territory of the three main cerebral arteries; the middle, posterior, and anterior arteries. Because these three major arteries terminate so close to one another, neoplastic emboli have a great tendency to develop there. In the majority of cases, tumor cells spread to the brain via the arterial pathway described.

The individual at greatest risk for metastatic CNS involvement has widespread systemic disease when neurologic symptoms develop.[4] Tumors that metastasize to the brain present in many ways and involve every portion of the brain. A metastatic brain tumor may mimic the presentation of any primary brain tumor. The major symptoms of metastatic brain tumors arise as a result of increased ICP. Early complaints include headache, nausea and vomiting, and personality changes. Destruction of neurologic structures, cerebral edema, and seizures lead to additional symptoms.

Meningeal carcinomatosis is rare and occurs with widespread dissemination of tumor cells throughout the meninges and ventricles. Adams and Victor[25] identify approximately 4% of neurologic metastases as meningeal carcinomatosis, arising from adenocarcinoma of breast, lung, gastrointestinal tract, melanoma, and childhood leukemia. Principal manifestations include headache, backache, radiculopathies, cranial nerve palsies, and dementia. Hydrocephalus may occur. Diagnosis includes examination of the CSF, with elevated protein and low glucose levels. Treatment includes radiation therapy to symptomatic areas, followed by intraventricular administration of methotrexate. Reports of median survival range from 43 days to 5.8 months following diagnosis.[25]

Another form of metastasis is described as occurring from seeding within the spinal canal. This has been identified as a late effect of glioblastoma that may present with paraplegia.[28] Such spinal canal seeding may be diagnosed by myelography, CSF cytology, and MRI.

CLINICAL MANIFESTATIONS

The signs and symptoms of brain tumors are variable. Clinical manifestations vary depending on the site, size, method of expansion, and other factors related to the nature of the tumor. The clinical manifestations can be classified into three major categories: generalized effects of increased ICP, secondary effects due to shifts or displacement of brain structures, and focal effects. Any one of these mechanisms may predominate throughout the course of an individual's illness. More often several of these mechanisms are producing effects simultaneously (Figure 39-7).

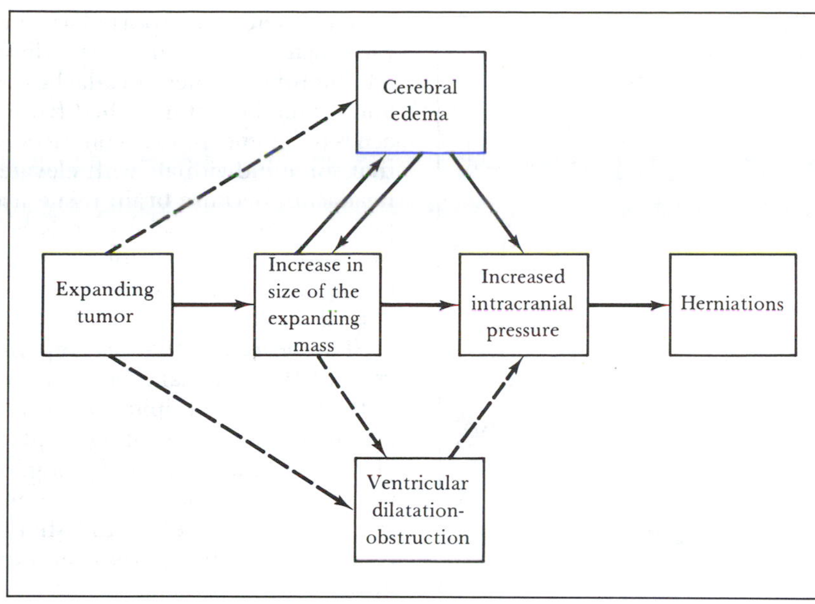

FIGURE 39-7 Mechanisms responsible for the clinical manifestations of intracranial tumors.

Increased Intracranial Pressure

In adults the skull acts as a rigid sphere. Its contents are fixed in total volume. The cranium encases the three normal components of the intracranial cavity: brain, cerebrospinal fluid, and blood. Each of these components is displaceable. To maintain normal ICP, an increase in the volume of one component must be accompanied by a proportional decrease in the volume of one or both of the other components. Compensatory mechanisms for accommodating a volume increase include decreased cerebral blood volume, decreased CSF production, increased CSF absorption, and brain fluid shifts from the head to the spinal cavity. The compensatory changes are limited, especially when a volume increase is too large or too sudden. Beyond a certain point, additions of any further volume result in large increases in ICP. Once all the compensatory mechanisms are exhausted, relatively small increases in volume create large increases in ICP.

Brain tumors increase ICP by their size, cerebral edema, or obstruction of CSF pathways. A combination of tumor bulk and peritumoral edema usually is responsible for an increase in ICP. In the area of the third and fourth ventricles, a comparatively small tumor can block CSF flow. In contrast, extensive tumors can sometimes exist without causing an immediate increase in ICP. These are tumors in the frontal or temporal lobes (such as meningiomas) and diffusely infiltrative tumors (glioblastomas), which only partially damage structures during infiltration.

Clinical manifestations are produced by the effects of increasing ICP on nerve cells, blood vessels, and dura. Prolonged increase in ICP ultimately produces nerve cell damage and cell death. An expanding tumor mass can create a vicious cycle of intracranial hypertension (Figure 39-8). Once all the normal compensatory mechanisms have been used, increased ICP is compensated for by a decrease in cerebral blood flow (total blood volume in the brain). A decrease in the supply of oxygen and glucose to the brain leads to tissue hypoxia and a decreased blood supply impedes the removal of carbon dioxide and lactic acid. These two products of metabolism are potent vasodilatators. Vasodilatation of cerebral blood vessels creates further vasogenic edema. The total volume within the cranium is increased, intracranial pressure again rises, and the cycle repeats itself.

Cerebral blood flow is relatively constant in the healthy brain; blood flow to the brain is independent of changes in arterial blood pressure. This autoregulation of cerebral blood flow ensures a constant blood supply to the brain between the limits of mean systemic arterial pressures of 60–145 mm Hg.[1] In the normal autoregulating brain, changes in systemic blood pressure have no effect on ICP. When ICP rises to very high levels, however, the autoregulatory system fails and the cerebral blood flow drops. The total blood supply to the brain is decreased. Lack of autoregulation means that cerebral blood flow fluctuates passively with the systemic arterial blood pressure. Increases in systemic blood pressure directly affect ICP. If the cycle of increasing pressure and decreasing cerebral blood flow

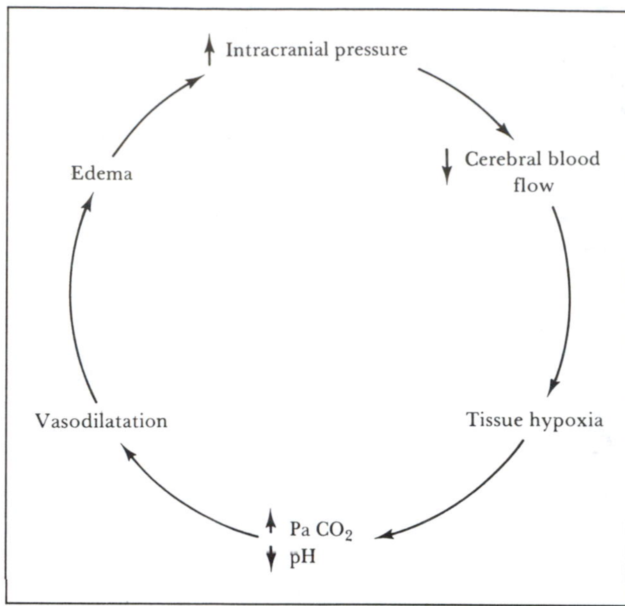

FIGURE 39-8 Cycle of intracranial hypertension.

continues, the brain tissue no longer receives an adequate blood supply and brain death eventually occurs.

The clinical manifestations of generalized increased ICP include mental changes, papilledema, headache, vomiting, and changes in vital signs. These signs and symptoms are nonspecific or nonlocalizing. Increased ICP can cause secondary effects by displacing brain tissue.

Changes in mental status include alterations in the level of consciousness, confusion, short-term memory loss, and personality changes. Each individual may show a wide variety of mental changes. These changes are frequently gradual in onset. Subtle initial changes may be evident only to the family or a skilled observer. In the early states of increasing ICP, individuals may complain of drowsiness, a decreased attention span, and memory loss. Families may report behavior and personality changes, mood changes, poor judgment, or blunting of intellectual functions. If the increased ICP is not treated, basic levels or states of consciousness are affected. The individual can change from a state of alertness (awake, fully aware of normal internal and external stimuli) to one of lethargy or somnolence. As ICP increases over time, the level of consciousness deteriorates from full alertness to somnolence, stupor, and finally coma.

Papilledema is considered a cardinal sign of increased ICP. An increase in CSF pressure around the optic nerve impairs the outflow of venous blood. Edema or swelling of the optic disk results. Blurred vision and visual field defects may accompany papilledema, especially in the presence of longstanding increased ICP. Papilledema may be an early or late finding, depending on the nature and location of the brain tumor.

Headaches are reported as an early symptom in approximately one-third of the individuals presenting with a brain tumor. These headaches are variable in nature and should be distinguished from other types of headaches (migraine, muscle contraction). It should be noted that some individuals with elevated ICP never report headache. Because brain tissue itself does not contain pain sensors, headache pain is believed to be a result of pressure or traction on the pain-sensitive structures of the dura, venous sinuses, surface blood vessels, and cranial nerves.

The headache that accompanies a generalized increased ICP is usually bilateral; it generally is located in the frontal or occipital regions. Individuals may give a history of early morning headache that subsides on arising. Bending over, coughing, or performing a Valsalva maneuver may aggravate or initiate a headache. Pain may be reported as dull, sharp, or throbbing. Over time the headaches increase in severity, frequency, and duration.

Vomiting is part of the classic triad of increased ICP (vomiting, papilledema, and headache). It appears unrelated to food ingestion. Vomiting may be preceded by nausea, or it may be sudden, unexpected, and forceful (projectile). Increased pressure on the vomiting center of the medulla is believed to precipitate this symptom.

Changes in vital signs are a late finding of increased ICP. They result from increased pressure on the vasomotor centers of the medulla. As ICP increases, circulatory and respiratory responses to intracranial hypertension occur. Systolic blood pressure rises, diastolic blood pressure drops, and the pulse pressure widens. Bradycardia and slowed, irregular respirations are seen. The combination of hypertension, bradycardia, and respiratory slowing is called the Cushing triad and is not always seen in individuals with elevated ICP. When this response is seen, it is a late finding; the individual is usually already comatose.

Secondary Effects: Displacement of Brain Structures

The cranial cavity is divided into compartments by the rigid dura mater surrounding the cerebral hemispheres (falx cerebri) and the cerebellum (tentorium cerebelli). Pressure is normally distributed equally throughout the compartments of the cranial cavity (Figure 39-9a). A growing tumor mass and the associated edema cause increased pressure within a cranial compartment. An increase in pressure in any one compartment can cause brain tissue to protrude from one compartment into another. Brain tissue shifts or herniates from the high-pressure compartment into a lower-pressure compartment. The resulting brain damage is life-threatening.

Herniation is a neurologic emergency. Shifting brain tissue causes compression damage, cerebral edema, and

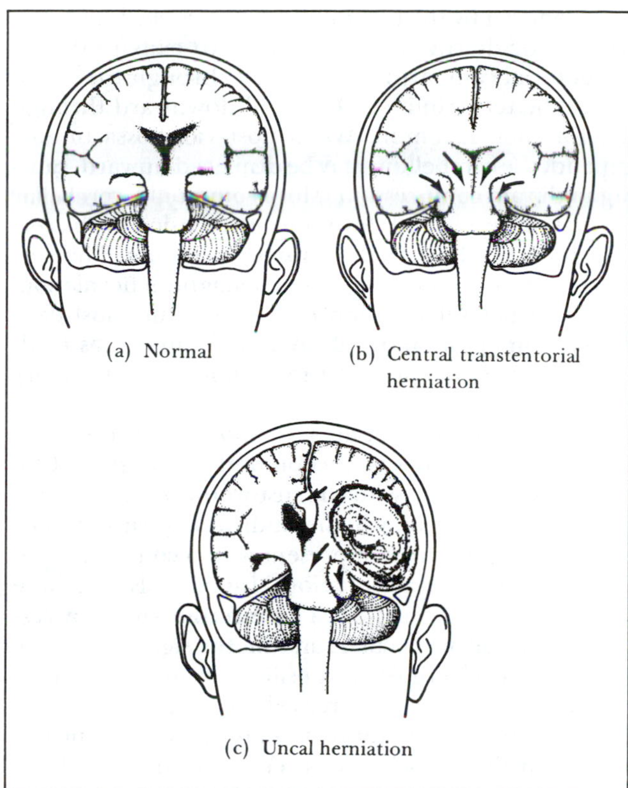

FIGURE 39-9 Displacement of brain structures.

ischemia. Blood vessels may be damaged by stretch and angulation pressures, which may produce an obstruction in blood flow or vessel rupture. Displaced brain tissue can obstruct CSF pathways, causing an obstructive hydrocephalus. These compressive, ischemic, vascular, and obstructive changes all add to and aggravate the original problem of increased ICP. The potentially reversible complications of an expanding tumor become irreversible.

An expanding tumor mass can displace tissue distant from the tumor site. The neurologic signs and symptoms accompanying these shifts may have true or false localizing value. There are two major classifications of herniations: supratentorial brain shifts and infratentorial brain shifts. The clinical manifestations of the two types differ. Supratentorial herniations cause changes in the level of consciousness and ocular, motor, and respiratory signs. Infratentorial herniations cause loss of consciousness and respiratory and cardiac changes. There is an orderly rostral-to-caudal progression of abnormal clinical signs. However, sudden changes in intracranial dynamics will rapidly precipitate medullary compression (as in hemorrhage or performance of a lumbar puncture).

Supratentorial tumors, lesions above the tentorium cerebelli, displace brain structures in the anterior and middle fossae. An expanding tumor eventually takes up so much space that the supratentorial compartment can no longer tolerate the volume it displaces. The pressure of the tumor mass and its edema push the brain downward. The only outlet for this pressure is the opening at the tentorial notch (incisura). As pressure forces brain structures downward, the tissue becomes ischemic and edematous. Blood vessels may rupture. These reactions add to the problem of increasing ICP. Additional increases in pressure displace the swollen brain tissue further downward.

Central or transtentorial herniation occurs when the cerebral hemispheres, basal ganglia, diencephalon, and adjacent midbrain are displaced downward. The final result is a protrusion of the diencephalon and adjoining midbrain through the tentorial notch (Figure 39-9b). The first signs of impending central herniation are those of diencephalic dysfunction. A change in behavior or level of consciousness may signal early dysfunction. The individual may become agitated, drowsy, inattentive, or forgetful. As the tumor continues to displace tissue downward, the individual passes from alertness to stupor and then coma. Pupil size is reduced. Depending on the degree of diencephalic impairment, eye movements may be roving, conjugate, slightly disconjugate, or unmoving. Oculocephalic and oculovestibular responses may be impaired, and upward gaze palsy may be seen. Motor signs include a bilateral Babinski's sign, contralateral hemiparesis, and ipsilateral paratonic resistance.

Uncal herniation occurs when the medial part of one of the temporal lobes is forced toward the midline and downward through the tentorial opening (see Figure 39-9c). This characteristically occurs when the expanding tumor is in the temporal lobe. The pressure of the tumor shifts the medial aspect of the temporal lobe (the uncus) over the edge of the tentorial notch. The uncus compresses the midbrain laterally; the midbrain (cerebral peduncle) becomes compressed against the opposite tentorial notch. The herniated rim of the temporal lobe compresses the third cranial nerve, the cerebral peduncle, and the posterior cerebral artery. The downward pressure may also result in the stretching of blood vessels, resulting in secondary brain stem hemorrhages.

In uncal herniation the early signs of compression of the third nerve and lateral midbrain (cerebral peduncle) may precede changes in the level of consciousness. The third nerve passes through the tentorial notch on its way to the eye and is vulnerable to compression. The third nerve ipsilateral to the brain tumor is affected. Initially the pupil contracts sluggishly to direct light. With further compression on the third nerve, pupillary dilation results. With midbrain compression, the motor pathways of the cerebral peduncle are compromised. Compression of the cerebral peduncle produces a contralateral hemiparesis. Sometimes uncal herniation pushes the opposite cerebral peduncle against the tentorial notch opposite the side of herniation. This is referred to as Kernohan's notch. A hemiparesis ipsilateral to the third nerve palsy is produced; this may cause confusion in determining the side of a unilateral brain tumor. The important thing to remember is that the tumor is ipsilateral to the third nerve palsy.

Babinski's sign is seen with hemiparesis. Decerebrate or decorticate rigidity is a later finding. In the early states, oculocephalic and oculovestibular responses are conjugate; later, they are disconjugate due to impaired ipsilateral eye movement (third nerve). Third nerve function, motor signs, and changes in level of consciousness are early clinical manifestations of uncal herniation.

Both central and uncal herniation cause changes in the respiratory pattern. Irregular depth and rhythm often are more significant than changes in respiratory rate alone. Respiration in the initial stages may be irregular with occasional pauses, sighs, or gasps. Later respiratory changes include Cheyne-Stokes breathing; sustained hyperventilation; slow, irregular (ataxic) breathing; apnea; and, finally, arrest.

The classic signs of Cushing's triad (rising systolic blood pressure, decreasing diastolic blood pressure, and bradycardia) do not occur with most supratentorial herniations. These changes in vital signs are seen during the terminal phase of herniation. The important clinical manifestations of supratentorial herniation are changes in level of consciousness, pupillary size and reaction to light, ocular movement, motor strength and response, and respiratory pattern.

Infratentorial herniations involve displacement of the cerebellum (see Figure 39-10). Neurologic deficits are produced by the protrusion of the cerebellum either upward or downward. There are two exits to the infratentorial compartment: upward through the opening in the tentorium cerebelli and downward through the foramen magnum. When posterior fossa tumors expand, the cerebellum may be displaced upward, causing midbrain compression. More commonly, cerebellar herniation results in a downward protrusion of the cerebellar tonsils through the foramen magnum. This cerebellar pressure cone, or foramen magnum herniation, results in medullary compression. It is the most dangerous complication of infratentorial tumors, as medullary compression produces respiratory and circulatory arrest.

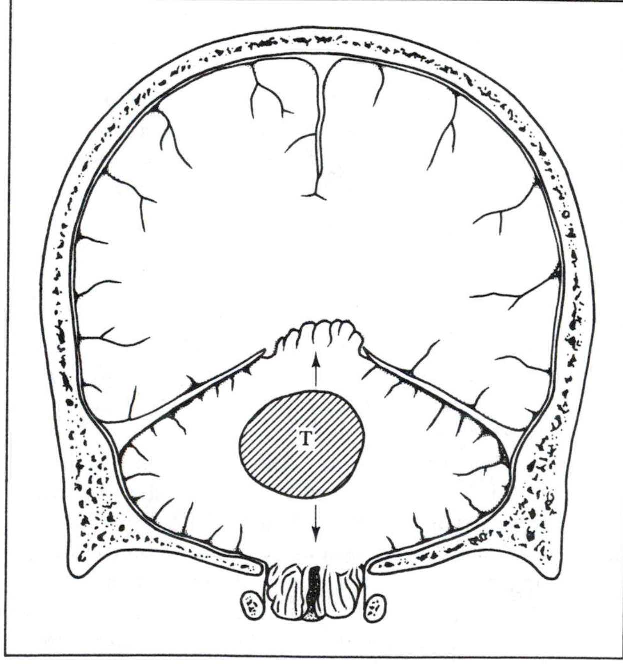

FIGURE 39-10 An infratentorial tumor causing upward and downward shifts of the cerebellum.

Upward transtentorial herniation compresses the midbrain. Vascular obstruction and blockage of CSF pathways can occur with the distortion of brain structures. It is not certain whether individuals with upward transtentorial herniation present with a consistent syndrome of clinical manifestations. Individuals often lose consciousness immediately. This is accompanied by respiratory, pupillary, ocular, and motor signs.

Downward cerebellar tonsillar herniation can be caused by generalized, increased intracranial pressure, midline tumor, or posterior fossa tumors. The outflow of the fourth ventricle is blocked by protrusion of the tonsils into the foramen magnum. The downward pressure also compresses the vasomotor centers of the medulla, causing respiratory changes. Sudden respiratory and circulatory arrest can occur. These may be precipitated by events causing a sudden rise in intracranial pressure, such as sneezing, coughing, or performing a Valsalva maneuver. Individuals with early signs of herniation may complain of a suboccipital headache and neck pain. The head may be held stiffly or to one side or the neck may be arched. Vomiting and cranial nerve palsies (cranial nerves VII–XII) may be seen. Altered consciousness with resulting coma is an early sign. Later signs of medullary dysfunction include respiratory irregularity (cluster breathing, gasping, ataxia), cardiac dysrhythmia, bradycardia or tachycardia, increased systolic blood pressure, and decreased diastolic blood pressure. Frequently, individuals with cerebellar-foramen magnum herniation have a sudden loss of consciousness followed by a respiratory arrest.

Focal Effects

Intracranial tumors produce a wide variety of neurologic symptoms due to their direct focal effects on brain tissue. The focal effects of brain tumors are caused by direct compression of nerve tissue or destruction and invasion of brain tissue through infiltration. Neurologic deficits are directly related to the damaged area of the brain; the accompanying signs and symptoms therefore have localizing value (Table 39-2). Cranial nerve function may be affected by tumors as the nerves pass

TABLE 39-2 Clinical Manifestations of Intracranial Tumors

Location	Function	Abnormality
Frontal lobes	Intellect	Intellectual deterioration
	Personality	Personality changes
	Judgment	Impaired judgment
	Abstract thinking	Bowel and bladder incontinence
	Mood and affect	Emotional lability
	Memory	Memory loss
	Motor activity (contralateral)	Muscle weakness or paralysis
		Babinski's sign
		Decreased deep tendon reflexes
	Expressive speech (left hemisphere)	Expressive aphasia
Parietal lobes	Sensory input (contralateral)	Decrease or loss of sensation (pain, temperature, pinprick, light touch, proprioception, vibration, two-point discrimination, double simultaneous stimulation, stereognosis, graphesthesia)
Occipital lobes	Sight	Visual field defects, hallucinations, inability to identify objects or symbols
	Visual identification of objects	
Temporal lobes	Hearing	Hearing changes, hallucinations
	Memory	Memory loss
	Receptive speech	Receptive aphasia
Cerebellum	Coordination	Ataxia, action tremor
		Nystagmus
	Balance (ipsilateral)	Loss of balance, wide-base gait
		Decreased deep, tendon reflexes

through the intracranial compartments. Individual cranial nerves are associated with certain structures of the brain. Cranial nerve dysfunction may therefore have localizing value.

Cerebral tumors of the motor and sensory strip cause deficits contralateral to the side of the tumor, whereas cerebellar tumors cause ipsilateral neurologic deficits. In the majority of individuals, the left side of the brain is the dominant hemisphere for speech representation. It is involved in the processing of information regarding language. The right hemisphere (nondominant in the majority of individuals) processes spatial-temporal information. A right-handed individual with a left hemisphere tumor may have problems with reading, arithmetic, writing, initiation of speech, or comprehension of speech, in addition to some degree of motor loss. An individual with a right hemisphere tumor is more likely to have problems with right-left discrimination, body image (neglect of one side or part of the body), stereognosis, and other processing of sensory information.

Seizures are a major manifestation of cerebral brain tumors. In many adults a seizure is the first clinical manifestation of a brain tumor. The focal effects of a tumor change normal nerve cells into abnormal, epileptogenic cells. These cells are highly excitable and fire repetitively; focal or generalized seizures are produced. In some cases a generalized seizure is initiated focally and spreads rapidly to involve the entire brain. A careful description of the onset of the seizure, the seizure activity, and postictal phase may have localizing value.

Seizures may be described as partial, general, or unclassified. Low grade or slow growing tumors, such as well-differentiated gliomas, are most likely to produce seizures.[29] Seizures may also be caused by metastases to the leptomeninges or dura. Also, treatment of CNS malignancies may contribute to seizure activity.[29]

Patients with intracerebral metastases represent a subgroup of individuals with CNS tumors who may be at increased risk for development of late seizures. Yet even with the known risk of postseizure sequelae, Cohen et al.[30] recommended withholding prophylactic anticonvulsant therapy, until the time of first seizure. Determination of this etiology of the seizure ensures proper therapy and management.[29]

ASSESSMENT

Patient assessment includes documentation of the presence and severity of both focal and generalized symptoms. The individual's response to the symptoms is identified, and a baseline measurement of neurologic dysfunction is made.

Posner[27] identifies the following symptoms of metastatic brain tumors in order of presentation: headache, focal weakness, mental disturbances, seizures, and other presenting symptoms such as aphasia and visual abnormalities. The evaluation of headache therefore assumes a major focus in the patient interview. The assessment will ascertain information regarding the location, onset, and duration of headache. Episodic effects of headache also must be explored. Headaches caused by brain tumors are discussed in detail in the section on clinical manifestations.

Other presenting symptoms such as mental changes and sensory loss need to be explored with the patient. Seizures represent an important area that warrants attention. The nurse determines whether the patient has had seizures or seizurelike activity, as well as the frequency and extent of such activity.

The physical examination includes a thorough neu-

TABLE 39-3 Examination of Cranial Nerves

Cranial Nerve	Method of Testing	Desired Response
I Olfactory	Inhalation of commonly recognized aromatic substance such as cloves; avoid the use of ammonia or alcohol because these stimulate the trigeminal nerve and evoke a pain response	Identification of the substance with each nostril
II Optic	Direct ophthalmoscopy; use finger movement and eye charts to test visual acuity and fields	Note the appearance of the optic disk macula, vessels, and retina; correct eye movement and chart identification with each eye separately
III Oculomotor IV Trochlear VI Abducens	Individual follows the examiner's finger with the eyes to test eye movement; check pupil response to light; observe for ptosis of the eyelid, which indicates destruction of cranial nerve III	Movement of eyes should be equal in six cardinal directions of gaze; pupils react to direct and consensual response to light; eyes are symmetric at rest and move conjugatively
V Trigeminal	Individual clamps the jaw, opens the mouth against resistance and masticates to check motor division of the nerve; touch both sides of the person's face, checking for pain, touch, and temperature response; gently touch the person's cornea with a cotton wisp to check the corneal reflex	Correct identification of sensations; rapid blinking
VII Facial	Observe for facial symmetry and the person's ability to contract muscles to check motor division; individual tastes sweet, sour, salty, and acidic flavors	Person smiles and frowns with symmetry, correct identification of tastes
VIII Acoustic	Test hearing ability with the use of whispered voice and tuning fork at various distances from the ear to check the cochlear nerve; check the vestibular nerve by having the person stand on one foot with eyes closed	Recognition of sound; maintain balance
IX Glossopharyngeal	Check the gag reflex by touching the pharynx with a tongue depressor	Gag response
X Vagus	Check the individual's swallowing ability; ask the person to cough and speak; glossopharyngeal and vagus nerves are easily examined together because of overlapping innervation of the pharynx	Speak without hoarseness or weakness
XI Spinal accessory	Ask the individual to elevate the shoulders, turn the head, and resist the examiner's attempts to pull the chin back to midline; check the symmetry of the trapezius and sternocleidomastoid muscles	Equal bilateral muscle strength; atrophy may indicate nerve dysfunction
XII Hypoglossal	Ask the individual to protrude the tongue	Absence of deviations, atrophy, or tremors

rologic examination, which involves an evaluation of the cranial nerves, the motor nervous system, the sensory nervous system, and cerebellar function and may also include extensive laboratory testing.

Testing of cranial nerve function is the most involved part of the neurologic examination. Table 39-3 represents the 12 cranial nerves, the methods of testing them, and the expected normal reactions.

DIAGNOSTIC STUDIES

Numerous diagnostic measures have been designed to determine the presence of CNS tumors. All of these measures require direct nursing intervention to help the individual understand the procedures.

Many metastatic lesions are relatively vascular. They are demonstrable only by their mass effect in displacing normal cerebral arterial patterns. Cerebral arteriography allows the circle of Willis and the large blood vessels that penetrate the cerebrum to be visualized by serial imaging of the transit of a contrast medium through the brain's vascular bed. Cerebral arteriography is used most often to confirm metastatic tumor in the individual with a positive brain scan but with doubtful diagnosis. This procedure can cause seizures, facial weakness, and decreased hand grip on the side opposite the injection of the contrast medium. The individual is observed for changes in pulse rate, blood pressure, and respiration after this procedure.

Evaluation of the central nervous system has been profoundly affected by contemporary imaging, and the diagnosis of brain tumors has been greatly facilitated by computed tomography (CT) and magnetic resonance (MRI).[31] CT scanning views one plane of the cranium over a period of seconds, and lesions are seen as nodules of varying size. Exact determination of location and size is possible from the photographs produced for diagnostic purposes. CT scanning also demonstrates the extent of accompanying soft tissue masses, both intracranially and beneath the scalp. Edema surrounding a tumor may be discerned by CT scanning.[32] CT scanning generally is less expensive than MRI and is available at more facilities. CT scanning can be conducted more rapidly than MRI, an important consideration in situations where sedation may be contraindicated.[31]

MR imaging has a multiplanar capability and offers several advantages over CT scanning. It is possible to determine more about the chemistry of the tissue being examined by MRI. This imaging provides superior definition of the borders of a CNS neoplasm, and the extent of the tumor and its invasiveness can be demonstrated better by MRI than CT.[31] Figure 39-11 illustrates an MRI scan of an intracranial mass.

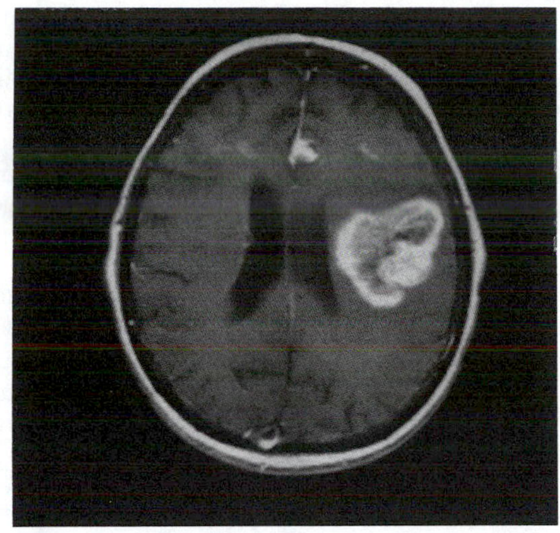

FIGURE 39-11 Brain MRI with Gadolinium showing a large glioblastoma. (Courtesy Rush-Presbyterian-St. Luke's Department of neuroradiology, Chicago)

MRI also demonstrates an increased sensitivity for small (<1 cm) tumors. This is helpful in detecting deep, medially located tumors involving the skull base or the posterior fossa. MRI is effective at demonstrating secondary features of tumors, such as degree of edema, cyst formation, and presence of calcium aggregates. Particularly with meningiomas, MRI can provide a clear histologic basis and offer crude predictions of pathologic subtype.[33]

Another noninvasive nuclear imaging technique used for diagnostic purposes is positron-emission tomography (PET). This technique combines properties of conventional nuclear scanning with physical characteristics of positron-emitting radionuclides. Mathematical logarithms are applied that provide quantitative data to delineate the biochemistry in relation to the overall structure of the tissue in vivo.

While CT scanning is useful in discerning structures, the value of PET scanning is that metabolic processes may be quantified. "Time of flight" information is obtained by measuring the difference in arrival time of two annihilation photons following positron annihilation. This eliminates blurring in the final reconstructed image and improves the spatial resolution of an existing tumor. PET also provides information on tumor metabolism through the study of blood flow and oxygen and glucose utilization.[34]

Francavilla et al.[35] found that fluorodeoxy-glucose (FDG) PET (with contrast) was helpful in the evaluation of malignant degeneration of low-grade gliomas. FDG-PET permits testing for ischemia, with resulting tissue degeneration. Identifying degeneration assists the physician in choosing the appropriate treatment modality.

Further research with PET in patients with glioma demonstrates the ability to study glucose metabolism in hypometabolic and hypermetabolic tumors. Alavi et al.[36] have determined that PET distinguishes tumors with a good prognosis (hypometabolic) from those with poor prognosis (hypermetabolic) and suggest that glucose metabolic studies may provide an independent measure of the aggressiveness of a brain tumor, as well as supplement the pathologic grading.

The use of PET in brain tumor diagnosis remains limited in comparison to CT and MRI. However, CT, MRI, and PET have produced a new era in the study of in vivo brain chemistry. Innovations in neuroradiology, including CT, PET, and MRI have contributed greatly to the diagnosis and precise localization of brain tumors. The ultimate diagnosis and subsequent treatment arise from histopathologic findings.[36]

Single photon emission tomography (SPECT) is a physiologic study that uses radionuclides with longer half-lives, such as 201 thallium. This diagnostic approach helps mitigate biopsy sampling errors by pinpointing areas of actively growing tumor. PET and SPECT represent physiologic measures of response that may supplement the anatomic changes seen with MRI or CT.[31]

CLASSIFICATION AND STAGING

Beahrs et al.[37] indicate that the most critical feature in the classification of CNS tumor is histopathology. Staging of such tumors, particularly intracranial tumors, has clinical and prognostic implications. Anatomic staging for tumors in general includes primary site, regional lymph nodes, and metastatic sites. There are no lymphatic structures draining the brain, but metastases from brain tumor may occur through seeding into the subarachnoid space.

Clinical staging of brain tumors is based on neurologic signs and symptoms, as well as diagnostic tests. Pathologic staging is based on histopathology, grade, and microscopic evidence of completeness of removal of resected tumor. The histologic staging of brain tumors is found in Table 39-4.

TREATMENT

The treatment of CNS malignancies is determined by a number of factors, including primary site, tumor grade, tumor type, and overall condition of the patient. For purposes here, treatment is discussed in general terms for any tumor of the CNS.

TABLE 39-4 Definition of TNM Classification of Brain Tumors

PRIMARY TUMOR (T)	
TX	Primary tumor cannot be assessed
TO	No evidence of primary tumor
SUPRATENTORIAL TUMOR	
T1	Tumor 5 cm or less in greatest dimension; limited to one side
T2	Tumor more than 5 cm in greatest dimension; limited to one side
T3	Tumor invades or encroaches upon the ventricular system
T4	Tumor crosses the midline, invades the opposite hemisphere, or invades infratentorially
INFRATENTORIAL TUMOR	
T1	Tumor 3 cm or less in greatest dimension; limited to one side
T2	Tumor more than 3 cm in greatest dimension; limited to one side
T3	Tumor invades or encroaches upon the ventricular system
T4	Tumor crosses the midline, invades the opposite hemisphere, or invades supratentorially
REGIONAL LYMPH NODES (N)	
This category does not apply to this site.	
DISTANT METASTASIS (M)	
MX	Presence of distant metastasis cannot be assessed
MO	No distant metastasis
M1	Distant metastasis
HISTOPATHOLOGIC GRADE (G)	
GX	Grade cannot be assessed
G1	Well-differentiated
G2	Moderately well-differentiated
G3	Poorly differentiated
G4	Undifferentiated

STAGE GROUPING

Stage IA	G1	T1	MO
Stage IB	G1	T2	MO
	G1	T3	MO
Stage IIA	G2	T1	MO
Stage IIB	G2	T2	MO
	G2	T3	MO
Stage IIIA	G3	T1	MO
Stage IIIB	G3	T2	MO
	G3	T3	MO
Stage IV	G1,2,3	T4	MO
	G4	Any T	MO
	Any G	Any T	M1

Source: Data from Behars OH et al.[37]

Surgery

The surgical treatment of brain tumors has improved with the use of the operating microscope and medical treatment to combat cerebral edema. Individuals with a primary brain tumor are usually candidates for surgical excision as the initial treatment. Surgery may be performed on metastatic brain tumors as a palliative measure aimed at increasing quality of life and possibly overall survival. In rare cases, long-term survival and even cure can be achieved.

Several factors are considered in the evaluation of an individual for surgery: tumor location, size, method of spread, general condition of the individual, and the individual's neurologic status. For example, an encapsulated tumor that occupies a pole of the nondominant cerebral hemisphere lends itself to extensive resection. Complete excision of a rapidly growing glioblastoma in the center of the brain that has necrotic and hemorrhagic cysts may not be possible. Rather, internal decompression may be performed by removing the main bulk of the tumor.

Fadul et al.[38] explored factors that influence morbidity and morality of craniotomy for excision of supratentorial gliomas. They found that patients with the highest morbidity and mortality were those with moderate to severe preoperative disabilities and deep midline lesions, persons over 55 years of age, and those receiving high doses of preoperative dexamethasone. These researchers also found that complete resection entailed no greater risks than biopsy or less extensive surgical procedures.

There are several approaches to the surgical management of the individual with a brain tumor: (1) surgery as the primary treatment, (2) surgery to facilitate nonsurgical therapy, (3) radiosurgery for metastases, and (4) no surgery at all. The aim of surgery as the primary treatment is complete removal of the tumor. The recent use of lasers and related approaches on eligible individuals permits more complete tumor excision. Partial tumor resection also may improve the individual's neurologic condition. Debulking the tumor may relieve symptoms by decreasing local compression and decreasing intracranial pressure. Small frontopolar, temporopolar, or occipitopolar tumors in the nondominant hemisphere are easier to resect. Resection is more difficult when the tumor is deep within the brain or in an area that controls vital human activities (brain stem, motor area). The surgical procedure must be technically possible and the projected quality of life for the individual worthwhile. The advantage of surgical therapy in carefully selected cases is increased survival time and an improved quality of survival.

Postoperative radiotherapy and/or chemotherapy is considered when tumor recurrence is likely. These treatments are indicated especially when excision is only partial. The aim of adjunctive therapy is to prevent or delay recurrence of the tumor.

Surgery may facilitate subsequent nonsurgical treatments, such as postoperative radiation. Surgery may be used to place radioactive substances within the tumor mass or to confirm the histologic or cytologic identification of a mass by biopsy. Stereotactic surgery was popular in the 1960s when it was used in the treatment of pain, movement disorders, epilepsy, and Parkinson's disease. More recently, stereotactic surgery with CT has been used in neurosurgery.[39] CT- and MRI-directed volumetric tumor removal by laser is feasible with computer-generated visual displays referenced to the patient's anatomy using sterotactic instrumentation.[40] Coffey et al.[41] propose stereotactic biopsy followed by radiation instead of surgical resection, especially for patients with malignant gliomas located in functionally important or inaccessible locations.

Surgical manipulation of a brain tumor may be inadvisable in individuals with invasive, rapidly growing tumors situated in critical areas of the brain who are in poor general health and have major neurologic deficits. Surgery or biopsy must be seriously evaluated and discussed with the patient and the family when the expected quality of survival is poor.

In the case of metastatic brain tumors, other factors should be considered. Factors favorable for surgery include a long interval between treatment of a primary extracranial neoplasm and diagnosis of an intracranial tumor, a single brain metastasis with no metastases to other parts of the body, an extracranial tumor that is responsive to therapy, a significant improvement in neurologic status with the administration of steroids, and minimal neurologic deficit with increased intracranial pressure being the major problem. Tumors that are favorably situated and are not radiosensitive can be removed surgically. Good general health and neurologic status and a projected functional survival time of 6 months are strong indications for surgery.

Although there are many exceptions, depending on each individual's circumstances, factors considered unfavorable for surgical intervention include the presence of multiple small intracranial tumors, a major neurologic deficit that is unresponsive to steroid therapy, or a rapidly growing and disseminated tumor. Because of potential harm to future rehabilitation endeavors, it is more difficult to operate on tumors in the dominant hemisphere, basal ganglia, speech centers, or motor areas.

The most serious postoperative complications of neurosurgery are intracranial bleeding, cerebral edema, and water intoxication. The signs and symptoms of these complications may be the same: decreasing level of consciousness, increased ICP, progressive hemiparesis, or other neurologic deficit, and possibly signs of herniation or seizures.

Hemorrhage into the operative cavity may take place within hours after surgery. Bleeding also may occur from traction on the bridging veins between the brain and the dura. Rupture of these vessels produces a subdural hematoma.

Postoperative cerebral edema frequently is severe

after the excision of malignant tumors. In anticipation of brain swelling, the dura may be left open. Cerebral edema is treated with corticosteroids and osmotherapy. The effects of osmotic diuretic therapy on ICP are best determined by use of an intracranial pressure monitor. Other techniques for controlling intracranial hypertension include hyperventilation, hypothermia, and the use of anesthetic agents.

Other complications may follow a craniotomy. Wound infection, cerebral spinal fluid infection, or aseptic meningitis may develop within 3 or 4 days. Seizures may be an early or late postoperative problem and are controlled with anticonvulsant medication. Individuals undergoing neurosurgery also are susceptible to all of the systemic complications that can follow any period of immobility (i.e., venous thrombosis and pulmonary embolism).

Surgery generally is the immediate treatment choice for tumors that cause spinal cord compression. Shaw et al.[42] discuss a one-stage posterolateral decompression-stabilization procedure for patients with thoracolumbar intraspinal tumors. These authors demonstrated surgical success, with return to previous function, in their small ($n = 9$) sample. However, a rapid surgical approach was found to be less effective in the treatment of malignant astrocytomas of the spinal cord in the presence of hydrocephalus and dissemination of disease.[30]

Radiosurgery

Stereotactic radiosurgery is a noninvasive technique that delivers a single, large fraction of ionizing radiation to a small, well-defined intracranial target. This approach has become increasingly available in the United States and is used extensively for brain metastases.[43] This approach is particularly effective for treatment of tumor in or near sensitive target structures, such as the optic nerve. Results are reported to be excellent, and this approach is considered to be cost-effective.[44]

Stereotactic radiosurgery has also been found to be effective in well-defined malignant gliomas. When used as an adjunct to other modalities, initial management of patients with small gliomas appears to produce long-term tumor control and survival.[45]

Radiotherapy

The use of radiotherapy in the treatment of primary malignant brain tumors depends on the radiosensitivity of the particular tumor type. For example, glioblastoma is considered to have a negligible response to radiation. In contrast, medulloblastoma is considered to be highly radiosensitive, and radiotherapy may be initiated immediately after histologic confirmation of this tumor. Other primary brain tumors may be treated with radiation after surgical resection.

Radiotherapy is also used in the treatment of metastatic brain tumors. Typically, individuals have multiple cerebral metastases and are not considered to be candidates for surgical resection. When the presence of multiple intracranial tumors is documented, cranial radiotherapy is initiated. As with primary tumors, response rates vary with the histologic characteristics of the primary tumor. For example, metastases from breast and lung tumors respond better to irradiation than metastases from melanoma or sarcoma. Individuals with metastatic brain tumors also may undergo more than one course of cranial irradiation in conjunction with chemotherapy or in the presence of recurring metastases.

Radiation dosages to the brain vary according to tumor type and bulk and the individual's general condition. Initial irradiation may be delivered over a period of 2–4 weeks. The delivery of 20 Gy within 1 week or 3 Gy in 2 weeks for palliation of metastatic brain cancer is acceptable practice. Higher doses of radiation delivered in shorter schedules are slightly superior in both promptness and duration of symptom relief.

Patients undergoing cranial radiotherapy may receive corticosteroids to promote more rapid improvement; however, this regimen does not contribute to overall survival or duration of improvement.

The problem of decreased radiosensitivity of hypoxic malignant cells has been identified. Malignant brain tumors are composed of a large portion of such cells, and hypoxia is believed to be a factor that limits the effectiveness of radiation. Treatment with fast neutron therapy in addition to conventional megavoltage therapy may be advantageous in the treatment of hypoxic brain tumors. Response to treatment is in part measured by the degree to which the individual is able to perform activities of daily living.

Irreversible radiation necrosis may develop following cranial radiotherapy.[46] This reaction is not considered common, but when it occurs, the necrosis is not distinguishable, clinically or by CT scan, from a neoplastic lesion, causing potential confusion in the diagnosis of recurrence of tumor growth.

Radiation therapy is also used in conjunction with surgery for some tumors. Following surgical exposure of the tumor site, high-dose fractionated radiotherapy is delivered via a cone-shaped lucite radiation applicator. This applicator protects healthy tissue from radiation, while maintaining the integrity of the radiation fields, either during delivery of radiation in the operating room or during patient transport between OR and radiation room.[47]

Whole-brain cranial irradiation remains a treatment option for childhood malignancy, with continuing concerns about effect on IQ decline. It has been determined that older age at time of irradiation results in less decline in subsequent IQ score. Further, it is possible to predict final IQ score based on initial IQ score, dose of irradiation, and age at time of irradiation.[48]

Chemotherapy and Related Drugs

An understanding of the blood-brain barrier is valuable for understanding the effect of chemotherapeutic agents on brain tumors. The blood-brain barrier (BBB) consists of a continuous lining of endothelial cells that are connected by tight junctions (Figure 39-12). Transendothelial vesicular transport is not facilitated by the endothelial cells, and the junctions restrict intercellular diffusion. This barrier limits blood-brain exchange of water-soluble drugs, ions, and proteins at the growing regions of a tumor edge but permits transport of lipid-soluble agents that can permeate the lipid membranes of the endothelial cells. Furthermore, permeability of the BBB varies within the tumor and is believed to be greater in or near the central tumor bulk, where blood flow is reduced.[19,46]

The presence of openings between the vascular compartments of brain tumors and the parenchyma hold promise for chemotherapy. Certain agents may have access to tumor tissue through bulk flow. Molecular size, lipid solubility, and degree of ionization are perhaps not the most crucial attributes of chemotherapeutic agents for brain tumors.

Research suggests that malignant oligodendroglioma is a uniquely chemosensitive glial tumor.[23] Unfortunately, this is not true of other intracranial tumors, and, within the accepted treatment methods for brain tumors, chemotherapy represents a limited approach. Most chemotherapeutic agents do not cross the BBB easily. However, the group of drugs classified as nitrosoureas are successful in penetrating the BBB. These drugs include carmustine (BCNU), and lomustine (CCNU), both of which are lipid soluble. Most commonly, carmustine is used in combination with 5-fluorouracil. Chemotherapy is indicated for patients who have a histologic grade III or grade IV neoplasm.

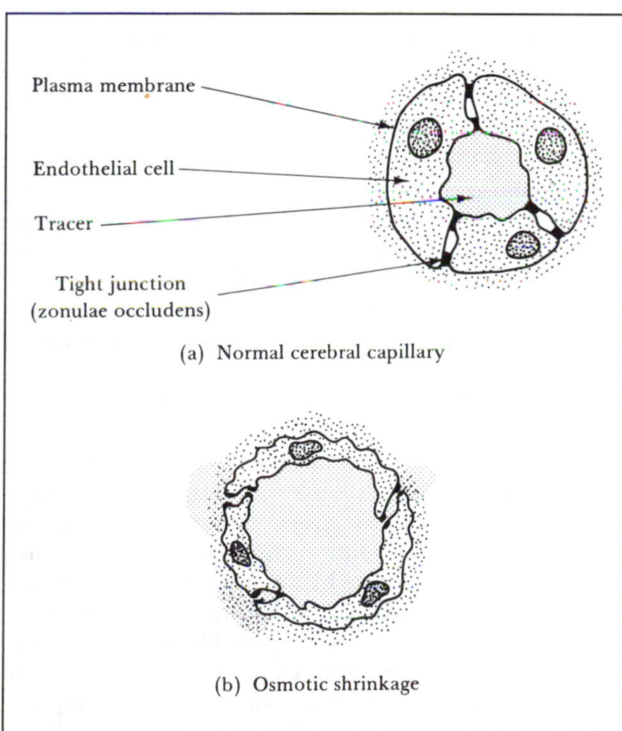

FIGURE 39-12 Schematic representation of the blood-brain barrier. (a) Normal cerebral capillary showing tight junctions. (b) Blood-brain barrier opening by widening of the interendothelial tight junctions. When the endothelial cells shrink in a hypertonic environment, the permeability of the junctions is increased.

Other means of delivering chemotherapy to brain tumors have been explored. For example, meningeal carcinomatosis either breaks down the BBB or permits neovascularization and thereby circumvents the barrier. This has implications for the use of such agents as intravenous methotrexate, cis-platinum, 5-fluorouracil, and interferon.

Hypertonic mannitol causes loss of fluid from the capillary endothelial cells, causing the endothelial cells to shrink and the tight junctions (Zonulae occuludens) to break, resulting in osmotic shrinkage (Figure 39-12b). Materials of large molecular size may then diffuse through the junctions into the surrounding brain.

Transitory osmotic disruption of the BBB, by perfusing the brain capillaries with a hypertonic solution of 25% mannitol, opens the tight junctions for 15–30 minutes.[49] Neuwalt[49] describes a protocol of combination chemotherapy, in conjunction with barrier disruption, at 28-day intervals. Intraarterial methotrexate, with citrovorum rescue, followed by intravenous cyclophosphamide, are used. To date, the best results have been achieved in primary CNS lymphomas.[49]

The use of liposomes as drug carriers is a recent approach in chemotherapy administration. This permits penetration of the BBB with prolonged tissue concentrations of systemically administered drugs entrapped in lipisomes such as cholesterol.[19]

Various other methods of drug administration attempting to circumvent the BBB have been described. These include intraarterial,[19] intrathecal, and intratumoral administration. Indeed, intratumoral injections of interleukin lymphoid effector cells have proven advantageous. However, such intracerebral injections are avoided in areas of the brain where small amounts of edema may prove life-threatening, such as the thalamus, hypothalamus, and brain stem.[49]

Several other uses of chemotherapy are undergoing investigation. Autologous bone marrow transplantation in conjunction with high-dose etoposide has demonstrated activity in the treatment of malignant primary brain tumors and metastatic tumors from small-cell lung carcinoma.[51] Hidalgo et al.[52] are finding enhanced responses to the treatment of brain metastases with weekly intravenous or intraarterial administration of cis-platinum during whole-brain irradiation. Palliative and enhanced survival responses have been noted following osmotic BBB modification to enhance drug delivery to tumor and surrounding brain.[53,54]

Intraarterial chemotherapy administration has been used for regionally confined malignancies, including intracranial tumors. An intraarterial catheter is placed, with fluoroscopic or angiographic visualization prior to infusion. A drug pump is used to deliver a high concentration at the tumor site.

Floxuridine is one drug successfully used for intraarterial infusion for various tumors considered incurable, such as certain metastatic and primary melanomas. Complications from such infusions include arterial aneurysm, arterial ischemia, arterial thrombosis, bleeding of catheter site, displaced or leaking catheter, infection of catheter site, and thrombophlebitis.[55]

The use of intraarterial chemotherapy for recurrent brain tumors remains experimental but continues to be an area of interest.[56] However, documentation of its benefits continues to be cloudy. Johnson et al.[57] studied the use of intracarotid BCNU dissolved in 5% D5W and reported an 11%–60% reduction of primary glioma in 8 of their 20 patients. Stewart et al.[58] used intraarterial mitomycin-C for recurrent brain metastases and reported a response in 6 of 13 patients. Both studies require clarification of the definition and significance of these response rates. This method of administration is not without its problems. Those of particular interest include direct toxicity to the ipsilateral eye and leukoencephalopathy.

The use of a combination of intraarterial and systemic chemotherapy was studied by Stewart et al.[59] It was found that a combination of systemic and regional drug therapy did not provide more effective therapy than the use of intraarterial drugs alone.

Further developments in chemotherapeutic approaches have been directed toward the treatment of meningeal malignancies. These include placement of a subcutaneous reservoir (Ommaya reservoir) to circumvent the BBB. Chemotherapeutic agents used include methotrexate and cytarabine.

This method ensures delivery of drug into the ventricular system, with less discomfort to the patient than via lumbar puncture.[60] High-dose systemic drug administration is also being used. Benefits of this approach include better penetration of drug into brain tissue and deep perivascular spaces, with the recognized potential for severe systemic toxicity.[60]

One final investigational drug therapy discussed involves an antibody-toxin conjugate.[61] A genetically engineered toxin, CRM 107, is structurally similar to diptheria toxin, with deviation in two amino acid chains. Intrathecal administration of CRM 107 demonstrated selective destruction of glioblastoma- and medulloblastoma-derived cell lines in humans. This therapy offers a wide therapeutic window, with extreme potency, and general applicability against CSF-borne primary and metastatic tumors and warrants further clinical trial.

Advances continue to be made in all areas of treatment for CNS malignancies. Further chemotherapeutic advances include the use of platinum-based agents in conjunction with radiation therapy.[62,63] Current research with diaziguone (AZQ), administered intrathecally, indicates that this regimen is safe, well tolerated, and highly active against refractory meningeal malignancies.[64]

GENERAL SUPPORTIVE MEASURES

The individual with a brain tumor may experience symptoms that drastically affect his or her ability to function normally. Furthermore, the prognosis for malignant CNS tumors has not changed greatly in the last 10 years, despite significant advances in therapeutic modalitics.[19] Supportive nursing measures assume importance in all areas of patient care.

CNS malignancies produce effects, often within the closed compartment of the cranium, that resemble traumatic head injuries. Furthermore, the daily care of these individuals continues to shift to the home and community, regardless of prognosis. Preparation of the family and home environment must become a discharge planning goal for the nurse.[65] Additionally, developments in rehabilitation for the traumatically brain-injured patient provide guidelines for family-managed care of the individual with CNS malignancy[66] and are explored for hospital-based nursing care and adaptation at home. Table 39-5 describes anticipated problems, the cause of the problem, and suggested solutions for the care of these individuals.

Brain tumors increase ICP by their size, cerebral edema, or obstruction of CSF pathways. When CSF pathways are blocked, a hydrocephalus can develop, necessitating a shunting procedure. The tumor bulk and accompanying peritumoral edema are usually responsible for an increase in ICP. Therapeutic measures are aimed at controlling cerebral edema, cerebral blood flow, and other factors affecting ICP.

Chronic cerebral edema may be managed with corticosteroids such as methylprednisolone. A reduction of peritumoral edema may occur over a period of hours or days. Corticosteroids are less helpful in the prompt reduction of acutely increased ICP. Osmotherapy is used to reduce the amount of fluid in the brain tissue. A hyperosmolar agent such as mannitol is administered intravenously. The drug creates an osmotic gradient across a semipermeable membrane. Fluid is drawn into the circulating bloodstream. Diuresis is achieved when the fluid is removed from the intravascular compartment by the kidneys. Osmotic diuretics remove fluid from normal brain cells (because they have an intact semipermeable cell membrane). The cerebral edema surrounding damaged cells is not directly removed by osmotherapy. Corticosteroids are administered concurrently because they are believed to have a direct

TABLE 39-5 Assessment Guidelines for the Care of Individuals with CNS Malignancy

Problem	Cause	Solution
Increased ICP	Tumor size Cerebral edema Obstruction of CSF pathways	Corticosteroid administration
	Increased systematic arterial blood pressure	Avoid Valsalva maneuvers, isometric muscle contractions, coughing, emotional arousal
	Decreased cranial venous outflow	Elevate head of bed, avoid head rotation, neck flexation, and extension
	Increased intraabdominal and inthrathoracic pressure	Avoid sneezing, coughing, straining Avoid hip flexion, prone position Monitor ICP level
Seizures	Disturbance of intracranial contents	Prophylactic anticonvulsants Safe environment Prevent harm during seizure activity Skin and oral hygiene following seizure activity
Personality changes	Frontal lobe involvement Cerebral edema	Maintain normal function Maintain orientation Acceptance of subtle change Avoid perilous behavior Encourage use of remaining cognitive functions Encourage social activities
Loss of sensation	Parietal, occipital, temporal lobe involvement	Monitor for visual disturbances Monitor for hearing loss Maintain orientation Safe environment, clothing
Disturbances in coordination	Cerebellum involvement	Ongoing assessment Intervention in physical surroundings Safety devices (bed rails, walker) Close off stairway Protect access to outdoors
Poor nutrition and hydration	Decreased activity GI effects of medications Overall deterioration	Small, attractive, frequent meals Dietary supplements Frequent oral fluids Use of alternative feeding routes, if necessary
Need for supportive care	Breakdown of patient/family social network	Assessment of Priorities Environment Resources Roles and family functioning

effect on vasogenic brain edema. Fluid intake is also restricted to prevent intracellular swelling. Cellular edema adds to and aggravates increasing ICP.

Many activities affect cerebral blood flow and thus ICP. Suctioning reduces $PaCO_2$, which creates a transient rise in ICP. Poor respiratory exchange can also elevate ICP. This is accomplished by an increased $PaCO_2$, which increases blood volume. Activities that increase systemic arterial blood pressure will also increase ICP. These include Valsalva maneuvers, isometric muscle contraction, coughing, and emotional arousal.

The venous outflow of blood from the cranial cavity affects ICP. A decrease in outflow increases the total blood volume in the cranium. Intracranial pressure arises when the total volume within the cranium is increased. The outflow of venous blood is impeded by jugular compression, head rotation, neck flexion, and neck extension. These head and neck positions should be avoided. Elevating the head of the bed promotes venous drainage and is used as a therapeutic measure when increased ICP is present.

Intraabdominal and intrathoracic pressures affect ICP. This is due to the transmission of increased pressure along the venous system to the intracranial veins. Intracranial venous pressure is increased, and total blood volume increases with positive end-expiratory pressure (PEEP), sneezing, coughing, straining, and Valsalva maneuvers. Intraabdominal pressure increases with hip flexion and pressure on the abdomen (such as lying in the prone position). These activities should be avoided because they may produce dangerously high elevations in ICP.

Several nursing measures involve the performance of activities that affect ICP (turning, pulmonary hygiene, positioning, range-of-motion exercises, suctioning). Although certain activities cannot be avoided, it is recommended that activities be spread out over time. When turning individuals in bed, the head and neck should be maintained in a neutral position. Alert individuals should be asked to permit themselves to be turned passively. Many individuals inadvertently perform a Valsalva maneuver or grab the side rails tightly (isometric muscle contraction) when turning.

Intracranial hypertension that is unresponsive to conventional treatment requires additional therapeutic measures. Levels of ICP must be determined by an intracranial pressure monitor. Intubation and hyperventilation may be used to control $PaCO_2$ and PaO_2. The vasoconstrictor effect of hyperventilation also reduces cerebral blood volume. Steroids, osmotic diuretics, and fluid restriction are used as usual. The head of the bed is elevated to promote venous drainage. Anesthetic agents such as barbiturates may be used to decrease cerebral blood flow and metabolism. Hypothermia also may be used to reduce the cerebral metabolic rate.

The use of steroids in the treatment of metastatic brain cancer has been discussed. Symptoms are ameliorated in 60%–75% of individuals treated with adrenocorticosteroids. Dexamethasone (Decadron) is used frequently in neurologic settings to decrease cerebral edema. However, one out of every six hospitalized individuals receiving corticosteroids develops side effects, particularly individuals with low serum albumin levels and those who are receiving high doses of the drug. Individuals receiving steroids should be observed for the following symptoms:

1. acute adrenal insufficiency, as evidenced by fatigue, muscular weakness, joint pain, fever, anorexia, nausea, and orthostatic hypotension
2. cardiovascular and renal problems, as evidenced by increased cardiac output and atrioventricular node conduction rate and sodium retention
3. gastrointestinal disturbances, as evidenced by induction or aggravation of peptic ulcers and melena with resulting anemia
4. metabolic problems, as evidenced by gluconeogenesis that leads to hyperglycemia and glucosuria, polydipsia, and polyuria
5. musculoskeletal problems, as evidenced by muscular atrophy and osteoporosis in immobilized individuals, petechiae, and decubiti

Ongoing assessment of patients receiving steroids will alert the nurse to the development of steroid side effects. Steroid dosages are decreased immediately in the presence of side effects and are tapered slowly, to prevent problems of hasty withdrawal.

Individuals receiving phenobarbital or phenytoin may need higher dosages of corticosteroids because these drugs stimulate hepatic corticosteroid metabolism. Individuals who receive dosages that are too high for a prolonged period of time may develop a steroid psychosis. Such individuals must be observed for personality changes and paranoid behavior, which tend to develop suddenly and dramatically.

Planning for discharge from the hospital for individuals who have been treated for a brain tumor encompasses an accurate assessment of existing limitations. Rehabilitation potential is always viewed with hope and optimism, and the attitude of realistic hope must be conveyed to the individual and family. Discharge goals include assisting the individual to attain realistic goals and directing the family to appropriate resources. Table 39-6 identifies points for family teaching and home care guidelines for these individuals.

TABLE 39-6 Family Teaching and Home Care Guidelines

Potential Problem	Care Guidelines
Physical injury due to unsteady gait	Call local ACS to obtain equipment (wheelchair, bedside commode, walker, three-prong cane, guard rail for bathroom, stool for shower) Take up throw rugs to prevent tripping Wear nonskid shoes when out of bed Eliminate the need to ambulate up and down steps Obtain assistance with physical care through home health aide and visiting nursing service
Decreased mobility due to physical disability	Obtain hospital bed if necessary to change position and assist with care needs Range of motion exercises four times daily Physical therapy consult Occupational therapy consult Change position in bed every 4 hours
Skin breakdown due to immobility and chronic steroid use	Bathe every 2–3 days using a nondeodorant soap Apply aloe-based or Eucerin cream daily, especially to pressure points Massage pressure points daily to stimulate blood flow Change position every 4 hours Keep perineum dry

(continued)

TABLE 39-6 Family Teaching and Home Care Guidelines (continued)

Oral fungal infections due to chronic steroid use	Oral hygiene three times daily Inspect oral cavity for white plaque build-up Mycostatin mouth wash
High blood sugar due to steroid use	Medical Management: Sliding scale insulin administration may be used Test blood sugar as directed: Record testape values as instructed Fingerstick glucose monitoring may be initiated Report appropriate levels to doctor or nurse: Testape urine values over 200 should be reported Phone number: ____________________ Report unusual symptoms to your doctor such as: Increased thirst Dry mouth Flushed skin Polyuria Nausea and vomiting
Stomach irritation and possible ulcer formation due to chronic steroid use	Eat small meals frequently Riopan or Maalox are useful to minimize stomach upset Avoid caffeine if possible Eat foods that are soft, easy to eat, and easy to digest Soft feeding tube may be necessary to maintain nutrition
Fatigue, dizziness, muscle weakness, and joint pain due to chronic steroid use and immobility	Conserve energy for activities individual enjoys Be out of bed as much as possible Walk out of doors daily as tolerated Nonsteroidal anti-inflammatory agent as needed for joint pain Vary activities to combat fatigue Avoid sleeping during the day if possible Removable splinting may be used for weakened muscles Slide items rather than lifting and carrying
Difficulty with dressing and personal hygiene due to decreased mobility and/or perception	Assess basic functional abilities to identify effective assistance devices Provide garments that are easy to put on, with large fasteners in easily accessible areas Nonskid shoes with velcro closings may be used Assess need for raised toilet seat, shower stool, tilted mirrors, and large faucets Lower closet rods Store frequently used items within easy reach, in consistent places
Memory impairment, perceptual deficits and cognitive processing impairments due to tumor growth or cerebral edema	Establish habitual use of safety devices and routines Provide compensatory cognitive devices: Labels Written instructions Reminders Memory logs
Urinary incontinence due to confusion, loss of muscle control	Note patterns of incontinence Establish habit retraining, based on time intervals Assess need for mechanical methods of urine collection Maintain positive attitude and recognize incontinence as a symptom, not a disease
Impending death related to anticipated cardiopulmonary failure and advanced disease	Family assessment of: Diminishing level of consciousness Decreased oral fluid intake Oliguria Labored, irregular breathing Bubbling in throat and chest Progressive cyanotic mottling in lower extremities Encourage participation in home hospice program Determine unfinished business Encourage worship and prayer that are consistent with family beliefs

TABLE 39-7 Factors for Consideration in Postacute Brain Injury Rehabilitation

Cognitive rehabilitation
Community reentry
Diagnostic evaluations
Long-term living
Neurobehavorial
Outpatient
Transitional living
Vocational rehabilitation

Source: Data from Centre for Neuro Skills.[67]

In the past 10 years, rehabilitation for the CNS-impaired individual has undergone tremendous growth and change. This is particularly true for the traumatically brain-injured individual.[66] Principles from rehabilitation programs for these individuals are applicable to the patient with CNS malignancy and are presented in Table 39-7.

Life expectancy at home generally is not of long duration. The patient may or may not be bedridden, but he or she requires a safe environment, regardless of activity level. Alteration in balance and confusion warrant housing the patient on the ground floor, when possible. When ambulating, the patient should wear sturdy footwear, and obstacles should be cleared from the pathway. Reality orientation devices (clocks, calendars, etc.) should be readily available.

The patient with progressive CNS involvement generally is in a terminal state, and death at home may occur slowly, through progression of disease (e.g., cardiac arrest, rapid systemic infection). A resource available to patient and family is hospice care, to ease the terminal process and facilitate hope and integrity for all involved.

REFERENCES

1. Fishman RA: *Cerebrospinal fluid in the Diseases of the Nervous System.* Philadelphia: Saunders, 1980, pp. 1–15.
2. Mitchell PH, Mauss NK: Intracranial hypertension: Implications for research for nursing care. *J Neurosurg Nurs* 12:145–154, 1980.
3. Silverberg E, Lubera J: Cancer statistics. *CA* 41:19–53, 1991.
4. del Regato J, Spjut H, Cox JD: *Cancer Diagnosis, Treatment and Prognosis* (6th ed). St. Louis, MO: Mosby, 1985, pp. 149–155.
5. Wilson CB, Fulton DS, Seager ML: Supportive management of the patient with malignant brain tumor. *JAMA* 244:1249–1251, 1980.
6. Kornblith PL, Walker MD, Cassady RR: *Neurologic Oncology.* Philadelphia: Lippincott, 1987.
7. Gilman S: Advances in neurology (II). *N Engl J Med* 326:167–176, 1992.
8. Amendola B, Amendola M, McClatchey K: Radiation-induced malignant fibrous histiocytoma: A report of five cases including two occurring post whole brain irradiation. *Cancer Inves* 3:507–513, 1985.
9. Rimm I, Li F, Tabell N, et al: Brain tumors after cranial irradiation for childhood ALL. *Cancer* 59:1506–1508, 1987.
10. Salvati M, Artico M, Caruso R, et al: A report on radiation induced gliomas. *Cancer* 67:392–397, 1991.
11. Penn I: Cancer is a complication of severe immunosuppression. *Surg Gynecol Obst* 162:603–609, 1986.
12. Jones RD: Epidemiology of brain tumors in man and their relationship with chemical agents. *Ed Chem Toxic* 24:99–103, 1986.
13. Thomas T, Stewart P, Stemhagen A, et al: Risk of astrocytic brain tumors associated with occupational chemical exposure. *Sc J Work, Env, Health* 13:417–423, 1987.
14. Wilkinson G, Tietjen G, Wiggs L, et al: Mortality among plutonium and other radiation workers at a plutonium weapons facility. *Am J Epidemiol* 125:231–247, 1987.
15. Axelson O: Cancer and combined exposures to occupational and environmental factors. *Rec Res Cancer Research* 122:60–67, 1991.
16. Goldberg RB, Creosey WA: A review of cancer induction by extremely low frequency electromagnetic fields. Is there a plausible mechanism? *Medical Hypothesis* 35:265–274, 1991.
17. Krause M, Westneat D: Possible link to cancer fuels debate regarding effects of magnetic fields. *Occ Health Safety* 1992, pp. 28–30.
18. Zulch KJ: Principles of the new World Health Organization (WHO) classification of brain tumors. *Neuroradiology* 19:59–66, 1980.
19. Jellinger K: *Therapy of Malignant Brain Tumors.* New York: Springer-Verlag, 1987.
20. Levin VA: Chemotherapy of primary brain tumors. *Neurol Clin* 3:855–865, 1985.
21. Schoenberg BS: The epidemiology of CNS tumors. In Walker MD (ed), *Oncology of the Nervous System.* Boston: Nijhoff, 1983, pp. 1–311.
22. Popp JA, Horton J: Primary tumors of the brain. *Cur Concepts Oncol* 2:3–11, 1980.
23. Cairncross, JG, MacDonald DR: Successful chemotherapy for recurrent malignant oligodendroglioma. *Ann Neurol* 23:360–364, 1988.
24. MacArthur JH, Palenicek JG: Human immunodeficiency virus and the nervous system. *Nurs Clin North Am* 23:823–841, 1988.
25. Adams RD, Victor M: *Principles of Neurology* (3rd ed). New York: McGraw Hill, 1985, pp. 487–493.
26. Levine A: Non-Hodgkin's lymphomas and other malignancies in the acquired immune deficiency syndrome. *Semin Oncol* 14(2):34–39, 1987.
27. Posner JB: Brain metastases: A clinician's view. In Weiss L, Gilbert HA, Posner JB (eds), *Brain Metastsis.* Boston: Hall, 1980.
28. Schwaninger M, Pott S, Henningsen P, Schmidt D: Spinal canal metastases: A late complication of glioblastoma. *J Neurol Oncol* 12:93–98, 1992.
29. Stein DA, Chamberlain MC: Evaluation and management of seizures in the patient with cancer. *Oncology* 5:33–40, 1991.
30. Cohen AR, Wisoff JH, Allan JC, et al: Malignant astrocytomas of the spinal cord. *J Neurosurg* 70:50–54, 1989.
31. Jaeckle KA: Neuroimaging for central nervous system tumors. *Semin Oncol* 18:150–157, 1991.

32. Wagner HM: Images of the brain; past as prologue. *J Nuc Med* 27:1929–1937, 1987.
33. Elster AD, Challa VR, Gilbert TH, et al: Mengiomas: MR and histological features. *Radiology* 170:857–862, 1989.
34. Thomas D, Brooks D, Jones T: Metabolic studies of the brain tumors by P.E.T. In Chatel M, Darval F, Pecker J (eds), *Brain Oncology*. Boston: Nijhoff, 1987, pp. 175–177.
35. Francavilla TL, Miletich RS, Di Chiro G, et al: Positron emission tomography in the detection of malignant degeneration of low-grade gliomas. *Neurosurgery* 24:1–5, 1989.
36. Alavi JB, Alavi A, Chawluk J, et al: Positron emission tomography in patients with glioma. *Cancer* 62:1074–1078, 1988.
37. Behars OH, Henson DE, Hutter R, et al: *Manual for Staging of Cancer* (3rd ed). Philadelphia: Lippincott, 1988, pp. 249–254.
38. Fadul C, Wood J, Thaler H, et al: Morbidity and mortality of craniotomy for excision of supratentorial gliomas. *Neurology* 38:1374–1379, 1988.
39. Glidenberg PL: Whatever happened to stereotactic surgery? *Neurosurgery* 20:983–987, 1987.
40. Powers SK: Current status of lasers in neurosurgical oncology. *Semin Surg Oncol* 8:226–232, 1992.
41. Coffey RJ, Lunsford LD, Taylor FH: Survival after stereotactic biopsy of malignant gliomas. *Neurosurgery* 22:465–471, 1988.
42. Shaw B, Mansfield FL, Borges L: One-stage posterolateral decompression and stabilization for primary and metastatic vertebral tumors in the thoracic and lumbar spine. *J Neurosurg* 70:405–410, 1989.
43. Mehta MP, Mackie TR, Levin AB, et al: Radiosurgery for brain metastases. *Contemp Oncol* 1991, pp. 12–19.
44. Wilson CB, Larson DA, Gutin PH: Radiosurgery: A new application? *J Clin Oncol* 10:1373–1374, 1992.
45. Loeffler JS, Alexander E, Shea WM, et al: Radiosurgery as a part of the initial management of patients with malignant gliomas. *J Clin Oncol* 10:1379–1385, 1992.
46. Shewmon DA, Mosdeu JC: Delayed radiation necrosis of the brain contralateral to original tumor. *Arch Neurol* 37:592593, 1980.
47. Haibeck SV: Intraoperative radiation therapy. *Oncol Nurs Forum* 15:143–148, 1988.
48. Silben JH, Radcliffe J, Peckham V, et al: Whole–brain irradiation and decline in intelligence: The influence of dose and age on IQ score. *J Clin Oncol* 10:1390–1396, 1992.
49. Neuwalt ER: *Implications of the Blood-Brain Barrier and Its Manipulation*. New York: Plenum Press, 1989.
50. Merchant R, Grant A, Merchant P, et al: Adoptive immunotherapy for recurrent glioblastoma multiforme using LAK cells and RIL 2. *Cancer* 62:665–671, 1988.
51. Leff RS, Thompson JM, Daly MG, et al: Acute neurologic dysfunction after high-dose etoposide therapy for malignant glioma. *Cancer* 62:32–35, 1988.
52. Hidalgo V, Cy C, Fernandez-Hidalgo O, et al: Simultaneous radiotherapy and cis-platinum for the treatment of brain metastases: A pilot study. *Am J Clin Oncol* 10:205–209, 1987.
53. Neuwalt EA, Howieson J, Frenkel EP, et al: Therapeutic efficancy of multiagent chemotherapy with drug delivery enhancement by BBB modification in glioblastoma. *Neurosurgery* 19:573–580, 1986.
54. Rama B, Jansen J, Mennel HD, et al: Renaissance of intratumoral chemötherapy. In Chatel M, Darcel F, Pecker J (eds), *Brain Oncology*. Boston: Nijhoff, 1988, pp. 433–435.
55. Frost DB, Patt YZ, Mavligit G, et al: Arterial infusion of dacarbazine and cisplatin for recurrent regionally confined melanoma. *Arch Surg* 120:478–480, 1985.
56. Morantz RA: Comments to intracarotid chemotherapy with 1,3-bis-(2-chloroethyl)-1-nitrosourea (BCNU) in 5% dextrose in water in the treatment of malignant glioma. *Neurosurgery* 20:583, 1987.
57. Johnson DW, Parkinson D, Wolpert SM, et al: Intraarterial Chemotherapy with 1,3-bis-(2-chloroethyl)-1-nitorsureia (BCNU) in 5% dextrose in water in the treatment of malignant glioma. *Neurosurgery* 20:577–582, 1987.
58. Stewart DJ, Grahovac Z, Hugenholtz H, et al: Intraarterial mitomycin-C for recurrent brain metastases. *Am J Clin Oncol* 10:432–436, 1987.
59. Stewart DJ, Grahovac Z, Hugenholtz H, et al: Combined intraarterial and systemic chemotherapy for intracerebral tumors. *Neurosurgery* 21:207–213, 1987.
60. Blaney SM, Balis FM, Poplak DG: Pharmacologic approaches to the treatment of meningeal malignancy. *Oncology* 5:107–127, 1991.
61. Johnson VG, Wrobel C, Wilson D, et al: Improved tumor-specific immunotoxins in the treatment of CNS and leptomeningeal neoplasia. *J Neurosurg* 70:240–248, 1989.
62. Douek E, Kingston JE, Malpas JS, Plowman PN: Platinum-based chemotherapy for recurrent CNS tumors in young patients. *J Neurol Neurosurg Psychiatry* 54:722–725, 1991.
63. Potel SR, Buckner JC, Smithson WA, et al: Cisplatin-based chemotherapy in primary central nervous system glrm cell tumors. *J Neurol Oncol* 12:47–52, 1992.
64. Berg SL, Bales RM, Zimm S, et al: Phase I/II trial and pharmacokinetics of intrathecal diaziquone in refractory meningeal malignancies. *J Clin Oncol* 10:143–148, 1992.
65. Wegmann JA: CNS tumors: Supportive management of the patient and family. *Oncology* 5:109–112, 1991.
66. Ashley MJ, Krych DK: Considerations in the purchase of post-acute rehabilitative services for the head injured. *J Ins Med* 22:230–234, 1990.
67. Centre for Neuro Skills (CNS). Bakersfield, CA 1992.

Chapter 40

Endocrine Cancers

Michele Girard Donehower, RN, MSN

INTRODUCTION

The endocrine system controls many of the body's most important physiologic functions through the release of hormones by endocrine organs. Hormones then initiate activities at the cellular level that permit target tissues to make the adaptive changes necessary to maintain homeostasis. When tumors arise in endocrine glands, the ability of these cells to perform their specific endocrine functions is altered. Although some endocrine tumors are not histologically malignant in that they do not have cellular changes characteristic of neoplastic transformation, they can, through hyperplasia and expansion of the tumor, result in significant morbidity or death. Because these cells are not subject to the normal regulatory feedback processes that control hormonal secretion, hyperplasia of the gland can result in excessive hormonal secretion. In some cases, localized growth of the tumor can also cause compression of vital structures. The clinical presentation of these tumors depends on their anatomic location and their ability to produce excess hormone secretion.

THYROID CANCER

Epidemiology

Although the incidence of thyroid cancer has risen slightly over the past 40 years, this neoplasm remains relatively rare.[1] It accounts for just over 1% of the total cancer incidence and approximately 0.2% of cancer deaths.[2] Women are more than twice as likely as men to develop a thyroid malignancy, with the majority of cases occuring between the ages of 25–65.[1] Thyroid tumors in children and adolescents without a history of prior irradiation are relatively uncommon.[3]

Etiology

The only well-documented etiologic factor in the development of thyroid cancer is head and neck irradiation given during early childhood and adolescence.[4,5] Prior to the 1950s, radiotherapy was commonly used for treating benign conditions such as enlarged tonsils and adenoids, mastoiditis, sinusitis, hemangiomas, acne, tinea capitis, and eczema. The association between this widespread practice and the development of thyroid cancer was first reported by Duffy[6] and later confirmed by other investigators.[4,5,7,8] The incidence of postirradiation thyroid cancer is a linear function of the dose received with risk increasing up to 12 Gy.[1] The risk declines with doses over 20 Gy because the thyroid gland becomes sterilized. Most cases of postirradiation thyroid cancer occur in patients receiving doses between 6.5 and 12 Gy.[1,4] There is generally a latency period of 5–10 years between radiation exposure and development of thyroid cancer, but an increased risk for development of these malignancies persists for at least 35 years in exposed subjects.[4] For this reason, persons at risk for developing thyroid cancer because of childhood irradiation to the head and neck require lifelong follow-up.

Treatment of thyroid malignancies with radioactive isotopes does not appear to have the same carcinogenic effect as external irradiation. Isolated reports of thyroid cancer[10–12] following ^{131}I therapy for hyperthyroidism have not been substantiated by studies of larger populations of patients receiving ^{131}I therapy.[13,14]

The relationship between thyroid-stimulating hormone (TSH) and the development of thyroid cancer is unclear. Although thyroid cancer in animals can be induced by prolonged TSH stimulation, the role of TSH as a causative factor in man has not been established.[15] Nevertheless, TSH is thought to function as a growth factor for well-differentiated thyroid malignancies,[16] and interventions to block TSH with administration of exogenous thyroxine are used in patients with documented thyroid malignancies.

The role of genetics in the etiology of thyroid cancers is not well defined except in the case of medullary thyroid cancer, where approximately 25% of cases occur as part of a genetically transmitted multiple endocrine neoplasia (MEN) syndrome.[17,18] (Refer to a discussion of MEN syndromes later in the chapter.) Because these syndromes are transmitted genetically in an autosomal dominant fashion, screening of family members of individuals with medullary carcinoma of the thyroid is recommended to increase the early detection of tumors and prevent the morbidity and mortality associated with these syndromes.[19]

Pathophysiology

Thyroid cancers demonstrate a wide range of biologic behavior depending on the histology of the tumor. Four types of primary thyroid carcinomas account for approximately 95% of all thyroid neoplasms: papillary, follicular, medullary, and anaplastic. The incidence and clinical characteristics of these types are outlined in Table 40-1.

The majority of thyroid tumors arise from the follicular and parafollicular cells (C-cells) of the gland. Tumors arising from the follicular cells can be further subdivided into differentiated and undifferentiated types. Papillary and follicular carcinomas are well differentiated in that they are histologically similar to their tissue of origin. Undifferentiated, or anaplastic, carcinomas bear little resemblance to their tissue of origin and lack the functional and histologic characteristics of normal thyroid tissue. Medullary carcinoma of the thyroid (MCT) is the only tumor of parafollicular, or C-cell origin. Although MCT is generally well differen-

TABLE 40-1 Clinical Characteristics of Thyroid Carcinomas

Tumor Type (Cell of Origin)	Incidence	Survival*	Metastatic Pattern
Papillary (follicular cells)	33%–73%	93%–20 years‡	Cervical lymph nodes involved early in disease; metastasizes to lung and less frequently to bone
Follicular (follicular cells)	14%–33%	78%–10 years†	More locally invasive than papillary, but less likely to have lymph node involvement; propensity for hematogenous spread to bone and, occasionally, lung
Anaplastic (follicular cells)	5%–10%	3.6%–5 years‡	Rapid invasion and compression of adjacent structures early in disease; lung is most common site of metastases
Medullary (parafollicular or C-cells)	10%	61%–10 years‡	50% have lymph node involvement at diagnosis; metastasizes to bone, liver, and lung

* With treatment.
† Disease-free survival.
‡ Total survival.
Source: Incidence data from McHenry et al,[30] survival data from Saad MF et al,[18] McConahey WM et al,[22] Harness JK et al,[32] Nel CJC et al.[38]

tiated, poorly differentiated variants have been reported.[18] Thyroid tumors also vary in their ability to concentrate iodine. This has therapeutic implications in that treatment with ^{131}I is effective only in tumors that are able to concentrate this radioisotope.

Papillary carcinoma

Papillary carcinoma generally follows a relatively indolent course, with survival measured in decades, even in patients with evidence of distant metastases.[20–25] It occurs in all age groups, but the biologic behavior and overall prognosis varies according to age. Older patients (>40 years) appear to have a more aggressive, rapidly growing form of the disease, with a significant decrease in survival.[23,24] As mentioned earlier, thyroid malignancies in children and adolescents without a prior history of head and neck irradiation are uncommon but are frequently associated with early nodal or pulmonary metastases.[26] Other important prognostic factors include sex, size of tumor, and extent of disease at the time of diagnosis.[22–25] Men have a poorer prognosis than women, as do patients with tumors >3 cm, extrathyroidal extension of their tumor, or distant metastases. Symptoms indicative of advanced local disease (e.g., dysphagia, dyspnea, dysphonia) have also been shown to confer a worse prognosis.[27]

Occult papillary carcinomas are small (<1.5-cm diameter), nonpalpable lesions that are detected incidentally after thyroidectomy or while searching for a primary site of a nodal neck metastasis. Pelizzo et al.[28] report that approximately 10% of patients resected for apparent benign thyroid disease will have occult disease after pathologic examination is completed. Occult papillary carcinomas are extremely benign even in the presence of nodal metastasis and highly curable when treated by conservative surgical approaches and postoperative thyroxine suppression.[28,29]

Cervical lymph node involvement occurs early in the course of papillary carcinoma and is present in approximately 24%–32% of cases at the time of diagnosis, with more than 50% of patients having involvement at some time in the course of their disease.[22–24,30] The implications of lymph node involvement with regard to recurrence and overall survival remain controversial. McHenry et al.[30] report that a higher rate of nodal and distant metastases is seen in patients with cervical node involvement, but that the impact of this on survival remains uncertain. Tubiana et al.[24] found the reverse to be true and suggest that the relatively good prognosis of patients with lymph node involvement may be due to the influence of age since lymph node metastases is more common in young patients. Several studies have reported no influence of lymph node involvement on long-term survival.[20,22,23]

The lung is the most common site of distant metastases, occurring in approximately 6% of cases at diagnosis.[23,31] Pulmonary metastases can remain clinically dormant for years. Bone involvement is present in approximately 3% of cases.[23]

Papillary carcinoma has a very prolonged natural history, which accounts for the frequency of late relapses and the prolonged interval between relapse and death.[24] Death is usually due to recurrent or uncontrolled local disease, even in patients with distant metastases.[23]

Follicular carcinoma

Follicular cancers tend to be more locally invasive than the papillary form. The average age at diagnosis is 45–50,[32,33] and it is rarely seen in children.[34] Compared with papillary carcinoma, follicular forms have a decreased likelihood of metastasizing to regional lymph nodes. When it occurs, cervical involvement is more likely to be a result of direct extension of a locally invasive tumor. Bone metastases occur more frequently because of the propensity for hematogenous spread.[29,30] Unlike other forms of thyroid malignancies, follicular carcinomas are more likely to retain their ability to produce the thyroid hormones, T3 and T4, and occasionally cause hyperthyroidism.[35]

Hurthle cell cancer of the thyroid is sometimes considered a distinct histologic entity, but for practical purposes it can be classified as a variant of follicular carcinoma since the clinical course and treatment recommendations are similar for both tumor types.[34]

Follicular tumors with capsular or vascular invasion are associated with a poorer prognosis.[32,33] Although most patients have metastatic disease at the time of death, death generally results from growth of local recurrences.

Medullary carcinoma

MCT develops spontaneously in about 80% of cases, with the remaining 20% occurring as part of genetically transmitted multiple endocrine neoplasia syndromes.[34] It occurs equally in both sexes. The average age for the sporadic form is 45–50,[18,34] while the familial forms have been detected in patients ranging in age from 1–80 years.[34] MCT follows a relatively indolent course in the majority of patients. Fifty percent of patients have lymph node involvement at diagnosis. Hematogenous spread occurs later to lung, bone, and liver.[18] Survival is highly variable, ranging from months to 30 years[18] and is significantly correlated to age, sex, and stage of disease, with the best prognosis seen in women younger than 40 years with an early stage of disease.[36] The familial form of MCT can occur as a component of MEN IIA or MEN IIB. Because the familial form that occurs as part of MEN IIB may be particularly virulent, every effort should be made to screen family members of affected individuals for the presence of disease.[37] Identification of families at risk permits early detection of medullary thyroid cancer, ultimately improving prognosis.[17,19]

Anaplastic carcinoma

Anaplastic carcinomas of the thyroid are among the most rapidly growing, lethal neoplasms. Death usually occurs within months of diagnosis, regardless of therapy, with median survival approximately 12 months.[38–40] The majority of patients are elderly individuals, with a mean age of 65 years,[34] and females are affected more than males. Most of the patients also have a history of goiter or previously diagnosed differentiated thyroid carcinoma.[40] The tumor rapidly invades surrounding structures and metastasizes early. Death usually occurs secondary to local invasion and tracheal encroachment.[35]

There is some evidence to suggest that well-differentiated papillary thyroid cancers may evolve histologically to a more anaplastic variety.[20] This may reflect end-stage behavior in the natural history of papillary tumors, although prior irradiation may also be involved in the transformation process. For this reason, Demeter et al.[40] recommend a more aggressive approach to the management of patients with well-differentiated thyroid malignancies, suggesting that total or near-total thyroidectomy may preclude subsequent histologic progression in patients left with occult residual disease.

Clinical Manifestations

Clinical presentation may vary according to the type of thyroid malignancy. Incidental discovery of an otherwise asymptomatic thyroid mass on routine physical examination is frequently the first indication of disease in patients with papillary carcinoma. Palpable cervical lymphadenopathy is also present in a large number of patients. Other symptoms occur with significantly less frequency and are related to compressive effects of the enlarging mass on adjacent structures. These complications are more commonly associated with the undifferentiated, anaplastic forms of the disease. Patients may experience a sensation of tightness or fullness in the neck that could progress to dyspnea or stridor if the trachea is compressed or infiltrated.[35] Esophageal compression will generally cause dysphagia, and hoarseness can result from malignant infiltration or destruction of the recurrent laryngeal or vagus nerves. Pain is uncommon and usually indicative of advanced disease. It may be localized to the thyroid gland or reported as referred ear pain.

Osseous metastases are more likely in follicular carcinoma, and patients may present with signs of bone involvement (e.g., bone pain, pathologic fractures).

Approximately 20%–30% of patients with medullary thyroid cancer experience persistent diarrhea related to excessive production of prostaglandins, vasoactive intestinal peptide, and serotonin by the tumor.[16,17]

Diagnostic Evaluation

Assessment

Patient history/physical exam A comprehensive patient history may provide clues to making the diagnosis. Information regarding growth rate of the tumor, associated symptoms, prior irradiation, and a family history of thyroid-related problems should be elicited.

On physical examination, the thyroid, adjacent neck structures, and surrounding lymph nodes are inspected for symmetry and palpated for masses. Diffusely enlarged thyroid glands can be attributed to a variety of nonmalignant causes and require further evaluation. Individuals presenting with thyroid nodules in whom thyroid cancer is suspected should be systematically evaluated. The head and neck exam should include indirect laryngoscopy in all patients with a history of voice changes to assess the possibility of vocal cord paralysis and laryngeal nerve invasion.

Although altered hormonal secretion is unusual, patients may exhibit systemic manifestations of thyroid hormone excess or deficiency. Clinical symptoms of hyperthyroidism include fine tremors, lid lag, brisk tendon reflexes, increased appetite and weight loss, tachycardia, heat intolerance, proptosis, irritability, and muscle weakness. In thyroid hormone deficiency, patients may experience dry skin, hair loss, cold intolerance, weight gain, slowed speech, bradycardia, decreased reflexes, and constipation.

Fine-needle aspiration Fine-needle aspiration biopsy is the most widely used technique in the evaluation of nodular thyroid diseases since it is the only diagnostic tool used in the work-up of thyroid cancer that can differentiate benign from malignant nodules with a high degree of accuracy.[41] Hawkins et al.[42] reported a false-negative rate of 2.4% and a false-positive rate of 6.5% when interpreting specimens categorized as suspicious. Cystic lesions should also be evaluated by this method since they are nearly as likely to be malignant as solid nodules, and, contrary to popular belief, the physical characteristics of the cyst are not necessarily predictive of malignancy.[43] A suggested approach to the evaluation of thyroid nodules is depicted in Figure 40-1.[41]

TSH suppression Because of the influence of TSH on the growth of thyroid nodules, suppression of TSH is done by administering exogenous thyroid hormone (thyroxine) to reduce the size of nodules and prevent prolonged TSH stimulation of the thyroid.[44] If, after several months of suppressive therapy, the size of the nodule increases or remains the same, surgery is indicated. Because there is a small possibility that nodules responding to suppression may be malignant, patients should continue to be followed for changes in the size of the nodule.[44]

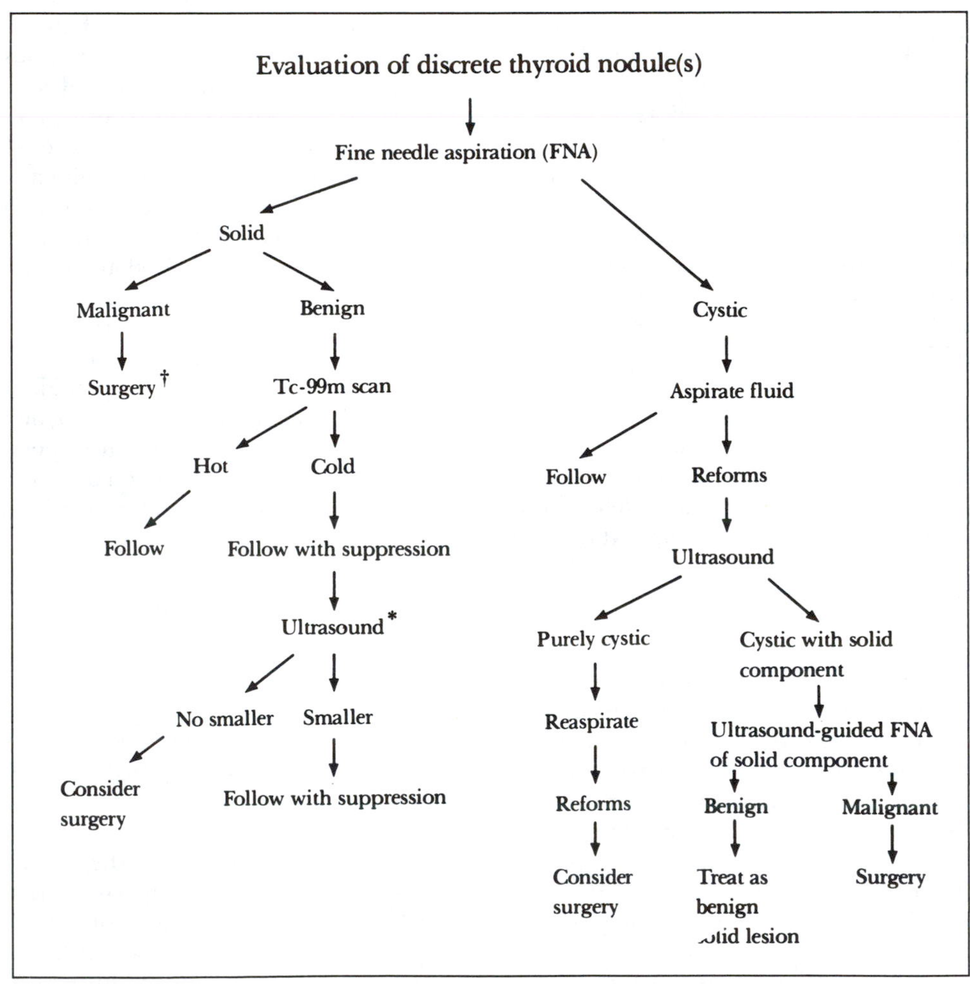

FIGURE 40-1 Evaluation of solitary thyroid nodules. Protocol for work-up and management. Asterisk (*) indicates one prominent nodule in a multinodular gland; dagger (†) indicates ultrasonography only if the mass is difficult to palpate. *FNA,* Fine needle aspiration; *Tc-99m,* technitium-99n. (Source: Friedman M, Toriumi DM, Mafee MF: Diagnostic imaging techniques in thyroid cancer, *Am J Surg* 155:215-223, 1988.)

Radionucleide imaging Thyroid scans provide useful information regarding the functional status of thyroid nodules. Normal thyroid tissue is functional in that it concentrates iodine for use in the production of thyroid hormones. Radioactive isotopes are used to classify nodules according to their ability to concentrate iodine. Nodules may do this to the same, greater, or lesser extent than normal thyroid tissue.[45] Nonfunctioning nodules are "cold," normal thyroid tissue is "warm," and hyperfunctioning nodules are "hot." Unfortunately, this technique is limited because it cannot distinguish benign from malignant nodules.[44]

Laboratory tests If thyroid dysfunction is suggested by history or physical exam, routine thyroid function tests (RAI, T3 uptake, total T4, free T4, and TSH) should be obtained, although these tests may be nonspecifically elevated in patients with other thyroid disorders.[44]

Serum calcitonin is an important tumor marker in the diagnosis and evaluation of treatment response in patients with MCT.[17,18] It is routinely used in screening for the familial forms of medullary thyroid cancer.[17]

Staging

The staging system proposed by the American Joint Committee on Cancer is widely used because it incorporates the important prognostic factors of age and histologic type into the classification (Table 40-2).[46]

TABLE 40-2 Staging Classification of Thyroid Carcinomas

PRIMARY TUMOR (T)	
All categories may be subdivided: (a) solitary; (b) multifocal—measure the largest for classification	
TX	Primary tumor cannot be assessed
T0	No evidence of primary tumor
T1	Tumor 1 cm or less in greatest dimension limited to the thyroid
T2	Tumor more than 1 cm but not more than 4 cm
T3	Tumor more than 4 cm in greatest dimension limited to the thyroid
T4	Tumor of any size extending beyond the thyroid capsule
LYMPH NODE (N)	
Regional nodes are the cervical and upper mediastinal lymph nodes	
NX	Regional lymph nodes cannot be assessed
N0	No regional lymph node metastasis
N1	Regional lymph node metastasis
N1a	Metastasis in ipsilateral cervical lymph nodes
N1b	Metastasis in bilateral, midline, or contralateral cervical or mediastinal lymph nodes
DISTANT METASTASIS (M)	
MX	Presence of distant metastasis cannot be assessed
M0	No distant metastasis
M1	Distant metastasis
STAGE GROUPING	
Separate stage groupings are recommended for papillary and follicular, medullary, and undifferentiated.	
Papillary or Follicular	
Under 45 Years	
Stage I	Any T, Any N, M0
Stage II	Any T, Any N, M1
45 years and Over	
Stage I	T1, N0, M0
Stage II	T2, N0, M0
	T3, N0, M0
Stage III	T4, N0, M0
	Any T, N1, M0
Stage IV	Any T, Any N, M1
Medullary	
Stage I	T1, N0, M0
Stage II	T2, N0, M0
	T3, N0, M0
	T4, N0, M0
Stage III	Any T, N1, M0
Stage IV	Any T, Any N, M1
Undifferentiated	
All cases are Stage IV	
Stage IV	Any T, Any N, Any M

Source: Beahrs OH et al: *Manual for Staging of Cancer* (4th ed). Philadelphia: Lippincott, 1992.

Treatment

Surgery

Early detection of disease before intraglandular or extraglandular invasion occurs maximizes the potential for cure in patients with thyroid cancer. Because of the indolent nature and prolonged natural history of well-differentiated thyroid cancers and the lack of large prospective clinical trials, controversy continues regarding the best treatment for papillary and follicular carcinomas. Consequently, most recommendations regarding surgical intervention are based on data obtained from retrospective analysis of large series of patients.

In general, a relatively aggressive approach in the management of patients with thyroid malignancies has been advocated.[20,22,25,47,48] Near-total or total thyroidectomy is widely utilized as the initial treatment for all differentiated thyroid cancers. Although ipsalateral total lobectomy may be performed in selected cases of occult papillary carcinoma where the lesion is <1.5 cm and confined to one lobe, higher rates of recurrence with this approach have been observed.[20] In all cases where a lobectomy is performed for occult disease, patients should be placed on lifelong thyroxine suppression following surgery.[29]

Several large studies have reported that total thyroidectomy decreases the incidence of local recurrences and increases the effectiveness of treatment with ^{131}I because of total surgical ablation of the gland.[34,47,50] Complications are higher with this approach but have decreased in recent years when the procedures are performed by skilled surgeons.[47,50,51] Other investigators have suggested reserving total thyroidectomy for patients with adverse prognostic factors (age >40, extracapsular extension of tumor, and follicular histology).[1,24,32] Sometimes initial surgery is inadequate because the frozen section at the time of surgery may not confirm a diagnosis of malignancy. In patients with subsequent confirmation of differentiated thyroid carcinomas >1 cm, second operations to complete adequate resection are justified because approximately 40% of these patients could be expected to have residual cancer.[25]

Proponents of more conservative surgical procedures (near-total thyroidectomy, subtotal thyroidectomy) report that patients are less likely to experience complications postoperatively.[1,52,53] In these studies, higher rates of recurrence have not been observed in patients followed for up to 30 years following initial therapy, and survival rates have been comparable with patients undergoing total thyroidectomy.[1,23,52,53]

Total thyroidectomy is recommended for patients with medullary thyroid cancer due to the high incidence of bilateral involvement of the thyroid gland.[16,17] Patients with anaplastic carcinoma who have resectable lesions are generally treated with lobectomy, because more radical surgery results in an increased complication rate and does not alter the outcome of the disease.[38] In patients with unresectable lesions, palliative surgery is done to locally debulk the tumor. Tracheostomy and gastrostomy may be required and performed at the time of the initial surgery.

Management of nodal metastases remains controversial because of conflicting data regarding survival in patients with lymph node involvement.[22–25,30,54] Generally, lateral lymph node dissection is not performed unless nodes are clinically enlarged or take up radioactive iodine on preoperative scanning.[55] Naguchi et al.[54] reported lymph node involvement in 70% of patients with papillary carcinoma who underwent bilateral modified neck dissection at the time of total or near-total thyroidectomy. Bilateral metastasis was frequently observed when the tumor involved both lobes or the isthmus. In patients with positive contralateral paratracheal nodes, a contralateral modified neck dissection is recommended.[54]

Postoperative complications

Although individuals scheduled for surgery are usually given thyroid suppressive therapy for several weeks preoperatively to induce thyroid atrophy and reduce vascularity, hemorrhage is possible due to the highly vascular nature of the gland. Postoperatively, patients are placed in a semi-Fowler's position. Bleeding is assessed by checking under the neck and shoulders as well as inspecting the anterior dressing over the wound. Complaints of a sensation of pressure or tightness over the operative site may also be indicative of hemorrhage. A Penrose drain or other suction-type apparatus is used to prevent hematoma formation or accumulation of fluid at the operative site.

The integrity of the parathyroid glands is threatened during resection of the thyroid because of their position on the posterior surface of the thyroid. Although every effort is made to preserve parathyroid tissue, the extent of surgery may not permit salvaging of these glands. If the parathyroid glands can be resected and are not involved with disease, they may be autotransplanted.[57] With this technique the gland is minced at the time of surgery and then embedded into muscle tissue, usually the sternocleidomastoid muscle. This process permits the preservation of sufficient functioning parathyroid tissue to avert permanent hypoparathyroidism. Because the transplanted tissue does not become functional immediately, hypocalcemia resulting from parathyroid hormone loss can occur. Patients should be observed for signs of hypocalcemia and tetany in the immediate postoperative period. Symptoms include: numbness, tingling, cramps in the extremities, stiffness, twitching, and a positive Chvostek's or Trousseau's sign. Serum calcium is monitored daily and calcium replacement is given until levels return to normal. If some parathyroid tissue has been preserved, normal function will gradually return. The duration of temporary hypoparathyroidism varies, with reports ranging from 6 weeks[41] to 1 year.[50] Permanent hypoparathyroidism occurs in 0.8%–11% of patients undergoing total thyroidectomy.[50,51]

Because the recurrent laryngeal nerves travel along the posterior surface of the thyroid, surgical resection of the thyroid may damage these nerves, resulting in temporary or permanent vocal cord paralysis. This can lead to respiratory obstruction necessitating emergency tracheostomy. A tracheostomy set should be kept at the patient's bedside at all times. Transient nerve injury lasts from a few days to several months.[47,50] The incidence of permanent recurrent laryngeal nerve injury has decreased in recent years when procedures are performed by surgeons skilled in thyroid surgery, occurring in less than 1% of cases.[47,50] It is more likely to occur in patients undergoing secondary procedures for re-resection of residual carcinoma.[58]

Recurrent laryngeal nerve damage and postoperative local edema also contribute to alterations in vocal quality. With near-total thyroidectomy, the nerve on one side can be salvaged, and patients will experience only hoarseness.[50] If damage to both laryngeal nerves is present, aphonia will result. Speech therapy may assist the individual to develop better vocal quality.

Patients undergoing total or near-total thyroidectomy require postoperative administration of exogenous thyroid hormone to prevent clinical effects of hypothyroidism and to suppress endogenous TSH, which may serve as a growth factor for differentiated thyroid tumors. Patients are maintained permanently on suppressive therapy with withdrawal only in preparation for ^{131}I.

Radiotherapy

Use of ^{131}I is recommended for the treatment of residual and metastatic disease in certain patients with well-differentiated cancer following surgical resection of the thyroid.[34,45,59] Well-differentiated cancers retain, to a variable extent, their ability to concentrate radioiodine. This characteristic makes them optimal candidates for treatment with ^{131}I after removal of normal thyroid tissue and the bulk of the primary tumor.

Prior to administration of ^{131}I, thyroid hormone must be discontinued. Initiation of therapy is delayed for 4–6 weeks to permit thyroid hormone blood levels to fall and previously suppressed TSH levels to rise.[45] Radioiodine uptake depends on TSH levels. Increasing TSH levels augments uptake of ^{131}I into well-differentiated cancers. In patients with poor uptake, TSH stimulation may increase uptake and can be accomplished with injections of bovine TSH or administration of an antithyroid drug such as methimazole or carcimazole to induce endogenous TSH stimulation.[60] The use of bovine TSH is controversial because it is associated with a high incidence of sensitivity reactions with repeated doses. If TSH levels cannot be raised sufficiently by these means, uptake of ^{131}I may be inadequate for the destruction of malignant tissue.[45]

^{131}I can be given for ablation and/or treatment following surgical resection. Ablation is done prior to treatment with ^{131}I for the purpose of totally eradicating any remaining normal thyroid tissue left in the neck after near-total thyroidectomy. Even after total thyroidectomy, residual functional thyroid tissue is detected on radionucleide scans.[60] It optimizes the effectiveness of ^{131}I treatment so that the isotope will be concentrated in functional tumor tissue.[45] Ablation is generally done in all patients with residual thyroid tissue, but McHenry et al.[59] have recently explored a more selective approach in the use of postoperative ^{131}I. Only patients with extrathyroidal extension or nodal or distant metastases were scanned following thyroidectomy. In this group, only 9% of patients had >3% uptake on ^{131}I scanning and went on to ^{131}I ablation. Only one recurrence has occurred in the group that did not undergo ablation, with a mean follow-up of 9 years. Further studies are needed to confirm this as an alternative approach to standard practice in the postoperative management of well-differentiated thyroid malignancies.

Two to 3 months after ablation, a whole-body scan is done to detect metastatic disease or evidence of residual functioning tissue in the thyroid bed.[34] Treatment with ^{131}I should not be given sooner than 6 months after ablation because of residual radioactivity in the neck.[45] Treatment with ^{131}I requires dosimetry calculations to determine the dose needed to deliver the maximal dose to metastases of thyroid carcinoma, while minimizing systemic exposure.[35] Therapy doses are given at 4–6 month intervals until there is no evidence of functioning tumor on whole-body imaging studies.

Patients selected for ^{131}I therapy must be alert and capable of self-care activities. Inpatient admission in a private room for administration of ^{131}I treatment is required since radiation precautions must be instituted.[34] ^{131}I is administered orally and is present in all body secretions. No children or pregnant women are allowed in the patient's room after the isotope is administered. Patients may be discharged when radiation dose emission readings show less than 30 mCi ^{131}I—about 48–72 hours after 100 mCi is given.[34] (Refer to Chapter 13 for other considerations for patients receiving brachytherapy.)

Complications of ^{131}I therapy include nausea and vomiting, fatigue, headache, sialadenitis (inflammation of the salivary glands), bone marrow suppression, and rarely, pulmonary radiation fibrosis and leukemia.[45]

Symptoms of fatigue, headache, and nausea and vomiting may be related to radiation sickness and can occur as early as 12 hours after ^{131}I administration. Premedication with antiemetics may be helpful.

Sialadenitis occurs within 24 hours of administering ^{131}I and may be due to the concentration of radioisotope in the salivary glands.[60] Stimulation of salivary flow using hard candy may avert this problem.

Transient bone marrow suppression is seen in almost all patients receiving ^{131}I therapy. More severe aplasia may be seen in patients with extensive metastatic disease or in those who have had repeated doses of ^{131}I.

External beam irradiation is used either alone or in combination with ^{131}I for patients with incompletely excised tumors. Tubiana et al.[61] report achieving local control of disease in approximately 90% of patients with inoperable differentiated cancers with high-dose external beam therapy to the thyroid, neck, and superior mediastinum.

Anaplastic and medullary thyroid cancers are unable to concentrate ^{131}I, which precludes its effectiveness with these tumors.[18,38,39]

Treatment of anaplastic carcinomas with external irradiation as a single modality has not been effective due to the radioresistance of this type of thyroid neoplasm, but Kim and Leeper[62] reported excellent results with local control by combining external beam radiation with low-dose doxorubicin as a radiosensitizer for hypoxic, radioresistant tumor cells. Dose reduction should be considered when administering chemotherapy and external radiation concurrently because of the potentiation of bone marrow suppression and local toxicities affecting the oral mucosa and esophagus.

External beam irradiation may also be helpful in the palliation of painful bony metastases.

Chemotherapy

The role of chemotherapy in the treatment of advanced differentiated medullary and anaplastic thyroid cancer has been disappointing, with low response rates.[1,39,63] As a single agent, only doxorubicin has demonstrated any significant antitumor activity.[1] Shimaoka[64] reports a 26% overall response rate in advanced differentiated and anaplastic thyroid carcinomas with combination doxorubicin and cisplatin.

Follow-up

Long-term follow-up is an integral part in the management of patients with thyroid malignancies due to incidence of late recurrences, particularly in patients with papillary carcinomas.

Because serum thyroglobulin is a sensitive indicator of recurrent disease in well-differentiated thyroid malignancies, this should be monitored in conjunction with serial isotope scanning.[65] Measurement of basal and stimulated calcitonin levels in medullary thyroid carcinoma is also helpful in the detection of early recurrence, although the impact of early detection of recurrent disease on subsequent treatment decisions and survival is uncertain.

PITUITARY TUMORS

The diagnosis and management of patients with pituitary tumors has changed significantly over the past 20 years due to the refinement of microsurgical and radiotherapy techniques, advances in laboratory evaluation of hormonal activity, and pharmacologic developments in the management of tumor-related hormonal abnormalities.

Epidemiology

Pituitary tumors make up approximately 10%–15% of all known intracranial neoplasms, although asymptomatic tumors are identified in 6%–23% of unselected autopsies.[66] The majority of these are benign pituitary adenomas, which arise from the adenohypophyseal cells in the anterior portion of the gland. The other tumor types observed are craniopharyngiomas, which occur primarily in children, and pituitary carcinomas. The incidence of pituitary carcinoma is exceedingly rare.[67] This discussion will be limited to pituitary adenomas.

Although adenomas have been reported in all age groups, they are rarely seen before puberty and occur primarily in middle-aged and older patients.[66]

Etiology

No definitive causative factors in the development of pituitary adenomas have been established. Although it has generally been believed that these tumors arise de novo as a result of hypothalamic dysfunction,[68] recent evidence supports the role of somatic cell mutation with clonal expansion.[69]

It has also been suggested that adenomas of the prolactin-secreting cells may result from disorders of dopamine synthesis and secretion. Because prolactin is inhibited by dopamine, disturbances in dopamine metabolism may result in an unopposed rise in prolactin secretion.[70]

There does not appear to be any genetic influence in the development of pituitary adenomas.[1]

Classification

Pituitary adenomas are categorized according to hormone activity and size. The major hormones secreted by the anterior pituitary gland are prolactin, growth hormone (GH), adrenocorticotropin hormone (ACTH), thyroid-stimulating hormone (TSH), follicle-stimulating hormone (FSH), and luteinizing hormone (LH) (Table 40-3).

Adenomas smaller than 10 mm in diameter are referred to as *microadenomas*, while those greater than 10 mm are termed *macroadenomas*. Microadenomas are associated with a better overall prognosis because they are generally confined to the pituitary gland and are more easily resectable.[71]

Pathophysiology

Although most pituitary adenomas do not exhibit the characteristic histologic changes indicative of malignant transformation, they are "malignant" by virtue of their ability to produce morbidity through growth in a confined space and mediation of hormonal dysfunction. Many adenomas are slow growing, noninvasive tumors confined to the sella turcica. Others are more aggressive in their clinical behavior, exhibiting rapid growth rates, invading adjacent tissues, and causing symptoms indicative of compression of vital structures.[66,71,72] Invasion occurs more frequently in macroadenomas than micro-adenomas.[71]

Pituitary carcinomas, although rare, are true malignant tumors in both their histologic appearance and biologic behavior and uniformly result in distant metastases.[67]

The majority of pituitary tumors arising from adenohypophyseal cells are well differentiated and retain their hormone-producing capabilities, but the tumor cells are not subject to the normal regulatory mechanisms of the body and produce hormones regardless of feedback from target organs.[66]

Clinical Presentation

The most common manifestations of pituitary adenomas are alterations in hormonal patterns and symptoms indicative of compression from a growing tumor.

Patients with functional tumors will exhibit symp-

TABLE 40-3 Hormonal Classification of Pituitary Adenomas

Classification	Prevalence (approximate)	Hormone Secreted	Clinical Manifestations
Lactotroph	27%	Prolactin	Women: amenorrhea, infertility, galactorrhea Men: decreased libido, impotence
Somatotroph	14%	GH	Acromegaly, gigantism
Corticotroph	14%	ACTH	Cushing's disease (approximately 6% have increased ACTH without endocrine symptoms)
Gonadotroph	6.5%	FSH/LH	Frequently are clinically silent with only elevated blood hormone levels
Thyrotroph	1%	TSH	Hyperthyroidism
Plurihormonal	10%	Two or more adenohypophyseal hormones (GH, prolactin are most common)	Depends on type of hormone secreted
Null cell	25%	None	Localized symptoms—headache, visual disturbances, dysfunction of cranial nerves

Source: Data taken in part from Scheithauer BW et al.[71]

toms of hormonal excess. Clinical effects of hypersecretion of the anterior pituitary hormones may be observed in these patients, although endocrine abnormalities have been reported in a high proportion of patients undergoing surgery for nonsecreting pituitary adenomas.[73] In this group, hypogonadism, adrenal insufficiency, hypothyroidism, and hyperprolactinemia were confirmed with laboratory evaluation preoperatively but were not manifest clinically.

Infrequently, tumor expansion will cause a clinical picture of hypopituitarism. This does not necessarily reflect irreversible damage to the gland but is more likely due to compression of the portal vessels and the pituitary stalk.[74] Recovery of function can be expected in the majority of patients postoperatively.[75]

An expanding pituitary neoplasm can cause compression of surrounding critical structures, resulting in headache, visual disturbances, and functional impairment of cranial nerves (Figure 40-2).[76] Headache occurs when the expanding tumor distends the diaphragma sellae. Suprasellar extension may also compress the optic nerves and chiasm. The most frequent ophthalmologic finding is a unilateral or bitemporal field defect.[77] Lateral tumor extension can also involve oculomotor nerves, causing oculomotor paresis. Occasionally, penetration into the sphenoid sinus is associated with a spontaneous CSF rhinorrhea.[77]

Diagnostic Evaluation

Although the histologic diagnosis of a pituitary adenoma cannot be confirmed prior to surgery, the anatomic extent of the pituitary mass and its functional status can be validated with appropriate endocrine and neuroradiologic studies.

Complete endocrine evaluation should include baseline and stimulated testing of the pituitary-gonadal, pituitary-adrenal, and pituitary-thyropidal axes.[73] Inferior petrosal sinus sampling to measure adrenocorticotropin hormone (ACTH) levels has been described as a method to identify a pituitary source of ACTH causing Cushing's disease.[78] With this technique, bilateral catheterization of the inferior petrosal sinuses is done and blood is sampled for ACTH levels. This method may also be helpful in localizing ACTH-secreting microadenomas since the anatomy of pituitary venous drainage is such that a laterally located microadenoma would preferentially secrete hormone to the ipsilateral sinus.[79]

Inferior petrosal sinus sampling may also be valuable in the early diagnosis of GH-producing adenomas when peripheral GH levels and radiographic studies are nondiagnostic.[80]

High-resolution MRI is the most sensitive imaging technique in diagnosing pituitary adenomas because it provides the most precise information regarding tumor margins, effect of tumor on adjacent structures, location of vascular structures, the optic apparatus and cavernous sinus, consistency of the tumor, and presence of normal pituitary tissue.[79,81] Angiography may also be done to further define the lumen of blood vessels and is indicated if there is a question of an aneurysm.

Information obtained during the diagnostic workup may aid in the selection of a therapeutic approach, as well as provide baseline data for assessing response to therapy.[77,81] Diagnostic tests are repeated following initial therapy to assess adequacy of treatment and the need for additional management.

Treatment

The goals of treatment are removal or eradication of the tumor, restoration of normal hormonal function,

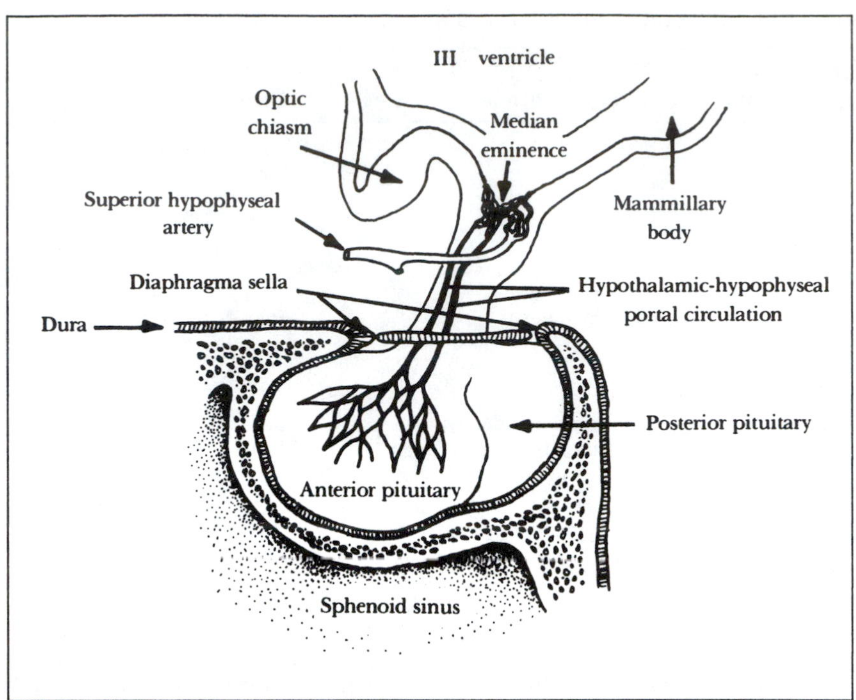

FIGURE 40-2 Anatomic relationship of pituitary gland to surrounding structures. (Source: Boyd AE III, Jordan RM, Kohler PO: Disorders of the hypothalamus and anterior pituitary, in Kohler PO (ed), *Clinical Endocrinology* [New York; Wiley, 1986], pp. 11–51. Used with permission from Churchill Livingstone, New York.)

and elimination of mass effects without residual morbidity.

Surgery

Prompt surgical intervention is indicated in patients with pituitary apoplexy (hemorrhage into the tumor and precipitous deterioration of neurologic status) and in patients with clinical manifestations of a progressive mass effect.[82]

Surgical resection is performed in the majority of patients with nonsecreting macroadenomas because of the frequency of visual impairment at the time of diagnosis.[73,83,84] Complete resection is not always possible in these patients, but subtotal resection followed by postoperative radiation yields recurrence rates in the range of 21%–27%, which is lower than that achieved with surgery alone.[73,84,85]

Surgical excision remains the primary treatment for most hypersecreting pituitary adenomas as well and is the most effective method for achieving rapid durable responses and normalization of hormone levels.[86–88]

Selection of the surgical technique depends on the size of the tumor, extent of suprasellar extension, and involvement of the cavernous sinus. Approximately 96% of adenomas are resected using the transsphenoidal route,[82] with the remainder requiring craniotomy. The transsphenoidal approach permits selective removal of the tumor with preservation of normal pituitary tissue. Disadvantages of this technique are visual limitations in the surgical field, including inability to visualize the optic nerves. Craniotomy permits complete visualization of the pituitary gland and surrounding intracranial structures but is associated with higher morbidity. Whenever possible, normal pituitary tissue is preserved.

Diabetes insipidus, cerebrospinal fluid (CSF) leak, and meningitis are the most frequently reported complications following transsphenoidal surgery.

Transient diabetes insipidus lasting 12–36 hours occurs in up to one-third of patients and is managed with desmopressin.[73,88] This complication is usually temporary even in patients with complete hypophysectomy since antidiuretic hormone (ADH) can be secreted directly from the hypothalamus without pituitary storage.[82]

CSF rhinorrhea is observed in approximately 5% of patients.[73] This is managed with bed rest, elevation of the head of the bed, and fluid restrictions. Activities that increase intracranial pressure, such as sneezing, coughing, and blowing the nose, should be avoided.

Because of the increased risk of meningitis following surgery, patients are frequently placed on prophylactic antibiotics and should be monitored for symptoms of meningitis, which include fever and stiff neck.[89]

Other possible surgical risks include damage to the hypothalamus, optic nerves, and carotid arteries.[84] Additional nursing considerations during the immediate postoperative period pertain to the care of the operative site. Nasal mucosa takes approximately 1 month to heal following surgery. Sneezing and nose blowing are contraindicated during this period to minimize pressure on the operative site. Because the surgical incision is located in the upper gingiva, oral inspection and meticulous mouth care are needed to maintain integrity of the mucous membranes and prevent infection.[89]

Postoperatively, measurement of pituitary hormone levels is done to assess the effectiveness of surgery in removing hypersecreting tumor tissue. As a result of surgery, normalization of hormonal levels occurs in approximately 80% of patients with acromegaly[86] and 85% of patients with Cushing's disease.[90] In patients with prolactinomas, postoperative hormone levels are strongly correlated with tumor size and preoperative hormone levels.[91–93] Randall et al.[91] report normalization of prolactin levels following surgery in 88% of cases with microadenomas and preoperative prolactin levels <100 ng/ml compared with 43% of patients with large, but noninvasive macroadenomas and preoperative levels of >100 ng/ml. In patients with invasive adenomas, normal levels were achieved in only 19%.

Radiotherapy

Because of recent advances in microsurgical techniques, external beam irradiation is seldom used as the primary treatment of pituitary adenomas except in patients who refuse surgery or are deemed inoperable.[83,85,87,94,95] Postoperatively, it is used in the management of patients with incompletely resected or recurrent tumors and in some patients with persistent hyperfunctioning endocrinopathies. Several large studies have reported a reduction in the local recurrence rate when surgery is followed by radiation therapy.[87,94,95] The usual radiation dose required is ≥45 Gy to produce long-term control.

Some debate surrounds the timing of the administration of radiation therapy following surgery. McCullough et al.[95] suggest that treatment be given immediately to decrease the expense and inconvenience associated with close surveillance and to avoid the possible need for additional surgical resection, but Chun et al.[94] report that comparable local control can be achieved when salvage radiation therapy is given after actual recurrence has been demonstrated. They recommend that treatment with external beam be deferred in those patients who do not have persistent symptoms or residual tumor that is at risk for regrowth in critical areas.[94]

Radiation therapy is less effective in controlling persistent endocrine hypersecretion following surgery. Irradiation progressively lowers GH in approximately 80% of patients with acromegaly and lowers glucocorticoids in 50%–80% of patients with Cushing's disease, but full effects may take months to years.[85] Because of the delay in radiation effect, this form of therapy alone is impractical in normalizing hormone levels in patients with hypersecreting tumors.

The major complication of irradiation of pituitary adenomas is hypopituitarism, which may become evident years after treatment has been given.[94,96] Although hypopituitarism can occur with surgery or radiation therapy alone, it is seen most frequently in patients treated with combined modality therapy.[96] Deficiencies of adrenal, thyroid, and gonadal hormones have been observed, and patients are placed on lifelong supplementation of the deficient hormone. Because of the prolonged interval between treatment and the development of hypopituitarism, patients need continued monitoring of endocrine function.

Pharmacotherapy

Several pharmacologic agents have been used in the medical management of hypersecreting pituitary adenomas. Bromocriptine, a dopamine agonist, has been shown to be effective not only in reducing hormone levels in patients with prolactin-secreting tumors but in reducing tumor size as well.[98,99] It acts by binding to dopamine receptors and inhibits the synthesis and release of prolactin. Side effects include nausea, orthostatic hypotension, and headaches. This approach is often used as first-line therapy for patients with prolactinomas. Bromocriptine as a single agent is not curative, and discontinuation results in rapid regrowth of tumor and hypersecretion of prolactin,[83] although long-term control of prolactin secretion has been reported in patients receiving postoperative bromocriptine.[97]

It has also been suggested that preoperative treatment of prolactinomas with bromocriptine may adversely affect surgical outcome in that it increases risk for interstitial fibrosis.[88,100] While it can make surgical resection technically more difficult, this fibrosis has not been found to affect the surgical outcome in patients receiving short-term (<6 weeks) preoperative therapy.[101] Bromocriptine has also been used, but less successfully, in the treatment of acromegaly, with normalization of growth hormone levels in approximately 20% of patients.[102]

A long-acting somatostatin analog, SMS 201-995, is more widely used in the preoperative treatment of GH-producing macroadenomas by suppressing GH-hypersecretion as well as reducing tumor size.[103] Maximal tumor reduction occurs after 8–12 weeks of treatment and GH levels remain within the normal range in 80% of patients postoperatively.[103] This compound has also been used in the postoperative treatment of TSH-producing adenomas and controls excess production of TSH.[83] It is given subcutaneously and can induce severe gastrointestinal distress in a large proportion of patients.

ADRENAL TUMORS

Adrenal tumors can arise from the cortical or medullary portions of the adrenal gland, with presentations differing significantly due to the physiologic diversity of these two types of tissues. In adults the majority of cancers involving the cortex are adrenocortical carcinomas, and those involving the adrenal medulla are pheochromocytomas.

Adrenocortical Carcinomas

Epidemiology

The incidence of adrenal cortical carcinoma is rare, occurring in approximately 1 in 1,000,000 people.[104] In several of the larger series of patients with adrenocortical carcinomas, the overall incidence was equal between the sexes, although women had a much higher proportion of functional neoplasms.[105–110] Approximately 60%–70% of patients have functional tumors that produce excess amounts of corticosteroids. Nonfunctional carcinomas occur most commonly in patients 40–70 years, with men predominating by 2 to 1. All series reported more frequent involvement of the left adrenal, with bilateral occurrence rarely seen.

Pathophysiology

Adrenocortical carcinomas are aggressive malignancies, with 70%–90% of patients presenting with either locally advanced or metastatic disease.[105–110] The delay in detecting disease is thought to be due to (1) difficulty in detecting retroperitoneal masses, (2) nonspecific symptoms of patients with nonfunctional tumors, and (3) gradual onset of symptoms in patients with functional tumors.

The most common sites of metastasis are lung, liver, and lymph nodes. Over 50% of patients in one series died of pulmonary insufficiency (from multiple lung metastases) and sepsis.[105] Local tumor extension can involve the kidneys, liver, vena cava, pancreas, and diaphragm. Median survival with treatment ranges from 1 month to 5 years.[105–110]

Clinical presentation

Patients with nonfunctional tumors commonly present with a palpable abdominal mass that may be associated with abdominal or back pain. Fever, weight loss, weakness, and lethargy are primarily seen in patients with advanced disease.[96]

Patients with functional tumors will have excessive production of one or more of the hormones secreted by the adrenal cortex. The five major steroid hormones are: cortisol, aldosterone, progesterone, testosterone, and estradiol. The majority of functional tumors result in Cushing's disease, virilization and feminization syndromes, and hyperaldosteronism.[111]

Clinical features of Cushing's disease include weight gain; obesity of the trunk, face, and neck; hirsutism; hypertension; and muscle wasting.[112] In females, androgen-secreting tumors result in a virulization syndrome characterized by amenorrhea, hirsutism, increased muscle mass, and deepening of the voice.[112] In men, estrogen-secreting tumors result in gynecomastia, testicular atrophy, and impotence. Estrogen-secreting tumors are difficult to detect until far advanced in premenopausal women. The incidence of aldosterone-secreting tumors is rare. Hypersecretion of aldosterone leads to hypertension and hypokalemia.

Diagnostic evaluation

Immunoassays of hormone precursors and mature hormones and their metabolites detect the presence of functional adrenal tumors. Patients with adrenocortical carcinoma commonly excrete large amounts of 17-ketosteroids and 17-hydroxycorticosteroids if excessive glucocorticoid or sex steroid production is present, and these compounds can be detected in the urine.[104]

Computerized tomography (CT) is the most common method used to localize adrenal tumors, and it provides information regarding hepatic, renal, and vena caval involvement.[113] Widespread use of CT has resulted in increasing numbers of incidentally discovered adrenal masses. These masses warrant careful evaluation to identify appropriate treatment interventions. Recent reports regarding the ability of MRI to discriminate benign adenomas from adrenocortical carcinomas and pheochromocytomas make this an invaluable diagnostic tool.[114,115] MRI may be particularly useful in the screening of asymptomatic masses. With earlier detection the prognosis for patients with adrenocortical carcinomas may improve.[114]

Treatment

Surgery is the primary treatment for adrenocortical carcinoma and can be curative for patients with small localized tumors.[108] Unfortunately, many are unresectable at the time of diagnosis because of local extension, lymphatic metastases, or distant metastases to the liver or lungs. In patients with locally advanced and invasive disease, maximal debulking should be undertaken before additional therapy is initiated. Results of treatment with conventional surgery, radiation therapy, and chemotherapy have been poor, with 5-year survival less than 30%.[105,116] Resection of locally recurrent as well as metastatic disease has been advocated because it is associated with a slight prolongation of survival and control of hypercortisolism.[108,116]

Because tumor hypersecretion may diffusely suppress adrenal hormone activity, causing atrophy of the uninvolved gland, glucocorticoids are administered pre- and postoperatively until normal function of the unaffected gland returns. In patients with bilateral involvement, ablation of both adrenals necessitates permanent replacement therapy of the mineralocorticoids and glucocorticoids. Exogenous administration of catecholamines is not required because of the ectopic sources at nerve endings and other ganglia in the sympathetic nervous system.[117]

The adrenocorticolytic drug o,p'-DDD (mitotane), which causes selective necrosis of the adrenal cortex, has a limited role as adjuvant therapy or in the treatment of inoperable disease.[109,111,118,119] In a series of 60 patients with residual disease postoperatively who received o,p'-DDD, objective tumor regression was seen in 34% of patients, but the mean duration of response was approximately 10 months.[118] Treatment with o,p'DDD is associated with disabling side effects that include nausea, vomiting, anorexia, diarrhea, lethargy, and profound depression that can significantly affect a patient's quality of life.[91] This toxicity is seen with therapeutic doses of 8–10 g/day.[111] Patient tolerance has been improved with reduced doses.[119] Also, many of the side effects seen with o,p'-DDD may reflect adrenal insufficiency rather than drug toxicity and can be corrected by increased doses of replacement corticosteroids.[120]

Aminogluthethimide, which blocks corticosteroid secretion, can also be used for palliation of excess hormone production in patients with recurrences, but this drug does not inhibit further growth of the tumor.[117]

Evaluation of the efficacy of cytotoxic chemotherapy is limited because of the rarity of this neoplasm. Anecdotal reports of combination o,p-DDD/streptozotocin, cisplatin/VP-16, and 5-fluorouracil/doxorubicin/cisplatin have shown limited activity.[121–123]

Radiation therapy following surgical resection does not improve survival but can be effective in palliating patients with painful bone metastases.[107,108]

Pheochromocytomas

Epidemiology

Pheochromocytomas are rare catecholamine-secreting tumors that arise from chromaffin cells of the sympathoadrenal system. Chromaffin cells, found not only in the adrenals but in other ectopic sites along the sympathetic chain, possess the enzymatic properties to synthesize amine hormones. Tumors that share these common biochemical characteristics for *a*mine *p*recursor *u*ptake and *d*ecarboxylation are referred to as *APUD* tumors.[124] APUD cells have been detected in the thyroid, adrenal medulla, sympathetic nervous system, and gastroenteropancreatic organs.

Pheochromocytomas are extremely rare, occurring in fewer than 0.1%–1% of hypertensive patients.[125]

Malignant pheochromocytomas occur in approximately 10% of patients with pheochromocytomas and can only be differentiated from benign tumors by their capacity for invasiveness and distant metastases.[125] Pheochromocytomas are occasionally associated with other endocrine tumors as part of a multiple endocrine neoplasia syndrome (Table 40-4). A genetic predisposition to development of pheochromocytomas in conjunction with other APUD-derived tumors is known to exist.[126]

TABLE 40-4 Multiple Endocrine Neoplasia Syndromes

Type	Clinical Pattern
MEN-1 (Wermer's syndrome)	Parathyroid hyperplasia Pituitary tumors Pancreatic islet cell tumors
MEN-2a (Sipple's syndrome)	Medullary thyroid carcinoma Parathyroid hyperplasia Pheochromocytoma
MEN-2b (Multiple mucosa neuroma syndrome)	Medullary thyroid carcinoma Pheochromocytoma Mucocutaneous neuromas Skeletal abnormalities (Marfanoid habitus, pes cavus, scoliosis and pectus excavatum) Parathyroid hyperplasia

Clinical presentation

Excess production of catecholamines accounts for most of the clinical manifestations of this tumor. Nearly all symptomatic patients with pheochromocytomas have sustained or paroxysmal diastolic hypertension, although, in one study, 35% of patients with autopsy-proven pheochromocytomas had no previously documented hypertension.[127] Other symptoms include headache, sweating, nausea and vomiting, palpitations, and anxiety.

Diagnostic evaluation

Measurement of urinary and circulating catecholamines or their metabolites (metanephrine, normetanephrine, and vanyl mandelic acid) confirms the diagnosis of pheochromocytoma in 98% of cases.[128]

CT is routinely used to localize tumors prior to surgery in all patients with abnormal urinary tests.[125] The metaiodobenylguanidine scan (MIBG) is also helpful in localizing pheochromocytomas. MIBG is a noninvasive technique that uses an agent that mimics norepinephrine. In this procedure, MIBG labeled with radioactive ^{131}I is injected and taken up by catecholamine-producing cells. Serial scintigraphic images are then obtained, and dense areas of activity identify any sites of pheochromocytomas.[129,130]

Treatment

Following biochemical confirmation of an existing pheochromocytoma, patients are pretreated with alpha adrenergic blocking agents to minimize the possibility of uncontrolled catecholamine release during invasive localization procedures and surgery.[131]

The goal of surgery is removal of all accessible disease and metastases, although resection of all functional catecholamine-secreting tissue may not be possible.[125,130] Prolonged exposure to the beta-adrenergic effect of circulating catecholamines may result in myocardial hypertrophy, thereby placing the patient at higher risk for cardiovascular complications during surgery.[131] Postoperatively, patients require rigorous monitoring for signs of shock related to the profound decrease in available catecholamines.

The role of cytotoxic therapy in the management of this tumor has not been fully ascertained. Averbuch et al.[132] reported an overall response rate of 57% in 14 patients with malignant pheochromocytoma treated with combined cyclophosphamide, vincristine, and dacarbazine.

PARATHYROID TUMORS

Epidemiology

Malignant tumors of the parathyroid gland are extremely rare, accounting for only 1%–4% of all cases of primary hyperparathyroidism.[133,134] The incidence is distributed equally between the sexes, with the majority of patients clustered between 30–60 years.[134] Parathyroid tumors are frequently seen in association with familial cancer syndromes. New molecular genetic techniques have isolated a chromosomal defect in patients with parathyroid tumors occurring as part of MEN I.[137]

Although no definitive causative factors have been identified, there is some evidence to suggest that head and neck irradiation, especially in childhood, increases the risk of developing hyperparathyroidism as a result of hyperplasia and adenoma formation.[135,136]

Pathophysiology

Generally, parathyroid carcinoma is an indolent, noninvasive tumor with the potential for metastases to regional nodes, liver, and lung late in the course of disease.[133,134,138,139] Although the 5-year overall survival rate reported in two of the largest series was 29% and 44%,[133,134] prolonged survival has been observed even when metastatic disease is present.[133,139,140]

Most parathyroid carcinomas are biochemically functional, causing clinical effects of hypercalcemia from hypersecretion of parathyroid hormone (PTH). Metabolic complications of hypercalcemia are frequently the cause of death.[117]

Clinical Presentation

A large proportion of patients with hyperparathyroidism are asymptomatic but have had an elevated serum calcium detected on routine laboratory evaluation or incidentally during the work-up of other unrelated problems.[133,138,139] Patients with carcinoma of the parathyroid are more likely to have higher calcium levels than those with benign tumors. Common clinical features in symptomatic patients include bone pain, urolithiasis, and neuropsychiatric and gastrointestinal symptoms related to hypercalcemia (e.g., confusion, drowsiness, nausea, anorexia, constipation, and pancreatitis).[138,139] Palpable neck masses are rarely seen with benign parathyroid adenomas, and when present are highly suggestive of carcinoma.

Diagnosis

Parathyroid tumors are most frequently detected by the presence of hypercalcemia on routine laboratory examination. Detection of hypercalcemia is a nonspecific finding and requires further evaluation to determine etiology. Temporary control of hypercalcemia can be achieved with conservative medical therapy until adequate preoperative evaluation is complete. Nuclear scanning, CT, and ultrasound are the most useful methods in localizing a parathyroid mass. By combining nuclear scanning with either CT or ultrasound, the sensitivity of detecting a mass improves to 85%–90%.[141] On x-ray, approximately one-half of patients with hyperparathyroidism have evidence of bony disease due to increased bone resorption that occurs with elevations in PTH levels.[133]

Treatment

Standard treatment consists of *en bloc* resection of the abnormal parathyroid tissue. Radical neck dissection is performed only if there are cervical lymph nodes or evidence of locally invasive disease. Aggressive initial surgery that includes parathyroidectomy and partial resection of the thyroid or thymus has also been advocated in patients with carcinoma.[139] Even if complete resection of macroscopic tumor is done, a high proportion of patients will eventually develop recurrent disease either locally or at distant sites.[133,142] Patients with recurrent disease are rarely cured, but since parathyroid carcinomas are slow growing, surgical resection of recurrent local disease or functioning metastases is recommended because palliation of symptoms and management of hypercalcemia can be achieved for prolonged periods of time with this approach.[139,142,143]

Ultrasound-guided percutaneous chemical parathyroidectomy is currently being evaluated as an alternative to traditional forms of surgery in patients with parathyroid tumors, but this technique remains investigational.[144] With this procedure, ethanol is injected into the parathyroid under ultrasound guidance, resulting in tissue destruction. Karstrup[144] reports that approximately 40% of patients became normocalcemic following injection.

Postoperative complications include hypoparathyroidism, recurrent laryngeal nerve damage, and hemorrhage. Residual normal parathyroid tissue may have atrophied due to suppressive effects of high circulating levels of PTH;[143] therefore, following removal of the hyperactive tissue it may take 1–2 weeks for normal function to return. During this period of hypoparathyroidism, patients may experience tetany and require temporary administration of calcium replacements.[142] The postoperative nursing management of patients with parathyroid tumor is similar to that of individuals undergoing thyroidectomy.

Neither radiation therapy nor chemotherapy has been effective in the treatment of primary or metastatic disease.[140]

MULTIPLE ENDOCRINE NEOPLASIA SYNDROMES

The term *multiple endocrine neoplasia* (MEN) has been used to describe the synchronous or metachronous development of hyperplasia or neoplasia in multiple different endocrine glands or tissues. These disorders occur in distinct clinical patterns and are characterized by familial inheritance of specific endocrine tumors. To date, three MEN syndromes have been described (Table 40-4).

Familial inheritance results from an autosomal dominant mutation.[145] The clinical expression of this varies, accounting for the fact that some patients may not have multiple organ involvement. Recent studies have identified a loss of alleles at chromosome 11 that occurs in patients with MEN I[136,146] and a defect close to the centromere in chromosome 10 has been linked to the MEN IIa locus and has been used to predict inheritance patterns for this syndrome with a high degree of accuracy.[147]

Identification of the specific genetic abnormalities involved in MEN syndromes has been helpful in providing a basis for screening family members of affected kindred. Early detection and appropriate surgical intervention can decrease morbidity and mortality associated with these syndromes.

Treatment for tumors occurring as part of a MEN syndrome is the same as when these tumors occur sporadically.

CONCLUSION

Progress in the treatment of endocrine tumors has generally been slow because of the lack of prospective, randomized clinical trials to evaluate new treatment approaches. This is due, in large part, to problems with accruing patients because of the rarity of these tumors.

Surgery remains the mainstay of treatment for the majority of endocrine malignancies, but pharmacologic agents have been used in select cases to control hypersecretion syndromes and the morbidity associated with these. Advances in the field of molecular genetics that permit identification of high-risk groups and new diagnostic techniques enabling early detection of disease may also improve the overall outcome of patients with endocrine tumors.

REFERENCES

1. Norton JA, Doppman JL, Jensen RT: Cancer of the endocrine system. In DeVita VT Jr, Hellman S, Rosenberg SA (eds): *Cancer: Principles and Practice of Oncology* (3rd ed). Philadelphia: Lippincott, 1989, pp. 1269–1344.
2. Boring CC, Squires TS, Tong T: Cancer statistics, 1992. *CA* 42(1):19–38, 1992.
3. Schlumberger M, DeVathaire F, Travagli JP, et al: Differentiated thyroid carcinoma in childhood: Long term follow-up of 72 patients. *J Clin Endocrinol Metab* 65:1088–1094, 1987.
4. Favus MJ, Schneider AB, Stachura ME, et al: Thyroid cancer occurring as a late consequence of head and neck irradiation: Evaluation of 1056 patients. *N Engl J Med* 294:1019–1025, 1975.
5. Refetoff S, Harrison J, Karanfilski BT, et al: Continuing occurrence of thyroid carcinoma after irradiation to the neck in infancy and childhood. *N Engl J Med* 292:171–175, 1975.
6. Duffy BJ, Fitzgerald PJ: Cancer of the thyroid in children: A report of 28 cases. *J Clin Endocrinol* 10:1296–1308, 1950.
7. Wilson SM, Platz C, Block GM: Thyroid carcinoma after irradiation: Characteristics and treatment. *Arch Surg* 100:330–337, 1970.
8. Hempleman LH, Pifer JW, Burke GJ, et al: Neoplasms in persons treated with x-rays in infancy for thymic enlargement, a report of the third follow-up survey. *JNCI* 38:317–341, 1967.
9. Schneider AB, Favus MJ, Stachura ME, et al: Incidence, prevalence and characteristics of radiation-induced thyroid tumors. *Am J Med* 64:243–52, 1978.
10. McDougall IR: Thyroid cancer after iodine-131 therapy. *JAMA* 227:438–440, 1974.
11. McDougall IR, Nelsen TS, Kempson RL: Papillary carcinoma of the thyroid seven years after I-131 therapy for Grave's disease. *Clin Nucl Med* 6:368–371, 1981.
12. Adamson AS, Gardham JRC: Post ^{131}I carcinoma of the thyroid. *Postgrad Med J* 67:289–290, 1991.
13. Holm LE, Dahlquist I, Israelsson A, et al: Malignant thyroid tumors after iodine-131 therapy. *N Engl J Med* 303:188–191, 1980.
14. Spencer RP, Chapman CN, Rao H: Thyroid carcinoma after radioiodine therapy for hyperthyroidism: Analysis based on age, latency, and administered dose of I-131. *Clin Nucl Med* 8:216–220, 1983.
15. Williams ED: The aetiology of thyroid tumours. *Clin Endocrinol Metab* 8:193–207, 1979.
16. Clark OH: TSH suppression in the management of thyroid nodules and thyroid cancer. *World J Surg* 5:39–47, 1981.

17. Baylin SB, Wells, SA: Management of hereditary medullary thyroid carcinoma. *Clin Endocrinol Metab* 10:367–377, 1981.
18. Saad MF, Ordonez NG, Rashid RK, et al: Medullary carcinoma of the thyroid: A study of the clinical features and prognostic factors in 161 patients. *Medicine* 63:319–342, 1984.
19. Gagel RF, Tashjian AH, Cummings T, et al: The clinical outcome of prospective screening for multiple endocrine neoplasia type 2a: An 18-year experience. *N Engl J Med* 318:478–484, 1988.
20. Mazzaferri EL, Young RL, Oertel JE, et al: Papillary thyroid carcinoma: The impact of therapy in 576 patients. *Medicine* 56:171–196, 1977.
21. Schlumberger M, Tubiana M, DeVathaire F, et al: Long-term results of treatment of 283 patients with lung and bone metastases from differentiated thyroid cancer. *J Clin Endocrinol Metab* 63:960–967, 1986.
22. McConahey WM, Hay ID, Woolner LB, et al: Papillary thyroid cancer treated at the Mayo Clinic, 1946 through 1970: Initial manifestations, pathologic findings, therapy, and outcome. *Mayo Clin Proc* 61:978–996.
23. Carcangiu ML, Giancarlo Z, Pupi A, et al: Papillary carcinoma of the thyroid: A clinicopathologic study of 241 cases treated at the University of Florence, Italy. *Cancer* 55:805–828, 1985.
24. Tubiana M, Schlumberger M, Rougier P, et al: Long-term results and prognostic factors in patients with differentiated thyroid cancer. *Cancer* 55:794–804, 1985.
25. DeGroot LJ, Kaplan EL, McCormick M, Straus FH. Natural history, treatment, and course of papillary thyroid carcinoma. *J Clin Endocrinol Metab* 71:414–424, 1990.
26. Merrick Y, Hansen HS: Thyroid cancer in children and adolescents in Denmark. *Eur J Surg Oncol* 15:49–53, 1989.
27. Kerr DJ, Burt AD, Boyle P, et al: Prognostic factors in thyroid tumours. *Brit J Cancer* 54:475–482, 1986.
28. Hubert JP, Kiernan PD, Beahrs OH, et al: Occult papillary carcinoma of the thyroid. *Arch Surg* 115:394–399, 1980.
29. Pelizzo MR, Piotto A, Rubello D, et al. High prevalence of occult papillary thyroid carcinoma in a surgical series for benign thyroid disease. *Tumori* 76:225–251, 1990.
30. McHenry CR, Rosen IB, Walfish PG. Prospective management of nodal metastases in differentiated thyroid cancer. *Am J Surg* 162:353–356, 1991.
31. Samaan NA, Schultz PN, Haynie TP, Ordonez NG: Pulmonary metastasis of differentiated thyroid carcinoma: Treatment results in 101 patients. *J Clin Endocrinol Metab* 65:376–380, 1985.
32. Harness JK, Thompson NW, McLeod MK, et al: Follicular carcinoma of the thyroid gland: Trends and treatment. *Surgery* 96:972–978, 1984.
33. Schmidt RJ, Wang C: Encapsulated follicular carcinoma of the thyroid: Diagnosis, treatment, and results. *Surgery* 100:1068–1075, 1986.
34. Greenfield LD: Thyroid tumors. In Perez CA, Brady LW (eds): *Principles and Practice of Radiation Oncology.* Philadelphia: Lippincott, 1987, pp. 1126–1156.
35. Leeper RD: Thyroid cancer. *Med Clin North Am* 69:1079–1096, 1985.
36. Schroder S, Bocker W, Baisch H, et al: Prognostic factors in medullary thyroid carcinomas. *Cancer* 61:806–816, 1988.
37. Kakudo K, Carney JA, Sizemore GW: Medullary carcinoma of thyroid: Biologic behavior of the sporadic and familial neoplasms. *Cancer* 55:2818–2821, 1985.
38. Nel CJC, VanHeerden JA, Goellner JR, et al: Anaplastic carcinoma of the thyroid: A clinicopathologic study of 82 cases. *Mayo Clin Proc* 60:51–58, 1985.
39. Carcangiu ML, Steeper T, Zampi G, et al: Anaplastic thyroid carcinoma: A study of 70 cases. *Am J Clin Pathol* 83:135–158, 1985.
40. Demeter JG, DeJong SA, Lawrence AM, Paloyan E: Anaplastic thyroid carcinoma: Risk factors and outcome. *Surgery* 110:956–963, 1991.
41. Friedman M, Toriumi DM, Mafee MF: Diagnostic imaging techniques in thyroid cancer. *Am J Surg* 155:215–223, 1988.
42. Hawkins F, Gellido D, Bernal C, et al: Fine needle aspiration in the diagnosis of thyroid cancer and thyroid disease. *Cancer* 59:1206–1209, 1987.
43. De los Santos ET, Keyhani-Rofagha S, Cunningham JJ, Mazzaferri EL: Cystic thyroid nodules: The dilemma of malignant lesions. *Arch Intern Med* 150:1422–1427, 1990.
44. Rojeski MT, Gharib H: Nodular thyroid disease: Evaluation and management. *N Engl J Med* 313:428–436, 1985.
45. Freitas JE, Gross MD, Ripley S, et al: Radionucleide diagnosis and therapy of thyroid cancer: Current status report. *Semin Nucl Med* 15:106–131, 1985.
46. Beahrs OH, Henson DE, Hutter RVP, Myers MH (eds): *Manual for Staging of Cancer* (4th ed). Philadelphia: Lippincott, 1992, pp. 53–56.
47. Clark OH, Levin K, Zeng Q, et al: Thyroid cancer: The case for total thyroidectomy. *Eur J Cancer Clin Oncol* 24:305–313, 1988.
48. Powell S, Harmer C. Thyroid cancer causing death after 40 years: Rationale for intensive treatment. *Eur J Surg Oncol* 16:457–461, 1990.
49. DeGroot LJ, Kaplan EL: Second operations for "completion" of thyroidectomy in treatment of differentiated thyroid cancer. *Surgery* 110:936–940, 1991.
50. Harness JK, Fung L, Thompson NW, et al: Total thyroidectomy: Complications and technique. *World J Surg* 10:781–786, 1986.
51. McHenry C, Jerosz H, Lawrence AM, Paloyan E: Improving postoperative recurrence rates for carcinoma of the thyroid gland. *Surg Gynecol Obstet* 169:429–434, 1989.
52. Schroder DM, Chambors A, France CJ: Operative strategy for thyroid cancer: Is total thyroidectomy worth the price? *Cancer* 58:2320–2328, 1986.
53. Rossi RL, Cady B, Silverman ML, et al: Current results of conservative surgery for differentiated thyroid carcinoma. *World J Surg* 10:612–622, 1986.
54. Noguchi M, Kumaki T, Tamija T, Miyazaki I. Bilateral cervical lymph node metastases in well differentiated thyroid cancer. *Arch Surg* 125:804–806, 1990.
55. Attie JN: Modified neck dissection in treatment of thyroid cancer: A safe procedure. *Eur J Cancer Clin Oncol* 24:315–324, 1988.
56. Kenady DE, Sloan DA, Schwartz RW: Diagnosis and treatment of thyroid, adrenal and thymic tumors. *Curr Opin Oncol* 4:89–98, 1992.
57. Wells SA Jr, Ross AJ III, Dale JK, et al: Transplantation of the parathyroid glands: Current status. *Surg Clin North Am* 59:167–177, 1979.

58. Herranz-Gonzalez J, Gavilan J, Marinez-Vidal J, Gavilan C: Complications following thyroid surgery. *Arch Otolaryngol Head Neck Surg* 117:516–518, 1991.
59. McHenry C, Jarosz H, Davis M, et al. Selective postoperative radioactive iodine treatment of thyroid carcinoma. *Surgery* 106:956–959, 1989.
60. Goolden AWG: The use of radioactive iodine in thyroid carcinoma. *Eur J Cancer Clin Oncol* 24:339–343, 1988.
61. Tubiana M, Haddad E, Schlumberger M, et al: External radiotherapy in thyroid cancers. *Cancer* 55:2062–2071, 1985.
62. Kim JH, Leeper RD: Treatment of anaplastic giant and spingle cell carcinoma of the thyroid gland with combination adriamycin and radiation therapy: A new approach. *Cancer* 52:954–957, 1983.
63. Wells SA, Dilley WG, Farndon JA, et al: Early diagnosis and treatment of medullary thyroid carcinoma. *Arch Intern Med* 145:1248–1252, 1985.
64. Shimaoka K, Schoenfeld DA, DeWys WD, et al: A randomized trial of doxorubicin versus doxorubicin plus cisplatin in patients with advanced thyroid cancer. *Cancer* 56:2155–2158, 1985.
65. Szanto J, Vincze B, Sinkowics I, et al. Postoperative thyroglobulin level determination to follow up patients with highly differentiated thyroid cancer. *Oncology* 46:99–104, 1991.
66. Kovacs K, Horvath E: Pathology of pituitary tumors. *Endocrinol Metab Clin* 16:667–683, 1987.
67. Nudleman KL, Choi B, Kusske JA: Primary pituitary carcinoma: A clinical pathological study. *Neurosurgery* 16:90–95, 1985.
68. Molitch ME: Pathogenesis of pituitary tumors. *Endocrinol Metab Clin* 16:503–527, 1987.
69. Herman V, Fagin J, et al: Clonal origin of pituitary adenomas. *J Clin Endocrinol Metab* 71:1427–1433, 1990.
70. Camanni R, Ghigo E, Caccarelli, et al: Defective regulation of prolactin secretion after successful removal of prolactinomas. *J Clin Endocrinol Metab* 57:1270–1276, 1983.
71. Scheithauer BW, Kovacs K, Laws ER Jr, et al: Pathology of invasive pituitary tumors with special reference to functional classification. *J Neurosurg* 65:733–744, 1986.
72. Landolt AM, Shibata T, Kleihues P: Growth rate of human pituitary adenomas. *J Neurosurg* 67:803–806, 1987.
73. Comtois R, Beauregard H, Somma M, et al: The clinical and endocrine outcome to transsphenoidal microsurgery of nonsecreting pituitary adenomas. *Cancer* 68:860–866, 1991.
74. Arafah BM: Reversible hypopituitarism in patients with large nonfunctioning pituitary adenomas. *J Clin Endocrinol Metab* 62:1173–1179, 1986.
75. Selman WR, Arafah BM. Commentary (Leavens et al article review). *Oncology* 6(6):79–80, 1992.
76. Boyd AE III, Jordan RM, Kohler PO: Disorders of the hypothalamus and anterior pituitary. In Kohler PO (ed): *Clinical Endocrinology*. New York: Wiley, 1986, pp. 11–51.
77. Ciric I: Pituitary tumors. *Neurol Clin* 3:751–766, 1985.
78. Oldfield EH, Nieman L, Chrousos G, et al. Petrosal sinus sampling with and without corticotropin-releasing hormone for the differential diagnosis of Cushing's syndrome. *N Engl J Med* 325:987–995, 1991.
79. Maroldo TV, Dillon WP, Wilson CB: Advances in diagnostic techniques of pituitary tumors and prolactinomas. *Curr Opin Oncol* 4:105–115, 1992.
80. Doppman JL, Miller DL, Patronas N, et al. The diagnosis of acromegaly: Value of inferior petrosal sinus sampling. *Am J Roentgenol* 154:1075–1077, 1990.
81. Kaufman B, Kaufman BA, Arafah BM, et al: Large pituitary gland adenomas evaluated with magnetic resonance imaging. *Neurosurgery* 21:540–546, 1987.
82. Laws ER Jr: Pituitary surgery. *Endocrinol Metab Clin* 16:647–665, 1987.
83. Leavens ME, McCutcheon IF, Samaan NA: Management of pituitary adenomas. *Oncology* 6(6):69–78, 1992.
84. Ebersold MJ, Quast LM, Laws ER Jr, et al: Long-term results in transsphenoidal removal of nonfunctioning pituitary adenomas. *J Neurosurg* 64:713–719, 1986.
85. Halberg FE, Sheline GE: Radiotherapy of pituitary tumors. *Endocrinol Metab Clin* 16:667–683, 1987.
86. Ross DA, Wilson CB: Results of transsphenoidal microsurgery for growth hormone-secreting pituitary adenoma in a series of 214 patients. *J Neurosurg* 68:854–867, 1988.
87. Ciric I, Mikhael M, Stafford T, et al: Transsphenoidal microsurgery of pituitary macroadenomas with long-term follow-up results. *J Neurosurg* 59:395–401, 1983.
88. Bevan JS, Adams CBT, Burke CW, et al: Factors in the outcome of transsphenoidal surgery for prolactinoma and non-functioning pituitary tumour, including preoperative bromocriptine therapy. *Clin Endocrinol* 26:541–556,1987.
89. Resio MJ: Nursing diagnosis: Alteration in oral/nasal mucous membranes related to trauma of transsphenoidal surgery. *J Neurosci Nurs* 18:112–115, 1986.
90. Mampalam TJ, Tyrell JB, Wilson CB: Transsphenoidal microsurgery for Cushing's disease. A report of 216 cases. *Ann Intern Med* 109:487–493, 1988.
91. Randall RV, Laws ER, Abboud CF, et al: Transsphenoidal microsurgical treatment of prolactin producing pituitary adenomas. Results in 100 patients. *Mayo Clin Proc* 58:108–121, 1983.
92. Rodman EF, Molitch ME, Post KD, et al: Long term follow up of transsphenoidal selective adenomectomy for prolactinoma. *JAMA* 252:921–924, 1984.
93. Schlechte JA, Sherman BM, Chapler FK, VanGilder J: Long term follow up of women with surgically treated prolactin-secreting pituitary tumors. *J Clin Endocrinol Metab* 62:1296–1301, 1986.
94. Chun M, Masko GB, Hetelekisis S: Radiotherapy in the treatment of pituitary adenomas. *Int J Radiat Oncol Biol Phys* 15:305–309, 1988.
95. McCollough WM, Markus RB, Rhoten AL, et al: Long term follow-up of radiotherapy for pituitary adenoma: The absence of late recurrence after ≥4500 cGy. *Int J Radiation Oncology Biol Phys* 21:607–614, 1991.
96. Snyder PJ, Fowble BF, Schatz NJ, et al: Hypopituitarism following radiation therapy of pituitary adenomas. *Am J Med* 81:457–462, 1986.
97. Moberg E, Trampe E, Wersall J, Werner S: Long term effects of radiotherapy and bromocriptine treatment in patients with previous surgery for macroprolactinomas. *Neurosurgery* 29:200–205, 1991.
98. Molitch ME, Elton RL, Blackwell RE, et al: Bromocriptine as primary therapy for prolactin-secreting macroadenomas: Results of a prospective multicenter study. *J Clin Endocrinol Metab* 60:698–705, 1985.

99. Luizzi A, Dallabonzana D, Oppizzi G, et al: Low doses of dopamine agonists in the long-term treatment of macroprolactinomas. *N Engl J Med* 131:656–659, 1985.
100. Weiss MH, Wycoff RR, Yadley R, et al: Bromocriptine treatment of prolactin-secreting tumors: Surgical implications. *Neurosurgery* 12:640–642, 1983.
101. Hubbard JL, Scheithauer BW, Abboud CF, et al: Prolactin-secreting adenomas: The preoperative response to bromocriptine treatment and surgical outcome. *J Neurosurg* 67:816–821, 1987.
102. Barkan AL: Acromegaly diagnosis and therapy. *Endocrinol Metab Clin North Am* 18:277–310, 1989.
103. Barkan AL, Lloyd RV, Chandler WF, et al: Preoperative treatment of acromegaly with long-acting somatostatin analog SMS-201-995: Shrinkage of invasive pituitary macroadenomas and improved surgical remission rate. *J Clin Endocrinol Metab* 67:1040–1048, 1988.
104. DeAtkine AB, Dunnick NR: The adrenal glands. *Semin Oncol* 18(2):131–139, 1991.
105. Didolkar MS, Besche RS, Elias EG, Moore RH: Natural history of adrenocortical carcinoma: A clinicopathologic study of 42 patients. *Cancer* 47:2153–2161, 1981.
106. Schteingart DE, Matazedi A, Noonan RA, et al: Treatment of adrenal carcinomas. *Arch Surg* 117:1142–1146, 1982.
107. Karakousis CP, Rao U, Moore R: Adrenal adenocarcinomas: Histologic grading and survival. *J Surg Oncol* 29(2):105–111, 1985.
108. Cohn K, Gottesman L, Brennan M: Adrenocortical carcinoma. *Surgery* 100:1170–1177, 1986.
109. Decker RA, Kuehner ME: Adrenocortical carcinoma. *Am Surg* 57:502–513, 1991.
110. Hutter AM, Kayhoe DE: Adrenal cortical carcinoma: Clinical features of 138 patients. *Am J Med* 41:572–580, 1966.
111. Brennan MF: Adrenocortical cancer. *CA* 37:348–365, 1987.
112. Loriaux DL, Cutler GB Jr: Diseases of the adrenal glands. In Kohler PO (ed): *Clinical Endocrinology.* New York: Wiley, 1986, pp. 167–238.
113. Thompson NW, Cheung PSY: Diagnosis and treatment of functioning and nonfunctioning adrenocortical neoplasms including incidentalomas. *Surg Clin North Am* 67:423–436, 1987.
114. Doppman JL, Reinig JW, Dwyer AJ, et al: Differentiation of adrenal masses by magnetic resonance imaging. *Surgery* 102:1018–1025, 1987.
115. Chang A, Glazer HS, Lee JKT, et al: Adrenal gland: MR imaging. *Radiology* 163:123–128, 1987.
116. Jensen JC, Pass HI, Sindelar WF, Norton JA: Recurrent or metastatic disease in select patients with adrenocortical disease. *Arch Surg* 126:457–461, 1991.
117. Henley DJ, vanHeerden JA, Grant CS, et al: Adrenal cortical carcinoma—A continuing challenge. *Surgery* 94:926–931, 1983.
118. Plager JE: Carcinoma of the adrenal cortex: Clinical description, diagnosis and treatment. *Int Adv Surg Oncol* 7:329–353, 1984.
119. Jarabak J, Rice K: Metastatic adrenal cortical carcinoma: Prolonged regression with mitotane therapy. *JAMA* 246:1706–1707, 1981.
120. Robinson BG, Hales IB, Henniker K, et al: The effect of o,p'-DDD on adrenal steroid replacement therapy requirements. *Clin Endocrinol* 27:437–444, 1987.
121. Eriksson B, Oberg K, Curstedt T, et al: Treatment of hormone-producing adrenocortical cancer with o,p'DDD and streptozocin. *Cancer* 59:1398–1403, 1987.
122. Johnson DH, Greco FA: Treatment of metastatic adrenal cortical carcinoma with cisplatin and etoposide (VP-16). *Cancer* 58:2198–2202, 1986.
123. Schlumberger M, Buigieres L, Gicquel C, et al: 5-fluorouracil, doxorubicin and cisplatin as treatment for adrenal cortical carcinoma. *Cancer* 67:2997–3000, 1991.
124. Pearse AGE: The diffuse neuroendocrine system and the APUD concept: Related endocrine peptides in brain, intestine, pituitary, placenta and anuran cutaneous glands. *Med Biol* 55:115–125, 1977.
125. Samaan NA, Hickey RC, Schutts PE: Diagnosis, localization and management of pheochromocytoma: Pitfalls and follow-up in 41 patients. *Cancer* 62:2451–2460, 1988.
126. Bravo EL, Gifford RW: Pheochromocytoma: Diagnosis, localization and management. *N Engl J Med* 311:1298–1303, 1984.
127. St John Sutton MG, Sheps SG, Lie JT: Prevalence of clinically unsuspected pheochromocytoma: A review of a 50-year autopsy series. *Mayo Clin Proc* 56:354–360, 1981.
128. Samaan NA, Hickey RC: Pheochromocytoma. *Semin Oncol* 14:297–305, 1987.
129. Sisson JC, Frager MS, Valk TW, et al: Scintigraphic localization of pheochromocytoma. *N Engl J Med* 305:12–17, 1981.
130. Sheps SG, Jiang NS, Klee GG, Heerden JA: Recent developments in the diagnosis and treatment of pheochromocytoma. *Mayo Clin Proc* 65:88–95, 1990.
131. Hull CJ: Pheochromocytoma: Diagnosis, preoperative preparation and anesthetic management. *Br J Anaesth* 58:1453–1468, 1986.
132. Averbuch S, Steakley CS, Young RC, et al: Malignant pheochromocytoma: Effective treatment with a combination of cyclophosphamide, vincristine, and dacarbazine. *Ann Intern Med* 109:267–273, 1988.
133. Wang C, Gaz RD: Natural history of parathyroid carcinoma, diagnosis, treatment and results. *Am J Surg* 149:522–527, 1985.
134. Schantz A, Castleman B: Parathyroid carcinoma: A study of 70 cases. *Cancer* 31:600–605, 1973.
135. Ireland JP, Fleming SJ, Levison EA, et al: Parathyroid carcinoma associated with chronic renal failure and previous radiotherapy to the neck. *J Clin Pathol* 38:1114–1118, 1985.
136. Hickey RC, Jong PA, Merrell R, et al: Parathyroid adenoma in a cancer center patient population. *Am J Surg* 161:439–442, 1991.
137. Friedman E, Sakaguicki K, Bale A: Clonality of parathyroid tumors in familial multiple endocrine neoplasia type 1. *N Engl J Med* 321:213–218, 1989.
138. Cohn K, Silverman M, Corrado J, Sedgewick C: Parathyroid carcinoma: The Lahey Clinic experience. *Surgery* 98:1095–1100, 1985.
139. Shortell CK, Andrus CH, Phillips CE, Schwartz SI: Carcinoma of the parathyroid gland: A 30-year experience. *Surgery* 110:704–708, 1991.
140. Shane E, Bilezidian JP: Parathyroid carcinoma: A review of 62 patients. *Endocrinol Rev* 3:218–226, 1982.
141. Krubseck AJ, Wilson SD, Lawson TL, et al: Prospective comparison of radionucleide, computed tomographic sonographic and magnetic resonance localization of parathyroid tumors. *Surgery* 106:639–646, 1989.
142. Sandelin K, Thompson NW, Bondeson L: Metastatic

parathyroid carcinoma: Dilemmas in management. *Surgery* 110:978–988, 1991.

143. Flye MW, Brennen MF: Surgical resection of metastatic parathyroid carcinoma. *Ann Surg* 193:425–435, 1981.
144. Karstrup S, Transbol IB, Holm HH, et al: Ultrasound-guided chemical parathyroidectomy in patients with primary hyperparathyroidism: A prospective study. *Br J Radiol* 62:1037–1042, 1989.
145. Caruso DR, O'Dorisio TM, Mazzaferri EL: Multiple endocrine neoplasia. *Curr Opin Oncol* 3:103–108, 1991.
146. Thakker RV, Bouloux P, Wooding C, et al: Association of parathyroid tumors in multiple endocrine neoplasia type 1 with loss of alleles on chromosome 11. *N Engl J Med* 321:218–224, 1989.
147. Telenius H, Mathew CG, Nakamura Y, et al: Application of linked DNA markers to screening families with multiple endocrine neoplasia type 2a. *Eur J Surg Oncol* 16:134–140, 1990.

Chapter 41

Gastrointestinal Cancer: Esophagus, Stomach, Liver, and Pancreas

Margaret Hansen Frogge, RN, MS

INTRODUCTION

Of all the organ systems in the body, the gastrointestinal tract accounts for the highest incidence of malignant tumors—more than 25% of cancer deaths annually in the United States. There are approximately 236,900 new cases of gastrointestinal cancer and 120,325 deaths from cancer of the gastrointestinal tract each year in the United States.[1] The incidence of cancer at different sites along the gastrointestinal tract presents an intriguing pattern when incidence among men is compared with that among women (Table 41-1). Incidence in men decreases from the esophagus to the large intestine, whereas the opposite is true for women. No clear explanations exist for this bidirectional pattern, but researchers are studying the question.

Most tumors of the gastrointestinal tract are adenocarcinomas, with the exception of tumors of the esophagus and anus, where squamous cell carcinomas predominate. Gastrointestinal tumors proliferate insidiously and extend locally, presenting signs and symptoms that can be misdiagnosed or self-treated for lengthy periods. As the tumor grows, it can exceed the distensible capacity of the gastrointestinal lumen and result in obstruction. The metastasis of gastrointestinal tumors typically occurs by local spread, blood vessel invasion, and dissemination via the lymphatic system. Prognosis depends on the tumor size, degree of cellular differentiation, extent of metastases, treatment efficacy, and the individual's general health status. The

TABLE 41-1 Gastrointestinal Tumors—Percentage Distribution by Sex

Site	Total Cases	Percentage of Males	Percentage of Females
Esophagus	11,300	72	28
Stomach	24,000	62	38
Pancreas	27,700	49	51
Liver	15,800	54	46
Small intestine	3,600	56	44
Colon-rectum	152,000	51	49

Source: Boring CC, Squires TS, Tong T: Cancer Statistics, 1993. *CA* 43(1):7–26, 1993.

prognosis for persons with gastrointestinal tumors varies according to site.

ESOPHAGEAL TUMORS

Many people with esophageal cancer mistakenly attribute its signs and symptoms to more common disorders that affect older adults (e.g., indigestion, heartburn, decreased appetite). If the person has delayed seeking medical attention, the tumor may be advanced and obstruct the esophageal lumen. The person can be dehydrated, malnourished, and debilitated as a result of inadequate nutrition and inappropriate self-treatment. Esophageal tumors that obstruct the lumen can cause a spillover of food, fluid, and saliva into the tracheobronchial tree resulting in aspiration pneumonitis. The physician and nurse are faced with the challenge of a candidate at poor risk for aggressive therapy. Because cancer of the esophagus grows rapidly, metastasizes early, and is diagnosed late, survival rates are poor.

EPIDEMIOLOGY

Esophageal cancer is uncommon in the United States as compared to other parts of the world, constituting only 1% of all forms of cancer and being responsible for a mere 2% of total deaths from cancer. There are approximately 11,300 new cases and 10,200 deaths from cancer of the esophagus in the United States annually.[1] The most alarming fact about esophageal cancer is that only 7% of those affected will be alive 5 years after diagnosis; this is one of the poorest survival rates among malignant diseases. In the United States the age-adjusted mortality rate from carcinoma of the esophagus per 100,000 persons is higher among white men (5.7) than among white women (1.5)[2] and is significantly increased among black men (16.4) and black women (4.1).[2] Carcinoma of the esophagus develops at a younger age in black persons than in white persons.[3] Overall, the average age of onset is 62 years. Most persons with this disease are 50–70 years of age.

A puzzling feature of esophageal cancer is the remarkable difference in incidence according to geographic location, sometimes varying more than 100-fold.[4] No other tumor demonstrates such variation, and there is no unifying concept that explains the intriguing differences. There are countries in which the incidence of esophageal cancer is 400 to 500 times that of the United States.[5]

ETIOLOGY

Although a variety of relationships yields clues to the etiology of esophageal cancer, the factors are complex and not well understood. Variations in incidence by geographic location point to nutritional and environmental factors. Individuals with esophageal cancer typically have a history of heavy alcohol intake, heavy tobacco use, and poor nutrition.[6,7] Cirrhosis, micronutrient deficiency, anemia, and poor oral hygiene may be contributing etiologic factors. Nitrosamines in food and vitamin deficiencies are among the factors associated with the high incidence of esophageal cancer in different regions of the world.[4]

Medical conditions of chronic irritation have been cited as possible etiologic factors: hiatal hernia, reflux esophagitis, and diverticula. In some cases, esophageal cancer has developed in individuals with longstanding injuries such as lye-induced strictures. The cancer usually appeared 40 or more years after the agent was ingested.[8] Extremes of temperatures in food are suggested as a possible contributory factor, especially hot tea and coffee.

Persons with untreated achalasia have a sevenfold to eightfold greater risk of developing esophageal cancer. Plummer-Vinson syndrome has been associated with esophageal cancer.[9] Barrett's esophagus, which develops as a sequela of chronic esophageal reflux, is considered a precursor to esophageal cancer.[10,11] Because dysplasia is the only reliable indicator of early malignant changes, periodic endoscopy of Barrett's esophagus is recommended for early detection.[12] Tylosis palmaris et plantaris, a rare inherited syndrome characterized by hyperkeratosis of the palms or soles and papillomata of the esophagus, has a strong association with esophageal cancer.[13] Approximately 95% of persons with tylosis develop esophageal cancer by the age of 65.

Dietary deficiencies of certain mineral elements are considered risk factors for esophageal cancer. In areas with a high incidence of esophageal cancer, dietary deficiencies of selenium were correlated with esophageal cytologic changes. Because selenium potentially increases resistance to cancer, a deficiency may signal a high-risk person.[14]

PATHOPHYSIOLOGY

Malignant lesions occur at all levels of the esophagus. The site of esophageal tumors is an important factor in detection and prognosis. The distribution of occurrence generally follows this pattern:

cervical esophageal	25%
upper thoracic esophagus	50%
lower thoracic esophagus	25%

Cellular Characteristics

Squamous cell carcinoma (>85%) and adenocarcinoma (<10%) are the two major histologic types of esophageal cancer.[4,10] In an organ lined almost entirely with squamous epithelium, it follows that squamous cell carcinoma would dominate the area from the pharynx to within a few centimeters of the esophagogastric junction. In the distal few centimeters of the esophagus, adenocarcinomas and squamous cell carcinomas appear equally. However, tumors in the area of the esophagogastric junction usually are primary gastric adenocarcinomas that have extended from the stomach into the lower esophagus. The occurrence of adenocarcinoma of the esophagus is rapidly increasing in the United States, with some reports indicating a shift upward to 20% of esophageal cancers.[10,11]

Carcinoma of the esophagus may be grossly classified as polypoid, ulcerative, or infiltrative.[15] An infiltrative pattern of tumor growth encircles and thickens the wall, thus leading to marked luminal narrowing. Most often the tumor has a polypoid mass projecting into the esophageal lumen. When tumor proportions exceed the distensible capacity of the esophageal wall, complete obstruction occurs. The ulcerative lesion is elevated and has irregular, nodular edges. Because the ulcerative lesion expands in the submucosa, the lesion can be elevated to such an extent that it obstructs the lumen. Some lesions will remain localized, whereas others will extend over a wide area of the esophagus.

Squamous cell carcinomas and adenocarcinomas exhibit a range of cellular differentiation. Some lesions are so poorly differentiated that it is difficult to ascertain cellular origin. At present, studies are being conducted to determine if there is a correlation between the degree of differentiation and factors such as rapidity of growth, invasiveness, metastases, response to therapy, and prognosis. Histopathologic characteristics,[16] flow cytometric analysis of DNA content,[17] epidermal growth factor receptors,[18] and karyometric measurements of cell contents[19] are some of the parameters being studied as possible predictors of extent of disease and response to therapy.

Progression of Disease

Squamous cell carcinomas extend beyond the lumen wall to invade contiguous structures in about 60% of cases.[20] Tumors of the cervical esophagus may directly involve the carotid arteries, pleura, recurrent laryngeal nerves, trachea, or larynx. Tumors of the upper thoracic esophagus may involve the left mainstem bronchus, thoracic duct, aortic arch, or pleura. In the lower portion of the thoracic esophagus, tumors may invade pericardium, pleura, descending aorta, and diaphragm. If the phrenic nerve is involved, paralysis of the diaphragm can result. Tumor invasion of contiguous structures may be extensive enough to prevent surgical resection, thereby necessitating alternative therapies.

Tumors of the esophagus metastasize principally via the lymphatic system. The rich intramural plexus of lymphatic vessels and the lack of a serosal barrier permit early regional extension and dissemination of esophageal carcinoma before clinical signs appear. Lesions of the cervical and upper thoracic esophagus usually metastasize to the anterior jugular chain and high peritracheal nodes in the supraclavicular region. In the middle thoracic esophagus, tumor cells may metastasize to the mediastinum and subdiaphragmatic lymph nodes. Tumors in the lower part of the esophagus will disseminate to the abdominal lymph nodes and the gastric and celiac lymph channels.

Hematogenous spread of tumor cells or tumor emboli is another mode of metastases. Tumor emboli may dislodge into the caval system and become embedded in the lung or liver. Distant metastases to the lung, liver, adrenal glands, bone, brain, and kidney are common with advanced disease.

CLINICAL MANIFESTATIONS

Early symptoms of esophageal carcinoma may be nonspecific and cause little concern. Symptoms may be present for only weeks or a few months, yet the esophageal carcinoma can be advanced. Initial symptoms include a vague sense of pressure, fullness, indigestion, and occasional substernal distress.

Dysphagia is the classic symptom in almost 90% of cases.[21] A significant characteristic of esophageal cancer is the progressive nature of the dysphagia. Because the esophagus initially will distend to allow liquid or food to pass the tumor, the individual will unconsciously masticate solid food more thoroughly and substitute soft and liquid foods to relieve the dysphagia. When tumor size exceeds a critical luminal circumference, saliva, food, and liquids may spill over into the lungs, causing aspiration pneumonitis. Pain on swallowing occurs in about 50% of patients with esophageal cancer.[2]

Weight loss, which inevitably follows, is a dramatic symptom, equaled in frequency only by pancreatic cancer. A loss of 10%–20% of initial body weight is common. Anorexia, anemia, and dehydration may add to a debilitated state.

The tumor is locally aggressive and produces symptoms that suggest invasion. A characteristic cough-swallow sequence at swallowing may indicate aspiration of food or a tracheo-esophageal fistula. Substernal and epigastric pain often will mimic heartburn. Fever can signal pulmonary involvement by tumor or aspiration pneumonia. Superior vena cava obstruction, pleural effusion, and hepatomegaly may also occur. Tumor involvement of the recurrent laryngeal nerve can result in laryngeal paralysis and hoarseness.[22]

ASSESSMENT

The nurse's role in the prevention and detection of esophageal cancer can influence early identification of this aggressive tumor. Any person with risk factors for esophageal cancer should be instructed both on the importance of health care follow-up and on ways to reduce or eliminate risk factors. Counseling on nutrition and alcohol or smoking abuse are important measures for prevention. Chronic users of over-the-counter home medications for gastrointestinal upsets should be encouraged to seek medical attention promptly.

The diagnosis of esophageal cancer depends on a thorough patient history, with particular attention to the sequelae of symptoms and nutritional alterations. The most definitive diagnostic procedures are routine and special radiologic examinations, endoscopic examinations, endoluminal ultrasound, biopsy, cytology, and exploratory surgery.[23]

Physical Examination

Physical examination reveals few findings for the definitive diagnosis, except in cases of advanced disease in which enlarged lymph nodes are palpable, organs are enlarged or displaced, dysphagia and weight loss are profound, and systemic manifestations such as aspiration pneumonia are present.

Diagnostic Studies

Radiologic examination

In addition to routine radiologic examination, the double-contrast barium study is useful for diagnosis. The typical changes noted with a barium esophogram or swallow are mucosal irregularity, displacement, narrowing, and stricture. Advanced lesions produce a characteristic annular apple-core pattern. Ulceration is difficult to visualize but is indicated by irregularity, angulation, and distortion of the linear mucosal folds. In cases of near-complete obstruction, antispasmodics are used to enhance visualization. Barium will leave the stomach within 2–6 hours. In consideration of the person's poor nutritional state, the nurse should be certain that laxatives or an enema are given after the test to prevent a barium impaction.

Computed tomography (CT scan) is an excellent modality for staging but is not appropriate to screen for esophageal cancer. Magnetic resonance imaging (MRI) does not offer a diagnostic advantage over CT for detection of this disease.

Endoscopy and biopsy

Endoscopic visualization plays an important role in the differential diagnosis of esophageal tumors. Most commonly the esophagoscope and tracheobronchoscope are used to identify the visible extent of the tumor. Following instrumentation, the individual will receive nothing to eat or drink and will remain with head elevated until the anesthetic dissipates. Nursing observations should be directed toward signs of esophageal perforation, fluid aspiration, and laryngospasm. Visualization of lesions by endoscopy has limitations and is therefore complemented by cytologic examination. A diagnosis can be made by cytologic study with an accuracy rate of 90%.[2] During endoscopy, samples for cytology are obtained by washings or by brushing the tumor directly. In China, cytologic examination is being used on a mass screening basis to detect early lesions and to monitor high-risk persons.[24]

Endoscopic ultrasound also has an important role in determining the stage of the tumor.[25] The endoscopic ultrasound enables direct visualization of the tumor and the determination of the depth of invasion and the presence of adenopathy. For the diagnosis of recurrent tumor following surgical resection, the endoscopic ultrasound is a technique that can produce detailed images.[26]

Biopsy of lymph nodes is a definitive diagnostic tool; however, nodes are not always accessible. If a laparotomy is performed as part of the therapeutic approach, extensive biopsy of the entire area is done, since the rich networks of lymph nodes often are metastatic sites.

CLASSIFICATION AND STAGING

Unlike the situation with more accessible cancers, clinical staging of esophageal cancer is difficult to accomplish without invasive measures. The extent of tumor growth (T) cannot be fully assessed by radiographic or endoscopic examination. The lymph node status (N) can be evaluated noninvasively only in cervical esophagus lesions. By the time a diagnosis is established, disease frequently has metastasized (M) to liver, lungs, or bone. The aggressiveness of the therapeutic approach is based on an evaluation of the individual and the extent to which the disease has progressed.

For purposes of classification and end results, the American Joint Committee for Cancer Staging and End-Results Reporting has developed a standardized classification system (Table 41-2).

TREATMENT

Treatment Planning

Selection of the treatment plan

In view of the biologic nature and poor prognosis of esophageal carcinoma, the goal of interdisciplinary planning is to select the therapies most appropriate for the extent of the tumor and for the individual. Despite advances in surgery, radiotherapy, and chemotherapy, esophageal carcinoma has a poor outcome, with approximately 7% of individuals surviving 5 years.[1] Careful interdisciplinary planning is needed to define the extent of the disease, to assess the individual's physiologic status, and to discuss alternatives completely with the individual before the course of treatment is selected. The nurse is in a valuable position to assess the person's understanding and reaction to the anticipated therapy.

TABLE 41-2 TNM Classification System for Cancer of the Esophagus

PRIMARY TUMOR (T)	
TX	Primary tumor cannot be assessed
T0	No evidence of primary tumor
Tis	Carcinoma in situ
T1	Tumor invades lamina propria or submucosa
T2	Tumor invades muscularis propria
T3	Tumor invades adventitia
T4	Tumor invades adjacent structures
REGIONAL LYMPH NODES (N)	
NX	Regional lymph nodes cannot be assessed
N0	No regional lymph node metastasis
N1	Regional lymph node metastasis
DISTANT METASTASIS (M)	
MX	Presence of distant metastasis cannot be assessed
M0	No distant metastasis
M1	Distant metastasis

STAGE GROUPING			
Stage 0	Tis	N0	M0
Stage I	T1	N0	M0
Stage IIA	T2	N0	M0
	T3	N0	M0
Stage IIB	T1	N1	M0
	T2	N1	M0
Stage III	T3	N1	M0
	T4	Any N	M0
Stage IV	Any T	Any N	M1

Source: Beahrs OH, Henson DE, Hutter RV, et al (eds): *American Joint Committee on Cancer: Manual for Staging of Cancer* (4th ed). Philadelphia: Lippincott, 1992.

Surgical resection, radiotherapy, and chemotherapy are used to treat esophageal cancer, but it is a combination of these treatment methods that appears to offer the greatest hope of cure or control. The most effective combination or sequence of therapies has yet to be established. Preoperative irradiation and chemotherapy have been shown to improve resectability rates but not long-term survival rates. Progress in surgical approaches and care has markedly reduced operative mortality rates to 5%–10%.[28,29] In light of the nature of this disease, aggressive efforts aimed at either cure or palliation are justifiable and constitute the only hope in many cases.

The optimal candidate for curative treatment should be free of concomitant renal, cardiac, and pulmonary diseases, be relatively well nourished, and have a tumor that is localized, responsive, and accessible to treatment (i.e., stage I or II). The interdisciplinary team will develop a plan that can include single or combined modalities of surgery, radiation, or chemotherapy.

The historical trend has been to treat lesions of the cervical esophagus initially with radiotherapy (4500–6000 cGy). Surgery is undertaken 3–4 weeks later.[2] Surgical resection is limited by the location of the tumor and problems with reconstruction. Improvements in restoring the continuity of the cervical esophagus have been reported.[28]

Although controversial, certain findings usually will preclude an individual from consideration for curative treatment:

- fixed lymph nodes (N3)
- a fixed tumor mass (T3)
- extension of the tumor outside the esophagus (T3,M1)
- recurrent laryngeal nerve involvement (T3, M1)

In cases of advanced disease, the quality of life can be improved by restoration or maintenance of a patent alimentary tract. Treatment can be radiotherapy, surgical resection or bypass, dilation, prosthetic device implants, or systemic chemotherapy. Although long-term survival is rarely affected, aggressive therapy can be tolerated by many patients and results in an improvement in the individual's quality of life.

Preparation for treatment

If an aggressive treatment plan has been selected, ideally the patient will undergo pretreatment preparation to improve general health and nutrition. If the disease is advanced and the symptoms and manifestations are severely debilitating, palliative therapy may need to be initiated immediately and supportive measures introduced whenever possible.

Progressive dysphagia affects about 90% of individuals with esophageal tumors.[2] The degree of weight loss a person experiences can be correlated with prognosis.[2] Because of difficulty with swallowing, protein calorie malnutrition, cachexia, muscle wasting, and negative nitrogen balance may be present. Intensive nutritional therapy that can include total parenteral nutrition (TPN), enteral tube feedings, or high-calorie protein liquid supplements may be given to improve therapeutic outcome.

The high incidence of aspiration that occurs in individuals with esophageal cancer dictates that pulmonary hygiene be a priority in pretreatment care. Since many are heavy smokers, this will further necessitate intensive chest physiotherapy. The person is taught to breathe deeply and cough, with careful attention to expectorating secretions. As an aid to achieving pulmonary toilette, the individual is instructed to bend forward when coughing and expectorate into a tissue, cloth, or basin. Expectorants, antibiotics, or bronchodilators can be used to facilitate pulmonary hygiene. Esophageal lavage via a nasogastric tube placed above the obstruction may be necessary to prevent aspiration of accumulated food or secretions.

The individual with a large esophageal tumor usually cannot swallow saliva and thus will drool and spit frequently. The nurse must be acutely aware of the psychologic impact of this embarrassing problem and change in body image. Assist the person to establish an acceptable method for controlling secretions (e.g., basin nearby, oral suction equipment, abundant tissues, room air filter).

The period of treatment preparation is an excellent time to begin teaching the patient and family about the proposed therapy and anticipated course of the disease and to establish supportive relationships.

Radiotherapy

Squamous cell carcinoma of the esophagus is more responsive than adenocarcinoma to radiotherapy. Radiation can result in rapid relief of an obstruction. Radiotherapy can be used alone, as preoperative, intraoperative, or postoperative therapy, or as palliative therapy. Radiotherapy alone is not being used often now because few patients are being diagnosed in the early stages when radiation can be effective for cure. Methods of therapy combining chemotherapy, radiation, and surgery are providing better results than radiation alone.[30] Radiation is an excellent therapeutic alternative for a person with advanced disease or for an elderly or severely debilitated person who could not withstand the rigor of aggressive therapy.

The most important factor in determining the appropriateness of radiation is whether the patient is potentially curable or whether palliation is the only option. Small localized lesions (<5 cm) with no evidence of metastases can be treated for cure with radiotherapy alone or in combination.[31] Tumoricidal doses of 5000–7000 cGy are administered over 6–8 weeks.

Unfortunately, about 60% of early cancers are beyond potential curability at diagnosis because of distant spread.[32] Radiotherapy is the treatment favored by many clinicians for stage I and II cervical esophageal lesions since surgical mortality rates are high and the larynx can be preserved with irradiation. Tumors located in the cervical esophagus are complex to treat because of their proximity to the spinal cord. Tumors located in the upper thoracic esophagus respond well to radiotherapy. Lesions of the lower thoracic esophagus usually are treated with multimodal therapy.

Complications and side effects of radiotherapy relate to tissue tolerance, site and amount of radiation, and adjuvant therapy. Esophageal fistula, stricture, hemorrhage, radiation pneumonitis, and pericarditis are possible problems. Side effects expected during therapy are swallowing difficulties (burning, pain, dryness) and skin reactions. Nursing management should be aimed at anticipating and preventing complications of the radiation therapy and concomitant therapies, maintaining adequate nutritional intake, and minimizing the discomfort of esophageal and skin irritation. (Nursing care of individuals who receive radiotherapy is discussed in detail in Chapter 13.) The nurse or dietitian must plan an intensive dietary program based on the constraints of an obstructive tumor, the degree of nutritional deficit, and the person's preferences.

Preoperative radiotherapy

Preoperative radiotherapeutic doses of 3000–6000 cGy can reduce tumor bulk and improve surgical resectability. It can also enable individuals with esophageal tumors to swallow and significantly improve nutritional status and reduce operative risk. Preoperative radiation therapy can potentially eradicate local microscopic disease and reduce the risk of dissemination of tumor cells during surgery.

Clinical studies lend credibility to the effectiveness of the combination of preoperative radiation and surgery.[33–36] Increased resectability rates and decreased operative mortality rates occur when combination therapy is used. The limitation to the aggressiveness of preoperative radiation or preoperative chemoradiation is toxicity.

Postoperative radiotherapy

Postoperative radiotherapy is administered to eradicate residual tumor cells in the area of the surgical site. These cells may have been implanted during surgery or could be residual in the unresected tumor or adjacent tissue. If the tumor is an unresectable advanced esophageal cancer, postoperative radiotherapy can be effective for local control. The surgeon can mark the involved area with radiopaque clips to enable more precise delivery of the radiation. If the tumor is resected and the stomach or colon is used to restore intestinal continuity, there will need to be a more limited radiation dose (4000–5000 cGy) delivered in order to avoid tissue injury.[2]

Postoperative radiotherapy does not affect surgical mortality, but it may not be as effective as chemoradiation prior to surgical resection. Further investigation is needed to determine the most effective sequence of radiation therapy in the treatment pattern.

Intracavitary radiation

Through the use of intraluminal brachytherapy, it is possible to provide a therapeutic boost to the local area involved. Implants are placed via an endoscope or through high-dose afterloading techniques. Intracavitary radiation can be useful for the purpose of retreatment after external beam therapy.[37]

Surgery

Surgical intervention is employed selectively for lesions at all three levels of the esophagus. The goal of surgery may be to cure or palliate, depending on the stage of the tumor and the overall condition of the patient. Curative surgery attempts to eradicate the tumor and reestablish esophageal continuity, whereas palliative surgery may aim at maintaining esophageal patency. Surgery can be used alone or in combination with chemotherapy or radiation.

Preoperative indications for curative surgery include a satisfactory nutritional state, a resectable tumor without evidence of invasion of contiguous structures (stages I and II), no distant metastases, and no serious concomitant disease. Age is not an issue, unless the person's general health is unsatisfactory. Curative surgery can be attempted if it is expected that the tumor will be removed completely and esophageal patency reestablished. If possible, blood, fluid, electrolyte, and nutritional balance should be established before aggressive surgical resection is done. Impaired wound healing and increased incidence of infection are associated with hypoalbuminemia.[38] Before surgery, chest physiotherapy includes respiratory exercise with intermittent positive pressure breathing and incentive spirometry. The patient is requested to refrain from smoking for 2–3 weeks before surgery. Improved perioperative care measures have significantly reduced operatively mortality.

Surgical approaches

The surgical technique and approach to esophageal resection depend on the location of the tumor. The cervical esophagus is approached in a radically different way and will be discussed separately. Four surgical approaches are currently being used: left transthoracic approach, combined right thoracotomy with laparotomy, transhiatal approach, and *en bloc* resection.[2,39] For cancers of the lower third of the esophagus, the left transthoracic approach facilitates esophageal dissection and esophagogastric anastomosis. For cancer of the upper and middle third of the esophagus, the right thoracotomy with laparotomy is the approach used by most surgeons. The laparotomy allows evaluation of the lower celiac nodes for tumor involvement. Cancer located in the lower esophagus and cardia usually is surgically removed via the standard transthoracic esophagogastrectomy.[40] The transhiatal esophagectomy can be used for cancer at all three levels of the esophagus (upper, middle, lower). The theoretic, but not proven, advantage of transhiatal esophagectomy is the avoidance of a thoracotomy and reconstruction via a cervical esophageal anastomosis rather than an intrathoracic anastomosis. The *en bloc* resection is used mostly for tumors of the lower esophagus and cardia. It involves removal of a tissue block that is completely surrounded by normal tissue and incorporates the submucosal lymphatics of the esophagus and stomach. Potentially involved lymph nodes are also removed.[41]

Esophagectomy is the most widely accepted procedure for surgical resection aimed at potential cure. Because lymph node involvement can occur at a distance from the primary esophageal cancer, complete removal of the esophagus and adjacent lymph nodes is considered the procedure of choice.[29] Vital structures in the area (heart, aorta, mainstem bronchus) make complete resection of the esophagus and nodes difficult; hence the rationale for adjuvant therapies. Whenever there is evidence that cure is a strong possibility, a more extensive *en bloc* excision is performed.

Reconstruction following esophagectomy can be achieved via various procedures. Elevating the stomach to create an esophagogastrostomy is the most widely used reconstructive procedure (Figures 41-1 and 41-2). If a gastrectomy has previously been performed or the stomach is not suitable as a reconstructive organ, a colon interposition may be done (Figure 41-3). A gastric tube sometimes is created from the greater curvature of the stomach, reversed, and elevated to reconstruct the esophagus (Figure 41-4).

Special considerations: cervical esophagus

Tumors of the cervical esophagus are the least common. Resection of lesions and reconstruction of the cervical esophagus require careful planing because of the difficulties imposed by its location. Surgery usually is extensive; therefore, it is recommended only if cure is the goal. Tumors of the cervical esophagus that do not have laryngeal involvement can sometimes be resected completely without removing the larynx. The surgical procedure consists of a radical neck dissection

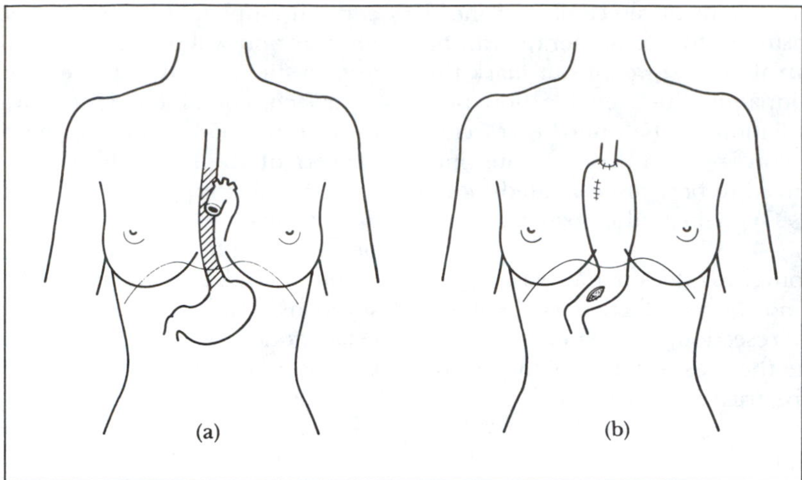

FIGURE 41-1 The technique of esophagectomy for cancers involving the mid-esophagus. (a) The extent of esophagus removed is shown by the darkened area. (b) The esophagogastrostomy above the aortic arch and pyloroplasty is illustrated.

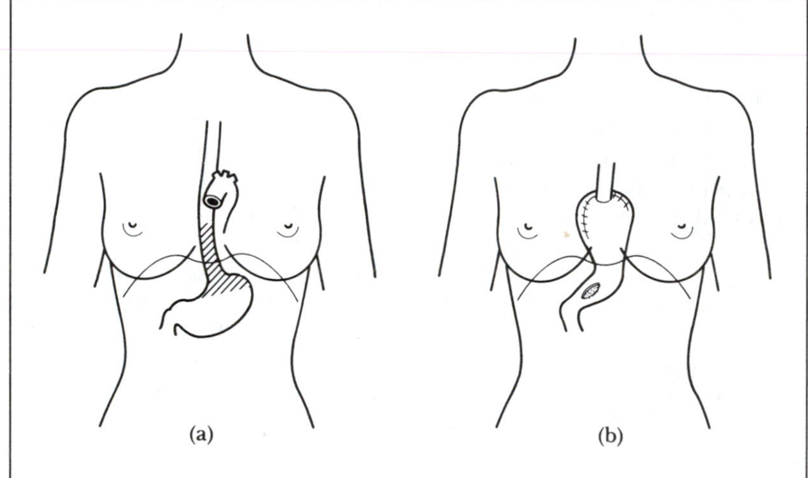

FIGURE 41-2 Esophagectomy for lesions of the lower esophagus. In most cases the procedure can be performed through the left thoracic incision. The midline abdominal incision is used when the duodenum must be mobilized to permit the esophagogastrostomy to be performed. (a) The extent of esophagus and stomach removed is shown by the darkened area. The lymph nodes at the celiac axis are removed with the specimen. (b) The esophagogastrostomy is illustrated. A pyloroplasty is also done.

and partial cervical esophagectomy. However, most tumors of the cervical esophagus are first detected at a more advanced stage and require more extensive surgery. Usually, resection of cervical esophagus lesions involves removing all or part of the pharynx, larynx, thyroid, and proximal esophagus.[2]

Reconstruction of intestinal patency is a major consideration, especially with irradiated tissue. The reconstructive procedure may be done at the time of the initial resection or later as a second-stage procedure. At present, cervical esophageal continuity usually is reestablished by anastomosing the stomach via the subcutaneous, substernal, or mediastinal route. In some instances the colon is interposed and anastomosed to the pharyngeal stump.

A satisfactory, functional result can be achieved with these procedures, but the postoperative period is plagued with complications of fistulas, anastomotic leaks, strictures, respiratory insufficiency, pulmonary embolism, obstruction, and infection.[2] Postoperative mortal-

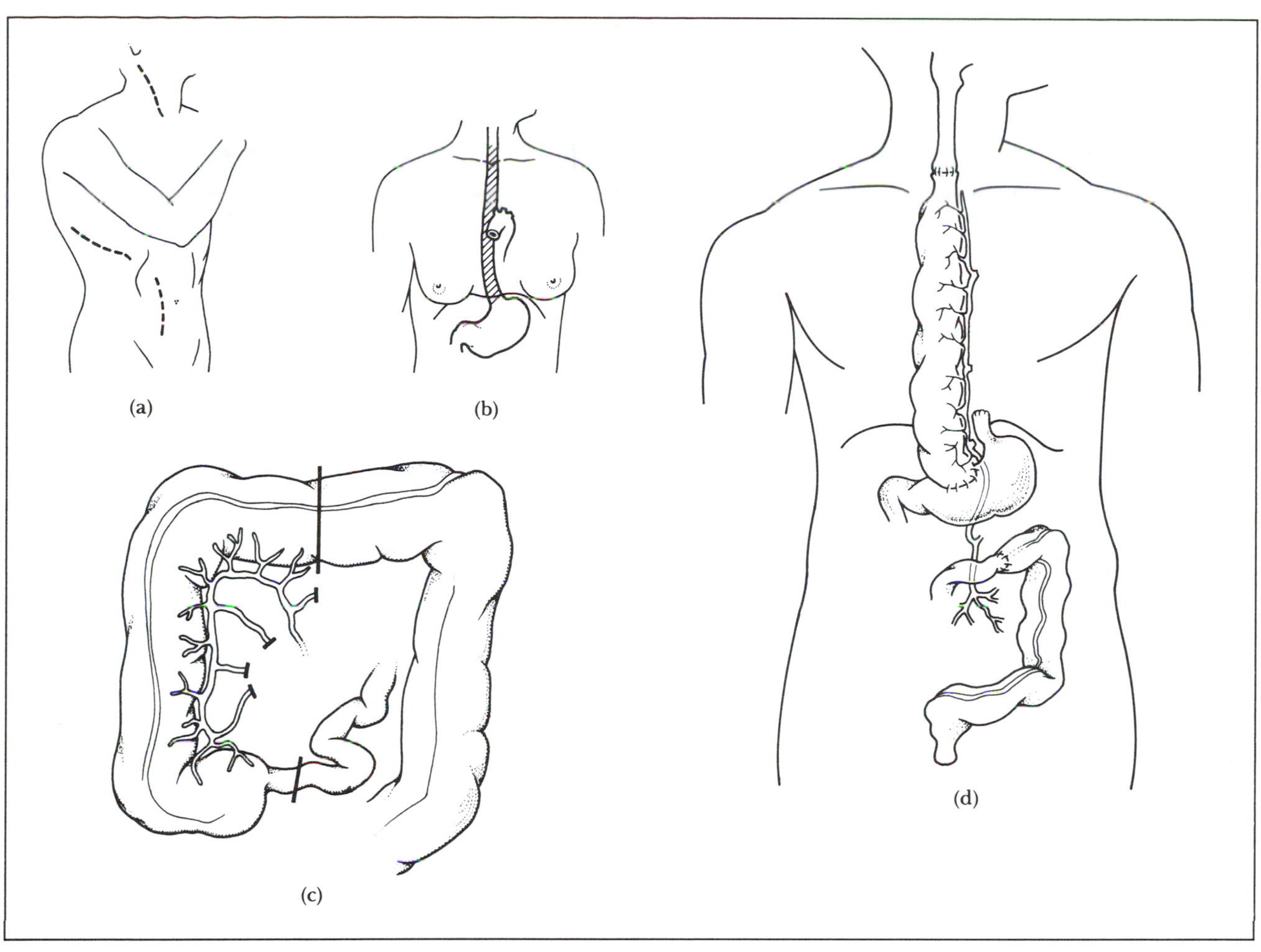

FIGURE 41-3 A right colon substernal transplant and total esophagectomy. (a) The cervical and abdominal incisions are made at the first stage of the operation. The right thoracic incision is used at the second stage to remove the esophagus. (b) The extent of esophageal resection is shown. (c) The right colon on a pedicle consisting of the midcolic artery and vein is illustrated. (d) The completed operation is shown.

ity ranges from 3%–26%,[28,31] with higher rates occurring among patients whose surgeons have less frequent experience with esophageal cancer surgeries.

Postoperative care

Respiratory complications, fistulae, and anastomotic leaks compose the bulk of complications following surgical resection for carcinoma of the esophagus.[42] Severe atelectasis, pneumonia, pulmonary edema, and adult respiratory distress syndrome contribute to postoperative morbidity and mortality.[28] Lengthy surgical procedures (5–8 hours) and a compromised preoperative pulmonary condition can precipitate problems, such as hypothermia and hypovolemia. Because most individuals who undergo surgery for an esophageal tumor are in a precarious nutritional state, protein depletion and generalized muscle weakness are common. Ability to breathe deeply and cough is compromised by weakness and incisional pain. Aggressive respiratory care can include tracheal intubation, chest physiotherapy, tracheobronchial aspiration, prevention of fluid overload, and antibiotic therapy. Early ambulation and mild exercise will improve respiratory status.

The esophagus is a thin-walled organ drawn upward with each swallow, so an anastomosis involving the esophagus has more of a tendency toward dehiscence and anastomotic leak than any other area of the gastrointestinal tract.[40,43] Decompression tubes, nasogastric or gastrostomy, must be patent at all times to prevent pressure or tension on the anastomotic site. Chest tubes may be placed to facilitate full reexpansion of the lungs and extraesophageal drainage. Bloody, purulent, or brown, malodorous drainage from the chest tubes would indicate leakage. Fever or pain usually are the earliest signs.[44] The nurse should routinely auscultate the patient's chest to identify any changes in lung expansion or accumulation of fluid. Six or 7 days after surgery, contrast studies can be done to evaluate anastomotic healing. Small leaks usually close spontaneously if

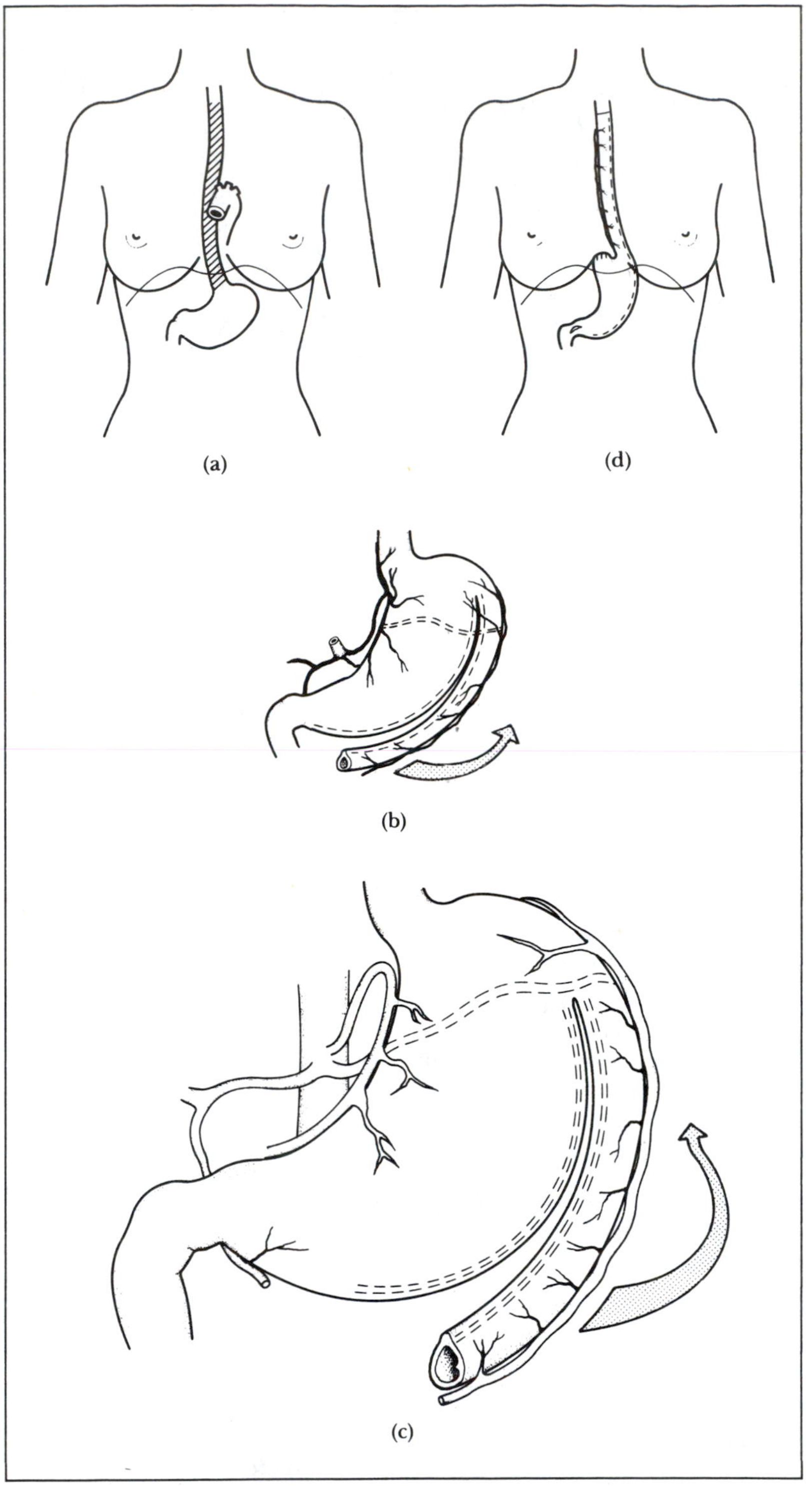

(a)

(d)

(b)

(c)

FIGURE 41-4 Reversed gastric tube and total esophagectomy. (a) The extent of esophageal resection is shown. (b) The reversed gastric tube created from two parallel rows of staples is shown. (c) The gastroepiploic vessels are carefully preserved and vascularize the gastric tube. (d) The completed operation, with gastrostomy and pyloroplasty, is shown.

decompression is adequate, whereas large leaks will require surgical approximation before mediastinitis or empyema occur. Intrathoracic anastomotic leaks usually are managed with chest tube drainage, aggressive antibiotic therapy, cessation of oral intake, and open thoracotomy if the disruption is large.[45]

Infections are a serious threat to recovery. Virulent mouth organisms and overgrowth of pathogenic bacteria on ulcerating lesions may be a source for wound and intracavitary infections. If the individual has had previous radiotherapy, the risks of tissue breakdown, poor wound healing, and fistulas are greatly increased. Nursing assessments for signs of infection and fistula include inspection of incision lines, monitoring of vital signs (particularly temperature), pulmonary auscultation, and close attention to drainage, urinary output, and hematologic factors.

Meticulous suture line care and constant monitoring for signs of inflammation, drainage, and edema are necessary. Esophagocutaneous fistulas usually appear in raised, reddened, or necrotic areas along the suture line. The individual should be observed carefully during swallowing because a leak may occur at the suture line. Chylous fistulas produce a milky white secretion that gradually increases in amount. Systemic signs of fistula are fever, malaise, and increased respirations and pulse rate. The individual is maintained in proper body alignment to reduce tension on the anastomosis. Suction catheters are not introduced into the oropharyngeal cavity without knowledge of the location of the suture line because the suture line may be disrupted. The nasogastric tube should be advanced or manipulated only with the aid of fluoroscopy.

If the individual had a cervical esophagectomy in conjunction with a laryngectomy, the nursing care needs are complex. The nursing care of the individual with a laryngectomy is discussed in detail in Chapter 44.

The postoperative nursing care of the individual with an esophagogastrectomy includes anticipation and prevention of reflux aspiration and esophagitis. The head of the bed should be elevated at all times. After the patient is discharged, a foam rubber wedge or multiple pillows correctly aligned will work well at home. Snacks or liquids after the evening meal should be avoided so the stomach will be relatively empty at bedtime. The person should ingest all food and liquids in small amounts in an upright position and should remain upright for 20–30 minutes after eating.[45,46] The person should be instructed to avoid bending over from the waist and especially to avoid any exercise or lifting that would increase intraabdominal and thoracic pressure and cause reflux.[47] Squatting to lift objects will displace the stress to the legs rather than to the abdomen.

When a segment of colon is used to reconstruct or bypass part of the esophagus, the individual will have complex nursing care needs in addition to those discussed previously for esophagectomy. Pulmonary hygiene, prevention of infection, prevention of reflux, control of odor, and nutrition are nursing priorities.

Prior to surgery for colon interposition, a regimen of antibiotics and sulfonamides is begun to suppress bacterial flora in the intestine. Despite efforts to sterilize and prepare the bowel for transposition, contamination of the peritoneal cavity and infection leading to fistula formation are common and serious complications. Gram-negative bacteria can produce endotoxic shock, evidenced by rapid pulse, decreased blood pressure, increased respirations and temperature, warm, dry skin, and confusion. The suture lines should be observed for signs of infection, vital signs monitored regularly, and careful lung assessments performed to detect an anastomotic leak or extraesophageal accumulation of fluid.

Foul-smelling breath is a distressing consequence of having used a segment of bowel to reconstruct the esophagus. The extensive program of preoperative bowel preparation will reduce but not eliminate fecal odor. Frequent, meticulous oral care is necessary in the postoperative period and after discharge. The individual should be instructed to avoid foods that cause belching, because the eructated air will have a fecal odor that could embarrass the person. The person can prepare a small, discreet travel kit that includes such items as a toothbrush, toothpaste, mouthwash, mint candies, and charcoal carbonate tablets. Some people find that commercially available breath sprays are useful. Charcoal carbonate tablets taken regularly will help to control odor.

Chemotherapy

Chemotherapy in the treatment of esophageal tumors has assumed an increasingly important role. Many agents have demonstrated activity with esophageal cancer. Two recent developments have stimulated a resurgence of interest: increased usage of cisplatin and enhanced effectiveness with infusional 5-fluorouracil (5-FU).[48] Cisplatin, 5-FU, mitomycin-C, mitoguazone (MGBG), doxorubicin, bleomycin, and vindesine have demonstrated cytotoxic activity with esophageal tumors.[49] Combination regimens are more effective than single-agent therapy.[50–52]

Sequenced chemotherapy and its use in multimodal treatment approaches offer the most promising areas to explore at this time. Theoretically, neoadjuvant chemotherapy exposes micrometastatic cells at a time of maximum sensitivity and minimal resistance. Preoperative chemotherapy could enable a surgical resection with less chance of metastatic disease recurrence. Current clinical trials of preoperative chemotherapy include various combinations of active agents.

Preoperative chemoradiation therapy delivers local and systemic therapy simultaneously. The radiation therapy component will improve resectability, and the chemotherapy is expected to reduce systemic micrometastases. Together, a higher rate of tumor sterilization is induced. Protocols include combination chemotherapy (usually cisplatin and 5-FU) and fractionated radiation doses that total 3000–5000 cGy before surgery.[53–55] Tumor regression is effected in most cases. Cisplatin and 5-FU may also act as radiosensitizers to improve the therapeutic effect. The toxicities associated with the extensive combination of chemotherapy, radiation therapy, and surgery are compounded and may be intolerable for some patients, but most appear to tolerate the therapy.[53] Severe mucositis and myelosuppression are the major toxicities noted. Operative morbidity and mortality have not been increased.[53] Some chemotherapeutic agents (doxorubicin, actinomycin D, and daunorubicin) can produce radiation-recall esophagitis and skin reactions in individuals who have received previous irradiation. Therefore, to reduce the severity of this effect, chemotherapy should not be initiated for several weeks after radiotherapy. It is not yet known whether this approach to esophageal cancer will improve long-term disease-free intervals.

Chemoradiation alone, without surgery, has received attention.[56,57] Results with early-stage cancers indicate that a better response is achieved with chemoradiation alone than with surgery or radiation alone. Optimal management of esophageal cancer is an unanswered question that will require further study.

Palliative Therapy

The objective of palliative therapy is to relieve the distressing symptoms of esophageal cancer, thereby improving the quality of the individual's life. Progressive dysphagia is probably the most debilitating of the symptoms, occurring in about 90% of the patients with advanced disease. Selection of a particular form of palliative therapy will depend on the individual's preference, nutritional status, hematologic status, and ability to tolerate palliative therapy.

Palliative radiotherapy provides rapid symptomatic and objective relief. Usually, 3000–5000 cGy will be given to decrease the size of the tumor or reduce bleeding or both.[58] Intracavitary brachytherapy has also been used. Because of its noninvasive nature, many oncologists will select palliative radiotherapy over other forms of supportive treatment.

Laser therapy is being used more frequently today to alleviate esophageal obstruction or severe dysphagia. The laser photocoagulation process is delivered via endoscope. It is generally well tolerated, and rapidly alleviates tumor blockage.[59–61] The patient may need to be rescoped 2 or 3 days after therapy to debride the necrotic material, and if necessary retreated with the laser.

In selected individuals with advanced disease, palliative resection with reconstruction or surgical bypass of the esophagus will be done to relieve severe symptoms of the disease or reduce the size of the tumor. Limited resection or bypass of the tumor can be achieved by elevation of the stomach, substernal or subcutaneous colon interposition, or a tube formed from the greater curvature of the stomach.[2] In some instances, esophagectomy may be performed as a palliative procedure for esophageal disruption.

A number of synthetic endoesophageal prosthetic tubes have been designed to create an open passage for swallowing when the esophagus is obstructed by an inoperable tumor. The two methods used most commonly to place the tube are the push-through method and the pull-through method. With the *push-through* method, the tube is placed blindly or with the aid of an esophagoscope.[62] The *pull-through* method involves pulling the tube into place by means of a guide wire or gastrostomy. Radiologic dilation before tube placement can reduce complications of tube placement. Esophageal perforation is a technical complication that occurs in about 5%–10% of individuals.[62] Dislodgement and/or obstruction with food occurs frequently. Satisfactory palliative results achieved with either type of tube are limited; however, increased food intake after tube placement occurs in about 80% of patients.[62] Overgrowth of the tube with cancer can occur but can be relieved with laser ablation.[63]

Nursing care of the individual with an endoprosthesis is aimed at preventing complications and maintaining tube patency. Individuals need to understand the purpose, function, and care of the endoesophageal prosthesis. With the prosthesis in place, reflux of gastric contents can lead to aspiration pneumonia. Nursing care measures to prevent reflux include elevating the head of the bed at all times, ensuring patency of decompression tubes, and pursuing aggressive pulmonary hygiene.[64] When the individual is able to begin eating, usually the day following placement, is the time to develop strategies to prevent reflux. The individual is instructed to take all meals and liquids in an upright position. The first attempts at swallowing may be uncomfortable, but encouragement by the nurse can greatly increase the person's confidence. Smaller amounts of liquid or food with each swallowing may be necessary. If food becomes lodged in the tube because it is too large or inadequately chewed, it usually can be dislodged carefully with a nasogastric tube. Discharge teaching should include instructions to drink at least a half glass of water or carbonated beverage at the end of a meal to clear the tube completely.

Other palliative treatment measures include hyperthermochemoradiotherapy,[65] high-dose photoirradiation,[66] and laser therapy to reduce the obstructive mass. Laser therapy is also used to reduce esophageal stricture caused by tumor.[67]

Gastrostomy and jejunostomy are alternative palliative procedures for individuals with esophageal cancer. Although they permit nutritional maintenance, they do not relieve the debilitating problem of inability to swallow solids, liquids, or saliva. Nursing measures to increase tolerance of tube feedings are discussed in Chapter 27. Nursing management of the individual with advanced esophageal cancer includes control of pain, nutritional support, and psychologic support. Because esophageal cancer grows rapidly and disseminates early, the nurse can be most helpful by anticipating problems and providing support to the individual and family.

In light of the dreary outlook on esophageal cancer, it is important to consider what the future may hold for persons with this disease. Is it possible to identify biologic markers or definitive risk factors that would be helpful in detecting esophageal cancer at an early stage or even in predicting the onset of esophageal cancer? In China, mass screening programs for esophageal cancer have proven successful in detecting early cases of esophageal carcinoma. Unfortunately, the present detection techniques are expensive, inefficient, and prohibitive for sustained use on a large scale.

The roles of multimodal therapy in the treatment of esophageal carcinoma are emerging. At present, numerous controlled studies are based on the use of multimodal therapy. It is hoped that these studies will lead to the development of a definitive set of guidelines for the treatment and management of esophageal tumors.

STOMACH TUMORS

INTRODUCTION

For reasons unknown at this time, the incidence of gastric cancer is decreasing in some parts of the world and increasing steadily in others. In the United States the incidence has progressively declined since 1930, when it was the leading cause of cancer mortality.[1] Gastric cancer continues to take a significant toll among inhabitants of Japan, Iceland, and portions of Central and South America.[68,69]

If detected at an early age and treated aggressively, cancer of the stomach can be cured.[70] Overall 5-year survival rates are reported to be about 16%–92%.[1,71,72] The Japanese report much higher survival rates than in the United States.[73] This is most likely due to aggressive screening programs and national efforts toward early detection of a disease that is a serious problem for the Japanese. Gastric cancer is insidious in its onset and can be disseminated throughout the body before overt signs are manifested. Gastric cancer mimics several other gastrointestinal maladies and diseases, such as polyps, ulcers, dyspepsia, and gastritis. The most challenging aspects of prevention and early detection are the informing and motivating of people at risk for developing gastric cancer to seek medical attention for chronic "stomach problems." Inappropriate use of home remedies, self-medication, and misdiagnosis are major hurdles to overcome.

EPIDEMIOLOGY

Japan has the highest incidence in the world of gastric cancer for both men and women; it is the major cause of death in Japan.[70,74] On the other hand, the incidence of gastric cancer is low in the United States.[1] The dramatic differences in geographic patterns of incidence throughout the world remain an enigma to epidemiologists.[75]

The United States has approximately 24,000 new cases and 13,600 deaths from gastric cancer each year.[1] This reflects a 65% decrease in incidence within the past 35 years, with the greatest decline occurring among white persons. In the United States, African Americans, Japanese, Chinese, and native Hawaiian individuals have a higher incidence and mortality rate than do white persons.[76] There is also great variation of incidence among the Native Americans of New Mexico, Hispanic Americans, and non-Hispanic whites.[75]

ETIOLOGY

Factors believed to contribute to or to be associated with gastric cancer are largely environmental and genetic. The fact that immigrants exhibit incidence rates similar to those of their country of origin has led researchers to accept exogenous influences such as environment and diet. A number of dietary factors are associated with gastric cancer, such as ingestion of large amounts of pickled and salted foods. Controversy exists over the role of nitrites found in soil-grown foods, drinking water, and prepared foods. Because refrigeration and a high intake of ascorbic acid inhibit the formation of nitrates, it is postulated that the presence of these factors may account for the decrease in gastric cancer in the United States. Decreases in incidence may also be due to the ingestion of greater amounts of fresh fruits, vegetables, and grains.[69]

Those at greatest risk for developing gastric cancer are older than 40 years of age and possess one or several of the following risk factors:[79]

- low socioeconomic status
- poor nutritional habits[77]
- vitamin A deficiency
- family history[78]
- pernicious anemia
- achlorhydria
- chronic gastritis
- gastric polyps
- benign peptic ulcer disease

People whose occupations appear to place them at risk for gastric cancer are coal miners, nickel refiners, rubber and timber processors, and asbestos workers.[69] Although rare, gastric cancer does occur in children.

PATHOPHYSIOLOGY

Cellular Characteristics

More than 90% of gastric cancers are adenocarcinomas.[69,80,81] Leiomyosarcoma and lymphoma are less common types of gastric tumors. Most gastric cancers arise in the antrum, the distal third of the stomach. Tumor involves the lesser curvature of the stomach much more often than the greater curvature.[69]

Adenocarcinomas that arise in the esophagocardia are considered to be a different disease for purposes of classification. Usually, adenocarcinomas of the esophagocardia are primary cancers of the stomach that have extended to the esophagus. There are different male/female and ethnic distribution ratios.[69,82] Gastric tumors may be grossly classified as polypoid, scirrhous, ulcerative, or superficial.

Progression of Disease

Because initial symptoms are vague, gastric cancer usually is locally advanced or metastatic when symptoms first appear. Gastric tumors can cause ulceration, obstruction, hemorrhage, or manifestations of metastatic involvement. There are several characteristic routes by which gastric carcinoma will progress and metastasize: (1) by extension and infiltration along the mucosal surface and stomach wall or lymphatics; (2) via lymphatic or vascular embolism, probably to regional lymph nodes; (3) by direct extension into adjacent structures such as the pancreas, liver, or esophagus; and (4) via the bloodstream. The pattern of metastatic spread of gastric cancer correlates with the size and location of the tumor. Lesions of the distal portion of the stomach usually will metastasize to infrapyloric, inferior gastric, and celiac lymph nodes. Tumors in the proximal portion often metastasize to pancreatic, pericardial, and gastric lymph nodes. With advanced gastric cancer, involvement of the left supraclavicular nodes may occur. Distant metastatic sites are the lung, adrenals, bone, liver, pancreas, and peritoneal cavity.

CLINICAL MANIFESTATIONS

Persons with gastric cancer have vague, nonspecific symptoms of variable duration. Individuals usually will delay several months between the onset of symptoms and initial medical consultation. Pain in the epigastric, back, or retrosternal area is often cited as an early symptom that was ignored or that responded temporarily to symptomatic treatment. The individual will complain of a vague, uneasy sense of fullness, a feeling of heaviness, and moderate distention after meals. Antacids and home remedies are employed successfully for a while until more definitive signs and symptoms appear. As the disease advances, progressive weight loss can result from disturbances in appetite, nausea, and vomiting. Weakness, fatigue, and anemia are common findings. Dysphagia may occur with tumors of the proximal portion of the stomach. Hematemesis, melena, or a change in bowel habits is sometimes reported. Unfortunately, definitive clinical signs occur mostly with advanced disease.[69,80]

ASSESSMENT

The use of radiography, endoscopy, and laparotomy may be necessary to establish a diagnosis of gastric carcinoma. Because the initial symptoms are vague, it is not unusual for misdiagnosis or treatment delay to occur. Although the incidence of gastric cancer is decreasing, aggressive preventive health care in high-risk individuals is necessary to ensure that this decline continues.

Patient and Family History

To establish a clinical picture, a complete assessment of the individual's nutritional status, physical examination, and social and family history should be done. An in-depth nutritional assessment and history will aid in identifying subtle changes in dietary habits or contributory signs such as pain or bowel changes. Areas to include in a nutritional history/assessment are as follows:

1. food and fluid intake patterns (types, amount, number, calories)
2. symptoms associated with eating (pain, eructation, dysphagia, nausea, fullness, reflux)
3. change in dietary habits or appetite (food intolerance, aversions, volume, types of food)
4. weight (actual, usual, ideal)
5. bowel patterns and habits (frequency, consistency, color, flatulence)
6. medications (over-the-counter, home remedies, prescriptions)
7. previous/concurrent illness (childhood, adult, transient maladies)

Physical Examination

The physical examination includes palpation of the abdomen and lymph nodes, particularly the supraclavicular and axillary lymph nodes, because they are possible metastatic sites. An abdominal mass and/or hepatomegaly may be palpated. Enlarged lymph nodes and hepatomegaly indicate the need for biopsy. A rectal examination could reveal a shelf of metastatic deposits. If an obstruction exists in the pyloric area, peristaltic activity moving in a left-to-right direction may be detected. Advanced gastric cancer can result in anemia and jaundice.

Diagnostic Studies

Any signs and symptoms suggestive of gastric cancer should be investigated by diagnostic procedures to identify their source. A double-contrast upper gastrointestinal series will reveal the mucosal pattern, character of mobility, distensibility, and flexibility of the walls. Filling defects and rigidity of walls suggest malignant involvement. Following radiologic examinations involving barium, care must be taken to administer laxatives to prevent barium impaction. Computerized tomographic (CT) scanning is useful in defining metastases and tumor extension.

Accuracy of diagnosis has been enhanced by endoscopic gastroscopy, which allows the clinician to view the lesion directly and to obtain multiple biopsies and brushings for cytology.[80] Flexible endoscopic gastroscopy is more comfortable for the individual and less traumatic to the gastrointestinal tissue and provides a diagnostic accuracy rate of greater than 90% when combined with biopsy and cytology.[80,83] Topical anesthetics, analgesics, or sedatives are administered to facilitate the endoscopic instrumentation and to make the patient comfortable. For 2–4 hours following the procedure, nursing measures should be employed to prevent aspiration or trauma. The patient receives nothing to eat or drink until a gag reflex returns. Hoarseness from throat irritation can be relieved by lozenges or warm saline gargles after the effects of anesthesia dissipate, and the patient should be observed periodically for signs of perforation (i.e., fever, abdominal pain or distention, dyspnea, cyanosis, subcutaneous crepitus).

Laboratory analyses include hematologic profiles, which may reveal anemia resulting from gradual blood loss in both gastric cancer and chronic gastric ulcer. Malignancy is highly probable when there is a chronic unresponsive gastric ulcer, gastric ulcer on the greater curvature of the stomach, obstruction in the presence of ulcer, or achlorhydria and positive cytologic findings. Karyometric studies of DNA content have correlated high-ploidy gastric tumors with a higher incidence of lymphatic and vascular invasion.[84] Several tumor markers are being investigated (CA50, CEA, TPA [tissue polypeptide antigen]).[85] To date, none has proven to be significant for clinical practice.

TABLE 41-3 TNM Classification for Gastric Carcinoma

PRIMARY TUMOR (T)	
TX	Primary tumor cannot be assessed
T0	No evidence of primary tumor
Tis	Carcinoma in situ: intraepithelial tumor without invasion of the lamina propria
T1	Tumor invades lamina propria or submucosa
T2	Tumor invades the muscularis propria or the subserosa
T3	Tumor penetrates the serosa (visceral peritoneum) without invasion of adjacent structures
T4	Tumor invades adjacent structures

REGIONAL LYMPH NODES (N)	
NX	Regional lymph node(s) cannot be assessed
N0	No regional lymph node metastasis
N1	Metastasis in perigastric lymph node(s) within 3 cm of the edge of the primary tumor
N2	Metastasis in perigastric lymph node(s) more than 3 cm from the edge of the primary tumor, or in lymph nodes along the left gastric, common hepatic, splenic, or celiac arteries

DISTANT METASTASIS (M)	
MX	Presence of distant metastasis cannot be assessed
M0	No distant metastasis
M1	Distant metastasis

STAGE GROUPING			
Stage 0	Tis	N0	M0
Stage IA	T1	N0	M0
Stage IB	T1	N1	M0
	T2	N0	M0
Stage II	T1	N2	M0
	T2	N1	M0
	T3	N0	M0
Stage IIIA	T2	N2	M0
	T3	N1	M0
	T4	N0	M0
Stage IIIB	T3	N2	M0
	T4	N1	M0
Stage IV	T4	N2	M0
	Any T	Any N	M1

Source: Beahrs OH, Henson DE, Hutter RV, et al (eds): *American Joint Committee on Cancer: Manual for Staging of Cancer* (4th ed). Philadelphia: Lippincott, 1992.

CLASSIFICATION AND STAGING

Treatment planning ensues once a diagnosis is confirmed and the extent of involvement is delineated. The prognosis and treatment plan depend on the stage of the disease and general well-being of the individual. The American Joint Committee for Cancer Staging and End-Results Reporting has established and adopted the TNM classification system listed in Table 41-3.

TREATMENT

Prior to the initiation of a treatment plan, the patient and family should receive a thorough explanation of the anticipated course and expected outcomes. The overall plan of therapy for gastric cancer depends on the stage of the disease and current techniques in surgery, radiotherapy, and chemotherapy.

Localized gastric carcinomas are treated with curative intent with aggressive surgery alone or in combination with chemotherapy or radiotherapy. Approximately 50% of patients will be candidates for curative resection.[86]

Advanced tumors that are partially resectable, unresectable, or disseminated are treated with combination therapy using surgery and chemotherapy, with or without radiotherapy, and palliative surgery. Palliative procedures such as esophagojejunostomy or partial gastric resection alleviate obstructive tumors and restore intestinal continuity. If the individual cannot withstand or elects not to have such a procedure, a less traumatic palliative procedure may be done, such as insertion of a synthetic tube or a gastrojejunostomy. Combinations of chemotherapeutic agents have produced transient improvements with advanced tumors.[80]

Surgery

A controversy exists among proponents of radical surgical approaches to gastric cancer and those who support a more conservative resection. The cure rates with both surgical approaches are comparable, but differences exist in operative mortality and surgical mortality that warrant ongoing investigation.[87,88]

In many cases, resectability for cure or palliation can only be definitively assessed on abdominal exploration. Operability rates are high, usually around 80%,[86,87] whereas resectability rates are lower, around 60%.[87] The choice of surgical procedure is based on the location and extent of disease.

Measures to prepare a patient for surgery include correction of fluid and electrolyte imbalances, correction of anemia from chronic blood loss, and attention to nutritional status. Weight loss, emaciation, and malnutrition can adversely affect therapy and require aggressive intervention.

Total gastrectomy

If the lesion is resectable and located in the midportion or body of the stomach, a total gastrectomy usually is performed. Linitis plastica usually is treated with total gastrectomy because of the extensive involvement of the gastric wall. The entire stomach is removed *en bloc*, along with supporting mesentery and lymph nodes. The esophagus is anastomosed to the jejunum. A thoracic approach sometimes is necessary to perform the esophagojejunostomy. Pneumonia, infection, anastomotic leak, hemorrhage, and reflux aspiration are frequent complications. Overall mortality rates are 10%–15% for persons who undergo total gastrectomy.[88] In Japan an even more radical approach, with extended lymph node dissection and extended regional resection including the pancreas, is common.[70]

Radical subtotal gastrectomy

Lesions located in the middle and distal portions of the stomach are treated by radical subtotal gastrectomy. A Billroth I or Billroth II will be done. A Billroth I, or gastroduodenostomy, involves resecting the first portion of the duodenum, the distal stomach, pylorus, and supporting circulatory and lymph vessels. The remaining stomach is anastomosed to the duodenum. (See Figure 41-5.) The Billroth I is the procedure of choice in elderly or debilitated individuals, when limiting intraoperative time is of paramount importance. Because the procedure limits the scope of resection, the Billroth I is not as desirable as the Billroth II for gastric cancer.

The Billroth II is the surgery of choice for a person who requires and can tolerate a more radical procedure. This wider resection includes about 75% of the stomach, thereby decreasing the possibility of nodal or metastatic recurrence. A Billroth II involves removal of the antrum, pylorus, first portion of the duodenum, supporting circulatory structures, and all visible and palpable lymph nodes. With this procedure the remaining stomach is anastomosed end-to-side to the jejunum. The duodenal stump is closed with sutures. (See Figure 41-6.)

Gastric emptying is altered by the Billroth I and II procedures. The potential complications and resultant sequelae are the same as with all postgastrectomy syndromes: steatorrhea, dumping syndrome, nausea, vomiting, weight loss, diarrhea, vitamin deficiency, and anastomotic leak.

Subtotal esophagogastrectomy

If a resectable tumor is located in the proximal portion of the stomach or cardia, the disease has characteristic patterns and usually a subtotal esophago-

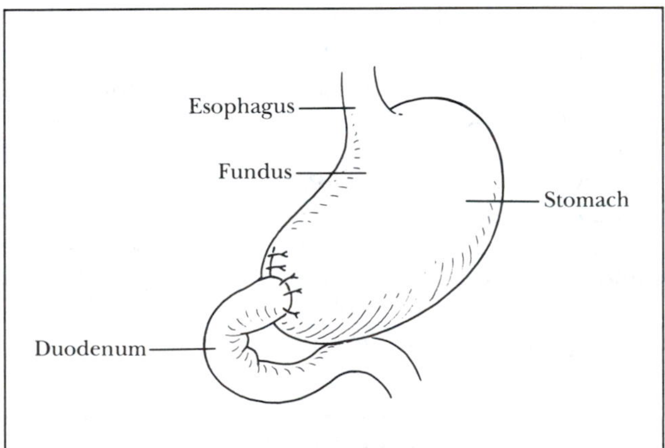

FIGURE 41-5 A Billroth I, or gastroduodenostomy, involves resection of the proximal duodenum, distal stomach, pylorus, and supporting structures.

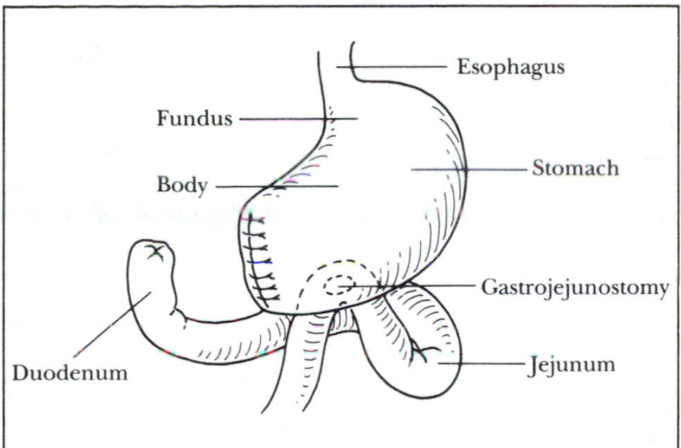

FIGURE 41-6 A Billroth II, or gastrojejunostomy, is a wider resection than the Billroth I. Up to 75% of the stomach can be resected. The remaining stomach is then anastomosed end-to-side to the jejunum.

gastrectomy is performed.[81,89] In some cases a total gastrectomy and distal esophagectomy will be selected for more extensive resection. This entails *en bloc* removal of the lower portion of the esophagus and supporting circulatory and lymphatic structures, removal of most of the greater and lesser omenta, and resection of the cardia, fundus, and body (sometimes a total gastrectomy). The esophagus is sutured to the duodenum or jejunum. A thoracoabdominal approach may be required. Potential complications include pneumonia, anastomotic leak, infection, reflux aspiration, and esophagitis.[86]

Postoperative care

Nursing measures for the person with gastric cancer who undergoes surgical resection do not differ from those for other individuals who undergo gastric surgery. The nurse must be acutely aware of the preoperative status of the individual and employ the nursing measures necessary to maintain or improve the person's preoperative condition. Pneumonia, infection, anastomotic leak, hemorrhage, and reflux aspiration are frequent complications following radical gastric surgery.[90] Occasionally, a patient will experience bezoar formations (ingested fibrous food clumping), causing gastric outlet obstruction. These can be dissolved with enzymes, such as papain, or may require surgical removal.

Dumping syndrome is a potential sequela of subtotal gastrectomy and total gastrectomy that affects many but not all individuals. Small, frequent feedings of low-carbohydrate, high-fat, high-protein foods are recommended. It is important to restrict liquids for 30–40 minutes before and after a meal to avoid the effects of dumping syndrome.[91] Antispasmodics and antiperistaltics can reduce diarrhea. Vitamin B_{12} deficiency will occur; thus, monthly parenteral replacement therapy is necessary to prevent pernicious anemia.

Radiation Therapy

Gastric adenocarcinomas generally are radiosensitive but are deep in the abdomen and often widely disseminated. In the abdomen are dose-limited organs (stomach, liver, kidney, spinal cord) that restrict the use of radiotherapy. Radiation therapy can be administered as adjuvant therapy in conjunction with chemotherapy or surgery. It is particularly useful for treating locally advanced or recurrent disease. Patients seem to tolerate 4000–5000 cGy administered in fractionated doses over 4–5 weeks.[87] Transient effects on the rapidly proliferating epithelial cells of the gastrointestinal tract may lead to abdominal cramps, diarrhea, anorexia, nausea, vomiting, or weight loss.

Radiotherapy is used to augment loco-regional control of residual or unresectable gastric cancer. Multimodal approaches using radiation and chemotherapy for patients with unresectable disease have been documented to improve survival, versus either radiotherapy or chemotherapy alone.[80,92] The sequence of administering chemotherapy and radiotherapy could take advantage of any radiosensitization effect, diminished repopulation between treatments, or synergistic effect.[93]

Intraoperative radiotherapy (IORT) is being used most extensively in Japan.[92,94] The advantages of delivering radiotherapy intraoperatively are the direct visualization of the site to be irradiated and the opportunity to manually move dose-limited tissues out of the field during the radiation.[94] Hemorrhage and fistula are potential complications.[92] The disadvantages of this treatment approach are the special equipment, operating room, and extensive professional collaboration required. IORT is provided by only a few institutions in the United States. Its role in the management of gastric cancer has not been studied well enough to know the full impact of this approach.

Chemotherapy

Interest in chemotherapy has increased in recent years, since a number of therapy regimens appear to have significant activity in gastric cancer. No specific chemotherapeutic regimen alone has been able to establish a clear impact on patient survival of gastric cancer. Single agents (5-FU, doxorubicin, cisplatin, etoposide, and mitomycin-C) have been studied, but combination-drug therapy appears to be superior. Single agents typically produce response rates in 20% of cases, whereas combination chemotherapy can result in 30%–50% response rates.[95,96]

The combination regimens used most commonly are FAM (5-FU, doxorubicin (Adriamycin), mitomycin-C), FAP (5-FU, doxorubicin, platinol), FAMTX (5-FU, doxorubicin, leucovorin), and EAP (etoposide, doxorubicin, cisplatin).[96–98] Other drugs used in combination regimens include cisplatin, its analogs, and nitrosoureas.[99,100] Toxicities depend on the drug and the dose.

Alternative methods of delivery are being investigated, such as intrahepatic and intraperitoneal administration[95,101,102]

Combining chemotherapy and biotherapy has little therapeutic benefit.[103] Survival time is increased somewhat when chemotherapy is used with surgical resection or radiotherapy.[104] At present, objective response rates of gastric tumors treated with chemotherapy are low and have not substantiated chemotherapy as a standard clinical treatment.

Supportive Therapy

Advanced gastric cancer can result in the individual's rapid deterioration. Medical and nursing management is aimed at controlling symptoms and maintaining optimal function. As gastric cancer advances, nutrition becomes a serious problem, either because of disruption of gastric continuity or gastric dysfunction. Lack of gastric secretory function leads to both enzyme and nutrient deficiencies. The resulting malnutrition decreases the individual's ability to withstand therapy, fight infection, and perform self-care activities. Nutritional surveillance and aggressive approaches to maintaining a high level of nutrition are nursing priorities. The reader is referred to Chapter 27 for suggestions for management of nutritional problems. From the time of diagnosis until death due to gastric cancer, nutrition will present one of the most challenging management problems.

When gastric cancer spreads to the most common metastatic sites (regional lymph nodes, intraperitoneal, liver, pancreas, lung, and bone), the manifestations of disease in those areas will require the anticipatory and symptomatic nursing measures discussed in the chapters on specific manifestations of cancer. Individuals with gastric cancer commonly die from bronchopneumonia or lung abscess secondary to malnutrition or immobility. Other causes of death seen with gastric cancer are deep-vein thrombosis, pulmonary emboli, anastomotic rupture, or a second primary tumor.[87]

Many patients and their families feel a strong sense of guilt and negligence if the patient has delayed seeking medical attention or self-medicated for any length of time. The nurse can support the individual and family by dispelling misconceptions and promoting a realistic sense of hope.

LIVER CANCER

INTRODUCTION

Liver cancer continues to be a serious problem in many areas of the world. In Africa and Asia, primary liver cancer is one of the leading causes of death from cancer.[105] In the United States, experience with liver tumors in children and adults is limited by the small number of cases. Many critical questions about this disease remain unanswered. Liver cancers have unusual clinical and pathologic features. At present, no specific treatment effectively controls this aggressive malignancy. Liver cancer disseminates within the liver early and is frequently associated with cirrhosis. Early detection and diagnosis are critical.

EPIDEMIOLOGY

An unusual epidemiologic aspect of liver cancer is its geographic distribution. Primary liver cancer is uncommon in North America, but it is a major problem in some of the more populous areas of the world, including South Africa, Asia, and the Pacific areas.[105] The United States has approximately 15,800 new cases and 12,600 deaths from primary liver cancer each year.[1] In some areas of the world, liver cancer is up to five times more prevalent among males than among females.[105] The average age of onset is 60–70 years; however, liver tumors are encountered in persons of all ages. Liver cancer among children in Western countries is rare, yet it is the fifth most common malignancy of children in Taiwan.[106]

ETIOLOGY

Hepatocellular carcinomas are associated with alcohol-induced, nutritional, or posthepatic cirrhosis. A rare form of cirrhosis called *hemochromatoses* (a genetic disorder of iron deposits in parenchymal cells) in combination with cirrhosis is associated with primary liver tumors. It is suggested that the chronic liver injury and subsequent continuous regeneration associated with cirrhosis precipitates a loss of normal cellular controls leading to liver neoplasia.

A close relationship has been identified between liver cancer and infection with hepatitis B or hepatitis C. Viral hepatitis infection causes liver damage and cirrhosis and appears to increase the risk of developing liver cancer.[107–110] There is a suggested carcinogenic interaction between hepatitis B virus and transforming growth factor-alpha, which is expressed at high levels in persons with liver cancer.[111]

Malnutrition has been cited as an etiologic factor, because many of the geographic areas with a high incidence of liver cancer are replete with food shortages, poverty, and malnutrition.[107] No particular nutrient deficiency has been identified, although the incidence of kwashiorkor (a form of protein-calorie malnutrition) closely parallels that of liver cancer. There is also a high incidence of liver cancer in tropical climates and areas where mold spoilage is significant.

Aflatoxins, mycotoxins derived from the fungus *Aspergillus flavus* and *A. parasiticus,* are among the naturally occurring substances that have become suspect as etiologic agents.[107,112,113] In Africa and Taiwan, researchers have found a correlation between the incidence of liver cancer and areas where food sources are heavily contaminated by aflatoxin.[113]

Thorotrast, a drug formerly used as a biliary contrast medium, may have produced progressive liver damage, which after a latent period of approximately 20 years may develop into liver cancer.[112] An increased incidence of liver damage and liver tumors has been reported among those working with vinyl chloride.

Ingestion of estrogen, androgens, or oral contraceptives has been reported to be associated with liver tumors; however, mostly benign tumors were involved.[114] Short-term use appears to have no association.[115] The relationship of oral contraceptives to liver tumors is unclear and the evidence scanty.

The association between etiologic factors and the development of liver cancer is not strong at this time, mostly because of the limited number of cases of primary liver cancer. Environmental, clinical, and genetic factors have all been suggested. It is hoped that further investigation will provide definitive explanations.

PATHOPHYSIOLOGY

Tumors in the liver may be a primary cancer of the liver or secondary tumors that have metastasized from other sites. One of the most critical issues in the diagnosis and treatment of liver cancer is to differentiate whether the cancer is a primary liver tumor or a metastatic growth.

Cellular Characteristics

Primary liver carcinoma

Most primary tumors of the liver are adenocarcinomas of two cell types: about 90% are hepatocellular carcinomas arising from liver cells; about 7% are cholangiocarcinomas arising from the bile duct cells; and a very small proportion are hepatoblastomas, angiosarcomas, or sarcomas.[105,107]

The macroscopic appearance of primary hepatocellular carcinoma is either nodular, massive, or diffuse. The *nodular* type consists of multiple, similarly sized, widely dispersed clusters of cells. The *massive* type often has a single dominant large mass from which there are associated satellite nodules. The *diffuse* form is characterized by an extensive pattern of infiltration that may involve the entire liver. All three forms of hepatocellular carcinoma originate mainly in the right lobe. The tumor may be multicentric in origin, as commonly seen in cirrhotic livers, or it may start with a single focus that subsequently develops satellite lesions. Hepatocellular carcinomas generally are soft, highly vascular, and diffluent with stroma. Parts of the liver may be dull gray or green as a result of the presence of bile. There may also be areas of necrosis and hemorrhage. Cholangiocarcinomas also exhibit nodular or diffuse forms but usually appear as a solitary grayish white mass. This firm, fibrous tumor may secrete mucin but does not form bile. Cholangiocarcinoma tends to invade surrounding parenchyma in a disorderly, irregular manner and to metastasize late.

Liver tumors are often well-differentiated lesions with clearly defined margins and cells that are larger than normal parenchymal cells. About 50% of patients with primary liver cancer will not develop extrahepatic spread of tumor.[105] When it occurs, it is usually to the diaphragm and neighboring tissues or the portal and/or hepatic veins. Regional lymph node metastasis is uncommon—a definitive characteristic of liver cancer. Tumor encapsulation and longer doubling time may be used as indicators of survival.[116,117]

Secondary liver carcinoma

The liver is a repository for metastatic deposits from nearly all sites and is 20 times more likely to harbor a metastatic deposit than a primary liver cancer.[118] Metastases to the liver usually are from the following high-incidence sites: lung, breast, kidney, and the intestinal tract (gallbladder, extrahepatic bile ducts, pancreas, stomach, colon, and rectum).[119] Metastasis may occur as a single mass, but metastatic deposits more often are multiple masses in the liver. Spread within the rest of the liver is through the extensive venous system. Metastatic tumors in the liver usually indicate that the primary carcinoma is incurable. However, if a localized metastasis in the liver can be resected or controlled with chemotherapy, then the primary tumor can be aggressively pursued. It is uncommon for a cancer to metastasize to a cirrhotic liver, possibly because the tissue damage precludes a favorable environment for metastases.[120]

Progression of Disease

Liver cancer tends to advance by direct extension within and around the liver. The tumor will enlarge within the lobules that have been weakened by pressure and derangement of the blood supply. Venous invasion commonly accounts for the multinodular appearance of hepatocellular carcinoma. The tumor grows along the veins as a solid mass to distal parts of the liver.[107] About 50% of individuals with liver cancer will have distant metastases to regional lymph nodes, lungs, bone, adrenal glands, and brain.[107,112]

Normal liver tissue receives its blood supply from both the hepatic artery and the portal vein and drains via the hepatic vein. Liver tumors typically alter the pattern of bloodflow within the liver. Tumors receive their blood supply almost exclusively from the hepatic artery and drain via the hepatic vein.[121] Within the liver the tumor may spread by emboli or by direct permeation of the hepatic and portal vein, resulting in rapid spread of the tumor throughout the liver. Portal vein occlusion is common.[107]

As liver cancer advances, serious complications arise and multiple body systems become affected. Liver failure and hemorrhage have been cited as the cause of death of about 50% of individuals with liver cancer.[122] It is postulated that if the portal vein becomes obstructed rapidly, as occurs with tumor emboli, there is insufficient time for the collateral branches of the hepatic circulatory system to compensate. As a result, the tamponade effect can lead to necrosis, rupture, and hemorrhage. Esophageal varices and unrelenting ascites are common sequelae of either primary or secondary liver cancer.

Because of the late onset of definitive signs, liver cancer can be far advanced by the time of diagnosis. The prognosis is poor, with an overall 5-year survival rate of about 5%.[1] If the disease is untreated, death usually occurs within 6–8 weeks following diagnosis.[123] The cause of death from liver cancer most often is pneumonia, malnutrition, thromboemboli, hepatic failure, or hemorrhage.[112]

CLINICAL MANIFESTATIONS

The natural history of carcinoma of the liver is insidious. The tumor can grow to huge proportions before symptoms appear. In adults the most common clinical manifestation is right upper quadrant abdominal pain that is not severe but, rather, dull and aching. The pain may radiate to the right scapula. The continuous pain may become more troublesome, prevent sleep, and be aggravated if the patient lies on the right side or experiences jolting movements. Profound, progressive weakness and fatigue are characteristic of liver cancer. Fullness in the epigastrium, especially after meals, and constipation or diarrhea are common manifestations. Anorexia and loss of weight are indicators of advanced disease.

Mild jaundice is present in some cases. Cirrhosis is found in 30%–70% of persons with hepatocellular carcinoma.[112] On palpation, the liver is an enlarged, hard, nodular mass; a pedunculated tumor occasionally can be felt. Enlargement may be either diffuse or limited to one lobe (usually the right). Liver cancer should be suspected in all persons with cirrhosis who experience sudden or unexpected deterioration in health.

Ascites and signs of portal hypertension that result from portal vein compression frequently accompany advanced disease. Hematemesis secondary to esophageal varices or tumor invasion of the stomach can occur. Paraneoplastic complications may occur, such as erythrocytosis, hypercalcemia, hypoglycemia, leukocytosis, carcinoidlike syndrome, porphyria, and coagulation abnormalities.[105]

ASSESSMENT

Primary liver cancer is silent for a long period before it produces signs and symptoms that prompt the individual to seek medical attention. The person may be treated initially for a disorder that mimics liver cancer, such as gastritis. Primary liver cancer must be distinguished from secondary liver cancer due to metastases. The only definitive diagnostic tool is tissue diagnosis. Unfortunately, the risk of hemorrhage following needle biopsy is significant; therefore, noninvasive measures are relied on heavily. The choice of therapy will be based on the location and extent of tumor involvement, whether extrahepatic spread has occurred, and the individual's general condition.

Physical Examination

A complete physical examination usually will reveal a painful, enlarged liver and such manifestations as ascites, edema, circulatory disorders, esophageal varices, jaundice, and hematemesis.[112] Endocrine changes, such as menstrual disorders, testicular atrophy, and gynecomastia, may be observed.

Diagnostic Studies

A simple radiograph of the abdomen may establish hepatomegaly and displacement or deformity of contiguous structures. An upper gastrointestinal series may evidence organ displacement. Plain films are useful in advanced disease but cannot be used for early diagnosis.

Ultrasound of the abdomen, CT of the abdomen and lungs, and MRI are noninvasive techniques used in the diagnostic evaluation of liver cancer. Ultrasound can detect masses and help determine the extent of invasion of the vasculature of the liver. Periodic ultrasound has been used as a screening measure for high-risk individuals.[105] CT, particularly with contrast, is able to demonstrate small lesions and vascular rearrangements. The CT scan is effective for detecting metastatic disease. MRI is as effective as CT for imaging liver tumors, but experience with the equipment is limited in certain areas of the country.

Radionuclide scanning is an effective noninvasive technique for outlining primary and metastatic tumors of the liver. Small lesions (<2.5 cm in diameter) may be missed by the photoscanning device. The SPECT imaging equipment has increased the rate of detection. The difference between a malignant and a benign tumor cannot be discerned with a scan; therefore, these findings should be correlated with the biopsy, laboratory studies, and hepatic arteriogram.

Selective hepatic arteriography is the single most useful procedure for identifying tumor vasculature and showing any abnormalities in the liver's blood supply.[124] This information will serve as the "road map" for ligation of vessels during hepatic resection, chemotherapy administration, or therapeutic diversion of bloodflow. For 24 hours following the procedure, the individual undergoing arteriography should be observed carefully for signs of hemorrhage from a perforated or weakened vessel.

Laboratory studies

The hematologic profiles and liver function tests of individuals with localized primary cancer who do not have cirrhosis will show normal findings. In the absence of cirrhosis, tumor growth can extensively involve parenchyma before liver function is impaired. Liver enzyme levels and liver function tests are not definitive diagnostic aids but can alert the clinician to a possible tumor.

Alpha-fetoprotein (AFP) is a tumor marker that is elevated in the serum of 70%–90% of persons with primary hepatocellular carcinoma.[105,107,112,125] AFP disappears 1–2 weeks after a hepatocellular carcinoma is successfully resected. A reappearance of AFP can indicate recurrence. Serial monitoring of AFP levels is being evaluated for definitive use as a measure of the effectiveness of therapy.

Serum alpha-L-fucosidase is a new serum marker being investigated with liver cancer.[126] Not all liver cancers secrete AFP, so other early indicators are needed. Elevated levels of carcinoembryonic antigen (CEA) are not indicative of primary liver cancer but may signify metastatic involvement. Colon cancer often metastasizes to the liver and will produce elevated CEA levels.

Biopsy

Biopsy is required to establish a histologic diagnosis. Many clinicians feel strongly that needle biopsy should be avoided at all cost if there is any chance for curative resection. They believe that the needle violates the tumor capsule, thereby potentially seeding and spreading the cancer. If a tumor appears to be resectable, tissue can be obtained during surgery, thus avoiding potential problems with bleeding.[127] If the tumor appears to be unresectable, a percutaneous needle biopsy can be performed with ultrasound or CT guidance. Needle biopsy should be done only on cooperative individuals with normal hemostatic function. The individual must be monitored closely for intraabdominal hemorrhage following needle biopsy. Potential complications following liver biopsy are hemorrhage, shock, peritonitis, and pneumothorax.

STAGING

A staging system has been developed for liver cancer that incorporates tumor size, location within the liver, extent of disease within and external to the liver, and metastatic sites.[27] The staging system has not been universally accepted but is available for use. See Table 41-4.

TABLE 41-4 TNM Classification System for Liver Cancer

PRIMARY TUMOR (T)	
TX	Primary tumor cannot be assessed
T0	No evidence of primary tumor
T1	Solitary tumor 2 cm or less in greatest dimension without vascular invasion
T2	Solitary tumor 2 cm or less in greatest dimension with vascular invasion, *or* Multiple tumors limited to one lobe, none more than 2 cm in greatest dimension without vascular invasion, *or* A solitary tumor more than 2 cm in greatest dimension without vascular invasion
T3	Solitary tumor more than 2 cm in greatest dimension with vascular invasion, *or* Multiple tumors limited to one lobe, none more than 2 cm in greatest dimension, with vascular invasion, *or* Multiple tumors limited to one lobe, any more than 2 cm in greatest dimension, with or without vascular invasion
T4	Multiple tumors in more than one lobe *or* Tumor(s) involve(s) a major branch of portal or hepatic vein(s)

REGIONAL LYMPH NODES (N)	
NX	Regional lymph nodes cannot be assessed
N0	No regional lymph node metastasis
N1	Regional lymph node metastasis

DISTANT METASTASIS (M)	
MX	Presence of distant metastasis cannot be assessed
M0	No distant metastasis
M1	Distant metastasis

STAGE GROUPING			
Stage I	T1	N0	M0
Stage II	T2	N0	M0
Stage III	T1	N1	M0
	T2	N1	M0
	T3	N0, N1	M0
Stage IVA	T4	Any N	M0
Stage IVB	Any T	Any N	M1

Source: Beahrs OH, Henson DE, Hutter RV, et al (eds): *American Joint Committee on Cancer: Manual for Staging of Cancer* (4th ed). Philadelphia: Lippincott, 1992.

TREATMENT

Treatment Planning

Treatment of liver cancer provides a twofold challenge. First, the limited number of cases of primary liver cancer makes prospective systematic investigation of therapy difficult. Second, the dismal outlook for persons with liver cancer has led to misconceptions about the effectiveness of various treatments, which have taken years to dispel. Surgery, radiotherapy, and chemotherapy play a significant role in the treatment of both primary and secondary liver cancer. At present, biotherapy has a more limited clinical role.

The 5-year survival rate for persons with primary liver cancer is low, less than 2%.[112] However, for individuals with solitary, localized liver cancer, advances in surgery, radiotherapy, and chemotherapy offer hope of cure or extended control. The choice of treatment depends on a number of factors: type and extent of the tumor, concomitant diseases, liver function and reserve, patient/family preference, hematologic status, nutritional status, age, and skill of the principal clinicians. Assessment of the patient's learning ability, coping mechanisms, and compliance potential are of great importance, especially if long-term therapy is anticipated.

Pretreatment therapy

Prior to the initiation of any therapeutic modality, physiologic parameters are examined carefully. Most individuals with primary liver cancer have some degree of anemia, which should be corrected. Efforts are made by the nurse and other health care workers to conserve the individual's energy and to begin instruction on appropriate measures to help minimize the anemia.

Depending on the extent of liver dysfunction produced by tumor involvement, deficits in clotting mechanisms can exist. Vitamin K is administered, fluid and electrolyte imbalances are corrected, and measures to prevent trauma or bleeding are taken.

Vitamins A, C, D, and B complex can be given to reduce the effect of jaundice. Pruritus, which frequently accompanies jaundice, is precipitated by irritation of the cutaneous sensory nerve fibers by accumulated bile salts. Meticulous skin hygiene and efforts to reduce itching are instituted. The use of deodorant soaps should be avoided, since they tend to dry the skin and intensify the pruritus. Relief is sometimes obtained with oil-based lotions, antihistamines, or cholestyramine. Side effects of cholestyramine are nausea, vomiting, constipation, and bleeding tendencies.[22] The only effective measure for relief of pruritus is resolution of the jaundice.

Most individuals with liver cancer are in a poor nutritional state and benefit greatly from a diet high in proteins and carbohydrates and moderate in fats. If weight loss has been significant (more than 7 kg/mo), enteral feedings or total parenteral nutrition may be used to correct the nutritional imbalance. If the treatment is expected to affect nutritional status adversely, aggressive nutrition regimens must begin early.

Objectives of treatment

Primary liver cancer Cure is the objective of therapy if the primary liver tumor is a localized, solitary mass without evidence of regional lymph node involvement or distant metastases. Aggressive efforts toward eradicating the tumor and possible micrometastases will be planned. Surgical excision of the primary liver cancer is the only definitive treatment for cure. Only about 25% of patients with primary liver cancer are candidates for radical resection.[107] Adjuvant chemotherapy and radiotherapy usually are initiated to eliminate residual cancer cells or micrometastases.

If the tumor is multicentric, involves a large portion of the liver, or involves extrahepatic areas, control of tumor growth is the objective of therapy. Control can be achieved by surgical resection to remove or debulk the tumor, by radiotherapy, or by specific vascular ligation or cannulation followed by aggressive use of chemotherapeutic agents.

Palliation of the disabling effects of liver cancer may be the objective of treatment for advanced disease. Surgery, chemotherapy, and radiotherapy are used selectively to increase the individual's comfort and quality of life.

Secondary liver tumors When metastatic deposits occur in the liver, cure of the primary cancer is difficult. Aggressive therapy is employed if the metastatic deposit is a solitary or well-defined mass in a single lobe of the liver. Treatment of metastatic tumors to the liver may be surgical excision, arterial infusion of chemotherapeutic agents, ligation or embolization of the hepatic artery, or radiotherapy.[124,128] The aim of aggressive treatment of metastatic tumors in the liver is to control the tumor, increase survival time, and palliate debilitating symptoms (such as jaundice, anemia, and pain). An individual with colorectal carcinoma that has metastasized to the liver is the typical candidate for resection, since the liver usually is the first metastatic site for colorectal tumors. The primary colon cancer can be subsequently eradicated in some cases.

Surgery

Surgical excision is the most definitive treatment for primary liver tumors.[124,129] If cirrhosis is present, the surgical risk is directly proportional to the degree of cirrhosis. If the noncancerous lobe of the liver is macroscopically normal or only mildly cirrhotic, lobectomy can be undertaken safely. If cirrhosis is moderately advanced, left lobectomy can be considered; however, right hepatic lobectomy would be difficult and potentially life-threatening. Local resection, ultrasound-guided cryosurgery, or laser surgery may be possible.[129,130] Patients with severe cirrhosis are not candidates for surgery.

Extensive assessment must be done prior to hepatic resection to identify any possible contraindications. In addition to severe cirrhosis, contraindications to major hepatic resection include:[105,112]

1. Distant metastases in the lung, bone, or lymph nodes indicate that an attempt at cure or control would likely be futile. Multiple discrete tumor nodules throughout both anatomic lobes would rule out surgery as the treatment of choice.
2. Although not always the case, jaundice could indicate tumor extension or obstruction of the common bile duct. Palliative resection of the tumor can be done to relieve the progressive jaundice.
3. Ascites usually indicates liver failure and inability to tolerate a surgical procedure. The ascites may result from tumor cell seeding in the peritoneal cavity and/or cirrhosis. In either case it is preferable to control the ascites medically; surgery could be considered but is risky.
4. Poor visualization on angiographic studies jeopardizes the certainty with which the surgeon resects the tumor. Because the liver is a highly vascular organ, intraoperative hemorrhage is a great risk in all hepatic surgical procedures.
5. Biochemical changes that indicate poor liver function lower the probability of survival.
6. Involvement of the inferior vena cava or retrograde intraluminal growth within and to the portal vein bifurcation makes surgical excision hazardous.

Therefore, if the tumor is localized, solitary, and can be defined anatomically, a wide *en bloc* surgical excision is the initial treatment of choice for both primary and secondary liver tumors. From 80%–85% of the noncirrhotic liver can be removed safely unless the tumor is in the posterior segment of the right lobe, where the hepatic veins are embedded. Because the hepatic veins can be difficult to isolate, resection is considered a dangerous procedure.[105] Hepatic lobectomy includes all the vessels involved with the lobe and requires extensive operative time. Partial resections (segmentectomy, wedge resection) are used with mildly cirrhotic patients.[131] Cryosurgery with liquid nitrogen has been employed for local excision of tumors in patients with nonresectable liver cancer.[130,132] The reader is referred to specific references for detailed information about the techniques of hepatic surgical procedures.[119,133,134] Liver transplantation is still in the experimental stage and fraught with a high incidence of recurrent cancer in the transplanted liver.[135]

Primary cancers of the liver develop a neovascular network arising exclusively from the hepatic artery. Hepatic artery occlusion or embolization is used to deprive the tumor of its blood supply and thereby necrose the tumor.[136] In some cases an occluder with an inflatable cuff is inserted and periodically inflated to interrupt the bloodflow and induce tumor regression.[105] Embolization can be induced with injection of nondegradable particles such as polyvinyl alcohol and cellulose. Degradable products such as starch microspheres and Gelfoam cubes are used for temporary occlusion. Several trials are under way to evaluate the effect of using chemotherapeutic agents adsorbed onto Gelfoam cubes or microspheres.[137] Ethanol injections under ultrasound guidance are a recently developed therapeutic option that takes advantage of selective diffusion of the cytotoxic ethanol into liver cancer cells.[138] Other approaches include suspensions of chemotherapy mixed in an oily contrast medium to enhance retention of the drug in the microvasculature of the liver for prolonged tumor-drug exposure.[139] Repeated transcatheter arterial embolization has been used to produce focal necrosis of the tumor.[107,112] These approaches are considered experimental and have not yet been proven superior to other treatment methods.

Postoperative care

Overall surgical mortality (individuals who do not survive the hospitalization period) is less than 15% with hepatic resection.[112,140–142] Individuals who have had hepatic resection require intensive medical and nursing support. The principal concerns in the care of an individual undergoing hepatic surgery are control of hemorrhage, replacement of blood loss, prevention of infection and pneumonia, and appropriate supportive care. The individual with cirrhosis will have greater difficulty in the postoperative period than the individual who is not cirrhotic. Knowledge of the potential complications, expected reactions, and anticipatory nursing care will aid immeasurably in the postoperative period. The major complications following liver resection include:

- hemorrhage
- biliary fistula
- infection
- transient metabolic consequences
- subphrenic abscess
- pneumonia
- atelectasis
- portal hypertension
- clotting defects

Postoperative complications

Hemorrhage The abundant vascularity of the liver cannot be overemphasized. Despite preventive measures to control bleeding, intraabdominal hemorrhage must be recognized early, i.e., before the condition is irreversible. Hemorrhage usually will appear within the first 24 hours following surgery. Nursing observations and assessments should include: frequent monitoring of vital signs; CVP monitoring; examination of the skin and extremities for perfusion; accurate measurement of abdominal girth; frequent checks for bleeding from incision sites, urine, and stool; and close attention to fluid and electrolyte levels and blood profiles. In addition, cirrhotic individuals should be watched closely for overt and subclinical signs of bleeding disorders, due to their predisposition to hematologic complications.

Biliary fistula In most individuals undergoing hepatic resection, a T-tube is placed in the common bile duct for drainage. A subhepatic drain also may be placed in the area of the surgical resection. A small amount of bile is expected to drain through the subhepatic drain from the necrosis on the edge of the liver. However, an excessive drainage of bile through the subhepatic drain could indicate a biliary fistula pouring large amounts of bile into the subhepatic space. The T-tube also can slip outside the common bile duct. The dislodged T-tube may continue to drain small amounts of bile, thus masking its malposition, but the properly positioned T-tube normally will drain about 400 ml of bile per day. Fever, pain, and altered vital signs accompany biliary fistula.

Subphrenic abscess Incomplete or insufficient drainage of the surgical defect can precipitate a subphrenic abscess. Close attention to vital signs and to the function and output of the drainage tubes should continue for an extended period, because the abscess will appear later in the postoperative course. Auscultation of the base of the lungs could signal the presence of the abscess and fluid accumulation. Development of sharp, piercing right upper quadrant pain later in the postoperative course and a low-grade fever are other warning signs.

Infection Individuals with cirrhosis are more prone to infection following hepatic resection than individuals without cirrhosis. The mortality associated with serious infection is high. Frequent monitoring of vital signs and assessment of the wound and drainage will provide early clues of impending infection. Constant, intermittent, or remittent hyperthermia or hypothermia secondary to infection requires aggressive intervention.

Pneumonia and atelectasis Nursing care directed toward prevention of respiratory complications is similar to that for any other person with abdominal or thoracic surgery. Aggressive pulmonary hygiene is especially important. These individuals will be reluctant to comply because respiratory exercises cause significant incisional pain. Early ambulation, administration of analgesics prior to pulmonary exercise, incisional support, and avoidance of contact with persons with respiratory infections are important nursing care measures.

Transient metabolic consequences Jaundice is common during the first postoperative week. Jaundice may result from the temporary inability of the remaining liver to handle bile, but the condition usually subsides by the third week, when the remaining liver regenerates. More often, however, jaundice results from the multiple transfusions and anoxia of the hepatocytes caused by vascular occlusion during surgery. If the jaundice in an individual without cirrhosis does not subside after 10 days, mechanical obstruction should be suspected. Nursing measures to relieve the discomforts of jaundice are discussed earlier, in the section on pretreatment planning.

Portal hypertension Another transient postoperative consequence of hepatic resection that the nurse should anticipate is portal hypertension. Portal hypertension is the result of the surgical rerouting of portal venous flow through a small remnant of liver, which leads to splanchnic circulatory sequestration. Fortunately, the liver has a great potential for increasing bloodflow if it is given adequate time to compensate. Central venous pressure monitoring is a good indicator of blood volume. Bleeding episodes from any cavity, wound, or puncture site require immediate intervention.

Clotting defects The prothrombin time may be delayed during the first week. Severe coagulopathies generally develop during the operative period and usually are not a concern postoperatively. The nurse should take measures to prevent and/or detect complications from deficiencies in the clotting mechanisms, such as applying pressure to injection sites, monitoring abdominal girth, and testing urine and stool for blood.

Chemotherapy

The majority of individuals with primary liver cancer are not candidates for curative or palliative surgery; therefore, chemotherapy may be the treatment of choice. Metastatic tumors to the liver also can be treated with chemotherapeutic agents, but surgical excision is the preferred therapy. Systemic administration of single-agent therapy has produced poor results; however, current trials of combination therapy are producing more promising results. Chemotherapeutic agents can be administered by two approaches: systemic administration of single or combination drug regimens, and regional infusion via hepatic artery or portal vein.[112] Chemotherapeutic agents used with primary and secondary liver cancer include doxorubicin, FUDR, 5-FU, cisplatin, streptozotocin, etoposide, mitomycin-C, folinic acid, mitoxantrone, epirubicin, methyl CCNU, and teniposide.[143–146] Significant interest in the role of biotherapy has spurred a number of investigations that have not yielded better results than current treatment approaches.[147,148]

Because a significant number of patients with liver cancer have bulky, unresectable disease that does not extend beyond the liver, regional therapy becomes a viable treatment alternative. The premise on which regional therapy is based is the ability to provide a high concentration of the drug directly and continuously to the tumor, with minimal systemic exposure.[149,150] Dose limitations are related to hepatic toxicity and upper gastrointestinal toxicity (ulcer, gastritis).[149,151,152] Continuous infusion pumps and the totally implantable pumps have renewed clinicians' interest in regional therapy.[144] Development of selective angiography has greatly aided the clinician in determining the pattern of bloodflow to the tumor and to normal liver tissue. In addition, advances in surgical technique for catheter placement have improved outcomes. Infections are an uncommon experience.[153] Catheters are placed into the specifically defined vessels identified as the major source of blood supply to the tumor.[151] Drugs that have been used for regional chemotherapy administration include 5-FU, cisplatin, doxorubicin, mitomycin-C, nitrogen mustard, and methotrexate.[154]

In general, regional infusion is considered superior to systemic chemotherapy.[151] A study by Safi et al.[155] indicates that the combination of both regional infusion and systemic therapy actually may prolong survival. Regional infusions have been combined with radiotherapy. However, if more than 50% of the liver is involved with tumor or if the major vessels to the liver are narrowed or nonfunctional, systemic chemotherapy usually is the route of administration selected.

Intraperitoneal administration of 5-FU has been well tolerated by patients and produces results comparable to those with regional infusion therapy.[156] Further investigation is needed to explore the role of intraperitoneal chemotherapy in liver cancer.

Radiotherapy

To date, because of the poor tolerance of normal liver tissue, the role of radiotherapy in liver cancer therapy is limited to palliation. Many questions still are unanswered regarding how high a dose of radiation normal liver can tolerate. Relief of pain, improvements in strength, increased appetite, and increased liver function have been reported with doses ranging from 1900 cGy to 3100 cGy over a period of 2–20 days.[112] A recent development to enhance the effectiveness of radiation therapy without damage to the normal parenchyma is the use of 131 I-Lipidiol, a radio-labeled iodinated contrast medium. When injected intraarterially, the agent is trapped selectively in the microvasculature and has been reported to produce up to a 40% objective response.[157,158] Razoxane, a radiosensitizing agent, has been administered for 3 days before external beam therapy.[159] Prospective, randomized trials are needed to determine the full impact of radiosensitizing agents on liver cancer.

In conjunction with surgery or chemotherapy, radiotherapy is used to palliate symptoms or to eradicate micrometastases. Researchers are investigating the effectiveness of concurrent chemotherapy and radiotherapy and are finding that such regimens have been well tolerated.[160] The major side effects of radiotherapy to the liver are nausea, vomiting, anorexia, and fatigue. These effects usually are compounded when two or more treatment modalities are combined.

Supportive Therapy

The prognosis for the person with liver cancer is dismal. Most individuals die within 6 months of diagnosis. The tumor proliferates rapidly and is difficult to detect and to treat. Individuals in advanced stages of the disease will experience hepatic failure, severe ascites, infection, bleeding diathesis, pain, weight loss, weakness, and pneumonia. The patient and family should be kept informed of the treatment plans and assured that efforts will be made to provide relief of symptoms.[161]

Pain is one of the most difficult problems to manage. In later stages the pain is severe, worsens at night, and often radiates to the right scapular or subscapular area. Position, activity, coughing, and deep breathing make the pain worse. Pulmonary hygiene can be attempted only when pain relief measures are most effective.

Ascites can become severe in advanced disease. Palliative measures to control ascites include fluid and sodium restriction, diuretic therapy, paracentesis, and albumin administration.

Anorexia and vomiting may be late-stage manifestations in liver cancer. Antiemetics, vitamin supplements, antidepressants, and tranquilizers have helped some individuals. Relief sometimes is afforded by manipulating the environment, food presentation, and distraction techniques.[162]

Significant weakness, muscle atrophy, and immobility eventually lead to pulmonary congestion, atelectasis, pneumonia, and death. Anticipatory management of the rapidly developing symptoms and patient and family support are the major goals of nursing care in advanced disease.

PANCREATIC CANCER

INTRODUCTION

Cancer of the pancreas is presently the fourth most frequent cause of death from cancer in the United States. It is ninth among all cancers in incidence, which is a remarkable change from a few years ago, when pancreatic cancer was believed to be rare.[1] However, the trend in 5-year relative survival is shifting upward toward 5%.[1] The National Cancer Institute established the National Pancreatic Cancer Project to determine the contributory factors, evaluate the effectiveness of present therapies, and establish guidelines for prevention, detection, and treatment.

Pancreatic cancer is one of the most difficult tumors

to detect or diagnose because of the anatomic location and biologic nature of the tumor. Its onset is insidious, with signs and symptoms that occur late, are vague and misleading, and mimic other diseases. The person with pancreatic cancer typically will ignore or rely on self-treatment of the initial signs and symptoms for months. The prognosis is poor, and the outlook for the person with this disease is guarded but improving. Fewer than 5% of individuals with pancreatic cancer are alive at 5 years.[1]

Future improvements in detection, diagnosis, and treatment of pancreatic cancer depend on systematic investigation of traditional and innovative therapeutic approaches and a willingness of practitioners to treat the disease aggressively.

EPIDEMIOLOGY

Cancer of the pancreas accounts for approximately 2% of all cancers in American men and women and results in 5% of all cancer deaths.[1] Cancer of the pancreas occurs at all ages, but peak incidence is between the ages of 60 and 70. It is rare before the age of 45 and rarely affects children.[163,164] Pancreatic carcinoma demonstrates a male dominance, with a male-to-female ratio of 1.3:1.0.[163,164]

The incidence of pancreatic cancer is two times higher in blacks than in native whites.[163] Japanese immigrants to the United States exhibit a higher incidence of pancreatic cancer than native whites.[163,165] Epidemiologic studies demonstrate some clustering in parts of Louisiana, a higher incidence in urban areas, and a higher incidence in American counties with many residents of Scandinavian or Russian descent.[165]

ETIOLOGY

An analysis of reported cases of pancreatic cancer yields relatively few etiologic factors for this disease. Increased risks attributed to environmental factors have been suggested. Persons occupationally exposed in aluminum milling or to gasoline derivatives, naphthylamine, and benzidine are considered to have a higher risk of pancreatic cancer.[163,165]

Blot and colleagues[166] found a correlation in the geographic pattern in the United States for lung cancer and pancreatic cancer, which suggests that tobacco may be a contributing factor. People who smoke more than two packs of cigarettes per day are at much higher risk for pancreatic cancer than are nonsmokers.[167] It has been hypothesized that carcinogenic elements in tobacco, such as nitrosoamines, or chemicals excreted by the liver may be refluxed into the pancreatic duct and result in cancer.

A diet that is high in fat, meat, or both has been associated with the development of pancreatic cancer. Dietary fat may act as a promoter of carcinogenesis. Likewise, diets high in fresh fruits and vegetables appear to provide a protective effect.[164]

A person with a history of peptic ulcer surgery also has a higher risk. Even 15–20 years after surgery, a twofold to fivefold increased risk exists.[164] Diabetes mellitus and chronic pancreatitis have an association with cancer of the pancreas.[168–170] Knowledge of specific risk factors and carcinogens associated with pancreatic cancer is limited by accessibility of epidemiologic data.

PATHOPHYSIOLOGY

Tumors in the pancreas develop in both the exocrine and endocrine parenchyma. Approximately 95% of pancreatic tumors arise from the exocrine parenchyma.[165,171] Islet cell tumors, which can develop in any part of the pancreas as functioning insulinomas or nonfunctioning carcinomas, are rare, constituting 5% of the cases of pancreatic cancer.[172] Adenocarcinoma of ductal cell origin, the predominant (75%–92%) morphologic type, is twice as frequent in the head of the pancreas as in the body or tail.[164]

Cellular Characteristics

Cancer most commonly arises in the proximal areas of the gland, which includes the head, neck, and uncinate process. Adenocarcinomas of the pancreas usually are hard, nodular, firm masses with a large amount of fibrosis. Adenocarcinomas commonly invade the entire pancreas, obliterate the lobulated tissue, and obstruct the common bile duct and Wirsung's canal. Exocrine functions of the gland are interrupted. As tumor growth advances within the pancreas or in lymph nodes along the biliary tree, complete obstruction and compression of the bile duct can result. The gallbladder becomes distended and the liver enlarges.

Pancreatic carcinomas may eventually infiltrate the duodenal musculature, stomach, transverse colon, portal vein, and superior mesenteric vein. Venous invasion or encirclement by tumor growth results in obstruction, thrombosis, ascites, and portal hypertension.

At the time of detection, large tumor masses may be fixed to the retropancreatic tissues or to the vertebral column. The tumor may directly invade the spleen, kidney, or diaphragm. Invasion of the celiac nerve plexus may account for the unrelenting pain associated with carcinoma of the body and tail of the pancreas. Obstruction of the portal vein and tributaries can lead to esophageal varices.

Although uncommon (<5%), islet cell tumors can arise from the endocrine parenchyma. The tumors usually occur as small, well-circumscribed, reddish tissue that rarely extends beyond the pancreas. On microscopy, islet cell tumors are well vascularized and encapsulated and usually compress adjacent parenchyma. Fibrosis and calcification may be seen. Islet cell tumors are difficult to distinguish as malignant because they closely resemble normal islet cells and retain secretory or synthetic functions. This leads many to believe that metastasis is the most reliable criterion for establishing malignancy. Chapter 40 presents a more detailed discussion of endocrine cancers.

Progression of Disease

Characteristically, tumors of the pancreas grow rapidly, with late signs or symptoms of pathology. At the time of diagnosis the cancer has invaded locally or metastasized in 90% of individuals.[173,174] Tumor growth frequently extends or spreads to the common bile duct and perineural and celiac nerve plexus. Metastatic spread initially involves regional and paraduodenal lymph nodes and later develops in mesocolic, parapancreatic, para aortic, mesenteric, and posterior mediastinal nodes and the hilum of the liver as the disease progresses. Supraclavicular nodes may be involved more frequently with carcinoma of the body and tail than with tumors of the head of the pancreas. Metastatic deposits reach the liver through the bloodstream in later stages of the disease. Peritoneal seeding by metastatic deposits can occur. Metastases to the lung, pleura, abdominal viscera, adrenal glands, and bone are common.[164]

Ascites can develop late in the course of the disease. Localized effects of the tumor may be the cause of rapid decline or death. Individuals with advanced pancreatic cancer usually die in a short time of cachexia, infection, or liver failure. Fewer than 15% of persons diagnosed with cancer of the pancreas are alive within 1 year of diagnosis.[164]

CLINICAL MANIFESTATIONS

The early signs and symptoms of pancreatic cancer are vague and are often referred to other organs or systems. Careful assessment and extensive inquiry into the character, onset, duration, and modulators of presenting signs and symptoms will greatly aid definitive diagnosis. Manifestations of disease differ according to the location of the tumor in the pancreas.

Head of Pancreas

When carcinoma involves the head of the pancreas, the signs and symptoms often will appear earlier than with a tumor in the body or tail of the pancreas. A classic triad of symptoms is apparent with cancer of the head of the pancreas: pain, profound weight loss, and progressive jaundice.

Most individuals initially experience pain in the epigastric region, dull and intermittent in nature, and shrug it off as indigestion or gaseous distention. The pain later becomes much more distinctive in nature, possibly as a result of celiac plexus and perineural invasion by tumor. The pain often is continuous and radiates to the right upper quadrant of the abdomen or dorsolumbar area. It may be colicky, dull, or vague in nature. The intensity of the pain is affected by activity, eating, and posture. The pain often is ameliorated if the person lies supine or sits up and bends forward.

Jaundice, precipitated by common bile duct obstruction, is the presenting symptom in 80%–90% of cases of cancer of the head of the pancreas.[174] Regardless of whether jaundice is the initial symptom or follows the onset of pain, it is the symptom that inevitably leads individuals to seek medical assistance. Contrary to previously held beliefs, pain with jaundice is far more common than painless jaundice.[164,165] The evolution of jaundice in pancreatic cancer is distinctive. It appears first on the mucous membranes, then on the palms of the hands, and gradually becomes generalized. The face, genitals, and linea alba are more discolored than other areas. The jaundice is progressive and persistent and leads to severe pruritus, dark urine, and clay-colored stools. Jaundice does not always indicate extensive disease and unresectability.

Weight loss and clinical wasting are classic symptoms of cancer in the head of the pancreas. The weight loss initially may not cause concern and can be attributed to gastric maladies. As the disease advances, weight loss of 20–30 pounds in a few weeks is common and often is accelerated by pain, anorexia, flatulence, nausea, and vomiting. Tumor involvement of the pancreas or common bile duct prevents secretion of digestive enzymes and often diminishes insulin production. Malabsorption can lead to diarrhea, constipation, steatorrhea, and muscle weakness. Metabolic disturbances such as hyperglycemia, glycosuria, and hypoalbuminemia may occur.[164]

Individuals with pancreatic cancer complain of emotional disturbances, such as irritability, depression, and personality changes. Considering the sudden onset of symptoms, severity of pain, and inability to eat or sleep, it is not surprising to find such emotional reactions.

Hemorrhage and bleeding disorders can result from liver involvement. Portal hypertension, hepatomegaly, and gallbladder enlargement are found in a large number of patients.

Body of Pancreas

Tumors in the body of the pancreas produce signs and symptoms late in the disease process, rendering early detection virtually impossible. By the time it is brought to the attention of a physician, the tumor may be large enough to be palpated. Severe epigastric pain usually is the first and predominant symptom. The individual may experience intense epigastric pain 3–4 hours after a meal. The pain often is excruciating and accompanied by vomiting. Relief is brought about by sitting up, leaning forward, or lying on the right side with both knees drawn up to the chest. These episodes of pain are short in duration and are most severe at night. The individual commonly fears that death is imminent and can become extremely anxious.

Hepatomegaly and splenomegaly may be found on palpation. Unexplained thrombophlebitis may be a clinical manifestation of cancer in the distal portion of the pancreas.[165] Jaundice occurs rarely.

Tail of Pancreas

Carcinoma in the tail of the pancreas mimics several other diseases. Metastases to liver, bone, lungs, peritoneum, and other organs may cause the first symptoms of carcinoma in the tail of the pancreas. Individuals with cancer of the tail of the pancreas complain of generalized weakness, gripping upper abdominal pain, vague indigestion, anorexia, and unexplained weight loss. Jaundice is an unusual finding. Pain radiates to the back left hypochondrial area. Pain is not encountered as often with tumors of the tail as with cancer of the head and body. Upper gastrointestinal bleeding, splenomegaly, and signs of portal hypertension or ascites may result from thrombosis of the portal system or extensive liver damage. In a few individuals, a bruit may be auscultated in the left upper quadrant of the abdomen because of splenic artery compression or involvement by tumor.

ASSESSMENT

Physical Examination

Physical examination of the pancreas itself is difficult, because it is an inaccessible organ. In many persons with cancer of the head of the pancreas, however, physical examination may demonstrate an enlarged gallbladder and a palpable, smooth liver. With tumors of the body and tail of the pancreas, a hard and well-defined mass may be palpated in the subumbilical or left hypochondrial region. The mass can adhere to the vertebral column or large vessels and may produce a pulsation. An abdominal bruit may be heard on auscultation of the left hypochondrium if the tumor has compressed or has involved the splenic artery.

Diagnostic Studies

A variety of diagnostic measures are available to assist in the identification of pancreatic carcinoma. If definitive diagnosis cannot be made with these studies, exploratory laparotomy and biopsy may be necessary.

Radiologic examination

When pancreatic cancer is suspected, abdominal ultrasonography is used as an initial diagnostic test. It provides an outline of the pancreatic mass, dilated biliary ducts, liver metastases, and extrapancreatic spread. Some centers are now using endoscopic ultrasonography for direct imaging via the intestinal lumen.[175] It has proven to be a significant tool for establishing a differential diagnosis. CT scanning affords similar but more explicit detailing of the mass and extent of disease. CT scan in combination with ultrasonography can detect tumors as small as 2 cm.[176] CT-guided fine-needle biopsy is a reliable tool for differentiating malignancy.[177] MRI is being evaluated as a diagnostic tool in pancreatic cancer but offers no advantage over CT.

Single-photon-emission computed tomography can enable the clinician to differentiate between pancreatic cancer and chronic pancreatitis. Radio-labeled antibodies are also useful for imaging purposes. Liver and bone scans are done to determine metastatic involvement.

Endoscopic retrograde cholangiopancreatography (ERCP) is a useful test for differential diagnosis. During endoscopy, biopsy specimens for cytologic analysis are obtained. If the bile duct has been abruptly terminated by an obstruction, ERCP will demonstrate the alteration. Because this invasive procedure involves the risk of infection and rupture, it should be performed only by skilled clinicians.[171]

If surgery appears to be an option, selective arteriography and angiography can define the vasculature of the pancreas and delineate involvement or deviation of major vessels. Percutaneous transhepatic cholangiography (PCTC) is useful in determining whether the distal common bile duct is obstructed. The nurse should thoroughly explain these procedures to the patient and family beforehand. Following these invasive procedures, catheter insertion sites and vital signs are monitored carefully to detect bleeding, peritonitis, and infection.[178]

Laboratory tests

The use of laboratory tests is limited because early disease produces few alterations that laboratory tests demonstrate definitively. Transaminase, serum bilirubin, and alkaline phosphatase levels will be high and prothrombin time prolonged, particularly if jaundice or liver involvement is present. In the presence of pancreatitis secondary to obstructive tumor, serum and urine amylase concentrations will be elevated.[179] Islet cell tumors are diagnosed by plasma insulin immunoassay and markedly abnormal fasting blood glucose levels. The DNA content of pancreatic tumors is being studied to determine if the ploidy characteristics could be used as prognostic indicators to guide the aggressiveness of therapeutic interventions.[180]

Tumors markers

Biologic markers are on the frontier of cancer research. The carbohydrate antigen CA 19-9, carcinoembryonic antigen (CEA), and pancreatic oncofetal antigen (POA) are the tumor-associated markers being extensively studied in relation to pancreatic cancer.[164] With the carbohydrate antigen CA 19-9, approximately 80% of the pancreatic cancer cases have been correctly diagnosed.[165,181] Unfortunately, the levels of CA 19-9 usually are normal in early pancreatic cancer, so it is not useful for screening. After a tumor is resected, however, it can be used as a specific indicator of response to therapy. CEA levels are elevated in pancreatic cancer (>2.5 ng/ml). CEA levels are not elevated in early pancreatic cancer and are not specific to pancreatic cancer.[165] POA can be significantly elevated in some individuals with pancreatic cancer. As with CEA, POA is not specific to pancreatic cancer; it also has been found to be elevated in persons with bronchogenic and breast cancer. POA levels will decrease after effective therapy and increase with tumor recurrence or progression. The limitations to serial monitoring of tumor markers pertain to cost, sensitivity, reliability, and overall risk versus benefit.

TABLE 41-5 TNM Classification System for Cancer of the Pancreas

PRIMARY TUMOR (T)	
TX	Primary tumor cannot be assessed
T0	No evidence of primary tumor
T1	Tumor limited to the pancreas
	T1a Tumor 2 cm or less in greatest dimension
	T1b Tumor more than 2 cm in greatest dimension
T2	Tumor extends directly to any of the following: duodenum, bile duct, or peripancreatic tissues
T3	Tumor extends directly to any of the following: duodenum, stomach, spleen, colon, or adjacent large vessels

LYMPH NODE (N)	
NX	Regional lymph nodes cannot be assessed
N0	No regional lymph node metastasis
N1	Regional lymph node metastasis

DISTANT METASTASIS (M)	
MX	Presence of distant metastasis cannot be assessed
M0	No distant metastasis
M1	Distant metastasis

STAGE GROUPING			
I	T1	N0	M0
	T2	N0	M0
II	T3	N0	M0
III	Any T	N1	M0
IV	Any T	Any N	M1

Source: Beahrs OH, Henson DE, Hutter RV, et al (eds): *American Joint Committee on Cancer: Manual for Staging of Cancer* (4th ed). Philadelphia: Lippincott, 1992.

CLASSIFICATION AND STAGING

Treatment and prognosis of pancreatic cancer are greatly aided by careful definition of the tumor classification and staging. The specific stage and classification system for pancreatic cancer being used by the Cancer of the Pancreas Task Force of the American Joint Committee on Cancer Staging and End-Results Reporting is illustrated in Table 41-5.

TREATMENT

Treatment Planning

The poor prognosis of persons with pancreatic cancer indicates that the extent of the tumor and its effect on the host should be carefully evaluated prior to initiation of therapy. If the disease is believed to be potentially curable, the therapy will be radical. Therefore, the individual must be physically and psychologically capable of withstanding radical therapy. Many clinicians have an extremely dismal outlook and are reluctant to treat the disease aggressively.[171] Recent reports on surgical outcomes are encouraging and should change the current perspectives.

Surgery, radiotherapy, and chemotherapy are the major treatment modalities used for pancreatic cancer. Surgery offers the only hope for cure at this time. Multimodal therapy that combines surgery, radiation therapy, and chemotherapy is being extensively studied to determine if survival periods can be lengthened. Palliation can be achieved with surgery, radiotherapy, chemotherapy, or combined modalities.

Once a diagnosis has been made, the extent of tumor involvement established, and complete assessment of the person's physiologic status undertaken, the interdisciplinary team will decide on a treatment plan. A number of factors contribute to the choice of therapy, including age, nutritional status, hematologic status, liver function, concomitant disease, and skill of the principal clinicians.

Cure is the objective of therapy if the tumor is localized and not fixed to other structures and if there is no evidence of regional or distant metastases (T1–T3, N0, M0). Radical surgical extirpation of the tumor will be performed and supplemented with adjuvant radiation or chemotherapy.

Control or palliation is the goal of therapy if the tumor is large and not localized, is fixed to other structures, or has metastasized to regional or distant nodes (T4, N1–N4, M0–M1). Approximately 40%–70% of all cases of pancreatic carcinoma are diagnosed when the tumor is unresectable.[174,182] Surgical bypass procedures, radiotherapy, chemotherapy, or combined-modality treatment aimed at palliating devastating symptoms will be selected.

Despite the urgent nature of initiating therapy, the patient must be adequately prepared physiologically and psychologically. Pretreatment biliary decompression may be needed to relieve obstruction and pressure, while also reducing operative risk.[183] Prior to initiation of therapy, baseline assessments of lung capacity, blood pressure, blood volume, hematologic status, and liver function are completed. Bleeding and prolonged clotting time usually are corrected with vitamin K administration and blood component replacement. Nutritional supplementation to achieve adequate total protein levels can decrease surgical risk.[164,182] At the outset, patterns of family support, coping, and communication are important to understand.

Surgery

Current surgical approaches for pancreatic cancer are plagued by low rates of resectability and limited prospective research experience evaluating the surgical procedures. In recent years, reports of increasing survival periods following resection have been encouraging, particularly when the patients are stratified according to extent of disease.[164] Most surgical results report aggregated outcomes, whereas patients with small (<2 cm) tumors experience 30% 5-year survival rates, and the figures trend upward for those with no residual disease or without lymphatic involvement.[164] The crux of the problem is late detection of pancreatic tumors. Until such time as improvements in early detection and diagnosis are made, curative surgery will be limited to very few candidates, and palliative procedures will continue as the mainstay of therapy.

The surgical approaches most used when cure is the objective are total pancreatectomy and pancreatoduodenectomy (Whipple procedure). Regional pancreatectomy and distal pancreatectomy also are done. Controversy exists over the advantages, disadvantages, and long term results with each of the surgeries. (See Table 41-6.) Proponents of total pancreatectomy and regional pancreatectomy believe that, although both procedures invariably induce exocrine insufficiency and brittle diabetes, the risk of leaving behind microscopic disease is greatly reduced by the more extensive procedures.[165,182,185] Proponents of pancreatoduodenectomy (Whipple procedure) believe that this procedure

TABLE 41-6 Comparison of Types of Pancreatic Resections for Malignancy

	Pancreatico-duodenectomy (Whipple)	Total Pancreatectomy	Regional Pancreatectomy	Distal Pancreatectomy
Indications	Periampullary or small carcinoma of head	Large carcinoma of head or diffuse carcinoma	Carcinoma involving portal system	Carcinoma localized to body or tail
Tissues removed	Head of pancreas Duodenum Gastric antrum Bile duct Gallbladder	Whole pancreas Duodenum Gastric antrum Bile duct Gallbladder Spleen Peripancreatic nodes	Whole pancreas Duodenum Gastric antrum Bile duct Gallbladder Spleen Peripancreatic, celiac, mesenteric nodes	Distal pancreas Spleen
Anastomoses	Choledochojejunostomy Gastrojejunostomy Pancreaticojejunostomy	Choledochojejunostomy Gastrojejunostomy	Choledochojejunostomy Gastrojejunostomy Portal vein	None
Potential advantages	Pancreatic remnant may prevent diabetes and malabsorption.	Excision of pancreas may remove multifocal tumor. Complete peripancreatic nodal dissection No pancreatico-jejunostomy	Wide excision may remove microscopic residual tumor. Complete regional nodal dissection No pancreatico-jejunostomy	Pancreatic remnant may prevent diabetes and malabsorption. No pancreatico-jejunostomy
Potential disadvantages	Limited resection may leave residual tumor. Pancreaticojejunostomy may fail.	Diabetes and malabsorption result.	Diabetes and malabsorption result. Technically complex Venous anastomosis may fail.	Limited resection may leave residual tumor.

Source: Sindelar WF, Kinsella TJ, Mayer RJ: Cancer of the pancreas, in DeVita VT, Hellman S, Rosenberg SA (eds); *Cancer: Principles and Practice of Oncology* (2d ed). Philadelphia: Lippincott, 1985, pp.691–739.

removes the cancer without creating another disease (diabetes) and that it is technically easier and reduces operative time.[173,185] Overall operative mortality rates range from 5%–50%.[164,173] Interestingly, survival rates are similar with all three procedures.[164,182,186] Whether this is due to the surgeon's expertise, the extent of resection, or the tumor cell characteristics can only be determined after more cases are systematically evaluated.

During the surgical procedure the pancreas and lymph nodes are biopsied and inspected before proceeding with further resection. The mesentery is examined and mobility of the duodenum and pancreas assessed. The vena cava, portal vein, and mesenteric veins also are checked for possible tumor involvement.

Total pancreatectomy

A total pancreatectomy is an *en bloc* resection in which a large number of lymph nodes (about 50) are removed. The antrum, common duct, gallbladder (if involved), pancreas, spleen, duodenum, proximal jejunum, and regional lymph nodes are resected *en bloc*. The biliary tract is anastomosed to the remaining jejunum proximal to a gastrojejunostomy (Figure 41-7). A vagotomy is done to decrease the risk of peptic ulcer. Biliary drains and a gastrostomy tube are inserted for drainage.

Pancreatoduodenal resection (Whipple procedure)

Pancreatoduodenal resection (Whipple procedure) entails removal of the distal portion of the stomach, pancreas to the right of the superior mesenteric vein, duodenum, proximal jejunum, distal portion of the common bile duct, and gallbladder (Figure 41-8). Gastrointestinal continuity is restored by anastomosing the common bile duct and the remaining pancreas to the jejunum proximal to the gastrojejunostomy. A gastrojejunostomy is formed to allow the alkaline bile and pancreatic juices to enter the jejunum before acidic gastric secretions. This decreases the potential of ulceration at the gastrojejunostomy. Some surgeons will also perform a bilateral vagotomy to minimize ulceration. Postoperative complications are infection, anastomotic leakage, fistulas, thrombophlebitis, abscess, and pneumonia.

Regional pancreatectomy

Regional pancreatectomy is an extensive *en bloc* surgery that includes the entire pancreas; duodenum; gastric antrum; bile duct; gallbladder; spleen; the parapancreatic, celiac, and mesenteric nodes; and a sleeve resection of the portal vein.[173,182,187] Controversy regarding this surgical procedure relates to its technical complexity, higher mortality rates, and limited experience to substantiate improved survival rates. Proponents believe that the high rate of failure in controlling pancreatic cancer supports the need to explore fully any promising methods to manage this lethal disease.

Distal pancreatectomy

In rare cases, tumors of the body or tail of the pancreas are detected early enough to be considered curable.

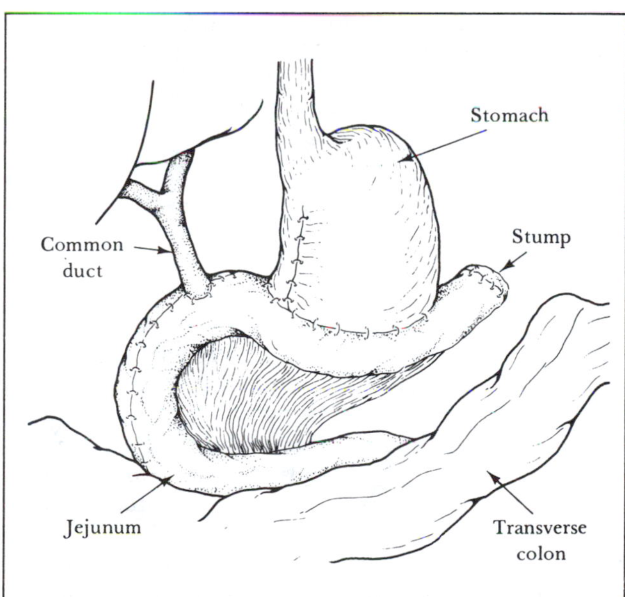

FIGURE 41-7 Total pancreatectomy. After resection of the pancreas, the biliary and gastrointestinal tracts are reconstructed by gastrojejunostomy and hepaticojejunostomy.

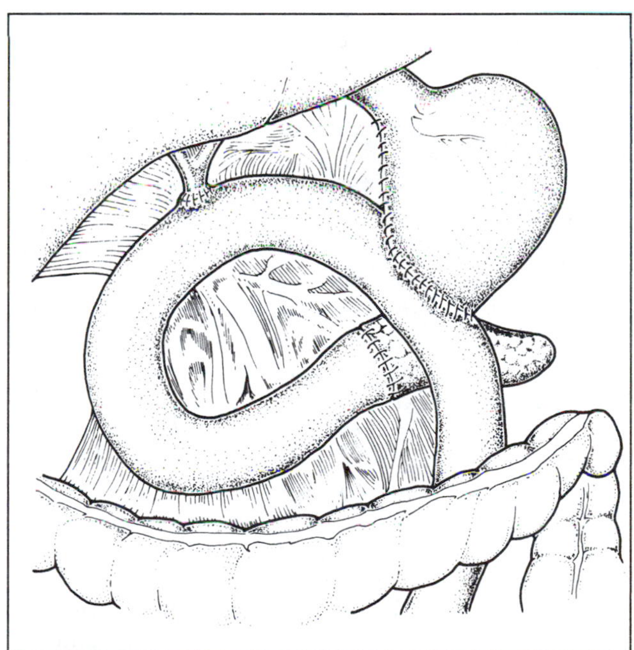

FIGURE 41-8 Whipple procedure. After resection of the head of the pancreas, reconstruction is achieved by pancreatojejunostomy, hepaticojejunostomy, and gastrojejunostomy. Vagotomy is performed to inhibit ulceration.

In such cases a distal pancreatectomy is performed. The entire tumor-bearing area plus a margin of safety is resected. The remaining pancreas is anastomosed to the duodenum and usually is capable of providing adequate exocrine and endocrine function.

Palliative surgical procedures

Palliative surgical procedures are used to remove tumor, relieve jaundice and obstruction, and decompress or bypass involved organs. Decompression procedures, including cholecystojejunostomy or choledochojejunostomy, are used for biliary tract obstruction; or pancreatojejunostomy is used for pancreatic duct obstruction.[174,188] Biliary bypass procedures (gastroenterostomy) will restore intestinal continuity if the duodenum has become obstructed or invaded by tumor. Delayed gastric emptying may be a serious postoperative problem for some patients.[189] Some surgeons have begun studying ways to minimize the trauma of surgery by using laparoscopic approaches for performing cholecystojejunostomy and other palliative surgeries.[190,191]

Postoperative care

Intensive postoperative medical and nursing management of individuals who undergo pancreatic resection is critical for reducing surgical mortality.[164,173,192] Careful assessment, anticipatory management, and complete patient/family teaching will greatly enhance recovery and rehabilitation. In the immediate postoperative period, hemorrhage, hypovolemia, and hypotension pose the greatest threats. Fistula, infection, and anastomotic leak are other potential problems.

Hemorrhage may occur from leakage at the surgical anastomosis or from generalized coagulopathy. Abdominal distention, shock, hematemesis, bloody stool, bloody drainage, or bleeding from the incision site warrant immediate attention. Retroperitoneal bleeding will manifest as a bluish-brown discoloration of either or both flanks. Prothrombin times are monitored frequently, and vitamin K and blood component therapy is administered as needed. There have been reports of disseminated intravascular coagulation occurring in the postoperative period.

Hypovolemia can develop from fluids lost during extensive surgery, through decompression tubes and drains, or from "third spacing" (the shift of fluid from the vascular space to the interstitial space). Low levels of circulating plasma proteins secondary to malnutrition and hypoalbuminemia usually account for the third-spacing syndrome. The first phase of fluid compartment shifting begins immediately after surgery and can last 48–72 hours. Signs of fluid shift are decreased blood pressure, increased pulse rate, low central venous pressure, decreased urine output, increased specific gravity, low levels of serum albumin, and hemoconcentration. When the plasma protein is replaced and levels return to normal, fluid reabsorption follows. Urine output will suddenly and dramatically increase, sometimes to as much as 200 ml/hr. Urine output will greatly exceed intake. The individual is monitored closely for signs of circulatory overload. The reabsorption phase will reach equilibrium within 24–48 hours.

Hypotension is a potential postoperative complication that is believed to result from severance of the sympathetic nerve fibers of the mesenteric complex.[22] Vital signs and urine output should be monitored frequently to detect alterations. Vasopressor drugs and liberal intravenous fluids may be administered.[22]

Pulmonary complications following surgery are common, possibly due to immobility and inadequate lung expansion secondary to pain and splinting. In addition, those individuals who are malnourished and protein-deficient are susceptible to pneumonia. The importance of vigorous pulmonary hygiene and progressive ambulation cannot be overemphasized. Total parenteral nutrition (TPN) often is needed to correct nutritional deficiencies.

Following resection of the pancreas, exocrine and endocrine functions will be temporarily or permanently altered, depending on the amount of viable pancreatic tissue remaining. In the immediate postoperative period, laboratory tests will be useful for monitoring protein, fat, and glucose levels. Prior to discharge, the patient and family must become familiar with and able to recognize the signs of exocrine and endocrine abnormalities such as hyper/hypoglycemia, steatorrhea, stupor, and lethargy.

Endocrine function (secretion of insulin and production of glucagon) most often is altered by resection involving the head of the pancreas. Serum and urine glucose levels are monitored at least every 6 hours, and insulin therapy is initiated. Most individuals can be controlled with about 25 units of NPH insulin each morning and a sliding scale of insulin dosages that maintain a mild hyperglycemia to prevent a precipitous drop in serum glucose.[178] Discharge teaching and home therapy programs are the same as for individuals with diabetes. Inability to control glucose levels could indicate a recurrence of disease.

Alteration of exocrine function by removal of pancreatic tissue results in a malabsorption syndrome characterized by an inability to use ingested forms of fat and protein. The caloric requirement of an individual following surgery exceeds 3000 calories per day; adequate nutritional intake is essential to recovery. In the immediate postoperative period, nutritional maintenance is difficult. Parenteral hyperalimentation solutions contain approximately 1000 calories per liter; however, one of the major components is hypertonic dextrose. Serum and urine glucose levels are monitored at least every 6 hours, and insulin is administered as needed.

As soon as possible following pancreatectomy, the

person is advanced to an oral diet. The aim of nutritional therapy is to replace calories lost as a result of the surgically induced inability to use ingested fats and proteins. Pancreatic enzymes are replaced with oral enzyme supplements. The two most reliable and frequently used forms are pancreatin (Viokase) and pancrelipase (Cotazym). Pancreatic enzyme supplements contain lipase, amylase, and trypsin.[22] Pancreatin and pancrelipase supplements are made from extracts of hog or beef pancreas enriched with bile salts and plant and fungal enzymes. The pancreas normally excretes 100,000 units of lipase per hour. Enzyme replacements contain about 4000 units of lipase per tablet. The usual therapeutic dose is eight tablets with each meal or 24 tablets (96,000 units) per day. It may require several approaches before the most appropriate dosage for each patient is determined, because eating patterns and individual responses vary.[178] The individual should be informed that steatorrhea will decrease but may not be eliminated, because oral pancreatic extracts are partially inactivated by acidic peptic fluids whereas bile salts are activated by acidic duodenal contents.[193]

Most oral pancreatic enzyme supplements are enteric-coated. There are conflicting reports regarding the efficacy of administering antacids with enzyme supplements. If diarrhea, steatorrhea, or weight loss persists with the administration of oral enzyme replacements, cimetidine, a potent gastric acid inhibitor, can be used.[194]

The second aim of nutritional therapy is to supply fats and proteins in a usable form. In most regular diets, 98% of dietary fat consists of long-chain triglycerides that are difficult to break down into usable form. Administration of lipase is necessary so that the individual who has had a pancreatectomy can hydrolyze naturally occurring fats (i.e., long-chain triglycerides). When lipase is administered in conjunction with pancreatic enzyme supplements, long-chain triglycerides can be broken down into medium-chain triglycerides (MCT). Food supplements that contain MCTs also can be ingested. Medium-chain triglycerides are easily absorbed directly into the portal venous system, and bile salts or lipase are not required for absorption. Unfortunately, supplemental MCTs are unpalatable and expensive.

After a pancreatectomy, individuals are placed on a diet of bland, low-fat foods high in carbohydrate and protein. Several small feedings are tolerated better than large meals. Restrictions include overindulgence (which places a great demand on the pancreas), caffeine, and alcohol. It is advantageous for the clinical dietitian to consult with the individual to select the most agreeable diet plan based on individual needs and lifestyle. The patient and family should be instructed on how to monitor the patient's tolerance to the diet and pancreatic enzyme replacement therapy. The stool should be examined daily for the characteristic sign of steatorrhea: frothy, floating, foul-smelling stool with fat particles floating in the water. If observed, this should be reported to the physician or nurse.

Chemotherapy

Chemotherapy as adjuvant treatment for pancreatic cancer is still being explored. The high rate of mortality associated with metastatic disease indicates that systemic therapy is needed; however, current applications of chemotherapy have failed to produce significant results. Perhaps, new approaches in sequencing therapies or new drug combinations will improve the outcome.

Only a few agents have been determined to be effective as single agents: 5-FU, mitomycin-C, streptozotocin, ifosfamide, and doxorubicin.[165,195] Continuous intravenous infusion of 5-FU is being studied to determine if there is a therapeutic advantage to continuous exposure.[195] It is hoped that combinations of chemotherapeutic agents will produce higher response rates, but few studies have substantiated this. The combination regimens used most often are SMF (streptozotocin, mitomycin-C, 5-FU) and FAM (5-FU, doxorubicin, mitomycin-C). Cisplatin, somatostatin, and cytosine arabinoside are among other agents being studied.[196–198]

Chemotherapy alone has made no significant difference in survival periods, although it has provided palliation of pain in some cases. When both chemotherapy and radiation therapy are administered to individuals who have had pancreatic resection, the survival period may be increased slightly.[199–201]

Radiotherapy

External irradiation has been used for both palliative and curative therapy of pancreatic cancer. If the cancer is unresectable, local control of tumor growth and relief of debilitating symptoms are accomplished in about 40% of individuals.[164] Several specialized methods of radiotherapy have been used, such as interstitial implants, intraoperative radiotherapy, high-linear-energy transfer radiation, and charged-particle irradiation. These methods have resulted in a slight increase in short-term survival, but 5-year survival rates are unaffected.[202] The major limitation to radiotherapy appears to be the large volume of tumor that usually is present at diagnosis.

Combinations of radiotherapy and chemotherapy have resulted in increases in survival time as compared to patients treated with radiation or chemotherapy alone.[199,200,203] The average survival time with radiotherapy alone is 6 months, but it is 11 months with combination radiotherapy and chemotherapy. It is postulated that chemotherapeutic agents may reduce tumor burden and act as intrinsic radiation sensitizers, increasing the impact of radiotherapy.

Supportive Therapy

Cancer of the pancreas is an aggressive and unrelenting invasive disease in the advanced stages. The obstructive process will begin to manifest itself fully and lead to hepatic failure, ascites, severe jaundice, hemorrhage, infection, and pain. The goal of palliative therapy is to reduce the debilitating symptoms of the disease.

Relief of pain is a primary objective, since pancreatic tumors usually invade the celiac plexus and cause excruciating pain. The most effective approach to pain therapy is to prevent it from peaking by routinely administering the selected relief measures. Narcotics, sedatives, nerve blocks, relaxation therapy, and proper positioning may provide pain relief. Surgery, radiotherapy, and chemotherapy have also been used selectively to reduce pain.

As a result of the obstructive nature of advanced pancreatic cancer, nutritional support is a serious problem. Oral feedings should be maintained as long as caloric requirements can be met. Frequent, small feedings and supplemental mixtures may be tolerated better than larger meals. Antiemetics prior to eating will assist in controlling nausea or vomiting. A feeding tube may be inserted below the point of obstruction if the individual can tolerate a surgical procedure. If exocrine function is disturbed, pancreatic enzyme replacements must be administered with oral or enteral feedings.

Jaundice due to ductal obstruction or liver damage is a debilitating symptom that occurs in 40%–70% of patients.[204] It causes severe pruritus and dry, friable skin. Cholestyramine, which combines with and promotes excretion of excess bile acids, may provide some relief of pruritus. The patient and family should be instructed to use soap sparingly, preferably using mild soaps such as Ivory. Oil-based lotions, calamine lotion, cocoa butter, or bathing in sodium bicarbonate may help to relieve pruritus.[22]

Nonsurgical procedures are used to relieve obstructive jaundice in the patient with advanced cancer. Percutaneous transhepatic biliary drainage (PTBD) is performed under fluoroscopy, with the patient receiving mild sedation and prophylactic antibiotics.[205] Endoscopic endoprosthesis placement can be done immediately following ERCP. Successful placement of the endoprosthesis or biliary stent occurs in 90% of the cases attempted.[164,206] Palliative percutaneous transhepatic biliary drainage produces modest relief; however, care of the drainage apparatus generally is tedious for the family.

Liver damage may lead to ascites, hemorrhage, and confusion. Almost 90% of persons with pancreatic cancer die within a year of diagnosis. The course of the disease is rapid, and supporting the individual and family through the process is critical. It is important that the patient and family understand that some form of treatment or another medication will always be available to make the individual as comfortable as possible.

REFERENCES

1. Boring CC, Squires TS, Tong T: Cancer statistics, 1993. *CA* 43(1):7–26, 1993.
2. Rosenberg JC, Lichter AS, Leichman LP: Cancer of the esophagus. In DeVita VT, Hellman S, Rosenberg SA (eds): *Cancer: Principles and Practice of Oncology* (3d ed). Philadelphia: Lippincott, 1989, pp. 725–764.
3. Blot WJ, Fraumeni JF: Trends in esophageal mortality among US blacks and whites. *Am J Public Health* 77:296–298, 1987.
4. Klumpp TR, Macdonald JS: Esophageal cancer: Epidemiology and pathology. In Ahlgren JD, Macdonald JS (eds): *Gastrointestinal Oncology*. Philadelphia: Lippincott, 1992, pp. 71–80.
5. Qui S, Yang G: Precursor lesions of esophageal cancer in high risk populations in Henan Province, China. *Cancer* 62:551–557, 1988.
6. Ziegler RG: Alcohol-nutrient interactions in cancer etiology. *Cancer* 58:1942–1948, 1986.
7. Gray JR, Coldman AJ, MacDonald WC: Cigarette and alcohol use in patients with adenocarcinoma of the gastric cardia or lower esophagus. *Cancer* 69:2227–2231, 1992.
8. Applequist P, Salmo M: Lye corrosion carcinoma of the esophagus. *Cancer* 45:2655–2658, 1980.
9. Mizroch S: Epidemiology of esophageal carcinoma. *JAMA* 239(22):2340, 1978.
10. Hesketh PJ, Clapp RW, Doos WG, Spechler SJ: The increasing frequency of adenocarcinoma of the esophagus. *Cancer* 64:526–530, 1989.
11. Blot WJ, Devasa SS, Kneller RW, Fraumeni JF: Rising incidence of adenocarcinoma of the esophagus and gastric cardia. *JAMA* 265:1287–1289, 1991.
12. Nishimaki T, Holscher AH, Schuler M, et al: Histopathologic characteristics of early adenocarcinoma in Barrett's esophagus. *Cancer* 68:1731–1736, 1991.
13. Helm F: *Cancer Dermatology*. Philadelphia: Lea & Feibiger, 1979, pp. 48–49.
14. Jaskiewicz K, Marasas WF, Rossouw JE, et al: Selenium and other mineral elements in populations at risk for esophageal cancer. *Cancer* 62:2635–2639, 1988.
15. Sasajima K, Takai A, Taniguchi Y, et al: Polypoid squamous cell carcinoma of the esophagus. *Cancer* 64:94–97, 1989.
16. Goseki N, Koike M, Yoshida M: Histopathologic characteristics of early stage esophageal carcinoma. *Cancer* 69:1088–1093, 1992.
17. Jin-Ming Y, Li-Hua Y, Guo-Qian, et al: Flow cytometric analysis of DNA content in esophageal carcinoma. *Cancer* 64:80–82, 1989.
18. Ozawa S, Ueda M, Ando N, et al: Prognostic significance of epidermal growth factor receptor in esophageal squamous cell carcinomas. *Cancer* 63:2169–2173, 1989.
19. Stephens JK, Bibbo M, Dytch H, et al: Correlation between automated karyometric measurements of squamous cell carcinoma of the esophagus and histopathologic and clinical features. *Cancer* 64:83–87, 1989.
20. Anderson LL, Lad TE: Autopsy findings in squamous cell carcinoma of the esophagus. *Cancer* 50:1587–1590, 1982.
21. Moses FM: Squamous cell carcinoma of the esophagus. *Gastroenterol Clin North Am* 20:703–716, 1991.

22. Given B, Simmons SJ: *Gastroenterology in Nursing*. St. Louis, MO: Mosby, 1979.
23. Germanov AB, Spivack PB, Lukjanchenko AB, Mazneva NL: Preoperative diagnosis of esophageal spread. *Semin Surg Oncol* 8:50–54, 1992.
24. Huang CJ: Esophageal cancer. *Japanese J Surg* 11:399, 1981.
25. Ziegler K, Sanft C, Friedrich M, et al: Evaluation of endosonography in TN staging of oesophageal cancer. *Gut* 32:16–20, 1991.
26. Lightdale CJ, Botet JF, Kelsen DP, et al: Diagnosis of recurrent upper gastrointestinal cancer at the surgical anastomosis by endoscopic ultrasound. *Gastrointest Endosc* 35:407–412, 1989.
27. American Joint Committee on Cancer. Beahrs O, Meyers M (eds): *Manual for Staging of Cancer* (4th ed). Philadelphia: Lippincott, 1992.
28. Gomes MN: Esophageal cancer: Surgical approach. In Ahlgren JD, Macdonald JS (eds): *Gastrointestinal Oncology*. Philadelphia: Lippincott, 1992, pp. 89–121.
29. Davydov MI, Akhvlediani GG, Stilidi IS, et al: Surgical aspects in the treatment of esophageal cancer. *Semin Surg Oncol* 8:4–8, 1992.
30. Forastiere AA, Orringer MB, Perez-Tamayo C, et al: Concurrent chemotherapy and radiation therapy followed by transhiatal esophagectomy for local-regional cancer of the esophagus. *J Clin Oncol* 8:119–127, 1990.
31. Ellis FH: Esophageal carcinoma. In Steele G, Cady B (eds): *General Surgical Oncology*. Philadelphia: Saunders, 1992, pp. 87–106.
32. Harter KW: Esophageal cancer: Management with radiation. In Ahlgren JD, Macdonald JS (eds): *Gastrointestinal Oncology*. Philadelphia: Lippincott, 1992, pp. 123–134.
33. Petrovich Z, Lam K, Langholz B, et al: Surgical therapy and radiotherapy for carcinoma of the esophagus. *J Thorac Cardiovasc Surg* 98:614–617, 1989.
34. Mamontov AS, Kiseleva ES, Kucharenko VM, Zimina HS: Combined therapy of thoracic esophageal cancer. *Semin Surg Oncol* 8:21–26, 1992.
35. Pirogov AI, Krasnitisky YN: Successive radiation and surgical treatment of esophageal cancer. *Semin Surg Oncol* 8:37–40, 1992.
36. Gill PG, Denham JW, Jamieson GG, et al: Patterns of treatment failure and prognostic factors associated with the treatment of esophageal carcinoma with chemotherapy and radiotherapy either as sole treatment or followed by surgery. *J Clin Oncol* 10:1037–1043, 1992.
37. Sur RK, Singh DP, Sharma SC, et al: Radiation therapy of esophageal cancer: Role of high dose rate brachytherapy. *Int J Radiat Oncol Biol Phys* 22:1043–1046, 1992.
38. Naini AB, Dickerson JW, Brown MM: Preoperative and postoperative levels of plasma protein and amino acid in esophageal and lung cancer patients. *Cancer* 62:355–360, 1988.
39. Orringer MB, Stirling MC: Esophagectomy for esophageal disruption. *Ann Thorac Surg* 49:35–43, 1990.
40. Mathisen DJ, Grillo HC, Wilkins EW, et al: Thoracic esophagectomy: A safe approach to carcinoma of the esophagus. *Ann Thorac Surg* 45:137–143, 1988.
41. Bremner RM, DeMeester TR: Surgical treatment of esophageal carcinoma. *Gastroenterol Clin North Am* 20(4): 743–763, 1991.
42. Tsutsui S, Moriguchi S, Morita M, et al: Multivariate analysis of postoperative complications after esophageal resection. *Ann Thorac Surg* 53:1052–1056, 1992.
43. Patil PK, Patel SG, Mistry RC, et al: Cancer of the esophagus: Esophagogastric anastomotic leak—a retrospective study of predisposing factors. *J Surg Oncol* 49:163–167, 1992.
44. Hoebler L, Irwin MM: Gastrointestinal tract cancer: Current knowledge, medical treatment, and nursing management. *Oncol Nurs Forum* 19:1403–1415, 1992.
45. Medvec BR: Esophageal cancer: Treatment and nursing interventions. *Semin Oncol Nurs* 4(4):246–256, 1988.
46. Morton KA, Karwande SV, Davis RK, et al: Gastric emptying after gastric interposition for cancer of the esophagus or hypopharynx. *Ann Thorac Surg* 51:759–763, 1991.
47. Cameron M: What patients need most before and after thoracotomy. *Nursing* 8(5):28–36, 1978.
48. Leichman L, Berry BT: Experience with cisplatin in treatment regimens for esophageal cancer. *Semin Oncol Nurs* 18:64–72, 1991.
49. Ahlgren JD: Esophageal cancer. In Ahlgren JD, Macdonald JS (eds): *Gastrointestinal Oncology*. Philadelphia: Lippincott, 1992, pp. 135–147.
50. Vikram B, Malamud S, Gold J, et al: Chemotherapy rapidly alternating with accelerated radiotherapy for advanced carcinomas of the hypopharynx and upper esophagus: A feasibility study. *Head Neck* 13:415–419, 1991.
51. Ajani JA, Roth JA, Ryan B, et al: Evaluation of pre- and postoperative chemotherapy for resectable adenocarcinoma of the esophagus or gastroesophageal junction. *J Clin Oncol* 8:1231–1238, 1990.
52. Kelsen D, Lovett D, Wong J, et al: Interferon alfa-2 and fluorouracil in the treatment of patients with advanced esophageal cancer. *J Clin Oncol* 10:269–274, 1992.
53. Stewart FM, Harkins BJ, Hahn SS, et al: Cisplatin, 5-fluorouracil, mitomycin C, and concurrent radiation therapy with and without esophagectomy for esophageal carcinoma. *Cancer* 64:622–628, 1989.
54. Orringer MB, Forastiere AA, Perez-Tamayo C: Chemotherapy and radiation therapy before transhiatal esophagectomy for esophageal carcinoma. *Ann Thorac Surg* 49:348–355, 1990.
55. Urba SG, Orringer MB, Perez-Tqamayo C, et al: Concurrent preoperative chemotherapy and radiation therapy in localized esophageal adenocarcinoma. *Cancer* 69:285–291, 1992.
56. Herskovic A, Martz K, Al-Sarraf M, et al: Combined chemotherapy and radiotherapy compared with radiotherapy alone in patients with cancer of the esophagus. *N Engl J Med* 326:1593–1598, 1992.
57. Rotman MZ: Chemoirradiation: A new initiative in cancer treatment. *Radiology* 184:319–327, 1992.
58. Reed CE, Marsh WH, Carlson LS, et al: Prospective, randomized trial of palliative treatment for unresectable cancer of the esophagus. *Ann Thorac Surg* 51:552–556, 1991.
59. Siegel HI, Laskin KJ, Dabezies MA, et al: The effect of endoscopic laser therapy on survival in patients with squamous-cell carcinoma of the esophagus. *J Clin Gastroenterol* 13:142–146, 1991.
60. McCaughan L: Lasers in photodynamic therapy. *Nurs Clin North Am* 25:725–738, 1990.
61. Isaac JR, Sim EK, Ngoi SS, Goh PM: Safe and rapid palliation of dysphagia for carcinoma of the esophagus. *Am Surg* 57:245–249, 1991.

62. Cusumano A, Ruol A, Segalin A, et al: Push-through intubation: Effective palliation in 409 patients with cancer of the esophagus. *Ann Thorac Surg* 53:1010–1014, 1992.
63. Sargeant IR, Loizou LA, Tulloch M, et al: Recanalization of tube overgrowth: A useful new indication for laser in palliation of malignant dysphagia. *Gastrointest Endosc* 38:165–169, 1992.
64. Mackety CJ: Caring for cancer patient who has an esophageal endoprosthesis. *RN* 40:51–53, 1977.
65. Maehara Y, Kuwano H, Kitamura K, et al: Hyperthermochemoradiotherapy for esophageal cancer. *Anticancer Res* 12:805–810, 1992.
66. Karanov S, Shopova M, Getov H: Photodynamic therapy in gastrointestinal cancer. *Lasers Surg Med* 11:395–398, 1991.
67. Loizou LA, Rampton D, Atkinson M, et al: A prospective assessment of quality of life after endoscopic intubation and laser therapy for malignant dysphagia. *Cancer* 70:386–391, 1992.
68. Dupont BJ, Cohn I: Gastric adenocarcinoma. *Curr Probl Cancer* IV(8):1–35, 1980.
69. Macdonald JS, Hill MC, Roberts IM: Gastric cancer: Epidemiology, pathology, detection, and staging. In Ahlgren JD, Macdonald JS (eds): *Gastrointestinal Oncology*. Philadelphia: Lippincott, 1992, pp. 151–158.
70. Maruyama K, Okabayashi K, Kinoshita T: Progress in gastric cancer surgery in Japan and its limits of radicality. *World J Surg* 11:418–425, 1987.
71. Lawrence M: Early gastric cancer. *Ann Surg* 213(4):327–334, 1991.
72. Soga J, Ohyama S, Miyashita K, et al: A statistical evaluation of advancement in gastric surgery with special reference to the significance of lymphadenectomy for cure. *World J Surg* 12:398–405, 1988.
73. Vezerdis MP, Wanebo HJ: Gastric cancer: Surgical approach. In Ahlgren JD, Macdonald JS (eds): *Gastrointestinal Oncology*. Philadelphia: Lippincott, 1992, pp. 159–170.
74. Nakamura K, Ueyama T, Yao T, et al: Pathology and prognosis of gastric carcinoma. *Cancer* 70:1030–1037, 1992.
75. Wiggins CL, Becker TM, Key CR, Samet JM: Stomach cancer among New Mexico's American Indians, Hispanic Whites, and non-Hispanic Whites. *Cancer Res* 49:1595–1599, 1989.
76. Horm JW, Asire AJ, Young JL, Pollack ES (eds): *SEER Program: Cancer Incidence and Mortality in the United States 1973–1981,* NIH Publication No. 85-1837. Bethesda, MD: National Cancer Institute, 1984.
77. Risch HA, Jain M, Choi NW, et al: Dietary factors and the incidence of cancer of the stomach. *Am J Epidemiol* 122(6):947–959, 1985.
78. LaVecchia CL, Negir E, Frannceschi S, Gentile A: Family history and the risk of stomach and colorectal cancer. *Cancer* 70:50–55, 1992.
79. Moller H, Toftgaard C: Cancer occurrence in a cohort of patients surgically treated for peptic ulcer. *Gut* 32:740–744, 1991.
80. MacDonald JS, Steele G, Gunderson LL: Cancer of the stomach. In DeVita VT, Hellman S, Rosenberg SA (eds): *Cancer: Principles and Practice of Oncology* (3d ed). Philadelphia: Lippincott, 1989, pp. 765–799.
81. Blomjous JG, Hop WC, Langenhorst BL, et al: Adenocarcinoma of the gastric cardia. *Cancer* 70:569–574, 1992.
82. MacDonald WC, Mac Donald JB: Adenocarcinoma of the esophagus and/or gastric cardia. *Cancer* 60:1094–1098, 1987.
83. Olearchyk A: Gastric carcinoma. *Am J Gastroenterol* 70:25–45, 1978.
84. Ohyama S, Yonemura Y, Miyazaki I: Proliferative activity and malignancy in human gastric cancers. *Cancer* 69:314–321, 1992.
85. Wobbes T, Thomas CM, Segers MF, Nagengast FM: Evaluation of seven tumor markers (CA 50, CA 19-9, TruQuant, CA 72-4, CA 195, carcinoembryonic antigen, and tissue polypeptide antigen) in the pretreatment sera of patients with gastric carcinoma. *Cancer* 69:2036–2041, 1992.
86. Vezeridis MP, Wanebo HJ: Gastric cancer: Surgical approach. In Ahlgren JD, Macdonald JS (eds): *Gastrointestinal Oncology*. Philadelphia: Lippincott, 1992, pp. 159–170.
87. Cady B: Gastric cancer. In Steele G, Cady B (eds), *General Surgical Oncology*. Philadelphia: Saunders, 1991, pp. 139–147.
88. Monson JR, Donohue JH, McIlrath DC, et al: Total gastrectomy for advanced cancer. *Cancer* 68:1863–1868, 1991.
89. Okamura T, Korenga D, Baba H, et al: Thoracoabdominal approach for cure of patients with an adenocarcinoma in the upper third of the stomach. *Am Surg* 55:248–251, 1989.
90. Salo JA, Kivilaakso E: Failure of long limb Roux-en-Y reconstruction to prevent alkaline reflux esophagitis after total gastrectomy. *Endoscopy* 2265–2267, 1990.
91. Wang JF: Stomach cancer. *Semin Oncol Nurs* 4(4):257–264, 1988.
92. Caudry M: Gastric cancer: Radiotherapy and approaches to locally unresectable or recurrent disease. In Ahlgren JD, Macdonald JS (eds): *Gastrointestinal Oncology*. Philadelphia: Lippincott, 1992, pp. 181–187.
93. O'Connell MJ, Gunderson LL, Moertel CG, et al: A pilot study to determine clinical tolerability of intensive combined therapy for locally unresectable gastric cancer. *Int J Radiat Oncol Biol Phys* 11:1827, 1985.
94. Abe M, Shibamoto Y, Takahashi, et al: Intraoperative radiotherapy in carcinoma of the stomach and pancreas. *World J Surg* 11:459–464, 1987.
95. MacDonald JS, Gohmann JJ: Chemotherapy of advanced gastric cancer: Present status, future prospects. *Semin Oncol* 15(3):42–49, 1988(Suppl.).
96. Havlin KA, Macdonald JS: Gastric cancer: Chemotherapy of advanced disease. In Ahlgren JD, Macdonald JS (eds): *Gastrointestinal Oncology*. Philadelphia: Lippincott, 1992, pp. 171–179.
97. Kelsen D, Atiq OT, Saltz L, et al: FAMTX versus etoposide, doxorubicin, and cisplatin: A random assignment trial in gastric cancer. *J Clin Oncol* 10:541–548, 1992.
98. Lerner A, Gonin R, Steele GD, Mayer RJ: Etoposide, doxorubicin, and cisplatin chemotherapy for advanced gastric adenocarcinoma: Results of a phase II trial. *J Clin Oncol* 10:536–540, 1992.
99. Epelbaum R, Haim N, Stein M, et al: Treatment of advanced gastric cancer with DDP (cisplatin), adriamycin, and 5-fluorouracil (DAF). *Oncology* 44:201–206, 1987.
100. Allum WH, Hallissey MT, Kelly KA: Adjuvant chemotherapy in operable gastric cancer. *Lancet* (March): 571–574, 1989.

101. Schlag P: Adjuvant chemotherapy in gastric cancer. *World J Surg* 11:473–477, 1987.
102. Raab K: Intraperitoneal techniques offer daring alternative for abdominal cancer. *Oncol Biotech News* (August):19, 1989.
103. Pazdur R, Ajani JA, Winn R, et al: A phase II trial of 5-fluorouracil and recombinant alpha-2a-interferon in previously untreated metastatic gastric carcinoma. *Cancer* 69:878–882, 1992.
104. Maehara Y, Emi Y, Moriguchi S, et al: Postoperative chemotherapy for patients with advanced gastric cancer. *Am J Surg* 163:577–580, 1992.
105. Ahlgren JD, Wanebo HJ, Hill MC: Hepatocellular carcinoma. In Ahlgren JD, Macdonald JS (eds): *Gastrointestinal Oncology*. Philadelphia: Lippincott, 1992, pp. 417–436.
106. Ni YH, Chang MH, Hsu HY, et al: Hepatocellular carcinoma in childhood. *Cancer* 68:1737–1741, 1991.
107. Wanebo HJ, Falkson G, Order SE: Cancer of the hepatobiliary system. In DeVita VT, Hellman S, Rosenberg SA (eds): *Cancer: Principles and Practice of Oncology* (3d ed). Philadelphia: Lippincott, 1989, pp. 836–874.
108. Lee SD, Lee FY, Wu JC, et al: The prevalence of anti-hepatitis C virus among Chinese patients with hepatocellular carcinoma. *Cancer* 69:342–345, 1992.
109. Lancaster WD: Viral role in cervical and liver cancer. *Cancer* 70:1794–1798, 1992.
110. Leung NW, Tam JS, Lai JY, et al: Does hepatitis C virus infection contribute to hepatocellular carcinoma in Hong Kong? *Cancer* 70:40–44, 1992.
111. Hsia CC, Axiotis CA, Bisceglie AM, Tabor E: Transforming growth factor-alpha in human hepatocellular carcinoma and coexpression with hepatitis B surface antigen in adjacent liver. *Cancer* 70:1049–1056, 1992.
112. Oberfield RA, Steele G, Gollan JL, Sherman D: Liver cancer. *CA* 39(4):206–218, 1989.
113. Linsell A: Primary liver cancer: Epidemiology and etiology. In Wanebo HJ (ed): *Hepatic and Biliary Cancer*. New York: Dekker, 1987, pp. 3–15.
114. Palmer JR, Rosenberg L, Kaufman DW, et al: Oral contraceptive use and liver cancer. *Am J Epidemiol* 130:878–882, 1989.
115. World Health Organization Collaborative Study of Neoplasia and Steroid Contraceptives. *Int J Cancer* 43:254–259, 1989.
116. Ng IO, Lai EC, Ng MM, Fan ST: Tumor encapsulation in hepatocellular carcinoma. *Cancer* 70:45–49, 1992.
117. Okazaki N, Yosshino M, Yoshida T, et al: Evaluation of the prognosis for small hepatocellular carcinoma based on tumor volume doubling time. *Cancer* 63:2207–2210, 1989.
118. Saddler D: Focus on the patient with metastatic disease. Hepatic metastasis: A nursing perspective. *Dimens Oncol Nurs* 1(2):4–6, 1985.
119. Ong GB: Techniques and therapies for primary and metastatic liver cancer. *Curr Probl Cancer* 2(6):1977.
120. Melato M, Laurino L, Mucli E, et al: Relationship between cirrhosis, liver cancer, and hepatic metastases. *Cancer* 64:455–459, 1989.
121. Bierman HR, Byron RL, Kelley KH, et al: Studies on blood supply of tumors in man. Vascular patterns of liver by hepatic arteriography in vivo. *JNCI* 12:107–131, 1951.
122. Case record of the Massachusetts General Hospital. *N Engl J Med* 302:1132, 1980.
123. Shepherd FA, Rostein LE, Houle S, et al: A phase I dose escalation trial of Yttrium-90 microspheres in the treatment of primary hepatocellular carcinoma. *Cancer* 70:2250–2254, 1992.
124. McDermott WV, Jenkins RL, Cady B, Steele G: Primary and metastatic cancer of the liver. In Steele G, Cady B (eds): *General Surgical Oncology*. Philadelphia: Saunders, 1992, pp. 185–194.
125. Tremolda F, Benevegnu L, Drago C, et al: Early detection of hepatocellular carcinoma in patients with cirrhosis by alphaprotein, ultrasound and fine-needle biopsy. *Hepatogastroenterology* 36:519–521, 1989.
126. Giardina MG, Matarazzo M, Varriale A, et al: Serum alpha-L-fucosidase. *Cancer* 70:1044–1048, 1992.
127. McGill DB, Zinsmeister AR, Ott BJ: Liver biopsy: Increased risks in patients with cancer. *Gastroenterology* 89:1396–1400, 1990.
128. Adson MA: Resection of liver metastases—When is it worthwhile? *World J Surg* 11:511–529, 1987.
129. Zhuo X, Tang Z, Yu Y, et al: Long-term survivors after resection for primary liver cancer. *Cancer* 63:2201–2206, 1989.
130. Onik G, Rubinsky B, Zemel R, et al: Ultrasound-guided cryosurgery in the treatment of metastatic colon carcinoma. *Cancer* 67:901–907, 1992.
131. Li GH, Zhu SL, Li JQ, Zhan YQ: Evaluation of partial hepatectomy for primary liver carcinoma. *J Surg Oncol* 41:5–8, 1989.
132. Zhou XD, Tang ZY, Yu YQ, Ma ZC: Clinical evaluation of cryosurgery in the treatment of primary liver cancer. *Cancer* 61:1889–1892, 1988.
133. Wanebo HJ: *Hepatic and Biliary Cancer*. Philadelphia: Saunders, 1987.
134. Cady B, Stone MD, McDermott WV, et al: Technical and biological factors in disease-free survival after hepatic resection for colorectal cancer metastases. *Arch Surg* 127:561–569, 1992.
135. Yokoyama I, Carr B, Saitsu H, et al: Accelerated growth rates of recurrent hepatocellular carcinoma after liver transplantation. *Cancer* 68:2095–2100, 1991.
136. Ikeda K, Kumada H, Saitoh S, et al: Effect of repeated transcatheter arterial embolization on the survival time in patients with hepatocellular carcinoma. *Cancer* 68:2150–2154, 1992.
137. Beppu T, Ohara C, Yamaguchi Y, et al: A new approach to chemoembolization for unresectable hepatocellular carcinoma using aclarubicin in combination with cisplatin suspended in iodized oil. *Cancer* 68:2555–2560, 1992.
138. Livraghi T, Bolondi L, Lazzaroni S, et al: Percutaneous ethanol injection in the treatment of hepatocellular carcinoma in cirrhosis. *Cancer* 69:925–929, 1992.
139. Raoul JL, Heresbach D, Bretagne JF, et al: Chemoembolization of hepatocellular carcinomas. *Cancer* 70:585–590, 1992.
140. Staryl T: Right trisegmentectomy for hepatic neoplasms. *Surg Gynecol Obstet* 150:208, 1980.
141. Vetto JT, Hughes KS, Rosenstein R, Sugarbaker PH: Morbidity and mortality of hepatic resection for metastatic colorectal carcinoma. *Dis Colon Rectum* 33:408–413, 1990.
142. Steele G, Bleday R, Mayer RJ, et al: A prospective evaluation of hepatic resection for colorectal carcinoma metastases to the liver: Gastrointestinal Tumor Study Group Protocol 6584. *J Clin Oncol* 9:1105–1112, 1991.
143. Kemeny N, Seiter K, Niedzwiecki D, et al: A randomized

trial of intrahepatic infusion of fluorodeoxyuridine with dexamethasone versus fluorodeoxyuridine alone in the treatment of metastatic colorectal cancer. *Cancer* 69:327–334, 1992.

144. Atiq OT, Kemeny N, Niedzwiecki D, Botet J: Treatment of unresectable primary liver cancer with intrahepatic fluorodeoxyuridine and mitomycin C through an implantable pump. *Cancer* 69:920–924, 1992.
145. Schober C, Kohne-Wompner CH, Schmoll HJ, et al: A 3-day schedule of 5-fluorouracil and folinic acid in metastatic progressive colorectal cancer and its impact in terms of palliation. *Semin Oncol* 19:136–140, 1992.
146. Steinke B, Gunther E, Hirschmann WD, et al: Fluorouracil versus folinic acid/fluorouracil in advanced colorectal cancer—Preliminary results of a randomized trial. *Semin Oncol* 19:141–147, 1992.
147. Bernhard H, Klein O, Meyer KH, et al: Treatment of refractory colorectal carcinomas with fluorouracil, folinic acid, and interferon alfa-2a. *Semin Oncol* 19(2):204–207, 1992.
148. Wadler S, Lembersky B, Atkins M: Phase II trial of fluorouracil and recombinant interferon alfa-2a in patients with advanced colorectal carcinoma: An Eastern Cooperative Oncology Group study. *J Clin Oncol* 9(10):1806–1810, 1991.
149. Niederhuber JE, Grochow LB: Status of infusion chemotherapy for the treatment of liver metastases. *PPO Updates* (3):1–9, 1989.
150. Patt YZ, Mavligit GM: Arterial chemotherapy in the management of colorectal cancer: An overview. *Semin Oncol* 18(5):478–490, 1991.
151. Sterchi JM, Richards F, White DR, et al: Chemoinfusion of the hepatic artery for metastases to the liver. *Surg Obstet Gynecol* 168(4):291–295, 1989.
152. Pozniak MA, Babel SG, Trump DL: Complications of hepatic arterial infusion chemotherapy. *Radiographics* 11:67–79, 1991.
153. Wong E, Khardori N, Carrasco CH, et al: Infectious complications of hepatic artery catheterization procedures in patients with cancer. *Rev Infect Dis* 13:583–586, 1991.
154. Rougier P, Laplanche A, Huguier M, et al: Hepatic arterial infusion of floxuridine in patients with liver metastases from colorectal carcinoma: Long term results of a prospective randomized trial. *J Clin Oncol* 10:1112–1118, 1992.
155. Safi F, Bittner R, Roscher R, et al: Regional chemotherapy for hepatic metastases of colorectal carcinoma (continuous intraarterial versus continuous intraarterial/intravenous therapy). *Cancer* 64:379–387, 1989.
156. Andersson R, Holmberg A: Intraperitoneal 5-fluorouracil in the management of colorectal liver cancer. *Eur J Surg Oncol* 18:152–155, 1992.
157. Yoo HS, Lee JT, Kim KW, et al: Nodular hepatocellular carcinoma. *Cancer* 68:1878–1884, 1991.
158. Raoul JI, Bretagne JF, Caucanas JP, et al: Internal radiation therapy for hepatocellular carcinoma. *Cancer* 69:346–352, 1992.
159. Hellman K, Goold M, Higgins N, Phillips RH: Responses of liver metastases to radiotherapy and razoxane. *J R Soc Med* 85:136–138, 1992.
160. Miller RL, Bukowski RM, Anderson S, et al: Phase II evaluation of sequential hepatic artery infusion of 5-fluorouracil and hepatic irradiation in metastatic colorectal carcinoma. *J Surg Oncol* 37:1–4, 1988.
161. O'Mary SS: Liver cancer: Primary and metastatic disease. *Semin Oncol Nurs* 4(4):265–273, 1988.
162. Welch D: Nursing the patient with advanced liver metastases. *Cancer Nurs* 2(4):297–303, 1979.
163. Fontham ET, Correa P: Epidemiology of pancreatic cancer. *Surg Clin North Am* 69(3):551–567, 1989.
164. Warshaw AL, Castillo CF: Pancreatic carcinoma. *N Engl J Med* 326(7):455–465, 1992.
165. Brennan MF, Kinsella T, Friedman M: Cancer of the pancreas. In DeVita VT, Hellman S, Rosenberg SA (eds): *Cancer: Principles and Practice of Oncology* (3d ed). Philadelphia: Lippincott, 1989, pp. 800–835.
166. Blot W: Geographic correlates of pancreas cancer in the United States. *Cancer* 42:373–380, 1978.
167. Hiatt RA, Klatsky AL, Armstrong MA: Pancreatic cancer, blood glucose and beverage consumption. *Int J Cancer* 41:794–797, 1988.
168. Ishikawa O, Ohhigashi H, Wada A, et al: Morphologic characteristics of pancreatic carcinoma with diabetes mellitus. *Cancer* 64:1107–1112, 1989.
169. DiMagno EP: Early diagnosis of chronic pancreatitis and pancreatic cancer. *Med Clin North Am* 72(5):979–992, 1988.
170. LaVecchiaa C, Negri E, D'Avanzo B, et al: Medical history, diet and pancreatic cancer. *Oncology* 47:463–466, 1990.
171. Ahlgren JD, Hill MC, Roberts IM: Pancreatic cancer: Patterns, diagnosis, and approaches to treatment. In Ahlgren JD, Macdonald JS (eds): *Gastrointestinal Oncology*. Philadelphia: Lippincott, 1992, pp. 197–208.
172. Yamada T: Secretory tumors of the pancreas. In Sleisenger NH, Fordtran JS (eds): *Gastrointestinal Disease* (3d ed). Philadelphia: Saunders, 1983.
173. Sindelar WF: Clinical experience with regional pancreatectomy for adenocarcinoma of the pancreas. *Arch Surg* 124:127–132, 1989.
174. Singh SM, Reber HA: Surgical palliation for pancreatic cancer. *Surg Clin North Am* 69(3):599–611, 1989.
175. Lightdale CJ, Botet FN, Woodruff JM, Brennan MF: Localization of endocrine tumors of the pancreas with endoscopic ultrasonography. *Cancer* 68:1815–1820, 1991.
176. Ross CR, Sharp KW, Kaufman AJ, et al: Efficacy of computerized tomography in the preoperative staging of pancreatic carcinoma. *Am Surg* 54:221–226, 1988.
177. DelMaschio A, Vanzulli A, Sirioni S, et al: Pancreatic cancer versus chronic pancreatitis: Diagnosis with CA 19-9 assessment, US, CT, and CT-guided fine needle biopsy. *Radiology* 178:95–99, 1991.
178. Spross JA, Manalatos A, Thorpe M: Pancreatic cancer: Nursing challenges. *Semin Oncol Nurs* 4(4):274–284, 1988.
179. Fabris C: Urinary enzymes excretion in pancreatic diseases. *J Clin Gastroenterol* 14(4):281–284, 1992.
180. Yoshimura T, Manabe T, Imamura T, et al: Flow cytometric analysis of nuclear DNA content of duct cell carcinoma of the pancreas. *Cancer* 70:1069–1074, 1992.
181. Satake K, Chung YS, Umeyama K, et al: The possibility of diagnosing small pancreatic cancer (less than 4.0 cm) by measuring various serum tumor markers. *Cancer* 68:149–152, 1991.
182. Manabe T, Ohshio G, Baba N, et al: Radical pancreatectomy for ductal cell carcinoma of the head of the pancreas. *Cancer* 64:1132–1137, 1989.
183. Wanebo HJ, Koness RJ: Pancreatic cancer: Surgical approach. In Ahlgren JD, Macdonald JS (eds): *Gastroin-*

testinal Oncology. Philadelphia: Lippincott, 1992, pp. 209–214.

184. Sindelar WF, Kinsella TJ, Mayer RJ: Cancer of the pancreas. In DeVita VT, Hellman S, Roseman SA (eds): *Cancer: Principles and Practice of Oncology* (2d ed). Philadelphia: Lippincott, 1985, pp. 691–739.
185. Merrick HW, Dobelbower RR: Aggressive therapy for cancer of the pancreas. *Gastroenterol Clin North Am* 19(4):935–962, 1990.
186. Miyata M, Nakao K, Takao T, et al: An appraisal of pancreatectomy for advanced cancer of the pancreas based on survival rate and postoperative physical performance. *J Surg Oncol* 45:33–39, 1990.
187. Jordan GL: Pancreatic resection for pancreatic cancer. *Surg Clin North Am* 69(3):569–597, 1989.
188. McGrath PC, McNeill PM, Neifeld JP, et al: Management of biliary obstruction in patients with unresectable carcinoma of the pancreas. *Ann Surg* 209(3):284–288, 1989.
189. Doderneck RC, Berndt GA: Delayed gastric emptying after palliative gastrojejunostomy for carcinoma of the pancreas. *Arch Surg* 122:827–829, 1987.
190. Rosemurgy AS, Burnett CM, Wasselle JA: A comparison of choledochoenteric bypass and cholecystenteric bypass in patients with biliary obstruction due to pancreatic cancer. *Am Surg* 55(1):55–60, 1989.
191. Shimi S, Banting S, Cuschieri A: Laparoscopy in the management of pancreatic cancer: Endoscopic cholecystojejunostomy for advanced disease. *Brit J Surg* 79:317–319, 1992.
192. Mannell A, Weiland LH, Heerden JA, Ilstrup DM: Factors influencing survival after resection for ductal adenocarcinoma of the pancreas. *Ann Surg* 203(4):403–407, 1986.
193. Regan PT, DiMagno EP: The medical management of malabsorption. *Mayo Clin Proc* 54:267–274, 1979.
194. Moosa AR: *Tumors of the Pancreas*. Baltimore, MD: Williams & Wilkens, 1980.
195. Tajiri H, Yoshimori M, Okazaki N, Miyaji M: Phase II study of continuous venous infusion of 5-fluorouracil in advanced pancreatic cancer. *Oncology* 48:18–21, 1991.
196. Scheithauer W, Funovics J, Mueller C, Ludwig H: Sequential high-dose methotrexate, 5-fluorouracil, and doxorubicin for treatment of advanced pancreatic cancer. *J Cancer Res Clin Oncol* 116:132–133, 1990.
197. Canobbio L, Boccardo F, Cannata D, et al: Treatment of advanced pancreatic carcinoma with the somatostatin analogue BIM 23014. *Cancer* 69:648–650, 1992.
198. Kelsen D, Hudis C, Niedzwiecki D, et al: A phase III comparison trial of streptozotocin, mitomycin, and 5-fluorouracil with cisplatin, cytosine arabinoside, and caffeine in patients with advanced pancreatic carcinoma. *Cancer* 68:965–969, 1991.
199. Douglass HO, Stablein DM, Thomas PR: An organized multi-institutional interdisciplinary evaluation of role of radiation therapy alone or combined with chemotherapy in treatment of adenocarcinoma of the gastrointestinal tract. *Natl Cancer Inst Monographs* 1988, pp. 253–257.
200. Gastrointestinal Tumor Study Group: Treatment of locally unresectable carcinoma of the pancreas: Comparison of combined-modality therapy to chemotherapy alone. *JNCI* 80:751–755, 1988.
201. Komaki R, Wadler S, Peters T, et al: High-dose local irradiation plus prophylactic hepatic irradiation and chemotherapy for inoperable adenocarcinoma of the pancreas. *Cancer* 69:2807–2812, 1992.
202. Bagne FR, Dobelbower RR, Milligan AJ, et al: Treatment of cancer of the pancreas by intraoperative electron beam therapy: Physical and biological aspects. *Int J Radiat Oncol Biol Phys* 16:231–242, 1989.
203. Mohiuddin M, Rosato F, Barbot D, et al: Long-term results of combined modality treatment with I-125 implantation for carcinoma of the pancreas. *Int J Radiat Oncol Biol Phys* 23:305–311, 1992.
204. Brandabur JJ, Kozarek RA, Ball TJ, et al: Nonoperative versus operative treatment of obstructive jaundice in pancreatic cancer: Cost and survival analysis. *Am J Gastroenterol* 83(10):1132–1139, 1988.
205. McGrath PC, McNeil PM, Neifeld JP, et al: Management of biliary obstruction in patients with unresectable carcinoma of the pancreas. *Ann Surg* 209:284–288, 1989.
206. Cotton PB: Nonsurgical palliation of jaundice in pancreatic cancer. *Surg Clin North Am* 69:613–627, 1989.

Chapter 42

Gastrointestinal Cancer: Colon, Rectum, and Anus

Beverly Hampton, RN, MS, ET

INTRODUCTION

In spite of extensive research advances in molecular biology, colon and rectal cancers remain a significant problem within the United States and other Westernized countries. In the United States it is estimated that in 1993 there will be a total of 152,000 new cases of colorectal malignancies; 109,000 of these will occur within the colon and 43,000 will develop in the rectum.[1] It is also estimated that an infant born within the United States has a 5% chance of developing either a colon or rectal tumor during his or her lifetime. Though incompletely understood, the mechanisms for the development of colorectal cancer are considered to be the result of both environmental and genetic factors.

EPIDEMIOLOGY

Incidence

Colorectal cancer accounts for 15% of all malignancies in both men and women. In men, prostate and lung cancer exceed colorectal cancer incidence, and among women only breast cancer exceeds colorectal cancer incidence.[1] In the United States a higher incidence is seen in the northeastern states than in the western and southern areas. However, within urban localities the incidence is higher than in rural settings.[3]

Death Rate

The 1993 estimated deaths from colorectal cancer are expected to be 25,000 male and 25,000 female and 7000 from rectal cancer.[1] Survival rates for whites and blacks are suggested at 58% and 47%, respectively. About 11% of the total deaths due to cancer are associated with colorectal malignancies.

Sex and Age

The rate of occurrence of colorectal cancer within the United States appears to be the same for males as for females. The rate increases after age 40, with a mean age at the time of diagnosis of 63 years for men and 62 years for women.[2] A decline in the occurrence of colorectal cancer is seen after the age of 75. Colorectal cancer can be diagnosed at any age and has even been reported in a 9-month-old infant.[4] Malignancies occurring in individuals 20–30 years of age are difficult to control and usually indicate a poor prognosis.[5]

Race and Religion

African Americans and white Americans within each region and each community of the United States display similar patterns of occurrence. In contrast to this, there is a low incidence of colorectal cancer among Native Americans, which is reported as less than half that for white Americans.[6]

Certain populations in specific countries, such as Africa and Japan, display a lower incidence of colorectal cancer as compared to white Americans; however, this low risk decreases once these persons migrate to Western countries. This change in incidence may be a result of both dietary and environmental factors.[7]

Studies of religious groups, e.g., Mormons and Seventh Day Adventists, have demonstrated a lower cancer mortality than that of the general population.[8,9] This is felt to be related to vegetarian diets or restricted meat and meat product consumption. These two groups also place restrictions on use of tobacco, alcohol, and caffeine-containing products. While specific studies do not implicate any of these individual products as carcinogenic, the products may act in combination with other factors that are not yet identified. In sharp contrast, Jews demonstrate a higher incidence than people of other religious groups.[2] Causative factors are not known.

ETIOLOGY

Diet

During the past 20 years, dietary factors have received considerable research and even generated controversy regarding their role in the pathogenesis of colorectal cancer.[10] A possible explanation of the etiology involves the fact that ingested foods come into contact with the bowel mucosa; thus, certain foods and/or the time that they are in contact with a specific bowel area may be the initiating factor for a malignancy by altering the environment of the gut. Another reason for suggesting diet as a factor is the difference in the incidence rates in various populations throughout the world.[11] Burkitt et al.[11] postulate from observations of native Africans and their low cancer incidence as compared to the higher colorectal cancer incidence in Western countries that a diet high in fiber reduces the incidence of cancer. The basis of this theory is that with an increased stool transit time there is a reduction in the time that the gastrointestinal (GI) tract is exposed to carcinogenic food substances.[12,13]

Selenium, a trace element, has been found to inhibit carcinogenesis by deactivating carcinogens and protecting cells from free-radical formation.[14] While it is unclear how substances could act within the GI tract to initiate a carcinogenic process, certain foods, such as fats, are regarded as agents that promote cellular changes in the bowel mucosa, whereas fiber products and calcium are believed to reduce the carcinogenic process.

Fat and protein

Dietary fat increases the risk of colon cancer through several possible mechanisms. First, when large amounts of dietary fat are present, there is an increase in the amount of fecal bile acid coming into contact with the GI mucosa.[14,15] Metabolites of fecal bile acid and sterol conversion products may be carcinogenic or may enhance or promote other cancer-causing agents that are present. The transit of food through the GI tract is slowed with the presence of fat, thus extending the time interval that the bile acid or any other carcinogenic substance may be in direct contact with the bowel lining. Persons in Western countries demonstrate a higher concentration of bile acids as well as a higher cancer rate than populations in Eastern and African countries.[16,17]

A high intake of protein is also linked to colon cancer.[15] People who ingest large amounts of beef are reported as having a higher incidence of colorectal cancer.

Fiber

Fiber, the indigestible component of plants, is composed of cellulose, hemicellulose, lignin, and pectin. When fiber is increased in the diet, it results in a larger stool volume, a softer stool, and an increased frequency of defecation. The increased intestinal transit time is important, since there will be a decrease in the contact time in the large bowel for any carcinogenic agents either endogenous or exogenous. Other protective roles of dietary fiber may include altering colonic pH, binding potentially cancer-causing agents, and decreasing the concentration of ammonia in the gut.[17]

Other investigators question the role of a high-fiber diet alone as a protection against colorectal cancer and suggest that high fiber intake, as seen in an animal model, is only effective when the fat content remains low. From their studies they suggest a 10% reduction in fat consumption, the addition of 25 g of dietary fiber per day, and plant steroids as possible preventions for colorectal cancer.[18]

Calcium

Calcium is being examined as a substance that may decrease the risk of colon cancer in general or in individuals who are asymptomatic yet kindreds of someone with hereditary colon cancer.[20] Calcium has been examined alone or in combination with vitamin D as well as in combination with vitamin D and low-fat diets.

The protective role of calcium is derived from its effect on the proliferative activity on the colonic mucosa. In pre- or neoplastic colon lesions, the proliferation of abnormal mucosal cells seem to be modified in laboratory animals with an oral intake of calcium.[19]

While the mechanism for reduction in cellular proliferation is not completely known, it is suggested that the calcium binds to free, ionized fatty acids and bile salts and then converts these acids and salts into calcium soaps, thus reducing their possible toxicity and cancer-promoting tendencies.[20] A decreased proliferation rate of the cells was noted when colon biopsies obtained from high-risk patients were cultured in vitro with high levels of calcium. A definite role of calcium in preventing colon cancer is yet to be determined.

Bacteria, Viruses, and Parasites

Carcinoma of the colon and rectum may develop as a result of the action of fecal bacteria on metabolites or the ingested fats. It is hypothesized that the fecal bacteria act on bile salts and thus produce metabolites that initiate malignant changes either as carcinogens or as co-carcinogens. Burkitt et al.[11] proposed that distal bowel carcinoma was more frequent, because of the increased amount of bacteria in this location. There is evidence of an increased amount of secondary bile acids in persons with cancer. Experimental studies show that secondary bile acids induce chemical carcinogenesis. Recently, cholecystectomy has been implicated as a precipitating event that introduces bile acids into the circulation. Although controversial, elderly women 10 years postcholecystectomy have an increased incidence of right-sided colon cancer.[21,22]

There is some evidence that colorectal cancer risk increases following infection with schistosomiasis, such as occurs in China, where the infection is endemic and the colorectal cancer rate is increased.[23] Schistosomiasal cysts have been identified with colorectal cancer. Dysplasia occurs following infections with schistosomiasis.

Chemoprotective Agents

Chemoprotective agents are potential inhibitors of carcinogenesis. Ascorbic acid is being investigated, as are the flavones and indoles, substances found in cruciferous vegetables such as Brussels sprouts, cauliflower, broccoli, and cabbage. Incidence of colon cancer is inversely related to the intake of these vegetables.[24]

Predisposing Conditions

Familial adenomatous polyposis (FAP), or *familial polyposis coli* as it was previously termed, is an autosomal dominant inherited disease. While the specific gene for FAP has not been identified, it has been demonstrated that the gene is located on the long arm of chromosome 5.[25] The disease is characterized by multiple (>100) colorectal adenomatous polyps, with a high risk that these polyps will develop into adenocarcinoma. The number of polyps in a macroscopic familial polyposis specimen averages 1000.[26] The polyps may develop at any age; however, they usually appear after puberty, with an average age at onset of 25 years, and symptoms occur around age 36. Adenocarcinoma usually develops before the person reaches age 40. FAP can develop in individuals with a negative family history and may represent new mutations.[27]

The development of carcinoma from these polyps is an extremely high risk. Surgical procedures are used to remove diseased bowel as well as any other tissue that could result in additional sites for the polyps to occur. Historically, the surgical procedure to treat familial polyposis was protocolectomy followed by the creation of an ileostomy. Today there are many advocates of (1) an abdominal colectomy with ileorectal anastomosis and (2) a proctocolectomy with ileoanal anastomosis and creation of a rectal pouch, thereby preserving bowel continuity.[28] Because carcinoma can develop in any retained unresected rectal area, these individuals require close surveillance, routine proctoscopic examination every 6 months, and a willingness to comply with close monitoring.[29]

As well as following family members at risk, patients with FAP are being followed by large registries throughout the world to determine specific recurrence rates related to age, the selected surgical procedures, and time intervals from diagnosis to any tumor appearance.

Gardner's syndrome, also an inherited autosomal dominant trait, is a variation of FAP and results in not only gastrointestinal polyps with a malignant potential but also osteomas of the long bones, mandible, and skull; polyps of the gastric and duodenal areas; as well as various cysts, keloids, cutaneous fibromas, peritoneal adhesions, and retroperitoneal fibrosis. There is debate regarding whether Gardner's is a separate syndrome or merely a different expression of familial polyposis coli.

Turcot's syndrome, or glioma-polyposis, is another type of hereditary disorder associated with adenomatous colorectal polyps. The condition is rare and may be transmitted as an autosomal recessive genetic disease that results in colorectal polyps, malignant central nervous system tumors, and an even earlier development of colorectal malignancies than among persons with FAP.[30]

Peutz-Jeghers syndrome, also a polyposis syndrome, is associated with multiple harmatomas within the GI tract, mucocutaneous pigmentation, and an increased cancer incidence. Malignant degeneration is less; however, an increased cancer risk of 16 times that of the normal population is seen, and lifetime risk exceeds 2%.[31]

Hereditary nonpolyposis colorectal carcinoma

Hereditary nonpolyposis colorectal cancer (HNPCC), originally called "cancer family syndrome," is known to account for 4%–6% of the total number of colorectal cancers. The name of the syndrome is confusing, since there actually are polyps present, but not in the numbers seen with FAP. There are two types of HNPCC: Lynch I site-specific and Lynch II nonsite-specific.[32] Site-specific HNPCC is colon-specific and includes those who are young at the time of colon cancer onset, whose cancer is located proximal to the splenic flexure, and who have synchronous and metachronous tumors. In nonsite-specific HNPCC the same characteristics are included, as well as extracolonic adenocarcinomas, such as endometrial, stomach, small intestine, renal, pelvis, ovary, and ureter. These polyps are genetically autosomal dominant and include a higher incidence of mucinous carcinomas.[33,34] The two types are seven times more common than FAP and account for 7% of all colon cancers.

Other terms, such as *cancer family syndrome* (Lynch I) and *hereditary colon cancer* (Lynch II), are used to identify HNPCC. For both types, subtotal colectomy and ileorectal anastomosis (possible hysterectomy, bilateral salpingo-oophorectomy) is the preferred treatment.[29]

Family history of colon cancer

Individuals with a first-degree relative with colon cancer are at three-times-greater risk of developing colon cancer than other persons in the general population.[35,36] When counseling high-risk families, it is important to assure the spouses in any familial or genetic situation that they are not at an increased cancer risk.

Inflammatory Bowel Disease

Ulcerative colitis

Patients with a history of inflammatory bowel disease (IBD), and particularly of ulcerative colitis (UC), develop colorectal cancer at significantly higher rates than the general population. Once UC develops, there is an approximate 3% risk of developing malignancy. This risk increases about 20% with each following decade of life, to as high as 60%–100% with 30 years of active total bowel disease.[29] Individuals with only ulcerative proctitis are felt to have a negligible risk of developing a malignancy. In this group, colorectal cancer is often preceded by dysplasia.[37] There is a similarity between the pathological features of UC and those of schistosomiasal infections.[23]

Indications for colectomy in patients with UC include active disease that is unresponsive to medical management, massive hemorrhage, toxic megacolon, and the development of dysplasia or carcinoma. Various surgical procedures are available for the individual with UC who develops carcinoma and may include any of the following: early prophylactic proctocolectomy, total proctocolectomy with creation of an external ileostomy, total proctocolectomy with creation of an internal reservoir (Koch pouch), and removal of the large bowel and rectum followed by the creation of an internal rectal pouch from a segment of ileum that is anastomosed to the anus and thus preserves continence.

Crohn's colitis

Crohn's colitis may result in the development of dysplasia and then a colorectal cancer. The risk is 4 to 20 times that of the general population, yet less than for persons with UC. Cancer among persons with Crohn's colitis arises at a younger age. The cancer can be present in bowel segments that have been bypassed during a previous surgical procedure. Mucosal dysplasia is present in 25% of cases prior to finding cancer, and an endometriosis-like invasion of gut stroma is evident in 40% of the cases.[38]

Any patients and families with familial or genetic risks should receive counseling from health care providers. They need to be aware of how the risk affects them, the detection tests that should be done, and the preventive measures that should be taken. (See Table 42-1.)

Other Factors

An additional documented association for colorectal cancer, although not clearly understood, is prior pelvic irradiation. Individuals who have undergone an appendectomy or cholecystectomy also may be at risk. Nulliparity is being examined, since a decreased incidence of colorectal cancer occurs in women with two (30%) or three (50%) children. Reduced physical activity and exposure to asbestos have also been noted.[39–41]

A relationship exists between creation of a ureterosigmoidostomy and colon carcinoma that is significant enough that various authorities suggest the procedure be abandoned, particularly in young persons with benign disease.

TABLE 42-1 Clinical Risk Factors for Colorectal Cancer

Genetic:
- Familial adenomatous polyposis syndrome
- Gardner, Oldfield, or Turcot syndrome
- Peutz-Jegher syndrome

Familial:
- Familial colorectal cancer syndrome
- Hereditary adenocarcinomatosis syndrome
- Family history of colorectal cancer

Preexisting disease:
- Inflammatory bowel disease
- Colorectal cancer
- Pelvic cancer postirradiation
- Neoplastic colorectal polyps

General:
- All men and women over age 40

Source: Data from DeVita VT, Hellman S. Rosenberg SA (eds): *Cancer: Principles and Practice of Oncology* (3d ed). Philadelphia: Lippincott, 1989.

PATHOPHYSIOLOGY

Cellular Characteristics

Adenocarcinoma is the major histologic type of neoplasm occurring in the colorectal area. (See Table 42-2.) Adenocarcinoma accounts for 94% of the malignancies, of which 7.8% are mucin-secreting. These tumors arise from glandular epithelium and can provide variable amounts of mucin and display varying degrees of differentiation. Adenocarcinomas extend into adjacent organs or spread by way of the lymphatics to regional lymph nodes, then into the bloodstream.[27]

Mucinous tumors produce large amounts of mucus, differ both epidemiologically and clinically from other colorectal tumors, appear in persons under 30 years of age, occur frequently in blacks, and have a poor prognosis. When large amounts of mucoid material accumulate within the cell, the cytoplasm displaces the nucleus and the cell takes on a segmented or ringed appearance.[42] This variant of the adenocarcinoma, like the mucin-producing tumor, signals a less favorable prognosis. Signet ring tumors metastasize early and can extend along the bowel. They cause minimal mucosal distortion but produce significant bowel rigidity.

TABLE 42-2 Classification of Cancer of the Large Bowel and Anus

Large Bowel
- Carcinoma
  1. Adenocarcinoma
  2. Squamous cell carcinoma
  3. Carcinoid
- Sarcoma
  1. Lymphoma
  2. Leiomyosarcoma
  3. Rhabdomyosarcoma
  4. Liposarcoma

Anus
- Carcinoma
  1. Squamous
  2. Basaloid carcinoma
  3. Small-cell carcinoma
  4. Adenocarcinoma
  5. Adenocanthoma
  6. Basal cell epithelioma
- Sarcoma
  1. Lymphoma
  2. Leiomyosarcoma/rhabdomyosarcoma/liposarcoma
  3. Melanoma

Source: Kirschner JB, Shortner RG, (eds): *Diseases of the Colon, Rectum, and Anal Canal.* Baltimore: Williams & Wilkens, 1989.

Another histologic variant and poorly differentiated cancer is the scirrhous carcinoma, or "leathery" tumor. Again, prognosis is less favorable for scirrhous or stenosing type versus nonscirrhous.[43]

Tumor types

Adenocarcinomas may be characterized macroscopically into polypoid or annular constricting lesions.[44] Polypoid tumors, the second most frequent type, may appear throughout the colon; however, they appear more frequently on the right side, whereas annular constricting lesions are associated with the left colon. Polypoid tumors usually are a large mass that only occasionally constricts the bowel lumen. Annular constricting lesions present as nodular infiltrating lesions that may ulcerate; appear on the left side, sigmoid, or rectum; and have a characteristic "apple core" appearance evident on barium enema.[43]

There are other colon tumors, such as lymphoma, carcinoid, leiomyosarcoma, Kaposi's carcinoma, squamous cell carcinoma, and melanoma, all of which are encountered infrequently, are difficult to treat, and have a guarded prognosis.[45] Within the rectum, the adenocarcinomas include sessile or polypoid lesions, which have the potential to ulcerate and extend into adjacent organs.

Anal cancer

Carcinomas of the anus are rare, accounting for less than 4% of distal GI neoplasms.[46] The incidence of anal cancer increases with age. The tumor occurs more frequently among females; however, there has been an increase in men, particularly those who are homosexual or bisexual or have a history of anal condylomata acuminata.[46–48]

While the etiology of anal carcinoma has not been identified, there appears to be an association with human papilloma virus, condylomata, HIV, immunosuppression in renal transplant, prior radiation, and cigarette smoking.[46,49]

The histological types of anal cancer include squamous cell carcinoma, transitional-cell carcinoma, adenocarcinoma, Paget's disease, basal cell carcinoma, and melanoma. Squamous cell carcinoma is the most prevalent of the cell types (63%). It originates from the stratified squamous epithelium, is usually well differentiated and slow growing, and may appear to be a fistula, benign lesion, hemorrhoid, or as a fissure.[46]

These lesions can occur in the anal canal as well as on the perianal skin, perineum, and vulvar area. There may be small nodules with ulcerations, and thickening if the lesion appears in the perianal area. The most frequent symptom of an anal cancer is spontaneous bright-red bleeding, alone or in conjunction with a bowel movement.[34] Individuals will also describe anal pressure or pain, pruritus, a change in stool caliber as the anal lumen decreases in size, and inguinal node enlargement.

Progression of Disease

Evidence suggests that invasive colorectal cancer actually transitions from benign polyps to cancer.[45] Support for this theory is listed in Table 42-3. It is unusual to find a small cancer in normal bowel mucosa.[50] Villous-type polyps carry the greatest risk of malignant transformation, about ten times that of tubular polyps. It is also known that malignant potential of polyps correlates with the grade, stage, size, and degree of dysplasia.

The progression of colorectal neoplasms depends on factors such as the histological classification, degree of differentiation, and local and distant metastases. This information is used to estimate survival times. The earlier the malignancy is identified, the greater the chances of long-term survival. The 5-year disease-free rates using Dukes' classification from several reported series indicate the following: Dukes' A, 67%–81%; Dukes' B, 51%–64%; and Dukes' C, 32%–44%.[2] Primary cancers of the large bowel grow slowly, with doubling times greater than 600 days, or 1.6 years. However, once metastases occurs, the doubling rate increases.

The duration of symptoms does not appear to relate to the degree of tumor advancement. The diagnosis of colorectal cancer in asymptomatic individuals has been shown to be related to improved survival, probably indicative of earlier diagnosis. Lesions that obstruct the

TABLE 42-3 Arguments for an Adenomatous Polyp-to-Cancer Transition

1. Residual adenomatous tissue is observed quite commonly in small cancers.
2. Patients from whom polyps are removed remain cancer-free.
3. Small foci of intramucosal cancer are commonly seen in polyps but are extremely rare in normal mucosa.
4. Some apparently benign adenomatous polyps have developed into cancer.
5. The incidence of cancer increases as the size of the adenomatous polyp increases.
6. There is an increasing incidence of cancer as the number of adenomatous polyps increase.
7. There are no good criteria by which adenomatous polyps can be classified as a different biologic entity from villous adenomas, a lesion with definite malignant potential.
8. The adenomatous polyp-to-cancer transition has been seen in familial polyposis.
9. The adenomatous polyp-to-cancer transition has been seen in experimental animals.
10. A presumed transition from a precancerous state to invasive malignancy is seen in several other epithelial tissues.
11. Polyps are usually diagnosed two years before cancer.
12. There are similar distributions of polyps and cancer within the large bowel.

Source: Sugarbaker PH, MacDonald, JS, Gunderson LL: Colorectal cancer, in DeVita VT Jr, Hellman S, Rosenberg SA (eds): *Cancer: Principles and Practice of Oncology* (3d ed). Philadelphia: Lippincott, 1989, p. 643.

continuity of the GI tract or perforate the bowel usually carry a poor prognosis, as do tumors in the younger age group.[2] Other factors affecting the progression of the disease are tumor location, indeterminate host factors, age and sex of the person, and complications due to metastases.

Lymph node involvement may be present in 50% of individuals with colorectal cancer at the time of diagnosis.[2] Lymphatic involvement occurs once the tumor invades the muscularis propria, and then the cancer spread follows a fairly predictable pattern. The number of lymph nodes involved has been shown to be a more accurate predictor of survival than the depth of penetration.

Venous invasion is an indicator of poor prognosis. The embolization of tumor cells through the vascular system leads to widespread dissemination of the disease. Surgical resection is ineffective once venous invasion has occurred, and other treatment modalities, such as chemotherapy and radiotherapy, are also ineffective in prolonging survival. Sites for metastasized venous invasion include the liver (75%), the lungs (15%), and the bones and brain (5%), with other organs occasionally involved.[45]

Implantation is another mode of tumor spread. Tumor cells freed from the primary site float to other receptor surfaces and grow. Peritoneal implants develop in 10% of those with colon cancer with or without vascular or lymphatic spread. Implantation at the suture line is rare in colon cancer surgery, but may be possible with low anterior resection for rectal cancer.[51]

Direct extension of colorectal and anal tumors is also possible. When the bowel wall is penetrated and adjacent organs are involved, there is a decreased survival rate. Any surgical intervention will be more radical. Cancer of the colon can grow into adjacent perirectal fat or the muscular side walls of the pelvis, prostate, vagina, bladder, ureters, duodenum, pancreas, or retroperitoneum. Anteriorly, the tumor can grow into bowel loops or the bladder dome. The omentum can twist and wrap itself over the inflamed areas; an extensive *en bloc* resection of the diseased area is required to remove the total mass.

Tumor growth along the nerves is also possible and sometimes results in pain so severe that it requires astute and careful management if any type of control is to be accomplished.

Cancer of the perianal area usually spreads by direct extension, with inguinal node involvement ranging from 20%–25%. Anal canal carcinomas may involve the anal muscles and metastasize to the prostate, urethra, bladder, vagina, sacrum, and ischial tuberosity.[52]

CLINICAL MANIFESTATIONS

The presentation of colorectal carcinoma is related to the location of the neoplasm within the colon. Individuals are asymptomatic in the early stages, then develop minor changes in their bowel patterns and experience occasional rectal bleeding. These early symptoms are not alarming, seem to be infrequent, and usually can be interrupted by the individual through changes in diet or through symptomatic treatment of the hemorrhoids. As the tumor increases in size, symptoms develop that reflect characteristics of lesions of a particular anatomical site.

Carcinomas of the right side of the colon may become large and fungating tumors prior to producing symptoms. Because the lumen of the cecal and ascending colon is large and distensible, it is capable of accommodating a bulky tumor. At the time of diagnosis, as many as 75% of patients will have a palpable abdominal mass.[38] Pain experienced prior to the identification of this mass is described as a vague cramping or an aching-pressure sensation. When the pain is acute, it is often indistinguishable from that of cholecystitis or acute appendicitis, yet there may be bowel perforation. Even though gross GI bleeding is not present, there can be chronic blood loss resulting in fatigue and shortness of breath secondary to the development of an iron deficiency anemia. If the patient's stool is examined for occult blood, the test will be positive. Mahogany-colored stools may be present when there is blood mixed with the stool; however, this is a less common finding.[53,54] Tumors of the right colon may obstruct the cecal and ascending colon and cause appendicitis-like symptoms.[2]

Cancers of the transverse colon may result in blood in the stool and changes in bowel patterns or possibly a bowel obstruction. Obstruction is possible in this portion of the bowel because the lumen is smaller and there is further narrowing at the hepatic and splenic flexures. The increasing consistency of the stool versus the liquid content found in the ascending and cecal area also contributes to the potential for obstruction.[2]

Cancer on the left side of the colon tends to be constricting due to lesions that can progressively reduce the lumen of the bowel. It produces identifiable symptoms and tends to be diagnosed earlier. Initially, sensations of fullness or cramping are identified, progressing to changes in bowel habits as the tumor increases in size. Obstipation and constipation result, and acute abdominal pain is experienced from either an intestinal obstruction or perforation. Bleeding with bright-red blood is more common with a carcinoma of the left side.[2]

Cancer of the rectum manifests as changes in bowel habits, particularly in increased frequency of evacuation in the morning. As the tumor grows, a sense of incomplete evacuation and tenesmus develop, along with rectal pressure and/or fullness. Stool caliber decreases and is described as "pencil-like" by the patient.[38] There will be frequent GI bleeding that is bright red, either mixed with or on the surface of the stool. Pain is a less prominent feature with early rectal carcinoma. However, as the tumor enlarges and invades perirectal tissues, a sensation of rectal fullness develops and may progress to dull, aching, perineal or sacral pain that can radiate down the legs. A patient may complain of mucus-laden diarrhea, since some tumors produce large amounts of mucus.

Less common symptoms of colorectal cancer include weight loss and fever. Fifty percent of patients with other symptoms will also report weight loss; however, this cannot be used alone as a definitive diagnostic indicator. The cause of fever is not specific but may be from an infectious process that develops following tumor penetration of an adjacent organ. Any fever of unknown origin should include evaluation for the presence of cancer.[2]

Nonmetastatic cutaneous manifestations of colorectal cancer can develop, such as acanthas nigrisams, dermatomyositis, and pemphigoid, among others.[55] These may occur most frequently with advanced disease. Nonresponsive skin lesions should be carefully evaluated to identify the need for biopsy and further therapy.

While colorectal tumors may present with specific symptoms, there are examples of asymptomatic persons who seek treatment related to pruritus and jaundice. Following their diagnostic evaluation, a liver metastasis can be identified as well as other metastatic complications, such as lung involvement, ascites, or enlarged ovaries.[38]

ASSESSMENT

The colon can be examined in a number of ways: by direct visualization with the use of various scopes, by the insertion of a finger, by various radiological techniques, and with a number of laboratory studies. Unfortunately, 50% of patients will have positive lymph nodes at the time of initial medical presentation.[53]

Physical Examination

As part of the diagnostic work-up, the examiner should seek information regarding general complaints and specific GI symptoms as well as about prior cancerous or precancerous conditions. A personal medical history includes questions related to risk factors for colorectal cancer, a review of prior medical conditions related to colorectal cancer, familial or hereditary conditions, as well as questions regarding family members with a positive cancer history that would indicate inclusion in a high-risk group. Physical findings depend on the patient's tumor site and stage and the individual's nutritional status.

Physical examination of the abdomen proceeds with inspection to detect distension, visible masses, or visible and enlarged veins that may be indicative of portal hypertension and metastatic disease. Auscultation includes evaluation in all four quadrants for presence or absence of peristaltic sounds. Palpation and percussion are useful in determining the presence of abdominal masses, liver enlargement, and the occurrence and location of pain.

A right-sided tumor may first be found on palpation and be the first indication of cancer within the area. Tumor masses in the transverse and descending area are more easily located and palpated. Notation is made of the size, quadrant location, shape, tenderness, and mobility of any identified mass.

Examination of the rectal area includes visual inspection of the anal and perianal area, since a malignancy may be present in this location. A digital rectal examination is important in any physical examination, since it is simple, without risk, bears no additional cost, and is capable of detecting 15%–20% of colorectal carcinomas within a 7-cm area from the anal verge.[45] Currently the American Cancer Society recommends a digital rectal examination yearly for persons over 40 years of age.[56]

Vaginal examinations in females are important when the complaint indicates a fistula, with stool being expelled from the vagina. Rectal cancer extending to the abdominal side walls can be evaluated better via vaginal exam.[34]

Diagnostic Studies

The diagnosis of colorectal cancer includes procedures to provide direct visualization of polyps or tumors and also laboratory tests and other techniques that are helpful in making a correct diagnosis.

Endoscopic examination may be performed with a rigid proctosigmoidoscope, a flexible fiberoptic sigmoidoscope, or a colonoscope. The rigid proctosigmoidoscope is employed as a diagnostic tool less frequently, since lesions proximal to the rectosigmoid area may not be detected because of the difficulty of complete insertion of a rigid scope.[45] Additionally, colorectal cancers occur more frequently on the right side of the colon and will not be visualized with this instrument.[57] It is reported that 50% of colorectal tumors are located in the distal 50 cm of the large bowel.[58]

Flexible sigmoidoscopes 60 cm in length allow for visualization of most of the left colon and are safe as well as more comfortable for the patient. A 30-cm flexible sigmoidoscope has been developed that produces similar detection rates for polyps and cancer yet is less expensive and less time-consuming to use.

Colonoscopy enables visualization of the entire large bowel, from rectum to cecum, in 85%–95% of patients. The procedure is highly sensitive. This scope, along with other fiberoptic instruments, enables tissue to be removed for histological examination and allows endoscopic polypectomy to be performed.[58] Biopsy is the best technique to establish a tissue diagnosis. It is advised to examine the colon segments beyond the identified cancer, since synchronous lesions may be identified.

A barium enema commonly is used to evaluate large-bowel cancers; however, the procedure may be diag-

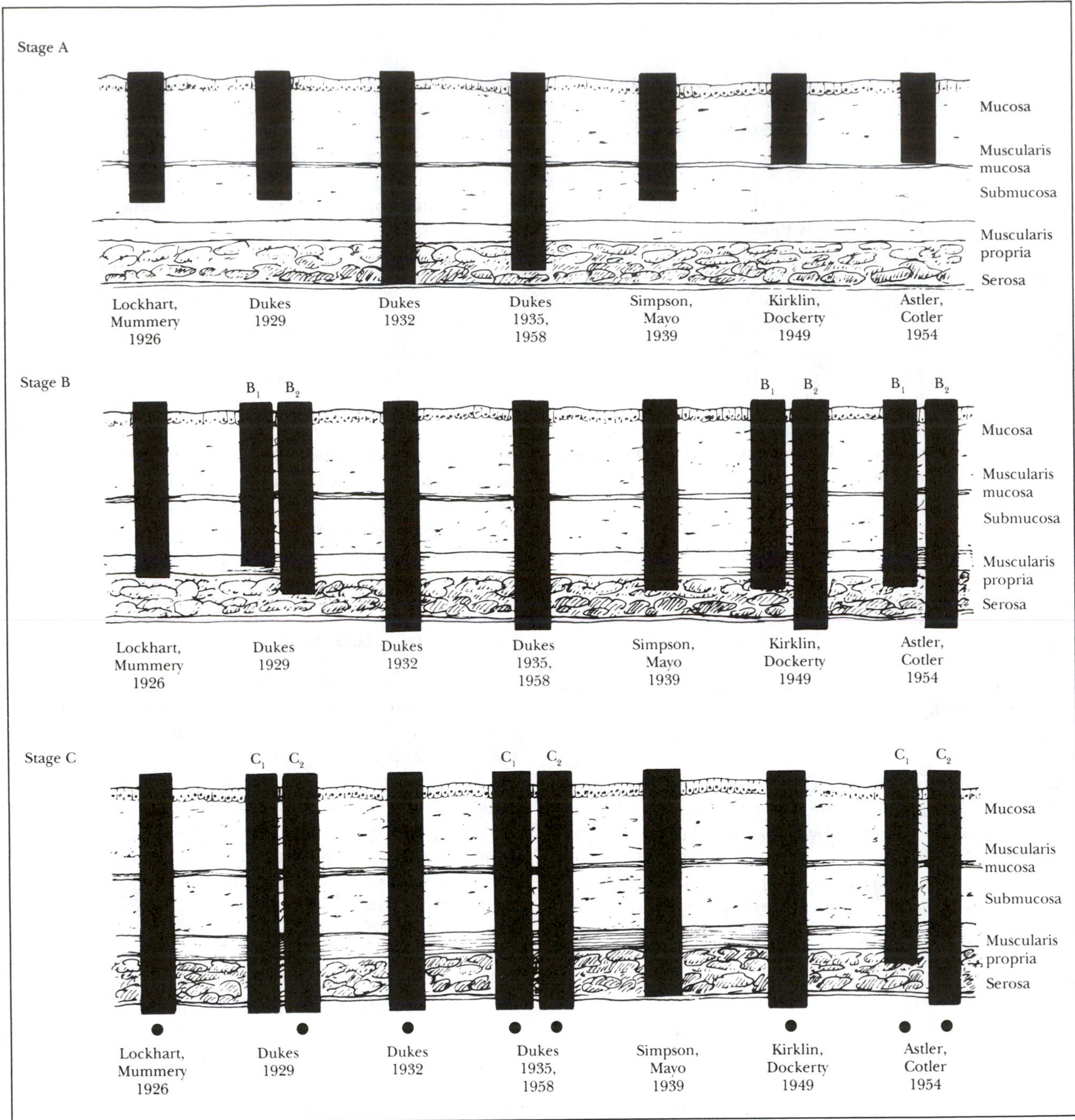

FIGURE 42-1 Modifications of Dukes' classification. The Astler-Coller modification of 1954 (furthest right on this schema) is the system most widely used today. (Source: Ahlgren JD, Macdonald JS (eds): *Gastrointestinal Oncology*. Philadelphia: Lippincott, 1992, Figure 26-7. Reprinted with permission.)

nostic in only 70% of cases when used alone. Optimally, the procedure is combined with sigmoidoscopy or with colonoscopy. Double-contrast studies are preferred to detect adenomas, particularly those less than 1 cm in size. Comparative studies have shown that colonoscopy is more accurate as a single diagnostic tool than are other procedures.[45,58]

Although its usefulness is questioned, fecal occult blood testing has been used as an indicator of GI malignancies for a number of years. Problems incurred are false-positive and false-negative tests. Patient compliance in following the dietary restriction (i.e., failure to avoid high-residue diet prior to specimen collection) and home testing techniques cause additional problems (specimen drying, outdated Hemoccult cards/reagent).[58] While the use of the Hemoccult test has limitations when used in mass screening, it can be useful for earlier detection of colorectal cancers in an initial screening situation. Currently the American Cancer Society recommends a fecal occult blood test every year after age 50.

Carcinoembryonic antigen (CEA) may be useful as a prognostic tool in the pretreatment phase for evaluating the effectiveness of various treatment protocols, surgery, chemotherapy, or radiation and to determine the presence of residual tumor or recurrence. Currently there is no indication for including this tumor marker in mass screening programs, since it is neither sensitive nor specific enough.[59,60]

A new radioimmunoassay is the CA 19-9 test, which measures a carbohydrate determinant of circulating antigen. The CA 19-9 assay appears to have some usefulness in predicting recurrence among persons who have undergone curative resection of a colorectal tumor.[61]

Routine abdominal films, both flat and upright, are suggested to evaluate those with an intestinal obstruction. The films may facilitate distinguishing between large- or small-bowel involvement. An intravenous pyelogram may be needed to evaluate the genitourinary tract and to evaluate further organ involvement. Liver function studies are initiated to identify liver metastasis, serum alkaline phosphatase, serum gamma-glutamyl transpeptidase (SGGT), lactic dehydrogenase (LDH), serum glutamic oxaloacetic transaminase (SGOT), and serum glutamic pyruvic transaminase (SGPT).[33]

Staging Studies

Computerized tomography (CT) scanning is useful in determining the spread of tumor to various adjacent organs, to assess lymph node involvement, and to detect liver, lung, or other distant metastasis. A CT scan is most reliable for lesions of ≥3-cm diameter. Doubtful but suspicious lesions should be biopsied with a needle.[58] About 2–3 months following definitive surgery, a baseline CT scan is obtained, since fiberoptic changes that occur in the postoperative period may mimic changes one would see with residual or recurrent tumor.

Magnetic resonance imaging (MRI) is used more successfully for staging rectal cancer than for staging colon cancer. MRI studies demonstrate direct tumor spread to structures of the pelvis and can be used to distinguish postoperative fibrosis from recurrent tumor.[58]

Endoluminal ultrasonography is important in staging of rectal tumors and determining lymphadenectomy. Currently the procedure is the most accurate means for evaluating the depth of penetration of a tumor into the bowel wall and is helpful in verifying or altering impressions formulated during a rectal examination.[59]

Specific diagnostic studies for anal cancer include primarily biopsy of suspicious areas and physical examination. Testing for human immunodeficiency virus (HIV) is indicated, since anal cancers are associated with acquired immunodeficiency disease syndrome (AIDS).[58]

CLASSIFICATION AND STAGING

The first classification system for rectal cancer was developed by Dukes in the 1930s and has since been modified to include colon cancer. The classification system has been modified further by Astler-Collier.[62] (See Figure 42-1) The tumor-node-metastases staging (TNM) system was developed in 1954 and was adopted by the American Joint Committee for Cancer (AJCC) Staging and End-Results Reporting. In 1987 the AJCC and the International Union Against Cancer (UICC) merged their respective staging systems and included elements to recognize the number of lymph nodes involved.[2] (See Figure 42-2.)

PRIMARY TUMOR (T)

Tis	Carcinoma *in situ:* intraepithelial or invasion of the lamina propria*
T1	Tumor invades the submucosa
T2	Tumor invades the muscularis propria
T3	Tumor invades through the muscularis propria into the subserosa or into nonperitonealized pericolic or perirectal tissues
T4	Tumor directly invades other organs or structures and/or perforates the visceral peritoneum**

REGIONAL LYMPH NODES (N)

N0	No regional lymph node metastasis
N1	Metastasis in one to three pericolic or perirectal lymph nodes
N2	Metastasis in four or more pericolic or perirectal lymph nodes
N3	Metastasis in any lymph node along the course of a named vascular trunk and/or metastasis to apical node(s) (when marked by the surgeon)

DISTANT METASTASIS (M)

M0	No distant metastasis
M1	Distant metastasis

STAGE GROUPING

AJCC/UICC				DUKES
Stage 0	Tis	N0	M0	—
Stage I	T1	N0	M0	A
	T2	N0	M0	
Stage II	T3	N0	M0	B
	T4	N0	M0	
Stage III	Any T	N1	M0	C
	Any T	N2	M0	
	Any T	N3	M0	
Stage IV	Any T	Any N	M1	—

FIGURE 42-2 Colon & rectum staging criteria. (Source: Beahrs OH, Henson DE, Hutter RV, et al (eds): American Joint Committee on Cancer: Manual for Staging of Cancer, 4th ed. Philadelphia: Lippincott, 1992.)

Factors that affect staging systems include the evaluation of the extent of local invasion, invasion of the lymphatics and vascular channels, and histological grade, as well as preoperative CEA levels. Consideration of these factors and individual patient characteristics will direct the clinical decisions regarding types of surgery, chemotherapy, radiation therapy, and any combinations of these treatment modalities. Meticulous planning is needed prior to initiating a definitive treatment approach.

TREATMENT

Surgery

The treatment of choice for colorectal carcinoma is surgery. The extent of the surgical resection is determined by the tumor location, vascular supply, and distribution of the lymph nodes in the region (Figure 42-3). While most resections include a margin of 2–5 cm on either side of the tumor, wider resections may be required to achieve necessary ligation of the arterial blood supply.[53,63]

Surgical procedures include *en bloc* removal of the neoplasm and segments of major arterial and venous supply to the diseased area and resection of the mesentery associated with the primary lymphatic drainage of the colon segment. The surgical procedure is designed to avoid intraoperative tumor implantation and damage to bowel vasculature.

Right hemicolectomy

A right hemicolectomy is indicated for neoplasms of the appendix, cecum, ascending colon, and hepatic flexure. Since the ileocolic and right colic arteries provide the blood supply to this area, they will be ligated and removed to prevent metastases. The terminal ileum, cecum, ascending colon, and right transverse colon are removed and the mesentery is resected. An end-to-end or end-to-side anastomosis of the remaining large bowel to the small bowel is then performed.[2,63]

Transverse colectomy

Tumors in the transverse colon are resected based on their location (right, middle, or left portion), the blood supply involved, and the probability of creating an adequate anastomosis. In certain instances it may be necessary to remove the right colon as well, with anastomosis of the remaining large bowel to the ileum.

Left hemicolectomy, left partial colectomy

When the splenic flexure and descending colon are involved, a left hemicolectomy may be the procedure of choice; however, there are significant technical problems for the surgeon. The left branch of the middle colic artery, along with the left colic artery, must be located and ligated. The transverse colon is then anastomosed to the sigmoid colon. In particular, the vascular supply and integrity of the ureter, spleen, and pancreas must be protected during this entire procedure. A partial left hemicolectomy is preferred for tumors of the distal transverse colon, splenic flexure, and descending colon that are not within the sigmoid ara.

Sigmoid colectomy

In the past, tumors of the sigmoid area were treated with an extended left colectomy. However, based on current data indicating that survival rates are not improved with this type of wide resection, now a sigmoid colectomy is performed, and the colon end is anastomosed to the upper rectum.

Subtotal or total colectomy

A subtotal or total colectomy involves removal of the majority of or the entire colon. This extensive procedure is indicated for large tumors found in either the left or right colon. The major limitation of this particular procedure is the potential for nutritional problems and skin management problems around the stoma.

Surgical Procedures for Rectal Cancer

The surgical procedure selected for rectal tumors is based on the location of the tumor and the probability of preserving bowel continuity. While preservation of continence is an advantage for the patient, the surgical procedure ultimately will be directed toward obtaining cure; therefore an external ostomy may be required. For rectal cancer, sphincter-saving procedures are an option that most surgeons will attempt to perform. These generally are not performed as a palliative procedure.[2]

The rectum is approximately 15 cm in length; thus, obtaining a tumor-free margin of 2–5 cm and preserving continence are important factors in the selection of the surgical approach. The tumor's degree of differentiation and the patient's age, sex, and physical condition are also considered in selecting a surgical approach. The final decision on the type of surgical procedure may be reserved until the time of surgery, when the tumor area can be observed directly.

Low anterior resection

A low anterior resection (LAR) will be the surgical procedure selected for a tumor lying in the distal sigmoid and upper rectum (6–11 cm from the anal verge). Either a temporary or permanent colostomy may be required. The development of the circular stapler has facilitated the surgeon's ability to perform a low anastomosis and thus avoid permanent colostomy while maintaining margins free of tumor. Recurrence of disease usually will develop 2 years after the resection and indicates a poor prognosis.[63] Complications associated with LARs include hemorrhage, anastomotic leak, stricture, abscess, irregular bowel function, and wound infection.

Abdominal perineal resection

When a rectal cancer or anal cancer is adjacent to the sphincter, an abdominal perineal resection (APR) is indicated. An APR requires a combined surgical approach through both the abdomen and the perineum. It is a physically altering procedure associated with a high morbidity rate and requires patient adaptation to a permanent colostomy. This has been the standard procedure for tumors 8 cm from the anal verge.

Various complications from the procedure include possible injury to the ureters, urinary dysfunction, perineal and abdominal wound infections, and stomal complications. Sexual dysfunction in males is also a significant outcome of this surgical procedure.

Perineal wounds The perineal wound may be closed immediately following the removal of the rectum, anus, muscle, and fatty tissue, or it may be left open for healing by secondary intention.

Primary closure of the perineal wound site is the preferred technique, because it is more comfortable for the patient and requires less care. Closed suction drains are inserted at the time of surgery and exit either through the incisional area or through a separate stab wound in the buttocks. The drains are removed on the third to fifth postoperative day. Primary closure is contraindicated when fecal spillage occurs, the bowel is perforated, an infected hematoma is present, or there is perineal disease such as abscess or fistula.[2]

Perineal wound healing by secondary intention prolongs the healing process, which may take as long as 4 months. The wound requires packing and meticulous care to promote granulation and to avoid infections or sepsis. Wound healing is facilitated by irrigations or sitz baths. The drainage and healing process must be carefully monitored.

Sexual dysfunction The wide excision required for an APR includes anatomical structures related to sexual functioning. The pelvic resection is extensive, and injury results to the parasympathetic and sympathetic nerves. Since colon cancer occurs most frequently in an older population, there may be preexisting medical conditions or medications that have already affected sexual functioning and resulted in the loss of erectile capacity for the male. Presurgery treatment with radiation is damaging to the blood vessels needed for erection.

The APR can impair erectile function, but recovery rates of erectile function are higher than those associated with radical prostatectomy or cystectomy. Dry ejaculations will occur due to damage of presacral parasympathetic nerves; however, the sensation of orgasm with mild loss of intensity remains. Sexual desire based on hormones and the capacity for pleasure from genital touch remain.[64]

Female sexual functioning following an APR remains relatively unchanged, because the sexual response is controlled by different and higher nerve centers not subject to dissection during APR. The posterior wall of the vagina may require repair due to the location of the tumor, and thus a decrease in the size of the vaginal area can occur.[64] Reproductive status can be affected if the uterus, cervix, ovaries, or fallopian tubes are removed. However, colorectal disease usually occurs in older women, who are postmenopausal; therefore, reproductive issues are not an issue. Among younger women, reproductive issues will pose significant concern.

Sexual functioning involves more than the act of intercourse and can encompass perceptions of the partner's acceptance, the individual's body image, and self-identity, as well as attitudes and feelings toward the partner. A negative emotional response to the cancer diagnosis, the surgery, the stoma, or the appliance that contains the effluent from the bowel may cause problems requiring professional counseling.[65]

Any potential effect on sexual functioning that could be caused by a surgical procedure for colorectal cancer should be discussed preoperatively by the physician with the patient and his or her partner. Nurses need to be involved in this process of informed consent and treatment in order to answer questions and provide education.

Colostomy

A colostomy can be created in any anatomic segment of the bowel, being thus identified as cecal, ascending, transverse, descending, or sigmoid colostomy.[66] Additionally, the stoma may be identified by the type of surgical construction: end, loop, or double barrel (Figure 42-4).[66] It is important to know the anatomic segment of the colon that has been exteriorized as well as the technique of surgical construction, since this affects the type of ostomy equipment that will be selected and patient self-care issues. Anatomic location is indicative of the type of effluent, either liquid or semiformed. Stomas on the right side of the colon produce a stool that is more liquid in content, while the consistency of the stool becomes more formed from the left transverse and descending colon toward the rectal area.

One type of surgical construction, the *end stoma,* is created by dividing the bowel and suturing the proximal colon segment onto the abdominal surface. The distal colon generally is removed; however, it may be oversewn and remain in the abdominal cavity, with the mesentery remaining intact. When the segment used for the end stoma is located in the low descending or sigmoid area, the oversewn rectal segment often is referred to as "Hartmann's pouch." The removal of the distal colon is an irreversible procedure.

A *loop colostomy* usually is created in the transverse bowel. A segment of bowel is exteriorized and secured to the abdomen over some type of supporting device, rod, or commercially available stoma bridge to prevent it from recessing into the abdominal cavity. Once the bowel adheres to the abdominal wall, usually in 7–10

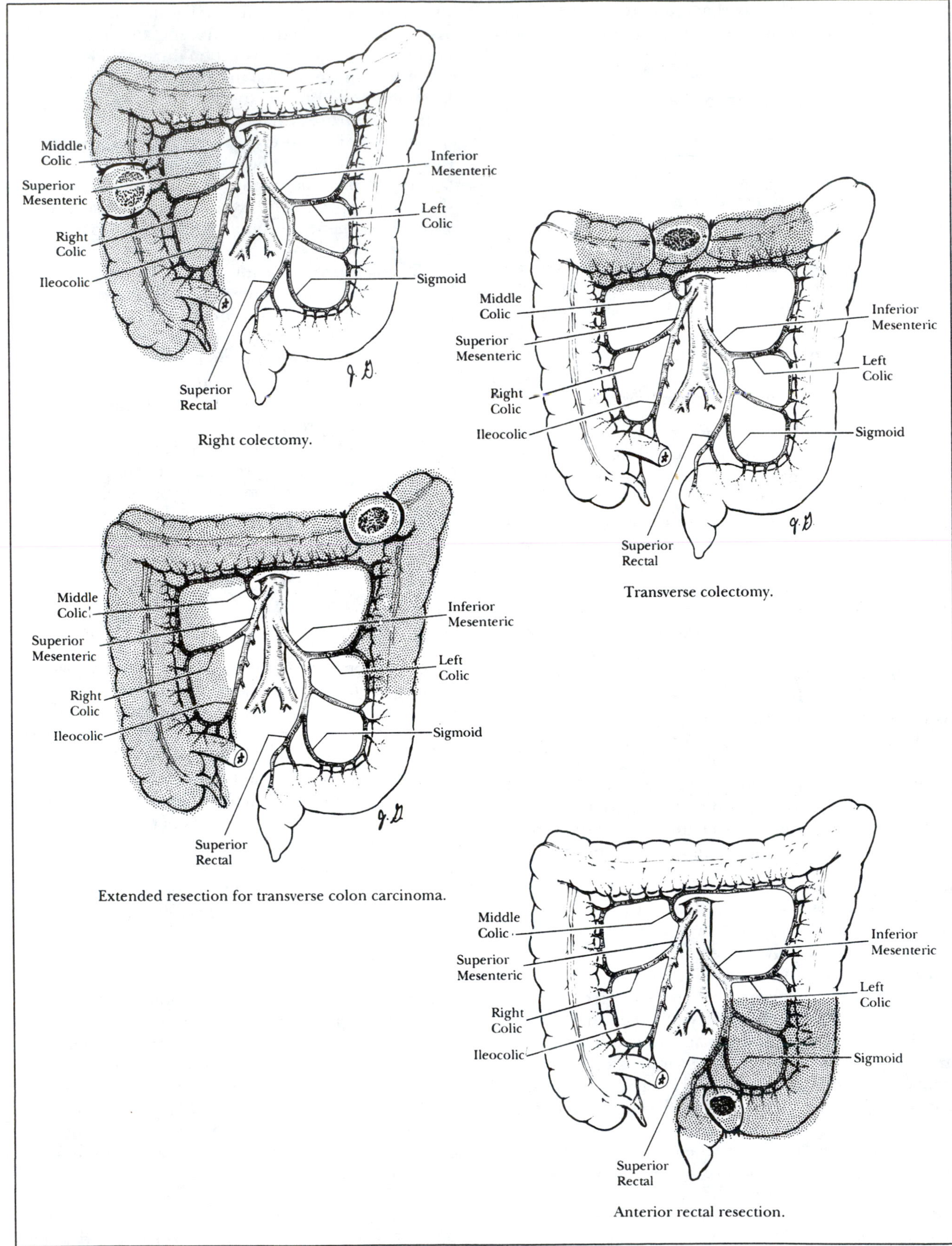

FIGURE 42-3 The choice of surgical procedure relates to the location and extent of the tumor. (Source: Ahlgren JD, Macdonald JS (eds.): *Gastrointestinal Oncology*. Philadelphia: Lippincott, Co, 1992.)

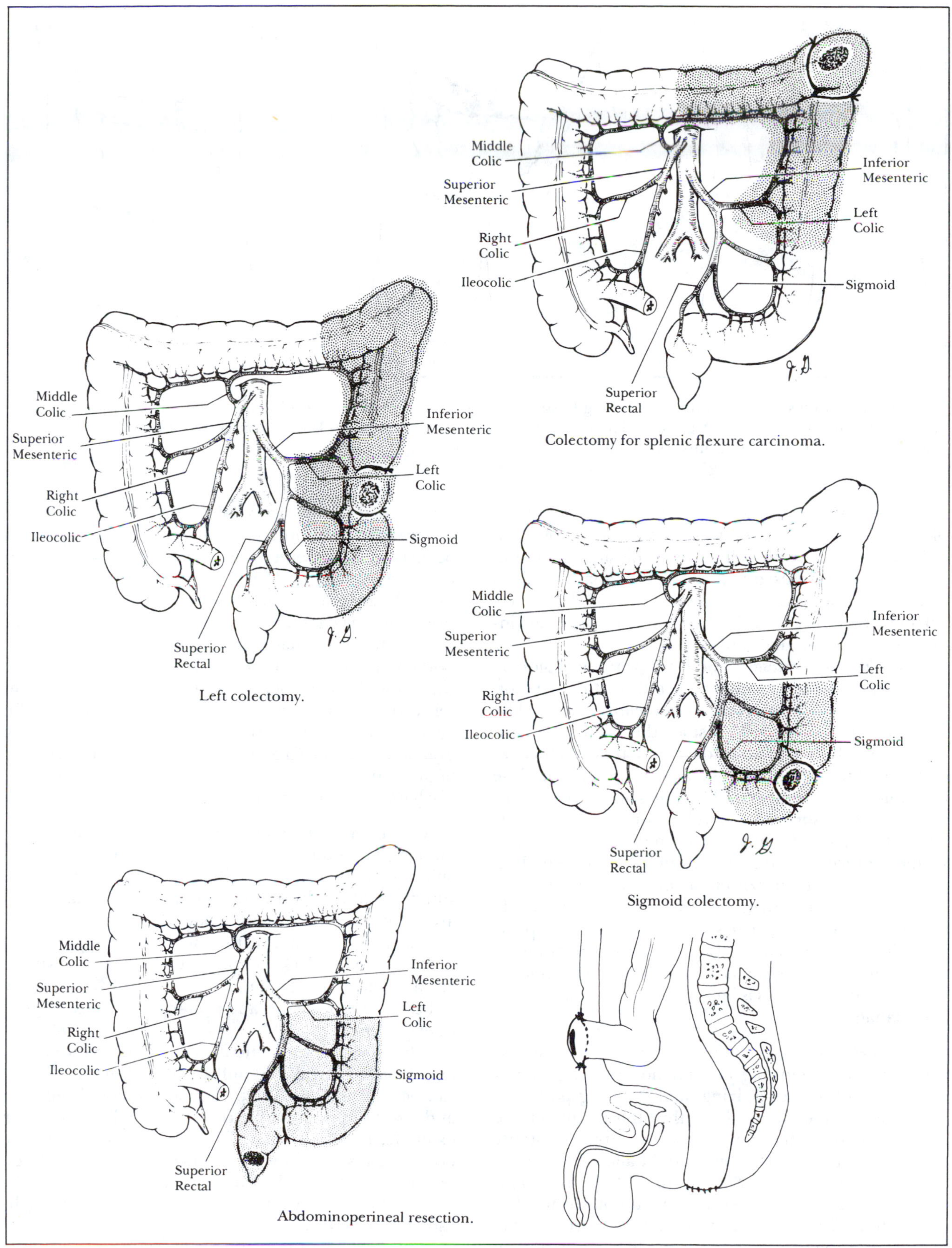

FIGURE 42-3 (continued)

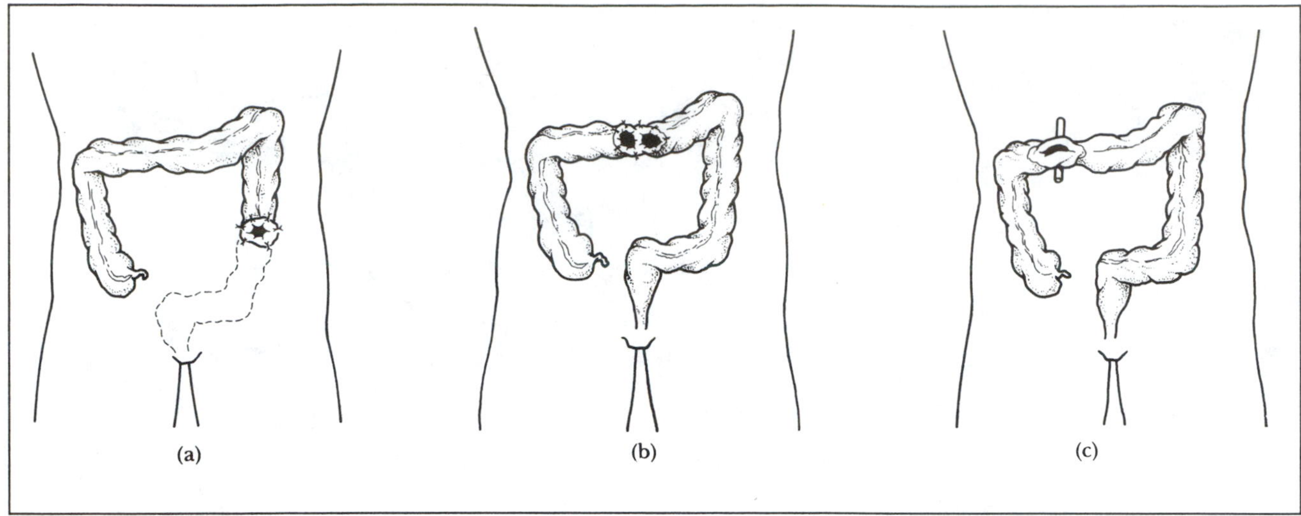

FIGURE 42-4 Colostomies identified according to structure. (a) End or single barrel colostomy. Abdominoperineal resection has been performed. Siginoid colon and rectum have been removed. (b) Double barrel colostomy in transverse colon. (c) Loop colostomy in transverse colon.

days, the device is removed. An alternative to the use of a supporting device is surgical construction of a fascial (skin) bridge. Generally, a loop colostomy is a temporary procedure used to allow a distal anastomosis to heal, but the loop ostomy may serve as a palliative diverting procedure to relieve an obstruction in an individual with terminal cancer.

A *double barrel colostomy* indicates two stomas side by side or apart from one another. In this latter situation the distal stoma is referred to as a *mucous fistula.* The proximal stoma will produce stool, the distal stoma mucus. A double barrel colostomy may be contained in one appliance when the stomas are situated in close proximity. However, when the stomas are located apart, only a gauze absorbent pad will be used on the mucous fistula to absorb the mucous drainage from the distal segment mucous fistula. The drainage may be high in mucus content if the bowel has previously been damaged by disease or radiation therapy. If a mucous fistula is planned, an appropriate site should be selected prior to the surgical procedure. Large amounts of drainage from some bowel segments may require using a pouch; therefore, site selection is important for patient comfort and management.

Stoma site selection Stoma sites need to be selected preoperatively following examination of the patient's abdomen in the sitting, lying, and standing positions. The selected site should be within the rectus muscle and in an area that can physically support ostomy equipment. The selected site should allow the patient to visualize the stoma.[67] Scars, skin folds, bony prominences, belt and waist lines, and the umbilicus need to be avoided. These characteristics can interfere with the seal of an appliance and result in stool leakage. The anatomical location of the stoma influences the abdominal quadrant placement as well as the surgical techniques. For example, deviations necessitated by the disease or by complications during the surgical procedure may result in a stoma of the descending bowel being located in another area as opposed to being placed in the left lower quadrant. Consultation with an ET nurse is suggested, since these nurses are trained in stoma site selection and management techniques.

It is suggested that individuals who use braces, supports of any type, or other assistive devices wear these when a stoma site is being selected. Later difficulties in self-care and/or maintaining an appliance seal on the abdominal surface can be avoided with a preoperative evaluation. This also assures the patient that there will not be interference of these items with the stoma after discharge from the hospital.

Colostomy management In the immediate postoperative period the stoma needs to be evaluated for viability, condition, size, and shape and to ensure that all sutures holding the everted stoma onto the abdomen are secure. An inadequate blood supply or tension on the bowel segment may cause the stoma to appear pale, dusky, or even black in color. A viable stoma will be red and shiny in appearance. Deviations from this may indicate early problems and require additional surgical intervention.

The first time the patient views the stoma usually is emotionally painful. Not only the color but also the size can be alarming. Size depends on the bowel segment and also the preoperative condition of the bowel. For example, the large dilated bowel segments that may occur as a result of bowel obstruction will be quite large postoperatively. The initial bowel edema gradually subsides following surgery, with the size becoming established in 6–8 weeks.

The time when the stoma will begin to function is variable. This depends on preoperative bowel cleansing and any prior obstruction, in which case stool is present almost immediately. Once peristalsis returns and flatus is passed, food is introduced. Stool will soon be expelled from the stoma. Usually, the more proximal a stoma is in the bowel, the sooner it functions and the more liquid the stool content.

Peristomal skin should resemble the skin on the abdominal surface. While ecchymoses and bruising appear in the postoperative period, this condition will disappear, and normal skin condition will return. Skin barriers are routinely used with the containment appliance for additional protection from stool leakage and subsequent denuding of the skin. Various skin products, barriers, and appliances are available to prevent skin irritation and to promote healing.[67,68]

Appliance selection Pouches are specifically evaluated and selected to accommodate the consistency of the stool output, to provide peristomal skin protection, to enable ease of client use and lifestyle, and to minimize profile beneath clothing. Fortunately, there are many styles of ostomy equipment to select from that assist in returning the individual to daily living activities.

Equipment costs vary but are reimbursable to some degree by Medicare and most private insurers. Certain agencies help with costs for those who have particular needs; however, these groups differ across the country. An enterostomal therapist (ET) nurse generally is aware of various groups who are of assistance in a specific region.

Teaching patients Preoperatively, the patient needs to understand the surgery and its rationale, understand the planned creation of a stoma and its function, and see and handle the containment equipment. Family members or those the patient requests should be included in all the teaching sessions if possible. They will learn how they can provide assistance while enabling the person to again become independent. Illustrations, written materials, and a visit with a volunteer with an ostomy from the United Ostomy Association can enhance the educational process and facilitate adjustment.

Postoperative teaching begins immediately. Early activities progress from small areas such as removing or applying the pouch closure clamp to looking at and cleansing the stoma to applying and emptying the appliance. Optimally, the patient can manage pouch changing prior to discharge. (See Figure 42-5.) Individuals with adequate bowel length postsurgery may learn to perform colostomy irrigation and thus regulate evacuation. (See Figure 42-6.)

Since discharge these days is accomplished at a more rapid pace, it has become important to provide educational materials that the patient can refer to once at home. Discharge planning also entails referral to home health agencies and to nurses who are sensitive to the needs of the ostomy patient. Chapter 32, "Altered Body Image and Sexuality," may be helpful with patient education and support.

Patients need to leave the hospital not only with detailed instructions but also with ostomy supplies adequate for 2–3 weeks, the names of the items to be used, and the name of community vendors as well as

APPLICATION OF ONE-PIECE FECAL POUCH*

1. Gather all supplies.
2. Gently remove soiled pouch by pushing down on skin while lifting up on pouch. Discard soiled pouch in odorproof plastic bag. *Save tail closure.*
3. Clean stoma and peristomal skin with water; pat dry. *If indicated,* shave or clip peristomal hair.
4. Use stoma-measured guide or established pattern to determine size of stoma.
   Presized pouch. Check to be sure pouch opening is correct size. Order new supplies if indicated.
   Cut-to-fit pouch. Trace correctly sized pattern onto back of barrier or pouch surface, and cut stomal opening to match pattern.
   NOTE: Once stoma shrinkage is complete, this step may be omitted and preparation of clean pouch may be completed before soiled pouch is removed.
5. Apply skin barrier paste around stoma if needed. (*Tip:* Wet finger to facilitate paste application.) An alternative approach is to apply skin barrier paste to aperture in prepared pouch or barrier. Allow paste to dry.
   Optional: Apply skin sealant to skin that will be covered by tape.
   Allow to dry.
6. Remove paper backing from pouch or barrier to expose adhesive surface; center pouch opening over stoma and press into place. Attach closure.
   Optional: Apply tape strips to "picture-frame" pouch-skin junction.
7. If two piece: Snap pouch onto flange of barrier wafer. Attach closure.

FIGURE 42-5 Patient instructions for fecal pouch application. (Source: Adapted from Hampton BG, Bryant RA (eds): *Ostomies and Continent Diversions.* St. Louis: Mosby Year Book, 1992.)

**Universal precautions* must be followed when this procedure is performed.

a catalog from a mail order vendor. Mail order vendors can be helpful with insurance forms and record keeping, and some provide items at a lower cost. The American Association for Retired Persons (AARP) provides this service.

The nurse may wish to provide a contact name for a local chapter of the United Ostomy Association (UOA), since this group can provide needed emotional support once a person is back in the community. The UOA can put the family in contact with an ET nurse in the vicinity and can provide a number of patient education aids, magazines, and a local support group. The American Cancer Society offers assistance with educational materials related to sexuality and ostomy care as well as to colorectal cancer, chemotherapy, radiation, and nutrition.

Surgical Procedures for Anal Cancer

Surgery alone or in conjunction with other treatment modalities may be selected to treat anal cancer. The

COLOSTOMY IRRIGATION*

1. Gather supplies. Explain procedure to patient, and provide for privacy and comfort.
2. Remove pouch or stomal covering.
3. Attach irrigation sleeve; place bottom of sleeve into toilet to direct returns, *or* close bottom of sleeve with rubber band, binder clip, or commercial tail closure. NOTE: Irrigation sleeves for two-piece systems are snapped onto the two-piece wafer with flange; other reusable sleeves are belted into place. Disposable adhesive sleeves also are available.
4. Prepare irrigating solution. Volume to be given is titrated for the patient and is based on the patient's tolerance and feelings of colonic distention ("fullness"). Initial irrigations usually are performed with 500 ml of solution or less to prevent overdistention and cramping. Routine irrigation for the average adult is performed using approximately 500–1000 ml of solution.
   Close clamp on irrigating bag, and fill bag with desired amount of tepid water or prescribed irrigant. Open clamp, and allow irrigating solution to flow to clear tubing of air. Suspend irrigating bag at approximately shoulder height or slightly higher.
5. Lubricate the cone tip; insert cone tip gently into stoma, and hold tip securely in place to prevent backflow. Use water soluble lubricant.
6. Open clamp, and allow irrigation solution to flow in steadily; the desired time frame for instillation of fluid is 5 to 10 minutes.
7. When desired amount of irrigant has been delivered *or* when the patient senses colonic distention, close the clamp and remove the cone.
8. Wait approximately 30 to 45 minutes for returns. After initial returns are complete (usually 10 to 15 minutes), the individual has the option to close the bottom of the sleeve and move around.
9. When returns are complete, rinse and remove the irrigation sleeve.
10. Clean peristomal skin, and apply pouch or desired stomal covering.
11. Prepare equipment for repeat use.

FIGURE 42-6 Instruction for patient teaching in colostomy irrigation. (Source: Adapted from Hampton BG, Bryant RA (eds): *Ostomies and Continent Diversions.* St. Louis: Mosby Year Book, 1992.)

**Universal precautions* must be followed when this procedure is performed.

tumor size, stage, and depth of penetration determine the treatment approach. Small, distal anal lesions or lesions of the perianal skin may be treated with local excision, although locoregional recurrence is possible. Locoregional recurrence rates of 20%–50% are reported, with 5-year survival of 21%–73%.[69,70]

The standard therapy for anal cancer has been an APR; however, other therapies are now being incorporated or used alone (radiation therapy), with similar or improved 5-year survival rates.[71]

The inability of surgery alone to cure is due in part to the anatomy of the anal region, which makes it difficult to remove adequately the lateral and distal zones of the lymphatic spread. If the anal margin is involved, a wider excision of perianal skin is required than in adenocarcinoma of the rectum.

Radiation Therapy

While advances in surgical techniques and an emphasis on colorectal detection and screening have occurred, the mortality rates have remained unchanged for the past 20 years. The primary reason for failure of disease control after surgery alone is a result of both local and/or regional recurrence. Thus, adjuvant radiation therapy has been investigated to determine if better cure rates could be achieved.

Preoperative radiation

Radiation therapy (RT) prior to surgery is proposed as advantageous for the following reasons: the rate of surgical resectability would improve, there would be a reduction in the viability of malignant cells, the number of positive lymph nodes would be reduced, and the chance of local recurrence would be lessened without compromising cure rate.[38] Once preoperative radiation is completed, an operation can be performed within 2–3 weeks.

Initial studies suggested an improved survival rate with low-dose RT followed by an APR for rectal cancer. Later trials have been unable to confirm this finding. However, the use of higher-dose RT (3000–5000 cGy) preoperatively has been shown to reduce local recurrence of rectal tumors and in one study demonstrated an increased survival rate.[72,73]

Also noted are disadvantages with the use of preoperative RT. It is felt that some patients may be treated unnecessarily with radiotherapy if they have early-stage disease, which could have been removed with surgery alone. Also, the histopathology of the tumor can be altered by preoperative radiation, thus making comparisons of treatment outcomes difficult.

Combined pre- and postoperative radiotherapy

Use of pre- and postoperative adjuvant treatment is referred to as the "sandwich" technique. The benefit is that there will be a decrease in tumor dissemination prior to surgery. In addition, there would not be an alteration in the ability to stage the tumor histologically at surgery.[74] Postoperative high-dose radiation is then used to treat those persons with pathologically confirmed advanced disease. Results have been encouraging in a limited number of studies with the use of low-dose preoperative and high-dose postoperative radiation therapy, which suggests further trials.[75]

A suggested disadvantage of the sandwich approach is the potential for repopulation by residual malignant cells if slow wound healing occurs following the surgical procedure and delays the delivery of postoperative RT. Higher-dose postoperative radiation cannot be used to eradicate repopulation because of the limitations on tissue tolerance imposed by the preoperative administration of radiation.[74] Chemotherapy may be indicated for some patients who receive both pre- and postsurgery radiation.

Postoperative radiation

Postoperative radiation is used primarily for those individuals at high risk of local recurrence. Individuals whose tumor has penetrated the bowel wall and who have positive lymph nodes are candidates for postoperative radiotherapy. Local tumor recurrence is decreased by radiation, but distant metastasis remains a problem. It is unclear if survival rates are altered.[74]

Patients with colon cancer are less likely to have locoregional disease than are those with a rectal malignancy. Data from studies of colon cancer being treated with RT are stage- and site-specific and retrospective rather than prospective. Treatment techniques for colon cancer may involve therapy to the whole pelvis and a boost to the tumor bed and/or the draining lymphatics.[74] There are dose limits of RT to the pelvis related to tissue tolerance of the surrounding organs and structures in a treatment field. (See Chapter 13 for a discussion of the management of the side effects of radiation therapy.) It may also be useful to select certain subgroups of patients who not only benefit from postoperative radiation but also benefit if chemotherapy is added.

Palliative radiation

Palliative radiotherapy is effective in treating symptoms of advanced rectal cancer. Pain and bleeding with rectal tumors can be controlled, and symptomatic control of metastasis to the bone, brain, and liver can be achieved.[74]

Other radiotherapy techniques

Endocavitary radiation is used as local treatment for rectal tumors. An endoscope is placed directly against the lesion, followed by the administration of a minimally penetrating dose of high-intensity irradiation. Endocavitary radiation can be administered on an outpatient basis, with three to five insertions every 6–7 weeks to reach a total dose of 2000–3000 cGy. Exophytic lesions less than 5 cm in size and less than 12 cm from the anal verge are most appropriate for this therapy.[75,76]

Locally advanced, recurrent, or inoperable rectal cancer may be treated with intraoperative radiotherapy. Because high doses of external-beam RT to a large area of the abdomen or pelvis are not feasible due to the damage that can occur to nearby organs, intraoperative radiation is a potential alternative for a select number of individuals with locally advanced or recurrent disease.[77] In some cases a suitable dose of external-beam therapy combined with an intraoperative dose can provide local control.[74,78]

Brachytherapy is accomplished by inserting radioactive sources into a body cavity or implanting sources into a tumor. Implanting radioactive seeds or afterloading a catheter inserted into an area are common brachytherapy techniques. This therapy may be selected for pelvic recurrence of rectal cancer, local tumor control, palliation of symptoms, and treatment of liver metastasis.

Hyperthermia may be used as adjunct therapy with RT and chemotherapy. Hyperthermia enhances the cytotoxic effects of the other modalities, principally by interfering with the repair of intracellular damage caused by radiation and chemotherapy.[74]

Laser therapy

Laser therapy may be useful for treating inoperable rectal and descending colon tumors in selected patients. The benefits include relief of bleeding, diarrhea, mucus drainage, and tenesmus.[79] Fulguration by laser has a low morbidity, usually does not require anesthesia, and can be done on an outpatient basis.

Chemotherapy

Chemotherapy is used as adjunct therapy for colorectal cancer that is residual, advanced, or metastatic. It may be used with surgery or combined with surgery and radiation therapy. Unfortunately, colorectal carcinomas are extremely resistant to most antineoplastic agents. Results from the various trials have indicated limited response or survival times for those with advanced lesions or metastatic disease. When chemotherapy is used as the only therapy for colorectal tumors, it has been found to be inadequate.[38]

The most researched single agent, 5-fluorouracil (5-FU), has been used to treat different stages of the disease with various dosage schedules and by different routes. Studies using continuous infusions of 5-FU for protracted times have shown response rates of 17%–40%. The definition for continuous infusions over protracted periods needs further clarification to ensure appropriate application of the treatment protocols. Oral administration of 5-FU has been studied in an attempt to reduce the drug's toxicity and improve its benefits and delivery, yet no other route of delivery of the agent appears to surpass the efficacy of intravenous delivery.[38]

Other single agents that have been tested for use with colorectal tumors as single agents include mitomycin-C, nitrosoureas (BCNU, CCNU, and methyl CCNU), cyclophosphamide, methotrexate, melphalan, doxorubicin, actinomycin D, and trizinate. None of these agents demonstrated a response rate greater than 20% in any of the reported studies. As a result of the limited effectiveness of single agents, combination chemotherapy has been investigated. The use of combinations as well as the addition of vincristine in certain trials show conflicting data. Also, trials with colorectal cancer have attempted to modify the metabolism of 5-FU and thus increase its therapeutic efficiency. To do this, folinic acid, leucovorin, thymine, phosphono-N-acetyl-L-aspartic acid (PALA), and methotrexate have been tried in combination with 5-FU. Currently there is insufficient data to determine long-term survival or benefit.

Levamisole, available for human use since 1968, became of interest to researchers after it was demonstrated that the drug was able to increase production of cytokines and increase response rate of T-cells to mitogens. The immunorestorative activity and mechanisms of levamisole remain unknown. Due to its immunorestorative activity, levamisole has been included with 5-FU and other agents for treatment of advanced colorectal carcinoma. When levamisole was tested as adjuvant therapy following surgery, it showed limited benefit; yet combination with 5-FU following surgery provided evidence to support findings of reduced rates of relapse in patients with Dukes' C colon cancer. However, after several extensive trials, it now appears that the drug plays a limited role in the treatment of colorectal cancer.[80]

Rectal tumors are associated with high rates of local recurrence felt to be related to the fact that cells that penetrate the bowel wall or rectum are unable to obtain immediate access to the peritoneal cavity. Preoperative and postoperative radiation therapy decreases local recurrence of rectal tumors but does not increase survival; thus, it was felt that the addition of antineoplastic agents would be beneficial. Trials are now in progress to explore the effectiveness of various chemotherapy agents, radiation, and surgical combinations for rectal cancer.

Intraarterial or intraportal chemotherapy has been developed based on the knowledge that hepatic metastasis from colorectal tumors occurs via the portal circulation. Based on this information, it was speculated that if regional chemotherapy could be administered early enough it could eliminate metastases to the liver. Initially, 5-FU and heparin infusions were used with promising results; later, 5-FU and other agents (FUDR) were evaluated, but again a limited response rate was noted. A major factor affecting intraarterial administration of chemotherapy is the high incidence of chemical hepatitis.[79] See Chapter 41 for additional information on treatment of hepatic metastases.

Anal cancer is most effectively treated with a combination of radiation therapy and chemotherapy. Surgery is advised for excision of local or residual disease following treatment or as a salvage procedure when there is a recurrence. A multimodal treatment approach has been shown to improve cure rates and lessen the number of patients undergoing radical surgical procedures. Commonly used chemotherapy agents include 5-FU and mitomycin-C. Other agents with demonstrated activity against anal cancer include adriamycin, cisplatin, CCNU, vincristine, and bleomycin.

Side effects from chemotherapeutic agents are drug-specific and may include bone marrow suppression (thrombocytopenia, leukopenia, anemia), gastrointestinal changes (nausea, vomiting, stomatitis, strictures, ulcers), and radiation-induced skin reactions.

Alternative Therapies

Biological response modifiers (BRMs) have also received attention in treating colorectal carcinomas. Studies of alpha-interferon, interleukin-2, and monoclonal antibodies have demonstrated varying degrees of activity and response rates. Tumor vaccines and Bacillus Calmetts-Guerin (BCG) seem also to effect no increase in long-term survival.[80]

Treatment of solid tumors with autologous bone marrow transplant (AuBMT) is being examined. This treatment, along with high-dose chemotherapy for colon cancer, shows only short periods of regression of the disease.

CONCLUSION

Colorectal and anal carcinomas continue to be a significant health problem within the United States. Although treatment modalities are researched continuously and surgical techniques have improved and are more discriminately selected in relation to location, stage, and metastasis, overall survival rates have not improved.

Prevention and detection techniques must become important to the public and to health providers. Dietary changes may be helpful in reducing the incidence; however, there are enough unanswered questions regarding nutritional patterns that overemphasis in this area may produce limited results that are difficult to research. Sigmoidoscopy examination is not an inexpensive or easy procedure, which would discourage persons from seeking the examination. Since home testing is a viable self-care technique, it is hoped that occult screening tests can become refined enough so that true positives will increase in number.

Nurses can utilize the available information to encourage individuals to recognize symptoms and to practice self-care and personal lifestyle changes that can diminish risk factors, as well as modeling positive health behaviors themselves.

REFERENCES

1. Boring CC, Squires TS, Tong T: Cancer statistics, 1993. *Cancer* 43(1):7–26, 1993.
2. Corman ML: Carcinoma of the colon. In Corman ML (ed): *Colon and Rectal Surgery*. Philadelphia: Lippincott, 1989, pp. 469–578.
3. Doll R: The geographical distribution of cancer. *Br J Cancer* 23:1–8, 1969.
4. Kern WH, White WC: Adenocarcinoma of the colon in a 9-month-old infant. *Cancer* 11:855–857, 1985.
5. Beart RW: Colorectal cancer. In Holleb AI, Fink DJ, Murphy GP (eds): *Clinical Oncology*. Atlanta, GA: American Cancer Society, 1991, pp. 213–219.

6. Creagan ET, Fraomen JF Jr: Cancer mortality among American Indians. *JNCI* 49:959–967, 1972.
7. Smith RL: Recorded and expected mortality among the Japanese of the United States and Hawaii with special reference to cancer. *JNCI* 17:459–473, 1956.
8. Phillips RL: Role of life-style and dietary habits in risk cancer among Seventh-Day Adventists. *Cancer Res* 35:3513–3522, 1975(suppl 2, part 2).
9. Enstrom JE: Cancer mortality among Mormons. *Cancer* 36:825–841, 1975.
10. Potter JD, McMichael AJ: Diet and cancer of the colon and rectum. A case-control study. *JNCI* 76:557–569, 1986.
11. Burkitt DP, Walder AR, Painter NS: Effect of dietary fibre on stools and transit-times and its role in the causation of disease. *Lancet* 2:1408–1412, 1962.
12. Boyle P, Zaridze DG, Smans M: Descriptive epidemiology of colorectal cancer. *Int J Cancer* 36:9–18, 1985.
13. Fleiszer D, MacFarlane J, Murray D, et al: Protective effect of dietary fibre against chemically induced bowel tumors in rats. *Lancet* 2:552–553, 1978.
14. Jacobs MN, Jansson B, Griffin AC: Inhibitory effects of selenium on 1, 2 dimethyhydrozine and methylazoxymethanol acetate induction of colon tumors. *Cancer Lett* 2:133–138, 1971.
15. Armstrong B, Doll R: Environmental factors and cancer incidence and mortality in different countries with special reference to dietary practices. *Int J Cancer* 15:617–631, 1975.
16. Kashton H, Stern HS, Jenkins DJ, et al: Manipulation of fecal pH by dietary means. *Prev Med* 19:607–613, 1990.
17. Burkitt DP: Etiology and prevention of colorectal cancer. *Hosp Pract* 19(2):67, 1984.
18. Nigro ND: A strategy for prevention of cancer of the large bowel. *Dis Colon Rectum* 25:755–758, 1982.
19. Buset M, Lipkin M, Winawer S, et al: Inhibition of human colonic epithelial cell proliferation in vivo in calcium. *Cancer Res* 46:5426–5430, 1986.
20. Liplein M, Newmark H: Effect of added dietary calcium on colonic epithelial cell proliferation in subjects at high risk for familial colonic cancer. *N Engl J Med* 33:1381–1384, 1985.
21. Turumen MJ, Kiuilaasko EO: Increased risk of colorectal cancer after acute cholecystectomy. *Ann Surg* 27:299–304, 1981.
22. Moorehead RJ, Kernohan RM, Patterson CC, et al: Does cholecystectomy predispose to colorectal cancer? A case control study. *Dis Colon Rectum* 29:36–38, 1982.
23. Chen MC, Chang PY, Chuang CY, et al: Colorectal cancer and schistosomiasis. *Lancet* 1:971, 1981.
24. Graham S, Dayal H, Swanson M, et al: Diet and epidemiology of cancer of the colon and rectum. *JNCI* 61:709–715, 1978.
25. Utsonomiya J, Iwana T, Hirayama R: Familial large bowel cancer. In De Cosse JJ (ed): *Large Bowel Cancer.* New York: Churchill Livingston, 1981, p. 16.
26. Flotte CT, O'Dell FD Jr, Coller FA: Polyposis of colon. *Ann Surg* 144:165, 1956.
27. Alabaster O: Colorectal cancer: Epidemiology, risks, and prevention. In Ahlgren JD, Macdonald JS (eds): *Gastrointestinal Oncology.* Philadelphia: Lippincott, 1992, pp. 243–259.
28. Jagelman DG: Choice of operation and familial adenomatous polyposis. *World J Surg* 15:47–49, 1991.
29. Yeatman TJ, Bland KI, Copeland EM: Malignant lesions of the colon, rectum, and anus. In Moody FG (ed): *Surgical Treatment,* 1990, pp. 799–816.
30. Turcot J, Defres JP, St. Pierre F: Malignant tumors of the central nervous system associated with familial polyposis of the colon. *Dis Colon Rectum* 2:465–568, 1959.
31. Dozois RR, Jodd ES, Dahlin DC, et al: The Peutz-Jeghers syndrome: Is there a predisposition to the development of intestinal malignancy? *Arch Surg* 98:509, 1969.
32. Lynch HT, Lanspa S, Smyrk T, et al: Hereditary nonpolyposis colorectal cancer (Lynch syndromes I and II). *Cancer Genet Cytogenet* 53:143–160, 1991.
33. Fitzsimmons ML: Hereditary colorectal cancers. *Semin Oncol Nurs* 8:252–257, 1992.
34. Fry RD, Fleshman JW, Kodner IJ: Cancer of colon and rectum. *Clin Symposia* 41(5), 1989 (New Jersey, CIBA-GEIGY).
35. Anderson DE, Romsdahl M: Family history: A criterion for selective screening. In Mulvihill JJ, Miller RW, Fraumeni J (eds): *Genetics of Human Cancer.* New York: Raven Press, 1977.
36. Jagelman DG: Proctocolectomy with ileostomy or colectomy with ileorectal anastamosis for familial polyposis coli. In Kodner IJ, Fry RD, Roe JP (eds): *Colon, Rectal, and Anal Surgery.* St. Louis, MO: Mosby, 1985.
37. Weisburger JH: Colorectal cancer: Etiologic factors and their mode of action as an effective approach to prevention. In Kuschner JB, Shortner RG (eds): *Diseases of the Colon, Rectum, and Anal Canal.* Baltimore, MD: Williams & Wilkins, 1988, pp. 371–394.
38. Faintuch JS, Levin B, Kirsner JB: Inflammatory bowel diseases and their relationship to malignancy. *Crit Rev Oncol Hematol* 2:222:1985.
39. Sinopolous AP: Energy imbalance and cancer of the breast, colon, and prostate. *Med Oncol Tumor Pharmacother* 7:109–120, 1990.
40. Kwale G, Heuch I: Is the incidence of colorectal cancer related to reproduction? A prospective study of 63,000 women. *Int J Cancer* 47:390–395, 1991.
41. Weiss NS, Daling JR, Chow WH: Incidence of cancer of the large bowel in women in relation to reproductive and hormonal factors. *JNCI* 67:57, 1981.
42. Symonds DA, Vickery AL: Mucinous carcinoma of the colon and rectum. *Cancer* 37:1891–1900, 1976.
43. Woolam GI, Jackman RT, Ramirez RJ: Scirrhous carcinoma of the lower intestine. *Surg Gynecol Obstet* 121:753–755, 1965.
44. Bonfiglio TA, Roger T: The pathology of cancer. In Rubin P (ed): *Clinical Oncology: A Multidisciplinary Approach.* Atlanta, GA: American Cancer Society, 1983, pp. 20–30.
45. Faintuch JS, Levin B: Clinical aspects of malignant tumors of the large intestine and anal canal, including therapy. In Kirschner JB, Shortner RG (eds): *Diseases of the Colon, Rectum, and Anal Canal.* Baltimore, MD: Williams & Wilkins, 1988, pp. 395–414.
46. Hartner KW, Ahlgren JD: Cancer of the anal canal. In Ahlgren JD, Macdonald JS (eds): *Gastrointestinal Oncology.* Philadelphia: Lippincott, 1992, pp. 437–443.
47. Wexner SD, Milsom JW, Dailey TH: The demographics of anal cancers are changing: Identification of high-risk population. *Dis Colon Rectum* 30:942–946, 1987.
48. Biggar RJ, Burnett W, Miki J, et al: Cancer among New York men at risk of acquired immunodeficiency syndrome. *Int J Cancer* 43:979, 1989.
49. Daling JR, Weiss NS, Hiolop TG, et al: Sexual practices, sexually transmitted diseases, and the incidence of anal cancer. *N Engl J Med* 317:973, 1987.
50. Fenoglio CM, Lane N: The anatomical precursor of colorectal carcinoma. *Cancer* 3:819–823, 1974.

51. Umpleby HC, Williamson RCN: Anastomotic recurrences in large bowel cancer. *Br J Surg* 74:878, 1987.
52. Hussain M, Al-Sarraf M: Anal carcinoma: New combined modality treatment approaches. *Oncology* 2:42–47, 1988.
53. Bresalier RS, Kim YS: Malignant neoplasms of the large and small intestine. In Sleisenger MN, Fordtran JS (eds): *Gastrointestinal Disease*. Philadelphia: Saunders, 1989, pp. 1519–1560.
54. Jones RS, Sleisenger M: Cancer of the colon and rectum. In Sleisenger MH, Fordtran JS (eds): *Gastrointestinal Disease*. Philadelphia: Saunders, 1989, pp. 1784–1800.
55. Rosato FE, Shelley WB, Fitts WT Jr, et al: Non-metastatic cutaneous manifestations of cancer of the colon. *Am J Surg* 117:277–281, 1969.
56. Fink DJ: *Guidelines for the Cancer Related Checkup*. Atlanta, GA: American Cancer Society, 1991.
57. Greene FL: Distribution of colorectal neoplasms. A left to right shift of polyps and cancer. *Am Surg* 49:62–65, 1983.
58. Siegel RS, Hill MC, Smith LE: Colorectal cancer: Diagnosis and staging. In Ahlgren JD, Macdonald JS (eds): *Gastrointestinal Oncology*. Philadelphia: Lippincott, 1992, pp. 285–292.
59. Go VLW, Zamcheck N: The role of tumor markers in the management of colorectal cancer. *Cancer* 50:2618–2623, 1982.
60. Gromberg C, Bury JN, Sezeur A: Preoperative assessment of the extension of rectal carcinoma: Correlation of MR, surgical, and histopathologic findings. *J Comput Assist Tomogr* 12:209, 1988.
61. Kuusela P, Jalanko M, Roberts P: Comparison of CA 19-9 and CEA levels in serum of patients with colorectal disease. *Br J Cancer* 49:135–139, 1984.
62. Astler VB, Collier FA: The prognostic significance of direct extension of carcinoma of the colon and rectum. *Ann Surg* 129, 1954.
63. Smith L: Colorectal cancer: Surgical approach. In Ahlgren JD, Macdonald JS (eds): *Gastrointestinal Oncology*. Philadelphia: Lippincott, 1992, pp. 299–377.
64. Schover LR, Jensen SB: *Sexuality and Chronic Illness—A Comprehensive Approach*. New York: Guilford Press, 1988.
65. Smith DB: Psychosocial adaptation. In Hampton BG, Bryant RA (eds): *Ostomies and Continent Diversions*. St. Louis, MO: Mosby Year Book, 1992, pp. 1–22.
66. McGarity WC: Gastrointestinal surgical procedures. In Hampton BG, Bryant RA (eds): *Ostomies and Continent Diversions*. St. Louis, MO: Mosby Year Book, 1992, pp. 349–369.
67. Erwin-Toth, Doughty DB: Principles and procedures of stomal management. In Hampton BG, Bryant RA (eds): *Ostomies and Continent Diversions*. St. Louis, MO: Mosby Year Book, 1992, pp. 29–104.
68. Hampton BG: Peristomal and stomal complications. In Hampton BG, Bryant RA (eds): *Ostomies and Continent Diversions*. St. Louis, MO: Mosby Year Book, 1992, pp. 106–123.
69. Frost DB, Richards PC, Montague ED, et al: Epidermoid cancer of the anorectum. *Cancer* 53:1285, 1984.
70. Greenall NJ, Quan SHQ, Urmacher C, et al: Treatment of epidermoid carcinoma of the anal canal. *Surg Gynecol Obstet* 161:509, 1985.
71. Eschwege F, Lasser P, Chavey A, et al: Squamous cell carcinoma of the anal canal: Treatment by external beam irradiation. *Radiother Oncol* 3:145, 1985.
72. Gerard A, Buyse M, Nordittinger B, et al: Preoperative radiotherapy as adjuvant treatment in rectal cancer: Final results of a randomized study of the European Organization for Research and Treatment of Cancer (EORTC). *Ann Surg* 208:606, 1988.
73. Stockholm Rectal Cancer Study Group: Preoperative short-term radiation therapy in operable rectal carcinoma. *Cancer* 66:49, 1990.
74. Rostock RA, Zajac AJ, Gallagher MJ: Radiation therapy in the treatment of colorectal cancer. In Ahlgren JD, Macdonald JS (eds): *Gastrointestinal Oncology*. Philadelphia: Lippincott, 1992, pp. 359–381.
75. Mohiuddin M, Derdel J, Mards G, et al: Results of adjuvant radiation therapy in cancer of the rectum: Thomas Jefferson University Hospital experience. *Cancer* 55:350 (updated at ASTRO, 1990), 1985.
76. Papillon J: *Rectal and Anal Cancers*. Berlin: Springer-Verlag, 1982.
77. Wang CC, Schultz MD: The role of radiation therapy in the management of carcinoma of the sigmoid, rectosigmoid, and rectum. *Radiology* 79:1–5, 1962.
78. Gunderson LL, Shipley WV, Suit H: Intraoperative irradiation: A pilot study combining external beam photons with "boost" dose intraoperative electrons. *Cancer* 49:2259–2266, 1982.
79. McGowan I, Barr H, Krasner N: Palliative laser therapy for inoperable rectal cancer, does it work? A prospective study on quality of life. *Cancer* 63:967–969, 1989.
80. Macdonald JS, Axelrod R: Adjuvant therapy of colon and rectal cancer. In Ahlgren JD, Macdonald JS (eds): *Gastrointestinal Oncology*. Philadelphia: Lippincott, 1992, pp. 383–395.

Chapter 43

Gynecologic Cancers

Janet Ruth Walczak, RN, MSN

Paula R. Klemm, RN, DNSc, OCN

INTRODUCTION

Gynecologic cancers account for about 13% of all cancers in women. In 1993 there will be approximately 71,500 new cases of invasive female genital cancer and 55,000 new cases of carcinoma in situ or intraepithelial neoplasia in the United States (Table 43-1). Approximately 24,400 women will die of gynecologic malignancies in 1993.[1] This constitutes about 9% of cancer deaths in women. Although the gynecologic cancers can occur at any age, the majority occur in the middle years (cervical), perimenopausal years (ovarian), and postmenopausal years (endometrial, vulvar, and vaginal). Like many other malignancies, cancers of the female genital tract can be cured if diagnosed in early stages. Unfortunately, only cervical cancer has a specific and sensitive screening tool that can be applied to large numbers of women safely and inexpensively. As a result, many women, particularly those with ovarian cancer, are diagnosed in later stages when the ability to achieve cure is limited by the lack of effective therapy.

TABLE 43-1 Gynecologic Cancer in the United States—1993

Cancer Site	Estimated New Cases	Estimated Deaths
Cancer of the cervix	13,500	4,400
Cancer of the endometrium	31,000	5,700
Cancer of the ovary	22,000	13,300
Other gynecologic cancers	5,000	1,000

Source: Boring CC, Squires TS, Tong T: Cancer statistics, 1993. *CA* 43(1):7–26, 1993.

The major gynecologic cancers are reviewed in this chapter. Cancer of the uterine corpus, or endometrial cancer, is the predominant cancer of the female genital tract and usually occurs in the postmenopausal years. Regular gynecologic visits that include a screening endometrial biopsy in high-risk women could increase early detection of curable adenocarcinoma of the endometrium. Ovarian cancer is usually disseminated at diagnosis. Localized disease is asymptomatic in the vast majority of cases and routine pelvic examinations frequently fail to detect ovarian tumors in this group. Efforts to define methods of detection are still in progress. Because ovarian cancer is usually diagnosed in late stages, it is the fifth leading cause of cancer death.

Cervical cancer predominantly occurs during the reproductive years when women are more likely to receive regular gynecologic care, including Pap smear testing. Therefore, the majority of cervical lesions are diagnosed in the preinvasive stages of intraepithelial neoplasia when the disease is curable. Vulvar and vaginal cancers usually occur in the postmenopausal years when many women feel that they no longer need to be seen by a gynecologist. These cancers are frequently preceded by preinvasive intraepithelial neoplasia and are readily curable if diagnosed in early stages.

ENDOMETRIAL CANCER

Epidemiology

Cancer of the endometrium is the predominant cancer of the female genital tract. While there will be an estimated 31,000 new cases of endometrial cancer diagnosed in the United States in 1993, only approximately 5700 women will die of the disease in 1993. This low

This chapter is dedicated to the memory of Linda M. Arenth, RN, MS, vice president for Nursing and Patient Services at The Johns Hopkins Hospital and first director of nursing at The Johns Hopkins Oncology Center. Linda was a source of inspiration and a mentor, innovator, and pioneer in oncology nursing.

mortality rate reflects the fact that 79% are diagnosed with localized disease.[1] Survival rates for endometrial cancer by stage are 76% for stage I, 50% for stage II, 30% for stage III, and 9% for stage IV.[2]

Endometrial cancer is primarily a disease of postmenopausal women. This median age at diagnosis is 61 years, with the majority of women diagnosed between 50 and 59 years of age. Only about 5% of women will be diagnosed before 40 years of age, and 20%–25% will be premenopausal.[3]

Etiology

Multiple risk factors have been associated with the development of endometrial cancer. These include obesity (>20 pounds overweight), nulliparity, late menopause (after age 52), diabetes, hypertension, infertility, irregular menses, failure of ovulation, a history of breast or ovarian cancer, adenomatous hyperplasia, and prolonged use of exogenous estrogen therapy. An obese, nulliparous woman who experiences menopause after 59 years of age appears to have a 5-fold greater risk of developing endometrial cancer.[3,4]

Excessive endogenous estrogen metabolism or production has been implicated in the development of endometrial cancer. Several hormonal aberrations can be linked to obesity. Increased body size plays a role in androgen conversion to estrogen.[4–6] Additionally, obese women with an upper body fat pattern have a 5.8-fold increase in risk over women who are nonobese or have lower body fat pattern.[7] Fat cells are an excellent storage depot for estrogen, and the chronic slow release of estrogen from these cells may account for the increased risk. In obese postmenopausal women, secretion of serum sex hormone–binding globulin (SHBG) is depressed, leaving higher concentrations of free estradiol in the blood. Obese women have endocrine malfunctions that cause anovulatory cycles with irregular menses. This results in failure of progesterone to oppose chronic estrogen effects on the endometrium. Another source of endogenous estrogen can be feminizing ovarian tumors (e.g., granulose cell tumors).[4–6]

Use of unopposed exogenous estrogens has been linked to an increased incidence of endometrial cancer since the mid-1970s.[8] This problem can be virtually eliminated by cycling estrogen and progesterone and by histologically sampling the endometrium for early detection.[3,9]

Either exogenous or endogenous estrogen may lead to endometrial hyperplasia. While adenomatous hyperplasia is considered a risk factor of endometrial cancer, it is unclear if it is a precursor, unless atypia accompanies the hyperplasia.[3]

Two factors appear to have a protective effect in preventing the development of endometrial cancer: oral contraceptives and cigarette smoking. Oral contraceptive usage for at least 12 months decreases the woman's risk of developing endometrial cancer, and this protection seems to persist for up to 15 years in nulliparous women. Similarly, smoking has demonstrated a reduction in risk, especially in women over 50 years old. However, the risks of developing lung cancer and other health problems well outweigh any protection gained against endometrial cancer.[3, 10–12]

Pathophysiology and Cellular Characteristics

The uterine corpus is a muscular, hollow, pear-shaped organ with an endometrial lining composed of ciliated epithelial cells. Throughout the epithelium are small, tubular glands that extend to the myometrium, or muscle wall of the corpus. Endometrial cancer develops in the epithelial layer. Tumors that arise in the lower uterine segment involve the cervix sooner and have a higher incidence of pelvic and paraaortic lymph node involvement than do tumors that arise higher in the fundus. Similarly, tumors that have deep myometrial invasion tend to be more aggressive and have a poorer survival rate.[3]

Over 90% of endometrial cancers are adenocarcinomas. Three types of adenocarcinomas account for 88% of histologic patterns: pure adenocarcinomas, adenoacanthoma (adenocarcinoma with a benign squamous component), and adenosquamous (where both components are malignant). The less frequent patterns include clear cell (mesonephroid) carcinoma, undifferentiated carcinoma, and the papillary carcinomas, which include the endometrioid and serous types. The clear cell and serous patterns are more aggressive than the other carcinomas.[3,12]

Natural History

Multiple factors affect the natural history and prognosis of endometrial cancer. These include histologic type and differentiation, uterine size, stage of disease, myometrial invasion, peritoneal cytology, lymph node metastasis, and adnexal metastasis.[3,13]

Cancer usually starts in the fundus and may spread to involve the entire endometrium. Through direct extension and infiltration, the cancer spreads to the myometrium, endocervix, cervix, fallopian tubes, and ovaries. Adnexal spread is infrequent but is found at surgery in about 10% of women with clinical stage I. Recurrence appears in 38% of women with adnexal spread versus 11% of those without such involvement.[3]

Metastatic spread is usually to pelvic and paraaortic lymph nodes and has been positively correlated with tumor differentiation, stage of disease, and amount of myometrial invasion. Pelvic and paraaortic lymph node metastases can be present, even in women with stage I disease (Figure 43-1) when about 10% will have positive pelvic nodes, and stage II disease when 36% will have positive nodes.[3,14]

Less common sites of metastases include the vagina, peritoneal cavity, omentum, and inguinal lymph nodes.

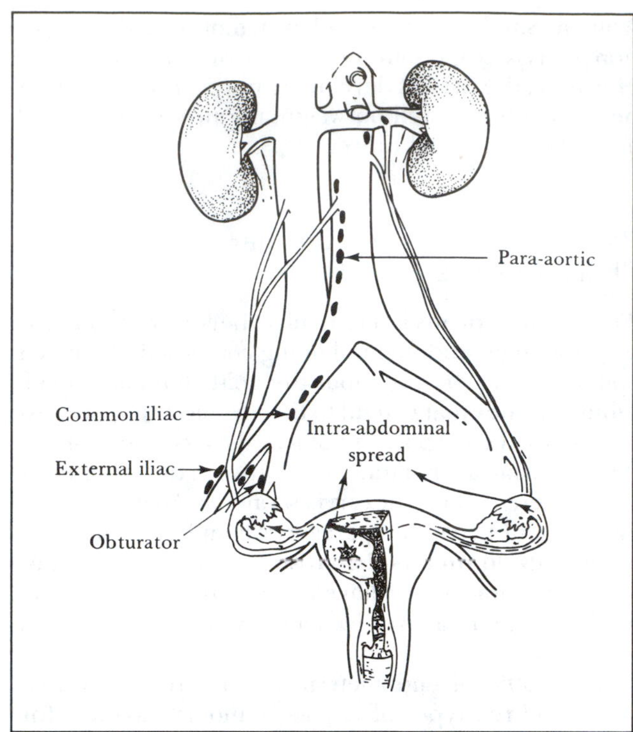

FIGURE 43-1 Spread pattern of endometrial cancer, with particular emphasis on potential lymph node spread. Pelvic and paraaortic nodes are at risk, even in stage I disease. (Source: DiSaia PJ, Creasman WT: *Clinical Gynecologic Oncology*. St Louis, MO: Mosby, 1989.)

Hematogenous spread often involves the lung, liver, bone, and brain. The size of the uterus, measured by uterine sound, has been an indicator of survival. However, since large uterine size can be secondary to intercurrent disease, such as fibroids, this factor is no longer included in the staging and prognosis of endometrial cancer. Even so, the 5-year survival rate for women with a normal-sized uterus is 84%, whereas that for women with an enlarged uterus is 67%.[15]

Histologic differentiation is one of the most sensitive indicators of metastases and prognosis. The less differentiated the tumor, the poorer the prognosis. Grade 1 tumors are highly differentiated, grade 2 tumors are moderately differentiated, and grade 3 tumors are mostly solid or undifferentiated carcinomas.[16] Overall 5-year survival rates for stage I are 96% for patients with grade I tumors, 79% for those with grade II tumors, and 70% for those with grade III tumors.[2,3]

Another prognostic indicator, the degree of myometrial invasion, is generally classified as: none (localized to the endometrium), superficial (invasion <50%), or deep (>50%).[2] The greater the invasion, the poorer the prognosis. Additionally, the less differentiated the tumor, the greater the chance of myometrial invasion. Thus, the grade of the tumor is combined with the degree of myometrial invasion to estimate survival.

During laparotomy, samples of peritoneal fluid or washings of the peritoneal cavity are obtained for staging purposes, but the results also have prognostic significance. Women with positive washings are at a higher risk for pelvic recurrence. DiSaia and Creasman[3] reported a 15% rate of positive washings in women with stage I disease. Recurrence developed in 34% of these individuals, compared with 10% among patients showing negative cytologic change.

Clinical Manifestations

Fortunately, the abnormal vaginal bleeding associated with endometrial cancer causes women to seek medical attention promptly. Postmenopausal bleeding should always be evaluated, even though only 20% of women with this symptom will have cancer. Any serosanguinous vaginal discharge or new heavy bleeding also needs evaluation. Premenopausal onset of irregular or heavy menstrual flow may be significant, especially if the patient is infertile with anovulatory cycles. Other more infrequent symptoms are pyometria and hematometria, particularly in the older woman, and lumbosacral, hypogastric, or pelvic pain in women with more advanced disease.[16]

Assessment

In women suspected of having endometrial cancer, a thorough pelvic examination is performed. A Pap smear will only occasionally detect an endometrial cancer.[16] A more reliable technique is endometrial biopsy, which allows histologic rather than cytologic examination. This procedure is 90% effective in detecting endometrial cancer and can be performed in the outpatient setting.[3] The American Cancer Society recommends endometrial sampling every 1–2 years for women taking exogenous estrogens and at high risk for the development of endometrial cancer at menopause.[17] If the endometrial biopsy is negative and symptoms persist, a fractional dilatation and curettage (D & C) is performed.[3]

Other diagnostic tests include chest radiograph, intravenous pyelogram (IVP), complete blood count (CBC), and blood chemistry profiles. Cystoscopy, barium enema, and proctoscopy are performed if bladder or rectal involvement is suspected. Other studies that may be used to evaluate pelvic, abdominal, and nodal disease status include hysterography, hysteroscopy, lymphangiography, and computerized axial tomogram scan.[18] Although magnetic resonance imaging (MRI) cannot distinguish benign from malignant neoplasms, it is used to detect degree of myometrial invasion in about 85% of cases.[19,20]

Treatment, Results, and Prognosis

Primary

Endometrial cancer is staged surgically (Table 43-2) in patients who are surgical candidates, that is, if medical condition and intraabdominal disease permit. Staging helps to define primary tumor size and location as well as extent of spread beyond the uterus. Approximately 75% of tumors are diagnosed in stage I, 13% in stage II, 9% in stage III, and 3% in stage IV.[2]

Surgical staging and treatment involve an extensive evaluation of the abdomino-pelvic cavity and the following procedures: bimanual examination under anesthesia, peritoneal cytology, inspection and palpation of all peritoneal surfaces, biopsy of suspicious areas, selective pelvic and paraaortic lymphadenectomy, total abdominal hysterectomy (TAH), bilateral salpingo-oophrectomy (BSO), and possible omentectomy and resection of tumor implants. Tissue from the primary tumor is obtained for analysis of estrogen and progesterone receptors. Surgical staging prior to any radiation therapy is advantageous since many women with early-stage disease will not need additional postoperative therapy and thus can avoid the time, effort, and morbidity associated with pelvic radiation therapy. Also, the pathologist is better able to evaluate untreated tissue for the histologic indicators of prognosis (histologic type, grade, and myometrial invasion).

Selection of adjuvant radiation therapy for early endometrial cancer is determined by stage, histology, and cytopathology. In patients with positive peritoneal cytology, intraperitoneal radioactive colloidal phosphorous (^{32}P) may be helpful in preventing or delaying recurrence if no other therapy is indicated. However, prospective data are not available to support or refute this approach. Patients with stage I, grade 1 disease and no myometrial invasion require no further treatment after TAH, BSO. Patients with stage I, grade 2 disease and less than 50% myometrial invasion require intravaginal radiation to reduce the risk of central recurrence. Indications for pelvic external beam radiation therapy include disease localized to the pelvis, a high-

TABLE 43-2 Corpus Cancer Staging

CARCINOMA OF THE UTERINE CORPUS

The Committee decided that corpus cancer should be surgically staged and as a result additional factors of prognostic importance are included in the staging. The Committee also decided to change the current definitions of tumour grading to coincide with the new recommendations of the International Society of Gynaecological Pathologists. The recommended staging is as follows:

STAGE

IA	G123	Tumour limited to endometrium
IB	G123	Invasion to <1/2 myometrium
IC	G123	Invasion to >1/2 myometrium
IIA	G123	Endocervical glandular involvement only
IIB	G123	Cervical stromal invasion
IIIA	G123	Tumour invades serosa and/or adnexa and/or positive peritoneal cytology
IIIB	G123	Metastases to pelvic and/or para-aortic lymph nodes
IVA	G123	Tumour invasion of bladder and/or bowel mucosa
IVB		Distant metastases including intra-abdominal and/or inguinal lymph nodes

HISTOPATHOLOGY: DEGREE OF DIFFERENTIATION

Cases of carcinoma of the corpus should be grouped with regard to the degree of differentiation of the adenocarcinoma as follows:

G1 5% or less of a non-squamous or non-morular solid growth pattern

G2 6%–50% of a non-squamous or non-morular solid growth pattern

G3 More than 50% of a non-squamous or nonmorular solid growth pattern

NOTES ON PATHOLOGICAL GRADING

(1) Notable nuclear atypia, inappropriate for the architectural grade, raises the grade of a grade I or grade II tumour by one.

(2) In serous adenocarcinomas, clear-cell adenocarcinomas, and squamous-cell carcinomas, nuclear grading takes precedence.

(3) Adenocarcinomas with squamous differentiation are graded according to the nuclear grade of the glandular component.

RULES RELATED TO STAGING

(1) Since corpus cancer is now surgically staged, procedures used previously for the differentiation of stages are no longer applicable, such as using dilatation and curettage findings to differentiate between stage I and stage II. (It is appreciated that there may be a small number of patients with corpus cancer who will be treated primarily with radiation therapy. If that is the case, the clinical staging adopted by FIGO* in 1971 would still apply but designation of that staging system would be noted.)

(2) Ideally, the thickness of the myometrium should be measured along with the depth of tumour invasion.

*FIGO, International Federation of Gynecology & Obstetrics.

Source: FIGO News, *Int J Gynecol Obstet* 28:189–193, 1989. Elsevier Science Publishers.

grade tumor, or greater than 50% myometrial invasion. Whole-pelvis radiation, in contrast to intravaginal radiation, allows treatment of all pelvic tissue including nodes and lymphatics. The role of whole-abdominal radiation in the treatment of serous and clear cell carcinomas and advanced adenocarcinomas is still under investigation.[3,12,13,22,23]

Adjuvant hormonal therapy in endometrial cancer is considered unproven and remains controversial.[16] Kauppila et al.[24] reported on over 1100 patients who received adjuvant progestin therapy for 2 years after primary treatment for endometrial cancer; recurrence occurred even in women with stage I disease.

Advanced or recurrent disease

Endometrial cancer is one of the most difficult cancers to treat if metastasis or recurrence has occurred.[25] Women with vaginal recurrences can be treated successfully with surgery or radiotherapy. These individuals do well and usually are long-term survivors.[3] However, women with recurrences outside the upper vagina (pelvis or distant) are not easily treated. Radiotherapy has a limited role in recurrent disease, although palliative radiation can be employed to control heavy vaginal bleeding in patients who present with advanced, incurable disease. Hormonal therapy or chemotherapy is essential to treat recurrent and advanced disease.[3]

Hormonal therapy The most commonly used systemic therapy for recurrent endometrial cancer has been synthetic progestational agents. Response rates range from 30%–37%, and response seems to be related to histologic grade of the tumor, length of the disease-free interval, the woman's age, and presence of areas of squamous metaplasia within the primary tumor.[16] Receptor status can also predict which tumors will respond to progestins. Positive estrogen and progesterone receptor status correlates with a better response to progestin therapy regardless of the grade of the tumor. If both receptors are positive, there is a 77% response rate associated with progestin therapy, compared with only a 9% response rate if both receptors are negative.[26]

Side effects of progestational agents include fluid retention, phlebitis, and thrombosis. Side effects are usually minimal unless high doses are employed. Patients have reported feelings of well-being as well as weight gain while taking progestins.[16]

Oral preparations of megestrol acetate or intramuscular medroxyprogesterone acetate are effective agents against endometrial cancer.[16] The progestins are continued until the disease progresses. At that time, chemotherapy is considered.

The antiestrogen tamoxifen, which can cause hot flashes, vaginal dryness, and infrequently emotional lability, has been used to treat advanced endometrial cancer in an attempt to induce progesterone receptor positivity. No improvement in length of response was seen, although the drug was shown to increase the number of receptors per tumor.[27] The use of tamoxifen is still experimental.[2] Quinn and Campbell[28] suggested using a combination of tamoxifen and progestogen as the first choice of hormonal therapy.

Chemotherapy Cytotoxic agents have a limited role in advanced endometrial cancer since only a few agents have demonstrated activity equal to or greater than progestin therapy. In single-agent trials, the most promising results were obtained by Thigpen et al.[29] using 60 mg/m^2 of doxorubicin every 3 weeks. These researchers reported a 37% response rate, with 26% complete responses. Prognostic factors did not correlate with the probability of response.

Administration of high doses (100 mg/m^2) of cisplatin has achieved response rates of 46% in women with no prior chemotherapy.[30] However, when cisplatin was used as a second-line treatment, the results were not impressive (4% response rate).[31] Thigpen et al.[32] studied 49 women with advanced or recurrent endometrial carcinoma who had not received prior chemotherapy and who were no longer controllable with other treatment modalities. Patients were treated with cisplatin, 50 mg/m^2 intravenously, every 3 weeks. Forty-five percent exhibited stable disease for at least 2 months, while 35% had disease progression in less than 2 months after beginning chemotherapy.

Combination therapy has been studied to a limited degree; however, cisplatin, doxorubicin, and cyclophosphamide resulted in an overall response rate of 45% in 209 patients.[33] Other studies have shown little improvement over response rates seen with single agents. In addition, the profile of side effects experienced with single agents is more limited.

There is little evidence at present to support the use of combination chemotherapy in the management of endometrial carcinoma.[32] Further well-controlled clinical trials examining the role of combination chemotherapy in patients with advanced or recurrent endometrial carcinoma are needed.[2]

Nursing Management

The care of the patient with endometrial cancer includes those issues discussed in the chapters devoted to the specific treatment modalities such as surgery, radiation therapy, and chemotherapy. The other major area for assessment and intervention is knowledge related to health maintenance behaviors, therapeutic interventions, and psychosocial concerns. These issues are summarized in Table 43-3.

Future Trends

While the majority of women are diagnosed with early-stage disease, women still die from recurrent or advanced disease. Ongoing efforts strive to define adjuvant therapy to further improve survival and reduce recurrence. The role of ^{32}P in early-stage disease with

TABLE 43-3 Information Needs Related to Endometrial Cancer

Topic	Information
Health maintenance issues that affect risk	
Estrogen replacement therapy (ERT)	Indications: Vaginal atrophy with infection or sexual dysfunction Loss of pelvic support with incontinence Postmenopausal osteoporosis Perimenopausal emotional lability Early surgical or radiation castration Vasomotor instability Lowered morbidity and mortality for cardiovascular disease Estrogen cycled with progesterone Annual pelvic exam Regular histologic sampling of endometrium Annual mammogram Seek medical attention if any abnormal vaginal bleeding occurs including postmenopausal bleeding (PMB)
Breast self-examination (BSE)	Importance of BSE in conjunction with ERT Determine schedule to aid in compliance Technique for performing BSE and demonstration of skill
Diet and weight control	Low-fat, calcium-rich diet Maintain weight within normal range Large amounts of caffeine and fiber may decrease calcium absorption Weight-bearing exercises to decrease bone loss, eg, walking
Abnormal vaginal bleeding	Seek medical attention for new onset of abnormal bleeding, including intramenstrual and PMB PMB and abnormal bleeding in the infertile patient with anovulatory cycles must be evaluated, even though only 20% of PMB is associated with malignancy Evaluation of abnormal bleeding includes pelvic exam and endometrial biopsy
Therapeutic interventions	
Surgery	Types of surgery planned, what will be removed, change in anatomy and function anticipated Clarify, reinforce informed consent Role in postoperative care to facilitate recovery, eg, progressive ambulation, respiratory care Discharge planning related to self-care issues, need for assistance, and appointment for postoperative follow-up
Radiation	Type of therapy planned Inpatient versus outpatient therapy Associated morbidity, eg, GI, GU Appointments for follow-up
Hormonal	Schedule for medications Expected side effects
Chemotherapy	Types of drugs and regimen planned Side effects and toxicities of drugs Inpatient versus outpatient versus home chemotherapy Duration of therapy Need for venous access device Regular appointments to monitor response
Psychosexual concerns	
Role functioning	Dispel myths related to perceived loss of femininity due to removal of uterus, tubes, and ovaries, eg, weight gain, loss of sexual interest/enjoyment, aging, mental deterioration[185] Help redefine self in terms other than reproduction
Sexual functioning	Review anatomy, physiology, and sexual functioning preoperatively Complete sexual assessment Alteration in sexual response secondary to hysterectomy: Cervix contributes to but is not essential for orgasm Uterus elevates during excitement phase and contracts rhythmically during orgasm[192] Alteration in sexual functioning secondary to radiation: Vaginal dryness and stenosis may result in patient who is not sexually active, unless vaginal dilators and lubricants are employed. Use of water-soluble lubricants during intercourse, such as Astroglide® or nonhormonal moisturizers used three times a week, such as Replens®

positive pelvic cytology needs to be defined in a prospective clinical trial. However, as better methods for control of central disease are achieved, patients who then fail to respond to primary therapy will recur outside of the pelvis. The role of whole-abdominal radiation therapy in preventing or treating recurrences is not yet defined; however, the Gynecologic Oncology Group has prospective clinical trials in progress.[22,34] Also, prospective clinical trials to identify cytotoxic drugs and drug regimens with improved response and survival rates continue.

The role of estrogen and progesterone receptor status in the choice of therapy and as a predictor of response needs to be defined. With the availability of assays for receptors, more information can be collected. Preliminary studies show a positive correlation between the presence of progesterone receptors and clinical response to progestin therapy.[35] This information also could be correlated with other prognostic factors to pinpoint more specifically those women who will respond. Theoretically, women with positive estrogen receptors should respond to anti-estrogen therapy. If both estrogen receptors and progesterone receptors are positive, future trials could employ combination hormonal therapy. Utaaker et al.[36] concluded that steroid receptors were found in more than 85% of primary endometrial carcinomas. Highly differentiated tumors were more often estrogen receptor and progesterone receptor rich than were poorly differentiated ones, but receptor status was not significantly associated with surgical stage.

Estrogen replacement therapy (ERT), while historically contraindicated in women with endometrial cancer, also needs further investigation in order to identify the appropriate candidate for ERT. For women with stage I disease, low-grade tumors, and no myometrial invasion, the benefits of ERT in decreasing the risk of cardiovascular disease and osteoporosis may outweigh the associated risk of breast cancer and recurrent endometrial cancer. Finally, as younger women develop endometrial cancer, conservative therapy for early-stage, low-grade disease needs to be prospectively evaluated for long-term outcomes.

OVARIAN CANCER

Epidemiology

In 1993 there will be approximately 22,000 new cases of ovarian cancer diagnosed in the United States and over 13,000 deaths from the disease. Ovarian cancer accounts for approximately 29% of all gynecologic cancers and 54% of deaths from cancer of the female genital tract. It is the most common cause of death from gynecologic cancers and the fifth leading cause of cancer death in women in the United States.[1] Ovarian cancer is a leading cause of death in industrialized countries (except Japan) but is rare in developing nations.[18]

It is estimated that 1 of every 71 women will develop ovarian cancer, with most cases seen in women between 55 and 59 years of age.[37,38] Only 7%–8% of ovarian carcinomas occur in women under 35 years of age.[39]

The overall 5-year survival rate for women with ovarian cancer is between 30% and 35% and has not changed over the past 30 years. The poor survival rate is due in part to several factors: (1) it is difficult to diagnose ovarian cancer early (60% to 70% of tumors are stage III or IV at diagnosis); (2) treatment, although intensive, has not been curative; (3) a high-risk population has not been clearly defined; and (4) the etiology is essentially unknown.

Etiology

Little is known regarding the etiology of ovarian cancer, but multiple risk factors have been identified including environmental, hormonal, menstrual, reproductive, dietary, and hereditary indicators. Environmental factors seem to play an important role since the industrialized nations, except Japan, have the highest incidence of ovarian cancer. The relationship between educational level, socioeconomic level, childbearing practices, and environment cannot be ignored. Women with higher educational and socioeconomic levels tend to delay childbearing, have fewer children, and have a higher incidence of ovarian cancer.[40] Additionally, the incidence of ovarian cancer in Japanese immigrants to the United States approaches that of white women in the United States by the second generation.[3]

Reproductive issues associated with ovarian cancer include age at first pregnancy, number of pregnancies, and use of oral contraceptives. Increased risk has been identified in nulliparous women and to a lesser degree in women who first became pregnant after age 35. Risk seems to be inversely related to the cumulative time that ovulation is suppressed during the childbearing years due to pregnancy, lactation, or oral contraceptives. The use of oral contraceptives not only has a protective effect against ovarian cancer, but this effect seems to persist for at least 15 years after use has stopped.[41] These factors support the theory that "incessant ovulation" produces chronic irritation to the ovarian epithelium. Gonadotropin levels, which are low during pregnancy and with the use of oral contraceptives, become elevated in the postmenopausal years and may be a factor in the increased incidence in women over 45 years of age.[11,42,43]

Recently other hormonal or endocrine abnormalities have been reported. Whittemore et al.[44] found that it was not the time over which ovulation occurred but the inability to conceive in ovulating women that increased risk. Early menarche, late menopause, and hormonal therapy have also been identified as impacting the risk for ovarian cancer. However, conflicting data exist so that the actual risk, if any, still needs to be defined.

Talc has been examined as a potential etiologic agent.

It has been suggested that talc may act as a tumor promotor by direct contact with the ovaries and peritoneal cavity after retrograde flow through the reproductive tract from the vagina.[38,45]

The relationship of ovarian cancer to diet is controversial. Some authors state that there is no relationship between ovarian cancer and dietary practices,[45] while others state that ovarian cancer is associated with a diet high in fats.[37,38]

Women with a family history of ovarian cancer are at an increased risk of developing the disease, though only 5%–10% of women with ovarian cancer have a genetic predisposition. Women with two or more first-degree relatives with ovarian cancer have a threefold increase in risk.[37,38] However, familial cancer may be more common than was previously indicated, and further data are needed to quantify the risk in daughters of women with ovarian cancer.[46] In addition, a family history of breast cancer doubles the risk of ovarian cancer,[45] as does a history of cancer of the colon, particularly in conjunction with breast cancer.[47]

Pathophysiology and Cellular Characteristics

Epithelial ovarian cancers arise from a malignant transformation of the ovarian surface epithelium. How this transformation occurs is not known, but there have been hypotheses suggested by the analysis of phenotypically malignant cells. Alterations in DNA quantities and structure have been demonstrated with the study of ovarian cancer cells by cytogenetics. These changes may correlate with alterations in cellular oncogene activities (including c-*myc,* H-*ras,* and K-*ras* and *neu* oncogenes) and growth factor signal transformations. Study of cytogenetics, oncogenes, and growth factor regulation has occurred in cultured tissue from patients with advanced ovarian cancer, but information about the early phases of the malignant transformation of the ovarian surface epithelium is not defined. Current knowledge of abnormal chromosomes and oncogenes associated with ovarian cancer indicates that carcinogenesis in ovarian cancer is a complex, multistage process that requires further investigation to define.[48]

Ovarian cancer includes several histologic types that may occur in different age groups, exhibit different methods of spread, and respond to different therapeutic regimens. Epithelial, stromal, and germinal cells give rise to the major subsets of ovarian cancer: epithelial, germ cells, and stromal tumors.

Epithelial tumors constitute 80%–90% of all malignant ovarian neoplasms.[37,45,49] The histologic categories of these tumors include serous, mucinous, endometroid, clear cell (mesonephroid), Brenner, and undifferentiated carcinomas. Epithelial histologic cell types have similar presentation and dissemination patterns. Histologic type itself has little prognostic value except for the clear cell type, which is more aggressive.[45]

Epithelial ovarian tumors of low malignant potential (LMP) constitute a separate clinical and pathologic entity between benign and invasive disease and represent about 15% of epithelial tumors. These tumors are described as neoplasms with no invasion of the ovarian stroma, yet they have greater cellular proliferation than the benign cystadenomas.[37,38] Tumors of LMP usually occur in women less than 40 years of age and have a favorable prognosis regardless of stage.[42]

Malignant germ cell tumors account for 4% of ovarian malignancies and are most often encountered in children and premenopausal women. The remaining 6% of ovarian malignancies are sex cord or stromal tumors. This chapter focuses only on the epithelial ovarian cancers.

Histologic grade is an important predictor of treatment response and survival.[29] Although important in all stages of disease, grade seems to be of greater prognostic significance in stage I and II disease, where the more differentiated tumors respond better to treatment.[49]

Natural History

Knowledge of the natural history of ovarian cancer is essential to appreciate the difficulties in staging and treatment. Most ovarian malignancies originate from the epithelial surface of the ovary. As the tumor grows, it invades the stromal tissue and penetrates the capsule of the ovary. The most common mechanisms of spread are by direct extension and peritoneal seeding. Direct extension occurs when tumor cells on the surface of the ovary invade the adjacent structures, including fallopian tubes, uterus, bladder, and rectosigmoid and pelvic peritoneum. Peritoneal seeding occurs when cells exfoliate into the peritoneal cavity, where they are carried in fluid via the posterior paracolic spaces to the subdiaphragmatic surfaces. Tumor nodules or seeds may be found on the peritoneal surfaces of the liver, diaphragm, bladder, and large and small bowel. The diaphragmatic and substernal lymphatics that drain the peritoneal cavity may become obstructed, and peritoneal fluid subsequently accumulates in the abdominal cavity.[49]

Although intraperitoneal spread is the most common method of dissemination, ovarian lymphatics may also have a role. The ovary contains an extensive lymphatic network that flows cephalad toward the aortic nodes. Piver et al.[50] found a 10% incidence of aortic and pelvic lymph node metastasis in stage I and II ovarian cancer. These nodes must be sampled during surgery to ensure proper staging. Hematogenous spread of disease is the least common method of dissemination. The most frequently encountered distant sites are the liver, lung, and pleura.[49]

Death is usually secondary to intraabdominal tumor dissemination. Bowel and mesentery are most commonly involved, producing multiple areas of malfunction, malabsorption, varying degrees of alteration in peristalsis, and eventually obstruction. Women with intraabdominal tumor dissemination gradually deteriorate and eventually die of electrolyte imbalance, sepsis, or cardiovascular collapse. Other contributory causes of death include toxicities of treatment, intercurrent medical problems, and pulmonary embolus.[47]

Clinical Manifestations

Unfortunately, there are typically no early manifestations of ovarian cancer. Localized disease limited to the ovary is asymptomatic in the majority of women. As the mass enlarges, the woman may experience abdominal discomfort, dyspepsia, indigestion, flatulence, eructations, loss of appetite, pelvic pressure, or urinary frequency. These vague complaints are often attributed to personal stresses and midlife changes and may precede other symptoms by months.[38] A physician examining a 40–70-year-old woman with these persistent symptoms should include ovarian cancer in the differential diagnostic work-up. Unfortunately, because these nonspecific complaints are not disabling, physicians may not initially pursue the search for ovarian cancer. Often evaluation does not occur until the woman has a palpable mass or ascites. As a result, the cancer has spread beyond the ovary in 75% of patients at the time of diagnosis.[3,49]

Assessment

Routine pelvic examination will detect 1 ovarian carcinoma in 10,000 examinations of asymptomatic women. Despite this, pelvic examinations remain the most usual method for detecting early disease. The use of transvaginal ultrasound in conjunction with CA-125, a tumor-associated antigen, is gaining popularity but needs further investigation as a screening method.[51–53] The use of transvaginal color flow imaging to identify malignant ovarian neoplasms is also being investigated and shows promise as a specific and sensitive technique for detecting ovarian cancer.[54,55] Any ovary that can be palpated in a woman more than 3–5 years after menopause should raise suspicions of an early ovarian neoplasm,[3] referred to as the "postmenopausal palpable ovary syndrome."[38]

Routine diagnostic tests are not of great value in the diagnosis of ovarian cancer, but they may help rule out another primary tumor as the source of the pelvic mass. A complete physical examination is carried out, with careful attention to the pelvis, abdomen, and breasts. A barium enema may be done to rule out primary rectosigmoid cancer, which can metastasize to ovaries. A proctosigmoidoscopy and gastrointestinal series can also be useful if the woman has intestinal symptoms.

Chest radiography helps to determine the presence of pleural effusion or parenchymal metastases. An IVP aids in determining the location of the pelvic mass relative to the ureters. Ultrasound (US) and computed tomography (CT) scans are used to evaluate the size and location of the mass. Also, MRI may be helpful to detect lesions smaller than either US or CT can identify. MRI will probably be most helpful for monitoring response to therapy.[38] Paracentesis is avoided because of the risk of rupturing an encapsulated ovarian mass and causing malignant cells to spill into the peritoneal cavity. Tumor cells can also seed along the needle tract. Whether or not the ascitic fluid is malignant, a laparotomy is necessary to confirm the diagnosis and to adequately determine the stage or extent of disease.

The staging of ovarian cancer is based on surgical evaluation and forms the basis for planning subsequent therapy.[56] Approximately 15%–20% of patients present as stage I, 10%–15% as stage II, 60%–70% as stage III, and 10%–15% as stage IV.[2] Table 43-4[57] summarizes the surgical staging for ovarian cancer.

The initial surgical exploration enables the surgeon to determine the precise diagnosis and accurate stage and to perform optimal debulking. Careful evaluation of all peritoneal surfaces is required to ensure accurate staging. The subdiaphragmatic surfaces need to be evaluated and scraped for cytopathology if no tumor is palpable. Similarly, all intraabdominal organs, surfaces, and retroperitoneal nodes are palpated to determine extent of disease. The surgeon then attempts cytoreduction of the tumor volume. Size of residual disease is an important prognostic factor. Maximally reducing the tumor size to <1 cm in diameter offers the patient a better chance of response with additional therapy.[37,45,57,58]

Unfortunately, accurate surgical staging is not obtained in all patients presenting with early ovarian cancer.[45] Only about 25% of women in the United States with stage I and II disease have a surgical incision adequate to allow evaluation of the entire pelvis and abdominal cavity. Often a lower abdominal transverse incision is used, particularly if ovarian cancer is not the preoperative diagnosis. Understaging is common. Thirty-three percent of patients thought to be free of disease following initial surgery actually have persistent, residual disease, and about 75% have disease that has spread intraabdominally.[59]

Treatment, Results, and Prognosis

Initial ovarian cancer therapy includes thorough evaluation, staging, and cytoreduction. A TAH-BSO, omentectomy, selected pelvic and paraaortic lymph node sampling, and maximal cytoreduction are performed when surgically feasible[3] (Figure 43-2).[60] Because the majority of women with epithelial ovarian cancer are diagnosed in the late stages, additional therapy is indicated. Selection of the appropriate therapy is based on stage, grade, size and location of residual tumor, and presence of ascites or peritoneal washings that contain malignant cells.[61]

Stage I

Patients with stage I, grade 1 tumors have a greater than 90% survival with surgery alone.[62] If fertility is a

TABLE 43-4 Staging Classification of Malignant Ovarian Tumors

PRIMARY TUMOR (T)

TNM	FIGO	Definition
T1a	IA	Tumor limited to one ovary; capsule intact, no tumor on ovarian surface, no malignant cells in ascites or peritoneal washings
T1b	IB	Tumor limited to both ovaries; capsules intact, no tumor on ovarian surface, no malignant cells in ascites or peritoneal washings
T1c	IC	Tumor limited to one or both ovaries with any of the following: capsule ruptured, tumor on ovarian surface, malignant cells in ascites or peritoneal washings
T2	II	Tumor involves one or both ovaries with pelvic extension
T2a	IIA	Extension and/or implants on the uterus and/or tube(s); no malignant cells in ascites or peritoneal washings
T2b	IIB	Extension to other pelvic tissues; no malignant cells in ascites or peritoneal washings
T2c	IIC	Pelvic extension (2a or 2b) with malignant cells in ascites or peritoneal washings
T3 and/or N1	III	Tumor involves one or both ovaries with microscopically confirmed peritoneal metastasis outside the pelvis and/or regional lymph node metastasis
T3a	IIIA	Microscopic peritoneal metastasis beyond the pelvis
T3b	IIIB	Macroscopic peritoneal metastasis beyond the pelvis 2 cm or less in the greatest dimension
T3c and/or N1	IIIC	Peritoneal metastasis beyond the pelvis more than 2 cm in the greatest dimension and/or regional lymph node metastasis
M1	IV	Distant metastasis (excludes peritoneal metastasis

REGIONAL LYMPH NODES (N)

NX	Regional lymph nodes cannot be assessed
N0	No regional lymph node metastasis
N1	Regional lymph node metastasis

DISTANT METASTASIS (M)

TNM	FIGO	Definition
MX	—	Presence of distant metastasis cannot be assessed
M0	—	No distant metastasis
M1	IV	Distant metastasis (excludes peritoneal metastasis)

STAGE GROUPING

AJCC/UICC				FIGO
Stage IA	T1a	N0	M0	Stage IA
Stage IB	T1b	N0	M0	Stage IB
Stage IC	T1c	N0	M0	Stage IC
Stage IIA	T2a	N0	M0	Stage IIA
Stage IIB	T2b	N0	M0	Stage IIB
Stage IIC	T2c	N0	M0	Stage IIC
Stage IIIA	T3a	N0	M0	Stage IIIA
Stage IIIB	T3b	N0	M0	Stage IIIB
Stage IIIC	T3c	N0	M0	Stage IIIC
	Any T	N1	M0	
Stage IV	Any T	Any N	M1	Stage IV

Source: Reprinted from American Joint Committee on Cancer: *Manual for Staging of Cancer* (4th ed). Chicago: AJCC, 1992.

concern, conservative surgical treatment may be acceptable in this select population.[3] There is no standard adjuvant therapy for other stage I ovarian cancers; therapies vary and are still under investigation. The therapies used include: no therapy, chemotherapy, intraperitoneal radioisotopes, and external radiotherapy. A platinum-based chemotherapy regimen is considered beneficial for patients with stage IC, grade 3 tumors who are at high risk for recurrence.[62–64]

Early studies of localized ovarian cancer did not always include careful surgical staging and thus were not conclusive in determining optimum treatment.[45] Generally, after the initial surgery, patients received no additional therapy, although pelvic irradiation or intermittent chemotherapy was occasionally given. Relapse after pelvic irradiation was 30%, while relapse with observation alone was 17%, and with intermittent oral melphalan was 6%.[45] Carefully controlled studies are now being performed to determine the best approach for treating stage I ovarian cancer patients, since

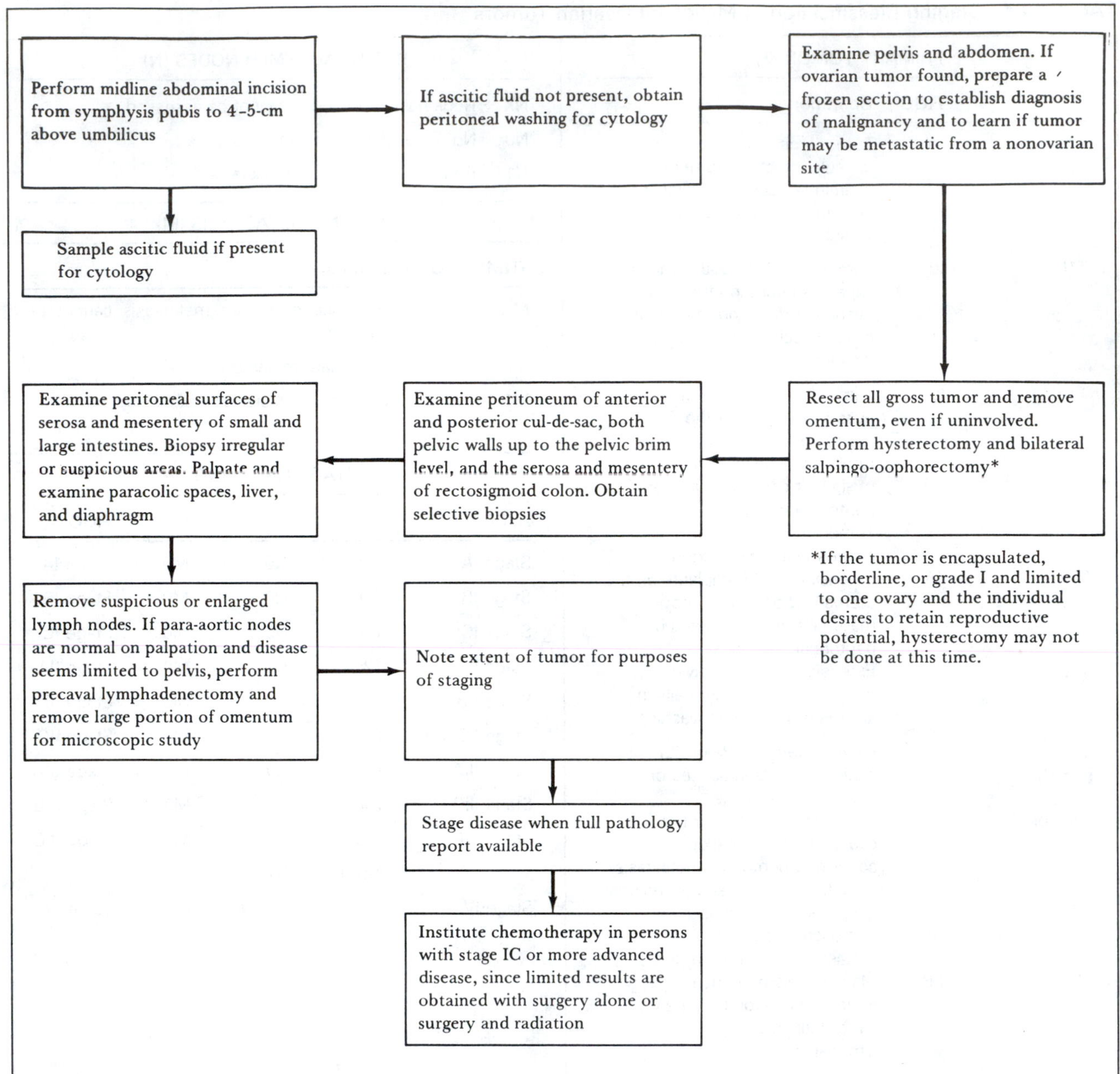

FIGURE 43-2 Surgery for ovarian carcinoma. (Source: Bristol Laboratories, Division of Bristol-Myers Co: Platinol: Effective palliation therapy in metastatic ovarian cancer. Syracuse, NY: Bristol Laboratories, 1982.)

approximately 20% of patients with early-stage disease still relapse and die.[2,65]

Stage II

Following the surgical staging and cytoreduction, intraperitoneal ^{32}P, whole-abdominal radiation, single-agent chemotherapy, or platinum-based combination chemotherapy may be employed.[3,38] Data on the therapy of stage II ovarian cancer are sparse because few women are diagnosed at this stage.

Stage III, IV

When the patient is a surgical candidate, aggressive staging and cytoreductive surgery are advocated to reduce the tumor burden and amount of residual disease. This debulking may involve dissection of multiple masses and the creation of a colostomy to prevent intestinal obstruction. If the tumor is cytoreduced and the patient has no area of residual disease greater than 1 cm in diameter, she may be treated with platinum-based chemotherapy or whole-abdominal and pelvic radiation. While survival rates are comparable for chemotherapy and radiation, morbidity is significantly greater with radiation therapy.[3]

Platinum-based combination chemotherapy is administered for stage III with residual disease greater than 1 cm and for stage IV disease. The use of neoadjuvant chemotherapy and subsequent cytoreductive surgery remains controversial. At the current time, survival is unchanged regardless of the timing of the surgical intervention relative to the institution of chemotherapy.[45,66]

Recurrent or persistent disease

Once a woman has persistent or recurrent disease following initial therapy, the benefits of salvage therapy are limited. Many chemotherapeutic agents have been used, with varying responses and limited duration of response. High-dose chemotherapy with autologous bone marrow rescue has been used in this population but remains investigational.[67–69] Other treatment modalities employed include immunotherapy, intraperitoneal chemotherapy, and biologic therapy.

Second-look surgery A second-look operation is performed on patients who have a complete clinical response following the full course of chemotherapy (usually 6 to 12 cycles) as evidenced by a negative tumor marker (CA-125) and negative CT scan or US. This surgery is advocated for the following reasons: (1) to determine if the patient had a complete remission and therapy can be stopped, (2) to assess the response and determine whether a change in the therapy is indicated, and (3) to perform secondary cytoreductive surgery to attempt to prolong survival. Controversy exists over the actual therapeutic value in doing a second-look laparotomy and when it should be done.[37,45,70,71] Sonnendecker[72] challenged whether second-look laparotomy was justified, especially in patients with initial stage I disease, since he found that 71.8% of patients had no gross or microscopic evidence of disease at the time of second-look surgery. He proposed that second-look surgery should be limited to clinical trials to define either optimum or minimum doses of chemotherapy or to assess new single or combination chemotherapeutic agents.[72] Barber[38] suggests that patients live longer and more comfortably, even though there are no prospective randomized clinical studies demonstrating that second-look surgery adds to long-term survival.

A second-look operation is performed through a vertical abdominal incision. The surgeon evaluates whether there is more or less tumor than was present at the initial laparotomy. If gross tumor is found, it is resected. If no gross disease is present, a thorough staging evaluation is performed, including peritoneal washings, biopsies of any irregularities or adhesions, multiple biopsies of areas where residual tumor was located at the initial operation, precaval lymphadenectomy, and thorough evaluation of the intestine. TAH-BSO and omentectomy should be performed if not done previously. Usually, 26 to 30 biopsy specimens are obtained.[63] Use of the Nd:YAG laser or the ultrasonic surgical aspirator is helpful for resecting tumors that are retroperitoneal, or fixed to the diaphragm, sacrum, pelvic side wall, or pubic symphysis.[73–75] If the second-look operation yields negative results, the woman is followed regularly for signs of recurrence. Further therapy is indicated if the second-look operation is positive for tumor. If the disease is microscopic, whole-abdominal and pelvic irradiation may be considered. If gross disease remains, second-line chemotherapy or investigational treatment is initiated. Additional controlled clinical trials will further delineate the role of second-look surgery. Peritoneoscopy may also be used in certain situations rather than laparotomy.[49]

Tumor-associated antigens If tumor-associated antigens specific for epithelial ovarian cancer could be detected in the bloodstream, they would provide a means for diagnosis at an early stage when patients could be cured. Tumor-associated antigens would also provide a means of monitoring tumor response during therapy and potentially allow discrimination between benign and malignant pelvic masses.[76] One monoclonal antibody that reacts with epithelial ovarian cancer cells has been developed and studied extensively.[77] It can detect an antigen (CA-125) in the blood of women with ovarian cancer. However, CA-125 is not specific for ovarian cancer alone and can be elevated from other conditions that produce inflammatory responses, such as endometriosis. Approximately 83%–96% of ovarian cancer patients have elevated serum CA-125 levels.[78]

Elevations of CA-125 have preceded clinical disease recurrence by 1–11 months.[76,79,80] A negative CA-125 value does not indicate that the patient is disease-free, since almost half will have persistent disease.[45] CA-125 is being used to supplement standard methods of disease monitoring. Jager et al.[81] propose that second-look surgery be done when serum CA-125 levels have fallen or returned to normal and also that patients with rising serum CA-125 levels should not undergo second-look surgery. However, Potter et al.[82] studied 45 women and found that CA-125 levels were not predictive of the potential for resection of disease at second-look.

CA-19-9 is another tumor marker used in combination with CA-125. It is a monosialoganglioside originally isolated from a colonic tumor cell.[83] Fioretti et al.[84] studied CA-125 and CA-19-9 levels in 21 patients receiving both surgical and chemotherapeutic treatment of ovarian carcinoma. They found an 89.7% correlation of CA-125 levels with disease status and a 72.2% correlation with CA-19-9. Rising values may precede the clinical and ultrasonographic detection of recurrence by several months. They think that measuring CA-19-9 in addition to CA-125 could offer some benefit in monitoring patients. Neunteufel and Breitenbecher[78] also advocated using more than one tumor marker, but this remains controversial and requires further study.

Chemotherapy

Single-agent therapy The mainstay of adjuvant therapy for stage III and IV epithelial ovarian cancer is chemotherapy. Historically, standard therapy consisted of single-alkylating agents: melphalan, chlorambucil, thiotepa, cyclophosphamide, and the nitrosoureas. In the United States the agent of choice was usually melphalan because it could be given orally and rarely caused alopecia or nausea.[85] Response rates seen with alkylating agents varied from 33%–65%.[49] A small number of women (5%–10%) were cured with single-alkylating agent therapy.[49] Because of the risk of leukemia from alkylating agents, other drugs were evaluated. No improvement in response was realized with other single agents such as hexamethylmelamine and doxorubicin, with response rates of 20%–35%. Cisplatin is now considered the single most active agent for treatment of ovarian cancer, with response rates reported as high as 55% depending on dose.[40,49] Other single agents that may have some activity in advanced ovarian cancer include ifosfamide, AZQ, VP-16 (etoposide), Peptichemio, and low-dose mitomycin C (Table 43-5).

TABLE 43-5 Single Agents Active in Advanced Ovarian Adenocarcinoma

Alkylating agents	Plant alkaloids
Melphalan	Vinblastine
Chlorambucil	VP-16
Thiotepa	Taxol
Cyclophosphamide	Miscellaneous
Mechlorethamine	Hexamethylmelamine
Ifosfamide	Cisplatin
AZQ	Carboplatin
Antimetabolites	Dianhydrogalacticol
5-fluorouracil	Peptichemio
Methotrexate	
Antitumor antibiotics	
Doxorubicin (adriamycin)	
Mitomycin C	

AZQ, Aziridinyl benzoquinone; *VP-16,* etoposide.

Source: Adapted from Young R, Fuks Z, Hoskins WJ: Cancer of the ovary, in DeVita VT, Hellman S, Rosenberg SA (eds): *Cancer: Principles and Practice of Oncology* (3d ed). Philadelphia: Lippincott, 1989, p. 1179.

Combination chemotherapy Combination chemotherapy for advanced ovarian cancer has been studied extensively. It is difficult to compare the studies because of great variation in patient selection, prognostic factors, and response criteria. However, the studies generally compared single agents to combination chemotherapy and to salvage chemotherapy regimens for those women who did not respond to previous therapy.[49]

The overall response rates for combination chemotherapy vary, with clinical complete remission seen in up to 40%–50% of women. Selected regimens for combination chemotherapy are summarized in Table 43-6. Half of the women who have a complete clinical remission demonstrate residual disease at second-look laparotomy.[29] The optimal combination regimen and duration of therapy remains elusive.[86]

The first study that demonstrated significantly improved survival using combination chemotherapy compared HexaCAF (hexamethylmelamine, cyclophosphamide, methotrexate, and 5-fluorouracil [5-FU]) with melphalan alone. The four-drug combination yielded better results, with an overall response rate of 75% versus 54%, a complete response rate of 33% versus 16%, and median survival of 29 months versus 17 months.[49,87] Several studies followed, showing that combination therapy is more beneficial than single-agent therapy in advanced ovarian cancer. The addition of cisplatin into combination chemotherapy regimens markedly improved response rates.[88,89] It appears that the platinum-based combination regimen given without dose modification offers the best chance for response (up to 80%) and for achieving a complete remission (20%–50%) in women with advanced ovarian carcinoma.[49,90]

In a recent meta-analysis of data from 1194 patients in four clinical trials comparing cisplatin-doxorubicin-cyclophosphamide (CAP) with cisplatin-cyclophosphamide (CP), a survival advantage was demonstrated with the CAP regimen ($P = 0.02$), as well as significant improvement in the number of negative second-look laparotomies with the CAP (CAP = 30%, CP = 23%; $P = 0.01$). It was unclear whether the improvement in survival and response at second-look was due to the addition of doxorubicin or to the dose intensity in three of the four trials.[91]

A number of studies with cisplatin have demonstrated the important relationship of response rate being proportional to the dose administered. Patients who were refractory to initial therapy or had recurrent disease, and those patients not previously treated, have received various schedules and ranges of high-dose cisplatin. The major dose-limiting toxicity of high-dose cisplatin is neurotoxicity. Results of these studies are not clear in terms of survival, but it does appear that the high-dose chemotherapy regimen is markedly effective in rapidly debulking tumors in patients who present with advanced-stage disease and large abdominal tumors.[45]

Carboplatin, a platinum analog, is an alternative to cisplatin. Pharmacologic techniques to decrease some of the toxicities associated with the platinum compounds are being investigated. A randomized trial comparing a CHAP-5 regimen (cisplatin 20 mg/m^2 daily × 5; doxorubicin 35 mg/m^2 on day 1, hexamethylmelamine 150 mg/m^2; cyclophosphamide 100 mg/m^2 orally on days 14 to 28) with CHAC-1 (carboplatin 350 mg/m^2 on day 1; all other drugs the same as CHAP-5) showed that antitumor activity did not appear to have any statistical differences between the two regimens but that the toxicity pattern observed in patients treated with CHAC-1 was much milder and more tolerable.[92] Like

TABLE 43-6 Selected Regimens for Combination Chemotherapy in Advanced Ovarian Cancer

Regimen	Schedule	Response	Reference
HexaCAF		CR and PR = 75%	49, 87
Hexamethylmelamine	150 mg/m² orally days 1–14		
Cyclophosphamide	150 mg/m² orally days 1–14		
Methotrexate	40 mg/m² IV day 1, 8		
5-fluourouracil	600 mg/m² IV day 1, 8		
CAP		pCR = 33%	91
Cisplatin	50–70 mg/m² IV		
Doxorubicin	30–60 mg/m² IV		
Cyclophosphamide	500–600 mg/m² IV		
CP		pCR = 23%	91
Cyclophosphamide	500–1000 mg/m² IV		
Cisplatin	50–70 mg/m² IV		
CHAP-5		pCR = 30% cCR = 23.5%	49, 92, 99
Cyclophosphamide	100 mg/m² orally days 15–28		
Hexamethylmelamine	150 mg/m² orally days 15–28		
Doxorubicin	35 mg/m² IV day 1		
Cisplatin	20 mg/m² IV days 1–5		
CHAC-1		CR = 24.4%	92, 99
Cyclophosphamide	100 mg/m² orally days 15–28		
Hexamethylmelamine	150 mg/m² orally days 15–28		
Doxorubicin	35 mg/m² IV day 1		
Carboplatin	350 mg/m² IV day 1		
TC		Results pending	100
Taxol	135 mg/m² IV over 24 hours day 1		
Cisplatin	75 mg/m² IV day 2		

CR = complete response; PR = partial response; pCR = pathologic complete response; cCR = clinical complete response.
Source: Adapted from Young R, Fuks Z, Hoskins HJ: Cancer of the ovary, in DeVita VT, Hellman S, Rosenberg SA (eds): *Cancer: Principles and Practice of Oncology* (3d ed). Philadelphia: Lippincott, 1989, p. 1181.

cisplatin, carboplatin has a significant dose-response relationship and can be given to patients who are not platinum refractory yet can no longer tolerate the neurotoxicity or nephrotoxicity associated with cisplatin. As a result, carboplatin has become an important drug in the treatment of ovarian cancer.[93] Diethyldithiocarbamate (DDTC) may protect against the myelosuppression of carboplatin and the dose-limiting neurotoxicity of cisplatin without changing the antitumor effect. If this is so, dose escalation could be achieved without increased toxicity.[45] Rothenberg et al.[94] studied 21 patients with relapsed or refractory ovarian cancer who were treated with high-dose carboplatin followed 3 hours later with DDTC (4g/m²). The overall response rate was 19%; however, the regimen was associated with clinically significant hematologic and autonomic toxic effects.

Colony stimulating factors (CSF) may allow higher doses of myelosuppressive drugs and are currently being incorporated into treatment regimens.[95] Another approach to enable the administration of high doses of myelosuppressive drugs is the use of autologous bone marrow rescue. Drugs used with the bone marrow rescue include cyclophosphamide, melphalan, and carboplatin. This approach remains investigational but has been used in patients with persistent disease.[69,96]

Since the majority of patients suffer disease recurrence despite response to initial chemotherapy, efforts continue to identify active new second-line agents. Current single-agent response rates range from 0%–6% in women who have received prior cisplatin therapy. Generally the responses are partial and of short duration.[97]

Alberts et al.[97] treated 25 relapsed ovarian cancer patients with mitomycin C 10 mg/m² intravenously on day 1 every 6 weeks and 5-FU 500 mg/m² intravenously daily on days 1–3 every 3 weeks. The overall objective response rate was 40%, and the most prevalent toxicity was bone marrow suppression. They suggest further trials of this combination. They also recommend the addition of cisplatin for first-line therapy in patients with clinically measurable diseases.[97]

A new drug, taxol, has demonstrated a 30% response in previously treated patients. Taxol, a diterpene plant product, is a unique antimicrotubule agent that acts by shifting the equilibrium between tubulin dimers and microtubules toward polymerization, which has the effect of creating overly stable and nonfunctional microtubules. Taxol has quickly gained popularity and is under investigation in phase III trials to define its role in the treatment of ovarian cancer.[98–101]

Drug resistance The development of multidrug resistance severely limits the effectiveness of chemotherapy. Patients with ovarian cancer die from chemotherapy-refractory disease. Drug resistance is likely due to multiple factors, including: (1) alterations in drug transport across cell membranes, (2) presence of the MDR-1 gene with its protein product, (3) the P-170 glycoprotein, (4) the elevation of sulfhydryl molecules such as intracellular glutathione (GSH), and (5) increased DNA repair.[49] It may be possible to pharmacologically reverse drug resistance,[49,102] and clinical trials using verapamil and buthionine sulfoximine (BSO) are underway to determine this.[49]

Debulking surgery to reduce tumor burden to aggregates of 1 cm or less improves the response to postoperative chemotherapy by reducing the potentially refractory disease. Moreover, complete responses are associated with significant increases in survival. Combination chemotherapy is associated with higher overall response rates and, more importantly, with an increase in complete responses. New combinations, alternate dosing schedules, and sequential and continuous infusion administration techniques to reduce drug resistance continue to be investigated.[103,104]

Intraperitoneal chemotherapy Because ovarian cancer usually remains confined to the abdominal cavity, one approach to chemotherapy administration is the intraperitoneal (IP) method. Intraperitoneal chemotherapy has been used for many years to control malignant ascites;[49] however, the aim of the IP approach currently is to increase cytotoxic drug levels to the tumor sites. Patients who will benefit most from IP therapy are those with: (1) minimal residual disease (microscopic or $\leq$0.5 cm in diameter) following systemic therapy with or without secondary surgical cytoreduction, (2) high-grade tumors with a surgically defined complete response, (3) high-grade stage I/II with the risk of covert disease in the upper abdomen, (4) advanced disease with all or some drugs administered IP, and (5) advanced disease with IP therapy following a limited course of intravenous therapy with or without secondary surgical debulking.[105–107]

Researchers have used methotrexate,[108] doxorubicin,[109] 5-FU,[110] cisplatin with systemic thiosulfate protection,[111] mitomycin-c,[112] mitoxantrone,[113] cytarabine,[114] and recombinant alpha-interferon.[115] Aclacinomycin (an analog of adriamycin) and carboplatin are also being evaluated to determine their efficacy as IP drugs.[106] Intraperitoneal combination chemotherapy approaches are also being studied in clinical trials.[45,116] Investigations of IP use of biologic agents including gamma-interferon, tumor necrosis factor, interleukin-2, and monoclonal antibodies have been conducted.[117–119] Intraperitoneal delivery of antineoplastic agents in 10% dimethyl sulfaoxide (DMSO) may also be useful with certain ovarian cancers.[120]

The technique for IP administration includes placement of a semipermanent Tenckhoff dialysis catheter or implanted port system into the abdominal cavity so that a large volume of fluid can be instilled. A volume of up to 2 liters of fluid is instilled intraperitoneally to ensure optimal distribution throughout the abdomen. The chemotherapeutic agent and fluids in the abdominal cavity are slowly absorbed into the general circulation. When daily treatments are required, alteration in the volume of fluid infused may be necessary in order to minimize the discomfort experienced by the patient from the volume of residual fluid left from the previous treatment.[107]

The Tenckhoff dialysis catheter and the infusion port both have problems associated with their use. In approximately 20% of cases a fibrin sheath forms that will not allow outflow and occasionally inhibits delivery of the drug.[45,105,106,116] A new catheter, designed specifically for IP chemotherapy, would allow improvement in drug administration and distribution and removal of any ascites prior to the IP chemotherapy infusion.[119,121]

Concerns persist about IP therapy related to the delivery of the drug to the tumor sites, toxicities specific to the IP route (such as infection secondary to bowel perforation), and the risk of chronic and long-term consequences (such as adhesions and bowel obstruction).[105] Ozols and Young[45] point out some unresolved clinical issues related to IP chemotherapy: (1) Can IP chemotherapy produce a significant objective response rate? (2) In what clinical situations should it be used? (3) What is the optimum drug to use? (4) What role do drug combinations have? and (5) What is the optimum technique to deliver IP drugs? While the use of IP cisplatin or carboplatin in selected patients who responded to an initial intravenous platinum-based regimen is appropriate, other applications of this method of administration do not have adequate data to support its use. Randomized trials are needed to demonstrate that the theoretical and pharmacologic advantages also correlate with survival advantages for this patient population.[107]

Hormone therapy

Hormone therapy for ovarian cancer has resulted in uneven responses.[122] Tamoxifen has been investigated as a second-line drug in individuals who have failed combination chemotherapy.[18,123] Belinson et al.[124] randomly treated 33 patients with either megestrol acetate alone or megestrol acetate and tamoxifen. Doses were 160 mg/day of megestrol and 20 mg/day of tamoxifen. There was no demonstrated tumor regression, but 39% of patients showed stabilization of disease from 4 to more than 16 months. Kavanagh et al.[122] used leuprolide acetate (1 mg subcutaneously daily for a minimum of 8 weeks) for patients with refractory epithelial ovarian cancer and found better responses in patients with grade 1 disease. Further clinical trials are needed to define the role of hormonal therapy in ovarian cancer.

Radiotherapy

Radioactive chromic phosphate (^{32}P) and radioactive gold (^{198}Au) have been used as adjuvant therapy in women with stage I ovarian cancer (Figure 43-3).[3] Colloidal gold is not presently available for therapy. Complications of ^{32}P can include small bowel obstruction and stenosis[49] and are higher in women who have uneven distribution of the radioactive material in the peritoneal cavity.[42,49,125] Prior to instilling ^{32}P, even distribution is verified by infusing radiopaque technitium sulfur colloid.[3]

Potter et al.[126] treated 59 patients with intraperitoneal chromic phosphate and concluded that it is an alternative to chemotherapy or external radiation in the primary treatment of early-stage ovarian lesions. It may also be useful for second-line therapy of early-stage or low-grade ovarian lesions after a positive second-look surgery, but only if microscopic disease remains. In general, reported cure rates with chromic phosphate in stage I tumors have been in the range of 90%, but there is no evidence that these results are better than those that might be achieved in the same patients without radiotherapy.[42]

The role of external beam radiotherapy in advanced disease has also been explored, and its effectiveness is directly related to the volume of disease at the time radiation is administered.[2,45] Patients who have less than 2 cm of disease have an approximately equivalent result with either combination chemotherapy or total abdominal radiation. Whole-abdominal radiation (WAR) appears to be most effective in those selected individuals with little or no gross residual disease.[70,127]

The use of WAR as salvage therapy for patients with persistent or progressive disease after combination chemotherapy who have been explored and have residual cancer (<2 cm) has also been studied.[70,127–130] Associated morbidity has been significant.[129] Schray et al.[128] found that patients with well- to moderately differentiated tumors or those with small-volume residual disease after the initial operation had a significantly better outcome from salvage radiation therapy. They suggest further randomized study to determine the best option for patients with poor prognostic factors.

Biologic therapy

The role of chemoimmunotherapy has been investigated by two cooperative groups. The Gynecologic Oncology Group[131] compared melphalan with melphalan plus *Corynebacterium parvum*. The response rate with melphalan alone was 55%, whereas the response rate with melphalan plus *C. parvum* was 65%. The Southwest Oncology Group[132] compared doxorubicin-cyclophosphamide alone and in combination with bacillus Calmette-Guerin (BCG). The response rates were 43% and 51%, respectively. In contrast, Alberts et al.[133] reported that the use of BCG did not add to the efficacy of a doxorubicin, cyclophosphamide, and cisplatin (DCP) regimen in patients with measurable stage III or IV disease.

Immunotherapy, including monoclonal antibodies, adoptive cellular immunotherapy, and interferon, may soon become the fourth modality of therapy for ovarian cancer (in addition to surgery, radiation, and chemotherapy).[117] These promising agents have cytotoxic mechanisms that are probably unrelated to the other treatment modalities and are most likely different enough from each other to enable sequential use. They can remain in the peritoneal cavity for prolonged periods when administered intraperitoneally, are most likely not mutagenic, and have manageable toxicities.[117] Immunotherapy using IP lymphokine-activated killer cells (LAK), interferons, and interleukin-2 (IL-2) is being examined in the treatment of women with minimal residual disease ovarian cancer.[2,45,117] Since immunother-

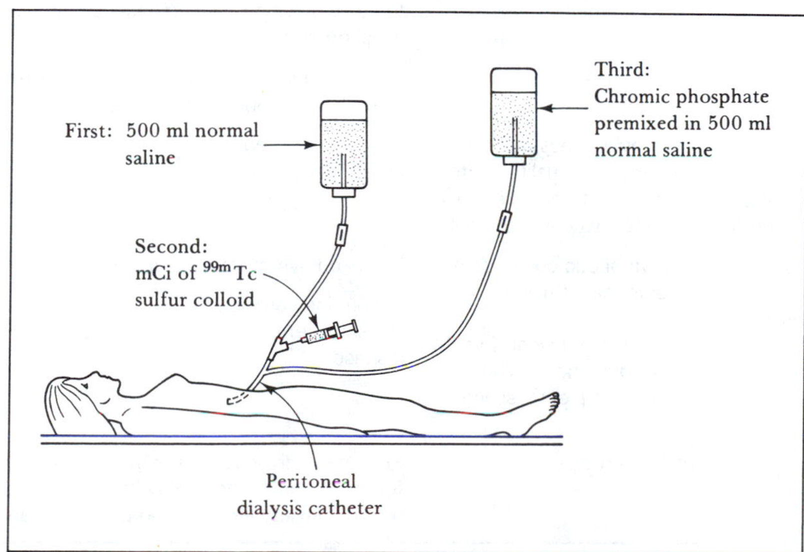

FIGURE 43-3 Method of administration of radioactive colloidal chromic phosphate into the peritoneal cavity. (Source: DiSaia PJ, Creasman WT: *Clinical Gynecologic Oncology*. St Louis, MO: Mosby, 1989.)

TABLE 43-7 Nursing Issues in the Care of the Woman with Ovarian Cancer

Treatment/Disease	Physical, Psychosocial Issues	Interventions
Diagnosis/staging laparotomy	Preoperative testing	Give information regarding preoperative testing
	Operative procedure planned	Reinforce information regarding operative procedure
	Facing extensive exploratory and cytoreductive surgery	Role in postoperative care, including promoting respiratory function, progressive ambulation, careful monitoring of vital signs, intake and output, electrolytes, GI function, renal function
	Facing potentially terminal disease	Encourage verbalization of fears, concerns from patient, family; clarify misconceptions; discuss additional therapy planned
Chemotherapy	Combination platinum-based regimen is therapy most ovarian cancer patients receive. Side effects include nausea, vomiting, diarrhea, bone marrow depression, alopecia, neurotoxicity, liver/renal toxicity	Instruct patient about types of therapy (standard or investigational), method of administration, drugs, side effects, frequency, and duration
	Most side effects can be managed	Monitor side effects and develop plan to minimize effects, including antiemetic regimen, colony stimulationg factors, hematologic monitoring
		Nutritional needs may require small frequent meals, dietary supplements, and continued antiemetics to overcome nausea, vomiting, anorexia
	Routine for blood testing, scans, and physical examinations	Develop schedule for appointments and follow-up
	Roles and relationships within the family may change due to therapy	Assist in coping with disease and treatment; assess need for referrals for additional support, eg, to other cancer patients, support groups, psychotherapy
Radiation therapy	^{32}P: acute side effects, IP route of administration, follow-up	Instruct patient about planned regimen, method of administration, side effects, duration of therapy, follow-up
	Whole-abdominal radiation: schedule, treatment ports, side effects (acute and chronic), and follow-up	Monitor side effects and develop plan to minimize effects; medication can help reduce side effects; nutritional support with antiemetics, antidiarrheals, antispasmodics, small frequent low-fiber meals, dietary supplements
	Roles and relationships within the family may change due to therapy	Assist in coping with disease and treatment Assess need for referrals for additional support, eg, to other radiation patients, support groups, psychotherapy
Progressive disease	Salvage therapy offers little response in chemotherapy-refractory disease	Instruct patient about salvage therapy: regimen, side effects, hope for response
	Parenteral hyperalimentation may address nutritional needs of patient but may not improve quality of life due to progressive disease; inability to eat is a great source of fright and frustration for patient and family	Nutritional support with dietary supplements or enteral feedings
	Disease progression leads to lymphatic obstruction, edema, anasarca, massive peritoneal effusions, and pleural effusions Ascites/pleural effusions are source of discomfort, respiratory compromise, and GI dysfunction (Table 43-8); effusions may be drained and pleural space sclerosed	Focus on symptom control, comfort measures Encourage verbalization by patient and family of fears/concerns regarding progressive/terminal disease
	Women often remain mentally alert despite deteriorating physical status	Encourage diversional therapy to enable patient to focus on other means of comfort that may reduce tension/anxiety experienced by patient and family

apy is nonspecific, results have been unpredictable. It is hoped that nonspecific immunotherapy will soon be replaced by specific vaccines.[38]

A phase II study with human leukocyte interferon suggested possible antitumor activity in epithelial ovarian cancer.[134] Recombinant alpha-interferon has shown some promise in patients with small-volume residual disease who were given the drug intraperitoneally.[117] Combination therapy of alpha-interferon and doxorubicin produced complete and partial responses with acceptable toxicity in 7 of 24 ovarian cancer patients with recurrent disease.[135] Lichtenstein et al.[136] conducted a phase I study using IP recombinant alpha-interferon for 11 patients with persistent epithelial ovarian cancer at second-look surgery and found that 45% experienced a surgically documented antitumor response. Further study is needed to more clearly define the role of biologics in the treatment of ovarian cancer.

Nursing Management

The patient with ovarian cancer has many diverse needs. Some are no different than what other cancer patients experience while undergoing extensive surgery and toxic chemotherapy or radiation therapy. The nursing management of patients receiving surgery, radiation, or chemotherapy for cancer is reviewed in previous chapters. Table 43-7 and Table 43-8 summarize some common nursing management issues as well as those specific to the woman with ovarian cancer. The overwhelming issue in caring for these women is that the majority are diagnosed in late stages when the hope for cure is grim. Although some women will have long-term responses to their initial therapy, most will not. Because of the generally poor survival rates and the ongoing need for treatment and support, the patient and her family will become well known to the health care team. Their emotional needs as well as the woman's physical problems will need to be addressed. A caring, comprehensive approach that focuses on continuity of care will enable the patient and her family to achieve optimal quality of life.

Future Trends

Despite aggressive multimodality therapy, the overall survival rate of ovarian cancer remains poor. Efforts to define new and more effective means of treating this disease continue. One area of ongoing research is new drug development and testing.

In addition to taxol, which was discussed previously, two other agents, topotecan and tetraplatin, are being tested to determine their activity in ovarian cancer. Topotecan, or hycamptamine, inhibits the enzyme topoisomerase I and leads to DNA cleavage. Drugs that are active with topoisomerase seem to be so in levels proportional to the target enzyme available. This is the opposite effect of other drugs, such as the antimetabolites, that effect target enzyme systems. Activity of topotecan in a phase I trial has led to the initiation of a phase II trial in ovarian cancer.[137]

Tetraplatin is an organoplatinum (IV) compound that is not cross-resistant with cisplatin. Preclinical results suggest that tetraplatin has greater antitumor activity than either cisplatin or carboplatin. A phase II study is anticipated.[138]

Biologic therapies are also being pursued. Mullerian

TABLE 43-8 Nursing Care of the Patient with Malignant Ascites

Symptom/Distress	Assessment	Intervention
Abdominal distension	Bulging abdomen and flanks; everted umbilicus; shiny skin	Daily abdominal girths, weights; palpate for fluid wave; percuss for sounds of shifting dullness.
Respiratory compromise	Dyspnea; shortness of breath; tachypnea; use of accessory muscles	Elevate head of bed; provide rest periods; restrict activities as tolerated; oxygen as needed; analgesics as ordered.
Fluid and electrolyte imbalance	Signs and symptoms of dehydration; lymphedema of lower extremities; signs of hypokalemia, hyponatremia, hypomagnesia	Monitor serum protein, albumin, electrolytes, fluid replacements as ordered; daily weight, abdominal girth; monitor intake and output, vital signs; high-protein diet; minimize sodium and fluid intake; diuretics as ordered; compression stockings, boots; assist patient in maintaining mobility.
Peritoneovenous shunting	Pain; infection; bleeding; skin integrity at operative site; DIC, tumor embolus	Teach patient and family about surgical procedure, operating room routine, methods of maintaining patency of shunt; provide shunt care; monitor fluid, electrolytes, and coagulation profile.

Source: Reprinted with permission from Eriksson, JH, Walczak, JR: Ovarian cancer, *Semin Oncol Nurs* 6(3):225, 1990.

inhibitory substance (MIS) is a growth factor that has inhibited in vitro clonogenic growth of some ovarian cancer cells. Further study is needed to determine if MIS has potential as an anticancer agent.[48] Radiolabeled antibodies may be able to demonstrate the presence of tumor, thus avoiding second-look laparotomy. Immunotoxins, antitumor antibodies conjugated to potent plant or bacterial toxins, are also under clinical trial. Antibodies conjugated to cytotoxic chemotherapeutic agents may improve the therapeutic index.[117,139]

Another investigational approach is to define methods of overcoming intrinsic or acquired drug resistance. Buthionine sulfoximine and ethacrynic acid are currently being studied.[140,141] However, other means of overcoming drug resistance, such as gene therapy, must be pursued. Biologics and gene therapy are exciting treatment modalities that are developing and will be further investigated in ovarian cancer.[139]

The areas of prevention and early detection cannot be ignored. Efforts need to continue to define sensitive and specific screening methods that can be widely applied. Research to further define risk factors, etiology, and carcinogenesis will be the only comprehensive means of reducing the morbidity and mortality from ovarian cancer.

There are also nursing management issues to be investigated. Certainly the issue of defining toxicities for new treatments and interventions to reduce morbidity will be addressed. Quality-of-life issues related to the aggressive nature of the disease and physically and emotionally demanding therapies also need to be pursued.

CERVICAL CANCER

Epidemiology

According to the American Cancer Society, 13,500 new cases of invasive cervical cancer will be diagnosed in 1993, and approximately 4400 women will die of the disease.[1] The incidence of invasive cervical cancer has steadily decreased as a result of the Pap smear, which can diagnose the disease in a preinvasive state. However, cervical cancer is a significant health problem for elderly women, since 24% of new cases and 40% of deaths from cervical cancer occur in women age 65 years and older.[142] Even so, the number of deaths from cervical cancer has decreased in women over age 45, while mortality in women under 35 years has increased.[3,143]

While the incidence of invasive cancer has decreased by nearly 50%, the incidence of carcinoma in situ (CIS) has climbed dramatically since 1945. More than 55,000 new cases of CIS will be diagnosed in 1993.[1] Women in their 20s are most often diagnosed with cervical dysplasia; those 30 to 39, with in situ cancer; and those over age 40, with invasive cancer.[1,144]

Etiology

Many personal risk factors have been associated with precancerous lesions of the cervix (Table 43-9).[145] A higher incidence of the disease occurs in lower socioeconomic groups; smokers; blacks; Hispanics; and women who become sexually active prior to age 17, have many sexual partners, and are multiparous. Conversely, cervical carcinoma is infrequent in women who are nulliparous, and those who are lifetime celibates or lifetime monogamous.[146–148] Females exposed to diethylstilbestrol (DES) in utero have a higher incidence of clear cell adenocarcinoma of the cervix and vagina.[149,150]

Certain sexually transmitted infectious oncogenes have been suggested as possible etiologic agents associated with cervical cancer. Herpes simplex virus type 2 (HSV2) has been shown to be carcinogenic in animals. Women with cervical cancer usually have higher HSV2 specific antibody titers than controls, but several prospective studies have failed to show an association between development of HSV2 antibodies and development of cervical cancer.[151,152]

Human papillomavirus (HPV) can cause a variety of warty infections. In women, the genital variety is called *papilloma acuminata* and is sexually transmitted. More than 46 distinct subtypes of the virus have been identified, but only some types of HPV are associated with genital warts, precancerous lesions, or invasive cervical carcinoma.[153–158]

Both HPV 16 and 18 are associated with high-grade cervical intraepithelial lesions or invasive cancer.[158,159] There is evidence linking HPV 6 and 11 to intraepithelial neoplasia of the cervix.[151,160] HPV 18 is associated with 15%–50% of invasive cervical cancer lesions.[160–163] The prevalence of HPV 16 appears to increase with the severity of the lesion.[162] One group of researchers, utilizing a DNA hybridization technique, indicated that HPV 18 is the most common papillomavirus found in women with adenocarcinoma of the cervix, while HPV 16 was more commonly associated with squamous carcinomas.[164,165]

The male plays a role in the etiology of cervical cancer. Women married to men whose previous spouses had cervical cancer seem to be at a higher risk of developing cervical cancer, but the cause for this apparent relationship has not yet been determined.[166] The male partner's age at first coitus, smoking habits, visitation of prostitutes, and number of sexual partners also may affect relative risk.[145,160,166] In addition, wives of men with cancer of the penis are at increased risk in the development of cervical cancer.[151] Several factors may lower a woman's risk. These include barrier-type contraception, vasectomy, recommended daily allowances of vitamin A, beta carotene, and vitamin C,[145] limiting the number of sexual partners, and initiating sexual activity at a later age.[151]

TABLE 43-9 Malignancies of the Lower Genital Tract: Risk Factors and Preventive Measures

Risk Factors	Preventive Measures
CERVICAL CANCER	
HSV2	Pap smears per ACS guidelines
HPV	Pelvic examinations
Abnormal transformation zone	Barrier contraception
Sex prior to age 17	Limit number of sexual partners
Multiple sexual partners	Sex after age 17
History of smoking	Stop smoking
Spouse whose previous wife had cervical cancer	
Maternal use of DES	
Immunosuppression	
Multiparous	
Lower socioeconomic status	
African American/Hispanic	
Spouse with cancer of the penis	
VULVAR CANCER	
HSV2	Routine vulvar examination
HPV	Pap smear
Condyloma	Barrier contraception
Immunosuppression	
Chronic vulvar disease	
Exposure to coal tar derivatives	
History of breast, cervical, endometrial malignancies	
VAGINAL CANCER	
Cervical CIN	Pap smear
HPV	Barrier contraceptives
Vaginal trauma	Limit number of sexual partners
Previous abdominal hysterectomy for benign disease	
Radiotherapy for cervical cancer	
Increased age	
African American	
Lower socioeconomic status	
Education	

HSV2, herpes simplex virus type 2; HPV, humanpapilloma virus.

Pathophysiology

The cervix, the lower part of the uterus, extends from the isthmus into the vagina and is divided into two major parts: the endocervix and the exocervix. The endocervix is contiguous to the exocervix, which includes the external os and extends to the vaginal fornix. The *squamocolumnar junction* refers to the area where the columnar epithelium of the endocervix joins the squamous epithelium of the exocervix at the os.[167]

Cancer of the cervix is the culmination of a progressive disease that begins as a neoplastic alteration of the squamocolumnar junction. Over time, these abnormal cells can progress to involve the full thickness of epithelium and invade into the stromal tissue of the cervix. The initial preinvasive or premalignant changes are called cervical intraepithelial neoplasia.

The term *cervical intraepithelial neoplasia (CIN)* was introduced in the mid-1960s to better define epithelial cervical abnormalities. CIN classification demonstrates the progression of the disease process rather than delineating distinctly different abnormalities. As such, each step in the cervical disease spectrum merges imperceptibly into the next.[143,150] CIN is divided into three categories: CIN I, CIN II, and CIN III (Figure 43-4).

The term *CIN I* is used to describe dysplasia or atypical changes in the cervical epithelium involving less than one-third the thickness of the epithelium. *CIN II* describes neoplastic changes involving up to two-thirds the thickness, and *CIN III* or *carcinoma in situ* describes a lesion that has neoplastic changes involving up to full thickness of the epithelium with no areas of stromal invasion or metastases.[3,168,169] Once the disease progresses beyond the basement membrane and invades the cervical stroma, the disease is considered invasive or malignant.

In 1988 a workshop sponsored by the National Cancer Institute was held to address problems inherent in

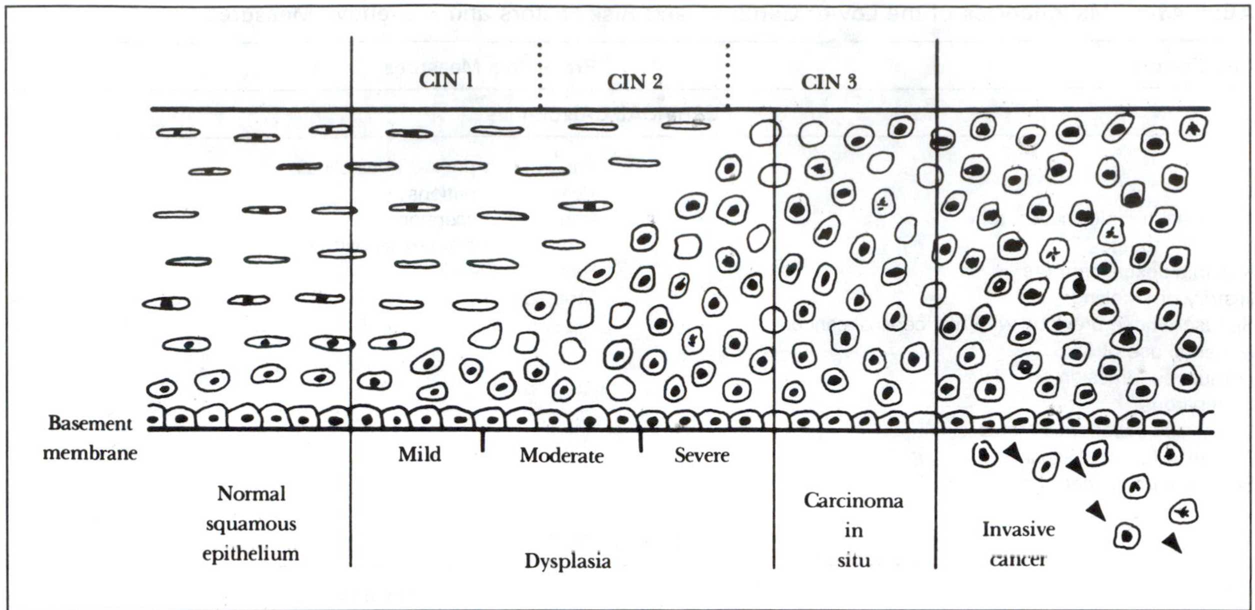

FIGURE 43-4 Schematic representation of precancerous cervical lesions. CIN = cervical epithelial neoplasia. (Source: Jones HW, Jones GS: *Novak's Textbook of Gynecology*. Baltimore, MD: Williams & Wilkins, 1981. © 1981, The Williams & Wilkins Co., Baltimore, MD.)

the Papanicolaou system. Clinical experts felt that the PAP system, introduced in the 1930s, did not: (1) reliably communicate information relevant to the clinician, (2) include diagnostic histopathic terminology, (3) provide diagnoses for noncancerous lesions, or (4) afford uniformity in reporting diagnostic interpretations.[170,171] The goal was to review existing terminology and make recommendations for a more effective method of reporting. The outcome of this conference was the Bethesda System, which is used today to report cervical/vaginal cytological diagnoses.[170–173]

The Bethesda System (Table 43-10) addresses the following elements: (1) a statement of the adequacy of the cytologic specimen (satisfactory, less than optimal, unsatisfactory), (2) a general categorization of the diagnosis (within normal limits, other), and (3) a descriptive diagnosis that includes two new terms: low-grade and high-grade squamous intraepithelial lesions (SIL). The descriptive diagnosis allows cytopathologists to list reactive and reparative changes (e.g., changes secondary to inflammatory processes, treatment [chemotherapy, radiotherapy], or contraceptive devices).

Low-grade SIL includes cellular changes associated with HPV or mild dysplasia (CIN I). High-grade SIL includes lesions formerly designated as moderate dysplasia (CIN II) and severe dysplasia or CIS (CIN III). The use of the word *grade* as it is utilized with the SIL terminology does not imply invasive carcinoma.[170,173]

Although use of the Bethesda System is becoming more widespread, there is still significant opposition to it. Some clinicians argue against using only one diagnostic category (SIL) with two subcategories (low-grade and high-grade SIL) for all intraepithelial lesions, even though qualifying terms may be added to the cytologic reports.[174,175] Bottles et al.[175] questioned the inclusion of CIN II and CIN III in the high-grade SIL category. They felt that lumping CIN II and III together implied similar management, which is not necessarily the case. Others have expressed the fear that women may be overdiagnosed and given unnecessary treatment.[174,176] The editorial board of *Obstetrics and Gynecology* voted unanimously not to accept the new terminology and continue to use the CIN nomenclature instead.

Due to a lack of consensus on a system for reporting cervical/vaginal cytologic diagnoses, the terms *CIN* and *SIL* are both seen in the literature, although the CIN terminology is most prevalent at this time. Therefore, the CIN nomenclature will be utilized to describe cervical abnormalities, although the reader is encouraged to refer to Table 43-10 for the SIL terminology.

Cervical cancer develops in one of three types of lesions: exophytic, excavating (or ulcerative), or endophytic (Figure 43-5). Exophytic lesions[177] are the most common and appear as cauliflowerlike, fungating cancers that are friable and bleed easily. The lesions may involve a small area of the cervix, or be quite extensive, involving the entire cervix and upper vagina.

The excavating or ulcerative lesion[177] is a necrotic lesion that replaces the cervix and upper vagina with an ulcer or crater that bleeds easily. These are often associated with local infection and purulent discharge.

The endophytic lesion[177] is located within the endocervical canal and is without visible tumor or ulceration. The cervix appears normal or enlarged and

TABLE 43-10 The 1988 Bethesda System for Reporting Cervical/Vaginal Cytologic Diagnoses

Statement on Specimen Adequacy

Satisfactory for interpretation
Less than optimal
Unsatisfactory

Explanation for less than optimal/unsatisfactory specimen:

- Scant cellularity
- Poor fixation or preservation
- Presence of foreign material (eg, lubricant)
- Partially or completely obscuring inflammation
- Partially or completely obscuring blood
- Excessive cytolysis or autolysis
- No endocervical component in a premenopausal woman who has a cervix
- Not representative of the anatomic site
- Other

General Categorization

Within normal limits
Other:
See "Descriptive Diagnoses"
Further action recommended

Descriptive Diagnoses

INFECTION

Fungal
- Fungal organisms morphologically consistent with *Candida* species
- Other

Bacterial
- Microorganisms morphologically consistent with *Gardnerella* species
- Microorganisms morphologically consistent with *Actinomyces* species
- Cellular changes suggestive of *Chlamydia* species infection, subject to confirmatory studies
- Other

Protozoan
- *Trichomonas vaginalis*
- Other

Viral
- Cellular changes associated with cytomegalovirus
- Cellular changes associated with herpesvirus simplex
- Other
- (Note: for human papillomavirus (HPV), refer to "Epithelial Cell Abnormalities, Squamous Cell")

Other

REACTIVE AND REPARATIVE CHANGES

Inflammation
- Associated cellular changes
- Follicular cervicitis

Miscellaneous (as related to patient history)
- Effects of therapy
- Ionizing radiation
- Chemothrapy
- Effects of mechanical devices (eg, intrauterine contraceptive device)
- Effects of nonsteroidal estrogen exposure (eg, diethylstilbestrol)
- Other

EPITHELIAL CELL ABNORMALITIES

Squamous Cell
- Atypical squamous cells of undetermined significance (recommended follow-up and/or type of further investigation: specify)
- Squamous intraepithelial lesion (SIL) (comment on presence of cellular changes associated with HPV if applicable)
  - Low-grade squamous intraepithelial lesion, encompassing:
    - Cellular changes associated with HPV
    - Mild (slight) dysplasia/cervical intraepithelial neoplasia grade 1 (CIN I)
  - High-grade squamous intraepithelial lesion, encompassing:
    - Moderate dysplasia/CIN II
    - Severe dysplasia/CIN III
    - Carcinoma in situ/CIN III
- Squamous cell carcinoma

Glandular Cell
- Presence of endometrial cells in one of the following circumstances:
  - Out of phase in a menstruating woman
  - In a postmenopausal woman
  - No menstrual history available
- Atypical glandular cells of undetermined significance (recommended follow-up and/or type of further investigation: specify)
  - Endometrial
  - Endocervical
  - Not otherwise specified
- Adenocarcinoma
  - Specify probable site of origin: endocervical, endometrial, extrauterine
  - Not otherwise specified
- Other epithelial malignant neoplasm: specify

NONEPITHELIAL MALIGNANT NEOPLASM: SPECIFY

HORMONAL EVALUATION (APPLIES TO VAGINAL SMEARS ONLY)

- Hormonal pattern compatible with age and history
- Hormonal pattern incompatible with age and history: specify
- Hormonal evaluation not possible
  - Cervical specimen
  - Inflammation
  - Insufficient patient history

OTHER

Source: Adapted from *JNCI* 82(12):989, 1990.

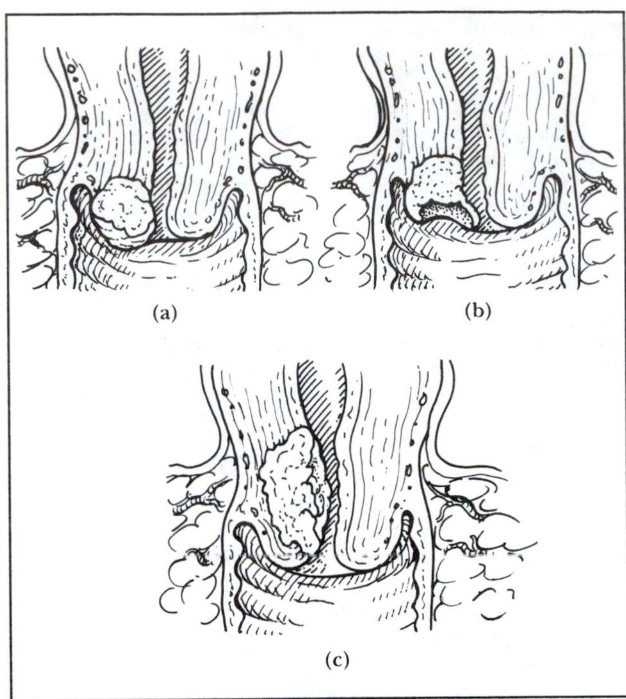

FIGURE 43-5 (a) Exophytic lesion. (b) Excavating or ulcerative lesion. (c) Endophytic lesion. (Source: Adapted from Caputo TA: *Uterine Cervical Cancer: The Current Approach to Diagnosis and Treatment.* Syracuse, NY: Bristol Laboratories, 1979.)

barrel-shaped and is hard to the touch. If there is parametrial involvement, the parametrium may also be hard and nodular.

Cellular Characteristics

Histologically, 80%–90% of cervical tumors are squamous, 10%–20% are adenocarcinomas, and a very small number are mixed adenocarcinomas, verrucous carcinoma, melanoma, adenocystic, or sarcoma.[145] Adenocarcinomas, generally in younger women, impose a greater risk because the tumor is within the cervix and can become quite bulky before becoming clinically evident. The bulkiness makes the tumor harder to treat and thus has a high rate of local recurrence.[3,178] Adenocarcinomas appear to be increasing in prevalence.[178]

Natural History

Each type of CIN lesion can regress, persist, or become invasive. CIN III is more likely to progress than the milder forms, which may regress spontaneously to normal. Because there is no way to predict which lesions will become invasive and which will not, all patients should be treated as soon as lesions are discovered. Most authorities believe that CIN is a venereal disease that has a prolonged incubation period.[150]

Once invasive, cervical cancer spreads by three routes: direct extension, via lymphatics, and by hematogenous spread. Direct extension is the most common route. The lesion begins on the endocervix and spreads throughout the entire cervix, into the parametrium, and through the vesicovaginal and rectovaginal septae into the bladder and rectum. The vagina and corpus of the uterus can also become involved.

The primary nodes involved in the spread of cervical cancer include the parametrial, paracervical, obturator, hypogastric, external iliac, and sacral. The secondary group of lymph nodes involved are the common iliacs, inguinal, and paraaortic. Lymph node involvement can be correlated with stage of disease. The prevalence of positive nodes is 15%–20% in stage I, 25%–40% in stage II, and at least 50% in stage III.[3]

Hematogenous spread through the venous plexus and the paracervical veins occurs less frequently than lymphatic spread but is relatively common in the more advanced stages. Carlson et al.[179] reviewed 2220 cases of squamous cell cervical cancer and found that only 15% of women developed distant metastases during the course of their disease. The majority of these individuals had stage III and IV disease. The most common sites of metastasis are the lungs, liver, bone, and mediastinal and supraclavicular nodes.

Clinical Manifestations

Cervical cancer is usually asymptomatic in the preinvasive and early stage, although women may notice a watery vaginal discharge. In the majority of cases the disease is discovered by PAP smear during routine examination. The later symptoms in cervical cancer that often prompt the woman to seek medical attention are postcoital bleeding, intermenstrual bleeding, or heavy menstrual flow. If this bleeding is chronic, the woman may complain of symptoms related to anemia. A common complaint in advanced cervical malignancy is foul-smelling vaginal discharge.

Other late symptoms that are indicative of advanced disease include pain in the pelvis, hypogastrium, flank, or leg. This is secondary to involvement of the pelvic wall, ureters, lymph nodes, or sciatic nerve roots. Urinary and rectal symptoms can indicate invasion of these structures by tumor. End-stage disease can be characterized by edema of the lower extremities due to lymphatic and venous obstruction. Massive vaginal hemorrhage and development of renal failure can result from local invasion of blood vessels and bilateral ureteral obstruction by tumor.

Assessment—CIN

The Pap smear is an effective, accurate, and economical screening technique to detect cervical neoplasia. Accuracy of the examination depends on the sampling method, staining, and microscopic examination.[180,181]

Computerized microscope systems can prescreen Pap smears at a lower false-negative rate than can human screeners. However, the cost-benefit relationship still remains a limiting factor with the automated method.[181,182]

The American Cancer Society recommends that women who are or have been sexually active or who are 18 years or older should have an annual Pap test and pelvic examination. After a woman has had three or more consecutive normal annual examinations, the Pap test may be performed less frequently at the discretion of her physician.[183] The American College of Obstetricians and Gynecologists recommends annual examination that begin with the onset of sexual activity or at 18 years of age.

Sexually active women should have annual Pap smears. Those who have any pelvic symptoms such as pain, vaginal discharge, or abnormal bleeding should be evaluated by their physician promptly. False-negative Pap smears occur and are thought to be due to sampling inefficiency.[184] A negative Pap smear offers no guarantee that the woman is free of cervical cancer.[184]

The correlation between cytologic diagnosis and subsequent histologic examination is over 90%.[185] Although *CIN* is used as the standard terminology for cervical intraepithelial lesions, some cytology laboratories still use the old I–V class system for reporting. The relationship between the two is depicted in Table 43-11.

If the Pap smear report shows CIN, referral for colposcopy, biopsy, and/or treatment is indicated.[186] Colposcopy is a diagnostic test usually done on an outpatient basis to evaluate the cervix after an abnormal PAP smear. A colposcope is a stereoscopic, binocular microscope that illuminates and magnifies the view of the cervix.[150,187] During this procedure the cervix is swabbed with 3% acetic acid solution, which accentuates the abnormalities and differentiates between normal or metaplastic areas.[180] The epithelium of the cervix is visualized and the abnormal areas biopsied.

TABLE 43-11 Cytologic Report Correlations

Class	CIN Terminology	Description
I		Smear normal, no abnormal cells
II		Atypical cells present below the level of cervical neoplasia
III	CIN I, CIN II	Smear contains abnormal cells consistent with dysplasia—mild: CIN I; moderate: CIN II
IV	CIN III	Smear contains abnormal cells consistent with carcinoma in situ—severe: CIN III
V		Smear contains abnormal cells consistent with invasive carcinoma of squamous cell origin

CIN, cervical intraepithelial neoplasia.

Source: Adapted from Nelson JH, Averette HE, Richare RM: Cervical intraepithelial neoplasia (dysplasia and carcinoma in situ) and early invasive cervical carcinoma, *CA* 39:157–178, 1989.

Treatment, Results, Prognosis—CIN

It is critical that the extent of the disease be evaluated as accurately as possible before treatment begins. The Pap smear, colposcopy, and biopsy determine the extent and severity of the cervical lesion, differentiating between CIN and invasive carcinoma of the cervix. Treatment for CIN may include a direct cervical biopsy, electrocautery/cryosurgery, laser surgery, electrosurgery, cone biopsy, or hysterectomy.[180,187]

Cryosurgery, the most commonly used method for treatment of CIN in the United States, involves using a portable probe to induce freezing of cervical tissue. It is a cost-effective, painless treatment with low morbidity that can be performed in the office. Patients most often complain of a watery discharge for 2–4 weeks after treatment.

Research studies[188–190] show that approximately 80%–90% of CIN can be eradicated by laser. The laser is mounted on the colposcope, and the laser beam is directed under colposcopic control. With the laser, significantly less disease-free tissue is removed with the entire lesion. Patients may experience a little more discomfort than with cryosurgery, but there is usually less vaginal discharge and complete healing occurs in about 2 weeks.[3,187,191] One disadvantage of the laser is that it may cause thermal damage to tissue, making it difficult to rule out invasive cancer.

Treatment of CIN using the loop electrosurgical excision procedure (LEEP) is an increasingly popular alternative. In selected patients this approach may allow for diagnosis and treatment of CIN during one outpatient visit. The LEEP utilizes a thin wire loop electrode that allows excision of lesions with minimal tissue ablation. The advantage of LEEP is that there is less likelihood of tissue ablation than with the use of other procedures such as the laser. Complications of LEEP are similar to those seen with laser treatment.[192]

Conization involves removal of a cone-shaped piece of tissue from the exocervix and endocervix (Figure 43-6).[3,187] This procedure, performed under general anesthesia as an outpatient, can be used as a diagnostic or therapeutic technique. The exact size of the cone depends on the colposcopic findings. Conization is performed in specific situations: (1) for diagnosis, if no lesion of the cervix is noted and an endocervical tumor is suspected; (2) to determine extent of the lesion if microinvasion is diagnosed on biopsy, or if the entire lesion cannot be seen with the colposcope; (3) if there are discrepancies between the cytologic report (PAP smear) and the histologic appearance of the lesions on

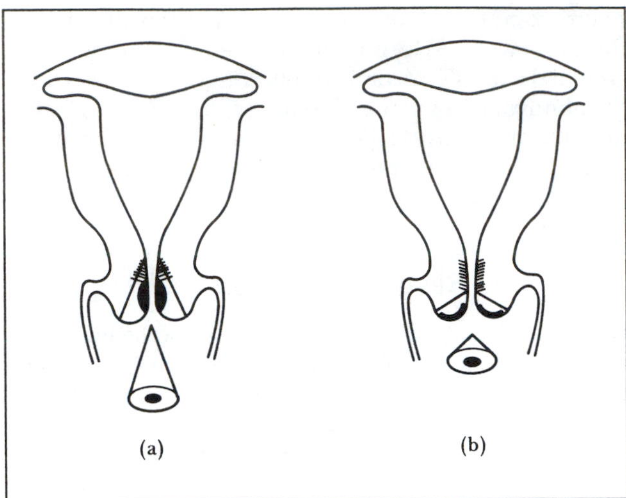

FIGURE 43-6 (a) Cone biopsy for endocervical disease. (b) Cone biopsy for CIN of the exocervix. CIN = cervical epithelial neoplasia. (Source: DiSaia PJ, Creasman WT: *Clinical Gynecologic Oncology.* St Louis, MO: Mosby, 1989.)

biopsy; and (4) if the patient cannot be relied upon for long-term follow-up.[193] Major immediate complications of conization include hemorrhage, uterine perforation, and complications of anesthesia. Delayed complications include bleeding, cervical stenosis, infertility, cervical incompetence, and increased chances of preterm (low birth weight) delivery. In general, complications of conization are related to the amount of endocervix removed.[187–191]

Total vaginal hysterectomy (TVH) may be employed for treatment of individuals with CIS. Total abdominal hysterectomy is appropriate for individuals with CIN who have completed childbearing. These individuals are followed as closely for recurrence as those treated with more conservative measures.[3]

Ultimately, the therapy selected is based on the extent of the disease, the patient's wishes to preserve ovarian and reproductive function, and the physician's experience. Women with CIN I or II who wish to maintain optimum fertility can be considered for electrocautery, laser therapy, or cryosurgery. CIN III also can be treated in this manner as long as the woman is aware that there is a slightly higher incidence of recurrence with this treatment method.[3]

Yliskoski et al.[194] studied the efficacy of interferon cream (IFN) in treating genital HPV-16 infections associated with CIN and/or vaginal intraepithelial neoplasia. Utilizing DNA hybridization techniques, they found that in two-thirds of the sample, HPV-16 infection was eradicated. However, the sample size was small and future work needs to be done to further support this finding. Iwasaka et al.[195] administered perilesional injections of interferon-γ to a group of eight women and found that dysplastic lesions resolved in five of the eight. The use of IFN for the treatment of CIN is inferior to surgical methods when cure rate is considered. However, the advantage of using IFN is that it does not deform the cervix nor interfere with a normal pregnancy. Therefore, it may be appropriate for use in selected females during the childbearing years.

Figure 43-7 summarizes the appropriate management of a patient with an abnormal Pap smear.[3] Re-

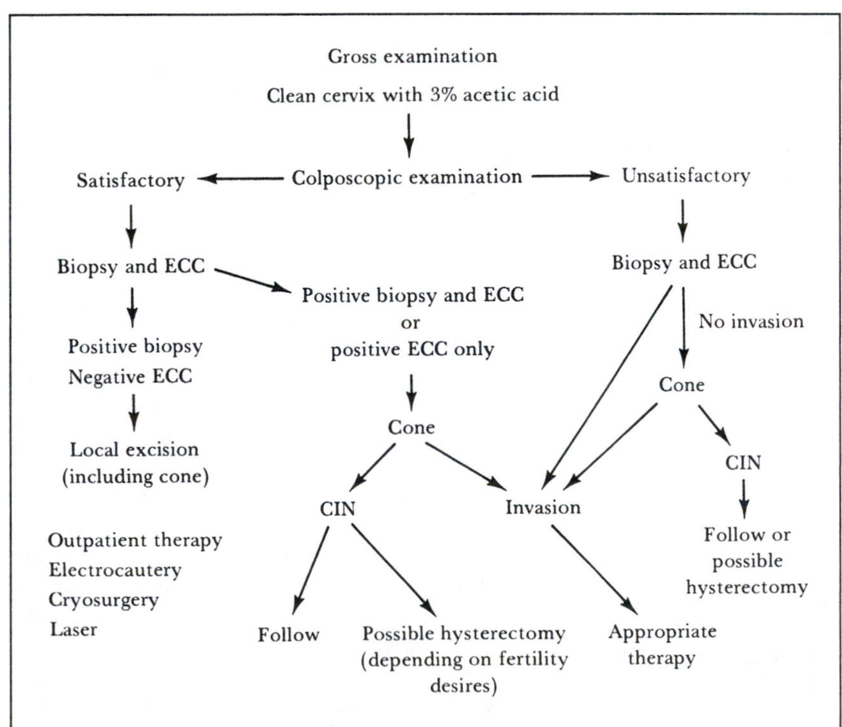

FIGURE 43-7 Evaluation and management schema for individual with abnormal Pap smear. (Source: DiSaia PJ, Creasman WT: *Clinical Gynecologic Oncology.* St. Louis, MO: Mosby, 1989.)

gardless of the type of treatment selected for CIN, frequent follow-up is essential.

Nursing Management—CIN

The primary nursing responsibilities for women with CIN focus on education. This educational process includes defining the disease, explaining treatment, and stressing the importance of close follow-up.

If the biopsy indicates CIN, the woman may erroneously think that she has invasive cancer. The nurse assures the patient that she does not have cancer and that CIN is an easily treated premalignant condition. McDonald[196] found that in women treated for CIN, self-esteem was lowest and anxiety highest during the initial and postsurgical visits. In addition, women expressed fear of losing sexual functioning. The nurse helps the woman to understand the type of treatment recommended. The nurse explains the nature, purpose of treatment, and side effects of the therapy.

Following treatment, the nurse instructs the woman on how to care for herself at home. Douching, tampons, and sexual intercourse are prohibited for at least 2–4 weeks, depending on the treatment. A return visit is scheduled for 2–4 weeks, then every 3 months for a year, and every 6 months thereafter. The importance of follow-up must be stressed because there is a possibility of treatment failure or recurrence of the CIN. Minimal bleeding and vaginal discharge may be present for a week or longer after biopsy, cryosurgery, or laser and for several weeks following conization.

Information concerning sexual functioning and fertility are discussed with women undergoing treatment for CIN, although electrocautery, cryosurgery, laser therapy, and conization rarely cause physiologic sexual dysfunction.[197] Most women report no change in libido, orgasm, coital frequency, or overall satisfaction with their sex life. Fertility is usually maintained, but difficulty with conception may occur. Table 43-12 summarizes issues specifically related to the nursing management of women diagnosed with cervical, vulvar, or vaginal cancer.

TABLE 43-12 Nursing Management of the Woman with Cervical, Vulvar, or Vaginal Cancer

Disease/Therapeutic Modality	Treatment Issues	Psychosocial Concerns
Preinvasive disease (CIN, VIN, VAIN) treated by:		
Local therapies (eg, laser, cryosurgery, electrocautery, electrosurgery, conization, interferon cream	Prepare patient by explaining the disease	Assure patient that CIN, VIN, VAIN are *not* cancer
	Explain treatment to patient	Educate patient on possible complications of the treatment
	Instruct patient in self-care after treatment (no douching, tampons, sexual intercourse for 2–4 weeks)	Address patient concerns related to sexual functioning, changes in libido, orgasm, coital frequency, fertility
	Stress importance of follow-up	Discuss possibility of treatment failure or recurrence
		Assess for anxiety, depression, changes in self- or body image
Invasive disease treated by:		
Surgery	Preoperative testing	Assess level of understanding
	Operative procedure planned	
	Review bowel preparation procedure	
	Instruct patient in use of incentive spirometer; importance of turning, coughing, deep breathing, abdominal splinting, and use of antiemboletic stockings	Have patient give a return demonstration as indicated
	Review need for IV, urinary catheter, colostomy, ileal conduit as indicated	Begin ostomy teaching preoperatively as indicated and involve family or significant others in teaching sessions
	Stress availability of pain medication	Review use of patient-controlled analgesia pump as indicated
	Stress importance of early ambulation	Explore with patient nonpharmacologic pain relief measures
	Provide wound care postoperatively	Encourage patient to participate in wound care
		Assess for changes in self- or body image
	Assess religious and cultural beliefs as related to treatment (eg, no blood transfusions, avoidance of drugs, dietary restrictions, etc.)	Assess spiritual needs/concerns

(continued)

TABLE 43-12 Nursing Management of the Woman with Cervical, Vulvar, or Vaginal Cancer (continued)

Disease/Therapeutic Modality	Treatment Issues	Psychosocial Concerns
	Monitor: Vital signs Respiratory function Cardiac function Circulatory function Neurologic function Renal function Fluid and electrolytes Assess: Nutritional status, lymphedema, skin integrity, hazards of immobility, alteration in sleep and rest patterns Assess for deep vein thrombosis	Preoperatively assess woman's knowledge of anatomy, physiology, and sexual function Preoperatively assess information on support systems, coping strategies, attitudes about self Assess for anxiety, depression Assess usual coping mechanisms; mutually devise ways to deal with current stress
	Assess for alteration in sexual functioning	Assess preoperative expectations of sexual outcome Assist patient to realize her intrinsic worth and dignity Assess effects of treatment on quality of life Assess psychological effects of loss of reproductive function Assess psychological response to loss of sexually responsive tissue Assist patient to redefine self-concept in ways other than reproduction Initiate a comprehensive counseling approach involving the patient and her sexual partner and make referrals as needed
Radiotherapy	Review treatment procedure (external beam, intracavitary, interstitial, etc.) Review side effects of therapy Assess skin integrity Assess G.I. function Monitor hemotologic values Assess for deep vein thrombosis	Assess level of understanding Assess information on support systems Encourage patient to express fears, concerns Begin teaching about prevention of vaginal stenosis as indicated
	Explain mobility restrictions with intracavitary, interstitial radiotherapy Assess pain related to radiation applicators Assess for placement of radiotherapy applicators	Encourage diversional activities to relieve boredom Emphasize availability of traditional pain relief measures Explore with patient nonphrmacologic pain relief measures (music, T.V. massage, etc.)
	Assess religious and cultural beliefs as related to treatment (eg, no blood transfusions, avoidance of drugs, dietary restrictions)	Assess spiritual needs/concerns Assess for anxiety, depression Assist woman to realize her intrinsic worth and dignity Encourage patient to express concerns related to fertility, sexuality, body/self-image Assess effects of treatment on quality of life Initiate a comprehensive counseling approach involving the patient and her sexual partner and refer as needed
Chemotherapy	Explain the treatment to the patient: rationale, name of drug(s), mechanism of action, dose, frequency of administration, nadir, method of administration, side effects	Assess evidence of learning Address patient concerns about side effects and treatment of side effects Assess emotional status of patient and family Encourage patient to express fears, concerns Assess information on support systems Assess for anxiety, depression, changes in self- or body image Assess usual coping mechanisms; mutually devise ways to deal with current stress Assess effects of treatment on quality of life
	Assess religious and cultural beliefs as related to treatment (eg, no blood transfusions, avoidance of drugs, dietary restrictions, etc.)	Assess spiritual needs/concerns

Assessment—Invasive Disease

Cervical cancer is staged clinically, with confirmation obtained from examinations completed with the patient under anesthesia. The clinical stage is not changed at surgery or when disease recurs. The initial staging is one of the best prognostic indicators. Approximate 5-year survival rates are: stage I, 80.5%; stage II, 59%; stage III; 33%; and stage IV, 7%.[2,198,199] Unfortunately, when clinical and surgical stage are compared, 30%–40% are understaged.[2,178]

A thorough clinical work-up includes cervical biopsies, endocervical curettage, cystoscopy, and proctosigmoidoscopy. Additional diagnostic tests may include chest radiograph, IVP, barium enema, CBC, and blood chemistries. If liver enzymes are elevated, a liver scan (or CT scan) is indicated.[3,187,199,200]

Lymphangiogram may be indicated in selected individuals. The use of lymphangiography has been controversial due to a high false-negative rate. Twenty-one percent of patients with lymphangiograms interpreted as normal are found to have histologically positive nodes at laparotomy.[2] If enlarged nodes are seen on lymphangiogram, fine-needle aspiration may be done. Lymph angiogram may also be valuable in outlining abnormal lymph nodes to be included in radiotherapy ports.[16,201]

Additional studies that are helpful in defining the extent of disease but do not alter clinical staging include CT and MRI. Computerized axial tomograms may be used to determine the extent of pelvic disease, define radiotherapy portals, and evaluate lymph node status; however, there is no evidence that this is a reliable procedure to evaluate nodes for the initial staging of cervical cancer.[202] Magnetic resonance imaging holds promise for defining tumor extent and tissue characterization more accurately than CT and US. It is hoped that MRI eventually will be used to determine the presence of both pelvic and retroperitoneal nodes more accurately than CT. Unfortunately, at present, differentiation between benign and malignant nodes cannot be determined with MRI.[202,203] Verification of tumor volume (the most important prognostic factor for survival of the patient with cervical cancer) by MRI may help the physician determine the best treatment modality.[204]

Clinical staging is not changed on the basis of surgical findings, but treatment may be altered. In selected cases where lymphangiogram or CT are equivocal, a selected pelvic and periaortic lymphadenectomy may be performed. Surgical staging is included in some investigational chemotherapy/radiation protocols to better define extent of disease and select appropriate radiation therapy.[205,206]

Supraclavicular node biopsy is done if one of these nodes is palpable or if paraaortic nodes are positive. The left node is most often positive because this is where the thoracic duct enters into the subclavian vein. Positive supraclavicular nodes are often associated with a positive aortic node. In such cases a blind scalene node biopsy is recommended. If this is positive, systemic therapy is necessary. Following a thorough evaluation, the clinical stage is determined (Table 43-13).[56,207]

Treatment, Results and Prognosis—Invasive Disease

Once invasive cervical cancer is diagnosed and the stage established, treatment is based on the woman's age, general medical condition, extent of the cancer, and the presence of any complicating abnormalities. Either surgery or radiation therapy can be used equally effectively for patients with early-stage disease. Radiotherapy can be used for all individuals, whereas surgery is indicated only for women who are considered good surgical candidates.[3,208] Key components include being treated in an institution with the appropriate personnel and equipment for either type of treatment and multidisciplinary planning.[16] In general, patients with stage IIb to IV are treated with radiotherapy.

Stage Ia

Stage Ia disease (microinvasive carcinoma) has been divided into Ia1 and Ia2. Stage Ia1, microinvasive disease too small to be measured, is treated by TAH or TVH if the patient is healthy and does not desire further childbearing. Conization can be done for those who are poor surgical risks or who wish to preserve fertility, as long as the biopsy margins are free of disease and the patient is followed closely.[16] Intracavitary radiation may also be utilized to treat cervical cancer in this stage.[209,210]

Stage Ia2 disease is treated by TAH or TVH if invasion is less than 3 mm and there is no lymphovascular space involvement. If the invasion is greater than 3 mm or there is lymphovascular invasion, the disease is managed the same as Stage Ib.[16] Five-year survival in patients with properly staged Ia cervical cancer is close to 100%.[16,187,210]

Stage Ib and IIa

The choice of therapy for patients with stage Ib and IIa disease remains controversial. The preference of one treatment over another depends on the gynecologist and radiation oncologist involved as well as the woman's condition and the characteristics of the lesion.

Stage Ib and Stage IIa disease can be treated with radical abdominal hysterectomy and pelvic lymphadenectomy or with external beam radiotherapy to the whole pelvis with one or two intracavitary insertions (5000–8000 cGy) of radiation.[3,210,211]

Surgery is preferred to radiotherapy by some gynecologic oncologists because ovarian function can be preserved. The vagina usually remains more pliable after surgery than with radiation. The overall treatment time is shorter. Long-term radiation complications to pelvic tissue can be avoided. Using radiation therapy has the advantage of avoiding major intra-

TABLE 43-13 Staging Classification for Cervical Cancer

PRIMARY TUMOR (T)

TNM	FIGO	Definition
TX		Primary tumor cannot be assessed
T0		No evidence of primary tumor
Tis	0	Carcinoma in situ
T1	I	Cervical carcinoma confined to uterus (extension to corpus should be disregarded)
T1a	Ia	Preclinical invasive carcinoma, diagnosed by microscopy only
T1a1	Iaa1	Minimal microscopic stromal invasion
Tla2	1a2	Tumor with invasive component 5 mm or less in depth taken from the base of the epithelium and 7 mm or less in horizontal spread
Tlb	1b	Tumor larger than T1a2
T2	II	Cervical carcinoma invades beyond uterus but not to pelvic wall or to the lower third of vagina
T2a	IIa	Without parametrial invasion
T2b	IIb	With parametrial invasion
T3	III	Cervical carcinoma extends to the pelvic wall and/or involves lower third of vagina and/or causes hydronephrosis or nonfunctioning kidney
T3a	IIIa	Tumor involves lower third of the vagina, no extension to pelvic wall
T3b	IIIb	Tumor extends to pelvic wall and/or causes hydronephrosis or nonfunctioning kidney
T4	IVa	Tumor invades mucosa of bladder or rectum and/or extends beyond true pelvis

LYMPH NODES (N)

NX	Regional lymph nodes cannot be assessed
N0	No regional lymph node metastasis
N1	Regional lymph node metastasis

DISTANT METASTASIS (M)

MX	—	Presence of distant metastasis cannot be assessed
M0	—	No distant metastasis
M1	IVb	Distant metastasis

STAGE GROUPING

AJCC/UICC				FIGO
0	Tis	N0	M0	
IA	T1a	N0	M0	I A
IB	T1b	N0	M0	I B
IIA	T2a	N0	M0	II A
IIB	T2b	N0	M0	II B
IIIA	T3a	N0	M0	III A
IIIB	T1	N1	M0	III B
	T2	N1	M0	
	T3a	N1	M0	
	T3b	Any N	M0	
IVA	T4	Any N	M0	IV A
IVB	Any T	Any N	M1	IV B

Source: Reprinted from American Joint Committee on Cancer: *Manual for Staging of Cancer* (4th ed). Chicago: AJCC, 1992.

operative and postoperative complications, and the patient can receive the therapy as an outpatient.[16]

Patients with bulky disease (barrel-shaped cervix) have a higher incidence of central recurrence, pelvic and paraaortic lymph node metastases, and distant dissemination. An increased dose of radiation to the central pelvis or radical hysterectomy, or both, has been advocated in patients with bulky disease.[16,210] The use of combined radical surgery followed by radiation remains controversial.

Stage IIb, III, and IV

Women with stage IIb, III, and IV cervical cancer are usually treated with high doses of external pelvic radiation, with parametrial boosts, intracavitary radiation, or a pelvic exenteration.[16] Radiation doses of 5500–6000 cGy to the whole pelvis over 5 or 6 weeks are recommended.[2] Interstitial parametrial implants may also be used to supplement standard radiation techniques.[16,210] The 5-year survival rates of patients with stage IIb cancer are 60%–65% while those with stage III have survival rates of 25%–48%, and those with stage IV have less than 10%.[16,212]

The role of surgery in the management of patients with advanced cervical cancer has expanded. Exenteration is employed as primary therapy only in a selected group of patients. Candidates for pelvic exenteration include those with centralized disease not adherent to pelvic side walls and not involving lymph nodes and those who are psychologically able to adjust to the change in body functioning and body image.

Surgical staging of advanced disease before initiating treatment is being advocated in an attempt to gain a more precise evaluation of the extent of the disease.[205,206,213] Arguments for pretreatment staging laparotomy include the following: (1) the extent of the disease can be ascertained, (2) patients who have disease not curable by radiation may be offered palliative therapy, and (3) those patients most likely to benefit from extended-field radiation are identified. Arguments against pretreatment staging laparotomy are: (1) surgical staging has associated morbidity and mortality, (2) many patients with paraaortic nodal metastases also have systemic disease not detected by surgery, (3) there is only minimal improvement in net survival, and (4) surviving patients have high morbidity. This procedure warrants further study and is not recommended for routine use.[213] Chemotherapy alone has not proven useful as initial therapy for women who are at high risk for recurrence but continues to be investigated for use as a radiation sensitizer in protocols.[205,206]

Complications of surgery Radical hysterectomy involves removal of the uterus, upper third of the vagina, entire uterosacral and uterovesical ligaments, the entire parametria, and pelvic node lymphadenectomy. This is a complex procedure because the organs removed are proximal to many vital body structures: the bladder, ureters, rectum, and great vessels of the pelvis.[3] The major complications of radical hysterectomy include ureteral fistulas, bladder dysfunction, pulmonary embolus, lymphocysts, pelvic infection, bowel obstruction, rectovaginal fistulas, and hemorrhage.[188,212]

Complications of radiotherapy Complications resulting from properly administered radiotherapy for cervical cancer are usually manageable. There are reported adverse reactions if poor technique is used, but reactions occur infrequently in properly treated women. The higher the dose of radiation, the greater the rate of complications. Some morbidity attributed to radiation is secondary to uncontrolled tumor or compounded effects of multiple therapies and not a direct result of radiation alone. Major complication rates for stage I and IIa disease range from 3% to 5%, respectively, and are 10% to 15%, respectively, for patients with stage IIb and III disease.[210,214]

The major complications related to radiotherapy include vaginal stenosis, fistula formation, sigmoid perforation or stricture, rectal ulcer or proctitis, intestinal obstruction, fistula, ureteral stricture, severe cystitis, pelvic hemorrhage, and pelvic abscess.

Sexual dysfunction secondary to vaginal atrophy, stenosis, and lack of lubrication is a known effect of radiation therapy. Women who are not sexually active experience a greater degree of atrophy and stenosis than do sexually active women. The use of vaginal dilators and water-soluble lubricants can minimize the radiation effects.

Recurrent or persistent disease

Approximately 35% of women with invasive cervical cancer will have recurrent or persistent disease.[3] Therefore, regular follow-ups after treatment are critical to early detection of recurrence.[3] Recurrent cervical cancer is difficult to diagnose. Clinical and cytologic evaluation of an irradiated cervix is difficult because the cells and configuration of the cervix are distorted from the radiation. Therefore, histologic confirmation of recurrence is essential.[3]

Most recurrences occur within 2 years following therapy. The signs and symptoms may be subtle and varied and include unexplained weight loss, leg edema (excessive and often unilateral), pelvic or thigh and buttock pain, serosanguinous vaginal discharge, progressive ureteral obstruction, supraclavicular lymph node enlargement (usually of the left side), cough, hemoptysis, and chest pain. If the woman presents with the triad of weight loss, leg edema, and pelvic pain, the outlook is grim. Evaluation after histologic confirmation will usually include chest radiograph, IVP, CBC, and blood chemistries. Some physicians will include a CT scan, lymphangiography, or fluoroscopically directed needle biopsies to evaluate the status of the regional lymph nodes, liver, and kidneys. These procedures have replaced more elaborate operative procedures to provide histologic confirmation of recurrence.[3] Tumor recurrence and radiation fibrosis may also be differentiated with fine-needle CT-guided aspiration.[203]

Following surgery or radiotherapy as primary treatment for cervical cancer, about 75% of recurrences are local (cervix, uterus, vagina, parametrium, and regional lymph nodes). The remaining 25% involve distant metastases to the lung, liver, bone, or mediastinal or supraclavicular lymph nodes.[215]

The prognosis for patients with persistent or recurrent carcinoma of the cervix is dismal. One-year survival rates are 10%–15%.[3] Survival averages 6–10 months once recurrent cervical cancer is diagnosed.[178] The aim of treatment in recurrent disease is palliation.

Surgery If cervical cancer recurs centrally following radiotherapy, pelvic exenteration may be considered. Total pelvic exenteration includes radical hysterectomy, pelvic lymph node dissection, and removal of the bladder and rectosigmoid colon. Occasionally, a posterior exenteration (preserves the bladder) or anterior exenteration (preserves the rectum) can be performed[3,216] (Figure 43-8). Partial pelvic exenteration is usually not done because the bladder and rectum may have residual radiation effects and be prone to complications.

Because the goal of surgery is curative, only a small percentage of women with recurrence will be candidates for pelvic exenteration. Women who are not candidates for pelvic exenteration have disease outside the pelvis or have the triad of unilateral leg edema, sciatic pain, and ureteral obstruction. Obesity, severe medical problems, and advanced age may also be reasons that this surgery is contraindicated.

Extensive preoperative evaluation is done to ensure that there is no disease outside the pelvis and that renal function is adequate. Studies usually performed include chest radiography, IVP, blood chemistries, cre-

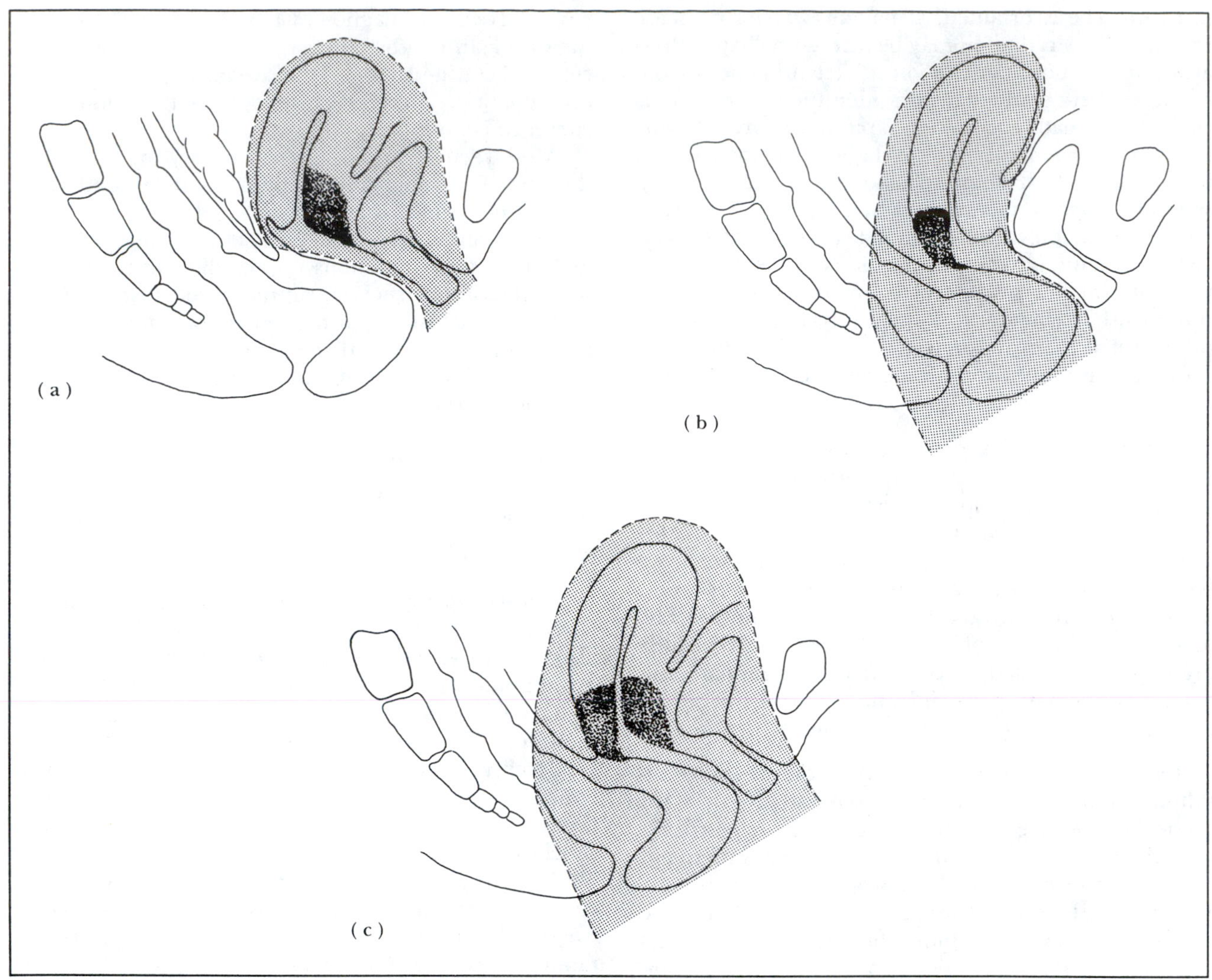

FIGURE 43-8 Total pelvic exenteration. (a) Anterior exenteration involves the surgical removal of the bladder, uterus, and cervix and is considered in patients with a deep cul de sac. It is imperative that frozen sections be obtained at the time of exploration. If tumor is present in the posterior vaginal margin, total exenteration is the preferred operation. (b) Posterior exenteration involves the surgical removal of the rectum, uterus, and cervix. Following radiation therapy, urinary complications are high. (c) Total exenteration involves the removal of bladder, urethra, cervix, uterus, vagina, and rectum. The anal canal may be preserved in some women, allowing reanastomosis of the sigmoid colon. (Source: Shingleton HM, Orr JW: *Cancer of the Cervix: Diagnosis and Treatment.* Edinburgh: Churchill Livingstone, 1987, pp. 225–226.)

atinine clearance, CT scan, bone scan, and liver-spleen scan. Some clinicians also order lymphangiography to evaluate the regional lymph nodes. If lymphadenopathy is present, a needle aspiration of the nodes may be done. If the aspirate is positive for malignancy, the woman may be spared an unnecessary laparotomy. A blind scalene node biopsy may be recommended to complete the evaluation.

At laparotomy the entire abdomen and pelvis are explored for metastases. A selective paraaortic lymphadenectomy, bilateral pelvic lymphadenectomy, and biopsies of the pelvic side walls are done and examined by frozen section. If any of these is positive, the exenteration is usually aborted because the disease is considered incurable.[3] However, some surgeons support the use of pelvic exenteration for patients with recurrent disease complicated by pelvic lymph node metastases.[213]

The use of the end-to-end anastomotic (EEA) stapling device has resulted in patients' not needing a permanent colostomy after pelvic exenteration.[216] The EEA also reduces the risk of anastomotic leak, fistula formation, and late strictures. Permanent colostomy can also be avoided by using a segment of sigmoid colon as a rectal substitute.[217,218]

Immediate postoperative problems include pulmonary embolism, pulmonary edema, cardiovascular accident, hemorrhage, myocardial infarction, sepsis, and small bowel obstruction. Long-term problems include fistula formation, urinary obstruction, infection, and sepsis. The use of pelvic exenteration had been limited to a highly select group of candidates, since reports indicate a 5-year survival of 23% and an operative mortality of approximately 9.8%.[16] Psychosexual and social rehabilitation of surviving patients is a major challenge.[213] Vaginal reconstruction at the time of exenteration and psychological support in the postoperative period can help patients adjust.

Chemotherapy Chemotherapy for patients with cervical carcinoma is complicated because these patients frequently have decreased pelvic vascular perfusion, a limited bone marrow reserve, and poor renal function related to previous radiation or surgery, and ureteral obstruction from tumor or scarring.[2,3,26]

Response rates for patients with recurrent squamous cell cervical cancer treated with single-agent and investigational chemotherapy range from 10%–40%[16,219] (see Table 43-14). In general, there is not long-term benefit, with responses lasting 4–8 months and variable lengths of survival. Response rates are higher in patients who have received no prior radiotherapy or chemotherapy. Documented activity has been shown for dibromoducitol, ifosfamide, CHIP (iproplatin), and carboplatin.[16,208,220] Of the single agents, cisplatin remains the drug with the greatest antineoplastic activity.[16,208,219,220] Even so, response rates with this drug only range between 17%–21% and effect no increase in survival time for patients.

Combination chemotherapy has not been proven more effective than single agents. Complete response rates of 10%–29% suggest some enhancement of effect by using a combination of drugs.[16] Many clinical trials using combination chemotherapy have been relatively small sample sizes, making it difficult to determine their usefulness in treating advanced cervical cancer.[219] (See Table 43-15.)

Pelvic intraarterial infusion of bleomycin, vincristine, and mitomycin-C has been studied in women with recurrent cervical cancer. Toxicity was significant and included pulmonary fibrosis from bleomycin and infectious or embolic complications from the catheterization. Response rates were low.

Kim et al.[221,222] used a regimen of vinblastine, bleomycin, and cisplatin initially in 54 patients (stages Ib and II with bulky tumors) followed by radical hysterectomy and found that it was effective in reducing tumor volume, the stage of disease, and lymph node involvement and in improving the 2-year survival rate. Kredentser et al.[223] utilized etoposide (VP-16), ifosfamide/mesna, and cisplatin in a phase II study of 14 women diagnosed with advanced or recurrent cervical cancer. They found an overall response rate in 8 of the 14 patients (57%), and 3 were disease-free up to 24 months posttreatment.

Chemotherapy can be used as a radiation sensitizer, particularly hydroxyurea and cisplatin.[210,224] Several studies have shown improved survival rates from the

TABLE 43-14 Single-Agent Activity in Squamous Cell Carcinoma of the Cervix

Drug	Response (%)
Alkylating agents	
Cyclophosphamide	38/251 (15%)
Chlorambucil	11/44 (25%)
Melphalan	4/20 (20%)
Ifosfamide	7/46 (15%)
	3/27 (11%)
	25/84 (29%)
Dibromodulcitol	16/55 (29%)
	7/47 (15%)
Galactitol	7/36 (19%)
Methyl CCNU	7/94 (7%)
CCNU	3/63 (5%)
Yoshi 864	0/18 (0%)
Heavy metal complexes	
Cisplatin	182/785 (23%)
	8/30 (27%)
Carboplatin	27/175 (15%)
Iproplatin	19/177 (11%)
Antibiotics	
Doxorubicin	12/61 (20%)
	33/205 (16%)
Mitoxantrone	2/26 (8%)
Esorubicin	0/28 (0%)
Piperazinedione	5/38 (13%)
Echinomycin	2/28 (7%)
Porfiromycin	17/78 (22%)
Antimetabolites	
5-fluorouracil	29/142 (20%)
Methotrexate	17/96 (18%)
6-mercaptopurine	1/18 (5%)
Dichloromethotrexate	3/37 (8%)
Baker's Antifol	5/32 (16%)
Plant alkaloids	
VP-16	0/31 (0%)
VM-26	3/22 (14%)
Vincristine	10/55 (18%)
Vinblastine	0/33 (0%)
	2/20 (10%)
Vindesine	5/21 (24%)
Maytansine	1/29 (3%)
Other Agents	
Hydroxyurea	0/14 (0%)
ICRF-159	5/28 (18%)
Aminothiadiazole	1/21 (5%)
AMSA	1/25 (4%)
PALA	0/36 (0%)
Diaziquone	1/26 (4%)
N-methylformamide	0/20 (0%)
Spirogermanium	0/18 (0%)
Hexamethylmelamine	12/64 (19%)

Source: Adapted from Thigpen JT: Chemotherapy of cancers of the female genital tract, in Perry MC (ed): *The Chemotherapy Sourcebook*. Baltimore, MD: Williams & Wilkins, 1992, p. 1048.

TABLE 43-15 Cisplatin-Based Combination Chemotherapy Used to Treat Squamous Cell Carcinoma of the Cervix

Regimen	No. of Patients/Response (%)
Cisplatin + 5-FU	55 (22%)
Cisplatin + adriamycin	19 (32%)
Cisplatin + cyclophosphamide	12 (42%)
Cisplatin + bleomycin	17 (59%)
	24 (54%)
Cisplatin + mitomycin C	49 (18%)
	30 (43%)
Cisplatin + dichloromethotrexate	13 (76%)
Cisplatin + galactitol	18 (39%)
Cisplatin + bleomycin	23 (65%)
+ vinblastine	10 (60%)
Cisplatin + bleomycin	9 (89%)
+ methotrexate	19 (53%)
Cisplatin + bleomycin	21 (38%)
+ adriamycin	
Cisplatin + adriamycin	23 (30%)
+ methyl CCNU	
Cisplatin + cyclophosphamide	20 (20%)
+ adriamycin	
Cisplatin + bleomycin	13 (78%)
+ vincristine	14 (50%)
+ mitomycin C	14 (43%)
	14 (21%)
	48 (17%)
Cisplatin + bleomycin	15 (67%)
+ vincristine	
+ methotrexate	
Cisplatin + bleomycin	5 (0%)
+ vinblastine	
+ methotrexate	

Source: Adapted from Thigpen JT: Chemotherapy of cancers of the female genital tract, in Perry MC (ed): *The Chemotherapy Sourcebook*. Baltimore, MD: Williams & Wilkins, 1992, p. 1050.

concurrent administration of radiation and hydroxyurea.[224,225] Results have also indicated that patients experienced an increased incidence of hematologic toxicity with hydroxyurea.[225] Weekly low-dose cisplatin with radiation has been associated with a modest improvement in disease-free survival without any significant increases in toxicity.[16] Kuske[225] utilized cisplatin and 5-FU as radiosensitizers and reported that 52% of patients in the study were disease-free 1–3 years after treatment, while 39% experienced pelvic recurrence.

Chemotherapy has not been shown to be useful as adjuvant therapy after definitive treatment in high-risk women (e.g., women with positive nodes, bulky lesions, or adenocarcinomas). However, Weiner et al.[227] suggested that a combination of mitomycin, vincristine, bleomycin, and cisplatin (MOBP) given before radiation therapy to patients with early disease and positive nodes may be beneficial in reducing recurrence.

Radiotherapy In previously irradiated individuals, metastatic disease outside the initial radiation field may be treated cautiously with radiation to provide local control and relieve symptoms. In selected cases, radiation within previously treated areas may be used.[3,16] For women treated initially with surgery, full-dose radiotherapy using a combination of external and intracavitary implants may afford excellent palliation or even cure.[16]

Nursing Management—Invasive Disease

General management of the patient receiving treatment for cancer is covered in Part III of this text. Table 43-12 summarizes issues related to the nursing management of women with malignancies of the lower genital tract.

Future Trends

Chemotherapy as part of the initial treatment of patients with cervical cancer is being investigated. Vogl[228] proposed its use in tumor debulking as a radiation sensitizer and as adjuvant therapy. Because radiotherapy is more effective with a smaller tumor volume, induction chemotherapy can be given to debulk the tumor before other therapies are started. This might also reduce the incidence of pelvic recurrence. As a result of the debulking process by chemotherapy, normal cervical size and architecture may be restored before radiotherapy.[229] If the cervix is of normal size and configuration, intracavitary radiotherapy is more effective and less toxic.

Recombinant alpha-2b-interferon is also being investigated as a treatment modality for advanced cervical cancer. Because cervical carcinoma is closely associated with HPV and premalignant lesions of the female genital tract appear to be sensitive to interferon, it is hoped that this will be a helpful approach.[230] However, despite the use of biologic response modifiers (BRMs) such as interferon, interleukin, and monoclonal antibodies in the treatment of other cancers, little is known thus far about their efficacy in the treatment of cervical cancer.[208]

The use of growth factors such as granulocyte-colony stimulating factor (G-CSF) and granulocyte/macrophage-colony stimulating factor (GM-CSF) may have a role in adjunctive therapy. Growth factors may allow for higher and more frequent doses of chemotherapy, while reducing myelosuppressive effects of therapy.[231]

Because cervical cancer can be treated successfully with radiotherapy, research with hyperbaric oxygen, hypoxic sensitizers, and hyperthermia is being investigated to increase the benefits of traditional radiotherapy. The results using hyperbaric oxygen are mixed, with some studies showing improvement in survival for women below the age of 55, while others do not show any significant benefit. Increased morbidity has been noted with patients treated with hyperbaric oxygen.[16] Outcomes using misonidazole as a hypoxic cell sensitizer have been equivocal. Morbidity is comparable to that of radiation alone, with the addition of misonidazole neurotoxicity. Thus far, no overall increase in tumor control or survival has been noted.

Use of hyperthermia is limited because it is difficult to deliver heat to a large part of the body such as the pelvis.[16] Interstitial brachytherapy and the use of intraoperative radiation therapy with electron beam are innovative procedures that may help the patient with recurrent disease.[232] The use of accelerated hyperfractionation may also hold promise.[233]

The availability of the Pap smear as a reliable screening device makes cervical cancer a potentially preventable disease. Health education and easy access to screening, especially for women in lower socioeconomic groups, would help decrease the morbidity and mortality associated with this disease. In addition, emphasis should be placed on health education to help women reduce the risk of contracting CIN (e.g., smoking cessation, use of barrier contraception, limiting the number of sexual partners).

VULVAR CANCER

Epidemiology

Vulvar carcinoma is a disease of the elderly, with peak incidence occurring in the seventh decade of life. It rarely occurs in women under 40 years of age and accounts for only 3%–4% of all gynecologic cancers.[5,234–236]

Vulvar intraepithelial neoplasia (VIN) is a term that describes epithelial abnormalities of the vulva. Like CIN, VIN is divided into three grades that differentiate the degree of epithelial involvement by neoplastic cells.[237] Preinvasive vulvar lesions account for about 1% of all vulva disease. Peak incidence is between 48–51 years of age, although it may affect females from adolescence well into the 90s. Even so, it appears to be increasing in younger women.[238–240]

A variety of premalignant vulvar conditions can progress over time to intraepithelial carcinoma or CIS. These lesions may vary clinically (e.g., papules or macules, coalescent or discrete, single or multiple) and can present as white epithelium or as areas with pink, red, or brown hyperpigmentation.[3,241]

Etiology

The etiology of VIN is unclear. Some connection with venereal disease, including herpes simplex virus type 2 and condylomata acuminatum, has been suggested.[3,16,239] Barbero[240] studied 60 patients with VIN and found that HPV infections were present in 51% of the sample, but the relationships between HPV and vulvar neoplasia remains unclear. Other potential factors in the development of VIN are immunosuppression and a history of genital or extragenital malignancies.[241,243]

Clinical characteristics of the woman with vulvar carcinoma are described in Table 43-16.[244] Vulvar dystrophies and VIN may occur in the presence of invasive vulvar cancer but rarely progress to vulvar cancer. A history of chronic vulvar disease and previous malignancies of the lower genital tract are also seen in women diagnosed with vulvar cancer. Medical problems associated with vulvar cancer may include hypertension, cardiovascular disease, obesity, and diabetes, but these are probably related to the advanced age of most women who present with vulvar cancer rather than to the cancer etiology. Chronic irritation and exposure to coal tar derivatives are also suspected.[5] Herpes simplex type 2 and HPV have been identified in women with vulvar cancers.[2,245] HPV in conjunction with an irritating physical, chemical, infectious, or immunological factor may act as a co-carcinogen in the formation of vulvar cancer.[245] A history of breast, cervical, or endometrial malignancy is associated with invasive vulvar carcinoma[244] (see Table 43-9).

Pathophysiology and Cellular Characteristics

Although primary disease can develop anywhere on the vulva, the labia is the site of vulvar cancer in 70% of cases, with the labia majora involved three times more often than the labia minora. The clitoris, Bartholin's glands, and perineum can also be the site of initial involvement.[246] Vulvar cancer usually remains a localized disease with well-defined margins.

Squamous cancer accounts for about 90% of vulvar malignancies;[27,247] melanoma accounts for 5%; and the remaining 10% are Bartholin's gland, sarcoma, basal cell, Paget's, and verrucous cancer.[18,237,239]

TABLE 43-16 Clinical Features of the Patient with Vulvar Cancer

Clinical Features
Advanced age (>60 years)
Chronic vulvar disease
Previous malignancy of lower genital tract
History of breast cancer
HPV
HSV2
Chronic irritation
Exposure to coal tar derivatives

HPV, humanpapilloma virus; HSV2, herpes simplex virus type 2.

Natural History

The most common routes of metastatic spread are through direct extension; lymphatic dissemination to regional lymph nodes; and, rarely, hematogenous spread to distant sites including the lungs, liver and bone.[248] Squamous vulvar cancer can spread to involve the vagina, urethra, and anus. Once the lymphatics are involved, vulvar cancer spreads rapidly to femoral and pelvic nodes. The overall incidence of positive lymph node involvement (both inguinal and pelvic) is 40%. For lesions smaller than 2 cm, the incidence of positive lymph nodes is 21%, and for lesions larger than 2 cm, the incidence of positive nodes is 45%.[249]

Clinical Manifestations

The symptoms of both VIN and invasive vulvar carcinoma are variable and insidious. With VIN, 50% of women are asymptomatic, whereas others may complain of vulvar pruritus or burning (vulvodynia).[241] Up to 20% percent of women with vulvar cancer are asymptomatic, with lesions detected only during routine pelvic examination. The most common complaint associated with vulvar cancer is the presence of a mass or growth in the vulvar area. Other symptoms include vulvar bleeding and pain.[16,247] The woman with vulvar cancer may delay seeking assistance because she is embarrassed due to the intimate area of the body that is involved. As a result, a woman may have symptoms for 2–16 months before seeking medical attention.[250] Even then, proper treatment may be delayed by misdiagnosis, with symptomatic topical treatment for vulvar lesions continuing for up to 12 months or longer before a biopsy is done for definitive diagnosis.[3,247] Fortunately, vulvar cancer is commonly indolent, extends slowly, and metastasizes fairly late.

Assessment—VIN

The most important diagnostic tool available is methodical inspection. Colposcopy is helpful in detecting multicentric lesions. A 1% toluidine blue solution can be used to stain suspicious areas but has a 20% false-positive rate.[3,16] To diagnose the underlying condition, multiple vulvar biopsies should be done when lesions are noted.[3]

Treatment—VIN

Some controversy exists about the treatment of choice in patients with VIN. Currently, wide local excision using either primary-closure skin flaps or skin graft is recommended, with close follow-up for localized lesions.[16] For multicentric disease, a skinning vulvectomy (Figure 43-9) is performed in which the vulvar skin is excised while conserving the fat, muscle, and glands below the skin. A split-thickness skin graft reconstruction is performed. This procedure produces excellent cosmetic and functional results.[241] DiSaia and Creasman[3] report that of 50 women treated with skinning vulvectomy, none had complaints of dyspareunia or diminished sexual responsiveness. A simple vulvectomy may be indicated in elderly women with chronic medical problems since healing of the skin graft after skinning vulvectomy requires prolonged bed rest.

Lesions of VIN may also may be treated locally by electrocautery, cryosurgery, or laser. These procedures can result in painful ulcers that may take up to 3 months to heal.[251] Some clinicians use the carbon dioxide laser rather than simple vulvectomy and split-graft skinning vulvectomy to treat patients with vulvar intraepithelial neoplasia. The advantages of the CO_2 laser are precision, sparing effect of surrounding tissue, promotion of rapid recovery, little postoperative edema, and minimal scarring.[252] Rader et al.[253] utilized ultrasonic surgical aspiration of vulvar tissue for treatment of VIN. They indicated that this approach had several advantages over laser treatment, including rapid healing, decreased postoperative discomfort, adequate tissue for histopathologic documentation, and excellent cosmetic results.

Other local therapies utilized include topical 5% 5-FU and dinitrochlorobenzene (DNCB) and bleomycin.[16,242,253,254] However, these medications require repeated daily applications and often cause painful, slow-healing ulcers that increase the likelihood of noncompliance.[3]

Assessment—Invasive Disease

Vulvar cancer is diagnosed by local excisional biopsy of the lesions. Colposcopy is useful for defining areas to biopsy. Pap smear of the cervix is essential since 10% of women with vulvar neoplasia also have cervical CIN or invasive cancer. Examination under anesthesia may be needed to fully evaluate the cervix, vagina, and pelvis. Careful physical examination with attention to the inguinal lymph nodes is mandatory. Metastatic evaluation includes chest radiograph, proctosigmoidoscopy, cystoscopy, barium enema, IVP, and biochemical profile. Computerized axial tomography or MRI of the pelvis may help to evaluate retroperitoneal nodal areas.[3,16]

A new FIGO staging for vulvar cancer based on surgical findings was adopted in 1988 (Table 43-17).[248] There is some evidence to suggest that the depth of stromal invasion may relate to node positivity and therefore to prognosis, even though this is not currently part of the staging classification.[2]

Treatment—Invasive Disease

The traditional treatment for women with cancer of the vulva has been surgical: *en bloc* dissection of the tumor, contiguous skin, subcutaneous fat, regional in-

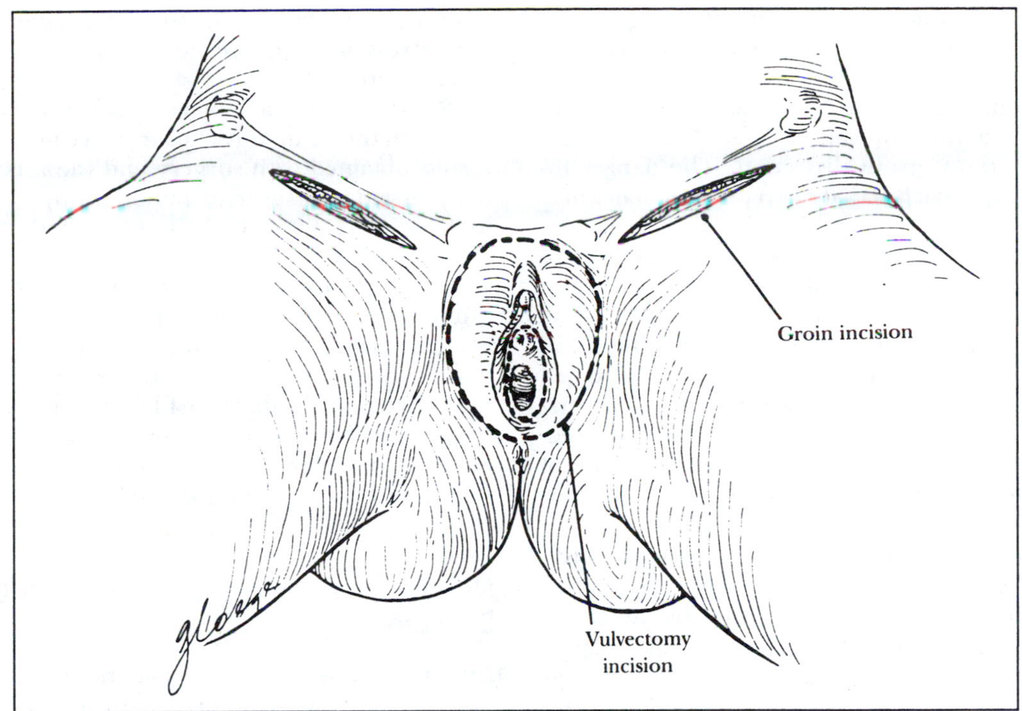

FIGURE 43-9 Skin incision for groin dissection through a separate incision. A line is drawn 1 cm below and parallel to the groin crease and a narrow ellipse of skin is removed. (Source: Hacker NF: Vulvar cancer, in Berek JS, Hacker NF (eds): *Practical Gynecologic Oncology*. Baltimore, MD: Williams & Wilkins, 1989, p. 404. © 1989, the Williams & Wilkins Co., Baltimore, MD.)

guinal and femoral nodes and vulva (labia minora, labia majora, clitoris, perineal body). Some physicians recommend routine pelvic node dissection; however, this procedure has essentially been reserved for women with positive groin nodes, large lesions, melanomas, sarcomas, and adenocarcinomas.[199,255–257] Many surgeons have abandoned the *en bloc* approach and are now performing the nodal dissections through separate groin incisions. See Figure 43-9.

Traditionally, stage I lesions were treated with radical vulvectomy and bilateral groin dissection,[16,256,258] but this has been associated with disturbances in sexual function and body image.[248,259] Recently the trend has been away from radical surgery to more emphasis on

TABLE 43-17 FIGO* Staging of Vulvar Cancer

TNM	Stage	Description
T1 N0 M0	I	Tumor confined to vulva or perineum, 2 cm or less in diameter
T2 N0 M0	II	Tumor confined to vulva or perineum, more than 2 cm in greatest dimension
T3 N0 M0 T3 N1 M0 T1 N1 M0 T2 N1 M0	III	Tumor of any size that spread to (1) any of the following: lower urethra, vagina, anus, and/or (2) unilateral regional lymph metastasis
T1 N2 M0 T2 N2 M0 T3 N2 M0 T4 any N M0	IVa	Tumor invades any of the following: upper urethra, bladder or rectal mucosa, pelvic bone and/or bilateral regional lymph node metastasis
Any T any N M1	IVb	Tumor of any size, location with distant metastasis

*FIGO, International Federation of Gynecology and Obstetrics.
Source: FIGO news, *Int J Gynecol Obstet* 28:189–193, 1989. Elsevier Science Publishers.

individualized treatment of the patient, taking into account age, location of disease, extent of disease, and psychosocial consequences.[235,236,260]

Early lesions under 2 cm in diameter with less than 5 mm of stromal invasion can be treated with a simple vulvectomy without groin dissection. The danger inherent in this approach is that deep femoral nodes may be positive even when superficial nodes are negative.

Stage II and III lesions may require more extensive surgery. This usually involves a radical vulvectomy and bilateral inguinal-femoral lymphadenectomy.[261] If the lesion involves the urethra, vagina, or anus, resection of these organs may be necessary to remove adequate tissue to allow for tumor-free margins. In selected patients with locally advanced disease adjacent to the rectum, a radical vulvectomy, with a tailored anal and rectal resection and temporary colostomy, may be considered.[262]

Patients with stage IV disease may require pelvic exenteration in addition to radical vulvectomy if the bladder or rectum is involved. If the disease is advanced, conservative surgery and radiotherapy may be used.[248,261] Operative mortality is only 1%–2%. This figure is low considering the age of most women who develop vulvar cancer.

Table 43-18 describes reported complications after radical surgery.[244] Wound breakdown occurs in nearly 50% of patients. Varying degrees of lymphedema of the lower extremities occur in about 30% of patients. The use of elastic stockings is recommended for 12 months after surgery to allow development of collateral pathways for lymph drainage.[3,28] Other complications include femoral nerve damage during surgery, causing paraesthesia of the anterior thigh (some recovery usually occurs with time), lymphocyst formation in the groin area, stress incontinence, genital prolapse, and femoral vessel rupture.[235,247]

Radiotherapy has not generally been used as primary treatment in vulvar cancer because of the good results obtained with surgery and the relative insensitivity of vulvar cancer to radiotherapy.[247] Moderately high doses (4500–5500 cGy) of radiotherapy can be used preoperatively to reduce the size of bulky tumor and increase the resectability rate.[16,263,264] Irradiation often causes major surgical problems, especially with wound healing. Patients who have undergone a resection of the primary lesion and are considered at high risk for recurrence due to inadequate resection margins or positive nodes may be good candidates for postoperative irradiation.[16] Radiotherapy may be useful for the patient who is a poor surgical risk.

TABLE 43-18 Reported Complications After Radical Surgery for Vulvar Cancer

Complication	Percentage of All Cases
Wound breakdown or infection	54%
Chronic leg edema	30%
Lymphocyst	10%
Genital prolapse	7%
Stress incontinence	5%
Thrombophlebitis	3.5%
Grafting of skin flaps	1.7%
Hernia (femoral, inguinal)	1.5%
Pulmonary embolus	1.2%
Ruptured femoral artery	1.9%
Hospital deaths	3.3%

Source: Adapted from Morrow CP, Townsend DE (eds): *Synopsis of Gynecologic Oncology* (3d ed). New York: Wiley, 1987, pp. 57–89.

Nursing Management—VIN and Invasive Disease

Nursing considerations for patients receiving chemotherapy, radiation, surgery, or biological therapy are covered in Part III of this text. Nursing management issues related specifically to VIN and invasive vulvar cancer are outlined in Table 43-12.

Results and Prognosis

The 5-year survival rate for vulvar cancer can be correlated with stage and nodal involvement. Overall 5-year survival rate is between 70% and 75% for all stages;[170,249] for women with stage I and II disease, the survival rate is 90%; and for those with stage III disease, 44%. About 25% of women with vulvar cancer will recur. Size of tumor, stage, pattern and depth of invasion, and vascular channel involvement by tumor is prognostically significant in predicting nodal metastases.[237] The survival rate for women with negative nodes is 80%–90%. Survival for women with positive groin nodes is 30%, and 20% with positive pelvic nodes.[261]

Recurrence

About 80% of recurrences will develop within the first 2 years after initial treatment. Patients with less than three positive nodes generally exhibit a low incidence of recurrence, while high recurrence rates are correlated with patients who have more than three positive nodes.[261] Over half recur locally and are usually in close proximity to the original lesion.[3]

Surgery using wide local excision with adequate margins is the treatment of choice in recurrent disease. Occasionally, surgery, radiation, and/or chemotherapy will be utilized if recurrence occurs at a different site than the original malignancy. Groin recurrence may be treated with local radiotherapy, but surgery should be considered if the lesion is small and easily resectable.[3,265] A combination of radiation and chemotherapy may be considered as a palliative measure in metastatic disease.[264,265]

Future Trends

Interferon has been utilized in the treatment of condylomatous vulvitis and HPV-associated VIN.[241,266] It has the potential to offer safe, economical, and effective therapy.[242]

Further investigation is needed to define the population for whom a conservative surgical approach will not compromise cure. A growing body of knowledge suggests that certain early lesions could be placed in a microinvasive category.[16,257] This might allow for a more conservative treatment approach and still provide acceptable results. The term *microinvasion* remains controversial, as does the appropriate treatment for this stage of the disease.[16,267] Studies defining microinvasive carcinoma and those investigating methods to reduce the radical extent of surgical procedures are especially important.[16]

The use of chemoradiotherapy for debulking large vulvar tumors prior to surgical excision needs to be prospectively studied. The Gynecologic Oncology Group has a trial underway to determine this.[268]

To date, chemotherapy has not been effective in the treatment of this disease. Further research needs to be conducted to uncover effective chemotherapy protocols for use in the treatment of vulvar cancer.

VAGINAL CANCER

Epidemiology

Carcinoma of the vagina, a rare malignancy, accounts for 1%–2% of gynecologic malignancies.[5,16,269–272] Usually, vaginal tumors are secondary sites of malignant dissemination from primary cancers of the cervix or other sites.[272,273] The peak incidence of squamous carcinoma of the vagina, the most common cell type, occurs in women between 50 and 70 years of age. In contrast, the peak incidence for clear cell adenocarcinoma of the vagina occurs in women 18–19 years of age.

Vaginal intraepithelial neoplasia (VAIN) is much less common than cervical intraepithelial neoplasia or vulvar intraepithelial neoplasia, with incidence being only 3%–4% of CIN. However, incidence is climbing due to better diagnostic tools and cytologic screening.[274] VAIN is usually seen in women who have been treated for CIN or after radiotherapy for invasive cervical cancer. Up to 30% of patients with a primary vaginal malignancy have had prior cervical CIS.[243,272] Like CIN, VAIN is divided into three categories (I, II, III), with each higher number indicative of increasing epithelial involvement. Unlike CIN, VAIN is generally multifocal in nature.[3]

Etiology

Incidence of squamous cell cancer of the vagina increases with age. Rates are higher in the black population and persons with limited education and income. Other related risk factors include a history of HPV, vaginal trauma (douching with preparations other than water or vinegar), previous abdominal hysterectomy for benign disease, and absence of regular PAP smears[194,274,275] (Table 43-9).

Like squamous cell carcinoma, adenocarcinoma is usually a disease of older women. However, since 1971 the study of adenocarcinoma of the vagina has focused on young women exposed to diethylstilbestrol (DES) in utero, who seemed to have an unusual incidence of vaginal cancer. DES was used in the management of diabetic pregnancy, threatened abortion, habitual abortion, and other high-risk obstetric problems. From the late 1940s to 1970, an estimated 2 million pregnant women received DES.[276] For women exposed to DES in utero, the risk of developing vaginal cancer is about 1 in 1000. Of greater risk is the development of cervicovaginal dysplasia, which has been estimated to be as high as 18% in this population.[277]

Pathophysiology and Cellular Characteristics

Vaginal cancers occur most commonly on the posterior wall of the upper third of the vagina. The second most common site is the anterior wall in the lower one-third of the vagina.[272,273] The tumor may spread along the vaginal wall to involve the cervix or vulva. However, if the cervix is involved, the tumor is considered a primary cervical lesion.

Squamous cell carcinoma makes up 75%–95% of the cases.[270] Other histologic types include adenocarcinoma, melanoma, sarcoma, and verrucous carcinoma.[3,274,275,278]

Natural History

Anterior vaginal lesions penetrate into the vesicovaginal septum during early stages. Posterior lesions can invade the rectum, but this is usually in the late stages. The tumor spreads by direct extension into the obturator fossa, cardinal ligaments, lateral pelvic walls, and uterosacral ligament.[16]

The lymphatic drainage of the vagina consists of a vast, interconnecting network that facilitates drainage into any of the local nodal groups regardless of the location of the vaginal lesion. The incidence of lymph node metastasis is directly proportional to the stage of the vaginal cancer. The overall incidence of positive nodes is about 21%. Metastasis to the lungs or supraclavicular nodes in squamous cell carcinoma tends to occur in more advanced stages.[246] However, in clear cell carcinoma, metastasis to the lungs and supraclavicular nodes occurs more frequently.[16]

Extension or metastasis of other malignancies to the vagina occurs more often than primary cancer of the vagina. Spread of cervical cancer to the vagina is most common, but cancer of the endometrium, ovary, urethra, bladder, rectum, and malignant trophoblastic disease may also metastasize to the vaginal area.[3]

Clinical Manifestations

An abnormal Pap smear is usually the event that initiates the search for a definitive diagnosis since many lesions are asymptomatic. Colposcopic examination is done and biopsies taken. If left untreated, VAIN lesions may spontaneously regress, persist, or progress to vaginal cancer.[279]

The most common initial symptoms of invasive vaginal cancer are abnormal vaginal bleeding, foul-smelling discharge, and dysuria. Even in early-stage disease, urinary symptoms are more common when vaginal tumors are in close proximity to the bladder neck and compress the urethra.[3,273]

Assessment

Clinical diagnosis of a vaginal neoplasm is made by careful visual examination and palpation of the vagina. Pap smear is helpful for assessing squamous carcinoma, but not for adenocarcinoma because it is often subepithelial. Colposcopy is particularly useful for directed biopsies of abnormal vaginal areas.[16]

Women with invasive vaginal cancer should be investigated in the same way as those with cervical cancer. All patients should have a history and physical examination, chest radiograph, biochemical profile, IVP, barium enema, cystoscopy, and proctosigmoidoscopy. Optional, but often helpful, are CT, MRI, and lymphangiogram.[16,280]

Colposcopic exam allows visualization and determination of location, number, and size of lesions and is essential for planning appropriate therapeutic management.[274] The disease may then be evaluated and staged under anesthesia by the gynecologic oncologist and radiation therapist, and additional vaginal and cervical biopsies taken. Negative biopsies of the cervix are necessary to rule out cervical cancer and confirm the diagnosis of primary vaginal carcinoma. Vaginal cancer is staged clinically using one of the staging classification systems shown in Table 43-19.[56]

TABLE 43-19 Staging Classification for Carcinoma of the Vagina

PRIMARY TUMOR (T)

TNM	FIGO	Definition
TX		Primary tumor cannot be assessed
T0		No evidence of primary tumor
Tis	0	Carcinoma in situ
T1	I	Tumor confined to vagina
T2	II	Tumor invades paravaginal tissues but not to pelvic wall
T3	III	Tumor extends to pelvic wall
T4	IVa	Tumor invades mucosa of bladder or rectum and/or extends beyond the true pelvis
M1	IVb	Distant metastasis

LYMPH NODES (N)

NX Regional lymph nodes cannot be assessed
N0 No regional lymph node metastasis

Upper two-thirds of vagina:
N1 Pelvic lymph node metastasis

Lower one-third of vagina:
N1 Unilateral inguinal lymph node metastasis
N2 Bilateral inguinal lymph node metastasis

DISTANT METASTASIS (M)

TNM	FIGO	Definition
MX		Presence of distant metastasis cannot be assessed
M0		No distant metastasis
M1	IVb	Distant metastasis

STAGE GROUPING

Stage 0	Tis	N0	M0
Stage I	T1	N0	M0
Stage II	T2	N0	M0
Stage III	T1	N1	M0
	T2	N1	M0
	T3	N0, N1	M0
Stage IVA	T1	N2	M0
	T2	N2	M0
	T3	N2	M0
	T4	Any N	M0
Stage IVB	Any T	Any N	M1

Source: Reprinted from American Joint Committee on Cancer: *Manual for Staging of Cancer* (4th ed). Chicago: AJCC, 1992.

Treatment—VAIN

Location of the lesion, the size of the lesion, and whether it is a single focus or multiple foci are considered in determining the treatment option.[16] Local excision is appropriate for single lesions or for several lesions clustered in a single portion of the vagina.[16] Surgery for diffuse multiple lesions may result in a shortened or absent vagina.[243] Total vaginectomy with reconstruction should be reserved for the woman in whom more conservative therapy has failed.

Local application of 5-FU cream can be effective, but care must be taken to ensure direct contact with the entire lesion.[243,274,281] Laser therapy can cure between 69% and 80% of patients with vaginal intraepithelial lesions.[274] Results are especially good for single lesions or multifocal lesions clustered in one area of the vagina.[282] The use of intravaginal radiotherapy for the treatment of VAIN has been disappointing, with marked recurrences and vaginal morbidity including stenosis, fibrosis, fistula formation, dyspareunia, and precocious menopause.[243,274,283]

Treatment—Invasive Disease

Radiotherapy is the treatment of choice for most invasive vaginal cancers, especially for patients with stage I and II disease.[3,280] Small lesions may be treated with local irradiation, while larger lesions can require both local and regional treatment. In general, radiation treatment provides good control of tumor with limited morbidity.[280] The use of hyperfractionated, high-dose local radiotherapy concomitantly with chemotherapeutic drugs with both cytotoxic- and radiation-sensitizing properties is being explored.[284]

Surgery may be used in early-stage adenocarcinoma of the vagina. This may involve partial or total vaginectomy for stage I lesions in the lower vagina, or radical hysterectomy and upper vaginectomy plus pelvic lymphadenectomy for lesions in the upper vagina.[270] Lesions in the middle or lower vagina may require either anterior or posterior exenteration as the primary surgical therapy.[16]

A combination of surgery and radiation may be useful. Davis et al.[270] compared treatment with radiation alone, surgery alone, or surgery plus radiation in 89 women diagnosed with stage I or stage II disease. In this study the 5-year survival rate for women with stage I disease who received a combination of radiation and surgery was 100%. This fell to 69% for women with stage II disease.

Lesions that fail to respond to radiation can be treated effectively with surgery. Depending on the extent of disease, surgery for recurrence may range from wide local excision to total pelvic exenteration. With advanced disease in older women, surgery is often impossible if adjacent structures have been invaded and disease is too extensive.[261] In these cases, radiation may be the best treatment option. In stage IV, surgery is usually palliative, while radiation has not proven to be effective.[270]

Nursing Management—VAIN and Invasive Disease

General nursing care for the patient undergoing treatment for a malignancy is reviewed in Part III of this text. Refer to Table 43-12 for specific issues related to the nursing management of women diagnosed with VAIN or invasive vaginal cancer.

Results and Prognosis

The overall 5-year survival rate for all stages of squamous vaginal carcinoma is between 40% and 50%. The survival rate is 80% for patients with stage I, 48% for those with stage II, 30% for those with stage III, and 6% for those with stage IV.[270,272,280] The 5-year survival rate for patients with adenocarcinoma is 75%. This may be related to the fact that females exposed to DES in utero have been followed closely due to their risk for developing adenocarcinoma and are often diagnosed early in the disease.[3]

Clinical stage is the most important prognostic indicator in vaginal cancer. A better prognosis is associated with early diagnosis, small tumor burden, and negative nodal involvement. Other prognostic factors include age of the patient, location of the lesion, and differentiation of tumor. Well-differentiated tumors respond better to treatment and overall survival is improved.[280] Eighty percent of women who recur have pelvic recurrences within 2 years of primary treatment.[3]

Future Trends

Primary vaginal cancer is one of the rarest malignancies of the female genital tract. The number of cases seen in any one institution is usually limited; thus, there is little consensus on treatment. Radiotherapy is the most common form of treatment, with surgery utilized in selected cases.[285] Treatment of primary vaginal cancer remains a challenge. An individualized approach to treatment is the best option at this time.[272,286]

CONCLUSION

Gynecologic cancer represents about 12% of all cancers in women and results in 9% of all female cancer deaths.[1] The potential for cure is enhanced when the disease is diagnosed in early stages. Only cervical cancer has an effective screening method for early detection. Continued research is essential in order to identify sensitive and specific screening methods for early detection and to decrease the incidence of endometrial and ovarian cancers. Treatment modalities for women with gynecologic malignancies are often very aggressive regardless of whether the approach is surgery, radiotherapy, chemotherapy, or biologic therapy. This may result in profound physical, sexual, and psychosocial demands on the woman and her family. When recurrences appear, expectations for cure are unrealistic and effective palliation becomes a challenge. Until improved methods of screening for early detection are developed to reduce the incidence of gynecologic cancers, the search for more effective treatment to reduce mortality is a priority.

Finally, nursing management issues related to the care of the woman with gynecologic cancer need to be investigated. A study conducted by the Oncology Nursing Society[207] indicated that quality of life and symptom management were the top research priorities identified by oncology nurses. These were followed by outcome measures for interventions, pain control and management, cancer survivorship, prevention and early detection, research utilization, cancer rehabilitation, cost containment, and economic influences. Certainly, these issues are relevant to the care of the woman with gynecologic cancer. In addition, a survey of research priorities was conducted by the Gynecologic Oncology Group Nursing Research Subcommittee. The top-ranked categories for nursing research included identifying means of enhancing the patient's control of the illness and treatment, and quality-of-life issues.[288,289] The issues of defining toxicities for new treatments and interventions to reduce morbidity need to be studied. Quality of life related to the aggressive nature of the disease and the physically and emotionally demanding therapies also need to be pursued. Finally, women with gynecologic malignancies may need to address changes in body image, alterations in sexuality, and coping and stress management. These issues are important for the nurse researcher to pursue and are relevant to preventing cancer or assisting women and their families to live with the disease and its treatment.

REFERENCES

1. Boring CC, Squires TS, Tong T: Cancer statistics, 1993. *CA* 43(1):7–26, 1993.
2. Young RC: Gynecologic cancers. In Wittes RE (ed): *Manual of Oncologic Therapeutics: 1989/1990.* Philadelphia: Lippincott, 1989, pp. 270–291.
3. DiSaia PJ, Creasman WT: *Clinical Gynecologic Oncology.* St. Louis, MO: Mosby, 1989.
4. MacMahan B: Risk factors for endometrial cancer. *Gynecol Oncol* 2:122–129, 1974.
5. Smith DB: Gynecological cancers: Etiology and pathophysiology. *Semin Oncol Nurs* 2:270–274, 1986.
6. Ewertz M, Schou G, Blice JD Jr: The joint effect of risk factors on endometrial cancer. *Eur J Cancer Clin Oncol* 24:189–194, 1988.
7. Elliott EA, Matonoski GM, Rosenshein NB, et al: Body fat patterning in women with endometrial cancer. *Gynecol Oncol* 39:253–258, 1990.
8. Persson I, Adami HO, Bergkvist L, et al: Risk of endometrial cancer after treatment with oestrogens alone or in conjunction with progestogens: Results of a prospective study. *Br Med J* 298:147–151, 1989.
9. Hulka BS: Replacement estrogens and risk of gynecologic cancers and breast cancer. *Cancer* 60:1960–1964, 1987.
10. Franks AL, Kendrick JS, Tyler CW Jr: Postmenopausal smoking, estrogen therapy, and the risk of endometrial cancer. *Am J Obstet Gynecol* 156:20–23, 1987.
11. The Cancer and Steroid Hormone Study of the Centers for Disease Control and the National Institute of Child Health and Human Development. *JAMA* 257:796–800, 1987.
12. Hubbard JL, Holcombe JK: Cancer of endometrium. *Semin Oncol Nurs* 6:206–213, 1990.
13. Hacker NF: Uterine Cancer. In Berek JS, Hacker NJ (eds): *Practical Gynecologic Oncology.* Baltimore, MD: Williams & Wilkens, 1989, pp. 285–326.
14. Morrow CP, DiSaia PJ, Townsend DE: Current management of endometrial carcinoma. *Obstet Gynecol* 42:399–406, 1973.
15. Jones HW: Treatment of adenocarcinoma of the endometrium. *Obstet Gynecol Surg* 30:147–169, 1975.
16. Hoskins WJ, Perez C, Young RC: Gynecologic tumors. In DeVita VT Jr, Hellman S, Rosenberg SA (eds): *Cancer: Principles and Practice of Oncology* (3d ed). Philadelphia: Lippincott, 1989, pp. 1099–1161.
17. American Cancer Society: Summary of current guidelines for the cancer-related health check-up: Recommendations. New York: American Cancer Society, 1988.
18. Beecham JB, Helmkamp BF, Rubin P: Tumors of the female reproductive organs. In Rubin P (ed): *Clinical Oncology: A Multidisciplinary Approach.* New York: American Cancer Society, 1983, pp. 428–480.
19. Yazigi R, Cohen J, Munoz AK, et al: Magnetic resonance imaging determination of myometrial invasion in endometrial carcinoma. *Gynecol Oncol* 34:94–97, 1989.
20. Belloni C, Vigano R, delMaschio A, et al: Magnetic resonance imaging in endometrial carcinoma staging. *Gynecol Oncol* 37:172–177, 1990.
21. Shepherd JH: Revised FIGO staging for gynaecological cancer. *Br J Obstet Gynaecol* 96(8):889–892, 1989.
22. Axelrod JH, Roy T, King M: A phase II study of the treatment of stage III and IV disease of advanced endometrial carcinoma and all stages of papillary serous carcinoma and clear cell carcinoma of the endometrium with total abdominal radiation therapy. A Gynecologic Oncology Group (GOG) Study No. 94, Philadelphia, 1984.
23. Piver MS, Hempling RE: A retrospective trial of postoperative vaginal radium/cesium for grade 1–2 less than 50% myometrial invasion and pelvic radiation therapy for grade 3 or deep myometrial invasion in surgical stage I endometrial adenocarcinoma. *Cancer* 66:94–97, 1989.
24. Kauppila A, Gornroos N, Nieminen U: Clinical outcome in endometrial cancer. *Obstet Gynecol* 60:473–480, 1982.
25. Edmonson JH, Krook JE, Hilton JF, et al: Randomized phase II studies of cisplatin and a combination of cyclo-

phosphamide-doxorubicin-cisplatin (CAP) in patients with progestin-refractory advanced endometrial carcinoma. *Gynecol Oncol* 28:20–24, 1987.
26. Thigpen T, Vance R, Lambuth B, et al: Chemotherapy for advanced or recurrent gynecologic cancer. *Cancer* 60:2104–2116, 1987.
27. Weintraub NT, Freedman ML: Gynecologic malignancies of the elderly. *Clin Geriatr Med* 3:669–696, 1987.
28. Quinn MA, Campbell JJ: Tamoxifen therapy in advanced/recurrent endometrial carcinoma. *Gynecol Oncol* 32:1–3, 1989.
29. Thigpen T, Buchsbaum HJ, Mangan C, et al: Phase II trial of adriamycin in treatment of advanced or recurrent endometrial carcinoma. *Cancer Treat Rep* 63:21–27, 1979.
30. Seski JC, Edwards CL, Herson J, et al: Cisplatin chemotherapy for disseminated endometrial cancer. *Obstet Gynecol* 59:225–228, 1982.
31. Thigpen T, Shingleton H, Homesley H, et al: Phase II trial of cisplatinum in the management of advanced or recurrent endometrial carcinoma. *Proc Am Soc Clin Oncol* 22:469, 1981.
32. Thigpen JT, Blessing JA, Homesley H, et al: Phase II trial of cisplatin as first-line chemotherapy in patients with advanced or recurrent endometrial carcinoma: A Gynecologic Oncology Group Study. *Gynecol Oncol* 33:68–70, 1989.
33. Turbow MM, Thornton J, Ballon S, et al: Chemotherapy of advanced endometrial cancer with platinum, adriamycin and cyclophosphamide. *Proc Am Soc Clin Oncol* 1:108, 1982.
34. Randall ME, Spertos N, Dvoretsky P, et al: Whole abdominal radiotherapy versus circadian-timed combination doxorubicin-cisplatin chemotherapy in advanced endometrial carcinoma. A Gynecologic Oncology Group Study No. 122, Philadelphia, 1992.
35. Creasman WT, McCarty KS Sr, McCarty KS Jr: Clinical correlation of estrogen, progesterone binding proteins in human endometrial adenocarcinoma. *Obstet Gynecol* 55:363–370, 1980.
36. Utaaker E, Iversen OE, Skaarland E: The distribution and prognostic implications of steroid receptors in endometrial carcinomas. *Gynecol Oncol* 28:89–100, 1987.
37. Runowicz CD: Ovarian cancer. *Mediguide Oncol* 7:1–5, 1987.
38. Barber HRK: Ovarian cancer. *CA* 36:149–184, 1986.
39. Hubbard SM: Ovarian carcinoma: An overview of current concepts in diagnosis and management. *Cancer Nurs* 1:115–128, 1978.
40. Barber HRK: *Ovarian Carcinoma: Etiology, Diagnosis, and Treatment* (2d ed). New York: Masson, 1982.
41. Parazzini F, Franceschi S, LaVecchia C, et al: Review: The epidemiology of ovarian cancer. *Gynecol Oncol* 43:9–23, 1991.
42. Richardson GS, Scully RE, Nikrui N, et al: Common epithelial cancer of the ovary. *N Engl J Med* 312:474–483, 1985.
43. Heintz APM, Hacker NF, Lugasse LD: Epidemiology and etiology of ovarian cancer: A review. *Obstet Gynecol* 66:127–135, 1985.
44. Whittemore AS, Wu ML, Paffenbarger RS, et al: Epithelial ovarian cancer and the ability to conceive. *Cancer Res* 49:4047–4052, 1989.
45. Ozols RF, Young RC: Ovarian cancer. *Curr Probl Cancer* 11:57–122, 1987.
46. Piver MS, Baker TR, Piedmonte M, Sandecki AM: Epidemiology and etiology of ovarian cancer. *Semin Oncol* 18(3):177–185, 1991.
47. McGowan L: Ovarian cancer. In McGowan L (ed): *Gynecologic Oncology*. New York: Appleton-Century-Crofts, 1978.
48. Perez RP, Godwin AK, Hamilton TC, et al: Ovarian cancer biology. *Semin Oncol* 18:270–291, 1991.
49. Young R, Fuks Z, Hoskins WJ: Cancer of the ovary. In DeVita VT, Hellman S, Rosenberg SA (eds): *Cancer: Principles and Practice of Oncology* (3d ed). Philadelphia: Lippincott, 1989, pp. 1162–1196.
50. Piver MS, Barlow JJ, Lele SB: Incidence of sub-clinical metastasis in stage I and II ovarian carcinoma. *Obstet Gynecol* 52:100–104, 1978.
51. Higgins RV, VanNagell JR, Woods CH, et al: Interobserver variation in ovarian measurements using transvaginal sonography. *Gynecol Oncol* 39:69–71, 1990.
52. Higgins RV, VanNagell JR, Woods CH, et al: Interobserver variation in ovarian measurements using transvaginal sonography. *Gynecol Oncol* 34:402–406, 1989.
53. Campbell S, Bhan V, Royston J, et al: Screening for early ovarian cancer. *Lancet* 1:710–711, 1988.
54. Weiner Z, Thaler I, Beck D, et al: Differentiating malignant from benign ovarian tumors with transvaginal color flow imaging. *Obstet Gynecol* 79:159–162, 1992.
55. Kawai M, Kano T, Kikkawa F, et al: Transvaginal doppler ultrasound with color flow imaging in the diagnosis of ovarian cancer. *Obstet Gynecol* 79:163–167, 1992.
56. American Joint Committee on Cancer: *Manual for Staging of Cancer* (3d ed). Chicago: AJCC, 1988.
57. Eriksson JH, Walczak JR: Ovarian cancer. *Semin Oncol Nurs* 6:214–227, 1990.
58. Smith JP, Day TG: Review of ovarian cancer at the University of Texas Systems Cancer Center, M.D. Anderson Hospital and Tumor Institute. *Am J Obstet Gynecol* 135:984–993, 1979.
59. Young RC: Initial therapy for early ovarian carcinoma. *Cancer* 60:2042–2049, 1987.
60. Bristol Laboratories, Division of Bristol-Myers Co: Platinol: Effective palliation therapy in metastatic ovarian cancer. Syracuse, NY: Bristol Laboratories, 1982.
61. Stanhope CR, Smith JP: Ovarian cancer: The current approach to diagnosis and treatment. Syracuse, NY: Bristol Laboratories, 1981.
62. Young RC, Walton LA, Ellenberg SS, et al: Adjuvant therapy in stage I and stage II epithelial ovarian cancer. *N Engl J Med* 322:1021–1027, 1990.
63. Dottino PR, Plaxe SC, Cohen CJ: A phase II trial of adjuvant cisplatin and doxorubicin in stage I epithelial ovarian cancer. *Gynecol Oncol* 43:203–205, 1991.
64. Monga M, Carmichael JA, Shelley WE, et al: Surgery without adjuvant chemotherapy for early epithelial ovarian carcinoma after comprehensive surgical staging. *Gynecol Oncol* 43:195–197, 1991.
65. Gallion HH, van Nagell JR, Donaldson ES, et al: Adjuvant oral alkylating chemotherapy in patients with stage I epithelial ovarian cancer. *Cancer* 63:1070–1073, 1989.
66. Jacob JH, Gepshenson DM, Morris M, et al: Neoadjuvant chemotherapy and interval debulking for advanced epithelial ovarian cancer. *Gynecol Oncol* 42:146–150, 1991.
67. Dauplat J, Legros M, Condat P, et al: High dose melphalan and autologous bone marrow support for treatment of ovarian carcinoma with positive second look operation. *Gynecol Oncol* 34:294–298, 1989.

68. Shpall EJ, Clarke-Rearson D, Soper JT, et al: High-dose alkylating agent chemotherapy with autologous bone marrow support in patients with stage III/IV epithelial ovarian cancer. *Gynecol Oncol* 38:386–391, 1990.
69. Bruckner HW, Cohen CJ, Goldberg JD, et al: Improved chemotherapy for ovarian cancer with cis-diamminedichloroplatinum and adriamycin. *Cancer* 47:2288–2294, 1981.
70. Solomon JH, Atkinson KH, Coppleson JVM, et al: Ovarian carcinoma: Abdominopelvic irradiation following reexploration. *Gynecol Oncol* 31:396–401, 1988.
71. Lawton FG, Redman CW, Luesley DM, et al: Neoadjuvant (cytoreductive) chemotherapy combined with intervention debulking surgery in advanced, unresected epithelial ovarian cancer. *Obstet Gynecol* 73:61–65, 1989.
72. Sonnendecker EWW: Is routine second-look laparotomy for ovarian cancer justified? *Gynecol Oncol* 31:249–255, 1988.
73. Brand E, Wade ME, Lagasse LD: Resection of fixed pelvic tumors using the Nd: YAG laser. *J Surg Oncol* 37:246–251, 1988.
74. Deppe G, Malviya VK, Doike G, et al: Use of cavitron surgical aspirator for debulking of diaphragmatic metastases in patients with advanced carcinoma of the ovaries. *Gynecol Obstet* 168:455–456, 1989.
75. Deppe G, Malviya VK, Malone JM, et al: Debulking of pelvic and para-aortic lymph node metastases in ovarian cancer with the cavitron surgical aspirator. *Obstet Gynecol* 76:1140–1142, 1990.
76. Bast RC Jr, Hunter V, Knapp RC: Pros and cons of gynecologic tumor markers. *Cancer* 60:1984–1992, 1987.
77. Bast RC, Klug TL, St. John E, et al: A radioimmunoassay using a monoclonal antibody to monitor the course of epithelial ovarian cancer. *N Engl J Med* 309:883–887, 1983.
78. Neunteufel W, Breitenbecker G: Tissue expression of CA 125 in benign and malignant lesions of ovary and fallopian tube: A comparison with CA 19-9 and CEA. *Gynecol Oncol* 33:297–302, 1989.
79. Niloff JM, Bast RC Jr, Schaetzl EM, et al: Predictive value of CA 125 antigen levels at second look procedures in ovarian cancer. *Am J Obstet Gynecol* 151:981–986, 1985.
80. Berek JS, Knapp PC, Malkasian GD, et al: CA 125 serum levels correlate with second-look operations among ovarian cancer patients: A prospective multi-institutional study. *Obstet Gynecol* 67:685–689, 1986.
81. Jager W, Adam R, Wildt L, et al: Serum CA-125 as a guideline for the timing of a second-look operation and second-line treatment in ovarian cancer. *Arch Gynecol Obstet* 243:91–99, 1988.
82. Potter ME, Moradi M, To ACW, et al: Value of serum CA 125 levels: Does the result preclude a second look? *Gynecol Oncol* 33:201–203, 1989.
83. MacDonald F, Bird R, Stokes H, et al: Expression of CEA, CA 125, CA 19-9 and human milk fat globule membrane antigen in ovarian tumours. *J Clin Pathol* 41:260–264, 1988.
84. Fioretti P, Gadducci A, Ferdeghini M, et al: Correlation of CA 125 and CA 19-9 serum levels with clinical course and second-look findings in patient with ovarian carcinoma. *Gynecol Oncol* 28:278–283, 1987.
85. Tobias JS, Griffiths CT: Management of ovarian carcinoma. *N Engl J Med* 294:818–823, 1976.
86. Gershenson DM, Taylor Wharton J, Copeland LJ, et al: Treatment of advanced epithelial ovarian cancer with cisplatin and cyclophosphamide. *Gynecol Oncol* 32:336–341, 1989.
87. Young RC, Chabner BA, Hubbard SM: Prospective trials of melphalan (L-PAM) versus combination chemotherapy (Hexa-CAF) in ovarian adenocarcinoma. *N Engl J Med* 299:1261–1266, 1978.
88. Bruckner HW, Cohen CJ, Feuer E, et al: Prognostic factors: Cisplatin regimens for patients with ovarian cancer after failure of chemotherapy. *Obstet Gynecol* 69:114–120, 1987.
89. Vogl SE, Pagano M, Kaplan BH, et al: Cis-platin based combination chemotherapy for advanced ovarian cancer. *Cancer* 51:2024–2030, 1983.
90. Thigpen JT, Blessing JA, Vance RB, et al: Chemotherapy in ovarian carcinoma: Present role and future prospects. *Semin Oncol* 16:58–65, 1989.
91. Ovarian Cancer Meta-Analysis Project: Cyclophosphamide plus cisplatin versus cyclophosphamide, doxorubicin, and cisplatin chemotherapy of ovarian carcinoma: A meta-analysis. *J Clin Oncol* 9:1668–1674, 1991.
92. ten Bokkel Huinink WW, van der Berg MEL, van Oosterom AT, et al: Carboplatin in combination therapy for ovarian cancer. *Cancer Treat Rev* 15:9–15, 1988(suppl B).
93. Yarbro CH: Carboplatin: A clinical review. *Semin Oncol Nurs* 15:63–69, 1989(suppl).
94. Rothenberg ML, Ostchega Y, Steinberg SM, et al: High-dose carboplatin with diethyldithiocarbamate chemoprotection in treatment of women with relapsed ovarian cancer. *JNCI* 80:1488–1492, 1988.
95. Reed E, Janik J, Bookman M, et al: High-dose chemotherapy and rGM-CSF in refractory ovarian cancer. *Proc Am Soc Clin Oncol* 9:157, 1990.
96. Mulder PO, Willemse H, Aalders JG, et al: High dose chemotherapy with autologous bone marrow transplantation in patients with refractory ovarian cancer. *Eur J Cancer Clin Oncol* 25:645–649, 1989.
97. Alberts DS, Garcia-Kendall D, Surwit EA: Phase II trial of mitomycin C plus 5-FU in the treatment of drug-refractory ovarian cancer. *Semin Oncol* 15:22–26, 1988(suppl 4).
98. McGuire WP, Rowinsky EK, Rosenshein NB, et al: Taxol: A unique antineoplastic agent with significant activity in advanced ovarian epithelial neoplasms. *Ann Intern Med* 111:273–279, 1989.
99. McGuire WP, Rowinsky EK: Old drugs revisited, new drugs and experimental approaches in ovarian cancer therapy. *Semin Oncol* 18:255–269, 1991.
100. McGuire WP, Hoskins WJ, Woodward J: A phase III randomized study of cyclosphosphamide and cisplatin versus taxol and cisplatin: A Gynecologic Oncology Group study No. 111, Philadelphia, 1990.
101. Muggia F, Braly PS: A phase III randomized study of cisplatin versus taxol versus taxol and cisplatin in patients with suboptimal stage III and IV epithelial ovarian cancer: A Gynecologic Oncology Group study No. 132, Philadelphia, 1992.
102. Fojo A, Hamilton TC, Young RC, et al: Multidrug resistance in ovarian cancer. *Cancer* 60:2075–2080, 1987.
103. Donehower RC, Rosenshein NB, Rotmensch J, et al: Sequential methotrexate and 5-fluorouracil in advanced ovarian carcinoma. *Gynecol Oncol* 27:90–96, 1987.
104. Goodman HM, Dottino PR, Kredenster D, et al: Continuous infusion fluoropyrimidines as salvage therapy for patients with advanced ovarian carcinoma. *Gynecol Oncol* 29:348–355, 1988.

105. Markman M: Intraperitoneal chemotherapy as treatment of ovarian carcinoma: Why, how and when? *Obstet Gynecol Survey* 42:533–539, 1987.
106. Ozols RF: Intraperitoneal chemotherapy. *Mediguide Oncol* 5:1–5, 1986.
107. Markman M: Intraperitoneal chemotherapy. *Semin Oncol* 18:248–254, 1991.
108. Jones RB, Collins JM, Myers CE, et al: High volume intraperitoneal chemotherapy with methotrexate in patients with cancer. *Cancer Res* 41:55–59, 1981.
109. Ozols RF, Young RC, Speyer JL, et al: Phase I and pharmacological studies of adriamycin administered intraperitoneally to patients with ovarian cancer. *Cancer Res* 42:4265–4269, 1982.
110. Speyer J, Collins JM, Dedrick RL, et al: Phase I and pharmacological studies of 5-FU administered intraperitoneally. *Cancer* 40:567–572, 1980.
111. Howell SB, Pfeifle CL, Wung WE, et al: Intraperitoneal cisplatin with systemic thiosulfate protection. *Ann Intern Med* 97:845–851, 1982.
112. Monk BJ, Surwit EA, Alberts DS, et al: Intraperitoneal mitomycin C in the treatment of peritoneal carcinomatosis following second-look surgery. *Semin Oncol* 15:27–31, 1988.
113. Loeffler T, Freund W: Pharmacokinetics of mitoxantrone intraperitoneal. *Proc Am Assoc Cancer Res* 27:175, 1986.
114. King ME, Pfeifle CE, Howell SB: Intraperitoneal cytosine arabinoside in ovarian carcinoma. *J Clin Oncol* 2:662, 1984.
115. Berek JS, Hacker NF, Lichtenstein A, et al: Intraperitoneal recombinant alpha-interferon for "salvage" immunotherapy in stage III epithelial ovarian cancer: A Gynecologic Oncology Group study. *Cancer Res* 45:4447–4453, 1985.
116. Piccart MJ, Abrams J, Dodion PF, et al: Intraperitoneal chemotherapy with cisplatin and melphalan. *JNCI* 80:1118–1124, 1988.
117. Hamilton TC, Ozols RF, Longo DL: Biologic therapy for the treatment of malignant common epithelial tumors in the ovary. *Cancer* 60:2054–2063, 1987.
118. Chapman PB, Hakes T, Gabrilove JL, et al: A phase I pilot study of intraperitoneal rIL-2 in ovarian cancer. *Proc Am Soc Clin Oncol* 5:23, 1986.
119. Smith LH, Tend NNH: Clinical applications of monoclonal antibodies in gynecologic oncology. *Cancer* 60:2068–2074, 1987.
120. Pommier RF, Woltering EA, Milo G, et al: Synergistic cytotoxicity between dimethyl sulfoxide and antineoplastic agents against ovarian cancer in vitro. *Am J Obstet Gynecol* 159:848–852, 1988.
121. Rubin SC, Hoskins WJ, Markman M, et al: Long-term access to the peritoneal cavity in ovarian cancer patients. *Gynecol Oncol* 33:46–48, 1989.
122. Kavanagh JJ, Roberts W, Townsend P, et al: Leuprolide acetate in the treatment of refractory or persistent epithelial ovarian cancer. *J Clin Oncol* 7:115–118, 1989.
123. Weiner SA, Alberts DS, Surwit EA, et al: Tamoxifen therapy in recurrent epithelial ovarian carcinoma. *Gynecol Oncol* 27:208–213, 1987.
124. Belinson JL, McClure M, Badger G: Randomized trial of megestrol acetate vs megestrol acetate/tamoxifen for the management of progressive or recurrent epithelial ovarian carcinoma. *Gynecol Oncol* 28:151–155, 1987.
125. Pezner RD, Stevens KR Jr, Tong D, et al: Limited epithelial carcinoma of the ovary treated with curative intent by intraperitoneal instillation of radiocolloids. *Cancer* 42:2563–2571, 1978.
126. Potter ME, Partridge EE, Shingleton HM, et al: Intraperitoneal chromic phosphate in ovarian cancer: Risks and benefits. *Gynecol Oncol* 32:314–318, 1989.
127. Weiser EB, Burke TW, Heller PB, et al: Determinants of survival of patients with epithelial ovarian carcinoma following whole abdomen irradiation (WAR). *Gynecol Oncol* 30:201–208, 1988.
128. Schray MF, Martinez A, Howes AE, et al: Advanced epithelial ovarian cancer: Salvage whole abdominal irradiation for patients with recurrent or persistent disease after combination chemotherapy. *J Clin Oncol* 6:1433–1439, 1988.
129. Bolis G, Zanaboni F, Vanoli P, et al: The impact of whole abdominal radiotherapy on survival in advanced ovarian cancer patients with minimal residual disease after chemotherapy. *Gynecol Oncol* 39:150–154, 1990.
130. Linstach DE, Stern JL, Quirey JM, et al: Salvage whole abdominal irradiation following chemotherapy failure in epithelial ovarian carcinoma. *Gynecol Oncol* 36:327–330, 1990.
131. Creasman WT, Yale SA, Blessing JA, et al: Chemoimmunotherapy in the management of primary stage III ovarian cancer: A Gynecologic Oncology Group study. *Cancer Treat Rep* 63:319–323, 1979.
132. Alberts DS, Moon TE, Stephens RA, et al: Randomized trials of chemoimmunotherapy for advanced ovarian carcinoma: A preliminary report of a Southwest Oncology Group Study. *Cancer Treat Rep* 63:325–331, 1979.
133. Alberts DS, Mason-Liddil N, O'Toole RV, et al: Randomized phase III trial of chemoimmunotherapy in patients with previously untreated stages III and IV suboptimal disease ovarian cancer: A Southwest Oncology Group study. *Gynecol Oncol* 32:8–15, 1989.
134. Einhorn N, Cantell K, Einhorn S, et al: Human leukocyte interferon therapy for advanced ovarian cancer. *Am J Clin Oncol* 5:167–172, 1987.
135. Welander CE: Use of interferon in the treatment of ovarian cancer as a single agent and in combination with cytotoxic drugs. *Cancer* 59:617–619, 1987.
136. Lichtenstein A, Spina C, Berek JS, et al: Intraperitoneal administration of human recombinant interferon-alpha in patients with ovarian cancer: Effects on lymphocyte phenotype and cytotoxicity. *Cancer Res* 48:5853–5859, 1988.
137. Rowinsky E, Grochow L, Hendricks C, et al: Phase I and pharmacologic study of topotecan: A novel topoisomerase I inhibitor. *Proc Am Soc Clin Oncol* 10:240, 1991.
138. Alberts DS, Garcia D, Roe D, et al: Lack of tetraplatin cross resistance with cisplatin against epithelial ovarian cancers obtained from more than 70 patients with advanced disease. *Proc Am Assoc Cancer Res* 32:2434, 1991.
139. Bookman MA, Bast RC: The immunobiology and immunotherapy of ovarian cancer. *Semin Oncol* 18:270–291, 1991.
140. Hamilton T, O'Dwyer P, Young R, et al: Phase I trial of buthionine sulfoximine (BSO) plus melphalan (L-PAM) in patients with advanced ovarian cancer. *Proc Am Soc Clin Oncol* 9:73, 1990.
141. Shilder RJ, Nash S, Tew KD, et al: Phase I trial of thiotepa (TT) in combination with the glutathione transferase inhibitor ethacrynic acid (EA). *Proc Am Assoc Cancer Res* 31:177, 1990.
142. Celentano DD, Shapiro S, Weisman CS: Cancer: Pre-

ventive screening behavior among elderly women. *Prev Med* 11:454–463, 1982.

143. Anderson M: The pathology of tumors of the cervix. In Blackledge GRP, Jordan JA, Shingleton HM (eds): *Textbook of Gynecologic Oncology*. Philadelphia: Saunders, 1991, pp. 265–283.
144. Spano, WJ, King A, Keeney E, et al: Age as a prognostic factor in carcinoma of the cervix. *Gynecol Oncol* 35:66–68, 1989.
145. Lovejoy NC: Precancerous lesions of the cervix: Personal risk factors. *Cancer Nurs* 10:2–14, 1987.
146. Hildesheim A, Reeves WC, Brenton LA, et al: Association of oral contraceptive use and human pappillomaviruses in invasive cervical cancers. *Int J Cancer* 45:860–864, 1990.
147. Parazzini P, La Vecchia C, Negri E, et al: Oral contraceptive use and invasive cervical cancer. *Int J Epidemiol* 19:259–263, 1990.
148. Herrero R, Brinton LA, Reeves WC et al: Risk factors for invasive carcinoma of the uterine cervix in Latin America. *Bulletin of PAHO* 24:263–283, 1990.
149. Cuzick J, Boyle P: Trends in cervix cancer mortality. *Cancer Surv* 7(3), 1988.
150. Burke L, Antonioli DA, Ducatman BS: *Colposcopy: Text and Atlas*. Norwalk, CT: Appleton & Lange, 1991.
151. Meanwell CA: The epidemiology and etiology of cervical cancer. In Blackwell GRP, Jordan JA, Shingleton HM (eds): *Textbook of Gynecologic Oncology*. Philadelphia: Saunders, 1991, pp. 250–264.
152. Vonka V, Kanka J, Jelinek J, et al: Prospective study on the relationship between cervical neoplasia and herpes simplex type-2 virus. I. Epidemiology characteristics. *Int J Cancer* 33:49–60, 1984.
153. Koss LG: Cytologic and histological manifestations of human papillomavirus infection of the female genital tract and their clinical significance. *Cancer* 60:1942–1950, 1987.
154. Syrjanen K, Vayrynen M, Saarikoski S, et al: Natural history of cervical human papillomavirus (HPV) infections based on prospective follow-up. *Br J Obstet Gynaecol* 92:1086–1092, 1985.
155. Meanwell CA, Blackledge G, Cox MF, et al: HPV 16 DNA in normal and malignant cervical epithelium: Implications for the aetiology and behaviour of cervical neoplasia. *Lancet* 1:703–707, 1987.
156. Howley PM, Schlegel R: The human papillomaviruses. *Am J Med* 85:155–158, 1988(suppl 2A).
157. Richart RM: Causes and management of cervical intraepithelial neoplasia. *Cancer* 60:1951–1959, 1987.
158. Lorincz AT, Reid R, Jenson AB, et al: Human papillomavirus infection of the cervix: Relative risk associations of 15 common anogenital types. *Obstet Gynecol* 79:328–337, 1992.
159. Pao CC, Lin CY, Chang YL, et al: Human papillomaviruses and small cell carcinoma of the uterine cervix. *Gynecol Oncol* 43:206–210, 1991.
160. Wright TC, Richart RM: Role of human papillomavirus in the pathogenesis of genital tract warts and cancer. *Gynecol Oncol* 37:151–164, 1990.
161. Boshart M, Gissmann L, Ikenberg H, et al: A new type of papillomavirus DNA, its presence in genital cancer biopsies and in cell lines derived from cervical cancer. *EMBO J* 3:1151–1157, 1984.
162. McCance DJ, Campion MJ, Clarkson PK, et al: Prevalence of human papillomavirus type 16 DNA sequences in cervical intraepithelial neoplasia and invasive carcinoma of the cervix. *Br J Obstet Gynaecol* 92:1101–1105, 1985.
163. Yoshikawa H, Matsukura T, Yamamoto E, et al: Occurrence of human papillomavirus type 16 and 18 DNA in cervical carcinoma from Japan: Age of patients and histologic type of carcinomas. *Jpn J Cancer Res* 76:667–671, 1985.
164. Hadjimichael O, Janerich D, Lowell DM, et al: Histologic and clinical characteristics associated with rapidly progressive invasive cervical cancer: A preliminary report from the Yale Cancer Control Research Unit. *Yale J Biol Med* 62:345–350, 1989.
165. Tase T, Okagaki T, Manias DA, et al: Human papilloma virus types and localization in adenocarcinomas and adenosquamous carcinoma of the uterine cervix: A study by in situ DNA hybridization. *Cancer Res* 48:993–998, 1988.
166. Eddy DM: Screening for cervical cancer. *Ann Intern Med* 113:214–226, 1990.
167. Anthony CP: *Textbook of Anatomy and Physiology*. St. Louis, MO: Mosby, 1983.
168. Jones HW, Jones GS: *Novak's Textbook of Gynecology*. Baltimore, MD: Williams & Wilkins, 1981.
169. Hopkins MP: Diseases of the vulva. In Wilson JR, Carrington LR (eds): *Obstetrics and Gynecology*. St. Louis, MO: Mosby Year Book, 1991, pp. 550–563.
170. Lundberg GD: The 1988 Bethesda System for reporting cervical/vaginal cytological diagnoses. *JAMA* 262:931–934, 1989.
171. Koss LG: The New Bethesda System for reporting results of smears of the uterine cervix. *JNCI* 82:988–991, 1990.
172. Soloman D: The 1988 Bethesda System for reporting cervical/vaginal cytologic diagnoses. *J Reprod Med* 34:779–783, 1989.
173. Kurman RJ, Malkasian GD, Sedlis A, et al: From Papanicolaou to Bethesda: The rationale for a new cervical cytologic classification. *Obstet Gynecol* 77:779–782, 1991.
174. Herbst AL: The Bethesda System for cervical/vaginal cytologic diagnoses: A note of caution. *Obstet Gynecol* 76:449–450, 1990 (editorial).
175. Bottles K, Reiter RC, Steiner AL, et al: Problems encountered with the Bethesda System: The University of Iowa experience. *Obstet Gynecol* 78:410–413, 1991.
176. Vooijs GP: Does the Bethesda System promote or endanger the quality of cervical cytology? *Acta Cytol* 34:455–456, 1990.
177. Caputo TA: Uterine cervical cancer: The current approach to diagnosis and treatment. Syracuse, NY: Bristol Laboratories, 1979.
178. Brand E, Berek JS, Hacker NF: Controversies in the management of cervical adenocarcinoma. *Obstet Gynecol* 71:261–269, 1988.
179. Carlson V, Delclos L, Fletcher GH: Distant metastases in squamous-cell carcinoma of the uterine cervix. *Radiology* 88:961–966, 1967.
180. Cashavelly BJ: Cervical dysplasia: An overview of current concepts in epidemiology, diagnosis, and treatments. *Cancer Nurs* 10:199–206, 1987.
181. Shy K: Concepts in the application of cervical cytology. In Greer BE, Berek JS (eds): *Gynecologic Oncology: Treatment Rationale and Techniques*. New York: Elsevier, 1991, pp. 13–32.
182. Stenkvist B, Bergstrom R, Brinne U, et al: Automated

analysis of Papanicolaou smears by digital image processing. *Gynecol Oncol* 27:1–14, 1987.

183. Fink DJ: Change in American Cancer Society checkup guidelines for detection of cervical cancer. *CA* 38:127–128, 1988.
184. Schwartz PE, Merino MJ, McCrea Curnen MG: Clinical management of patients with invasive cervical cancer following a negative Pap smear. *Yale J Biol Med* 61:327–338, 1988.
185. Kern WH, Zivolich MR: The accuracy and consistency of the cytologic classification of squamous lesions of the uterine cervix. *Acta Cytol* 21:519–523, 1977.
186. Learmonth GM, Durcan CM, Beck JD: The changing incidence of cervical intra-epithelial neoplasia. *SAMJ* 77:637–639, 1989.
187. Hatch K, Helm CW: Cancer of the cervix—surgical treatment. In Blackledge GRP, Jordan JA, Shingleton HM (eds): *Textbook of Gynecologic Oncology.* Philadelphia: Saunders, 1991, pp. 313–327.
188. Masterson BJ, Krantz KE, Calkins JW, et al: The carbon dioxide laser in cervical epithelial neoplasia: A five-year experience in treating 230 patients. *Am J Obstet Gynecol* 139:565–567, 1981.
189. Burke L: The use of carbon dioxide laser in the therapy of cervical intraepithelial neoplasia. *Am J Obstet Gynecol* 144:337–340, 1982.
190. Anderson MC: Treatment of cervical intraepithelial neoplasia with the carbon dioxide laser: Report of 543 patients. *Obstet Gynecol* 59:720–725, 1982.
191. Reid R: Preinvasive disease. In Berek JS, Hacker NF (eds): *Practical Gynecologic Oncology.* Baltimore, MD: Williams & Wilkins, 1989, pp. 195–239.
192. Tabbara S, Saleh ADM, Andersen WA, et al: The Bethesda classification for squamous intraepithelial lesions: Histologic, cytologic, and viral correlates. *Obstet Gynecol* 79:338–346, 1992.
193. Nelson JH, Averette HE, Richart RM: Cervical intraepithelial neoplasia (dysplasia and carcinoma in situ) and early invasive cervical carcinoma. *CA* 39:157–178, 1989.
194. Yliskoski M, Cantell K, Syrjanen K, et al: Topical treatment with human leukocyte interferon of HPV 16 infections associated with cervical and vaginal intraepithelial neoplasias. *Gynecol Oncol* 36:353–357, 1990.
195. Iwasaka T, Hayashi Y, Yokoyama M, et al: Interferon *y* treatment for cervical intraepithelial neoplasia. *Gynecol Oncol* 37:96–102, 1990.
196. McDonald TW, Neutens JJ, Fischer LM, et al: Impact of cervical intraepithelial neoplasia diagnosis and treatment on self-esteem and body image. *Gynecol Oncol* 34:345–349, 1989.
197. Lamb MA: Sexual dysfunction in the gynecologic oncology patient. *Semin Oncol Nurs* 1:9–17, 1985.
198. Young RD: Gynecologic cancers. In Wittes RE (ed): *Manual of Oncologic Therapeutics: 1989/1990.* Philadelphia: Lippincott, 1989, pp. 270–291.
199. Hernandez E, Rosenshein NB: *Manual of Gynecologic Oncology.* New York: Churchill Livingstone, 1989.
200. Chan KK: The presentation of carcinoma of the cervix. In Blackledge GRP, Jordan JA, Shingleton HM (eds): *Textbook of Gynecology Oncology.* Philadelphia: Saunders, 1991, pp. 306–312.
201. Greer BE, Berek JS (eds): *Gynecologic Oncology: Treatment Rationale and Techniques.* New York: Elsevier, 1991.
202. Walsh JW, Amendola MA, Konerding KF, et al: Computed tomographic detection of pelvic and inguinal lymph node metastases from primary and recurrent pelvic malignant diseases. *Radiology* 137:157–166, 1980.
203. Lewis E: The use and abuse of imaging in gynecologic cancer. *Cancer* 60:1993–2009, 1987.
204. Burghardt E, Hofmann HMH, Ebner F, et al: Magnetic resonance imaging in cervical cancer: A basis for objective classification. *Gynecol Oncol* 33:61–67, 1989.
205. Rose PG, Watkins E, Amyot K, et al: A randomized comparison of hydroxyurea *versus* hydroxyurea, 5FU infusion, and bolus cisplatin *versus* weekly cisplatin as adjunct to radiation therapy in patients with stage IIb, III, IVa carcinoma of the cervix and negative paraaortic nodes. Philadelphia: Gynecology Oncology Group, 1992.
206. Varia MA, Remmenga S, Evers C, et al: Extended field radiation therapy with concomitant 5FU infusion and cisplatin chemotherapy in patients with cervical carcinoma metastatic to para aortic lymph nodes. Philadelphia: Gynecology Oncology Group, 1992.
207. Hatch KD: Cervical cancer. In Berek JS, Hacker NF (eds): *Practical Gynecology Oncology.* Baltimore, MD: Williams & Wilkins, 1989, pp. 241–284.
208. Omura GA: Chemotherapy of cervix cancer. In Blackledge GRP, Jordon JA, Shingleton HM (eds): *Textbook of Gynecologic Oncology.* Philadelphia: Saunders, 1991, pp. 361–368.
209. Kolstad P: Follow-up study of 232 patients with stage 1a1 and 411 patients with stage 1a2 squamous cell carcinoma of the cervix (microinvasive carcinoma). *Gynecol Oncol* 33:265–272, 1989.
210. Perez CA: Radiation treatment of carcinoma of the uterine cervix. In Blackledge GRP, Jordan JA, Shingleton HM (eds): *Textbook of Gynecologic Oncology.* Philadelphia: Saunders, 1991, pp. 328–360.
211. Kinney WK, Alvarez RD, Reid GC, et al: Value of adjuvant whole-pelvis irradiation after Wertheim hysterectomy for early-stage squamous carcinoma of the cervix with pelvic nodal metastasis: A matched-control study. *Gynecol Oncol* 34:258–262, 1989.
212. Clarke-Pearson DL, Soisson AP, Wall LL: Surgical treatment of early-stage cervical cancer. In Greer BE, Berek JS (eds): *Gynecologic Oncology: Treatment Rationale and Techniques.* New York: Elsevier, 1991, pp. 187–206.
213. Jones WB: Surgical approaches for advanced or recurrent cancer of the cervix. *Cancer* 60:2094–2103, 1987.
214. Perez CA, Breaux S, Bedwinek JM, et al: Radiation therapy alone in treatment of the uterine cervix. II. Analysis of complications. *Cancer* 54:235–246, 1984.
215. Henriksen E: The lymphatic spread of carcinoma of the cervix and the body of the uterus. *Am J Obstet Gynecol* 58:924–942, 1949.
216. Osborne RJ, Murphy KJ, DePetrillo AD: Pelvic exenteration. In Greer BE, Berek JS (eds): *Gynecologic Oncology: Treatment Rationale and Techniques.* New York: Elsevier, 1991, pp. 207–226.
217. Lagasse LD, Johnson GH, Smith ML, et al: Use of sigmoid colon for rectal substitution following pelvic exenteration. *Am J Obstet Gynecol* 116:106–110, 1973.
218. Hatch KD, Shingleton HM, Potter ME, et al: Low rectal resection and anastomosis at the time of pelvic exenteration. *Gynecol Oncol* 31:262–267, 1988.
219. Thigpen JT: Chemotherapy of cancers of the female genital tract. In Perry MC (ed): *The Chemotherapy Sourcebook.* Baltimore, MD: Williams & Wilkins, 1992, pp. 1039–1067.
220. Hannigan EV, Dinh TV, Doherty MG: Ifosfamide with

Mesna in squamous carcinoma of the cervix: Phase II results in patients with advanced or recurrent disease. *Gynecol Oncol* 43:123–129, 1991.

221. Kim DS, Moon H, Kim KT, et al: Two-year survival: Preoperative adjuvant chemotherapy in the treatment of cervical cancer stage 1b and II with bulky tumor. *Gynecol Oncol* 33:225–230, 1989.
222. Kim DS, Moon H, Hwang YY, et al: Preoperative adjuvant chemotherapy in the treatment of cervical cancer stage 1b, IIa, and IIb with bulky tumor. *Gynecol Oncol* 29:321–332, 1988.
223. Kredentser DC: Etoposide (VP-16), ifosfamide/mesna, and cisplatin chemotherapy for advanced and recurrent carcinoma of the cervix. *Gynecol Oncol* 43:145–148, 1991.
224. Piver MS, Barlow JJ, Vongtama V, et al: Hydroxyurea and radiation therapy in advanced cervical cancer. *Am J Obstet Gynecol* 120:969–972, 1974.
225. Hreshchyshyn MM, Aron BS, Boronow RC, et al: Hydroxyurea or placebo combined with radiation to treat stage IIIB and IV cervical cancer confined to the pelvis. *Int J Radiat Oncol Biol Phys* 5:317–322, 1979.
226. Kuske RR, Perez CA, Grigsby PW, et al: Phase I/II study of definitive radiotherapy and chemotherapy (cisplatin and 5-fluorouracil) for advanced or recurrent gynecologic malignancies. *Am J Clin Oncol* 12:467–473, 1989.
227. Weiner SA, Aristizabal S, Alberts DS, et al: A phase II trial of mitomycin, vincristine, bleomycin, and cisplatin (MOBP) as neoadjuvant therapy in high-risk cervical carcinoma. *Gynecol Oncol* 30:1–6, 1988.
228. Vogl SE: Chemotherapy of squamous cell carcinoma of the uterine cervix: Progress and potential. *Curr Concepts Oncol* 5:10–11, 15–17, 1983.
229. Stuart GCE, Robertson DI, Fedorkow DM, et al: Recurrent and persistent squamous cell cervical carcinoma in women under age 35. *Gynecol Oncol* 30:163–172, 1988.
230. Dutcher JP, Wadler S, Wiernik PH: Biologic response modifiers in gynecologic malignancies. *Yale J Bio Med* 61:367–378, 1988.
231. Berchuck A, Rodriguez G, Bast RC: Recent advances in immunodiagnosis and immunotherapy. In Greer BE, Berek JS (eds): *Gynecologic Oncology: Treatment Rationale and Techniques.* New York: Elsevier, 1991, pp. 33–56.
232. Brady LW, Markoe AM, DeEulis T, et al: Treatment of advanced and recurrent gynecologic cancer. *Cancer* 60:2081–2093, 1987.
233. Wang CC: Altered fractionation radiation therapy for gynecologic cancers. *Cancer* 60:2064–2067, 1987.
234. Crum CP: Carcinoma of the vulva: Epidemiology and pathogenesis. *Obstet Gynecol* 79:448–454, 1992.
235. Cavanagh D, Fiorica JV, Hoffman MS, et al: Invasive carcinoma of the vulva. *Am J Obstet Gynecol* 163:1007–1014, 1990.
236. Husseinzadah N, Wesseler T, Schneider D, et al: Prognostic factors and the significance of cytologic grading in invasive squamous cell carcinoma of the vulva: A clinicopathologic study. *Gynecol Oncol* 36:192–199, 1990.
237. Rollason TP: Vulva and vagina: Pathology of malignant tumors. In Blackledge GRP, Jordan JA, Shingleton HM (eds): *Textbook of Gynecologic Oncology.* Philadelphia: Saunders, 1991, pp. 390–411.
238. Husseinzadeh N, Newman NJ, Wesseler, TA: Vulvar intraepithelial neoplasia: A clinicopathological study of carcinoma in situ of the vulva. *Gynecol Oncol* 33:159–163, 1989.
239. Woodruff JD: Pathology. In Berek JS, Hacker NF (eds): *Practical Gynecologic Oncology.* Baltimore, MD: Williams & Wilkins, 1989, pp. 109–166.
240. Barbero M, Micheletti L, Preti M, et al: Vulvar intraepithelial neoplasia: A clinicopathologic study of 6 cases. *J Reprod Med* 35:1023–1027.
241. di Paola GR, Belardi MG: Squamous vulvar intraepithelial neoplasia. In Knapstein PG, diRe F, Disaia P, et al (eds): *Malignancies of the Vulva.* New York: Thieme Medical Publishers, 1991, pp. 57–72.
242. Green TH: Carcinoma of the vulva: A reassessment. *Obstet Gynecol* 50:462–468, 1978.
243. Nolte S, Hanjani P: Intraepithelial neoplasia of the lower genital tract. *Semin Oncol Nurs* 6:181–189, 1990.
244. Morrow CP, Townsend DE (eds): *Synopsis of Gynecologic Oncology* (3d ed). New York: Wiley, 1987.
245. Baker VV: The etiology and epidemiology of vulvar and vaginal neoplasms. In Blackledge GRP, Jordan JA, Shingleton HM (eds): *Textbook of Gynecologic Oncology.* Philadelphia: Saunders, 1991, pp. 383–389.
246. Plentl AA, Friedman EA: *Lymphatic System in the Female Genitalia.* Philadelphia: Saunders, 1971.
247. Monaghan JM: Presentation of carcinoma of the vulva. In Blackledge GRP, Jordan JA, Shingleton HM (eds): *Textbook of Gynecologic Oncology.* Philadelphia: Saunders, 1991, pp. 412–418.
248. Hacker MF: Vulvar cancer. In Berek JS, Hacker NF (eds): *Practical Gynecologic Oncology.* Baltimore, MD: Williams & Wilkins, 1989, pp. 391–424.
249. Morley GW: Infiltrative carcinoma of the vulva: Results of surgical treatment. *Am J Obstet Gynecol* 124:874–880, 1976.
250. Rubin D: Gynecologic cancer: Cervical, vulvar, and vaginal malignancies. *RN* May:56–63, 1987.
251. Baggish MS, Dorsey JH: CO_2 laser for the treatment of vulvar carcinoma-in-situ. *Obstet Gynecol* 57:371–375, 1981.
252. Heinzl S: Vulvar intraepithelial neoplasia: Diagnosis and laser therapy. In Knapstein PG, diRe F, DiSaia, et al: *Malignancies of the Vulva.* New York: Thieme Medical Publishers, 1991, pp. 50–56.
253. Radar JS, Leuke JF, Dillon MB, et al: Ultrasonic surgical aspiration in the treatment of vulvar disease. *Obstet Gynecol* 77:753–756, 1991.
254. Raaf JH, Krown SE, Pinsky CM, et al: Treatment of Bowen's disease with topical dinitrochlorobenzene and 5-fluorouracil. *Cancer* 37:1633–1642, 1976.
255. Curry SL, Wharton JT, Rutledge F: Positive lymph nodes in vulvar squamous carcinoma. *Gynecol Oncol* 9:63–67, 1980.
256. Berman ML, Soper JT, Creasman WT, et al: Conservative surgical management of superficially invasive stage I vulvar carcinoma. *Gynecol Oncol* 35:352–357, 1989.
257. Atamdede F, Hoogerland D: Regional lymph node recurrence following local excision for microinvasive vulvar carcinoma. *Gynecol Oncol* 34:125–128, 1989.
258. Ball B: Easing the shock of radical vulvectomy. *Nursing* 5:27–31, 1975.
259. Andreasson B, Visfeldt J, Bock JE: Value of four models for selecting patients for local excision of invasive squamous cell carcinoma of the vulva. *J Reprod Med* 35:1041–1043, 1990.
260. Hacker NF: Management of stage I vulvar cancer. In Knapstein PG, diRe F, DiSaia P, et al (eds): *Malignancies of the Vulva.* New York: Thieme Medical Publishers, 1991, pp. 80–95.
261. Durrant KR: Tumors of the vulva and vagina: Treat-

ment of advanced disease. In Blackledge GRP, Jordan JA, Shingleton HM (eds): *Textbook of Gynecologic Oncology.* Philadelphia: Saunders, 1991, pp. 426–431.

262. Remmenga S, Barnhill D, Nash J: Radical vulvectomy with partial rectal resection and temporary colostomy as primary therapy for selected patients with vulvar carcinoma. *Obstet Gynecol* 77:577–579, 1991.
263. Schreer I, Bahnsen J, Frischbier H-J: Radiotherapy of vulvar carcinoma. In Knapstein PG, diRe F, Disaia P, et al (eds): *Malignancies of the Vulva.* New York: Thieme Medical Publishers, 1991, pp. 143–152.
264. Greer BE, Berek JS: Evolution of the primary treatment of invasive squamous cell carcinoma of the vulva. In Greer BE, Berek JS (eds): *Gynecology Oncology: Treatment Rationale and Techniques.* New York: Elsevier, 1991, pp. 227–238.
265. Monaghan JM: Radical surgical treatment of cancer of the vulva: The Gateshead experience, 1974–1989. In Knapstein PG, diRe F, Disaia P, et al (eds): *Malignancies of the Vulva.* New York: Thieme Medical Publishers, 1991, pp. 124–132.
266. Horowitz B: Interferon therapy for condylomatous vulvitis. *Obstet Gynecol* 73:446–448, 1989.
267. Averette HE, Donato DM, Lovecchio JL, et al: Surgical staging of gynecologic malignancies. *Cancer* 60:2010–2020, 1987.
268. Moore D, Marshall R, Thomas GM: A phase II evaluation of preoperative chemoradiation for advanced vulvar cancer. Philadelphia: Gynecologic Oncology Group, 1989.
269. Podczaski E, Herbst AL: Cancer of the vagina and fallopian tube. In Knapp RS, Berkowitz RS (eds): *Gynecologic Oncology.* New York, MacMillan, 1986, pp. 339–424.
270. Sulak P, Barnhill D, Heller P, et al: Nonsquamous cancer of the vagina. *Gynecol Oncol* 29:309–320, 1988.
271. Davis KP, Stanhope CR, Garton GR, et al: Invasive vaginal carcinoma: Analysis of early-stage disease. *Gynecol Oncol* 42:131–136, 1991.
272. Hacker NF: Vaginal cancer. In Berek JS, Hacker NF (eds): *Practical Gynecologic Oncology.* Baltimore, MD: Williams & Wilkins, 1989, pp. 425–440.
273. Chamorro T: Cancer of the vulva and vagina. *Semin Oncol Nurs* 6:198–205, 1990.
274. Audet-Lapointe P, Body G, Vauclair R, et al: Vaginal intraepithelial neoplasia. *Gynecol Oncol* 36:232–239, 1990.
275. Binton LA, Nasca PC, Mallin K, et al: Case-control study of in situ and invasive carcinoma of the vagina. *Gynecol Oncol* 38:49–54, 1990.
276. Auclair CA: Consequences of prenatal exposure to diethylstilbesterol. *J Gynecol Nurs* 8:35–39, 1979.
277. Robboy SJ, Noller KL, O'Brien P, et al: Increased incidence of cervical and vaginal dysplasia in 3980 diethylstilbestrol-exposed young women. Experience of the National Collaborative Diethylstilbestrol Adenosia Project. *JAMA* 252:2979–2983, 1984.
278. Rollason TP: Vulva and vagina: Pathology of malignant tumors. In Blackledge GRP, Jordan JA, Shingleton HM (eds): *Textbook of Gynecologic Oncology.* Philadelphia: Saunders, 1991, pp. 390–411.
279. Aho M, Vesterinen E, Meyer B, et al: Natural history of vaginal intraepithelial neoplasia. *Cancer* 68(1):195–197, 1991.
280. Kucera H, Vavra N: Radiation management of primary carcinoma of the vagina: Clinical and histopathological variables associated with survival. *Gynecol Oncol* 40:12–16, 1991.
281. Cagler H, Hertzog R, Hreshchyshyn M: Topical 5-FU treatment of vaginal intraepithelial neoplasia. *Obstet Gynecol* 58:580–583, 1981.
282. Ferenczy A: Laser treatment of patients with condylomata and squamous carcinoma precursors of the lower female genital tract. *CA* 37:334–347, 1987.
283. Hernandez-Linares W, Puthawala A, Nolan JF, et al: Carcinoma in situ of the vagina: Past and present management. *Obstet Gynecol* 56:356–360, 1980.
284. Reddy S, Lee MS, Graham JE, et al: Radiation therapy in primary carcinoma of the vagina. *Gynecol Oncol* 26:19–24, 1987.
285. Manneta A, Pinto JL, Larson JE, et al: Primary invasive carcinoma of the vagina. *Obstet Gynecol* 72(1):77–81, 1988.
286. Gallup DG, Talledo OE, Shah KJ, et al: Invasive squamous cell carcinoma of the vagina: A 14-year study. *Obstet Gynecol* 69:782–785, 1987.
287. Mooney KH, Feukell BR, Nail LM, et al: 1991 Oncology Nursing Society Research Priorities Survey. *ONS* 18:1381–1388, 1991.
288. Walczak JR, Nolte S, Eriksson JH: A survey of research priorities in gynecologic (GYN) nursing. Poster of NAACOG Ninth National Meeting, Minneapolis, MN, 1992.
289. Nolte S, Walczak JR, Eriksson JH: A model for developing a nursing research program in a national cooperative group. *Proc Oncol Nurs Soc 17th Congress,* 1992.

Chapter 44

Head and Neck Malignancies

Connie Yuska Bildstein, RN, MS

INTRODUCTION

The challenges presented by a diagnosis of head and neck cancer for the patient are significant. No other tumor site is exposed so completely to society's view. The patient not only must cope with extreme physiologic changes in structure and function but also must incorporate changes in body perception as well. In addition, nurses need to understand the magnitude of the rehabilitation needs based on the structural and functional changes that result. It is important to understand the normal anatomical and functional relationships that exist in the head and neck area so that the extent of subsequent deficits created by surgery or tumor can be predicted and rehabilitation planned.

The challenge for the nurse caring for the head and neck cancer patient is to understand the disease process and available treatment options. In addition, the ability to clearly predict and support rehabilitation needs is paramount. The purpose of this chapter is to provide a comprehensive review of the disease process as it presents in various anatomical sites in the head and neck area and to discuss treatment options and care.

EPIDEMIOLOGY

Approximately 67,000 new cases of head and neck cancer are diagnosed in the United States each year. This is an annual incidence rate of approximately 17 per 100,000 and represents approximately 5% of the 660,000 newly diagnosed cancers in the United States per year. The frequency of distribution of primary tumors in the anatomic sites are as follows: 40% oral cavity, 25% larynx, 15% oro/hypopharynx, 7% major salivary glands, and 13% in remaining sites. The ratio of male to female incidence remains 3:1, although that ratio may change as the trend of more women smoking continues. The incidence increases markedly after age 50, averaging about 45 in 100,000 during the sixth decade and 65 in 100,000 during the seventh and eighth decades. For males the incidence increases to 70 in 100,000 in the seventh decade and 100 in 100,000 during the eighth decade.[1]

In some locations in the head and neck, pain occurs very late, causing a delay in medical treatment. On initial presentation, 80%–90% of oral cancers are 2 cm or more in diameter. More than 60% of the 67,000 individuals in whom head and neck cancer is diagnosed each year in the United States will have advanced disease. Complicating this picture is the fact that the development of head and neck tumors is associated with the personal habits of smoking and drinking alcohol. Although the intake of these substances is under the control of the individual, the presentation of a patient who has a history of addiction to cigarettes and alcohol is consistent with the denial of symptoms and a subsequent delay in seeking medical treatment.

RISK FACTORS

Tobacco use remains the primary risk factor in the development of head and neck cancer. This includes not only cigarette use but the use of smokeless tobacco as well. The sites at greatest risk for developing cancer from tobacco use are the areas in which direct contact with tobacco and tobacco smoke occur. Those sites are the oral cavity, pharynx, larynx, and esophagus. The relative risk and development of disease will vary according to the daily consumption, type, and manner of tobacco use.[2]

The use of smokeless tobacco increased significantly during the 1970s because it was promoted as a "safe" alternative to smoking. The group of users changed from men over 50 years of age and older women living primarily in the South to white, male adolescents and young adults in the age range of 14–29 years.[3]

It is felt that there is a synergistic effect between alcohol and tobacco, when consumed in large amounts, in the development of head and neck cancers. The combination of alcohol and tobacco potentiates carcinogenesis and creates a significantly higher risk than does either one alone.[4] Some studies have also shown an association with exposure to wood, metal, leather, or textile dust. In addition, poor oral hygiene and possibly chronic mechanical irritation from ill-fitting dentures and plates or sharp, jagged teeth have been predisposing factors in the development of carcinoma of the tongue as well as the gingiva and other sites in the oral cavity. The Epstein-Barr virus has long been associated with the development of nasopharyngeal cancers. The high incidence of nasopharyngeal cancer among people of Cantonese descent and the presence of a specific HLA antigen profile suggest a genetic predisposition.[5]

Nutritional deficiencies are also seen in patients with head and neck cancer. Plummer-Vinson syndrome, in which iron deficiency anemia occurs, has been associated with cancers of the tongue, hypopharynx, and esophagus. This syndrome is characterized by generalized nutritional deficiencies, anemia, achlorhydria, chronic dysphagia, and splenic enlargement. Atrophy of the mucous membranes in the mouth and pharynx may also be presenting symptoms. Vitamin A deficiencies and retinoids may play a role in the development of disease as well. Other associated risk factors are listed in Table 44-1.

TABLE 44-1 Risk Factors in the Development of Head and Neck Cancer

Risk Factor	Associated Site
Tobacco use (cigarettes, snuff)	Oral, pharyngeal, laryngeal
Heavy alcohol intake	Oral, pharyngeal, laryngeal
Poor oral hygiene	Oral
Jagged teeth	Oral
Improperly fitting dentures	Oral
Exposure to wood dust	Nasopharyngeal
Leather manufacturing	Oral, pharyngeal, laryngeal
Mustard gas	Oral, pharyngeal, laryngeal
Betel nut chewing	Oral
Exposure to metals (nickel, chromium)	Oral, pharyngeal, laryngeal
Exposure to the sun	Lip

PRIMARY PREVENTION

Avoiding use of tobacco and alcohol is key to prevention of head and neck cancer. As public awareness of the dangers of tobacco use grows and a negative image of smoking is portrayed in the media, it is anticipated that the incidence of head and neck cancer will decrease. Nurses can play an active role in community education by participating in health fairs and corporate health-related events and by contacting the media to emphasize the dangers of tobacco use. In 1989 a coordinated, nationwide campaign was launched by the American Academy of Otolaryngology–Head and Neck Surgery, Inc., and the National Cancer Institute to persuade our nation's youth from using smokeless tobacco. The campaign is titled "Through with Chew" and is primarily directed toward young boys aged 11–17. Nurses and other health professionals can participate in this and other community awareness programs by presenting lectures at local area schools.

DETECTION

Early Detection

Early detection remains the key to successful control of disease. Five-year disease-free cure rates remain about

30%–40%, regardless of tumor site. These poor results are related to size of tumor at diagnosis as well as the presence of regional lymph node disease and distant metastases.[1] More than 60% of individuals diagnosed each year with head and neck cancer have advanced disease upon presentation. Diagnosis may be delayed because pain may not be present and denial of symptoms and a fear of treatment are common.

Often, metastasis to regional lymph nodes has already occurred when the patient first seeks medical care. Head and neck cancers typically are very aggressive locally and spread initially to anatomic sites within the head and neck area. This pattern of spread makes treatment more complex and the subsequent course of rehabilitation more challenging. The role of the nurse in early detection clinics is becoming even more important as health care institutions and payors emphasize "wellness care." This includes periodic screening of high-risk individuals. Nurses in early detection clinics can perform thorough head and neck exams and collect comprehensive patient histories. Referrals can be made to smoking-cessation programs to decrease the chance of individuals developing head and neck malignancy.

Retinoids

Isotretinoin has shown some activity in suppressing oral premalignancies and in preventing second primary tumors in patients with squamous cell cancer of the head and neck. One hundred three patients who received prior treatment for oral cavity carcinoma were either randomized to placebo or to 50–100 mg/m²/d of isotretinoin orally for 1 year. Although there was no significant difference in recurrence rate of primary cancers, 4% of patients in the isotretinoin group had second primaries at 32 months, compared with 24% of those in the placebo group. Despite these promising results, further clinical trials are needed to identify the ideal chemopreventive approach to treating oral cancers.[6]

History and Symptoms

A thorough review of the patient's medical history should be done, with particular emphasis on exposure to carcinogens as well as a positive family history of cancer. A review of lifestyle habits and occupation should also be included. In addition, a thorough review of current symptomatology should be included. The following symptoms are all significant: unilateral nasal obstruction or discharge, persistent ulceration, persistent hoarseness, odynophagia, dysphagia, sore throat, and cervical adenopathy. Persistent symptoms lasting longer than 3 weeks should be promptly reported to a physician.[3]

A thorough assessment should be performed using inspection and palpation techniques. The following equipment will be necessary: a good light source, gloves, tongue blade, nasal speculum, laryngeal mirror, and otoscope. Bimanual examination is essential in assessing the oral cavity and neck. Careful attention must be directed toward the exam of the oral cavity. The buccal mucosa should be retracted and the U-shaped floor of the mouth should be closely inspected. The areas of the oral cavity and oropharynx are generally considered high-risk areas and should be assessed carefully. Regional metastasis in the neck is the *only* presenting symptom in more than one-third of patients with head and neck cancers. The most common lymph node groups involved will be the jugular and posterior cervical chains and the submandibular lymphatics. In particular, the subdigastric nodes including the upper jugular and tonsillar nodes will most frequently be involved.[7]

In addition to a thorough history and physical exam, an indirect mirror examination of the pharynx and larynx will be performed. Advances in optics technology have allowed greater visualization of the hypopharyngeal and laryngeal areas with flexible fiberoptic endoscopes. This exam is easily performed in the physician's office using local anesthetics.

An even more thorough exam of the entire head and neck area is next performed under either local or general anesthesia in the operating room. Biopsies of suspicious areas are obtained to confirm a histologic diagnosis. In addition, conventional radiography, computerized tomography (CT) and magnetic resonance imaging (MRI) are valuable tools in performing a comprehensive evaluation. Open biopsy of a neck mass should be considered only as a last resort when a primary cannot be identified. Normal anatomical relationships and structural function of specific sites in the head and neck area will be discussed individually.

CLASSIFICATION AND STAGING

Head and neck tumors are classified and staged according to the TNM classification system as outlined by the American Joint Classification of Cancer guidelines. The *T* (tumor) indicates the extent of the primary tumor. The *N* (node) indicates regional lymph node involvement. The *M* (metastasis) indicates spread outside the head and neck region. Because of anatomic considerations, the specific details for each site differ; however, the general interpretations remain the same. An overview of the distinctions in the TNM method is outlined in Table 44-2.

PATHOPHYSIOLOGY

Approximately 95% of all head and neck carcinomas are squamous cell in origin. Arising from the epithe-

TABLE 44-2 TNM Classification System for Head and Neck Tumors: Nodal and Distant Sites

NODAL INVOLVEMENT (N) CLASSIFICATION FOR ALL HEAD AND NECK MALIGNANT NEOPLASMS	
NX	Nodes cannot be assessed
N0	No clinically positive nodes
N1	Single clinically positive homolateral node 3 cm or less in diameter
N2	Single clinically positive homolateral node 3–6 cm in diameter
N2a	Single clinically positive homolateral node 3–6 cm in diameter
N2b	Multiple clinically positive homolateral nodes, none more than 6 cm in diameter
N3	Massive homolateral node(s), bilateral nodes, or contralateral node(s)
N3a	Clinically positive homolateral node(s), none more than 6 cm in diameter
N3b	Bilateral clinically positive nodes (each side of the neck is clinically staged separately)
N3c	Contralateral clinically positive node(s) only
DISTANT METASTASIS (M) CLASSIFICATION FOR ALL HEAD AND NECK MALIGNANT NEOPLASMS	
MX	Not assessed
M0	No known distant metastasis
M1	Distant metastasis present; specify site and degee of organ impairment
STAGE GROUPING	
Stage I	T1, N0, M0
Stage II	T2, N0, M0
Stage III	T3, N0, M0 T1 or T2 or T3, N1, M0
Stage IV	T4, N0 or N1, M0 any T, N2 or N3, M0 any T, any N, M1

Source: Beahrs OH, Henson DE, Hutter RV, et al (eds): American Joint Committee on Cancer: Manual for Staging of Cancer, 4th ed. Philadelphia: Lippincott, 1992.

lium that lines the upper aerodigestive tract, the typical mucosal lesion can appear as an ulceration, roughened or thickened area, cauliflowerlike lesion, or a combination of all of these. Submucosal lesions can begin in epithelial invaginations such as the tonsils or tongue base, or from the ducts of minor salivary glands. Early lesions generally have either a reddish (erythroplasia) or whitish (leukoplakia) color. As the tumor grows, infection, necrosis, or bleeding may occur.

The majority of head and neck tumors invade locally, deep into underlying structures as well as along tissue planes (including perichondrium or periosteum) or nerves. Direct invasion into bone occurs late in the course of the disease, through preexistent anatomic openings. Perineural and lymphatic spread contribute to the metastasis of malignant cells beyond the primary site.

Lymphatic spread occurs both locally at the primary site and regionally through lymphatic channels when tumor implantation into the lymph nodes occurs. Enlarged cervical lymph nodes combined with a diagnosis of a head and neck malignancy reflects this implantation and may be the presenting symptom. Poorly differentiated tumors tend to metastasize early to regional lymph nodes and beyond. Lymphatic drainage of the head and neck area is depicted in Figure 44-1.

The presence or absence of histologically proven lymph node metastasis is an important factor in determining prognosis. As the number of nodes involved with tumor increases, the degree of lymph node involvement and the presence of soft tissue spread after

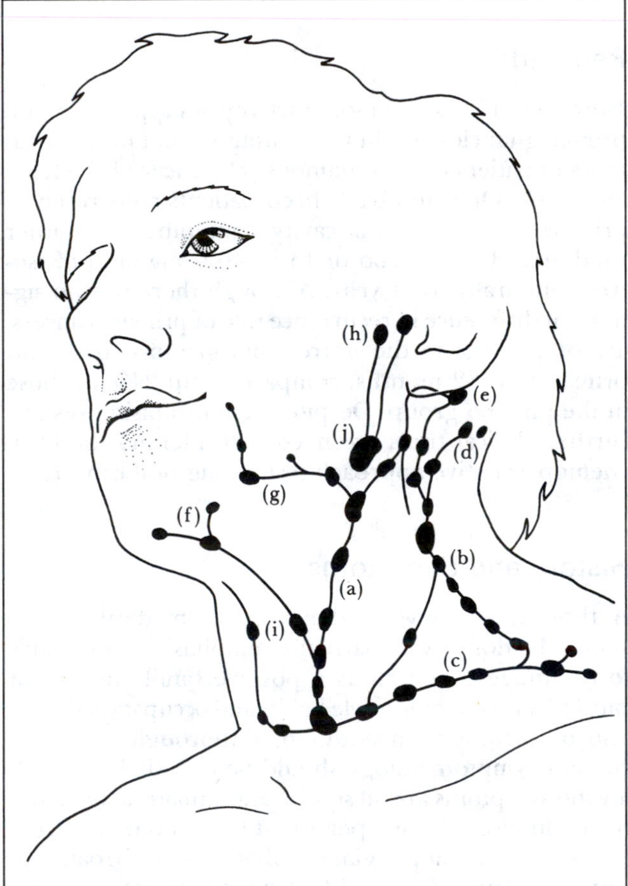

FIGURE 44-1 Lymphatic drainage of the head and neck. (a) Lateral cervical midjugular. (b) Midposterior cervical. (c) Supraclavicular. (d) Occipital. (e) Posterior auricular. (f) Submental. (g) Submandibular. (h) Preauricular. (i) Anterior cervical. (j) Subdigastric.

penetration of the lymph node capsule are other factors that affect prognosis. As tumor spreads to lower nodes in the neck, there appears to be a related reduction in the 5-year survival rate. The prognosis and survival rates are the lowest for individuals with involvement in the lower third of the neck and with three or more positive nodes.

The greatest risk of a second primary tumor occurs within the initial 3-year period following treatment for primary cancer. Approximately 30% of individuals with head and neck cancer will have a second primary cancer; in many cases the lung will be the site of second primary. For this reason it is recommended that the patient be examined at regular intervals for the first 3–5 years following treatment.

MULTIDISCIPLINARY MANAGEMENT

A diagnosis of head and neck cancer makes a significant impact on the patient's emotional as well as physical health. Multimodality therapy consisting of chemotherapy, radiotherapy, and surgery results in a number of health professionals participating at different intervals in the provision of care. A multidisciplinary approach is essential to provide quality care throughout the course of treatment as well as during the rehabilitation period. Optimally, the following members of the health care team should approach the diagnostic phase jointly: surgeon, radiation oncologist, and medical oncologist. The clinical case can be reviewed and a treatment plan outlined in a comprehensive manner. It may be helpful to structure a system that allows for all three physicians to evaluate the patient in a clinic setting prior to treatment planning as well as at predetermined intervals following each phase of treatment. This approach ensures a comprehensive approach to diagnosis and treatment planning throughout the patient's course of treatment. Ideally, appropriate members of the health care team should meet the patient and family prior to admission to the hospital. This often can be incorporated into the multidisciplinary clinic appointment. Additional members of the multidisciplinary team include: the nurse, social worker, chaplain, pharmacist, speech and swallowing therapist, discharge planner, dietitian, and prosthodontist.

Successful multidisciplinary teams find that regular meetings facilitate implementation of the plan of care as well as assist in preparing the patient and family for discharge. If major surgery that results in loss of speech or changes in facial contour is planned, the individual and family will have to adjust to these changes. In addition, the basic functions of eating and talking must often be relearned. It is not uncommon for the patient to experience feelings of anger and frustration during the immediate postoperative period. The members of the multidisciplinary team can assist the patient and family during this readjustment period.

CARCINOMA OF THE NASAL CAVITY AND PARANASAL SINUSES

Eighty percent of cancers in the nasal cavity and paranasal sinus area are squamous cell in origin. The remainder are adenocarcinomas. The maxillary sinus is the most commonly afflicted site in this area and most tumors are squamous cell in origin. Adenocarcinoma is more commonly diagnosed in the ethmoid sinus, which accounts for the remainder of tumors in the area. Primary carcinomas are rarely seen in the frontal or sphenoid sinuses. Most patients are over the age of 40 at diagnosis, and there is a 2:1 male predominance over females.[1]

The incidence of nasal cavity carcinoma is increased in persons with occupations in nickel plating, furniture manufacturing, and leather working. In addition, exposure to chromate compounds, hydrocarbons, nitrosamines, and dioxane has proven to be a risk. Other occupational exposures include mustard gas, isopropyl alcohol, and petroleum.

Symptoms may be similar to those of chronic sinusitis, although in the early stages of disease the patient may be asymptomatic. Other symptoms include a stuffy nose, history of sinus headache, dull facial pain, rhinorrhea, epistaxis, cheek hypoesthesia, trismus, and loose teeth. Physical findings may include diplopia, proptosis, a submucosal palatal mass, maxillary fullness, or a cranial nerve deficit. General prognosis is more favorable if tumors are located anterior and inferior to a plane connecting the medial canthus to the angle of the mandible. Tumors that are posterior and superior to this plane, such as those that are closer to the orbit and cranium, carry a less favorable prognosis. Cervical adenopathy is also an unfavorable finding that occurs in 10% of patients at diagnosis.[1]

Anatomy

The nasal cavity is separated into two chambers by the nasal septum. This area communicates with four pairs of sinus cavities: sphenoid, ethmoid, frontal, and maxillary. The lateral margin is formed by the frontal sinus, cribiform plate, and sphenoid sinus. The cavity is divided internally into the vestibule, septum, floor, roof, cribiform, and lateral wall or turbinates (Figure 44-2).

The triangular-shaped maxillary sinus forms the floor of the orbit superiorly and the palate inferiorly. Together, the right and left maxilla form the upper jaw. The ethmoid sinus forms a portion of the medial wall of the maxillary sinus and the entire medial wall of the orbit. The medial wall of the sinus is the middle turbinate and the roof is the fovea ethmoidalis. Symp-

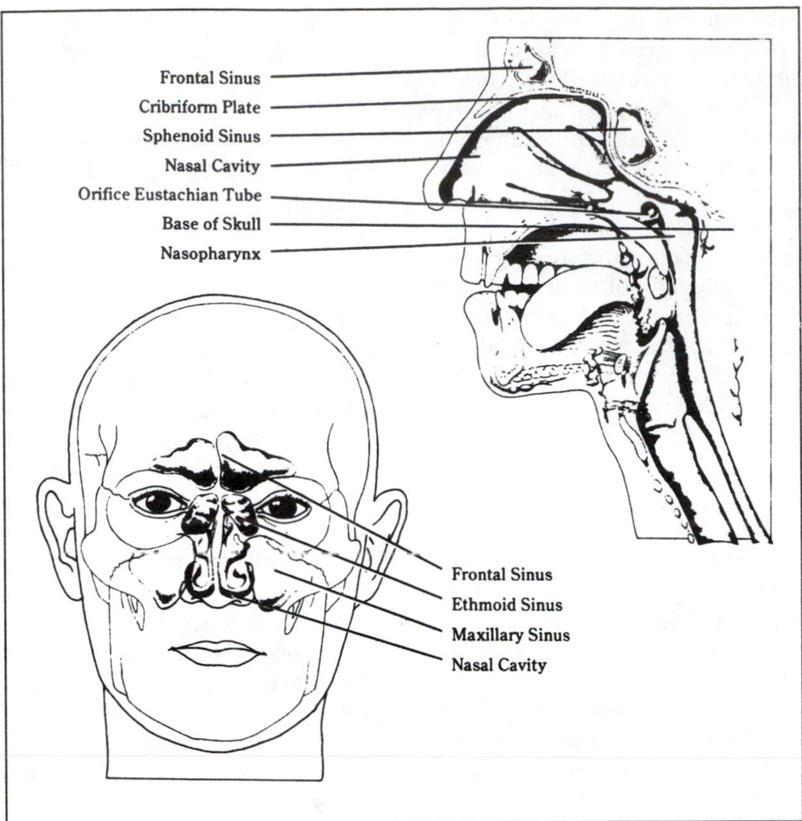

FIGURE 44-2 The nasal cavity and the paranasal sinuses.

toms of ethmoid sinus involvement can include decreased vision, epiphora (excessive tearing), medial orbital swelling, and olfactory changes. Distant metastasis from the paranasal and nasal cavity area can occur, but death is usually caused by tumor extension to the brain. The frontal sinus is an extension of the ethmoid sinus into the frontal bone. The anterior portion is the medial forehead, while the posterior portion separates the sinus from the anterior cranial fossa. The floor of the frontal sinus forms the medial roof of the orbit to the midline.

The sphenoid sinus is in the sphenoid bone and consists of a cubicle body in the center of the skull. Three processes extend from the body of the sphenoid—the lesser wing, greater wing, and pterygoid process. The optic canal passes through the root of the lesser wing.[8] Tumor extension in the area of the sphenoid sinus can cause compression of the third, fourth, and sixth cranial nerves, resulting in diplopia. In addition, pressure on the optic nerve can result in gradual loss of vision.

Treatment

Early carcinomas of the nasal cavity and paranasal sinuses can be effectively treated with either surgery or radiation therapy. However, most tumors are not discovered until they are advanced. In those situations, loco-regional control may be best achieved by a combination approach of surgery and radiation therapy.

Maxillectomy remains the treatment of choice for tumors in the maxillary sinus. More extensive disease with invasion into the floor of the orbit may necessitate combining radical maxillectomy with orbital exenteration.

Before surgical excision the maxillofacial prosthodontist will take an impression of the hard and soft palate to create an obturator, which is placed following resection and before the patient leaves the operating room suite. The obturator restores oronasal continuity and allows the patient to speak and eat immediately following surgery. Moreover, the obturator enhances the patient's comfort by protecting the wound from irritation and debris. Approximately 5 days after surgery, the packing that was placed in the defect is removed and the obturator is replaced.

The patient is instructed about meticulous wound care before discharge from the hospital. Mucosal drying and atrophic changes will occur in the maxillectomy cavity following surgery. The skin grafts that line the defect are subject to crusting and drying. The problems of drying, crusting, and superficial infection are increased if the patient has had prior irradiation. It is imperative that the defect be kept clean. An oral irrigating device with controlled pressure of the jet stream will effectively cleanse the cavity. A solution that has an alkaline base is recommended to increase ciliary action and prevent drying. A solution of saline and baking soda can provide adequate cleansing and will not burn. After irrigation, the patient can instill a solution containing the following: 5 ml of mineral oil, 2 drops of camphor, 2 drops of eucalyptol, and 2 drops of menthol. This will help loosen crusts and decrease oral odors. Irrigation of the defect should be done after each meal and at bedtime. The patient who is receiving chemotherapy, radiotherapy, or both should be particularly alert for mucositis and report this to both the oncologist and the prosthodontist. The patient should not remove the obturator for prolonged periods because atrophic changes may occur. A permanent obturator is usually made 6 months after the initial surgery to allow time for complete healing and consolidation of scar tissue.

There is minimal facial deformity following maxillectomy because the incision along the nose generally blends in with facial lines and fades over time. However, if an orbital exenteration is performed, the patient loses the eyeball and orbital contents. A skin flap is generally used to provide coverage and reconstruct the area. If the orbit has been removed and the cheek is intact, the patient may choose to wear a patch or be fitted with an external orbit prosthesis, which is cosmetically acceptable, especially when worn with glasses.

Cranial Base Surgery

Tumors located in the skull base were once believed inaccessible to surgical intervention and were treated only with radiation therapy. Today, advances in surgical techniques combined with technological advances offer new hope to what once was considered a very dismal situation.

The craniofacial approach, one of the most challenging areas of head and neck surgery, is used to resect tumors involving the skull base. Benign intracranial tumors and low-grade malignant tumors of the skull base with extension to the nasal cavity, paranasal sinuses, orbit or infratemporal fossa may be reached by the intracranial approach. In addition, benign and malignant diseases of the nose and paranasal sinuses, nasopharynx, or infratemporal fossa may be resected via the craniofacial approach. Other potential candidates include patients whose disease has failed to respond to radiation therapy or to limited surgical resection such as esthesioneuroblastoma and ethmoid and nasopharyngeal carcinoma.[9]

Cranial base surgery often combines the talents of the otolaryngologist, microvascular surgeon, and neurosurgeon to offer a comprehensive approach to the treatment of skull base tumors. The cranial or skull base is divided into three regions: the anterior, middle, and posterior regions. The ethmoid sinuses, frontal sinuses, and superior hemisphere of the orbits are included in the anterior region. The greater and lesser wings of the sphenoid bone, the infratemporal fossa, the optic apex, and chiasm are contained in the middle region. Finally, the clivis, posterior fossa, jugular foramen, and internal auditory canal are included in the posterior cranial base.

The surgical approach depends upon the location of the tumor. The transpalatal and transoral approaches are often employed, as well as the subtemporal-infratemporal approach.[10]

The patient and family must understand the potential dangers and complications of cranial base surgery. In addition, any expected functional sequelae should be explained. Expected outcomes will depend upon the surgical approach, anatomic location of the tumor, and the biologic behavior of the tumor being treated. For example, orbital exenteration may be necessary and will result in loss of vision. Temporary facial paralysis resulting from dissection in the infratemporal fossa can commonly occur. Anesthesia of the middle or lower face can occur as well. Loss of smell will result from transection of olfactory nerves. If midface or maxillary defects are created by the resection, preoperative plans need to be made for postoperative rehabilitation. Although the potential for central nervous system complications is great, the incidence should approach zero when surgical techniques are carefully executed. When surgical intervention, anesthesia, and postoperative care have been carefully planned, craniofacial resection may be no more stressful than a standard maxillectomy.[9]

Nursing Considerations

Following cranial base surgery the patient is on bed rest with the head of the bed elevated 20–30 degrees. A lumbar subarachnoid drain is left in place 24–48 hours postoperatively with the drainage bag suspended at the level of the orbit to maintain a low-normal cerebrospinal fluid pressure.[9] Typically, these patients are monitored very closely in the neurosurgical intensive care unit. Intravenous antibiotics are given as long as the cavity packing is in place. The cavity packing is removed on post-op day 5–8 if split thickness skin grafts were done. The packing may be removed in 4–5 days if no skin graft has been applied.

Careful monitoring of fluid balance must be done because of the effects of extreme fluctuations in blood pressure on cerebral blood flow, such as inadequate cerebral perfusion and vasoconstriction.[11]

A thorough neurologic assessment is performed preoperatively to establish a baseline for the frequent monitoring that occurs postoperatively. In addition to careful monitoring of the neuro status, another nursing concern is the monitoring and maintenance of the lumbar spinal drain. The purpose of a lumbar drain is to relieve pressure at the operative site through cerebral spinal fluid decompression. Typically, 50 cc of spinal fluid are ordered to be drained from the patient every 8 hours. The cerebrospinal fluid must be monitored closely, and any changes in appearance of the fluid, lack of drainage, or disruption in drainage system sterility should be promptly reported. Management of headache pain that can accompany the presence of a lumbar drain is generally controlled with a mild narcotic that does not interfere with monitoring the patient's level of consciousness.[10]

Radiation Therapy

Overall, 30%–40% of patients with nasal cavity and paranasal disease develop local recurrence. Local recurrence rates for patients with maxillary sinus cancer are even higher, at 60%.[12] These high local recurrence rates accentuate the need for early diagnosis and for delivering adequate radiation doses to bulky disease as well as generous margins of normal tissue. For this reason, treatment doses well above 60 Gy are often needed to achieve the best results. When radiation therapy is the definitive modality, many physicians prefer to debulk the lesion and create a large nasoantral window that facilitates drainage of necrotic tissue. Elective irradiation of the clinically negative neck is usually not done.[1] Despite advances in treatment approaches and diagnostic imaging, the prognosis for patients with paranasal sinus tumors remains bleak. The 5-year survival rate for patients diagnosed early and receiving combined therapy is 40%. Patients with unresectable tumors treated with aggressive radiation therapy have a 5-year survival rate of 15%–19%.[9]

CARCINOMA OF THE NASOPHARYNX

Epidemiology and Etiology

The incidence of nasopharyngeal carcinoma in the United States is only 0.6/100,000. The incidence in males compared to females is 3:1. On the average, the disease strikes men in the 40–44 age group and women between the age of 60–64.[1] Squamous cell carcinomas account for approximately 98% of all malignancies in the nasopharynx. Most often these tumors are poorly differentiated or undifferentiated. The incidence of nasopharyngeal cancer increases to approximately 18% in Eastern populations with the exception of the Japanese.[13] Factors postulated to account for the increase include genetic predisposition, an increased size of the nasopharynx in South Chinese, and an environmental relationship to the ingestion of salted fish. There appears also to be a viral association with the Epstein-Barr virus.[1]

Anatomy

The nasopharynx is cuboidal shaped and continuous with the nasal cavities, lying just posterior to the nasal passages. This area is called the posterior choanae. The superior portion is attached to the base of the skull and slopes downward to become the posterior pharyngeal wall. The orifice of the eustachian tube is the most prominent landmark on the lateral wall. Between the cartilaginous medial end of this tube and the posterior wall is the fossa of Rosenmueller. This is a cleftlike space whose apex reaches the anterior margins of the carotid canal. A rich, capillary lymphatic system drains into ipsilateral and contralateral nodes. Metastasis occurs most often to the cervical triangle, the entire jugular chain, and the supraclavicular nodes.

Symptoms

Symptoms of nasopharyngeal carcinoma may include nasal obstruction (with or without epistaxis), hearing impairment and tinnitus secondary to obstruction of the eustachian tube, and otitis media. An enlarged node in the neck may be the first indication of nasopharyngeal carcinoma in many patients. Poorly localized headache and facial pain are symptoms that occur late in the course of disease and can signify bony erosion and pressure on the fifth cranial nerve. Invasion of tumor through the base of the skull results in cranial nerve involvement; therefore, cranial nerve abnormalities provide important diagnostic information (Table 44-3). Double vision will occur when the third, fourth, and sixth cranial nerves are involved. The presence of Horner's syndrome represents tumor invasion of the sympathetic nerve fibers accompanying the carotid artery as it passes intracranially. The syndrome is characterized by ptosis, miosis, and anhidrosis.[13] Epistaxis may occur with necrosis of the tumor and vessel walls. Malignant tumors of the nasopharynx are one of the few tumors in the head and neck that metastasize widely. Frequent sites of metastasis include the lung, liver, and bone.

Assessment

The diagnosis of nasopharyngeal carcinoma is made by careful examination of the area using a head mirror, tongue depressor, and laryngeal mirror to visualize the area. CT scans and other radiologic evaluations can determine extensiveness of spread. Angiography can assist in determining potential collaterizations in the cerebrovascular tree.

Treatment

Radiotherapy remains the primary treatment for nasopharyngeal carcinoma; however, surgical treatment following radiation is gaining credibility.[13] The course of radiation usually involves laterally opposed fields through which a dose of 60–75 Gy is delivered to the primary site over a 6–9-week period. Special care must be taken to provide a minimal dose to the brain and

TABLE 44-3 Symptoms of Cranial Nerve Compression from Nasopharyngeal Carcinoma

Nerve	Symptoms
Olfactory (I)	Seldom occurs; difficult to assess unilateral deficiency to olfaction
Optic (II)	Complete unilateral blindness
Oculomotor (III)	Paralysis of the upper, lower, and inner rectus muscle of the eye; complete fixation of the eye except for its lateral movement
Trochlear (IV)	Paralysis of the superior oblique muscles of the eye
Trigeminal (V)	Neurologic pain of supraorbital and superior maxillary regions; painful anesthesia of half of the tongue, floor of the mouth, and buccal mucosa; compression of the mandibular branch results in paralysis of the temporal, internal pterygoid, and masseter muscles; lack of corneal reflex
Abducens (VI)	Paralysis of the external rectus muscle of the eye and diplopia
Facial (VII)	Peripheral facial paralysis; seldom occurs
Acoustic (VIII)	Loss of hearing and vertigo; seldom occurs
Glossopharyngeal (IX)	Difficulty swallowing, partial loss of taste, hoarseness, hemi-anesthesia of the soft palate
Vagus (X)	Anesthesia of the soft palate, pharynx, and larynx; tachycardia and tachypnea
Spinal accessory (XI)	Paralysis and atrophy of the trapezius and sternocleidomastoid muscles; hemiparesis of the soft palate and larynx
Hypoglossal (XII)	Rapid atrophy of the affected side of the tongue, which, when protracted, deviates toward the affected side
Cervical sympathetic nerve	Constriction of the pupil, retraction of the eye into the orbit, and narrowing of the palpebral fissure (Horner's syndrome)

spinal cord. Radioactive implants may also be used to boost the dosage.

Information about the efficacy of chemotherapy for patients with recurrent or metastatic carcinoma of the nasopharynx is scarce. However, recent retrospective reviews of patients treated with cisplatin-based combinations suggest the following: (1) Carcinoma of the nasopharynx should be considered a malignant neoplasm that is distinct from squamous cell cancer of the head and neck, and (2) selected patients with recurrent or metastatic carcinoma of the nasopharynx should receive aggressive combination chemotherapy.[14]

The patient with advanced disease often has severe pain and headaches resulting from bony invasion and erosion. In addition, the patient may experience multiple cranial nerve palsies, visual problems, sensory losses, anorexia, severe weight loss, respiratory difficulty secondary to vagal nerve paralysis, and laryngopharyngeal edema.

CARCINOMA OF THE ORAL CAVITY

Pathophysiology

If diagnosed early when tumor size is small, cure rates for cancer of the oral cavity improve dramatically. Unfortunately, cancer of the oral cavity will develop in approximately 29,000 people in the United States each year, and approximately 9500 of those will succumb to the disease.[15] Cancer of the oral cavity and oropharynx account for 4% of all cancers in men and 2% of all cancers in women.[16]

The assessment and finding of oral cavity lesions are frequently first made in the dentist office and are then referred to the otolaryngologist/head and neck cancer surgeon. The following positive findings in the history should alert the clinician to the possibility of an oral malignancy: history of smoking (cigarettes, cigars, and pipes), alcohol abuse, use of smoking tobacco (chewing tobacco and snuff), and systemic syphilis. Other potential factors include a history of poor oral hygiene; poorly fitting dentures and dental appliances; and, particularly in India (or among persons of Indian descent), a habit of chewing betel nuts. Also, a custom in India that is associated with a higher incidence of hard palate carcinomas is the habit of reverse smoking of cigarettes, or "chuttas," in which the lighted end is placed in the mouth.[17]

Alcohol also acts as an irritant to the oral mucosa. In combination with tobacco, alcohol is thought to act synergistically in causing oral cavity cancers. In addition, it may act indirectly by promoting malnutrition and cirrhosis. These two side effects may indirectly stimulate activity of oral carcinogens.

Field cancerization is the development of multiple primary cancers that occur either concurrently or subsequently in the same patient. The mechanism of action is unclear; however, it is suggested that groups of cells are stimulated to form lesions in an appropriate tissue environment. The continuance of the habits of smoking and alcohol consumption contribute to the provision of a suitable environment for the development of cancer. As many as 37% of patients with oral cavity cancers have been reported to develop multiple tumors. Tumors can involve separate organ systems; however, most seem to involve the same organ area. The initial 3-year period following therapy for the primary lesion is the period of greatest risk for the development of a second primary.[18]

More than 90% of oral cavity tumors are squamous cell carcinomas. Adenocarcinomas rank second in frequency. Squamous cell cancers are more often seen in men and older age groups, while adenocarcinomas predominate in younger aged women.[19] However, it is important to remember that oral cavity carcinomas are neither age- nor sex-specific.

Anatomy

The anatomical boundaries of the oral cavity are outlined in Table 44-4 and Figure 44-3. The following discussion is limited to the behavior of squamous cell tumors in the oral cavity. Squamous cell carcinomas generally grow along mucosal surfaces. They can first appear as a white, patchy lesion or an oral ulcer that fails to heal. In advanced lesions, infiltration into deeper structures is seen. Due to their surface friability, some lesions ulcerate easily and suffer trauma from mechanical actions such as chewing. Figure 44-4 illustrates a tumor in the posterior oral cavity.

A steady, persistent growth pattern is demonstrated by most squamous cell tumors. As deep invasion occurs, spread may be evident along preformed pathways of muscle fascia or nerves. In addition, as the tumor grows, regional lymph node metastasis frequently occurs. Generally, the upper cervical nodes are affected, with the submandibular and upper jugular nodes most commonly involved. Contralateral cervical metastases can frequently result from lesions in the floor of the mouth and tongue. The mechanism of action is that tumor cells from oral lesions pass through lymphatics that cross the midline from the primary tumor. A second route of spread can occur from ipsilateral regional nodes via collateral lymph flow resulting in contralateral node involvement.

In general, tumor metastases occur when a primary lesion has been present for some time. However, when primary tumors are poorly differentiated and clinically aggressive, metastases occur in relatively short periods of time.[17] Distant metastases occur from cancer cells spreading through the lymphatic system or by blood vessel embolization.[20] When underlying bone is affected, the destruction is secondary to tumor invasion.

Treatment

One may postulate that diagnosis of oral tumors would occur expeditiously since the area is immediately ac-

TABLE 44-4 The Oral Cavity

Site	Anatomical Borders
Lip	Begins at the junction of vermillion border. Well defined into upper and lower lip, which are joined laterally at the commissure of the mouth.
Buccal mucosa	Membranous lining of the inner surface of the cheeks and lips from the line of contact of the opposing lips to the line of attachment of mucosa of the alveolar ridge.
Lower alveolar ridge	Includes alveolar process of the mandible and its covering mucosa. Extends from the line of attachment of mucosa in the buccal gutter to the line of free mucosa of the floor of the mouth. Posteriorly ascends to the ascending ramus of the mandible.
Upper alveolar ridge	Upper ridge is the alveolar process of the maxilla and covering mucosa. Extends from upper gingival-buccal gutter to junction of hard palate. Posterior margin is upper end of pterygopalatine arch.
Retromolar trigone	Attached mucosa overlying the ascending ramus of the mandible from the level of the posterior surface of the last molar tooth to the apex superiorly. Adjacent to the tuberosity of the maxilla.
Floor of the mouth	Semilunar space of the mylohyoid and hypoglosses muscles. Extends from inner surface of lower alveolar ridge to undersurface of the tongue. Posterior boundary forms base of anterior pillar of the tonsil. Anterior portion divided into two sides by frenulum of the tongue. Contains the ostia of the submandibular and sublingual salivary glands.
Hard palate	Semilunar area between the upper alveolar ridge and the mucous membrane covering the palatine process of the maxillary palatine bones. Extends from inner surface of superior alveolar ridge to posterior edge of palatine bone.
Oral tongue	Anterior two-thirds is freely mobile and extends anteriorly from line of circumvallate papilla to the undersurface of the tongue at the junction of the floor of the mouth. Composed of four areas: tip, lateral borders, dorsum, and undersurface.

Source: Rice D, Spiro R: *Current Concepts in Head and Neck Cancer.* New York: American Cancer Society, 1989.

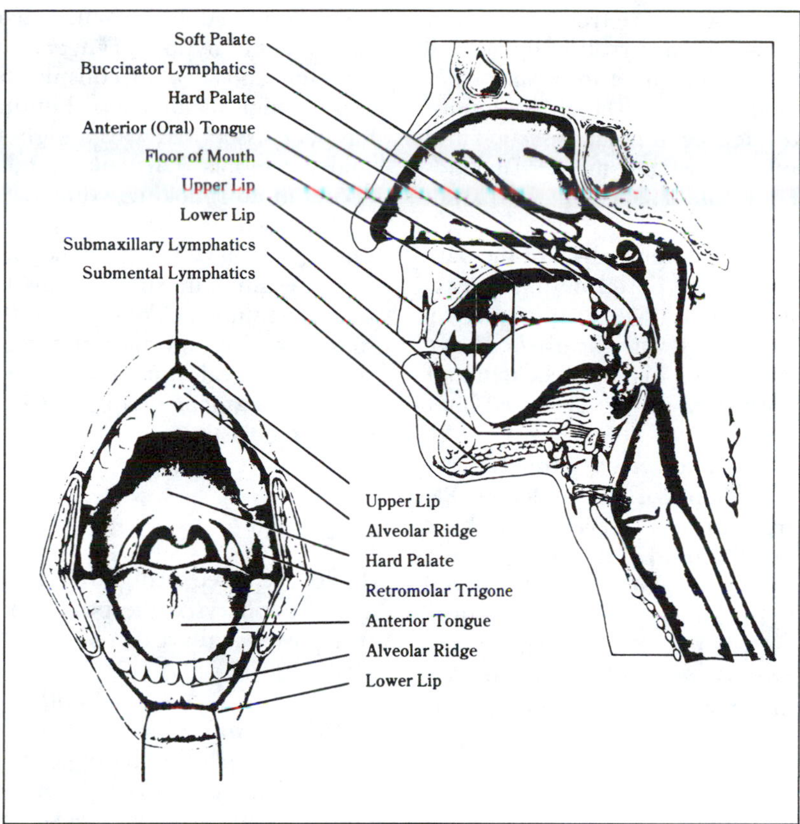

FIGURE 44-3 The oral cavity.

cessible to the examiner. However, delays in treatment may occur if the lesion is treated initially as benign. In the past, such treatment has included topical medications, antibiotics, dental extractions, and dental adjustment. Fortunately, over the past two decades the dental community has become keenly aware of the hazards of delaying a diagnosis of oral cancer and now includes a screening exam in routine visits.

Unfortunately, many patients will delay seeking treatment due to denial of symptoms. The most common historical complaint may be a painless lesion that has existed for some time. Pain may or may not be present at the primary site. It is commonly reported as referred pain to the ear or jaw. Referred pain is an important sign that can indicate induration, ulceration, or pressure affecting adjacent nerves. As the lesion increases in size, the individual may experience difficulty chewing foods and swallowing.

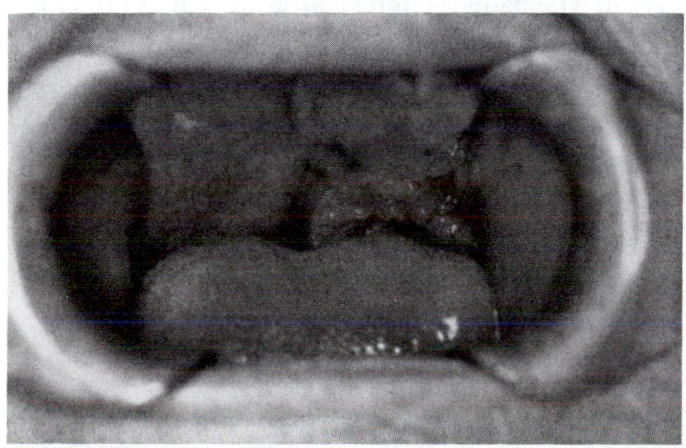

FIGURE 44-4 Posterior oral cavity tumor.

Treatment options will be determined by the size of the tumor. Surgery and radiation alone have comparable cure rates in early-stage lesions. The choice of treatment in early-stage lesions depends on functional and cosmetic results, the patient's general health, and patient preference. While chemotherapy alone cannot cure oropharyngeal cancer, complete and partial response rates as high as 90% have been demonstrated for platinum-based combinations. However, these responses are rarely of long duration, and studies continue to investigate the effect of combination therapy on survival.[21]

Surgical Resection

Surgical resection in this area involves a neck dissection in continuity with the tumor and regional tissues. An ipsilateral neck dissection is often done because there is a high frequency of metastasis to ipsilateral nodes.[22–24] If the mandible is involved, the appropriate portion is included in the resection.[25] The guiding principle of surgical resection is removal of the primary tumor with adequate margins that are free from tumor involvement. Resection of 2 cm of surrounding normal tissue is usually considered adequate to ensure clear margins. Surgical treatment of stage III and IV lesions often results in a greater degree of tissue resection and thus greater dysfunction and disfigurement.[22] Depending on the location of the tumor, speaking and swallowing can be greatly affected.

A typical resection may include removal of the base of the tongue, a portion of the posterior pharyngeal wall, and a segment of the mandible. In this case, reconstruction would be completed with the use of a large tissue flap such as a pectoralis major myocutaneous flap. Reconstructive techniques will be discussed later in this chapter.

The individual's rehabilitation needs after surgery are dependent upon the extent of the resection. Patients who have had large surgical resections will have a temporary tracheostomy for approximately 7–10 days. In addition, an enteral feeding tube will be placed and the patient will be NPO for 10 days to 2 weeks or until all intraoral suture lines are healed. The patient and family will need assistance coping with any alterations in facial contour that may have occurred with the surgical resection.

Use of the Laser

One of the single most important advances in the treatment of head and neck lesions over the past decade has been the increasing use of the laser in surgical excision of early-stage oral cavity, pharyngeal, and laryngeal cancers. The CO_2 laser has the advantage of being very precise, and it contributes to decreased possibility of tumor spread by sealing lymphatics as tissue is removed. The use of the laser has resulted in reduced patient morbidity, decreased hospital stay, and an improved recovery.[26]

Another advancement in surgical technology that has contributed to decreased morbidity is the use of preoperative internal carotid occlusion with placement of intraluminal balloons. The use of this technology results in relatively safe ligation and excision of the common and internal carotid artery, decreasing the rate of stroke to less than 5%.[26]

CARCINOMA OF THE HYPOPHARYNX

Etiology

The incidence of hypopharyngeal cancer is approximately 8 per 100,000. The ratio of male to female occurrence is 2:1. The specific site within the hypopharynx area that is most commonly afflicted is the pyriform sinus (70%), followed by the postcricoid (15%), and the posterolateral wall (15%).

Common etiologic factors that contribute to the development of hypopharyngeal cancer include excessive smoking and alcohol consumption. In northern Europe, a high incidence of Plummer-Vinson syndrome has been associated with a higher incidence of postcricoid carcinoma, particularly noteworthy because this occurs in nonsmoking women.

Most lesions in the hypopharynx are squamous cell in origin. There is a tendency for submucosal spread, often resulting in what appears to be multiple separate primary tumors. Carcinoma of the hypopharynx tends to metastasize superiorly to the base of the skull via the parapharyngeal lymphatics. Inferiorly the spread is seen toward the tracheo-esophageal lymph nodes and then to the mediastinum.

Anatomy

There are three distinct regions in the hypopharynx—the hypopharynx, the posterior surface of the larynx (the postcricoid area), and the lower posterior pharyngeal wall.

The two recesses on both sides of the larynx are called the *pyriform sinuses*. The superior border of each sinus is the pharyngo-epiglottic fold, and the inferior border is the upper border of the cricoid cartilage. On either side of the pyriform sinuses lie the aryepiglottic fold and the arytenoid cartilages. The postcricoid area extends from the posterior aspect of the arytenoid cartilages and their connecting folds to the inferior limit of the cricoid cartilage. The area is bounded laterally by the pyriform sinuses.[1] The remaining portion of the hypopharynx consists of the posterior and lateral walls (Figure 44-5).

Assessment

Patients with cancer of the hypopharynx typically present with: odynophagia (painful swallowing), referred otalgia (usually unilateral), and dysphagia (difficulty swallowing). Advanced tumors of the pyriform sinus and pharyngeal wall with extension into the larynx may have the associated symptoms of hoarseness or aspiration. The patient often reports a history of difficulty swallowing even liquids and has a sensation of a foreign body in the throat as evidenced by repeated attempts to clear the throat. If these symptoms have persisted for some time, there is often an accompanying weight loss and an alteration in the nutritional status.

The physical examination includes visualization of the pharyngeal wall and pyriform sinus area using a laryngeal mirror and a tongue depressor. The pyriform sinuses are best visualized during phonation. When the mirror is angled against the soft palate, adequate visualization of the posterior and lateral pharyngeal wall is possible. It is seldom possible to visualize the inferior tip of the pyriform sinus and the area below the superior aspect of the postcricoid area. This area is best

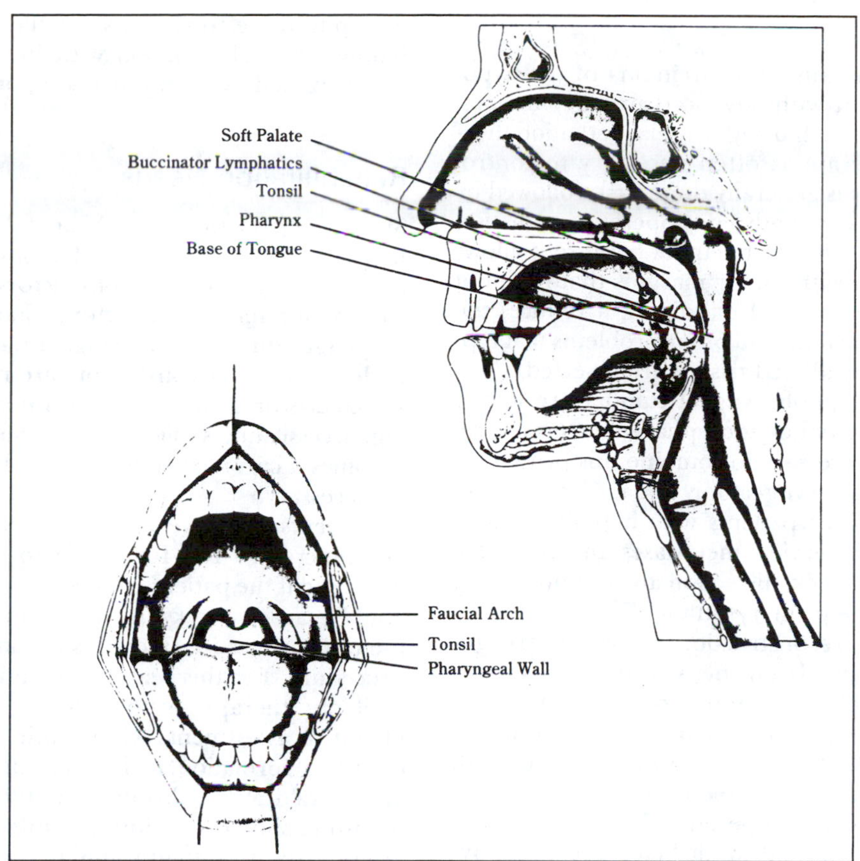

FIGURE 44-5 The hypopharynx.

examined with a flexible laryngoscope. A flexible laryngoscope is also helpful to examine a patient with a hyperactive gag reflex.

Diagnostic studies include CT, which can help to define the extent of the primary tumor and may demonstrate nonpalpable metastases in the lateral or retropharyngeal cervical lymph nodes. Direct laryngoscopy and biopsy are performed to confirm a tissue diagnosis. Because pyriform sinus tumors tend to be necrotic, multiple deep biopsies may be necessary to ensure an adequate tissue sample. Esophagoscopy with biopsy may be necessary if posterior invasion of the esophagus appears evident on pharyngoscopy.

Pertinent findings that may indicate cervical esophageal extension and thereby influence treatment planning include the following:

1. *Presence or absence of laryngeal involvement by tumor.* If both cords are mobile, invasion by tumor has not occurred, and the lesion is exterior to the larynx. If one cord is fixed, the individual may be a candidate for a partial laryngectomy in continuity with the primary site.

2. *Tumor invasion and mucosal involvement of the posterior wall of the pharynx.* The posterior pharynx is often used to reconstruct the site after resection, but involvement by tumor would obviate its use for reconstruction, and alternate tissues would need to be used.

3. *Pooling of saliva in or around the pyriform sinus and pharynx.*

These findings could indicate cervical esophageal extension or obstruction of the opening of the cervical esophagus, which would require aggressive treatment.

Treatment planning is based on the stage of disease, as outlined in Table 44-5.

TABLE 44-5 TNM Classification System for Carcinoma of the Hypopharynx

T1	Tumor confined to the site of origin
T2	Extension of tumor to adjacent region or site, without fixation of the hemilarynx
T3	Extension of tumor to adjacent region or site, without fixation of the hemilarynx
T4	Massive tumor invading bone or soft tissue of the neck

Source: Beahrs OH, Henson DE, Hutter RV, et al (eds): American Joint Committee on Cancer: Manual for Staging of Cancer, 4th ed. Philadelphia: Lippincott, 1992.

Treatment

The majority of patients with carcinoma of the hypopharynx will present with advanced primary tumors. A combination approach using surgery, radiation therapy, and chemotherapy is often necessary to control the disease. Surgery is generally done first, followed by radiation therapy. Currently, postoperative radiation therapy is preferred in most centers because it allows the surgeon to deal with tumor margins that have not been altered by treatment. In addition, it reduces the chance of delayed healing and other problems that typically occur when irradiated tissues are resected.

Because most hypopharyngeal tumors are locally advanced, either partial or total pharyngectomy is required. It may be necessary to combine this procedure with a partial or total laryngectomy and neck dissection. Approximately 75% of patients with hypopharyngeal cancer present with cervical metastases and require a radical or bilateral neck dissection to be done along with resection of the primary tumor.

The method of reconstruction following laryngopharyngectomy depends on the amount of tissue removed from the pharynx and esophageal areas. If sufficient pharyngeal tissue remains, direct closure is the easiest method. If primary closure is performed, great care must be taken to avoid tension on the suture line in order to avoid a postoperative fistula. If a greater amount of tissue is needed to facilitate closure, a myocutaneous flap from either the pectoralis major or latissimus dorsi areas can be utilized to close the pharyngeal defect. If the full circumference of the pharyngeal wall must be resected to achieve adequate margins, alternative reconstructive procedures may include the following: posterior tongue flap with dermal graft; tubed pectoralis major or latissimus dorsi myocutaneous flap; or gastric pull-up, colon interposition, free jejunal interposition, or other free flaps.[27]

Pfister et al.[28] recently reported results using combined chemotherapy and radiation therapy in 40 patients with advanced, resectable squamous cell carcinoma of the larynx, oropharynx, or hypopharynx. These patients would have required total laryngectomy due to the extent of disease. They were treated with one to three cycles of cisplatin-based chemotherapy before local therapy. The goal was preservation of the larynx. Sixty-five percent of the patients achieved either a clinical complete response or partial response. The disease-free survival rate was 42% and 33% at 2 and 5 years, respectively. This approach demonstrated that larynx preservation with combined chemotherapy and radiation is feasible and effective in patients with advanced but resectable disease.[28]

Radiation Therapy

The total dose of radiotherapy that is effective in hypopharyngeal tumors is at least 60 Gy. Currently, there is much interest in delivering radiation in daily fractions of two to three treatments per day. In addition, combining external radiation with interstitial radiation is being studied as an adjunct component of therapy.

Rehabilitation Needs

Swallowing is often a problem following surgery for hypopharyngeal carcinoma. The surgical resection may involve the pharyngeal constrictors, which assist with control of a food bolus with resultant delivery into the esophagus during swallowing. If more than half of the middle and lower constrictors are resected and reconstructed, scar contracture can interfere with swallowing, necessitating swallowing rehabilitation. If aspiration becomes a chronic problem, a total laryngectomy may be necessary.

Patients who have undergone surgical resection will be at increased risk for fistula formation. The risk is increased if the patient has had previous radiation therapy. Because surgery in this area involves opening of the upper digestive tract, this becomes a contaminated procedure. For this reason, the individual will receive antibiotic therapy postoperatively. In addition, postoperative assessments will include observing for signs of fistula formation such as an elevated temperature and saliva draining through the suture line. If infection or fistula should develop, the integrity of the carotid artery is severely compromised.

Postoperatively these patients will have a temporary tracheostomy, enteral feedings, and wound care consisting of suture line care. If an orocutaneous fistula develops, the area may be packed with betadine-soaked or iodoform gauze and be allowed to close spontaneously. Large fistulas are generally repaired with flap reconstruction.

Speech rehabilitation will depend on the clinical status of the patient. Patients who have had a pharyngolaryngectomy will rarely be able to learn esophageal speech. This may be due in part to the method of reconstruction, which can interfere with the muscular vibratory activity necessary to produce sound. The options for these patients may be the electrolarynx or a tracheo-esophageal puncture procedure.

CARCINOMA OF THE LARYNX

Etiology

The incidence of laryngeal carcinoma in the United States is 4.2/100,000. The male to female ratio is 9:1. Approximately 80% of laryngeal carcinomas are found in persons over 50 years of age, with the highest incidence occurring in the sixth decade of life. Over 90% of laryngeal cancers are squamous cell in origin, ranging from well-differentiated to undifferentiated tumors. The majority of tumors are moderately well-differentiated. Tobacco and alcohol use as well as a history of exposure to ionizing radiation have been implicated as etiologic factors. The incidence of multiple primary tumors is 5%–10%.

Cancer of the larynx cannot be considered one disease, but, rather, as cancer involving different areas within the larynx such as the glottis (space between the true cords), supraglottis (area and structures above the glottis), and subglottis (area and structures below the glottis). Tumors in each region involve distinct signs and symptoms, treatment regimens, and, most important, rehabilitation measures.

Glottic Carcinoma

The glottic area includes the upper surface of the vocal fold (horizontal plane at the floor of the ventricle) and extending 1 cm below this plane. This area includes the true vocal folds and the anterior and posterior glottic commissures. Tumors in this area tend to be well-differentiated, grow slowly, and metastasize late. Because there are limited lymphatics in the cord, metastasis usually occurs only when the disease infiltrates muscle or has spread beyond the limits of the true cord. The lesion may extend across the midline to the opposite cord or may invade the thyroid cartilage. In addition, spread may occur superiorly into the ventricles, ventricular bands, and aryepiglottic fold. Inferior extension may occur into the subglottic space. If vocal cord motion is impaired, it may indicate extension of posteriorly situated cord lesions into the cricoarytenoid articulation and arytenoid region. Important diagnostic information includes the mobility of the cords, evidence of fixation of the cord, involvement of the anterior commissure, and involvement of cervical lymphatic vessels.

Staging guidelines for glottic carcinoma are outlined in Table 44-6.

TABLE 44-6 TNM Classification System for Glottic Carcinoma

TIS	Carcinoma in situ
T1	Tumor confined to the vocal cord(s) with normal mobility (includes involvement of anterior or posterior commissures)
T1a	Tumor limited to one vocal cord
T1b	Tumor involves both vocal cords
T2	Supraglottic and/or subglottic extension with normal or impaired cord mobility
T3	Tumor confined to the larynx with cord fixation
T4	Massive tumor with thyroid cartilage destruction and/or extension to other tissues beyond the larynx (eg, oropharynx, soft tissues of the neck)

Source: Beahrs OH, Henson DE, Hutter RV, et al (eds): American Joint Committee on Cancer: Manual for Staging of Cancer, 4th ed. Philadelphia: Lippincott, 1992.

Treatment

T1 lesions of the membranous cord are treated with equal success by both radiotherapy and conservation surgery. The advantage of radiation therapy in the treatment of early glottic lesions is preservation of excellent vocal quality. Early lesions have also been successfully treated with microlaryngoscopy and vocal cord stripping as well as laser excision. When there is no evidence of cord fixation, a conservative laryngeal resection is usually the treatment of choice. Conservative surgery for glottic cancer includes laryngofissure, partial laryngectomy, or hemilaryngectomy.

Early disease (T1 or T2)

When tumor extends forward to the anterior commissure or posteriorly to or beyond the vocal process, the surgery that is most effective is hemilaryngectomy. The anatomical limits of the surgery are outlined in Table 44-7.

Following hemilaryngectomy, the individual will have a temporary tracheostomy and receive enteral feedings. Decannulation will occur between the 10th and 14th postoperative days. The nasogastric tube is removed and the patient is started on feedings by mouth following healing of all incisions, usually 10–14 days after surgery. Postoperatively the patient will have a hoarse but serviceable voice. Vocalization is accomplished by the adduction of the remaining cord against the scar tissue that eventually takes the place of the resected cord. Damage to the superior and recurrent laryngeal nerves can lead to persistent aspiration. In this case a total laryngectomy may be indicated to prevent recurrent aspiration pneumonia.

Radiotherapy is utilized as an option for cure in early lesions. The usual dosage is 55–70 Gy over 6–7 weeks. If there is no response after 40 Gy, the therapy may be discontinued and surgery may be indicated.

Advanced disease (T3 to T4)

A total laryngectomy is reserved for patients who have persistent or recurrent disease after radiotherapy or present with advanced disease. In either case, vocal cord mobility is impaired. The procedure of total laryngectomy involves removal of all laryngeal structures

TABLE 44-7 Hemilaryngectomy (Vertical Partial Laryngectomy)

Structure Removed	Structures Remaining	Postoperative Outcome
One vocal cord and underlying cartilage, false vocal cord	Epiglottis set of vocal cords on unaffected side	Hoarse but serviceable voice
Arytenoid on affected side		Minimal swallowing problems

between and including the thyroid bone, thyroid cartilage, cricoid cartilage, and two to three tracheal rings. Radical neck dissection is indicated for any patient who presents with obvious metastasis to the lateral neck nodes. This is most frequently seen in patients with larger, high-grade tumors or vocal cord fixation. The major effects of removal of the larynx are permanent loss of voice and alteration in the airway. Because these losses are considerable, the patient and family should be provided every opportunity to express their fears and anxieties. In addition, coping strategies that have been successful in the past should be identified and a multidisciplinary plan established to assist the patient and family in the coping process.

Preoperative counseling with a speech therapist is essential to review potential methods of speech rehabilitation. Approaches that may be used to facilitate communication in the immediate postop period range from writing and use of communication boards to the use of artificial larynges. The patient should be an active participant in selecting the method that seems most comfortable.

Use of an electrolarynx, esophageal speech, and esophageal prosthetic voice restoration are three options for communication on a long-term basis.[29] Each method produces a vibration that is introduced as sound into the vocal tract. The sound is then shaped by tongue and lip movements into intelligible speech.[29]

In the early postoperative period the speech-language pathologist may give the patient an electrolarynx to use while in the hospital. Following a period of healing, the patient may choose to learn esophageal speech. This requires that the patient learn to produce sound by injecting air into the esophagus by movements of the tongue and lips. The air is trapped in the esophagus, causing tissue at the top of the esophagus to vibrate. Through practice of specific exercises, the patient learns to prolong the esophageal voice, refine it, and ultimately produce esophageal speech. This process can take as long as a year or more. If the patient has scarring in the area of the pharynx or tumor recurrence, it may be impossible to ever learn intelligible esophageal speech.

In some centers, tracheoesophageal (TE) puncture is done in combination with total laryngectomy. As a result of this procedure the patient can divert exhaled pulmonary air through a surgically constructed fistula tract directly into the esophagus. The exhaled air causes the cricopharyngeus muscle at the top of the esophagus to vibrate producing sound. There is not as much effort exerted to learn the often complicated method of air injection required by esophageal speech; however, the patient must learn to insert, clean, and replace the small prosthesis that fits into the fistula tract, preventing food and fluid from back-flowing into the trachea.

It is ideal if patients are given an opportunity to see and learn about all three types of communication that can be used. It is important for the patient to have choices concerning different methods of speech rehabilitation at a time when he or she may feel the situation is uncontrollable. Many patients may ultimately use all three methods at different times in the rehabilitation period: artificial larynx immediately after surgery; esophageal voice therapy a month or so after surgery; and, after a few months, surgical voice restoration or TE puncture.[30]

Postoperative care

In the immediate postoperative period, most patients will have a laryngectomy tube placed. The decision to place a tube will depend on the surgical technique used to create the stoma and the amount of contracture that occurs as healing progresses. The tube will help prevent trauma to the tracheal mucosa due to suctioning and, most importantly, will maintain an adequate stoma size. Since the laryngectomy stoma is permanent, the tube may be removed and cleaned without fear of stomal closure. The stoma area underneath the tube should be kept clean and free of crusting. The presence of crusts due to drainage from the stomal incision can lead to infection and increased scar formation. If the patient continues to experience stomal stricture over a period of time, the laryngectomy tube will need to be placed at night to help prevent further stricture.

The provision of adequate humidity will remain a life-long concern for the laryngectomized patient. Because the airway is diverted and the patient no longer has the ability to warm, moisten, and filter the air through the nose, supplemental humidity will need to be provided, especially in dry climates. Generally a large room humidifier is recommended for use in the home. A small bedside humidifier may also be necessary. The humidity level in the home should be kept above 50%.

In addition, the patient should be aware of changes in secretions that could signal insufficient humidity, including blood-tinged sputum, an increase in thickness or tenacity of secretions, or increased difficulty mobilizing secretions. The patient should be taught how to instill 1–3 cc of normal saline into the stoma to keep secretions thin, moist, and easy to cough out. The frequency of instillation will depend on environmental humidity. For example, in the winter months the frequency of instillation may be hourly, while in the summer months when the humidity level is higher it may only be necessary three times a day. The goal of instruction should be an understanding of the concept of lack of humidity and the subsequent effect on the tracheal secretions. Another method to ensure rapid mobilization of secretions is to fill a room with steam from a shower and stand in the room for approximately 15 minutes. The patient should also be instructed to wear a stoma covering, especially in the winter. The covering will assist to warm, moisten, and filter dry, cold air. In addition, adequate fluid intake will assist in hydration, prevent changes in secretions, and prevent tracheitis. The oral ingestion of potassium iodine is also helpful in increasing the volume and viscosity of secretions. Cough effectiveness is significantly reduced because the laryngeal sphincter is absent and thus intrabronchial pressure cannot be elevated, making adequate mobilization of secretions even more of a challenge.

Hyposmia occurs to some degree in every laryngectomized patient. This is a permanent loss recognized early on by the patient. Some limited odor detection and recognition will develop in the accessory olfactory areas over time. The ability to taste is closely related to stimulation of olfactory cells and is also reduced. This combination of factors may affect the patient's appetite, indicating a need for early intervention and nutritional counseling to prevent long-term weight loss.

An enteral feeding tube is placed during surgery to allow for nutritional support until the suture lines have healed. Because the feeding tube rests on the incision line, it should not be manipulated in any way. If it should become dislodged or pulled out, the possibility of its being replaced without perforation of the suture line is limited. The tube remains in place for approximately 7 days in the nonirradiated patient and for 10 days in the previously irradiated patient.

If the patient has had previous irradiation, the potential for fistula formation is increased. This usually extends the hospital stay. In addition, increased scarring in the suture line will contribute to later problems with esophageal stricture and dysphagia. Strictures can be treated effectively with periodic dilation, although occasionally a secondary surgical procedure is necessary. Other conditions that may interfere with swallowing may be pseudodiverticuli that develop at the base of the tongue. In addition, submucosal masses on the posterior pharyngeal wall caused by contraction of the detached constrictor muscles can interfere with swallowing. Finally, dysphagia can also occur in the absence of stricture as a result of the uncoordinated contractions of the detached inferior constrictor muscles.

Most laryngectomy patients resume their preoperative lifestyle, with only a few limitations. Due to the absence of thoracic fixation after laryngectomy, the patient's ability to lift heavy objects is compromised. The patient is instructed not to lift more than 10 pounds for 4 months after surgery. Heavy lifting and strenuous exercise may be performed gradually. A second precaution involves the avoidance of water sports. The laryngectomy patient cannot protect the airway during activities such as swimming and boating, and these activities should be avoided. Special precautions must be taken to avoid getting dust or dirt in the airway when performing activities such as gardening or housework. If the patient's occupation depends on communication, the pressure to communicate effectively using an alternate method increases. However, even executives who deliver speeches have returned to their positions and through perseverance in learning either esophageal speech or another method have been successful communicators.

Supraglottic Carcinoma

Lesions that lie superior to a horizontal plane passing through the floor of the ventricles and including the epiglottis, aryepiglottic folds, arytenoids, and ventricular bands (false cords) are classified as supraglottic tumors. Supraglottic tumors account for 35% of laryngeal cancers and are characterized by aggressive growth patterns, both by direct extension and lymph node metastases. Approximately one-half of these patients will present with lymph node involvement, which occurs because lymphatic channels drain into the jugulodigastric, mid, and inferior levels of the internal jugular chain.[1]

Clinical manifestations

Supraglottic cancer is often advanced when first detected because there are few early symptoms. The patient may complain of pain and poorly defined throat and neck discomfort that occurs during swallowing. Many patients complain of referred otalgia in combination with throat pain. Glottic hoarseness may occur in advanced disease and usually means that vocal cord fixation has occurred from tumor extension. The presence or absence of vocal cord fixation is an important factor in deciding on therapy (Table 44-8).

Assessment

The diagnosis of supraglottic cancer is usually made through indirect laryngoscopy, with direct laryngoscopy used for obtaining a biopsy specimen. Radiographs, CT, and MRI scans are helpful in determining the inferior extent of disease.

Treatment

In some institutions, supraglottic tumors are treated initially with radiation therapy. This approach remains controversial because some clinicians believe that a number of larynges could have been saved with supraglottic laryngectomy as the primary treatment approach. If radiation fails, total laryngectomy will usually be required as a salvage procedure.

The standard supraglottic laryngectomy consists of resection of the following structures: the hyoid bone, epiglottis, pre-epiglottic space, thyrohyoid membrane,

TABLE 44-8 TNM Classification System for Supraglottic Carcinoma

TIS	Carcinoma in situ
T2	Tumor confined to one subsite of supraglottis or glottis with normal cord mobility
T3	Tumor limited to the larynx with vocal cord fixation and/or invades the postcricoid area, medial wall of the pyriform sinus, or preepiglottic space
T4	Tumor invades through thyroid cartilage and/or extends to other tissues beyond the larynx (eg, to oropharynx, soft tissues of the neck)

Source: Beahrs OH, Henson DE, Hutter RV, et al (eds): American Joint Committee on Cancer: Manual for Staging of Cancer, 4th ed. Philadelphia: Lippincott, 1992.

superior half of the thyroid cartilage, and the false vocal cords. The sucess of supraglottic laryngectomy is limited by the following: fixation of the arytenoid, thyroid cartilage invasion, pyriform fossa apex involvement, postcricoid involvement, impaired vocal cord mobility, glottic extension, bilateral arytenoid involvement, cricoid cartilage involvement, and extensive involvement of the base of the tongue.[31]

Postoperative airway obstruction is common following supraglottic laryngectomy due to edema in the surgical area. For this reason, patients will have a temporary tracheostomy tube placed at the time of surgery. The tube will be removed following successful swallowing without aspiration in 10–14 days after surgery. Some patients may be sent home with the tube in place until they are able to learn how to protect the airway during swallowing.

Aspiration during swallowing is one of the major complications following supraglottic laryngectomy. Because the epiglottis, which is a protective mechanism during swallow, has been removed, the chances for chronic aspiration are increased. The patient must relearn to swallow without aspirating. A thorough evaluation and treatment plan is identified by the speech and swallowing therapist and is reinforced by the nursing staff. The mechanisms of action in the supraglottic swallow are outlined in Table 44-9. It is important to remember that the approach to the supraglottic swallow is individualized for each patient according to the extent of the resection. Further complicating the ability to swallow without aspirating is the fact that sensation of the area is destroyed when the supraglottic larynx and the internal laryngeal nerve are resected. In addition, if the arytenoid or a portion of the vocal cord is included in the resection, the aspiration rate increases significantly.

During normal swallowing, aspiration is prevented by three major sequential events: The epiglottis closes over the laryngeal inlet, the true vocal cords close, and the larynx elevates to oppose the base of the tongue. The procedure of supraglottic laryngectomy interferes with one or all of these variables. In some institutions, cricopharyngeal myotomy is performed in order to prevent failure of relaxation of the cricopharyngeal sphincter during swallowing. This allows food to pass more easily through this sphincter. Laryngeal suspension is another surgical technique that may be performed to decrease aspiration. This is accomplished by suturing the thyroid cartilage remnant to the mentum of the mandible. This results in lifting the larynx superiorly and tilting it posteriorly. There are conflicting reports regarding the ultimate success of this technique in improving the swallow. If the arytenoid or a part of it is included in the surgical resection, the remaining vocal cord should be fixed in the midline. If this is not done, the posterior glottic area will be incompetent during adduction of the vocal cords and aspiration will consistently result. Because of the difficulties associated with aspiration, elderly individuals or those with chronic bronchitis or decreased lung compliance may not be candidates for supraglottic laryngectomy. If aspiration becomes severe, meal times can become a period of frustration and anxiety for the patient and family. If pneumonia develops and aspiration persists, the patient may need to undergo total laryngectomy as a life-saving procedure.

A cine-esophogram and videofluoroscopy are usually obtained before the tracheostomy tube is removed to evaluate the patient's ability to swallow without aspirating. Commonly referred to as a "cookie swallow," this exam is often repeated at specified intervals to determine the progress of the swallowing therapy.

Liquids are the most difficult thing for the patient to swallow without aspirating. For this reason the patient should be started on foods that have a soft consistency such as mashed potatoes, applesauce, or baby food. The patient should be in a sitting position with minimal distractions during meal times. Small bites should be taken initially. The cuff of the tracheostomy tube should be deflated because it will inhibit elevation of the laryngeal remnant against the base of the tongue. If aspiration during meals is severe, the cuff will need to be inflated to protect the airway. Generally, in this situation the cuff will be inflated for meals and for

TABLE 44-9 Standard Supraglottic Laryngectomy and Supraglottic Swallow

Structure Removed	Structures Remaining	Post-operative Problem	Rehabilitation Outcome
Epiglottis Hyoid bone False vocal cords Superior half of thyroid cartilage	True vocal cords Arytenoids	Aspiration	Minimal aspiration

SUPRAGLOTTIC SWALLOW SEQUENCE*

Action	Effect
Cough or clear throat	Clears airway of secretions
Inhale	Closes vocal cords
Valsalva maneuver Place food in the mouth Swallow	Forces food into esophagus
Cough or clear throat again	Vibration causes excess food to clear from vocal cords
Swallow again	Remaining food enters esophagus

*Note: This sequence is modified by the speech therapist following a thorough swallowing assessment.

Source: Thawley SE, Panje WR, Batsakis JG, Lindberg RD (eds): *Comprehensive Management of Head and Neck Tumors.* Philadelphia: Saunders, 1987.

approximately one-half hour following the meal. The swallowing therapist should initiate the swallowing plan and be present with the patient for the first meal and for following meals as indicated.

The nursing role in swallowing therapy is one of support and collaboration. The nursing staff should be familiar with the specifics of the swallowing therapy so they can reinforce the steps of the swallow when the therapist is unable to be present. It is helpful to have the sequential steps written clearly on a large card that can be kept at the bedside and referred to by the patient during meal times. In addition, clinicians should remember that many patients are "silent aspirators" and will not cough during swallowing if aspiration occurs.

Relearning a basic function like swallowing is frustrating and often humiliating. The patient must be treated with patience and dignity during this process. Specific strategies may need to be outlined for the family to be supportive in this process as well. Often, in their quest to be helpful, they unknowingly can exert undue pressure on the patient to be successful. As swallowing therapy progresses, the patient gradually learns to swallow solid foods, semisolids, and finally liquids.

Tracheal suctioning is especially important after supraglottic laryngectomy. There are an abundance of secretions caused by increased edema in the laryngeal area. Generally, the tracheal secretions are extremely thin and liquid. For this reason, more frequent tracheal suctioning may be necessary to prevent aspiration and pneumonia. The patient should also be encouraged to cough and deep breathe every few hours and should be encouraged to ambulate outside the room at least four times a day.

METHODS OF RECONSTRUCTION

The goal of reconstructive procedures in the head and neck are to restore function while simultaneously retaining socially acceptable cosmesis. There are a variety of reconstructive options available today for the head and neck cancer patient. The decision regarding which option to employ will depend on the location and extent of tissue resected. The decision regarding the method of reconstruction should be discussed with the patient and family prior to surgery; however, the precise outcome may not be known because the extent of tumor may not be able to be precisely identified preoperatively.

Myocutaneous Flap

The advent of the pectoralis major myocutaneous flap in 1977 was a major breakthrough in reconstruction of the head and neck. Major surgical resections are now possible in which vital organs such as brain dura and the carotid artery are exposed without risking a high rate of meningitis, brain abscess, and carotid hemorrhage.

The myocutaneous flap is especially useful when large amounts of tissue have been resected and bulk is needed to reconstruct the defect. These flaps consist of muscle, skin, and blood supply and, in some cases, even contain bone or cartilage. The muscles most often used to reconstruct defects in the head and neck area include the pectoralis major, sternocleidomastoid, trapezius, and latissimus dorsi.

Another major breakthrough occurred with the use of the trapezius osseomyocutaneous flap for one-stage reconstructive procedures requiring reconstruction of a mandibular bony defect associated with a large soft tissue defect.[32] These flaps rely on well-vascularized muscles that receive their blood supply from a major arterial vessel. The pectoralis myocutaneous flap can be simply elevated from the anterior chest wall. The blood supply is provided by the pectoral branch of the thoracoacromial artery. In some cases an island of pectoral skin can be transported upon the pectoralis muscle to reach the oral cavity, and the vascularized muscle pedicle is placed beneath the neck skin. This flap is best utilized for reconstruction of larger defects of the oral cavity.

Free Flap

First used in the early and mid-1970s, the microvascular free flap was the first successful attempt at one-stage reconstruction in the head and neck.[33] The free flap is completely removed from its donor site and placed into the recipient site using microvascular anastomosis. Donor sites that have been used successfully include the groin and the radial forearm. Some of the major advantages of the free flap are that immediate functional reconstructive replacement of removed tissue is possible, the donor site is not exposed, and bulky exposed pedicles are avoided. Disadvantages of using this technique include prolonged operating time and the need for microsurgical expertise and two teams of operating surgeons.

Deltopectoral Flap

Popularized during the 1960s, the deltopectoral flap had the advantage of bringing well-vascularized tissue to a previously irradiated surgical bed from an area that had not been treated with radiation. There is no muscle included in the deltopectoral flap. It maintains its blood supply from its base and consists of skin and the blood supply only. The disadvantages of this flap include strictures, fistulas, and the fact that several stages are necessary. Due to its thinness, the deltopectoral flap is still useful today in the reconstruction of circumferential defects.[3]

Nursing Care of Flaps and Grafts

The goal of nursing care of any type of flap is to ensure flap viability. This is accomplished through frequent and thorough observation and assessment of the flap area. In addition, if a skin graft has been placed, both the donor and recipient site are observed closely for signs of adequate healing.

Skin grafts

Split-thickness skin grafts are used frequently to reconstruct a primary defect or to protect a major structure such as the carotid artery. Skin grafts are composed of a thin layer of epidermis and a small amount of dermis. The skin graft is resected completely from the donor site and sutured into the recipient site. A commonly used donor site is the anterior thigh on the operative side. Nursing assessment and care will include both the donor and recipient sites. The patient usually returns from the operating room with a protective covering placed over the donor site. This covering may differ from institution to institution depending upon the preference of the surgeon. If a transparent covering is used, observation of the area for complications such as bleeding can be easily done. If bleeding does occur, the physician may order small slits to be placed in the covering to release the pressure and allow the blood to escape. If a nontransparent covering is used, the area will be wrapped with a circular gauze dressing. This dressing generally stays in place for 1–2 days after surgery. Re-epithelialization occurs in the donor site area as the healing process takes place. The area must be kept free from infection during this process. This is accomplished by using sterile technique when caring for the wound and remaining alert for any signs of infection.

The patient will complain of pain in the donor site area. This is due to exposure of nerve endings and bruising of the underlying muscle during resection of the graft. It is helpful to avoid mechanical contact with the donor site area from pajama bottoms or other articles of clothing. In addition, the patient may require a mild analgesic every 3–4 hours to alleviate discomfort.

The donor site is often exposed to air while healing occurs. A heat lamp may be used to dry the area if excess drainage is present. The heat lamp is generally applied once every shift for one-half hour with care taken to avoid overexposure. This can be accomplished by positioning the heat lamp approximately 2–3 feet from the area. Once the donor site heals and the protective dressing dries, the dressing will come off on its own. If it is not easy to remove the dressing, saline-soaked gauze may be applied to the area to help loosen the dressing. Frequent application of saline soaks should assist in loosening the dressing until it can be easily pulled off. It is important, however, not to use force in removing the dressing because this can interfere with the healing process. If the dressing continues to adhere to the donor site, the patient is instructed to soak in the bathtub several times a day until the dressing is easily removed.

The recipient site should also be observed for signs of infection. The skin graft is sutured in place and a bolus of gauze impregnated with bismuth tribromophenate (XeroForm®) is placed over the graft. The bolus packing generally remains in place for 5 days. During this time, if the graft has been placed in the oral cavity, oral hygiene is avoided. The area is observed for odor and drainage. Once the packing is removed, oral hygiene can be performed four times a day using a solution of one-quarter hydrogen peroxide and three-quarters water.

Skin flaps

The following principles should guide nursing assessments and interventions in performing flap care.

Circulation is very important. The viability of any flap depends on adequate vascularization. The blood supply coming into the flap area must be adequate, and, concurrently, the blood flowing out of the flap must not be obstructed. More flap deaths occur from venous blood that is unable to flow out of the flap than from not enough blood flowing into the flap. The following indicators should be assessed every 2 hours through postop day 2 and then every 4 hours until postop day 5:

1. *Color:* Color is usually the best indicator of adequate blood supply. The flap color is usually a pale pink in Caucasians. The color may not match surrounding skin exactly but should be close to the color of the skin at the donor site. A white color indicates a dearterialized flap that has lost its blood supply, and a blue color indicates venous congestion has occurred or the input of blood exceeds output. It may be more difficult to detect subtle changes in color in African Americans.

2. *Temperature:* The flap should feel warm to the touch. Because the pads of the fingers can be less sensitive to temperature, the back of the fingers should be used to touch the flap area to assess the temperature. A flap that is cool to the touch indicates that arterial inflow is decreased.

3. *Capillary refill:* The tissue of the flap should blanche with gentle pressure applied to the flap and return to normal color quickly.

The criteria of temperature and capillary refill are not applicable to the assessment of intraoral flaps. The color of the flap is one assessment that may be used as an indicator of viability. In addition, a doppler can be used to detect aberrations in blood flow that may signal danger to the viability of the flap.

Significant changes in any of the above indicators should be reported promptly to the physician. Flaps can only tolerate approximately 4 hours of ischemia before irreversible tissue necrosis occurs. Figures 44-6 through 44-10 (Plates 13 through 17) illustrate the sequence of flap failure and repair.

External factors can also compromise flap viability. Care must be taken to avoid any circumferential pressure on the flap from either dressings or tracheostomy ties. It is for this reason that the physician may suture a tracheostomy tube and avoid neck tapes to secure the tube until flap viability is ensured. Proper positioning of the patient is essential to prevent tension or kinking of the pedicle of the flap. The proper position is dependent on flap location. This should be discussed with the surgeon and communicated clearly to all health care workers caring for the patient. It is also helpful to include the patient and family in these discussions, so the proper position can be maintained at all times.

Surgical drains are placed in the flap area for approximately 4–6 days after surgery. The drains will remove any accumulation of blood or fluid from underneath the flap area that could interfere with healing. When the drainage decreases to 50 cc or less in a 24-hour period, the drains are usually removed. After removal of the drains, the area should be inspected closely for any accumulation of blood or serum. If a hematoma occurs, the area may be drained at the bedside, or, depending on the size, the patient may need to return to the operating room for evacuation of the hematoma.

Incision lines in the flap area and in other areas should be cleansed with a solution of half-strength hydrogen peroxide and normal saline at least once a shift. An accumulation of dried blood and serum on the suture line can interfere with healing and provide an environment for infection.

The patient should be placed in a semi-Fowler's to high-Fowler's position. This position will help to decrease edema by gravitational drainage and will prevent hyperextension of the neck, which could place excessive tension on neck flaps and compromise wound healing.[34]

CHEMOTHERAPY

In the late 1960s and early 1970s, chemotherapy was reserved for the palliative setting and was administered with single agents only. More recently, various centers have studied the effects of administering chemotherapy in the neoadjuvant (primary chemotherapy) and adjuvant settings in combination with radiation therapy and surgery.

Modalities

Primary chemotherapy

There has been an increased interest in the use of induction combination chemotherapy before definitive treatments with surgery or radiation in previously untreated patients with stage III or IV disease. The rationale of this approach is that patients will be in optimal general medical condition and better able to tolerate aggressive chemotherapy. In addition, because tumor vascularity has not yet been altered by surgery or radiation, there is adequate drug delivery to tumor tissues. Moreover, the efficacy of surgery or radiation will be increased by reducing the tumor bulk with chemotherapy.

The regimen that has been most frequently used is a combination of cisplatin at 100 mg/m^2 followed by 5-day continuous infusion of fluorouracil (5-FU) at 1000 mg/m^2/d. Reported response rates from this regimen are generally good, ranging from 88%–94% of patients achieving at least a partial response. However, survival data are not as good. One center reported a median survival of 22 months and a 5-year survival rate of only 25%. The median time to progression of disease was 14 months, with 57% having documented progression of their head and neck cancer and 16% having progression of a second neoplasm.[35]

Single-agent chemotherapy

Methotrexate, cisplatin, bleomycin, and other agents have demonstrated cytotoxic effects when used as single agents in the treatment of head and neck cancer. However, they produce only partial responses in 20%–40% of patients treated.[36] The overall survival impact of single-agent chemotherapy has been negligible, but it can serve an important role in palliation by reducing tumor bulk and promoting comfort in the patient's final days.

Single-agent chemotherapy is generally administered in the outpatient or home setting. Generally, there are minimal side effects and the patient can maintain normal activities.

Chemotherapy used sequentially with radiation

In selected situations, chemotherapy has been used sequentially with radiation therapy. It has been speculated that reducing tumor volume with chemotherapy prior to receiving radiation will increase control of the disease. In addition, some investigators have observed that response to chemotherapy in previously untreated patients predicts a further response to radiation therapy and may predict conversion to complete disease remission status after subsequent radiation.[37] This combination of therapies is attractive for advanced stage head and neck cancer patients because functional problems associated with large surgical resections are avoided, the patient does not experience a long hospitalization, and, in some cases, results have been promising.

Organ Preservation

Although there have been advances in treatment of head and neck cancer over the past 10 years, the need remains for more effective treatment. Despite undergoing standard treatment, 50%–60% of patients will develop local recurrence, 20%–30% will develop distant metastases, and 10%–40% will develop a second primary.[38] This, combined with the fact that squamous cell cancer of the head and neck is sensitive to chemotherapy, makes systemic therapy an attractive treatment option. The quality-of-life issues that result from extensive surgery can leave functional as well as cosmetic defects and cannot be ignored. Therefore, patients who experience complete response to induction chemotherapy may be candidates for organ preservation. The objective of organ preservation is to prevent loss of organ function or severe disfigurement without compromising survival.[39]

Biologic Response Modifiers

There has been recent interest in the role that biologic response modifiers may play in the treatment of head and neck cancer. That interest has been rather slow due to the fact that head and neck cancer is responsive to surgery, radiation therapy, and chemotherapy. However, the efficacy of these treatment modalities is limited, as discussed earlier. Studies have demonstrated that the immune system plays a role in response to cancer, and biologic response modifiers may have therapeutic potential in head and neck cancer.

Interferon

Although the precise mechanism of antineoplastic effect is yet to be determined, interferons have been used with varying success in a number of different tumors.[40] Recent studies focus on the role that combination chemotherapy and interferon may play in the treatment of nasopharyngeal cancer. Phase I trials have demonstrated some activity in the combination of interferon with 5-FU.

Interleukin-2

Interleukin-2 has been used in a pilot clinical trial reported by Forni et al.[41] After the treatment course, a partial or complete response was noted in four of the five patients evaluated.

Future directions

Although exploration of the role played by biologic response modifiers in head and neck cancer is just beginning, responses in even heavily pretreated patients have been demonstrated following administration of interferon. Because the disease of head and neck cancer is a locally aggressive one, regional administration of biologics may play a greater role in control of the disease than in other malignancies. Newer biologic agents such as tumor necrosis factor, interleukin-4, and interleukin-6 are just beginning to be explored. The route of administration, dosage, and combination with chemotherapy are components of future trials that warrant further study.

Chemotherapy as a Primary Treatment Modality

Recently the role of chemotherapy as a primary treatment modality was studied in a large cooperative group trial that investigated preservation of the larynx. Although the results did not show a difference in survival between surgically treated patients and those who received induction chemotherapy, the larynx was preserved in two-thirds of the patients. These and other randomized trials have indicated that induction chemotherapy can change the expected pattern of recurrence by decreasing the rate of distant metastases. It is theorized that this early systemic treatment of micrometastases may also reduce the mutation rate of the tumor for the development of drug resistance. In this study, 64% of patients were histologically disease-free after three courses of cisplatin and 5-FU therapy in an area of the head and neck that historically was treated with surgery as the primary treatment modality.[42]

Various platinum analogs have been developed in an attempt to minimize or eliminate side effects of chemotherapy while retaining the antitumor activity of the drug. The most active and successful of these analogs is carboplatin. Myelosuppression was the dose-limiting side effect evidenced in phase I trials. Response rates of 22% have been observed in phase II trials.[43] In one study a combination of carboplatin 350 mg/m^2 and cisplatin 50 mg/m^2 were administered every 28 days to patients with recurrent or metastatic disease of the head and neck. None of these patients had received prior chemotherapy. Twenty-four percent achieved a partial response; no complete responses were observed. Hematologic toxicity required a decrease in dosage. Nonhematologic toxicities were infrequent and easily controlled. Results especially in terms of limited side effects were promising and warrant further study.[44]

RADIATION THERAPY

Radiation therapy has an important role as a treatment modality in head and neck cancer. Used as primary treatment in early lesions, radiation therapy can effect a cure. When radiation is combined with surgery for advanced lesions, control of disease and decrease of subsequent recurrence are often achieved.

The mode of delivery can vary and will depend on the treatment plan. The following methods of treatment are most frequently seen: external beam, interstitial implantation, and intraoperative therapy. The ultimate goal of any radiation treatment is to eradicate tumor while preserving function and cosmesis.

Dosage decisions for planning external beam therapy are dependent upon the size and location of the tumor as well as neck node involvement. Standard radiation therapy consists of five daily treatments per week for 5–7 continuous weeks. The dose usually prescribed for treatment of microscopic disease is a total of 45–50 Gy delivered over a period of 4–5 weeks. To adequately treat gross disease that is visible, a dose of at least 65 Gy and up to 75 Gy depending on the size of the tumor may be needed. The spinal cord is usually protected at doses of approximately 45 Gy.[45]

The success of radiation therapy depends on cell death during division. The damage occurs in the DNA during cell division. Head and neck tumors are in the middle range of sensitivity to radiation. They can be controlled with radiation but will require a higher dose than other tumors such as lymphomas that are more radiosensitive.[46]

Implant Therapy (Brachytherapy)

Implant therapy is the use of radioactive sources placed directly into the tumor. These low-energy sources deliver the radiation dose to the tumor bed while causing minimal morbidity to the surrounding tissues. The sources are placed using a procedure called *after-loading*. Under general anesthesia, hollow catheters are inserted in the tumor bed. These hollow catheters will hold the radioactive source, which is placed following the patient's return to his or her room. The radioactive material usually used is iridium 192 or cesium 137. The implant is usually left in place for 3–5 days. This will deliver a total dose of 30–70 Gy.[47]

Implants may be used as a curative therapy for early-stage lesions in the floor of the mouth and anterior tongue or may be used to boost a tumor that has received prior external beam therapy. Lesions that can effectively be treated with interstitial implants include those on the lip, floor of the mouth, buccal mucosa, nasal vestibule, and skin.

Radioactive seeds may also be implanted permanently at the time of surgery. Generally, seeds will be used at positive margins, neck nodes, or extension of the tumor into the base of the skull. The seeds have a low-level activity, with radiation being absorbed within the tumor with little or no exposure at the skin surface.[47]

Hyperthermia with Radiation

Hyperthermia may be combined with radiation to enhance tumor response. Heating the tumor superficially with ultrasound or microwave increases blood flow in the area and subsequently increases oxygen in the tumor bed, enhancing the radiation response. The area is generally heated to 41°–45°C for 45–60 minutes. The treatment is given once or twice weekly and is delivered through temperature sensors that are held in catheters that have been placed directly into the site. Patients may complain of a burning sensation, and blisters may appear in the treated area. The efficacy of this technique to enhance radiation response in head and neck cancers continues to be evaluated.

Intraoperative Radiation Therapy

A treatment that shows some promise and may soon be used on a wider scale is intraoperative radiation therapy (IORT). This treatment consists of delivery of a single, large dose of radiation therapy to either gross disease or a tumor bed after the surgical resection and during the operative procedure. One advantage of this approach is that the tumor site can be exposed in such a way that the radiation therapy can be delivered without going through vital structures that are not involved with tumor. This is in contrast to conventional external beam radiation, which affects all overlying structures whether affected with disease or not. Although the experience with this treatment modality has been limited to date, it has been delivered to control close margins of resection, for microscopic disease, and for gross residual disease. Total doses delivered can range from 10 Gy to 100 Gy. Results have been varied, and the approach warrants further study before definitive assumptions can be made regarding effectiveness.[45]

Concomitant Radiation Therapy and Chemotherapy

Head and neck cancer is a locally aggressive disease, with few patients presenting with clinically overt distant metastases at the time of diagnosis. Therefore, standard therapies have been aimed at control of local disease. However, there is a high regional recurrence rate even when surgery and radiotherapy are used together. The goal of therapy is to control regional disease, thereby decreasing the high incidence of persistent disease. The rationale for using radiotherapy with concomitant chemotherapy meets this goal. Chemotherapy can be successful at eliminating systemic micrometastases while concurrently enhancing the activity of radiotherapy in the irradiated field.[48]

The use of concomitant chemoradiotherapy has been studied in patients with head and neck cancer since the 1960s. Recently, studies have used combination chemotherapy schedules with split-course radiotherapy.

Cisplatin, 5-FU, and bleomycin have all been used as single agents in combination with radiotherapy. Results from trials using intermittent single-agent chemotherapy with concomitant radiotherapy have been promising; however, the numbers of patients that have received benefit from this approach do not at this time warrant making any of these approaches standard therapy.[48]

Combination chemotherapy with concomitant radiotherapy has also been studied. Some of the drug regimens that have been used include cyclophosphamide and bleomycin; vincristine, bleomycin, and methotrexate; cisplatin and 5-FU; and 5-FU, hydroxyurea (HU), and leucovorin. Although the approach of combining neoadjuvant chemotherapy and concomitant chemoradiotherapy seems promising, further study is warranted to justify the approach.[48]

Nursing Management of Patients Undergoing Radiation Therapy

Nursing interventions in caring for the patient undergoing radiation therapy are aimed at helping the patient understand the goal of therapy, as well as dealing with both acute and long-term side effects. The patient is making daily trips during the week to receive treatments at the radiation facility. This often results in a 5–7 week daily disruption in normal activities combined with increased fatigue as the course progresses.

The following side effects are usually experienced by any patient who receives radiation therapy to the head and neck area: mucositis, xerostomia, loss of taste, anorexia, fatigue, and local skin reaction. Nursing assessments and interventions can be extremely successful in abating and controlling symptoms during and after the treatment course.

Mucositis

Mucositis is an inflammatory response of the oral mucosa to radiation therapy. The soft palate, tonsilar pillars, buccal mucosa, pharyngeal walls, and lateral tongue are most susceptible to the development of mucositis. It can appear as early as the first week of treatment and generally will resolve within 3 weeks after the treatment is completed. The oral cavity will appear reddened and inflamed, and white patchy areas may be noted on oral exam. In addition, the patient will complain of a sore mouth and throat.

Oral care is essential during this time to alleviate discomfort and prevent infection. Commercial mouthwashes should be avoided because of their high alcohol content, which acts as a mucosal irritant. A mouthwash consisting of 1 teaspoon of salt and 1 teaspoon of soda in a glass of warm water will effectively rinse debris and soothe oral membranes. Viscous lidocaine may be prescribed to decrease discomfort. In addition, the patient should be instructed to avoid spicy foods, citrus juices, and fruits and vegetables such as grapefruit and tomatoes.

Xerostomia

Xerostomia is a drying of the oral mucosa that results from loss of saliva from damage that occurs to the salivary glands subsequent to radiation therapy to the head and neck. Studies have demonstrated that a decreased quantity of saliva is reported by the second week of treatment. In addition, salivary changes include a thicker saliva by the third week of treatment. These salivary changes are reported to persist for 3 months after treatment is completed in 43% of patients.[49]

To prevent dental caries, which can occur as a result of loss of the protective mechanisms of saliva, meticulous oral hygiene and prophylactic dental care should be initiated. A dental consult is indicated prior to the initiation of radiation therapy. Daily fluoride treatments that the patient performs at home can help to prevent dental caries. Artificial saliva products exist and can be recommended to the patient; however, the effect is only temporary and patients report equally satisfying relief from drinking frequent small sips of water. Although some salivary function can return following the cessation of treatment, the patient should understand that salivary return will never reach the preradiated level.

Loss of taste

A side effect that frequently occurs with radiation to the head and neck is loss of or alteration in taste. This symptom occurs when the taste buds are included in the radiated field and is compounded by mucositis and xerostomia. Patients will find eating very difficult at a time when maintenance of good nutritional status is paramount. Frequent meals that include high-protein, high-calorie foods should be encouraged. Because the patient may experience taste changes associated with favorite foods, bland foods may be better tolerated. High-calorie, high-protein malts and shakes generally are soothing to the oral mucosa and are not associated with any taste changes. Anorexia is an accompanying symptom that can interfere with an optimal nutritional status. Nutritional interventions will be discussed later in this chapter.

Fatigue

Fatigue is a frequently reported side effect of radiation therapy. Patients should be aware that this is a normal side effect that can occur at any time during the treatment course. Daily activities should be planned to include frequent rest periods for conservation of energy. In addition, depression and poor nutritional intake can also contribute to fatigue.

Skin reactions

Wet and or dry desquamation can occur in the tissues of the radiated site. This is frequently observed in areas of the neck that are subjected to frequent irritation, like the collar line. A variety of protocols exist for treatment of skin reactions. The radiation therapy department should determine the specific treatment approach. Generally, the patient should be instructed to avoid using harsh creams, lotions, or soaps in the radiated area. The area should be protected from the sun both during and after treatment. If the patient has a metal tracheostomy tube, it should be changed to a plastic one during treatment to prevent an enhanced reaction at the tracheostomy site.

The patient and family should understand the importance of radiation therapy in the treatment plan. Often, the symptoms experienced will be very difficult to endure and may affect the patient's ability to persevere to complete the treatment course. However, with support from family and health care workers and with information and suggestions for symptom control, the radiation course can be successfully completed.

MANAGEMENT OF THE ALTERED AIRWAY

If the treatment plans include compromise of the upper airway or if the tumor affects the patient's ability to breathe, a temporary tracheostomy will be placed. The accompanying nursing care is a large portion of both caring for and teaching the head and neck cancer patient. Tracheostomy is effectively used in situations where airway obstruction or compromised pulmonary function is anticipated or already exists. In the postoperative head and neck cancer patient, the massive edema that develops after oropharyngeal procedures necessitates tracheostomy at the time of surgery.

The procedure is usually performed under general anesthesia in the operating room. The patient is positioned with the neck hyperextended. A horizontal skin incision is made about 1½ mm below the level of the cricoid cartilage. A vertical incision (one of several types of incisions) is made through the second and third tracheal rings. A cuffed tracheostomy tube is then placed into the trachea and sutured into place. If the incision is made below the level of the third ring, the end of the tracheostomy tube can erode the innominate or right common carotid arteries and can result in massive hemorrhage.[50]

The Tracheostomy Tube

The type of tracheostomy tube utilized will depend on the surgical procedure performed and the clinical objectives to be achieved. A cuffed tracheostomy tube is the tube of choice for postoperative management of the patient. The standard parts of any tracheostomy tube and their functions are outlined in Table 44-10.

TABLE 44-10 The Standard Tracheostomy Tube

Part	Function
Obturator	Provides smooth tapered end during insertion to avoid tearing tracheal mucosa. Only used during insertion of outer cannula.
Outer cannula	Rigid structure inserted into tracheostoma. Curved between 70 and 95 degrees.
Inner cannula	Removed and cleaned (nondisposable) type or changed (disposable) to prevent accumulation of mucous plugs in outer cannula. Locks into outer cannula.
Cuff	Bonded to outer cannula. When inflated, provides seal between the tracheostomy tube and sides of tracheal wall.

Tracheal Suction

The tracheal suctioning procedure is an important part of postoperative nursing care of the head and neck cancer patient. The procedure itself is often one of the most frightening procedures for the patient; however, with adequate preoperative teaching and discussion, fears and anxiety can be minimized. If the procedure is performed correctly, the patient should not experience pain. The suction catheter should be passed gently into the trachea and a small "pill-rolling" motion should occur on removal of the catheter. Controversy surrounds the recommendation of sterile versus a clean procedure for suctioning. This author believes that sterile procedure should be employed until self-care teaching begins. Clean technique is always used in the home environment, and the patient is taught good hand washing and a procedure for cleaning and reusing suction catheters.

Each institution will have an approved procedure for suctioning the trachea, but all procedures should follow the same basic sequence:

1. Wash hands thoroughly.
2. Open sterile suction kit and/or tracheostomy tray.
3. Apply sterile gloves.
4. Attach catheter to source of negative pressure.
5. Fill basin with sterile water or saline solution.
6. Quickly insert catheter without pressure.
7. Apply suction and slowly withdraw catheter using a rotating motion.
8. Rinse saline or water through lumen of catheter.
9. Repeat procedure if secretions are profuse.

Some points to remember regarding suctioning a tracheostomy include the following:

- Only suction after a thorough respiratory assessment reveals the patient cannot clear the airway effectively. Routine suctioning can produce tracheal trauma and irritation.
- Limit suctioning to 10 seconds or less at 120 mm Hg or less.[51]
- Hyperoxygenation and hyperinflation of the lungs are advised both before and after the procedure to prevent suction-induced hypoxemia and subsequent arrhythmias. The optimal amount of oxygen and best method of hyperinflation remain in question and warrant further study.[51]

Inner Cannula Care

The inner cannula allows for removal and cleaning to maintain patency of the tracheostomy tube. The inner cannula should be removed and cleaned as needed but should be checked at least every 4 hours in the immediate postoperative period. Tubes that are constructed of a polyvinyl chloride or other plastic material can be cleaned with hydrogen peroxide and saline. Inner cannulas from metal tracheostomy tubes should be cleaned with saline or sterile water only. If metal tubes are cleaned with hydrogen peroxide, the oxidizing properties will tarnish the metal quickly.

Tracheostomy Site Care

The tracheostomy site should be treated like any other surgical wound. The nurse must be alert to signs and symptoms that can signal infection such as erythema and purulent drainage from the site. The site should be cleansed with a cotton swab that has been dipped in half-strength hydrogen peroxide and then should be rinsed with a swab dipped in sterile water. Generally, site care is performed once every 8 hours in the immediate postoperative period. The tracheostomy ties should be threaded through the slots in the flange of the tube and tied in a double knot on the uninvolved side of the neck. The ties should be secured at a tension that allows one finger to slip easily between the ties and the neck. The ties should be changed whenever they become soiled. The new ties should be in place before the soiled ties are cut and removed to prevent accidental dislodgement of the tube. The tracheostomy dressing should be placed under the flange of the tube and should also be changed whenever it becomes soiled. The dressing is always a gauze dressing that will absorb secretions and help to keep the tracheostomy area dry. If wound breakdown occurs at the tracheostomy site, care is directed toward promoting healing and preventing infection. It may be helpful to apply an occlusive material such as Stomahesive® to the skin adjacent to the tracheostomy site to promote healing. If there are flaps or grafts or a large amount of edema in the area, breakdown can occur at pressure points of the neck flange of the tube. Meticulous site care, relieving pressure by not tying the ties too tightly, and changing the tracheostomy dressing whenever it becomes soiled will help promote wound healing.

Humidity

The concept of providing adequate humidity to the patient with an altered airway is one of the most important points for the patient and family to understand. It is important to remember that the patient has lost the functions of the nose in warming, moistening, and filtering the air when breathing through a tracheostomy site. If supplemental humidity is not provided, the tracheal secretions become thick, tenacious, and difficult to clear from the airway. In the immediate postoperative period, high humidity (100%) with oxygen if indicated, or room air if oxygen is not indicated will prevent drying of the tracheal mucosa. In addition, the mucociliary transport process is not interrupted, and crusting of mucus along the airway passages is prevented.[50] The most commonly used device to provide supplemental humidity in the immediate postoperative period is the tracheostomy high-humidity collar. In the home setting the patient should have a large, 9–10-gallon room humidifier in the living area of the home and a small bedside humidifier during the nighttime.

Instillation of Normal Saline

Up to 5 ml of sterile normal saline may be instilled directly into the tracheostomy tube if secretions are tenacious and difficult to remove.[51] The action of the saline is to lavage and irritate the trachea and bronchi; coughing is precipitated and secretions are mobilized.[52] In addition, a nasal atomizer may be filled with saline and four or five "puffs" of saline sprayed into the tracheostoma on a regular basis to keep secretions thin and moist.

Cuffed Tracheostomy Tubes

The purpose of a cuff on a tracheostomy tube is to protect the airway from aspiration of blood or secretions. A cuff should only be used if indicated and should not be overfilled. Cuffs on tracheostomy tubes are high volume and low pressure, exerting less than 25 mm Hg on the tracheal wall.[53] Inflating a cuff beyond its maximal resting volume can cause tracheal necrosis and damage. The recommended procedure for cuff inflation, the "minimal leak technique," is performed as follows:

1. Using a hand-held resuscitation bag, simultaneously ausculate the neck.
2. Slowly inflate the cuff until a seal is obtained.
3. Withdraw 0.1 ml of air to create a small leak.

This procedure will ensure safe use of the tracheostomy cuff. Indications for use of a cuff may be the following:

- chronic aspiration
- bleeding in the head and neck area
- cardiopulmonary resuscitation
- positive pressure respiratory treatments
- emesis

A sample teaching plan that summarizes specifics of preparing a patient to go home with a tracheostomy can be found in Table 44-11.

Laryngectomy Care

Care of the altered airway of the laryngectomy patient includes all of the respiratory care mentioned previously. If the patient has a laryngectomy tube, it will have an inner cannula that can be cleaned as previously described. If there is no tube in place, the edges of the laryngectomy stoma are kept clean and free from crusting with the same procedure indicated for

TABLE 44-11 Teaching Plan for Tracheostomy Care

OBJECTIVE: To prepare the patient and family for performing tracheostomy care in the home.

	Activity	Expected Outcome
DAY 1 *Equipment:* Clean basin with H_2O_2 and water Soft, lint free cloth to dry inner cannula Trach brush	1. Teach removal and cleaning of inner cannula: If patient is going home with a *reusable* inner cannula, it will need to be removed and cleaned at least three times a day or as indicated by accumulation of secretions. Clean cannula in hydrogen peroxide using trach brush to remove secretions. Rinse with tap water. Replace.	Patient/significant other (S.O.) is able to unlock and remove cannula, stabilize neck plate during removal, and successfully clean cannula.
	If patient has a *disposable* inner cannula, it will need to be checked for secretions at *least* three times a day. If secretions have accumulated, discard soiled cannula and replace with clean cannula.	Patient/S.O. uses snap-lock mechanism; removes and changes inner cannula.
	If patient has metal tube, use water instead of hydrogen peroxide, which will tarnish the metal.	
DAY 2 *Equipment:* Suction machine Suction catheters Mirror Small cup of saline Small basin with soap and water Lint free towel to dry catheter	SUCTIONING THE TRACHEOSTOMY 1. Clean technique may be used. 2. Wash hands prior to performing procedure. 3. Attach appropriate-sized suction catheter to portable suction machine. 4. Turn machine on. 5. Occlude suction port; test suction in small cup of saline. 6. Introduce catheter into tracheostoma, keeping suction port *open*. 7. Occlude suction port to apply suction. 8. Slowly withdraw catheter using "pill-rolling" motion to facilitate suction of all secretions. 9. Suction saline through catheter to clear. 10. Catheter may be washed in mild liquid soap and stored in a clean, covered container for reuse.	Patient/S.O. will perform suction technique correctly and will understand indications for performing suction technique.
	INDICATIONS FOR SUCTIONING 1. Suction technique should be used whenever secretions become thick, tenacious, and difficult to mobilize by coughing.	
Equipment: H_2O_2 Cotton-tipped applicator Saline in small cup Clean gauze dressing	TRACHEOSTOMY SITE CARE 1. Tracheostomy site should be cleaned at least daily and more frequently as indicated by accumulation of secretions. 2. Use hydrogen peroxide–soaked applicator to clean skin under neck plate close to stomal edges.	Patient/S.O. will carefully perform trach site care. He or she will understand rationale for frequency of cleaning as indicated by drainage. He or she will know signs and symptoms of infection to be reported.

(continued)

TABLE 44-11 Teaching Plan for Tracheostomy Care (continued)

	Activity	Expected Outcome
	TRACHEOSTOMY SITE CARE (continued)	
	3. Follow by cleansing skin with saline-soaked applicator. 4. Report any signs of infection: erythema, purulent drainage, fever. 5. Change tracheostomy dressing whenever it becomes soiled. Tracheostomy dressing consists of a gauze dressing (noncotton back).	
DAY 3	IMPORTANCE OF SUPPLEMENTAL HUMIDITY	
	1. Supplemental humidity is required for any patient with a tracheostomy or laryngectomy. 2. Methods of administration of supplemental humidity include: instilling 1½–2 cc of normal saline into tracheostomy tube *or* using saline-filled nasal atomizer (four or five puffs to tracheostomy tube). 3. The humidity level in the home should be kept at least at 40%. A large 9–10 gallon room humidifier and a bedside humidifier will usually provide adequate humidity.	Patient/S.O. will understand the need to provide supplemental humidity. He or she will be able to manually perform instillation procedures and will be able to verbally relate signs and symptoms of inadequate humidity as well as actions to correct situation in which additional humidity is required.
	CARE OF EQUIPMENT IN THE HOME	
	1. Suction catheters may be rinsed in mild soap and water and stored in a clean, covered container. They may be reused until discoloration in the catheter appears. 2. Follow manufacturer's recommendations for care of suction machine and humidifer. Generally, weekly cleaning is recommended. 3. One-quarter-inch seam binding, purchased from a fabric store, may be substituted for tracheostomy ties. 4. A second tracheostomy tube of the same size should be sent home with the patient. All parts to the tube should be kept together and not interchanged with second tube.	The patient/S.O. will understand that equipment may be reused in the home if cared for properly. Not only does this decrease cost, but it is safe in the home environment.
	CHANGING THE TRACHEOSTOMY TUBE	
Equipment: New trach tube with ties Water-soluble lubricant Cotton-tipped swabs Hydrogen peroxide quarter strength Scissors Mirror	1. Change tracheostomy tube once a week or as directed by physician. 2. Tracheostomy tubes are only changed once the track is firmly established. (Usually 2–3 weeks postoperatively) 3. Assemble equipment. Place clean trach tube with tie on clean cloth surface. Place obturator inside trach tube. Lubricate tip with water-soluble lubricant. Snip trach tie. Remove trach with downward curved motion.	Patient/S.O. will demonstrate trach change on a model or patient as directed by physician.

(continued)

TABLE 44-11 Teaching Plan for Tracheostomy Care (continued)

Activity	Expected Outcome
CHANGING THE TRACHEOSTOMY TUBE (continued)	
Cough—Wipe stoma with gauze. Inspect stoma. Cleanse with hydrogen peroxide and saline-soaked gauze. Insert clean trach tube into stoma. Lead with obturator tip in an upward curved motion into stoma. Immediately remove obturator. Secure with trach ties. Take a moment to catch your breath. Suction if necessary.	
PRECAUTIONS	
1. The patient should avoid swimming and water sports and exercise care in the shower to prevent water from entering the tracheostomy tube. 2. If difficulty breathing is experienced, the first action should be to remove the inner cannula—a mucous plug in the cannula could be obstructing the airway. If not relieved, suctioning should be performed. Finally, emergency assistance should be summoned and transportation to a local emergency room should be arranged.	The patient/S.O. will verbalize an understanding of precautions and potential emergency situations.

tracheostomy site care. Suctioning occurs directly through the stoma in this instance as well.

The provision of adequate humidity is a lifelong concern for the laryngectomy patient. Seasonal variances and geographic location will affect the amount of humidity needed to keep secretions moist and easy to mobilize. In addition, the laryngectomy patient should take care to protect the stoma from dirt, dust, and other particulate matter. A variety of stoma covers that are attractive and effective in protecting the airway are available. The local branch of the American Cancer Society can be helpful in recommending vendors who supply laryngectomy appliances.

GENERAL NURSING CONSIDERATIONS

Nutritional Management

Cancers of the head and neck by virtue of their location often impair the patient's ability to take nourishment by mouth. Often this results in a 15–20-pound weight loss that prompts the patient to seek medical treatment, presenting initially in a nutritionally compromised state. The discussion here will focus specifically on the interventions commonly utilized to improve the nutritional status in the head and neck cancer patient. (See Chapter 27 for a complete discussion on nutritional disturbances.)

Enteral therapy

The primary goal of nutritional support in the patient with head and neck cancer is to correct nutritional imbalances and to maintain an adequate weight. Patients who undergo surgical resections will have compromised oral intake necessitating placement, at least temporarily, of a feeding tube.

Most head and neck patients have a gastrointestinal tract that is intact and functioning. The obstruction in the GI tract is usually seen in the head and neck cancer patient in the upper area of the tract, therefore requiring enteral support to be delivered below the level of the obstruction. The type of feeding tubes that are most comfortable for the patient are small-bore, weighted tubes that are sized from 7–12 French. These tubes are flexible and have a low incidence of nasopharyngeal and nasogastric irritation. In addition, there is a decreased risk of reflux aspiration compared to large-bore tubes.[54] Small-bore tubes may be inserted with or without a stylet. Because there are inherent risks of esophageal perforation and pulmonary intubation with lung puncture, it is recommended that only experienced personnel place the tubes with a stylet. In addition, proper placement of the tube should be verified radiographically prior to the first feeding.[55]

The feeding tube is placed during surgery for the surgical patient. Following return of bowel sounds, the patient is started on a continuous slow feeding of an isotonic commercial formula. Usually, feedings are started slowly at 25 cc/hour and gradually increased to 100 cc/hour or as tolerated. When the patient is more active and mobile, the feeding may be changed to intermittent feedings every 4 hours. The dietitian monitors the patient's nutritional status closely and makes appropriate changes in either the method of delivery or the formula.

If enteral support is anticipated to be necessary for a prolonged period of time, a feeding gastrostomy tube may be recommended. Gastrostomy tubes are frequently seen in the head and neck cancer patient in the palliative setting. They are easily cared for in the home and can deliver nutrients that will increase the patient's comfort.

Oral feeding

Prior to initiating oral feedings for the postoperative head and neck cancer patient, an assessment of the patient's oral competence is necessary. Assessing a patient's ability to swallow is discussed in the swallowing rehabilitation section of this chapter. In addition, nutritional counseling should include an evaluation of dietary intake and an explanation of the patient's requirement for calories and proteins. The teaching should include suggestions for dietary changes that will be necessary as the patient begins to experience difficulty in ingestion such as during radiation therapy. The movement from a regular to soft to blenderized diet may be gradual as the patient begins to experience dysphagia.[56]

The psychosocial aspects of long-term enteral nutrition or even an altered method of eating should not be overlooked. The isolation that occurs from an inability to participate in meals and the body image changes associated with an alteration in eating pattern affect the quality of life for many patients.

Oral Care

The provision of regular and thorough oral care is imperative in the head and neck cancer patient. Not only can halitosis be a significant problem, but, more importantly, the surgical site of the oral cavity should be kept clean to prevent infection.

The method of oral care will depend upon the extent of surgical resection and the method of reconstruction. Generally, due to a compromise of competence, oral care via lavage or power spray is most effective. A solution of hydrogen peroxide and water will adequately cleanse debris from the area and will not interfere with healing. Oral care should be delivered every 4 hours in the early postop period. As wound healing occurs, it can be performed once every 8 hours to prevent odors and promote healing. A foul-smelling odor from the oral cavity could signal an infection in the area and should be investigated further. To avoid disruption of the suture line when using an oral power spray, the lowest setting on the machine should be used to deliver the treatment.

Swallowing Rehabilitation

The act of swallowing involves transporting a bolus of food or liquid from the mouth to the stomach. During swallowing, food that has been placed in the mouth is broken down in preparation for the swallow. The act of swallowing is one that is taken for granted until impairment from surgery or neurological disease occurs.

The four phases of the normal swallow include: the oral preparation phase, the oral phase, the pharyngeal phase, and the esophageal phase.[30] The sequence of events in a normal swallow is outlined in Table 44-12.

There are two primary components of the swallowing evaluation: the bedside evaluation and the radiographic evaluation. Completed by the swallowing therapist, the bedside evaluation can alert the practitioner to alterations in the oral preparatory and oral stages of swallowing. This portion of the assessment process evaluates the labial, lingual, and palatal range of movement during both speech and swallowing exercises. The bedside exam will not provide accurate information on the pharyngeal stage of swallow. In addition, it will not indicate why a patient aspirates if there is clinical evidence of material entering the airway. During the bedside evaluation it is important to remember that the patient can aspirate material and show no evidence of it by coughing. Many patients who have problems with aspiration never cough.

TABLE 44-12 The Normal Swallow

Phase	Action
Oral preparation phase	Food prepared for processing. Chewing occurs. Lip closure occurs to prevent drooling.
Oral phase	Bolus of food is propelled into pharynx.
Pharyngeal phase	Velopharyngeal valve closes to prevent nasal reflux. Soft palate retracts and elevates. Food enters pharynx. Tongue base retracts into pharynx.
Esophageal phase	Bolus approaches pyriform sinuses and enters esophagus. Cricopharyngeus muscle opens to allow entry. Larynx moves upward and forward. Peristalsis assists transport into the stomach.

Source: Logemann J: Swallowing and communication rehabilitation, *Semin Oncol Nurs* 5:205–207, 1989.

The assessment of the oral and pharyngeal stages of swallow are completed by a modified barium swallow, or "cookie swallow," in which the patient ingests small amounts of liquid, paste, and semisolid materials that have been coated with barium. The modified barium swallow will detect aspiration. From this study the etiology of the problem can be defined and swallowing therapy can be initiated.

Wound Care

The nursing responsibility in wound management lies initially in observation of dressings or the surgical site for any signs of infection or dehiscence. External suture lines are cleansed with cotton swabs soaked in a solution of half-strength hydrogen peroxide followed by sterile water or saline. This will help to loosen and remove crusting that accumulates following surgery. The use of an antibiotic or other ointment has been controversial and the physician should be consulted for preference.

A wound that requires debridement will be treated with wet to dry dressings. Gauze packing that has been soaked in saline is applied slightly wet, followed by application of a dry dressing as the outer dressing. Within 3–4 hours the packing will dry and it is gently removed, pulling necrotic tissue from the wound during the removal process. This procedure is repeated until all necrotic tissue is removed and evidence of tissue growth in the wound is seen. If an increased length of time for wound healing is projected, this procedure can be taught to the family and performed in the home.

Wound breakdown

Wound breakdown with subsequent exposure of the carotid artery is one of the most serious and life-threatening sequelae of either the disease process itself or of surgical therapy. Rupture of the carotid artery or any other major artery in the head and neck is a medical emergency. All health care workers who interact with head and neck cancer patients should be familiar with the procedures that are necessary to save a patient's life after carotid hemorrhage. The patient who is at risk for carotid hemorrhage should be identified to all as soon as there is evidence of wound breakdown in the area. In addition, emergency equipment should be placed at the bedside to manage the patient effectively until transport to the operating room for ligation can be arranged. An example of equipment needed is included in Table 44-13.

TABLE 44-13 Carotid Precautions: Equipment

Sterile cotton dressings (6 packages 4 × 4s)
2 cotton bath towels
Sterile bowl and normal saline solution
Ringer's lactate
Albumin
Type and crossmatch equipment (Vacutainer, holder, needle)
Completed requisitions for 2 units of blood
Two 20-ml syringes
Alcohol swabs
1 cuffed tracheostomy tube if indicated
Suction equipment

Source: Adapted from Schwartz SS, Yuska CM: Common patient care issues following surgery for head and neck cancer, *Semin Oncol Nurs* 15(3):191–194, 1989.

The nursing actions during a carotid hemorrhage focus on maintenance of the airway and control of bleeding. If the patient has a tracheostomy, the cuff should be inflated to prevent aspiration. The pressure from the cuff can also provide additional pressure internally to slow bleeding. The head of the bed should be elevated to facilitate drainage of secretions. The airway should be suctioned to maintain patency. Firm pressure should be applied to the neck using a towel or dressing material. If an internal carotid bleed is suspected, a vaginal pack or fluff dressing should be used to tightly pack the oral cavity and oropharynx. The pressure should not be released during preparation and transport of the patient to the operating room. Hemorrhagic shock is avoided by rapid infusion of intravenous fluids. Preparation for administration of blood should emergently occur. The patient is then transported to the operating room for ligation of the carotid artery. Unfortunately, patients generally remain conscious throughout this ordeal and are extremely frightened, not only by the sight of a large amount of blood but also by the intense level of activity that occurs rapidly around them. Measures to decrease the level of anxiety include speaking to the patient in a calm voice while explaining the activities that are occurring and emphasizing the goal to stop the bleeding.

The patient should be observed closely for subsequent hemorrhage or neurologic deficits following a carotid artery ligation. Numbness or tingling of the extremities on the ipsilateral side, diplopia, blindness, progressive motor loss, and changes in the level of consciousness will alert the nurse to possible cerebral ischemia secondary to carotid artery ligation.[57]

Carotid hemorrhage in the terminal patient

The goal following carotid hemorrhage in the terminal patient will not be ligation but providing an atmosphere that minimizes anxiety and ensures death with dignity. All of the previously mentioned precautions should be observed for the terminal patient, with the exception of transportation of the patient to the operating room for ligation. Narcotics should be administered to relieve discomfort and distress. The patient and family should be aware of the activities that will occur during carotid hemorrhage. If the plan includes discharging the patient to home, the nurse should discuss precautions to prepare the patient and family for the event of carotid hemorrhage at home. The realization of the eminence of death will make the patient and family apprehensive, but an open and frank discussion regarding the goal of treatment and an empathetic and knowledgeable approach by the nurse can facilitate a calm atmosphere at the time of death.

Pain Management

The management of pain following surgery for head and neck cancer or in the palliative setting requires an understanding of the physiology involved as well as utilization of keen assessment skills. Nicolson and colleagues[58] reported that head and neck cancer patients report less pain than do other cancer patients. In the immediate postoperative period this can be attributed to the severing of superficial nerves in the neck area, which results in a feeling of numbness in the surgical area rather than overt pain.

The type of pain usually experienced by the head and neck cancer patient is described as "throbbing, pounding, or pressurelike." The rise in spinal fluid pressure that occurs with occlusion or ligation of the jugular vein contributes to this description.

As with any pain management regimen, the goal is to provide adequate relief while simultaneously allowing the patient to function at an optimum level or to die with minimal discomfort. There are a variety of products available that can achieve this goal. It is preferable to use an oral or enteral route for pain management on a long-term basis. In addition, concentrated doses can be administered to patients with dysphagia so there is a smaller volume of liquid to swallow.[59]

Psychosocial Issues

In addition to coping with a diagnosis of cancer and its subsequent treatment, the head and neck cancer patient must also cope with an alteration in facial appearance and possible loss of speech, sight, taste, smell, and ability to swallow. This combination of adjustments is an enormous threat to the self-image. In addition, the patient's very identity and confidence are often threatened. Survival and adequate coping require great emotional strength. It is imperative that the practitioner working with the head and neck cancer patient understand the process of reintegrating the alterations that have resulted from surgery and identify a plan to assist the patient in the process.

Anxiety and depression are commonly reported both prior to surgery and during the rehabilitative period. The psychological investment in the head and neck area is greater than that in any other part of the body. This is because social interaction and emotional expression depend greatly on the integrity of the face, especially the eyes.[60] This is of even greater concern for the head and neck cancer patient who cannot hide the structural changes that result from treatment and must therefore deal with constant exposure to others. It is expected that the patient will have fears regarding the reaction of family, friends, and strangers to the alteration in appearance.

Two parameters must be considered in the adjustment process: disfigurement and dysfunction. Although both may vary from minor to major, the health care worker must be sensitive to both issues. The degree of body image change required of the patient in adapting to the loss correlates with the extent of dysfunction and disfigurement. This can predict the severity of emotional response and can be helpful in constructing a plan of care.

Dropkin[61] has extensively studied the process of coping with disfigurement and dysfunction following head and neck cancer surgery. Regulations that limit the time a cancer patient may stay in the hospital have made it imperative to recognize maladaptive coping immediately and initiate appropriate interventions quickly. The Dysfunction/Disfigurement Scale developed by Dropkin and others at Memorial Sloan-Kettering Cancer Center can assist the nurse in developing a treatment plan to address these issues.[61] The results of Dropkin's study revealed important information about the way patients cope with disfigurement and dysfunction after head and neck cancer surgery. It was found that, generally, postoperative days 4–6 are pivotal in the recovery process in terms of acceptance of the defect. The measurements included assessment of self-care and amount of social affiliation that occurred between the patient and others. Acceptance of the defect, as demonstrated by the performance of self-care tasks, usually preceded social affiliative behaviors. Patients who do not cope effectively should receive more intensive interventions prior to discharge to prevent noncompliance with care at home. Moreover, failure to adequately cope with disfigurement and dysfunction can lead to pathological obsession with or denial of the defect, depression, or social isolation.[62]

CONCLUSION

There have been significant advances in the treatment of head and neck cancer over the past decade. The disease process as well as the treatment regimen present significant challenges to the patient as well as health care providers. Government regulations have resulted in a decreased length of stay in the hospital, which in turn mandates a multidisciplinary approach that addresses the patient's physical and psychosocial needs in a comprehensive and timely manner. Providing quality care to the head and neck cancer patient in the next century will require a system that transcends institutional boundaries and extends into the home and community setting. The opportunity for expansion of the role that nursing plays in providing preventive education and assessment will become even more important in the years to come.

REFERENCES

1. Spiro R, Rice D: *Current Concepts in Head and Neck Cancer.* New York: American Cancer Society, 1989, p. 1.
2. Rothman KJ, Cann CI, Flanders D, et al: Epidemiology of laryngeal cancer. *Epidemiol Rev* 2:195–209, 1980.
3. Schleper JR: Prevention, detection, and diagnosis of head and neck cancers. *Semin Oncol Nurs* 5:139–149, 1989.
4. Wynder EL, Mushinski M, Spivak J: Tobacco and alcohol consumption in relation to the development of multiple cancers. *Cancer* 40:1872–1878, 1977.
5. Simons MJ, Chan SH, Wee GB, et al: Nasopharyngeal carcinoma: Significance of changes in Epstein-Barr virus related antibody patterns following therapy. *Int J Cancer* 20:663–672, 1977.
6. Ryan D, Starr B: Vitamins in prevention and treatment of cancer. *Contem Oncol* 2:45–65, 1992.
7. Lindberg R: Distribution of cervical lymph node metastases from squamous cell carcinoma of the upper respiratory and digestive tracts. *Cancer* 29:1446–1450, 1972.
8. Thawley SE, Panje WR, Batsakis JG, Lindberg RD (eds): *Comprehensive Management of Head and Neck Tumors.* Philadelphia: Saunders, 1987.
9. Schramm V: Craniofacial surgery for sinus tumors. In Thawley SE, Panje WR, Batsakis JG, Lindberg RD (eds): *Comprehensive Management of Head and Neck Tumors.* Philadelphia: Saunders, 1987, pp. 390–407.
10. Nestler A: Integral nursing interventions for cranial base surgical patients. *ORL-Head Neck Nurs* 10:7–10, 1992.
11. Guyton AC: *Physiology of the Human Body.* Philadelphia: Saunders, 1979, pp. 145–146.
12. Moss WT: Radiation therapy for tumors of the nasal cavity and paranasal sinuses. In Thawley SE, Panje WR, Batsakis JG, Lindberg RD (eds): *Comprehensive Management of Head and Neck Tumors.* Philadelphia: Saunders, 1987, pp. 344–352.
13. Panje WR, Gross CE: Treatment of tumors of the nasopharynx: Surgical therapy. In Thawley SE, Panje WR, Batsakis JG, Lindberg RD (eds): *Comprehensive Management of Head and Neck Tumors.* Philadelphia: Saunders, 1987, pp. 662–683.
14. Chao R, Tannock I: Chemotherapy for recurrent or metastatic carcinoma of the nasopharynx. A review of the Princess Margaret Hospital experience. *Cancer* 68(10): 2120–2124, 1991.
15. Crawford BE, Callihan MD, Cario RL, et al: Oral pathology. *Otolaryngol Clin North Am* 12:29, 1979.
16. Hannon L: Cancer of the oral cavity. *Semin Oncol Nurs* 5:150–159, 1989.
17. Kornblut A: Clinical evaluation of tumors of the oral cavity. In Thawley SE, Panje WR, Batsakis JG, Lindberg RD (eds): *Comprehensive Management of Head and Neck Tumors.* Philadelphia: Saunders, 1987, pp. 460–479.
18. Richardson MF: The problem of multiple primary tumors in patients with oral malignant disease. *Otolaryngol Clin North Am* 12:155, 1979.
19. Adams G, Haselow R: Oral and pharyngeal cancer—Early diagnosis for optimal treatment. Part I. *Hosp Med* 19:173, 1983.
20. Robbins SL, Angell M, Kumar V: *Basic Pathology* (3d ed). Philadelphia: Saunders, 1981.
21. Oken MM: Chemotherapy in the treatment of head and neck cancer. In McQuarrie DG, Adams GL, Shons AR, et al (eds): *Head and Neck Cancer: Clinical Decisions and Management Principles.* Chicago: Year Book Medical, 1986, pp. 133–143.
22. Sessions DG: Composite resection and reconstruction with skin grafts for oral cavity and oropharynx cancer. In Chretien PB, John ME, Shedd DP, et al (eds): *Head and Neck Cancer: Proceedings of the International Conference,* July 22–24, 1984. Philadelphia: Dekker, 1985, pp. 187–193.
23. Shah J, et al: Buccal mucosa, alveolus, retromolar trigone, floor of mouth, hard palate, and tongue tumors. In Thawley SE, Panje WR, Batsakis JG, Lindberg RD (eds): *Comprehensive Management of Head and Neck Tumors.* Philadelphia: Saunders, 1987, pp. 551–563.
24. Jesse RH, Ballantyne AJ, Larson RL: Radical or modified neck dissection: Therapeutic dilemma. *Am J Surg* 136:516, 1978.
25. Lingeman R, Shellhamer R: Surgical management of tumors of the neck. In Thawley, SE, Panje WR, Batsakis JG, Lindberg RD (eds): *Comprehensive Management of Head and Neck Tumors.* Philadelphia: Saunders, 1987, pp. 1325–1350.
26. Scher N, Panje W: New concepts in head and neck surgery. *Hemol Oncol Clin North Am* 5:627–634, 1991.
27. Thawley S, Sessions D: Surgical therapy of hypo-pharyngeal tumors. In Thawley S, Panje WR, Batsakis JG, Lindberg RD (eds): *Comprehensive Management of Head and Neck Tumors.* Philadelphia: Saunders, 1987, pp. 774–812.
28. Pfister D et al: Larynx preservation with combined chemotherapy and radiation therapy in advanced but resectable head and neck cancer. *J Clin Oncol* 9(5):850–859, 1991.
29. Edels Y (ed): *Laryngectomy: Diagnosis to Rehabilitation.* Rockville, MD: Aspen, 1983.
30. Logemann J: Swallowing and communication rehabilitation. *Semin Oncol Nurs* 5:205–212, 1989.
31. Thawley S, Sessions D: Surgical therapy of supraglottic tumors. In Thawley S, Panje WR, Batsakis JG, Lindberg RD (eds): *Comprehensive Management of Head and Neck Tumors.* Philadelphia: Saunders, 1987, pp. 959–991.
32. Panje WR: Myocutaneous trapezius flap. *Head Neck Surg* 2:206–212, 1980.
33. Ackland RD, Flynn MB: Immediate reconstruction of oral cavity and oropharyngeal defects using micro-vascular free flaps. *Am J Surg* 136:419, 1978.
34. Sigler BA: Nursing care for head and neck tumor patients. In Thawley S, Panje WR, Batsakis JG, Lindberg RD (eds): *Comprehensive Management of Head and Neck Tumors.* Philadelphia: Saunders, 1987, pp. 79–99.
35. Vokes EE et al: Cisplatin and fluorouracil chemotherapy does not yield long-term benefit in locally advanced head and neck cancer: Results from a single institution. *J Clin Oncol* 9:1376–1384, 1991.
36. Carter SK: The chemotherapy of head and neck cancer. *Semin Oncol* 4:413–424, 1977.
37. Ensley JF, Jacobs JR, Weaver A, et al: Correlation between response to cisplatin-combination chemotherapy and subsequent radiotherapy in previously untreated patients with advanced squamous cell cancer of the head and neck. *Cancer* 54:811–814, 1984.

38. Hong WK, Bromer R: Current concepts: Chemotherapy in head and neck cancer. *N Engl J Med* 3308:70–75, 1983.
39. Urba LS, Wolf G: Organ preservation in multimodality therapy of head and neck cancer. *Hemol Oncol Clin North Am* 5:713–724, 1991.
40. Vlock D: Immunobiologic aspects of head and neck cancer. *Hemol Oncol Clin North Am* 5:797–821, 1991.
41. Forni G, Cavallo GP, Giovarelli M, et al: Tumor immunotherapy by local injection of interleukin 2 and nonreactive lymphocytes. Experimental and clinical results. *Prog Exp Tumor Res* 32:187, 1988.
42. Forastiere AA: Randomized trials of induction chemotherapy. A critical review. *Hemol Oncol Clin North Am* 5:725–736, 1991.
43. Eisenberger M, Hornedo J, Silva H, et al: Carboplatin (NSC-241–240): An active platinum analog for the treatment of squamous-cell carcinoma of the head and neck. *J Clin Oncol* 4:1506–1509, 1986.
44. Dimery I, Brooks B, Winn R, et al: Phase II trial of carboplatin plus cisplatin in recurrent and advanced squamous cell carcinoma of the head and neck. *J Clin Oncol* 9:1939–1944, 1991.
45. Awan A, Vokes E, Weichelbaum R: Recent advances in radiation therapy for head and neck cancer. *Hemol Oncol Clin North Am* 5:635–655, 1991.
46. Sutherland R, Mulcahy R: Basic principles of radiation therapy. In Rubin P (ed): *Clinical Oncology for Medical Students and Physicians: A Multidisciplinary Approach* (6th ed). New York: American Cancer Society, 1983, pp. 40–57.
47. Strohl R: Radiation therapy for head and neck cancer. *Semin Oncol Nurs* 5:166–173, 1989.
48. Vokes E, Awan A, Weichselbaum R: Radiotherapy with concomitant chemotherapy for head and neck cancer. *Hemol Oncol Clin North Am* 5:753–767, 1991.
49. King KB, Nail LM, Kreamer KK, et al: Patients' descriptions of the experience of receiving radiation therapy. *Oncol Nurs For* 12:55–61, 1985.
50. Martin L: Management of the altered airway in the head and neck cancer patient. *Semin Oncol Nurs* 5:182–190, 1989.
51. Shekelton ME, Nield M: Ineffective airway clearance related to artificial airway. *Nurs Clin North Am* 22:167–178, 1987.
52. Ackerman MH: The use of bolus normal saline instillations in artificial airways: Is it useful or necessary? *Heart Lung* 14:505–506, 1985.
53. Hoffman (Kiriloff) LA: Airway management for the critically ill patient. *Am J Nurs* 87:40–53, 1987.
54. Whatley K, Turner LW, Dey M, Meier M: Transpyloric passage of feeding tubes. *Nutr Supp Serv* 3:18, 1983.
55. Martyn-Nemeth P, Fitzgerald K: Tube feeding in the elderly. *J Geront Nurs* 18:30–36, 1992.
56. Grant M, Rhiner M, Padilla G: Nutritional management in the head and neck cancer patient. *Semin Oncol Nurs* 5:195–204, 1989.
57. Carini E, Owens G: *Neurological and Neurosurgical Nursing* (6th ed). St. Louis, MO: Mosby, 1980, p. 232.
58. Nicholsen BA, McGuire DB, Maurer VE: Assessment of pain in head and neck cancer patients using the McGill questionnaire. *J Soc Otorhino Head/Neck Nurs* 6:8–12, 1988.
59. Levy MH: Pain management in advanced cancer. *Semin Oncol* 12:394–410, 1985.
60. Breitbart W, Holland J: Psychosocial aspects of head and neck cancer. *Semin Oncol* 15:61–63, 1988.
61. Dropkin M: Coping with disfigurement and dysfunction after head and neck cancer surgery: A conceptual framework. *Semin Oncol Nurs* 5:213–219, 1989.
62. Nordlicht S: Facial disfigurement and psychiatric sequelae. *NY State J Med* 9:1282, 1384, 1979.

Chapter 45

Leukemia

Debra Wujcik, RN, MSN, OCN

INTRODUCTION

Leukemia is the name given to a group of hematologic malignancies affecting the bone marrow and lymph tissue. First described by the German pathologist Virchow in 1847 as simply "white blood," the term *leukemia* now includes abnormalities of proliferation and maturation in lymphocyte and myeloid (nonlymphocyte) cell lines. The acute leukemias are marked by an abnormal proliferation of immature blood cells with a short natural history (1–5 months), while the chronic leukemias have an excessive accumulation of more mature-appearing but still ineffective cells and a slower, progressive course (2–5 years). The excessive proliferation of the leukemia cells results in an overcrowding of the bone marrow, causing a decreased production and function of normal hemopoietic cells.

EPIDEMIOLOGY

Leukemia represents 3% of the cancer incidence, with an estimated 29,300 new cases and 18,600 deaths expected in 1993[1,2] Approximately one-half of the cases are acute and the remaining cases are chronic, but the number of new cases per year is greater in adults (26,700) than in children (2600). The most common types of leukemia in adults are acute myelogenous leukemia (AML) and chronic lymphocytic leukemia (CLL), while acute lymphocytic leukemia (ALL) accounts for 80% of all childhood leukemias.[3,4] The incidence of leukemia rose steeply from 1900 to the 1940s. Since then the incidence of AML has continued to increase steadily, both in the United States and developing countries, suggesting the influence of occupational and environmental exposure.[5]

ETIOLOGY

The cause of leukemia is not known. The etiologic factors most commonly considered are genetic predisposition, radiation, chemicals, drugs, and viruses.

Genetic Factors

The relationship of genetic factors to the incidence of leukemia has been suggested in certain high-risk families and specific hereditary syndromes. There is evidence of familial clustering with a four- to sevenfold increased risk in individuals with a family member diagnosed with leukemia.[6,7] Additionally, 10%–20% of monozygous twins of individuals with leukemia develop the disease.[6–8]

Certain genetic disorders are associated with increased incidence of leukemia. Children with Down's syndrome (trisomy 21) have an 18-fold to 20-fold increased incidence of acute leukemia.[9,10] Other disorders with chromosome abnormalities or fragilities also associated with acute leukemia are Bloom's syndrome, Fanconi's anemia, Kleinfelter's syndrome, and Ellis-Van Creveld syndrome.[3,11,12]

Diseases such as ataxia telangiectasia and congenital agammaglobulinemia are also prone to terminate in acute leukemia.[6,8] Although chromosomal abnormalities in these diseases are not detectable, deficiencies exist in humoral and cellular immunity. Whether congenital chromosomal defects cause or coexist with leukemia remains unclear; evidence of chromosomal abnormality and/or fragility appears to favor progression to a malignant state. In addition to certain genetic factors being associated with the development of leukemia, new techniques in chromosome analysis allow investigators to correlate chromosomal aberrations with survival rates.[12] This should allow the modification of therapy to include intensive or investigational therapy to improve outcome for those with low response rates.

Radiation

Populations exposed to ionizing radiation have an increased incidence of leukemia, especially AML. Japanese survivors of the atomic bomb experienced a 20-fold increased incidence of AML and chronic myelogenous leukemia (CML). There appeared to be a direct relationship with the distance the individual was from the center of the explosion. The peak incidence was at 5–7 years following exposure, and increased risks continued for 20 years.[13,14] In addition, early radiologists exposed to excessive irradiation experienced a higher incidence of leukemia.[15] Also, patients who were diagnosed with ankylosing spondylitis and treated with 2000 cGy had a 14-fold increase of AML when compared with similar patients who were not irradiated.[16] Radiation remains the most conclusively identified leukemogenic factor in human beings.

Chemicals

Chronic exposure to certain chemicals has been associated with an increased incidence of pancytopenia and subsequent AML. Benzene, an aromatic hydrocarbon, is produced by natural processes and by industry (unleaded gasoline, rubber cement, cleaning solvents).[17] It was first implicated in the development of acute leukemia in Turkish cobblers in the early 1900s. Since then other populations have been identified as being at risk, including workers with explosives, distillers, dye users, painters, and shoemakers.[18,19]

TABLE 45-1 Characteristics of Treatment-Induced Acute Nonlymphocytic Leukemia (ANL) Compared to "Spontaneous" ANL

Treatment-Related ANL	"Spontaneous" ANL
Related to prior exposure to alkylating agents and/or radiotherapy	Etiology largely unknown; small % related to chemical exposure (eg, benzene)
Prolonged pancytopenia/preleukemia prior to onset	Approximately 30% present with preleukemia; rest have sudden onset
Latency period 2–5 years postexposure, with peak in incidence approximately 5 years	Latency period unknown
Dysplasia of one or more cell lines on marrow biopsy	May show dysplasia of cell lines
Specific cytogenetic abnormalities of chromosomes 3, 5, 7, 17. Approximately 90% have abnormalities of 5 and/or 7. 11q abnormalities are associated with epipodophyllotoxin exposure.	Specific cytogenetic abnormalities of chromosomes 5, 7, 8, 11, 15, 16, 17, 21, (rarely 3, 4). Less than 5% have abnormalities of 5 and/or 7.
Refractory to treatment	Responsive to combination chemotherapy
Poor survival; almost uniformly fatal within a few months	Approximately 50% 1-year survival with some long-term survivors following BMT
Peak age varies depending on primary tumor, age of onset, about 5 years after treatment for first cancer	Peak age onset in 50s

Source: Reprinted from the *Oncology Nursing Forum* with permission from the Oncology Nursing Press. Fraser MC, Tucker MA: Late effects of cancer therapy: Chemotherapy-related malignancies. *Oncol Nurs Forum* 15(1):70, 1988.

Drugs

Drugs that have demonstrated a relationship to the etiology of acute leukemia include certain alkylating agents, the antibiotic chloramphenicol, and phenylbutazone. AML is the most frequently reported second cancer following aggressive chemotherapy and is associated with treatment for Hodgkin's disease, multiple myeloma, ovarian cancer, non-Hodgkin's lymphoma, and breast cancer. Recently the epipodophyllotoxin etoposide has also been implicated as a leukemogen.[20–22]

Characteristics that distinguish therapy-related and *de novo* (with no known causative factors) leukemia are summarized in Table 45-1.[23] Secondary leukemias induced by alkylators are characterized by chromosome translocations such as t(9;22) or t(4;11), while leukemias arising after epipodophyllotoxin therapy are identified by 11q abnormalities. Therapy-related leukemia now represents 10%–15% of all AML patients,[24] and overall median survival is 4–8 months.[25,26] The time of greatest risk appears to be the first 10 years after treatment. Chloramphenicol and phenylbutazone are known to cause aplastic anemia and chromosomal breaks that eventually terminate in AML.[27,28]

Viruses

The role of viruses in the etiology of human leukemia is unclear. The enzyme reverse transcriptase is present primarily in C-type viruses, a group of RNA viruses that can cause leukemia in animals. This enzyme reverses the usual transcription of genetic information from DNA to RNA, allowing the RNA tumor virus to produce oncogenic DNA within the host cells.[29] There is evidence of horizontal transmission of this leukemogenic virus from cat to cat.[30] Reverse transcriptase has been detected in human leukemic blood cells, but not in normal blood cells.

Adult T-cell leukemia in Japan and the Caribbean is associated with the human T-cell leukemia virus (HTLV-I). There is evidence for a role of HTLV-1 in the etiology of adult T-cell leukemia in the United States.[31] HTLV-II has been identified in a rare form of hairy cell leukemia and is also prevalent in intravenous drug addicts.[32,33]

CLASSIFICATION

Leukemias are classified as either chronic or acute and as either myeloid or lymphoid. In chronic leukemia the predominant cell is mature-appearing although it does not function normally. The disease has a gradual onset, prolonged clinical course, and a relatively longer survival time. The predominant cell in acute leukemia is undifferentiated or immature, usually a "blast" cell. The abrupt onset and rapid disease progression result in a short survival time. However, as progress is made in the treatment of children with acute lymphocytic leukemia and longer survival occurs, it may no longer be appropriate to describe acute leukemia as having a short survival.

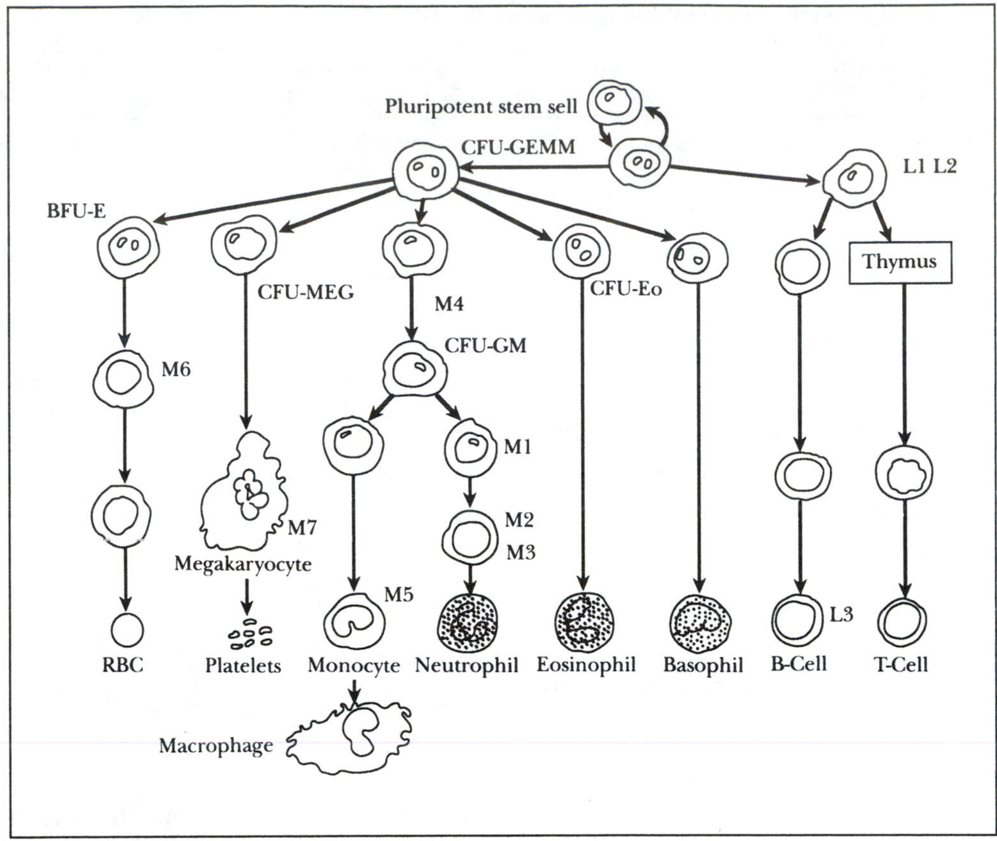

FIGURE 45-1 Hematopoietic cascade with FAB classifications of acute nonlymphocytic leukemia and acute lymphocytic leukemia at proposed levels of arrested cell maturation. BFU, burst-forming unit; CFU, colony-forming unit; GM, granulocyte, macrophage; GEMM, granulocyte, erythrocyte, macrophage, megakaryocyte; Epo, erythropoietin; MEG, megakaryocyte; Eo, eosinophil; E, erythrocyte; M1, undifferentiated myelocytic; M2, myelocytic; M3, promyelocytic; M4, myelomonocytic; M5, monocytic; M6, erythroleukemia; M7, megakaryocytic; L1, childhood; L2, adult; L3, Burkitt's type.

Figure 45-1 presents the major classification of leukemia according to the type of cell that predominates and the location of arrested cellular maturation. All cell lines arise from the same totipotent stem cell. From this cell, which has the potential to differentiate into a variety of cells, the myeloid and lymphocyte series are derived. The myeloid stem cell is pluripotent and gives rise to erythrocyte, thrombocyte, granulocyte, and monocyte progenitors or committed cells. These are immature forms that mature into fully functional red blood cells, platelets, and white blood cells. The lymphoid stem cell matures in the thymus to form T-cell progenitors, or in the bone marrow to form B-cell progenitors.

The type of leukemia is named according to the point at which cell maturation is arrested. Although the terms *lymphocytic* and *myelogenous* (nonlymphocytic) leukemia are most commonly used, further specification within each class (for example, *promyelocytic, myelocytic*) describes the exact point at which arrest of maturation seems to occur.

In 1976 the French-American-British (FAB) Cooperative Group developed criteria for the classification of the acute leukemias[34] (Table 45-2). The purpose was to provide a systematic, objective system that would be feasible in most hematologic laboratories. The system, based on morphology and number of cells, has

TABLE 45-2 French-American-British (FAB) Classification of Acute Leukemia

Myeloid		Lymphocytic
M1	Undifferentiated myelocytic	L1, childhood (Pre B- and T-cell)
M2	Myelocytic	L2, adult (Pre B- and T-cell)
M3	Promyelocytic	
M4	Myelomonocytic	L3, Burkitt's type (B-cell)
M5	Monocytic	
M6	Erythroleukemia	
M7	Megakaryocytic	

Source: Data from Bennett JM et al.[34–36]

been revised and updated.[35,36] The additional information obtained through cytogenetics, identification of surface markers, and histochemical staining provides important therapeutic and prognostic information.

PATHOPHYSIOLOGY

In the normal bone marrow, efficient regulatory mechanisms ensure that cell proliferation and maturation are adequate for the needs of the individual. In leukemia, control is missing or abnormal. The results are (1) arrest of the cell in an early phase of its maturation process, causing the accumulation of immature cells; (2) an abnormal proliferation of these immature cells; and (3) crowding of other marrow elements, resulting in inhibited growth and function of these elements and eventual replacement of the marrow by leukemic cells.

Manifestations of leukemia are related to three factors: (1) excessive proliferation of immature leukocytes within blood-forming organs such as the bone marrow, spleen, and lymph nodes, resulting in destruction of tissue; (2) infiltration of proliferating leukocytes into various organs of the body; and (3) decrease in the number of normal leukocytes, erythrocytes, and thrombocytes as a result of crowding of the bone marrow by proliferating leukemic cells. Table 45-3 summarizes possible leukemic manifestations, although these vary considerably with each type of leukemia.[37] The presenting manifestations, complications, course of disease, and treatment for each major type are discussed separately (Table 45-4).

TABLE 45-3 Manifestations of Leukemia

	Organ	Manifestations
	PRIMARY MANIFESTATIONS	
Result from the proliferation of leukocytes within blood-forming organs	Bone marrow	Hyperplasia of abnormal cells Hypoplasia of all normal cellular components Thrombocytopenia leads to bleeding Erythrocytopenia leads to anemia Granulocytopenia leads to infection
	Spleen and liver	Hepatosplenomegaly Changed consistency: Acute leukemia—soft Chronic leukemia—hard Infarction causes pain Hypersplenism leads to pancytopenia
	Lymph nodes	Lymphadenopathy May be painful Obstruction of adjacent organs or structures
	SECONDARY MANIFESTATIONS	
Result from the infiltration of leukemic cells into body tissues *or* consequences of bone marrow suppression	Liver	Hepatomegaly May be painful or tender
	Bones, joints, and muscle	Enlargement of the cortex of the long bones in children with acute lymphoblastic leukemia Osteolytic lesions Goutlike symptoms Pain Swelling
	Central nervous system	Thrombosis } paralysis Hemorrhage } Increased intracranial pressure Headache Vomiting
	Skin	Purpura Petechiae Ecchymoses Infection

(continued)

TABLE 45-3 Manifestations of Leukemia (continued)

Organ	Manifestations
SECONDARY MANIFESTATIONS	
Gastrointestinal system	Ulceration Hemorrhage Infection
Mouth, throat, and nose	Bleeding gums Epistaxis Ulceration Necrosis Infection
Lungs	Infarction Infection Pleural effusion
Eyes	Retinal hemorrhage Subconjunctival hemorrhage Papilledema Visual disturbances
Kidneys	Bilateral asymmetric enlargement Hyperuricemia Rare pyelonephritis leads to renal failure

TABLE 45-4 Comparative Features of the Leukemias at Presentation

Description	Median Age	Initial Remission Rate	Median Survival with Treatment	Splenomegaly	Infection	Adenopathy	Hemoglobin	White Blood Cell Count	Platelets
Acute myelogenous leukemia	50–60	60%–70%	10–15 mos	No	Yes	No	Low	Variable	Low
Acute lymphoblastic leukemia	4	Adult 70%; children 90%	Adult 2 years; children 5 years	Yes	Yes	Yes	Low	Variable	Low
Chronic myelogenous leukemia	49	90%	3 years	Yes	No	No	Low	100,000–300,000 granulocytes	Normal or low
Chronic lymphocytic leukemia	60	90%	4–6 years	Yes	Yes	Yes	Low	20,000 lymphocytes	Low

ASSESSMENT OF ACUTE LEUKEMIA

Factors that influence the symptoms and physical findings are: (1) the type of leukemic cell, (2) the degree of leukemic cell burden (early-stage or advanced disease), (3) the involvement of organs or systems outside of the bone marrow or peripheral circulation, and (4) the depression of normal marrow elements by the leukemic process. Since the presenting symptoms of AML and ALL are similar, the assessment parameters of acute leukemia will be combined first. The classification and treatment of AML and ALL will be discussed individually. The chronic leukemias, CML and CLL, will be discussed separately.

Patient History

Acute leukemia presents with a large and rapidly growing population of leukemic cells. Usually, signs and symptoms have been present for less than 3 months, and perhaps for only a few days. Although the diagnosis cannot be made by history taking alone, many of the findings are typical and essential in guiding the diagnostic work-up.

The most common complaints of the patient are nonspecific—that is, fatigue, malaise, weight loss, and fever. The presenting symptoms are the manifestations of the effects of leukemic cells on the normal marrow elements. Infections are recurrent in the common sites such as the skin, gingiva, perianal tissue, lung, and urinary tract. The patient may complain of sore throat and describe fever with or without signs of localized infection. Unexplained bleeding may occur with nosebleeds, gingival bleeding, mid-cycle menstrual flow, or heavy bleeding with menses. Symptoms of progressive anemia include fatigue, palpitations, shortness of breath, and anorexia. Pain may arise from several sources: bones such as the sternum, enlarged lymph nodes, and hepatosplenomegaly.

Neurologic complaints are frequent and may signal either leukemia infiltration (especially in ALL) or intracerebral hemorrhage. These include a history of headache, vomiting, visual disturbances, or seizures.

Review of the individual's past medical history may be noncontributory. However, it is of etiologic importance to note a history of recurrent infections or bleeding tendencies as well as the type and time of any drug exposure to try to document the approximate onset of leukemia. Similarly, the occupational (especially chemical and radiation) exposure and family history of genetic abnormalities or cancer contribute to the total epidemiologic picture.

An essential part of the initial history that serves as a baseline for understanding the individual and planning care is the psychosocial profile. Questions that elicit details concerning past and present coping strategies with illness or other crises should be asked. Determination of significant others can be made by asking such questions as, "Who can you talk to most easily about your illness?" Finally, the nurse must ascertain how the patient and family perceive the illness and what their previous experience with hospitalization has been.

Physical Examination

The physical findings of acute leukemia usually relate directly to the effects of pancytopenia. Vital signs may demonstrate fever, tachycardia, and tachypnea. The skin and mucous membranes generally appear pale, with readily apparent ecchymoses or petechiae. Generalized or localized adenopathy may be present due to leukemic infiltration or infection.

A comprehensive physical examination serves to validate findings elicited in a complete history and review of symptoms. Ophthalmoscopic examination may reveal retinal capillary hemorrhage or papilledema due to leukostatic or thrombocytopenic-induced bleeding and/or increased intracranial pressure. An oral infection with *Candida albicans* may be present. Examination of the lungs and heart may reveal the effects of anemia (cardiac murmurs) or infection (abnormal lung sounds). Abdominal palpation may demonstrate hepatosplenomegaly or enlarged kidneys due to leukemic infiltration, especially in children with ALL. Perirectal tissue may be tender and swollen and the only evidence of an abscess or a fistula. Finally, gentle palpation of bones and joints may reveal swelling and elicit pain.

Diagnostic Studies

Laboratory and radiographic studies are essential for proper diagnosis. It is important to separate AML and ALL, since the treatment and prognosis differ markedly. An ongoing explanation to the patient and family of the plan and purpose of the exhaustive diagnostic work-up will facilitate cooperation, decrease anxiety, and create an atmosphere of confidence and trust.

The diagnosis is suggested by the peripheral smear but requires a full examination of the bone marrow. The white blood cell count may be low, normal, or high, and 90% of patients have blast cells present in the peripheral blood. Neutropenia (absolute granulocyte count less than 1000 cells/mm^3) is frequent, and thrombocytopenia is present in 40% of patients. Blood chemistry studies may reveal hyperuricemia and increased lactic dehydrogenase as well as altered serum and urine muramidase (greatly increased with monocyte and myelomonocytic leukemia, but normal to low in lymphoblastic leukemia). If acute promyelocytic leukemia (M_3) is suspected, laboratory evaluation should include plasma fibrinogen, fibrin split products, and prothrombin time.

Bone marrow contents are usually hypercellular, with 60%–90% blasts in the differential blood count. Auer rods are diagnostic of AML, and so are special stains (Sudan Black and peroxidase).

Improved techniques of cytogenetics (chromosome analysis) can provide information confirming the diagnosis and specific classification of the leukemia. Approximately half of patients with de novo acute leukemia exhibit nonrandom chromosome abnormalities,[12] and 40% of adults with leukemia have some cytogenetic translocations. Translocations are an adverse feature in ALL, while some translocations in AML indicate a better prognosis. These abnormalities in the leukemic cells serve as tumor markers that disappear during remission and reappear with recurrence of the leukemia.[38]

Cytogenetic analysis is performed at the time of diagnosis. Cells from the bone marrow or peripheral blood are collected and placed in culture for 24–72 hours. Cells are stimulated chemically to divide, then stopped in metaphase by the addition of drugs such as vinblastine or colchicine. After special stains are applied, the cells are examined for abnormalities in number and shape. These abnormalities are described as translocations, inversions, or loss or gain in chromosome number. Specific aberrations are related to a favorable or unfavorable outcome (see Table 45-5). The results of chromosome analysis are usually available within 4 weeks. Since this is also the time the patient is recovering from induction therapy, this information is useful in planning further treatment.

Further information is obtained from immunologic studies. Monoclonal antibodies reactive to immature cells can identify the predominant cell type and stage of arrested development in the leukemic cell line.[39] The use of surface marker antigens in patients with ALL has revealed the presence of markers for both lymphoid and myeloid cells. Mixed lymphoid and myeloid surface markers are found in 21% of patients with de novo ALL.[40] In general, patients with mixed lineage leukemia have a poor response to treatment and should be considered for other investigational therapies.

TABLE 45-5 Prognostic Factors in Acute Leukemia

	Poor Prognosis	Favorable Prognosis
Acute myelogenous leukemia	Age > 60 yr FAB: M5, M6 Chromosome abnormalities: −5/5q−; −7/7q− t(6;9); t(4;11); t(9;22) Prior radiation/chemotherapy Prior MDS Infection at diagnosis	Age < 60 yr FAB: M3 Chromosome abnormalities: t(15;17); t(8;21); inversion 16
Acute lymphocytic leukemia	Age > 10 yr FAB: L3 WBC > 25,000/mm³ Male Immunophenotype: T-cell with tumor bulk Pre-B, B-cell cALLa − Cytogenetics: hypodiploidy chromosome abnormalities: t(9;22); t(4;11); t(8;14) CNS involvement Late achievement of CR	Age < 10 yr FAB: L1, L2 WBC < 10,000/mm³ Female Immunophenotype: Pre pre B-cell cALLa + Cytogenetics: hyperdiploidy

Source: Data from Champlin R;[45] Keating MJ et al;[61] Priesler HD et al;[62] Foon KA, Todd RF;[68] Clarkson B et al;[74] Hoelzer D, Gale RP.[76]

ACUTE MYELOGENOUS LEUKEMIA

Classification

Acute myelogenous leukemia (AML), also referred to as acute nonlymphocytic leukemia (ANLL), is a disease of the pluripotent myeloid stem cell. The malignant clone arises in the myeloid, monocyte, erythroid, or megakaryocyte lines. The exact event that triggers the malignant transformation is not known.

The leukemic cells have more abundant cytoplasm and granulation in the cytoplasm is usually but not always present. Auer rods, which are abnormal lysosomal granules, are present and pathognomonic for AML. Multiple nucleoli are present and tend to vary in size.

As previously stated, the type of leukemia is named for the predominant cell. The most common myeloid leukemia is acute myelocytic leukemia (M_1). Acute promyelocytic leukemia (APL) (M_3) is associated with an increased risk of disseminated intravascular coagulation. This is due to the release of procoagulants from granules within the leukemic promyelocyte, especially during remission induction therapy.[25] Patients with acute monocytic (M_5) or myelomonocytic (M_4) leukemia often exhibit extramedullary leukemic infiltration with gingival hypertrophy, cutaneous leukemia, and liver, spleen, and lymph enlargement.[10]

Erythroleukemia (M_6), which was first described by DiGugliolmo, has both a chronic and acute form.[3] As the erythroleukemia progresses, the morphologic picture resembles that of myelocytic or myelomonocytic leukemia. Megakaryocytic leukemia (M_7) is quite rare and less responsive to chemotherapy.[41]

By the time an individual is diagnosed with AML, the bone marrow and peripheral blood contain up to 10^{12} leukemic cells.[42] The accumulation within the bone marrow space results in inhibition and crowding out of normal marrow stem cells and infiltration of other organs by myeloblasts. Anemia, thrombocytopenia, and neutropenia result. If the disease is left untreated, death occurs within a few months due to infection or uncontrolled bleeding.

Treatment

The goal of antileukemic treatment for AML is the eradication of the leukemic stem cell. Complete remission is defined as the restoration of normal peripheral counts and <5% blasts in the bone marrow.[43] Treatment regimens capable of inducing a complete remission are composed of several drugs, each of which is known to be effective against leukemic myeloblasts. The course of therapy is divided into two stages: (1) induction and (2) postremission therapy.

Induction therapy

The goal of induction therapy is to cause severe bone marrow hypoplasia. At diagnosis the leukemic cells are proliferating more slowly than normal myeloid precursors. Therefore, the myeloid stem cells repopulate the depleted marrow faster than leukemic cells. The cornerstone for remission induction is the cell-cycle specific antimetabolite cytosine arabinoside plus an anthracycline (daunorubicin, doxorubicin, mitoxantrone, amsacrine, or idarubicin).[44–46] It is theorized that a drug that is non–cycle-specific will have a synergistic effect when given sequentially with a cell cycle-specific drug by causing proliferating cells to enter the cell cycle concurrently. Cytosine arabinoside is administered continuously for 7 days and the anthracycline is given for 3 days. The continuous infusion of cytosine arabinoside ensures that slowly cycling leukemia cells are adequately exposed to the drug during the synthesis phase of the cell cycle.[47] This protocol is called "7 + 3,"[48] but variations include 5-day or 10-day infusions of cytosine arabinoside. Gale and Foon,[49] in a review of the results of eight clinical studies, reported a complete response rate of 50%–75%, with the best results in the protocols with 7 days of cytosine arabinoside.

The impact of the chemotherapy is assessed at 1 week after the completion of therapy with a bone marrow biopsy and aspiration on the 14th day. If residual leukemia is present, a second course is begun. Bone marrow recovery usually takes 14–21 days after the end of the chemotherapy with median time to complete recovery at 28–32 days. Complete response rates are now observed in 65%–80% of patients.[50,51] Unfortunately, in spite of improving remission rates, only 20% of patients remain in complete remission. Relapse occurs in the remaining cases within 1–2 years.[52,53] Thus, postremission therapy is essential.

Postremission therapy

By the addition of postremission therapy, the median duration of remission can be increased from 4–8 months to 10–15 months.[50] Wolff et al.[54] have used high-dose cytosine arabinoside to increase the continuing complete remission rate to 51%. The goal of further therapy is to prevent leukemic recurrence related to undetectable, resistant disease, also called *minimal residual disease*. Postremission therapies include consolidation, intensification, maintenance, and allogeneic or autologous bone marrow transplant.[55,56] None has emerged as the clear-cut, optimal therapy. (See Figure 45-2.)

Consolidation therapy consists of one or two courses of very high doses of the same drugs used for induction. Up to 30 times induction doses of cytosine arabinoside are used to consolidate the remission.[53] Although the patient is in a healthier state for this part of the treatment, the toxicities are substantial, with extended myelosuppression, cerebellar dysfunction, dermatitis, hepatic dysfunction, and conjunctivitis. The longest remissions appear to occur after two or more courses of consolidation therapy, with a median remission of 1–2 years.[45]

Intensification may be initiated right after remission induction (early intensification) or several months later (late intensification). Different drugs are used with the hope that they will be non–cross-resistant with the induction drugs. Mitoxantrone is less cardiotoxic and has less extramedullary toxicity than daunorubicin. With a steep dose-response curve, mitoxantrone is good for dose intensification.[56] The terminology is somewhat confusing in various clinical investigations.

Maintenance therapy is treatment with lower doses of the same or other drugs given monthly for a prolonged period of time. Maintenance therapy is not currently recommended in the treatment of AML.[50,55]

Because microscopic disease is being treated in postremission therapy, it is difficult to know how much treatment is enough. Investigation continues to determine the optimal curative treatment.

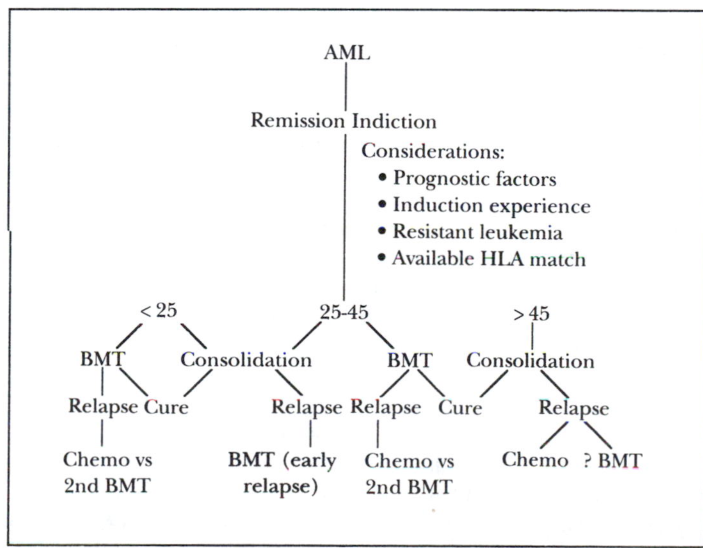

FIGURE 45-2 Treatment considerations and options for patients with acute myelogenous leukemia.

Patients who relapse after induction and postinduction chemotherapy have a 30%–60% likelihood of achieving a second remission.[49,57,58] Leukemic cells acquire increasing resistance to chemotherapy. The cellular kinetics change due to an increased growth fraction and shortened generation time, resulting in a decreased doubling time.[43] The second and subsequent remissions are influenced by prior treatment, length of remission, and the initial response to therapy. Patients who relapse quickly or who have resistant leukemia should be considered for clinical trials or bone marrow transplant.[58]

The role of bone marrow transplant (BMT) in the treatment of AML remains controversial.[59,60] Approximately 40% of patients with AML are less than 40 years of age. Of those, approximately 40% have an HLA-matched donor. Therefore, only 16% or fewer of patients with AML are eligible for an allogeneic transplant.[43] Other options may include a matched unrelated donor BMT obtained through the National Marrow Donor Program. There are increased risks of graft-versus-host disease (GVHD) and lack of engraftment from these histocompatible but unrelated cells. A purged autologous BMT may be performed in a young patient with no HLA match. In patients less than 30 years of age, BMT may offer a higher cure rate than standard treatment. In patients in the fourth decade, the results of chemotherapy versus BMT vary. Transplant centers usually do not admit patients over the age of 50. Because allogeneic BMT carries the risk of GVHD, interstitial pneumonia, and infection with cytomegalovirus, the decision for BMT is not easy. The question of the optimal timing for transplant remains unanswered. (See Chapter 18 for an in-depth discussion of bone marrow transplantation.)

Another consideration in the treatment of AML is the significance of prognostic indicators, which may be useful in determining the best course of therapy (Table 45-5).[4,45,61,62] For example, patients with unfavorable factors such as older age or multiple chromosomal abnormalities may be treated with high-dose or investigational drugs. A patient who had a poor response to initial therapy and other medical problems is unlikely to benefit from reinduction therapy. Such patients may benefit from a less aggressive approach, with transfusion support and oral hydroxyurea to control the WBC count. In a younger patient with an unfavorable morphologic subtype, BMT may be preferred to consolidation therapy.

A newer strategy being applied to patients with risk factors, early relapse, or resistant leukemia is drug therapy to overcome multidrug resistance (MDR). MDR is the phenomenon by which a cancer becomes resistant to multiple drugs that have little similarity in their chemical structure and mechanism of action.[63] MDR can be kinetic in origin, meaning the malignant cells are resistant at the onset of the disease. MDR is also acquired when drugs that were initially effective are no longer effective. Acquired MDR is associated with P-glycoprotein, which acts as a pump to transport drugs in and out of malignant cells. P-glycoprotein is associated with the MDR phenotype. The MDR1 message or its P-glycoprotein product is expressed in 10%–20% of cases of newly diagnosed AML. In addition, more than 50% of cases with relapsed AML express P-glycoprotein.[64,65]

The anthracyclines, specifically daunomycin and doxorubicin, are associated with acquired MDR. One strategy to overcome P-glycoprotein resistance is to use cyclosporine, a lipophilic endoecapeptide with immunosuppressive properties. Cyclosporine restores daunorubicin sensitivity in drug-resistant tumor cell lines.[65]

Strategies altering cellular kinetics to overcome de novo MDR are being explored. High-dose therapy with etoposide by continuous infusion for 29–69 hours along with cyclophosphamide on 3–4 days produced a complete remission (CR) in 42% of 40 patients with AML, including 6 patients with resistance to high-dose cytosine arabinoside.[66] Hematopoietic colony stimulating (CSF) factors such as granulocyte (G-CSF), granulocyte-macrophage (GM-CSF), and interleukin 3 (IL3) can enhance recruitment of cells into synthesis phase and optimize the cytotoxicity of cytosine arabinoside.[38,47,67,68]

A new therapeutic option is available for patients with APL. During the past several years, all-trans retinoic acid (RA), a derivative of vitamin A, has been used to induce remissions in some patients.[69,70] The break point for the chromosome region abnormality characteristic in APL (15;17) is clustered near the location of the retinoid acid receptor-alpha. The administration of RA seems to induce terminal differentiation and subsequent death of the previously arrested leukemic cells. Warrell[71] summarized the current use of RA in European trials. The most commonly used dosage is 45 mg/m^2/day administered orally BID for remission induction. About one-half of patients experience the complications of disseminated intravascular coagulopathy, but few hemorrhagic deaths occur. Common side effects include headache, dry skin, xerostomia, cheilitis (cracking at the corners of the lips), and bone pain.

The current use of RA is in patients with resistant or recurrent APL and patients unable to tolerate conventional chemotherapy (older or with concomitant illness). The European studies are continuing and, as of 1991, the United States National Cancer Institute was conducting an intergroup study to evaluate the use of RA in remission induction and maintenance in APL patients.

ACUTE LYMPHOCYTIC LEUKEMIA

Acute lymphocytic leukemia (ALL) is a malignant disease of the lymphoid progenitors. The abnormal clone originates in the marrow, thymus, and lymph nodes, but the exact etiologic event is unknown. The leukemic lymphoblast is nongranular, with little cytoplasm. The round nucleus resembles a normal lymphoblast. Although the defect does not involve the myeloid cell lines, the secondary effect of the high leukemic cell burden on the bone marrow interferes with normal hematopoietic activity.

Classification

The FAB classification for ALL is based upon several cell properties: size ratio of nucleus to cytoplasm; number, size, and shape of nucleoli; and amount and basophilia of the cytoplasm (Table 45-2).[34–36] In childhood ALL, 85% have L1 morphology, whereas the majority of adults with ALL have L2 morphology. Patients with L3 ALL, which resembles Burkitt's lymphoma, are rare.

Another classification system for ALL is based upon immune features.[68,72] Four subtypes are identified by the presence of certain markers on the cell surface. Common ALL (cALL) is the most frequent and least differentiated ALL.[73] It is identified by the common ALL antigen (cALLa). T-cell markers such as sheep erythrocyte receptors and T-cell–specific antigens identify T-ALL. Both cALLa and T-cell antigens contain another marker, terminal deoxynucleotidyl transferase (TdT). Other surface and cell immunoglobulins denote the rare B-cell ALL. Finally, about one-fourth are pre pre B (formally null) leukemias, which do not have any identifiable surface markers.

Lymphoblasts have a propensity for organ infiltration and may remain sequestered in sanctuary sites even after remission has been achieved. Leukemic cells infiltrate into the central nervous system (CNS) early in the disease.[74] Because drugs used for treatment penetrate poorly into the cerebrospinal fluid, the leukemic cells are sheltered from the cytotoxic effects of the drugs. Over time, the leukemic cells proliferate and cause relapse. Cells can also be harbored in the testes.[4] In addition, 80% of patients have lymphadenopathy and/or splenomegaly at the time of diagnosis due to the infiltration of these organs by leukemic cells.[10]

The prognosis for long-term survival is more favorable for individuals with ALL than AML since drugs are available that are uniquely effective against lymphocytes—for example, prednisone. CNS prophylaxis is used in ALL and has proven successful.

As with AML, long-term survival and cure for individuals with ALL is possible only if a complete remission is achieved. This is documented by a bone marrow aspirate containing <5% lymphoblasts and the disappearance of all peripheral manifestations of the disease.

Treatment

In contrast to AML, current chemotherapeutic regimens proven effective against ALL contain drugs that are selectively toxic to lymphoblasts and relatively sparing of normal hematopoietic stem cells. Therefore, the patient experiences hypoplasia that is less severe and of shorter duration with greater leukemic cell kill. In addition, relapses may be more effectively treated because the marrow is better able to recover.

The focus of therapy for ALL is to eradicate all leukemic cells from the marrow and lymph tissue and eliminate any residual foci of disease within the CNS. Treatment is divided into three stages: (1) induction, (2) CNS prophylaxis, and (3) postremission therapy. (See Figure 45-3.)

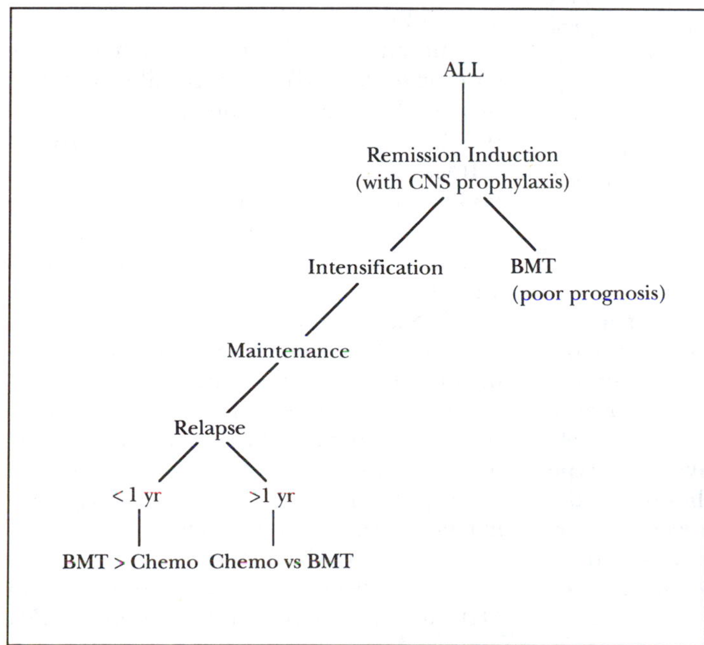

FIGURE 45-3 Treatment considerations and options for patients with acute lymphocytic leukemia.

Induction therapy

Although it is possible to achieve complete remission in 93% of children with ALL by using a combination of vincristine, prednisone, and L-asparaginase,[75] the same drugs even with the addition of an anthracycline produce remission rates of only 70%–75% in adults with ALL.[75,76] About 35% achieve long-term disease-free survival.[74] Therapy usually begins in the hospital, but hypoplasia is shorter than with AML treatment. Once remission is documented, the therapy is completed on an outpatient basis.

CNS prophylaxis

Meningeal leukemia is present at diagnosis in about 2% of patients and is known to occur in up to 50% of patients with ALL in the absence of CNS prophylaxis.[73,77] By comparison, in patients with AML the incidence is less than 5%. Leukemic lymphoblasts enter the leptomeninges either by direct extension from the blood of the meningeal vessels or by seeding from thrombocytopenic bleeding. The cells extend deeply into the cerebral sulci and nerve sheaths, causing a mechanical obstruction of the cerebral spinal fluid (CSF). If unchecked, hydrocephaly and death occur. Several factors may explain the increased incidence of CSF infiltration with ALL.[78] There is a selective tendency for lymphoblasts rather than myeloblasts to enter the CNS. Drugs used in ALL enter the CSF slowly or in concentrations too low to be cytotoxic. The slower proliferation of lymphoblasts in the CSF may require longer drug exposure. Signs and symptoms of CNS leukemia include headache, blurred vision, nausea/vomiting, and cranial nerve palsies.[73]

CNS prophylaxis should start within a few weeks of the initiation of therapy. Treatment usually includes intracranial radiation and intrathecal methotrexate.[45,74,79] Cranial radiation delivered in fractionated doses of 200 cGy up to a total dose of 2400 cGy produces predictable penetration of leukemic cells regardless of CSF dynamics. This therapy can also kill or sterilize cells not undergoing cell division. However, this therapy has recognized side effects, including somnolence, chemical meningitis, paraparesis, and leukoencephalopathy.[73]

Postremission therapy

As in AML, even after complete remission, patients with ALL harbor remaining leukemic cells. Relapse occurs in 2–3 months if there is no continuing therapy. Prolonged chemotherapy may lead to a 40% overall cure rate, but the type and duration are not completely defined.[74] Currently many patients receive some type of intensification with high-dose chemotherapy or the use of multiple new drugs.[4,80] Methotrexate and 6-mercaptopurine may be added to the drugs used during induction. Maintenance therapy often continues for 2–3 years.

The outlook for patients in whom relapse occurs during therapy is quite poor, and younger patients with an HLA-matched donor should be immediately referred for BMT.[79] If relapse occurs after the completion of therapy, treatment is continued with high-dose methotrexate, tenoposide, and cytarabine, or high-dose cytosine arabinoside with an anthracycline or amsacrine. Second remission can be achieved in up to 50% of cases.[76] An analysis of eight studies using high-dose cytosine arabinoside in relapsed patients with ALL revealed a mean CR of 38%.[81] This same researcher reviewed 19 other studies that combined high-dose cytosine arabinoside (HDCA) with anthracyclines, vincristine, and/or prednisone and determined the CR rates to be 36%–63%.[81] Idarubicin and HDCA induced second remissions in 65% of adults with ALL.[56]

Prognostic factors (summarized in Table 45-5) are also important in planning treatment for ALL.[74,76] Because patients treated with allogeneic BMT show a trend toward longer survival if the transplant is performed during the first remission,[59] it is important to identify patients with an unfavorable prognosis in the early stages of disease.

MYELODYSPLASTIC SYNDROMES

Myelodysplastic syndromes (MDS) are a group of hematologic disorders with an increased risk of transformation to AML. They are characterized by a change in the quantity and quality of bone marrow products. Hematologic disorders that preceded acute leukemia were first reported in the late 1940s and referred to as *preleukemia anemia*.[82] Other terms used are *preleukemia, hematopoietic dysplasia, refractory anemia with excessive myeloblasts, subacute myeloid leukemia, oligoblastic leukemia,* and *dysmyelopoietic syndromes*.[83]

Currently MDS are divided into five subtypes according to the FAB group classification: refractory anemia (RA), refractory anemia with ringed sideroblasts (RARS), refractory anemia with excessive blasts (RAEB), refractory anemia with excessive blasts in transformation (RAEB-t), and chronic myelomonocytic leukemia (CMML).[84] Table 45-6 lists each type, along with diagnostic criteria, risk of evolution into acute leukemia, and average survival time.[83,84]

MDS are believed to occur as the result of an altered stem cell. The cause is unknown. Chromosome abnormalities are present at the level of the totipotent hematopoietic stem cell. Since MDS can progress to AML, ALL, or a mixed cell leukemia, it is thought that both myeloid and lymphoid progenitors are involved.[85]

Approximately 30% of patients diagnosed with AML initially present with preleukemic syndrome.[10] MDS may be considered to be different stages of the same disease. Cases have been noted of transition from one type of MDS to another before transition to AML.[85] Even if

TABLE 45-6 Classification of Myelodysplastic Syndrome with Percentage of Blast Cells, Leukemia Risk, and Average Survival

Category	Blasts (%)		Risk of Evolution to Acute Leukemia (%)	Survival (months)
	Blood	Bone Marrow		
RA	<1	<5	0–25	18–71
RARS	<1	<5	8	14–76+
RAEB	<5	≥5	20–44	7–16
RAEB-t	>5	20–30	27–60	2.5–20
CMML	<5 >10^9 Monocytes	1–20	14	9–60

RA, refractory anemia; RARS, refractory anemia with ringed sideroblasts; RAEB, refractory anemia excess blasts; RAEB-t, refractory anemia with excess blasts in transformation; CMML, chronic myelomonocytic leukemia

Source: Data from Buzaid AC et al;[83] Bennett JM et al.[84]

the evolution to acute leukemia never occurs, life-threatening anemia, thrombocytopenia, and/or neutropenia invariably occur. The defect is usually noted in the erythrocyte line first, then in the granulocytes and megakaryocytes.

Twenty percent of patients diagnosed with MDS are older than 50 years of age, with a median age of 60. The incidence is slightly higher in males than females.[86] A bone marrow biopsy and aspirate usually reveal dyshematopoiesis in all cell lineages. Ringed sideroblasts, abnormal nuclear shapes, cytoplasmic abnormalities, and maturation defects of RBCs indicate dyserythropoiesis. Evidence of dysmegakaryocytopoiesis includes atypical shapes; multiple, small nuclei; and increased or decreased numbers of platelets. Dysgranulocytopoiesis is seen with hypogranular cells, nuclear abnormalities, and maturation defects of granulocytes. A hypocellular bone marrow with one or more of these lineage defects provides a diagnosis of MDS.

About half of patients with MDS develop AML. Historically patients with MDS do not respond as well from antileukemic therapy as do those with de novo AML. Survival for MDS ranges from several months to years, with median survival of 28 months. Poor prognostic indicators include excessive blast cells in the bone marrow, small clusters of immature myeloid precursors, pancytopenia, and complex chromosome abnormalities.[85] Death usually occurs within 2 years from complications related to bone marrow depression or transformation to acute leukemia.

Treatment for MDS is as aggressive as the course of the disease.[83] Serial bone marrow and peripheral blood examinations allow the physician to monitor the pace of the disease.[87] Supportive therapy includes replacement of RBCs or platelets and antibiotics for infection. Continuous infusion of low-dose cytosine arabinoside (20 mg/m²/day) is thought to induce differentiation of immature myeloid cells in 25%–35% of patients with MDS.[85] Other differentiation inducers include retinoic acid, dimethyl sulfoxide (DMSO), and vitamin D derivatives.[88] A synthetic androgen, danazol, is sometimes used to elevate platelet levels.[89] For the rare group of patients less than 40 years of age with an HLA-matched donor, BMT is the treatment of choice.[83]

CHRONIC MYELOGENOUS LEUKEMIA

Chronic myelogenous leukemia (CML), also called chronic granulocytic leukemia, is a disorder of the myeloid stem cell characterized by marked splenomegaly and an increased production of granulocytes, especially neutrophils.[90] Approximately 90% of patients with CML have a diagnostic marker, the Philadelphia chromosome (Ph^1). The G group chromosome, number 22, is missing a portion of the long arm (q), which has been translocated to the long arm of number 9.[91,92] The significance of the marker is that a proto-oncogene is activated. When the proto-oncogene *c-abl* is translocated from chromosome 9 to 22, a new oncogene, *bcr-abl,* is formed. This gene produces a protein that is associated with triggering growth factor receptors.[93,94] It is speculated that this gene may induce uncontrolled growth of leukemic cells. Patients with Ph^1-negative CML have been found to have activation of this same gene even though no visible chromosome change is present.[95] In addition, as long as the marker is present, the patient is not cured of the disease.

There is no known specific cause for CML, except exposure to ionizing radiation.[92] The peak incidence is in the third and fourth decades, and both sexes are affected equally.[90]

The natural course of CML is divided into a chronic and terminal phase. The initial chronic phase is characterized by excessive proliferation and accumulation of mature granulocytes and precursors. There is an absence of lymphadenopathy, but 90% of patients have palpable splenomegaly.[90] Within 30–40 months the disorder transforms into a terminal phase consisting of accelerated and blastic phases. The accelerated phase includes progressive leukocytosis with increasing myeloid precursors (including blasts), increasing basophils, splenomegaly, weight loss, and weakness. There is increasing resistance to therapy, and serial cytogenetic studies indicate progressive chromosomal abnormalities.[92]

The blastic phase resembles AML, with 30%–40% of the bone marrow cells being blasts or promyelocytes. A crisis occurs as blast cell counts rise rapidly, often exceeding 100,000/dl. Leukostatic lesions caused by the high cell count result in occlusion in the microvasculature of the CNS or lungs.[90] The majority of patients have myeloblastic transformation, but some have lymphoblastic transformation, evidenced by the presence of TdT or cALLa. Median survival after the onset of the terminal phase is 3 months.[91]

Assessment

CML in up to 20% of affected individuals is diagnosed in the absence of any symptomatology.[92] Most patients, however, present with a history that reflects the gradual accumulation of a white blood cell mass that is 10–150 times normal.

Patient history

The initial symptoms of illness typically include symptoms related to massive splenomegaly due to infiltration of the spleen by leukemic cells: left upper quadrant pain, early satiety, and vague abdominal fullness may be the presenting complaints. Leukemic infiltration of joints may also cause bone and joint pain. A history of malaise, fatigue, weight loss, and fever caused by a gradually worsening hypercatabolic state may precede more acute symptoms of anemia.[96]

To a lesser extent than with acute leukemia, epidemiologic clues may be provided by a complete past medical and family history, such as a history of exposure to ionizing radiation or a positive family history for leukemia.

Physical examination

The vast majority of people are diagnosed during the chronic phase of their disease. The anemic individual appears pale. Examination of the eyes, ears, nose, and throat may reveal leukemic infiltration. Splenomegaly and hepatomegaly are common.

The physical examination of the patient in blast crisis is similar to that for the patient with acute leukemia. In blast crisis, blastic transformation of the leukemic granulocytes has replaced the bone marrow, causing an acute illness with pancytopenia, infection, and hypercatabolism. Rapid diagnosis and treatment to reduce the number of proliferating blasts are essential.

Diagnostic studies

A complete blood count in the chronic phase reveals anemia and severe leukocytosis (WBC >100,000 mm^3). The differential count of the leukocytes demonstrates WBCs in every stage of maturation, with a predominance of more mature cells. The presence of functional but leukemic granulocytes in these individuals accounts for the low incidence of infection during the chronic phase. There is usually moderate anemia and thrombocytosis. The anemia is normocytic and normochromic with a median hemoglobin of 9–10 gm/dl.[92]

Other laboratory studies reveal high serum B_{12} levels and a low leukocyte alkaline phosphatase level (LAP).[91,97] Both may return to normal with successful therapy.[90] Bone marrow biopsy demonstrates hyperplasia, with a myeloid to erythroid ratio of 15:1 and normal to increased megakaryocytes (platelet precursors). If the abnormal Ph^1 chromosome is found in the granulocytic, erythrocytic, and megakaryocytic series of the marrow, the diagnosis of CML is confirmed.[98]

Treatment

The only chance for cure of CML is with ablation of the Ph^1 chromosome. Currently this occurs after high-dose therapy followed by allogeneic BMT. CML is a chronic disease and is usually suppressed by chemotherapy with hydroxyurea or busulfan. Late in the disease or at blastic crisis, investigational drugs are used. Recently, interferon has been found useful in early disease.[99,100]

Chronic phase

The standard therapy during the chronic phase is single-agent oral chemotherapy.[97,98] Busulfan, an alkylating agent, is active against primitive hematopoietic stem cells. The WBC count begins to drop 10–14 days after starting therapy. To prevent prolonged or severe myelosuppression, treatment is stopped if the WBC is less than 20,000/mm^3. Long-term side effects include skin hyperpigmentation and pulmonary or retroperitoneal fibrosis. Hydroxyurea is cytostatic to cycling cells and inhibits ribonucleotide reductase. It acts on late progenitor stem cells causing rapid disease control, but it requires frequent monitoring of blood levels. Since hydroxyurea does not have the long-term toxicities on pulmonary and bone marrow tissue, it may be a better choice if a future BMT is a possibility.[99] Although both of these drugs decrease the leukemic cell mass and improve the quality of life, the progression to a terminal, refractory stage is not altered.

Terminal phase

CML is a chronic neoplasm with a 100% incidence of blastic transformation.[101] This transformation, also described as a metamorphosis, is a gradual failure of response to treatment and failure of production of erythrocytes and platelets. Serial cytogenetic analyses can reveal signs of blastic transformation 3–4 months before clinical signs are evident. However, bone marrow aspirations are required, which are costly and uncomfortable for the patient.[91] The current trend is to treat the accelerated phase by continuing chronic phase therapy until evidence of the blastic phase appears. Because the transformation from benign to malignant appears to be random in length, it is difficult to predict survival, although life expectancy is less than 1 year.[96]

Blast crisis requires intensive chemotherapy, similar to that used in the treatment of AML. If the transformation is myeloblastic, therapy includes cytosine arabinoside, an anthracycline, and thioguanine. If lymphoblastic transformation has occurred, vincristine and prednisone are added. Patients who develop lymphoblastic transformation are more responsive to treatment and live longer.[102]

In a review of 18 clinical investigations, Talpaz et al.[99] concluded the median survival from diagnosis has increased from 19 months for untreated patients to a range of 30–45 months for those receiving conventional, single-agent therapy. The range for those treated with intensive therapy (during the chronic phase) is 50–65 months.

Although BMT remains the only chance for cure, it is an option for only 25% of patients.[97] The best results have been obtained in patients receiving allogeneic BMT during the chronic phase, with 55%–70% being disease-free at 3–5 years.[103] With the availability of the National Marrow Donor Program, unrelated HLA-matched marrow provides another option for BMT.[104]

Alpha-interferon when used alone in patients with early disease appears to produce a complete hematologic response (CHR) in 30%–70% of patients. The time to CHR is at least 4–6 months.[93,100] Interferon is not usually helpful in patients with advanced disease. However effectiveness is noted in patients with advanced disease when interferon is given after cytotoxic therapy has decreased the tumor load.[105]

CHRONIC LYMPHOCYTIC LEUKEMIA

A progressive accumulation of morphologically normal but functionally inert lymphocytes is found in chronic lymphocytic leukemia (CLL).[106] As the disease progresses, the abnormal lymphocytes accumulate in the bone marrow, spleen, liver, and lymph nodes. In 95% of the cases, there is clonal (from a single cell) expansion of neoplastic B-lymphocytes.[107] The median age at diagnosis is 60 years; the majority of cases are male.[92,108]

The pathological cells are usually small lymphocytes with markers of B-lymphocytes and surface IgM or IgD.[42] Approximately one-half of individuals with CLL experience frequent viral and fungal infections due to hypogammaglobulinemia.[107,108] For more than 25% of patients the diagnosis is an incidental finding during routine examination. Anemia, lymphadenopathy, or infection may be present. Coomb's positive autoimmune hemolytic anemia occurs in 25% of patients.[42]

The clinical course is variable, and, as with other hematologic malignancies, many attempts have been made to correlate a staging system with prognosis.[109–112] The two most commonly used systems are Rai and Binet. The Rai staging system has five levels based on the extent of tissue involvement and compromise of bone marrow function.[106] The Binet system identifies three groups, each with a subsequently worsening prognosis.[106] The International Workshop on CLL (IWCLL) attempted to combine the two systems (Table 45-7).[113] Binet et al.[110] reviewed numerous systems and concluded that all staging systems defined a high-risk group of patients with anemia and/or thrombocytopenia.[110] In general, treatment is withheld until the patient shows evidence of hemolytic anemia, cytopenia, disfiguring or painful lymphadenopathy, symptomatic organomegaly, or marked systemic symptoms.[42]

Assessment

One-fourth of individuals with CLL are diagnosed during a routine physical examination. Clues that alert the clinician early on, however, may be provided by a complete health history.

Patient history

Early CLL may be asymptomatic. However, because CLL is a disease of immunoglobulin-secreting cells, a history of recurrent infections, especially of the skin and respiratory tract, may be elicited. The onset, location, duration, and response to treatment for infection should be documented.

Progressive infiltration and accumulation in nodal structures and the bone marrow gradually produce the symptoms that are typical of more advanced disease. Vague complaints of malaise, anorexia, and fatigue are common, as is noticeable and bothersome lymphade-

TABLE 45-7 Three Systems for the Classification of Chronic Lymphocytic Leukemia

Rai	Binet	IWCLL*	Prognosis
0	A	A(0), A(I), A(II)	Good: >10 yr
I	B	B(I), B(II)	Intermediate: <7 yr
II	C	C(III), C(IV)	Poor: <2 yr
III			
IV			

*IWCLL: International Workshop on Chronic Lymphocytic Leukemia

Source: Data from Binet JL et al.[113]

nopathy. Splenomegaly may cause early satiety and abdominal discomfort. The past medical history should focus on the documentation of any underlying autoimmune or immune-deficiency diseases, bleeding tendencies, and infectious episodes.

Physical examination

The individual with early CLL appears well. Splenomegaly may be the only clinical finding. In advanced disease there may be evidence of infection, fever, and rashes. Lymphadenopathy occurs in 60% of patients, especially in the cervical, axillary, inguinal, and femoral nodes. The nodes are described as mobile, discrete, and nontender.[107]

Diagnostic studies

Peripheral blood examination reveals lymphocytosis with normal or immature lymphocytes. The lymphocyte count is greater than 20,000/mm^3 in early disease and may be over 100,000/mm^3 in advanced disease. Protein electrophoresis documents the hypogammaglobulinemia that occurs in approximately 50% of patients. Bone marrow aspirate reflects the lymphocytosis seen peripherally, with varying degrees of infiltration. The severity of infiltration depends on the severity of the disease. Although early CLL causes patchy or focal infiltrates of the mature-appearing lymphocytes, progressive disease leads to a "packed marrow" with few normal hematopoietic cells. Lymph node biopsy may be interpreted as well-differentiated lymphocytic lymphoma if the blood count and bone marrow findings are unknown to the pathologist.

Treatment

In general, treatment consists only of observation until the patient is symptomatic with cytopenias or organomegaly.[107,108] The rate of progressive lymphocytosis directs the frequency of observation and start of therapy. Patients may show a fluctuating moderate lymphocytosis for many years with no treatment at all.

Chlorambucil and cyclophosphamide are two alkylating agents used to treat CLL.[108,114] Chlorambucil is most effective in suppressing growth of well-differentiated, small lymphocytes. Cyclophosphamide suppresses growth of less mature lymphocytes with relative sparing of neutrophils and platelets. These drugs provide a response rate of 60%, with complete remission in 10%–20% of patients. There is a concern, however, that prolonged use of alkylating agents may induce secondary development of AML.[114,115]

Corticosteroids are used to control leukocytosis and immune-mediated cytopenias. When the patient no longer responds to steroid therapy, splenectomy may provide relief of symptoms.[114]

Radiation therapy may be used to treat lymphadenopathy or painful splenomegaly. Total body irradiation (TBI) and extracorporeal irradiation of blood to reduce lymphocyte counts are treatment options that may induce a temporary remission. TBI causes severe bone marrow depression, which limits usefulness.[107,108]

For patients with advanced disease (stage III or IV) and anemia or thrombocytopenia, combination therapy is recommended.[110] This includes cyclophosphamide, vincristine, doxorubicin, and prednisone. Fludarabine is the newest agent approved for use in B-cell CLL and is especially promising in patients refractory to alkylator therapy. Fludarabine is given as a daily 30-minute infusion for 5 days and is generally well tolerated.[116] Future studies include the use of interferon and monoclonal antibodies in the treatment of CLL.[114,117]

HAIRY CELL LEUKEMIA

Etiology

An unusual variant of the chronic leukemias is *hairy cell leukemia (HCL),* so named for the prominent cytoplasmic projections on circulating mononuclear cells. Golomb[118] suggested that these cells share a common stem cell origin with histiocytes or monocytes and that the malignant cell is an immunoglobulin-bearing B-lymphocyte. HCL is also called *leukemic reticuloendotheliosis.*

Clinically, HCL may be difficult to distinguish from CLL or malignant lymphoma. The distinguishing characteristics are massive splenomegaly and little or no adenopathy. The characteristic hairy cells stain positively for tartrate-resistant acid phosphatase.[42] Two-thirds of individuals with HCL have pancytopenia, with symptomatic anemia, bleeding, and infection.

Treatment

The goal of therapy in HCL has progressed from palliation to cure with the use of nucleoside analogs and interferon. Historically, patients without cytopenias required no immediate treatment. However, since infection is the primary cause of death, patients with HCL are monitored closely. Splenectomy is the treatment of choice for patients with marked pancytopenia, recurrent infections, massive splenomegaly, or rapid disease progression and may allow prolonged survival of up to 15 years.[118,119] Recently, complete remissions have been obtained in HCL with 2′-deoxycoformycin and 2-chlorodeoxyadenosine. Normalization of pheripheral blood counts occurs with absence of hairy cells in the bone marrow.[120,121] Recombinant alpha-interferon is considered the treatment of choice for those in whom disease progresses either before or after splenectomy.[118,122,123] Administered daily by intramuscular or subcutaneous injection, alpha-interferon decreases the need for transfusions, reduces risk of infection, and improves overall quality of life.

SUPPORTIVE THERAPY

The increase in the length and quality of survival experienced by most individuals with leukemia is due not only to advances in antileukemic therapy but also to improved blood product and antimicrobial support and specialized nursing care. The complex means of providing effective supportive care include medical management to maintain physiologic homeostasis as well as an interdisciplinary approach to the health care plan.

Effective nursing participation in the supportive care of any patient with leukemia depends on an understanding of the staging and natural history of each of the leukemias. From this base of knowledge the nurse contributes to the care of the patient with leukemia in each of the areas of education, physical care, symptom management, and psychosocial adaptation.

Education

Providing information related to the disease process and treatment is clearly a standard in oncology nursing.[123,124] The nurse caring for the patient with AML has the unique opportunity of providing information to the patient and family because the patient is usually hospitalized throughout the course of therapy. The teaching plan for all patients includes pertinent information about the diagnosis, strategies for self-care in the prevention and treatment of side effects both in the hospital setting and at home, and methods to facilitate coping and adaptation to the illness.

For all patients with leukemia it is helpful to include the basic physiology of the bone marrow in the teaching plan. A hematologic malignancy is not as easy to understand as the concept of a solid tumor. Describing the bone marrow as the center of the bone where all blood products are made is a simple start. Further explanation includes the type, function, and abnormalities of the blood cells (see Figure 45-4). From this base, individualized instruction related to the specific leukemia is given. Educational materials can be obtained from the Leukemia Society, American Cancer Society, and the National Cancer Institute. Information for contacting the organizations is found in the "Yellow Pages" at the end of this book.

Physical Care

The physical care needs of patients with leukemia require nurses who are skilled in physical assessment. Patients with AML receive intensive therapy aimed at producing bone marrow aplasia for several weeks. Those with ALL have defective lymphocytes producing al-

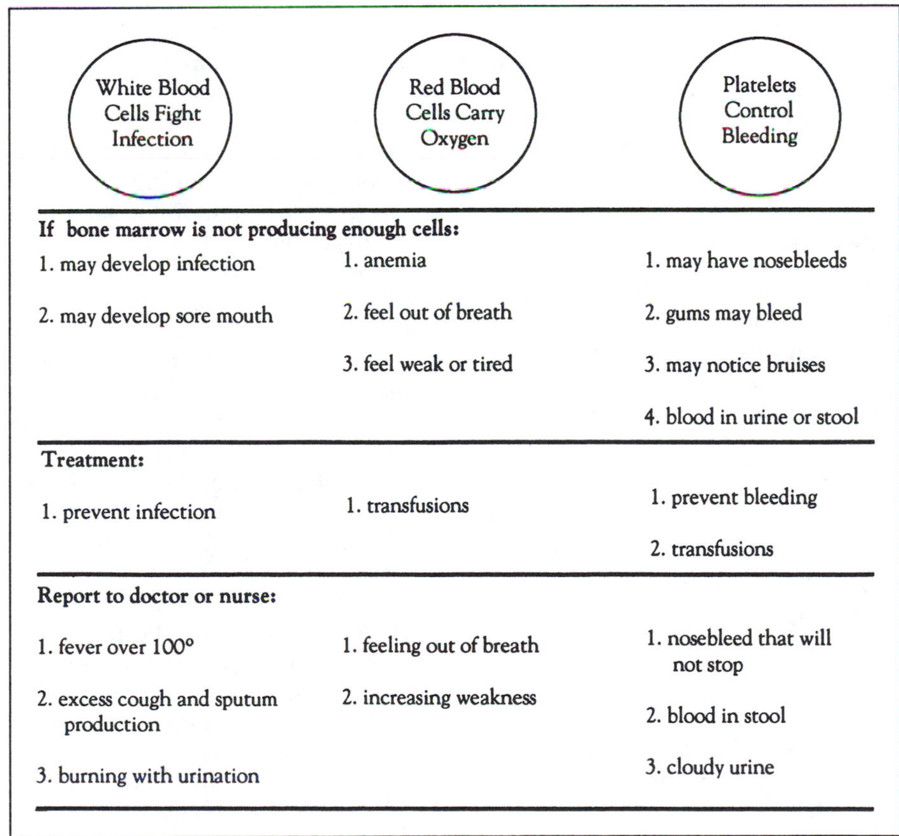

White Blood Cells Fight Infection	Red Blood Cells Carry Oxygen	Platelets Control Bleeding
If bone marrow is not producing enough cells:		
1. may develop infection	1. anemia	1. may have nosebleeds
2. may develop sore mouth	2. feel out of breath	2. gums may bleed
	3. feel weak or tired	3. may notice bruises
		4. blood in urine or stool
Treatment:		
1. prevent infection	1. transfusions	1. prevent bleeding
		2. transfusions
Report to doctor or nurse:		
1. fever over 100°	1. feeling out of breath	1. nosebleed that will not stop
2. excess cough and sputum production	2. increasing weakness	2. blood in stool
3. burning with urination		3. cloudy urine

FIGURE 45-4 Patient teaching sheet for blood cell function.

tered immunocompetence. The drugs received are cytotoxic. The hypogammaglobulinemia associated with CLL increases the patient's susceptibility to viral and fungal infections. In any type of leukemia the incidence of infection is high, but the usual signs and symptoms of infection are diminished or absent. Therefore, the nurse must regularly conduct a thorough physical examination in order to detect any evidence of infection. Subtle changes in vital signs and mentation may indicate early sepsis. Oozing of blood from gums and intravenous sites may be the first sign of disseminated intravascular coagulation. Cerebellar toxicity related to chemotherapy may be manifested as slightly altered responses in the neurologic examination. Each of these situations may be life-threatening, and the astute skills of the experienced nurse may be the crucial factor in initiating appropriate treatment.

In addition to having good assessment skills, the nurse caring for the patient with acute leukemia must be experienced in the use of right atrial catheters (RACs) and vascular access devices (VADs). Patients undergoing aggressive induction therapy in the hospital often have a double or triple lumen RAC placed prior to the start of therapy. The RAC is used for blood sampling as well as for the infusion of fluids, chemotherapy, antibiotics, total parenteral nutrition, and blood products.[125] Patients who require ongoing treatment but less frequent blood sampling and no simultaneous infusion of multiple fluids may have a VAD placed subcutaneously.[126] The advantages, disadvantages, and nursing procedures associated with RAC and VAD are beyond the scope of this chapter. However, since most patients with acute leukemia have one of these devices, it is important for the nurse to become familiar with them.

Symptom Management

Certain side effects associated with antileukemic therapy and disease-related complications can best be ameliorated if detected early and treated promptly. Knowing which side effects are expected and when they may occur allows the nurse to focus care appropriately.

Bone marrow depression

The desired effect of cytotoxic therapy is bone marrow hypoplasia. The duration of pancytopenia is variable, depending on the type of therapy and the person's ability to recover. However, individuals with acute leukemia in the induction phase or individuals with CML in blast crisis may remain severely hypoplastic for months.

Neutropenia It takes 9–10 days for immature cells formed in the bone marrow to become mature granulocytes. Because granulocytes circulate for only 6–10 hours, any interruption in their production quickly places the patient at risk for developing an infection. Infection is the major complication for leukemia patients, with up to 20%–30% mortality.[52,127,128] Neutropenia is commonly defined as an absolute neutrophil count less than 1000/mm^3. Since the neutrophils are responsible for phagocytosis, neutropenia eliminates one of the body's first lines of defense against infection. The patient with leukemia is particularly at risk due to a rapid drop in WBC with the initiation of therapy, a continuing decrease until the nadir (lowest point) is reached, and a prolonged time for recovery.[127]

Approximately 60% of neutropenic individuals develop infection. One-third have documented bacteremia, another third have documented infection without bacteremia, and the final third have apparent infection with no microbiologically documented pathogen. The risk of infection rises as the neutrophil count decreases, with 100% incidence of infection, if the neutrophil count remains <100/mm^3 for 3 weeks.[129,130] Other factors that add to the risk of infection are corticosteroids, hospital environment, antibiotic usage leading to increased col onization, and mucosal alteration.[129,131]

Adrenal corticosteroids are frequently used as part of the chemotherapeutic regimen or as supportive therapy. Steroids cause lysis of lymphocytes, suppression of antibody production, protein malnutrition, and suppression of inflammatory responses. As a result, the use of corticosteroids predisposes the patient to infection.

Most infections are due to organisms endogenous to the host or present in the environment.[129] The most common sites of infection are the alimentary tract (pharynx, esophagus, anorectum), sinuses, lungs, and skin.[129,132,133] The alimentary mucosa is directly damaged by the chemotherapy and the neutropenia allows colonization with yeasts and/or gram-negative bacilli. Perianal infection occurs in 25% of patients with AML. The only signs may be induration, erythema, and pain on defecation. Pneumonia can be caused by gram-negative organisms such as *Pseudomonas aeruginosa, Klebsiella pneumonia,* or *Escherichia coli.* The most common gram-positive organism causing infection is *Staphylococcus epidermidis.*[129,133]

More serious infections associated with prolonged neutropenia are fungal infections with *Candida* species or *Aspergillus* or protozoa such as *Pneumocystis carinii.* When these infections occur during severe aplasia and immune depression, recovery of the blood counts is the best hope for survival.

Empiric antibiotic therapy is used to treat high-risk (neutropenic and febrile) patients until an infecting organism is identified. Early empiric antibiotic therapy includes drugs to cover both gram-negative and gram-positive organisms. The usual combinations include an aminoglycoside plus an extended-spectrum cephalosporin or a broad-spectrum antipseudomonal penicillin.[129,131,133] There is currently a trend toward initial broad-spectrum monotherapy.[134]

Amphotericin B is used to treat life-threatening fungal infections in myelosuppressed, immunosuppressed individuals. It is indicated if fever continues for 5–7 days after the start of antibiotic therapy, if there is no identified source of infection, and continued neutropenia is expected.[130,135] Side effects of this toxic therapy include fever, chills, and rigors (80%–90%); nephrotoxicity (90%); headache (45%); anorexia (50%); vomiting (20%); and anemia.[135,136] Because anaphylaxis is a risk, a test dose of 1 mg is administered over 30 minutes. If the patient does not experience cardiopulmonary or mental changes, the starting dose is given. Fever is not a contraindication when the patient has recurrent fevers prior to the therapy. The dose is escalated daily until the desired dose is reached, and therapy continues for weeks to months, depending on the organism being treated and the patient's response.

Symptom management includes the following interventions to prevent or treat fever, chills or rigors: premedication with corticosteroids, acetaminophen, or diphenhydramine, and adding 10–15 mg hydrocortisone sodium succinate to the infusion. Intravenous meperidine 25–50 mg is given at the onset of chills or as a premedication.[136,137] Increasing room temperature, adding extra covers, using relaxation and hypnosis, and isometric leg and arm movements are other suggested comfort measures.[137] Potential nephrotoxicity due to a decreased glomerular filtration rate requires close monitoring of blood urea nitrogen, creatinine, sodium, and magnesium as well as evaluation of fluid balance. Peripheral phlebitis can be avoided by adding heparin to the solution. The anemia associated with amphotericin B is reversible and problematic only in that it compounds the existing myelosuppression.

Some centers now place patients on prophylactic fluconazole to prevent disseminated infections in patients expected to have prolonged neutropenia.[138]

Because the neutropenic patient does not produce an adequate inflammatory response to infection, the usual signs and symptoms are absent. Fever is usually the first sign of infection that leads to closer inspection of high-risk areas (perirectal area, oral mucosa, IV sites). Patients are often unable to produce sputum; thus, the early indications of pneumonia are shortness of breath or cough. Vital signs are assessed every 4 hours. At the onset of fever over 100°F in the neutropenic patient, blood, urine, and sputum cultures are obtained and empiric antibiotic therapy is initiated. The importance of prompt reporting of fever and initiation of therapy cannot be overemphasized since delay of only a few hours can allow the patient to go into septic shock.

Prevention of infection focuses on restoring host defenses, decreasing invasive procedures, and decreasing colonization of organisms. Treatment and remission induction will restore normal defenses against infection. Decreasing invasive procedures includes avoiding the use of Foley catheters. If catheterization is necessary, the smallest lumen possible should be used, and the catheter should be anchored. Other measures are meticulous care of IV or RAC exit sites and aseptic technique for any invasive procedures.

To decrease the number of gram-negative organisms, uncooked fruits and vegetables are avoided, especially salads. *P. aeruginosa* can be decreased by removing aerators from faucets, using ice machines in which the ice falls directly into the cup, and by frequently changing stagnant water sources such as oxygen humidifiers. Proper hand-washing techniques by everyone in contact with the patient can eliminate the main source of gram-positive organisms. Fungi that are found in food or the air can also be decreased by cooking foods and eliminating live plants or flowers from the patient's room. A private room is necessary, and visitors are restricted. All of these measures are to be practiced by the health care team and taught to the patient and family.[129,139,140] Further information is provided in Chapter 24, "Infection."

In certain circumstances such as BMT, total reverse isolation may be used. The patient is kept in a sterile laminar air-flow room. Nonabsorbable antibiotics are used to sterilize the alimentary canal. Normal skin flora is decreased by frequent cleansing with hexachlorophene or an iodine-base soap.[3,52]

Granulocyte transfusions may be indicated for patients with profound neutropenia and documented infections not responding to antibiotics.[133,141] However, the hazards of this therapy (increased alloimmunization and refractoriness to platelet transfusions) and its high cost make it a controversial therapy.

Colony stimulating factors have been used in the treatment of patients with leukemia. Both granulocyte (G-CSF) and granulocyte-macrophage (GM-CSF) have been administered to patients after completion of standard induction therapy to shorten the period of neutropenia.[142,143] Because myeloid leukemia cells have receptors for CSFs and have demonstrated increased growth in response to CSFs in vitro,[143] there is concern about administering myeloid CSFs to patients with AML. There is, however, some evidence of decreased myelosuppression and infection.

Erythrocytopenia Individuals undergoing intensive chemotherapy develop a tolerance for chronic low-grade anemia. However, in severe cases of hypoplasia, sudden blood loss due to bleeding, or symptomatic anemia, support with transfusions of RBCs is provided. Premedication with acetaminophen and diphenhydramine can decrease the febrile response to antibodies to white cells that occurs after multiple transfusions. Leukocyte-poor RBCs may be used to decrease the antibody production against antigens on the leukocytes.[144,145]

Thrombocytopenia *Thrombocytopenia* is the abnormal decrease in the number of circulating platelets. The potential for bleeding occurs when levels reach ≤50,000 platelets/mm^3, and spontaneous bleeding occurs at levels of ≤20,000 platelets/mm^3.[146] The first evidence of bleeding may be petechiae or ecchymoses on the skin of dependent limbs or on mucous membranes or oozing from gums, nose, or IV site.

Random donor platelets are given to keep the platelet count above 20,000/mm^3. Once antibodies to the platelets develop, refractoriness to random donor platelets occurs. When blood counts 1 hour posttransfusion reveal poor increments, the patient may require HLA-matched single-donor platelets.[132] Because chills and fever can destroy circulating platelets, the patient is premedicated with acetaminophen and diphenhydramine.[133] Additional measures used to prevent bleeding include maintaining skin integrity, preventing trauma, and avoiding medications that have the potential to induce or prolong bleeding.[146] Stool softeners will prevent the Valsalva maneuver and rectal tears. Further detail is given in Chapter 25, "Bleeding."

Complications

Certain complications of the specific leukemic process or therapy may be singled out as untoward but not unexpected side effects. Knowledge of these occurrences assists the nurse in anticipating problems in high-risk individuals. These complications include leukostasis, disseminated intravascular coagulation, oral complications, and cerebellar toxicity.

Leukostasis Individuals with extremely high numbers of circulating blasts are at risk of leukostatic-induced hemorrhage. This occurs most often in patients with ALL. Leukostasis occurs as leukemic blasts accumulate and invade vessel walls, causing rupture and bleeding. Because of the extensive capillary network and the limited vasculature space of the brain, intracerebral hemorrhage is the most common and most lethal manifestation of this complication. Therefore, early detection of patients at risk (WBC >50,000 cells/mm^3) and immediate efforts to reduce the number of circulating cells are imperative. Treatment consists of high doses of cytotoxic drugs to reduce the burden of circulating cells. Leukapheresis and cranial irradiation may be used to provide immediate treatment.[3]

Disseminated intravascular coagulation Disseminated intravascular coagulation (DIC) is most frequently associated with acute promyelocytic leukemia, although it may occur with any acute leukemia.[52] During induction therapy there is excessive release of procoagulants from granules within the leukemic promyelocyte. (See Chapter 25 for a discussion of the pathophysiology of DIC.)

Correction of the coagulopathy in DIC depends on the successful treatment of the leukemia. Therapy usually includes heparin and replacement of plasma factors and platelets. Nursing care focuses on the prevention of injury, administration of prescribed therapy, and monitoring of the appropriate laboratory results.[146–148]

Oral complications Oral complications of leukemia may be the result of the disease or the therapy. Gingival hypertrophy due to massive infiltration by leukemic cells is associated with acute myelomonocytic and monocytic leukemia.[10,41] The gingiva may be swollen, necrotic, and/or superinfected. The most effective treatment is therapy for the leukemia. Stomatitis due to the direct toxicity of chemotherapeutic agents such as the anthracyclines or methotrexate, combined with prolonged neutropenia and antibiotic therapy, renders the patient at high risk for oral infection.

Oral care consists of regular cleansing with a solution of one quart of water with one teaspoon each of salt and sodium bicarbonate, treatment of infection with nystatin mouth rinses, and appropriate analgesia as needed.[148]

Cerebellar toxicity Cerebellar toxicity is a CNS toxicity associated with the administration of high-dose cytosine arabinoside (HDCA). Conventional dosages are 100–200 mg/m^2, whereas HDCA is ≥3 g/m^2. The incidence of neurotoxicity is 11%–28% at dosages of 3 g/m^2 and as high as 67% in dosages up to 4.5 g/m^2.[149,150] This toxicity is also age-related, with an increased risk in patients over 50 years of age.[151] The syndrome may begin with signs of ataxia and nystagmus and progress to dysarthria (difficulty in articulating words) and adiadochokinesis (inability to perform rapid alternating movements). This toxicity may be irreversible if not detected early. Therefore, it is essential that prior to each dose of HDCA the nurse completes a full neurological assessment.[152] Any changes are reported and the dosage is held until the physician evaluates the patient.

PSYCHOSOCIAL SUPPORT

Individuals and their significant others are at risk for ineffective coping during the diagnostic work-up for malignancy and during subsequent treatments.[153] A primary objective of supportive care must be to facilitate the most effective coping mechanisms for the individual and family as well as to enable the patient to live as full and normal a life as possible. Several factors should be taken into consideration as the nurse coordinates the care plan for psychologic and physical rehabilitation.

The age of the individual at the time of diagnosis may vary from infancy to old age. Issues may range from concern about fertility or the risk of a second malignancy in the young adult to fear of job stigma in the middle-aged individual. The elderly patient may be dealing with increasing physical decline in addition to the debilitating effects of cancer. Assessment of the individual's needs and degree of stress will facilitate the planning of suitable intervention.[154]

The stage and "curability" of the disease are other factors to be considered. It is imperative that the nurse understand the implications of the planned therapy and assist the patient in making appropriate decisions. For example, a young mother undergoing intensive chemotherapy for AML may need to make the necessary arrangement for child care and housekeeping for 6–8 weeks. A patient undergoing BMT may need to discuss with his or her employer the need to be on extended sick leave. The emotional ups and downs related to multiple remission inductions and relapses are exhausting to the patient and family.[155] As survival with leukemia increases, patients must deal with many issues such as fear of relapse, return to an independent state, and an uncertain future.[156] Ongoing support from the health care team is essential to overcome these fears. Education and reassurance by consistent nursing staff can help the individual regain a sense of control and hopefulness.

CONCLUSION

The care of the individual with a diagnosis of leukemia requires a multidisciplinary approach that considers many factors. The classification of acute or chronic and myeloid or lymphoid determines diverse treatment plans and prognoses that are quite variable. The age of the patient and the stage of the disease determine the aggressiveness of therapy. Newer diagnostic studies allow the identification of both favorable and high-risk subsets of patients. As research continues, more durable cure rates may be achieved.

The role of the nurse providing direct care for patients with leukemia includes education, physical care, symptom management, and psychosocial support. In addition, contributions to research studies are essential. Although the nurse has an indirect impact on the prognosis through correct administration of therapy and management of side effects, the direct result of continuous support and education is an improved quality of life.

REFERENCES

1. *Cancer Facts and Figures 1992*. New York: American Cancer Society, 1992, p. 12.
2. Boring CC, Squires TS, Tong T: Cancer Statistics, 1993. *CA* 43: 7–26, 1993.
3. Henderson ES: Acute leukemia: General considerations. In Williams WJ, Beutler E, Erslev AJ, Lichtman MA (eds), *Hematology*. New York: McGraw-Hill, 1983, pp. 221–253.
4. Maguire ME: Leukemia. In Ziegfeld, C (ed), *Core Curriculum for Oncology Nursing*. Philadelphia: Saunders, 1987, pp. 173–192.
5. Sandler OP: Epidemiology of acute myelogenous leukemia. *Semin Oncol* 14:359–364, 1987.
6. Miller RW: Relation between cancer and congenital defects: An epidemiological evaluation. *J Natl Cancer Inst* 40:1079, 1968.
7. Keating MJ, Freireich EJ, McCredie KB, et al: Acute leukemia in adults, 1977. *CA* 27:2–25, 1977.
8. Gunz FW: Genetic factors in human leukemia. In Gunz FW (ed), *Leukemia*. New York: Grune & Stratton, 4th ed., 1983, pp. 313–328.
9. Rosner F, Lee SL: Down's syndrome and acute leukemia: Myeloblastic or lymphoblastic? *Am J Med* 53:203–218, 1972.
10. Wiernik PH: Acute leukemias. In DeVita VT, Hellman S, Rosenberg SA (eds), *Cancer: Principles and Practice of Oncology* (3d ed.). Philadelphia: Lippincott, 1989, pp. 1809–1835.
11. Zuelzer WW, Cox DE: Genetic aspects of leukemia. *Semin Hematol* 6:228, 1969.
12. Bloomfield CD, de la Chapelle A: Chromosome abnormalities in acute nonlymphocytic leukemia: Clinical and biological significance. *Semin Oncol* 14:372–383, 1987.
13. Brill AB, Tomonaga M, Heyssell RM: Leukemia in man following exposure to ionizing radiation: Summary of findings in Hiroshima and Nagasaki and a comparison with other human experience. *Ann Intern Med* 56:590–609, 1962.
14. Bizzozero OJ, Johnson KG, Crocco A: Radiation-related leukemia in Hiroshima and Nagasaki. *N Engl J Med* 274:1095–1097, 1966.
15. Matanowski GM, Seltser R, Sartwell PE: The current mortality rates of radiologists and other physician specialists: Specific causes of death. *Am J Epidemiol* 101:199–210, 1975.
16. Court-Brown WM, Doll R: Leukemia and aplastic anemia in patients irradiated for ankylosing spondylitis. Medical Research Council Special Reports Series No 295. London: Her Majesty's Stationery Office, 1957.
17. Rinsky RA, Smith AB, Horning R, et al: Benzene and leukemia. *N Engl J Med* 316:1044–1050, 1987.
18. Thorpe JJ: Epidemiologic survey of leukemia in persons potentially exposed to benzene. *J Occup Med* 16:375–382, 1974.
19. Yin SN, Li G, Tain FD, et al: Leukemia in benzene workers: A retrospective cohort study. *Br J Ind Med* 44:124–128, 1987.
20. Whitlock JA, Greer JP, Lukens JN: Epipodophyllotoxin-related leukemia. *Cancer* 68:600–604, 1991.
21. Pedersen-Bjergaard J, Daugaard G, Hansen SW, et al: Increased risk of myelodysplasia and leukaemia after etoposide, cisplatin, and bleomycin for germ-cell tumours. *Lancet* 338:359–363, 1991.
22. Levine EG, Bloomfield CD: Leukemias and myelodysplastic syndromes secondary to drug, radiation, and environmental exposure. *Semin Oncol* 19:47–84, 1992.
23. Fraser MC, Tucker MA: Late effects of cancer therapy, chemotherapy related malignancies. *Oncol Nurs Forum* 15:67–77, 1988.
24. Keating M, Cork AL, Broach Y, et al: Towards a clinically relevant cytogenetic classification of acute myelogenous leukemia. *Leuk Res* 11:119–133, 1987.
25. Foon KA, Gale RP: Controversies in the therapy of acute myelogenous leukemia. *Am J Med* 72:963–978, 1982.
26. Kantarjian HM, Keating M: Therapy related leukemia and myelodysplastic syndrome. *Semin Oncol* 14:435–443, 1987.
27. Dougan L, Woodleff AJ: Acute leukemia associated with phenylbutazone treatment. *Med J Aust* 1:217–219, 1965.
28. Brauer MJ, Dameshek W: Hypoplastic anemia and myeloblastic leukemia following chloramphenicol therapy. *N Engl J Med* 277:1003–1005, 1967.
29. Gallagher RE, Gallo RC: Type of C RNA tumor virus isolated from cultured human acute myelogenous leukemia cells. *Science* 187:350–353, 1975.
30. Jarrett W, Essex M, Mackey L, et al: Horizontal trans-

mission of leukemia virus and leukemia in the cat. *J Nat Cancer Inst* 51:833–841, 1973.

31. Heath CW: Epidemiology and hereditary aspects of acute leukemia. In Wiernick PH, (ed), *Neoplastic Diseases of the Blood* (vol. 1). New York: Churchill Livingstone, 1985, pp. 183–200.
32. Kalyanaraman VS, Sarngadharan MG, Robert-Guroff M, et al: A new subtype of human T-cell leukemia virus (HTLV-II) associated with a T-cell variant of hairy cell leukemia. *Science* 218:571–573, 1982.
33. Rosenblatt JD, Plaeger-Marshall S, Giorgi JV, et al: A clinical, hematologic, and immunologic analysis of 21 HTLV-II-infected intravenous drug users. *Blood* 76:409–417, 1990.
34. Bennett JM, Catovsky D, Daniel MT, et al: Proposals for the classification of the acute leukemias. *Br J Haemat* 33:451–458, 1976.
35. Bennett JM, Catovsky D, Daniel MT, et al: Criteria for the diagnosis of acute leukemia of megakaryocyte lineage (M7). *Ann Intern Med* 103:460–462, 1985.
36. Bennett JM, Catovsky D, Daniel MT, et al: Proposed revised criteria for the classification of acute myeloid leukemia. *Ann Intern Med* 103:626–629, 1985.
37. Johnson BL: Leukemias. In Groenwald S (ed), *Cancer Nursing: Principles and Practice.* Boston: Jones and Bartlett, 1987, pp. 654–670.
38. Arlin ZA, Heddeman W, Feldman E, et al: Further thoughts on "cell kill" in acute leukemia. *Acta Haematol* 85:1–5, 1991.
39. Griffin JD, Davis R, Nelson DA: Use of surface marker analysis to predict outcome of adult myeloblastic leukemia. *Blood* 68:1232–1241, 1986.
40. Sobel RE, Mick R, Royston I: Clinical importance of myeloid antigen expression in adult acute lymphoblastic leukemia. *N Engl J Med* 316:1111–1117, 1987.
41. Peterson BA, Ellis EG: Uncommon subtypes of acute nonlymphocytic leukemia: Clinical features and management of FAB M^5 M^6 M^7. *Semin Oncol* 14:425–434, 1987.
42. Champlin R, Golde DW: The leukemias. In Braunwald E, Isselbacher KJ, Petersdorf RG, et al (eds), *Harrison's Principles of Internal Medicine* (11th ed). New York: McGraw-Hill, 1987, pp. 1541–1550.
43. Cassileth PA: Adult acute nonlymphocytic leukemia. *Med Clin North Am* 68:675–695, 1984.
44. Larson RA, Daly KM, Choi KE, et al: A clinical and pharmacokinetic study of mitoxantrone in acute nonlymphocytic leukemia. *J Clin Oncol* 5:391–397, 1987.
45. Champlin R: Acute myelogenous leukemia: Biology and treatment. *Mediguide Oncol* 8:1–9, 1988.
46. Berman E, Heller G, Santorsa J, et al: Results of a randomized trial comparing idarubicin and cytosine arabinoside with daunorubicin and cytosine arabinoside in adult patients with newly diagnosed acute myelogenous leukemia. *Blood* 77:1666–1674, 1991.
47. Brach MA, Henschler R, Martelsman R, et al: To overcome pharmacologic and cytokinetic resistance to cytarabine in the treatment of acute myelogenous leukemia by using recombinant interleukin-3. *Semin Hematol* 28:39–43, 1991.
48. Preisler H, Davis RB, Kirshner J, et al: Comparison of three remission induction regimens and two postinduction strategies for the treatment of acute nonlymphocytic leukemia: A cancer and leukemia Group B study. *Blood* 69:1441–1449, 1987.
49. Gale RP, Foon KA: Therapy of acute myelogenous leukemia. *Semin Hematol* 24:40–54, 1987.
50. Mayer RJ: Current chemotherapeutic treatment approaches to the management of previously untreated adults with de novo acute myelogenous leukemia. *Semin Oncol* 14:384–396, 1987.
51. Arlin ZA, Hagenbeek A, Feldman E, et al: Implications of leukemia "cell kill" for the treatment of acute myelogenous leukemia (AML): Can the cure rate be increased? *Acta Haematol* 82:175–178, 1989.
52. Foon KA, Gale RP: Controversies in the therapy of acute myelogenous leukemia. *Am J Med* 72:963–978, 1982.
53. Wolff SN, Marion J, Stern RS, et al: High dose cytosine arabinoside and daunorubicin as consolidation therapy for acute nonlymphocytic leukemia in first remission: A pilot study. *Blood* 65:1407–1411, 1985.
54. Wolff SN, Herzig RH, Phillips CL, et al: High dose cytosine arabinoside and daunorubicin as consolidation therapy for acute nonlymphocytic leukemia in first remission: An update. *Semin Oncol* 14:12–17, 1987 (suppl).
55. Bloomfield CD: Post remission therapy in acute myeloid leukemia. *J Clin Oncol* 3:1570–1572, 1985 (editorial).
56. Arlin ZA, Feldman ET, Finger LR, et al: Short course high dose mitoxantrone with high dose cytarabine is effective therapy for adult lymphoblastic leukemia. *Leukemia* 5:712–714, 1991.
57. Cassileth PA, Begg CB, Bennett JM, et al: A randomized study of the efficacy of consolidation therapy in adult acute nonlymphocytic leukemia. *Blood* 63:843–847, 1984.
58. Grever MR: Treatment of patients with acute nonlymphocytic leukemia not in remission. *Semin Hematol* 14:416–424, 1987.
59. Champlin R, Gale RP: Bone marrow transplantation for acute leukemia: Recent advances and comparison with alternative therapies. *Semin Oncol* 24:55–67, 1987.
60. Applebaum FR, Fisher LD, Thomas ED, et al: Chemotherapy versus marrow transplantation for adults with acute nonlymphocytic leukemia: A five year follow-up. *Blood* 72:179–184, 1988.
61. Keating MJ, Gehan EA, Smith TL, et al: A strategy for evaluation of new treatments in untreated patients: Application to a clinical trial of AMSA for acute leukemia. *J Clin Oncol* 5:710–721, 1987.
62. Priesler HD, Raza A, Barcos M, et al: High dose cytosine arabinoside as the initial treatment of poor risk patients with acute nonlymphocytic leukemia: A leukemia intergroup study. *J Clin Oncol* 5:75–82, 1987.
63. Dalton WS, Miller TP. Multidrug resistance. *PPO Updates* 5(7):1–13, 1991.
64. Herweijer H, Sonneveld P, Baas F, et al: Expression of *mdr1* and *mdr3* multidrug-resistence genes in human acute and chronic leukemias and association with stimulation of drug accumulation by cyclosporine. *J Natl Cancer Inst* 82:1133–1140, 1990.
65. Nooter K, Sonneveld P, Oostrum R, et al: Overexpression of the *mdr1* gene in blast cells from patients with acute myelocytic leukemia is associated with decreased anthracycline accumulation that can be restored by cyclosporine. *Int J Cancer* 45:262–268, 1990.
66. Brown RA, Herzig RH, Wolff SN, et al: High dose etoposide and cyclophosphamide without bone marrow transplantation for resistant hematologic malignancy. *Blood* 76:473–479, 1990.
67. Cannistra SA, Groshek P, Griffin JD: Granulocyte-macrophage-colony-stimulating factor enhances the cyto-

toxic effects of cytosine arabinoside in acute myeloblastic leukemia and in the myeloid blast crisis phase of chronic myeloid leukemia. *Leukemia* 3:328–334, 1989.

68. Foon KA, Todd RF: Immunologic classification of leukemia and lymphoma. *Blood* 68:1–31, 1986.
69. Castaigne S, Chomienne C, Daniel MT, et al: All-trans retinoic acid as a differentiation therapy for acute promyelocytic leukemia. I. Clinical results. *Blood* 76:1704–1709, 1990.
70. Warrell RP, Frankel S, Miller WH, et al: Differentiation therapy of acute promyelocytic leukemia treated with tretinoin (all-trans retinoid acid). *N Engl J Med* 324:1385–1393, 1991.
71. Warrell RP: Retinoic acid and acute promyelocytic leukemia. *Biologic Ther Cancer Updates* 1(3):1–12, 1991.
72. Foon KA, Gale RP, Todd RF: Recent advances in the immunologic classification of leukemia and lymphoma. *Semin Hematol* 23:257–283, 1986.
73. Henderson ES: Acute lymphocytic leukemia. In Williams WJ, Beutler E, Ersler AJ, Lichtman MA (eds), *Hematology*. New York: McGraw-Hill, 1983, pp. 970–978.
74. Clarkson B, Elles S, Little C, et al: Acute lymphoblastic leukemia in adults. *Semin Oncol* 12:160–179, 1985.
75. Ortega JA, Nesbit ME, Donaldson MH, et al: L-asparaginase, vincristine and prednisone for induction of first remission in acute lymphocytic leukemia. *Cancer Res* 37:535–540, 1977.
76. Hoelzer D, Gale RP: Acute lymphoblastic leukemia in adults: Recent progress, future directions. *Semin Hematol* 24:27–39, 1987.
77. Law IP, Blum J: Adult acute leukemia—Frequency of CNS involvement in long-term survivors. *Cancer* 40:1304–1306, 1977.
78. Kuo AH, Yataganas X, Galicich YY, et al: Proliferative kinetics of central nervous system leukemia. *Cancer* 36:232–239, 1975.
79. Chessells JM: Acute lymphoblastic leukemia. *Semin Hematol* 19:155–171, 1982.
80. Hoelzer D: Acute lymphoblastic leukemia in adults. In Hoffman R, Benz EJ, Shattel SJ, et al, (eds), *Hematology: Basic Principles and Practice*. New York: Churchill Livingstone, 1991, pp. 793–804.
81. Hoelzer D: High-dose chemotherapy in adult acute lymphoblastic leukemia. *Semin Hematol* 28:84–89, 1991.
82. Hamilton-Paterson JL: Pre-leukemia anemia. *Acta Haematol* 2:309–316, 1949.
83. Buzaid AC, Garewal HS, Greenberg BR: Management of myelodysplastic syndromes. *Am J Med* 80:1149–1157, 1986.
84. Bennett JM, Catovsky D, Daniel MT, et al: The French-American-British (FAB) Co-operative Group: Proposals for the classification of the myelodysplastic syndromes. *Br J Haematol* 51:189–199, 1982.
85. Tricot GJ, Lauer RC, Appelbaum FR, et al: Management of the myelodysplastic syndromes. *Semin Oncol* 14:444–453, 1987.
86. Greenberg PL: The smoldering myeloid leukemic states: Clinical and biologic features. *Blood* 61:1035–1044, 1983.
87. Koeffler HP: Myelodysplastic syndromes (preleukemia). *Semin Hematol* 23:284–299, 1986.
88. Yoemans AC, Harle MT: Myelodysplastic syndromes. *Semin Oncol Nurs* 6:9–16, 1990.
89. Cines DB, Cassileth PA, Kiss JE: Danazol therapy in myelodysplasia. *Ann Intern Med* 103:58–60, 1985.
90. Adamson JW: The myeloproliferative diseases. In Braunwald E, Isselbacher KJ, Petersdorf RG, et al (eds). *Harrison's Principles of Internal Medicine* (11th ed). New York: McGraw-Hill, 1987, pp. 1527–1533.
91. Coleman M, Allen SL: Chronic myelogenous leukemia: Evolving concepts in diagnosis and treatment. *Mediguide Oncol* 3(4):1–5, 1983.
92. Canellos GP: Chronic leukemias. In Williams WJ, Beutler E, Erslev AJ (eds), *Hematology*. New York: McGraw-Hill, 1983, pp. 221–253.
93. Eisbruch A, Blick M, Evinger-Hodges MJ, et al: Effect of differentiation-inducing agents on oncogene expression in a chronic myelogenous leukemic cell line. *Cancer* 62:1171–1178, 1988.
94. Fitzgerald PH, Morris CM: Ph-negative chronic myeloid leukemia: The nature of the breakpoint junction and mechanism of ABL transposition. *Leukemia Lymphoma* 6:277–287, 1992.
95. Cannellos GP: Chronic leukemias. In DeVita VT, Hellman S, Rosenberg SA (eds), *Cancer: Principles and Practice of Oncology* (2d ed). Philadelphia: Lippincott, 1985, pp. 1739–1752.
96. Spiers AS: Chronic granulocytic leukemia. *Med Clin North Am* 68:713–727, 1984.
97. Griffin JD: Management of chronic myelogenous leukemia. *Semin Hematol* 23(suppl 1):20–26, 1986.
98. Haines ME, Goldman JM, Worsley AM, et al: Chemotherapy and autografting for chronic granulocytic leukemia in transformation: Probable prolongation of survival for some patients. *Br J Haematol* 58:711–721, 1984.
99. Talpaz M, Kantarjian HM, Kurzrock R, et al: Therapy of chronic myelogenous leukemia: Chemotherapy and interferons. *Semin Hematol* 25:62–73, 1988.
100. Morra E, Lazzarino M, Alimena G, et al: The role of interferon in the treatment of chronic myelogenous leukemia: Results and prospects. *Leukemia Lymphoma* 6:305–315, 1992.
101. Sokal JE, Baccaran M, Russo D, et al: Staging and prognosis in chronic myelogenous leukemia. *Semin Hematol* 25:49–61, 1988.
102. Kantarjian HM, Smith TL, McCredie KB, et al: Chronic myelogenous leukemia: A multivariate analysis of the associations of patient characteristics and therapy with survival. *Blood* 66:1326–1335, 1985.
103. Champlin RE, Goldman JM, Gale RP: Bone marrow transplantation in chronic myelogenous leukemia. *Semin Hematol* 25:74–80, 1988.
104. Beaty PG, Anasetti C: Marrow transplantation from donors other than HLA identical siblings. *Hematol Oncol Clin North Am* 4:677–688, 1990.
105. Shalrid M, Lugussy G, Berrebi A: High response rate to recombinant interferon alpha in chronic myeloid leukemia after intensive cytoreductive chemotherapy. *Blood* 74:370A, 1989.
106. Rai KR, Montserat E: Prognostic factors in chronic lymphocytic leukemia. *Semin Hemat* 24:252–256, 1987.
107. Rai KR, Sawitsky A, Jagathambal K, et al: Chronic lymphocytic leukemia. *Med Clin North Am* 68:697–711, 1984.
108. Silbar R, Stahl R: Chronic lymphocytic leukemia and related diseases. In Williams WJ, Beutler E, Erslev AJ, Lichtman MA, (eds), *Hematology*. New York: McGraw-Hill, 1990, pp. 1005–1025.
109. Lipshutz MD, Mu R, Rai KR, et al: Bone marrow biopsy

and clinical staging in chronic lymphocytic leukemia. *Cancer* 46:1422–1427, 1980.
110. Binet JL, Chastang C, Dighiero G, et al: Prognostic and therapeutic advances in CLL management: The experience of the French Cooperative Group. *Semin Hematol* 24:275–290, 1987.
111. Lee JS, Dixon DO, Kantarjian HM, et al: Prognosis of chronic lymphocytic leukemia: A multivariate regression analysis of 325 untreated patients. *Blood* 69:929–936, 1987.
112. Mandelli F, DeRossi G, Mancini P, et al: Prognosis in chronic lymphocytic leukemia: A retrospective multicenter study from the GIMEMA Group. *J Clin Oncol* 5:398–406, 1987.
113. Binet JL, Cavotsky D, Chandra P, et al: Chronic lymphocytic leukemia: Proposals for a revised prognostic staging system. *Br J Haemat* 48:365–367, 1981.
114. Foon KA, Gale RT: Staging and therapy of chronic lymphocytic leukemia. *Semin Hematol* 24:264–274, 1987.
115. Pape LH: Therapy related acute leukemia: An overview. *Cancer Nurs* 11:295–302, 1988.
116. Cheson BD: New modalities of therapy in chronic lymphocytic leukemia. *Crit Rev Oncol Hematol* 11:167–177, 1991.
117. Foon KA, Bunn PA: Interferon treatment of cutaneous T cell lymphoma and chronic lymphocytic leukemia. *Semin Oncol* 13(suppl 5):35–39, 1986.
118. Golomb HM: Hairy cell leukemia: An unusual lymphoproliferative disease. *Cancer* 42:946–956, 1978.
119. Steis RG, Longs DL: Update on the treatment of hairy cell leukemia. *PPO Updates* 2(6):1–12, 1982.
120. Piro LD, Carrera CJ, Carson DA, et al: Lasting remissions in hairy-cell leukemia induced by a single infusion of 2-chlorodeoxyadenosine. *N Engl J Med* 322:1117–1121, 1990.
121. Spiers AS, Moore D, Cassileth PA, et al: Remissions in hairy-cell leukemia with pentostatin (2′-deoxycoformycin). *N Engl J Med* 316:825–830, 1987.
122. Quesada JR, Reuben J, Manning JT, et al: Alpha interferon for induction of remission in hairy-cell leukemia. *N Engl J Med* 310:15–18, 1984.
123. Fanslow J: Knowledge deficit related to disease process. In McNally JC, Stair JC, Somerville ET, (eds.), *Guidelines for Cancer Nursing Practice.* Philadelphia: Saunders, 1985, pp. 39–45.
124. Somerville ET: Knowledge deficit related to chemotherapy. In McNally JC, Stair JC, Somerville ET (eds), *Guidelines for Cancer Nursing Practice.* Philadelphia: Saunders, 1985, pp. 39–45.
125. Wilson JM: Right atrial catheters (Broviac and Hickman): Indications for insertion, maintenance, and protocol for home care. *Natl Int Ther Assoc J* 6:23–27, 1983.
126. Goodman MS, Wickham R: Venous access devices: An overview. *Oncol Nurs Forum* 11:16–23, 1984.
127. Bodey GP: Infection in cancer patients: A continuing association. *Am J Med* 81(suppl 1A):11–26, 1986.
128. Oniboni AC: Infection in the neutropenic patient. *Semin Oncol Nurs* 6:50–60, 1990.
129. Bodey GP: Infection in cancer patients. *Cancer Treat Rev* 2:89–129, 1975.
130. Carlson AC: Infection prophylaxis in the patient with cancer. *Oncol Nurs Forum* 12:56–64, 1985.
131. Reheis CE: Neutropenia: Causes, complications, treatment, and resulting nursing care. *Nurs Clin North Am* 20:219–225, 1985.
132. Scheffer CA, Wade JC: Supportive care: Issues in the use of blood products and treatment of infection. *Semin Oncol* 14:454–467, 1987.
133. Young LS: Management of infections in leukemia and lymphoma. In Ruben RH, Young LS (eds), *Clinical Approach to Infection in the Compromised Host.* New York: Plenum Medicare Book, 1981, pp. 461–497.
134. Hathorn JW, Ruben M, Pizzo PA: Empirical antibiotic therapy in the febrile neutropenic cancer patient: Clinical efficacy and impact of monotherapy. *Antimicrob Agents Chemother* 31:971–977, 1987.
135. Bodey CP: Topical and systemic antifungal agents. *Med Clin North Am* 72:637–659, 1988.
136. Mahon SM: Taking the terror out of amphotericin B. *Am J Nurs* 88:961–966, 1988.
137. Rutledge DN, Holtzclaw RJ: Amphotericin B-induced shivering in patients with cancer: A nursing approach. *Heart Lung* 17:432–440, 1988.
138. Freifeld A, Pizzo P: New developments in the antimicrobial supportive care of the immunocompromised patient. *PPO Updates* 5:1–14, 1990.
139. Brandt B: A nursing protocol for the client with neutropenia. *Oncol Nurs Forum* 11:24–28, 1984.
140. Spross JA: Protective mechanisms. In Johnson BL, Gross J (eds), *Handbook of Oncology Nursing.* New York: Wiley, 1985, pp. 229–302.
141. Nusbacher J: Preservation and clinical use of leukocytes. In Williams WJ, Beutler EJ, Erslev AJ (eds), *Hematology.* New York: McGraw-Hill, 1983, pp. 1549–1555.
142. Ohno R, Tomonoage M, Kobayaski T, et al: Effect of granulocyte colony stimulating factor after intensive induction therapy in relapsed or refractory acute leukemia. *N Engl J Med* 323:871–877, 1990.
143. Karp JE, Gruke DH, Donehower RC: Effects of the rhGM-CSF on intracellular ara-c pharmacology in acute myelocytic leukemia: Comparability with drug induced humorol stimulatory activity. *Leukemia* 4:553–556, 1990.
144. Masauredis SP: Preservation and clinical use of erythrocytes and whole blood. In Williams WJ, Beutler EJ, Erslev AJ (eds), *Hematology.* New York: McGraw-Hill, 1983, pp. 1529–1549.
145. Erickson JM: Blood support for the immunocompromised patient. *Semin Oncol Nurs* 6:61–66, 1990.
146. Gannon CT: Bleeding due to thrombocytopenia. In Yasko JM (ed), *Guidelines for Cancer Care: Symptom Management.* Reston, VA.: Reston Publishing, 1983, pp. 25–32.
147. Rooney A, Hawley C: Nursing management of disseminated intravascular coagulation. *Oncol Nurs Forum* 12:15–22, 1985.
148. Ziga SE: Stomatitis/mucositis. In Yasko JM (ed), *Guidelines for Cancer Care: Symptom Management.* Reston, VA: Reston Publishing, 1983, pp. 219–229.
149. Sylvester RK, Fisher AJ, Lobell M: Cytarabine-induced cerebellar syndrome, case report and literature review. *Drug Intel Clin Pharm* 21:177–179, 1987.
150. Herzig RH, Lazarus GP, Herzig PF, et al: Central nervous system toxicity with high dose cytosine arabinoside. *Semin Oncol* 12:233–236, 1985 (suppl).
151. Herzig RH, Hines JD, Herzig GP, et al: Cerebellar toxicity with high dose cytosine arabinoside. *J Clin Oncol* 5:927–932, 1987.
152. Conrad KJ: Cerebellar toxicities associated with cytosine arabinoside: A nursing perspective. *Oncol Nurs Forum* 13:57–59, 1986.

153. Doublsky J: Ineffective individual coping. In McNally JC, Stair JC, Somerville ET (eds), *Guidelines for Cancer Nursing Practice*. Philadelphia: Saunders, 1985, pp. 66–72.
154. Smith K, Lesko LM: Psychosocial problems in cancer survivors. *Oncol* 2:33–40, 1988.
155. Scott DW, Goode WL, Arlin ZA: The psychodynamics of multiple remissions in a patient with nonlymphoblastic leukemia. *Cancer Nurs* 6:201–206, 1983.
156. Levinson JA, Lesko LM: Psychiatric aspects of adult leukemia. *Semin Oncol Nurs* 6:76–83, 1990.

Chapter 46

Lung Cancer

Ellen Heid Elpern, RN, MSN

INTRODUCTION

Lung cancer has a devastating impact on our nation's health. It is our most serious cancer problem and most common cancer killer. In recent years, improvements have been made in diagnostic and staging techniques, but there have been no consistent advances in therapies. Five-year survival for individuals with bronchogenic cancer remains poor. Ironically, yet hopefully, it has been estimated that 85% of lung cancers are preventable if cigarette smoking could be eliminated. Clearly, our best hope in controlling this disease lies in its prevention.

EPIDEMIOLOGY

Examination of epidemiologic studies related to lung cancer reveals alarming trends. The first significant monograph on lung cancer was published by Adler in 1912.[1] He described lung cancer as among the rarest of diseases, with only 374 cases reported worldwide. Today lung cancer is the most frequent cause of death in people who die of malignant disease. While the peak incidence in males is 50–60 years of age, it is no longer unusual to diagnose lung cancer in individuals under or near 40 years of age. Although lung cancer occurs predominantly in males, the rate of incidence in

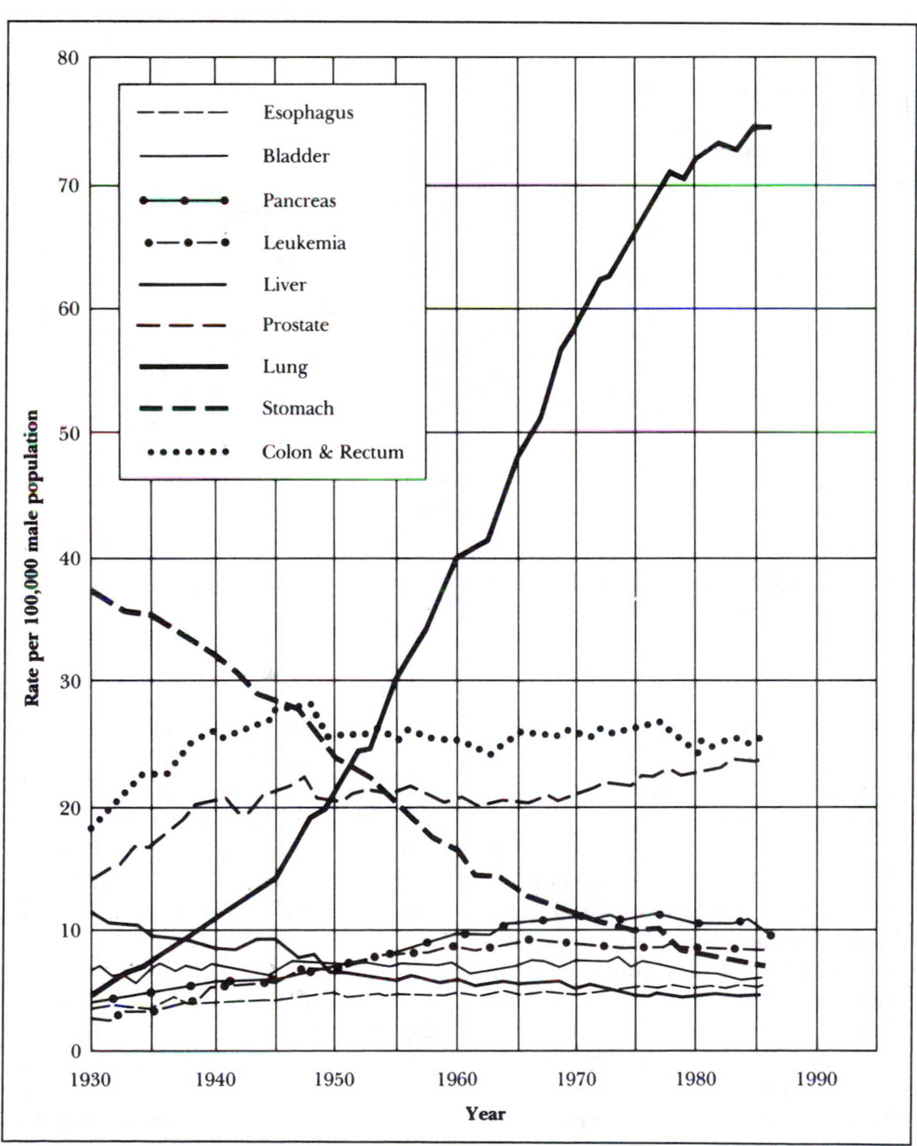

FIGURE 46-1 Age-adjusted cancer death rates, for selected sites, males, United States, 1930–1988.

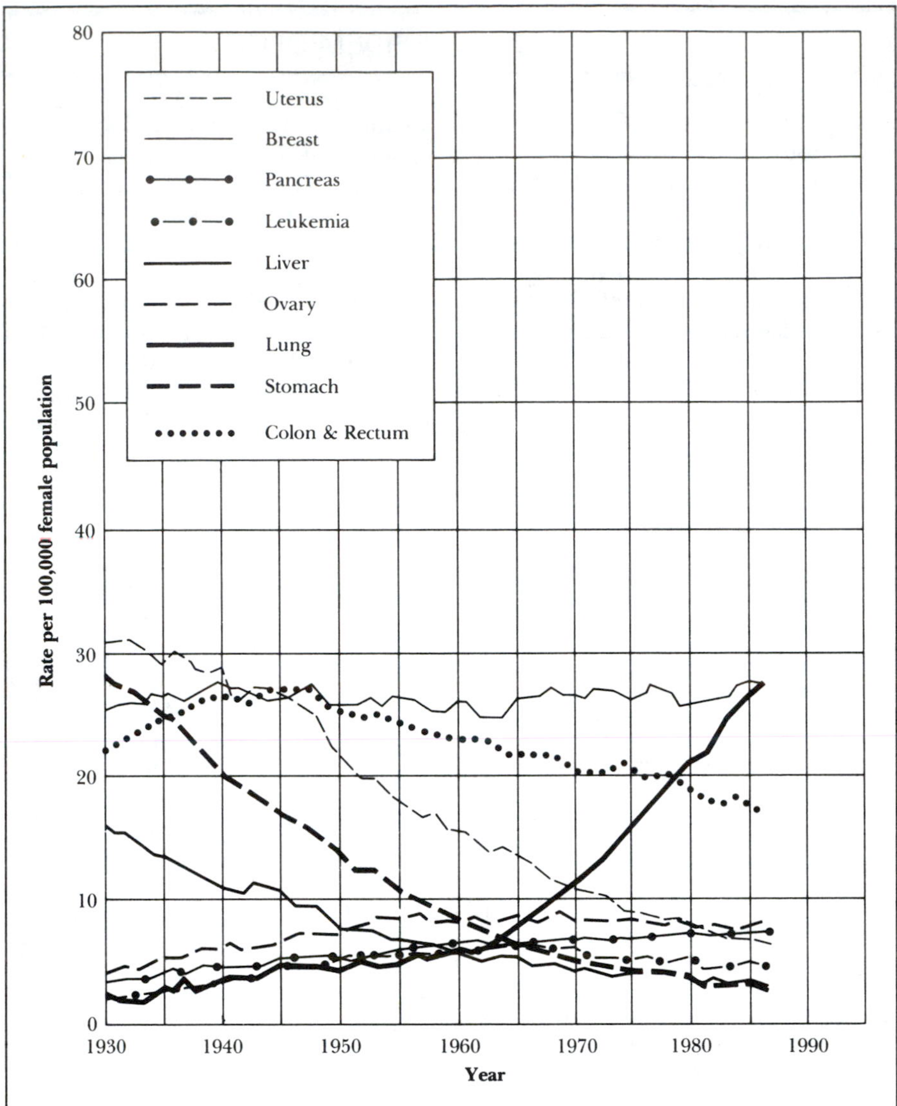

FIGURE 46-2 Age-adjusted cancer death rates for selected sites, females, United States, 1930–1988.

females is rising dramatically. As a result, the sex ratio has steadily decreased in the United States and is likely to continue to decline. Already the source of most male cancer deaths (Figure 46-1), in 1986 lung cancer became the leading cause of cancer death in women (Figure 46-2). In the United States the mortality rate for women due to lung cancer increased over 400% since the mid-1950s. Although the lung cancer mortality rates are higher for blacks than for whites, lung cancer incidence rates have been declining for black males since the mid-1980s, and the incidence in black women appears to be leveling off in the younger age groups.[2]

The highly virulent and rapidly fatal nature of lung cancer is obvious when data on incidence and mortality are examined. There is a close relationship between incidence and death rates, indicating that most individuals diagnosed with lung cancer die of the disease. Both incidence and death rates from lung cancer are highest in large industrial cities, emphasizing the environmental factors implicated in this disease. In the United States, 168,000 new cases of lung cancer and 146,000 deaths from lung cancer were estimated for 1992. The 5-year survival for individuals diagnosed with lung cancer is 13% for whites and 11% for blacks.[3]

ETIOLOGY

Lung cancers most commonly occur following repeated exposure to substances that cause tissue irritation and inflammation. Lung tissues are exposed to these substances primarily as they are inhaled with ambient air.

Tobacco smoke, air pollutants, and exposure to certain metals, fibers, and gases are major risk factors in the development of lung cancer. For many single agents a direct cause-and-effect relationship has not been firmly established. The interactive and synergistic effects of exposure to more than one carcinogenic agent have been recognized and must be emphasized in a discussion of the etiologies of lung cancer. A future challenge lies in determining the degree to which multiple-factor interactions in the genesis of lung cancer can be identified and ultimately prevented.

Tobacco Smoke

European explorers were introduced to tobacco smoking in the 1600s by the Native Americans and quickly popularized the practice in Europe. The automatic roller, patented in 1880, allowed for the mass production of cigarettes. In the past century, changes in tobacco growing and curing methods altered the quality of tobacco smoke so that it became less caustic and more "inhalable." The mass production and marketing of cigarettes, along with the practice of repetitive inhalation of cigarette smoke, have had a devastating impact on the incidence of lung cancer. There is a strong and irrefutable causal relationship between cigarette smoking and lung cancer. This conclusion has been confirmed by an abundance of epidemiologic studies beginning in the 1950s and continuing to the present. In addition to a strong statistical relationship between lung cancer and smoking, Spencer[4] summarized further evidence for this association:

- the finding of benzopyrene and other carcinogens in combusted tobacco
- the finding of precarcinomatous histologic changes in the bronchial epithelium of heavy smokers
- the increased incidence of other diseases associated with smoking in individuals with lung cancer
- the experimental production of tumors in animals following the internal and cutaneous application of tobacco condensates

The evidence that has accumulated suggests that the relationship of smoking to lung cancer has a dose–response nature, where the relative risk of lung cancer increases with the quantity of cigarettes smoked. Fortunately, there is also a reduced risk of lung cancer over time for exsmokers, eventually approaching that for lifetime nonsmokers. Although improvements begin shortly after the cessation of smoking, it appears to take approximately 15 years for an exsmoker's risk of lung cancer to approximate that of a lifetime nonsmoker.[5] In determining risk, the number of pack years (packs of cigarettes consumed per day multiplied by the number of years of smoking) appears to be a crucial factor. Age at onset of smoking is also an influential factor. Individuals who start smoking at an early age (15 years) have a greater risk than do individuals who start smoking later (25 years or older). Other factors that are influential to cancer risk are smoking practices (size of puff, depth of inhalation, time of breath holding, amount of cigarette smoked) and type of cigarette smoked (tar content, filtered vs nonfiltered).

Although the incidence of lung cancer clearly corresponds to smoking habits, the mechanisms by which tobacco smoke causes cancer are less clear. Cigarette smoke contains more than 3600 chemicals, many of which are carcinogens or mutagens. The potential interactive effects of inhalation of these chemicals with environmental or genetic factors in the causation of lung cancer are unclear. The correlation between cigarette smoking and lung cancer differs among the specific tumor cell types. Squamous cell and small cell cancers occur almost exclusively in smokers and are generally dose-related. The influence of cigarette smoking on other histologic types of bronchogenic cancer is less dramatic.

Passive Smoking

Passive smoking refers to the involuntary exposure of nonsmokers to tobacco combustion products in the indoor environment. Oleske[6] has summarized the evidence for an increased risk for lung cancer among nonsmokers with spouses who smoke. The 1986 Report of the Surgeon General[7] presented evidence that sidestream smoke is qualitatively similar to mainstream smoke inhaled by the smoker and that both act as carcinogens. The report concluded that involuntary smoking can cause lung cancer in nonsmokers. The number of lung cancers due to passive smoking is much less than those due to active smoking. The magnitude of increased lung cancer risk that results from passive smoking has yet to be clearly determined, but a dose–response relationship between exposure and risk is expected. One of the most important methodological issues to be addressed in this emerging field of research relates to quantification of tobacco smoke exposure in passive smokers.

Air Pollution

There are three major sources and types of air pollution: (1) the sulfur oxide/particulate complex arising from the combustion of sulfur-containing fuels, (2) photochemical oxidants related to motor vehicle emissions, and (3) miscellaneous pollutants from localized sources such as refineries and manufacturing plant [illegible] Known carcinogens have been identified in a[illegible] pheric pollution, and it has been hypothesize[illegible] peated exposure to these pollutants causes [illegible] At this time, this hypothesis remains [illegible] nor disproved. There is evidence th[illegible] lung cancer increases in pollute[illegible] separate and/or interactive contributions of cigarette smoking, occupational exposure, and indoor air pollution to the development of lung cancer confuse the relationship. Some inhaled irritants may be more important as tumor promoters than as direct carcinogenic agents. Air pollutants most probably contribute little risk in themselves but exert a powerful effect in determining lung cancer occurrences in smokers.

Occupational Factors

A substantial number of chemicals are associated with lung cancer in humans. These chemicals and the occupations that result in exposure are listed in Table 46-1. Occupational exposure to such substances offers opportunities for tumor induction, usually after a long latency period. About 12% of the overall annual lung cancer deaths result from chronic exposure to industrial carcinogens. The interactive effects of smoking and occupational exposure must again be stressed. For example, smoking clearly compounds the risk of lung cancer for asbestos and uranium workers. Asbestos workers who actively smoke are up to 50 times more likely to develop lung cancer than are nonexposed nonsmokers.[9] The enhanced carcinogenic potential of certain agents in combination is a recurrent theme in lung cancer causation.

TABLE 46-1 Occupational Risk Factors to the Development of Lung Cancer

Cancer-Causing Substance	Occupations
Arsenic	Oil refining; copper smelting; mining; using pesticides; tanning; working in the chemical industry
Asbestos	Asbestos milling and manufacture; working with insulation; shipyard work; brake and clutch repair; asbestos mining
Bischloromethyl ether and mustard gas	Working in the chemical industry; making ion exchange resins
Chromates	Glass making; potting; acetylene and aniline manufacturing; bleaching; battery making; spray painting
Coke oven fumes	Steel mill, foundry, and petroleum workers
[illegible]	Nickel refining
[illegible]	Working with lubricating oils, paraffins, [illegible] wax oils or coke and rubber filler
[illegible]	[illegible] in the atomic energy industry; [illegible]iology; uranium mining

Radon

Radon from uranium ore has long been recognized as a cause of lung cancer in uranium miners. Radon is now recognized as a cause of lung cancer in the general population as well. Radon is a naturally occurring radioactive gas that is colorless, odorless, and tasteless. It is found in variable concentrations in soil and rocks, formed by the natural decay of uranium and thorium. Radon can migrate up through porous soils and enter homes through basement or foundation cracks, sumps, drains, or deep private wells. Radon levels vary by geographic location, climate, season, and type of heating and ventilation system. It has been estimated that indoor radon may be responsible for 9000–13,000 lung cancer cases per year.[10] A synergistic effect exists between radon exposure and cigarette smoking. The longer the period of radon exposure, the greater the risk. Cancer risk decreases with time after cessation of exposure. Radon is measured in picocuries per liter (pCi/l). The EPA has set 4 pCi/l as the level above which action to lower radon levels is recommended. Detection devices are available for home monitoring.

Vitamin A

Because vitamin A is known to play a role in the regulation of cell differentiation, the association between vitamin A and cancer risk has been investigated. Studies compiled in the last 20 years suggest an inverse relationship between lung cancer and dietary intake of vitamin A.[11] These studies demonstrated consistently that patients with lung cancer consumed smaller quantities of foods rich in vitamin A or had lower blood levels of retinol and/or beta carotene than did matched controls. Although not all studies controlled for cigarette smoking, the association between low vitamin A levels and lung cancer held when smoking history was considered. It is not yet clear whether or how dietary interventions can modify lung cancer risk, but the available epidemiologic evidence points to dietary intervention as an encouraging area for further study.

Constitutional Factors

Some researchers[12,13] have claimed that an individual's genetic makeup may predispose him or her to lung cancer. Certain individuals are believed to be genetically predisposed to lung cancer, and the finding of multiple cases of lung cancer within the same family has been used as supportive data. Strong evidence to confirm this hypothesis is lacking, and no conclusions can be drawn from available data.

Several studies[14,15] suggest that the presence of chronic obstructive pulmonary disease is a risk factor for the development of lung cancer independent of smoking history. The mechanisms for this risk are not known but may relate to impaired mucociliary transport with enhanced deposition of carcinogens, chronic inflammation and scarring, and genetic predisposition to mucosal injury. Smokers with bullous emphysema may be at particular risk for lung cancer, presumably attributed to poor clearance of carcinogens from areas of destroyed lung.

An association between progressive systemic sclerosis (PSS) and lung cancer has also been suggested.[16] The increased incidence of lung cancer with PSS may be associated more with the presence of pulmonary fibrosis in these patients than with cigarette smoking.

Both focal lung scars and more diffuse parenchymal fibrosis can become sites of lung malignancies. These so called "scar cancers" of the lung probably occur when regenerative hyperplasia becomes excessive and develops into malignant changes. Scar cancers are usually adenocarcinomas.

PREVENTION

Smoking-Related

Lung cancer is a common and particularly lethal disease. Ironically, it is also a condition that could be readily controlled with the elimination of its major causative factor—cigarette smoking. Efforts aimed at lung cancer prevention must focus on changing smoking behaviors.

In 1990, 25% of adult Americans were smokers.[17] The numbers of adult smokers peaked at 40% in the early 1960s and has declined since publication of the first Surgeon General's Report on Smoking and Health in 1964. Likewise, the per capita consumption of cigarettes has declined by 20% in the past 20 years. Despite these encouraging overall statistics, smoking remains a major health concern generally and for certain populations in particular. The decline in smoking among teenagers over the past 10 years has been insignificant. In a 1991 survey, 70% of students in grades 9–12 reported having tried cigarette smoking, and 12.7% reported frequent cigarette use.[18] The prevalence of adolescent smokers has been higher for females than for males. In the adult population there is a higher percentage of black than of white smokers. Blacks are also less likely to quit smoking than are whites. Men and women in blue-collar professions have higher smoking rates than professional workers.

Research increasingly supports the conclusion that multiple factors influence the initiation and maintenance of smoking. Generally, the reasons why an individual starts to smoke are entirely different from those that lead him or her to continue smoking. It follows, therefore, that activities aimed at reducing the development of smoking behaviors will be different from those designed to assist smokers to quit. The social and psychological factors that influence the initiation or maintenance of smoking must be considered in such programs.

Horn[19] has concluded that smoking behaviors are usually initiated at a fairly young age and in response to opportunity, curiosity, and a need for self-expression. Several steps to reduce the development of smoking behavior have been proposed:

1. Reduce the easy availability of cigarettes to young people.
2. Encourage parents and important role models to set the example of not smoking.
3. Reduce the intensity of emotionally-charged proscriptions against smoking, which serve to stimulate contrary action.
4. Stress the costs associated with smoking without denying the benefits. Encourage the achievement of these benefits in less damaging ways.
5. Avoid stereotyping smoking and smokers in ways that turn youth away from antismoking "do-gooders."
6. Help young people develop insight into their perception of smoking as attractive. Encourage them to seek alternate means of satisfying this need.

Past efforts to influence young people not to smoke have not been effective. The number of preadolescent and teenage smokers has steadily increased, particularly among females. Programs aimed at preventing youngsters from starting to smoke are of particular importance to lung cancer control and should be initiated as early as the first grade.

Whereas initiation of smoking is largely socially determined, maintenance of smoking involves other factors. The regular use of cigarettes leads to behavioral and pharmacologic dependence. Smoking becomes not only a habitual, conditioned response, but necessary to satisfy a chemical dependence on nicotine. Nicotine is a drug with powerful physiologic and psychoactive effects that lead to its compulsive use.

Changing smoking habits is a complex and difficult task. Despite the growing awareness of the serious health hazard that cigarette smoking represents, about one person out of four in this country continues to smoke. Although the majority of these people indicate a desire to quit smoking, only one of three smokers remains abstinent 1 year after attempting to quit smoking.

Ninety-five percent of those who quit smoking do so without the aid of an organized program.[20] Success at quitting increases with the number of attempts made. Clearly, successful self-help programs require attention to techniques to first achieve and then maintain abstinence. Many program formats are available, includin[illegible] self-help manuals and broadcast media programs [illegible] tensive individual programs utilizing thera[illegible] antismoking specialists are also available. N[illegible] placement products are available to con[illegible] of nicotine withdrawal during sm[illegible]

Nicotine delivery systems used in combination with counseling sessions can increase smoking cessation rates, at least in the short term (6 months).[21]

Nurses may play a prominent role in reducing smoking and lung cancer risk. Risser[22] has suggested strategies that include example setting, limiting smoking in the workplace, identification of high-risk individuals, counseling or referral of smokers motivated to quit, and reinforcement of cessation attempts. Colleagues as well as patients may benefit from such efforts. Ten percent of physicians smoke; 20% of registered nurses are active smokers.[23–26]

It is likely that a large number of individuals will take up smoking and/or continue to smoke despite all contrary efforts. To reduce the risk of lung cancer in smokers, an additional research thrust has been the development of less harmful cigarettes. Such cigarettes would have to contain considerably less particulate matter and lower levels of those components known to be carcinogens or tumor promoters. There is evidence that reducing the levels of tar and nicotine in cigarettes, as has been done in the last 20 years, can favorably affect lung histopathology in smokers. Smokers who died in the 1970s had less metaplasia and atypia on autopsy than did smokers who died in the 1950s, when the tar content of cigarettes was twice as great.[27] Although it is now possible to manufacture cigarettes that are less hazardous than those currently available, their tastelessness makes them unacceptable to most smokers. Smokers may offset the potential benefits of switching to lower tar and nicotine cigarettes by adjusting their smoking habits (smoke more cigarettes, take deeper puffs) to maintain a certain intake of nicotine.

Government initiatives to control tobacco use can be summarized[28] under the following headings:

Regulatory Activities

- laws restricting smoking in public places
- policies restricting smoking in government buildings
- prohibitions on access to tobacco products
- restrictions on tobacco advertising
- warning label requirements

Community Education/Information

- public information campaigns
- smoking cessation programs

Economic Incentives/Deterrents

- differential benefits packages for nonsmokers
- excise taxes

mo... citize... and the...

In rece... ...king activist groups at a com... garding the ... ...are available for concerned ...lly oriented than others, ...y considerably.

...ncern has arisen re... ...r involuntary smoking, that is, the exposure of nonsmokers to tobacco combustion products in the indoor environment. Health risks include an increased incidence of lung cancer in nonsmokers who have lived with smokers and an increased frequency of respiratory infections and symptoms in children whose parents smoke. Concern over the effect of passive smoking is reflected in ongoing studies to ascertain its health consequences and in the proposal of laws and regulations restricting smoking in public places. Enthusiasm is growing for a tobacco-free society in the United States. Many cities have passed legislation requiring employers to regulate or, if necessary, ban smoking in the workplace. In 1988 a federal bill was passed banning smoking on commercial airline flights of 120 minutes or less. All hospitals that wish to be accredited by the Joint Commission of Healthcare Organizations must comply with a rule requiring them to be smoke-free.

A joint project of the National Cancer Institute and the American Cancer Society entitled the American Stop Smoking Intervention for Cancer Prevention (ASSIST) will commence in 1993. ASSIST is the largest cancer control project ever undertaken. This demonstration project aims to rapidly reduce smoking prevalence by the turn of the century. It is expected to reach 50 million people and will cost approximately $125 million.

Occupation-Related

The prevention of occupational lung diseases is dependent upon eliminating or reducing lung exposure to toxic substances. Although the number of cases of lung cancer caused by occupational exposure alone is relatively small, job-related lung cancer is potentially entirely preventable. The risk of lung cancer from occupational exposure is multiplied greatly if the worker also smokes cigarettes.

As summarized by Landrigan and Selikoff,[29] prevention of occupational lung cancer may be achieved by a combination of techniques including premarket toxicologic testing of new chemical compounds, application of industrial hygiene techniques, legal and regulatory approaches, and epidemiologic surveillance. The federal government has taken some steps to ensure safer working conditions (Occupational Safety and Health Act, Federal Mine Safety and Health Act, Toxic Substances Control Act), but the response of industry has been generally slow and often controversial. Special-interest groups continue to debate the degree of carcinogenic risk for workers exposed to certain substances, as well as the potential economic hardships imposed by stringent regulations. Governmental commitment to the control of job-related hazardous exposure has also been variable. An increased awareness of the health hazards of certain occupations on the part of labor, management, and government and voluntary compliance with exposure-reduction methods, although potentially costly and difficult to effect, would substantially reduce the incidence of job-related lung cancer.

Chemoprevention

In light of the epidemiologic data suggesting a relation between vitamin A deficiency and lung cancer incidence, the National Cancer Institute has undertaken study of preventive research in nutrition and lung cancer. Vitamin A and its precursor, beta-carotene, are among the agents to be tested. The potential benefits of chemoprevention are conceptually exciting but await confirmation by intervention trials.

EARLY DETECTION

The natural history of lung cancer usually includes years of tumor growth prior to clinical presentation. The potential benefits of the earliest possible detection of a lung malignancy seem straightforward. The earlier the disease is detected, the more probable it is that the cancer is localized and the better the chances for cure. Unfortunately, occult or localized lung cancers are diagnosed infrequently. It is probable that this frequency could be significantly increased through mass screening programs for the detection of lung cancers.

The screening tests currently available for the diagnosis of asymptomatic lung cancers are sputum cytologies and chest radiographs, which are generally used in combination. Cancerous lesions may be present that are radiographically undetectable because of their small size or because their presence is obscured by other chest structures or abnormalities. Sputum cytologies are necessary for the detection of such lesions. Chest radiographs are more effective in detecting peripherally located lung tumors, and sputum cytologies more often detect lung tumors located in the central airways. Sputum cytologies are sensitive detectors of lung cancer only if multiple specimens are evaluated. Both sputum studies and chest radiographs are costly and require special facilities and personnel. The cost of performing these screening measures on the general adult population is considered excessive, and mass screening for lung cancer is considered to be unwarranted. Screening programs do exist but are applied only to individuals considered at high risk for lung cancer.

In the early 1970s the National Cancer Institute initiated a cooperative program of lung cancer screening. Objectives of this screening program were to determine: (1) whether detection of lung cancer could be improved by adding modern sputum cytologic screening techniques to the examination at regular intervals by chest radiolography, and (2) whether the mortality from lung cancer could be reduced significantly with this type of screening program followed by newer localizing methods and appropriate treatment.[30] Enrollment was limited to individuals considered at risk: males, age 45 years or older, who chronically smoked at least one package of cigarettes per day. Approximately 10,000 men have been enrolled at each of the three centers. Conclusions supported by analysis of current results[31] are that the two screening modalities are effective and complementary in the detection of lung cancer. Tumors are more frequently detected by chest x-ray than by sputum cytology. However, sputum cytology is the most effective detector of early resectable tumors. Unfortunately, although screening programs achieved earlier diagnoses and longer survival, no significant reduction in lung cancer mortality was demonstrated. Earlier detection appears to lengthen the interval between diagnosis and death without increasing total life span. In light of the cost of even selective radiographic screening, many authorities have revised their recommendations in this regard. Most scientific societies (including the American Cancer Society) do not recommend routine screening for lung cancer in asymptomatic persons.

It has been repeatedly demonstrated that substances not produced by normal cells can be elaborated by cancer cells. If such ectopic substances could be identified and detected in human tissues, important new methods for screening for cancer and measuring the effects of therapy would become available. Neither serologic testing nor breath analysis has as yet proved useful as screening tests to distinguish diagnostic markers for localized lung cancer. Some of the agents that have been tested as possible markers include ferritin, sialic acid, beta-2-microglobulin, lipotropin, human chorionic gonadotropin, calcitonin, parathyroid hormone, adrenocorticotropic hormone, and carcinoembryonic antigen. Although some of these substances seemed to have some value for detecting localized lung cancer, they are too nonspecific to be considered for screening. The potential use of these and other substances as tumor markers is receiving intensive study, and future developments could have significant clinical implications.

HISTOGENESIS

Bronchogenic tumor cells differ in appearance and behavior from normal bronchial epithelial cells. Carcinogenic-induced alterations in chromosomes cause the aberrations seen in cancer cells. It is believed that early tumor cells retain many of the morphologic and metabolic features of the tissue of origin and such tumors are described as "well-differentiated." With rapid multiplication and growth, tumor cells become dedifferentiated and less recognizable in morphology and arrangement from normal bronchial epithelial cells.

Over 90% of all primary lung tumors arise from the bronchial epithelium. Normal bronchial epithelial cel
serve a lining and protective function. They are de
from the endodermal cell layer of the human
Pseudostratified columnar epithelial cells
cheobronchial tree from the trachea
bronchioles. The columnar cells
membrane. Some of these colu
while others are mucus-sec

Interspersed between the columnar cells but not reaching the bronchial lumen are the smaller, shorter basal cells. Some of these basal cells are the reserve or stem cells that can differentiate to become mature columnar lining cells. Other basal cells (called *Kulchitsy cells*) contain secretory granules. It is speculated that these basal cells have a neurosecretory or endocrine function of some kind.

Abnormalities occur in the bronchial epithelium as it is chronically exposed to irritating substances inhaled with ambient air. Chief among such irritants are those contained in inhaled cigarette smoke. As a protective layer between the body and the outer environment, the bronchial epithelium is continually damaged, shed, and replaced. Inhaled irritant substances are most commonly deposited in the airways at points of major bronchial bifurcation. Short-term exposure to cigarette smoke may change ciliary structure or reduce ciliary beating but is principally associated with mucous cell hyperplasia and hypersecretion of mucus. With continued years of smoking, ciliated cells are repeatedly damaged and shed from the basement membrane. More rapid loss of these cells stimulates an increase in the cell turnover rate in the basal cell layer (basal cell hyperplasia). With basal hyperplasia the epithelium appears more stratified or layered. With repeated insult, the rapidly proliferating basal cells have less energy available for differentiation, and squamous cell metaplasia is a frequent occurrence. Not only is the number of epithelial cells increased, but the cells assume the more primitive, flattened and rounded appearance of squamous cells.

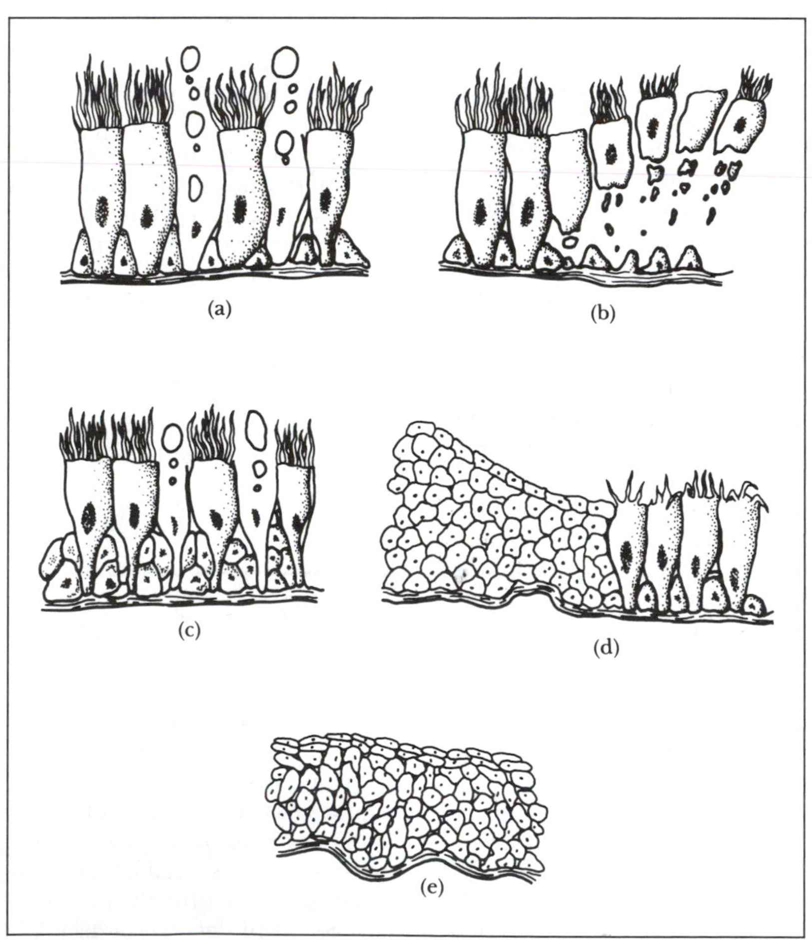

FIGURE 46-3 Response of bronchial epithelium to chronic irritation. (a) Normal bronchial epithelium; (b) ciliated airway cells are continuously shed and replaced in response to irritant exposure; (c) ciliated cells regenerate from basal cells; (d) chronic irritation results in an increased ·rnover of cells, damaged cilia, and basal cell proliferation; ·tinuation of irritation may produce bronchial epithelial dysplasia ·oma-in-situ. (Source: Adapted from Kotin P: Carcinogenesis of ·Liebow AA, Smith DE (eds), *The Lung*. Baltimore, MD: ·ilkins, 1968.)

The protective ciliated and mucus-producing cells are replaced by these dysplastic cells, allowing easier access of irritants and carcinogens. Even at this point of squamous metaplasia, epithelial injury is not irreversible if the cause is removed. With the continuation of heavy smoking, atypia of the epithelial cells progresses to nuclear enlargement, nuclear variability, hyperchromatism, and mitotic activity. Several sites of fully developed intraepithelial carcinomas that do not invade the basement membrane (carcinoma-in-situ) can develop, located in the bronchi of both lungs. Not all foci of carcinoma-in-situ will progress to become invasive tumors. Over time, invasion through the basement membrane may occur with downgrowth of the tumor. Figure 46-3 illustrates the response of the bronchial epithelium to chronic irritants.[32]

The transformations of the bronchial epithelium just described occur over extended periods of time, usually several decades. The developmental period probably depends on the duration and degree of exposure to lung irritants and/or carcinogens.

HISTOLOGY

Bronchogenic tumors are classified according to recognized variations in histology as squamous cell carcinomas, adenocarcinomas, large-cell carcinomas, and small-cell carcinomas. Histologic classifications are important to the organization of data on incidence, natural history, etiology, and treatment. Due to significant differences in presentation, natural history, and treatment response, lung tumors are usually referred to simply as *small-cell lung cancer (SCLC)* or *non–small-cell lung cancer (NSCLC)*.

Histologic classification depends on the identification of the distinct morphology of tumor cells. Unfortunately, many lung tumors contain more than one cellular element, or the cell type identified at diagnosis may evolve to a different type with treatment. The presence of multiple cell types in a single tumor mass, as well as the possibility of conversion to other cell types, suggests a common progenitor cell for all lung carcinomas. This unitary theory of histogenesis is a relatively new concept, as SCLC was thought historically to originate from a cell line different from other lung tumors. All tumors probably arise not from mature epithelial cell types but from proliferating simple pleuropotential reserve cells and differ only in their degree of differentiation. Yesner[33] suggests a spectrum of lung cancer ranging from poorly differentiated small-cell cancer that evolves into more differentiated adenocarcinomas and squamous cell tumors, with large-cell undifferentiated tumors as intermediate (Figure 46-4). Characteristics of the various cell types of lung tumors are discussed below.

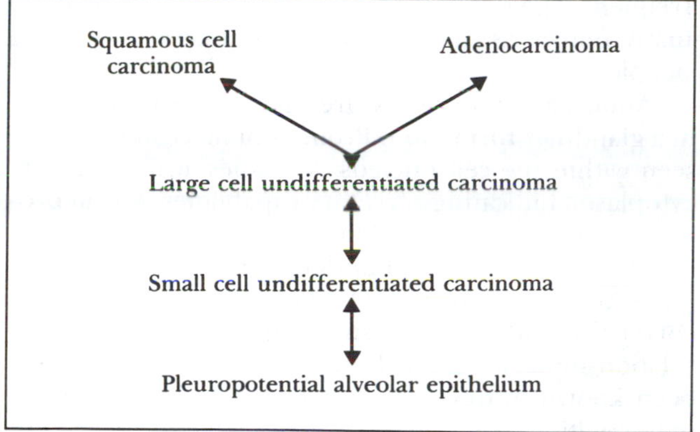

FIGURE 46-4 Proposed histological schema of lung cancer. (Source: Adapted from Yesner R, Carter D: Pathology of carcinoma of the lung, *Clin Chest Med* 3:257–289, 1982.)

Non–Small-Cell Lung Cancers

Squamous cell carcinomas

Squamous cell cancers show a very strong dose-response association with cigarette smoking, that is, the greater the quantity of cigarettes smoked, the higher the incidence of squamous cancer. Currently, squamous cell cancers are more common in males than females, probably as a function of sex differences in smoking history. This sex ratio is changing as the incidence of female smokers increases. Squamous tumors account for about 30% of all bronchogenic cancers.

Histologically these tumor cells can be elongated, spindle shaped, tadpole shaped, oval, or round. Well-differentiated cells have the ability to produce keratin. Tumor cells are often arranged in a whorling pattern, and intracellular bridges are often seen.

Squamous cell tumors most often occur in the major bronchi or their primary divisions. Grossly, these tumors appear as grey, white, or yellowish masses. Tumors that arise in the central airways may invade, encircle, and compress the bronchi from which they originate. Others may grow into the bronchial lumen. In both instances, signs and symptoms of bronchial obstruction would result. Other lesions may be seen as tumor plaques extending along the airway surface. Central necrosis and cavitation are common. Squamous cell tumors remain more localized than other cell types. Metastases to structures within the thorax commonly occur. Patients with squamous cell cancer survive longer than those with other cell types, probably as a function of slower growth rate, the possibility of surgical res-
tion, and late metastasis.

Adenocarcinomas

Adenocarcinomas are the mo
lung cancers (30%–35% incid

frequent type of lung cancer found in women (with as many female as male cases), nonsmokers, and young people.

Adenocarcinoma cells are characteristically found in a glandular formation. Prominent macronucleoli are seen within the cell nucleus. Vacuoles are seen in the cytoplasm, indicating secretory capabilities. Mucin production is frequently evident. The pathogenesis of adenocarcinoma is not well understood. Unlike other cell types, the occurrence of adenocarcinomas shows poor correlation with cigarette smoking. Although no causal relationship can be concluded, adenocarcinomas have been known to develop after longstanding parenchymal irritation, scarring, or fibrosis. These tumors generally present as slow-growing peripheral masses. Hematogenous spread occurs frequently and relatively early in the course of the disease. Adenocarcinomas demonstrate a particular predilection to metastasize to the brain.

A variant of the adenocarcinoma classification is the bronchioloalveolar tumor. As with other adenocarcinomas, these tumors usually present in the periphery of the lung and are characteristically slow growing. Bronchioloalveolar tumors may vary widely in presentation from solitary nodules to diffuse interstitial infiltrates. Well-differentiated bronchioloalveolar tumor cells resemble peripheral respiratory epithelial cells.

Large-cell carcinomas

Large-cell carcinomas are a heterogenous group of lung cancers, constituting 10%–15% of all bronchogenic malignancies. Tumors of this type often show almost no differentiated histological features. Some clinicians refer to this category as a "wastebasket" for lesions that do not clearly fit into the other three categories.

Large-cell carcinomas show prominent macronucleoli and are usually mucin negative, with no glandular pattern to the cytoplasm. Peripheral lesions are more common than central ones. Patterns of metastasis are similar to those of adenocarcinomas, with an additional tendency to metastasize to the gastrointestinal tract. Survival rates are generally poor.

Small-Cell Lung Cancer

Small-cell tumors are strongly associated with cigarette smoking, with an increasing incidence of small-cell tumors associated with increased amount of smoking. About 25% of lung cancers are of the small-cell variety, [illegible] are histologically identified as cells containing [illegible] and very little cytoplasm. Cells are often [illegible]ibed as resembling lymphocytes even [illegible] or three times larger than lym[illegible]ally located in central regions [illegible]. Tumors typically grow [illegible]phatic invasion. Be[illegible] early lymphatic metastases, small-cell tumors often present as hilar or perihilar masses. Rapidly growing central tumors can cause bronchial obstruction and pneumonia.

In past years, small-cell cancers were believed to be derived from Kulchitsky cells, which have neurosecretory capabilities. The finding of neurosecretory granules in small-cell tumor cells and the frequent production of ectopic hormones by these tumors were considered supportive evidence. Such occurrences are now recognized as not exclusive to small-cell cancers, and they are thought not to have a unique histogenesis.

Small-cell cancers carry a poor prognosis because of their high growth rate and tendency to metastasize early and widely. Although these tumors are the most sensitive of the histologic types to radiation and chemotherapy, short-term relapses are common.

METASTATIC PATTERN

As with any solid tumor, lung cancers spread by direct extension, lymphatic invasion, and blood-borne metastases. Tumors can spread within the bronchus of origin by direct invasion. Growth can occur such that the lumen is partially or completely filled and occluded. Other tumors extend in a flattened, plaquelike fashion along the inside of the lumen. Others may invade the bronchial wall and encircle and obstruct the airway. Intrapulmonary spread may lead to compression of lung structures other than airways, such as blood or lymph vessels. alveoli, and nerves. Direct extension through the pleura can result in spread over the surface of the lung, chest wall, or diaphragm. Most centrally located tumors spread to the hilar lymph structures, either by direct extension or lymphatic spread. When lymphatic structures are invaded by tumor, the pattern of subsequent spread depends on the tumor cell type and the anatomic location of the tumor. The central hilar, mediastinal, and paratracheal glands are most commonly affected by lung tumors, although supraclavicular, cervical, and abdominal channels may be invaded. Tumors originating in the lower lobes tend to spread more widely by lymph channels than do those located elsewhere in the lung.

The widespread pattern of hematogenous metastases in lung cancer is due to the invasion of the pulmonary vascular system and is associated with a poor prognosis. Once tumor cells enter the pulmonary venous system, they can be carried through the heart and disseminated systemically. Tumor emboli can become lodged in areas of organ systems where vessels become too narrow for their passage and/or where blood flow is reduced. Invasion of branches of the pulmonary arteries occurs less commonly, but is not infrequent with small-cell carcinomas and adenocarcinomas. Metastatic lesions outside the thorax frequently involve the liver, adrenals, bone, and brain.

PROGRESSION OF DISEASE

Cures in lung cancer are very rare. Even in cases of the slower-growing types of lung cancer, three out of four individuals will not be alive 5 years after diagnosis, with or without intensive therapy. The 5-year survival rate for all types of bronchogenic cancer is about 11%. At the time of diagnosis, most tumors have probably progressed through the majority of their life spans. As mentioned previously, metastatic spread occurs via the lymph and vascular routes, often before the primary site is detectable. Survival time can be extended by surgical, chemotherapeutic, and radiotherapeutic interventions. These and other forms of therapy are also of critical importance in palliation. The prognosis and selection of appropriate treatment protocols are generally based on the anatomic extent or stage of the cancer at diagnosis.

CLINICAL MANIFESTATIONS

The presence and nature of symptoms in lung cancer depend on the location and extent of the tumor. Systemic symptoms such as anorexia, weight loss, and fatigue may suggest cancer. Presenting pulmonary symptoms may include cough, chest pain, hemoptysis, dyspnea, and wheezing. Because most of these symptoms are also associated with cigarette smoking and chronic obstructive pulmonary disease, their significance as indicators of an oncologic process may be unappreciated initially. Symptoms of local metastases may include hoarseness (recurrent laryngeal nerve involvement), chest or shoulder pain (chest wall, pleural, or brachial plexus involvement), dysphagia (esophageal compression or invasion), or head and neck swelling (superior vena caval obstruction). Tumors of the superior sulcus or the apical cap of the lung may invade the brachial plexus, causing shoulder and arm pain. If the cervical nerves are involved, unilateral exopthalmos, pupillary constriction, and lack of perspiration (Horner's syndrome) may also be seen. Extrathoracic symptoms appear with tumor metastasis and depend on the site and extent of metastatic tumor growth.

Symptoms related to the systemic syndromes that can be associated with lung cancers are numerous and diverse. The ectopic hormone syndromes described in Chapter 29 are one set of syndromes that may occur. Numerous paraneoplastic syndromes are associated with lung cancer. These phenomena represent the release by tumor cells of hormones or other biologically active substances. Although ectopic hormone syndromes may occur with other carcinomas, they are seen most frequently with lung cancer. SCLCs are more often associated with paraneoplastic syndromes than are NSCLCs. Exceptions to this are the hypercalcemic and ectopic parathyroid hormone syndromes that are seen with squamous cell tumors. Hypertrophic pulmonary osteoarthropathy and dermatomyositis are also more common in NSCLC. The appearance of these syndromes may precede any other symptoms of lung cancer and may provide the impetus for establishing the diagnosis. Treatment of the lung tumor may result in the remission of symptoms.

CLASSIFICATION AND STAGING

Non–Small-Cell Lung Cancer

The staging of lung cancer is based on the TNM system recommended by the American Joint Committee on Cancer. This system provides standardized descriptors of the anatomic extent of disease, which is the crucial determinant of treatment and ultimate survival. Numerical suffixes under *T* describe increasing size and/or involvement of the primary tumor. *N* suffixes describe regional lymph node metastases. *M* suffixes describe the presence or absence of metastases to distant sites (Table 46-2).

Subsets of the TNM categories have been combined into stages that describe growth, dissemination, and prognosis for tumors in each stage. The International Staging System for Lung Cancer illustrated in Table 46-3 describes six levels of tumor progression that are related to therapeutic options and to estimates of prognosis for NSCLC. Survival according to cell type and clinical staging criteria is illustrated in Figures 46-5 and 46-6.[34]

Small-Cell Lung Cancer

In SCLC the TNM staging system has little prognostic significance, as illustrated in Figure 46-7.[34] SCLCs are aggressive tumors that disseminate rapidly and widely and carry a poor prognosis regardless of stage classification. The anatomic extent of disease in SCLC is most often described as "limited" or "extensive" using stages proposed by the Veteran's Administration Lung Cancer Study Group (VALG). Limited disease can be treated within a single radiotherapy portal and is generally defined as tumor confined to one hemithorax and regional lymph nodes without pleural effusion. Extensive disease refers to spread beyond this area. This two-stage system does provide significant prognostic information. Long-term survival (>2 yrs) in SCLC occurs almost exclusively in the limited disease category.

Multiple factors are known to influence prognosis in SCLC.[35] Extent of disease is the most important prognostic factor. Although patients with limited disease usually have a better initial performance status than those with extensive disease, performance status at the time of diagnosis has been shown to be an important

TABLE 46-2 TNM Definitions

	PRIMARY TUMOR (T)
TX	Tumor proven by the presence of malignant cells in bronchopulmonary secretions but not visualized by imaging or bronchoscopy
T0	No evidence of primary tumor
TIS	Carcinoma in situ
T1	A tumor 3 cm or less in greatest dimension, surrounded by lung or visceral pleura, and without evidence of invasion proximal to a lobar bronchus at bronchoscopy
T2	A tumor more than 3 cm in greatest dimension, or a tumor of any size that either invades the visceral pleura or has associated atelectasis or obstructive pneumonitis extending to the hilar region. At bronchoscopy, the proximal extent of demonstrable tumor must be within a lobar bronchus or at least 2 cm distal to the carina. Any associated atelectasis or obstructive pneumonitis must involve less than an entire lung
T3	A tumor of any size that directly invades into the chest wall (including superior sulcus tumors), diaphragm, or the mediastinal pleura or pericardium without involving the heart, great vessels, trachea, esophagus or vertebral body, or a tumor in the main bronchus within 2 cm of the carina without involving the carina, or associated atelectasis or obstructive pneumonitis of entire lung
T4	A tumor of any size that invades the mediastinum, heart, great vessels, trachea, esophagus, vertebral body or carina or presence of malignant pleural effusion
	NODAL INVOLVEMENT (N)
N0	No demonstrable metastasis to regional lymph nodes
N1	Metastasis in the peribronchial or the ipsilateral hilar lymph nodes, or both, including direct extension
N2	Metastasis in ipsilateral mediastinal lymph nodes and/or subcarinal lymph nodes
N3	Metastasis in contralateral mediastinal, contralateral hilar, ipsilateral or contralateral scalene or supraclavicular lymph nodes
	DISTANT METASTASIS (M)
M0	No distant metastasis
M1	Distant metastasis

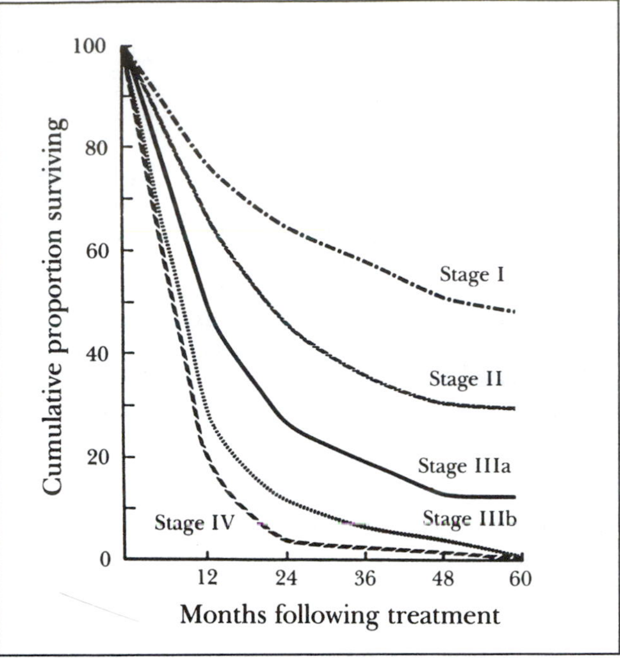

FIGURE 46-5 Proportion of patients with squamous cell lung cancer expected to survive 5 years according to clinical stage of disease. (Source: Mountain CF: Prognostic implications of the International Staging System for Lung Cancer, *Semin Oncol* 15:236–245, 1988.)

TABLE 46-3 Stage Grouping

Occult Carcinoma	TX	N0	M0
Stage 0	TIS Carcinoma in situ		
Stage I	T1	N0	M0
	T2	N0	M0
Stage II	T1	N1	M0
	T2	N1	M0
Stage III-a	T3	N0	M0
	T3	N1	M0
	T1-3	N2	M0
Stage III-b	Any T	N3	M0
	T4	Any N	M0
Stage IV	Any T	Any N	M1

independent determinant of treatment response and survival. Similarly, weight loss, independent of performance status, has been shown to have prognostic significance. Poor response to chemotherapy, defined as either poor initial response or relapse after treatment, is an additional adverse prognostic sign.

DIAGNOSTIC/STAGING TESTS

When an individual presents with symptoms that might indicate a lung malignancy, a battery of examinations

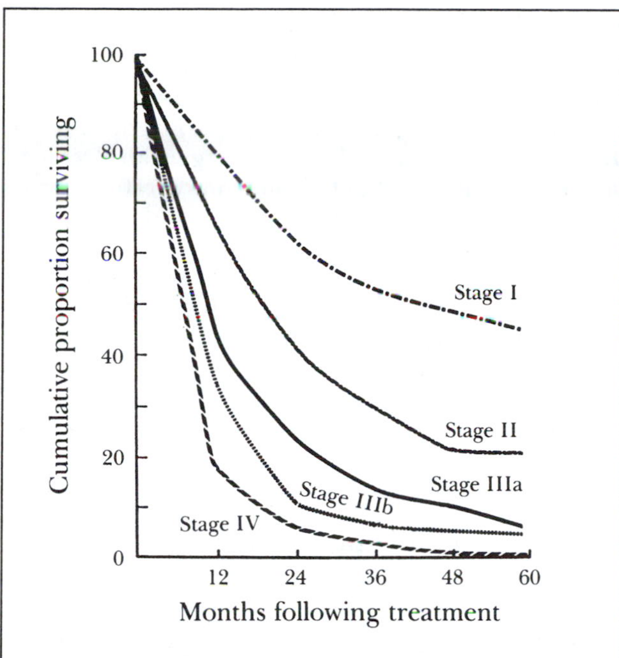

FIGURE 46-6 Proportion of patients with adenocarcinoma; large-cell lung cancer expected to survive 5 years according to clinical stage of disease. (Source: Mountain CF: Prognostic implications of the International Staging System for Lung Cancer, *Semin Oncol* 15:236–245, 1988.)

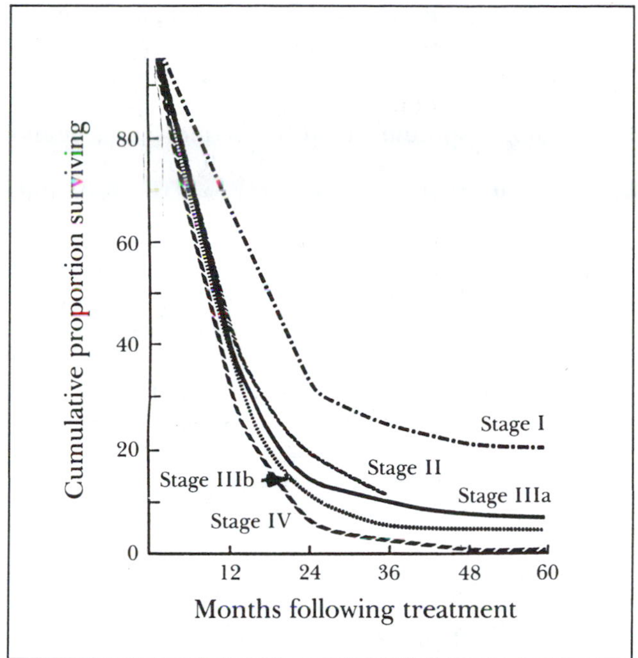

FIGURE 46-7 Proportion of patients with undifferentiated small-cell lung cancer expected to survive 5 years according to clinical stage of disease. (Source: Mountain CF: Prognostic implications of the International Staging System for Lung Cancer, *Semin Oncol* 15:236–245, 1988.)

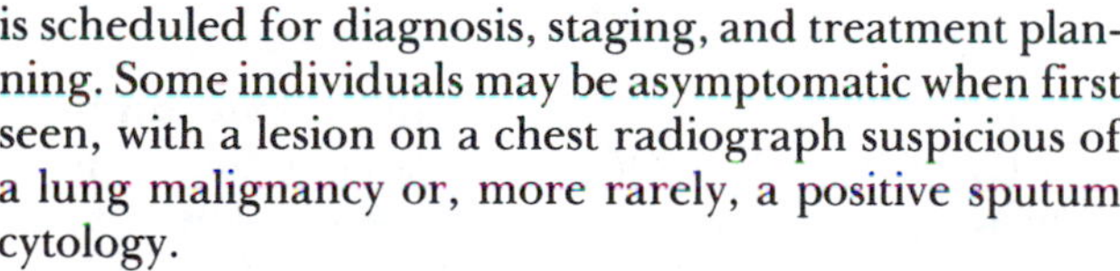

is scheduled for diagnosis, staging, and treatment planning. Some individuals may be asymptomatic when first seen, with a lesion on a chest radiograph suspicious of a lung malignancy or, more rarely, a positive sputum cytology.

The initial evaluation will include an assessment of the presence, duration, and severity of pulmonary and extrapulmonary symptoms. The history will include questions regarding prolonged exposure to and inhalation of carcinogenic substances. A past medical history of tuberculosis or pulmonary inflammatory processes may suggest the development of tumors from pulmonary scars. Also of significance would be any apparent familial clustering of lung cancer, suggesting the possibility of an inherited susceptibility to bronchogenic carcinoma.

A number of procedures are available for use in investigating a possible lung tumor and for staging purposes. The following discussion of applications of the available techniques is organized according to the TNM system.

T (Tumor) Sites

A diagnosis of lung cancer is ultimately established by cytologic examination of secretions and/or biopsied tissue. The method of choice for obtaining tissue depends on the location of the suspected tumor. Centrally located endobronchial tumors are most likely to yield positive sputum cytologies. Nurses are usually responsible for instructing and assisting in sputum collection and can increase the efficiency of this method of cancer detection by collecting and handling the specimen appropriately. The recommended procedure for outpatient collection of pooled sputum specimens for cytologic examination is as follows:

1. The individual is given three to five containers, each containing 2 oz of fixative. Each container is labeled to indicate consecutive days of collection. The probability of detecting malignant cells is approximately 75% with three daily specimens and 90% with five consecutive daily specimens.
2. The person is instructed to cough and expectorate into one of the containers according to the following procedure:
   - **a.** Specimens should be obtained on arising in the morning. This provides the best specimen of secretions from deep in the lungs.
   - **b.** No mouth care, eating, or drinking of fluids other than water should be done prior to obtaining the specimen.
   - **c.** The person should breathe deeply and cough to raise sputum. Saliva specimens have no benefit in cancer detection. Heated hypertonic aerosol,

ultrasonic mist, and postural drainage may be used to assist in sputum induction.
   d. The person should expectorate directly into the specimen container.
3. Additional sputum raised by the individual should be added to the same container during the day.
4. A separate container is used for each day's sputum.

Centrally located tumors are also accessible for bronchoscopic visualization and washing, brushing, and biopsy. More peripherally located tumors may be reached by percutaneous needle biopsy of the lung. Pleural effusions may result from tumor extension to the pleural surface. Examination of pleural fluid and biopsied pleura may confirm the diagnosis of lung cancer. The presence of malignant cells in pleural fluid is usually considered a contraindication to surgical resection.

N (Node) Status

Approximately 70% of all individuals with lung cancer have regional lymph node involvement at the time of diagnosis. Evaluation of the presence and extent of regional lymph node metastases is critical to determining surgical resectability and prognosis. Individuals with mediastinal node metastases are usually considered to have unresectable disease, although this depends on the tumor cell type and location of the affected nodes.

Computerized tomographic (CT) scanning is the standard noninvasive method used to evaluate thoracic structures in patients with carcinoma of the lung. CT scanning is useful for distinguishing small differences in tissue density and in detecting nodal enlargement that cannot be appreciated on the radiograph. CT scanning is more sensitive than conventional tomography in the detection of mediastinal adenopathy. There is no significant difference between the yield of CT and magnetic resonance imaging (MRI) scans in the evaluation of lymph node metastasis. Neither method can distinguish malignant from nonmalignant adenopathy; histological confirmation is required.

Regional nodes can be sampled by transbronchial needle aspiration, mediastinoscopy, and mediastinotomy. Transbronchial needle aspiration is accomplished through a flexible bronchoscope and allows tissue from the paratracheal, hilar, and subcranial regions to be obtained. Mediastinoscopy is a more invasive procedure and is done under general anesthesia because of the coughing and pain that result from manipulation of the trachea. Some clinicians routinely employ mediastinoscopy in all cases of bronchogenic tumor without distant metastases to assess operability. Others rely on CT scanning to define nodal involvement. A left anterior mediastinotomy through the left second intercostal space can be used to evaluate pre- and subaortic mediastinal modes, a common site of tumor spread from the left upper lobe and left hilum.

M (Metastasis) Status

A careful history and physical examination, along with routine blood chemistries, are the most useful techniques in evaluating metastatic spread. In the absence of signs or symptoms of specific organ involvement, organ scanning is of limited value in detecting unsuspected disease. Metastatic disease not detectable by physical examination or biochemical screening is rarely encountered. Also, the incidence of false-positive scans can be significant. Organ scans and biopsies may be employed for assessment of stage and/or operability.

TREATMENT

Non–Small-Cell Lung Cancer

Surgery

With rare exceptions, complete surgical resection of a lung tumor offers the only chance for cure. Only 20%–25% of patients with lung cancer qualify for curative resectional surgery. Patients who are considered surgical candidates are those with NSCLCs with occult, stage I, or stage II disease. Occasionally, some patients with localized stage IIIa disease may be considered for surgery, particularly in instances of squamous cell tumors.

Occult and Stage I Cancer If the individual has an occult cancer or a tumor that is not detectable on chest radiograph, it is necessary to locate the source of the malignant cells seen in the sputum prior to surgery. Localization may be achieved by search of the tracheobronchial tree by fiberoptic bronchoscopy. The flexible fiberoptic bronchoscope allows visualization and biopsy down to the fourth or fifth branchings of the bronchial tree. Cancerous lesions may not appear as discrete and easily recognizable from surrounding mucosa, and any suspicious site is brushed and biopsied. This procedure may be repeated at frequent intervals (3–6 months) if localization is initially unsuccessful.

An alternative method has recently been developed for locating occult malignancies that arise from the trachea or central bronchi. This technique, bronchoscopic laser photoirradiation, depends on the use during bronchoscopy of the chemical hematoporphyrin derivative (HpD) as a tumor marker. Parenterally administered HpD selectively accumulates in malignant tissue and produces a red fluorescence when photoirradiated with a laser light source. Laser photoirradiation may establish a diagnosis of lung cancer in individuals whose tumors have not been diagnosed by means of radiography or conventional fiberoptic bronchoscopy.

The nurse is in a position to provide information and support during the process of localizing the tumor. It is likely to be a difficult time for the individual and family. The person must adjust to the fact that he or she has a serious disease despite being entirely or largely asymptomatic. There is a realistic basis for optimism, however, in light of improved survival statistics following surgical treatment of localized lung cancer. Accurate information presented in realistically optimistic terms is recommended in dealing with individuals with occult or stage I cancer and their families.

Several surgical procedures may be considered for resection of localized cancer, including wedge resection, segmentectomy, lobectomy, or pneumonectomy. Figure 46-8 illustrates three of the more common surgical procedures. Opinions as to the most appropriate procedure differ, but in general the most conservative procedure that will encompass all of the known tumor is selected. The anatomic location and extent of the tumor are crucial factors in the selection of the surgical approach. In all instances the risks of surgery are weighted against the purposes and realistic outcomes of the procedure. The results of surgery vary by TNM category and cell type. Five-year survival for stage I disease is 50% or more. Survival statistics for squamous tumors are better than those for adenocarcinomas or large-cell cancers.

Thorough discussions of the nursing care of individuals before and after thoracotomy are available and will not be reiterated here. Several of the most important considerations are highlighted in the discussion that follows.

Preoperatively, all individuals scheduled for resectional surgery will undergo testing to evaluate operative

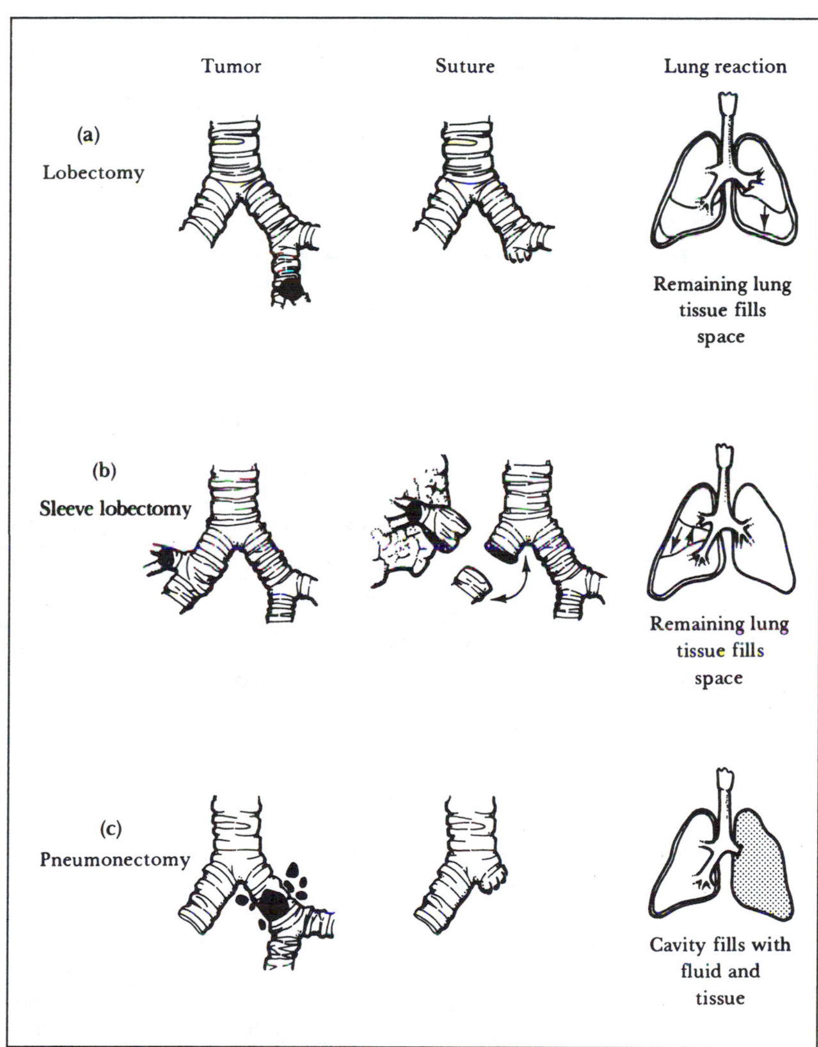

FIGURE 46-8 Appoaches to lung resection. (a) Lobectomy: A single pulmonary lobe is resected. (b) Sleeve lobectomy: The tumor-bearing lobe is resected together with a segment of the main bronchus, followed by an end-to-end anastomosis. Classic indication is a carcinoma of the right upper lobe bronchus. (c) Pneumonectomy: The lung alone is removed (simple pneumonectomy) or the lung and involved adjacent nodes are removed (radical pneumonectomy).

risk and to predict postoperative pulmonary function. In general, postresection changes in pulmonary function and hemodynamics depend on the amount of functional lung tissue resected. The decision to operate may be complicated by the fact that individuals often present with two diseases related to cigarette smoking: lung cancer and chronic obstructive lung disease. Operative morbidity and mortality vary greatly. Individual recommendations must be formulated with consideration to such factors as age, overall constitutional status, the type of surgery contemplated, and the type of anesthesia to be used.

General screening tests prior to lung resection include chest radiography, spirometry, and arterial blood gas analysis. Individuals with spirometric limitations or evidence of ventilatory failure are always at higher risk than those with normal pulmonary functions, and the greater the decline the greater the risk. Measurement of the forced expiratory volume in 1 second (FEV_1) has been particularly relied on as a predictor of postoperative pulmonary impairment. A predicted postoperative FEV_1 of 0.8–1 liter has been defined as the lower limit of acceptable pulmonary function, below which there is great risk of postoperative ventilatory insufficiency and intolerance of exertion.

In individuals with marginal pulmonary functions, more extensive tests may be ordered to assess tolerance for the degree of anticipated resection. Radioisotopic lung scanning techniques (quantitative ventilation-perfusion lung scan) are commonly used to ascertain regional lung function and predict postoperative values. Individuals with pulmonary hypertension may undergo temporary balloon occlusion of either the right or left pulmonary artery to help determine the adequacy of the pulmonary vasculature remaining after resection.

To maximize ventilatory capacities, particularly in individuals identified as at risk before surgery, airway clearance measures are employed. These include postural drainage, inhalation of aerosol solutions, and deep breathing and coughing techniques. Bronchodilators are indicated in instances of reversible airways obstruction. Pathogens identified by sputum culture are treated with appropriate antibiotics.

Cigarette smoking, which predisposes to oxygen desaturation, increased secretions, and pulmonary infection, should be curtailed before surgery. This prescription may be difficult for the individual to follow. In caring for such individuals, the nurse would do well to examine his or her feelings about smoking and lung cancer. For the most part, cancer is considered to be a disease that "attacks" unsuspecting victims. Lung cancer is notably at odds with this portrayal. The causal relationship between smoking and lung cancer has been widely publicized. Smokers who develop lung cancer may be seen less as innocent victims than as active participants in causing their cancer. Although blaming the person serves no useful purpose, it is difficult to avoid ambivalence in dealing with such individuals. Particularly troubling may be those individuals who continue to smoke after diagnosis, as about 20%–30% of patients will.[36,37] A judgmental approach by the nurse can increase the person's anxiety, discourage an open and therapeutic relationship, and deter cooperation toward important goals. It may be helpful to remember that compulsive cigarette smoking is an addictive behavior, not one that results from a lack of willpower.

After surgery, individuals generally undergo mechanical ventilatory assistance for a brief period of time. In resective lung surgery it is desirable to discontinue positive pressure ventilation as soon as feasible to minimize the risk of barotrauma to the sutured airway. Analgesics will be necessary to control incisional pain. Morphine or fentanyl are often administered through an epidural catheter in the initial postoperative period. Atelectasis is the most frequent complication of lung surgery. After extubation, deep breathing and coughing exercises are crucial to mobilize secretions and prevent atelectasis. These activities should be coordinated with times of analgesic administration to minimize the person's discomfort. The incision line should be splinted during deep breathing and coughing exercises. It is important to realize that many individuals forget their preoperative instructions regarding coughing and deep breathing. It may be necessary to repeat instructions from session to session because carryover of teaching may be poor. Other postoperative nursing care is specific to the operative procedure performed and is outlined in Tables 46-4, 46-5, and 46-6.

Stage II Cancer Surgical resection is usually the treatment of choice for stage II bronchogenic carcinomas other than those of the small-cell variety. The

TABLE 46-4 Nursing Care of Individuals after Lobectomy

Discussion	Nursing Implications
Ventilation—perfusion relationships are disrupted by lobe removal	Gas exchange status must be monitored carefully, particularly through arterial blood gas analysis; supplemental oxygen is usually administered
After lobe removal, the remaining lobe(s) expand to fill the space created by removal	Position the person to foster expansion; avoid leaving the individual lying on the operative side for prolonged periods of time
The bronchus leading to the resected lobe is stapled or sutured closed	Suction only as necessary; suction returns should be carefully inspected for evidence of bleeding, necrosis, or infection of the stump
Closed chest-tube drainage is employed to remove air and fluid from the pleural space	The water seal must be maintained at all times; drainage collection devices must be below chest level at all times; chest tubes must be kept patent and free of leaks

TABLE 46-5 Nursing Care of Individuals after Pneumonectomy

Discussion	Nursing Implications
All pulmonary volumes and capacities are reduced by approximately one-half as compared with the preoperative state	Volume and pressure settings on the mechanical ventilator must be determined accordingly; supplemental oxygen is usually administered; avoid positions that compress the remaining lung (Trendelenburg, lying on the unoperated side)
Blood flow to the remaining lung is increased	Carefully monitor individual for signs of pulmonary hypertension; fluid intake and output must be calculated carefully to avoid fluid overload; use of a volumetric pump for the administration of intravenous fluids is recommended
The thoracic cavity left after lung removal must be filled to prevent mediastinal shift of the heart and remaining lung	Chest tubes are not inserted or placed, but clamped; clamps should be left in place and labeled to prevent removal; the position of the trachea should be monitored closely and the physician notified immediately of a shift from the midline position; a shift toward the unoperated side may indicate hemorrhage or a bronchopleural fistula
The bronchial stump is stapled or sutured after lung removal	Intermittent positive-pressure breathing is generally not used postoperatively; vigorous, deep suctioning should be avoided to prevent suture line trauma or perforation; at the physician's discretion, suctioning may be contraindicated and secretions removed via a flexible bronchoscope; positioning the person on the unoperated side may be initially restricted to prevent fluid from leaking through the stump and into the remaining lung
If intrapericardial node dissection is done during pneumonectomy, herniation of the heart through the pericardial sac is a rare but lethal complication	Individuals must be monitored closely for the development of hypotension, tachycardia and central venous obstruction; immediate thoracotomy is essential to reposition the heart and correct the defect

goal is cure, although the incidence of cure in stage II disease is low. The probability of residual tumor after resection is great, as is the probability of occult distant metastasis. Accordingly, some types of adjuvant therapy or combinations of therapies are being used and studied. Most protocols involve the use of preoperative radiation and/or chemotherapy to improve resectability and survival. Such additions to the surgical procedure have not been impressive in influencing survival.

Preoperative radiotherapy (RT) may be employed to debulk the primary tumor, to control lymph node metastasis not accessible for removal, and to reduce local and systemic dissemination of viable tumor cells during the operative procedure. If preoperative irradiation is employed, surgery may be postponed for 4–6 weeks. Postoperative irradiation is designed to kill any cancer cells not resected. Although postoperative radiation therapy has been effective in reducing local recurrences, there is no evidence that survival is prolonged.

Adjuvant systemic chemotherapy may be employed to control occult metastasis and cancer recurrence. To date, survival rates have not been significantly affected, although older protocols often tested single agents or agents now known to have only limited activity in lung cancer.

Stage III Some cancer patients with advanced NSCLC may benefit from surgical resection in combination with radiation and/or chemotherapy. Patients who may benefit are those in whom the primary tumor and local metastases can be completely resected (stage IIIa). Patients selected for surgery are usually younger individuals with good cardiopulmonary reserve. Postoperative RT and/or chemotherapy may provide a modest prolongation of life in completely resected patients.

Radiation

In instances where curative resection is impossible either because of tumor extent or other disease, radiation therapy is standard treatment. Although RT is capable of eradicating NSCLC, impact on overall survival is equivocal.[38] Guidelines for radiation therapy have been summarized as follows:[39]

1. Radiation for cure in patients with intrathoracic but inoperable NSCLC is appropriate in those who are in good physical condition without extrathoracic metastases.

2. Curative radiation in clinically operable patients who are at increased risk because of advanced age or medical illness is an appropriate therapeutic approach.

3. Preoperative radiation can sterilize tumor and make inoperable patients operable, but overall survival is not improved and may be worse than with operation alone.

TABLE 46-6 Discharge Planning of Individuals after Thoracotomy

Discussion	Nursing Implications
Painful or fatiguing coughing can occur following exposure to bronchial irritants	The importance of smoking cessation should be emphasized; the person should be instructed to avoid situations where exposure is likely (air pollution alerts, crowded or smoke-filled rooms); vocational counseling may be necessary
After resectional surgery, individuals are at risk for the development of pulmonary hypertension	Individual should be monitored for the development of right-sided heart failure
The development of pulmonary infection can threaten gas exchange status	Individual should be assessed to ensure that he or she is free of pulmonary congestion prior to discharge; instruct the person to avoid contact with persons with known infections; provide the person with information to monitor for the development of symptoms of a respiratory tract infection; the person may be vaccinated against influenza at the physician's discretion
Easy fatigability may persist after thoracotomy	A progressive activity regimen may be prescribed
Individuals with a previous lung cancer are at risk of cancer recurrence	Postdischarge follow-up will generally include semiannual chest radiographs and sputum cytologies; any new symptoms should be reported immediately to the physician

4. Postoperative irradiation is indicated in patients with mediastinal nodes removed at operation. In such circumstances, irradiation can reduce local recurrences but does not necessarily increase overall survival.

5. Poor general condition, distant metastases, inadequate pulmonary reserve, malignant pleural effusion, and tumor size greater than 6 cm are contraindications to curative radiation. Palliative radiation can improve symptoms, often dramatically. Tumor shrinkage with relief of pressure on adjacent structures may help relieve dyspnea, cough, hemoptysis, and symptoms associated with superior vena caval obstruction, airway compression, paralysis of the recurrent laryngeal nerve, or pleural effusion. Bone and brain metastases are also managed by irradiation.

Most NSCLCs demonstrate poor radiosensitivity, and high doses of radiation (50–60 Gy) are necessary for cure. These doses of radiation therapy exceed normal lung tissue tolerance levels, and some degree of damage to the airways and parenchyma is inevitable. The severity of the resulting inflammatory reaction depends on the dose of radiation received and the size of the treatment field. Acute radiation pneumonitis usually produces symptoms within 1–3 months after treatment. Symptoms include dyspnea, fever, night sweats, and thick sputum. Pulmonary infections are an associated risk. Radiation fibrosis may develop 6 months or more after completion of radiation therapy and is discussed subsequently as a late complication of treatment.

Other structures in the irradiated field may also evidence tissue destruction. Radiation-induced pharyngitis and esophagitis with dysphagia are particularly common. During treatment, individuals may need to be placed on a high-protein, soft diet and monitored for signs of gastrointestinal bleeding. More serious complications such as radiation carditis, radiation myelitis, and bronchoesophageal fistulae occur in less than 3% of patients.

Prophylactic brain irradiation may be given to patients with NSCLC, particularly those with adenocarcinoma where brain metastases are frequent. Prophylactic brain irradiation would be given as part of curative therapy to prevent the CNS from becoming a site of relapse.

The use of radiotherapy for individuals diagnosed with NSCLC lung cancer has not had a major impact on overall survival, although several techniques to improve the response of lung tumors to radiotherapy have been suggested and are under investigation. It is hoped that dosage and fractionation schedules may be adjusted to be optimally effective in relation to the various cell types and stage groups of lung cancer. Hyperfractionation, short-course, and split-dose techniques are being studied for their effects on various tumors at various stages. Also, methods to increase the sensitivity of lung tumor cells to radiation using such agents as oxygen and vitamin K are being tested.

Some clinicians have attempted to provide concentrated localized radiotherapy through brachytherapy. Radioactive sources are placed in or adjacent to tumor-bearing tissues, either during resective surgery or through a bronchoscope in nonoperated patients. Brachytherapy may be used as an adjuvant to resectional surgery, as a boost component of initial radiotherapy, or for palliation at the time of recurrent endobronchial disease.

Chemotherapy

The role of chemotherapy in localized NSCLC is strictly as an adjuvant to radiotherapy or surgery. The role of chemotherapy in nonresectable NSCLC has been seriously debated. Compared to most tumors, NSCLCs are less sensitive to chemotherapeutic agents. Many of the drug regimens employed in early tests of the impact of chemotherapy on survival contained agents now known to be inactive against NSCLC. More effective agents have recently emerged. Current investigations in NSCLC include evaluation of drug regimens composed of platinum analogs (cisplatin, carboplatin), mitomycin C, newer alkylating agents (ifosfamide), vinca alkaloids (vindesine, vinblastine), and etoposide (VP-16). With combination chemotherapy the tumor response rates are around 20%–25%, but improvement in prognosis is modest and has not been consistently produced. It is not known if or how chemotherapy in NSCLC may affect quality of life.

At present, chemotherapy is not considered to be standard treatment for NSCLC but may be undertaken in a research setting. Because toxicities are considerable, only patients who have a reasonable chance to tolerate and respond to chemotherapy should be selected. This includes people with good performance status and minimal weight loss. Treatment should be discontinued if tumor shrinkage is not evident or if performance status or quality of life deteriorate during treatment.

The limited benefits of chemotherapy in NSCLC have provided impetus to researchers seeking to improve tumor response. Strategies have included the use of lung cancer cell lines to identify new chemotherapy agents that are active specifically against lung tumors. A related approach has been the use of in vitro drug sensitivity testing using fresh tumor specimens to select agents for use in vivo. The laboratory techniques necessary for the success of these drug screening efforts are under development.

Chemotherapy combined with radiation therapy

Although no striking benefit to the use of chemotherapy in NSCLC has been demonstrated, recent evaluations focus most often on chemotherapy combined with radiation therapy. Because of its demonstrated efficacy against NSCLC as well as its action as a potentiator of radiation therapy, cisplatin is the chemotherapy agent most often selected for combination therapy. There is evidence from randomized trials that patients with inoperable NSCLC treated with cisplatin and chest irradiation survive longer than patients treated with RT alone. The survival increase is generally on the order of 4–6 months.[40]

Small-Cell Lung Cancer

Regardless of the findings at the time of diagnosis, small-cell cancer is considered a systemic disease. As such, the mainstay of treatment is combination chemotherapy, with or without radiotherapy. SCLC is a highly responsive neoplasm and the most sensitive of all lung tumors to both chemotherapy and radiotherapy.

The role of surgery as an adjunctive treatment in SCLC is not clear. Surgical resection combined with preoperative and/or postoperative chemotherapy may be considered in the rare patient with a small peripheral tumor without apparent nodal involvement.

Chemotherapy

Combination chemotherapeutic regimens can dramatically influence survival. Major advances in chemotherapy in SCLC occurred in the 1970s, with only limited gains since then. The results of clinical trials have demonstrated several principles that guide current therapy.

1. Multiple, simultaneously administered chemotherapeutic agents are preferable to single agents in both limited and extensive disease. A regimen is continued if a complete response occurs. A second-line regimen is tried if a lesser response is obtained. Drug regimens frequently used against SCLC are listed in Table 46-7.[41] Etoposide (VP-16) has demonstrated such high activity against SCLC that it is included in most new drug regimens. Ifosfamide has also been found to be active against SCLC and is under evaluation in clinical trials.

2. Maximum results require high-dose therapy sufficient to produce serious toxicity. To a point, more intensive regimens appear to produce higher response rates. However, there is a limit to this dose response above which increased toxicity occurs without improved survival.

3. Tumor regression in response to chemotherapy often occurs quickly. Unfortunately, most responders relapse

TABLE 46-7 Frequently Used Chemotherapy Regimens for SCLC

Regimen	Agents
CAV	Cyclophosphamide Doxorubicin (adriamycin) Vincristine
CCM	Cyclophosphamide Semustine (CCNU) Methotrexate
RANDOMIZED TRIALS CONTAINING ETOPOSIDE (VP-16)	
CAE	Cyclophosphamide Doxorubicin (adriamycin) Etoposide
CAVE	Cyclophosphamide Doxorubicin (adriamycin) Vincristine Etoposide
CEV	Cyclophosphamide Etoposide Vincristine
EP	Etoposide Cisplatin
ECP	Etoposide Carboplatin
VIP	VP-16 (etoposide) Ifosfamide Cisplatin

within a short time, frequently at the initial intrathoracic site. The optimal duration of chemotherapy has not yet been determined.

4. The development of drug resistance is a common problem. Alternating chemotherapy regimens to prevent the development of drug resistance is a proposed but not confirmed strategy.

5. Median survival times are in the order of 14 months for limited disease and 7–9 months for extensive disease. Less than 20% of patients achieve long-term (>2 years) survival after initiation of treatment. Typically, there are patients with limited disease who achieve a complete response to therapy. Relapses in long-term survivors are often related to the appearance of NSCLC.

It may be possible to significantly improve the prognosis of SCLC if synergistic drugs can be combined in therapy, more effective modes of administration and schedules of administration developed, and appropriate combinations of multimodal approaches to therapy established. Several centers are attempting to achieve cures in SCLC by utilizing autologous bone marrow transplantation to individuals after megadose chemotherapy and total body irradiation. Survival data are not significantly improved with this regimen.

Radiation therapy

The role of localized radiotherapy in the treatment of SCLC is still being formulated. Since thoracic recurrence is the most significant treatment failure, chest irradiation has been combined with chemotherapy to reduce the frequency of intrathoracic relapse after chemotherapy alone. A reduced frequency of tumor recurrence in the chest and an increased 2-year survival have been reported from combined modality therapy in patients with limited disease. Combination therapy is associated with increased toxicity, particularly to the skin, esophagus, and lung parenchyma. The availability of colony stimulating factors may improve tolerance for combined modality treatment. Combined therapy is reserved for patients with limited disease, as patients with extensive disease have not been shown to benefit from the addition of RT.

Many patients with SCLC have brain metastasis at the time of diagnosis or develop signs of brain metastasis sometime before death. The longer the patient with SCLC survives, the greater is the likelihood of the development of detectable cerebral metastases. Prophylactic brain irradiation has been recommended for patients who have achieved a complete response to chemotherapy to eliminate the CNS as a site of early relapse. Although only small numbers of patients have been studied, no great survival advantage has been demonstrated from the use of brain irradiation, and clinically significant neurotoxicity frequently occurs.

Smoking Cessation

Smokers who develop lung cancer may believe that, since the worst danger of smoking has been realized, there is no compelling reason to quit smoking. There is evidence that cigarette smoking adversely affects prognosis in individuals with lung cancer. Investigations of patients with SCLC demonstrated that patients who discontinued smoking either prior to diagnosis or at the time of diagnosis survived longer than individuals who continued to smoke.[42] The reasons underlying the relationship between cigarette smoking and survival were hypothesized to relate to impaired host defenses against tumor growth associated with smoking. Additionally, patients who continue to smoke during therapy for SCLC had a greater risk of developing NSCLCs than did those who discontinued smoking. These findings illustrate the probable immunodepressive effects of cigarette smoking in terms of tumor development and growth. The potential benefits of smoking cessation after the diagnosis of lung cancer is made should be recognized and efforts should be directed toward assisting patients to stop smoking.

Phototherapy

Phototherapy using a neodymium yttrium-aluminum-garent (YAG) laser has been applied as palliation in individuals with far advanced obstructing airway tumors. Applied through a bronchoscope, the neodymium-YAG laser can produce thermal necrosis and tumor shrinkage, allowing pieces of the tumor to be removed through biopsy forceps. Heating also reduces blood supply and may help control bleeding, although hemorrhage is a recognized complication of neodymium-YAG laser therapy.

COMPLICATIONS OF TREATMENT

The discussion of treatments rendered to patients with lung cancers, particularly SCLCs, has emphasized the intensity of therapy and the likelihood of serious side effects. Toxicities associated with radiation therapy and chemotherapy are discussed next.

Radiation Therapy

Pulmonary fibrosis is a common late effect of chest irradiation, occurring months to years after radiation to the thorax. The severity of this condition is related to the total dose of radiation and the size of the treatment portal. Injury to lung tissue is markedly enhanced when chemotherapy and radiation are combined in treatment.

Effects on pulmonary function include a progressive decline in lung volumes and a decrease in lung compliance and diffusing capacity. Clinical manifestations include dry cough, dyspnea, weakness, hypoxemia, and perhaps cor pulmonale. Pericarditis and myelitis can follow curative-dose RT to the heart or spinal cord. The frequency of complications increases with increasing doses. Because of the poor survival generally seen in lung cancer, patients often die of their cancer before these complications develop.

In cases of cranial irradiation, particularly when combined with chemotherapy, a "central nervous system syndrome" of neurologic abnormalities has been seen. Memory loss, tremor, slurred speech, and somnolence can occur acutely. A similar syndrome with abnormalities on CT scan has been described in long-term survivors who received prophylactic cranial irradiation.

Chemotherapy

The aggressive multiagent chemotherapy regimens often used in lung cancer, particularly when combined with chest irradiation, can cause serious toxicities. An increased incidence of preleukemia and leukemia posttherapy has been seen and is indicative of long-term bone marrow toxicity. Patients aggressively treated with cytotoxic agents, particularly with alkylating agents, are at high risk for this hazard.

Many pharmacologic agents are associated with pulmonary parenchymal damage. Risks of pulmonary toxicity from cytotoxic drugs may increase with cumulative drug dose, age, use of chest radiotherapy, and concurrent oxygen therapy.[43] The agents that can cause lung injury are listed below.

- bleomycin
- mitomycin
- busulfan
- cyclophosphamide
- chlorombucil
- melphalan
- carmustine
- semustine
- methotrexate
- azathioprine
- mercaptopurine
- cytosine arabinoside
- procarbazine
- VM-26
- vinblastine
- vindasine
- chlorozotocin

Lung injury in the form of pneumonitis and fibrosis most commonly occurs. Treatment involves withdrawal of the offending agent and administration of corticosteroids. Some syndromes of injury are self-limited, but progressive disease is more often encountered.

SYMPTOM MANAGEMENT

Distressing physical symptoms associated with the tumor and/or its treatment are encountered in virtually all individuals with lung cancer. Degree of symptomatic distress influences physical performance, subjective well-being, and quality of life. Oncology nurses are most often responsible for managing the side effects of tumor growth, spread, and therapy. Management of toxicities related to cancer therapies are covered elsewhere in this text. The following discussion addresses potential interventions for symptoms commonly experienced by individuals with lung cancer.

Cough

A chronic cough may result from stimulation of irritant receptors in the bronchial mucosa through tumor infiltration. Hypersecretion of mucus also may cause coughing. The dry, irritating cough must be distinguished from the productive cough. Although it may be appropriate to suppress a dry, persistent, and debilitating cough, this should not be attempted at the expense of secretion retention. Narcotic medications, specifically codeine preparations, are generally used for cough suppression. In addition, inspired air should be warmed and humidified and cigarette smoking discouraged. Deep breathing and effective coughing techniques should be taught and reinforced as necessary. Tracheal suctioning should be used only if the person's cough is ineffective in removing secretions. A chronic nonproductive cough in a patient with underlying chronic obstructive lung disease may respond to inhaled bronchodilators.

Pain

Pain associated with lung cancer varies in its characteristics and etiologies. Chest pain due to a bronchogenic tumor is usually dull, poorly localized, and described as an ache. The mechanism of pain production is not clear, but the pain itself is seldom severe. A more sharp and severe type of chest pain can occur with tumor involvement of the bony thorax or parietal pleura. Pain may increase in intensity and duration with advancing metastatic disease and cancer treatment.

Pain control measures often require input from multiple disciplines. If standard cancer therapies fail to relieve or control pain, pharmacologic agents are usually ordered. If agents such as hydromorphone hydrochloride (Dilaudid) or morphine are ultimately necessary to control pain, such drugs should not be withheld because of fear of addiction. Individuals in pain generally have significant disease and a short life expectancy and should be made as comfortable as possible.

Dyspnea

Dyspnea is a complex reaction that involves physiologic and psychologic processes. Dyspnea is a common presenting symptom in individuals with lung cancer and develops in others after diagnosis. The presence and severity of dyspnea may relate to multiple factors including airway obstruction, fibrosis, edema, tumor infiltration, pleural effusion, inspiratory muscle fatigue, anxiety, and depression.

In lung cancer patients the presence of dyspnea is often associated with fatigue and decreased energy.[44] Emotional stress may contribute to the production of dyspnea and may also result from the experience of dyspnea. Nurses should assess the events that appear to stimulate dyspnea, the individual's description and interpretation of the experience, and self-management strategies. Such evaluation may suggest possible interventions to limit the frequency or severity of dyspneic episodes or to increase tolerance of this symptom. Depending on the cause, dyspnea may improve following thoracentesis, irradiation, chemotherapy, diuretics, steroids, or supplemental oxygen. Activity limitation, bronchial hygiene measures, a bedside fan, appropriate positioning, and systematic relaxation training may help control persistent dyspnea.

Although sometimes useful in controlling dyspnea in individuals with chronic airway obstruction, breathing retraining should not be automatically prescribed for lung cancer patients with dyspnea. Diaphragmatic breathing with slow exhalation through pursed lips may not be appropriate for patients whose dyspnea relates to restrictive pulmonary disorders and may, in fact, cause greater distress. In patients with intractable dyspnea, narcotics or anxiolytics may be of benefit in symptom reduction. Potential side effects, including hypoventilation, are considered acceptable risks in selected patients.

Hemoptysis

Hemoptysis is caused by tumor erosion into pulmonary blood vessels, usually bronchial arteries or their branches. Bleeding may appear as streaks or dots or as gross blood loss. The therapeutic approach to the lung cancer patient with hemoptysis is generally determined by the time course and volume of bleeding.

Persons with mild hemoptysis (less than 50 ml in 24 hours) are usually treated as outpatients using conservative measures. The frequency and amount of bleeding are monitored on an ongoing basis. Patients are advised to refrain from any activities that tend to aggravate bleeding. Cough suppressants may help if hemoptysis is associated with significant coughing. Because blood provides an excellent medium for bacterial growth, antibiotics may also be prescribed. Bleeding episodes are likely to be frightening, and the individual should be reassured if the blood loss is not significant. Most bleeding will stop within several days.

Patients with significant bleeding or respiratory compromise are hospitalized and monitored carefully for increasing blood loss, changes in blood pressure and pulse, and respiratory distress. Although infrequent, major bleeding (200 ml in 24 hours) requires immediate attention if asphyxiation and shock are to be avoided. As soon as bleeding is encountered the patient should be positioned on one side so that the lung most probably containing the bleeding site is dependent. Such positioning is undertaken to prevent spillover of blood into the nonbleeding lung. Aggressive measures to control massive bleeding may include angiographic embolization of the bronchial artery source of the bleed or emergency surgery.

Wheezing

Unilateral persistent wheezing occurs if a tumor partially obstructs a bronchus. This troublesome symptom can generally be relieved by tumor shrinkage through irradiation. Wheezing may be more severe when the individual lies on one side, and positioning should be undertaken to protect bronchial patency. Diffuse wheezing may represent underlying chronic airways obstruction. Standard pharmacologic therapies for chronic obstructive pulmonary disease (e.g., inhaled bronchodilators, corticosteroids, mucolytics) may provide relief.

PSYCHOSOCIAL ISSUES

Quality of Life Assessment

The intent of treatment in lung cancer is more often palliation than cure. The primary goal of palliative treatment is improving quality of life, a multidimensional construct that includes physical function, disease- and treatment-related symptoms, psychologic functioning, and social activity. Emphasis is placed on assessing the individual's subjective experience. Despite its importance, quality of life has been only recently considered as a variable in assessing patient needs and responses to treatments for lung cancer. Use of quality-of-life measures and evaluations in patients with lung cancer has been recently reviewed.[45] Although data are insufficient at present to support general conclusions and recommendations for treatment, this is an important developing area of research. Areas to be addressed include: development of a systematic database on the psychosocial concerns of lung cancer patients, development and evaluation of quality-of-life instruments in lung cancer patients in all phases of disease and treatment, and longitudinal description of quality-of-life patterns during the course of treatment.[46]

Sources of Distress

Psychosocial issues and concerns of individuals with malignancies have been discussed elsewhere in this text. Certain responses or dilemmas that may relate particularly to individuals with lung cancer are discussed below.

Social isolation

Individuals with lung cancer are usually symptomatic at the time they present for diagnosis. Presenting symptoms commonly include dyspnea, cough, weight loss, and fatigue. These symptoms may worsen as a result of treatment and/or disease progression. Social isolation is a coping strategy frequently used to deal with distressing symptoms, particularly dyspnea and fatigue.[47] Patients may find it necessary to curtail previously important social contact to prevent physical decompensation and social embarrassment.

Individuals who continue to smoke beyond diagnosis and treatment may feel vulnerable to criticism and consequently avoid or limit contact with others. This behavior may prove to be an additional stressor for the patient or the family, who feels isolated from social supports at a time when they are especially needed. To the extent possible, patients should be assisted to balance their need to avoid disabling emotional and physical activity against the reduced quality of life associated with psychosocial isolation.

Limited survival

Individuals with cancer have indicated their need for caregivers to deal with them honestly and hopefully. This need can be of greater importance than the need to discuss issues related to death and dying.[48] Given the typically limited prognosis of most patients with lung cancer, this may seem to pose a dilemma of balancing optimism with realism. To prevent undue distress it is important to keep several factors in mind. First, hope and honesty are not incompatible. Patients hope not only for a cure or an extension of life but to preserve the quality of their life. Second, needs of patients may vary in importance according to changing phases of illness. Fortunately, most patients provide cues, some overt and some subtle, regarding when and how much information they are prepared to handle. Nurses who are sensitive to such cues can help provide timely information and support.

While it is not helpful to give early and frequent reminders to patients that their days are limited, it is also a disservice to ignore disease progression and impending death. Patients often appreciate help in anticipating and planning how to spend their remaining days. Patients with lung disorders sometimes express fear of a "smothering" type of death and are relieved to hear that dyspnea can be controlled and that such an experience is unlikely.

Patients also need accurate information about the use of life-sustaining technologies in order to formulate their desires regarding the use of these treatments. Discussions should take place with the attending physician well before a medical crisis necessitates urgent decisions about the use of life supports. Planning for end-of-life care is a process rather than an event and usually requires substantial time and discussion. Anticipatory discussions should occur with patients and family members about the realities, outcomes, and alternatives to critical care. For example, lung cancer patients who develop respiratory failure and are placed on mechanical ventilatory assistance rarely survive the hospitalization.[49] Knowing this, patients may elect to forgo or limit use of ventilator treatment unless a clearly reversible cause for the respiratory failure can be identified. In any event, it is extremely important that everyone involved in decision making about the use of life-sustaining technologies understand that the decision is not one of treatment versus no treatment, but rather deciding among forms of treatment. Lest the patient and family fear abandonment by caregivers, emphasis should be on care that the patient will receive (e.g., comfort measures such as positioning, analgesics, sedatives, oxygen) no matter what other decisions are made.

Patients and/or family members should be informed of the availability of advance directives such as the Living Will and Durable Power of Attorney for Health Care to document their treatment preferences. This step in care planning is essential for two reasons. First, committing hopelessly ill patients to mechanical ventilation and other resuscitative measures simply because no one has specifically ascertained and documented their preferences is insupportable morally, ethically, and economically. Second, patients' actual preferences for treatment and life-supportive care often differ from what family members and caregivers infer them to be.[50,51] When decisions about care are made without patient participation, treatment may be more or less aggressive than the patient would have desired.

Family disruptions

Disease progression may be especially rapid in individuals with lung cancer. Major shifts in family roles and dynamics may occur in a short time period, possibly straining family resources and aggravating conflicts predating the cancer diagnosis. With the shift in management of lung cancer from the inpatient to the outpatient setting, family coping may become more compromised and stressed by the need to manage tumor- and treatment-related problems at home. Crises within the family may be controlled by the experienced nurse who anticipates problems, rehearses approaches and solutions with the family, and initiates early referrals to appropriate support systems and personnel.

CONCLUSION

The challenges to those involved in the care of individuals with lung cancer are significant. Given the high potential for prevention and the low probabilities for cure, the oncology nurse's role assumes special prominence. Nurses may have particular opportunities and competencies for supporting individual efforts to avoid or cease smoking. In individuals with lung cancer for whom curative measures are impossible or unsuccessful, the nurse often becomes a principal coordinator and practitioner of interventions aimed at palliation. Practice in these areas is as much art as science. There is much to be learned from scientists, clinical colleagues, patients, and families. We know of many interventions that do not benefit patients; the challenge of the future is to develop and perfect more that do. Nurses who are willing to be educated and guided by experience and who remain open to investigating innovative and creative approaches are essential to all such efforts.

REFERENCES

1. Adler I: *Primary Malignant Growths of the Lung and Bronchi.* New York: Longman, Green, 1912.
2. Boring CC, Squires, TS, Heath CW: Cancer statistics for African Americans. *CA* 42:7–17, 1992.
3. Boring CC, Squires TS, Tong T: Cancer statistics, 1992. *CA* 42:19–38, 1992.
4. Spencer H: *Pathology of the Lung,* (Vol 2) (4th ed). Oxford: Pergamon Press, 1985.
5. Wynder EL, Stellman SD: Impact of long term filter cigarette usage on lung and laryngeal cancer risk. *J Natl Cancer Inst* 62:471–477, 1979.
6. Oleske DM: Epidemiology of lung cancer. *Semin Oncol Nurs* 3:165–173, 1987.
7. Report of the Surgeon General: The health consequences of involuntary smoking. US Dept of Health and Human Services, 1986.
8. American Thoracic Society Scientific Assembling on Occupational and Environmental Health: Health effects of air pollution. *ATS News* 4:22–63, 1978.
9. Hammond EC, Selikoff IJ, Seidman H: Asbestos exposure, cigarette smoking and death rates. *Ann N Y Acad Sci* 330:473–490, 1979.
10. Samet JM: Radon and lung cancer. *J Natl Cancer Inst* 81:745–757, 1989.
11. Willett WC: Vitamin A and lung cancer. *Nutritional Reviews* 48:201–211, 1990.
12. Birrer MJ, Minna JD: Molecular genetics of lung cancer. *Semin Oncol* 15:226–235, 1988.
13. Mulvihill JJ, Bale AE: Ecogenetics of lung cancer. In Mizell M, Correa P (eds.), *Lung Cancer: Causes and Prevention.* Deerfield Beach:Verlag Chemie International, 1984, pp. 141–152.
14. Skillrud DM, Offord KP, Miller RD: Higher risk of lung cancer in chronic obstructive pulmonary disease. *Ann Intern Med* 105:503–507, 1986.
15. Filderman AE, Carter DC, Baue AE, et al: Lung cancer. In Matthay RA, Matthay MA, Wiedemann HP (eds.). *Annual Review of Pulmonary and Critical Care Medicine.* Philadelphia: Hanley & Belfur, 1988, pp. 53–75.
16. Baumm AD, Medsger TA: Cancer and systemic sclerosis: An epidemiologic study. *Arthritis Rheum* 28:1336–1340, 1985.
17. ———: Cigarette smoking among adults—United States, 1990. *MMWR* 41:355, 1992.
18. ———: Selected tobacco use behaviors and dietary patterns among high school students—United States, 1991. *MMWR* 41:417–420, 1992.
19. Horn D: Social and psychologic aspects of starting smoking. In Nieburgs HE (ed), *Prevention and Detection of Cancer* (vol 1). New York:Dekker, 1977, pp. 739–746.
20. Report of the Surgeon General: The health consequences of smoking. US Dept. of Health and Human Services, 1982.
21. Transdermal Nicotine Study Group: Transdermal nicotine for smoking cessation. *JAMA* 266:3133–3138, 1991.
22. Risser NL: The key to prevention of lung cancer. *Semin Oncol Nurs* 3:228–236, 1987.
23. Garfinkel L, Stellman SD: Cigarette smoking among physicians, dentists and nurses. *CA* 36:2–8, 1986.
24. ———: Smoking-related mortality decline among physicians—Rhode Island. *MMWR* 39:656–658, 1990.
25. Gritz ER, Kanim L: Do fewer oncology nurses smoke? *Oncol Nurs Forum* 13:61–64, 1986.
26. Haughey BP, Mattewson MK, Dittmat SS, Wu YB: Smoking practices of critical care nurses. *Heart Lung* 18:29–35, 1989.
27. Auerbach O, Hammond EC, Garfinkel L: Changes in bronchial epithelium in relation to cigarette smoking, 1955–1960 vs. 1970–1977. *N Engl J Med* 300:381–386, 1979.
28. ———: State tobacco prevention and control activities. *MMWR* 40:1–7, 1991.
29. Landrigan PJ, Selikoff IJ: Primary prevention against occupational carcinogens. In Bannasch P (ed), *Cancer Risks.* New York:Springer-Verlag, 1986, pp. 94–100.
30. Berlin NI, Buncher CR, Fontana RS, et al: The National Cancer Institute cooperative early lung cancer detection program. *Am Rev Respir Dis* 130:545–549, 1984.
31. Early Lung Cancer Cooperative Study: Early lung cancer detection. *Am Rev Respir Dis* 130:565–570, 1984.
32. Kotin P: Carcinogenesis of the lung. In Liebow AA, Smith DE. (eds), *The Lung.* Baltimore, MD: William & Wilkins, 1968.
33. Yesner R, Carter D: Pathology of carcinoma of the lung. *Clin Chest Medicine* 3:257–289, 1982.
34. Mountain CF: Prognostic implications of the International Staging System for Lung Cancer. *Semin Oncol* 15:236–245, 1988.

35. Abrams J, Dole LA, Aisner J: Staging, prognostic factors and special considerations in small cell lung cancer. *Semin Oncol* 15:261–277, 1988.
36. Sridharks KS, Raub WA: Present and past smoking history and other predisposing factors in 100 lung cancer patients. *Chest* 101:19–25, 1992.
37. Knudsen N, Schulman S, VanDenHoek J, et al: Insights on how to quit smoking: A survey of patients with lung cancer. *Cancer Nurs* 8:145–150, 1985.
38. Hazuka MB, Bunn PA: Controversies in the nonsurgical treatment of stage III non-small cell lung cancer. *Am Rev Respir Dis* 145:967–977, 1992.
39. Hande KR, Des Prez RM: Chemotherapy and radiation therapy for non-small cell lung carcinoma. *Clin Chest Med* 3:399–414, 1982.
40. Dillman RO, Seagren SL, Propert KJ, et al: A randomized trial of induction chemotherapy plus high dose radiation versus radiation alone in stage III non–small-cell lung cancer. *N Engl J Med* 323:940–945, 1990.
41. Feld R, Ginsberg RJ, Payne DG: Treatment of small cell lung cancer. In Roth JA, Ruckdeschel JC, Weisenburger TH (eds.): *Thoracic Oncology*. Philadelphia: Saunders, 1989, pp. 229–262.
42. Johnston-Early A, Cohen MH, Minna JD, et al: Smoking abstinence and small cell lung cancer survival. *JAMA* 244:2175–2179, 1980.
43. Cooper JA, White DA, Matthay RA: Drug induced pulmonary disease: Cytotoxic drugs. *Am Rev Respir Dis* 133:321–340, 1986.
44. Foote M, Sexton DL, Pawlik L: Dyspnea: A distressing symptom in lung cancer. *Oncol Nurs Forum* 13:25–31, 1986.
45. Fergusson RJ, Cull A: Quality of life measurements for patients undergoing treatment for lung cancer. *Thorax* 46:671–675, 1991.
46. Bernhard J, Ganz PA: Psychosocial issues in lung cancer patients (pt 2). *Chest* 99:480–485, 1991.
47. Brown ML, Carrieri V, Janson-Bjerklie S, et al: Lung cancer and dyspnea. *Oncol Nurs Forum* 13:19–24, 1986.
48. Young-Brockopp D: Cancer patients' perception of five psychosocial needs. *Oncol Nurs Forum* 9:31–35, 1982.
49. Ewer MS, Ali MK, Atta MS, et al: Outcome of lung cancer patients requiring mechanical ventilation for pulmonary failure. *JAMA* 256:3364–3366, 1986.
50. Uhlmann RF, Pearlman RA, Cain KC: Physicians' and spouses' predictions of elderly patients' resuscitation preferences. *Arch Intern Med* 145:235–239, 1985.
51. Slevin ML, Stubbs L, Plant HJ, et al: Attitudes to chemotherapy: Comparing views of patients with cancer with those of doctors, nurses, and general public. *Br Med J* 300:1458–1460, 1990.

Chapter 47

Malignant Lymphomas

Mary Ellen McFadden, RN, MLA, OCN

INTRODUCTION

The malignant lymphomas constitute a diverse group of neoplasms that arise from the uncontrolled proliferation of the cellular components of the lymphoreticular system. This complex network of specialized cells and organs defends the body against infection. Malignancies of the immune system may present locally; however, the majority are often widespread at the time of diagnosis, presumably because of the natural ability of the immune cells to circulate. Based on histologic characteristics, the lymphomas are divided into two major subgroups—Hodgkin's disease (HD) and non-Hodgkin's lymphoma (NHL). Some references suggest that the term *lymphocytic lymphoma* be ascribed to the latter because it emphasizes the essential role that lymphocyte transformation has in its ontogeny.[1] However, both terms are equally acceptable, and since *NHL* is used most frequently in practice and in literature, it is selected for this chapter.

Lymphomas are among the most studied human tumors, and determination of their immunophenotypes, gene rearrangements, cytogenetic abnormalities, and oncogene activation are providing valuable clues about the inherent mechanisms of the neoplastic process itself. Also, some are considered to be among the most curable of all malignancies. Impetus for this clinical success is provided by therapeutic advances using combination chemotherapy, chemotherapy plus radiation therapy, and ablative chemotherapy followed by bone marrow transplantation in patients with refractory disease.[2]

Despite a number of shared superficial similarities, the distinctions between HD and NHL are important because their clinical courses, prognoses, and treatment modalities are substantially different. Indeed, controversy truly begins at the cellular level with an unresolved debate about their respective cells of origin. Although several distinct T-cell lymphomas have been identified, B-cell neoplasms account for the majority of non-Hodgkin's lymphomas.[3] A variety of candidates have been proposed for the originating cell in HD, including lymphocytes (T and B), monocytes-macrophages, and interdigitating reticulum cells.[4] Although monocyte-macrophage origin is currently favored, experimental support remains conflicting and inconclusive.[5]

The clinical behavior of the malignant lymphomas is highly variable. Some patients follow a rapid downhill course, with progressive generalized adenopathy, fever, night sweats, splenomegaly, and infiltration of the bone marrow, lungs, liver, and other organs with proliferative neoplastic cells. Death often occurs within 1–2 years of diagnosis and usually results from infection, hemorrhage due to tumor-induced destruction of the bone marrow, or systemic failure of vital organ function. Other individuals follow a more indolent course in which the disease is apparently limited to the lymph nodes for many years. Eventually the malignant process becomes more aggressive, and invasion of extranodal organs requires a revision in management strategies.[6]

Recent statistical analysis indicates that the incidence of lymphomas, particularly NHL, is escalating, and it has now become the fifth most common cancer in the United States. Incidence in 1993 is estimated at nearly 43,000 newly diagnosed cases, and the annual mortality rate is expected to reach nearly 20,500.[7] A major factor contributing to this increase is the established association between NHL and the acquired immunodeficiency syndrome (AIDS) caused by the retrovirus known as human immunodeficiency virus (HIV). Before 1986, the median survival after AIDS diagnosis was less than 1 year, and most patients died before the presence of NHL could be confirmed. However, advances in antiviral therapy and treatment or prophylaxis against opportunistic infections have resulted in the prolonged survival of AIDS patients. Thus, since 1986, a substantial increase in secondary NHL has been noted in the AIDS population. Gail et al.[8] estimate that between 8% and 27% of all 1992 cases of NHL will be attributable to this syndrome. Considering the fact that the incidence and death rate from NHL had shown noteworthy increases even before the AIDS epidemic, this malignancy truly has the potential to become an increasing burden and challenge to health care systems well into the twenty-first century.[9]

In an effort to help oncology nurses effect optimal patient care and education, this chapter will provide comprehensive information about the etiology, classifications, clinical manifestations, staging, diagnosis, and therapeutic management of HD and NHL. Treatment and disease-related complications as well as important issues related to survivorship also will be addressed.

THE IMMUNE SYSTEM AND NEOPLASIA

The immune system is a highly integrated, complex mechanism that has evolved to help the body protect itself against foreign tissues and invading microbes such as viruses, bacteria, fungi, and parasites. It distinguishes such threats from normal tissue by recognizing invasive antigens or foreign molecules as "nonself" and seeks to eliminate or destroy them by mounting an appropriate response via the formation of antigen-specific protein antibodies.[10] The organs of the immune system are scattered throughout the body and are generally referred to as *lymphatic* or *lymphoid* organs because they are concerned with the growth, development, and deployment of T- and B-lymphocytes. These white blood cells are the key operatives of immune function and the primary cellular component of malignant lymphomas. The lymphoid organs as illustrated in Figure 47-1 include the spleen, bone marrow, thymus, lymph nodes, tonsils, adenoids, appendix, and clumps of lymphoid

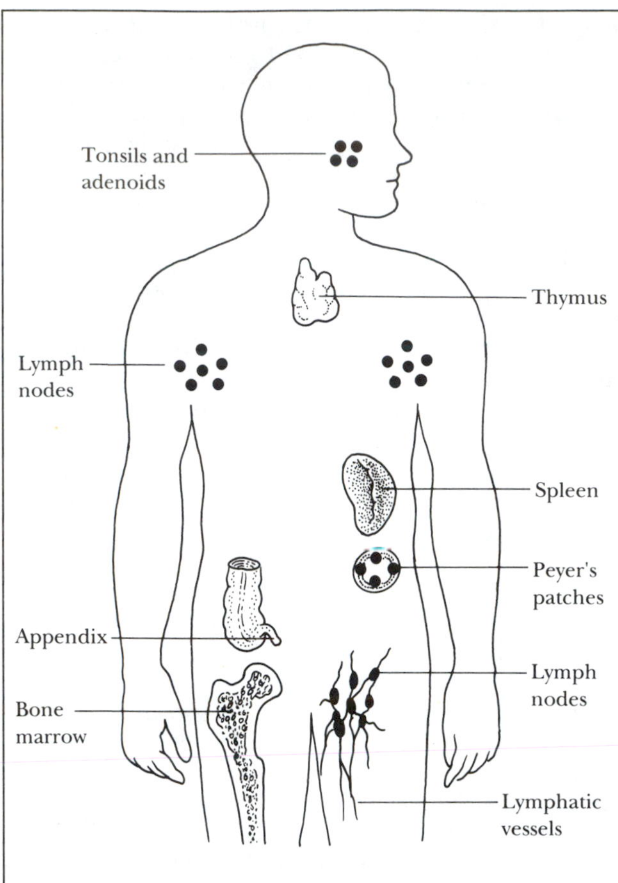

FIGURE 47-1 Organs of the immune system. (Illustrated by J. Thommen.)

tissue in the small intestine known as Peyer's patches. The blood and lymphatic vessels that transport lymphocytes also can be considered part of this system.

Lymph is derived from interstitial fluid and flows through lymphatic vessels transporting immune cells and foreign antigens to the circulatory system via the thoracic duct. Along its course, lymph is filtered of detritus by the lymph nodes. These small, encapsulated clusters in the neck, axilla, abdomen, and groin (Figure 47-2) have a very specific structure and contain specialized compartments that facilitate lymphocyte maturation and differentiation. T-lymphocytes are selectively concentrated in the paracortical regions of the lymph node and within the periarterial lymphoid sheaths of the spleen. Small numbers of T-cells are also found within the follicles, where they facilitate B-cell differentiation. On the other hand, B-lymphocytes are concentrated in the follicles and medullary cords of the lymph nodes and in the follicles of the spleen. The lymphoid follicles represent the proliferative site of the B-cell system, and the medullary cord region represents its secretory component. Monocytes circulate in the peripheral blood, while histiocytes are preferentially found in the subcapsular and medullary sinuses of the lymph nodes and the red pulp of the spleen.[9] Figure 47-3 depicts normal lymph node architecture and the areas associated with lymphoid localization and malignant transformation.

Lymphomas are preeminently a malignancy of the lymphocyte, and the process by which a lymphoid neoplasm is generated may be thought of as a series of cellular changes whereby a once normal lymphoid cell (or cell clone) becomes refractory to the regulation of its differentiation and proliferation. These changes are, of necessity, genetic, whether induced by mutation, chromosomal translocation/deletion, or insertion of foreign genes (e.g., viral genes) into the cell. Translocations generally result in altered expression of an adjacent gene. Deletions may cause loss of genes necessary for appropriate cellular regulation and differentiation. Mutations could stimulate either of these effects, while viruses are likely to enhance modification of adjacent genes by viral promotion/enhancement or of distant genes via viral transactivation.[10]

Once transformed, the new clone of malignant cells follows the behavior pattern of the stage at which lymphocyte alteration took place. For example, if the function of the maturing lymphocyte is secretion of an antibody protein, the tumor cells will continue to secrete the normal protein, albeit in abnormal quantities. In this case a faulty regulatory mechanism and not abnormal cell proliferation is responsible for the neoplastic change. However, if the function at the time of transformation is for the lymphocytes to form maturing nodules in the lymph nodes, their excessive production will result in nodular lymphoma.[6]

The association of certain malignancies with congenital or acquired immunodeficiency diseases and the bimodal distribution of cancer in the very young and the very old suggests that an immature or debilitated immune system predisposes to neoplasia.[11] Malignant lymphomas are linked strongly with congenital immunodeficiency disorders such as Wiskott-Aldrich syndrome, Klinefelter syndrome, and ataxia telangiectasia. The chronic inflammatory process activated by many autoimmune diseases (e.g., rheumatoid arthritis, systemic lupus erythematosus, and Sjögren syndrome) predisposes an individual to lymphomas of extranodal origin. Renal, cardiac, and other organ transplants also have been found to increase risk. Such tumors usually occur in the first year following transplant; they are rapidly progressive and frequently involve the central nervous system. Definitive cause of these lymphomas is unknown, but viral infection, drug-induced immunosuppression, and chronic antigenic stimulation from the graft may be contributing factors.[4]

MATURATION OF THE LYMPHOCYTE

The origin of the lymphocyte can be traced to a pluripotent stem cell in the bone marrow that has the potential to develop into any of the cells that normally

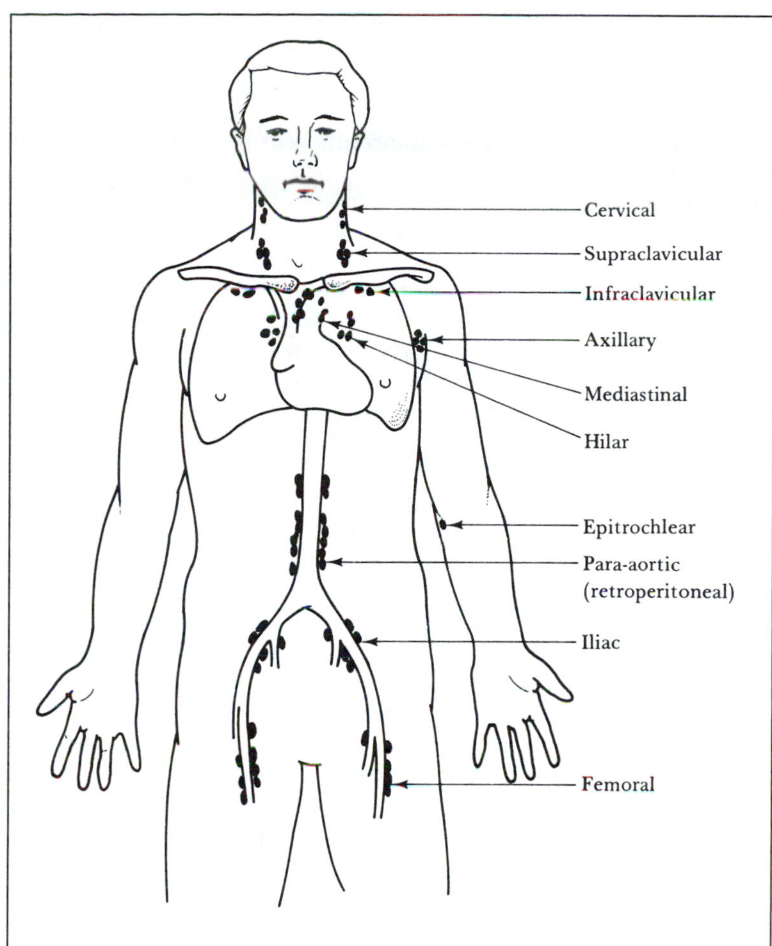

FIGURE 47-2 Major lymph node groups. (Source: Yarbro CH: Lymphomas. In Groenwald SL, Frogge MH, Goodman M, Yarbro CH [eds]: *Cancer Nursing: Principles and Practice* [2d ed]. Boston: Jones and Bartlett, 1990. Reprinted with permission.)

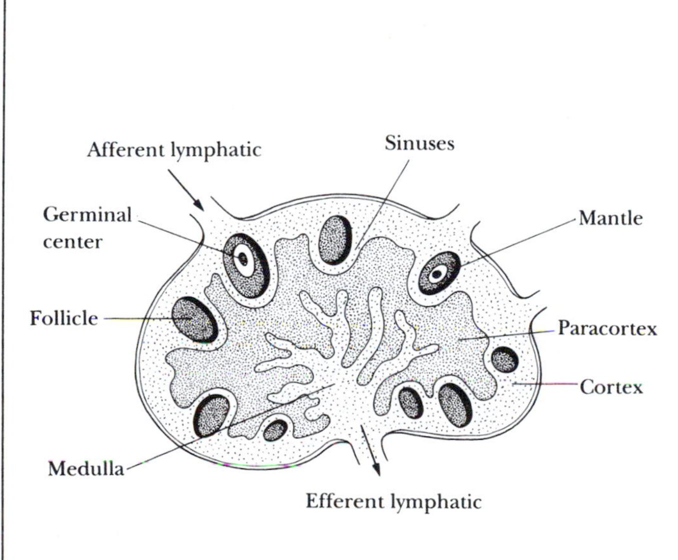

B-CELL LYMPHOMAS

Follicle
- Nodular lymphoma
- Large-cell lymphoma (sonic)
- Burkitt's lymphoma

Germinal Center/Mantle Zone
- Lymphocytic lymphoma
- Mantle zone lymphoma (intermediate differentiation)

Medulla
- Chronic lymphocytic leukemia
- Well-differentiated lymphocytic lymphoma
- Waldenström's macroglobulinemia

T-CELL LYMPHOMAS

Paracortex
- Peripheral T-cell lymphoma
- Mycosis fungoides
- Sézary syndrome
- Acute lymphoblastic leukemia
- T-cell lymphoblastic lymphoma

Miscellaneous Malignancies

Sinus Region
- Malignant histiocytosis
- Kt-1 large-cell lymphoma

FIGURE 47-3 Sites of lymphocyte transformation in the lymph node (illustrated by J. Thommen)

circulate in the blood. At each step along the path of differentiation, a cell loses its capacity to proceed along an alternate route. In the first step, the stem cell matures so that it is either the precursor of the lymphocyte series or of all the other cellular series of the blood (erythrocyte, megakaryocyte, polymorphonuclear neutrophil, or monocyte). The lymphocyte precursor then develops into one of a number of types of mature lymphocytes. Figure 47-4 demonstrates the maturation sequence of the immunocompetent lymphocyte.[6]

Lymphocytes are responsible for the two arms of the immunologic defense system: the humoral arm, which consists of plasma cells that produce circulating antibodies against foreign antigens, and the cellular arm, which consists of circulating lymphocytes that have developed specificity against foreign antigens. These two arms of the immune process are distinct, but they function jointly in defending the host against foreign proteins. An early step in the differentiation of the maturing lymphocyte occurs when the cell is programmed either by the bone marrow (bursa equivalent) or by the thymus to become a B-lymphocyte or a T-lymphocyte respectively. Humoral immunity is provided by the B-lymphocytes, which, when exposed to an appropriate foreign antigen, mature into plasma cells and produce antibodies against that antigen. T-lymphocytes, when similarly exposed to a foreign antigen, develop into killer lymphocytes that will attack and destroy the foreign antigen without benefit of an antibody intermediary, thus providing cellular immunity. In addition, some T-lymphocytes develop specific regulator roles in which they either suppress or stimulate immune functions (suppressor cells and helper cells).[6]

Eighty percent of lymphomas manifest B-cell origin, and most patients initially present with disease involving bone marrow or lymph nodes. Non-lymphoid tissue extension is also common, particularly in the thyroid, gastrointestinal tract, salivary glands, and conjunctiva. Diagnosis is usually straightforward because of characteristic monoclonal immunoglobulin elevations and/or distinct morphologic features. In general, B-cell neoplasms tend to follow a more indolent course than those induced by T-cell transformation.[12]

Lymphomas derived from T-lymphocytes are a complex group of diseases with marked biologic and clinical heterogeneity. These neoplasms usually arise in bone marrow, thymus, lymph nodes, and skin. They may produce abnormal amounts of lymphokines or may markedly activate histiocytes (macrophages) throughout the body. These activated cells often destroy normal blood cells, causing anemia, thrombocytopenia, and/or leukopenia.[13] T-cell lymphomas are generally more aggressive and grow more rapidly than their B-cell counterparts.

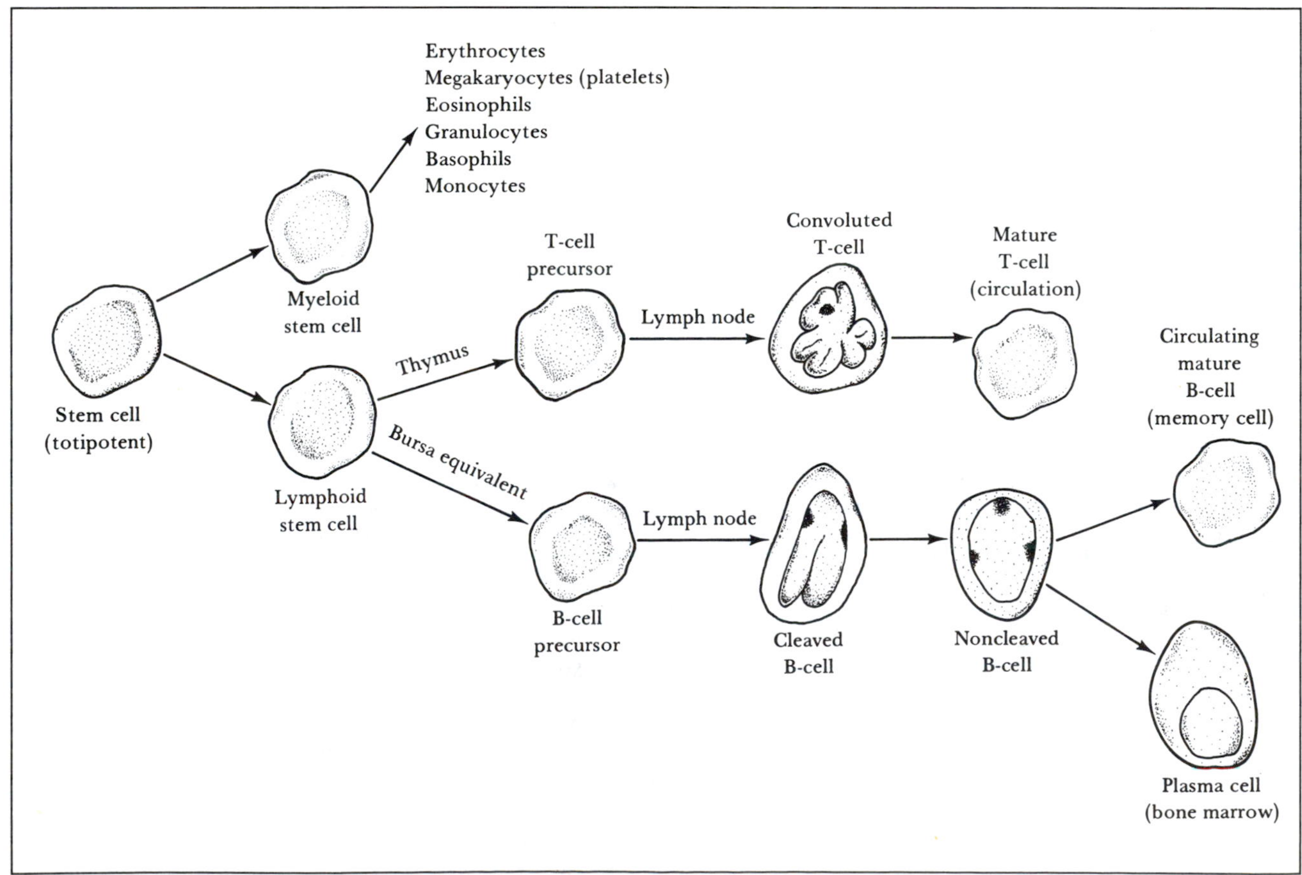

FIGURE 47-4 Maturation sequence of the lymphocyte. (Illustrated by J. Thommen.)

HODGKIN'S DISEASE

Historical Perspective

In 1832, Dr. Thomas Hodgkin, an English physician, described clinical data and postmortem findings of seven patients with a relentlessly progressive, ultimately fatal tumorous enlargement of the lymph nodes, liver, and spleen.[14] His recognition that these pathologic changes represented a primary proliferation inherent in the nodal tissues themselves rather than a reactive, inflammatory process was extremely important and insightful. Prior to that time, lymphomas often had been mistaken for a common infectious disease, tuberculosis of the lymph nodes. Modern-day analysis of the high frequency of mycobacterial and fungal infections in patients with HD now identifies an underlying defect in cellular immunity as the likely causative factor.[15]

More than three decades after Hodgkin's paper was presented, Samuel Wilks rediscovered the original manuscript and, after further clinical clarification and elaboration, he attached the eponym "Hodgkin's disease" in 1865.[16] A review of the original tissues nearly 100 years later demonstrated that Hodgkin's cases actually represented examples of what we now call Hodgkin's disease as well as non-Hodgkin's lymphoma. All lymphomas were called HD until around the turn of the century when the giant, multinucleated cells in the nodal material of HD patients were characterized by Reed[17] and Sternberg,[18] and their names have been associated with the pathognomonic cell of HD ever since. Subsequently, those lymphomas demonstrating the Reed-Sternberg cell were classified as HD and those in which the cell was absent were called lymphosarcoma or reticulum cell sarcoma and later NHL. Although the nature and origin of the Reed-Sternberg cell remain uncertain, it is clear that this cell is useful in prognosis since lymphocytic malignancies that are similar in pathologic appearance behave differently according to the presence or absence of this cell.[6] Today, diagnosis of HD requires two components. First, the presence of Reed-Sternberg cells must be verified. Second, the diagnostic cells must be identified within an appropriate cellular background that is composed of a polymorphous mixture of apparently normal inflammatory cells in various proportions.[19]

Epidemiology

Hodgkin's disease currently accounts for approximately 15% of the malignant lymphomas and less than 1% of all cancers. However, because a disproportionate number of HD victims are young adults, it is viewed as a particularly serious problem. The American Cancer Society estimates that in 1993, 7900 new cases (4500 male, 3400 female), and 1500 deaths will occur.[7] The disease has a worldwide distribution, and its most prominent epidemiologic feature pertains to the distinct age-related incidence patterns that have been observed. In developed countries the incidence of HD is clearly bimodal. In these areas the disease is infrequent in children under 10 years old. Incidence rises rapidly in adolescence and has its first peak among young adults ages 20–30. Subsequently, it falls until after age 45; then the incidence of new cases begins to climb steadily. This second upslope continues throughout the seventh and eighth decades.[20] Similar bimodality appears to exist in less developed countries except that the young adult age peak is shifted closer to childhood. Of interest is the fact that as underdeveloped geographic areas become increasingly progressive, their incidence patterns of HD change as well. Histologic category and anatomic distribution also vary with age. The nodular sclerosis form of the disease predominates in young adults, while mixed cellularity is more common in middle age and lymphocyte-depleted HD is the predominant histology in the elderly.

It has been suggested that HD is really two separate entities and that the first incidence peak may represent a disease of viral etiology, more common in middle-class than in lower-class families and more common in developed than in undeveloped countries.[21] These characteristics are consistent with a virus that is widely disseminated under conditions of poor hygiene and which, if contracted, rarely leads to severe illness. Such a pattern favors the evolution of a subclinical or asymptomatic process in low socioeconomic groups and undeveloped countries because children in such circumstances are antigenically exposed at a very early age, when they are resistant and able to develop immunity. In middle-class families and developed nations, however, improved hygiene delays such exposure until adolescence or young adulthood.[6] Indeed, the general level of home hygiene has been found to correlate inversely with incidence—the better the general sanitation, the higher the risk of HD among children in the household. The second incidence peak of HD in those over 45 years of age appears to be relatively similar across all societal groups.[20]

Etiology

Although many theories have been proposed, the etiology of HD remains unclear. Because of clinical manifestations such as fever, chills, and leukocytosis and because of histologic similarity to a granulomatous process, an infectious source has long been a topic of speculation. Although only indirect evidence currently exists in support of this concept, several key factors have been identified. First, a herpes virus, originally described by Epstein-Barr and referred to as *Epstein-Barr virus* or *EBV*, is now recognized as the likely cause of one form of NHL, Burkitt's lymphoma.[22] In addition, EBV is the known etiologic agent of infectious mononucleosis. Even though laboratory evidence to date does not directly implicate EBV in the etiology of HD, it has been confirmed that among large populations of patients with infectious mononucleosis there is an increased risk of subsequently developing HD.[20]

Recent information concerning HD in HIV-infected patients reveals that the AIDS population is subject to a much more aggressive neoplastic process and exhibits distinct alterations in clinical features. Safai et al.[23] report that 80% of evaluated patients present with stage III or IV disease compared to an expected rate of only 40% in the non–HIV-infected population. Ninety percent of the patients manifest constitutional symptoms of fever, night sweats, and weight loss. In addition, unusual extranodal sites of involvement such as central nervous system, gastrointestinal tract, and skin frequently are diagnosed.[23]

Genetic and occupational predispositions for HD may also exist. Familial patterns have been documented, and HD clearly occurs with increased frequency in first-degree relatives of HD patients.[24,25] Although such findings might also be expected to lend support to the notion of an infectious vector, increased incidence has not been documented in marital partners or health care professionals caring for HD patients.[26] In contrast to other forms of cancer, evidence is sparse that chemical exposures are a significant factor in the development of HD. Persons employed in woodworking and using benzene compounds may be at increased risk, but current data are not convincing.[24]

Cellular Abnormalities

Although humoral immunity appears to remain relatively intact, patients in all stages of HD exhibit a molecular defect characterized by markedly reduced cellular immunity. This deficit is manifested by impaired delayed hypersensitivity skin reactions and reduced T-cell proliferation following antigenic stimulation. They also display increased susceptibility to infectious complications from opportunistic pathogens such as herpes zoster, cytomegalovirus, and *Pneumocystis carinii*.[27]

Despite recent advances in the understanding of the cellular origin of the NHLs, the delineation of cytogenetic abnormalities in HD has been very sluggish. Specific problems in HD include a lower mitotic index and a paucity of malignant Reed-Sternberg cells in the tissues of HD patients in comparison to the normal lymphoid components. Among recent studies, cytogenetic analysis suggests that the oncogene *bcl-2* has a role in the pathogenesis of HD.[28] In addition, chromosomal analyses indicate that 70% of HD tumors have an abnormal karyotype. Hyperdiploidy is a characteristic feature, and structural rearrangements of chromosome 1 are frequently observed. However, the overall clinical and biologic significance of these aberrations remains to be determined.[29]

Clinical Manifestations

A typical HD patient presents with a slow, insidious, superficial lymphadenopathy. Characteristic nodes of variable size (from 1 cm to several centimeters) are firm, rubbery, and freely movable. Occasionally their size varies spontaneously over a period of several days. The enlarged nodes may be unilateral or bilateral, and most are located in the cervical and supraclavicular areas. Axillary and inguinal involvement is reported in less than 10% of the patients. A second common presentation, mediastinal adenopathy, is often recognized during routine chest roentgenogram. Overall, the adenopathy is usually painless unless lymph node growth is rapid. However, pain does occur in about 20% of the cases following ingestion of alcohol.

Constitutional symptoms of fever, malaise, night sweats, weight loss (>10% of normal body weight), and pruritus appear in about 40% of affected individuals. A classic clinical sign of HD is the Pel-Ebstein fever, in which cyclical bouts of high fevers become increasingly frequent and nearly continuous.[30] These manifestations, called *B symptoms,* are more common in patients with advanced disease.

The spread of HD is via contiguous nodal groups, and the pattern is quite predictable. In general, symptomatology and prognosis are related to the location and number of disease sites. Local pressure symptoms may arise from enlarged mediastinal nodes causing cough, dyspnea, dysphagia, pleural effusions, and, in extreme situations, superior vena cava syndrome. An enlarged spleen will result in left upper quadrant pain. Jaundice may evolve due to hepatic extension or extrahepatic bile duct obstruction. Retroperitoneal adenopathy often induces gastrointestinal and genitourinary dysfunction, abdominal pain, and ascites. Bone pain and fractures may be caused by secondary skeletal involvement of the vertebrae, ribs, and sternum. Herpes zoster infections are a relatively frequent finding and usually indicate impending epidural involvement. Exfoliative dermatitis and intense pruritus develop when the lymphatics of the skin are involved; indeed, they are often the first subjective symptoms to be reported.[31]

Assessment

The diagnosis of HD can be established only by biopsy of involved tissue, usually a lymph node. Cervical nodes are preferable to axillary and inguinal nodes because the latter often reveal evidence of chronic inflammatory changes. Occasionally, multiple biopsies are necessary for proper evaluation since reactive hyperplasia of nodes adjacent to those involved with tumor may provide equivocal results. It is important to remember that there are many causes of lymphadenopathy, especially in younger individuals. These include upper respiratory infections (bacterial or viral), infectious mononucleosis, allergic reactions, and other nonspecific causes. Older persons with cancers of the head and neck also may present initially with enlarged cervical nodes.

When an abnormal node is palpated during routine physical examination or when the patient reports such a complaint, a careful history and physical examination should be performed. If there is evidence of a recent infection or other nonmalignant process, the physician may choose to delay biopsy and observe the clinical course. In most cases, lymphadenopathy of infectious origin will usually resolve in a few days or weeks. When the adenopathy persists or the etiology is not apparent, a biopsy is generally indicated. Because a family history of HD increases the risk to other siblings, this, too, may be a factor in the decision process. In the absence of fever or overt systemic complaints, the detection of an enlarged lymph node in the neck of an older person is an indication that a careful search of the mouth, pharynx, and larynx for the presence of a malignant process should be made. Once a diagnosis is confirmed, it is necessary to obtain accurate histologic typing and staging of the disease in order to determine the precise prognosis and selection of therapy.[6]

Histopathology

Hodgkin's disease is distinguished from other lymphomas by the presence of the Reed-Sternberg cell. This is a large, bizarre cell with two or more mirror-image nuclei, each containing a single prominent nucleolus. Unlike most cancers, this characteristic cell represents only a small fraction of the cells in a malignant lymph node. Normal lymphocytes, plasma cells, and fibrous stroma comprise the bulk of palpable tissue. Although Reed-Sternberg cells are essential for the diagnosis of HD, they also have been reported in other conditions such as lymphoid hyperplasia, infectious mononucleosis, nonlymphoid malignancies (carcinomas and sarcomas), and phenytoin (Dilantin) therapy.[32]

The current histopathologic classification of HD was established in 1966 by an international conference in Rye, New York.[33] Four distinct subtypes of HD were enumerated: nodular sclerosis, lymphocyte-predominant, mixed cellularity, and lymphocyte-depleted. Each category has well-defined characteristics and manifests certain features of natural history (Table 47-1). Prior to the availability of highly curative chemotherapy and radiation therapy, these subtypes also implied notable differences in expected survival. However, recent therapeutic advances have rendered each of them potentially curable.

TABLE 47-1 Rye Classification of Hodgkin's Disease

Histology	Frequency (%)	Features
Nodular sclerosis	30–70	Stage I and II disease Young females predominate
Lymphocyte-predominant	10–15	Middle-age peak Males predominate Localized stage I and II disease
Mixed cellularity	20–40	Males predominate Intermediate prognosis B symptoms common
Lymphocyte-depleted	5–15	Older males predominate Widespread dissemination Poor prognosis

Nodular sclerosis (NS), with its unique age incidence (between ages 15 and 34) and its different sex incidence (females more commonly than males), has a singular histologic makeup that does not fit into the spectrum presented by the other three types. In NS-HD, the lymph node is divided into nodules by sclerosing bands of collagen. Lymphocytes within these collagen-bound nodules may be of various types, from predominantly small lymphocytes to large histiocytic forms. A variation of the Reed-Sternberg cell, the lacunar cell, is an identifiable feature of this subtype. Most patients are asymptomatic at presentation and exhibit stage I or II disease. They also tend to be clustered in the urban areas of developed countries. Anterior mediastinal involvement is exceedingly common and ultimately may involve cervical, supraclavicular, and upper abdominal lymph nodes as well as the spleen. Bulky mediastinal disease often contributes to metastatic infiltration of the lung parenchyma.

The other three histologic types of HD exhibit a range of prognoses from good to poor. The *lymphocyte-predominant (LP)* is characterized by sheets of mature-appearing small lymphocytes and few Reed-Sternberg cells. Patients usually present with localized stage I or II disease, primarily in the cervical lymph nodes. Peak incidence occurs in the fourth or fifth decades, and B symptoms are uncommon. Its natural history is usually indolent. Outcome is quite favorable.

Mixed cellularity (MC) HD is intermediate between lymphocyte-predominant and lymphocyte-depleted in terms of histology and prognosis. Disorderly fibrosis may be seen, but the broad fibrous bands indicative of the NS subtype are absent. There is a wide age range that peaks in the 30–40-year-old age group, and male cases predominate. More than 50% of the patients have stage III or IV disease and the majority manifest B symptoms. Extranodal abdominal extension is common.

Lymphocyte-depleted (LD) HD is the most aggressive of the four Rye classifications. It is marked by a paucity of small lymphocytes and an increased number of Reed-Sternberg cells. Two slightly different variants have been identified—reticular and diffuse fibrosis. Reticular LD-HD patients often present with bone marrow infiltration and peripheral lymphadenopathy. Those with diffuse fibrosis are more likely to exhibit lymph node and visceral involvement. Patients in this group are usually elderly males with advanced-stage disease and B symptoms. Prior to the advent of combination therapy, it carried a very poor prognosis. It is interesting to note that in some retrospective histologic studies, up to one-third of LD-HD tumors have been reclassified as NHL.[19]

Staging

After the diagnosis of HD has been established on the basis of lymph node biopsy and the histologic type has been determined in accordance with the outlined criteria, the next step in patient management is the careful determination of the extent of the disease. This process is referred to as *staging* and it indicates the degree of systemic progression and the intensity of treatment that will be required; it also allows the clinician to draw an inference with regard to the disease process.

Beginning in 1970, most HD patients were staged according to the Ann Arbor Classification System.[34] Over time, however, adherence to its guidelines became less strict due to: (1) new features of recognized prognostic importance, (2) questions concerning the need for staging laparotomy, and (3) advances in diagnostic imaging techniques that facilitated recognition of occult disease sites. In an effort to address these issues, a meeting was convened in Cotswolds, England, in 1989. Specialists in attendance approved criteria for a new system that retained the original Ann Arbor framework but included modifications incorporating designations for number of sites and bulk of disease.[35] Figure 47-5 provides a schematic representation of the new Ann Arbor–Cotswolds classification system created for both HD and NHL.

Lymph node involvement in just one area is designated as stage I disease. Involvement of two or more areas confined to one side of the diaphragm constitutes stage II. In stage III, lymph node groups above and below the diaphragm are affected. The spleen may be involved (stage IIIs), and this often precedes widespread hematogenous dissemination. In HD, stage III is subdivided further into stage III_1 for disease limited to the upper abdomen (spleen and splenic, hilar, celiac, and/or porta hepatis nodes), and stage III_2 for disease involving the lower abdomen (periaortic, pelvic, or inguinal nodes). Stage IV is marked by diffuse extralymphatic progression that may affect, for example, the liver, bone marrow, lung, and skin. A subscript *E* in stages I, II, and III indicates localized extranodal ex-

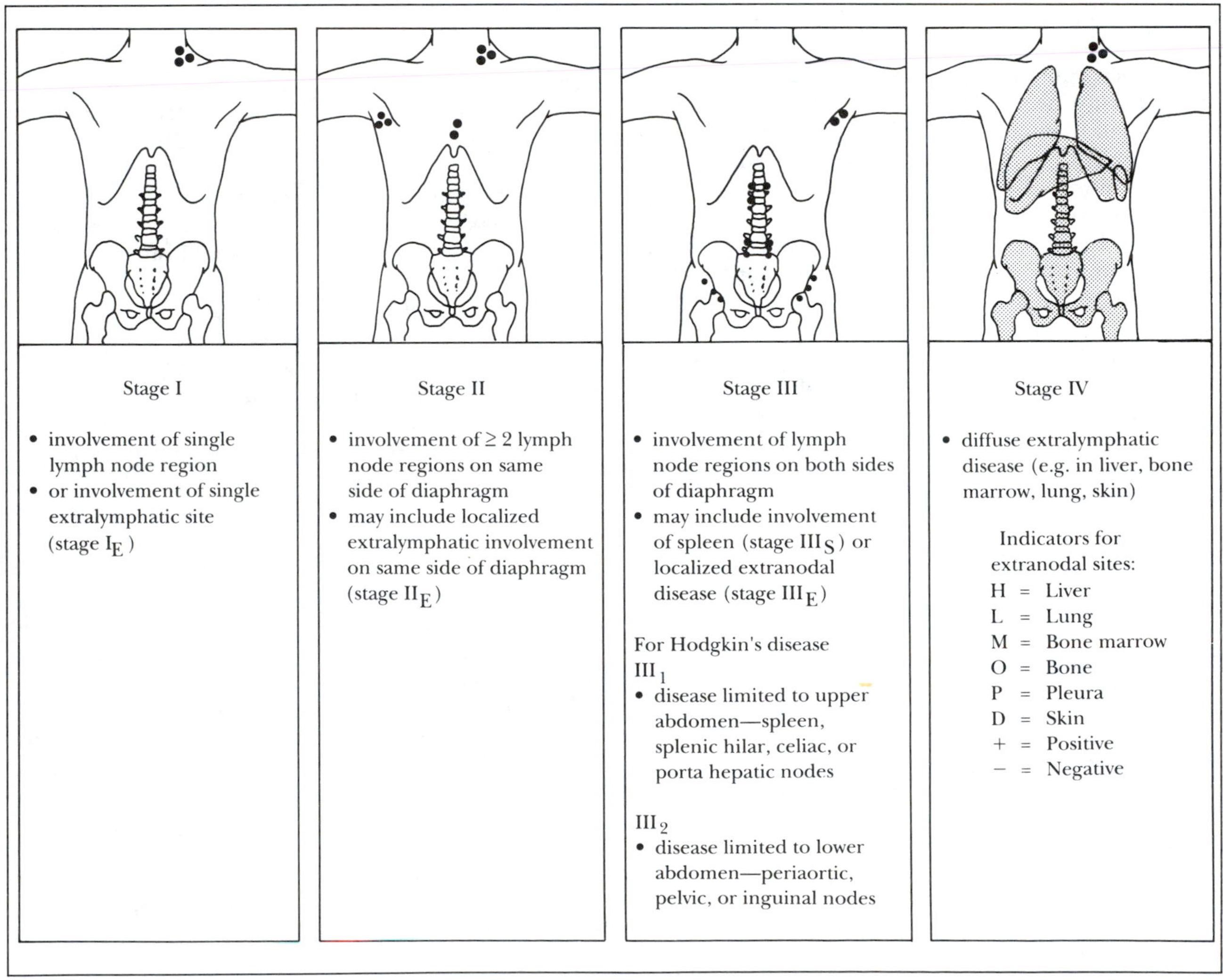

FIGURE 47-5 Ann Arbor–Cotswolds staging system for Hodgkin's disease and non-Hodgkin's lymphoma. (Source: Skarin AT [ed]: *Dana Farber Cancer Institute Atlas of Diagnostic Oncology*. Philadelphia: Lippincott, 1991. Reprinted with permission.)

tension from a nodal mass, and designation of a stage as either *A* or *B* indicates the absence *(A)* or presence *(B)* of unexplained weight loss greater than 10% of body weight in the preceding 6 months and/or fever of greater than 38°C and/or night sweats. Subscript *X* is indicative of bulky disease.

The adoption of this classification schema implies a dual system of stage designation according to both clinical and pathologic criteria. Clinical staging (CS) rests on history, physical examination, initial diagnostic biopsy, laboratory tests, and radiographic evidence. Pathologic staging (PS) adds definitive histopathologic information obtained through biopsy of strategic sites.[36] It is customary to specify whether a stage is determined on the basis of clinical signs alone (e.g., an abdominal lymphangiogram) or on the basis of pathologic examination of a biopsy section. Thus, a patient may be referred to as having "clinical" stage III (CS III) or "pathologic" stage III (PS III), depending on the strength of the evidence.[6] The nurse should be familiar with the essential procedures and terms used in diagnostic staging (Table 47-2) in order to help a patient follow the sequence and understand the significance of the evaluative work-up.

A controversial component of the staging process is the exploratory laparotomy, an extensive surgical procedure that includes splenectomy, wedge and needle liver biopsies, anterior iliac crest bone marrow biopsy, and extensive biopsy and dissection of abdominal lymph nodes. Although surgical mortality is quite uncommon, morbidity may include wound infection, subphrenic abscess, pulmonary embolus, stress ulcer, gastrointestinal bleeding, and wound dehiscence. In addition, splenectomy patients face the lifelong risk of a septic event from encapsulated organisms. Removal of the spleen may also be a factor in the development of secondary acute myeloid leukemia or myelodysplasia.[19] Current recommendations advocate that staging laparotomy be utilized only when the surgical findings will either (a) alter the extent of radiation therapy to be administered or (b) make chemotherapy rather than radiation therapy the primary treatment modality. With more recent movement toward a combined modality approach, especially in patients with bulky stage II disease or confirmed stage III_2 A disease, the need for laparotomy to define possible sites of occult intraabdominal disease has become limited.[20]

TABLE 47-2 Staging Procedures for Hodgkin's Disease

CLINICAL STAGING (CS)
Adequate surgical biopsy reviewed by an experienced hemopathologist. In primary extranodal lymphomas, biopsy should also include a lymph node when palpable.
Detailed history with special attention to the presence or absence of systemic symptoms
Careful physical examination, emphasizing node chains, size of liver and spleen, Waldeyer's ring inspection, and bony tenderness
Routine laboratory tests: complete blood count, erythrosedimentation rate, liver function tests, serum uric acid, serum copper
Chest roentgenogram (posteroanterior and lateral) with measurement of mass/thoracic ratio
Bilateral lower extremity lymphogram
Chest and abdominal computed CT scan or MRI
Radioisotopic evaluation with gallium 67 when the results of other conventional diagnostic procedures are inconclusive
PATHOLOGIC STAGING (PS)
Core needle biopsy of bone marrow from posterior iliac crest. Biopsy should be bilateral, especially in the presence of CS III and in patients with systemic symptoms.
Needle or surgical biopsy of any suspicious extranodal (eg, hepatic, splenic, osseous, pulmonary, cutaneous) lesion(s)
Cytologic examination of any effusion
Staging laparotomy with splenectomy, needle and wedge biopsy of liver, and biopsies of para-aortic, mesenteric, portal, and splenic hilar lymph node remains indicated after negative bone marrow biopsy in initial stages (CS I to II) only if therapeutic decisions will depend on the identification of occult abdominal involvement

Source: Bonadonna G, Wiernik PH, Santoro A: Clinical treatment of Hodgkin's disease. In Wiernik PH, Canellos GP, Kyle RA, Schiffer CA (eds): *Neoplastic Diseases of the Blood* (2d ed). New York: Churchill Livingstone, 1991. Reprinted with permission.

Treatment

The initial treatment plan for HD is crucial in determining eventual outcome because the overwhelming majority of patients, even those in the most advanced disease stages, are potentially curable if optimal therapy is employed. A comprehensive approach is essential and requires input from a variety of disciplines (radiology, surgery, pathology, medical oncology) working together collaboratively as an interdisciplinary team.

Association with multiple physicians and the complexity of the staging procedures often cause a patient to feel confused and overwhelmed. In many cases the nurse may be the only constant contact this individual has with the diagnostic and treatment teams. Therefore, it is essential that psychological support be provided as the individual adjusts to the full ramifications of a malignant diagnosis. The diverse procedures to which the patient will be subjected may require clarification and repeated explanations. These should be given with understanding, empathy, compassion, and tact.[6,37]

Current treatment recommendations are relatively noncontroversial and guidelines for stage-specific ther-

TABLE 47-3 Guidelines for Treatment of Hodgkin's Disease

Stage	Recommended Therapy	Alternative Therapy
I, II (A or B, negative laparotomy)	Subtotal lymphoid irradiation	Irradiation to involved field with combination chemotherapy
I, II (A or B, with mediastinal mass >⅓ diameter of the chest)	Combination chemotherapy followed by irradiation to involved field	Subtotal lymphoid irradiation followed by chemotherapy
III A_1, (minimal abdominal disease)	Total lymphoid irradiation	Combination chemotherapy with irradiation to involved sites
III A_2, (extensive abdominal disease)	Combination chemotherapy with irradiation to involved sites	Total lymphoid irradiation or combination chemotherapy alone
III B	Combination chemotherapy	Combination chemotherapy with irradiation to involved sites
IV (A or B)	Combination chemotherapy	Combination chemotherapy with irradiation to involved sites

Source: Eyre HJ, Farver ML: Hodgkin's disease and non-Hodgkin's lymphoma. In Holleb AI, Fink DJ, Murphy GP (eds): *Textbook of Clinical Oncology.* Atlanta, GA: the American Cancer Society, 1991. Reprinted with permission.

apies are outlined on Table 47-3. In all instances, the primary objective is to cure the most patients with the least therapy in order to avoid complications to the greatest extent possible. Since nearly one-third of all HD patients die without evidence of lymphoma at autopsy, the prevention of iatrogenic complications must be of paramount importance.[36]

Radiation therapy is curative in most patients with limited disease. Several important factors impact upon its effectiveness—skilled use of linear accelerators, careful field simulation, administration of tumoricidal doses, and comprehensive follow-up. The radiation fields commonly employed in HD may be divided into three volumes: the mantle, the paraaortic, and the pelvis (Figure 47-6). In order to achieve high cure rates, each of these fields generally must be extended to include adjacent, clinically negative nodal sites. Carefully constructed field shapes and blocks are used to protect the lungs, heart, spinal cord, larynx, kidneys, iliac crests, and gonads. All standard radiation treatments employ an opposed field, usually anterior-posterior, technique to provide homogenous dose distribution and to minimize potential radiation damage.[2]

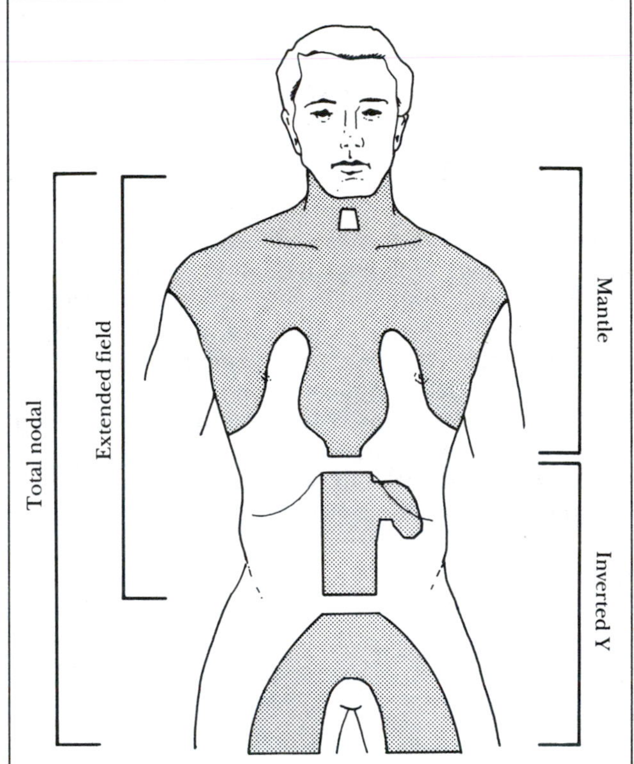

FIGURE 47-6 Standard radiation fields for Hodgkin's disease. Mantle—from mandible to diaphragm. Lungs, heart, spinal cord, and humeral heads are shielded. Inverted Y—from diaphragm to ischial tuberosities, including the spleen if not removed; spinal cord, kidneys, bladder, rectum, and gonads are shielded. Extended Field—involves mantle zone and uppermost inverted Y zone; does not include the pelvic, inguinal, or femoral nodes. Total Nodal—mantle zone and complete inverted Y zone.

For stage I A and II A disease above the diaphragm, without bulky mediastinal extension, mantle irradiation to a total dose of 3500–4400 cGy over a period of 4–6 weeks is advocated. Para-aortic lymph nodes are usually included except in those with mediastinal involvement or those with lymphocyte predominant histology. Stage III_1 A patients having only splenic involvement may be treated with total or subtotal nodal irradiation. Generally, total nodal irradiation is considered inappropriate for stage III_2 A individuals.[38] If careful laparotomy staging has been conducted, patients with stage II B disease may receive total or subtotal nodal radiotherapy; otherwise, chemotherapy is indicated. When bulky mediastinal disease is known to be present, combination radiation and chemotherapy are unequivocally required. In addition, the combined approach is usually indicated for patients with adverse prognostic factors such as B symptoms, bulky masses, or disease involving nodes in the lower abdomen.

Therapeutic advances in HD have provided much of the foundation of modern medical oncology. Single-agent therapy produces complete and partial responses, but the remissions are usually of limited duration. However, individual drugs can be useful in palliating advanced disease in the elderly and in managing patients with severe myelosuppression who are unable to tolerate combination chemotherapy due to prior intensive treatment.[2] An alkylating agent such as mechlorethamine or cyclophosphamide is generally selected, and therapy is continued until the patient relapses or excessive toxicity occurs. Once an initial response is obtained, an oral alkylating agent is required for maintenance.[36]

Because of their high response and durable remission rates, the MOPP regimen (Table 47-4) and the ABVD regimen (Table 47-5) have become the benchmarks for combination chemotherapy in HD. Both regimens are routinely administered in 28-day cycles for a minimum of six cycles. As a rule, chemotherapy is continued for two cycles after complete remission is documented.[19] Each combination can be expected to produce remissions in more than 80% of previously untreated patients, and 60%–70% of those who achieve complete remission will be alive with no evidence of disease after 10 years, presumably cured.[6] No relapses have been seen beyond 42 months after induction of a complete response with MOPP.[39]

Overall, either MOPP or ABVD can be expected to produce a complete remission in more than half of the patients who have recurrent disease after treatment with the other combination. At present, there is no evidence that maintenance therapy adds to cure for patients in remission.[6] It is important to note that recent studies indicate ABVD may actually be superior to MOPP because it eliminates the leukemogenesis and permanent male sterility associated with regimens containing alkylating agents.[40,41]

The combined use of MOPP and ABVD, in three alternating cycles of each, shows evidence of being superior to either regimen alone.[41] Underlying principles contributing to this success are based on the Goldie-Coldman hypothesis and include avoidance of drug cross-resistance, prevention of overlapping organ toxicity, and maintenance of full dosage and optimal administration schedules.[42] Other combinations that seek to reduce known complications such as infection, gastrointestinal disturbances, and hemorrhagic cystitis are also under investigation.[43,44]

The success of aggressive chemotherapeutic regimens is quite dependent on the dosage and timing of drug administration because even minor alterations can have a substantial impact on efficacy. The reduction of doses and omission of drugs to avoid nausea and vomiting, with its attendant loss of curative potential, is truly a poor bargain for any patient.[19] Nursing can play a pivotal role in promoting patient compliance by providing emotional support, effective symptom management, and reassurance about the finite nature of the treatment program.

Refinements in treatment protocols have led to the identification of specific subsets of patients who appear to benefit from combined chemotherapy and radiation therapy.[45] These patients present with what has been called "bulky" disease, usually defined as adenopathy greater than one-third the width of the chest on x-ray examination. This pattern of disease has a high recurrence rate after radiotherapy alone and poses some risk in exploratory laparotomy because the mediastinal mass may complicate anesthesia.[46,47] It is probably best for chemotherapy to be used as an adjunct after radiotherapy in these patients.[6,48]

Residual or recurrent disease poses a unique challenge. For patients with a favorable prognosis (e.g., limited disease at recurrence, good performance status, absence of B symptoms, age <60 years, slow-growing residual tumor), salvage therapy is a potential option.[36,49] Those who relapse following irradiation can be treated with chemotherapy, and, under certain cir-

TABLE 47-4 The MOPP Regimen for Hodgkin's Disease

Drug	Dosage	Schedule
Nitrogen mustard	6 mg/m² IV	Days 1 and 8
Vincristine (Oncovin)	1.4 mg/m² IV	Days 1 and 8
Procarbazine	100 mg/m² PO	Days 1 through 14
Prednisone (cycles 1 and 4 only)	40 mg/m² PO	Days 1 through 14

Repeat cycle every 28 days for a minimum of six cycles. Complete remission must be documented before discontinuing therapy.

TABLE 47-5 The ABVD Regimen for Hodgkin's Disease

Drug	Dosage	Schedule
Doxorubicin	25 mg/m² IV	Days 1 and 15
Bleomycin	10 units/m² IV	Days 1 and 15
Vinblastine	6 mg/m² IV	Days 1 and 15
Dacarbazine (DTIC)	375 mg/m² IV	Days 1 and 15

Repeat cycle every 28 days for a minimum of six cycles. Complete remission must be documented before discontinuing therapy.

cumstances, additional radiation may be possible. When relapse occurs after chemotherapy, the extent of the disease-free interval is very important. If relapse takes place more than 12 months after initial therapy, the patient can be retreated with the same agents and the probability of long-term survival remains high.[50]

When relapse transpires less than 12 months after initial remission, patients are seldom cured with conventional salvage therapies. A host of exciting approaches are currently under investigation that offer hope to this population. Recently, autologous bone marrow transplantation has become a viable treatment choice for an expanding number of individuals. About 30% of HD patients whose disease is not eradicated with conventional therapy experience long-term, disease-free survival with this modality. Depending on prior exposure to radiation therapy, patients receive either high-dose cytoreductive chemotherapy or chemotherapy plus total body irradiation. Both have been used with success.[51–53] Although current data are limited, patients with prior bone marrow damage or infiltration may have a promising alternative in transplantation with autologous peripheral blood stem cells.[54] Future efforts to reduce morbidity and mortality in this population must focus on identifying the optimal high-dose therapy, decreasing nonmarrow toxicity, and shortening the post transplant period of aplasia. Progress in achieving the latter goal is indicated by recent clinical trials that reveal that morbidity due to infection is likely to be reduced when granulocyte-macrophage colony stimulating factor is used to enhance hematopoietic recovery following transplantation.[52]

NON-HODGKIN'S LYMPHOMAS

Historical Perspective

The non-Hodgkin's lymphomas are a diverse group of neoplasms derived from the different developmental and functional subdivisions of the lymphoreticular system.[15] Although these malignancies have many features in common, they also reflect the diversity of their normal counterpart cells and exhibit a wide range of immunologic and biologic characteristics. There is no precise definition of NHL that is universally accepted, and although many meet the criteria that have been proposed for neoplasia, others lurk in a nebulous arena between benign lymphoproliferation and true malignancy.[55]

Throughout the nineteenth century, scientists used a variety of terms (e.g., *giant follicle lymphoma, lymphosarcoma,* and *reticulum cell sarcoma*) to categorize these tumors, and "pseudoleukemia" became a catchall for a host of conditions that exhibited lymphadenopathy and splenomegaly. Use of these designations persisted into the twentieth century and did much to obscure the delineation and subclassification of NHL.[56]

Recent technological refinements have enabled pathologists and clinicians to classify NHL according to a number of individual determinants including their ability to reproduce the same cytoarchitecture (follicular versus diffuse), cell size (small or large), nuclear characteristics (cleaved or noncleaved, convoluted or cerebriform), and immunological ontogeny (T-cell or B-cell lymphocytes).[55] Today the most accurate definition of lymphoma type is one that includes each of these elements. Further differentiation appears to be on the horizon, and future designations will likely include genetic markers as well.

Epidemiology

In the United States, NHL is diagnosed nearly 6 times as often as HD, and its death rate is 13 times greater. American Cancer Society statistics for 1993 indicate that 43,000 new cases and 20,500 deaths will occur.[7] Age-adjusted incidence is somewhat higher in males than in females (24,000 to 19,000), and the white population is affected more than the black population. Data suggest that environmental factors are mainly responsible for the differences in racial incidence rates; thus, it seems likely that a continuing increase of NHL will be seen in blacks as variations in lifestyle are lessened. Age-specific analyses reveal a preadolescent peak, a late teenage drop, and then a logarithmic rise with increasing age that persists into the eighth decade. The current mean is in the fifth decade. Like HD, higher mortalities are associated with higher socioeconomic status and urban residence.[57]

Because of the many available classification schemes for NHL, it is difficult to compare the incidence or frequency of the histological subtypes of lymphoma in different parts of the world. However, a rising incidence appears to be noted internationally; there has been a one- to twofold increase in most Western countries since 1960.

Etiology

The heterogeneity of NHL suggests that a variety of factors including viral infections, genetic abnormalities, and immune disturbances interact in the pathogenesis. The most convincing evidence of a viral etiology of malignant lymphoma has come from the studies of adult T-cell leukemia/lymphoma (ATL). A unique RNA retrovirus, human T-cell leukemia/lymphoma virus type I (HTLV-I), has been isolated from lymphocytes of patients with ATL in endemic areas of southwestern Japan, the Caribbean, and southeastern United States. ATL is primarily a disease of adults over 40 years old. Its manifestations include a high frequency of cutaneous infiltration, hepatosplenomegaly, lymphadenopathy, and hypercalcemia.[58]

Epstein-Barr virus (EBV), a DNA herpes virus, is the most likely etiologic agent for another form of NHL,

Burkitt's lymphoma (BL). This neoplasm is confined almost exclusively to endemic areas of Africa and New Guinea, and, indeed, evidence of EBV infection is found in 96% of African cases of BL. In Africa, BL is a malignancy of childhood. The mean age at presentation is 7 years, and males are affected twice as often as females. The children usually present with large extranodal tumors involving the bones of the jaw (72%) and abdominal organs (56%), particularly the ovaries, kidneys, and retroperitoneum. Although the etiology of BL is unknown, a current hypothesis focuses on an acute malarial infection as the environmental factor that interacts with a susceptible host immune system to predispose an individual to EBV-induced lymphoma.[59,60] Recently, EBV has been linked to neoplastic proliferation in a variety of congenital, iatrogenic, and acquired immunodeficient conditions.[61,62]

Environmental factors and exposure to chemicals in the workplace also are implicated in the pathogenesis of NHL. Pesticides and fertilizers have been suspected because of increased lymphoma incidence among midwestern farmers born after 1900 and dying before age 65 years. Vinyl chloride workers in the U.S. tire manufacturing industry exhibit increases, as do anesthetists, chemists, and workers in petroleum refining, asbestos, and herbicide industries. Japanese survivors of the atomic bomb and patients receiving ionizing radiation for congenital disorders and HD also face increased neoplastic potential.[63]

Cellular Abnormalities

A consideration of the molecular pathogenesis of both B- and T-cell origin in NHL reveals several consistent features. In most cases, chromosomal translocations facilitate the identification of the genetic lesion responsible for oncogenesis. Nearly all individuals with BL have one of three translocations involving the *c-myc* proto-oncogene. These include chromosomes 8 and 14 (t 8;14), chromosomes 2 and 8 (t 2;8), and chromosomes 8 and 22 (t 8;22). The *bcl-1* oncogene (t 11;14) is seen in nearly 50% of low-grade lymphocytic lymphomas, while the majority of follicular lymphomas involve the *bcl-2* oncogene (t 14;18).[64,65]

Cytogenetic analysis of lymphoma cells has identified other abnormalities as well. Deletions on chromosome 6 are found in a significant portion of patients with large-cell lymphoma. Such a loss of chromosomal material may lead to deleterious effects via the elimination of functional suppressor or growth inhibitory genes. Gains of one or more whole chromosomes are common, and trisomy of chromosomes 2,3,7,18, and 21 have been described.[66] At present the sequence of events that explains the transformation of a normal lymphocyte into a lymphomatous cell is unknown. Optimally, a better understanding of the genetic mechanisms of malignancy will translate eventually into new strategies of treatment based on the biology of the disease.[57,67]

Clinical Manifestations

The non-Hodgkin's lymphomas encompass a spectrum of neoplasms ranging from indolent tumors, which can occasionally undergo spontaneous regression, to rapidly progressive tumors, which may be fatal within weeks if untreated. They are usually generalized diseases and can involve almost any organ or tissue, thus resulting in a wide array of systemic manifestations (Table 47-6). Some of the clinical features may be caused by chemical

TABLE 47-6 Systemic Alterations in Non-Hodgkin's Lymphoma

System	Manifestations
Lymphoid system	Lymphadenopathy—peripheral or central Hepatosplenomegaly Thymic (anterior superior mediastinal) mass Waldeyer's ring involvement Bone marrow involvement
Gastrointestinal system	Abdominal or pelvic mass Upper or lower gastrointestinal bleeding Malabsorption Intussusception Perforation Fistula Biliary obstruction Pancreatic mass Ascites Salivary gland swelling
Genitourinary system	Renal mass, ureteric obstruction Testicular mass Ovarian mass Vaginal bleeding
Nervous system	Meningeal involvement Cranial nerve palsies Intracranial mass (extradural or intracerebral) Paraspinal mass Intraorbital, periorbital or ocular mass Peripheral neuropathy Progressive multifocal leucoencephalopathy
Endocrine system	Thyroid mass Adrenal mass
Other	Bone involvement Paranasal sinus involvement Jaw involvement Skin infiltration Venous or (rarely) arterial obstruction Pericardial effusion Pulmonary infiltration
General	Pyrexia/night sweats Weight loss Lethargy

Source: Magrath IT, Wilson W, Horvath K, et al: Clinical features and staging. In Magrath IT (ed): *The Non-Hodgkin's Lymphomas.* Baltimore, MD: Williams & Wilkins, 1990. Reprinted with permission.

mediators produced by the lymphoma cells, by metabolic changes resulting from a high rate of cell death in the tumor, or by secondary events such as opportunistic infections, immunosuppression, and paraneoplastic electrolyte abnormalities.[68] In contrast to HD, 80% of patients with NHL present to their physicians with advanced disease (stage III or IV). This is usually reflected by painless, generalized lymphadenopathy. Systemic B symptoms (fever, night sweats, and/or weight loss) are the initial complaint in as many as 20% of the cases.[69] Although their presence signifies advanced disease, it is not as predictive of prognosis as in HD.

Extranodal lymphoma is seen in nearly 20% of individuals during initial evaluation and it generally is confirmed in more than 50% of cases at autopsy.[57] Gastrointestinal involvement is fairly common at presentation; the most frequent sites of infiltration are the stomach and small intestine. Malignancies originating in Waldeyer's ring of the nasopharynx have a particular propensity for gastric extension. Common clinical signs are pain, abdominal mass, and anorexia and, less commonly, nausea, vomiting, bleeding, diarrhea, or obstruction.

Pulmonary parenchymal disease is related most often to lymphatic tumor spread from hilar and mediastinal nodes, and cough, dyspnea, and chest pain are quite indicative of lung infiltration. Central lymphatic obstruction or pleural seeding with tumor may result in superior vena cava syndrome or pleural effusion. Lytic bone lesions are seen in the femurs, pelvis, vertebrae, ribs, and skull. Lymphomas occasionally infiltrate the skin as red or purplish nodules, primarily in the head and neck region, while tumorous replacement of the bone marrow can result in a leukemia-like picture in the peripheral blood. Liver involvement often occurs without signs or symptoms, and, unlike the situation in HD, splenic extension need not occur concomitantly. Solitary brain lymphomas are being reported with increasing frequency. They are often associated with AIDS or iatrogenic immunosuppression. These mass lesions may induce headaches, seizures, and changes in mental status. Another common central nervous system manifestation is leptomeningeal spread, which results in cranial nerve palsies, meningeal irritation, and increased intracranial pressure.[69]

Assessment

Because every enlarged lymph node does not necessarily represent NHL, careful histologic evaluation is the most important first step toward initiating proper care of the patient. When a lymphoma is suspected, the pathologist should be notified so that special processing procedures including cytogenetics, surface markers, immunohistochemistry stains, and molecular biologic studies can be used in addition to routine histology of biopsied specimens. Since NHL occurs more commonly in extranodal sites than HD, needle biopsies may be more diagnostically helpful; widespread visceral extension or occult retroperitoneal disease may require open biopsy or laparotomy for confirmation.

A careful history and physical examination should be precise in evaluating abnormal clinical manifestations and the length of time they have been present. This is particularly important in patients who present with vague constitutional complaints or with derangements referable to more than one organ system. In general, the principles governing assessment of NHL are the same as those previously identified for HD.

Histopathology

Few areas of pathology have evoked as much controversy and confusion as the classification of NHL, and the lack of consistent standardization makes international analysis and comparison extremely difficult.[69] The first widely accepted classification was proposed by Rappaport[70] in 1956. This scheme separates lymphomas on the basis of two morphologic features: (1) pattern of growth (nodular or diffuse depending on the macrostructure of the lymph node); and (2) the degree of cytologic differentiation of the predominant malignant cell. Tumors composed of cells similar in size and morphology to normal lymphocytes are considered *well-differentiated,* whereas those composed of irregularly shaped lymphocytes are referred to as *poorly differentiated.* If tumor cells are two to three times larger than small lymphocytes and have abundant cytoplasm, they are called *histiocytes* because of their resemblance to macrophages. *Undifferentiated* lymphomas are composed of intermediate-sized cells that fail to demonstrate evidence of either lymphoid or histiocytic origin. *Mixed lymphomas* are tumors formed by poorly differentiated lymphocytes and histiocytes.[71] Over the years, the Rappaport classification has been popular with clinicians because it is reproduced easily and correlates well with clinical observations. However, it gives little insight into the underlying pathophysiology.

As knowledge accumulated, additional categories were added. Lukes and Collins[72] proposed an immunologic classification system that provides important correlations with the pathophysiology of the lymphoreticular system. Their approach relates lymphoma cell morphology to the sequential stages in the histogenesis of normal B- and T-lymphocytes (Figure 47-3), and the observations are reinforced by the identification of specific T- or B-cell markers on the cell surfaces.

By the late 1970s, in addition to the schemes of Rappaport and Lukes and Collins, four other classifications were in use throughout the world. The alternatives included those of the British National Lymphoma Group, Dorfman, the World Health Organization, and Kiel. Recently, a study funded by the National Cancer Institute developed what is hoped will become an international standard of classification for NHL. The Working Formulation[73] was proposed as a means of translation among the various systems to facilitate clinical comparisons and therapeutic trials. The major classifications in the Working Formulation and their pathologic counterparts in the Rappaport and Lukes-Collins systems are compared in Table 47-7. The low-grade lymphomas are predominantly B-cell tumors; intermediate-grade lymphomas include B-cell and some T-cell neoplasms; immunoblastic malignancies are predominantly B-cell in origin, while the lymphoblastic group usually is composed of T-cell tumors. Burkitt's and non-Burkitt's lymphomas manifest B-cell origin, and the rare, true histiocytic lymphomas most likely are derived from the monocyte/macrophage line. Mycosis fungoides is a T-cell neoplasm.[2]

Although the diagnosis of NHL in the Working Formulation is based solely on morphologic features, it has predictive value for survival. Tumors with a good prognosis include all the low-grade NHLs and some of the intermediate-grade tumors with long natural histories. Tumors with a poor prognosis include the rapidly progressive high-grade tumors as well as the diffuse large-cell malignancies from the intermediate-grade group. However, because of their biologic behavior and clinical course, most treatment protocols recognize only two major groups—low-grade and high-grade.

Low-grade lymphomas

The low-grade category includes three tumors: small lymphocytic lymphoma; follicular, predominantly small cleaved cell lymphoma; and follicular mixed (small cleaved and large-cell) lymphoma. These malignancies occur predominantly in older individuals (median age is 55 years), and they affect males and females equally. The majority of patients are asymptomatic. The usual presenting problems are connected with a painless, progressive, often symmetrical generalized lymphadenopathy. Except for liver and bone marrow involvement, extranodal extension is uncommon. Tumor cells in the follicular lymphomas reveal a characteristic translocation of chromosomes 14 and 18. The breakpoint on chromosome 18 involves the locus where the proto-oncogene *bcl-2* has been mapped.[74]

Like normal lymphocytes, low-grade B-cell lympho-

TABLE 47-7 Non-Hodgkin's Lymphoma Nomenclature: Comparative Classifications

Working Formulation	Rappaport System	Lukes-Collins System
	LOW-GRADE	
A Small lymphocytic	Diffuse, well-differentiated lymphocytic	Small lymphocytic B-cell or T-cell
B Follicular, small cleaved	Nodular, poorly differentiated lymphocytic	Follicular, small cleaved FCC
C Follicular, mixed small cleaved, and large-cell	Nodular, mixed lymphocytic and histiocytic	Follicular, mixed small cleaved and large FCC
	INTERMEDIATE-GRADE	
D Follicular, large-cell	Nodular histiocytic	Follicular, large cleaved and/or non-cleaved FCC
E Diffuse, small cleaved	Diffuse, poorly differentiated lymphocytic	Diffuse, small cleaved FCC
F Diffuse, mixed small and large	Diffuse, mixed lymphocytic and histiocytic	Diffuse, mixed small and large cleaved or noncleaved FCC
G Diffuse, large-cell	Diffuse histiocytic	Diffuse, large cleaved or noncleaved FCC
	HIGH-GRADE	
H Immunoblastic, large-cell	Diffuse histiocytic	Immunoblastic sarcoma, B-cell or T-cell
I Lymphoblastic	Lymphoblastic	Convoluted T-cell
J Small, noncleaved Burkitt's	Undifferentiated, Burkitt's and non-Burkitt's	Small, noncleaved FCC
	MISCELLANEOUS	
Composite Mycosis fungoides Histiocytic Extramedullary plasmacytoma Unclassifiable Other		

FCC = follicular center cell.

mas often circulate; thus, patients generally present with widespread stage III or IV disease. Some patients describe a history of lymph nodes that wax and wane in size for many years prior to diagnosis. Host immunity has been invoked to explain this phenomenon, and, in some cases, clinical regression has been preceded by a viral or bacterial infection.[69]

Most low-grade lymphomas have a long natural history (median survival is 7–9 years) that appears to be largely unaffected by treatment. As the disease progresses, patients may complain of increasing fatigue, malaise, low-grade fever, night sweats, and weight loss. Eventually the general pace of the disease accelerates and the majority of indolent lymphomas convert from low-grade to intermediate- or high-grade malignancies. Treatment strategies must then be modified to be appropriate for aggressive lymphomas. Death usually results from progressive growth and eventual tumorous replacement of hematopoietic and lymphoid tissues, thereby producing multiple systemic dysfunctions. Although the overall picture for these lymphomas seems optimistic, the disease is usually fatal; median survival generally is less than 1 year after such transformation.[78]

Intermediate-grade lymphomas

There are four neoplasms under the intermediate-grade category in the Working Formulation—an uncommon tumor with a follicular architecture and three others with a diffuse pattern. The follicular, predominantly large-cell NHL has a more aggressive clinical course than that of the other more indolent subtypes of follicular lymphomas. Most patients have advanced disease at the time of diagnosis. Peripheral blood involvement is unusual. Immunologically, these are neoplasms of B-lymphocytes, and almost all cases exhibit translocations of chromosomes 14 and 18.

Because they share similar clinical, histologic, and immunologic features, the three diffuse subgroups in the Working Formulation can be grouped together. These lymphomas occur mainly in adults, and, unlike follicular NHL, patients with diffuse neoplasms often present with disease limited to one side of the diaphragm. Although nodal presentation is common, these subtypes frequently involve extranodal progression to the gastrointestinal tract, skin, and bone. Privileged sites such as the testes and central nervous system also may be involved. If left untreated, diffuse NHLs are invariably fatal and survival is less than 2 years. However, these malignancies are responsive to chemotherapy and a significant chance for cure exists, particularly in patients with localized disease.

High-grade lymphomas

High-grade lymphomas consist of three quite distinct diseases that are grouped together in the Working Formulation because of their aggressive clinical behavior and poor prognosis. The first of this group are immunoblastic lymphomas. The term *immunoblast* refers to an activated lymphocyte. Under the influence of mitogens and/or antigens to which the individual has been previously exposed, T- and B-cells transform from small or dormant lymphocytes to large, metabolically active, dividing forms.[71] The majority of immunoblastic tumors are of B-cell origin, although a small percentage with T-cell ontogeny are related to peripheral T-cell lymphomas. These neoplasms usually occur in adults over 50 years old. Anemia, B symptoms, and advanced stage are common at presentation, and a high incidence of cutaneous disease has been reported. It is of interest to note that approximately 50% of B-immunoblastic lymphomas are associated with a previous history of immunologic impairment such as that seen in Sjögren's syndrome or with states of immunosuppression as in transplant recipients or patients with AIDS.[74] Poor responses to chemotherapy and poor survival are characteristic of this group.

Lymphoblastic lymphoma is a high-grade, usually T-cell malignancy that is closely related to T-cell acute lymphocytic leukemia. Adolescents and young adults account for the majority of cases; 40% of childhood lymphomas fall into this category. Males outnumber females by a 2:1 ratio. Approximately two-thirds of the patients present with a prominent anterior mediastinal mass suggestive of a thymic origin. There is usually widespread involvement of lymph nodes, and lytic bone lesions are not uncommon. Unless effectively treated, patients have a rapidly progressive, downhill course with dissemination of tumor to the bone marrow, blood, cerebrospinal fluid, and central nervous system. Recent attempts to treat this malignancy with aggressive leukemic protocols and bone marrow transplantation offer new encouragement.[75]

Within the category of small, noncleaved cell lymphomas are two distinct subtypes. Burkitt's lymphoma occurs endemically in tropical Africa and New Guinea, where it is associated with the Epstein-Barr virus. As previously noted, this lymphoma is more common in males than females, and the average age at onset is 7 years. Massive involvement of the jaw, ovaries, kidneys, liver, mesentery, and central nervous system is a prominent feature. U.S. cases of BL are not associated with EBV and arise in slightly older children (11 years). Involvement of the ileocecal region of the bowel is common and often results in obstruction and intussception. Children older than 13 years of age at onset have a poorer prognosis. In general, Burkitt's tumors are highly sensitive to chemotherapeutic agents, and their response is often dramatic and enduring.

Non-Burkitt's lymphoma is a relatively uncommon malignancy. The median age is 34 years, and incidence is equal for males and females. Peripheral lymphadenopathy is a common clinical manifestation, and bone marrow, liver, central nervous system, and gastrointestinal tract are major sites for extranodal progression. In patients who have undergone treatment for HD and in those with AIDS, this type of lymphoma often occurs as a complicating factor.[76] Because the disease disseminates rapidly, even multiagent chemotherapy is generally ineffective, and the median survival is approximately 1 year.

Typically, aggressive lymphomas exhibit rapid tumor growth and a high mitotic index. Without treatment, survival is usually less than 18 months. However, because these neoplasms respond better to chemotherapy than the indolent, low-grade lymphomas, they have a greater potential for cure, especially if complete remissions are sustained for at least 2 years.[13] From a prognostic perspective, clinical evaluation of NHLs at the National Institutes of Health has revealed that the following features independently have an adverse effect on survival: male sex, poor performance status, B symptoms, anemia (hemoglobin <12 g/dl), high serum lactate dehydrogenase (>500 U), bone marrow involvement, liver involvement, large (>10 cm) abdominal mass, and age greater than 65 years.[71]

Mycosis fungoides (cutaneous T-cell lymphoma)

Among the miscellaneous group of lymphomas, the best characterized is a rare disorder referred to in older literature as *mycosis fungoides* and in current reviews as *cutaneous T-cell lymphoma (CTCL)*. Involvement of the skin is a hallmark of this malignancy that results from the clonal proliferation of T-lymphocytes. CTCL tends to be initially indolent, but it may evolve into a widely disseminated malignancy. The disease occurs in middle age, and males are affected more often than females. Histologically, there is infiltration of the epidermis and upper dermis with neoplastic T-cells, which have an extremely unusual cerebriform nucleus. Clinically, the lesions exhibit three distinct cutaneous stages. The initial premycotic stage is characterized by superficial inflammatory skin eruptions and generalized pruritus. In this stage, CTCL may be confused with other dermatologic disorders such as psoriasis and eczema. Eventually the disease progresses through an aggravated plaque stage to one with nodular tumors. In most patients with extensive disease, extracutaneous manifestations and visceral dissemination develop and ultimately lead to a fatal outcome. A variant of CTCL, the Sézary syndrome, presents with generalized exfoliative erythroderma and circulating leukemia-like cerebriform lymphocytes. The full implication of detecting circulating neoplastic cells has not been fully determined. In general, however, CTCL patients with a high percentage of circulating Sézary cells have a shorter survival compared to those with a lower percentage.[77]

Staging

Once a histologic diagnosis of NHL has been confirmed by biopsy, a careful, comprehensive staging work-up is essential to determine the extent of the disease, the bulk of the tumor mass, and the imminence of potential complications. The work-up enables the physician to provide an accurate prognosis and to plan effective treatment. Both the condition of the patient and the histopathologic classification of the tumor direct the type and speed of staging procedures to be performed. For example, an individual with a rapidly progressive, high-grade lymphoma whose natural history can be measured in weeks requires immediate initiation of therapy with only essential procedures performed beforehand. On the other hand, an indolent, low-grade lymphoma can be staged at the convenience of the patient and physician.[78]

Baseline studies for all patients should include complete history and physical examination with particular emphasis on all lymphoid tissue including liver, spleen, Waldeyer's ring, and lymph nodes. Also required are complete blood counts, blood chemistries including liver and kidney function tests, erythrocyte sedimentation rate, uric acid, serum immunoglobulins, and bone marrow biopsy. The latter is an important evaluative component because there is an high incidence of marrow involvement in stage III and IV disease in the low-grade lymphomas and an equal distribution of stage I and II versus stage III and IV with less marrow involvement in the intermediate- and high-grade groups.[2]

Unlike HD, where the disease sites are more predictable and orderly, the multiplicity of potential NHL locations and the variety of their clinical presentations forestall the adoption of a single radiologic scheme. All patients require a chest x-ray to facilitate detection of hilar adenopathy, mediastinal mass, parenchymal lung infiltration, or pleural/pericardial effusions. Computed tomography (CT) of the chest is advised when the X ray is suspicious. Abdominal and pelvic CT should be performed on all individuals because nodal and extranodal masses in these regions occur frequently in some subgroups.[68] The CT scan is replacing lymphangiography (LAG) in many patients because of its usefulness in detecting upper retroperitoneal and mesenteric nodes, as well as hepatic and splenic extension. These are important areas of assessment in most cases of NHL. LAG does have one distinct advantage: The dye often remains in nodal tissues for 6 months or more, so abnormal nodes can be closely monitored during treatment and follow-up.

Additional studies that may be appropriate in certain circumstances include multiple biopsies of the liver, removal of the spleen for pathologic study, and exploratory laparotomy for biopsy of multiple lymph node groups. As a rule, surgical evaluation of the abdomen should be undertaken only if it clearly makes a major difference in the treatment selection. However, in patients with extensive gastrointestinal disease, a staging laparotomy can be helpful in reducing the risk of perforation and/or bleeding complications.[2] A recent study indicates that refinements in endoscopic technology may eliminate the need for gastrectomy and its associated sequelae during the initial treatment phase of gastric lymphomas.[79] Table 47-8 outlines the current suggestions for staging procedures in NHL.

After the clinical evaluation is complete, patients are classified according to the criteria previously outlined for HD in the Ann Arbor–Cottswolds staging system

TABLE 47-8 Staging Procedures for Non-Hodgkin's Lymphoma

REQUIRED

1. Adequate surgical biopsy, reviewed by an experienced hematologist
2. A detailed history recording duration and the presence or absence of fever, unexplained sweating and its severity, unexplained pruritus, and unexplained weight loss
3. A careful and detailed physical examination; special attention to all node-bearing areas, including Waldeyer's ring (indirect laryngoscopy is the procedure of choice) and determination of size of liver and spleen
4. Necessary laboratory procedures
   a. Complete blood count, including an erythrocytic sedimentation rate
   b. Serum alkaline phosphatase
   c. Evaluation of renal function
   d. Evaluation of liver function
5. Radiologic studies include
   a. Chest roentgenogram (posteroanterior and lateral)
   b. Bilateral lower extremity lymphogram
   c. Abdominal-pelvic computed axial tomographic scan
6. Bilateral bone marrow needle biopsies (not just aspirates; biopsy should be performed before aspirate, if both are done together)

VARIABLE

1. Whole-chest tomography if any abnormality is noted or suspected on the routine chest roentgenogram
2. Abdominal ultrasonogram, inferior cavography, intravenous pyelogram or upper and lower GI contrast studies to supplement lymphographic findings or investigate sites of unexplained symptoms
3. Plain bone radiographs of symptomatic or tender areas
4. Head or spinal CT for neurologic signs or symptoms
5. Exploratory laparotomy and splenectomy, if management decision will depend on the identification of abdominal involvement. Note: Decision to proceed with laparotomy requires knowledge of treatment plan used at institution of record

ANCILLARY

1. Magnetic resonance imaging (under investigation)
2. Gallium whole-body scans
3. Skeletal scintigrams
4. Hepatic and splenic scintigrams
5. Serum chemistries to include serum calcium and uric acid for overall management of patient
6. Estimates of the patient's delayed hypersensitivity of the tuberculin type

Source: DeVita VT, Jaffe ES, Mauch P, et al: Lymphocytic lymphomas. In DeVita VT, Hellman S, Rosenberg SA (eds): *Cancer: Principles and Practice of Oncology,* (vol 2) (3d ed). Philadelphia: Lippincott, 1989. Reprinted with permission.

(Figure 47-5). It is important to note that this system is not as useful in directing the management of NHLs because these malignancies are characterized by early hematogenous dissemination and their natural history is poorly described by staging criteria based primarily on anatomical distribution. However, the clinical stage within each histologic subtype does appear to carry reliable prognostic significance.[78]

Treatment

The treatment of NHL usually requires a multidisciplinary approach to effect an optimal cure rate. This approach is determined by several key factors: histology of the tumor, stage of the disease, and physiologic performance status of the patient. The histologic grades of the Working Formulation represent a spectrum of survival in untreated patients that ranges from just weeks in the highly aggressive lymphomas to years in the indolent grades. Thus, the primary determinant in any treatment program is the natural history of the histologic subtype.

The second major consideration is the extent of disease. Unlike HD, with its organized progression via contiguous nodal groups, most NHLs are widely disseminated at diagnosis. Therefore, in order to be of any practical use, their staging must always be modified according to histology.

Evaluation of individual performance status is the final component in treatment planning. Because the primary goal for many lymphomas is cure, the majority of therapeutic regimens are quite toxic. However, the observed toxicities are nearly always dose-related and predictable. Although the patient's physical status, age, and underlying medical problems should be taken into consideration when planning aggressive therapy, it is important to remember that advanced age per se is not a contraindication to using an effective program. "Patients with aggressive lymphomas will have a short and unpleasant life because of the lymphoma. Those with potentially curable disease should therefore not be treated gently out of fear of causing toxicities. The alternative to effective therapy—gentle palliation—has a uniformly fatal outcome."[69] Table 47-9 delineates the recommended guidelines for treatment of NHL.

Indolent lymphomas

There is no area of lymphoma treatment that is more controversial than what, if any, approach, can alter the natural history of indolent or low-grade NHLs and induce their long-term, disease-free survival. This concern is quite understandable because the natural history of these malignancies has been such that, despite any therapeutic intervention, most patients live with their disease and eventually die from it. Although some physicians advocate a policy of "watchful waiting" until systemic symptoms require intervention, evidence is growing that radiation therapy is potentially curative in early-stage disease and intensive combined regimens may be beneficial in some of the advanced stages.

Up to 50% of individuals with low-grade, nonbulky stage I, I_E, or limited stage II lymphoma have survived 10 years relapse-free when treated with radiation therapy (RT).[80] Curative RT consists of 4000 cGy administered over 4 weeks to the entire tumor and adjacent

TABLE 47-9 Guidelines for Treatment of Non-Hodgkin's Lymphoma

Grade	Recommended Therapy		Alternative Therapy
	Stage I, II_1*	Stages II_2†, III, IV	
Low	Localized irradiation	Observation until disease progression, then palliative irradiation or single-agent or combination chemotherapy	Initial combination chemotherapy for stages III, IV
Intermediate	Combination chemotherapy with localized irradiation	Combination chemotherapy	Initial radiation followed by combination chemotherapy for stages I, II
High	Combination chemothrapy with localized irradiation	Combination chemotherapy	

*Stage II_1 = nonbulky disease.

†Stage II_2 = bulky disease >10 cm or ⅓ diameter of chest.

Source: Eyre HJ, Farver ML: Hodgkin's disease and non-Hodgkin's lymphoma. In Holleb AI, Fink DJ, Murphy GP (eds): *Textbook of Clinical Oncology.* Atlanta, GA: American Cancer Society, 1991. Reprinted with permission.

nodal areas. Good control rates generally are achieved with doses in excess of 3000 cGy. Suspected involvement of Waldeyer's ring and distant nodal groups often requires that treatment fields be extended.

In the majority of cases, low-grade NHL is diagnosed as a systemic disease. Newer staging techniques are revealing more frequent bone marrow, liver, spleen, and peripheral blood dissemination, and approximately 90% of all cases present in stages III and IV. Few in these advanced categories are ever cured with either RT or chemotherapy. Although generally regarded as indolent neoplasms, they are ultimately fatal. Given the lengthy, benign course experienced by most patients (median survival is 7–9 years), a conservative approach may be best. For those exhibiting systemic symptoms, administration of single oral alkylating agents such as chlorambucil or cyclophosphamide is often beneficial. Total body irradiation induces complete remissions in a large number of patients, but the average duration is only 2–3 years, and it is doubtful that any will remain disease-free at 10 years. To date there has been little study in this group of the more modern combination regimens that are effective in aggressive lymphomas.

A prospective study at the National Cancer Institute[69] may cause a change in "watchful" strategies. In a comparison of conservative treatment (no initial therapy) with aggressive combined modality use of PROMACE/MOPP flexitherapy followed by low-dose total lymphoid RT, results seem to indicate that aggressive interventions may be curative for a subset of indolent lymphoma patients with good prognostic indicators.[69] A new antimetabolite, fludarabine, also shows promise in similar patient populations.[81]

Aggressive lymphomas

Patients with unfavorable histology (intermediate- and high-grade lymphomas) have a much more aggressive disease process, which usually results in a rapid, downhill progression. Thus, there is no place for administration of single agents in the primary treatment plan. Historically, RT has been used with moderate success in those with stage I and II disease. Recently, the course of these malignancies has been significantly improved by the introduction of a combined modality approach.

The recognized treatment of choice for advanced-stage aggressive NHL is combination chemotherapy.[82] Over the past 20 years, therapeutic regimens of increasing intensity have evolved (Table 47-10). The initial combination of an alkylating agent, a vinca alkaloid, and a corticosteroid (CVP or COP) has been enhanced by the addition of doxorubicin and other agents, resulting in such protocols as CHOP, BACOP, and C-MOPP. These are usually given as monthly cycles for 6–9 months and produce long-term remissions in 35%–45% of cases.[69] The major problems associated with these combinations involve tumor regrowth between cycles and central nervous system relapse.[83]

Because of their ability to cross the blood-brain barrier, second-generation regimens such as M-BACOD, m-BACOD, PROMACE/MOPP, and COP-BLAM have been designed. These combinations use methotrexate with leucovorin rescue or cytosine arabinoside to prevent lymphomatous extension to the central nervous system. In an attempt to defeat the intrinsic drug resistance of tumor cell populations, they also utilize a staggered dose schedule for myelotoxic and nonmyelotoxic agents. Such protocols have been shown to enhance long-term survival.[70]

Attempts to refine programs with even more intense protocols have led to third-generation combinations such as MACOP-B, PROMACE/CYTABOM, and COP-BLAM III. The two major principles that have influenced their design are the Goldie-Coldman[42] hypothesis and the Hryniuk[84] dose-intensity hypothesis. The former theory estimates that a larger fraction of

TABLE 47-10 Chemotherapeutic Regimens for Aggressive Lymphomas

Regimen	Dose and Route	Day	Frequency
CVP			
C—cyclophosphamide	400 mg/m² PO	1–5	Repeat every 21 days
V—vincristine (Oncovin)	1.4 mg/m² IV	1	
P—prednisone	100 mg/m² PO	1–5	
C-MOPP			
C—cyclophosphamide	650 mg/m² IV	1, 8	Repeat every 28 days
O—vincristine (Oncovin)	1.4 mg/m² IV	1, 8	
P—procarbazine	100 mg/m² PO	1–14	
P—prednisone	40 mg/m² PO	1–14	
BACOP			
B—bleomycin	5 u/m² IV	15, 22	Repeat every 28 days
A—doxorubicin (Adriamycin)	25 mg/m² IV	1, 8	
C—cyclophosphamide	650 mg/m² IV	1, 8	
O—vincristine (Oncovin)	1.4 mg/m² IV	1, 8	
P—prednisone	60 mg/m² PO	15–28	
CHOP			
C—cyclophosphamide	750 mg/m² IV	1	Repeat every 21 days
H—doxorubicin (Adriamycin)	50 mg/m² IV	1	
O—vincristine (Oncovin)	1.4 mg/m² IV (max 2.0 mg)	1	
P—prednisone	100 mg PO	1–5	
COMLA			
C—cyclophosphamide	1500 mg/m² IV	1	Repeat every 91 days
O—vincristine (Oncovin)	1.4 mg/m² IV (max 2.0 mg)	1, 8, 15	
M—methotrexate	120 mg/m² IV (bolus)	22, 29, 36, 43, 50, 57, 64, 71	
L—leucovorin	25 mg/m² PO × 4	24 hours after methotrexate	
A—cytarabine	300 mg/m² IV	Same as methotrexate	
COP/BLAM			
C—cyclophosphamide	400 mg/m² IV	1	Repeat every 21 days
O—vincristine (Oncovin)	1 mg/m² IV	1	
P—prednisone	40 mg/m² PO	1–10	
BL—bleomycin	15 u/m² IV	15	
A—doxorubicin (Adriamycin)	40 mg/m² IV	1	
M—procarbazine	100 mg/m² PO	1–10	
M-BACOD			
M—methotrexate*	3000 mg/m² IV (over 40–60 minutes)	14	Repeat every 21 days
B—bleomycin	4 u/m² IV	1	
A—doxorubicin (Adriamycin)	45 mg/m² IV	1	
C—cyclophosphamide	600 mg/m² IV	1	
O—vincristine (Oncovin)	1 mg/m² IV	1	
D—dexamethasone (Decadron)	6 mg/m² PO	1–5	
m-BACOD			
m—methotrexate*	200 mg/m² IV (over 15 minutes)	8, 15	Repeat every 21 days
B—bleomycin	4 u/m² IV	1	
A—doxorubicin (Adriamycin)	45 mg/m² IV	1	
C—cyclophosphamide	600 mg/m² IV	1	
O—vincristine (Oncovin)	1.4 mg/m² IV	1	
D—dexamethasone (Decadron)	6 mg/m² PO	1–5	
ProMACE-MOPP			
Pro—prednisone	60 mg/m² PO	1–14	Repeat every 28 days
M—methotrexate*	1500 mg/m² IV (over 12 hours)	15	
A—doxorubicin (Adriamycin)	25 mg/m² IV	1, 8	
C—cyclophosphamide	650 mg/m² IV	1, 8	
E—etoposide	120 mg/m² IV	1, 8	

(continued)

TABLE 47-10 Chemotherapeutic Regimens for Aggressive Lymphomas (continued)

Regimen	Dose and Route	Day	Frequency
Followed by MOPP after maximal response			
M—mechlorethamine	6 mg/m² IV	1, 8	Repeat every 28 days
O—vincristine (Oncovin)	1.4 mg/m² IV	1, 8	
P—procarbazine	100 mg/m² PO	1–14	
P—prednisone	40 mg/m² PO	1–14	
ProMACE-CytaBOM			
Pro—prednisone	60 mg/m² PO	1–14	Repeat every 21 days
A—doxorubicin (Adriamycin)	25 mg/m² IV	1	
C—cyclophosphamide	650 mg/m² IV	1	
E—etoposide	120 mg/m² IV	1	
Cyta—cytarabine	300 mg/m² IV	8	
B—bleomycin	5 u/m² IV	8	
O—vincristine (Oncovin)	1.4 mg/m² IV	8	
M—methotrexate*	120 mg/m² IV bolus	8	
ProMACEd1/MOPPd8			
Pro—prednisone	60 mg/m² PO	1–14	Repeat every 28 days
M—methotrexate*	500 mg/m² IV (over 1 hour)	15	
A—doxorubicin (Adriamycin)	25 mg/m² IV	1	
C—cyclophosphamide	650 mg/m² IV	1	
E—etoposide	120 mg/m² IV	1	
M—mechlorethamine	6 mg/m² IV	8	
O—vincristine (Oncovin)	1.4 mg/m² IV	8	
P—procarbazine	100 mg/m² PO	8–14	
MACOP-B			
M—methotrexate*	400 mg/m² IV (100 mg/m² IV bolus, then 300 mg/m² IV over 4 hours)	8, 36 64	Repeat every 84 days
A—doxorubicin (Adriamycin)	50 mg/m² IV	1, 15, 29, 43, 57, 71	
C—cyclophosphamide	350 mg/m² IV	1, 15, 29, 43, 57, 71	
O—vincristine (Oncovin)	1.4 mg/m² IV (max. 2.0 mg)	8, 22, 36, 50, 64, 78	
P—prednisone	75 mg/m² PO	1–84	
B—bleomycin	10 u/m² IV	22, 50, 78	

*Leucovorin rescue is given for 24 hours after each methotrexate dose.

IV, intravenously; PO, by mouth.

Source: Gaynor ER, Fisher RI: Diffuse aggressive lymphomas in adults. In Magrath IT (ed): *The Non-Hodgkin's Lymphomas.* Baltimore, MD: Williams & Wilkins, 1990. Reprinted with permission.

patients will be cured if they are exposed to the largest number of agents at full doses as early as possible in the treatment course. The latter predicts that the best results will occur when a maximum rate of drug delivery is maintained. Although these regimens may lead to toxic deaths in up to 5% of patients and are clearly not suitable for those who are elderly or incapacitated, disease-free survival and cure may be possible for the majority of individuals treated.[57,85–87]

Salvage Therapy

Relapsed indolent lymphomas are rarely resistant to treatment unless they undergo histologic progression. Thus, retreatment with the same induction program often produces additional responses. In contrast, however, the outlook for nonresponsive or relapsed aggressive lymphomas is dismal. Despite the fact that most of the tumors originally are sensitive to chemotherapeutic combinations at the time of relapse, refractoriness to treatment is the rule rather than the exception; thus, cure is rarely possible with recurrent aggressive NHL. Patients who relapse generally have a reduced bone marrow reserve as a result of primary therapy (whether radiotherapy or chemotherapy) and tolerate secondary treatment poorly. These individuals require platelet transfusions as the chemotherapy drives their platelet counts into the danger zone below 20,000/mm³. Some institutions use granulocyte transfusions for bacterial infection or fever of unknown origin in the presence of their significantly reduced white cell count. Overall, sepsis is a major cause of morbidity and mortality.

With the advent of high-dose therapy followed by autologous bone marrow transplantation (ABMT), a substantial number of relapsed patients with aggressive lymphoma are achieving durable second complete remissions.[88,89] The induction regimen usually consists of high-dose cyclophosphamide followed by total body irradiation, and it appears that other agents such as cytosine arabinoside and etoposide can be added without significant increase in toxicity.[90] It has been suggested that for individuals with especially poor-risk lymphoma, ABMT might be used earlier in the course of treatment.[91] Clinical trials seem to indicate that allogeneic bone marrow transplantation may provide an alternative to conventional chemotherapy for those with poor-prognosis Burkitt's lymphoma.[92] In patients with positive marrow disease, a new technique for collecting stem cells from peripheral blood provides a viable transplant option.[93,94]

Biological response modifiers have shown initial promise in the treatment of select malignancies and presumably work by boosting an endogenous antitumor immune response. In an attempt to provide better treatment outcomes for patients with lymphoma, a number of these agents (e.g., interferons, monoclonal antibodies, interleukin-2, and colony stimulating factors) have been used.[95,96] Current results from clinical trials, although promising in some instances, remain generally inconclusive. Longo[97] is quite emphatic in stating that at present "biologic therapy has no role in the primary treatment of any stage of any histologic subtype of lymphoma."

COMPLICATIONS OF TREATMENT

Radiotherapy often causes complications during treatment (acute) or following the completion of treatment (subacute or late). The most common reactions associated with mantle irradiation are loss of taste, dry mouth, redness of skin, dysphagia, loss of hair at the nape of the neck, nausea, and vomiting. Because the amount of saliva is decreased, these individuals are at increased risk of dental caries. Therefore, instructions in proper dental hygiene, which includes routine examination and cleaning every 4–6 months, should always be given.[6]

Inverted-Y port irradiation usually results in nausea, vomiting, anorexia, diarrhea, and malaise. Bone marrow depression may occur and must be monitored by frequent complete blood counts. Total nodal irradiation leads to all the side effects noted previously and particularly to severe bone marrow depression.[6]

The various combinations of chemotherapy used in the treatment of HD and NHL will invariably result in acute and chronic side effects. The nature of these responses depends on the drugs used, but many are common to most anticancer agents. The most frequent side effect is nausea and vomiting. Although the severity of this reaction varies from one individual to another, it is generally transient and can often be effectively controlled by antiemetics. Depending on the particular drug regimen administered, other reactions can include alopecia, myalgia, chills, fever, euphoria, fluid retention, stomatitis, gastrointestinal disturbances, hemorrhagic cystitis, and mental depression. The most serious side effect produced by all combination regimens is bone marrow suppression, which renders the individual susceptible to infection and hemorrhage. Specific aspects of nursing care related to these side effects are covered elsewhere in this text.

CONSEQUENCES OF SURVIVAL

Oncologic advances in diagnostic technology, therapeutic regimens, and supportive interventions have shown great progress in the past two decades, and many lymphoma patients face a future in which long-term survival is a reasonable expectation. However, the cost of such progress is yet to be determined. While acute toxicities of established treatment modalities are well documented, clinical evaluation studies are just beginning to investigate the delayed effects and iatrogenic risks associated with surgery (splenectomy/laparotomy), radiation therapy, and chemotherapy. The delayed toxicities tend to produce lifelong problems and may vary in severity from relatively minor to potentially fatal.[98] Table 47-11 highlights a number of long-term complications that may develop in those cured of malignant lymphomas.

It is important to stress that no organ system is immune to alteration. An extension of injury to the lungs is common in mantle irradiation, and it may develop as early as 1–3 months after RT is completed. Resulting complications can include pneumothorax, radiation pneumonitis, pulmonary fibrosis, and superimposed pulmonary and parenchymal infections. In addition, nitrosoureas, high-dose busulfan, and bleomycin are known to induce fibrotic lung damage.[99]

Tumors on the right side of the superior mediastinum have the potential to obstruct the return of blood to the heart from the superior vena cava. This produces a characteristic syndrome of edema in the upper half of the body that is associated with prominent collateral circulation. Lung cancer, especially the oat cell variety, is the most common cause of this complication, but the lymphomas represent the second most common precipitating factor. This is an oncologic emergency that necessitates prompt therapy aimed at relieving pressure on the superior vena cava. External beam radiation therapy has been the traditional approach, especially in the management of an acute-onset syndrome.[6,100]

Both RT and chemotherapy promote toxic effects on the heart and peripheral blood vessels. Acute and chronic pericarditis are not uncommon, and a patient often presents with a spectrum of symptoms ranging

TABLE 47-11 Long-Term Complications in Patients Cured of Malignant Lymphoma

Complication	Etiology and Risk Factors	Management and Prevention
Immunologic dysfunction	Underlying disease, therapy	Appropriate vaccinations
Herpes zoster-varicella	Underlying disease, therapy	Systemic antiviral therapy, zoster immune globulin
Pneumococcal sepsis	Splenectomy Functional asplenia post radiation therapy (RT)	Pretherapy pneumonococcal vaccine, selected antibiotic prophylaxis, avoid unnecessary staging splenectomy
Nonlymphocytic leukemia	Therapy, age above 40	Avoid combined modality therapy for HD; supportive care; low-dose chemotherapy; aggressive therapy +/− bone marrow transplant
Myelodysplastic syndromes	Therapy, age above 40	Same as above
Non-Hodgkin's lymphoma	Therapy	Aggressive combination CT (eg, MACOP-B)
Solid tumors	Direct or indirect RT exposure	Conventional management
Thymic hyperplasia	Underlying disease, therapy	Resection
Hypothyroidism	Direct or indirect RT exposure	Hormone replacement, thyroid suppression during therapy (?)
Thyroid cancer	Direct or indirect RT exposure, chronic thyroid stimulation	Thyroid suppression
Male infertility	Therapy, underlying disease	Attempt sperm storage, testicular shielding during RT, suppression of spermatogenesis during CT (?), alternative chemotherapy regimens
Male impotence	Therapy, underlying disease	Counseling, trial of testosterone
Female infertility	Therapy	Oophoropexy, ovarian suppression during therapy (?), cyclic estrogen replacement
Female impotence	Therapy, underlying disease	Counseling, cyclic estrogen replacement
Pericarditis, acute	Mediastinal RT, recall with chemotherapy (CT) post-RT	Appropriate RT shielding and technique; avoid doxorubicin post-RT; anti-inflammatory medication; pericardiocentesis
Pericarditis, chronic	Mediastinal RT	Appropriate RT shielding and technique, pericardiectomy
Cardiomyopathy	Mediastinal RT, doxorubicin, recall with CT post-RT	Appropriate RT shielding and technique; avoid doxorubicin post-RT; monitor for early signs of toxicity; limit cumulative doxorubicin dose; supportive medical management
Pneumonitis, acute	Direct or indirect RT, bleomycin, nitrosoureas, recall with CT post-RT	Appropriate RT shielding and technique, monitor for early signs of toxicity, avoid known toxic drugs, avoid excessive pO_2
Pneumonitis, chronic	Same as above	Supportive management
Avascular necrosis	Steroid therapy, underlying disease (?)	Anti-inflammatory medications, joint surgery
Growth retardation	Pediatric RT	Minimize RT, use symmetric RT fields
Dental caries	Salivary change post-RT	Maintain good oral hygiene, daily fluoride treatment

Source: Hellman S, Jaffe CS, DeVita VT:Hodgkin's disease. In DeVita VT, Hellman S, Rosenberg, SA (eds): *Cancer: Principles and Practice of Oncology*. Philadelphia: Lippincott, 1989. Reprinted with permission.

from cough and chest pain to edema, paradoxical pulse, cardiac tamponade, and hemodynamic compromise. Coronary artery disease and cardiomyopathy are also seen following extensive mediastinal radiation. Similar risks have been noted with doxorubicin, whose cumulative dose effect often is potentiated when drug administration follows RT.[101]

The multiagent regimens used most in HD (MOPP and ABVD) appear to induce little nephrotoxicity. However, glomerulonephritis is considered a paraneoplastic syndrome of this malignancy. Despite improvements in shielding techniques, radiation damage to the kidneys is possible in retroperitoneal NHL. Limiting the radiation dose to 2000 cGy or less may minimize the risk of a functional deficit.[37] Cyclophosphamide induces topical damage to the bladder, and hemorrhagic cystitis is a potentially serious complication of all chemotherapeutic regimens using this drug.[102]

Because both chemotherapy and radiotherapy are immunosuppressive, bacterial as well as other unusual infections may occur. The most common gram-negative organisms in individuals with lymphoma are *Escherichia coli, Pseudomonas aeruginosa,* and *Klebsiella.* Various species of *Staphylococcus* are also becoming increasingly prevalent infectious agents in these patients. Although fever as a presenting complaint may be attributable to the lymphoma itself, fever in a patient who has been treated (especially one who is neutropenic) must always be considered a sign of potentially life-threatening sepsis until proven otherwise. Thus, appropriate cultures should be obtained and empiric antibiotic therapy must be started immediately.[6]

The two fungal infections diagnosed most often are candidiasis and aspergillosis. *Pneumocystis carinii* is a rare protozoal infection in immunologically normal individuals, but it is frequently pathogenic in lymphoma patients. Currently it is recognized as one of the leading causes of death in the AIDS population.

Herpes zoster is a troublesome complication that is often seen in individuals with HD and NHL. It results from the reactivation of latent foci of chickenpox virus, presumably secondary to the immunosuppression caused by the lymphoma and/or its treatment. The virus is usually localized, but on occasion a life-threatening fulminant process may occur.[6] This infection may be seen at any time during the course of illness, from initial treatment to relapse. In addition, patients who have undergone splenectomy face a lifelong risk of activation by encapsulated organisms.

Chronic progressive radiation myelopathy is a disabling neurological problem associated with mantle radiation. Symptoms include paresthesias, weakness, and bowel/bladder dysfunction. Peripheral neuropathies are associated with vincristine and vinblastine, and the incidence of central nervous system lymphoma is increasing dramatically in the AIDS population.

Rare as a presenting symptom but commonly seen in progressive lymphoma, compression of the spinal cord represents a complication that is dreaded because of its potential to cripple with paraplegia a person who might otherwise have many productive years remaining. This oncologic emergency develops swiftly, with weakness of the lower extremities, increased tendon reflexes, positive Babinski signs, and the development of a sensory "level" below which sensation is lost. Precise localization of the compression by myelogram is essential. Recently, MRI has offered the promise of a noninvasive diagnostic technique, but myelography remains the current diagnostic standard. Early diagnosis is critical to prevention of neurologic impairment. Patients who have already developed compromised neurologic *status* usually do not have a return of function after treatment.[103] Consequently the nurse must be sensitive to complaints of leg weakness or bowel and bladder dysfunction, especially in patients with back pain.[6]

Two of the most devastating complications associated with lymphoma treatment are sterility and carcinogenesis. Because many of the patients are less than 40 years old when initially diagnosed, these tragic consequences not only confer physical alterations; they also create severe psychological distress as the individual is forced to face a lack of procreative potential and another malignant threat to life.

During RT, men will experience transient aspermia, but recovery of spermatogenesis has been documented when careful testicular shielding is employed. Women who have not had an oophoropexy or shielding of the ovaries may undergo artificial menopause. At the time of exploratory laparotomy, surgical fixation of the ovaries to the uterus is often performed in young female patients to preserve their ovarian function.[6]

Transient and sometimes permanent male sterility is a recognized complication of induction chemotherapy for lymphoma. As a group, the alkylating agents are the most toxic to the testicular germ cells. In general, reversible changes occur up to a given threshold level; irreversible germinal aplasia develops once that threshold has been exceeded. Individuals with HD who are treated with MOPP have a greater than 80% likelihood of developing germinal aplasia, azoospermia, and testicular atrophy with elevated serum follicle-stimulating hormone levels.[104] Chapman and colleagues[105] reported 100% infertility during the first 12 months after therapy in 74 men who received this regimen. Return of active spermatogenesis was seen in only 4 of 64 men 15–51 months after therapy stopped. ABVD, an alternative chemotherapy program for HD, may be as effective as MOPP, but it is less toxic to germinal epithelial cells.[40] The use of combination chemotherapy in women also produces ovarian dysfunction, with those older than 35–40 years of age being the most susceptible. In the case of MOPP therapy, only 40%–50% of the women experienced ovarian failure.[104] Clearly, the complications of gonadal dysfunction may result in considerable psychosocial problems in both men and women being treated for cure.[6] Thus, reproductive counseling and procreative alternatives are essential components of nursing care to consider for this patient population.[106]

Second malignancies may develop after curative treatment for lymphoma.[107] Acute nonlymphocytic leukemia is the most common and well-recognized long-range complication of exposure to radiation or alkylating anticancer drugs. Cumulative risk varies according to the intensity and nature of the treatment and the period of observation. It may range from less than 1% to well over 10%.[108] If both radiation and chemotherapy are used, the risk of subsequent leukemia is greatest. It is generally believed that the alkylating agents are more leukemogenic than other anticancer drugs; thus, a regimen such as ABVD might be associated with a lower rate of leukemia than MOPP and CHOP.[6]

SUPPORTIVE CARE

Supportive care of the lymphoma patient begins at diagnosis with an explanation of the disease, a description of the steps that will be taken for staging and treatment, and a generation in the patient of a feeling of confidence in the multidisciplinary team responsible for care. Regardless of whether the primary treatment is radiotherapy or chemotherapy, it is certain that the clinical course will be lengthy and highly toxic. The individual must be prepared to cope with this reality.[6] The person who presents with constitutional symptoms and receives several cycles of chemotherapy often becomes completely asymptomatic. Because symptoms are relieved, the patient might question why he or she should proceed with a treatment program that causes adverse side effects. This follow-up period is crucial if a positive outcome is to be achieved. The nurse can play a major role by providing the understanding and emotional support the patient needs and by making sure the patient understands that although small foci of disease cause no symptoms, they will, if untreated, lead to recurrence.[6]

After the primary treatment there will be a prolonged period (months to years) during which the patient must be observed for a recurrence of disease. This is a particularly trying period because the individual has already, in his or her own mind, been very close to death by virtue of having dealt with the diagnosis of cancer. The treatment has (as a rule) produced complete remission, but each visit to the clinic now carries with it the threat that the disease may have relapsed and the nightmare must begin all over again. The nurse must be aware that whereas the treatment team views this as a "routine" visit for a patient who has responded very well to therapy, the individual perceives every word or facial expression as a potential clue that the cancer has recurred.[6] The reader is referred to Chapter 22 for a comprehensive review of the psychosocial dimensions of cancer survivorship.

CONCLUSION

The lymphomas comprise more than a dozen separate neoplasms that exhibit a wide gamut of clinical presentations ranging from slow, indolent growth to rapidly fatal progression. Some lymphomas are highly curable with appropriate therapy, while others show no increase in survival following treatment. These malignancies are separated from each other on the basis of subtle differences and require expert interpretation and evaluation. Megavoltage radiotherapy and combination chemotherapy have provided improved management techniques, leading to the expectation of cure in well over 50% of all individuals with lymphoma. However, the skillful application of the complex and toxic treatments requires a precise delineation of histologic type and extent of disease in accordance with rigorously established principles of staging.[6]

Although the etiology of the lymphomas remains elusive, tantalizing hints are provided by the strong suggestion of Epstein-Barr virus–induced Burkitt's lymphoma in Africa, the viruslike epidemiologic pattern of nodular sclerosing Hodgkin's disease, and the clear association between malfunction of the immune defense system and the development of non-Hodgkin's lymphoma.[6]

Effective diagnosis, staging, and multimodal management of the lymphomas require the collaborative efforts of multiple health care disciplines. The contributions of the nurse are vital to the achievement of a positive outcome. It is the nurse who, to a greater extent than others on the team, must respond to the patient's deepest need for support and understanding; it is the nurse who must meet the patient's need for careful explanation of the complex diagnostic and therapeutic methods designed to deal with a life-threatening malignancy; and it is the nurse who must be constantly alert to the possible complications of both the disease and its treatment.

The ultimate goal of any therapeutic regimen should be to return the individual to as healthy a lifestyle as possible. Because the cohort of cancer survivors continues to increase, the scope of nursing practice must expand as well. Now that cure is no longer beyond our grasp, emphasis must shift to the rehabilitation arena, where attention that complements the goals of the acute care setting can be directed toward the individual's functional, psychological, vocational, and economic limitations. Although many iatrogenic effects cannot always be anticipated or reversed, early identification of rehabilitation issues and timely intervention by an expert caregiver can help minimize potential disability and enhance overall quality of life. Patients who have struggled to overcome their cancer experience and those who supported them make such efforts meaningful and worthwhile.

REFERENCES

1. DeVita VT: Hematologic malignancies: Non-Hodgkin's lymphomas. *Hosp Pract* 21:103–118, 1986.
2. Eyre HJ, Farver ML: Hodgkin's disease and non-Hodgkin's lymphoma. In Holleb AI, Fink DJ, Murphy GP (eds), *Textbook of Clinical Oncology*. Atlanta: American Cancer Society, 1991, pp. 377–396.
3. Foon KA, Schroff RW, Gail RP: Surface markers on leukemia and lymphoma cells: Recent advances. *Blood* 60:1–19, 1982.
4. Keegan P, Ozer H: Immunology of the lymphomas. In Wiernik PH, Canellos GP, Kyle RA, Schiffer CA (eds), *Neoplastic Diseases of the Blood* (2d ed). New York: Churchill Livingstone, 1991, pp. 663–688.
5. Pinkus GS, Thomas P, Said JW: Leu-M1-A marker for Reed-Sternberg cells in Hodgkin's disease: An immunoperoxidase study of paraffin-embedded tissues. *Am J Pathol* 119:244–252, 1985.
6. Yarbro CH: Lymphomas. In Groenwald SL, Frogge MH, Goodman M, Yarbro CH, (eds), *Cancer Nursing: Principles and Practice* (2d ed). Boston: Jones and Bartlett, 1990, pp. 974–989.

7. American Cancer Society: *Cancer Facts and Figures—1993.* Atlanta: American Cancer Society, 1993, pp. 7–26.
8. Gail MH, Pluda JM, Rabkin CS, et al: Projections of the incidence of non-Hodgkin's lymphoma related to acquired immunodeficiency syndrome. *J Natl Cancer Inst* 83:695–701, 1991.
9. Foucar K: Pathology of nodal and extranodal lymphoma: Non-Hodgkin's and Hodgkin's disease. In Allison JG, (ed), *Pathology and Management of Lymphoma.* Mount Kisco, NY: Futura, 1984, pp. 1–49.
10. Magrath IT: Lymphocyte ontogeny: A conceptual basis for understanding neoplasia of the immune system. In Magrath IT, (ed), *The Non-Hodgkin's Lymphomas.* Baltimore, MD: Williams & Wilkins, 1990, pp. 29–48.
11. Appelbaum JW: The role of the oncogene in the pathogenesis of cancer. *Semin Oncol Nurs* 8:51–62, 1992.
12. Parker JW, Lukes RJ: Neoplasms of the immune system. In Stites DP, Terr AI (eds), *Basic and Clinical Immunology* (7th ed). Norwalk, CT: Appleton and Lange, 1991, pp. 599–631.
13. Rahr VA, Tucker R: Non-Hodgkin's lymphoma: Understanding the disease. *Cancer Nurs* 13:56–91, 1990.
14. Hodgkin T: On some morbid appearances of the absorbent glands and spleen. *Med Chir Tran* 17:68–114, 1832.
15. Owens AH: The malignant lymphomas. In Harvey AM, Johns RJ, McKusick VA, et al (eds), *The Principles and Practice of Medicine* (22d ed). Norwalk, CT:Appleton and Lange, 1988, pp. 419–429.
16. Wilks S: Cases of enlargement of the lymphatic glands and spleen, or Hodgkin's disease. *Guy's Hosp Rep* 11:56–67, 1865.
17. Reed DM: On the pathological changes in Hodgkin's disease, with especial reference to tuberculosis. *Johns Hopkins Rep* 10:133–196, 1902.
18. Sternberg C: Über eine eigenartige unter dem Bilde der Pseukoleukamie verlaufende: Tuberculose des lymphatischen apparates. *Z Heilkd* 19:21–90, 1898.
19. Hellman S, Jaffe E, DeVita VT: Hodgkin's disease. In DeVita VT, Hellman S, Rosenberg SA (eds), *Cancer: Principles and Practice of Oncology,* (vol 2) (2d ed). Philadelphia: Lippincott, 1989, pp.1623–1709.
20. Parker BA, Green MR: Hodgkin's disease. In Moosa AR, Schimpff SC, Robson MC (eds), *Comprehensive Textbook of Oncology,* (vol 2) (2d ed). Baltimore, MD: Williams & Wilkins, 1991, pp. 1257–1267.
21. Cole P, MacMahon B, Aisenberg A: Mortality from Hodgkin's disease in the United States: Evidence for the multiple etiology hypothesis. *Lancet* 2:1371–1376, 1968.
22. Poplack DG, Kun LE, Cassady JR, et al: Leukemias and lymphomas of childhood. In DeVita VT, Hellman S, Rosenberg SA (eds), *Cancer: Principles and Practice of Oncology* (vol 2) (3d ed). Philadelphia: Lippincott, 1989, pp. 1671–1695.
23. Safai B, Diaz B, Schwartz J: Malignant neoplasms associated with human immunodeficiency virus infection. *Cancer* 42:74–95, 1992.
24. Grufferman S, Delzell E: Epidemiology of Hodgkin's disease. *Epidemiol Rev* 6:76–106, 1984.
25. Robertson SJ, Lowman JT, Grufferman S, et al: Familial Hodgkin's disease. *Cancer* 59:1314–1319, 1987.
26. Haskell CM, Parker RG: Hodgkin's disease. In Haskell CM (ed), *Cancer Treatment* (2d ed). Philadelphia: Saunders, 1985, pp. 758–788.
27. Slivnick DJ, Nawrocki JF, Fisher RI: Immunology and cellular biology of Hodgkin's disease. *Hematol Oncol Clin North Am* 3:205–220, 1989.
28. Stevenson MA, Stanton SC, Cossman J: Involvement of the *bcl-2* gene in Hodgkin's disease. *J Natl Cancer Inst* 82:855–858, 1990.
29. Thangavelu M, LeBeau MM: Chromosomal abnormalities in Hodgkin's disease. *Hematol Oncol Clin North Am* 3:221–236, 1989.
30. Longo DL, Broder S: Lymphoproliferative disorders. In Samter M (ed), *Immunologic Diseases* (vol 1) (4th ed). Boston: Little, Brown, 1988, pp. 553–595.
31. Griffiths MJ, Murray KH, Russo PC: Leukemia and lymphoma. In *Oncology Nursing—Pathophysiology, Assessment, and Intervention.* New York: Macmillan, 1984, pp. 241–257.
32. Strum SB, Dark JK, Rappaport H: Observations of cells resembling Sternberg-Reed cells in conditions other than Hodgkin's disease. *Cancer* 26:176–190, 1970.
33. Craver LF, Hall TC, Rappaport H, et al: Report of the nomenclature committee. *Cancer Res* 26:1311, 1966.
34. Carbone PP, Kaplan HS, Musshoff K, et al: Report of the committee on Hodgkin's disease staging. *Cancer Res* 31:1860–1861, 1971.
35. Lister TA, Crowther D, Sutcliffe SB, et al: Report of a committee convened to discuss the evaluation and staging of patients with Hodgkin's disease: Cotswolds meeting. *J Clin Oncol* 7:1630–1636, 1989.
36. Bonadonna G, Wiernik PH, Santoro A: Clinical treatment of Hodgkin's disease. In Wiernik PH, Canellos GP, Kyle RA, Schiffer CA (eds), *Neoplastic Diseases of the Blood* (2d ed). New York: Churchill Livingstone, 1991, pp. 701–727.
37. Marino LB, Kooser JA: The psychosocial care of cancer clients and their families: Periods of high rise. In Marino LB (ed), *Cancer Nursing.* St. Louis, MO: Mosby, 1981, pp. 53–66.
38. Lister TA, Dorreen MS, Faux M, et al: The treatment of Stage III A Hodgkin's disease. *J Clin Oncol* 1:745–759, 1983.
39. DeVita VT, Simon RM, Hubbard SM, et al: Curability of advanced Hodgkin's disease with chemotherapy: Long-term follow-up of MOPP treated patients at the National Cancer Institute. *Ann Intern Med* 92:587–595, 1980.
40. Santoro A, Bonadonna G, Valagussa P, et al: Long-term results of combined chemotherapy-radiotherapy approach in Hodgkin's disease: Superiority of ABVD plus radiotherapy versus MOPP plus radiotherapy. *J Clin Oncol* 5:27–37, 1987.
41. Bonadonna G, Valagussa P, Santoro A: Alternating non–cross-resistant combination chemotherapy or MOPP in Stage IV Hodgkin's disease. *Ann Intern Med* 104:739–746, 1986.
42. Goldie JH, Coldman AJ, Guaduskus GA: Rationale for the use of alternating non-cross resistant chemotherapy. *Cancer Treat Rep* 66:439–449, 1982.
43. Bakemeier RF, Anderson JR, Costello W, et al: BCVPP chemotherapy for advanced Hodgkin's disease: Evidence for greater duration of complete remission, greater survival, and less toxicity than with a MOPP regimen. *Ann Intern Med* 101:447–456, 1984.
44. Canellos GP: Can MOPP be replaced in the treatment of advanced Hodgkin's disease? *Semin Oncol* 17 2:2–6, 1990, (suppl).

45. Henkelmann GC, Hagemester FB, Fuller LM: Two cycles of MOPP and radiotherapy for Stage III_1 A and III_1 B Hodgkin's disease. *J Clin Oncol* 6:1293–1302, 1988.
46. Schomberg PJ, Evans RG, O'Connell MJ, et al: Prognostic significance of mediastinal mass in adult Hodgkin's disease. *Cancer* 53:324–328, 1984.
47. Prakash U, Abel MD: Mediastinal mass and tracheal obstruction during general anesthesia. *Mayo Clin Proc* 63:1004–1011, 1988.
48. Leopold KA, Canellos GP, Rosenthal D, et al: Stage IA-IIB Hodgkin's disease: Staging and treatment of patients with large mediastinal adenopathy. *J Clin Oncol* 7:1059–1065, 1989.
49. Fisher R, DeVita VT, Hubbard S, et al: Prolonged disease-free survival in Hodgkin's disease with MOPP reinduction after first relapse. *Ann Intern Med* 90:761, 1979.
50. Jotti GS, Bonadonna G: Prognostic factors in Hodgkin's disease: Implications for modern treatment. *Anticancer Res* 8:749–759, 1988 (review).
51. Jones RJ, Piantadosi S, Mann RB, et al: High-dose cytotoxic therapy and bone marrow transplantation for relapsed Hodgkin's disease. *J Clin Oncol* 8:527–537, 1990.
52. Taylor KM, Jagannath S, Spitzer G, et al: Recombinant human granulocyte colony-stimulating factor hastens granulocyte recovery after high-dose chemotherapy and autologous bone marrow transplantation in Hodgkin's disease. *J Clin Oncol* 7:1791–1799, 1989.
53. Williams SF, Bitran JD: The role of high-dose therapy and autologous bone marrow reinfusion in the treatment of Hodgkin's disease. *Hematol Oncol Clin North Am* 3:319–330, 1989.
54. Korbling M, Holle R, Haas R, et al: Autologous blood stem-cell transplantation in patients with advanced Hodgkin's disease and prior radiation to the pelvic site. *J Clin Oncol* 8:978–985, 1990.
55. Magrath IT: The non-Hodgkin's lymphomas: An introduction. In Magrath IT (ed), *The Non-Hodgkin's Lymphomas.* Baltimore, MD: Williams & Wilkins, 1990, pp. 1–14.
56. Aisenberg AC: A historical overview of malignant lymphoma. In Wiernik PH, Canellos GP, Kyle RA, Schiffer CA (eds), *Neoplastic Diseases of the Blood* (2d ed). New York: Churchill Livingstone, 1991, pp. 597–607.
57. Lester EP, Ultmann JE: Lymphoma. In Williams WJ, Beutler E, Erslev AJ, Lichtman MA (eds), *Hematology* (4th ed). New York: McGraw-Hill, 1990, pp. 1067–1087.
58. Purtilo DT, Stevenson M: Lymphotropic viruses as etiologic agents of lymphoma. *Hematol Oncol Clin North Am* 5:901–923, 1991.
59. Urba WJ, Longo DL: Burkitt's lymphoma. In Moosa AR, Schimpff SC, Robson MC (eds), *Comprehensive Textbook of Oncology* (vol 2) (2d ed). Baltimore, MD: Williams & Wilkins, 1991, pp. 1296–1301.
60. Wright DH: Pathogenesis of non-Hodgkin's lymphoma: Clues from geography. In Magrath IT (ed), *The Non-Hodgkin's Lymphomas.* Baltimore, MD: Williams & Wilkins, 1990, pp. 122–134.
61. Shapiro RS: Epstein-Barr virus-associated B-cell lymphoproliferative disorders in immunodeficiency: Meeting the challenge. *J Clin Oncol* 8:371–373, 1990 (editorial).
62. Joncas JH, Russo P, Brochu P, et al: Epstein-Barr virus polymorphic B-cell lymphoma associated with leukemia and with congenital immunodeficiencies. *J Clin Oncol* 8:378–384, 1990.
63. Urba WJ, Longo DL: Lymphocytic lymphomas: Epidemiology, etiology, pathology, and staging. In Moosa AR, Schimpff SC, Robson MC (eds), *Comprehensive Textbook of Oncology* (vol 2) (2d ed). Baltimore, MD:Williams & Wilkins, 1991, pp. 1268–1276.
64. Hardy R, Horning SJ: Molecular studies in the clinical evaluation of non-Hodgkin's lymphoma. *Hematol Oncol Clin North Am* 5:891–900, 1991.
65. Haluska FG, Tsujimoto Y, Croce CM: The molecular genetics of non-Hodgkin's lymphomas. In Magrath IT (ed), *The Non-Hodgkin's Lymphomas.* Baltimore, MD: Williams & Wilkins, 1990, pp. 96–108.
66. Levine EG, Bloomfield CD: Cytogenetics of malignant lymphomas. In Wiernik PH, Canellos GP, Kyle RA, Schiffer CA (eds), *Neoplastic Diseases of the Blood* (2d ed). New York: Churchill Livingstone, 1991, pp. 689–700.
67. Peng JW, Lee EC: Cytogenetics. In Magrath IT (ed), *The Non-Hodgkin's Lymphomas.* Baltimore, MD: Williams & Wilkins, 1990, pp. 77–95.
68. Magrath IT, Wilson W, Horvath K, et al: Clinical features and staging. In Magrath IT (ed), *The Non-Hodgkin's Lymphomas.* Baltimore, MD: Williams & Wilkins, 1990, pp. 180–199.
69. DeVita VT, Jaffe ES, Mauch P, et al: Lymphocytic lymphomas. In DeVita VT, Hellman S, Rosenberg SA (eds), *Cancer: Principles and Practice of Oncology* (vol 2) (3d ed). Philadelphia: Lippincott, 1989, pp. 1741–1798.
70. Rappaport H, Winter WJ, Hicks EB: Follicular lymphoma: A reevaluation of its position in the scheme of malignant lymphomas, based on a survey of 253 cases. *Cancer* 9:792, 1956.
71. Medeiros LJ, Jaffe ES: Pathology of malignant lymphomas. In Wiernik PH, Canellos GP, Kyle RA, Schimpff CA (eds), *Neoplastic Diseases of the Blood* (2d ed). New York: Churchill Livingstone, 1991, pp. 631–661.
72. Lukes RJ, Collins RD: Immunologic characterization of human malignant lymphomas. *Cancer* 34:1488–1503, 1974.
73. Horning SJ, Rosenberg SA: The natural history of initially treated low-grade non-Hodgkin's lymphomas. *N Engl J Med* 311:1471–1475, 1984.
74. Ziegler JL: Cancer in the immunocompromised host. In Stites DP, Terr AI, (eds), *Basic and Clinical Immunology* (7th ed). Norwalk, CT: Appleton and Lange, 1991, pp. 588–598.
75. Sandlund J, Magrath IT: Lymphoblastic lymphomas. In Magrath IT (ed), *The Non-Hodgkin's Lymphomas.* Baltimore, MD: Williams & Wilkins, 1990, pp. 240–255.
76. Skarin AT (ed): *Dana Farber Cancer Institute Atlas of Diagnostic Oncology.* Philadelphia: Lippincott, 1991.
77. McFadden ME: Cutaneous T-cell lymphoma. *Semin Oncol Nurs* 7:36–44, 1991.
78. Vose JM, Bierman PJ, Armitage JO: Non-Hodgkin's lymphoma. In Wiernik PH, Canellos GP, Kyle RA, Schiffer CA (eds), *Neoplastic Diseases of the Blood* (2d ed). New York: Churchill Livingstone, 1991, pp. 739–751.
79. Maor MH, Velasquez WS, Fuller LM, et al: Stomach conservation in Stages IE and IIE gastric non-Hodgkin's lymphoma. *J Clin Oncol* 8:266–271, 1990.
80. Paryani SB, Hoppe RT, Cox RS, et al: Analysis of non-Hodgkin's lymphomas with nodular and favorable histologies, stages I and II. *Cancer* 52:2300–2307, 1983.
81. Hochster HS, Kim K, Green MD, et al: Activity of fludarabine in previously treated non-Hodgkin's low-grade

lymphoma: Results of an Eastern Cooperative Oncology Group Study. *J Clin Oncol* 10:28–32, 1992.
82. Gaynor ER, Fisher RI: Diffuse aggressive lymphomas in adults. In Magrath IT (ed), *The Non-Hodgkin's Lymphomas*. Baltimore, MD: Williams & Wilkins, 1990, pp. 317–329.
83. Urba WJ, Longo DL: Lymphocytic lymphomas: Clinical course and management. In Moosa AR, Schimpff SC, Robson MC (eds), *Comprehensive Textbook of Oncology* (vol 2) (2d ed). Baltimore, MD: Williams & Wilkins, 1991, pp. 1277–1295.
84. Hryniuk W, Bush H: The importance of dose intensity in chemotherapy of metastatic breast cancer. *J Clin Oncol* 2:1281–1287, 1984.
85. Sweetham JW, Mead GM, Whitehouse JA: Intensive weekly combination chemotherapy for patients with intermediate-grade and high-grade non-Hodgkin's lymphoma. *J Clin Oncol* 9:2202–2209, 1991.
86. Zuckerman KS, LoBuglio AF, Reeves JA: Chemotherapy of intermediate- and high-grade non-Hodgkin's lymphomas with a high-dose doxorubicin-containing regimen. *J Clin Oncol* 8:248–256, 1990.
87. Vitolo U, Bertini M, Brusamolino E, et al: MACOP-B treatment in diffuse large-cell lymphoma: Identification of prognostic groups in an Italian multicenter study. *J Clin Oncol* 10:219–227, 1992.
88. Phillip T, Armitage JO, Spitzer G, et al: High dose therapy and ABMT after failure of conventional chemotherapy in one hundred adults with intermediate or high grade non-Hodgkin's lymphoma. *N Engl J Med* 316: 1493–1498, 1987.
89. Freedman AS, Takvorian T, Anderson KC: Autologous bone marrow transplantation in B-cell non-Hodgkin's lymphoma: Very low treatment-related mortality in 100 patients in sensitive relapse. *J Clin Oncol* 8:784–791, 1990.
90. Gribben JG, Goldstone AH, Linch DC, et al. Effectiveness of high-dose combination chemotherapy and autologous bone marrow transplantation for patients with non-Hodgkin's lymphomas who are still responsive to conventional-dose therapy. *J Clin Oncol* 7:1621–1629, 1989.
91. Gulati SC, Shank B, Black P, et al: Autologous bone marrow transplantation for patients with poor-prognosis lymphoma. *J Clin Oncol* 6:1303–1313, 1988.
92. Troussard X, Leblond V, Kuentz M, et al: Allogeneic bone marrow transplantation in adults with Burkitt's lymphoma or acute lymphoblastic leukemia in first complete remission. *J Clin Oncol* 8:809–812, 1990.
93. Takaue Y, Watanabe T, Kawano Y, et al: Isolation and storage of peripheral blood hematopoietic stem cells for autotransplantation into children with cancer. *Blood* 74:1245–1251, 1989.
94. Bitran JD, Williams SF, Moormeier J, et al: High-dose combination chemotherapy with thiotepa and autologous hematopoietic stem cell reinfusion in the treatment of patients with relapsed refractory lymphomas. *Semin Oncol* 17:39–42, 1990.
95. Weber JS, Yang JC, Topalian SL, et al: The use of interleukin-2 and lymphokine-activated killer cells for the treatment of patients with non-Hodgkin's lymphoma. *J Clin Oncol* 10:33–40, 1992.
96. Gianni AM, Bregni M, Siena S, et al: Recombinant human granulocyte-macrophage colony-stimulating factor reduces hematologic toxicity and widens clinical applicability of high-dose cyclophosphamide treatment in breast cancer and non-Hodgkin's lymphoma. *J Clin Oncol* 8:368–378, 1990.
97. Longo DL: Biologic agents and approaches in the man agement of patients with lymphoma: A critical appraisal. *Hematol Oncol Clin North Am* 5:1067–1087, 1991.
98. Ruccione K, Weinberg K: Late effects in multiple body systems. *Semin Oncol Nurs* 5:4–13, 1989.
99. Wickham R: Pulmonary toxicity secondary to cancer treatment. *Oncol Nurs Forum* 13:69–76, 1986.
100. Baker GL, Barnes HJ: Superior vena cava syndrome: Etiology, diagnosis, and treatment. *Am J Crit Care* 1:54–64, 1992.
101. Kaszyk LK: Cardiac toxicity associated with cancer therapy. *Oncol Nurs Forum* 13:81–88, 1986.
102. Lydon J: Nephrotoxicity of cancer treatment. *Oncol Nurs Forum* 13:68–77, 1986.
103. Wilson JK, Masaryk TJ: Neurologic emergencies in the cancer patient. *Semin Oncol* 16:490–503, 1989.
104. Yarbro CH, Perry MC: The effect of cancer therapy on gonadal function. *Semin Oncol Nurs* 1:3–8, 1985.
105. Chapman R, Rees L, Sutcliffe SB, et al: Cyclical combination chemotherapy and gonadal function: Retrospective study in males. *Lancet* 1:285–289, 1979.
106. Kaempfer SH, Wiley FM, Hoffman DJ: Fertility considerations and procreative alternatives in cancer care. *Semin Oncol Nurs* 1:25–34, 1985.
107. Jacquillat C, Khayat D, Desprez-Curely JP, et al: Occurrence of non-Hodgkin's lymphoma after therapy for Hodgkin's disease. *Cancer* 53:459–462, 1984.
108. Fraser MC, Tucker MA: Second malignancies following cancer therapy. *Semin Oncol Nurs* 5:43–55, 1989.

Chapter 48

Multiple Myeloma

Carol A. Sheridan, RN, MSN, OCN

INTRODUCTION

Plasma cell disorders are a group of diseases characterized by the overproduction of immunoglobulins.[1] In these diseases the malignant cell is the plasma cell, the functional mature cell that differentiates and develops from the B-lymphocyte.[2,3] Multiple myeloma is the most common malignant plasma cell disorder. It has the ability to affect the hematologic, skeletal, renal, and nervous systems.[4]

EPIDEMIOLOGY

Within the United States, multiple myeloma represents 1% of all hematologic malignancies.[1] Although the incidence of multiple myeloma appears to be increasing in the United States, there is some evidence that the increased incidence may be due to earlier and improved diagnosis in older, high-risk populations.[5] The onset of multiple myeloma is late, with peak occurrence between the fifth and seventh decade of life.[6] Differences in disease incidence can be noted based on sex and race. Within the United States, multiple myeloma is more common among blacks than among whites by 14 to 1.[1] For all groups there is a male predominance, although black females have a higher incidence than white males. Worldwide, some Asian populations have the lowest incidence rates.[5] These rates reflect both male and female populations from tumor registries in Osaka, Japan, Shanghai, Singapore, China, and Japanese individuals living in Hawaii.[5]

ETIOLOGY

The exact etiology of multiple myeloma is unknown, although a variety of factors have been associated with the development of the disease. In an attempt to better understand the etiologic factors, Potter[7] used an animal model and demonstrated that only specific strains of mice developed plasmacytomas following mineral oil injections. An analogous case for genetic linkage was made by Maldonado and Kyle,[8] who documented an increased frequency of plasma cell disorders among close relatives of individuals with multiple myeloma. Chromosomal abnormalities have also been documented in mice that underwent experimentally induced plasma cell disease. Although a specific chromosomal abnormality involving the immunoglobulin loci has not been detected in humans with multiple myeloma, frequent chromosomal abnormalities have been observed.[1,6] Chronic low-level exposure to radiation has been associated with a two- to sixfold increase in the incidence of multiple myeloma, which may develop as late as 20 years after the radiation exposure.[4,6] Chronic antigenic stimulation, such as recurrent infections and drug allergies, may be part of the medical history in individuals who develop multiple myeloma. No clear evidence demonstrating a common environmental or chemical etiologic factor has been established. In all such instances, further study is warranted to demonstrate a definitive risk relationship.

PATHOPHYSIOLOGY

The pluripotent stem cell resides within the bone marrow and has the ability to either self-replicate or differentiate into either the myeloid or lymphoid stem cell. The lymphoid stem cell is the earliest lymphoid cell. It resides within the bone marrow and retains the ability to self-replicate or differentiate into either T-lymphocytes or B-lymphocytes. T-lymphocytes regulate the immune response and participate in cell-mediated immunity. B-lymphocytes mature into plasma cells that manufacture and secrete large quantities of immunoglobulins. B-lymphocytes are responsible for humoral immunity. Five classes of immunoglobulins are secreted: IgG, IgA, IgM, IgD, and IgE. IgM is the first immunoglobulin produced during a primary immune response and is the first immunoglobulin produced in infants.[1] IgA is the primary immunoglobulin in saliva, tears, and the secretions of the gastrointestinal and respiratory tract. IgA plays a primary role in protecting these mucous membranes and vital organ systems by maintaining the first line of defense.[4] IgD and IgE are trace immunoglobulins found in the plasma. IgD acts as a cell-surface receptor that binds with antigen and triggers further B-lymphocyte differentiation and production. IgE can be elevated in response to parasitic infections and allergic response such as hay fever and asthma. It is thought that IgE binds to receptors on basophils and mast cells and may stimulate these cells to release vasoactive substances as part of the allergic response.[1,4] IgG is the primary immunoglobulin in the serum. It has four subclasses (IgG 1–4) with slightly different physiologic properties. IgG_1 and IgG_3 bind complement and mononuclear cells better than IgG_2 and IgG_4. When IgG_1 and IgG_3 are overproduced in multiple myeloma, the hyperviscosity syndrome may result. IgG is the only immunoglobulin that can cross the placenta and therefore confers passive immunity to newborns. In adults, IgG constitutes the largest proportion of immunoglobulin, followed by IgA and IgM.

In multiple myeloma there is abnormal overproduction of one immunoglobulin called the M protein; the *M* refers to monoclonal antibody, myeloma protein, or malignant protein. Although an excessive amount of immunoglobulin is being produced, the M protein is unable to effectively produce antibody necessary for maintaining humoral immunity. Approximately 80%–90% of all multiple myeloma patients will show evidence of the aberrant M protein in the serum.[6]

DIAGNOSIS/STAGING

Once symptoms are present, untreated individuals with multiple myeloma have a median survival of 7 months.[2] This can be extended with standard therapy to a median survival of 2–3 years.[2,6,9] Individuals with multiple myeloma may have a long prodromal, indolent, or asymptomatic period. However, once symptoms occur, systemic therapy becomes necessary. Patients may eventually enter a period where their disease becomes refractory or unresponsive to conventional therapy; then experimental therapies are warranted.[10,11]

The most frequent symptom at presentation is bone pain. The clinical course of the disease is complicated by pathologic fractures, hypercalcemia, spinal cord compression, anemia, thrombocytopenia, recurrent bacterial infections, and renal failure. The diagnosis of multiple myeloma can be confirmed by bone marrow biopsy with histologic confirmation of increased (>10%) numbers of plasma cells and the presence of the monoclonal (M) protein in either the serum or the urine. Osteolytic "punched-out" lesions may or may not be present at initial diagnosis. The diagnostic work-up for multiple myeloma is designed to determine the extent of involvement of other organs (Table 48-1). Serum B_2 microglobulin, platelet count, and the presence of either renal failure and/or infection have been identified as having a role in predicting prognosis when diagnosing, staging, and treating myeloma patients.[9–15]

Since 1975 the Durie/Salmon system has been proposed for use in staging multiple myeloma. (See Table 48-2).[16] This staging system integrates clinical and laboratory findings associated with multiple myeloma. In-

TABLE 48-1 Diagnostic Work-up for Multiple Myeloma

Diagnostic Exams	Purpose
Bone marrow aspirate/biopsy	Check % of plasma cells
Serum protein electrophoresis (SPEP) Immunoelectrophoresis (IEP)	Check for the presence of M protein
Serum chemistry	Check for evidence of hypercalcemia, renal dysfunction
Complete blood count (CBC)	Check for evidence of anemia, thrombocytopenia
Skeletal survey	Check for evidence of osteolytic bone lesions

TABLE 48-2 Myeloma Staging System

Criteria	Measured Myeloma Cell Mass (Cells × $10^{12}/m^2$)
Stage 1	
All of the following: Hemoglobin value >10 g/dL Serum calcium value normal (<12 mg/dL) On roentgenogram, normal bone structure (scale 0) or solitary bone plasmacytoma only Low M-component production rates IgG value <5 g/dL IgA value <3g/dL Urine light chain M-component on electrophoresis <4g/24 hr	<0.6 (low)
Stage II	
Overall data not as minimally abnormal as shown for stage I and no single value as abnormal as defined or stage III	0.6-1.20 (intermediate)
Stage III	
One or more of the following: Hemoglobin value <8.5 g/dL Serum calcium value >12 mg/dL Advanced lytic bone lesions (scale 3) High M-component production rates IgG value >7g/dL IgA value >5 g/dL Urine light chain M-component on electrophoresis >12 g/24 hr	>1.20 (high)
Subclassification A = relatively normal renal function (serum creatinine value >2.0 mg/dL) B = abnormal renal function (serum creatinine value ⩾2.0 mg/dL)	
Examples Stage IA = low cell mass with normal renal function Stage IIIB = high cell mass with abnormal renal function	

IgA, Immunoglobulin A; *IgG,* immunoglobulin G.

Source: Salmon SE, Cassady JR: Plasma cell neoplasms, in DeVita VT, Hellman S, Rosenberg SA (eds): *Cancer: Principles and Practice* (ed 3). Philadelphia, JB Lippincott, 1989.

vestigational approaches to staging and treating multiple myeloma include the use of flow cytometry analysis, in vitro drug testing, and radionuclide bone scanning. As clinical studies progress, the ability to apply new technologies to treatment regimens may improve clinical outcomes.[17]

CLINICAL MANIFESTATIONS

Skeletal Involvement

From 68% to 80% of individuals with multiple myeloma present with destructive, painful osteolytic lesions at the time of diagnosis.[6,18] Symptoms associated with these lesions include hypercalcemia (20%–40% of patients), pathological fractures with acute and chronic pain, decreased mobility, and an inability to fully participate in activities of daily living.[19,20] The bone lesions can be of three distinct types: (1) a solitary osteolytic lesion, (2) diffuse osteoporosis, and (3) multiple discrete osteolytic "punched-out" or "cannon-ball" lesions. The pathophysiology of the bone destruction is thought to be myeloma cell production of osteoclast-activating factor (OAF). Once thought to be a single substance, OAFs have now been identified as a class of bone-resorbing factors produced by lymphocytes and monocytes. Several OAFs have been purified and molecularly cloned, including lymphotoxin, tumor necrosis factor (TNF), the interferons, and interleukin (IL-1).[18] If untreated, myeloma-induced osteolytic lesions can lead to compression fractures of the spine with irreversible neurological sequelae, refractory hypercalcemia compromising renal function, and possibly death.

Infection

As with most cancer, 50%–70% of all multiple myeloma patients will die as a result of bacterial infection.[6,21] The two most common sites of infection are the respiratory and urinary tracts.[22] Common infectious organisms include *S. aureus, S. pneumoniae, E. Coli, Pseudomonas,* and *Klebsiella.* In the 1980s, Savage and associates[23] demonstrated a biphasic pattern of infection in the person with multiple myeloma. Streptococcus pneumoniae and Haemaphilus influenza occurred early in the disease (within 8 months of diagnosis) or in patients who responded early to chemotherapy, whereas infections caused by nonencapsulated gram-negative bacilli typically occurred in patients with unresponsive or refractory disease.

A number of mechanisms have been identified as responsible for the immunosuppression and infection associated with multiple myeloma. These include a deficiency in the normal amount of immunoglobulins, neutropenia associated with plasma cell replacement in the bone marrow, qualitative defects in neutrophil and complement system functioning, and decreased physical activity as a result of symptoms/syndromes caused by the disease.

Bone Marrow Involvement

A normocytic, normochromic anemia clinically manifested by fatigue and weakness occurs in over 60% of patients at initial diagnosis.[4,6] The anemia is initially caused by the excessive replacement of erythrocyte precursors with plasma cells in the bone marrow. Anemia can also be caused by increased red blood cell destruction. The M protein can coat normal erythrocytes, causing the red cells to line up similar to a roll of coins (rouleau formation). This formation results in capillary sludging with associated hemolysis.[1,24] As the myeloma cell burden increases or if the patient is treated with systemic chemotherapy, qualitative as well as quantitative defects in neutrophil and platelet function can occur. Bleeding can be caused by a decrease in the number of circulating platelets, by the M protein's effect on clotting factors, or by nonspecific coating of platelets with immunoglobulins.[1] The final result is platelet dysfunction and bleeding.

Renal Insufficiency

At initial diagnosis, renal insufficiency is present in 29% of patients with multiple myeloma. During the course of the disease and its treatment, 50% of these individuals will experience renal failure, and 15% will die as a result of renal insufficiency.[6] The presence of renal insufficiency as a negative prognostic indicator in multiple myeloma has been well established.[2,12,14] Multiple myeloma can cause intrinsic renal lesions as well as renal failure precipitated by the sequelae of the disease (infection, hypercalcemia, and dehydration).[25]

"Myeloma kidney" is the principal type of lesion associated with renal failure. In myeloma kidney, the renal tubules are filled with damaging, dense casts surrounded by multinucleated giant cells. These large dense tubular casts lead to the formation of precipitates in the tubules that can obstruct and rupture the tubular epithelium. In addition, interstitial inflammation, fibrosis and tubular degeneration may occur, resulting finally in renal failure.[1,26] The tubular casts have been shown to contain characteristic light chain immunoglobulins (Bence Jones proteins). Bence Jones proteins may be directly toxic to the renal tubular epithelium regardless of the presences of tubular casts.[6] The excretion of large amounts of Bence Jones proteins in the face of clinical dehydration with a low urine pH contributes to the risk of precipitation of light chain proteins in the renal tubule and possible co-precipitating with calcium, further exacerbating acute renal failure.

Another renal lesion that occurs in approximately 10%–30% of myeloma patients is caused by amyloid deposits.[1,26] Amyloid deposits can be found in the tubular basement membranes, renal blood vessels, the interstitium, or glomerulus. Evidence of albuminuria and nephrotic syndrome strongly suggests amyloidosis. Amyloidosis is an adverse prognostic factor and can occur in up to 10% of myeloma patients.[6]

Sequelae

Hypercalcemia as a clinical sequela of multiple myeloma has been described earlier. Untreated hypercalcemia in multiple myeloma patients can precipitate renal insufficiency by reducing the glomerular filtration rate, altering renal blood flow, changing the kidney's ability to concentrate urine, and precipitating calcium in the tubules or renal interstitium.

Hyperuricemia occurs in multiple myeloma patients as a result of a large tumor burden with an increased rate of cell death. Uric acid–induced nephropathy is caused by precipitation and crystallization of uric acid in the distal tubules, where the urine pH is low and the concentration of uric acid is high.[26] This syndrome can be exacerbated in patients who are dehydrated. If untreated, elevated uric acid levels will lead to further kidney damage.

Infection is the leading cause of death in multiple myeloma patients. Any episode of sepsis associated with hypotension or the use of nephrotoxic antibiotics (aminoglycosides with or without concurrent cephalosporins) should alert the clinician to closely monitor the individual for signs and symptoms of renal insufficiency.[26]

The treatment of renal insufficiency associated with multiple myeloma should be directed toward preventing or correcting the predisposing factors (dehydration, hypercalcemia, infection, hyperuricemia) and reducing the concentration and/or risk for precipitation of light chain proteins in the renal tubules. A recent study demonstrated that aggressive approaches to treatment resulted in 51% of the patients achieving normal renal function.[15] The prognosis for multiple myeloma patients with renal insufficiency has clearly improved.

Hyperviscosity Syndrome

Although rare (<5% of multiple myeloma patients), hyperviscosity syndrome can occur in individuals with IgM myeloma and occasionally in those with IgA, IgG_1 and IgG_3 myeloma.[1,4,26] It is caused by a high concentration of proteins that increase serum viscosity and result in vascular sludging. Initial clinical signs (blurred vision, irritability, headache, drowsiness, confusion) may indicate neurological impairment. Vascular sludging may also occur within the kidney, further compromising renal perfusion and increasing the risk for renal insufficiency. Plasmapheresis can be life-saving and is the treatment of choice for hyperviscosity syndrome.

TREATMENT

Chemotherapy

Patients with indolent, asymptomatic multiple myeloma are typically not treated with systemic therapy until clinical symptoms occur. There is widespread agreement that with the onset of symptoms (bone pain, hypercalcemia, anemia, renal failure), systemic antineoplastic therapy consisting of melphalan and prednisone is the first line of therapy.[1,3,4,27] The response rate is 30%–60%, with a median survival of 24–36 months.[28] Melphalan is usually administered on an intermittent schedule (0.25 mg/kg/day × 4 days) along with prednisone (2 mg/kg/day × 4 days). The treatment cycle is repeated every 4 weeks. This intermittent schedule allows patients to recover from the immunosuppresive effects of the drugs, is associated with fewer acute toxicities, and requires fewer blood counts. This chemotherapy protocol can be safely administered on an outpatient basis and allows the myeloma patient to remain in the community. Patients are monitored closely for signs of renal impairment (increased BUN and creatinine, proteinuria), and the dose of melphalan may need to be reduced based on the severity of renal toxicity. It is also important to closely monitor serial blood counts because the bone marrow suppressive effects of melphalan may be cumulative in older patients. Although the addition of prednisone increases the response rate, it does not confer any benefit toward long-term survival; it is useful, however, in preventing bone resorption that could lead to hypercalcemia and pathological fractures.[1,4] More recently, Samson and associates[29] demonstrated that VAD—vincristine (0.4 mg/24 hour continuous infusion × 4 days), doxorubicin (adriamycin 9 mg/m^2/continuous infusion × 4 days), and dexamethasone (odd-number cycles 40 mg PO days 1–4, 9–12, 17–20; even-number cycles 40 mg PO days 1–4 only)—could be safely administered as first-line therapy, with an improved response rate (84%) and improved median survival (44 months). VAD is administered every 28 days.

Clinicians must monitor the total dose of doxorubicin and treat patients to a maximum tolerated dose of 450 mg/m^2. Patients will most likely require an implantable intravascular device to enable safe administration of these vesicants and close monitoring of blood counts. Patients are closely monitored for signs and symptoms of steroid toxicity: severe dyspepsia, fluid and sodium retention, corticosteroid myopathy, acute pancreatitis, insulin-dependent hyperglycemia, and steroid psychosis. Any one of these toxicities mandates at least a 50% reduction, if not complete discontinuation, of dexamethasone. Severe neurologic toxicities (paresthesias or constipation) require at least a 50% reduction in the vincristine dose. In the face of progressive toxicity (paralytic ileus), vincristine must be discontinued. Prolonged thrombocytopenia and granulocytopenia requires 50%–100% reduction in the dose of adriamycin. If the adriamycin cannot be administered due to prolonged bone marrow suppression, the entire cycle may be delayed for 1 week and therapy resumed once the platelet count is above 50,000/mm^3 and the absolute neutrophil count (ANC) is over 750. Hepatic toxicity characterized by a bilirubin greater than 2.0 requires reduction or discontinuation of both adriamycin and vincristine depending on the severity. If the bilirubin is greater than 5.0, both adriamycin and vincristine are discontinued. If drug resistance emerges, cyclophosphamide (cytoxan) is another, structurally different alkylating agent that is cross-resistant with melphalan. Cyclophosphamide is also administered orally on an intermittent schedule. Patients are encouraged to increase their oral intake to avoid possible exacerbation of underlying renal dysfunction. Carefully monitor patients who may be concurrently receiving allopurinol, as this agent may enhance bone marrow suppression in patients receiving cytoxan.

Thirty percent to 40% of myeloma patients will not respond to first-line therapy, while those who initially respond will eventually relapse.[1,30] Consequently, second-line combination chemotherapy regimens have been developed. The most consistently effective second-line therapy, resulting in a 70% response rate with projected survival greater than 1 year, is the combination of vincristine, doxorubicin (adriamycin), and dexamethasone (previously described).[30,31] In an effort to minimize toxicity, increase response rates, and improve overall survival, investigators continue to combine agents such as doxorubicin and carmustine (BCNU); vincristine, carmustine, doxorubicin, and prednisone (VBAP); and etoposide, dexamethasone, cytarabine and cisplatin (EDAP).[11,30,32] To date, these clinical trials have been equivocal; further studies are warranted.

Interferon

In view of the equivocal results with combination chemotherapy for refractory multiple myeloma, it is not unreasonable for investigators to examine alternatives, such as alpha-interferon (IFNα).[33] The specific mechanism of action of IFN in multiple myeloma is unknown but is thought to be multifactorial. Interferon exerts its biologic effects by stimulating the host cells to indirectly affect tumor cells.[34] Despite this indirect effect on tumor cells, clinical investigators have demonstrated "minimal" to "no effect" in previously treated myeloma patients.[10,35] One study identified thrombocytopenia as a treatment-related toxicity that required transfusion support.[36] More recently, investigators have begun to use interferon for maintenance therapy in patients who have responded to 12 courses of induction chemotherapy. The investigators concluded that they were able to prolong response and survival with minimal toxicity (flulike syndrome).[37] The patient is closely monitored for evidence of interferon toxicity: anorexia, fatigue, hepatic toxicity (increased SGOT/bilirubin), and neurological changes. The dose reduction schedule (50%–100%) and plan to discontinue interferon are dependent on the severity of the toxicity. Nurses play a key role in assessing and grading treatment-related toxicities and in assisting patients and their families in managing side effects. Tumor burden and responsiveness to induction therapy appear to influence response rates, though further investigation with IFN is warranted.

Radiation

Radiation has been consistently used in the treatment of multiple myeloma for palliation of bone lesions and control of pain.[4,19,20] Fractionated doses (2000–2400 cGy) over a 2-week period can rapidly relieve pain, decrease local tumor growth, be effective in preventing pathological fractures and maintaining the patient's functional capacity. Over the course of the disease, patients and families require preparation and education regarding the local effects of radiation therapy and the possible need for multiple treatment fields (e.g., humerus, femur, spine).

Multiple myeloma is highly radioresponsive. Hemibody irradiation is a sequential technique in which the upper body is irradiated followed by a 4- to 6-week rest period and then by treatment to the lower body. In most cases, 750–850 cGy are given at a low-dose rate (25 cGy/min) to the hemibody.[4] Hemibody irradiation has been used for refractory myeloma and has been reported to decrease total myeloma cell mass and relieve pain.[30] Toxicities such as nausea, bone marrow suppression, and pneumonitis may be severe and limit the use of this technique. Nursing preparation for hemibody irradiation includes extensive patient and family education and the administration of corticosteroids and antiemetics. Although radiation therapy has demonstrated objective responses hemibody in the reduction of total myeloma cell mass, acute toxicities and treatment-related deaths may limit its utility.[30]

Bone Marrow Transplantation

Bone marrow transplantation (syngeneic, allogenic, autologous) has been attempted in the treatment of multiple myeloma.[30] Age restrictions of donors (syngeneic and allogeneic) may limit the availability of transplant to myeloma patients. Additionally, the technical difficulty in purging myeloma from the bone marrow limits the usefulness. One investigator demonstrated that a myeloma patient's autologous bone marrow could be purged with monoclonal antibodies.[38] No unexpected toxicity occurred, and 4 of 11 patients are disease-free posttransplant at 12.3, 17.5, 18.9, and 29 months.[38] The use of colony stimulating factors (GM-CSF, G-CSF, erythropoietin, and IL-1) to shorten the duration and severity of bone marrow suppression may be incorporated into future studies. Several clinical trials will be required to determine whether this costly and ambitious approach to myeloma will alter the natural history of the disease or affect long-term survival.

Treatment-Related Leukemia

A long-term sequela of treatment for multiple myeloma is the development of acute leukemia. Treatment-related leukemia is thought to result from prolonged exposure to alkylating agents and has been reported at a frequency of 20% after 50 months of follow-up.[1] The first signs of treatment-related acute leukemia may be signs of myelodysplastic syndrome. Bone marrow examination may show karyotypic abnormalities on chromosomes 5 and 7. Although treatment-induced acute leukemia can be treated with standard induction therapy for acute nonlymphocytic leukemia (ANLL), it has a lower response rate than de novo ANLL.

NURSING MANAGEMENT

Multiple myeloma is a chronic disease with no known cure. The patient may experience indolent periods as well as acute episodes. In planning the nursing care it is imperative that the physician and nurse agree on the treatment goals, and share these with the patient and family. Goals can encompass preventing/delaying life-threatening complications, prolonging survival, palliation or terminal care. A symptom management approach to nursing care with a review of systems is presented in Table 48-3.

Neurologic

The most frequent symptom that myeloma patients present with is pain. Bone destruction from the myeloma results in osteoporosis and pathologic fractures of long bones and vertebrae that require aggressive assessment and management of both acute and chronic pain.[19,20] Acute pain is characterized by a specific trauma (fracture) and is of short duration (less than 6 months), whereas chronic pain has no specific initiation point that is obvious. Interventions for pain include assessment, proper positioning of affected limbs, use of supports and braces (cervical collar, back brace, sling) to prevent additional stress on bones, and consultation with physical and occupational therapists. The effective and appropriate utilization of narcotics and nonnarcotic analgesics, massage, heat, and/or cold where appropriate should be included.[40,41]

Mental status changes can be an initial sign of hypercalcemia, hyperviscosity syndrome, or drug toxicity. Any change in mental status requires closer assessment to determine etiologic factors so the appropriate treatment can be promptly initiated. The nurse also plans for prevention of injury and maintaining the patient in a safe environment.[42] Depression, anxiety, and insomnia are but a few of the psychological responses that patients may exhibit in response to their disease and treatment.[43,44] Guidelines for care of patients with these psychological responses to their disease are provided in Chapters 19–22.

Protective Mechanisms

Infection is the leading cause of death in patients with multiple myeloma. The supportive care of cancer pa-

TABLE 48-3 Nursing Care of the Patient with Multiple Myeloma

System	Signs/Symptoms	Patient Education
Neuromuscular	Hypercalcemia Hyperviscosity syndrome Pathological fractures Cord compression Pain Depression	Signs and symptoms of hypercalcemia Prevention of pathological fractures Pain control measures Distraction therapy, hopeful attitude
Protective mechanisms	Anemia Neutropenia Thrombocytopenia	Conservation of energy Prevention of infection Prevention of bleeding
Respiratory	Pneumonia	Prevention of pooling of pulmonary secretions Increasing gas exchange
Gastrointestinal	Constipation	Prevention Change in fluid/dietary intake, meds Increase activity
Genitourinary	Renal insufficiency (hyperuricemia, hypercalcemia, infection)	Increase fluid intake Allopurinal administration Recognition of signs of UTI

tients with anemia, thrombocytopenia, and neutropenia is well documented in the nursing literature.[45-47] Guidelines for the care of neutropenic patients are principally aimed at the early recognition and/or prevention of infection; care of the thrombocytopenic patient is directed toward preventing bleeding. Blood product support will mainly consist of packed red blood cell and platelet transfusions. Although hematopoietic growth factors are available for the treatment of anemia and neutropenia (e.g., erythropoietin-EPO®; Neupogen®, G-CSF), none of the agents is specifically FDA-approved for use with multiple myeloma.

Respiratory

The respiratory system is the most frequent site of infection in myeloma patients. As a result, nursing care is directed toward teaching patients and their families activities that decrease pooling of pulmonary secretions and increase gas exchange (e.g., coughing and deep breathing exercises, use of incentive spirometers, avoiding family members with signs and symptoms of URI). Patients and families are instructed about the symptoms that are important to report to the physician immediately, such as fever, cough, sore throat, and sputum production.[4] Due to the underlying defect in humoral immunity induced by multiple myeloma, patients should be instructed not to receive vaccines with live organisms or be in close contact with others who may have received live organism vaccines that may be shedding organisms.[4]

Gastrointestinal

Multiple myeloma patients are at risk for constipation as a result of decreased physical activity due to bone pain/pathological fractures, treatment of pain with narcotic analgesics, dehydration, and the use of vincristine. Although not considered a life-threatening clinical problem, this condition can influence nutritional intake, comfort, and quality of life.[20] Nursing management includes the assessment of past and present bowel habits, changes in fluid and dietary intake, medication administration, activity changes, and patient and family education.[48]

Genitourinary

Renal insufficiency or failure can be exacerbated as a result of the primary disease, fluid and electrolyte abnormalities (hyperuricemia, hypercalcemia), dehydration, and/or infection. Nursing care is directed at preventing or quickly reversing renal insufficiency. Maintaining adequate hydration along with the administration of allopurinol will protect the kidneys from uric acid nephropathy.[4,26] The nurse closely monitors the patient for early signs and symptoms of UTI (fever, dysuria, frequency, urgency) and educates patients and families to recognize these symptoms and report them promptly to the physician.

CONCLUSION

The last decade has witnessed dramatic improvements in the overall response rates for patients with multiple myeloma. The utilization of combination chemotherapy, earlier recognition of complications, and appropriate utilization of support therapies have all contributed to increasing patient survival.

In the next decade, we will witness increasing utilization of new technologies to better determine etiologic factors contributing to the development of multiple myeloma.

The nursing care of multiple myeloma patients and their families offers the nurse an opportunity to care for patients experiencing both the acute and chronic sequelae of disease. Nursing care can have a direct effect in early recognition of complications and managing toxicity. Patient and family education can lead to the early recognition and identification of complications, contributing to overall improvement in quality of life. Future areas for nursing research include studying specific nursing interventions aimed at symptom distress.

REFERENCES

1. Bubley GJ, Schnipper LE: Multiple myeloma. In Holleb AI (ed), *American Cancer Society Textbook of Clinical Oncology*. Atlanta, GA: ACS, 1991, pp. 397–409.
2. Jacobs P: Myeloma. *Dis Mon* 36(6):317–371, 1990.
3. Barlogie B, Epstein J, Selvanayagam P, et al: Plasma cell myeloma—New biological insights and advances in therapy. *Blood* 73(4):865–879, 1989.
4. Barton Cook M: Multiple myeloma. In Groenwald SL et al (eds), *Cancer Nursing: Principles and Practice* (2d ed). Boston: Jones and Bartlett, 1990, pp. 991–998.
5. Riedel DA: Epidemiology of multiple myeloma. In Wiernik PH (ed), *Neoplastic Diseases of the Blood*. New York: Churchill Livingston, 1991, pp. 347–372.
6. Oken MM: Multiple myeloma. *Med Clin North Amer* 68(3):757–787, 1984.
7. Potter M: Plasmacytomas in mice. *Semin Oncol* 13:275–281, 1986.
8. Maldonado JE, Kyle RA. Familial myeloma: Report of eight families and a study of serum proteins in their relatives. *Am J Med* 57:875–884, 1974.
9. Durie BG, Stock-Novack D, Salmon SE, et. al: Prognostic value of pretreatment serum beta 2 microglobulin in myeloma: A Southwest Oncology Group study. *Blood* 75(4):823–830, 1990.
10. Alexanian R, Barlogie B, Gutterman J. Alpha interferon combination therapy of resistant myeloma. *Am J Clin Oncol* 14(3):188–192, 1991.

11. Friedenberg WR, Kyel RA, Knospe WH, et al: High-dose dexamethasone for refractory or relapsing multiple myeloma. *Am J Hematol* 36(3):171–175, 1991.
12. Cherng NC, Asal NR, Kuebler JP, et al: Prognostic factors in multiple myeloma. *Cancer* 67(12):3150–3156, 1991.
13. Cavo M, Galieni P, Zuffa E, et al: Prognostic variables and clinical staging in multiple myeloma. *Blood* 74(5):1774–1780, 1989.
14. San Miguel JF, Sanchez J, Gonzalez M: Prognostic factors and classification in multiple myeloma. *Br J Cancer* 59(1):113–118, 1989.
15. Alexanian RJ, Barlogie B, Dixon D: Renal failure in multiple myeloma pathogenesis and prognostic implications. *Arch Intern Med* 150(8):1693–1695, 1990.
16. Durie BGM, Salmon SE: A clinical staging system for multiple myeloma. *Cancer* 36:842–854, 1975.
17. Durie BGM: Staging and kinetics of multiple myeloma. *Semin Oncol* 13(3):300–309, 1986.
18. Mundy GR, Bertolini DR: Bone destruction and hypercalcemia in plasma cell myeloma. *Semin Oncol* 13(3):291–299, 1986.
19. Anderson MG: The lymphomas and multiple myeloma. In Baird SB et al (eds), *A Cancer Source Book for Nurses.* Atlanta, GA: American Cancer Society, 1991, pp. 286–295.
20. Farrant C: Multiple myeloma: Controlling pain, prolonged survival. *RN* 50:38–42, 1987.
21. Jacobson DR, Zolla-Pazner S: Immunosuppression and infection in multiple myeloma. In Wiernik PH (ed), *Neoplastic Diseases of the Blood.* New York: Churchill Livingston, 1991, pp. 415–426.
22. Jacobson DR, Zolla-Pazner S: Immunosuppression and infection in multiple myeloma. *Semin Oncol* 13(3):282–290, 1986.
23. Savage DG, Lindenbaum J, Garrett TJ: Biphasic pattern of bacterial infection in multiple myeloma. *Ann Intern Med* 96:47–50, 1982.
24. Duffy TP: The many pitfalls of diagnosis of myeloma. *N Engl J Med* 326(6):394–396, 1992.
25. Cohen DJ, Sherman WH, Osserman EF, et al: Acute renal failure in patients with multiple myeloma. *Am J Med* 76:247–256, 1984.
26. Ellison DH, Johnson Bia M: Renal, fluid, and electrolyte disorders in the critically ill immunosuppressed patient. In Parrillo JE (ed), *The Critically Ill Immunosuppressed Patient: Diagnosis and Management.* Rockville MD: Aspen 1987, pp. 81–118.
27. Boccadoro M, Marmont F, Tribalto M, et al: Multiple myeloma: VMCP/VBAP alternating combination chemotherapy is not superior to melphalan and prednisone even in high-risk patients. *J Clin Oncol* 9(3):444–448, 1991.
28. Ahre A, Bjorkholm H, Mellstedt G, et al: Human leukocyte interferon and intermittent high-dose melphalan-prednisone administration in the treatment of multiple myeloma. *Cancer Treat Rep* 68(11):1331–1338, 1984.
29. Samson D, Gaminara E, Newland A, et al: Infusion of vincristine and doxorubicin with oral dexamethasone as first-line therapy for multiple myeloma. *Lancet* (2):882–885, 1989.
30. Kyle RA, Greipp PR, Gertz MA: Treatment of refractory multiple myeloma and considerations for future therapy. *Semin Oncol* 13(3):326–333, 1986.
31. Barlogie B, Smith L, Alexanian R: Effective treatment of advanced multiple myeloma refractory to alkylating agents. *N Engl J Med* 310:1353–1356, 1984.
32. Barlogie B, Velasquez WS, Alexanian R, et al: Etoposide, dexamethasone, cytarabine, and cisplatin in vincristine, doxorubicin, and dexamethasone-refractory myeloma. *J Clin Oncol* 7(10):1514–1517, 1989.
33. Kirkwood JM, Ernstoff MS: Interferons in the treatment of human cancer. *J Clin Oncol* 2(4):336–352, 1984.
34. Cooper MR, Welander CE: Interferons in the treatment of multiple myeloma. *Semin Oncol* 13(3):334–340, 1986.
35. Wagstaff J, Lyonds P, Scarffe JH: Phase II study of rDNA human alpha-2 interferon in multiple myeloma. *Cancer Treat Rep* 69:495–498, 1985.
36. Rtodjer S, Vikrot O, Wahlin A, et al: Effect of interferon alpha-2b in advanced multiple myeloma. *J Intern Med* 227(1):45–48, 1990.
37. Mandelli F, Avvisati G, Amadori S, et al: Maintenance treatment with recombinant interferon alpha-2b in patients with multiple myeloma responding to conventional induction chemotherapy. *N Engl J Med* 322(20):1430–1434, 1990.
38. Anderson KC, Barut BA, Ritz J, et al: Monoclonal antibody-purged autologous bone marrow transplantation therapy for multiple myeloma. *Blood* 77(4):712–720, 1991.
39. Donovan MI: Acute pain relief. *Nurs Clin North Amer* 25(4):851–861, 1990.
40. Paice J: Alteration in comfort: Acute pain. In McNally JC et al (eds), *Guidelines for Oncology Nursing Practice.* Philadelphia: Saunders, 1991, pp. 125–130.
41. Willoughby SJ: Alteration in comfort: Chronic pain. In McNally JC et al (eds), *Guidelines for Oncology Nursing Practice.* Philadelphia: Saunders, 1991, pp. 131–142.
42. Kanak MF: Interventions related to patient safety. *Nurs Clin North Amer* 27(2):371–395, 1992.
43. Kline PM: Reactive depression in the client with cancer. In Chernecky CC (ed), *Critical Nursing Care of the Client with Cancer.* Norwalk, CT: Appleton-Century-Croft, 1984, pp. 265–271.
44. Buckwalter KC, Babich KS: Psychologic aspects of depression. *Nurs Clin North Amer* 25(4):945–954, 1990.
45. McNally JC, Stair J: Potential for infection. In McNally JC et al (eds), *Guidelines for Oncology Nursing Practice.* Philadelphia: Saunders, 1991, pp. 191–202.
46. Alexander EJ: Potential for injury related to thrombocytopenia. In McNally JC et al (eds), *Guidelines for Oncology Nursing Practice.* Philadelphia: Saunders, 1991, pp. 203–207.
47. Rostad M: Potential for injury related to anemia. In McNally JC et al (eds), *Guidelines for Oncology Nursing Practice.* Philadelphia: Saunders, 1991, pp. 208–215.
48. French M, Rostad M, Wroblewski SK: Alteration in bowel elimination: Constipation. In McNally JC et al (eds), *Guidelines for Oncology Nursing Practice.* Philadelphia: Saunders, 1991, pp. 297–301.
49. Hull AR: Complications of uremia. *Urol Clin North Amer* 9(2): 275–278, 1982.

Chapter 49

Skin Cancers

Marsha Ketcham, RN, OCN

Lois J. Loescher, MS, RN

INTRODUCTION

Cancers of the skin consist of basal cell carcinoma (BCC), squamous cell carcinoma (SCC), and malignant melanoma. BCC and SCC are often grouped together and referred to as nonmelanoma skin cancer (NMSC). Most melanomas are cutaneous (CM); others, which are rare, originate in the eye or viscera. Although cutaneous cancers share common etiologic factors, they vary in other regards. NMSCs have a higher incidence but have a low metastatic potential and mortality rate. The associated morbidity is of concern, as NMSC often requires costly, extensive, and repeated treatments that may result in cosmetic and functional damage. Conversely, melanoma has a much lower incidence but a mortality rate triple that of the NMSC. The increased mortality from melanoma is directly related to its high potential for metastasis. An understanding of the associated epidemiologic, etiologic, and pathophysiologic factors will help oncology nurses recognize the subtle and major differences among these skin cancers. Knowledge of assessment, treatment, and prevention of nonmelanoma and melanoma skin cancers enables nurses to provide quality care for individuals with the disease and those at high risk.

EPIDEMIOLOGY

The rising incidence of skin cancers has been called an "emerging epidemic."[1] Over 700,000 new skin cancers are reported annually, with most of those being BCC or SCC.[2] The incidence of NMSC among whites in the United States is about 165/100,000 persons. BCC is the most common form of skin cancer in whites and outnumbers SCC by a ratio of 3:1.[3] BCC occurs twice as often in men as in women; similarly, SCC occurs two to three times more often in men.[4,5] One study found that over a 20-year period, SCC increased 2.6 times in men and 3.1 times in women.[1] Figure 49-1 shows the age-specific, increasing incidence rates for NMSC for white males and females.[6] BCC and SCC are associated with an overall 5-year survival rate of 95% but still account for an estimated 2300 deaths per year.[2] One recent study estimated an age-adjusted NMSC mortality rate of 0.44/100,000 per year.[7]

Approximately 32,000 melanoma cases are reported annually.[2] Since 1973 the incidence of CM in whites has increased more than that of any other major cancer, except lung cancer in women.[8] There has been an overall increase of 80% from 1973 to 1987, and a yearly increase of about 4%. CM is largely confined to

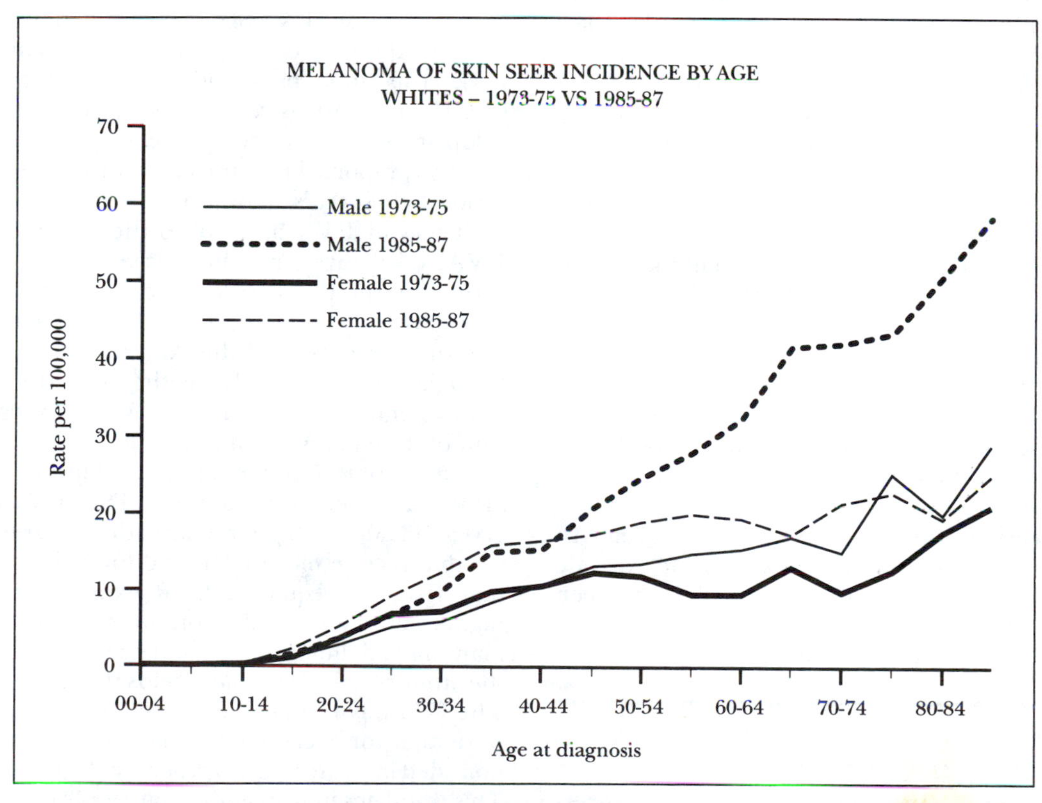

FIGURE 49-1 Melanoma of skin. SEER incidence by age in whites 1973–1975 vs 1985–1987.

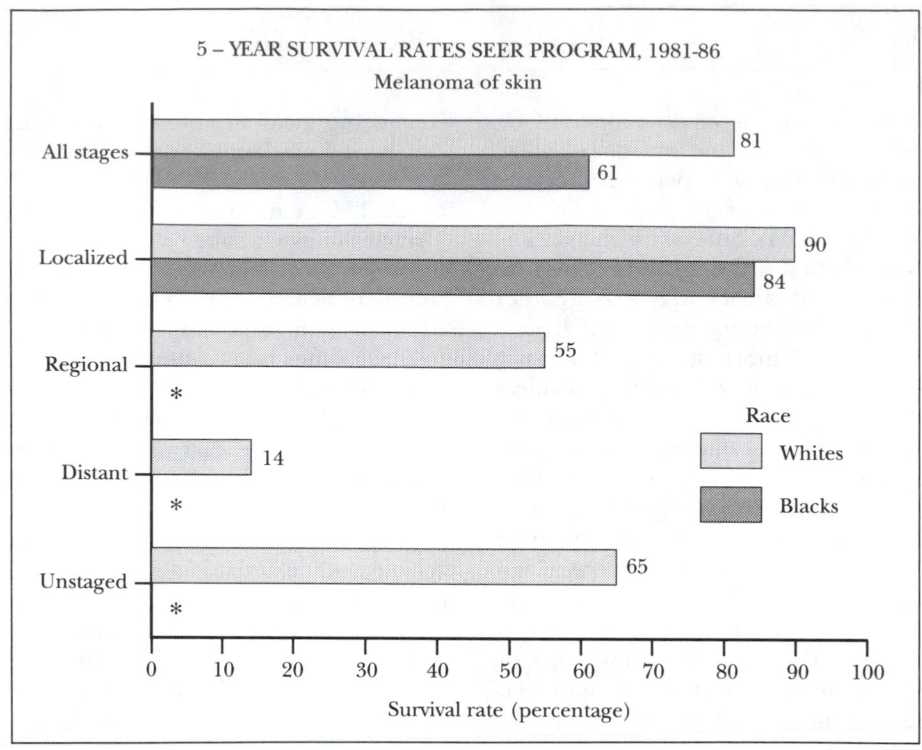

FIGURE 49-2 Five-year survival rates, SEER program, 1981–1986.

whites, who have an incidence of about 10/100,000.[8] Age-adjusted CM incidence rates among white males are higher than those for white females, being approximately 11.9 and 8.9 per 100,000 respectively.[6] Glass and Hoover[1] found that over 20 years, men had a 3.5-fold and women a 4.6-fold increase of CM.

Although CM represents only about 4% of skin cancers, its malignant potential must not be underestimated, as it accounts for an estimated 6700 cancer deaths annually.[2] In the age-adjusted cancer mortality rates reported by the SEER (Surveillance, Epidemiology, and End Results) program in 1990, the percent increase in mortality for both sexes and all races from 1973 to 1987 was 29.8%.[6] Early detection and treatment, however, increased the overall relative 5-year survival rate for whites from 60%–68% during 1960–1973 to about 80% from 1974–1986. The relative 5-year survival rate for blacks ranged from 49%–60% during 1974–1986.[6,9] Figure 49-2 shows the CM 5-year survival rates in whites and blacks based on disease stage.

Skin cancers of any type are rare in children. Although the incidence rate increases with each decade of age, skin cancers generally occur in adults between 30 and 60 years of age.[5]

ETIOLOGY

Multiple etiologic factors associated with skin cancers were recently reviewed by Fraser et al.[10] These are summarized in Table 49-1. Ultraviolet radiation (UVR) is the probable cause of the majority of skin cancers, although other etiologic factors also are involved. UVR is a major cause of NMSCs, which are commonly found on sun-exposed areas of the body such as the head and neck, arms, upper back, and legs. The direct association of CM with UVR is controversial, as CM can also develop in non–sun-exposed areas. Scotto and Fears,[11] however, reported that the effect of UVR exposure on incidence of CM is significant.

Types of UVR harmful to the skin are UVB and UVA. UVB rays have short wavelengths and are absorbed by the top skin layer, causing sunburn. UVA rays have long wavelengths and can penetrate deeply into the lower levels of the skin, causing damage. The biologic effects of UVR on the skin are most likely photochemical alteration of DNA and partial suppression of T-cell and B-cell immunity.[3,12,13]

Geographic, environmental, and lifestyle factors all affect human exposure to UVR. The incidence of both CM and NMSC is higher in latitudes closer to the equator that receive more UVR and lower in latitudes farther from the equator. UVR exposure increases at higher altitudes.[3,14] Chlorofluorocarbons (CFCs) are man-made pollutants that deplete stratospheric ozone, the atmospheric layer that shields the earth from UVR. The U.S. Environmental Protection Agency (EPA) reports that for every 1% decrease in ozone, a 2% compounded increase in UVB reaching the earth will result. This translates into an additional 1%–3% increased skin cancer incidence per year.[15] The type of clothing worn,

TABLE 49-1 Examples of Etiologic Factors for Basal Cell Carcinoma, Squamous Cell Carcinoma, and Cutaneous Melanoma

Factor	Examples
Host factors	
Pigmentation/Phenotype	Light skin, hair, and eyes; easily sunburned
Precursor lesions	Actinic keratosis,* arsenical keratosis,* Bowen's disease,* chronic radiation keratosis*
Hereditary conditions	Nevoid basal cell syndrome,† xeroderma pigmentosum, dysplastic nevus syndrome,‡ congenital nevi,‡ lentigo maligna‡
Immunosuppression	Organ transplant recipients*
Environmental factors	
Ultraviolet (UV) radiation	Solar UVA and UVB rays; tanning devices
Pollutants	Chlorofluorocarbons (CFCs)
Chemicals	Polycyclic hydrocarbons,*† inorganic arsenic,*† psoralens†
Ionizing radiation	X-ray therapy for tinea capitis,*† enlarged thymus; radon,*† radium*†
Viruses	Human papilloma virus*
Physical trauma	Cutaneous damage following burns

*Only squamous cell carcinoma.
†Only basal cell carcinoma.
‡Only cutaneous melanoma.

as well as the time of day also affect the amount of UVR exposure.

Most individuals have many pigmented lesions on their bodies (moles, freckles, birthmarks), and the average white adult averages 10–40 lesions.[16] A few of these lesions may be present at birth, while others develop throughout life. Almost all are normal; however, a change in any pigmented area can be indicative of skin cancer.[17,18] A persistently changed or changing mole or presence of irregular pigmented precursor lesions (dysplastic nevi, congenital nevi, lentigo maligna) represents a major high-risk situation for CM. Dysplastic nevi (atypical moles) are cutaneous markers that identify family members who are at extremely high risk for CM. Individuals with familial dysplastic nevi are several hundred times more likely to develop melanoma than controls in the general population.[16] Dysplastic nevi are discussed in more detail in the "Cutaneous Melanoma" section of this chapter.

Skin pigmentation is clearly important in the etiology of skin cancers in that American blacks and persons of African, Asian, or Mediterranean descent are known to have a lower incidence.[6] When these individuals do develop CM, it usually originates on the less densely pigmented areas of the body such as the palms, soles, and fingernails.[14] Whites with red hair and fair complexions who tend to sunburn or freckle easily have higher relative risks for all skin cancers, ranging from 1.4 to 20.1.[18–20]

Other possible risk factors for CM include age, hormonal factors, immunosuppression, and a previous history of melanoma.[8,18] Family history of CM increases its relative risk in the range of two to eight times.[21,22] No conclusive evidence exists regarding the use of oral contraceptives and the increased risk of CM;[23–25] however, some physicians recommend that women with a history of melanoma use a nonhormonal contraceptive.

NONMELANOMA SKIN CANCERS

Basal Cell Carcinoma

Pathophysiology

BCC is the least aggressive type of skin cancer. BCC is an epithelial tumor with a disputed site of origin, believed to arise either from cells in the basal layer of the epidermis that have an impaired ability to mature and keratinize or from cells in the surrounding dermal structures.[3,26] BCC usually grows slowly by direct extension and has the capacity to involve and destroy local tissue, including nerves, lymphatics, blood vessels, cartilage, and bone.[27,28]

Assessment

Differences in BCC classifications are determined clinically and histologically. Common classifications include nodular (also called nodulo-ulcerative), superficial, pigmented, morpheaform, and keratotic[27] (Table 49-2). Nodular BCC is the most common type. Histologically, nodular BCC consists of masses of tumor cells that have large oval nuclei, are uniform in appearance, and resemble basal cells of the epidermis. These cells descend from the epidermis and fill the dermis, with the peripheral cells resembling a picket fence pattern.[26,29] Clinically, nodular BCC begins as a small, firm, well-demarcated, dome-shaped papule. The color can be pearly white, pink, or skin-colored, with telangiectases often evident on the surface. As the lesion enlarges, it ulcerates peripherally or centrally and develops raised, pearly, well-circumscribed borders. Nodular BCC most commonly occurs on the face, head, and neck.[3,29–31] (See Figure 49-3/Plate 18).

TABLE 49-2 Comparisons of the Classifications of Nonmelanoma Skin Cancers

Type	Site	Clinical Description	Histologic Factors
Nodular BCC (most common)	Face, head, neck	Small, firm, well-demarcated dome-shaped papule; pearly, white, pink, or flesh colored with telangiectases; may ulcerate	Uniform masses of cells with large oval nuclei; resemble, epidermal basal cells
Superficial BCC (2nd most common)	Trunk, extremities	Flat, erythematous or pink scaling plaques or papules; well-defined margins; occasional shallow erosions or crusts	A bud of irregular proliferating tumor attached under the epidermis
Pigmented BCC (less common)	Head, neck, face	Melanin-pigmented center; shiny, pearly, papulary border with well-defined margins and telangiectases; resembles melanoma	Similar to nodular
Morpheaform BCC (rare)	Head, neck	Flat, ivory-colored or colorless; scarlike, ill-defined margins	Many roots with branching strands embedded in collagen and elastic fibers
Keratotic BCC (basosquamous)	Pre- and postauricular sulcus	Similar to nodular BCC	Contains basal cells and squamous-appearing cells that keratinize
Squamous cell carcinoma	Areas exposed to UV radiation; common sites: nose, forehead, ear, back of hands, lower lip	Flesh-colored or erythematous; raised, firm papule; may ulcerate, indurate crust and bleed	Well differentiated (similar to normal squamous epithelium, keratin pearls common); anaplastic (distorted nuclei, numerous mitoses, bizarre cells)

BCC; basal cell carcinoma.

Superficial BCC is the second most common type, histologically exhibiting a bud of irregular proliferating tumor tissue attached to the undersurface of the epidermis. Clinically, it is flat and has erythematous or pink scaling plaques or papules with well-defined margins and occasional shallow erosions or crusts.[29–31] Superficial BCC usually develops on the trunk and extremities.

Pigmented BCC is less common and may be nodular or superficial. It has a melanin pigment concentrated in the center of a nest of BCC cells, causing a brown, black, or blue color that can be clinically mistaken for melanoma.[27] Also present is a shiny, pearly, papulary border with well-defined margins, and telangiectases.[29,30] Biologically, the behavior of pigmented BCC is similar to that of nodular BCC.[29] Pigmented BCC most commonly occurs on the head, neck, and face.

Morpheaform BCC is the rarest type. Histologically, this tumor has many roots with branching strands embedded in dense fibrous stroma of collagen and elastic fibers.[29–31] Clinically, it is flat and ivory-colored or colorless, resembles a scar, lacks translucency, and has ill-defined margins. This lesion is more aggressive than nodular BCC, having increased invasiveness and destructiveness of surrounding tissues, particularly, muscle, nerve, and bone. Morpheaform BCC develops primarily on the head and neck.

Keratotic (or basosquamous) BCC contains basal cells and squamoid-appearing cells that keratinize. Unlike the other BCCs, this tumor grows aggressively, recurs locally, and is more likely to metastasize. Keratotic BCC develops in the pre- and postauricular sulcus.[27]

Squamous Cell Carcinoma

Pathophysiology

SCC is a tumor that may arise in any epithelium. Its behavior in the skin is similar to that of neoplasms arising from stratified squamous epithelium in other organ sites. The cells of SCC vary from well-differentiated to completely anaplastic. The well-differentiated tumor cell has a histologic appearance similar to that seen in normal squamous epithelium, in that it is a large polygonal cell with intercellular bridges and round nuclei. Some individual cell keratinization exists, and formation of keratin pearls is common. Keratinization and keratin pearl formation diminish as the tumor becomes less well-differentiated and disappears with high-grade tumors. As the tumor cells become more anaplastic, the nuclei become distorted in shape, mitosis become more numerous, cell shapes become more bizarre, and cell numbers increase.[3,32] SCC is more aggressive than BCC as it has a faster growth rate, less well-demarcated margins, and a greater metastatic potential.[3,30,33] The depth of SCC plays an important role in determining metastatic potential. SCC that is involved at the level of the sweat gland is more malignant.[27] In addition, the metastatic potential of SCC is increased in patients receiving immunosuppressive agents.[3,30,32–34] Metastatic disease is usually first noted in the regional lymph nodes.

Assessment

SCC appears as a flesh-colored or erythematous raised firm papule. It may be crusted with keratin products and in its early or late stages may ulcerate and bleed, becoming tender and painful. Infiltration of the tumor into normal surrounding skin produces induration around the nodule (Figure 49-4—Plate 19). SCC is usually confined to areas exposed to UVR. The most highly exposed areas of skin, such as the top of the nose, the forehead, the ear helices, the back of hands and the lower lip, tend to be more affected. With the exception of the lower lip site, SCC on these areas is less likely to metastasize than lesions located on areas not exposed to UVR.[30,35] SCC can also arise in old radiation, thermal, or chemical burn scars; in areas of chronic inflammation or increased cell proliferation; and in mucous membranes. Tumors originating in these areas are more aggressive and have a high frequency of metastasis.

Several preexisting conditions may lead to invasive SCC. Intraepidermal SCC, also called carcinoma in situ, may develop in existing cutaneous lesions such as scar tissue, solar keratoses, radiation keratoses, and Bowen's disease. Intraepidermal SCC remains in the epidermis for an extended time but unpredictably passes through the basement membrane and extends into the dermis. These lesions appear as slightly raised erythematous plaques with varying amounts of scaling and well-defined margins. Other conditions include keratoacanthomas, which are hyperkeratotic lesions morphologically similar to SCC, and epidermodysplasia verruciformis, characterized by multiple flat, wartlike lesions containing oncogenic type 5 human papillomavirus.[36]

Treatment of Nonmelanoma Skin Cancers

Standard treatment for NMSC includes surgical excision, chemosurgery, curettage and electrodesiccation, radiation, and cryotherapy. Factors to consider when choosing a treatment are tumor type, location, size, growth pattern, and whether the tumor is primary or secondary. The patient's age and general health also should be considered. No single therapy is applicable to all tumors; however, the primary goals of treatment are cure, preservation of tissue and function, minimal operative risk, and optimal cosmetic results.

The four types of biopsy techniques used for NMSCs are the shave biopsy (a superficial part of the tumor is sliced with a scalpel), the punch biopsy (a deeper specimen is punched out by an instrument placed into the reticular dermis or subcutaneous tissue), the incisional biopsy (a portion of the tumor is removed with a scalpel), and the excisional biopsy (the entire lesion is removed for histologic analysis). The biopsy technique should be individually selected to yield the optimum specimen for determining correct diagnosis.[3]

Surgical excision

Surgical excision can be performed for any NMSC and may be simple or complex, depending on tumor size and location. An elliptical excision with suture closure of a small to moderate lesion using local anesthesia usually can be done on an outpatient basis. Surgical excision facilitates healing of large carcinoma sites where thin layers of subcutaneous tissue overlie bony areas such as the forehead, scalp, and distal extremities. Surgical excision also is beneficial in treating residual tumor and large carcinomas presenting in conjunction with late radiation dermatitis and those arising in scars and ulcers, as these areas cannot tolerate radiation therapy. In addition, excision of large carcinomas of the eyelid and lip preserves function and allows reconstruction by graft or flap.[32]

A skin graft or flap may be performed as an adjunct to surgical excision. A graft or flap is indicated when a lesion is large or located in an area where insufficient tissue for primary closure would result in deformity. A skin flap consists of skin and subcutaneous tissue transferred from one area of the body to another. A flap contains its own blood supply, whereas a graft is avascular and depends on the blood supply of the recipient site for its survival. Skin grafting or flapping requires hospitalization, and possible complications include graft failure, hematoma, scarring, and infection.

The advantages of surgical excision as a treatment are rapid healing, the fact that an entire specimen for histologic examination can be obtained, and favorable cosmetic results. Disadvantages are that the procedure is time-consuming and requires a skilled physician to judge the exact extent of the tumor and risk of infection.[29–31,35]

Mohs micrographic surgery

Another type of surgical treatment available for select tumors is Mohs micrographic surgery (also called chemosurgery). This procedure involves horizontal shaving and staining of tissue in thin layers with careful histologic mapping of all specimen margins. This is the most accurate technique of assessing the actual extent of NMSC. Mohs microsurgery is most often used as a first line of treatment for cancers in high-risk areas such as the nose and nasolabial folds, the medial canthus, and pre- and postauricular locations.[37] It is also used for lesions with unclear margins, recurrent lesions, aggressive tumors, and extensive lesions (usually larger than 2 cm). Skin grafting may need to accompany this treatment. The advantages of Mohs microsurgery include preservation of the maximum amount of tissue for easier reconstruction, the ability to histologically map tumor margins, and performance of the procedure on an outpatient basis using a local anesthetic.[29,35,37,38] The disadvantages are the requirement of specialized training and equipment, the time-consuming nature of the procedure (4–6 hours), the need for daily wound care postoperatively, and the possibility of graft rejection and wound dehiscence.[37–39]

Curettage and electrodesiccation

Curettage and electrodesiccation treatment is used only for BCC skin cancers that are small (<2 cm), superficial, or recurrent because of poor margin control. The tumor is destroyed by scraping out the tumor mass through curettage and treating the tumor base with electrodesiccation, or a low-voltage electrode. The physician uses the curettage to determine the tumor edges. As tumor tissue is softer and more friable than normal tissue, electrodesiccation maintains hemostasis and softens normal tissue so a safe margin can be curettaged.[3,30–32] Advantages of this treatment are its rapidity, good cosmetic results, preservation of normal tissue, and the opportunity to obtain a tissue specimen for histopathology. Disadvantages include no margin control, prolonged healing, the need for physician skill to seek out the tumor tissue by "feel," and persistent tumor in some anatomical areas.[3,29] In place of the low-voltage electrode physicians may use a carbon dioxide laser to vaporize tumor. When used with curettage, this treatment is beneficial for superficial BCC and non-aggressive BCC. Advantages of this alternative treatment are minimal thermal injury to adjacent cells, faster healing, and minimal pain.[27]

Radiotherapy

Radiotherapy generally is recommended only for lesions that are inoperable; lesions located in sites such as the corner of the nose, eyelid, lip and canthus; and those greater than 1 cm but less than 8 cm.[27] Patients who are poor surgical candidates may benefit from radiotherapy, but the treatment is not recommended for younger patients (less than age 45) since the irradiated area becomes more atrophic, erythematous, and irregular over the years.[3,29–31,35,40] Radiation is administered in fractional doses because increased skin tolerance may enhance its effectiveness.[32] Advantages of radiotherapy are painless treatment, preservation of normal anatomic contours, and the ability to extend treatment into areas surrounding the tumor if desired. Disadvantages include lack of histologic tissue for margin control, long treatment periods (3–4 weeks), the danger that the treatment itself may lead to BCC or SCC, and the need for clinical facilities with persons trained in radiotherapy.

Radon moulds, the direct application of radioactive sources to the lesion have been used since 1975. Ashby et al.[41] reported that published experiences and results of the use of radon moulds are lacking. Radon moulds are mainly indicated for use in the treatment of superficial lesions (not >4-mm depth) at sites of poor radiation tolerance (e.g., the dorsum of the hand and the anterior lower leg).

Cryotherapy

Cryotherapy involves tumor destruction by using liquid nitrogen to freeze and thaw tumor tissue. The tumor is locally anesthetized; then liquid nitrogen is applied to the lesion by open spray, causing a quick, intense freezing of the tissue, which is then allowed to thaw slowly. This cycle is repeated, and tumor necrosis and erosion follow.

Cryotherapy can be used for small to large primary tumors, for certain recurrent lesions such as those in areas of prior radiation, for multiple superficial BCC, and for lesions needing palliative treatment. Only lesions with well-defined margins (both lateral and depth) benefit from this treatment.[31,39] A minimum of 3-mm margins should be used.[42] Cryotherapy is not recommended for the medial canthal area and the rim of the ears as frozen cartilage buckles during healing and recurrence rates are high.[31,35] Advantages to this treatment include the fact that it produces minimal discomfort (a burning or hot sensation is usually experienced), can be done on an outpatient basis, and can be performed quickly with good cosmetic results. Disadvantages include the need for wound care, prolonged healing time, possible temporary nerve damage, bleeding, and the lack of a specimen for pathology.[39,42,43] Careful follow-up is suggested for 2 years postoperatively to detect secondary tumors, which usually occur within 18 months.[42]

Other treatments

Investigational studies for NMSCs are currently ongoing. Those showing encouraging results for the preexcisional treatment of superficial or nodular BCC and SCC are intralesional alpha-2 interferon[27,44] and photodynamic therapy.[45] Topical application of photosensitizers such as tetraphenylprophenosulphonate (TPPS) to superficial BCC, followed by exposing the tumors to the dye laser, has produced a complete response rate as high as 94%.[46,47]

MELANOMA

Cutaneous Melanoma

Pathophysiology

CM arises from melanocytes, which are cells specializing in the biosynthesis and transport of melanin. These pigment-producing cells migrate from the neural crest to the skin, uveal tract, meninges, and ectodermal mucosa by the third month of gestation.[8,48] Melanocytes are most commonly found in the basal layers of the epidermis and in the eye but are also found in the meninges, in the alimentary and respiratory tracts, and in the lymph nodes.[8] Melanocytes contain a melanosome, the specific organelle that synthesizes the melanin pigment. Melanin is synthesized using the tyrosinase enzyme in the melanin synthetic pathway.[8] The melanosome-melanin package migrates upward from the basal layer through the epidermis and may be visible in the skin as pigmented melanin granules[48] (Figure 49-5—Plate 20). In melanomas, the melanosomes may be abnormal or even absent in amelanotic clones.[48] Melanocytes produce receptors for growth factors (e.g., nerve growth factor, epidural growth factor) that may have a critical role in the pathogenesis of melanoma.[8] Three specific precursor lesions of CM include dysplastic nevi, congenital nevi, and lentigo maligna.

Dysplastic nevi (DN) Dysplastic nevi are possibly the most controversial lesions in the practice of dermatology and pathology. Critics question their actual existence, whereas proponents suggest they may represent a paradigm for the evolutionary sequence of all cancer.[49] Also known as B-K moles and atypical moles, DN may occur in both familial (familial atypical multiple mole–melanoma syndrome) and nonfamilial (sporadic dysplastic nevi) settings. The histologic and clinical findings are similar for both.[50] In members of families with familial DN, even though these families are uncommon, the risk of developing CM approaches 100%. The risk of nonfamilial DN in the general population is estimated at 5%–10%; however, the upper range of some risk estimates have been 50% or more. The magnitude of this risk is still under discussion.[51–55] One study of persons with sporadic DN indicated they have a 6.8-fold risk of developing CM.[56]

DN are absent at birth. An early clinical indication may be the presence of an increased number of histologically normal nevi between the ages of 5 and 8 years, with dysplastic changes occurring after puberty.[16]

DN generally have one or more of the clinical features of CM (i.e., asymmetry, border irregularity, color variegation, and a diameter greater than 6 mm). A patient with "classic" DN has a triad of more than 100 moles, at least one mole 8 mm or larger in diameter, and at least one mole with CM features.[50] DN appear on the face, trunk, and arms but also may be seen on the buttocks, groin, scalp, and female breast. Pigmentation is irregular with mixtures of tan, brown, and black, or red and pink. A distinctive feature is a "fried egg" appearance with a deep pigmented papular area surrounded by an area of lighter pigmentation. The surface is pebbly, and the border is indistinct and irregular[18,57–59] (Figure 49-6—Plate 21).

Individuals with DN or suspected DN should be thoroughly questioned about family or personal history of melanoma, atypical pigmented lesions, and prior lesion excisions of any kind. Results of any prior skin biopsies should be obtained, if possible. The entire skin surface should be examined, including the scalp, axilla, genitalia, and between the toes and fingers. The first line of treatment is excisional biopsy of the most atypical lesions to document the presence of histologic dysplasia and to rule out melanoma.[58,60,61] Once a diagnosis of a DN has been established, the individual should receive periodic skin examinations by a dermatologist, with accompanying total body photographs every 3–6 months. Changing or new lesions suspicious for melanoma should be removed and biopsied. Individuals with dysplastic nevi and their first-degree relatives should be taught to examine their entire body every 1–2 months and should be educated about melanoma risk factors and preventive behaviors.[18,58,62]

Congenital nevi Congenital nevi are present at birth or shortly thereafter. They are classified as large or small and range in size from 1.5–3.0 cm to large lesions covering extensive body surfaces such as the trunk, arm, or a hand. They have a lifetime risk of malignant transformation of 6%–7%.[51] The color of a congenital nevus ranges from brown to black, and lesions may be slightly raised, and have an irregular surface and a fairly regular border. Larger lesions may contain areas of nodularity. A careful history and examination of congenital nevi are essential to management and should include dates of first appearance and subsequent changes. A biopsy should be obtained from any abnormal-appearing lesion to confirm its exact histology. Treatment primarily consists of surgical excision. Some debate exists as to whether smaller congenital nevi should be surgically removed as a preventive measure.[9,57] Larger lesions may require several surgeries, which can be disfiguring depending upon their location and size. After treatment, regular follow-up examinations are essential.

Lentigo maligna Lentigo maligna is detailed in a following section describing its very similar counterpart, lentigo maligna melanoma. Treatment of this precursor lesion is discussed in the melanoma treatment section.

Assessment

A thorough patient history and physical examination are essential to identify individuals at high risk and for early detection of CM and suspicious lesions. Comments and complaints about a pre-existing nevus or a new lesion should be investigated. Important questions to ask patients include:

1. When was the lesion first noted?
2. Is the lesion new or pre-existing? How long has it been there?
3. What caused you to notice the lesion: change in color, size, or texture; bleeding; a different sensation such as burning, itching, tingling, etc.?
4. How long has the lesion been changing and over what time period?
5. Do you have a history of frequent or intense sun exposure, chemical or thermal injury, or skin trauma?
6. Do you have a family history of dysplastic nevus syndrome or melanoma?

Physical recognition of CM by practitioners and those at risk can be initiated by using the "ABCD" rule.[51] In this rule, A = asymmetry, B = border irregularity, C = color variation or dark black color, and D = diameter greater than 0.6 cm (pencil eraser size). The initial step of the physical examination includes a complete visual examination of the cutaneous surface, the questionable lesion(s), and the area surrounding the lesion to determine the presence of satellite lesions or in-transit metastases. All accessible lymph nodes, particularly those in the regional drainage sites, are palpated. A review of systems is obtained. The skin assessment is described in detail in the "Nursing Management" section of this chapter.

Melanoma can metastasize to virtually every organ in the body, and individuals with the diagnosis should undergo the recommended examinations for metastatic disease. Initially, a chest x-ray, a complete blood count, and serum chemistries with liver function tests are performed postdiagnosis. Liver function tests have proven to be most useful in determining liver metastasis.[63–65] The combination of an elevated LDH, SGOT, and alkaline phosphatase suggests the possibility of liver involvement and indicates that a computerized tomography (CT) scan of the liver is necessary.[63] If clinical findings indicate possible involvement of other common metastatic sites such as skin, subcutaneous tissue, lymph nodes, lung, brain, and bone, a more extensive metastatic work-up is performed. This may include skin or lymph node biopsy for new lesions; a chest x-ray for increased shortness of breath, new cough, or hemoptysis; a CT scan of the brain for neurologic abnormality, headaches, mental deficits, or seizures; and a bone scan for undetermined bone pain.[66] Magnetic resonance imaging (MRI) scans offer clearer images and detect different characteristics of lesions than does a CT scan. Since the cost of MRI is high, it may be reserved for special situations.

Research is being done in the areas of cytogenetics and computer use to help with the diagnosis of CM. Cytogenetic analyses of patients with a hereditary predisposition for CM formation have demonstrated slightly increased levels of spontaneous chromosome abnormalities in both peripheral blood lymphocytes and human skin fibroblasts. Abnormalities of chromosomes 1 and 6 are frequent in CM.[67] Little is known at this time about the effect these abnormalities will have clinically, and much research remains to be done. Melanoma Analysis and Graphic Imaging by Computer (MAGIC) is a new computer imaging project that reconstructs a lesion three-dimensionally using the ABCD rules defining asymmetry, border, color, and diameter. MAGIC could become a cost-effective tool for diagnosis because all that is needed beyond the personal computers in most offices is the software. The use of this technique has shown that tumor volume is a better predictor of survival than is tumor thickness.[68]

Classification

Melanoma has been classified into several types: lentigo maligna (LMM), superficial-spreading (SSM), nodular, acral lentiginous (mucocutaneous), those in which the radial growth phase is not characteristic of SSN or LMM, those arising from congenital nevi, those arising from blue nevi, visceral, and ocular. The four major types of CM described here include lentigo maligna, superficial-spreading, nodular, and acral lentiginous (Table 49-3). Each of these is characterized by a radial and/or vertical growth phase. In the radial growth phase, tumor growth is parallel to the surface of the skin. This phase may last several years. The propensity for the tumor to metastasize is very small, and surgical excision may be curative. In the vertical growth phase, however, there is focal, deep penetration of atypical melanocytes into the dermis and subcutaneous tissue. This penetration occurs rapidly, increasing the risk of metastasis.[8,60,69–71]

Lentigo maligna melanoma constitutes 4%–10% of all CM and is the least serious type.[51] It occurs on body areas heavily exposed to UVR, such as the face, neck,

TABLE 49-3 Comparisons of the Four Major Types of Cutaneous Melanoma

Type	Site	Radial Growth Phase	Vertical Growth Phase	Characteristics
Lentigo maligna melanoma	Face, neck, dorsal hands, lower legs; areas chronically exposed to sun	Yes (10–25 yr)	Yes (less aggressive)	Size: Large (10 cm) Color: Tan/brown Radial phase: Irregular mottling with regression Vertical phase: Raised nodules on surface
Superficial-spreading	Men: trunk, back Women: legs	Yes (1–5 yr)	Yes (aggressive)	Radial phase: Flat with fine crust/scaly surface; tan/brown color Vertical phase: Shiny surface; tan/brown/black to red/white/blue color; borders irregular; raised nodules; ulceration
Nodular	Head, neck, trunk (may or may not be exposed to sun)	No	Yes (aggressive, 2–18 mo)	Vertical phase: Raised, dome-shaped blue-black/red color; ulcerations/bleeding may be present
Acral lentiginous	Palms, soles, nail beds, mucous membranes	Yes (2–5 yr)	Yes (aggressive)	Radial phase: Flat, tan/brown/black color similar to lentigo maligna Nail bed: Tan/brown stain/streaking Vertical phase: Elevated areas of nodularity

and occasionally the dorsal hands and lower legs. Early premalignant, in situ lesions often precede lentigo maligna melanoma and are termed *lentigo maligna*. Both lentigo maligna and lentigo maligna melanoma are large in size and are primarily a tan color with different shades of brown throughout (Figure 49-7—Plate 22). The predominant histologic feature of lentigo maligna is proliferation of atypical melanocytes along the basal layer of the epidermis. This early radial growth phase usually lasts between 10–25 years, with the lesion growing as large as 10 cm. As soon as these melanocytes invade the dermis, the lesion becomes malignant. With increased growth of the lentigo malignant melanoma, irregular mottling or freckling may occur, along with regression in some areas. A portion of the lesion may begin a vertical growth phase, with accompanying raised nodules over the surface.[19,60,62,69,71]

Superficial-spreading melanoma accounts for approximately 70% of CM.[51] In men, this lesion is most commonly seen on the trunk, and in women, on the legs. Superficial-spreading melanoma usually arises in a pre-existing nevus. Early lesions are generally flat with a fine crust or scaly surface. The radial growth phase lasts between 1–5 or more years. As the lesion enters the vertical phase, a rapid increase of growth occurs, with a change in color ranging from a mixture of tan, brown, and black to a characteristic red, white, and blue appearance. As the lesion continues to grow, the borders become irregular and notched and the surface becomes shiny and irregular, with raised nodules and ulceration[8,62,69,71,72] (Figure 49-8—Plate 23). A 35%–85% chance of metastasis exists in the vertical growth phase.[5]

Nodular melanoma constitutes 15%–30% of CM.[51] This lesion appears as a raised, dome-shaped blue-black or red nodule on areas of the head, neck, and trunk that may or may not be exposed to the sun. Ulcerations and bleeding may be present (Figure 49-9—Plate 24). Nodular melanoma only has a vertically invasive component, making early diagnosis difficult. It is more aggressive than the other melanoma types and has a shorter clinical onset. Commonly, these lesions begin de novo in uninvolved skin rather than from a pre-existing lesion. Because this lesion lacks a radial phase and is difficult to detect in early stages, there is an increased chance of metastasis being present at diagnosis.[19,71,72]

Acral lentiginous or mucocutaneous melanoma is found in 35%–60% of dark-skinned persons, particularly blacks, Asians, and Hispanics, and in only 2%–10% of whites.[19,62] This lesion occurs on the palms, soles, nailbeds, and mucous membranes. Acral lentiginous melanoma exhibits both a radial and vertical growth phase. The radial growth phase may last for years and resembles an early lentigo maligna. In this phase the lesion is flat, with nonpalpable margins, and is haphazardly pigmented with tan, brown, and black colors. In subungual areas the radial growth phase appears as an irregular tan-brown stain of streaking in the nailbed (Figure 49-10—Plate 25). Acral lentiginous melanomas in the vertical phase become elevated, with areas of nodularity. A small percentage are flesh-colored. In the vertical phase, acral lentiginous melanomas are more aggressive and can metastasize.

Juvenile melanomas occur before puberty. They are similar in appearance to CM of adults; however, they can be distinguished histologically by the presence of giant cells. Juvenile melanomas rarely metastasize; therefore, conservative surgery is appropriate treatment. There is, however, a rise in the ability of juvenile melanomas to metastasize after puberty, an event possibly related to hormonal activity.[73]

Staging and prognostic factors

Microstaging is a term used to describe the level of invasion of the CM and maximum tumor thickness. Two systems are used in assessing the depth of invasion of melanoma (Figure 49-11). The first is the anatomic level of invasion, or the Clark level, and the second is the thickness of tumor tissue, or the Breslow level. The Clark system categorizes CM into five histologic levels based on vertical depth of tumor invasion, with the deeper lesions having the worst prognosis for metastases and survival. When using the Clark system, subjective difficulties in classifying certain melanomas may occur, such as those located in thin-skinned areas (e.g., elbow, under the eye) and lead to poor reproducibility of classification among pathologists. To eliminate these problems, the Breslow system modified the Clark system by using an ocular micrometer to measure, in millimeters, the maximum vertical tumor thickness. This measurement is made from the top of the granular cell layer of the tumor to the deepest level of invasion of the melanoma.

The traditional three-stage system (Table 49-4) is still used, even though it does not include important disease criteria such as tumor thickness. The American Joint Committee on Cancer (AJCC) four-stage system for CM is preferable because it divides patients more evenly and allows for more consistent exchange of information[51,74] (Table 49-5). This staging system includes level of invasion and nodal involvement using the tumor-node-metastasis (TNM) nomenclature.

It is well documented that as CM thickness increases, survival rates decrease. Thus, the Breslow level has consistently proved to be a significant prognostic variable in stage I CM.[69,70,75–77] Other factors that predict survival are age, sex, clinical, and histologic factors. Younger patients and women have a somewhat better prognosis. Clinically, survival related to the anatomical site of the CM is still controversial. With equivalent thicknesses, lesions on the hands, feet, and scalp may have a poorer prognosis.[51] One difficulty in determining prognosis related to feet and scalp lesions is that these lesions are not easily visible and are usually detected later. Histologic factors that predict an unfavorable prognosis are the presence of microscopic satellites of tumor, high miotic activity, ulceration, vertical growth phase, and large tumor volume.[51]

Koh[51] reported that stage I lentigo maligna and

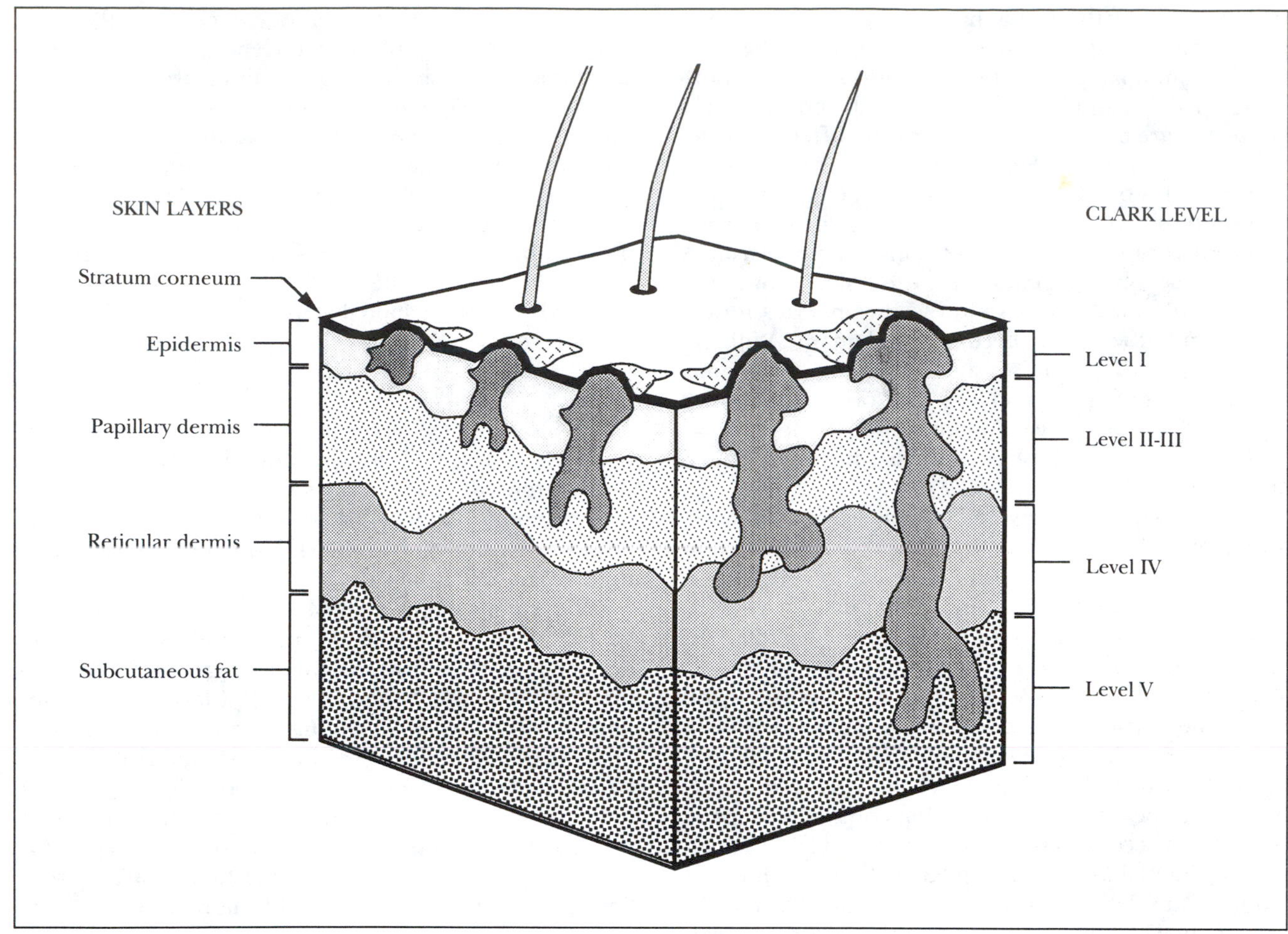

FIGURE 49-11 Corresponding thicknesses of Clark and Breslow levels.

superficial-spreading melanomas have better 5-year survival rates (85%–90%) than do nodular (about 60%) and acral lentiginous melanomas. In stage II disease the 5-year survival rates are 36%, but these rates vary according to the clinical status of nodes, the number of nodes involved, and the presence or absence of ulceration in the primary tumor. Stage III (AJCC stage IV) disease is generally incurable secondary to metastases. Median survival is approximately 6 months.[51]

TABLE 49-4 The Traditional Three-Stage System for Cutaneous Melanoma

Stage	Extent of Disease
I	Localized primary melanoma
IA	Local recurrence (satellite lesions)
II	Regional lymph node involvement or in-transit metastases
III	Distant metastases

Treatment

Surgery The initial surgical procedure for suspected CM is a biopsy. An excisional biopsy that removes a few millimeters of normal tissue surrounding the lesion is preferable since it provides a definitive diagnosis along with microstaging information. An incisional biopsy can be used for lesions located in cosmetically sensitive areas or for large lesions. The incisional site should include any areas of change, particularly suspicious raised or nodular-appearing areas. Both techniques should remove full thickness of the skin and some underlying subcutaneous fat.[78,79] Electrocoagulation, curettage, shaving, and burning should never be used to remove a suspicious mole.

For stage I CM the standard treatment is a wide excision. Debate exists as to the extent of the excision needed to achieve optimal control.[8,62,79–81] The common margin standard has been 3–5 cm of normal skin, but increasing evidence has shown that the risk of local recurrence correlates with the thickness of the lesion and that margin size dose not influence survival.[78–80] Since a minimal risk of local recurrence exists for thin melanomas (<0.76 mm), only a 1cm-margin of clini-

TABLE 49-5 The AJCC's* Four-Stage System for Cutaneous Melanoma

PRIMARY TUMOR (pT)	
pTX	Primary tumor cannot be assessed
pTO	No evidence of primary tumor
pTis	Melanoma in situ (Clark's level 1)
pT1	Tumor ≤0.75 mm thick, invading papillary dermis (Clark's level II)
pT2	Tumor 0.76–1.50 mm thick, invading papillary-reticular dermal interface (Clark's level III), or both
pT3	Tumor 1.5–4.00 mm thick, invading reticular dermis (Clark's level IV), or both
pT3a	Tumor 1.51–3.00 mm thick
pT3b	Tumor 3.01–4.00 mm thick
pT4	Tumor >4.00 mm thick, invading subcutaneous tissue (Clark's level V), or both, or satellites within 2 cm of primary tumor
pT4a	Tumor >4.00 mm thick, invading subcutaneous tissue, or both
pT4b	Satellites within 2 cm of primary tumor
REGIONAL LYMPH NODES (N)	
NX	Regional lymph nodes cannot be assessed
N0	No regional lymph node metastasis
N1	Metastasis ≤3cm in greatest dimension in any regional lymph node
N2	Metastasis >3 cm in greatest dimension in any regional lymph node or in-transit metastasis
N2a	Metastasis >3 cm in greatest dimension in any regional lymph node
N2b	In-transit metastasis
N2c	Both (N2a and N2b)
DISTANT METASTASIS (M)	
MX	Presence of distant metastasis cannot be assessed
M0	No distant metastasis
M1	Distant metastasis
M1a	Metastasis in skin, subcutaneous tissue, or lymph node beyond the regional lymph nodes
M1b	Visceral metastasis
STAGES	
I	pT1 or pT2, N0, M0
II	pT3, N0, M0
III	pT4, N0, M0 Any pT, N1 or N2, M0
IV	Any pT, any N, M1

*AJCC, American Joint Committee on Cancer.

Source: Beahrs OH, Henson DE, Hutter RV, et al (eds): *American Joint Committee on Cancer: Manual for Staging of Cancer,* 4th ed. Philadelphia: Lippincott, 1992.

cally normal skin around the lesion, along with removal of underlying subcutaneous tissue down to the fascia, is recommended.[71,78,80,82] An excision margin 1-cm wide is also suitable for lentigo maligna melanoma, which has a low metastatic potential. Thicker lesions require a 3–5-cm margin of normal skin with a split thickness graft.[78] For lesions in areas of sensitivity or where cosmesis is an issue, the surgeon determines the safest wide excision margin. Subungual lesions are treated by amputation.

Controversy exists over the use of elective lymph node dissection (ELND) in the treatment of stage I disease. ELND has a high degree of morbidity, and use of this procedure is debatable when no clinical evidence of nodal involvement exists. There is agreement that neither a primary CM lesion less than 0.76 mm nor a lentigo maligna melanoma requires an ELND. In addition, patients with large lesions (>4 mm) do not benefit from ELND because they most likely have microscopic metastases.[79,83,84] Proponents of ELND argue that 20%–30% of the clinically normal nodes contain malignant cells and that managing these nodes while the tumor burden is low will decrease the incidence of distant metastases. Opponents maintain that since nodal metastases are rare in patients with thinner melanomas, 70%–80% of these individuals will undergo unnecessary surgery.[79,83,84] Reviews of some nonrandomized, prospective studies have demonstrated improved survival in patients with intermediate-thickness extremity lesions treated with ELND.[80,84–86] Prospective randomized studies, however, have shown no survival benefit.[83–85] No prospective randomized trials have been performed addressing the use of ELND for CM of the trunk, head, and neck.[84,85] Retrospective studies are also inconclusive; however, there are some that suggest some patients with stage I CM of intermediate thickness (1–3.99 mm) may benefit from ELND.[8,79,86]

Standard surgical therapy of clinical stage II (clinical, but not histologic, evidence of draining lymph node involvement) disease includes excision of the primary lesion, along with surgical dissection of the involved nodes.[8] In cases where the index of suspicion is low for metastatic disease, a palpable node may be biopsied by either the open or fine-needle approach.[87]

Surgery is also useful for palliation of disease and symptomatic involvement. Surgical removal of a solitary metastatic lesion is recommended if the lesion is easily accessible and if removal will enhance quality and duration of survival. For example, craniotomy is indicated for removal of a solitary brain metastasis, and thoracotomy for removal of an isolated lung lesion.[88]

Chemotherapy Metastatic malignant melanoma is highly resistant to systemic chemotherapeutic agents currently available, indicating the need for further research in this area. Dacarbazine (DTIC) is the most active agent, with an overall response rate of 15%–28%.[8,62,69,89,90] Other single agents with activity include the nitrosoureas (BCNU, CCNU, methyl-CCNU, and chlorozotocin) and cisplatin, all having response rates no greater than that of DTIC and more toxicities.[51,91] Drug combinations that show some promise for treatment of metastatic disease are DTIC, BCNU, cisplatin, and tamoxifen (DBPT); bleomycin, vindesine, CCNU, and DTIC (BELD); DTIC, CCNU, bleomycin and vincristine (BOLD); and combinations of cisplatin and DTIC with or without vinblastine. Responses of 40%–50% are primarily seen in patients with lung or soft tissue metastases. These regimens are still investigational, and more information is needed to support their efficacy.[91] The toxicities of the most frequently used chemotherapeutic agents are discussed in detail elsewhere in this text.

Isolated limb perfusion is a controversial adjuvant therapy for advanced melanoma confined to a limb or for disease involving melanoma satellites, in-transit metastasis, and poor-prognosis extremity lesions. The treatment consists of hyperthermia plus vascular perfusion of chemotherapy through an isolated region, enabling high concentrations of chemotherapeutic agents to be administered with minimal systemic toxicities. The agent most commonly used for this procedure is melphalan. Others used alone and in combination include thiotepa, dacarbazine, carmustine, cisplatin, and doxorubicin.[89,92–94] Complications of treatment include tissue necrosis, transient or persistent edema of the treated extremity, neurologic disorders, wound infection, pain, and deep vein thrombosis.[92,93,95] Although isolated limb perfusion has been used since 1957, it remains expensive, investigational, and extremely controversial, since a limited number of control groups have been utilized in reported studies.[69,92,95,96]

Another technique that has been used is intraarterial infusion chemotherapy without hyperthermia. This involves applying a tourniquet proximally and infusing the chosen chemotherapy agent intraarterially. This method is simpler than the perfusion technique, but drug levels may not be as high or as evenly distributed.[91,97]

A newer approach is the use of high-dose chemotherapy followed by autologous bone marrow transplantation. This can obtain up to 48% response rates but is complicated by several treatment-related toxicities and significant morbidity, and the responses are usually short-lived. Its role in the treatment of CM requires further study.[91,98,99]

Radiotherapy Radiotherapy is most effective when tumor volume is low and when a high dose per fewer fractions radiation level is used (>4 Gy per fraction). Response rates range from a low of 0%–25% to a high of 45%–71%.[91] Radiotherapy is often used for palliation in disease with subcutaneous, cutaneous, and nodal metastases that are inaccessible for surgical removal.[100–102] Palliative radiation to the brain in conjunction with steroids offers considerable relief of neurologic symptoms. Pending bone fractures and bone pain can also be reduced with the use of radiotherapy. Radiotherapy cannot be used to treat liver or lung metastases because of resultant loss of function.[102]

Hyperthermia may enhance the effect of radiation. Recent studies have shown that when heat (42°–43° C) is applied to lesions for 30–45 minutes before or during radiotherapy, the complete response rate may increase by a factor of 1.5 to 2. These results have created new interest in this treatment.[91]

Hormonal therapy A hormonal influence on melanocyte and melanoma cell proliferation has been suggested by the usual occurrence of CM following puberty, increased incidence during menopause, and increased or decreased CM growth during pregnancy or after parturition.[24,103,104] Hormonal effects are also evidenced by the presence of estrogen and progesterone receptor sites on some CM cells, suggesting that endocrine therapy may be beneficial. Clinically, steroid hormones may directly affect CM growth or may indirectly be mediated by gonadotropins or other pituitary or hypothalamic factors modulated by steroids.[103] A high incidence of steroid binding in melanoma tissue has led to clinical trials demonstrating some tumor response with tamoxifen, diethylstilbestrol, estramustine phosphate, progesterone, and antiandrogens.[103] Another strategy in hormonal therapy is to use melanocyte stimulating hormone (MSH) to target chemotherapeutic agents toward melanocytes.[91] Trials utilizing endocrine therapy still remain inconclusive.[8,90]

Immunotherapy Immunotherapy is a recent form of melanoma treatment with the rationale for use paralleling the natural history of CM, indicating that immunologic intervention by the host may alter the growth pattern of CM. This immunologic interaction is demonstrated by the occurrence of more spontaneous remissions in CM than in other adult tumors. In addition, specific tumor antigen antibodies have been found in melanoma patients. Patients who have lymphocytic infiltrates at the tumor site have a more favorable prognosis.[105]

Immunotherapy is currently being investigated as adjuvant therapy and as treatment for metastatic disease. Agents such as interferons, interleukins, levamisole, tumor necrosis factors, monoclonal antibodies, and Bacillus Calmette-Guerin (BCG) are being studied either singly, in combination with each other, or in combination with chemotherapy (chemoimmunotherapy). The frequently used DTIC and BCG combination has better responses than when either drug is used alone.[91]

Adoptive immunotherapy involves obtaining lymphocytes from patients via leukapheresis, incubating the cells with interleukin-2 (IL-2) to generate and expand lymphokine-activated killer (LAK) cells, and then reinfusing the LAK cells along with IL-2 into the patient. Response rates range between 15% and 25%. Unfortunately, the toxicities of this treatment, mainly capillary leak syndrome, hypotension, respiratory distress, anemia, and liver and renal dysfunction, have limited its use. Current research is striving to improve the remission rate and limit its toxicity.[51]

Interferon use in CM remains a palliative measure

with a chance of stabilization. Interferons can be used alone or in combination with chemotherapy after tumor removal in cases of high-risk melanoma or CM with early metastatic spread.[106–109]

Other treatments Topical 5-FU has shown desirable results for extensive facial lentigo maligna melanomas. In lentigo maligna CM with poor prognosis, preoperative treatment with topical 5-FU has been improving surgical results.[110] One small study indicated that topical tretinoin (Retin-A) solution applied to dysplastic nevi may have a biologic effect.[111]

Melanoma vaccines have been reported to slow the progression of metastatic lesions in some patients and delay recurrence after surgical excision in stage II disease.[50,112] They appear to be toxicity-free, with the exception of localized swelling. Ongoing trials with melanoma vaccines are being done to test efficacy; however, preliminary results are encouraging.[50,113]

Uveal Melanoma

Uveal melanoma affects the iris, ciliary body, and choroid portions of the eye and arises from uveal melanocytes that have a common embryologic origin with melanocytes of the conjunctiva and skin. The frequency of uveal melanomas in the right and left eye is equal, but bilateral incidence is rare. Only one in five million whites develop a choroidal melanoma each year,[114] but overall, uveal melanomas are fatal in more than 50% of cases.[115] Most melanomas of the choroid and ciliary body are diagnosed after age 50; iris melanomas can be diagnosed earlier. Uveal melanomas exhibit no familial tendency, although there is some controversy as to whether they have an association with dysplastic nevi.[114,116–118] Predisposing factors for uveal melanomas include ocular melanocytosis (congenital hyperpigmentation of the sclera and uvea), ocular nevi, and neurofibromatosis. Exposure to UVR may be an important risk factor.[119,120] Shields et al.[121] reported that women with a history of pregnancy or estrogen replacement therapy were at increased risk for uveal melanoma.

Choroidal melanoma is the most common type of uveal melanoma in adults. Large lesions left untreated can extend locally, metastasize, and inevitably become fatal. Metastasis is primarily to the liver or lung.[114] The treatment for small melanomas, particularly those affecting the choroid, may be observation, as these lesions have little potential to produce local extension or metastasis.[114] Tumors affecting the iris and ciliary body may be surgically removed. Choroidal melanomas may also be treated with photocoagulation (xenon arc or laser). Treatment for larger choroidal melanomas remains controversial. For many years, standard therapy has been enucleation; however, some investigators have hypothesized that intraoperative manipulation causes tumor cell dissemination and metastases.[122] Others, however, believe that post-enucleation mortality is due to pre-existing dormant or subclinical metastases.[123,124] Five-year mortality rates range from 16% (small tumors) to 53% (large tumors).[125]

Radiotherapy is also a widely used treatment that has the potential advantage of preserving both life and vision. Radiotherapy is most commonly administered via external beam or plaque methods. Tumor regression and survival rates (40% survival at 10 years) following radiotherapy are comparable to those for enucleation; however, more prospective research needs to be done in this area.[122,126,127] With severe extrascleral involvement, exenteration may be performed, involving removal of the eye and orbital contents or structures.[114]

PREVENTION

Primary Prevention

Many skin cancers can be prevented by reducing exposure to avoidable risk factors. Primary prevention of skin cancers involves the avoidance of excessive UVR exposure. The harmful effects of this exposure begin in childhood, and as UV-induced damage is cumulative, severe effects may be seen by young adulthood.[5] For example, Weinstock et al.[128] found a significant association between blistering sunburns in young women age 15–20 and increased melanoma risk after age 30. Holman et al[129] suggested that the type of swimsuit worn by young women age 15–25 affects their later risk of developing CM. They estimated a 13-fold increased CM risk in women who wore bikinis or were nude bathers, compared with women who wore conservative, one-piece suits. Stern et al.[130] estimated that using a sunscreen with a sun protection factor (SPF) of 15 during the first 18 years of life would reduce the lifetime incidences of NMSC by 78%. Thus, prevention behaviors for reducing exposure must start early in life. Specific behaviors recommended by the Skin Cancer Foundation[131] and the Arizona Sun Awareness Project[132] include:

1. *Minimize sun exposure* during the hours of 10 AM to 3 PM, when UVR is the strongest.

2. *Cover up* with a wide-brimmed hat, long-sleeved shirt and long pants (made out of tightly woven material), and protective sunglasses.

3. *Use a waterproof or water-resistant sunscreen with an SPF of 15 or more* before every exposure to the sun. Reapply after the protection time is up. Suncreen should be applied on overcast days because 70%–80% of UVR can penetrate cloud cover. Individuals with any risk factors for skin cancer should get into the habit of applying sunscreen on a daily basis. If an allergic reaction to a particular product develops, another brand with different active ingredients can be tried (e.g., PABA-free products). Sunscreens specially formulated for children can be used on children as early as 6 months of age, but perform a "patch test" to determine whether the child's skin is sensitive to the product.

4. *Be aware of photosensitivity* caused by certain medications (e.g., tetracycline, oral contraceptives) and cosmetics.

5. *Be protected when on or near surfaces such as sand, snow, concrete, or water,* which can reflect more than half the UVR onto the skin. Sitting under a shade tree or beach umbrella near these surfaces does not guarantee any added protection from UVR.

6. *Avoid tanning parlors* as UVA emitted by tanning booths damages the deep skin layers, causing early skin aging and wrinkling.

7. *Keep infants well-protected* when outdoors.

Individuals who work with substances known to cause skin cancer should wear protective clothing and use protective equipment to reduce their exposure.

Secondary Prevention

Secondary prevention of skin cancers involves reduction of morbidity and mortality through early detection, diagnosis, and treatment of high-risk individuals having a changing or changed pigmented lesion, a precursor lesion, a previous history of skin cancer, or a family history of CM.[18] These people should receive periodic skin examinations by a qualified dermatologist. Ophthalmic examinations should also be performed for those at risk for uveal melanomas.

Early detection and diagnosis of skin cancers is of utmost importance. Most changes on the skin are easily visible and can be detected early, thereby improving chances for cure. Both the general public and health care professionals must be made aware of the need for early evaluation of an unusual skin lesion. Figure 49-12 is an example of a patient education poster that describes these early changes.

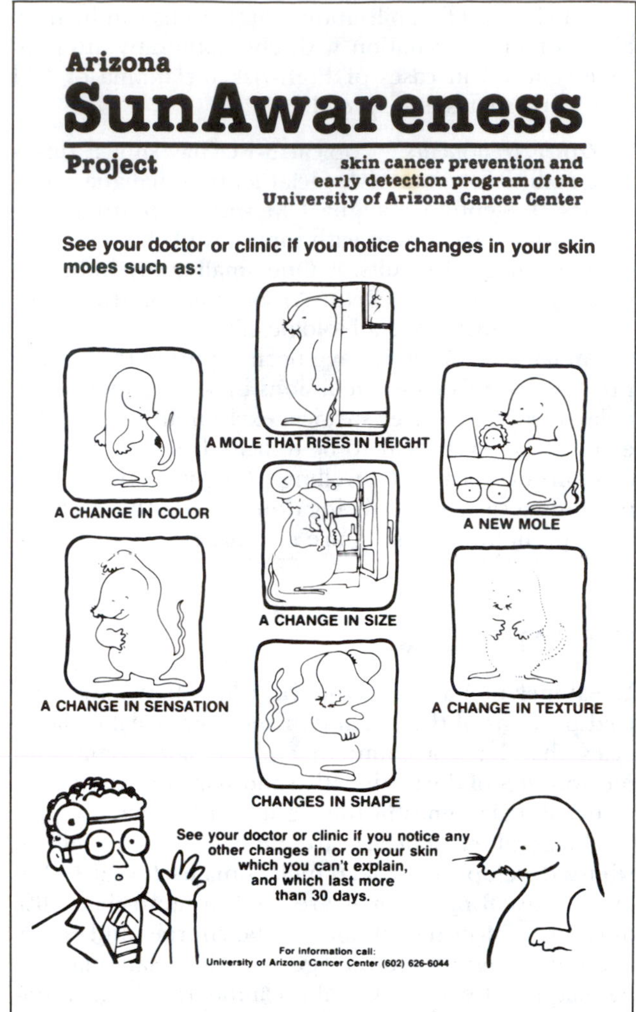

FIGURE 49-12 Patient education poster describing mole changes that should be reported to a physician. (Printed by permission from the Arizona Cancer Center.)

Tertiary Prevention

Randomized, controlled clinical trials that involve treatment of humans with precursor lesions for cutaneous cancers are ongoing. Retinoids (vitamin A and its derivatives) used as biologic treatment agents have shown some effect as chemopreventive agents in persons with BCC, actinic keratosis, keratoacanthoma, epidermodysplasia verruciformis, and dysplastic nevi.[36,133] Retinoids used as dietary agents also exhibit potential anticancer effects.[134] Carotenoids (β-carotene) are also being studied as chemoprevention agents; however, in persons with recurrent NMSC, treatment with β-carotene did not reduce the occurrence of new skin cancers over a 5-year follow-up period.[135] The mineral selenium may have some protective benefit against skin cancers.[136] The role of α-difluoromethylornithine (DFMO) in skin cancer prevention is currently being investigated.[136] Definitive results from these and other chemoprevention studies will take several years.

NURSING MANAGEMENT

Because skin cancers are reaching epidemic proportions, the involvement of the nurse in prevention, early detection education, screening, and management of these cancers continues to escalate. Important components of nursing management include interview, skin assessment, education, and posttreatment management.

Interview

All individuals with skin cancer or those at risk should be questioned about their knowledge of skin cancers, past medical history, and exposure to risk factors. Familiarity with the etiologic factors and clinical manifestations described throughout this chapter is an essential prerequisite for prevention and early detection education and screening. The diagnosis of skin cancer can be frightening for the patient and family members, and the interview elicits information about their knowledge and attitudes, potential fears, and coping mechanisms. Attitudes toward the disease can influence health practices; thus, the patient and family are provided with the opportunity to discuss any concerns or issues and are given appropriate information and reassurance.[137,138] Information about environmental factors such as exposure to UVR, ionizing radiation, and chemicals is routinely collected during the interview. A review of systems may reveal information about changes in moles or an overlooked cancer-related symptom.[139,140] Finally, a family pedigree is completed to ascertain family history of skin cancers. The history and exposure to risk factors will determine how detailed a skin assessment should be.[141]

Skin Assessment

Nurses working in hospitals, nursing homes, clinics, schools, and home care settings all have an opportunity to examine a person's skin.[140] A thorough nursing skin assessment can initially identify suspicious lesions. Good lighting (preferably bright, natural light) and magnification are essential for the examination. Formal skin assessment is usually performed with the individual seated, although any opportunity such as bathing, dressing changes, or back rubs can be used to check a hospitalized patient's skin. Skin assessment consists of inspection and palpation to identify obvious lesions; visible swellings; adenopathy; alterations in normal borders and contour of nevi; discoloration in skin or mucosa; and areas of ulceration, scaling, crusting, and erosion. Tightly stretching the skin during the examination helps identify nodular and scaly lesions, as well as those within the dermis.[27]

Before the examination the person should undress totally or to his or her underpants, which can easily be pulled away from the body for inspection of the skin underneath.[142] The examination begins with the head and neck, including the entire scalp; eyelids; external ear and auditory canal; external and interior surfaces of the nose; the oral cavity; and the parotid, submaxillary, and sublingual glands. If the nurse is trained to do indirect ophthalmoscopy, an eye examination should also be performed. Next, the thyroid is palpated along with the regional lymph nodes of the neck. The examination then progresses to the chest, abdomen, back, and extremities, with special attention to intertrigous areas such as under pendulous breasts, between the buttocks, the chin, an obese abdomen, hairy areas, axillae, nail beds, webs between fingers and toes, and soles of the feet. External genitalia are also examined. The location and descriptive characteristics of suspicious lesions should be recorded on an anatomical chart.[139,141] Warts, moles, scars, vascularities, and birthmarks should also be documented.

Education

Nurses have the opportunity to educate about skin cancer in many professional and social settings. Berwick et al.[142] summarized educational models that could be used by nurses. In one model the nurse is an educator and support person for the dermatologist. Another model uses the nurse as an educator and "prescreener" who conducts the first assessment of the patient, then alerts the physician to the clinical findings and the potential need for referral to a dermatologist.

Numerous educational brochures describing various aspects of skin cancers and prevention are available from the American Cancer Society, American Academy of Dermatology, National Cancer Institute, Skin Cancer Foundation, pharmaceutical companies that manufacture sunscreens, and other agencies.[143] These teaching aids are usually free of charge.

Education for those at high risk for or diagnosed with skin cancers begins with an initial assessment of their knowledge deficit related to skin cancers. Assessment of educational background, readiness to learn, and patient and family response to education is performed. Clear and accurate information related to the diagnosis is then given to the patient and repeated several times, if necessary. Photographs of normal moles and birthmarks compared with photographs of skin cancers can be used as teaching aids. Patients are taught systematic self-skin assessment and encouraged to examine their skin monthly.[137] Family members may assist in checking hard-to-see areas such as the scalp, back, ears, and soles. Examinations should be scheduled at least twice yearly with a dermatologist or oncologist specializing in skin cancers. It is important for the nurse to emphasize that with attentive self-care and medical management, most patients can lead relatively normal lives.[137] At the conclusion of any educational session, the nurse documents patient and family response to instruction, including comprehension and ability to perform skin self-examination.

Posttreatment Management

Surgical excision is still the most common treatment for skin cancers, and nursing management postoperatively is determined by the extent of the procedure. Patients who have had surgical excision only should be instructed to limit environment insults to the surgical site and to protect the site against exposure to irritants and mechanical trauma. Patients who have undergone skin grafting or flapping require careful and frequent observation for signs of infection and hemorrhage in both donor and recipient sites. The recipient site should be immobilized to prevent separation, and involved limbs should be elevated to minimize edema. Some sloughing of a graft site may occur but can be controlled by use of mineral oil or lanolin.[144]

Nursing management of patients receiving chemotherapy, radiotherapy, or immunotherapy is determined by the specific treatment regimen administered. General nursing care for patients receiving these therapies is described in Part III of this text.

All patients diagnosed with melanoma should be evaluated at regular intervals for recurrence or metastatic disease. This evaluation should occur every 3–4 months for the first 2 years, every 6 months up to 5 years, and yearly thereafter. These intervals should be adjusted according to the risk of metastatic disease in any individual patient.[62,63] It is imperative that patients understand the importance of these follow-up visits and of informing the physician or nurse of any physical or mental changes that occur.

CONCLUSION

This chapter has described three primary forms of skin cancer: basal cell carcinoma, squamous cell carcinoma, and cutaneous malignant melanoma (including uveal melanoma). The best known treatment to date for most skin cancers is prevention, and oncology nurses are in an ideal position to educate the public and other professionals about primary and secondary preventive behaviors. By practicing early detection, screening, and preventive behaviors themselves, oncology nurses can serve as role models for the general population and for those at high risk.

REFERENCES

1. Glass AG, Hoover RN; The emerging epidemic of melanoma and squamous cell skin cancer. *JAMA* 262:2097–2100, 1989.
2. *Cancer Facts and Figures.* Atlanta, GA: American Cancer Society, 1993.
3. Patterson JAK, Geronemus RG: Cancers of the skin. In DeVita VT, Hellman S, Rosenberg SA, eds, *Cancer: Principles and Practice of Oncology* (2d ed). Philadelphia: Lippincott, 1989, pp. 1469–1498.
4. Scotto J, Fears TR, Fraumeni JF Jr: Incidence of nonmelanoma skin cancer in the United States. Publication No. 83-2433. Bethesda, Md: National Institutes of Health, 1983.
5. National Cancer Institute: Nonmelanoma skin cancers: Research report. NIH Publication No. 88-2977. Bethesda, MD: National Institutes of Health, 1988.
6. Ries LAG, Hankey BF, Edwards BK (eds.): Cancer statistics review 1973–87. Publication No. 90-2789. Bethesda, Md: National Institutes of Health, 1990.
7. Weinstock MA, Bogaars HA, Ashley M, et al: Nonmelanoma skin cancer mortality: A population-based study. *Arch Dermatol* 127:1194–1197, 1991.
8. Balch CM, Houghton A, Peters L: Cutaneous melanoma. In: DeVita VT, Hellman S, Rosenberg SA eds., *Cancer: Principles and Practice of Oncology* (3d ed). Philadelphia: Lippincott, 1989, pp. 1499–1556.
9. Boring CC, Squires TS, Tong T: Cancer statistics, 1993. *CA* 43:7–26, 1993.
10. Fraser MC, Hartge P, Tucker MA: Melanoma and nonmelanoma skin cancer: Epidemiology and risk factors. *Semin Oncol Nurs* 7:2–12, 1991.
11. Scotto J, Fears TR: The association of solar ultraviolet and skin melanoma incidence among Caucasians in the United States. *Cancer Invest* 5:275–283, 1987.
12. Scotto J, Fears TR, Fraumeni JF Jr: Solar radiation. In Schottenfeld D, Fraumeni JF Jr, (eds), *Cancer Epidemiology and Prevention.* Philadelphia: Saunders, 1982, pp. 254–276.
13. Kripke ML: Immunoregulation of carcinogenesis: Past, present, and future. *J Natl Cancer Inst* 80:722–727, 1988.
14. Lee JAH: The causation of melanoma. In Balch CM, Milton GW, Shaw HM, Soong SJ, (eds), *Cutaneous Melanoma.* Philadelphia: Lippincott, 1985, pp. 303–311.
15. National Institutes of Health Consensus Development Conference: Sunlight, ultraviolet radiation, and the skin. Bethesda, MD: National Institutes of Health, 1991.
16. Greene MH, Clark WH, Tucker MA, et al: Acquired precursors of cutaneous malignant melanoma: The familial dysplastic nevus syndrome. *N Engl J Med* 312:91–97, 1986.
17. Friedman RJ, Rigel DS, Kopf AW: The ABCD's of moles and melanomas. New York: Skin Cancer Foundation, 1985.
18. Rhodes AR, Weinstock MA, Fitzpatrick TB, et al: Risk factors for cutaneous melanoma. *JAMA* 258:3146–3154, 1987.
19. Milton GW, Balch CM, Shaw HM: Clinical characteristics. In Balch CM, Milton GW, Shaw HM, Soong SJ (eds), *Cutaneous Melanoma.* Philadelphia: Lippincott, 1985, pp. 13–28.
20. Evans RD, Kopf AW, Lew RL, et al: Risk factors for the development of malignant melanoma—I: Review of case-control studies. *J Dermatol Surg Oncol* 14:393–408, 1988.
21. Holman CDJ, Armstrong BK: Pigmentary traits, ethnic origin, benign nevi, and familial history as risk factors for cutaneous malignant melanoma. *J Natl Cancer Inst* 72:257–266, 1984.
22. Green A, MacLennon R, Siskind V: Common acquired nevi and the risk of malignant melanoma. *Int J Cancer* 35:297–300, 1985.
23. Rampen FHJ: Sex differences in survival from cutaneous melanoma. *Int J Dermatol* 23:444–452, 1984.
24. Holly EA: Melanoma in pregnancy. In Gallagher RP (ed), *Recent Results in Cancer Research: Epidemiology of Malignant Melanoma.* New York: Springer-Verlag, 1986, pp. 118–125.
25. Schwartz BK, Zashin SJ, Spencer SK, et al: Pregnancy and hormonal influences on malignant melanoma. *J Dermatol Surg Oncol* 13:276–281, 1987.
26. Grimwood RE, Siegle RJ, Ferris CF, et al: The biology of basal cell carcinomas: A revisit and recent developments. *J Dermatol Surg Oncol* 12:805–808, 1986.

27. Vargo N: Basal and squamous cell carcinomas: An overview. *Semin Oncol Nurs* 7:13–25, 1991.
28. Howat AJ, Levick PL: Metastatic basal cell carcinoma. *Dermatologica* 174:132–134, 1987.
29. McKinney P, Robinson JK: Basic principles in management of basal cell epithelioma. *Ill Med J* 173:105–111, 1988.
30. Edwards L, Levine N: Skin cancer: The best route to early diagnosis. *Mod Med* 54:42–54, 1986.
31. Tobinick EL: Basal cell carcinoma. *Am Fam Phys* 36:219–224, 1987.
32. Stoll HL, Scwartz RA: Squamous cell carcinoma. In Fitzpatrick TB, Eisen AZ, Wolff K, Freedberg IM, (eds), *Dermatology in General Medicine*. New York: McGraw-Hill, 1987, pp. 746–758.
33. Marks R: Squamous cell carcinoma. *Aust Fam Phys* 15:937–938, 1986.
34. Friedman HI, Cooper PH, Wanebo HJ: Prognostic and therapeutic use of microstaging of cutaneous squamous cell carcinoma of the trunk and extremities. *Cancer* 56:1099–1105, 1985.
35. Stegman SJ: Basal cell carcinoma and squamous cell carcinoma: Recognition and treatment. *Med Clin North Am* 70:95–107, 1986.
36. Lippman SM, Kessler JF, Meyskens FL: Retinoids as preventive and therapeutic anticancer agents (parts 1 and 2). *Cancer Treat Rep* 71:391–405, 493–515, 1987.
37. Roenigk RK: Subspecialty clinics: Dermatology—Moh's micrographic surgery. *Mayo Clin Proc* 63:175–183, 1988.
38. Crawfort E, Girouard M, Johnson S, et al: Moh's chemosurgery: Day surgery for cutaneous malignancies. *AORN J* 43:464–468, 1986.
39. Torre D: Cryosurgery of basal cell carcinoma. *J Am Acad Dermatol* 15:917–929, 1986.
40. Levine HL, Ratz JL, Bailin P: Squamous cell carcinoma of the head and neck: Selective management according to site and stage-skin. *Otolaryngol Clin North Am* 18:499–503, 1985.
41. Ashby M, Pacella J, deGroot R, et al: Use of a radon mould technique for skin cancer: Results from the Peter MacCallum Cancer Institute (1975–1984). *Brit J Radiol* 62:608–612, 1989.
42. Holt PJA: Cryotherapy for skin cancer: Results over a 5-year period using liquid nitrogen spray cryosurgery. *Brit J Dermatol* 119:231–240, 1988.
43. Wheeland RG, Bailin PL, Ratz JL, et al: Carbon-dioxide laser vaporization and curettage in the treatment of multiple superficial basal cell carcinomas. *J Dermatol Surg Oncol* 13:119–125, 1987.
44. Greenway H, Cornell R, Tanner D et al: Treatment of basal cell carcinoma with intralesional interferon. *J Am Acad Dermatol* 15:437–443, 1986.
45. McCaughan J, Guy J, Hicks W, et al: Photodynamic therapy for cutaneous and subcutaneous malignant neoplasms. *Arch Surg* 124:211–216, 1989.
46. Sacchini V, Melloni E, Marchesini R, et al: Preliminary clinical studies with PDT and TPPS administration in neoplastic skin lesions. *Lasers Surg Med* 7:6–11, 1987.
47. Santoro O, Bandieramonte G, Melloni E, et al: Photodynamic therapy by topical meso-tetraphenylporphinesulfonate tetrasodium salt administration in superficial basal cell carcinomas. *Cancer Res* 50:4501–4503, 1990.
48. Worth AJ: Growth patterns in melanoma and its precursor lesions. In Gallagher RP (ed), *Epidemiology of Malignant Melanoma*. Berlin: Springer-Verlag, 1986, pp. 1–7.
49. Murphy GE, Halpern A: Dysplastic melanocytic nevi: Normal variants or melanoma precursors? (editorial). *Arch Dermatol* 126:519–522, 1990.
50. Friedman R, Rigel D, Silverman M, et al: Malignant melanomas in the 1990's: Continued importance of early detection and role of physician examination and self-examination of the skin. *CA* 41:201–226, 1991.
51. Koh H: Cutaneous melanoma. *N Engl J Med* 325:171–182, 1991.
52. Kraemer K, Greene M, Tarone R, et al: Dysplastic naevi and cutaneous melanoma risk. *Lancet* 2:1076–1077, 1983.
53. Rigel DS, Rivers JK, Kopf AW, et al: Dysplastic nevi: Markers for increased risk for melanoma. *Cancer* 63:386–389, 1989.
54. Piepkorn M, Meyer LJ, Goldgar D, et al: The dysplastic melanocytic nevus: A prevalent lesion that correlates poorly with clinical phenotype. *J Am Acad Dermatol* 20:407–415, 1989.
55. Ackerman AB: Pathobable: Confusing terminology in the language of melanocytic neoplasia. In Cascinelli N, Santinami M, Veronesi U (eds), *Cutaneous Melanoma Biology and Management*. Milan, Italy: Masson, 1990, pp. 127–132.
56. Halpern AC, DuPont G IV, Elder DE, et al: Dysplastic nevi as risk markers of sporadic (nonfamilial) melanoma. *Arch Dermatol* 127:995–999, 1991.
57. Rhodes AR: Benign neoplasias, hyperplasias, and dysplasias of melanocytes. In Fitzpatrick TB, Eisen AZ, Wolff K, Freedberg IM (eds), *Dermatology in General Medicine*. New York: McGraw-Hill, 1987, pp. 877–946.
58. Barnhill RL, Hurwitz S, Duray PH: The dysplastic nevus: Recognition and management. *Plast Reconstr Surg* 81:280–288, 1988.
59. Landow KR: Differential diagnosis and treatment of pigmented skin lesions. *Comp Ther* 14:25–32, 1988.
60. Wade TR, White CR: The history of malignant melanoma. *Med Clin North Am* 70:57–69, 1986.
61. Bergman W, Ruiter DJ, Scheffer E, et al: Melanocytic atypia in dysplastic nevi. *Cancer* 61:1660–1666, 1988.
62. Kibbi AG, Mihm MC, Sober AJ, et al: Diagnosis and management of malignant melanoma. *Comp Ther* 12:23–31, 1986.
63. Berdeaux DH, Moon TE, Meyskens FL: Management of stage I cutaneous melanoma. *Arizona Med* 40:768–772, 1983.
64. Finck SJ, Giuliano AE, Morton DL: LDH and melanoma. *Cancer* 51:840–843, 1983.
65. Balch CM: Cutaneous melanoma: A review of clinical management. *Texas Med* 83:70–78, 1987.
66. Balch CM, Milton GW: Diagnosis of metastatic melanoma at distant sites. In Balch CM, Milton GW, Shaw HM, Soong SJ (eds), *Cutaneous Melanoma*. Philadelphia: Lippincott, 1985, pp. 221–250.
67. Trent JM: Cytogenetics of human malignant melanoma. *Cancer Metastasis Rev* 10:103–113, 1991.
68. Greenberg A: MAGIC helps in diagnosing melanoma. *Oncol Times* pg. 5, 1990.
69. MacKie RM, Young D: Human malignant melanoma. *Int J Dermatol* 23:433–443, 1984.
70. Chanda JJ: The clinical recognition and prognostic factors of primary cutaneous malignant melanoma. *Med Clin North Am* 70:39–53, 1986.
71. Stal S, Loeb T, Spira M: Melanoma of the head and neck. *Otololaryngol Clin North Am* 19:549–564, 1986.
72. Briele HA, Walker MJ, Das G, et al: Melanoma of the

head and neck: Update and perspective. *Clin Plast Surg* 12:495–502, 1985.
73. Spitz S: Classics in oncology: Melanoma of childhood. *CA* 41:40–51, 1991.
74. Beahrs OH, Henson DE, Hutter RP, Kennedy BJ (eds): *Manual for Staging of Cancer: American Joint Committee on Cancer* (4th ed.). Philadelphia: Lippincott, 1992, pp. 143–148.
75. Balch CM, Soong SJ, Shaw HM, Milton GW: An analysis of prognostic factors in 4000 patients with cutaneous melanoma. In Balch CM, Milton GW, Shaw HM, Soong SJ (eds), *Cutaneous Melanoma*. Philadelphia: Lippincott, 1985, pp. 321–352.
76. Ketcham A, Balch CM: Classification and staging systems. In Balch CM, Milton GW, Shaw HM, Soong SJ (eds), *Cutaneous Melanoma*. Philadelphia: Lippincott, 1985, pp. 55–62.
77. Kopf AW, Welkovich B, Frankel RE, et al: Thickness of malignant melanoma: Global analysis of related factors. *J Dermatol Surg Oncol* 13:345–420, 1987.
78. Urist MM, Balch CM, Milton GW: Surgical management of the primary melanoma. In Balch CM, Milton GW, Shaw HM, Soong SJ (eds), *Cutaneous Melanoma*. Philadelphia: Lippincott, 1985, pp. 71–90.
79. Meyer KL, Kenady DE, Childers SJ: The surgical approach to primary malignant melanoma. *Surg Gynecol Obstet* 160:379–386, 1985.
80. Roses DF, Harris MN, Gumport SL: Surgery for primary cutaneous malignant melanoma. *Dermatol Clin* 3:315–326, 1985.
81. Veronesi U, Cascinelli N: How wide and deep is wide and deep enough? *Am J Dermatopathol* 7:123–126, 1985.
82. Goldberg KB, Boyd JD (eds): NIH Consensus Panel find narrower margins curative for early melanoma. *Cancer Letter* 18(6):5, 6, 1992.
83. Sim FH, Taylor WF, Pritchard DJ, et al: Lymphadenectomy in the management of stage I malignant melanoma: A prospective randomized study. *Mayo Clin Proc* 61:697–705, 1986.
84. Veronesi U: Delayed node dissection in stage I malignant melanoma: Justification and advantages. *Cancer Invest* 5:47–53, 1987.
85. Balch CM: The role of elective lymph node dissection in melanoma: Rationale, results, and controversies. *J Clin Oncol* 6:163–172, 1988.
86. Day CL, Lew RA: Malignant melanoma prognostic factors 7: Elective lymph node dissection. *J Dermatol Surg Oncol* 11:233–239, 1985.
87. Balch CM, Urist MM, Maddox WM, et al: Management of regional metastatic melanoma. In Balch CM, Milton GW, Shaw HM, Soong SJ (eds), *Cutaneous Melanoma*. Philadelphia: Lippincott, 1985, pp. 93–130.
88. Wornon IL, Smith JW, Soong SJ, et al: Surgery as palliative treatment for distant metastases of melanoma. *Ann Surg* 204:181–185, 1986.
89. Golumb FM: Chemotherapy of melanoma. *Dermatologic Clinics* 3:335–340, 1985.
90. Coates AS, Durant JR: Chemotherapy for metastatic malignant melanoma. In Balch CM, Milton GW, Shaw HM, Soong SJ (eds), *Cutaneous Melanoma*. Philadelphia: Lippincott, 1985, pp. 275–282.
91. Ho V, Sober A: Therapy for cutaneous melanoma: An update. *J Am Acad Dermatol* 22:159–176, 1990.
92. Klein ES, Ben-Ari GY: Isolation perfusion with cisplatin for malignant melanoma on the limbs. *Cancer* 59:1068–1071, 1987.
93. Krementz ET, Ryan RF, Carter RD, et al: Hyperthermic regional perfusion for melanoma of the limbs. In Balch CM, Milton GW, Shaw HM, Soong SJ (eds), *Cutaneous Melanoma*. Philadelphia: Lippincott, 1985, pp. 171–195.
94. Muchmore JH, Carter RD, Krementz ET: Regional perfusion for malignant melanoma and soft tissue sarcoma: A review. *Cancer Invest* 3:129–143, 1985.
95. Ghussen F, Kruger I, Groth W, et al: The role of regional hyperthermia cytostatic perfusion in the treatment of extremity melanoma. *Cancer* 61:654–659, 1988.
96. Franklin HR, Koops HS, Oldhoff J, et al: To perfuse or not to perfuse? A retrospective comparative study to evaluate the effect of adjuvant isolated regional perfusion in patients with stage I extremity melanoma with a thickness of 1.5mm or greater. *J Clin Oncol* 16:701–708, 1988.
97. Clark WH Jr, Elder DE, Guerry D IV, et al: Model predicting survival in stage I melanoma based on tumor progression. *J Natl Cancer Inst* 81:1893–1904, 1989.
98. Cascinelli N, Fontana V, Cataldo I, et al: Multiple primary melanoma. *Tumori* 61:481–486, 1975.
99. Rogers GS, Kopf AW, Rigel D, et al: Hazard-rate analysis in stage I malignant melanoma. *Arch Dermatol* 122:999–1102, 1986.
100. Rofstad EK: Radiation biology of malignant melanoma. *ACTA Radiol* 25:1–10, 1986.
101. Overgaard J: The role of radiotherapy in recurrent and metastatic malignant melanoma: A clinical radiobiological study. *Int J Radiat Oncol* 12:867–872, 1986.
102. Brascho DJ: Radiotherapy for metastatic melanoma. In Balch CM, Milton GW, Shaw HM, Soong SJ, (eds), *Cutaneous Melanoma*. Philadelphia: Lippincott, 1985, pp. 283–293.
103. Meyskens FL: The endocrinology of malignant melanoma. *Rev Endocrine-Related Cancer* 9:5–13, 1981.
104. Reintgen DS, McCarty KS, Vollmer R, et al: Malignant melanoma and pregnancy. *Cancer* 55:1340–1344, 1985.
105. Johnson BL: Malignant melanoma. In Groenwald SL (ed), *Cancer Nursing: Principles and Practice*. Boston: Jones and Bartlett, 1987, pp. 684–692.
106. Stadler R, Mayer-da-Silva A, Bratzke B, et al: Interferons in dermatology. *J Am Acad Dermatol* 20:650–656, 1989.
107. Creagan ET, Ahmann DL, Frytak S, et al: Recombinant leukocyte A interferon in the treatment of disseminated malignant melanoma. *Cancer* 58:2576–2578, 1986.
108. Kokoschka EM, Sommerbegger K: Alpha 2-recombinant interferon therapy bei patienten mit malignem melanoma. *Hautarzt* 38:176–181, 1987.
109. Bratzke B, Stadler R, Garbe C, et al: Interferon (rIFNaZa, BIFN) for postsurgical adjuvant treatment in stage II malignant melanoma. *Seventh World Congress in Dermatology, Berlin,* Abstracts vol. II:164, 1987.
110. Ryan R, Krementz E, Litwin M: A role for topical 5-Fluorouracil therapy in melanoma. *J Surg Oncol* 38:250–256, 1988.
111. Edwards L, Jaffe P: The effect of topical tretinoin on dysplastic nevi. *Arch Dermatol* 126:494–499, 1990.
112. Dugan M, Oratz R, Bystryn JC: Immunotherapy in the treatment of malignant melanoma. In Friedman RJ, Rigel DS, Kopf AW, et al (eds), *Cancer of the Skin*. Philadelphia: Saunders, 1991.
113. Goldberg KB, Boyd JD (eds): Melanoma vaccine nearing phase 3: Other potential therapies discussed. *Cancer Letter* 16:3–4, 1990.

114. Shields JA: *Diagnosis and Management of Intraocular Tumors.* St. Louis, MO: Mosby, 1983.
115. Jensen OA, Prause JA: Malignant melanomas of the human uvea in Denmark: Incidence and a 25-year follow-up of cases diagnosed between 1943 and 1952. In Lommatsch PK, Blodi FC, (eds), *Intraocular Tumors.* New York: Springer-Verlag, 1983, pp. 85–92.
116. Bellet RE, Shields JA, Soll DB, et al: Primary choroidal and cutaneous melanomas occurring in a patient with the B-K mole syndrome phenotype. *Am J Ophthalmol* 89:567–570, 1980.
117. Greene MH, Sanders RJ, Chu FC, et al: The familial occurrence of cutaneous melanoma, intraocular melanoma, and the dysplastic nevus syndrome. *Am J Ophthalmol* 96:238–245, 1983.
118. Vink J, Crijns MB, Mooy CM, et al: Ocular melanoma in families with dysplastic nevus syndrome. *J Am Acad Dermatol* 23:858–862, 1990.
119. Tucker MA, Shields JA, Hartge P, et al: Sunlight exposure as a risk factor for intraocular malignant melanoma. *N Engl J Med* 313:789–792, 1985.
120. Seddon JM, Gragoudas ES, Glynn RJ, et al: Host factors, UV radiation, and risk of uveal melanoma. *Arch Ophthalmol* 108:1274–1280, 1990.
121. Shields CL, Shields JA, Eagle RC, et al: Uveal melanoma and pregnancy. *Ophthalmology* 98:1667–1673, 1991.
122. Zimmerman LE, McLean IW: Do growth and onset of symptoms of uveal melanomas indicate subclinical metastasis? *Ophthalmology* 91:685–691, 1984.
123. Shammas HF, Blodi FC: Prognostic factors in choroidal and ciliary body melanomas. *Arch Ophthalmol* 95:63–69, 1977.
124. Wilhelm JL, Zakov AN: Choroidal melanoma with liver metastasis before enucleation. *Ann Ophthalmol* 14:789–796, 1982.
125. Diener-West M, Hawkins BS, Markowitz JA, et al: A review of mortality from choroidal melanoma. II. A meta-analysis of 5-year mortality rates following enucleation, 1966 through 1988. *Arch Ophthalmol* 110:245–250, 1992.
126. Packer S, Rotman M, Salanitro P: Iodine-125 irradiation of choroidal melanoma: Clinical experience. *Ophthalmology* 91:1700–1708, 1984.
127. Augsburger JJ, Gamel JW, Sardi VF, et al: Enucleation vs cobalt plaque radiotherapy for malignant melanomas of the choroid and ciliary body. *Arch Ophthalmol* 104:655–661, 1986.
128. Weinstock MA, Colditz GA, Willet WC, et al: Nonfamilial cutaneous melanoma incidence in women associated with sun exposure before 20 years of age. *Pediatrics* 84:199–204, 1989.
129. Holman CDJ, Armstrong BK, Heenan PJ: Relationship of cutaneous malignant melanoma to individual sunlight exposure habits. *J Natl Cancer Inst* 76:403–414, 1986.
130. Stern RS, Weinstein MC, Baker SG: Risk reduction for nonmelanoma skin cancer with childhood sunscreen use. *Arch Dermatol* 122:537–545, 1986.
131. Simple guidelines to help protect you from the damaging rays of the sun. New York: Skin Cancer Foundation, 1988.
132. Living well in Arizona. Tucson: Arizona Cancer Center, 1992.
133. Bertram JS, Kolonel LN, Meyskens FL: Rationale and strategies for chemoprevention of cancer in humans. *Cancer Res* 47:3012–3031, 1987.
134. Ritenbaugh CK, Meyskens FL: Analysis of dietary associations of vitamin A with cancer. In Bland J (ed), *The Year in Nutritional Medicine.* New Canaan, CT: Keats, 1986, pp. 263–291.
135. Greenberg ER, Baron JA, Stukel TA, et al: A clinical trial of beta carotene to prevent basal-cell and squamous-cell cancers of the skin. *N Engl J Med* 323:789–795, 1990.
136. Loescher LJ, Meyskens FL: Chemoprevention of human skin cancers. *Semin Oncol Nurs* 7:45–52, 1991.
137. Fraser MC: The nurse's role and malignant melanoma. *Cancer Nurs* 5:351–360, 1982.
138. Fraser MC, McGuire DB: Skin cancer's early warning system. *Am J Nurs* 84:1232–1236, 1984.
139. White LN, Cornelius JL, Judkins AF, et al: Screening of cancer by nurses. *Cancer Nurs* 1:15–20, 1978.
140. Lawler PE, Schreiber S: Cutaneous malignant melanoma: Nursing's role in prevention and early detection. *Oncol Nurs Forum* 16:345–352, 1989.
141. Schulmeister L: Screening for skin cancer: A necessary part of your assessment routine. *Nursing* 11:42–45, 1981.
142. Berwick M, Bolognia JL, Heer C, et al: The role of the nurse in skin cancer prevention, screening, and early detection. *Semin Oncol Nurs* 7:64–71, 1991.
143. Grossman DJ: Public and professional educational materials on skin cancer. *J Am Acad Dermatol* 21:1012–1018, 1989.
144. Stern C: Melanoma: The most lethal skin cancer. *RN* 50:53–57, 1987.

Chapter 50

Urologic and Male Genital Malignancies

Julena Lind, RN, MN, PhD cand.

Kathy Kravitz, RN, MA

Betty Greig, RN, CETN

INTRODUCTION

Cancer of the prostate gland is one of the most prevalent male cancers in the world. Bladder and kidney tumors are common in both adult men and women. Testicular tumors, although rare, are important because they are associated with a high risk of cancer death in men between 29 and 35 years of age.[1] Tumors of the urethra, penis, scrotum, epididymis, and seminal vesicles are rare and are not discussed in this chapter.

Figure 50-1 gives an overview of the sites of genitourinary tumors and metastases in men. Figure 50-2 represents the sites and routes of genitourinary tumor metastases in women.

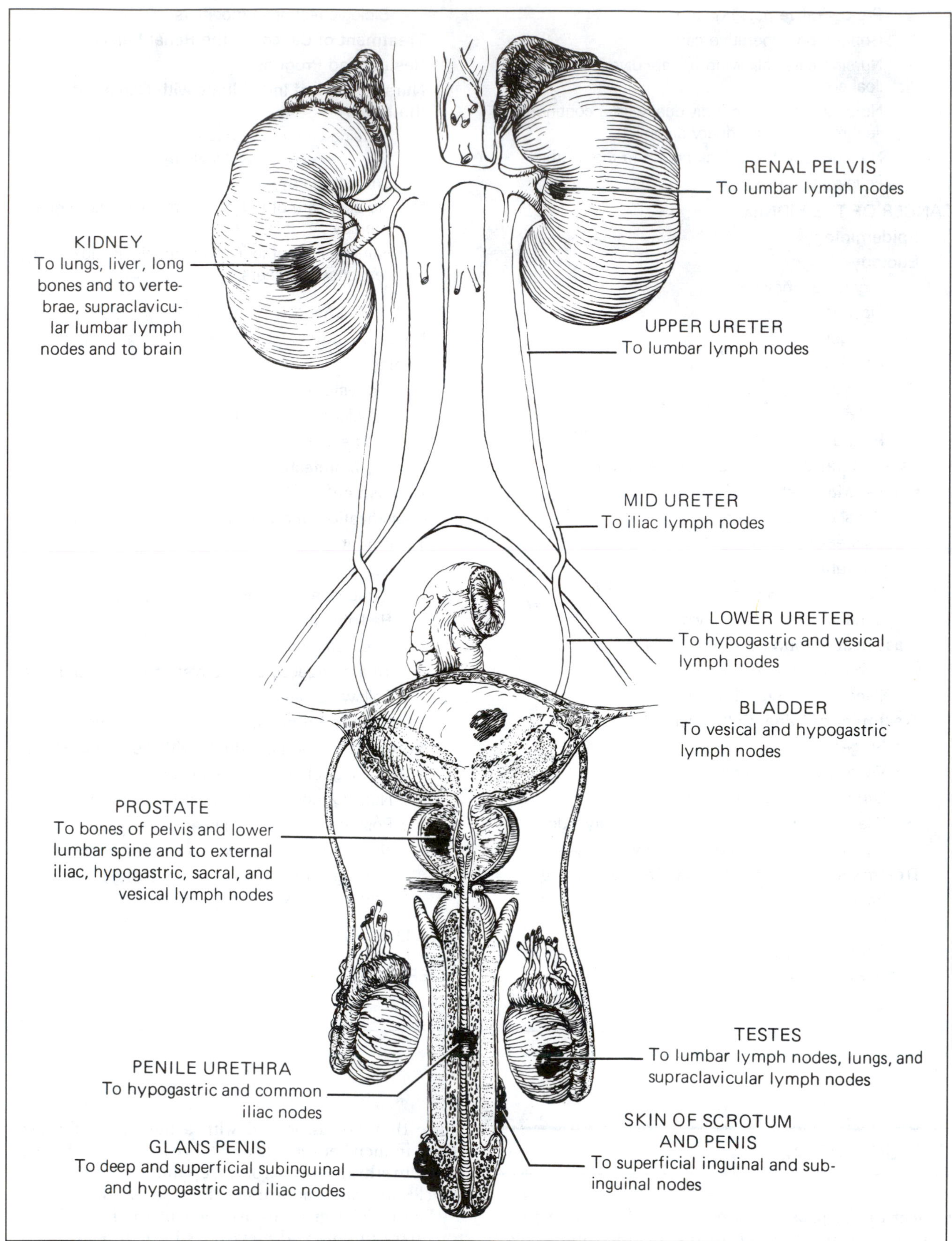

FIGURE 50-1 Sites of tumor origin and metastasis in the male. (Source: Adapted from Johnson DE, Swanson DA, von Eschenbach AC: Tumors of the genitourinary tract, in Tanagho EA, McAninch JW, (eds), *Smith's General Urology*.[12th ed]. San Mateo, CA: Appleton & Lange, 1987, p. 332.)

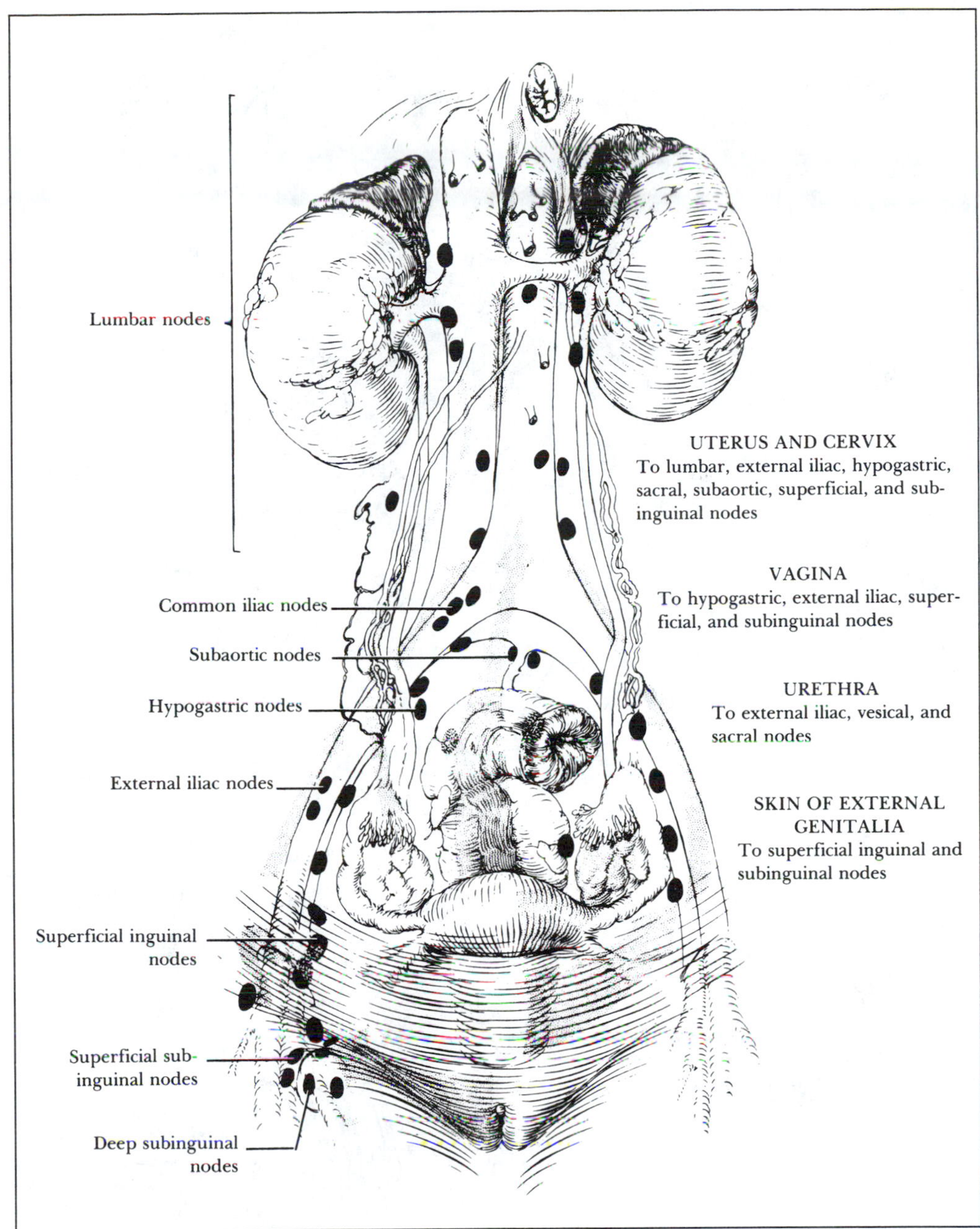

FIGURE 50-2 Sites and routes of tumor metastasis in the female. (Source: Adapted from Johnson DE, Swanson DA, von Eschenbach AC: Tumors of the genitourinary tract, in Tanagho EA, McAninch JW (eds), *Smith's General Urology* [12th ed]. San Mateo, CA: Appleton & Lange, 1987, p. 333.)

PROSTATIC CANCER

Anatomy and Physiology

The prostate is a small, firm organ that is shaped like an inverted and flattened pyramid. It is made up of glands and musculature enclosed in a fibrous capsule. In the adult male the prostate is usually about the size of a walnut (4–6 cm long). It lies posterior to the symphysis pubis, just inferior to the bladder and in front of the rectum (Figure 50-3). The prostate gland is inverted so that its base is at the neck of the bladder. A segment of the urethra runs through the prostate and is known as the prostatic urethra.

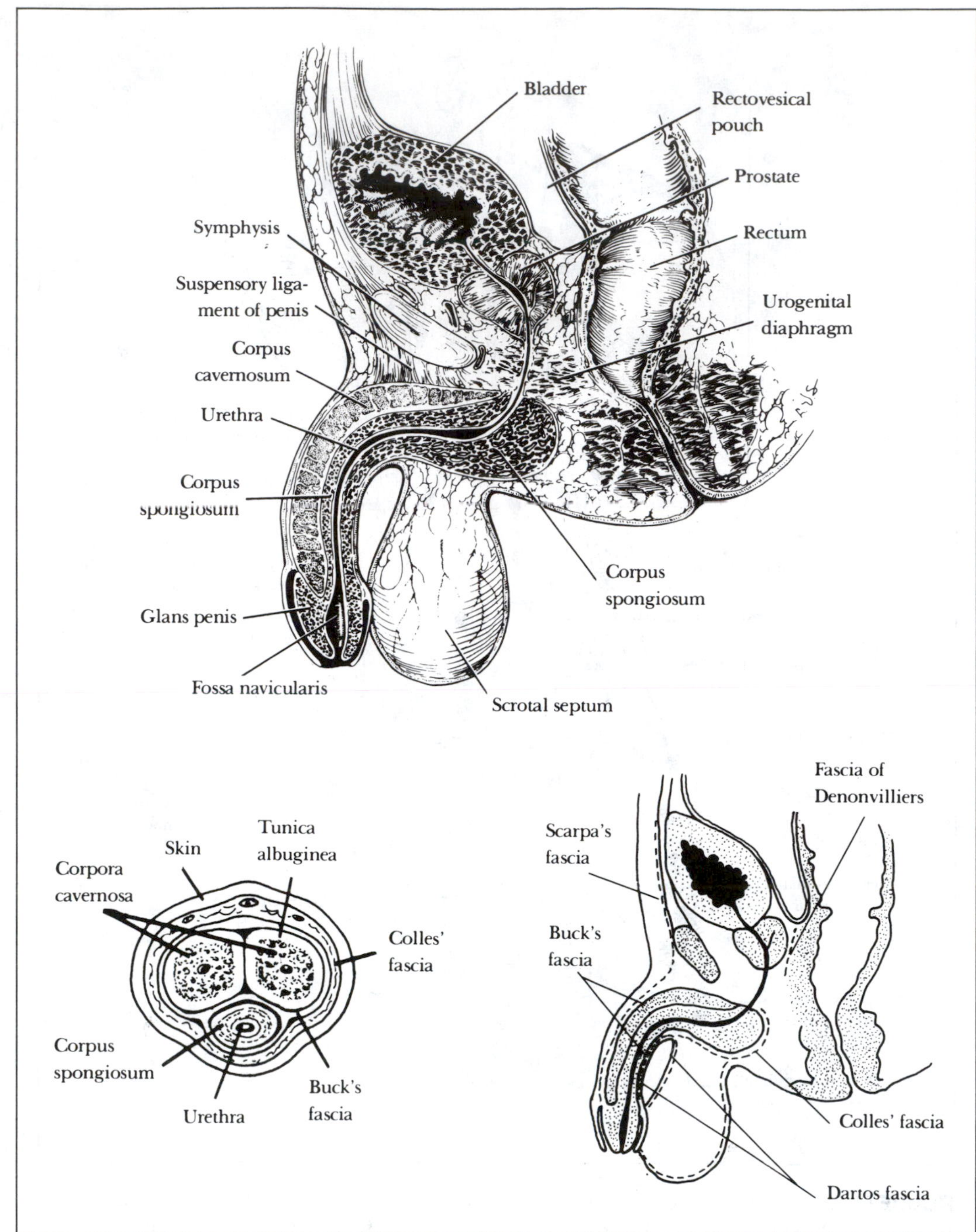

FIGURE 50-3 Relation of the bladder, prostate, seminal vesicles, penis, urethra, and scrotal contents. (Source: Tanagho EA: Anatomy of the genitourinary tract, in Tanagho EA, McAninch JW (eds), *Smith's General Urology* [12th ed]. San Mateo, CA: Appleton & Lange, 1987, p. 10.)

Epidemiology

There are approximately 132,000 new cases of prostate cancer and 34,000 deaths from the disease in the United States each year. Prostate cancer accounts for approximately 23% of all cancer in men in the United States and 12% of cancer deaths.[2] It is the second most common cancer in American men.

The highest rate of prostatic cancer in the world is among black Americans. The higher incidence in blacks appears not to be associated with social class, since the higher age-adjusted rate in blacks as compared to whites is the same across all social classes.[3] However, the disease is reportedly less common in African blacks, which suggests more than a genetic basis to the disease. Japan has the lowest prostatic cancer rate among countries with reliable reporting. When Japanese men migrate to the United States, the incidence of prostate cancer rises but remains only about half that of American whites.[3]

Many recent studies suggest the prevalence of clinically occult prostatic cancer found at autopsy is similar throughout the world and racial groups.[3] Nevertheless, there are differences in clinical presentation of the disease in different ethnic groups. Migration studies indicate that if individuals migrate from a host population with a low rate of prostatic cancer to an area with a high rate, the migrants develop a substantially higher rate of prostate cancer in the new country.[3] These studies suggest the possible role of environmental factors in the development of prostate cancer.[4] In addition, it is important to note that the rate of clinically apparent disease and prostatic cancer mortality differ widely.[3] In general, the currently available epidemiologic trends data are conflicting and difficult to interpret.[4]

The other important demographic variable is age. Prostatic cancer is rare in men under 40 years of age, and the risk increases with age. The peak incidence is in men between 60 and 70 years of age. There has been a significant relative rise in the incidence of prostatic cancer in asymptomatic American males ranging in age from 55–70.[5] Histologic data obtained from autopsy studies demonstrating prostatic cancer indicates that 40% of men whose death occurs in their ninth decade have evidence of the disease.[3]

Etiology

Age, infectious agents, and endocrine factors are the three main etiologic factors hypothesized to be related to prostatic cancer. In addition, there is emerging evidence that familial patterns and dietary factors may play a role in the development of the disease.[6] The role of vasectomy in the incidence of prostate cancer has also been questioned.

Infectious agents, transmitted through sexual activity, have been suggested as possible etiologic factors in prostate cancer. The sexual transmission hypothesis was tested by the University of Southern California Cancer Surveillance Program. This study examined death rates and cancer death rates in celibate men (Catholic priests in the Archdiocese of Los Angeles) and compared those rates with the expected number of cancer deaths in white males in the United States for the same years. They found that cancer mortality in celibate men was 79% of what was expected, but the incidence of prostatic cancer deaths was higher in these men than would be expected. The relatively high cancer mortality rate among celibate men argues against the theory of sexual transmission of this disease.[7] Other researchers argue that the hypothesis of infectious etiology for prostatic cancer needs to be reexamined in the light of the current understanding of viral oncology. Herpesvirus, SV-40 virus, cytomegalovirus, and RNA viruses have been implicated in the origins of prostatic cancer along with others, although no causal relationship has been established.[3]

The prostate's growth and function are controlled by hormones. Adenocarcinoma of the prostate appears difficult to induce in animal models. But testosterone alone, given subcutaneously, can produce this cancer in rats,[8] thus lending support to the theory that prostatic cancer has a hormonal basis. A few human epidemiologic studies focus on this hypothesis. One study of 77 subjects showed that individuals with prostatic cancer had higher levels of serum testosterone than healthy controls of the same age.[9] Another study looking at the circulating steroid hormone levels in white and black college students found that the mean testosterone level in blacks was 15% higher than that of whites, which might explain the twofold increased risk of prostatic cancer in American blacks.[10]

Certain case-controlled studies have looked at the consumption of dietary fat and its association with the incidence of prostatic cancer and have found that persons whose fat intake was above the median were at higher risk for prostate cancer.[11] The hypothesis is that dietary fat in some way changes the hormonal environment.

Emerging evidence indicates that familial patterns also play a role in the development of the disease. Steinberg and colleagues[6] studied 691 men who underwent radical prostatectomy. Their research demonstrated that men with a positive family history were twice as likely to have cancer of the prostate. Despite some limitations of the study design, a significant correlation between family history and the development of the disease is clearly evident.[6]

Historically, the relationship between vasectomy and prostate cancer has been questioned. In a recent study by Rosenberg[12] a relationship between the disease and vasectomies has again been suggested. The investigation was designed as a "hypothesis-hunting" study. The study alone is not powerful enough to demand any change in current policy. However, the possibility that a relationship exists is important to investigate in precisely designed research.

Pathophysiology

Cellular characteristics

Prostatic cancers are almost always adenocarcinomas that vary in appearance and differentiation. They arise most commonly in the posterior lobe and are usually multifocal.[13] The prostate has been shown to be composed of discrete zones based on morphology, ductal patterns, and embryonic origin.[13] Peripheral, central, and transitional zones compose most of the prostate. Carcinoma develops most often in the peripheral zone but can originate in the transition and central zones as well.[13]

Progression of disease

Prostatic tumors grow and spread locally to the seminal vesicles, bladder, and peritoneum. Despite the fact that many prostatic tumors are extremely slow growing and indolent, it appears that there is an unusually wide range of biologic malignancy. Some prostatic tumors are rapidly progressive and fatal, some have intermediate behavior, and others are detected only accidentally and never grow and spread.

Adenocarcinoma of the prostate spreads via the blood vessels and lymphatic system. It spreads in the perineural lymphatics, involving the seminal vesicles and the sacral, external iliac, and lumbar lymph nodes. One-third of men with early cancer have evidence of metastases to the pelvic lymph nodes.[14] From the pelvis the lymphatic fluids travel to the thoracic duct and then dump into the venous system at the junction of the left internal jugular and the left subclavian veins. Because the supraclavicular nodes lie adjacent to the veins that communicate with the thoracic duct, patients with widespread cancer often have scalene or supraclavicular node involvement.

Hematogenous spread of prostatic cancer typically involves the lungs, liver, kidneys, and bones. Up to half of the men who die of prostate cancer demonstrate lung metastases on autopsy, and 66% have bone metastases.[14] The vertebrae, pelvis, femur, and ribs are often involved.

Clinical Manifestations

Prostatic cancer is usually asymptomatic in its early stages. Detection occurs as a result of routine rectal examination that reveals a nodule or mass. Because the posterior surface of the prostate is in close contact with the rectum, it is the only portion that can be palpated. Tumors also may be discovered during examination of transurethral resection specimens.

A common presenting picture is an elderly man with weight loss, back pain, and prostatism. Other symptoms include urinary frequency and nocturia, dysuria, slow urinary stream, or hematuria. Unfortunately, many of these symptoms are similar to those of other disorders, particularly benign prostatic hypertrophy.

More than half (56%) of patients present with localized disease, 19.5% with regional involvement, and 23.7% have distant metastases.[15] Signs related to spread of the disease are anemia and weight loss, lumbosacral pain (which may radiate to the hips or down the legs), and hematuria if the bladder or urethra has been invaded.

Assessment

Screening

Of the many prostatic cancer controversies, screening techniques and their value are among the most hotly contested. Screening of asymptomatic males for prostatic cancer by any means has not shown true benefit to date.[16] There are, however, several areas of disagreement surrounding that assertion. Three mechanisms currently exist to aid in earlier detection of prostatic cancer: digital rectal examination; transrectal ultrasonography (US); and biochemical markers, particularly prostatic acid phosphatase and prostate specific antigen. An optimal screening test should be safe, inexpensive, widely available, accurate, and reasonably specific for the disease. The goal of effective screening in prostatic cancer should be to diagnose more stage A and B1 lesions and to improve survival. There has been no satisfactory study of a true high-risk group of asymptomatic men that has met all the preceding requirements and detected more early cancers.[16]

Rectal palpation has been the most important step in detecting carcinoma of the prostate; there is an increased incidence of early detection when digital rectal exam is done routinely.[17,18] However, the value of the rectal examination in screening an asymptomatic population is controversial. First, optimal age to begin screening has not been determined; second, many hard nodules are benign disorders, and several studies have shown little correlation between the clinical impression during rectal examination and the biopsy results. Only 30%–40% of cancers detected by screening using digital rectal examination can be expected to be localized to the prostate.[17] It is currently estimated that the positive predictive value of an abnormal rectal examination ranges from 11%–26%.[17]

Transrectal US was initially thought to be a very useful screening modality. Today, evaluation of this technique is being weighed in light of the expense of the equipment, the steep learning curves for both the imager and the clinicians,[19] the fact that the positive predictive value of a transrectal US is in the range of 30%–35%, and studies that indicate false-positive and false-negative rates that are unacceptably high.[17] Others argue that the future of early detection and improved survival depends on finding those 70% of cancers that lie in the peripheral zone and which can be visualized by transrectal US.[16,19] A recent study by Lee and colleagues[20] concludes that transrectal US is more sensitive than digital rectal examination in the detection of prostate cancer, and they advocate its broader implementation. Others counter that the study supports the concept of "case finding" and not screening in the true sense.[19]

Transrectal US may be combined with needle biopsy. Once a suspect area is identified on US, the needle may be guided into that area for sampling. This technique has high specificity but is obviously invasive and is expensive.[21,22]

Prostate specific antigen

Various markers including serum acid phosphatase, prostatic acid phosphatase, and serum and bone alkaline phosphatase have been used in the diagnosis and staging of prostatic cancer. However, none of these markers has been reliable in detecting early cancer.[23] A new serum marker, prostate-specific antigen (PSA), has recently been identified.

This antigen is made exclusively by prostatic tissue, and it is immunologically distinct from prostatic acid phosphatase. It is not cancer-specific, however, as it is present in both healthy, benign hyperplastic and malignant prostatic tissue.[23] PSA is a single-chain glycoprotein, elaborated by the prostate, that has a half-life of 2–3 days. Therefore, 2–3 weeks may be necessary for the serum PSA to return to baseline after manipulation, diagnostic intervention such as cystoscopy or transrectal US, or various treatments to the prostate, and therefore these procedures can cause spurious elevations of the PSA.[24]

Concentrations of PSA per gram of tissue do not differ significantly among healthy, hyperplastic, and cancerous tissue. Several researchers have attempted to establish normal ranges for a given volume of prostatic tissue. However, no such reliable range has been identified, and, because a diagnostically reliable measurement that denotes the presence of cancerous tissue is not available, it is unlikely that PSA by itself will become an effective screening tool for the early diagnosis of prostate cancer. However, many argue that if it is combined with digital rectal examination and/or transrectal US, it could be part of an effective early detection program.[24] It appears much more promising than the other markers, which all have high false-positive rates.[17,24]

In addition to the clinical considerations involved in developing a reliable screening strategy, the cost-effectiveness of the process must also be considered in this era of cost containment.

Many feel that early detection is still probably done best and most cost effectively with routine yearly digital examination beginning at age 50. A study of 1807 patients in which digital examination, US, and PSA determinations were used found a cancer detection rate of 14.6% as compared with a digital examination plus digitally guided biopsy detection rate of 1.3–1.7%. Digital examinations plus PSA levels are often recommended for initial screening to be followed by rectal US if there is a suspicious finding.

In conclusion, to date there is not a consensus on a single, effective screening test for prostatic cancer. There are several contributing factors, including:

1. Because of the puzzling natural history of prostate cancer, no test currently in use can reliably separate potentially aggressive tumors from those that will remain indolent.

2. The wide variations in applying screening techniques, from digital rectal examinations to transrectal US, prohibit accurate comparisons of results.

3. Two important biases confound the interpretation of screening study findings. Lead-time bias happens when earlier diagnosis results in a greater duration of life (after diagnosis and treatment) without extending survival. The other bias is length bias, where cancers that are not progressing or are progressing very slowly are included in statistical calculations. This automatically improves survival rates but actually dilutes the real impact of screening techniques.[26]

Diagnosis

Common procedures used to diagnose prostatic cancer include rectal examination, biopsy, chemical studies, cytologic examination of urine and prostatic fluid, excretory urogram, bone scans, computerized tomography (CT), and magnetic resonance imaging (MI).

On rectal examination the consistency of the prostate normally feels rather rubbery. Early cancer presents as a nonraised, firm lesion that often has a sharp edge. Advanced cancer is hard and stonelike. The difficulty is differentiating the firm areas of the prostate that might be cancer from infection, tuberculosis, and prostatic calculi.

Every suspected prostatic mass should be biopsied.[27] Various techniques are used. Transrectal or transperineal needle biopsy is most commonly used in the United States. Needle aspiration consists of inserting a fine needle into the prostate and aspirating cells with a syringe. Open biopsy is probably the most accurate technique, but a high degree of morbidity is associated with this procedure.

Because of the difficulty in diagnosing prostate cancer, some researchers have argued for the use of flow cytometry to help in confirming a cytopathological diagnosis.[28] Flow cytometry can examine prostatic needle biopsy aspirate for DNA content and help to predict the malignant potential of the disease based on changes in the DNA. The detractors of flow cytometry use in prostate cancer contend that ploidy data alone are not enough on which to base treatment decisions. The champions of assessing DNA ploidy as a predictive tool believe that, along with other clinical factors, it is helpful in making day-to-day clinical decisions in patients with prostate cancer.[28]

Serum prostatic acid phosphatase can now be distinguished via a radioimmunologic technique. Eighty percent of men with stage D cancer have an increased serum prostatic acid phosphatase level.[27] An elevation of this enzyme is considered to indicate advanced disease regardless of whether the metastatic sites are obvious. This test is generally inexpensive, and it is fairly accurate when in the high range, but it is difficult to interpret when the acid phosphatase is in the normal or near normal range.[29]

PSA has been shown to be a good tumor marker, but it does not correlate well enough with tumor mass to reflect tumor stage accurately. PSA may be most valuable in monitoring response to therapy.[30] Residual disease should be suspected in any patient with detectable PSA levels 3 weeks or more after radical prostatectomy.[30]

Other serum factors also may be elevated. The isoenzyme of lactic dehydrogenase has been elevated in men with prostatic cancer. An increase in serum creatinine and urea nitrogen values occurs if the cancer is causing an obstruction associated with renal back pressure or ureteral occlusion.

Additional diagnostic studies may include cytologic examination of urine and expressed prostatic fluid, which is positive in as many as 85% of men with prostate cancer. An excretory urogram may be done to demonstrate hydroureteronephrosis as a result of obstruction (caused by metastases to the pelvic lymph nodes) or direct invasion by the primary tumor. Bone scans have demonstrated metastases in 75% of patients with advanced disease.[27] CT scans can help to diagnose pelvic lymph node involvement, and MRI can demonstrate involvement of the seminal vesicles and changes in the contour of the prostate.[27,31]

Classification and Staging

The staging system for prostatic cancer most commonly used in the United States was developed in the mid-1950s and gradually evolved into the familiar stage A through D clinical staging system that has widespread use. Other staging systems have been proposed by the American Joint Committee on Cancer (AJCC) and the UICC (International Union Against Cancer), but these have never been received enthusiastically by American urologists. Because of the staging confusion in the literature and the inability to agree on the preferred use of one of the existing systems, the Organ Systems Coordinating Center (OSCC) of the National Cancer Institute (NCI) has recently proposed a new staging system[32] (Figure 50-4). A comparison of the various staging systems is seen in Table 50-1.

A staging work-up to determine the presence of metastases should be done. The tests that might be included are chest radiography to show hilar nodes and involvement of lungs and ribs; bone scans to show areas of bony metastases; and pelvic CT scans to show extraprostatic extension, including enlarged lymph nodes.

In some centers, staging pelvic lymphadenectomies have been advocated to aid in treatment selection. The rationale is that the pelvic lymphadenectomy will more accurately define the anatomic extent of spread. In men who are free of bony disease and who have a negative acid phosphatase level and no other signs of metastases, it is important to accurately define whether there is nodal involvement.[33] Treatment will differ and will be less surgically aggressive if nodal involvement is present.

The Gleason classification system is also widely incorporated into today's staging profiles.[34] This is a system of histopathological grading based on the glandular pattern of the tumor at relatively low magnification[35] (Figure 50-5). Combining clinical staging and histopathological grading helps predict the biologic potential of prostate cancer. The Gleason system is unique in that histologic grade is determined from the majority of the specimen and not the most undifferentiated portion.[15]

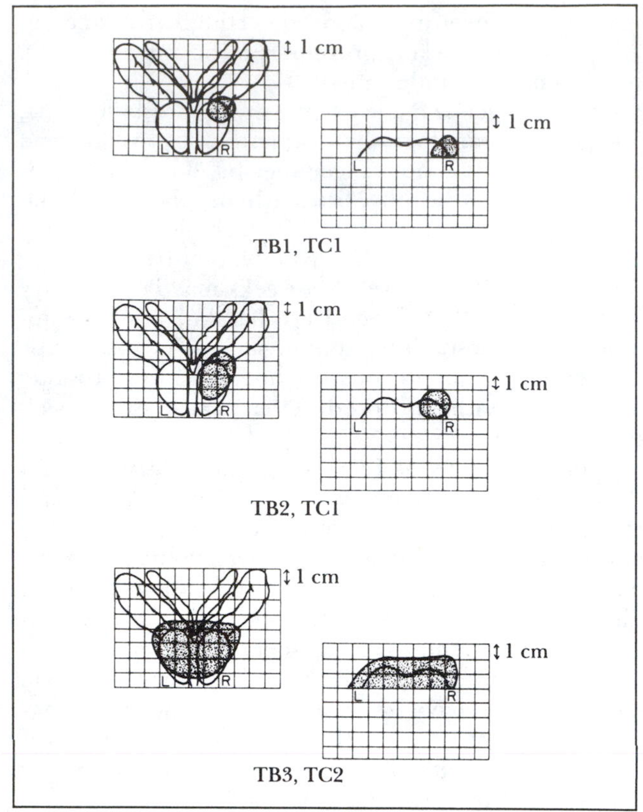

FIGURE 50-4 Staging diagram for patients with prostate cancer illustrating the Organ Site Coordinating Center (OSCC) staging system for quantifying both intracapsular and extracapsular extent of the primary tumor. (Source: Catalona WJ, Whitmore WF Jr: New staging systems for prostate cancer. *J Urol* 142:1302–1304, 1989.)

Treatment

The treatment of prostatic cancer remains controversial. Four methods have been applied alone or in combination: surgery, radiotherapy, endocrine manipulation, and chemotherapy. Each method plays a role in the treatment of prostate cancer.

Surgery

Radical prostatectomy The term *radical prostatectomy* refers to the surgical removal of the entire prostate, including the true prostatic capsule, the seminal vesicles, and a portion of the bladder neck. Total prostatectomy may involve taking only a portion of the attached seminal vesicles. In the radical prostatectomy,

TABLE 50-1 Summary of Clinical Staging Systems for Prostatic Adenocarcinoma

Modified Whitmore-Jewett	TNM		OSCC	
A No clinical neoplasm	Tx	Primary tumor cannot be assessed	Tx	Anatomic relationship undefinable
A_1 <5% total tissue	T0	No evidence primary tumor	TA	Digitally unrecognizable neoplasm
A_2 >5% total tissue	T1a	≤3 micro foci	TA1	≤5% total specimen and/or high grade
	T1b	>3 micro foci	A2	>5% total specimens and/or high grade
B Palpable neoplasm	T2a	Focal, 1 lobe	TBx	Palpable tumor but not characterized
B_1 ≤1.5 cm, 1 lobe	T2b	Diffuse	TB	Palpable tumor, not beyond capsule
B_2 >1.5 cm, >1 lobe			TB1	Not more than ½ lobe
			TB2	More ½ lobe, <1 lobe
			TB3	>1 lobe or more than 1 tumor
C Local invasion	T3	Invasion bladder, seminal vesicles or prostatic capsule	TCx	Extension but not characterized
C_1 Invasion one or both sulci	T4	Fixed tumor or adjacent structures	TC1	Extension beyond margin unilaterally
C_2 Base of seminal vesicle			TC2	Extension beyond margin with involvement of bladder base and/or rectum, and/or levator, and/or pelvic side wall
C_3 More seminal vesicle involvement and/or adjacent structures				
D Metastasis	NX	Regional nodes cannot be assessed	N0	No regional node metastasis
D_0 Elevated PAP	N0	No nodal metastasis	N1	Microscopic lymph node metastasis
D_1 Regional lymph node metastasis	N1	≤p2 cm regional nodes	N2	Gross regional lymph node metastasis
D_2 Distant metastasis	N2	2–5 cm regional nodes	N3	Extra regional lymph node metastasis
	N3	>5 cm regional nodes	Nx	Requirements not met
	MX	Distant metastasis cannot be assessed	M0	No evidence of metastasis
	M0	No distant metastasis	M1	Elevated acid phosphatase
	M1	Distant metastasis	M2	Visceral and/or bone metastasis
			Mx	Requirements not met

Source: Catalona WJ, Whitmore WS: New staging systems for prostate cancer, *J Urol* 142:1302–1303, 1989 (editorial).

removal is from the bladder neck to just beyond the apex of the prostate gland (Figure 50-6). The remaining portion of the bladder neck is then reanastomosed to the urethra.

Radical perineal prostatectomy is a common surgical method of choice.[36] Although this approach prohibits simultaneous pelvic lymphadenectomy, many authorities feel that it permits better visualization and better vesicle neck reconstruction and reanastomosis of the bladder to the urethra.[36] The individual is placed in an exaggerated lithotomy position for this surgery. Possible complications include infection and fecal incontinence from sphincter injury.

Radical retropubic prostatectomy provides for a simultaneous pelvic lymphadenectomy and may make a high-riding prostate gland more accessible. The retropubic approach is preferred by some authorities, who feel that it provides more urinary control and less stricture formation.[37] Complications of this approach include thromboembolism (which can be prevented by administering anticoagulants postoperatively), infection (the risk of which is greater if a penile prosthesis is implanted at the time of surgery), and rare later lymphedema.[37]

Sexual dysfunction is a common sequela of radical prostatectomy. All men undergoing radical prostatectomy will have absence of emission and ejaculation because of removal of the seminal vesicles and transection of the vas deferens. Loss of the ability to achieve an erection also occurs. An impotency rate of 90% has been reported following radical prostatectomy.[38] Erectile potency, however, does not depend on ejaculatory potency but on a combination of other factors. Psychologic aspects, blood supply, and nerve supply all work together to determine erectile potency.

The internal pudendal artery is the major blood supply for the erectile tissue and should not be significantly damaged during surgery.[39] The nerves responsible for potency are much more at risk. The autonomic nerve fibers that supply the area are susceptible to damage during the dissection of the prostate, prostatic capsule, and seminal vesicles. If a pelvic lymph node

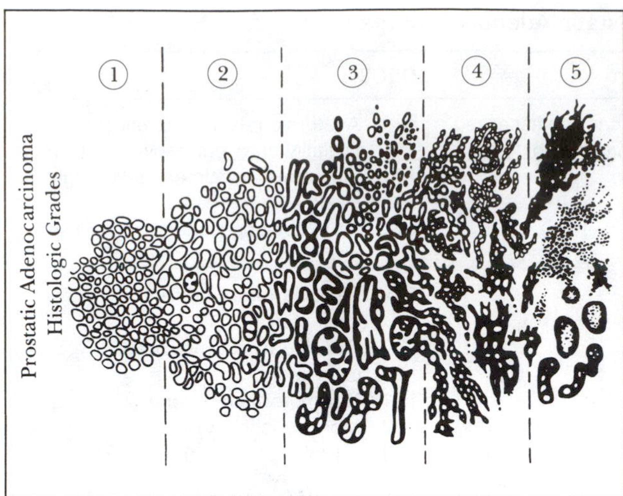

FIGURE 50-5 Gleason grading system. (Source: Gleason DF: The Veterans Administrative Cooperation Urologic Research Group: Histologic grading and clinical staging of prostatic carcinoma. In Tannenbaum M (ed), *Urologic pathology: The prostate.* Philadelphia: Lea & Feibiger, 1977, pp. 171–198.)

dissection is included, the risk of damage is even greater. Patients undergoing a radical retropubic prostatectomy with limited pelvic lymph node dissection will almost certainly experience erectile impotence.[37] Anatomic differences may influence which men retain erectile potency. In some men, some nerves may simply escape surgical damage.

Walsh and Donker[40] suggested in 1982 that post-prostatectomy impotence was caused by damage to the pelvic nerve plexus that innervate the corpora cavernosa. Subsequently, Walsh modified the technique for radical retropubic prostatectomy to carefully avoid injury to the pelvic nerves by visualizing and preserving the nerves bundles intraoperatively. This approach has saved sexual function in a large majority of patients—up to 72% potency in some reports.[41] It has also shown fewer problems with incontinence.[42]

Recent studies have investigated the role of nerve-sparing radical prostatectomy in different stages of the disease. Bigg and colleagues[43] examined its usefulness and associated risk in patients with clinical stage B2 disease. They found that its value in that context is questionable due to the increased risk of extracapsular

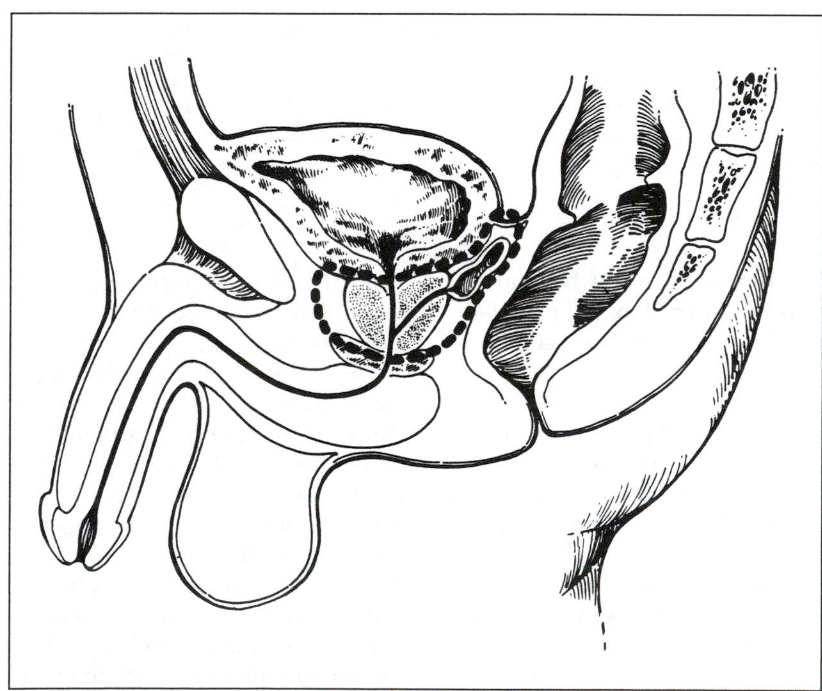

FIGURE 50-6 Surgical boundaries of a radical prostatectomy. The specimen includes the prostate with the true prostatic capsule and the seminal vesicles. (Source: Swanson D: Cancer of the bladder and prostate: The impact of therapy on sexual function, in von Eschenbach AC, Rodriguez D (eds), *Sexual Rehabilitation of the Urologic Cancer Patient.* Boston, Hall, 1981, p. 93.)

extension.[43] Catalona and Bigg[44] studied another 250 patients with stage A or B prostate cancer and corroborated the findings of the earlier studies by concluding that completeness of tumor excision correlated with tumor stage. Therefore, while the benefit of this procedure for preserving potency is clearly documented, the stage of the tumor must be considered in the decision to use it.[44]

Subtotal prostatectomy Subtotal prostatectomy can be either an open enucleative procedure or a transurethral resection. In a transurethral resection a resectoscope is inserted through the urethra and the prostatic tissue is scraped out with a movable loop of metal that cuts tissue with a high-frequency current. A resectoscope has an insulated sheath that protects the urethra from damage. This approach is not used as a curative surgical technique for prostatic cancer.[4]

In the transurethral process the bladder neck is altered anatomically, virtually destroying the competence of the internal bladder sphincter. The closure of this physiologic sphincter is necessary for the ejaculation of seminal fluid. The destruction of the sphincter allows the seminal fluid to pass retrograde (back into the bladder) rather than antegrade (out through the penis). This is known as *retrograde ejaculation* and almost always happens after transurethral resection. Some men equate ejaculation with normal sexual functioning. The loss of the sensation of ejaculation may be confused with the loss of sexual interest or potency.[39] Patient education is essential.

Reports about the incidence of actual erectile dysfunction after transurethral prostatectomy (TURP) are conflicting. Psychologic factors may play a large part in this type of impotence.[39]

Radiotherapy

External beam radiotherapy Radiotherapy as a cure for prostatic cancer is relatively new. The usual dose is 60–70 Gy for cure and 40–50 Gy for palliation. One example of a curative radiotherapy treatment regimen includes local and extended field irradiation of both the primary tumor and the first-echelon lymphatic drainage.[45] A four-field technique is used for anterior, posterior, left lateral, and right lateral fields. In this example a dose of 70 Gy is delivered in 7 weeks to the prostate at 2 Gy/day. A dose of 45–50 Gy in 7 weeks is delivered to the pelvic lymph nodes at 2 Gy/day. This is accomplished by giving 26 Gy (at 2 Gy/day) through the four-field technique. Another 20 Gy are given to the prostate and the periprostatic tissue over a 2-week period, and then the four-field technique is reinstituted for another 24 Gy.[45]

Common side effects of radiotherapy to the prostate are proctitis, diarrhea, and urinary frequency. These side effects usually develop toward the end of treatment, and complications requiring hospitalization are infrequent (only 6% of all men treated with curative radiotherapy).[46] Impotency rates following external beam radiotherapy vary from 20%–40%.[45,46] The reason for the erectile dysfunction is unknown, but in most series, age is a critical variable, and the higher potency rates usually apply to men under 60 years of age.[45]

When determining the overall efficacy of a treatment, it is important to consider survival, tumor-free survival, and quality of life. Tumor-free survival is linked to quality of life by the absence of symptoms that could otherwise occur if the disease continued to progress. Only limited data exist at this time comparing treatments and their associated tumor-free survival rates.[4]

Internal radiotherapy Interstitial radioactive gold (198Au) and radioactive iodine implantation (125I) have both been used as treatment methods in prostatic cancer. The radioactive gold grains have a half-life of 2.7 days and are inserted via a needle implanter after the prostate is surgically exposed. After implantation the wound is irrigated and closed without drainage. This method delivers approximately 30–35 Gy directly to the prostate, thereby sparing normal local tissue. After 2 weeks a course of external beam radiotherapy is begun, with 40–50 Gy delivered to the prostate and the periprostatic area.[47]

Radioactive iodine has a half-life of 60 days and is implanted under anesthesia with the patient in a modified lithotomy position. In one protocol, hollow 17-gauge needles 15 cm long are placed in the prostate, parallel to one another about 1 cm apart in an anteroposterior direction. The radioactive iodine seeds, which are 4.5 mm in length, are inserted through these hollow needles at intervals of 0.5–1.0 cm, and the needle is then withdrawn. The crossing of the prostatic urethra or bladder neck by the hollow needles is inevitable but does not seem to present later complications.[48]

The most common problem associated with 125I implantation is delayed, irritative voiding symptoms. Proctitis, rectal ulceration, or fistula have also occurred.[47] Complications of gold seed implantation are similar to those of 125I. In both of these methods, sexual function is preserved in 70%–90% of individuals potent before treatment.[47]

Endocrine manipulation

About 85% of prostatic cancers are androgen-dependent. Approximately 50% of patients have metastases at the time of diagnosis, and the mainstay of treatment of advanced prostate cancer is to decrease the circulating androgens. Androgen-dependent tissues get androgen from the testes and/or from the adrenal glands. Figure 50-7 demonstrates the normal androgen feedback mechanism. The testes produce 90%–95% of the circulating testosterone, which is the most powerful androgen. Normally a low level of testosterone signals the hypothalamus, via a negative feedback mechanism, to secrete gonadotropin-releasing hormone (GnRH) which stimulates the pituitary to

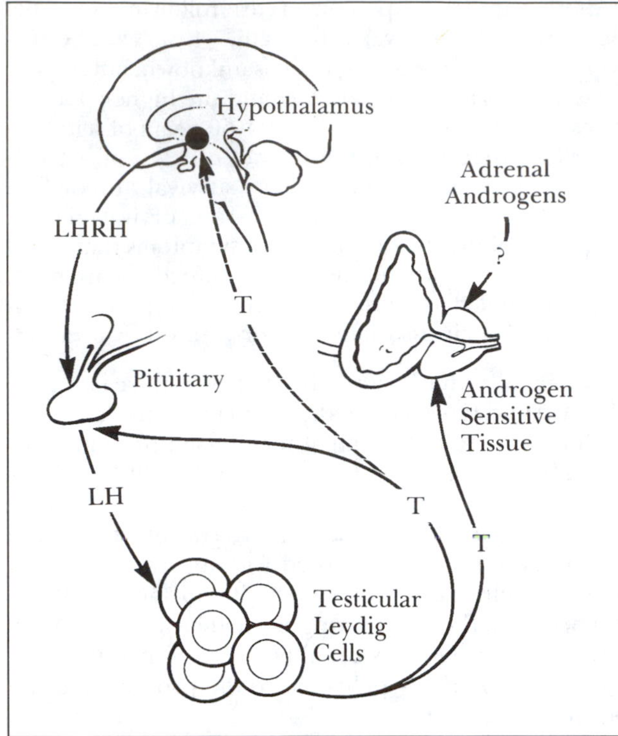

FIGURE 50-7 Pituitary luteinizing hormone (LH) is regulated by the pulsatile release of LH-releasing hormone (LHRH or gnRH) from the hypothalamus. Subsequently, LH stimulates production of testosterone (T) by testicular Leydig cells; T regulates both LH and LHRH release by negative feedback mechanisms. (Source: McConnell JD: Androgen ablation and blockade in the treatment of benign prostatic hyperplasia, *Urol Clin North Am* 17:661, 1990.)

release luteinizing hormone (LH). The LH stimulates the Leydig cells in the testes to synthesize testosterone. The testosterone secreted by the Leydig cells enables the spermatogenesis at the Sertoli cells in the testicular seminiferous tubules. The adrenals also produce the weak androgens, androstenedione and dihydroepiandrosterone, which account for 5% of all androgens. By the same negative feedback mechanism the hypothalamus signals the pituitary gland to release ACTH, which stimulates the adrenal glands to secrete androstenedione and dihydroepiandrosterone. If testosterone production via the testes has been inhibited for any reason, the adrenals will also produce testosterone.

Inhibition of testosterone secretion occurs via a negative feedback on the hypothalamus producing direct suppression of LHRH and corticotropin-releasing hormone (CRH) and resulting in decreased secretion of LH and ACTH. Hydrocortisone may directly inhibit adrenal androgen production at the level of the pituitary. Most testosterone is converted into dihydrotestosterone (DHT). DHT, the most common intracellular androgen, binds to receptors in the nuclei of prostate cells and stimulates normal and neoplastic prostatic cellular growth.[15] For the hormone to have an effect within the cell, it must bind with a receptor protein.

Since the prostatic cancer cell appears to be dependent on androgens for its growth, treatment attempts to block androgen formation or utilization at some point in the cycle. The major methods of endocrine manipulation in the treatment of prostate cancer are as follows:[49]

1. Surgical castration:
   - Bilateral orchiectomy, which removes the organs that primarily produce androgens and rapidly and directly lowers plasma testosterone levels
2. Medical castration:
   - Administration of estrogen (in the form of diethylstilbestrol), which has been used for over 40 years to block the release of LH
   - Administration of gonadotropin-releasing hormone (GnRH) analogs, which if given in large doses over time disrupt the pulsatile release of GnRH and cause a paradoxical suppression of gonadotropins and testosterone levels
   - Administration of ketoconazole, which blocks testicular and adrenal androgen synthesis
3. Adrenal suppression:
   - Administration of aminoglutethimide, which blocks adrenal androgen production
   - Administration of glucocorticoids, which decrease adrenal androgen production by suppressing ACTH
4. Pure antiandrogens:
   - Administration of antiandrogen drugs, which interfere with intracellular androgen activity
5. Mixed action drugs:
   - Administration of progestins (e.g., megestrol acetate, hydroxyprogesterone caproate), which inhibit pituitary LH secretion
   - Administration of cyproterone acetate, which inhibits pituitary LH secretion and androgen receptors
6. Total androgen ablation, which simultaneously blocks both adrenal and testicular androgens

Surgical castration Orchiectomy, or removal of the testes, is a brief surgical procedure with little morbidity or mortality that immediately stops the production of testicular androgens. Bilateral orchiectomy will reduce plasma testosterone levels by 90%. Advantages of orchiectomy over a medical approach include immediate response, elimination of cardiac complications, and no problems with patient compliance.[50] A disadvantage of this procedure is the psychological trauma that the patient experiences as the result of surgical castration. For some men this perception of the procedure makes it an unacceptable treatment option.[15]

Medical castration Diethylstilbestrol (DES), 1–3 mg/day orally, is the estrogen most commonly used and is the least expensive. Examples include premarin, estradiol, stilphostrol (given IV in high doses), and estramustine phosphate, which is a combination of nitrogen mustard and estrogen. Major complications of diethylstilbestrol are cardiogenic and include cardiac failure and edema. Other side effects are gynecomastia, loss of libido, and impotency. Individuals are also at increased risk of thrombophlebitis, especially if the dosages are high.[51]

Administration of GnRH analogs is one of the latest attempts at managing advanced prostate cancer through endocrine manipulation. The literature often confusingly describes specific drugs as *luteinizing hormone-releasing hormones (LHRH)* rather than using the broader, more generic term *GnRH*. The most current usage has been of LHRH analogs such as Lupron, Leuprolide, Zoladex, and Buserelin. Therefore, in this chapter the term *LHRH* will be used.

Normally, a GnRH like LHRH is released in pulse fashion from the hypothalamus and stimulates the pituitary gland to release luteinizing hormone (LH) in men. LH subsequently controls the release of testosterone. Administration of LHRH initially causes an abrupt increase in LH release and subsequent testosterone release. However, after the acute "flare" period, testosterone levels paradoxically fall to castration level.[49] The exact mechanism is not clear, but it probably involves changes and confusion in the central feedback control of LH release and/or desensitization of the gonad to high levels of LH by reducing the number of gonadal LH receptor sites.[49] Ultimately the biologic effect is medical castration, with fewer toxic side effects than with estrogen therapy.

Although three drugs have been studied in clinical trials (LHRH [Lupron, Leuprolide], Buserelin, and Zoladex), in the United States the two LHRH agonists approved for the treatment of advanced prostate cancer are goserelin acetate (Zoladex) and leuprolide acetate (Lupron, Leuprolide). LHRH has been tested the most extensively in the United States. Leuprolide can be given subcutaneously every day or as a depot formulation given intramuscularly every 4 weeks. Side effects include loss of libido and hotflashes.[52]

Buserelin is a compound that can be given intranasally or subcutaneously, with results similar to LHRH. One study reported a high frequency of durable objective and subjective responses in patients with advanced prostate cancer. Side effects are hotflashes, loss of libido, and impotence.[53]

Zoladex is a simple monthly injection given subcutaneously in the upper abdomen. Side effects include gynecomastia, nausea and vomiting, edema, thromboembolic, and cardiovascular sequelae.[15] At present, Zoladex is slightly less expensive than the bioequivalent of Leuprolide.

Both Zoladex and Leuprolide produce a transitory elevation in testosterone for approximately 1–2 weeks. Subsequently, testosterone levels fall to castration levels in 1 month. This initial testosterone flare may produce a worsening of symptoms. Since most prostatic metastases affect the bone or lymph nodes, common indications of flare phenomena are an increase in bone pain and/or urinary difficulties seen shortly after beginning treatment. Pretreatment with 1 week of flutamide has been shown to block testosterone flare.[15]

Several studies have recently been conducted to evaluate the efficacy of the addition of flutamide to LHRH agonist therapy. Flutamide (Eulexin) is a pure antiandrogen that blocks DHT from binding with androgen receptors in the cytoplasm. Flutamide is used to achieve a more complete androgen blockage and thus to further inhibit the stimulation and growth of tumor cells. A common protocol uses flutamide 250 mg orally three times a day in combination with either the daily or the monthly LHRH agonist. It is recommended that to achieve the adjunctive benefit of the flutamide, it must be started in conjunction with the LHRH agonist. The results of these studies are mixed in regards to the long-term benefit of this drug combination.[54] The side effects of combination flutamide/LHRH agonist treatment can include hotflashes, loss of libido, impotence, gynecomastia, and diarrhea. However, the first four of these side effects are known to be associated with LHRH agonist treatment alone.

Ketoconazole is an antifungal agent that given in high doses will inhibit androgen production. Its use has been limited by the gastrointestinal intolerance experienced by recipients of the drug.[50]

Adrenal suppression Adrenalectomy (either surgical or medical with aminoglutethimide or other drugs) blocks adrenal androgens and has been proposed for individuals who originally responded to hormonal therapy but have since relapsed. Surgical adrenalectomy has a significant mortality rate associated with it and is not commonly used today.[51] Aminoglutethimide may help one-third of those who have relapsed after primary endocrine therapy (with orchiectomy or estrogen).[55] Side effects of aminoglutethimide therapy include lethargy, ataxia, hypotension, nausea, and hypothyroidism.[50] Other drugs that produce a medical adrenalectomy are ketoconazole, spironolactone, and glucocorticoids. Spironolactone inhibits adrenal and testicular precursors. Glucocorticoids suppress ACTH and provide only rare responses, with significant side effects.[50]

Pure anti-androgens Antiandrogens peripherally inhibit the action of dihydrotestosterone, usually by interfering with receptor steroid binding at the intracellular level. Flutamide, Anadron, Casodex, and 5-alpha reductase inhibitors (e.g., Finasteride) are antiandrogen drugs that have been used in endocrine manipulation.

Flutamide (Eulexin) is a potent antiandrogen without estrogenic activity and without cardiopulmonary complications. It works by inhibiting the binding of testosterone and DHT to the androgen receptor in target tissues. It seems to be more effective in patients who have received no prior endocrine therapy. Although flutamide has been given alone in small studies, its use generally has been in combination either with surgical or medical castration (total androgen blockade).[49]

Anadron is a nonsteroidal antiandrogen with receptor-binding properties similar to flutamide. Like flutamide, it leads to an increase in plasma testosterone secondary to LH increases. In clinical trials it has shown efficacy similar to flutamide, both alone and in combination with medical or surgical castration.[49]

5-alpha reductase inhibitors act to prevent conversion of testosterone to DHT. Currently, clinical trials with finasteride are under way.[49]

Mixed-action drugs Cyproterone acetate is a steroidal antiandrogen that not only competes with testosterone and DHT for the androgen receptor but also possesses progestational and glucocorticoid properties, leading to partial suppression of LH secretion. It has fewer cardiac complications than DES or megestrol acetate. Side effects include mild gynecomastia and peripheral edema. Outside of clinical trials, this drug is not available in the United States.[49]

Megesterol acetate decreases LH release, but studies show that there is an "escape" phenomenon after 6 months of treatment, when the androgen production is no longer totally blocked.[49]

Total androgen ablation Total androgen ablation has been proposed for first-line endocrine treatment as an alternative to testicular androgen ablation alone. This can take various forms: antiandrogen drugs, such as flutamide combined with estrogen; orchiectomy plus adrenalectomy; or GnRH plus antiandrogens. It is difficult to measure the impact of this modality on survival, and at present this therapy and its efficacy require further study.[49]

Evaluation of hormone manipulation In general, 70%–85% of patients with advanced prostatic tumors respond to hormonal manipulation. This response is demonstrated by a definite regression in size of tumor, lessening of the degree of urinary obstruction, disappearance of or decrease in bone pain, and weight gain. The duration of response is from 1–3 years. Only 10% survive 10 years after the start of endocrine therapy. The palliative role of hormonal therapy therefore is significant. It has not been possible, however, to establish whether orchiectomy and/or estrogen therapy can increase overall survival.[52]

Controversy exists concerning timing of treatment. Few would argue against the initiation of treatment in symptomatic patients with advanced metastatic disease. However, in the absence of evidence, some clinicians are uncomfortable beginning therapy in the asymptomatic patient. Those who are included towards early treatment use as their rationale:

1. Survival of patients with metastatic disease is greater in the postendocrine period than in the preendocrine period.
2. Patients with stage C and D disease who are treated with radical prostatectomy and orchiectomy appear to have delayed progression and prolonged survival.
3. Animal models support early androgen deprivation.

Early initiation of hormonal therapy in asymptomatic patients is appealing; however, its efficacy remains unproven.[15]

Chemotherapy

There is a limited role for chemotherapy in the treatment of advanced, hormonally unresponsive prostatic cancer. Both single-agent and combination protocols have been attempted. Numerous clinical studies have shown that chemotherapy has an acceptable risk–benefit ratio in the treatment of advanced prostatic cancer.[57]

The response rates observed in clinical trials of single agents and combination therapies are disappointing.[61] Single agents used include cyclophosphamide, methotrexate, doxorubicin, mitomycin, vinblastine, 5-fluorouracil, cisplatin, and dacarbazine. Of those, mitomycin C, weekly doxorubicin, and continuously infused vinblastine have produced significant objective responses.[56] Drugs that have been used in combination include doxorubicin, 5-fluorouracil, and mitomycin C (DMF); and vinblastine, doxorubicin, and mitomycin C (VAM). Other agents that combine a hormonal agent with an antineoplastic agent such as estramustine phosphate have been combined in protocol with cyclophosphamide.[57]

The results of an important animal study[58] demonstrate the relationship between tumor burden and curability. Cures were obtained only when cyclophosphamide and hormonal deprivation were combined at a time of minimal tumor burden. The researchers argue for combining surgery and adjuvant cyclophosphamide chemotherapy in the treatment of metastatic prostate cancer to minimize the total tumor burden and, optimally, to improve the cure rate.[58]

Recent studies have suggested a correlation between androgen action and growth factors. It is possible that androgens may stimulate cell proliferation by autocrine and paracrine mechanisms as well as by direct endocrine mechanisms.[4] Suramin, a B-naphthyl urea, is antagonistic to several growth factors. Clinical trials of this agent were begun in 1988. More than two-thirds of treated patients had a reduction in PSA levels and a decrease in bone pain. This agent is associated with significant toxicity, including demyelinating neuropathy and nephrotoxicity.[4]

Treatment According to Stage

Stage A

In Stage A disease, clinically occult cancer is detected incidentally. The tissue is described according to the degree of differentiation present. If the tumor is well differentiated, follow-up may be the only treatment recommendation, as most tumors have a slow growth potential. However, this approach may cause difficulties because it is common for prostatic tumors to have multiple foci, and the single-needle biopsy might have missed the more aggressive cells in the neoplastic clone.

The common treatment for Stage A tumors that are not well differentiated is radical perineal or retropubic prostatectomy. Some centers also recommend pelvic lymph node dissection.[37] Selected patients, such as those who are very old or those with small volume tumors or poor medical status, may be managed best by surveillance.[4]

Stage B

Stage B is defined as a palpable tumor in one or more lobes that has not extended through the prostatic capsule. Although radical prostatectomy is the standard treatment for these tumors, characteristics of the individual are important. A younger man or one who is more physically capable of tolerating surgery, with no evidence of metastases by bone scan and no increased level of prostatic acid phosphatase, is a much more likely surgical candidate. Pelvic lymphadenectomy might be included for those men at higher risk for metastases (i.e., those with more than one lobe involved or with diffuse involvement of the prostate). The problems associated with this procedure are pulmonary embolus, sepsis, wound infection, and hematoma.

Paulson and colleagues[59] conducted a long-term study of 441 patients with T1-2NOMO disease. This study supports other observations that patients with high Gleason grades, positive surgical margins, and increased prostatic acid phosphatase levels have a poor prognosis.[59]

Modified radical prostatectomy certainly has a place in the therapy of prostate cancer patients. However, its role in patients with more advanced stages of the disease is unclear. A study evaluating the role of this procedure in stage B2 disease seems to indicate that since cancer cure is the goal of the surgery, the procedure may be appropriate for patients with smaller clinical stage B2 lesions that are not poorly differentiated, and that wide excision with sacrifice of the neurovascular bundle should be considered for patients with bulky B2 disease.[43]

Radiotherapy for stage B prostatic cancer has been used more in the last 10 years. In the few studies available on Stage B cancer, the long-term outcome for radical prostatectomy and radiation therapy is similar. For the 10% of prostate cancers detected at this stage, it appears that either radiation therapy or surgery have equally curative results, with fewer complications reported for radiation therapy.[46]

Stage C

Forty to fifty percent of men present clinically with stage C disease, which extends through the prostatic capsule and/or involves the bladder neck or seminal vesicles. Many men with this stage disease already have occult bone or pelvic lymph node metastases. However, a well-differentiated stage C tumor is less likely to have occult metastases. The acid phosphatase level may be elevated, but there should be no evidence of metastases on bone scan.[27]

A variety of treatment options have been recommended for stage C prostatic cancer: radical prostatectomy with or without pelvic lymph node dissection, preoperative radiotherapy (to convert stage C to stage B) followed by radical prostatectomy and lymph node dissection, external beam radiotherapy alone, internal implants (125I or 198Au) with lymphadenectomy, and hormonal therapy as a postsurgical or postradiotherapy adjunct. There are conflicting studies about whether lymph node dissection added to radical prostatectomy improves long-term survival.

Reports on external beam radiotherapy (as an alternative to radical surgery) also have interpretation problems. There are inconsistencies in the grading and staging of stage C tumors, which make it difficult to compare survival statistics. Aggressive external beam radiotherapy of the prostate and potential regional adenopathy is recommended by some as the best hope for cure with the fewest side effects for men with stage C prostatic cancer.[45] The major deficiency of radiation therapy is that not all localized prostate cancers can be destroyed by therapeutic doses of radiation. Radiation therapy works by fractional cell kill. If not all the cells are killed, then they proliferate and treatment fails.[4]

The results of interstitial implant treatment may well be comparable with external beam radiotherapy and offer fewer side effects.[47,48]

The addition of hormonal therapy to either surgery or radiotherapy has not been proven to add years to survival time.[45,50]

The choice of therapy depends on the person's physical condition, actual spread of cancer, degree of differentiation or grade of the tumor, and the person's preference.

Stage D

Stage D disease involves metastases, either confined to the pelvis, including pelvic lymph nodes (D1); or distant metastases (D2). Stage D is the most common presenting clinical stage. There is no surgical cure for this stage. Men with D1 lesions who have only limited nodal involvement might benefit from pelvic lymph dissection, but in individuals with extensive nodal disease a biopsy is probably enough. Treatment options for men with advanced prostatic cancer include hormonal manipulation, interstitial or external beam radiotherapy, and/or chemotherapy. At one research center a common treatment plan for stage D disease might include interstitial or external beam radiotherapy followed by hormonal therapy and possibly chemotherapy and then second-line hormonal manipulation followed by chemotherapy if the hormonal therapy fails.

Results and Prognosis

Survival rates for prostatic cancer have increased significantly for both whites and blacks.[2] Approximate survival rates after prostatectomy are shown in Table 50-2. Clearly, the survival rates for stage D disease are less encouraging.

Nursing Care

Nursing role in early detection

The American Cancer Society recommends an annual rectal examination for all men over 40 years of age. Even though other evaluation procedures such as transrectal US are being used in the initial evaluation, the digital examination is still the most efficient means of detecting early prostate cancer.[17] It is important to impress on men that regular rectal prostatic examination is the best way to detect prostatic cancer early enough for effective treatment.

As mentioned previously, black males in the United States have the highest incidence of prostate cancer in the world. The American Cancer Society statistics revealed a significantly poorer outcome for blacks with prostate cancer. Poor cancer awareness has been cited as a major cause of poorer survival and higher mortality rates in the black population. Poorer awareness leads to poorer outcomes, probably because persons present themselves to the medical care system when their cancer is already at a later stage. Health care providers for the black community will want to target prostatic cancer patient education and early detection programs that will meet their special needs.

Patients undergoing rectal prostatic examination

Having a rectal prostatic examination may be uncomfortable for the patient. The nurse can minimize the patient's discomfort by informing him about the procedure. Immediately before the rectal prostatic examination, ask the man to empty his bladder. Explain to him that this will make the examination more accurate and comfortable. The nurse should also inform the patient that the examiner will ask him to "bear down" during the insertion of the examining finger. Reassure the patient that it is normal to experience sensations of having to urinate or defecate during the procedure. Inform him that there are two possible positions he may be asked to take during the examination: (1) knee-chest position with buttocks elevated or (2) bending from the hips with elbows either on the knees or on the examining table.[60]

TABLE 50-2 Approximate Survival Rates after Prostatectomy

Stage	5 Years	10 Years
A	88%	57%
B	73%	53%
C	62%	28%

Source: Boring CC, Squires TS, Tong T: Cancer statistics, 1992. *CA* 42:19–45, 1992.

Nursing care of individuals undergoing treatment for prostate cancer

The major treatments for prostate cancer include surgery, radiotherapy, endocrine therapy, and cytotoxic chemotherapy. The nurse should be aware that these treatments may produce loss of libido, impotence, loss of fertility, or urinary incontinence. These possibilities and suggestions for management should be presented and discussed by the physician with the patient and his family prior to any treatment. The discussion should include alternate ways to achieve sexual gratification. Many individuals and their spouses have been unprepared for the loss of sexual function after cancer treatment.

Preoperative nursing care Because most patients will have their diagnostic and staging work-up as an outpatient, a patient teaching guide describing the type of tests to be done and the rationale for each is an important nursing tool. Table 50-3 can be given to the patient and his family to help in their understanding of the preliminary work-up. Reading about the disease can be an important way to cope. The American Cancer Society publishes two booklets: "Facts on Prostate Cancer" and "For Men Only: Prostate Cancer." The National Cancer Institute also publishes a guide entitled "What You Need to Know About Prostate Cancer." These materials can be obtained by calling the local American Cancer Society office or the NCI's toll-free Cancer Information Service at 1-800-4-CANCER.

Surgical approaches to removing the prostate include retropubic, perineal, and transurethral. (See the section entitled "Treatment" for indications for each approach.) The person undergoing prostate surgery is usually extremely anxious. The emotional implications of this surgery involve both the patient and his mate. The major concerns usually focus on sexual competence and urinary control. The nurse must encourage expressions of concern, assess the individual's needs and knowledge, and give information accordingly. The preoperative regimen is similar to that for other abdominal surgery. Preoperative bowel preparation consists of cathartics, enemas, antibiotics, and a low-residue diet. The person should be taught how to deep breathe, cough, and turn properly to minimize postoperative pulmonary complications. Leg exercises should be taught to avoid thrombophlebitis. A general description of what may be expected after surgery should be given. The person's fluid, electrolyte, and nutritional status should be optimum. If the individual has renal problems such as urinary retention or urinary obstruc-

TABLE 50-3 Patient Teaching Guide for Prostate Cancer Work-Up

DIAGNOSIS AND STAGING TESTS FOR PROSTATE CANCER	
In order to determine the size and extent of the spread, or stage, of your prostate cancer, your doctor will perform tests that involve seeing internal parts of the body, measuring the levels of substances in the blood, and examining samples of prostate cells. Specific tests are described in the chart below.	
Visualizations:	
Chest x-ray	To determine whether cancer has spread to the lungs
Lymphangiogram	Another x-ray that makes use of a special dye to determine whether the cancer has spread to the lymph nodes
Bone scan	A picture that shows whether cancer has spread to the bone
Transrectal ultrasonography	A picture that shows sound waves, made by an instrument inserted into the rectum, as they echo from the prostate and nearby structures
Computerized tomography (CT)	A picture produced by a computer from x-rays, showing the prostate and nearby structures
Intravenus pyelogram (IVP)	An x-ray of the kidneys, ureter, and bladder that is taken after the patient is injected with a special dye
Magnetic resonance imaging (MRI)	A picture produced by a computer and a high-powered magnet that shows the prostate and nearby structures
Blood Tests:	
Prostatic acid phosphatase (PAP)	A blood substance that rises above normal in many patients when the prostate cancer has spread
Prostate specific antigen (PSA)	A blood substance that rises in cases of prostate cancer and other prostate disease
Tissue Samples:	
Prostate biopsy	The removal and examination under a microscope of a small sample of a prostate tumor to determine whether it contains cancer cells
Pelvic node dissection (also called lymphadenectomy)	This procedure is used to help identify the stage of prostate cancer; the procedure is typically done during surgery for removal of the prostate

Source: Adapted from ICI Pharma: Prostate cancer, what it is and how it is treated, Wilmington, DL: ICI Americas, 1990.

tion, insertion of an indwelling urinary catheter may be necessary. Because the average age of the person diagnosed with prostate cancer is over 50, other co-existing diseases such as hypertension, cardiovascular disease, diabetes, and pulmonary disease may be present. Concurrent drug therapy for the coexisting diseases should not be overlooked.

Postoperative nursing care

Radical prostatectomy The person who has had a radical prostatectomy usually returns from surgery with a three-way indwelling urethral catheter. Monitoring the type and amount of urinary output and maintaining catheter patency are major nursing responsibilities. During the first 24 hours after surgery, frank bleeding rarely occurs. Hematuria is common during the first 3–4 days after surgery. The nurse must be alert for signs and symptoms of hemorrhage and shock. Vital signs need to be monitored accurately and as frequently as indicated by the patient's clinical status. A normal blood pressure reading may be a significant drop for a person with hypertension. Thus, baseline data must be available for assessment. The amount and color of the urinary drainage should be observed.

Bladder irrigation after radical prostatectomy is common. The irrigation can be continuous or intermittent according to the patient's need and the physician's choice. The purpose of irrigation is to avoid clot formation and promote adequate drainage of the bladder. Obstruction of urinary flow must be prevented because it can cause secondary hemorrhage by stretching the coagulated vessels. Catheter obstruction can be caused by kinked tubing, mucus plugs, or blood clots and can lead to uncomfortable bladder distention and painful bladder spasms.

Other nursing responsibilities include preventing infection and maintaining placement of the catheter. Urinary catheter, drainage tubing, and collecting bag must remain as a closed system to avoid urinary tract infection. Catheter care must be carried out diligently using aseptic technique to prevent the instillation of bacteria. Precautions should be taken to prevent accidental removal of the catheter. The individual should be encouraged to refrain from pulling on the catheter. Premature removal of the catheter can interfere with the patient's recovery, and surgical replacement may be required. Taping the drainage tubing to the inner thigh can prevent traction to the bladder and keep the tubing secure. With a radical prostatectomy the urethral catheter serves as a splint for urethral anastomosis, as well as for urinary drainage.

Bladder spasms may occur after prostatectomy. They can be caused by the presence of the urethral catheter or by bladder distention. These spasms have a rapid onset and usually subside in a few minutes. They can be quite painful, and antispasmodics may be required.

The nurse should keep in mind that antispasmodics should not be given to individuals with cardiac problems or glaucoma because these drugs can increase heart rate and intraocular pressure. If antispasmodics are used, stool softeners should be administered concurrently to avoid constipation.

The urethral catheter usually stays in place for 2–3 weeks after radical prostatectomy depending on the person's progress. After the urethral catheter is removed, the patient should be advised to note the amount and frequency of voiding. The person should be informed that his urine may be cloudy for several weeks after surgery and that it will clear up as the wound heals.

There may be some dribbling and urgency for several weeks. For most individuals this is transient and will gradually improve. But urinary incontinence is common after any type of prostate surgery, occurring in up to 15% of patients. Incontinence is often a disturbing problem for the adult and may have several etiologies. In patients with prolonged outlet obstruction, the bladder's detrusor muscle gradually loses function because of the repeated attempt to contract and empty the bladder against the obstruction.[61] Table 50-4 describes various types of urinary incontinence.

In patients with postprostatectomy incontinence, treatment options vary from behavioral techniques to surgery. Promising success rates have been reported by nurses who teach pelvic floor muscle exercises to men with postprostatectomy incontinence, especially among those with sphincteric damage.[61] Pelvic floor muscle exercise programs usually teach patients to contract the muscles on a regular basis: five times per hour, 15 sets of exercises per day. Table 50-5 is a patient teaching guide for strengthening pelvic muscles. Regular contraction of the sphincter muscles leads to strengthening of those muscles, which, alone, can significantly improve incontinence symptoms over time. Some regimens also include visual or auditory feedback. If patients continue to use the exercises permanently, they can resolve postprostatectomy incontinence problems.[61]

TABLE 50-4 Urinary Incontinence

Type	Description
Stress	Leakage of urine during physical activity, usually during an increase in intraabdominal pressure, such as laughing, coughing, or exercising
Urge	Leakage of urine immediately following an initial urge to urinate. The patient cannot "hold it" long enough to get to the bathroom.
Total	Continuous leakage of urine in the absence of any sensation or urge to urinate.
Overflow	Leakage of urine that is intermittent; it occurs when the bladder is so full of urine that leakage from the urethra occurs.
Functional	Leakage of urine that is related only to the patient's inability to get to the bathroom or to other toileting facilities.

Note: Some patients suffer from a combination of the above types of incontinence and do not fall into any one category.

Source: Reilly NJ: Urinary incontinence: New attitudes and treatment options, *Innov Urol Nurs* 3(2):1–13, 1992.

TABLE 50-5 Patient Teaching Tool for Strengthening Exercises

HOW TO FIND THE PELVIC MUSCLE

To find the muscle, imagine you are at a party and the rich food you have just consumed causes you to have gas. The muscle that you use to hold back gas is the one you want to exercise. Some people find this muscle by voluntarily stopping the stream of urine. Another way to find the muscle is by pulling your rectum and urethra up inside.

EXERCISING THE MUSCLE

Begin by emptying your bladder. Then try to relax completely. Tighten this muscle and hold back for a count of 10 for 10 seconds, then relax the muscle completely for a count of 10 for 10 seconds. You should feel a pulling sensation around your rectum.

WHEN TO EXERCISE

Do 10 exercises in the morning, 10 in the afternoon, and 15 at night. Or, you can set your kitchen timer and exercise for 10 minutes, three times a day. Initially, you may not be able to hold this contraction for the complete count of 10. However, you will slowly build to 10-second contractions over time. The muscle may start to tire after six or eight exercises. If this happens, stop and go back to exercising later. If you have a "Bladder Exercise" tape, listen to it twice a day and do what it says.

WHERE TO PRACTICE THESE EXERCISES

These exercises can be practiced anywhere, anytime. Most people seem to prefer exercising lying on their bed or sitting in a chair.

COMMON MISTAKES

Never use your stomach, legs, or buttocks muscles. To find out if you are also contracting your stomach muscles, place your hand on your abdomen while you squeeze your pelvic muscle. If you feel your abdomen move, then you are also using these muscles. In time, you will learn to practice effortlessly. Eventually, work these exercises in as part of your lifestyle—tighten the muscle when you walk, before you sneeze, as you stand up, and on the way to the bathroom.

WHEN WILL I NOTICE A CHANGE?

After 4 to 6 weeks of constant daily exercise you will begin to notice fewer urinary accidents, and after 3 months you will see an even bigger difference.

CAN THESE EXERCISES HURT ME?

NO! These exercises cannot harm you in any way. Most patients find them relaxing and easy. If you get back pain or stomach pain after you exercise, then you are probably trying too hard and using stomach muscles. Go back and find the pelvic muscle, and remember, this exercise should feel easy. If you experience headaches, then you are also tensing your chest and probably holding your breath.

Source: Reilly NJ: Urinary incontinence: New attitudes and treatment options, *Innov Urol Nurs* 3(2):1–15, 1992.

Pharmacologic agents are also used for incontinence problems. Anticholinergic and antispasmodic drugs can help decrease urgency incontinence associated with uninhibited bladder contractions. Alpha-blocker medications are used in combination with pelvic floor muscle exercises to improve stress incontinence. Drugs are not useful with overflow incontinence, but intermittent catheterizations will relieve the problem.[61] For overflow incontinence, timed voiding schedules can also aid in reducing the impact of incontinence on daily activities.

Individuals who have a radical prostatectomy also may have a suprapubic cystotomy catheter inserted to provide additional security against catheter obstruction. It is inserted directly into the bladder and may have some drainage around the tube, even though it is connected to gravity drainage. If the drainage is copious, the position of the tube should be checked for patency and displacement. This catheter may be removed 2–3 days after surgery and a simple dry dressing applied.

Wound care for the person who has had a radical prostatectomy depends on the surgical approach used during surgery. For retropubic prostatectomy, a Penrose-type rubber drain is inserted deep into the incision, advanced gradually, and removed in about 5 days. Because drainage is common, sterile dressing changes should be carried out every 4–8 hours and as needed. Individuals who have had perineal prostatectomy are prone to wound infection because of the location of the incision. About 1–2 days after surgery, the perineal area should be meticulously cleansed and a heat lamp treatment applied to promote healing. To preserve skin integrity, it is advisable to use a T-binder rather than tape to hold the dressing in place integrity. Sitz baths usually begin after the drain is removed. A low-residue diet is ordered to minimize bowel activity. Rectal tubes, rectal thermometers, and enemas should be avoided until the wound is healed.

Sexuality The incidence of sexual impotence following radical prostatectomy is about 90%.[38] The sexual dysfunction is usually caused by damage done during surgery to the nerves and muscular tissue surrounding the prostate capsule. Sexual dysfunction includes the loss of erectile potency and absence of emission and ejaculation. Recently, the insertion of a penile prosthesis has made it possible for some men who are unable to achieve erection to have penile–vaginal intercourse.

It is of utmost importance that the nurse thoroughly assess the individual and his partner regarding their feelings about sexual activities after surgery. A brief sexual assessment may include such questions as:[62] Has being ill interfered with your being a husband? Has your surgery changed the way you see yourself as a man? Has your disability affected your sexual function? Assessment should include learning about the couple's physical and emotional states, what they want to know, and what they need to know.[63] Nursing intervention depends on the person's level of need. The nurse may suggest to the individual alternative ways to achieve sexual gratification such as touching and caressing or masturbation. However, the nurse must recognize that some alternative sexual behaviors may not be acceptable to the individual and/or his significant other for personal or religious reasons. The individual and his partner need to be reminded that there is no right or wrong way to achieve sexual gratification. Only they can determine what is fulfilling for them. Referral to a qualified therapist may be beneficial to those who desire it.

Transurethral resection Transurethral resection (TUR) requires no incision. The tumor is removed transurethrally with a resectoscope. When the patient returns from the operating room, he will have a three-way indwelling urethral catheter inserted in his bladder with continuous irrigation. The purpose of the irrigation is to reduce blood clot formation and promote drainage. The most important nursing responsibilities after TUR are to watch carefully for any hemorrhage and to maintain catheter patency. Catheter care is similar to that described for individuals who have had radical prostatectomy. The urethral catheter is usually removed 3–5 days after surgery, at which time the urine should be clear. After the catheter is removed, the nurse should monitor the person's ability to void and observe any signs of bladder distention. Patients may be unable to void because of urethral edema, which may necessitate reinsertion of the urinary catheter. If the external sphincter has been injured during surgery, the person may experience urinary incontinence. Straining, dysuria, or a decrease in the size of the urinary stream may indicate urethral stricture. The physician should be notified of these symptoms, and the discharge teaching plan should include instructions to report these symptoms.

Nursing care of individuals receiving radiotherapy In recent years the curative potential of radiotherapy for prostatic cancer has been recognized. The incidence of impotence following radiation treatment is about 20%–40%, roughly half that associated with radical prostatectomy, and incontinence rarely occurs.[45,46]

Radiotherapy may be a frightening experience. Occasionally people mistakenly believe that the person receiving external radiation is radioactive and can cause harm to others. Answering questions and correcting any misconceptions is the first step in nursing care planning.

External radiotherapy Some of the common complications of external radiotherapy are cystitis, proctitis, skin reaction, and radiation syndrome.

Cystitis usually occurs during the first 1–3 weeks of therapy and may not subside for 3–4 months.[4] The use of antispasmodics and analgesics can alleviate some of the symptoms. The patient should be encouraged to drink at least 2 quarts of fluid per day.

Proctitis is mainly due to damage of the intestinal lining. Antidiarrheal medication may decrease this symptom. Patients should be on a low-residue diet. The use of steroid enemas or suppositories also may alleviate the symptoms. Acute GI complications include diarrhea in 30%–40% of the patients. Symptoms usually subside in 3–4 months. However, problems requiring surgery occur in 2%–3% of the patients.[4]

Skin reaction is one of the most common acute effects of radiation, although it is much less common now than it was 20 years ago. Radiodermatitis usually begins about 2 weeks after the beginning of treatment and reaches its peak during the fifth or sixth week. Skin reactions include epilation, erythema, and/or dry or wet desquamation. Patients need to be educated about proper skin care to maintain skin integrity. The irradiated area should be kept clean and dry. Direct exposure of the irradiated area to the sun should be avoided, and the skin should not be exposed to extreme heat or cold. Commercial skin creams or lotions should be avoided because some contain metal bases, which can cause further burning. Some of the water-based lotions, such as Aquaphor, may be used with special approval from the radiologist. Treatment of skin side effects differs. The nurse should assess the skin and report changes to the physician. See Chapter 13 for detailed information on care of the person receiving radiotherapy.

Internal radiotherapy Interstitial implants can deliver relatively high radiation doses to the diseased area with minimal damage to the surrounding tissues. Nursing care of the individual with interstitial implants is based on the penetration energy level of the radioactive substance and its half-life.[64] For those few individuals receiving 198Au implants, the length of time the nurse spends with each patient should be determined by a physicist. Nursing care must be done quickly and efficiently, but the patient should not be made to feel abandoned. The allotted time for patient contact does not need to be used all at once. The nurse can divide the time over the entire shift and utilize the principles of distance, time, and shielding to dictate care. Some of the person's feelings of rejection may be alleviated by explaining the need for shortened contact. The person also must be reminded that he is no longer radioactive after the radiation substance has decayed. The person who has had 125I implants should have his urine and bed linen monitored. Nursing care of individuals with radioactive implants is discussed further in Chapter 13.

Nursing care of individuals receiving hormonal therapy Diethylstilbestrol (DES) is the drug of choice for hormonal treatment of prostatic cancer. One major side effect of DES is sodium retention, which can adversely affect a person with cardiovascular disease and may induce pulmonary edema and congestive heart failure. The concurrent use of diuretics may be necessary. Serious hypercalcemia may occur during the initial period of therapy, manifested by polyuria, general weakness, and mental disorientation. Other side effects of DES include nausea, hypertension, feminization, gynecomastia, loss of libido, and impotency. Individuals taking DES are also at higher risk for thromboembolic complications such as pulmonary embolus and strokes. Nurses should be aware of the potential side effects of estrogen therapy and pay special attention to individuals with a history of cardiopulmonary disease.

LHRH agonists are used in hormonal treatment of advanced prostatic cancer. These drugs do not cause gynecomastia. The patient may experience frequent high-intensity hotflashes, decreased libido, and erectile impotency. LHRH agonists do not produce the metabolic side effects of estrogen.[65]

Leuprolide acetate for depot suspension (Lupron Depot) is packaged as a kit with a vial containing lyophilized microspheres, a glass ampule containing a special diluent, a syringe with hypodermic needle, and alcohol swabs. The vial of microspheres is to be reconstituted with 1 ml of the accompanying diluent to form a depot suspension that is given monthly. After reconstitution, the vial should be shaken well to thoroughly disperse the particles and to obtain a uniform suspension, which will appear milky. Saline or sterile water should not be substituted for the diluent that is provided. This solution does not currently contain a preservative. Intramuscular injection sites should be rotated.[66]

Zoladex is given as a monthly subcutaneous injection into the upper abdomen. Figure 50-8 shows directions for injecting Zoladex. The Zoladex "pellet" is delivered into the subcutaneous tissue via a large-gauge needle, and although most patients deny the need for a local anesthetic, lidocaine or ethyl chloride spray can be used to numb the skin before injection.[66]

For patients with hormonally refractive metastatic prostate cancer, ketoconazole has been used combined with orchiectomy, estrogens, or LHRH agonists to achieve total androgen ablation. Because of ketoconazole's short duration of action, it is imperative that the nurse administer this drug on a strict 8-hour schedule. Hepatotoxicity has been reported in about 50% of patients.[67]

Nursing care of individuals undergoing orchiectomy Bilateral orchiectomy, surgical removal of the testes, is another method of hormonal manipulation. Orchiectomy can provoke a high degree of anxiety for many men because of its connotation of castration. Some men mistakenly believe that removal of the testes will leave them with feminine voices and enlarged breasts. Having the testicles removed during adulthood has no impact on masculinity. Discussion of these side effects with patients is critical.

The immediate postorchiectomy nursing care plan includes pain management with analgesics, prevention of wound infection through aseptic care of the incision site, and maintenance of overall physiologic functions.

Nursing care of individuals receiving chemotherapy Disseminated prostatic cancer has demonstrated var-

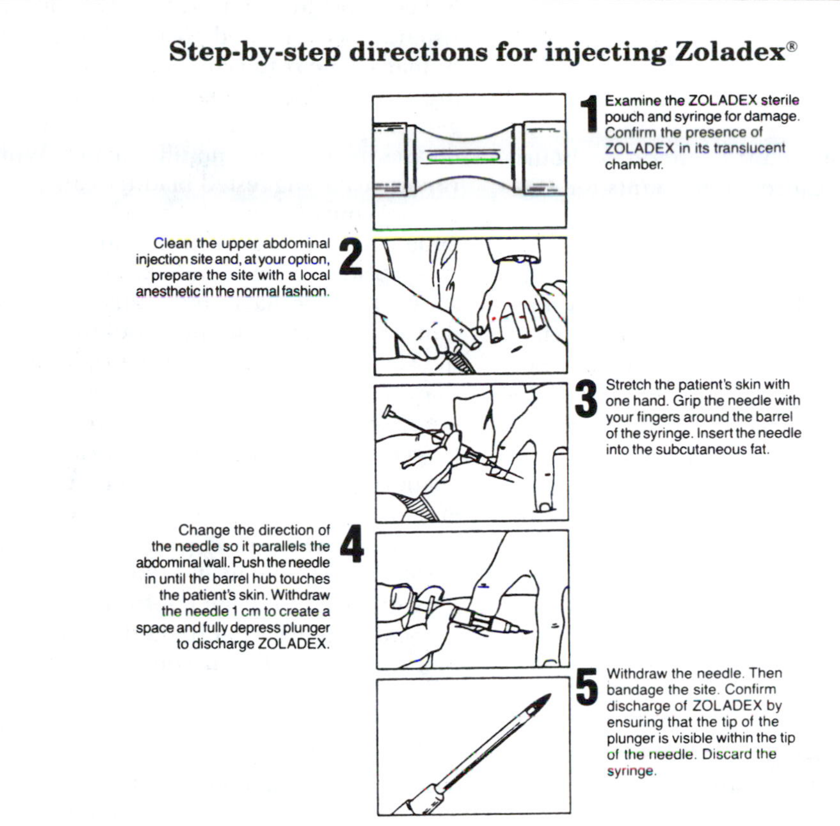

1. Examine the ZOLADEX sterile pouch and syringe for damage. Confirm the presence of ZOLADEX in its translucent chamber.
2. Clean the upper abdominal injection site and, at your option, prepare the site with a local anesthetic in the normal fashion.
3. Stretch the patient's skin with one hand. Grip the needle with your fingers around the barrel of the syringe. Insert the needle into the subcutaneous fat.
4. Change the direction of the needle so it parallels the abdominal wall. Push the needle in until the barrel hub touches the patient's skin. Withdraw the needle 1 cm to create a space and fully depress plunger to discharge ZOLADEX.
5. Withdraw the needle. Then bandage the site. Confirm discharge of ZOLADEX by ensuring that the tip of the plunger is visible within the tip of the needle. Discard the syringe.

FIGURE 50-8 Directions for injecting Zoladex. (Source: Taylor TK: Endocrine therapy for advanced stage D prostate cancer, *Urol Nurs* Sept:22–26, 1991.)

ious responses to cisplatin, cyclophosphamide, methotrexate, doxorubicin, 5-fluorouracil, and vinblastine, used singly and in combination. The nurse should be aware of the major toxicities of these drugs. Nephrotoxicity, severe nausea and vomiting, and ototoxicity are the major side effects of cisplatin. Cyclophosphamide can cause hemorrhagic cystitis and myelosuppression. Methotrexate induces myelosuppression, stomatitis, and nephrotoxicity. Doxorubicin can cause myelosuppression and cardiotoxicity. 5-fluorouracil induces myelosuppression, stomatitis, and diarrhea. Vinblastine causes delayed myelosuppression. Extramustine, an investigational combination of estradiol and nitrogen mustard, has no hematologic toxicity but causes gastrointestinal disturbances such as nausea and vomiting, which can be alleviated by antiemetics.

BLADDER CANCER

Epidemiology

Bladder cancer is the second most common genitourinary cancer after prostate cancer. It accounts for 4%–5% of cancers in the United States.[2]

The four major variables related to bladder cancer incidence are race, gender, age, and geographic location. In the United States the most outstanding epidemiologic feature is the high incidence among white men. The age-adjusted bladder cancer rate in white men is twice the rate for black men.[68] In whites the bladder cancer ratio of men to women is 4:1.[68] Most of these cancers occur in men over 50 years of age. There is a high incidence of squamous cell carcinoma of the bladder in certain areas of the world, notably Egypt. This is linked to the parasite *Schistosoma haemotobium (S. haemotobium).*

Etiology

There are four etiologic hypotheses related to bladder cancer: cigarette smoking, occupational exposure to industrial chemicals, ingestion of other physical agents, and exposure to *S. haemotobium.*

In the United States, only cigarette smoking and occupational exposure to aromatic amines are well-established risk factors.[68] Cigarette smoking was first associated with bladder cancer in 1956.[69] Since that time, most case-controlled studies report a twofold relative risk for cigarette smokers as compared with nonsmokers.[70] However, there are apparent inconsistencies between the case-controlled studies and supporting demographic evidence. For example, the incidence of smoking in women is increasing, while the incidence of bladder cancer in women is decreasing. Certain populations that have been studied for bladder cancer incidence, such as Polynesian men and American blacks, have a very high rate of cigarette smoking and a low incidence of bladder cancer.[68] Despite the inconsistencies, the overwhelming statistical evidence points to cigarette smoking as a prime epidemiologic factor, accounting for as much as 50% of all bladder cancer in American men.[68] The effect of cigarette smoking on bladder tissue seems to be different from that on lung cancer and is likely to be influenced by metabolic and genetic factors.

Among occupational exposure agents, arylamine(s), used in the synthetic textile dye industry, the rubber industry, hair dyes, and as paint pigment, is the class of chemical most strongly related to bladder cancer.[68] Beta-naphthylamine and benzidine are two examples of this chemical class. Occupations with relative risk estimates for bladder cancer of 2 or greater include janitors and cleaners, mechanics, miners, and printers.[70]

Ingestion of other physical agents, such as coffee, alcohol, saccharin, and phenacetin, have been weakly linked to bladder cancer. None of these agents has consistently been related to bladder cancer incidence in humans. The results of studies looking at coffee drinking as a possible etiologic factor in bladder cancer have generally been inconsistent, and the associated increases in risk are generally small.[68] While some recent reports have suggested bladder cancer association with alcohol consumption,[71,72] a 1987 study of 823 men and 2469 age-matched controls showed no association between bladder cancer and alcohol.[70] Animal studies have shown that saccharin may cause bladder cancer in rodents.[68] However, if the dose–incidence curve in rodents is extrapolated to humans, it has been calculated that saccharin users would experience only a 4% increase in bladder cancer occurrence. That level is not detectable by epidemiologic studies. Furthermore, diabetics (who consume a large quantity of artificial sweeteners) do not have a high incidence of bladder cancer.[68] Heavy regular use of phenacetin has also been suggested as an etiologic link; however, the results of various studies have been confusing.[68]

Schistosomiasis is rare in the United States but common in many African countries, especially Egypt. In areas where schistosomiasis is endemic, the incidence of squamous cell carcinoma of the bladder is much higher. In these areas a high percentage of the individuals with squamous cell bladder cancer are found to have *S. haemotobium* ova in the bladder wall.[68]

Pathophysiology

Cellular characteristics

The urinary bladder is lined by transitional epithelium, often called the urothelium. About 90%–95% of bladder tumors in North America are transitional cell carcinomas that arise in the epithelial layer of the bladder. The epithelial layer rests on the basement membrane. Approximately 7% are squamous cell (associated with *S. haemotobium*), and 2% are adenocarcinomas.[73]

Bladder cancer is a multifaceted problem. Major variables in the systems of classification are patterns of growth (in situ versus papillary versus solid), the presence or absence of invasion (the stage), and the degree of differentiation (the grade).[74]

Grading of bladder tumors is commonly done to predict the speed of recurrence and the progression to invasion and metastases. The more well-differentiated bladder tumors (low-grade) generally have a slower growth rate and therefore a better prognosis. Progression is noted in 10%–20% of grade I, 19%–37% of grade II, and 33%–67% of grade III tumors.[75]

Papillary tumors, although they may have a low cytologic grade and be noninvasive, have a propensity for recurrence. Carcinoma in situ is usually multifocal and is associated with high recurrence rate and multicentricity, which necessitate aggressive follow-up after initial diagnosis and treatment.[74]

Progression of disease

Many of these tumors arise on the floor of the bladder and may involve one or both of the ureteral orifices.[73] The growth rate varies depending on the histologic type and grade of the tumor. The most important growth feature is the depth of penetration into the bladder wall.

Some tumors spread rapidly to the regional lymph nodes, which are the pelvic nodes just below the bifurcation of the common iliac arteries. Others grow more slowly and spread directly into pelvic tissues.

Growth occurs inward into the hollow aspect of bladder (in papillary tumors) and outward from the urothelial mucosa to the submucosa and to the detrusor muscle.

Metastasis takes place via direct extension out of the muscle of the bladder into the perivesicle fat (or serosa). Depending on the location of the tumor, it may obstruct the ureters or bladder neck and prostatic urethra. Figure 50-9, which shows the staging of bladder cancer, also depicts the anatomic spread within the bladder. Cancer can also spread by direct extension to involve other adjacent structures, particularly the sigmoid colon, the rectum, and/or the prostate, as well as the uterus and vagina. Hematogenous spread occasionally occurs to the bones, liver, and lungs.[74]

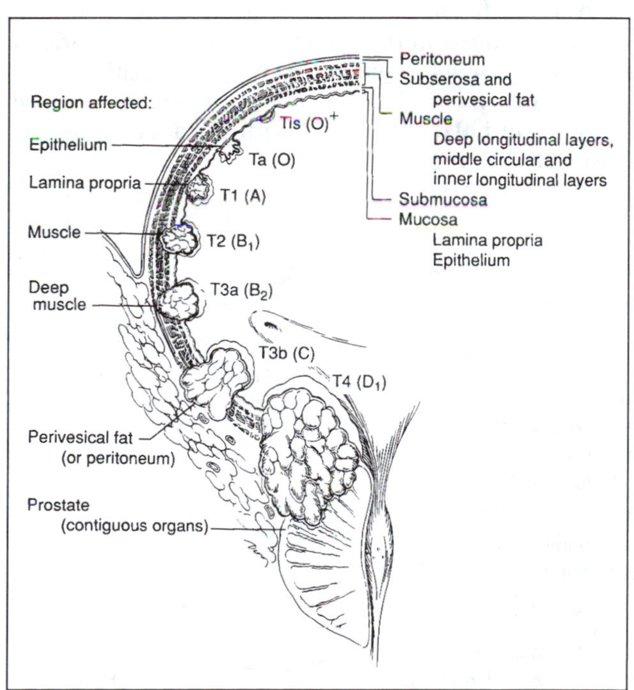

FIGURE 50-9 Staging of bladder cancer. (Source: Caroll PR: Urothelial carcinoma: Cancers of the bladder, ureter, and renal pelvis, in Tanagho EA, McAninch JW (eds), *Smith's General Urology* [13th ed]. Norwalk, CT: Appleton & Lange, 1992, p. 343.)

Clinical Manifestations

Gross hematuria is the most common presenting symptom of bladder cancer. Painless hematuria is usually present through the entire stream of urine. This bleeding is rarely profuse, often microscopic, and usually intermittent.

Another symptom is irritability of the bladder. This manifests itself as dysuria, urinary frequency, and urgency and burning on urination if infection is present.

Symptoms associated with large tumor growth or metastasis also may be present. If the tumor is pushing on the internal urethral orifice, symptoms of bladder neck obstruction may be present including urinary hesitancy and decrease in the force and caliber of the stream. Obstruction of the ureters can cause flank pain and results in hydronephrosis.

Pain in the suprapubic region, rectum, or back, as well as symptoms of lung, bone, or liver metastasis, occurs occasionally in individuals with advanced disease.

Assessment

Physical examination

There are no early signs of bladder cancer on physical examination. An invasive mass in the trigonal area occasionally may be revealed by rectal examination.

Diagnostic studies

Cytology Exfoliative urinary cytology is a relatively simple diagnostic tool in the assessment of bladder cancer. Many experts recommend the collection of a total voided specimen obtained late in the morning or early afternoon and sent immediately for cytology to reduce the chance of obscuring the results. Bladder washings obtained through saline irrigation of the bladder produce even more reliable results.[76]

Flow cytometry For superficial transitional cell bladder cancer, identification of patients who are at risk of recurrent disease and/or of progression to a higher stage is critical to assessment. Flow cytometry, which is a technique used to examine the DNA content of urine cells, has been useful in providing prognostic information beyond grading and staging. In this technique the interaction of fluorochromes or dyes with DNA causes the emission of light on exposure to high-intensity light (like a laser). Machines are able to analyze large numbers of urine samples, sort the urine cells by size, and indirectly measure the DNA content. This procedure can also be done on biopsy specimens and bladder washings.[77] Aneuploidy, or large numbers of DNA per cell, is an indication of high-grade, high-stage transitional cell tumors.[77]

Excretory urogram (intravenous pyelogram) Excretory urogram (intravenous urogram) should be done prior to cystoscopy to help in evaluating the upper tracts at the same time.[73] Although it is not a conclusive diagnostic tool, excretory urography can help evaluate a suspected bladder tumor by possibly showing the tumor itself or by showing evidence of ureteral obstruction (hydronephrosis). Urethral obstruction also may be demonstrated with excretory urography.

Cystoscopy Although initial diagnosis of bladder cancer is usually made using office cystoscopy and topical anesthesia, definitive evaluation requires general or spinal anesthesia.[76] Cystoscopic examination can serve several purposes: tumor visualization, an opportunity for biopsy, and an opportunity for bimanual examination of the bladder.

Once the tumor is visualized, a deep biopsy specimen is taken from the center of the tumor and its outside border. The goal of these biopsies is to assess the presence or absence of muscle invasion. Multiple biopsy specimens of the rest of the bladder wall, the bladder neck, and the trigone also may be taken to diagnose carcinoma in situ or atypia. Selected mucosal biopsy can also be an effective adjunct to the management of superficial bladder cancer.[74]

The development of the flexible fiberoptic cystoscope has made outpatient cytoscopy easier, reduced the morbidity, and made possible the use of local or regional anesthesia.[76]

Bimanual palpation performed under anesthesia may detect a palpable tumor or induration, which could indicate deep muscle invasion, inflammation of the tumor site, or extension of the tumor into the serosa.

Tumor markers Serum carcinoembryonic antigen (CEA) levels are moderately elevated in 50% of late-stage (T3 and T4) bladder cancer patients.[77] A larger CEA elevation is seen in tumors that are metastasizing.[78]

The expression of blood-group antigens on the surface of bladder cancer cells has proved to be a useful prognostic determinant. Tumors that elaborate A, B, or H antigens are often associated, stage for stage, with a better prognosis than tumors that do not express antigens.[74]

Computerized tomography, ultrasound, magnetic resonance imaging Advocates of using CT scans in staging bladder cancer feel that they aid in defining the extent of the local tumor and in identifying pelvic lymph node metastasis.[73]

Transurethral US has been used to define the local extension and the degree of involvement of the bladder wall.[79] The exact role of both US and CT scanning remains to be determined.[73]

MRI has been successful in distinguishing cancer from the normal bladder wall, as the tumor generates a higher signal intensity.[80] It has also been used to identify the presence of pelvic lymph node involvement.[81]

Classification and Staging

Several attempts have been made to develop a universal staging system for bladder cancer, but the most common systems used in the United States are the Jewett-Strong system (modified by Marshall) and the TNM system developed by the American Joint Committee for Cancer Staging and End Results Reporting.[73] A compilation of these systems is depicted in Figure 50-9 and described in Table 50-6. Table 50-7 describes the distinction between superficial and invasive bladder cancer according to staging systems.

Another factor sometimes considered in treatment but not included in the staging systems is the grade of the tumor, or its degree of cell differentiation. The grades for cancer of the bladder are usually referred to as grade I, II, III, or IV, with IV designating the least well differentiated.

TABLE 50-6 Staging Systems for Bladder Cancer

1946 Jewett-Strong	1952 Jewett	1952 Marshall		1978, TNM Clinical	1978, TNM Pathologic
			No tumor, definitive specimen	T0	P0
		0	Carcinoma in situ	TIS	PIS
A	A		Papillary tumor with invasion	Ta	Pa
		A	Invasion of the lamina propria	T1	P1
B	B1	B1	Superficial muscle invasion	T2	P2
	B2	B2	Deep muscle invasion	T3	P3A
C	C	C	Invasion of perivesical fat		P3B
			Invasion of prostate, vagina, or uterus	T4	P4A
		D1	Fixed to pelvic or abdominal wall		P4B
			Pelvic nodes		N1-3
		D2	Distant metastases		M1
			Nodes above the aortic bifurcation		N4

Source: Lieskovsky G, Ahlering T, Skinner DG: Diagnosis and staging of bladder cancer, in Skinner DG, Lieskovsky G (eds), *Diagnosis and Management of Genitourinary Cancer.* Philadelphia: Saunders, 1988, p. 267.

TABLE 50-7 Staging Descriptors of Superficial and Invasive Bladder Cancer

Extent of Tumor	TNM System	Modified Jewett System
Superficial		
Carcinoma in situ	Tis	O
Noninvasive papillary	Ta	O
Invasion into lamina propria	T1	A
Invasive		
Superficial muscle	T2	B_1
Deep muscle	T3a	B_2
Perivesical fibroadipose tissue	T3b	C
Prostate, uterus, cervix, or vagina	T4a	D_1
Pelvic or abdominal wall	T4b	D

Source: Raghavaan D, Shipley WU, Garnick MB, et al: Biology and management of bladder cancer, *N Eng J Med* 322:1131, 1990.

Treatment

Carcinoma in situ

Transurethral resection, electrocautery followed by intravesicle thiotepa, or radical cystectomy with urinary diversion are three common treatment options for carcinoma in situ of the bladder. Radiotherapy has no proven value in the treatment of carcinoma in situ.[74]

Superficial, low-grade tumors

More than 70% of the patients with bladder cancer present initially with superficial tumors (stages Tis, Ta, and T1).[74] Superficial tumors of the bladder remain in the epithelium and lamina propria. In 80% of these patients, invasive tumors do not develop.[74] Standard treatment of these tumors is transurethral surgery with resection and fulguration (if there are multiple small lesions), laser therapy, or cystectomy. The overall 5-year survival rate of patients with superficial bladder cancer treated with transurethral resection alone is approximately 80%.[74] Because the chance of recurrence is so great, intravesical chemotherapy following surgery has been investigated.

Intravesical treatment Several agents have shown some effectiveness when instilled into the bladder, including thiotepa, mitomycin C, Epodyl (triethylene glycol diglycerol ether, ethoglucid), doxorubicin, VM-26 (teniposide or epipodophyllotoxin), and bacillus Calmette-Guerin (BCG). These agents are typically instilled into the bladder through a urethral catheter for 2 hours weekly for 6 weeks.[82] The most widely used drug for this purpose in the United States has been thiotepa. Dosages vary from 30–60 mg diluted in equal amounts of sterile water. It is generally instilled and retained for 1–2 hours every week for 6–8 weeks and in some instances at monthly intervals for 2 years thereafter. The drug's side effects include severe bladder irritability, myelosuppression, and renal failure if there is reflux.[82]

Mitomycin C also has been used in the treatment of superficial disease. Because it has limited intravesical absorption, myelosuppression is rare, and the major side effects are chemical cystitis and skin reactions from contact with the drug.[82] If, as some believe, the benefits of mitomycin C and thiotepa are comparable, the deciding factor might be the greater expense of using mitomycin C.

The use of intravesical BCG has gained renewed attention and recently demonstrated efficacy. BCG is a live, attenuated culture preparation of the bacillus Calmette-Guerin strain of mycobacterium bovis. Unlike conventional intravesical chemotherapeutic agents that attack tumor cells directly, BCG is a biologic response modifier that is believed to exert its antitumor effect by stimulating various immune responses in the host. While the exact mechanism of action is unknown, it appears that direct contact between tumor cells and BCG is essential.[83] Complete responses of up to 79%, reduction in the rate of relapse, and prolonged disease-free survival have been reported.[74,83–85] This treatment is considered both safe and effective in treating superficial bladder cancer and in reducing transitional cell recurrences. It is considered the most successful adjuvant treatment for superficial recurrent bladder cancer.

A typical regimen begins 1–2 weeks after biopsy or transurethral resection of tumor and is repeated once a week for six treatments. For some patients a single 6-week course of intravesical BCG is not sufficient and an additional 6-week course is given.[85] Other protocols require BCG intravesically weekly for 6 weeks, then every other week times three, again at 6 months, and every 6 months for up to 4 years.[86] Most patients tolerate BCG instillation reasonably well, although side effects are expected as the patient becomes sensitized to the BCG. Side effects include dysuria, frequency of urination, and urgency, which occur 3 or 4 hours after the instillation. Mild hematuria associated with cystitis happens in about 50% of the patients and tends to occur after the third or fourth treatment.[86] Occasional influenzalike symptoms happen in about 25% of patients.[86]

Laser therapy Small superficial bladder tumors have also been treated by laser beams. One of the most useful lasers is the neodymium yttrium-aluminum-garnet laser (Nd:YAG). This outpatient photodynamic therapy can be done through a small cystoscope, without causing bleeding or the stimulation of the obturator nerve, while the patient is under local anesthesia.[82] However, photodynamic therapy can be associated with quite severe side effects, including inflammation of the bladder mucosa, and it is not clear whether it offers substantial advantage over more conventional treatment.[74] Patients with recurrent superficial papillary tumors (Ta), who are at low risk for tumor progression, are good candidates for laser therapy.[82]

Partial (or segmental) cystectomy is advocated by some authorities but only for individuals with diffuse unresectable tumors or tumors that have not responded to intravesical therapy.[82] The success of partial cystectomy is much higher with stage A, grade I or II lesions. The greatest disadvantage of partial cystectomy is a high tumor recurrence rate.

Invasive tumors

Because of invasion of the bladder muscle, high-stage, high-grade tumors have dramatically altered prognoses. High-stage tumors are generally described as stages T2 to T4 or B1 to D1. Common treatment options for these bladder tumors include definitive irradiation (that is, radiation alone with the intent to cure), radical cystectomy with urinary diversion with or without pelvic lymph node dissection, or a combination of preoperative irradiation followed by surgical excision.[97] From the available data, it is clear that the conventional treatment of muscle-invasive bladder cancer offers a 5-year survival rate of only 50% or less, whatever therapy is used.[74]

Definitive radiotherapy Historically, definitive radiotherapy involved approximately 60 Gy delivered to the pelvis in 7–8 weeks, along with 50 Gy delivered to the pelvic lymph nodes. There has been controversy about the effectiveness of this treatment. In comparing several studies of radiotherapy versus cystectomy versus radiotherapy plus cystectomy, it appears that in stage T2 (B1) and T3 (B2, C) the 5-year survival for radiotherapy was 20%–58% and for cystectomy was 16%–88%.[74] Some recent studies contend that radiotherapy can produce results comparable to surgery if there are certain prognostic factors present: the absence of ureteral obstruction, a complete transurethral resection, and a papillary rather than a sessile lesion; with the use of "salvage cystectomy" for those cancers that have local recurrence.[74] The use of radiotherapy with salvage cystectomy for failures of local treatment has improved survival rates for radiotherapy.[74]

Several retrospective studies on definitive radiotherapy demonstrate clinically useful information. First, fewer than half the treated patients will have a complete response to conventional external beam radiation, and, second, only one-third to two-fifths will have permanent control of their local bladder tumor.[87] Those who argue against definitive radiotherapy emphasize that to achieve comparable survival rates, those with local treatment failure must be treated with cystectomy anyway and that radical surgery following radiation therapy to the surgical area poses greater risk of morbidity.

While radiation therapy does not appear to offer all the advantages of the surgical approach, study of radiation treatment is important. Medical or tumor-related factors may prevent some patients from being eligible for chemotherapeutic or surgical intervention. For these patients, definitive radiotherapy is an option that may eradicate disease in some.[88]

There has been considerable debate about preoperative radiotherapy as an adjunct to cystectomy for invasive bladder cancer. In comparing the results of radical cystectomy versus radiotherapy plus cystectomy, most studies have failed to demonstrate a statistically significant survival benefit from such combined treatment.[74]

Primary chemotherapy In primary chemotherapy, cytotoxic drugs are given as the first step of treatment, followed by radiotherapy, cystectomy, or both. It is currently an investigative approach for invasive (T2 to T4) transitional cell carcinoma of the bladder, and it is not a substitute for definitive surgery.[89] An initial transurethral resection of the tumor is done to obtain tissue for adequate staging, followed by a minimum of two courses of chemotherapy. Definitive surgery after chemotherapy includes partial or total cystectomy or in some cases radiotherapy. This treatment approach is a reasonable therapeutic option for selected patients, particularly those who have a strong desire to retain their bladders.[89]

Radical cystectomy The term *radical cystectomy* in men is usually synonymous with prostatocystectomy. The procedure includes excision of the bladder with the pericystic fat, the attached peritoneum, and the entire prostate and seminal vesicles (Figure 50-10).

In women, radical cystectomy includes removal of the bladder and entire urethra, the uterus, ovaries, fallopian tubes, and the anterior wall of the vagina (Figure 50-11).

Including pelvic lymphadenectomy with this surgery is controversial. The evidence that it improves survival is sparse and inconclusive. Some surgeons have demonstrated that adding a meticulous lymph node dissection has resulted in a low incidence of pelvic recurrence compared with results for simple total cystectomy without dissection or preoperative radiation therapy.[87]

Complications of this surgical procedure include uretero-cutaneous fistula, wound dehiscence, partial small bowel obstruction, wound infection, and small bowel fistula.

Cystectomy with urinary diversion Until the 1980s, nearly all men who underwent radical cystectomy became impotent. To help patients overcome the problem of impotence after pelvic surgery, Walsh[41] described the neurovascular anatomy of the bladder and prostate more clearly and developed a surgical approach in which nerves crucial to the mechanisms of penile erection are spared. Although the majority of published experience relates to the management of prostate cancer, the removal of bladder cancer has also been performed in this way, and erectile potency has been preserved in 80% of young men.[41,74]

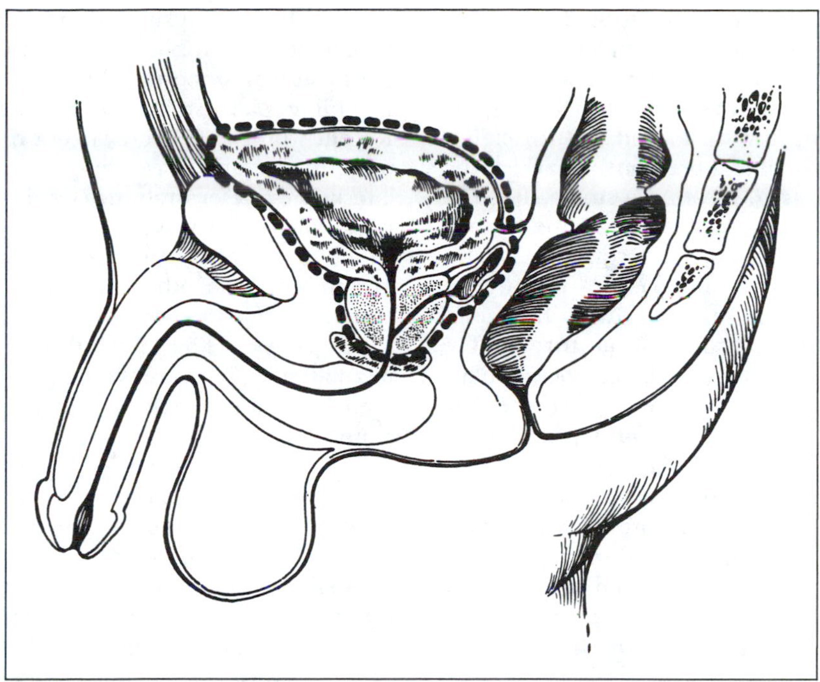

FIGURE 50-10 Surgical boundaries of radical cystectomy in a man. The specimen includes bladder, the prostate, and the seminal vesicles. (Source: Swanson D: Cancer of the bladder and prostate. The impact of therapy on sexual function, in von Eschenbach AC, Rodriguez D, (eds), *Sexual Rehabilitation of the Urologic Cancer Patient.* Boston: Hall, 1981, p. 102.)

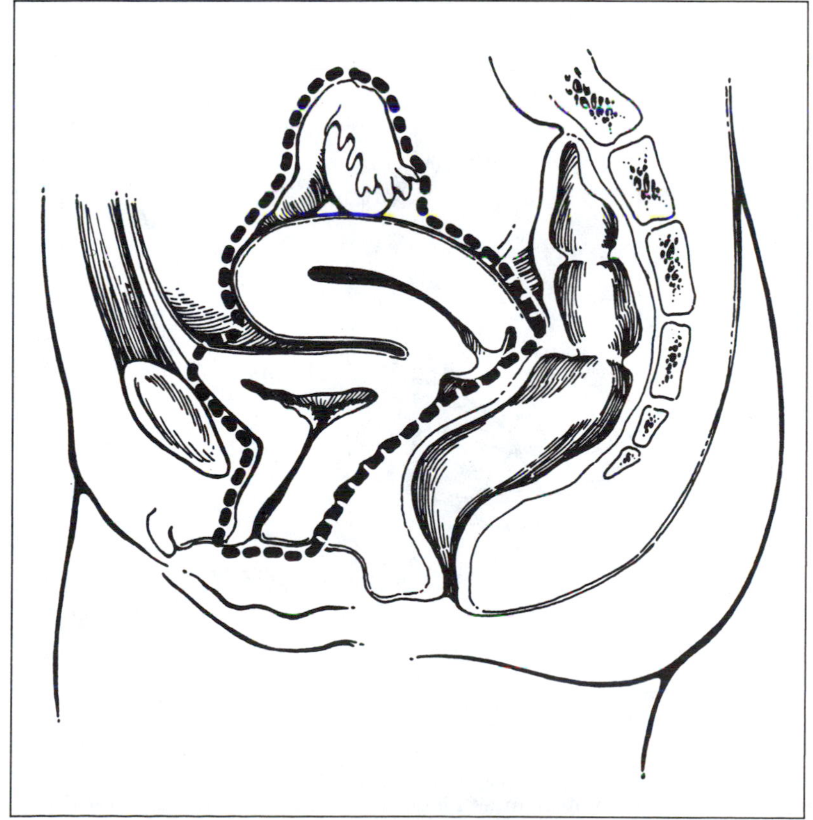

FIGURE 50-11 Surgical boundaries of a radical cystectomy in a woman. The specimen includes the bladder and entire urethra, uterus, ovaries, fallopian tubes, and the anterior wall of the vagina. (Source: Swanson D: Cancer of the bladder and prostate. The impact of therapy on sexual function, in von Eschenbach AC, Rodriguez D (eds), *Sexual Rehabilitation of the Urologic Cancer Patient.* Boston: Hall, 1981, p. 103.)

Ileal conduit Since the early 1950s the Bricker ileal conduit has been a popular method of diverting urinary flow in the absence of bladder function. This procedure involves isolating a piece of terminal ileum, closing the proximal end, bringing the distal end out through a hole in the abdominal wall at a previously marked site, and suturing it to the skin, creating a stoma. It is important for proper functioning that the segment reach from the retroperitoneum to the skin comfortably and without tension on the distal (stoma) end.[86] The ureters are implanted into the ileal segment, urine flows into the conduit, and peristalsis propels it out through the stoma (Figure 50-12). Urinary stents may occasionally be threaded into the ureters to allow for free-flowing urine in the early postoperative period. Urinary stents are usually left in place for 7–10 days, but may be left in longer at the physician's discretion.[86] Other portions of the bowel also have been used to divert the urine. Portions of the sigmoid colon are used infrequently as conduits in urinary diversions associated with bladder cancer. Construction of any of these conduits necessitates that the person wear an external collection appliance.

Complications are related to stoma construction and placement and to the possibility of long-term kidney damage. Stomas placed in skin creases, scars, or bony prominences have difficulty with appliance adherence. Stomas that are flush with the skin and recessed have problems with appliance fit. Other complications include stomal stenosis, which has a host of sequelae, including pain, stones, and potential pyelonephritis. Recent studies have indicated a high incidence of ureteral reflux and ascending infection that results in late kidney deterioration. Despite the long-term complications, the Bricker ileal conduit is still the most widely used form of urinary diversion and the standard to which all other diverting procedures must be compared.[90]

Loop stoma The Turnbull loop stoma has been used in an attempt to decrease the problems of stoma placement and stomal stenosis. In this technique,[91] an ileal conduit is constructed, and both the distal and proximal ends are sutured closed. A loop of the conduit is pulled out through the abdominal wall, and the ureters are implanted into the proximal portion (Figure 50-13). The loop is anchored to the skin, and the conduit is opened, creating a mucous fistula at the distal end of the conduit and a urinary diversion at the proximal end. The major complication is parastomal hernia.

Ureterosigmoidostomy Ureterosigmoidostomy involves implanting the ureters into the sigmoid colon utilizing an antirefluxing anastomosis. The urine is then excreted through the rectum. Before Bricker described the ileal conduit in 1950, the ureterosigmoidostomy was the most popular form of urinary diversion. The early

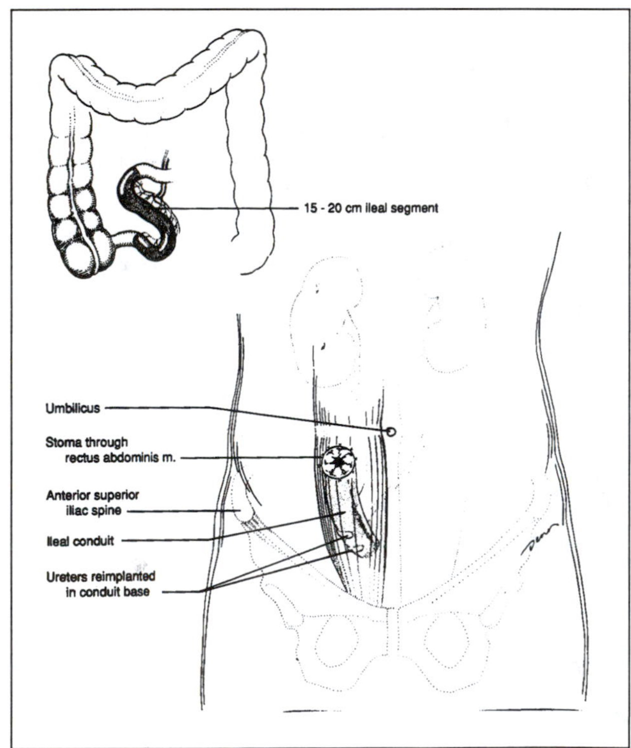

FIGURE 50-12 Ileal conduit. (Source: Caroll PR, Barbours S: Urinary diversion and bladder substitution, in Tanagho EA, McAninch JW (eds), *Smith's General Urology* [13th ed]. Norwalk, CT: Appleton & Lange, 1992, p. 427.)

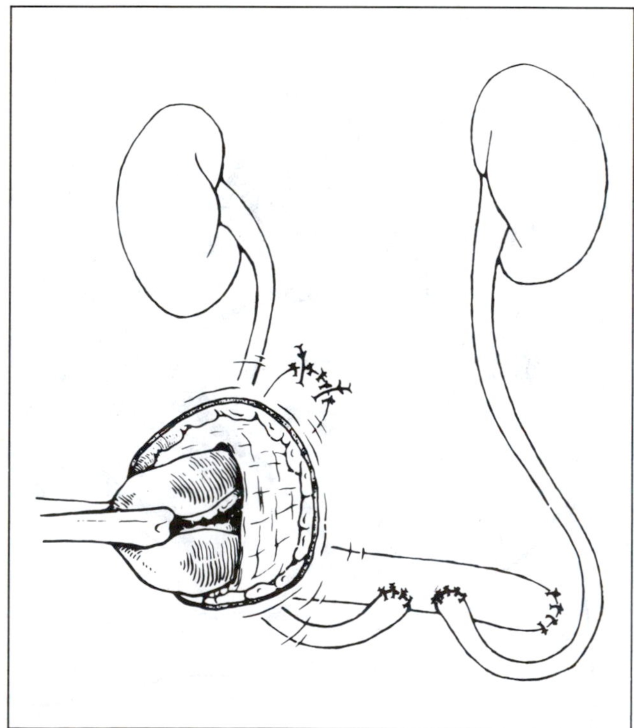

FIGURE 50-13 A Turnbull loop is pulled through an abdominal wall defect using a small Penrose drain as a tractor. (Source: Bloom DA, Lieskovsky G, Rainwater G, et al: The Turnbull loop stoma, *J Urol* 129:716, 1983.)

and late complications include metabolic acidosis because of the absorptive quality of the sigmoid colon, potassium depletion, anastomotic stenosis, and ascending infection, particularly in individuals with impaired renal function. This surgical procedure is rare today.

Continent urinary diversion In recent years there has been a surge of enthusiasm for continent urinary diversions. Continent urinary diversions were created in an attempt to better substitute for the functions of the lower urinary tract. Ideally, voiding of urine should be under voluntary control at convenient intervals, and the upper renal tract should be protected from both obstruction and urine reflux. Continent diversions offer the patient opportunity for control of voiding and urinary reflux by the creation of low-pressure reservoirs and the use of one-way valves.[90]

There are several types of continent urinary diversions currently being performed. They differ, largely, in the portion of intestine used to create the pouch; the presence, absence, and/or number of valves; and the location of the urinary outlet. Nursing care for each type of diversion differs.[92]

Kock pouch Figure 50-14 illustrates a type of continent reservoir technique originated by Nils Kock in Sweden.[93] Urinary diversion through a continent ileal reservoir provides an intraabdominal pouch for storage of urine and two nipple valves that maintain continence and prevent ureteral reflux. One procedure for constructing the urinary pouch describes using a 60–70cm-segment of ileum, isolated approximately 50 cm from the ileocecal valve. The ureters are anastomosed to a short segment of the ileum that leads into an ileal nipple, which prevents reflux of the urine to the kidneys. Proximal to this segment, two 22-cm segments are used to create the reservoir pouch itself. The remaining segment is used for the continence nipple and the stoma.[94]

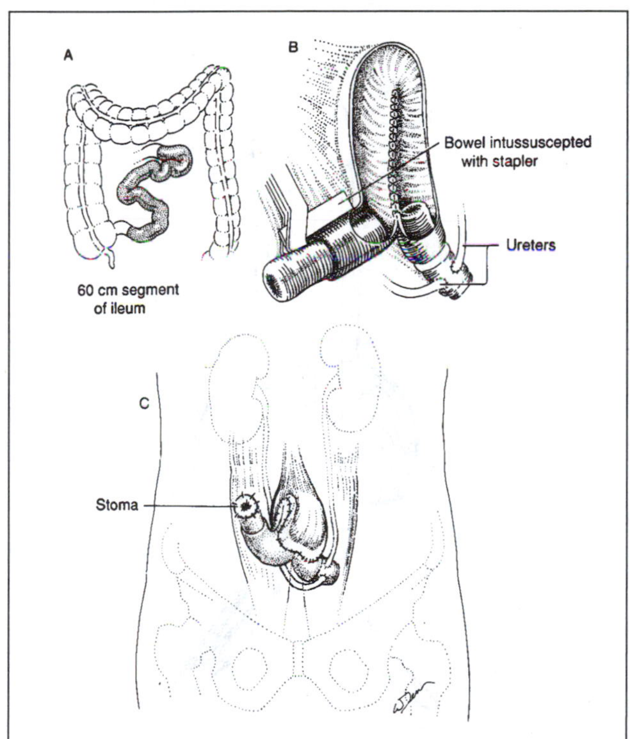

FIGURE 50-14 Kock Pouch urinary reservoir. (A) 60 cm of small intestine selected. (B) Afferent (nonrefluxing) limb or ureteral reimplantation and efferent limb for stoma fashioned using stapling devices. (C) Completed reservoir. (Source: Caroll PR, Barbour S: Urinary diversion and bladder substitution, in Tanagho EA, McAninch JW (eds), *Smith's General Urology* [13th ed]. Norwalk, CT: Appleton & Lange, 1992, p. 432.)

The outlet for the reservoir may be brought to the skin, urethra, and/or rectum. Male patients are the only candidates for a Kock to the urethra because of the limitations of the female urologic anatomy. Kock pouches to the rectum have been utilized in other countries with success.[93]

When the lengthy surgical procedure is almost complete, a number 30 Medena tube is passed into the pouch and positioned so that the drainage holes are several centimeters beyond the efferent nipple. This tube is sutured in place to secure it for 3 weeks. A 1-inch Penrose drain is passed through a separate stab incision and sutured to the muscle or peritoneum to keep it from moving into the pouch.

To prevent mucus obstruction postoperatively, the Medena tube should be irrigated every 4 hours or more with 30–60 ml of normal saline. Three weeks following surgery the reservoir is checked radiographically for any signs of extravasation. If the reservoir is patent the Medena tube is removed and the patient is taught self-catheterization technique, beginning at 2- to 3-hour intervals.

Late complications usually involve problems with continence or catheterization, such as urinary leakage at the stoma, difficult catheterization, electrolyte abnormalities, pyelonephritis, hydronephrosis, and stone formation.

Indiana reservoir The Indiana reservoir is another type of continent diversion. It is constructed from the cecum, the ascending colon, the ileocecal valve, and the terminal ileum. The colon is opened for its entire length in order to eliminate the normal peristaltic motion of the intestine and to create the pouch. The ureters are tunneled into the wall of the bowel. The ileocecal valve and the terminal ileum are fashioned into a structure that serves as a natural continence mechanism, preventing the outflow of urine.[95] The creation of an Indiana reservoir is technically less difficult than the Kock pouch because it does not require the creation of nipple valves from bowel.[96]

Other continent urinary reservoirs There are many other reservoirs being constructed that are modifications of the Indiana reservoir. Some of these modifications include the Mainz pouch (right colon, cecum, and adjacent ileum) and the Florida pouch (right colon, distal ileum, ileocecal valve). These reservoirs differ

TABLE 50-8 Continent Urinary Diversions

	Cutaneous Kock Reservoir	Kock Reservoir to Urethra	Indiana Reservoir
Structure	Ileum	Ileum	Ileum, ileocecal valve, cecum, ascending colon
Valves	Two	One	Ileocecal
Construction	Intussuspeted and stapled	Intussuspeted and stapled	Ileocecal
Advantages	Continence; prevents ureteral reflux	Continence and natural voiding through urethra	Continence; prevents uretheral reflux

from the Kock pouch in that they use different segments of the bowel to construct the pouch and to fashion the continent valves.[90] Table 50-8 illustrates the differences in construction of the pouches.

The Camey procedure is a technique of bladder substitution that uses a 40-cm segment of the ileum that is anastomosed directly to the urethra and to the ureters above the iliac vessels.[97]

Sexuality A radical cystectomy with urinary diversion, performed in the traditional manner, particularly if accompanied by a lymphadenectomy, can affect many aspects of sexual functioning. The etiology of physiologic sexual dysfunction in men is similar to that associated with treatment for prostatic cancer. In addition, the psychologic impact of a stoma and external appliance may contribute to changes in body image and libido.[98]

Erectile impotence that results after radical cystectomy (or radical prostatectomy) may be helped by the insertion of a penile prosthesis. Three categories of devices are currently used. The Jonas prosthesis is an example of a malleable, semirigid, plastic rod that is inserted into the bodies of the corpora cavernosa (Figure 50-15). The result is a permanent semierection that is not painful and does not interfere with daily activities.

The Scott prosthesis, an example of various types of inflatable prostheses (Figure 50-16), makes it possible to control erectile function. When the man wishes to have an erection, he squeezes and repeatedly releases the pump bulb in the scrotum to pump fluid from the reservoir into both of the penile cylinders until an erection is achieved. To deflate the erection, finger pressure is exerted on the valve that holds the fluid under pressure.[99] A third and the newest type of prosthesis consists of a self-contained inflatable cylinder.[100]

In women, removal of the ovaries and uterus will result in sexuality changes similar to those following hysterectomy and oophorectomy for gynecologic malignancies. Psychologic problems may occur as a result of the external urinary stoma and/or perceived losses related to hysterectomy and oophorectomy or may result from hormonal changes that occur as a result of surgery. A more direct physiologic effect, however, involves removal of the anterior wall of the vagina. The vagina is closed after surgery and therefore retains its original shape. However, if more than the anterior third of the vaginal wall is removed, the diameter of the introitus and the vaginal barrel can be severely compromised, and intercourse may be restricted. In addition, because of its close proximity to the urethral meatus, the clitoris may be injured or have compromised function because of scarring and fibrosis after surgery.[98] The physiologic changes can result in an alteration in sensation and potential for orgasm and impairment of the ability to permit insertion of the penis into the vagina.

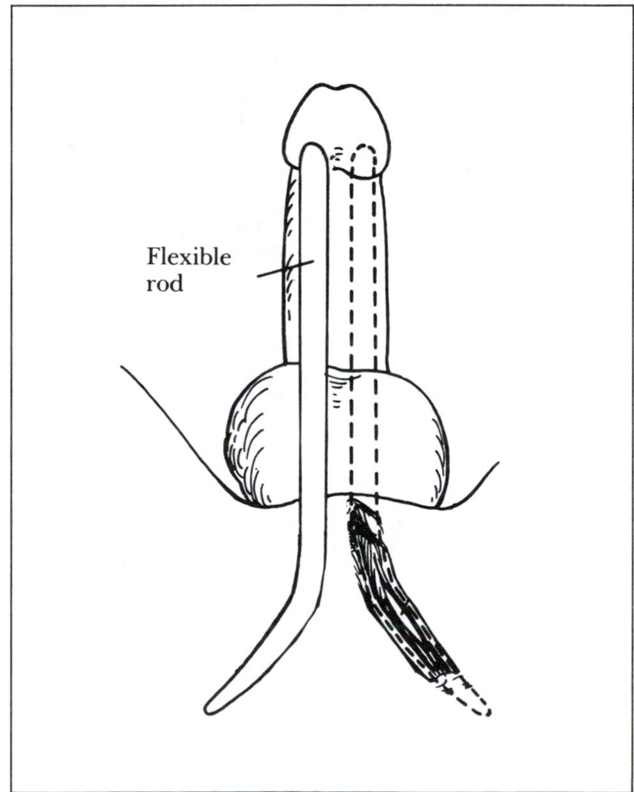

FIGURE 50-15 Penile prosthesis. Semirigid prosthesis consisting of flexible rods. (Source: Adapted from Luckmann J, Sorenson K: *Medical-Surgical Nursing—A Psychophysiologic Approach.* Philadelphia: Saunders, 1978, p. 1843.)

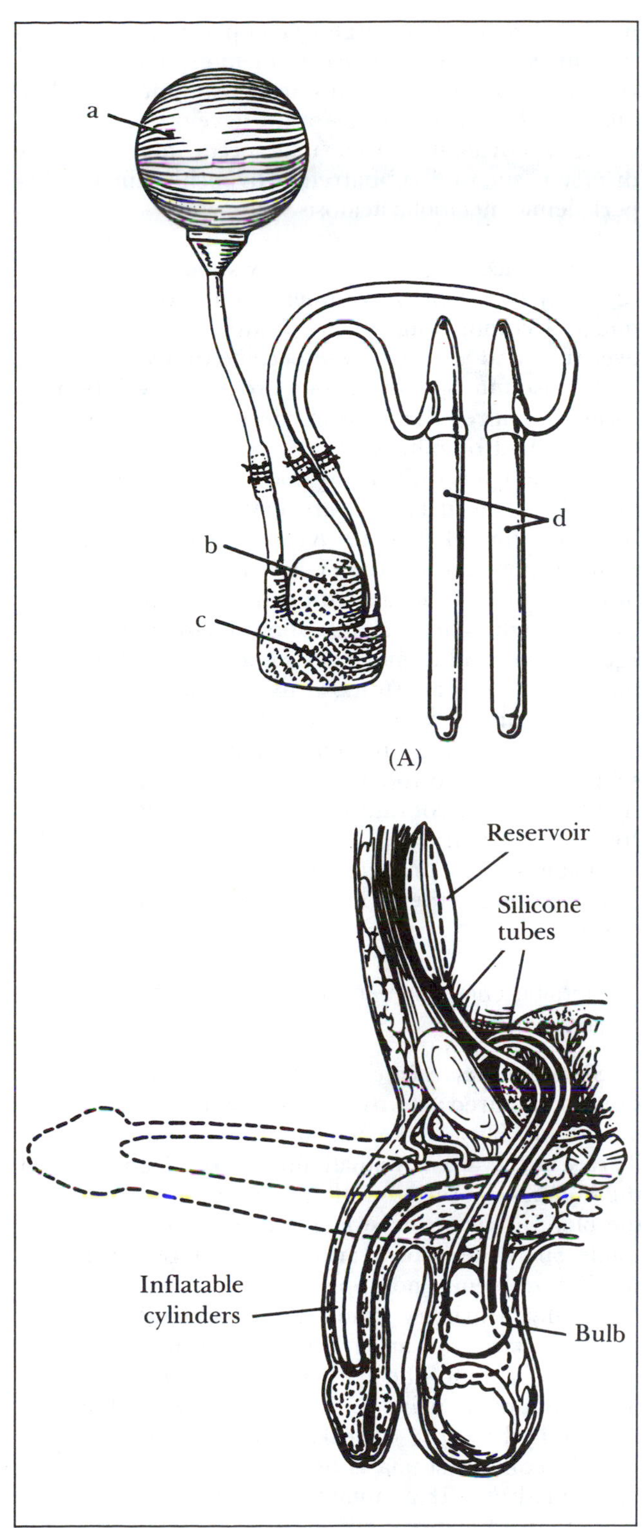

FIGURE 50-16 Inflatable penile prosthesis. (A) The apparatus: (a) spherical reservoir, (b) pump, (c) release valve, and (d) penile cylinders. (B) Prosthesis in place. (Source: Adapted from Scott FB, Kantzavelos D: Erectile impotence after urologic cancer surgery treated with the inflatable penile prosthesis, in von Eschenbach AC, Rodriguez D (eds), *Sexual Rehabilitation of the Urologic Cancer Patient.* Boston: Hall, 1981, p. 243.)

Advanced bladder cancer

In spite of improvements in the diagnosis and treatment of bladder cancer, 50% of individuals with high-stage, high-grade tumors will eventually relapse.[101] Because by then it is a systemic disease, attempts have been made to treat it with chemotherapy but with limited success. Complete responses have been seen in 40%–50% of patients, with a 1-year median duration of response.[101] Single agents and combinations have been attempted. Single agents that have been used in bladder cancer include doxorubicin, bleomycin, methotrexate, cisplatin, and vinblastine. A review of the results of various studies indicates that, in general, single agents produce only partial responses of short duration and that cisplatin and methotrexate have demonstrated significant activity.[101]

The highest response rates documented have been observed with combination regimens that include cisplatin, methotrexate, and vinblastine, with or without doxorubicin.[74] These have been called the CMV or M-VAC regimens. The M-VAC regimen has produced frequent and lasting remissions in patients with invasive and/or metastatic bladder cancer.[76] There is a suggestion that intensive combination chemotherapy that includes cisplatin produces a higher complete response rate than single-agent chemotherapy.

Surgical treatment is seldom used to palliate symptoms of advanced bladder cancer. An individual with severe irritative symptoms due to a bladder tumor occasionally may have an improved quality of life if urinary diversion alone is performed.[101]

Radiotherapy can improve the problem of hemorrhage in the person with advanced bladder cancer and certainly plays an important role in treating bony metastases. But local irritative symptoms can be made worse by radiotherapy.

Results and Prognosis

The American Cancer Society reports 5-year survival rates (adjusted for normal life expectancy) to vary between American whites and blacks (Table 50-9).[2]

TABLE 50-9 Approximate 5-year Survival Rates for Bladder Cancer

Stage	Whites (%)	Blacks (%)
Localized	88	80
Disseminated	41	25
All stages	79	59

Source: Boring CC, Squires TS, Tong T: Cancer statistics, 1992, *CA* 42:19–45, 1992.

Nursing Care of Individuals with Bladder Cancer

Preoperative nursing care

When a diagnosis of bladder cancer has been confirmed and the treatment of choice includes urinary diversion, the type of diversion best suited for the individual must be chosen. The decision is based on each person's needs, anatomy, history, and prognosis. Most urinary diversions that will utilize a segment of the bowel and require an external stoma for the excretion of urine have similar preoperative nursing considerations.

A low-residue diet is given 2 days before surgery, followed by a clear liquid diet on the day before surgery. Bowel preparation using antibiotics, cathartics, and low-residue and liquid diets is necessary as before any intestinal bowel surgery.

Emotional support is extremely important. The procedure to be performed should be explained to the person. It is important if possible to involve another family member or significant other. If indicated, the nurse can arrange for a preoperative visit by someone who has had similar surgery and has adjusted well.

The selection of a stoma site is an important preoperative consideration; the type of urinary diversion to be performed will dictate to some extent the stoma site selected. Any diversion that requires the wearing of an external appliance for the collection of urine must have an adequate surface for the adherence of the appliance.

Ideally, the stoma site is selected and marked before surgery. It is of utmost importance that an appropriate site be chosen only after discussing with the person his or her personal habits pertaining to work and recreational activities. The abdomen is examined and the individual observed while standing, sitting, and reclining. This is done to find an area at least 3 inches in diameter that is free of wrinkles and slightly convex. The site chosen should be visible to the individual and away from bony prominences, old scars or creases, and belt lines.

The Kock pouch, a continent ileal reservoir, needs no external collecting device, but the stoma must be placed for easy catheterization access by the person.

There are several methods of marking the site selected. After the site is cleansed with alcohol, an insoluble dye such as gentian violet or methylene blue can be applied subdermally, or the dye can be tattooed into the midpoint of the selected site. Any method of marking the site that will remain visible after the surgical scrub is acceptable.

General postoperative care

Postoperative care will vary depending on the method of urinary diversion or bladder substitution. As with all patients who have undergone major abdominal surgery, early ambulation, use of elastic stockings, and incentive spirometry may be used to prevent pulmonary emboli or respiratory complications. Nasogastric tubes are left in place until intestinal peristalsis resumes. Serum electrolytes and creatinine should be monitored postoperatively for the development of metabolic abnormalities that may occur after urinary diversion, such as hyponatremia, hypochloremia, or hyperkalemic metabolic acidosis.[97]

Continent urinary reservoirs and bladder substitutes produce much mucus. They should be irrigated regularly in the early postoperative period to prevent mucus accumulation. Mucus production will decrease over time and irrigation will become unnecessary.

Ultrasound or intravenous urography will be performed on a regular basis to check the upper urinary tract for hydronephrosis.[97]

Unlike a fecal diversion that is subject to an adynamic ileus, the urinary diversion should produce urine from the time of surgery. As mentioned in the treatment section, the continent ileal reservoir will be intubated with a Medena silastic catheter, which has been sutured to the skin line and connected to gravity drainage. An ileoconduit may have stents threaded through the ureteral ileo anastomosis to provide for adequate urinary drainage while the anastomosis heals. If ureteral stents have been placed, they are usually removed sometime after postoperative day 5. The urinary flow should be rather continuous, and, in the case of an ileal conduit, a urinary appliance is needed to contain the drainage and to provide for accurate measurement. The appliance is then connected to the bedside gravity drainage.

Nursing care following urinary diversion with an ileal conduit

Stoma characteristics The intestinal stomal tissue can be compared with the mucosal lining of the mouth. The stoma may bleed when rubbed because of the capillaries in the area. A small amount of bleeding from the stoma is not serious, but it must be determined that the blood is from the stoma and not from the urine. Table 50-10 describes various stoma types and their specific problems and appliances.

Ideally, a urinary stoma should protrude one-half to three-quarters of an inch above the skin to allow the urine to drain into the aperture of an appliance. Flush stomas allow the urine to drain at skin level. This frequently is the cause of leakage and skin breakdown. The ileoconduit stoma is usually placed in the lower right quadrant. If a suitable area is not available to support an appliance there, it can be placed on the right side (within the confines of the rectus muscle to support the stoma).

Viability of the stoma is assessed by its color. This should be checked regularly, especially in the early postoperative period. Normal color of the stoma is deep pink to dark red. A dusky appearance ranging from purple to black may develop if circulation is seriously impaired. The appearance of a necrotic stoma may occur immediately after surgery or as late as 5–7 days

TABLE 50-10 Stoma Types and Their Specific Problems and Appliances

Stoma Type	Appliance Needed	Problems Seen
Nipple or bud	Any pouch	Minimal
Flush	May need convex skin barrier with belt	Skin irritation and insecurity Inability to see stoma when applying the pouch Occlusion of the stoma by the pouch Decreased wearing time causing higher costs
Retracted	Rigid faceplate or convex skin barrier with belt	As above
Prolapsed	Flexible skin barrier so as to not constrict base of stoma	Ischemia or erosion of exposed bowel

Source: Carroll MD, Barbour S: Urinary diversion and bladder substitution, in Tanagho EA, McAninch JW (eds), *Smith's General Urology* (13th ed), Norwalk, CT: Appleton & Lange, 1992, p. 436.

after surgery.[102] The dusky appearance of the stoma immediately after surgery may change in a few hours and appear viable. Sustained color change of the stoma should be reported to the surgeon.

A necrotic stoma may develop from abdominal distention causing tension on the mesentery, from twisting of the conduit at the time of surgery, or from arterial or venous insufficiency.[91] To determine the depth of the necrosis, a clear test tube can be inserted into the stoma with the use of a small flashlight directed into the tube. The viable bowel will transilluminate the level of the necrosis. If the tissue at skin level is viable, surgical revision may be unnecessary. However, if necrotic, the tissue will slough, leaving a flush, retracted, or stenotic stoma. This leads to difficult management problems.

Stoma edema is normal in the early postoperative period as a result of surgical manipulation. This should not interfere with stoma functioning, but a larger opening will need to be cut in the appliance to prevent pressure or constriction of the stoma. Most stomas continue to shrink down over the next several months, and some will continue to decrease in size slightly for a year. Teaching the individual to continue to measure the stoma with a weekly change of appliance should alleviate the problem of the person wearing an appliance with an aperture too large for the stoma. The stoma needs only a space of one-eighth to one-sixteenth of an inch to allow for expansion during peristalsis.

Mucus production The intestine normally produces mucus, and mucus will be present in all diversions using segments of the bowel for a conduit or continent pouch. The amount of mucus produced varies with individuals and will cause the urine to appear cloudy. Excessive mucus also may be produced by an inflamed mucosa if infection is present. Some urinary appliances provide larger outlets to assist with the free flow of urine. Increasing fluid intake to 2 liters/day also will help by acting as a natural irrigant.

Pouching a urinary stoma The fairly continuous flow of urine from a conduit requires the person to wear an appliance at all times. In the early postoperative period, any one of the many clear, disposable urinary pouches may be used. The selection of a particular type of pouch may be governed by the availability of supply in the facility or the surgeon's choice.

The skin around the stoma should be clean and thoroughly dry before positioning the appliance over the stoma. The importance of dry skin cannot be emphasized enough. Very small amounts of moisture may cause adherence problems and leakage. The pouch should initially be positioned to the person's side so that it can be attached to bedside drainage without placing stress on the seal. The flange can then be "picture framed" with microporous tape to enhance the seal.

Many of the urinary pouches today are manufactured with an antireflux valve. This is double thickness of the pouch, which prevents the urine from returning to the stoma. If stents are used to maintain patency, it may be necessary to thread them through the antireflux valve. The stoma should be clearly visible through the pouch.

Although not always possible, an effective urinary pouch should adhere at least 3 days. If no leakage occurs, the same pouch can remain adhered to the skin for 10 days. It should then be changed for hygienic reasons and to observe the peristomal area. Table 50-11 describes common stoma problems and their management.

Today there is a constant and ever-changing supply of new appliances. Materials and design are being updated rapidly to provide the consumer with the best protection and easiest care.

Patient teaching for continuing care of a conduit The initial care rendered to the person with a new conduit is extremely important both physiologically and psychologically. Before the individual is able to actively participate in self-care, the nurse or enterostomal therapist can teach by example. Procedures are "talked" through as they are being performed. Applied pouches should remain in place without leakage for 3–5 days. Peristomal skin should remain intact without irritation. This reinforces the attitude that a normal life is possible

TABLE 50-11 Common Stoma Problems and Their Management

Problem	Cause	Management
Poor technique	Opening too large/too small	Reeducation and follow-up
Fungal infections	Urine accumulating under barrier, frequently with diabetes mellitus and concurrent antibiotic use	Nystatin powder Dry skin (hair dryer) Prevent leakage under wafer
Contact dermatitis	Sensitivity to solvents, adhesives, detergents	Identify reagent (skin patch test and exchange or discontinue offending product Hydrocortisone cream around periphery if affected (avoid prolonged use) Avoid solvents and soaps in general Properly fitting pouch
Mechanical trauma	Frequent or "excessive" pouch changing leading to skin stripping Pressure from belts Overuse of adhesive strips around the faceplate	Minimize pouch changes Gentle skin care Consider nonadhesive (belt) pouches Minimize use of sealants and pastes

Source: Carroll MD, Barbour S. Urinary diversion and bladder substitution, in Tanagho EA, McAninch JW (eds), *Smith's General Urology* (13th ed), Norwalk, CT: Appleton & Lange, 1992, p. 436.

with a conduit. As the individual's condition improves, he or she should be encouraged to verbalize concerns and fears. A visit from a person who has been rehabilitated with a similar diversion may be arranged to give reassurance. The patient should be given the opportunity to handle the equipment and do as much of the needed care as possible. All the procedures necessary for continuing care of the stoma should be written down. Names and addresses where future supplies may be purchased should be included. Names and telephone numbers of resource people to call if emergencies arise are a source of reassurance to the person. The United Ostomy Association is an excellent resource for the patient in need of information and support.

Follow-up nursing care Many complications of a urinary diversion can be averted by a periodic reevaluation of both the stoma and the function of the conduit. The stoma may continue to decrease in size for several months or more. The size of the appliance opening should reflect this change. An opening too large for the stoma will permit peristomal skin to be exposed to urine, causing maceration and denudation of the skin. Openings that are too large also can permit the formation of hypertrophic lesions, which are referred to as *epitheliomatous hyperplasia*. Epitheliomatous hyperplasia can appear as smooth epithelium that extends onto the stoma mucosa or as a rough keratosis that is warty in appearance.[103] It can be painful to the individual and lead to poor adherence of the appliance because of the weeping or oozing, which in turn will cause continued leakage.

Alkaline encrustations around the stoma can lead to stoma stenosis as a result of skin contact with alkaline urine. Because bacteria thrive in an alkaline environment, infections can develop more readily when the pH of urine is allowed to become alkaline and is accompanied by serious weeping of the skin. Nurses have traditionally recommended that patients increase the intake of cranberry juice to help maintain a more acetic urine. However, research has not been able to support the efficacy of this intervention. Currently, patients in some settings are advised to take 500–2000 mg of vitamin C per day, along with at least a quart of acetic fruit juice such as orange, grapefruit, or cranberry juice to lower bacteria counts in urinary diversions.

Stenosis, or narrowing, can occur in the stoma at the level of the skin, muscle, fascia, or any level of the ileal segment. Stenosis interferes with drainage and can lead to stasis, dilatation of the intestine, and infection.

The urinary component of a conduit is formed by the kidneys and their collecting systems, the renal pelvis and ureters. Ureteral angulation, stenosis, obstruction, or lithiasis leads to hydronephrosis, or irreparable renal damage. Periodic evaluation by means of excretory pyelography or loopography can detect this before irreparable damage occurs. Urine for analysis and culture should not be collected from the external appliance because the specimen collected will show bacteria and will not reflect the true conditions in the conduit.

Nursing care of the individual with a continent ileal reservoir for urinary diversion

The patient remains in the hospital for 8–10 postoperative days. It is during this period that initial recovery and teaching begins. Discharge instructions for a Kock pouch with Medena tube are found in Table 50-12.

Three weeks after surgery, the individual will be readmitted to the hospital. A radiographic picture of the pouch will be taken to confirm that there is no extravasation or reflux of urine from the pouch, and then the Medena tube and ureteral stents will be removed. The patient is taught to intubate/catheterize the pouch using a #20 French or #22 French Coudé red-rubber catheter every 2 hours during the day and every 3 hours at night during the first week after it is removed. This is increased gradually (by 1 hour each week) until the pouch is being intubated and drained approximately three or four times in 24 hours. In approximately 6 weeks the patient should be able to do catheterization every 6 hours during the day and not at all at night. The method of draining the pouch is simple, there is no need to wear an external appliance, and the time intervals between emptying the pouch can duplicate normal bladder function. Table 50-13 describes patient instructions for home care of a Kock urinary reservoir.

Patient teaching accompanied by written instruction and periodic reevaluation of all components of the urinary diversion should facilitate the rehabilitation of the individual with minimal complications. The nurse's teaching efforts should focus on catheterization of the pouch, stoma care, and care of the catheter.

TABLE 50-12 Discharge Instructions for Patients with Kock Pouch with a Medena Tube

DISCHARGE INSTRUCTIONS
"Kock Pouch with a Medena Tube"

PURPOSE:

Irrigations are done to maintain patency of the catheter. Mucus and small blood clots can obstruct the catheter.

SUPPLIES:

Discharge pack for Kock pouch with Medena catheter:

1. 20 Fr Coudé-tip red-rubber catheter.
2. Small package of Lubafax.
3. One roll cloth adhesive tape.
4. One roll paper adhesive tape.
5. Urinary leg bag.
6. Six ABD/wet proof dressing.
7. Irrigation set.
8. Two quarts normal saline.

RECIPE FOR NORMAL SALINE:

Mix two teaspoons of table salt to one quart of distilled water.

INSTRUCTIONS:

You will be discharged with a Penrose drain and Medena catheter sutured in place.

PENROSE DRAIN CARE:

1. If drainage from Penrose drain is minimal, cut wet proof ABD pad in half and cover drain. Hold in place with paper tape.
2. When preparing for a shower, remove the dressing from the drain site and cover drain with a piece of plastic wrap taped in place.
3. The area around Medena catheter can be cleaned gently with soap and water when in the shower.
4. After the shower re-dress drain with ABD/wet proof pad.

TABLE 50-12 Discharge Instructions for Patients with Kock Pouch with a Medena Tube (continued)

INSTRUCTIONS FOR IRRIGATION OF THE MEDENA CATHETER:

You will be discharged with your Medena tube sutured in place.

1. The Medena catheter should be irrigated with 30 cc normal saline every 4 hours during the day only, following the method taught in the hospital.
2. If you experience problems with the Medena catheter drainage, or pain, you should irrigate to make sure catheter is not plugged with mucus.
3. Sutures around the Medena tube might dry out and may result in the Medena tube slipping out of the pouch. If this should happen:
   A. Remove the sterile catheter from the package.
   B. Lubricate the catheter with Lubafax.
   C. Slip the catheter through the stoma into the pouch. You may notice bleeding when you pass the catheter through the stoma—this is normal and will stop on its own. The catheter is into the pouch when you see some mucus and urine return.
   D. Tape the catheter in place to the skin securely. Reconnect it to the continuous gravity drainage.
   E. Call the physician for further orders, or earlier if you have any problems passing the catheter into the pouch.

HOSPITAL PHONE NUMBER:

Source: USC/Kenneth Norris Jr. Cancer Hospital, Department of Nursing Services.

TABLE 50-13 Patient Home Care Instructions for Patients with Kock Urinary Diversion without a Medena Catheter

HOME CARE INSTRUCTIONS
"Kock Urinary Reservoir without a Medena Catheter"

EQUIPMENT:

1. Three resealable plastic sandwich bags
2. Four Coudé-tip red-rubber catheters, 20 or 22 Fr.
3. Clean paper towels
4. Stoma coverings (*Nice & Natural Maxi Shields* or *Always* panty liner ½ or ⅓'s)
5. Povidone-iodine solution (Betadine)

CATHETERIZATION TECHNIQUE:

1. Wash hands prior to catheterizing.
2. Swab stoma with povidone-iodine solution on tissue or wipes to remove mucus.
3. Insert the catheter into the stoma of the Kock pouch and drain completely. If the catheter drains slowly or not at all, remove the catheter and run it under hot water to remove mucus plugs and reinsert it into the stoma to drain pouch of urine.
4. The mucosal lining of the stoma stays moist, so most patients do not need lubricating jelly. If lubrication is needed, use only water-soluble types such as K-Y Jelly or Lubafax. Never use Vaseline.
5. Tape your preferred stoma covering over stoma. Always have a waterproof covering to protect clothing.

(continued)

TABLE 50-13 Patient Home Care Instructions for Patients with Kock Urinary Diversion without a Medena Catheter (continued)

Catheterization Schedule:

1. 1st Week: Catheterization should be done every 2 hours during the day and every 3 hours at night.
   2nd Week: Catheterize every 3 hours during the day and every 4 hours at night.
   3rd Week: Catheterize every 4 hours during the day and every 5 hours at night.
   4th Week: Catheterize every 5 hours during the day and every 6 hours at night.
   5th Week: Catheterize every 6 hours during the day and not at all during the night.
2. Irrigate the Kock pouch once a day, following your catheterization procedure, for 2 months after your discharge from the hospital. Use a 60cc syringe full of normal saline or tap water and attach to the catheter to remove excess mucus. If a 60cc syringe is not available, use a turkey or meat baster.
3. After two months, you can irrigate if you notice an increase in mucus or a change in the odor of your urine.
4. Pressure or discomfort can be felt when the pouch is overdistended. If this happens, catheterize your pouch. Never go longer than 7 hours, except at night, without catheterization.
5. To make your own normal saline solution: Add 2 teaspoons of table salt to 1 quart of distilled water.

Catheter Care:

1. Cleanse used catheters in warm, soapy water. Use a syringe or turkey baster to push water through the catheter. Repeat this procedure, using clear water to rinse the catheter. Pour a small amount of Betadine solution through the inside of the catheter. Do not rinse the solution out.
2. Place catheter on a clean paper towel to air dry.
3. Place the clean, air-dried catheter in a clean, covered plastic container. A Tupperware celery container is perfect.
4. Make a kit up to use away from home.
   Female patients use a cosmetic bag; male patients use a pipe tobacco pouch.
   Place two dry, clean catheters into double-bagged resealable sandwich bags. In the outer bag keep extra stoma dressings and Betadine pledgets. Place this equipment into the cosmetic or tobacco pouch. Strips of paper tape may be adhered to the outer plastic bag to eliminate carrying a roll of tape.
5. When catheterizing in a public restroom:
   a. Remove old dressing from stoma.
   b. Swab stoma off with Betadine pledget.
   c. Insert catheter and drain reservoir completely.
   d. Dry catheter off with toilet tissue and place dirty catheter into the outside resealable sandwich bag to be cleaned when returning home.
   e. Cover the stoma with dressing of choice.

NOTE:

Patients with a urinary diversion need to wear a Med-Alert band with the following inscription:

"My stoma is a Continent Urinary Kock Pouch, catheterized every 4 to 6 hours with a 20Fr—*NON* Foley type catheter"

Source: USC/Kenneth Norris Jr. Cancer Hospital, Department of Nursing Services.

Basic principles of care for the continent diversions are similar. However, the nurse must have a thorough understanding of the method used to construct the continent valve. In the case of the Kock pouch, the valve is made of intussepted bowel. The structure of this valve allows the patient to digitally locate the tract should catheterization become difficult.[92] This is not the case with the Indiana reservoir or its modifications. The use of the ileocecal valve to form the continent valve mandates that a much smaller catheter be used to access the pouch and prohibits digitalization.[95] Table 50-8 describes the differences in the procedures. Under no circumstances are Foley catheters ever to be used with continent diversions. Patients are instructed to wear medical alert identification to inform health care personnel of care needed in case of emergency.[92]

TABLE 50-14 Discharge Instructions for Patients with a Kock Pouch to the Urethra

DISCHARGE INSTRUCTIONS
"Patients with a Kock Pouch to the Urethra"

PURPOSE:

Irrigations are done to keep the temporary Foley catheter open and functioning well (mucus and small blood clots can obstruct the catheter).

Equipment:

1 roll paper tape	Large package of 4 × 4 sterile dressing
2 quarts normal saline solution	Irrigation set
4 ABD dressings	Bedside gravity drainage set-up
Urinary leg bag	

Recipe for Normal Saline Solution:

To every quart of distilled water, add 2 teaspoons of table salt. Mix thoroughly.

Instructions:

You will be discharged with the catheter and Penrose drain sutured in place.

1. The Foley catheter should be irrigated at home every 4 hours during the day only. Follow the instructions taught to you in the hospital.
2. Wash your hands.
3. Fill a 60cc catheter tip syringe with normal saline solution.
4. Disconnect the Foley catheter from the gravity drainage tubing.
5. Insert the catheter tip syringe into the catheter and slowly push in normal saline.
6. Aspirate with syringe and dispose of the returned solution.
7. Repeat these steps immediately.
8. Irrigations with normal saline solution should be done every 4 hours until bedtime. This procedure may be repeated at any time if you feel discomfort or if a decrease in drainage occurs.

Source: USC/Kenneth Norris Jr. Cancer Hospital, Department of Nursing Services.

Nursing care for a Kock pouch to the urethra

The male patient who has chosen the continent urinary Kock reservoir to be anastomosed to the urethra following a radical cystectomy is cared for in much the same way postoperatively as the patient who has had a continent reservoir procedure. The difference is that he has a #24 French Foley catheter inserted through the urethra into the reservoir for 3 weeks. Irrigations are done to keep the temporary Foley catheter open and functioning well. Table 50-14 describes discharge instructions for the patients. Three weeks postoperative he will be readmitted for Kock pouch training. After his radiographic study, if the reservoir is negative for extravasation, the Foley catheter and stents will be removed. Then the patient will be taught Kegal exercises and to stop and start his stream. He will void on a schedule night or day until the reservoir has expanded and continence is obtained. It takes a very motivated man 3–6 weeks to obtain total control during the day. It may take longer for him to have good control at night. Discharge instructions after removal of the Foley catheter are included in Tables 50-15 and 50-16.

TABLE 50-15 Discharge Instructions for Patients with a Kock Pouch to the Urethra without a Foley Catheter

DISCHARGE INSTRUCTIONS
"Kock Pouch to the Urethra, without a Foley Catheter"

PURPOSE:

Instructing continent ileourethrostomy diversion patients to regain control of urinary elimination and return to a state of continency.

DISCHARGE PACK INCLUDES:

1. Incontinent pads—Attends—Chux
2. 18 Fr Red Robinson catheter
3. Urinal
4. Measuring container

INSTRUCTIONS:

Your catheter has been removed. Now your new urinary reservoir (Kock pouch) has to be trained:

1. You will start to leak urine after removing the catheter. Try to empty the reservoir by bearing down and/or using gentle pressure over the lower abdomen with your hands. Empty the reservoir as completely as possible.
2. Urinate on a schedule of every 2 hours during the day and every 3 hours at night. Try to increase the time between urination every week by 1 hour. If leaking starts before that scheduled time, try to empty the reservoir as instructed.
3. Kegal exercises are also of help with improving muscle tone.
   A. Kegal exercise:
      Isometric exercise involving a series of voluntary contractions of the pelvic muscles and perineum to improve the retention of urine.
   B. Directions:
      1. Relax abdominal muscles when doing the exercises.
      2. Contract pelvic muscles in three sets of 17 contractions.
      3. Do the contractions while sitting, standing, and lying.
      4. 1st week hold contractions for 3 seconds.
         2nd week hold contractions for 5 seconds.
         3rd week hold contractions for 7–10 seconds.

      Do these exercises every other hour during the day until continence has been obtained.
4. Your Kock pouch has to learn to expand and hold adequate amounts of urine. IT TAKES TIME AND PATIENCE TO RETURN TO A STATE OF CONTROL AND CONTINENCY.

Source: USC/Kenneth Norris Jr. Cancer Hospital, Department of Nursing Services.

Follow-up care

Radiological studies are used to confirm the integrity of the pouch, to test the competence of the nipple valves, and to ensure complete emptying of the reservoir.[92] Intravenous pyelogram is performed to view the upper tracts. Renal function can be checked by the usual laboratory tests. The evaluations of the urea

TABLE 50-16 Discharge Instructions for Self-Catheterization

DISCHARGE INSTRUCTIONS
"Self-Catheterization"

PURPOSE:

Three weeks after surgery the Foley catheter is removed and you begin voiding through your urethra. The urethra could become plugged with mucus and cause problems when you urinate. If this should occur, you would have to pass a catheter into the Kock pouch to drain it.

Self-catheterization is taught before surgery so that you will know how to pass a catheter into your urinary reservoir (Kock pouch).

STEP I: Preparing penis and catheter

A. Swab penis with Betadine (generic name: povidone-iodine) solution.
B. Lubricate the catheter heavily with a water soluble lubrication such as K-Y jelly or Lubafax.

STEP II: Catheter insertion

Insert the catheter slowly. There may be slight discomfort when it passes through the prostatic area. This is normal. Continue inserting with gentle pressure until urine flows freely. Using the same instructions that you were taught in the hospital, empty the pouch completely and irrigate it through the catheter with normal saline to remove mucus from the Kock pouch.

STEP III: Catheter care

A. After using the catheter, wash it with warm soapy water.
B. Rinse the catheter thoroughly with clear water.
C. Dry the catheter and store it in a clean resealable sandwich bag.

Source: USC/Kenneth Norris Jr. Cancer Hospital, Department of Nursing Services.

nitrogen, serum creatinine, urinary pH, and specific gravity or osmolality are the most useful tests of renal function. If urine is to be tested for culture, it is important to remember that continent diversions are not closed, sterile systems as the bladder is. The diversions are often colonized with bacteria, and the presence of bacteria does not necessarily indicate pathology.

CANCER OF THE KIDNEY

Epidemiology

There are two major types of kidney cancer. *Renal cell cancer* is the most common form. It occurs in the parenchyma of the kidney and also has been known as *renal cell carcinoma, renal adenocarcinoma, cancer of the kidney, renal parenchymal neoplasm,* and *hypernephroma.* The diversity of nomenclature reflects the early confusion regarding the histopathology of renal cell cancer.[104] The second major type is *cancer of the renal pelvis.*

Kidney cancer is not a common cancer in the United States, accounting for only about 3% of all cancers. Renal cell carcinoma accounts for about 85% of kidney cancers.[105]

There is a 2:1 male predominance in kidney cancer, especially in renal cell cancer.[105] The incidence of renal cancer is equivalent between whites and blacks. However, Hispanic men and women have kidney cancer rates more than one-third higher than those of white Americans.[105]

There seem to be striking geographic differences, with the rate of kidney cancer being quite high in Scandinavian countries (about 11% of all cancers).[106] Japan has a low incidence, and the United States and most western European countries appear to have an intermediate risk. Interestingly enough, Scandinavians who migrate to Los Angeles do not have higher than expected rates of either cancer of the kidney or cancer of the renal pelvis.[105]

One of the most important demographic risk factors for both renal cell cancer and cancer of the renal pelvis is age. Both are rare in people under 35 years of age, and thereafter the incidence increases with age. Renal cell cancer occurs most frequently in the fifth to sixth decade.[104]

Etiology

Cigarette smoking

The causes of kidney cancer remain obscure. The only risk factor that has been linked persistently to kidney cancer by both cohort studies[107–109] and epidemiologic case-controlled studies[110–112] is cigarette smoking. For renal cell cancer, a consistent relationship between the number of cigarettes consumed and the risk of cancer has not been established. But for cancer of the renal pelvis there does appear to be a strong association between the number of cigarettes smoked and the risk for cancer.[105] It is not clear how cigarette smoking might induce kidney cancer, but studies have shown numerous mutagenic chemicals in the urine of cigarette smokers.[109]

Occupation

Kidney cancer seems to be associated with certain occupational exposures. Exposures to cadmium,[110] asbestos,[113] and lead (pigment in colored printing ink)[114] have each demonstrated a slightly increased risk for renal cell cancer than might otherwise be expected. But currently, occupational exposure is associated with only a very small proportion of all renal cancers.[105]

Analgesic use

Heavy use of analgesics, specifically aspirin, phenacetin or acetaminophen-containing products, has been shown to increase the risk of cancer of the renal pelvis. A possible association between analgesics and renal cell cancer has been reported but not conclusively substantiated.[111]

Other factors

A strong association between renal cell cancer and obesity in women was first identified in 1974.[112] Others have found similar associations,[111] but there remains the question of whether the increased incidence in women is related to obesity or to hormonal (estrogen) influences.[105]

Although often mentioned speculatively, studies have failed to establish a uniform association between coffee drinking and kidney cancer.[114]

An increased incidence of acquired cystic disease of the kidney and of renal cell carcinoma has been reported in patients undergoing dialysis. A recent study reported the risk of renal cell cancer in patients undergoing dialysis to be 57–134 times higher than in the general population.[116]

Pathophysiology

Cellular characteristics

Renal cell carcinoma is the most common form of kidney cancer and accounts for about 75%–85% of kidney cancers. Although the histology is diverse from tumor to tumor, renal cell carcinoma can be separated into two broad groups: clear cell tumors and granular cell tumors.

Renal cell carcinoma arises from tubular epithelial cells that are found in the parenchyma of the kidney. Tumors of the renal pelvis generally arise from epithelial tissue anywhere in the renal pelvis and are often papillary. These tumors often have independent, multifocal origins.[117]

Cancer of the renal pelvis accounts for about 5%–9% of all kidney cancers. The mucosal lining of the renal pelvis and ureter is similar to that of the urinary bladder, being composed of transitional epithelium.[117] Thus, the two major cell types in tumors of the renal pelvis are transitional cell cancer (most common) and squamous cell cancer. Grading is similar to that of bladder cancer. Papillomas account for 15%–20% of cases.[117]

Progression of disease

Renal cell cancers tend to grow toward the medullary portion of the kidney, whereas tumors of the renal pelvis often grow at the ureteropelvic junction and invade the underlying submucosa and muscular coats.

Cancer of the renal pelvis and renal cell carcinoma spread through the venous and lymphatic routes. Hematogenous spread most often involves the lungs, bones, and liver. Lymphatic drainage of the kidneys is to the nodes in the ipsilateral renal hilus. These nodes then drain into the regional lymph nodes.

Renal cell carcinoma also spreads by direct extension to the renal vein and sometimes farther into the vena cava. It can also extend by growing up through the renal capsule into the perinephric fat or the adjacent visceral structures.[104]

Cancer of the renal pelvis grows by extension, as mentioned, down into the ureter and out through the muscular coats. Although the majority of upper urinary tract transitional cell cancers are localized at diagnosis, the most common metastatic sites are regional lymph nodes, bone, and lung.[117]

Exact numbers vary, but somewhere between 30% and 50% of individuals with kidney cancer have metastasis at diagnosis.[118]

Paraneoplasia and Renal Cell Carcinoma

Renal cell carcinoma has a considerable association with certain paraneoplastic syndromes. The term *paraneoplastic syndrome* is used to describe systemic effects of a tumor on the host. The effects are not directly related to the tumor presence (such as compression or obstruction from a solid tumor) or to a particular metastatic lesion (for example, brain or bone metastasis). Rather, paraneoplastic syndromes are thought to be associated with compounds that the malignant cells synthesize that are not normally synthesized by cells of that type (see Chapter 29). Although uncommon in general, renal cell carcinomas seem to have a higher association with paraneoplasia, particularly that which is related to the endocrine system.[119] Some of the ectopic (or inappropriately secreted) hormones that have been ascribed to tumors of renal origin are parathyroid hormone, erythropoietin, renin, gonadotropins, and adrenocorticotropic hormone.[119,120]

Clinical Manifestations

Renal cell carcinoma

In 40% of individuals diagnosed with renal cell carcinoma the initial symptom is gross hematuria. The hematuria appears uniform throughout the urinary stream, and lower tract discomfort is not present. Pain (which is usually dull and aching) is also a common presenting symptom, as is a palpable abdominal mass.[120] These three symptoms—hematuria, pain, and a palpable abdominal mass—represent the classic triad of symptoms of renal cell carcinoma. However, their simultaneous appearance on presentation is infrequent. Because of the well-protected anatomic position of the kidney, the presence of a tumor is unfortunately often concealed until advanced stages. Other more generalized symptoms also have been described with cancer of the kidney, including fever, weight loss, an elevated erythrocyte sedimentation rate (ESR), or anemia.

Cancer of the renal pelvis

Only a few individuals with cancer of the renal pelvis present with the classic triad of symptoms. Most tumors of the renal pelvis originally present with hematuria (gross or microscopic). Some individuals may have both hematuria and flank pain, which is probably caused by the passage of blood clots or by obstruction of the ureteropelvic junction.[117] A palpable mass in a tumor of the renal pelvis is almost always either because the tumor has extended outside the kidney or because of massive hydronephrosis (resulting from a ureteropelvic junction obstruction).

Techniques for early detection have not been identified for either renal cell carcinoma or cancer of the renal pelvis.

Assessment

Renal cell carcinoma

Tests used in the diagnosis and staging of renal cell carcinoma include kidney, ureter, and bladder (KUB) radiographs; nephrotomograms; excretory urogram; retrograde urogram; renal US; renal CT; and renal angiography. MRI examinations help to identify renal cysts more readily, and solid renal masses can be distinguished from normal renal parenchyma by MRI. While some claim that the diagnosis of renal cancer has not been improved by MRI,[91] others believe it to be similar or slightly greater in accuracy than CT and maintain that its role in the systematic evaluation of kidney cancer is complementary to the CT evaluation and is particularly sensitive and useful for evaluation of adjacent organ invasion and major vascular involvement.[121–123]

Excretory urograms have traditionally been known as *intravenous pyelograms*. The prefix *pyelo* implies, however, that only the renal pelvis is shown. *Excretory urogram* is probably a more apt name because the test does show the entire urinary tract. Excretory urogram and renal tomography are considered by most to be the screening tests of choice for suspected renal mass lesions, although they are only 70%–75% accurate in differentiating benign cysts from malignant lesions.[121]

Renal US, which is generally the next step in the assessment of a renal mass, has the apparent advantage of being easy to do, noninvasive, relatively inexpensive, and requiring a minimal physical expenditure on the person's part. It can generally differentiate solid from cystic masses. Individuals who have solid or questionable masses should undergo further tests.

Renal US coupled with CT makes it possible to diagnose small tumors suggestive of malignancy. A CT scan can accurately evaluate a questionable lesion, determine the local extent of the cancer, identify the presence of enlarged regional lymph nodes, and describe the presence of tumor within the main renal vein and the inferior vena cava.[104,122] A CT scan of the abdomen, chest, and brain also can aid in detecting distant metastases.

The value of renal angiography has decreased with the advent of US and CT. In most cases the superiority of a technically adequate CT scan with US makes diagnostic angiography a last resort.[123]

Recently, DNA flow cytometry has added information in predicting the prognosis of renal cell cancer. Aneuploid tumors were found to be more likely to develop to invasive lesions than diploid tumors.[124]

Cancer of the renal pelvis

Excretory urogram, retrograde urogram, and urinary cytology are the most useful techniques for establishing a diagnosis of cancer of the renal pelvis. Angiography has been unsuccessful with these tumors. Routine use of US and CT scanning does not appear to have the same major impact on cancer of the renal pelvis as with renal cell cancer.[125] However, US may show a mass density in the central region of the kidney, and a CT scan might detect the presence of a soft tissue mass in the renal hilum. Using MRI with CT aids in the detection of regional lymph node involvement.[117]

20%–30% of low-grade renal pelvic cancers and 60% of higher-grade lesions can be detected on urinary cytology.[117] Urinary cytology can be done on a freshly voided urine specimen or on washings from the renal pelvis obtained during a retrograde urogram.

Classification and Staging

Renal cell carcinoma

Staging for renal cell carcinoma, as with all cancers, is founded on those aspects that influence survival, including regional lymph node involvement, invasion through the renal capsule, extension to contiguous organs, and distant metastases.[126] Extension into the renal veins or the inferior vena cava is thought by some authorities to have no influence on prognosis if properly managed.[120] Likewise, the size of the primary tumor is not strongly correlated with survival and may not be a significant factor in staging.

The system used most often for classifying renal cell carcinoma is a modification of the system of Flocks and Kadesky[127] originally proposed, a staging system based on gross physical characteristics of the tumor. Robson proposed modifications of the system that took into account the degree of vascular involvement, and it is that system that is most widely used (Figure 50-17). The TNM system (Table 50-17) more accurately classifies the magnitude of tumor involvement.

Cancer of the renal pelvis

Staging of both renal pelvic and ureteral cancers is based on an accurate assessment of the degree of tumor infiltration and parallels the staging system developed for bladder cancer.[117] Table 50-18 outlines the TNM system for staging cancer of the renal pelvis.

Treatment of Renal Cell Carcinoma

Surgery

Renal cell carcinoma is treated by surgical removal. A radical nephrectomy routinely includes removal of the kidney, its enveloping fascia, the ipsilateral adrenal,

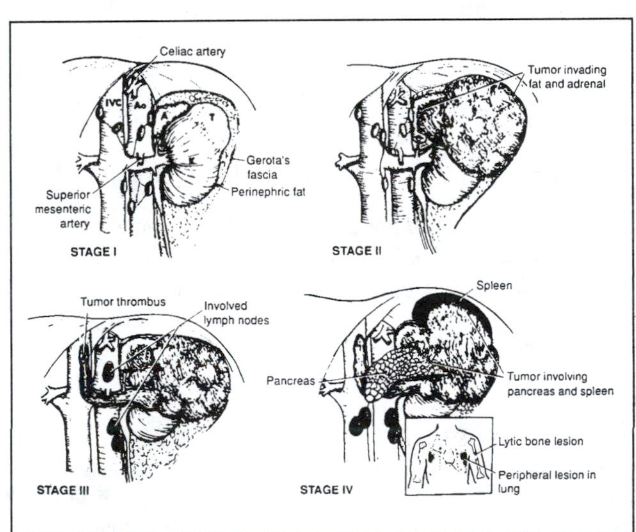

FIGURE 50-17 Robson staging system for renal cell carcinoma. In stage A, IVC is inferior vena cava; Ao, aorta; A, left suprarenal gland; T, tumor; K, left kidney. (Source: Dreicer R, Williams RO: Renal parenchymal neoplasms, in Tanagho, EA, McAninch JW (eds), *Smith's General Urology* [13th ed]. Norwalk, CT: Appleton & Lange, 1992, p. 363.)

TABLE 50-17 TNM Staging System for Cancer of the Kidney

PRIMARY TUMOR (T)	
TX	Primary tumor cannot be assessed
T0	No evidence of primary tumor
T1	Tumor 2.5 cm or less in greatest dimension limited to the kidney
T2	Tumor more than 2.5 cm in greatest dimension limited to the kidney
T3	Tumor extends into major veins or invades adrenal gland or perinephric tissues but not beyond Gerota's fascia
T3a	Tumor invades adrenal gland or perinephric tissues but not beyond Gerota's fascia
T3b	Tumor grossly extends into renal vein(s) or vena cava
T4	Tumor invades beyond Gerota's fascia
LYMPH NODE (N)	
NX	Regional lymph nodes cannot be assessed
N0	No regional lymph node metastasis
N1	Metastasis in a single lymph node, 2 cm or less in greatest dimension
N2	Metastasis in a single lymph node, more than 2 cm but not more than 5 cm in greatest dimension, or multiple lymph nodes, none more than 5 cm in greatest dimension
N3	Metastasis in a lymph node more than 5 cm in greatest dimension
DISTANT METASTASIS (M)	
MX	Presence of distant metastasis cannot be assessed
M0	No distant metastasis
M1	Distant metastasis
SITES OF DISTANT METASTASIS	
Pulmonary	PUL
Osseous	OSS
Hepatic	HEP
Brain	BRA
Lymph nodes	LYM
Bone marrow	MAR
Pleura	PLE
Peritoneum	PER
Skin	SKI
Other	OTH

Source: Beahrs OH, Henson DE, Hutter RV, et al (eds): *American Joint Committee on Cancer: Manual for Staging of Cancer* (4th ed). Philadelphia: Lippincott, 1992.

the proximal one-half of the ureter, and lymph nodes in the renal hilar area.[117]

Various surgical approaches have been used for radical nephrectomy. The abdominotransperitoneal approach can be performed with a midline or subcostal abdominal incision. The thoracoabdominal approach may also be used. Figure 50-18 displays the boundaries of a left radical nephrectomy.

TABLE 50-18 TNM Staging System for Cancer of the Renal Pelvis and Ureter

PRIMARY TUMOR (T)			
TX	Primary tumor cannot be assessed		
T0	No evidence of primary tumor		
Tis	Carcinoma in situ		
Ta	Papillary noninvasive carcinoma		
T1	Tumor invades subepithelial connective tissue		
T2	Tumor invades beyond muscularis into periureteric or peripelvic fat or renal parenchyma		
T4	Tumor invades adjacent organs or through the kidney into perinephric fat		
LYMPH NODE (N)			
NX	Regional lymph nodes cannot be assessed		
N0	No regional lymph node metastasis		
N1	Metastasis in a single lymph node, 2 cm or less in greatest dimension		
N3	Metastasis in a lymph node more than 5 cm in greatest dimension		
DISTANT METASTASIS (M)			
MX	Presence of distant metastasis cannot be assessed		
M0	No distant metastasis		
M1	Distant metastasis		
STAGE GROUPING			
0	Tis	N0	M0
	Ta	N0	M0
I	T1	N0	M0
II	T2	N0	M0
III	T3	N0	M0
IV	T4	N0	M0
	Any T	N1	M0
	Any T	N2	M0
	Any T	N3	M0
	Any T	Any N	M1

Source: Beahrs OH, Henson DE, Hutter RV, et al (eds): *American Joint Committee on Cancer: Manual for Staging of Cancer* (4th ed). Philadelphia: Lippincott, 1992.

Vena caval involvement

About 5%–9% of individuals with renal cell carcinoma have varying degrees of tumor extension into the vena cava. Because of the shorter right renal vein, tumor thrombus occurs more often on the right side. To prevent tumor embolization, a tumor thrombus in the vena cava is removed in continuity with the renal tumor. Tumor invasion of the wall of the vena cava is no longer thought to be a completely incurable situation, and while the surgical treatment is complicated, published experience indicates a positive outcome for many of these patients if they are free of distant metastases.[128,129]

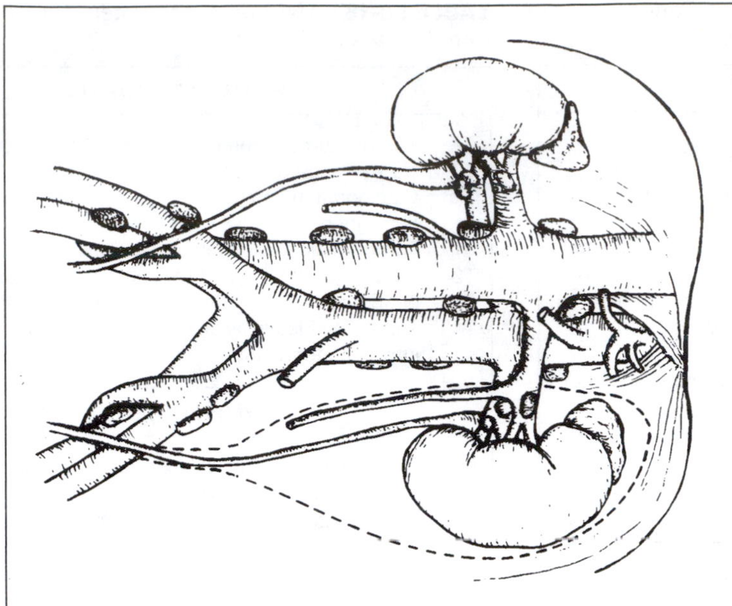

FIGURE 50-18 Boundaries of a left radical nephrectomy. Dotted line represents both the surgical margin and Gerota's fascia. (Source: Drecier R, Williams RO: Renal parenchymal neoplasms, in Tanagho, EA, McAninch JW (eds), *Smith's General Urology* [13th ed]. Norwalk, CT: Appleton & Lange, 1992, p. 368.)

Classically, individuals with vena cava tumor thrombus have been classified as having stage III renal cell carcinoma and have been grouped along with individuals who have regional lymph node metastasis. This may be an inappropriate staging. Individuals who have vena caval extension (without capsular invasion, perinephric fat invasion, or regional lymph node metastases) have a prognosis comparable to individuals with stage I tumors.[130]

Lymphadenectomy

Regional lymphadenectomy remains controversial.[104] Lymphatic metastases have been found (by lymph node dissection) in 8%–22% of individuals without other evidence of metastasis.[131] Those who argue against lymphadenectomy feel that it does not improve survival; its staging value in terms of predicting survival is limited because the cancer can spread via the venous system alone; and that because there is as yet no effective adjuvant therapy, identification of lymph node metastases is not important.[131,132] There are no controlled clinical trials demonstrating that this procedure impacts the disease-free or overall survival of patients.[104]

Those who favor lymphadenectomy feel that it adds to a more comprehensive and meaningful staging using the TNM system.[133] Some settings routinely perform lymphadenectomy on all patients with stage I, II, or III disease. It is argued that this offers the best chance of survival to those for whom radical nephrectomy is potentially curative.[134]

Bilateral tumors or tumors in a solitary kidney

In the unusual case of bilateral tumors or cancer in a solitary kidney, two treatment options are available. In bilateral tumors where there is a larger tumor in one kidney than in the other, partial nephrectomy is performed on the kidney with the smaller tumor, and several weeks later radical nephrectomy is carried out on the kidney with the larger tumor. In cases where there is a tumor in a solitary kidney with no evidence of metastasis, partial nephrectomy or radical nephrectomy with subsequent chronic hemodialysis or renal transplantation are treatment alternatives. A surgical alternative to a radical or partial nephrectomy is the enucleation of multiple lesions.[135]

Radiotherapy and Chemotherapy

Renal cell carcinomas and their metastases are usually radio-resistant, and radiotherapy's treatment role is controversial. Adjuvant chemotherapy has not demonstrated any improvement in survival rates than may be accomplished without chemotherapy.[120] Vinblastine is generally believed to be the most active single agent, with response rates reported in the 15% range.[104]

Treatment of Advanced Renal Cell Carcinoma

About 30% of individuals with renal cell carcinoma present with metastases at the time of diagnosis. Another 50% will develop metastases after radical nephrectomy.[118] The mean survival rate in patients with metastases at the time of diagnosis is approximately 4 months, and only about 10% survive 1 year.[136] Radiotherapy, surgery, chemotherapy, hormonal therapy, and immunotherapy have all been suggested as means of managing the disease.

Radiotherapy

Radiation therapy is an important modality in the palliation of patients with metastatic renal cell cancer. Despite the belief that this is a radio-resistant tumor, effective palliation of metastatic disease to the bone, brain, and lungs is reported in up to two-thirds of patients. External beam radiation therapy has occasionally been used to palliate patients with gross hematuria pain, but without significant efficacy.[104] Metastatic bone pain can be palliated by irradiating the area involved with significant doses up to 40–50 Gy.[137]

Surgery

Adjunctive or palliative nephrectomies have been described as approaches for individuals with metastatic renal cell carcinoma. Adjunctive nephrectomy is done to improve survival, whereas palliative nephrectomy is done to relieve symptoms of the primary renal tumor.

Individuals whose survival is improved by adjunctive nephrectomy are those who have the best performance status and least amount of tumor before surgery.[118]

Palliative nephrectomy may be justifiable for individuals who have severe disabling symptoms such as local pain, bleeding, or endocrinopathy but who otherwise have a reasonable life expectancy of greater than 6 months.[118] Radiotherapy might relieve these symptoms equally well.

Angioinfarction of the primary tumor with a subsequent radical nephrectomy has been used in an aggressive, but unsuccessful attempt to improve survival.[138]

Chemotherapy

Chemotherapy has had no great impact on metastatic renal cell carcinoma.[131] Some clinicians, however, feel that chemotherapeutic trials might be appropriate for certain individuals because metastatic renal cell carcinoma presents so few options. Vinblastine (Velban) is one chemotherapeutic agent that has demonstrated some success in achieving tumor responses.[104,118] Several clinical trials have tested chemotherapy combinations that include vinblastine. Better responses have been achieved than with vinblastine alone, but the response duration is short and the toxicity significant.[128]

Hormonal therapy

Because progestational agents have proven useful in diethylstilbestrol-induced renal tumors in hamsters, several clinical trials in humans have been conducted in the last 20 years. Response rates vary from 2%–15%. Drugs most often used have been progesterones such as medroxyprogesterone acetate (Depo-Provera) or megesterol acetate (Megace), testosterone, and anti-estrogens such as tamoxifen. The infrequent responses to hormonal therapy have not significantly improved survival. There are a few individuals, however, who may be helped by this relatively benign therapy.[120]

Biologic response modifiers

Although renal cell cancer has been resistant to chemotherapy and hormonal therapy, in 1985 Rosenberg and associates[139] first demonstrated antitumor responses after adoptive immunotherapy with high doses of interleukin-2 (IL-2) and large numbers of lymphokine-activated killer (LAK) cells in metastatic renal cancer. Interleukin-2 has been used alone in patients with advanced disseminated disease, but complete and partial responses have been much higher when IL-2 is combined with LAK cells.[140]

Treatment with biologic response modifiers is complicated, toxic, and expensive.[141] At this time, several phase II clinical studies are under way to confirm treatment effectiveness and to determine whether the complicated technology required can be transferred outside a pure research setting.[154] One current protocol gives recombinant interleukin-2 (rIL-2) by bolus intravenous injection three times per week, in high doses, preceded by oral indomethacin for a total of 16 doses.[142] An older study required a 16-day treatment cycle with patients initially being primed with 5 days of IL-2 to stimulate LAK cell precursors. After a 2-day rest, patients have five consecutive daily leukaphereses. The lymphocytes are incubated with IL-2 for 3–4 days. After the last leukapheresis, patient cells are reinfused along with additional IL-2, during the last 4 days of the cycle.[143] Response rates vary from 11%–35%.[104]

IL-2 toxicities include fever, GI bleeding, rash and pruritus, hepatic dysfunction, thrombocytopenia, somnolence, disorientation, and pulmonary edema.[143]

Alpha-interferon has shown modest activity in the treatment of advanced renal cancer. It has been shown to directly inhibit the division of a variety of cells in vitro and in vivo. Interferon treatment allows some renal cell cancer patients to experience an objective response, frequently of prolonged duration with a tolerable level of side effects that are considerably milder than those associated with chemotherapy.[144]

Treatment of Cancer of the Renal Pelvis

Treatment of renal pelvic cancers should be based on tumor grade, stage, and position. The standard treatment has been nephroureterectomy. To avoid recurrence in this segment, a radical nephrectomy, including the kidney, all perinephric tissue, regional lymph nodes, the ureter, and a small cuff of the bladder, is performed. Proponents of this radical procedure feel it is necessary to treat the secondary ureteral and vesical tumors that may be present.[104] Others who argue for more conservative kidney-sparing approaches to surgical treatment of this cancer stress the poor prognosis associated with advanced lesions and the mortality risks of radical procedures.[125]

Radiation therapy has not proven to be an effective adjunct for the control of residual tumor, local recurrence, or unresectable disease.[125] Although controversial, postoperative radiotherapy is believed by some to decrease recurrence rates and improve survival in patients with deeply infiltrating cancer. Chemotherapeutic agents that have been used with limited results include doxorubicin, cisplatin, methotrexate, and vinblastine.[145]

Results and Prognosis

Survival rates for renal cell carcinoma and cancer of the renal pelvis are shown in Table 50-19.

The prognosis for cancer of the renal pelvis is relatively poor and is closely correlated with the degree of differentiation and extent of the tumor. While the overall survival rates are approximately 40%, the reported 5-year survival rate for individuals with differentiated transitional cell carcinoma of the renal pelvis is approximately 60%, whereas for undifferentiated carcinomas it is only 14%.[195] Extension outside the kidney indicates a very poor prognosis.

Nursing Care of Individuals with Cancer of the Kidney

Individuals who are undergoing diagnostic procedures or treatments for kidney malignancy are extremely anxious. Some individuals equate the loss of a kidney with imminent death. Others worry that the remaining kidney will not be able to meet the body's total need for total urine elimination. The alert nurse can help by providing correct information to the individual and family. The nurse should assess the individual's knowledge and feelings about the disease and its treatment to help the patient set realistic goals for dealing with the malignancy.

Nursing care of individuals undergoing surgery

In general, the principal treatment of primary renal carcinoma is surgical excision. Radical nephrectomy is performed on all resectable lesions in stage I to III and is sometimes done palliatively for symptoms such as pain and bleeding for individuals with advanced disease. The pre- and postoperative nursing management of the person undergoing radical nephrectomy is similar to that of the individual undergoing laparotomy.

Preoperative nursing care A renal infarction may be done 2–3 days prior to surgery in an attempt to decrease surgical hemorrhage by decreasing tumor vascularity. Following this procedure, the individual may experience considerable pain, fever, nausea, and vomiting. Those symptoms may persist for up to 36 hours. Analgesic and antiemetic medications should be administered for symptomatic control. Intravenous fluid supplement may be necessary if the individual has a severe fluid loss. Emotional support and reassurance during this time can be comforting to the patient and family.

Postoperative nursing care

Pain relief The primary objectives during the postoperative period are the management of pain and the prevention of postoperative complications. Pain can be quite severe after nephrectomy. For lower pole renal tumors, the flank incision (retroperitoneal) approach is generally used, and the individual is placed in a hyperextended side-lying position. The thoracoabdominal incision approach is generally used for larger and upper pole lesions. In this approach the person is placed in an oblique position with rolled towels situated to elevate the flank.

As a result of the position on the operating table, the individual undergoing nephrectomy experiences not only incision pain but also muscular aches and pains. The nurse should administer adequate pain medication on a regular schedule for the first 48 hours after surgery and only gradually decrease the frequency and strength of analgesics according to the person's needs per the physician's order. When establishing an effective pain management program postnephrectomy, it is important to remember that this is a painful surgery.

The use of moist heat, massage, and pillows to support the back while the person is on his or her side also can provide relief. The individual should be turned from side to side at least every 2 hours or whenever desired.

Prevention of atelectasis and pneumonia Because of the close proximity of the incision to the diaphragm, deep breathing and coughing can be extremely uncomfortable. The person needs to be taught how to splint the incision while coughing. Use of analgesics at proper intervals will help the person perform deep breathing and coughing more effectively. The nurse should instruct the individual to take at least ten deep breaths each hour while awake. The use of an incentive spirometer also may be beneficial. Intermittent positive pressure ventilation is not indicated for the average patient.

Monitoring renal function If an indwelling catheter is in place, urine output should be monitored every hour immediately after surgery. The urine will be slightly blood-tinged for the first few hours after surgery. Urine output should be greater than 30 ml/hr. If

TABLE 50-19 5-Year Survival Rates for Renal Cell Cancer (RCC) and Cancer of the Renal Pelvis (CRP)

RCC		CPR	
Stage I	88%–100%	Low-grade Low-stage	60%–90%
Stage II, IIIa	60%		
Stage IIIb	15%–20%	High-grade or penetration into ureteral wall	0%–33%
Stage IV	0%–20%		

Source: Data from Dreicer R, Williams RD.[104]

the individual does not have a urinary catheter and has not voided within 8–10 hours after surgery, catheterization must be done to determine renal status. Accurate recording of fluid intake and output and weight should be done daily to determine the person's overall fluid balance status.

Paralytic ileus Paralytic ileus is fairly common following renal surgery. It is thought to be due to a reflex paralysis of intestinal peristalsis. The individual is usually allowed nothing to eat or drink by mouth for the first 24–48 hours after surgery. Oral food and fluids are avoided until bowel sounds are heard and gas is passed. The symptoms of paralytic ileus are abdominal distension, pain, and absence of bowel sounds. Nothing is given by mouth, and a nasogastric tube and/or rectal tube is used to relieve abdominal distention. Other measures such as ambulation, turning the person, and use of a heating pad on the abdomen may also assist the individual in expelling flatus.

Hemorrhage Although not a frequent complication, postnephrectomy hemorrhage is a danger, because the kidney is a highly vascular organ. Acute massive hemorrhage manifests itself by profuse drainage and distention at the suture line or internally. It can be reflected in an elevation of pulse rate and a drop in blood pressure. However, slow bleeding may not manifest itself in such obvious changes in vital signs. The nurse should observe the individual closely for symptoms of hemorrhage and shock. The person should be turned and the underlying sheet examined for blood when the nephrectomy dressing is checked.

Wound care Wound care after nephrectomy is fairly routine. Frequently no drain is inserted. The frequency of dressing changes depends on the condition of the incision and the amount of drainage.

Potential for pneumothorax When the thoracoabdominal incision approach has been used for nephrectomy, the individual will have a chest tube placed during surgery to remove air and fluid from the thoracic cavity and to reexpand the lung. The nurse must maintain the chest tube under water drainage and keep it free of kinks.

Discharge planning Discharge planning begins as soon as the individual is admitted to the hospital and is frequently updated. At the time of discharge, the nurse needs to discuss with the individual the importance of continued liberal oral intake of fluids (at least 2500 ml/day) and the need to avoid any fad diets, which may result in excess protein catabolism. Individuals who are prone to hypertension should be encouraged to have frequent blood pressure checks because the nephrotic pressure gradient may change when only one kidney is present. Individuals who have had surgery to remove a renal tumor should be advised to have a complete physical examination and chest radiograph annually to rule out lung metastasis and to have an intravenous pyelogram yearly to check for contralateral tumors. The person also should be educated to report any symptoms of respiratory distress, hemoptysis, pain, or fracture of an extremity. These symptoms may signify metastasis. Last but not least, the person should be reassured that life with one kidney can be normal.

Nursing care of individuals receiving chemotherapy

Antineoplastic chemotherapeutic agents have generally not had a significant effect on metastatic renal carcinoma. Vinblastine is a commonly used agent. The major toxicity of vinblastine is dose-related myelosuppression. Other infrequent side effects are nausea, vomiting, stomatitis, neurotoxicity, and paralytic ileus. This drug is administered intravenously. The nurse must ensure vein patency prior to drug administration because extravasation can cause local skin and tissue necrosis.

The general nursing responsibilities regarding chemotherapy include familiarity with the normal dosage ranges and routes of administration and potential acute and delayed side effects.

Nursing care of individuals receiving hormonal therapy

Progesterone and testosterone agents (for example, Depo-Provera and Megace) have been used in hormonal therapy for the treatment of metastatic renal cell carcinoma. They are generally well tolerated except for mild fluid retention and body weight gain. Testosterone (androgens) such as fluoxymesterone (Halotestin) and testolactone (Teslac) are also well tolerated. Acute side effects may include some nausea, vomiting, and edema.

Nursing care of individuals receiving biological response modifiers

Numerous clinical trials using a variety of biologic response modifiers (BRMs) such as interferon (INF), recombinant interleukin-2 (rIL-2) and lymphokine-activated killer cells (LAK) are being conducted in patients with metastatic renal cell carcinoma. Among the BRMs, interferons have had the broadest therapeutic experience in clinical oncology.[146] There are three distinct antigenic species identified as alpha-, beta-, and gamma-interferons. The alpha-interferons have demonstrated positive response in metastatic renal cell carcinoma, while gamma-interferon showed minimal activity in this disease.[157] Alpha-interferon is usually administered by intramuscular (IM) or subcutaneous (SC) injection. Nurses should know the proper route of drug administration for each particular agent. Some of the common side effects of alpha-interferon are malaise, weakness, fever, chills, pancytopenia, nausea, vomiting, and diarrhea.

Interleukin-2 can be administered by various routes, including intravenous bolus, continuous infusion, SC injection, and peritoneal infusion. The optimal administration route and dosing schedule have not been established.[148] Some of the major toxicities are fluid retention, hypotension, confusion, oliguria, nausea, vomiting, diarrhea, hepatoxicity, skin rash, chills, fever, and malaise. The major dose-limiting toxicity of interleukin-2 is the fluid imbalance caused by capillary permeability—leaks allowing intravascular fluids to shift into extravascular space. This is manifested as peripheral edema, abdominal ascites, or pulmonary infiltrates.[149] The nurse must monitor the patient's cardiovascular and pulmonary status carefully. Management of hypotension may require colloid solutions such as 5% human albumin. Fluid replacement must be carefully monitored to avoid fluid overload.

Lymphokine-activated killer cells (LAK) are generally given as a part of the IL-2 treatment. LAK is given intravenously using a tubing without filter over about 30 minutes after a test dose is given.[149] The patient may experience shaking chills, fever, nausea, vomiting and other toxicities induced by IL-2.

In caring for patients undergoing BRM therapy, the nurse needs to assess the patient's anxiety and expectation and attempt to maintain a balance between hope and the possibility of negative clinical response. Severe toxicities may require reduction of the dose or discontinuation of the treatment. Patient and family need to be educated about the potential side effects and when to seek help.

TESTICULAR CANCER

Epidemiology

Testicular cancer is an uncommon cancer, accounting for only 1%–2% of all cancer in men and less than 0.5% of all cancer deaths in men.[150] It is a striking type of cancer, however, for three reasons. First, it is the most common solid tumor in men between 29 and 35 years of age. Second, its incidence has been increasing over the last 50 years in whites, whereas the incidence in young black males is low. Third, the dramatic improvement in the management of this disease has been one of cancer's real success stories.

Age, race, and geographic location are all significant in the epidemiology of testicular cancer. The peak age is between 20 and 40 years of age. From 40–60 years of age the incidence declines, and then the incidence increases slightly. The rate in blacks is less than one-third the rate in whites. Scandinavian countries have the highest incidence of testicular cancer. In Denmark it accounts for 6.7% of all cancers. But there is an increase in incidence among young white males in all of Europe and North America. Asian and African countries have the lowest rate. Japan's testicular cancer incidence is 0.8%.[150]

The other epidemiologic factor of note is that the incidence of testis cancer is highest in men of the highest socioeconomic classes. Regardless of ethnicity, there is an association between higher incidence and higher economic status.[150]

Etiology

Two factors have been associated with an increased incidence of testicular cancer: cryptorchidism and exogenous estrogens. Cryptorchidism (undescended testicle) has a relative 3- to 14-fold risk for testicular cancer.[151,152] Normal descent of the testicle is under hormonal control. Whites have a three times greater risk of undescended testes than do blacks.[150]

Exogenous estrogens given to women as birth control pills or as diethylstilbestrol (to prevent spontaneous abortion) have been hypothesized to influence the incidence of testicular cancer in subsequent male children. Case-controlled studies have examined the relationship between risk of testicular cancer of the testis and exogenous estrogen administration during pregnancy and found an increased risk of testicular cancer ranging from 2.8–5.3 over the expected incidence in the male children of women exposed to diethylstilbestrol, estrogen, or estrogen-progestin combinations.[150]

Henderson and colleagues[150] propose a unifying etiologic hypothesis that describes the initial carcinogenic event occurring in utero in response to free estrogen. Subsequent factors combine throughout the boy's development and culminate in "abnormal" primitive germ cells producing a neoplastic cell line.[150]

Pathophysiology

Cellular characteristics

Cell types of testicular cancer are classified in terms of embryonal tissue. Almost all of these tumors arise from the primordial germ cell, a multipotent cell in the yolk sac of the embryo.[153] *Multipotent* refers to a cell that will have many varieties of cell types as its "offspring." This can explain why one primary testicular tumor may have a wide variety of cell types. It also explains why there are so many different types of primary testicular tumors. Several classification systems have been proposed for germ cell tumors. The following is a common grouping of the various histologic types of testicular cancer that separates the various types as seminomas or nonseminomas:

Arising from Germ Tissue (Germinal) (97%)

- Seminoma (also called germinoma)
  - typical (most common testicular tumor)
  - anaplastic
  - spermatocytic

Nonseminomatous germ cell tumors (NSGCT)

embryonal (including yolk sac)

teratocarcinoma

teratoma

choriocarcinoma

Arising from Stromal Tissue (3%)

Interstitial cell tumors (Leydig cell tumors)

Gonadal-stromal tumors

This chapter focuses only on germinal tumors, that is, the seminomas and nonseminomas.

Most testicular tumors arise from germ tissue. They can arise either focally from a single cell or multifocally.[153] Malignant growth is fairly rapid. This cancer usually appears in only one testis.

Progression of disease

Metastases of germinal testicular cancers occur either by extension or via the lymphatics. Testicular germ cell tumors almost always spread lymphatically first and hematogenously later. Choriocarcinoma is the exception and spreads primarily by the hematogenous route. Lymphatic spread occurs in a step-wise fashion in the retroperitoneal lymph nodes. It spreads from the right testis to the interaortocaval, precaval, preaortic, paracaval, right common iliac, and right external iliac lymph nodes, in that order; from the left testis to the paraaortic, preaortic, left common iliac, and left external iliac lymph nodes.[154] Because of the complicated lymphatic network that surrounds the testes, metastasis can occur while the primary tumor is still small. Seminomas can spread to the mediastinal or supraclavicular nodes, but this usually occurs later. Lymph node invasion may cause displacement of the ureters or kidneys and occasionally may obstruct the ureters.

Testicular cancer also spreads via direct extension. The tumor may invade the epididymis, extend up the spermatic cord, or extend through the tunica vaginalis to the scrotum.

Germinal tumors of the testes ordinarily do not metastasize by hematogenous spread. Metastatic spread to the lung, liver, adrenal gland, or bone occasionally may occur as a late manifestation of the disease.

Clinical Manifestations

Painless enlargement of the testicle is the most common presenting symptom of testicular cancer. This can be discovered accidentally, or a dragging sensation, sometimes described as a "heaviness" in the scrotum (caused by the weight of the tumor) may call attention to the tumor's presence.

Lumbar pain, abdominal or supraclavicular masses, pain from obstruction, or a cough could all be symptoms related to metastases.

Trauma, which is often associated with the discovery of a lump, is not an etiologic factor but rather calls attention to an already present problem. Local signs of testicular cancer include a firm, diffuse enlargement; an inability to transilluminate the testis; and a lack of pain on palpation.[154] Any painless lump in the testis that does not respond promptly to antibiotics should be thought of as cancer until proven otherwise.

Assessment

The following is a list of the diagnostic procedures used for testicular cancer:

Radical inguinal orchiectomy (as biopsy)

Radiologic techniques

- Chest radiograph
- Full-lung tomograms or chest CT scan
- Lymphangiogram and/or abdominal CT scan (to detect retroperitoneal nodes)
- Intravenous pyelogram
- Testicular US (to help distinguish between epididymitis and tumor)

Laboratory studies

- Serum alpha-fetoprotein (AFP)
- Serum lactic acid dehydrogenase
- Serum beta human chorionic gonadotropin (HCG)

Physical examination includes palpation of the testes, abdominal palpation to exclude bulky abdominal disease, and supraclavicular lymph node palpation.

A high inguinal orchiectomy (with removal of the entire specimen) is done for biopsy purposes. A transcrotal testicular biopsy or exploration should not be done because of the risk of tumor seeding.[155]

Radiologic techniques include chest radiographs with full-lung tomograms or chest CT scan to detect the presence of pulmonary metastases. Excretory urograms (intravenous pyelograms) are needed to determine any displacement by tumor of the ureters or kidneys, and they also indicate ureteral stenosis or obstruction.

Lymphangiograms and/or abdominal CT scans are important to demonstrate whether and to what extent the retroperitoneal lymph nodes are involved. These procedures, when used in individuals with later-stage disease, not only can help assess response to therapy but also can help plan for retroperitoneal lymphadenectomy.

Laboratory studies in testicular cancer have become important diagnostic aids in the last few years. Two radioimmunologic assays, alpha-fetoprotein (AFP) and beta human chorionic gonadotropin (HCG), have contributed to improved survival in individuals with testicular cancer.[154] These two tumor markers aid in detecting whether a germ cell tumor is present, marking the response to treatment, detecting the presence of residual tumor, and perhaps in differentiating between seminomas and nonseminomas.

Alpha-fetoprotein is a glycoprotein produced in the liver, yolk sac, and gastrointestinal tract of the fetus. Normal adult levels are less than 16–30 ng/ml. AFP is not elevated in patients with pure seminoma but is elevated in approximately 75% of those with nonseminomatous germ cell tumors.[156] High levels of AFP may indicate an aggressive biologic tumor.

Lactic acid dehydrogenase (LDH) is a cellular enzyme that is normally found in muscle (smooth, cardiac, skeletal), liver, kidney, and brain. Elevation of total serum LDH has been shown to be elevated in NSGCTs and in seminomas.[155]

Human chorionic gonadotropin is also a glycoprotein and is normally only produced in pregnant women. There are two subunits, alpha and beta. The beta subunit is the type that more specifically has been associated with testicular tumors. At present, 50%–60% of individuals with nonseminomatous germ cell tumors will have an elevated level of beta HCG.[157] With a short half-life of less than 24 hours, the HCG falls rapidly after successful treatment and is thus an excellent tumor marker. One study reported that up to 30% of men with pure seminoma also will have an elevated beta HCG level;[158] other researchers find elevated HCG levels in only 7% of seminomas.[155]

The clinical significance of AFP and HCG is to (1) corroborate initially the presence of a germinal testicular tumor, (2) determine whether treatment is effective (if the markers go down, the treatment is theoretically working), and (3) predict the prognosis and thereby aid in the choice of treatment both by helping to differentiate between seminomas and nonseminomas and by possibly indicating the biologic aggressiveness of the tumor.

It is important to determine the most appropriate interval of marker measurement. Factors to be considered are (1) the relationship between marker levels and disease, (2) cost, and (3) impact on the patient. Some researchers have argued for weekly testing of marker levels, particularly for patients with stage I disease or those at risk of recurrence. However, it is impractical to consider weekly testing in the face of the cost (procedural and lost wages necessitated by weekly appointments), impact on patient compliance and quality of life, and the effectiveness of current surveillance protocols.[159]

Classification and Staging

Numerous classification systems have been developed and many are in use today. A common staging system is presented in Table 50-20. Table 50-21 outlines the TNM classification system as described by the American Joint Committee for Cancer Staging and End Results Reporting.

Treatment

Surgery

Surgical treatment for testicular cancer includes high radical inguinal orchiectomy, which is considered a diagnostic step as well as the first phase of treatment; and possibly a radical retroperitoneal lymphadenectomy. Radical inguinal orchiectomy removes the testis, epididymis, a portion of the vas deferens, and portions of the gonadal lymphatics and blood supply. The remaining organ undergoes hyperplasia and produces enough testosterone to maintain sexual capacity, sexual characteristics, and libido.[160] After orchiectomy alone the potential for fertility theoretically remains the same. However, some studies have shown that a large percentage of men with testicular cancer had a low sperm count and/or reduced sperm motility after unilateral orchiectomy and before any other treatment.[161] The reason for the poor semen quality after orchiectomy is unclear. It is possibly attributed to the stress of surgery or abnormality of the remaining testis. Clinical experience has shown that semen with a sperm count below 40 million per milliliter and sperm motility under 60% has only a remote chance of inducing pregnancy by artificial insemination. As a result, banking sperm or preserving semen after surgery may be of no benefit.[161] The individual should be informed about the limitations of sperm preservation. Pretreatment fertility eval-

TABLE 50-20 Staging System for Testicular Carcinoma

Stage	Description
Stage A	Tumor is confined to the testicle; there is no evidence of spread beyond the confines of the scrotum
Stage B1	Evidence of *minimal* retroperitoneal lymph node metastases, determined either by retroperitoneal lymph node dissection or lymphangiogram (less than six positive nodes, well encapsulated)
Stage B2	Evidence of moderate retroperitoneal lymph node spread (more than six nodes)
Stage B3	Massive retroperitoneal lymph node involvement, usually a palpable mass on physical examination but without evidence of spread above the diaphragm (may directly invade contiguous structures)
Stage C	Metastatic tumor noted above the diaphragm or to solid visceral organs (liver, brain, or bone)

Source: Smith RB: Testicular cancer, in Hasdkell C (ed), *Cancer Treatment* (2d ed). Philadelphia: Saunders, 1985, p. 397.

TABLE 50-21 TNM Classification System for Testicular Cancer

PRIMARY TUMOR (T)	
The extent of primary tumor is classified after radical orchiectomy.	
TX	Primary tumor cannot be assessed (in the absence of radical orchiectomy, TX is used)
T0	Histologic scar or no evidence of primary tumor
Tis	Intratubular tumor: preinvasive cancer
T1	Tumor limited to testis, including rete testis
T2	Tumor invades beyond tunica albuginea or into epididymis
T3	Tumor invades spermatic cord
T4	Tumor invades scrotum
REGIONAL LYMPH NODES (N)	
NX	Regional lymph nodes cannot be assessed
N0	No regional lymph node metastasis
N1	Metastasis in a single lymph node, 2 cm or less in greatest dimension
N2	Metastasis in a single lymph node, not more than 5 cm in greatest dimension
N3	Metastasis in a lymph node more than 5 cm in greatest dimension
DISTANT METASTASIS (M)	
MX	Presence of distant metastasis cannot be assessed
M0	No distant metastasis
M1	Distant metastasis

Source: Beahrs OH, Henson DE, Hutter RV, et al (eds): *American Joint Committee on Cancer: Manual for Staging of Cancer* (4th ed). Philadelphia: Lippincott, 1992.

uation should be done for the person who wishes to father a child at a later time.

Lymphadenectomy

Retroperitoneal lymphadenectomy Retroperitoneal lymphadenectomy removes all perivascular tissue from the anatomic area that is bounded superiorly by the renal arteries and veins, laterally by both ureters, and inferiorly by the common iliac arteries to their bifurcation. This procedure is usually unilateral unless there is a large mass. Many autonomic nerves necessary for erectile potency and for ejaculation are located in this area, and surgery may damage the nerve supply to the prostate, seminal vesicles, vasa, and bladder neck. Therefore, ejaculatory ability may be altered, even if erectile potency is maintained. Bracken[160] reported that 90% of men who had undergone postretroperitoneal lymphadenectomy had a reduction in or total loss of ejaculate.

Modified retroperitoneal lymphadenectomy The effectiveness of treatment for stage I nonseminomatous germ cell cancer has allowed a focus on treatment strategies that offer maximum disease control with minimum treatment morbidity, including the issue of ejaculatory dysfunction after standard retroperitoneal lymphadenectomy.[1]

Lumbar sympathetic fibers have been determined to be important in the preservation of normal emission and subsequent antegrade ejaculation postoperatively.[162] For normal antegrade ejaculation to occur, neurologic pathways must coordinate three separate events: (1) closure of the bladder neck, (2) seminal emission, and (3) antegrade ejaculation.[1] The efferent impulses that promote constriction of the seminal vesicles travel down the spinal cord via the anterolateral columns. Emission is mediated by sympathetic fibers emanating from T12 to L3 thoracolumbar spinal cord. These fibers mingle to form the hypogastric plexus and then travel from the plexus via the pelvic nerves to innervate the seminal vesicles, prostate, and bladder neck.[1]

Modified retroperitoneal lymphadenectomy is a technique that limits the boundaries of lymph node resection in those patients determined to be without detectable lymph node metastasis. While various boundaries are used at different centers, most preserve the superior hypogastric plexus at and immediately below the bifurcation of the great vessels. This leaves the sympathetic nerve pathways necessary for ejaculation in place.

In one study of 75 patients who were treated with nerve-sparing lymphadenectomy to preserve antegrade ejaculation, all 75 were disease-free after 2 years and able to ejaculate normally.[163] Additional studies have supported these findings and establish modified retroperitoneal lymphadenectomy as a viable treatment option in low-stage nonseminomatous testis tumor.[164]

The advantages of the modified retroperitoneal lymphadenectomy include the preservation of ejaculatory ability, fewer complications, and aid in accurate staging of the disease. Critics point out that the modified procedure is only applicable to a limited number of patients. About 20% of men with NSGCT will have positive nodes on frozen section and will have to undergo radical lymphadenectomy. In addition, the relatively short follow-up after modified lymphadenectomy in most series may not yet demonstrate the true rate of local recurrence, which may increase with extended follow-up.

Radiotherapy

External beam radiotherapy is aimed at the lymph node areas. In the pelvic (retroperitoneal) region the ipsilateral inguinal, iliac, and bilateral paraaortic nodes are irradiated. In the chest the mediastinal and/or supraclavicular nodes are irradiated. The amount of radiation ranges from 20 to 35 Gy. (See the following section entitled "Treatment According to Histologic Type and Stage" for a discussion of how and when each of these two techniques is employed.)

Complications of radiotherapy are related to the port and dose of irradiation and vary from individual to individual. Side effects of radiation to the pelvic region may be fatigue, bone marrow suppression, and diarrhea. Even with testicular retraction and shielding, there may be radiation "scatter" to the remaining testicle. Rowley and colleagues[165] have determined that the degree of damage to sperm production depends on the amount of radiation exposure. A single testicular dose of 8–50 cGy could induce oligospermia (scant numbers of sperm), and 80–300 cGy can cause azoospermia (no sperm production). The recovery of spermatogenesis is also dose-related. At doses up to 100 cGy, sperm recovery requires 9–18 months, doses of 200 cGy require 30 months for sperm recovery, and doses of 600 cGy require 5 years or more to bring the sperm count back to preradiation levels.[160]

Chemotherapy

Chemotherapy has been used as an adjunct to other treatments, for disseminated disease, and for recurrences. Adjuvant chemotherapy has been attempted with both seminomas and nonseminomas. However, the experience with chemotherapy in the treatment of seminomas has more typically been limited to recurrent disease.[162] Chemotherapy as an adjunct to retroperitoneal lymphadenectomy for patients with stage B NSGCT is recommended by some. These experts feel that even though recurrent disease can be cured with an appropriate cisplatin combination regimen, prophylactic use of less-toxic outpatient chemotherapy can substantially reduce the recurrence rate and spare the patient the toxicities of a more aggressive regimen.[166]

The major role of chemotherapy in testicular cancer is in disseminated disease. In August 1974, early studies were begun at Indiana University on men with disseminated testicular cancer, combining cisplatin, vinblastine, and bleomycin (PVB).[167] An example of this original regimen includes cisplatin, 20 mg/m2/day for 5 days every 3 weeks; bleomycin, 30 units on days 2, 9, 16; and vinblastine, 0.2 mg/kg on days 1 and 2 every 3 weeks. This cycle is repeated three to four times.[167]

The result of this chemotherapy combination on nonseminomatous tumors has been remarkable. Einhorn[167] reports a regularly achieved 80% disease-free status and a relapse rate of approximately 10%, with approximately 70% long-term survivors. This chemotherapeutic regimen has essentially revolutionized the treatment of disseminated testicular cancer.

The toxicity of the PVB regimen, however, is considerable. The incidence of leukopenia and sepsis is high in these individuals. Other side effects reported include nausea, vomiting, and cisplatin-induced nephrotoxicity. Pulmonary fibrosis is an uncommon complication, but one associated with bleomycin. Myalgias, constipation, and paralytic ileus are all side effects associated with vinblastine. After having established an effective regimen, studies looked at reducing the morbidity associated with vinblastine.[157]

A recently completed study of 244 patients compared the effectiveness of the PVB combination of agents to the use of bleomycin, etoposide, and cisplatin (BEP). The difference in results was not found to be statistically different.[168] In addition, the incidence of neuromuscular toxicity was decreased with BEP.[168]

Chemotherapy also has been used in those approximately 30% of men who have relapsed or who were refractory to chemotherapy initially. A variety of treatment programs have been tried,[168] as follows:

- cisplatin plus doxorubicin
- cisplatin plus doxorubicin plus vincristine plus bleomycin
- cisplatin plus vincristine plus bleomycin (PVB)
- PVB plus actinomycin D plus cyclophosphamide
- cisplatin plus VP-16 (etoposide) plus bleomycin (BEP)
- cisplatin plus VP-16 plus ifosfamide

As mentioned previously, cure rates for testis tumors are very good, and as a result, attention is now focused on reducing morbidity. A body of data is developing to suggest that three cycles of chemotherapy may be used instead of four, thereby reducing exposure. Wozniak and colleagues[169] have conducted a study that indicates that VP-16 may be used instead of bleomycin with reduced morbidity and equivalent cure rates.

In the mid-1980s, ifosfamide emerged as the only drug other than etoposide to have single-agent activity against cisplatin-refractory germ cell tumors.[170] As a single agent, this drug failed to produce a durable cure. Ifosfamide and cisplatin demonstrate a preclinical synergy. Therefore, etoposide, ifosfamide, and cisplatin (VIP) and vinblastine, ifosfamide, and cisplatin (VeIP) were evaluated as salvage therapy. These regimens were able to produce a 15%–20% cure rate.[170] The dose-limiting toxicity of ifosfamide is hemorrhagic cystitis. Now that mesna is available for rescue, this side effect can be managed effectively.

Other agents are being assessed for their usefulness in testicular cancer. Carboplatin, an analog of cisplatin, is showing promise. Its dose-limiting toxicity is myelosuppression, but it shows a much lower rate of gastrointestinal, renal, and neurologic toxicities than its parent compound.[170]

Treatment according to histologic type and stage

Seminomas Stage A, B1, and B2 seminomas are very radio-sensitive. If there is no evidence of metastases and if retroperitoneal node involvement is not bulky, radical orchiectomy followed by radiotherapy of 25–30 Gy over 3 weeks is the primary treatment.[155] Men with evidence of retroperitoneal disease may receive additional 10 Gy to the involved nodal areas.

A recent study compared stage 1 seminomas treated with orchiectomy and adjuvant radiotherapy to those treated with orchiectomy and surveillance alone.[171] They found orchiectomy with surveillance worrisome because the natural history of the disease warrants close follow-up for at least 3 years after surgery and patient compliance over a long period of time was problematic. Therefore, these researchers support the current standard of management of this disease as orchiectomy and adjuvant radiotherapy.[171]

It is recommended that patients with bulky disease and any seminoma with an elevated AFP (high-stage seminoma—IIB, III) should receive primary chemotherapy. Seminomas, like NSGCT, are also sensitive to platinum-based regimens. Some of the successful regimens[155] include cisplatin, vincristine, and bleomycin (PVB); vinblastine, cyclophosphamide, dactinomycin, bleomycin, and cisplatin (VAB-16); and cisplatin and etoposide. Ninety percent of patients with stage III disease will achieve a complete response with chemotherapy.[155]

Nonseminomas With the revolutionary changes in management, stage A, B1, and B2 tumors now have the highest cure rate of any solid tumor. Historically, NSGCT had been treated with radiotherapy, retroperitoneal lymphadenectomy, and chemotherapy after orchiectomy. Today the most common approach to early-stage NSGCT is retroperitoneal lymphadenectomy and chemotherapy.[1] Postoperative radiotherapy, which prior to 1973 had been used routinely, has now been replaced for the most part by postoperative chemotherapy.

Einhorn[167] currently describes cisplatin plus VP-16 (100 mg/m2 × 5) plus bleomycin as standard therapy. The VP-16 protocol results in less neurotoxicity. Others recommend postoperative chemotherapy that is less toxic.[166] A "mini-VAB" combination is used that includes vinblastine, actinomycin D, and bleomycin. There is no cisplatin in this regimen.

Because 75% of the patients with clinical stage A disease will be cured by orchiectomy alone and the morbidity of RPLND can be significant, other alternatives have been explored. Beginning in the late 1970s, clinical trials were begun to evaluate the effectiveness of orchiectomy and surveillance for the initial management of nonseminomatous germ-cell cancer.[1] Patient selection is of the utmost importance in the success of this regimen, with accurate staging facilitated by the use of serum tumor markers, lymphangiography, and CT scan. One surveillance protocol consists of monthly serum tumor markers, chest radiography, and abdominal plain films and quarterly abdominal and pelvic CT scans for the first 2 years; during the third year, patients are examined quarterly with CT scans; during the fourth year, the patients are seen every 4 months and thereafter at 6-month intervals. If relapse is identified, then further treatment with chemotherapy or retroperitoneal lymphadenectomy, or both, is given.[1] In case of massive metastases to the retroperitoneal nodes or to other organs (stage B3 and C), preradiation chemotherapy typically using cisplatin, vinblastine, and bleomycin with or without doxorubicin is commonly used.[162]

Stage B3 and C testicular cancer generates the most treatment controversy. Aggressive primary chemotherapy using a cisplatin-based combination protocol is generally accepted as standard therapy. The controversy is usually over what drugs to combine with the cisplatin and whether or not retroperitoneal lymph node dissection should be done. Most centers advocate lymph node dissection for any residual disease after chemotherapy.[167] In other settings, surgery is only recommended in men who do not achieve a complete response from chemotherapy and in whom persistent retroperitoneal disease is suspected.[167]

Follow-up care

Patients with testicular cancer require follow-up care. Visits should include careful examination of the remaining testis, the abdomen, and lymph areas. Laboratory tests include AFP, HCG, and LDH levels. A chest x-ray and abdominal film should also be included. This follow-up usually continues for at least 5 years.[155]

Results and Prognosis

During the last few years the survival rate for individuals with testicular cancer has improved significantly, especially for the nonseminomas. The advent of tumor markers and the use of sophisticated chemotherapy accounts for this improvement. For nonseminomatous testicular tumors treated by orchiectomy plus retroperitoneal lymph node dissection, or radiotherapy plus chemotherapy for bulky disease, the average reported 5-year survival rates are approximately 96%–100% for stage A, 90% for stage B, and 55%–80% for patients with bulky retroperitoneal or disseminated disease treated with chemotherapy followed by surgery.[155]

For seminomatous testicular cancers treated by radiotherapy, the reported 5-year survival rates are 98% for stage I, 92%–94% for stage II A, and approximately 71% for stage B3 and C.[155]

Nursing Care of Individuals with Testicular Cancer

Surgery, radiation, and chemotherapy are all important components of testicular cancer treatment and play significant roles in the curative or palliative treatment of this disease.

Nursing role in early detection

The only routine recommended screening methods for early detection of testicular cancer are monthly testicular self-examination (TSE) and the annual physical examination by a physician. Various research studies have revealed that very few men practice TSE. Blesch[172] studied 233 professional men and found that only 9.5% practiced TSE. Reno[173] studied 126 male college students and found that only 13% had heard about TSE prior to the survey. Many men stated that vague discomfort and heaviness of the testicles alone would not seem serious enough for them to seek medical attention. This delay in consulting a physician probably accounts for the fact that 25% of seminomas[162] and 66% of nonseminomatous[166] testicular cancer has metastasized by the time it is diagnosed.

There is a need for nurses to provide information on testicular cancer and on the benefits of practicing TSE. The technique and importance of TSE should be taught to young men so that they can practice this health behavior regularly.

Nursing role prior to diagnostic tests and surgery

Orchiectomy is usually the first diagnostic and curative step for all primary testicular tumors. Further treatment is based on the type of cells found in the tumor. Orchiectomy has tremendous psychologic impact on many individuals. It may carry the connotation of castration and a sense of loss or reduction of masculinity. The nurse has a responsibility to provide psychological support for these men and to teach them the implications of the diagnostic procedures and the phases of treatment.

Several diagnostic procedures (previously discussed in "Assessment") assist in determining disease type and extent. To minimize the man's anxiety and fear, the nurse should provide easily understandable information about each test.

Orchiectomy is a relatively minor operation, but it may present great emotional trauma for the man and his family. Before surgery the nurse should assess the patient's knowledge and encourage the expression of fears and concerns. Preoperative patient teaching should include such matters as the location of the incision, intravenous infusions, coughing and deep breathing, and the availability of analgesics to control pain. Because of the location of the disease, patients may need a basic review of the anatomy and physiology of the surgical site and how the treatment will affect them.

Postoperative nursing care

For orchiectomy the individual generally has a high inguinal incision. The nursing emphasis during the immediate postoperative period is primarily on the alleviation of pain. Drainage tubes are uncommon for this type of surgery. A simple dry, sterile dressing is applied to the incision. The nurse should watch for excessive bleeding and should use aseptic technique in wound care. Perhaps the greatest postoperative complication is altered body image. Although a unilateral orchiectomy will not alter a man's potency, some individuals may feel that they are less than whole with only one testis. These men need to be assured that clinical experience has shown that men have normal sexual function after unilateral orchiectomy. The potential for fertility after unilateral orchiectomy is presumably unchanged if the remaining testis is normal. The actual fertility of these men may be eventually threatened by the treatments that follow orchiectomy such as lymphadenectomy, radiotherapy, and/or chemotherapy.

Retroperitoneal lymphadenectomy, if indicated, is generally performed a few weeks following orchiectomy. A transabdominal approach is commonly used. No drainage tube is necessary for the wound. A nasogastric tube is usually placed for stomach decompression the first few days after surgery. Because the abdominal organs are handled during this surgery, bowel inertia may result. The man receives nothing to eat or drink by mouth until bowel sounds are noted. The person also may have an indwelling urinary catheter to monitor urinary output. Hemorrhage is a major (but uncommon) complication after retroperitoneal lymphadenectomy because many of the lymph nodes resected are located around the large abdominal vessels. Accurate monitoring of vital signs will detect any signs of hemorrhage and shock. The incisional dressing should be checked often to assess any excessive drainage. Pain and nutritional status also should be assessed. Nutritional status is important for wound healing and for preparing the individual for further therapy. About 10 days after surgery, the man may start radiotherapy and/or chemotherapy.

Another major and more common side effect of retroperitoneal lymphadenectomy is the loss of ejaculatory ability. It is important to assure the man that his ability to have an erection and experience orgasm is usually not permanently impaired by the surgery.

Nursing care of individuals receiving radiotherapy

External beam radiotherapy is frequently the treatment of choice following orchiectomy for seminoma. Overall, individuals generally tolerate radiotherapy to the retroperitoneal regions very well. Some of the common side effects are mild nausea and vomiting, diarrhea, myelosuppression, and azoospermia. The transient nausea and vomiting may be controlled with antiemetics. Bone marrow suppression is usually mild unless the mediastinal and supraclavicular regions are also included in the treatment field. Azoospermia may result from inadvertent radiation scatter to the testis. To avoid unnecessary radiation exposure, a lead cup can be utilized to shield the remaining testis.

Nursing care of individuals receiving chemotherapy

Testicular tumors have responded to a variety of cytotoxic agents, including cisplatin, vinblastine, and bleomycin (PVB). If the patient does not respond to combination chemotherapy, the physician may initiate a salvage chemotherapy strategy that combines cisplatin with other active agents not previously used in the patient, such as VP-16 or ifosomide.[174]

The major side effects of cisplatin are severe nausea and vomiting, ototoxicity, and dose-related nephrotoxicity. Antiemetics should be given before the infusion and on a regular basis or as needed during drug infusion to control nausea. Prior to drug administration the nurse must be certain that the man has been well hydrated and has adequate renal function. Mannitol and furosemide are commonly given with cisplatin to maintain adequate urinary output. The nurse must administer this drug with needles and intravenous sets free of aluminum because the aluminum causes drug precipitation and subsequent loss of drug potency.

The major side effects of vinblastine are dose-related myelosuppression, neurotoxicity (constipation and paralytic ileus), mild nausea and vomiting, alopecia, and stomatitis. Because of the extravasation potential of this drug, the nurse must ensure vein patency prior to drug administration. Prophylactic stool softeners may be of help in preventing constipation.

The nurse should be aware that there is a potential for an anaphylactoid reaction with bleomycin, the third agent in the PVB regimen. A test dose should be given to individuals who have not previously received this agent. Emergency medications such as epinephrine, hydrocortisone, and diphenhydramine should be available at the bedside. The person may experience fever and sweats after receiving bleomycin. The nurse should obtain a baseline temperature prior to drug administration and monitor the temperature at least every 4 hours during the 24-hour period after chemotherapy. The other side effects of bleomycin are mild nausea and vomiting, mild myelosuppression, stomatitis, alopecia, and delayed pulmonary toxicity from an accumulated dose in excess of 300 U/m^2. Pulmonary fibrosis is by far the most serious side effect of bleomycin. Some of the manifestations are dry cough, dyspnea, rales, and pulmonary infiltrate.

Etoposide is incompatible with D5W and should be diluted in at least 20 equivalent volumes of sodium chloride injection. It is given intravenously over at least 30 minutes. Hypotension may occur if the drug is administered too fast. Be sure to ensure vein patency prior to drug administration because of potential tissue necrosis from drug extravasation.

Ifosfamide is given intravenously by slow intravenous push or continuous infusion over about 5 days. The patient should be well hydrated during the therapy to minimize the potential for hemorrhagic cystitis. Placement of a Foley catheter with continuous irrigation may be necessary to prevent this complication. The patient may experience some urinary frequency and dysuria. Nausea, vomiting, lethargy, and a mild degree of leukopenia may occur in most patients.

In general, treatment of testicular tumors can be lengthy and require surgery, radiation, and chemotherapy. The major nursing concern with this type of cancer is to anticipate the anxiety these young men will probably experience. There is a perceived and sometimes real threat to their sexual potency and fertility. Education, encouragement, and emotional support are essential nursing functions if these men are to cope fully with testicular cancer and its treatment.

REFERENCES

1. Sogani P: Evolution of the management of stage 1 nonseminomatous germ-cell tumors of the testis. *Urol Clin North Am* 18:561–572, 1991.
2. Boring CC, Squires TS, Tong T: Cancer statistics, 1992. *CA* 42:19–45, 1992.
3. Meikle AW, Smith JA: Epidemiology of prostate cancer. *Urol Clin North Am* 17:709–718, 1990.
4. Catalona WJ: Prostate cancer. In Wells SA (ed), *Current Problems in Surgery*. St. Louis, MO: Mosby Year Books, 1990, pp. 395–461.
5. Fowler JE Jr, Mills SE: Operable prostatic carcinoma: Correlations among clinical stage, pathological stage, Gleason histological score and early disease-free survival. *J Urol* 133:40–42, 1985.
6. Steinsberg GD, Carter BS, Beaty TH, et al: Family history and the risk of prostate cancer. *Prostate* 17:337–347, 1990.
7. Ross RK, Paganini-Hill A, Henderson BE: Epidemiology of prostatic cancer. In Skinner D, Lieskovsky G (eds), *Diagnosis and Management of Genitourinary Cancer*. Philadelphia: Saunders, 1988, pp. 40–45.
8. Noble RL: Production of Nb rat carcinoma of the dorsal prostate and response of estrogen-dependent transplants to sex hormones and tamoxifen. *Cancer Res* 40:3574–3580, 1980.
9. Ghanadian R, Puah CM, O'Donoghue EPN: Serum testosterone and dihydrotestosterone in carcinoma of the prostate. *Brit J Cancer* 39:696–699, 1979.
10. Ross RK, Bernstein L, Judd H, et al: Serum testosterone levels in healthy young black and white men. *J Natl Cancer Inst* 76:45–48, 1986.
11. Graham S, Haughey B, Marshall J, et al: Diet in the epidemiology of carcinoma of the prostate gland. *J Natl Cancer Inst* 70:687–692, 1983.
12. Rosenberg L, Palmer JR, Zauber AG, et al: Vasectomy and the risk of prostate cancer. *Am J Epidemiol* 132:1051–1055, 1990.
13. Morse RM, Resnick MI: Detection of clinically occult prostate cancer. *Urol Clin North Amer* 17:567–574, 1990.
14. Waisman J: Pathology of neoplasms of the prostate gland. In Skinner D, Lieskovsky G (eds), *Diagnosis and Management of Genitourinary Cancer*. Philadelphia: Saunders, 1988, pp. 150–194.
15. Badalament RA, Drago JR: Prostate cancer. In Bone RC (ed), *Disease-a-Month*. St. Louis, MO: Mosby Year Books, 1991, pp. 199–268.
16. Murphy GP: Screening for prostatic carcinoma—useful or not? EORTC Genitourinary Group Monograph 5: Progress and Controversies in Oncological Urology II. New York: Alan R. Liss, 1988, pp. 131–137.
17. Resnick MI: Background for screening—epidemiology and cost effectiveness. EORTC Genitourinary Group Monograph 5: Progress and Controversies in Oncological Urology II. New York: Alan R. Liss, 1988, pp. 111–120.
18. Thompson IM, Rounder JB, Teague JL, et al: Impact of routine screening for adenocarcinoma of the prostate on stage distribution. *J Urol* 137:424–426, 1987.
19. McClennan BL: Transrectal US of the prostate: Is the technology leading the science? *Radiology* 168:571–575, 1988.

20. Lee F, Littrup PJ, Torp-Pedersen ST, et al: Prostate cancer: Comparison of transrectal US and digital rectal examination for screening. *Radiology* 168:389–394, 1988.
21. Friedland GW, Change P: The role of imaging in prostate cancer. *Radiol Clin North Amer* 29:581–589, 1991.
22. Muldoon L, Resnick MI: Results of ultrasonography of the prostate. *Urol Clin North Amer* 16:693–702, 1989.
23. Brawer MK: Laboratory studies for the detection of carcinoma of the prostate. *Urol Clin North Amer* 17:759–768, 1990.
24. Oesterling JE: Prostate specific antigen: A critical assessment of the most useful tumor marker for adenocarcinoma of the prostate. *J Urol* 145:907–923, 1991.
25. Cooner WH, Mosley BR, Rutherford CL Jr, et al: Prostate cancer detection in a clinical urological practice by ultrasonography, digital rectal examination and prostate specific antigen. *J Urol* 143:1146–1154, 1990.
26. Whitmore WF Jr: Background for screening: Natural history and treatment. EORTC Genitourinary Group Monograph 5: Progress and Controversies in Oncological Urology II. New York: Alan R. Liss, 1988, pp. 123–130.
27. McCullough DL: Diagnosis and staging of prostatic cancer. In Skinner D, Lieskovsky G (eds), *Diagnosis and Management of Genitourinary Cancer.* Philadelphia: Saunders, 1988, pp. 405–416.
28. deVere White RW, Deitch AD: Flow cytometry in urologic cancer. In Williams RD (ed), *Advances in Urologic Oncology* (vol 1). New York: MacMillan, 1987, pp. 25–42.
29. Cooper EH, Siddall JK, Newling DWW, et al: Acid phosphatase, alkaline phosphatase and prostate specific antigen: Which markers should we choose? EORTC Genitourinary Group Monograph 5: Progress and Controversies in Oncological Urology. New York: Alan R. Liss, 1988, pp. 43–53.
30. Hardeman SW, Wake RW, Soloway MS: Two new techniques for evaluating prostate cancer. *Postgrad Med* 86:197–208, 1989.
31. Poon PY, McCollum RW, Henkelinan MM: Magnetic resonance imaging of the prostate. *Radiology* 154:143–150, 1985.
32. Catalona WJ, Whitmore WS: New staging systems for prostate cancer. *J Urol* 142:1302–1303, 1989 (editorial).
33. Beahrs OH, Henson DE, Hutter RVP, et al (eds): *Manual for Staging of Cancer* (3d ed) Philadelphia: Lippincott, 1988, pp. 177–179.
34. Kramer SA, Spahr J, Brendler C, et al: Experience with Gleason's histopathologic grading in prostatic cancer. *J Urol* 124:223–225, 1980.
35. Gleason DF, Mellinger GT, et al: Prediction of prognosis for prostatic adenocarcinoma by combined histological grading and staging. *J Urol* 111:58–64, 1974.
36. Paulson DF: Technique of radical perineal prostatectomy. In Skinner D, Lieskovsky G (eds): *Diagnosis and Management of Genitourinary Cancer.* Philadelphia: Saunders, 1988, pp. 721–734.
37. Lieskovsky G: Technique of radical retropubic prostatectomy (Campbell's procedure) with limited pelvic lymph node dissection. In Skinner D, Lieskovsky G (eds): *Diagnosis and Management of Genitourinary Cancer.* Philadelphia: Saunders, 1988, pp. 735–752.
38. Perez CA, Fair UR, Ihde DC: Carcinoma of the prostate. In DeVita VT, Rosenberg SA, Hellman S (eds), *Cancer: Principles and Practice of Oncology* (3d ed). Philadelphia: Lippincott, 1989, pp. 1044–48.
39. Lue TF: Male sexual dysfunction. In Tanagho EA, McAninch JW (eds), *Smith's General Urology* (12th ed). San Mateo, CA: Appleton & Lange, 1987, pp. 663–678.
40. Walsh PC, Donker PJ: Impotence following radical prostatectomy: insight into etiology and prevention. *J Urol* 128:492–497, 1982.
41. Walsh PC: Technique of radical retropubic prostatectomy with preservation of sexual function—an anatomic approach. In Skinner D, Lieskovsky G (eds): *Diagnosis and Management of Genitourinary Cancer.* Philadelphia: Saunders, 1988, pp. 753–778.
42. Walsh PC, Mostwin JC: Radical prostatectomy and cystoprostatectomy with preservation of potency. Results using a new nerve-sparing technique. *Br J Urol* 56:694–699, 1984.
43. Bigg SW, Kavoussi LR, Catalona WJ: Role of nerve-sparing radical prostatectomy for clinical stage B2 prostate cancer. *J Urol* 144:1420–1424, 1990.
44. Catalona WJ, Bigg SW: Nerve-sparing radical prostatectomy: Evaluation of results after 250 patients. *J Urol* 143:538–544, 1990.
45. Bagshaw MA: Radiation therapy for cancer of the prostate: In Skinner D, Lieskovsky G (eds), *Diagnosis and Management of Genitourinary Cancer.* Philadelphia: Saunders, 1988, pp. 425–445.
46. Hanks GE: Radical prostatectomy or radiation therapy for early prostate cancer. *Cancer* 61:2153–2160, 1988.
47. Carlton CE: Radioactive isotope implantation for cancer of the prostate. In Skinner D, Lieskovsky G (eds), *Diagnosis and Management of Genitourinary Cancer.* Philadelphia: Saunders, 1988, pp. 446–453.
48. Whitmore WF Jr: Experience with 125 iodine implantation in the treatment of prostate cancer. In Skinner DG (ed), *Urological Cancer.* New York: Grune & Stratton, 1983.
49. McConnell JD: Physiologic basis of endocrine therapy for prostatic cancer. *Urol Clin North Amer* 18:1–13, 1991.
50. Crawford ED: Hormonal therapy of prostatic carcinoma. *Cancer* Suppl 66:1035–1038, 1990.
51. Paulson DF: Role of endocrine therapy in the management of prostatic cancer. In Skinner D, Lieskovsky G (eds), *Diagnosis and Management of Genitourinary Cancer.* Philadelphia: Saunders, 1988, pp. 464–472.
52. Sogani PC, Fair WR: Treatment of advanced prostatic cancer. *Urol Clin North Am* 14:353–371, 1987.
53. Presant CA, Soloway MS, Klioze SS, et al: Buserelin treatment of advanced prostatic carcinoma: Long-term follow-up of antitumor responses and improved quality of life. *Cancer* 59:1713–1716, 1987.
54. Lunglmayr G: A multicenter trial comparing the luteinizing hormone releasing hormone analog Zoladex, with Zoladex plus Flutamide in the treatment of advanced prostate cancer. *Eur Urol* 18 (suppl 3):28–29, 1990.
55. Trachtenberg J: Hormonal management of stage D carcinoma of the prostate. *Urol Clin North Am* 14:685–694, 1987.
56. Einhorn LH: An overview of chemotherapeutic trials in advanced cancer of the prostate. In Skinner DG (ed), *Urological Cancer.* New York: Grune & Stratton, 1983, pp. 89–200.
57. Huben RP, Murphy GP: Management of advanced cancer of the prostate. In Skinner D, Lieskovsky G (eds), *Diagnosis and Management of Genitourinary Cancer.* Philadelphia: Saunders, 1988, pp. 473–482.
58. Henry JM, Isaacs JT: Relationship between tumor size and the curability of metastatic prostatic cancer by sur-

gery alone or in combination with adjuvant chemotherapy. *J Urol* 139:1119–1128, 1988.

59. Paulson DF, Moul JW, Walther PJ: Radical prostatectomy for clinical stage T1-2NOMO prostatic adenocarcinoma: Long-term results. *J Urol* 144:1180–1184, 1990.
60. Luckmann J, Sorenson K: *Medical-Surgical Nursing—A Psychophysiologic Approach* (3d ed). Philadelphia: Saunders, 1987, p. 1703.
61. Reilly NJ: Urinary incontinence: New attitudes and treatment options. *Innov Urol Nursing* 3(2):1–13, 1992.
62. Lamb M, Woods N: Sexuality and the cancer patient. *Cancer Nurs* 4:137, 1981.
63. Shipes E, Lehr S: Sexuality of the male cancer patient. *Cancer Nurs* 3:375–381, 1982.
64. Hilderly LJ: Radiotherapy. In Groenwald SL, Frogge MH, Goodman M, et al (eds), *Cancer Nursing: Principles and Practice* (2d ed). Boston: Jones and Bartlett, 1990, pp. 199–229.
65. Lukkarinen O, Kontturi M: Treatment of advanced prostatic carcinoma with a slow release depot LHRH analogue (Zoladax depot r). *Scand J Urol Nephrol* 110:109–112, 1988.
66. Taylor TK: Endocrine therapy for advanced stage D prostate cancer. *Urol Nurs* Sept: 22–26, 1991.
67. Johnson D, Babaian R, Von Eschenbach A, et al: Ketoconazole therapy for hormonally refractive metastatic prostate cancer. *Urology* 31:132–134, 1988.
68. Ross RK, Paganini-Hill A, Henderson BE: Epidemiology of bladder cancer. In Skinner D, Lieskovsky G (eds): *Diagnosis and Management of Genitourinary Cancer.* Philadelphia: Saunders, 1988, pp. 23–31.
69. Lillienfeld AM, Levin ML, Moore GE: The association of smoking with cancer of the urinary bladder in humans. *Arch Intern Med* 98:129–135, 1956.
70. Brownson RC, Chang JC, Davis JR: Occupation, smoking, and alcohol in the epidemiology of bladder cancer. *Am J Public Health* 77:1298–1300, 1987.
71. Claude J, Kunze E, Frentzel-Beyme R, et al: Life-style and occupational risk factors in cancer of the lower urinary tract. *Am J Epidemiology* 124:578–589, 1986.
72. Mommsen S, Aagaard J, Sell A: An epidemiological case-control study of bladder cancer in males from a predominantly rural district. *Eur J Cancer Clin Oncol* 18:1205–1210, 1982.
73. Lieskovsky G, Ahlering T, Skinner DG: Diagnosis and staging of bladder cancer. In Skinner D, Lieskovsky G (eds), *Diagnosis and Management of Genitourinary Cancer.* Philadelphia: Saunders, 1988, pp. 264–280.
74. Raghavan D, Shipley WU, Garnick MG, et al: Biology and management of bladder cancer. *N Engl J Med* 322:1129–1138, 1990.
75. Caroll PR: Urothelial carcinoma: Cancers of the bladder, ureter, and renal pelvis. In Tanagho DA, McAninch JW (eds), *Smith's General Urology* (13th ed). Norwalk, CT: Appleton & Lange, 1992, pp. 341–350.
76. Badalament RA, Drago JR: Bladder cancer. *Postgrad Med* 88:63–70, 1990.
77. Badalament RA, Fair WR, Whitmore WF, et al: The relative value of cytometry and cytology in the management of bladder cancer: The Memorial Sloan-Kettering Cancer Center experience. *Semin Urol* 6:22–26, 1988.
78. Mostofi FK: Markers of bladder cancer. *J Natl Cancer Inst* 80:1184, 1988.
79. Marini F, Signori GB, Valente R: The relationship between transurethral ultrasound and pathological findings in 16 cases of tumors of the bladder. *Prog Clin Biol Res* 260:271–274, 1988.
80. Javadpour N, Lalehzarian M: Magnetic resonance imaging (MRI) in bladder cancer. *Prog Clin Biol Res* 260:265–270, 1989.
81. Williams RD: Magnetic resonance in the diagnosis and staging of urologic cancer. In Williams RD (ed), *Advances in Urologic Oncology* (vol 1). New York: Macmillan, 1987, pp. 69–88.
82. Catalona WJ, Dresner SM, Haaff EO: Management of superficial bladder cancer. In Skinner D, Lieskovsky G (eds), *Diagnosis and Management of Genitourinary Cancer.* Philadelphia: Saunders, 1988, pp. 281–294.
83. Morales A, et al: Treatment of residual non-infiltrating bladder cancer with bacillus Calmette-Guerrin. *J Urol* 125:649, 1981.
84. Lamm DL, Thorde, Harris SC, et al: Bacillus Calmette-Guerin immunotherapy of superficial bladder cancer. *J Urol* 124:38–40, 1980.
85. Coplen DE, Marcus MD, Myers JA, et al: Long-term follow-up of patients treated with 1 or 2, 6 week courses of intravesical bacillus Calmette-Guerin: Analysis of possible predictors of responses free of tumor. *J Urol* 144:652–657, 1990.
86. Skinner DG, Lieskovsky G: Management of invasive and high-grade bladder cancer. In Skinner D, Lieskovsky G (eds), *Diagnosis and Management of Genitourinary Cancer.* Philadelphia: Saunders, 1988, pp. 295–312.
87. Richie JP, Shipley WU, Yagoda A: Cancer of the bladder. In DeVita VT, Hellman S, Rosenberg SA (eds), *Cancer: Principles and Practice of Oncology* (3d ed). Philadelphia: Lippincott, 1989, pp. 1013–1021.
88. Greven KM, Solin LJ, Hanks GE: Prognostic factors in patients with bladder carcinoma treated with definitive irradiation. *Cancer* 65:908–912, 1990.
89. Herr HW, Whitmore WF, Morse MJ, et al: Neoadjuvant chemotherapy in invasive bladder cancer: The evolving role of surgery. *J Urol* 144:1083–1088, 1990.
90. Webster GD, Khoury JM: Continent urinary diversion. In Devita VT, Hellman S, Rosenberg SA (eds), *Important Advances in Oncology 1992.* Philadelphia: Lippincott, 1992, pp. 137–155.
91. Bloom DA, Lieskovsky G, Rainwater G, et al: The Turnbull loop stoma. *J Urol* 129:715–718, 1983.
92. Greig BJ: Interventions of the ET nurse with the continent urinary Kock pouch patient. *J Enterostomal Ther* 13:226–231, 1986.
93. Kock NG, Nilson AE, Nilsson LO, et al: Urinary diversion via a continent ileal reservoir: Clinical results in 12 patients. *J Urol* 128:469–475, 1982.
94. Skinner DG, Boyd SD, Lieskovsky G: Creation of the continent Kock ileal reservoir as an alternative to cutaneous urinary diversion. In Skinner D, Lieskovsky G (eds), *Diagnosis and Management of Genitourinary Cancer.* Philadelphia: Saunders, 1988, pp. 653–674.
95. Heneghan GM, Clark N, Hensley BJ, et al: The Indiana pouch: A continent urinary diversion. *J Enterostomal Ther* 17:231–236, 1990.
96. Ahlering TE, Weinberg AC, Razor B: A comparative study of the ileal conduit, Kock pouch, and modified Indiana pouch. *Urology* 142:1193–1196, 1989.
97. Carroll PR, Barbour S: Urinary diversion and bladder substitution. In Tanagho EA, McAnnich JW (eds), *Smith's General Urology* (13th ed). Norwalk, CT: Appleton & Lange, 1992, pp. 426–438.
98. Swanson D: Cancer of the bladder and prostate: The

impact of therapy on sexual function. In von Eschenbach A, Rodriguez D (eds), *Sexual Rehabilitation of the Urologic Cancer Patient*. Boston: Hall, 1981, pp. 88–109.

99. Scott FB, Kantzavelos D: Erectile impotence after urologic cancer surgery treated with the inflatable penile prosthesis. In von Eschenbach A, Rodriguez D (eds), *Sexual Rehabilitation of the Urologic Cancer Patient*. Boston: Hall, 1981, pp. 240–249.
100. Boyd SD: Management of male impotency, including technique of penile prosthesis placement. In Skinner DG, Lieskovsky G (eds), *Diagnosis and Management of Genitourinary Cancer*. Philadelphia: Saunders, 1988, pp. 675–683.
101. Daniels JR, Skinner DG, Lieskovsky G: Chemotherapy of carcinoma of bladder. In Skinner D, Lieskovsky G (eds), *Diagnosis and Management of Genitourinary Cancer*. Philadelphia: Saunders, 1988, pp. 313–322.
102. Phipps WJ, Long BC, Woods NF: *Medical Surgical Nursing: Concepts and Clinical Practice*. St. Louis, MO: Mosby, 1987, pp. 212–230.
103. King A: Nursing management of stomas of the genitourinary system. In Broadwell D, Jackson B (eds), *Principles of Ostomy Care*. St. Louis, MO: Mosby, 1982, pp. 290–320.
104. Dreicer R, Williams RD: Renal parenchymal neoplasms. In Tanagho EA, McAnnich JW (eds), *Smith's General Urology* (13th ed). Norwalk, CT: Appleton & Lange, 1992, pp. 359–377.
105. Paganini-Hill A, Ross RK, Henderson BE: Epidemiology of renal cancer. In Skinner D, Lieskovsky G (eds), *Diagnosis and Management of Genitourinary Cancer*. Philadelphia: Saunders, 1988, pp. 32–39.
106. Waterhouse J, Muir C, Shanmugaratnom K, et al: *Cancer Incidence in Five Continents* (vol 4). Lyon, France: IARC Scientific Publications, 42:1–807, 1982.
107. Hammond EC: Smoking in relation to death rates of 1 million men and women. In *Epidemiological Approaches to the Study of Cancer and Other Chronic Diseases*. National Cancer Institute Monograph 19. Washington, DC: Government Printing Office, 1966.
108. Weir JM, Dunn JE: Smoking and mortality. A prospective study. *Cancer* 25:105–112, 1970.
109. Doll R, Peto R: Mortality in relation to smoking: 20 years' observations on male British doctors. *Br Med J* 2:1525–1536, 1976.
110. Kolonel LN: Association of cadmium with renal cancer. *Cancer* 37:1782–1787, 1976.
111. McLaughlin JK, Mandel JS, Blot WJ, et al: A population-based case-control study of renal cell carcinoma. *J Natl Cancer Inst* 72:275–284, 1984.
112. Wynder E, Mabuchi K, Whitmore W: Epidemiology of adenocarcinoma of the kidney. *J Natl Cancer Inst* 53:1619–1634, 1974.
113. Selikoff IJ, Hammond EC, Seidman HP: Mortality experience of insulation workers in the United States and Canada, 1943–1976. *Ann NY Acad Sci* 330:91–116, 1979.
114. Paganini-Hill A, Glazer E, Henderson BE, Ross RK: Cause-specific mortality among newspaper web pressmen. *J Occup Med* 22:542–544, 1980.
115. FingerKantor AI, et al: Epidemiology of renal cell cancer in Connecticut. *J Natl Cancer Inst* 57:495, 1976.
116. Ishikawa I, Saito Y, Shikura N, et al: Ten-year retrospective study on the development of renal cell carcinoma in dialysis patients. *Am J Kidney Dis* 16:452–458, 1990.
117. Carroll PR: Urothelial carcinoma: Cancers of the bladder, ureter and renal pelvis. In Tanagho EA, McAnnich JW (eds), *Smith's General Urology* (13th ed). Norwalk, CT: Appleton & Lange, 1992, pp. 351–358.
118. deKernion JB: Treatment of advanced renal cell cancer: Traditional methods and innovative approaches. *J Urol* 130:2–7, 1983.
119. Sufrin G, Chasan S, Golio A, et al: Paraneoplastic and serologic syndromes of renal adenocarcinoma. *Semin Urol* 7:158–161, 1989.
120. Pritchett TR, Lieskovsky G, Skinner DG: Clinical manifestations and treatment of renal parenchymal tumors. In Skinner D, Lieskovsky G (eds), *Diagnosis and Management of Genitourinary Cancer*. Philadelphia: Saunders, 1988, pp. 337–361.
121. Boswell WD: Diagnostic imaging in genitourinary cancer. In Skinner D, Lieskovsky G (eds), *Diagnosis and Management of Genitourinary Cancer*. Philadelphia: Saunders, 1988, pp. 237–263.
122. McClennan BL: Oncologic imaging-staging and follow up of renal and adrenal carcinoma. Cancer 67:1199–1208, 1991.
123. Graham TE, Rockey KE: Renal masses in adults. *Postgrad Med* 87:111–126, 1990.
124. deVere White RW, Deitch AD, West B, et al: The predictive value of flow cytometric information in the clinical management of stage O (Ta) bladder cancer. *J Urol* 139:279–282, 1988.
125. Richie JP: Carcinoma of renal pelvis and ureter. In Skinner D, Lieskovsky G (eds), *Diagnosis and Management of Genitourinary Cancer*. Philadelphia: Saunders, 1988, pp. 313–322.
126. deKernion JB: Renal cell carcinoma. In Haskell C (ed), *Cancer Treatment* (2d ed). Philadelphia: Saunders, 1985.
127. Flocks RH, Kadesky MC: Malignant neoplasms of the kidney: An analysis of 353 patients followed 5 years or more. *J Urol* 79:196–198, 1958.
128. Schefft P, Novick AC, Sheaffon RA, et al: Surgery for renal cell carcinoma extending into the inferior vena cava. *J Urol* 120:28–31, 1978.
129. Skinner DG, Lieskovsky G, Pritchett TR: Management of renal cell carcinoma involving the vena cava. In Skinner D, Lieskovsky G (eds), *Diagnosis and Management of Genitourinary Cancer*. Philadelphia: Saunders, 1988, pp. 694–703.
130. Cherrie RJ, et al: Prognostic implications of vena caval extension of renal cell carcinoma. *J Urol* 128:910–912, 1982.
131. McDonald M: Current therapy for renal cell carcinoma. *J Urol* 127:211–217, 1982.
132. deKernion JB: Lymphadenectomy for renal cell cancer: Therapeutic implications. *Urol Clin North Am* 7:697–703, 1980.
133. Marshall F, Powell K: Lymphadenectomy for renal cell cancer: Anatomical and therapeutic considerations. *J Urol* 128:677–681, 1982.
134. Skinner DG, Lieskovsky G, Pritchett TR: Technique of radical nephrectomy. In Skinner D, Lieskovsky G (eds), *Diagnosis and Management of Genitourinary Cancer*. Philadelphia: Saunders, 1988, pp. 684–693.
135. Stephens R, Graham SD: Enucleation of tumor versus partial nephrectomy as conservative treatment of renal cell carcinoma. *Cancer* 665:2663–2667, 1990.
136. deKernion JB, Ramming K, Smith R: The natural history of metastic renal cell cancer: A computer analysis. *J Urol* 120:148–152, 1978.

137. Brady LW Jr: Carcinoma of the kidney—the role for radiation therapy. *Semin Oncol* 10:417–421, 1983.
138. Swanson DA, Johnson DE, von Eschenbach AC, et al: Angioinfarction plus nephrectomy for metastatic renal cell carcinoma—an update. *J Urol* 130:449–452, 1983.
139. Rosenberg SA, Klotze MT, Muul LM, et al: Observations on the systematic administration of autologous lymphokine-activated killer cells and recombinant interleukin-2 with metastatic cancer. *N Engl J Med* 313:1485–1492, 1985.
140. Belldegrun A, Uppenkamp I, Rosenberg SA: Antitumor reactivity of human lymphokine activated killer (LAK) cells against fresh and cultured preparations of renal cell cancer. *J Urol* 139:150–155, 1988.
141. Fowler JE: Adoptive immunotherapy using lymphokine-activated killer cells. *J Urol* 139:148–149, 1988.
142. Bukowski RM, Goodman P, Crawford ED, et al: Phase II trial of high-dose intermittent interleukin-2 in metastatic renal cell carcinoma: A Southwest Oncology Group study. *J Natl Cancer Inst* 82:143–146, 1990.
143. Fisher RI, Coltman CA, Doroshow JH, et al: Metastic renal cancer treated with interleukin-2 and lymphokine-activated killer cells. A phase II clinical trial. *Ann Intern Med* 108:518–523, 1988.
144. Horoszewicz JS, Murphy GP: An assessment of the current use of human interferons in therapy of urologic cancers. *J Urol* 142:1173–1180, 1989.
145. Yagoda A: Chemotherapy for advanced urothelial cancer. *Semin Urol* 1:60–74, 1983.
146. Figlin RA: Biotherapy with interferon in solid tumors. *Oncol Nurs Forum* 14:23–26, 1987.
147. Irwin MM: Patients receiving biological response modifiers: Overview of nursing care. *Oncol Nurs Forum* 14:32–37, 1987.
148. Jassak PF, Sticklin LA: Interleukin 2: An overview. *Oncol Nurs Forum* 13:17–22, 1986.
149. Seipp C, Simpson C, Rosenberg S: Clinical trials with IL-2. *Oncol Nurs Forum* 13:25–29, 1986.
150. Henderson BE, Ross RK, Pike MC: Epidemiology of testicular cancer. In Skinner D, Lieskovsky G (eds), *Diagnosis and Management of Genitourinary Cancer.* Philadelphia: Saunders, 1988, pp. 46–52.
151. Mostofi FK: Testicular tumors: epidemiological, etiologic and pathologic features. *Cancer* 32:1186–1188, 1978.
152. Henderson BE, Benton B, Jing J, et al: Risk factors for cancer of the testis in young men. *Intl J Cancer* 23:598–602, 1979.
153. Friedman NB: Pathology of testicular tumors. In Skinner D, Lieskovsky G (eds), *Diagnosis and Management of Genitourinary Cancer.* Philadelphia: Saunders, 1988, pp. 215–234.
154. Johnson, Swanson D, von Eschenbach A: Tumors of the genitourinary tract. In Tanagho EA, McAninch JW (eds), *Smith's General Urology* (12th ed). San Mateo, CA: Appleton & Lange, 1987, pp. 330–434.
155. Presti JC, Herr HW: Genital tumors. In Tanagho EA, McAninch JW (eds), *Smith's General Urology* (13th ed). Norwalk, CT: Appleton & Lange, 1992, pp. 413–421.
156. Messing EM: Tumor antigens in the diagnosis, staging, and prognosis of urologic cancer. In Williams RD (ed), *Advances in Urologic Oncology* (vol 1). New York: Macmillan, 1987, pp. 43–68.
157. Higgs DJ: The patient with testicular cancer: Nursing management of chemotherapy. *Oncol Nurs Forum* 17:243–249, 1990.
158. Lange PH, et al: Serum alpha fetoprotein and human chorionic gonadotropin in patients with seminoma. *J Urol* 124:472–475, 1980.
159. Seckl MJ, Rustin GJS, Bagshawe KD: Frequency of serum tumor marker monitoring in patients with non-seminomatous germ cell tumors. *Br J Cancer* 61:916–918, 1990.
160. Bracken RB: Cancer of the testis, penis and urethra: The impact of therapy on sexual function. In von Eschenbach A, Rodriguez D (eds), *Sexual Rehabilitation of the Urologic Cancer Patient.* Boston: Hall, 1988, pp. 108–127.
161. Bracken RB, Smith KD: Is semen cryopreservation helpful for the patient with testicular cancer? *Urology* 15:581–583, 1980.
162. Smith RB: Testicular seminoma. In Skinner D, Lieskovsky G (eds), *Diagnosis and Management of Genitourinary Cancer.* Philadelphia: Saunders, 1988, pp. 508–515.
163. Donohue JP, Foster RS, Rowland RG, et al: Nerve-sparing retroperitoneal lymphadenectomy with preservation of ejaculation. *J Urol* 144:287–292, 1990.
164. Richie JP: Clinical stage I testicular cancer: The role of modified retroperitoneal lymphadenectomy. *J Urol* 144:1160–1163, 1990.
165. Rowley MJ, et al: Effect of graded doses of ionizing radiation in the human testes. *Radiation Res* 59:665, 1974.
166. Skinner DG, Lieskovsky G: Management of early stage nonseminomatous germ cell tumors of testis. In Skinner D, Lieskovsky G (eds), *Diagnosis and Management of Genitourinary Cancer.* Philadelphia: Saunders, 1988, pp. 516–525.
167. Einhorn LH: Chemotherapy of disseminated testicular cancer. In Skinner D, Lieskovsky G (eds), *Diagnosis and Management of Genitourinary Cancer.* Philadelphia: Saunders, 1988, pp. 526–531.
168. Williams SD, Birch R, Irwin L, et al: Disseminated germ cell tumors: Chemotherapy with cisplatin plus bleomycin plus either vinblastine or etoposide. *N Engl J Med* 316:1435–1440, 1987.
169. Wozniak AJ, Samson MK, Shah NT, et al: A randomized trial of cisplatin, vinblastine and bleomycin versus vinblastine, cisplatin, and etoposide in the treatment of advanced germ cell tumors of the testis: A Southwest Oncology Group study. *J Clin Oncol* 9:70–76, 1991.
170. Loehrer, PJ: Etoposide therapy for testicular cancer. *Cancer* 67:220–224, 1991 (suppl).
171. Duchesne GM, Horwich A, Dearnaley DP, et al: Orchidectomy alone for stage I seminoma of the testes. *Cancer* 65:1115–1118, 1990.
172. Blesch KS: Health beliefs about testicular cancer and self-examination among professional men. *Oncol Nurs Forum* 13:29–33, 1986.
173. Reno DR: Men's knowledge and health beliefs about testicular cancer and testicular self-examination. *Cancer Nurs* 11:112–117, 1988.
174. Einhorn LG: Complicated problems in testicular cancer. *Semin Oncol* 15:9–15, 1988.

PART VII

Delivery Systems for Cancer Care

Chapter 51

Development of Cancer Programs and Services

Luana Lamkin, RN, MPH, OCN

INTRODUCTION

The explosion of technology in cancer treatment, the economic constraints imposed by payers, and the growing sophistication of consumers have coalesced to form an unprecedented impetus for integrating cancer care programs. Most consumers are unwilling to accept fragmented care that causes them to traverse the country or even their communities to access the complex services they require. They are seeking full-service centers recognized for excellence in cancer care in their communities.

In addition, health care facilities that have historically provided acute care on a fee-for-service basis are now faced with declining bottom lines from prospective payment systems and a desire to capture the ever-increasing ambulatory-based care market. Most oncology physicians have been educated in major university cancer treatment facilities that offer a wide variety of cancer services under one roof. These oncology physicians want a similar scope of services to be available in the communities where they now practice.

During the 1970s the United States saw the beginning development of "cancer programs" in communities. This development accelerated in a piecemeal, one-service-at-a-time fashion in many acute care facilities. Today's emphasis has shifted to development of well-integrated, full-service, highly technical cancer care programs of high quality.

Scope of Cancer Programs in the United States

The Association of Community Cancer Centers (ACCC) is an organization founded in the late 1970s by a group of administrators and physicians who wished to improve cancer care in the community setting. The membership of ACCC has quadrupled in the last ten years to 779.[1] In 1988 the American Hospital Association's (AHA) Division of Ambulatory Care and Health Promotion conducted a survey of 1779 hospitals to ascertain the scope and developmental plans for outpatient oncology services.[2] Thirty-two percent had programs and 50% intended to expand oncology programs in the next 2 years, particularly those hospitals in the size range of 100 to 300 beds. Sixty-one percent of all cancer programs were initiated after 1981. The surveyors also found a delivery system that is seriously fragmented, reporting little, if any, interface between inpatient and outpatient oncology services.[3] The surveyors also found that data regarding the scope of services, numbers, and types of cancer patients being treated in different departments and the financial rewards of such care are frequently not available or not obtainable from a central data source. Though this particular survey focused on ambulatory oncology program development, it points to a growing desire on the part of hospitals to develop broader-scope oncology programs.

The Nurse's Role in Program Development

The nurse, as a cancer patient advocate, is in an excellent position to influence administrators to provide a full range of services to patients. Since 50% of hospitals have or will develop broader cancer programs, most oncology nurses have an opportunity to shape those programs and ensure that the programs respond to the voiced needs of patients, meet quality standards, and fulfill financial goals. Because nurses clearly understand the clinical needs of cancer patients, they should be integral members of planning teams for program development.

Frequently, nurses are called upon to become oncology program developers. In a recent survey of cancer program administrators, 53% of the respondents held nursing degrees.[4] The nursing process prepares nurses to be planners, implementors, and evaluators, not just of nursing care but also of broad programs. The nurse chosen for a development role generally has well-established relationships with pivotal physicians who can form vital coalitions of health care providers. Clinical nurses sought for such roles are cautioned to carefully define the new responsibilities and ensure that enough time is allotted for new administrative functions. Frequently, an outstanding clinical nurse is asked to accept an additional program-planning role while maintaining current patient responsibilities. An overwhelming work load can result in frustration for the nurse, the patients, and other program staff.

Every nurse who works in a setting where cancer program development and implementation is in progress can have a positive impact. Nursing staff and managers have the responsibility for keeping the program's development patient- or client-centered. They also become the day-to-day communication links between departments so the integration of patient care and program development flourishes.

Motivations for Developing Cancer Services

There are many varying reasons for developing an integrated oncology program. Program development can be capital-intensive and technology-driven; therefore, hospitals should be clear about their objectives for expansion. Typical motivations are listed in Table 51-1.

Some hospitals are part of communities that are changing. Either a growth in total population or the aging of a constant population will result in a higher volume of cancer patients to be served. Failing competitors may leave a vacuum in the oncology services available to a community. The community may also desire to have quality services close at hand rather than traveling long distances to a regional center.

Nearly every community can be assured of an aging population. The U.S. Census Bureau projects that by the year 2030, 21% of the population will be 65 years or older; today, only 12% of the population falls into that age category.[5] Coupled with the fact that the incidence of cancer among those over 79 years is one in

TABLE 51-1 Motivating Factors for Developing a Cancer Program

Meet a community need
Population growth
Population aging
Quality of competitors
Distance to other centers
Create a service niche
Distinguish hospital's services from competitors'
Develop significant expertise
Positively impact financial success
Maintain current market share
Gain new market share
Ensure continuity of care
Enhance communication
Multidisciplinary team planning
Integrate quality, cost containment, and databases
Shared services and supports

ten, it is clear that the volume of elderly cancer patients will grow significantly.

Oncology services provide an excellent way for a facility in a competitive environment to distinguish itself. Cancer has broad emotional appeal (unlike sports medicine, for example), and will affect nearly every family in the community (unlike trauma care, for instance). One hospital executive points out that if a facility has an excellent reputation for cancer care, which requires a high level of technology in the hands of caring professionals, its reputation for other services is also enhanced (Pritchard, personal communication, Sept. 1992).

From a financial perspective, oncology is not considered one of the highest-ranking service lines in health care delivery. Most facilities in the AHA survey reported at least breaking even in oncology.[2] The utilization of outpatient services for cancer care is high. If outpatient diagnostic records were coded to reflect the patient's primary diagnosis, most facilities would find that their overall oncology revenue is positive.[6] Even if oncology inpatient care is at the break-even level, expansion of outpatient cancer care services will help maintain market share as care shifts to the ambulatory setting. A thorough market analysis may also uncover an underserved oncology market or market that presently travels long distances for cancer care they would prefer to have closer to home if the scope and quality of services were equal.

Physicians are usually motivated by a desire for fuller services at one location for themselves and their patients. They may also project that their referral base will increase if they are associated with a facility known for its oncology programs. The hospital that can provide a broad range of services and a solid base of referring primary care physicians will have less difficulty recruiting oncology specialists.

The key to continuity of care is communication. Oncology patients are confronted with a highly complex health care system, which can mean numerous and changing care givers, physical surroundings, and forms of treatment. Our ability to prevent additional dysfunction and inconvenience for the patient is highly dependent upon a coordinated multidisciplinary program.[7] Our ability to communicate with other health team members is greatly enhanced if the program is structurally and organizationally bound.

Finally, the development of an integrated cancer program can help an organization meet its goal of providing quality care in an environment of cost containment. The ability to measure quality in a "systems" integrated approach is easier because it is not hampered by individual department loyalties and data keeping. Regulatory agencies and health care insurers are seeking measures that combine quality of care and cost competitiveness. By integrating the complex service delivery departments of an oncology program, systemwide quality data and cost data can be combined. Insurers are also now searching for centers of excellence for their clients. An integrated program can respond to the multiple needs for cost management, revenue management, and quality management.[8]

Defining a Cancer Program

A confusing list of descriptive titles for cancer programs exists. The National Cancer Institute (NCI) classifies cancer centers as comprehensive, clinical, basic science, or consortium programs.[9] As of August 1992, there were 57 cancer centers.[10] The NCI restricts the use of the term *NCI-designated* to those centers that have been awarded funding through a core grant award and meet eight major criteria. There are currently 28 designated NCI comprehensive cancer centers.[11]

In 1976 the NCI began a program to enlist patients cared for in community hospitals into clinical trials: the Cooperative Group Outreach Program (CGOP). The success of that program led to the initiation of the Community Clinical Oncology Program (CCOP) in 1983 to provide support for physicians to enter community-based patients into clinical research protocols. During its first 3 years, 62 community programs were designated in 34 states.[12] Each CCOP is required to enter a certain number of patients annually into clinical treatment and cancer control trials. Many community cancer programs choose to make their NCI affiliation part of their marketing strategy.

Many facilities without NCI designation have chosen titles to distinguish themselves in their geographic areas, such as *comprehensive cancer center, cancer center, oncology center, cancer institute, regional cancer center,* and *freestanding cancer center.* For the purpose of this chapter, the terms *cancer centers* and *cancer programs* are used interchangeably and are defined as hospital-based integrated cancer programs that offer the three major treatment modalities, diagnostic and screening services, in- and outpatient treatment units, and clinical research trial opportunities.

PROGRAM DEVELOPMENT

Most cancer programs have grown one department or service at a time. Each department has a manager who reports through a chain of hierarchy. As new departments are initiated, the reporting structure may or may not coincide with that of existing oncology departments. Because cancer care is so complex, the departments frequently have divergent reporting relationships and may or may not be guided by the same principles, goals, and mission. They may or may not communicate about these goals or even about the patients they jointly serve. Such scenarios frequently lead to piecemeal planning, competition, isolation, and poor continuity of care. It may seem that bringing together all the varied components into an integrated cancer center is at worst impossible or at best an arduous task.

The developmental process takes more than just hard work. Leadership, the ability to motivate individuals and groups to work for a greater good for the organization and ultimately the patients, is a necessity. Perhaps the ideal is the complementary leadership of a physician and an employee. The leadership team that has experience in the health care community, knows the stakeholders, has the ear of the top executives, and can envision the future of health care delivery will be successful in planning for a comprehensive program. The team that can address both the need to provide quality clinical care outcomes and the need to provide cost-effective care will succeed in implementing a program and maintaining its viability and growth.

Excellent programs can be designed and implemented without these leadership prerequisites if the team recognizes their shortcomings and seeks assistance. No blueprints exist for the perfect program, but successful programs developed across the country provide an excellent resource for those embarking upon this process.

Strategic Planning

A major frustration for many oncology managers is finding that just when they think they know their strategic direction, some internal or external factor changes the priorities. This generally is the result of not knowing the target, not appreciating the organization's mission, or not taking political factors into consideration. Because no plan is static, the process of developing a strategic plan requires the planners to assess these fundamental variables and develop a clear picture of the target.

Strategic planning is the process used to determine and evaluate alternatives for an organization to achieve its mission and objectives.[13] Generally, a strategic plan spans 3–5 years and sets out the major initiatives that will absorb the bulk of human and financial resources over the time frame. The plan identifies the priorities for future decision making and also defines what initiatives will not be pursued. There are a variety of methods for developing a strategic plan.[13–20] Perhaps the single most important element in the strategic planning process is knowing the process and adhering to it.

Planning process—the mission

Johnson[16] simplifies the planning process into three phases: (1) clarify values and aspirations, (2) analyze information, and (3) develop a strategy to create the image. The central focus of a strategic plan relies upon shared values.[21] Generally, an organization undertaking a strategic planning process begins by evaluating and, perhaps, revising its mission. This is usually done by a heterogeneous group of staff, physicians, and board members. The mission spells out the organization's intent (e.g., "Provide the highest-quality, most cost-effective health care"), whom it serves (e.g., "to the people of Hawaii regardless of their ability to pay"), and through what means (e.g., "through inpatient and outpatient care, education, and research"). The mission statement clearly spells out the basis upon which indigent care policy will be established, defines the market as a specific geographic area, and prioritizes patient care, education, or research. The strategic plan will be based upon these few critical phrases.

The next stage is to identify what service lines will be the cornerstones of future development. Most facilities have many services vying for resources. The bar graph in Figure 51-1 depicts inpatient volume by service line and payer at a hypothetical community hospital. Data such as this combined with an external assessment of growth potential will determine which services the organization will pursue. Strategic goals of the organization may be to develop centers of excellence in oncology and cardiology and to increase referrals from outlying geographic locations. It is not imperative that the entire organization embark upon a major planning effort for one service line to pursue its own strategic planning.

Planning process—data analysis

Identifying who will be involved in the planning process and who will serve as interim and final decision makers is imperative. The involvement of maximum numbers of staff and physicians is ideal for future commitment but not practical for working meetings. An alternative is to include a broad representation of professionals, administrators, patients, and community agencies in focus groups to gather information and ideas and to designate a small working group of six to eight people to actually evaluate data and develop a plan.[20]

One well-utilized framework for data gathering is the SWOT analysis to identify *S*trengths, *W*eaknesses, *O*pportunities, and *T*hreats.[19] In general, an internal assessment results in a list of strengths and weaknesses,

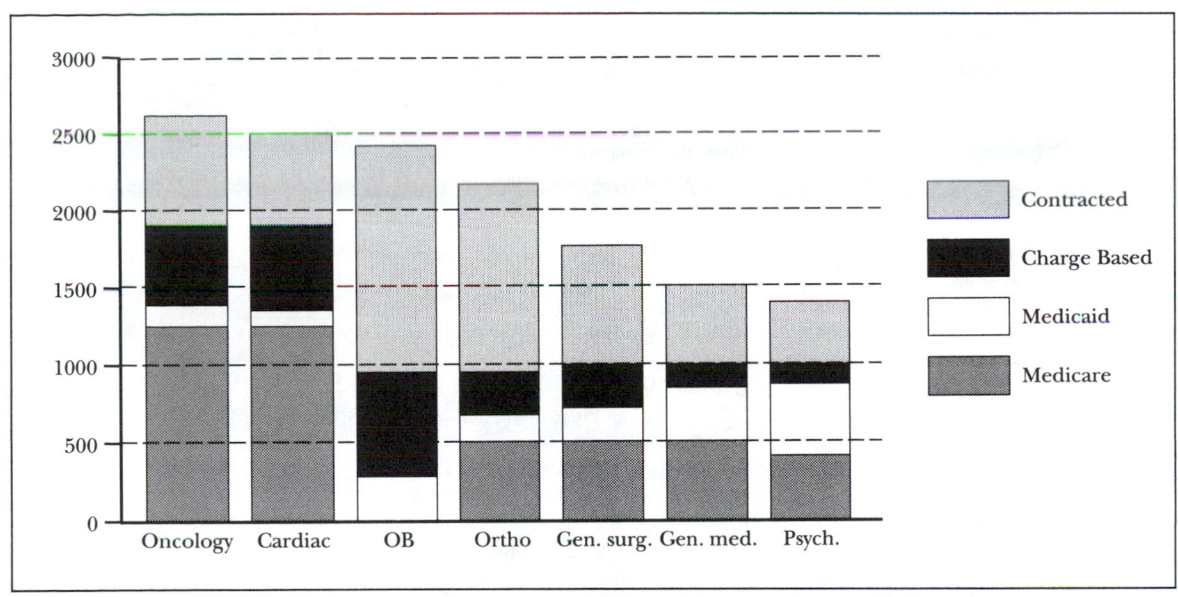

FIGURE 51-1 Inpatient admissions by payer by service line FY 1991. (Source: Reprinted from *Semin Oncol Nurs,* February 1993, Vol. 9, No. 1, p. 18, Saunders. Used with permission.)

while the external assessment results in a list of opportunities and threats.

Internal assessment data for an oncology program includes an evaluation of present services such as nursing care areas, surgery, laboratory, pharmacy, diagnostics, radiation therapy, and patient education. Human resources are evaluated including availability, general reputation, and skill level. Assessment of current physician strengths and weaknesses using these same criteria is of great importance. An assessment is also made of the physical facilities including condition, technological ability, location, accessibility, visibility, parking, and potential for renovation or expansion. Waterman[21] suggests further evaluation of the systems through which work is accomplished, such as the admitting process. He also suggests that the style or culture of the service area and the organizational structure under which it is managed should be evaluated.

A careful evaluation must be conducted with the financial department regarding present workload, payer mix, cost, charges, and revenue for oncology care.[14] Few organizations are capable of providing these details for analysis for both in- and outpatient services. If estimates or extrapolations are made, they should be developed with the financial and planning personnel who can attest to their validity.

An assessment is made of the present cancer market in the service area, demographics, the number of patients, where they are treated, and by whom. Patient satisfaction with the present care and services and other major providers' current programs and plans for expansion should be taken into consideration.

Projections for future work load and revenue are as difficult to develop as they are imperative. Anticipated changes in practice patterns, reimbursement policies of third-party payers, technology, personnel policies, shifts to managed care, and changes in physicians practicing at the facility should all be detailed as footnotes to market projections. Figure 51-2 depicts the progression of analysis for strategic planning.

Planning process—the strategic plan

The compiled list of strengths, weaknesses, opportunities, and threats will probably be long and require significant pondering. Can a strong reputation for inpatient nursing care be translated to an outpatient clinic to meet the growing shift to ambulatory care? Can the recruitment of a surgical oncologist meet the needs for specialized care of an aging population without alienating the general surgeons? The list of potential plans requires careful prioritization. One method of organizing these issues is to develop a position statement on each major issue and match the ideas to the full range of considerations. One list of major issues might be:

- mission and objectives
- physical plant
- education
- research
- human resources
- technology
- reimbursement
- organizational structure

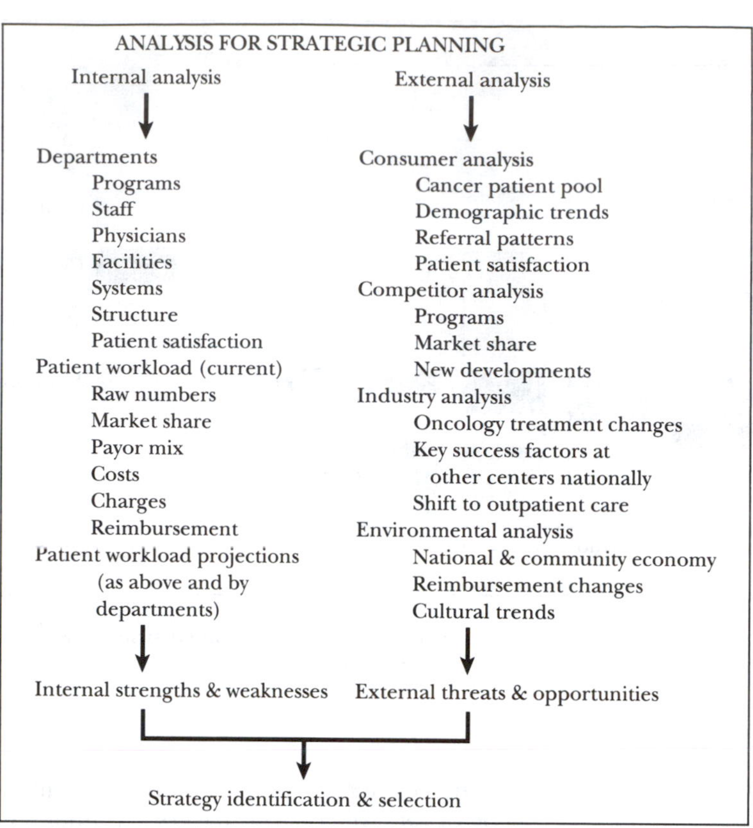

FIGURE 51-2 Analysis for strategic planning.

For each issue, develop a philosophical statement and long-range goals. The strategic plan is then presented to the focus groups who provided initial input, to the hospital administration, to the medical executive committee, and, finally, to the board of trustees for approval.

The development of a strategic plan requires considerable time and the cooperation of a variety of people, many of whom care more about the organization as a whole than they do about any specific service. Garnering cooperation from associated departments and ultimately making the plan advantageous to the entire medical staff and board challenges the leadership of the oncology team.

The strategic plan defines the long-range target and the sequence of development. To realize the strategic goals—for example, to increase outpatient oncology revenue by 12% in 2 years—specific programs such as a breast health center may be developed. These specific plans are called *business plans.*

The strategic planning process is an opportunity for groups from divergent oncology departments to become a multidisciplinary team and develop a shared vision. The process itself can enable the oncology service to see itself as a united group that will work together to implement its plans. The process serves as the basis for integrating oncology services. The team must now begin planning for individual business units while not losing track of the overall mission and goals. The group should continue to meet regularly to evaluate progress and reevaluate internal and external projections.

Planning process—the business plan

After a list of potential business plans has been developed from the strategic plan's goals, it is wise to establish a small working group to design very specific business plans. Include the staff and physicians who will ultimately manage or utilize the service. Business plans generally have a time frame of 1 year or less and are specific in terms of financial projections, milestones for development, and evaluation criteria. A sample business plan outline is shown in Table 51-2.

Most hospitals have criteria for the development and approval of new plans. For instance, a new program requiring greater than $25,000 initial outlay and/or greater than one full-time equivalent (FTE) requires rigorous financial assessment, as shown in Table 51-2. Criteria for approval might include positive cash flow in 24 months.

A similar but more focused assessment of internal and external environment is required to identify market share. Data for the assessment can be difficult to assemble. Some states have requirements for reporting data to health departments or health care associations. If the specific data required do not exist and estimates must be made by extrapolating the information, document the assumptions initially made so trends can be followed over time using the same assumptions. For most oncology services, market share can only grow by capturing a competitor's market or by identifying an unserved or underserved market component.

Part of a business plan's report should be quality

TABLE 51-2 Sample Business Plan Outline

1. Description
   A. Title
   B. Description of proposal
   C. Service objectives
2. Relationship to strategic plan
3. Assessment of competition in service area
4. Degree of risk
   A. Financial
   B. Liability
5. Implementation
   A. Time line of major planning and implementation milestones
   B. Responsibility and authority
   C. Resources required:
      - human resources
      - capital expense (one-time expense over $500 for items with a life greater than 2 years, such as computers, furniture)
      - operational expense (ongoing annual expenses such as personnel, office supplies, medical supplies)
      - space
6. Evaluation
   A. Measures of success
   B. Reporting requirements
7. Financial analysis
   A. Projected workload
   B. Projected market share
   C. Projected payer mix
   D. FTE requirements
   E. Supplies and expenses
   F. Capital expense—equipment
   G. Renovations
   H. Overhead cost (eg, housekeeping)
   I. Impact on other services (eg, admissions)
   J. Rate setting, reimbursement forecast
8. Pro forma income statement (3–5 years)
9. Net present value analysis (3–5 years)
10. Recommendation

Source: Reprinted from *Seminars in Oncology Nursing*, February 1993, Vol. 9, No. 1, p. 22, Saunders. Used with permission.

related and part should be financially based. Quality improvement will be discussed later in this chapter. Financial indices are most easily tracked if a new cost and revenue center is established at the time a new program is established. If, however, the new service will become part of an existing cost center (for instance, if a new breast health center's workload, revenue, and expense are reported as part of an x-ray department's aggregate budget) the type of data, frequency of reporting, and responsibility for collection should be identified before initiation of the service.

Frequently oncology services will include nonchargeable or undercharged services such as nutritional counseling and public education and screening programs that cannot financially support themselves independently. Be certain to identify ancillary charges that a new service will produce that can support these nonchargeable services. For example, a breast health center can result in additional localizations, biopsies, and surgery or radiation oncology care. It can be useful to establish systems to track subsequent care.

Even if a method for measuring additional referrals is not feasible, occasionally the development of a loss-leader service is advisable. Support groups may not generate revenue, but they do help establish the facility as a full-service oncology center. Without support groups, clients may be lost to other facilities that do provide such services. Nonrevenue or low-revenue services may be approved as pilot programs.

Organizational Structures and Options

A variety of structures for oncology services can function actively within an existing organization.[22] One's zeal for a perfectly functioning oncology program without the bureaucracy of a large organization may sway the program's creators to lobby for a product line management structure that can result in the greatest autonomy. Autonomy may compare favorably to a structure that has oncology services reporting to many different vice-presidents—for instance nursing, ambulatory care, ancillary services, and community relations. Consider those benefits the program's departments gain from the overall organization—for instance, billing services, night supervisor coverage, planning department activities, housekeeping, and the overall reputation of the organization. It is difficult for a single service line to be restructured to a product line management form while the rest of the organization maintains a functional arrangement. Because product line management structures have advantages and disadvantages, a number of variations have been implemented.

External pressures have forced nurses and administrators to view care from the client's perspective and not merely from that of the health care provider's perspective or convenience. Medicare initiated Diagnosis Related Groups (DRGs) in 1983, which aggregated all the services the patient receives during one hospitalization into one payment category. Since then, hospitals have examined all that a patient encounters in a hospital stay. This systemwide focus has led to new approaches to managing care. The Joint Commission on Accreditation of Healthcare Organizations (JCAHO) and others are advocating (and will soon require) continuous quality improvement of the systems and processes involved in providing care. We no longer point to a medication error as one person's mistake but search to find how we can reduce the chances of error in the system, and how we can avoid the extra hospital days such an error can cause. JCAHO is also studying oncology outcome indicators that will require tracking the cancer patient's outcome through the spectrum of health care interventions.[23] Critical pathways are a method of ensuring timely care and a tool for viewing a total health care experience from emergency room to discharge.

Finally, insurers who offer managed care policies are now seeking centers of excellence consisting of inpatient and ambulatory services for their clients. These external forces providing high-quality, cost-efficient, timely care to cancer patients support the idea that oncology services must be structurally integrated.

One option for integrating oncology services is product line management (PLM). "Options for implementation are so numerous that when a health care organization says it is implementing PLM, it conveys neither its goals nor corporate responses."[24] One sweeping definition of PLM is a structure where one single administrator is responsible for strategy formation, coordination of resources, monitoring of production and marketing, budgeting, and measuring results for each product line within the hospital.[52] A broader, more appealing definition is the bundling together of systems and services related to cancer management to enhance market success.[26] One consistent theme is that PLM includes the functions of planning, managing, and marketing one service line to some degree or other.[27]

In general, PLM, or as many health care administrators prefer to call it, *service* line management requires that one individual be responsible for developing, maintaining, and ensuring the quality and financial viability of a group of patients. Zelman and Parham[24] developed a typology of decentralization alternatives to implement PLM: traditionalist, market-driven, product-driven, and czar approach. With the czar approach, every department and function related to the product (oncology care) reports to the PLM manager. The other options are matrix organizations where the manager has responsibility for outcome but specific departments (nursing, pharmacy, laboratory) maintain their functional relationships. A hybrid of these, with some oncology-related departments reporting to the oncology manager, was most frequently reported in a survey of oncology managers in 1990.[28] Regardless of structure, PLM requires that the manager be the central focus of all information relative to the product line. This manager plans, motivates and controls, develops and markets new products, and continually reviews the growth and strength of the service.[22]

Figures 51-3, 51-4, and 51-5 illustrate three optional structures. Nursing units that report to a nonnurse oncology manager can lose their ability to maintain professional ties and stimulation. They frequently also lose those support services that can only be provided by a larger organization, such as float staff, supervisory coverage, and non–oncology-related continuing education. Many resourceful oncology managers have proven that they can successfully create a multidisciplinary team of oncology professionals who plan, budget, and support priorities for oncology together without having reporting control over nursing units. The greatest advantage to direct-line authority is the ability to implement change more quickly.[22]

In a survey of hospital executives, 58% reported that they had or were likely to adopt PLM in their institutions. However, only 4.2% were willing to delegate human and financial resources utilization to the PLM manager.[24]

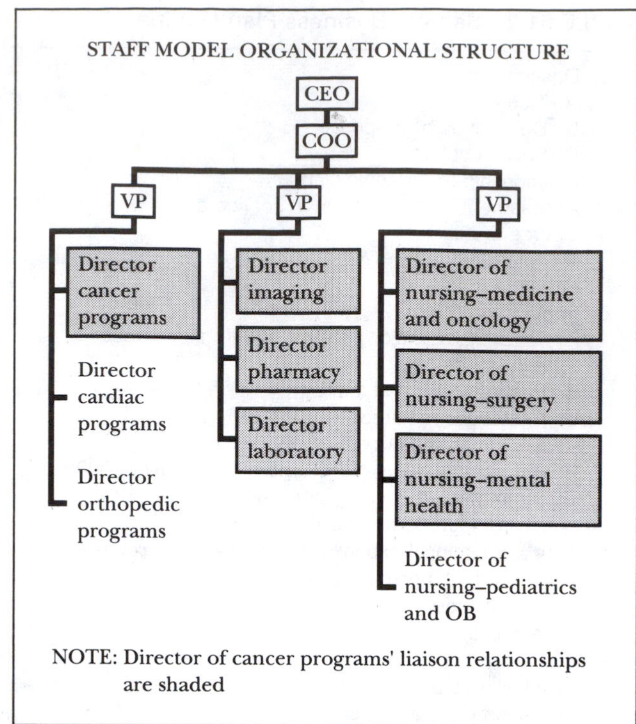

FIGURE 51-3 Staff model organizational structure option.

Management Personnel

The success of an oncology program depends not just on an array of services but also upon the ability of the leader to envision the future and be prepared to move quickly to meet changing needs. Many cancer programs are built around the reputation and dynamic leadership of one individual, frequently a physician. Ideally, leadership for a program is shared by a physician director and an administrative director.

Administrative director

In Fountain's 1990 survey of cancer program administrators,[28] she found a variety of titles and reporting structures. "Administrative Director" or "Cancer Program Director" was the most popular title. Fifty-one percent reported to either the CEO or a vice president; 12% reported to the oncology medical director. Over 50% of the following departments reported to the administrative director: marketing, education, research, tumor registry, hotline, outpatient clinics, and tumor board. Primary duties of the administrative director included marketing, education, program planning, and construction and renovation. Major challenges

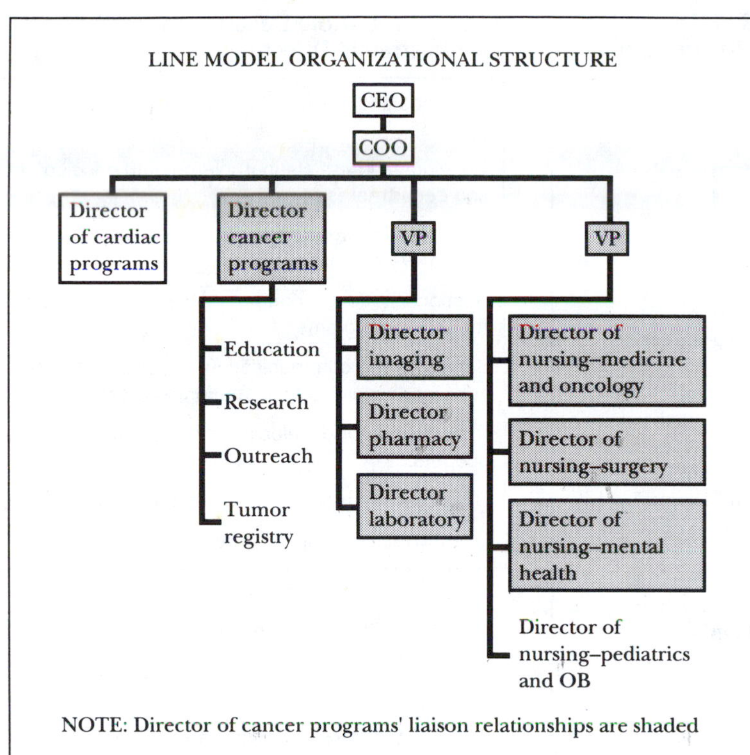

FIGURE 51-4 Line model organizational structure option.

were competition for market share and relationships with oncology physicians.

Table 51-3 lists typical duties of an administrative director. Depending upon the organizational structure, some duties will be in cooperation with others. Final authority should be clear in the director's job description. Folger and Gee[29] suggest in their chapter titled "Finding the Miracle Worker: The Hospital Product Manager" that the manager or director should be a combination of Lee Iacocca, Alexander Haig, Henry Kissinger, and Rodney Dangerfield.

Medical director

In general, the medical director of a cancer program is the liaison between physicians and administration.[30] The physician who accepts this challenge should be respected for clinical expertise and planning and administrative ability. Controversy continues regarding the advisability of a part-time medical director position. In a nonuniversity setting where the private physicians' livelihood depends upon patient referrals, a part-time medical director may have an advantage or a perceived advantage in gaining referrals. This can be ameliorated by a carefully written contract that is widely communicated to attending physicians. Full-time positions must be compensated well enough to allow a physician to abandon a medical practice. A full-time medical director has time to devote to planning, research, and quality assurance activities, but many programs are not large enough to require full-time attention.

In a brief survey of four oncology medical directors in community hospitals, the Health Care Advisory Board found that their time was divided thus: 15% administrative, 50% clinical, 20% research, 10% quality assurance, and 5% teaching. The duties of the administrator and medical director overlap, but clear job descriptions and role expectations and continuous communication can help distinguish the responsibilities (see Table 51-4).

In facilities where service line management does not include direct reporting relationships of nursing units or other oncology departments, it helps to develop an executive committee structure that includes the directors of nursing, radiation therapy, and others. This facilitates communication about problems and keeps the problem-solving process jointly managed.

Standards for Management

Fortunately, one embarking upon the development of an integrated cancer program has many resources to tap for defining quality and program development. JCAHO identifies seven major characteristics of quality health care: efficacy, appropriateness, accessibility, acceptability, effectiveness, efficiency, and continuity.[31] JCAHO is also defining specific oncology patient outcome standards that monitor primary medical care and are being beta tested by JCAHO (Table 51-5).

The American College of Surgeons' Commission on Cancer is the only agency that specifically "accredits"

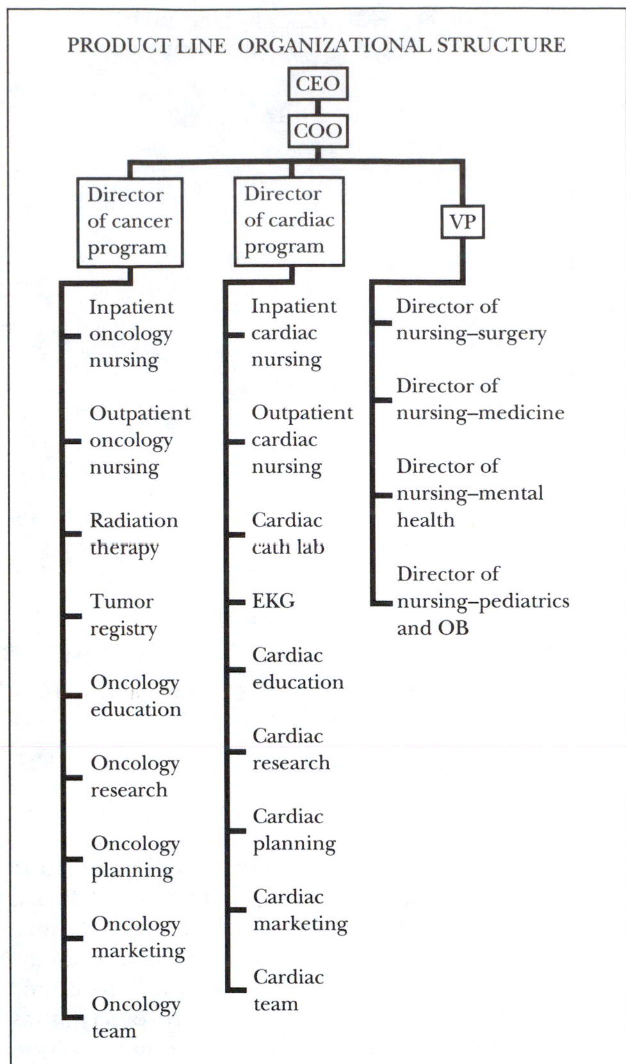

FIGURE 51-5 Product line management organizational structure.

TABLE 51-3 Role Description: Administrative Director

Develops and implements oncology strategic and business plans.
Develops and assists in implementing oncology programs and departments.
Responsible for information systems, analysis, and reporting of quality and financial data.
Responsible for marketing, education, and research activities for cancer programs.
Serves as the communication link between oncology services, hospital administration, and community agencies.
Responsible for developing and maintaining cancer program budgets.
Develops and monitors product pricing and contracts.
Directly manages specific departments.

TABLE 51-4 Role Description: Medical Director

Establishes a positive alliance between physicians and administration.
Develops, implements, and monitors quality improvement programs; ensures the quality of medical care.
Oversees oncology-related research.
Oversees or provides education for physicians and staff.
Plans new oncology programs and ensures adequate human and financial resources.

cancer programs. Their approval is based upon services available, medical staff qualifications, residency programs, research, tumor conferences, and the presence of a multidisciplinary cancer committee and tumor registry.[33] The College recognizes a vast array of cancer programs and approves eight separate categories.

The Association of Community Cancer Centers (ACCC) has developed standards and a self-assessment guide for the many facets of an oncology program.[34] The specificity of assessment criteria varies widely, but the guide is an excellent document to use as a comprehensive blueprint for developing goals and evaluation measures. The standards are presently being revised.

The Oncology Nursing Society has published many useful documents to assist in planning and monitoring individual programs. The *Resource Manual for Oncology Nurse Managers*[35] provides a brief update on 57 topics and an extensive bibliography.

COMPONENTS OF A CANCER PROGRAM

There is no specific answer to the question "How big must a hospital be to have a cancer program" and "What are the necessary components of a hospital-based oncology program?" Across the country, hospitals from 100 beds to well over 1000 beds have varying components based upon the organizations' strategic plans, internal and external assessments, and human and financial resources. Table 51-6 lists some of the hundreds of components program designers may consider. The ability to move from "small" to "large" depends upon the market to be served, the resources available, and the emphasis to be placed upon oncology as a whole or upon a specific component. Certainly, there are internationally recognized cancer centers that have few of the components listed because they have chosen to focus on one area. A long list of services or components should not be construed to imply quality.

TABLE 51-5 Joint Commission on the Accreditation of Healthcare Organizations' Oncology Indicators for Beta Testing

1. Surgical pathology consultation reports (pathology reports) containing histological type, tumor size, status of margins, appropriate lymph node examination, assessment of invasion or extension as indicated, and AJCC/PTN classification for patients with resection for primary cancer of the lung, colon/rectum, or female breast
2. Patients undergoing treatment for primary cancer of the lung, colon/rectum, or female breast with AJCC stage of tumor designated by a managing physician
3. Survival of patients with primary cancer of the lung, colon/rectum, or female breast by stage and histologic type
4. Female patients with invasive primary breast cancer undergoing initial biopsy or resection of a tumor larger than 1 centimeter in greatest dimension who have presence of estrogen receptor analysis results in medical record
5. Female patients with AJCC stage II pathologic lymph node positive primary invasive breast cancer treated with systemic adjuvant therapy
6. Patients with non–small-cell primary lung cancer undergoing thoracotomy with complete surgical resection of tumor
7. Patients undergoing pulmonary resection for primary lung cancer with postoperative complication of empyema, broncopleural fistula, reoperation for postoperative bleeding, mechanical ventilation greater than 5 days postop, or intrahospital death
8. Patients with resections of primary colorectal cancer whose preoperative evaluation by a managing physician includes examination of the entire colon, liver function tests, chest x-rays, and carcinoembryonic antigen (CEA) levels
9. Patients with resection of primary colorectal cancer whose preoperative reports include location of primary tumor, local extent of disease, extent of resection, and assessment of residual disease
10. Patients with primary rectal cancer undergoing abdominoperineal resections with 6 cm or more of free distal surgical margin present on specimen, as documented in surgical pathology gross description
11. Patients with AJCC stage II or III primary rectal cancer with documentation of referral to or treatment by a radiation or medical oncologist

Source: *1992 Accreditation Manual for Hospitals.*[23]

Inpatient Oncology Units

In a recent survey of 398 cancer programs approved by the American College of Surgeons' Commission on Cancer, 39% had dedicated medical oncology units and 33% combined medical and surgical oncology units.[36] Over 65% of respondents were from community hospital units varying in size from 6 to 60 beds. Hospitals strive to develop nursing units that will accommodate at least 90% of their average daily census for a particular patient population.

If the average daily census of oncology patients approaches 20, the argument to establish a dedicated nursing unit is strong. By centralizing the patients, nursing and support staff who prefer to care for cancer patients can be recruited. Daily experience with oncologic nursing problems increases the potential for expert nursing assessment and intervention. A specialized oncology nurse can devote continuing education time to oncology care. A dedicated unit also enables cancer team members to interact with each other continuously; therefore, they can appreciate the skills of each team member and use them appropriately. Daily contact raises the trust level and ability to work collaboratively toward quality patient care.

There are no set staffing standards for an oncology nursing unit. The Oncology Nursing Society's survey of inpatient nursing practice, however, details the state of the art for staffing, staff mix, acuity systems, and a myriad of other indicators for eight different types of oncology nursing units.[36]

In designing an oncology inpatient unit, Goldsmith's prediction that inpatient hospital use will decline by 20%–30% over the next 10 years should be taken into account.[37] He also predicts that the need for critical care beds and general beds with sophisticated monitoring will increase, while the need for general medical, and especially general surgical, beds will decrease. Creating an ICU within an oncology unit or transforming an ICU into an oncology ICU is widely debated. Either decision will require extensive training for nursing staff. The physical space available and the skill of the personnel in an individual setting will help shape the decision.

The decision to develop a bone marrow transplant program is major. The nursing unit where patients are to be cared for is an important factor, but not the sole driving criterion. The American Society of Clinical Oncologists and American Society of Hematology have recommended minimum criteria for the performance of bone marrow transplantation.[38] The criteria state that at least a two-bed unit be designated and that there be a patient isolation policy and a plan for air handling, either via HEPA filters or laminar air flow. In addition, the nursing staff should be full time, with a ratio of one nurse to two patients 24 hours per day. They should be committed oncology nurses with appropriate training in the care of immunosuppressed patients. The criteria also address additional facilities, personnel, volume, and reporting results.

Ambulatory Clinics

Oncology care, like health care in general, is shifting to the outpatient arena due to technology changes, cost constraints, and quality issues. Sixty percent of hospital-based oncology ambulatory clinics were developed after 1981.[2] During the first 7 months of 1990, hospital-based ambulatory revenues grew by 18.2%, compared with a 9.1% growth from inpatient revenues.[39] The strategic

TABLE 51-6 Potential Components of a Cancer Program by Hospital Size or Stage of Development

Component	Small	Medium	Large
Inpatient oncology units	Scattered oncology beds	Dedicated medical oncology and hematology unit or Dedicated medical-surgical oncology unit	Dedicated medical oncology and hematology unit Surgical oncology unit Pediatric oncology unit Bone marrow transplant unit Oncology ICU
Ambulatory clinics	Chemotherapy infusion center	Chemotherapy and biotherapy center Symptom management clinic Day hospital Breast health center	Chemotherapy and biotherapy center Symptom management clinic Day hospital Breast health center Risk assessment center Screening clinics Disease-specific clinics Treatment planning clinic 24-hour clinic Rehabilitation center Pain management
Radiation therapy	External beam therapy Simulation Medical physics Brachytherapy	External beam therapy Simulation Medical physics Brachytherapy Hyperthermia High-dose afterloader brachytherapy	External beam therapy Simulation Medical physics Brachytherapy Hyperthermia High-dose afterloader brachytherapy Intraoperative therapy Conformation
Surgery	Inpatient surgery Outpatient surgery	Inpatient surgery Outpatient surgery Laser surgery	Inpatient surgery Outpatient surgery Laser surgery Stereotactic radiosurgery
Laboratory	Clinical and anatomical pathology FNA cytology	Clinical and anatomical pathology FNA cytology Flow cytometry Immunology Cell analysis	Clinical and anatomical pathology FNA cytology Flow cytometry Immunology Cell analysis Cytogenetics Monoclonal antibody Cryopreservation Histocompatibility
Imaging	Mammography Fluoroscopy Ultrasound Nuclear medicine	Mammography Fluoroscopy Ultrasound Nuclear medicine CT MRI	Mammography Fluoroscopy Ultrasound Nuclear medicine CT MRI PET
Physicians	Medical oncologist Radiation oncologist	Medical oncologists Radiation oncologists Hematologists Surgical oncologist Immunologist	Medical oncologists Radiation oncologists Hematologists Surgical oncologists Immunologists GYN oncologist ENT oncologist Specialized pathologists
American College of Surgeons	Accreditation	Accreditation	Accreditation

(continued)

TABLE 51-6 Potential Components of a Cancer Program by Hospital Size or Stage of Development (continued)

Component	Small	Medium	Large
Support services	Social services Nutritionist Clinical nurse specialist Clergy Financial counselor Pharmacists	Social services Nutritionists Clinical nurse specialists Clergy Financial counselors Pharmacists Enterostomal therapists Pain management Psychologists Protocol nurses	Social services Nutritionists Clinical nurse specialists Clergy Financial counselors Pharmacists Enterostomal therapists Pain management Psychologists Protocol nurses Data managers Patient educators Group counselors
Home care and hospice care	Contracted home care and hospice services	Hospital-based home care including chemotherapy Hospital-based outpatient hospice	Hospital-based oncology homecare including chemotherapy Hospital-based inpatient and outpatient hospice
Rehabilitation services	Rehabilitation services with oncology focus	Oncology team of rehabilitation specialists	Expanded oncology team of rehabilitation specialists
Research	Cooperative group treatment protocols Nursing research to practice forum	Cooperative group treatment protocols Cancer control protocols Original treatment protocols Nursing research to practice forum Original nursing research	Cooperative group treatment protocols Cancer control protocols Original treatment protocols Nursing research to practice forum Original nursing research Epidemiologic research Basic science research
Oncology database	Tumor registry Inpatient financial data	Integrated quality outcome and cost data—inpatient and outpatient	Integrated quality outcome, cost and research data—inpatient and outpatient
Professional education	Staff competency-based continuing education Team education programs	Staff competency-based continuing education Team education programs Outreach education University affiliation	Staff competency-based continuing education Team education programs Outreach education University faculty appointments Regional conferences National conferences
Community education	Speakers bureau Focused education to employees and families	Speakers bureau Focused education to employees and families Work site program	Speakers bureau Focused education to employees and families Work site program School outreach efforts Mass media Cancer information hotline
Cancer screening	National screening participation annually	Continuing screening programs Mobile vans	Ongoing cancer screening and risk assessment clinics Mobile vans

decision to develop or expand outpatient oncology services hinges heavily upon the needs of the practicing physicians. Recent resource-based relative value system (RBRVS) legislation regarding physician payment has caused many physicians to attempt to capture a larger share of ambulatory care within their offices. Creative arrangements can be made with private physicians so that both the hospital and the physician can benefit from use of ambulatory hospital-based chemotherapy clinics.

The scope of ambulatory services for cancer care is broad, as depicted in Table 51-6. An ambulatory chemotherapy clinic requires an environment that is homelike, can accommodate both treatment beds and chairs, and is staffed by a team of registered nurses who are experts in oncology and outpatient care as well as trained in the safe handling of antineoplastic drugs. The ability to provide not just chemotherapy but also hydration, blood products, research protocol management, expanded hours, and an organized patient education program makes an ambulatory care setting advantageous to patients and physicians. Typically, oncology clinics offer patient and family education, patient assessment, direct administration of intermittent or continuous-infusion chemotherapy, symptom management, antiemetic and antibiotic therapy, and care of vascular access devices. According to guidelines of the Oncology Nursing Society, only specially trained registered nurses should administer chemotherapy regardless of clinical setting.[40]

Ambulatory settings should be physically situated so they are easily accessible to cancer patients. The challenges of ambulatory care also include the future of reimbursement and our ability to prepare patients and families for self-care. Patient education is especially important in the ambulatory setting, where a patient must learn how to become self-reliant after a brief clinic stay. Because teaching time is not usually billable time, less than adequate attention to patient teaching is frequently observed.

Chapter 54 explores a variety of ambulatory settings. One setting that is gaining popularity is the 24-hour clinic, where patients can receive routine treatment or seek urgent care at a time most convenient to them.[41] These clinics usually offer supportive care, urgent procedures such as thoracentesis, and a telephone triage nurse. The day hospital clinic is another type of ambulatory setting that offers similar services during expanded hours, but not 24 hours a day. Some centers have patient volume that supports the development of site-specific, symptom management, and/or pain management clinics. These clinics may be nurse-managed with physician back-up or may be physician-run. Outpatient rehabilitation services are available in most hospitals, but few have developed oncology-specific outpatient rehabilitation centers to provide exercise classes, support groups, and nutritional counseling in addition to physical, occupational, and vocational therapies.

Breast health centers have developed in many centers as a way to provide "one-stop shopping" for patients and clients.[42] These generally include screening and diagnostic services, risk assessment and risk reduction counseling, multidisciplinary treatment planning panels, and outreach education programs. The success of breast health programs in increased patient satisfaction and securing new patients for ongoing therapy will probably result in the proliferation of other site-specific or general cancer screening and risk analysis clinics.

No staffing or equipment standards currently exist for ambulatory centers. Surveys including staffing, staffing mix, salary, procedures performed, and reporting relationships are reported in two Oncology Nursing Society publications.[43,44]

Radiation Therapy

More than the other treatment modalities, radiation therapy requires a major commitment in terms of equipment and facilities. External beam radiation requires a minimum of 4000 square feet of partially lead-shielded space and equipment including a linear accelerator, simulator, and computerized treatment planning systems costing $1.0 to $1.5 million. The capital investment can prove profitable if a need for services exists. The American Hospital Association (AHA) survey of outpatient oncology programs found that the vast majority of hospitals offering radiation therapy reported oncology to be a financially sound service line.[3] The decision to initiate or expand radiation therapy services must be part of a well-developed strategic plan and a detailed business plan. A rule of thumb widely circulated purports that a volume of 20 to 25 patients per day will result in at least a break-even business venture.

Staffing a radiation department has become more problematic over the last few years. The radiation oncologist is a pivotal position for the success of a program. According to a recent AHA survey, radiation technologists (now known as radiation therapists) are in shorter supply than registered nurses.[45] Training for radiation technology requires 1 year in addition to diagnostic radiology training. Physicists and dosimetrists are also in short supply in many areas of the country.

Nine organizations collaborated to develop *Radiation Oncology in Integrated Cancer Management,* commonly known as "The Blue Book."[46] This publication describes criteria for the population base necessary to develop services, staffing recommendations, and quality improvement measures.

Technology continues to expand the capabilities of radiation therapy. Many programs include department-based computerized tomography machines to aid in treatment planning and high-dose afterloading brachytherapy (HDR) equipment. HDR allows patients who previously would have been admitted for implanted radiation to be treated on an outpatient basis. Hyperthermia technology is still a popular treatment in some areas of the country. Intraoperative radiation is generally limited to large university oncology programs since it requires the development of an operating room within the radiation department.

The Oncology Nursing Society published results from a national survey, "Salary, Staffing and Professional Practice Patterns in Radiation Therapy-Based Oncology Nursing."[47] The 1991 survey data are an excellent resource for establishing staffing patterns, mix, nursing responsibilities, and reporting structures.

Surgery

Nearly every cancer patient will undergo surgery during the course of the disease. Jako[48] reports that 62% of 5-year cancer cures (disease-free intervals) are provided by surgery alone. Future improvements in surgical success will relate more to the technical ability of the surgeon to locate and remove tumor growth than to equipment or technology breakthroughs.[49]

The cancer program administrator wishing to enhance surgical treatment looks to recruiting and retaining skilled specialists. The hypothesis that surgeons who frequently perform specific oncologic surgical procedures have greater success has been validated by Munoz et al.[50] In their study of 2627 elective surgical oncologic admissions, low-volume surgeons utilized greater hospital resources (resulting in losses instead of profits) and had a greater patient mortality than did high-volume surgeons.

Thus, the development of surgical expertise is part of the overall strategic plan. Goldsmith[37] estimates that by 2002, ambulatory surgery will account for 85% of all surgery. He advises providers contemplating expansion of surgical capacity to carefully evaluate their community's specific surgical demand curve adjusted for age before committing capital. Expansion funds might be better spent on organized perioperative teaching programs and home care visits as part of a same-day surgery package.

Surgery continues to be a profitable service even in a prospective payment environment. A patient's initial surgical experience may also be a deciding factor in where the patient prefers to have continuing care.

Diagnostics

Predictions are that the revolution in health care during the next 15 years will originate in the clinical laboratory and the pharmacy.[37] We will progress from the ability to diagnose cancer to the ability to do genetic screening for the future growth of cancer. Most community hospitals are not prepared to be involved in genetic research. All health care managers should, however, be prepared to rethink health care in terms of predictive tools, genetic counseling, and risk reduction classes in lieu of the present acute care model.

Clinical laboratory science offers a vast array of opportunity and support to oncologists. Basics for a cancer program include excellent pathologists, timely turnaround for routine blood work, and cytology on minute products (e.g., fine-needle aspirates). Many would argue that flow cytometry and cell analysis systems are standard oncology requirements. The cytogenetic laboratory is extremely helpful in a fairly narrow range of diseases. Reimbursement for these and other procedures is changing rapidly. Third-party payers make it their business to keep up with what is considered research. A technique that is classified as research for some diseases may be highly acceptable state of the art for another disease. These techniques require moderately expensive equipment and highly skilled physicians and technologists, who are also in short supply. Specific programs such as bone marrow transplant require significant laboratory support. Histocompatibility laboratories are necessary for allogeneic transplant, and cryopreservation capabilities are required for autologous transplant.[38]

With the exception of radiation therapy, imaging technology is the most expensive equipment-related component of oncology care. Most oncologists feel that computerized tomography (CT) and magnetic resonance imaging (MRI) capability is essential for diagnosis and follow-up of oncologic diseases. Positron-emission tomography (PET) is the next generation of high-tech diagnostic armaments.

Because the cost of imaging technology is so extraordinary, many administrators look to regional planning to meet their patients' needs.[51] Careful evaluation of the market expansion and volume projections for a region compared with projections for a community can provide direction for investments in expensive technology. Again, skilled physicians and technologists are necessary to appropriately utilize the new technology. A facility's geographic location and oncology patient volume will help determine if these experts should come from training existing staff, recruiting new staff at usually significant expense, or developing contractual relationships or joint ventures with competing regional facilities.[52]

A multidisciplinary team of oncology specialists is necessary to provide quality patient care. The team can be immeasurably helpful in determining what technology is necessary for a particular program. When a team understands the financial constraints for equipment and facility expansion, they can make valuable recommendations regarding expenditure priorities.

Physicians

It is imperative for a hospital wishing to excel in cancer care to have a cadre of oncology physicians who are board-certified clinical experts with good interpersonal relations skills. These physicians cannot just be medical staff members; they must be involved in priority setting and program development and feel that they are part of the hospital's oncology team.

Consumers are accepting more responsibility for decisions regarding their care and frequently have an impact upon which facility will be involved in their care. Most American patients seek a physician first, and that physician plays the major role in deciding where care is provided. Providing physician office space specifically for oncologists on the hospital grounds is the one way to meet physicians' convenience needs when deciding where to admit a patient. Physicians report that a skilled and caring staff and available technology are the other reasons they choose one facility over another.

The decision to recruit specialists is difficult. The Munoz study[50] implies that oncologic surgeons are more efficient and competent in performing oncologic surgery than general surgeons who occasionally perform cancer surgery. The recruitment of an oncologic surgeon must, however, be weighed against the potential of negatively impacting a group of general surgeons, particularly in a smaller community or facility.

Clearly, it is most advantageous if oncology physicians recruit partners to their practice or if a group of physicians and hospital administration joins forces to recruit a new specialty physician. For instance, most obstetricians-gynecologists do not welcome the idea of caring for ovarian cancer patients. If the patient volume is large enough, they are usually eager to recruit a gynecologic oncologist to their hospital.

The medical director of a cancer program can have a significant impact upon recruiting and retaining skilled physician specialists. The medical director can identify existing or new patients to support an additional specialist. The role of the medical director includes garnering support for additional specialists among colleagues for the benefit of patients.

American College of Surgeons Accreditation

More than 70% of patients newly diagnosed with cancer receive their initial care at an institution that is accredited by the American College of Surgeons' (ACOS) Commission on Cancer; 1200 hospitals are accredited nationally.[33] ACOS identifies eight categories of programs depending upon available resources. Two categories of community hospitals are distinguished by greater or lesser than 300 new cancer patients per year.

At a minimum, ACOS requires[33]:

- JCAHO accreditation
- a multidisciplinary cancer committee that is deemed a standing committee by institutional or medical staff bylaws
- a prospective patient-oriented multidisciplinary cancer conference on a scheduled basis (also known as tumor conference or tumor board)
- a cancer registry to monitor all types of cancer diagnosed and treated in the institution, staffed by at least one certified tumor registrar
- two patient care evaluation studies annually, one of which must include survival and comparison data
- an annual report to the medical staff regarding program goals and accomplishments and patient treatment and outcome data

Each of these requirements is imperative for an integrated cancer program. The existence of all criteria does not necessarily reflect successful integration of physicians and departments that have a common strategic goal, but they do help in moving toward that end.

Building a cancer program around ACOS accreditation criteria will urge employed staff and physicians to interact for the good of patient care (via tumor conferences) and for the good of the overall program (via cancer committee). This collaboration is the basis for patient care teams that provide multidisciplinary care on a daily basis. The National Joint Practice Commission[53] identifies five essential factors for collaboration among team members: communication, competence, accountability, trust, and administrative support. Kerstetter[54] describes a step-by-step process for developing a functional multidisciplinary oncology team and addresses the sensitive issue of potential lack of trust among team members.

The tumor registry is a cornerstone of the broad oncology data base necessary for an integrated cancer program. In many hospitals the only comprehensive patient outcome data base for any group of patients may be via the tumor registry. Because the registry is entirely overhead expense, it requires administrative support and frequently does not receive the attention it deserves for staffing and computerization. The need to link this information with financial data will be addressed later in this chapter.

ACOS also requires cancer programs to do the minimum of internal marketing through an annual report. The annual report can serve as an excellent tool for internal (and external) visibility. Besides providing data comparing the program's relative treatment success, it offers an opportunity to highlight the many support services for cancer patients.

Support Services

Standards of the Association of Community Cancer Centers describe the rationale for providing a myriad of services for cancer patients.[34] The decision to include specific services and the staffing required for each is dependent upon the volume of patients served and the mission of the organization but there are some basic services that are necessary. Ideally, support services are provided by team members who have special education in oncology and devote 100% of their time to oncology, but that is not always practical for a small program. Even a small program with a designated unit, radiation oncology, and ACOS accreditation can usually provide social services, nutritional counseling and intervention, spiritual counseling, financial counseling, pharmacy services, and an oncology clinical nurse specialist. ACCC identifies staffing standards for dietitians (one full-time oncology nutritionist for every 50 oncology inpatients) but not for other disciplines.[33] The hospital may not have a full-time cleric on staff, but even a small program can recruit volunteer clergy to become part of the oncology team. Financial counseling is of utmost importance to patients and families; they need to understand

and develop plans for the financial implications of their treatment decisions. This should be considered part of informed consent.

In larger centers, all team members usually devote 100% of their time to oncology. The reasons for developing a designated oncology nursing unit apply to each team member as well: Experience leads to expertise, continuing education is focused, team collaboration is enhanced, and improved-quality patient care results. If research is a part of the program, protocol or research nurses, data managers, and oncology pharmacists are required. A pain management team can be the most important support a patient experiences.

Chapter 62 details the rationale for and development of patient teaching. Patients undergoing cancer diagnosis and treatment require extensive education. In smaller facilities this may be the purview of the staff nurse in the inpatient and outpatient settings. Larger facilities may choose to establish a patient education department to assist in selecting adult and pediatric teaching methods, develop useful understandable materials, and schedule and provide group teaching programs to be followed by individual sessions. A program to assist clients going through diagnostic evaluation and diagnosis before initial entry to the hospital can be of great importance to the patient, family, and physician and will impact the patient's future choice of treatment facilities. A patient education department is in the best position to manage a resource center where patients and others can seek information on an as-needed basis.

Support groups and wellness groups are other services that can be offered regardless of size or complexity of the cancer program. These can be directed by oncology nurses, clinical specialists, clergy, social workers, or volunteers. In larger programs, a patient education department can schedule and staff programs and groups to meet the needs of specific clients. The "Yellow Pages" for the cancer nurse in this text (Part IX) lists contacts for national groups who assist in developing programs locally.

Support programs for cancer survivors help clients become maximally functional again. Long-term survivorship comes with a myriad of physical and psychosocial manifestations. See Chapter 22 of this text for information on the issues that support programs may need to address.

The list of additional support services to benefit patients and distinguish a program is limited only by imagination. Boutiques, weekend retreats, 24-hour hotlines, patient transportation, and family risk analysis programs are but a few of the many ideas. Patients and families cannot always articulate the services they would like, but they can describe the difficulties they are facing, which can lead to innovations. Accurate data collection and analysis can usually prove that nonrevenue services will be paid for by the excess revenues over expenses for the total oncology program. A skilled administrative director can use revenue analysis, cost containment trends, and the potential of new patients to obtain support for a nonrevenue service.

Home Care and Hospice Services

As cancer treatment has advanced and cost containment has become an everyday fact of life, the need for home care and hospice services has exploded. Chapters 55 and 56 deal with the philosophy of care, components of care, organizational structure, and reimbursement for these programs.

The question for the hospital-based cancer team is not whether home care and hospice programs are required but whether the hospital chooses to provide the service itself. Any program that wishes to provide the full continuum of care must incorporate home care and hospice either through contracting services or developing its own. The strategic plan should spell out this choice based upon patient need, existing programs, and existing resources.

The advantages to developing in-house programs are continuity of care and a broad philosophical base in holistic care. A home care nurse should be part of a hospital-based multidisciplinary cancer team regardless of organizational relationship. It may be easier to provide continuity between home and hospital care if, for instance, documentation forms and other communication tools are coordinated within the entire health care system. The continuum of care will be strengthened if the home care nurses have experienced the same chemotherapy education and certification as the outpatient clinic and inpatient nurses. Since experience generally leads to expertise, then the larger the oncology home care workload, the better prepared the home care staff will be to handle oncologic emergencies. A hospital that contracts home care services may choose to offer free education to home care and hospice staff.

The closer the relationship is between all care providers, the more the hospital-based team and the patient will benefit. The holistic health care philosophy of living while dying that emanates from the hospice staff can bring a more humanistic approach to the acute care setting. A close relationship between hospice and inpatient care providers also can help providers transfer their patients to another level of care with a minimum of anxiety and territorialness.

Rehabilitation Services

Most hospitals have basic physical and occupational therapy services available. An oncology program or cancer center can develop a team of oncology-focused rehabilitation specialists. Just as many nurses shy away from specializing in orthopedic or ICU nursing, many rehabilitation therapists choose not to deal with cancer patients. A rehabilitation team, including a physiatrist and physical, occupation, speech and hearing, and enterostomal therapists who have specialized training in oncology can help a cancer patient become a person with cancer. Art, music, recreational, and vocational therapists are integral team members. The question is not whether to provide rehabilitation as a part of the cancer program but how to integrate these services for each patient and how to best train rehabilitation specialists in the care of cancer patients. Chapter 53 contains a thorough review of cancer rehabilitation.

Research

The purpose of cancer research is to improve the survival and quality of life of cancer patients by providing care and documenting it so that others will benefit from our experience. Research is conducted in many arenas, from molecular biology to chemoprevention. It is a serious decision for a community hospital to engage in research.

Many agree that until we can consistently cure cancer we must conduct prospective randomized clinical trials of treatment options to determine efficacy. If one believes that clinical trials offer not only the method of determining efficacious treatments for future patients but also the best in state-of-the-art therapy randomized against new, potentially better therapy, then one would expect the majority of patients to be treated in such trials. However, the institution and key medical personnel must be committed to the rigorous clinical research process.

The humanitarian reason for participating in clinical trials is obvious. Borzo[55] identifies these additional advantages: increased patient referrals, marketing opportunities, early access to advanced treatment, facilitation of staff recruitment and retention, and program prestige. However, the cost of conducting research is escalating and community hospitals involved in cancer research should not plan on more than breaking even financially.

Clinical research can be conducted through cooperative groups, the Community Clinical Oncology Program, pharmaceutical companies, and other agencies such as the American Cancer Society (ACS). From 1971 to 1991 the number of research grant applications reviewed by the ACS more than doubled to 3000, while the number funded remains fairly constant at 500 to 600 per year. In 1991, ACS devoted nearly $90 million to research.[55] The only growing source of research funds is the pharmaceutical industry. Corporate studies are usually narrow in scope, testing only one drug, and the hospital may derive limited application.

In 1990, more than 23,000 patients were entered into cooperative group clinical treatment trials, representing about 20% of potentially eligible adults.[11] The 13 national cooperative groups include 4700 individual investigators from 1300 institutions and have over 500 protocols available for treatment. The "Yellow Pages" of this text list the cooperative groups and how to contact them. Cooperative groups have minimal accrual requirements and absorb some costs for pathology studies, radiology exams, and data management.

The National Cancer Institute's Community Clinical Oncology Program (CCOP) makes national clinical trials available at the community hospital level. During its first 3 years of operation, 14,000 patients were entered onto trials.[12] In 1991, 52 programs were ongoing in 27 states. CCOP members are required to enter 50 patients annually into treatment protocols and 50 patients into cancer control protocols. NCI approval for CCOP status and funds is highly competitive.

A community hospital that provides the opportunity for patients to be entered onto clinical trials must be prepared to develop an infrastructure to oversee the process. Engleking[56] suggests a protocol review process that projects the impact a study will have upon resources in the institution. The review process includes evaluating the case mix of patients the study would attract, the suitability of physical space available to care for patients, any additional workload, and a variety of operational issues.

Small facilities and programs can accommodate cooperative clinical trials if they commit to providing the diagnostic imaging and laboratory procedures necessary and the personnel to manage the protocols and data. Expanding involvement into original treatment studies requires a new level of commitment in terms of researchers, scientific review committees, and funding for nonreimbursable studies. To embark upon basic science or epidemiologic research requires further commitment to develop a solid research team.

Nursing research should be a part of every oncology nurse's practice. Even in small settings, a clinical specialist can assist nurses in evaluating published studies and translating the results into new procedures and daily practice. Most university schools of nursing are glad to assist an inexperienced nursing staff in developing research methodologies to incorporate into practice. A hospital-based nurse researcher is advantageous for growing programs.

Oncology Database

Throughout this chapter, reference has been made to planning based upon past performance and future projections internally and externally. During strategic planning and business planning, one usually finds some data lacking. This deficit may inspire the systematic development of an oncology database, such as the tumor registry.

Many software packages exist for capturing data to meet strategic requirements—ELM, Oncolog, Cancernet, to name a few. The data from such packages are patient-specific and generally relate to treatment and outcome over time. They do not provide the details of patient treatment that clinical trials require, nor the financial information required to evaluate present services or to plan for the future.

Insurers' requirements, particularly those of prospective payment insurers, have resulted in the proliferation of financial software packages that generally report patient charges by admission. These software programs may provide detail by DRGs, which does little to assist the oncology program manager[8] because these programs lack specificity for outpatient encounters and for tracking patient costs over time.[39] The cost of providing care by department may be included, but the data rarely detail the cost of care for oncology patients versus other categories of patients.

Clinical trial reporting requirements focus on the process and outcome of a particular treatment. Exhaustive data are collected regarding dosages, laboratory results, and side effects, but not regarding cost, charges, or reimbursement.

Ultimately, hospitals find themselves with three or four databases for cancer patients that cannot be integrated as useful planning tools. Developing the linkages between data sets can require expensive programming time and frequently does not match organizationwide data processing priorities.

An integrated product or service line defines more clearly the full scope of data that needs be identified. (See Table 51-6.) The leaders of the cancer program should identify the electronic data needs, platforms, and software that best meet their needs without requiring a revamp of the entire medical center's information system and without creating an abstracting and management nightmare. Data necessities, reporting formats, and product analysis formats will vary among institutions.[29]

Professional Education

Providing professional education programs can meet a variety of goals for a hospital-based cancer center. Such education increases the skills and knowledge of the program's physicians and staff and optimally leads to a better quality of day-to-day care. Involvement in educational activities increases the potential for physician and staff recruitment and retention and provides the center recognition on a national or regional basis.

The oncology team can develop a menu of basic classes to be offered to departments who care for cancer patients such as radiology, financial counseling, and housekeeping. The team may want to offer oncology education to affiliated agencies that provide continuing care to the facility's cancer patients such as home care, hospice, or physicians' offices.

Regional conferences or outreach education programs establish the center as a referral center for a geographic area. Many satellite arrangements are begun with the provision of basic oncology education by the referral center. Outreach education programs also give the center's staff an opportunity to develop teaching skills and can be used to recognize exceptional staff. National or regional conferences sponsored by the center not only bring experts to the community to share their knowledge but also expose national experts to the services that the community can provide. This may be the beginning of excellent cooperative relationships. Association with university schools of medicine, nursing, social work, and other health professions is ideal. Many professionals can only be recruited to a community hospital if a university clinical faculty appointment can be arranged.

Community Education

The purposes of health education are to provide the public with health information and to inspire them to adopt new health practices. The National Cancer Institute[51] has identified eight barriers to the public's acceptance of health messages, particularly cancer-related messages. The public is looking for easy, convenient, absolute answers to their health behavior questions, yet we have few to offer. This makes our jobs difficult, but far from impossible.

If a cancer center aspires to be comprehensive in its scope, community education must be an integral part of the program. Morra[58] describes an educational program development sequence, target populations, and examples of public education activities. Communication strategies can be interpersonal and mass-mediated and should be carefully sequenced.[59]

The hospital-based cancer program that chooses to embark upon public education should be clear about goals before developing target markets and methods. The AHA[60] suggests six possible benefits to hospitals:

- fulfills a mission to improve the overall health of the community
- generates new revenue sources (e.g., mammographies)
- increases patient referrals to hospital services (e.g., inpatient admissions)
- better utilizes hospital resources (increases outpatient care while decreasing emergency admissions)
- develops stronger relationships with employers
- enhances public image and community relations

Community education strategies are wide-ranging and should be linked to the target population and goals. A method may be as simple as providing a speakers bureau on types of cancer, cancer risk reduction, and nutrition. Highly successful specific programs are reported in work site cancer prevention programs.[60–63] Work sites, comprising 62% of the U.S. population over 16 years of age, provide the potential to interact over the long term with a fairly stable population.[61] Programs in smoking cessation, nutrition, and mammography are particularly popular. Interventions range from incentive programs, physician or nurse advice, behavior modification, group and individual education, and employer policy changes.[61] Beck et al.[64] describe a prevention and education program aimed at high-risk families identified through health education programs for senior high school students.

Families of cancer patients are another population that is eager for health promotion and cancer prevention information. This education can be integrated as part of more patient-centered education the family is receiving in the inpatient or outpatient hospital-based center. Formats such as that described by Love and Olsen[63] for patient education in the primary health setting could easily be altered to meet these needs.

Mass media offer a different level of community education. The disadvantage to the use of mass media is the lack of a target audience and the lack of control over the timing of message delivery. The advantage is the wide dissemination of information and potential to deliver a health message associated with the particular facility offering it. Public service announcements for radio and television are a popular option. Creative approaches include cancer risk reduction messages displayed free through a local grocers' association on paper grocery bags and by signage on public buses (Iwahashi, personal communication). In this situation the cancer program provided only camera-ready copy or fully produced placards.

The degree to which public education can be emphasized is dependent upon the program goals and resources. Small programs may concentrate on providing speakers from staff ranks. Larger programs may develop entire departments whose function is to provide public health education and screening programs.

Screening Programs

Closely related to community education are direct screening and early detection programs for the public. Screening programs offer an added benefit because they actually engage clients in a positive behavior that results in new knowledge about their health. The provider reaps the benefit of having potential clients actually enter the cancer program's doors and make judgments about the care and expertise they observe for future health care choices.

A broad scope of programs exists for developing cancer programs. The National Prostate Cancer Awareness program, co-sponsored by the American Urological Association and Prostate Cancer Education Council, supports hundreds of local facilities that offer free prostate cancer screening with a nationally produced public media campaign, standard forms, and standard results reporting. Many local units of the American Cancer Society assist in screening programs at many facilities by offering group advertising and aggregate results reporting.

The facility choosing to participate in mass screenings should carefully evaluate the medical evidence supporting the efficacy of screening, their ability to follow up with individuals regarding results, and their moral obligation to provide continuing care if disease is detected. Some cancer programs have elected to participate in free or low-cost screenings only if both the client and the client's primary physician are notified of the results. This decreases the perception that the facility or its physicians is more interested in gaining new patients than in serving a community need.

Many facilities have established ongoing screening clinics for cancers of the breast, colon and rectum, cervix, skin, testes, and oral cavity.[60] Well-established cancer risk analysis programs at major centers are often managed by nurses.[62]

Mobile vans equipped to provide cancer screening can now provide this service at work sites, shopping centers, and health fairs. The convenience to the client and active participation by employers who allow paid time for screening make these programs particularly appealing.

MAINTAINING PROGRAM PROMINENCE

There is a tendency among hospital managers to add programs and services, watch them grow, measure their activity in terms of volume, but rarely eliminate or completely refocus them. Perhaps the greatest attribute of PLM is that it holds one person, or perhaps jointly the medical and administrative directors, responsible for monitoring all oncology functions and revising them annually. Many cancer programs that held national prominence 10 years ago are now rarely heard from. To maintain market position, vigilance and vision are necessary. Product lines are intended to be based on strategic and business plans that can be measured and should be organized so that bureaucracy is held to a minimum and new opportunities can be grasped readily.

Ongoing Evaluation and Reprioritization

The director(s) is responsible for establishing monitoring criteria and ensuring that data are collected. A small executive team periodically (usually quarterly) analyzes the results of the data and revises the course of action as necessary. This group also updates the strategic plan annually and determines new business plans. Program evaluation in terms of quality and cost are intertwined; decisions to relinquish one program or develop a different one are based upon a combination of shifting external and internal environments.

Quality evaluation

Hundreds of pages have been written on quality assurance, total quality management, and continuous quality improvement, yet little has been written on improving the quality of an integrated program. Integrated cancer programs have an excellent opportunity to be the leaders in their facilities to establish system-oriented quality improvement. Because a team is already functioning, they are prepared to launch into quality improvement team projects and the groundwork has been set for a multidisciplinary systems approach in contrast to finger pointing. The team is prepared to test quality indicators throughout the system. The active involvement of physicians is integral to successful quality improvement, and the cancer team's medical director can play a major role.[65] Finally, most cancer teams are familiar with the research process and appreciate that significant fact finding must take place before system improvement solutions are identified.

It is ideal to have one quality manager responsible for assisting the oncology team and its components to develop and monitor their quality improvement strategies. Problem areas such as pain control, patient education, and continuity of care involve more than one department, and the solutions are frequently available from within the team membership. Critical paths and standard treatment protocols span many departments and are more easily put into place via previously organized teams. Fiengold et al.[66] report expected new profits of $600,000 for their 375-bed hospital after implementing oncology standard treatment protocols.

In Chapter 57, Dorsett describes cancer program studies completed or under way in the areas of comfort, nutrition, coping, information, and prevention and detection. Many studies could be replicated using patients from inpatient, outpatient clinic, radiation therapy, and support group settings from one cancer program. Dorsett[67] also lists oncology-related indicators, predictors, and guidelines for care from the literature. The quality of programs is judged differently by different audiences. The organized oncology program also has the opportunity to conduct patient satisfaction surveys that relate to the entire system that impacts the patient, not just one department or service. Such a questionnaire can inquire about continuity of care in a complex organization from the patients' perspective. Wiggers et al.[68] tested a 60-item satisfaction scale to assess the perception of 232 ambulatory cancer patients about the importance of and satisfaction with nine dimensions of patient care that cut across departments. Their data can be used to select questions that best meet the needs of the individual institution.

The results of the cancer program's evaluation should be reported not only to the oncology team but also to the cancer committee and general hospital administration. Selected data should be included in the program's annual report.

Financial evaluation

The cancer program's strategic plan sets overall goals for volume and income growth. Individual departments and services will have similar growth projections or goals. One method for ensuring support for nonreimbursable services is to ensure that aggregated oncology revenue and expenses are reported. Tumor registries, community education, and support groups are important qualitatively but result in no revenue. To collate aggregated data, cancer programs should be able to show by ICD-9 code: inpatient volume, inpatient length of stay, inpatient cost, inpatient charges, inpatient revenue, payer mix, productivity measure, and percent of change in all of these.

Outpatient data, especially comparable outpatient data, are much more difficult to determine in most facilities. By using a relative value scale to assign cost weights to services and procedures regardless of whether they were provided on an inpatient or outpatient basis, Young et al.[69] developed a framework for integrating inpatient and ambulatory payment systems. As another approach, Ford[70] created the composite patient encounter to equate outpatient care to inpatient care by measuring the production cost associated with each. He found the production cost per outpatient visit was about 10% of similar costs for one inpatient discharge in a 338-bed community hospital.

An integrated information system should be able to identify that a patient having an outpatient procedure (e.g., laboratory blood work or x-ray) is part of the cancer service line. Only by combining inpatient and outpatient data for an individual patient can actual resource consumption be measured and the actual profitability of the service line be judged.

Ideally, outpatient statistics should include by ICD-9 code: outpatient visit volume, outpatient visit cost, outpatient visit charge, outpatient visit revenue, payer mix, productivity measure, and percent change in all of these.

When tracking resource utilization, it is helpful to sort data by attending physician and by procedure. However, since many physicians are involved in each patient's care, these data may not accurately reflect only cancer care, especially for outpatient encounters.

Each cancer center will choose the data most important to its particular program. A sample annual tracking form is shown in Figure 51-6. If revenue per inpatient discharge is declining, additional reports regarding payer mix, revenue per payer, and/or revenue per ICD-9 code may become relevant. Because outpatient procedures vary so greatly by charge and complexity (e.g., MRI versus complete blood count), aggregate outpatient figures may not mean much by themselves but will uncover trends in patient volume and profit. Individual outpatient department oncology data are required to accurately track changes in volume and profit. A grand total for all oncology care revenue in excess of cost is probably the critical figure that will allow for future program development or will necessitate that the program determine what services are to be eliminated.

Plotting volume growth and income for oncology services can be enlightening. Figure 51-7 is an example in which in a hypothetical hospital, support group volume is growing but contributes negatively to the overall income, while surgical oncology admissions are growing slightly in volume and are profitable. Folger and Gee[29] provide formulas to develop such a graph and suggestions for strategies for each quadrant. For instance, a high-growth, high-income program may develop a strategy to invest additional capital, market the program further, and identify markets outside the service area. A high-growth, low-income service (e.g., research in this scenario) may cause the oncology

	Patient discharges or visits	Average LOS (inpatient only)	Average cost per visitor discharge	Average charge per visit or discharge	Average revenue per visitor or discharge	Total cost	Total charges	Total reim-bursement	Average revenue over expense	Total revenue over expense
Total cancer inpatient discharge FY ______										
% change from prior year										
Total cancer outpatient visits FY ______										
% change from prior year										
Chemotherapy clinic visits FY ______										
% change from prior year										
Radiation therapy outpatient treatments										
(Repeat for remaining departments)										

FIGURE 51-6 Sample annual oncology service line form.

management to rethink their commitment to research, identify new funding sources, concentrate on cost-cutting measures, or consider an increase in prices for other services to support research.

Shifts in reimbursement

Changes in payer mix and revenue from specific payers can significantly impact a program's strategy. DRGs, resource-based relative value system (RBRVS), and managed care have combined to provide an ever-changing basis for reimbursement. Predictions about future changes are risky at best. The prudent oncology manager is well versed in upcoming legislation and local market shifts so quick action can be taken. For instance, RBRVS legislation was debated for months before it was passed and quickly put into practice. The RBRVS payment change directly affected what many oncologists did in their offices and what they chose to send to the outpatient oncology department of a hospital. Astute managers dealt directly with their medical oncologists to determine what impact the physicians felt RBRVS may have on their referral patterns and to develop mechanisms that would favor both the hospital's and the physicians' incomes.

A cancer program's database, again, can assist it in preparing to negotiate with managed and contracted care. How large a volume must the hospital serve to grant a significant discount? How much revenue will be lost if the contract for care is given to a competitor? How much risk is the facility willing to share with a health maintenance organization? What other service lines are impacted? These questions will require a larger percentage of the program manager's time in the future.

Demographic shifts

We tend to focus our annual review of the strategic plan on internal strengths and weaknesses. It is wise to also evaluate shifts in the service area's demographics. Earlier decades saw mass migration from city centers to suburbs, which left intercity hospitals caring for a primarily indigent population. Similar changes have been felt as the population ages faster than it grows in

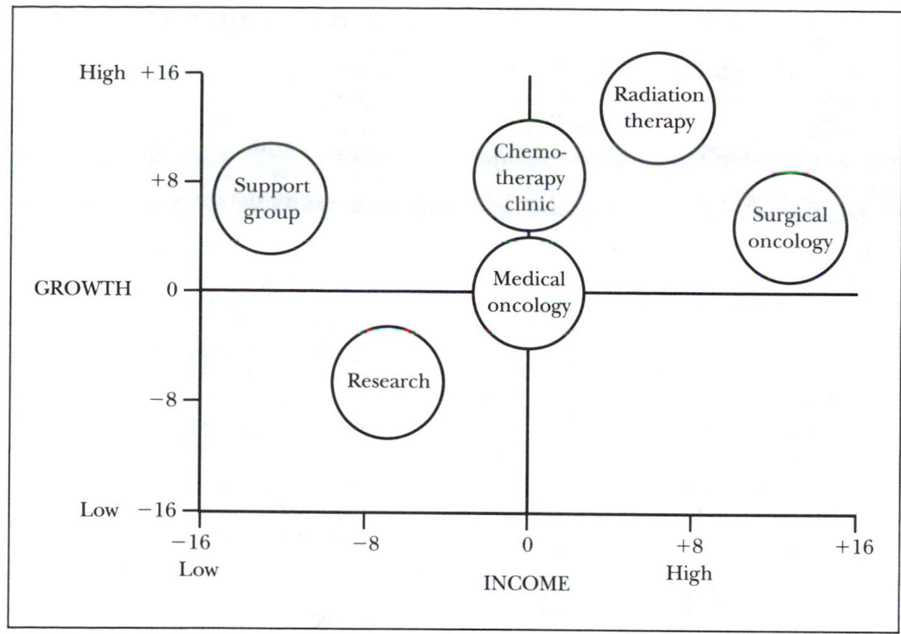

FIGURE 51-7 Sample graph measuring growth and income of oncology services.

volume. It is also wise to evaluate neighboring service areas to determine if a market segment elsewhere can be encouraged to travel for integrated services or if a satellite can be established.

Changes in technology

There is apparently a never-ending list of clinical innovations and new technology being developed in oncology. The more dynamic the oncology program team is, the more innovations they will be eager to implement. Because cancer itself, its diagnosis, treatment, and care are so complex, the innovations come from a variety of sources, and requests to the oncology program leadership are wide ranging. Most programs are not in a position of unlimited resources, either human or financial, and must make difficult and careful choices.

It helps to have a process and people in place to evaluate the relative merits of new technology. In most settings the oncology leadership recommends adoption of new technology, but final resource allocation is made at the administrative or board of trustees level of the organization.

Table 51-7 describes a process of evaluating new technology that has five basic steps: determining decision makers, oncology team evaluation, oncology team recommendations, business planning, and organizational approval. It is advantageous to build consensus among the oncology stakeholders before organizational approval is sought. The oncology leadership may be required to evaluate and prioritize a list of technology improvements. Most facilities have criteria determining when a business plan and financial analysis are required, for example, any program requiring greater than 1.0 full-time equivalent employee or greater than $25,000 capital expense. Before the financial analysis is undertaken, the oncology leadership should have evaluated its scientific merit, fit with the strategic plan, resources required, and relative benefit. The process for evaluating and adopting new technology or clinical innovations should be rigorous enough to ensure that funds are being wisely allocated, without being such a tedious process that team members are reluctant to suggest new ideas.

TABLE 51-7 Process for Evaluating New Technology

1. Selection of interim and final decision makers
2. Oncology team determines:
    - scientific merit
    - "fit" with the oncology strategic plan and mission
    - financial resources required
    - human resources required, necessary education
    - space necessary
    - timing, how urgent is the need, can it be incrementally implemented
    - barriers to implementation
    - relative yield
3. Oncology team or leadership consensus and recommendation
4. Business plan
5. Organizational approval

Physical Facilities

Perhaps the biggest undertaking for any oncology program is the development of new or renovation of existing facilities. A physical facility that is modern, visible, accessible, and has a comfortable ambience is advantageous in recruiting patients, physicians, and employees. The decision to develop or renovate is based upon the need for new space to meet projected volume of patients, new technology being introduced, or the need to consolidate present services in contiguous space.

After it is determined that new areas will be designed, small work groups are established to work with architects to perform functional analysis and help design the structure. The clinician's role is to tell the architect what will be done in the space (function), so the architect can design the space (form) in which to do the work safely and efficiently.[71] Work groups may include inpatient nursing unit, ICU or bone marrow transplant unit, outpatient infusion service, radiation therapy, medical physics, 24-hour clinic, physician office space, research laboratory, and support space. As functions within the spaces become defined, integration of some services such as outpatient reception and medical records, or patient teaching may be considered. Functional issues to address are listed in Table 51-8.

A matrix is frequently used to determine how closely adjacent new departments must be to each other and to existing departments within the facility.[20] For example, is it more important for the outpatient infusion center to be adjacent to the inpatient nursing unit, the pharmacy, or patient parking? Discussions regarding adjacent location will help determine if areas can be functionally related by use of computers or pneumatic tube systems in lieu of spatial contiguity.

It is important to not become so mired in space details that systems planning is neglected. The systems by which people, medical records, supplies, food, and drugs are moved, ordered, and returned are critical to the smooth functioning of all areas. There is no better time to realign systems and traffic flow than when planning new facilities.

Clinicians from each work group have the opportunity to design details within their areas. The nurse is in the best position to determine where the intravenous fluid control pump will stand, where oxygen can best be accessed, and where bathroom access is necessary. A friendly, comfortable environment and ambience are important to patients, visitors, and staff. Combining comfort and technology is a challenge, especially with constraints such as infection control and cost containment.

TABLE 51-8 Functional Issues in Facility Planning

Department Description
Purpose
Services
Population served
Educational programs
Anticipated changes
Current deficiencies
Statistical activity
Historical (3 years)
Workload
Inpatient days or outpatient visits per day
Average length of stay
Number of discharges
Number of special procedures (eg, total body irradiation)
Staff
FTEs by job description
Total number of people
Greatest number of people on duty at one time, including students, physicians, etc.
Projected (3 years)
Workload
Inpatient days or outpatient visits per day
Average length of stay
Number of discharges
Number of special procedures
Staff
FTEs by job description
Total number of people
Greatest number of people on duty at one time
Relationships (spatial and communication)
Intradepartmental
Interdepartmental
Planning considerations
Operational system (eg, cart exchange, pneumatic tube)
Major equipment and technology needs
Unique design requirements

Source: Reprinted from *Semin Oncol Nurs,* February 1993, Vol. 9, No. 1, p. 20, Saunders. Used with permission.

Marketing

Throughout this chapter a number of topics have been covered that many define as *marketing*—for example, community education, physician recruitment, and the annual report. Developing a marketing strategy and planning specific activities are increasingly important in this time of escalating health care competition. Perhaps the most important issue in marketing health care is to avoid promoting anything that cannot be delivered.

Many service line managers come from a school of thought where the sequence of events is: plan, market, manage.[29] Others believe that marketing follows the sound development and quality testing of a cancer program. Cancer care is generally an unwanted service. Gilden[72] points out that "cancer care marketing requires scrupulous sensitivity to even implied promise of the one real sought after benefit from cancer care—cure for the disease."

Developing the marketing plan is a four-step process. The first step is to conduct an internal and external assessment annually. The second step is to define the products (what services are to be provided) and marketing objectives. Third, identify target audiences. Target audiences in this case may be the patient, the physician, the internal hospital community, the external community, and purchasers of services such as managed care buyers. And, finally, plan specific activities to implement the strategy.

Most facilities have some kind of marketing or community relations department staffed by professionals who can guide clinicians in developing and implementing plans. They are important members of the team who can help avoid public or political blunders. For instance, they are expert at assisting clinicians to define the audience for specific publications. The American College of Surgeons accrediting body requires that the annual report be circulated to physicians. A marketing expert can assist in making such a publication serve a broader community market. One audience frequently overlooked is the internal hospital community who can serve as ambassadors of the cancer program if they know enough about it to describe it to their friends and neighbors.[72]

Table 51-9 lists examples of marketing activities for specific target audiences.

TABLE 51-9 Potential Marketing Activities by Target Audience

PATIENTS
Calendars imprinted with the facility logo for patients on research protocols with blood work and treatment dates highlighted
Annual picnic for former radiation therapy or bone marrow transplant patients in conjunction with National Cancer Survivors' Day
PHYSICIANS
Annual report with special letter of thank you to key referrers
Monthly or quarterly newsletter of new programs and new priority research protocols
Oncology classes at a discount rate for physician office staff
HOSPITAL COMMUNITY
First opportunity to participate in screening programs
First opportunity to tour new facility or program or preview new advertising
List every oncology employee in the annual report
EXTERNAL COMMUNITY
Low-cost or free cancer risk analysis or screening
Public forums on timely topics
Newspaper or television coverage of opening of new service
HEALTH CARE PURCHASERS
Luncheon presentations and tour of facilities
VIP receptions before public open house for new services
Annual report to managed care buyers and major employers

Satellites and Management Contracts

Depending upon size and sophistication, a cancer program may look for a large center with which to affiliate or may develop a network of smaller referring facilities.

A smaller program may establish an affiliation with a large, well-known cancer treatment center for a variety of reasons. The Healthcare Advisory Board surveyed a small number of programs in 1990 to determine why such agreements are helpful. They found that affiliations positively impact the image of a smaller facility, make new research protocols or treatment plans available, allow attendance at educational programs, provide consultation at a reduced rate, and create confidence that patients referred for specialized treatment will be returned to the referring physician.

Larger centers may establish agreements with smaller programs to ensure that patients needing specialized care will be referred to them, to gain accruals to research protocols, and to expand their geographic name recognition. Major centers such as Duke University and M.D. Anderson Cancer Center have recently established extensive linkages.[73]

Due to physical constraints or shifting demographics, opening satellite treatment facilities may meet a program's strategic goals. Freestanding cancer centers usually provide radiation therapy, chemotherapy, some diagnostics, and patient education. Lokich et al.[74] propose that freestanding centers must be involved in clinical trials but not in on-site basic research. These centers are usually advantageous to the sponsoring home facility because they capture a new market for tertiary care.

Another option for expansion is to offer management services to smaller community hospitals. A center could contract to provide chemotherapy for a community hospital including pharmaceutical agents, staff, procedure development, and day-to-day management or any combination of these. Major centers may also consider temporary or long-term staffing arrangements for difficult-to-fill positions such as tumor registrars, chemotherapy-certified registered nurses, or oncology rehabilitation specialists. Facilities that offer radiation therapy may be interested in contracting for medical physics with a large, more comprehensive center.

The decision to expand should be based upon sound strategic and financial planning. Expansion of services, whether the introduction of new technology in the center or development of a freestanding center, should not be allowed to detract from the basic quality of care upon which the center is built. Care must be taken to not expand at such a rate that resources, human and financial, are strained to the point of deterioration of basic services.

CONCLUSION

As nurses move from clinical roles to program development roles, they have the opportunity to affect a greater number of patients with their skill and knowledge. Nurses are in an excellent position to shape the future of integrated, full-service, highly technical yet caring comprehensive cancer programs. Nurses must work with administrators and physicians using the planning and communication skills they have developed. Many will be challenged to gain new knowledge in strategic and business planning and financial analysis so that they are as well respected in the board room as at the bedside.

This chapter suggests planning guidelines, possible cancer program components, and expansion ideas to maintain prominence. Each nurse must evaluate the present situation, internally and externally, and the potential for growth in a particular setting. With the nurse rests the responsibility to ensure that planning and implementation, at whatever level, remains patient-centered.

REFERENCES

1. Association of Community Cancer Centers: *Community Cancer Programs in the United States 1989–1990.* Rockville, MD: Association of Community Cancer Centers, 1990.
2. Sandrik K: Who's managing outpatient programs? *Hospitals* 64(3):33–36, 1990.
3. Nathanson SN, Lerman D: Directions in cancer care. In Nathanson SN (ed): *Outpatient Cancer Centers Implementation and Management.* Chicago: American Hospital Publishing, 1988, pp. 1–16.
4. Association of Community Cancer Centers: *Community Cancer Programs in the United States 1988–1989.* Rockville MD: Association of Community Cancer Centers, 1989.
5. Frank-Stromborg M: Population changes in the coming decade: Healthcare implications. In *Issues in Cancer Care Economics, Proceedings of the Sixth National Conference on Cancer Nursing.* Atlanta, GA: American Cancer Society, 1992, pp. 1–19.
6. Palmer P, Steiger N, Engleberg C: The cost of oncology care in a small community hospital. *Proc Am Society Clin Oncol* 5:241, 1986(abstr).
7. Conklin VK: Continuity of care issues for cancer patients and families. *Cancer* 64(1):290–294, 1989.
8. Alfirevic J, Kroman B, Ruflin P: Informational needs for a product line management system. *Healthcare Financial Management* 3(3):60–66, 1987.
9. Yates JW, Lyons C: The delivery of cancer care services: Resources and referral systems. In Baird SB (ed): *Cancer Nursing, A Comprehensive Textbook.* Philadelphia: Saunders, 1991, pp. 993–999.
10. National Cancer Institute: *National Cancer Institute Cancer Centers Program.* Washington, DC: National Cancer Institute Office of Communication, 1992.
11. Cheson B: Clinical trials program. *Semin Oncol Nurs* 7(4):235–242, 1991.
12. Fall-Dickson JM: Clinical trials and research in the community. *Semin Oncol Nurs* Vol. 9, No. 1, pp. 38–43.
13. Nash MG, Opperwall BC: Strategic planning: The practical vision. *J Nurs Admin* 18(4):12–18, 1988.
14. Bookbinder NF: Strategic planning. In Nathanson SN (ed): *Outpatient Cancer Centers Implementation and Management.* Chicago: American Hospital Publishing, 1988, pp. 17–32.
15. Henderson JC: Aligning business and information technology domains: Strategic planning in hospitals. *Hosp Health Svcs Admin* 37(1):71–87, 1992.
16. Johnson L: Strategic management: A new dimension of the nurse executive's role. *J Nurs Admin* 20(9):7–10, 1990.
17. Buller PF, Timpson L: The strategic management of hospitals: Toward an integrative approach. *Health Care Manage Rev* 11(2):7–13, 1986.
18. Beckman JD: Strategic thinking and the road to relevance. *Healthcare Forum J* 34(6):37–43, 1991.
19. Aaker DA: *Developing Business Strategies.* New York: Wiley, 1988.
20. Lamkin L: Assessment, development and evaluation of cancer programs. *Semin Oncol Nurs* Vol. 9, No. 1, pp. 17–24.
21. Waterman RH: The seven elements of strategic fit. *J Bus Strategy* Winter:69–73, 1982.
22. MacDonald, SA: Organizational approaches to cancer program development. *Semin Oncol Nurs* Vol. 9, No. 1, pp. 8–16.
23. *1992 Accreditation Manual for Hospitals.* Chicago: Joint Commission on the Accreditation of Healthcare Organizations, 1992, pp. 137–138.
24. Zelman WN, Parham DL: Strategic, operational and marketing concerns of product line management in healthcare. *Health Care Manage Rev* 15(1):25–35, 1990.
25. Fottler, MD, Repasky LJ: Attitudes of hospital executives toward product line management: A pilot survey. *Health Care Manage Rev* 13(3):15–22, 1988.
26. Charns MP, Smith LJ: Product line management and continuity of care. *Health Matrix* 7(1):40–49, 1989.
27. MacStravic RS: Product line administration in hospitals. *Health Care Manage Rev* 11(2):35–43, 1986.
28. Fountain M: A survey of cancer program administrators. *Oncol Issues* 6(1):20–22, 1991.
29. Folger JC, Gee EP: *Product Management for Hospitals, Organizing for Profitability.* Chicago: American Hospital Publishing, 1987.
30. Cancer care in the 1990's: Expected advances, potential problems. *Oncol Issues* 5(2):8–10, 1990.
31. *Quality Assurance in Ambulatory Care* (2d ed). Chicago: Joint Commission on the Accreditation of Healthcare Organizations, 1990, p. 8.
32. Ogorzalek LL: Quality management issues. *Semin Oncol Nurs* Vol. 9, No. 1, pp. 32–37.
33. American College of Surgeons Commission on Cancer: *Cancer Program Manual 1991.* Chicago: American College of Surgeons, 1991.
34. Association of Community Cancer Centers: *Standards Self-Assessment Guide.* Rockville, MD: Association of Community Cancer Centers, 1989.
35. Oncology Nursing Society: *Resource Manual for Oncology Nurse Managers and Administrators.* Pittsburgh, PA: Oncology Nursing Press, 1991.
36. Oncology Nursing Society: Salary, staffing and profes-

sional practice patterns in oncology nursing. Pittsburgh, PA: Oncology Nursing Press, 1989.
37. Goldsmith J: The reshaping of healthcare, part 2. *Healthcare Forum J* 35(3):34–41, 1992.
38. Vose JM, Armitage JO: Developing a bone marrow transplant unit. *Oncol Issues* 5(2):17–19, 1990.
39. Anderson HJ: Outpatient planning: Still more art than science? *Hospitals* 64(24):26–32, 1990.
40. Oncology Nursing Society: Cancer chemotherapy guidelines module III: Recommendations for nursing practice in the outpatient setting. Pittsburgh, PA: Oncology Nursing Press, 1988.
41. Lamkin L: The new oncology ambulatory clinic. In Yarbro C (ed): *Oncology Nursing in Ambulatory and Outpatient Care Settings*. Boston: Jones and Bartlett (in press).
42. Brady AM, Foster J: Development of site-specific centers: The breast clinic. *Oncol Issues* 7(1):12–14, 1992.
43. Oncology Nursing Society: Salary, staffing and professional practice patterns in oncology-related infusion units. Pittsburgh, PA: Oncology Nursing Press, 1992.
44. Oncology Nursing Society: Salary, staffing and professional practice patterns in ambulatory oncology clinics. Pittsburgh, PA: Oncology Nursing Society, 1992.
45. U.S. hospitals are still short of allied health personnel. *Am Hosp Assoc News* 28(3):3, 1992.
46. Inter-Society Council for Radiation Oncology: *Radiation Oncology in Integrated Cancer Management*. Philadelphia: Inter-Society Council for Radiation Oncology, 1991.
47. Oncology Nursing Society: Salary, staffing and professional practice patterns in radiation therapy-based oncology nursing. Pittsburgh, PA: Oncology Nursing Press, 1991.
48. Jako GJ: New strategies and initiatives in cancer treatment. *Lasers Surg Med* 7:217–218, 1987.
49. Winchester DP: The challenges facing the surgeon in caring for cancer patients. *Am Coll Surg Bull* 70(9):18–25, 1985.
50. Munoz E, Mulloy K, Goldstein J, et al: Costs, quality and the volume of surgical oncology procedures. *Arch Surg* 125:360–362, 1990.
51. Berkowitz DA: Medical technology in a competitive market. *Healthcare Exec* 6(1):18–20, 1991.
52. Boxerman SB, Gribbins RE: Technology management in the '90s. *Healthcare Exec* 6(1):21–23, 1991.
53. National Joint Practice Commission: *Guidelines for Establishing Joint or Collaborative Practice in Hospitals*. Chicago: Neely Printing, 1981.
54. Kerstetter NC: A stepwise approach to developing and maintaining an oncology multidisciplinary conference. *Cancer Nurs* 13(4):216–220, 1990.
55. Borzo G: Pursuing cancer research despite limited funds. *Healthcare Strat Manage* 10(4):1, 19–22, 1992.
56. Engleking C: Clinical trials: Impact evaluation and implementation considerations. *Semin Oncol Nurs* 8(2):148–155, 1992.
57. National Cancer Institute: Making health communications programs work: A planner's guide. NIH Publication No. 89-1493. Bethesda, MD: Office of Cancer Communications, National Cancer Institute, 1989.
58. Morra M: Teaching strategies: The public. In Groenwald SL, Frogge MH, Goodman M, Yarbro CH (eds): *Cancer Nursing: Principles and Practice* (2d ed). Boston: Jones and Bartlett, 1990, pp. 1228–1245.
59. Buller DB, Buller MK: Approaches to communicating preventive behaviors. *Semin Oncol Nurs* 7(1):53–63, 1991.
60. Kernaghan SG, Jones LD: *Preventive Strategies in Ambulatory Care: A Manager's Guide*. Chicago: American Hospital Association Press, 1992.
61. Haynes SG, Odenkirchen J, Heimendinger J: Worksite health promotion for cancer control. *Semin Oncol Nurs* 7(4):463–484, 1990.
62. Frank-Stromborg M: Nursing's role in cancer prevention and detection. *Cancer* 62:1833–1838, 1988.
63. Love RR, Olsen SJ: An agenda for cancer prevention in nursing practice. *Cancer Nurs* 8(6):329–338, 1985.
64. Beck S, Breckenridge-Potterf S, Wallace S, et al: The family high risk program: Targeted cancer prevention. *Oncol Nurs Forum* 15(3):301–306, 1988.
65. Koska M: CEOs say hospitals must learn from each other for TQM success. *Hospitals* 66(12);42–50, 1992.
66. Feingold MG, Meyer JW, Briggs DS: Controlling cost and quality through clinical pathways: One cancer center's experience. *Oncol Issues* 6(4):24–28, 1991.
67. Dorsett DS: Quality of care in Groenwald SL, Frogge MH, Goodman M, Yarbro CH (eds): *Cancer Nursing: Principles and Practice* (2d ed). Boston: Jones and Bartlett, 1990, pp. 1151–1177.
68. Wiggers JH, O'Donovan KO, Redmen S, et al: Cancer patient satisfaction with care. *Cancer* 66:610–616, 1990.
69. Young WW, Joyce DZ, Bivens GD, et al: Incorporating the cost of ambulatory care into case mix-based hospital reimbursement. *J Amb Care Manage* 11(3):54–67, 1988.
70. Ford RL: What we do and how we measure it. *Hosp Health Serv Admin* 32(3):399–407, 1987.
71. Davis PB: Facility design. In Nathanson SN (ed): *Outpatient Cancer Centers Implementation and Management*. Chicago: American Hospital Publishing, 1988, pp. 63–91.
72. Gilden KM: The challenge of cancer care marketing. *Semin Oncol Nurs* Vol. 9, No. 1, pp. 51–58.
73. Cancer center beats odds. *Profiles Healthcare Marketing* July:54–57, 1991.
74. Lokich JJ, Silvers SS, Brereton H, et al: Freestanding cancer centers: A rationale for improving cancer care delivery. *Am J Clin Oncol* 12(5):402–406, 1989.

Chapter 52

Continuity of Care

Betty R. Ferrell, RN, PhD, FAAN

Edith O'Neil-Page, RN, BS

INTRODUCTION

Standards of Oncology Nursing Practice[1] emphasizes the importance of providing continuity of care throughout the span of diagnosis, treatment, rehabilitation, and terminal illness for the person with cancer. Part VII of this book addresses the major delivery systems for cancer care. This chapter discusses the concept of continuity of care, care setting alternatives and issues, selecting and recommending settings, and the transition from hospital to the community. The three chapters that follow focus on the major delivery systems in the community: ambulatory care, home care, and hospice care.

CONTINUITY OF CARE—AN OVERVIEW

The eighties (1980–1990) was the decade for the initiation of drastic health care reforms and major alterations in systems of care. This trend will continue through the turn of the century. Although the full impact of these changes is yet to be realized, on the positive end of the continuum are alternative delivery systems that provide improved care. On the negative extreme is the potential for fragmentation of care and compromised outcomes for the patient. Interestingly, this same decade witnessed significant advancement in the specialty of oncology nursing. Oncology nurses will maintain the standards of oncology nursing practice within this rapidly changing environment by understanding the meaning and process of continuity of care.

Definition

While there is general agreement that *continuity of care* is a desirable goal,[2,3] few people have a clear definition of the term. The concept of continuity of care is often used interchangeably with the terms *discharge planning* or *continuing care.* Discharge planning can be considered the process of preparing the patient for transfer from one system and entry into the next phase of care.[2] Because patients' needs exist after discharge, there is generally continuing care, whether it is provided by the patient, the family, or another organized health care system. Continuity of care, however, implies a standard of care in which there is planned coordination of care that results in improved outcomes for the patient, irrespective of care setting or provider.

Several social and health care factors have stimulated increased emphasis on the concept of continuity of care. The most significant factor has been the implementation of diagnostic related groupings (DRGs), resulting in restricted use of acute care settings and reliance on alternative care systems. Shortened hospital stays, combined with more complex "high-tech" care, have also precipitated the concern and attention given to continuity of care. Cancer patients and their families are asked to assume nursing procedures at home that only a few years ago were limited to intensive care settings.

Another influence has been the evolution of cancer care delivered in multiple health care settings. Over the course of diagnosis and treatment, the cancer patient may experience a number of systems, including diagnostic clinics, physicians' offices, community hospitals, major cancer centers, ambulatory care centers, rehabilitation programs, home care, and hospice or nursing home care. The patient's experience will not be a linear progression from one system to another but, rather, a trajectory with multiple transitions between systems.

Therefore, continuity of care is much more than an empty phrase; it is a standard of care to be achieved. The outcome of continuity of care is efficient, optimum care over time. Studies have documented benefits of continuity of care that include decreased hospital stays, fewer hospital admissions, and increased patient satisfaction.[4–9] Figure 52-1 presents a model of continuity of care that illustrates the relationship of the patient and health care settings.

Principles Underlying Effective Continuity of Care

Since continuity of care has come to be uniformly valued, many health care agencies blindly assume that their settings are providing continuity. However, evaluation of the care in many instances would indicate that the concept is more idealistic than realistic. Table 52-1 lists the major characteristics of continuity of care. These characteristics are cited in the literature as referents of continuity of care.[2,10] This table can be used as a checklist by nurse managers or clinicians to evaluate their own settings.

Organizational philosophy is considered to be a prerequisite for achievement of continuity of care.[2,11,12] The philosophy of patient care, for example, is an organization that values family-centered care and interdisciplinary care is more likely to foster continuity. Well-defined standards of care may be used as a guide to achieve continuity of care.

It is important to consider the rationale behind the current emphasis on continuity. Beyond our acceptance of continuity as a desirable goal, positive outcomes have been identified as a result of patients receiving continuity of care. The most commonly cited outcomes include quality of care, patient satisfaction, nurse and physician satisfaction, and a decrease in complications or unnecessary hospital admissions.[13–16]

Standards of Oncology Nursing Practice indicates that achievement of any standard is contingent on continuity in the care provided. The standards emphasize the use of an interdisciplinary approach and identify

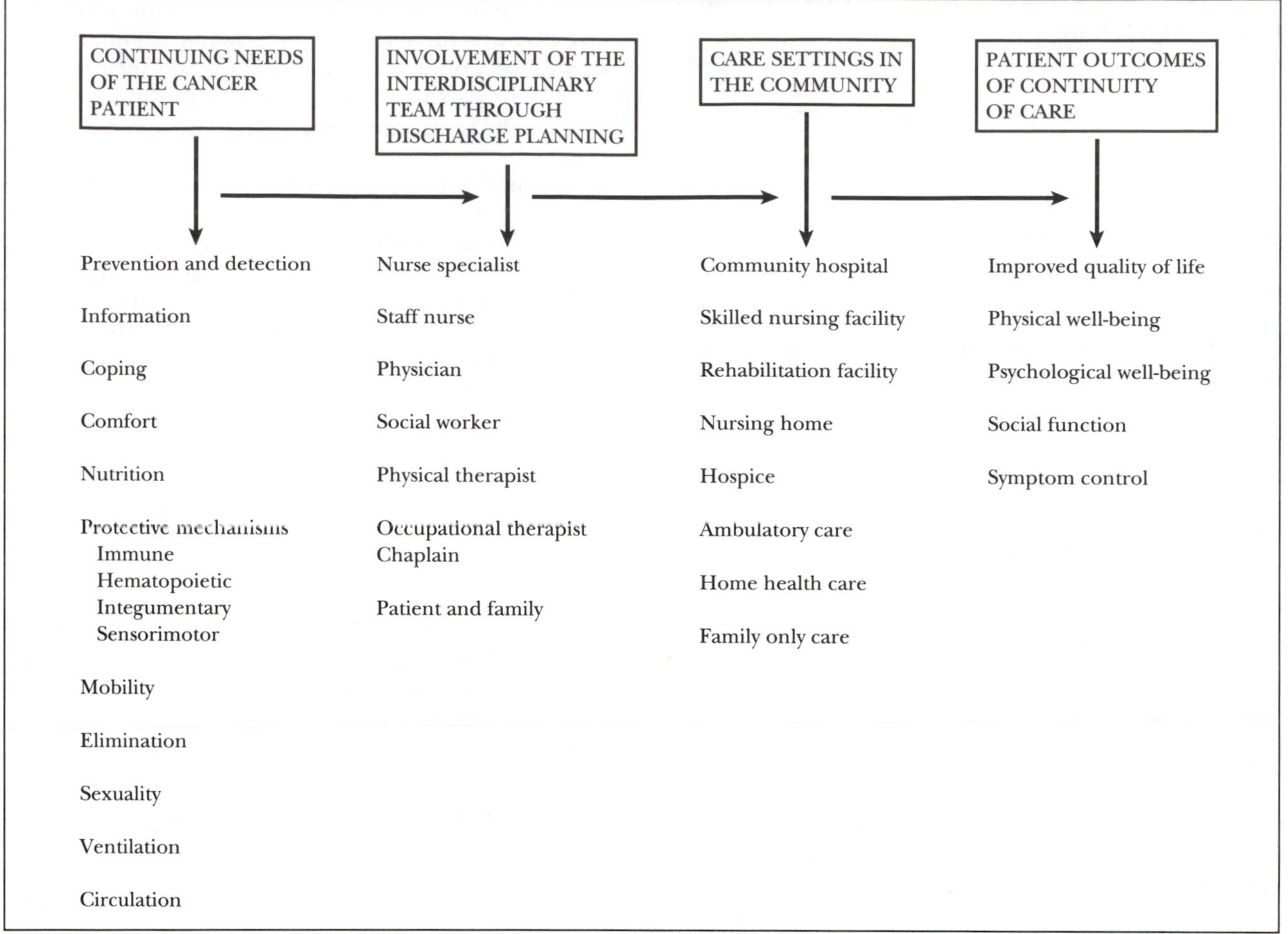

FIGURE 52-1 Model of continuity of care for the cancer patient. This model illustrates the continuing needs of cancer patients as derived from the *Standards of Oncology Nursing Practice*. Through involvement of an interdisciplinary team in discharge planning, care continues in community settings. The outcomes of effective continuity of care are dimensions of quality of life.

TABLE 52-1 Characteristics of Continuity of Care

C	Communication exists between settings
O	Organization exists in the form of policies, procedures, or standards of care
N	Nursing care is delivered at a level consistent with the patient's needs
T	The patient and family are informed and involved in care
I	Interdisciplinary care is provided
N	Nursing care is efficient
U	Unplanned and unavoidable events are minimal
I	Individual goals are established for each patient
T	There is adequate written documentation of care
Y	Your discharge-planning process begins prior to or at the time of admission.

patient needs to include issues such as comfort, coping, mobility, and elimination. To practice excellence in oncology nursing, therefore, is not to question the need for continuity of care but, rather, to question how cancer care can exist without continuity.

Specific Concerns Related to the Person with Cancer

Continuity of care is being emphasized by all areas of health care and among disciplines. The concept has particular significance for oncology. Although often perceived as a terminal diagnosis, cancer is, in fact, a chronic disease. Patients with cancer are now living longer with this illness, and many achieve long-term survival and cure.

Patients with cancer can develop complex problems during the course of their disease. It is not uncommon for patients with cancer to experience disruption of several major body systems. Current technology and therapy can enable patients to overcome these disruptions; however, there may be residual effects to cope with.

Treatment of cancer involves various modalities: surgery, radiation, chemotherapy, biotherapy, and multiple support therapies. The number of health care providers interacting with the cancer patient is reason alone for concern about continuity. An individual with newly diagnosed colon cancer, for example, may receive direct care provided by a medical oncologist, a radiation oncologist, the surgical oncology staff, an oncology nurse clinical specialist, staff nurses, an enterostomal therapist, and a dietitian. This is without mention of the additional encounters with the hospital chaplain, volunteer services, patient support groups, and other medical consultants.

Many characteristics of cancer patients' experiences place them at increased risk of compromised continuity of care. Coupled with complex physical needs is the intense psychologic impact of a diagnosis of cancer. Responses commonly cited in association with cancer include shock, fear, anxiety, depression, and hopelessness.[17,18] These psychologic responses can be barriers to the patients' participation in care.

Cancer patients are frequently elderly individuals with special needs for continuity of care.[19] Coupled with the burdens of a cancer diagnosis are the factors associated with aging, including decreased social supports, diminished financial resources, and multiple medical problems.

Continuity of care, therefore, is an essential element in achieving quality of care. The oncology nursing profession must evaluate current systems and devise strategies for enhancing continuity of care. This is best accomplished through careful evaluation of the specific settings used by cancer patients and planning of the transition from the acute care hospital to those settings.

CARE SETTING ALTERNATIVES AND ISSUES: FROM HOSPITAL TO COMMUNITY

Hospital to Hospital

Transition between hospitals is often necessary at the time of cancer diagnosis if the patient is referred from a community hospital to a more comprehensive cancer center. Other common transition points are at the completion of treatment, when the patient resumes care closer to home or when a terminally ill patient prefers to be closer to home during the final stage of illness.

The most effective tool for continuity of care between hospitals is written communication. Most hospitals have discharge-planning tools that document the patient's status and anticipated needs after discharge. Written care instructions are essential between settings but are particularly important when the patient will continue to receive acute care and complex treatments.

Verbal communication between nurses is an effective avenue for exchanging pertinent information about the patient. Some cancer centers have established systems for nurses in community hospitals to telephone the patient's primary nurse from the cancer center to discuss care issues verbally.

Nursing Home or Skilled Nursing Facility

Since they have approximately three times as many beds as hospitals have in the United States, nursing homes represent a major segment of the health care system.[20] Contrary to popular beliefs, nursing homes care for a dynamic population of patients constantly in transition between settings, including home, hospitals, and other long-term care institutions.[20] Eighty percent of residents in nursing homes are admitted from acute care hospitals, 13% are admitted from home, and another 7% are transferred from other nursing homes.[20] Patients admitted to the nursing home are likely to be older, poorer, sicker, mentally impaired, and to have fewer family members or friends than those discharged to their own homes.[20] Discharges from the nursing home include 50% to the hospital, 40% to the patients' homes, and 10% to other nursing homes.[21]

With the increase in long-term survival of patients with cancer, the nursing home and the skilled nursing facility will likely be common settings for many patients with cancer. A major limitation to continuity of care in these settings is the reliance on a predominantly nonprofessional staff of nursing assistants and medication aides. Certain patients, such as those who require aggressive management of pain or continuous parenteral infusions, require highly skilled care, and the average nursing home, convalescent setting, or skilled nursing facility may not be appropriate. Patients at particular risk in this setting include those who have recently completed chemotherapy. Delayed complications of chemotherapy, such as myelosuppression or neurotoxicity, require careful assessment and early intervention by skilled professionals.

Oncology nurses from the acute care hospital can greatly enhance care in the nursing homes and skilled nursing facilities by offering education programs related to cancer care. Teaching basic principles of oncology nursing, such as nutrition needs, oral care, and pain management, can contribute to improved care and increased communication among staff.[22]

A major problem in care for nursing home or skilled nursing residents is inadequate documentation in the medical record. All too frequently, patients arrive from the hospital for admission to the nursing home or skilled nursing facility with little or no medical history. Patients in this setting are often not able to provide this information because of communication deficits, dementia, or poor memory. Miller et al.[23] documented that as many as 60% of primary diagnoses and 80% of secondary diagnoses were inaccurate in the nursing home record. Adverse drug reactions and inappropriate prescriptions have been associated with inaccurate diagnosis and poor medical records.[24]

In contrast, excellent care is available in some nursing homes. Many skilled nursing facilities can provide highly technical procedures for nursing, pharmacy, respiratory, and rehabilitation therapy. With the variable availability of technology and quality of care in nursing homes and skilled care facilities, there is no substitute for a thorough knowledge of individual facilities within the community.

As with all settings, basic patient information is important on transfer to and from the nursing home or the skilled nursing facility. Specific information, in addition to the nursing care plan, includes mental status information, for example, to determine the risk of falls. Other specific information needed on transfer to a nursing home would include the time of last medication administration, functional status, mental status, specific nutritional needs, and skin condition.[25]

Hospice

The transition from acute care to the hospice setting raises several important issues. The first issue is the psychologic impact on the patient and family of transfer to a hospice. While the hospice is usually considered a positive setting desired by patients and families, admission to a hospice can signify a transition from active treatment to terminal illness. Patients and families may be facing the reality of death for the first time as goals of care shift from cure to palliative care.[26] This transition requires careful attention to the psychologic needs of the patient and the family.

Another area of concern for continuity of care during a transfer to a hospice is the need for continuous symptom control. Primarily a home-based service, hospice care usually means that the family assumes responsibility for providing relief of symptoms. Studies have documented that symptom control is a chief concern of family members and that the ability to manage symptoms such as pain will influence the family's adjustment during bereavement.[27–30]

A national survey by Lauer et al.[31] examined home-based hospice services for terminally ill children. Major challenges reported were the need for hospice programs with pediatric expertise, the need for a cohesive working relationship between family and hospice staff, and the need for continued pain management.

Ambulatory Care

Increasing costs of care for the cancer patient and decreasing financial resources have influenced the utilization of ambulatory care facilities as a major setting for oncology practice. Effective continuity of care provided in an ambulatory care setting can greatly reduce the need for hospitalization.

The major issues in the ambulatory setting are teaching patients and families self-care measures and preparing patients to detect an adverse reaction early enough to avoid serious sequelae or hospitalization. Outpatient radiation therapy is an example of a setting in which nurses can ensure continuity of care. Patients may experience many acute and chronic symptoms related to radiation therapy, including skin alterations, gastrointestinal symptoms, fatigue, and potential disruption of major organ systems.[32] (See Chapter 13.) Intervention by the nurse is critical to prepare the patient for self-management of symptoms that may not occur until the conclusion of treatment or later. Dodd[14] has documented that patients who receive adequate education are more capable of self-care activities.

Other examples in which nurses can impact continuity of care include the bone marrow transplant patient, the patient receiving high-dose chemotherapy with stem cell rescue, and the patient receiving drugs that stimulate rapid hematologic recovery. These patients are in particular need of high-quality continuing care. In order to meet this need, many institutions are developing outpatient discharge coordinators or utilizing a case management care delivery method. Since inadequate symptom management places a patient at high risk for inpatient readmission, coordinators or case managers are responsible for providing the patient and family with post therapy instruction regarding home care, coordinating community services, and referring the patient to outside agencies for assistance as necessary. The result is an efficient use of health care dollars with the provision of high-tech, high-quality care.[7]

Tighe et al.[33] conducted a comparative study of the roles of oncology nurses and nononcology nurses in ambulatory care. Their findings indicate that oncology nurses have a greater role in interdisciplinary communication and in direct physical care of cancer patients.

Nail et al.[8] studied the delivery of nursing care by telephone for ambulatory oncology patients. Results of this study indicate that nurses provide care by telephone either independently or in consultation with another nurse. Nurses use the calls as an opportunity to assess the patients' responses to treatments and to provide information related to symptom management and self-care activities.

Home Care

One of the primary areas for continuity of care in the home is symptom control. The author's research[34,35] indicates that management of cancer pain is not effectively provided in the home. Family members tend to undermedicate patients for pain because of their fears of drug addiction and respiratory depression and their general misunderstanding of pain relief.

Continuity in the management of symptoms is strongly correlated with the patient's ability to function and his or her overall quality of life.[36] Few home health agencies specialize in cancer care, and therefore home care providers may not be skilled in the special needs of the cancer patient. One approach to provision of that expertise has been the integration of oncology services into home care agencies. The pain management team at Mercy Health Center in Oklahoma City has a pain team nurse provide consulting visits through the hospital home health agency to ensure continuity and adequacy in pain management.[37]

Family members may be so overwhelmed by their own emotional response to having a loved one with cancer that they are less able to provide direct care. Yet social influences have encouraged families to provide care at home rather than to seek institutional care. Studies in geriatrics have indicated that home care is often immensely burdensome on family members.[38–40]

The impact of cancer on the family is multifocal. The authors' research in the area of home care for the dying patient[29] indicates that while family members want to care for the dying patient at home, the experience may have deleterious effects on the physical and psychological health of surviving family members. While family caregiving in the home can be a demanding responsibility, it can be enhanced through accurate assessment of the family prior to implementing home care, management of symptoms, assessment of psychological needs and moods, provision of continuity of care, and appropriate use of technology in the home care setting.[41] These activities enhance the quality of life for the patient and caregiver at home.

Another issue of concern for continuity of care is the increase in high-tech home care for oncology patients, including such procedures as tube feedings; epidural catheters; intravenous infusions for total parenteral nutrition (TPN), hydration, and antibiotics; or blood transfusions.[7,42,43] It is imperative that the family be involved throughout the hospitalization to learn the skills necessary to provide care when the patient goes home. Instructions given to families in the final hours before discharge are often not adequately learned and can result in compromised care for the patient and feelings of inadequacy for the family.

Home care has been cited as a valuable asset in the transition from care in a major hospital setting to eventual resumption of primary care by the community physician.[44]

Rehabilitation Facility

Many patients will be discharged from the hospital with continuing acute care needs that are more appropriately met through a skilled nursing facility or a rehabilitation setting. Both settings are designed as interim care facilities to help in the patient's transition from acute care to home or alternate care.

The diagnosis of cancer once carried the stigma of certain and immediate death. Patients may live for long periods after diagnosis, however, and will need time and skills to adjust to the deficits or changes they have incurred. Cancer is a chronic disease that necessitates rehabilitation measures as an integral part of therapy for some patients.[45] Rehabilitation is the action taken to return the patient to a maximum level of function and, as such, implies the need for continuity of care across settings. Mutual goal setting by the patient and the staff and interdisciplinary collaboration are particularly important for the achievement of continuity of care in cancer rehabilitation.[46,47]

Cancer rehabilitation includes not only the traditional areas of physical rehabilitation and mobility but also psychologic and social recovery.[48] Even today, patients with cancer may find it difficult to return to work or to social activities because of misconceptions and fears by employers or friends. A woman undergoing bilateral radical mastectomies could require both occupational therapy and vocational counseling to adjust to physical and social deficits. On discharge of the patient from the hospital setting to the rehabilitation setting, it is important to communicate information regarding the patient's psychologic status and social concerns.

The Patient with No Follow-Up Care

Alternative care settings have become such a common part of the health care system that it is often assumed that all patients will receive ongoing care after hospital discharge. This is not the case; moreover, the majority of cancer patients are discharged from hospital settings to self-care or family care only.[2] Financial constraints, geographic location, and resource limitations are the primary barriers to continuing services. Oncology nurses are often uneasy about discharging the patient, realizing that while the DRG demands discharge, the patient may be inadequately prepared for or incapable of meeting the care demands. One innovative way to enhance care at home when families are the only care providers is to designate a primary care provider at home. This person can be targeted to receive instructions and can be involved in actual care during the hospitalization.

Patients and their families may elect discharge without community referral, assuming that they can meet the patient's needs. It is not until the reality of being alone in the home sets in that they are aware of the scope of care needed. For this reason, all families should be advised on how to obtain services at a later time if arrangements are not made before hospital discharge.

Because of financial constraints or third-party reimbursement limitations, many patients are ineligible for home or hospice care, even though they have definite needs for care. Nurses should be particularly alert to the patient and family who are resistant to being discharged. Requests for "just one more day" in the hospital usually indicate hesitancy and feelings of inadequacy to assume care. Additional support and teaching may be helpful.

The concerns regarding caregiver burden are crucial in the instances of care by family alone. The nursing staff can help the family to realistically address the

NAME: ______________ PHYSICIAN: ______________ PHONE: ______________

PATIENT GOALS:
1. To be able to remain at home while I get my radiation therapy treatments.
2. To gain my strength back and gain some weight.

MEDICATIONS:
1. Metamucil—take one teaspoon two times a day.
2. Doxidan—take one capsule every day.
3. Tylenol #3—take one tablet every 4 hours if needed for pain. Contact your physician if your pain increases or if the medicine isn't working.

ACTIVITY RESTRICTIONS:
1. Take a short walk each day if weather permits.
2. Do not lift anything heavier than 1 pound for the next 4 weeks.

DIET:
1. Eat 3 meals a day and continue your Ensure®, one can two times a day.
2. Use the suggested foods list from the dietician.
3. Weigh yourself once a week. Report any weight loss to the home health nurse.

TREATMENTS:
Clean your suture site two times a day with peroxide for the next week. After that time, clean your suture site with warm water only during shower.

NOTES:
1. The American Cancer Society will provide your transportation for radiation therapy. Call them at ______________ to make arrangements.
2. The Hospital Home Health Care nurse will visit 3 times a week on Monday, Wednesday, and Friday. The first visit will be tomorrow. Their number is ______________.
3. Your Radiation Therapy will begin on ______ and is scheduled once a day for 2 weeks at _____ a.m./p.m. Call the Radiation Therapy Department with any questions at ______________.
4. You may also call the Hospital Oncology Patient Hot Line for any questions about your care. The number is ______________.

FIGURE 52-2 Family care plan. A family care plan will enhance continuity of care at home. Note that the instructions are clearly written for family understanding on the basis of patient goals.

responsibilities that await them and to plan for assumption of care at home. Volunteer groups may be able to offer some relief or assistance.

Preparation of families to assume care at home centers around family involvement during the hospitalization with ample opportunity to demonstrate procedures, such as dressing changes or tube feedings, before discharge. Responsibilities should be assumed gradually (e.g., from first having the family care provider perform a single procedure to eventually assuming all the care during a shift). Another strategy is to plan the first 24 hours after discharge in great detail to assist with this critical time period. Family "care plans" and a "cardex" can be used. An example of such a plan is included in Figure 52-2.

SELECTING AND RECOMMENDING SETTINGS

Assessment of Patient and Family Needs

The importance of the patient's involvement in the process of discharge planning cannot be overstated. Continuity of care must be based on a comprehensive nursing assessment specific to the needs of the patient with cancer. There are model tools available that provide an excellent assessment base for oncology nursing.[2,43,49]

It is essential to first identify who is "family" for the patient. Family is broadly interpreted to include whomever is identified as such by the patient.[50] Assessment includes evaluation of the normal family routine, normal roles in the family, and the health status of the family members. Rose[51] has identified a number of excellent tools for the assessment of families with school-age children. Wright and Leahey[52] have identified effective interviewing methods to assess families as well as intervention strategies for enhancing family care. They present the use of interviewing skills to assess relationships within the family and interventions that maximize family strengths. Our clinical experiences have included arriving for a home visit to find the patient in better health than the family members.

The best approach to assessment of family and patient needs is one characterized by individuality. It is a tremendous challenge to balance both the patient's and the family members' best interests. Accurate assessment of patient and family needs is a prerequisite to effective intervention.

Collaborative Planning and Roles of the Health Care Team

The benefits of collaborative practice and its impact on improved outcomes have been documented.[53–55] Patients benefit from clear communication between health care providers and from consistent goals of care. Patients experience a sense of support and reduced conflict when care is based on collaborative planning.

Multidisciplinary care is not necessarily interdisciplinary care.[56] While there may be many disciplines involved, it is critical that these multiple care providers interact to avoid conflict. Territorial struggles and political battles can greatly impede continuity of care for the patient and may result in either duplication and conflicting goals or the absence of planning as the patient falls through the system.

Discharge-planning teams exist in most acute care settings, either in a formal structure or often in an informal sense. Models of discharge planning include formal teams who develop coordinated plans of care through conferences, discharge planners functioning as consultants to staff, and staff nurses or social workers who assume discharge-planning functions within their normal roles.[2]

The nurse has the central role in the discharge-planning team.[2,57] As the provider with the greatest amount of interaction with the patient and the most comprehensive view of the total needs, the nurse is best suited to coordinate the team approach. The nurse member of the discharge-planning team can be an advanced practitioner, a clinical specialist, or the staff nurse. As the primary provider of inpatient care, the staff nurse generally is best informed of the patient's care and response. Rusch[57] has presented a model program in which staff nurses are educated about community resources and discharge-planning principles to enhance their role in discharge planning. This includes knowledge of the specific resources as well as procedures for making these resources available to a patient.

The social worker also has an important role in discharge planning.[56] Nurses and social workers collaborate to provide a comprehensive approach to discharge planning. This is facilitated by clear delineation of responsibilities.

Communication among the discharge team members greatly influences achievement of continuity of care. Written documentation is essential as discharge plans are made. Methods to promote communication include weekly discharge-planning conferences, walking rounds for discharge planning, or daily communication among team members.

Case management is a care-delivery method that is emerging and being refined.[58–60] Developed during the 1970s in the area of psychiatric and geriatric care, case management is now being extended to other areas of health care. Wesley and Easterling[60] describe the project management techniques utilized at St. Joseph Mercy Hospital in Pontiac, Michigan to implement a nursing case management model. They found that this approach promoted maximum input from everyone affected by the change and promoted communication through all levels of staff. The program utilizes nurses with advanced clinical expertise as case managers.[61] Selection of case managers is based on clinical practice and interpersonal skills, leadership ability, and previous performance appraisals.

Zander et al.[59] have developed the concept to include a primary nurse/case manager who uses a production plan process to organize, direct, revise, and evaluate care. The case manager model emphasizes the need for interdisciplinary collaboration while maintaining the central role of the nurse as case manager.

Case management uses specific outcome criteria and predicted time frames to monitor the patient's hospital stay and discharge. This nursing delivery system uses standards or critical paths to map out the patient's expected progress.[62] The nurse case manager is responsible for the total management of the patient and collaborates with other disciplines to achieve the outcomes. Schwab and Pierce[63] evaluated the case management system in an ambulatory pediatric setting and reported that it was useful in achieving desirable patient outcomes.

This concept has potentially a great deal to offer oncology, particularly as a method to ensure continuity of care. Since this is a new service delivery method, research is warranted to evaluate the use of case management in other areas such as oncology.

Evaluation of Alternatives

Individualized attention to the needs and goals of the patient is a critical part of the evaluation and selection of alternative care arrangements. Discharge from the hospital setting can become a routine with little attention given to careful identification of the most appropriate alternatives. It is not uncommon for a patient to be admitted to home health care when his or her needs would have more appropriately been met by hospice care.

Cost is a critical consideration in the evaluation of alternatives. If applicable, insurance coverage and benefits should be thoroughly checked for important information on alternative care choices. If insurance coverage is not available, the patient and the family should receive realistic estimates of potential expenses. Example: When a patient with leukemia was admitted to the home health agency, the nurse calculated the cost of necessary supplies for the management of a central line catheter. Both the patient and the nurse were distressed to learn that the costs of supplies exceeded the patient's total income. The hospital social worker had assumed that the cost of supplies in the home would be covered by insurance but, in fact, no coverage was available.

To make appropriate referrals, health care providers must be well informed of the services provided by the alternative care settings or agencies. For example, when one is referring a patient for home chemotherapy, it is necessary to know the qualifications of the home care nurse who will administer the chemotherapy and the availability of on-call services for help with potential problems. A patient discharged to nursing home care after administration of chemotherapy will require laboratory services for follow-up blood work. Since cancer patients may move among multiple settings, the referring agency must carefully evaluate the services available in the potential setting.

To ensure continuity, the referring nurse should be aware of the quantity of services needed and the ability of the alternative agency to provide those services. Knowing that the home health nurse will be available to visit only once a week will indicate the need for intense family teaching, since the family will assume responsibility for most of the patient's care.

Choices

When the assessment and evaluation of alternatives are completed, an informed choice can be made and the specific arrangements can begin. Patients should be advised that choices may be flexible and that alterations can be made at any time. A patient who finds that return trips to the hospital ambulatory care center are too exhausting may need reevaluation for possible change to a closer community clinic or to in-home chemotherapy.

In most instances there is a wide variety of services for the patient to select. The nurse, functioning in a patient-advocacy role, should encourage the patient and the family to be assertive consumers in their choices of care. A family selecting a nursing home setting should inquire specifically into the experience of that facility in caring for cancer patients. The family preparing for transfer of the patient to hospice care should be informed of the extent or limit of emergency on-call services so that an informed choice between home care and hospice can be made.

Assessment of the Care Setting

Continuity of care requires integration of the patient's past, present, and future in the planning and provision of care.[3] Nurses must remember that some of the patient's current needs could have existed before admission to a health care service. The nurse determines how the patient's needs were met before the current hospitalization in order to evaluate future plans. An effective approach for assessment of the proposed transfer setting includes a visit to the setting before the patient's hospital discharge. A visit to the patient's home by the home health nurse prior to discharge can provide valuable insight into specific needs for continued care. Another assessment strategy is to have the patient describe the environment and routines that existed before the present hospitalization.

If the patient is not going home, the family should be encouraged to visit the alternative care setting in advance of the discharge. If the patient is going to be transferred to a hospice, a visit from the hospice nurse may greatly allay the patient's and family's anxiety regarding discharge.

Hospital staff members may fall into a pattern of discharge planning that does not adequately assess individual needs. Settings that routinely refer cancer patients for home care may fail to recognize that some patients may best be served through a short stay in a skilled nursing facility. Some discharge-planning programs have home care nurses to assist in appropriate referrals.

TRANSITION

Coordination

Regardless of the amount of prior planning, transfer from one setting to another evokes anxiety for the patient, the family, and the health care staff. It is common to find that the patient who had been eagerly awaiting discharge is quite hesitant when the actual day arrives.

The stress of transition may be greatly reduced by active involvement of the staff nurse. The primary nurse is in the best position to assess the patient's status and to provide instruction to patient and family in a timely and coordinated manner. The staff nurse coordinates the involvement of specialists and support staff to help the patient during the transition. In addition, discharge instruction given over a period of time will most likely be more effective than teaching that occurs on the day of discharge when anxiety is at a peak.[64,65]

The case management care delivery method also facilitates the exchange of information between inpatient and outpatient services. The model stresses the patient and family as the primary focus.[61] It promotes a cooperative relationship among the patient and family, nurse case manager, physician, and other members of the interdisciplinary health care team.

Communication Process and Tools

Providing continuity of care requires complex interactions between the patient, family, and health care team. The need for shared information is well substantiated in the literature.[6,7,9,12,66–68] Several continuing care models identify the need for a specific professional manager.[7,9,61,69] However, final decisions regarding care should rest with the patient after open interaction and sharing of information with the family and all members of the health care team.

Since cancer patients are now receiving their care in multiple settings throughout the course of their disease, innovative strategies to improve and facilitate communication will be needed. Preuss et al.[70] developed a model program that includes a statewide telecommunication system to facilitate communication between nurses at a tertiary referral center and a community hospital. The project, entitled CHILD (Continued Help in Lending Direction), has resulted in improved patient outcomes, increased patient satisfaction, and continuity of care.

A comprehensive patient-assessment tool is invaluable during the transition from the hospital to any community setting. Miaskowski and Nielson[49] developed a cancer nursing assessment tool that provides a comprehensive database from which to plan care. Another tool, developed by O'Neil-Page for use in discharge planning is included in Figure 52-3.

While the format of information has traditionally been verbal or written, electronic technology, such as facsimile machines, has accelerated the timing of communication. The sharing of data among multiple treatment areas within a single facility is evolving with the use of computer-based information systems.[66]

Acceptance and Adjustment

The concept that discharge planning begins on admission to the hospital has changed from a desirable process to a required process. Family members and patients must understand the need for early discharge planning and must be involved from the time of admission. New models for better utilization of health care resources are beginning the discharge-planning process before the patient's admission to the hospital.

Experience has shown that gradual transition from the acute care setting to the community is best accomplished through transfer to a day hospital, respite care, or gradual assumption of care by the family during hospitalization. Unfortunately, it is often assumed that the transition is over and continuity of care has been achieved when the patient is discharged and all the appropriate forms have been completed. The characteristics for continuity of care (see Table 52-1) can be a useful checklist for evaluation of ongoing care.

The previous decade has witnessed a movement away from acute care settings. However, there is interest in the idea that the acute care setting should be the center of care for the patient amid the multiple alternative settings. Model programs, such as the Supportive Care Program at Memorial Sloan-Kettering Cancer Center,[13] have demonstrated the ongoing role of the hospital in coordinating continuity of care. This program emphasizes the central role of nursing in the extension of the acute care setting into the community. The Supportive Care Program provides expertise to ensure that standards of care, particularly in the area of patient comfort, are met after hospital discharge.

EVALUATION AND FOLLOW-UP

Evaluation to determine the effectiveness of health care is based on patient outcomes, which are individualized and derived from the patient assessment. For example, a priority in the care of a patient after radical surgery for a neck tumor is continued nutritional support. To determine the status of care at home, evaluation of outcomes would be based on measures of nutrition, such as intake, weight gain, and wound healing.

Hospitals have used follow-up questionnaires or surveys of the primary physician to obtain information regarding the patient's status after discharge. To fully appreciate the cancer patient's experience, one would need to evaluate every care setting and service encountered by that person. Further research is needed to determine the quality of transitions of cancer patients among settings and to evaluate such settings according to standards of care.

CONCLUSION

Evaluation of services is clearly a challenge amid the constraints of the health care system at present. Evaluation is essential to ensuring the quality of services but is undoubtedly time-consuming. One innovative evaluation program, which has been reported by Siegel et al.,[71] uses a computer-automated telephone outreach system to follow up chemotherapy outpatients.

One implication of continuity of care relates to the education of future health care providers. Students in nursing and other health disciplines need curricula that include knowledge of continuity of care.[3,16] Nursing students need to evaluate patients in a broad spectrum of care rather than only in their current care setting. Nursing education can incorporate knowledge and experience in continuity of care into student experiences by exposure to advanced practitioners, oncology clinical specialists, and nurse managers who are familiar with nursing roles in interdisciplinary discharge-planning teams. Such concepts as case management should be included in continuing education in oncology.

Continuity of care provides nurses with greater professional satisfaction.[72] Oncology nurses are characterized by concern and involvement with the cancer patient. The inpatient nurse can become frustrated without follow-up contact with the patient after discharge from the hospital. Communication channels made available through continuity-of-care systems can provide feedback to inpatient nurses. It is hoped that when a complete feedback loop exists for care providers to communicate and evaluate outcomes of continuity of care, cancer patients will achieve an improved quality of life.

PLAN OF CARE
DAY HOSPITAL/PHYSICIANS OFFICE

Day Hosp.

DATE INITIATED: 8/1/92

PRIMARY DISEASE PROCESS(S): CA breast (L)
s/p mastectomy —

SECONDARY DISEASE PROCESS(S): Bone mets
ribs + spine

NURSING DIAGNOSIS(ES): Alt. in comfort; alt in skin integrity: oral mucosa; alt in mobility deficit 2° exertion

NURSING PROBLEMS: ① Pain control. ② oral hygiene ③ Instruction in pacing activities, seek outside assist early.

SOCIAL SERVICE CONSULT: Jane Doe MSW @ Community hosp – con't c̄ F/u via home care.

TREATMENT PLAN: Pt. adm q 28d. for chemo to hosp. F/u in Day Hosp. for transfusion support.

SHORT TERM GOALS: ① Prevent infection @ nadir ② Assist c̄ pain control ③ Assist c̄ management of stomatitis + diarrhea.

LONG TERM GOALS: ① Assist c̄ life style changes to maximize independence.

CHEMO RECEIVED/RECEIVING: 5 FU q 28d

PRE MEDS: Zofran

ADVANCED DIRECTIVES: (Y/N) Yes
(Identify)
John Smith – Spouse durable power of attorney

NAME OF DESIGNATED DECISION MAKER
Same as pt.
Phone Number

VENOUS ACCESS DEVICE
Hickman
Type
Blood Type: O+
Irradiated (Yes/No) — Yes circled
CMV Neg. (Yes/No) — Yes circled
Antibodies Identified:
ID. Antibodies None

Platelets:
CMV Neg. (Yes/No) — Yes circled
HLA Matched (Yes/No) — No circled
Irradiated (Yes/No) — Yes circled
(Please Circle Yes/No)

DATE	PLACE	TREATMENT	DATE	PLACE	TREATMENT
8/1	DH.	2 U PRBC's			
8/19	DH.	PLT's			
8/24	O	F/u			

KEY:
O – MD Office
H – Hospital
DH – Day Hospital
HC – Home Care
C – Convalescent
B – Blood Product
CH – Chemotherapy

(Please have your nurse complete this information when you receive treatment.)

FIGURE 52-3 Self-care nursing discharge tool. Careful assessment is critical to continuity of care after hospital discharge. This comprehensive assessment will enhance continuing care.

DISCHARGE SUMMARY TOOL

DATE	COMMENT/QUESTION	INSTRUCTION	TO WHOM
8/15	Diarrhea — Lomotil doesn't work —	Diet changed To Liquid only — x 24° Call to MD	Mary Smith by Nancy Nurse RN (Home Care) N.N. Rn
8/20	Diarrhea controlled. Stomatitis better (grade II improving)	Cont c̄ Saline mouth wash	

PATIENT NAME: Mary Smith
ADDRESS: 1234 Central St.
Any Town, CA 92400
PHONE: (555) 555-2222
PRIMARY LANGUAGE: English
DC DATE: Community Hosp. 8/14/92 TIME: AM M.D. J. Smythe
DX: CA Breast Ⓛ

ALLERGIES: PCN
HOSPITALIZATION: 8/9 — 8/14 —

TX: Chemo x 5d. 5 FU

MEDICATIONS:

DATE:	AGENT	DOSE	FREQUENCY
	Compazine	10 mg.	q 6° (Every 6 hrs.) + as needed
	Lomotil		

PHYSICAL FINDINGS UPON DISCHARGE:

SELF CARE STATUS: 80% Independent - Tires easily

CARDIOPULMONARY: Stable
NUTRITIONAL/FLUID STATUS: Nutritional deficit due to poor appetite from N/V
ELIMINATION: Diarrhea — episodic
ACTIVITY/REST: Rest pds. every 2-3 hrs.
SAFETY: Ambulation slow but safe.

FAMILY SUPPORT SYSTEMS: Married — supportive spouse, 3 grown children who live locally.

COMFORT MEASURES/PAIN CONTROL: M.S. Contin 30 mg. every 12 hrs.
COPING/PATIENT CONCERNS: Fear — loss of independence.
REFERRALS: Home care; Wellness Group "CAN DO" Support group
HOME CARE AGENCY: Best Care-Centerville TEL (555) 555-2438

of care, cancer patients will achieve an improved quality of life.

REFERENCES

1. *American Nurse's Association and Oncology Nursing Society: Standards of Oncology Nursing Practice.* Kansas City, MO: ANA, 1987.
2. O'Hare P, Terry M: *Discharge Planning: Strategies for Assuring Continuity of Care.* Rockville, MD: Aspen, 1988.
3. Ruane T, Brody H: Understanding and teaching continuity of care. *J Med Educ* 62:969–973, 1987.
4. Wasson J, Sauvigne A, Mogielnicki P: Continuity of outpatient medical care in elderly men. *JAMA* 252:2413–2417, 1984.
5. Magill M, Senf J: A new method for measuring continuity of carc in family practice residencies. *J Fam Pract* 24:165–168, 1987.
6. Ophof J, Leucht R, Frohmuller S, et al: Experiences in home care of cancer patients: A new approach in cancer nursing. *Acta Oncol* 1:35–38, 1989.
7. Chielens D, Herrick E: Recipients of bone marrow transplants: Making a smooth transition to an ambulatory care setting. *Oncol Nurs Forum* 17:857–862, 1990.
8. Nail LM, Greene D, Jones LS, Flannery M: Nursing care by telephone: Describing practice in an ambulatory oncology center. *Oncol Nurs Forum* 16:387–395, 1989.
9. Ventafridda V: Providing continuity of care for cancer patients. *J Psychosoc Oncol* 8:3–10, 1990.
10. Rehr H: Discharge planning: An ongoing function of quality care. *QRB* 12(2):47–50, 1986.
11. Notkin MS: Collaboration and communication. *Nurs Admin Q* 7:1–7, 1983.
12. Staff: Restructuring care: Patient focus is key to innovation. *Hospitals* August:26–33, 1991.
13. Coyle N: A model of continuity of care for cancer patients with chronic pain. *Med Clin North Am* 71:259–270, 1987.
14. Dodd M: Patterns of self-care in patients receiving radiation therapy. *Oncol Nurs Forum* 11(3):23–30, 1984.
15. Feetham S: Hospitals and home care: Inseparable in the 80s. *Pediatr Nurs* 12:383–386, 1986.
16. Klingbeil G, Fiedler I: Continuity of care: A teaching model. *Am J Phys Med* 67:77–81, 1988.
17. Welch-McCaffrey D: Cancer: Anxiety and quality of life. *Cancer Nurs* 8:151–158, 1985.
18. Meyerowitz BE, Heirich RL, Coscarelli-Schag CA: Helping patients cope with cancer. *Oncology* 3:120–129, 1989.
19. King F, Figge J, Harman P: The elderly coping at home: A study of continuity of nursing care. *J Adv Nurs* 11:41–46, 1986.
20. Kane RL, Matthias R: From hospital to nursing home: The long term care connection. *Gerontologist* 24:604–609, 1984.
21. Lewis MA, Shan C, Kane RL: The natural history of nursing home patients. *Gerontologist* 25:382–388, 1985.
22. Goldman L, Miller D, Moeller T: Hospital-nursing home collaboration. *QRB* 12(6):215–217, 1986.
23. Miller MB, Elliot F, Elliot DF: Errors and outcomes in diagnostic records on admission of patients to nursing homes. *J Am Geriatr Soc* 34:108–116, 1976.
24. Segal JL, Thompson JF, Floyd RA: Drug utilization and prescribing patterns in a skilled nursing facility: The need for a rational approach to therapeutics. *J Am Geriatr Soc* 27:117–122, 1979.
25. Wright H, Lancot A: From hospital to nursing home. *QRB* 6(8):7–10, 1980.
26. Martocchio B: *Living While Dying.* New York: Brady, 1983.
27. Hine V: Dying at home: Can families cope? *Omega* 10:175–187, 1979.
28. Martinson I: Care for the dying child. *Nurs Clin North Am* 1:467–475, 1979.
29. Ferrell BR: Home versus hospital cancer deaths and bereavement outcomes. *Am J Hospice* (July–August): 18–23, 1985.
30. Scanlon C: Creating a vision of hope: The challenge of palliative care. *Oncol Nurs Forum* 16:491–496, 1989.
31. Lauer M, Mulhern R, Hoffmann R, et al: Utilization of hospice/home care in pediatric oncology. *Cancer Nurs* 9:102–107, 1986.
32. Strohl R: The nursing role in radiation oncology: Symptom management of acute and chronic reactions. *Oncol Nurs Forum* 15:429–434, 1988.
33. Tighe M, Fisher S, Hastings C, et al: A study of the oncology nurse role in ambulatory care. *Oncol Nurs Forum* 12:23–27, 1985.
34. Ferrell BR, Schneider C: Experience and management of cancer pain at home. *Cancer Nurs* 11(2):84–90, 1988.
35. Ferrell BR, Patterson B: Pain at home. *Caring* 6(11):22–25, 1987.
36. Ferrell BR, Ferrell BA: Comfort. In Corr D, Corr C (eds): *Nursing Care in an Aging Society.* New York: Springer, 1990.
37. Ferrell BR, Wisdom C, Wenzl C: Evolution and evaluation of a pain management team. *Oncol Nurs Forum* 15(3):285–289, 1988.
38. Litman T: Health care and the family. *Med Care* 9:67–81, 1971.
39. Zarit S: Subjective burden of husbands and wives as caregivers: A longitudinal study. *Gerontologist* 26(3):253–259, 1986.
40. Hinds C: The needs of families who care for patients with cancer at home: Are we meeting them? *J Adv Nurs* 10:575–581, 1985.
41. Ferrell BR, Grant MM, Rhiner M, Padilla GV: Home care: Maintaining quality of life for patient and family. *Oncology* 6(suppl):136–140, 1992.
42. Birmingham J: *Home Care Planning Based on DRGs.* Philadelphia: Lippincott, 1986.
43. Bulau J: *Clinical Policies and Procedures for Home Health Care.* Rockville, MD: Aspen, 1986.
44. Mor G, Joseph A, Carel C, et al: Evaluation of the annual activity of a continuing medical and home care unit. *Soc Sci Med* 24:967–972, 1987.
45. Broadwell D: Rehabilitation needs of the patient with cancer. *Cancer* 60:563–568, 1987.
46. Dudas S, Carlson C: Cancer rehabilitation. *Oncol Nurs Forum* 15:183–188, 1988.
47. Gruca J: Oncology rehabilitation. *Rehabil Nurs* 9(3):27–30, 1984.
48. Dietz J: Adaptive rehabilitation in cancer. *Cancer Rehabil* 68:145–153, 1980.
49. Miaskowski C, Nielson B: A cancer nursing assessment tool. *Oncol Nurs Forum* 12:37–42, 1985.
50. Leahey M, Wright L: *Families and Life Threatening Illness.* Springhouse, PA: Springhouse, 1987.
51. Rose D: Assessing families of school aged children with

cancer. In Leahey M and Wright L (eds): *Families and Life Threatening Illness.* Springhouse, PA: Springhouse, 1987.

52. Wright L, Leahey M: *Families and Chronic Illness.* Springhouse, PA: Springhouse, 1987.
53. Crowley S, Wollner I: Collaborative practice: A tool for change. *Oncol Nurs Forum* 14:59–63, 1987.
54. Anderson DJ, Finn MC: Collaborative practice: Developing a structure that works. *Nurs Admin Q* 7:19–25, 1983.
55. Ryan LS, Edwards R, Rickles F: A joint practice approach to the care of persons with cancer. *Oncol Nurs Forum* 7:8–11, 1980.
56. Blumenfield S: Discharge planning: Changes for hospital social work in a new health care climate. *QRB* 12(2):51–54, 1986.
57. Rusch S: Continuity of care: From hospital unit into home. *Nurs Management* 17:38–41, 1986.
58. McIntosh L: Hospital based case management. *Nurs Econ* 5:232–236, 1987.
59. Zander K, Etheredge M, Bower R: *Nursing Case Management: Blueprints for Transformation.* Boston, MA: Winslow, 1987.
60. Wesley ML, Easterling A: Improving clinical care through project management. *Nurs Admin Q* 15:22–28, 1991.
61. Staff: On the scene. *Nurs Admin Q* 15:50–53, 1991.
62. Weisman E: Practical approaches for developing a case management program. *QRB* 13(1):380–382, 1987.
63. Schwab S, Pierce P: Assessment of clinical nursing practice in a rural decentralized case-management system. *Public Health Nurs* 3:111–119, 1986.
64. Knowles M: *The Modern Practice of Adult Education.* New York: Association Press, 1970.
65. Rankin S, Duffy K: *Patient Education: Issues, Principles, and Guidelines.* Philadelphia: Lippincott, 1983.
66. Case C, Jones L: Continuity of care development and implementation of a shared patient data base. *Cancer Nurs* 12:332–338, 1989.
67. Conkling V: Continuity of care issues for cancer patients and families. *Cancer* 64:290–294, 1989.
68. Lauria M: Continuity of cancer care. *Cancer* 67:1759–1766, 1991(suppl).
69. Shegda L, McCorkle R: Continuing care in the community. *J Pain* 5:284–285, 1990.
70. Preuss N, Perez N, Randall J, et al: Continued help in lending direction: A proposed nurse to nurse communication system. *Issues Comprehensive Pediatric Nurs* 9:229–237, 1986.
71. Siegel K, Mesagno F, Chen J, et al: Computerized telephone assessment of the concrete needs of chemotherapy outpatients: A feasibility study. *J Clin Oncol* 6:1760–1767, 1988.
72. Rulin M, Havashi T, Badway D: Continuity of ambulatory care in an obstetrics and gynecology residency program. *Obstet Gynecol* 71:787–790, 1988.

Chapter 53

Rehabilitation of the Person with Cancer

Sue L. Frymark, RN, BS

Deborah K. Mayer, RN, MSN, OCN

INTRODUCTION

Cancer and the treatments required to cure or control it have significant impacts on individuals and their families. Helping an individual learn how to adapt to the effects of this disease and its treatment is the purpose of cancer rehabilitation. *Rehabilitation* refers to "the process by which individuals, within their environments, are assisted to achieve optimal functioning, within the limits imposed by cancer."[1] The basic principles of cancer rehabilitation include: using an interdisciplinary team approach, emphasis on maximizing strengths, focus on practical day-to-day issues, facilitation of coping with loss, family care, and focus on prevention in areas of high risk for complications. The goals of rehabilitation are to improve the quality of life for those experiencing cancer and to assist the individual to regain "wholeness." This chapter reviews identified patient needs, nursing assessment of the patient's rehabilitation needs, goals of cancer rehabilitation, and organizational issues that arise in providing these services.

REHABILITATION GOALS

The overall goal of rehabilitation is to help the individual reach an optimal level of independence while preventing disabilities that might limit the individual's potential.[2] Four categories for rehabilitation goals were defined originally by Dietz[3]:

1. *Preventive:* To prevent or reduce the impact of expected disabilities. Example: An individual with leukemia is instructed in an exercise program to minimize weakness that may occur with decreased activity due to fatigue during treatment.

2. *Restorative:* To return the individual to optimal functional status with expected complete medical recovery. Example: The laryngectomized person is taught esophageal speech.

3. *Supportive:* To maximize function and prevent secondary disabilities while the disease persists and the possibility of progressive disability exists. Example: The woman with metastatic breast cancer receiving chemotherapy and experiencing fatigue and weakness is instructed in energy-conservation techniques and the use of assistive devices to maintain her daily routine as much as feasible.

4. *Palliative:* To assist the dying person and his or her family in maximizing their independence, while providing comfort. Example: The family of a semi-bedbound man dying of metastatic prostate cancer is taught to do passive range-of-motion exercises to minimize stiffness of the joints and promote comfort. In addition, family members are instructed in bedside transfers of the patient to a wheelchair or commode.

Initial rehabilitation goals can be established once a baseline assessment has been conducted. Over the course of a person's cancer history, these goals are continually defined, reached, and modified. The goals could include returning to work, staying as active as possible through cancer treatments, or being independent enough to attend a daughter's graduation. The individual, family, and health care team should remain flexible; goals may need to change if medical status changes, coping skills fluctuate, or reduced energy level slows progress. Goals are a balance between having a hopeful vision of tomorrow and being realistic about current limitations.

REHABILITATION NEEDS

The rehabilitation needs of those with cancer fall into a variety of categories that include physiological, functional, emotional, spiritual, and social (Table 53-1). A number of studies have found these needs to be related to the type of cancer site and stage of disease, type of treatment and side effects experienced, length of illness, coping skills, family and other medical history, social issues, and the individual's response. Of all these factors, severity or duration of disease is most related to the cancer patient's rehabilitation needs.[4] Lehmann et al.[5] studied the type and frequency of rehabilitation problems that occur in a general cancer population and found that psychosocial needs were the most common, whether or not accompanied by physical disabilities, and were the most severe in the presence of physical disabilities. The physical needs frequently occurring with a variety of cancers included general weakness, limited activities of daily living, and issues related to limited mobility. Other needs included pain control, adequate nutrition, and dealing with financial and family issues.

Houts et al.[6] studied the psychological, social, and economic needs of cancer patients and found that 59% had at least one unmet need in these areas. Communication and information were common needs identified in other studies.[7,8] Health care professionals can help to identify unmet patient needs and enhance the individual's ability to adjust to cancer and comply with the treatment plan.

Some problems are more chronic or long-term than others. For example, fatigue, anorexia, and weakness may be associated with recovery from surgery and be of short duration, while at other times these symptoms are associated with metastatic or advancing disease and are of longer duration. A multidisciplinary cancer rehabilitation team or service may be the most prepared with the resources and skills to deal with the challenges of addressing the changing and varying rehabilitation needs of patients.

TABLE 53-1 Areas of Rehabilitation Needs

PHYSIOLOGICAL
Skin care
Bowel and bladder dysfunction
Ostomy and wound care
Fatigue
Symptom control
Lymphedema
Nutrition
Cognitive skills
Sleep
EMOTIONAL
Coping defenses
Fear of recurrence
Fear of death
Change in body image
Self-esteem
Intimacy
Fear of losses
FUNCTIONAL
Mobility
ADL-activities of daily living
Gait/balance
Strength and endurance
Swallowing
Speech
Sexual
Prosthesis
Stair climbing
Transfers: chair, bathroom, auto
Upper extremity function: fine motor skills
SOCIAL
Communication
Family relationships
Workplace
Legal/financial
Leisure
Transportation
Social isolation
Role changes
Insurance coverage
SPIRITUAL
Why me?
Disharmony: God, self, others
Forgiveness
Love
Meaning of life
Peace

Physiological Needs

Many physiologic needs of individuals with cancer related to alterations in mobility are best addressed with preventive measures. These needs include skin breakdown or constipation. Adequate symptom control will provide the patient with sufficient comfort to enable mobilization. Teaching the patient both preventive measures and self-care measures minimize physiological distress.

Functional Needs

This category includes the problems related to day-to-day practical issues of living that may be temporary or permanent. Functional needs of the cancer patient are often unrecognized or not appreciated by acute care providers.[5,10] For the patient, physical dependence can be a constant reminder of life-threatening illness. The rehabilitation goal may be to maintain acceptable function while receiving cancer treatment. For example, individuals recovering from surgery, radiation, or a bone marrow transplant may experience short-term changes in their activity level. Rehabilitation therapists can instruct the individual in a progressive activity program. Assistive devices such as a walker or a raised toilet seat may be needed. For individuals receiving chemotherapy, functional needs issues may continue for some months until they are able to work on a recovery program. Individuals with progressive metastatic cancer may also focus on maintaining an optimal level of independence within the limits imposed by their disease; for example, their independence may diminish as their disease progresses. For the person with progressive disease, rehabilitation is often an ongoing process of learning and adapting to new levels of disability.

Long-term cancer survivors also have changing rehabilitation needs. The person with a prosthesis may experience body weight changes requiring adjustments in the prosthesis. The person with a laryngectomy may experience stoma stenosis and need a revision of the stoma. The woman who received pelvic irradiation may require instruction about vaginal dilation to continue sexual intercourse. Functional rehabilitation needs can arise at any time during the course of a person's cancer experience.

Emotional Needs

The emotional needs of those with cancer and their families can be dynamic. Young-Brockopp[11] identified five major emotional needs: hope, honesty, information, emotional expression, and discussion of issues related to death. In addition, cancer patients face many issues related to real or anticipated loss, such as loss of hair, loss of a limb, loss of organs, loss of loved ones, loss of life, and so on. These emotional issues may be affected by the patient's prognosis or change in status as well as functional and physical limitations. Psychological needs may be in response to a new event or may be related to coping with the chronic uncertainty about the future. The rehabilitation care team needs to remain sensitive to the emotional needs of the patient.

Cancer is also an emotional experience for the family. Family members may each be coping with different fears and concerns. The stress of family role changes, whether temporary or permanent, can compound concerns about the future. If family relationships were strained in the past, they may be strained further with cancer-related issues. Although rehabilitation focuses on fostering the independence of the individual with cancer, the family is viewed as the individual's major support system. It is critical, therefore, to be responsive to the family's needs regarding role changes and added responsibility. Many patients and families learn to adjust and cope well with the support of their care team and others. Some patients and families may benefit from referrals to specific counseling services.

Spiritual Needs

Patients with cancer will frequently reexamine their priorities and their beliefs and values throughout their experience with cancer. Confronting the thought of suffering and dying raises many existential concerns.[12] Assessing spiritual needs can be emotionally difficult for the health professional. It can be done as an extension of a psychosocial assessment, as beliefs, values, and faith can be the foundation for coping.[13,14] For an individual to retain wholeness, a variety of spiritual needs[13,15] may need to be addressed. Issues surrounding spiritual needs often arise during support group sessions.

Social Needs

Like other chronic illnesses, cancer can have an impact on family, friends, and co-workers. Problems that existed before diagnosis are often compounded by the illness. Many cancer patients fear withdrawal of their family, friends, and colleagues. This fear is often enhanced if there are any noticeable physical changes as a result of the cancer. While assessing the social network, the nurse must also assess the patient's attitude about cancer. Early in the rehabilitation process, social assessment is important to understanding the extent and depth of the person's social and support network and resources.[14] Although rehabilitation focuses on restoring an individual's independence, certain areas of limitation or disability may need the assistance of family, friends, colleagues, or the community. Northouse and Sivcun[9] found that a partner's distress is equally as intense as that of the one experiencing the cancer. Special effort may be needed to initiate contact with the family, to assess their needs, and to inform them that the services of the cancer rehabilitation team are available for them as well.

Separate support groups for family members or caregivers may help them openly acknowledge their own needs. Providing family, friends, or co-workers the freedom to openly discuss cancer within the setting of a support group often allays their fears. One does not need to discuss with the support group the details of the person's cancer; rather, it is valuable to correct cancer myths and sort past experiences from current experiences. Some individuals with cancer have a limited social network. For those in rural communities, distance can be a factor. For the elderly, it may be that their circle of friends has diminished due to health changes or death. Individuals with a continuing history of substance abuse may have already withdrawn from social and family relationships. The social assessment process must consider all of these factors and identify community resources that may be assistive. Local social service agencies change frequently, so a systematic approach is needed to maintain an effective referral network.[17]

Social needs may have an impact on the individual's ability to continue treatment. Transportation, financial, and work-related problems must be assessed early so appropriate referrals can be made and resources utilized. A variety of financial issues confront the person with cancer. The individual may have difficulty maintaining income or paying health care costs and expenses related to nonskilled home services, such as a homemaker or attendants. Policies regarding public assistance vary according to state and degree of disability. Teamwork is required among the patient, family, physician, nurse, social worker, and vocational counselor to explore options and identify available resources.[18]

NURSING ASSESSMENT OF REHABILITATIVE NEEDS

Careful assessment of the patient's needs is critical since each individual has unique needs and may not require all the resources of a cancer rehabilitation team. Because it is unrealistic to postpone rehabilitation services in order to ascertain the future, rehabilitation assessment should begin at the onset of a cancer diagnosis. A systematic assessment should occur early in the person's care and be repeated regularly and when changes in status occur.[7] The initial assessment may be global, followed by a more detailed evaluation by the appropriate health care discipline. The global assessment and coordination of services is usually done by a nurse, social worker, or rehabilitation counselor who is knowledgeable in both the acute and rehabilitation aspects of cancer care.[8] The assessment process may occur in phases since the individual may be too fatigued, be experiencing symptoms, or be emotionally uncomfortable discussing his or her cancer and subsequent issues to complete the assessment in one visit. The assessment process continues as new issues arise or past issues reoccur.

Assessment Tools

Although there is no universally accepted cancer rehabilitation assessment tool, most cancer rehabilitation services use some type of instrument—an informal inventory of needs, a survey, or a specially designed self-assessment tool—as a systematic way to gather information and identify the need for assistance. When evaluating the effectiveness of an assessment tool, consider:

- whether the patient can understand the questions
- restrictiveness of the form (limited problems)
- state of health, influencing one's ability to complete the tool
- willingness to acknowledge and confront needs openly

It may not be easy for an individual who has functioned independently to acknowledge his or her needs, yet it is a first step toward obtaining help. An inventory of needs can be used by the assessor as a checklist so that actual or potential problems frequently experienced are not overlooked. This is probably of most value to newer cancer rehabilitation team members or for use in a newly developed program. An inventory of needs can also serve as an informal record or data form.

A self-assessment tool (the Oncology Clinic Patient Checklist) was developed by Romsaas and colleagues[19] for use in an outpatient clinic. It is designed to be completed by the patient on each visit to the clinic. The assessment categories list many common problems such as fatigue, mobility, pain, information, and home care. Once completed, the tool is followed up by an interview with an oncology nurse.

Initiated in 1948, a frequently used tool in oncology and clinical trials is the Karnofsky Performance Status (KS),[20] a quantitative measure of the individual's functional level. The KS is limited for identifying rehabilitation needs because it measures only global functional activity. It can, however, indicate to the assessor the need for a more detailed clinical evaluation by the rehabilitation team. Another functional tool is the Inventory of Functional Status—Cancer (IFS-CA).[21] Based on the Roy Adaptation Model, it provides a baseline and compares the individual's current status to it. This 39-item questionnaire explores three realms of function: (1) personal care, (2) household and work activities, and (3) community and social activities.

Henrich et al.[22] studied the use of an inventory of 92 potential problems that someone with cancer could experience, the CIPS (Cancer Inventory of Problem Situations). This tool's scope is broader than the IFS-CA's. It covers psychosocial, physiologic, and functional issues and is completed by the individual with cancer. The CARES (Cancer Rehabilitation Evaluation System) tool was developed from this work.[23] The CARES tool also is completed by the individual and has items assessing psychosocial, functional, vocational, sexual, and informational needs. It allows the person to indicate the severity of the need and whether he or she is interested in help with that particular problem.

Assessment Process

The use of an assessment tool is optimally followed by observation or a more detailed assessment of particular problems. As a screening process, the assessor can interview the patient and family to identify needs. Depending on the severity of the problem and the degree to which the person wants the problem addressed, other team members are involved. This flexibility allows the interviewer to encourage and guide the person to express needs he or she may feel hesitant to share. An open, accepting style of assessment allows feelings such as anger, frustration, or guilt to be aired and then dealt with productively.[8] Some of the patient's greatest needs often are not easily expressed and therefore can go overlooked. An interview style of assessment allows not only the needs to be identified but also the severity and the importance with which the individual perceives them. Limitations of this approach include the time involved and the skill of the interviewer. When individuals are referred to a specific service (e.g., physical therapy for lymphedema), the initial comprehensive assessment may be inadvertently bypassed. This omission could lead to fragmented rather than comprehensive, coordinated care. Therefore, it is important that each team member be skilled in initial assessment.

As needs are identified, a more detailed evaluation and development of a treatment plan are initiated by the appropriate rehabilitation team member.[24] Table 53-2 provides a sample rehabilitation plan. In working with the patient and family, the rehabilitation team members can observe and monitor any problems that might have a negative impact on treatment efforts. The team's ongoing assessment of patient rehabilitation needs promotes a quality of life for the individual that is realistic in terms of health status and relevant in terms of desired goals. Ongoing assessment also demonstrates to patients and their families that the rehabilitation team wants to help them maintain the highest level of independence possible. A comprehensive rehabilitation approach provides individuals with the support, courage, and ability to do what they desire most with their lives.

REHABILITATION RESOURCES

Organization of Care

Although the design of a cancer rehabilitation service is dependent upon the institution's resources, flexibility, and interest of various nursing and medical specialties, each includes basic elements: a comprehensive approach addressing needs (emotional, social, spiritual, physiologic, functional); an interdisciplinary team knowledgeable about cancer, family care, and coordinated services integrated into the acute care of the cancer patient. The tumor registry can help to identify the

TABLE 53-2 Rehabilitation Plans

Problem	Rehabilitation Goals	Rehabilitation Program
Loss of joint mobility. Example: postsurgery, postradiotherapy, secondary to soft tissue tightness.	Increase range of motion. Promote normal musculoskeletal movement patterns.	Stretching and strengthening exercises Instruction in proper posture, movement, and functional patterns Joint mobilization techniques
Loss of muscle strength or coordination. Example: secondary to surgery, radiotherapy, immobility, deconditioning, etc.	Increase strength. Maximize functional independence.	Strengthening exercises Functional and ADL training Adaptive equipment as indicated
Central or peripheral nervous system (PNS) dysfunction. Example: primary or metastatic brain tumors, lesions of the PNS, chemotherapy reactions.	Maintain normal range of motion. Strengthen weakened musculature. Maximize independence in ambulation and activities of daily living. Minimize abnormal muscle tone. Evaluate for necessary splints, braces, assistive devices. Facilitate normal swallowing, voice, and articulation.	Range of motion, strengthening, endurance, and balance exercises Facilitation/inhibition techniques Gait training with or without assistive devices Functional and ADL training Braces, splints, self-help devices Perceptual motor training Speech therapy
Bone instability. Example: primary or metastatic bone tumor.	Minimize stress and pain in involved bone. Maintain maximal independence in ambulation and self-care.	Instruction in protective functional techniques Splinting, bracing Pain reduction modalities
Pain. Example: secondary to tumor nerve irritation, soft tissue	Decrease pain. Facilitate normal movement patterns.	Use of modalities such as Hubbard tank, TENS, relaxation exercises, biofeedback
Difficulty in ambulation. Example: secondary to neurological or orthopedic lesions, deconditioning, tightness, etc.	Maximal independence in ambulation. Normalize gait pattern.	Gait training and/or use of assistive devices and adaptive equipment
Edema. Example: following surgery or pelvic hympadenectomy secondary to metabolic imbalances.	Decrease and control edema.	Positioning Exercise and/or gentle massage Patient education Pneumatic pump and elastic supports
Generalized deconditioning. Example: secondary to disease or chemotherapy.	Increase general strength and endurance. Maximize independence in ambulation, self-care, and activities of daily living (ADL).	Exercises for strengthening and endurance Gait training with or without assistive devices ADL training and education in energy conservation, work simplification techniques
Respiratory compromise with functional limitation. Example: lung cancer, deconditioning, chemotherapeutic reaction.	Promote maximum efficiency in breathing patterns during functional activities. Mimimize problems secondary to excessive secretions.	Breathing exercises and retraining Education in energy conservation, work simplification techniques Instruction in postural drainage, coughing, etc.
Speech and/or swallowing dysfunction. Example: post–head and neck surgery; laryngectomy.	Optimal speech intelligibility. Maximum normalization of swallowing patterns.	Articulation, voice, respiration, and communication technique training Swallowing evaluation and training
Loss of limb or body part. Example: amputation, mastectomy.	Independence in ADL Restoration of strength, range of motion (ROM), and functional abilities. Assist with restoration of good self-images and feelings of self-worth.	Exercises for ROM, strengthening, endurance, and balance Transfer, gait, ADL, training Evaluation for necessary assistive/prosthetic devices
Emotional reactions.	Provide ongoing support and reassurance regarding patient's physical abilities/disabilities and his/her response. Facilitate and assist with patient integration into normal social and vocational opportunities.	Ongoing emotional support and sensitivity toward the patient's reaction and responses to his/her disease and disability Leisure activity group to facilitate interpersonal interaction, normal leisure opportunities, fine motor skills, and emotional release

Source: From Boyd-Walton J: The role of rehabilitation services in oncology, *Clin Manage Phys Ther* 5:24–28, 1985. Reprinted from *Clinical Management* with the permission of the American Physical Therapy Association.

largest cancer populations being served and therefore potential referrals for rehabilitation services. The most successful cancer rehabilitation programs have a broad base of support and interdepartmental teamwork in the assessment and planning of a program or service. As the number of team members and referral sources expands, the ability to add new services also occurs. Growth and expansion require ongoing evaluation of current services and education of those who are potential referral sources. A mission or goal statement is needed initially since it encourages the team's planning processes to be more focused.

The delivery of cancer rehabilitation services is dependent upon the coordinating structure, but there are various organizational models, ranging from informal to formal structures. Each model requires a team that is knowledgeable in both oncology and rehabilitation fields. The interdisciplinary team may work from individual departments or may be organized in one department. The coordinator of the team's services may be a nurse responsible for the individual's acute care, or the coordinator may be a specialty nurse focused only on cancer rehabilitation services.

Another issue to consider when developing a rehabilitation service is whether there should be a unit affiliation and, if so, whether it should be based on the oncology or rehabilitation unit. Some programs, however, serve individuals dispersed throughout an institution including the various medical/surgical inpatient and ambulatory areas. There are many options to consider when developing a cancer rehabilitation service that best meets the needs of the community served (see Table 53-3).

Cancer Rehabilitation Team

The cancer rehabilitation team is a cohesive group of interdisciplinary members who apply their professional expertise to the benefit of individuals with cancer (Table 53-4). Many of these disciplines have oncology or-

TABLE 53-3 Organizational Options for a Rehabilitation Service

Identify Team Members:
Are the members department based or cancer program based?

Patient Coordinator:
Is this a specialty role or a role performed by the acute care nurse?

Area of Service:
Where will individuals be treated—oncology unit, rehabilitation unit, any nursing unit, radiation, other outpatient or home settings?

Population Served:
Will the team see patients with all cancer types and stages of cancer or focus on subgroups?
Who are the supportive referring physicians and nurses?

TABLE 53-4 Cancer Rehabilitation Team Members

Nurse: Assists with assessment, care planning, coordination of services. Provides patient/family education relevant to medical and rehabilitation needs, particularly issues of the bed-bound patient—skin care, bowel and bladder needs. Contributes to and/or coordinates discharge planning needs and services between care settings.

Social Worker: Assists with assessment, social service/financial planning, coordination of community and team services. Provides emotional guidance and counseling. Contributes to and/or coordinates discharge planning needs and services between care settings.

Rehabilitation Counselor: Assists with the assessment, care planning, counseling, and coordination of rehabilitation services.

Physical Therapist: Addresses issues of strength and endurance, range of motion, ambulation skills, transfer skills, need for assistive devices, family training, lymphedema management, use of modalities for pain management.

Occupational Therapist: Addresses issues of upper extremities, fine motor skills, activities of daily living, energy conservation, homemaking and work skills, need for assistive devices, family training, and cognitive and perceptual assessment.

Dietitian: Provides nutritional assessment, counseling, and planning, including alternate routes of nutritional intake and use of supplements.

Recreational Therapist: Addresses issues of diversion, leisure skills, social and community resources, and stress management through relaxation.

Speech-Language Pathologist: Addresses issues of speech, language, chewing, sucking, and swallowing skills.

Enterostomal Therapist: Assists in management and teaching of ostomy, wound, and skin care.

Chaplain: Provides spiritual support and care, which may include counseling, referrals, and religious traditions of prayers, readings, and sacraments.

Psychologist/Counselor: Helps identify the emotional issues and coping skills needed, particularly for those with complex family and personal histories.

Pharmacist: Serves as a resource to team, patient, and family regarding medication uses, particularly symptom control.

Physiatrist: Provides consultation regarding chronic and rehabilitation needs, particularly issues related to bracing, splinting, and control of contractures and muscle spasms.

Vocational Rehabilitation Counselor: Addresses issues of returning to work through retraining, education, and workplace accommodation.

Volunteer: Complements the team's role by creating a pleasant/warm atmosphere, a friendly sounding board, help with practical needs, and role model as a cancer survivor.

Source: Reprinted with permission from Frymark S: Rehabilitation resources within the team and community, *Semin Oncol Nurs* 8(3):213, 1992.

ganizations (or sections within their professional associations) such as the Oncology Nursing Society, National Association of Oncology Social Workers, and the Oncology Section of the American Physical Therapy Association. The professionals within the rehabilitation team are skilled in addressing the wide array of needs individuals and their families may experience. However, it is not simply the utilization of rehabilitation resources that creates a cancer rehabilitation team. Members from all disciplines involved need to be interested in cancer and capable of modifying traditional methods to be applicable to individuals with cancer. For example, the dietitian must have an understanding of the effect of chemotherapy on taste and appetite as well as the feelings of sadness and apathy that may accompany anorexia. Although each team member has his or her own professional knowledge base, together the team develops a common knowledge base of: cancer pathophysiology, cancer treatments and side effects, emotional responses to cancer, coping styles, family dynamics, and symptom control.[25] Rehabilitation team members must be familiar with the skills and resources contained within the team itself so appropriate referrals can be made. The individual with cancer will have a variety of needs at once, requiring a variety of resources within the team simultaneously.

Teamwork does not happen automatically. It is not simply the utilization of resources but rather how they work together that influences their effectiveness. A team's effectiveness is related to its capabilities to do the work and its ability to manage itself as an interdependent group of people.[26] Four barriers to team effectiveness are: (1) goal conflicts, (2) organizational structure, (3) interprofessional conflicts, and (4) lack of communication.[27]

Goal conflicts can arise for several reasons—frequently from failure to communicate relevant information among team members. Since medical goals, social support systems, and available resources can change frequently, team members must be alerted to changes so their treatment goals are modified appropriately.

Since many teams may consist of disciplines accountable to their departments as well as to the team itself, it is likely that organizational conflicts will arise. A strong commitment to the rehabilitation services is needed from the various departments, and communication between the managers of these departments is essential.

Interprofessional conflicts arise when roles are unclear. This is especially true when there is overlap in expertise—for example, physical therapists, nurses, recreational therapists, and psychologists all teach relaxation techniques. Other disciplines that may overlap in skills are physical and occupational therapy addressing functional issues. Conflictual issues must be discussed openly while considering individual professional interests and skills, local standards of practice, and reimbursement for services.

Poor communication, the most common barrier to the team's efficiency, is frequently an issue of accessibility of one team member to another. Strategies for prevention of communication problems include defining clinical communication methods such as documentation, team log books, scheduling boards, and care plans. There are several critical areas for effective team communication:

- assessment
- rehabilitation plan and referrals
- further assessment
- progress notes
- interdisciplinary conferences
- discharge plans

In addition, informal communication becomes important as changes occur in day-to-day patient care. The team environment must allow freedom to express new ideas as well as acknowledge problems that affect the common goal. Many rehabilitation services utilize a team meeting format with each discipline reporting on the case presented. In cancer rehabilitation a more effective format may be to focus the discussion around the problem list of each client. This allows any team member to respond to any issue. Multidisciplinary meetings are organized according to which clients and their particular needs will be reviewed. Complete information is given concisely, with time prioritized for group problem solving. Although it is important that all team members contribute, it is also important to have a meeting facilitator. Issues that require extensive discussion should be referred to a special session.

A designated leader, whether formal or informal, is needed to monitor the team's needs and facilitate its effectiveness. This requires awareness of all team members' strengths and weaknesses, their knowledge base and need for growth, and their working style, as well as sensitivity to their emotional comfort and stress level as they work. The leader not only advocates for team members' individual needs but also for the group. The team must continuously strive to improve as a group by identifying issues and ways to address them. This may be achieved by planning an annual evaluation of the team and an opportunity for the team to "renew" itself emotionally and socially. Teams develop their own identity, pride, and culture. As new members affiliate, orientation to the team members and the various procedures becomes as important as clinical orientation. New team members working in cancer care may have some fears about cancer that can be addressed within the team.[26]

Coordination of Care

A key to an effective, cohesive cancer rehabilitation program is coordination of care. Following the assessment and development of a plan, a coordinator involves the necessary team members. For the woman who has had a mastectomy, coordination of care may mean involving a physical therapist for arm and shoulder mobility, a nurse for education related to wound care and hand and arm care, and a Reach to Recovery volunteer for support and consumer advice in breast forms. The individual with metastatic disease may need almost all team members to address the numerous practical issues of mobility, self-care, nutrition, and related emotional issues. The individual newly diagnosed with melanoma may need support through the adjustment of a cancer diagnosis and coping with an uncertain future. Each situation requires a unique subset of team members that needs to be carefully coordinated. Coordination of care includes ongoing monitoring with input from the primary nurse as to the status of each problem area and the identification of new areas of need. Over time, this process allows the coordinator to develop a rapport with the individual and the family and to acknowledge and address new concerns and fears.

The coordinator is the hub for providing updated information to the team members[28] (Figure 53-1). Any changes in medical status, caregiver issues, and discharge planning are important communications for team members so that their interventions can be relevant and timely. This requires the coordinator to have frequent communication with the acute care team and the family, who along with the rehabilitation team depend on the coordinator for information relevant to the rehabilitation status, assessment of the individual and family's ability to function independently, and availability of community resources.

In partnership with the acute care oncology nurse, the coordinator is central to the interdisciplinary conference, which is usually held weekly. This conference may be the only time the team is together to discuss the progress and goals of each client. For maximal learning and the broadest perspective, the entire rehabilitation team and some of the acute oncology team should be represented. Some teams invite the individual and family, depending on the time and goal of the session. Other teams have separate client and family conferences with the team as needed. This is particularly helpful when there is a complexity of needs and/or a large family involved. The interdisciplinary cancer rehabilitation conference provides: an update on patient status, review and revision of goals and strategies, interdisciplinary team support, finalization of discharge plans, and education of team members.

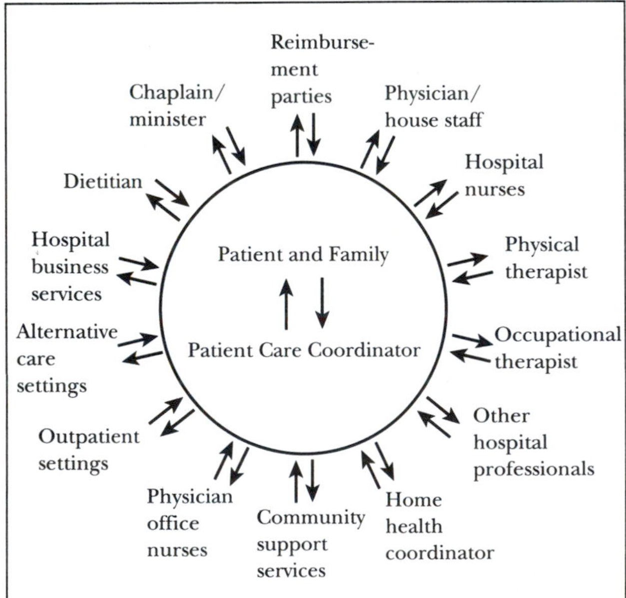

FIGURE 53-1 A coordinator model of cancer rehabilitation service. (Source: Reprinted with permission from Frymark S: Cancer rehabilitation in the outpatient setting, *Oncol Issues* 5:12–17, 1990.)

Outpatient Needs and Continuity of Care

With hospitalization periods shortening, there is an increasing need for pre- and posthospital rehabilitation. Many individuals are only hospitalized for major surgeries or treatment complications. If rehabilitation is to be involved early in the cancer care, outpatient rehabilitation is required. Although the issues can be the same in the outpatient setting as in the inpatient setting, some are more dominant than others. Individuals continuing to have acute medical problems that limit their activity are followed by the home health team, preferably a cancer team if available. Individuals who are sufficiently medically and functionally independent can receive care in the outpatient setting, which allows them to be part of the support network of others receiving treatment and rehabilitation.

Access to rehabilitation services prior to hospitalization allows the individual to become familiar with the team and resources that can help through this time of change and uncertainty. Prehospitalization contact also allows the team to gain an understanding of the social and family issues, coping skills, and premorbid functional level. The team's subsequent involvement during the hospitalization period becomes one of continuation rather than introducing another new service. The individual and health care team can proceed through this period of cancer care with a foundation based on familiarity and clarity in goals for the rehabilitation process. The same is true for posthospital rehabilitation. The rehabilitation team can enhance continuity of care by coordinating and providing services in most care settings.

Although physiological and functional issues may continue to exist for the individual in the outpatient setting, individuals often find more energy and freedom to address emotional, family, social, and vocational needs as well. Longer-term issues related to survival become more central in order to reintegrate from an illness to a wellness approach to living with cancer. During the survival period or posttreatment phase of care, long-term issues can arise, such as lymphedema, stoma stenosis, prothesis problems, and vocational issues. The services of a rehabilitation team can help the person address these issues.

Outpatient rehabilitation services require consideration of several factors. The first is easy access to services. Individuals receiving or recovering from treatment often experience fatigue. If the rehabilitation services are provided near the acute care delivery site, compliance with the program is easier. Scheduling rehabilitation activities between late morning and early afternoon can allow time for those who fatigue greatly to fulfill their morning self-care routine but not have activities too late in the day, when fatigue may be increasing. Since individuals may come for rehabilitation services alone, team interaction with the family may be more limited than during hospitalization.

Cancer rehabilitation services can complement outpatient chemotherapy clinics and radiation oncology centers. Whether it is nutritional counseling, strengthening programs, energy-conservation instruction, relaxation (especially prior to the first treatment), or social services, the cancer rehabilitation team has much to offer to the person receiving outpatient care.

Education and Support Groups

An advantage of education and support groups is that the individual can choose to participate to the degree desired. When the acute care team and the rehabilitation staff facilitate and teach these sessions together, individuals become familiar with not only the acute and chronic issues but with the resources that can help as well. Groups provide an opportunity for those with cancer and their families to meet others who confirm their progress or offer a new perspective on their diagnosis. The American Cancer Society offers "I Can Cope" and other support groups. Specialty support groups are also gaining popularity, such as "Y-Me" for women with breast cancer or "US-TOO" for men with prostate cancer.

Exercise Groups

Modified exercise classes accentuate the value of physical activity and support combined. Some classes focus on stretching, strengthening, and relaxation, while others focus on reaching an aerobic state. Exercise groups can serve a wide range of people with various types of cancers. Winningham's research and clinical work[29] has enhanced the awareness of the need for exercise. She refers to an energetic rehabilitation program that recognizes the limitations imposed by cancer and its treatment but also the importance of preventing further loss. An exercise program focuses on the physiologic and psychosocial issues of living through energy conservation, energy utilization, and restoration strategies. Exercise can be either a group event offering peer support, or it may involve an individual activity such as walking.

Survivor Needs

As individuals survive longer with cancer, a whole new spectrum of needs may be arising.[30] In the outpatient setting, patients and families discuss the transitional issues of reintegration from an illness to wellness orientation. Issues include workplace concerns, sexuality and intimacy, issues related to body image and self-esteem, and a reexamination of one's values and beliefs. (See Chapter 22 for a discussion of issues in survivorship.)

While the long-term physical effects of cancer treatment have been studied more extensively with pediatric populations, adult needs are only more recently being identified.[31,32] As cancer treatments become more sophisticated, the long-term effects may change. For example, with earlier diagnosis, less radical surgery is needed for breast and head and neck cancers. Many of the late effects of cancer treatment, such as neuropathies, cardiomyopathy, and pulmonary fibrosis, may have significant functional effects that pose new rehabilitation needs.

It is usually difficult for those who have received cancer treatment to adjust emotionally to the thought they are no longer receiving therapy.[33] With the support network at the treatment center gone, outpatient rehabilitation services, particularly support groups and counseling services, can continue to facilitate emotional independence. Survivors and transition groups for those who have completed treatment are becoming more common.

Workplace issues include both emotional and functional factors. Of persons with cancer, 80% will return to work, and 25% will have problems in the workplace.[33] The issues may be difficulties peers and supervisors have; withdrawal; facing questions one would rather not discuss; or fatigue, which impairs ability to work a full shift or presents specific functional limitations. The American Disabilities Act, however, requires employers to accommodate, within reason, those with medical, emotional, and mental limitations. There are many opportunities for the acute care and rehabilitation team and employer to work together with the cancer survivor to facilitate reentry into the workplace.

CONCLUSION

Cancer rehabilitation services are a vital care component for improving the quality of life for those experiencing and surviving cancer. Cancer rehabilitation services can be an efficient way to organize and utilize already existing services. Research is still needed to identify and evaluate various models of delivery and outcomes of these services.[34] Enhanced reimbursement for rehabilitation services will facilitate their development. The complexity of needs of those with cancer and the variance from one individual to another make a team approach invaluable. For many diagnosed with cancer, the cancer rehabilitation service provides continuity in care from diagnosis into the years of survival.

REFERENCES

1. Mayer D, O'Connor L: Rehabilitation of persons with cancer: An ONS position statement. *Oncol Nurs Forum* 16(3):433, 1989.
2. Gruca JK: Oncology rehabilitation. *Rehabil Nurs* 3:27–30, 1984.
3. Dietz JH: Adaptive rehabilitation in cancer. *Postgrad Med* 68:145–153, 1980.
4. Mor V, Guadagnoli E, Wool M: The role of concrete service in cancer care. *Adv Psychosoc Med* 18:108–118, 1988.
5. Lehmann JF, DeLisa JA, Warren CG, et al: Cancer rehabilitation: Assessment of need, development, and evaluation of a model of care. *Arch Phys Med Rehabil* 59:410–419, 1978.
6. Houts P, Yasko J, Kahn B, et al: Unmet psychological, social and economic needs of persons with cancer in Pennsylvania. *Cancer* 58:2355–2361, 1986.
7. Dietz JH: Rehabilitation of the cancer patient. *Med Clin North Am* 53:607–624, 1969.
8. Romsaas EP, McCormick JM: Assessment and resource utilization for cancer patients. *Arch Phys Med Rehabil* 67:459–462, 1986.
9. Northouse PG, Northouse LL: Communication and cancer: Issues confronting patients, health professionals, and family members. *J Psychosoc Oncol* 5:17–46, 1988.
10. Arenth LM, Mamon JA: Determining patient needs after discharge. *Nurs Manage* 16:20–24, 1985.
11. Young-Brockopp D: Cancer patients' perceptions of five psychosocial needs. *Oncol Nurs Forum* 9:31–35, 1982.
12. Olson S: Ministry and hospice care. *Lutheran Partners* 2:8–10, 1987.
13. Stoll RI: Guidelines for spiritual assessment. *Am J Nurs* 9:1574–1577, 1979.
14. Cluff CB: Spiritual intervention reconsidered: *Top Geriatr Rehabil* 1:77–82, 1986.
15. Highfield MF, Cason C: Spiritual needs of patients: Are they recognized? *Cancer Nurs* 6:187–192, 1983.
16. Ganz PA: Current issues in cancer rehabilitation. *CA* 65:742–751, 1990.
17. Polinsky ML, Ganz PA, Rofessart-O'Berry J, et al: Developing a comprehensive network of rehabilitation resources for referral of cancer patients. *J Psychosoc Oncol* 5:1–10, 1987.
18. Kudsk EG, Hoffman GS: Rehabilitation of the cancer patient. *Primary Care* 14:381–390, 1987.
19. Romsaas EP, Juliani LM, Briggs AL, et al: Method for assessing the rehabilitation needs of oncology outpatients. *Oncol Nurs Forum* 10:17–21, 1983.
20. Yates JW, Chalmer B, McKegney FP: Evaluation of patients with advanced cancer using the Karnofsky performance status. *CA* 45:2220–2224, 1980.
21. Tulman L, Fawcett J, McEvoy MD: Development of the inventory of functional status—cancer. *Cancer Nurs* 14:254–260, 1991.
22. Heinrich RL, Coscarelli-Shag C, Ganz P: Living with cancer: The cancer inventory of problem situations. *J Clin Psychol* 40:972–980, 1984.
23. Coscarelli-Schag CA, Henrich RL: Developing of a comprehensive quality of life measurement tool: CARES. *Oncology* 4:135–138, 1990.
24. Boyd-Walton J: The role of rehabilitation services in oncology. *Clin Manage Physical Ther* 5:24–28, 1985.
25. Frymark SL: Rehabilitation resources within the team and community. *Semin Oncol Nurs* 8(3), 212–218, 1992.
26. Taylor CM, Crisler JR: Concerns of persons with cancer as perceived by cancer patients, physicians, and rehabilitation counselors. *J Rehabil* 1:23–28, 1988.
27. Ducanis AJ, Golin AK (eds): *The Interdisciplinary Health Care Team.* Germantown, MD: Aspen Systems Corporation, 1979.
28. Frymark S: Cancer rehabilitation in the outpatient setting. *Oncol Issues* 5:12–17, 1990.
29. Winningham ML: How exercise mitigates fatigue: Implications for people receiving cancer therapy. *The Biotherapy of Cancer V.* ONS Monograph. Pittsburgh: Oncology Nursing Press, 1992.
30. Dow KH: The growing phenomenon of cancer survivorship. *J Prof Nurs* 7:54–61, 1991.
31. Loescher L, Welch-McCaffrey D, Leigh S: Surviving adult cancers. Part 1: Physiologic effects. *Ann Intern Med* 111:411–432, 1989.
32. Welch-McCaffrey D, Hoffman B, Leigh S, et al: Surviving adult cancers. Part 2: Psychological implications. *Ann Intern Med* 111:517–524, 1989.
33. Brown H, Tai-Seale, M: Vocational rehabilitation of cancer patients. *Semin Oncol Nurs* 8(3):202–211, 1992.
34. Mayer D: The healthcare implications of cancer rehabilitation in the twenty-first century. *Oncol Nurs Forum* 19:23–27, 1992.

Chapter 54

Ambulatory Care

Diane M. Otte, RN, MS, ET

AMBULATORY CARE OVERVIEW

Ambulatory services increasingly play a major role in the provision of care to individuals with cancer. It is not anticipated that this role will diminish in the 1990s.[1] Ambulatory care is synonymous with outpatient care and includes services such as diagnostic testing; screening and detection; treatment modalities such as chemotherapy, biotherapy, radiation therapy, and minor surgical procedures; as well as psychosocial intervention.[2]

Advances in cancer treatment and technology and the influences of economics and quality of life issues have promoted ambulatory services as a method for providing cancer patient and family care.[1] The increasing interest in health promotion practices, demographics of advancing age, and a greater number of cancer survivors will force the development of even more outpatient oncology care in the future.[3]

Ambulatory care has evolved to be available to people of all socioeconomic levels through a variety of settings.[4] Already, 80%–90% of all cancer care is delivered in outpatient settings, such as physicians' offices, freestanding oncology centers, and hospital outpatient departments.[5] *Nursing's Agenda for Health Care Reform*[6] calls for a restructured health care system that would enhance consumer access by delivering care in community-based settings, foster consumer responsibility for self-care and informed decision making, and facilitate utilization of the most cost-effective providers in appropriate settings.

Ambulatory Care Settings

A wide variety of ambulatory care settings are available. These settings include comprehensive cancer centers, community cancer centers, freestanding cancer centers, 24-hour clinics, chemotherapy and blood therapy infusion centers, day hospital clinics, physicians' offices, outreach and network programs, and other specialty centers that focus on screening, rehabilitation, and symptom management.

Cancer centers can be classified according to stated purpose, organizational structure (freestanding, joint venture, departmental, matrix, consortium) or source of funding (federal, state, private).[7] However, there is no consensus about what constitutes a cancer center. Shingleton defines a cancer center in the following way:

> . . . composed of a multidisciplinary group of research scientists and/or physicians who are bound together with a unity of purpose, who share concepts, facilities, and other resources, and who have developed an organizational structure that fosters effective management practices to achieve the desired goals of the group.[7,p.44]

The distinction between models or types of cancer centers and ambulatory settings is not always clear. A variety of services are generally provided by all settings.

Comprehensive cancer centers, authorized by the National Cancer Act of 1971 and designated by the National Cancer Institute (NCI), are dedicated to conducting clinical research, training physicians in oncology subspecialties, maintaining data for new diagnoses, and providing clinical care to cancer patients.[2,7] Since the passage of the National Cancer Act, 28 comprehensive cancer centers have been established. A majority of these centers are allied with university medical schools and have an emphasis on the multidisciplinary approach to cancer research and patient care. The centers also provide a focal point for public awareness about the cancer problem, act as a regional base for cancer control and prevention, and develop organized support programs for patients with cancer. Each comprehensive cancer center must meet a number of requirements to be classified as such. These requirements mandate that the centers should: (1) have an NCI-funded Cancer Center Support Grant; (2) possess a research program that is collaborative among basic and clinical disciplines and participate in regional and national clinical trials; (3) serve as a local and regional cancer control focal point through research activities in prevention, detection, diagnosis, treatment, and rehabilitation; (4) serve as a local and regional information center, provide lay and professional education programs, and train professional and support personnel; (5) have a formal commitment of support from the parent institution, with the director having control of space, equipment, staff appointments, beds and ambulatory facilities, and responsibility for planning, preparation of budgets, and sound management; and (6) have a geographic impact to assist the national capability to conduct regional cancer-related activities.[7]

Community cancer centers have mushroomed over the last decade and are found in many areas. They may have been established as part of a university system or as part of a community hospital. Lokich et al.[8] describe three components that comprise a cancer center. First, there must be a multiplicity of services including chemotherapy, radiation therapy, and some surgical services (usually limited to biopsies and placement of venous access devices); programs for patient and staff education; support services and diagnostic services. Second, such centers should provide access to clinical trials that make new therapies available; and finally, cancer centers offer programs not typical to the traditional office setting such as blood transfusions and prolonged chemotherapy infusions.[8] These community cancer centers have provided a way for patients to receive care "close to home" with a "one-stop shopping" approach. Many patients no longer need to travel long distances to see an oncologist or receive treatment.

Freestanding centers

A freestanding cancer center (FSCC) may be a facility separate from an existing medical care delivery building such as a hospital, or it may be contiguous with or within a hospital facility. Freestanding centers may be joint ventures between hospitals or a hospital(s) and a group of community oncologists or they may be physician-owned and -operated. The movement toward FSCCs resulted from the shift in medical care delivery from inpatient to outpatient settings and from patient demand for sophisticated therapies in the local community. FSCCs are usually based within the community, do not incorporate training of oncologists, and are not involved with on-site basic research. The establishment of a quality assurance program is an essential component of any FSCC.[8] The FSCC may provide a multitude of services or may be focused only on one service, for example, radiation oncology. Freestanding radiation oncology practices often are located within close proximity (across the street) to a hospital to enable easy transport of hospitalized patients for treatment. The center may also provide service to a number of hospitals in the area.

Affiliation of community programs with university-based cancer centers is emerging. Outreach Corporation, a separate, not-for-profit group, has been formed by M.D. Anderson Cancer Center (MDACC) at the University of Texas to develop, market, and operate programs in partnership with community institutions around the country.[9] Orlando Regional Medical Center has entered into a formal agreement with MDACC to construct and operate a freestanding cancer center in central Florida. This prototype is expected to expand to other areas of the country. MDACC will select the management team but will not provide the medical staff. It has not yet been determined which patients will be referred to MDACC. The joint venture is expected to increase the volume of patients at the Florida facility as well as in Houston.[9]

Twenty-four–hour clinics

The need for ambulatory services on a continuous basis has precipitated the development of a number of 24-hour services across the country. Lamkin[10] describes two categories of service: urgent oncology care and traditional infusion therapies given during expanded hours. Salick Health Care, Inc. operates several 24-hour centers for the provision of diagnostic services, chemotherapy, radiation therapy, and psychosocial support programs. Even though the centers may not be open 24 hours a day initially, health care professionals are on call to meet the needs of patients seeking therapy during nontraditional hours.[10] The Ambulatory Treatment Center (ATC) of the University of Texas MDACC operates an acute care unit 24 hours per day. Urgent care visits and outpatient procedures as well as chemotherapy and blood product therapy are available.[10,11]

Such settings are specifically designed to deal with side effect management and unpredictable changes in the patient's condition following therapy. Many visits to the emergency rooms of hospitals can be avoided since the patient has access to highly trained individuals to manage the specific oncologic-related problems and implement the necessary interventions.

Day hospitals

The day hospital concept has been widely incorporated into cancer centers and community settings.[12] The day hospital provides a system of partial hospitalization—individualized care, treatments, and diagnostic tests are provided for extended periods. Hours of operation vary depending on the location. The day hospital is designed to provide a care setting for more prolonged or acute interventions that exceed office setting capabilities but are less intensive than those interventions necessitating hospitalization.[13] Generally, chemotherapy, blood products, antiemetics, antibiotics, and intravenous hydration are administered in these settings. Patient education, patient assessment, placement of central lines, symptom management related to therapy, and a variety of supportive services are also provided.[10]

Outreach and satellite centers

Since patients often want to remain in their own communities to receive cancer treatment, linkages between tertiary and rural hospitals are being developed. Harvey and Walker[14] describe a successful networking program in South Carolina. Through this pilot program, patients are treated by oncologists at a tertiary setting and then return to rural or community hospitals for continued treatment. Staff in the rural setting were trained to provide the specialized care. Physician, patient, and family satisfaction with care in the outreach area was consistently evaluated as high.[14]

Indiana Community Cancer Care (ICCC) is another example of a networking program, with 24 network cancer clinics throughout Indiana. These clinics are established in hospitals to provide chemotherapy. A medical oncologist from ICCC makes the visits and is available to the local site clinic coordinator. ICCC also provides education for the satellite nurses and assists in the development of standards, procedures, protocols, quality assurance activities, and documentation systems.[10]

Many community oncologists also perform outreach services through satellite centers in clinics within 20–50 miles from their base office practice. Communication and professional relationship skills are critical factors for successful care in outreach service arrangements.

Physician office practices

Physician office practices continue to expand the scope of services provided. Many office practices administer chemotherapy and perform a number of other care services for patients. These services may be similar to what a hospital provides, that is, laboratory, x-ray, nutritional counseling, education, and support groups. In the future, changes in reimbursement may be the factor determining where the patient will receive the bulk of care.

Other ambulatory centers (screening, rehabilitation)

Individuals participating in cancer screening programs prefer convenient, nonhospital facilities with a warm, friendly atmosphere.[15] The basic focus of these newly developing programs is directed low-cost cancer detection services. Many centers established initially for cancer screening and detection are being redesigned without rebuilding to add screening programs for other diseases, including heart disease. One obstacle to the establishment of these centers is physician support. Involvement and investment by primary care physicians in the formation of the center is ideal; otherwise, physicians typically view screening centers as competitive entities and refrain from referrals or support. Among the factors contributing to a successful screening center are convenience and visibility, adequate volume to keep the cost affordable, and an approach directed at screening programs outside the usual programs.[15]

With more than five million cancer survivors in America, a great potential exists for interventions and programs to meet the needs of this group. Promoting new behaviors that enhance early detection of recurrent disease and reduce risk factors for second malignancies should be addressed as part of the rehabilitation of patients with cancer.[16]

Cancer rehabilitation services, symptom control clinics, pain management centers, and cancer psychosocial clinics are also offered through a variety of settings.[10] Satterwhite et al.[17] describe the development of a primary care HIV/AIDS clinic within a large university teaching hospital to meet the growing needs of this patient population. As certain patient care needs become more complex, specialized centers designed to meet these needs will likely develop.

Another recent trend is the development of site-specific cancer centers, such as breast clinics or centers. Brady and Foster[18] suggest that a breast clinic may be an ideal choice for a site-specific program because of the increasing utilization of breast cancer screening services, the large number of breast cancer patients seen in most programs, and the amount of revenue generated during treatment. Lee et al.[19] provide an overview of the development of a comprehensive breast cancer. Table 54-1 highlights the operational and programmatic components. Site-specific programs have a number of advantages: patient convenience, improved medical decision making and, ultimately, improved quality of care.[18] Services not generally available in the community can be offered in these site-specific centers. These services include risk assessment, screening for the disadvantaged and minorities, and educational programs for both professionals and the public.[18] The American Hospital Association[20] has recently issued a publication that describes components for organizing and operating breast centers.

Specialized programs for all major cancers (breast, lung, prostate, gastrointestinal, gynecologic) may soon be developed, most likely in larger institutions due to the cost of setting up the programs and the need for large populations of patients.[18]

Planning Issues

Detailed discussions about planning ambulatory care services and facility design are available in the litera-

TABLE 54-1 Components of a Hospital-based Comprehensive Breast Center

Operational	Programmatic
ACR accreditation	Breast self-examination instruction
Dedicated clinical, technical, and clerical staff	Clinical history and breast exam
Ongoing training/inservice: physicians, technologists, nurses	Sophisticated breast imaging/diagnostic procedures with dedicated equipment
Criteria-based physician-referral panels and physician-approved triage protocols for "unassigned" women; primary care (asymptomatic) and surgeons (symptomatic)	Fine-needle aspiration for both palpable and nonpalpable masses if appropriate cytopathology available (otherwise large-core biopsy)
Quality assurance protocols: procedures, equipment, patient flow, and follow-up	Second opinion and breast consultation service
Effective relationships with hospital-based tumor registry, finance, medical records, information systems, and diagnostic/therapeutic departments	Interdisciplinary pretreatment planning conferences: weekly sessions for all diagnosed patients
	Risk analysis and counseling
Well-researched marketing plan/evaluation: internal and external	Psychosocial assessment, crisis intervention, support group, and referral for long-term care
Computer-based information and tracking system: financial and clinical	Access to local, regional, and national clinical and behavioral research trials
Clearly defined charge codes for all procedures: screening and diagnosis	Community outreach: public, professional, and patient education

Source: Reprinted from the *Journal of Oncology Management* with permission from Lee CZ, Coleman C, Link J: Developing comprehensive breast centers. Part one: Introduction and overview. *J Oncol Manage* 1:20–23, 1992.

ture.[10,21,22] Consideration should be given to space, staffing, equipment needs, management support, and how the services will be delivered.

A functional development plan should be written using information elicited from both external and internal surveys. Determination of present services, physician referral patterns, the patient population, financial and human resources, as well as local reimbursement policies are critical elements of the plan.[10]

Space requirements are primarily determined by the services that will be provided. If all treatment modalities will be administered, space is provided for each area as well as room for education of the public, patients, and health professionals. Space for the oncologists' office practices is often contained within the facility and leased to physicians.[10]

Provisions are made in all areas to ensure privacy of the patient while undergoing treatment. Careful consideration is given to the nursing station, support space, and waiting areas. Overall, the goal is to provide a friendly, warm atmosphere. Easy access to parking is essential. Equipment decisions will be based upon the services provided.

Increased competition has changed the focus of ambulatory care to be more responsive to the patient and family's requests. Providing individualized, prompt, and high-quality care is the major goal of cancer programs.[4]

THE ROLE OF THE NURSE IN AMBULATORY CARE

The role of the nurse in ambulatory care is complex and varied. Inherent in the role is provision of direct nursing care, education and counseling, health maintenance and preventive care, coordination of services, and continuity of care.[10] Three elements make the role of the ambulatory care nurse unique: the scope of practice, the use of the telephone in delivery of care, and the nurse's role in continuity of care.[12]

Ambulatory Care Standards

The American Academy of Ambulatory Nursing Administration describes the philosophy of ambulatory care nursing as follows: "Ambulatory care nurses participate in a comprehensive, coordinated, interdisciplinary approach to health care."[23] The standards developed by this group are in the process of being revised and should be available later in 1993. They can be obtained by contacting The American Academy of Ambulatory Nursing Administration, North Woodbury Road/Box 56, Pitman, NJ 08071. These standards can be adopted in most ambulatory care settings. Other professional groups have also defined standards. The American Nurses' Association and the Oncology Nursing Society (ANA/ONS) Standards of Oncology Nursing Practice were developed for the generalist in oncology nursing and have applicability to the ambulatory care nurse.[24] The Joint Commission on Accreditation of Healthcare Organizations (JCAHO) requires that ambulatory care meet the same standards of quality as the inpatient setting.[25] The Association of Community Cancer Centers (ACCC) also has standards (currently in the process of being revised) that address the role and qualifications of the oncology nurse in a cancer program.[26]

Ambulatory Care Responsibilities

The responsibilities of the nurse in the ambulatory care setting are multiple. Several research studies have been conducted to more clearly delineate these responsibilities[27,28] (Table 54-2). Tighe[28] studied 68 nurses representing both oncology and nononcology settings in ambulatory care with respect to the frequency with which they performed certain tasks and activities. Oncology nurses reported most frequent involvement in (1) health care maintenance activities, followed by (2) counseling and (3) communication. There was also a statistically significant finding of greater involvement in communication and therapeutic care by the oncology nurses.[28]

Hastings and Muir-Nash[29] surveyed 33 ambulatory nursing administrators about the roles and responsibilities of nurses in ambulatory care settings. This study involved a revision of Verran's[27] original taxonomy that resulted in nine responsibility areas and 61 activities (in contrast to the seven areas and 47 activities of Verran's original taxonomy). All nine areas of responsibility were confirmed as components of nursing practice in ambulatory care by over 50% of the sample, with the exception of three activities—"forms preparation," "transporting," and "maintenance."[29] Continued research is needed to develop a consistent vocabulary to describe the practice of ambulatory nursing and to develop a consensus about the role of the nurse.[29] Defining the contribution of ambulatory care nurses to patient care outcomes and institutional revenues will be an important task of the 1990s.[29]

Two recently completed surveys by the Oncology Nursing Society add to this body of knowledge by addressing salary, staffing, and professional practice patterns in ambulatory oncology clinics (N = 244)[30] and oncology-related infusion units (N = 135).[31] Results of the surveys show that 85% of clinics reported that staff nurses in ambulatory oncology clinics were paid the same salary as other hospital nurses. Eighty-two percent indicated their first-line manager was a registered professional nurse. Social workers were available in 94% of these clinics, and a dietitian was available in 87%. Primary nursing was utilized in 53.19% of the clinics. Eight-hour shifts were worked in almost 80% of the clinics. Telephone activities constituted a major percentage of time, with 66% reporting up to 25% of time spent in telephone work.[30]

Similar responses were seen with the oncology-

TABLE 54-2 Classification of Ambulatory Care Nursing (Adapted from Verran, 1981)

I. PATIENT COUNSELING
The provision of professional guidance and support to patients in regard to general reassurance on health status or disease state and support during clinic visit.
-client advocacy
-general support
-clinic procedures
-terminal/chronic illness
-screening/counseling by phone
-counseling regarding research process and informed consent

II. HEALTH CARE MAINTENANCE
Nursing assessment directed toward continuing a state of wellness including follow-up monitoring of status and instruction on general health care needs.
-general assessment
-preventive care instruction
-follow-up assessment
-provide information
measure physiologic indices

III. PRIMARY CARE
The responsibility for physical assessment and follow-up of medical and broader health care needs including general screening for specialized referral, physical diagnosis, and treatment.
-referral
-triage
-protocol care
-physical
-history
-expanded nursing role
-referred to within NIH

IV. PATIENT EDUCATION
Planned education given to an individual or a group of patients regarding specific health or illness self care.
-health care maintenance program
-home care
-illness/condition program
-plan of care
-group educational programs

V. THERAPEUTIC CARE
The delivery of direct physical care to patients following the direction of a health care team member, and the observation and measurement of the results of that care, or of the care of others.
-surgical preparation
-respiratory treatments
-irrigations
-applications
-specimens
-recovery
-invasive
-noninvasive
-dressings
-medications
-IV medications
-blood and IV therapy
-collecting research specimens

VI. NORMATIVE CARE
The delivery of services received by most clinic patients involving traditional entry and exit procedures, provision of assistance in the preparation for and during a primary care visit, and general direction or transportation to another care provider.
-directing
-transporting
-communication
-chaperoning
-assisting
-preparation
-documentation
-system
-comfort
-coordination
-appointments

VII. NON-CLIENT-CENTERED CARE
Nursing functions that do not involve contact with a specific patient, but are required for clinic maintenance and staff development.
-maintenance
-training
-materials
-nursing research
-searching for room space
-requesting service by phone
-checking stock
-answering telephones

VIII. COMMUNICATION
The provision of information to and interaction with other health professionals regarding specific patient-centered issues.
-inpatient staff
-physicians
-other health professionals
-referring physician

IX. DOCUMENTATION
The provision of written factual material for the purpose of authentication and/or supportive evidence of health care.
-documenting/revising care plans
-care provided

X. PLANNING
The mental formulation of a systematic method for achieving particular patient care outcomes.
-care based on assessment
-nursing diagnosis from assessment

Source: Reprinted from the *Oncology Nursing Forum* with permission from the Oncology Nursing Press. Tighe MG, Fisher SG, Hastings C, et al: A study of the oncology nurse role in ambulatory care. *Oncol Nurs Forum* 12(6):23–27, 1985.

related infusion unit survey. Nurses in these units were paid the same salaries as other hospital nurses 90% of the time. Ninety-five percent had a first-line manager who was a registered professional nurse. Availability of social workers and dietitians was almost identical at 95% (social worker) and 88% (dietitian). Primary nursing was used slightly less (51.54%) and 8-hour shifts continued to be the norm at 76.74%. Once again, telephone activities required a great deal of time.[31] Procedures performed, including approximate times and personnel performing the procedure, are highlighted in both surveys.[30,31]

Office-Based Nursing

The role of the oncology nurse in the office practice has expanded greatly with the shift of health care to the outpatient area. Choosing the office for oncology care may be a result of increasing health care costs, consumer demand, and the chronicity of the disease.[32] The office-based oncology nurse must possess sharp assessment skills in order to handle the large patient population in which patient care is intermittent and brief. These assessments must be ongoing and include treatment-specific, nutritional, pain, psychosocial, home care, and resource assessments. Patients can be asked to fill out questionnaires themselves while waiting for appointments, thus making them part of the assessment team.[33]

Barhamand[34] surveyed 192 office-based nurses about their roles, responsibilities, salaries, and benefits. A high level of job satisfaction was reported by 87% of the respondents. The opportunity to work with patients throughout the entire disease process was identified as the most gratifying aspect of their job. Table 54-3 is a summary task profile with the number of nurses performing each task on a routine and expected basis as well as those tasks done routinely but extending beyond role expectations.[34] The survey demonstrated the multifaceted role of the nurse in the office setting.

Triaging phone calls appropriately and efficiently is a major role of the office-based oncology nurse.[35] Phone calls may relate to symptom complaints, clarification of information, prescription refills, crisis management, reporting and interpreting lab tests, referrals to community resources, assistance with reimbursement, and counseling. Phone calls may also be made for follow-up purposes and provide an opportunity to reinforce symptom management and preventive actions.[35] Barhamand suggests the use of a reference file of standardized protocols to provide a systematic approach to handling these phone calls. Confidentiality must also be considered when dealing with patients' diagnoses, test results, and treatment decisions. Keeping a log of tests ordered is a way of tracking patients and written reports.[35] Documentation of phone calls and interventions must be done as a minimum standard of care. Figures 54-1 and 54-2 are examples of two different forms that can be used for this purpose. It is also critically important to document prescription refills.[35]

The office-based oncology nurse frequently acts as the liaison between providers of each phase of the pa-

TABLE 54-3 Task Profile for Sample of Office-Bfased Oncology Nurses (N = 192)

	No. (%) of Nurses Reporting Routine Tasks Within Job Description	No. (%) of Nurses Reporting Routine Tasks Beyond Job Description
NURSING-RELATED ACTIVITIES		
Receive phone calls from patients	184 (96%)	2 (1%)
Provide psychological support	184 (96%)	1 –
Teaching chemotherapy/side effects	183 (95%)	1 –
Call prescriptions to pharmacies	180 (94%)	5 (3%)
Administer chemotherapy	176 (92%)	– –
Teaching: dietary interventions	177 (92%)	2 (1%)
Renew prescriptions to pharmacies	175 (91%)	5 (3%)
Access venous access devices	175 (91%)	1 –
Teaching: pain control	174 (91%)	3 (2%)
Reconstitute chemotherapy	161 (84%)	1 –
Assist with medical procedures	155 (81%)	– –
Take vital signs	155 (81%)	6 (3%)
Intervene with orders to home/hospice nurses	153 (80%)	3 (2%)
Interview patient/register chief complaint	149 (78%)	5 (3%)
Dressing changes	140 (73%)	2 (1%)
Prescribe medications according to protocol	135 (70%)	7 (4%)
Intervene with orders to hospital nurses	132 (69%)	5 (3%)
Escort patients to exam rooms	132 (69%)	7 (4%)
Initiate chemo with infusion pump	130 (68%)	1 –
Weigh patients	130 (68%)	6 (3%)
Venipuncture for lab specimens	120 (63%)	19 (10%)
Bereavement counseling	105 (55%)	16 (8%)
Teaching: breast self-exam	90 (48%)	12 (6%)
Perform EKGs	58 (30%)	5 (3%)
Facilitate support group	35 (19%)	9 (5%)
Transfuse blood/blood products	25 (13%)	– –

(continued)

TABLE 54-3 Task Profile for Sample of Office-Based Oncology Nurses (N = 192) (continued)

	No. (%) of Nurses Reporting Routine Tasks Within Job Description	No. (%) of Nurses Reporting Routine Tasks Beyond Job Description
ADMINISTRATIVE DUTIES		
Train other nurses	48 (25%)	13 (7%)
Supervise other nurses	45 (24%)	7 (4%)
Precept other nurses	40 (21%)	10 (5%)
Supervise non-nursing employees	40 (21%)	15 (8%)
Act as office manager	23 (12%)	10 (5%)
Hire other nurses	23 (12%)	5 (3%)
Hire/train non-nursing employees	16 (8%)	9 (5%)
Issue payroll	8 (4%)	– –
CLERICAL-RELATED ACTIVITIES		
Order medical supplies	132 (69%)	12 (6%)
Maintain patient records/file reports	109 (57%)	21 (11%)
Schedule tests/hospital admissions	99 (52%)	21 (11%)
Intervene for meds for indigent patients	86 (45%)	23 (12%)
Update reports for tumor registry	70 (37%)	15 (8%)
Order office supplies	63 (33%)	16 (8%)
Data collection for research	62 (32%)	13 (7%)
Problem solve for insurance reimbursement	37 (19%)	31 (16%)
Explain/justify medical charges	23 (12%)	20 (10%)
Bill patients and present statements	13 (7%)	6 (3%)
Pay invoices	10 (5%)	1 –
Work with delinquent accounts	6 (3%)	3 (2%)
Make bank deposits	6 (3%)	2 (1%)
ANCILLARY ACTIVITIES		
Clean work station	144 (75%)	10 (5%)
Stock supplies	134 (70%)	8 (4%)
Meet with pharmaceutical representatives	123 (64%)	19 (10%)
Clean/maintain general office space	58 (30%)	23 (12%)
Attend tumor conferences	52 (28%)	20 (10%)
Perform CBCs/centrifuge blood	42 (22%)	13 (7%)
Be on-call for technical assistance	42 (22%)	7 (3%)
Travel to satellite offices	34 (18%)	2 (1%)
Make hospital rounds with MD	29 (15%)	9 (5%)
Run errands for office	18 (10%)	14 (7%)
Make home visits for MD	9 (5%)	4 (2%)
Make nursing home visits	7 (4%)	5 (3%)

Source: Reprinted from the *Oncology Nursing Forum* with permission from the Oncology Nursing Press. Barhamand BA: A survey of the role, benefits, and realities of the office-based oncology nurse. *Oncol Nurs Forum* 18(1):31–37, 1991.

tient's care.[36] Communication among all concerned is critical and facilitates the exchange of information. Figure 54-3 is an example of an interagency referral form that can be used to promote continuity. Shuster[36] also suggests that in an ideal situation the office-based nurse would make hospital rounds. Implementation of a "nurse exchange" program where a hospital outpatient-department nurse and an office-based nurse trade places for a period of time may lead to increased cooperation and coordination between the two settings.[36]

The office nurse also plays a key role in long-term follow-up planning, management, and education. Cancer survivors have many concerns, and the office nurse is in the unique position of addressing how the survivor is adapting to life after treatment. Psychosocial assessments are particularly critical. The nurse's role is that of educator, supporter, counselor, coordinator, and referral source.[37]

The Oncology Nursing Society[38] also surveyed 329 office-based oncology nurses to provide a comparative database of oncology nurses' salaries and benefits, provide information on practice patterns, and determine

PATIENT CALL-IN RECORD

Date:	Patient name:	Patient phone:
Diagnosis:	Current therapy: Chemo ☐ Rad ☐	Being seen at: ☐ E ☐ N ☐ S IRCC
Next appt:	Physician:	
Reason for call:		
Instructions:		
Nurse signature:		Time:
Physician comments:		
Physician signature:		

FIGURE 54-1 Patient call-in record. (Source: Reprinted with permission from the Oncology Nursing Press, Barhamand BA: Optimizing the use of the telephone for oncology nurses in office practices, in Carroll-Johnson RM (ed): *Meeting the Expanding Needs of the Office-Based Oncology Nurse.* Pittsburgh, PA: Oncology Nursing Press, 1992, pp. 8–14.)

PHONE CALL DOCUMENTATION FORM

(Patient Name, etc.)

Additional notes:

Nurse signature Date

Allergies ______

Time of call ______

Time call returned ______

Length of call ______

Purpose of call

☐ Pt problem ______

☐ Drug refill

Test results ______

☐ Questions about appt/tests

☐ Update on pt status

☐ Special instructions ______

☐ Other

Call Initiated by:

☐ PT

☐ Family ______

☐ MD ______

Phone # ______

☐ Pharmacy # ______

☐ Visiting RN # ______

Name ______

Urgency:

☐ Emergency

☐ ASAP

☐ Today

Disposition of call

☐ See orders

☐ Drug refill

☐ TLH

☐ Called

☐ Script mailed

☐ Medication change

☐ Test results given:

☐ By RN per MD OK

☐ To be given by MD

Notified ______

☐ F/U required ______

Phone call documentation

FIGURE 54-2 Phone call documentation form. (Source: Reprinted with permission from the Oncology Nursing Press. Barhamand BA: Optimizing the use of the telephone for oncology nurses in office practices, in Carroll-Johnson RM (ed): *Meeting the Expanding Needs of the Office-Based Oncology Nurse.* Pittsburgh, PA: Oncology Nursing Press, 1992, pp. 8–14.)

OUTPATIENT CHEMOTHERAPY/AMBULATORY INFUSION PATIENTS
ST. LUKE'S HOSPITAL
Referral Form

Name ______________________

Address ______________________

City ______________________

Phone ______________________

Caregiver ______________________

Notify in case of emergency ______________________

Attending MD ______________________

Diagnosis ______________________

Prognosis ______________________

____

____

Patient/family aware ______________________

Access device ______________________

Date of insertion of access device ______________________

Type of pump ______________________

Treatment protocol ______________________

____

____

____

Additional medications: ______________________

____

____

Additional comments:

____
Signature of nurse

____
Date

FIGURE 54-3 Referral form—ambulatory infusion patients. (Source: St. Luke's Cancer Center, Davenport, Iowa.[92])

staffing patterns. The survey respondents reported specifics related to telephone activities. Billing practices were also reported, with 23% of the respondents indicating that patients were billed separately for nursing services and 78% indicating that patients were billed if they were seen only by a nurse.[38] Detailed information was also obtained regarding procedures performed in the office setting. Nurses performed patient assessments; patient teaching; and catheter, port, and pump care. Nurses conducted patient support groups and performed most infusion therapy procedures.[38]

Radiation Oncology Practice Nursing

Hilderley[39] recently described the role of the clinical nurse specialist in a radiation oncology private practice. She emphasizes the importance of "mutual trust, understanding, open communication, flexibility, common goals, competence, independence as well as interdependence, and a strong desire to make it work" as essential components of a nurse–physician collaborative practice.[39]

The Oncology Nursing Society's *Manual for Radiation Oncology Nursing Practice and Education*[40] delineates the scope of practice and makes recommendations for practice. Patient outcomes based on 11 high-incidence problem areas are identified and can be used as quality improvement indicators. Course content recommendations for nurses within the radiation oncology department are also included.[40]

A survey of salary, staffing, and professional practice patterns in radiation-therapy–based oncology nursing was also recently completed by the Oncology Nursing Society. The survey, completed with data from 219 respondents, offers a comparative database of staffing, salary, benefits, and practice patterns in radiation therapy settings.[41] Primary nursing was utilized in 48.11% of centers responding to the survey. Eighty-eight percent of the respondents indicated that the administrative manager was not a registered professional nurse. Nurses performed patient assessments; patient teaching; and care of catheters, ports, and pumps.[41] The reader will find an extensive discussion of radiation therapy inclusive of the role of the nurse and management of care in Chapter 13.

NURSING ISSUES

Nurses face a variety of issues in the ambulatory care setting. These include models of nursing care delivery, patient classification and productivity, reimbursement, quality improvement, occupational hazards, and continuity of care.

Models of Nursing Care Delivery

Several models of nursing care delivery are utilized in the ambulatory setting. The evolution of the role of the ambulatory nurse and the complexity of care requirements have resulted in several models, including primary nursing, multidisciplinary teams, and collaborative practice. Regardless of the model chosen, maintaining a consistent approach over the long periods of time the patients are seen in this setting and meeting the needs of the particular setting are crucial.[12]

Primary nursing is designed to improve the quality of nursing care; recognize the patient and family as the unit of care, with the care designed accordingly; improve coordination of care between specialties; and ensure continuity of care between settings.[42] The primary nurse is accountable for coordinating a comprehensive plan of care that is continually reassessed, evaluated, modified, and implemented.[42]

The reality of high patient to low staff ratios in a complex and sophisticated environment makes the primary nursing model even more of a challenge today. Elements necessary to implement primary nursing include a decentralized system with authority vested in a primary nurse who is comfortable in an expanded role, availability of experts throughout the system for consultation and referral, and adequate staffing for the provision of quality care. Selection of the primary nursing model will depend on the philosophy and resources of the particular setting. The adaptability of this model makes it desirable for ambulatory care. Creativity in adapting the model to a particular setting is encouraged.[12]

The multidisciplinary team model emphasizes the important element of teamwork necessary to address patient and family needs in the ambulatory setting. A collaborative and respectful approach between team members ensures a more successful and functional team. The nurse is but one member of this team, which includes but is not limited to physicians, dietitians, pharmacists, social workers, rehabilitative services, pastoral care, research nurses, et cetera. The particular services of the setting will dictate who is part of the multidisciplinary team.[12]

The collaborative nurse–physician model has been implemented in all types of ambulatory settings.[1,10] This model usually has five components: (1) primary nursing, (2) increased clinical decision making by the nurse, (3) a collaborative practice committee of nurses and physicians, (4) joint record review, and (5) an integrated medical record.[43] This model allows nurses to manage resources so that triage occurs appropriately and there are designated appointment systems, easy access, and long-term follow-up.[43] Case management models, with critical paths throughout hospitalization, ambulatory care, and shared governance, have also been reported in the literature.[10,44] Case management models are being developed to address both quality-of-care issues and effective utilization of health care resources.

Patient Classification and Productivity

The increasing scope and intensity of nursing care provided in the ambulatory setting have resulted in the recent development and use of classification systems/tools.[45] Patient classification systems are used extensively in the inpatient setting and can be useful in the ambulatory area, with some adaptation. Developing a system for ambulatory care is complex due to the many variables affecting the nursing role as well as the variety of facilities and types of clinics. Patients are classified based on medical diagnosis and treatment plans, nursing requirements, and the purpose of the visit.[46]

Hastings[46] describes an urgent need for tools appropriate to the ambulatory setting that reflect the variables affecting nursing workload. Workload is generally influenced by three factors: (1) patient characteristics, (2) nursing role characteristics, and (3) the actual number of patients who require care. A workload analysis can be used to develop the staffing plan by classifying workload variables so they can be assigned a numerical value that is then converted into hours of staff time.[46]

Giovannetti[47] has identified two types of patient classification instruments: factor and prototype. Factor classification requires the nurse to rate the patient based on specific characteristics such as independence in activities of daily living, medications, treatments, and psychological needs. The prototype instrument requires an evaluation of the overall status of the patient and placement into a defined category. The resulting score is then computed to reflect the amount of nursing time and effort required.[45] Hastings[46] discusses the development of a simple prototype system in which patients are placed into one of six categories based on the nurse's estimate of time used at the visit. The system is used to make broad comparisons between areas and to identify overload or underutilization.

Classifying activities are often done as an adjunct to other measurements of workload such as time studies. Henninger and Daily[48] describe a nursing workload measurement system using the concept of relative value units (RVU). The RVUs per procedure are calculated by measuring the time spent in each nursing activity.[48] Johns Hopkins Oncology Center has implemented this type of classification system. Ashley[45] describes the development of a system through an operational review as well as a functional and facility analysis. An operational review is a comprehensive analysis of the specific department or area including a functional analysis to identify the types of activities conducted in the department, a facility analysis to evaluate the size and layout of the physical space, a material analysis to evaluate supplies and equipment, an organizational analysis to evaluate the organizational structure, and a staffing analysis to determine the time required to perform the activities in the department.[49]

When considering a classification system, it is important to account for time spent in indirect care and in telephone activity.[46] Recognition of the greater amount of time spent engaged in these activities in the ambulatory setting is critical. Prospective planning for staffing is the primary purpose of a classification system.[46] However, in the outpatient setting, classification systems are typically used for retrospective trending of patient characteristics, justification of resources, use of monitored trends for program planning, nursing workload analysis, patient care charges, validation of nursing care provided, and quality assurance.[45]

A major concern in the ambulatory area is maximizing productivity. Effectively utilizing resources can result in improved profitability. Budd[49] discussed five techniques to improve productivity. These techniques are:

1. improving scheduling
2. staffing only for current workload
3. improving functional design of facilities
4. ensuring employee motivation
5. increasing patient volume

It requires great skill to improve productivity without sacrificing quality.

Parrinello and Witzel[50] conducted a descriptive study using a modified version of Verran's Ambulatory Care Client Classification Instrument (ACCCI)[27] to examine and quantify nursing care requirements in four ambulatory care areas of a large university teaching facility. This study demonstrated wide variability in the average nursing care time for patient visits even among patient groups with the same medical diagnosis. Further study is suggested to determine how nursing care time and patient characteristics are related.[50]

The ideal ambulatory care classification system has yet to be developed. The importance of these systems will not be fully realized until a prospective payment system for outpatient visits is implemented. A number of different outpatient payment systems have been proposed and examined. They include ambulatory patient related groups (APGs),[51] ambulatory visit groups (AVGs),[52] products of ambulatory care (PACs),[53] ambulatory care groups (ACGs),[54] isoresource consumption groups,[55] ambulatory services weighting system (ASWS),[56] and the ambulatory severity index (ASI).[57] Lion et al.[52] state there are three motives for redesigning the reimbursement system for ambulatory care: "(1) the need for a rational system that is consistent, (2) cost containment, and (3) the need to shift the focus of patient care to a primary ambulatory setting and away from excessive use of hospitals and costly subspecialty services."[52] An outpatient prospective payment system has not yet been implemented, even though it seems inevitable. Administrators of ambulatory settings will need to be alert to developments in this area and become proficient with appropriate coding to maximize reimbursement.[58]

Additional questions about patterns of reimbursement and health care delivery are addressed in Griffith and Miller's recent exploratory study[59] of 43 oncology nurses performing services listed in the *Physicians Current Procedural Terminology (CPT) Manual.* The study indicated that oncology nurses regularly perform at least 68 CPT-coded services. This study has many implications for reimbursement of nursing practices. If the nurse in many of these settings is the only individual performing the services, one could argue that the nurse should be reimbursed. Obviously, many questions have been generated that require further study before an equitable payment structure can be implemented.[59]

Quality Assurance/Improvement

The goal of a quality assurance/improvement program is to ensure that care is provided according to established standards and procedures. The outcome of this care should improve the health status of the patient.[60] Standards of care mentioned previously can serve as the basis for developing a program in an ambulatory setting. It is essential to identify major aspects of care and critical indicators to monitor and evaluate. Anderson et al.[60] feel that one of the greatest impediments to the development of effective quality assurance programs in ambulatory care has been the lack of consensus regarding critical components or parameters that reflect quality care and their generalizability to diverse practice settings. One approach is the development of AmbuQual, a computer-supported ambulatory quality assurance system, based on ten parameters that define quality health care in diverse ambulatory settings. Each parameter is divided into *aspects* of ambulatory care and *indicators* to evaluate each aspect. Each indicator has its own *standard. Parameters, aspects,* and *indicators* are all weighted. Basic audits of peer review performance, clerical procedures, and patient satisfaction are completed. The computer program emphasizes any indicator with a score below a certain level that has been predetermined by the organization.[60] Main et al.[61] surveyed physicians and staff at two group practices prior to and 1 year after introducing AmbuQual at each site. The system led to an increase in knowledge about quality assurance for some participants, but the program will need to be studied further to determine its potential.

With an emphasis on "total quality management" or "continuous quality improvement," interest has been renewed in identifying problems/deficiencies from a systems approach. It is no longer acceptable to assign the sole responsibility for quality to the quality assurance coordinator. This model lends itself well to the oncology population. Careful examination and improvement of care practices between inpatient and ambulatory settings will benefit patients. Brachytherapy and venous access devices are examples of aspects of care that involve multiple departments.

Another approach to quality improvement may be the development of indicators standard to all oncology settings, with reports given to the hospital or clinic cancer committee.[10] Clinical indicators for oncology developed by JCAHO are being beta tested for possible implementation within 2–3 years.[25,62] There are indicators for breast, colon, and lung cancer, with a primary focus on the diagnosis and treatment of the primary tumor. These indicators are not inclusive of many other important aspects of care but are important in defining quality care for the patient with cancer.[62] Reporting data regarding these indicators would be mandated and would allow for comparison of cancer programs across the state, region, and country. Lamkin[10] suggests that a major focus for quality measures in ambulatory settings should be geared toward an examination of the effectiveness of education since that is a primary function of the ambulatory care nurse.[10]

Wiggers et al.[63] completed a study of 232 ambulatory cancer patients that assessed the importance of and satisfaction with several aspects of care. Sixty questionnaire items included physicians' technical competence and interpersonal and communication skills, accessibility and continuity of care, hospital and clinic care, nonmedical care, family care, and finances. Results of the study showed that greater importance was given to technical quality of care, the interpersonal and communication skills of physicians, and accessibility of care. Table 54-4 lists the ten items with the highest and lowest ratings of satisfaction for patients and their categorization into a priori care dimensions.[63] Replication of this study examining specific disease stages and other settings would be beneficial.

It is obvious that the emphasis on quality is here to stay and that the task of determining how best to demonstrate quality is still being developed. The completion of testing of the JCAHO oncology clinical indicators and implementation throughout the country is sure to have a significant impact.

TABLE 54-4 Patient Satisfaction with Care

	Proportion Agreeing/ Strongly Agreeing (%)	Proportion Rating Item as Very or Moderately Important (%)	A Priori Care Dimension
	MOST SATISFIED		
Cancer specialist competence	96	100	Technical competence
Nursing care in hospital	96	94	Hospital and clinic care
Correctness of treatment	90	100	Technical competence
Honesty of general practitioner	89	97	Communication skills
Opportunity to ask questions of doctor	88	99	Communication skills
Inclusion of family when discussing cancer	86	93	Communication skills
Diagnosis disclosed in a private place	86	97	Communication skills
General practitioner support	85	97	Interpersonal skills
Willingness of GP to discuss fears/worries	84	97	Interpersonal skills
Information from specialist about progress	84	91	Communication skills
	LEAST SATISFIED		
Insurance cover of cost of care	5	87	Finances
Choice of own doctors (Medicare)	6	92	Finances
Support for caregivers at home	9	93	Family care
Home care services for cancer patients	11	85	Accessibility of care
Help for patients and families to support each other	16	86	Family care
Information about symptom control at home	17	90	Communication skills
Provision of information in hospital	19	95	Communication skills
Information about treatment benefits/side effects	22	93	Communication skills
Patient control of life	23	91	Communication skills
Support for relatives and friends	24	90	Family care

Source: Reprinted from *Cancer* with permission from J.B. Lippincott Co. Wiggers JH, Donovan KO, Redman S, et al: Cancer patient satisfaction with care. *Cancer* 66:610–616, 1990.

Occupational Hazards

Oncology nurses working in ambulatory settings are involved with occupational hazards—specifically, the safe handling of antineoplastic agents, radioactive materials, and blood and body fluids. Guidelines for protection in handling antineoplastic agents were issued by the Occupational Safety and Health Administration (OSHA) in 1986.[64] In addition, the Oncology Nursing Society published guidelines specific to the ambulatory setting.[65] Unfortunately, the subject remains controversial, and wide variations in practice exist. Ambulatory oncology nursing administrators are challenged to establish protective measures in their settings.

The growth of continuous infusion administration of chemotherapy in the home setting necessitates considering these same issues for the home. Many patients receiving continuous infusions at home are not referred to home health agencies for in-home evaluations. One should question if patients have received adequate instruction about how to change drug cassettes or handle drug spills.

Implementation of a facility-wide chemotherapy and radiotherapy task force to establish standards, protocols, procedures; recommend protective equipment purchases; and evaluate compliance with the accepted standards is highly desirable. This group should represent all departments involved with chemotherapy or radiotherapy preparation, handling, and administration. Physicians' offices and home care agencies should be included in this task force to encourage consistent approaches and continuity of care.

The Occupational Safety and Health Administration (OSHA) recommendations published in the Federal Register in 1991 reinforce previous recommendations about protective guidelines related to blood-borne pathogens. Exposure of staff to patients' blood and body fluids is common in all oncology settings, and strict adherence to the guidelines is essential for protection of both staff and patients.[66] To comply with the recommendations, personal protective equipment is to be provided at no cost to the employee. This includes but is not limited to gloves, gowns, laboratory coats, face shields or masks, eye protection and similar items.[66]

Nurses in ambulatory oncology settings have a responsibility to be informed and adhere to current practices to avoid occupational hazards. Patients and families should also be protected from unnecessary exposure to hazardous situations. Education and compliance are critical factors for safe care.

Continuity of Care

The oncology nurse in the ambulatory setting is the person who frequently maintains continuity of care with the patient and family. This results because hospitalization is utilized only for acute care and home or hospice care is usually only required for a limited time. Ambulatory nurses may follow patients for weeks, months, or even years. As third-party payers scrutinize care and consumers demand more, the necessity for continuity is even greater. The question remains as to how this continuity can best be accomplished. One might also ask the question: How do we define continuity of care in oncology? Lauria[67] offers the following definition:

> the systematic assurance of uninterrupted, integrated medical and psychosocial care of the patient, in accord with the patient's wishes, from assessment of symptoms in the prediagnostic period, throughout the phase of active treatment, and for the duration of posttreatment monitoring and/or palliative care.

The definition reflects the multifaceted processes requiring mutual patient, family, and professional planning as well as advocacy, coordination, and implementation necessary to achieve an optimal outcome.[67]

Issues impacting continuity of care include economic forces, health care provider concerns, patient interests, family involvement, and demographic factors. Lauria[67] offers six key components necessary for quality continuity of care planning and implementation; see Table 54-5.

Several models of providing continuity of care have been implemented, including creation of a Director of Continuing Care position,[68] a continuing care team,[69] and "patient navigators."[70] Other strategies to enhance

TABLE 54-5 Key Components of Continuity of Care Planning and Implementation

Key Components
Uniform access
Access for all patients to all services
Affordability of care
Inclusive of screening and education about early detection/prevention
Comprehensive medical and psychosocial planning
Inclusive of social, psychologic, and environmental needs
Multidisciplinary team delivery of care
Responsiveness to patient/family needs
Provision of social and psychologic services in all settings
Assistance to negotiate systems and agencies
Recognition of deficits in personal and family strengths
Support for family members in caregiving roles
Establishment of self-help groups and volunteer efforts
Availability of resources and services
Identification of resources and services needed
Change in reimbursement patterns and allocation of dollars
Coordination of medical and psychosocial care
Coordination among all segments of the system
Identification of a coordinator (individual or team)
Monitoring and Accountability
Incorporation of evaluation and monitoring
Development of criteria and standards

Source: Adapted with permission from *Cancer* with permission from J.B. Lippincott Co. Lauria MM: Continuity of cancer care. *Cancer* 67:1759–1766, 1991.

continuity of care have been reported in the literature. Case and Jones[71] describe an Inpatient/Outpatient Data Flow Sheet that was developed and converted into a computerized program that could be initiated and/or accessed by oncology nurses in multiple areas to obtain and update information on shared patients. Most nurses questioned after the implementation of the system could give examples of how continuity of care had been improved.

Use of the computer for information flow and retrieval of clinical databases is just one example of the future potential. The technical capability of the computer to integrate information from multiple sources, store, and then later transmit the data to another location is especially advantageous for care of patients with cancer.[72] Bedside terminals promote timely documentation. Discharge planning and decision-support capabilities are also available with more advanced computer systems. This is an ideal way to enhance continuity; thus, it is essential that oncology nurses become familiar with computers.

Another approach to enhancing continuity of care is through multidisciplinary patient care conferences. Kerstetter[73] reported on the oncology multidisciplinary conference as a tool to increase communication and knowledge among departments providing oncology services. The Association of Community Cancer Centers (ACCC) Standard I emphasizes the importance of collaboration through a multidisciplinary team approach.[26] The goals of multidisciplinary conferences are twofold:

1. to provide a forum for education and communication among those involved in the care of the patient
2. to develop and evaluate individualized multidisciplinary care plans for oncology patients[73]

Team members attending the conference include oncologists, oncology staff nurses, the oncology dietitian, social worker, the home health care coordinator, hospice nurse, oncology clinical nurse specialist, pharmacist, research nurse, radiation therapist, pastoral care coordinator, pain management specialist, oncology director and rehabilitation services.[73] The particular setting may suggest others who should be part of the team.

Another important aspect of continuity of care involves defining who the patient should call if a question or concern comes up after traditional working hours. The answer to this question probably varies according to setting. However, the patient and family must clearly understand who should be called and when to call.

Another method for ensuring improved continuity of care is the daily morning conference to discuss new patients coming on a given day, problems that have arisen, or general issues. This short meeting can include only the physician and the nurse or can be expanded to include the research nurse, radiation oncology/chemotherapy nurse, pharmacist, and others.

In summary, continuity is critical to providing quality care to patients with cancer and will continue to be an essential component of a cancer program. The ambulatory oncology nurse is a key player in facilitating this continuity.

NURSING CARE DELIVERY

Nursing care delivered in the ambulatory setting follows the constructs of the nursing process. Several aspects of the role of the nurse in the ambulatory setting require more research and definition. These include patient teaching, telephone triage/counseling, and documentation.

Admission and Assessment

The patient's first visit to the ambulatory setting provides an opportunity to establish what may be a long-term relationship. Every attempt is made to help the patient and accompanying significant other feel welcome and comfortable. The homelike, warm atmosphere present in many ambulatory settings attempts to do this. A hospital visit or phone call by the ambulatory primary nurse prior to the first visit can ameliorate anxiety.[10] The first visit is a time that can be utilized to give important details of parking facilities, how to find the department, the routine at the time of the visit, and how long to plan to be there. Giving this information can demonstrate concern and caring on the part of the health care team and may alleviate some of the fear and anxiety associated with the experience since many patients are newly diagnosed and still in shock and denial.[10]

Knowing as much as possible about the patient prior to the first visit is ideal. Obtaining reports and old charts is helpful. Most ambulatory settings require that the patient complete the routine admission procedure, at least on the first visit. Thereafter, patients may be "part of the system" and additional, time-consuming stops in the admitting area are not necessary. For some patients, entering a door clearly marked "Cancer Center" (or some equivalent) is very difficult, thus immediately putting the patient at ease is critical. Welcoming the patient and introducing the team and staff members is a common courtesy too often overlooked in the busy pace of the ambulatory setting. Simple things like offering refreshments or something to read while waiting are much appreciated.

Many excellent assessment forms exist, and most ambulatory settings have developed one specific to their setting. These forms should be brief but inclusive of pertinent physical, social, and psychological data and contain an indication of where detailed information can be found in the medical record.[10] A discussion with the patient about the financial implications of the treatment plan is initiated and appropriate referrals are made to the oncology social worker or patient financial services representative.

A thorough explanation of future visits is reviewed with the patient and family. Accompanying the patient to the laboratory, other departments of the hospital, or other pertinent settings is ideal.

Patient Education

Patient education is a key component of the nurse's role in the ambulatory setting. Challenges involve determining the appropriate time to teach and having specific materials available. Each patient and family requires an individualized approach. In an extremely busy ambulatory setting, this may be difficult to accomplish.

Nurses in the ambulatory setting are fortunate that there is a great deal of printed material available related to cancer, cancer treatment, and management of side effects. Educational materials can be obtained from the American Cancer Society, National Cancer Institute, the Leukemia Society, pharmaceutical companies, and many other related organizations. In addition, some hospitals and health care organizations have developed their own materials, many of which are available for purchase. This written material can be used to reinforce or supplement patient education efforts. A variety of audiovisual materials are also available for purchase, but, unfortunately, many videotapes or slide programs are too expensive for many ambulatory departments to purchase. It is important to assess the patient's desired method of learning, rather than use the same approach for all patients. Some patients prefer to see a demonstration, while others prefer a one-to-one teaching approach. Still others may find a videotape that can be taken home, watched at leisure, and reviewed many times advantageous.

Nurses should be involved with the planning, development, and testing of educational materials. It is important to pay special attention to the reading level of materials distributed to patients or available in display areas. The SMOG formula can be used to calculate reading levels.[74] Printing the reading level on the printed material has been suggested.[75]

The readability of cancer patient education materials has recently been addressed in the literature. A discrepancy exists between the reading level of the average adult and the reading level of many printed materials.[74–77] Meade et al.[75] evaluated 51 booklets produced by the American Cancer Society. Using the SMOG formula, the reading level of the booklets ranged from grade 5.8–15.6 ($SD = 2.2$) with a mean reading level of grade 11.9. The median reading level of most Americans is closer to grades 8–10. Only six of the 51 publications sampled were written at a grade nine or lower reading level.[75] Another interesting finding in this study was that more than half of the materials had not been revised in over 5 years. A lack of non-English publications was also noted.[75]

Michielutte et al.[76] did a similar analysis of the readability level of educational literature on cancer prevention and early detection. Reading level (SMOG) scores were computed for 159 brochures and pamphlets obtained from the American Cancer Society, the National Cancer Institute, private companies, public nonprofit agencies, and state health departments. The average reading level found was between 10th and 11th grade.[76] Since low-income, low-education subgroups are at high risk for cancer, much of the available literature may be of limited value in providing information.[76]

Suggestions for improving readability include determining the medical terms that need definition and substituting simpler terms whenever possible. Correcting typographical errors and eliminating extraneous material is also important. Illustrations may improve understanding of the material.[76]

More intensive one-on-one discussions or use of picture cards, flipcharts, and videos rather than the written material may help in the education process.[75] It is also important to assess the patient's reading level using informal cues. A lack of interest in the material, lack of reading speed, expressions of frustration, inability to answer questions about the material, or the desire to let another person read the text may all be cues to the patient's inability to read at the needed level.[75] Another important fact is that reading ability will not necessarily predict how well a patient understands what he or she has read.[77]

Houts et al.[78] did a literature review of information needed by family members of cancer patients and suggested strategies for meeting their needs (see Table 54-6). The increasing movement of patient care to the ambulatory setting has resulted in the family playing an increasingly important role in the patient's care. Family members find themselves in shock and unfamiliar with who to ask and what to ask.[78] Unfortunately, many family members' needs for information are not being met. Family members can be confused by the complexities of today's health care system. Limited contact with health care professionals, uncertainty about when to contact physicians, what questions to ask and how to ask them, and fear that they will not understand the answer compounds problems of obtaining information.[78]

Nurses are an important source of information for family members. Lovejoy[79] suggests three ways nurses can provide important information to families:

1. serving as a guide through vocabulary and procedures common to the cancer setting
2. treating family members as part of the treatment team
3. offering assurance that the patient is being well cared for

Patients do not always understand that the nurse can give them information. Frequently, family members receive filtered information, either from the patient or another health care professional. Strategies for meeting

TABLE 54-6 Information Needs of Families of Cancer Patients

Understandable medical information about cancer
Specific information about: Patient's current medical status Ongoing and future treatment plans Expected side effects Intended results
Best way to meet patient's physical and emotional needs
Emotional reactions to anticipate during various stages of treatment
Physical caregiving skills
Services available to help with coping

Source: Adapted with permission from *Journal of Cancer Education* 6: 255–261, Houts PS, Rusenas I, Simmonds MA, et al: Information needs of families of cancer patients: A literature review and recommendations, 1991, Pergamon Press.

TABLE 54-7 Strategies for Meeting Families' Information Needs

Use of generic information sources including booklets, tapes, and group education programs
Individualized communication of information
Demonstration of skills needed to care for the patient at home
Greater use of the nurse to convey information about the patient's medical status
Greater assertiveness by family members
Willingness of health care professionals to be available and provide needed information

Source: Adapted with permission from *Journal of Cancer Education* 6: 255–261, Houts PS, Rusenas I, Simmonds MA, et al: Information needs of families of cancer patients: A literature review and recommendations, 1991, Pergamon Press.

information needs of families are described in Table 54-7.

Another approach to meeting patient education needs has been suggested by Berg et al.,[80] who constructed a "generic guide," a comprehensive assessment form of individual patient education needs to be used as a tool for staff inservice training about patients' needs, to guide staff regarding individual patient education needs, and as a strategy for determining program development. Use of this lengthy guide has not yet been evaluated in the literature.[80]

Patient teaching in the ambulatory setting has changed over the years.[81] There is an increased emphasis on prevention and management of problems as well as therapeutic goals. Factors affecting patient education include the patient variables of acuity; psychosocial issues and resources; and the institutional variables of time, money, and environment.[81]

The level of illness of patients often presents a learning barrier. Education can only be accomplished after the patient has achieved symptom relief. Psychosocial issues may either help or hinder the patient's ability to learn about the disease, treatment, and self-care. With more complicated therapies such as continuous infusion pumps and total parenteral nutrition comes the need for more indepth patient education. One must determine the patient's financial and personal resources prior to beginning these therapies.[81] Finding time to develop teaching materials or actually teach the patient is a daily challenge to the nurse in the ambulatory setting. Difficulties with using printed material and the cost of purchasing commercially available materials may inhibit education. The appropriate location for teaching is also constrained in most settings due to space limitations and overcrowding.[81]

Promoting effective patient education includes active involvement by the nurse in planning and presenting material and evaluating learning. A trusting relationship is built on effective communication skills, such as introducing one's self, a firm handshake, good eye contact, and a friendly demeanor.[81]

Rimer et al.[82] studied the improvement of cancer patients' pain control through a planned patient education program. Patients in the experimental group who received nurse counseling over a 1-month period and printed materials were more likely to have taken pain medication correctly (schedule and dosage) and were less worried about tolerance and addiction than were those in the control group.[82]

Newsletters can be valuable for patient education.[83,84] Hagopian's[83] study of subjects reading a weekly radiation therapy newsletter showed that these individuals scored significantly higher on the knowledge test, but no significant differences were seen in the helpfulness or number of self-care behaviors or the severity of side effects.[83] She suggests further study to determine the benefits to be derived from a newsletter. Ventura et al.[84] studied the effect of a series of newsletters for patients with peripheral vascular disease and found that 65% of the respondents receiving the newsletter reported that the information prompted a positive change in behavior. Nurses in ambulatory settings may want to explore implementing this tool.

Group teaching is another approach utilized in a variety of settings. One MDACC ambulatory treatment center holds a 2-hour class on chemotherapy prior to the patient starting treatment.[10] Many other settings offer structured, ongoing weekly or monthly educational sessions for patients. Group classes provide opportunities for patients to interact with each other and share common experiences. It is also a time-efficient approach for the health professional. However, the opportunity for one-to-one consultation should always be available to supplement group classes.[10]

The Oncology Nursing Society standards provide a guideline for patient and family education as well as for public education.[85] Teaching guides can assist in patient education.[86] Table 54-8 is an example of an ambulatory continuous infusion chemotherapy teaching plan that delineates teaching activities as well as expected patient/family outcomes. Teaching guides are handy references that provide a source of security and control to families and patients when unexpected questions or anticipated side effects eventually occur.

Still another approach is the development of a "learning center" or lablike environment for learning, practicing, and demonstrating skills necessary for self-care.[87] A variety of learning or skill units can be offered, including administration of IV or IM medications, caring for ostomies and wounds, providing home intravenous nutrition, placing feeding tubes and administering feedings, caring for venous access devices, et cetera.[87] Goldstein[87] reports that attendance at a learning center resulted in patients and families achieving more learning outcomes as well as fewer hospital readmissions for reinsertion or treatment of complications of right atrial catheters.[87]

Telephone Triage/Counseling

The amount of time spent on the telephone is a unique feature of ambulatory nursing practice.[12,34] Telephone activities include assessing patients' responses to the treatment given, providing information about prevention of side effects and symptoms, and evaluating patient outcomes.[88] Patient care–oriented calls can have multiple purposes: communication of changes in the care plan, reassurance of the patient and family about side effects, instructions to lessen the severity of the side effect, and assessment of supportive services.[88] Nail et al.[88] studied 1844 patient calls over a 6-month period. The mean length of calls was 6.65 minutes. Nurses handled 48.4% of the calls without consultation from another care provider. Information, coping, and comfort were the three major purposes of the calls.[88] Many nursing hours are consumed by the time spent on each telephone call, the time necessary to obtain and review the chart and then write a note, and the time to locate and discuss a problem with the consultant (physician, nurse, etc.). This time is important to take into consideration during budget planning. Establishing specific times for nurses to make and receive routine phone calls may be helpful.[88] Standard protocols for frequently occurring problems may facilitate nursing care delivery by telephone. Educational programs on the use of the telephone for care delivery may also be useful for the ambulatory nurse new to the setting.

A high potential for liability exists when medical advice is provided over the telephone to patients and families.[89] The implementation of protocols for telephone management as well as nursing educational programs and precise documentation are recommended. It is important to maintain a record of phone calls with specific data about the purpose, duration, and outcome of each call.[35,88]

Another use of the telephone in ambulatory oncology care is the "hotline." The hotline may be established through a toll-free 800 number that patients can call to make appointments or ask questions about their

TABLE 54-8 Ambulatory Continuous Infusion Chemotherapy Teaching Plan

Topic	Teaching Session Activities	Patient/Family Outcomes
		Upon completion of the teaching session(s), the patient and/or family will be able to:
Care of Vascular Access Device	Review and demonstration of institution's guidelines for care of vascular access device. Return demonstration by patient or family of vascular access home care.	Demonstrate the following skills consistent with the institution's guidelines and appropriate to the patient's vascular access device: –flushing –dressing change –cap change
	Review procedures for: –flushing –dressing change –cap change	Describe frequency of vascular access device care.
	Review signs/symptoms of infection, occlusion, extravasation.	Describe signs and symptoms of vascular access device infection, occlusion, or extravasation.
	Provide appropriate written information and homecare supplies.	Describe plan for management of vascular access device by homecare agency if necessary.

(continued)

TABLE 54-8 Ambulatory Continuous Infusion Chemotherapy Teaching Plan (continued)

Topic	Teaching Session Activities	Patient/Family Outcomes
Introduction to Continuous Infusion Therapy	Discussion and pre-treatment assessment:	
	• Patient's treatment plan –drugs to be infused –start/stop times –monitoring/follow-up	Identify the period of continuous infusion.
	• Patient's responsibilities during infusion –monitor for pump problems –discontinue or adjust if necessary	List primary responsibilities during infusion.
	• Display pump and how it is worn by patient	Verbalize concerns about responsibilities related to monitoring the infusion at home.
Toxicities and Side Effects of Medication	Review written information (e.g., NIH Publication #88-1139 *Chemotherapy and You*).	
	• Chemotherapy names	State the name(s) of medication to be infused.
	• Potential side effects	List possible side effects associated with medication to be infused.
	• Self-care measures (specific to each medication administered)	Describe appropriate self-care behaviors to prevent/alleviate side effects.
	• Toxicities to report	List toxicities of medication which necessitate contacting the physician.
Infusion Pump Operation	Demonstration using pump and equipment.	
	• Pump Anatomy Review written and verbal pump operation information.	Identify the following components of the infusion pump: • on-off switch • drug reservoir • power source (battery) • pump tubing • pump pouch
	• Review alarm system	State when pump alarms (when available) will go off.
	• Power Source	State how long the power source lasts. Rechargeable power source. • State minimum amount of time required to recharge the power source. • Demonstrate connection of power source to charger. Disposable battery • State how frequently the battery needs to be charged. • Demonstrate connection of battery to the pump.
	Changing the Drug Reservoir	
	• Review safety precautions (non-sterile gloves) when handling drug reservoir and disposing of used equipment.	Describe proper storage conditions for drug reservoir containing medication. List the safety precautions necessary to prevent skin contact with medication during reservoir change. Describe disposal procedure for used equipment.
	• Review when drug reservoir should be replaced.	State day and time when drug reservoir will be replaced.
	• Review ways to check when the reservoir is empty.	Describe how to verify that the drug reservoir is empty.
	• Review and demonstrate how to re-program pump after drug reservoir change if necessary.	Demonstrate change procedure and pump program adjustment.

(continued)

TABLE 54-8 Ambulatory Continuous Infusion Chemotherapy Teaching Plan (continued)

Topic	Teaching Session Activities	Patient/Family Outcomes
Daily Monitoring	Assessment Review written instructions about where assessment should occur and appropriate interventions. (These may be adapted from manufacturer's guidelines.)	Discuss ways to assess for problems in the vascular access device site, power source, tubing, alarms. State frequency of assessment for problems during infusion.
	Indicate where to inspect for the following potential problems: • Vascular access device site –infiltration –dressing/needle dislodgement –redness, swelling, tenderness, shoulder pain –leakage of medication –bleeding • Pump –power source disconnection dead battery –tubing kinked tubing leaks –pump display screen indicates no drug given –alarms low reservoir volume low battery occlusion completion of infusion pump dysfunction	
	Special Considerations Discuss with patient adjustments required in lifestyle during infusion:	Describe the adjustments which may be required in the following areas during the infusion:
	• loose fitting clothes best conceal pump	• clothing
	• vascular access device and pump must be protected during bathing	• bathing
	• pump can be safely placed under patient's pillow while asleep	• sleeping
	• heavy lifting, working with hazardous equipment and contact sports should be avoided	• sports/strenuous activity • work
	• pump may cause metal detectors in airports to alarm.	• travel
Discontinuing the Infusion	Indicate expected infusion completion time.	State the day and time when infusion is to be completed.
	Demonstrate and practice procedure using pump and equipment.	Demonstrate procedure for discontinuing infusion.
Follow-Up	Review names and telephone numbers of medical personnel for advice and emergency contact.	State procedure for contacting physician and nurse.
	Provide patient with physician and nurse's business cards, telephone number, and location of emergency facility.	State procedure for reporting to emergency facility.
	Review ongoing follow-up plans.	Describe plan for ongoing home care and follow-up with nurse at next outpatient visit.

Source: Reprinted from the *Oncology Nursing Forum* with permission from the Oncology Nursing Press. Reville BB, Almadrones L: Continuous infusion chemotherapy in the ambulatory setting: The nurse's role in patient selection and education. *Oncol Nurs Forum* 16(4):529–535, 1989.

treatment or side effects. The hotline also lends itself to calls from the general public about screening or educational programs being offered in the community or general questions about problems or symptoms a person may be experiencing. Unless a particular staff member is identified to take these calls, it may be difficult to incorporate this activity into the daily routine. Before implementing such a program, consider this staffing issue as well as the expense of the toll-free number. In larger ambulatory settings, it is common for a telephone triage nurse to be identified.[10]

Siegel et al.[90] developed a system whereby routine assessment of the needs of chemotherapy outpatients is done with a computer-automated telephone outreach system. The computer is programmed to call each of the 99 patients participating in the study at a preset convenient time. Answers to 12 survey questions about their concrete needs are recorded. Over time, the computer survey has achieved broad-based acceptance, and patients comply accurately with the instructions. This method may offer a cost-efficient, timely, and ongoing means of assessing patient needs.[90]

Recent surveys conducted by the Oncology Nursing Society specific to nurses in offices, radiation therapy settings, oncology-related infusion units, and ambulatory oncology clinics provide interesting information about telephone activities (see Table 54-9). Even though there are some differences, the primary telephone activities of all groups include symptom management, follow-up, physician contact to discuss patient-care issues, and patient education.[30,31,38,41]

Providing patients with instructions and a way to reach someone after routine hours is critical and can be accomplished in a variety of ways. Arrangements can be made to have the inpatient unit take phone calls from patients after routine hours and on weekends. In most situations, however, this is not desirable. Even though the patients may be known to the inpatient nurses, it is unlikely that these nurses will be thoroughly informed about the latest treatment, problem, and so forth that the patient is experiencing. An answering machine on the ambulatory setting telephone can provide a detailed message about how to handle a problem or to reach someone. An example of this might be a patient who calls to report a fever or another side effect. The patient would call the department phone and get a message directing him or her to contact the physician on call through the physician's answering service. Often, patients are calling to check on blood work, reschedule appointments, and so forth. In this case, they are able to leave a message that the nurse can respond to on the next working day.

Hagopian and Rubenstein[91] studied the effects of telephone call interventions on 55 subjects undergoing radiation therapy. No significant differences were noted between the experimental group (who received the weekly telephone call) in anxiety, severity of side effects, helpfulness of self-care strategies, and coping strategies. The telephone calls did, however, demonstrate a caring attitude toward patients and allowed patients to talk about any concerns.[91]

Follow-up phone calls after treatment has been completed are a routine practice in many settings. This practice provides an excellent opportunity for patient

TABLE 54-9 Average Percentage of Time Nurses Spent in Specific Telephone Activities

	Office-based Nurses		Radiation Therapy–Based Nurses		Ambulatory Clinic Nurses		Oncology-Related Infusion Unit Nurses	
Telephone Activities	Percentage of Nurses Who Indicated They Perform This Activity	Mean Percentage of Total Telephone Time in This Activity	Percentage of Nurses Who Indicated They Perform This Activity	Mean Percentage of Total Telephone Time in This Activity	Percentage of Nurses Who Indicated They Perform This Activity	Mean Percentage of Total Telephone Time in This Activity	Percentage of Nurses Who Indicated They Perform This Activity	Mean Percentage of Total Telephone Time in This Activity
Triage	74.5	15.79 ± 15.5	52.27	7.79	59.05	10.18	34.65	5.08
Follow-up	93.9	14.89 ± 11.64	83.52	14.61	86.21	17.11	73.27	12.71
Symptom management	98.8	32.15 ± 16.86	90.34	25.32	90.09	23.69	76.24	17.62
Patient education	86.8	13.21 ± 9.73	81.25	14.02	79.31	13.08	65.35	10.34
Scheduling appointments, tests	70.9	9.17 ± 11.40	75.00	19.16	71.12	11.70	78.22	14.31
MD contact to discuss patient-care issues	74.2	10.05 ± 11.76	76.70	12.25	87.93	20.09	92.08	32.27
Other	23.6	5.05 ± 12.77	23.43	5.39	22.08	3.93	22.77	5.89

Source: Adapted with permission from the Oncology Nursing Society: The National Survey of Salary, Staffing, and Professional Practice Patterns in Office-based Oncology Nursing and The National Survey of Salary, Staffing and Professional Practice Patterns in Radiation-Therapy–based Oncology Nursing. Pittsburgh, PA: Oncology Nursing Press, 1991; The National Survey of Salary, Staffing, and Professional Practice Patterns in Oncology-Related Infusion Units and The National Survey of Salary, Staffing, and Professional Practice Patterns in Ambulatory Oncology Clinics. Pittsburgh, PA: Oncology Nursing Press, 1992.

assessment and further self-care instructions. Phone calls to patients may be perceived as supportive. When patients know they have someone to call, anxiety may be relieved.

Patients receiving chemotherapy through an ambulatory infusion pump should be given precise instructions about how to handle a problem after routine office hours. The clinic/office might contract with a local home health agency to provide that service. The home health agency may be willing to troubleshoot any minor problems with patients over the phone and if necessary make a home visit. Not every patient will need or want a specific home care referral, but many are reassured to know that someone to handle a problem is "only a phone call away." A key component of successful implementation of this approach is communication of important and current information about the patient. A form can be utilized for this communication (see Figure 54-4). It is completed when the patient is started on chemotherapy that will continue at home and is transmitted to the home health agency and updated when any changes occur. The home health agency's "on call" nurse carries a notebook of these forms at all times. If a problem occurs, the referring ambulatory oncology nurse receives feedback on the next working day. In the meantime, the situation is handled by the home health agency nurse. This particular arrangement has the potential for meeting patients' and families' needs as well as ensuring continuity of care.

Conference calls can enable discussions of cases with family members or colleagues.[93] The telephone is an important communication tool that will continue to play an integral role in the care of ambulatory oncology patients.

Documentation

Documentation is a major challenge facing nurses in ambulatory settings because greater complexity of care and higher patient–nurse ratios demand accurate, concise, clear, and objective documentation.[94] Documentation includes the nursing process, fulfills legal requirements, describes the nursing care delivered, and reflects the quality of nursing care. Documentation of initial nursing assessments does not usually pose the same difficulty as documentation of ongoing assessment, teaching, problem intervention, and evaluation.[94]

In many settings, flowsheets have been developed to fulfill a number of patient care needs. Specific to the oncology settings are flowsheets to record side effects, laboratory data, chemotherapy administration information, and patient teaching. A number of flowsheets have been developed and reported in the literature.[31,94,95] Figure 54-5 is an example of a flowsheet specific to therapy side effects. It is completed by the patient.

Moore and Knobf[94] developed a practical and efficient documentation tool designed to limit narrative notes. The tool also functioned as a means of obtaining quantifiable and objective data that could be followed over time.[94] Staff members using this tool found it practical, easy to use and not excessively time consuming. The structured format also prompted more comprehensive assessments. The authors suggest ways to improve the form and to adapt it to inpatient settings.[94]

Lynch and Yanes[95] report on the implementation of a flowsheet designed to document chemotherapy administration, patient teaching, and symptom management.[95] After using the form for more than a year, the authors found decreased documentation time, and improved consistency of charting the details of chemotherapy administration. Initial and ongoing patient teaching and management of side effects documentation were also simplified. The patient signs the form to acknowledge initial patient teaching.[95]

Another approach to documentation is a patient self-assessment tool described by Hirshfield-Bartek et al.[96] Along with the tool is a flowsheet containing frequently used nursing diagnoses and potential interventions.[96] This tool can be used with outpatients beginning a course of radiation therapy as primary or adjunct treatment. Patients are asked to complete the tool at home and bring it on the first day of treatment. The nurse then reviews the self-assessment, identifies concerns, and discusses interventions. Patients felt that completing the form gave them something constructive to do and allowed them to share concerns in their own words. Nurses using the forms found that documentation was less time-consuming and that objective assessments improved[96] (see Figures 54-6 and 54-7).

Mikos and Finn[97] developed a flowsheet to document and monitor routine management of vascular access devices. After a year of implementation, less time was spent on documentation, continuity of care was enhanced, and a concise and comprehensive overview of venous access devices provided a database for monitoring quality assurance.

Use of point-of-care computer terminals has the potential for simplifying documentation issues.[93] These systems enable the nurse to immediately enter data into the computer, thus decreasing documentation time and improving accuracy. Many inpatient settings are already using such systems, but descriptions of use in the ambulatory setting are limited. Using the computer in the ambulatory setting may decrease paper flow; allow for greater efficiency in documentation and more timely retrieval of patient information, and decrease frustration over inaccessible charts.[45]

A frequent omission in ambulatory care is the nurse's documentation of behavioral expectations for patients providing their own care.[89] Careful assessment and documentation of the patient's and family's ability to successfully provide treatment independent of the nurse is important.

For assessing quality of care, complying with regulations, and a multitude of other reasons, documentation will remain a significant challenge to the oncology nurse in the ambulatory setting. The expanding use of

INTERAGENCY REFERRAL FORM

Patient name ______________ Primary caretaker ______________ Insurance ______________
Address ______________ Relationship ______________ SS # ______________
Phone ______________ Pharmacy ______________ DOB ______________

Primary MD ______________ Phone ______ Surgeon ______________ Phone ______
Oncologist ______________ Phone ______ Oncology nurse ______________ Phone ______

Diagnosis ______________ Onset ______ Primary hospital ______________ Treatment modalities ______________
Secondary DX ______________ Last hospitalization ______________ Last chemo ______________
______________ Last XRT ______________
Mets ______________ Referral to ______________ Date ______________

SERVICES REQUESTED: SN__ PT__ OT__ ST__ ET__ MSW__ HHA__ Chaplain ______ Other ______

ABILITY TO MAINTAIN VENTILATION & CIRCULATION

BP		SOB		Edema		MEDS
P		DOE				
WBC		Cough		Fatigue		
CRIT		Chest pain		Trans-fusion		
PLT		Breath sounds		VAD		Last flush ____

ABILITY TO MAINTAIN COMFORT

Pain description	Mild Mod Severe	PAIN REGIMEN
Location		
Control	Good Poor	
Bone mets		
XRT	Calcium ____	

ABILITY TO MAINTAIN FLUID STATUS

Oral intake		Skin	MEDS
Mucosa		Wound ____	
Thrush		Drainage	
Stomatitis		NG tube	
BUN ____	Creat ____	Fistulae	

ABILITY TO PREVENT HAZARDS & ACHIEVE SAFETY

Mental status		MEDS
Ambulation		
Sensory status		
Brain mets		

ABILITY TO MAINTAIN FOOD INTAKE

Current weight		Nausea		MEDS
Weight change		Vomiting		
Appetite		Dysphagia		
Diet		Dry mouth		
Dentures				

ABILITY TO COPE WITH ILLNESS & TREATMENT

Anxiety		MEDS
Depression		
Self-esteem		
Role changes		
Family support		

ABILITY TO MAINTAIN ELIMINATION

Bowel habits		Colostomy		MEDS
Constipation				
Diarrhea				
Bladder habits		Foley		
Incontinent				

ANTICIPATED TEACHING NEEDS

1. Dressing
2.
3.
4.

ANTICIPATED DME NEEDS Co ______

1. Hospital bed
2. Oxygen @ ____ L/m oximetry ____ PO2 ____
3. Wheelchair
4.

OTHER:

FIGURE 54-4 Interagency referral form. (Source: Reprinted with permission from the Oncology Nursing Press. Shuster SA: The oncology office nurse's role in the coordination and continuity of care, in Carroll-Johnson RM (ed): *Meeting the Expanding Needs of the Office-Based Oncology Nurse*. Pittsburgh, PA: Oncology Nursing Press, 1992, pp. 15–20.)

THERAPY SIDE-EFFECT FLOW CHART

Please put the number (0-3) that best describes the severity of the need/problem you are currently experiencing in the space provided. A score of 0 indicates absence of the problem, while a rating of 3 indicates that the problem is severe in intensity.

Physical/Emotional Status

I am experiencing	Date __/__/__	__/__/__	__/__/__	__/__/__	__/__/__	__/__/__	__/__/__
1. Change in appetite a. Decrease b. Increase							
2. Change in weight during past week a. Loss b. Gain							
3. Change in taste a. Describe taste change							
4. A sore mouth							
5. A dry mouth							
6. A sore throat							
7. Difficulty swallowing							
8. Indigestion							
9. Nausea							
10. Vomiting							
11. Bloating							
12. Diarrhea							
13. Constipation							
14. Difficulty urinating							
15. Difficulty breathing							
16. A cough							
17. Skin changes a. Location of skin change b. Redness c. Soreness d. Peeling e. Blistering f. Rashes g. Dryness							
18. Itching a. Location							
19. Bleeding a. Location							
20. Fever							
21. Chills							

FIGURE 54-5 Therapy side effect flowsheet. (Source: Reprinted with permission from the Oncology Nursing Press. Holton-Smith D: Enhancing nursing assessments in the oncology office practice, in Carroll-Johnson RM (ed): *Meeting the Expanding Needs of the Office-Based Oncology Nurse*. Pittsburgh, PA: Oncology Nursing Press, 1992, pp. 1–7.)

	Date __/__/__	__/__/__	__/__/__	__/__/__	__/__/__	__/__/__	__/__/__
22. Joint pain/soreness							
23. Muscle soreness							
24. Pain a. Location							
25. Headache							
26. Numbness							
27. Dizziness/light headedness							
28. Changes in vision							
29. Change in hearing							
30. Feeling tired or fatigued							
31. Difficulty feeding/dressing self							
32. Difficulty walking							
33. Difficulty climbing stairs							
34. Difficulty getting in/out of bed							
35. Changes in sexual activity or functioning							
36. Changes in rest/sleep patterns							
a. Unable to fall asleep b. Waking up too soon c. Nightmares d. Sleeping longer than usual							
37. Feeling anxious/nervous							
38. Feeling discouraged/blue							
39. Feeling out of control							
40. Difficulty with family relationships							
41. Difficulty with friendships							
42. Difficulty thinking clearly							
43. Difficulty in decision making							
44. Feeling confused/disoriented							

45. Please list other problems or needs in the space below

______________________________ Date ________

______________________________ Date ________

46. Of all the problems/needs you are experiencing, list the three of greatest concern to you:							
47. Please note your overall feeling or state of health today on a scale of 0-3, with 0 meaning "good as I have ever felt" and 3 meaning "worse than I have ever felt"							

FIGURE 54-5 (continued)

FUNCTIONAL HEALTH PATTERN PATIENT SELF-ASSESSMENT*

Health Perception/Health Management*
Who provides your health/dental care?
How often do you see your doctor?
Dentist?
List the medications you take.
How much? How often?
How much alcohol do you drink in a week?
Do you smoke cigarettes/cigars?
If so, how much?
What allergies do you have?
What happens when you have an allergic reaction?
What other medical problems do you have?

Nutritional/Metabolic Pattern
Are you on any special diet?
What did you eat yesterday (over the last 24 hours)?
How much fluid do you drink a day?
List the vitamins that you take each day.
Have you noticed any changes in your appetite?
If yes, describe.
Have you noticed any changes in your weight?
If yes, describe.
What foods do you avoid?
Who cooks your meals?
Do you wear dentures? Partial plates?
How do you take care of your skin? (What creams, lotions, or powders are you using?)
What soaps do you use?
Do you take baths or showers? How often?

Elimination Pattern
How often do you move your bowels?
Do you have problems with diarrhea?
Constipation?
Loss of control?
What foods/medications do you use to regulate your bowels (laxatives, prunes, bran, other)?
How many times a day do you urinate?
Have you had any changes such as loss of control, burning, frequency, or difficulty urinating?

Activity/Exercise Pattern
Do you feel tired during the day?
Is this new?
What changes have you noticed in your energy level?
What exercises do you do? How often?
What do you do for relaxation and fun?
Do you need help with: ambulating? bathing? toileting? dressing? grooming? feeding? cooking? food shopping? housecleaning? food preparation?

Sleep/Rest Pattern
What time do you go to bed?
What time do you get up?
Do you have any problems sleeping?
How do you feel when you wake up?
Do you take any medications to help you sleep?

Cognitive/Perceptual Pattern
Are you having problems hearing?
Have you noticed any recent changes in your hearing?
Do you use any hearing aids?
Have you noticed any changes in your vision?
How often do you have your eyes examined?
Do you wear glasses/contact lenses?
Are you experiencing any pain?
If yes, where is the pain located?
Describe it.
What do you do to manage your pain?
How does the pain affect your life-style?
What is your occupation?

Roles/Relationships Pattern
What is your marital status?
Do you have children/grandchildren?
Who do you live with?
What changes in your family roles or relationships have you noticed since your illness?
How do you anticipate that the radiation treatment will affect your daily routine?
What is the best time for your radiation treatment?

Self-Perception/Conceptual Pattern
How would you describe yourself?
What are your strengths/weaknesses?

Sexual/Reproductive Pattern
Are you sexually active?
Do you use any form of birth control?
Have you had any changes in your sexual relations?

Coping/Stress Management Pattern
How do you handle major problems/stresses in your life?
How are you coping with your life now?
Your diagnosis?
What do you do to relax?
What are your concerns regarding your treatment?

Value/Belief Pattern
What is important in your life?
Describe your spiritual needs.
What part does religion play in your life-style?

Life Patterns/Life-style Patterns
Describe your usual day.
What means of transportation do you have?

*On the actual form, space is provided for patients' responses.

FIGURE 54-6 Functional health pattern patient self-assessment. (Source: Reprinted from the *Oncology Nursing Forum* with permission from the Oncology Nursing Press. Hirshfield-Bartek J, Dow KH, Creaton E: Decreasing documentation time using a patient self-assessment tool. *Oncol Nurs Forum* 17(2):251–255, 1990.)

FLOW SHEET OF COMMONLY USED NURSING DIAGNOSES IN RADIATION THERAPY

OBJECTIVE ASSESSMENT	NURSING DIAGNOSIS	POTENTIAL INTERVENTION	DATE	INITIALS	EVALUATION
	1. Health perception/management A) Knowledge deficit 1) Treatment 2) Preventative health behaviors 3) Risk factors	 Discuss treatment plan Review dose/fractionation Arrange daily treatment time Orient to unit/routines on treatment visit Discuss: BSE, TSE, and Smoking			
	2. Nutritional/metabolic A) Alterations in nutritional status secondary to 1) Disease 2) Treatment B) Fluid volume deficit C) Altered skin integrity D) Impaired protective mechanisms	 Nutritional counseling Give patient written teaching guide Weekly weight check Refer to nutritional services Counsel dietary modification Discuss antiemetic therapy Discuss methods of relaxation Teach nondrug therapy Discuss antidiarrheal medication Review normal changes in skin secondary to treatment Provide patient with written skincare instructions Review processes of bone marrow depression Discuss weekly blood checks Discuss protective precautions for bone marrow depression			
	3. Elimination A) Altered bowel elimination B) Altered urinary elimination	 Review treatment-related changes in bowel elimination Counsel on dietary modification Discuss drug therapy Review changes in urinary pattern Counsel on dietary modification Discuss drug therapy			
	4. Activity/exercise A) Fatigue B) Altered ADL's	 Review factors that contribute to fatigue Discuss scaling of fatigue levels Seek assistance in activities of daily living			
	5. Sleep/rest A) Sleep pattern disturbance	 Discuss factors affecting sleep disturbance Discuss relaxation methods Discuss sleep medication			
	6. Cognitive/perceptual A) Altered comfort B) Knowledge deficit C) Sensory deficit D) Impaired verbal communications	 Discuss scaling of pain Discuss relaxation techniques Discuss positioning techniques Discuss pain medication options			
	7. Roles/relationships A) Altered family dynamics				
	8. Self-perception/conceptual A) Altered body image				
	9. Sexuality/reproductive A) Sexual dysfunction B) Reproductive dysfunction	 Birth control counseling			
	10. Coping/stress management A) Altered coping pattern	 Refer to social services Refer to Mind/Body Group			
	11. Value/belief A) Spiritual distress	 Refer to pastoral counseling			
	12. Life patterns/life-styles A) Altered life-styles				

FIGURE 54-7 Flowsheet of commonly used nursing diagnoses in radiation therapy. (Source: Reprinted from the *Oncology Nursing Forum* with permission from the Oncology Nursing Press. Hirshfield-Bartek J, Dow KH, Creaton E: Decreasing documentation time using a patient self-assessment tool. *Oncol Nurs Forum* 17(2):251–255, 1990.)

computers in this setting may simplify and expedite the process during the next decade.

PATIENT-RELATED ISSUES

A number of patient-related issues are dominant in the ambulatory care setting. Self-care, ethical issues, and care of the socially disadvantaged are among the major issues that will be addressed in this section.

Self-Care

Transition of patient care from the hospital to ambulatory and home settings has resulted in a shift in responsibility for family members caring for patients receiving treatment. *Self-care* is defined as how individuals care for themselves or alter conditions or objects in their environment in the interest of their own lives, health, or well-being.[98] Applying this definition to oncology, actions initiated by patients and families to prevent, detect, and manage side effects of radiation and chemotherapy can be defined as self-care. Instead of the nurse being the sole provider managing these side effects, the patient and family are expected to participate. Since the vast majority of oncology patients now receive treatment in the ambulatory care setting, there are a number of considerations for the health care provider.

Dodd[99] conducted research examining self-care behaviors of patients receiving chemotherapy that supported the belief that self-care activities can be learned. More self-care behaviors were performed by individuals who received specific information on side effect management techniques, enabling them to act promptly and knowledgeably.[99]

Nail et al.[100] developed a self-care diary that was used with 49 adult patients with cancer. The patients recorded their side effects, rated the severity of each, and reported the use and efficacy of self-care activities 2 and 5 days after chemotherapy. Most frequently reported side effects received a moderate severity rating. A variety of self-care activities were used to manage the side effects, resulting in little to some relief.[100] This diary mechanism was effective for obtaining patients' reports of the side effects experienced and the usefulness of self-care activities. This method of reporting can be used routinely beginning with the first cycle of chemotherapy. Diary entries can form the basis for evaluating the effectiveness of self-care activities and adjusting as necessary for future treatments.[100]

Hiromoto and Dungan[101] developed and implemented a chemotherapy learning needs assessment tool and contract. The learning contracts may instill a sense of responsibility and control for the patient during a time of uncertainty. Four of the five study patients were able to recognize symptoms, identify options, initiate self-care behaviors, and evaluate the effectiveness of self-care activities.[101]

Brandt[102] conducted a study with 22 patients undergoing brachytherapy to determine informational needs, the degree to which patients preferred to be informed and participate in their medical care, and the relationship between informational needs and selected variables. More than 86% of patients desired maximum information about their illness. Frequently identified learning needs included: (1) how to manage side effects, (2) activity restrictions during implant, (3) pain management and comfort measures, (4) cause of current symptoms, and (5) how the implant could affect symptoms.[102] Nurses caring for this population of patients should be aware of the benefits of patients' knowledge and active participation in their own care to help alleviate anxiety. Self-care is an important behavior for cancer survivors also, since they need to be motivated to take an active role in their own health care. Participating in health-promoting activities may help to lessen their feeling of hopelessness.[16]

An exploratory study of 49 family caregivers of patients receiving chemotherapy showed that giving emotional support was the most time-consuming and difficult task for family members.[103] Assisting with household tasks, errands, and transportation was also reported as time-consuming. Dependency was identified as the main contributor to caregiver burden.[103] These results point out the importance of the ambulatory care nurse establishing a relationship with the family caregiver as well as the patient in order to facilitate assessment, intervention, and support. A baseline of information about communication patterns, caregiver health, and family resources is critical.[103]

The ambulatory care setting is increasingly being utilized for follow-up care after major cancer treatments, such as for bone marrow transplant patients who are discharged earlier yet have to face long, stressful, and expensive recovery periods. An outpatient discharge coordinator can enable a smoother transition and improve continuity of care from the inpatient to outpatient setting.[104] The coordinator reinforces self-care teaching and provides written guidelines for patients and families. Patients and families are taught to care for venous access lines, to administer parenteral fluids, and to manage symptoms.[104]

For optimal self-care behavior, patients and families need to be adequately taught about the specific treatment modality and side effect management. Safety issues, safe handling of drugs, and infection control are addressed. Lifestyles, distance, and financial and family issues may make compliance with treatment regimens difficult or impossible. Often, the patient will turn to the nurse to discuss the situation. Encouraging and supporting self-care is a critical component of the nurse's role in the ambulatory oncology setting.

Ethical Issues

Ethical issues encountered in ambulatory care are similar to those that arise in other settings. Whether patients are making informed decisions and how best to provide high-quality care are ever-present issues. Unfortunately, even today some patients sign informed consents for participation in clinical trials or other research without having a good understanding of what they will be experiencing. The ambulatory care nurse faced with this dilemma should alert other health team members. At times, decisions may have to be referred to administrators or an ethics committee. In an office or small setting, discussion and resolution of ethical dilemmas can be particularly difficult. Open and honest professional dialogue is usually an effective approach.

Economic Issues

Access to health care has become a major concern for many Americans. Poverty has been shown to correlate with poor prognosis for all types of cancer.[70,105] In the past, any person meeting established criteria for research was eligible to participate and have the cost borne by the sponsor, government, or other funding agency.[105] However, current reimbursement to health care institutions as well as physicians is increasingly being scrutinized. Refusal by insurers to pay for research treatments tends to limit participation in studies.[105] Rationing policies for health care have also become a reality with Oregon's Medicaid program for life-saving medical care.[106] Unfortunately, poor people are being denied care, not only because they cannot afford to pay but also because they do not have input into the politically controlled decision-making systems in society.[106] As health care professionals, we have a responsibility to help economically disadvantaged individuals. Bal[106] suggests adaptation of programs, materials, and methods of care as well as a commitment to help the poor at both the organizational and individual levels. Nurses should advocate for more accessible cancer care for everyone.

CONCLUSION

The ambulatory care setting will continue to grow as a provider for oncology services. To remain competitive in the marketplace and to meet the growing needs of health care consumers, ambulatory care centers will need to provide a multitude of cancer services. The eventual implementation of prospective payment for ambulatory care will present challenges for health care organizations. Increased computer capabilities will positively impact the ambulatory setting by simplifying documentation as well as assisting in decision making.

The impact of large numbers of cancer survivors will be especially felt in the ambulatory care area. Preparing patients and family members to assume 24-hour responsibility for self-care with intensive treatment regimens will continue to challenge the health care team. The inclusion of nurses as providers of Medicare-reimbursed services offers impetus and support to nurses in a variety of ambulatory settings.[107]

Implementation of clinical pathways, standard treatment protocols, and algorithms[108–110] will become a reality and result in more thorough patient assessment,[110] decreased costs, enhanced quality care, improved communication,[108] and greater autonomy for nurses.[109]

Nurses in all settings must consider the special needs of the elderly. The ambulatory care setting provides an ideal setting to sponsor age-specific cancer prevention and early detection activities, perform age-specific assessments, evaluate treatment side effects, refer to established support networks, ensure continuity of care, modify patient education programs and strategies, serve as patient advocates, and influence health care policy.[111]

Issues in ambulatory care that will challenge all nurses include: "growth, reimbursement, managing volumes, greater patient acuities, care standards, fewer dollars, billing and coding, delivery systems, managing margins, physician and employee compensation systems, recruitment and retention, incentives, governance, and coordination of multi-disciplinary providers and support staff."[112] These issues and others present tremendous opportunities to impact the care of cancer patients for nurses in ambulatory care settings.

REFERENCES

1. Brown JK: Ambulatory services: The mainstay of cancer nursing care. *Oncol Nurs Forum* 12:57–59, 1985.
2. Nathanson SN, Lerman D: Directions in cancer care. In Nathanson SN, Lerman D (eds): *Outpatient Cancer Centers.* Chicago: American Hospital Publishing, 1988, pp. 1–13.
3. Sandrik K: Oncology: Who's managing outpatient programs. *Hospitals* February 5, 1990, pp. 32–37.
4. Esparza D: Ambulatory care. In Groenwald SL, Frogge MH, Goodman M, Yarbro, CH (eds): *Cancer Nursing: Principles and Practice* (2d ed). Boston: Jones and Bartlett, 1990, pp. 1089–1105.
5. Sandrik K: Outpatient programs for oncology. *Trustee* April, 1990, p. 19.
6. *Nursing's Agenda for Health Care Reform.* Kansas City, MO: American Nurses Association, 1991.
7. Shingleton WW: Cancer centers—Origins and purpose. *Arch Surg* 124:43–45, 1989.
8. Lokich JJ, Silvers S, Brereton H, et al: Free-standing cancer centers: Rationale for improving cancer care delivery. *Am J Clin Oncol* 12:402–406, 1989.
9. Mannisto MM: The emergence of cancer specialty centers. *Oncol Issues* 5:11–14, 1990.

10. Lamkin L: The new oncology ambulatory clinic. In Buchsel PC, Yarbro CH (eds): *Ambulatory*. Boston: Jones and Bartlett (in press).
11. Rubenstein E, Moreland B, Stewart C: Ambulatory care of the cancer patient. *Nurs Interven Oncol* 3:6–8, 1991.
12. Farley BA: Ambulatory care services. In Baird SB, McCorkle R, Grant M (eds): *Cancer Nursing: A Comprehensive Textbook.* Philadelphia: Saunders, 1991, pp. 1011–1022.
13. Clark M: A day hospital for cancer patients: Clinical and economic feasibility. *Oncol Nurs Forum* 13:41–45, 1986.
14. Harvey CD, Walker JR: Clinical linkages: A model for providing cancer care in a rural setting. *Oncol Issues* 5:11–12,17, 1990.
15. Humphrey LJ, Lester P: Cancer prevention and detection centers: An overview and critique. *Semin Surg Oncol* 5:211–218, 1989.
16. Rose MA: Health promotion and risk prevention: Applications for cancer survivors. *Oncol Nurs Forum* 16:335–340, 1989.
17. Satterwhite BE, Settle JT, Cushnie PB, et al: Ambulatory care for patients with HIV/AIDS: Creating a specialty clinic. *Oncol Nurs Forum* 18:555–558, 1991.
18. Brady AM, Foster J: The development of site-specific centers: The breast clinic. *Oncol Issues* 7:12–14, 1992.
19. Lee CZ, Coleman C, Link J: Developing comprehensive breast centers. Part one: Introduction and overview. *J Oncol Manage* 1:20–23, 1992.
20. American Hospital Association: *Why Care About Breast Care.* Chicago: AHA, 1992.
21. Bookbinder NF: Strategic planning. In Nathanson SN, Lerman D (eds): *Outpatient Cancer Centers.* Chicago: American Hospital Publishing, 1988, pp. 17–31.
22. Davis PB Jr: Facility design. In Nathanson SN, Lerman D, (eds): *Outpatient Cancer Centers.* Chicago: American Hospital Publishing, 1988, pp. 63–91.
23. American Academy of Ambulatory Nursing Administration: *Ambulatory Care Nursing Administration and Practice Standards.* Pitman, NJ: Janetti, 1987.
24. American Nurses Association, Oncology Nursing Society: *Standards of Oncology Nursing Practice.* Kansas City, MO: American Nurses Association, 1987.
25. Joint Commission on the Accreditation of Healthcare Organizations: *Accreditation Manual for Hospitals.* Chicago: JCAHO, 1992.
26. Association of Community Cancer Centers: *Community Cancer Programs in the United States 1988–1989.* Rockville, Md: ACCC, 1989.
27. Verran JA: Delineation of ambulatory care nursing practice. *J Ambulatory Care Manage* 4:1–13, 1981.
28. Tighe MG, Fisher SG, Hastings C, et al: A study of the oncology nurse role in ambulatory care. *Oncol Nurs Forum* 12:23–27, 1985.
29. Hastings C, Muir-Nash J: Validation of a taxonomy of ambulatory nursing practice. *Nurs Econ* 7:142–149, 1989.
30. Oncology Nursing Society: *The National Survey of Salary, Staffing, and Professional Practice Patterns in Ambulatory Oncology Clinics.* Pittsburgh, PA: Oncology Nursing Press, 1992.
31. Oncology Nursing Society: *The National Survey of Salary, Staffing, and Professional Practice Patterns in Oncology—Related Infusion Units.* Pittsburgh, PA: Oncology Nursing Press, 1992.
32. Behrend SW, Schulmeister L: Introduction. In Carroll-Johnson RM (ed): *Meeting the Expanding Needs of the Office-Based Oncology Nurse.* Pittsburgh, PA: Oncology Nursing Press, 1992, p. ii.
33. Holton-Smith D: Enhancing nursing assessments in the oncology office practice. In Carroll-Johnson RM (ed): *Meeting the Expanding Needs of the Office-Based Oncology Nurse.* Pittsburgh, PA: Oncology Nursing Press, 1992, pp. 1–7.
34. Barhamand BA: A survey of the role, benefits, and realities of the office-based oncology nurse. *Oncol Nurs Forum* 18:31–37, 1991.
35. Barhamand BA: Optimizing the use of the telephone for oncology nurses in office practices. In Carroll-Johnson RM (ed): *Meeting the Expanding Needs of the Office-Based Oncology Nurse.* Pittsburgh, PA: Oncology Nursing Press, 1992, pp. 8–14.
36. Shuster SA: The oncology office nurse's role in the coordination and continuity of care. In Carroll-Johnson RM (ed): *Meeting the Expanding Needs of the Office-Based Oncology Nurse.* Pittsburgh, PA: Oncology Nursing Press, 1992, pp. 15–20.
37. Deming P: Survivors of cancer: Meeting their needs in the office setting. In Carroll-Johnson RM (ed): *Meeting the Expanding Needs of the Office-Based Oncology Nurse.* Pittsburgh, PA: Oncology Nursing Press, 1992, pp. 21–26.
38. Oncology Nursing Society: *The National Survey of Salary, Staffing, and Professional Practice Patterns in Office-based Oncology Nursing.* Pittsburgh, PA: Oncology Nursing Press, 1991.
39. Hilderly LJ: Nurse-physician collaborative practice: The clinical nurse specialist in a radiation oncology private practice. *Oncol Nurs Forum* 18:585–591, 1991.
40. Oncology Nursing Society: *Manual for Radiation Oncology Nursing Practice and Education.* Pittsburgh, PA: Oncology Nursing Society, 1992.
41. Oncology Nursing Society: *The National Survey of Salary, Staffing and Professional Practice Patterns in Radiation Therapy-based Oncology Nursing.* Pittsburgh, PA: Oncology Nursing Press, 1991.
42. Farley B: Primary nursing in the oncology ambulatory setting. *Nurs Adm Q* Summer:44–53, 1981.
43. Koerner BL: Clarifying the role of nursing in ambulatory care. *J Ambulatory Care Manage* 10:1–7, 1987.
44. Zander K: Nursing case management: Resolving the DRG paradox. *Nurs Clin North Am* 23:503–520, 1988.
45. Ashley BW, Cross-Skinner S: Oncology nursing care delivery issues in the ambulatory setting. In Hubbard SM, Greene PE, Knobf MT (eds): *Current Issues in Cancer Nursing Practice* vol. 1, no. 1. Philadelphia: Lippincott, 1992, pp. 1–10.
46. Hastings CE: Classification issues in ambulatory care nursing. *J Ambulatory Care Manage* 10:50–64, 1987.
47. Giovannetti P: Understanding patient classification systems. *J Nurs Adm* 9:4–9, 1979.
48. Henninger D, Dailey C: Measuring nursing workload in an outpatient department. *J Nurs Adm* 13:20–23, 1983.
49. Budd GB: Productivity: The challenge for ambulatory services. *J Ambulatory Care Manage* 11:1–12, 1988.
50. Parrinello KM, Witzel PA: Analysis of ambulatory nursing practice. *Nurs Econ* 8:322–328, 1990.
51. Fetter RB: Ambulatory patient related groups. Unpublished manuscript, Yale University, 1980.
52. Lion J, Henderson MG, Malbon A, et al: Ambulatory visit groups: A prospective payment system for outpatient care. *J Ambulatory Care Manage* 7:30–45, 1984.

53. Tenan P, Fillmore H, Caress B, et al: PACS classifying ambulatory care patients and services for clinical and financial management. *J Ambulatory Care Manage* 11:36–53, 1988.
54. Starfield B, Weiner J, Mumford L, et al: Ambulatory care groups: A categorization of diagnoses for research and management. *Health Serv Res* 26:53–74, 1991.
55. Stimson DH, Charles G, Rogerson CL: Ambulatory care classification systems. *Health Serv Res* 20:683–703, 1986.
56. Young W, Joyce D, Blivens G, et al: Incorporating the cost of ambulatory care into case mix-based hospital reimbursement. *J Ambulatory Care Manage* 11:54–67, 1988.
57. Horn S, Buckle J, Carver C: Ambulatory severity index: Development of an ambulatory case mix system. *J Ambulatory Care Manage* 11:53–62, 1988.
58. Dougherty E, Hagin D: Move quickly but cautiously in outpatient cancer care. *Health Care Strategic Manage* 7:2, 18–20, 1989.
59. Griffith H, Miller I: Performance of current procedural terminology codes by oncology nurses: A report to the ONS Board of Directors. *Oncol Nurs Forum* 18:1391–1397, 1991.
60. Anderson JG, Benson DS, Schweer HM, et al: AMBUQUAL: A computer-supported system for the measurement and evaluation of quality in ambulatory care settings. *J Ambulatory Care Manage* 12:27–37, 1989.
61. Main DS, Fried RA, Benson DS, et al: Changes in knowledge and attitudes following implementation of a structured ambulatory quality assurance system. *J Ambulatory Care Manage* 15:71–76, 1992.
62. Marder RJ: Measuring the quality of care for the cancer patient. *Cancer* 67:1753–1758, 1991.
63. Wiggers JH, Donovan KO, Redman S, et al: Cancer patient satisfaction with care. *Cancer* 66:610–616, 1990.
64. OSHA: Work practice guidelines for personnel dealing with cytotoxic (antineoplastic) drugs. OSHA Instruction Pub. 8-1.1. Washington, DC: Office of Occupational Medicine, OSHA, 1986.
65. Oncology Nursing Society: *Cancer Chemotherapy Guidelines: Module III—Recommendations for Nursing Practice in the Outpatient Setting*. Pittsburgh, PA: Oncology Nursing Press, 1988.
66. Occupational Safety and Health Administration: Occupational exposure to bloodborne pathogens, final rule. Federal Register 56: 29 CFR Part 1910.1030, Dec. 6, 1991.
67. Lauria MM: Continuity of cancer care. *Cancer* 67:1759–1766, 1991.
68. Conkling VK: Continuity of care issues for cancer patients and families: Proceedings of the workshop on quality assurance in cancer care. *Cancer* 64:290–294, 1989(suppl).
69. Mellette SJ: Rehabilitation issues for cancer survivors: Psychosocial challenges. *J Psychosoc Oncol* 7:93–110, 1989.
70. Freeman HP: Cancer in the socioeconomically disadvantaged. *CA* 39:266–288, 1989.
71. Case CL, Jones LH: Continuity of care. Development and implementation of a shared patient data base. *Cancer Nurs* 12:332–338, 1989.
72. Hendrickson G, Kelly JB, Citrin L: Computers in oncology nursing: Present use and future potential. *Oncol Nurs Forum* 18:715–723, 1991.
73. Kerstetter NC: A stepwise approach to developing and maintaining an oncology multidisciplinary conference. *Cancer Nurs* 13:216–220, 1990.
74. Stephens ST: Patient education materials: Are they readable? *Oncol Nurs Forum* 19:83–85, 1992.
75. Meade CD, Diekmann J, Thornhill D: Readability of American Cancer Society patient education literature. *Oncol Nurs Forum* 19:51–55, 1992.
76. Michielutte R, Bahnson J, Beal P: Readability of the public education literature on cancer prevention and detection. *J Cancer Educ* 5:55–61, 1990.
77. Estey A, Musseau A, Keehn L: Comprehension levels of patients reading health information. *Patient Educ Couns* 18:165–169, 1991.
78. Houts PS, Rusenas I, Simmonds MA, et al: Information needs of families of cancer patients: A literature review and recommendations. *J Cancer Educ* 6:255–261, 1991.
79. Lovejoy NC: Family responses to cancer hospitalization. *Oncol Nurs Forum* 13:33–37, 1986.
80. Berg BK, Eckhoff-Biagi P, Hebert P, et al: Patient education needs assessment: Constructing a generic guide. *Patient Educ Couns* 9:199–207, 1987.
81. DeMuth JS: Patient teaching in the ambulatory setting. *Nurs Clin North Am* 24:645–654, 1989.
82. Rimer B, Levy MH, Keintz MK: Enhancing cancer pain control regimens through patient education. *Patient Educ Couns* 10:267–277, 1987.
83. Hagopian GA: The effects of a weekly radiation therapy newsletter on patients. *Oncol Nurs Forum* 18:1199–1203, 1991.
84. Ventura MR, Todd K, Burch K, et al: Patient newsletter: A teaching tool. *Patient Educ Couns* 15:269–274, 1990.
85. Oncology Nursing Society: *Standards of Oncology Education. Patient/Family and Public.* Pittsburgh, PA: Oncology Nursing Press, 1989.
86. Reville B, Almadrones L: Continuous infusion chemotherapy in the ambulatory setting: The nurse's role in patient selection and education. *Oncol Nurs Forum* 16:529–535, 1989.
87. Goldstein NL: Patient learning center reduces patient readmissions. *Patient Educ Couns* 17:177–190, 1991.
88. Nail LM, Greene D, Jones LS, et al: Nursing care by telephone: Describing practice in an ambulatory oncology center. *Oncol Nurs Forum* 16:387–395, 1989.
89. Chamorro T, Tarulli D: Strategies for risk management in cancer nursing. *Oncol Nurs Forum* 17:915–920, 1990.
90. Siegel K, Mesagno FP, Chen JY, et al: Computerized telephone assessment of the "concrete" needs of chemotherapy outpatients: A feasibility study. *J Clin Oncol* 6:1760–1767, 1988.
91. Hagopian GA, Rubenstein JH: Effects of telephone call interventions on patients' well-being in a radiation therapy department. *Cancer Nurs* 13:339–344, 1990.
92. Otte DM: Referral Form—Ambulatory Infusion Patients. Davenport, IA: St Luke's Cancer Center.
93. Adamski MG, Hagan BR: Using technology to create a professional environment for recruitment and retention. *Nurs Adm Q* 14:32–37, 1990.
94. Moore JM, Knobf MT: A nursing flow sheet for documentation of ambulatory oncology. *Oncol Nurs Forum* 18:933–939, 1991.
95. Lynch M, Yanes L: Flowsheet documentation of chemotherapy administration and patient teaching. *Oncol Nurs Forum* 18:777–783, 1991.
96. Hirshfield-Bartek J, Dow KH, Creaton E: Decreasing documentation time using a patient self-assessment tool. *Oncol Nurs Forum* 17:251–255, 1990.
97. Mikos KA, Finn TR: Quality assurance monitoring

through use of a vascular access device flowsheet. *Oncol Nurs Forum* 17:427–432, 1990.

98. Orem DE: *Nursing: Concepts of Practice* (3d ed). New York: McGraw-Hill, 1985.
99. Dodd MS: Self-care in patients with cancer. In McCorkle R and Hongladarom G (eds): *Issues and Topics in Cancer Nursing.* Norwalk, CT: Appleton-Century-Crofts, 1986, pp. 225–238.
100. Nail LM, Jones LS, Greene D, et al: Use and perceived efficacy of self-care activities in patients receiving chemotherapy. *Oncol Nurs Forum* 18:883–887, 1991.
101. Hiromoto BM, Dungan J: Contract learning for self-care activities. *Cancer Nurs* 14:148–154, 1991.
102. Brandt B: Informational needs and selected variables in patients receiving brachytherapy. *Oncol Nurs Forum* 18:1221–1229, 1991.
103. Carey PJ, Oberst MT, McCubbin MA, et al: Appraisal and caregiving burden in family members caring for patients receiving chemotherapy. *Oncol Nurs Forum* 18:1341–1348, 1991.
104. Chielens D, Herrick E: Recipients of bone marrow transplants: Making a smooth transition to an ambulatory care setting. *Oncol Nurs Forum* 17:857–862, 1990.
105. Merrill JM: Access to high-tech health care. *Cancer* 67:1750–1752, 1991.
106. Bal DG: Prevention and changing demographics: The underserved and cancer. *Cancer* 67:1814–1816, 1991.
107. Maraldo PJ: The nursing solution. *HMQ* 2:18–19, 1989.
108. Feingold MG, Meyer JW, Briggs DS: Controlling cost and quality through clinical pathways: One cancer center's experience. *Oncol Issues* 6:24–28, 31, 1991.
109. Rudolf VM: Oncology nursing protocols: A step toward autonomy. *Oncol Nurs Forum* 16:643–647, 1989.
110. Shackelford-Akers PA: An algorithmic approach to clinical decision making. *Oncol Nurs Forum* 18:1159–1163, 1991.
111. Boyle DM, Engelking C, Blesch KS, et al: Oncology Nursing Society position paper on cancer and aging: The mandate for oncology nursing. *Oncol Nurs Forum* 19:913–933, 1992.
112. Curran CR: An interview with Mary Ann Moore. *Nurs Econ* 10:87–93, 1992.

Chapter 55

Home Care

Joan C. McNally, RN, MSN, OCN

OVERVIEW OF HOME HEALTH CARE

The dramatic change in the health care delivery system that has occurred during the past decade has significantly impacted home health care. Home health care is one of the most rapidly growing and changing fields in health care. The Health Care Financing Administration (HCFA) reports that 392,700 persons (16 per 1000 enrollees) received an average of 21 covered Medicare home health visits in 1974. In 1986, 1.6 million persons (50 per 1000 enrollees) received an average of 24 home visits. During the same 12 years, Medicare program expenditures increased at an average annual rate of 23.6%, and the number of home health agencies increased from 2250 in 1975 to approximately 5700 in 1990.[1] The National Association for Home Care (NAHC) confirmed this growth and reported home care expenditures by all payers in 1990 at $16.2 billion, or 2.48% of total home health care expenditures.[2]

Many factors have influenced the consumption of health care services, including the increase in our elderly population and their increased life span. In addition, changes in family structure, the increase in women working outside the home, and the mobility of our society have decreased the support from family members who traditionally have provided the care needed to enable the elderly to remain in their home. The political factor that significantly impacted use of home health care services was the enactment in 1982 of the prospective payment system (PPS) for hospital care as an effort to curb Medicare spending.[3] PPS resulted in shortened hospital stays, discharge of acutely ill patients, and the shift from hospital to community-based care.

As defined by insurance eligibility guidelines, care at home can be preventive, diagnostic, therapeutic, rehabilitative, or long-term maintenance care. Home health care is an extension of the medical care system in which a physician oversees the care and the nurse is a primary provider and care manager through collaboration with the patient's physician. From the patient's point of view, home care seems to be the most efficient, effective, and least traumatic form of care, supported by the full range of multidisciplinary services.[4]

Home Care Service

The goals of home health care are to promote, maintain, or restore health; to minimize the effects of illness and disability; or to allow for a peaceful death. Home health care provides short-term intermittent services to enhance the knowledge and skill of the patient and family in managing care. The services provided depend on the needs of the individual and the family. The traditional services covered by Medicare reimbursement and provided by certified home health agencies include nursing, physical therapy, speech and language pathology, medical social work, occupational therapy, home health aide services, and nutrition therapy.

Nursing

Nursing is the foundation of home health care. Historically, nursing was the first health service to be provided in the home and remains the one most frequently utilized. Federal legislation has reinforced the position of nursing in home health care by requiring that nursing services be available in all home health agencies certified to receive Medicare or Medicaid funds. The nurse is the coordinator of all care provided to the patient. Home care nursing responsibilities include assessment, direct physical care, evaluation of patient progress, patient and family teaching, supervision and coordination of patient care, and provision of psychosocial support.

Home health care nursing differs from private duty nursing in that care is provided on an intermittent basis rather than daily or for extended time periods. Previously, home nursing care was available only during daytime hours; however, this has changed because home care demands have increased. Twenty-four–hour availability of home nursing care is now the norm.

Homemaker–home health aide

The availability of homemaker–home health aide service is often the factor that determines whether a patient and family can opt for home care. The National Council for Homemaker–Home Health Aide Services defines responsibilities of the home health aide to include assistance with personal hygiene and homemaking tasks. The home health aide must have successfully completed a home health aide training course or have passed the home health aide competency evaluation written and skills test. The aide is supervised by the home health nurse, who is responsible for developing a care plan for the aide.

Under the direction of the nurse, the home health aide may assist the patient and family to perform treatments (e.g., wound care or ambulation exercises). The aide may perform personal care activities for the individual such as feeding, bathing, and grooming.

Physical therapy

Physical therapists provide maintenance, preventive, and restorative treatment for individuals at home to promote patient functioning to the optimal level. For example, physical therapy can be effective in restoring function compromised by brain tumor or pathological bone fracture. This emphasis on restorative therapy is reinforced by the present interpretation of Medicare regulations, which basically restrict reimbursement to restorative physical therapy.

Occupational therapy

Occupational therapists assist individuals to achieve their highest functional level and to be as self-reliant as possible. They can teach the individual adaptive techniques and use of adaptive equipment to perform tasks essential to daily living. Occupational therapists provide preprosthetic and prosthetic training. They also assist in the selection or construction of splints to correct or prevent a deformity.

Speech and language pathology

Speech pathologists provide therapy to individuals with communication problems of speech, language, or hearing or those with swallowing disorders. A major treatment goal is to facilitate maximum speech and language recovery and to enable the person to use to the optimal level whatever speech ability is present.

Social work

Social workers in the home care setting have traditionally been considered referral agents who have knowledge of and access to the available community resources, particularly those involving money. Although this is one aspect of their role, equally important in home health are the social worker's roles as counselor and patient advocate.

Nutrition services

The role of the nutritionist in home health care encompasses direct patient care through diet counseling and indirect care through staff consultation and education about dietary practices. In most instances, direct care is often secondary to consultation and staff education because few third-party insurers will reimburse for direct patient counseling by the nutritionist at home.

Additional care services

In addition to the traditional services provided by certified home health agencies, a diverse assortment of services for the patient in the home are provided by physicians, dentists, chiropodists, respiratory therapists, vocational rehabilitation personnel, barbers, hairdressers, in-home companions and homemaker/chore workers. Laboratory specimens can be obtained, radiographs taken, meals delivered, and transportation provided for the patient in the home. Home maintenance and repair services are also usually available.[5]

Some supplemental services may require payment by the individual requesting them. However, some may be available from community service organizations at a reduced rate (e.g., Meals on Wheels from church groups, transportation from cancer societies) or covered by the patient's insurance if approved by the case manager.

Types of Home Care Agencies

In a similar context, many types of organizations provide home care service. Selection of the most appropriate type of home care agency is based primarily on patient and family needs, the patients' financial arrangement or type of health care insurance coverage, availability of family and community support, as well as the type of home care services available in the patient's community.

Three classifications of agencies provide home care services: the official agency of the public health departments, Medicare-certified home health agencies, and private duty agencies. However, many large home care organizations have combined agencies within the parent organization (e.g., the public health department has a certified Medicare home health agency division).

Official public health agencies

Official agencies are organized and administered within city, county, or multicounty health departments. Historically, the major focus of official health agencies has been preventive health care and infectious disease control. As such, home nursing care consists of biweekly or monthly home visits for patient teaching and supervision rather than direct physical care. State and local tax revenues fund the health department's traditional health promotion and disease prevention programs.

A number of official public health departments have expanded the scope of their services and have developed Medicare-certified home health agencies. These operate as separate entities within their organizations.

Medicare-certified home health agencies

Home health agencies, structured and operating within the specific guidelines defined by the HCFA in the Conditions of Participation, may be certified to participate in the federal health insurance program.[6] When certified, the home health agency is reimbursed for services provided to Medicare patients if those services are provided within their guidelines.

Medicare certification also authorizes the home health agency to provide and be reimbursed for services to Medicaid patients if those services are provided within the guidelines defined by each state for home care for the indigent. Medicare certification of a home health agency is also usually required by private insurance companies before reimbursement for home care services will be considered.

It is essential that the home care nurse be aware of the type of insurance coverage for each patient in the nurse's caseload and the guidelines defined by each reimbursement source in order to obtain the necessary approvals for care, complete the required forms, and provide services within the guidelines for reimbursement of home care services.

Private duty agencies

Private duty agencies provide nursing care in the home by Registered Nurses, Licensed Practical Nurses, home health aides, or companions for specific periods of time (e.g., 4, 8, 12, or 24 hours per day). The services may be contracted and paid by the patient or family or arranged through a case manager from the patient's health insurance company. These private duty agencies are often large, national, for-profit organizations.

Other agencies

As home care agencies have become more comprehensive in scope, other agencies have emerged, such as durable medical equipment (DME) companies and infusion therapy agencies. DME companies provide medical equipment and supplies including respiratory equipment, ostomy appliances, and parenteral feedings and supplies. Many DME companies have professional staff who teach and monitor the patient's ability to use equipment appropriately. Infusion therapy agencies provide parenteral medications (e.g., antibiotics, antineoplastics), total parenteral nutritional feedings, parenteral solutions, infusion devices, and equipment necessary for provision of infusion therapy at home. Most agencies maintain a pharmacy and professional nursing staff to administer the medications and fluids and teach the patient and family self-administration. Frequently the complex care requirements of the patient with cancer necessitate collaboration between the home health nurse and infusion therapy nurse to avoid fragmentation of care and to ensure comprehensive home care services.

Continuity of Care

Continuity of care has been described as a complex interaction of the patient with a variety of health professionals, clinics, institutions, agencies, and systems with the objective of restoring bodily and psychosocial functions to an optimum potential and preventing additional dysfunction and inconvenience.[7] This multidisciplinary coordinated care must be provided throughout the continuum of disease if quality care is to be achieved. The most frequently used processes to ensure a comprehensive multidisciplinary approach to patient care are case management and discharge planning.

Case management

Case management is a multidisciplinary approach to the process of identifying patient needs and coordinating the appropriate use of services and the health care system. The case manager may be a nurse from the hospital, clinic, insurance company, or home health agency who may follow the patient through the continuum of his or her illness.[8]

Discharge planning

Discharge planning is an interdisciplinary approach that centers on the family or significant other to facilitate the transition of the patient from one level of care to another. Discharge planning can enhance continuity of care through appropriate use of health care and community resources.[9]

A continuing care program begins with a comprehensive assessment of patient needs and the patient's and family's ability to comply with the treatment plans and cope with the disease. The patient's and family's perspective should be included as well as the observations and evaluations of professionals who have provided care to the patient. Assessment parameters include diagnosis, age, treatments, care requirements, functional limitations, cognitive abilities, interpersonal relationships with family members, concurrent illness of the patient or family members, usual coping mechanisms, financial and insurance resources, knowledge of disease and treatments, cultural factors, and social support systems.[7] The patient's diagnosis alone may not reflect the degree of illness, the complexity of care, or the number of support personnel required to assist the person at home.[10] In some cases the physical facilities may be adequate and the family supportive, but the emotional adjustments and 24-hour commitment to provide care may overwhelm the patient and family, thus necessitating admission to an extended care facility. For others, caring for a loved one at home may be a positive experience that enables the family to function in their natural environment while providing ongoing patient care.

The majority of individuals diagnosed with cancer whose situations are appropriate for home care have advanced disease that is metastatic and incurable but not imminently terminal.[11] Palliation of symptoms and pain control are major home care issues. Home care is also indicated for patients with self-care difficulties (either temporary or long-term), those who lack knowledge in managing the direct effects and side effects of cancer treatments, or patients who are homebound and require treatments (e.g., chemotherapy, antibiotics, or total parental nutrition). Slevin[12] reported that patient problems requiring posthospital care include inadequate or no support system, inadequate financial resources, poor environmental conditions, inability to carry out treatment and medication regimen, inability to carry out activities of daily living, poor socialization, or anticipated problems resulting from one of these factors.

The potential for success in home care is increased if the types of home health services necessary to assist with the supervision and management of the patient are available. A family can usually manage well if they know that a home care nurse will be accessible to provide direction and assistance. The degree of informal support available also affects the family's ability to manage home care.[13] *Informal support* refers to support systems such as friends, neighbors, and church groups.

Assistance may range from check-in phone calls or running errands to providing the caregivers with respite by staying with the ill person. Continuity of care can be enhanced through the appropriate use of community resources.[9]

The continuing care plan developed by the discharge planner or case manager in the acute care setting includes goals based on essential assessment data and interventions that address the patient's overall care needs. To promote continuity of care, it is essential to have effective communication between the referring professionals (e.g., discharge planner, case manager, clinic nurse) and the community service agency staff (e.g., home health nurse) who are caring for the patient during the next phase of care. In addition, timely reports of the patient's status promote quality patient care as the patient moves through the health care system.

Until recently the critical factor in determining whether a person was cared for at home or not was the degree of family/caregiver support and willingness to take on the task.[14] However, recent changes in insurance coverage have impacted discharge planning and community care. The Medicare diagnosis-related group (DRG)-based prospective payment system significantly changed discharge planning activities of hospitals. One study investigating the influence of DRGs on discharge planning reported that patients with certain medical diagnoses, including cancer, were most affected. They tended to exceed the DRG length of stay because they were not able to manage their care independently.[15]

Shortened hospital stays have resulted in the early discharge of cancer patients with highly complex treatment plans that must be managed in the home. It is expected that families will assume a significant increase in responsibility for the patient's care. Thus, in the current health care environment, patient and family involvement is essential for developing a plan for posthospital care and critical to the successful implementation of posthospital treatment.[16]

Unique Characteristics of the Home

The home is an important setting of care for the chronically or terminally ill, as well as for patients requiring sophisticated technologic services. The home presents the nurse with conditions unlike those encountered in other health care settings. The protective environment and control the clinic/hospital provides the professional are absent. In the home the patient and family determine when and how the patient's plan of care will be implemented.

The patient and family are encouraged to assume responsibility for the care of the patient; this is the overall goal of home care. When an individual or family member states how things will be done, it reflects a desire to maintain independence. Lewis[17] examined the association between personal control and quality of life for individuals with late-stage cancer and demonstrated that greater personal control over an individual's life was associated with higher levels of self-esteem, lower self-reported anxiety, and more purpose in life.

It is critical that the home health nurse evaluate the physical and financial conditions to support the care required by the patient at home. Environmental barriers to safe care, including lack of utilities and equipment to provide for hygiene and the storage and preparation of food, or the presence of vermin are within the scope of the home health nurse's assessment. Inadequate health care coverage and financial limitations may prohibit leasing modern medical equipment or purchasing adequate medical supplies and pharmaceuticals. The nurse can assist the family in obtaining wheelchairs, walkers, and electric beds from community loan closets and teach the family aseptic techniques and proper handling of reusable medical supplies such as glass syringes and feeding tubes.

ROLE OF THE NURSE IN HOME HEALTH

When home care nursing began in the 1890s, the role of the nurse was to provide nursing care to the sick and teach families cleanliness, proper care of the sick, and measures to promote health.[18] The advances in treatment of disease and changes in reimbursement of health care services have shifted the focus of home care nursing in the 1990s to one that emphasizes care of the acutely ill patient in the home.[4] Nursing remains in the unique position to contribute to the care of the home health patient and the caregiver through advocacy, counseling, teaching, and direct care.[19]

The Patient and Family as the Unit of Care

The cancer patient at home is an integral member of a unique system—the family. For home health nursing care to be successful, the nurse assesses the family's structure and processes, develops a plan of care that is congruent with the family's values and lifestyle, and includes the patient and family in the decision-making process.[20]

Speece-Owens[21] identified three types of family units: supportive, ambivalent, and hostile. The way a family functioned in the past is generally the way they will confront the current crisis of cancer. When a family member is faced with the threat of a potentially fatal disease, it is thought that people will forgive old behaviors, forget past misunderstandings, and band together for a common cause. This may occur in some families, but not in many. Knowledge of the family's response to previous crises can provide insight into the family's basic coping patterns.[22]

Family behavior can be described in terms of cohesion, adaptability, and communication. Family cohesion is the emotional bonding that members have toward one another. Family adaptability is the ability of the system to change its power structure, role relationships, and relationship rules in response to situational and developmental stress. Family communication is a facilitator; it can enhance or restrict movement on the cohesion and adaptability dimensions.[23] Family organization is influenced by communication processes, such as decision making and problem solving. Family coping is an indicator of family health. Health family systems adjust to life changes and transitions by implementing functional strategies to utilize internal and external resources.

Family assessment

Assessment of family organization begins with the patient's family of origin to obtain a history of family functioning. Their ages, geographic location, socioeconomic status, cultural and ethnic background, roles, relationship to patient, developmental level, major stressors, alliances, and frictions are identified.[24]

The present living group, if different from the family of origin, is then assessed. In addition to the previous criteria, the assessment includes patterns of authority, level of family development, values, behavior, coping ability, health and functional status, stressors, support systems, and knowledge of the illness and health practices.

As the communication link with the health care system, the home health nurse has the opportunity and responsibility to assess family structure and processes and design interventions that mobilize a family's internal resources and facilitate receptivity to and utilization of external informal and formal resources.

The following questions should be addressed during assessment of the family:

1. *Structure:* What is the composition of the family? Who is living in the household, and how are the household activities distributed? What family members live outside the home? Are there young children at home? Is the caregiver's role that of parent, requiring time and energy? The nurse can assist the family to redefine roles and redistribute household tasks or responsibilities.

2. *Pattern of authority:* Who is the decision maker? It is important to identify the persons in authority to facilitate patient care.

3. *Level of family development:* What is the level of family development that is being interrupted or affected? Families have certain developmental tasks that, if successfully completed, confer a sense of accomplishment and growth. For example, a young couple addresses the developmental tasks of establishing a household and planning for a family. A cancer diagnosis for either spouse disrupts the ability of the couple to achieve the identified tasks. Understanding and acknowledging the larger impact of a cancer diagnosis on the family can assist in the development of alternate acceptable goals for an intervening time period.

4. *Values:* What are the family's health care values? The caregiver who values health promotion is more likely to perform tasks to prevent problems than the individual whose orientation is that of illness or problem management. To promote optimal functioning of the patient, determine family activities that are important and will provide direction for care. For instance, if dinner taken together as a family is valued, nursing interventions are directed at facilitating this goal (e.g., obtaining necessary ambulation aids to enable the individual to get to the dining room).

5. *Behavior:* Do coordination and cohesion exist between various family members? Which members work together? What is the general pattern of family activities? Do family members do things together?

6. *Coping ability:* What are the strengths of the family and its individual members? What is the meaning of the cancer event to the family? How vulnerable is the family unit to a crisis event (such as cancer) related to the ability of family members to modify their respective roles, perform tasks essential for the continuity of family life, and redefine personal expectations and goals?[22] If a mother's cancer interferes with her adolescent daughter's autonomy and peer relationships because the teenager is depended upon to participate in care, the daughter may become a resentful or unwilling caregiver. The complexity of patient and family problems can sometimes overwhelm and immobilize the family. The nurse can assist members to identify measures to alter the experience and cope more effectively.

7. *Health and functional status:* What is the health and functional status of the caregiver(s)? Because 24-hour care of a loved one is physically and emotionally taxing, attention to the health of the caregiver(s) is imperative. Assessment also includes the caregiver's physical ability to perform the necessary tasks or procedures (such as lifting, moving, or transferring).

8. *Stressors:* Are there stressors outside of the individual's illness that may affect the family? Additional burdens that the family may be carrying are often overlooked by health care professionals in the face of a potentially fatal illness of one family member. However, these outside stressors may interfere with the delivery of care to the patient (e.g., a daughter who relieves the caregiver on weekends becomes ill) or with the energy level and emotional ability of the family to cope with the cancer experience.

9. *Support systems:* What outside support systems or assistance are available to the family? Patients and families are reluctant to ask for help or may not be aware of community support or resources available. The nurse can help the family identify and gather support in an attempt to prevent or diminish caregiver fatigue.

10. *Knowledge of illness and health practices:* What is the family's level of comprehension related to health practices? Because the family provides the majority of care, an assessment of their cognitive skills is necessary for the nurse to develop strategies to appropriately teach the caregivers the necessary patient care.

Demands on caregivers

In several studies exploring the demands on primary caregivers of adult cancer patients, most caregivers reported that the patient's daily physical needs were being met by immediate relatives and close friends.[25–27] The problem most often identified was a lack of knowledge in management of the patient's physical symptoms such as pain, and nutritional and elimination problems.

A pilot investigation of home health care needs of cancer patients and their families found that family members who serve as primary caregivers are often themselves in a state of unsatisfactory health.[28] The study also identified problems with extra financial burdens and stress. Caregivers have reported a decrease in their abilities to cope when changes occur in the patient's health status. In addition, feelings of despair, isolation, vulnerability, and helplessness often negatively affect their coping abilities. Table 55-1 lists the home care situations that have been identified as evoking the greatest stress for families and caregivers.

To enhance the family's ability to care for a patient at home, the home health nurse must function in two significant areas: nursing care that contributes to the physical well-being of the patient and nursing care that provides the patient and family with reassurance and practical and emotional support.[29] Nursing interventions that foster cohesion of the family and strengthen interaction, communication, cooperation, and emotional involvement will decrease isolation and enable the family to increase its autonomy and stability. Directing nursing intervention toward daily problem solving decreases the helplessness that families feel. Welch[30] reported that patients cared for by a home health agency perceived their care as satisfactory and they reported less disruption in family functioning than was indicated in other investigations.[30]

The nursing intervention most often cited by patients and caregivers as the most helpful is for the nurse to give excellent, knowledgeable, skilled, and personalized nursing care to the patient.[30–33] Other interventions reported to be helpful are listed in Table 55-2.

TABLE 55-1 Situations That Evoke the Greatest Stress for Caregivers

Managing the patient's physical care and treatment regimen
Managing their own home and the patient's home and finances
The need to be available 24 hours/day, 7 days a week
The fear of leaving the patient alone when the caregiver must leave the home
A change in the relationship or communications between the patient and caregiver
Disruption in the household routines; preparing different meals
Inability to spend time with their own spouse and children causing a strain in relationships
Often trying to balance the need to work outside the home with the care of the patient
The inability to meet the expectations of the health care system due to lack of time, knowledge, skill, or just being overwhelmed

Implementation of the Nursing Process

Today's home health nurse is expected to apply knowledge of the biological, social, and behavioral sciences to the nursing process, including a systematic assessment of patient and family needs, defining the characteristics of patient problems, formulating nursing diagnoses, developing and implementing the plan of care, and evaluating the outcomes of care.[34] The home health nurse often serves as the communication link in coordinating components of care.

Assessment

The assessment of health problems in the home setting includes the patient's actual and potential health problems as well as relevant characteristics of the family and the environment (social, economic, and physical). The parameters for assessment of patients with cancer and their families at the time of admission to home care are listed in Table 55-3. The planning of interventions and the identification of patient outcomes should include the impact of the family and environment on the patient's health status and care needs.

A systematic approach to assessment of the specific

TABLE 55-2 Most Helpful Nursing Interventions as Identified by Patients and Caregivers

1. To give excellent, knowledgeable and skilled, personalized nursing care to the patient
2. Providing the patient with the necessary emergency measures if the need arises
3. Assuring the patient that nursing services will be available 24 hours a day, 7 days a week
4. Allowing the patient to do as much for himself/herself as possible
5. Teaching family members how to keep the patient physically comfortable
6. Answering questions honestly, openly, and willingly
7. Supporting the cohesion of the family by initiating and promoting interaction, communication, cooperation, and social and emotional involvement
8. Directing nursing intervention toward daily problem solving

TABLE 55-3 Assessment Parameters on Admission of Cancer Patients to Home Care

A. Patient History:
1. Primary tumor site and histology
2. Metastatic site(s)
3. Previous and current treatments
4. Use of medications, vitamins not prescribed by physician
5. Family cancer history
6. Other health problems
7. Patient's chief concern

B. Physical Assessment:
All body systems (integumentary system; eyes, ear, nose, and throat; hematopoietic/lymphatic systems; respiratory system; cardiovascular system; gastrointestinal/abdominal areas; genitourinary system; nervous system; and musculoskeletal system)

C. Functional Status—ability to perform:
1. Activities of daily living
2. Instrumental activities of daily meal preparation, shopping, housekeeping, medication administration, communication

D. Physical Care Requirements of Patient (see Table 55-5)

E. Psychosocial Assessment:
1. Patient's mood state or affect
2. Causative factors/associated problems affecting the patient's mood state
3. Impact of mood on the person's functioning (role performance, sexual functioning, functional performance status [IADL])
4. Coping mechanisms
5. Social supports
6. Diversional activities

F. Caregiver Assessment:
1. Health problems
2. Functional status and physical stamina
3. Knowledge of patient's illness, course of disease, and prognosis
4. Knowledge of patient's physical care requirements
5. Emotional ability to provide care
6. Communications and relationship with patient
7. Availability (caregiver's other roles and responsibilities)

G. Family Assessment:
1. Structure (composition of members, roles, and responsibilities)
2. Pattern of authority (who and how are decisions made)
3. Level of development
4. Values (important activities, characteristics)
5. Behavior (cohesion, coordination, communication)
6. Coping ability
7. Health and functional status of members
8. Stressors
9. Support systems
10. Knowledge of illness and health practices

H. Equipment and Supply Needs (see Table 55-5)

I. Environment:
1. Heat, ventilation, water
2. Sanitation (waste disposal, vermin present)
3. Safety factors in home (portable heaters, scatter rugs, lack of support rails)
4. Barriers in home (bulky furniture, clutter)
5. Safety of location

J. Financial Assessment:
1. Health insurance(s) for coverage of services, supplies, and equipment
2. Family income available for out-of-pocket expenses

physical tasks involved in the care of the patient will identify all potential aspects of care and will facilitate planning and delegating responsibilities among caregivers.

Planning

The high-incidence problem areas defined in the ANA/ONS Standards of Oncology Nursing Practice[35] provide the framework for assessment and planning for the patient's physical care requirements. These problem areas include comfort, nutrition, protective mechanisms, mobility, elimination, sexuality, ventilation, and circulation.

An assessment identifies specific care requirements to maintain the individual in the home setting; the assistance needed by the person who performs the identified care tasks; the equipment, assistive devices, and/or supplies required; and any associated factors that have an impact on the individual's ability to carry out identified care. These special care requirements are listed in Table 55-4.

Nursing interventions

Nursing interventions in home health assist the patient and family by providing direct care and treatment, supervision of patient care, health and disease management teaching, counseling, and coordination of health care services. The home health nurse is responsible for observing and reporting changes to the patient's physician or other health care team members. The typical interventions, functions, and activities of the nurse in a cancer home health agency are listed in Table 55-5.

Evaluation

Outcome measures can be used to assess the quality of nursing care in specific areas based on predictable results. Outcome measures may be based on the adequacy of patient teaching (e.g., patient/caregiver demonstrates Hickman catheter flush and dressing change), improvement in physiological status (e.g., pain controlled, wound healing), improvement in functional status (e.g., patient transfers from bed to chair independently), improvement in compliance with treatments (e.g., medications are given as scheduled), and satisfaction with care as reported on patient and family surveys.[36,37]

However, outcomes are influenced by the multifactoral aspects of a patient's care environment and the natural history of the disease, which are beyond the nurse's control. Therefore, the potential limitations must be considered when outcome measures are used for quality assessment of home health care.[38]

TABLE 55-4 Patient Assessment—Physical Care Requirements

Common Problem Areas	Specific Care Tasks (examples)	Assistance Required (examples)	Equipment/Supplies (examples)	Associated Factors
Comfort	Medication administration (oral, suppositories, injections, IV); positioning; odor control methods; distraction; massage	To what degree is the person able to meet comfort needs? Self-medication vs. minimal, moderate, or total assistance?	Hospital bed; medications; syringes; IV supplies	Anxiety; family conflict
Nutrition	Preparation of special diets; management of nausea/vomiting; preparation/administration of tube feedings; hyperalimentation administration; measures to manage anorexia	To what degree is the person able to meet nutritional needs? Needs assistance with food purchase, preparation, feeding?	Blenders; food supplements, special foods; infusion pumps; gavage equipment; hyperalimentation supplies	Urine testing
Protective mechanisms	Personal hygiene needs; general measures to promote skin integrity; management of impaired skin/mucosal integrity (stomatitis, decubitus ulcers, wounds, radiation dermatitis); prevention/management of infection (medication administration, cleansing/care of equipment)	To what degree is the person able to accomplish activities of daily living; independent in activities of daily living vs. moderate or total assistance? Degree of assistance required with measures to maintain skin integrity?	Shower equipment (bars, chairs); dressings; irrigating syringes	Individual's mobility status
Mobility	Active/passive range-of-motion exercises; transferring, turning, positioning, application of braces; management of edema	To what degree is the person able to ambulate, turn, move, or transfer independently? How many assistants are needed?	Wheelchair; walker; trapeze; Hoyer lift; splints; braces	Individual's pain; fatigue; fractures; bone metastases; edema/ascites; altered respiratory status
Elimination	Foley catheter care; self-catheterization; suprapubic catheter care; stoma management; ostomy bag changes; irrigations; skin care; management of constipation/diarrhea; use of bedpans; administration of enemas	To what degree is the person able to manage elimination needs? How much and what type of assistance is required?	Bedpan; urinal; bedside commode; enema equipment; laxatives; ostomy supplies	Individual's nutritional status; hydration; use of narcotic analgesics
Sexuality	Measures to maintain vaginal integrity (eg, dilator); douching; intermittent catheterization	To what degree is the person able to perform tasks related to sexuality needs?	Foley catheters; straight catheters; douche equipment	Urinary elimination needs
Ventilation	Oxygen use; suctioning; tracheostomy care; postural drainage; chest percussion and vibration; medication administration	To what degree is the person able to perform tasks related to respiratory care?	Oxygen; suction catheters/machine; humidifier; tracheostomy care sets	Modification of environmental temperature and humidity; removal of pollutants (smoke, chemicals, exhaust, dust)
Circulation	Increase fluid intake; prevent falls, injury, skin breakdown; encourage energy saving; perform activities of daily living; elevate extremities	To what degree is patient able to perform activities of daily living? What amount of assistance is needed? What activities are important to patient?	Hospital bed; wheelchair; walker; bedpan; shower rails and stool	Edema; ascites; postural hypotension; electrolyte imbalance

Source: McNally JC, Sumerville ET, Miaskowski C, et al: *Guidelines for Oncology Nursing Practice.* Philadelphia: Saunders, 1991.

TABLE 55-5 Nursing Functions and Activities in Home Health

The Home Care Program nurse is especially prepared to offer the following services and support for patients with cancer and their families:

Direct nursing care
- Completes physical examination of the patient during each home visit
- Demonstrates all nursing care procedures being taught to the caregivers in the home
- Performs all procedures requiring the skill of a nurse (administration of intravenous fluid, insertion of a feeding tube, etc.)
- Administers chemotherapy prescribed by the physician
- Obtains laboratory specimens requested by the physician to monitor effects of the disease or disease treatment (specimens of blood, urine, sputum, or wound cultures)

Observation and reporting
- Assesses and reports signs and symptoms of an emergency medical problem resulting from side effects of medical treatment of the disease (eg, bone marrow depression following chemotherapy)
- Assesses and reports potential signs and symptoms of an emergency medical problem resulting from the tumor (eg, hypercalcemia)
- Assesses and reports signs and symptoms of disease progression
- Evaluates patient's response to prescribed medications and therapies
- Assesses patient's and family's emotional response to the course of the disease and/or the course of treatment of the disease

Supervision of patient care
- Identifies current and potential problems influencing the patient's care, including ability of patient to obtain needed care in the home
- Plans nursing care to correct, improve, or manage the identified patient problems
- Provides written instructions of medication schedules or patient care procedures for caregivers in the patient's home
- Supervises the care given to the patient in the home by the family, friends, volunteers, or home health aides
- Coordinates admission to the hospital if the need arises

Health and disease management teaching
- Instructs regarding actual and potential effects of the disease process based on the patient's or caregiver's readiness and ability to learn
- Teaches actual and potential effects of the disease treatment on the patient
- Teaches signs and symptoms requiring immediate notification of the nurse or physician
- Teaches purpose, side effects, amount, frequency and method of administering each medication and treatment prescribed (eg, analgesics, colostomy care, decubitus ulcer care, etc.)
- Instructs regarding nutrition and hydration requirements, including methods appropriate for the individual patient
- Instructs regarding rehabilitation and self-care techniques (eg ambulation with walker, range-of-motion exercises for lymphedema, energy saving, comfort measures)
- Instructs regarding prevention of complications and infections, including environmental safety and hygiene

TABLE 55-5 Nursing Functions and Activities in Home Health (continued)

- Instructs regarding health promotion and maintenance, with emphasis on prevention and early detection of disease

Counseling
- Identifies emotional, spiritual, or social problems experienced by the patient and family
- Assists the patient and family to identify and express their feelings about effects of the disease or treatments
- Facilitates referral to appropriate resources for extended counseling

Coordination and collaboration
- Assists the patient and family to utilize formal and informal support services within the community
- Assesses and prioritizes patient and family needs; integrates and coordinates appropriate home health services into the plan of care (eg, home health aide, medical social work, occupational therapy, physical therapy, speech therapy, nutrition consultation)

Source: Michigan Cancer Foundation Services, Inc. Home Care Program, 110 E. Warren, Detroit MI 48201.

Coordination of Services

Coordination and collaboration skills are essential to promote continuity of care from the acute care setting, coordination of services in the home setting, and achievement of rehabilitation goals.[7,8] A multidisciplinary group of health care professionals from a variety of health care institutions and community service agencies may be involved with the home care of the person with cancer. The responsibility for coordinating these interventions and teaching the patient and family about the multitude of services is frequently undertaken by the home health nurse.[39] It is not unusual for the patient with cancer to be receiving care from an oncologist, radiologist, and family physician concurrently, in addition to having phlebotomists from laboratories, technicians from infusion therapy agencies, equipment vendors from medical equipment agencies, and therapists and home health aides visits to provide specific services. People with cancer may become alarmed and anxious about the number of "strangers" who enter their homes to provide care services. The nurse can provide reassurance to the patient and family by explaining the purpose of each service and coordinating the visits. The nurse also maintains and shares an awareness of the goals for rehabilitation for each patient in order to provide direction to the service providers.

A study by Shuster and Cloonan[40] of 24 home health agencies determined that nursing activities related to coordination of services (clinical case management) accounted for 13% of the nurse's time. Care coordination and collaborative activities of the home health nurse often expand to become case management, especially when caring for the patient with advanced metastatic disease or severe functional limitations. The home health nurse assumes responsibility for ongoing patient assessment, care planning, referrals for services, monitoring for appropriateness of services provided, routinely communicating the patient status with all services providers and payers, and evaluating the care provided based on patient and family goals and patient care outcomes.[41,42] Incorporating case management into the role of the home health nurse will achieve better patient care as described by the American Nurses Association, whose goals for case management are "the provision of quality health care along a continuum, decreased fragmentation of care across many settings, enhancement of the client's quality of life, and cost containment."[19]

Documenting Nursing Care

Legal responsibilities of the home health oncology nurse include knowledge of and compliance with the nursing role as defined in the state Nurse Practice Act, the regulations that govern home health, and the standards of nursing practice for the nurse's community. The best evidence that the nurse has complied with these regulations and standards is the documentation of patient care.[43,44] Documentation must be complete, clear, accurate, objective, and timely to fulfill federal and state certification requirements and Medicare and third-party reimbursement requirements.[45] The written report of nursing activity provides the only concrete evidence of what occurred and can provide legal protection for the nurse and the home health agency. The guiding principle should be "more is better."[46]

Principles of documentation include a comprehensive, accurate, and objective description of assessments, nursing actions, and the responses of the patient, family, and caregivers to interventions. The date and time of the occurrence and complete signature of the nurse must be included. Late entries are labeled as an "addendum," signed, and dated.[44] Inadequate documentation implies inadequate nursing care and it will impact negatively on the agency's fulfillment of state licensure and certification requirements, delay or prohibit third-party reimbursement, place the agency at risk of a legal suit, and reflect a negative image of the agency and the quality of care provided.[43]

Warling[45] notes that legally correct records include objective and subjective observations that are pertinent but avoid general terms (e.g., "patient doing well"), value judgments (e.g., "the change in the dose of Dilantin (phenytoin sodium) apparently was not noted by nurse on previous visit"), opinions (e.g., "the confusion appears to be increasing"), or conclusions (e.g., "apparently the patient has bone metastasis").

The legal criteria for timeliness is the recording of an event at the time the care is given.[43] In the home health setting, this is within a day of the visit. Timely documentation is an essential component of nursing care. In addition to being a permanent record of the actions of the health care providers, the patient's clinical record communicates the patient's progress and health care services to other members of the health care team, quality assessment reviewers, and third-party payers.

Rehabilitation Nursing

As treatment advances lead to increased survival for persons with cancer, rehabilitation has become a more important aspect of comprehensive cancer care. Cancer rehabilitation involves assisting the person with cancer to attain maximum physical, social, psychological, and vocational functioning within the limits of treatment and disease. The goal of cancer rehabilitation is to improve the quality of life by maximizing functional ability and independence regardless of life expectancy and, when appropriate, reintroduction into the socioeconomic life of the community.[5] The underlying concepts of rehabilitation focus on interdisciplinary collaboration, comprehensive services, self-care, maximum function, prevention, family and cultural values, and the patient and family as a unit of care in the community.[47]

The impact of cancer is experienced by everyone involved in the life of the patient. Effective intervention requires the participation of the family in planning and implementing care.[48] When patients and families become co-partners with the rehabilitation team, they contract mutually agreeable goals, foster empowerment, educate for self-care, and enhance positive coping behaviors.[47]

Education is the key to enhancing patient independence and promoting self-care. Teaching plans should correlate with the patient and family's learning needs and abilities. The plans incorporate interventions that emphasize activities the patient can perform. If patients cannot perform self-care activities themselves, they may benefit from learning techniques for directing others to perform the care according to their preferences. These teaching plans would include practical skills, assertiveness, and techniques for both giving instructions and problem solving.

The greatest needs of patients with cancer and their caregivers have been found to be primarily psychological and informational.[49] Teaching stress reduction methods, communication and problem-solving skills, and information on disease process and care principles may facilitate patient and family coping.

The debilitating sequelae of cancer and treatment often necessitate the use of adaptive equipment to maintain the optimal level of independence and meaningful activity. Equipment such as ramps, rails, grab bars, and enlarged doorways can be constructed or modified for the home. Assistive devices, such as universal cuffs for holding grooming devices, promote patient independence and self-care.

Encouraging the patient and family to develop networks and supports in the community fosters independence and facilitates patient discharge from the home health agency. The discharge plan provides information on community agencies and services; the patient's health insurance coverage and contact persons; transportation services; vocational rehabilitation programs; and support groups identified by the rehabilitation nurse, patient, and family. To prevent fragmentation of care, referrals to appropriate agencies are carefully timed so they can begin their services when the patient is discharged from home health care. Insurers often limit payment for services to patients with chronic, debilitating disease and may terminate benefits before the patients have achieved their rehabilitation potential and are educated about self-care. Introducing the discharge plan at time of admission to home care and revising it as needed may avert the negative effects of a premature discharge.

As the disease advances and ability to maintain activities for independent functioning wanes, it is important to recognize that cancer patients are likely to need services such as personal care, meal preparation, shopping, housekeeping, and transportation. Failure to obtain these services may precipitate a family crisis. Recognizing these needs and initiating appropriate referrals will increase the quality of life for the patient and family.[50] In the home setting, the patient and family are in control; the family is an integral part of the patient's achievement of maximum rehabilitation potential.

Role of the Oncology Clinical Nurse Specialist

The complex care requirements of persons with cancer who are referred to home care coupled with the need for highly specialized, cost-efficient, quality care has created a need for the skills and education of the Oncology Clinical Nurse Specialist (OCNS). Several home health agencies have successfully integrated the OCNS to improve the quality of care provided, but the literature has few articles addressing the role of the OCNS in the home health setting.[51]

Hamric[52] has defined the role of the Clinical Nurse Specialist (CNS) as an expert practitioner in a specific area of clinical nursing and as change agent within the health care system to improve the quality of patient care. The nursing activities associated with the change agent role include education, consultation, research, supervision, communication, and innovation. Studies of CNSs in a hospital setting indicate that CNSs spend 47% of their time in direct care activities.[53,54] In home health care, the percentage of time spent in these activities will vary with the agency's needs and resources.

Practitioner role

Direct care activities provided by the OCNS in home health care include advanced services and skills not usually available from the general nursing staff. The OCNS is particularly adept in management of complex physical and psychological care requirements such as infusion therapy, extensive wounds, parenteral nutrition, intractable pain, and counseling and problem solving.

The home health agency must consider the cost-effectiveness of the OCNS's provision of direct nursing care. Experienced community health nursing staff have been providing competent nursing care to patients with cancer prior to the advent of the OCNS. Staff nurses may feel frustrated by the loss of challenging cases, lack of freedom to select cases, and the absence of recognition for services they have provided in the past.[55] Restructuring the OCNS's role to include sharing complex cases with staff nurses provides the opportunity for the OCNS to increase the knowledge of agency staff in the new complex skills, fosters patient and family confidence when the OCNS is not available, and increases the availability of the OCNS to additional patients. Although this approach is more cost-effective over time for the home health agency, it can diffuse the bonding that occurs between patient and the OCNS or staff nurse, and it can lessen rewards and satisfaction in nursing.[55]

Educator role

Educational activities for both individual and group instruction of staff are usually included in the OCNS role. The OCNS has expertise in developing and implementing staff orientation, continuing education programs for the agency and community, and presenting patient care conferences to enhance staff knowledge and improve patient care.

Consultant role

Consultative activities of the OCNS vary according to focus and goal. Consultation may include assisting staff with managing difficult cases or providing information to improve their skills, knowledge, self-assurance, or objectivity. The administration may ask the OCNS to develop or revise agency programs or assist with counseling problem staff.[56] Frequent personal contact between the OCNS and staff will enhance the perception of the OCNS as a colleague with advanced knowledge and skills, it will facilitate sharing of goals and values in nursing, and it promotes collaboration between the OCNS and staff nurse in the provision of quality nursing care.

Researcher role

Research activity for the OCNS varies from the basics of interpreting, evaluating, and communicating research findings to caregivers to the advanced level of research collaboration and actively generating or replicating research projects. The research activities of the OCNS in home health care are usually limited to reviewing research reports, communicating relevant data to agency staff, and incorporating research findings into nursing practice standards. Occasionally the opportunity arises for the OCNS to collaborate with colleagues in other settings on the implementation of relevant research studies and projects.

Evaluation of the OCNS role in home health

Evaluation of the OCNS role is limited;[57] however, how CNSs spend their time has been examined,[54] as well as staff and unit leaders' perception of the importance of specific CNS activities in job descriptions and rating of CNS performance. Boyd et al.[53] reported that the merit of the CNS role was demonstrated in publications, revenue production, submission and acceptance of grant proposals, and positive patient outcomes. The significance was demonstrated by decrease in errors after the CNS's review of serious occurrences/incidents. Further study is needed to evaluate the impact of the CNS on patient outcomes.

In some home health agencies, OCNSs have provided education and support to staff nurses by sharing complex cases, presenting and participating in case conferences, developing and teaching orientation and inservice programs, distributing pertinent educational and research reports, and being available for consultation. The OCNSs have produced revenues through home visits; participated in revisions of policies, procedures, and charting forms; developed and conducted nursing process audits; served as home health liaisons to community health care organizations; and participated in professional oncology nursing activities in the community. As such, they have increased the credibility and recognition of the home health agency and improved quality of home care services.

ECONOMIC ISSUES

Financing Home Health Care

In the current environment of cost containment, home health nurses struggle with issues such as who should have access to their care, what the quality of care should be, and who is worthy of care at the public's expense.[58] Advocates of home health care can demonstrate its desirability and potential cost-effectiveness in answering these questions. If comprehensive patient care is to be provided in a financially responsible manner, home health nurses need to be familiar with reimbursement guidelines. Knowledge of the services, equipment, and supplies covered by the individual's insurance is essential.

The Medicare Act of 1965 included a home health benefit for the Medicare beneficiary living at home. Home health services available to Medicare recipients include nursing, physical therapy, speech therapy, occupational therapy, home health aid, and social work services. Eligibility requirements state that the beneficiary must be homebound and require skilled nursing, physical therapy, or speech and language pathology services ordered by a physician. *Homebound* means that leaving the home requires considerable effort. Services must be provided on a part-time, intermittent basis.[59] *Part-time* currently is defined as nursing and home health aide time totaling less than 8 hours per day or 35 hours per week. *Intermittent* currently is defined as services required at least every 60 days and daily visits limited to 21 consecutive days or having a predictable and finite end if daily visits extend beyond 21 days. Many health insurance payers have incorporated portions of the Medicare regulations into their policies.

Medicare reimburses at the lower end of reasonable cost or agency charge, up to a limit that is set annually by the U.S. Health Care Financing Administration (HCFA). The home health agency bills the Medicare program its established charges and is reimbursed a predetermined percentage of those charges. At the end of the agency's fiscal year, the agency files a cost report, from which a reasonable cost for providing services to Medicare beneficiaries is determined. A final settlement is determined based on the agency's costs for providing the service and the amounts billed by the agency and paid by the Medicare program.[60,61]

Medicaid funding for home health services is a joint federal–state assistance program for the poor of all ages.[62] Federal regulations require states to provide a minimum range of home health services including part-time nursing care, home health aides, medical supplies, and equipment. States receive matching funds for their expenditures and are allowed extensive flexibility in determining eligibility, services, and reimbursement. States may opt to provide additional services (e.g., physical, occupational, or speech therapy) or to reimburse home health agencies on a flat fee for service or agency cost. States may also offer waiver programs that are partially funded with federal funds and cover a broader range of services such as case management, long-term nursing, personal care, and homemaker or chore services. Lack of available state funds has limited state participation in these programs.

Private insurance carriers (e.g., Blue Cross/Blue Shield, Aetna) vary significantly in their coverage for home health services. Individual plans may require partial payment (co-payments) by the beneficiary and may cover only specific services (e.g., nursing, home health aide services). Prior to admission, the home health agency will contact the carrier to determine the patient's specific coverage.

The oncology home care nurse must be aware of the services covered for each patient by the reimbursement source in order to avoid nonpayment of services. A referral to the agency's social worker may be helpful in locating a community agency that will provide noncovered but needed service.

Documenting for Reimbursement

Accurate descriptive documentation of home health nursing care is vital to reimbursement and continuation of home health services. Completing timely, appropriate documentation consumes a significant amount of staff time; a study of nursing activities in home health care showed that paperwork, charting, and completing recertifications accounted for 19% of nursing time.[40] Many articles have been published describing methods of documentation to ensure successful reimbursement,[63–65] and conferences on documentation techniques are usually well attended.

The adage "If it wasn't charted, it wasn't done" has been expanded to "and if it wasn't charted in keeping with the regulations, it will not be reimbursed." It has been postulated that the rise in health care expenditures, including home health care, has led the government and fiscal intermediaries to enact regulations requiring specific documentation and has increased focused review in an effort to decrease costs by denial of payment for services designated as "noncovered" by the reviewer.[65]

If the nurse is able to document changes in the patient's physical status and changes in the treatment plan that correspond to the identified goals and outcomes, nursing service should be viewed as reasonable and necessary and therefore reimbursable.[63] Accurate and comprehensive nursing documentation, although time-consuming and requiring thoughtful deliberation, is essential for procuring reimbursement.

Home Care for the Socially Disadvantaged

Health care expenditures for 1990 reached $666.2 billion and absorbed 13.3% of the gross national product.[66] Despite these expenditures, Americans are not healthier than citizens of other countries of similar or lesser wealth.[67] Approximately 15% of Americans or 37 million are not covered by any insurance plan, and another 20% have inadequate health insurance.[68] The United States is one of only two large, industrialized nations that does not have a plan of universal health care for all citizens.[67]

Concern over the rapid increases in health care spending, the serious financial difficulties of the government health care programs, and the crisis in employer-paid private financing of health care coupled with the fact that more than one-third of the population has minimal or no health care insurance protection has raised the call for health care reform of the U.S. health care system.[68] Leaders in health care reform are debating this issue; more than 30 proposals by various organizations and legislators have been designed.[69] One plan, the Oregon Plan, is an attempt by the State of Oregon to ensure equitable and universal access to health care by prioritizing types of care.[70] Criticized as a dangerous rationing scheme by some, its progress is being closely watched by health care reform leaders, ethicists, health care providers, and insurers.

Since home health reimbursement by payers is computed on the cost per visit, most home health agencies have limited funds available for services to persons without home health insurance. In some communities the United Way has allocated funds for home health care of the indigent that are usually granted to voluntary home health organizations (e.g., the Visiting Nurses Association). The Medicare home health benefit does not cover long-term or chronic care. However, there are a growing number of elderly persons with cancer with functional limitations and chronic health problems who live alone or with a spouse or sibling who may also be frail and elderly. During an acute exacerbation of an illness, these patients are admitted to home health care usually after hospitalization. When the acute episode is resolved, the chronic problems continue. If a patient is kept beyond the need for skilled care, the home health agency faces a denial of payment for services provided. When a patient has a limited income, the oncology home care staff are faced with the problem of locating a community service agency that provides follow-up monitoring and support services for personal care or homemaking without cost. Currently there are few publicly financed long-term care programs available for the needy.[62] The Omnibus Reconciliation Act (OBRA) of 1990 approved an optional Medicaid home health benefit that would allow states to add a new program for the elderly and disabled.[62] However, states have been slow to expand home care services because soaring costs have strained the state Medicaid budget. Several bills to provide long-term personal care and support services to the elderly have been introduced in Congress, but to date none has passed.[71]

In 1989 the HCFA published revisions to the *Health Insurance Manual-II* that recognize "management and evaluation of a beneficiary's plan of care" as skilled nursing care and thus reimbursable. To be reasonable and necessary the plan of care must include complex "necessary, unskilled services which are a necessary part of the medical treatment."[72] Notably, this benefit expanded reimbursable home health services to include assessment, monitoring, teaching, and revisions of the plan of care for persons whose condition have stabilized but who are at risk for complications or require frequent unskilled care from caregivers. This service should provide additional support needed by chronically ill persons for prevention or early detection of complications and prevention or delay of hospitalization.

Implementation of this benefit has been limited as agencies begin to interpret its "management and evaluation" terms, identify categories for patient selection, determine appropriate criteria to be included in documentation, and evaluate extent of Medicare reimbursement. Carr[73] proposes that patients who have severely limited mobility, are at risk for complications, and are very dependent on caregivers should meet the requirements for "management and evaluation."

Oncology home health nurses traditionally focus on interactive services such as teaching and performing hands-on nursing procedures as means to qualify care to meet reimbursement guidelines. It will require nursing reeducation and clearly written guidelines to expand the oncology home care nurse's practice and make the needed service of "management and evaluation" more widely available.

ETHICAL CONCERNS

The rapid growth and increased complexity of home health care have generated an increase of ethical concerns unique to the home care setting. Homes are shaped by the personal lifestyle and financial means of the cancer patient. Possessions, routines, and family structures may not be conducive to the provision of health care in the home.[74] For example, dirt or clutter in the home may create a safety hazard, obstruct movement, or impede provision of patient care. Family routines may not include accepted hygienic practices, and family activities may occur at any time of the night or day. Family structure may include aged parents, dependent spouses, young children, or estranged relatives with varied capabilities and motivation to learn and perform necessary treatments for patient care. Frequently, the cancer patient has been the primary caregiver of the family.

There is little documented evidence of the type and incidence of ethical problems in home health care.[75] A study by Young et al.[76] demonstrated that the ethical concerns of home health providers were primarily maintaining agency solvency while not denying care to indigent patients, responding to conflicts between patients and families, providing care to abused or neglected patients, and candidly addressing decisions about treatment with the terminally ill. In another study, Aroskar[77] surveyed 319 home health nurses and identified their most frequently cited ethical problems as: (1) patient decisions regarding treatment and health care that conflict with the health care provider's goals, (2) truth telling that reveals patient confidences or would deny needed patient care, and (3) provisions of health care benefits that are based on insurance reimbursement rather than patient need. Haddad[75] surveyed 30 health care providers to identify ethical concerns that are troublesome to role performance. Their concerns were categorized as problems with regulations that restricted services; incompetence of co-workers; and a broad category of various problems including elder abuse, incompetent caregivers, abandonment, and racism.

Home health nurses are usually familiar with the ethical principles of advocacy for patient autonomy (e.g., the right to make an informed decision regarding treatment and services) and the patient's right of self-determination to refuse treatment when incapacitated.[78,79] The OBRA of 1989 and 1990 mandated home health agencies to inform patients of their rights and specifically of the right to be informed of advance directives and to have information about each patient's advance directives recorded in the patient's clinical record.

Moral Values

Moral values are beliefs that are of ultimate importance to oneself, apply to all persons, guide our actions, and focus on promoting humankind. Values important to health care providers are respect for persons, patient advocacy, and accountability.[80] Respect for persons is to respect another person as one who shares the same human destiny as oneself.[81] Patient advocacy is the active support of the patient to be informed of his or her rights and options. Accountability is answerability for one's actions when one has agreed to provide a service. Moral values are described in the American Nurses Association (ANA) *Code for Nurses with Interpretive Statements*.[82]

The values of the patient, family, and caregiver are not usually known when a patient is admitted to home care nor easily assessed during the initial visit. Their values have sometimes been formulated by cultural and societal beliefs different from those held by the nurse and may not include respect for handicapped, elderly, terminally ill, or mentally retarded persons. Families may be unwilling to purchase medical supplies or equipment needed by the patient because for them the value of money supersedes the value of new and sometimes expensive equipment for a terminally ill person. The nurse's efforts to advocate for the patient may also be rejected by the dependent patient who relies heavily on the family and caregivers to provide care. Thus, ongoing assessment of the values of the patient, family, and caregivers is essential to identify potential ethical conflicts and plan for nursing care that is compatible with their needs and values.

Ethical Principles

The ANA Code for Nurses identifies six principles that the nurse should use as moral guides to action. They are autonomy, beneficence, justice, veracity, confidentiality, and fidelity.[81,82]

Autonomy is the principle that gives patients the right to determine their actions based on their own decisions and implies that patients are independent and self-reliant. Conflicts arise in the home setting if a patient's decisions are detrimental to his or her health (e.g., refusing medications that are effective treatment for illness, choosing to remain at home when the care provided by the family/caregivers is substandard).

The principle of beneficence directs the nurse to do good, to promote the welfare or well-being of others. A conflict may occur for the home care nurse if the patient lives in an apartment or neighborhood that is a risk to the personal safety of the nurse or when threats or attempts to do bodily harm may necessitate closing or not opening a case to home care service.

The principle of justice guides the nurse to treat all persons equally and give individuals what is owed to them by another person or society. However, limited health care coverage restricts compliance with this principle if needed services are not covered or partially covered and the patient does not have personal resources to purchase the service and supplies.

The principle of veracity obligates the nurse to be truthful with the patient, peers, and other professionals and avoid lying or deception. Conflicts may arise when the family or caregivers insist that the patient not be informed of specific information because it may distress the patient. Truthfulness also requires the nurse to report a peer for poor performance that may not be observed by supervisors in the home care setting.

The principle of confidentiality requires the nurse to respect and hold confidential all information shared by the patient. However, when innocent parties are in jeopardy, public law requires disclosure of this information, as in suspected cases of child abuse.

Lastly, the principle of fidelity requires the nurse to be faithful to his or her commitments and profession. When an agency is short-staffed, overtime work may create conflicts between the nurse's professional and personal life.

Ethical Decision Making

When conflict occurs, the nurse uses a decision-making process to assess the problem and potential courses of action and to consider what is right or good based on the values of the persons involved and ethical principles. Guidelines, similar to the nursing process, have been developed to assist the nurse.[81,83–85] (See Table 55-6.)

In the home care setting, potential conflicts arise as the patient becomes increasingly dependent on caregivers and multiple caregivers are involved. Frequently, a primary caregiver has not been designated as decision maker to manage the case. Patient autonomy is no longer the primary ethical principle guiding nursing care. The nurse must consider the patient, family, and caregivers as the unit of care and identify the moral values held by each person involved in the cooperative tasks of home care (i.e., the ethical value of accommodation).[74] Also, the nurse assists the family in designating the decision maker for patient care.

TABLE 55-6 Process for Ethical Decision Making

1. Identify the ethical problem. Clarify the issues, including conflicting moral claims, the values of the involved persons, and their emotional responses.
2. Collect data from all involved in the problem. Identify the decision makers, listen to each person's perspective, and separate facts from emotions.
3. Identify all possible actions, the ethical principles that will be enhanced or negated by each action, and the projected outcome for each action.
4. Evaluate each action thoroughly. Consider the consequences of each action and its effect on each person. Attempt to prioritize the positive and negative outcomes for each action.
5. Make the decision. Select the action that most agrees with the values involved and has the most positive consequences. Inform all involved persons.
6. Act and then evaluate all aspects of the outcome.

Source: Adapted with permission from DeWolf MS: Ethical decision-making, *Semin Oncol Nurs* 5:77–81, 1989; Andrew Jameton: *Nursing Practice: The Ethical Issues*, © 1984, pp. 66–69. Adapted by permission of Prentice-Hall, Englewood Cliffs, NJ.

INFUSION THERAPY IN THE HOME

Infusion therapy is one of the most rapidly growing segments of home care. The National Association for Home Care reports a 31.5% annual growth rate from 1986 to 1991 for home antibiotic and chemotherapy services and a 17.3% annual growth rate for parenteral and enteral nutrition programs.[2] The growth of home infusion therapy has been stimulated by cost-containment pressure from third-party payers; the increase in the aging population; and advances in technology that have increased the safety, effectiveness, and availability of home infusion therapies.[86,87]

Advanced technology has produced an array of long-term central venous access devices (VADs) and infusion pumps that simplify parenteral administration of drugs in the home and have less risk for complications. The most frequently used central VAD for cancer therapies in the home are venous access ports. Infusion pumps have become smaller, more lightweight, simpler to program and adjust, and therefore easier to operate and maintain in the home.

The peripherally inserted central catheter (PICC), a soft, flexible silicone or polymer catheter, is used frequently in the home because it can be inserted by a nurse who is certified in the procedure.[86,88] Because the PICC is biocompatible and flexible, it can often remain in place for weeks or months. The PICC is inserted in the antecubital fossa and advanced until the catheter tip is in the axillary, subclavian, or brachiocephalic vein. Radiograph verification is required for placement beyond the axillary vein.[89] PICC lines require frequent flushing with heparin and dressing changes every 3–7 days. The advantages of the PICC as an alternative to a central VAD are the possibility of insertion in the home by a certified home health nurse, decreased cost, comfort to the patient, and long-term placement.

Home health management of the cancer patient receiving infusion therapy that incorporates sophisticated infusion pumps and VADs focuses on caring for the patient and family rather than on management of the equipment. Teaching self-care procedures for flushing a long-term central catheter is ineffective if the patient or caregiver is overwhelmed by a beeping infusion pump or manipulating a syringe and needle. An elderly spouse may expect the nurse to care for the VAD and refuse to learn the procedures. Counseling the patient, caregiver, and family regarding high-technology home care becomes the first priority. The home health nurse may need to discuss alternatives of nursing home or private duty nursing care if the spouse or caregiver is unwilling or unable to care for the patient.[87]

Communication between the infusion therapy personnel and the home health nurse for coordination of services and delineation of responsibilities will also decrease patient and family confusion and anxiety. A joint visit by the home health and infusion therapy nurses at the patient's home when home infusion therapy is initiated to review medical orders, set up and test equipment, review schedules and procedures for ordering supplies, and define each nurse's specific responsibilities promotes coordination of services. An Infusion Therapy/Home Health Coordination Record (see Table 55-7) can be helpful in decreasing confusion and false expectations. After it is signed by both nurses, each agency receives a copy. A copy is left in the patient's home.

If risk of exposure to blood or other potentially infectious materials occurs during care of the patient receiving infusion therapy in the home, the nurse must comply with federal regulations for prevention of occupational exposure issued December 6, 1991.[90] In general, for home care these regulations mandate observation of universal precautions.

Chemotherapy Administration

The demand for more cost-effective methods of treating cancer patients has stimulated the development of comprehensive services including administration of chemotherapy. For patients whose physical conditions preclude travel to an outpatient setting, administration of chemotherapy in the home has become a viable option. Advanced technology not only has produced sophisticated drugs but has also provided methods to control the clinical side effects, promoting safe administration at home. In addition to cost reduction, home chemotherapy reduces the risk of complications from nosocomial infections, is convenient for the patient and caregiver, and provides psychological benefits to patients who desire the comfort of their homes.

Criteria for patient selection

Specific criteria must be met for administration of chemotherapy in the home. These include:

1. The patient meets the requirements for admission to home care as determined by the agency's licensing or certification agency.
2. The patient is stable and free of symptoms that preclude the safe administration of antineoplastic drugs.
3. The patient desires chemotherapy and is willing to pay for that portion of drugs and services not covered by medical insurance.
4. The patient has received the initial course of chemotherapy prior to administration in the home with no untoward effects.
5. The patient and family are willing and able to assume related caregiving activities.
6. Resources are available in the community for medications, supplies, laboratory services, and additional nursing or caregiving services.

Insurance reimbursement for antineoplastic drugs, equipment, supplies, and nursing services varies. The patient's medical insurance must be reviewed to determine coverage prior to referring a patient for home chemotherapy since it may not be feasible for the patient to assume the costs.

Policies for chemotherapy administration

Home health agencies that offer chemotherapy as a service must develop specific policies and procedures.[91] These usually include:

- patient eligibility requirements
- antineoplastic drugs approved for administration at home
- acceptable parameters of laboratory profiles and the schedule for obtaining laboratory studies
- procedures for each route of administration that include preparation, administration, and disposal of the drugs[92,93]
- specific criteria for withholding antineoplastic drugs
- educational requirements for nurses who administer antineoplastic drugs

Some agencies limit approved antineoplastic agents given at home to those that are nonvesicant[92] or noncaustic.[93] Many home health agencies will only administer drugs that can be infused within 1–2 hours. Home infusion therapy companies may administer antineoplastic drugs that require hydration and infusion over several hours, such as cisplatin. Investigational drugs should only be considered for home administration if the side effects have been identified and written information describing the drug's action and side effects has been provided to the agency. Although this information is readily available to the hospital or clinic nurse, it is more difficult for home care agencies to obtain.

The use of VADs has facilitated the administration of chemotherapy at home. However, not all patients receiving chemotherapy have an existing intravenous line. An agency must determine whether the nurses will perform venipunctures. Some agencies require a patient to have an existing line if chemotherapy is to be given at home. Others include the mandatory establishment of a free-flowing IV through which chemotherapy is administered rather than direct intravenous push administration. This ensures venous access and facilitates the flushing of the tubing.

TABLE 55-7 Infusion Therapy/Home Health Coordination Record

Patient Name ______________________ Date ____________ ☐ Initial ☐ Update

I.D. No. ______________________ H.I.T. Agency Involved ____________

Start of H.I.T. Service ______________________ H.I.T. Contact ____________

Type of H.I.T. ______________________ H.I.T. Phone ____________

Pump Type ______________________

RESPONSIBILITIES FOR SERVICE

Activity	H.I.T. Agency	MCFSI
1. Initial assessment of infusion therapy (Date ___________)		
2. Initial teaching of infusion therapy (Date ___________)		
3. Supplies management (ordering/delivery)		
4. Pharmaceuticals (preparation/delivery)		
5. Provision of medical equipment, pumps, supplies		
6. Ongoing assessment of equipment, supplies, etc.		
7. Ongoing assessment of patient's response to therapy		
8. Clinical monitoring, laboratory studies		
9. Catheter management		
10. Restarting I.V.		
11. Catheter repair		
12. Tubing/cassette changes If MCFSI responsible, H.I.T. contact demonstrated procedure with MCFSI nurse ☐ Yes ☐ No (If no, explain below)		
13. Dosage adjustment/pump reprogramming If MCFSI responsible, H.I.T. contact demonstrated procedure with MCFSI nurse ☐ Yes ☐ No (If no, explain below)		
14. Troubleshooting problems with pump		
15. Replacement of pump		
16. Pump Operations manual in home		
17. Physician contacts/reports		
18. 24-hour availability		
19. Other		

COMMENTS:

____
H.I.T. Representative (if available) Date

____
MCFSI Home Care Program Nurse Date

☐ Duplicate copy sent to agency

____
Beeper Number

H.I.T. = Home Infusion Therapy; *MCFSI* = Michigan Cancer Foundation Services, Inc.
Source: Michigan Cancer Foundation Services, Inc. Home Care Program, Detroit, MI 48201.

Specific hematologic parameters must be designated for white blood cell (WBC) and platelet levels at which chemotherapy will or will not be administered. A complete blood cell count (CBC), differential, and platelet counts are obtained 36–48 hours prior to administration of each series of drug(s), and the physician is contacted to confirm, adjust, or withhold the dose of the antineoplastic agent. The Michigan Cancer Foundation Home Care Program's policy states that chemotherapy will not be administered when the WBC is below 3000 mm^3 or the platelet count is below 75,000/mm^3. In the home, serial laboratory testing that may indicate bone marrow recovery is generally not available.

Staff education

As in any setting, the nurse administering chemotherapy must have the theoretical knowledge base and technical skills necessary to ensure the safety of the patient. Many agencies have developed a chemotherapy certification course based on the Cancer Chemotherapy Guidelines developed by the Oncology Nursing Society.[94] To be eligible to administer chemotherapy at home, the nurse should demonstrate:

- knowledge of administration procedures and the purpose, action, and side effects of drugs as well as measures to manage untoward effects
- the ability to administer IV drugs via VADs, catheters, ports, pumps, and peripheral lines
- knowledge of appropriate preparation, transportation, and disposal of antineoplastic agents (a comprehensive review of this information is included in Chapter 15).

Safety considerations

Several studies have determined that mutagenic changes may occur in persons who handle chemotherapy drugs.[95–97] Potential hazards associated with the administration of antineoplastic agents have prompted the Occupational Safety and Health Administration (OSHA) to set guidelines for compounding, transporting, administering, and disposing of toxic chemotherapy agents.[98] These guidelines can be found in Chapter 16.

Potential risks to persons who come into contact with chemotherapy drugs and associated safety measures should be discussed with the patient and family prior to the initial home chemotherapy treatment.

Safety considerations include:

1. *Transport of drugs:* In the home setting the antineoplastic drugs may be obtained from the pharmacy by the family or nurse. The drugs should be labeled as cytotoxic, securely capped or sealed, and packaged in an impervious packing material for transport. The family is cautioned to protect the package from breakage and is taught the necessary procedures should a spill occur.

2. *Preparation of drugs:* An area of the patient's home that is apart from frequent family activity and food preparation should be selected to prepare the drugs. If present, ceiling fans should be turned off. A work surface area that can be cleaned should be utilized (e.g., a card table). All family members should remain outside the rooms where the drugs are prepared and administered. If possible, the family should make arrangements for children to be cared for outside the home on the day of chemotherapy.

Supplies are assembled on a disposable, absorbent, plastic-backed pad that is taped over the work surface area. Only syringes, needles, and IV sets with Luer-lock fittings should be used. A plastic or metal tray can be lined with sterile gauze squares to catch and collect excess solution. A closable, puncture-resistant, shatter-resistant container is necessary for the disposal of contaminated sharp or breakable materials. Appropriate containers can be purchased from medical supply companies. Sealable 4-mil polyethylene or 2-mil polypropylene plastic bags with wire ties and labeled as "Biological Hazard" must be used for disposal of all supplies used in the preparation and administration of antineoplastic drugs.

Before donning the protective nonpenetrable gown, surgical latex gloves, mask, and goggles, the nurse reminds the patient and caregiver of the need for protection from exposure to the drugs. The patient or caregiver who participates in administering the drug should also wear protective garments.[91] While preparing and administering the drugs, care is taken to prevent aerosolization; for example, sterile gauze should be wrapped around ampules prior to breaking and around needle tips while expelling air from syringes, priming IV lines, or inserting needles into vials or IV lines. While administering antineoplastic drugs, universal precautions for preventing transmission of HIV, hepatitis B virus, and other blood-borne pathogens must be followed.[90]

In many parts of the country, the drugs may be prepared in an appropriate laminar-flow hood in a licensed pharmacy and then delivered to the home. In the home the drugs (which usually require refrigeration) must be stored away from food, cosmetics, and frequently used household areas.[91]

3. *Spills:* Spills and breakages must be cleaned up immediately by a person wearing a protective gown, gloves, mask, and goggles. Liquids and solids are wiped up with absorbent pads or gauze and the area is cleaned three times with detergent solution and rinsed with clean water. All contaminated materials should be placed in the plastic bag labeled "Biological Hazard."

4. *Patient care:* Blood, emesis, and excreta from patients who have received antineoplastic agents within 48 hours may be contaminated. The health care providers and caregivers must be informed of the need to wear protective garments if the potential exists to become contaminated, for example, when caring for the bedbound or incontinent patient. All contaminated linens should be prewashed separately once and then laundered again with the family laundry. All disposable bed pads, tissues, gowns, and gloves must be sealed in a plastic bag for disposal. Children should be discouraged from visiting the patient while chemotherapy is being administered.

5. *Disposal:* When administration is completed, all items that have been in contact with the drug are wrapped in an absorbent pad (including unused portions of the drug unless they are to be used in the future) and placed into the plastic bag labeled "Biological Hazard."

A reusable drug vial should be cleaned with an alcohol pad, placed in a plastic bag, and stored according to the packaged directions regarding environmental temperature. The patient and family are warned that all persons must avoid contact with the drug (especially children). The nurse will transport the bag of contaminated waste to the home care agency for disposal. OSHA[98] recommends that all hazardous waste be disposed of in a licensed sanitary landfill. Therefore, home care agencies that administer antineoplastic drugs must have a contract for disposal of the hazardous wastes.

Patient and family responsibilities

If the family assumes responsibility for obtaining the drugs, solutions, and equipment, they will need a list of specific items required and places where they can be purchased. Some agencies require a caregiver to be present on the day(s) chemotherapy is administered to observe for problems and assist the patient to manage side effects. Written information about potential side effects is provided along with the descriptions of symptoms that need to be reported immediately to the physician or nurse. It is helpful to include the phone number of the health care providers on the written instructions. Patient and family education regarding management of side effects is an obvious need. Many institutions have developed appropriate patient teaching guidelines. An excellent guideline, "Chemotherapy and You" is available without cost from the National Cancer Institute by phoning 1-800-4-CANCER.

Nontraditional methods of chemotherapy administration, such as continuous infusion and regional infusion of antineoplastic drugs, are being used more frequently today since these methods can increase exposure of tumor cells to higher total dose of drug, theoretically increasing tumor cell kill.[99] Nursing responsibilities may include changing the pump cassette containing the antineoplastic drugs, reprogramming the infusion pump, and monitoring and evaluating side effects of the therapy.

Reimbursement for chemotherapy administration in the home varies according to the reimbursement policies of the third-party payers.[100] Neither Medicare nor most Medicaid programs cover antineoplastic drugs for home health administration. Blue Cross/Blue Shield and several health maintenance organizations (HMOs) usually cover most of the cost. Prior approval is typically necessary to ensure insurance coverage.

Home Parenteral Nutrition

The administration of parenteral nutrition at home is a rapidly growing option for cost-effective and beneficial therapy for the malnourished patient with cancer.[101–103] In 1968 the first person in the United States received parenteral nutrition at home,[102] and by 1970 the University of Washington developed a system to permit home administration of parenteral nutrition.[103]

Criteria for patient selection

Certain criteria are recommended for acceptance of a patient into a home parenteral nutrition (HPN) program:[104]

1. The patient's physical status is sufficiently stable to allow hospital discharge and safe home care for a reasonable period of time.
2. The patient has received parenteral nutrition for a minimum of 1 week prior to discharge from the acute care facility.
3. The patient and/or family is willing and able to learn and maintain the procedures necessary for HPN.
4. The amount and types of care requirements as well as the benefits, risks, and financial considerations have been evaluated and explained to the patient and caregiver prior to discharge.
5. Adequate resources are available in the community for obtaining medications and supplies as well as troubleshooting on a 24-hour basis. Additionally, laboratory services and home nursing care must be accessible. Most areas in the United States are currently serviced by home infusion therapy companies that provide the supplies, medications, and equipment needed.
6. The home environment is conducive to providing safe HPN, including running water, electricity, and a telephone.

The patient and family must assume primary responsibility for the administration of HPN. If the patient lives alone, a caregiver must be identified who will stay with the patient and administer the HPN until the patient is able to manage this care. Private duty nurses may be considered if a family member or willing caregiver is not available. Frequently the patient with cancer who requires HPN has additional complex care requirements, and the total amount of care required, especially at night, can impose a severe burden on the caregiver,[30] who will therefore need occasional respite.

The financial costs of HPN vary according to locale and patients' needs. In 1986 the Oley/American Society for Parenteral and Enteral Nutrition Information System reported that 5500 persons received HPN at a cumulative annual cost of $170 million,[105] which included solutions and supplies, home nursing visits, and cost of clinical follow-up with laboratory tests. The patient's medical insurance must be reviewed by the discharge planner or home infusion company to determine HPN coverage. Handy[87] reports that many third-party payers have extended their coverage to include intravenous administration of drugs and solutions in the home because of the substantial savings involved. Frequently, the patient's insurance will cover 80% of the cost, as will Medicare Part B coverage, with the other 20% becoming the patient's responsibility. Infusion therapy companies usually bill the patient's medical insurance agency directly.

Initial home assessment

The initial visit by the home care nurse should occur soon after the patient's arrival at home and coincide with the arrival of the supplies, equipment, medication, and home infusion therapy company personnel. This will allow time to review the medical orders for HPN with the patient and caregiver, test the infusion pump, review the schedule and procedures for ordering supplies, and define the specific responsibilities of the home care nurse and infusion therapy company personnel. It is essential that agencies administering HPN provide 24-hour service. Since HPN is usually infused at night, most problems occur at this time.

Completing a patient assessment may take several visits because of the many essential activities required during the initial home visit related to the HPN. The initial assessment includes:

1. The type and status of the venous access device. VADs currently used include the single, double, and triple lumen catheters, right atrial catheters, and implanted ports.
2. The patient's and family's knowledge of the management of HPN and other caregiving needs.
3. Evaluation of the home environment for safety and cleanliness factors required for HPN (e.g., running water, electricity, working telephone).

Most acute care facilities have developed complete teaching programs that include catheter care, home monitoring techniques, solution preparation (if applicable), administration techniques, and emergency care.[103] However, because the prospective payment system results in earlier discharges, patients may be sent home before they are fully knowledgeable of HPN management.

Adequate refrigeration must be available in the home to store the 2–4-week supply of solutions. Most infusion therapy companies will provide a small refrigerator if needed. An electric infusion pump is necessary for safe administration of HPN.[103–106] Most infusion pumps have a battery back-up that can operate the pump for several hours during an electrical outage. Thick carpeting or steps in multilevel homes may impede the patient's mobility during the infusion since the pumps are attached to portable IV poles.

Nursing management

Twice-a-day home nursing visits are usually required initially. The nurse starts the infusion of HPN in the evening and discontinues it in the morning. The role of the nurse encompasses ongoing assessment and evaluation of the patient's status, direct patient care (e.g., HPN administration), supervision of the patient/family management of HPN, and patient/family education.

Written instructions for HPN procedures are usually given to the patient at time of discharge from the acute care setting. It is helpful to adjust the HPN infusion time to the family's routine. HPN is often administered over 10–16 hours including the patient's sleeping time. The infusion rate for the first and last hours is decreased to prevent hyperglycemia upon initiation and rebound hypoglycemia upon withdrawal of the HPN. A typical 10-hour schedule will start 80–100 ml/hour, increase to 200 ml/hour over 8 hours, and then decrease to 80–100 ml for the last hour.

A flowsheet for documenting monitoring tasks is necessary. The patient and family are instructed to record the date, time, and results of the following:

- time of initiation/completion of HPN infusion
- daily temperature, pulse, respirations
- weight
- urine fractionals
- intake (HPN, additional IV fluids, oral fluids)
- output
- medications added to HPN; other medications given
- catheter care (heparin flush, cap change, dressing change)
- blood draws for laboratory tests

Although complications occur less frequently in the home than in the inpatient setting,[103] the patient and caregiver need oral and written instructions regarding symptoms requiring notification of the nurse or physician. The caregiver(s) and nurse should also observe the patient for depression or anxiety, which can occur with long-term HPN.[107]

Intravenous Antibiotic Therapy

Antibiotic therapy is the most commonly used IV therapy at home.[108,109] Home parental antibiotic therapy (HPAT) is a preferred method for delivering a course of therapy for many infectious diseases because of the significant cost savings as compared with hospitalization costs.[110] It is the most appropriate therapy for infectious diseases that require either prolonged, repeated, or short-term antibiotics with infrequent administration of drugs that are relatively safe.[111,112]

Criteria for patient selection

Criteria for patient selection for HPAT include:[109,112]

1. Medical status is stable.
2. Other aspects of the patient's treatment plan can be monitored or performed at home; hospitalization continues for IV therapy only.
3. The patient and family understand and agree with the plan for home therapy.

4. The patient is psychologically stable with no history of drug abuse.
5. The patient or caregiver has manual dexterity, basic mathematical and reading skills, ability to comprehend and follow instructions, and the motivation to be educated to administer antibiotics.[113]
6. The patient has a caregiver or support person available in the home to assist the patient.
7. The patient has peripheral veins suited for repeated cannulizations or has a central venous catheter in place.
8. The patient has a suitable home environment for therapy (e.g., refrigerator, freezer, telephone, transportation).
9. The arrangement of payment for supplies, medication, skilled nursing visits, laboratory tests, and clinic appointments is agreeable to the patient and family.

Nursing management

As with any type of parenteral therapy, before the patient is discharged from the hospital, arrangements need to be made for the preparation and delivery of pharmaceutical supplies to the home. Infusion therapy agencies with pharmacies will prepare and deliver the antibiotics and the supplies on schedule. The patient is usually given enough supplies to last a week. If antibiotics are prepared in batches and sent to the patient for storage, frequent deliveries may be required depending upon the stability of the specific antibiotic agent.[114]

During the active treatment phase, nursing visits may vary in frequency from three times a day to once a week. On each visit the nurse monitors vital signs, laboratory tests, equipment operation, supplies, adverse drug effects, and signs/symptoms of complications. Although the patient may prepare, store, and administer the HPAT, the home care nurse is responsible for ensuring that specific pharmaceutical guidelines are followed during the course of therapy (e.g., storage and mixing of drugs).

By far the simplest and least costly drug delivery system is gravity infusion adapted to the home. In those cases where the infusion rate is a critical factor in administration, it is preferable to use a mechanized infusion pump. The development of portable, programmable infusion pumps (such as the CADD-Plus® [Pharmacia Deltec]) that deliver a prescribed amount of drug intermittently over a 24-hour period have made HPAT feasible for persons who were ineligible in the past because of lack of caregiver support or dexterity.[115]

Factors such as dosing interval or adverse effects profile are important in selecting a drug. The antibiotic of choice for home administration would be the safest, most effective, cost-efficient, and easily administered antibiotic available. A drug that needs to be administered only once or twice daily is especially well suited for the home setting.[112]

Consideration must be given to the stability of the medication and type of storage required. Recommended refrigeration temperature of 2°–8°C (36°–44°F) can be achieved in most home and commercial refrigerators.[114] To prevent unnecessary freezing or warming, the temperature should be pretested before placing a supply of prepared parenteral bags in the refrigerator. It is advisable to purchase a refrigerator thermometer to monitor the temperature during active storage. Since some antibiotics have a stability of 30 days or more, they are available as commercially frozen piggyback solutions as well as solutions prepared and frozen by pharmacies. If antibiotics are frozen, it is necessary to use proper thawing techniques to prevent inactivation or degradation. The antibiotic needs to be left at room temperature until it is completely thawed (approximately 1–3 hours and 4–6 hours for 50-ml and 100-ml bags respectively[114]). Except for certain drugs, a 24-hour supply of frozen, small-volume parenteral bags can be thawed in advance and then refrigerated to meet the next day's needs.

Patient education is the key to safe administration of antibiotics in the home. Content areas include venous access site care, signs/symptoms of drug side effects and recurrent infection, proper drug preparation procedures, drug administration techniques, catheter flushing and care, infusion pump operation (if applicable), and the identification and resolution of problems. Instructions for patients in administration of antibiotics in the home are listed in Table 55-8.

Reimbursement for HPAT varies according to the reimbursement policies of the individual third-party payer.[100] Medicare covers equipment and supplies, but not medications that are administered in the home un-

TABLE 55-8 Patient Teaching for Self-Administration of IV Antibiotics Without a Pump

1. Remove bag with antibiotic solution from refrigerator and thaw according to directions (if applicable).
2. Wash hands thoroughly.
3. Insert needle with syringe attached into vial of heparin solution and withdraw prescribed amount. Replace needle on syringe. Keep capped.
4. Hang bag of antibiotic solution above arm on IV pole.
5. Fill chamber of IV tubing with fluid and purge air from tubing.
6. Cleanse venous access catheter cap with alcohol swab.
7. Connect IV tubing to catheter.
8. Establish IV flow rate as determined by physician.
9. When antibiotic is infused, disconnect tubing and inject heparin and flush venous access catheter.
10. Discard syringe and needles into a nonpenetrable container labeled "Infectious Wastes" for appropriate disposal.
11. Discard remaining used materials into double plastic bags. Seal and dispose with wastes.

Source: Adapted from Brown RB: Selection and training of patients for outpatient intravenous antibiotic therapy. *Rev Infect Dis* 13:s147–s151, 1991 (suppl 2).

der the supervision of a nurse. Medicaid, Blue Cross/Blue Shield, commercial insurers, and HMOs usually cover HPAT. Pretreatment approval from the insurer is usually necessary.

A quality assurance instrument for at-home IV antibiotic care has been developed that identifies outcome criteria in six areas:[109] infusion-related complications, drug-related complications, home care management, psychosocial response of patient/caregiver, cost, and recovery (cure).

Pain Management

Principles of pain management in the home setting include:

- an analgesic regimen that is the simplest to administer and provides sufficient pain relief to allow optimal functioning of the patient
- pain medications given around the clock, not PRN (continuous pain requires continuous treatment)
- measures other than analgesics to decrease pain employed consistently and effectively (e.g., relaxation techniques)
- interventions to prevent potential side effects of a narcotic analgesic regimen initiated concurrently (e.g., anticonstipation medications)
- ongoing comprehensive assessment of the patient's pain (identify the source of pain whenever possible and do not assume that the patient's pain is due to the malignant process)
- patient and family misconceptions about the use and abuse of narcotic analgesics identified and dispelled

Oral analgesics or analgesic combinations should, when possible, be used in the management of chronic cancer pain. The oral route is preferable for long-term cancer pain management for a number of reasons: comfort, ease of administration, increased compliance, no restriction of movement, and no equipment requirement.[116] Oral administration is as effective as parenteral routes once serum equilibration has been achieved.[117] Medications with high oral potency and long duration of action permit longer dosing intervals that allow uninterrupted sleep.

Chapter 23 provides an in-depth review of medications for mild, moderate, and severe pain. Morphine is the prototypic agent for cancer pain and is often the analgesic of choice. It is easy to use, safe, versatile, effective, and well tolerated.[117,118] Newer preparations, such as concentrated solution and sustained-release tablets, have facilitated home pain control for the patient with cancer.

Intermittent or continuous infusion therapy is being utilized in the home setting via a variety of routes: subcutaneous, intravenous, epidural, subarachnoid.[119–122] For continuous infusions, use of ambulatory infusion pumps offers unimpeded mobility.[119]

The epidural or subarachnoid route is indicated for pain that is refractory to analgesics administered by conventional means or analgesics that have produced severe, intolerable side effects that cannot be modified by alterations in drug therapy.[120] The use of epidural analgesia permits control or alleviation of severe pain with less opioid-mediated side effects because a smaller absolute dose of drug is utilized.[120,123,124] The analgesic most frequently prescribed is preservative-free morphine.

Patients and families are taught preparation and administration procedures, dressing change procedures, and emergency administration of naloxone for severe respiratory depression. Catheter site care is accomplished using clean rather than aseptic technique.[123] The nurse is usually responsible for filling the analgesic infusion pump.

Patient-controlled analgesia (PCA) is an intravenous drug delivery system that allows patients to administer predetermined doses of analgesic. The ability to self-administer medication and manage their pain produces a sense of control for patients that seems to decrease feelings of powerlessness and vulnerability.[125,126] Several studies have examined the efficacy of utilizing PCA with cancer patients. Keeri-Szanto[127] studied a small number of patients and found PCA provided effective pain relief and reduced total dose requirements. Citron et al.[128] reported that PCA-administered morphine produced significant pain relief without undue sedation in severe cancer pain episodes.

PCA pumps that deliver continuous and incremental dosing are particularly useful. Small, portable, computerized PCA pumps are available for home use. The pump is lightweight, easy to use, and delivers a continuous amount of medication along with an incremental dose that is self-administered for breakthrough pain. The caregiver is taught to attach the pump to the long-term venous catheter and to change the medication cassette as needed.

Difficulty in obtaining narcotics for home use must be considered. Community pharmacies do not routinely stock potent narcotics and may require 1 or 2 weeks to obtain the drugs. Telephone-ordered prescriptions for potent narcotics are not accepted by a pharmacy. Therefore, analgesic requirements must be anticipated and methods of obtaining prescriptions planned. New prescriptions can be obtained from the hospital outpatient pharmacy until arrangements can be made with local pharmacies to order certain narcotics for the cancer patient.

Measures other than narcotic analgesics to decrease pain may be more effective in the comfort of the patient's home. Behavioral coping strategies and noninvasive techniques can be taught to patients and families. These include distraction, relaxation,[129–131] and cutaneous stimulation. Diversions such as music, hobbies, visitors, and television may be useful for the patient at home. Ensuring a quiet environment for relaxation exercises is often more easily achieved at home. Cutaneous stimulation can be achieved through the use of cold packs, hot packs or heat pads, massage and backrubs, warm baths, topical ointments, and anesthetics. Patients and caregivers can also be taught other comfort measures such as repositioning with pillow supports or range-of-motion exercises.

Other types of medications may be considered as adjunctive therapy. The emotional and psychological component of pain must be recognized. Tricyclic antidepressants are one group of drugs that most clinicians agree can play a role in pain management.[132] Other categories of medications include anticonvulsants (especially carbamazepine) and steroids for nervous system involvement.[132] Over-the-counter medications such as hypnotics for insomnia, antitussives for cough, and antacids for dyspepsia are frequently found in home medicine cabinets and may be helpful.

Assessment of pain is ongoing. A change in the location, severity, or type of pain may indicate an acute problem that requires other interventions. Little clues that may signal a change can go unheeded if all pain is attributed to the malignant disease. For example, a home care patient with cancer of the prostate and diffuse bony metastases complained to the nurse that his pain was getting worse. A detailed pain assessment determined that the pain was now sharp versus dull, localized to the center of his back, and became excruciating when he attempted to sit. He previously described his pain as more diffuse, regardless of position. No neurologic deficits were noted. After a conference with the physician, the patient went by ambulance to the hospital where radiologic studies confirmed the presence of three vertebral compression fractures.

Patients and caregivers often negatively influence the treatment of pain as a result of their fears about potent narcotics. They may increase the dose interval, withhold doses, or refuse certain medications or certain routes as they attempt to prevent dependence, addiction, somnolence, or sedation. Physiologic dependence and tolerance are anticipated, but particular problems in the home can be managed by both adjusting dose upward according to need or, conversely, by slowly decreasing the dose over time before discontinuing the narcotic.[117] Twycross and Lack[133] note that experience with morphine and other opioidlike drugs shows that the dose usually increases over time, indicating the development of tolerance. However, similar experiences and studies have shown that the longer a patient receives morphine therapy: (1) the rate at which the dose rises is slower; (2) the intervals between dose increases are longer; and (3) the chance that the dose will be reduced is greater, especially when optimal pain control has been achieved through combination methods.[133] Addiction (that is, psychological craving for a drug's psychic effects) is a phenomenon so rarely seen in cancer pain management that concern is needless.[117] This information is helpful to share with patients and families as they struggle to manage cancer pain at home.

DISCHARGE FROM HOME HEALTH CARE

Critics of home health care often express concern that individuals will receive care for longer than necessary and therefore that the cost-effectiveness of home health care may not be achieved. This is rarely the case since the overall goal of home health care is to facilitate the patient's and family's independence in managing daily life within the constraints imposed by the malignant disease. Furthermore, guidelines for reimbursable services are specific and services are monitored so that home health services are discontinued or modified when the level of care required by the person changes.

The obvious reason for discontinuing home health services occurs when the patient and family have achieved the identified outcomes developed by the nurse, patient, and family. For example, a person who is being followed for wound care may be discharged from services when it is apparent that the individual and family are demonstrating safe wound care and can identify signs/symptoms of potential problems. This does not necessarily mean that the wound is healed, but rather that the patient can manage independently and safely. This is particularly true in the case of severely disrupted tissue integrity that is not anticipated to heal.

Patients will be discharged from home health care when an exacerbation of the disease process produces symptoms that require management in an inpatient setting or when service needs change. For instance, when professional nursing is no longer required but assistance with household tasks or personal care is still necessary, the nurse should make a referral to a community service agencies for homemaker/chore provider or personal care services.

Another reason for discharge is when the person's health status declines so that family members are physically, mentally, or emotionally unable to provide care at home. Sometimes just informing the family that they have options can enable them to maintain the person at home longer. Patients and families need to be assisted and supported in their decision to move the patient to a long-term care setting. With increased emphasis on the home as the "ideal" (and financially advantageous) setting for care, families can often feel like failures when they decide to place the person in an extended care facility or to return the patient to the hospital. Guilt occurs even when families have provided excellent care for long periods of time.

An area of concern in patient discharge from home health care occurs when the patient and family desire to continue services but the nurse must discharge the patient because his or her physical status has changed and no longer meets the requirements for reimbursable home health care. Potential liability may occur if the patient is subsequently injured as a result of precipitous termination of care.[134] The home health nurse may reduce the potential for liability with a thorough assessment of the patient's health status, nursing and health

TABLE 55-9 Planning for Discharge from Home Care

1. Assess patient's physical, functional, psychosocial status prior to discharge and compare and evaluate with assessment at time of admission.
2. Identify patient outcomes and evaluate with goals identified at time of admission or as revised while receiving home health care.
3. Discuss plans and rationale for discharge with patient and family at time of admission, periodically during service, and 3 weeks prior to discharge.
4. Identify continuing patient care needs.
5. Assess patient and family knowledge and skill in performing continuing care needs.
6. Assist the patient and family to identify and form networks in the community.
7. If patient care needs exist, provide the patient and family with the names and addresses of community resources and assist with the referral if needed.

Source: Adapted from Brent NJ: Avoiding patient abandonment charges: Balancing the legal and ethical issues. *Home Healthcare Nurse* 7:7–8, 1989.

care needs, and the family and home situation prior to admission. If the nurse determines that the agency and staff cannot manage the patient and family service needs, the case should not be admitted to home health care. If the case is admitted to home health care, risk may be reduced by developing and implementing a comprehensive discharge plan at the time of admission. Table 55-9 lists the components of a discharge plan.

When evaluating the discharge process, important points to consider and document are: (1) the patient's status on discharge, (2) evidence of planning for discharge, and (3) timeliness of the decision to discharge.

QUALITY ASSESSMENT IN HOME CARE

Quality assessment as an evaluation strategy is essential in home health care in light of recently enacted federal regulations; the increased risks associated with expanded, highly technological services; and a growing industry's need to quantify credibility.[135] Quality assessment is a formal and systematic exercise that requires a usable definition of quality; standards and criteria against which quality can be judged; collection, analysis, and dissemination of relevant data and findings; and implementation of methods to initiate and evaluate subsequent planned changes.

A quality assessment program begins with identification and adoption of standards for home health care. The home health care regulatory bodies (e.g., Department of Public Health, HCFA), professional organizations (American Nurses Association, Oncology Nursing Society), credentialing organizations (National League for Nursing and Joint Commission on Accreditation of Health Organizations), and national organizations for home care have developed standards. Home health care agencies should incorporate these standards in the development and revision of their philosophy, purpose, goals, and objectives as well as their policies and procedures for operations. Standards that are pertinent to home care for persons with cancer include the Oncology Nursing Society's and American Nurses Association's *Standards of Oncology Nursing Practice*[35] and the American Nurses Association's *Standards of Home Health Nursing Practice*.[19]

Donabedian's[136] model for evaluation of quality embodies the home health agency's organizational structure, process of service delivery, and the outcomes of care as interrelated dimensions of a system of care. Quality is evaluated by the level of achievement of each identified standard of care. Evaluation of the home health agency's organizational structure includes review of the agency's philosophy, goals, objectives, organizational chart, financial resources, human resources, staff education, and the community served.

The process of service delivery is routinely evaluated by most home health agencies in quarterly utilization review committees, periodic process audits, and routine clinical record review by supervisors.[137] Comprehensive documentation is essential to evaluation of the quality of care.

Currently there is a move to shift the measurement focus from structure or process toward examining the links between processes of care and the desired, defined outcomes.[136] Health care providers, recipients, payers, and the general public are attempting to design new models to define quality and effective systems to assess, monitor, and improve the care provided to patients.[137] A provider's success in meeting a patient's values and expectations may be reflected in the patient's satisfaction with the care received, compliance with recommended treatment modalities, and subsequent outcomes.[137] A sampling of quality indicators are listed in Table 55-10. Additional studies and measures of quality of care are discussed in Chapter 57.

TABLE 55-10 A Sampling of Quality Indicators

Indicator	Example
Physiologic status	Stable BP, controlled pain
Functional status	Increased strength, steady gait
Health-related knowledge	Demonstrates wound care procedure
Treatment compliance	Follows medication schedule
Satisfaction	Care consistent with family values

SUMMARY

The home is an appropriate health care setting for individuals with cancer and other chronic or long-term illnesses. Home care agencies are expanding in numbers and variety of services. Advances in technology and cost-containment measures have shifted the focus of care from inpatient facilities to alternate delivery sources such as home care. Society's awareness of the scope of patient needs is increasing, as evidenced by the hospice movement, and families are becoming more willing to care for their members in the home. Individuals are living longer with a cancer diagnosis because of earlier detection and more effective treatment modalities. Today the majority of the life of a person diagnosed with cancer is spent in the home setting. The person and family living with cancer at home require a range of health care and social services to maintain optimal levels of physical, psychologic, and social functioning. They also need help to support the patient through the continuum of illness. The nurse in the home setting is challenged to expand the quality of care provided to the patient and support for the family.

Speaking on a very human level, the nurse has the privilege of entering the homes of individuals and families living with cancer at extremely critical times. The home setting provides an opportunity to fully understand the impact of the cancer experience on the lives of those involved and allows the nurse the opportunity to interact with patients and families on a level that is often difficult to achieve in other settings.

REFERENCES

1. Dept. of Health and Human Services Health Care Financing Administration: Medicare program: Medicare coverage of home health service, Medicare conditions of participation and home health aide supervision. *Federal Register* 56:49155, 1991.
2. National Association for Home Care: Basic statistics about home care—1991. *NAHC Bulletin,* 1991.
3. Yasko JM, Fleck A: Prospective payment (DRGs): What will be the impact on cancer care. *Oncol Nurs Forum* 11(3):63–72, 1984.
4. Rose MA: Home care nursing practice: The new frontier. *Holistic Nurs Pract* 3:1–5, 1989.
5. Council on Scientific Affairs, American Medical Assoc: Home care in the '90's. *JAMA* 263:1241–1244, 1990.
6. Department of Health and Human Services Health Care Financing Administration: *Health Insurance for the Aged Home Health Agency Manual.* Baltimore, MD: DHHS, 1966.
7. Conkling VK: Continuity of care issues for cancer patients and families. *Cancer* 64:290–294, 1989.
8. Peters DA: A concept of nursing discharge. *Holistic Nurs Pract* 3:18–25, 1989.
9. Koch MW: Synergy: Utilization management and discharge planning. *Continuing Care* 10:12–15, 1991.
10. Tolkoff-Rubin NE: Coordinated home care, the Massachusetts General Hospital experience. *Med Care* 16: 453–464, 1978.
11. Rosenbaum E. Rosenbaum I: Home care of patients with advanced cancer. *Your Patient and Cancer* 2(7):86–91, 1982.
12. Slevin AP, Roberts AS: Discharge planning: A tool for decision making. *Nurs Manage* 18(12):47–50, 1987.
13. Hays A: Family care: The critical variable in community-based long-term care. *Home Healthcare Nurse* 6:26–31, 1988.
14. Baird SB: Nursing roles in continuing care: Home care and hospice. *Semin Oncol* 7:28–38, 1980.
15. Bull MJ: Influence of diagnosis-related groups on discharge planning, professional practice, and patient care. *J Prof Nurs* 4:415–421, 1988.
16. Simmons WJ: Planning for discharge with the elderly. *Quality Review Board* 12:68–71, 1986.
17. Lewis FM: Experienced personal control and quality of life in late-stage cancer patients. *Nurs Res* 31:113–119, 1982.
18. Kalish PA, Kalish BJ: *The Advance of American Nursing.* Boston: Little, Brown, 1986, pp. 259–289.
19. American Nurses' Association: *Standards of Home Health Nursing Practice.* Kansas City, MO: ANA, 1986.
20. Presznecker BL, Zerwekh JV, Horn BJ: The mutual-participation relationship: Key to facilitating self-care practices in clients and families. *Public Health Nurs* 6:197–203, 1989.
21. Speese-Owens N: Psychological components of cancer nursing. In Bouchard-Kurtz R and Speese-Owens N (eds): *Nursing Care of the Cancer Patient* (4th ed). St. Louis, MO: Mosby, 1981.
22. MacVicar MG, Archbold P: A framework for family assessment in chronic illness. *Nurs Forum* 15:180–194, 1976.
23. Olsen DH, McCubbin HL: *Families: What Makes Them Work.* Beverly Hills, CA: Sage, 1983, pp. 47–80.
24. DuFault K Sr, Firsich SC, Gardner A, et al: Ineffective family coping. In McNally JC (ed): *Guidelines for Oncology Nursing Practice.* Philadelphia: Saunders, 1991, pp. 103–107.
25. Stetz KM: Caregiving demands during advanced cancer: The spouse's needs. *Cancer Nurs* 10:260–268, 1987.
26. Wingate AL, Lackey NR: A description of the needs of noninstitutional cancer patients and their primary caregivers. *Cancer Nurs* 12:216–225, 1989.
27. Rose MA: Problems families face in home care. *Am J Nurs* 75:416–418, 1975.
28. Googe MC, Varricchio CG: A pilot investigation of home health care needs of cancer patients and their families. *Oncol Nurs Forum* 8:24–28, 1981.
29. Goldstein V, Regnery G, Wellin E: Caretaker role fatigue. *Nurs Outlook* 29:24–30, 1981.
30. Welch D: Planning nursing intervention for family members of adult cancer patients. *Cancer Nurs* 4:365–369, 1981.
31. Hull MM: Hospice nurses: Caring support for caregiving families. *Cancer Nurs* 14:63–70, 1991.
32. Skorupka P, Bohnet N: Primary caregiver's perceptions of nursing behaviors that best meet their needs in a home care hospice setting. *Cancer Nurs* 5:371–374, 1982.
33. Giaquinta B: Helping families face the crisis of cancer. *Am J Nurs* 77:1585–1588, 1977.

34. Van Ort S, Woodtli A: Home health care: Providing a missing link. *Gerontol Nurs* 15:4–9, 1989.
35. American Nurses' Association and Oncology Nursing Society: *Standards of Oncology Nursing Practice*. Kansas City, MO: ANA, 1987.
36. Shiber S, Larson E: Evaluating the quality of caring: Structure, process, and outcome. *Holistic Nurs Pract* 5:57–66, 1991.
37. Leming T: Quality customer service: Nursing's new challenge. *Nurs Admin Q* 15:6–12, 1991.
38. Kramer AM, Shaughnessy PW, Baumen MK, et al: Assessing and assuring the quality of home health care: A conceptual framework. *Milbank Q* 68:413–443, 1990.
39. Cloonan PA, Shuster GF: Care coordination: A resource-intensive component of home health nursing practice. *Public Health Nurs* 7:204–208, 1990.
40. Shuster GF, Cloonan P: Nursing activities and reimbursement in clinical case management. *Home Healthcare Nurse* 7:10–15, 1989.
41. O'Hare PA, Terry MA: Community-based care management: A framework for delivery of services. *Home Healthcare Nurse* 9(3):26–32, 1991.
42. Knollmeuller RN: Case management: What's in a name? *Nurs Manage* 20(10):38–42, 1989.
43. Creighton H: Legal significance of charting—Part 1. *Nurs Management* 18:17–22, 1987.
44. Connaway N: Documenting patient care in the home: Legal issues for home health nurses. *Home Healthcare Nurse* 3:6–8, 1985.
45. Warling M: Legal aspects of the client's record: A guide for community health nurses. *Caring* 1:14–17, 1982.
46. Keating G: Documentation: The key to avoiding liability. *Oncol Bull* 4:4–5, 1986.
47. Hoeman SP: Community-based rehabilitation. *Holistic Nurs Pract* 6:32–41, 1992.
48. Habeck RV, Romsaas EP, Olsen SJ: Cancer rehabilitation and continuing care. *Cancer Nurs* 7:315–319, 1984.
49. Hileman JW, Lackey VR: Self-identified needs of patients with cancer at home and their caregivers: A descriptive study. *Oncol Nurs Forum* 17:907–913, 1990.
50. Mor V, Guadagnoli E, Wool M: An examination of the concrete service needs of advanced cancer patients. *J Psychosoc Oncol* 5:1–7, 1987.
51. Cyr LB: The clinical nurse specialist in a home health care setting. *Home Healthcare Nurse* 8:34–39, 1990.
52. Hamric AB: Role development and functions. In Hamric AB, Spross J (eds): *The Clinical Nurse Specialist in Theory and Practice*. Orlando, FL: Grune & Stratton, 1986, pp. 39–58.
53. Boyd NS, Stasiowski SA, Catoe PT, et al: The merit and significance of the clinical nurse specialist. *J Nurs Admin* 21:35–43, 1991.
54. Robichaud AM, Hamric AB: Time documentation of clinical nurse specialist activities. *J Nurs Admin* 16:31–36, 1986.
55. Felder LA: Direct patient care and independent practice. In Hamric AB, Spross J (eds): *The Clinical Nurse Specialist in Theory and Practice*. Orlando, FL: Grune & Stratton, 1983, pp. 59–72.
56. Barron AM: The CNS as consultant. In Hamric AB, Spross J (eds): *The Clinical Nurse Specialist in Theory and Practice*. Orlando, FL: Grune & Stratton, 1983, pp. 91–113.
57. Girouard S, Spross J: Evaluation of the CNS: Using an evaluation tool. In Hamric AB, Spross J (eds): *The Clinical Nurse Specialist in Theory and Practice*. Orlando, FL: Grune & Stratton, 1983, pp. 207–218.
58. Pera MK, Gould EJ: Home care nursing: Integration of politics and nursing. *Holistic Nurs Pract* 3(2):9–17, 1989.
59. Puig L: Health care comes home for savings. *Business Health* 7:10–20, 1989.
60. Reif L: Making dollars and sense of home health policy. *Nurs Economics* 2:382–388, 1984.
61. Simione WJ: Reimbursement for home care services. *Caring* 5:22–26, 1986.
62. Keenan JM, Fanale JE, Ripsin C, et al: A review of federal home-care legislation. *J Am Geriatrics Soc* 38:1041–1048, 1990.
63. Della Monica E, Yuan J: Documentation in home care: Skilled observation. *Home Healthcare Nurse* 6:39–40, 1988.
64. Galten R: Documentation: The key to reimbursement. *Caring* 6:68–70, 1987.
65. Omdahl DJ: Preventing home care denials. *Am J Nurs* 87:1031–1033, 1987.
66. Health Care Financing Administration: National health expenditures, 1990. *Health Care Finan Rev* 13:29–58, 1991.
67. Rooks JP: Let's admit we ration health care—then set priorities. *Am J Nurs* 90(5):39–43, 1990.
68. Health Care Financing Administration: Projections of national health expenditures through the year 2000. *Health Care Finan Rev* 13:1–15, 1991.
69. Operation: Health care reform. *Continuing Care* 11:12–16, 1992 (editorial).
70. Capuzzi C, Garland M: The Oregon plan: Increasing access to health care. *Nurs Outlook* 38:260–286, 1990.
71. National Association for Home Care: Oakar reintroduces long-term care bill. NAHC Report No. 396. Washington DC, 1991.
72. Dept. Health and Human Services HCFA: Medicare home health agency manual. Transmittal No 235. Baltimore, MD: DHHS, June 1990.
73. Carr P: Management and evaluation. *Home Healthcare Nurse* 8:51–53, 1990.
74. Collopy B, Dubler N, Zuckerman C: The ethics of home care: Autonomy and accommodation. *Hastings Cen Rep* 20:1–16, 1990(suppl).
75. Haddad AM: Ethical problems in home health care. *J Nurs Admin* 22(3):46–51, 1992.
76. Young A, Pignatello CH, Taylor M: Who's the boss? Ethical conflicts in home care. *Health Prog* 69(11):59–62, 1988.
77. Aroskar MA: Community health nurses: Their most significant ethical decision-making problems. *Nurs Clin North Am* 24:967–975, 1989.
78. Veatch RM, Fry ST: *Case Studies in Nursing Ethics*. Philadelphia: Lippincott, 1987.
79. Gadow S: An ethical case for patient self-determination. *Semin Oncol Nurs* 5:99–101, 1989.
80. Beauchamp TL, Childress JF: *Principles of Biomedical Ethics* (2d ed). New York: Oxford University Press, 1983.
81. Fry ST: Ethics and cancer care. In Baird S, McCorkle R, Grant M (eds): *Cancer Nursing: A Comprehensive Textbook*. Philadelphia: Saunders, 1991, pp. 31–37.
82. American Nurses' Association: *Code for Nurses with Interpretive Statements*. Kansas City, MO: ANA, 1985.
83. DeWolf MS: Ethical decision-making. *Semin Oncol Nurs* 5:77–81, 1989.
84. Flaherty G: Ethics in nursing practice. *Today's Prof Nurse* 1:10–12, 1990.

85. Jameton A: *Nursing Practice: The Ethical Issues.* Englewood Cliffs NJ: Prentice-Hall, 1984.
86. Brown JM: Home care models for infusion therapy. *Caring* 9(5):24–26, 1990.
87. Handy CM: Patient-centered high-technology home care. *Holistic Nurs Pract* 3(2):46–53, 1989.
88. Massoorli S, Angeles T: PICC lines: The latest home care challenge. *RN* 1:44–51, 1990.
89. Rountree D: The PIC catheter. *Am J Nurs* 91(8):22–26, 1991.
90. Department of Health and Human Services Care Financing Administration Part II, 29 CRF 1910, 1030. Occupational exposure to bloodborne pathogens; Final rule. *Federal Register* 56(235):64175–64182, December 6, 1991.
91. Weinstein SM: Biohazards of working with antineoplastics. *Home Healthcare Nurse* 5(1):30–34, 1987.
92. Gullo SM: Safe handling of antineoplastic drugs: Translating the recommendations into practice. *Oncol Nurs Forum* 15:595–601, 1988.
93. Barry LK, Booher RN: Promoting the responsible handling of antineoplastic agents in the community. *Oncol Nurs Forum* 12:(5)41–46, 1985.
94. Oncology Nursing Society: *Cancer Chemotherapy Guidelines.* Pittsburgh, PA: ONS, 1988.
95. Gross J, Johnson BL, Bertino JR: Possible hazards of working with cytotoxic agents: A review of the literature. *Oncol Nurs Forum* 8(4):10–12, 1981.
96. Cloak M, Connor TH, Stevens KR, et al: Occupational exposure of nursing personnel to antineoplastic agents. *Oncol Nurs Forum* 12(5):33–39, 1985.
97. Rogers B, Emmett EA: Handling antineoplastic agents: Urine mutagenicity in nurses. *Image: J Nurs Schol* 19:108–113, 1987.
98. Occupational Safety and Health Administration: Work practice guidelines for personnel dealing with cytotoxic (antineoplastic) drugs. OSHA Instruction Pub 8–11, Office of Occupational Medicine, Jan. 29, 1986.
99. Graves T, Proemer J: New methods of chemotherapy administration-selected routes. *J Pharm Pract* 4:49–63, 1991.
100. Balinsky W: Reimbursement for outpatient antibiotic therapy: Update. *Rev Infect Dis* 13:s193–s195, 1991 (suppl 2).
101. Blackburn G: Home TPN: State of the art. *Am J Intraven Ther & Clin Nutr* 11:20–32, 1984.
102. Konstantinides NW: Home parenteral nutrition: A viable alternative. *Oncol Nurs Forum* 12(1):23–29, 1985.
103. Dudrick SJ, O'Connell JJ, Englert DM et al: 100 patient years of ambulatory home total parenteral nutrition. *Ann Surg* 199:770–781, 1984.
104. Steinborn PA: Total parenteral nutrition: The transition from hospital to home. *J Home Health Pract* 1(4):39–50, 1989.
105. Orr ME: Nutritional support in home care. *Nurs Clin North Am* 24:437–445, 1989.
106. Gulledge AD, Gipsom WT, Steiger E, et al: Home parenteral nutrition for the short bowel syndrome: Psychological issues. *Gen Hosp Psychiatry* 2:271–281, 1980.
107. Bloch AS, Brown P: Methods of nutritional support in the home. *J Pain Symp Manage* 2(5):297–306, 1990.
108. Barfoot KR, Ross KL: Intravenous therapy at home: An overview: *Home Healthcare Nurse* 6(4):11–13, 1988.
109. Dolbee SF, Creason NS: Outcome criteria for the patient using intravenous antibiotic therapy at home. *Home Healthcare Nurse* 6(4):22–29, 1988.
110. Grizzard MB, Harris G, Karns H: Use of outpatient parenteral antibiotic therapy in a health maintenance organization. *Rev Infect Dis* 13:s174–s179, 1991 (suppl 2).
111. Kasmer RJ, Hoisington LM, Yukniewicz S: Home parenteral antibiotic therapy, part I: An overview of program design. *Home Healthcare Nurse* 5(1):12–18, 1987.
112. Brown RB: Selection and training of patients for outpatient intravenous antibiotic therapy. *Rev Infect Dis* 13:s147–s151, 1991 (suppl).
113. Gorski LA: Effective teaching of home IV therapy. *Home Healthcare Nurse* 5(5):10–17, 1987.
114. Kasmer RJ, Hoisington LM, Yukniewicz S: Home parenteral antibiotic therapy, Part II: Drug preparation and administration considerations. *Home Healthcare Nurse* 5(1):19–29, 1987.
115. Williams DN: Home intravenous antibiotic therapy: New technologies. *Recent Results Cancer Research* 121:215–222, 1991.
116. Stoll HR: Effective pain control in cancer patients in the home care setting. *Recent Results Cancer Research* 121:36–42, 1991.
117. Tartaglia MJ: The management of chronic cancer pain, principles and practices. *J Intrav Nurs* 11:79–87, 1988.
118. Stephany T: Oral medication for pain relief. *Home Healthcare Nurse* 7:44–45, 1989.
119. Dennis EMP: An ambulatory infusion pump for pain control: A nursing approach for home care. *Cancer Nurs* 8:309–313, 1984.
120. Patt RB: Interventional analgesia: Epidural and subarachnoid therapy. *Am J Hospice Care* (March/April):11–14, 1989.
121. Hensley JR: Continuous S C morphine for cancer pain. *Am J Nurs* 91(3):98–101, 1991.
122. Storey P, Hill HH, St. Louis RH, et al: Subcutaneous infusions for control of cancer symptoms. *J Pain Sympt Manage* 5:33–41, 1990.
123. Lonsway RA: Care of the patient with an epidural catheter: An infection control challenge. *J Intrav Nurs* 11: 52–55, 1988.
124. Wild L, Coyne C: The basics and beyond: Epidural analgesia. *Am J Nurs* 92(4):26–34, 1992.
125. Panfilli R, Brunckhorse L, Dundon R: Nursing implications of patient-controlled analgesia. *J Intrav Nurs* 11(2):75–77, 1988.
126. Enck RE: Parenteral narcotics for pain control in the home care environment. *Caring* 9:38–41, 1990.
127. Keeri-Szanto M: Demand analgesia for the relief of pain problems in terminal illness. *Anesth Rev* 2:29–31, 1987.
128. Citron ML, Early AJ, Boyer M, et al: Patient controlled analgesia for severe cancer pain. *Arch Intern Med* 146:734–736, 1986.
129. Mast D, Meyers J, Urbanski A: Relaxation techniques: A self-learning module for nurses, Unit I. *Cancer Nurs* 10(3):141–147, 1987.
130. Mast D, Meyers J, Urbanski A: Relaxation techniques: A self-learning module for nurses, Unit II. *Cancer Nurs* 10(4):217–225, 1987.
131. Mast D, Meyers J, Urbanski A: Relaxation techniques: A self-learning module for nurses, Unit III. *Cancer Nurs* 10(5):279–285, 1987.
132. Enck RE: Adjuvant analgesic drugs. *Am J Hospice Care* (March/April):9–10, 1989.
133. Twycross R, Lack S: *Oral Morphine in Advanced Cancer.* Beaconsfield, Bucks, England: Beaconsfield, 1984.
134. Brent NJ: Avoiding patient abandonment charges: Bal-

ancing the legal and ethical issues. *Home Healthcare Nurse* 7:7–8, 1989.
135. Daniels K: Planning for quality in the home care system. In Fishen K and Gardner R (eds): *Quality and Home Care: Redefining the Tradition.* Chicago: Joint Commission on Accreditation of Healthcare Organizations, 1987.
136. Donabedian A: Quality assessment and assurance: Unity of purpose, diversity of means. *Inquiry* 25:173–192, 1988.
137. Sorgen LM: The development of a home care quality assurance program in Alberta. *Home Health Care Svcs Q* 7(2):13–28, 1986.

Chapter 56

Hospice Care

Jeanne Martinez RN, MPH

Steven Wagner RN, BSN

INTRODUCTION

Hospice care was developed to meet a simple objective: to facilitate a comfortable and natural death. However, the concept of a natural death runs counter to our society's values on youth, health, and technology, including medical technology. In our modern society, death is a taboo topic.[1] This has been reinforced by our current complex medical system, which errs on the side of technological intervention and overtreatment to prevent death.

Development of Hospice Concept

Developers of the hospice concept recognized that allowing a "natural death" requires preparation of the patient and family, changes in medical practice, and redesign or circumvention of some aspects of the existing health care system.[2] An analogy can be made to birthing and medical care in American society. In the 1960s birthing was treated primarily as a medical problem. Change in obstetrics was instituted largely by consumer demand from the women's movement, which sought to view birth as a life process that involved the individual woman's right of control over her body and childbirth, as well as the importance of family participation. In response to this demand, obstetric medical practice changed to focus more on prenatal preventive care and education.[2] Attempts to deinstitutionalize the process were made by creating birthing centers that are more homelike and can facilitate family participation.

Hospice care in America was also influenced by consumer groups. Initially, hospice was most likely to be described as a movement or as an "alternative" to mainstream medical care. When hospices first began to appear as organized programs, they were commonly volunteer programs with lay volunteers and a few nurses, organized from a church basement or around someone's dining room table. Today this model is all but extinct, except that hospice has kept the tenet of lay volunteers as part of the core team of interdisciplinary hospice services. The ideas for the American hospice were adapted directly from the English model at St. Christopher's Hospice, the world's first hospice, developed by Dame Cicely Saunders in 1968.

Role of Nurses in the Development of Hospice

The word *hospice,* or *hospitia,* was used during the crusades in the Middle Ages to designate a place of temporary shelter for travelers or sick pilgrims.[2,3] In the late nineteenth century *hospice* was applied to the care of the dying by Sister Mary Aikenhead, a colleague of Florence Nightingale, who opened Our Lady's Hospice, in Dublin,[2,3] the first facility dedicated to care of the terminally ill.

Although Dame Cicely Saunders is best known as the medical director and founder of St. Christopher's Hospice, she began her career as a nurse and went on to become a medical social worker prior to attending medical school. Dame Saunders developed many of the current concepts in palliative care, including oral narcotic administration on a regular rather than PRN basis (the British use the term "regular giving").[2]

It was Dame Saunders' visit to Yale University in 1963 that precipitated the interest of Florence Wald, Dean of the Yale School of Nursing, in the concept of hospice care. Florence Wald subsequently resigned as dean to participate in the development of the first American hospice, Connecticut Hospice Inc. Connecticut Hospice began serving home care patients in 1974, and in 1979 opened an independent 44-bed inpatient facility, the first to be designed as a hospice.[3]

In 1984 the Joint Commission on Accreditation of Hospitals (JCAH) published its first standards manual for hospice programs.[4] Anne Rooney, R.N., a former hospice director of Proviso-Leyden Hospice in Illinois and a former president of the Illinois State Hospice Organization joined the JCAH in 1985 as Associate Director of Hospice and Home Care, to facilitate the nationwide accreditation process. This separate accreditation was eliminated in 1990, but some of the original hospice standards have now been incorporated into the 1992 Joint Commission on Accreditation of Healthcare Organizations (JCAHO) standards applied to dying patients.[5] Dame Cicely Saunders, Florence Wald, and Anne Rooney are among the many who have made history and continue to make contributions in the area of palliative care.

Another factor influencing the development of palliative care was the ground-breaking work in the 1960s of Elisabeth Kübler-Ross, a psychiatrist at the University of Chicago. Dr. Kübler-Ross pointed out that health care professionals, due largely to their own ineffectual coping with the subject of death, isolated dying patients.[1] She helped to demystify the dying process by devising the radical teaching technique of interviewing dying patients in front of a group of health care professionals.[1] This not only provided an opportunity to learn first-hand from patients themselves, but also provided role modeling for professionals on *how* to talk to patients. More than anyone else, Elisabeth Kübler-Ross opened the debate on care of the dying, not only for the lay public but for health care professionals as well.

PALLIATIVE CARE APPROACHES

Hospice care pivots around the idea of palliative medical management. *Palliative management* involves a shift in treatment goals from curative toward providing relief from suffering.[2] And relief of suffering in dying patients goes beyond merely identifying and treating physical symptoms. The emotional, spiritual, and existential cocomponents of suffering and pain must also be addressed. Our current health system consists largely of fragmented, specialized care episodes for specific problems, rather than a holistic approach to illness.[2] Therefore, management of a patient via palliative care will differ from that via acute care.

Principles of Palliative Care

- The overall goal of treatment is to optimize quality of life; that is, the hopes and desires of a patient are fulfilled.
- Death is regarded as a natural process, to be neither hastened nor prolonged.
- Diagnostic tests and other invasive procedures are minimized, unless likely to result in the alleviation of symptoms.
- Use of "heroic" treatment measures is discouraged.
- When using narcotic analgesics, the right dose is the dose that provides pain relief without unacceptable side effects.
- The patient is the "expert" on whether pain and symptoms have been adequately relieved.
- Patients eat if they are hungry, and drink if thirsty; fluids and feeding are not forced.
- Care is individualized and based on the goals of the patient *and* family, as the unit of care.

Palliative Versus Acute Care

The following example of a patient with shortness of breath illustrates the differences in approach if the goals of treatment are palliative versus curative.

> In an *acute care* situation, a patient with shortness of breath will have diagnostic studies to determine the etiology of the problem. These commonly include blood gas studies, a chest x-ray, CBC, and pulmonary function tests. The patient usually will be given oxygen for comfort.
>
> When the goal of care is *palliation,* the etiology generally is either already known or unimportant if the patient has a short time to live. The diagnostic procedures for acute care result in some discomfort, but chest x-ray and pulmonary functions demand that a considerable amount of energy be expended by the patient. Results of such studies still may not provide the information needed to determine which intervention will provide relief from shortness of breath. For example, a patient with chronic lung disease and abnormal blood gas studies may have symptomatically compensated, and not feel as distressed as a patient with borderline blood gas studies, for whom shortness of breath is a new symptom.
>
> When symptom management is the primary goal, first-line palliative treatment for shortness of breath is low-dose oral morphine given at regular intervals.[6,7] This can be used concurrently with oxygen if needed, but often is effective alone. Another important palliative measure is positioning the patient to maximize lung expansion. Many patients report that the use of a room fan provides significant relief.[8] Like pain, shortness of breath may be as closely related to psychological and social problems as it is to physical ones. These issues need to be identified, addressed, and treated. When anxiety is a significant factor, low-dose anxiolytic (e.g., a benzodiazepine) can be effective.[6,7]

Patient Criteria for Hospice Care

Each program determines its own criteria for selecting patients to receive hospice care. To qualify for the Medicare Hospice Benefit, two physicians must certify that a person is terminally ill and has less than 6 months to live.[9] This latter criterion is controversial, for a number of reasons. Professionals who work with the dying know that accurate predictions of time of death cannot be made. It could be detrimental for physicians or nurses to attempt to give predictions about time of death to patients.[1] Another criterion under Medicare and most state hospice regulations is that the patient sign a consent form or election statement declaring that hospice and palliative care are their choice of treatments and that they have the right to elect out of hospice at any time.[9] The following are additional criteria required by most hospice programs.

- The patient must have a primary caregiver; that is, friend or family member willing to be responsible for the patient's overall care.
- For home care, the patient needs to reside in the hospice program's geographic area.
- The patient must agree to palliative, not curative, treatment.
- Some programs require that the patient have a "Do not resuscitate" (DNR) status prior to admission to the hospice program.[2,3]

HOSPICE CARE IN THE PRESENT

Development of a hospice program is not as simple as it was in the early phases of the hospice movement. Hospice programs have been affected by mandated guidelines of federal and state legislation. Currently, 26 states have their own licensing regulations. In some states, these regulations include a certificate of need review that can limit the number of hospices in a given area. Federal guidelines define the Hospice Medicare Benefit Plan used today. These guidelines were developed by hospice program planners to include cost incentives for encouraging home hospice care rather than hospitalization, and cost control via a financial cap for all hospice care provided. These cost incentives were proposed for the federal legislature prior to the implementation of Medicare diagnostic related groups (DRGs).

Models of Hospice Care

The present models for hospice care vary greatly in size and means by which they provide care. A recent National Hospice Organization (NHO) study indicated that 40% of all hospices were independent, community-based programs.[10] Though these independent hospices contract with hospitals for inpatient care, their primary focus is care in the home. Funding, boards of directors, and policy decisions are independent of the hospital or agencies they contract with. Thirty percent of hospices are owned by hospitals. The caseload is made up primarily of patients referred by physicians or staff from within the parent hospital. Funding is integrated into the existing system.

Beds in the hospital for hospice patients may be scattered in the medical or oncology units. Other hospitals may have a unit specifically designed for care of hospice patients. These units attempt to simulate a comfortable, homelike atmosphere. Care is focused on symptom management and limiting invasive or painful procedures. Visiting hours are less restricted, and pets may be allowed to visit. Inpatient admission is principally for acute care management of pain or other symptoms that cannot be controlled easily in the home, or is used for short-term respite care. Often patients return home after symptoms have been alleviated and they are medically stable.

According to Medicare guidelines, at least 80% of an individual hospice's *aggregate* patient days of care under the Hospice Benefit must be provided at home. A maximum of 20% of aggregate days of care can be provided in the inpatient setting. If the maximum aggregate inpatient ratio is exceeded, the hospice can be denied reimbursement for excess days.

Similarly, the annual per-patient reimbursement cap (which for 1992 was a little more than $11,000) is applied on an aggregate basis. For example, a hospice program can be reimbursed $14,000 within a year for one patient if this can be balanced out with another patient whose hospice reimbursement does not exceed $8,000 in the same year.

Twenty-four percent of hospices are operated as part of a home health agency. The agency usually has a separate hospice component with at least one nurse coordinating hospice home care. Visiting nurses from home care may function as part-time hospice nurses. In effect, the hospice component contracts for their services. The remaining 7% of hospices are coalition programs or operated in a nursing home setting.[10]

The 1991 NHO study found that two of every three hospice programs were Medicare certified (approximately 1125). The annual growth rate for programs being newly certified is 13%.[10] The Medicare guidelines dictate that a full-service hospice be a medically directed, nurse-coordinated program that incorporates social services along with pastoral counseling and trained volunteers to complete the nucleus of its core services. Beyond these core services, the following may be included: dietary counseling, occupational therapy, physical therapy, speech therapy, art therapy, home health aide/homemaker, and psychologist, as well as volunteer and bereavement coordinator (see Figure 56-1). Under the Hospice Medicare Benefit, medical supplies, durable medical equipment, and medications are paid for by the hospice. Since the aim of care is to keep patients at home, nursing and physician services, as well as medications, must be available 24 hours a day. In addition, the hospice must provide bereavement counseling to the patient's family after death has occurred. The nurse assesses the needs and facilitates the hospice services and supplies for individual patients. Hospice care was a prototype for what many now would term "case management." Consistent with this case management approach is the Medicare Hospice Benefit's per diem reimbursement structure.

Reimbursement and Funding Methods

Per diem is a system of reimbursement that pays a flat daily rate for all services provided to a patient, rather than paying for the individual services or items. The advantages of the per diem system are that it allows the hospice to provide a comprehensive approach to assess needs and prevent problems, and to provide additional team services as the patient's condition changes. This case management approach is the most efficient and effective way to keep a patient at home.

The per diem for the Medicare Hospice Benefit is reimbursed on four levels, as defined by the Health Care Finance Administration (HCFA): a routine rate, a continuous rate for home care, an inpatient rate for acute care, and an inpatient rate for respite care.[3]

For a patient to qualify for the Hospice Medicare Benefit, certification by two physicians of a prognosis of 6 months or less is required. Recertification of the patient's appropriateness for hospice care is required three times under the benefit. The first and second recertification periods are 90 days each. The third period is 30 days. The fourth benefit period is unlimited, so that after 210 days of care the patient does not need to be recertified for hospice services to continue. Only hospital care, pharmacy, or home care services contracted with the hospice program will receive reimbursement under the benefit. At any time, the patient has the option to rescind the hospice benefit and return to regular Medicare Part A coverage.[9]

Eighty-nine percent of current hospices are operated not for profit.[10] Many hospice programs have made a commitment to provide basic hospice service of nursing visits, physician follow-up, social services, and volunteers, despite the inability to be reimbursed for it. While the majority of hospice programs are Medicare

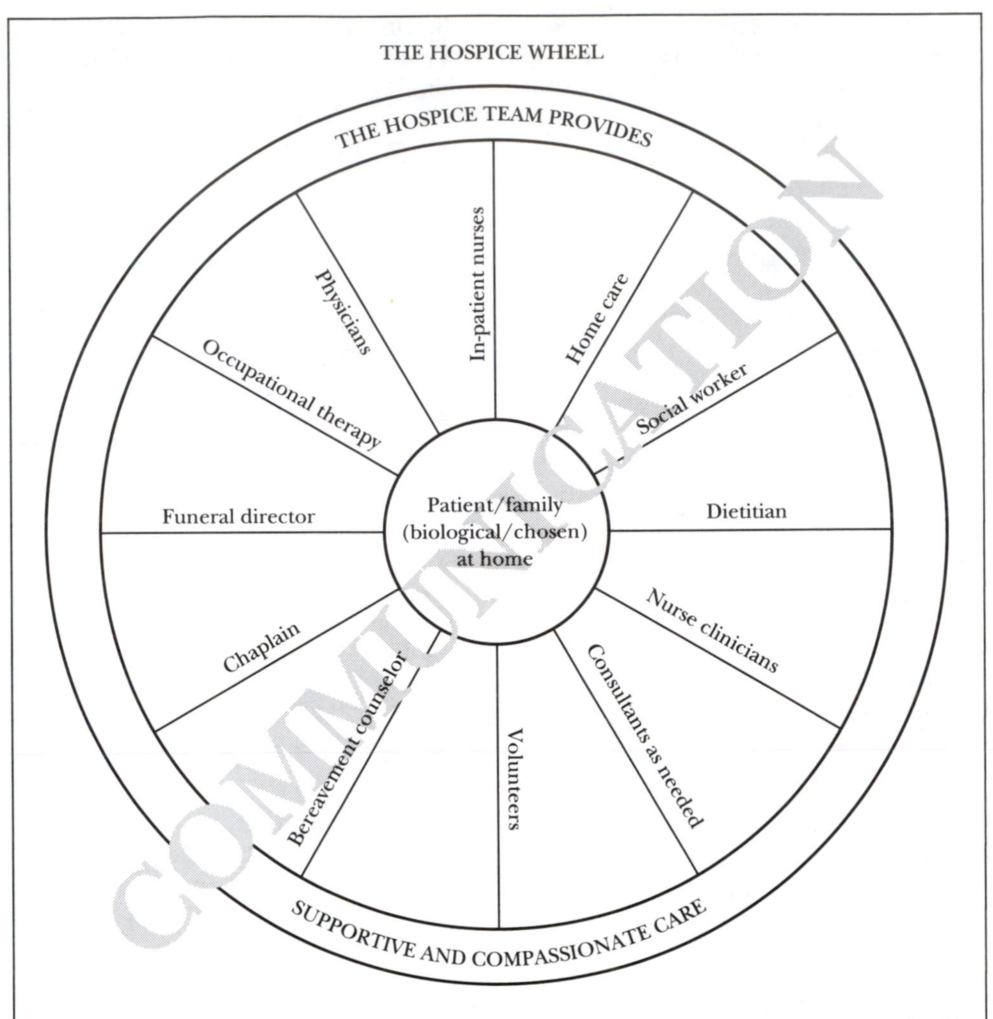

FIGURE 56-1 Many disciplines are involved in a coordinated effort to provide supportive and compassionate hospice care to the patient and family. (Source: Reprinted with permission of Northwestern Memorial Hospice Program, Chicago. Used by permission of John DeBerry.)

certified, one-third continue to operate with funds received from donations, contracts with health maintenance organizations (HMOs), and/or reimbursement from private insurance companies. Hospices have been successful in introducing per diem billing as the preferred means of reimbursement for private insurance hospice benefits.

Patient Population

Over 206,000 patients and families received hospice care in 1990 according to an NHO study. Eighty-four percent were diagnosed with cancer: 4% had AIDS; 3% had cerebral vascular disease.[10] The remaining 9% had other terminal conditions, such as end-stage heart and lung disease and Alzheimer's disease. Of all these diagnoses, AIDS presents the greatest challenge to the health care system, including hospice programs.[2]

The principles of palliative care were originally developed by hospice to meet the needs of the elderly cancer patient. Hospice care is evolving to include patients of differing age groups who have more complex physical and psychosocial concerns. The case study presented in Tables 56-1 and 56-2 demonstrate some of the unique challenges presented by a young patient with AIDS whose case follows the multidisciplinary care management hospice model.

TABLE 56-1 Case Study and Interdisciplinary Team Care Plan

Addie is a 31-year-old woman with acquired immune deficiency syndrome (AIDS). She has three children, ages 11, 7, and 5. She contracted the disease through having unprotected sex with her late husband, Sam, who was an intravenous drug abuser. Sam died a year and a half ago. Addie is now living with her boyfriend, Ted. They have been together for 1 year. Ted has refused to be tested for the human immunosuppressive virus (HIV). He reports having recurrent nightmares with a religious theme. Addie is living on disability insurance from her former job. She was diagnosed with cytomegalovirus (CMV) retinitis 9 months ago. Within the past month she has experienced increased forgetfulness, which her physician diagnosed as AIDS dementia. It is difficult for Addie to walk because she has severe neuropathy and Kaposi's sarcoma lesions on her feet. She has shooting pains up her leg when she bears weight on her leg. She is on Elavil, 75 mg every night, and Tylenol #3 every 4 hours as needed for her neuropathy pain. In addition Addie is receiving Foscarnet for the CMV. Burrows soaks are applied three times a day to her feet to help control drainage from the Kaposi's sarcoma lesions. In addition, combination chemotherapy is being given to attempt to control the Kaposi's sarcoma foot lesions. Addie's referral to hospice was initiated by the oncology nurse who was giving her the chemotherapy. The following is an example of some of the problems included in her care plan.

INTERDISCIPLINARY CARE PLAN

Problem	Persons Responsible	Goals/Outcome	Plan
Knowledge deficit related to home death and infection control	Nurse	Patient and family to express understanding of home death protocol, ie, no heroic measures, no paramedics, no police; call hospice Patient and family to demonstrate compliance with home infection control instructions	Family meeting to discuss home death. Provide both written and verbal instructions as to signs and symptoms of home death and hospice protocol. Reinforce availability of hospice on 24-hour call. Provide written and verbal instructions regarding home infection control. Observe the family for compliance with instructions.
Maintaining continuity of care	Nurse, hospice team	Hospice coordinates patient's home care	Weekly multidisciplinary meeting to review hospice plan of care. Supervisor from high-tech agency to attend weekly meeting. Hospice nurse to make combined visit with high-tech nurse to discuss coordination of care with family on monthly basis. Send written plan of care to patient's physician on regular basis.
Altered comfort level related to neuropathy, Kaposi's sarcoma on feet	Nurse, physician	Patient to express satisfaction with comfort level, ie, describes pain as 2 or less on 0–5 comfort scale, with 0 being no pain and 5 being severe pain	Assess comfort level with each visit, at least twice weekly. Provide written and verbal instruction regarding analgesic regimen. Instruct family to contact hospice if discomfort increases. Hospice physician to visit monthly if patient is unable to visit clinic.
Alteration in physical mobility and safety related to neuropathy, weakness, change in mental status	Physical or occupational therapist	Patient will be injury-free at home	Assess safety and mobility status at home. Promote activities of daily living. Assess need for assistive devices. Address work simplification and energy conservation measures.

(continued)

TABLE 56-1 Case Study and Interdisciplinary Team Care Plan (continued)

Problem	Persons Responsible	Goals/Outcome	Plan
Alteration in psychosocial status related to loss of independence, change in parenting role	Social worker, occupational therapist, volunteer, nurse	Patient will demonstrate adaptation to partial independence Patient will complete legal arrangements for her children prior to death	Social worker visits every week to assess patient's psychosocial status and provide emotional support. Facilitate discussion and plans regarding choice of legal guardian for children after patient's death. Occupational therapist and volunteers to assist patient in creating a lasting remembrance that she can leave for her children after her death.
Alteration in family psychosocial status related to altered family process roles; anticipatory grieving of Addie, Ted, and children	Social worker, nurse, volunteers	Family to express feelings of increased support, ability to manage care at home Patient and family will be able to verbalize good-byes to each other Children will be able to express their feelings through verbal and/or nonverbal methods (ie, art, play or writing)	Notify school counselor of the stress the children are under so that the school can be helpful in providing support. Volunteers visit 8 hours per week to provide respite support. Social worker to visit every week and address anticipatory grieving based on the developmental age of each child. Nurse and social worker to meet with Ted to help him identify his needs, encourage testing to determine HIV status. Social worker to address financial concerns. Team visits regularly to provide opportunity for family to express feelings.
Alteration in value/belief pattern related to spiritual distress	Chaplain	Patient and family to express feelings of enhanced spiritual support	Assess patient and family spiritual needs. With family permission, identify community clergy and notify them of hospice involvement. Offer chaplain home visit to enhance spiritual support. Encourage Ted to write the details of his dream so it may be discussed with chaplain and/or community clergy.

NURSING AND HOSPICE CARE

Nurse's Role

The nurse has a pivotal role on the multidisciplinary hospice team. It is imperative that the nurse be an experienced practitioner who develops skill in the specialized area of care for the terminally ill. The nurse works cooperatively and communicates effectively within a multidisciplinary framework actively to promote holistic palliative care for hospice patients and their families. The nurse demonstrates self-direction and initiative in the role as practitioner, educator, and consultant. The nurse coordinates the care and services provided to the hospice patients and their families.[2] The education and experience required for hospice nurses vary among hospice programs. Many programs stipulate that nurses have a baccalaureate degree in nursing and have practiced for at least 2 years. Experience in oncology

TABLE 56-2 Aspects of Spiritual Care

The spiritual aspects of care encompass a person's relationship to things larger than the self: causes, principles, art, history, values, a higher power

- **Spiritual issues** include an individual's values, beliefs, religious practices, and concerns with the meaning of life.
- **Spiritual distress** may cause emotional or physical suffering.
- **Spiritual concerns** greatly affect the way someone grieves and the way someone dies.
- **Spiritual peace** leads to reconciliation with others and one's own self in the time of dying.

nursing, home care, or hospice-related fields is a definite advantage for a nurse considering a position in hospice.

The nurse has a strong leadership role within the multidisciplinary hospice team. Good communication skills, both verbal and written, enable the nurse to foster cooperation within the team and to fulfill federal and state medical record documentation requirements adequately. As well as being technically competent, each nurse in hospice needs to be mentally healthy to provide adequate psychosocial care, support, and counseling.[11] The nurse individualizes the plan of palliative care to maximize the patient's physical and emotional comfort. When goals of care conflict, the nurse prioritizes care issues after consultation with the physician and team. Weekly team conferences help in resolving conflicts and developing a consistent approach.

The ability of the nurse to foster a relaxed, warm, personal relationship with the patient, family, and other team members helps to promote confidence in achieving the goals of care. Interpersonal skills are invaluable in enabling the nurse to discuss such difficult issues as preparation for home death and funeral arrangements. The stressful nature of terminal illness tends to bring out the best and the worst in ourselves and the patient and families we care for. An unhurried approach to care gives the patient and family time and encouragement to address their concerns. When hospice nurses were compared with nonhospice nurses, nurses involved with hospice care were found to be higher in self-actualization, i.e., self-directing, possessing healthier internal values, demonstrating flexibility in the application of their values, exhibiting sensitivity to their own needs and feelings, and being able to express their needs and feelings freely to the hospice team.[12]

Management of Care Issues

Direct patient care and physical assessment skills are important to the hospice nurse's role. The nurse often provides basic nursing care, such as skin care, care of central venous lines, checking compliance with medication regimens, and indwelling catheter management.

Ongoing assessment of pain is an activity best accomplished with a formal assessment tool. Some hospice nurses use a pain-intensity scale numbered 0–5 with 0 indicating no pain and 5 denoting maximum pain. Some nurses also utilize a visual analog scale, with faces demonstrating emotional responses corresponding to the 0–5 number scale. A general rule of thumb is that pain intensity of 0–2 represents adequate pain control. Pain intensity of 3 or above indicates a need for adjustment in the analgesic dosage. The nurse performs a general assessment of body systems with each home visit. It takes particular skill to make the assessment less obvious or less mechanical, not interfering with the therapeutic rapport developed with the patient.

The goal of hospice is to provide palliative care in the home; therefore, effective physical assessment skills can make a difference in identifying a potential problem early enough for timely intervention to occur. A nurse on the hospice team is available to the patient on call 24 hours, 7 days a week, to address questions or concerns that developed between visits by the team. A physician also is available on a 24-hour basis to assist in consultation on medical issues. (See Tables 56-3 and 56-4 on selected principles for symptom management in palliative care.)

Once the knowledge base and experience needed to function comfortably in the role of hospice nurse has been developed, the role of educator and consultant becomes more prominent. Initially, the nurse instructs the patient and family in the skills needed to provide safe and comfortable home care. Teaching tools include both written and verbal material. The patient and family's knowledge base is assessed, information is provided, and then understanding of the new information is confirmed. The experienced nurse also has the opportunity to educate peers and members of other disciplines in topics such as: general hospice information, pain and symptom management, and the hospice approach to such terminal diseases as AIDS, Alzheimer's, end-stage heart and lung disease. The consultative role comes into play when a patient is referred to hospice to be assessed for potential admission into the hospice program. The attending physician is contacted to determine reason for referral, do-not-resuscitate status, expected prognosis, and appropriate medical information. Other disciplines involved in patient care may also be contacted to obtain information on financial status, family dynamics, or home care support network. After eliciting the important referral information, the nurse approaches the patient and family to discuss the option of hospice care. Many hospice nurses find it takes about 2 years for a nurse to develop full expertise in the specialized assessments and skills needed to provide excellent care for a hospice patient.

DEATH IN THE HOME

The hospice care philosophy is uniquely characterized by its approach to facilitating a person's death at home.

TABLE 56-3 Selected Principles and Approaches for Symptom Management

Problem	Principles	Management Approaches
Pain	• Pain has both a sensory and an emotional component. • Pain perception escalates with anxiety. • Respiratory depression can be avoided by careful dose titration. Pain is a natural antagonist to narcotics. (Even patients with severe lung disease can tolerate large doses of narcotics if the dose is escalated gradually.)[7] • Tolerance is rarely a problem due to the wide therapeutic range of narcotics. • Addiction is extremely rare and unimportant in the terminally ill. • Placebos are never appropriate.	• Explore patient and family perceptions of pain and usage of pain medication. • Ask the patient how pain changes mood or contributes to fear and anxiety. Consider cultural influences on pain and its management. • Instruct patient and family on positive effects of pain management, ie, control of pain, improved mood and activity. • Reinforce that addiction is not an issue.
	Constant pain requires constant medication: • Most short-acting narcotic analgesics are given every 4 hr. • Sustained-release morphine is given every 12 hr, ie, (MS Contin). • Medicate to prevent pain. It takes less pain medication to keep pain away than to break acute pain cycles. • Adequate pain control requires adequate dosing • Oral route is preferable: easy to administer, economical, maintains therapeutic level of drug in blood plasma with regular dosing.	• Assess/document patient's goal for pain management. • Monitor/document pain level using 0–5 pain scale or visual analog scale. 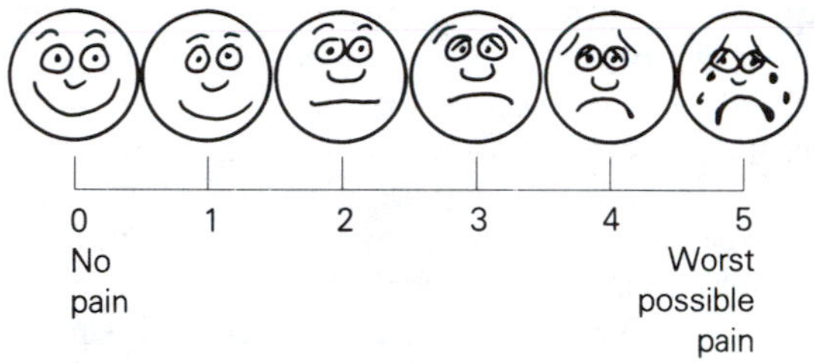 0 No pain — 1 — 2 — 3 — 4 — 5 Worst possible pain • Analgesic ladder I. *Mild pain:* Start with nonopioids (acetaminophen, aspirin, or NSAIDs), with or without adjuvant (see Table 56-4). II. *If pain persists:* Try weak opioid (codeine, oxycodone hydrocodone) with or without nonopioids, with or without adjuvant. III. *If pain still persists:* Try strong opioid, with or without nonopioid, with or without adjuvant.[6,7] • **Avoid:** –meperidine (Demerol)—very low oral potency; toxic metabolite accumulation –pentazocine (Talwin)—no more potent than codeine; high incidences of hallucinations and agitation (30% in cancer patients) –methadone (Dolophine)—extremely long half-life (48–72 hr); short duration of analgesia (6–8 hr); makes dose titration difficult in severely ill patients; however, may be the only affordable long-acting agent for your patient –IM/SC injections—morphine 30 mg PO is as potent as 10 mg IM/SQ; can avoid pain and expense of injections with PO or SC morphine

(continued)

TABLE 56-3 Selected Principles and Approaches for Symptom Management (continued)

Problem	Principles	Management Approaches

• **Commonly used drugs:** (Published tables vary in their suggested equianalgesic (equiv.) doses. Clinical response is the criterion that must be applied for each patient.)

Drugs	Oral (approx. equiv. dose, mg)	Parenteral (approx. equiv. dose, mg)	Dosing interval (hr)
Morphine	30	10	3–4
Hydromorphone (Dilaudid)	4–6	1.5–2	4
Levorphanol (Levo-Dromoran)	4	2	6–8
Codeine	130†	75	4–6
Fentanyl patch (Duragesic)	50 μg on skin	N/A	72
Methadone (Dolophine)	20	10	6–8
Meperidine* (Demerol)	150–250	75–100	2.5–3.5

*Avoid use for chronic pain.

†Codeine doses above 65 mg usually are inappropriate due to diminishing incremental analgesia.

Problem	Principles	Management Approaches
	• According to WHO, morphine is the drug of choice for severe cancer pain. There is no ceiling to effective narcotic dosage.[7] • If PO medications are not possible, narcotics can be given by buccal, sublingual, rectal, or subcutaneous routes without resorting to IV or IM administration. • Continuous subcutaneous infusions can be initiated at home with the help of home health or hospice nurses. • If central line access is *already* established, intravenous infusion may be the route of choice and usually can be initiated at home.	• Titrate dose as needed. • Utilize noninvasive comfort measures as appropriate, eg, applications of ice, heat, gentle massage, relaxation techniques. • See Chapter 23, "Pain," for specific guidelines. • Evaluate effectiveness of analgesia at regular intervals. Teach the patient and family about the medications and alternate measures.
Dyspnea	• Defined as unpleasant awareness of increased need to ventilate. • Avoid high-dose bronchodilators. • Theophylline toxicity is common as patients approach death. • Adrenergic agonists (metaproterenol, etc) may exacerbate anxiety more than they help with dyspnea.	• Oral morphine in low doses 5–10 mg every 4 hr. helps to decrease air hunger.[7] • Help patient decrease anxiety through use of an anxiolytic, eg, a benzodiazepine. • Position patient for maximum comfort by elevating head of bed. • Advise patient in methods to modify environment or activity to decrease physical exertion. • Oxygen may be effective but more expensive than oral narcotics.
Seizures	• Patients with *recent history* of seizures should receive therapeutic doses of phenytoin, phenobarbital, carbamazepine or valproic acid.	Options • If patient cannot swallow phenytoin: –midazolam—5–10 mg/day by sc infusion –phenobarbital—20–60 mg oral, sublingual BID –carbamazepine (Tegretol)—600 mg per rectum or SC BID-TID –valproic acid—250 mg QID per rectum • Instruct caregiver on seizure precautions. Protect patient from injury in event of seizure. Remove or pad objects near head of body. Instruct patient and family regarding needs for regular dosing and side effects of seizure medication.
Diarrhea	• Rule out fecal impaction, bowel obstruction, laxative overuse, and other drug side effects.[7]	• Maintain hydration according to patient's comfort level and tolerance of fluids. Bland low-residue diet. Protect skin with barrier cream. –Immodium—2–4 mg QID PRN –Lomotil—2.5–5 mg QID PRN –Metamucil—1–3 tsp BID[7]

(continued)

TABLE 56-3 Selected Principles and Approaches for Symptom Management (continued)

Problem	Principles	Management Approaches
Constipation	• Nearly all patients on narcotics require a maintenance laxative regimen to prevent constipation. • As the dose of narcotic is increased, the dose of laxative must be increased. • Patients who are not eating still may require laxatives as waste continues to be produced in the bowel in form of secretion, bacteria, and desquamation. • Avoid –bulk laxatives—difficult for anorexic patients to take, and cause impaction if fluid intake is inadequate; *not* effective unless a patient is active and eating –frequent enemas—useful for severe cases of constipation; however, oral medications are better tolerated for prophylaxis.	• "Ladder" of increasing potency of laxatives: a. Senokot-S or Pericolace—1–2 tabs at hs b. Senokot-S or Pericolace—2 tabs BID c. Senokot-S or Pericolace—3 tabs BID d. Lactulose—15cc BID e. Lactulose—30cc BID f. Lactulose—30cc TID-QID or along with b or c above. If a patient has not had a bowel movement in 24 hr, increase the laxative dose to the next higher level. If a patient has not had a bowel movement in 3 days, check for impaction and consider one of the following treatments once or twice daily until results are obtained: a. MOM 30cc at bedtime b. 2 bisacodyl suppositories c. lactulose or sorbitol 30cc q 1 hr until results

It is common, if not universal, for patients and families to respond initially to the idea of death at home with fear and anxiety. Many adults have never seen anyone die.[13] In a society in which death has been regarded as a medical problem requiring technologic support, hospitalization, and professional care, we have lost the basic idea of death as a natural life event.[2] Patients' overriding concerns about death at home often revolve around being a burden to their family.[1] Family caregivers are concerned about their emotional ability to cope with a home death and the potential effects on other family members, particularly when children are in the home. After someone has died at home, families initially may be concerned about being able to live in the home, sleep in a room, etc.[13]

For most families, the ability to provide care for a home death will require teaching them about the death event itself, immediate signs of death, how to relieve symptoms and suffering, and how to access professional help if needed. When given enough time to work with a patient and family, hospice care is ideally structured to provide this support, education, and preparation. It is most satisfying for hospice nurses to begin care with a family that expresses much anxiety about caring for a patient at home through the death event, and end with family members in bereavement who cannot say enough about what a wonderful experience it was for them. In her book *Dying at Home,* Andrea Sanker relates her experience with the home death of her mother: "Home death is a powerfully significant ex-

TABLE 56-4 Adjuvant Pain Therapy—Promote a Co-Analgesic

Pain Source	Pain Character	Drug Class	Examples
Bone or soft tissue	Tenderness over bone or joint; pain on movement	NSAID	Ibuprofen 400 mg q4hr
Nerve damage or dysaesthesia	"Burning" or "shooting" pain radiating from spinal root or plexis	Tricyclic Anticonvulsant	Amitriptyline (Elavil) 10—50 mg q hs Carbamazepine (Tegretol) 200 mg q 6–12hr
Smooth muscle spasms	Colic-cramping, abdominal pain, bladder spasms	Anticholinergic	Diclomine (Bentyl) 10 mg q 4–8hr Oxybutynin (Ditropan) 5–10 mg q 8hr
Anxiety	Generalized restlessness and discomfort	Antihistamine Benzodiazepine	Hydroxyzine (Atarax or Vistaril) 10–50 mg q 4hr Lorazepam (Ativan) 0.5–1 mg q 6hr
Intracranial pressure	Headache	Steroids	Dexamethasone (Decadron) 6–10 mg q 6hr

perience despite the strain, exhaustion, and conflict that sometimes accompanies it. Its power lies in the fact that in the face of certain death, the caregiver can give the person life—that is, the continuation of life as a social being."[13]

Advantages of Home Death

The approach of death evokes feelings of loss in a dying person.[14] Loss of control may be the most overwhelming and distressing feeling. This loss can be further intensified by hospitalization. Terminal care and death at home can afford the patient and family control over their own environment, as well as the comfort of being in the midst of familiar surroundings. The patient at home maintains the opportunity to interact with neighbors, children, and pets. If children are living in the same home as the dying person, there is often concern that this will be detrimental to them. However, the opposite is often true. Rather than being protected from the illness and death, children can benefit from being involved in very concrete ways to understand the dying process better and facilitate their own grief.[2,13]

Another major loss for patients is diminishment of their role as a contributing, social being. Individuals may have several roles that make up their identity. Loss of role in the workplace is one of the first major adaptations for a chronically or terminally ill person. However, being cared for at home can afford the opportunity for an alert patient to maintain his or her family role. When possible, this person will continue to be included in family events and in decision making as was previously the norm.[13]

A final and obvious advantage of home death is that it is much less likely that unwanted medical intervention will be ordered for a terminally ill person at home than for one in a hospital or nursing home setting. The greatest potential risk for a home patient to receive unwanted medical intervention arises if the Emergency Medical System (EMS) is accessed, since this can result in unplanned and unwanted resuscitation and, ultimately, ventilator care.

Disadvantages of Home Death

Caregivers, particularly those lacking social outlets or family support, may find the physical and emotional task of home care and home death too difficult. Home death must be prepared for within the context of a realistic plan of care.

A patient may be too acutely ill at the end of life to be comfortably cared for at home. For example, a patient with uncontrolled hemorrhage may require hospitalization. Lack of resources to provide adequate home care is another reason home death can prove too burdensome.

When hospice care is initiated, a psychosocial assessment is completed by interviewing the patient and family in the home environment. This assessment should address the emotional and physical health of the caregiver as well as the exploration of social and financial resources. Social resources include other family, friends, or neighbors willing to assume some of the patient care or other tasks. Financial resources include eligibility for the Medicare benefit or benefits available from commercial insurance plans. Often, life insurance policies can be cashed in *before* death for a terminally ill patient to assist with the cost of home care or other needs.

This information, together with the nursing assessment of the patient, provides the basis for planning care and determining patient/family needs. However, even an in-depth assessment by experienced staff may not provide a reliable predictor for whether a patient will remain home to die. Hospices have seen a wide spectrum of families, from those with every resource who at the last minute access the Emergency Medical System, to those with limited finances and inadequate coping histories that are able to provide good care at home through the death event. Therefore, the hospice team generally will present the option of hospice home care to every patient and family if a safe plan of care can be established. At the same time, hospice staff should also discuss any other options for care available (e.g., extended care facility). At each subsequent home visit, the hospice staff must reevaluate the patient/family situation and revise plans as necessary.

Preparation of the Patient and Family

Once home death has been established as a desired goal, an individualized home care plan is developed with the patient and family. They need to know specifically what the hospice team can and will provide. Friends and other resources are also identified. The patient's primary caregiver may need specific permission and encouragement to ask for help from these other resources. It is emphasized with the primary caregiver that when a person is terminally ill, friends and neighbors may have difficulty coping with their feelings. This may be due to their discomfort with knowing how to help. Many people are grateful to a patient or family caregiver who can give specific ideas and assign specific tasks, enabling them to respond in a concrete way that is helpful.

The primary caregiver is continually and carefully assessed as to what he or she wants to and is capable of doing for direct care. Support to the primary caregiver and other family members includes acknowledging how physically and emotionally exhausting caring for someone ill at home can be. There are times when caregivers also need permission to take a break and to delegate care. The most effective hospice worker facilitates a series of informed choices and, as much as possible, allows patients and families to make their own decisions.

Knowledge and preparation for the death event

Families need to be prepared for the actual time of the patient's death and the time immediately preceding it. The most difficult aspect of preparation is that each patient is an individual and each death occurs in a way that may not be totally predictable. However, there are some universal signs that families can anticipate and on which they can receive instruction. Table 56-5 is an example of a patient/family instruction sheet that lists many of the common signs seen in patients who are imminently dying. For family members who have cared for an ill person for a long time or are health care professionals themselves, it is important to emphasize that laboratory results and vital signs are unreliable indicators of the time of death.

Emotional care of the patient and family around the time of death occurs as the opportunity arises. The family is instructed to listen to the patient carefully, even if it appears that the patient is confused. Many times dying patients will speak in symbolic language.[15] A common example is a patient who talks about "going home." It may seem that the patient is confused if he or she already is home. Further conversation may indicate that "going home" refers to dying. It is not unusual for patients to report actually seeing or having conversations with a loved one who has died. Family members may be the most capable of interpreting some symbolic language for the patient. Patients may indicate when they feel they are ready to die. If this occurs, family members can be encouraged to allow the patient to "let go," that is, give the patient permission to die.[15] Although no one can be sure how much an individual has control over the time of his or her own death, having a family member tell the patient that it is all right to "let go" can add to the patient's peace of mind.[2]

Funeral arrangements

In most situations a home death will go more smoothly if the patient and/or family chooses a funeral home before the death occurs. Although it can be most helpful for complete funeral arrangements to be made prior to the death of the patient, family members may find this action premature. Beyond choosing a funeral home, no other arrangements need be made prior to death.

The hospice team should be a resource to families as to different types of funeral homes available in their area. Important factors that differentiate funeral homes are religious affiliation, financial considerations, and policies about home death. The hospice team can also be a resource for information on organ and body donation and on autopsy as it relates to home death. These procedures usually are compatible with home death, as long as the wishes of the patient and/or family are known in advance so arrangements can be made with the funeral home.

Availability of the Hospice Team

Of utmost importance in supporting families through a patient's home death is instructing them on how to access the hospice team at any time on any day as needed. Families should be encouraged to call about any changes in the patient's status or for what may seem like minor questions to them. For the hospice team, emotional

TABLE 56-5 Hospice Home Care Instruction Sheet: Signs and Symptoms of Approaching Death

The hospice team's goal is to help prepare you for some things that might occur close to the time of death. Although we can never predict exactly when a terminally ill person will die, we know when the time is getting close by a combination of signs and symptoms. Not all of these signs will appear at the same time, and some may never appear at all. All of the signs described are ways the body prepares itself for the final stages of life.

1. Your loved one may sleep more and might be more difficult to awaken. Hearing and vision may decrease.
   What to do: Plan your time and activities for times when he/she is more alert. Always talk as if the person can hear you, even if he/she appears to be in a coma. When providing care, explain what you are doing as you do it.
2. There may be a gradual decrease in need for food and drink. Your loved one will say he/she doesn't have an appetite, isn't hungry. This is the body's natural response to the dying process. It is telling the person that eating and drinking are no longer helpful—that the body can't use food and fluid properly anymore.
   What to do: Allow your loved one to choose when and what to eat or drink, even if this means little or nothing will be taken in. Liquids often are more easily tolerated than solid food.
3. Your loved one may become more confused or restless or experience visions of people and places.
   What to do: Remind him/her of the time and the day and who is there with them. Be calm and reassuring when talking to him/her.
4. Hands, arms, feet, and legs may become cooler, and the skin may turn a bluish color with purplish splotches.
   What to do: Use blankets for warmth. Do *not* use an electric blanket or heating pad.
5. Irregular breathing patterns may occur. There might be a space of time (10–30 seconds) when there will be no breathing at all. This is called *apnea.* There may be phlegm in the throat that is difficult to cough.
   What to do: Position the person on his/her side with head elevated.

Contact hospice team at any time for questions, or to discuss changes.

support to exhausted and anxious family members is just as important an intervention as a change in pain medication for the patient. Family members also need to be instructed to call the hospice immediately should a home death occur. The time of instruction regarding accessing the hospice team is also a good time to remind families not to call the emergency medical system, and to inform them of the possible consequences of such an action. This instruction often needs to be repeated because many people call 911 as a natural reaction to an "emergency."

Facilitating Grief

As family members prepare for the death of a loved one at home, they are also preparing themselves for the loss. We often refer to this as *anticipatory grief.*[16] Family members who can give a dying person permission to "let go" are at the same time letting go themselves. Part of the hospice team's care is assisting loved ones in this grief phase. First, it may be helpful to explore with family members previous losses and coping mechanisms used. The family is encouraged to identify and discuss unresolved issues with the dying person. This can be a time of opportunity to resolve certain issues, so that after death there are no regrets on the part of the family. Even when conflict does not exist, family members can say things to the dying person that they may not have said or feel that they have not said enough previously.[2] The dying person and family members can honor the meaning of their relationship and their life together.[1] Asking a couple how they met or going through a family photo album with them is a good way to facilitate grieving and therapeutic review of life. What follows is an example of one family's preparation for the death of their baby daughter and how it helped them work through their grief.

> Mr. and Mrs. S were referred to a hospice program by their daughter's pediatric oncologist when they were told there was no more treatment available for the 2-year-old's cancer. The hospice nurse and a hospice volunteer were able to establish a good rapport with the parents early. The parents were concerned that their daughter no longer suffer, and they wished to care for her at home as long as possible. The parents had support from grandparents, friends, neighbors, and their local minister, who visited them at home. The parents described feeling much strength and love from all this support, *until* the hospice nurse talked to them about choosing a funeral home. Mrs. S was devastated. "I was *so* angry with that nurse. I thought, 'How dare she talk about such a horrible thing?' My daughter was still alive, and I wanted her with us as long as possible. I was so angry I almost called the hospice and told them never to send anyone out to see us again."
>
> However, after a few days, Mr. and Mrs. S talked for the first time about the inevitable death of their child. Rehearsing it in her mind, Mrs. S began to think about how she might feel if a stranger (the funeral director) would come into their home and remove her baby. She wondered if there was any reason she and her husband could not take the body to the funeral home themselves when death occurred. Mrs. S researched this and discovered there was no law in her state that would preclude this action. Mrs. S eventually was able to talk to the hospice nurse about her idea. The nurse contacted several area funeral homes to discuss the situation and gave Mr. and Mrs. S the names of the ones that would comply with this arrangement. The baby lived for another 2 months before she died quietly at home in her mother's arms. Mrs. S later recalled: "The nurse was wonderful. She came out and helped us wash and dress the baby and wrap her in a blanket. She understood that we needed time to do this. Our daughter died without any tubes or shots and we were able to take her to the funeral home ourselves. I think we did the best for her that we could."

This family had the time needed to experience the death event on their own terms. Preparing family members for the death of their loved one often means discussing issues the nurse assesses they may not yet be ready to hear. As in this situation, the nurse was not sure how much time was left prior to death. Ultimately, the family was able to process their feelings and exert some choice and control in a very difficult situation.

BEREAVEMENT CARE

Bereavement support is a required component of hospice care under Medicare and most state licensing regulations.[9] However, the specific structure of an individual hospice's bereavement program is not well defined. Each program develops its own policies and mechanism for follow-up.

Grieving is a normal reaction to loss, with a wide variety of physical and emotional manifestations. Some of these are loss of appetite, sleeplessness, heart palpitations, lack of energy, sadness, and anger. J. William Worden[14] describes the following four tasks as necessary for the normal grief process to progress:

1. to accept the reality of the loss
2. to experience the pain of grief
3. to adjust to the environment in which the deceased is missing
4. to withdraw emotional energy, and replace it in another relationship

The goal of bereavement care or counseling is to assist and support survivors to move through the loss and towards resolution.[14,16] Hospice programs generally follow survivors for 1 year, although there is no mandated standard time for follow-up. This period should be understood as a period in which the most acute grief can occur, *not* for mourning to be completed; for grief resolution is a very individualized process that takes place gradually over time.

Methods of bereavement follow-up can vary, but generally include a bereavement assessment, contact of survivors at regularly scheduled intervals, and, as necessary, additional referrals for professional counseling for those with complicated or abnormal grief reactions. Bereavement support can also take the form of support groups, "socials" or "teas," classes on specific topics, and/or memorial services conducted by the hospice program.[2]

Abnormal Grief

Survivors unable to progress through the tasks of mourning will develop some form of abnormal or complicated grief.[14] Generally, complicated grief will manifest itself in one of three ways: First, the grief reaction may be prolonged. Second, the grief reaction may be masked in behavioral or physical symptoms, even such seemingly unrelated symptoms as pain, sexual impotence, and behavioral "acting out." Finally, abnormal grief may manifest itself in exaggerated or excessive expressions of normal grief reactions, such as excessive anger, sadness, or depression.[14] For most hospice programs, therapy for abnormal grief extends beyond the scope of the bereavement care services provided. However, the hospice program staff should be able to identify and recommend competent referrals for abnormal grief syndromes.

Unresolved grief has been associated with multiple physical and emotional illnesses, including increased risk of suicide.[14,16] Therefore, facilitation of anticipatory grieving and bereavement can be viewed as preventive health care for survivors. Collin Murray Parkes, psychiatrist and consultant to St. Christopher's Hospice, came to the following conclusion after a review of the literature on the effectiveness of grief counseling: "The evidence presented here suggests that professional services and professionally supported voluntary and self-help services are capable of reducing the risk of psychiatry and psychoanalytic disorders resulting from bereavement."[16]

STRESS AND THE HOSPICE NURSE

Providing compassionate care to the terminally ill and their loved ones can create unique stressors for the hospice team. Studies have shown that nurses and other hospice staff members tend to identify with younger patients, those under 40, and feel a greater sense of injustice when these patients die. Staff attitudes towards death can be greatly influenced by unresolved grief issues in their own personal or professional life. Stress can be increased due to unrealistic expectations of ourselves, our co-workers, or the therapy we use to manage symptoms. The inability to relieve totally such symptoms as intractable pain and nausea can evoke feelings of impotence or helplessness. Supportive interactions with patients and their families can be emotionally draining, especially when long-standing problems in their interpersonal relationships are involved.[11]

Caregivers with high-stress jobs who cope successfully are able to recognize when signs of stress are de-

TABLE 56-6 Useful Methods for Coping with Stress

- Take responsibility for caring for yourself. Allow at least 15–20 minutes each day for quiet introspection. Assess your body for signs of stress, for example, muscle tension, headaches, insomnia, G.I. distress, and frequent illness. The body systems showing stress should be the focus for rejuvenation. For example, muscle tension may indicate a need for relaxation therapy.[17]
- Reduce stress by prioritizing work. Make a conscious choice between those events worth your energy and those you need to delegate or otherwise not take on at all.
- Promote training and education not only for new staff but also for experienced team members. The continual development of our knowledge base promotes confidence. Special attention should be placed on identified stresses. If you are feeling overwhelmed, then dealing with family dynamics, reading, or attending a seminar on that subject could give you additional tools to improve future interactions.[17]
- Take time off! Whenever possible get out of town, away from reminders of work.
- Take time for your hobby. Creative self-expression through arts, crafts, or hobbies can provide an additional outlet for release of stress.
- Focus on maintaining a healthy body through regular exercise and eating a balanced diet. Leave the clinical setting during lunch, and go for a long walk or do something not work-related.
- Seek supportive interactions with individuals or in a group. Regular involvement with a support group can be helpful in providing an environment to share with others on the team who are under similar pressures. Such interactions serve to promote team building and problem identification. For a group to be successful, trust and an open, nurturing environment must be established. An experienced facilitator can be invaluable in attaining this goal. Group members make a contract with each other to be supportive and nonjudgmental and to keep all conversation in strict confidence.
- Give yourself permission to find the humor in certain situations that otherwise may be tragic or depressing. Share this humor with other members of the hospice team, being careful to keep it respectful of patient and families involved.
- Focus on the positive satisfying aspects of the role of hospice caregiver. Assisting a patient in the last few days of life can be very rewarding. Promoting comfort and quality-of-life issues involves nursing skills and principles of the highest order.

veloping within themselves, acknowledge their own limits, and initiate self-help techniques or seek the help of others. Several methods for coping with stress have been used successfully by hospice staff members (see Table 56-6).

LEGAL AND ETHICAL ISSUES SURROUNDING HOSPICE CARE

Due to the population characteristics and specialized nature of terminal care, hospice programs have been innovators in encouraging patients to identify their own goals, particularly goals related to cardiopulmonary resuscitation (CPR), invasive procedures, and identification of family or friends to assist in decision making if the patient becomes incapacitated. However, the hospice nurse and other members of the team are directly affected by recent legislative and court decisions that can either hinder or enhance the ability to assist the family in meeting those goals.

Advance Directives

The federal Patient Self-Determination Act enacted in December 1991 requires hospices, hospitals, and other health care agencies to provide patients, on admission, with written information about two key areas: (1) their right to accept or refuse treatment under state law and (2) ways to execute advance directives such as a living will and a durable power of attorney for health care.[18] The purpose of this legislation is to ensure that patients' wishes are carried out in the event they become mentally incapacitated or are incapable of making or communicating their decisions. As with all other health care organizations receiving federal funds, hospice programs are mandated to provide information to facilitate completion of a living will or a durable power of attorney for health care. The nurse provides whatever information is needed to assist the patient in making an informed decision, especially when it affects the patient's decision not to have CPR, intravenous fluids, or tube feedings.

Patients with malignancy, sepsis, pneumonia, renal failure, diabetes, or advanced age have a low chance of survival after CPR. An average of 4% of patients receiving CPR in a general acute care setting survive. For those who do survive, quality of life afterwards is compromised.[19] Hospice patients and families may need reassurance that their focus on comfort and quality of life is being reinforced by their decision not to have CPR. This same approach holds true when the decision not to have intravenous fluids or tube feedings is challenged. As death approaches, the patient may lose the ability to drink. Dehydration often occurs if death does not soon follow the inability to drink. However, fluid depletion has the following benign effects on quality of life:

- Urine output is decreased, so there is less incontinence.
- Gastric secretions lessen, therefore episodes of vomiting decrease.
- Pulmonary secretions lessen, resulting in less congestion.
- Peripheral edema secondary to tumor subsides, resulting in decreased pain from nerve compression.
- Although the sensation of dry mouth and thirst may increase, this can be relieved by good mouth care and small amounts of oral fluids.[20]

The U.S. Supreme Court's 1990 decision in the *Cruzon* case made it clear that life-and-death decisions depend on the availability of written evidence of the patient's wishes. Under the current Patient Self-Determination Act, individuals are not required to enact an advanced directive. However, failure to do so may compromise their ability later to limit aggressive medical treatment. In general, the power of attorney for health care is more useful than the living will. A living will may be applicable only when it pertains to a terminal illness but not for a patient whose health is declining for medical reasons other than those that can be classified as terminal or if the patient is in a permanent vegetative state. The living will does not identify another person who can act as the agent for a disabled patient.[18]

Through the power of attorney for health care, the patient chooses an agent to act on the patient's behalf if the patient is no longer competent to make decisions. This is especially important for individuals who have diagnoses such as AIDS, cancer metastases to the brain, or other medical problems where eventual confusion or other mental status changes are an expected complication of the disease. By electing to use a power of attorney, the patient is able to make a statement as to his or her wishes regarding: degree of removal of life support in the event of irreversible coma, use of artificial feeding if unable to swallow, and any limitation on the decision-making powers of the agent. A patient may also identify restrictions to care, such as those prohibiting blood transfusions for religious reasons.

The health care team caring for the patient in accordance with these documents usually is protected from liability if it follows the patients wishes. A copy of the living will or health care power of attorney needs to be placed in the patient's medical record.

Euthanasia and Suicide

The moral, ethical, and legal questions surrounding terminal illness and methods used to hasten death have their origins in ancient times. The English word *euthanasia* is taken from the Greek *euthanasias,* meaning "good or easy death." For the Greeks and other ancients, euthanasia did not necessarily denote an act or method of hastening death. It was important to the ancients that a person meet death voluntarily, with peace of mind and minimal suffering. This "good death" meant that the ill individual was meeting death in a condition of self-control. Towards this end, it was permissible to shorten a person's life intentionally.[21]

In modern times euthanasia has come to mean the intentional taking of the life of a terminally ill person for purposes of compassion. The modern concept is more accurately described as *active* euthanasia, for it is achieved by "doing something," such as giving the patient a lethal injection. *Passive* euthanasia can be described as "not doing something" that would preserve life, yet without being significantly burdensome.[21] Therefore, passive euthanasia has little bearing on our discussion of suicide and active euthanasia.

Suicide is derived from the Latin word for "self-kill." In many states suicide is not against the law; however, encouraging or aiding suicide is a criminal act. It is known that terminally ill patients contemplate suicide or consider being a voluntary subject of active euthanasia. The hospice nurse's appropriate first response to an expression of suicide is a listening and caring attitude to learn of the concerns that prompt such despair in a patient. For many, the fear of pain or suffering associated with dying or the burden it places on others can stimulate thoughts of ways to hasten death.[22] The focus of hospice is toward a natural death with a minimum of pain and a maximum of patient and family support. This is the hospice view of a "good death."

Euthanasia is quite different from refusing to receive medical treatment that will not contribute reasonably to improved quality of life and/or that proves to be gravely burdensome. Additionally, pain medication or other symptom management measures that are used in unusual quantity to improve comfort but could lead to an early death should not be considered euthanasia.[21] The operative concept is *intent.* If the intent is to relieve pain or manage symptoms and not to cause death, then the unintentional hastening of death is not euthanasia. Hospice philosophy does not promote involvement in either the act of suicide or euthanasia. Hospice promotes treatment for the cause of the despair and support during the process of dying.

FUTURE TRENDS AND CHALLENGES FOR HOSPICE CARE

Underserved Populations

African American and Hispanic populations historically have been underserved by health care agencies and hospice. The earliest hospices in Connecticut, California, New Jersey, and Arizona were founded by and served a predominantly middle-class, white population. The African American population is better served than Hispanics, but not in proportion to their cancer-related death rates. Both of these minority populations are underrepresented, or totally lacking, among hospice staff and volunteers, even in urban hospice programs.[23] The reasons for this are complex, but they include the fact that African American and Hispanic populations have less access to health care in general and are less likely to have medical insurance. Some religious beliefs and cultural values may also be a factor.[24]

Children represent another nationally underserved population. In the United States, only 14 of approximately 1700 hospice programs are dedicated to pediatric care. The 1990 NHO survey of hospice providers indicated that although most hospices will provide pediatric services, actual representation of children cared for by hospice was less than 1% of total patients served.[10] In the Chicago metropolitan area, which is served by more than 20 hospice programs and four large children's hospitals, there are no dedicated pediatric hospice services.

Patients with AIDS represent a tremendous challenge to hospice, on a number of levels. It is difficult to find a hospice program that will acknowledge denying services to those with an AIDS diagnosis. However, there remains the opinion among some in hospice leadership that AIDS does not "fit in" to current hospice practice. This is in spite of the evidence from the urban programs that successfully care for patients with AIDS, and from NHO support for AIDS care in hospice.[25]

AIDS patients utilize more resources than have been the norm for hospice patients. Their care is more complex and requires longer and more frequent nursing and social work visits. They require more attendant or custodial care due to the lack of primary caregivers and limited finances. The medications and supplies used are more varied and expensive.

With AIDS, a more flexible interpretation of symptom management and a creative approach to quality-of-life issues are needed. Hospice programs differ as to what constitutes palliative care for AIDS patients. Treatments for AIDS often are double edged—providing for comfort while also extending life. No accepted standards for AIDS care in hospice have been firmly established. The course of AIDS is less predictable than that of most cancers, making prognostication within the 6-month criterion difficult. The combined physical, psychosocial, spiritual, and financial needs of those with AIDS can greatly tax the hospice team. Hospices, because of their commitment to compassionate care to all with a terminal disease, have a moral and ethical obligation to provide care to those who request it.[26]

There are others who are considered "outliers" confronting hospice care. The Medicare Hospice Benefit was designed for the elderly cancer patient with an intact family available to provide most of the home care, supplemented by the support and resources of the hospice team.[2] For that population, hospice works well. However, we are rapidly facing an aging population with either no primary caregivers or immediate support persons too frail to provide care. The challenge for hospice is to broaden its scope to create effective care models for divergent populations. Residential and day care hospice components are two models currently being explored around the country.

Research Issues

Empirical research is still needed in all areas of hospice and palliative care. Research that exists focuses on pain and symptom management. Areas least studied are volunteerism and spiritual care, the features most unique to hospice.[27] Other palliative care research topics could include: suicidal ideation in the terminally ill, emotional factors hindering pain management, and long-term effectiveness of bereavement care. Both hospice models and hospice patient populations inherently make research difficult.[27] Limited funding and the relative lack of hospice and palliative care programs associated with academic institutions provide additional barriers to research.

Integration into Health Care Practices

For years, Dame Cicely Saunders has believed that rather than creating a segregated system for the dying, hospice principles should be diffused throughout the health care system.[2]

Hospice in the United States began as an anti–medical establishment and antiphysician movement. This antagonistic bias has unfortunately been a major factor preventing hospice and palliative care principles from being applied to terminally ill patients on a wider scale. Terminal care should be integrated into all health care practice, particularly in the areas of oncology, geriatrics, and AIDS. The JCAHO has already begun to foster such integration with the revision of its standards for 1992, which address needs of the dying patient under the Patient Rights section[5] (see Table 56-7). The federal Patient Self-Determination Act should also play a role in furthering the ability of patients to forego unwanted heroic treatment in the face of terminal illness.

In its short history, hospice has led the way on many health care trends, including case management, cost containment, home care utilization, and advance directives. Hospice now needs to integrate and adapt to the challenges facing our ever-changing health care system.

CONCLUSION

Hospice is a program that is coordinated by nurses and staffed by professionals and volunteers all striving to promote comfort and quality of life to those with a limited life span who wish such support. The thrust of this chapter has been to dispel the notion that hospice is a place for a dying person to spend their last hours without hope of enjoying life. The hope changes from that for a cure and a long life to hope for care and living for the moment. Death is no longer something

TABLE 56-7 JCAHO 1992 Standards: Patient Rights

Preamble

The organization respects the rights of the patient, recognizes that each patient is an individual with unique health care needs, and, because of the importance of respecting each patient's personal dignity, provides considerate, respectful care focused upon the patient's individual needs.
The organization affirms the patient's right to make decisions regarding his/her medical care, including the decision to discontinue treatment, to the extent permitted by law.
The organization assists the patient in the exercise of his/her rights and informs the patient of any responsibilities incumbent upon him/her in the exercise of those rights.

R1.1 The organization supports the rights of each patient.

R1.1.1 Organizational policies and procedures describe the mechanisms by which the following rights are protected and exercised:
- *R1.1.1.1* the right of the patient to the hospital's reasonable response to his/her requests and needs for treatment or service, within the hospital's capacity, its stated mission, and applicable law and regulation;
- *R1.1.1.2* the right of the patient to considerate and respectful care;
  - *R1.1.1.2.1* The care of the patient includes consideration of the psychosocial, spiritual, and cultural variables that influence the perceptions of illness.
  - *R1.1.1.2.2* The care of the dying patient optimizes the comfort and dignity of the patient through:
    - *R1.1.1.2.2.1* treating primary and secondary symptoms that respond to treatment as desired by the patient or surrogate decision maker;
    - *R1.1.1.2.2.2* effectively managing pain; and
    - *R1.1.1.2.2.3* acknowledging the psychosocial and spiritual concerns of the patient and the family regarding dying and the expression of grief by the patient and family.

Source: Excerpted from the *Accreditation Manual for Hospitals.* Oakbrook Terrace, IL: Joint Commission on Accreditation of Healthcare Organizations, 1992. Copyright 1991; reprinted with permission.

to be avoided at all costs; rather, it is something as natural as birth, a doorway out of the suffering of this world. Home, family, and friends are not left behind, but are included as an important part of the plan of care. It is a privilege for health care professionals to be involved with human beings during the end of their lives. We hear their stories about what life was like for them. We help them towards what they would like the natural end of life to be.

REFERENCES

1. Kübler-Ross E: *On Death and Dying.* New York: Macmillan, 1974.
2. Amenta MO, Bohnet NL: *Nursing Care of the Terminally Ill.* Boston: Little, Brown, 1986.
3. Paradis LF: *Hospice Handbook.* Rockville, MD: Aspen, 1985.
4. Joint Commission on Accreditation of Hospitals: Chicago: The Commission, 1986.
5. Joint Commission on Accreditation of Healthcare Organizations: *Accreditation Manual for Hospitals.* Oakbrook Terrace, IL: The Commission, 1992, pp. 103–105.
6. Kaye P: *Notes on Symptom Control.* Essex, Eng.: Hospice Education Institute, 1991.
7. Johanson G: *Symptom Relief in Terminal Care* (ed. 3). Santa Rosa, CA: Home Hospice of Sonoma County, 1988, pp. 18.1–18.4
8. Kerr D: A bedside fan for terminal dyspnea. *Am J Hospice Care* 6:23, 1989.
9. *Hospice Surveyor Operation Manual.* Washington, DC: Hospice Association of America, 1989.
10. National Hospice Organization: 1990 hospice statistics. *NHO Newsline* 1, 1991.
11. Alexander D, Ritchie E: Stressors and difficulties in dealing with the terminal patient. *J of Palliative Care* 6:28–33, 1990.
12. Vincent PA: Do hospice nurses differ from non-hospice nurses? *Am J Hospice Care* 3:41–42, 1986.
13. Sankar A: *Dying at Home.* Baltimore: John Hopkins Publ., 1991, pp. 1–15.
14. Worden JW: *Grief Counseling and Grief Therapy.* New York: Springer, 1982.
15. Pflaum MC, Kelley P: Understanding the final messages of the dying. *Nursing '86* 16(6):26–29, 1986.
16. Parkes CM, Weiss RS: *Recovery from Bereavement.* New York: Basic Books, 1983.
17. Daleo RE: Nursing aspects taking care of the caregivers. *Am J Hospice Care* 4:33–38, 1986.
18. Wadill G: Advanced directives. *Hospice* 2:10–11, 1991.
19. VonGunten C: CPR in hospitalized patients. When is it futile? *Am Fam Phys* 4:2130–2134, 1991.
20. Musgrave C: Terminal dehydration. *Cancer Nurs* 13:62–66, 1990.
21. O'Connell L: *Active Euthanasia, Religion and the Public Debate.* Chicago: Park Ridge Center Publ., 1991, pp. 18–22.
22. Kliban M: Suicide and the hospice patient. *Am J Hospice Care* 4:15–21, 1987.
23. Machuca M: Marketing and minorities: Hospice in the Hispanic community. *Am J Hospice and Palliative Care* 7:21–22, 1990.
24. Gorden AK: Hospice and minorities: A national study. Unpublished doctoral thesis. University of Illinois, 1992.
25. Beresford L: The challenge of AIDS. *Calif Hospice Report* 7:3–5, 1989.
26. Amento MO, Tahan CB: AIDS and the hospice community. *Hospice Journal* 7:1–2, 1991.
27. Dush D: Trends in hospice research and psychosocial palliative care. *Hospice Journal* 4:13–27, 1988.

PART VIII

Professional Issues for the Cancer Nurse

Chapter 57

Quality of Care

Diane Scott Dorsett, RN, PhD, FAAN

CONCEPTUAL FOUNDATIONS OF QUALITY CARE

Historical Context and Origins

Well over a century ago, Nightingale[1] said that the prime objective in nursing was "to put the patient(s) in the best condition for nature to act." Since then, both conceptually and operationally, care has become the essence of nursing. Over the past 15 years, a science of caring has emerged as a discrete theme in the nursing literature,[2–6] but only recently has care been accorded the importance recognized by Nightingale so long ago.

The relevance of care to society's health is becoming increasingly evident as demographic trends, such as an expanding elderly population, accelerate the incidence of chronic disease and as an increasingly advanced treatment technology extends life. Cure, once an important concept in the history of illness, when disease was primarily acute and infectious, has been replaced by the notion of prolonged remission with maximal quality of life. As modern science ushers in a biologic wave of modalities influencing prevention, detection, and treatment, clinical health care providers will continue to face the reality of increasingly rigorous treatments and more critically acute, morbid episodes superimposed on the chronic illness itself. Thus, as Benner[2] eloquently states, "In health care, caring sets up the possibility for cure."

As physicians attempt to master the rapidly changing complexities of cancer treatment in an increasing number of sicker patients, nursing care becomes a central issue. Quality of care is challenged by a health care system that contracts hospital stay time and health care cost coverage and by a health care environment in which large segments of the most vulnerable members of society (nonwhite, poor, less educated), who have greater than average health care needs, also have less than equal access to health care. Furthermore, those disadvantaged who do gain access often receive health care of lower quality—especially when measured in terms of appropriateness, timeliness, comprehensiveness, and continuity.[7] Documented in a publication of the President's Commission for the Study of Ethical Problems in Medicine and Biomedical and Behavioral Research, *Securing Access to Health Care,*[8] cancers of white Americans are detected earlier than those of nonwhites, and those of paying patients are found earlier than those of nonpaying ones.

Although the reasons for these trends are complexly interwoven into the social, political, and economic fabric of American society, the outcome places a heavy burden not only on the underserved population but on all other segments of the society as well. Given today's challenges of specialization, complex technology, patterns of chronic illness, and restrictive health care environment, the quality care of cancer patients and their families demands an interdisciplinary team approach and the extension of the role of nursing in its total management.

By the end of 1988, the Oncology Nursing Society had revised and expanded its scope-of-practice statement on the basis of a philosophic recognition that persons with cancer and their families need to be fully informed and to participate actively in their care and treatment and, further, that competent, humane care demands a complementary team of specialty practitioners who communicate with one another and augment one another's efforts. Increasingly, the notion of the patient as the owner-manager of his or her total health, with the need for a head coach and a qualified, well-coordinated health care team, has been gaining acceptance.[9]

Recognizing the emerging health care system as possessing an ever-expanding place for the nurse as direct caregiver, educator, administrator, and researcher, the Oncology Nursing Society statement emphasized the importance of the oncology nurse as a *coordinator* of care, collaborating with other health care team members to make the best use of resources available to patients and families and, as their *advocate,* assessing and communicating the uniqueness of each patient's response to cancer, thereby promoting maximum independence and autonomy. In short, oncology nurses, by virtue of their knowledge, skills, and holistic (biopsychosocial) perspective of persons with cancer, are often viewed as the most qualified practitioners to assume the head coach role.

Care and caring

To care is to respond to another in need because of pain, illness, or distress. Caring involves a sense of commitment and responsibility and, when taken to higher levels, can be considered a body of knowledge and skill known tacitly, empirically, or scientifically to accomplish change for the good. Although caring behavior is central to most public and private human activity, when defined for nursing, caring becomes a set of meaning-laden actions.[2,10] To wit, early in the education of most nursing students, Virginia Henderson's classic definition of nursing is introduced:

> Nursing is primarily assisting individuals (sick or well) with those activities contributing to health, or its recovery (or to a peaceful death) that they perform unaided when they have the necessary strength, will or knowledge; nursing also helps individuals carry out prescribed therapy and be independent of assistance as soon as possible.[11]

The definition of nursing as a profession, a discipline, and a practice, through such theaters of relevance, becomes public domain through the Nurse Practice Act. Nurse practice acts are state determined but are remarkably similar in wording throughout the country. Most legislate nursing as the diagnosis and treatment of human responses in health and illness—a broad definition, further operationalized in the interest of public safety by a regulated and standardized system of education, registration, certification, standards of practice, and quality assurance.

Following the broad, formative brushstrokes of Nightingale,[1] who recognized "the fundamental needs of the sick and principles of good care," a concise, comprehensive definition of nursing by Harmer and Henderson,[11] and the more recent revisions that modernized nurse practice acts in this country, nursing began the establishment of a taxonomy of nursing diagnoses.[12–14] Nursing diagnoses operationalize the nurse practice act terminology, "human responses to an actual or potential health problem."[15]

Diagnostic taxonomies generally allow for a clear definition of professional purpose and for faster communication among the practitioners of a discipline, and they become the basis for a profession's research and development activity. As Herberth and Gosnell[13] advise, the next step is the integration of standards of practice and nursing diagnoses (Table 57-1) to foster relevant research, promote therapeutic interventions, and, ultimately, advance the quality of care.

TABLE 57-1 Functional Health Pattern Categories and Nursing Diagnoses

Health perception—health management pattern
Health maintenance alteration
Health management deficit (total)
Health management deficit (specify)
Health seeking behavior
Noncompliance (specify)
Potential noncompliance (specify)
Potential for infection
Potential for physical injury
Potential for poisoning
Potential for suffocation

Nutritional-metabolic pattern
Alteration in nutrition: potential for more than body requirements or potential obesity
Alteration in nutrition: more than body requirements or exogenous obesity
Alteration in nutrition: less than body requirements or nutritional deficit (specify)
Ineffective breast feeding
Impaired swallowing
Potential for aspiration
Alterations in oral mucous membranes
Potential fluid volume deficit
Fluid volume deficit (actual) (1)
Fluid volume deficit (actual) (2)
Fluid volume excess
Potential or actual impairment of skin integrity or skin breakdown
Decubitus ulcer (specify stage)
Impaired skin or tissue integrity
Altered body temperature
Ineffective thermoregulation
Hyperthermia
Hypothermia

Elimination pattern
Alteration in bowel elimination: constipation or intermittent constipation pattern
Alteration in bowel elimination: diarrhea
Alteration in bowel elimination: incontinence or bowel incontinence
Altered urinary elimination pattern
Urinary incontinence: functional, stress, urge or total
Stress incontinence
Urinary retention

Activity-exercise pattern
Potential activity intolerance
Activity intolerance (specify level)
Fatigue
Impaired physical mobility (specify level)
Potential for disuse syndrome
Total self-care deficit (specify level)
Self-bathing—hygiene deficit (specify level)
Self-dressing—grooming deficit (specify level)
Self-feeding deficit (specify level)
Self-toileting deficit (specify level)
Self-care skills deficit
Diversional activity deficit
Impaired home maintenance management (mild, moderate, severe, potential, chronic)
Potential joint contractures
Ineffective airway clearance
Ineffective breathing pattern
Impaired gas exchange
Decreased cardiac output
Altered tissue perfusion
Dysreflexia
Altered growth and development

Sleep-rest pattern
Sleep-pattern disturbance

Cognitive-perceptual pattern
Pain
Chronic pain
Pain self-management deficit
Uncompensated sensory deficit (specify)
Sensory-perceptual alterations: input deficit or sensory deprivation
Sensory-perceptual alterations: input excess or sensory overload
Unilateral neglect
Knowledge deficit (specify)
Uncompensated short-term memory deficit
Potential cognitive impairment
Impairment of thought processes
Decisional conflict (specify)
Altered parenting
Parental role conflict
Impaired verbal communication
Altered growth and development: communication skills
Potential for violence

(continued)

TABLE 57-1 Functional Health Pattern Categories and Nursing Diagnoses (continued)

Self-perception—self-concept pattern	**Sexuality-reproductive pattern**
Fear (specify focus)	Sexual dysfunction
Anticipatory anxiety (mild, moderate, severe)	Altered sexuality patterns
Anxiety	Rape trauma syndrome
Mild anxiety	Rape trauma syndrome: compound reaction
Moderate anxiety	Rape trauma syndrome: silent reaction
Severe anxiety (panic)	**Coping—stress tolerance pattern**
Reactive depression (situational)	Coping, ineffective (individual)
Hopelessness	Avoidance coping
Powerlessness (severe, low, moderate)	Defensive coping
Self-esteem disturbance	Ineffective denial
Body image disturbance	Impaired adjustment
Personal identity confusion	Posttrauma response
Role-relationship pattern	Family coping: potential for growth
Anticipatory grieving	Ineffective family coping: compromised
Dysfunctional grieving	Ineffective family coping: disabling
Disturbance in role performance	**Value-belief pattern**
Unresolved independence-dependence conflict	Spiritual distress (distress of human spirit)
Social isolation	
Social isolation (rejection)	
Impaired social interaction	
Altered growth and development: social skills (specify)	
Translocation syndrome	
Altered family process	
Weak mother-infant attachment or parent-infant attachment	
Potential altered parenting	

Source: Reproduced by permission from Gordon M: *Manual of Nursing Diagnosis 1988–1989*. St. Louis, MO: Mosby.

Caring actions cannot be separated from intent, however, if the outcome is to be effective. It is not enough to practice according to a guiding set of rules and regulations. To achieve even an acceptable level of quality of care, one must have commitment, creativity, and a willingness to innovate at reasonable risk. Knowing one's craft well is not enough. Caring requires knowing our patients and their beliefs, values, and cultural norms and tailoring care accordingly. Thus understanding and defining quality of care in terms of practices that enable health promotion and recovery from illness requires that caring be intrinsic to the process. Leininger[5] defined caring as behavioral attributes characterized by empathy, support, compassion, protection, succor, and education, firmly grounded in a comprehension of the needs, problems, values, and goals of the person or group being assisted.

Quality

The nature of quality is multifaceted and difficult to define, especially in relation to nursing care. Yet quality has emerged as the most important issue in patient care services in the final two decades of the twentieth century. The 1980s witnessed an integration of quality management, control, and assurance in nursing practice. To some observers, this integration has changed practice habits and promoted the individuation of care in innovative ways. These new ways of practice have led to the development of standards of care as the basic unit of analysis in the evaluation of quality in practice.[16]

Quality has become the focus of all cancer service provider groups, including the Commission on Cancer of the American College of Surgeons, the National Cancer Institute, the American Cancer Society, the College of American Pathology, the American College of Radiology, and, in joint affiliation, the American Nurses' Association and the Oncology Nursing Society.[17] Quality was, as Beyers[16] stated, "the banner of the 1980s" and will be the established base for the next major advance in clinical nursing during the 1990s and beyond.

Quality, by definition, is a set of properties, attributes, and capacities that are essential and unique to the focus of evaluation, be it nursing or a work of art. In a generic sense, quality connotes a degree of excellence as measured by recognized standards. Standards are characterized by utility, durability, stability, flexibility, and aesthetics and, in the health care environment, require the definition of correlates related to both clinical and organizational qualities. Beyers[16] defines these correlates of quality as cost, productivity, and risk.

Historically, approaches to quality management in the United States have gone through several "eras," from inspection and statistical accounting measures (time and motion studies), to quality assurance processes and procedures (chart audit), to the newest era of "strategic quality management."[18] Strategic quality management is based on the realities of market share and fiscal viability since health care is big business and the driving force has become patient satisfaction. The "new" approach to quality recognizes four important factors: (1) recognition of consumer need and response, (2) integrated service teams, (3) standards of practice, organization, and professional performance, and (4) data management systems that document structure, process, and outcome elements.[16]

Beyers[16] views these factors as interactive and as having the potential for a positive effect. When patient needs are understood, recognized, and met by a well-coordinated team of clinicians who are guided by high standards, the associated documentation will allow clinical outcomes to be "known," ultimately modifying patient response for the better.

Thus quality embraces the dimensions of structure (patient and environment norms), process (strategies of quality management), and outcome (documentation of clinical outcomes and patient satisfaction). For many experts, quality is driven by the profit motive. For nursing, quality must be powered both by its value as a public service and by the caring ethic for maximal effect.

The concept of quality of care is grounded in the integration of a sound body of knowledge and skill, standards of practice and performance that promote excellence, a coordinated team approach, and a built-in capacity for innovation (research), with all components fired by a deep sense of caring.

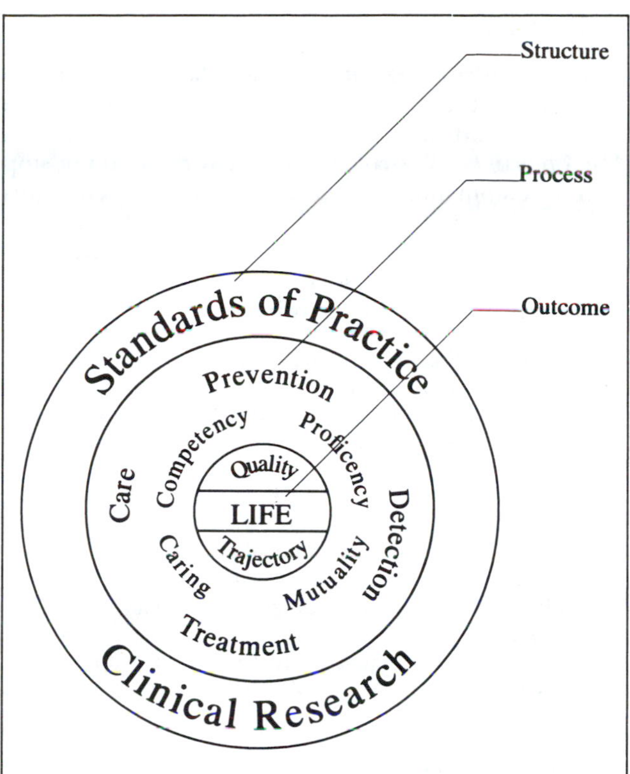

FIGURE 57-1 This model represents the major goals in cancer care and those structural factors that ensure quality of care in terms of process and outcome.

Quality of Care Model

A model of quality of care (Figure 57-1) has been designed to represent the major goals in cancer care and treatment and those structural factors that ensure quality in terms of process and outcomes.

Structure

In the 1980s, several critical components were set in place that allowed for a guiding definition of quality in cancer care. These structural elements include overall *standards for oncology nursing practice and for the professional performance of the nurse* who cares for patients with cancer and their families. These standards currently are undergoing integration with the classification of nursing diagnoses and further categorization into Gordon's 11 functional health pattern categories.[14] Another major structure that promotes quality of care is clinical research and the development of nursing technology to test and improve interventions and maximize positive results. Nursing research in cancer care can be built into every patient care environment on some level. For some, this might mean keeping up with the nursing research literature or participating in a journal club, or it might involve undertaking a small study of one's own or participating in a larger multisite research project. Research allows for the development of nursing technology as well: Audiovisual patient teaching programs, drug dispensers that allow for safer self-administration of the many medications that cancer patients take at home, or measures that aid mobility, protect the skin and mucous membrane, or improve ventilation are examples of methods that achieve practical purposes toward the improvement or refinement of care. As these innovations are developed, they need to be tested and the results shared with others.

Process

The second dimension of the quality of care model is represented by the process variables of cancer prevention, detection, treatment, and nursing care. This dimension brings together the nursing care–medical treatment complex because the components of this complex are mutually dependent in achieving the desired outcome. More often than not, nursing care revolves around medical treatment but, in the best sense, extends itself beyond the immediate goals of interest to the physician. Cell kill and reduced tumor size are important, but without attention to management of side effects and promotion of functional recovery, the effect is diminished at best and ineffective at worst. In this sense, cure and care are not dichotomous. Care augments and enhances cure and in the process humanizes the total outcome.

Outcome

On a structural bed of sound standards and research innovation, the processes of prevention, detection, treatment, and care lead to patient outcome variables. The objectives of oncology care providers do not stop with the elimination of disease. Given the current status of cancer treatment, with a documented 50% cure rate in all patients with a diagnosis of cancer,[19,20] Paul Marks, president of Memorial Sloan-Kettering Cancer Center, placed the current climate in perspective:

> The implication of this [sic, cancer biologic revolution] massive research effort is not that cancer will fade away in the next few years, or even decades. The discovery of oncogenes suggests that cancer may be an integral part of living, the result of interaction of our genes with the environment. Certainly, an understanding of the fundamental nature of carcinogenesis will transform the nature of clinical care. But it will not yield a magic bullet to cure the disease, nor a vaccine to prevent it. Cancer will not be eradicated like smallpox or polio. Rather, what seems likely to emerge are new approaches to early diagnosis of cancers and new techniques to treat them, providing steady gains in our ability to cure and, more important, to prevent cancer.[20]

The bottom-line results of 30 years of massive biomedical scientific effort has been an extension of life for many patients with a diagnosis of cancer. Paralleling the work on this frontier, the biopsychosocial scientific effort in nursing has promoted advances in the quality of the lives that medical science has extended. The amalgamation of life extension and quality of life makes clear the ultimate and optimal outcome of cancer care: maximal quality of life for cancer patients and their families.

Standards of Care

Nursing, as a science of caring, is based on a theoretical foundation for practice, continuously tested, refined, and verified by research, and a clearly articulated set of principles guiding that practice. Central to the concept of quality care is a set of standards that exists to guide practice by operationalizing its essence.

The publication of *Outcome Standards for Cancer Nursing Practice*[21] in 1979 and of its integration into the *Standards of Oncology Nursing Practice*[22] in 1987 were joint ventures of the Oncology Nursing Society (ONS) and the American Nurses' Association (ANA). Although the revision, *Standards of Oncology Nursing Practice*,[22] is rooted in the ANA published standards of nursing practice,[23] the former is a separate statement developed in recognition of cancer as a major health problem and of the importance of oncology nursing as a specialty practice devoted to the care of cancer patients and their families.

There are 11 Standards of Oncology Nursing Practice,[22] 6 that address professional practice and 5 that concern professional performance (Table 57-2). Practice standards focus on the process involved in patient care (theory, data collection, diagnosis, planning, intervention, and evaluation), with emphasis on 11 commonly occurring problem areas. Performance standards, in contrast, are criteria for professional development, interdisciplinary collaboration, quality assurance, ethics, and research in nursing as a discipline. To com-

TABLE 57-2 Standards of Oncology Nursing Practice

Standards of Professional Practice

I. *Theory:* The oncology nurse applies theoretical concepts as a basis for decisions in practice.

II. *Data collection:* The oncology nurse systematically and continually collects data regarding the health status of the client. The data are recorded, accessible, and communicated to appropriate members of the interdisciplinary team.

III. *Nursing diagnosis:* The oncology nurse analyzes assessment data to formulate nursing diagnoses.

IV. *Planning:* The oncology nurse develops an outcome-oriented care plan that is individualized and holistic. This plan is based on nursing diagnoses and incorporates preventive, therapeutic, rehabilitative, palliative, and comforting nursing actions.

V. *Intervention:* The oncology nurse implements the nursing care plan to achieve the identified outcomes for the client.

VI. *Evaluation:* The oncology nurse regularly and systematically evaluates the client's responses to interventions in order to determine progress toward achievement of outcomes and to revise the data base, nursing diagnoses, and the plan of care.

Standards of Professional Performance

VII. *Professional development:* The oncology nurse assumes responsibility for professional development and continuing education and contributes to the professional growth of others.

VIII. *Multidisciplinary collaboration:* The oncology nurse collaborates with the multidisciplinary team in assessing, planning, implementing, and evaluating care.

IX. *Quality assurance:* The oncology nurse participates in peer review and interdisciplinary program evaluation to assure that high-quality nursing care is provided to clients.

X. *Ethics:* The oncology nurse uses the *Code for Nurses** and *A Patient's Bill of Rights*† to guide ethical decision making in practice.

XI. *Research:* The oncology nurse contributes to the scientific base of nursing practice and the field of oncology through the review and application of research.

*American Nurses' Association: *Code for Nurses with Interpretive Statements.* Kansas City, MO: The Association, 1985.

†American Hospital Association: *A Patient's Bill of Rights.* Chicago: The Association, 1972.

Source: Reprinted with permission from *Standards of Oncology Nursing Practice,* © 1987, American Nurses' Association, Kansas City, MO.

plement practice standards, ONS published *Outcome Standards for Cancer Nursing Education,*[24] *Cancer Patient Education,*[25] *and Public Cancer Education.*[26] A summation of the oncology nursing practice standards follows.

Standards of oncology nursing practice

I. The central core of oncology nursing is a logically articulated theoretical framework derived from the biologic, social, behavioral, and physical sciences. There are at least a dozen major nursing theories that have been constructed to guide practice, but two of the most frequently used in oncology nursing are Orem's self-care deficit theory[27] and the Johnson behavioral system model.[28] With a sound theoretical base, the nursing process is firmly grounded in established knowledge that can be constantly tested, evaluated, modified, and shared with colleagues.

II. Effective communication, assessment, and analytic skills are necessary to enable the oncology nurse to plan appropriate interventions for clients. The result is a sound database, available to the multidisciplinary team, that is maintained to reflect the most current and accurate clinical status of the patient.

III. The ability to make nursing diagnoses from the theoretical framework and the patient's database is essential to the plan of care. The diagnoses may emerge from actual or potential problems in 11 parameters: (1) prevention-detection, (2) information, (3) coping, (4) comfort, (5) nutrition, (6) protective mechanisms, (7) mobility, (8) elimination, (9) sexuality, (10) ventilation, and (11) circulation. Nursing diagnoses enable nurses to document problems and risks, planning, evaluation, and ultimately the research in care and collegial sharing that fosters continuity of care.

IV. Planning care is the first step in actively ensuring quality of care. During the planning process, goals are established and methods addressing the 11 parameters are decided.

V. The implementation of the plan uses independently and interdependently determined actions to achieve its goals. In most cases, however, the nurse should function autonomously but collaboratively with others. Intervention should be flexible and documented and should provide measurable evidence of effect in light of the plan.

VI. Finally, the evaluation of the plan and its outcomes allows for continuous update, revision, improvement, and refinements in the database and diagnoses and for resulting modifications in intervention. This evaluation is done in collaboration with the patient and family and the health care team, is fully documented, and ultimately leads to scholarly, scientific analysis through research.

Standards of professional performance

VII. The first standard for professional performance makes clear (1) that the nurse is accountable for keeping abreast of advances in the field, maintaining current knowledge and skill, and incorporating them into practice and (2) that there is a commitment to the betterment of self, patients, colleagues, and the profession.

VIII. The complexity of cancer care today requires a multidisciplinary approach. Learning how to communicate effectively and to collaborate with team members is another indicator of professional development. There is considerable latitude in this standard in that the nurse may function effectively as participant, coordinator, and leader.

IX. Peer review and program evaluation have become mandated mechanisms in today's health care structure. Actively participating with an open, inquiring, and creative mind maximizes the possibility of quality improvement on individual, unit, and organizational levels.

X. The cancer care experience provides ample opportunity for ethical judgments. The rationale for the ethics standard spells out the profound ethical concerns in oncology nursing: right of self-determination, surrogate decision making, informed consent, treatment options, nontraditional treatment modalities, decisions about quality of life, confidentiality, distribution of resources, and matters of economics and value. Involvement with these issues can be demanding and challenging as well as stressful and exhausting. Continuing education and peer support are important vehicles for professional growth in this area.

XI. The 1970s and 1980s ushered in a new era of research-based practice in nursing. Oncology nursing practice must be kept therapeutically effective through research. The latitude in this performance standard is substantial. Minimally, the practitioner should keep abreast of research-based studies published in the most relevant specialty journals and incorporate findings into practice. Through expanded education, the nurse might ultimately become the principal investigator of his or her own study and might cultivate a scholarly interest in research that becomes a lifelong pursuit and vehicle for the enhancement of quality care.

The most recent (1987) revisions of the *Standards of Oncology Nursing Practice* incorporated the separately published *Outcome Standards for Cancer Nursing Practice* published in 1979. The original outcome standards reflected ten high-incidence problem areas (Table 57-3) common to cancer as a major chronic disease with "intermittent acute episodes." When integrated with the 1987 revised practice standards concerned with data collection (II), nursing diagnoses (III), planning (IV), and evaluation (VI), the outcome assumes a patient-family-community focus, cuts across all phases of the cancer experience from prediagnosis to death, and recognizes the multiplicity of settings where patients are cared for today. These ten high-incidence areas provide an essential link between the operating practice standard and quality assurance.

TABLE 57-3 High-Incidence Problems in Cancer Nursing Practice

I.	*Prevention and early detection:* Client and family possess adequate information about cancer prevention and detection.
II.	*Information:* Client and family possess knowledge about disease and therapy in order to attain self-management, participate in therapy, optimal living and peaceful death.
III.	*Coping:* Client and family manage stress optimally according to their individual capacity and in accord with their value system.
IV.	*Comfort:* Client and family manage factors that influence comfort.
V.	*Nutrition:* Client and family manage nutrition and hydration optimally.
VI.	*Protective mechanisms:* Client and family possess knowledge to prevent or manage alterations in protective mechanisms.
VII.	*Mobility:* Client and family maintain optimal mobility.
VIII.	*Elimination:* Client and family manage problems with elimination.
IX.	*Sexuality:* Client and partner can manage threats to sexual function and satisfaction and maintain their sexual identity.
X.	*Ventilation:* Client and family can anticipate factors that impair ventilatory function and maintain optimal ventilatory capacity.

Source: Adapted from Oncology Nursing Society: *Outcome Standards for Cancer Nursing Practice.* Pittsburgh, PA: The Society, 1979.

RESEARCH AND EVALUATION IN QUALITY OF CARE

Background and Context

Research-based clinical practice and quality care are the hallmarks of professional nursing. These important processes are based on a theoretical body of knowledge, standards for practice, and valid and reliable measurements that allow for the evaluation of care and the expansion of the scientific foundation of practice.

The nursing literature of the 1970s saw a significant expansion in standardized approaches to measuring the quality of nursing care. As early as 1966, Donabedian[29] identified structure, process, and outcome variables in medicine as the three classic approaches to patient care evaluation.

One of the earliest studies of quality in nursing additionally tested the research tool "Patient Indicators of Nursing Care."[30] Seven physiologic indicators reflecting nursing care–related complications were assessed. This study was a prototype of today's research evaluating patient outcome standards and nursing diagnosis–specific interventions. Majesky et al.[30] chose three broad functional categories from Dorothy Johnson's theoretical framework—infection, immobility, and fluid imbalance—and operationalized them using 27 measurable indicators. The overall goal was to establish a reliable, valid, easy-to-use, clinically useful instrument to evaluate quality of nursing care.

Oncology nursing literature came of age with the beginning publication of two journals, *Cancer Nursing* and *Oncology Nursing Forum.* In a review[31] of research-based articles published in these journals through 1984, a total of 15 were found to evaluate nursing care programs. All interventions tested were educative or of a supportive, counseling nature, perhaps reflecting Herberth and Gosnell's finding[13] that over 40% of diagnoses involve knowledge deficit. Most of the studies did not allow for control group comparisons. Nine articles described tools designed to evaluate patient outcomes. Rarely was care measured directly, and most measures were constructed by the investigator because of the lack of sound instrumentation at that time. Few were tested for accuracy or consistency.

A distinct shift in the cancer nursing literature, noted from 1985 onward, seemed to coincide with the establishment of oncology nursing standards and their clinically useful format (patient outcome standards and functional health classification). Clearly, more authors attempted schema that integrated patients' clinical problems and deficits, nursing diagnoses, assessment parameters, causes, and interventions into plans for care that provided a useful guide for the practicing nurse and a methodical approach for quality assurance programs.

The following review of methods for measuring quality of cancer nursing care recognizes the seminal work of early researchers[32–36] but concentrates on studies published in the cancer nursing literature since 1985 that reflect more recent trends in the field (i.e., standards, nursing diagnoses, quality assurance, and measurement methods).

Approaches to Measuring Quality of Care

There are three major approaches to measuring quality of care: (1) quality assurance programs, (2) clinical research that includes both program evaluation and experimental studies of interventions, and (3) measurement tool or instrument development that includes the construction of quantitative scales, questionnaires, and inventories and qualitative measures that include the establishment of clinical indicators, predictors, and guidelines for assessment.

Quality assurance

The Joint Commission on Accreditation of Health Care Organizations publishes standards used in the accreditation of hospitals and five other types of health care organizations (long-term care, psychiatric care, ambulatory health care, hospice care, and home care organizations) in this country.[37] These standards are concerned with the structures, processes, and outcomes of patient care activities in all services provided by the organization, including nursing services. There are eight standards that address the provision, management, and monitoring of nursing services regardless of location or institutional type. Four of the eight standards are concerned directly with the quality of nursing care: NR3 requires maintenance of established standards of nursing practice; NR5 mandates the use of the nursing process; NR7 delineates written documentation that care reflects optimal standards of practice; and NR8 provides for the monitoring and evaluation of care and the identification and resolution of problems.

The Joint Commission on Accreditation of Health Care Organizations distinguishes between standards of care and standards of practice.[37] Whereas standards of care reflect expected patient outcomes of care activities, standards of practice are concerned with "the structure and process elements used by the nurse and nursing service to provide patient care."[38] Thus a standard of care focuses on the patient, and a standard of practice focuses on the nurse. Patterson[38] differentiates the two concepts further by explaining that a standard of care is what the patient outcome should be and what the patient can expect from nursing service, whereas standards of practice relate to what and how the nurse provides care to achieve the patient outcome. The outcomes of care generally are based on clinical criteria or well-defined indicators that are measurable and that reflect the quality and appropriateness of intervention. Quality, in this sense, depicts the degree of adherence between the standard of care and actual patient outcome, and appropriateness reflects the degree of congruence between what the patient needed to achieve in terms of a desired outcome and what the nurse provided.

Therefore, to operationalize a quality assurance program, the health care institution must maintain a sound system for documentation of nursing care activities and patient outcomes and must establish a system to review and assess regularly both quality and appropriateness. In addition to evaluation, there is need for a system to rectify or resolve problems or breeches of quality in all aspects of care: diagnostic, preventive, therapeutic, rehabilitative, supportive, and palliative.

Depending on the nature and specialization of the nursing care unit, there may be need for a more precise definition of both patient outcomes and nursing practices to achieve those outcomes, or what is known as clinical functions. Oncology nursing is a prime example of the need for care and practice standards to be tailored to the unique needs and problems of the cancer patient and for more precise operationalization of clinical functions such as assessment, evaluation of learning needs, provision of physical care, teaching, goal setting, nursing interventions based on nursing diagnosis, implementation of the medical plan of care and required medications and treatments, and the coordination of nursing goals and plans for care with those of other professional team members.[38]

In these specific cases, both health care institutions and accrediting organizations look to the professional specialty group to establish and promulgate those standards of nursing practice. Quality assurance structures look to organizations such as ONS for current, state-of-the-art research-based standards.[38] On the basis of these published specialty guides, the hospital or agency customizes the standards further to be in line with the nature and character of its own care-giving environment. For example, nursing practice standards at one of the nation's five major cancer centers might differ from those in a small community hospital, where there may or may not be a discrete oncology unit or where there may or may not be a department of nursing research that focuses on oncology care. However, no matter how specialized or how large or small the institution might be, mandated quality assurance accords the *right* to quality of care as defined by the ONS standards of nursing practice to every oncology patient.

The literature is sparse in studies evaluating the quality of cancer nursing care by using patient outcomes as evidence. However, several articles stand out in their effort to improve the quality assurance process. This small body of literature reflects the complexities involved in studying quality and the many dimensions in focus and approach. Five issues important to quality assurance (QA) were examined in nine studies reported in the period from 1985 to 1988: (1) QA audit results for specific areas of care, (2) oncology patient classification systems, (3) Occupational Safety and Health Administration (OSHA) guidelines, (4) clinical database development, and (5) methods to identify and measure oncology nursing competencies and practice proficiency.

Oleske et al.[39] conducted a controlled study that measured the effects of both nurse specialist consultation and continuing education on the home care of cancer patients, using an audit measure documenting assessment, intervention, and evidence of outcomes for patients with breast and colon cancers. Findings revealed that improvement in nursing assessment and management performance occurred over time in all three intervention groups. However, only half the criteria for optimal nurse performance were achieved, with little increase in patient outcome scores. The greatest improvements were noted in patients' nutrition, and little improvement was noted overall in the management of pain and physiologic complications. The authors recommend replication and offer the complete set of audit forms on request.

Similarly, Stephany[40] tested the reliability and validity of the Hope Hospice Quality Assurance Tool (HQAT), which assesses physical concerns, patient and caregiver education, and emotional and spiritual support, using operationally defined criteria. Test-retest stability and internal consistency of the tool were established. Content, criterion-related, and construct validities were tested and found to be high in the nurse group but only moderate for lay volunteers. The tool was modified, with subsequent improvement in reliability and validity scores. The report provides detailed descriptions of the QA program, standards, and criteria of the assessment form. The rigor of the study produced an effective audit tool to measure the quality of hospice care.

Arenth[41] developed and validated an acuity classification of oncology patients based on the definition of four categories of emergent status. The system has served as the basis for calculating nursing hours per patient day, patient volumes, nursing utilization or productivity, and variable staffing in a large medical center.

Dudjak[42] described the Radiation Therapy Nursing Care Record, comprising six flowsheets designed to document the nursing care of patients undergoing radiation therapy. The record allows for baseline assessment of risk factors and problems and for nursing practices in assessment, teaching, and other interventions. The record has been used to justify staff needs and cost of nursing care and to establish standards of practice further.

Because safety is a cornerstone of quality assurance for both patients and health care providers, periodic updates such as Gullo's review[43] of safe handling of antineoplastic drugs are essential to the application of the OSHA guidelines to practice. Recommendations for avoiding exposure, for safe disposal, and for health evaluation and monitoring are given clearly according to a well-articulated knowledge framework. Gullo estimated that more than 60% of nurses were not using safe handling techniques, an important factor in quality assurance. Two articles by Williamson et al.[44,45] reviewed the occupational risks of infection, musculoskeletal injury, exposure to antineoplastic agents, stress in the work environment, shift work, and reproductive health concerns of nurses. Their articles call for a greater intensity of clinically oriented research efforts in this area.

Two articles suggest methods of establishing a clinical database to provide a structured framework for the collection of critical data with which to formulate nursing diagnoses. Miaskowski and Nielsen[46] developed the Cancer Nursing Assessment Tool to evaluate the integrity of 15 functional systems at high risk because of cancer and its treatment. The assessment included teaching needs and discharge planning. Gray et al.[47] published a clinical database that provides description and analysis of age, metastatic sites, diagnoses, and associated symptoms of hospitalized patients with advanced cancer. Their study of 1103 patients generated more than 400 variables and provided important information on problem areas related to cancer metastasis. Since symptom management is the "cornerstone of care" in this patient group, the database facilitated the identification of relevant nursing diagnoses and related nursing practices that improved the measurement of quality of care.

On another level, two separate studies by Moore et al.[48] and McGee et al.[49] sought to establish nurse competencies and to measure proficiency in cancer nursing practice. The Moore team constructed the Appraisal of Practice Behaviors Instrument, based on the five dimensions of the theoretical framework used by ONS to develop the Standards of Oncology Nursing Practice. Three classes enrolled in a master's level oncology nursing graduate program were tested before and after each of the 2 years of their educational program for both frequency and self-assessed proficiency in achieving the ONS outcome standards of oncology practice. The instrument consists of 92 items divided among six subscales. Findings revealed that frequency of practice and proficiency were positively related and that students significantly increased in self-assessed proficiency as their educational program progressed. The investigators suggest further evaluation of the instrument in both academic and clinical settings to expand the database.

In contrast, McGee et al.[49] conducted a two-round Delphi survey to identify oncology clinical nurse specialist (OCNS) competencies. The initial pilot study amassed 363 competencies, which the investigators further divided into knowledge, skill, attitude, and human trait categories. Ranking by means for each category revealed that attitude and human traits were ranked highest in importance by the 47 respondents. Attitudes of greatest importance had to do with ethical practice, respect for humanity, responsibility for behavior, and commitment to continued learning. Identifying nursing diagnoses and commitment to cost-effective practices were ranked lowest in the category. The human traits most valued included accountability, common sense, caring, flexibility, and resourcefulness. Of lower importance were sympathy and abstract thinking. The highest number of competencies, 173, were amassed in the "skills" category, and knowledge ranked second in number of competencies, totaling 137. The investigators, in interpreting their results, concluded that attitudes and human traits concerned with caring, commitment, and professionalism were ranked as those most important to OCNS functioning. They considered their results to be consistent with Yasko's survey[50] of 185 OCNSs, who reported a decided "care orientation" described as "keeping the client comfortable, maintaining a therapeutic environment, providing emotional support, personalized care, friendliness, emotional acceptance and ensuring that clients understand their medical problems."

The information generated from these key studies helps to expand and facilitate attempts to improve quality of care. By integrating findings from these and future studies on acuity, audit assessment tools, safety guidelines, clinical databases, and nursing competencies and practice proficiency, quality assurance will move into the era of strategic quality management predicted by Garven[18] and Beyers.[16]

Clinical research

Research offers a means of improving and refining practice to ensure optimal outcomes. The desired result of practice usually is defined as a valuable change in the patient for the better. In most institutional settings, this means cost-effective patient outcomes and consumer satisfaction.

Clinical research, in the context of evaluating quality of care, includes two major categories: (1) experimental studies of nursing interventions and (2) evaluations of programs of care. The program of research in most disciplines is shaped by the intellectual and practical problems and challenges encountered in carrying out its objectives and by the diagnostic and functional categories that constitute its focus. For nursing, these areas for investigation can best be illustrated by the results of two Delphi surveys conducted during the past decade to examine research priorities in cancer nursing.

Oberst[51] polled a group of 575 oncology nurses throughout the United States, asking them what they thought was important to investigate systematically in order to improve their clinical practice. From those nurses giving the most direct care to cancer patients, Oberst's goal was to capture a heuristic force that would have an impact on patient welfare by using the research process as a catalyst. She asked nurses to identify the problems they confront every day in practice, the problems cancer patients have from the time of diagnosis, and how these problems arrange themselves in priority.

The results of Oberst's study determined ten priorities for cancer nursing research: (1) chemotherapy- or radiation-induced nausea and vomiting, (2) pain, (3) discharge needs, (4) grief, (5) stomatitis, (6) venipuncture in long-term therapy, (7) comfort and dignity of the terminally ill patient, (8) effective analgesia, (9) assistance with providing effective pain management, and (10) understanding the nurses' own attitudes toward pain and how it affects their ability to provide effective pain management. In addition, the oncology nurses responding to Oberst's survey reported that patient- and nurse-related research needs parallel one another. Optimal patient outcomes were inextricably tied to the reduction of deficits in nurse knowledge and skill in the ten patient-focused research priority areas.

Ten years later, a partial replication of Oberst's work was conducted with 143 practicing oncology nurses from the four western provinces of Canada.[52] Results were similar but were expressed by requests for studies of specific interventions. Of the top 15 research priorities, the following areas emerged as most important: relaxation, imagery, and biofeedback techniques in the reduction of anticipatory nausea and vomiting and other side effects of treatment and in the enhancement of quality of life; ways to increase effectiveness of patient teaching in areas of patient compliance, self-care, and coping; approaches to improve discharge planning programs; methods of communicating diagnosis and prognosis to patients and families; approaches to strengthen effectiveness in primary care; ways to improve preceptorship programs; and therapeutic approaches to the relief of treatment- and disease-related symptoms and side effects. The emphasis of the Canadian results was clearly on studying nursing practices that improve the patient's condition, rather than on the problem itself. This shift may reflect the result of descriptive nursing research efforts and a more sophisticated practice during the past 10 years after Oberst's survey.[51]

In a review of research-based articles appearing in the cancer nursing literature between 1976 and 1984, Scott[31] found 122 articles representing 25% of all articles published. More than 60% of the studies were published after 1981, most concerned with side effects of treatment (26%) or with oncology nurses themselves (24%). Approximately 15% examined the impact of cancer on the family, and another 16% described phenomena about cancer patients. Only 12% were intervention-management studies, and fewer (7%) offered assessment-measurement approaches to evaluate care.

In a developmental sense, the era before 1985 may be viewed as a descriptive phase when the rich database that exists today was established. Clinical research, comprising both program evaluation and experimental studies of interventions, began slowly between 1980 and 1985, marked by the seminal work of Satterwhite et al.,[53] Edlund,[35] Dodd and Mood,[54,55] Johnson,[56] Miller and Nygren,[57] Marty et al.,[58] Watson,[59] and Henrich and Schag.[60] Since 1985, there has been an expansion of the cancer research literature addressing the priorities in the two Delphi surveys and testing the therapeutic effect of larger-scale programs of care.

Twenty experimental studies published since 1984 (Table 57-4)[61–74,166–171] addressed four of the ten (40%) outcome standards for cancer nursing practice. More than half tested interventions to promote patient comfort and reduce treatment-related side effects. Seven studies (35%) tested interventions to optimize protective mechanisms by preventing infection or reducing skin and mucous membrane integrity deficits. Two studies (1%) evaluated educational programs to promote early cancer detection practices. As a whole, these studies reflected a growing sophistication in research design and measurement. Most were randomized, controlled investigations of the effect of a clearly defined intervention on a small, homogeneous sample. The instruments used to measure patient outcomes generally had been tested for reliability and validity or consisted of well-defined clinical indicators rated for construct validity by a panel of experts. All reports discussed study limitations, the generalizability of results, and implications for further research. Moreover, practically all made useful contributions to clinical knowledge.

From 1984 to 1992, a total of 16 program evaluation reports (Table 57-5)[75–88,172,173] covering a wider range of outcome standards were published. The largest number (6, or 38%) evaluated programs designed to assist patients and families to cope with cancer. The next largest category (4, or 25%), comfort, described multidisciplinary pain management programs. The rest were divided among prevention-detection (1, or 6%), information (1, or 6%), nutrition (1, or 6%), protection (1, or 6%) and two economic feasibility studies (13%) of an adult day care hospital and a home transfusion program.

The therapeutic programs generally were well defined, as was the patient population. Most were service

TABLE 57-4 Experimental Studies of Oncology Nursing Interventions and Patient Outcomes by Functional Pattern Category

Author	Problem	Method	Findings	Implications
		PREVENTION AND EARLY DETECTION		
Rudolf and Quinn[61]	Education to promote TSE	*N* = 64 college men; Health Beliefs Survey for Testicular Cancer and Testicular Self-Examination Survey (modified by authors); pretest and posttest; educational program with film and silicone practice model	• Subjects lacked knowledge about testicular cancer and TSE • Increased perception in benefits and decrease in barriers to TSE resulted • Of "never performers," 63% did TSE at least once after program • Perception of susceptibility and disease seriousness did not increase	• Need for education and for research testing of a variety of educational approaches • Nurses should take lead • Replication with time between testing and more controlled methods • Further testing of instrument
Coleman et al.[166]	BSE proficiency in older women (>50 years)	*N* = 79 women; random assignment 2-group design to compare women who were taught BSE using self-modeling as well as breast model methods with women taught by use of breast model only. Subjects evaluated using pre- and posttesting method. First posttest immediately after the teaching; second posttest 3 months later	Women taught by both methods performed BSE significantly more proficiently than those taught by model only	• Performance is not always related to a woman's reported self-confidence • Patients need to be evaluated directly to determine proficiency in BSE
		INFORMATION		
Hagopian[167]	Effect of weekly radiation therapy newsletter on knowledge, self-care, and severity of side effects	*N* = 103 radiation patients were assigned to experimental (51) and control (52) groups. Experimentals had opportunity to read newsletter during treatment; controls did not. *Instruments:* Radiation Side Effects Profile, a knowledge test, and a demographics form; posttest-only design.	• Subjects who read newsletter scored significantly higher on knowledge test • All other correlations nonsignificant	• Majority of patients found newsletter to be helpful source of information • It cannot replace a caring professional
		COMFORT		
Beck[168]	Effect of music in decreasing cancer pain	*N* = 15 outpatients with cancer receiving scheduled analgesics for pain; experimental repeated measures cross-over design	• When listening to music, 75% had <20% response, 50% had <40% or >40% responses	Music therapy has promise as a pain reducing modality, but further refinements in methods and research required

(continued)

TABLE 57-4 Experimental Studies of Oncology Nursing Interventions and Patient Outcomes by Functional Pattern Category (continued)

Author	Problem	Method	Findings	Implications
		COMFORT		
Beck[168] (continued)		using McGill Pain Questionnaire and analog scales to measure mood and pain; from a menu of 7 types of music, subjects chose type of music preferred; controls listened to tape with low-frequency hum; tapes were 45 min in length; study conducted in 4 phases: baseline data for 3 days, randomized to E or C group for 3 days, cross-over to alternate group for 3 days, baseline repetition for all subjects for 3 days; pain ratings taken before and after listening to tape	• When listening to hum, 20% had <40% and >40% responses and 53% had no change in pain • 60% listening to music reported some improvement in mood with music, with ⅓ responding with moderate to great improvement • Mood and pain were found to be unrelated • Although not statistically significant, overall music decreased pain 22%; hum decreased pain 11%	
Broome et al.[169]	Effect of distraction and imagery on reducing pain during painful procedures in children and on reducing anxiety in child's mother	N = 14 children receiving lumbar punctures and their mothers; multiple case study design; children videotaped for first 3 visits to obtain baseline; distraction and imagery program not described; *instruments (child):* Child Medical Fear Scale, Observation of Behavioral Stress Scale, Baker-Wong FACES Scale; *instruments (mother):* Spielberger's State-Trait Anxiety Inventory (STAI), Parent Behavior Tool	• No change in children's fears or behavioral distress; children's pain ratings decreased significantly over time • Mothers' state anxiety did not change • Mothers' behaviors were nondistressed and stable over time	• Research control of ability of child to relax and use distraction and frequency of parent–child practice need to be improved • Decrease in children's pain reports an important finding and corresponds with previous reports
Cotanch et al.[62]	Self-hypnosis as antiemetic therapy	N = 20 children, ages 9–18 years, receiving chemotherapy; experimental and control groups; investigator-constructed visual analog scale, self-report, nurse's charting; experimental subjects trained in relaxation and self-hypnosis	• Decrease in intensity and severity of nausea and vomiting in experimental group • Increased oral intake in experimental group • No difference in antiemetic administration between groups	Further research in other age groups
Frank[63]	Music and guided imagery as antiemetic therapy	N = 15 adults on variety of chemotherapy regimens—13 women, 2 men; single group; pretest and posttest STAI; Nausea and	• Decreased anxiety (STAI) • Decreased intensity of vomiting • No difference in perception of nausea,	Test intervention in other stressful, threatening situations (ie, crisis and pain)

(continued)

TABLE 57-4 Experimental Studies of Oncology Nursing Interventions and Patient Outcomes by Functional Pattern Category (continued)

Author	Problem	Method	Findings	Implications
		COMFORT		
		Vomiting Questionnaire; *intervention:* musical tapes and poster images during and after chemotherapy	but duration showed nonsignificant downward trend	
Scott et al.[64]	Progressive Muscle Relaxation (PMR), guided imagery, and slow-stroke back massage vs drug regimen as antiemetic therapy	*N* = 17 women with gynecologic cancer receiving chemotherapy; relaxation and drug groups; drug group received high-dose metaclopramide; Emetic Process Rating Scale (EPRS); relaxation group received 1-hr educational program with slide tape and were coached by nurse in relaxation	• Relaxation group had reduced total duration • Drug group had reduced peak vomiting phase • No difference in intensity or amount of emesis between groups • Drug group experienced significantly increased diuresis unexplained by intake • Content validity of EPRS established • Verification of phase periodicity	• Testing interventions combining both methods • Replication in other populations • Continued testing of EPRS • Data on norm phase periodicity for other chemotherapy regimens
Cotanch and Strum[65]	PMR as antiemetic therapy	*N* = 60; *3-group design:* experimental, placebo control (music), true control (no intervention); Dukes Descriptive Scale; Diary of Food Intake; STAI; upper skin-fold size; blood pressure; admission-discharge assessments	PMR most effective in reducing frequency and duration of vomiting, general anxiety, and physiologic arousal and in improving caloric intake in patients 48 hr after chemotherapy	Replication
Parker[66]	Scalp hypothermia to reduce alopecia	*N* = 12 subjects receiving cyclophosphamide randomly assigned to 2 groups; experimental and control; SPENCO Hypothermia Cap; samples of hair loss for 7 days after treatment; scalp photographs	Control subjects have significantly more hair loss than experimental subjects	Clinical use
Dudjak[67]	Mouth care for mucositis therapy	*N* = 15 subjects receiving radiation therapy to head and neck area; random assignment of experimental and control groups; experimental subjects received hydrogen peroxide solution;	• Increase in perceived comfort in experimental group • No difference in mouth condition between groups • Hydrogen peroxide treatment judged more effective	• Replication • Test other interventions • Clinical use

(continued)

TABLE 57-4 Experimental Studies of Oncology Nursing Interventions and Patient Outcomes by Functional Pattern Category (continued)

Author	Problem	Method	Findings	Implications
		COMFORT		
Dudjak[67] (continued)		control subjects received baking soda and water; oral examination guide; Oral Comfort Guide; subjects evaluated 8 times: once before radiation therapy and then once weekly for 5 weeks, at completion, and 1 month after completion	• Both groups at lower incidence than published norms • Rate of infection equal in both groups	
Winningham and MacVicar[68]	Aerobic exercise as antiemetic therapy	$N = 42$ breast cancer patients; matched age and functional capacity; *3-group design:* experimental (stationary bike), placebo control (mild stretching), control (no treatment); *Treatment:* supervised 10-wk 3×/wk aerobic training on cycle ergometer; Symptom-Limited Graded Exercise Text (SLGXT); Symptom Checklist 90—Revised; Somatization Subscale; all tests given before and after treatment	• Marked improvement in experimental compared with other groups in patient reports of nausea • Increase in somatization scores in experimental groups	Studies of other types of exercise, emetic treatment protocols, and studies to determine difference between exercise and relaxation
Giaccone et al.[69]	Scalp hypothermia to reduce alopecia	$N = 39$ patients receiving doxorubicin; randomly assigned to experimental (scalp hypothermia) or control (no treatment) group; SPENCO Hypothermia; evaluations after 2 full chemotherapy cycles; hair loss evaluated by nurse and physician using an operationalized scale	• Control subjects, 100% alopecia • Experimental subjects, 37% prevention of hair loss • No or slight hair loss in 7 of 19 • No instances of scalp metastasis in either group	Clinical use
		PROTECTIVE MECHANISMS		
Shivnan et al.[170]	Comparison of transparent adherent dressing (TAD) and dry sterile gauze dressing (DSGD) in preventing infection in long-term central catheters	$N = 98$; TAD (51); DSGD (47); randomized, stratified design with assignment to DSGD changed daily or TAD changed every 4 days; data collected with investigator-designed demographic and assessment forms for	• DSGD group had significantly more skin irritation and wet dressings after showering, and had more exudate • Exit site infection occurred in 2 TAD and 1 DSGD subjects	TADs provide a safe, comfortable, and cost-effective alternative to DSGDs

(continued)

TABLE 57-4 Experimental Studies of Oncology Nursing Interventions and Patient Outcomes by Functional Pattern Category (continued)

Author	Problem	Method	Findings	Implications
		PROTECTIVE MECHANISMS		
Shivnan et al.[170] (continued		skin irritation and intactness, dryness of dressing, erythema, swelling, pain, and exudate; dressing comfort, ease of application, safety, change frequency, and satisfaction recorded	• No systemic infection occurred • One catheter-related sepsis occurred in TAD group • TADs required significantly fewer dressings and less nursing time and were significantly less costly • Subjects reported greater satisfaction and comfort with TADs	
Yeoman et al.[171]	Effect of chlorhexidene gluconate (CHG) in reducing perirectal infections in patients with acute leukemia	*N* = 40 acute or chronic leukemia patients; 16 randomized to CHG group, 24 to nonmedicated skin cleanser group; chi-square and *t*-tests used to analyze (1) incidence of skin breakdown and rectal infections, and their correlation, (2) positive history of rectal infections, fissures, hemorrhoids, (3) presence of hemorrhoids, (4) severity of diarrhea, and, (5) duration and severity of granulocytopenia; *instruments:* Perirectal Skin Assessment Tool (PSAT), perirectal clinical examinations conducted by blinded evaluators for duration and severity of granulocytopenia, presence of hemorrhoids, severity of GI mucositis, signs of perirectal infection	• Treatment did not influence development of perirectal infections or degree or incidence of skin breakdown • Severity and duration of granulocytopenia significantly related to development of rectal infections • No other variable a statistically significant influence	• Due to small sample size, replication is advisable • PSAT has some demonstrated validity and reliability • Need for strategies to prevent rectal infection in immunocompromised patients is clear
Shell et al.[70]	Dressings to treat radiation therapy skin reactions	*N* = 16 patients with moderate to severe radiodermatitis; comparison of moisture-permeable to conventional hydrous	Healing time for MVP: 19 days vs 24 days for lanolin gauze	Warrants further study

(continued)

TABLE 57-4 Experimental Studies of Oncology Nursing Interventions and Patient Outcomes by Functional Pattern Category (continued)

Author	Problem	Method	Findings	Implications
		PROTECTIVE MECHANISMS		
		lanolin gauze; evaluation of healing time by use of 4 visual inspection parameters in number of days		
Harwood and Bachur[71]	DMSO vs local cooling in extravasation therapy	Animal study using 4 pigs; posttest-control experimental design; micromeasurements by primary investigator; measured time to healing DMSO vs local cooling with ice vs no-treatment control	• Local cooling more highly effective in preventing tissue necrosis after extravasation • No difference between DMSO and control groups • Time to healing increased with DMSO • DMSO not recommended for treatment	More studies to determine optimal schedule of cooling
Jones[72]	Catheter care procedures in central venous catheter infection	Evaluation of 2 catheter care procedures, one using fewer supplies and less time; assessment of observable evidence of infection, neutrophil count, and blood cultures	• No difference • Only common factor connected with likelihood of infection: low neutrophil count at time of positive blood culture	Conduct further studies to refine predictive risk factors
MacGeorge et al.[73]	Mixing vs reinfusion methods in drawing blood from Hickman catheter	N = 18 bone marrow transplant patients; hematocrit (Coulter counter); visual determination of hemolysis by expert laboratory technician	• No statistical difference in accuracy of laboratory values between 2 methods • Mixing has advantage of less infection	Replication in pediatric population with larger sample in variety of clinical settings
Petrosino et al.[74]	Dressing to reduce central venous catheter infection	N = 52 patients with central venous catheters; random assignment to 4 dressing groups: Tegaderm transparent, Op-Site, gauze, no dressing; observation at 7 and 30 days for 5 indicators: skin culture, oral temperature, erythema, tenderness, drainage	• No difference among groups • No dressing option seems simpler and less costly	Further research on skin cleansing techniques

TSE, testicular self-examination; *STAI,* State-Trait Anxiety Inventory; *PMR,* progressive muscle relaxation; *DMSO,* dimethyl sulfoxide.

innovations based on the institution's database of patient needs and problems. In a majority of these studies, evaluation methods proved to be the weakest component. Although all programs were judged as valuable by the investigators, only half employed evaluation criteria developed before program initiation. Some measured quality by the number of clients seen or by unsolicited patient feedback. Others, however, made use of standardized surveys, questionnaires, interviews, and preprogram and postprogram comparisons of knowledge tests or needs assessments with baseline findings. Almost all investigative teams communicated willingness to share their programs with others but advised tailoring them to the unique needs of the institutions and their patient populations. Most suggested the need for further study and program modifications or refinements.

Although the program evaluations reflected significant effort in planning and execution by hard-working teams, it must be remembered that program evaluation is a mature methodology, generally requiring an expert team of outside investigators to conduct the study. Two noteworthy examples include the Brown University evaluation of the Adult Day Care Hospital, Memorial Sloan-Kettering Cancer Center[89] and the as-yet-unpublished University of Washington study of the effect of the Planetree Unit, a primary-nursing, family-centered care facility at California Pacific Medical Center (Pacific campus), San Francisco.

The overall picture of 36 studies published over a 8-year period suggests the beginning establishment of a clinical scientific base for practice. Clearly, much more research is needed in all standards-of-practice domains. Research that replicates or builds on the work of others and that refines established interventions may be the most economic ventures. However, to address meaningfully the issue of quality of care, longitudinal studies expanding the clinical database and testing effects of nursing intervention over time are critically needed. The oncology nursing research program, to have an impact on quality of care, will need not only to continue building the growing knowledge base in symptom management and patient education but also to turn attention to the issues of quality of life, recovery, transition, and the effect of a host of new modalities on patients' lives and health.

Measurement tool development: Quantitative

As psychometric theory advances and the results of nursing research build over time, better methods for measuring quality of care will emerge. Hartshorn,[90] Duffy,[91] and Lynn[92] emphasize the importance of using reliable and valid instruments in clinical research. Duffy said that research-based practice should be precise enough to be replicable and to produce predictable patient outcomes. Hartshorn warned that results from studies employing poor instruments cannot be accepted or implemented. Indeed, many nursing studies that have required considerable time and effort conclude with a long list of limitations to the generalizability of their findings and with an underdeveloped interpretation of important data because of faulty design, inadequate sampling technique, and use of untested measurement tools.

The basic ingredients of sound quantitative measurement techniques include adequate reliability and validity of the instrument. Reliability tests both the stability (test–retest correlations) and the internal consistency (intercorrelations among items or alpha coefficient) of an instrument. Correlations of at least .8 in internal consistency and test–retest correlations ensure that the instrument is reliably measuring the construct it purports to measure and is stable in its ability to reproduce results in repeated testing of the sample. A third type of reliability, interrater reliability, is also important to ensure that all persons using a set of evaluation criteria have closely correlated results.[93]

Validity testing offers a way to assess the ability of the instrument to measure the construct of interest accurately and objectively. The three most important types of validity include construct, content, and criterion related (predictive or concurrent).[90,93] One of the most definitive signs of increasingly improved and sophisticated cancer nursing research is growing evidence that reliable and valid instruments were used.

Table 57-6 provides a partial list of cancer nursing measurement tools* grouped by functional category, including the construct measured and whether evidence of reliability and validity testing are given.[94–114] Note that most of these instruments quantify patient attributes. The aim is to establish further a normative database or to measure the qualitative outcomes of nursing practice, or both.

Measurement tool development: Qualitative

During the past 10 years, an increasing interest in qualitative methods of research has become evident in the nursing literature. Measuring quality of care quantitatively does not readily capture the contextual nature and natural richness of the situational and interpersonal data that compose the nursing care environment.

Nursing literature generally reflects attempts at establishing patient databases composed of qualitative sets of indicators, predictors, and assessment parameters that form the etiologic foundations of patient concerns and nursing practices. For example, if we review the available quantitative tools, most are based on the iden-

*For a current, inclusive discussion of clinical research tools in nursing, consult Frank-Stromborg's *Instruments for Clinical Nursing Research.*[94]

TABLE 57-5 Care Program Evaluation Studies

Program	Author	Method	Results
		I. PREVENTION AND DETECTION	
Family High Risk Program	Beck et al.[75]	Health Family Tree Questionnaire; Family health survey to assess satisfaction with program, health practices, health history, and behavior; includes retrospective data	• Evaluation ongoing • No results as of publication
		II. INFORMATION	
Patient Education Program	Nieweg et al.[76]	Comparison of patient self-care of chemotherapy port infection rates with literature-based norms; weekly clinical assessments; no standardized evaluation methods used	• Empirically judged effective • Takes considerable time • Required teaching materials • Greater social support involvement • Less need for hospitalization • Greater patient freedom
		III. COPING	
Living with Cancer	Pillon and Joannides[172]	Based on anecdotal statements and empirical observation of a program conducted since 1979	• Program needs to be comprehensive, addressing problems of the entire family from diagnosis to disease-free state or death • Facilitators should include an oncology nurse and mental health clinician
We Can Weekend	Lane and Davis[77]	Postprogram participant evaluation; staff feedback; director-evaluation of training sessions, staff, facilities, schedule, public relations, and supplies	• Recommended use of preprogram questionnaires to enable advance custom planning • Also use a postprogram questionnaire
Living With Cancer	Fredette and Beattie[78]	Precourse and postcourse knowledge test; precourse and postcourse personal needs assessment; postcourse interviews; written comments of specialist-observer; end-of-class and end-of-program evaluations	• Coping skills can be taught • Profiles "good coper" as one who pursues information and seeks opportunities to learn • Adaptive, resilient, optimistic, and assertive • Need further exploration into program design for those who desire less or differently structured programs • Teaching skills of coping was primary value of program
Cancer Caregivers Program	Cawley and Gerdts[79]	Committee-constructed evaluation tool: evaluates 8 dimensions of care in terms of time, instructor, handouts	• Provides steps in establishment of program • Evaluation tool developed and provided • Ongoing evaluation • No results

(continued)

TABLE 57-5 Care Program Evaluation Studies (continued)

Program	Author	Method	Results
		III. COPING	
I Can Cope	Diekmann[80]	Postprogram mail questionnaire	• Demographic characteristics • Overall evaluation: valuable to help people learn about cancer • More research to improve impact on coping
Bereavement Outreach Program	Mosely et al.[81]	No formal means of evaluation	• Excellent client response • Need to tailor program to institution
		IV. COMFORT	
Home Pain Management Program	Coyle et al.[82]	Evaluated 123 patients with advanced disease for pain management at home	• Nurse becomes primary liaison • Successful pain management at home with use of analgesic and behavioral modes • Team as expert information resource in community
Continuous SC Infusion Pain Management Program	Coyle et al[83]	Evaluated 15 patients for quality of pain management	Avoids repeated injection, need for intravenous access, analgesia delay, pain breakthrough
Pain Management Team	Ferrell et al.[84]	No evaluation of effect of interventions on pain	• Patients visits: 7500 (750 patients) over course of 5 years • Community presentations: 300
Patient-controlled Analgesia (PCA) Service	Kane et al.[85]	Patient questionnaire on discharge; nurse evaluation of two pumps regarding safety, ease of use, saving of time; bedside flowsheets to rate pain and sedation; daily patient evaluation by PCA team	• Use of pump gives excellent control of pain in postsurgical patients, has few problems, and frees nurse to care for patient • Further studies in chronic pain populations needed • Choice of one pump over another
		V. NUTRITION	
Home Parenteral Nutrition Program	Konstantinides[86]	Patient teaching flowsheet; no formal evaluation methods presented	• Cost estimated between $55,000 and $70,000 for nutritional solutions, supplies, home visits, clinic follow-up, and laboratory costs • Guides for patient teaching, discharge planning, laboratory monitoring, and follow-up given
		VI. PROTECTION	
Protocol for Venous Access Port	Long and Ovaska[173]	N = 26 outpatients with venous access devices	• After 6 months, no documented infection in

(continued)

TABLE 57-5 Care Program Evaluation Studies (continued)

Program	Author	Method	Results
VI. PROTECTION			
		randomly assigned to sterile (12) or clean (14) group; sterile group used commercially prepared kit; compared occurrence of infection assessed by increase in WBC, febrile episode (>100.4), drainage, pain, redness, swelling, warmth at port site	either group • Institution changed to nursing protocol based on its cost effectiveness
VII. GENERAL FOCUS			
Day Hospital for Cancer Patients	Clark[87]	Economic feasibility measures	• One-year pilot project • Ongoing as of publication
Home Care Transfusion Program	Pluth[88]	Cost comparisons with patients receiving transfusions in different settings; client satisfaction; difficulties in implementation	Cost-effective and beneficial to patients' quality of life

tification of indicators grouped to facilitate diagnostic reasoning. However, less precision is found in scoring instrument results. Few scoring systems are based on large amounts of normative data, particularly those established in healthy populations that allow clear comparisons and interpretation of new data.

The most recognized qualitative approaches include case study, grounded theory, phenomenology, and ethnography, among others (Ammon-Gaberson and Piantanida).[115] Qualitative research begins with carefully conceptualized and clearly articulated research questions to guide data collection and later interpretation. The motive is to understand an aspect of human experience and to shape a representation of it from the data. The results of the qualitative method may include (1) operationalizing a single concept, (2) developing a conceptual framework, (3) establishing guidelines for practice, (4) creating portraits, paradigm cases, or typologies, and (5) forming theory.

Although reliability testing and validity testing in the conventional sense do not have a place in the qualitative process, there are sound principles and methods to guide study design, data gathering, data analysis and management, data interpretation, and paradigm construction. These processes are no less rigorous than those of the quantitative approach. In many areas of quality-of-care research, the qualitative paradigm or a combination of the qualitative and quantitative paradigms may be the best approach.

The qualitative cancer nursing research literature represents a mixed bag of clinically relevant information that, for the purposes of a quality-of-care discussion, may be categorized according to format and content considerations. The research articles have been grouped as either indicators, predictors, or guidelines for care.

Indicators are sets of variables that describe empirically an important clinical manifestation. These sets are derived generally from a review of published work on the subject or a descriptive exploratory or qualitative study, or both. For example, Saunders and Valente's article[116] on suicide in cancer patients brings together their wealth of empirical knowledge as well as general information about depression and suicide. One outcome is a useful "Brief Suicide Assessment Guide" for practitioners. In contrast, Thorne[117] reported the results of her phenomenologic study of the family cancer experience, providing important insights into family perceptions and coping strategies when a member has cancer. Therefore information in a wide variety of content areas produced sets of clues to facilitate better understanding of many common clinical issues.

Predictors are variables that have been tested to determine their ability to predict a future event with some degree of accuracy. Predictors are critical to nursing's role in health promotion and prevention. For example, Hays's article[118] on predictors of hospice utilization identified specific patient and family parameters that, when taken into consideration early enough in the nursing plan of care, have a good chance of strengthening the family unit so that the patient can be maintained at home under quality care conditions for longer periods. Another illustration of the establishment of predictors is the research that has identified clusters of variables predicting the occurrence of anticipatory nausea and vomiting.[119,120]

TABLE 57-6 Tools to Measure Patient Outcomes

Tool	Author	Construct	Findings	Implications
Quality of Life Index (QLI)	Ferrans and Powers[95]	Quality of life	Likert scales (2) to determine importance and satisfaction in 18 life areas: life goals, general satisfaction, stress, physical health; reliability established; validity established; versions for normal, healthy adults and for kidney transplant, heart transplant, kidney dialysis, and cancer patients	Establishing norms in different populations
Cancer Malaise Scale	Kobashi-Schoot et al.[96]	Physical fatigue, mental fatigue, malaise, psychologic complaints in radiotherapy cancer patients; validity established	Malaise increased during course of treatment; physical symptoms increased late in course of treatment; malaise correlates with "feeling ill" or "not well"	Further correlation stratified by treatment level of radiation exposure
Quality of Life Index (QLI)	Padilla and Grant[97]	Linear analog: psychologic well-being, physical well-being, symptom control; 14 items; reliability established; validity established		Further testing in variety of subject populations; use to test intervention effectiveness
Information Preference Questionnaire (IPQ)	Hopkins[98]	Information seeking; 5-point scale measuring preference for treatment information	Information seeking negatively related to age and severity of disease; reliability established; validity established	Needs additional testing to establish criterion and construct validities
Emetic Process Rating Scale (EPRS)	Scott et al.[64]	Analog scale: nausea, retching, vomiting, intake, output, vital signs, treatment; validity established	Evaluated antiemetic effect of clinical relaxation vs drug intervention; scale found clinically useful	Further reliability and validity testing
Sexual Adjustment Questionnaire (SAQ)	Waterhouse and Metcalf[99]	Desire, activity level, relationship, arousal, techniques, orgasm	Persons with cancer significantly reduced scores on activity level, relationships, and techniques	Continued refinement and larger sample testing
Derdiarian Informational Needs Assessment (DINA)	Derdiarian[100]	Informational needs related to disease: personal, family, and social parameters		Further instrument assessment and use in patient referral and follow-up
Patient Care Needs Survey	Fleming et al[101]	Comfort needs in advanced cancer patients: physiologic, spiritual, psychosocial, patients' rights, dignity, self-worth	Identified 7 themes of comfort; decreased with severity of illness; calls for social support approach, including multidisciplinary	Further development and testing
Human Needs Assessment Scale	Lilley[102]	Likert scale of 35 human needs based on work by Yura and Walsh; modified to a 4-point scale; reliability established; evaluates importance of need	Instrument easy to use; nurses perceived patients' human needs similarly to patients' own assessment	Suggest development of nursing diagnosis and evaluation of nursing care to be based on this Human Need Model
Quality of Life Questionnaire (QLQ)	Young-Graham and Longman[103]	Likert-type brief scale: social dependency, symptom distress, behavior-morale, direction of life change; reliability established	Pilot study of patients with melanoma to test model of major hypothesized factors in quality of life	Further use in other populations; internal consistency confirmed
Derogatis Sexual Functioning Inventory (DSFI) (modified)	Blackmore[104]	Affect, body image, symptoms, drive, satisfaction, activity	Reduction in sexual activity postoperatively in orchidectomy cancer group	More research on sexuality of cancer patients

(continued)

TABLE 57-6 Tools to Measure Patient Outcomes (continued)

Tool	Author	Construct	Findings	Implications
McGill Pain Questionnaire	Camp[105]	Location, quality, pattern, increase, intensity, verbal-nonverbal symptoms; reliability established; validity established	Compared patient perceptions and nurse documentation; less than 50% of patients' pain perceptions were documented	Replication and assessment of pain management protocols
Hypercalcemia Knowledge Questionnaire (HKQ)	Coward[106]	Hypercalcemia risk factors and knowledge		Need for educational program to evaluate
Derdiarian Behavioral System Model	Derdiarian[107]	Achievement, affiliation, aggressive-protective, dependence, elimination, ingestion, restoration, sexuality; based on Johnson Behavioral Symptom Model; reliability established; validity established	Defines imbalance in behavioral subsystems caused by illness; predicts direction and quality of change; sensitive to age, site of cancer, and stage of cancer	Further studies in larger samples
Oral Assessment Guide	Eilers et al.[108]	Stomatitis or oral mucositis and mucosal changes in radiotherapy and chemotherapy patients: voice, swallow, lips, tongue, saliva, mucous membranes, gingivae, teeth, and dentures	Clinical guide to evaluate oral care protocols and toxic effects of treatment protocols and persons at risk	Further clinical use
Breast Self-Examination (BSE) Belief and Attitude Questionnaire	Lauver[109]	Remembering, competence, comfort, interference, efficacy; reliability established	Positive relationship between frequency of BSE and competence, remembering, and comfort	Replication in larger, heterogeneous population with test–retest reliability; further testing for methods to promote competence and remembering
Pain Assessment Tool (PAT) and Pain Flow Sheet (PFS)	McMillan and Williams[110]	Ongoing assessment of pain and its management	Pain intensity and level of sedation documented in 2-group study	Further research with both tools
Self-care and Symptom Report Interview	Rhodes et al.[111]	Symptom distress, self-care activities, coping strategies regarding fatigue and weakness; based on Orem's self-care deficit theory	Lays foundation for tool to measure symptom occurrence and distress and to assess self-care efficacy	Ongoing development and testing
Linear Analogue Modification (LAM) of Profile of Mood States (POMS)	Sutherland et al.[112]	Emotional distress; fatigue, anxiety, confusion, depression, energy, anger	Significant correlation between LAM and POMS in 29 subjects	To evaluate patients' ongoing emotional status as base for psychosocial interventions over time
Cancer Knowledge Test	Weinrich and Weinrich[113]	Belief in cancer myths, recall of American Cancer Society 7 warning signals, recognition of disease symptoms	Overall significant difference in cancer knowledge based on race, education, and income	Evaluation of health teaching on elderly, less educated, and low-income black persons
Champion's Instrument and Williams's Breast Inventory	Williams[114]	Likert scale of 5 constructs of Health Belief Model, health history, and personal knowledge	Health motivation represents 18% of variance; barriers, 8%; age differences	Further testing of variables

Guidelines for care are organized, integrated schemata for practice. These presentations are readily identifiable by title descriptors such as nursing care, nursing interventions, nursing implications, the nursing role, nursing assessments, nursing management, and nursing plans for a variety of patient problems, specialized treatments, or situations. In most cases, guidelines are in tabular format, resembling the traditional nursing care plan (problem, care, scientific rationale) with updated language such as nursing diagnoses, nursing etiology, nursing interventions, and nursing evaluations by outcome criteria.

TABLE 57-7 Indicators, Predictors, and Guidelines for Quality of Care

Indicators

Hypnosis for pain management in children[174]
Self-care and chemotherapy side effects[175]
Postchemotherapy quality of life in sarcoma patients[176]
Self-care and symptom distress in HIV seropositive men[177]
Quality of life after BMT[178]
Pain and psychological distress during ABMT[179]
Restrictions and obstacles in home care[180]
Quality of life and care during biological therapy[181]
Pain in children with cancer[182]
Family caregivers' descriptions of patients' pain[183]
Support and caring[184]
Maintaining hope during BMT[185]
Quest for meaning after BMT[186–188]
Treatment effect on male fertility and sexuality[189]
Breast self-examination techniques[190]
Nursing diagnosis in an oncology population[191]
Use of topical anesthetic to reduce pain in pediatric oncology patients[192]
Spiritual health of oncology patients[193]
Patient/significant other's response to detection program[194]
Nurse knowledge/teaching/performance of breast exams[195]
Fever patterns in neutropenic patients[121]
Psychologic model of adjustment in gynecologic cancer patients[122]
Family cancer experience[117]
Sexual and reproductive issues for women with Hodgkin's disease[123,124]
Cancer-induced hypercalcemia[125]
Primary caregiver's perception of the dying trajectory[126]
Alterations in taste during cancer treatment[127]
Family responses to cancer hospitalization[128]
Characteristics of pain in hospitalized cancer patients[129]
Sexual changes after gynecologic cancer treatment[130]
Cisplatin-related peripheral neuropathy[131]
Weakness, fatigue, and self-care abilities[111]
Suicide in cancer patients[116]
Cancer pain control behavior[132]

Predictors

Informational needs of patients receiving brachytherapy[196]
Impact of cancer pain on family caregivers[197]
Burdens of family members caring for chemotherapy patients[198]
Effect of granulocyte colony stimulating factor on quality of life[199]
Biopsychosocial effects of interleukin-2[200]
Breast cancer detection behavior[201]
Amphotericin-B-induced rigors[202]
Aerobic exercise and quality of life in women with breast cancer[203]
Life satisfaction and illness distress[204]
Protein deficiency, pressure sores, and cancer mortality[205]
Needs of home caregivers[206]
Fatigue mechanisms: tumor necrosis factor and exercise[207]
Sources of hope in chronic illness[208]
ARDS during interleukin-2 immunotherapy[209]
Precursors of cervical cancer[210]
Flushing protocols for central venous catheters[211]
Information seeking in HIV-positive homosexual/bisexual men[212]
Factors influencing successful return to workplace for cancer patients[213]
Effect of alkylating agent in acute nonlymphocytic leukemia[214]
Patterns of lung cancer dyspnea[133]
Anticipatory nausea and vomiting associated with cancer chemotherapy[119]
Patterns of hospice utilization[118]
Radiotherapy symptom profile[134]
Carotid artery rupture[135]
Colorectal cancer[136]
Glucocorticosteroid-induced depression[137]
Needs of family members of cancer patients[138]
Anticipatory nausea and vomiting[120]
Patterns of nausea, vomiting, and distress with antineoplastic drug protocols[139]

Guidelines for Care

Nursing implications for photodynamic therapy[215]
Care of patients with esophageal cancer[216]
Nursing of patients with multisystem organ failure[217]
Care of families[218]
Nursing care of irradiated skin[219]
Neurologic assessment of cerebral edema[220]
Spinal cord compression surgical care[221]
Care of patient with malignant ascites[222]
Care of patient with occult primary malignancy[223]
Care of patient with Von Hippel-Lindau disease[224]
Nursing management of cancer recurrence[225]
Documentation of chemotherapy administration and patient teaching[226]
Chemotherapy flow sheet[227]
Management of hypomagnesemia[228]
Nursing during high-dose-rate brachytherapy[229]
Diversion activity to enhance coping[230]
Home care resources for rural families[231]
Nursing of patient receiving antimitotics in chemotherapy[232]
Bereavement care[233]
Handling of antineoplastic drugs[234]
Prevention of chemotherapy-associated pneumonia in non-Hodgkin's lymphoma[140]
Primary, secondary, and tertiary interventions for lymphedema[141]
Management of disseminated intravascular coagulation[142]
Care of patients treated with intrapleural tetracycline for malignant pleural effusion[143]
The compromised host[144]
Management of venous access ports[145]
Morphine infusion for intractable cancer pain by implanted pump[146]
Care of head and neck cancer patients receiving myocutaneous flap reconstructive surgery[147]
Care of patients receiving radiation therapy for rectal cancer[148]
Care of patients receiving third-generation cephalosporins[149]
Assessment of gynecology patients[150]
Needs of the spouse of the patient with advanced cancer[151]
Care of the family with cancer[152]
Skin care during radiotherapy[153]

Table 57-7 provides a list of indicators, predictors, and assessment guidelines used in recent studies addressing quality of care.[121–153] These articles report studies of cancer-related disease and treatment problems, psychosocial adjustment, risk factors, and family response and coping.

QUALITY IN PERFORMANCE: APPLICATIONS IN PRACTICE

No discussion of care is complete without a look at process—the performance of nursing care and its meaning for both patient and nurse. Although patient outcome has become the basis for care evaluation, the multiple forces impinging on a patient's condition often make this method partially precise at best. Outcomes are relative, and frequently are only partly related to the quality of nurse performance. More often, quality is deeply embedded in the rich mutual interpretations of care and caring that constitute the nurse–patient bond. Measuring quality of care by documented patient outcome is only one aspect of the multipronged approach demanded, an important indication that evaluation must go beyond the standard.

Determining the quality of a process is tricky, and yet critical to the search for excellence. There are four important patterns to the process of giving and receiving care. The first is *mutuality*. Care behavior and the caring attitude forge a mutuality of response between two people that is characterized by reciprocity and complementarity. The experience is shared and cooperative, and the roles of caregiver and care receiver are complementary in that there is a degree of dissimilarity in the nature of the role relationship that works in a nondissonant way, allowing for harmony. However, the degree of dissimilarity is important in that the effect of care can be compromised if patient–nurse perceptions are either too much alike or radically different.

The nature of the mutual experience of caregiver and care receiver and their interacting perceptions are central to the quality of care. A growing literature focused on the congruity of nurse and patient perceptions reflects this phenomenon. In an early study by Jennings and Muhlenkamp,[154] caregivers' perceptions of their patients' affective states and the patients' self-reports of their anxiety, hostility, and depression were significantly different. Caregivers (i.e., physicians, nurses, nursing assistants) assessed patients as feeling significantly worse than patients reported feeling. Findings were interpreted in light of "Wright's requirement-of-mourning hypothesis" that caregivers may perceive patients as having negative feelings so that the caregivers' own value systems, which place emphasis on health, will be supported.[155]

In 1987, Verron et al.[156] hypothesized that attitudes of health care providers, grounded in their values, influence the quality of patient care. The authors cited work linking learning, experience, and consequent changes in attitude with positively modified behavior that endured for long periods.[157] Further, they attempted to identify and measure attitude themes pertinent to caring for oncology patients. The "Ideas About Oncology Patient Care Scale" (IAOPC) resulted, generating four attitude-related factors: therapy, future outlook, terminality, and drug use. Through repeated instrument testing, the attitudes were found to be multidimensional, another indication of the complexities of measuring human responses to caregiving and care receiving.

Larson[3,158,159] laid a foundation for unraveling the intricacies involved in giving and receiving care. She interviewed two separate samples of patients and nurses to determine what nurse behaviors were most and least important in making cancer patients feel "cared for." Her assumption was that the optimal expectation of nursing care is for patients to feel cared for as a result of nursing actions. Feeling cared for was defined as a sensation of well-being and safety linked to the behavior of the nurse. Nurses and patients were asked to rank, in order of importance, 50 nurse caring behaviors categorized by six action themes: anticipation, accessibility, explanation-facilitation, provision of comfort, establishment of trust, and monitoring with follow-through. Findings revealed that patients and nurses held very divergent opinions of what was most important. The highest-ranked behaviors reported by patients were those demonstrating competency, actions mostly concerned with monitoring and follow-through and with accessibility. Actions rated highest by nurses were more focused on meeting comfort and psychosocial needs, such as listening and touch. In an examination of the top ten responses of both groups, however, several mutual choices appeared: being quickly accessible, giving good physical care, putting the patient first, and listening. These choices indicated several important shared values.

Mayer[160] replicated Larson's study and found similar results. There was 100% agreement between samples of nurses in both studies regarding the most and least important caring behaviors. Comparisons of the two patient groups revealed 40% agreement for the most important behaviors and 80% for the least important. Across both studies and all samples, conventions of professional etiquette, such as appearance, cheerfulness, and polite social behavior, were viewed as least important. In Mayer's study, listening was again rated highest by nurses, and knowing how to give injections and intravenous infusions, and managing technical equipment remained most important to patients. Mayer concluded that patients seem to value the instrumental, technical caring skills and that nurses are more attuned to expressive caring behaviors.

These results might reflect understandable differences in perception between the two groups. Patients seemed to value those competencies and skills most concretely apparent and directly linked to their welfare. Nurses, on the other hand, may have perceived expressive and instrumental dimensions of care as inextricably connected, similar to the mutuality of care and cure. Who can deny the effect when patient preparation, technical skill, and gentleness are integrated during administration of an uncomfortable, intrusive procedure? To emphasize one aspect without the others decontextualizes care and strips it of its healing quality.

Several other comparison reports have documented discrepancies between patients' self-reports and their nurses' knowledge and understanding of patients' needs. Sodestrom and Martinson[161] found that 76% of a sample of nurses caring for hospitalized terminally ill patients considered spiritual needs low on the list of priorities because of the lack of time to incorporate spiritual assessment into care. Although the nurses correctly identified the meaning and purpose of their patient's relationship with God and the patient–nurse definitions of the term *spiritual* did not differ significantly, the nurses in this study did not view themselves as essential in meeting the spiritual needs of their terminally ill patients.

As the location of cancer care increasingly moves into the home, the concept of caregiver expands to include family members and others in charge of the patient's welfare. In light of this trend, congruence between caregiver and care recipient perceptions of quality of life was examined in 23 care dyads in a home hospice program.[162] The overall trend, although not statistically significant, was for patients to report a higher quality of life for themselves in comparison with their caregivers' assessments. Patients reported better sleeping and pain control than did caregivers, but much less fun and sexual satisfaction. Thus nurse caregivers are not alone in their struggle to interpret the patient's situation accurately.

The needs of family members as they care for their loved ones with cancer are emerging as an important dimension in quality of care. Dyck and Wright[163] found that almost half of their sample of next-of-kin said that nurses did not do anything for them as family members, nor did they expect anything. Their expectation, however, seemed to be a function of limitations in their knowledge of the role of the nurse and what was thought to be the appropriate focus—the patient. If the patient was competently cared for and the nurse kept the family accurately informed, families said they could not expect more. Yet a parallel analysis of their needs documented acceptance, support, and comfort as being very important to them. Furthermore, their rank-order of traits looked for in nurses differed depending on the stage of the patient's illness. Competence was number one in the early diagnostic stage, friendliness when the disease recurred, and compassion during the terminal stage. The authors concluded that appropriate emphasis of a trait is contextually determined and a significant way that nurses may express "caring for" patients.

The second major pattern in the caregiving and care-receiving process is *contextuality*. The contextual aspects of care have been highlighted repeatedly in these studies, with location of care and phase of illness emerging as two important determinants of the most appropriate clinical approach. Often, phenomenologic studies provide the best look at contextuality.

For example, Thorne,[117] in studying helpful and unhelpful communications in care, refers to cancer as "a modern metaphor for human confrontation with existential uncertainty." She found that communication is important in shaping the illness experience. Patients in Thorne's study were able to recall communication with health care providers during their illness and distinguish between styles that were more and less helpful. She found that the more uncertain a patient's situation, the greater was the vulnerability to communication characterized by lack of concern. On the other hand, the providers' feelings of failure, vulnerability, and hopelessness were part of the total picture as well. Nurses did not figure prominently into this compilation of opinions about helpful and unhelpful communicators, although study subjects reported that physicians communicated more about the disease and nurses provided advice about treatment and the illness. More often, a communication was perceived to be helpful if it was thought to be intentionally supportive. The most frequent unhelpful type was described as advice that was intentionally unhelpful, when the person withheld information or abused his power. Moreover, most important to the caring process was content, style, and a manner perceived by the patient as intentionally designed to be useful, encouraging, and supportive.

As a unit, these studies highlight the importance of mutuality and contextuality in determining the quality of nursing care performance. Yet two other patterns have emerged as major influences on quality of performance; these patterns are so mutually dependent that they must be considered as one: *competence and proficiency*.

Benner[164,165] says that the practical knowledge embedded in expert nursing needs to be understood and yet has not been fully elucidated. Since clinical practice involves constant interpretation and prediction based on complex, contextual information, expertise increases as the nurse becomes intuitively able to read the situation as a whole as a result of past experience. The experience of the nurse is central to proficiency, which Benner views as having five levels: novice, advanced beginner, competent nurse, proficient nurse, and expert. Experience is the vehicle by which the nurse passes through these phases.

Progress in the movement from novice to expert is reflected by three gradual changes in performance. Initially, rather than relying solely on abstract principles and procedures to guide nursing practice, the nurse acquires a personal knowledge rich in "paradigms" of various care issues. The paradigms emerge from past experience that not only challenges previously held perceptions but is powerful enough to change and refine those preconceptions and understandings. Later, as the nurse gains experience, situations are viewed holistically, with the nurse focusing only on the most relevant elements and having a deep sense of confidence in intuitive interpretations. Finally, there is full involvement in the situation as a confident, effective performer.

The fourth major pattern of the care process is *intentionality of caring.* Intentionality of caring represents the connecting pattern or matrix holding together mutuality, contextuality, and competence with proficiency. Intentionality of caring requires awareness and a determined effort to provide quality care in any setting or to facilitate others as they provide care for cancer patients. Intentionality of caring serves to enhance quality in practice by the following:

- recognizing that care is mutual—a cooperative venture between two human beings, based on a balanced complement of perceptions
- considering the context of the care environment on the basis of an understanding of the shared meaning of the circumstances
- encouraging pride in one's acquired competencies (knowledge, skills, attitudes, and traits) and having a desire to increase proficiency and become expert

Overall, intentionality of caring links the science and the art of nursing knowledge and skill. Its most overt manifestation in practice is known as clinical judgment.

CONCLUSION

Every health care provider group today is struggling with the definition, provision, and evaluation of quality care. Nursing comes to the task from a long tradition of empirically established caring skills and a more recent scientific knowledge based on clinical research.

For two decades, experts in the quality assurance field have advocated a three-dimensional approach to the quality question based on structure, process, and outcome variables and their relatedness (see Figure 57-1). Structural elements are those grounding fundamentals that provide a sense of shared purpose and criteria against which effect can be measured. The structural elements include nursing's direction, definition, education, legislation, diagnostic taxonomy, standards of practice, research and technology, and programs of peer review and quality assurance.

Process is a much more elusive phenomenon in that it represents the individualized enactment of competencies characterized by knowledge, skills, human traits, and attitudes[49] under diverse and unique environmental conditions (contextuality) where the mutuality of caregiver and care receiver is central. Process is most manifest in the intentionality of caring of the care provider and in the proficiency with which competencies are revealed. Therefore process is much more difficult to evaluate in comparison with the components of structure and outcome.

Oncology nursing has come closest to evaluating the process dimension by defining standards of performance that recognize several critical determinants of quality: continuously working to perfect the art, science, and skill of practice; participating as a contributing, valued member of the health care team; utilizing the problem-solving process in the planning, organization, and execution of care and in its evaluation through the conduct or utilization of research; and providing a health care service to patients on the basis of a host of both independent and interdependent interventions conducted in an autonomous way. The measurement of process is based generally on written documentation and periodic peer evaluation. Some attempts have been made to categorize[164] and to measure[48] proficiency, and the literature on caring as a science is expanding rapidly.

Outcome criteria have been defined in terms of patient outcomes, quality of life, and, for nursing to some degree, maximum life extension. These criteria are best represented by patient outcome standards and by a burgeoning literature focused on the quality of life of the person with cancer and his or her family. As we gain knowledge about the quality of life, the purpose of nursing as a science of caring will more clearly be understood, and will further enable us to foster, nurture, and strengthen its quality.

REFERENCES

1. Nightingale F: *Notes on Nursing.* New York: Appleton-Century-Crofts, 1859.
2. Benner P: Nursing as a caring profession. Working paper for the Academy of Nursing Annual Meeting, October 16–18, 1988, Kansas City, MO.
3. Larson P: Cancer nurses' perceptions of caring. *Cancer Nurs* 9:86–92, 1986.
4. Gaut DA: A philosophic orientation to caring. In Leininger MM (ed.): *Care: The Essence of Nursing and Health.* Thorofare, NJ: Slack, 1984, pp. 17–26.
5. Leininger MM: *Care: The Essence of Nursing.* Thorofare, NJ: Slack, 1984.
6. Watson J: *Nursing: The Philosophy and Science of Caring.* Boston: Little, Brown, 1979.
7. Dougherty CJ: *American Health Care: Realities, Rights, and Reforms.* New York: Oxford University Press, 1988.
8. President's Commission for the Study of Ethical Problems in Medicine and Biomedical and Behavioral Research: *Securing Access to Health Care,* vol. I. Washington, DC: U.S. Government Printing Office, 1983.
9. Oncology Nursing Society: Board approves revised scope of practice statement. *ONS News* 3:1–2, 1988.
10. Taylor C: *Philosophic Papers,* vols. I and II. Cambridge, Eng.: Cambridge University Press, 1985.
11. Harmer C, Henderson V: *Principles and Practices of Nursing.* New York: Macmillan, 1956.

12. Mundinger L: Nursing diagnoses for cancer patients. *Cancer Nurs* 1:221–226, 1978.
13. Herberth L, Gosnell DJ: Nursing diagnosis for oncology nursing practice. *Cancer Nurs* 10:41–51, 1987.
14. Gordon M: *Nursing Diagnoses: Process and Application.* New York: McGraw-Hill, 1982.
15. American Nurses' Association: *Nursing: A Social Policy Statement.* Kansas City, MO: The Association, 1980.
16. Beyers M: Quality: The banner of the 1980s. *Nurs Clin North Am* 23:617–623, 1988.
17. Winchester DP: The assurance of quality for the cancer patient. Paper presented at the American Cancer Society Symposium on Advances in Cancer Management. Hilton Towers, Los Angeles, CA, December 1988.
18. Garven DA: *Managing Quality: The Strategic and Competitive Edge.* New York: Free Press, 1988.
19. National Cancer Institute: Five-year survival rates. *SEER Program.* Washington, DC: U.S. Government Printing Office, 1983.
20. Henderson M: Introduction. In Roberts L (ed.): *Cancer Today: Origins, Prevention, and Treatment.* Washington, DC: National Academy of Sciences Press, 1984.
21. Oncology Nursing Society: *Outcome Standards for Cancer Nursing Practice.* Pittsburgh, PA: The Society, 1979.
22. Oncology Nursing Society and American Nurses' Association: *Standards of Oncology Nursing Practice.* Kansas City, MO: The Association, 1987.
23. American Nurses' Association: *A Plan for Implementation of Standards of Nursing Practice.* Kansas City, MO: The Association, 1979.
24. Oncology Nursing Society: *Outcome Standards for Cancer Nursing Education.* Pittsburgh, PA: The Society, 1982.
25. Oncology Nursing Society: *Cancer Patient Education.* Pittsburgh, PA: The Society, 1982.
26. Oncology Nursing Society: *Public Cancer Education.* Pittsburgh, PA: The Society, 1983.
27. Orem DE: *Nursing Concepts of Practice.* New York: McGraw-Hill, 1987.
28. Johnson DE: The behavioral system model for nursing. In Riehl JP, Roy C (eds.): *Conceptual Model for Nursing Practice* (ed. 2). New York: Appleton-Century-Crofts, 1980.
29. Donabedian A: Structure, process and outcome standards. *Am J Public Health* 59:1833, 1969.
30. Majesky SJ, Brester MH, Nishio KT: Development of a research tool: Patient indicators of nursing care. *Nurs Res* 27:365–371, 1978.
31. Scott DW: *The Research Connection: Practice, Research, Theory.* Keynote Address: American Cancer Society Nursing Research Conference, Honolulu, Hawaii, June 1985. Proceedings. Denver, American Cancer Society, 1986.
32. Brown MH, Kiss ME: Cancer audit. *Cancer Nurs* 2:1–6, 1979.
33. Legge JS, Reilly BJ: Assessing the outcomes of cancer patients in a home nursing program. *Cancer Nurs* 3:357, 1980.
34. Valencius JC, Packard R, Widiss T: The ONS-ANA Outcome Standards for Cancer Nursing Practice: Two models for implementation—Implementation of the Nutrition Standard at City of Hope National Medical Center. *Oncol Nurs Forum* 7:137–140, 1980.
35. Edlund BJ: Patient education: Determining the effectiveness of an ostomy care guide in facilitating comprehensive patient care. *Oncol Nurs Forum* 8:43–46, 1981.
36. Wood HA, Ellerhorst JM: Using site-specific nursing algorithms as an adjunct to oncology nursing guidelines. *Oncol Nurs Forum* 10:22–27, 1983.
37. Joint Commission on the Accreditation of Hospitals: *Accreditation Manual for Hospitals* (AMH/88). Chicago: The Commission, 1987.
38. Patterson CH: Standards of patient care: The Joint Commission focus on nursing quality assurance. *Nurs Clin North Am* 23:625–638, 1988.
39. Oleske DM, Otte DM, Heinze S: Development and evaluation of a system for monitoring the quality of oncology nursing care in the home setting. *Cancer Nurs* 10:190–198, 1987.
40. Stephany TM: Quality assurance for hospice programs. *Oncol Nurs Forum* 12:33–40, 1985.
41. Arenth LM: The development and validation of an Oncology Patient Classification System. *Oncol Nurs Forum* 12:17–27, 1985.
42. Dudjak LA: Radiation Therapy Nursing Care Record: A tool for documentation. *Oncol Nurs Forum* 15:763–777, 1988.
43. Gullo SM: Safe handling of antineoplastic drugs. Translating the recommendations into practice. *Oncol Nurs Forum* 15:595–601, 1988.
44. Williamson KM, Selleck CS, Turner JC, et al: Occupational health hazards for nurses: Infection. *Image* 20:48–53, 1988.
45. Williamson KM, Turner JG, Brown KC, et al: Occupational health hazards for nurses. Part II. *Image* 20:162–168, 1988.
46. Miaskowski CA, Nielsen B: A cancer nursing assessment tool. *Oncol Nurs Forum* 12:37–42, 1985.
47. Gray G, Adler D, Fleming C, et al: A clinical data base for advanced cancer patients: Implications for nursing. *Cancer Nurs* 11:77–83, 1988.
48. Moore IM, Piper B, Dodd MJ, et al: Measuring oncology nursing practice: Results from one graduate program. *Oncol Nurs Forum* 14:45–49, 1987.
49. McGee RF, Powell ML, Broadwell DC, et al: A Delphi survey of oncology nurse specialist competencies. *Oncol Nurs Forum* 14:29–34, 1987.
50. Yasko JM: A survey of oncology clinical nursing specialists. *Oncol Nurs Forum* 10:25–30, 1983.
51. Oberst MT: Priorities in cancer nursing research. *Cancer Nurs* 1:281–290, 1978.
52. Western Consortium for Cancer Nursing Research: Priorities for cancer nursing research. *Cancer Nurs* 10:319–326, 1987.
53. Satterwhite BA, Pryor AS, Harris MB: Development and evaluation of chemotherapy fact sheets. *Cancer Nurs* 3:277–284, 1980.
54. Dodd MJ, Mood DW: Chemotherapy: Helping patients to know the drugs they are receiving and their possible side effects. *Cancer Nurs* 4:311–318, 1981.
55. Dodd MJ: Self-care for side effects in cancer chemotherapy: An assessment of nursing interventions. Part II. *Cancer Nurs* 6:63–67, 1983.
56. Johnson J: The effects of a patient education course on persons with a chronic illness. *Cancer Nurs* 5:117–123, 1982.
57. Miller MW, Nygren C: Living with cancer: Coping behaviors. *Cancer Nurs* 1:297–302, 1978.
58. Marty PJ, McDermott RJ, Gold RS: An assessment of three alternative formats for promoting breast self-examination. *Cancer Nurs* 6:207–211, 1983.
59. Watson PJ: The effects of short-term postoperative

counseling on cancer/ostomy patients. *Cancer Nurs* 6:21–29, 1985.
60. Heinrich RL, Schag CC: A behavioral medicine approach to coping with cancer: A case report. *Cancer Nurs* 7:243–247, 1984.
61. Rudolf VM, Quinn KL: The practice of TSE among college men: Effectiveness of an educational program. *Oncol Nurs Forum* 15:45–48, 1988.
62. Cotanch P, Hockenberry M, Herman S: Self-hypnosis as antiemetic therapy in children receiving chemotherapy. *Oncol Nurs Forum* 12:41–46, 1985.
63. Frank JM: The effects of music therapy and guided visual imagery on chemotherapy-induced nausea and vomiting. *Oncol Nurs Forum* 12:47–52, 1985.
64. Scott DW, Donahue DC, Mastrovito RC, et al: Comparative trial of clinical relaxation and an antiemetic drug regimen in reducing chemotherapy-related nausea and vomiting. *Cancer Nurs* 9:178–187, 1986.
65. Cotanch P, Strum S: Progressive muscle relaxation as antiemetic therapy for cancer patients. *Oncol Nurs Forum* 14:33–37, 1987.
66. Parker R: The effectiveness of scalp hypothermia in preventing cyclophosphamide-induced alopecia. *Oncol Nurs Forum* 14:49–53, 1987.
67. Dudjak LA: Mouth care for mucositis due to radiation therapy. *Cancer Nurs* 10:131–140, 1987.
68. Winningham ML, MacVicar MG: The effect of aerobic exercise on patient reports of nausea. *Oncol Nurs Forum* 15:447–450, 1988.
69. Giaccone G, DiGuilio F, Morandini MP, et al: Scalp hypothermia in the prevention of doxorubicin-induced hair loss. *Cancer Nurs* 11:170–173, 1988.
70. Shell JA, Stanutz F, Grimm J: Comparison of moisture vapor permeable (MVP) dressings to conventional dressings for management of radiation skin reactions. *Oncol Nurs Forum* 13:11–16, 1986.
71. Harwood KVS, Bachur N: Evaluation of dimethylsulfoxide and local cooling as antidotes for doxorubicin extravasation in a pig model. *Oncol Nurs Forum* 14:39–44, 1987.
72. Jones PM: Indwelling central venous catheter–related infections and two different procedures of catheter care. *Cancer Nurs* 10:123–130, 1987.
73. MacGeorge L, Steeves L, Steeves RH: Comparison of the mixing and reinfusion methods of drawing blood from a Hickman catheter. *Oncol Nurs Forum* 15:335–338, 1988.
74. Petrosino B, Becker H, Christian B: Infection rates in central venous catheter dressings. *Oncol Nurs Forum* 15:709–717, 1988.
75. Beck S, Breckenridge-Patter S, Wallace S, et al: The Family High-Risk Program: Targeted cancer prevention. *Oncol Nurs Forum* 15:301–306, 1988.
76. Nieweg R, Greidanus J, de Vries EGE: A patient education program for a continuous infusion regimen on an outpatient basis. *Cancer Nurs* 10:177–182, 1987.
77. Lane CA, Davis AW: Implementation: We Can Weekend in the rural setting. *Cancer Nurs* 8:323–328, 1985.
78. Fredette S, La F, Beattie HM: Living with cancer: A patient education program. *Cancer Nurs* 9:308–316, 1986.
79. Cawley MM, Gerdts EK: Establishing a cancer caregiver's program: An interdisciplinary approach. *Cancer Nurs* 11:266–273, 1988.
80. Diekmann JM: An evaluation of selected "I Can Cope" programs by registered participants. *Cancer Nurs* 11:274–282, 1988.
81. Mosely JR, Logan SJ, Tolle SW, et al: Developing a bereavement program in a university hospital setting. *Oncol Nurs Forum* 15:151–155, 1988.
82. Coyle N, Monzillo E, Loscalzo M, et al: A model for continuity of care for cancer patients with pain and neuro-oncologic complications. *Cancer Nurs* 8:111–119, 1985.
83. Coyle N, Mauskop A, Maggard J, et al: Continuous SC infusions of opiates for cancer patients with pain. *Oncol Nurs Forum* 13:53–57, 1986.
84. Ferrell BR, Wenzl C, Wisdom C: Evolution and evaluation of a pain management team. *Oncol Nurs Forum* 15:285–289, 1988.
85. Kane NE, Lehman ME, Drugger R, et al: Use of patient-controlled anesthesia in surgical oncology patients. *Oncol Nurs Forum* 15:29–32, 1988.
86. Konstantinides NI: Home parenteral nutrition: A viable alternative for patients with cancer. *Oncol Nurs Forum* 12:23–29, 1985.
87. Clark M: A day hospital for cancer patients: Clinical and economic feasibility. *Oncol Nurs Forum* 13:41–45, 1986.
88. Pluth NM: A home transfusion program. *Oncol Nurs Forum* 14:43–46, 1987.
89. Lewis PM: Implementing practice and organizational models. *Cancer Nurs* 8:75–78, 1985 (suppl. 1).
90. Hartshorn JC: Research-based practice: The need for, use and reporting of instrument reliability and validity. *Heart Lung* 16:100–101, 1987.
91. Duffy ME: Research in practice: The time has come. *Nurs Health Care* 6:127, 1985.
92. Lynn MR: Reliability estimates: Use and disuse. *Nurs Res* 34:254–256, 1985.
93. Nunally JC: *Psychometric Theory.* New York: McGraw-Hill, 1978.
94. Frank-Stromborg M (ed.): *Instruments for Clinical Nursing Research.* Norwalk, CT: Appleton & Lange, 1988.
95. Ferrans C, Powers M: Quality of Life Index: Development and psychometric properties. *Adv Nurs Sci* 8:15, 1985.
96. Kobashi-Shoot JAM, Gerrit JFPH, Frits SAM et al: Assessment of malaise in cancer patients treated with radiotherapy. *Cancer Nurs* 8:306–313, 1985.
97. Padilla G, Grant M: Quality of life as a cancer nursing outcome variable. *Adv Nurs Sci* 8:45, 1985.
98. Hopkins MB: Information seeking and adaptational outcomes in women receiving chemotherapy for breast cancer. *Cancer Nurs* 9:256–262, 1986.
99. Waterhouse J, Metcalf MC: Development of the sexual adjustment questionnaire. *Oncol Nurs Forum* 13:53–59, 1986.
100. Derdiarian AK: Informational needs of recently diagnosed cancer patients. *Cancer Nurs* 10:156–163, 1987.
101. Fleming C, Scanlon C, D'Agostino NS: Patient care needs survey. *Cancer Nurs* 10:237–243, 1987.
102. Lilley LL: Human need fulfillment alteration in the client with uterine cancer: The registered nurse's perception versus the client's perception. *Cancer Nurs* 10:327–337, 1987.
103. Young-Graham K, Longman AJ: Quality of life and persons with melanoma: Preliminary model testing. *Cancer Nurs* 10:338–346, 1987.
104. Blackmore C: The impact of orchidectomy upon the sexuality of the man with testicular cancer. *Cancer Nurs* 11:33–40, 1988.

105. Camp LD: A comparison of nurses' recorded assessments of pain with perceptions of pain as described by cancer patients. *Cancer Nurs* 11:237–243, 1988.
106. Coward DD: Hypercalcemia knowledge assessment in patients at risk of developing cancer-induced hypercalcemia. *Oncol Nurs Forum* 15:471–476, 1988.
107. Derdiarian AK: Derdiarian Behavioral System Model (DBSM). *Scholarly Inquiry for Nursing Practice* 2(2):103–121, 1988.
108. Eilers J, Berger AM, Petersen MC: Development, testing and application of the oral assessment guide. *Oncol Nurs Forum* 15:325–330, 1988.
109. Lauver D: Development of a questionnaire to measure beliefs and attitudes about breast self-examination. *Cancer Nurs* 11:51–57, 1988.
110. McMillan SC, Williams FA, Chatfield R, et al: Validity and reliability study of two tools for assessing and managing cancer pain. *Oncol Nurs Forum* 15:735–741, 1988.
111. Rhodes VA, Watson PM, Hanson BM: Patients' descriptions of the influence of tiredness and weakness on self-care abilities. *Cancer Nurs* 11:186–194, 1988.
112. Sutherland HJ, Walker P, Till JE: The development of a method for determining oncology patients' emotional distress using linear analogue scales. *Cancer Nurs* 11:303–308, 1988.
113. Weinrich SP, Weinrich MC: Cancer knowledge among elderly individuals. *Cancer Nurs* 9:301–307, 1987.
114. Williams RD: Factors affecting practice of BSE in older women. *Oncol Nurs Forum* 15:611–616, 1988.
115. Ammon-Gaberson KB, Piantanida M: Generating results from qualitative data. *Image* 20:159–161, 1988.
116. Saunders JM, Valente SM: Cancer and suicide. *Oncol Nurs Forum* 15:575–581, 1988.
117. Thorne SE: Helpful and unhelpful communications in cancer care: The patient perspective. *Oncol Nurs Forum* 15:167–172, 1988.
118. Hays JC: Patient symptoms and family coping. *Cancer Nurs* 9:317–325, 1986.
119. Duigon A: Anticipatory nausea and vomiting associated with cancer chemotherapy. *Oncol Nurs Forum* 13:35–40, 1986.
120. Coons HL, Leventhal H, Nerenz DR, et al: Anticipatory nausea and emotional distress in patients receiving cisplatin-based chemotherapy. *Oncol Nurs Forum* 14:31–35, 1987.
121. Henschel L: Fever patterns in the neutropenic patient. *Cancer Nurs* 8:301–305, 1985.
122. Krouse HJ: A psychological model of adjustment in gynecologic cancer patients. *Oncol Nurs Forum* 12:45–49, 1985.
123. Cooley ME, Cobb SC: Sexual and reproductive issues for women with Hodgkin's disease. I. Overview of issues. *Cancer Nurs* 9:188–193, 1986.
124. Cooley ME, Yeoman AC, Cobb SC: Sexual and reproductive issues for women with Hodgkin's disease: Application of PLISSIT Model. *Cancer Nurs* 9:248–255, 1986.
125. Coward DD: Cancer-induced hypercalcemia. *Cancer Nurs* 9:125–132, 1986.
126. Holing EV: The primary caregiver's perception of the dying trajectory: An exploratory study. *Cancer Nurs* 9:29–37, 1986.
127. Huldij A, Giesbers A, Poelhuis EHK, et al: Alterations in taste appreciation in cancer patients during treatment. *Cancer Nurs* 9:38–42, 1986.
128. Lovejoy N: Family responses to cancer hospitalization. *Oncol Nurs Forum* 13:33–37, 1986.
129. Donovan MI, Dillon P: Incidence and characteristics of pain in a sample of hospitalized cancer patients. *Cancer Nurs* 10:85–92, 1987.
130. Jenkins B: Patients' reports of sexual changes after treatment for gynecological cancer. *Oncol Nurs Forum* 15:349–354, 1988.
131. Ostchega Y, Donahue M, Fox N: High-dose cisplatin-related peripheral neuropathy. *Cancer Nurs* 11:23–32, 1988.
132. Wilkie D, Lovejoy N, Dodd M, et al: Cancer pain control behaviors: Description and correlation with pain intensity. *Oncol Nurs Forum* 15:723–731, 1988.
133. Brown ML, Carrieri V, Janson-Bjerklie S, et al: Lung cancer and dyspnea: The patient's perception. *Oncol Nurs Forum* 13:19–24, 1986.
134. King KB, Nail LM, Kreamer K, et al: Patients' descriptions of the experience of receiving radiotherapy. *Oncol Nurs Forum* 12:55–61, 1986.
135. Lesage C: Carotid artery rupture: Prediction, prevention, preparation. *Cancer Nurs* 9:1–7, 1986.
136. Messner RL, Gardner SS, Webb DD: Early detection: The priority in colorectal cancer. *Cancer Nurs* 9:8–14, 1986.
137. Post-White J: Glucocorticosteroid-induced depression in the patient with leukemia or lymphoma. *Cancer Nurs* 9:15–22, 1986.
138. Tringali CA: The needs of family members of cancer patients. *Oncol Nurs Forum* 13:65–70, 1986.
139. Rhodes VA, Watson PM, Johnson MH, et al: Patterns of nausea, vomiting and distress in patients receiving antineoplastic drug protocols. *Oncol Nurs Forum* 14:35–44, 1987.
140. Foote M: Nursing care of the patient with non-Hodgkin's lymphoma: Prevention of pneumonia associated with combination chemotherapy. *Cancer Nurs* 8:263–271, 1985.
141. Getz DH: The primary, secondary and tertiary nursing interventions of lymphedema. *Cancer Nurs* 8:177–184, 1985.
142. Rooney A, Haviley C: Nursing management of disseminated intravascular coagulation. *Oncol Nurs Forum* 12:15–22, 1985.
143. Rossetti AC: Nursing care of patients treated with intrapleural tetracycline for control of malignant pleural effusion. *Cancer Nurs* 8:103–109, 1985.
144. Gurevich I, Tafuro P: The compromised host: Deficit-specific infection in the spectrum of prevention. *Cancer Nurs* 9:263–275, 1986.
145. Moore CL, Erickson KA, Yanes LB, et al: Nursing care and management of venous access ports. *Oncol Nurs Forum* 13:35–39, 1986.
146. Paice JA: Intrathecal morphine infusion for intractable cancer pain: A new use for implanted pumps. *Oncol Nurs Forum* 13:41–47, 1986.
147. Rodzwic D, Donnard J: The use of myocutaneous flaps in reconstructive surgery for head and neck cancer: Guidelines for nursing care. *Oncol Nurs Forum* 13:29, 1986.
148. Hassay KM: Radiation therapy for rectal cancer and the implications for nursing. *Cancer Nurs* 10:311–318, 1987.
149. Link DL: Antibiotic therapy in the cancer patient: Focus on third generation cephalosporins. *Oncol Nurs Forum* 14:35–41, 1987.

150. Moreland BJ: A nursing form for gynecology patient assessment. *Oncol Nurs Forum* 14:19–23, 1987.
151. Stetz KM: Caregiving demands during advanced cancer: The spouse's needs. *Cancer Nurs* 10:260–268, 1987.
152. Lewandowski W, Jones SL: The family with cancer: Nursing intervention throughout the course of living with cancer. *Cancer Nurs* 11:313–321, 1988.
153. Strohl RA: The nursing role in radiation oncology: Symptom management of acute and chronic reactions. *Oncol Nurs Forum* 15:429–434, 1988.
154. Jennings BM, Muhlenkamp AF: Systematic misperception: Oncology patients' self-reported affective states and their care-givers' perceptions. *Cancer Nurs* 4:485–489, 1981.
155. Wright BA: *Physical Disability: A Psychological Approach.* New York: Harper & Row, 1960.
156. Verron JA, Longman A, Clark M: Development of a scale to measure undergraduate students' attitudes about caring for patients with cancer. *Oncol Nurs Forum* 14:51–55, 1987.
157. Robb S: Attitudes and intentions of baccalaureate nursing students toward the elderly. *Nurs Res* 28:43–50, 1979.
158. Larson P: Important nurse caring behaviors perceived by patients with cancer. *Oncol Nurs Forum* 11:46–50, 1984.
159. Larson P: Comparison of cancer patients' and professional nurses' perceptions of important nurse caring behaviors. *Heart Lung* 16:187–192, 1987.
160. Mayer DK: Oncology nurses' versus cancer patients' perceptions of nursing care behaviors: A replication study. *Oncol Nurs Forum* 14:48–52, 1987.
161. Sodestrom KE, Martinson IM: Patients' spiritual coping strategies: A study of nurse and patient perspectives. *Oncol Nurs Forum* 14:41–46, 1987.
162. Curtis AE, Fernsler JI: Quality of life of oncology hospice patients: A comparison of patient and primary caregiver reports. *Oncol Nurs Forum* 16:49–53, 1989.
163. Dyck S, Wright K: Family perceptions: The role of the nurse throughout an adult's cancer experience. *Oncol Nurs Forum* 12:53–56, 1985.
164. Benner P: *From Novice to Expert: Excellence and Power in Clinical Nursing Practice.* Menlo Park, CA: Addison-Wesley, 1984.
165. Benner P, Wrubel J: *The Primacy of Caring: Stress and Coping in Health and Illness.* Menlo Park, CA: Addison-Wesley, 1989.
166. Coleman EA, Riley MB, Fields F, Prior B: Efficacy of breast self-examination teaching methods among older women. *Oncol Nurs Forum* 18:561–566, 1991.
167. Hagopian GA: The effects of a weekly radiation therapy newsletter on patients. *Oncol Nurs Forum* 18:1199–1203, 1991.
168. Beck SL: The therapeutic use of music for cancer-related pain. *Oncol Nurs Forum* 18:1327–1337, 1991.
169. Broome ME, Lillis PP, McGahee TW, Bates T: The use of distraction and imagery with children during painful procedures. *Oncol Nurs Forum* 19:499–502, 1992.
170. Shivnan JC, McGuire D, Freedman S, et al: A comparison of transparent adherent and dry sterile gauze dressings for long-term central catheters in patients undergoing bone marrow transplant. *Oncol Nurs Forum* 18:1349–1356, 1991.
171. Yeoman A, Davitt M, Peters CA, et al: Efficacy of chlorhexidene gluconate use in the prevention of perirectal infections in patients with acute leukemia. *Oncol Nurs Forum* 18:1207–1213, 1991.
172. Pillon LR, Joannides G: An 11-year evaluation of a Living with Cancer program. *Oncol Nurs Forum* 18:707–711, 1991.
173. Long MC, Ovaska M: Comparative study of nursing protocols for venous access ports. *Cancer Nurs* 15:18–21, 1992.
174. Valente SM: Using hypnosis with children for pain management. *Oncol Nurs Forum* 18:699–704, 1991.
175. Nail LM, Jones LS, Greene D, et al: Use and perceived efficacy of self-care activities in patients receiving chemotherapy. *Oncol Nurs Forum* 18:883–887, 1991.
176. Arzouman JMR, Dudas S, Ferrans CE, Holm D: Quality of life of patients with sarcoma postchemotherapy. *Oncol Nurs Forum* 18:889–894, 1991.
177. Lovejoy NC, Paul S, Freeman E, Christianson B: Potential correlates of self-care and symptom distress in homosexual/bisexual men who are HIV seropositive. *Oncol Nurs Forum* 18:1175–1185, 1991.
178. Belec RH: Quality of life: Perceptions of long-term survivors of bone marrow transplantation. *Oncol Nurs Forum* 19:31–37, 1992.
179. Gaston-Johansson F, Franco T, Zimmerman L: Pain and psychological distress in patients undergoing autologous bone marrow transplantation. *Oncol Nurs Forum* 19:41–48, 1992.
180. Maloney CH, Preston F: An overview of home care for patients with cancer. *Oncol Nurs Forum* 19:75–80, 1992.
181. Rieker PP, Clark EJ, Fogelberg PR: Perceptions of quality of life and quality of care for patients with cancer receiving biological therapy. *Oncol Nurs Forum* 19:433–440, 1992.
182. Sutters KA, Miaskowski C: The problem of pain in children with cancer: A research review. *Oncol Nurs Forum* 19:465–471, 1992.
183. Ferrell BR, Cohen MZ, Rhiner M, Rozek A: Pain as a metaphor for illness. Part II: Family caregivers' management of pain. *Oncol Nurs Forum* 18:1315–1321, 1991.
184. O'Berle K, Davies B: Support and caring: Exploring the concepts. *Oncol Nurs Forum* 19:763–767, 1992.
185. Ersek M: The process of maintaining hope in adults undergoing bone marrow transplantation for leukemia. *Oncol Nurs Forum* 19:883–889, 1992.
186. Steeves RH: Patients who have undergone bone marrow transplantation: Their quest for meaning. *Oncol Nurs Forum* 19:899–905, 1992.
187. Ferrell B, Grant M, Schmidt GM, et al: The meaning of quality of life for bone marrow transplant survivors. Part 1: The impact of bone marrow transplant on quality of life. *Cancer Nurs* 15:153–160, 1992.
188. Ferrell B, Grant M, Schmidt GM, et al: The meaning of quality of life for bone marrow transplant survivors. Part 2: Improving quality of life for bone marrow transplant survivors. *Cancer Nurs* 15:247–253, 1992.
189. Smith DB, Babaian RJ: The effects of treatment for cancer on male fertility and sexuality. *Cancer Nurs* 15:271–275, 1992.
190. Murali ME, Crabtree K: Comparison of two breast self-examination palpation techniques. *Cancer Nurs* 15:276–282, 1992.
191. MacAvoy S, Moritz D: Nursing diagnoses in an oncology population. *Cancer Nurs* 15:264–270, 1992.
192. Zappa SC, Nabors SB: Use of ethyl chloride topical anesthetic to reduce procedural pain in pediatric oncology patients. *Cancer Nurs* 15:130–136, 1992.

193. Highfield MF: Spiritual health of oncology patients. Nurse and patient perspectives. *Cancer Nurs* 15:1–8, 1992.
194. Vranicar-Lapka D, Barbour-Randall L, Trippon M, et al: Oncology patients' and their significant others' responses to a proposed cancer prevention/detection program. *Cancer Nurs* 15:47–53, 1992.
195. Ludwick R: Registered nurses' knowledge and practices of teaching and performing breast exams among elderly women. *Cancer Nurs* 15:61–67, 1992.
196. Brandt B: Informational needs and selected variables in patients receiving brachytherapy. *Oncol Nurs Forum* 18:1221–1229, 1991.
197. Ferrell BR, Rhiner M, Cohen MZ, Grant M: Pain as a metaphor for illness. Part I: Impact of cancer pain on family caregivers. *Oncol Nurs Forum* 18:1303–1309, 1991.
198. Carey PJ, Oberst MT, McCubbin MA, Hughes SH: Appraisal of caregiving burden in family members caring for patients receiving chemotherapy. *Oncol Nurs Forum* 18:1341–1348, 1991.
199. Fazio MT, Glaspy JA: The impact of granulocyte colony-stimulating factor on quality of life in patients with severe chronic neutropenia. *Oncol Nurs Forum* 18:1411–1414, 1991.
200. Jackson BS, Strauman J, Frederickson K, Strauman TJ: Long-term biopsychosocial effects of interleukin-2 therapy. *Oncol Nurs Forum* 18:683–690, 1991.
201. Champion VL: The relationship of selected variables to breast cancer detection in women 35 and older. *Oncol Nurs Forum* 18:733–739, 1991.
202. Carney-Gersten P, Giuffre M, Levy D: Factors related to Amphotericin-B-induced rigors (shivering). *Oncol Nurs Forum* 18:745–750, 1991.
203. Young-McCaughan S, Sexton DL: A retrospective investigation of the relationship between aerobic exercise and quality of life in women with breast cancer. *Oncol Nurs Forum* 18:751–757, 1991.
204. Coward DD: Self-transcendence and emotional well-being in women with advanced breast cancer. *Oncol Nurs Forum* 18:857–863, 1991.
205. Waltman NL, Bergstrom N, Armstrong N, et al: Nutritional status, pressure sores and mortality in elderly patients with cancer. *Oncol Nurs Forum* 18:867–873, 1991.
206. Hileman JW, Lackey NR, Hassanein RS: Identifying the needs of home caregivers of patients with cancer. *Oncol Nurs Forum* 19:771–777, 1992.
207. St. Pierre BA, Kasper CE, Lindsey AM: Fatigue mechanisms in patients with cancer. Effects of tumor necrosis factor and exercise on skeletal muscle. *Oncol Nurs Forum* 19:419–425, 1992.
208. Raleigh EDH: Sources of hope in chronic illness. *Oncol Nurs Forum* 19:443–448, 1992.
209. Farrell MM: The challenge of Adult Respiratory Distress Syndrome during interleukin-2 immunotherapy. *Oncol Nurs Forum* 19:475–480, 1992.
210. Yoder L, Rubin M: The epidemiology of cervical cancer and its precursors. *Oncol Nurs Forum* 19:485–493, 1992.
211. Kelly C, Dumenko L, McGregor SE, McHutchion ME: A change in flushing protocols of central venous catheters. *Oncol Nurs Forum* 19:599–605, 1992.
212. Lovejoy NC, Morgenrath BN, Paul S, et al: Potential predictors of information seeking behavior by homosexual/bisexual (gay) men with a human immunodeficiency virus seropositive health status. *Cancer Nurs* 15:116–124, 1992.
213. Berry DL, Catanzaro M: Persons with cancer and their return to the workplace. *Cancer Nurs* 15:40–46, 1992.
214. Uhlenhopp MB: An overview of the relationship between alkylating agents and therapy-related acute nonlymphocytic leukemia. *Cancer Nurs* 15:9–17, 1992.
215. Dachowski LJ, DeLaney TF: Photodynamic Therapy: The NCI experience and its nursing implication. *Oncol Nurs Forum* 19:63–67, 1992.
216. Held JL, Peahota A: Nursing care of patients with esophageal cancer. *Oncol Nurs Forum* 19:627–634, 1992.
217. McFadden ME, Sartorius SE: Multiple system organ failure in patients with cancer. Part II: Nursing implications. *Oncol Nurs Forum* 19:727–737, 1992.
218. Jassack PF: Families: An essential element in the care of the patient with cancer. *Oncol Nurs Forum* 19:871–876, 1992.
219. Sitton E: Early and late radiation-induced skin alterations: Part II: Nursing care of irradiated skin. *Oncol Nurs Forum* 19:907–912, 1992.
220. Saba MT, Magolan JM: Understanding cerebral edema: Implications for oncology nurses. *Oncol Nurs Forum* 18:499–505, 1991.
221. Dyck S: Surgical instrumentation as a palliative treatment for spinal cord compression. *Oncol Nurs Forum* 18:515–521, 1991.
222. Kehoe C: Malignant ascites: Etiology, diagnosis and treatment. *Oncol Nurs Forum* 18:523–530, 1991.
223. Yeomans AC, Washington JB. Occult primary malignancies. *Oncol Nurs Forum* 18:539–544, 1991.
224. Martz CH: Von Hippel-Lindau Disease: A genetic condition predisposing tumor formation. *Oncol Nurs Forum* 18:545–551, 1991.
225. Mahon SM: Managing the psychosocial consequences of cancer recurrence: Implications for nurses. *Oncol Nurs Forum* 18:577–583, 1991.
226. Lynch M, Yanes L: Flowsheet documentation of chemotherapy administration and patient teaching. *Oncol Nurs Forum* 18:777–783, 1991.
227. Moore JM, Knobf MT: A Nursing Flow Sheet for documentation of ambulatory oncology. *Oncol Nurs Forum* 18:933–939, 1991.
228. McDermott KC, Almadrones LA, Bijorunas DR: The diagnosis and management of hypomagnesemia: A unique treatment approach and case report. *Oncol Nurs Forum* 18:1145–1152, 1991.
229. Jordan LN, Mantravadi RVP: Nursing care of the patient receiving high-dose-rate brachytherapy. *Oncol Nurs Forum* 18:1167–1171, 1991.
230. Radziewicz RM, Schneider SM: Using diversional activity to enhance coping. *Cancer Nurs* 15:293–298, 1992.
231. Buehler JA, Lee HJ: Exploration of home care resources for rural families with cancer. *Cancer Nurs* 15:299–308, 1992.
232. Lobert S: Antimitotics in cancer chemotherapy. *Cancer Nurs* 15:22–33, 1992.
233. Cooley ME: Bereavement care. A role for nurses. *Cancer Nurs* 15:125–129, 1992.
234. Valanis B, McNeil V, Driscoll K: Staff members' compliance with their facility's antineoplastic drug handling policy. *Oncol Nurs Forum* 18:571–576, 1991.

Chapter 58

Cancer Economics

Arlene E. Fleck RN, MNEd

INTRODUCTION

In the past, the ability to apply clinical expertise to solve patient care problems was the major focus of the cancer nurse specialist. However, in today's health care arena the challenge is to integrate this clinical expertise and apply it in a cost-effective manner, that is, balancing cost requirements and standards of excellence.

Cancer care is rapidly changing because of new technology, innovative therapy, and current economic and health care policy issues. Nurses specializing in oncology must be prepared to adapt to this constant change. This chapter will explore the economic environment, which is a major influencing factor in the practice of oncology nursing. The discussion begins with a review of basic economic theory and the historical and current issues that have an impact on health care economics. The remainder of the chapter emphasizes how these economic changes are affecting cancer care.

SCOPE OF THE PROBLEM

Since the early 1980s, revolutionary changes have occurred in the health care economics of this country. Before that time, the word *economics* did not have the strong association with health care that it does today. In today's health care environment, nurses are affected daily by economic issues: cost justification, *more* does not mean *better,* limited access to care, quality versus cost, and lack of resources, just to name a few. These issues represent dramatic changes introduced when expenditures on health care reached 9.4% of the U.S. gross national product (GNP), or $147 billion, in 1982; this figure was in sharp contrast to the 1960 health care expenditures, which were only 4.5% of the GNP. The United States currently devotes 12.3% of GNP to health care. Medical costs, for the federal government, have become the fastest-growing major budget item, increasing at an annual rate of 8% at a time when the U.S. inflation rate is only about 5%.[1] At this pace, within 20 years Americans will be spending a third of their resources on medical care. It has been estimated that health care will account for 17%–18% of the GNP by the turn of the century. These rising costs are being scrutinized by government officials, who are continually trying to trim the federal budget, and by business leaders and consumers as well. Pressure by these groups has been applied to constrain the use of health care resources. To accomplish the task of meeting the demands of the public, nurses and other health care professionals must continue to deliver quality, cost-effective patient care, doing more with less.

ECONOMICS THEORY

In the past, economics was not a popular elective course among student nurses, nor was there a demand for the ability to apply economic principles to the health care field. However, with the current major emphasis on the high costs of health care and national health policy changes, an introduction to economics could become not only beneficial but also essential. Because of the increasing scarcity of health care resources in the 1990s, the need to understand economic issues has become more critical. The ability to analyze economic issues could provide important insights into the operation of health care systems and the evaluation of health care policies.

Economics is the science that deals with the production, distribution, and consumption of wealth or resources and the consequence of resource scarcity. Economics describes, explains, and evaluates the problems that contribute to resource scarcity.[2] In simple words, economics is the study of supply and demand. Figure 58-1[3] illustrates a normal, or balanced, economic environment. Two parties are involved in the exchange of money. One party, the supplier, provides the good or service to the other party, the consumer. The consumer is responsible for the demand for the goods or services. Pricing is established to balance the supply of and demand for goods and services, making for an important equilibrium:

Supply = Demand
and
Demand = Supply

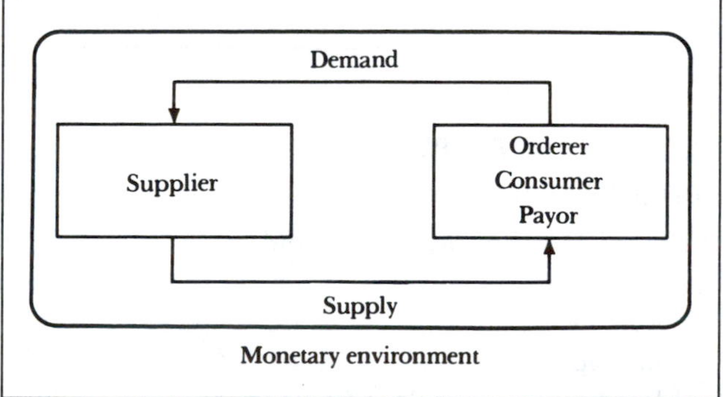

FIGURE 58-1 Normal economic environment. In a normal economic environment, there are essentially two parties—supplier and consumer (also referred to as payer and orderer). The former supplies goods and services, the latter demands goods and services. Money, or the promise of it, is exchanged between the two parties, thus establishing a market price for the goods and services. (Source: Ward WJ Jr: *An Introduction to Health Care Financial Management.* Baltimore, MD: National Health Publishing, 1988, p. 5.)

The ability of price to act as a balance mechanism between the supply of and demand for a good or service is referred to as *price elasticity* or *price sensitivity*. This concept is illustrated in Figure 58-2. When the price of a good or a service falls, the quantity demanded will rise.

The significance of the law of supply and demand is readily apparent in health care of the late 1960s and early 1970s. For employed Americans, health insurance coverage was a standard part of virtually every employee benefit package; most Americans believed health care services to be their "right," not a privilege. The cost for health care was not an issue, since only insurance companies saw the bill or charges. The ready access to health care coverage as an employee benefit often encouraged indiscriminate use of high-cost services. The prevailing attitude was that of getting the best and most sophisticated care regardless of cost. This health care behavior caused costs to spiral. Persons who were unemployed or retired, and who therefore lacked employer health care insurance coverage, were often eligible for federal health insurance programs (i.e., Medicare or Medicaid). The method of federal payment for services was retrospective and cost-based. Hospitals were reimbursed by the government for their costs of treating patients, after the treatment and care was delivered. The incentive for hospitals (where 70% of all Medicare dollars were spent[4]) was to spend as much money as possible on the care of each patient. The more money a hospital spent, the more the government paid. This system of payment for services provided resulted in overutilization of resources, extended hospitalization, duplication of equipment, and more treatments and diagnostic tests prescribed than were actually necessary.

The health care economic environment of the late 1960s and early 1970s is depicted in Figure 58-3, which illustrates why problems arose in the U.S. health care economic system.[3] Because neither the consumer, the physician, nor the health care professional was concerned with the price of the goods or services, the demand became unlimited. Consumers came to expect a health care system that provided everything possible. Physicians, nurses, and other health care professionals continued to use all available technology and resources to care for the patient, often in excess of what was required. The increased number of malpractice lawsuits led physicians to practice defensive medicine, ordering more tests than usual and thereby driving costs up. Moreover, costs rose because people were living longer and thus contributing to the increasing number of elderly citizens, many with chronic health care needs. Thus in the 1980s, there was a resultant demand for more health care resources than could be satisfied.

To address and sustain these increasing demands Congress enacted two laws. The first law, introduced in August 1982, was the Tax Equity and Fiscal Responsibility Act (TEFRA). This introduced a change in the manner of providing inpatient services for Medicare beneficiaries, from a retrospective, cost-based payment system to a prospective payment system. Then in 1989, the Omnibus Budget Reconciliation Act instituted the Resource-Based Relative Value Scale (RBRVS), which set a timetable for the elimination of the customary/reasonable charge–based system for physician services under Medicare Part B.

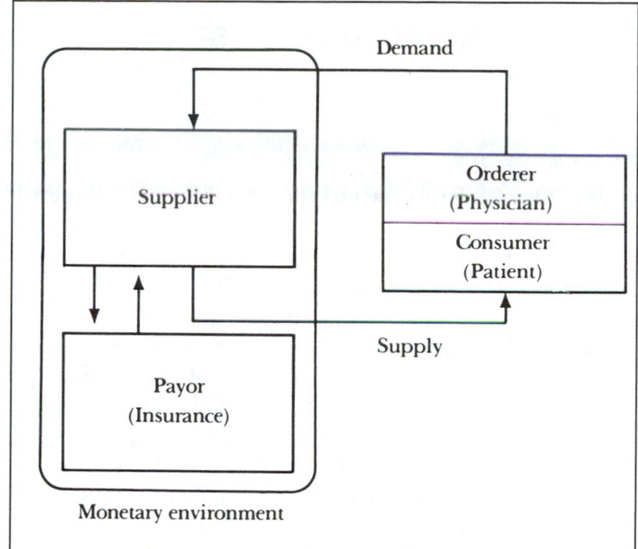

FIGURE 58-3 Health care economic environment. The economic environment as applied to health care is significantly different than in other areas of the economy. There are now four parties instead of two, and the supply of and demand for health care services no longer include the payer for those services. Because the monetary environment does not include the orderer (consumer), price is unable to establish a balance between supply and demand. (Source: Ward WJ Jr: *An Introduction to Health Care Financial Management.* Baltimore, MD: National Health Publishing, 1988, p. 8.)

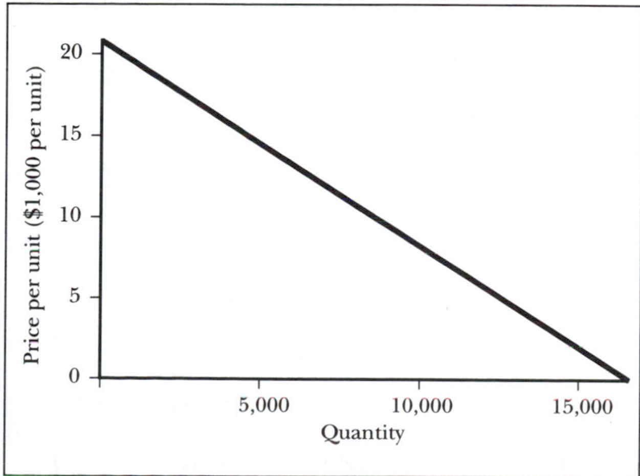

FIGURE 58-2 Price sensitivity. As the price for goods and services goes down, the demand goes up.

PROSPECTIVE PAYMENT SYSTEM

History

The Prospective Payment System (PPS) was signed into Public Law 98-21 as part of the Social Security Amendment of 1983. This system reimburses hospitals with a fixed payment based on the complexity of the problems that precipitated during the patient's hospitalization. The exact amount is determined by using one or more of the 492* diagnostic related groups (DRGs). Each DRG is assigned a specific, fixed cost, for which the hospital is reimbursed regardless of the actual cost of the patient's care. The individual DRGs originally were developed by a group of researchers at Yale University as a hospital management tool; they were adapted for use as a federal payment system after being field-tested in New Jersey. In the pilot study, the major factor observed was the number of days a patient stayed in the hospital.[5] It was hypothesized that if the number of days a patient stayed in the hospital was decreased, the overall hospital bill would decrease. By 1982, all acute care hospitals in New Jersey were reimbursed according to the PPS; a 6% reduction compared to national hospital costs was observed.[6]

To help standardize hospital costs throughout the country, researchers assigned a specific weight to each DRG. This weighting factor reflects the estimated relative costs of hospital resources used (i.e., laboratory tests, medications, medical and surgical supplies, room, ancillary services) per patient discharge. The principal sources of data to compile the cost weights originally were based on the Medicare cost reports for 1981 and a national representative sample of inpatient Medicare claims.

The Health Care Financing Administration (HCFA), an agency of the federal government, now assigns the appropriate weighting factor for each DRG. An average standardized cost for each of the original 468 DRGs was developed from the cost data received; the statistical method of regression was used to establish a variance for each DRG. It can be estimated statistically that 95% of the patients assigned to a specific DRG actually will incur the cost allocated within the parameter of the DRG.[7]

This system was integrated gradually over the first 5 years following its inception (1983–1987); hospitals were reimbursed for each discharge at a prospective payment rate that was a blend of national and regional data and the respective hospital's historic cost per case. The current method for determining payment rates for each DRG is no longer based on the individual hospital's costs but rather on a national standardized payment amount, which differs according to hospital location. Location classification categories include: *large urban area* (a metropolitan statistical area, or MSA, with a population of over 1 million); *other urban area* (an MSA with a population of 1 million or fewer); and *rural area* (outside of any MSA).

*In 1982, when DRGs were first used in hospitals, there were 470 of them. As the need for other DRGs was established, the number increased. In 1992 there were 492 DRGs; however, DRGs 109, 438, 469, 470, and 474 are no longer valid for Medicare reimbursement.

Calculation

An example of a 1992 prospective payment calculation is shown in Figure 58-4. An understanding of how a payment is calculated for a hospital is important for nurses because it provides a basis for understanding many of the current and future trends of health care economics. For a more extensive history on the DRGs or calculation details, see References 8–12.

Exemptions

All hospitals that participate in the Medicare system are reimbursed by the PPS, with the following exceptions:

1. long-term hospitals: average length of inpatient stay is more than 25 days
2. psychiatric hospitals and units: engage primarily in treatment of mentally ill persons
3. rehabilitation hospitals and units: meet federally established criteria for a rehabilitation center
4. children's hospitals
5. hospitals located in states with state-regulated PPS plans (Maryland)
6. Veterans' Administration hospitals
7. cancer hospitals: those recognized by the National Cancer Institute as comprehensive cancer centers or as clinical cancer research centers. The entire facility must be organized primarily for the treatment of, and research on, cancer. As of 1992 the hospitals recognized under this exemption included M.D. Anderson Cancer Center, Houston, TX; Fox Chase Cancer Center, Philadelphia, PA; Kenneth Norris, Jr., Cancer Center, University of Southern California, Los Angeles, CA; City of Hope National Medical Center, Duarte, CA; Fred Hutchinson Cancer Center, Seattle, WA; Memorial Sloan-Kettering Cancer Center, New York, NY; Roswell Park Memorial Institute, Buffalo, NY; Dana-Farber Cancer Institute, Boston, MA; and Ohio State University–Arthur G. James Cancer Hospital, Columbus, OH.

DRGs were developed with a primary orientation toward the short-term, acute care hospitals. Their applicability in specialty (exempt) hospitals is limited. PPS-excluded hospitals still have limitations and incentives for reimbursement that were established in the 1982 TEFRA. These restrictions are updated annually.

PROSPECTIVE PAYMENT CALCULATION

Base line data

1. Fiscal year 1992
2. 600 bed acute care hospital
3. Large urban (population of more than one million)
4. Principal diagnosis example DRG #82, respiratory neoplasms

Formula

[Adjusted labor component = Labor component x Wage index $2,526.80 x 1.0962 = $2,769.88][1] + Non-labor component[2] $1,041.01 x DRG weight[3] 1.2453

Payment rate to hospital = $4,066.25
Hospital costs for Patient "A" = 3,200.00
Profit for hospital $ 866.25

[1]*Adjusted labor component*—is determined by the mean urban or rural cost per discharge then adjusted to reflect regional differences in hospital wages. This figure is derived from regional and national aggregate data of cost reports submitted by hospitals and reflects the labor intensive costs (i.e., wages, salaries, employee benefits, professional fees).

[2]*Non-labor component*—is adjusted to the appropriate regional or national standardized figure. The geographic location and urban/rural designation of the hospital is also considered. This figure accounts for all other resource consumption used for patient care (i.e., pharmaceuticals, food, energy, malpractice insurance, surgical and medical instruments).

[3]*DRG weights*—are based on a nationwide random sample study. The variables reviewed in hospitals to arrive at a cost reimbursement figure per case includes length of stay, per diem cost in routine and special care, estimated cost of ancillary services (laboratory, radiology, drugs, medical supplies).[(4)] From these reports each DRG is assigned relative weights, reflecting the resources needed to care for a patient with a specific diagnosis. PROPAC annually recommends to the Congress the appropriate annual percentage change in payment for hospital inpatient discharges. This report is due by March 1st of each year.

FIGURE 58-4 Prospective payment calculation. Specific details for calculating a prospective payment reimbursement are outlined. Although there is no need to memorize this calculation, it is important to understand which components are used to compute the reimbursement. This will help to clarify many of the dilemmas encountered by the prospective payment system.

Hospital Cost-per-Case Comparisons

To establish a set price per DRG for every acute care hospital in the United States is virtually impossible. A variety of variables can cause fluctuations in the federal payment amount. The variables used to compare one hospital's cost per case to another's include case mix (a classification by diagnosis of a hospital's caseload or patient population), number of low-income patients served (disproportionate share), labor costs, urban versus rural location, teaching intensity, and outlier cases (cases with an extremely long length of stay [day outliers] or extraordinarily high costs [cost outliers] when compared with other cases classified in the same DRG). These adjustment factors, which were incorporated into the PPS, explain an estimated 65% of the variation in average cost per case.[13] Teaching intensity was originally a "pass through" reimbursement (i.e., the total costs for education were reimbursed). However, in the past several years the system has been adjusted so that only a percentage of teaching costs are reimbursed.

The current PPS assumes that variations in cost per case that are not accounted for by the allowed adjustment factors are due to differences in hospital efficiency. As hospitals become more efficient (i.e., produce targeted health care outcomes with the least costly input), these additional variations in cost should be significantly reduced.[14]

Monitoring Activities

The PPS legislation requires close monitoring of costs. Each hospital is required to contract with a peer review organization (PRO) established by the U.S. Department of Health and Human Services. The purpose of the PROs is to conduct required medical reviews to ensure that quality patient care is provided and maintained and that the duration of hospital stay is appropriate to the required level of care. The HCFA also will review periodically the records of each hospital for compliance to the PPS regulations and will deny payment if the regulations are not followed.

To update and maintain the new Medicare payment system, Congress established the Prospective Payment Assessment Commission (ProPAC).* A 15-member commission of experts was appointed by the Office of Technology Assessment (OTA) in 1983.†[15] The PPS law mandates that ProPAC make recommendations annually to the Congress in two primary areas:[16] the annual percentage increase in Medicare expenditures on a per-case basis (the update factor), and the DRG patient classification categories and weights. However, ProPAC's responsibilities have expanded over time to include analyzing and developing prospective payment policies for all facility services under Medicare. Congress has also asked ProPAC to examine and report on broader issues regarding the effectiveness and quality of health care delivery in the United States. In recent years, ProPAC has been reviewing several other areas: the hospital market-basket structure (figure used to estimate inflation rates in the price of patient-utilized goods and services purchased by hospitals); improvements in case-mix index (average DRG weight for all cases paid under PPS, which reflects the severity of illness or resource needs); capital expenditure policy (outlay made by a hospital to purchase a fixed asset, such as a piece of equipment, for a period greater than a year;[3] the effects of PPS on rural hospitals; outpatient payment reform; and uncompensated care, which includes both charity cases and bad debts.

Impact of PPS

The change in hospital reimbursement method from costs incurred to fixed rates has resulted in drastic restructuring of health care incentives. If the actual cost of a patient's care is less than the fixed or assigned DRG rate, the hospital retains the excess amount. These DRGs are known as "winners." If the hospital's costs exceed the fixed payment scale, the hospital must absorb the excess costs. These DRGs are known as "losers." Hospitals are striving to reduce costs to an efficient and effective level. Adaptation to prospective reimbursement has led to changes in the health care environment. The following section will first review the impact PPS had on the hospital industry over the decade from 1982 to 1992,‡ and then discuss several key trends that have resulted from implementation of PPS, including decreasing length of stay in the hospital, restraining technological advances, and limiting access to health care. Each trend will be discussed in terms of its history or development, current issues, and impact on nursing.

Changes in the hospital industry

The major objectives of PPS were to reduce the rates of increase in the Medicare inpatient payments and to decrease hospital costs overall. In the first 2 fiscal years of PPS (1984 and 1985), most hospitals had positive operating margins (profits). However, this initial gain was followed by more than one-half of all hospitals having negative PPS operating margins (losses) by 1989.[17] After the first few years of implementation, changes in policy became more stringent. Congress mandated periodic updating, including changes in DRG rates, and Medicare payments were no longer tied to a hospital's actual costs or regional rates rather than national rates.

As hospital operating margins became tighter, other significant changes in the hospital industry developed. Soon after the implementation of PPS, hospital inpatient admissions declined. This continued until about 1987, when such admissions stabilized.[17] Despite a 1% yearly increase in the U.S. population, in 1989 there were 4 million fewer hospital admissions than in 1979, a drop of 11.3%. This decline in admissions particularly affected smaller hospitals (fewer than 100 beds), rural hospitals, and urban hospitals that had inefficient operations or had high costs per patient case. Financial difficulty for these hospitals resulted in their closure. Approximately 500 hospitals closed their doors between 1980 and 1991.[11] The number of closures 4 years after PPS inception was double the number of closures in the 4 years prior to the implementation of PPS.[17]

By contrast, the utilization of hospital-based outpatient services has grown steadily. From 1979 to 1989 outpatient surgical operations and visits increased by 44%.[11] Ambulatory surgical services are now available in 95% of all community hospitals.[11] In recent years, a large number of new for-profit ambulatory sites of care have emerged that compete directly with hospital out-

*Any individual interested in keeping abreast of ProPAC's latest recommendations to the Congress can be added to the mailing list to receive these reports by calling (202) 401-8986 (Office of the Prospective Payment Assessment Commission).

†The OTA was created in 1972 as an analytic arm of Congress. OTA's basic function is to help legislative policymakers anticipate and plan for the consequences of technologic changes. OTA provides Congress with independent and timely information about the potential effects of the change. The board is composed of members of the U.S. House of Representatives, U.S. Senate, and the OTA director.

In 1992 a total of 17 members (16 males and 1 female, a nurse) were appointed to ProPAC.

*For a concise review of literature regarding the impact of PPS refer to the Extramural Technical Report (E-91-06) prepared for ProPAC; An examination of winners and losers under Medicare's Prospective Payment System: A synthesis of the evidence. October 1991.

patient services. Examples of these free-standing centers include diagnostic imaging centers, cancer centers, women's centers, pain centers, outpatient psychiatric clinics, and sports medicine clinics.

This shift to outpatient services has allowed patients with less complex cases to be treated in outpatient facilities. However, those patients that continue to need inpatient care frequently are severely ill and in need of complex services. The severity of illness or amount of services provided to patients is measured by the case-mix index (CMI), which is the average DRG weight for all cases paid under PPS. The CMI index has been increasing each year since the implementation of PPS, which reflects the fact that resource needs of patients are also continually increasing. Hospitals try to meet the challenge of having to do more for patients with less money.

Medicare spending continues to rise, despite a decade of intensified attempts to control costs. Medicare Part B expenditures for physicians and other ambulatory services have grown much faster than spending under Part A, which covers hospitals and some other facility services (skilled nursing, hospice). Between 1980 and 1990 total Medicare spending per enrollee increased by 147%. However, the Medicare costs per enrollee increased at a slower rate than the national health care costs per person during the late 1980s.[11] This is an indication that government cost containment is more effective than cost containment efforts in the private sector. Hospitals that have done well under Medicare's PPS are those that reduced their length of stay, controlled their labor costs in relation to other hospitals in their market area, and offered more services to attract patients.

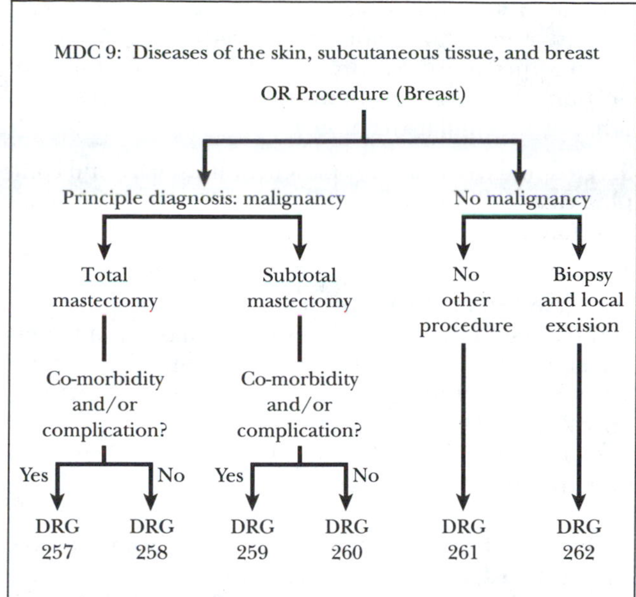

FIGURE 58-5 This is an example of the splitting of a major diagnostic category, MDC 9. This decision tree, or algorithm, helps the medical records department classify a patient's discharge status under a particular DRG. The criteria, or splitting variables, used to select the appropriate DRGs include the use of an operating room (OR procedure), the principal diagnosis, the type of OR procedure, and the type or severity of comorbidity and/or complication.

Decrease in length of stay

History The original studies at Yale University that provided the methodology for the DRGs used length of stay (LOS) as the dependent variable. This variable was chosen because the initial purpose of developing DRGs was to improve utilization review activities, which consisted of reviewing the appropriateness of patient care services by a single-diagnosis method.[5] Before the Yale study, a single-diagnosis patient classification system (International Classification of Disease Adopted, 8th revision [ICDA-8]) was used for the review of patient care. This scheme was limited to classifying patients only by similar ailments. Yale researchers adjusted the classification system by adding the LOS variable. After reviewing the results of their work, the Yale researchers concluded that the LOS variable was not entirely appropriate, because variations were too wide. They therefore found it necessary to consider several other classification factors in addition to ICDA-8 codes and LOS. The revisions included classifying diseases on the basis of 23 major diagnostic categories (MDCs), based on human anatomy. These 23 MDCs were divided further by factors that have an impact on a patient's LOS: the patient's age, the presence of comorbidities (i.e., the presence of disease conditions concurrent with the patient's principal condition), disease complications, and the use of surgical procedures (see Figure 58-5). These additional factors still are not an inclusive list for determining a patient's LOS. The assumed homogeneity* of each particular DRG needs to be examined critically, because many other factors can contribute to variations in a patient's LOS, including the following:

1. The severity index reflects the stage of the patient's illness within each DRG, which significantly influences the extent of resource consumption. Take, for example, a patient with cancer who has just been informed of disease progression and who is undergoing 5 days of a new inpatient chemotherapy. It is also discovered, on admission, that the patient's venous access device (VAD) is malfunctioning. Chemotherapy DRG 410 is used, which gives no consideration to special services needed by the patient, such as information about side effects of the new drug regimen, X rays used to correct the problem with the VAD, or the increased demand for psychosocial support.

**Homogeneity:* the assumption that the variances in patient cases classified under the same DRG are equal.

2. The socioeconomic status of the patient is a concern, because the socioeconomically disadvantaged patient may require more resources, such as nursing care, education, discharge planning, and social services, than others with similar diagnoses.

3. Hospitals that care for patients with severe and complex cases will likely be underpaid relative to hospitals that have less complex cases.

4. A physician's or surgeon's practice that is unique may affect the patient's resource consumption. For example, one patient with a simple mastectomy performed by Doctor A stays in the hospital 5 days; a second mastectomy patient, Doctor B's patient, stays only 2 days. Doctor A's patient is not discharged until her surgical drain is taken out; Doctor B's patient, however, is taught to care for the drain at home.

ProPAC has begun studies of variations in resource use with DRGs across individual hospitals. These studies are critical to an understanding of variations in medical practices and appropriateness of services furnished to Medicare beneficiaries. As payments have been constrained, hospitals are examining closely their practices and eliminating inappropriate or ineffective services. Many hospitals have concentrated their resources in a few specialties (e.g., oncology, cardiology). This specialization of services can help hospitals to increase their profitability and quality of patient care.

Current trends A great emphasis in hospital care management is on decreasing the length of hospital stays, which strongly affects the utilization of resources. Consequently, there is a powerful incentive to discharge patients earlier than before. The average LOS was decreasing slowly before the implementation of PPS. In 1980, prior to PPS, the average LOS was 7.18 days for all adults (10.37 days for adults age 65 and over). Compare this to 1984, the initial year of PPS, when the average LOS was 6.66 days for all adults (8.95 days for adults age 65 and over). The length of stay has remained relatively stable for all groups of patients since 1985.[11] Trends in LOS reflect combinations of changes in medical technology and the shift of inpatient care to outpatient care.

In the early years of PPS, one of the greatest concerns was that LOS would be inappropriately shortened, especially for the elderly patient. In October 1990 the RAND Quality of Care Study was published.[17] The study compared pre- and post-PPS outcomes of care, process of care, and impairment at discharge for nearly 17,000 Medicare patients hospitalized for five common medical conditions (congestive heart failure, acute myocardial infarction, pneumonia, cerebral vascular accidents, and hip fracture).[19] The RAND study found evidence to support the fear that patients were discharged more quickly and sicker. Before the implementation of PPS, 10% of medicare beneficiaries were discharged to home in an unstable condition as compared to 15% after PPS. Patients in an unstable condition at discharge were 1.5 times more likely to die within 90 days of discharge than patients discharged in stable condition.[11] However, extending the length of stay for these patients would not necessarily have reduced their mortality rate.

Peer Review Organizations continue to be responsible for monitoring quality of care. These have conducted several types of reviews over the past few years. Of the 2 million records reviewed in 1990, only about 1% had quality care problems.[11]

Nursing implications Nurses have a greater need than ever to increase patients' knowledge and skills related to their self-care. Rather than being a specific nursing intervention, teaching about self-care is an attempt to provide a model of care, to teach an individual how to manage his or her own care throughout a lifetime.[20]

Coordinating discharge planning is a vital role for the nurse. Continuity of care between the hospital and home must be ensured. A greater emphasis has been placed on hospital discharge planning, since this phase of the hospital admission was identified by the RAND study as a weak link in patient care after the implementation of PPS. With patients leaving the hospital setting sooner, the number of home care agencies has multiplied, and technology for the home care setting has quickly advanced to meet acute patient care needs. Careful research on hospital discharge protocols and the management of discharged patients is needed. Nursing can be instrumental in this important endeavor.

Nursing case management models have been developed to maximize resources and expertise needed in the care of hospitalized patients who have similar diagnoses. One of the first hospitals in the country to develop a case management model was New England Medical Center's Department of Nursing. A strategy was initiated that formally joins together a specific group of nurses into a group practice. Each group practice was then linked to a specific physician. Together the nurses and physicians care for patients throughout the continuum of hospitalization. Case management assignments can be aligned with caseloads in a variety of ways. For example, a nurse may be assigned to a physician and all of his or her patients, assigned to manage cases within a geographic unit, or assigned to cases on the basis of diagnosis. Collectively, the nurses and physicians are responsible for developing standards, management tools, and designs for delivery of care.[21] This plan can be very effective because nurses and physicians together are responsible for more than 80% of all the resources expended during each hospitalization.[22] A case management plan at the New England Medical Center is used to discuss possible cause-and-effect relationships in commonly encountered patient problems. The plan also results in the development of intermediate patient goals that outline nursing and physician interventions appropriate to achieve the specific desired clinical outcomes. The entire plan is designed to function within the DRG-LOS framework.[23]

Through these strategies, this center was able to reduce the LOS for patients undergoing induction therapy for leukemia from 48 days to 32 days.[24]

With the watchword of the 1990s being *managed care,* many other case management models have been identified in the literature, including the model from the American Nurses Association.[25,26] Case management concepts shared among many models include patient care delivery systems, quality care, achievement of outcomes, effective time frames, collaboration, and rationalization of resources.

One tool for case management and managed care is the *critical pathway* (CP), which is an abbreviated version, usually a one-page outline, of the clinical practices for the physicians and nurses involved in the case management plan of a particular DRG. Critical pathways show key incidents that occur in a predictable and timely order to achieve the shortest length of stay possible with efficient utilization of resources. An example of a critical pathway for a patient with a lumpectomy/axillary node dissection is shown in Figure 58-6.

The development of a critical pathway starts as a collaborative effort between physicians, nurses, and other supportive services. A specific DRG in the institution that is high volume, high cost, and problem prone (complications or length of stay too long) is targeted. When developing critical pathways, it is easier to prepare surgical DRGs than medical DRGs, which have

CRITICAL PATHWAY
LUMPECTOMY WITH AXILLARY NODE DISSECTION

DRG 260
HCFA LOS 2.4 days

Patient: ____________ Primary nurse: ____________ Physician: ____________

	Pre-hospital	**Day of admission** **OR day**	**Post-op #1** **Day 2**
Tests	Pre-op labs EKG Chest x-ray		
Activity		Out of bed w/assistance	Ambulate Instructions given for discharge No heavy lifting with affected arm Driving permitted upon discharge Bathing permitted but dressing to stay dry
Diet	NPO prior to surgery	Advance as tolerated	As tolerated
Medications			Analgesic Antiemetic Prescriptions given
Treatments	Two consents signed	v.s. q 4hr IVs, Jackson-Pratt drain q 2hr Coughing and deep breathing exercises I & O	Dressing care
Teaching	NCI booklets given	Drain care	Occupational therapy R.O.M. exercises Drain care with return demonstration
Psychosocial resources	Breast health center RN coordinator Patient/family assessment Consult Reach to Recovery (ACS)	Social worker referral, breast health center RN coordinator	Reach to Recovery (ACS) volunteers List of support groups given
Other	Second opinion clearance if needed	Sign above bed for arm restrictions (No IVs, vena punctures, or BP)	Emergency number given Follow-up appointment made for 7 days

FIGURE 58-6 Example of a critical pathway. This critical pathway lists the clinical practices to be followed by the physicians and nurses who are caring for patients receiving a lumpectomy with an axillary node dissection.

less variability and are therefore easier to use. If a critical pathway for DRG 410, chemotherapy, is developed, it is best to design it specific to a one-drug regimen so there is a commonality of drug administration and side effects.

Next, a retrospective chart review is done of patients with the targeted DRG, and an outline of current clinical practices is established. A collaborative team then considers adding, excluding, or adjusting tasks in the critical path that might help to reach patient goals sooner.

Case management requires the nurse to be prepared at a bachelor's or master's degree level of education, since the nurse in this role must define and facilitate clinical and financial outcomes.[25] Critical pathways would be helpful in nursing shift reports. Variances in the order or occurrence of the daily interventions outlined (e.g., "Regular diet not started on day 2") must be justified (e.g., "Regular diet not started because patient had no bowel sounds") or rectified.

Restraining technologic advances

History Information in the literature regarding the cost of new technology is scarce prior to the birth of the PPS in the early 1980s. At that time, when industry introduced a new product to the health care market, feasibility and cost studies were not a priority for the purchasing hospital. Since PPS inception, when a request is made for an item that uses new technology, administrators want documentation of its cost effectiveness or a feasibility report before approving the purchase. The literature now overflows with information about technology costs, and educational conferences usually have abundant workshops related to economic issues.

There have been significant scientific and technologic advances in the treatment of illness since the birth of PPS. Technologic advances are evidenced in the development of new drugs, devices, diagnostics equipment, and any equipment needed for medical and surgical procedures that prevent, diagnose, and treat disease. It is estimated that 20%–50% of the growth in health care costs can be attributed to new technology.[14]

Initially under the PPS, capital expenditures were reimbursed on the basis of actual costs. The initial cost of the purchase was not the major concern; rather, the indirect costs of operation, maintenance, and salary for trained personnel were the issues. These indirect costs are accounted for in the DRG calculation under the labor and nonlabor components. If a hospital's indirect figures are not in line with the standard DRG calculation, the hospital loses money for the specific DRG.

Not only are the indirect costs a concern, but Congress continues to mandate percentage reductions in hospital capital payments. In fiscal year 1992, hospitals started receiving capital payments based on a prospective per-case payment. The capital payment method will be phased in over a 10-year transitional period and will be based on a national average payment rate.[27]

The government uses different avenues to influence the development and utilization of technology. Some of these avenues include the following:[14]

- *National Institutes of Health:* supplies financial support for both basic and applied research related to the development of new medical technologies.
- *Food and Drug Administration (FDA):* reviews the safety and efficacy of the new medical technologies, drugs, and medical devices.
- *State government:* regulates, in many states, the purchase of new equipment through a certificate of need (CON) program.
- *Medicare and Medicaid:* influence indirectly the availability of new technology through decisions regarding reimbursement.
- *Office of Technology Assessment (OTA):* provides Congressional committees with objective analysis of the emerging, difficult, and often highly technical issues of our time; also indicates the beneficial and adverse impacts of the applications of technology.
- *Patent Law:* provides manufacturers a monopoly for a period of several years.

In addition to the federal government's historic involvement, third-party payers (insurance companies) have developed techniques to control costs. This involvement is in response to the soaring health care costs and high insurance premiums. Some of the mechanisms include:[14]

- *Technological assessment:* Many third-party payers have established formal processes for evaluating the clinical and economic effects of new technology.
- *Utilization review:* Insurers are constantly reviewing the course of treatment provided and establishing protocols for appropriate treatment. If their protocols are not followed, payment is not given.
- *Case management:* Insurers are using case management techniques to direct patients to efficient providers.
- *Selective contracting and price discounting:* Some health care systems have developed contracting mechanisms with suppliers of drugs, medical supplies, and equipment. These mechanisms provide patient care at a fixed, discounted price.

In response to the rapid proliferation of new technology and to the expanding use of existing technologies, attempts to evaluate, regulate, and advise on its usage have been developed. In 1989 the Public Health Service Department of Health and Human Services (DHHS) created the Agency for Health Care Policy and Research. This agency was formed as part of the requirements contained in the Omnibus Budget Reconciliation Act (P.L. 101-239). It was charged with enhancing quality and promoting appropriate and effective health care services through a broad program of scientific research and information dissemination. Three components were developed to support the work of this agency: the Office of Health Technology Assessment (OHTA), the Medical Treatment and Effectiveness Program (MEDTEP), and the Office of the Forum for Quality and Effectiveness in Health Care (the Forum).

OHTA evaluates the safety and effectiveness of new or unestablished medical technologies that are being considered for coverage under Medicare. These assessments are performed at the request of the HCFA. They are the basis for recommendation to the HCFA regarding coverage under Medicare. The assessment process includes a comprehensive review of the medical literature and emphasizes participation from within and outside the federal government. After information is gleaned from experts and the scientific literature, the results are analyzed and developed into an assessment report. The reports are referred to as the *Health Technology Assessment Reports*. Each report presents a detailed analysis of the safety, clinical effectiveness, and uses of new or unestablished medical technology for Medicare coverage. These reports are available free to the public once the HCFA has made a decision regarding Medicare's coverage of the subject technology.*

The MEDTEP is involved in four major activities: data development, outcomes of research, clinical guideline development, and dissemination of research findings and practice guidelines. Integrating these activities provides scientific information about the most effective medical strategies for practitioners, consumers, employers, educators, and insurers.[28] MEDTEP research is focused on patient outcomes and generation of scientific information on alternative strategies for the prevention, diagnosis, treatment, and management of patient conditions.

The development and review of clinical practice guidelines are facilitated by the Office of the Forum for Quality and Effectiveness in Health Care. Multidisciplinary expert panels were created to develop guidelines initially in seven priority areas of clinical practice. Some of the priorities included: diagnostics and treatment of benign prostatic hyperplasia, management of acute postoperative pain, and urinary incontinence in adults. Guidelines are developed by a panel of about 15 members plus numerous consultants. Guidelines are written after vigorous reviews of scientific evidence, meetings of the panel members, and open forums where testimonies are heard regarding the clinical practice issues.[29] The Center for Research Dissemination and Liaison coordinates the dissemination of MEDTEP information.

Current trends High tech has become synonymous with everyday medical practice in the United States, and America is the world's acknowledged high-tech leader.[30] Technology development is considered to be the main force underlying the rapidly escalating costs in health care.[31] Schwartz, in an analysis of American Hospital Association data, found "that half the increases in real hospital costs (costs after adjusting for the effect of inflation) came from the need to develop and apply even better diagnostic and therapeutic resources."[32]

As the economy and median income in our nation rise, Americans tend to spend more on health care, demanding more and different kinds of health services. The relationship between income and health care spending has been quantified in two major studies. In a study by Schleber and Poullier,[33] 20 member countries of the Organization for Economic Cooperation and Development (OECD) were found to have a 10% increase in their real gross domestic product accompanied by a 19% rise in health care spending. The other study by Getzen[30] found a 16% rise in health care spending for each 10% gain in real national income in the United States.

Americans expect nothing but the best in health care and react negatively to any efforts to slow technologic advancement. In fact, Americans continue to believe that everyone should have the right to "the best possible health care—as good as a millionaire gets."[34] It will be hard to retard technologic development if it means sacrificing the quality of health care.

Since the beginning of PPS, ProPAC has been examining the impact of prospective payment on the diffusion of new technologies in conjunction with estimating the appropriate increase in PPS payments.[11] Project Hope, under contract to ProPAC, studies technologies that significantly increase inpatient operating costs. Eighteen cost-increasing, quality-enhancing technologies were studied for 1993. The estimated incremental impact of these technologies on inpatient operating costs is $532 million, increasing Medicare inpatient operating payments almost 1%.[18] Monoclonal antibodies, advances in computer technology, and automatic implantable cardiovascular defibrillators are expected to have the largest impact on costs.[18]

The state-of-the-art cancer therapies increasingly drive the development and rapid changes in technology. The 1990s have witnessed an explosion in highly sophisticated, new treatment modalities. Some examples of new modalities include colony stimulating factors, genetic engineering, monoclonal antibodies, new antiemetic and chemotherapy agents, and revolutionary bone marrow transplants. Excellent cost-effectiveness studies have been done in these areas.[35-38] Yarbro states, "There is a tendency for both doctors and patients to want to use dramatic and potentially effective, but unproven treatments outside of clinical trials."[39, p.1725] He believes that expensive, high-tech treatments should be restricted to clinical trials unless they have demonstrated prolonged survival or improvement in quality of life.

*To receive copies of these reports, contact the Publication Clearing House at 1-800-358-9295.

Nursing implications No longer is it appropriate for nurses to base decisions regarding patient care on the assumption that resources are unlimited. In any economy or organization, there are more demands on resources than can be satisfied. As a result of these demands, output must be rationed. The objective of rationing is to use available resources to maximize social welfare or institutional well-being.[41] As health care expenditures continue to take a large share of our society's total resources, pressure on the industry will continue to increase to justify outcomes relative to their costs.

Nurses must be able to justify the resources needed to improve patient care. This can be accomplished through the use of financial management tools or techniques. Some examples of these techniques include feasibility studies and cost analysis studies. A *feasibility study* is a documentation process to determine whether a new program within a health care agency should be developed and implemented.[41] Such studies provide a comprehensive economic and financial forecast for a new idea or program. The basic steps of a feasibility study include:

- *Prepare an executive summary:* Write an abbreviated overview of the proposed plan. This section of the proposal usually is the one that most decision makers of the management team review. It should therefore be as brief and concise as possible—usually one page.
- *Define objectives:* List the goals the study is to achieve.
- *List assumptions:* Discuss the existing conditions the reader of the feasibility study would otherwise not be familiar with if he or she had not read it. This section allows the reader to understand the writer's global perspective on the situation or problem.
- *Describe the current situation:* Answer the question "Why is this project possible?" then present relevant background data on the project, list who or what is in competition, and discuss the macroenvironment (e.g., government, legal issues).
- *Develop a plan of action:* List what will be done, assign a person or persons to act, provide a time line or framework, and document the cost.
- *Record the projected profit and loss:* Discuss the expected financial gains or losses of the project. Enlist the assistance of the institution's finance department for the coordination of this section.
- *Describe controls:* Present a plan for monitoring the study.

Cost analysis techniques generally are classified as one of two types: cost–benefit analysis (CBA) or cost-effective analysis (CEA). Larson and Peters define each of these techniques: "Cost–benefit analysis assigns monetary value to all costs and benefits of a potential program, practice, or product, resulting in a cost–benefit ratio"[42,p.2] (e.g., a decision needs to be made on whether an outpatient oncology unit will be designed anew or whether an outpatient department will be expanded). Cost-effective analysis is defined as follows: "All the costs measured in dollars necessary to achieve a certain effect (benefit) are calculated and expressed as cost/unit of effectiveness".[42,p.3] This technique compares relative costs of several alternatives. All of the alternatives are designed to have the same outcomes (e.g., inserting an indwelling catheter for a chemotherapy regimen versus individual dosing via venipuncture). Steps used in conducting either analysis also have been delineated by the OTA. Larson and Peters[42, p.3] reviewed the OTA analysis:

1. Define the problem.
2. State the objective of the proposed program, practice change, or product.
3. Identify alternatives.
4. Define the perspective of the analysis. (For example, does it represent costs and benefits to the patient or to employees? If it represents more than one viewpoint, each should be analyzed separately.)
5. Analyze costs (include both direct and indirect costs).
6. Evaluate benefits (in dollars for CBA, in effects for CEA).
7. Determine the present value of any future costs and benefits by calculating a discount. This is called discounting. Formula:

$$\text{Present value} = \frac{\text{Future value}}{(1 + \text{Interest rate})^{\text{interval, in years}}}$$

8. Analyze uncertainties. Substitute different values from within the range of possible values for costs and benefits calculated to determine whether changes in the values will alter the conclusions of the analysis. (This is called a sensitivity analysis.)
9. Address ethical issues (e.g., the appropriate distribution of limited resources in the population, the accessibility of programs and resources, the extent to which the analysis can be influenced by bias).
10. Interpret results.

Another important contribution that nurses can make to an evaluation of new technology is to organize a product evaluation committee (PEC) or to serve as a member of such a committee. The PEC is responsible for controlling which product or service will be used in a health care agency. Larson and Maciorowski[43] describe a four-step process to be utilized by a PEC:

Step 1: Any requests for new products or changes in the use of existing products are directed to the PEC.

Step 2: Product options are explored in depth by potential users and the PEC.

Step 3: Product options are carefully evaluated on the basis of a review of the literature (historical and research perspectives), consultation with other experts, and field testing of products. Methods of field testing should be consistent for everyone involved. The PEC should use objective criteria (e.g., quality of product compared with that of others, safety, serviceability, cost, standardization, prevention of duplication of products).

Step 4: Summarize findings in a comparison chart.

With the creation of the Clinical Practice Guidelines by AHCPR, nurses have an opportunity to inform patients about their development and use. These practice guidelines were systematically developed to help physicians, nurses, other health professionals, and patients make decisions about appropriate care. If patients utilize these guidelines, they will become better-informed health care consumers, working as partners with their health care providers. When nurses increase their understanding and utilization of these processes, cost effectiveness will no longer be just a buzz word but rather a significant approach for the justification of resources needed to care for patients and their families.

Nurses involved with the updating of products or the purchase of new products should collaborate with many hospital departments: materials management, biomedical engineering, central supply, and research and development. Once a product is selected, information should be shared with hospital committees, such as policy and procedure, safety, and quality assurance and improvement. In order to deal with the increasing pressure stemming from the problem of decreasing resources, one hospital developed a position and job description for a product nurse specialist, whose role is to coordinate new product evaluations in collaboration with all the departments just mentioned.[44]

Besides the internal health care system's serving as a resource for nurses responsible for product changes, an external nonprofit agency, Emergency Care Research Institute (ECRI), can be contacted.* This agency began its initial work approximately 20 years ago in the area of emergency equipment. However, over the years their mission has changed to that of testing and evaluating all aspects of health care technology. Nurses can ask their employing agency if they are a member of the Health Device System. This membership brings numerous newsletters and consultations with a variety of health specialists, including biochemists, engineers, and nurses. The Health Device System develops reports that compare products as to their advantages and disadvantages.

Nursing input is a vital link in helping to control costs and providing quality care. The profession of nursing continues to gain interest in and knowledge about the important area of cost containment.

Limiting access to health care

History *Access to care* refers to a person's ability to pay for provided health care services. Before the early 1980s, few patients had financial burdens from medical expenses; their health care insurance paid any bills, and the burden of health care expenses was therefore on the third-party payer. With the implementation of PPS, the issue of access to care has gained prominence.

The following brief history of health care coverage in the United States should help give perspective on this issue.[45]

- *Before the 1930s:* Ninety percent of the money spent on medical bills came directly from the patient's own pocket.
- *During the Great Depression, beginning in 1929:* The cost of medical care rose sharply, and people had less money to spend on medical bills. Doctors were collecting only 40% of the fees they charged.
- *1935:* The American Hospital Association, which represented hospitals throughout the United States, promoted Blue Cross insurance to pay for hospital stays.
- *During World War II, beginning in 1941:* Although the federal government halted price and wage increases, health insurance was not counted as a wage. This enabled labor unions to negotiate for better health care coverage.
- *1950:* The high cost of national health care was beginning to gain attention by the politicians. The cost per person was $80.
- *1965:* Medicare and Medicaid federal health insurance programs started. Medicare is a program for people 65 or older and certain disabled people; Medicaid is a program for people with very low income (federal regulations mandate that each state be responsible for administering the program and establishing income levels for cash assistance). Health insurance coverage became a common employee benefit. Federal and state governments paid about 26% of all monies spent for health care in the United States. National health care costs rose to $141 per person.
- *1970:* Medical costs went up faster than the general rate of inflation. In this era of explosive growth for medical technologies and services, intensive care units became very popular. The cost of national health care continued to climb, until it had reached $340 per person.
- *1980:* The early 1980s were regarded as a time of economic recession. The government's share of the national medical bill rose to 43%, and national health care costs rose to $1054 per person. Health care costs consumed one-fourth of the corporate profits left after paying taxes. As a result, government and industry (the employers) started paying closer attention to the health benefits package.
- *1983:* TEFRA was passed. Prospective reimbursement was implemented for the national Medicare program; however, each state had the responsibility

*ECRI is an international agency located in Plymouth Meeting, PA. They can be reached at (215) 825-6000.

for establishing its own reimbursement process for the Medicaid program.

- *1992:* The Resource-Based Relative Value System (RBSVS) was implemented. This reimbursement system for Medicare recipients establishes national rates for each physician procedure, activity, and patient visit.

Throughout the approximately 60-year period from 1930 to the 1990s, many uninsured, indigent Americans were ineligible for employee or government assistance benefits. Hospitals provided charity care to these patients by *cost shifting,* the practice of charging higher rates to those patients whose care is paid through an insurance plan and using the extra income to compensate for the cost of care for those patients unable to pay their bills. As a result of this cost shifting practice, insurance premiums rose. For example, in some states the cost of insuring a family of four rose about 400% between 1980 and 1989.[46] With these enormous increases, corporations reduced their health care benefits. Today it is becoming more difficult, with cutbacks from the government and big business, for hospitals to afford to provide nonreimbursed care to the more than 37 million uninsured Americans.[14] To do so would require an increase in a hospital's gross revenue, which is not the focus of cost containment efforts.[47]

Current trends The demand for charity care is steadily increasing at a time when many hospitals have negative operating margins. A significant reason for the increased need for charity care is the increased number of persons who do not receive health insurance as an employee benefit. Approximately 60% of the uninsured are employed in companies that do not offer health insurance.[11] These small companies cannot afford to offer health coverage benefits. Average annual costs per employee for employer-sponsored group health plans increased from $1645 in 1984 to $2748 in 1989[30] and averaged a 25% increase each year from 1989 to 1992. As our nation continues the transition from a manufacturing to a service economy, this category of uninsured persons will increase. Service companies frequently are small and nonunionized, and both of these characteristics are associated with limited employer-sponsored insurance plans. Part-time work, which is less likely to include health insurance, has expanded. Today about one in six jobs is part-time.[30] Almost half of the uninsured are under age 25, and one-third of this group are children or other dependents.[14]

Many employers are changing their traditional health plan insurance benefits, in which the worker chooses his own physician and receives reimbursement for all or part of the incurred expenses. Instead, employers are adopting programs that restrict both the extent of coverage and physician selection. As recently as 1984, a total of 96% of insured workers were covered by the traditional plan, compared to 28% of workers enjoying such plans in 1989.[46] Newly organized care delivery systems have been introduced.

Alternative care delivery systems An array of acronyms, such as *HMO, IPA,* and *PPO* have emerged in the literature. They represent models of health care coverage in which companies offer employee health benefits and at the same time monitor and evaluate the "appropriateness" of medical care prescribed by physicians. A term that is used to summarize this activity is *managed care.*

One of the most popular alternatives is the *health maintenance organization (HMO).* HMOs are membership organizations that provide health care, ranging from prevention to treatment, for a prenegotiated price over a fixed time period. Members may solicit care from only those doctors and hospitals designated by the HMO. This type of alternative care delivery system is the oldest alternative to the traditional health insurance plan. Prepaid group practices, as they were first called, started in farming communities in the 1800s.[45] In the 1940s, Henry Kaiser, an industrialist, founded the HMO known as Kaiser-Permanente, in California. Kaiser believed in the preventive approach to medicine rather than just curing the sick.[48] He encouraged people to visit a physician before illness developed—and these visits were paid for by the HMO. This preventive health maintenance was distinctly different from traditional health care benefits (e.g., Medicare, Blue Shield), which would only pay if the patient had a problem that needed treatment. Today, Kaiser-Permanente represents one of the biggest corporation-backed HMO chains in the United States.

HMOs first gained national prominence in the 1970s during President Nixon's administration, when Congress passed the Health Maintenance Organization Act, a national policy designed to control escalating health care costs. Federal loans and other incentives were provided to increase HMO growth. HMOs provide corporations the financial advantage of fixed rates of reimbursement rather than steadily increasing health insurance premiums. Under this plan, physicians are salaried employees of the HMO.

The *individual practice association (IPA)* is a type of HMO in which the participating physician accepts patients who are HMO members as well as those who are fee-for-service patients. The physician is reimbursed for care provided to the HMO patients according to a set fee schedule. This fee includes the cost of diagnostic tests and the fee for referral to a specialist if needed. The physician who does not spend all the money allotted by the set fee schedule can keep some portion or all of the balance. However, if costs exceed the predetermined rates, the physician must absorb the difference.

A *preferred provider organization (PPO)* is another alternative plan for health care coverage. This is a negotiated business arrangement between an industry or business (the buyer) and a hospital or physician (the seller). A limited number of physicians and hospitals join a network and offer a discounted fee for service.

In PPO plans, members pay a reduced fee or nothing at all when they are seen by a PPO physician. The physician and hospitals in the PPO are able to discount their fees in return for a guaranteed volume of patients. The PPO offers the employer cost control mechanisms through a claims review process that provides prospective review of recommended diagnostic tests, surgery, and hospitalizations. Any care considered unnecessary is not approved. PPOs usually offer a wider selection of doctors and hospitals than do HMOs.

It is estimated that before the year 2000 up to 80% of the insured population will be enrolled in HMOs or PPOs.[46] The greatest controversy surrounding these alternative health care systems is in the implications of the strong incentive to reduce overall spending. Some persons believe that these alternative delivery systems result in fewer tests and procedures or in delays in their being prescribed, to the detriment of the patient's health. Moreover, strong ethical concerns are raised when physicians have the authority to approve or disapprove patient referrals to specialists and at the same time are permitted to keep a percentage of the money they save by not referring patients to specialists. One questions whether such a system can produce unbiased judgment. There are few data available to confirm or deny these concerns.

In defense of the alternative care delivery system, results of two studies showed that there were no statistical differences between the HMO and fee-for-service populations in the care provided for the diagnosis and treatment of patients with breast cancer or colorectal cancer.[48,49] Variables analyzed for these studies included the mean age of diagnosis, the duration of symptoms before diagnosis, the number of physician visits for symptoms due to cancer before diagnosis, the stage of diagnosis at which diagnosis was made, the methods of diagnosis and treatment, the length of hospital stay, the severity and type of complications, and survival rates. Further research is needed to explore the pros and cons of managed care and to validate data and conclusions.

National health care Many Americans have been spoiled by having been able to receive immediate access to almost any kind of medical treatment. However, health care is not a constitutional right, a fact that has become more apparent as the impact of PPS continues to be felt. Because U.S. citizens have come to view health care as a right, the role played by government in paying for medical services has increased. Legislators continue to debate health care reform and struggle to find a consensus. Many members of Congress believe controlling health care costs could be a major factor in balancing the national budget. But controlling costs is not the only factor driving change; the need to expand access to medical care is also part of the challenge.

The American health care system was founded on the principle of universal access, but runaway health costs have eroded the system's ability to deliver care to all.[51] A growing number of individuals in this country are arguing that the American health care system has failed and that the nation needs some kind of nationalized health insurance system. A 1991 poll showed that 91% of Americans believed the nation's health care system to be in need of fundamental changes.[52] However, individuals are reluctant to give up the perks of a private system that includes choice of doctor and health care setting. Whenever limits are introduced, such as PPS, an army of lobbyists and special interest groups descend on Congress to object to the restrictions.

In an effort to respond to the ailing American health care system, approximately 40 different reform proposals that discuss possible solutions have been developed by either individuals or organizations. Three of these proposals will be highlighted here: (1) American Medical Association's (AMA) "Health Access America," (2) Nursing Agency for Health Care Reform, and (3) American Hospital Association's (AHA) "National Health Care Strategy: A Starting Point for Debate."

1. AMA Plan. This plan proposes to achieve universal access through reform of the existing system of health care. Several major points are emphasized in the proposal.[53,54] The first point is reform of the Medicaid program, requiring the use of only one national formula for eligibility, in place of the existing method of state discretion in setting the economic level for eligibility. Added coverage for prescription drugs, rehabilitative services, and emergency services will be provided. Medicaid reimbursement levels are increased to the Medicare level. Second, this reform requires employer provision of health insurance for all full-time employees and their families, with tax help to employers. Third, the plan would create state-level risk pools in all states, that is, a legislatively created insurance program that extends coverage to individuals who are not covered and cannot afford health insurance. Last, the plan would expand long-term care for senior citizens. Financial incentives such as income tax deductibility and tax-free withdrawals from individual retirement accounts are proposed for the purchase of this insurance.

2. Nursing Plan. This proposal calls for a basic core of essential health care services to be made available to everyone.[55] Nursing's "core of care" includes several key ideas. All United States citizens would be provided a standard package of essential services. Employers that did not offer private coverage would be required to pay into the public plan for their employees. Financial relief would be made available to small businesses. The Medicare and Medicaid systems would be replaced by a single public program administered by the state but based on federal guidelines and eligibility requirements. Government subsidies would be extended to individuals earning less than 20% of the federally designated poverty level. The plan encourages managed care, private plans through lower deductibles, and copayments. Case management services would be used to integrate, coordinate, and advocate for people requiring extensive services. For long-term care coverage, individuals would be expected to assume personal sponsibility through strengthened insurance programs and a variety of innovative financial arrangements. Such strategies include privately purchased long-term insurance, new savings, tax incentives, and home equity conversion opportunities.

3. AHA Plan. This reform discusses a basic benefit that would cover preventive care, inpatient and outpatient care, and long-term care. It sets no fixed limits on the types or quantities of service; rather, coverage is based on medical necessity and reasonableness. Medicare and Medicaid would be replaced by a public plan financed through federal taxes and premium contributions. Individuals earning less than 150% of the federally designated poverty level would pay no premiums but would pay nominal copayments and deductibles. All employers would be required to offer a basic benefit package with additional coverage options. The plan would be financed half by employers and half by employees. If employees did not want this option, they would be covered by the public plan. State insurance pools would be established to help small businesses and self-employed individuals. Quality of care would be ensured by establishing medical practice parameters, and by providing to the public information on the practices of individual practitioners, costs of services, and quality outcomes. Guidelines on the cost-effective use of health care technology and specialty services would be established. Incentives to increase collaboration between hospitals and physicians would be developed. A private advisory commission would be established to provide Congress with the information it needs to set the budget targets.

In addition to national proposals, several states have initiated legislation in response to the struggle related to access of care and allocation of resources. Hawaii has succeeded in legally requiring that most people working more than 19 hours per week be covered by employer-subsidized insurance.[57] The state of Massachusetts passed legislation requiring most employers to provide a certain level of coverage to workers or else pay an assessment.[57] Residents of Florida, New York, Michigan, Maine, and Wisconsin subsidize health insurance coverage for some of their poorest citizens, and South Carolina sponsors physician house calls for pregnant women.[52]

The state of Oregon has gained the most visibility by asking the U.S. government to approve changes in Medicaid rules to provide a limited list of medical services to all people below the poverty level, regardless of their current Medicaid status. Oregon has a comprehensive health plan that requires all employers to provide health insurance for full-time employees. The plan obliges insurance companies to renew policies without exclusion criteria for individuals considered too risky. The most controversial feature of the plan is the establishment of the priority list. This list ranks medical conditions and treatments according to their seriousness and the likelihood that treatment will restore the patient to long-term good health. In June 1987 the Oregon legislature voted to stop using Medicaid funds to pay for heart, liver, bone marrow, and pancreas transplants.[58] In December 1987, the media alerted the public to the fact that a 7-year-old Portland, Oregon, boy with leukemia died. His mother was on welfare (Medicaid), and the state refused to pay for a bone marrow transplant.

As Oregon makes difficult choices about resource allocation, it gains recognition as a model for other state initiatives. Many Congress members are observing carefully the outcomes of Oregon's program before submitting or supporting national reform recommendations. Oregon has created a citizen-based, nonprofit educational foundation—Oregon Health Decisions—to increase public awareness and build consensus on bioethical issues.[59] Through the Citizens Health Care Parliament, this organization has developed principles for health care resource allocations (Table 58-1).[60] These principles can help direct anyone involved in the serious problem of allocating health care resources in today's economic crunch.

In addition to poor persons, elderly persons, who generate 29% of this nation's health care expenses, are suffering.[58] Physicians who care for frail elderly persons are penalized for having patients who require longer hospitalization. Prior to the federal budget reconciliations of 1991, Medicare recipients were not covered for routine mammograms, even though most breast cancers are diagnosed in the later years of life. Proposed legislation such as this is an attempt to assist the elderly. However, at the current time, little has been accomplished to help this struggling segment of the population.

Our national health care system is only beginning to feel the impact of our aging society. It is estimated, by the U.S. Census Bureau projection, that people age 65 years and over, currently 12% of the population, will increase to 21% by the year 2030.[61] Also, Americans age 85 years and older, the old-old, are now the fastest-growing segment of the population. This group is expected to double by the year 2020.[30] It is the old-old American who consumes the most health care resources. An individual 65–74 years old has an average annual Medicare cost of $2017; this jumps nearly 65% to $3215 for people 85 and over.[30]

Under the existing tax rates, future escalations in Medicare spending will not be matched by the tax revenues from the working class. Such tax revenues from the individual worker are deposited in the Hospital Insurance Trust Fund, which supports the Medicare Program. The ratio of retired 65-year-old individuals to those under 65 who are working is expected to be 1:3 in the year 2025.[62] The Hospital Insurance Trust Fund is projected to run out of money by the turn of the century. Another fact that has an impact on the elderly's health care is that $50 billion a year is spent on patients during the last 6 months of their life.[58] Our country will be faced with tough choices; some form of health care rationing will be difficult to avoid. For ex-

TABLE 58-1 Principles for Health Care Resource Allocation Adapted by the 1988 Citizens Health Care Parliament

PURPOSE OF HEALTH SERVICES

- The responsibility of government in providing health care resources is to improve the overall quality of life of people by acting within the limits of available financial and other resources.
- Overall quality of life is the result of many factors, health being only one of these. Others include economic, political, cultural, environmental, aesthetic, and spiritual aspects of life.
- Health-related quality of life includes physical, mental, social, cognitive, and self-care functions, as well as a perception of pain and a sense of well-being.
- Allocations for health care have a claim on government resources only to the extent that no alternative use of these resources would produce a greater increase in overall quality of life of the people.
- Health care activities should be undertaken to increase the length of life or the health-related quality of life during one's life span, or both.
- Quality of life should be one of the ethical standards when allocating health care resources involving insurance and government funds.

WHY PRIORITIES NEED TO BE SET

- Every person is entitled to adequate health care.
- It is necessary to set priorities in health care so long as health care demands and needs exceed society's capacity, or willingness, to pay for them. Thus an "adequate" level of care may be something less than an "optimal" level of care.

HOW TO SET HEALTH PRIORITIES

- Setting priorities and allocating resources to health care should be done explicitly and openly, taking careful account of the values of the broad spectrum of the Oregon population. Value judgments should be obtained in such a way that the needs and concerns of minority populations are not undervalued.
- Both efficiency and equity should be considered in allocating health care services. *Efficiency* means the greatest amount of appropriate and effective health care benefits for the greatest number of persons is provided with a given amount of money. *Equity* means that all persons have an equal opportunity to receive available health services.
- Allocation of health care resources should be based, in part, on a scale of public attitudes that quantifies the trade-off between length of life and quality of life.
- In general, a high-priority health care activity is one where the personal and social health benefits-to-cost ratio is high.

WHO SETS WHAT PRIORITIES?

- The values of the general public should guide planning decisions that affect the allocation of health services resources. As a rule, choices among alternative treatments should be made by the patient, in consultation with the health care provider.
- Planning or policy decisions in health care should rest on value judgments made by the general public and those who represent the public and on factual judgments made by appropriate experts.
- Private decision makers, including third-party payers and health care providers, have a responsibility to oversee the allocation of health care resources to ensure that their use is consistent with the values of the general public.

Source: Oregon Health Decisions: *Quality of Life in Allocating Health Care Resources.* Portland, Oregon, 1988.

ample, should an elderly person with a diagnosis of incurable adenocarcinoma of the lung be given chemotherapy? If so, for how long?

The United States is one of only two industrialized countries (South Africa being the other) that does not have some kind of national health financing program. In the United States, per capita health care cost is 41% higher than in Canada, 61% higher than in Sweden, 85% higher than in France, 131% higher than in Japan, and an astounding 171% higher than in Great Britain.[63]

An organization that compares the health care of 24 wealthy countries is the Organization for Economic Cooperation and Development (OECD). The OECD reveals that medical practice is similar everywhere and that physicians are quick to learn about the medical advances in other countries; however, the biggest differences between wealthy countries and poorer ones is in the organization and financing of health care.[64] The OECD has also addressed the phenomenon that although countries have much different health systems, they share the same problems: how to restrict financially the practices of hospitals and physicians, and how to control an apparently infinite demand for health care.[64]

The next question that comes to mind is whether the quality of care in the United States is better than in other countries. Measured by quality indicators such as life expectancy and infant mortality, the United States ranks low. In a report by Meyer[30] it is noted that U.S. life expectancy (71.5 years, males; 78.3 years, females) is about the same or slightly shorter than in other industrial nations, such as Canada (73.0 years, males; 80.3 years, females), France (72.0 years, males; 80.3 years, females), and Japan (75.6, males; 81.4, females). Also, the U.S. infant mortality rate ranked 18th out of 20 OECD nations.

This report further suggests that these quality indicators may say more about lifestyles and social problems than about health care. Today, the United States is struggling with social problems of drug use and saving babies of crack-addicted mothers. The increasing number of teenage pregnancies affects our infant mortality rate. Our homicide rate is far higher than that of other countries, which, in turn, affects life expectancy.

In the United States, however, rationing of medical care through waiting lists is not yet the norm (as it is in countries with nationalized health care systems). In Great Britain, waiting lists for elective procedures such as hip replacements and cataract surgery can stretch out to 2 years.[48] Moreover, kidney dialysis ordinarily is not provided for anyone over 55 years of age,[58] whereas in the United States this procedure is available to anyone. The fact that the United States has the highest health care costs but produces the most sophisticated care is an outcome that must not be dismissed. In all industrialized nations, the aging population has increasing long-term care needs. Sophisticated advances in technology are increasing the public's demand for it, at high costs. With these trends, it is predicted that eventually the spending in health care across industrialized nations will equalize.

As our country is pondering the idea of a nationalized health care plan, a great concern regarding assessment and the definition of quality of care is exploding. Reports such as "Quality of Medical Care Information for Consumers"* have been prepared by The OTA for Congressional review. Dr. Paul M. Elwood, Jr., founder of InterStudy, a Minnesota-based health care policy think tank, is generally credited with coining the term *health maintenance organization.* He pioneered the theory known as *outcome management,* whereby a collection of objective criteria helps providers, payers, and purchasers define the relationship between medical interventions and health outcomes.[65]

Outcome management draws on four techniques: selection of physician interventions from standards or guidelines; systematic measurement of patient functioning and quality of life; collection of clinical and outcome data; and dissemination of results that continually modify the outcome management system.[66] To collect these data, a quality-of-life scale was designed and tested. It is a 5-minute, self-administered test that measures patients' ability to function, via questions about roles, social interventions, physical functioning, emotions, and perceptions of health and pain.[66]

Many managed health care organizations are using similar survey tools to negotiate contracts. Measuring medical outcomes by means of patient surveys is a new endeavor. The public's current perception of quality hospital care often is based on satisfaction, convenience, cost, and anecdotal medical information.[67] Whichever survey tool is chosen, it must be valid and reliable. Data comparison should only be made between similar groups of patients.

In the 1990s, cost-effective quality care will be a dominant theme. Keeping abreast of the latest information and research is imperative.

Nursing implications There has not been a more important time period than the present for nurses to become proactively involved in helping formulate our nation's health care policies related to access to care. A variety of directions can be taken.

1. Initiate an educational program to increase the knowledge and skills of the public related to decision-making ability, weighing quality with cost. According to competitive theory, the cost and quality of care will be guided by the consumers who weigh price and quality levels in the selection of health insurance and medical care providers.[14]

2. Develop clinical nursing research methodology that investigates strategies to reduce health care costs without compromising care. According to Fuch,[68] "10% of delivered care may be considered harmful and another 10% is delivered with marginal benefits. If funding cuts were concentrated on this 20% the overall negative effect on health care would be minimal." The results from nursing research can be presented to legislators to assist them in deciding about cutbacks. Nursing research can answer questions about which cutbacks have serious health implications versus those that will have no adverse clinical effects.

3. Engage in political activities. As drastic changes continue to appear on the horizon, nurses must take a proactive stance in health care decisions, rather than being reactive and merely trying to justify or rectify the current changes. There is a political, bioethical movement in this country for organizing grass-roots health care organizations. To date, 19 states, including Oregon, have organized groups of concerned citizens who tell their legislators how they want their tax dollars spent on health care issues such as rationing and biomedical ethics.

4. Nurses are advocates of patient care and should assist consumers in selecting the alternative care system that is the best for their needs. Millensen[45] identified

*A copy of this report can be purchased through National Technical Information Services, Springfield, VA; PB 89-102-180 is the order number.

several questions to help people who are considering health care through an HMO.

a. What do comments from friends or acquaintances indicate about the reputation of the physicians and hospitals that belong to the HMO?
b. How are the HMO physicians paid? Is there a financial incentive to withold certain kinds of services on specialist referrals?
c. What happens if an individual gets sick away from home or outside his HMO service area? Does the HMO pay for care if treated elsewhere?
d. Can consumers choose their primary physician, or is the primary physician assigned?
e. Are all the physicians listed as members of the HMO actually available? (Sometimes a popular physician is unable to accept referrals for new patients.)
f. What are the benefits of the particular HMO? For example, are home prescription drugs and home care visits available?

For consumers considering a PPO, it is appropriate to consider the following questions:

a. Do the participating physicians and hospitals meet the individual's specific needs for medical care? For example, are specialized services for certain illnesses or treatments, pediatric facilities, maternal care, prescriptions, and home care services available?
b. How much will the PPO pay toward the care provided by a physician who is not participating in the discounted fee arrangement?
c. Are financial incentives given to physicians that would motivate them to increase the number of office visits and prescribed tests in order to make up for discounted fees?
d. Will the PPO pay for a second opinion if it is sought before consumers undergo any tests or treatment that might be unwarranted?

5. Understand the basic types of health care insurance, insurance terminology, and regulatory agencies, to help patients cope with the newly evolving reimbursement restrictions. Insurance coverage varies from state to state, procedure to procedure, and case to case. When denial of an insurance claim becomes an issue for a patient, develop a systematic team approach to solve the problem. Members of the team can include nurses, patient-billing account office, hospital-based utilization review staff, medical record coders, the reimbursement or financial department, physicians, and legal counsel if appropriate. Individuals in these departments usually are not well known by nurses. However, if nurses are true patient advocates, this team of individuals should become acquainted.

6. Develop mechanisms to document, in financial terms, the nursing care needed for indigent patients. Reports show that the acuity level of indigent patients is higher than average.[69,70] This information should be directed to members of ProPAC and Congress, the persons responsible for recommending reimbursement amounts for indigent care.

7. Read *In Search of Excellence* by Peters and Waterman.[71] This book provides insights into how companies have arrived at strategies for cost savings, cost effectiveness, and quality services and thus offers the nurse an added perspective on how to influence such changes in the future. A major theme of the book, which can serve as a caution for the hospital industry, is that low-cost providers are not the winners in terms of quality or profit over the long term.

8. Keep abreast of the Joint Commission on Accreditation of Healthcare Organizations (the agency responsible for accrediting health care organizations) for the Study of Change. This study is a major research and development project intended to improve the commission's ability to evaluate health care organizations and generate greater attention to the quality of patient care. Clinical indicators are developed to evaluate specific areas of patient care (e.g., obstetrics, oncology). Organizations such as the American College of Surgeons, the Association of Community Cancer Centers (ACCC), the American Society of Clinical Oncology, and the Oncology Nursing Society usually provide updated reports on the status of this study.

RESOURCE-BASED RELATIVE VALUE SYSTEM

History

In 1965 the Medicare program established the physician payment policies, Part B, which was modeled after plans developed by private insurers. Payments were based on what the law considered to be the usual, customary, and reasonable (UCR) charge. The amount of the government's payment was based on the lowest of the following: (1) the physician's actual charge, (2) the physician's customary charge (the charge most frequently made by the doctor for his or her service), and (3) the prevailing charge (based on all the customary charges in the locality for each type of service). Medicare beneficiaries would then pay 20% of the approved charges after meeting the annual deductible. Medicare pays the doctor 80% of the approved charge.

Reasonable charges were established to try to rectify the problem of the aging population in the 1960s, for many of these individuals lacked health insurance. The retired elderly wanted comparable physician services to be enjoyed by all. Within a short period, spending for physician services under Medicare began to rise, jumping by more than double-digit rates each year. In 1972 the laws changed and the government would pay no more than what 75% of the practitioners in the geographic area were charging for the same services. Medicare payment was also based on the difficulty of the procedures performed by the physician.

Over the years, Medicare began delaying recognition of physician fee increases, and payment amounts lagged behind market value. Physicians tired of this treatment, played a game with the government by rapidly inflating their fees, believing that if they asked for more, they eventually would get a higher share.[72] Politicians became upset and established through Congress the Physician Payment Review Commission (PPRC) in 1986.[73] In 1988 the commission reported to Congress that the current "reasonable charge"-based system for the reimbursement of Medicare Part B payment needed to be replaced.

The PPRC recommended a payment schedule based on resource costs. Their recommendations were based on the Harvard University study by William Hsiao: the National Study of Resource-Based Relative Value Scales for Physician Services. The following year, President Bush signed into law the Omnibus Reconciliation Act of 1989, Public Law 101-239, which announced three new major elements: (1) establishment of Medicare Volume Performance Standard (MVPS) rates of increase for physician services, (2) replacement of the "reasonable charge" payment mechanism with a fee schedule for physician services, and (3) replacement of the maximum actual allowable charge (MAAC) with a new limiting charge. The MAAC is the total amount that nonparticipating Medicare physicians could charge Medicare patients for their services. A nonparticipating physician is an individual who chooses not to accept the charge approved by Medicare for payment. Patients must pay out of pocket and then apply for Medicare reimbursement. Medicare will pay 80% of the approved charge after subtracting any part of the individual's remaining annual deductible. The MVPS was developed with the intent to moderate the rate of increase in costs of physician services. The secretary of Health and Human Services had to recommend to Congress a target rate of growth based on several factors: general inflation, number of Medicare beneficiaries, the aging population, and changes in technology.[74]

On November 25, 1991, the HCFA issued its final rules to implement the new Medicare physician fee schedule, RBRVS, by January 1992. A 4-year timetable was set to phase in the program, eliminating the current/customary/reasonable charges. The new scale is based on resources such as the time, mental effort, judgment, technical skill, and physical effort involved in the patient procedure or treatment. Allowances are given for differences among geographic locations. The intent of this new system is to raise reimbursement for primary care physicians, who evaluate and manage patient care, and to offer less reimbursement to procedure-oriented physicians, pathologists, radiologists, ophthalmologists, and thoracic surgeons. The limiting charges on nonparticipating Medicare physicians was phased in over 2 years, from January 1991 to January 1993. Initially, the limiting charge reflected a physician's historical charges. Beginning in 1993, the limiting charge became 115% of the fee schedule amount for nonparticipating physicians.

Calculation

A relative value for each Current Procedural Terminology (CPT) code has been established. These codes were developed by the American Medical Association and other specialty societies to reimburse for Medicare Part B payments. CPT provides a list of descriptive terms and numeric identifying codes and modifiers for reporting medical services and procedures performed by physicians. Medicare Part B pays for doctor's services, outpatient hospital care, diagnostic tests, durable medical equipment, ambulance services, and supplies not covered by Medicare Part A. The total relative value unit (RVU) is based on three separate units: the amount of physician work, practice expenses (such as rent, staff salaries, equipment, and supplies), and professional liability insurance or malpractice costs. The physician work must reflect the physician's resources, time, and intensity of required effort to provide a patient service. The practice overhead and malpractice expenses are based on historical data. The initial historical data used for the RVUs was from the 1989 AMA Socioeconomic Monitoring Survey for physician specialists.

The relative value for each of the three separate units is multiplied by a conversion factor (CF) and a geographic adjustment factor (GAF). A conversion factor can be viewed as a multiplier that transforms RVUs into payment amounts. For the year 1992, the CF was 31.001. The GAF is developed from Medicare localities (in 1992 there were 240 different ones). These localities are based on local medical practices and economic conditions. The products of each of the three separate units and geographic areas are multiplied by the conversion factor (CF), and the end result is the dollar amount of Medicare payment.

An example computation of an estimated payment amount for a specific service in 1992 is presented in Figure 58-7. Several transitional rules may be quickly instituted because of RBRVS's newness and lack of experience with it. For detailed information regarding this payment plan refer to the Federal Register for November 1991.[75]

Another important element of the new system is the CPT codes used by physicians for reporting evaluation and management (E/M) services. Every time a physician visits a patient in a hospital or an outpatient setting, a CPT code must be selected that reflects the care the patient received from the physician. As previously mentioned, one of the major aims of the new RBRVS is to raise reimbursement for primary care physicians who evaluate and manage patient care. Patient-visit CPT codes have been revised to become E/M codes, and now reflect, through clearer descriptions, the types of physician visits. Table 58-2[76] presents a tool designed to help physicians determine the appropriate code for the services provided to their patients. These new descriptive codes will increase consistency in reporting by physicians across all specialties.

TABLE 58-2 Tool for Coding Patient Visits: Medicare Revised Coding System for Evaluation/Management (E/M) Services

Key to Content Descriptors* of E/M Codes:

Your History and Exam are:
PF = Problem focused
E = Expanded
D = Detailed
C = Comprehensive

Your Medical Decision Making Is:
S = Straightforward
LC = Low complexity
MC = Moderate complexity
HC = High complexity

The Severity of Presenting Problems is:
MI = Minor severity
LS = Low severity
MS = Moderate severity
HS = High severity
SR = Stable, recovering
RP = Responding poorly
SC = Significant complication(s), unstable
UE = Urgent evaluation required
LT = Life-threatening problem(s)

Service	CPT Code #	History and Physical Exam	Medical Decision Making	Severity	Average Physician Time (min)*
Office visit (new)	99201	PF	S	MI	10
	99202	E	S	LS-MS	20
	99203	D	LC	MS	30
	99204	C	MC	MS-HS	45
	99205	C	HC	MS-HS	60
Office visit (established)	99211	—	—	MI	5
	99212	PF	S	MI	10
	99213	E	LC	LS-MS	15
	99214	D	MC	MS-HS	25
	99215	C	HC	MS-HS	40
Initial hospital care (new or established)	99221	C	S-LC	LS	30
	99222	C	MC	MS	50
	99223	C	HC	HS	70
Subsequent hospital care	99231	PF	S-LC	SR	15
	99232	E	MC	RP	25
	99233	D	HC	SC	35
	99238	Final hospital care for discharge			
Critical care	99291	Critical care, first hour			
	99292	Critical care, each additional 30 min			
Office consultations (new or established)	99241	PF	S	MI	15
	99242	E	S	LS	30
	99243	D	LC	MS	40
	99244	C	MC	MS-HS	60
	99245	C	HC	MS-HS	80
Initial hospital consultations (new or established)	99251	PF	S	MI	20
	99252	E	S	LS	40
	99253	D	LC	MS	55
	99254	C	MC	MS-HS	80
	99255	C	HC		110
Follow-up consultations (established)	99261	PF	S-LC	SR	10
	99262	E	MC	RP	20
	99263	D	HC	SC	30
Emergency department (new or established)	99281	PF	S	MI	—
	99282	E	LC	LS-MS	—
	99283	E	LC-MC	MS	—
	99284	D	MC	UE	—
	99285	C	HC	LT	—

*History, Exam and Medical Decision Making are considered the KEY components in selecting a visit code. *These service descriptors, NOT TIME, are used to select the correct level of code.* Time becomes a key consideration in selecting a level of code only when counseling or coordination of care accounts for over 50% of the time spent with the patient.

Source: Association of American Medical Colleges. All CPT codes and descriptors copyright 1991 AMA.

RESOURCE-BASED RELATIVE VALUE SYSTEM CALCULATION

BASELINE DATA

1. Fiscal year 1992
2. Philadelphia medical school hospital
3. CPT code for skin biopsy: 11100

Payment formula

[(RVUw × GPCIw) + (RVUpe × GPCIpe) + (RVUm × GPCIm)] × CF
= [(0.65 × 1.014) + (0.55 × 1.014) + (0.04 × 1.552)] × 31.001

RVUw = Physician-work relative value units for the service
RVUpe = Practice-expense relative value units for the service
RVUm = Malpractice relative value units for the service
GPCIw = Geographic-practice-cost-index value for physician work applicable in the fee schedule area
GPCIpe = Geographic-practice-cost-index value for practice expense applicable in the fee schedule area
GPCIm = Geographic-practice-cost-index value for malpractice applicable in the fee schedule area
CF = Uniform national conversion factor

Payment rate to the hospital: $39.65.

Find the CPT code for a skin biopsy. Make a note of the corresponding relative value units (RVUs) for work, practice expense, and malpractice for the service. Next, look up the geographic practice cost index (GPCI) and make note again of the corresponding work practice expense and malpractice figures. Use the 1992 value of 31.001 as the uniform national conversion factor. The result of the computation will be the Medicare payment received for a skin biopsy in a Philadelphia medical school hospital.

FIGURE 58-7 Resource-Based Relative Value System calculation. Formula for calculating a Medicare payment for the physician's outpatient care of a skin biopsy is outlined. This new Medicare reimbursement system will equalize physician payments received throughout the country.

SPECIFIC ECONOMIC ISSUES IN CANCER CARE

Economics has a major effect on the outcome and delivery of today's patient care. Unfortunately, the specialty of oncology did not escape the PPS regulations. During the 1970s and early 1980s, cancer care had a reputation as a sacred cow, with an "ask and you shall receive" aura. However, this honeymoon has come to an end in the eyes of today's insurance providers and federal officials. The specialty must now justify all of its resource costs. For some hospitals and administrators, cancer is not a winner from a cost perspective; consequently, resources such as specialized personnel and state-of-the-art technology are scarce.

However, with the AHA prediction that oncology will overtake cardiology as the dominant medical specialty in the 1990s, many hospitals are scurrying to get in the business of cancer care.[77] With this increasing demand for oncology care, hospitals are trying to develop competitive programs of high quality but low cost. In this section of the chapter current issues posing threats to the specialty of oncology will be addressed.

Oncology as a specialty embodies several unfavorable economic conditions: increasing patient volume; increasing number of socioeconomically disadvantaged patients in need of care; hospital-intensive, high acute care needs; chronicity; a need for intensive monitoring throughout treatment; growth of high-tech care at extensive costs; and the abundant need for psychologic interventions. The specific details of the problems change frequently, but the overall picture of cancer care is that it is expensive, in need of budgetary cuts, and under the scrutiny of the legislators. Markman, in an editorial in the *Journal of Clinical Oncology*, noted that any individuals "interested in the welfare of patients with malignant disease have an obligation to understand the current crisis in the funding of health care and to appreciate the importance of the future decision-making process."[78, p. 938]

Cancer-Specific DRGs

Since the inception of DRGs, updates have occurred yearly regarding the weights, and occasionally new DRGs are added. Cancer DRGs have been affected by these changes. Currently there are 81 cancer or cancer-related DRGs. Forty-six DRGs, or 9.3% of all DRGs, are designated as "pure" cancer DRGs, for most of their titles include the word *cancer*. In Table 58-3 these are indicated by a "P".

TABLE 58-3 Cancer and Cancer-Related DRGs

DRG No.	DRG Title
"P" 10	Nervous System Neoplasms, w/complications
"P" 11	Nervous System Neoplasms, w/o complications
46	Other Disorders of the Eye, Age >17 w/ complications
47	Other Disorders of the Eye, Age >17 w/o complications
48	Other Disorders of the Eye, Age 0–17
"P" 64	Ear, Nose, Mouth, and Throat Malignancy
73	Other Ear, Nose, Mouth, and Throat Diagnoses, Age >17
"P" 82	Respiratory Neoplasms
145	Other Circulatory System Diagnoses w/o complications
164	Appendectomy w/Complicated Principal Diagnosis, w/complications

TABLE 58-3 Cancer and Cancer-Related DRGs (continued)

DRG No.	DRG Title
165	Appendectomy w/Complicated Principal Diagnosis, w/o complications
"P" 172	Digestive Malignancy, w/complications
"P" 173	Digestive Malignancy, w/o complications
185	Dental and Oral Disease Except Extraction and Restoration, Age >17
187	Dental Extractions and Restorations
188	Other Digestive System Diagnoses, Age >17 w/ complications
189	Other Digestive Diagnoses, Age 17 w/o complications
190	Other Digestive System Diagnoses, Age 0–17
"P" 199	Hepatobiliary Diagnostic Procedure for Malignancy
"P" 203	Malignancy of Hepatobiliary System or Pancreas
"P" 239	Pathologic Fractures and Musculoskeletal and Connective Tissue Malignancy
256	Other Musculoskeletal System and Connective Tissue Diagnoses
"P" 257	Total Mastectomy for Malignancy, w/ complications
"P" 258	Total Mastectomy for Malignancy, w/o complications
"P" 259	Subtotal Mastectomy for Malignancy, w/ complications
"P" 260	Subtotal Mastectomy for Malignancy, w/o complications
261	Breast Procedure for Nonmalignancy Except Biopsy and Local Excision
262	Breast Biopsy and Local Excision for Nonmalignancy
272	Major Skin Disorders, w/complications
273	Major Skin Disorders, w/o complications
"P" 274	Malignant Breast Disorders, w/complications
"P" 275	Malignant Breast Disorders, w/o complications
276	Nonmalignant Breast Disorders
284	Minor Skin Disorders, w/o complications
300	Endocrine Disorders, w/complications
301	Endocrine Disorders, w/o complications
"P" 303	Kidney, Ureter, and Major Bladder Procedure for Neoplasm
"P" 318	Kidney, Urinary Tract Neoplasms, w/complications
"P" 319	Kidney and Urinary Tract Neoplasm, w/o complications
334	Major Male Pelvic Procedures w/complications
"P" 336	Transurethral Prostatectomy, w/complications
"P" 338	Testes Procedure for Malignancy
"P" 344	Other Male Reproductive System OR Procedure for Malignancy
345	Other Male Reproductive System OR Procedure Except for Malignancy
"P" 346	Malignancy, Male Reproductive System, w/ complications
"P" 347	Malignancy, Male Reproductive System, w/o complications
352	Other Male Reproductive System Diagnoses
"P" 353	Pelvic Evisceration, Radical Hysterectomy, and Radical Vulvectomy
"P" 357	Uterine and Adnexa Procedures for Ovarian or Adnexal Malignancy
"P" 363	D&C, Conization, and Radioimplant for Malignancy
"P" 366	Malignancy, Female Reproductive System, w/ complications
"P" 367	Malignancy, Female Reproductive System, w/o complications
368	Infections, Female Reproductive System
369	Menstrual and Other Female Reproductive System Disorders
395	Red Blood Cell Disorders, Age >17
396	Red Blood Cell Disorders, Age 0–17
398	Reticuloendothelial and Immunity Disorders, w/ complications
399	Reticuloendothelial and Immunity Disorders, w/o complications
"P" 400	Lymphoma or Leukemia w/Major OR Procedure
"P" 401	Lymphoma Nonacute Other OR Procedure, w/ complications
"P" 402	Lymphoma and Nonacute Other OR Procedure, w/o complications
"P" 403	Lymphoma and Nonacute Leukemia, w/ complications
"P" 404	Lymphoma and Nonacute Leukemia, w/o complications
"P" 405	Acute Leukemia w/o Major OR Procedure, Age 0–17
"P" 406	Myeloproliferative Disorder or Poorly Differentiated Neoplasm w/Major OR Procedure, w/complications
"P" 407	Myeloproliferative Disorder or Poorly Differentiated Neoplasm w/Major OR Procedure, w/o complications
"P" 408	Myeloproliferative Disorder or Poorly Differentiated Neoplasm, w/Other OR Procedure
"P" 409	Radiotherapy
"P" 410	Chemotherapy w/o Acute Leukemia as Secondary Diagnosis
"P" 411	History of Malignancy, w/o Endoscopy
"P" 412	History of Malignancy, w/Endoscopy
"P" 413	Other Myeloproliferative Disorder or Poorly Differentiated Neoplasm diagnosis, w/ complications
"P" 414	Other Myeloproliferative Disorder or Poorly Differentiated Neoplasm diagnosis, w/o complications
"P" 465	Aftercare w/History of Malignancy as Secondary diagnosis
467	Other Factors Influencing Health Status
"P" 473	Acute Leukemia w/o Major OR Procedure, Age >17
475	Respiratory System Diagnosis w/Ventilator Support
481	Bone Marrow Transplant
488	HIV w/Extensive OR Procedure
489	HIV w/Major Related Condition
490	HIV w/ or w/o Other Related Conditions
492	Chemotherapy with Acute Leukemia as Secondary Diagnosis

"P," "pure" cancer DRG; *OR,* operating room; *w/,* with; *w/o,* without.

One of the leaders in reporting information specific to cancer DRGs is the Association of Community Cancer Centers (ACCC). This organization gathered information in 1991 from 116 of its affiliated hospitals. Information of interest from the compilation and analysis of these data includes the following.[79]

- The ten DRGs with the highest total reimbursement or relative income for each cancer DRG have been identified by calculating the total reimbursement, or overall income, for each of the specified cancer or cancer-related DRGs in the 116 institutions surveyed by the ACCC (Table 58-4).[79] These are reported in rank order. Please note that these high reimbursement DRGs do not necessarily constitute "winning" DRGs for hospitals. In fact, many of the DRGs that have the highest reimbursement are "losers" (unprofitable) for hospitals. For example, the type of cancer with the highest incidence in this country is lung cancer; thus the highest number of cancer patients are categorized under DRG 82 (Respiratory Neoplasms). Hospital care for these patients usually is more expensive than the allowed DRG reimbursement. If a hospital's largest number of cancer patients are in DRG 82, its highest reimbursement will be from this DRG. However, each time a hospital seeks reimbursement through Medicare for patients with lung cancer it loses money, making this DRG unprofitable for the hospital.

- Variations in cancer-DRG profit and loss are also related to regional location. Patterns of care vary throughout the United States and include recommended types of treatment and average length of stay in a hospital setting. In this ACCC study, 15 cancer DRGs were selected for review. It was noted that the smallest average loss was for institutions located in the northeast region of the country (Maine, South Carolina, New York, Pennsylvania, West Virginia). The largest average loss for institutions was in the southeast geographical area (Mississippi, Tennessee, Alabama, Georgia, Florida).

A copy of similar reports can be requested from a hospital's finance department. An oncology clinical nursing specialist (OCNS) examines this institutional list to identify which DRGs are "winners" and which are "losers." Individual hospitals can compare their data to national studies such as the one completed by the ACCC. If there is a negative difference between a hospital's financial DRG data and regional or national data, measures to improve this status should be investigated. (For example, can length of stay be decreased? Are procedures such as intravenous chemotherapy administration, dressing changes, mouth care protocols, and antibiotic protocols too costly?) If there is a significant difference between the hospital's DRG data and the regional or national data, this information should be shared with other OCNSs.

TABLE 58-4 The Ten Cancer or Cancer-Related DRGs with the Highest Total Reimbursement

DRG 82	DRG 395
DRG 410	DRG 188
DRG 239	DRG 172
DRG 403	DRG 203
DRG 303	DRG 400

Source: Adapted from Drilea S, Mortenson L, Clune C, Evans M: *Cancer DRGs—A Comparative Report on Key Cancer-Related DRGs* (ed. 5). Rockville, MD: Association of Community Cancer Centers, 1991.

When an institution's profit-or-loss-DRG list is reviewed, the variability of volume must be considered. It is important to ensure that those DRGs with the highest volume are monitored to produce "winning" DRGs for the hospital. If a DRG is a "loser," the hospital, with the assistance of an OCNS, must find ways to improve their profit margins via strategies such as reducing the length of inpatient stays; by reviewing the necessity and appropriateness of tests, procedures, and drugs that are prescribed; and by determining other variable costs that might be financially draining.

In an analysis of the profit-and-loss nature of a cancer program, it is important to avoid two major pitfalls. First, the patient with cancer should not be used as the unit of analysis. This practice ignores the importance of multiple admissions for patients with cancer. Instead, the unit of analysis should be total number of cancer admissions. A report from the ACCC revealed that half of all cancer patients' admissions are generated by one-fourth of the cancer patients.[80] Second, a limit should not be set on the number of DRGs analyzed for the entire oncology product line. For example, if one is interested in assessing the hospital's profitability in the treatment of lung cancer, data from numerous DRGs (e.g., 82, 75, and 76, or a total of 26 others) should be used to analyze the profitability rather than limiting data to only DRG 82 (Respiratory Neoplasms). The combined DRG list best reflects the true profit-or-loss figure. If these two mistakes are made, a significant portion (up to 40%) of the cancer program revenues are likely to be missed.[80]

With more than a decade of PPS experience, more studies specifically related to oncology have been published.[81–84] One study by Munoz et al.,[81] tested the hypothesis that hospital costs and outcomes (mortality) would differ for each surgical oncologist by the volume of patients he or she treated per DRG. The study demonstrated that patients of higher-volume surgeons had lower hospital costs and a shorter hospital stay, compared with patients of lower-volume surgeons. This study helps to support the growing trend in oncology of site-specific cancer centers.[85] A site-specific cancer center is a program that specializes in one type of cancer (e.g., breast, colon, lung). A unique expertise is developed by the various medical specialties involved in the program. Patients who visit the site-specific center can be seen by a variety of doctors, depending on the problem, all in one visit. These centers operate under the notion that quality of care and outcomes are affected by the volume of patients treated for the same condition or by the number of high-tech procedures performed.

Clinical Trials

The future of clinical trials has been a major concern since the inception of DRGs. In 1983, a study was done to illustrate that the cost of conducting clinical research was too great. The results of this New Jersey–based study concluded that the average loss for each patient on a clinical trial was $1057, or 30 times greater than the loss for patients not in a clinical trial.[86] Additional costs for clinical trials occur because of the increased use of laboratory and radiology tests, the need for an environment conducive to safe, high-quality care (e.g., a special unit, an educated interdisciplinary team, higher staff/patient ratios, nutritional support), and data management. The HCFA's response to this inflated figure was that "the Medicare program has always been prohibited from paying the research costs and for items or services that are either experimental in nature or that are paid for by another government entity."[87] The HCFA also commented, "There is substantial federal support through NCI's programs."[87]

This issue became most problematic as a result of work done by researchers at Yale University in assigning weights to the cancer-related DRGs. Patients in clinical trials were not differentiated from others. Thus, when hospitals conducting research (e.g., in community clinical oncology programs [CCOPs]) were reimbursed under PPS, they lost money. Ironically, before PPS, Medicare did pay for the costs of research, such as the patient's care on specialized oncology units, services provided by the interdisciplinary team, and laboratory and radiology services.[12]

One potential solution to this problem is the suggestion by ACCC to create DRG 471, for patients in clinical trials. This strategy initially was rejected by the HCFA. In the spring of 1983, an amendment was passed by Congress to provide exemption or adjustment for hospitals involved in cancer treatments or engaged in cancer research. Congress limited the amendment by including only three comprehensive cancer centers: M.D. Anderson Cancer Hospital, Houston, TX; Fox Chase Cancer Center, Philadelphia, PA; and City of Hope National Medical Center, Duarte, CA. Since then six more hospitals have been added (refer to DRG-cancer hospital exemptions on page 1488). This amendment, however, still did not solve all the problems. Thus many patients who were eligible to receive investigational drugs through clinical trials (e.g., patients whose cancer is refractory to all known forms of standard therapy) would not be covered, because they were receiving care in a hospital that was not exempt. Thus the cost of receiving investigational drugs was prohibitive to such patients.

To intensify the problem, many insurance companies are following the HCFA's policy. An NCI report to the U.S. Senate, "Remedies and Cost of Difficulties Hampering Clinical Research," noted that Medicare policy excludes coverage for investigational therapy because treatment with agents not yet approved by the FDA does not satisfy the "reasonable and necessary" criterion included in the legislative language relating to Medicare.[88] In addition, this same report pointed out that many third-party insurance contracts are excluding payments for patient care costs associated with investigational drugs. Although this exclusion has been a part of most insurance contracts for many years, it was not enforced until recently because of the growing emphasis on cost containment. Thus, some insurance companies are denying claims whenever an investigational agent clearly is a part of the therapy. Claims that are denied may include the entire costs of the hospitalization, regardless of what the cost would have been without the investigational treatment.[88] The NCI and other health-related organizations are attempting to convince third-party carriers that the treatment received by patients in clinical trials represents the best medical approach that can be offered.[85]

To draw the attention of Congress to the need for change in this reimbursement trend, factual data documenting the scope of the problem must be presented. The Agency for Health Care Policy and Research, Hospital Study Program, and the NCI conducted a retrospective research study: "Cancer Research in U.S. Hospitals: Extent, Cost, and Incentives." The principle objectives of the study were: (1) to determine whether there are cost differences between protocol and nonprotocol patients; and (2) to estimate the extent to which incentives for hospitals to participate in clinical trials may have changed after the implementation of PPS.[89] The results of this study have not yet been released.

The most frightening concern expressed occasionally by third-party payers is that living longer can waste resources because new technology does not prevent or cure disease but, rather, prolongs the course of illness, especially for patients who are near death. This disturbing concept surfaces at times when budget problems in health care are being discussed. Treating cancer patients with stage III and/or stage IV disease is viewed by some as a financially ineffective use of national resources. Reese[90] discussed the cost effectiveness of cancer treatment in the United Kingdom, which has a national health program, and reported that patients with cancer are being denied the best available treatment because of the spending limits imposed by the National Health Service. For example, treatment to reduce pain and improve the quality of life was not always available, and some hospitals could not afford to give chemotherapy because of the costs. Costs were determined by dividing a measure of the effectiveness of intervention in avoiding death or long-term disability into the cost of treatment for one patient.[90] An equivalent of $22,000 was documented as the amount available to save a life or to avoid severe disability (a bone-marrow transplantation would exceed this figure).

Fortunately, these cost assessment procedures are not the primary source for making decisions about what care to provide. The thought of calculating the worth of a person's life by a formula is astounding. Yet Reese[90] concludes that the rationing of resources for cancer patients is inevitable and that cost assessment is a means of enabling hospitals and physicians to make optimal use of resources.

Changes in reimbursement policies occur almost daily. Medicare, Medicaid, and private insurers presently handle reimbursement on a case-by-case basis and usually require a written narrative (a preauthorization) of the patient's diagnosis, prognosis, treatment plan, effectiveness of prior treatment, and supporting data on the efficacy of the drugs to be used.[91] Studies cited to demonstrate efficacy must be well designed, appear in refereed scientific journals, and be applicable to community settings. In addition, the treatment study must show a positive tumor effect and cost–benefit comparison with conventional therapy and be the acceptable medical practice in the specified geographic area.[91] Policies and regulations vary from state to state.

Information, questions, and complaints regarding reimbursement or denial of reimbursement should be sent to the appropriate insurance carrier and/or regulatory agency. A list of common insurers and their regulatory body can be seen in Table 58-5.[92] Free reimbursement hotlines have been established by companies releasing new, costly treatments or products. The hotline usually provides information regarding reimbursement policies, billing procedures, codes, and claims appeals related to new releases. The ACCC publishes a listing of current reimbursement assistance programs once a year.

TABLE 58-5 Insurance Contact Information

If Your Insurer Is . . .	It Is Regulated By . . .
A private company (e.g., Blue Cross, Prudential)	Your state department of insurance
A licensed health care services plan (e.g., Kaiser and other HMOs)	Your state department of corporations, division of health care service plans
Federally qualified health maintenance organization	U.S. Department of Health and Human Services, Division of Compliance
Private employer or union self-insurance or self-financed plans	U.S. Department of Labor, Office of Pension and Welfare Benefits
Medicaid (sometimes called other names: e.g., in California it's known as MediCal)	Your state department of social services
Medicare Supplemental Security Income Social Security benefits	U.S. Social Security Administration
Veterans Benefits C.H.A.M.P.U.S.	Department of Veterans Affairs

Source: National Cancer Institute: *Facing Forward—A Guide for Cancer Survivors,* no. 90-2424, 1990.

Cancer treatment in the past decade has become highly sophisticated because of experimental trials in areas such as bone marrow transplantation, genetic engineering, colony stimulating factor therapy, and biologic response modifier therapy. The FDA's approval for selective use of colony stimulating factors has been a double-edged sword. Patients on these factors have had decreased length of hospital stays, with decreasing costs, yet insurance coverage for this expensive product has been denied for many patients. In a 1991 National Gallup Poll commissioned by Lederle Laboratories with the cooperation of the National Cancer Institute,[93] oncologists were asked to label specific new cancer treatment modalities as having a high, medium, or low impact on cancer care. Sixty-two percent of the oncologists believed that colony stimulating factors have a high impact on cancer care. Approximately one in four oncologists (23%) reported bone marrow transplants would have a high impact. About the same proportion (22%) said biologic response modifiers would have a high impact on cancer treatment. Genetic engineering was viewed by 38% as having a high impact on cancer care.

The biggest controversy over reimbursement denials for new, experimental treatment modalities has been autologous bone marrow transplantations (ABMT). Continuous denials of reimbursement for this extremely costly yet state-of-the-art therapy in the treatment of breast cancer has led to lawsuits. Because patients have been winning the suits, the National Blue Cross/Blue Shield Association agreed to participate in a 5-year program with the NCI to fund phase III randomized clinical trials for ABMT.[94]

Pharmaceutical companies often assist in funding clinical trials, because the trials provide a means of testing their products. Companies usually pay an agreed-upon dollar figure per accrued patient, with funding for laboratory tests, clinical coordination, data management, and physician fees. But rarely does the budget allocate money for the costs of routine patient care and clinical management, including the cost of hospitalization.[91]

Funds from the NCI are available for clinical trials. However, the designated budget is not adequate to support the current explosion in scientific discovery and biotechnology. For example, the President's budget request in 1993 for the NCI was \$2 billion; yet an additional \$764 million is needed to sustain the existing level of services.

To add further confusion to the reimbursement scenario, new institutions or corporations are being developed outside the auspices of NCI to deliver advanced technologic care to patients whose cancer is refractory to standard therapy. An example is the

Biologic Therapy Institute, Biotherapeutics, Inc., of Franklin Tennessee, where patients paid their own medical expenses to receive experimental therapy. Unfortunately, financial difficulties caused Biotherapeutics to close. Such delivery systems, considered patient sponsored, promulgate the notion that care is available for those who can pay. In addition, consumers of the "baby boom" generation are willing to pay extra for high-quality services.[95] The future for patient-sponsored research is not well defined, but already the National Academy of Sciences Institute of Medicine is proposing guidelines for responsible behavior in research.[96]

Through self-education, patients, legislators, and nurses can have an impact on the issue of reimbursement for clinical trials. Barbara Hoffman, JD, past vice president of the National Coalition for Cancer Survivorship, summarized the predicament of clinical trials:[97]

> The current lack of adequate health insurance coverage for experimental clinical trials and newly developed treatment bodes poorly for improving cure rates in the near future. The costs that society is paying now for cancer treatments is slight when compared with the cost of productive lives lost to oncology care that is dictated by M.B.A.s rather than M.D.s.

Unlabeled Use of FDA-Approved Chemotherapy Agents

The government and insurance companies began in the late 1980s to deny reimbursement for drugs used for indications that do not fall within the drug-package-insert guidelines approved by the FDA (unlabeled drugs). Some insurers are denying reimbursement for unlabeled indications of chemotherapy, calling this experimental use.[98]

The ACCC conducted an audit of 3500 patients' records from 1986 in 165 oncologists' offices. The audit concluded that of the eight most frequently used chemotherapy drugs (adriamycin, cyclophosphamide, fluorouracil, methotrexate, mutamycin, vincristine, cisplatin, and Vepesid), 46% were being used for unlabeled indications.[99] The impact of this conclusion for the third-party payers who can deny payment is an annual savings of \$150–\$200 million; for patients with cancer it means that 372,000 were denied reimbursement for treatment with vincristine, 218,000 were denied reimbursement for treatment with cyclophosphamide, 88,000 were denied reimbursement for treatment with cisplatin, and 121,000 were denied reimbursement for treatment with methotrexate.[98] All these treatments are considered standard medical practice. In addition, approximately 90% of chemotherapy is given in standard combination regimens, and none of these combinations has ever had FDA approval.[98]

Insurers are asking drug manufacturers to obtain FDA approval for indications not listed on the label. Pharmaceutical representatives say that this process of supplemental application is very time-consuming and costly, ranging from \$500,000 to \$5 million per drug.[100] In addition, the burden on the FDA would be astronomical. However, "under Section 502 of the Federal Drug and Cosmetic Act, the FDA must support the policy that an approved drug must be labeled, promoted and administered only for uses for which its safety and efficacy have been established." This guideline has not always been followed, however. In the past, the package inserts were used mainly as a guide for physicians.

In 1988, a joint Senate/House conference committee recommended that the Department of Health and Human Services consult three specific drug compendia when establishing standards for drug coverage under the outpatient drug amendment of the Medicare Catastrophic Coverage Act of 1988.[101] These compendia, published by the U.S. Pharmacopeia, the American Hospital Formulary Service, and the American Medical Association, present evidence of a drug's effectiveness that extends beyond its labeled indications. In 1989, the Federal Register announced a change in Medicare policy for off-label drug use, which did little to change the denial patterns. Two major insurance trade associations (Blue Cross/Blue Shield and Health Insurance Association of America) revised their recommendations also, but neither had an impact on changing the off-label drug denial pattern.

Finally, in February 1991, after much public awareness and pressure from lobbyists, the Senate Committee on Labor and Human Resources asked the General Accounting Office (GAO) to examine off-label drug use in the treatment of cancer.[102] The committee requested information in three specific areas: (1) the extent to which approved anticancer drugs were prescribed for off-label uses, and how this varied by patient characteristics, therapeutic intent, and type of cancer; (2) the extent to which physicians have altered the way they treat cancer patients because of difficulties in obtaining reimbursement for off-labeled drug use; and (3) the extent to which third-party payers are reimbursing physicians for off-label usage. The findings were that off-label drug use among oncologists is widespread; more than half (56%) of the patients studied had at least one off-label drug as part of their chemotherapy drug regimen (Figure 58-8).[102]

The GAO review covered drugs used for treatment of 11 different types of cancer. The reports from oncologists showed that the extent of off-label drug use was low for disease that had standard regimens of chemotherapy (breast cancer and Hodgkin's disease) and high for cancer for which there was little agreement about the best way to treat patients (non-small-cell lung cancer, hormone-refractory prostate cancer). Costs of drugs did not seem to be a prime factor for denial. The drugs most frequently denied reimbursement for off-label uses were interferon and carboplatin, which are not the most expensive drugs.

The reimbursement problems for off-label drug treatments seem to be increasing today. Approximately half of the oncologists who responded to the GAO sur-

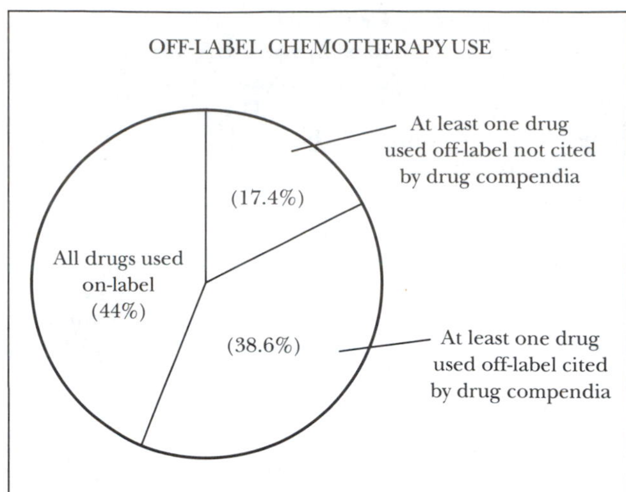

FIGURE 58-8 The results of the GAO report that examined the patterns of off-label drug use in the treatment of cancer. Notice that 56% of patients were prescribed at least one off-label drug in their chemotherapy regimen. (Source: U.S. GAO: *Off-Label Drugs: Reimbursement Policies Constrain Physicians in Their Choice of Cancer Therapies.* Washington, DC: U.S. General Accounting Office, GAO/PEMD-91-12, 1991.

vey reported problems; of these same respondents, 76% thought the rate of denials was getting worse. Attempts are continually being made to challenge payment denials for chemotherapy off-label drug use. Legislative initiatives have been introduced in many states, including California, Massachusetts, Hawaii, Illinois, Indiana, Minnesota, and New Jersey. The ACCC is very active in helping to support legislation through the efforts of their director of public policy. Consumer involvement is also being emphasized. Two free pamphlets that outline specific consumer actions are: "Cancer Treatment your Insurance Should Cover," available through the ACCC, and "Facing Forward: A Guide for Cancer Survivors," from the NCI.

As the reader can surmise, we are just beginning to see cost-cutting warfare. Nurses must keep abreast of the most current information for creating profitable strategies for oncology programs. Keeping well informed will also enable nurses to react quickly as advocates for patients who are being denied payment for their health care.

Outpatient Cancer Care

Implementation of the PPS caused a major shift in the treatment environment from inpatient care to outpatient care. Patients receiving treatment for cancer, especially chemotherapy, felt the impact most heavily. The DRG limit for reimbursement, pressure for early patient discharge, and patient preference have been strong incentives for the accelerated growth of outpatient cancer care facilities. The delivery of quality outpatient care has quickly become possible through advanced technologic support (e.g., vascular access devices, ambulatory infusion pumps), the results of pharmacology research (e.g., oral chemotherapeutic agents), and the specialized knowledge and skills of oncology nurses and physicians. Management of toxic effects has become possible on an outpatient basis by increasing the education and responsibility of patients and their families. Moreover, triage by telephone has become an important monitoring modality in outpatient cancer care (see Chapter 54, Ambulatory Care).

Shifting chemotherapy to the outpatient setting has not sheltered it from the scrutiny of insurance coverage. To ensure payment from an insurance company, the health care provider must contact the company to determine whether it will pay for outpatient treatment, which billing codes to use, and which limitations are applicable to a particular patient. However, by asking these questions many times, a red flag is waved causing oncologists to alter their preferred patient treatment setting. The GAO off-label report stated that approximately 2% of oncologists surveyed admitted patients to hospitals for chemotherapy solely to circumvent reimbursement problems. The final outcome of this practice is escalation of health care costs.

One of the most unstable factors in outpatient care is the billing procedures. Physician payments are based on diagnostic codes. There have been four different types of coding for physician insurance payments.

- Current Procedural Terminology (4th ed.) (CPT-4) codes developed by the AMA and utilized by the HCFA for reimbursement of Medicare Part B
- Health Care Financing Administration Common Procedure Coding System (HCPCS) codes developed by the HCFA as a supplement to CPT-4 codes
- local codes for local Medicare problems
- insurance company codes created by individual carriers

In 1989, oncologists working in group practice in a hospital outreach clinic were ordered to return $75,000 in chemotherapy supervision fees charged over the preceding 2 1/2 years.[103] The ruling was based on a longstanding Medicare regulation by which only the entity that owns or leases the space in which outpatient chemotherapy is delivered and that pays the employees can charge for the office visit, drug charges, and the administration and supervision for chemotherapy.[103] In 1990 the CPT-4 codes changed, disallowing the charge for supervision of chemotherapy. Physicians moved their patients receiving chemotherapy from the outpatient departments of hospitals to their private offices. By 1991 the AMA had convinced the HCFA to change the code book again, allowing a physician fee for the supervision of chemotherapy administration.[104] Moreover, because the HCFA regulates only Medicare, individual insurance companies can continue to disallow this fee if they choose. The current RBRVS regulations state that if the chemotherapy administered is provided in the outpatient hospital setting, the oncologist will not be reimbursed for the administration, but the hospital will receive payment. In a hospital outpatient setting, the physician will only be able to bill the appropriate EM code.[105] If, on the other hand, the physician is in leased or rented office space and employs the nurse, the chemotherapy administration will be reimbursed to the oncologist through the fee schedule of the RBRVS.

All these continual changes have caused a great deal of turmoil. Anyone involved in the development of a cancer program must keep abreast of these changes.

Preventive Cancer Care

The concept of *wellness* has been part of nursing and medicine for years and is reflected in the old adage "An ounce of prevention is worth a pound of cure." However, not until the medical world convinced the industrial world through profitable financial data reports did industry understand that this advice was both medically and economically sound. A report from the National Cancer Health Statistics indicates that $10.3 million was spent for medical care for cancer in 1985.[106] Care for male patients with lung cancer accounted for $1 million of this (48% of these patients were younger than 62 years of age, and 52% were 65 and older); $900,00 was spent on female lung cancer patients (74% were under 65 years of age, and 26% were 65 and over). The investment in smoking cessation programs has the potential for effecting great savings for industry.

Another federal study demonstrated that hospital care expenditures account for roughly 60%–75% of the total direct cost of cancer, compared with about 35%–50% spent on hospital care for all other diseases.[107] A study by Brown[84] estimated that the cost of cancer from 1985 to 1990 in this country increased by 45%. For the approximate $700 billion being spent nationwide on health care, only a tiny fraction has been invested in disease prevention and health promotion. Yet nine preventable chronic diseases are responsible for more than half of all deaths among Americans each year.[108]

It takes an act of Congress for Medicare to begin coverage for preventive services. In 1991 final regulations were issued for Medicare coverage and reimbursement of screening mammography. The HCFA estimates this new budget will cost $440 million in fiscal year 1995.[109]

HMOs such as Kaiser-Permanente have increasingly advocated for health promotion and preventive medicine. This HMO has developed guidelines for preventive medicine based on epidemiologic information research and cost containment efforts.[109] Blue Cross and Blue Shield in 1991 announced a plan to offer periodic preventive and screening services for healthy adults. Now individual employees are deciding on what they will include in their employer plan. One study at the University of Pennsylvania's Wharton School, Institute of Health Economics, found that companies can save more than 40% in hospitalization costs by implementing wellness programs for employees.[46] Wellness programs are increasingly popular; two of every three firms with 50 or more employees now offer some health promotion activity.[110]

Worried about the skyrocketing costs of caring for employees with cancer, industry has also started cancer screening programs. Lately, more insurance providers are investigating mammography screening. However, data reviewing cost effectiveness of breast cancer screening have not been optimistic. In a review article by Mushlin and Finton,[111] nine breast cancer screening studies were reviewed; all indicated that the screenings were not a cost-saving tool. The article also emphasized that caution be exercised when attempting to make policy decisions based on these findings. Based on the current findings, the cost benefits of screening younger women may be outside the range that society and third-party payers can afford. Emphasis is directed to screening older women, with whom there is a greater certainty about favorable cost effectiveness.

For future changes in cancer prevention and screening to be positive, many cost–benefit studies must be initiated that produce evidence of an overall cost savings.

Cancer and the Socioeconomically Disadvantaged

Since the early 1970s, studies have investigated cancer incidence in African Americans. Conclusions are that overall 5-year cancer survival among African Americans is 38%, compared to 50% among Caucasians. African American men have the highest cancer mortality and lowest survival rates, and higher overall cancer incidence than Caucasians. Research in the areas of minorities and cancer has concluded that the racial differences in cancer statistics are due primarily to differences in socioeconomic status, not to racial differences per se. Poor Americans, regardless of race, have a10%–15% lower 5-year cancer survival rate, as well as a higher overall incidence, compared to other Americans.

Basic features of the poor that affect the problems of early cancer detection, treatment, and survival are unemployment, inadequate education, substandard housing, chronic malnutrition, and diminished access to medical care. Of the 39 million people in this country who live below the poverty level, 23 million are Caucasian, 9.6 million are African American, and 6.4 million are other races. (Living below the poverty level in 1992 meant having $13,950 or less annual income for a family of four.)[112] The expanding number of legal and illegal immigrants entering the United States is a major factor contributing to the increased number of people living below the poverty line. Asian Americans are now the country's fastest-growing minority, and by the year 2000, they will probably represent 4% of the population.[113] Hispanic Americans are expected to outnumber African Americans and become the largest minority group by the year 2000.[113]

The ACS and NCI both prioritized activities to eliminate this gap in cancer survival between the economically disadvantaged and other Americans. In a 1986 ACS report, "Cancer in the Economically Disadvantaged," it was concluded that both cancer incidence and survival are related to socioeconomic status (SES), and that at least 50% of the survival difference (based on African American/Caucasian comparison) is due to late diagnosis in the economically disadvantaged. Late diagnosis usually is related to limited treatment options, and overall prognosis is poorer. The problem is due in part to a low awareness of cancer warning signs and the inability to pay for recommended preventive health care. This is certainly the case for cervical cancer. In the years 1980–1987, the mortality rate for African American women was 2.5 times that of Caucasian women.[114] Another factor is a reflection of inadequacies in the U.S. health care system. Those with a symptom of cancer who are unable to pay a private physician are often seen first in an emergency room. They are then referred to a clinic, where long waiting periods and complex registration procedures are common. Emergency rooms are geared toward treating acutely ill people. Poor people with an early cancer are triaged, later reappearing with advanced stages of the disease. The U.S. medical system does little to encourage preventive health care for the poor.

To understand better the dimensions of these problems and to identify possible solutions, the ACS sponsored a series of hearings across the country in 1989. Sixty-eight disadvantaged people and 94 professionals who worked with the disadvantaged presented testimony at seven regional hearings (Georgia, Mississippi, New Jersey, Missouri, Texas, California, Arizona). The five most critical issues related to cancer and the poor outlined in the compelling "Cancer and the Poor: Report to the Nation" were:[115]

1. Poor people endure greater pain and suffering from cancer than other Americans.
2. Poor people and their families must make extraordinary personal sacrifices to obtain and pay for care.
3. Poor people face substantial obstacles in obtaining and using health insurance and often do not seek care if they cannot pay for it.
4. Current cancer education programs are culturally insensitive and irrelevant to many poor people.
5. Fatalism about cancer is prevalent among the poor and prevents them from seeking care.

After reflecting on these key issues, the ACS responded by identifying ten specific challenges that address the problems poor people encounter when seeking cancer education, prevention, detection, and treatment services.[115]

1. Ensure that cancer prevention, detection, treatment, and rehabilitation services are accessible and available to all who need them, regardless of their ability to pay.
2. Improve cancer prevention and early detection among poor Americans to eliminate unnecessary pain, suffering, and death.
3. Undertake aggressive educational efforts to counteract fatalism, overcome fears, and enable poor people to reduce cancer risk.
4. Improve and expand public and private assistance for the poor, including health insurance.
5. Develop cancer education materials and outreach programs that are culturally sensitive, understandable, and relevant to poor people.
6. Establish patient advocate and referral services to help poor patients navigate the health system and manage personal problems that result from cancer treatment.
7. Involve community organizations serving the poor and poor people themselves in cancer education and patient advocacy programs.
8. Train health care providers to be sensitive to the needs of poor patients and to serve their needs more effectively.
9. Expand the availability of and accessibility to health services for poor people of rural areas, which are now underserved.
10. Conduct research to further document the scope of the problem and identify effective interventions.

The ACS authorized $1.8 million in grants to initiate demonstration programs. One such pilot project was in West Oakland, CA.[116] The project's goal was to provide a full spectrum of cancer prevention services (risk assessment, behavior modification, state-of-the-art early-detection tests, such as mammography and sigmoidoscopy) to persons who are not normally receiving such services. Initial results show that the poor are interested in receiving cancer-prevention-related services and will use them if they are made available to them. Second, there are professionals extremely interested in working with the poor to help them prevent cancer.

Another demonstration site was Dade County, FL.[117] Cancer screening for three major sites—breast, cervical, and prostate—were made available to community health care centers located in low-income neighborhoods. This study revealed that many cancer education programs are insensitive and irrelevant to poor people, who often have little formal education; people who cannot afford to pay for health care do not seek care; and a major impediment to providing services to the socioeconomically disadvantaged is the unresponsiveness of the health care system to the problems faced by this particular population. The ACS has made cancer control and the socioeconomically disadvantaged a priority for their divisions and units. Health professionals interested in working with this population should request the booklet "Successful Activities in Reaching and Serving the Socioeconomically Disadvantaged" (No. 24550.07) from their local ACS.

NURSING'S FUTURE IN THE ECONOMICS OF HEALTH CARE

Changes in health care policy and economics are not new. In each decade there has been a different focus—in the 1960s it was access to care; in the 1970s, technologic advancements; in the 1980s, cost containment; and in the 1990s, cost containment with quality care. The birth of the prospective payment system has offered nursing the chance to change from a reactionary, follow-the-textbook, nostalgic approach and to become a proactive, creative, open-minded economically aware profession. It is important to retain the successes and values that nursing has achieved throughout the years while also being ready to advance to a new era of influence and power.[4]

An initial impact of PPS on nursing was to uncouple nursing services from hospital per diem charges along with charges for housekeeping, dietary, and laundry services. The effort to make this change began in 1977, when the New Jersey Health Department initiated development of a model for nursing allocation of resources that was DRG-specific; the model was called relative intensity measures (RIMs) of nursing.[12] The RIMs have been criticized for methodologic failure; the time necessary for planning care, obtaining patient care resources, and evaluating care was not allocated.[12, 118] These daily nursing activities often are more time-consuming than nursing assessments or interventions. In the RIMs study, however, emphasis was given to these components of assessment and intervention. Also criticized was the assumption that care delivered equals care required.[119]

Various other schemes have been used to determine the cost of nursing services or to estimate nursing resource utilization. In 1985 a report from the American Nurses Association Center for Research entitled "DRGs and Nursing Care" was submitted to the HCFA.[120] The project was funded through an HCFA grant. The pilot study examined the relationship between DRGs and both nursing resource utilization and nursing costs. This report noted that the DRGs were developed without explicit attention to nursing resource use or nursing costs in hospitals, which is a significant component of overall hospital activities and costs. Data from the study consisted of approximately 1600 patient records from two hospitals in Wisconsin. Twenty-one DRGs, selected because of the high frequency with which they were encountered among the hospitalized Medicare beneficiaries, were examined. The principle findings outlined in the study follow.[121]

- DRG relative-cost weights generally appear to reflect differences in nursing resource requirements among the DRGs in the study.
- Some DRGs in the study are interpretable groupings of patients both in terms of nursing care by DRG and in terms of the daily pattern of nursing resource consumption during the course of hospitalization.
- Even though nursing care was not given explicit attention when the prospective pricing was developed, nursing costs as defined in the study have been shown to account for between 20% and 28% of hospital costs for two-thirds of the DRGs in the study.
- Sufficient variations in nursing resources utilization patterns and in nursing costs were found to suggest further study in the refinement of prospective pricing. This study clearly defines the need for nursing to be identified in prospective pricing. However, to date the Prospective Payment Commission has not acknowledged this fact. The only concern related to nursing that the Commission discussed in its June 1989 report to Congress was the shortage of registered nurses.

Although there has been great interest in and concern about determining nursing care costs for separate billing in the past several years, rapid movement in that direction has been limited because of the lack of financial or hospital administration support. Unfortunately, some of the nursing literature even suggests that such cost assessments may not be helpful and may not be effective unless the professional nursing staff is salaried.[118] Even with these restraints, success has been achieved in many hospitals toward the goal of billing patients directly for nursing costs. Hospitals in Arizona, Connecticut, New York, and Miami have been noted for their achievement in this area.[4]

Professional nursing has made great strides during the past decade, clinically and in the public policy arena. In a 1990 study conducted by the Office of Technology Assessment it was concluded that professional nursing provides care of a quality equivalent to that provided by physicians, and in a highly cost-effective manner.[122] In 1991 the Treasury Postal Service and General Government Appropriations Bill modified the "freedom of choice" provisions of federal employees' health benefits to accord nurse midwives, nurse practitioners, and nurse clinical specialists, the same independent recognition as accorded their colleagues in optometry, psychology, and clinical social work.[123] Federal employees and their families could receive their health care from these specialists. Medicaid requires all state Medicaid plans to reimburse for the service of certified nurse midwives and certified pediatric and family nurse practitioners.[123] Legislation has been proposed to expand Medicaid mandated coverage for all categories of advanced nurses throughout rural America. The Omnibus Budget Reconciliation Act of 1991 provides reimbursement for all categories of advanced-practice nurses under Medicare Part B within nursing facilities and rural America.

CONCLUSION

The Prospective Payment System will not be static: Changes will occur over time and will further restrict health care payments. A significant opportunity for nurses will be to conduct or participate in the clinical research needed to determine which nursing interventions are most beneficial from a cost–benefit perspective. Although nurses traditionally have developed a variety of interventions to manage patient care problems, there has been minimal research to determine which approach produces the best results. It is important to determine not only which approaches are the best, but also which are the best at the lowest possible cost. When nurses collaborate in this type of research, they will have an impact on the cost of health care and consequently will gain recognition from health care and policy leaders. Nurses are beginning to be appointed to advisory committees involved in research studies with a direct influence on changing our nation's health policy. The nursing profession must strive for this recognition.

Perhaps the greatest impact of DRGs on nursing is in the systems for delivery of nursing care, which often have not kept pace with the rapid and complex changes in health care.[20] One current popular nursing delivery system is primary nursing, which is being monitored by nursing executives not only for its quality but also for its patient care costs. However, newer changes in nursing care delivery systems are on the horizon. O'Malley et al.[20] note that these delivery systems will have to be redesigned to: (1) integrate with hospital business plans, (2) be consumer driven, outcome focused, and flexible, and (3) define more clearly the practice of professional nursing that requires an advanced level of clinical and management skills at the bedside. One example of a redesigned system that has been discussed in this chapter is case management.

In the decade of the 1990s, the profession of nursing will continue to pursue recognition by health care leaders as the most vital link in successfully managing quality patient care at low cost. By unifying the large number of nurses in this country through professional nursing organizations, nurses can gain a strong and powerful voice in the health care arena.

Throughout the chapter it was made very evident that legislation plays an important role in the economics of cancer care. It is almost impossible, as a nurse, to be interested in cancer economics and not be involved in legislative activities. To keep updated on the legislative activities that directly or indirectly affect the costs of health care, contact the Government Relations Committee of the Oncology Nursing Society or the Public Issues Committee of the American Cancer Society.

The clinical nurse specialist will be in a pivotal position in the nursing organization structure. As Yasko and Fleck state:[12, p.71]

> The CNS, with the emphasis on the word *nursing* as the focus of their practice, will be needed to ensure the implementation of sophisticated patient care, which includes: the development, implementation, and evaluation of standards of care; systematic early-discharge programs; methods to document accurately the delivery of nursing care; systems to determine the cost/benefit of new supplies and equipment; methods to more effectively and efficiently teach patients and significant others self-care; and systems to determine the cost of planning, implementing, and evaluating nursing care.

REFERENCES

1. Castro J: Condition: Critical. *Time* 138(21):34–42, 1991.
2. Jacobs P: *The Economics of Health and Medical Care.* Rockville, MD: Aspen, 1987.
3. Ward W: *An Introduction to Health Care Financial Management.* Baltimore, MD: National Health Publishing, 1988.
4. Davis CK: Health care economic issues; projection for oncology nurses. *Oncol Nurs Forum* 12:17–22, 1985.
5. Ernst and Whinney: Diagnosis Related Groups, their evolution, current applications and future implications. Executive Series (No. J58341), Ernst and Whinney, 1980.
6. Bird S, Mailhot C: DRGs: A new way to reimburse hospital costs. *AORN J* 38:773–777, 1983.
7. Joel L: DRGs: The state of the art of reimbursement for nursing services. *Nurs Health Care* 4:560–563, 1983.
8. Medicare program: Final rules. *Federal Register* 43196, August 30, 1991.
9. Hunt K: DRG: What it is, how it works and why it will hurt. *Med Econ* September 5:262–272, 1983.
10. Shaffer F: DRGs: History and overview. *Nurs Health Care* 4:389–396, 1983.
11. Prospective Payment Assessment Commission: Report to Congress: Medicare and the American Health Care System. June 1991.
12. Yasko JM, Fleck AE: Prospective Payment (DRGs): What will be the impact on cancer care? *Oncol Nurs Forum* 11:63–72, 1984.
13. Department of Health and Human Services: *Report to Congress: DRG refinement: Outliers, severity of illness and intensity of care.* Washington, DC: The Department, 1987.
14. National Committee for Quality Health Care: An American health strategy: Ensuring the availability of quality health care. Washington, DC: The Committee, 1988.
15. Young D: Prospective Payment Assessment Commission: Mandate, structure and relationships. *Nurs Econ* 2:309–311, 1984.
16. Young D: PROPAC: Future directions. *Nurs Econ* 4:12–15, 1986.
17. Coulam R, Gaumer G: Medicare's prospective payment system: A critical appraisal. *Health Care Financing Rev* (Annual Supplement):45–77, 1991.

18. Prospective Payment Commission: Report and recommendations to the Congress, March 1992.
19. Rubenstein L, et al: Changes in quality of care for five diseases measured by implicit review, 1981–1986. *JAMA* 264:1974–1979, 1990.
20. O'Malley J, Loveridge C, Cummings S: The new nursing organization. *Nurs Manag* 20:29–33, 1989.
21. New England Medical Center: Definition. The Center for Nursing Case Management. pp. 1–3, 1988.
22. Tokarski C: Hospital inflation a recurring problem. *Mod Healthcare* 18:38–43, 1988.
23. New England Medical Center: Definition. The Center for Nursing Care Management. pp.1–4, 1987.
24. Zander K: Nursing case management: Strategic management of cost and quality outcomes. *J Nurs Admin* 18:23–30, 1988.
25. William B: The utility of nursing theory in nursing case management practice. *Nurs Admin Q* 15:60–65, 1991.
26. Case management: Reports from the field. Special section. *Nurs Manag* 22:30–64, 1991.
27. Grimaldi P: PPS for operating and capital costs. *Nurs Manag* 22:17–19, 1991.
28. Agency for Health Care Policy and Research: Report to Congress: Progress of research on outcomes of health care services and procedures (AHCPR Pub. No. 91-0004). Rockville, MD: The Agency, May 1991.
29. Jacox A, Carr D: Nursing and technology—Clinical practice guidelines. *Nurs Econ* 9:118–120, 1991.
30. Meyer J, Caroll-Silow S, Sullivan S: Critical choices—Confronting the cost of American health care. Report to the National Committee for Quality Health Care. Washington, DC: 1991.
31. Aaron H, Schwartz WB: Rationing health care: The choice before us. *Science* 247:418–422, 1990.
32. Schwartz W: The inevitable failure of current cost containment strategies. *JAMA* 257:222–224, 1987.
33. Schieber G, Poullier J: Recent trends in international health care spending. *Health Affairs* 6:105–112, 1987.
34. Making difficult health care decisions. *Business and Health* 7:11, 1989 (editorial).
35. Finley R: Measuring the cost effectiveness of hematopoietic growth factor therapy. *Cancer* May 15: 2727–2730, 1991 (suppl).
36. Welch H, Larson E: Cost effectiveness of bone marrow transplantation in acute nonlymphocytic leukemia. *N Engl J Med* 321:807–812, 1989.
37. Bedder M, Burchiel K, Larson A: Cost analysis of two implantable narcotic delivery systems. *J Pain & Symp Manag* 6:368–373, 1991.
38. Schulman K, Glick H, Rubin H, et al: Cost-effectiveness of HA-1A Monoclonal antibody for gram-negative sepsis—Economic assessment of a new therapeutic agent. *JAMA* 266:3466–3471, 1991.
39. Yarbro J: Changing cancer care in the 1990s and the cost. *Cancer* March 15 Suppl: 1718–1727, 1991.
40. Hicks L: Using benefit cost and cost effectiveness analysis in health care resource allocation. *Nurs Econ* 3:78–84, 1985.
41. Hochhauser M: A format for health care feasibility studies. *Health Marketing Q* 4:35–41, 1986.
42. Larson E, Peters D: Integrating cost analysis in quality assurance. *J Nurs Quality Assurance* 1:1–7, 1986.
43. Larson E, Maciorowski L: Rational product evaluation. *J Nurs Admin* 16:31–36, 1986.
44. Stahler-Wilson J, Worman F: A product nurse specialist: The complete clinical shopper. *Nurs Manag* 22:36–38, 1991.
45. Millenson M: New options in health insurance. In Zeleny RO, ed. *The World Book Health and Medical Annual*. Chicago: World Book, 1988, pp. 99–107.
46. Miller A, Bradburn E, Hager M, et al: Can you afford to get sick? *Newsweek* 113:45–51, 1989.
47. Murphy E: Health care: Right or privilege? *Nurs Econ* 4:66–68, 1986.
48. Easterbrook G: The revolution in medicine. *Newsweek* 109:40–74, 1987.
49. Hughes J, Heckel V, Vernon F et al: HMO versus FFS practice: A four year retrospective analysis of colorectal cancer diagnosis and treatment. Is there a difference in quality of care? Quality versus reimbursement and other conundrums. (Abstract). Proceedings of 15th National Association of Community Cancer Care, 1989.
50. Kulkarni PR, Vernon SW, Jackson GL, et al: Stage at diagnosis of breast cancer, comparison in a fee-for-service and health maintenance organization practice. *Medical Care* 27:608–621, 1989.
51. Kitzhaber J: Uncompensated care—The threat and the challenge. *West J Med* 148:711–716, 1988.
52. Castro J: Condition critical. *Time* 138:34–42, 1991.
53. Todd J, Seekins S, Krichbaum J, et al: Health access America—Strengthening the U.S. health care systems. *JAMA* 265:2503–2506, 1991.
54. Nutter D, Helms C, Whitcomb M, et al: Restructuring health care in the United States. *JAMA* 265:2516–2520, 1991.
55. National League for Nursing, American Nurses Association, et al: *Nursing's Agenda for Health Care Reform.* New York: National League for Nursing, 1991.
56. American Hospital Association: *National Health Care Strategy—A Starting Point for Debate.* Chicago: American Hospital Association, 1991.
57. Friedman E: The uninsured from dilemma to crisis. *JAMA* 265:2491–2495, 1991.
58. Robinson D: Who should receive medical aid? *Parade Magazine* May 28, 1989, pp. 4–5.
59. Crawshaw R, Garland M, Hines B, et al: Oregon health decisions, an experiment with informed community consent. *JAMA* 254:3213–3216, 1985.
60. Oregon Health Decisions: *Quality of Life in Allocating Health-Care Resources.* Portland, OR: 1988.
61. Goldsmith, J: The US health-care system in the year 2000. *JAMA* 256:3371–3375, 1986.
62. Waldman HB: Knowing more about the elderly can help if we want to provide need services. *Gerontology* 4:83–85, 1985.
63. Iacocca L: Not ready for national health insurance but. . . . *Houston Chronicle* April 16, 1989.
64. Sick health service. *Economist* July 16, 1988, pp. 19–22.
65. Ellwood explains his theory, terminology and outcomes method of managing care. *Modern Healthcare* 19:30, 1989.
66. Ellwood P: Shattuch Lecture—Outcomes management. *N Engl J Med* 318:1549–1556, 1988.
67. Boscarino J: The public's perception of quality hospitals, II: Implications for patient surveys. *Hosp & Health Svcs Admin* 37:13–35, 1992.
68. Fuch VR: The ratio of medical care. *N Engl J Med* 311:1572–1573, 1984.
69. Studnick J: Differences in length of stay of Medicaid and Blue Cross patients and the effect of intensity of services. *Public Health Report* 94:43845, 1979.

70. Presgrove M: Indigent patients: More nursing or less revenue. *Nurs Manag* 16:47–51, 1985.
71. Peters TJ, Waterman RH: *In Search of Excellence.* New York: Harper & Row, 1982.
72. Markus G: Considered approaches to physician payment in the 90s. *Nurs Econ* 6:63–66, 1988.
73. Hagland M: The RBRVS and hospitals: The physician payment revolution on our doorstep. *Hospitals* February 20, 1991.
74. Grimaldi P: Medicare reduces targets for physician payments. *Nurs Manag* 22:14–15, 1991.
75. Medicare program: Final rules. *Federal Register* 56:59502–59819, 1991.
76. Association of American Medical Colleges: *Medicare Revised Coding System for Evaluation/Management (E/M) Services.* Washington, DC: Association of American Medical Colleges, 1992.
77. American Hospital Association: *Meditrends in Cancer Care 1991–1992.* Chicago: American Hospital Association, 1992.
78. Markman M: An argument in support of cost-effectiveness analysis in oncology (Editorial). *J Clin Oncol* 6:937–938, 1988.
79. Drilea S, Mortenson L, Clune C, Evans M: *Cancer DRGs—A Comparative Report on Key Cancer-Related DRGs* (ed. 5). Rockville, MD: Association of Community Cancer Centers, 1991.
80. Katterhagen JG, Clarke RT, Mortenson LE: Understanding the economics of outpatient care. *Oncology Issues* 4:11–14, 1989.
81. Munoz E, Mulloy K, Goldstein J, et al: Costs, quality and the volume of surgical oncology procedures. *Archives Surgical* 125:360–363, 1990.
82. Iezzoni L, Henderson M, Bergman A, et al: Purpose of admissions and resources during cancer hospitalizations. *Health Care Financing Rev* 13:29–40, 1991.
83. Scheffler R, Andrews N: *Cancer Care and Cost: DRGs and Beyond.* Ann Arbor, MI: Health Administration Press Perspectives, 1989.
84. Brown M: The national economic burden of cancer: An update. *J Natl Cancer Inst* 82:1811–1814, 1990.
85. Brady A, Foster J: The development of site specific centers: The breast clinic. *J Cancer Prog Manag* 7:12–14, 1992.
86. Mortenson LE, Winn R: The potential negative impact of prospective reimbursement on cancer treatment and clinical research progress. *Cancer Prog Bull* 9:7–9, 1983.
87. Medicare regulations: Final report. *Federal Register* 49:234, 1989.
88. The Cancer Letter. 15(11):1–6, 1989.
89. Coffey R, Wallen J: *Hospital Cost and Clinical Research Project.* National Center for Health Services Research, National Cancer Institute, Public Health Service, U.S. Department of Health and Human Services, February, 1985.
90. Reese GJ: Cost effectiveness in oncology. *Lancet* 2:1405–1407, 1985.
91. Yasko J: Biological response modifier treatment: Reimbursement: Present status and future strategies. *Oncol Nurs Forum Suppl* 15:28–34, 1988.
92. National Cancer Institute: Facing forward—A guide for cancer survivors. NIH pub. no. 90-2424. Bethesda MD: NCI, 1990.
93. A Gallup Survey of Oncologists' Attitudes and Experiences with Cancer Treatment. Princeton, NJ: Gallup Organization, 1991.
94. Evan M: Trial testimony in a Maryland bone marrow transplant suit. *J Cancer Prog Manag* 6:13–15, 1991.
95. Jensen J: Consumers consider quality in deciding on a hospital, but measurements differ. *Mod Health Care* 19:88, 1989.
96. Report on the responsible conduct of research in the health sciences. *Cope Magazine* 3(6):12–13, 1989 (editorial).
97. Oncology Forum: Is the current system of reimbursement for experimental cancer treatment appropriate for the patient and/or oncologist? *Cope Magazine* 3(6):17–18, 1989 (editorial).
98. Mortenson LE: Insurers target chemotherapy payments. *Wall Street Journal* May 11, 1989.
99. Mortenson LE: Audit indicates half of current chemotherapy uses lack of FDA approval. *Oncol Issues* 3:21–25, 1988.
100. FDA review of new indications is lengthy, costly process. *Oncol Issues* 3:19, 1988 (editorial).
101. Johnson K, Proudfit C, McEvoy G: A guide to drug compendia. *J Cancer Prog Manag* 4:29–31, 1989.
102. United States General Accounting Office: Off-label drugs: Reimbursement policies constrain physicians in their choice of cancer therapies. Washington, DC: U.S. General Accounting Office, GAO/PEMD-91-12 BR, 1991.
103. Medicare demands supervision fee refunds in Indiana. *Oncol Issues* 4:5, 1989.
104. Yasko J, Verfurth M: Closing Comment: Economic trends. *Semin Oncol Nurs* 8:156–158, 1992.
105. Miller C: The impact of the final RBRVS rules on oncology practices. *J Cancer Prog Manag* 7:17–19, 1992.
106. U.S. Department of Health and Human Services: *Cancer Rates and Risks.* NIH Publication (ed. 3), 1985, pp. 33–35.
107. Baird S: Changing economics of cancer care, challenges, opportunities. American Cancer Society Proceedings from the Fifth National Conference on Cancer Nursing. New York: American Cancer Society, 1987, pp. 1–16.
108. Harkin T: Another pound of cure. *JAMA* 266:1692–1693, 1991.
109. Grimaldi P: Screening mammogram is back. *Nurs Manag* 22:20–22, 1991.
110. Lawrence D: A provider's view of prevention approaches in a prepaid group practice. *Cancer* 67:1767–1771, 1991.
111. Mushlin A, Fintor L: Is screening for breast cancer cost-effective? *Cancer* 69:1957–1962, 1992.
112. Medicare Program: Final Rules. *Federal Register,* vol. 57:54–55, 1992.
113. Frank-Stromberg M: Changing demographics in the US—Implications for health professionals. *Cancer* 67(Suppl): 1772–1778, 1991.
114. Steiner C: Access to cancer prevention, detection, and treatment. *Cancer* 67:1736–1740, 1991.
115. American Cancer Society: Report to the nation: Cancer in the poor. Atlanta: American Cancer Society, 1989.
116. Renneker M: An inner city cancer prevention clinic. *Cancer* 67:1802–1807, 1991.
117. McCoy C, Nielsen B, Chitwood D, et al: Increasing the cancer screening of the medically underserved in South Florida. *Cancer* 67:1808–1813, 1991.
118. Kramer M, Schmalenberg C: Magnet hospitals talk about

the impact of DRGs on nursing care. *Nurs Manag* 18:33–40, 1987.
119. Mowry M, Korpman R: Do DRGs reimbursement rates reflect nursing costs? *J Nurs Admin* 15:29–35, 1985.
120. American Nurses' Association, Center for Research: *DRGs and Nursing Care.* HCFA Grant No. 15-C-98421/7-02. Kansas City, Missouri, 1985.
121. Prospective Payment Commission: Medicare Prospective Payment and the American health care system. Report to the Congress. Washington, DC: The Commission, 1989.
122. Office of Technology Assessment: Nurse practitioners, physician assistants, and certified nurse-midwives: A policy analysis. Washington, DC: OTA, 1986.
123. DeLeon P: Nursing: Policy agenda for the future. *Nurs Econ* 10:137–139, 1992.

Chapter 59

Ethical Issues in Cancer Nursing Practice

David C. Thomasma, PhD

INTRODUCTION

Cancer care is challenging on many fronts. In addition to the many physical and emotional challenges faced by oncology nurses, many different ethical issues arise in caring for patients with cancer. Some of these issues are common to all branches of health care, some more specific to nursing, and some specific to cancer itself. This chapter will examine the issues in three broad categories: general issues, nursing issues, and cancer issues.

GENERAL ETHICAL ISSUES

It is customary in every review of ethical theories to sketch the ethical principles of autonomy, beneficence, nonmaleficence, and justice.[1] To these I will add alternative ethical analyses, including virtue theory, with a view toward suggesting the future of health care ethics.

Autonomy

Autonomy is shorthand for a principle that compels us to respect the self-command of the individual. Since *autonomy* means quite literally self-rule, respect for the individual therefore includes not only the free choice a competent patient might make, but also respect for the source of that freedom within the individual.[2] It would be contradictory to attempt to heal a patient while denying the patient's freedom and ability to make decisions about the healing process.

The idea of autonomy originated in the moral realm; that is, autonomy is part of what makes us moral. We are responsible for our own moral acts and must make our own moral rules. Therefore, autonomy should not be equated simply with patients' rights or even with the freedom to choose. It implies something deeper—that the core of what it means to be a person is moral responsibility to oneself and to others. This is not "pure" freedom, but rather freedom to take responsibility for one's own actions and their consequences. In response to that level of responsibility, caregivers have a duty to respect the moral origins of the person, not just to respect the choices the person makes, as will be clarified later.

The notion of autonomy is foreign to traditional health care practice. For centuries, health care practitioners governed by the Hippocratic ethic practiced a form of paternalism, acting in the best interests of others without asking their preferences, or even explicitly acting against their preferences. An example would be refusing to acknowledge the wish of an elderly, competent but somewhat depressed woman to be "left alone" and allowed to die. Caregivers are often reluctant to accept the wishes of individuals with serious disease, especially if they think something still might be done to improve either longevity or quality of life. Another example might be a patient who, fearing the outcomes of cancer, decides to forgo not only any interventionist chemotherapy but also even a biopsy. Despite the right of individuals to determine their own treatment, this scenario would create a conflict between the caregiver's sense of duty to protect and prolong life and the autonomy and privacy rights of the individual patient.

Beneficence

Beneficence is the principle of altruism, that is, to act in the best interests of others. It is the fundamental guiding force behind the helping professions, leading, for example, to the maxim "the patient comes first." Of course, it would be difficult to act at all times on the basis of this principle, since self-interest is a part of duty to oneself. Yet the principle creates an expectation in patients and in society as a whole that health professionals, who are often strangers to the patient, have promised and will take exceptional steps to place their patients' interests above their own.[3]

Sometimes a good thing like beneficence can run amok and lead to a paternalistic (maternalistic) form of "doing good" without attention to the wishes of the other person.[4] In some instances there is a necessary medical paternalism. For example, a patient may have executed the advance directive to refrain from putting her on a respirator due to advanced metastatic liver cancer but now finds herself in the emergency room due to an automobile accident. Her crushed rib cage is potentially treatable. Presumption would be to treat her, even with a respirator, for a reversible event she had not foreseen in her previous determinations about end-stage cancer. Most often, however, paternalism is regarded with moral opprobrium. Beneficence does not rule out trying to persuade patients and even sometimes to almost coerce them to overcome their fears and to help them choose what is in their best interests. But in the final analysis, it is unethical to act against the wishes of patients if they continue to refuse the offerings of modern health care.[5]

In cancer care it is frequently hard to determine what is in the patient's best interest. There may be conflicting courses of treatment, or only statistical or epidemiological information that may or may not apply to the circumstances.[6-8] Also, patients may become incompetent to speak for their own care in the later stages of the disease. In these instances, caregivers focus their efforts on trying to determine objective standards of care, avoiding making quality-of-life judgments by appealing to medical indications.[9] Yet these standards are not as objective as they might first appear. Often they are a combination of current practice, the best medical knowledge of the time, and attention to the context in which care is to be delivered. For instance, the patient's wishes are combined with a judgment about prognosis and weighed against the patient's condition, age, and reasons for treatment requests and refusals.

Nonmaleficence

The third principle governing general health care ethical concerns is the principle of *nonmaleficence.* This principle covers the famous Hippocratic aphorism, "To help, or at least, to do no harm." When caregivers find that there is confusion or disagreement about what is in the patient's best interest, they must fall back to a position of trying, according to the Hippocratic oath, "at least, to do no harm."

In a way, nonharm is a minimalist beneficence position. Respecting the personhood of the patient requires an attempt to honor autonomy *and* to act in his or her best interests. At the very least, however, it means never harming intentionally.

The problem is to define harm. The definition scale can run from physical to psychological and even spiritual harm. Some examples will be discussed later in the context of dying. Since most cancer patients recover or stay in remission, however, it is appropriate here to consider a different example: A 42-year-old woman develops breast cancer metastases while being tried in court for running a prostitution ring under the guise of a high-class escort service. Her cancer now involves her spine and causes her intense pain. But an even greater problem for her is that her son is dying of AIDS, and she wants to care for him before succumbing to her disease and to her trial sentence.[10] Harm for her is the spiritual pain of not being able to nurture her son, rather than her physiological concerns (the spinal involvement of the cancer), or even her likely incarceration ("If the government wants me to go to jail, so be it," she said, "I'd like to spend my time now with my son, and after that they can have my life. I don't care"). This example demonstrates how harms ideally are determined by the patient in conjunction with caregivers, so that a mutually agreed-upon treatment plan can be developed.

Justice

The principle of justice requires that we give each person his or her due. There are competing opinions of how to measure what is due.[11] Some thinkers argue for equity, trying to equalize the inequities of human life by taking from the rich and giving to the poor. Major social programs like Social Security, Medicare, Medicaid, and the income tax exemplify this method. Others argue that egalitarian methods are more appropriate; that is, everyone is entitled to exactly the same treatment (equality) regardless of the starting point.[12] Still others like libertarians argue that justice requires a fundamental respect for autonomy[13] and that one cannot alter the social situation of rich and poor without the consent of the governed. For example, one cannot charge paying patients and their insurance companies more for cancer care than nonpaying patients, thus taking from those who have to help those who do not, without the express consent of the paying patients and their third-party payers.

The different views of justice have little bearing on clinical decisions at this time, although they do influence various proposals for access to care, and hover in the background of most of our social programs, which, as nurses are often aware, can do damage to individuals. As part of the principles of beneficence and nonmaleficence, efforts must be made to provide a better health care delivery system than that currently in place.

Alternative Ethical Theories

The difficulty in clinical ethics is rooted in a confrontation between an abstracting tendency in the long and rewarding history of ethics and the concrete, individual problems encountered by professionals who must make quick decisions about very complex matters in order to benefit their patients. Ethical analysis must take careful note of numerous ethical theories, axioms, and other concerns in order to conduct a minimally decent conceptual and problematic analysis. This process takes time and, of necessity, becomes quite abstract. Health professionals and patients quickly lose interest in these abstractions and theoretical meanderings if they are not decisively and explicitly related to the realities of patient care. They must do ethics on the run.

Ethical principles appear abstract—or better, speculative—because they do not have as much social legitimacy as do the values of everyday life. Moral abstractions frequently are seen by nonphilosophers as devoid of the ingredients of moral concerns that people have in their day-to-day life. No doubt they can and do seep into that daily life, but the process of connecting theory to practice is long and subtle.[14] How often do we encounter physicians and patients who become impatient with "thinking" that has no practical consequence?[15]

Dissatisfaction with principle-based ethical theories has led to new proposals for moral analysis, such as casuistry, hermeneutics, and "ethics as story." *Casuistry* is an ancient methodology by which each case is analyzed on its own merits. No overarching principles will lead to a conclusion from one case to another. *Hermeneutics* is named after the Greek god Hermes, the messenger of the gods. It means interpreting the case in its whole context—the individual's life plans and values, the family's values, social and cultural factors, and the like. *Ethics as story* relies upon concrete narrative to ferret out the interests and values in each instance, especially with relationship to caregivers themselves. Each of these movements stresses the concreteness of the individual situation, the importance of interpreting values of those involved in the case, and the deeper moral drama and constraints that take place during the lives of individuals experiencing serious disease.

Virtue theory is also an alternative that may complement principle-based ethics. No principle could be implemented without the commitment of caregivers or patients to the good as they perceive it. Even the most rule-bound person must have virtues of interior committment to the rules. On the other hand, relying solely on the virtuous caregiver and patient, without a set of objective moral guidelines or principles, leads to follies and foibles and opportunity for abuse.

A nursing philosophy goal to act *as if* the nurse were the patient and *as if* the nurse's values became the patient's values would require some limits. Clearly, the nurse could not carry out actions that would compromise her or his conscience. Further, sometimes disputes about care, like instituting or withdrawing fluids and nutrition for the dying patient,[16,17] limit the ability of some nurses to accomplish this nursing philosophy goal. This dynamic reveals the need for a relation between objective standards (the goal of nursing in this instance) and the virtue of the nurse (his or her own conscience and personal standards).

Arguably the most important virtue for the nurse is compassion. This assertion is based on the view that of all the caregivers involved with the patient, the nurse is the one with the most "hands-on" duties. The implications of this virtue will be explored in the section on Nursing Ethical Issues.

Reconciliation Efforts

The emphasis on personal autonomy in medical ethics is coming under greater scrutiny today. Thinkers concerned about libertarian assumptions implied by this emphasis have countered autonomy with the need for beneficence as well.[18,19] The implications of conflicts about medical ethics and ethics theory include the increased role of the health provider's values in caring for the dying patient;[20] greater attention to the relation between physician and patient, rather than exclusive focus on the needs and wants of the patient alone; and questions about the kind of society we ought to be.[21]

Pellegrino and I have proposed that the goal of health care ought to be "beneficence-in-trust." By this we mean that the caregiver holds in trust the values of the patient in making joint decisions with the patient about best interests. It would not be appropriate to act in the best interests of the patient without paying attention to the autonomous decision making and values of the patient.[3] This is but one of a number of proposals to integrate the power of the healer's art with the autonomy of the patient.[22]

Another approach is that of libertarianism. Perhaps the most articulate spokesperson for a libertarian version of secular humanism is H. Tristram Engelhardt, Jr. In his *Bioethics and Secular Humanism,* he argues that secular humanism itself has no moral content. But as an ethical position it reigns supreme for moral argumentation among moral strangers, that is, individuals whose fundamental values are either unknown to one another, or, actually, whose moral values can be considered to be estranged from one another. Engelhardt bases his argument on a fundamental rationality all human beings share that can enlighten them in their pursuit of consensual agreements in bioethics.[23]

No matter what approach is taken, it is important that individual moral commitments are not separated from ethical decision making. Further, schema for resolving ethical dilemmas must remain exceptionally sensitive to the concrete situation and particularities of both patient and nurse.[24] Finally, any doctrine of human rationality must be met with reservation: Our own ineptitude at honoring others, our downright evil deeds, and the general violent nature of today's human society, in which individuals are treated as objects for the pleasure and good of others, call into question an unexamined view of human rationality. More important, a rationalistic approach to bioethical decision making ignores human beings' potentialities of nature and virtue to identify with a vulnerable, sick, or dying individual through compassion.

Let us look at two clinical management concepts in more detail, since they are closely related.

Casuistry

Casuistry can be used as the basic model for how the good decision emerges in health care. Put simply, casuistry is the theory that each case is unique, and from that case are developed certain norms that may or may not be applicable in analogous cases. The goal of casuistry is to establish the paradigm case, in which most analysts would agree that a certain norm predominates—say, truth telling as an obligation to a cancer patient whose family is trying to protect the individual from the devastating news. Other cases are then related to this one and analyzed for the extent to which they "match" or "do not match" the paradigm case. Continuing the example of truth telling, an analogous case would be one in which the patient has had two heart attacks already and is prone to panic when hearing bad news. The family's desire to protect this patient is based on a different reason than in the paradigm case.

More theoretical work needs to be done on the assumptions of casuistry, however. This becomes apparent when we begin to delve into the ways in which we use clinical judgment to interpret experience by "mining" the good. By this I mean that we pay particular attention to patient and caregiver value systems, as well as the hierarchy of those values. Which values outrank others in the minds of the parties of the healing relationship? The following discussion targets two major problems with casuistry.

The most difficult part of casuistry is that it presupposes a unified theory of human nature by which one case can be logically compared to another. This unified theory of human nature was provided by the *natural law* theory. But this theory, as it was employed in the past, is now as discredited as is traditional casuistry. Toulmin and Jonsen[25] argue that casuistry arose as a method at just that time in Western civilization when the metaphysical superstructure of Christianity began to collapse under the rise of the modern state, nationalism, and the age of reason.[27] They therefore make the case that casuistry is eminently suitable for modern times, times of pluralism, times without a moral consensus.[26] Yet it is difficult to ignore the need for some mode of comparison by which one case is at the very least analogous to the other. Meaning is not wholly and completely individual. It arises in a context beyond or encompassing the individual case. The very basis for analogous cases is some lasting "something" that crosses the boundaries of each case.

There is a second, and related, problem. Casuistry was discredited by those who held that ethical theory was very important. The method of ethical analysis changed from case orientation to deducing practical conclusions from principles. Reinstituting casuistry as the model for both ethical and medical decisions neglects the importance of ethical theory and, analogously, of the relationship of individuals within the case and their values to the emergence of the good.

Contextualism

Casuistry challenges the deductive model of ethical reasoning. It is closer to clinical judgment, it describes realistically (rather than ideally) how good decisions come about, and it is practical. Yet casuistry neglects the importance of theory and of the nexus of values that ethical theory seeks to protect. Is there a middle ground between deducing the good decision from abstract and theoretical principles that ignore clinical realities and educing the former entirely from the latter? Is there a middle ground between deduction and induction of the good?

A middle course between a generalist application of ethical theory and specialized case-by-case analysis is possible with a contextual grid for medical ethics.[27] Clinical ethics must address itself to contexts. Neither axioms nor standard moral rules are sufficient (although they are necessary, of course) to determine the validity of moral theory and ethical principles in resolving medical ethics problems.[28] Additional rules, or guidelines for relating theory and practice, must be developed according to this approach. Among these rules is that context serves as a way to analyze value hierarchies in concrete circumstances. Earlier I emphasized the importance of considering the particularities of a case, including its context, for a properly compassionate analysis (to be discussed in more detail in the next section).

Thus, according to the contextualism theory, what is needed is a means by which to locate a moral problem and to exhibit the likely values and principles at issue within that locus. The context having been established by such a "grid," the discussion can proceed toward means for resolving the case by protecting the interests and values of those affected by it. But that is not all. The grid not only locates and focuses the moral discussion; it also hints at the cross-case commonalities that legitimize the acts of organizing similar cases, comparing them, and drawing conclusions about the new case.

A variability of contexts in the clinical resolution of cases is noticeable to all who work in the medical setting. This variability does not so much describe the relativity of values and principles as it does how the weight they bring to bear on a case is partially determined by the medical specialty involved; the personal values of the patient, family, or social group; the personal and professional values of the health care professionals involved; and the institutional setting in which the problem arises. Some principles and axioms will be given more weight than others in such a scheme, and one important component of the weighting will stem from the contexts. The good will arise out of the mix of these components.

Such a contextual grid is only one aspect, then, of what might be called *context-variable moral rules.* Other examples could be examined that do not fit the contextual grid pattern but are moral rules that in other ways vary with the context. Further, the contextual grid cannot encompass all of the variables in a case, but only the ones most likely to be affecting the emphasis of some values or principles over others. This is precisely where deductive models of ethical reasoning fall short.

For example, the rule of protection of autonomy is more likely to be given prominent focus in a primary care context than in a tertiary care context, wherein one's autonomy is virtually always depressed and hence concern for autonomy is diminished in favor of a goal of preservation of life and/or restoration of health.[29] Furthermore, the rule of protection of autonomy is more likely to be emphasized in cases in which there is no threat to others than in cases wherein the common good must be considered. Finally, because the grid only *describes* most likely weights given to moral principles and rules in formulating an indicated course of action, one should not misconstrue the contextual grid as claiming that physicians in tertiary care settings do not care about protecting their patients' autonomy, or that public health officials stress social responsibility to the exclusion of individual well-being. All of these moral values bear upon a case. The grid only describes what values are most likely to take precedence over others.

The contextual grid theory rests on two distinctions. The first is the distinction between primary, secondary, and tertiary care settings, a standard distinction in medicine that forms one set of coordinates of the grid. Its importance for moral reasoning lies in the seriousness of the assault on personal wholeness brought about by the diseases in question.[30] Thus, a patient's wishes are more likely to be sought and respected in a primary care setting than in an emergency room after a pulmonary insufficiency attack, where a paternalistic response may be more appropriate. The second distinction or coordinate of the grid is that between the individual and the number of persons affected by the problem. A good example would be the difference in moral analysis between an individual who refuses chemotherapy and wishes to die from cancer without "any fuss" and a mother of four whose children might still need her to help them cope with her impending death. The former wish might be respected almost immediately, whereas the latter's wish should be balanced with other duties she has as a mother.

The moral significance of this distinction is based on the increasing complexity that occurs when the values of different persons whose interests are affected by the outcome of the case enter our consideration and on our increased tendency to protect the common good the greater the number of affected persons. Recall again the grid's purpose to describe context-variable rules, that is, which principles and axioms are likely to be given more weight than others in a given circumstance in formulating a moral policy or in developing an indicated course of action.

Ethical Work-up

An excellent tool developed for case analysis embodying the points raised so far is the Ethical Work-up. The aim of this tool is to try to examine as many values as possible in the case and to reach a resolution that respects as many of these as possible. This is done through critical reflection on the importance of some values and principles over others in the context of the particular circumstances of the case. Thorough consideration of each step of the work-up permits nurses and other health professionals to examine their own values as well as those of the patient, other caregivers, the hospital, and society as a whole. Furthermore, principles, rules, duties, and virtues also come into play in the later steps during the resolution process. I have developed the following six-step work-up for case-oriented bioethics courses. The health professional examining the case is addressed directly in the instructions:

ETHICAL WORK-UP GUIDE

The work-up is an attempt to distill from the discipline of ethics an essential process of moral reasoning that can be used to resolve cases. In other words, no attempt is made to force you to take one or another position in the history of ethical theory. Instead, you are asked to follow only one absolute: Come up with an ethically justifiable course of action for the patient. This meshes with your professional duty to act in the best interests of the patient.

Step 1. *What are the facts in the case?* Be sure to research any medical facts not presented in the case but possibly relevant to its outcome.

Step 2. *What are the values at risk in the case?* Describe all relevant values—that is, values of the physicians, patients, house staff, nurses, hospital administration, the institution, and society itself. This may not be an exhaustive listing of interests in the case.

Step 3. *Determine the principal conflicts between values and professional norms and between ethical axioms, rules, and principles.* Conflicts can occur among *prima facie* absolute values, norms, axioms, rules, and principles, and/or among each other. The principal clash, in the end analysis, is the one you determine it to be.

In determining this principal clash, you should explain if you think principles and values are absolute and whether to be ethical means to act on principles, or whether you hold that they are only at first glance, that is, *prima facie* absolute, and can yield to other important values and principles in the case. You should also note the difference between values, norms, axioms, rules, and principles.

Step 4. *Determine possible courses of action, and state which values and ethical principles each course of action would protect or infringe.* At this step you will grapple with fundamental moral theory. Are you willing to seek a solution that is based on a single principle? Or are you willing to note that each decision you might make will place some values, principles, etc., at risk? Would you then be satisfied with being utilitarian—that is, protecting as many values and principles as possible in the case?

Step 5. *Make a decision in the case.*

Step 6. *Defend this course of action. Why is X better than Y?* In defending this course of action, ask whether consensus ethics is appropriate. Does doing what most think is right necessarily right? Should the decision rest on a single value or principle? Instead, should it protect as many values as possible? Or should it rest on the virtue of the caregivers or institutions in which it takes place?

Please respond to each of the following:

- Were any values, principles, norms, axioms, or rules weighted more heavily than others? If so, which values, principles, etc., were most important to protect and why? If not, was the case decided by protecting as many of the values in the case as possible?
- Try to identify the type of moral reasoning applied in resolving the case (utilitarian, deontologic, virtue-ethic, care ethics, casuistic ethics, other) and state whether it was used because of your general preference in similar situations or because of its particular applicability to this specific case.
- Universality test: Would you be willing that your decision and its reasons become universal law and apply to every similar situation? To yourself? Is this test actually a valid way to determine what is ethical?
- What role does society play in making this decision palatable? Can you imagine a different society and different solution? Would the decision require you to change the political system or the way health care is delivered? Are social and political duties a feature of the nature of the profession and clinical judgment? Do you believe in cultural relativism?
- How does this decision relate to others you have made in your life, in courses, and in actuality as a professional?

NURSING ETHICAL ISSUES

As we have seen, beneficence must go well beyond the minimalistic interpretation of avoiding harm. It entails helping others even when that involves inconvenience, sacrifice, and risk to self-interest. Conflicts occur between the obligation to help others and self-interest. At risk is the primary obligation of advocacy of the patient's interest, which is at the heart of any compassion-based medical ethic. If, as Loewy[31] contends, the possibility of suffering is the basis of a beneficent community, the compassion for the sick is one of the highest forms of virtue.

The Virtue of Compassion

The community traditionally supported compassionate care of individuals by providing for individuals who were sick to be surrounded by those who loved them the most and knew their values. Decisions about health care were made within a context of compassion and respect for the values of the patient. Such care was impervious to marketplace economics. It was an act of mercy, not a commodity to be traded or delivered.

By contrast, today the community seems more concerned about the resources the sick divert from other projects. Rationing care appears to be more valued than providing it. The most vulnerable—the poor, the elderly, the chronically handicapped, the infants, the mentally ill, and the retarded—are the ones who will suffer the most from rationing. With concern about rationing comes a danger of shrinking from sacrifice—of time, emotions, energies, and money—that the care of the sick requires. So urgent has the economics of health care become that some traditional caregivers, like religious hospitals, contemplate withdrawing from this vital service.

But none of the changes in society or the technology of medical care can alter the call the sick themselves press upon caregivers so insistently, the call from fellow creatures in need.[32] Recognizing their need as persons can only be done if the caregiver's own self-perception is of being an agent of mercy and compassion. What is the meaning of this compassion within the context of biomedical decisions?

Compassion is more than pity or sympathy. It transcends social work, philanthropy, and government programs. It is the capacity to feel, and suffer with, the sick person—to experience something of the predicament of illness, its fears, anxieties, temptations, its assault on the whole person, the loss of freedom and dignity, the utter vulnerability, and the alienation every illness produces or portends. And true compassion is more than feeling. It flows over in a willingness to help, to make some sacrifice, to go out of one's way. "No one can help anyone without entering with her whole person into the painful situation; without taking the risk of becoming hurt, wounded, or even destroyed in the process."[33]

Compassion entails a comprehension of the suffering experienced by another. Individuals who have themselves suffered are sometimes better able to understand others' suffering. As De Unamuno[34] says, "Suffering is the substance of life and the root of personality, for only suffering makes us persons." Compassion for the suffering of others thus enriches self-understanding, especially of what we too must some day pass through. Compassion helps us realize that sick brothers and sisters are not aliens; they are still very much part of the human family and are vital to one's own spiritual growth. The healthy need the sick to "humanize" them as much as the sick need the healthy to humanize their sickness.

For health professionals and the family or surrogates, compassion is the quality that keeps them from operating solely on the basis of objectivity and rationality. It enables them to recognize that, effective as our science and technology can be, they do not remove suffering. The sick cannot escape the confrontation with mortality that even a minor illness may entail. Human illness is always illness of the whole person—body, mind, and spirit. Hence, the illness and/or dying process is more than some aberration in an organ system. The illness transcends the biological to encompass the whole person and his or her value system. Illness fractures self-image, upsets the balance the patient has struck between aspirations and limitations. Illness is nothing less than a deconstruction of the self.

Compassion enables decision makers to assist in healing, if by healing we can mean the reconstruction of the person. Involved here is an effort to put back together a ruptured self that has separated into an ego and a body that has betrayed that individual.[35] Nurses help defend against the attack on the spirit as well as the attack on the body. The particularities of culture, ethnicity, and language make illness a unique experience for each person. True healing and appropriate decision making can only take place when all of the particulars and values of the individual and all the parties involved in the process of caring for the sick person are taken into account.[36] Compassionate care also means that the patient who cannot be cured by medical sciences—especially the dying cancer patient—may still be "healed" if we help him or her to express the meaning of a life in the final days of that life by respecting, insofar as possible, the patient's values and commitments.

Clinical Ethics and the Relation to the Patient

Since the beginning of modern clinical ethics, it has been clear that the reasoning patterns of clinical judgment in medical care parallel those of ethical judgment. This realization is important for many reasons. For example, education programs in health professional schools have acquired a "clinical" focus of relevance and reality by stressing the similarities among nursing, medical, and ethical decision making.[37] Articles and books on the philosophy of health care have sometimes underscored the relation of the ethics of health care to clinical judgment.[38] More pointedly for our purpose, the nexus between clinical judgment and clinical ethics can help reveal structures of good decision making in patient care that are not simple products of contractual models of the provider–patient relationship. More is going on in that relationship than initially meets the eye.

Contrast a superficial view of the provider–patient relationship with one that digs more deeply into the humanity of caregiving. Some thinkers argue profoundly about traditional commitments to the value of human life within the patient care relationship as contrasted to respect for autonomy alone.[39] Thus, Leon Kass[40] presents a thoughtful articulation of what is owed a dying patient by health professionals. He argues that humanity is owed humanity, not just "humaneness" (i.e., being merciful by killing the patient). Kass suggests that the reason we are compelled to put animals out of their misery is that they are *not* human and thus demand from us some measure of humaneness. By contrast, human beings demand from us our humanity itself. This thesis, in turn, rests on the relationship "between the healer and the ill" as constituted, essentially, "even if only tacitly, around the desire of both to promote the wholeness of the one who is ailing.[40]

We might call the temptation to employ technology rather than one's personhood in the process of healing "the technological fix." The technological fix is not only easier to conceptualize and implement than the more difficult processes of human engagement but is also "suggested" by technology itself. The training and skills of modern health professionals are overwhelmingly nurtured within an environment of technological fixes. By instinct and proclivity, people in a modern civilization are tempted by technical rather than personal solutions to problems.

A responsible use of technological intervention with and for the sake of a patient requires not only rational analysis but also sensitivity to the particularities of the case and the emotional content of value commitments of the parties involved. The responsible use of power is a clinical ethics judgment about the best balance of interventions and outcomes. Such interactive concerns tend to present counterpressures to a straightforward honoring of patient wishes and autonomy.[41] The virtue of compassion requires an almost exquisite awareness of the physical condition of the patient (to assess outcomes) and the values of patients or of those speaking for them (to assess the quality of those outcomes measured against the patient's values).

The most dramatic examples of taking responsibility for the particularities of a case are culled from problems of withholding and withdrawing care from the dying. But compassion is also required to assess properly the interventions to be given to the weak and debilitated elderly, to the demented, to individuals with metastases, to other vulnerable persons, and to individuals who wish to exercise their autonomy in ways that are clearly self-destructive.

The Patient Self-Determination Act

The Patient Self-Determination Act went into effect in December, 1991. Essentially, the act requires all health care institutions, including home care and hospice, to notify patients upon admission to the institution or service of their rights under state law to execute an advance directive. Other provisions include asking patients whether they have issued an advance directive or wish to do so, asking for a copy if they have, putting that copy prominently in the patient record, and notifying the patient of the institution's commitment to honor the patient's wishes. Obtaining the wishes of individuals before they enter health care institutions or home health care should not be seen as yet another bureaucratic process. Instead, the Act should be used as an opportunity to evidence respect for the moral center of the person.

Part of the reason for the Act was surely to underscore the importance of patients' rights. But another was Congress's interest in controlling costs of health care, particularly during the last 6 months of a patient's life. Almost 40% of the Medicare budget covers this period. It would stand to reason that honoring patient wishes would not only show respect for persons but also would help save critical health care funds.

Difficulties arise when the wishes expressed do not anticipate future events. Sometimes a patient agrees to a "do not resuscitate" (DNR) order regarding the primary disease of progressive, metastatic cancer but then develops sepsis that might be reversible. If the patient also had said earlier that she did not want to "be on a respirator," but that treatment is required to treat the sepsis, can her wishes be disregarded in this instance? Many health professionals are concerned that advance directives will artificially tie their hands in treatment decisions. Many patients agree, avoiding advance directives in favor of "letting the doctor decide." Nurses are usually caught in the middle on issues like this, as they find it difficult to interpret the treatment plan if the physician chooses to ignore advance directives for any reason. In such cases an ethics consult or patient-care discussion is recommended.

Compassionate Analysis

The notion of "compassionate analysis" mentioned earlier embodies both the virtue of compassion and the various mechanisms available for protecting patient autonomy. Advances have occurred in emphasizing the rights of patients not only to determine the treatments they desire and do not desire during the dying process, but also to choose treatments at any time during life, not just while dying. The efforts of patient advocacy groups in sponsoring and supporting legislation and court deliberations have been outstanding. As the use of Living Wills and Advance Directives, including the Durable Power of Attorney, becomes more common, patient rights will be further clarified (e.g., how will they impact long-term care settings?).[42] What is important to note is that the underlying principle of such instruments is the prevention of suffering—that is, to increase the role of compassion in decisions about life-prolonging technology.[43] A logical extension of patient rights could be to allow even greater control over the dying process.

A Living Will gives advance directives for the final period of terminal illness. In most states where it has been approved, the Living Will covers only the terminal phase of an illness, interpreted to mean the last few weeks of a person's life. Most states explicitly rule out directives about fluids and nutrition. Consequently, the Living Will is a limited instrument. Much more favored is the Durable Power of Attorney. This instrument gives another person authority to make health care decisions for an individual who becomes incompetent to do so. Not only would this person know the patient's wishes, but also he or she could communicate with the caregivers to discern the best treatment or nontreatment options during the course of temporary or permanent incompetency. The disease course changes, as do options along the way. Unforeseen events may occur.

The Durable Power, unlike the Living Will, covers any treatment decisions, formally anticipated or not, and at any stage in life, not just in a terminal situation. This is important because medical technology gives health care providers enormous power at all levels of life, especially at the end. Most often health care providers are concerned about the ethical issues in active, direct euthanasia, instead of being concerned with meeting a person's physical and social needs. Tendency of the "technofix" society is to prolong suffering in conditions of what Braithwaite and I[44] have defined as "hopeless injury":

> a condition in which there is no potential for growth or repair; no observable pleasure or happiness from living . . . and a total absence of one or more of the following attributes of quality of life: cognition or recognition, motor activity, memory or awareness of time, consciousness, and language or other intelligent means of communicating thoughts or wishes.

Daily life is full of interactions with "things"—nonhuman and fundamentally incomprehensible to most persons. We sometimes get so used to technological processes that we behave as though they are substitutes for human and compassionate care. Eating for many elderly and dying patients has been replaced by tubes; participating in the spiritual and material values of human life has been replaced by "merely surviving," as a being subjugated to the products of human imagination. As Illich observes: "Medical civilization is planned and organized to kill pain, to eliminate sickness, and to abolish the need for acts of suffering and dying. . . . The new experience that has replaced dignified suffering is artificially prolonged, opaque, depersonalized maintenance."[45, p. 106]

"Beings" subjected to such depersonalized maintenance may no longer be as human as the rest of us. This is no way to respect the value of human life. Is a permanently unconscious being without any ability to relate to its environment a "person"? Part of taking responsibility for our technology is to avoid this subjugation of human life to machinery in the first place, through more thorough discussions of possible outcomes and patient values regarding them.

CANCER ETHICAL ISSUES

There is an increasing concern that medical technology impedes the search for meaning in life. This is especially true during serious illness, during its initial diagnosis, the hopeful process of recovery, and the anguished process of dying. Society's impediments to a search for meaning have been well described by thinkers such as MacIntyre.[26] The focus of this section will be on the concrete processes of decision making in caring for the cancer patient that reveal that same search for meaning. In other words, the primary ethical duty of compassionate cancer care is rooted in a mutual exploration of the human condition. The following are only a few of the specific ethical concerns related to cancer care.[46]

The Dynamics of Cancer

The *dynamics of cancer* refers to the spiritual struggle of the patient to come to terms with the diagnosis of cancer. The word *spiritual* is used deliberately to identify the intense inner realm of fundamental values each person possesses. The realm is often neglected in daily life because external matters and concerns so easily obscure it. Driving to the grocery store to select items for dinner, having the grandchildren at the house over the weekend, planning a vacation, and pursuing the myriad other events of daily living funnel our attention outside this spiritual dimension, though the values connected to the choices made in the external life are stored there. Periodically we may examine these values. Indeed, Socrates admonished that "the unexamined life is not worth living." But serious trauma in the external life is often necessary before people face their spiritual realm directly.

For a patient with cancer this spiritual struggle may be intensified by confusion about goals of treatment, longevity concerns, doubts about the most effective therapy, problems of cost and benefit, and the relation of these difficulties to the patient's longstanding system of values. Hence the examination of values that is forced on everyone with trauma and dreadful news is compressed in patients first hearing the news that they have cancer. Even though today advanced care can relieve the fear that to have cancer means to be sentenced to die, death is often the most immediate fear.

The dynamics of cancer has its own structure. At first, patients may feel guilty. Cancer is seen as self-destructive, almost as if the body is eating itself. One patient with colon cancer blamed herself, for example, because of her lengthy struggle with her son's alcoholism. She thought that she "took it out" on her own body, that she was bound to become seriously ill (and statistics bear her out). Another patient undergoing interleukin-2 therapy complained in tears that he could not spend another night with the nightmares he kept having, nightmares that acid he unleashed was destroying him and his family as it ate into the basement where they were hiding.

Later, patients usually arrive at a more peaceful stage. They come to see that they are not usually responsible for their cancer. Even if they risked cancer through smoking or other bad habits, they might forgive themselves. In this phase of the dynamic, cancer is made into an object, an "It,"[47] an invading army of cells. Because cancer, however, is an autocorporeal disease, conceptually it is inescapable to feel that one's own body has betrayed the person. For this reason, patients continue to view the body as a contributing factor to their disease, which contributes profoundly to the level of suffering they experience.

Depending on age and habits of resiliency, patients may choose to do battle with the "It" that is cancer. But the battle and the desire to fight it are complicated by the patient's own assessment of his or her life span. Regularly, patients refer to their own sense of impending end. Yet, as the data seem to indicate, caregivers treat cancer patients near the end of their lives more and more aggressively (and expensively).[48]

Guilt reemerges when individuals decide not to continue against the odds. This guilt is attached to the patient's worries about loved ones. Does my husband understand that I still love him, although I am no longer going to "fight" the cancer? Do my children perceive that I no longer find the odds of getting better while feeling worse on experimental therapy worth it? Families, in turn, seem to deny that their loved one could wind up like this, wasting away before their eyes.

The likelihood of participating in research therapies for cancer treatment may decline in elderly cancer patients due to lowered life span expectations; poorer prognosis due to more advanced stages of the disease; the body's inability to cope with the collateral effects; and, very importantly, a value hierarchy that places other factors, like the grandchildren's college education, over one's own continued life.

This then is the cancer dynamic: guilt, to objectification of the disease, to a sense of betrayal by the body, to struggles with the cancer, to relapse, and guilt about deciding to stop. The dynamic is a spiritual struggle. In the elderly it is compressed by their sense of the limitations on their life span. An important component at each step of the dynamic is the autonomous ranking of values, which is essential to grasp in the care of all patients, especially the elderly, who have had more opportunities to establish and hone their values through the challenges life has thrown their way.[49]

Cancer and Autonomy

Autonomy is often identified with decision making, but patients themselves seldom make this identification.[50] Given the complexity of the cancer dynamic, it is not surprising that caregivers might misjudge the role of autonomy in the spiritual struggles of their patients. The latter are engaged with at least three struggles:[51]

1. with the body, often leading to physical exhaustion
2. with the environment, their family, community, job, nursing home, etc.
3. with their own values, including their life plans, expectations, the hierarchy of their values, and so on

While the cancer dynamic continues, the patient identifies autonomy with reshuffling a hierarchy of values. These values are not communicated to caregivers as a general rule, and this is the challenge of creating a good therapeutic plan that does not deprive the patient of that which is most dear. The values can easily be missed in well-intentioned but ineffective efforts to respect the patient.

The importance of this value hierarchy for quality-of-life decisions cannot be overemphasized. By respecting this hierarchy we can best protect against paternalistic overtreatment against a patient's wishes[52] and any biased undertreatment of cancer patients. This point underlines the importance of finding out patients' values as part of the process of respecting them as persons. It is also the guiding principle in constructing a therapeutic plan.[53] If a patient chooses no therapy for prostate cancer in order to give his money to his grandchildren for their college education, this value is essential to the person he has chosen to become during his life. It makes no sense to strip his personhood from him.

Cancer and Suffering

Pain is a major consideration in caring for any cancer patient. It can so preoccupy caregivers that concomitant suffering is masked. Yet it is the suffering of the patient that should appeal most to our compassion. The first source of suffering is the bifurcation of the person into an ego, often isolated and alone, and the body that has betrayed that person, the object taken over by the disease. This betrayal is bad enough for a person at any age, but in the elderly it is compounded by what are euphemistically called "the indignities of age." There is a documented disparity between patient and physician evaluation of the quality of life.[54,55] The patient's own judgment of his or her quality of life influences and predicts the patient's term of survival. Involving patients in decisions about the therapeutic plan can help heal the suffering caused by the division of the self into ego and body. This is an irony because patients' efforts to reconstitute the self tempt them to abandon decisions about their traitorous body to the doctors, turning instead to the ego and its values.

Attention to quality-of-life concerns can breach the gap and center the decisions about patient care.[56] In other words, concern for patient values, both making the effort to discover them and using them to design a humane treatment plan, is fundamental. Paying attention to patient decision making per se is structurally correct, but it is not enough to make a difference. Decision making is only a door through which higher forms of respect for persons pass. A good example would be how a "difficult patient," dying of breast cancer metastases, becomes less belligerent as soon as she is involved in the decisions yet to be made about her care. Once the offer to participate is accepted, the patient not only "accepts" the illness, either explicitly or implicitly, but also, by that very participation, she becomes part of the healing relationship that was dysfunctional earlier.

The biggest danger a cancer patient faces is that of being stripped of his or her values in the face of the panoply of interventions we have available. The emotional roller coaster of promises and hopes versus outcomes and despairs can disrupt the relationships people have constructed all of their lives.[57] Letting go not only of one's life but also of one's social roles and relationships is part of this kind of care that only adds to the suffering the patient experiences. It is endemic to the goal of palliative medicine.

Suffering, then, is much more than personal disruption. Yet its base lies there, where the disease has shattered the human entity, at least for a time, until some synthesis can be effected. The primary task of caregivers is to aid in this synthesis as much as possible. Some recommendations are:

- Minimize suffering, not only through pain control efforts but also by confronting one's own blockages to meeting the suffering person as a person. Training in pain control is essential to this step, but so is training in avoiding withdrawal and fears we have ourselves about dying.
- Make every effort to understand the patient's value system, so that it can be respected and employed in the treatment plan. This may include using values assessment tools.
- Implement the care plan as a means to minimize suffering. There is nothing worse for patients who are dying than having to wrestle with caregivers over the treatment plan.
- Even when the patient can no longer feel pain and is in a comatose state near the end of life, respecting his or her values is still essential so that the person he or she was, despite the current condition, is nonetheless respected.

Termination of Treatment

All the preceding reflections are essential to a consideration of issues of termination of treatment. Such decisions involve the proportionality of the treatment to the expected and sometimes realized outcome for the individual in his or her specific circumstances.[58] The word *specific* is important. There is no absolute objective standard by which to measure this proportionality. Each instance must be judged on its own characteristics.

What might be deemed appropriate care for a younger patient, say an experimental chemotherapeutic regimen for a 36-year-old man newly diagnosed with pancreatic cancer, cannot be proposed for an older patient, for example a 93-year-old previously healthy widow. The reasons for this difference may be broader than physical condition of the body alone. They may also be related to the individual's life plans.[59] The younger person may wish to buy some time to put his affairs in order, for little hope can be offered for improvement for a significant length of time in the face of pancreatic cancer.[6] The elderly patient may have no such plans and may be quite willing to die despite any entreaties by the family to try to fight the disease. Her body may have given her so much pain by this point that she has come to consider it an impediment.

Withholding and withdrawing

Most caregivers today seem more willing to withhold and withdraw major interventions deemed "heroic," but their reasons appear somewhat confused. Should this action be done with the goal of bringing about the patient's death (an action I have called "death induction"[69])? In this analysis, death is seen as good and actions are taken to bring about that good.[61] Graber and I[62] have argued that we may be morally obligated to bring about what is perceived as the good in this regard. Or, instead, should the goal be to remove treatments that prolong the patient's suffering, while not intending the patient's death? This intent is entirely different from the first. It assumes that death is either neutral or an evil, and that one cannot will such an evil and still maintain purity of heart. The action of withholding or withdrawing will be the same in either case, however.

The distinction in intent between aiming at the patient's death and aiming at reducing suffering originally was used to distinguish between active and passive euthanasia. The distinction has recently become essentially moot, since most of those who pay attention to the distinction find that there is no moral difference between withholding and withdrawing on the one hand and actively bringing about death on the other, if the intent is that the patient's death would be a good thing.[63] This makes sense. If our intent in withdrawing care is to bring about death, then other more direct forms of euthanasia may seem much more appropriate. We do not want patients to suffer unduly, even if the pain itself is under control.

Currently Americans are hotly debating whether to legalize active euthanasia, aid in dying, and physician-assisted suicide.[64] In the majority of cases, pain control and addressing the suffering of patients as is done in hospice will be sufficient to properly care for patients. More effort must be made to confront and alleviate the patient's suffering, however. I have suggested that having more dialogue about values will honor and support dying cancer patients. Use an interview format around values assessment, but do not confine the process to a single conversation. A continuing dialogue would be most appropriate. Although values do not change, attitudes about values do as the disease progresses.

Planning for a good death would lead to restraint of our technological interventions at various stages in the course of disease, depending on the patient's values, willingness to trade possible severe side effects for the chance of an improved, albeit temporary quality of life, and the patient's self-definition.[65] Of major concern is allowing physicians to kill patients out of mercy in the context of a society that has so little respect for human life in other areas.

Control of dying and life support

Our concerns should not be confined to dispatching persons too early by injections, if simultaneously little or no attention is paid to meeting their physical and social needs. One "technofix" solution to patient anguish is to prolong suffering in conditions of hopeless injury.[66] A good example, unfortunately all too common, is putting an 80-year-old senile and incompetent patient, dying of cancer, on renal dialysis. No family members are left to protest. The patient is brought three times a week to the medical center from the nursing home.

Much of earlier technological intervention was not so much life-supporting but, as Albert Jonsen[67] suggests, organ-supporting. Now, increasingly, truly systematic efforts are made to prolong all the vital organ systems at once, getting the essential nutrients in and wastes out. Not only have we moved from organ-specific technologies to systemic ones, but also from temporary support to permanent support. Jonsen wonders just what exactly life support supports:

> We talk about the maintenance of life; we don't often talk about the maintenance of personhood. It interests me little, indeed, not at all, to be alive as an organism. In such a state I have no interests. It is enormously interesting for me to be a person . . . It is the perpetuation of my personhood that interests me; indeed, it is probably my major and perhaps my sole real interest.[67,p.67]

The effect of employing life-prolonging technology on the dying without patient involvement in its application is to increase patient and family suffering. It may prolong the suffering of dying, and it provides social suffering by wasting resources that might benefit those with potentially reversible diseases.[68]

In order to protect human dignity, societies must maintain constant vigilance about protecting persons from both undertreatment and abandonment and inappropriate overtreatment. But how? Undertreatment occurs when the "bottom line" predominates over benefit to the patient. Only a national health coverage plan would eliminate this injustice. Overtreatment occurs through the technological enthusiasms of caregivers, the fear of "letting go," or appeals for unreasonable treatments from patients. Only institutional policies about appropriate treatment decisions coupled with compassionate analysis, as suggested earlier, will answer these problems. In both instances, we will be shepherding our technology for good human aims. This shepherding can be focused on an obligation to attempt to eliminate pain and to address suffering.

Control over one's own dying ought to be the focus of our public policy efforts. Decisions and choices patients make in this regard arise out of the context of their relationships with their loved ones and caregivers and of their own value history. Every effort should be made to help the caregivers and the dying maintain a personal and professional relationship.

Nutrition and hydration

Those who oppose the withdrawal of nutrition and hydration do so on grounds that providing food and water to the dying is a special obligation not covered by our considerations so far, and that beneficence should overrule patient autonomy.[69,70] Specifically, they argue that such withdrawing or withholding leads directly to the death of the patient as much as does an injection, since the patient dies not of the underlying disease process but from starvation and dehydration.[71]

There are two problems with this contention. First, patients have a common law right and probably a constitutional right to refuse treatment even if they are not dying. Second, patients may request aid in dying on the grounds we have just examined, namely, that death is a good and others have a duty out of compassion to bring about such a good. "Bringing it about" does not necessarily entail active, direct euthanasia, or even physician-assisted suicide. But it does require that all interventions, including fluids and nutrition, be examined for their impact on the desired goal of treatment.[72] If an earlier and less painful death, with less suffering for the patient, is the desired goal, then how does it make sense to provide medically delivered food and water unless the patient specifically requests it?

Nonetheless, those who support withholding or withdrawing fluids and nutrition may miss a main concern of opponents, that in the absence of expressed wishes, vulnerable persons may be "put to death" by such actions. For this reason some ethicists think that only objective criteria (medical indications presumably), not the context, life plans, or values of the individual, can be used in all withholding and withdrawing decisions.[71] Furthermore, they argue that anything else cannot be used to bring about death in patients who have made no advance directives or who have left only vague statements about not using heroic measures to prolong their lives. The family's expression of the values of the patient are regarded as insufficient reasons to remove such therapy.

The role of the family

In light of the U.S. Supreme court decision in re *Cruzan*,[73] it is clear that the role of the family in speaking for patient values is confused. Recall that Nancy Cruzan was left in a permanent vegetative state after a car accident. For 7 years she was fed through a feeding tube. After 5 years her parents sought to have the tube removed on the grounds that Nancy had mentioned before the accident that she would not want to live in such a condition. The State of Missouri argued that it had a Living Will law that required advance directives of this sort in writing. It interpreted the need for evidence of patient wishes very strictly. When the case reached the U.S. Supreme Court (the first and only termination-of-life-support case to do so), the Court affirmed the right of patients to control their medical interventions but seemed to place more emphasis on the right of the state to require evidence of patient wishes than on the right of families acting as guardians to speak for the values of patients. Although the case does not apply directly to persons with cancer, it does demonstrate that guardianship and family issues are still being worked out for incompetent patients.

Thus, it is very important to obtain advance directives from all patients, especially seriously ill ones. The preferred instrument in most states is the Durable Power of Attorney for Health Care. This document names ahead of time an individual who will speak for the patient when the patient is incompetent to make decisions about health care. It is limited in time to the duration of incompetence and in scope to decisions about health care only. Such an instrument often designates a family member to speak for the patient. Despite the cautions noted by the Supreme Court about family surrogacy, most persons feel comfortable about naming a family member to make decisions, since such a person knows them and their values best.

Access to care

Callahan[74] proposes, when patients are competent and can speak for themselves about medical care, that their options be limited past 80 years of age. Some interventions would no longer be considered.[74] While we might conceivably agree with Callahan that there exists a certain point beyond which expensive medical technology should not be offered to elderly persons, this point should not be set by ageist limits, but rather by the limits of medicine to provide any meaningful change in the outcome for patients during their last years.[75]

It may not be necessary to set such limits on the basis of age if we first try to respect a patient's value system.[76] Elderly persons will usually choose highly technical interventions less often than will younger cancer patients. Statistics show that when patients approach 80 years of age, we spend less on their care. So age and patient wishes apparently begin at that time to be "factored in." Does this mean that physicians ignore the patient's calculation of life span until one reaches "old old" age? Do these data suggest instead that there is a natural life span of about 80 to 85 years, after which it makes no sense, as Callahan has suggested, to employ major technological interventions to save lives?

Many patients over 80 are more ready to die than to fight cancer. It is not an instance of wanting to die, necessarily. Quite the contrary. Life is still regarded as precious. Instead, it is a matter of proportion. Patients over 80 are more accustomed to thinking that they will soon die anyway. One woman, 92 years old, refused to see a doctor for her suppurating breast cancer. She figured she would die soon and did not want to do so in a hospital where her little bit of savings would almost immediately vanish. She still lived at home, where neighbors and friends looked in on her. Yet when finally convinced to enter a hospital and have the breast removed, she was relieved to learn from her doctors that she would live for some time. ("Let's face it," they said, "you will most probably die of something else than the cancer because it grows so slowly in the elderly.") She was very happy that she would return home. Her plan? To go on a tour of Alaska!

So the post-80 syndrome cuts both ways. It may lead patients to give up too early on their care when they could achieve a significant quality of life. Or it may lead to age bias in offering and withholding care. On the other hand, it also may lead caregivers to sell patients a "bill of goods" that may bankrupt other patient values. A person from the Association of American Retired Persons in Nebraska wrote about a friend in another state who lost two premier family farms that had to be sold to pay for his care during his dying months. He had intended to bequeath them to his grandchildren. The end-stage "battle" with his disease was orchestrated and managed by his oncologist without attention to these primary values.

Among other important issues regarding access to cancer care are the problem of the rights of all persons to expensive interventions, the right to request experimental therapy (if any),[77] allocating scarce resources like interleukin-2, large-scale distribution of health care among competing health needs (e.g., the drain of caring for persons with AIDS on state and local health care budgets), and the distribution of funding for other human needs versus health care needs.

Playing God

Modern medical technology empowers individuals beyond their normal capacities. Because technology is, by definition, an extension of human work, it tempts us to exceed the bounds of temperance. This leads to a kind of paternalism in which an individual comes to believe that he or she knows best what is good for another person due to superior technical knowledge. Medical technology adds to this traditional paternalism an even greater temptation, the temptation to "play God."[78] Usually a physician "god" is unrelenting in applying treatment interventions. Rarely, a pusillanimous abandonment of patients without sufficient intervention is found, as might occur when inappropriate judgments about either patient values or the patient's quality of life are made.[79]

It must be admitted that human beings have an incredible thirst for power. Surely this is one reason that humanity is perpetually dissatisfied with the *status quo* and constantly wants to change for the better. General Electric's slogan used to be "Progress is our most important product." Progress in what, one might ask? The answer cannot be just technological improvement. Leading a good life must include mastery of life's vicissitudes. There is nothing intrinsically wrong with our efforts to improve our lives; on the contrary, it is part of the mission of all human beings to use their facilities and propensities to bring about the good in their lives and in society. Yet it is important for health care that providers understand the risks and benefits of the technological interventions they propose.[80]

Euthanasia

The problem of euthanasia, as well as the incredibly difficult questions about human reproduction and all the others in between the origin of life and the final moment of death, involves the question of dominion over life. Our technology makes the temptation to take control over life itself almost overwhelming. Inappropriate withdrawal and withholding of care is also a kind of "playing God" since it involves one individual, entrusted with the care of another, making judgments about the value of that person's life. It is important to distinguish here between objective evaluation of interventions and outcomes on the well-being of the patient and subjective quality-of-life judgments in which the physician and other caregivers judge that the life the patient is now living is not worthwhile for that person.

The danger in the United States today is in the economic sphere.[81] Will it be easier to use a simple method of dispatching those persons whose care costs too much or who are now considered to be a burden on society, like patients with advanced stages of cancer who require extensive care, than to address their suffering, which sometimes is overwhelming even for the most dedicated caregivers? The issue focuses attention on the importance of maintaining compassionate respect for human life in our society. For some, actions to eliminate burdensome life, even if requested by the patient him- or herself, are a form of "privatizing life," denying its social and communal dimensions as both a private and public good. These persons would argue strongly against direct euthanasia or physician-assisted suicide.[82] Others argue that euthanasia and/or assisted suicide are appropriate and important forms of caring for persons whose lives, by their own assessment, have become too burdensome to continue.[83–86]

CONCLUSION

Some suggestions might therefore be:

1. Consider that the duty to protect a patient's life lies primarily in protecting his or her autonomy and value hierarchy. It makes little sense to prolong a life if one does not respect the biography of that life as "written" by the patient. For this reason, I recommend paying more attention to discovering the patient's value system, through a values assessment interview and through constant discussion with the patient and the family throughout the course of treatment.

2. Require advance directives before one receives the first retirement check, enter that advance directive on a central computer, and update it whenever one enters a health care institution, nursing home, or hospice in accordance with current Patient Self-Determination Act procedures.[87] This suggestion differs significantly from the Patient Self-Determination act of 1990 (implemented in December, 1991), in that the latter requires only information and education, while my proposal requires executing an advance directive itself.[88,89] Current procedures for informing patients of their right to issue advance directives could be used with sample forms attached for their implementation. Home care nurses should be recruited for discussing these instruments with all persons ready to retire as part of a national effort to prevent unnecessary and unwanted care.

3. Teaching guides should be developed for all health care professionals that would train them in the processes of implementing patient advance directives, since resistance to these directives is still encountered.

4. Change the current default mode of health care delivery in which it is assumed that everyone desires technological support of their life. Instead of assuming that during the last months of a patient's life everything possible should be done to prolong that life, the opposite assumption would be made unless the patient has issued advance directives to the contrary. Since some people's advance directive will be that they wish to make none, they will need to be warned that this means an assumption in favor of restraint rather than intervention.

5. Use a process like the Ethical Work-up Guide to analyze and discuss cases that arise in one's service. By doing this, one not only gains greater critical awareness of one's own assumptions and values, but also becomes more able to discuss the deepest commitments of one's profession.

REFERENCES

1. Graber GC: Basic theories in medical ethics. In Monagle J, Thomasma DC (eds), *Medical Ethics: A Guide for Health Professionals.* Rockville, MD: Aspen, 1988, pp. 462–475.
2. Beauchamp T, Childress J: *Principles of Biomedical Ethics* (3d ed.) New York: Oxford University Press, 1989.
3. Pellegrino ED, Thomasma DC: *For the Patient's Good: The Restoration of Beneficence in Health Care.* New York: Oxford University Press, 1988.
4. Thomasma DC: Beyond medical paternalism and patient autonomy: A model of physician conscience for the physician-patient relationship. *Ann Int Med* 98:243–248, 1983.
5. Thomasma DC: Some philosophical observations about autonomy in oncology. In *Autonomy and the Cancer Patient.* Utrecht, Netherlands: Department of Social Sciences and Medicine, Rijksuniversiteit Utrecht Medical School, 1985, pp. 29 38.
6. Thomasma DC: When healing involves risk to life: Risky medical procedures and experimentation. *New Catholic World* 230:163–167, July/August, 1987.
7. Thomasma DC: High technology and dying. *New World Outlook* 46:256–258, 1986.
8. Thomasma DC: Philosophical reflections on a rational treatment plan. *J Med Phil* 11:157–165, 1986.
9. Thomasma DC: Quality of life judgments and medical indications. *Qual Life Cardiovascular Care* 2:113–118, 1986.
10. Rossi R: Madam gets 1-yr house detention. *Chicago Sun-Times,* March 19, 1992.
11. MacIntyre A: *Whose Justice? Which Rationality?* Notre Dame, IN; University of Notre Dame Press, 1988.
12. Veatch R: *A Theory of Medical Ethics.* New York: Basic Books, 1981, pp. 301ff.
13. Engelhardt HT Jr: *The Foundations of Bioethics.* New York: Oxford University Press, 1986.
14. Graber G, Thomasma D: *Theory and Practice in Medical Ethics,* New York: Continuum, 1989.
15. Thomasma D: Applying general medical knowledge to individuals: A philosophical analysis. *Theor Med* 9:187–200, 1988.
16. Jansson L, Norberg A: Ethical reasoning concerning the feeding of terminally ill cancer patients: Interviews with registered nurses experienced in the care of cancer patients. *Cancer Nurs* 12:352–358, 1989.
17. Davidson B: Ethical reasoning associated with the feeding of terminally ill elderly cancer patients: An international perspective. *Cancer Nurs* 13:286–292, 1990.
18. Pellegrino ED, Thomasma DC: The conflict between autonomy and beneficence in medical ethics: Proposal for a resolution. *J Cont Health Law Policy* 3:23–46, 1987.
19. Loewy E: The restoration of beneficence. *Hastings Center Rep,* 19:42–43, 1989.
20. Thomasma DC: Ethical and legal issues in the care of the elderly cancer patient. *Clinics Ger Med* 3:541–547, 1987.
21. Thomasma DC: The basis of medicine and religion: Respect for persons. *Linacre Quart* 45:142–150, 1980.
22. Brody H: *The Healer's Power.* New Haven, CT: Yale University Press, 1992, p. 119.
23. Engelhardt HT Jr: *Bioethics and Secular Humanism.* London/Philadelphia: SCM/Trinity Press International, 1991.
24. Walker MU: Moral particularity. *Metaphilosophy* 18:171–185, 1987.
25. Toulmin S, Jonsen A: *The Abuse of Casuistry.* Berkeley, CA: University of California Press, 1988.
26. McIntyre A: After Virtue. Notre Dame, IN: University of Notre Dame Press, 1981.
27. Thomasma D: The context as moral rule in medical ethics. In Wright RA (ed), *Human Values in Health Care.* New York: McGraw-Hill, 1987, pp. 142–156.
28. Thomasma D: Decision making and decision analysis: Beneficence in medicine. *J Crit Care* 3:122–132, 1988.
29. Thomasma D: Beyond medical paternalism and patient autonomy: A model of physician's conscience for the doctor-patient relationship. *Ann Int Med* 98:243–248, 1983.
30. Bergsma J, Thomasma D: *Health Care: Its Psychosocial Dimensions.* Pittsburgh, PA: Duquesne University Press, 1982.
31. Loewy E: *Suffering and the Beneficent Community: Beyond Libertarianism.* Buffalo, NY: SUNY Press, 1991.
32. John Paul II Pope: Humanize hospital work. Address to the Sixty-First General Chapter of the Hospital Order of St. John of God. *L'Osservatore Romano,* January 24, 1983.
33. Nouwen H: *The Wounded Healer.* New York: Doubleday, 1972, p. 72.
34. De Unamuno M: *The Tragic Sense of Life,* Translated by Kerrigan A. Princeton, NJ: Princeton University Press, Bollingen Series, LXXXV, 4, 1972, p. 224.
35. Bergsma J, Thomasma DC: *Health Care: Its Psychosocial Dimensions.* Pittsburgh, PA: Duquesne University Press, 1983.
36. Pellegrino ED, Thomasma DC: *Helping and Healing.* Rome: Edizione Dehoniane, in press (Italian translation).
37. McElhinney T, Pellegrino ED (eds): *Teaching Ethics, the Humanities, and Human Values in Medical Schools: A Ten-Year Overview.* Washington, DC: Institute on Human Values in Medicine, Society for Health and Human Values, 1982.
38. Graber GC, Thomasma DC: *Theory and Practice in Medical Ethics.* New York: Continuum, 1989.
39. Gaylin W, Kass L, Pellegrino ED, Siegler M: Commentaries: Doctors must not kill. *JAMA* 259:2139–2140, 1988.
40. Kass L: Arguments against active euthanasia by doctors found at medicine's core. *Kennedy Institute of Ethics Newsletter,* 3:1–3, Jan. 6, 1989.
41. Marsden C: Care giver fidelity in a pediatric bone marrow transplant team. *Heart Lung* 6:617–625, 1988.
42. Rouse F: Living wills in the long-term care setting. *J Long-Term Care Adm* 17:14–19, Summer, 1988.
43. Mehling A: Living wills: Preventing suffering or a deadly contract? *State Government News* pp. 14–15, Dec. 1988.
44. Braithwaite S, Thomasma DC: New guidelines on foregoing life-sustaining treatment in incompetent patients: An anti-cruelty policy. *Ann Int Med* 104:711–715, 1986.
45. Illich I: *Medical Nemesis: The Expropriation of Health.* New York: Pantheon, 1976, p. 106.
46. Thomasma D: Ethics and professional practice in oncology. *Semin Oncol Nurs* 5:89–94, 1989.
47. Cassell E: Disease as an "It." *Soc Sci Med* 10:143–146, 1976.
48. Bried EM, Scheffler RM: The impact of healthcare financing on the quality of life of older cancer patients. *Oncology* 6(suppl):153–160, 1992.
49. Thomasma D: The ethics of caring for the older patient with cancer: Defining the issues. *Oncology* 6(suppl):124–130, 1992.
50. Thomasma DC, Bergsma J: Incurable and patients. Article submitted for publication.
51. Slevin ML, et al: Attitude to chemotherapy: Comparing views of patients with cancer with those of doctors, nurses, and general public. *Brit Med J* 300:1458–1460, 1990.

52. Cranford R: The care of the dying: A symposium on the case of Betty Wright—Going out in style, the American way, 1987. *Law, Med Health Care* 17:208–210, Fall, 1989.
53. Thomasma DC: Ethics and professional practice in oncology. *Semin Oncol Nurs* 5:89–94, 1989.
54. Thomasma DC: Ethical judgments of quality of life in the care of the aged. *J Am Ger Soc* 32:525–527, 1984.
55. Ganz P: Does (or should) chronological age influence the choice of cancer treatment? *Oncology* 6(suppl):45–49, 1992.
56. Walter JJ, Shannon TA (eds): *Quality of Life: The New Medical Dilemma.* New York and Mahwah, NJ: Paulist Press, 1990.
57. Ferrell BR, Grant MM, Padilla GV, et al: Home care. *Oncology* 6(suppl):136–140, 1992.
58. O'Rourke K: Should nutrition and hydration be provided to permanently unconscious and other mentally disabled persons? *Iss Law Med* 5:181–196, 1989.
59. Pellegrino ED, Thomasma DC: *For the Patient's Good: The Restoration of Beneficence in Health Care.* New York: Oxford University Press, 1988.
60. Thomasma DC: Caveat philosophus: Technology's abuse potential in the decision to terminate life. *J Am Ger Soc* 35:124–125, 1987.
61. Bayles MD: Euthanasia and the quality of life. In Bayles MD, High DM (eds), *Medical Treatment of the Dying: Moral Issues.* New York: Schenkman Books, 1978, pp. 128–152.
62. Thomasma DC, Graber GC: *Euthanasia: Toward an Ethical Social Policy.* New York: Continuum, 1990.
63. Rachels J: *Moral Problems.* New York: Harper & Row, 1971, pp. 42–66.
64. Doctor-aided suicide spurs ethics debate. *Chicago Tribune,* March 7, 1991, Sec. 1, 1.
65. Bujorian GA: Clinical trials: Patient issues in the decision-making process. *Oncol Nurs Forum* 15:779–783, 1988.
66. Luce EA, et al: Lingering death from squamous cell carcinoma of the face. *Hosp Prac* 24:60–61, 65–66, 71–72, 1989.
67. Jonsen A: What does life support support? In Winslade W (ed), *Personal Choices and Public Commitments: Perspectives on the Humanities.* Galveston, TX: Institute for the Medical Humanities, 1988, pp. 61–69.
68. Raffin TA, Shurkin JN, Sinkler W III: *Intensive Care: Facing the Critical Issues.* New York: Freeman, 1988, p. 185.
69. Callahan D: On feeding the dying. *Hastings Center Rep* 13:22–23, 1983.
70. Davidson B, Vander Laan R, Davis A, et al: Ethical reasoning associated with the feeding of terminally ill elderly cancer patients: An international perspective. *Cancer Nurs* 13:286–292, 1990.
71. May W, et al: Feeding and hydrating the permanently unconscious and other vulnerable persons. *Issues Law Med* 3:203–211, Winter, 1987.
72. Paris JJ, McCormick RA: The Catholic tradition on the use of nutrition and fluids. *America,* 356–360, May 2, 1987.
73. Thomasma DC: The Cruzan decision and medical practice. (Editorial). *Arch Int Med* 151:853–854, 1991.
74. Callahan D: *Setting Limits: Medical Goals in an Aging Society.* New York: Simon and Schuster, 1987, pp. 159–185, 241–242.
75. Thomasma DC: Moving the aged into the house of the dead: A critique of ageist social policy. *J Am Ger Soc.* 37:169–172, 1989.
76. Thomasma DC: Ethical and moral issues in access to cancer care. In Scheffler RM, Andrews NC (eds), *Cancer Care and Cost: DRGs and Beyond.* Ann Arbor, MI: Health Administration Press, 1989, pp. 211–223.
77. Thomasma D, Micetich K: The ethics of patient requests in experimental medicine. Reprinted as monograph by the American Cancer Society, Oct., 1984.
78. Taylor C: Ethics in health care and medical technologies. *Theor Med* 11:111–124, 1990.
79. Wilkes E: Ethics in terminal care. In Dunstan GR, Shinebourne EA (eds), *Doctors' Decisions: Ethical Conflicts in Medical Practice.* New York: Oxford University Press, 1989, pp. 197–204.
80. Melski JW: Prices of technology: A blind spot. *JAMA* 267:1516–1518, 1992.
81. Scitovsky AA, Capron AM: Medical care at the end of life: The interaction of economics and ethics. *Ann Rev Pub Health* 7:59–75, 1986.
82. Bernardin J Cardinal: Euthanasia: Ethical and legal challenge. Address to the Center for Clinical Medical Ethics, University of Chicago Hospital, May 26, 1988.
83. Kevorkian J: A fail-safe model for justifiable medically-assisted suicide. *Am J Forensic Psych* 13:7, 41, 1992.
84. Quill TE: Death and dignity—A case of individualized decision making. *N Engl J Med* 324:691–694, 1991.
85. Humphrey D: *Final Exit: The Practicalities of Self-Deliverance and Assisted Suicide for the Dying.* Eugene, OR: The Hemlock Society, 1991.
86. *Trends Health Care, Law Ethics* 7: Winter, 1992.
87. Thomasma DC: Advance directives and health care for the elderly. In Hackler C Jr, Moseley R, Vawter D (eds), *Advance Directives in Medicine.* New York: Praeger, 1989, pp. 93–109.
88. Thomasma DC: From ageism toward autonomy. In Binstock R, Post S (eds), *Too Old for Health Care?* Baltimore, MD: Johns Hopkins University Press, 1991, pp. 138–163.
89. PSDA well received in hospitals, despite early confusion. *Med Eth Advisor* 8:25–30, 1992 (editorial).

Chapter 60

Questionable Methods of Cancer Therapy

Connie Henke Yarbro, RN, BSN

INTRODUCTION

Each year more than a million Americans are diagnosed as having cancer, and more than half will be cured with scientifically sound therapies. Each year thousands of cancer patients and many others who merely fear they might develop it will devote countless hours and invest billions of dollars in the use of questionable cancer remedies outside the realm of mainstream medicine. Additionally, thousands will seek information about such treatments.[1] Whether labeled "unconventional," "unsound," "unproven," "unorthodox," or "alternative," these treatments range from those that are both fraudulent and dangerous to those that are hazardous mainly to the pocketbook. Often, these treatments offer individuals a chance to participate in their own care, reflecting the naturalistic approaches so popular with the public today.[2]

Questionable methods of cancer management include diagnostic tests or therapeutic methods that have not shown activity in tumor animal models or in scientific clinical trials but are promoted for general use in cancer prevention, diagnosis, or treatment. Such methods do not protect the consumer, since they have not met the requirements of the U.S. Food, Drug and Cosmetic Act. According to a 1984 report by the U.S. House of Representatives' Subcommittee on Health and Long-term Care, each year Americans spend $10 billion on unscientific remedies and $4 billion to $5 billion on fraudulent ones.[3,4] Questionable nutritional supplements alone are more than a $2 billion-a-year industry in the United States.[5] The exact number of cancer patients who try questionable treatments is unknown, but various studies have reported that 9%–50% of cancer patients admitted using an unproven remedy.[6–9]

HISTORICAL PERSPECTIVES

For thousands of years, individuals in need have turned to people offering what they hope will be an answer to their medical problems. Popular folk remedies for the treatment of cancer have been available for centuries. Only in relatively recent times has the scientific method, in conjunction with organized medicine and government, been able to provide a measure of confidence that a treatment is safe and effective.[10]

Legislation

Before the Food and Drug Act of 1906, thousands of unproven treatments were promoted to the American public. Often, the treatments were not harmful in themselves. But as an anonymous physician noted in a letter to the *National Quarterly Review* in 1861, "Quackery kills a larger number annually than the disease it pretends to cure."[11]

In 1906 President Theodore Roosevelt signed into law the Pure Food and Drug Act, which forbade misleading or false statements on the labels of remedies. However, Janssen[12] reported that in 1910, in a crucial test of the new law, the U.S. Supreme Court ruled that the law involved only truthful labeling of ingredients used in drugs, not the false therapeutic claims on the drug label. Justice Oliver Wendell Holmes, Jr., concluded that individuals could not be prosecuted for what he termed "mistaken praise" of their treatments, even though the claims were false.

Noting the dangers of permitting unsafe and ineffective drugs on the market, President Taft exhorted the Congress, in 1911, to pass tougher legislation:

> There are none so credulous as sufferers from disease. The need is urgent for legislation which will prevent the raising of false hopes of speedy cures of serious ailment by misstatements of facts as to the worthless mixtures on which the sick will rely while their disease progresses unchecked.[13]

In 1912 Congress passed the Sherley Amendment, which made it a crime to make false or fraudulent claims regarding the therapeutic efficacy of a drug. However, this legislation was limited, in that it was still necessary to prove that the promoter intended to defraud the public. Mistaken claims could still be made, and patients could continue to be defrauded. In 1938 Congress eliminated this difficulty by passing legislation that required scientific proof of safety before a drug could be marketed.

In 1962 Congress clarified some of the language of the previous legislation and further added that drugs must demonstrate efficacy in addition to safety before they could be marketed. Thus, the process was created by which a substance became approved for prescription use by the Food and Drug Administration (FDA). The Food and Drug Commissioner[14] noted that the Food and Drug Act of 1962 means that "the absolute freedom to choose an ineffective drug was properly surrendered in exchange for the freedom from danger to each person's health and well-being from the sale and use of worthless drugs." This is, in fact, the same decision made over the years by those in government who have decided that only persons certified by experts may practice medicine and are qualified to help the patients who would choose to seek their assistance. Although the Food and Drug Act of 1962 frequently has been challenged by those who promote questionable methods, the act was upheld by a decision of the U.S. Supreme Court in 1973.

Past Unproven Methods

Questionable approaches to cancer treatment have existed for centuries, but a popular new alternative suddenly seems to develop and thrive almost every decade.

TABLE 60-1 Popular Questionable Treatments in the United States

Era	Questionable Approaches and Treatments
1800–1850	Thompsonianism: emetics and hot baths
1850–1900	Homeopathy: use of highly distilled or diluted inorganic and organic substances
1890s	Naturopathy: diets, massages, colonic irrigation Early osteopathy and chiropractic: spinal manipulation
1900s	Tablet, ointment, and tonic cancer cures
1920s	"Energy" cancer cures: cosmic energy, radio waves, light therapy, psychic diagnoses and treatments
1940s	Koch's glyoxylide
1950s	Hoxsey's cancer treatment
1960s	Krebiozen
1970s	Laetrile
1980s	Metabolic therapies: diet, megavitamins, minerals, enzymes, colonic irrigation Macrobiotic diets Pharmacologic and biologic therapies: antineoplastons, cancell, dimethyl sulfoxide (DMSO), Greek cancer cure, live-cell therapy, megavitamins, herbal therapy, oxymedicine Immuno-augmentative therapy (IAT) Electronic devices Behavioral and psychologic: mental imagery; spiritual, faith, or mind healing

Examples of unorthodox approaches, arranged according to their eras of popularity, are identified in Table 60-1.[8] We have gone from the nineteenth century "holistic," or "natural," movement to the so-called drug approach of the early and mid-1900s, back to the holistic, natural, or diet-oriented regimens of today.[15] Many of the popular questionable methods of cancer treatment parallel the most promising developments in scientific clinical trials.[16] For example, during the 1960s and 1970s, when drugs were being developed as an effective treatment for cancer, spurious compounds (e.g., Krebiozen and laetrile) were being promoted to cancer patients. In the 1980s, the cancer clinical trials of immunotherapy and biologics corresponded with the unproven use of immunoaugmentative therapy and other compounds that purported to boost the immune system. The following discussion will review the alternative approaches from the era of the 1940s through the 1970s.

Koch antitoxin therapy: 1940s–1950s

Koch antitoxin therapy, first mentioned in 1919,[17] was a popular unproven cancer treatment during the 1940s and 1950s. The treatment consisted of pure distilled water mixed with one part per trillion of a chemical called glyoxylide, which is merely glyoxylic acid (a normal body constituent) with water removed. Koch proposed that cancer was caused by a microorganism susceptible to the differential poison in his antitoxins. He also prescribed enemas and a special diet. Over 3000 health practitioners in the United States employed this regimen, paying $25 per ampule for it and charging patients as much as $300 for a single injection.[12] In 1942 the FDA held hearings across the United States in an effort to gather information regarding the promotion and use of Koch antitoxins. In 1943 the Canadian Cancer Foundation reported that no patients on a clinical trial using the Koch method benefited from the treatment.[18] Subsequently, the Federal Trade Commission issued a court order forbidding the promotion of Koch antitoxins because of their lack of therapeutic value. Although Koch antitoxins are illegal in the United States, they can still be obtained through the underground medical community or in Mexico.

Hoxsey method: 1950s

The Hoxsey method has been around since the early 1920s. Hoxsey maintained that cancer was a result of a chemical imbalance in the body that caused healthy cells to mutate and become cancerous and that his therapy restored the chemical environment and killed the cancerous cells. Hoxsey's Herbal Tonic consisted of several different formulas: the "black medicine" was composed of cascara (a laxative) in an extract of licorice root, alfalfa, burdock root, red clover blossoms, buckthorn bark, barberry root, pokeweed, and prickly ash bark; the "pink medicine" contained potassium iodide and lactated pepsin.[19] Except for potassium iodide and the laxative, which are effective drugs but have no value in treating cancer, all the other ingredients have been discarded as medically ineffective.[12] Hoxsey also developed a tablet form of his medicines.

The FDA investigated nearly 400 cases of persons who claimed to be cured of cancer through use of the Hoxsey method, and no legitimate case of a cure was discovered. In 1960 a federal court injunction declared sale of the treatment illegal.[12] At the time the Hoxsey clinics in Dallas, Texas and Portage, Pennsylvania were closed, over 10,000 individuals were enrolled as patients. The FDA estimated that over $50 million was spent for the Hoxsey drugs.[20] Today, Hoxsey's medicines are available at the BioMedical Center in Tijuana, Mexico.[21–23] Mildred Nelson, Hoxsey's former head nurse at the Dallas clinic, is now the proprietor of the BioMedical Center. She has added a special diet and an attitudinal approach to Hoxsey's medicines.[22]

Krebiozen: 1960s

Krebiozen allegedly was first produced by a Yugoslavian physician named Steven Durovic, who developed the substance from blood extracted from horses. In the mid-1950s Andrew C. Ivy, professor emeritus at the University of Illinois, endorsed Krebiozen as an effective cancer therapy. In 1961 the National Cancer Institute (NCI) obtained a sample of Krebiozen, and the substance was identified as creatine monohydrate, an amino acid found in all animal tissue.[24] Pre-1960 samples of Krebiozen actually contained mineral oil and small amounts of amyl alcohol and methylhydantoin.[25] The Krebiozen Research Foundation submitted 504 case records to the NCI in an effort to demonstrate therapeutic efficacy in justification of a clinical trial. A panel of 24 scientists reviewed these records and unanimously concluded that Krebiozen was an ineffective drug.[26] Although no clear scientific evidence of efficacy has been brought forward, the treatment was available until 1977.[12]

Laetrile: 1970s

Laetrile is a general term for a group of cyanogenic glucosides, derived from several different seeds, e.g., apricot, peach, cherry, and almonds. It is also known as amygdalin and "vitamin B_{17}." Ernst T. Krebs, Sr., a physician, claimed to be the first individual to use a cyanogenic glucoside as an anticancer agent. In the 1940s he used amygdalin, derived from apricot kernels, and found it to be too toxic for use in humans, despite what he claimed were encouraging results. In 1952 his son, Ernst Krebs, Jr., reported that he had made an apricot formula that was safe for parenteral administration.

Laetrile's purported mechanism of action has changed over the years as scientific thinking has changed. Perhaps the most common hypothesis is that cancer cells possess an enzyme called β-glucosidase in larger quantities than healthy tissue, whereas normal tissue supposedly has greater quantities of the enzyme rhodanese, which is not present in cancerous tissue. The theory claims that the β-glucosidase in the cancerous tissues causes the laetrile to break down into glucose and mandelonitrile, which breaks down further into hydrogen cyanide (a toxic substance) and benzaldehyde (a mild anesthetic). The cyanide kills the cancer cells, so the theory goes, while the healthy tissue is protected by rhodanese, which converts cyanide into nontoxic sodium thiocynate. Manner et al.[27] expand this theory and suggest that the benzaldehyde may interfere with respiration in cancer cells. They also claim to have demonstrated a differentiation in quantities of rhodanese and β-glucosidase in the directions predicted by the theory. However, this result is inconsistent with other investigators.[28–30] Most likely, the majority of the injected laetrile probably is excreted intact in the urine.[30]

Claims have been made that laetrile is a nontoxic form of "vitamin B_{17}" and that taking this vitamin can prevent cancer. No reputable scientist accepts the existence of vitamin B_{17}. Laetrile does not fulfill the requirements of a vitamin, because no disease state exists in its absence.[31] Evidence suggests that laetrile has toxic effects. The gastric lumen has enzymes capable of breaking laetrile down into hydrogen cyanide and mandelonitrile.[32] There are numerous reports of cyanide toxicity with the ingestion of fruits or seeds containing cyanogenic glucosides, including amygdalin.[33–37] Ingestion of laetrile with certain other foods, such as sweet almonds, lettuce, certain fresh fruits, and mushrooms, can potentiate the toxic reaction. In addition, a number of deaths attributed to cyanide poisoning from oral laetrile have been reported,[38–40] and laetrile by enema is also poisonous.[41,42]

Laetrile in the United States is either imported illegally or brought in under court order (exempting the substance from FDA supervision). This means the product is not required to meet standards of purity. There have been reports of fungal contamination of parenterally formulated laetrile, variations in dosage, and mislabeling of contents of laetrile exported from Mexican manufacturers.[43] For the cancer patient, whose immune system may already be compromised, an infection resulting from contamination could be fatal.

It is noteworthy that laetrile has been the most extensively tested unproven method of all time. Numerous animal studies[44–48] and two retrospective studies have shown no therapeutic benefit.[49,50] In the 1970s there was a movement to legalize laetrile in many states, and approximately 75,000 U.S. cancer patients were seeking laetrile therapy, many of them while discontinuing effective conventional therapy.[51] Laetrile was a billion-dollar-a-year industry in 1979.[38] Thus, in 1980 the FDA gave approval to the NCI for the first prospective clinical trial of laetrile, and once again it was demonstrated that laetrile is ineffective against cancer.[52] The power of the proponent of questionable treatments over the public is illustrated by the fact that despite the proof published in 1982 that laetrile was worthless,[52] laetrile was still a billion-dollar-a-year industry in 1983.[53]

Laetrile's use as an anticancer drug has not ended. Today, many of the proponents of laetrile have changed their strategy of using it as a single agent and are combining it with vitamins, enzymes, or so-called metabolic therapy.[54]

POPULAR QUESTIONABLE METHODS OF TODAY

Questionable methods of cancer treatment during the 1980s and into the 1990s are primarily related to lifestyle, and as such cannot be regulated by the FDA. Many of the unproven methods place responsibility for a healthy lifestyle on the patient and have an aura of respectability in relation to conventional scientific medicine that is concerned with diet, environmental carcinogens, lifestyle, and relation between emotions and physiologic responses.[55]

In a study of contemporary unorthodox cancer treatments, Cassileth and colleagues[7] reported that 13%

of 304 patients being treated at the University of Pennsylvania Cancer Center have turned to practitioners of questionable methods at one time or another. An additional 365 patients who received questionable treatments were identified by contacting questionable practitioners and clinics. The total sample of 669 patients was interviewed. Among all the patients who had turned to questionable therapy, the most commonly used remedies were, in order, metabolic therapy, diet therapies, megavitamins, mental imagery, spiritual or faith healing, and "immune" therapy. The first three involved some form of nutritional therapy and were selected twice as frequently as the other regimens. This is supported by Read et al.,[56] who found a high rate of vitamin/mineral/herbal supplementation in a group of 32 patients with cancer.

Thus nutritional therapy represents a major type of questionable cancer treatments. In part this may reflect public perceptions of the relationship of nutrition to health; in part it may reflect the fact that the FDA cannot regulate foods and vitamins in the same way it regulates drugs. In addition, other pharmacologic and biologic approaches and herbal approaches have gained popularity.[1] The following discussion will review dietary/metabolic therapy, pharmacological and biologic approaches, immunoaugmentative therapy, and behavioral and psychological approaches as questionable methods of cancer management.

Dietary Therapy/Metabolic Therapy

The goals of questionable dietary therapy overlap the goals of conventional nutritional support for cancer patients, since both try to counteract the nutritional and metabolic effects of the disease and its treatment.[1] However, questionable dietary methods go beyond scientifically accepted nutritional measures in that they claim to reverse the course of disease.

Many questionable cancer therapies emphasize natural cure through dietary manipulation or "metabolic" approaches. There are approximately 20 different types of metabolic regimens for the prevention of cancer and for cancer treatment, including restricted diets, specific dietary modification, enzyme therapy, cellular therapy, megavitamins, detoxification with colonic irrigations, and the development of an appropriate mental attitude.[57] The concepts of metabolic therapy are based on the theory that cancer is a result of impaired metabolism that causes a buildup of toxins in the body. Detoxification and manipulation of diet can remove these toxins, reestablish metabolic balance, and build the immune system to accomplish cure.[15,23,57]

Gerson regimen

The Gerson treatment for cancer, developed by German physician Dr. Max Gerson in the 1920s, is the original "metabolic" therapy. It proposes that constipation or inadequate elimination of wastes from the body interferes with metabolism and healing.[58] Cure can be achieved through manipulation of diet and "detoxification," or purging the body of so-called toxins. There are many adaptations of Dr. Gerson's original program, but all have a consistent approach, which includes (1) avoidance of exposure to carcinogens, (2) positive mental outlook, and (3) eliminating wastes from the body. The daily schedule for the first 3–4 weeks includes 13 glasses of raw vegetable and fruit juices a day prepared in a specific way, five coffee enemas 4 hours apart, castor oil and castor oil enema every other day, and supplemental vitamins, minerals, and enzymes. Salt, drinking water, coffee, berries, nuts, fish, meat, and dairy products are forbidden.[23,58,59] Other components that have been added to the regimen are oral and/or rectal hydrogen peroxide; rectal ozone gas treatments; "live-cell" therapy; IV glucose, insulin, and potassium; laetrile, and vaccines.[1]

The Gerson regimen, administered at Hospital de Baja California in Mexico costs approximately $2000 a week and lasts from 3 to 6 weeks.[23,58] There is an additional cost for a companion, since the patient will require help with the food preparation and enemas. Several reports[1,58] have noted that promotional brochures from the Gerson Institute claim to cure 90% of patients with early cancer and 50% of patients with advanced cancer; however, these claims are not supported by data or statistics. What has been reported is that repeated enemas and purgatives are more likely to lead to metabolic imbalance than to correct it, and coffee enemas have killed people.[42,60,61]

Manner metabolic therapy

The late Harold Manner, PhD, a former professor of zoology at Loyola University, was another proponent of metabolic cancer therapy. He founded the Metabolic Research Foundation and supervised Clinica Manner in Tijuana, Mexico, up to his death in 1988. He claimed that "metabolic therapy" enhances the body's immune system so the tumor will disappear. The "Manner cocktail" consists of an intravenous solution of dimethyl sulfoxide (DMSO), and massive doses of vitamin C, vitamin A, and laetrile. There are various protocols for his metabolic therapy that may also include coffee enemas, fasting, a highly restricted diet that advocates raw milk, megavitamins, live-cell therapy, and enzymes.[62] The Manner regimen lasts 21 days and costs $6800.[23] More important, there is no objective evidence that the metabolic therapy of Harold Manner has any benefit in the treatment of cancer.[62]

Macrobiotic diets

Over the years, a variety of diet therapies have been purported to be useful in the treatment of cancer. Today, the macrobiotic diet probably is the most popular, both for curing cancer and for preventing cancer. This diet has its origin in Zen mysticism, which proposes two antagonistic and complementary forces, yin and yang, that govern all things in the universe. Each food is classified as yin or yang, whereas each tumor is classified as being caused by an imbalance of either yin or yang. The diet is matched to the tumor to restore the balance between yin and yang, resulting in a cure or prevention, as the case may be.[53] In addition to diet, balance is also achieved through cooking techniques and attitude toward life.[63]

The original version of the diet, developed by George Ohsawa (1893–1966), involved ten macrobiotic diets ranging from diet −3 to diet 7. As an individual progresses from diet −3 toward diet 7, more and more foods are forfeited, until in diet 7 the diet consists exclusively of cereal grains.[63] In the 1970s, Michio Kushi[64] recommended a more "standard macrobiotic diet" that was less restrictive than diet 7. This consisted of 50%–60% whole cereal grains, 20%–25% vegetables, 5%–10% soups, 5%–10% beans and sea vegetables, occasional fish and fruits, and liquids sparingly. Some foods are not allowed because they are excessively yin or yang: meat, animal fat, poultry, eggs, dairy products, bananas, citrus fruits, potatoes, tomatoes, spinach, coffee, sugar, and vitamin supplements. Thus, the macrobiotic diet uses only plant proteins and is high in bulk and low in fat. The result is that a large quantity of macrobiotic foods must be eaten to meet the daily recommended energy allowance. For example, a healthy male who requires 2700 kilocalories would need 17 cups in volume.[65] At one time Kushi[64] recommended that modern medicine should be avoided except for emergency life-saving techniques; however, he is no longer against cancer patients' combining mainstream treatment with the macrobiotic diet.[1] He encourages patients to believe that since they had the power to create their illness, they also have the power to recover from it.

With adequate planning, vegetarian diets may be nutritionally sound; however, the diet recommended by Kushi is unsound. Macrobiotic therapy can result in malnutrition and cause a variety of serious health problems.[66] Of special note, cancer patients who follow the macrobiotic regimen should ensure adequate intakes of vitamins B_{12} and D.[67] The American Cancer Society recently reviewed the literature and available information and found no objective evidence that macrobiotic diets are of benefit in the treatment of cancer.[67] There are also no valid data on the efficacy of the macrobiotic diet in the prevention of cancer.[66]

Pharmacologic and Biologic Approaches

Antineoplaston therapy

Antineoplastons were developed by Stanislaw R. Burzynski, MD, in the late 1960s. Burzynski originally isolated the antineoplastons from blood and then from the urine of individuals without cancer. He claims that antineoplastons are natural peptides and amino acid derivatives that cause cancer cells to change to normal cells, inhibit the growth of malignant cells, and are also useful in diagnosing cancer. However, his product is not a naturally occurring peptide. Also, he does not claim to cure cancer but reports complete remissions with minimal side effects.[1] He has numerous publications on antineoplastons in which he claims effectiveness; however, many of these publications are duplicates, published overseas and in non–peer-reviewed journals. Green[68] conducted an extensive review of Burzynski's publications between 1964 and 1990 and reported that none of the publications contained objective experimental evidence to support his hypothesis that a naturally occurring antineoplastic biochemical surveillance system exists in humans and that the urinary antineoplastons have not shown anticancer activity in experimental tumor systems. Yet other scientists believe that the compounds show some evidence of activity.[1,69]

Burzynski applied for an investigational new drug (IND) exemption in 1983, but it was put on "hold" because data were insufficient to justify its investigative use in humans. In 1989 the FDA released the hold to allow a study of the oral form (antineoplaston A10) in a small number of women with advanced refractory breast cancer. However, the study has not been initiated because the Burzynski staff reported that it is too costly to conduct a clinical trial in the United States.[1] To date, prospective, controlled clinical studies of antineoplastons have not taken place. Recently, an NCI site-visit team reviewed a best-case series of seven patients prepared for them by Burzynski. Based on their review, NCI plans to conduct a phase II study in patients with brain tumors.[68,69]

Meanwhile, Burzynski administers antineoplaston therapy at the Burzynski Research Institute in Houston, Texas, and uses different formulations for different forms of cancer. Duration of initial treatment is 2–4 weeks.[1] Antineoplastons are given orally or intravenously in regular, high, or megadoses.[70] A deposit of $3000–$5000 is required to start treatment, and this does not include the additional diagnostic tests or necessary equipment for administration.

Cancell

Cancell, also known as Entelev, Jim's Juice, Croinic Acid and Sheridan's Formula, is a mixture of synthetic chemicals created for their electrical properties. James Sheridan, a chemist, developed the formula as a result of what he describes as a dream and inspiration from God. In 1984 Edward J. Sopack acquired the formula for manufacturing Cancell after Sheridan was forced by the FDA to stop production;[71] however, they are both manufacturing and distributing the drugs today out of their homes in Michigan. The active ingredients include inositol, nitric acid, sodium sulfite, potassium hydroxide, sulfuric acid, and catechol, which are heated for most of the day, put in pint bottles, and refrigerated. According to Sopack,[72] the formula reacts with the body electrically and lowers the voltage of the cell structure. Because cancer cells are weak, they convert directly to waste material when the voltage is lowered by Cancell, and the body then eliminates this waste material. The cancer cells are replaced with normal cells, and the cancer no longer exists.

According to Sopack,[72] Cancell is more effective if taken internally and externally at the same time and must be taken for a minimum of 45 days. For internal usage, the liquid is given either orally (1/4 teaspoon every 6 hours, held under the tongue for 5 minutes, and then swallowed) or rectally (1/4 teaspoon injected into the rectum every 6 hours). For external usage, an area on the ball of the foot or the inside of the wrist is thoroughly cleaned with soap and water and several drops of DMSO are applied to that area. Then, one-eighth teaspoon of Cancell is placed on a cotton pad and the treated pad taped to the foot or wrist site. This process is repeated every 12 hours. In addition, Sopack recommends 3000 mg of Bromelain (pineapple enzyme) a day. If the patient has liver involvement, AIDS, or herpes virus, 1000 mg of glutathione should be taken before each meal. If the patient has AIDS, herpes, or EB virus, 2000 mg of butylated hydroxytoluline (BHT) should also be taken every night. Sopack advises patients that Cancell does not work if nicotine is in the blood; vitamins will interfere with function of Cancell; and it cannot be used with any other cancer therapy.[72]

Although the FDA obtained a permanent injunction prohibiting the distribution of Cancell in interstate commerce,[73] Sopack continues to distribute Cancell as "a gift" to anyone who requests it.

Dimethyl sulfoxide (DMSO)

DMSO is an agent that has been used as an industrial chemical solvent and as a preservative for culture cells. It is rapidly absorbed through the intact skin. The use of a 50% solution of DMSO for bladder instillations is the only FDA-approved use of this agent in humans. However, the industrial form has been used alone or in combination with laetrile and other forms of "metabolic" therapy (e.g., Manner cocktail), with claims that it will restore the cancer cell to being a normal cell. A review of the literature by the American Cancer Society revealed no evidence that DMSO results in objective benefit in the treatment of cancer patients.[70]

Live-cell therapy

Live-cell therapy—fresh-cell therapy, or cellular therapy—is the injection of cells from animal embryos or fetuses. The type of cells given supposedly matches the diseased tissue or organ in the patient. Proponents claim that the live cells contain active agents (not identified) that stimulate the immune system and repair and regenerate the host cells.[1,75] Cellular therapy is promoted for a variety of indications (e.g., menstrual disorders, premature aging, sterility, neoplastic conditions in early and advanced states).[76]

Live-cell therapy was developed by Dr. Paul Niehans of Switzerland. Currently, Dr. Wolfram Kuhnau, an associate of Dr. Niehans, heads the live-cell therapy program at the American Biologics Hospital in Tijuana, Mexico. Live-cell therapy is also offered at other Mexican clinics, usually is given in conjunction with metabolic therapy, and costs more than $20,000.[76] In a review of the literature, the American Cancer Society[75] found no scientific evidence that live-cell therapy was effective in the treatment of cancer. More important, serious side effects (brucellosis, encephalomyelitis, anaphylactic shock) have resulted from the injection of live-cell therapy.

Megavitamins

The use of supplemental vitamins is another unproven approach that has been promoted as a treatment for cancer. Whereas certain cancers have been associated with low intake of some vitamins (e.g., lung cancer and vitamin A), there is no clear-cut evidence that high doses of vitamins prevent cancer. Studies are under way using retinoids (analogs of vitamin A) to reduce the incidence of cancer, but these studies have not yet demonstrated statistically significant reductions in incidence. Meanwhile, megadoses of vitamin C, vitamin A, and pangamic acid ("vitamin B_{15}") have been alleged to have antitumor properties and usually are combined with the metabolic/dietary regimens discussed earlier. However, excessive vitamin intake is useless against cancer and, more important, may be toxic.

Vitamin C Megadose vitamin C probably is the most popular self-administered vitamin supplement. It has been promoted as a remedy for conditions ranging from the common cold to arthritis. It gained popularity when Cameron and Pauling[77] published a study claiming that terminal cancer patients who received massive doses of vitamin C survived much longer and had an improved quality of life. However, their study was not valid, because they selected the patients who received vitamin C whereas control subjects were selected from files, making the groups not comparable.[78] Widespread interest among cancer patients prompted a series of three NCI-funded randomized trials of vitamin C. These three prospectively randomized, placebo-controlled studies documented no consistent benefit from vitamin C in patients with advanced cancer.[79–81] There are theoretic reasons that ascorbic acid, acting as an antioxidant, might reduce the incidence of some cancers, and studies of the role of vitamin C in cancer continue.[82] However, megadoses of vitamin C can cause severe kidney damage,[83] release cyanide from laetrile,[84] and may cause death if administered intravenously.[85–87]

Vitamin A Megadoses of vitamin A have also become popular for the treatment of cancer, either alone or in combination with other agents. Doses of vitamin A supplements, as low as five times the recommended dietary allowance (RDA), may be toxic and have no clear value in the treatment of cancer.[88] Studies of retinoids in cancer prevention are under way.

Pangamic acid ("vitamin B_{15}") Pangamic acid, or "vitamin B_{15}," is not a vitamin. It has no standards for use and is not recognized by the FDA as a drug.[53] Even though it is illegal to sell it as either a drug or a food supplement in the United States, it is still available in many health food stores.[89–91] There is evidence that the chemicals in products labeled "B_{15}" or "pangamate" may promote the development of cancer.[92,93]

Oxymedicine

Oxygen treatments (hydrogen peroxide, ozone gas, antioxidant enzymes) have gained popularity among the promoters of questionable cancer regimens. Hydrogen peroxide is administered by various routes: oral, rectal, intravenous, and vaginal. It is used by Donsbach as a part of the cancer cure at the Hospital Santa Monica in Tijuana, Mexico, where patients receive dilute infusions of 35% food-grade hydrogen peroxide during their stay at the clinic.[1] Promoters claim that it stimulates immunity, oxidizes toxins, and kills bacteria and viruses.[1] Ozone gas can be administered by rectal infusion, intramuscularly, or in blood transfusion. Ozone enemas are a part of the Gerson regimen at the Hospital de Baja California in Tijuana. Published information on ozone therapy in the treatment of cancer is minimal. Oxidizing agents such as hydrogen peroxide and ozone can be harmful, causing oxygen emboli and death.[94–97]

Immunologic Approach: Immunoaugmentative Therapy (IAT)

Dr. Lawrence Burton, PhD (doctor of Zoology), is the originator of immunoaugmentative therapy (IAT) for cancer; treatment is given at his Immunology Research Centre located in the Bahamas. IAT is based on the theory that stimulation of the immune system will enable the body's normal defenses to destroy tumor cells. Several reviews of the therapy[1,16,98,99] describe the following theory of IAT:

> Normally the body produces "tumor antibody" that destroys tumor cells. There are two conditions where the protective system fails: if there is not enough "tumor complement" to signal the body to produce antibody, or if there is a "blocking protein" that blocks the antibody effect on the tumor. There is also a "deblocking protein" that opposes the action of the "blocking protein."

Burton's treatment regimens are based on the determination of the individual's daily or twice-daily blood levels of "tumor antibody," "tumor complement," "blocking protein factor," and "deblocking protein factor." Based on these results, Burton determines dosages for daily injections of "tumor complement," obtained from patients with cancer, and "tumor antibody" and "deblocking protein factor," which are obtained from the serum of persons without cancer.

Burton has not conducted any controlled trials of his treatment. An NCI analysis of the IAT materials revealed that the materials were dilute solutions of blood plasma, with no biologic activity and none of the components that Burton suggests.[100] Scientific documentation of this therapy is lacking.[1,15,99,101]

In addition to the Bahamas facility, Dr. Burton recently opened facilities in Mexico and Germany. IAT treatment lasts from 6 to 12 weeks. The basic cost of treatment is \$5000–\$5200 for the first 4 weeks and \$500 per week for additional weeks and \$50–\$85 for home maintenance.[99]

Safety concerns have arisen over the years: The unopened vials of treatment materials examined by NCI were found to be unsterile and contaminated with various bacteria;[102] skin abscesses at the injection site of IAT materials have been reported;[103] and in 1985 antibodies to hepatitis B and acquired immunodeficiency syndrome (AIDS) were found in the IAT serum.[100] Numerous attempts have been made to design a scientific clinical trial so IAT could be evaluated, but final agreements could not be reached.[1] IAT remains a hazardous approach to the treatment of cancer, with no documented clinical activity or scientific rationale.

Behavioral and Psychological Approaches

Mental imagery

The Simonton Method, a program of relaxation and imagery, is a self-help approach that has been popular since the 1970s. O. Carl Simonton, a board-certified radiologist, and Stephanie Simonton-Atchley, a psychotherapist, believe that attitude and stress are crucial in causation and cure of cancer and that relaxation and imagery will enhance the immune system and alter the course of malignancy.[104] It is their belief that a positive mental attitude can improve an individual's physiologic responses, resulting in improved results to standard therapy. Cancer patients and their partners are taught to use mental imagery and relaxation techniques to visualize cancer cells as weak and sick and to imagine body defenses as a powerful army that attacks and eliminates the cancer cells.[104] The Simontons strongly advocate that participants in their counseling sessions continue to receive conventional medical treatment.

Although the scientific and medical communities support the notion that a positive mental attitude can increase patient comfort and promote a sense of control and well-being, the following problems remain concerning the Simonton method:

1. There are no carefully controlled clinical studies that show objective benefit from the Simonton method for the treatment of cancer.
2. The method may be harmful, in that individuals may be made to feel guilty because their particular personality type was responsible for the development of cancer.
3. If individuals become overly reliant on the Simonton method, they may be encouraged to abandon standard medical therapy.

Holland[2] notes that the Simontons have softened their approach, so patients whose disease progresses may not feel guilty; however, their method still stresses the individual's responsibility for improvement.

Bernie Siegel also places responsibility on the individual by emphasizing a positive attitude toward survival.[105] He believes that medical treatment is only as effective as the patient's unconscious mind allows. Positive reinforcement and stress reductions can allow healing to take place.

Clearly, both these approaches allow individuals' participation in care; however, they suggest that those patients who do not survive may not have been strong enough or had a good attitude. The ethical implications of these approaches should be a major concern. Until the efficacy of the Simonton method is documented by carefully controlled clinical studies, the American Cancer Society has determined that the Simonton method should be listed as a questionable method of cancer treatment.[106] In counseling patients about available options, nurses can point out potential benefits of the Simonton program while stressing that the method has no scientific documentation of effectiveness in tumor reduction or increased survival.

Spiritual, faith, or mind healing

Many people find empowerment and comfort through various aspects of spiritual or faith healing. Cassileth and Brown[15] found that 71 of their 378 patients were attracted to this method of therapy, which involved use of prayer, "laying on of hands," incantation, or other ways of obtaining divine intervention to rid themselves of the disease. On the other hand, many patients resort to commercialized faith healers who defraud people of their money by claiming they can cure cancer. Other healers espouse self-love as a way to improve health.[107] Holland[108] notes that some methods that require patients to accept the idea that emotions contributed to their cancer may render patients vulnerable to guilt and depression. Thus, these methods may be more hazardous to the patients' well-being than is usually recognized.

QUESTIONABLE TREATMENT FACILITIES

Unorthodox clinics are flourishing in Tijuana, Mexico, which has become a haven for promoters who treat cancer patients with unconventional cancer therapies. Treatment for many other diseases as well as for AIDS are also promoted in many of these clinics. Most therapies are metabolic in nature, but combinations of numerous approaches exist.

Patients arriving at these clinics encounter not only dubious cancer treatments but also dubious diagnostic tests. Although most of the Tijuana clinics are unable to perform standard diagnostic biopsies and complicated tests, they often perform SMAC-24 and the carcinoembryonic antigen (CEA) test but use the tests inappropriately.[23,109] Useless tests that patients will encounter are the metabolic tolerance test and hair analysis, which are used to determine a patient's metabolic status. A "blood crystallization test" and "live-cell analysis" are others. There are tests to determine whether an individual is susceptible to or has cancer. These include Navarro Urine Test; Radionics analysis of energy from the blood; iridology, in which markings, discolorations, and textures of the iris reflect problems in the body; applied kinesiology, which involves testing various muscles to determine if the cancer is responding, improving, or gone; and Kirlian photography, which takes a picture of an individual's fingers.[23] Table 60-2 provides information on the major Tijuana clinics.[21,23,109]

PROMOTERS AND PRACTITIONERS OF QUESTIONABLE METHODS

Strategies Used by Promoters

Promoters of questionable cancer remedies survive, thrive, and grow rich. Much effort and money are devoted to public relations and media presentations that use scientific words or phrases in a misleading and deceptive manner while retaining their emotional impact. Not mentioned are the facts that their remedies have never been objectively tested and found valid. They never acknowledge that any patients have failed to benefit from their regimen. Instead, they rely heavily on testimonials and anecdotes that do not separate fact from fiction, coincidence, or the natural history of the disease.[53] They also claim that a conspiracy exists within organized medicine or the government to keep "cures" from the American public so the "establishment" does not lose the money and business generated from cancer patients.

As with all advertising, the strategies used by the promoters of questionable treatment methods have become very sophisticated. Their claims are attuned to the times: (1) At a time when nutrition and mental attitude are being emphasized by the public, this reasonable interest is being exploited for personal profit; (2) at a time when society is emphasizing prevention, prevention of cancer is represented by purveyors of questionable methods as achievable with their remedies; (3) there has been a tendency to combine many questionable methods to make objective evaluation difficult; and (4) a rising distrust of health professionals is being exploited.[53,110] It is a paradox that highly motivated and better-educated individuals are more likely

TABLE 60-2 Cancer Clinics in Tijuana, Mexico

Clinic	Type of Facility	"Special" Diagnostic Tests	Major Treatment Regimens
American Biologics—Mexico SA. Medical Center	Small, modern clinic; inpatient and outpatient	• *RLB blood test:* detects effects of "reactive oxygen toxic species" which signifies metabolic disruption • *Live-cell analysis:* cells and debris viewed by patient and practitioner • *Metabolic intolerance test:* blood on slide is mixed with food extracts; patient is allergic if white cells break	Individualized metabolic programs, "fresh" live-cell therapy injections; DMSO, oxymedicine, electromedicine
BioMedical Center	Large mansion; outpatient treatment		Hoxsey's herbal preparations, vitamins, dietary instructions
Hospital de Baja California (Gerson Therapy Hospital)	Converted motel; outpatient		Gerson therapy, coffee enemas, pressed liver juice, vegetable and fruit juices
Hospital Ernesto Contreras	Small, modern hospital; inpatient and outpatient	*Navarro Urine Test* (a chorionic gonadotrophin quantitative test): supposedly can find "precancer"	Laetrile, enzymes, detoxification, live-cell therapy, interferons, low-dose chemotherapy, iscador, bible study, sing-along sessions
Hospital Santa Monica	Hotel-like clinic; inpatient	Nutrient Deficiency Test	Hydrogen peroxide (intravenous, oral, ear drops, nasal spray, enemas); DMSO, live-cell therapy, colonics
Manner Clinic	Large, motel-like facility; inpatient	• *Kirlian photography:* patient's finger placed on film in a little black box, and a picture is taken • Manner Normal Blood Profile	Manner cocktail, colonics, special enzymes, DMSO, "electroacuscope 80" (patient hooked up via electrodes and machine electronically manipulates patient's tissue to boost regeneration process), live-cell therapy
St. Jude International Clinic	Three rooms in back of a rundown building, outpatient	• *Applied kinesiology:* pressing down on patient's arm and leg muscles to tell when cancer is gone or responding to treatment. • *Radionics:* various gadgets to detect cancer by analyzing energy radiating from blood, a picture of the person, or even a copy of patient's signature	Amino acid therapy, cobra venom, oxymedicine, herbal therapy

Source: Data from Kreiger L,[21] Lowell JA,[23] and the American Cancer Society.[109]

to turn to questionable methods because of the promise that "you control your disease."[7,111]

Organized Advocates of Questionable Cancer Therapy

The organizations most active in promoting questionable methods of cancer treatment are the International Association of Cancer Victors and Friends, Inc.;[112] the National Health Federation;[113] the Cancer Control Society; the Foundation for Advancement in Cancer Therapies (FACT); Coalition for Alternatives in Nutrition and Healthcare; American Quack Association; Project Cure and the Center for Alternative Cancer Research; Committee for Freedom of Choice in Medicine; and patient organizations associated with specific therapies (e.g., IAT).[1] Most of these organizations have journals or newsletters (which emphasize the antimedical establishment), hold seminars, and assist patients with information on unconventional treatments and provide lists of "recovered" patients. Some organizations take a more political stance by supporting legislation in deregulation of practitioners and promoting "freedom of choice."

WHO SEEKS QUESTIONABLE CANCER TREATMENTS, AND WHY

Limited studies have shown that patients who seek questionable therapies are more likely to be Caucasian and asymptomatic and to have localized disease.[6] They are also better educated.[6–8,114] In addition, many patients seek unconventional therapy after completing their mainstream treatment regimens, when they have no evidence of disease.[1,6] Most patients learn about unconventional treatments by word of mouth, through the mass media (books, newspapers, television, radio), from advocacy groups, and at health food stores.

Motivations and Reasons for Use

There are a variety of reasons why cancer patients pursue questionable therapy.

Fear

Cancer creates many fears: fear of treatment, of death, of an uncertain future, of pain, of disfigurement, of loss of family, of loss of self-control and independence, of alienation, and of costly medical care. Given these fears, it is not difficult to understand why many individuals with cancer are in great need of hope and may seek unproven therapies that are offered as "nontoxic" therapies that will "cure" their disease. Most individuals want a treatment without risks or pain and with a good probability of cure. Resorting to some dietary or enzyme therapy that promises no side effects or uses "the body's natural defenses" may coincide with the person's fantasies about being cured. That is, by utilizing unconventional therapy, the patient hopes for an unconventional cure.[10]

Desire for self-control

Use of an unproven method may provide an individual with a greater sense of self-control. This desire for control may result from feeling like a passive recipient of treatments designated by the health care team rather than like a partner in treatment decision making. Patients dissatisfied with their doctors and with conventional therapy feel they have control over their health, thus more confidence and a sense of well-being, since conventional therapy is often passive. Better-educated and highly motivated patients are more likely to turn to unproven methods, because the methods falsely promise to give the patient control over the disease.[7,53,111]

Isolation/antiestablishment

The promoters of questionable methods frequently suggest that the government and organized medicine are in a conspiracy against curing cancer. They often appear as the underdog in battling the medical system in order to make a new risk-free treatment available to individuals with cancer. The isolation that is projected by the purveyors of questionable treatment methods may be easy for the cancer patient to identify with, since they too feel isolated.

Social pressures

Other reasons to use unproven methods can come via pressures exerted by family or friends.[108] The family has many of the same fears as the patient, and they often assist the patient in making treatment decisions. This responsibility can be overwhelming and frightening in and of itself. The family may feel that the best course is to try everything, with the hope that something will work; and it may also help them feel less guilty if the treatment does not work or the patient does not recover. In turn, the patient may feel obligated to meet the family's expectation to submit to these treatments so as not to alienate his or her support system. On the other hand, cancer patients might want to try whatever treatments are available, and, thus, the family might feel pressured to discover "cancer cures." Friends are also a source of information and may influence the patient and family.

Even with the best intentions of all parties, the overall outcome can be torturous for those involved. How difficult these times will be depends greatly on the personalities and relationships that existed before the cancer was diagnosed, the quality of communication that takes place, the availability of accurate information on treatment options and outcomes, and the effects of disease and therapy.

CONTROL OF QUESTIONABLE METHODS

Any claim for a new method of cancer management in the United States must meet certain scientific standards and be capable of confirmation before it receives approval by the federal government for interstate distribution. The standards of scientific investigation are:[115] (1) examination of clinical evidence; (2) analysis of the drug/treatment on experimental animals and reproducibility; (3) observation of therapeutic effects of treatment under study on a sufficient number of patients with biopsy-proven cancer; (4) assessment of results; (5) examination of autopsy data on patients who die after treatment; and (6) consultation with researchers and other investigative groups. However, most unconventional approaches for the treatment of cancer lack scientifically interpretable data.[1]

Recently, the National Institutes of Health (NIH) were congressionally mandated to establish the NIH Office of the Study of Unconventional Medical Practices.[116] Hawkins and Friedman,[117] from the NCI Cancer Therapy Evaluation Program, Division of Cancer

Treatment, note that the pivotal question for the NCI in trying to improve cancer therapy is whether the treatment in question is effective, regardless of the source. Thus, the best way for NCI to resolve the controversies surrounding unconventional treatment approaches is to identify potential approaches for further evaluation by advising investigators in the preparation of best-case series and the conduct of pilot clinical trials.

The federal and state governments participate in the regulation of questionable treatment methods. The FDA has regulatory authority over the manufacturing and marketing of food, drugs, devices, and cosmetics so safety and efficacy are ensured. The FDA regulations do not apply to treatment regimens or practices but only to specific substances used in treatment (e.g., laetrile, antineoplastons, IAT). The Federal Trade Commission (FTC) monitors the advertising of foods and over-the-counter drugs and prohibits false or deceptive advertising. The U.S. Postal Service has authority to monitor for false advertising of mail order products. State laws regulate commerce within states (intrastate). For example, it is legal to manufacture and prescribe treatments that are not approved by the FDA, but only in the state in which the manufacture of the treatment takes place (e.g., Cancell in Michigan). It is illegal to transport unapproved drugs across state lines; however, such transport continues via underground networks. Some states have enacted laws that exempt questionable treatments from state regulation. For example, Oklahoma and Florida enacted provisions to legalize the use of IAT, although they later repealed the laws.

TABLE 60-3 Sources of Information on Questionable Cancer Remedies

American Cancer Society Committee on Questionable Methods of Cancer Management 1599 Clifton Road, N.E. Atlanta, GA 30329 (404) 329-7607
American Cancer Society (Cancer Response System) 1-800-ACS-2345
Consumer Health Information & Research Institute 3521 Broadway Kansas City, MO 64111 (816) 753-8850
Food and Drug Administration Office of Consumer Affairs—(301) 443-5006 Office of Health Affairs—(301) 443-5470 Rockville, MD
National Cancer Institute (Cancer Information Service) 1-800-4-CANCER
National Council Against Health Fraud, Inc. P.O. Box 1276 Loma Linda, CA 92354 (714) 824-4690

In addition to scientific investigation and legislative regulation, education plays a major role in the control of questionable cancer treatment. Private and government organizations provide information to health professionals and the public. The American Cancer Society maintains a continual, accurate record of questionable methods for cancer management with the support of their Committee on Questionable Methods of Cancer Management. The Cancer Response System, a telephone information service, allows the American Cancer Society to keep a record of inquiries regarding questionable methods. Other private organizations involved with the control of questionable methods are the American Society of Clinical Oncology, American Medical Association, and the National Council Against Health Fraud (NCAHF). The National Cancer Institute also receives inquiries through their Cancer Information Service and is in the process of developing a more detailed database on unconventional treatments. Table 60-3 identifies sources of information on questionable cancer remedies.

ROLE OF NURSES/NURSING INTERVENTIONS

The progress in cancer care as a result of advances in science and technology over the last 20 years has been tremendous. In fact, it has become a major challenge just to maintain one's knowledge on the numerous drug combinations, biologic therapies, and treatment protocols for the different types of cancer. Along with this progress has come the development of questionable cancer remedies and combinations of these treatment regimens. As nurses, we provide the support, care, and comfort for patients within a health care system with rapidly changing and complex scientific treatment modalities. How can we sort through the confusing array of facts and choices available? How can we separate fact from fiction?

Some nurses are vulnerable to the simplicity of "holistic" medicine. The movement away from high technology is evident in several recent articles[118–120] in which nurses in England discussed the use of reflexology, aromatherapy, massage, herbalism, and dietary practice—all "complementary therapies." Reflexology on the feet is supposed to correspond to specific organs and to balance the body's energy. The NCAHF newsletter considers it "fringe nursing" and notes that it is unfortunate that nurses undermine their credibility by promoting such therapies.[121] Several state boards of nursing even award continuing education credits for nonscientific seminars on such topics as crystal healing, firewalking, reflexology, therapeutic touch, applied kinesiology, and aromatherapy.[122,123]

Behavioral methods (mental imagery, biofeedback, and even humor, which some clinicians and patients are using more systematically) are of major interest to nurses. How does a nurse sort through the beneficial or detrimental aspects of something like the Simonton method? What about nutritional intervention, such as vitamin supplements? Many patients want to do something for themselves. How can nurses help them develop a plan of self-care, and when does that cross over into promoting ineffective cancer remedies?

Two recent articles highlight the problem that nurses face. Spiegel et al.[124] reported that psychosocial intervention significantly increased survival in patients with metastatic breast cancer. (Reportedly, Spiegel never conceived such an outcome when he began the study. In fact, the study was undertaken to disprove the effect.[125]) However, it must be noted that a larger randomized study is needed to verify their results. A second study, by Cassileth et al.,[114] further confuses the situation by providing convincing evidence that for patients with extensive cancer, there is no difference in survival between patients who received a particular unorthodox treatment regimen versus conventional therapy. However, they noted that quality of life was better among conventionally treated patients. Deprived of our conventional wisdom regarding unorthodox treatments, how are we to respond to patients who say, "Why not? It can't hurt, and it might help!"

The responsible position requires that nurses avoid simplistic cliches and deal realistically with the complexities and limitations of modern cancer care as well as the subtlety and seductiveness of the unorthodox cancer treatment industry. Four specific steps will assist in this difficult task.

Identification of Quackery (Legitimate vs. Fringe Care)

The health professional must be informed both regarding technical information on the most frequently encountered unproven methods and the particular aims of a given individual's therapy. The health professional should be able to explain the risks of unproven methods, such as toxicity, or, in instances where the unproven method is being used as a sole form of therapy, the risk of further progression of disease. For individuals using an unproven method in combination with standard therapy, it is still important to know what side effects to look for. A drug analysis may prove valuable for any substances the patient has been given by an unproven methods clinic. The risks of adverse effects can be increased when drugs are mixed with unorthodox substances, and the patient must be informed that all risks may not be known.

The Subcommittee on Unorthodox Therapies of the American Society of Clinical Oncology[126] has listed ten questions to ask in making a decision as to whether a treatment should be suspected of being questionable (Table 60-4). Although these questions were developed as a guide for the layperson, they are an excellent resource for the health professional.

TABLE 60-4 Ten Questions to Ask in Deciding Whether a Treatment is Questionable

1. Is the treatment based on an unproven theory?
2. Is there a purported need for special nutritional support?
3. Is there a claim for painless, nontoxic treatment?
4. Are claims published only in the mass media and not in reputable, peer-reviewed scientific journals?
5. Are claims for benefit merely compatible with a placebo effect?
6. Are the major proponents recognized experts in cancer treatment?
7. Do proponents claim benefit for use with proven methods of treatment? for prolongation of life? for use as a cancer preventative?
8. Is there a claim that only specially trained physicians can produce results with the drug, or is the preparation secret?
9. Is there an attack on the medical and scientific establishment?
10. Is there a demand by promoters for "freedom of choice" regarding drugs?

Source: Subcommittee on Unorthodox Therapies, American Society of Clinical Oncology: Ineffective cancer therapy: A guide for the layperson. *J Clin Oncol* 1:154–163, 1983.

Assessment of Communication Channels and Patient Motivations

Communication patterns between the patient and family must be evaluated. The family may become preoccupied with seeking different therapies as a means of coping with stress. Such a situation may be intense enough to cause the family to engage in a conspiracy to exclude the patient from the decision-making process. Thus the patient is separated from the family's communication system and from the psychologic and physical support that is so important. In this case, the family must be made aware of the impact of their actions on the patient. A social worker, chaplain, or patient-family support group might facilitate more effective intrafamily communication.

Maintenance of Positive Communication Channels

Cassileth et al.[7] noted that the majority of patients will inform their physicians they are using questionable methods, but only a small number of patients will discuss with their physicians whether they are considering the use of unproven methods. It is important for the physician and health care professional to discuss questionable methods of cancer management with patients, since patients are likely to hear about a variety of methods. By initiating such a discussion, the health care professional helps keep communication channels open for further inquiry by the patient and/or family. Table 60-5 identifies some potential questions to ask in order to assess a patient's risk and possible motivations for

TABLE 60-5 Questions That May Be Helpful in Assessing a Patient's Risk and Possible Motivation for Seeking Questionable Cancer Remedies

- Do you feel like an active participant in your health care?
  If not: How would you like to play a more active role?
- Are you having difficulty accepting your diagnosis?
- Do you feel a sense of helplessness and hopelessness?
- Do you feel depressed?
- Do you feel anxious?
- What type of diet do you follow?
- Do you take supplemental vitamins?
  If so: What kind?
- Do you frequent health food stores?
- Have you received any information regarding alternative methods of cancer treatment?
  If so:
  - Are you considering using this therapy?
  - What benefits do you perceive you will derive from this therapy?
  - Is your family encouraging you to pursue this therapy?
  - Would you like us to review the information?

seeking questionable methods of cancer therapy. These questions provide an opportunity to discover unmet needs of the patient and family, assess their understanding of the therapies they have been receiving, assess their potential interest in unproven methods, and provide reinforcement to the patient and family that discussion of questionable treatment methods will not cause rejection or impair their communication with the health care team. A nonjudgmental attitude facilitates the assessment of the patient's and family's motivations for wanting to try an unproven method. In turn, the patient and family will likely be more receptive to the information provided by a health care professional who offers no negative response or moral judgment.

Maintenance of Patient Participation in Their Health Care

Many patients turn to questionable cancer remedies because they do not feel like an active participant in their care and have lost hope that their conventional therapy will work. It is important for patients and family to participate in health care. Patients will be less likely to seek questionable cancer remedies if such needs are met.[2] Patient education can increase patient satisfaction, increase patient knowledge, and enhance self-care. For example, information on diet and nutrition provided in a positive context will help the patient feel a part of the therapeutic effort and may prevent the use of questionable dietary therapies. In the event of advancing illness or when conventional treatment modalities have been exhausted, hope and a sense of participation can sometimes be generated if we offer the patient participation in a clinical trial of investigative therapy.

If the patient pursues questionable methods, health care professionals should communicate that they will continue to provide care and would like to be kept informed of the treatments the patient is going to pursue. The patient should be urged to continue standard medical care.

CONCLUSION

The health professionals caring for patients with cancer must be kept informed of questionable methods. The terms *questionable, unconventional, quackery, alternative*, and *complementary* suggest that the substance or method is being promoted even though it has not been proven effective. Just because a therapy is being promoted that has not been proven effective does not necessarily mean that it has no therapeutic value. It must be tested to determine its safety and efficacy. The present system relies on the scientific method to determine what therapies will be on the market, and improvements are continually being made in methods of evaluation. In this way the health care consumer is protected from unsafe and fraudulent therapies. As nurses we have the responsibility to become informed; report any questionable methods to the health department, consumer protection agency, local medical society, or the American Cancer Society; and support legislation that will remove fraudulent methods of health care. The nurses' role as a patient educator provides one of the most powerful approaches towards controlling questionable cancer remedies.

REFERENCES

1. Office of Technology Assessment: *Unconventional Cancer Treatments.* OTA-H-405. Washington, DC: U.S. Government Printing Office, September 1990.
2. Holland JC, Geary N, Furman A: Alternative cancer therapies. In Holland JC, Rowland JH (eds.): *Handbook of Psychooncology.* New York: Oxford University Press, 1989, pp. 508–515.
3. House Subcommittee on Aging: *Quackery: A 10-Billion-Dollar Scandal,* (report). Committee publication no. 98-435. Washington DC: U.S. Government Printing Office, 1984, pp. 1–250.
4. House Subcommittee on Aging: *Quackery: A 10-Billion-Dollar Scandal,* (hearing). Committee publication no. 98-463. Washington DC: U.S. Government Printing OFfice, 1984.
5. Herbert V, Barnett S: *Vitamins and "Health" Foods: The Great American Hustle.* Philadelphia: George F. Stickley, 1981.
6. Lerner IJ, Kennedy BJ: The prevalence of questionable methods of cancer treatment in the United States. *CA* 42:181–191, 1992.

7. Cassileth B, Lusk E, Strouse T, et al: Contemporary unorthodox treatments in cancer medicine. *Ann Intern Med* 101:105–112, 1984.
8. Cassileth BR: Unorthodox cancer medicine. *Cancer Invest* 4:591–598, 1986.
9. Louis Harris and Assocs: Health information and the use of questionable treatments: A study of the American Public. U.S. Department of Health and Human Services, study number 833015, September, 1987.
10. Yarbro, CH: Unproven methods of cancer treatment. In Groenwald S, Frogge MH, Goodman S, Yarbro CH (eds.): *Cancer Nursing: Principles and Practice* (ed. 2). Boston: Jones and Bartlett, 1990, pp. 1216–1227.
11. Janssen WF: The cancer "cures": A challenge to rational therapeutics. *Analytical Chem* 50:197A–202A, 1978.
12. Janssen WF: Cancer quackery—The past in the present. *Semin Oncol* 6:526–536, 1979.
13. Message from President Taft. Congressional Record, 62 Cong., 1 Sess 2380 (June 21, 1911).
14. Kennedy D: Commissioner decision on status. *Federal Register* 42:39806–39967, 1977.
15. Cassileth B, Brown H: Unorthodox cancer medicine. *CA* 38: 176–186, 1988.
16. Curt GA: Unsound methods of cancer treatment. *PPO Updates.* 4(12):1–10, 1990.
17. Koch WF: A new and successful treatment and diagnosis of cancer. *Detroit Med J*, 1919.
18. Letter to the Editor: Senator Langer abuses franking privilege by circulation of propaganda for Koch's cancer quackery. *JAMA* 137:1333, 1948.
19. Hoxsey HM: *You Don't Have to Die—The Amazing Story of the Hoxsey Cancer Treatment.* New York: Milestone Books, 1956.
20. Food and Drug Administration: Press release HEW-020. Washington DC: U.S. Department Health, Education and Welfare, September 21, 1960.
21. Kreiger L: Unorthodox clinics flourishing in Tijuana. *Am Med News* 3:25–27, 1985.
22. American Cancer Society: Unproven methods of cancer management: Hoxsey method/BioMedical Center. *CA* 40:51–55, 1990.
23. Lowell JA: Mexican cancer clinics. In Barrett S, Cassileth BR (eds.): *Dubious Cancer Treatment.* Tampa, FL: American Cancer Society, Florida Division, 1991, pp. 53–62.
24. Holland JF: The Krebiozen story—Is cancer quackery dead? *JAMA* 200:213–218, 1967.
25. American Cancer Society: *Unproven Methods of Cancer Management.* New York: American Cancer Society, 1971.
26. Food and Drug Administration: Report of Director, National Cancer Institute, to Secretary Department of Health, Education and Welfare concerning decision of the Institute not to undertake clinical testing of Krebiozen. Washington DC: FDA Records, 539.1.PX, October 16, 1963.
27. Manner HW, DiSanti SJ, Michalsen TL: *The Death of Cancer.* Evanston IL: Advanced Century Publishing, 1978.
28. Conchie J, Findlay L, Levvy GA: Mammalian glycosidases. Distribution in the body. *Biochem J* 71:318–325, 1959.
29. Gal EM, Fung FH, Greenberg DM: Studies on the biological action of mandelonitriles. II. Distribution of rhodanese (transulfurase) in the tissues of normal and tumor-bearing animals and the effect of mandelonitriles thereon. *Cancer Res* 169:449–450, 1952.
30. Greenberg DM: The vitamin fraud in cancer quackery. *West J Med* 122:345–348, 1975.
31. Greenstein JP, et al: Quantitative nutritional studies with water-soluble chemically defined diets. I. Growth, reproduction and lactation in rats. *Arch Biochem Biophysics* 72:396–416, 1957.
32. Everly RC: Laetrile: Focus on the facts. *CA* 26:50–54, 1976.
33. Grabois B: Exposure to hydrogen cyanide in processing of apricot kernels. *Monthly Review: New York Department of Labor* 33:33–36, 1954.
34. Sayre JW, Kaymakcalan S: Cyanide poisoning from apricot seeds among children in central Turkey. *N Engl J Med* 270:1113–1115, 1964.
35. Gunders AE, Abrahamov A, Weisenberg E: Cyanide poisoning following the ingestion of apricot (*Prunas armeniaca*) kernel. *J Israel Med Ass* 76:536–538, 1969.
36. Humbert JR, Tress JH, Braico KT: Fatal cyanide poisoning: Accidental ingestion of amygdalin. *JAMA* 238:482, 1977 (letter).
37. Sadoff L, Fuchs K, Hollander J: Rapid death associated with laetrile ingestion. *JAMA* 239:1532, 1978.
38. Herbert V: *Nutrition Cultism: Facts and Fictions* (ed. 3). Philadelphia: George F. Stickley, 1981.
39. Herbert V: Laetrile: The cult of cyanide. Promoting poison for profit. *Am J Clin Nutr* 32:1121–1158, 1979.
40. Vogel SN, Sultan TR: Cyanide poisoning. *Clin Toxicol Exp Ther* 18:367–383, 1981.
41. Ortega JA, Creek J: Acute cyanide poisoning following administration of laetrile enemas. *J Pediatr* 93:1059, 1979.
42. Eisele JW, Reay DT: Deaths related to coffee enemas. *JAMA* 244:1608–1609, 1980.
43. Food and Drug Administration: Toxicity of laetrile. *FDA Drug Bulletin* 7:25–32, 1977.
44. Wodinsky I, Swiniarsky JK: Antitumor activity of amygdalin as a single agent and with beta-glucosidase on a spectrum of transplantable rodent tumors. *Cancer Chemo Rep* 59:939–950, 1975.
45. Hill GJ, Shine TE, Hill HZ, et al: Failure of amygdalin to arrest B16 melanoma and BW5147 AKR leukemia. *Cancer Res* 36:2102–2107, 1976.
46. Stock CC, Tarnowski GS, Schmid FA, et al: Antitumor tests of amygdalin in transplantable animal tumor systems. *J Surg Oncol* 10:81–88, 1978.
47. Stock CC, Martin DS, Suguira K, et al: Antitumor tests of amygdalin in spontaneous animal tumor systems. *J Surg Oncol* 10:89–123, 1978.
48. Ovejira AA, Houchens DP, Barker AD, et al: Inactivity of DL-amygdalin against human breast and colon tumor xenografts in athymic (nude) mice. *Cancer Treat Rep* 62:576–578, 1978.
49. California Medical Association, Cancer Commission: The treatment of cancer with "Laetriles". *Calif Med* 78:320–326, 1953.
50. Ellison NM, Byar DP, Newell GR: Special report on laetrile: The NCI laetrile review. *N Engl J Med* 299:549–552, 1978.
51. Henney JE: Unproven methods of cancer treatment. In DeVita VT, Hellman S, Rosenberg SA (eds.): *Cancer Principles and Practice of Oncology* (ed. 2). Philadelphia: Lippincott, 1985, pp. 2333–2342.
52. Moertel CG, Fleming TR, Tubin J, et al: A clinical trial of amygdalin (laetrile) in the treatment of human cancer. *N Engl J Med* 306:201–207, 1982.
53. Herbert V, Yarbro CH: Nutrition quackery. *Semin Oncol Nurs* 2:63–69, 1986.

54. American Cancer Society: Unproven methods of cancer management: Laetrile. *CA* 41:187–191, 1991.
55. Cassileth BR: Historical trends and patient characteristics. In Barrett S, Cassileth BR (eds.): *Dubious Cancer Treatment.* Tampa, FL: American Cancer Society, Florida Division, 1991, pp. 27–34.
56. Read MH, St. Jeor S, Seymour K, et al: Supplementation practices of a group of patients with cancer. *J Am Diet Assoc* 90:278–279, 1990.
57. Miller NJ, Howard-Ruben J: Unproven methods of cancer management. Part I: Background and historical perspectives. *Oncol Nurs Forum* 10:46–52, 1983.
58. American Cancer Society: Unproven methods of cancer management: Gerson Method. *CA* 40:252–256, 1990.
59. Gerson M: The cure of advanced cancer by diet therapy: A summary of 30 years of clinical experimentation. *Physiol Chem Physi* 10:449–464, 1978.
60. Istre GR, Kreiss K, Hopkins RS, et al: An outbreak of amebiasis spread by colonic irrigation at a chiropractic clinic. *N Engl J Med* 307:339–342, 1982.
61. Markman M: Medical complications of "alternative" cancer therapy. *N Engl J Med* 312:1640–1641, 1985 (letter).
62. American Cancer Society: Unproven methods of cancer management: The metabolic cancer therapy of Harold W. Manner, Ph.D. *CA* 36:185–189, 1986.
63. Ohsawa G: *Cancer and the Philosophy of the Far East.* Binghamton NY: Swan House Publishing, 1971.
64. Kushi M: *Macrobiotic Approach to Cancer.* Wayne, NJ: Avery Publishing, 1982.
65. Arnold C: The macrobiotic diet: A question of nutrition. *Oncol Nurs Forum* 11:50–53, 1984.
66. Bowman BB, Kushner RF, Dawson SC, et al: Macrobiotic diets for cancer treatment and prevention. *J Clin Oncol* 2:702–711, 1984.
67. American Cancer Society: Unproven methods of cancer management: Macrobiotic diets for the treatment of cancer. *CA* 39:248–251, 1989.
68. Green S: "Antineoplastons": An unproved cancer therapy. *JAMA* 267:2924–2928, 1992.
69. NCI plans trials of Burzynski's "Antineoplaston"; JAMA Report says no antitumor activity in tests. *Cancer Letter* 18(23):1–4, 1992.
70. Burzynski Research Institute: Patient brochure on antineoplaston treatment. Houston, TX: The Institute, 1989.
71. Lowell J: Cancell. *National Council Against Health Fraud Newsletter.* 14(2):3, 1991.
72. Sopack E: *Important Information About Cancell* (promotional literature). Howell, MI: November 1988.
73. *U.S. vs James V. Sheridan and Edward J. Sopack.* Complaint for permanent injunction filed in the U.S. District Court of the Eastern District of Michigan. February 21, 1989.
74. American Cancer Society: Unproven methods of cancer management: Dimethyl sulfoxide (DMSO). *CA* 33:122–125, 1983.
75. American Cancer Society: Unproven methods of cancer management: Fresh-cell therapy. *CA* 41:126–128, 1991.
76. Alvarez G: Live-cell therapy at the Manner Clinic. *Manner and Metabolic Research Foundation Newsletter* 1:2–3, 1992.
77. Cameron E, Pauling L: Supplemental ascorbate in the supportive treatment of cancer, prolongation of survival time in terminal human cancer. *Proc Natl Acad Sci USA* 73:3685–3689, 1976.
78. Sampson WI: When the big C is a vitamin. *Coping* 2:35, 1988.
79. Creagan ET, Moertel CG, O'Fallon JR, et al: Failure of high-dose vitamin C to benefit patients with advanced cancer. *N Engl J Med* 301:687–690, 1979.
80. Moertel CG, Fleming TR, Creagan ET, et al: High-dose vitamin C versus placebo in the treatment of patients with advanced cancer who have had no prior chemotherapy. *N Engl J Med* 312:137–141, 1985.
81. Tschetter L, Creagan ET, O'Fallon JR, et al: A community-based study of vitamin C (ascorbic acid) therapy in patients with advanced cancer. *Proc Am Soc Clin Oncol* 2:92, 1983 (abstr.).
82. Marwick C: Cancer institute takes a look at ascorbic acid. *JAMA* 264:1926, 1990.
83. Swartz RD, Wesley JR, Somermeyer MG, et al: Hyperoxaluria and renal insufficiency due to ascorbic acid administration during total parenteral nutrition. *Ann Int Med* 100:530–531, 1984.
84. Backer RC, Herbert V: Cyanide production from laetrile in the presence of megadoses of ascorbic acid. *JAMA* 241:1891–1892, 1979.
85. Herbert V: The rationale of massive-dose vitamin therapy. (Megavitamin therapy: hot fiction vs cold facts). In Whilte PL, Selvey N (eds.): *Proceedings: Western Hemisphere Nutrition Congress IV.* Acton, MA: Publishing Sciences Group, 1975, pp. 84–91.
86. Hodges RE: *Nutrition in Medical Practice.* Philadelphia: Saunders, 1980.
87. Marshall CW: *Vitamins and Minerals: Help or Harm?* Philadelphia: George F. Stickley, 1983.
88. Herbert V: Toxicity of 25,000 IU vitamin A supplements in "Health" food users. *Am J Clin Nutr* 36:185–186, 1982.
89. Herbert V: Pangamic acid (vitamin B_{15}). *Am J Clin Nutr* 32:1534–1540, 1979.
90. Herbert V, Herbert R: Pangamate (vitamin B_{15}). In Ellenbogen L (ed.): *Controversies in Nutrition.* New York: Churchill Livingstone, 1981, pp. 159–170.
91. McPherrin EW, Herbert V, Herbert R: *"Vitamin B_{15}": Anatomy of a Health Fraud.* New York: American Council on Science and Health, 1981.
92. Colman H, Herbert V, Gardner A, et al: Mutagenicity of dimethyglycine when mixed with nitrite: Possible significance in human use of pangamates. *Proc Soc Exp Biol Med* 164:9–12, 1980.
93. Gelernt MD, Herbert V; Mutagenicity of diisopropylamine dichloroacetate, the "active constituent" of vitamin B_{15} (pangamic acid). *Nutr Cancer* 3:129–133, 1982.
94. Sleigh JW, Linter SPK: Hazards of hydrogen peroxide. *Br Med J* 291:1706, 1985.
95. Bassan NM, Dudai M, Shaley O: Near-fatal systemic oxygen embolism due to wound irrigation with hydrogen peroxide. *Postgrad Med J* 58:448–451, 1982.
96. Danis RK, Brodeur AE, Shields J: The danger of hydrogen peroxide as colonic irrigating solution. *J Pediatr Surg* 3:131–133, 1967.
97. Giberson TP, Kern JD, Pettigrew DW III, et al: Near-fatal hydrogen peroxide ingestion. *Ann Emer Med* 18:778–779, 1989.
98. Zavertnik JJ: Immuno-augmentative therapy. In Barrett S, Cassileth BR (eds.): *Dubious Cancer Treatment.* Tampa, FL: American Cancer Society, Florida Division, 1990, pp. 63–72.
99. American Cancer Society: Questionable methods of cancer management: Immuno-augmentative therapy (IAT). *CA* 41:357–364, 1991.
100. Curt GA, Katterhagen G, Mahaney FX: Immunoaug-

mentative therapy: A primer on the perils of unproved treatments. *JAMA* 255:505–507, 1986.
101. Easy cures for cancer still find support. *JAMA* 246:714–716, 1981.
102. Curt GA: Warning on immunoaugmentative therapy. *N Engl J Med* 311:859, 1984.
103. Centers for Disease Control: Cutaneous nocardiosis in cancer receiving immunotherapy injections—Bahamas. *MMWR* 33:471–477, 1984.
104. Simonton OC, Simonton SM, Creighton JL: *Getting Well Again: A Step-by-Step, Self-Help Guide to Overcoming Cancer for Patients and their Families.* New York: Bantam, 1980.
105. Siegel B: *Love, Medicine & Miracles.* New York: Harper & Row, 1986.
106. American Cancer Society: Unproven methods of cancer management: O. Carl Simonton, MD. *CA* 32:58–61, 1982.
107. Irish AC: Maintaining health in persons with HIV infection. *Semin Oncol Nurs* 5:302–307, 1989.
108. Holland JC: Why patients seek unproven cancer remedies: A psychological perspective. *CA* 32:10–14, 1982.
109. American Cancer Society: Questionable cancer practices in Tijuana and other Mexican border clinics. *CA* 41:310–319, 1991.
110. King M: Falling victim twice. *Cancer News* 39:8–11, 1985.
111. Hiratzka S: Knowledge and attitudes of persons with cancer toward use of unproven treatment methods. *Oncol Nurs Forum* 12:36–41, 1985.
112. American Cancer Society: Unproven methods of cancer management: International Association of Cancer Victors and Friends, Inc. *CA* 39:58–59, 1989.
113. American Cancer Society: Unproven methods of cancer management: National Health Federation. *CA* 41:61–64, 1991.
114. Cassileth BR, Lusk EJ, Guerry D, et al: Survival and quality of life among patients receiving unproven as compared with conventional cancer therapy. *N Engl J Med* 324:1180–1185, 1991.
115. Grant RN, Bartlett I: Unproven cancer remedies: a primer. *CA* 16:42–59, 1966.
116. Senate gives NIH director authority to permit research by unconventional MDs. *Cancer Letter* 18(37):3–4, 1992.
117. Hawkins MJ, Friedman MA: Commentary: National Cancer Institute's evaluation of unconventional cancer treatments. *J Natl Cancer Inst* 84:1699–1702, 1992.
118. Passant H: A holistic approach in the ward. *Nurs Times* 86:26–28, 1990.
119. Evans M: Reflex zone therapy for mothers. *Nurs Times* 86:29–31, 1990.
120. Smith M: Healing through touch. *Nurs Times* 86:31–32, 1990.
121. National Council Against Health Fraud: Fringe nursing. *National Council Against Health Fraud Newsletter* 13(5):4, 1990.
122. National Council Against Health Fraud: Registered nurses get CE credit for crystal healing coursework. *National Council Against Health Fraud Newsletter* 13(3):3, 1990.
123. National Council Against Health Fraud: Colorado RN confronts pseudoscience in nurses continuing education. *National Council Against Health Fraud Newsletter* 15(4):3, 1992.
124. Spiegel D, Bloom JR, Kraemer HC, et al: Effect of psychosocial treatment on survival of patients with metastatic breast cancer. *Lancet* 2:888–890, 1989.
125. Barinaga M: Can psychotherapy delay cancer deaths? *Science* 246:448–449, 1989.
126. Subcommittee on Unorthodox Therapies, American Society of Clinical Oncology: Ineffective cancer therapy: A guide for the layperson. *J Clin Oncol* 1:154–163, 1983.

Chapter 61

Teaching Strategies: Public Education

Marion E. Morra, MA, ScD

INTRODUCTION

Communicating to and educating the public in the area of health has been a responsibility of nurses for many years. Health care professionals in the cancer field view themselves as role models, not only to the patients they serve but also to the public at large.

DEFINITION OF TERMS

There are many definitions of health education. Some relate to the field of education as a whole; others are based in the areas of communications, behavior, and marketing. The President's Committee on Health Education views health education as a way to bridge the gap between health information and health practices. Health education motivates the person to take information and do something with it—to keep healthier by avoiding actions that are harmful and by forming habits that are beneficial.[1] The World Health Organization (WHO) defines health education as any combination of planned activities leading to a situation where people want to be healthy, know how to obtain health information, do what they can individually and collectively, and seek help when needed.[2] Green at al.[3] have a broader definition: Health education is any combination of learning experiences designed to facilitate voluntary adoption of behavior conducive to health. Glanz et al.[4] widen the definition of the scope of health education, incorporating teaching activities directed at patients in the health care system as well as at people in the community, organizational efforts, policy directives, and economic supports. This increases the scope as well as the purpose of health education, allowing for a wide variety of programs, activities, and methods to enrich the field.

THEORIES AND MODELS

Health education embodies theories in the fields of education, psychology, and communications. Following are several theories relating to health education.

Health Belief Model

The Health Belief Model, often considered the basis for health behavioral research, was developed in the 1950s[5] and established a framework for explaining and predicting why people engage in specific preventive behaviors. The Health Belief Model provides insight into how an individual makes such a decision. Based on the tenet that the beliefs and values acquired over a lifetime affect a person's decisions, it combines variables such as the person's perception of being susceptible to that condition, the perceived seriousness of the problem, and the availability of specific actions that prevent or treat the condition. This model is discussed in detail in Chapter 6.

PRECEDE Model

The PRECEDE model of health education[3] provides an organizing framework within which more detailed theories might be integrated. The PRECEDE (an acronym for predisposing, reinforcing, and enabling causes in educational diagnosis and evaluation) framework is highly focused on intervention, be it with people whose health is in question or with those who control resources or rewards, such as community leaders, parents, peers, teachers, and health care professionals. PRECEDE has seven phases: (1) assessment of social problems of concern, (2) identification of specific health-related problems, (3) identification of specific health-related behaviors linked to the health problems, (4) categorization of factors that have direct impact on these behaviors (predisposing, enabling, or reinforcing factors), (5) assessment of relative importance of factors and resources available to influence them, (6) development and implementation of programs, and (7) evaluation.

Transtheoretical Model of Behavior Change

The Transtheoretical Model of Behavior change, introduced by Prochaska and DiClemente,[6] posits that people who are changing their health behavior move through a series of stages, including: *precontemplation* (people are not thinking seriously about changing, at least not in the next 6 months), *contemplation* (people are thinking seriously about changing an unhealthy behavior in the next 6 months), *action* (a 6-month period in which an overt modification of an unhealthy behavior occurs), *maintenance* (from 6 months after an overt behavior change until problem is finally terminated), and *termination* (a stable period of zero temptation and maximum confidence in ability to resist relapse). When this model is applied to smokers, for instance, the data from Prochaska show that approximately twice as many smokers in the contemplation stage took action during the first 6 months of a self-help intervention study as did those in the precontemplation stage.[7] Using national survey data, Prochaska et al. estimated that nearly 70% of smokers were not in a stage ready to take action on their smoking.

Communications Theory

In communications theory,[8] six basic elements are described as essential to any process of communications:

(1) a source (that constructs a message), (2) an encoder (that produces it), (3) the message itself, (4) a channel (that carries it), (5) a decoder (that translates it), and (6) a receiver (that gets the message). Within the source and the receiver, four factors impinge on the success of communications: communications skills, attitudes, knowledge level, and social or cultural systems.

McGuire[9] added to these traditional communications variables five behavioral steps in the processing of health information: attention, comprehension, yielding, retention, and action.

Social Marketing Theory

Social marketing theory introduces the principles and practices of marketing into social issues, causes, and ideas.[10] It takes the attitudes and needs of the target audience into account in planning programs and campaigns. A social marketer uses research as a basis for segmenting audiences, positioning the offering, and identifying audience needs, wants, expectations, satisfactions, and dissatisfactions. In addition to the offering, social marketing contains other essential elements, such as price strategies, channel strategies, and communications, It embraces classic health promotion models and other behavioral theories and disciplines. Social marketers believe in designing related products and services, making them available when and where consumers are, and using effective channels to promote the wares.

Since health behavior is caused and determined by many factors, education must incorporate different methods and channels to effect change in behaviors.

DEVELOPMENT OF PROGRAMS

The extent of the planning process of a health education program will depend on many factors. For example, a nationwide program will entail more extensive planning than will a program carried out in one community. However, several planning steps should be considered for every program, and a decision should be made on their applicability to each situation.

The Office of Cancer Communications of the National Cancer Institute (NCI) outlines six stages in developing health communications programs.[11]

Stage 1: Planning and Strategy Selection

Careful assessment is made of the problem to determine whether it can be addressed by communication strategies. During this phase, information is gathered and available data are reviewed to identify existing activities and any gaps that must be addressed. Goals and objectives are written to establish what the program will accomplish. Target audiences are defined and described. The direction the program will take and the strategy for reaching the target audiences are planned. Major obstacles and barriers are identified. Resources needed to carry out the strategies are identified. Finally, a program plan and timetable are produced.

Stage 2: Selecting Channels and Materials

In this stage, the decisions made in the planning process are used to select the kinds of materials needed to reach the target audience. An assessment is made about whether existing materials can be used or adapted or whether new materials must be produced. Decisions about how the target audience will be reached (channel to be used) are also made during this stage—whether it will be a face-to-face campaign, one delivered in a classroom or a work site, one using mass media or community groups, or a combination of more than one channel.

Stage 3: Developing Materials and Pretesting

If new materials are to be developed, this stage is essential. Pretesting is used to determine whether materials produced by you or by someone else will be suitable for use with a specific target audience. This stage ensures that all messages in the materials reinforce each other, are based on the strategies determined in stage 2, and are presented in a way that is understandable to the target audience. Both the written material and the illustrations are pretested to be sure they convey the proper response. For example, when NCI tested the term *cancer prevention,* with an apple substituted for the *o* in prevention, respondents failed to link apples to either good health or prevention and thus did not use it.[11]

Stage 4: Implementing the Program

During this stage, the program is introduced to the target audience. The promotion and distribution of the materials is begun. Before starting this stage, it is essential to ensure that all materials are ready in sufficient quantities, that promotion plans are in place, and that the methods of tracking progress (process evaluation) have been developed. The written program plan for this stage will also contain a strategy for informing and working with other organizations involved, as well as information on when resources are needed, when specific events are planned, and ways to identify potential problems. Specific periodic assessments are planned to determine whether some strategies are more successful than others, how the program is operating, whether the target audience is responding, and whether the resources are being used as planned. Written progress reports and modification of program components are important aspects of this stage.

Stage 5: Assessing Effectiveness

Assessment of the program's effectiveness is based on the goals and objectives planned in stage 1 and used throughout the life of the program. This stage determines the outcome or results of the program, that is, whether the target audience learned, acted, or made a change. Outcome evaluation usually consists of a comparison of target audience awareness, attitudes, or behavior before and after the program.

Stage 6: Feedback

Using the information gathered at each stage—about the audience, the messages, the channels of communication, and the program's intended effect—this stage prepares to improve an ongoing program, revise it, or plan a new cycle of program development. It is also a time for sharing what has been learned, such as writing an article, sending materials to a related clearinghouse or agency, or presenting a poster or an abstract at a professional meeting.

It is essential when planning programs to set priorities, developing those programs with the greatest need and the highest opportunity to make an impact. A system needs to be developed that periodically reviews the priorities and revises, deletes or adds to them as needs change. In addition, plans should be made for at least a 3-year period, so that some continuity will be ensured.

BARRIERS TO EDUCATING THE PUBLIC

The National Cancer Institute has defined several barriers to the public's acceptance of health messages.[11]

1. *Health risk is an intangible concept.* Many people underestimate their risk of common health problems, such as cancer, stroke, and diabetes. People believe a serious illness will not happen to them regardless of their actual risk.
2. *The public responds to easy solutions.* People are more likely to respond to simple actions (such as getting a blood test for cholesterol checking) than to a more complicated one (such as quitting smoking).
3. *People want absolute answers.* In the cancer field, there are not many firm answers from scientists.
4. *The public may react unfavorably to fear.* Frightening information may result in denial, hysteria, anxiety, and helplessness, which may be compounded if there are no immediate actions to take.
5. *The public doubts the verity of science.* People may not believe a scientist's prediction.
6. *The public has other priorities.* Many times, daily problems are more important than intangible health information.
7. *The public holds contradictory beliefs.* Even though an individual believes "it can't happen to me," he or she can still believe "everything causes cancer" and can find no need to alter behavior.
8. *The public lacks a future orientation.* Many Americans, especially lower socioeconomic groups, have trouble relating to the idea of changing their behaviors for something that may not happen to them.

It is important to take such barriers into consideration during the various phases of program development. It may be possible to turn barriers into opportunities, thus creating better programs.

OPPORTUNITIES AND CHALLENGES

The NCI, in establishing its Year 2000 goal to achieve a 50% reduction in the 1985 cancer death rate, has set a challenge for concentrated efforts by health organizations, voluntary and professional associations, government agencies, industry, and the media. The Year 2000 goal offers a framework for action and has been further enhanced by the setting of cancer control objectives[12] based on the goal. The prevention objectives center on the reduction of smoking—responsible for some 30% of all cancer deaths—and on diet, which is associated with several cancers, including colorectal cancer, the leading cause of cancer deaths after lung cancer. The screening objectives relate to detecting cervical and breast cancers in asymptomatic women. There are effective screening techniques available for both types of cancers, and women who are diagnosed early have excellent prognoses.

The U.S. Public Health Service has continued its practice of setting out agendas for 10-year periods. Its Health People 2000[13] is an expansion of its 1980 objective-setting document. A statement of national opportunities, this is the product of an effort involving 22 expert working groups, a consortium that has grown to include almost 300 national organizations, and all the state health departments. More than 10,000 people reviewed and commented on the objectives before the final report was published.

The American Cancer Society (ACS) has set its priorities for the decade of the 1990s, along with measures on which it will judge its success in the Year 2000.[14] Its priority setting involved a yearlong process, with thousands of volunteers and staff from across the country participating. The ACS set a narrowed agenda, with three cancer control core programs to be accomplished in each of its 3600 local units: comprehensive school health education, comprehensive year-round tobacco control, and breast cancer detection. It has also developed measures of nationwide success for these core

TABLE 61-1 Selected Cancer Control Objectives to Meet Year 2000 Goals

Action	NCI Year 2000 Goals and Objectives	Selected Objectives from Health People Year 2000 Goals	Selected ACS Measures of Nationwide Success
Prevention			
Smoking	Reduce percentage of adults who smoke from 43% to 15% or less. Reduce percentage of youths who smoke by age 20 from 36% to 15% or less	Reduce cigarette smoking to no more than 15% among people age 20 and older; also, specific objectives for 11 special target populations	Reduce overall cigarette smoking prevalence among adults age 20 and older to 15%; also, specific goals for high school students and specialized adult populations
Diet	Reduce average consumption of fat from 37% or 38% to 30% or less of total calories	Reduce dietary fat intake to an average of 30% of calories or less and average saturated fat intake to less than 10% of calories among people age 2 and older	Increase the proportion of high school students who daily eat no more than two servings of selected food typically high in fat content to 80% from 65%
	Increase average daily consumption of fiber from 8–12 g to 20–30 g	Increase complex-carbohydrate- and fiber-containing foods in the diets of adults to five or more daily servings of vegetables (including legumes) and fruits and to six or more daily servings of grain products	Increase the proportion of high school students who daily consume five or more servings of fruits and vegetables to 35% from 13%
Screening			
Breast	Increase the percentage of women ages 50 to 70 who have an annual physical breast examination coupled with mammography from 45% for physical examination alone and 15% for mammography to 80% for each	Increase to at least 80% the proportion of women age 40 and older who have ever received a clinical breast exam and a mammogram and to at least 60% those age 50 and older who received them within the preceding 1–2 years; additional objectives for ten special target populations	Increase the proportion of women age 40 and older who have ever had a mammogram to 75% from 40%; increase the proportion of women ages 40–49 who have had a mammogram within the past 2 years to 50% from 20%; increase the proportion of women age 50 and older who had a mammogram in the past year to 50% from 15%; increase the proportion of women age 65 and older who had a mammogram in the past year to 35% from 10%
Cervix	Increase the percentage of women who have a Pap smear every 3 years from 70% (ages 20–39) to 90% and from 57% (ages 40–70) to 80%	Increase to at least 95% the proportion of women age 18 and older with uterine cervix who have ever received a Pap test and to at least 85% those who have received a Pap test within the preceding 1–3 years	

Source: Adapted from National Cancer Institute: *Cancer Objectives for the Nation: 1985–2000.* NCI monograph no. 2, appendix B. Bethesda, MD: Division of Cancer Prevention and Control, The Institute, 1986; U.S. Department of Health and Human Services. *Healthy People 2000: National Health Promotion and Disease Prevention Objectives.* Washington, DC: U.S. Public Health Service, 1991, pp. 424–432; and American Cancer Society: *Priorities for the Decade of the 1990s.* Atlanta: The Society, 1991.

programs to serve as a benchmark for measuring progress in addressing the priorities. These objectives form a strong basis for program planning and offer widespread opportunities. Table 61-1 outlines selected prevention and screening objectives from these three institutions.

The Behavior Risk Factor Surveillance Survey (BRFSS), a system now used in 35 states to collect data through telephone surveys, gives comparable data on behavior risk factors such as smoking, dietary habits, and alcohol consumption.[15] It can be used in planning programs, designing marketing strategies, and evaluating trends.

These national programs offer many challenges to health education. A few of the tactics embodied in them will be discussed further: segmenting audiences, reaching the disadvantaged, and using the media as a gatekeeper.

Segmenting Target Audiences

A major challenge in public education is to identify the main audience for particular programs. The most basic way to segment audiences is by age, that is, into adult and child learners. Factors other than age, however, must be taken into account, including sex, education, income level, race and ethnic origin, attitudes, and beliefs. Audience segmentation has become so complex that it encompasses an entire new field of study called *psychographics.*[16]

Need for targeting

The NCI reinforces the need for segmenting audiences to increase the likelihood that the targeted learner is reached by the particular educational program. Several studies on the national level have detailed cancer prevention opportunities as well as the knowledge, attitudes, and behaviors of specific target groups. The NCI outlines several opportunities for health education in cancer prevention:[17]

1. The lung cancer rate for women is rising much faster than that for men and has surpassed the death rate for breast cancer. As a result of smoking, the lung cancer death rate among women, almost 110% greater today than it was in 1973 for women of all ages, has risen by 165% for women over 65.
2. Cigarette smoking among adolescent girls (ages 17–19) is now greater than among boys in the same age group. Young women are starting to smoke at an earlier age (50% before tenth grade). More than 3000 teenagers become regular smokers each day in the United States.[18]
3. Low-income Americans have a higher incidence of cancer as well as lower survival rates. Among low-income groups, many cancers are diagnosed at a later stage, when the cancer has already spread.
4. Since nearly 60% of all cancers occur in Americans age 65 and over, a group that represents only 12% of the U.S. population, this age group is a primary target for early-detection tests.
5. The proportion of women who have ever had a mammogram decreases with age, with only one-fourth of women over 75 having had one. Black and Hispanic women are less likely than white women to have ever had a mammogram.[19]

Using psychographics

Psychographics, sometimes referred to as attitudinal or lifestyle research, segments the United States into neighborhood types, personality types, media users, product and brand buyers, and benefit seekers. Its roots come from sociology, political science, and developmental psychology. Psychographics goes beyond demographics in identifying smaller, more targeted clusters in the population. One branch of psychographics is called *geodemographics.* Based on the theory that people in similar neighborhoods have similar lifestyles, geodemographics divides the country into neighborhoods with specific characteristics.[16] Using these techniques in the cancer field can give information about who the targeted learner is—who is at highest risk and who is most needy of learning about the particular issue—as well as what kind of message to deliver.

Databases are now available to give comprehensive multivariate demographic profiles of U.S. households, including specific information on health care practices. These databases link lifestyle information, consumer survey data, consensus data, media information, and demographics with the health care information. They offer a new vehicle to use in targeting audience segments.

Primary and secondary targets

In segmenting audiences, it may be useful to identify both primary and secondary audiences. A *primary* target audience is one that will be affected in some way by the messages given. A *secondary* target audience is one that has some influence on the primary audience or that must do something to help cause the change in the primary target audience. For instance, women over age 50 may be the primary audience for a mammography education program. Physicians serving this population can be a secondary target audience, to be reminded to refer these women for the screening test.

One of the steps to developing a successful education program is to get to know as much as possible about the target audience and to write as detailed a description as possible. Items that should be delineated include:[11]

- age, sex, ethnic background, area of residence or work
- knowledge, attitudes, and behavior as related to the patterns to be changed
- available health-related services and patterns of use
- media preference and habits
- information sources considered credible by the potential target group

Obtaining information about audiences

There are many sources of demographic information about potential target audiences: census data, reports from chambers of commerce, health departments and health system agencies, economic development agencies, and local hospitals. Advertising agencies, television and radio stations, newspapers, and media guides can provide data on the use of the media and the composition of the media's audiences. Information on the knowledge and attitudes of various groups is available from polling companies, voluntary health agencies, health professional organizations, and universities. Library searches can yield useful data for audience segmentation. As noted earlier, databases are now available that merge much of this information. In addition, databases such as the Combined Health Information Database (CHID) include subfiles related to cancer (Table 61-2).

New data may be needed to pinpoint specific information about the target audience. Focus group interviews are one of the methods often used to provide

TABLE 61-2 Government Agencies as Resources for Cancer Education

Agency	Major Functions/Programs	Special Features
Center for Health Promotion and Education Centers for Disease Control and Prevention Bdg 1 So, Rm SSB249 1600 Clifton Rd,. NE Atlanta, GA 30333 (404) 329-3492	Provides technical assistance to state and local health departments; coordinates Behavior Risk Factor Surveillance Systems (BRFS); implements School Health Education Program (SHED); maintains Health Education Database (HED)	Tracks risk factors in population with BRSF—telephone survey on smoking, alcohol, nutrition; SHED evaluates impact of program on student's health-related behaviors; HED gives on-line computer summary of health education efforts
Clearinghouse for Occupational and Health Information National Institute for Occupational Safety and Health Technical Information Branch 4676 Columbia Pkwy Cincinnati, OH 45226 (513) 684-8326	Provides technical information to institute's research programs; gives information to others on request	
Clearinghouse on Health Indexes National Center For Health Statistics Division of Epidemiology and Health Promotion 3700 East-West Hwy, Rm 157 Hyattsville, MD 20782 (301) 436-8500	Provides informational assistance in development of health measures for researchers, administrators, and planners	
Combined Health Education Information Database Box CHID 9000 Rockville Pike Bethesda, MD 20892	Computerized bibliographic database; includes cancer subjects	
Consumer Information Center General Services Administration Pueblo, CO 81009 (303) 948-3334	Distributes consumer publications on many topics, such as food and nutrition, health, and exercise	Provides *Consumer Information Catalog* from which to order publications
Consumer Product Safety Commission Washington, DC 20207 (301) 492-6800 (800) 638-2772 (hotline)	Sets standards and conducts information programs on potentially hazardous products, such as carcinogens	Independent federal regulatory agency; has jurisdiction over consumer products in and around home
Food and Nutrition Information Center U.S. Department of Agriculture National Agricultural Library Building, Rm 304 Beltsville, MD 20705 (301) 344-3719	Serves information needs of professionals interested in nutrition education, food services, and food technology	Acquires and lends books, journal articles, and audiovisual materials
National Audiovisual Center National Archives 8700 Edgeworth Dr Capitol Heights, MD 20743-3701 (301) 763-1896 (301) 763-4385 TDD)	Distributes more than 8000 programs on over 600 topics, including cancer and environment, cancer detection, smoking, specific cancer sites.	Central source for federally sponsored audiovisuals. Provides free catalogs. Charges for audiovisuals and accompanying materials.
Division of Cancer Prevention and Control National Cancer Institute National Institutes of Health Bethesda, MD 20892-4200 (301) 496-6616	Plans and conducts basic and applied research programs aimed at reducing cancer incidence, morbidity, and mortality; plans, directs, and coordinates the support of basic and applied research on cancer prevention and control at cancer centers and community hospitals; coordinates programs activities with federal and state agencies; establishes liaison with professional and voluntary health agencies, labor organizations, cancer organizations, and trade associations	Activities carried out across five phases of research: hypothesis development, methods testing controlled intervention, trials, defined population studies, and demonstrations relevant to the prevention and management of cancer

(continued)

TABLE 61-2 Government Agencies as Resources for Cancer Education (continued)

Agency	Major Functions/Programs	Special Features
Office of Cancer Communications National Cancer Institute National Institutes of Health Bethesda, MD 20892 (301) 496-6631	Provides information on all aspects of the cancer problem to physicians, scientists, educators, Congress, the executive branch, the media, and the public; fosters and coordinates a national cancer communications program designed to provide the public and health professionals with information they need to take more responsible health actions	The Cancer Information Service (1-800-4-CANCER) is centered at this office, with a network of locations across the country
Office of Prevention, Education and Control National Heart, Lung, and Blood Institute (NHLBI) National Institutes of Health 9000 Rockville Pike Bethesda, MD 20892 (301) 496-5437	Initiates educational activities for NHLBI, which fosters informational and educational activities designed to reduce preventable heart, lung, and blood disease morbidity and mortality	
National Clearinghouse for Alcohol Information National Institute on Alcohol Abuse and Alcoholism P.O. Box 2345 6000 Executive Blvd Rockville, MD 20857 (301) 468-2600	Gathers and disseminates current information on alcohol-related subjects; provides literature searches, referrals, a library and reading room, and summaries of current alcohol-related information	Responds to requests from the public, health professionals, scientists, and other professionals
National Library of Medicine National Institutes of Health 8600 Rockville Pike Bethesda, MD 20892 (301) 496-6308 (Public Information Office) (301) 496-6095 (Reference Station)	Collects, organizes and disseminates both printed and audiovisual materials, technical and scientific in nature, primarily for medical professionals; offers extensive computerized literature retrieval service	Listing of bibliographies, catalogs, and indexes, with specific ordering instructions, is available from the Public Information Office
National Center for Education in Maternal and Child Health National Maternal and Child Health Clearinghouse 38th and R St, NW Washington, DC 20057 (202) 625-8410 (202) 625-8400	Provides information and publications on maternal and child health and genetics, including topics such as smoking and pregnancy and nutrition and pregnancy	Provides materials to consumers and health professionals; free catalog lists materials according to topic
National Toxicology Program National Institute of Environmental Health Sciences M.D. B2-04, Box 12233 Research Triangle Park, NC 27709 (919) 541-3991	Develops and disseminates scientific information regarding potentially hazardous chemicals, including those that can cause cancer; coordinates research conducted by four agencies of the Department of Health and Human Services	Information in the form of technical reports is available free of charge to scientists and other health professionals
Office of Consumer Affairs Food and Drug Administration 5600 Fishers Lane Rockville, MD 20857 (301) 443-3170	Responds to consumer inquiries; serves as clearinghouse for consumer publications on a variety of topics, including pregnancy, food and nutrition, cosmetics, proper use of drugs, and health fraud	Over 250 publications available free of charge
National Rehabilitation Information Center 8455 Colesville Rd, Ste 935 Silver Spring, MD 20910-3319 (800) 346-2712 (301) 588-9284	Information and referral center and biographic database producer on rehabilitation, disabilities, and related issues	Over 33,000 abstracts on federally funded research, journal articles, and audiovisual materials

(continued)

TABLE 61-2 Government Agencies as Resources for Cancer Education (continued)

Agency	Major Functions/Programs	Special Features
National Health Information Clearinghouse Office of Disease Prevention and Health Promotion P.O. Box 1133 Washington, DC 20013-1133 (800) 336-4797 (202) 429-9091	Central source of information and referral for health questions from the public and health professionals; maintains computer database of government agencies, support groups, professional societies, and other organizations that can answer questions on specific health topics; offers library containing medical and health reference books, directories, information files, and periodicals; database development on organizations that provide health information; and a number of publications including resource guides and bibliographies	Among publications prepared are Prevention Abstracts, which summarize prevention-oriented findings in the scientific literature; Prevention Activities Calendar, which highlights major prevention events for the month; Healthfinder Series, which provides resource lists on specific health topics such as exercise for older Americans, health risk appraisals, health statistics, among many other issues; *Staying Healthy: A Bibliography of Health Promotion Materials,* which serves as a guide to current information on health promotion and disease prevention topics
Office on Smoking and Health U.S. Department of Health and Human Services National Center for Chronic Disease, Prevention and Health Promotion Mail Stop K-J0 1600 Clifton Rd, NE Atlanta, GA 30333 (404) 488-5705	Produces and distributes a number of informational and educational materials; offers bibliography and reference services to researchers and others; produces pamphlets, posters, and public service announcements containing various health messages	Materials and services are available free of charge
Public Information Center Environmental Protection Agency 820 Quincy St, NW Washington, DC 20210 (202) 829-3535	Provides information on programs and activities of the Environmental Protection Agency, including topics such as hazardous wastes, the school asbestos project, air and water pollution, pesticides, and drinking water	
Publication Distribution Office Occupational Safety and Health Administration U.S. Department of Labor 200 Constitution Ave, NW, Rm s4203 Washington, DC 20210 (202) 523-9667	Responds to inquiries about a limited number of job-related carcinogens and toxic substances	Single copies of materials available free to general public, health professionals, industry, educational institutions, and other sources
Information Office National Institute on Aging Federal Building, 6th Fl 9000 Rockville Pike Bethesda, MD 20892 (301) 496-1752	Distributes information for older Americans on many topics, including cancer and smoking	
Office of Minority Health Resource P.O. Box 37337 Washington, DC 20013-7337 (800) 444-MHRC (6472)	Provides minority health information and referrals; maintains computerized database of materials, organizations, and programs; provides network of professionals active in the field	Provides bilingually staffed, toll-free number.

Source: Adapted from National Cancer Institute: *Making Health Communications Programs Work: A Planner's Guide.* NIH pub. no. 92-1493. Bethesda, MD: Office of Cancer Communications, The Institute, 1992.

insight into the beliefs, perceptions, and feelings among a particular group of people. Usually consisting of 12–14 persons, a focus group is good for stimulating discussion of issues and for gathering opinions in a short time. However, it is not a representative sample of target populations, usually has too few participants for consensus or decision making, and depends greatly on a skilled moderator. Focus groups can be especially useful before production for testing materials in the areas of appropriate language, a message's appeal, or a particular spokesperson's appeal to a specified target population. For instance, the NCI, in planning a major national survey on public knowledge and attitudes surrounding breast cancer, conducted separate focus groups with white, black, and Hispanic men and women to help develop the wording for specific questions. Focus groups can also be used (1) to clarify the results of survey research (especially if the results are different from those expected), (2) to generate hypotheses, or (3) to give depth to feelings about health-related issues.

Personal interviews, either by mail, by telephone, or at home, are another method to gather vital data, but they are more expensive. If the questions that need answering are few, it may be possible to add them to an ongoing survey (such as polls that are conducted by newspapers or other enterprises to determine consumer attitudes). Mailed questionnaires are a relatively inexpensive way to reach large numbers of people. However, response rates can be low, respondents may not be representative of the whole sample, and only minimal information could result. Telephone interviews generally give a higher response rate but may limit the questionnaire length. Interviews in the home, although they may give the most information, also cost the most.

Whatever the method used, it is worth the time to identify the people who are most important to reach so that pertinent messages can be developed and communication channels established. In this process, decisions can be made about audiences that will not be targeted, ensuring that the available resources will be used in the most cost-effective manner.

Reaching the Disadvantaged

In 1987 and 1988, the NCI's National Advisory Board sponsored public hearings in Los Angeles, Atlanta, Miami, Dallas, and Philadelphia. As a result of these hearings, the board recommended intensified efforts to provide caller-information, prevention, and early-detection programs to special population groups for whom a combination of economic disadvantage and indigenous cultural factors impedes access to the health care system.[20] Disproportionately high cancer rates are found in minority groups and are theorized by experts as being heavily influenced by lifestyle risk factors, such as tobacco, alcohol, a diet high in fat and low in fiber, occupational risks, and patterns of care related to early detection, diagnosis, and treatment. Many of these issues are also associated with socioeconomic status, as represented by income and education. Many of the racial and ethnic minority groups in the United States have disproportionately large numbers of their members living in poverty, with low educational attainment and higher unemployment rates than the majority.[17] Thus, although racial and ethnic origins and economic status are two distinct variables, they combine to create an adverse impact on the risk of developing cancers for these populations. Groups included in the NCI special population category are the poor, older Americans, blacks, Hispanics, Asian Americans, and Native Americans.

Serious cancer problems have been defined in the disadvantaged populations.[17] For instance, black Americans have a 10% greater risk of developing cancer, a 5-year survival rate that is 30% lower than the general population's, and a mortality rate that is 30% higher than that for whites. Blacks experience higher incidence and mortality rates for cancers of the cervix, esophagus, oral cavity, lung, pancreas, prostate, and stomach. Hispanics have lower survival rates for all cancer sites combined and for cancers of the breast, corpus uteri, and prostate as compared to whites. There is also evidence of a relationship between low socioeconomic level and cancer incidence. For example, women of lower socioeconomic status are less likely to have regular examinations, such as Papanicolaou (Pap) tests for cervical cancer.[19] Black and Hispanic women are less likely than white women to have ever had a Pap test. Incidence rates for cervical cancer are higher among black, Hispanic, and Native American women than among white women.[19]

Other issues related to ethnic minorities create special requirements for cancer prevention information. On the average, blacks are less aware of cancer signs, available treatment options, and early-detection techniques and their importance than whites.[21] Both blacks and Hispanics underestimate the prevalence of cancer and have a fatalistic attitude about the disease.[22]

There are several strategies for implementing health education programs in communities where the socioeconomically disadvantaged live and work. It is useful, especially in the early planning stages, to make a list of leaders who can provide information about and access to the community. The list should include those who are respected and have personal contacts with the specific audience to be reached. The influentials can include any of the following categories:[8] church leaders, leaders in the school system, merchants and other members of the business community, members of the media, health care providers, government and civic leaders, officers of fraternal orders, and leaders in teenage communities. The influential leaders can help identify the needs of the community and assist with education programs where people live, work, and play.

Social service and health organizations are an important point of entry into these communities. A program's success can be increased by coordinating with these trusted and respected organizations and working through their existing programs. Creating special health events that address the concerns of the audience and adding them to established neighborhood-based efforts can also help ensure success.

Addressing cultural characteristics

Health education programs must take into consideration the many socioeconomic and cultural characteristics among minorities. The following considerations must be addressed during the development stage to ensure successful programs for reaching the socioeconomically disadvantaged audiences.

1. *The family.* The family is a dominant influence on many minority populations and can be a credible source of health-related information. On the other hand, depending on factors such as the disease being discussed and the type of program being planned, the family can also be a major barrier. For instance, in the Native American population, tribal elders may need to be used as role models to ensure program success.

2. *The community.* Many minority groups, especially those that have recently come to this country, strongly identify with neighborhood and community groups. In rural areas and in some urban neighborhoods, the community acts as an extension of the family and becomes the focus of social interaction. There may be a distinct microculture, such as a religious society, within a community, Knowing the community structure is essential. It can open up different locations for presenting health education messages—such as in churches, barber shops, libraries, malls, gyms, and bodegas (stores in Hispanic neighborhoods).

3. *The language.* Language may be a barrier, especially in areas where new settlers to the country are located. It is crucial, when producing materials in a different language, to involve persons who understand the nuances of the particular language. In some communities, language can be a major obstacle to conducting successful health education programming, and extra time and planning will be needed to ensure success.

4. *Folk beliefs and traditions.* Some minorities have strong beliefs and traditions in folk medicines, depending on cultural mores. Programming may need to incorporate these beliefs and traditions to enhance messages or at least to determine their potential impact.

5. *The influence of poverty.* Some people living in poverty develop a sense of powerlessness, a loss of control over the outcomes of day-to-day living. Self-esteem may be lost, along with the hope for a better life. In addition, some may have a short-term perspective on living. The day-to-day stresses of crime and drugs, of foraging for meals and an existence, make issues like cancer risk seem unimportant. These influences create serious obstacles to programming for health education on issues such as cancer prevention and behavioral change.

Reaching the Elderly

The elderly population provides different challenges and obstacles to anyone presenting health education messages. These individuals have beliefs and attitudes acquired over a lifetime that may significantly influence their health practices.

A study conducted at Fox Chase Cancer Center[23] showed that most of the older people surveyed did not realize they are at increased risk for cancer. In addition, more than 50% of the older people surveyed believed cancer treatments are worse than the disease and had negative attitudes about physicians (80% thought that physicians cause patients to worry because they do not explain everything). In general, older persons usually are not as aware of their risk of developing cancer, are less likely to participate in screening programs, and are less likely to practice self-examination. The elderly also are more apt to underreport significant symptoms and thus present to the health care system with more advanced disease. This may be due to the fact that aches and pains are seen as more normal occurrences among the elderly and are taken for granted rather than viewed as potential symptoms of disease.

Dellefield[24] defines several topics that must be addressed in educating older persons: (1) the increased risk of developing cancer with advancing age, (2) the seven warning signals of cancer, (3) normal versus abnormal changes of aging, (4) the health maintenance practices recommended by the ACS, (5) the benefits of early detection in relation to reduced morbidity and mortality, (6) the acceptability and management of cancer treatments, (7) the skills and coping strategies needed to make the elderly more successful as patients in the contemporary health care system, and (8) the community resources available to provide early-detection services and assistance in developing better self-care skills.

On average, the elderly do not learn as quickly and as easily as do younger persons. They may not see and hear as well. They may have had many negative lifetime experiences with cancer and cancer treatment. In preparing materials and in presenting programs to this target group, special attention must be paid to specific strategies to overcome these barriers. Self-paced learning may be a useful strategy for this population.

Socializing and social atmospheres are attractive to this target population. Taking advantage of already existing meetings, such as senior citizen groups, may add to a program's success. Using positive, wellness-related tactics is another strategy. A gastroenterologist in Connecticut found that entitling his program "The Care and Feeding of Your Digestive Tract" rather than "Cancer of the Colon" increased his audiences twofold. Older Americans are an important group to target. They present special problems and have distinct barriers that must be overcome if programming is to be successful. Table 61-3 summarizes the strategies for reaching special audiences.

Specific Barriers to Getting Mammography and Pap Test Among Special Populations

A recent study completed for the U.S. Centers for Disease Control and Prevention[19] reviewed 318 articles published from 1986 to 1991 on studies and programs related to breast and cervical screening and compiled a series of profiles on barriers to and use of mammography and Pap screening among several populations:

TABLE 61-3 Reaching Special Audiences

Production of Materials	Strategies for Older Learners	Strategies for Lower Socioeconomic Groups
Use language appropriate to different cultural groups (one word may have different meanings to different groups).	Keep learning sessions brief (10–15 min), and pace instructions.	Work through existing programs and agencies.
Understand values and customs for each cultural group.	Avoid rushing the learner.	Work through people already trusted in the community.
Identify channels that will be credible and most capable of reaching the different minority audiences.	Proceed from the simple to the complex.	Try to create programs incorporating agency's objectives into already-ongoing programs.
Use current information to choose the best channels and message strategies.	Focus and maintain attention on a single, well-defined piece of information.	Use concern for family as a motivator.
Develop separate message appeals for each different group, since perceived needs,values, and beliefs may differ.	Use concrete examples, short sentences, slow speech, and abundant repetition.	Stress payoffs for changing attitudes or beliefs.
Use simply written print materials, reinforced with graphics and pretested.	Use redundant or multiple cuing. Say it, draw it, write it.	Create simple, concrete messages.
Pretest both print materials and graphics; people perceive graphics and illustrations in different ways, just as words have different meanings.	Allow the initial learning task to proceed slowly.	Use visual materials—people learn more by seeing than by any other method.
Use bilingual materials to ensure that intermediaries and family members who are not comfortable with English can help readers understand content.	Do not present new information until earlier concepts have been mastered.	Use both visual and written materials to reinforce messages.
Do not simply translate print materials from the English; rewrite the material, since concepts and appeals may differ by culture just as the words do.	Allow ample time for learning tasks involving psychomotor skills.	Repeat the same message and some themes.
Consider audiovisual materials or interpersonal communication that may be more successful for certain messages and audiences.	Deemphasize tasks involving abstract reasoning.	Use television as a primary channel.
	Minimize the number of alternative responses available.	Use personalized, direct mail messages.
	Compensate for sensory changes by using nonglare lighting, large print, mid- to low-pitched speaking voice, and a quiet environment.	
	Reinforce learning with social support.	
	Provide positive feedback to make learner aware of progress.	
	Express warmth and respect.	

Source: Adapted from National Cancer Institute: *Making Health Communications Programs Work: A Planner's Guide,* NIH pub. no. 92-1493. Bethesda, MD: Office of Cancer Communications, The Institute, 1992; and Dellefield MD: Informational needs and approaches for early cancer detection in the elderly. *Semin Oncol Nurs* 7:156–168, 1992.

the female population as a whole; low-income black, Hispanic, and white women; older women; and middle- and upper-income women. The study concluded that the two major barriers causing underuse of mammography are: an absence of physician referrals, and a lack of perception that going without mammography involves risk. The strong influence of physicians is found across age, income, race, and education, and matters to women getting first-time mammograms as well as those getting repeat mammograms. Although women understand that early detection is beneficial, they perceive mammograms not as something they themselves need but rather as a service needed by other women. Cost is also a barrier for some women, though not as much as physician referral and perception of risk. Half the women in a national survey reported they would not pay $150 a year for mammograms, and nearly 40% reported they thought mammograms cost too much. Table 61-4 summarizes tactics to be used in overcoming the barriers found in this study.[19]

Low Literacy and Readability

One of the major problems facing those producing printed health communications materials is how to make them easy to read. About 20% of the adult American population reads at or below the fifth-grade level. An additional 35% reads at the fifth- to tenth-grade level.[25] Many high school graduates can be expected to read only at a seventh- to eighth-grade level.

In general, the problem of low literacy is more widespread in minority groups and in the elderly. There is also a relationship between level of education and in-

TABLE 61-4 Planning Programs on Breast and Cervical Cancer for Selected Audiences

Audience	Mammography	Pap Tests
Female population as a whole	• Use physicians as primary channels. Use media both for education as well as for publicizing screening sites. • Emphasize that all women are at risk. • Continually assess barriers to detect changes; for instance, cost may become a more significant barrier as more women get regular mammograms. • Make getting mammograms easier by providing low-cost screening at fixed or mobile sites.	• Emphasize awareness of individual risk and need for regular tests; address fears. • Provide supplementary community screening services as well as physician screening. • Assess barriers and customary uses of medical care among specific audiences. • Use multiple strategies to reach women with abnormal smears. • Provide clear guidelines for frequency of testing in public messages.
Low-income black women	• Use physician or health care giver as one of primary channels. • Deal with fear of pain and cost barriers.	• Highlight the prevention of cervical cancer as means of ensuring woman's continuing ability to care for her family. • Use television and radio as primary channels.
Low-income Hispanic women	• Spanish-speaking health professionals with cultural sensitivity are high priority. Understand value of polite agreement and probe beyond it. • Tailor messages to specific local populations, taking into account dialect, idioms, national origins, etc. Television messages in Spanish are preferable. • Use brief guidelines, written in simple Spanish. Repeat messages orally and in writting.	
	• Use radiologists and technologists to educate patients in screening guidelines and importance of regular mammography.	• Include male partners as decision makers in counseling and education regarding disease transmission, thereby invoking the traditional male role as protector.
	• Convenient access and transportation make a difference.	
Low-income white women	• Encourage physicians to provide mammography information when conducting clinical breast exams. Stress importance of physician encouragement. • Use radiologists and technologists to educate patients, particularly about screening guidelines and importance of mammography. Repeat information. • Design brochures to reach women with low literacy skills. Train personnel to recognize and assist patients who have difficulty reading or completing forms. • Train peers as educators for informing women about the risks of breast cancer and value of mammography.	
Older women	• Encourage physicians to use clinical opportunities, such as breast physicals, to recommend mammograms and educate patients about benefits of breast screening.	• Encourage physicians to use clinical opportunities to recommend Pap tests and to educate patients about the benefits of cervical cancer screening.

Source: Adapted from AMC Cancer Research Center: *Breast and Cervical Screening: Barriers and Use Among Specific Audiences.* Atlanta: U.S. Centers for Disease Control, 1992.

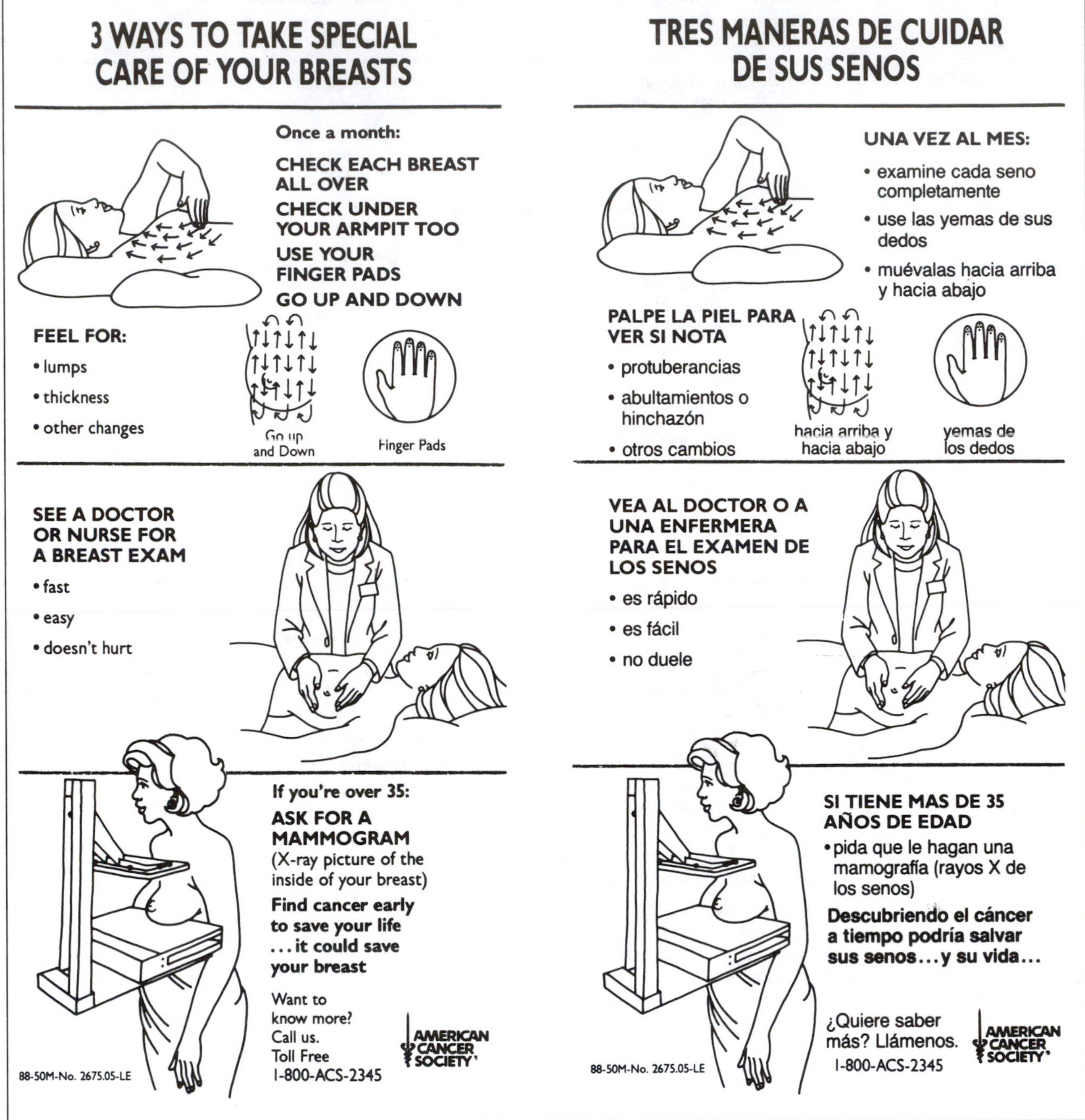

FIGURE 61-1 The American Cancer Society has published a series of educational cards, with English on one side and Spanish on the other, written at the fifth-grade level. (Source: American Cancer Society: *Three Ways to Take Special Care of Your Breasts.* Pub. no. 88-2675.05-LE. Atlanta: The Society, 1988.)

come and health-related behaviors. For instance, women over 39 with less than a high school education are about half as likely to have a mammogram as those with some college; those with family incomes of $35,000 or more are twice as likely to have ever had a mammogram as compared to women with family incomes of less than $10,000.[19]

Most printed materials being used for cancer prevention and early detection are written at levels that many segments of the population cannot understand. For instance, the NCI pamphlet "Good News for Blacks About Cancer" is written at the seventh-grade level. The ACS pamphlet "Fry Now, Pay Later," about skin cancer, is written at the eleventh-grade level. A *Readers Digest* article called "Why Can't We Get the Medicine We Need?" tests at the fourteenth-grade level. In the area of patient information, there is also a wide gap between the readability level of commonly used health-teaching materials and patients' reading comprehension skills. Much of the material is written at tenth-grade level. Average patients have word recognition skills at about the seventh-grade level, although they state that they are high school graduates.[25]

Both the NCI and the ACS are developing more materials in easy-to read language and are testing alternatives to traditional printed materials in order to communicate cancer information to people who have difficulty reading. A series of simple, one-page cards on each of the major cancer sites has been produced by the ACS (Figure 61-1),[26] with the message in English on one side and in Spanish on the other. These have a fourth- to fifth-grade readability level. The NCI has pretested and produced a series of fact sheets, with simple messages and practical guidelines, as well as pamphlets geared to low-literacy audiences (Figure 61-2).[27]

Performing readability tests

Readability testing measures the approximate level of education needed to understand printed materials.

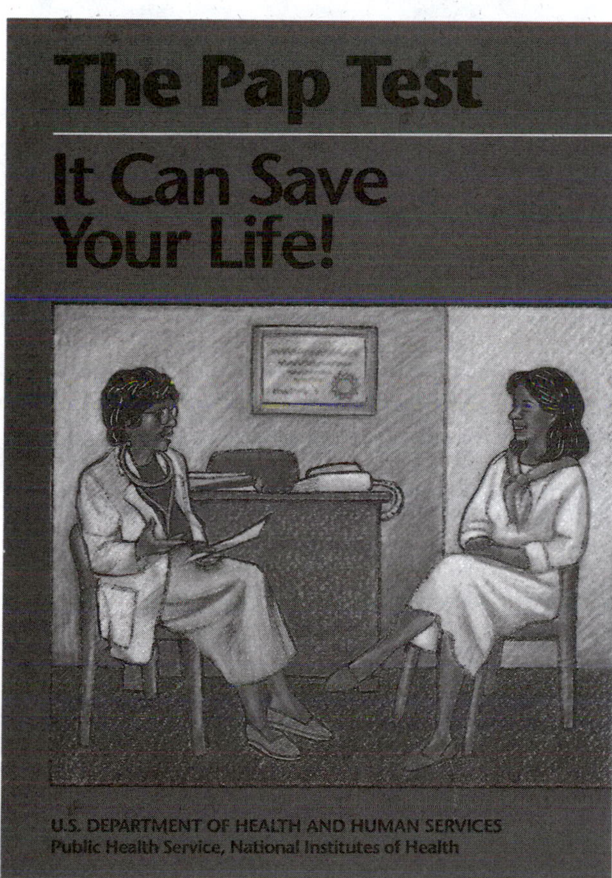

FIGURE 61-2 An NCI pamphlet on Pap tests, written for a low-literacy audience. (Source: National Cancer Institute: *The Pap Test: It Can Save Your Life*. NIH pub. no. 91-3212. Bethesda, MD: The Institute, 1991.)

Most of the formulas used to test how readable an item is take into account the difficulty of the words being used and the length of sentences. Short sentences and words of two syllables or fewer make materials easier to read. Adding illustrations alone will not automatically lower readability level; the text itself must be altered.

Several computer software packages now include readability testing as part of their writing packages (Grammatik^M, RightWriter®). Depending on the version used, the software gives the educational level, average sentence length, tense of verb, and length of words. It can aid in making changes by calling attention to grammar and style problems.

The Office of Cancer Communications of the NCI reviewed 12 readability formulas and chose the SMOG grading system for testing its own materials because it is both easy to use and accurate. Here is how the SMOG system is used:

1. Pick ten consecutive sentences near the beginning, in the middle, and at the end of the material (30 sentences total).
2. Count the words that have three or more syllables, including repeats of those words.
3. Using the following conversion numbers listed, find the approximate grade level that a person must have reached to understand fully the text being examined (the grade will be ±1.5 grades).

Word count	*Grade level*
0–2	4
3–6	5
7–12	6
13–20	7
21–30	8
31–42	9
43–56	10
57–72	11
73–90	12
91–110	13
111–132	14
133–156	15
157–182	16
183–210	17
211–240	18

Guidelines for producing simpler material

To produce materials that will be understandable to a general audience, use the following guidelines:

- Pick short words—two syllables or fewer.
- Create short sentences; this makes you write more simply.
- Use short paragraphs—limit each paragraph to one idea.
- Pick simple language.

- Write to one person, using action verbs and a conversational style.
- Use the same words to describe an item. For instance, do not say *cancer* one time and *tumor* the next.
- Use examples to illustrate important points.
- Do not use abbreviations.
- Repeat the same information in several ways: Write it, show a picture or sketch of it, make a chart out of it.
- Use subheads to tell the reader what is coming.
- Break up the text with graphics at key points, using boldface type, bullets, underlining, or boxed text.
- Summarize at the end of major points.
- Do a readability test; if the level is too high, go back and try again.

THE MEDIA AS GATEKEEPER

The media are an essential part of many programs for communicating with and educating the public. The mass media, which include radio, television, wire service, newspapers, and magazines, can also involve other channels, such as direct mail, billboards, and transit cards. Mass media transmit information quickly to a broad audience and are probably the public's main source of information. The media play an important role for some target audiences, since the average American has a television set turned on for almost 7 hours a day and individual family members watch television approximately 3 hours each. In addition, many Americans read a newspaper daily.

Drawbacks of Mass Media

Mass media have several drawbacks when used for public education about cancer: (1) their main purpose is to inform and entertain rather than to educate, (2) they are difficult to use for transmitting complex messages, (3) they have major constraints of space and time, and (4) they carry a high risk of miscommunication, particularly if the material is controversial (Table 61-5).

Public service announcements (PSAs), which the mass media will carry for free for nonprofit organizations, are often thought of as the major use of the mass media for public education purposes. Since deregulation, however, television and radio stations are no longer required to donate a specific amount of time to public service programming, and the number of PSAs being carried has diminished. Although well-planned and well-produced PSAs can be effective, many other opportunities exist in the mass media, such as news programs, public affairs programs, interview and talk shows, local television panel discussions, call-in programs, editorials, letters to the editors, and health and political columns.

There are professionals in the media ("media gatekeepers") who decide what material will be used and when it will be used. It is their responsibility to understand what the public wants. If the health information messages or programming do not fit into the gatekeepers' needs, they will not be used or they will be used at odd hours or, in the case of print media, will be placed in nonprominent positions. It is a challenge to produce materials that are appealing to media formats and relevant to media needs as well as to target audiences.

Beliefs Among Gatekeepers

Stuyck and Chilton[28] conducted a study to examine the role of mass media gatekeepers in disseminating cancer information. The study gathered information on the beliefs among gatekeepers of the major health problems, the perception of their roles, and their opinions on materials they received for cancer information. The following are observations and recommendations based on the information gained from the study.

1. Disease mortality and morbidity in themselves do not guarantee media interest. Cancer and acquired immune deficiency syndrome (AIDS) ranked highest as important health care issues. Cardiovascular disease was ranked by less than half to be among the three major health concerns (although heart disease annually kills more than twice as many Americans as does cancer). There was little correlation between the prevalence or impact of disease and related problems and their relative rank among health issues.

2. Health professionals should be armed with information before approaching the media. Most gatekeepers feel a responsibility to educate the public but consider themselves trained to report and write, and they expect health educators to be informed about the issues and about the needs of the media.

3. Health communicators should be aggressive if they wish to achieve results. In the Stuyck and Chilton survey[28] there was a correlation between how often the gatekeepers were contacted by persons in the cancer field and how often they covered cancer news. Since the gatekeepers did not consider reporting cancer news as a top priority for their media, health communicators must be knowledgeable and active advocates for their causes.

4. The media are more likely to pay attention to information from sources they perceive to be credible. Among seven factors with the potential for influencing news coverage, the credibility of the news source was ranked highest, significantly above others, such as management interests and audience or readership surveys. Gatekeepers also said they were most likely to cover a

TABLE 61-5 Characteristics of Mass Media Channels

	Television	Radio	Magazines	Newspapers
Audiences	Potentially largest/widest range of audiences, but not always at times when public service announcements (PSAs) are most likely to be broadcast Can reach low-income and other audiences not likely to turn to health sources for help	Various formats offer potential for more audience targeting than television (eg, teenagers through rock stations); may reach fewer people than television Can reach black and other audiences that do not use the health care system	Can target more specific segments of the public (eg, young women, people with an interest in health) Audience has chance to clip, reread, contemplate material	Can reach broad audiences rapidly Easy audience access to in-depth issue coverage is possible
Availability of public service announcements (PSAs)	Deregulation ended government oversight of station broadcast of PSAs, public affairs programming	Deregulation ended government oversight of station broadcast of PSAs, public affairs programming	No requirement for PSA use; PSAs more difficult to place	PSAs virtually nonexistent
Special opportunities	Opportunity to include health messages through broadcasts, public affairs/interview shows, dramatic programming	Opportunity for direct audience involvement through call-in shows	Can explain more complex health issues, behaviors	Can convey health news/breakthrough more thoroughly than television or radio and faster than magazines; feature placement possible
Visual and audio appeals	Visual as well as audio make emotional appeals possible; easier to demonstrate a behavior	Audio alone can make messages less intrusive	Visual effects can be intensified	Print can lend itself to more factual, detailed, rational message delivery
Convenience	Passive consumption by viewer; viewers must be present when message aired; less than full attention likely; message may be obscured by commercial "clutter"	Generally passive consumption; exchange with audience possible, but target audience must be there when aired	Permits active consultation; may pass along to others; read at reader's convenience	Short life of newspaper limits rereading, sharing with others
Flexibility	PSAs can be expensive to produce and distribute; feature placement requires contacts and may be time-consuming	Live copy is very flexible and inexpensive; PSAs must fit station format; feature placement requires contacts and may be time-consuming	PSAs are inexpensive to produce; ad or article placement may be time-consuming	Small papers may take public service ads; coverage demands a newsworthy item

Source: National Cancer Institute: *Making Health Communications Programs Work: A Planner's Guide.* NIH pub. no. 92-1493. Bethesda, MD: Office of Cancer Communications, The Institute, 1992.

news story from an institution with a reputation in the cancer field.

5. Media gatekeepers want information they consider useful to their audiences. Gatekeepers showed great interest in helping their audiences become informed consumers in the area of cancer, especially in advances in cancer treatment and risk reduction (tobacco and nutrition).

6. Media gatekeepers want information that is clearly written and brief. The main reason for not using materials sent to them by health professionals were: inappropriate format (43%), lack of space or time (28%), uninteresting material (18%). Complicated terminology and inability of physicians and scientists to discuss findings in simple language were also cited. Ways in which the information could be improved include tailoring the information to local audiences (29%), making information more concise (18%) or simple and clear (13%), and sending information on a regular basis (8%). Gatekeepers from all types of media were interested in receiving materials they perceived as relevant to their audiences and of help in doing their jobs.

This study emphasizes the importance of looking at material being produced and disseminated through the eyes of the people who control its use, be they news directors or public service directors at radio and television stations or medical reporters, science writers, lifestyle editors, or journalists in the print media.

EXAMPLES OF PUBLIC EDUCATION ACTIVITIES

If one were to consider all the activities that educate and inform the public about health in the media and in community sites of various descriptions around the country, they would number in the thousands per month. In the government arena alone, some 20 agencies directly offer information related to cancer prevention and detection (see Table 61-2). The activities range from a simple talk before a woman's group to complete curricula proposed for school systems in entire states, from an 8-second mention on a local television news program to the organization of a national 1-day event such as the Great American Smokeout. The evaluation of these programs also varies widely—from none at all to highly sophisticated. Two major activities have been selected and will be considered in this section—smoking-related programs and the Cancer Information Service.

Helping People to Stop Smoking

There have been programs in the United States to help people to stop smoking since the 1950s. Although more than 40 million Americans have stopped smoking since the first surgeon general's report on smoking and health in 1964, over 50 million Americans continue to smoke and last year consumed some 533 billion cigarettes.[29] There are more heavy smokers today than ever before.[17] To help these people quit and to reach the national Year 2000 goal will require a major effort by all the health groups in the country. It will also require knowledge of the most effective intervention strategies and widespread implementation of these strategies.

The NCI commissioned a comprehensive review and evaluation of smoking cessation methods in the United States and Canada for the years 1978–1985, as an update to a review carried out under the auspices of the Centers for Disease Control (CDC) for the years 1969–1977 (an earlier review of smoking control methods was support by the National Clearinghouse for Smoking and Health and published in 1969). The conclusions of this review are follows.[30]

1. Smokers prefer to quit on their own with the help of instructions, medicines, and guides. Less complex quit guides achieve higher success rates. Of people who select to quit on their own, 16%–20% are not smoking 1 year later. These data are supported by national studies that show that of those who try to quit, 20% report that they succeed. Self-quitting seems to involve cumulative learning over repeated efforts.

2. Many people who quit act on the advice or warning of a health professional. Physician advice and counseling encourage many individuals to attempt to break their cigarette habit. Where the physician adds a stronger message, gives tips on how to quit, or provides follow-up support, the results improve.

3. The nurse is an ideal person to counsel smokers, since the nurse is viewed as a credible health worker. The nurse involves the patient's family in the counseling process so that family members can provide support and encouragement.

4. The roles of other health professionals, such as dentists, dental hygienists, physician's assistants, nurse practitioners, inhalation therapists, paramedics, and pharmacists, have not been studied adequately in terms of their effects on influencing patients to quit smoking.

5. Nicotine chewing gum (Nicorette) can be an effective tool for persons who are motivated to quit. Longer use (6 months to 1 year) appears to improve quit rates. Other methods (counseling, support) should be used to supplement the gum.

6. Hypnosis and acupuncture are popular treatments, but evaluation has been inadequate. In general, counseling and support also are needed.

7. The media reaches a wide number of smokers with instructions on how to quit smoking. Long-term quit rates are low, but these programs could be more effective if combined with group or individual instructions. Use of the telephone to promote maintenance support is noteworthy.

8. Community studies have mixed results but suggest that a combination of mass media and intensive instruction is more successful than media alone.

9. Behavioral techniques reveal a wide range of success. Adversive therapy (e.g., electric shock, breath holding, unpleasant taste) showed poor results. Rapid smoking appears to be effective in the short term. Covert sensitization (use of subject's imagination) has failed to produce long-term results but, like rapid smoking, may be useful combined with other procedures.

10. The work site offers an excellent opportunity for implementing strategies that lead to cessation of smoking. There is a growing movement to restrict smoking in employee work areas. Some companies offer smoking cessation programs, such as educational programs, distribution of self-help kits, and physician advice during physical examinations and groups.

11. Maintenance support is the critical ingredient in the long-term success of smoking cessation. Successful quitters score higher than recidivists in personal security, ease of quitting on last attempt, expectation of success in giving up smoking, and social support. They had smoked fewer cigarettes the day before quitting and had lower levels of anxiety.

12. Leading causes of relapse are anxiety, stress, anger, frustration, social pressures, weight gain, and lack of inner resources. Being around other smokers, eating, and drinking alcohol or coffee also contribute to relapse.

13. The highest median quit rates for trials with 1-year follow-up were scored by physician intervention programs for patients with cardiac disease (these patients are highly motivated due to life-threatening illness). High quit rates were also scored by physician intervention with patients with pulmonary disorders, risk factor studies, and rapid smoking and satiation when each was combined with other procedures. Support groups and nicotine chewing gum, combined with behavioral treatment or therapy, came next.

14. A significant trend is the public's increased negative attitude toward cigarette smoking, as exemplified by the numerous regulations for nonsmoking sections in schools, restaurants, work sites, military areas, and other public places.

Smoking, Tobacco, and Cancer Program (STCP)

In 1982, the NCI launched an intervention research effort, the Smoking, Tobacco, and Cancer Program (STCP), the focal point for NCI's disease prevention and health promotion research activities related to tobacco use and cancer.[29] The primary thrust of the STCP is the development of intervention activities to reduce the incidence and/or prevalence of smoking and tobacco use. It includes research to determine the best intervention strategies to reduce smoking and tobacco use and research on dissemination methods to implement these strategies efficiently, particularly on a wide-scale population basis in order to achieve a broad public health impact. Also included is research that focuses on identifying and intervening with target populations in which the greatest tobacco-related cancer prevention and control gains can be expected.

The first set of large-scale community initiatives, Community Intervention Trial for Smoking Cessation (COMMIT) was launched by the STCP in 1984; the results are providing the rationale for the next step in the strategic plan—the American Stop Smoking Intervention Study for Cancer Prevention (ASSIST).

COMMIT trials

The COMMIT trials were conducted in several areas: adolescent tobacco use prevention; the use of the mass media; physician, dentist, and self-help/minimal interventions; smokeless tobacco use; and black, Hispanic, and women smokers. Some of the intervention trials have been completed; others are still under way. The published results of the trials[29] provide an invaluable tool for anyone working on public education programs. They cover the methods tested, the channels involved, key elements and materials used, factors influencing the effectiveness of programs, program results, and additional research needs.

In the area of self-help/minimal interventions, for instance, the results of 13 trials found

> little need to devote resources to changing or improving existing materials and programs. Rather, efforts need to be concentrated on using existing cessation approaches and materials more effectively, particularly in motivating far greater numbers of smokers to make serious attempts to stop. The most effective self-help intervention strategies do the following: (a) motivate more smokers to stop; (b) include a variety of program delivery modes; (c) target programs to smoking cessation stages and specific populations; (d) include content on basic smoking information and cessation/maintenance exercise; (e) make programs widely available; and (f) use adjunctive activities and procedures.[30]

The data from these and more than 100 controlled intervention trials sponsored by the NCI during the 1980s have been used to formulate a national smoking strategy.

The program has provided strategies that can be used by nurses, as well as physicians and dentists, to help patients change their smoking habits. The NCI has developed a nationwide training program for health professionals that teaches them brief intervention techniques for smoking cessation.

National smoking strategy

The national strategy recognizes that no single approach is best for all individuals, that no one intervention channel is capable of effectively reaching all smokers, and that no single time is best for individual smokers to attempt to quit. Persistent and inescapable messages to quit (or not to start smoking) need to be coupled with continuously available support for individual cessation attempts, and all need to be provided through multiple channels and reinforced by environmental incentives for nonsmokers.

The STCP research has shown that different programs have impact on different points in the press of initiation, maintenance, and cessation of smoking behavior. More than one program may simultaneously influence an individual to alter smoking behavior, and a single program may have different effects on individuals at different stages of smoking behavior (Table 61-6). In addition, individuals are greatly influenced by the social environment in which they act. A work break or the end of a meal can give the smoker a cue to smoke, while working in a designated no-smoking area can inhibit the smoker's behavior. This makes changing the environment that surrounds a smoker an important synergistic strategy for program planning.

The COMMIT trials are providing the scientific foundation for the largest, most comprehensive smoking control project ever undertaken—the American Stop

TABLE 61-6 Planning Smoking Cessation Programs for Selected Target Audiences

Audience	Barriers to Smoking Cessation	Channels for Reaching	Message Content
Women	• Tendency to underestimate health risks • Concern about weight gain • Identity with independence, success, and glamour • Using as a mechanism for coping with stress	• Health care system, since women are high utilizers of services • Prenatal period in public health clinics and neighborhood health centers • Counteradvertising in women's magazines • Supermarkets and food stores	• Smoking is as much a health risk for women as it is for men • Quitting smoking promotes health of children • Possibility of being slimmer not important enough to risk the health dangers of smoking • How to acquire social support from family members, friends, and co-workers
Blacks	• Reliance on cigarettes as way of coping with life stress and social disadvantages related to low SES • Limited access to health care in general and to smoking-related services and resources in particular • Limited confidence in ability to quit • Receipt of regular health care from hospitals, public health clinics, and emergency rooms; less physician advice to stop • Stronger smoking norms and tobacco advertising influences in black community	• Integrate program components into many existing communications channels, including black-focused mass media, churches, voluntary health organizations, health care system, fraternal and mutual aid organizations, workplaces, unemployment offices, job-training programs, retail establishments, families, and neighborhood and tenants' organizations • Families and social networks • Black rather than white sources for information about smoking risks for blacks; everyday people instead of celebrities as sources	• Include clear information about health consequences of smoking, health benefits, and other gains from quitting • Suggest how to quit smoking; reassure about overcoming common quitting barriers (concerns about weight gain and loss of smoking as a coping tactic) • Give information on health risks of second-hand smoke exposure; emphasize family life and economic burden of smoking-related illness for black families • Use counteradvertising as strategy
Hispanics	• Unemployment, little education, and lack of English • Little or no awareness of cessation services • Smoking as a part of social and machismo culture • Financial access to health care, and immigrant documentation status	• Spanish-language media, especially television and radio PSAs • Radio talk show with Hispanic experts, especially call-in shows • Printed media such as billboards and posters	• Use collective loyalty to extended family; it ranks higher than individual needs; use graphic presentation of adverse health effects on smokers and loved ones • In print media, aim at nonsmoking family members as well as smokers • Use authoritative figures such as physicians both for individual encounter and for public campaigns • Promote willpower with self-help methods • Include culturally appropriate ways to resist social pressures to smoke

Source: Adapted from National Cancer Institute: *Strategies to Control Tobacco Use in the United States: A Blueprint for Public Health Action in the 1990s.* NIH pub. no. 92-3316. Bethesda, MD: U.S. Department of Health and Human Services, 1991.

Smoking Intervention Study for Cancer Prevention (ASSIST).

ASSIST/2000 Program

ASSIST is a project designed to demonstrate that the widespread, coordinated application of the best available strategies to prevent and control tobacco use will significantly accelerate the current downward trend in smoking and tobacco. A collaborative effort between the National Cancer Institute and the American Cancer Society, working with state and local health departments and other voluntary organizations, ASSIST will develop comprehensive tobacco control programs in 17 states. Public health departments in Colorado, Indiana, Maine, Massachusetts, Minnesota, Missouri, New Jersey, New Mexico, New York, North Carolina, Rhode Island, South Carolina, Virginia, Washington, West Virginia, and Wisconsin were awarded contracts estimated to total $114 million over the life of the program. The ACS will support ASSIST with a matching 15% contribution of the total contract funding in each ASSIST site.

It is estimated that some 91 million Americans, including 18 million smokers, will be reached by ASSIST. More than 4.5 million extra adults will quit smoking and 2 million adolescents will be prevented from becoming addicted. Overall, it is expected that 1.2 million premature deaths will be averted, including 422,000 deaths from lung cancer.

The ASSIST interventions are based on proven smoking prevention and control methods developed within the NCI's intervention trials and other smoking and behavioral research. The primary objective of ASSIST is to demonstrate and evaluate ways to accelerate the decline in smoking prevalence, in all ASSIST sites combined, to less than 15% of adults by the year 2000. The secondary objective is to reduce by 50% the numbers of new smokers among adolescents, in all award sites, by the year 2000.

Groups with high smoking rates and groups that have displayed slower rates of decline will be targeted. These include women, youth, the medically underserved, the less educated, and several ethnic minority populations. Through ASSIST, media, policy, and cessation support will be delivered to target groups using the health care system, schools, the work site, and other community channels. Specific interventions include training health care providers to deliver brief cessation counseling, implementing smoke-free policies in schools and work sites, and enhancing media coverage of tobacco use issues. The program has two phases: as 24-month planning period that began in September 1991 (phase I), and a 5-year implementation phase, beginning September 1993 and continuing through 1998 (phase II).

California's experience

In 1988, Californians passed Proposition 99—an initiative to increase the excise tax on tobacco by 25 cents per pack, with tax monies earmarked for tobacco-related health, research, education, and environmental activities—58% of the voters supported the additional tax. The Assembly's bill earmarked 29% of the estimated $1.4 billion of Proposition 99 funds for the establishment of health education programs to reduce tobacco use in California. The program is simultaneously pursuing four strategies: First, it is striving to raise the priority of smoking as a public health issue. Second, it is improving the ability of communities to change smoking behavior. Third, it is striving to increase the influence of the existing legal and socioeconomic factors that discourage tobacco use. And fourth, it is strengthening social norms and values that discourage tobacco use.[31]

Cigarette consumption in California has gone down and stayed down since the passage of Proposition 99. This permanent drop is a departure from the typical pattern, in which sales fall initially after a tax increase and then rise again. The per capita consumption in California is down 7% and continues to drop. The decline is on track for reaching the goal of 75% reduction in smoking prevalence by the year 1999.[32]

Cancer Information Service (CIS)

CIS as public educator

The Cancer Information Service (CIS), a program of the NCI, is a toll-free telephone service that answers questions about cancer prevention and control, diagnosis, treatment, and rehabilitation. Begun in 1976, the CIS has a network of offices throughout the country based in comprehensive cancer centers, community cancer centers, and hospitals. Via a common number (1-800-4-CANCER), calls are routed automatically to CIS offices in local areas. Since 1976, when the CIS received 47,000 calls, the calls have grown steadily to over 500,000 a year; over 5 million calls have been taken since the service began.[33]

CIS counselors, after completing a standardized training program, provide accurate, up-to-date information tailored to the needs of individual callers. The NCI's computerized database, PDQ (Physicians' Data Query), which contains state-of-the-art treatment information and NCI-approved clinical trials, is a major resource for treatment information. Almost 50% of inquiries to the CIS are from cancer patients, their relatives, and their friends. The callers are predominantly white, female, over age 30, and with at least a high school education. A 1983 national user survey of a random sample of over 7600 CIS callers showed that the respondents found the information helpful (94%) and clear and easy to understand (96%). The CIS staff was seen as knowledgeable (95%), courteous (97%), and friendly (97%). Nearly 98% said they would call the service again if they had questions, and more than 50% had already recommended CIS to others. About 93% of the callers reported taking some kind of action, with 58% sharing the information with at least one other person (information from 4091 initial inquiries reached 11,386 people). In addition, 91% indicated the CIS was important in their decisions to take action following the call.[33] As one of the oldest continuously funded programs of the NCI, and its major outreach arm, the CIS has grown in size, in quality, and in the services it offers.

CIS as change agent

The CIS, in addition to its roles in public and patient information and education, is increasingly acting as a change agent in the area of cancer prevention and risk reduction. In CIS offices across the country, telephone counselors have been trained to help smokers who wish to quit, based on a research project conducted at the Roswell Park CIS[34] and on basic strategies for behavior change (using a protocol concentrating on steps that include precontemplation, contemplation, action, and maintenance). The counselors assess the individual's needs, identify roadblocks and facilitators to altering personal behavior, and give the appropriate advice, referrals, and written materials to help the caller make the change. A similar training program has been conducted to enable counseling about clinical trials.

A study currently being conducted at the University of California at Los Angeles and the University of Southern California uses the CIS as an instrument to increase breast screening among female callers. This project attempts to change the CIS from a passive system, which depends on a specific request from the caller, to an active one, which targets particular subgroups of high-risk callers for specific cancer control messages. All female CIS callers 40 years and older who are not currently being treated for cancer will be randomized within these groups: group I (information about mammography will be given only in response to a specific request by the caller); group II (information about breast screening and age-specific behavioral recommendations will be given, following a strict intervention protocol, to all callers regardless of their initial reason for calling the CIS). The intervention protocol is grounded in communications and persuasion theory. Assessment of the outcome (self-reported adherence to the mammography recommendations made by the CIS) will be by telephone interview 6 months after the initial call, along with measures of attitudes, barriers, beliefs, and intentions related to mammography.[34]

This new thrust of the CIS into the role of change agent has the potential for major impact. It uses in a new and different way an existing system with a proven track record for satisfying the needs of people who wish cancer information. These studies, showing that a telephone system can be used to reinforce positive health messages and stimulate encouraging behavioral change, could provide a new catalyst to altering knowledge and health practices.

CHALLENGES FOR THE FUTURE

There have been many changes in public information and education during the 1980s and early 1990s. The cancer field, led by the NCI and the ACS, has kept pace, using sophisticated marketing techniques. New opportunities will continue, and health professionals must join with colleagues in other areas to meet them. As health professionals work toward reaching the NCI's Year 2000 goals, a number of challenges present themselves: how to develop interventions to reduce cancer risk most effectively, how to implement those interventions to reach the greatest number of people at risk, how to plan public education programs that will use resources, both nationally and locally, to their greatest benefits, and how to plan and implement programs that will be sensitive to the needs of minority and other target audiences. These challenges demand new ways of thinking, new interrelationships, and new methods of operation. Nurses can assume a leadership role in providing innovative, research-based educational opportunities that will help meet these challenges.

REFERENCES

1. Gochman DS: *Health Behavior: Emerging Research Perspectives.* New York: Plenum Press, 1988.
2. Kolbe LJ: The application of health behavior and research: Health education and health information. In Gochman DS (ed.): *Health Behavior: Emerging Research Perspectives.* New York: Plenum, 1988, pp. 381–396.
3. Green LW, Kreuter MW, Deeds SG, et al: *Health Education Planning: A Diagnostic Approach.* Palo Alto, CA: Mayfield, 1980.
4. Glanz K, Lewis FM, Rimer BC: The scope of health education. In Glanz K, Lewis FM, Rimer BK (eds.). *Health Behavior and Health Education: Theory, Research and Practice.* San Francisco: Jossey-Bass, 1990, pp. 3–16.
5. Rosenstock IM: Historical origins of the health belief model. *Health Ed Monographs* 2:328–335, 1974.
6. Prochaska JO, DiClemente CC: Stages and processes of self-change of smoking: Toward an integrative model of change. *J Consul Clin Psych* 51:390–395, 1983.
7. Prochaska JO: Assessing how people change. *Cancer* 65:805–807, 1991.
8. Berlo DK: *The Process of Communication: An Introduction to Theory and Practice.* New York: Holt, Rinehart and Winston, 1960.
9. McGuire WJ: Personality and attitude change: An information processing theory. In Greenwald AG, Brock TC, and Ostrom TM (eds.): *Psychological Foundations of Attitudes.* Orlando, FL: Academic Press, 1968.
10. Kotler P, Andreasen AR: *Strategic Marketing for Nonprofit Organizations* (ed. 3). Englewood Cliffs, NJ: Prentice-Hall, 1987.
11. National Cancer Institute: *Making Health Communications Programs Work: A Planner's Guide.* NIH pub. no. 92-1493. Bethesda, MD: Office of Cancer Communications, The Institute, 1992.
12. National Cancer Institute: *Cancer Control Objectives for the Nation: 1985–2000.* NCI monograph no. 2, appendix B. Bethesda, MD: Division of Cancer Prevention and Control, The Institute, 1986.
13. U.S. Department of Health and Human Services: *Healthy People 2000: National Health Promotion and Disease Prevention Objectives.* Washington DC: U.S. Public Health Service, 1991, pp. 424–432.
14. American Cancer Society: *Priorities for the Decade of the 1990s.* Atlanta:The Society, 1991.
15. Centers for Disease Control: *The Behavioral Risk Factor Surveillance System 1984–87 in Perspectives on Prevention.* Atlanta: Centers for Disease Control, 1987, p. 34.
16. Weiss MJ: *The Clustering of America.* New York: Harper & Row, 1988.

17. National Cancer Institute: *NCI 1993 Budget Estimate.* Bethesda, MD: The Institute, 1991.
18. American Cancer Society: *Cancer Facts and Figures—1989.* Atlanta: The Society, 1989.
19. AMC Cancer Research Center: *Breast and Cervical Screening: Barriers and Use Among Specific Audiences.* Atlanta: U.S. Centers for Disease Control and Prevention, 1992.
20. National Cancer Institute: *Fighting Cancer in America: Findings and Recommendations of the 1987–88 Public Participation Hearings of the National Cancer Advisory Board on Cancer Prevention and Early Detection.* Bethesda, MD: Office of Cancer Communications, The Institute, 1989.
21. U.S. Department of Health and Human Resources: *Report of the Secretary's Task Force on Black and Minority Health (Vol III), Cancer, 1986.* Washington, DC: U.S. Government Printing Office, 1986.
22. U.S. Department of Health and Human Resources: *Report of the Secretary's Task Force on Black and Minority Health (Vol VIII), Hispanic Health Issues.* Washington, DC: U.S. Government Printing Office, 1986.
23. Wilson CM, Rimer BK, Bennett DJ, et al: Educating the older cancer patient: Obstacles and opportunities. *Health Ed Q,* 10:76–87, 1984.
24. Dellefield ME: Informational needs and approaches for early cancer detection in the elderly. *Semin Oncol Nurs* 7:156–168, 1988.
25. Doak CC, Doak LG, Root JH: *Teaching Patients with Low Literary Skills.* Philadelphia: Lippincott, 1985.
26. American Cancer Society: *Three Ways to Take Special Care of Your Breasts.* Pub. no. 88-2675.05-LE. Atlanta: The Society, 1988.
27. National Cancer Institute: *The Pap Test: It Can Save Your Life.* NIH pub. no. 91-3212. Bethesda, MD: The Institute, 1991.
28. Stuyck SC, Chilton JA: Examining the role of mass media gatekeepers in disseminating cancer information. *Cancer Bull* 40:334–343, 1988.
29. National Cancer Institute: *Smoking, tobacco, and cancer programs: 1985–1989 status report* NIH pub. no. 90-3107. Bethesda, MD: U.S. Department of Health and Human Services, 1990.
30. National Cancer Institute: *Strategies to control tobacco use in the United States: A blueprint for public health action in the 1990s.* NIH pub. no. 92-3316. Bethesda, MD: U.S. Department of Health and Human Services, 1991.
31. California Department of Health Services: *Toward a Tobacco Free California: A Status Report to the California Legislature on the First Fifteen Months of California's Tobacco Control Program.* Sacramento: State of California, December, 1990.
32. California Department of Health Services: *Tobacco Use in California, 1990–1991.* San Diego: University of California, 1991.
33. Morra ME, Van Nevel P, Nealon E, et al.: The history of the cancer information service. *JNCI* (in press).
34. Ward JD, Duffy K, Sciandra R, et al: What the public wants to know about cancer: The Cancer Information Service. *Cancer Bull* 40:384–389, 1988.

Chapter 62

Teaching Strategies: Patient Education

Judith (Judi) L. Bond Johnson, RN, PhD, FAAN

Barbara D. Blumberg, ScM

INTRODUCTION

Approximately 83 million Americans now living are expected to get cancer.[1] Given the complexity of the disease, along with the wide range of physiologic and economic accompaniments, one would expect the education of patients and their family members to be of prime concern. Within the broader context of cancer education itself, the education of those who are ill has been overshadowed by public and preventive efforts.[2]

HISTORICAL PERSPECTIVE

Patient education itself is not a new concept in health care. For years doctors and nurses, in the course of regular contact with patients, have explained illness and its consequences. As a rule, however, these efforts have been sporadic and lacking in consistency.[3]

Literary references to patient education first appeared in the 1950s. A prime factor responsible for increased attention to the field was the development of prepaid health care plans. A basic tenet of these plans was that informed self-care could reduce the costs of long-range patient care.[4] Patient education was viewed by some as a factor that facilitated such self-care.

At a 1964 conference on health education, the American Hospital Association took the position that it should act as the nationwide agency for stimulating the development of patient education programs. Their advocacy served as a milestone in the recognition of patient education within the health care system. Patient education was recommended as an integral part of patient care. This conference served as the impetus for *A Patient's Bill of Rights,*[5] which was approved by the association's House of Delegates in 1973.

Both the National Cancer Institute's document entitled *Adult Patient Education in Cancer*[6] and the Oncology Nursing Society's *Outcome Standards in Cancer Patient Education*[7] identify a number of tasks for patient education. These include helping patients and family members adjust to the disease, participate in treatment, carry out treatment regimens, manage stress, recognize and control side effects, prevent social isolation and strengthen relationships with significant others, mobilize and manage resources, and adapt to a life of uncertainty.

In addition to these efforts are several other factors that contribute both to the historical development of patient education and to its role in the future.

1. As the population of older Americans increases, so will the number of individuals who have chronic diseases and disabilities. The emergence of chronic illness as a major health problem has provided much stimulus for the development of patient education services.[8]
2. The consumer rights movement has resulted in more patients asking for greater amounts of information and in *A Patient's Bill of Rights.* This document outlines the patient's right to know. It states that "the patient has the right to obtain . . . complete, current information concerning his diagnosis, treatment, and prognosis in terms that he can be reasonably expected to understand . . . " and that "the patient has the right to refuse treatment to the extent permitted by law and to be informed of the medical consequences of his action."[5]
3. As a result of increasing health care costs and changing medical reimbursement policies, cost effectiveness of patient education has become a matter of concern.
4. Accountability by the health care provider has become more of a necessity and, as a result, issues related to informed consent are of greater concern. In addition, auditing of medical and nursing records, an attempt to document accountability, has become more of a routine practice.

Recent Literature

A review of articles on cancer patient education published between 1970 and 1985[9] cited growing evidence that cancer patient education can improve knowledge, attitudes, behavior, and health status. Additional review by the chapter authors of articles published through 1991 reinforce's and expands on these areas.

Specifically, Dodd's work with chemotherapy patients[10-15] provided evidence that patients who learned how to manage chemotherapy and radiation therapy side effects carried out self-care and initiated it sooner than their uneducated counterparts. In a study by Beck[16] that looked at the effect of an oral protocol on stomatitis after chemotherapy, patient education was credited with reducing infection and thus lowering financial as well as physiologic and psychologic costs of cancer. Other patient education programs have resulted in decreased anxiety and/or increased knowledge[17-20] as well as improved self-concept and self-esteem.

Johnson's work[21] demonstrated that patients who were informed of sensations involved in medical procedures experienced less stress than their uneducated cohorts. Later work[22] found reduced amounts of pain medication required by patients who received information on behavioral coping strategies.

The trend toward briefer hospital stays and outpatient therapy administration has resulted in greater need for information related to self-care management. Programs that can be carried out at home or in the outpatient setting have received more impetus as a result.[23,24]

Self-regulation theory as developed by Leventhal and Johnson[25] recognizes patients as active problem solvers. The educator attempts to enter the patients' problem-solving domain by providing corrective information, models, and support so they can achieve more accurate understanding and more effective regulation of both the illness and its treatment. Much of Johnson's work has been conducted with cancer patients. In collaboration with Lauver and Nail she carried out a study with men receiving radiation therapy for prostate cancer. Results supported self-regulator theory for explaining the effects of information on outcomes for coping with radiation therapy.[26] The self-regulation model also guided the content of a slide/tape program used as an intervention in a study examining the effects of social support and communication on self-esteem of patients undergoing chemotherapy.[27] With care trends being as they are, patient education needs more than ever to focus on self-care and self-regulation.

On the basis of their timely review, which still holds today, Rimer and colleagues[9] suggest that patient education programming include the following:

- use of a combination of education methods[11–14,19,28]
- enhancement of educational methods by combining them with behavioral modalities such as relaxation, guided imagery, and/or hypnosis[29–32]
- use of repetition to improve the generally compromised recall facilities of those with cancer[33]
- preparation of informed-consent forms at a reading level and in a format conducive to their use as educational vehicles
- development of programs with the objective of teaching self-care as part of treatment regimens[10,11,34]
- development of programs targeted at the special needs of the older patient as well as other high-risk patient audiences

Program Priorities

As a result of changing educational needs of cancer patients and their families, along with the American Cancer Society's emphasis on issues related to quality of life, in 1987 the National Cancer Institute Coping with Cancer Program broadened. Both the National Cancer Institute's Office of Cancer Communications and the National Office of the American Cancer Society provided more emphasis in cancer patient education by adding a patient education section and a national office staff position, respectively. These changes were due to historical events in the evolution of cancer patients and family needs, resulting in observers from both the NCI and ACS noting the following.[35]

- Patients wanted more technical information related to living with physical limitations imposed by the disease.
- Patients wanted more of a participatory, as opposed to passive, role in decision making related to their care and treatment.
- Patients were shopping around for information in order to make decisions related to their care and caregivers.
- Earlier discharge of sicker patients from hospitals necessitated additional care concern.
- Subsequent family responsibilities for care and management increased educational needs of this audience.
- Family members and patients, as well, were required as part of this home care phenomenon to perform very specialized medical care monitoring.
- The role of patients and family members in coordinating their care became greater.

Activities of the National Cancer Institute's (NCI) Patient Education Program[36] help shed light on extant national priorities in this area.

- The Third Cancer Patient Education Conference on March 28, 1992, addressed concerns of regional populations, cancer patient and survivor support groups, innovative educational programs, patient education research, and psychosocial issues.
- Development and expansion of the Cancer Patient Education subfile of the Combined Health Information Database (CHID) represents a computerized bibliographic database for lay and professional audiences. The CHID currently contains educational resources sponsored by NCI-designated comprehensive cancer programs and is being expanded.
- Projects related to cancer survivors include a training program on cancer survivor issues for the Cancer Information Service and a curriculum for cancer survivors.
- A Patient Information File (PIF) is included in the PDQ database.
- Activities designed to promote and educate patients and physicians about participation in clinical trials include videotapes, trial descriptions, exhibits and presentations, and reimbursement issues.
- A new initiative addressing cancer pain is in progress.
- Patient education publications are being revised and updated; new publications are also being developed as needed.

Since the 1950s, the American Cancer Society's (ACS) patient service programs have provided information to patients and their families. Over time, development of quality patient education materials has become an increasingly more important component, as evidenced by the adoption of the I Can Cope program in 1979.[37]

This 12-hour structured patient education course responded to the growing awareness that, with advances in cancer treatment, cancer was becoming a chronic, rather than a fatal, disease.[35] It has been estimated that approximately a half million people attended an I Can Cope course in the first 10 years of its existence.

A national survey in 1991 indicated that close to 1000 I Can Cope courses had been held the previous year. An evaluation of the existing programs was conducted as a first step in program revision. A carefully developed research design under the direction of Susan McMillan at the University of South Florida was implemented. Data from 400 programs nationwide was gathered and analyzed. Findings indicated that the goals and objectives of the I Can Cope program remain sound, and participant response is positive. Considerable variation existed in programs, such as number of hours offered and emphasis on content. As to audiovisual materials, there was a strong preference for videotapes. Program evaluation was inconsistent, and many of the respondents viewed the ACS role in the program as minimal.[38] A revised I Can Cope package of materials will incorporate these findings and be ready for distribution in 1993.

To further emphasize the importance of patient education, the American Cancer Society has established a Patient/Family Education Work Group under the direction of the Service and Rehabilitation Department. The goal of this group is to enable cancer patients and their families to gain needed information concerning cancer prevention, diagnosis, and care; prevent or minimize physical, psychologic, and social problems due to cancer or cancer treatment; and develop the needed coping skills that will assist in improving the quality of life. They have been charged with overseeing the review and revision of the existing materials and programs of the ACS. Their activities also include the development of materials and programs that are culturally sensitive, understandable, and relevant to the poor and underserved populations.[35]

Other current ACS projects include new materials on sexuality and information on insurance concerns and employment discrimination. A program called Look Good—Feel Better is directed at helping patients acquire skills that improve their appearances and maintain their lifestyles during treatment.

The Oncology Nursing Society (ONS) has addressed patient education through their special-interest-group structure. The mission of this group is to promote highly effective education for patients and families who are actually and/or potentially afflicted with cancer. Their activities include providing a centralized forum to facilitate networking among ONS members who have a strong interest in cancer patient education, to initiate and support research in patient education, and to exchange information and educational resources with the membership at large. They provide a newsletter for members and are intending to publish a directory of patient education tools.

As more people live longer, and as more of those who have cancer experience long-term control or cure, the needs of two specific audiences—the elderly and cancer survivors—take on greater importance. Specific needs of older audiences must be considered, including their peculiar beliefs, myths, and misconceptions about the disease, information style preference,[39] and concomitant medications and diseases. Although these variables are necessary considerations in the education of any audience, older persons have needs and predispositions that are unique to them and should be considered in any effort to reach them.

CANCER SURVIVORS

Fitzhugh Mullan,[40] a physician and cancer survivor, brought new light to the definition of the terms *patient* and *survivor*. He maintains that the lives of all those living with cancer are similar in concept, if not always in form, and views their needs and concerns along a continuum that he has referred to as "seasons of survival."

There are specific implications for patient education in this updated definition of *patient* as one who should be considered a "survivor" from diagnosis onward. Educational needs of the "survivor," however, change according to the specific point along the continuum that the patient inhabits at a particular point in time.

The first season—the medical or acute stage—commences with diagnosis and is focused on efforts, both diagnostic and therapeutic, to contain the illness. Educational efforts at this time should focus on the medical and psychosocial needs for information and self-care. The emphasis should be on maintenance of as good a quality of life as possible by fostering a "surviving" rather than "getting by" attitude.

The next season begins when the patient has gone into remission or has completed the primary course of treatment. This period, aptly termed "watchful waiting," has as its governing force the fear of recurrence. During this phase, the person with cancer reintegrates into the community; medical personnel do not play the major role that they did during the previous phase. Educational efforts should address both the need for continuing medical surveillance and ways to live as normal a life as possible. Teaching strategies incorporate health promotion behaviors and a wellness concept.

The final season is "permanent survival" or cure. Besides "victory over the disease," those who have entered this phase of the continuum have a very special comradeship with those in the previous seasons of survival. This phase is characterized by concerns about employability, insurability, and long-term effects of treatment. Educational concerns are similar to those previously mentioned. Teaching people to be their own advocates is a means of empowering them to speak up for their rights.

In recognition of the ever-growing network of cancer survivors, the American Cancer Society prepared a *Cancers Survivors' Bill of Rights* to call public attention to the 8 million Americans alive today who have a history of cancer.[1] The purpose of this document is to call attention to the specific needs of the cancer survivor in areas that include continued excellence in acute cancer care, as well as ongoing lifelong medical care, health insurance, job opportunities, and interpersonal happiness. In addition, 1986 saw the birth of the National Coalition for Cancer Survivorship, an organization dedicated to the needs of the survivor.

In summary, this emphasis on the patient as a survivor should be a major theme in patient education programming. Considering all who are diagnosed with cancer as survivors, with needs peculiar to the specific "season" they inhabit, appears to be more timely than using the more traditional medical model to delineate patient needs in the educational arena.

DEFINITIONS

In an earlier article,[41] a composite definition of patient education was developed. *Patient education* is a series of structured or unstructured experiences designed to help patients cope voluntarily with the immediate crisis response to their diagnosis, with long-term adjustments, and with symptoms; gain needed information about sources of prevention, diagnosis, and care; and develop needed skills, knowledge, and attitudes to maintain or regain health status.

Patient education is able to accomplish all of this by enabling patients and their families to plan strategies for change; interpret and integrate needed information for achieving the desired attitudes or behaviors; and meet patients' specific learning needs, interests, and capabilities.[42] Patient education, through a combination of learning experiences derived from joint planning by patients, significant others, and health care professionals, is considered part of total health care.[43]

RATIONALE FOR PATIENT EDUCATION

Teaching is integral to healing. It is a facet of cancer rehabilitation programs. Providing structured patient education courses and classes gives people an option for coping with their cancer diagnosis. Adaptation is enhanced by patient education efforts.[44]

First, a structured patient education program ensures that important medical and psychosocial information is made available in a consistent manner. The key word is *consistency*. When procedures or treatments are being explained as part of routine care, interruptions are certain to occur that lead to disruption in teaching time and inadvertent deletion of pieces of information. Distractions and lack of privacy inherent in the hospital environment also create a less-than-ideal learning environment. This can be remedied by providing a planned and scheduled time for patient education. This is not to say that the informal bedside exchange of information is not valuable. This approach should continue to be viewed as an integral part of patient care. Both approaches to providing patient education are incorporated into an overall plan. They work in concert, with each reinforcing information exchange.

Second, patient education addresses one of the major difficulties experienced by people with cancer—the loss of control over their disease and over their lives. In addition to providing information, patient education offers options, choices, and ways to engage self-care. It sets forth an expectation that people can be involved in their treatment decisions and obtain what they want and need from their health care providers. It promotes a proactive stance.

Patient education classes bring together people who have a common purpose or problem, providing opportunity for the exchange of ideas, problems, and solutions. Patients can learn from each other because of their similar situations. The educational setting is different from that of the neighborhood gathering or the doctor's waiting room. It provides a forum for exchange and constructive, guided direction for interaction among participants.

Finally, patient education broadens the opportunity for patient and provider to interact. Their roles in this setting are that of trainee and teacher, respectively. Patients gain a different perspective of their health care provider—that of facilitator and patient advocate. The relationship between patients and their health care providers can be strengthened by a broadening of the concept of partnership in health care.

DEVELOPING PATIENT EDUCATION MATERIALS AND PROGRAMS

Integral to the success of any patient education material or program is the extent to which the needs of the intended audience are met. Also called "social marketing," this perspective incorporates assessment of audience needs at particular points in program/material development and implementation.

Developing patient education materials and programs is viewed as a process whereby time and available resources are allocated in quantities sufficient to include concept, message, and actual resource development, along with attendant evaluations. This process is conceptualized in a six-part wheel (Figure 62-1).[45] Each

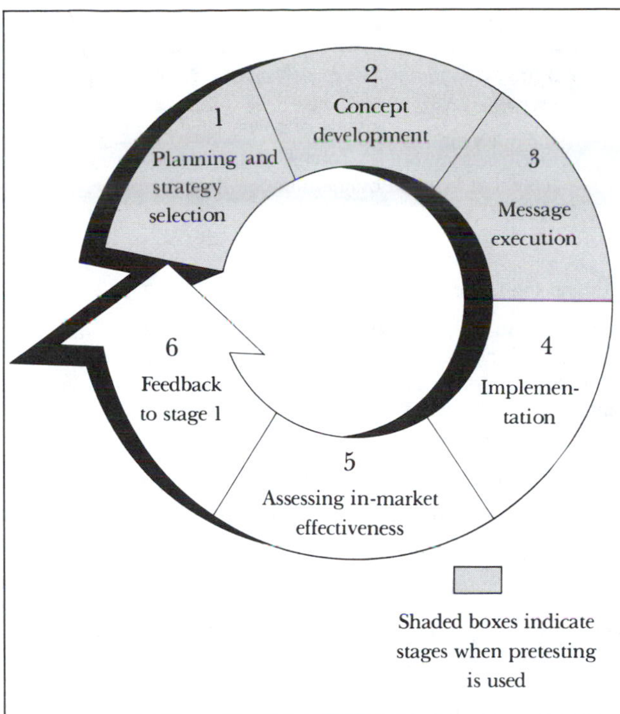

FIGURE 62-1 Stages in the development of patient education materials and resources. (Source: U.S. Department of Health and Human Services. *Pretesting in Health Communications.* NIH pub. no. 84-1493. Washington, DC: U.S. Government Printing Office, 1984.)

section of the wheel represents a stage in a circular process in which the last stage feeds back to the first in a continuous loop of replanning and improvement.

The key to the development process is pretesting, a qualitative research method executed during the development of materials and programs. The purpose of pretesting is systematically to gather target audience reactions to draft concepts and materials before final production and implementation. Pretesting is useful in determining which version of a concept, message, or material is most likely to meet stated objectives. In addition, pretesting is useful in identifying strengths and weaknesses of draft materials. Variables particularly amenable to pretesting are awareness and interest, comprehension, audience relevance, believability, acceptability, and gain in short-term knowledge.

Pretesting provides important diagnostic information that can lead to improvements in draft materials and programs before they are made widely available. It is important to recognize, however, that pretesting is a qualitative method and, as such, does not yield findings that are reportable in terms of their statistical significance. Results of pretesting are not absolutely predictive of potential success or failure of items in terms of variables pretested. Rather, pretesting provides direction on the basis of perception of needs of representative members of the target audience.

Pretesting Techniques

A host of research techniques can be usefully employed in pretesting. The particular method chosen depends on the target audience, the message or concepts being tested, objectives of the pretest, the best mode of access to the target audience, and time and resources available. In general, the techniques most conducive to pretesting of patient education materials and programs are the following: readability testing, focus group interviews, individual in-depth interviews, self-administered questionnaires, and gatekeeper review.

Readability testing is an easily employed technique used to predict the level of reading comprehension necessary to understand a particular written piece. After extensive review of 12 selected formulas,[33] the Office of Cancer Communications of the National Cancer Institute chose the SMOG grading formula for readability testing of its public and patient education materials.[46] SMOG was chosen because of the ease of its use and its accuracy in determining readability. This formula considers the number of words of at least three syllables in determining the grade level needed for comprehension. Table 62-1[45] describes how to apply this formula.

Focus group interviews are guided group discussions with a group of 8–10 individuals who share specific target audience characteristics. Interviews are led by a facilitator, who uses a list of open-ended questions to guide the discussion. This technique is particularly appropriate during the concept development stage and provides insight into audience beliefs and perceptions. Adapted from group therapy, focus group discussion encourages participants to converse about specific topics. Frequently, direct or paraphrased dialogue from focus groups can be incorporated into educational materials, making them more realistic and readable. Reactions to artwork and logos can also be gathered through use of this pretesting technique.

Individual in-depth interviews or one-on-one discussions are carried out by an interviewer, who uses a prepared questionnaire consisting of both open-ended and closed-end items. This technique is appropriate when the subjects addressed are sensitive or require in-depth probing.

Self-administered questionnaires that can be completed by the subject without the assistance of an interviewer are more widely used in gathering reactions to draft materials. Use of short, closed-end questions and a data collection technique that ensures return of completed questionnaires is advised when this technique is employed. Hand delivering and retrieving questionnaires, offering a small incentive for return of completed questionnaires, and/or including a postage-paid return envelope are techniques that have yielded higher return rates.

Since many health education materials and programs reach their audiences by way of health professionals, it is prudent to seek review and comment from such persons during the development of programs and materials. Because of their role in determining whether

TABLE 62-1 The SMOG Readability Formula

To calculate the SMOG reading grade level, begin with the entire written work that is being assessed, and follow these four steps:

1. Count off 10 consecutive sentences near the beginning, in the middle, and near the end of the text.
2. From this sample of 30 sentences, circle all of the words containing three or more syllables (polysyllabic), including repetitions of the same word, and total the number of words circled.
3. Estimate the square root of the total number of polysyllabic words counted. This is done by finding the nearest perfect square and taking its square root.
4. Finally, add a constant of 3 to the square root. This number gives the SMOG grade, or the reading grade level that a person must have reached if he or she is to fully understand the text being assessed.

A few additional guidelines will help to clarify these directions:

- A sentence is defined as a string of words punctuated with a period (.), an exclamation point(!), or a question mark (?).
- Hyphenated words are considered one word.
- Numbers that are written out should also be considered; and if in numeric form in the text, they should be pronounced to determine if they are polysyllabic.
- Proper nouns, if polysyllabic, should be counted too.
- Abbreviations should be read as unabbreviated to determine if they are polysyllabic.

Not all pamphlets, fact sheets, or other printed materials contain 30 sentences. To test a text that has fewer than 30 sentences:

1. Count all of the polysyllabic words in the text.
2. Count the number of sentences.
3. Find the average number of polysyllabic words per sentence as follows:

$$\text{Average} = \frac{\text{Total \# of polysyllabic words}}{\text{Total \# of sentences}}$$

4. Multiply that average by the number of sentences *short of 30.*
5. Add that figure on to the total number of polysyllabic words.
6. Find the square root and add the constant of 3.

Perhaps the quickest way to administer the SMOG grading test is by using the SMOG conversion table. Simply count the number of polysyllabic words in your chain of 30 sentences and look up the approximate grade level on the chart.

SMOG Conversion Table*

Total Polysyllabic Word Counts	Approximate Grade Level (± 1.5 Grades)
0–2	4
3–6	5
7–12	6
13–20	7
21–30	8
31–42	9
43–56	10
57–72	11
73–90	12
91–110	13
111–132	14
133–156	15
157–182	16
183–210	17
211–240	18

*Developed by Harold C. McGraw, Office of Educational Research, Baltimore County Schools, Towson, MD.

Source: U.S. Department of Health and Human Services: *Pretesting in Health Communications* (NIH pub. no. 84-1493). Washington, DC: U.S. Government Printing Office, 1984.

a particular material or program reaches its intended audience, such health professionals are referred to as "gatekeepers." Review of draft materials by gatekeepers can be carried out through short, self-administered questionnaires and can occur at the same time as the target audience review. If a discrepancy occurs between target audience needs and gatekeeper perception of these needs, deference should be made to the needs of the target audience. A memo announcing the availability of the program or material can summarize the extensive process and note that information ultimately included reflects the viewpoints of a number of persons.

The Development Process

Planning and strategy selection are the first activities in the development of patient education materials and programs. During this period, a concise definition of what the material or program will be about, objectives, and target audience identification are addressed. Planning and selection of educational strategies can be facilitated by conducting a needs assessment. Perusal of literature in the field and identification of other, analogous materials and programs are undertaken. In addition, it may be useful to conduct a more formal assessment to determine educational needs and strategies that have the greatest potential for meeting objectives.

Before development of the National Cancer Institute publication *What are Clinical Trials All About?*, a small-scale needs assessment survey was conducted, with patients, family members, and health professionals participating in clinical trials. This survey helped the staff determine that a booklet addressing specific topics would be most useful to the target audience, patient, and family members given the option of clinical trial participation.[47] Useful pretesting techniques during this stage are in-depth interviews, focus group interviews, and small-scale surveys.

During the concept development stage, draft educational resources are developed on the basis of concepts that appear to have the greatest potential for educating the target audience. Drafts can take a variety of forms, ranging from short manuscripts with rough artwork, to slides or storyboards with accompanying dialogue, to draft posters. During the message execution stage, draft educational resources are pretested before final production. Gatekeeper review takes place as part of pretesting to ensure that those responsible for disseminating the education to the target audience are familiar with it and have had a chance to submit comments. Self-administered questionnaires are the most unobtrusive method of pretesting to employ during this stage. Pretesting comments can then be incorporated before final production.

During the next stage—implementation—the educational material or program is used with the target audience, with initial reaction monitored closely. With both informal comments and observations, along with more formal methods, initial use and usefulness of materials and programs can be assessed. The number of copies distributed, how often the program is carried out, and the value of short evaluation forms accompanying a material or program are all to be considered during this period of process evaluation.[48]

During the next stage—assessment of in-market effectiveness—the effectiveness of materials and programs, in terms of meeting stated objectives, is assessed. Self-administered questionnaires completed before and after exposure to the material or programs and assessment of behavioral change targeted by the material or program are sample methods of assessment.

The final stage in the development of educational materials and programs involves critical assessment of information gathered during pretesting, process, and outcome evaluations for the purpose of replanning. Problems incurred in using the material or program, strengths of the material or program, and other feedback are assessed in terms of change necessitated by actual implementation.

CLIMATE FOR LEARNING

Considerable time, energy, and money can be committed to providing quality patient education programs. However, unless peoples' health beliefs, attitudes, cultural backgrounds, and personal values are considered, patient education efforts may be less than successful.

Chaisson[49] reports on past patient education efforts from which the following mistakes were discovered by default:

1. telling people what they should know rather than what they are ready and willing to learn
2. failure to individualize patient teaching content to accommodate the person's personal background, attitudes, and motivation
3. failure to assess a person's knowledge before beginning the teaching process
4. lack of coordination of patient teaching efforts across the continuum of care
5. expecting people to be effective teachers when they are not knowledgeable about educational principles, methods, and evaluation
6. use of an incidental, informal approach as a basis for a patient education program

Techniques of teaching are nearly as varied as people. Learners should be offered ways to participate actively throughout the entire educational process. To maximize readiness to learn, it is necessary to ascertain the concerns people have at that particular moment. Unless these concerns are addressed first, additional health teaching will not be heard.

A person's age will directly affect his or her ability to understand and master information and skills. Ability to learn depends on maturation. Growth and development of children is a crucial element of the teaching-learning process. Intellectual development moves from concrete to abstract. As children mature, they move toward a clearer distinction between what is internal and what is external to themselves.

Knowles[50] provides some valuable insights into the adult as a learner. He coined the word *andragogy,* the science of teaching adults, to distinguish the adult learner from the child. He proposes four assumptions about the adult learner. As people mature, (1) their self-concept moves from dependency to self-direction, (2) they accumulate life experiences that are an increasing resource for learning, (3) their readiness to learn is increasingly oriented to developmental tasks and social roles, and (4) time perspective changes and orientation to learning shifts to immediate application of knowledge and learning that is problem-centered rather than subject-centered.

Adult learners are motivated to learn when they recognize a gap between what they know and what they want to know. They accept a share of the responsibility for planning and carrying out a learning experience and therefore have a feeling of commitment to it. The learning process capitalizes on their past experiences.[51]

Changes brought on by aging need to be acknowledged when the learner is an older adult. Intellectual ability does not necessarily diminish with age; rather, it changes. The speed of learning declines, *not* the ability. Thus, factors other than age are more likely to be barriers to learning for the older adult.[52] Alford[53] identifies the following changes:

1. Slowed processing time requires that older persons have more time to think through and absorb new information.

2. Stimulus persistence means that older persons must be given time to explore each concept in its entirety and to ask questions.
3. Decreased short-term memory causes older persons difficulty in remembering new information. Learning can easily become frustrating if learning requires recent recall. Ways can be devised to reinforce learning, such as linking it with past experiences or providing written data to supplement the verbal information.
4. Test anxiety occurs because older persons sense they cannot remember as well. Taking tests would prove this fact. If tests are necessary, verbal ones should be considered. Elderly learners need confidence in their ability to maintain independence.

Material for older adults is printed in 10- or 11-point type on paper with a dull finish, and two-tone beige or green-tone colors are avoided. The print size used in written materials, the volume and speed of visual presentations, and the amount of information given at any one time are paced. Teaching is limited to three to five points. Older persons are accustomed to being in control, and teaching addresses this need whenever possible.

In addition to age, difference in culture, language, level of literacy, and physical impairment (for example, hearing and/or sight deficiencies) must be considered in providing the appropriate educational climate for each particular patient. Cultural differences significantly influence communication and subsequent education. Recognizing the importance of the person's family and even the immediate community as a support system is essential. Acknowledging culture-specific medical and religious beliefs and practices and attempting to incorporate them into educational opportunities is also advisable. Communicating in a language or dialect that is not the one most frequently used by a person can change both the expression of symptoms and the level of comprehension. When educating a patient with a different cultural background, it is wise to consider the use of a variety of methods both to convey and to understand messages. For example, the use of pictures to illustrate instructions, and/or materials that have been translated into the person's primary language, is helpful.[54]

Literacy level is also an important consideration in the education of any patient. Although concise communication can enhance the education of any patient, those with poor reading or comprehension skills require special consideration concerning their educational needs.

One implication of this challenge is to ensure that readability is addressed when developing and disseminating educational materials. It is important that people's reading levels be congruent with the reading levels of cancer education literature. A study was undertaken to estimate the reading level of 51 booklets printed by the American Cancer Society.[55] It was found that, according to the SMOG formula, the mean reading level was grade 11.9 and that 55% of the materials were written for people with grade-12-or-higher reading skills. However, booklets produced since 1985 were found to be written at significantly lower reading levels, which is a positive trend. To ensure that information is understood, educators must first be cognizant of the possible disparities between readability of cancer information and the reading skills of patients.

A major caveat in working with this audience is to simplify the language used. In addition, Chatham and Knapp[56] suggest the following: Speak and write in short sentences; as often as possible, use words of not more than two syllables; use nontechnical language that the patient understands in offering explanations of medical terms; speak or write in the active voice. An excellent reference by Doak, Doak, and Root,[57] entitled *Teaching Patients with Low Literacy Skills,* provides a variety of additional suggestions.

A second aspect to consider when establishing a climate for learning is the need for support from the organization or institution. Squyres[58] proposes a foundation for health education services. It requires integration of a person's personal philosophy and goals with those of the organization, along with the position statements of professionals, legal, and accrediting bodies. Often, patient education is given only lip service by an institution. Strategies for gaining support and recognition include knowing the state-of-the-art literature, supporting claims of effectiveness with research data, and presenting a cost-effective plan for implementing a program of quality patient care. Patient education addresses accreditation standards, requirements for informed consent, self-care interests of consumers, and trends for earlier discharge with home care collaboration. Quality patient education is nurtured by a supportive administrative and medical staff.

The physical component also must be considered in creating a climate conducive to learning. The environment can be used to focus people's attention on what is to be learned. A learning resource center facilitates self-initiated learning. Visual aids, such as anatomic charts and a human torso, heighten people's interest in their own body parts. A positive learning environment offers mutual respect, acceptance of differences, and freedom of expression. If patient education is valued as an integral part of patient care, then time and space should be allocated for carrying it out. It is less than ideal to teach when there are frequent interruptions, a lack of privacy, and interference by hospital routines. For group classes, chairs and tables should be arranged in advance; lighting and microphones adequate to group size and the availability of group leaders who are knowledgeable about audiovisual equipment are important factors. Otherwise, distractions will interfere with class interaction and the group process.

A final factor to consider is the choice of educational methods and materials. Consideration must be given to ways to present best the content to be taught. People learn better when more than one of their senses is involved in the learning process.[59] Hearing alone is a passive activity. Thus the use of only the lecture method to present information does not promote optimal learning. For each sense that is included, the more involved the learner and the more likely learning will occur.

The computer revolution has increased interest in the use of computers in patient education. A recent review of current literature by the Patient Education Office at M.D. Anderson Cancer Center[60] found that computer-based education and interactive videodiscs can benefit patient education in the following ways:

- reduces learning time by one-third
- offers privacy for user learning
- provides personal control in instructional pace
- accommodates a variety of learning styles
- reduces teaching time required by care providers
- offers options for teaching patients of low literacy

Audiovisual materials are the tools of patient education programs. However, their use alone is not considered adequate for providing patient education.[61] Education requires, human interaction. Appropriate materials enhance the teaching–learning process and are selected with that purpose in mind.

CONCLUSION

The rapid changes in health care technology as well as the complexities of the health care system present a challenge to both health care professionals and health care consumers. People enter the system, become patients, and find themselves faced with a life-threatening illness that requires multiple changes. They need assistance in the form of guidance and information. Facilitating adaptation to these changes comes in the form of patient education. The process begins before an illness is diagnosed and continues long after the acute phase of an illness is over. Patient education has as its ultimate goal the restoration of a person to his or her highest state of wellness and reentry into society.

In addition to rapid changes in health care technology, patient education in the future needs to be tuned into the following additional historical trends:[62]

- the aging of the population
- increasing numbers of cancer survivors
- special needs of minorities and the disadvantaged
- increasing illiteracy

The future of patient education depends on attention to these continuing trends and changes.

REFERENCES

1. American Cancer Society: *Cancer Facts and Figures.* Atlanta: The Society, 1992, p. 1.
2. Green LW: The future of cancer patient education. *Health Educ Q* 10:102–110, 1984 (special suppl.).
3. Brechon D: Highlights in the evolution of hospital-based patient education program. *J Allied Health* 3:35, 1976.
4. Shapiro I: The patient and control of quality in medical care. Proceedings Tenth Annual Group Health Association of America. Chicago, 1960.
5. American Hospital Association: *A Patient's Bill of Rights.* AHS Catalog No. 2415. Chicago: The Association, 1975.
6. National Cancer Institute: *Adult Patient Education in Cancer.* NIH pub. No. 83-2601. Washington, DC: The Institute, 1983.
7. Oncology Nursing Society: *Outcome Standards for Cancer Patient Education.* Pittsburgh, PA: The Society, 1982.
8. Simonds S: *Current Issues in Patient Education.* New York: American Group Practice Association and Core Communications in Health, 1974.
9. Rimer B, Keintz MK, Glassman B: Cancer patient education: Reality and potential. *Prev Med* 14:801–818, 1985.
10. Dodd M: Assessing patient self-care for side effects of cancer chemotherapy. Part I. *Cancer Nurs* 5:263–268, 1982.
11. Dodd M: Cancer patients' knowledge of chemotherapy: Assessment and informational interventions. *Oncol Nurs Forum* 9:39–44, 1982.
12. Dodd M: Self-care for side effects in cancer chemotherapy: An assessment of nursing interventions. Part II. *Cancer Nurs* 6:63–67, 1983.
13. Dodd M, Mood D: Chemotherapy: Helping patients to know the drugs they are receiving and their possible side effects. *Cancer Nurs* 4:311–318, 1981.
14. Dodd M: Patterns of self-care in cancer patients receiving radiation therapy. *Oncol Nurs Forum* 10:23–27, 1984.
15. Dodd M: Patterns of self-care in patients with breast cancer, *West J Nurs Res* 10:7–24, 1988.
16. Beck S: Impact of a systematic oral care protocol on stomatitis after chemotherapy. *Cancer Nurs* 2:185–199, 1979.
17. Cassileth BR, Heiberger RM, March V, et al: Effects of audiovisual cancer programs on patients and families. *J Med Educ* 57:54–59, 1982.
18. Jacobs C, Ross R, Walker IM, et al: Behavior of cancer patients: A randomized study of the effects of education and peer support groups. *Am J Clin Oncol* 6:347–350, 1983.
19. Johnson J: The effects of a patient education course on persons with a chronic disease. *Cancer Nurs* 5:117–123, 1982.
20. Watson PG: The effects of short-term postoperative counseling on cancer/ostomy patients. *Cancer Nurs* 6:21–29, 1983.
21. Johnson J: Effects of structuring patient's expectations on their reactions to threatening event. *Nurs Res* 21:499–504, 1972.
22. Johnson J, Christman N, Stitts C: Personal control interventions: Short and long term effects on surgical patients. *Res Nurs and Health* 8:131–143, 1985, and *Sem Oncol* 7:135–142, 1991.
23. Villejo L, Flynn V, Klucharich S, et al: Strategies for cancer patient education: Overcoming barriers. *Cancer Bull* 40:365–369, 1988.

24. Redman BK: Strengthening patient education programs in oncology. *J Psychosoc Oncol* 3:75–81, Winter 1985/1986.
25. Leventhal H, Johnson JE: Laboratory and field experimentation: Development of a theory of self-regulation. In Wooldridge PJ, Schmitt JK, Leonard RC, et al (eds.): *Behavioral Science and Nursing Theory.* St Louis: Mosby, 1983, pp. 189–262.
26. Johnson JE, Lauver DR, Nail LM: Process of coping with radiation therapy. *J Consult Clin Psychol* 57:358–364, 1989.
27. Ward S, Leventhal H, Easterling D, et al: Special support, self-esteem, and communication in patients receiving chemotherapy. *J Psychosoc Oncol* 9:95–116, 1991.
28. Green LW, Kreuter MW, Deeds SG, et al: *Health Education Planning.* Palo Alto, CA: Mayfield, 1980.
29. Burish T, Lyles J: Effectiveness of relaxation training in reducing the adversiveness of chemotherapy in the treatment of cancer. *Behav Ther Exp Psychiatry* 10:357–361, 1979.
30. Burish T, Lyles J: Effectiveness of relaxation training in reducing adverse reaction to cancer chemotherapy. *J Behav Med* 14:65–78, 1981.
31. Redd W, Andreasen G, Minagwa R: Hypnotic control of anticipatory emesis in patients receiving cancer chemotherapy. *J Consult Clin Psychol* 50:114–119, 1982.
32. Redd W, Hendler C: Learned aversions to chemotherapy treatment. *Health Educ Q* 10:57–64, 1984 (special suppl.).
33. Ley P: Towards better doctor-patient communications. In Bennett AE (ed.): *Communication Between Doctors and Patients.* London: Oxford University Press, 1976, pp. 75–98.
34. Thomas NP, Cloak M, Crosson K, et al: Preparing cancer patients to administer medication. *Patient Couns Health Educ* 3:137–143, 1982.
35. Stevenson E, Crosson K: Patient Education: History, Development, and Current Directions of the American Cancer Society and the National Cancer Institutes. *Semin Oncol Nurs* 7:134–142, 1992.
36. National Cancer Institute: Overview of current activities. Unpublished material. January 1992.
37. Johnson J, Klein L: *I Can Cope, Staying Healthy with Cancer.* Minneapolis, MN: DCI Publishing, 1988.
38. Black BL, Stevenson E: *I Can Cope Program Evaluation. (Summary of Evaluation Data and Analysis).* Atlanta: American Cancer Society, 1992.
39. Wilson CM, Rimer B, Kane-Williams E, et al: Educating the older cancer patient: Obstacles and opportunities. *Health Educ Q* 10:76–87, 1984 (special suppl.).
40. Mullan F: Seasons of survival: Reflections of a physician with cancer. *N Engl J Med* 313:270–273, 1985.
41. Johnson JL, Blumberg BD: A commentary on cancer patient education. *Health Educ Q* 10:7–18, 1984 (special suppl.).
42. DeJoseph J: Writing and evaluating educational protocols. In Squyres W (ed.): *Patient Education: An Inquiry Into the State of the Art.* New York: Springer, 1960.
43. Ulrich M, Kelley K: Patient care includes teaching. *Hospitals* 46:59–65, 1972.
44. Johnson J, Flaherty M: The nurse and cancer patient education. *Semin Oncol Nurs* 7:63–70, 1980.
45. National Cancer Institute: Pretesting in Health communications. NIH pub. no. 84-1493. Washington, DC: The Institute, 1984.
46. Rader LA: The SMOG grading readability formula. Unpublished dissertation. Michigan State University, 1980.
47. Blumberg B, Nealon E: Educational needs of the patient considering clinical trials. Paper presented at the Oncology Nursing Society Congress, Toronto, Canada, 1984.
48. Blumberg BD: Evaluating patient education programs. *Oncol Nurs Forum* 8:29–31, 1981.
49. Chaisson GM: Patient education: Whose responsibility is it and who should be doing it? *Nurs Admin Q* 4:1–11, 1980.
50. Knowles M: *The Modern Practice of Adult Education.* New York: Associated Press, 1975.
51. Woldum K, Ryan-Morrell V, Towson M, et al: *Patient Education Foundations of Practice.* Rockville, MD: Aspen, 1985.
52. Casserly D, Strock E: Educating the older patient. *Caring* 7:60–67, 1988.
53. Alford PM: Tips for teaching older adults. *Nurs Life* 2:60–64, 1982.
54. American Hospital Association, Center for Health Promotion: *Culture Bound and Sensory Barriers to Communication with Patient: Strategies and Resources for Health Education.* Chicago: The Association, 1982.
55. Meade C, Diekman J, Thornhill D: Readability of American Cancer Society patient education literature. *Oncol Nurs Forum* 19:61–55, 1992.
56. Chatham MAH, Knap BL: Teaching patient with low literacy skills. In Chatham MAH, Knap BL (eds.): *Patient Education Handbook.* Bowie, MD: Robert J Brady, 1982, pp. 145–150.
57. Doak CC, Doak LG, Root JH: *Teaching Patients with Low Literacy Skills.* Philadelphia: Lippincott, 1985.
58. Squyres W: *Patient Education and Health Promotion in Medical Care.* Palo Alto, CA: Mayfield, 1985.
59. Bille DA: *Practical Approaches to Patient Teaching.* Boston: Little, Brown, 1981.
60. Personal communication: Patient Education Office, M.D. Anderson Cancer Center, March 1992.
61. Monaco RM, Salfen L, Spratt J: The patient as an education participant in health care. *J Mo Med Assoc* 69:932–937, 1972.
62. Morra ME: Future trends in patient education. *Semin Oncol Nurs* 7:143–145, 1991.

Chapter 63

Cancer Nursing Education

Gloria A. Hagopian, RN, EdD

INTRODUCTION

In this chapter the history of cancer nursing education and some of the major influences on its development of cancer education will be discussed. The current state of cancer nursing education at the generalist, advanced, and continuing education levels will be highlighted. Critical issues facing cancer nursing education today and in the future will be discussed.

HISTORY OF CANCER NURSING EDUCATION

Specialized education in oncology nursing began in the 1940s. Day-long, then week-long continuing education programs were offered, often under the sponsorship of the American Cancer Society (ACS). Efforts to incorporate cancer nursing content at the baccalaureate level began in 1954 when the National Cancer Institute (NCI) funded four schools for this purpose.[1] There were several outcomes of this project, including the development by Diller of a cancer nursing test to measure student's knowledge, a cancer curriculum, and evaluation tools for faculty.[2] In 1982, *Outcome Standards for Cancer Nursing Education at the Fundamental Level* was written by the Oncology Nursing Society in cooperation with the American Nurses' Association, giving faculty guidelines for integrating oncology content into the curriculum at the fundamental or generalist level.[3] This document also served as the impetus to develop other guidelines for practice and graduate education.

The first graduate-level course with both theoretical and clinical components in cancer nursing was offered at Teacher's College in New York in 1946 by Nelson.[1,4,5] This course, two semesters in length, provided 16 credits toward a Master of Arts degree. The course focused on the nature of cancer as a biological phenomenon, patient needs, and nursing care measures. Public health aspects, such as early detection, home care, and community resources also were emphasized. The clinical part of the course was held at Memorial Hospital in New York. The program was supported in part by a grant from the ACS, New York Division. In 1950 a course for credit in cancer nursing and chronic disease was offered by the University of Minnesota School of Public Health.[1]

One of the first surveys of graduate programs to identify those that offered cancer nursing in the curriculum was done by the ACS in 1958.[1] Of the 22 programs responding to the questionnaire, only two indicated that cancer nursing was included. With specialization in nursing in other fields, such as coronary care, dialysis, burns, and intensive care, the interest in specialization in oncology nursing followed naturally, and university courses in oncology nursing soon developed. The first graduate oncology track leading to a master's degree was started at the University of Pittsburgh in 1968.[5]

Continuing education (CE) has always played an important part in cancer nursing and has been the most widely used method to increase knowledge and skill of nurses.[6] Because of the lack of consistent preparation of nurses at the generalist level, CE programs were the most convenient way to provide the expertise needed to practice cancer nursing. The ACS was an early provider of educational programs for practicing nurses. Several cancer centers also have offered CE programs for nurses through the years, including Memorial Sloan-Kettering Cancer Center, Roswell Park Memorial Hospital, Ellis Fischel State Cancer Center, and City of Hope National Medical Center.[4] One of the first institutional CE programs to teach nurses cancer screening procedures was developed by White at M.D. Anderson Hospital.[1] This unique program, sponsored by the NCI, still offers 1-week modules of site-specific cancer screening procedures.

IMPORTANT INFLUENCES ON CANCER NURSING EDUCATION

Organizations

Several very important cancer organizations have had a powerful impact on education in cancer nursing. They include the American Cancer Society, the Oncology Nursing Society (ONS), the National Cancer Institute, and the Association of Pediatric Oncology Nurses (APON).

American Cancer Society

The ACS, organized in 1913, is a nationwide voluntary health agency dedicated to eliminating cancer as a health problem by preventing cancer, saving lives, and decreasing suffering through research, education, and service. It has more than 3000 units and 2.5 million volunteers. Among its activities are publications, continuing education programs, conferences, scholarships, professorships, and programs for students.[7] It sponsors several publications, *CA: A Journal for Clinicians, Cancer, Cancer News, Cancer Nursing News,* and the newest, *Cancer Practice.* The *Cancer Source Book for Nurses,* first published in 1950, has undergone several revisions, the latest in 1991.[8] The ACS distributes thousands of publications and audiovisual materials to nurses each year. A national conference is held every 2–4 years, a nursing research conference is held every 2 years, and many continuing education programs are held at the local level.

The ACS professorship program was established to

improve the care of the patient and the quality of nursing education in cancer. ACS professors are doctorally prepared experts in cancer nursing engaged in teaching, practice, and research whose salaries and research are funded by local divisions of the ACS. The professorship program was initiated in 1981, and since that time eight ACS local divisions have funded 15 ACS professors.[9]

Oncology Nursing Society

The ONS was incorporated in 1975. It was conceived and organized under the leadership of Marino. It began because Marino, Yarbro, and others wanted to define their roles in cancer care, communicate with oncology nurses in similar roles, and develop continuing education programs.[1,10] Its mission today is to promote excellence in oncology nursing by setting standards, studying ways to improve oncology nursing, encouraging nurses to specialize in oncology nursing, fostering the professional development of oncology nurses, and maintaining an organizational structure responsive to the needs of its members.[11] Today the ONS has over 19,000 members in 148 chapters; over 6000 members attend the annual congress.[12] Activities of the ONS include the annual congress, the fall institute, coordination of 23 special interest groups (SIGs), and publication of *Oncology Nursing Forum* and *Oncology Nursing News*. In addition, there are a number of active committees, including Bylaws and Resolutions, Chapters, Clinical Practice, Congress, Finance, Legislation, Nominating, Nursing Administration, Membership and Public Relations, Education, and Research.

The Education Committee of the ONS has been active over the years in developing standards of education that have had a significant impact on cancer nursing education. The standards developed for the generalist and advanced levels have provided guidelines for curriculum development.

National Cancer Institute

The NCI, established in 1976, has made major contributions to oncology nursing education in a number of ways, including educational programs, work-study programs, fellowship programs, funding for research, predoctoral and postdoctoral research training grants, publications, and providing access to current reliable information through the Cancer Information Service (CIS).

Among some of the educational programs in cancer for nurses funded by the NCI are: a short course in research training for postmaster's, doctoral, and postdoctoral nurses engaged in research; a short course in cancer prevention, detection, and screening for minorities; regional workshops for African American, Hispanic and Native American nurses; and a short course for nurses in developing countries in prevention and early detection.

The NCI also has been instrumental in providing funding for faculty education. In 1950 a 3-week institute on cancer nursing was offered to 30 nursing instructors.[4] Later, surveys by Oberst,[13] Miller and Herbst,[14] and VanScoy-Mosher[15] indicated there was a shortage of programs to prepare nurses to teach in oncology education programs. Because the rapidly expanding knowledge in cancer care required strengthening of oncology programs and because there was concentration of educational programs in large urban areas, a unique project was funded by the NCI. This 5-year project to develop a model for postmaster's fellowship programs in oncology nursing education was intended to increase the number of oncology nurse educators.[16] San Jose State University and the University of Alabama at Birmingham were awarded funds to develop the model curriculum. Thirty-four fellows completed the yearlong program, which included clinical nursing, educator, and change agent roles.

Today, under the Cancer Nurse Training Program, the NCI offers a 9-month clinical traineeship for new baccalaureate graduates. The graduates work and attend classes on current cancer nursing practice and receive a monthly stipend.[17]

Association of Pediatric Oncology Nurses

Another important organization is the Association of Pediatric Oncology Nurses (APON), established in 1973. Among its objectives are to promote excellence in the care of children with cancer, provide communication for nurses, disseminate information about care of patients, encourage publication in professional and lay literature, and support research in pediatric oncology. The activities of the organization include the publication of the *Journal of the Association of Pediatric Oncology Nurses (JAPON)*, a newsletter, and an annual meeting. The organization has more than 900 members.[7]

Scholarships

The existence of a large number of scholarships, fellowships, and other forms of financial assistance has had an important influence on attracting qualified students into cancer nursing programs. In 1981 scholarships for master's-level preparation were established by the ACS.[5,18] Twenty $8000 scholarships are awarded yearly. In 1986 scholarship support at the doctoral level began, and three are awarded each year.[19] To date, 256 ACS scholarships have been awarded at the master's level, while 22 students have received doctoral scholarships. This scholarship program represents a significant investment in cancer nursing education.

The ONS also offers scholarships at both the bachelor's and the master's levels. Since this program has been in existence, many recipients have benefited from the opportunity to attend school.

As mentioned earlier, the NCI offers fellowships at the predoctoral, doctoral, and postdoctoral levels. In addition to scholarships and fellowships, there have been other efforts in the past by the NCI and ACS to encourage nursing students to enter cancer nursing. The ACS sponsored a 6-week summer course for senior students, and in 1971, the NCI in conjunction with the ACS offered a 10-week work-study program for baccalaureate students to increase their skills in caring for persons with cancer in the area of prevention, early detection, diagnosis, treatment, and rehabilitation.[20]

Many hospitals have tuition reimbursement programs that allow students to attend school and pay back the loan in work. If it were not for programs such as these, many nurses would have been unable to get advanced degrees.

Certification

Certification has had a positive influence on cancer nursing. Certification acknowledges nurses' additional education or experience. The level of knowledge of certified nurses is above the level required for licensure, thus protecting the public by demanding a certain level of excellence in those who are certified. The mission of the Oncology Nursing Certification Corporation (ONCC) is to advance oncology nursing through the certification process.[21] Ultimately, the goal of certification is to promote the health and well-being of those diagnosed with or at risk for experiencing cancer.

In 1984 the ONCC contracted with the Educational Testing Service (ETS) to develop a test to assess the general oncology knowledge of the professional nurse.[21] Questions were written by oncology nurses and reviewed by the ONCC Test Development Committee and staff of the ETS. Questions for the 1986–1990 examination were based on the Oncology Nursing Society Core Curriculum. The current examination was based on a study sponsored by the ONCC. This study defined the dimensions of practice of oncology nursing and identified the knowledge required for practice as a competent oncology nurse. This Role Delineation Study, based on the responses of 1297 oncology nurses, formed the blueprint for the new generation of certification examinations in oncology nursing.

The certification examination is open to nurses who have the following:

- a current license
- two and a half years of experience as a registered nurse over the 5-year period prior to application
- at least 1000 hours of oncology nursing practice within two and a half years prior to application

The 3-hour examination consists of 300 multiple-choice questions and covers seven subject areas: cancer nursing practice, major cancers, treatment, issues and trends in cancer care, prevention and detection, pathology, and epidemiology.[21]

Oncology-certified nurses have the opportunity to renew their certification at 4-year intervals. Since 1986, 12,674 nurses have taken the certification examination. To date, 10,158 nurses have passed the examination. Of the nurses who were due to renew their certification in 1990, 598 did not. At the end of 1990, there were 8774 oncology certified nurses. Of these, 77% were ONS members. Fourteen percent (14%) had diplomas, 23% had associate degrees, 45% had bachelor's degrees, 17% had master's degrees, and 1% had doctorates.[12]

CANCER NURSING EDUCATION TODAY

Conceptual Framework

A conceptual framework consistent with the *Outcome Standards for Cancer Nursing Practice* has been developed by the Education Committee of the ONS consisting of four concepts: individual and family, health–illness, health care system, and community–environment.[3] Central to oncology nursing practice is the individual–family concept. The health–illness concept is the adaptation of the individual and family along a continuum. The practice of cancer nursing occurs in the health care system. The community–environment concept provides the resources and support necessary for individuals with cancer. The methods used to organize the knowledge necessary for cancer nursing practice is the nursing process and the research process.

Standards of Oncology Nursing Education

The *Outcome Standards for Cancer Nursing Education at the Fundamental Level* were first published in 1982.[22] The ultimate outcomes of the standards are to enhance the quality of oncology nursing education and to improve the health care for the public. In 1987 the *Scope of Advanced Oncology Practice* was developed and laid the foundation for the development of *Standards for Oncology Nursing Education: Advanced Level.*[23,22] Guidelines for all levels of educational preparation are published in the *Standards of Oncology Nursing Education: Generalist and Advanced Practice Levels.* The purpose of the standards is to provide guidelines to:[22]

- plan and evaluate generalist education encompassing diploma, associate, and baccalaureate programs
- plan and evaluate advanced education at the master's, doctoral, and postdoctoral levels
- plan and evaluate continuing education programs at all levels
- assess individual knowledge of oncology nursing care

At both the generalist and specialist levels, five categories of standards with general descriptive statements relate to faculty, resources, curriculum, the teaching–learning process, and the learner.

Generalist level

The generalist level of cancer nursing, originally referred to as the fundamental level, provides a core of knowledge, skill, and attitudes for beginning practice in cancer nursing. Although the generalist level encompasses diploma, associate, and baccalaureate educational programs, the literature deals only with baccalaureate education.

There are several significant studies that have examined the oncology content at the undergraduate level and contributed to our understanding of existing problems. In 1983 Brown, Johnson, and Groenwald sent a questionnaire to determine the status of cancer education to 982 NLN-accredited schools of nursing.[24] The study was undertaken because of concern that the fundamental education for nurses in cancer care was inadequate. Questions pertained to the content included in the curriculum, educational resources, preparation of faculty, and areas needing improvement. Responses from 672 schools (68%) were obtained. The investigators found that an average of 14.5 classroom hours were devoted to cancer nursing. The content areas inadequately covered included prevention, detection, oncologic emergencies, late effects of treatment, unorthodox treatment, attitudes toward cancer, home care, social issues, political issues, resources, legal implications, and educational resources for nurses. The study suggested that an examination of the undergraduate curriculum was in order.

Pope reports on a similar study conducted in Switzerland by Stoll and Fellinger to identify the place of oncology education in basic programs.[25] Their questionnaire was sent to 50 schools, and 32 (64%) responded. The results were strikingly similar to the study by Brown and her colleagues. The average amount of time devoted to oncology nursing was 14 hours. The investigators concluded that cancer nursing education was inadequate in Switzerland in both quality and quantity. One of the recommendations of this study was to incorporate the practicing oncology nurse specialist into teaching.

Pope surveyed the wishes and needs of oncology students in six basic education programs in Switzerland. She questioned if some oncology content was too well integrated, thereby frustrating students. She suspected integration caused some students to forget that the programs had certain oncology content. Students responding to the survey could not agree as to what areas in oncology were most important in preparing them for care of patients with cancer. The students agreed that clinical experience is helpful and that content should be taught by an oncology nurse active in the field.[25]

Another European study, by Copp, reports the findings of the European commission about the state of cancer nursing in Western Europe. Again, the investigator came to the conclusion that cancer nursing education in Western Europe follows the medical model, the faculty is without oncology experience, there is a paucity of teaching materials, and there is little connection between theory and practice.[26]

Others have argued about the importance of the professional in developing a positive, empathetic attitude toward the patient and family. Fanslow suggested that a lack of educational preparation in oncology led to negative attitudes of both students and nurses.[27] Pope's study confirms the findings that suggest lack of oncology content leads to negative attitudes on the part of students.[25] Welch-McCaffrey[28] suggested that the development of an empathetic attitude toward the care of the patient with cancer is developed at the undergraduate level of nursing education.

Many creative ways to improve curricula in cancer nursing and promote positive attitudes about cancer care at the baccalaureate level have been attempted. Nevidjon and Deatrich offered an intensive 8-week elective course that included lecture, patient care, seminar, skills lab, and individual supervision for senior students. The ONS/ANA *Outcome Standards* provided the organizing framework for the course.[29] Horvitz and Trigg developed a 10-week in-depth cancer course for senior students that included content on the physiological and psychological impact of cancer on the patient, family, and nurse.[30] Mooney and Dudas offered a two-credit 10-week independent course in cancer nursing for eight selected students. Content included the roles and responsibilities of nurses, psychosocial reactions of patients, critical knowledge needed by the oncology nurse, the purposes and activities of the ONS and other cancer organizations, and specialized skills needed to care for patients. Classes were held for 2 hours each week. A field experience at an ACS office, a support group, or observation experience in a hospital was included.[31]

Quinn-Casper and Holgren, also believing that the highly specialized skills needed to care for patients with cancer were not consistently addressed at the baccalaureate level, tried a different approach.[32] Their belief that undergraduate curricula were deficient was based on the results of the survey by Brown and her colleagues.[24] Quinn-Casper and Holmgren developed a program with the ACS to provide supplementary cancer education programs for nursing students. After the first highly successful and well-attended 1-day workshop was held, yearly workshops were instituted. Over 800 students attended the annual 1-day sessions over a 4-year period. Local ACS chapters throughout the country now offer such programs for students.

Daly and Eardmann reported on the use of what they called an oncology search. A study guide consisting of 12 items was used to provide opportunities for students to learn about a variety of topics beyond their assigned readings in an undergraduate course. Participating students became more aware of oncology resources and more interested in cancer nursing.[33]

Although these efforts are commendable, these programs are scarce, and only limited numbers of students are able to benefit. In many other programs, glaring deficiencies still exist. Guidelines for curriculum content have been written, standards exist, teaching materials from the ONS and ACS are available, but many undergraduate curricula still are inadequate in content.

As part of a 5-year federally funded project to increase and improve oncology nursing content in undergraduate programs, Longman and her colleagues initiated several activities.[34] First was the development of two tools, an attitude inventory and a knowledge test. A 30-item test was developed based on the *Outcome Standards.* The results indicated that students in the first semester scored lower than in other semesters, but scores increased as the students progressed through the program. The improvement of scores suggested a better incorporation of essential oncology content by faculty and increased knowledge on the student's part due to participation in the activities of the project. Longman also offered an elective course on cancer care for students, provided opportunities for students to participate in ongoing oncology research, instituted a research symposium, and provided seminars to faculty about latest therapies and care to update their knowledge.[35]

Advanced level

The advanced level of cancer nursing education encompasses graduate education. Education at this level in concerned with the development of a broader scope of practice, coordination, continuity, and evaluation of care. Most of the literature at this level is concerned with master's programs.

The *Master's Degree with a Specialty in Oncology Nursing* is an invaluable tool for faculty of all graduate oncology programs.[36] Its purpose is to provide a role definition and curriculum guide for educators in planning educational offerings as well as a program selection guide for students. The guide encompasses the six content areas of clinical practice, education, consultation, administration, research, and professionalism. Each area is organized by steps of the nursing process, suggested content, and outcome objectives.

At the end of 1991, there were 45 graduate oncology programs listed by the Education Committee of the ONS.[37] Each program has its unique qualities, and any program should be carefully examined before an applicant selects a school.[38] Many questions need to be asked by potential students to assess and choose the appropriate program, including: What is the reputation of the school? Who are the faculty? What are the resources of the school? What will the clinical experiences be like? Will oncology clinical nurse specialists be clinical preceptors? What is the tuition? Are sources of funding or research or teaching assistantship positions available?

As part of a feasibility study to determine the need to develop new graduate programs in oncology nursing, Piemme identified the most significant problems of graduate oncology programs. Of the 21 programs responding, recruitment of students was listed by seven schools and was the most frequently cited problem. Six schools listed lack of financial support, four listed pressures on faculty time, and four listed a need for faculty prepared in oncology nursing as the most significant problem of their graduate oncology programs.[5] Although this study has not been replicated, many of these same problems continue to exist today.

There have been several reports of the development of instruments to test graduate student knowledge, attitudes, and skills. As part of their program evaluation, Piper, Moore, and Dodd studied changes in knowledge and attitudes in two cohorts of graduate students in oncology nursing.[39] Significant improvements were obtained in the knowledge domain, while there was lack of significant changes on the attitude instrument. The faculty also used the test scores to recommend remedial work.

A follow-up study evaluated the students' ability to apply their knowledge to clinical practice during the 2-year master's program.[40] Using the ONS Conceptual Framework as the basis for the Appraisal of Practice Instrument, 39 students were asked to rank the frequency of use and degree of proficiency of each clinical behavior on subscales of Individual and Family, Health and Illness, Health Care System, Community and Environment, Cancer Nursing Process, and Cancer Nursing Research Process. The results show that students rated themselves more proficient in the more frequently used behaviors, gained in proficiency over time, and were more proficient in subject matter that was emphasized in the program.

In a survey of 185 clinical nurse specialists (CNSs) who were ONS members employed in oncology, Yasko found that 69% of the specialists reported they did not have theoretical content or planned experiences in oncology nursing in their graduate programs.[41] Sixty percent (60%) of the sample did not have planned contact with a CNS role model in the curriculum. At first, this lack of preparation in oncology theory and practice during their master's program appears shocking, but it may be explained by the fact that the respondents received their master's degrees from 60 different colleges. Since there were only 45 oncology graduate programs in 1990 and far fewer in 1983, when the study was reported, many of the nurses in the sample must have graduated from schools that did not have oncology programs. In any event, one could question if these specialists met the qualifications for the job at the time they were hired.

Continuing Education

That nurses should participate in CE to maintain and enhance special knowledge and skills unique to oncology nursing seems to be universally accepted. Many CE programs are sponsored by the ONS and ACS, at both the national and the local levels. The content for CE programs in oncology nursing can be identified from many sources, including the ONS publications *Cancer*

Nursing Education at the Fundamental Level, Standards of Oncology Nursing Education, and *Scope of Advanced Oncology Practice.*[3,22,23]

The *Standards for Continuing Education,* published by the American Nurses Association (ANA), may be useful as a general guide for those who plan CE programs.[42] Since 1987 the ONS has been an ANA-accredited approver and provider of CE programs and can provide assistance for planning CE materials and programs. In 1990 the ONS reviewed more than 50 applications for approval of CE programs.[12] Annually the *Oncology Nursing Forum* publishes a list of long-term CE programs, prepared by the Education Committee of the ONS.

Another helpful resource is a series of articles by Fernsler, Volker, Itano, Belcher, and McMillan that describe how to develop and implement a CE program incorporating adult learning principles.[43–47] The articles take the novice through the steps of doing a needs assessment, developing objectives, defining content and methods, and evaluating a program.

The ONS has a responsibility to provide CE to its members to help them acquire the knowledge and skills necessary for competent practice. In order to ensure successful CE program planning, the ONS conducted a needs assessment of its membership to determine learning needs.[48] A questionnaire was developed and mailed to one-half of the membership, or approximately 6500, and 38% responded. The top five topics about which the members said they definitely would attend a seminar were the clinical practice issues of oncologic emergencies, pain, critical care, legal issues, and advanced practice roles.

Donaldson and his colleagues also tried to identify content areas as priorities for planning CE programs.[49] They developed an 87-item knowledge test based on the proposed core curriculum for certification examination. The results indicated that the topics labeled as the highest priority for CE program planning included nursing management of spinal cord compression, electrolyte imbalance, hypercalcemia, susceptibility to depression, treatment modalities such as chemotherapy and safe handling of drugs, prevention and early detection of cancer, characteristics of cancer, ONS standards, and patient advocacy. The nurses who participated in the study were nurses who provided cancer management care and did not designate themselves as oncology specialists.

Bushy and Kost confronted the issue of inaccessibility of CE programs in rural North Dakota and came up with a novel but successful model of delivering CE programs.[50] Recognizing that either hiring a consultant or bringing a prepared program to a small institution is a costly solution, the program planners decided to use Knowles' model of adult learning and place the responsibility for learning in the realm of the learners. The nurses decided on a topic they were interested in, listed objectives, and made active learning assignments. For a CE program on breast cancer the nurses gathered information by seeking out community resources, had mammograms, visited radiation therapy departments, interviewed patients about mastectomies, went to stores that sold prostheses, visited support groups, and participated in other action activities before reconvening to share their information in a CE program. The new CE model was thought to be successful, based on increased attendance and active participation of the nurses in attendance. The model encourages peer discussion and getting to know the community and its resources.

CRITICAL ISSUES AND CHALLENGES

Invitational Conference on the Clinical Nurse Specialist Role

There are a number of critical issues and challenges in cancer nursing that educators must consider and make decisions about. Some of these issues have been raised by clinical specialists. Two invitational conferences on the role of the oncology clinical nurse specialist have been held.[51,52] The first conference was held in 1984, and the recommendations, intended primarily for individuals, were widely read. A study on burnout among oncology clinical specialists was an outgrowth of the conference. The second conference was held in 1991. Among the recommendations for oncology education at the undergraduate level were the following.

- Cancer nursing content needs to be emphasized in classroom and clinical settings using the *Standards of Oncology Nursing Practice and Education.*
- Faculty need updates.
- Hospitals need to use the *Standards of Nursing Practice.*

Specific recommendations to achieve these goals included closer cooperation between the National League for Nursing and the ONS Education Committee; distribution of *Standards of Oncology Nursing Education* and *Standards of Nursing Practice* to all faculty; and identification of model programs. Elective course offerings were encouraged, along with work-study programs, and the use of innovative teaching strategies, including computer-assisted interactive video.

Recommendations also were made for oncology nursing education at the graduate level. It was suggested that the following be more strongly emphasized at the time of the next revision of the standards:

- physical assessment
- clinical decision making
- prevention, screening, and early detection
- care of high-risk and underserved clients, such as the elderly and socioeconomically disadvantaged
- public health policy
- basic sciences, especially immunology

- developing skills for proposal development
- role immersion
- state-of-the-art communication systems
- alternative health care settings
- marketing the role
- mandatory clinical component

Certainly, one cannot argue with the recommendations. However many schools already include this content or are working on the implementation of some of these ideas. Some of the recommendations warrant further consideration, discussion, and implementation by educators.

Continuing Education

The invitational conference on the role of the oncology clinical nurse specialist did not specifically address CE and its role in meeting some of the recommendations. Since baccalaureate and master's educational programs do not always have the time or the flexibility to include all things, continuing education must be relied on to provide some of the content that cannot be dealt with within the confines of a curriculum. It may be necessary to establish separate, more definitive standards for informal and formal educational levels.

Recruitment of Students

Much effort needs to go into recruitment of highly qualified students at all levels, especially at the master's and doctoral levels, to ensure an adequate supply of clinicians, specialists, teachers, and researchers in oncology nursing. Because admissions to nursing programs at both the undergraduate and graduate levels have decreased over the past few years, effort must be made to try to attract the traditional as well as the older, nontraditional student, an often untapped source. In order to do so, more flexibility may be needed in programs and course offerings, for more students may need to study part-time, due to high tuition costs and family responsibilities.

Also, recruitment of minority nurses is crucial. A critical mass of minority nurses who can work with minority populations to encourage prevention and early-detection practices is needed to make an impact on cancer care in this group of patients and reduce high mortality rates. Studies have suggested that someone from the same culture is the best provider for the socioeconomically disadvantaged.[53] Creative clinical placements and experiences may need to be explored in order to reach the target population of patients. Some nontraditional settings that might be used are screening programs in food pantries, feeding centers, or storefront free health clinics, and church- or school-sponsored screening programs. Once enrolled in nursing programs, financial, academic, and other supportive services must be provided to ensure student success.

More students from other countries are studying in schools in the United States. Many of these students need assistance with socialization and language skills and other types of support. It is important that resources be identified to help foreign students with the transitions needed.

Prevention and Early Detection

More emphasis must be placed on prevention, risk reduction, and early-detection activities. Most authorities believe that a large number of cancers can be prevented by choosing a healthier lifestyle. In addition, it is estimated that one in four persons could be saved through early detection. The NCI has proposed that cancer mortality be reduced by 50% by the year 2000. Currently, much of the activity in prevention and early detection is concentrated on breast, cervical, and lung cancer, with the majority of activity related to breast cancer. Nurses can have a powerful impact on patients in prevention and early-detection activities for the major sites of cancer. The nurse's role in primary and secondary prevention of cancer has been well documented by Frank-Stromborg and Rohan.[54]

Practitioner or Specialist

In order to provide the care necessary to meet the challenges of the twenty-first century, highly knowledgeable, highly skilled nurses who can function in multiple roles and settings are crucial. Certainly, a combined clinical nurse specialist and nurse practitioner role is essential to meet future challenges. Traditionally, most oncology programs have prepared clinical nurse specialists, who have provided exemplary care, made extraordinary contributions, and moved the nursing profession ahead. However, in today's health care arena, a clinical nurse specialist with practitioner skills is required to meet the varied needs of persons with cancer and their families in a variety of settings.

Standards and the Curriculum

Faculty should be familiar with the recommended curriculum and follow the guidelines set forth in the *Standards*. As mentioned earlier, efforts began in the 1950s to incorporate cancer nursing into the curriculum. Now, almost 40 years later, we are still struggling to incorporate cancer nursing content at the undergraduate level. It is crucial that basic information about oncology be included in baccalaureate programs. We have the tools and faculty, but curricula vary greatly in cancer content. Perhaps more definitive guidelines at the undergraduate level need to be written, similar to the master's degree guidelines.

While still in school students should be encouraged to share their knowledge, skills, and expertise with others. The nursing curriculum should include content on publishing. Practicing nurses at all levels need to share ideas to improve oncology nursing practice. Craytor reported that the *Nursing Studies Index* listed only three articles by nurses about oncology nursing between 1900 and 1930.[4] The first oncology nursing textbook was not published until 1967, by Bouchard.[55] Today there are several journals devoted to oncology nursing and numerous textbooks. Although there has been exponential growth in the numbers of publications by oncology nurses, still more creative work needs to be shared.

Students also need public-speaking skills and media awareness training and should be well-versed in the legislative process and public policy issues. A working knowledge of nursing informatics and hospital information systems is essential. *Nursing informatics* is the science of the properties, structure, storage, and transmission of nursing knowledge. Hospital information systems involve the dedicated use of computers to collect, store, process, retrieve, and communicate patient care and administrative information to support those who provide care. It is imperative that graduates of nursing programs be computer literate and knowledgeable about using information by way of electronic networks.

Students should be encouraged to participate in local and national ACS and ONS activities or, if in pediatrics, APON activities. Participation should be mandatory, particularly at the graduate level. The meetings and conferences held by these organizations offer many opportunities to participate on committees, speak at meetings, and hold office. The opportunities to network with others, share ideas, and interact with the leaders in oncology nursing abound in these organizations, and can enhance one's career.

Teaching Approaches

Adult learning principles must be employed in our curricula. Reed Ash reminds us that we live in an ever-changing health care environment that requires us to change not only the way patient care services are provided but also the way we educate nurses to provide these services.[56] She cites the rising cost of health care, the increasingly sophisticated technologies, the increase in complex treatment protocols, and the demand for more and better health care as catalysts for change in our educational approaches. It is essential to develop program content and structure learning experiences at all levels that acknowledge the nurse as an adult learner. Adult learning concepts—including problem-centered approaches to teaching, immediate application of knowledge, recognition of individual experience, flexible scheduling, and self-directed learning—must be incorporated into educational offerings. In addition, computer-assisted instruction (CAI) needs to be incorporated into curricula.

Faculty Competence

Faculty at all levels need to be prepared in oncology nursing. In addition, faculty need to be both knowledgeable in the latest trends and clinically competent. Attendance at oncology continuing education programs or required certification may help, but this will not completely solve the problem. The clinical doctorate (DNS and DNSc) is not a solution to clinical competence unless the graduates of these programs find ways to keep their skills and expertise current. Although some schools allow faculty to have joint appointments, this is not feasible for all faculty. New and different ways to ensure competency must be explored.

New forms of collaboration between faculty and clinical staff could be developed to provide faculty entrance and exposure to the clinical arena. A faculty consultation service in clinical sites could be developed that could provide benefits to all involved. Faculty have much theoretical knowledge that could be shared with clinical staff, while the faculty could get an update on current clinical practice. Another innovation might be joint research projects between faculty and clinical specialists that would allow faculty exposure to current clinical problems. Faculty collaboration with the nursing staff on clinical papers could also help keep faculty abreast of current practice issues. Faculty could assist staff with publication while keeping up to date on the latest in practice. Other ways to update faculty may already exist, but these need to be shared in the literature so others can benefit.

Program Evaluation

Evaluation of oncology programs should be an ongoing process. However, very few program evaluation studies have been published.[24–26,34,35,39,40] Results of studies and evaluation tools need to be shared so our programs can continue to develop.

Preceptors and Clinical Facilities

Nursing educators must continue to nurture clinical preceptors to act as role models for students in clinical agencies. Faculty need to assume responsibility for preparing clinical preceptors to work with students. Seminars devoted to adult learning principles, evaluation, and how to deal with the difficult student may be helpful in preparing preceptors for their roles. It is essential to recognize the contributions made by preceptors to our clinical programs and to give recognition for their time and commitment to student learning. Such recognition could be in the form of appointment as adjunct faculty, which will allow library privileges and attendance at school functions, or editorial assistance with manuscripts could be offered to encourage publication.[57] Close cooperation between teachers and clinicians is essential to belie the old dichotomy between education and practice.

Doctoral Education

Well-qualified students and graduates of master's programs should be encouraged to continue their education in doctoral programs. Doctorally prepared oncology nurses are needed to ensure high-quality education, research, and practice in the future.

Complex Care

Advances in technology and early-discharge practices have changed both inpatient and outpatient care. The use of ambulatory services has greatly escalated because of technological advances, changes in reimbursement, and consumer choice. It is estimated that nearly 90% of cancer care is delivered in the outpatient setting. Patients cared for in the home today are far sicker, with many more complex needs, than hospital patients of yesterday. This calls for changing roles and responsibilities of nurses in ambulatory and home settings, and more emphasis on these roles must be given in the curriculum.

Certification and Recertification

Certification offers many benefits to the individual: increased visibility, peer recognition, self-satisfaction, and sometimes an edge in the job market. Sixty percent of the nurses certified in 1986 took the recertification examination. This is comparable to other specialty organizations.[12] However, less than half of ONS members are certified. Efforts need to continue to increase the numbers of members who are certified. The question of recertification may need to be explored further to determine if reexamination is the best alternative for keeping the knowledge and practice of the membership current. In the near future the advanced-practice examination will be prepared. This will have to be evaluated as we have more experience.

Meeting New Health Care Challenges

Today more than 6 million Americans are survivors of cancer, and it is expected that by the twenty-first century over 65% of persons diagnosed with cancer will survive longer than 5 years. This will have an enormous impact on delivery of services, rehabilitation, and quality-of-life issues. While more people are living with cancer, more and more people are becoming infected with HIV and dying of AIDS. It is expected that 20,000 children will have AIDS by the year 2000. Nurses must be prepared to meet the challenges of a diverse spectrum of patients and problems. The content of our educational programs must reflect the current and future problems and concerns of the health care arena. We can never become complacent about what we do in cancer education or practice, for new challenges continually arise, requiring innovative solutions and application of new knowledge and skills.

As Craytor wrote in 1982, oncology nurses face complex problems.[4] It is necessary to nurture and support all members of the specialty, for competition and jealousy can interfere with a powerful, united front. She added that collaboration on the health care team is essential, and suggested that we focus on cost-effective practices and maintain adaptability to changing scientific, social, and economic conditions.

SUMMARY

Much has been accomplished in oncology nursing. Many fine educational programs exist at all levels of undergraduate, graduate, and continuing education. Oncology nursing has enjoyed strong support from many organizations. Many nurses have been certified in oncology nursing. A large number of highly motivated, highly effective, highly productive oncology clinical nurse specialists prepared at the master's level have made numerous contributions to the specialty. Many more doctorally prepared oncology nurses are now available than ever before, and they have made numerous contributions to practice, education, and research. Craytor said, "We owe much to the bold, intelligent, persuasive, and clinically able nurses who pioneered in the field. They were and are a truly remarkable group."[4,p.57]

Oncology nurses should be proud of their accomplishments, but at the same time they must recognize the continual need to update knowledge, skills, and competence. We cannot abandon the good things that have been achieved over the years, such as the certification program, the development of standards, curriculum guides, scholarships, ACS professorships, and high-quality meetings, conferences, and congresses; nor can we rest on our laurels. We need to continue to evaluate, change, improve, and think in new and creative ways and always be prepared to meet new challenges as they arise.

REFERENCES

1. Hilkemeyer R: A historical perspective in cancer nursing. *Oncol Nurs Forum* 9(2):47–56, 1982.
2. Diller D: *An Investigation of Cancer Learning in Ninety Se-*

lected Schools of Nursing. Third Report. Saratoga Springs, NY: Skidmore College, 1957.

3. Oncology Nursing Society: *The Outcome Standards for Cancer Nursing Education at the Fundamental Level.* Pittsburgh, PA: Oncology Nursing Society, 1982.
4. Craytor JC: Highlights in education for cancer nursing. *Oncol Nurs Forum* 9(4):51–59, 1982.
5. Piemme JA: Oncology clinical nurse specialist education. *Oncol Nurs Forum* 12(2):45–48, 1985.
6. Longman AJ: Cancer nursing education. In Groenwald SL, et al (eds.): *Cancer Nursing: Principles and Practice.* Boston: Jones and Bartlett, 1990, pp. 1256–1269.
7. Greene PA, Ades T: Cancer organizations. In Baird SB, McCorkle R, and Grant M (eds.): *Cancer Nursing: A Comprehensive Textbook.* Philadelphia: Saunders, 1991, pp. 1162–1172.
8. Baird SB (ed.): *A Cancer Source Book for Nurses* (ed. 6). Atlanta: American Cancer Society, 1991.
9. American Cancer Society: Three nursing professorships approved. *Cancer Nurs News* 10(2):3, 1992.
10. Yarbro CH: The history of cancer nursing. In Baird SB, McCorkle R, and Grant M (eds.): *Cancer Nursing: A Comprehensive Textbook.* Philadelphia: Saunders, 1991, pp. 10–20.
11. Oncology Nursing Society: ByLaws. May 1991.
12. Oncology Nursing Society, Oncology Nursing Certification Corporation, Oncology Nursing Foundation: 90/91 Annual Report. *ONS News* 6(7), 1991 (suppl.).
13. Oberst M: Priorities in cancer nursing research. *Cancer Nurs* 1:281–290, 1978.
14. Miller S, Herbst S: Summary of ONS membership survey. *Oncol Nurs Forum* 5:22–23, 1978.
15. Van Scoy-Mosher C: *Oncology Nursing Survey.* Pittsburgh, PA: Oncology Nursing Society, 1979.
16. Siegele D: Longitudinal evaluation of a model post-master's program in oncology nursing education. *Oncol Nurs Forum* 11:61–62, 1984.
17. National Cancer Institute: *Cancer Nurse Training Program.* Washington DC: National Institutes of Health, 1987.
18. American Cancer Society: *Master's degree students: Scholarships in cancer nursing.* #0306. Atlanta: American Cancer Society, 1992.
19. American Cancer Society: *Doctoral degree students: Scholarships in cancer nursing.* #0351. Atlanta: American Cancer Society, 1992.
20. Barckley V: Workstudy program in cancer nursing. *Nurs Outlook* 19:328–330, 1971.
21. Oncology Nursing Certification Corporation: *Oncology Nursing Certification Bulletin.* Pittsburgh, PA: Oncology Nursing Society, 1992.
22. Oncology Nursing Society Education Committee. Standards of Oncology Nursing Education: *Generalist and Advanced Practice Levels.* Pittsburgh, PA: Oncology Nursing Society, 1989.
23. Oncology Nursing Society: *Scope of Advanced Oncology Practice.* Pittsburgh, PA: Oncology Nursing Society, 1987.
24. Brown JK, Johnson, JL, Groenwald SL: Survey of cancer nursing education in U.S. schools of nursing. *Oncol Nurs Forum* 10:82–83, 1983.
25. Pope S: Fundamentals for a new concept of oncology nursing in the professional nursing education program. *Cancer Nurs* 15:137–147, 1992.
26. Copp K: Education and training in cancer: A European perspective. *Cancer Nurs* 11:255–258, 1986.
27. Fanslow J: Attitudes of nurses toward cancer and cancer therapies. *Oncol Nurs Forum* 12:42–45, 1984.
28. Welch-McCaffrey D: Promoting the empathetic development of nursing in the care of the patient with cancer. *J Nurs Ed* 23:37, 1986.
29. Nevidjon B, Deatrich, J: Oncology clinical elective. *Oncol Nurs Forum* 12:57–59, 1985.
30. Horvitz I, Trigg JM: Registered nurses and nursing students learn together in a cancer nursing course. *Nurs Educat* 12:6, 18, 42, 1987.
31. Mooney M, Dudas S: Undergraduate independent study in cancer nursing. *Oncol Nurs Forum* 14:51–3, 1987.
32. Quinn-Casper P, Holmgren C: Enhancing cancer nursing concepts in undergraduate curricula. *Cancer Nurs* 10:274–278, 1987.
33. Daly J, Eardmann W: Oncology search: An innovative teaching method. *Nurs Educat* 13:28–30, 1988.
34. Longman AJ, Verran JA, Clark M: Oncology knowledge inventory for undergraduate students. *Oncol Nurs Forum* 18:107–111, 1991.
35. Longman A, Verran J, Clark L: Improving oncology nursing content in an undergraduate program. *J Nurs Ed* 27:42–44, 1988.
36. Oncology Nursing Society, American Nurses Association: *The Master's Degree with a Specialty in Oncology Nursing.* Pittsburgh, PA: Oncology Nursing Society, 1988.
37. ONS Education Committee: Survey of graduate programs in cancer nursing. *Oncol Nurs Forum* 18:1402–1414, 1991.
38. ONS Education Committee: Assessing Masters' programs in oncology nursing. *Oncol Nurs Forum* 18:1401–1402, 1991.
39. Piper B, Moore I, Dodd M: Changes in cancer-related knowledge and attitudes: One graduate curriculum's experience. *Cancer Nurs* 8:272–277, 1985.
40. Moore IM, Piper B, Dodd MJ, et al: Measuring oncology nursing practice: Results from one graduate program. *Oncol Nurs Forum* 14:45–49, 1987.
41. Yasko J: A survey of oncology clinical nursing specialists. *Oncol Nurs Forum* 10:25–30, 1983.
42. American Nurses Association: *Standards for Continuing Education in Nursing.* Kansas City, MO: The Association, 1984.
43. Fernsler J: Developing continuing education programs in cancer nursing: An overview. *Oncol Nurs Forum* 14:59–60, 1987.
44. Volker DL: Learning needs assessment. *Oncol Nurs Forum* 14:60–62, 1987.
45. Itano J: Developing educational objectives. *Oncol Nurs Forum* 14:62–65, 1987.
46. Belcher A: Defining content and methods. *Oncol Nurs Forum* 14:65–67, 1987.
47. McMillan S: Program evaluation. *Oncol Nurs Forum* 14:67–70, 1987.
48. Itano J, Miller CA: Learning needs of Oncology Nursing Society members. *Oncol Nurs Forum* 17:697–706, 1990.
49. Donaldson WS, Glass EC, Helmick F, et al: Determining continuing education priorities in cancer management for nurses. *Oncol Nurs Forum* 15:625–630, 1988.
50. Bushy A, Kost S: A model of continuing education for rural oncology nurses. *Oncol Nurs Forum* 17:207–211, 1990.
51. Donoghue M, Spross J: Report from the First National Conference. *Oncol Nurs Forum* 12:35–73, 1985.
52. Spross JA, Gallagher J, Powel LL: Conference recommendations: Practice administration research education

and health care policy. *Oncol Nurs Forum* 19:32–41, 1992 (suppl.).

53. American Cancer Society: *Special Report on Cancer in the Economically Disadvantaged.* New York: The Society, 1986.
54. Frank-Stromborg M, Rohan K: Nursing's involvement in the primary and secondary prevention of cancer. *Cancer Nurs* 15:79–108, 1992.
55. Bouchard R: *Nursing Care of the Cancer Patient.* St. Louis: Mosby, 1967.
56. Reed Ash C: Education: A case for change. *Cancer Nurs* 8:A15, 1985 (editorial).
57. Hagopian GA, Ferszt GA, Jacobs LA, et al: Preparing clinical preceptors to teach master's level students in oncology nursing. *J Prof Nurs* 8:295–300, 1992.

Chapter 64

Cancer Nursing Research

Marcia Grant, RN, DNSc, FAAN, OCN

Geraldine Padilla, PhD

Betty Ferrell, PhD, RN, FAAN

INTRODUCTION

Research has provided critical knowledge concerning the care of cancer patients. Basic science, medical science, and nursing science all form the foundation important in the prevention, detection, treatment, and management of cancer. The focus of this chapter is the role of the cancer nurse in the implementation of medical research and in the development, implementation, dissemination, and application of cancer nursing research. An examination of the role of the nurse in each of these activities provides a basis for understanding the rapid development of nursing research in the provision of care for today's cancer patient.

RESEARCH DEFINED

Research involves a structured approach to answering questions or discovering new knowledge.[1] It is conducted for the broad purpose of increasing scientific knowledge. Research can be replicated, and is considered valid only when it is replicated. The process of research involves an orderly and standardized series of steps. These steps can be compared to the steps in the nursing process; that is, both processes are specialized forms of problem solving.[2] Differences between the two involve the amount of detail and the accuracy of measurement. In addition, research focuses on a group of patients and includes the obligation to disseminate the results for critique by others. A comparison of the research and nursing processes is found in Table 64-1.

In the developmemt of cancer treatment, medical research is used to describe the natural history of the diseases, to test new treatment approaches, and to evaluate the value of singular and multimodal approaches to cancer treatment. Through these endeavors have developed surgical, chemotherapeutic, radiation, biologic, and genetic approaches to cancer treatment, as well as the use of supportive care measures.[3–5]

TABLE 64-1 Comparison of Clinical Nursing and Research Processes

Steps Involved	Clinical Nursing	Nursing Research
Defining the problem	Individual patient assessment	Identify area of concern
	Nursing diagnosis	• Review literature and select a conceptual or theoretical framework • Conduct preliminary studies • Define methods • Select population • Define designs • Define samples • Operationally define variables • Describe procedures • Identify data analysis
Carrying out the action	Intervention implementation	• Implement study • Accrue consenting subjects • Administer standardized tools • Check reliability of data collection
Evaluating the results	Outcome evaluation	• Code and analyze data • Interpret findings • Publish results

CLINICAL TRIALS

The Clinical Trials Approach

The medical research approach to clinical investigation of cancer treatment methods has resulted in a specialized approach called the clinical trials approach.[6] Developed and encouraged under the influence of studies funded by the National Cancer Institute (NCI), this approach involves several phases of studies, each designed to answer specific clinical questions at a different time in the development of applied scientific knowledge. Each study, or research protocol, includes a well-written and detailed guide for implementation.

Clinical trials are divided into phase I, II, and III studies.[6] Each has a different purpose and design. After testing of medical treatment approaches (surgical, chemotherapeutic, or radiation) with appropriate animal or cell models, phase I studies are implemented as the first clinical tests of new treatments on human patients. The purpose of a phase I study is the determination of dose schedules and toxicities, and the focus is on the drug or treatment. Because new drugs and treatments are involved, the population eligible to participate in phase I clinical trials includes patients for whom standard therapy has failed. Since the determination of how to use a drug or treatment in a phase I clinical trial has not yet been made, patients for whom standard treatments can be issued are *not* eligible or enrolled in them.

Data in phase I clinical trials include determination of the maximum tolerated drug (MTD) and toxicities. Pharmacokinetic data on the medication being tested may be conducted as well. Thus the collection of timed specimens is common and demands precision of the nursing staff implementing the protocol. A current example of a phase I trial is the use of new, investigational

Partial support provided by NIH Cancer Support Grant CA-33572.

drugs for patients for whom standard chemotherapy has failed and who are not eligible for other treatments, such as radiotherapy. A phase I clinical trial requires the smallest number of patients needed to determine at what dose or schedule of treatments toxicities occur. Frequently, the only benefit to the phase I patient is the satisfaction of having contributed to scientific knowledge for treatment of other cancer patients. However, patients often view participation in a phase I study with hope—for prolongation of life for themselves or for others.

In phase II trials, the focus shifts to specific tumor types for which the treatment appears promising.[6] To be eligible for phase II trials, patients must either be unable to participate in standard therapy or have failed standard therapy. Specific tumors are selected that have shown some positive responses in preclinical or phase I trials. A current example of a phase II trial is the use of lymphokine-activated killer (LAK) cells and interleukin 2 for patients with colorectal cancer and renal cell carcinoma. Toxicities during phase II trials frequently are profound, and close monitoring of patients is necessary to provide data for evaluation of patient response and early detection of toxicities.

The focus shifts again for phase III studies,[6] which determine (1) the effects of a treatment relative to the natural history of the disease, (2) whether a new treatment is more effective than a standard therapy, and (3) whether a new treatment is as effective as a standard therapy but associated with less morbidity. In phase III trials, the focus is on comparing a new treatment with the standard treatment. These studies involve randomization of patients to the experimental or the standard treatment.

Phase I clinical trials are implemented only at NCI-designated cancer centers (Table 64-2). This is to ensure availability of the full spectrum of clinical support needed in studies in which toxicities are unpredictable and close monitoring of patients is critical. Depending on the nature of the treatment being tested, phase II trials may also be conducted in NCI-designated cancer centers. Phase III trials, which require the greatest number of subjects to answer the research question, are conducted in large medical centers, university hospitals, and community centers with qualified cancer researchers and needed clinical support resources.

Participation of cancer patients in all three kinds of clinical trials has been the critical element in the rapid development of current cancer treatment options. Through clinical trials we have developed options for primary breast cancer treatment involving either radiation therapy or surgery, and options for Hodgkin's disease involving either chemotherapy or radiation therapy. An interesting corollary to this approach to medical research is the increased participation and involvement of the patient in the selection of medical treatment. Today, an informed citizen may read about a new cancer treatment in the newspaper and seek out a physician who is able to provide that approach to treatment.

Settings for Cancer Research

Medical research related to cancer treatment may be conducted in a number of settings. Four types of cancer centers are defined by the NCI. Though together all four types provide a broad foundation of peer-

TABLE 64-2 NCI-Designated Cancer Centers

ALABAMA
University of Alabama
Comprehensive Cancer Center
Birmingham, AL

ARIZONA
Arizona Cancer Center
Comprehensive Cancer Center
Tucson, AZ

CALIFORNIA
Kenneth Norris Jr. Comprehensive Cancer Center
Los Angeles, CA

Jonsson Comprehensive Cancer Center
Los Angeles, CA

La Jolla Cancer Research Foundation
La Jolla, CA

University of California, San Diego, Cancer Center
San Diego, CA

Beckman Research Institute/
City of Hope Cancer Research Center
Duarte, CA

Armand Hammer Center for Cancer Biology
Salk Institute
San Diego, CA

COLORADO
University of Colorado Cancer Center
Denver, CO

CONNECTICUT
Yale Comprehensive Cancer Center
New Haven, CT

DISTRICT OF COLUMBIA
Lombardi Cancer Research Center
Comprehensive Cancer Center
Washington, DC

FLORIDA
Sylvester Comprehensive Cancer Center
Miami, FL

ILLINOIS
University of Chicago Cancer Research Center
Chicago, IL

(continued)

TABLE 64-2 NCI-Designated Cancer Centers (continued)

INDIANA
Purdue Cancer Center
West Lafayette, IN

MAINE
The Jackson Laboratory
Bar Harbor, ME

MARYLAND
Johns Hopkins Oncology Center
Comprehensive Cancer Center
Baltimore, MD

MASSACHUSETTS
Dana-Farber Cancer Institute
Comprehensive Cancer Center
Boston, MA

Worcester Foundation for Experimental Biology
Shrewsbury, MA

Massachusetts Institute of Technology
Center for Cancer Research
Cambridge, MA

MICHIGAN
Comprehensive Cancer Center of Metropolitan Detroit
Detroit, MI

University of Michigan Comprehensive Cancer Center
Ann Arbor, MI

MINNESOTA
Mayo Clinic Comprehensive Cancer Center
Rochester, MN

NEBRASKA
Eppley Institute
Omaha, NE

NEW HAMPSHIRE
Norris Cotton Cancer Center
Comprehensive Cancer Center
Lebanon, NH

NEW YORK
Cold Spring Harbor Laboratory
Cold Spring Harbor, NY

Memorial Sloan-Kettering Cancer Center
Comprehensive Cancer Center
New York, NY

Roswell Park Cancer Institute
Comprehensive Cancer Center
Buffalo, NY

Albert Einstein College of Medicine Cancer Research Center
Bronx, NY

Columbia University Comprehensive Cancer Center
New York, NY

Kaplan Comprehensive Cancer Center
New York, NY

NEW YORK (continued)

University of Rochester Cancer Center
Rochester, NY

PENNSYLVANIA
Wistar Institute Cancer Center
Philadelphia, PA

Fels Research Institute
Philadelphia, PA

Pittsburgh Cancer Institute
Comprehensive Cancer Center
Pittsburgh, PA

RHODE ISLAND
Roger Williams Medical Center
Cancer Center
Providence, RI

TENNESSEE
St. Jude Children's Research Hospital
Memphis, TN

Drew-Meharry-Morehouse Consortium Cancer Center
Nashville, TN

TEXAS
M.D. Anderson Cancer Center
Comprehensive Cancer Center
Houston, TX

Institute for Cancer Research & Care
San Antonio, TX

UTAH
Utah Regional Cancer Center
Salt Lake City, UT

VERMONT
Vermont Regional Cancer Center
Comprehensive Cancer Center
Burlington, VT

VIRGINIA
Massey Cancer Center
Richmond, VA

University of Virginia School of Medicine
Cancer Center
Charlottesville, VA

WASHINGTON
Fred Hutchinson Cancer Research Center
Comprehensive Cancer Center
Seattle, WA

WISCONSIN
University of Wisconsin Comprehensive Cancer Center
Madison WI

McArdle Laboratory for Cancer Research
Madison, WI

Source: NCI Cancer Centers Branch, Division of Cancer Biology, Diagnosis, and Centers. Bethesda, MD: NCI, 1993.

reviewed research activities, they differ from each other in the type of research conducted. *Basic science centers* conduct laboratory research (for example, research on the biology of cancer). *Clinical cancer centers* conduct a combination of basic and clinical research. *Comprehensive cancer centers* conduct the same kind of research as clinical cancer centers, plus cancer control research and community outreach activities. *Consortium centers* involve clinical and cancer control research, plus cancer control activities.

Cancer control research focuses on the reduction in incidence of cancer by primary and secondary disease prevention activities. Medical research related to cancer treatment may be conducted at any of these settings. Oncology nurses have been involved in all aspects of these studies, ranging from extravasation studies that use animal models, to clinical trials of experimental therapies, to research and activities on cancer prevention and early detection.

The conduct of phase I clinical trials is restricted to NCI-designated cancer centers. However, because of the low number of cancer patients proportionately treated at cancer centers, programs have been developed to allow patients at community agencies to participate in cancer treatment research. Thus, phase II and III clinical trials are conducted at institutions with cooperative arrangements with NCI-designated cancer centers. This not only means a larger number of patients is available for research accrual, it also provides patients with options unavailable in the practices of their own private physicians. As more patients become involved in phase II and III trials, results will accumulate more rapidly and new, successful treatments may be demonstrated earlier and made available to a wider spectrum of patients.

Studies on cancer treatment are also conducted by principal investigators not located at NCI-designated centers. Thus, nurses from a variety of settings may be involved in medical research and learn a variety of research skills useful in nursing studies as well.

The Cancer Research Team

Implementation of clinical trials for cancer is carried out by a multidisciplinary research team composed of: principal investigator, co-investigator, research or protocol nurse, data manager, investigational pharmacist, statistician, and clinical nursing staff. Clinical nurses are important members of this team.

Principal investigator The principal investigator, generally a physician, is responsible for the scientific integrity of the study. Responsibilities include development of the protocol, presentation of the study to the institutional review board for review of appropriate informed consent procedures, and implementation of the study.

Co-investigator Co-investigators may include other physicians whose patients may be eligible for the study and other scientists (e.g., molecular biologists, psychologists) interested in other aspects of cancer patients' responses.

Research or protocol nurse The research nurse is responsible for patient accrual, implementing the physician's orders as described in the protocol, and observing patient responses and toxicities. In implementing the role, the nurse is involved in informed consent issues, astute clinical care, and education of supporting nursing staff.

Although the principal investigator is legally responsible for obtaining informed consent from the patient, all members of the research team share this responsibility.[7] The research nurse ensures that patients understand what has been defined as the treatment, what the risks and benefits are, what alternative treatment approaches are available, and what the probability is that the patient will receive personal benefit from the treatment. This is especially important if the patient is participating in phase I or II clinical trials, wherein personal benefit to the individual patient is infrequent or nonexistent. Since many patients are reluctant to ask questions of the physician, the nurse frequently is in a position to answer patients' questions, explain further, define more clearly, and generally help the patient understand the research. Identification of patients who obviously do not understand either the treatment approach or the implications of the research in relation to personal benefits requires that the principal investigator be notified, so that before any treatment is administered further clarification of the patient's concerns is provided and any possibility of coercion is eliminated.

The nurse also carries out astute clinical care in implementing the study for the research patient. Since many of the patients on phase I and phase II trials may develop profound toxicities, the observation and reporting of these toxicities is critical for safe patient care. The nurse is in a key position to monitor the patient's symptoms and report toxicities that are a threat to the patient's comfort. For some studies, toxicities are unknown, and life-threatening complications are a possibility. Both anticipated and unanticipated toxicities occur, making it essential for the nurse to observe patients frequently and thoroughly.

The observation and evaluation of toxic responses to the research protocol are important priorities in clinical research trials. When the research or protocol nurse is not available, those responsibilities must be delegated to someone else. Thus a major responsibility of the protocol nurse is the education of the patient's caregiver. Education may involve the clinical nursing staff, the patient, and/or the family or significant other. Depending on the protocol, observations for specific reactions may be necessary. For example, nausea and vomiting may be an expected toxic response, but they need to be monitored and treated so that nutritional depletion does not occur. The patient and the caregiver need to know when to notify the physician or the research nurse of side effects. The use of one-on-one teaching followed by discussion of standard educational materials is a common and effective way to provide the patient with the information needed to recognize and report significant toxic effects.

Data manager The role of the data manager is to collect the information on toxicities from the chart and to enter these data into the computer for statistical analysis. Various forms in the chart are used. Laboratory responses, pathology reports, and physician's progress notes are frequent sources of data. The toxicity data usually are collected from standardized forms, including a grading system for rating various symptoms. The data manager does not have to be a nurse, and thus the job description generally does not include any clinical observations for which clinical nursing skills are needed.

Investigational pharmacist The investigational pharmacist is a part of the team when the focus of the clinical trial is chemotherapy. Many phase I and II trials involve investigational drugs, which are not available for public use and for which specific records need to be kept. The investigational pharmacist is responsible for dispensing these medications and for making sure that the records on the drugs are in order. This person also is usually the first to learn about changes in drug administration, dosage changes, problems reported by other research institutions, and reclassification of the medications. Once a drug moves from an investigational status to being a medication available for general use (usually with a physician's prescription), it is no longer available free of charge. This change could have a major impact on the patient's ability to continue the protocol.

Statistician The statistician is responsible for a variety of activities in relation to a clinical trial. These include determination of initial sample size, study design and protocol review, data evaluation and analysis, interpretation of findings and preparation of manuscripts. Frequently, data managers report to the statistician, and protocol tracking, randomization, data entry, and statistical analysis are carried out in the department of biostatistics. This support is vital to maintaining the integrity of the study design.

Clinical nursing staff Members of the clinical nursing staff make up the remainder of the research team. While most of the patients on medical research protocols are hospitalized, other settings may be involved as well. Thus, staff includes nurses in hospital units, ambulatory care settings, physicians' offices, and home care agencies. The protocol nurse frequently is involved in the education of clinical nursing staff, ensuring that patient assessments are relevant and charted. Introduction and explanation of toxicity rating forms frequently are needed. The clinical nursing staff have a major contribution to make in terms of patients' responses to the research therapy.

The Chemotherapy Research Nurse

Chemotherapy nurses assumed one of the first specialty roles in the development of the cancer nursing practice. These nurses were responsible for the administration and monitoring of chemotherapy They accrued patients to medical protocols, administered medications, counseled patients on management of side effects, collected data, and kept the physicians informed of the patients' conditions. Because of the complex nature of the medications and their potentially lethal side effects, chemotherapy nurses sought out and developed an extensive knowledge base about chemotherapeutic principles. Their involvement with accruing, monitoring, and teaching chemotherapy patients increased their familiarity with the clinical chemotherapy research process. These nurses were among the first nurses to participate as collaborators in cancer research.[7] With their research skills as background, many of them sought further education and developed into primary investigators, interested in either medical or nursing aspects of cancer care.

The first survey of research skills of Oncology Nursing Society (ONS) members conducted by the ONS Research Committee revealed that a large proportion of oncology nurses had participated in a variety of steps in the research process.[8] This has been confirmed in subsequent ONS research surveys.[9–11] These surveys also identified research activities and research support provided and projected by the Oncology Nursing Society. Research grants, needed publications, abstract sessions, and the success of the Advanced Research Special Interest Group and the research Mentorship Program of the ONS Research Committee all provide evidence of the rapid development of the independent research role for the oncology nurse.[11]

NURSING RESEARCH

The focus of nursing research differs from that of medical research. Nursing research is defined as the systematic investigation of the responses of patients to actual or potential health problems.[12] Nursing research focuses on the patient rather than on the disease, and may encompass biologic, psychologic, and social aspects.

Because of the profound effect of cancer and cancer treatment on the patient, cancer nursing care has provided a rich source of questions and problems for nursing research investigators. The inclusion of a large proportion of data-based articles in cancer nursing journals (e.g., *Oncology Nursing Forum* and *Cancer Nursing*) attests to the flourishing amount of nursing research relevant to cancer care. This discussion will examine the development of cancer nursing research by focusing on the role of the nurse in clinical research, emphasizing the increasing participation in research, and the priorities for research questions as identified by cancer nurses. A summary of major areas of cancer nursing research is used to exemplify recent activity. This is followed by a discussion of the resources available for cancer nurses.

Role of the Nurse in Clinical Research

Currently the nurse has several roles in the implementation of research for cancer patients. For the protocol nurse or the clinical staff nurse, the role is that of a member of the research team conducting medical research. Another role is as an initiator of a study conducted along with a medical protocol. This arrangement has been useful in testing a variety of nursing approaches. Advantages include the participation of patients already involved in another study and the provision of many of the basic demographic and treatment variables needed for study analysis. Cotanch's work on relaxation for chemotherapy-related nausea and vomiting provides a good example of such a study.[13]

The nurse may also act as a principal investigator, initiating the study, writing the protocol, selecting the subjects, and evaluating the results. The growing number of nurses participating as principal investigators is evident from one of the ONS Research Committee surveys.[10] The advantage of this trend is that study results can expand the knowledge basic to the development of nursing science. Several recent developments have made the expansion of cancer nursing research possible. Priorities have developed that reflect clinical needs. Resources for nursing research have increased and include financial as well as knowledge dissemination opportunities.

Priorities for Cancer Nursing Research

One method that has proved useful in the development of depth in the scientific foundation for nursing practice has been a systematic targeting of researchers and resources to areas of needed knowledge. The identification of priorities for studies has provided information useful in the development of a program for nursing research that leads to well-tested areas of study. With such an approach, the accurate information needed for development of clinical nursing practice is possible. The National Center for Nursing Research has been involved in identification of clinical nursing research priorities through the development of a national nursing agenda.[14] One aspect of this endeavor has been to seek out research priorities identified by various nursing groups.

Cancer nursing research priorities have been identified and revised over the years. One of the first reports was published by Oberst.[15] This list of priorities was developed through a Delphi survey technique in which 254 oncology nurses participated. The following five top-priority areas were identified:

1. relieving nausea/vomiting induced by chemotherapy/radiation
2. pain management
3. discharge planning and follow-up
4. grief and death
5. stomatitis

This study was followed by several others conducted through the Oncology Nursing Society, the Canadian Consortium, and the National Cancer Institute.[8–10,16,17] The most recent survey is that by Mooney and colleagues.[11] This survey was sent to a convenience sample of 429 ONS members, with a return of 310 (70% return rate). The educational distribution among respondents was diploma or associate degree 9%, baccalaureate degree 14%, master's degree 48%, and doctoral degree 19%. The survey revealed an average of 18 years of nursing experience, with nearly 12 years in oncology nursing. Researchers and ONS leaders were the only members selected for this survey. Thus this survey may not represent the Oncology Nursing Society membership. Table 64-3 compares the top ten cancer nursing research priorities for 1981–1991. Changes that have occurred include the rise of quality of life to first place in 1991, the persistence of symptom management, pain control and management, prevention and early detection, cancer rehabilitation, and economic influence on oncology. Newcomers to the top ten priorities for 1991 included quality of life, outcome measures for interventions, cancer survivorship, and cost containment. Another newcomer to the list was research utilization.

Factors that may contribute to changes in priorities are as follows. The emphasis on quality of life as a critical outcome of all cancer treatment occurred in response to the National Cancer Institute's policy to include quality of life as an outcome measure in all clinical trials.[18] Additionally, there is a growing awareness of the need to consider the quality-of-life costs of cancer treatment. Outcome measures for intervention reflect recognition of the shift from process-oriented to outcome-oriented research. Since the quality of a process is not always reflected in the effectiveness of the process, it is critical for nurses to focus on the effectiveness of interventions. Cancer survivorship reflects an ever-increasing awareness of the chronic nature of cancer and the recognition of the burden of cancer care on family and the health care system. Along that same vein is the issue of cost containment. The newcomer, research utilization, is appropriate to the current state of an expanding science of nursing. Nursing research has established a critical mass of studies in specific areas, giving rise to a focus and an interest in nursing research utilization. Persistence of some topics illustrates the continued need for research in those areas.

Major Areas of Current Cancer Nursing Research Activity

To provide an accounting of recent progress in cancer nursing research, a search of the *Cumulative Index for*

TABLE 64-3 Comparison of Top Ten* ONS Research Interests/Priorities, 1981–1991

1981 Survey		1984 Survey		1988 Survey		1991 Survey	
Rank	Interest	Rank	Interest	Rank	Priority	Rank	Priority
1	Patient/health education	1	Pain control and management	1	Prevention and early detection	1	Quality of life
2	Coping and stress management	2	Symptom management	2	Symptom management	2	Symptom management
3	Pain control and management	3	Patient/health education	3	Pain control and management	3	Outcome measures
4	Family support	4	Coping and stress management	4†	Patient/health education	4	Pain control and management
5	Symptom management	5	Role of the specialist	4†	Coping and stress management	5	Cancer survivorship
6	Nurse burnout	6†	Professional issues	5	Home care	6	Prevention and early detection
7	Prevention and early detection	6†	Patient support system	6	Economic influences	7	Research utilization
8	Hospice care	6†	Oncology nurse characteristics	7	Cancer rehabilitation	8†	Cancer rehabilitation
9	Nutrition	8	Counseling	8	AIDS	8†	Economic influences
10	Counseling	9	Home care	9	Compliance with treatment	9	Family issues

*Based on total number of votes.

†Tied for rank.

Source: Data from Grant and Stromberg,[8] McGuire et al,[9] Funkhouser and Grant,[10] and Mooney et al.[11]

Nursing and Allied Health Literature (CINAHL) was made for the 3 1/2 years from 1989 to 1992. The major focus was nursing research studies in the area of cancer; the key words used were *cancer* plus *nursing research.*

The most studies were found in the areas of pain (25 references), quality of life (15 references), patient education (33 references), coping (17 references), stress (11 references), home care (18 references), and self-care (15 references). Of the topics identified in the 1991 ONS Research Priorities Survey, quality of life and pain received attention, as evidenced by publications indexed in the Cumulative Index for Nursing and Allied Health.

Quality-of-life research

The 1980s and early 1990s witnessed a growing nursing interest in quality-of-life research. (In 1983, the CINAHL introduced the subject heading *quality of life* into its database.)[19] Interest in quality of life and cancer nursing culminated in 1992, with two requests for applications (RFAs) for research grants from the National Center for Nursing Research (NCNR) and the National Cancer Institute. One RFA addresses interventions to enhance adjustment to cancer risk or diagnosis;[20] the other addresses quality-of-life assessment in special populations.[21]

Oncology nursing investigators have provided conceptual definitions of quality of life. For example, Ferrans defined quality of life as "a person's sense of well-being that stems from satisfaction or dissatisfaction with the areas of life that are important to him/her." [22,p.15] Grant and colleagues defined quality of life as "a personal statement of the positivity or negativity of attributes that characterize one's life."[23,p.261] Young and Longman focused on the subjective dimensions of quality of life, i.e., individual aspirations, frustrations, attitudes, and perceptions.[24] Lewis equated personal control with quality of life.[25,26]

Cancer nursing researchers have examined the domains of the concept of the quality of life. Cain and Henke described attributes that influenced quality of life: pain, nausea, vomiting, work, leisure activity, dependency needs, future concerns, and religious beliefs.[27] Freidenbergs and colleagues interviewed cancer patients about problems with physical discomfort, medical treatment, hospital service, mobility, housework, vocational activities, finances, family, social, worry, affect, body image, and communication changes and the extremity of these changes.[28] Padilla and colleagues, via open-ended interviews with 40 patients with chronic pain from cancer, identified three dimensions of quality of life: psychologic, physical, and interpersonal well-being.[29] Others have focused on specific dimensions of quality of life, such as symptom distress (McCorkle and colleagues[30–32]) and social dependency (Benoliel, McCorkle, and Young[33]).

Oncology nursing has led the effort to develop reliable and valid instruments to measure quality of life. In 1981, a medical oncologist, Presant, together with a nurse and a social worker, Klahr and Hogan, developed a brief set of linear analog scales to measure quality of life.[34] Later, Padilla, Grant, and colleagues[35,36] and Ferrell and colleagues[37,38] expanded on this instrument, calling it the Quality of Life Index. Through different versions of the instrument, these investigators measured quality of life as a multidimensional construct characterized by psychologic well-being, physical well-being, symptom control, nutritional concerns, social concerns, and affective states.[52] This scale has been renamed the Multidimensional Quality of Life Scale[53] to distinguish the instrument from those of Ferrans and Powers[39] and of Spitzer and colleagues.[40]

Stromborg and Wright's Health Survey identifies the specific areas that are changed by the disease (cancer), the patient's perception of the severity of the change, and the patient's attitude toward the alteration in life style.[41] Content validity was established with 340 cancer patients.

Ferrans and Powers developed an instrument they called the Quality of Life Index.[39] The instrument measures satisfaction with various domains of life and the importance of these domains to the subject. Both parts of the instrument include 32 items that assess health care, physical health and functioning, marriage, family, friends, stress, standard of living, occupation, education, leisure, future retirement, peace of mind, personal faith, life goals, personal appearance, self-acceptance, general happiness, and general satisfaction. Subjects respond on a six-point Likert-type scale from "very satisfied" to "very dissatisfied" and from "very important" to "very unimportant." The instrument has appropriate levels of reliability and validity.[22,37,39]

Oncology nursing studies have focused on several significant clinical objectives related to quality of life. One important objective concerns the description of patient psychosocial and physical responses to specific diseases. For example, Young and Longman reported an inverse relationship of quality of life to symptom distress and social dependency, and a positive relationship of quality of life to behavior-morale in melanoma patients.[24] A second clinical objective examines symptom management responses to disease and treatment. Ferrell and colleagues showed that cancer pain was associated with quality-of-life indicators such as fatigue, nausea, appetite disturbance, anxiety, fear, and depression.[38,42] A third objective relates to comparisons of patient responses to treatment. Sarna described the effects of the initial cycle of chemotherapy on quality of life and functional status in adults over 65 years of age with non-small-cell lung cancer. She found that older adults were more severely limited in physical dimensions of quality of life, and had less psychosocial problems except in the areas of cognition and worries about family coping. Older adults had less disruption in marital function than younger adults. She also found that subjects with comorbid diseases had lower quality of life.[43] Lewis focused on families of cancer patients to determine the influence of disease and treatment on the family's quality of life.[44] A fourth objective demonstrates the effect of specific rehabilitative approaches. A fifth objective concerns the identification of vulnerable periods in the health–illness continuum. Grant and colleagues discussed the importance of tracking fluctuations in physical and psychologic distress throughout the course of the disease and treatment to anticipate the times when quality of life is at a low.[23] McCorkle and colleagues discuss home nursing care for lung cancer patients.[31]

Cancer nursing has played a prominent role in encouraging clinical interest in quality-of-life research. For example, nursing played an important role in the introduction of quality-of-life measures in cancer clinical trials in the Southwest Oncology Group in 1988.[45,46] In 1990, *Seminars in Oncology Nursing* dedicated an issue to quality-of-life assessment in clinical practice.[47] The issue includes discussions of single[19] and multiple measures[48] of quality of life. The first pre- and postdoctoral nursing research training program in health-related quality of life was launched in 1992 at the University of California, Los Angeles, School of Nursing. Research training focuses mainly on quality of life in cancer and other chronic disease populations.

Of the major nursing associations, the Oncology Nursing Society leads the way in support of research, with an annual Quality of Life Award and an annual Quality of Life Lecture at its Fall Institute. Through the ONS Research Committee, reviews of quality-of-life measures were undertaken and published in 1988, under the editorship of Dr. Frank-Stromborg, as *Instruments for Clinical Nursing Research*.[49] Quality-of-life instruments were discussed in two chapters, one dedicated to single measures of quality of life[50] and another to multiple measures.[51] This book has served to disseminate information about quality-of-life measures in nursing.

In summary, oncology nursing maintains a vital interest in quality-of-life issues, as reflected in numerous articles in scientific journals, only a few of which are listed here. The scope of cancer nursing's commitment to promoting quality-of-life research includes studies to describe quality of life, develop measures, and test interventions to promote it in different cancer populations; conferences to disseminate information; pre- and postdoctoral training programs to foster research interest; and awards for excellence in research.

Cancer nursing research on pain

Advances in pain management have undoubtedly been influenced by knowledge derived from nursing research. The nursing profession has developed as a scholarly discipline in recent years in concert with the development of oncology as a nursing specialty. Oncology nurses have made important contributions in the areas of pain assessment, interventions, and eradication of factors that impede pain relief. Nursing studies related to pain have been identified through a review of the oncology nursing literature. Investigators were invited to summarize their research and published work. These contributions were used to identify major areas of work. Table 64-4 lists but a few examples of the vast contributions nurses have made to the research on the topic of cancer pain.[55–107] The table has been organized into several categories: (1) pain as a component of oncology nursing, (2) pain assessment, (3) nursing knowledge and attitudes regarding pain, (4) pharmacologic interventions, (5) nursing models of pain intervention, and (6) other contributions.

TABLE 64-4 Examples of Nursing Contributions to Pain Research

Principal Nurse Investigator	Contribution
	PAIN AS A COMPONENT OF ONCOLOGY NURSING
McCaffery[55]	Established pain as a priority for nursing care, and the independent function of nurses in the assessment and management of pain; identified the patient as the expert in pain
Benoliel[56–57]	Recognition of pain as a critical issue in cancer nursing and as a major symptom in terminal illness
Copp[58,59]	Recognition of the nurse's role in chronic pain management; identified the suffering dimension of pain
Jacox[60]	Identified pain as a component of nursing care; independent nursing assessment and interventions for pain
McCorkle[30,61,62]	Development of Symptom Distress Scale; examined pain management outside of inpatient setting
Oncology Nursing Society[63,108]	Comfort is identified as a component of cancer nursing in the *Standards of Oncology Nursing Practice;* the ONS *Position Paper on Pain* provides a comprehensive statement on cancer pain, including nursing involvement in practice, education, and research
	PAIN ASSESSMENT
Hester[64,65]	Assessment of pain in children; evaluation of pain assessment tools for children; assessment of children's pain by health care providers
Dalton[66,67]	Role of biobehavioral and environmental factors and affective states in cancer pain; development of a scale to measure the range of cognitive, behavioral, and physiologic responses to pain
McGuire[68]	Assessment of pain in cancer inpatients; evaluation of McGill Pain Questionnaire
Eland[69,70]	The pain experience in children; assessment of children's pain
Donovan[71]	Incidence and characteristics of pain in cancer inpatients; problem of inadequate analgesic dosages
Wilkie[72–74]	Numerous studies related to pain assessment, validation of pain assessment scales, meta-analysis of McGill Pain Questionnaire; behavioral dimensions of pain, including pain expression, behaviors to control pain, and behaviors prevented by pain
Ferrell[75]	Pain assessment in the elderly, including special characteristics of the elderly and evaluation of instruments to assess pain in the elderly
McCaffery[76,77]	Explored factors influencing nursing assessment of pain, including patient behaviors, age bias, nurse and patient characteristics
Sheidler[78,79]	Correlations between patients' and professional caregivers' assessment of pain; validation of the Hopkins Pain Rating Instrument
Schmitt[80]	Perceptions of patients, family members, and health professionals of the meaning of pain and pain intensity ratings
	NURSING KNOWLEDGE AND ATTITUDES REGARDING PAIN
Dalton[81]	Nurses' perceptions of their pain assessment skills and pain management practices
Ferrell[82]	Pain content in nursing textbooks; faculty knowledge, attitudes on pain
McCaffery[83,84]	Nurses knowledge of opioids and addiction; factors influencing nurses' assessment of pain and decisions regarding pain medications; nurses' knowledge of equianalgesia
Sheidler[85]	Nurses' ability to recognize appropriateness and safety of analgesic orders written by physicians
Watt-Watson[86]	Lack of knowledge in nursing students and nurses related to pain assessment and narcotic administration
	PHARMACOLOGIC INTERVENTIONS FOR PAIN
Coyle[87–89]	Patterns of opioid use and routes of drug administration in terminal cancer patients; pain management using subcutaneous opiate administration; self-medication program for oncology inpatients

(continued)

TABLE 64-4 Examples of Nursing Contributions to Pain Research (continued)

Principal Nurse Investigator	Contribution
	PHARMACOLOGIC INTERVENTIONS FOR PAIN
Sheidler[90]	Comparison of intravenous methadone and morphine
Wilkie[91,92]	Use of continuous-infusion intraspinal analgesia for pain relief
Paice[93–95]	Intrathecal morphine for intractable cancer pain; long-term implanted pumps
Ferrell[42,96–98]	Pain management at home, including drug adherence and nondrug interventions; evaluation of controlled-release morphine and application of quality of life as an outcome variable in an analgesic clinical trial
McGuire[99]	Fixed-interval vs as-needed dosing; adherence to prescribed analgesics
	NURSING MODELS OF PAIN INTERVENTION
Coyle[100]	Model of care for cancer patients and families; demonstrated ability to manage complicated pain problems in the home setting
Ferrell[101]	Evaluation of a nurse-managed pain service
McCorkle[62]	Nursing care at home for patients in pain; survival analysis for comparison of symptoms predictive of patient survival
	OTHER CONTRIBUTIONS
Rhiner (in progress)	Needs of family caregivers related to use of PCA at home
Ferrell[102]	Pain management as a quality-assurance outcome
Grant (in progress)	Hospital readmissions related to uncontrolled pain and associated costs
Dalton[103]	Patient education regarding cognitive and behavioral strategies for pain control; locus of control related to pain
Williams (in progress)	Defining costs in pharmacologic management of cancer pain; comparison of costs associated with oral, parenteral, and intraspinal opioids
Ferrell[104–106]	Ethical issues and clinical decisions by nurses, patients, and family caregivers, related to pain; family factors in cancer pain management
McGuire[107]	Nondrug interventions used by cancer outpatients and their effectiveness

Pain as a component of oncology nursing The first important contribution to pain research by nurse investigators was the identification of pain as a component of oncology nursing. McCaffery provided a critical foundation for nursing research in pain by identifying the patient as the expert in pain assessment and the independent functions of the nurse in managing pain.[55] Oncology nursing pioneers included researchers such as Benoliel and Crowley.[56] Benoliel and McCorkle,[57] Copp,[58,59] and Jacox[60] made enormous contributions in early literature and emphasized the importance of symptom control for the person with cancer.

Another final important contribution that firmly established pain as a dimension of oncology nursing was the identification of comfort as a basic goal of cancer nursing. The ONS *Standards of Practice* identify 11 high-incidence problem areas for oncology, of which comfort is one.[108] These standards have directed the ONS to establish many activities related to pain management. This commitment to pain management by the profession was reinforced by the publication in 1991 of the comprehensive ONS *Position Paper on Pain*.[63]

Pain assessment A second major contribution has been made in the area of pain assessment, an area that has likely seen the most abundant contribution from nurse investigators. McGuire[68] and Donovan and colleagues[71] are examples of researchers whose work has identified the incidence and characteristics of pain in cancer patients and evaluated pain assessment tools. Pain assessment has been extended to special populations, such as children[64,65,69,70] and the elderly.[75]

Research in pain assessment has also been extended to more complex issues. Dalton and co-workers have explored the role of biobehavioral and environmental factors, and affective states associated with cancer pain.[66,67] Continued evaluation of the validity and reliability of assessment tools has been an important component in the progress of pain research.[72–74,78,79]

Nurse investigators such as McCaffery, Sheidler, and

Schmitt also have identified the discrepancy in pain assessment between the patient and others, such as nurses, physicians, and family members.[76–80] Their work has reinforced the importance of relying on the patient as the expert source of pain assessment.

Nursing knowledge and attitudes regarding pain A third contribution has been in the area of nursing knowledge and attitudes regarding pain and the resulting effect on pain relief. The first step in any change process is identification of the problem. Investigators such as Dalton and Watt-Watson have identified the gross lack of knowledge by nurses regarding basic principles of pain relief.[81,86] Recently, McCaffery et al.[83,84] and Sheidler et al.[85] extended this research to explore nursing knowledge specific to pharmacology in areas such as equianalgesia, opioid addiction, and appropriate dosing. Based on the inadequacies in nursing textbooks and in nursing faculty, nursing education about pain has been identified as an area requiring attention essential to the basic preparation of nurses.

Pharmacologic interventions A fourth major area of nursing research related to pain has been pharmacologic interventions. Although physicians prescribe analgesics, nurses have been intimately involved in all aspects of drug management of pain, including patient education, appropriate dosing, conversion between drugs, route of administration, and evaluating the impact of various drug interventions on the patient in pain. McGuire and co-workers conducted basic research evaluating fixed interval versus as-needed dosing and patient adherence to prescribed analgesics.[99] Ferrell et al. explored drug management by patients at home and the impact of morphine use on quality of life.[42,96–98]

Advances in pain management have led to the introduction of new routes of drug administration and the use of technology. These modalities have been tested by nurse researchers. Coyle and co-workers have explored self-medication for inpatients and subcutaneous infusions.[87–89] Sheidler and colleagues compared intravenous morphine with intravenous methadone use, which was important in establishing morphine as the optimum medication for pain.[90] Wilkie[91,92] has evaluated continuous infusion of intraspinal analgesia for pain relief, and Paice[93–95] examined the use of intrathecal morphine for intractable pain and the long-term use of implanted pumps.

Nursing models of pain intervention An important yet understudied area of pain research has been the evaluation of nursing models of pain intervention. Coyle et al. pioneered research that evaluates the role of the nurse in supportive care.[100] McCorkle and colleagues[62] and Ferrell and co-workers[101] also attempted to document the contributions of nurses in pain management. This is clearly an important area for future research and an essential component of the many emerging nursing roles in pain management.

Other contributions Several other contributions have occurred in recent years that explore significant issues related to pain. The role of the patient's family in pain management is a new area of exploration, as is the evaluation of patient education related to pain.[103–106] Although in the literature there are many discussions related to the use of nondrug interventions, unfortunately, few researchers have evaluated these interventions.[107]

Ethical issues related to pain and its treatment are also an emerging area of research.[104–106] Related to this topic is the evaluation of costs of pain treatment, which is in progress by Grant and by Williams.

In summary, nursing research has made major contributions to research on pain and pain management. Studies include identification of pain as a component of oncology nursing, pain assessment, nursing knowledge and attitudes regarding pain, pharmacologic interventions for pain, and nursing models for pain intervention. These studies provide a basis on which to build future studies.

Resources for Oncology Nursing Research

Financial support for oncology nursing research has expanded in the last few years, and is a major resource for the growth of cancer nursing research activities. While some research can be carried out with a minimum of expense, most research requires financial support for literature searches, proposal development time, supplies, space, data management, secretarial assistance, statistical analysis, and manuscript preparation. Support is available in both educational and clinical settings.

One source increasingly available to nurses is internal support at one's own institution. This is an especially valuable resource for the investigator with limited or no grant-writing experience. In educational institutions, seed money frequently is available through the school or college of nursing as well as from the general institutional budget. These funds are specifically focused toward increasing research productivity in faculty.

Biomedical support grants from the federal government are available for both educational and clinical institutions that have already achieved a specific level of research support from the government. These biomedical support monies are used to fund beginning or pilot studies that are expected to develop into large-scale projects submitted for outside funding. Each institution establishes criteria by which these funds are distributed.

External funds are available for individual investigators to apply to and can be divided into those available from the government and those available from private foundations. For cancer nursing research, two major sources for federal funds are the National Center for Nursing Research and the National Cancer Institute. Federal funds for research support, by far the biggest resource for research funding, are distributed through a well-defined application and review process. A valuable resource for cancer nurses seeking federal funds is the *NIH Guide for Grants and Contracts,* published by the National Institutes of Health. This document, mailed at regular intervals, lists grant programs and deadline dates for grants and contracts administered by the NIH, provides program descriptions, and calls for research proposals in specific problem areas. This free publication can be ordered from: NIH Guide, Distribution Center, National Institutes of Health, Room B4B-N-08, Bldg. 31, Bethesda, MD 20892.

Private funds for cancer nursing research have expanded. The Oncology Nursing Foundation funds a variety of research projects yearly. Sigma Theta Tau, both the national organization and local chapters, fund many research projects. Multidisciplinary private groups funding oncology nursing research include the American Cancer Society and the Robert Wood Johnson Foundation. Information about these funds is available from the Oncology Nursing Foundation. This financial support has increased through the last few years, as the educational background and experience of cancer nurses has increased and the demand for research support has risen.

Resources for oncology nursing research have changed over the last few years, and these changes have been positive. Increased financial support has become available. The education and experience of oncology nurses reflect increased academic preparation for research and increased involvement in a variety of research activities. These resources will continue to expand the knowledge base of cancer nursing care as studies become more sophisticated and are replicated.

Future Directions for Cancer Nursing Research

Review of the cancer nursing research conducted reveals areas where clusters of studies have begun, such as quality of life and pain, and areas where much work is still needed, such as prevention and early detection, management of symptoms such as fatigue and anxiety, and approaches to nursing care for special populations such as ethnic minorities, the young, and the elderly. Support for these areas, while limited and competitive, is available through the NIH and private organizations. Development of programs of research where studies build on one another provides for sequential scientific knowledge. Research utilization cannot be emphasized enough as the critical step to applying findings of studies to the daily care of patients. Utilization of the clinical trials approach to nursing research and multisite studies are ways that will provide efficient designs with large enough populations that generalization may become possible.

SUMMARY

Research continues to be an important aspect of the cancer nursing specialty. Both medical and nursing research activity are important in improving the care, treatment, and quality of life for patients with cancer. A review of the nature of research in cancer care and of nursing research activities provides ample evidence of the essential role that nurses play in this aspect of care. Recent review of cancer nursing research publications reveals a rapidly growing body of valuable studies. Nurses have made and will continue to make important contributions through research endeavors.

REFERENCES

1. Polit D, Hungler B: *Nursing Research: Principles and Methods* (ed. 3). Philadelphia: Lippincott, 1987.
2. Padilla GV: Incorporating research in a service setting. *JONA* 9:44–49, 1979.
3. Eilber FR: Principles of cancer surgery. In Haskell CM (ed.): *Cancer Treatment* (ed. 2). Philadelphia: Saunders, 1985, 7–13.
4. Rubin P: The emergence of radiation oncology as a distinct medical specialty. *Int J Radiat Oncol Biol Phys* 2:1247–1270, 1985.
5. Jenkins J: Biology of cancer: Current issues and future prospects. *Semin Oncol Nurs* 8:63–69, 1992.
6. Cassidy J, Macfarlane DK: The role of the nurse in clinical cancer research. *Cancer Nurs* 14:124–131, 1991.
7. Hubbard SM: Cancer treatment research: The role of the nurse in clinical trials of cancer therapy. *Nurs Clin North Am* 17:763–783, 1982.
8. Grant M, Stromborg M: Promoting research collaboration: ONS research committee survey. *Oncol Nurs Forum* 8(2):48–53, 1981.
9. McGuire D, Frank-Stromborg M, Varricchio C: 1984 ONS research committee survey of membership's research priorities. *Oncol Nurs Forum* 12(2):99–103, 1985.
10. Funkhouser SW, Grant MM: 1988 ONS survey of research priorities. *Oncol Nurs Forum* 16:413–416, 1989.
11. Mooney KH, Ferrell BR, Nail LM, et al: 1991 Oncology Nursing Society research priorities survey. *Oncol Nurs Forum* 18:1381–1388, 1991.
12. American Nurses' Association: *Nursing—Social Policy Statement.* Kansas City, MO: American Nurses' Association, 1980.
13. Cotanch PH: Relaxation training for control of nausea and vomiting in patients receiving chemotherapy. *Cancer Nurs* 6:277–283, 1983.
14. Hinshaw AS, Heinrich J, Bloch D: Evolving clinical nursing research priorities: A national endeavor. *J Prof Nurs* 4:398, 458–459, 1988.
15. Oberst M: Priorities in cancer nursing research. *Cancer Nurs* 1:281–290, 1978.
16. Degner L, Arcand R, Chekryn J, et al: Priorities for cancer nursing research. *Cancer Nurs* 10:319–326, 1987.

17. Dodd M: Problems approaches and priorities in oncology nursing research. *AARN Newsletter* 43(2):13–14, 1987.
18. National Cancer Institute: Measurement of progress against cancer. *J Natl Cancer Inst* 82:825–836, 1990.
19. Lockwood, D (ed.): *Cummulative Index for Nursing and Allied Health Literature*. Glendale, CA: CINAHL Information Systems, 1992.
20. National Cancer Institute: *Interventions to Enhance Adjustment to Cancer Risk or Diagnosis*. RFA CA/NR-92-26. Bethesda, MD: National Cancer Institute, 1992.
21. National Cancer Institute: *Quality of Life Assessment in Special Populations*. RFA CA/NR-92-27. Bethesda, MD: National Cancer Institute, 1992.
22. Ferrans CE: Development of a quality of life index for patients with cancer. *Oncol Nurs Forum* 17:15–19, 1990 (suppl.).
23. Grant M, Padilla GV, Ferrell BR, et al: Assessment of quality of life with a single instrument. *Semin Oncol Nurs* 6:260–270, 1990.
24. Young KJ, Longman AJ: Quality of life and persons with melanoma: A pilot study. *Cancer Nurs* 6:219–225, 1983.
25. Lewis FM: Attributions of control, experienced meaning, and psychosocial well-being in patients with advanced cancer. *J Psychosoc Oncol* 7:105–119, 1989.
26. Lewis FM: Experienced personal control and quality of life in late stage cancer patients. *Nurs Res* 31:113–119, 1982.
27. Cain M, Henke C: Living with cancer: A random sample of 50 patients in a hematology-oncology clinic. *Oncol Nurs Forum* 5:4, 1978.
28. Freidenbergs I, Gordon W, Hubbard M, et al: Assessment and treatment of psychosocial problems of the cancer patient: A case study. *Cancer Nurs* 3:111, 1980.
29. Padilla GV, Ferrell B, Grant MM, et al: Defining the content domain of quality of life for cancer patients with pain. *Cancer Nurs* 13:108–115, 1990.
30. McCorkle R, Young K: Development of a symptom distress scale. *Cancer Nurs* 1:373–378, 1978.
31. McCorkle R, Benoliel JQ, Donaldson G, et al: A randomized clinical trial of home nursing care for lung cancer patients. *Cancer* 64:1375–1382, 1989.
32. McCorkle R: The measurement of symptom distress. *Semin Oncol Nurs* 3:248–256, 1987.
33. Benoliel J, McCorkle R, Young K: Development of a social dependency scale. *Res Nurs Health* 3:3–10, 1980.
34. Presant CA, Klahr C, Hogan L: Evaluating quality-of-life in oncology patients: Pilot observations. *Oncol Nurs Forum* 8:26–30, 1981.
35. Padilla GV, Grant MM: Quality of life as a cancer nursing outcome variable. *Adv Nurs Sci* 8:45–60, 1985.
36. Padilla GV, Presant C, Grant MM, et al: Quality of life index for patients with cancer. *Res Nurs Health* 6:117–126, 1983.
37. Ferrell BR: Development of a quality of life index for patients with cancer: Critique of the study. *Oncol Nurs Forum* 17:20–21, 1990 (suppl.).
38. Ferrell BR, Wisdom C, Wenzl C, et al: Effects of controlled-release morphine on quality of life for cancer pain. *Oncol Nurs Forum* 16:521–526, 1989.
39. Ferrans CE, Powers MJ: Quality of life index: Development and psychometric properties. *Adv Nurs Sci* 8:15–24, 1985.
40. Spitzer WO, Dobson AJ, Hall J, et al: Measuring the quality of life of cancer patients. A concise QL-Index for use by physicians. *J Chronic Dis* 34:585–597, 1981.
41. Stromborg M, Wright P: Ambulatory cancer patients' perceptions of the physical and psychosocial changes in their lives since the diagnosis of cancer. *Cancer Nurs* 7:117, 1984.
42. Ferrell BR, Wisdom C, Wenzl C: Quality of life as an outcome variable in the management of cancer pain. *Cancer* 63:2321–2327, 1989.
43. Sarna LP: Impact of chemotherapy on the quality of life and functional states of older adults with non-small-cell lung cancer. University of California, San Francisco, 1989 (diss.).
44. Lewis FM, Ellison ES, Woods NF: The impact of breast cancer on the family. *Semin Oncol Nurs* 1:206–213, 1985.
45. Moinpour CM, Feigl P, Metch B, et al: Quality of life end points in cancer clinical trials: Review and recommendations. *J Natl Cancer Inst* 81:485–495, 1989.
46. Moinpour CM, Hayden KA, Thompson IM, et al: Quality of life assessment in Southwest Oncology Group trials. *Oncology* 4:79–89, 1990.
47. Varricchio CG, Ferrans CE: Quality of life assessment in clinical practice. *Semin Oncol Nurs* 6(4) (entire issue), 1990.
48. Jalowiec A: Issues in using multiple measures of quality of life. *Semin Oncol Nurs* 6:271–277, 1990.
49. Frank-Stromborg, M (ed.): *Instruments for Clinical Nursing Research*. Norwalk, CT: Appleton & Lange, 1988.
50. Frank-Stromborg M: Single instruments for measuring quality of life. In: Frank-Stromborg M (ed.): *Instruments for Clinical Nursing Research*. Norwalk, CT: Appleton & Lange, 1988, pp. 79–95.
51. Dean H: Multiple instruments for measuring quality of life. In: Frank-Stromborg M (ed.): *Instruments for Clinical Nursing Research*. Norwalk, CT: Appleton & Lange, 1988, pp. 97–106.
52. Padilla GV: Validity of health-related quality of life subscales. *Prog Cardiovas Nurs* 7(2):13–20, 1992.
53. Padilla GV, Mishel MH, Grant MM: Uncertainty, appraisal and quality of life. *Q Life Res* 1:155–165, 1992.
54. Ferrell BR, Rhiner M, Grant M: Pain management, nursing contributions through pain research presented at the Proceedings of the sixth national conference on cancer nursing. Seattle, WA: American Cancer Society, 1991.
55. McCaffery M: *Nursing Management of the Patient with Pain*. Philadelphia: Lippincott, 1979.
56. Benoliel JQ, Crowley DM: The patient in pain: New concepts. *Nurs Digest* 5:41–48, 1977.
57. Benoliel JQ, McCorkle R: A holistic approach to terminal illness. *Cancer Nurs* 1:143–149, 1978.
58. Copp L: The spectrum of suffering. *Am J Nurse* 74:63–67, 1974.
59. Copp L: The nurse's role in chronic pain management. In: Burrows GD, Elton D, Stanley GV (eds.). *Handbook of Chronic Pain Management*. Amsterdam: Elsevier, 1987, pp. 227–242.
60. Jacox AK: *Pain: A Source Book for Nurses and Other Health Professionals*. Boston: Little, Brown, 1977.
61. McCorkle R, Quint-Benoliel J: Symptom distress, current concerns and mood disturbance after diagnosis of life-threatening disease. *Soc Sci Med* 17:431–438, 1983.
62. McCorkle R, Benoliel J, Georgiadou F: The effects of home care on patient's symptoms, hospitalizations, and complications. In: Funk S, Tornquist EM, Champagne MT, et al (eds.): *Key Aspects of Comfort: Management of Pain, Fatigue and Nausea*. New York: Springer, 1989, pp. 303–317.
63. Spross JA, McGuire DB, Schmitt RM: *Oncology Nursing*

Society Position Paper on Cancer Pain. Pittsburgh, PA: Oncology Nursing Press, 1991.

64. Hester N, Barcus C: Assessment and management of pain in children. *Pediatr Nursing Update* 1:1–7, 1986.
65. Hester NO: Comforting the child in pain. In: Funk SG, Tornquist EM, Champagne MT, et al (eds.): *Key Aspects of Comfort: Management of Pain, Fatigue and Nausea.* New York: Springer, 1989, pp. 290–302.
66. Dalton J, Feuerstein M: Behavioral factors in cancer pain. *Pain* 33:137–147, 1988.
67. Dalton J, Feuerstein M: Fear, alexithymia and cancer pain. *Pain* 38:159–170, 1989.
68. McGuire DB: Assessment of pain in cancer inpatients using McGill Pain Questionnaire. *Oncol Nurs Forum* 11:32–37, 1984.
69. Eland J, Anderson J: The experience of children's pain. In: Jacox A: *Pain: A Source Book for Nurses and Other Health Professionals.* Boston: Little, Brown, 1977, pp. 453–473.
70. Eland J: The role of the nurse in children's pain. In: *Perspectives on Pain.* Edinburgh, Eng.: Churchill Livingstone, 1985, pp. 34–40.
71. Donovan M, Dillon P, McGuire L: Incidence and characteristics of pain in a sample of medical-surgical inpatients. *Pain* 30:69–78, 1987.
72. Wilkie D, Lovejoy N, Dodd M, Tesler M: Cancer pain intensity measurement: Concurrent validity of three tools—Finger dynamometer, pain intensity, number scale, visual analogue scale. *Hospice J* 6:1–13, 1990.
73. Wilkie D, Savedra M, Holzemeier W, et al: Use of the McGill Pain Questionnaire to measure pain: A meta-analysis. *Nurs Res* 39:36–41, 1990.
74. Wilkie D, Holzemeier W, Tesler M, et al: Measuring pain quality: Validity and reliability of children's and adolescents' pain language. *Pain* 41:151–159, 1990.
75. Ferrell BA, Ferrell BR: Pain in the nursing home. *J Am Geriatr Soc* 38:409–414, 1990.
76. McCaffery M, Ferrell BR: How would you respond to these patients in pain? *Nurs* 21:34–37, 1991.
77. McCaffery M, Ferrell BR: Pain control for the adult vs. elderly. Does age make a difference? *Nurs* 21:44–48, 1991.
78. Grossman S, Sheidler VR, Swedeen K, et al: Correlation of patient and caregiver ratings of cancer pain. *J Pain Symp Manag* 6:53–57, 1991.
79. Sheidler VR, Grossman SA, McGuire DB, et al: Validation of a new instrument to facilitate pain assessment in cancer patients. Presented to the American Society of Clinical Oncology Conference, San Antonio, 1991.
80. Schmitt R: A holistic approach to cancer pain. Denver: University of Colorado, 1979 (thesis).
81. Dalton J: Nurse's perceptions of their pain assessment skills, pain management practices and attitudes toward pain. *Oncol Nurs Forum* 16:225–231, 1989.
82. Ferrell BR, McCaffery M, Rhiner M: Pain addiction: An urgent need for change in nursing. *J Pain Symptom Manag* 7:117–124, 1992.
83. McCaffery M, Ferrell BR, Page EO, et al: Nurses knowledge of opioid analgesics and psychological dependence. *Cancer Nurs* 13:21–27, 1990.
84. McCaffery M, Ferrell BR: Opioid analgesics: Nurses' knowledge of doses and psychological dependence. *J Nurs Staff Dvlp* 8:77–84, 1992.
85. Sheidler VR, McGuire DB, Gilbert MR, Grossman SA: Nurses' inabilities to recognize safe narcotic orders. Presented at the Oncology Nursing Society Conference, San Francisco, May 1989.
86. Watt-Watson JH: Nurses' knowledge of pain issues: A survey. *J Pain Symp Manag* 2:207–211, 1987.
87. Coyle N: Analgesics at the bedside. *Am J Nurs* 79:1554–1557, 1979.
88. Coyle N, Adelhardt J, Foley K, Portenoy R: Character of terminal illness in the advanced cancer patient: Pain and other symptoms during the last four weeks of life. *J Pain Symp Manag* 5:83–93, 1990.
89. Coyle N, Mauskop A, Maggard J, Foley K: Continuous subcutaneous infusions of opiates in cancer patients with pain. *Oncol Nurs Forum* 13:53–57, 1986.
90. Grochow L, Scheidler V, Grossman S, et al: Does intravenous methadone provide longer-lasting analgesia than intravenous morphine? A randomized, double-blind study. *Pain* 38:151–157, 1989.
91. Krames ES, Wilkie DJ, Gershow J: Intrathecal D-Ala-D-Leu-enkephalin (DADL) restores analgesia in a patient analgetically tolerant to intrathecal morphine sulfate. *Pain* 24:205–209, 1986.
92. Krames ES, Gershow J, Glassberg A, et al: Continuous infusion of spinally administered narcotics for the relief of pain due to malignant disorders. *Cancer* 56:696–702, 1985.
93. Paice JA: Intrathecal morphine sulfate for intractable cancer pain. *Am Assn Neuroscience Nurs* 16:237–240, 1984.
94. Paice JA: Intrathecal morphine infusion for intractable cancer pain: a new use for implanted pumps. *Oncol Nurs Forum* 13:41–47, 1986.
95. Penn RD, Paice JA: Chronic intrathecal morphine for intractable pain. *J Neurosurg* 67:182–186, 1987.
96. Ferrell BR: Pain management at home: Implications for home care providers. *Caring: J Natl Assoc Home Care* November:22–25, 1987.
97. Ferrell BR, Schneider C: Experience and management of cancer pain at home. *Cancer Nurs* 11:84–90, 1988.
98. Ferrell BR, Wisdom C, Wenzl C, Brown J: Controlled-release vs. short-acting analgesia: Effects on pain and quality of life. *Oncol Nurs Forum* 26:521–526, 1989.
99. McGuire DB, Barbour L, Boxler J, et al: Fixed-intervals vs. as-needed analgesics in cancer outpatients. *J Pain Symp Manag* 2:199–205, 1987.
100. Coyle N, Monzillo E, Loscalzo M, et al: A model of continuity of care for cancer patients with pain and neuro-oncologic complications. *Cancer Nurs* 8:111–119, 1985.
101. Ferrell BR, Wenzl C, Wisdom C: The pain management team: Five years experience. *Oncol Nurs Forum* 15:515–516, 1988.
102. Ferrell BR, Wisdom C, Rhiner M, Alletto J: Pain management as a quality assurance outcome. *J Nurs Quality Assur* 5:50–58, 1991.
103. Dalton J: Education for pain management: A pilot study. *Patient Educ Counsel* 9:155–165, 1987.
104. Ferrell BR, Rhiner M: High tech comfort: Ethical issues in cancer pain management in the 1990s. *J Clin Ethics* 2:108–112, 1991.
105. Whedon M, Ferrell BR: Professional and ethical considerations in the use of high tech pain management. *Oncol Nurs Forum* 18:1135–1143, 1991.
106. Ferrell BR, Ferrell BA, Rhiner M, Grant M: Family factors influencing cancer pain management. *Post Grad Med J* 67:S64–S69, 1991 (suppl.).
107. Barbour LA, McGuire DB, Kirchoff KT: Nonanalgesic methods of pain control used by cancer outpatients. *Oncol Nurs Forum* 13:56–60, 1986.
108. American Nurses Association and Oncology Nursing Society: *Standards of Oncology Nursing Practice.* Washington DC: American Nurses' Association, 1987.

Chapter 65

Thriving as an Oncology Nurse

Mary Cunningham, RN, MS

STRESS

Stress is a pervasive human problem, one that is associated to some degree with all the major institutions with which we are involved daily. That stress is associated with work is almost a given in our society, and this is no less true for nurses than for anyone else. Indeed, as shown throughout this chapter, cancer nursing has the potential for very high levels of stress.

The cost of not dealing with stress effectively (coping) can be high. As will be shown, patient care may be compromised, job burnout can be experienced, and even physical and psychological deterioration can result. It is therefore important for the nurse to recognize potential sources of stress and to implement coping strategies that permit continued job and life effectiveness.

What is stress? *Stress* has been variously defined as a response, as a stimulus, and as a transaction. Selye[1] defined stress as a response to events in the environment, a response that is physiological and therefore unrelated to the nature of the stressor, the individual's thoughts and beliefs, or the situational context. Others have characterized stress as the potential residing within the stimulus or as something that results because of the event itself, again unmediated by personal factors or variations in the setting.[2–4]

Both of these definitions of stress can be criticized for being too simplistic and not reflecting what is known from empirical evidence. People respond differently to external events, both interpersonally (between people) and intrapersonally (within individuals at different times). Thus, stress does not reside solely in the event or in the response of the person; it must instead reflect some *transaction* between the two that is modified by a third factor or set of factors.

The transactional model on which the discussion in this chapter is based views stress as the tension that results when the perceived demands of a situation (whether imposed from within the person or by the environment) are out of balance with (particularly, exceeded by) the perceived resources (again, both internal and external) available to the individual.[5–6] The individual is the focal mediator between stimulus and response, for stress lies in the individual's appraisal of events and not necessarily in the events themselves.[5] The use of the word *perceived* is deliberate: In the case of stress it is not so important that the resources ("supplies," in economic terms) are inadequate for the demands as it is that the person experiencing the stress believes this to be true.

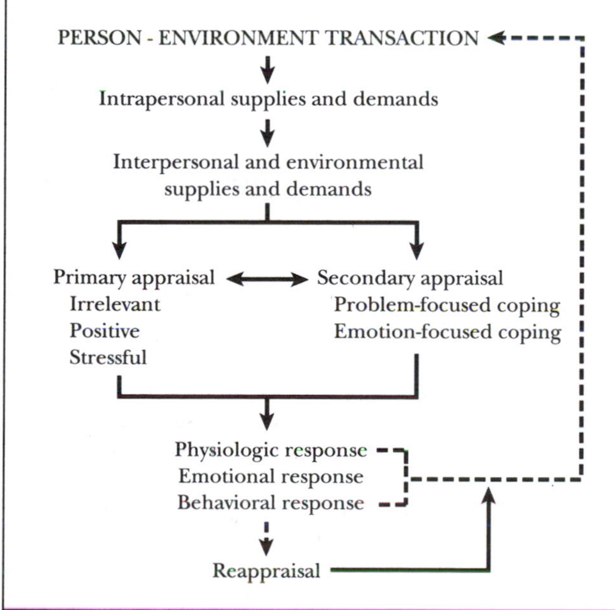

FIGURE 65-1 Lazarus' transactional model of stress.

INDIVIDUAL APPRAISAL

The central focus of Lazarus' transactional model of stress is the nature of the transactions between the person and the environment[5–7] (Figure 65-1). The individual appraises the events to which he or she is exposed as well as his or her own behavior in response to those events. An individual's appraisal of events and actions plays a determining role in the psychological stress experience. Stress arises from a transaction between the individual and the environment when the individual judges the stimuli as damaging, threatening, or challenging in relation to whether the demands tax or exceed appraised available resources.[6] Stress is the perceived imbalance between demands and abilities or resources. These appraisals and judgments determine stress reactions, the intensity and quality of the emotional response, and the outcomes of attempts to adapt to perceived stressors.[7] Therefore, stress lies in the perception of the event and not in the event itself.

Cognitive appraisal refers to evaluations and judgments of events and one's reactions to those events. Lazarus[5] described two types of cognitive appraisals: primary and secondary. *Primary* appraisal refers to a person's judgment about the significance of a stressor. It determines "what is at stake" in the situation and whether the person is in trouble or deriving benefit.[5] Primary appraisals of the transaction take three forms: irrelevant, positive (benign), or stressful.[5] The encounter is *irrelevant* if it carries no implications for a person's well-being, and it is *positive* if it preserves or enhances well-being. *Stressful* appraisals involve judgments of harm or loss, challenge, and threat. In *secondary* appraisal, judgments are made about resources and options available for coping, constraints on using these resources, and consequences. Primary and secondary appraisals differ in content but are interdependent processes. If the individual believes he or she can handle most stressful situations (secondary appraisal), then most transactions will be judged as nonthreatening (primary appraisal).[6]

The relationship between an individual and the environment is ever-changing. As a consequence, appraisals change. This process of changing judgments is called *reappraisal.* Reappraisal gives feedback in two forms: reappraisal of the person–environment relationship, and reappraisal of events.[5–6] The former attempts to reduce stress by reevaluating and changing perspective on supplies and demands. Such reappraisals typically are associated with coping and adaptation.

PERSON–ENVIRONMENT FIT

The transaction model of stress, which focuses on the relationship between the person and the environment, is furthered by the person–environment-fit model developed by French, Rodgers, and Cobb.[8] This model is based on a model of supplies and demands. French et al.[8] conceived of adaptation as a function of the "goodness of the fit" between the person and the environment. Fit is determined by the extent to which environmental supplies are available to meet individual needs (demands) as well as the ability (supplies) of the person to manage the demands imposed by the environment.[8–9] Fit is derived from the reality-based and perception-based assessment of demands and supplies, which is determined primarily by the person's appraisal of environment and self. This importance assigned to appraisal is rooted in the transaction-based approach to stress. If the demands exceed supplies, or vice versa, adjustment is required to create a good fit.[8]

The person–environment-fit model is useful in understanding the relation between job satisfaction and occupational stress and that between a person's interacting roles and the environment. "A job is stressful to the extent that it does not provide supplies to meet the individual's motives and to the extent that the ability of the individual falls below the demands of the job, which are prerequisite to receiving supplies."[10,p.178] The extent to which there is a discrepancy between supplies and demands is based in part on the individual's appraisal of self and environment. Clearly, it is important that individuals have an accurate understanding of their own personal resources and limitations as well as of environmental resources and demands.[7,9,11]

DEMANDS—SOURCES OF STRESS

How can you work with dying patients? How can you give so much of yourself to perfect strangers? How can you work in today's health care environment? How do you stay calm in an emergency? Is your caring codependent? Most cancer nurses have been asked variations of these questions. Perceptions of self, role, co-workers, recipients of care, and work situations are key to the answers. The supplies and demands inherent in each area influence the amount of stress the nurse experiences. In general, stress in nursing generates from mismatches between efforts and results,[11–12] mismatches between nurse and environment[13] leading to role ambiguity and conflict, and mismatches between people[11–12] leading to interpersonal conflict.

In the transactional model of stress, the stress experienced by cancer nurses (and, indeed, everyone) involves an interplay between intrapersonal (self-concept, motivations, and personal needs), interpersonal (relationships with recipients of care and co-workers and the nature of cancer care), and environmental factors. These factors provide the demands and supplies that are appraised as satisfying or discrepant.

Intrapersonal Factors

Lazarus,[5] Appley and Trumbull,[14] and McGrath[15] emphasized the personal equation in assessing reactions to stress, and noted that reactions vary from person to person. Individuals bring into relationships and situations personal characteristics that influence their perceptions of other people and events as well as their reactions. Assessing personal characteristics is not about placing blame; rather, examining personal variables aids in understanding an individual's transaction with other people and events. Self-concept, personal needs, and motivations have the potential both of providing interpersonal demands and supplies and of playing a significant role in the mediation of a stress response.

Self-concept

How we see ourselves plays an important role in our relationships with other people and our appraisal of events. Self-concept is developed through self-appraisal as well as through appraisal by others.[16] The self is made known by listening to self and listening to others. People think and engage in self-talk, which affects self-concept and self-esteem.[17] Negative self-talk ("People don't like me," "I'm incompetent," "I can't do that procedure," "She's better than me") can inadvertently encourage a person to meet the expectation of the negative statement. Pearlin and Schooler found that "freedom from negative attitudes toward self, the possession of a sense that one is in control of the forces impinging on oneself, and the presence of favorable attitudes towards oneself" were helpful in coping.[18,p.12] Likewise, self-concept can be threatened by the demands and negative input from co-workers and recipients of care as well as from the environment. In the supply-and-demand model of stress, people and environmental demands can be overwhelming if a person has little self-confidence or becomes too dependent on the explicit or implicit messages of others.

Personal needs

Most people want approval, praise for accomplishments, love, and respect.[16] These are basic human needs. The strength of an individual's motivation to fulfill these needs and where the individual looks to have them fulfilled have implications in helping relationships and work environments. Fulfillment of personal needs is a demand an individual brings to the environment.

Approval and affection Individuals with intense needs for approval and affection may work exceedingly hard to be pleasing and to satisfy the demands of recipients of care and co-workers.[9,11] Meeting the demands of others in order to gain approval and be liked can lead to a reluctance to say "no," the sabotage of self-needs, disappointment, a sense of betrayal, and resentment if one's efforts are not appreciated or approved.

Autonomy and control People vary in their expectations about the extent to which they have control over their lives. An *internal* locus of control is the tendency to perceive that actions and outcomes are correlated and that one is in control of one's life.[19] Individuals with an *external* locus of control tend to expect little control over events. This perception of control is created through interaction with the environment, where actions and outcomes are either related (producing a sense of control) or unrelated (producing a sense of powerlessness).[20]

Clearly, the need to be independent and self-determining is a hallmark of personal growth and maturity.[21] Yet an excessive need to control, to refuse to share or delegate power, or to take on responsibility for everything and everyone is a perfect setup for a *mea culpa* reaction,[11] that is, the sense that "It's me," "I'm responsible," "It's my fault," and then overlooking the interpersonal and situational factors that influence the outcomes. The externally controlled individual bends at the demands of other people and the environment. Disappointments, blaming, and resentments can develop as personal needs go unfulfilled and the individual feels no power in affecting outcomes. DuCette and Wolk[22] argued that the critical element in this perception is for the person to distinguish where control is possible and where it is impossible.

Personal motivations

Motivation has been defined as "the process of arousing or initiating behavior."[23,p.55] Behavior is incited by a desire for satisfaction of needs.[24] An individual's behavior is influenced by the expectation that behavior will bring about need fulfillment. One might question, for instance, "What leads people to enter a helping career?" or "Why did I choose cancer nursing?" Failure to fulfill the motivation that prompted the decision to enter a helping profession can generate a great amount of stress.[25] Vachon[25] explored the idea that motivation influences the nature of the stress experienced by professionals working with terminally ill patients. To illustrate: Individuals motivated out of past personal experiences with cancer may expose previous, unresolved guilt, resulting in an overidentification with dying patients that can lead to emotional depletion and conflicts with other staff. Vachon[25] found that if working with the dying happened by accident, emotional involvement with patients was minimal and the stress experienced stemmed from a lack of knowledge and feelings of professional impotence.

There are also self-centered reasons for choosing a helping profession.[11] Some may look for approval and affection through expressions of appreciation. Some may be involved in helping relationships to boost self-esteem and feelings of self-worth, or to fulfill the need for intimacy. Feeling good about oneself and feeling good about being helpful are reasonable outcomes in helping professions. Yet danger may rest in attempting to get personal needs met in a helping relationship, for often neither the recipients of care nor co-workers are able or expected to fulfill these needs.

Motivation or drive for need fulfillment influences how an individual appraises situations (whether or not needs will be fulfilled); so as a result, motivations influence stress reactions (behavior).[5] Motivations are modified by the expectations of self and others. These expectations influence appraisal.[17] If expectations are unrealistic, needs often go unmet. Smythe[26] identified unrealistic expectations stereotypically associated with nurses, such as: "A good nurse cares for all patients equally and is concerned about people all of the time," "A nurse's worth, whether or not she does a good job, is related to patient compliance, patient outcome, patient improvement, and patient happiness," and "Patients and supervisors and co-workers should appreciate us and our work."[p.30] Expectations modify motivations and influence appraisal; if expectations are unrealistic, then feelings of anger and hostility (external expressions of unmet needs) can result, as can depression, a sense of failure, and low self-esteem (internal expressions of unmet needs).

Interpersonal Factors

Cancer nursing is a person-to-person profession that at the same time involves deeply rewarding and very demanding work.[27] "It takes a lot of energy to be calm in the midst of crisis, to be patient in the face of frustrations and to be understanding when surrounded by fear, pain, anger, or shame."[11,p.17] To understand the interpersonal demands inherent in cancer nursing, one must understand the dynamics of nurse–patient relationships and the nature of cancer care.

Helping relationships

According to Maslach,[11] the very structure of the helping relationship can promote a negative view of people or a shift from a positive to a negative view. This shift tends to frustrate the helper, dampen the helper's sensitivity, diminish the helper's sense of accomplishment, and generate emotional and physical exhaustion. As well, the quality of the interaction with the recipient in the helping relationship suffers. Four aspects of the helping relationship are pivotal in this positive-to-negative shift: focus on the problem, lack of positive feedback, level of emotional stress, and perceived possibility of change or improvement.[11]

Focus on problems By definition, the recipient of care in a helping relationship has a problem (weakness, deficiencies, illness), which is the focus of the relationship.[11] The negative part of an individual or the individual's life is what the helper sees. Although most of us have been taught to evaluate the strengths and resources of patients and families, what is normal or healthy (supplies) is often ignored. The language or practices in most health care environments promote this problem-focused orientation: We make problem lists and nursing diagnoses such as "self-care deficit" and "knowledge deficit"; we use quality assurance measures that track deficiencies; we provide "salvage" treatment to cancer "victims." Helpers have no choice but to focus on the most urgent or acute problems in environments where time, money, and human resources (supplies) are scarce; as a result, supporting human assets necessarily becomes a secondary consideration. In most helping relationships, when the problem is resolved, the recipient goes away;[11] the relationship is over. It is easy to see how helpers can shift to a negative view of people in such settings.

Lack of positive feedback The motivation for helping is to make a difference. Most helpers want both feedback about the quality of their efforts and appreciation. If complaints or criticism from recipients and co-workers are the norm, a negative view of helping can result.[11] What kind of feedback is implied in the death of a patient? Do you hear from co-workers and managers when things go smoothly, or only when things go wrong?

Likewise, recipients may take for granted what the helper does well. Society, professional organizations, institutions, accrediting bodies, peers, and self can set up no-win situations by establishing very high standards that are difficult or nearly impossible to achieve. If the helper is able to meet these expectations, recognition and appreciation may still not be forthcoming because recipients may not feel the need to provide feedback when the caregiver is "merely doing her job." Feedback may only come if the expectations are not met. Lack of positive feedback is a source of stress, and helping relationships that offer no positive feedback over time are viewed negatively.

Level of emotional stress Society upholds the belief that cancer inevitably means pain, suffering, and death. As a consequence, the diagnosis of cancer often is regarded with more fear and viewed as more threatening than other diagnoses.[28] The diagnosis of cancer generates a great deal of emotional distress. Helpers may attempt to decrease the emotional distress of recipients by encouraging the disclosure of feelings, facilitating coping by providing for a catharsis of the tension and anxiety connected with emotions while allowing for feedback and enhancing problem solving.[29] Yet what is the consequence to the helper of being on the receiving end of emotional disclosure or catharsis?

Larson described the helper's pit: The person we are trying to help is in the pit, and the helper is standing above, on the edge of the pit, reaching in to help.[27] If the nature of contact with people is especially upsetting, depressing, or difficult, the helper may fall into the pit. To avoid this, the helper may develop a negative, even dehumanized, perception of the recipient.[11,27] Nurses may claim immunity in order to deal with the threatening realities of being confronted with extreme distress, the threat inherent in being confronted repeatedly with one's own mortality, the inhumanity of others, and the threat of pain and disfigurement.[21] Another way to handle the feelings is by distancing oneself emotionally and/or physically, creating a shelter by adding a layer of callus. This strategy, however, often only adds to the nurse's distress.[27,30]

Possibility of change or improvement The recipient's responsiveness to the helper influences the helper's view of the recipient. Lack of responsiveness dehumanizes. If the helper feels dehumanized, it is much easier to dehumanize the recipient and to view the recipient in a negative light. Helpers can react not only to a lack of personal responsiveness but also to a lack of change or improvement in the recipient's condition.[11] Evidence of making a difference often requires change or improvement. In its absence, the helper may have feelings of personal failure and ineffectiveness. Dealing with problems of a chronic nature, like cancer, where signs of change or improvement evolve slowly (or not at all) can magnify this sense of failure. To diminish these feelings, the helper may blame other people. The blame may be explicitly or implicitly expressed toward co-workers ("If you weren't so lazy," "Why didn't you give him a transfusion?") or patients ("You smoked cigarettes for 30 years and see what happened," "You ignored the lump"). This shift in blame to "it's you" contrasts with the *mea culpa* reaction, but both reactions place blame on people and fail to acknowledge the environment as a source of stress.[11,27]

Cancer trajectory

Cancer poses unique challenges to care providers as well as to patients. Each cancer diagnosis and resulting illness has a unique trajectory.[9,31] Some patients will be cured, others will live with a chronic illness with periods of remission and recurrence, still others will die quickly.[32] Trajectory variability creates demands on care providers as variability creates uncertainty.[33] The demands are magnified when the nurse has to juggle numerous trajectories simultaneously. To deal with uncertainty, care providers often develop expectations regarding a patient's trajectory.[32] Although intended to diminish uncertainty, this too can serve as a stressor if the predictions are incorrect. If a patient dies sooner than predicted or unexpectedly, a crisis ensues.[32] Stress is acute but short-lived. On the other hand, if a patient's death takes "too long," chronic stress develops. Anger and resentment can develop in response to a feeling of powerlessness at being unable to change the trajectory. The unpredictability of cancer leaves the cancer nurse with the dilemma of what messages to convey to patients and family members. The juxtaposition of hope and truth is stressful. The care provider may feel as though he or she is conspiring against the patient, feeling hypocritical by "seeing the handwriting on the wall" yet continuing to participate in providing treatment that is believed ineffective in changing the cure trajectory. "This helplessness is a product of the conflict between the helping person's concept of himself as a restorer and the patient's inability to be restored."[34,p.43]

Prolonged involvement

Cancer nurses often are involved with patients and their families for extended periods of time.[9] This is a double-edged sword, for prolonged involvement provides both rewards for and demands on cancer nurses. In general, nurses "live with" patients and their families, whereas other health care professionals merely make episodic visits. Strength of identification with the patient and family is directly proportional to the intensity and extent of contact.[35] During sustained relationships (in many cases, from diagnosis through death), patients and families may manifest a kaleidoscope of emotions, including anger, frustration, grief, and fear.[36] The demands increase exponentially as the nurse cares for multiple patients and families experiencing different emotions, for there is no reaction among patients that cannot also occur in caregivers.[37] This sense of emotional liability is stressful.[31,32,34,35]

Fagin and Diers[38] describe nursing as a metaphor for intimacy. "Nurses are involved in the most private aspects of people's lives, and they cannot hide behind technology or a veil of omniscience as other practitioners or technicians in hospitals may do. Nurses, as trusted peers, are there to hear secrets, especially the ones born of vulnerability."[38,p.117] Patients and family members may view the nurse as "safe" for the expression of fears and feelings of sadness, isolation, helplessness, anger, or profound grief. Being faced with human suffering and distress of the spirit places the listener in a vulnerable position. "To sympathize is to give part of ourselves to others, and in giving and sharing to become vulnerable."[39,p.69]

One way to lessen the intensity of the relationship is to withdraw physical and emotional support. Withdrawal can take many forms: "becoming emotionally distant, ignoring patients' needs, avoidance, holding a part of myself back, feeling cold and unsympathetic,"[30,p.24] and task orientation.[40] Paradoxically, these attempts to withdraw physical and emotional support tend to increase rather than reduce stress for the care provider. A stress-avoidance-guilt sequence develops, for distancing often leads to feelings of betrayal of the patient or family, doubt about one's helping ability and motivation, and guilt.[30]

Treatment sequelae

The nurse often is responsible for the administration of treatments that induce distress and illness,[35,41] creating iatrogenic illness. Feeling as though one, as a nurse, is contributing to the suffering of patients is distressing, because it is not in keeping with an idealized image of the nurse as a professional provider of comfort and help.[42]

An assortment of stressors emerge at the start of aggressive treatment.[32] If the treatment is curative, the staff may feel hopeful and rally to support patient compliance. Hope is felt by staff and patients. If the treatment fails, doubt surfaces. To deal with repetitive treatment failures, the caregiver may shift the responsibility for failure: from "the treatment failed" to "Mr. Smith failed treatment X" or "He's a treatment failure." If the therapies are causing significant morbidity, ambivalence or cynicism may develop[32] ("We may be trying to cure his sarcoma, but he'll need a heart transplant if he survives the treatment"). The nurse administering investigational therapies may feel incompetent in predicting and managing side effects. The values and ethics of research may be questioned, especially if the staff is exposed only to patients who die from the treatment or who experience intolerable side effects.[32]

Radical surgery often causes dramatic adverse changes in a patient's appearance and serves as a stressor to nurses. Radical neck dissections, hemipelvectomies, or radical vulvectomies were among the stressors categorized by nurses as disfiguring or difficult illnesses in a study conducted by Vachon.[32] The stress to the care provider associated with disfiguring surgeries stems from the disfigurement itself and, as with other therapies, questioning whether or not the surgery will actually have a positive impact on the quantity and/or quality of the individual's life.[32]

Lack of consensus among health providers and patients regarding treatment goals is a source of stress for cancer nurses.[33,35] Patients may request continuation of aggressive treatment, creating a dilemma for the nurse who believes palliation is the reasonable choice ("How can I support his decision when I know what's coming?"). When palliation is the goal, if caregivers are unable to provide the expected relief from symptoms, particularly if they view symptom management as a mandate ("It's the least we can do"), they experience great stress.[32] Staff may feel impotent, guilty, helpless, and even that they are part of a conspiracy that let the patient down.

Death

We are a death-denying society.[21] Yet in 1991 it was estimated that 514,000 Americans would die of cancer.[43] Cancer nurses will encounter physical death; and, in a broader context, loss of social worth, value, control, energy, relationships, role, life's work, or hopes for the future.

Death calls the living into action.[44] Confrontation or repeated exposure causes us to face our own fears about death and contemplate our own mortality. Zilboorg[45] suggests that continual consciousness of the fear of death impairs functioning; in defense, the fear is repressed. Repression is more than simply putting it away; it means "constant psychological effort to keep the lid on."[45,p.467] Continual psychological efforts to repress fear of death or feelings associated with death of a patient demands energy. Losses do not occur in a vacuum; rather, they interact with, modify, and augment the other stresses in our personal and professional lives.[46] And when we don't share each experience of death with significant others, the feelings or distress associated with each death accumulate.[30]

Nurses' realities—women's realities

Nurse is derived from the Latin word for "nourish." Caring is the essence, the core of nursing.[47] Fagin and Diers considered *nursing* a metaphor for "mothering," which shares links with "nurturing, caring, comforting, laying on of hands."[38,p.6]

Leininger states that "caring is one of the most crucial and essential ingredients for health, human development, human relatedness, well-being, and survival."[48,p.46] Caring includes "those assistive, supportive, or facilitative acts toward or for another individual or group . . . [meant] to ameliorate or improve a human condition or lifeway."[48,p.45] Caring and feeling cared for are basic human needs that promote personal and societal health.[21] Yet many of the activities associated with caring are seen in our society as essentially "mundane and hardly worth noticing."[21] Pearson wrote that "caregiving is, at this moment in history, humble and invisible work, often unappreciated or under-appreciated."[49,p.117]

Caring is devalued in our society in part because it is associated with "women's work" and subservience. American society is dominated by the constructs of a white male system in which individualism, independence, one-upsmanship, logic, and rational thought are prized.[50] Consequently, bonding, consensus-making, comforting, empowering of others, generativity, and caring are suspect and are subordinated to individual desires and needs.[21,50] If the essence of nursing is caring, a major source of stress in nursing lies in the devaluation of caring and the lack of recognition and rewards given to the caregiver.[21]

Another societal devaluation of caring stems from the proliferation of codependency theory that calls into question the motive for caregiving.[51] Caring may be perceived as an illness when popularized by definitions such as "any suffering and/or dysfunction that is associated with or results from focusing on the needs and behaviors of others."[52] The damage of such labeling may include viewing caring as a symptom of a disease, self-blame for the stress experienced in caring work, doubting caring motivations, and cutting off social support.[51]

Environmental Factors

Environmental factors that may be considered demanding include role stressors, organizational and work climates, and professional relationships. A discussion of these factors follows.

Role stressors

Role ambiguity An individual must understand the expectations that others have of a particular role, as well as the duties, rights, responsibilities, and activities of the role, in order to adequately perform the role.[32] Role ambiguity is the extent to which role expectations are not clearly communicated.[32] In part, role ambiguity experienced by nurses stems from a lack of clear definition of professional nursing as well as the diversity of roles currently enacted by nurses.[53] Lack of trust and respect in working relationships limits the flexibility often necessary to deal with role ambiguity. In general, the greater the perceived role ambiguity, the greater the perceived stress.

Role conflict Role conflict is the extent to which the expectations of various others are in conflict or incompatible.[32] Vachon[32] found role conflict to be a major stressor for nurses. The evolving role of the nurse may cause conflicts, particularly with physicians and social workers who feel that nurses are infringing on their traditional roles. Likewise, the evolving roles of other professionals can create conflict by infringing on the traditional roles of nursing, for example, pharmacists involved with patient teaching or social workers coaching patients regarding symptom management. Kahn found that "persons subjected to high role conflict report greater job-related tensions, lower job satisfaction, less confidence in the organization itself, and more intense experience of conflict."[55,p.5]

Role overload Role overload is the extent to which a person is incapable of meeting multiple expectations,[32] and may result in physical and emotional exhaustion, negative feelings about patients, co-workers, and the organization, and a diminished sense of accomplishment.[11] French and Kaplan[56] distinguished between quantitative and qualitative overload. *Qualitative* overload implies that the job skills and knowledge exceed those of the individual. *Quantitative* overload implies that there is more work than can be done in a given period of time.[12] As the size (quantitative) or acuity of overload (qualitative) increased, "burnout" manifested among health care professionals.[57,58] Larson[27,30] and Arena and Page[59] wrote about the stress of the "imposter phenomenon" experienced by nurses: the feeling of inadequacy and incompetence that can be attributed to both quantitative and qualitative role overload. Feelings of inadequacy and incompetence can evolve from rapidly changing medical technologies,[30] defining *competence* as "perfection,"[59] "terror of error" or accountability overload,[30] and excessive demands.[30]

The experience of overload can be aggravated by the imposition of tasks that have a high priority for the organization but a low priority for the worker (paperwork versus providing emotional support to a patient and family).[60] Role overload puts nurses in no-win situations, for if the nurse complies with the organizational demand for quantity service (one nurse for ten patients) the nurse may be unable to provide quality service ("It's impossible to provide quality care for ten sick patients on this unit!").[57] Rather than compromising quality of care, nurses may end up working overtime, often without compensation, and perpetuating the perceived stress.

Control issues: autonomy and authority

Job control is associated with autonomy and authority, that is, the sense that one has control of one's time and activities.[61] Pines and Aronson[12] found that stress increased as autonomy, a sense of control, and discretionary time decreased. Organizational characteristics such as "circumscribed authority, downward channels of commands, specialization, and formal accountability and hierarchy contribute to a sense of lack of autonomy and control."[12,p.106] A lack of autonomy engenders feelings of frustration, victimization, and helplessness.[7] Nurses are most prone to this experience, for they are charged with tremendous responsibility but are given no real power or authority.[7] Nursing carries with it a high-risk element in the delivery of service; this, coupled with limited authority, can result in a feeling of accountability overload or the dilemma of being accountable yet not having the requisite power or authority to balance the demand.

Nurses can develop feelings of powerlessness as they discover that what happens is independent of their input, expressed concern, or verbal complaint.[62] As a consequence, estrangement from the work environment can occur ("I am going to put in my 8 hours and then get the hell out of here!"). On the other hand, the need for autonomy can be so great that nurses will blame themselves for problems, errors, and the like just to maintain a sense of control.

Work environment

Research in organizational psychology has demonstrated that the physical quality of the work environment has an effect on performance.[7,p.84] Claus and Bailey[13] found that overcrowded units, noise, poor lighting, poor ventilation, and malfunctioning equipment were physical stressors identified by health care professionals. Noise in health care environments tends to be intermittent, unexpected, and reverberant. In response, stress accumulates via a constant low level of arousal of the autonomic nervous system.[13] Many work environments were not designed to accommodate the people, equipment, or supplies that are required to care for people today. Nurses can experience increased stress when care must be provided in cramped, confined areas. In addition, advances in health care technology have expanded the range of sophisticated equipment that nurses must master in order to care for patients. Given the plethora of technology, it is not uncommon for nurses to be responsible for using multiple pieces of equipment, each of which accomplishes the same goal ("I am expected to know how to use ten different types of large-volume, small-volume, ambulatory, and multichanneled parenteral infusion pumps. I am so afraid of making a mistake").

Intragroup and intergroup conflict

Conflict seems inevitable in the dealings of any two autonomous persons whose interests or relationships are interdependent.[54] Wise[63,p.73] said,

> It is naive to bring together a highly diverse group of people and expect that, by calling them a team, they will in fact behave as a team. It is ironic indeed to realize that a football team spends 40 hours a week practicing teamwork for the two hours on Sunday afternoon when their teamwork really counts. Teams in organizations seldom spend 2 hours per week practicing when their ability to function as a team counts 40 hours per week.

Factors that influence intragroup and intergroup conflicts are varied: scarcity of, or competition for, resources (time, money, people, skills), divergent goals, and group interdependence for work sequencing.[54] Where team concepts are employed, the greater the interrelatedness and dependence on one another, the greater the potential for conflict.[54] The size of the organization, levels of authorities, and specialized roles influence the amount of conflict: As each increases, so does the conflict. Group cohesiveness, compatibility, and group attitude about conflict influences whether and the means by which conflicts are addressed.[54,55]

Among the basic commitments for nurses who practice in accordance with generally accepted standards is that they participate as members of the health care team.[64] The Oncology Nursing Society's *Standards of Oncology Nursing Practice* state: "The oncology nurse collaborates with the multidisciplinary team."[65,p.18] This involves intergroup and intragroup relationships. Much has been written about physician–nurse conflict. Conflict is rooted in historical antecedent, power and status inequity, mutual lack of knowledge of and respect for unique contributions of each role, personality conflicts, and lack of communication regarding treatment goals.[26] Unresolved intragroup conflicts (nurse to nurse) seem to represent losing sight of the basic idea of nursing as a caring profession that includes care for and of not only patients but also fellow nurses.[64] Intragroup conflicts disrupt team stability, isolate team members, and lessen the likelihood that nursing staff will share feelings related to work experiences. Intragroup conflicts potentially rob the individual of the valuable resource of other nurses who can provide technical support and appreciation of one's work, facilitating the realization that one's feelings are not unique.[30,33,66] Maslach[60] showed that the incidence of burnout was lower for health care workers who actively expressed and shared their feelings with co-workers.

Organizational climate

Size, structure, goals, and organizational climate are organizational factors that can serve as sources of stress. Investigations reveal that the size of the organization is related directly to organizational tension.[61] Hospitals have inherent characteristics that foster stress: multiple levels of authority, heterogeneity of personnel, work interdependence, and specialization.[67] Ambiguity of organizational structure, procedures, and policies and, conversely, overregulation can both be perceived as stressful. Precise organizational charts, a chain of command, and detailed job descriptions and procedures can create stress due to perceived inflexibility and lack of individual control.[54] Organizational structure has been described as a major determinant of job performance, satisfaction, and burnout.[12]

Organizational goals may be in conflict with the goals of the individual. Weisbord[68] speculated that health care professionals may experience more conflict with institutional goals because health care professionals are socialized to value autonomy and personal achievement. The organizational goal may be to provide care at minimal cost, whereas the goal of the caregiver may be to do everything possible. Goals of the organization are both explicit and implicit. For instance, the organization may state explicitly that direct patient care services are top priority, yet only reward or recognize staff who excel in research or publishing. Consequently, the caregiver may experience stress when stated goals differ from reality.[46]

Menzies[69] found that organizational climate can support or diminish nurse–patient relationships. Matthews[70] rated hospital administrations on a continuum from technological orientation to social-process (person) orientation. The degree of patient-centered nursing increased as social-process orientation increased and decreased as technological orientation scores increased. How this translates into nursing, which is a people-oriented profession, is that nurses who work in an organization that places a higher value on technology would be expected to experience job stress due to the devaluation of their patient-centered orientation.[70]

Management strategies—rewards

Reward, recognition, praise, encouragement, expressions of appreciation, and clear feedback are extremely powerful incentives. Pines and Aronson[12] found that employees were better equipped to handle work stress when these kinds of rewards (supplies) were available. Health care professionals often experience increased stress when there is a noticeable lack of these rewards.[7,12,71]

Health care professionals gauge their relative worth in the organization by making inferences about the extent to which they are compensated for their contributions.[12] Lack of differentiation of rewards (everyone receives a merit increase regardless of efforts) encourages only average performance as the high-contributor concludes that there is no need to work harder. And the low-contributor, seeing that the high-contributor gets equal reward, concludes that hard work does not pay off. Bureaucratic organizations that fail to differentiate compensation based on effort serve as a source of stress.[11]

Recognition and appreciation often are more important than dollars. Feedback from managers regarding work performance, negative and positive, is vital. People who receive recognition, appreciation, satisfaction, and a sense of significance from their work are more likely to be content with their income.[58] Lack of feedback, as well as a mismatch of work performance expectations between nurses and managers, can create conflict. Managers' ideas about how to evaluate work performance may differ from the nurse's ideas.[9] Managers may base their judgments on quantitative criteria, such as number of care plans, size and acuity of patient caseload, number of publications, committee attendance, and quality assurance activities. On the other hand, the nurse may place a higher value on the quality of the care rendered. The nurse may believe the manager is using unimportant criteria to judge performance or that the manager is out of touch with what is really important.

SUPPLIES—STRESS MANAGEMENT STRATEGIES

Stress results from a mismatch or discrepancy between environmental demands and individual supplies or between environmental opportunities and individual needs and goals. Efforts to reduce stress then must alter one or both elements—environment or self—by either reducing demands or increasing supplies or altering one's interpretation of demands and supplies.[72] Coping embraces actions to reduce the mismatch between self and environment. Lazarus[5] suggested two general types of coping: problem-focused and emotion-focused. *Problem-focused* coping targets the environment or self for direct action by changing one's behavior or environmental conditions.[9] *Emotion-focused* coping attempts to palliate or eliminate distressing emotions elicited by the stressor.[73] Emotion-focused coping does not change the self or environment, only the way one feels. Both direct and indirect actions call for a reappraisal of environment and self.[72] When a situation is assessed as having the potential for change, a person typically will use problem-focused coping, whereas emotion-focused coping is employed if the harmful or threatening situation holds little potential for change. The challenge is to learn to manage effectively those things that can be controlled, to accept the things that cannot be controlled, and to recognize the difference.[7,18]

Caplan[74] identified characteristics of effective coping strategies. These characteristics can be useful criteria in evaluating coping behaviors.

1. *There is an active exploration of reality issues and a search for information.* Effective coping involves looking for realities without denial, repression, avoidance, or projection. The individual examines the role he or she plays in the situation as well as his or her response. Information is sought in order to gain an accurate appraisal.

2. *There is a free expression of positive and negative feelings. Feelings are mastered where possible; and where mastery is not possible, the inevitable is accepted.* Identifying what can be controlled decreases the frustration and energy drain in trying to control uncontrollable situations.

3. *There is an active effort to engage the help of others.* The individual realizes that it is okay to ask for information and support from other people.

4. *Problems are broken down into manageable bits and worked through one at a time.*

5. *There is a fundamental trust in oneself and others and a sense of optimism that something can be done to bring about a positive outcome.*

Because stress is a personal experience, stress prevention and management strategies begin with the person. This is not to suggest that the experience of work stress is a sign of weakness or deficiency. Rather, the effects of self-regulation enable nurses to reappraise self and environment, evaluate the supplies and demands of the work environment, and develop problem- or emotion-focused coping strategies. Self-regulation involves knowing one's self and one's personal values, priorities, and beliefs.

Pines and Aronson[12] suggested several concrete coping strategies to manage stress: reappraisal of goals, time management, acknowledging vulnerabilities, compartmentalizing life and work, self-reinforcement, change in attitudes, creating balance, accentuating the positive, adopting a wellness philosophy, relaxation, and establishing a sense of control over one's practice. Several of the strategies will be presented in the following section.

Intrapersonal Coping Strategies

Recognizing stress responses

"To thine own self be true." It is imperative that an individual begin to recognize the triggers and signs of physical, emotional, and mental stress (Figure 65-2). Self-understanding begins with self-observation.

PHYSICAL, BEHAVIORAL, AND INTELLECTUAL MANIFESTATIONS OF STRESS

Physical
Feelings of exhaustion and fatigue
Weight change
Insomnia
Gastrointestinal disturbances
Cool, clammy skin
Sweating
Trembling; tics; twitches
Muscle tension
Rapid, uncontrolled speech
Loss of libido; impotence
Frequent headaches
Increased use of food, nicotine, alcohol, tranquilizers
Repetitive accidents
Frequent illness

Behavioral/Emotional
Lability of mood; mood swings
Suspiciousness; mistrust
Anger; antagonistic attitude toward others; hostility
Depression
Defensive behavior; blaming; scapegoating
Feelings of helplessness, inadequacy
Loss of sense of humor
Irritability
Distancing from others; reduced personal involvement
Nail biting; habitual teeth gritting
Critical of self and others
Panic; feeling pressured
Increasing expression of dissatisfaction

Intellectual
Increased rigidity in thinking
Increased use of intellectualization as defense
Lack of initiative
Forgetfulness
Preoccupation
Lack of attention to detail
Diminished concentration
Increased depersonalization
Dreams laden with conflict
Absenteeism
Frequent job change or feeling stuck in job
Frequent excuse making

FIGURE 65-2 Source: Adapted from References 7, 11, 16, 32, 46, 60, and 67.

DAILY STRESS AND TENSION LOG

Daily incidents of stress are recorded using the following categories:

Description of Physical Signs of Stress	Time	Where? What? Who?	Thoughts? Feelings?	Response
Wake late; tired from working late on special project	6:30 AM	DK calls to invite me to dinner; DK sounds happy and care-free	DK never takes on extra projects; she knows I am under a deadline; I feel like she does not understand	Feel defensive; feel guilty about never initiating contact with DK; feel angry; refuse invitation; know I need some fun
Tight shoulder muscles, fatigue; grit teeth	1:30 PM	At work, in the middle of lunch and get paged with a new consult	I will never get home on time; feel anger and resentment at co-workers who all seemed to take vacations; I feel abandoned	Ate dessert; abrupt with secretary
Racing pulse; feel breathless; thoughts disorganized; difficult to concentrate	3:30 PM	At work, meeting with new section chief; I want him to like and respect me	Resent that he has not met with me and now only at my request; I do not feel heard	Last minute preparation; did not communicate clearly; beat myself up after meeting, with a lot of negative messages
Insomnia; cannot turn off thoughts	11:30 PM	At home, trying to fall asleep	Thinking about work day; fearing work load and what I need to get done in the next two days before vacation	Get up and make a list; decide to read

FIGURE 65-3 Source: Maslach C: *Burnout: The Cost of Caring.* Englewood Cliffs, NJ: Prentice-Hall, 1982.

Maslach suggests keeping a daily stress and tension log[11] (Figure 65-3). Recording this type of information can provide very helpful insight into emotional and cognitive responses, the precipitator of responses, and styles of coping. This exercise is not about enumerating faults; rather, it allows one to recognize patterns of behavior and self-talk and thus to become able to make choices about how one will think and feel or appraise self and the environment.

Setting realistic goals

Unrealistic self-expectations are a formula for defeat. Unrealistic expectations are a major cause of "self-doubt, self-blame, and lowered self-esteem."[30,p.25] It is imperative to examine self-expectations and goals. Reappraisal of goals involves knowing what your goals are (what you want from life and work), evaluating whether or not the goals are realistic, and redefining the goals as necessary. Establishment of goals involves values clarification, in which those things of greatest value are given highest priority. It involves knowing what can be changed and what cannot. Goals need to be specific, realistic, and measurable. Setting realistic goals improves the probability of success.

Time management

Time is a scarce resource. Time management is vital to self-management[75] and essentially involves structuring time in order to meet goals. The first step in time management is knowing how one spends time. A time log facilitates distinguishing time use from time waste or time problems. Time waste is caused by self, by others, and by the organization.[75] Self-generated time wasters include lack of self-discipline, worry, always saying "yes," procrastination, disorganization, and an unwillingness to delegate. Time problems generated by other people might include interruptions, phone calls, interdependency of work, and meetings that do not start or stop on time or where people arrive late or come unprepared. Steps can be taken to minimize other people's use of your time by documenting time in terms of cost (delay in supplies, phone calls that do not require nursing response, pattern of interruptions by a particular person, tracking the time wasted in starting meetings late). Time wasters generated by the organization and the nature of nurses' work include ambiguity of roles, lack of clarity regarding goals, redundancy of effort, frequent changes (mid-stream), failure to plan, and engaging nurses in nonnursing tasks.[75] The overriding principle in time management is knowing how time is spent and being methodical in planning time in order to accomplish goals. Keeping a record of how time is spent can be helpful.

Tuning into inner dialogue

A critical variable in what is experienced as stressful is one's perception or interpretation of the stressor.[5]

These perceptions and interpretations are given voice in an ongoing dialogue we have with ourselves. Our beliefs about reality and about ourselves underlie our self-talk. Self-talk can be rational or irrational. Self-talk based on rational thoughts promotes self-respect and goal attainment. Self-talk based on irrational thoughts tends to sabotage self-esteem, results in negative emotions, and inhibits the realization of goals.[26]

Ellis and Harper[17] developed the A-B-C model for examining the relationship between thoughts, feelings, and behaviors. Event A is the activating event. For example, a physician reprimands the nurse for not carrying out his or her orders for a patient. Following the reprimand, the nurse doubts his or her work performance, event C; the consequence represents feelings and behaviors. On being criticized, the nurse becomes defensive, stating "I didn't see it as a priority; if it was so important you should have called it to my attention." Many believe that A, the activating event, directly causes C, the consequence. But something happens between A and C: event B, our self-talk, which influences our feelings and behavior. After being reprimanded, the nurse may have said, "I failed; I'm dumb; I can't be trusted; my mistakes will someday result in a catastrophe."

The technique called *cognitive restructuring* involves learning to listen to self-talk and changing unwanted or irrational thoughts in order to change emotional response.[17,76] The first step in cognitive restructuring is to look at the event or persons as objectively as possible in order to gain a clearer perspective on the event and any irrational thinking and to consider different responses. Although it is unrealistic to expect to make a positive response to all stressful situations, a sense of mastery and control comes from knowing that one has a choice in how situations are perceived, in addition to choosing the response.

Accentuating the positive

Helping relationships often have a negative bias, for the recipients of care have problems for which they seek help from the caregiver.[11] The negatives in helping relationships can be countered by actively emphasizing what is good, pleasant, or satisfying about the helping relationship. The nurse asks for feedback from care recipients and peers. Larson recommends that nurses reflect on their "greatest moments"; those times "when you make a difference, when you see the real impact of your caring."[27,p.862] Keeping a journal, maintaining a file of letters from patients and families or simply sharing the "moment" with a colleague helps to lessen the negative bias that can creep into helping relationships (Figure 65-4).

Compartmentalizing work and life

Pines and Aronson[12] recommend making a clear distinction between home and work, including finding a balance between the energy expended at work and home activities. One form of compartmentalization is not discussing work-related issues at home, and vice versa. Although talking about work-related stress with family members or friends may provide catharsis and support, reliving work stress at home or with friends causes a reexperiencing of the distress.[7] Work-related stress is best discussed with someone who does the same kind of work, someone who can immediately empathize; colleagues provide technical support and technical challenge.[27,30] Another strategy to create a sense of separation between work and home is to allow for decompression time.[12] A decompression routine is a ritual that signals that one part of daily life is ending and another is beginning, that is, the passage from work life to personal life. One sequence of decompression activities might include: making a to-do list for the next day's activities before leaving work; listening to music on the way home; exercising, meditating, showering immediately on arriving home, or changing from work uniform into at-home clothes.

Creating balance

"Every helper needs to find a way to be involved emotionally as a caregiver without burning out. . . . Empathy is a double-edged sword; it is simultaneously [the nurse's] greatest asset and point of real vulnerability."[27,p.857] Most nurses move along a continuum between overinvolvement and underinvolvement. Creating a balance between overinvolvement and depersonalization involves finding a blend of compassion and objectivity: detached concern.[7,11,27,77] With detached concern, the nurse has an honest concern for the patient's well-being but is able to maintain emotional and psychological distance.

So how does one learn detached concern? Most nursing educational programs stress the importance of empathy, but few balance that recommendation with the importance of maintaining emotional and physical distance.[21] Experienced practitioners typically learn detached concern through experience, most likely only after experiencing both ends of the involvement continuum. Weisman[37] recommends making the least possible contribution, sharing concerns, or calling on an absent witness. Making the least possible contribution does not mean doing as little as possible; rather, it means making a contribution that has the best chance for success with the least amount of strain. Another way to learn about detached concern is through sharing of experiences and seeking the feedback of peers regarding involvements with patients and families. "Coping well is aided by having something to measure our efforts (involvements) against and someone to derive support from."[37,p.167] The absent-witness technique involves asking a former patient, in absentia, to evaluate the care received. Questions couched in pragmatic terms provide feedback as to whether expectations regarding the level of involvement were desired or unrealistic.[37]

Intellectualization is another way of trying to achieve detached concern. It involves dealing with emotionally

GREATEST MOMENTS

The following are examples of "greatest moments" shared by colleagues:

I have known Cindi for only one year. I did her initial assessment when she came to the brain tumor clinic for the first time. I knew that Dr. S. was going to tell Cindi that there wasn't anything else to do so. I went into the exam room with him. Cindi and her parents were devastated. I couldn't help it, but my eyes filled with tears. Her parents saw the tears in my eyes and later told me "We appreciate how much you care. You're really good at what you do." —*JB*

I was a brand new nurse and new to the unit. Nita was a 67-year-old woman with three or four primary malignancies. Nita was essentially living in the hospital. She had been labeled LTC, or long-term care. People treated her like she looked: bad body–bad brain. She was extremely dependent on the staff for physical care. I heard a lot of stories. She was very isolated. I began to question "What are we doing?" The tenured staff rolled their eyes at me, but my head nurse was very supportive. I went to Nita and told her that I was going to be her primary nurse and that I needed her help in developing a care plan. I will never forget coming out of report about 2 or 3 weeks later to find that Nita had showered, washed her hair, and made her own bed. Although she died at the hospital, she was able to make several visits home. I know that I had helped to make it possible.—*MS*

This is a card I got from Willard at Easter ("Happy Easter. God bless and watch over you. Your friend, Willard"). Willard is in a wheelchair and lives in a housing project. His girlfriend was a GYN patient. She died 12 years ago, and at Christmastime that year, several other staff and I took Willard fruit and gifts. We've been doing it ever since. In his own way, I know he loves us.—*DS*

Mr. Smith was being sent home to die, and he knew it. He had just spoken with his doctor. It was rough because he was such a fighter. He had trouble communicating because of the multiple head and neck surgeries. I will never forget this. He put on his call light and, in his garbled voice, asked the clerk to find me. He held my hand and told me how much it had meant to him that I had been part of his ammunition. We cried together.—*GW*

A patient was referred to the pain clinic. She questioned how she could continue in light of the amount of pain she was having. She had had radiation therapy and had terrible esophageal pain. As a consequence, she hadn't been able to eat. We gave her 10 mg of intravenous morphine, and it gave her complete relief. Only 10 mg! With the relief, she wanted to eat something. Someone had brought donuts to the clinic that morning, so I offered her one. I will never forget her saying: "Eating this donut is like having an orgasm." I think we all need to eat more donuts.—*DT*

Gloria is a 42-year-old woman diagnosed with breast cancer. At the time I met her, she had bone metastasis and had excruciating pain due to C4-C6 bone disease with cord compression. Gloria and I had developed a professional friendship. I went into her room to inquire about her degree of pain relief. She told me that her pain was under control, but she was quiet, not acting like herself, and looked really down. I took a risk by asking her if she wanted me to stay for a while. I told her that I thought she looked upset and sad. That was all the permission she needed. Up from the depths came pent-up anguish. It would have been easier to have been satisfied that her pain was relieved and not address the suffering. As she cried and I held her, my eyes filled with tears. The next day, as I walked by her room, Gloria called out to me. She asked me to come close to her bedside. There she was in her hard cervical collar reaching up to embrace me. She said, "I know you care. I saw the tears in your eyes. You really helped me." I needed to hear that because I was afraid that all I had done was contribute to her suffering by being the catalyst. It felt good to know that I had helped.—*MC*

FIGURE 65-4 Source: Larson D: The challenge of caring in oncology nursing. *Oncol Nurs Forum* 19:857–861, 1992.

stressful situations in the abstract or as technical realities.[7] It serves as a defense mechanism in creating psychological or emotional distance from distressing situations. Given the intensity and intimacy of contact nurses have with patients, this process of dealing with people and events in one's head rather than in one's heart can serve as a buffer. A word of caution: Exclusive use of intellectualization creates imbalance as one becomes increasingly underinvolved. This underinvolvement creates stress, since most nurses are dissatisfied with underinvolvement. Additionally, suppression of one's emotional experiences requires energy and at some point will require attention.

Creating control of one's practice

This coping strategy involves developing and maintaining competency, setting limits, and organizing one's work to minimize stress and enhance satisfaction.[32] Developing and maintaining competence evolves through a series of stages. Nurses gain competency by developing professional skills through formal education programs, establishing goals, and testing competencies in clinical situations.[32] Competency continues to be refined in ongoing professional experiences to the point that nurses feel secure in their work environment. Competency and control are nurtured through ongoing professional experiences, feedback, development of more complex skills through continuing education, refinement of personal and professional goals, and professional affiliations.[32]

Mount stated that "reasonable limits of personal giving must be established if sustained, effective functioning is to be ensured."[46,p.1132] Limit setting helps to create a sense of mastery over one's work. This involves knowing and respecting one's limits and deciding what one can and cannot do and what one will and will not do. Working overtime and being on call while off duty are prime examples of areas where limit setting is required.[32] Changing on-call status by rotating responsibility is another. The individual can do a lot to set limits, but individual effort can be greatly strengthened by organizational policies that establish limits for overtime, provide a mechanism for equal sharing of on-call responsibility, and give adequate compensation for overtime and on-call work.

Strategies to foster a sense of control over one's work include reorganization of work and development of specialized roles.[9] Organizing work assignments so the work is varied can counterbalance emotionally draining work with task-oriented work. Strategies to restructure work assignments could include job sharing (e.g., research nurse and staff nurse job sharing), changing the context of the contact with patients (e.g., cross-training staff to work in inpatient and outpatient settings), sharing responsibility for difficult patient care assignments (e.g., two to three staff nurses serve as patient's primary care nurses and rotate direct care responsibilities), and creating a balanced mix of patients (e.g., chemotherapy nurse cares for the newly diagnosed patient, the patient in remission, and the patient receiving relapse therapy). Developing specialized roles can give a sense of control and pleasure from one's work. Specialized roles might include developing an expertise in a particular aspect of care (e.g., mouth care, venous access devices, pain management) and taking on special assignments (e.g., developing patient-teaching materials, serving on a patient care products and equipment committee, coordinating the evaluation of a patient care protocol).

Relaxation

Chronic stress often produces tense muscles, increased blood pressure, and fatigue.[78] Relaxation brings mental and physical restoration. Relaxation is based on the mind–body connection and the premise that a relaxed body is the antithesis of a stressed mind. There are many forms of relaxation techniques: progressive deep-muscle relaxation, biofeedback, guided imagery, meditation, yoga, and autogenic training.[78] The key to the effectiveness of any technique is practice. Practice requires a commitment to self-care. Regular use of relaxation techniques can yield a state of relaxation that is incompatible with stress. Stress symptoms signal a warning; recognizing the symptoms requires learning to listen to one's body. Relaxation treats the symptoms, not the cause, but provides renewal to face the next challenge.

Adopting a wellness philosophy

A wellness philosophy promotes health behaviorally. Healthy choices include eating a balanced diet, limiting alcohol and caffeine intake, ceasing smoking, practicing preventive health care (e.g., mammograph, Pap smear, annual physical, dental care, eye exam), exercise, rest, recreation, socialization, and development of intimate relationships. The principal benefit of actively adopting a wellness philosophy is conditioning the body to withstand the deleterious effects of stress. Nurses are taught to train their minds for professional lives; likewise we must train and care for our bodies and spirits.

Environmental Strategies

Opportunities for personal achievement, recognition, growth, responsibility, and advancement mean work satisfaction. Organizations must be responsive to supplying these opportunities. Allen and Kraft[79] described six principles that lead to a more satisfying work environment: involvement with establishing work objectives and methods, clarity of organization and structure, feedback and information, orientation and training, rewards, and supportive culture. The initial organization-based stress management strategy requires an assessment of the nurse's perceptions of the following: discrepancies between accountability and authority, extent to which the job provides variety and challenge, extent to which the nurse's role is clearly defined, extent to which the nurse's role conflicts with purported roles of others of different status and position, opportunities for continued training and development, adequacy of supplies/equipment/space, amount of actual freedom and independence, and extent to which the nurse is receiving feedback concerning performance.[7]

Nurse–patient ratios

Nurses have a right to work in an environment that minimizes physical and emotional stress. Employers have a legal responsibility to provide sufficient staff to meet the care needs of patients.[80] The quality of nurse–patient interactions is influenced by the number as well as the acuity of the people for which the nurse is responsible.[12] As the number increases, so does role overload for the nurse. Staff–patient ratios that support the provision of quality patient care and equalization of demands with supplies decrease work load stress.[33] Unfortunately, in response to cost/benefit calculations or insufficient staffing, the norm in health care is the assignment of larger numbers of patients; yet, even if the numbers do not change, the complexity and acuity of care have increased. One organizational strategy to address nurse–patient ratios is to review the cost of staff turnover and staff burnout. Replacing an experienced nurse not only includes orientation training costs but the ongoing cost incurred until the novice nurse becomes expert. The measurement of patient care outcomes also serves as an index of the impact of nurse–patient ratios. In addition, time-and-motion studies provide information regarding nonnursing tasks that nurses are called on to do that could be handled by ancillary staff in order to free up nurses to be nurses.

Organizational flexibility

Kahn[55] wrote of organizational strategies to bring the organization more in line with the needs and abilities of the employee. A key strategy is organizational flexibility. Organizational flexibility implies concern for the individual. Often this involves giving the individual freedom, the permission to exert some control over her or his practice, and providing variability in routines.[32] Distrust and failure to recognize the needs and abilities of the individual employee create an inflexible system. A decentralized management system that puts the authority and responsibility for decision making at the level of the front-line practitioner is a means of providing flexibility and control. Decentralization also can serve to decrease the stress associated with feeling that those who make decisions are out of touch with the realities of providing care. Other areas in which organizations can provide flexibility include self-scheduling, job sharing, involvement with equipment selection, development of ongoing job descriptions that change with the individual's expertise and interests, and clinical ladders.

Creating opportunities for withdrawal

Pines and Aronson[12] emphasized the importance of time out from stressful situations. This concept of "time out" is important to any work that involves emotional, physical, or mental stress.[12] Time-out activities include providing not only for meal breaks but also for breaks from stressful work. Staff could share the direct care responsibilities for a particularly tedious or arduous patient care situation. A change in routine, perhaps working on a special project or attending continuing education programs away from the work site, could provide a needed time out. Strict attention must be paid to adhering to the rule that time away from work is truly time away from work. Organizations need to establish policies that guarantee protected time off and regular vacations. In addition, mental health days without penalty can provide emotional breathing space.

Social support

John Donne wrote, "No man is an island, entire to himself." The presence or absence of social support plays a major role in stress. Caplan[74] defined social support as "enduring interpersonal ties" to a group of people who can be relied on to provide emotional sustenance, assistance, and resources, who provide feedback, and who share standards and values. Social support systems serve a number of functions.[12] Most people need someone to listen actively to them, to listen without offering advice or making judgments. Technical appreciation and affirmation of competence can really only come from people who understand our work; nonexpert family members and friends are important for other types of emotional support and challenge that require someone who cares on a human-to-human level.[27]

Social support is crucial to nurses' well-being in today's complex health care system.[81] For nurses, receiving support often is difficult, for many nurses view themselves as caregivers, not as care receivers. Fear often keeps nurses from seeking support or expressing emotions: fear of not being accepted, fear of being seen as incompetent or inadequate, fear of being misunderstood, or fear of betrayal. Pines and Aronson[12] and Larson[30] refer to the phenomenon of the "fallacy of uniqueness," in which individuals falsely assume they are the only one feeling, thinking, or behaving in a particular way. By expressing feelings and experiences, nurses can learn that others share similar experiences—the nurse is no longer alone and isolated. These fears underscore the pivotal first step in the giving and getting of support: the development of trust and mutual respect. Larson[27,30] believes that, when helpers (nurses) talk about their stress and begin to see that much of how they feel, think, and behave is an inevitable part of their work, much of the distress in work can be ameliorated.

It is important to build work-based sources of support, because these seem to be more potent than individual efforts at reducing occupational stress.[81] In nursing, work-based supports not only provide for individual support but also provide a mechanism for institutional change through group problem solving. Staff meetings that give individuals opportunities to express themselves and to be involved with group problem solving can be a catalyst for the development of social support systems, as can task sharing and informal socialization.[12] Formalized support groups also can provide social support. They communicate a strong message of administrative support, for it is important for staff to feel that administration recognizes the stress that staff can experience and that it is willing to provide the extra resources necessary.[80,81]

Work team development

Vachon found that an important organizational coping mechanism was the "sense of belonging to a team that knew what it was doing, knew how to get members to work towards defined professional and personal goals, and knew how to support one another through professional and personal stressors."[32,p.212] Beckard[82] identified the characteristics of an effective team: clarity of objectives, goals, and priorities that are agreed on by team members; role expectations that are realistic and clearly defined; problem-solving and decision-making skills; group rules that support the objectives, goals, and priorities; concern for group members; and the ability to maximize group resources for the good of the group and the individual. These characteristics can be used as criteria for the periodic assessment of overall team functioning and effectiveness.

The organizational conditions of scarcity of or competition for resources, ambiguity (in procedures, policies, roles), overregulation, and exceptions ("The rules do not apply equally to everyone") provide rich fuel for conflict.[54] Effective group functioning can do much to manage or resolve conflict. When people in conflict are able to approach the conflict in an atmosphere of trust and mutual support, the energy that normally would be diverted to defensiveness is freed up for use in resolving the conflict.

CONCLUSION

Stress is pervasive to the human condition. Stress is the perceived imbalance between person–environment demands and abilities, or supplies. The reality-based and perception-based appraisals of intrapersonal, interpersonal, and environmental supplies and demands influence the amount and intensity of stress an individual experiences. The potential demands encountered and supplies available to cancer nurses have been described. Given the consequences to both person and environment, it is imperative that cancer nurses and the organizations that employ them be committed to decreasing demands and increasing supplies where possible.

REFERENCES

1. Selye H: *Physiology and Pathology of Exposure to Stress.* Montreal: ACTA Medical Publishers, 1950.
2. Derogatis L: Self-report measures of stress. In Goldberger L, Breznitz S (eds.): *Handbook of Stress: Theoretical and Clinical Aspects.* New York: Free Press, 1982, pp. 270–294.
3. Holmes T, Masuda M: Magnitude estimates of social readjustments. *J Psychosom Res* 11:219–255, 1966.
4. Holmes T, Rahe R: The social readjustment rating scale. *J Psychosom Res* 12:213–218, 1976.
5. Lazarus R: *Psychological Stress and Coping Process.* New York: McGraw-Hill, 1966.
6. Lazarus R, Folkman S: *Stress, Appraisal, and Coping.* New York: Springer, 1984.
7. Muldary T: *Burnout and Health Professionals: Manifestations and Management.* Norwalk, CT: Appleton-Century-Crofts, 1983.
8. French J, Rodgers W, Cobb S: Adjustment as person-environment fit. In Coelho GV, Hamburg DA, Adams JE (eds.): *Coping and Adaptation.* New York: Basic Books, 1974, pp. 213–222.
9. Vachon M, Stylianos S: Caring for the caregiver: A person-centered framework. In Baird S, McCorkle R, Grant M (eds.): *Cancer Nursing. A Comprehensive Textbook.* Philadelphia: Saunders, 1991, pp. 1084–1093.
10. Harrison R: Person-environment fit and job stress. In Cooper CL, Payne R (eds.): *Stress at Work.* New York: Wiley, 1979, pp. 175–205.
11. Maslach C: *Burnout: The Cost of Caring.* Englewood Cliffs, NJ: Prentice-Hall, 1982.
12. Pines A, Aronson E: *Career Burnout. Causes and Cures.* New York: Free Press, 1988.
13. Claus K, Bailey J: *Living with Stress and Promoting Well Being.* St. Louis: Mosby, 1980.
14. Appley M, Trumball R: On the concept of psychological stress. In Appley M, Trumball R (eds.): *Psychological Stress: Issues in Research.* New York: Appleton-Century-Crofts, 1967, pp. 1–13.
15. McGrath JE: Stress and behavior in organization. In Dunnette M (ed.): *Handbook of Industrial and Organizational Psychology.* Chicago: Rand McNally, 1976, pp. 1351–1396.
16. Haber J, Leach A, Schudy S, et al: *Comprehensive Psychiatric Nursing.* New York: McGraw-Hill, 1982.
17. Ellis A, Harper R: *A New Guide to Rational Living.* Hollywood:Wilshire Book, 1975.
18. Pearlin L, Schooler C: The structure of coping. *J Health and Soc Behavior* 19:2–21, 1978.
19. Rotter J, Seeman M, Liverant S: Internal vs. external locus of control of reinforcements: A major variable in behavior therapy. In Washburne N (ed.): *Decisions, Values and Groups.* London: Pergamon, 1962, pp. 76–99.
20. Keane A, DuCette J, Adler D: Stress in ICU and non-ICU nurses. *Nurs Res* 34:231–236, 1985.
21. Benner P, Wrubel J: *The Primacy of Caring. Stress and Coping in Health and Illness.* Menlo Park, CA: Addison-Wesley, 1989.
22. DuCette J, Wolk S: Cognitive and motivational correlates of generoleged expectancies for control. *J Personality Soc Psych* 22b:420–426, 1973.
23. Benton D, White D: Satisfaction of job factors for registered nurses. *J Nurs Admin* 11:55–63, 1972.
24. Maslow A: *Motivation and Personality.* New York: Harper & Row, 1954.
25. Vachon ML: Motivation and stress experienced by staff working with the terminally ill. *Death Ed* 2:113–122, 1978.
26. Smythe E: *Surviving Nursing.* Menlo Park, CA: Addison-Wesley, 1984.
27. Larson D: The challenge of caring in oncology nursing. *Oncol Nurs Forum* 19:857–861, 1992.
28. Northouse P, Northouse L: Communication and cancer: Issues confronting patients, health professionals and family members. *J Psychosoc Oncol* 5:17–46, 1988.
29. Silverman R, Wortman C: Coping with undesirable life events. In Garber J, Seligman M (eds.): *Human Helplessness: Theory and Applications.* New York: Academic Press, 1980, pp. 279–341.
30. Larson D: Helper secrets. *J Psychosocial Nurs* 25:20–27, 1987.
31. Larson P, Jennings B: The generation of stress in the provision of care. In Baird S, McCorkle R, Grant M (eds.): *Cancer Nursing. A Comprehensive Textbook.* Philadelphia: Saunders, 1991, pp. 1076–1083.
32. Vachon ML: *Occupational Stress in the Care of the Critically Ill, the Dying, and the Bereaved.* Washington, DC: Hemisphere Publishing, 1987.
33. McElroy A: Burnout—A review of the literature with application to cancer nursing. *Cancer Nurs* 5:211–217, 1982.
34. Holsclaw P: Nursing in high emotional risk areas. *Nurs Forum* 4:36–45, 1965.

35. Newlin N, Wellisch D: The oncology nurse: Life on an emotional roller coaster. *Cancer Nurs* 1:447–449, 1978.
36. Ehlke G: The psychological aspects of cancer. In Burkhalter P, Donley D (eds.): *Dynamics of Oncology Nursing.* New York: McGraw-Hill, 1976, pp. 211–226.
37. Weisman AD: Understanding the cancer patient: The syndrome of caregiver's plight. *Psychiatry* 44:161–168, 1981.
38. Fagin C, Diers D: Nursing as metaphor. *N Engl J Med* 309:116–117, 1983.
39. Travelbee J: "What's wrong with sympathy?" *Am J Nurs* 64:68–71, 1964.
40. Wegmann J: Avoidance behaviors of nurses as related to cancer diagnosis and/or terminality. *Oncol Nurs Forum* 6:8–14, 1979.
41. Stewart B, Meyerowitz B, Jackson L, et al: Psychological stress associated with outpatient oncology nursing. *Cancer Nurs* 5:383–387, 1982.
42. Steeves R, Kahn D, Benoliel J: Nurses' interpretation of the suffering of their patients. *West J Nurs Res* 12:715–731, 1990.
43. Boring C, Squires T, Tong T: Cancer statistics, 1991. *CA* 41:19–38, 1991.
44. Becker E: *Denial of Death.* New York: Macmillan, 1973.
45. Zilboorg G: Fear of death. *Psychoanal Q* 12:465–475, 1943.
46. Mount B: Dealing with our losses. *J Clin Oncol* 4:1127–1134, 1986.
47. Larson P: Important nurse caring behaviors perceived by patients with cancer. *Oncol Nurs Forum* 11:46–50, 1984.
48. Leininger M: Caring: A central focus of nursing and health services. In Leininger M (ed.): *Care: The Essence of Nursing and Health.* Thorofare, NJ: Slack, 1984, pp. 45–58.
49. Pearson C: *Awakening the Heroes Within.* San Francisco: HarperCollins, 1991.
50. Schaef A: *Women's Reality.* San Francisco: Harper & Row, 1985.
51. Larson D: The codependent caregiver: A dangerous myth? *Hospice* 6:17–19, 1991.
52. Whitfield C: *Healing the Child Within.* Deerfield Beach, FL: Health Communication, Inc., 1967.
53. Gunning C: The profession itself as a source of stress. In Jacobson S, McGrath H (eds.): *Nurses Under Stress.* New York: Wiley, 1983, pp. 113–126.
54. Pneuman R, Bruehl M: *Managing Conflict.* Englewood Cliffs, NJ: Prentice-Hall, 1982.
55. Kahn R: Conflict, ambiguity and overload: Three elements in job stress. *Occup Mental Health* 3:2–9, 1973.
56. French J, Kaplan R: Organizational stress and individual strain. In Marrow A (ed.): *The Failure of Success.* New York: AMACOM, 1973, pp. 89–103.
57. Maslach C, Pines A: The burnout syndrome in the daycare setting. *Child Care Q* 6:100–113, 1977.
58. Pines A, Kafry D: Occupational tedium in the social services. *Social Work* 23:499–507, 1978.
59. Arena D, Page N: The imposter phenomenon in the clinical nurse specialist role. *Image: J Nurs Scholar* 24:121–125, 1992.
60. Maslach C: The burn-out syndrome and patient care. In Garfield C (ed.): *Stress and Survival.* St. Louis: Mosby, 1980, pp. 43–56.
61. Kahn R, Wolfe D, Quinn R, et al: *Organizational Stress: Studies in Role Conflict and Ambiguity.* New York: Wiley, 1981.
62. Seligman M: *Helplessness: On Depression, Development and Death.* San Francisco: William Freeman, 1975.
63. Wise H: Preface. In Wise H, Beckhard R, Rubin I (eds.): *Making Health Teams Work.* Cambridge, MA: Ballinger, 1974, p. 73.
64. Curtin L, Flaherty M: The nurse-nurse relationship. In McCorkle R, Hongladarom G (eds.): *Issues and Topics in Cancer Nursing.* Norwalk, CT: Appleton-Century-Crofts, 1986, pp. 24–40.
65. American Nurses' Association and Oncology Nursing Society: *Standards of Oncology Nursing Practice.* Kansas City, MO: American Nurses' Association, 1987.
66. Cox A, Andrews P: The development of support systems on oncology units. *Oncol Nurs Forum* 8:31–35, 1981.
67. Calhoun G, Calhoun J: Occupational stress-implications for hospitals. In Selye H (ed.): *Selye's Guide to Stress Research* (vol. 3). New York: VanNostrand Reinhold, 1983, pp. 99–110.
68. Weisbord M: *Organizational Diagnosis: A Workbook of Theory and Practice.* Reading, MA: Addison-Wesley, 1978.
69. Menzies I: A case study in the function of social systems as a defense against anxiety. *Human Relat* 13:13–19, 1960.
70. Matthews P: A study of the effect of administrative climate on the nurses' psychological orientation toward the hospitalized patient. Unpublished doctoral dissertation. University of California, Berkley, 1962.
71. Lavandero R: Nurse burnout: What can we learn? *J Nurs Admin* 11:17–23, 1981.
72. Menaghan E: Individual coping efforts: Moderators of the relationship between life stress and mental health outcomes. In Kaplan H (ed.): *Psychosocial Stress.* New York: Academic Press, 1983, pp. 157–191.
73. Auerbach S: Stress management and coping research in the health care setting: An overview and methodological commentary. *J Consult Clin Psych* 57:388–395, 1989.
74. Caplan G: *Principles of Preventative Psychiatry.* New York: Basic Books, 1964.
75. Smith C: Principles in time management. In Jacobson S, McGrath H (eds.): *Nurses Under Stress.* New York: Wiley, 1983, pp. 226–236.
76. Ellis A: *Reason and Emotion in Psychotherapy.* New York: Lyle Stuart, 1962.
77. Lief H, Fox D: Training for "detached concern" in medical students. In Lief H, Lief V, Lief N (eds.): *The Psychological Basis of Medical Practice.* New York: Harper & Row, 1963, pp. 56–65.
78. Charlesworth E, Nathan R: *Stress Management.* New York: Atheneum, 1985.
79. Allen R, Kraft C: From burnout: Improving the quality of hospital work life. *Hospital Forum* 24:18–28, 1981.
80. Jacobson S, McGrath M: *Nurses Under Stress.* New York: Wiley, 1983.
81. Schmitt M: Social support, occupational stressors, and health in cancer nursing. In Baird S, McCorkle R, Grant M (eds.): *Cancer Nursing. A Comprehensive Textbook.* Philadelphia: Saunders, 1991, pp. 1065–1075.
82. Beckard R: Organizational implications of team building. In Wise H, Beckard R, Rubin I, Kyte A (eds.): *Making Health Care Teams Work.* Cambridge, MA: Ballinger, 1974, pp. 69–94.

PART IX

Yellow Pages: Cancer Nursing Resources

Marilyn Frank-Stromborg, RN, EdD, NP, FAAN

Barbara Barhamand, RN, MS, OCN

The "Yellow Pages" entries were compiled from a recent survey of a variety of health- and oncology-related organizations, which responded in varying lengths and formats. This compilation is the latest information the authors have received, but the accuracy and timeliness of membership information, prices for publications, and other data remain the responsibility of the respondents.

AUDIOVISUAL

Audiovisual Resources

1. American Cancer Society
1599 Clifton Road N.E.
Atlanta, GA 30029-4251
(404) 320-3333; (800) ACS-2345

The American Cancer Society has videos, filmstrips, audiotapes, and slides with accompanying text available for free loan. A catalogue listing of patient and professional education AV materials can be obtained by calling a local ACS unit. Availability may vary from unit to unit.

2. American Hospital Association
840 North Lake Shore Drive
Chicago, IL 60611
(312) 440-6800; (800) 242-2626

The AHA publishes an annual catalogue of monographs and AV products available, with a section designated for nursing resources.

3. National Audiovisual Center
Information Services SF
Washington DC 20409
(301) 763-1896; TDD: (301) 763-4385

This center distributes over 8000 U.S. government–sponsored productions at low prices. Contact the center for your specific area of interest and request free catalogues. Sample listing: *Diet and Cancer Prevention* (1986) Dr. Peter Greenwald, Director, Division of Cancer Prevention and Control, NCI, explores the effects of fat on breast and colon cancer, 58-minute videocassette.

4. National League of Nursing (NLN)
350 Hudson Street
New York, NY 10014
(800) 669-1656

In 1991 the Field Institute for Technology in Nursing Education (FITNE) and NLN published the fourth edition of the *Directory of Educational Software for Nursing*, which provides information for anyone interested in using a computer to teach nursing. There are complete descriptions and purchasing information for over 300 computer-assisted instruction (CAI) programs. Included are 100 new CAI programs for IBM and Apple Macintosh computers. Ratings were done by more than 2500 health care professionals; there are several oncology-related programs listed in this directory. Publication No. 41-2405 ($79.95).

Many universities and medical centers produce audiovisual material that can be purchased or rented. Their film libraries may also contain cancer-related audiovisuals that can be borrowed. Four examples are:

Carle Media
110 W. Main
Urbana, IL 61801
(217) 384-4838
Topics include AIDS, cancer, cancer survivorship, and hospice.

Lincoln Medical Education Foundation
4600 Valley Road
Lincoln, NE 68510
(402) 483-4581
Topics include chemotherapy, radiation therapy, and self-image.

University of Michigan Media Library
Dept. of Postgraduate Medicine & Health Professionals' Education
R4440 Kresge, Box 0518
Ann Arbor, MI 48109-0518
(313) 763-2074
Catalogue of medical and nursing audiovisuals, free upon request.

University of Wisconsin-Madison
Wisconsin Clinical Cancer Center
Cancer Prevention Program
1300 University Avenue—7C
Madison, WI 53706
(608) 263-6919
Title "Cancer Prevention: It's Up to You" can be rented or purchased; comes with corresponding public education materials.

Cancer Communications Pretesting

The National Cancer Institute's Office of Cancer Communications has published a booklet that provides information and guidance about measuring the effectiveness of the health message. It is provided free of charge and can be obtained by calling 1-800-4-CANCER.

One booklet, *Making Health Communication Programs Work: A Planner's Guide* (NIH Pub. No. 89-1493), discusses the purpose of pretesting, planning the health message, conducting pretesting research, conducting the pretest, and measuring the readability of the health message. It provides an extensive bibliography about pretesting and evaluating public service announcements and is provided free of charge.

ACADEMIC PROGRAMS AND CONTINUING EDUCATION OPPORTUNITIES

Master's Degree Oncology Nursing Programs

Several nursing schools offer graduate education in oncology, and the potential student can choose from several types of programs. Some programs offer separate, distinct, oncology clinical specialist master's curricula, whereas others offer the oncology component within the graduate program in medical–surgical nursing. Because curricula and programs change, the reader is advised to contact local universities to determine if the school of nursing offers a master's program in oncology nursing. In addition, the Oncology Nursing Society publication, "The Master's Degree With a Specialty in Oncology Nursing: Role Definition and Curriculum Guide" (1988), serves a dual purpose as a guide for (1) nursing educators in establishing new oncology programs or evaluating current ones and (2) prospective students in selecting a program. Another excellent source is the article "Survey of Graduate Programs in Cancer Nursing" in *Oncology Nursing Forum* 19:1417–1425, 1992. This article details specific information about each program (clinical focus, program length, application deadline, NLN accreditation, etc.).

Alabama
University of Alabama
School of Nursing
Judy Holcombe, RN, DSN
Associate Professor
Pediatric—Penelope Wright, RN, PhD
Assistant Professor
University of Alabama at Birmingham
University Station
Birmingham, AL 35294

Arizona
University of Arizona
Alice J. Longman, RN, EdD
Associate Professor
College of Nursing
Tucson, AZ 85721

California
University of California, Los Angeles
School of Nursing
Linda Sarna, RN, DNSc, OCN
Oncology Nursing Program Coord.
Los Angeles, CA 90024

University of California, San Francisco
Patricia Larson, RN, DNSc
School of Nursing
Department of Physiological Nursing
San Francisco, CA 94143

Connecticut
Yale University
School of Nursing
Wendy Holmes, RN, MSN
Assistant Professor/Coordinator
Medical-Surgical Nursing Program
New Haven, CT 06520

Delaware
University of Delaware
Jayne Fernsler, RN, DSN
Associate Professor
College of Nursing
University of Delaware
Newark, DE 19716

District of Columbia
Catholic University of America
Janice Hallal, RN, DNSc
Coordinator—Graduate Oncology Nursing
School of Nursing
Washington, DC 20064

Georgetown University
School of Nursing
Caroline Bagley-Burnett, ScD, RN
Assistant Professor
Washington, DC 20007

Florida
University of Miami
School of Nursing
Beverly Nielsen, RN, EdD
American Cancer Society Professor
of Oncology Nursing
Miami, FL 33124

University of South Florida
College of Nursing
Susan McMillan, RN, PhD
American Cancer Society Professor
of Oncology Nursing
Chairperson, Oncology Nursing
Tampa, FL 33612

Georgia
Emory University
Ann T. Foltz, RN, DNSc
Assistant Professor
Oncology Nursing
Marilyn Hockenberry-Eaton, MS, RNC, PNP
Associate Professor
Atlanta, GA 30322

Georgia State University
School of Nursing
Carolyn Kee, RN, PhD
Chairperson, Adult Health
Associate Professor, Nursing
Patricia Cotanch, RN, PhD
Research Liaison Professor, Nursing
College of Health Science
Atlanta, GA 30303

Illinois
Loyola University of Chicago
Niehoff School of Nursing
Esther Mattassarin, RN, PhD, OCN
Associate Professor
Medical Surgical Nursing
Chicago, IL 60626

Northern Illinois University
School of Nursing
Sara Berger, RN, PhD, FAAN
Professor
DeKalb, IL 60115

Rush University
College of Nursing
Judith Paice, RN, PhD
Assistant Professor
Graduate Program in Oncology Nursing
Chicago, IL 60612

Indiana
Indiana University
School of Nursing
Cheryl Bean, DSN, RN, CS, OCN
Associate Professor
Indianapolis, IN 46223

Maryland
University of Maryland
School of Nursing
Anne E. Belcher, RN, PhD
Associate Professor and
American Cancer Society Professor
of Oncology Nursing
Baltimore, MD 21201

Massachusetts
Massachusetts General Hospital Institute of Health Professions
Elizabeth M. Grady, PhD, RN
Program Director
Boston, MA 02108-9990

Missouri
- St. Louis University
  School of Nursing
  Ramona M. Wessler, RN, PhD
  St. Louis, MO 63104
- University of Missouri, Columbia
  Elizabeth A. Geden, RN, PhD
  Associate Dean for Research
  Director, Graduate Studies
  Columbia, MO 65211

Nebraska
- University of Nebraska
  College of Nursing
  Adult Health and Illness Department
  Lani Zimmerman, RN, PhD
  Omaha, NE 68105-1065

New York
- Columbia University
  School of Nursing
  Marianne Glasel, RN, MS, MA
  Director, Oncology Program
  New York, NY 10032
- The Sage Colleges
  Vaughn L. Nevin, RN, EdD
  Director, Graduate Program
  Troy, NY 12180
- State University of New York, Buffalo
  School of Nursing
  Katherine Wallace, RN, PhD
  Assistant Professor
  910 Kimball Tower
  Buffalo, NY 14214
- University of Rochester
  School of Nursing
  Jean Johnson, RN, PhD
  Associate Director/Professor
  Cancer Center Nursing
  Rochester, NY 14642

North Carolina
- Duke University
  School of Nursing
  Mary T. Champagne, RN, PhD
  Dean
  Durham, NC 27710
- University of North Carolina at Chapel Hill
  Inge Corless, PhD, FAAN
  Chairman, Secondary Care Nursing
  School of Nursing
  Chapel Hill, NC 27514

Ohio
- Frances Payne Bolton School of Nursing
  Case Western Reserve University
  M. Linda Workman, PhD, RN, OCN
  Associate Professor
  Cleveland, OH 44106
- Medical College of Ohio
  School of Nursing
  Joanne Guyton-Simmons, PhD, RN
  Medical–Surgical Nursing
  Toledo, OH 43699
- University of Cincinnati
  Jan S. Fulton, PhD, RN
  Assistant Professor
  College of Nursing and Health
  Cincinnati, OH 45221

Pennsylvania
- Gwynedd-Mercy College
  Patricia Bennett, RN, MA
  Oncological Nursing
  Graduate Nursing Division
  Gwynedd Valley, PA 19437
- University of Pennsylvania
  Ruth McCorkle, RN, PhD, FAAN
  American Cancer Society
  Professor, Oncology Nursing
  Nursing Education Building
  School of Nursing
  Philadelphia, PA 19104
- University of Pittsburgh
  School of Nursing
  Catherine Bender, RN, MN
  Assistant Professor
  Graduate Program Oncology Nursing
  Pittsburgh, PA 15261

South Carolina
- University of South Carolina
  College of Nursing
  Janet F. Nussbaum, RN, EdD
  Oncology Nursing
  Columbia, SC 29208

Tennessee
- University of Tennessee
  College of Nursing
  Dianne Greenhill, RN, EdD
  Associate Dean
  Memphis, TN 38163
- Vanderbilt University
  James C. Pace, RN, DSN, MDN
  Oncology Specialty
  Nashville, TN 37240

Texas
- University of Texas
  Health Science Center
  Jeanette Adams, RN, DrPH, OCN
  Division Head—Oncology
  School of Nursing
  Houston, TX 77030

Utah
- Brigham Young University
  Camilla Wood, RN, PhD
  Professor and Oncology Nursing Program Coordinator
  College of Nursing
  Provo, UT 84602
- University of Utah
  Kathi Mooney, RN, PhD
  Associate Professor
  College of Nursing
  25 South Medical Drive
  Salt Lake City, UT 84112

Virginia
- George Mason University
  Jeanne Sorrell, DAEd
  Coordinator

Advanced Clinical Nursing
Fairfax, VA 22030

Virginia Commonwealth University
Medical College of Virginia
Lorna Mill Barrell, PhD, RN
Interim Director, Master's Program
Richmond, VA 23298

Washington

University of Washington
Betty Gallucci, RN, PhD
Professor, Department of Physiological Nursing
Diana Wilkie
Assistant Professor, Department of Physiological Nursing
Seattle, WA 98195

University of Washington
Jane Cornman, RN, PhD
Assistant Professor
Department of Parent & Child
Nursing SC-74
Seattle, WA 98195

Wisconsin

University of Wisconsin
School of Nursing
Marilyn Oberst, RN, EdD
Clinical Science Center
Madison, WI 53792

Enterostomal Therapy Programs

Enterostomal therapy (ET) is an allied healthcare field specializing in the care of patients with all types of abdominal stomas as well as the management of patients with a wide variety of draining sinus tracts and fistulas. This nurse specialist is called an enterostomal therapist. Currently, an applicant must be an RN with a baccalaureate degree in nursing with 1 year of recent (within 5 years) clinical experience in medical–surgical nursing. Tuition varies among programs. Scholarships are available through the International Association for Enterostomal Therapy, Inc. (IAET), ACS, United Ostomy Association, and many of the individual ET nurse programs.

It is best to first obtain a list of IAET-approved professional education programs from:

IAET
27241 La Paz Road
Suite 121
Laguna Niguel, CA 92656

IAET is the professional association for ET nurses. "The mission is to provide education, research, certification and a collaborative atmosphere to support state of the art health care management for individuals with wounds, ostomies and incontinence." Membership includes: *Journal of ET Nursing*, Standards of Care, ET Nursing Education Programs, scholarships, research grants, professional practice manual.

IAET-Accredited ET Nurse Education Programs

Please contact individual programs for program dates, types of structure(s), and costs.

Abbott Northwestern ET Nursing
Education Program
800 E. 28th Street at Chicago Avenue
Minneapolis, MN 55407
Phone: (612) 863-4601
Program Director: Brenda M. Kerschbaum, RN, MS, CETN
Medical Director: Stanley Goldberg, MD

Emory University Enterostomal Therapy
Nursing Education Program
The Emory Clinic—Room 3525
1365 Clifton Road, N.E.
Atlanta, GA 30322
Phone (404) 248-4067
Program Director: Dorothy Doughty, RN, MN, CETN
Medical Director: William C. McGarity, MD

M.D. Anderson Hospital and Tumor Institute
ET Nursing Education Program
Department of Nursing
Box #82, 1515 Holcombe Blvd.
Houston, TX 77030
Phone (713) 792-7132
Program Director: Beverly Hampton, RN, MSN, CETN
Medical Director: Richard Martin, MD

R.B. Turnbull, Jr. School of ET
Cleveland Clinic Foundation
Cleveland Center Hotel—KK 501
9500 Euclid Avenue
Cleveland, OH 44195-5161
Phone (216) 444-5966
Program Director: Paula L. Erwin-Toth, RN, MSN, CETN, CS
Medical Director: Frank Weakely, MD

Harrisburg Area ET Nursing Education Program
Wicks Educational Associates, Inc.
423 N. 21st Street
Camp Hill, PA 17011
(717) 737-2770
Program Development: Lucy J. Wicks, MSN, RN, CETN
Program Coordinator: Peggy E. Fallen

Albany Medical Center ETNEP, A-149
Albany Medical Center
New Scotland Avenue
Albany, New York 12208
Program Director: Sharon Aronovitch, RN, MS, CETN

Board Certification: The graduate of an IAET-accredited ET Nurse Education Program is eligible to become Board Certified by taking the Enterostomal Therapy Board Certification Examination. A brochure and application for Board Certification can be requested from the IAET.

PRINT SOURCES

Library Retrieval Services

Library or electronic information services have become a convenient, timely, and cost-effective method of accessing information by computer. Most hospital and university libraries subscribe to specific online databases, or they can be accessed from personal computers via a modem.

1. National Library of Medicine
8600 Rockville Pike
Bethesda, MD 20894
(301) 496-6193; (800) 638-8480

The NLM's MEDLARS is a service that allows for cost-effective searching of specialized databases. Available 24 hours a day. The user pays only for the actual costs of searching the databases. Citations can be printed on the user's printer, or printed at the NLM and mailed ("offline"). An offline print costs $0.18 per page, with a typical page containing eight citations without abstracts and two or three citations with abstracts. Specific databases include:

MEDLINE (abstracts to journal articles)
CATLINE (records of books)
AVLINE (records of audiovisuals)
CHEMLINE (information about chemical substances)
HEALTH (information about health care services)
TOXLINE (toxicological information)
DIRLINE (directory of 15,000 information resources)
AIDSLINE (AIDS-related references)
PDQ (advances in cancer treatment and clinical trials)

The NLM developed GRATEFUL MED software to allow for easy access to the Library's vast collection of medical and health science information. Because it both formulates the search strategy and presents the results offline, computer time is brief, productive, and cost-effective. An average search costs less than $3.00. The software is IBM- or Macintosh-compatible, available on 5¼" floppy disks or 3½" diskette, and sells for $29.95.

2. BRS Search Services
Maxwell Online, Inc.
8000 Westpark Drive
McLean, VA 22102
(800) 289-4277

BRS Information Technologies is another comprehensive electronic information service. Nearly 200 databases are available in the areas of medicine/pharmacology, education, life sciences, physical/applied sciences, reference, business, and social sciences/humanities; costs are based on online time, document charges and telecommunications (if applicable). BRS After Dark is a menu-driven service offering the most popular BRS databases (including CANCERLIT, MEDLINE, PDQ and NURSING & ALLIED HEALTH) at reduced rates for evening and weekend users.

3. DIALOG Information Services, Inc.
3460 Hillview Avenue
Palo Alto, CA 94304
(800) 3-DIALOG; (415) 858-3785 in CA

The Dialog Retrieval Service has a scope of 380 databases in the subject areas of science, business, technology, chemistry, law, medicine, engineering, social sciences, economics, current events, and more. Average costs are $6.00 to $16.50 for a 10-minute search, plus printing charges, if done offline. MEDLINE, CIS, and NURSING & ALLIED HEALTH are all accessible with DIALOG Services.

4. CancerFax—National Cancer Institute
International Cancer Information Service
9030 Old Georgetown Road
Bldg. 82 Room 219
Bethesda, MD 20892
FAX: (301) 402-5874; for assistance: (301) 496-8880

CancerFax was created by the NCI to combine the computer and the fax machine. The NCI sends current data on cancer treatment to any health care professional with a fax machine free of charge utilizing the PDQ database. There are two types of summaries, one for health professionals and one for the general public; the service is available 24 hours a day, 7 days a week. There is no charge for the service itself; the user pays only for the cost of the call to the CancerFax computer in Maryland.

Oncology Periodicals and Books

There are a myriad of oncology-related journals and books available for reference. *Medical and Health Care Books and Serials in Print,* found in most medical libraries, is an excellent bibliographic resource. Each journal listing includes publisher, subscription price, frequency of publication, and indexing information. A partial list, from the headings Oncology or Hematology, includes:

Acta Haematologica
Acta Oncologica
Advances in Cancer Research
American Journal of Clinical Oncology
American Journal of Hematology
American Journal of Pediatric Hematology-Oncology
Annals of Oncology
Anticancer Research
Blood
Breast Cancer Research and Treatment
British Journal of Cancer
British Journal of Haematology
CA—A Cancer Journal for Clinicians
Cancer
Cancer Chemotherapy and Pharmacology
Cancer Forum
Cancer Genetics and Cytogenetics
Cancer Immunology and Immunotherapy
Cancer Letters
Cancer Nursing
Cancer Research
Cancer Review
Cancer Treatment Reviews
Carcinogenesis
Clinical Oncology Alert
Contemporary Hematology-Oncology
Critical Review in Oncology-Hematology
Current Problems in Cancer
European Journal of Cancer and Clinical Oncology
European Journal of Gynecological Oncology
European Journal of Surgical Oncology
Hematology-Oncology Clinics of North America
International Journal of Cancer
Journal of Cancer Education
Journal of Clinical Oncology
Journal of Experimental and Clinical Hematology
Journal of Neuro-Oncology
Journal of Psychosocial Oncology
Journal of Tumor Marker Oncology
Leukemia Research
Medical and Pediatric Oncology
Medical Oncology and Tumor Pharmacotherapy
National Cancer Institute (NCI) Monographs
National Cancer Institute Journal
Neoplasma
Nutrition and Cancer
Oncogene

Oncology
Oncology Nursing Forum
Pediatric Hematology and Oncology
Progress in Cancer Research and Therapy
Recent Results in Cancer Research
Seminars in Hematology
Seminars in Oncology
Seminars in Oncology Nursing
Seminars in Surgical Oncology
Yearbook of Oncology

Books for the Health Care Professional (Sample Listing)

American Cancer Society: *American Cancer Society's Complete Book of Cancer: Prevention, Detection, Diagnosis, Treatment and Rehabilitation.* Holleb AI, Fink D, Murphy G (eds.).

Baird S: *Decision Making in Oncology Nursing.* Decker, 1987.

Baird S, McCorkle R, Grant M: *Cancer Nursing: A Comprehensive Textbook.* Saunders, 1991.

Brager BL, Yasko J: *Care of the Client Receiving Chemotherapy.* Appleton-Century-Crofts, 1984.

Chabner BA, Collins JM: *Cancer Chemotherapy: Principles and Practice.* Lippincott, 1990.

Chesler MA, Barbarian OA: *Childhood Cancer and the Family: Meeting the Challenge of Stress and Support.* Brunner-Mazel, 1987.

DeVita VT, Hellman S, Rosenberg SA (eds.): *Cancer: Principles and Practice of Oncology.* Lippincott, 1989.

Donovan M, Girston S: *Cancer Care Nursing* (2nd ed.). Appleton-Century-Crofts, 1984.

Groenwald SL, Frogge MH, Goodman M, Yarbro CH (eds.): *Cancer Nursing: Principles and Practice* (2nd ed.). Jones and Bartlett, 1990.

Haskell CM: *Cancer Treatment* (3rd ed.). Saunders, 1990.

Maul-Mellott SK, Adams JN: *Childhood Cancer: A Nursing Overview.* Jones and Bartlett, 1987.

Priestman TJ: *Cancer Chemotherapy* (3rd ed.). Springer-Verlag, 1989.

Ramstack J: *Nutrition for the Chemotherapy Patient.* Bull, 1990.

Smith DB, Johnson DE (eds.): *Ostomy Care and the Cancer Patient: Surgical and Clinical Considerations.* Saunders, 1986.

Williams WJ (ed.): *Hematology* (4th ed.) McGraw-Hill, 1990.

Yasko J (ed.): *Care of the Client Receiving External Radiation Therapy.* Appleton & Lange, 1982.

Oncology Patient Education Materials

Many organizations offer patient education materials that emphasize their special interest. Most are free of charge and can be ordered in quantity.

1. American Academy of Dermatology
P.O. Box 681069
Schaumburg, IL 60168
(708) 330-0230

The American Academy of Dermatology offers a catalogue of brochures that are available by writing the above address and enclosing a self-addressed, stamped envelope. The brochures are free of charge unless requested in quantities. The Academy gives physician referrals for the patient in their geographic location. Sample brochure titles include:

The Sun and Your Skin
Melanoma/Skin Cancer

2. American Cancer Society
1599 Clifton Road, NE
Atlanta, GA 30029-4257
(404) 320-3333; (800) ACS-2345

Each local chapter or division has an extensive assortment of booklets, videos, slides, reprints, posters, audiotapes, programs, and proceedings available at no charge covering all aspects of the cancer experience. Many are also available in Spanish. Some states also have a computer response system for approved information. The caller can request information on most cancer-related topics (e.g., unproven methods of cancer treatment) and receive a written synopsis with the "ACS's official opinion." Sample pamphlet titles include:

First Aid for Laryngectomees
First Steps: Helping Words (for laryngectomees)
Your New Voice
Rehabilitating Laryngectomees
Finding a Lump in Your Breast
Back to School (for parents of children with cancer)
Caring for the Patient with Cancer at Home
Chemotherapy: What It Is, How It Helps
It Helps to Have Friends (when Mom or Dad has cancer)
Talking with Your Doctor
Talking with the Cancer Patient: Listen with Your Heart
When Your Brother or Sister Has Cancer
Colostomy—A Guide
Ileostomy—A Guide
Urostomy—A Guide
Sexuality and Cancer (for the woman who has cancer)
Sexuality and Cancer (for the man who has cancer)

3. American Lung Association
1740 Broadway
New York, NY 10019-4374
(212) 315-8700

Local chapters can provide a free catalogue of public education materials including:

Lung Hazards on the Job: Occupational Lung Cancer
Facts About Lung Cancer
Facts About Radon
Occupational Lung Diseases
Carcinogens in the School

4. Candlelighters Childhood Cancer Foundation
7910 Woodmont Avenue, Suite 460
Bethesda, MD 20814
(800) 366-2223
(301) 657-8401

Candlelighters is an organization for children and the parents of children with cancer. Their newsletter, *Candlelighters Childhood Cancer Foundation Youth Newsletter* is written by and for adolescent cancer patients and teenage siblings.

5. *Coping*
Media America, Inc.
2019 North Carothers
Franklin, TN 37064
(615) 790-2400

The magazine *Coping* is published quarterly for cancer patients and their families. It includes such categories as education, support, lifestyle, treatment, research, and progress reports. Cost is $17 for 1 year ($23 outside the U.S.) and $30 for 2 years.

6. Ellis Fischel Cancer Center
115 Business Loop 70 West
Columbia, MO 65203
(314) 882-2100

The booklet "Implant Therapy and You" is available for patient education.

7. Office of Cancer Communications
National Cancer Institute
Building 31, Room 10A 24
Bethesda, MD 20892
(800) 4-CANCER

NCI publications are available on a wide variety of topics including prevention and detection, treatment, survivorship and research. Many are also available for Spanish or pediatric clientele. All are free, but quantities may be limited per monthly order. Allow 4 to 6 weeks for delivery of large orders. A catalogue listing or specific booklets are available by phone order. Examples include:

Chemotherapy and You
Radiation Therapy and You
Eating Hints
Facing Forward
Taking Time
Advanced Cancer: Living Each Day
Talking with Your Child About Cancer
What Are Clinical Trials All About
When Cancer Recurs: Meeting the Challenge Again
When Someone in Your Family Has Cancer
Young People with Cancer
Cancer Survivorship: An Annotated Bibliography

Site-specific booklets address individual cancers in the series: What you need to know about . . .

Bladder
Bone
Brain and Spinal Cord
Breast
Cervix
Colon and Rectum
Esophagus
Hodgkin's Disease
Kidney
Larynx
Adult Leukemia
Childhood Leukemia
Lung
Melanoma
Multiple Myeloma
Non-Hodgkin's Lymphoma
Head or Neck
Ovary
Pancreas
Prostate
Skin
Stomach
Testis
Uterus

8. National Coalition for Cancer Survivorship (NCCS)
1010 Wayne Avenue, 5th Floor
Silver Springs, MD 20910
(301) 650-8868

The NCCS is dedicated to providing a voice and advocacy in the area of survivorship. Publications available include a free booklet, "Teamwork: Talking with Your Doctor," and a book, *An Almanac of Practical Resources for Cancer Survivors*, by F. Mullan and Barbara Hoffman ($14.95). *The Networker* is the NCCS's quarterly newsletter.

9. Patient Education Office
University of North Carolina Hospitals
101 Manning Drive
Chapel Hill, NC 27514
(919) 966-1091

Series of patient education booklets are available that cover a variety of topics. For example, the *Series of Home Health Care Procedures* includes booklets on wound drainage, tracheostomy care, intracavity radiation therapy, biliary catheter care, and turning and positioning a patient. Each booklet is illustrated, uses simple language, and has questions throughout to test the patient's understanding of the material. The cost of each booklet is $2; a list of series is available. Materials can be photocopied.

10. Skin Cancer Foundation
245 Fifth Avenue, Suite 2402
New York, NY 10016
(212) 725-5176

The Skin Cancer Foundation has a variety of booklets, posters, a slide presentation, and video available regarding a multitude of issues. A contribution of $25 pays for a 1-year subscription to *Sun & Skin News* (4 issues, for public education) or *The Melanoma Letter* (4 issues, for professional education). Write or call for a free catalogue, or send a self-addressed, stamped envelope for a sample of a specific brochure. Bulk orders for distribution are available for a fee. Their booklets include:

Sunproofing Your Baby
Basal Cell Carcinoma—The Most Common Cancer
The Many Faces of Malignant Melanoma
Squamous Cell Carcinoma
For Every Child Under the Sun: A Guide to Sensible Sun
The ABCD's of Moles and Melanomas
Dysplastic Nevi & Malignant Melanoma—A Patient's Guide
Sun Sense

The resource books *Medical and Health Care Book and Serials in Print* also list numerous books available on cancer-related topics for the public. Many deal with coping with the diagnosis and treatment of cancer; some are anecdotal in style. A sample of books from this bibliographic resource includes:

Bloch, Annette & Bloch, Richard. *Cancer . . . There's Hope.* Cancer Connection, 1986.
Bloch, Annette & Bloch, Richard. *Fighting Cancer.* Cancer Connection, 1987.
Borysenko, J. *Minding the Body, Mending the Mind.* Bantam, 1988.
Bruning, Nancy. *Coping with Chemotherapy.* Ballantine, 1986.
Cook, Jeffrey C. *Coping with Cancer One Day at a Time.* Woodland, 1988.
Doan Noyes, D. & Mellody, P. *Beauty & Cancer: A Woman's Guide to Looking Great While Experiencing the Side Effects of Cancer Therapy.* AC Press, 1988.
Dollinger, Malin, Rosenbaum, Ernest & Cable, Greg. *Everyone's Guide to Cancer Therapy.* Andrews & McMeel, 1991.
Dravecky, Dave & Stafford, Tim. *Comeback.* HarperCollins, 1990.
Gaes, J. *My Book for Kids with Cansur.* Melius Peterson, 1988.
Harwell, Amy & Tomasik, Kristine. *When Your Friend Gets Cancer: How You Can Help.* Shaw, 1987.

Johnson, Judy & Klein, Linda. *I Can Cope: Staying Healthy with Cancer.* DCI, 1988.
Kauffman, Danette G. *Surviving Cancer: A Practical Guide for Those Fighting to Win.* Acropolis, 1989.
MacDonald, John A. *When Cancer Strikes: A Book for Patients, Families & Friends.* Prentice-Hall, 1982.
Morra, Marion & Potts, Eve. *Choices: Realistic Alternatives in Cancer Treatment.* Avon, 1987.
Mullan, Fitzhugh. *Vital Signs: A Young Doctor's Struggle with Cancer.* FS & G, 1983.
Muraa, Andy & Stewart, B. *Man to Man: When the Woman You Love Has Breast Cancer.* St. Martin's Press, 1989.
Rollin, Betty. *First You Cry.* Lippincott, 1976.
Siegel, Bernie S. *Love, Medicine, & Miracles.* Harper & Row, 1986.
Siegel, Mary-Ellen. *The Cancer Patient's Handbook: Everything You Need to Know about Today's Care & Treatment.* Walker & Co. 1986.
Simonton, C., Matthews-Simonton, S., & Creighton, J. *Getting Well Again.* Bantam, 1988.
Snyder, M. *An Informed Decision: Understanding Breast Reconstruction.* Little, Brown, 1989.

ORGANIZATIONS: PROFESSIONAL AND CLIENT SELF-HELP

Self-Help and Patient-Oriented Oncology Organizations

1. American Brain Tumor Association
3725 North Talman Avenue
Chicago, IL 60618-4712
[formerly Association for Brain Tumor Research]
(312) 286-5571; (312) 549-5561 FAX
(800) 886-2282 Patient Services

The American Brain Tumor Association is a national organization that provides written information about brain tumors and their treatment. Services include patient education materials, listings of brain tumor support groups, referrals to support organizations, and information about treatment facilities. A triannual newsletter, the *Message Line,* describes research advances and announces updates to publications

Publications for American Brain Tumor Association:

Publications	Price @
Basic Series:	
AFBTR Dictionary (Booklet)	.75
A Primer of Brain Tumors (Booklet)	1.00
Coping with a Brain Tumor (Booklet)	.75
Living with a Brain Tumor: A Bibliography	.25
When Your Child Is Ready to Return to School	.25
Tumor Series:	
About Ependymoma	.25
About Glioblastoma and Malignant Astrocytoma	.25
About Medulloblastoma/PNET	.25
About Meningioma	.25
About Oligodendroglioma	.25
Treatment Series:	
Chemotherapy of Brain Tumors (Booklet)	.75
Immunotherapy of Brain Tumors (Booklet)	.75
Radiation Therapy of Brain Tumors, Part I: A Basic Guide	.25
Radiation Therapy of Brain Tumors, Part II: Background and Research Guide (Booklet)	.75
Shunts	.25
About the Association for Brain Tumor Research	No Charge

2. American Cancer Society: *I Can Cope*

This program addresses the educational and psychological needs of people with cancer and their families. A series of eight classes discusses the disease, coping with daily health problems, expressing feelings, living with limitations, and local resources. Through lectures, group discussions, and study assignments, the course helps people with cancer regain a sense of control over their lives.

American Cancer Society: Loan Closets and Transportation Services

Many ACS units have loan closets that supply sickroom equipment for home cancer patients. Equipment may include wheelchairs, walkers, surgical dressings, bedpans, hospital beds, shower chairs, etc. This equipment can be borrowed for as long as needed. Contact your local unit for this free service. In some communities the ACS offers patient transportation to physicians' offices, hospitals, or clinics for diagnosis and treatment. This service is run by ACS volunteers.

American Cancer Society: *Reach to Recovery*

Women with breast cancer today have a growing number of rehabilitation options to choose from. Reach to Recovery is one of the first and largest of the American Cancer Society's patient visitor programs.

Volunteers—women who already have adjusted successfully to their own breast surgery—visit new patients, with their physicians' consent. These visits are made both preoperatively and after surgery. One of the newer aspects of Reach to Recovery is to provide information to postmastectomy patients who are considering breast reconstruction. Updated materials also focus on the special needs of minority groups and single women who have had breast cancer treatment.

3. American Foundation for Urologic Disease, Inc.
1120 North Charles Street
Suite 401
Baltimore, MD 21201

"The Mission of the American Foundation for Urologic Disease is the prevention and cure of urologic disease through the expansion of medical research, and the education of the public and health care professionals concerning urologic diseases."

4. American Lung Association

Some of the smoking literature, posters, buttons, and smoking cessation materials are listed below. Contact your local American Lung Association.

Pamphlets:

How Not To Love Your Kids (English and Spanish)
Emphysema—The Facts About Your Lungs

Cigarette Smoking—The Facts About Your Lungs
Marijuana: A Second Look at Health Hazards
Is There a Safe Tobacco?
Facts About Second-Hand Smoke
A Guide to Smokeless Tobacco
A No-Smoking Coloring Book (coloring booklet for children)
Help a Friend Stop Smoking
Nonsmokers' Rights, What You Can Do
Me Quit Smoking? How?

Posters:

This Is a Smoke-Free Workplace
Thanks for Not Smoking
Almost 35 Million Americans Quit Smoking
Brooke Shields: Smoking Spoils Your Looks
Be Kind to Nonsmokers

Films:

Breathing Easy Film—film for fifth- and eighth-graders
As We See It—made for preteens
Everything You Always Wanted to Know About How to Stop Smokers but Were Afraid to Try—interviews with nonsmokers, filled with humor and imagination

Anti-smoking programs:

Freedom from Smoking Booklets—Freedom from Smoking in 20 Days—self-help book shows you how to quit smoking in 20 days
Freedom from Smoking Home Video Program "In Control"
Freedom from Smoking T-Shirt Iron-Ons
Freedom from Smoking in The Workplace Booklets
Freedom from Smoking buttons and posters and tent cards

Puzzles:

Have Fun!! Figure Out the Smoking Puzzle

5. American Self-Help Clearinghouse
St. Clares-Riverside Medical Center
Denville, NJ 07834
(201) 625-7101 group information; TDD (201) 625-9053
(201) 625-9565 Administrative

Self-Help Clearinghouse in Canada
Calgary (403) 262-1117
Halifax (902) 422-5831
Saskatchewan (306) 652-7817
Toronto (16) 487-4512
Vancouver (604) 731-7781
Winnipeg (204) 589-5500 or 633-5955
National newsletter, *Initiative* (613) 728-1865 (C.C.S.D. in Ottawa)

For information on any group, phone (201) 625-7101, or via TDD dial (201) 625-9053 any weekday between the hours of 9 AM and 5 PM Eastern time.

Staff and volunteers will seek to provide current information and contacts for any *national self-help groups* that deal with the caller's particular concern. If no appropriate national groups exist and the caller is interested in the possibility of joining with others to start a local group, they can often also provide information on *model groups* operating in other parts of the country, or *individuals who are attempting to start such networks.* They will also always provide information on any *state or local self-help clearinghouse* that may exist to serve the caller's area. Such clearinghouses can often advise of existing local groups that may not be part of a national self-help organization. Most clearinghouses can also provide varying degrees of assistance to individuals who want to start a local group.

For a *free listing of phone contacts for self-help clearinghouses* in the United States and Canada, please send them a stamped, self-addressed envelope with request.

Consultation Service

If there is *no group or support network that exists anywhere* for a problem and the individual is interested in starting one, the *Clearinghouse can help them* with suggestions, materials, and other possible support, e.g., listing the individual and their interest on its computer database that is used by over a dozen self-help clearinghouses in the United States and Canada.

In any case, for a *free handout on Ideas for Starting a Self-Help Group,* simply send a stamped, self-addressed envelope with request.

Other Helpful Organizations

O.D.P.H.P. National Health Information Clearinghouse (800) 336-4797 in U.S.
National Organization for Rare Disorders (800) 999-N.O.R.D. in U.S.
Alliance of Genetic Support Groups (genetic illnesses) (800) 336-GENE in U.S.

Also available from the Self-Help Clearinghouse:

The Self-Help Sourcebook
A comprehensive national guide to finding and forming mutual aid and self-help groups.

Updated contacts and descriptions for now over 600 national and model self-help groups, which cover a broad range of addictions, disabilities, illnesses, parenting concerns, bereavement, and many other stressful life situations. Includes an easy-to-use index.

Includes general ideas and suggestions for starting a mutual-aid self-help group.

Provides contacts for dozens of self-help clearinghouses worldwide and listing of over 100 national toll-free helplines.
Additional sections on resources for rare and genetic illnesses and home computer networks.

Cost per copy postage-paid is $9.00 book rate or $10.00 first-class mail. Prepayment required.

The *Self-Help Sourcebook* can be a valuable resource for community networkers as well as for professionals. It can prove especially helpful for those serving in the health, mental health, or social service fields; for reference librarians, information and referral helplines, or Employee Assistance Program staff; for clergy, self-help intergroups, or for others who help people to find or create the mutual support groups they seek. ISSN: 8756-1425. Paperback, 174 pages, printed September, 1990.

6. American Society for Parenteral and Enteral Nutrition (ASPEN)
8630 Fenton Street, Suite 142
Silver Spring, MD 20910
(301) 587-6315

7. Association for the Care of Children's Health
7910 Woodmont Avenue
Suite 300
Bethesda, MD 20814
(301) 654-6549; FAX (301) 986-4553

The Association for the Care of Children's Health (ACCH) is an educational and advocacy organization with a multidisciplinary membership structure. ACCH membership totals over 4,000, representing health and social service professionals, educators, researchers, parents, and community leaders. ACCH members work within their institutions, organizations, and communities to promote improved systems of health care for children and their families.

Beyond this service of advocacy, ACCH:

produces educational materials that provide greater understanding of psychosocially sound, developmentally supportive, family-centered care and practical knowledge to make it a reality;

holds an annual conference, bringing together members and others to share knowledge, skills, and experiences;

plans and coordinates Children and Hospitals Week each year to focus community attention on the unique needs of children and families as they interact with the health care system;

publishes *Children's Health Care,* a quarterly journal, along with five newsletters, *ACCH News, ACCH Network, Affiliate Update, Canadian Connections,* and *Child Health Design;*

assists a North American parent network in working collaboratively with professionals in shaping systems of health care;

convenes periodic meetings of families caring for children with HIV infection;

provides services to designers and architects to ensure that planning, space allocation, construction, renovation, and design are responsive to the unique needs of children, families, and other care providers; and

provides information, referral, and support through a clearinghouse for professionals and families of infants with disabilities and special health needs.

ACCH publishes many educational resources for professionals, children, and families. ACCH also educates and supports its members and others through an annual conference, Children and Hospitals Week, and several award and grant programs. Through four major program areas, the National Center for Family-Centered Care, Pediatric AIDS: Commitment to Caring, the Design Resource Center, and the National Information Clearinghouse for infants with disabilities and life-threatening conditions, ACCH offers significant support for greater understanding and improved systems of health care for children and their families.

Selected publications that are available from the Association for the Care of Children's Health include:

Parent Resource Directory (4th Edition; C. Schmitt, Ed., 1991)

A networking resource for those caring for children with chronic illnesses or disabilities. Listings by state/province of over 400 parents of children with special needs. Included addresses, child's condition, and parents' particular interests and skills. 121 pp. $7.00

Pediatric AIDS: The Challenge of HIV Infection in Infants, Children, and Adolescents (P. A. Pizzo & C. M. Wilfert, Eds., 1990)

Comprehensive, authoritative text on pediatric HIV infection covering many perspectives: evolving epidemiology; biology, pathogenesis, and transmission; diagnostic issues; clinical manifestations; treatment; and prevention, education, and public policy. 813 pp. $84.95

You and HIV: A Day at a Time (L.S. Baker, 1991)

This easy-to-read, illustrated book guides children with HIV and their families through the medical and psychological whats and whys of HIV—transmission, diagnosis, treatment, home care, and emotional responses. Strongly emphasizes living with the disease, with room to write personal notes or information. 258 pp. $16.95

Seasons of Caring (Film/Videotape; 1986)

Reveals the concerns and priorities of families caring for children with special health needs. Addresses issues encountered by parents, teachers, social workers, school administrators, physicians, nurses, and others caring for these children and their families. 40 minutes, color.
16 mm—$245.00
½" VHS—$140.00
Preview—$60.00

8. Association for Research of Childhood Cancer
P.O. Box 251
Buffalo, NY 14225-0251
(716) 689-8922

The Association for Research of Childhood Cancer is composed of parents who have lost children to cancer and of people who support cancer research. The association funds the expansion and continuation of research in pediatric cancer centers and provides money for pilot projects in cancer research. The association meets six times per year to support parents of children with cancer and also publishes a quarterly newsletter and the *Parent/Child Handbook.*

9. Cancer Care, Inc.
and the National Cancer Care Foundation
1180 Avenue of the Americas
New York, NY 10036
(212) 221-3300

Cancer Care is a nonprofit, nonsectarian, East Coast, social service agency founded in 1944 to help cancer patients and their families and friends cope with the impact of cancer. Cancer Care is separate and apart from any other cancer organization. They are the largest agency in the nation solely dedicated to providing psychological and financial support to cancer patients and their families and community education programs for the general public. They treat people at all stages of the illness and provide help to both patient and family.

Cancer Care provides the following services:

professional counseling for cancer patients and their families, both on an individual basis and in groups

supplementary financial assistance to help families meet certain home care costs such as homemakers, home health aides, housekeepers, and for transportation for radiation and chemotherapy treatments

bereavement counseling to help surviving family members cope with their loss

information and referral to homemaking services, hospices, child care services, hospitals, and other resources in the community guidance to develop a plan for care for the patient at home

volunteer program where volunteers act as friendly visitors to homebound or frail cancer patients

education and training regarding psychosocial aspects of cancer for professionals and allied health care providers

Cancer Care has offices in:

New York City
1180 Avenue of the Americas
New York, NY 10036
(212) 302-2400

Long Island
20 Crossways Park North
Suite 304
Woodbury, NY 11797
(516) 364-8130

New Jersey
Central office:
241 Millburn Avenue, Suite 241-C
Millburn, NJ 07041
(201) 379-7500

Bergen County office:
127 East Ridgewood Avenue
Ridgewood, NJ 07450
(201) 444-6630

Connecticut
120 East Avenue
Norwalk, CT 06851
(203) 854-9911

Services are available at other part-time offices in the tri-state area. For information call (212) 302-2400.

10. CAnCare
Cancer Partners: A Supportive Network
2929 Selwyn Avenue
Charlotte, NC 28209
(704) 372-1232

CAnCare is a one-on-one psychosocial support service for cancer patients and their families. Volunteers have experienced cancer either as patient or family member. After completing a required training course, volunteers are matched with cancer patients with whom they build supportive relationships that last throughout the trauma. Volunteers, men and women, represent some 30 different cancers, and range in age from the 20s to the 80s. Listening to the concerns of the cancer patient, they help defuse fears and build hope. The link between volunteer and patient is a win-win situation, helping both as healing energy flows between them. CAnCare has been in service for 9 years. It is supported by churches, corporations, and grass-roots contributions.

11. Cancer Support Network
802 E. Jefferson
Bloomington, IL 61701
(309) 829-2273

The Cancer Support Network is a not-for-profit organization formed to provide personal support and encouragement to cancer patients in a number of ways. They do not provide medical advice or make referrals. Although not funded by the American Cancer Society or the National Cancer Institute, they do network with them and a variety of support groups across the country to get answers to questions asked by people with cancer. Cancer Support Network has a lending library, support groups, and hotline manned by volunteers (309) 829-CARE.

12. Candlelighters Childhood Cancer Foundation
Suite 460
7910 Woodmont Avenue
Bethesda, MD 20814
(301) 657-8401
(800) 366-CCCF
(301) 657-8319 FAX

Candlelighters began in April 1970 as a group of parents of young cancer patients at local hospitals and clinics in the Washington, DC, area. The group's focus is children, adolescents, and teens. There are presently 250 chapters in the United States. Candlelighters have two primary goals: to obtain consistent and adequate federal support for cancer research and to help parents and other family members who share the particularly difficult experience of living with a child with cancer. A national newsletter is published quarterly, which serves as a communication link among parents and parents' groups and concerned professionals. A quarterly youth newsletter is also published to provide information to young cancer patients. The free newsletters include information about research in childhood cancer, bibliography materials, and group activities. Local groups usually have their own newsletter. Candlelighters also publishes a resource list of childhood cancer education materials. All the above information is available free on request.

13. Children's Hospice International
901 North Washington Street
Suite 700
Alexandria, VA 22314
(703) 684-0330
(800) 242-4453

Children's Hospice International provides a network of support for dying children and their families. It serves as a clearinghouse on research programs, support groups, and education and training programs for the care of terminally ill children. It also offers publications on topics such as home care for seriously ill children and on pain management.

14. Choice In Dying
250 West 57th St.
New York, NY 10107
[formerly Concern for Dying and Society for the Right to Die]

Choice In Dying provides members and nonmembers with a *Living Will Declaration* and a state-specific *Statutory Short Form Power of Attorney For Health Care.* A nominal annual membership fee provides the latest information on right-to-die developments, including any changes in the law; a subscription to the Choice In Dying newsletter, published three times a year; a wallet-size Living Will Membership Card to alert people that holder has a Living Will in the event of an emergency; and a discount on their publications, listed below:

General Publications

About Advance Medical Directives	$ 1.50
Spanish language version of About Medical Directives	$ 1.50
Medical Treatments and Your Living Will	$ 1.50
Nutrition and Hydration by Tube	$ 1.50

Stopping Unwanted Medical Treatment: Questions to Ask, People Who Can Help You	$ 1.50
The Complete Guide to Living Wills	$ 7.95
Options at the End of Life	
Study packet on assisted suicide	$ 15.00
Professional Education	
Talking about Advance Directives: A Guide for Health Care Providers	$ 1.50
Advance Directives and Community Education: A Manual for Institutional Caregivers	$ 30.00
Advance Directive Protocols and the Patient Self-Determination Act	$ 10.00
Refusal of Treatment Legislation: A State-by-State Compilation of Enacted Statutes	$100.00
Video: A Time To Choose (on advance directives)	$ 70.00
Video: In Sickness or in Health (about decision making in long-term care)	
Resident version	
Family version	$ 75.00
Staff version	each

15. Corporate Angel Network, Inc.
Westchester County Airport, Building One
White Plains, NY 10604
(914) 328-1313
(800) 328-4226 FAX

The Corporate Angel Network (CAN) is a nonprofit organization designed to arrange free air transportation for cancer patients. This nationwide program uses available seats on corporate aircraft being flown on business trips. CAN enables patients to obtain optimum treatment for their life-threatening disease. CAN permits patients to travel in comfort and dignity, spared the stresses of commercial air travel. CAN has already flown over 4300 patients through the cooperation and generosity of more than 500 participating corporations. Financial need is *not* a requirement.

Patient criteria:

Going to or from recognized treatment, consultation, or check-up.
Be able to walk onto the aircraft unassisted.
Not require life support systems or special services.
Provide doctor's name, address, and telephone number.
May be the bone marrow or blood platelet donor.
May be accompanied by someone, if space permits. Both parents may accompany a child patient.
Patients should make back-up commercial transportation plans.
CAN cannot guarantee to find an appropriate flight.

16. ENCORE
ENCORE Supervisor
National Board
YWCA
726 Broadway
New York, NY 10003
(212) 614-2827

ENCORE is the YWCA's discussion and exercise program for women who have had breast cancer surgery. It is designed to help restore physical strength and emotional well-being. A local branch of the YWCA, listed in the telephone directory, can provide more information about ENCORE.

17. The Gilda Radner Familial Ovarian Cancer Registry
Roswell Park Cancer Institute
New York State Department of Health
Elm and Carlton Streets
Buffalo, NY 14263
(716) 845-8063
(716) 845-3545 FAX

Individuals can register, and the registry has a newsletter.

18. Hospice Education Institute
Five Essex Square
P.O. Box 713
Essex, CT 06426
(800) 331-1620; (203) 767-1620; (203) 767-2746 FAX

The Hospice Education Institute is an independent, nonprofit organization founded in 1985.

The Hospice Education Institute serves a wide range of individuals and organizations interested in hospice and palliative care throughout the United States and around the world. Its toll-free referral service directs over 8000 callers a year to local hospice programs. Further, by working with health and caring professionals and with educators who teach courses on dying, grief, and bereavement, the Hospice Education Institute disseminates information about hospice care at many levels.

The services of the Hospice Education Institute include:

HOSPICELINK, which maintains a computerized and continually updated directory of hospice programs in the United States, and operates a toll-free telephone number (800-331-1620) to refer callers to local hospice and palliative care programs. HOSPICELINK also provides general information about the principles and practice of hospice care. Staff members will listen sympathetically and give limited, informal support to callers who wish to discuss immediate personal problems relating to terminal illness and bereavement. (HOSPICELINK does not offer medical advice or provide psychological counseling.) There is no charge for any HOSPICELINK service.

Regional seminars on many aspects of caring for dying and the bereaved are organized for health and caring professionals and qualified hospice volunteers. Since 1986, seminars have been offered in 24 states. Faculty members for these seminars are international multiprofessional experts on hospice care. The Institute also sponsors the annual Hospice Study Seminar in Britain—a 2-week workshop for hospice professionals from all over the world.

Advice and assistance are freely given to people working to begin or improve hospice care in their communities.

Books and pamphlets are available from the Hospice Education Institute on hospice-related subjects. The Hospice Education Institute's *Notes on Symptom Control in Hospice and Palliative Care* is the definitive work to date on symptom control. ($28.95)

Other publications are:

Loss and Bereavement (Cook/Phillips) ($12.95)
Communicating with Dying People and Their Relatives (Lugton) ($12.95)
Caring for Dying People of Different Faiths (Neuberger) ($11.95)

Being There: Pastoral Care in Time of Illness (Speck) ($13.95)
Letting Go: Caring for the Dying and Bereaved (Ainsworth-Smith/Speck) ($13.95)
Surviving Death (Meyer) ($9.95)
Terminal Care Support Teams: Hospice–Hospice Interface (Hockley) ($19.95)
Saying Goodbye Activity Book for Children (Boulden) ($4.95)
Life & Death: A Collected Wisdom (Boulden) ($14.95)

19. International Association of Laryngectomees
c/o American Cancer Society
Tower Place
1599 Clifton Road, NE
Atlanta, GA 30329-4251
(404) 320-3333

The International Association of Laryngectomees was founded in 1952 in affiliation with the ACS and consists of 270 domestic and 25 foreign clubs whose members are laryngectomees. For the location of the "Lost Chord," "New Voice," or "Anamile" club nearest you, write the IAL or contact your local ACS. The goal of these lost chord clubs is to assist newly laryngectomized persons to make early adjustments to loss of voice and to overcome psychosocial problems. They accomplish this by service as hosts for newly laryngectomized persons at club meetings and by collaborating with surgeons in preoperative and postoperative speech orientations. Members of the Lost Chord Club visit new laryngectomee patients in the hospital (at the invitation of the physician). The Lost Chord Club member discusses with both the spouse and the patient early home adjustment, speech therapy, the need for early return to normal work and recreation, required changes in the activities of daily living, and benefits of joining a Lost Chord Club. Meetings enable patients and their spouses to discuss common problems of caring for a laryngectomee and to offer moral support and encouragement and social confidence after similar surgery. Manuals and newsletters are available to members. A laryngectomy kit is available and contains an emergency identification card, various booklets (first aid, stoma care, tracheostomy care, speech, etc), and a directory of sources of supplies.

20. Johanna's On Call To Mend Esteem, Inc.
Cancer Rehabilitation Nurse Consultants
199 New Scotland Avenue
Albany, New York 12208
(518) 489-7233 (800) 866-SELF

Johanna's On Call To Mend Esteem is a nonprofit cancer rehabilitation nursing service that promotes preventive, restorative, supportive, and palliative nursing interventions for people with cancer. Educational services intended to enhance knowledge and promote the practice of self-examination are provided to the general public.

Educational booklets written for patients and for use as an educational tool by nurses:

Maintaining a Positive Image with Cancer Therapy (a wellness workbook/journal) $4.00

Maintaining a Positive Image with Breast Cancer Surgery $1.00

Maintaining a Positive Image with Hair Loss and Cancer Therapy $1.50

Hair Goes, Hair Grows After Cancer Therapy (for children, adolescents, and teens) $3.00

Breast Health Diary—A Monthly Reminder to Keep an Eye on Your Breast Health $1.00

Educational audiovisual tapes for combined audiences patients/families/community/professional):

Maintaining a Positive Image with Hair Loss and Cancer Therapy (15 minutes) loan $15.00
purchase $35.00

Maintaining a Positive Image with Breast Cancer Surgery (15 minutes) loan $15.00
purchase $35.00

It's Your Body Check Yourself Out—a teen breast self-exam program (6 minutes) loan $15.00
purchase $35.00

BSE Rap—an instructional music audio tape $8.00

Members will receive quarterly the newsletter *ESTEEM*, a catalogue of available educational resources, and a sample resource guide.

MEMBERSHIP FEE $25.00 per year

21. Let's Face It
A network for people with facial difference.
Box 711
Concord, MA 01742
(508) 371-3186

Let's Face It is the U.S. branch of an international mutual help organization dedicated to helping people with facial difference, their loved ones, the professionals who care for them, and the communities in which they live, to understand and to solve the problems of living with this disability.

The goals of our organization are:

To link and educate family, friends, and professionals.

To educate the public to value the person behind every face.

To assist facially different people to share their experiences, strengths, and hopes. Sharing experiences through a mutual help network often speeds adjustment to disabilities.

To educate and provide continuing education to medical, nursing, and allied health professionals.

The organization has an annual *Resource Directory* that provides information on a variety of organizations the individual with a facial difference could utilize.

22. Leukemia Society of America
National Headquarters
733 Third Avenue
New York, NY 10017
(212) 573-8484; (800) 955-4LSA (Hotline for Information)

The Leukemia Society of America, Inc. is a national voluntary health agency dedicated solely to seeking the cause and eventual cure of leukemia and allied diseases. The Society supports five major programs: research, patient aid, public and professional education, and community service.

Research:

The Society's research program is based on the belief that all medically sound approaches toward a cure or control of leukemia should be encouraged on a worldwide basis. To this end, over $6 million was allocated in 1991 to support about 200 researchers working at 80 accredited institutions in the United States and throughout the world. Since its establishment, the Society has awarded more than $67 million in research grants.

Education:

The Society pursues an aggressive program to provide current information on leukemia and related diseases to the general public. It alerts the public to disease danger, treatment, and therapy through literature and posters, films and other audiovisual materials, speaking engagements, seminars and educational programs, news and feature releases, and public service advertising in all media.

Information is available from each local chapter and from the Society's national headquarters in New York City.

Patient Aid:

Financial assistance up to $750 a year per person is given by the Society to outpatients being treated for leukemia, the lymphomas, multiple myeloma, and preleukemia. Outpatients are those not confined to a hospital, although they may be treated at various times at a hospital. They do not remain there for continuous management of their illnesses.

Community Service:

The Society conducts a two-way communications program established with the social service agencies and treatment facilities in the area. Information is collected for the benefit of patients and families who may need to know about resources available to them. Chapters interact with government health departments and many varied family assistance organizations. The compilation and maintenance of resource and referral material is a high-priority item on our list of services so that assistance is available to all leukemia patients at all times.

Publications from the Leukemia Society of America:

Facts About the Leukemia Society of America (English)
Facts About the Leukemia Society of America (Spanish)
Leukemia
Lymphomas
Hodgkin's Disease
Multiple Myeloma
Research
Patient-Aid Program (English)
Patient-Aid Program (Spanish)
What Everyone Should Know About Leukemia (English)
What Everyone Should Know About Leukemia (Spanish)
Leukemia—The Nature of the Disease
Leukemia Quiz
Pink Facts Sheet (mail stuffer)
Emotional Aspects of Childhood Leukemia
Bone Marrow Transplantation
Bone Marrow Transplantation (Spanish)

Update and Reprints

Facts About Leukemia
Radiation and Nuclear Power
Cat Leukemia: Research into Its Origins Hold Promise for Man
Forty Years of Progress: The Story of the Leukemia Society Research Report
Interleukin-2 and Society Research
Interferon and Hairy Cell Leukemia

Videotapes/Films (Specify Format)

A Sense of Hope — VHS or ¾″
You're Not Alone — VHS or ¾″
Must Win — VHS or ¾″
What It Is That I Have, Don't Want, etc. . . — VHS or ¾″

23. Look Good . . . Feel Better (LGFB)
The CTFA Foundation
1101 17th St., N.W.
Suite 300
Washington, DC 20036
(800) 395-LOOK

Look Good . . . Feel Better is a free public service program for women cancer patients who are undergoing chemotherapy or radiation treatments. LGFB is dedicated to teaching these women beauty techniques to help restore their appearance and self-image.

Look Good . . . Feel Better is sponsored by The Cosmetic, Toiletry & Fragrance Association (CTFA) Foundation, the American Cancer Society (ACS), and the National Cosmetology Association (NCA). The CTFA Foundation provides the complimentary makeup and free educational materials, such as videotapes and pamphlets, and secures financial support for LGFB. The ACS administers the program and the NCA organizes the volunteer cosmetologists.

Look Good . . . Feel Better is available to patients in one of two ways. The first, and most popular LGFB format, is a structured group session consisting of six to ten patients. This group session is usually offered in a hospital and includes a group of trained cosmetologists who instruct the patients in how to use makeup, wigs, scarves, turbans, and accessories to camouflage the appearance changes resulting from their treatments. Each patient receives a complimentary bag of assorted cosmetics that are used in the session, with guidance from the cosmetologists. The goal is to teach the patients cosmetic techniques they can take home and use every day, allowing them to gain some control over their lives.

The second format available is a free, private consultation with a trained cosmetologist in a salon or other private setting. The techniques taught are the same as in a group session. We have found that the group session is the more popular of the two formats, because it tends to serve as an informal support group for the women by allowing them to discuss a part of their treatment that no one else understands quite as well as other patients and cosmetologists.

24. Make-A-Wish Foundation of America
2600 North Central Avenue
Suite 936
Phoenix, AZ 85004
(602) 240-6060
(800) 722-9474

The Make-A-Wish Foundation of America is a nonprofit organization whose main purpose is to fulfill the favorite wish of a child with a life-threatening or terminal illness. The foundation will consider the wish of any child under the age of 18 anywhere in the world and covers all expenses related to granting the wish.

25. Medic Alert
Medic Alert Foundation International
2323 Colorado Ave.
Turlock, CA 95381-1009
(800) 344-3226 Implant Registry
(800) 736-3342 Links To Life

(800) ID ALERT Medic Alert
(800) 423-6333 MARS®

Medic Alert's three-part life-protecting system consists of:

1. A metal alerting emblem worn as a bracelet or necklace. The emblem bears the staff of Aesculapius, the internationally recognized insignia of the medical profession, and the words "Medic Alert" in red. On the reverse side are engraved the special medical conditions of the wearer such as "hypertension," "takes beta blocker," "allergic to penicillin," or "wearing contact lenses." Also engraved on the back are the member's identification number and the number for Medic Alert's Emergency Response Center.

2. The 24-hour-a-day Emergency Response Center provides detailed data to emergency personnel via a collect telephone call from anywhere in the world. Medic Alert's emergency hotline number engraved on the back of the emblem and printed on the wallet card provides vital information that aids diagnosis and spreads life saving treatments.

3. Each member receives a wallet card with personal and medical information in addition to that engraved on the emblem. Each year, the members receive a wallet card copy of the information listed on their computerized medical record. This serves as a reminder to members to keep their record up to date. The record may be updated at any time by phone or mail. Whenever the record is updated, a new wallet card is prepared with the new information and sent immediately to the member.

Medic Alert serves 38 countries from 21 affiliate offices worldwide—United Kingdom, Japan, Canada, Grenada, Switzerland, Sweden, Netherlands, Greece, Cyprus, Israel, Iceland, Australia (south and west), Malaysia, New Zealand, Fiji Islands, South Africa, Zambia, Zimbabwe, Jamaica.

Implant Registry:

A public service of the Medic Alert Foundation, the International Implant Registry is a computerized link between implant manufacturers, the United States Food and Drug Administration, implant patients, their doctors, and hospitals. It is a link whose prime objective is the maintenance of a current list of implant recipients that can be quickly accessed in the event of a device recall or safety alert. It also serves as an implant information resource for doctors, hospitals, and all others concerned with the latest statistics and information on implanted medical devices.

When an implant recall or safety alert is issued, the International Implant Registry computer is accessed for the names of affected recipients. This information is then quickly relayed to their physicians and/or hospitals. To ensure patient notification, the Registry currently contacts the patient directly only if the physician does not R.S.V.P. the Registry using the forms provided. This direct notification occurs 2 weeks following the physician notification.

As part of the patient tracking service, the Registry also strives to keep implant recipients up to date on the latest research via a semiannual newsletter in which device manufacturers, doctors, hospitals, and government agencies are encouraged to publish recent findings as well as future plans.

MARS®:

The Medic Alert Response Service (MARS 5000) offers greatly enhanced security and protection for the elderly or disabled person living alone. MARS ensures prompt emergency care at the touch of a button. When pressed, the button, worn as a neckchain, bracelet or belt clip, activates any home phone from up to 200 feet away (depending on the construction of the home) and automatically connects the caller to an emergency operator 24 hours a day at Medic Alert's Response Center. The Response Center representative accesses the caller's computerized medical records and within seconds notifies a predesignated neighbor or relative, or the representative may immediately dispatch rescue workers to the caller's home.

MARS 5000 is a three-pronged service, consisting of: a one-ounce waterproof personal help button worn by the user; a home communications box that, when activated by the help button, serves as a two-way speaker through which the caller can speak with Response Center representatives; and the traditional protection of a Medic Alert emblem, annually updated wallet card and a 24-hour emergency telephone hotline that protects subscribers when they are away from their home.

Links To Life:

The Links To Life program was the first of its kind in the nation. A trust fund of $10,000 was created to assist senior citizens who may not be able to afford Medic Alert's emergency medical identification service. Since the program began in 1987, hundreds of memory-impaired persons have been enrolled in Medic Alert's lifetime service.

Medic Alert has focused special attention on Alzheimer's patients who are prone to wandering or have medical conditions. Medic Alert not only ensures patients' confidential protection; it also provides relatives and caregivers the peace of mind and knowledge that the person they care about will be properly identified and taken care of in a crisis.

Medic Alert's Links To Life program is spreading nationwide as groups of seniors and agencies responsible for the aged are establishing local programs with the assistance of police, sheriff, emergency medical service personnel, fire fighters, local governments, media, and businesses.

26. National Alliance of Breast Cancer Organizations (NABCO)
1180 Avenue of the Americas
2nd Floor
New York, NY 10036
(212) 719-0154
(NABCO prefers written inquiries)

NCI
Office of Cancer Communications
National Cancer Institute
Building 31
Room 10A18
Bethesda, MD 20205
(301) 496-5583
(800) 4-CANCER

Komen Foundation
5005 LBJ Freeway
Suite 730
Dallas, TX 75240

The following is a list of publications developed from the 1992 edition of the National Alliance of Breast Cancer Organizations' (NABCO) Breast Cancer Resource List. NABCO is a central resource for information on breast cancer.

Breast Cancer Resources: General Information about Breast Cancer

Breast Cancer: Risk, Protection, Detection, and Treatment
DES Action 1615 Broadway
Oakland, CA 94612
31 pages
Cost: $2.50

Breast Cancer: Your Best Protection . . . Early Detection
Source: NABCO
Catalogue # GRP0278
Cost: Free (single copies)

Dr. Susan Love's Breast Book
Author: Susan M. Love
Publisher: Addison-Wesley
455 pages
Cost: $18.95 (hardcover)
$12.45 (paperback)

Every Woman's Guide to Breast Cancer
Author: Vicki L. Seltzer, MD
Source: Bookstores
Publisher: Penguin Books
196 pages
Cost: $7.95

If You've Thought About Breast Cancer . . .
Author: Rose Kushner
Source: Komen Foundation
44 pages
Cost: Free (single copies)

Make Sure You Do Not Have Breast Cancer
Author: Philip Strax, MD
Source: Bookstores
Publisher: St. Martin's Press
118 pages
Cost: $15.95

The Breast Cancer Digest: A Guide to Medical Care, Emotional Support, Educational Programs, and Resources
Author: NCI
Source: 84-1691
212 pages
Cost: Free

The Race Is Run One Step at a Time: My Personal Struggle and Every Woman's Guide to Taking Charge of Breast Cancer
Author: Nancy Brinker with Catherine McEvily Harris
Source: Bookstores or Komen Foundation
Publisher: Simon & Schuster
219 pages (hardcover)
Cost: $18.95
224 pages (paperback)
Cost: $10.00

What You Need to Know About Breast Cancer
Source: NCI
Catalogue # 91-1556
33 pages
Cost: Free

27. National Brain Tumor Foundation
323 Geary St., Suite 510
San Francisco, CA 94102
(415) 296-0404
(415) 296-9303 FAX

Research:

The National Brain Tumor Foundation has funded basic and applied laboratory research and clinical trials of new treatments at major institutions in the United States.

The Foundation has also supported research into quality-of-life issues that regularly face brain tumor patients.

Recovery:

The National Brain Tumor Foundation refers patients and family members to a network of support groups throughout the United States.

A volunteer-staffed SUPPORT LINE connects brain tumor patients with professional caregivers and those who have survived the disease. Further, the SUPPORT LINE serves as a link for friends, family members, and others involved in the lives of brain tumor patients.

Resources:

A comprehensive GUIDE is available for patients and families who want to learn about brain tumors, often in a very short period of time, in order to make informed decisions.

SEARCH, the Foundation's newsletter, keeps readers in touch with advances in treatment and psychosocial support.

Publications available from the National Brain Tumor Association:

Brain Tumors, *A Guide*

72 pages of up-to-date information on the diagnosis, treatment, and classification of brain tumors. Examples of current research into causes and cures. A special section on pediatric brain tumors. How to be a survivor; what are your rights as a patient; how to join a support group; and much much more.

1 copy to a patient or family member/review copy for organizations	FREE
2–10 copies	$6.50
11–50 copies	5.75
51 or more copies	5.50

Brain Tumor Support Groups in North America

Published annually by the American Association of Neurological Surgeons, Joint Section on Brain Tumors, and sponsored by NBTF, this is the most up-to-date listing of patient/family brain tumor support groups. This publication also includes a list of national resources for those with central nervous system neoplasms.

1 copy to a patient or family member/review copy for organizations	FREE
Additional copies	$1.50

Gathering a Life—A Journal of Recovery, by Jeanne Lohmann

When Jeanne Lohmann's husband was diagnosed as having a brain tumor, she responded as a wife and as a writer. These short prose pieces are a tribute to Hank's life and the manner in which he left it, and to their marriage. 61 pages.

Each copy $8.75

"Short and Long Term Disability Income Synopsis"

1 copy FREE with any order

28. The National Coalition for Cancer Research
Capitol Associates Incorporated
Stanton Park
426 C Street, NE
Washington, DC 20002
(202) 544-1880
(202) 543-2565 FAX

The NCCR was founded in 1986 to support the purposes of the National Cancer Act. Today, the Coalition is composed of nearly every organization in this country that is dedicated to the eradication of cancer.

The NCCR represents more than:

10,000 cancer survivors and their families
21,000 children with cancer as well as their parents and brothers and sisters
65,000 cancer researchers, nurses, physicians, and health care workers
76 cancer research centers

The watchwords of the NCCR epitomize its mission—Research Cures Cancer. The collaborative actions of the key organizations in the cancer community are designed to:

communicate the value of research to progress against cancer
make clear the contributions that the National Cancer Program has made to the reduction of cancer morbidity and mortality as well as to the quality of life experienced by cancer patients and survivors
ensure adequate funding for research that will improve cancer diagnosis, treatment, and prevention
cooperate with other organizations in support of public health policies that will lead to the eradication of cancer

The Coalition's main mission in life is to increase visibility for the issue of cancer funding with policy makers on Capitol Hill and within the administration. Therefore, membership comprises a diverse group of individuals that are patient-focused as well as research-focused. The bylaws of the organization stipulate that only an organization or institution is able to participate as members and therefore no individual members are accepted. The membership fee is a three-tiered structure with the professional research organizations at the top of the tier and the nonprofit advocacy organizations such as the National Coalition of Cancer Survivorship at the bottom of the tier.

29. National Coalition for Cancer Survivorship
1010 Wayne Ave.
5th Floor
Silver Springs, MD 20910
(301) 650-8868

The National Coalition for Cancer Survivorship (NCCS) represents grassroots organizations throughout the United States of over 10,000 cancer survivors. The NCCS was founded in 1986 by 24 cancer experts and Dr. Fitzhugh Mullan, a cancer survivor, to promote an understanding of cancer survivorship and provide advocacy to improve the quality of living for cancer survivors.

Through the national organization and a network of local organizations, the NCCS fosters the following goals:

to promote programs that will empower survivors as informed consumers;

to operate a clearinghouse that disseminates survivorship articles, literature, and information on local and national survivorship activities and programs; and

to act as a voice for cancer survivors to the media, medical establishment, and government.

NCCS publications highlight issues vital to survivors such as locating resources, communicating with the health care team, being a savvy consumer of medical services, and fighting job and insurance discrimination.

NCCS *Networker,* a quarterly publication offering the latest news of people, events, and issues that impact survivors' lives

Charting the Journey, an almanac of resources for survivors published by Consumer Reports Books

Facing Forward, a guide for those finishing treatment, published by the National Cancer Institute in collaboration with NCCS.

Teamwork: The Cancer Patient's Guide to Talking with Your Doctor. Published by NCCS through an educational grant from Lederle Laboratories.

30. National Hospice Organization
1901 North Moore Street
Suite 901
Arlington, VA 22209
(703) 243-5900

Established in 1978, NHO is a nonprofit organization, promoting quality care to the terminally ill and their significant others. NHO has worked over the past decade to establish hospice as a part of the health care delivery system in the United States. As a result of its efforts, hospice is now included as a Medicare/Medicaid benefit and as an employee benefit for 66% of American workers. The number of hospices has also increased from 1 in 1974 to over 1725 in 1990. Most hospices are members of NHO and receive NHO's technical assistance, education programs and events, publications, and advocacy and referral services. Membership has several categories and includes *The Hospice Journal* among numerous other publications and workshops.

31. National Leukemia Association, Inc.
585 Stewart Avenue
Suite 536
Garden City, NY 11530
(516) 222-1944

The National Leukemia Association, Inc. was founded in 1965 as a not-for-profit organization dedicated to raising funds to support research efforts into the causes and cure of leukemia and to provide patient aid to those families in need while meeting the expenses incurred in leukemia treatment. The Association is a voluntary agency that is totally supported by public contributions.

Patient Aid Services:

The National Leukemia Association provides aid to leukemia patients and their families. The Board of Trustees, in conjunction with its Patient Aid Committee, sets the policies and standards for administering this program.

The National Leukemia Association will assist patients not covered by existing medical policies in the following categories:

a. Laboratory fees
b. X-ray therapy treatment
c. Drugs
d. Blood replenishment
e. Unusual and extraordinary expenses not covered above will be considered based upon need and availability of funds.

32. National Marrow Donor Program
Coordinating Center
3433 Broadway Street, N.E.
Suite 400
Minneapolis, MN 55413
(612) 627-8140; (612) 627-5899 FAX
(800) 526-7809

The National Marrow Donor Program, which is funded by the federal government, was created to improve the effectiveness of the search for bone marrow donors so that a greater number of bone marrow transplants can be carried out. It keeps a registry of potential bone marrow donors and provides a free packet of information on bone marrow transplantation.

Patients who need resources in this area can obtain help from the office of patient advocacy within the National Marrow Donor Program.

For additional bone marrow donor information call:

Children's Leukemia Foundation (800) 825-CLFM
American Red Cross (313) 494-2787
National Bone Marrow Donor Registry, 100 S. Robert Street
St. Paul, MN 55107 (612) 291-6789 or (800) 654-1247

33. The Oley Foundation
A-23 Hun Memorial
Albany Medical Center
New Scotland Avenue
Albany, NY 12208
(518) 445-5079
(800) 776-6539 (OLEY)

The Oley Foundation is a nonprofit, tax-exempt organization affiliated with the Clinical Nutrition Division of Albany Medical College. It was established in 1983 to address the special needs of those involved in home parenteral–enteral nutrition (PEN). Since then, Oley has worked to build a home PEN community that fosters the cooperative efforts of consumers (patients), clinicians, home care services, and third-party payers. Within this context, Oley is committed to:

enhancing the quality of life and functional status of persons requiring home PEN.
improving the quality and cost-effectiveness of home PEN.
promoting the availability of home PEN for eligible persons.

Specific projects of the foundation include:

Maintenance of the home PEN national patient registry. Known as O.A.S.I.S., it is a cooperative project undertaken with the American Society for Parenteral and Enteral Nutrition that provides a research database for analyzing the outcomes and complications associated with home PEN.

Publication of the *LifelineLetter*. Written for the consumer, the *Letter* is published bimonthly and includes articles contributed by home PEN consumers, families, clinicians, researchers, and home care services. As part of Oley's education and outreach effort, it is provided at no charge to consumer/consumer families.

34. Ronald McDonald House
Kroc Drive
Oak Brook, IL 60521
(708) 575-7418

Ronald McDonald House is a "home away from home," a temporary lodging facility, for the families of seriously ill children being treated at nearby hospitals. The Houses provide an environment for emotional support to parents and siblings of sick children through a loving, caring, stable place they can call "home."

People helping people in times of serious need has made the Ronald McDonald House program what it is today. Each of the 150 Houses in nine countries is owned and operated by a local not-for-profit corporation composed of members of the medical community, McDonald's owner/operators, businesses and civic organizations, and parent volunteers. Each House raises money locally, as well as benefits from a general Ronald McDonald House fund.

Families staying at Ronald McDonald House are asked to make a donation ranging from $5 to $15 per day; if that is not possible, their stay is free.

35. The Skin Cancer Foundation
245 Fifth Avenue
New York, NY 10016
(212) 725-5176; (212) 725-5751 FAX

The Skin Cancer Foundation, a nonprofit foundation, is the only national organization concerned solely with the world's most prevalent malignancy—cancer of the skin. The Foundation conducts public and medical education programs and provides support for medical training and research to help reduce the incidence, morbidity, and mortality of skin cancer.

Medical Education:

The *Melanoma Letter* focuses on vital issues concerning this form of skin cancer.

Public Education:

The Foundation's national Public Information Program is implemented in the following ways:

A public awareness campaign conveys its messages by means of nationwide distribution of brochures, posters, pamphlets, and audiovisual materials to the public, to physicians' offices, and to screening clinics, health fairs, and corporate and community wellness programs throughout the country.

Audiovisual materials have been developed for use in physicians' offices and waiting rooms, schools, and community education programs. *Skin Cancer: Preventable and Curable* is available as a 15-minute VHS video presentation narrated by Dick Cavett or as a slide program with recorded narration on an audio cassette.

A new book published by the Foundation entitled *Sun Sense: A Complete Guide to the Prevention, Early Detection, and Treatment of Skin Cancer,* by Perry Robins, MD, offers detailed information in a highly readable style.

Sun & Skin News, a quarterly publication written in non-technical language, contains up-to-date information on the prevention, diagnosis, and treatment of skin cancer. *The Skin Cancer Foundation Journal,* published annually, features articles by leading physicians and scientists on recent developments in the field.

A Children's Sun Protection Program to promote the adoption of preventive measures early in life—when it counts the most—continues to expand. This national campaign is aimed at young people and those who care for them: parents and grandparents, babysitters and day-care center personnel, teachers, coaches, scout leaders, and camp directors. Brochures and posters are distributed to the public, the media, nurses, pediatricians, dermatologists, and family and general practitioners. The newest element of the Children's Program is "The Sun Day News," an educational poster that has been distributed to 60,000 elementary schools throughout the country and will be offered this year to summer camps as part of a comprehensive sun-safety package.

Publications from the Skin Cancer Foundation:

BROCHURES

Skin Cancer Brochure Sampler:
Includes the three brochures below, assembled in convenient folder.
50/$23 100/$40 300/$109 500/$178 1000/$300

It's Never Too Early to Stop Skin Cancer . . . Or Too Late:
100/$12 200/$23 300/$35 500/$58 1000/$98

Types & Descriptions of Skin Cancers:
100/$15 200/$30 300/$39 500/$65 1000/$110

The ABCD's of Moles and Melanoma:
100/$15 200/$30 300/$39 500/$65 1000/$110

The Many Faces of Malignant Melanoma:
50/$29 100/$46 200/$80 300/$104 500/$172

For Every Child under the Sun:
100/$26 200/$46 350/$80 500/$104 1000/$173

Basal Cell Carcinoma:
100/$26 200/$46 350/$80 500/$104 1000/$173

Dysplastic Nevi and Malignant Melanoma:
50/$23 100/$40 200/$69 300/$86 500/$115

Squamous Cell Carcinoma:
50/$23 100/$40 200/$69 300/$86 500/$115

Simple Guidelines on Sun Protection:
200/$12 300/$17 500/$29 1000/$58 2000/$104

Malignant Melanoma:
Guidelines and Early Warning System
50/$23 100/$40 200/$69 300/$103 500/$144

NEWSLETTERS

Sun & Skin News:
One-year subscription (4 issues) $25
Multiple copies 50/$10 100/$20 200/$35

The Melanoma Letter:
One-year subscription (4 issues) $25
Multiple copies 50/$10 100/$20 200/$35

AUDIOVISUALS

"Skin Cancer: Preventable and Curable":
15-minute slide presentation (111 color slides) $195

SLIDE SETS

Basal Cell Carcinoma: $20
10 color slides

Squamous Cell Carcinoma: $10
5 color slides

The Many Faces of Malignant Melanoma: $48
24 color slides

The ABCD's of Moles and Melanoma: $24
12 color slides

Poster Slide Set: $18
9 slides

JOURNAL

Skin Cancer Foundation Journal
1–20 copies $5/ea. 41–60 copies $3/ea.
21–40 copies $4/ea. 61–100 copies $2/ea.

OTHER PUBLICATIONS

Sun Sense: A Complete Guide $12.95 (Prepublication price)
Skin Cancer Screening Manual $5/ea.

POSTERS

When You Work on a Tan $3/ea.
If You Worship the Sun $3/ea.
It Takes Years $4/ea.
People Who Need the Most Sun Protection $5/ea.
When We Find a Better Way $4/ea.
Can You Spot a Killer? $5/ea.
For Every Child Under The Sun $5/ea.
People in High Places $5/ea.
Protect Your Most Important Assets $5/ea.

36. The Sunshine Foundation
4010 Levick Street
Philadelphia, PA 19135
(215) 335-2622 inside Philadelphia; (800) 767-1976 outside Philadelphia

The Sunshine Foundation reaches out to all children from throughout the country and the world suffering from terminal as well as chronic illnesses such as: spina bifida, muscular dystrophy, sickle cell anemia, cystic fibrosis, progeria, and many others too numerous to mention. The wishes and dreams of these children are fulfilled by the Foundation. The Sunshine Foundation is a registered, nonprofit organization with 32 chapters throughout the country.

37. Sunshine Foundation
Dream Village Site
5400 C.R. 547 North
P.O. Box 255
Loughman, FL 33858
(800) 457-1976

On a 21-acre site just 15 minutes from the Magic Kingdom, the Sunshine Foundation has constructed a fairy tale village where children and their families stay while fulfilling the child's dream of visiting Disney World.

Over 400 children have enjoyed this unique complex, which is specifically designed with them in mind. Each of the three cottages has a fantasy setting in the child's bedroom. Special features include a pool with a ramp for wheelchair-dependent children, a handicapped accessible playground, and a gameroom.

38. TOUCH
American Cancer Society (Alabama division)

The TOUCH program is a program for cancer patients, their families, and friends to help them better understand and cope with cancer. TOUCH is a support program for people who have had cancer or are living with cancer and are undergoing cancer treatment. Through others, understanding, caring, and hope are available to the cancer patients and the family members.

Emotional support is available from people who have undergone cancer treatment and have successfully coped with cancer. TOUCH volunteers are trained cancer patients, their family members, and other interested persons who visit in hospitals, outpatient clinics, physicians' offices, or in homes. Visits are made with the physician's approval.

The TOUCH program also offers support group meetings to discuss mutual problems and concerns encountered in coping with a diagnosis of cancer. Patients can talk alone with a counselor or meet in a group with other patients and their family members to share concerns, to receive help with personal or family problems, or to learn about services available to persons with cancer.

39. United Ostomy Association
36 Executive Park
Suite 120
Irvine, CA 92714
(714) 660-8624
(800) 826-0826

Local chapters are composed primarily of ostomates who provide aid, moral support, and education to those who have a colostomy, ileostomy, or urostomy surgery. The chapter supplements the work of the surgeon by offering rehabilitation through follow-up by people who have learned to live with an ostomy. Trained members make visits to homes and hospitals, on request, with the prior consent of the patient's physician. Chapters have medical advisory board consisting of nonsurgeon physicians, surgeons, and enterostomal therapists trained in ostomy care and the use of equipment. At regular monthly meetings, open to anyone who is interested, members can exchange practical, personal experiences about their ostomies, see ostomy equipment displayed, and hear speakers who are knowledgeable about ostomy. All local chapters are volunteer organizations. A list of the chapters is available on request from the UOA. Annual chapter dues vary from no fee to $30. Each member of the UOA receives the *Ostomy Quarterly* magazine and is eligible to participate in the UOA insurance programs. The UOA has both publications and slide programs, which cover every aspect of ostomies.

A sample of publications available from the United Ostomy Association are:

The Ostomy Book for Nurses
Coping with an Ostomy
Ostomy Dietary Guidelines
Anatomy of Ostomy Brochure
So You Have/Will Have an Ostomy
About Ostomy
Colostomy: A Guide (English)
Colostomy: A Guide (Spanish)
Colostomy: A Guide (French)
Colostomy: A Guide (Chinese)
Ileostomy: A Guide
Urostomy: A Guide
Transverse Colostomy: A Guide
Sex/Courtship/Single Ostomate
Sex and the Female Ostomate

40. The Wellness Community®
2200 Colorado Ave.
Santa Monica, CA 90404-3506
(310) 453-2200
(310) 315-9596 FAX

The Wellness Community provides free psychosocial support services for adults with cancer and their families. There are Wellness communities throughout the United States. The Wellness Community is a tax-exempt, charitable corporation. The following services are provided.

1. Sharing groups that are held twice a week. These are informal, drop-in groups led by people who have or had cancer.

2. Participant groups are ongoing 2-hour weekly groups led by licensed psychotherapists.

3. Family groups are ongoing 2-hour weekly groups led by licensed psychotherapists composed of significant others of people with cancer in a participant group.

4. Relaxation/Visualization: Twice per week there are sessions where participants are taught how to involve themselves in the self-help procedures.

5. Education: During the month, lectures and dialogues are presented by authorities in fields of interest to cancer patients.

6. Workshops: Each week, there are workshops presented by experts in matters such as voice dialogue, use of humor, moderate exercise, art therapy, journal writing, etc.

7. Special Groups: Special groups are presented on an ongoing basis to consider specific areas of concern to cancer patients such as breast, prostate, and brain cancer networking; problems of parents with cancer; groups for couples to look at the problems of intimacy brought on by cancer; etc.

8. The Wellness Connection: Twice during the month, members of The Wellness Community who wish to remain connected to the community come together for support and socializing.

9. Open Forum: Every 2 months, participants meet with staff members to present new ideas and suggestions for optimizing their use of the program.

10. Clubs: Groups of participants meet on their own at the facility to carry on activities such as the Nutrition Club, where a highly trained nutritionist leads discussions on selected topics of interest to the participants where diet can be used in the fight for recovery.

11. Social Events: At least once a month, there are social gatherings such as seasonal parties, potlucks, charade nights, joke fests, sing-a-longs, and other events that bring participants together to laugh and play.

41. Y-ME
18220 Harwood Avenue
Homewood, IL 60430
(708) 799-8338 Business; (708) 799-5937 FAX
(708) 799-8228 24-Hour Hotline; (800) 221-2141 National Hotline

Founded in 1978 by Ann Marcou and Mimi Kaplan, two mastectomy patients, Y-ME has become the largest breast cancer support program in the USA. It provides hotlines (staffed by volunteers who have personally experienced breast cancer), presurgery counseling, open door meetings, early detection workshops, speakers bureau, resource library, wigs and prosthesis bank, and inservice workshops for health care professionals. Volunteers are professionally supervised, and the information provided to patients is monitored by a medical advisory board. Contributing members receive a quarterly newsletter and an invitation to attend the Y-ME national conference at discounted rates.

AIDS-Related Organizations

1. AIDS Action Council
2033 M. Street, N.W.
Suite 802
Washington, DC 20036

A national organization dedicated solely to shaping federal AIDS policy was formed in 1984 to represent, in Washington, people with HIV and the organizations that serve them. AIDS Action speaks for over 500 community-based AIDS organizations from around the country—from rural networks and church-based groups to the largest New York and San Francisco service providers. Since the beginning, AIDs Action works to ensure that their voices are heard by Capitol Hill officials and policy makers in federal agencies. AIDS Action Council also convenes the national organizations responding to AIDS, a 150-member coalition of national health care, civil liberties, women's, minority, and gay groups involved in the fight against AIDS.

2. AmFAR
American Foundation for AIDS Research
1515 Broadway
Suite 3601
New York, NY 10036-8901
(212) 719-0033
and
5900 Wilshire Boulevard
2nd Floor East Satellite
Los Angeles, CA 90036-5032
(213) 857-5900

The American Foundation for AIDS Research is the nation's leading private-sector funding organization dedicated to AIDS research, education, and public policy. AmFAR serves as a catalyst to identify major gaps in AIDS biomedical and social science research and education, and provides funding to support innovative projects designed to fill the gaps.

Since it started in late 1985, AmFAR has awarded $32 million in seed or start-up grants to more than 530 research teams and education projects.

Eighty percent of AmFAR's grants underwrite a broad range of scientific research to find a vaccine and effective treatments for AIDS. Twenty percent of the grants go to experimental educational programs designed to prevent the spread of the disease.

AmFAR is dedicated to mobilizing the good will, energy, and generosity of caring Americans to end the AIDS epidemic.

AmFAR sponsors a number of major publications, including the *AIDS/HIV Experimental Treatment Directory,* published quarterly, which tracks the testing of promising AIDS Treatments; the *AIDS Information Resources Directory,* published annually, which lists and critically evaluates most AIDS-related educational materials available in the U.S.; *AIDS Clinical Care,* published monthly by the *New England Journal of Medicine,* which contains the latest AIDS clinical management information for physicians; and *AIDS Education, A Business Guide,* a blueprint for developing AIDS education; *AIDS Targeted Information Newsletter,* published monthly, which lists, with editorial comments, all major AIDS-related scientific, medical, social science, and public policy research papers published worldwide.

3. Association of Nurses in AIDS Care
704 Stony Hill Road
Suite 106
Yardley, PA 19069
(215) 321-2371

The Association of Nurses in AIDS Care is a national association with members all over the United States and Canada plus members in Australia, France, The Netherlands, Taiwan, Panama, England and The Philippines.

"The mission of ANAC is to promote the individual and collective professional development of nurses involved in the delivery of health care to persons infected or affected by the Human Immunodeficiency Virus (HIV) and to promote the health and welfare of infected persons by:

creating an effective network among nurses in AIDS care;

studying, researching, and exchanging information, experiences, and ideas leading to improved care for persons with HIV infection.

providing leadership to the nursing community in matters related to AIDS/HIV infection;

promoting social awareness concerning issues related to HIV/AIDS.

Inherent in these goals is the abiding commitment to the prevention of further HIV infection."

The Association of Nurses in AIDS Care was founded in September of 1987, held its first formal meeting in New York City in May 1988, and has now grown to a membership of over 1400 nurses.

Membership in ANAC entitles members to the following benefits:

Journal of the Association of Nurses in AIDS Care, which is published quarterly

Newsletter of the Association of Nurses in AIDS Care, which is also published quarterly

Monographs and position statements on issues affecting health professionals

Discounted educational meetings

4. Gay Men's Health Crisis (GMHC)
129 West 20th Street
New York, NY 10011-0022
(212) 807-6655 Hotline; (212) 645-7470 TDD for hearing impaired

GMHC offers many services (many are free) including the following:

1. Client services to help people with the emotional and practical aspects of living with AIDS, legal services to offer them advice and represent them in court, and ombudsman services to investigate and resolve the problems they have with health care delivery.
2. The education department is the largest nongovernmental distributor of AIDS education in the world. Educational materials include booklets, brochures, videos, manuals, posters, newsletters, buttons, T-shirts, and magnets. Materials are in English and Spanish. A selected list of materials are given below:

Booklets (01)	
Catalog of AIDS Educational Resources (49)	FREE
Client Services Directory (15)	.50
Legal Answers About AIDS (16)	2.00
Medical Answers About AIDS (17)	2.50
Brochures (02)	
Brothers Loving Brothers Safely (03)	.35
Cuando Un Amigo Tiene AIDS (04)	.35
HIV + AIDS : The Basics (86)	.35
I Can't Cope with My Fear of AIDS (05)	.35
I'm HIV Positive—What Next? (06)	.35
Infection Precautions for People with AIDS (07)	.25
La Mujer Debe Informarse Sobre El SIDA (08)	.35
Loving Sharing Caring (09)	.35
Overview of Psycho-Social Issues (10)	.25
The Safer Sex Condom Guide (11)	.35
When a Friend Has AIDS (13)	.35
Women Loving Women (84)	.35
Women Need to Know About AIDS (14)	.35
Videos (03)	
A Test of the Nation (19)	20.00
An Informed Approach to HIV Antibody Testing (96)	20.00
Bleach, Teach and Outreach (20)	20.00
Manuals (04)	
Eroticizing Safer Sex (55)	10.00
Facing the Future (100)	5.00
Living with AIDS: A Resource Guide to NYC (57)	15.00
Supporting People with AIDS (29)	10.00
Time Out (30)	10.00
Posters (05)	
Always Practice Safer Sex (31)	5.00
Cujelo Con Cuidado/Take It Safely (32)	5.00
A Rubber Is a Friend in Your Pocket/Un Condon Es un Amigo en el Bolsillo (33)	5.00
Once, Twice, Thrice (98)	5.00
Rubbers Are Bringing Men Together Again (34)	5.00
Safer Sex: How to Do It (35)	5.00
Safer Sex: Keep It Up! (87)	5.00
Newsletters (06)	
Treatment Issues	
Subscription (10 issues) (63)	30.00
Compilation (53)	30.00
Most recent issue (one only) (36)	FREE

5. National AIDS Clearinghouse
Post Office Box 6003
Rockville, MD 20849-6003
(800) 458-5231
Deaf Access (800) 243-7012 (TDD)

The National AIDS Clearinghouse was initiated in October 1987 by the U.S. Department of Health and Human Services, Public Health Service, Centers for Disease Control (CDC), as part of its national information and education plan to respond to the public health threat posed by the human immunodeficiency virus (HIV) and acquired immunodeficiency syndrome (AIDS).

The Clearinghouse is a centralized source providing current information on HIV infection and AIDS programs, materials, and services to professionals.

The National AIDS Clearinghouse:

identifies and responds to the information needs of professionals involved in the development and delivery of HIV-prevention programs

distributes selected HIV prevention-oriented publications.

coordinates an information network among organizations involved in the fight against AIDS.

disseminates information about ongoing federally and privately sponsored HIV and AIDS clinical trials through the AIDS Clinical Trials Information Service (ACTIS). For more information about ACTIS call (800) TRIALS-A (800) 874-2572.

provides information about funding opportunities for community-based and HIV and AIDS service organizations.

The *Catalog of HIV/AIDS Materials for Professionals* lists publications and audiovisual materials distributed by the National AIDS Clearinghouse. The Clearinghouse offers a comprehensive information service for people working in the field of HIV and AIDS prevention including public health professionals, educators, social service workers, attorneys, human resource managers, and employers. These professionals work in a variety of settings, including state AIDS programs, community-based organizations, service organizations, businesses, and associations.

The materials in the *Catalog of HIV/AIDS Materials for Professionals* are produced by the Centers for Disease Control, other U.S. Public Health Service agencies, and other organizations. Most publications are free of charge and can be ordered easily by calling (800) 458-5231 or by returning the order form in the centerfold of the *Catalog*.

6. The National Association of People with AIDS (NAPWA)
1413 K Street, N.W., 10th Floor
Washington, D.C. 20005
(202) 898-0414

The National Association of People With AIDS (NAPWA) is the only national organization directed by and primarily serving people with AIDS. NAPWA enables people with HIV disease to live fuller lives by helping them make informed choices and take positive, life-affirming actions. NAPWA accomplishes this mission by providing:

easily-understood INFORMATION enabling individuals to learn about HIV disease and more easily access treatments, social services, and financial and legal options

TRAINING and technical assistance to local People With

AIDS Coalitions (PWACs), AIDS service organizations (ASOs), and other support groups for people with AIDS

nationwide ADVOCACY for the needs of people with HIV disease, the organizations that serve them, and all people impacted by the AIDS epidemic

NAPWA's programs reflect these competency goals, with each program targeting a critical need facing HIV+ individuals, the organizations that serve them, and all people impacted by the AIDS epidemic:

NAPWA News: a bi-monthly journal/newsmagazine helping individuals understand social service, legal, financial, mental health and treatment options, and providing technical assistance to PWACs/ASOs.

NAPWA-Link: a computerized AIDS information bulletin board providing a wide range of information on many aspects of HIV/AIDS and the issues entailed within it.

National Speakers Bureau: over 110 speakers presenting the perspectives of HIV+ people through such forums as conferences, community organizations, media inquiries; and through program planning with PWACs/ASOs and local, state, and federal agencies.

Information and Referral: fulfilling an average of 200 requests per month from individuals and groups desiring AIDS statistics, medical information, prevention information, psychosocial service referrals, governmental resources, grant opportunities, and other information pertaining to HIV infection.

Staff/Volunteer Training/Technical Assistance: through a series of venues we are providing assistance in the various aspects of organizational and programmatic development for ASOs. We are currently co-hosting three training conferences and the National Skills Building Conference. In addition, we provide assistance through publications, phone, and one on one.

7. National Community AIDS Partnership
1726 M. Street, N.W.
Suite 501
Washington, DC 20036
(202) 429-2820; (202) 429-2814 FAX

The National Community AIDS Partnership is in its fourth year of making grants to local communities for planning and service provision in response to America's HIV epidemic. Begun in April 1988 as a challenge grant program by a consortium of private funding organizations, NCAP was intended to achieve the following goals.

1. To stimulate community planning both to reduce the spread of AIDS and to offer appropriate services to people who have the disease;
2. To strengthen the ability of community-based AIDS organizations to provide AIDS services and education programs;
3. To build interest among funders and to increase the dollars available for AIDS education and services; and
4. To provide a national mechanism through which communities and local agencies can share information and resources about effective work against AIDS.

In December 1990, the National Advisory Committee added a fifth goal:

5. To stimulate effective public policy responses to AIDS at all levels of government so as to (a) ensure adequate and ongoing funding of education, prevention, and treatment services; (b) ensure that medical advances will result in improved humane treatment and care for HIV-infected persons in as timely a manner as possible; and (c) integrate the AIDS and public policy agenda into those of other fields.

In its first 2 years of operations, the Partnership made grants in 8 communities around the country. Over the past year, 14 new communities have joined NCAP, bringing the total number of communities served to 22. These communities cover all regions of the U.S. and represent a diverse set of local strategies for addressing the prevention and care of HIV disease. Since its inception, NCAP has made 576 individual project grants totally $13,256,158 through June 30, 1991.

Overview of NCAP Grants: A fundamental principle within the NCAP model is local determination of needs and HIV funding priorities. This important autonomy is reflected in the Local Partners' established grant-making emphasis and in the breadth of the grants made to date. During the 3 years of the Partnership, funding priorities have remained fairly consistent. Local Partners have remained committed to investing in education and HIV prevention programs as a long-term strategy to reducing the level of new infections.

In the area of direct service, the most commonly supported type of intervention was case management. There is, however, increasing emphasis in other areas, such as the housing needs of the people living with AIDS, programmatic-specific support groups such as orphan bereavement, pediatric AIDS and mental health-related grantmaking. Although some Partners have historically made mental health projects an important component of their grantmaking, it is anticipated that there will be an increased emphasis in this area. During the past year, 10 of the 15 grant-making partners having grant cycles made as many mental health grants as were made during the first 2 years by the original eight Local Partners.

Within the preventive education area, a number of Local Partners have aggressively focused on populations that had not previously been targeted by HIV prevention efforts. Women are increasingly the focus of these programs, and programs for youth, always a high priority, continue to increase.

An emerging area of grantmaking is in public policy/advocacy. While the Partnership's efforts to raise and disburse funds at the local level have made a difference, the epidemic and its accompanying social issues have continued to grow. In response, the Partnership began to develop an influential role in HIV/health policy in order to have a sustained impact on the epidemic.

Structure: The National Community AIDS Partnership is administered by a national staff located in Washington, DC. The Partnership's programmatic and policy direction is established by its Board of Trustees composed of prominent funders, AIDS experts, and persons living with HIV and AIDS. The National Advisory Committee (NAC) advises the Board of Trustees, who are elected from its membership. The organization uses a subcommittee structure to develop program plans and monitor their implementation. Committees include representatives of the Board, NAC, National, and Local Partners.

8. Project Inform
(Legal title: San Francisco Project Inform, Inc.)
501 (C) (3) #94-3052723
1965 Market Street Suite 220
San Francisco, CA 94103
(415) 558-8669; (415) 558-0684 FAX

Fighting HIV/AIDS takes knowledge, strength, and dedication. Founded in 1985, Project Inform is an independent, nonprofit, community-based AIDS service organization, dedicated to providing direct services to person infected with HIV or at risk for infection. The Project has a singular national reputation for effectively providing the public with clear and trustworthy information about HIV testing, early intervention strategies, and treatments for HIV-related problems. Project Inform also advocates on behalf of those infected at the Food and Drug Administration and the National Institutes of Health. The Project's work has strongly influenced the direction of national AIDS policy.

Services include: a national tool-free hotline; fact sheets and bulletins; a periodic journal, *PI Perspective;* a local and national speakers bureau; and the Treatment Action Network.

Their hotline for HIV+, AIDS, and ARC is (415) 558-9051 (local and international), (800) 334-7422 (California) and (800) 822-7422 (USA).

Their in-depth discussion papers include: (1) Day One—After you've tested positive, Doctor, Patient and HIV: Building a cooperative relationship; (2) AZT-Retrovir; (3) Preventing PCP; (4) ddl-dideoxyinosine—(videx); (5) ddc—(dideorycytidine)-HIVID; and (6) Acyclovir.

9. Women's AIDS Network
c/o S.F.A.F.
P.O. Box 6182
San Francisco, CA 94101-6182
(415) 864-4376 Ext. 2004

The Women's AIDS Network (WAN) was established in June 1983, at the Second National AIDS Forum in Denver. In March 1984, women involved with AIDS services in the San Francisco Bay Area began meeting monthly. The membership includes women in medical, mental health, and social services, along with women with HIV, community activists, and social and political advocates.

Available from the organization are:

A catalogue of educational materials available through Impact AIDS, including some specifically related to women and children.

Copies of the following articles and other resources:

Women and AIDS in the United States (English and Spanish)

The Impact of AIDS on Women (Nancy Padian, MS, MPH)

Women, AIDs, and Public Policy (Janet L. Mitchell)

Antibody to Human Immune Virus in Female Prostitutes; Morbidity & Mortality Weekly Report CDC Vol. 36/no. 11 1987

Role of Prostitutes in Prevention of HIV Transmission (Priscilla Alexander)

Rape, Sexual Assault & AIDS (S.F. Dept. of Health Sexual Trauma Services)

Isolation of AIDS-Associated Retrovirus from Genital Secretions of Women with Antibodies to the Virus (Constance B. Wofsy, MD, et al.)

Male-to-Female Transmission of Human Immunodeficiency Virus (Nancy Padian, PhD, et al.)

Lesbians and AIDS: Still Invisible After All These Years (Karen Lee Erlichman)

Women & AIDS (Barbara Sartee, PhD)

Human Immunodeficiency Virus Infection in Women, *JAMA* Ed. 4-17-87 (Constance Wofsy, MD)

Women and the Acquired Immunodeficiency Syndrome (Constance Wofsy, MD)

Preventing AIDS Among Women: The Role of Community Organizing (Nancy Stoller Shaw, PhD)

The Challenge of Human Immunodeficiency Virus (HIV) and Acquired Immunodeficiency Syndrome (AIDS) in Women and Children (Thomas A. Peterman, MD, MSc et al.)

HIV Disease in Reproductive Age Women: A Problem of the Present, *JAMA* Ed. 3-3-89 (Sheldon H. Landesman, MD et al.)

Pregnancy and HIV Infection (Laurie B. Hauer, RN)

Pregnancy-Associated Deaths Due to AIDs in the United States (Lisa M. Koonin, MD, MPH et al.)

Prospective Study of Human Immunodeficiency Virus Infection and Pregnancy Outcomes in Intravenous Drug Users (Peter A. Selwyn, MD et al.)

Screen All Pregnant Women for AIDS; Johns Hopkins Medical Report Update, 6-21-90

AIDS in Children: A Review of the Clinical Epidemiological and Public Health Aspects (Martha F. Rogers, MD)

Caring for Children with HIV Infection (Ellen R. Cooper, MD)

Serving Your Patients in the Age of AIDS (Nancy Stoller Shaw, PhD)

AIDS and Women: Remaining Ethical Issues (Nora Kizer Bell, PhD)

AIDS and Women: Remaining Ethical Issues (Nora Kizer Bell, PhD)

The full packet of articles is available for $10 + $2 shipping and handling. Individual articles can be ordered for $1.00/article + 1.50 shipping and handling.

Organizations Devoted to Pain

1. American Academy of Pain Medicine
5700 Old Orchard Road, First Floor
Skokie, IL 60077-1057

AAPM is the official organization representing physicians in the field of pain in the United States. Our mission is to enhance the practice of pain medicine in the United States. In working to achieve this mission, AAPM's goals are to promote a socioeconomic and political climate conducive to the practice of pain medicine in an effective and efficient manner, and to ensure quality and comprehensive medical care by physicians specializing in chronic pain medicine to patients in need of such services.

The benefits of membership in AAPM include the following:

Membership directory, listing primary care and specialty physicians with an interest in pain medicine.

Subscriptions to *The Clinical Journal of Pain,* the official AAPM journal.

Special rates on all AAPM activities and products, such as annual meetings, regional seminars, and the *Directory of Pain Management Facilities* (not available to trainee members).

AAPM awards recognition program.

2. American Pain Society
5700 Old Orchard Road, First Floor
Skokie, IL 60077-1057
(708) 966-5595; (708) 966-9418 FAX

The American Pain Society, a national chapter of the International Association for the Study of Pain (IASP), is a multidisciplinary, not-for-profit educational and scientific organization comprising clinicians and researchers. The mission of APS is to serve people in pain by advancing research, education, treatment, and professional practice. We recognize that this goal can best be accomplished as a joint and interactive effort among basic scientists and healthcare professionals.

APS was founded in 1979 and has grown to more than 2000 members. Over the years, the American Pain Society has expanded its programming and publications to meet the needs of its membership.

Publications of the American Pain Society are:

APS Journal, a quarterly publication, provides a forum for the scholarly presentation and discussion of issues.

APS Bulletin offers feature articles on clinical and basic science topics, organizational news, and a calendar of events.

APS Membership directory features a complete listing of all APS members—geographically, alphabetically, and by specialty.

Principles of Analgesic Use (3rd edition) is a concise, compact, easily accessible reference guide. ($2.00/nonmembers)

Benefits of membership include reduced fees on education programs:

Annual Scientific Meeting features plenary sessions, workshops, symposia, posters, and exhibits—more than 200 presentations in all. Network with the 1000 people who attend.

Pain Update programs offer a series of in-depth half-day clinical sessions dealing with the latest in pain research and professional practice.

Educational programs offer continuing education credits.

3. International Association for the Study of Pain
909 NE 43rd St., Suite 306
Seattle, WA 98105
(206) 547-6409; (206) 547-1703 FAX; Telex: 265214

IASP was founded in 1973 and was incorporated in 1974 as a nonprofit organization:

To foster and encourage research of pain mechanisms and pain syndromes and to help improve the management of patients with acute and chronic pain by bringing together basic scientists, physicians, and other health professionals of various disciplines and backgrounds who have interest in pain research and management.

To promote education and training in the field of pain.

To promote and facilitate the dissemination of new information in the field of pain, including sponsorship of a journal, *PAIN.*

To promote and sponsor a triennial World Congress of the Association and such other meetings as may be useful or desirable for the advancement of the purposes of IASP.

To encourage formation of national associations for the study and treatment of pain

To encourage the adoption of a uniform classification, nomenclature, and definition regarding pain and pain syndromes.

To encourage the development of a national and international data bank and to encourage the development of a uniform records system with respect to information relating to pain mechanisms, syndromes, and management.

To inform the general public of results and implications of current research in the area.

To advise international, national, and regional agencies of standards relating to the use of drugs, appliances and other procedures in the therapy of pain.

To engage in such other activities as may be incidental to or in furtherance of the aforementioned purposes.

Regular Members: Active membership in IASP is open to all scientists, physicians, dentists, psychologists, nurses, physical therapists, and other health professionals actively engaged in pain research and those who have special interest in diagnosis and treatment of pain syndromes.

Publications

PAIN: The monthly journal *PAIN,* begun in 1975 and published by Elsevier, is the official journal of IASP and contains review articles, original research articles in both the clinical and basic sciences, book reviews, and letters to the editor.

Newsletter: Published bimonthly and mailed to all members.

Directory of Members: Published annually and mailed to all members.

Classification of Chronic Pain: (Description of Chronic Pain Syndromes and Definitions of Pain Terms). Prepared by the Committee on Taxonomy, this is a detailed, comprehensive classification of pain syndromes and a minimum standard vocabulary (terms and definitions) for the field of pain. Available for purchase. (226 pages) ($18.00) (1986).

Core Curriculum for Professional Education in Pain: Prepared by the Task Force on Professional Education to identify the core of common knowledge necessary to best serve the patient and to communicate across disciplinary lines. In outline form with an extensive bibliography. Available for purchase. (97 pages) ($20.00) (1991).

Ethical Guidelines for Investigations of Experimental Pain in Conscious Animals: (Free to members) (1983).

Curriculum on Pain for Medical Schools: An outline of a model pain course for a medical undergraduate curriculum. Curricula for dentistry, nursing and pharmacy are in preparation (Free to members) (1988).

Desirable Characteristics for Pain Treatment Facilities: Prepared by the Task Force on Guidelines for Desirable

Characteristics for Pain Treatment Facilities to serve as a guideline for both practitioners and governmental and professional organizations involved in the establishment of pain treatment facilities. (Free to members) (1990)

Standards for Physician Fellowship in Pain Management: Prepared by an IASP Task Force to serve as a guideline for physicians who seek further training in the pain field. Includes prerequisites for both trainee and training facility. (Free to members) (1990).

Refresher Course Syllabus: Refresher Courses are held at the time of IAS's triennial world congresses. A syllabus is available for purchase. (140 pages, approx.) ($15.00).

Congress Abstracts: Abstracts of all papers to be presented at an IASP Congress are mailed to all IASP members in advance of the Congress and are available for all registrants. Additional copies are available for purchase. (500 pages, approx.) ($15.00).

Congress Proceedings: Proceedings of all the IASP World Congresses have been published as hardbound books. These books contain the major invited plenary papers presented at IASP Congresses and selected free communication papers. At the time of a Congress they are offered to members at discounted prices. (600 pages, approx.).

4. National Chronic Pain Outreach Association, Inc.
7979 Old Georgetown Road, Suite 100
Bethesda, MD 20814-2429
(301) 652-4948; (301) 907-0745 FAX

The National Chronic Pain Outreach Association, Inc. (NCPOA) is a nonprofit organization established in 1980. Its purpose is to lessen the suffering of people with chronic pain by educating pain sufferers, health care professionals, and the public about chronic pain and its management.

The benefits of joining include:

NCPOA operate an information clearinghouse that offers books, pamphlets, cassettes, and videotapes for both pain sufferers and health care professionals. (Nonmembers can also purchase these pamphlets, books, cassettes, tapes, and videotapes.)
NCPOA publishes a quarterly magazine, *Lifeline,* which provides information on pain management and coping methods.
NCPOA sponsors lectures and seminars to increase public awareness of chronic pain.
NCPOA provides a "do-it-yourself kit" for people who want to start their own local chronic pain support groups.
NCPOA provides referrals to NCPOA member health care professionals and medical facilities nationwide.
NCPOA maintains a computerized registry of chronic pain support groups in the United States and Canada (although NCPOA does not directly sponsor any groups).

5. Nursing Pain Association
Pain Study Office, N411Y, Box 0606
School of Nursing
University of California
San Francisco, CA 94143
(415) 476-4040

The purpose of the organization is to foster and promote education, research, and high standards of practice in the care of patients with pain. To emphasize the application of pain research findings to nursing care by:

Improving the quality of nursing care provided to the patient in pain
Providing opportunities for members to continue their growth as pain specialists.
Providing a forum for networking among members.
Providing continuing pain education to nurse colleagues.
Promoting nursing research related to pain.

Membership Benefits:

Pain Education Programs
  Annual Bay Area Conference in California—reduced fee
Regular members' meetings—no charge
  Dinners (informal, social/professional, networking)

Referral Service
  Professional network—
    Identify local and national experts for a specific pain problem
  Direct individuals to current literature on a specific pain topic

Consultation Bureau
  Pain curricula, research, and client-based practice (fees negotiated by individual consultant)

Speakers Bureau
  Pain education programs for site-specific needs

Membership Directory

Newsletter

6. State Cancer Pain Initiatives

The state pain initiative movement is one primarily of education, advocacy, and creation of a positive regulatory climate. Pain initiatives are developed at the state level in order to tailor their programs to the unique geographic, cultural, and political characteristics of their region. The focus is on cancer relief because it is a pain syndrome easily recognized and described. It is hoped that progress toward relief of cancer pain will bring new awareness of and skill in relieving pain of other etiology and disease states.

State Contacts for Cancer Pain Initiatives

Arizona
Eugenie A. Obbens, MD
University Medical Center
1501 N. Campbell Avenue
Tucson, AZ 85724
(602) 626-4147

California*
Pamela J. Haylock, RN
220 Ware Road
Woodside, CA 94062
(415) 851-2881

Colorado
Albert Brady, MD
Cancer Care Center
Porter Memorial Hospital
2525 S. Downing Street
Denver, CO 80210
(303) 778-5741

Connecticut
Judith Floyd, RN, MSN
Radiation Oncology Dept.

Veterans Memorial Medical Center
1 King Place
Meriden, CT 06450
(203) 238-8433

Florida
Lisa O. Slenon, RN, OCN
Lee Moffitt Cancer Center
Pain Service
PO 280179
Tampa, FL 33682
(813) 972-8456

Hawaii
Hob Osterlund, RN, MS
The Queen's Medical Center
1301 Punchbowl Street
Honolulu, HI 96813
(808) 538-9011

Illinois*
Michael E. Frederich, MD
305 S. Illinois
Belleville, IL 62220
(618) 235-1703

Indiana*
Neil Irick, MD
Pain Resource Center
2020 W. 86th Street, Suite 310
Indianapolis, IN 46260
(317) 872-2332

Iowa
Wendy Gronbeck, RN
4-S GH U. of Iowa Hospitals & Clinics
Iowa City, IA 52242
(319) 356-2654

Massachusetts
Margaret Barton Burke, RN, MS, OCN
247 Commonwealth Avenue
Boston, MA 02114
(617) 469-9549

Michigan*
Josephina Magno, MD
International Hospice Inst.
Henry Ford Hospital
2799 W. Grand Boulevard
Detroit, MI 48202
(313) 876-9234

Minnesota*
Thomas E. Elliott, MD
The Duluth Clinic, Ltd.
400 E. Third Street
Duluth, MN 55805
(218) 722-8364

Missouri
Mary Ann Nalley, RN
Professional Education Director
3322 American Avenue
Jefferson City, MO 63131
(314) 893-4800

New Hampshire
Marion B. Dolan
Heritage Home Health
12 Summer Street, PO 127
Bristol, NH 03222
(603) 279-4700

New Mexico*
Walter B. Forman, MD
Clinical Director
U of New Mexico Cancer Center
900 Camino de Salud NE
Albuquerque, NM 87131
(505) 277-2858

New York
(New York does not have a state cancer pain initiative; the name of the contact person at Cancer Care is given here.)
Kim Calder, MPS
Cancer Care
1180 Avenue of Americas
New York, NY 10036
(212) 302-2400

North Carolina*
Faye W. McNaull, RN, OCN
Durham VA Medical Center
508 Fulton Street
Durham, NC 27705
(919) 286-0411

Ohio*
Warren Wheeler, MD
Hospice at Riverside
Kobacker House
c/o OH Cancer Pain Initiative
3595 Olentangy River Road
Columbus, OH 43214
(614) 459-0241

Oregon
Kelly Scott, PharmD
Good Samaritan Hosp.
1015 NW 22nd Avenue, #T010
Portland, OR 97210
(503) 229-7774

Pennsylvania*
Mary Simmonds, MD
Cowley Associates
Plaza 21, Suite 2-1
425 N. 21st Street
Camp Hill, PA 17011
(717) 761-7400

Rhode Island
Phoebe Fernald, RN, MS, OCN
Rhode Island Hospital
Department of Medical Oncology
593 Eddy Street
Providence, RI 02903
(401) 277-5013

Texas*
C. Stratton Hill, Jr. MD
Director, Pain Services
UTMD Anderson Cancer Center
1515 Holcombe Boulevard
Houston, TX 77030
(713) 792-2824

Utah*
Perry G. Fine, MD
Associate Professor
Department of Anesthesiology
U of Utah Health Sciences Center
50 N. Medical Drive
Salt Lake City, UT 84132
(801) 581-6393

Vermont
Amy Becker, RPH
Medical Center Hospital of Vermont
111 Colchester Avenue
Burlington, VT 05401
(802) 656-2880

Virginia
Thomas J. Smith, MD
Medical Director
Dalton Oncology Clinic
Box 230 MCV Station
Richmond, VA 23298
(804) 786-0450

Washington*
Linda Sandwich
1124 Columbia Street FB600E
Seattle, WA 98104
(206) 667-5162

Wisconsin
June L. Dahl, PhD
3675 Medical Sciences Center
1300 University Avenue
Madison, WI 53706
(608) 262-0978

Courtesy of Wisconsin Cancer Pain Initiative.

*State with more than one contact person. Contact the Wisconsin center for other listings.

(from Smith, J: State cancer pain initiatives: making pain relief a priority. *Problem-Solving in Office Oncology Nursing* 6(3): 1–3, 1992.

7. The Wisconsin Cancer Pain Initiative
3675 Medical Sciences Center
1300 University Avenue
Madison, WI 53706
(608) 262-0978

The Wisconsin Cancer Pain Initiative is a multidisciplinary effort aimed at improving the management of cancer pain. It is a cooperative effort of clinical care facilities, higher education, government and many health care professionals including physicians, nurses, pharmacists, social workers, and others throughout the state of Wisconsin. The Initiative is a World Health Organization demonstration program.

It is the goal of the Wisconsin Cancer Pain Initiative to:

help health professionals acquire and apply cancer pain information and management techniques,
promote the use of existing drug and nondrug methods to alleviate suffering,
change attitudes about cancer pain management,
dispel fears about medications that relieve pain,
educate patients and families on available treatments.

The Wisconsin Cancer Pain Initiative is working to improve the management of cancer pain in Wisconsin through the development of:

a handbook on cancer pain management for health professionals,
educational displays for the public and professionals,
educational booklets about cancer pain for adults and children,
a speakers' bureau,
a network of patient advocates and clinical consultants,
a clearinghouse of resource materials,
improved communication among health professionals,
media coverage to improve public information,
curriculum improvements in the schools of medicine, nursing, and pharmacy,
evaluation of laws and regulations that may be barriers to good pain management.

Resource material available from the Wisconsin Cancer Pain Initiative:

A Treatment Oriented Guide for Health Professionals

The Handbook of Cancer Pain Management ($3.00 per copy plus postage)

Patient Education Booklets (25 cents per copy plus postage)

Cancer Pain Can Be Relieved—a guide for adult patients and families

Children's Cancer Pain Can Be Relieved—for parents of children with cancer

Jeff Asks About Cancer Pain—a booklet for teens about cancer pain

Brochure

"The Wisconsin Cancer Pain Initiative: Helping Health Professional Help Cancer Patients in Pain"

This brochure presents the basic principles of cancer pain management and the goals of the Wisconsin Cancer Pain Initiative. It is available free of charge.

Displays

These are useful for showing at meetings and in clinics, hospitals and shopping malls. Borrowers are asked to pay the UPS shipping fee and to return the display to the Initiative.

Teaming Up to Fight Cancer Pain (for health professionals)

Helping Patients and Families Improve Cancer Pain Management (for the general public)

Video

Borrowers are asked to pay the UPS shipping fee to return these materials to the Initiative.

"Cancer Pain Can Be Conquered" (Slide/tape set)
An 11-minute slide tape set, produced by the Wisconsin Cancer Pain Initiative, is available to health professionals to show to lay groups. It emphasizes that cancer doesn't have to hurt and that addiction rarely if ever occurs when patients are given opioids for cancer pain. Also stressed is the importance of good communication among patients, families, and health care providers.

"Conquering Cancer Pain" (Videotape)
This is a video tape presentation of the slide tape set mentioned above.

"The Assessment and Management of Cancer Pain." This 28-minute color videotape has been developed in conjunction with the Wisconsin Cancer Pain Initiative and is moderated by Dianne Howser, RN, BSN, OCN.

Content includes: pathophysiology of cancer pain, types of cancer pain; basic analgesic pharmacology; opioid tolerance, dependence, addiction; a brief discussion of nondrug interventions; and an interview with a cancer patient with pain. This is available in either ¾″ U-Matic or ½″ VHS formation for $150.00. Check should be made to: Milwaukee County Medical Complex (check must accompany order). For more information contact: Mary K. Black, RN, MS, Program Director—Human Resources Development, Milwaukee County Medical Complex, 8700 W. Wisconsin Avenue, Box 139, Milwaukee, WI 53226. (414) 257-5950.

"Why Not Freedom from Cancer Pain?" 14-minute videotape from the World Health Organization. The tape is geared for health care professionals as well as the general public, and focuses on the fact that cancer pain can be relieved and that patients and families have the right to adequate medication. Highlights include a global perspective on the program of unrelieved cancer pain, an explanation of the WHO three-step pain control ladder, and moving testimonials from cancer patients and their families.

"My Word Against Theirs." M.D. Anderson Cancer Center. Several cancer patients describe the barriers they faced as they tried to get adequate relief of their pain. There is particular emphasis on concerns about addiction. To order, write Dr. C. Stratton Hill, Jr., M.D. Anderson Hospital, 1515 Holcombe Boulevard, Houston, TX 77030, (713) 792-2824.

"Winning the Battle" and "Control Your Cancer Pain": Both about 12 minutes. Produced in 1990 by the Marshfield Clinic. The first video addresses three common myths about cancer pain control; the second corrects common misconceptions about how pain medications work, $59 each; $99 the pair. Order from Marshfield Video Network, 1000 North Oak Avenue, Marshfield, WI 54449.

"Fighting Cancer Pain." McNeil-Lehrer, National Public Television; 1990, 12 minutes. The cancer pain problem, the Wisconsin Initiative, Congressman Stark's proposal to require triplicate prescription orders for all controlled substances. Borrow from the WCPI.

"When Pain Strikes." This film aired on the television program "10/10" on August 18, 1989. To get a copy of this program, send a $16.00 check or money order made payable to ABC Distribution Company at Capital Cities, ABC Video Enterprises, 825 7th Avenue, New York, NY 10019. Please indicate which tape format you require (½" VHS, ½" Beta, or ¾" U-Matic) along with the program's title and airdate as stated. Payment must accompany order. Orders will be filled within 2 to 3 weeks of the date orders are received. You may also get written transcripts of the program by sending $4.00 made payable to ABC News to: Journal Graphics, 267 Roadway, New York, NY 10007.

"Cancer: Freedom from pain" and "Cancer Pain: A Prescription for Compassion." Produced by Wisconsin Public Television in 1987 and 1988, respectively. Both 29 minutes. Borrow from the WCPI.

Oncology Nursing Organizations and Related Oncology Professional Organizations

1. American Association for Cancer Education, Inc.
   C. Michael Brooks, EdD
   Secretary
   University of Alabama
   School of Medicine
   UAB Station 401 CH19
   Birmingham, AL 35294
   (205) 934-3054; (205) 934-3278 FAX

   The purpose of the AACE has been "to provide a forum for those concerned with education of groups who attempt to advance the cause of early cancer detection, promote individualized multimodality therapy, or develop programs of rehabilitation for cancer patients." This multidisciplinary organization brings together basic scientists, surgeons, internists, oncology nursing educators, pediatricians, pathologists, gynecologists, dentists, and radiation oncologists. They hold an annual fall meeting.

   The official journal of the Association is the *Journal of Cancer Education,* which is listed in *Index Medicus.* The Association has occasionally sponsored other publications such as *Concepts in Cancer Medicine,* edited by S. Benham Kahn, MD et al., and *Self-Assessment of Current Knowledge in Oncology,* edited by John Foley, MD. The Association also distributes a President's Newsletter, and abstracts accepted for presentation at the annual meeting are published as a Supplement to the *Journal of Cancer Education.*

   The American Association for Cancer Education does not produce or distribute cancer education materials.

2. American Association for Cancer Research
   Margaret Foti, Executive Director
   Public Ledger Building
   620 Chestnut Street, Suite 816
   Philadelphia, PA 19106
   (215) 440-9313 FAX

   The American Association for Cancer Research (AACR) is the world's largest professional society of scientists specializing in both basic and clinical cancer research. Its 7600 members are experts in the areas of molecular biology and genetics of cancer, tumor biology, virology, carcinogenesis, toxicology and risk assessment, endocrinology, epidemiology and prevention, pharmacology and therapeutics, immunology, and all aspects of clinical investigations pertaining to human cancer. The publications of the association include: *Cancer Research, Cell Growth and Differentiation, Cancer Epidemiology, Biomarkers and Prevention, Directory of Members,* and *Proceedings of the American Association for Cancer Research.*

3. American Cancer Society
   Terri Ades, RN, BSN, OCN
   Director, Nursing Programs
   1599 Clifton Road, NE
   Atlanta, GA 30329-4251
   (404) 329-7617; (800) ACS 2345

   The American Cancer Society is the nationwide voluntary health organization dedicated to eliminating cancer as a major health problem by preventing cancer, saving lives from cancer, and diminishing suffering from cancer through research, education, and service.

   The Society offers scholarships to interested oncology nurses at both the Master's and Doctoral level. The scholarships provide a stipend of $8000 per year for a maximum of 2 years for a Master's degree in nursing and $8000 per year for a maximum of 4 years for a Doctoral degree in nursing or related area.

4. American Society of Clinical Oncology
   435 North Michigan Avenue, Suite 1717
   Chicago, IL 60611-4067

(312) 644-0828; (312) 644-8557 FAX
and
Director of Government Relations
American Society of Clinical Oncology
750 17th Street, NW, Suite 1100
Washington, DC 20006
(202) 778-2396; (202) 778-2330 FAX

The Society directs its effort to the promotion of cancer research. The publication of the society is *Journal of Clinical Oncology*.

5. American Society of Hematology
Michael Payne, Executive Director
1101 Connecticut Avenue, NW
Suite 700
Washington, DC 20036
(202) 857-1174; (202) 223-4579 FAX

The American Society of Hematology (ASH) is a professional organization that devotes its efforts to research and information dissemination about the blood and blood-forming tissues frequently related to the development of or the treatment of cancer.

The Society directs its efforts to the following objectives:

to promote and foster research and research collaboration; and
to encourage investigation of hematologic matters.

6. American Society for Therapeutic Radiology and Oncology
1892 Preston White Drive
Reston, VA 22092
(703) 648-3794; (703) 648-9176 FAX

The American Society for Therapeutic Radiology and Oncology (ASTRO) comprises American Board of Radiology certified physicians, radiation therapists, and radiation biologists whose professional practice is therapeutic radiology. The objectives of the Society are:

to extend the benefits of radiation therapy to cancer patients;
to advance the scientific basis of radiation therapy; and
to provide for the education and professional fellowship of its members.

7. Association of American Cancer Institutes
c/o Roswell Park Cancer Institute
666 Elm Street
Buffalo, NY 14263
(716) 845-3028; (716) 845-8178 FAX

The Association of American Cancer Institutes (AACI) was originally established in 1959 as the Association of Cancer Institute Directors. In 1973 the organization was incorporated as the AACI. Today, 71 cancer centers throughout the United States are members of the AACI; 5 cancer centers throughout the world are corresponding members.

The AACI provides an organization structure to carry out the following objectives:

to afford an opportunity for the leadership of cancer institutes and centers throughout the world to meet and discuss mutual problems;
to foster collaboration via state, regional, national, and international programs for the control of cancer through research, education, and service;
to support investigations into the causes, nature, prevention, and treatment of cancer and the rehabilitation of cancer patients by encouraging the exchange of ideas, information, personnel, and the provision of special facilities and training opportunities;
to foster educational and training opportunities in the related biomedical sciences; and
to provide guidance to federal, state, and local governments, private, and civic organizations concerning cancer research, diagnosis, treatment and prevention, and the rehabilitation of cancer patients.

8. Association of Community Cancer Centers
Lee Mortenson, Executive Director
11600 Nebel Street, Suite 201
Rockville, MD 20852
(301) 984-9496; (301) 770-1949 FAX

The ACCC acts as the national voice of community cancer care professionals. It serves as a forum on national issues and a source of information on clinical research organizations, new technology, and research results. Annual dues for individuals $100 (1992). Members include institutions and individuals.

The Association publishes *Oncology Issues: The Journal of Cancer Program Management,* a quarterly publication devoted to information on the economic and programmatic issues of community cancer programs and their components. The Association's Washington, DC office issues *Special Communiques* on federal legislation and regulation affecting cancer care providers' ability to deliver quality care.

In addition, the association publishes *Community Cancer Programs in the United States,* the annual ACCC Delegate Roster. This volume provides detailed information on each Delegate member institution, including program components, personnel, and history. The names and addresses of general members are also listed.

Each year, ACCC publishes the most recent comparative data on current cancer-related DRGs. These reports contain analyses of average reimbursement, average cost, average profit/loss, and total reimbursement by hospital size and region. The report is titled "Cancer DRGs: A Comparative Report on Key Cancer DRGs."

9. Association of Freestanding Radiation Oncology Centers
3960 Park Boulevard, Suite E
San Diego, CA 92103
(610) 692-1598

AFROC is a nonprofit organization composed of physicists, physicians, administrators, technicians, and clinical personnel working in freestanding, fully equipped radiation centers. It acts as a forum for addressing concerns and as an advocate for reimbursement and legislative policies affecting the centers. Full membership is $400, and benefits include a quarterly newsletter, *Source;* legislative information; reduced rates at the annual meeting; and current information on reimbursement, economic issues, practice development/marketing ideas, financial management, quality assurance, and more.

10. Association of Pediatric Oncology Nurses
11512 Allecingie Parkway
Richmond, VA 23235
(804) 379-9150; (804) 379-1386 FAX

APON has been in existence since 1973. Membership in the organization is open to all registered nurses who are either interested in or engaged in pediatrics or pediatric oncology. Annual dues are $55 (1992), which entitles the member to receive a copy of the quarterly journal, *J.A.P.O.N., A.P.O.N. Newsletter,* and other pertinent publications; attend all business meetings and programs at a reduced rate; and vote on all issues concerning the organization. The objectives of the organization are to promote excellence in the specialty of pediatric oncology nursing, provide opportunities for communication among all nurses who work with children who have cancer through quarterly newsletters and an annual seminar, encourage dissemination of information among nurses about the medical and nursing care of pediatric oncology patients that is used in various areas of the country, encourage members to update professional and lay literature with regard to the care of children with cancer, and encourage and support research in nursing care of children with cancer.

APON has several publications for purchase by both members and nonmembers: *Chemotherapy Book, Scope of Practice and Outcome Standards of Pediatric Oncology Nursing,* and *Patient/Family Annotated Bibliography.*

11. Commission on Accreditation of Rehabilitation Facilities
101 North Wilmot Road, Suite 500
Tucson, AZ 85711

The Commission on Accreditation of Rehabilitation Facilities' fundamental commitment is to an organized and productive national system of human services that is designed effectively and efficiently to be responsive to the needs of people with disabilities. Through the mechanism of standards setting and accreditation, the Commission is the recognized accountability authority for the wide range of rehabilitation/habilitation organizations and programs. The goal of these programs is to make a positive difference in the lives of people with disabilities as they strive to attain optimal self-sufficiency, independence, and productivity.

The Commission began in 1966. It is a private, not-for-profit organization that has had the benefit of a broad base of support and involvement on the part of consumers, providers, and purchasers of specialized services for people with disabilities. The Commission's success is directly attributed to the profound impact it has had on the provision of quality-oriented services to people with disabilities.

The following materials can be purchased from the Commission:

1. *Standards Manual for Organizations Service People with Disabilities*—$35
2. *Self-Study Questionnaire*—$25 (available only to those who purchase a *Standards Manual*)
3. A variety of resource publications in program evaluation—$14 each
4. *Directory of Accredited Organizations Serving People with Disabilities*—$25
5. Performance Evaluation and Accreditation Institutes: 1 and ½ day seminars designed to familiarize groups with the standards, their utilization in day-to-day operations, and how the standards are applied in the accreditation process.

12. Food and Drug Administration
Office for Consumer Affairs
HFE-88
5600 Fishers Lane
Rockville, MD 20857
(301) 443-3170

The FDA serves as a source for information regarding FDA regulations, cosmetics, foods, drugs, health fraud, and medical devices.

13. International Society of Nurses in Cancer Care
Mulberry House
The Royal Marsden Hospital
Fulham Road
London SW36JJ
071-352 8171 Ext. 2123; 071-351 2191 FAX

Established in 1984, this society's goal is "to enable cancer nurses to share their knowledge and problems on a worldwide basis." Members of the society are required to pay an annual fee based on the size of the active membership of their organization, institution, or agency. Societies, interest groups, and clinical or educational institutions are able to join the Society in their own right. The range of fees is from $100–250. Members receive the newsletter *International Cancer Nursing News.* The International Society of Nurses in Cancer Care have "A Core Curriculum for a Post-Basic Course in Palliative Nursing" that is available for purchase.

14. International Union Against Cancer
(Union Internationale Contre Le Cancer—UICC)
Rue de Conseil—General 3
1205 Geneva, Switzerland
(41-22) 20 18 11

UICC is composed of multidisciplinary cancer organizations. Its purpose is to encourage the fight against cancer worldwide, promoting communication internationally in cancer research, treatment, and prevention. It is also a certifying government of legitimate cancer-fighting organizations. Membership dues are based on an organization's ability to pay. Congresses are held biennially.

15. Intravenous Nurses Society
Two Brighton Street
Belmont, MA 02178
(617) 489-5205; (617) 489-0656

The Intravenous Nurses Society is the national nonprofit professional association for nurses involved in the delivery of intravenous therapies. Membership fee is $75 (1992). Founded in 1973, the purpose of the organization is to upgrade the intravenous therapy nursing practice through continuing education, professional certification, and the development of standards of practice. The Society provides a variety of national and local educational opportunities for I.V. nurses, in order to ensure a high level of quality of nursing care for the public. Membership benefits include:

Subscriptions to the Society's publications, including the *Journal of Intravenous Nursing* and the membership newsletter *Newsline*
Reduced registration fee at INS Annual Meeting
Reduced rate for *Intravenous Nursing Standards of Practice,* the nationally recognized standards of IV nursing care
Reduced rate for "Implantable Ports" videotape.

16. National Alliance of Breast Cancer Organizations (NABCO)
Amy J. Schiffman
Administrative Director

1180 Avenue of the Americas, 2nd Floor
New York, NY 10036
(212) 719-0154
(NABCO prefers written inquiries)

NABCO is a central resource formed to provide individuals and health organizations with accurate, up-to-date information on all aspects of breast cancer and to promote affordable detection and treatment. Annual membership in NABCO is available to individuals and organizations and includes a year's subscription to the quarterly *NABCO News,* which monitors new research and events related to breast cancer. Membership, which is tax-deductible, includes access to a constantly updated resource list of written materials and other information about breast cancer.

17. National Institute for Occupational Safety and Health
US Department of Health and Human Services
Directorate of Technical Support
200 Constitution Avenue, N.W.
Washington, DC 20210
(202) 523-7047

NIOSH is a federal research agency. Of interest is its research in the area of handling cytotoxic drugs and laminar airflow hoods. It also has developed guidelines for health care workers in preventing the transmission of hepatitis B virus and HIV.

18. National Tumor Registrars Association
11600 Nebel Street, Suite 201
Rockville, MD 20852
(301) 984-1748

The purpose of the NTRA is to provide support and promote tumor registry and its use. Both certified and noncertified tumor registrars may be members in this organization. The NTRA will assist certified members in maintaining their credentials. Information gathered from tumor registry is used for statistics, research, epidemiology, quality assurance, screening, etc., but its main focus is the patient and quality care.

19. Occupational Safety and Health Administration (OSHA)
US Department of Labor
200 Constitution Avenue, NW
Washington, DC 20210
(202) 523-7047

OSHA is a federal enforcement agency. It has published guidelines for handling antineoplastic drugs (currently being updated) and other information related to health care worker safety.

20. Oncology Nursing Society
501 Holiday Drive
Pittsburgh, PA 15220-2749
(412) 921-7373; (412) 921-6565 FAX

ONS was founded in 1975 to promote the highest professional standards of oncology nursing; study, research, and exchange information, experiences, and ideas leading to improved oncology nursing; encourage nurses to specialize in the practice of oncology nursing; identify resources within the group; and establish guidelines of nursing care for patients with cancer. Annual dues are $63 (1992), which entitles a member to the society's referred journal, *Oncology Nursing Forum,* and a newsletter, *ONS News,* which are published six times per year. Members are also entitled to reduced rates for the annual Congress, the annual Fall Institute, an opportunity to serve on society committees, and research and travel awards. In 1982 the Oncology Nursing Foundation, an allied organization of ONS, was established to enhance the quality of cancer nursing throughout the disease process. Annually, this national Foundation awards nursing research grants; presents undergraduate, graduate, and doctoral scholarships; and funds public education projects. Additional awards include the Mara Morgensen Flaherty Memorial Lecture and the Pearl Moore Career Development Award.

In 1984, ONS founded another allied organization, the Oncology Nursing Certification Corporation, whose purpose is to develop, administer, and evaluate a program for the certification of oncology nurses. The certification examination tests the general oncology nursing knowledge base of the professional nurse. The first exam, offered in 1986, resulted in 1384 Oncology Certified Nurses. Testing is offered each year at the ONS Congress and at five different locations throughout the United States in the fall. Presently, there are over 9000 oncology certified nurses.

ONS publishes guidelines and standards for various aspects of oncology nursing and makes these publications available through its national office. In 1992 there were more than 148 chapters of ONS across the country.

Partial list of publications:

The *Oncology Nursing Forum,* the Society's official journal
The Society's newsletter, the *ONS News*
Guidelines for Cancer Nursing Practice
Cancer Chemotherapy Guidelines (module format)—Course Content and Clinical Practicum, Acute Care Setting,
Outpatient Setting, Home Care Setting and Management of Extravasation of Anaphylaxis
Biological Response Modifiers Guidelines: Recommendations for Nursing Education and Practice
Access Device Guidelines (module format)—Catheters, Ports and Reservoirs and Pumps
Guidelines for Safe Handling of Cytotoxic Drugs: An Independent Study
Standards for Cancer Nursing Practice, Cancer Nursing Education, Cancer Patient Education, Public Cancer Education, and *Advanced Practice in Oncology Nursing Core*
Curriculum in Oncology Nursing
ONS Consultant and Research Interest Directories
The 1989 National Survey of Salary, Staffing, and Professional Practice Patterns in Oncology Nursing
The 1991 Bone Marrow Transplant Nursing Resource Directory
ONS Position Paper on Cancer Rehabilitation
ONS Position Paper on Cancer Pain
Oncology Nursing Review: A Computer Assisted Instruction Program

21. Radiation Research Society
1891 Preston White Drive
Reston, VA 22091
(703) 648-3780; (703) 648-9176 (FAX)

The Radiation Research Society (RRS) is a professional organization composed of basic and clinical researchers who have specialized expertise in the effects of environmental radiation exposure, including mutagenesis and oncogenesis. Research and clinical interests include the use of radiation in medicine and industry, mainly for the radiation therapy of cancer and for imaging in diagnostic tests.

The Radiation Research Society has set forth a number of objectives to meet the needs of its professional membership, such as:

encouraging in the broadest manner possible the advancement of radiation research in all areas of the natural sciences;

facilitating cooperative research between the disciplines of physics, chemistry, biology, and medicine in the study of the properties and effects of radiation; and

promoting the dissemination of knowledge in these and related fields through publications, meetings, and educational symposiums.

22. The Society of Gynecologic Oncologists
410 N. Michigan Avenue
Chicago, IL 60611
(312) 644-6610; (312) 527-6640 FAX

The Society of Gynecologic Oncologists (SGO) currently has over 550 members who devote their professional research and clinical expertise to cancers that affect the female reproductive organs. The SGO includes physicians from all over the United States and directs its efforts to the following objectives:

to improve the care of patients with gynecologic cancer;

to advance knowledge and raise standards of practice in gynecologic oncology;

to encourage research in gynecologic oncology; and to cooperate with other individuals and organizations interested in oncology and related fields.

23. The Society of Surgical Oncology
13 Elm Street
Manchester, MA 01944
(508) 526-8330; (508) 526-4018 FAX

The Society of Surgical Oncology (SSO) is composed of over 900 physicians whose mission is to ensure the highest quality of comprehensive cancer care possible. To carry out this mission, the Society endorses and supports the following objectives:

to develop and disseminate optimal standards for multidisciplinary cancer care, including screening, skilled operative management, adjuvant therapies, rehabilitation, and follow-up;

to promote the specialty of surgical oncology through continuing education and the training of medical students, surgical residents and fellows; and

to foster clinical and laboratory research and the dissemination of new information to its membership, the surgical and other professional cancer communities, and the public.

GOVERNMENT AGENCIES/PROGRAMS

Resources for Cancer Education

1. National Center for Chronic Disease Prevention & Health Promotion
Centers for Disease Control
1600 Clifton Road, Mailstop K13
Atlanta, GA 30333
(404) 488-5080

The Center provides assistance to state and local health departments in tracking risk factors/conditions in the population; coordinates a telephone-based survey, the Behavioral Risk Factor Surveillance System, on major risk factors such as smoking, alcohol, nutrition, hypertension, weight, and seat belt use; implements School Health Education Evaluation project, an extensive evaluation of the impact of school health education programs on students' health-related behaviors; and maintains a Health Education Database, a computer online summary of national health education efforts.

2. Consumer Information Center
General Services Administration
Pueblo, CO 81009
(303) 948-3334

The Consumer Information Center, a mail order operation, distributes consumer publications on topics such as children, food and nutrition, health, exercise, and weight control. The *Consumer Information Catalog* is available free from the Center and must be used to identify publications being requested.

3. Consumer Product Safety Commission
Washington, DC 20207
(301) 492-6800; (800) 638-2772 (hotline)

An independent federal regulatory agency with jurisdiction over consumer products used in and around the home, the Commission sets standards and conducts information programs on potentially hazardous products, among them carcinogens and other chronic hazards. Single copies of printed materials are available free of charge. The hotline number allows the caller via a touch tone system to obtain and report information on specific products. Written reports and information should be requested in writing.

4. Food and Nutrition Information Center
US Department of Agriculture
National Agriculture Library Building—Room 304
Beltsville, MD 20705-2351
(301) 504-5719

The Center is a resource for the informational needs of professionals interested in nutrition education, food service management, and food technology. They acquire and lend books, journal articles, and audiovisual materials to answer questions on the topics of food and nutrition.

5. National Audiovisual Center
National Archives
8700 Edgeworth Drive
Capitol Heights, MD 20743-3701
(301) 763-1896; TDD: (301) 763-4385

The National Audiovisual Center, a nonprofit public service is the central source for federally sponsored audiovisuals. The Center distributes more than 8000 programs on over 600 topics, including cancer and the environment, breast cancer, cancer detection, and smoking. Costs for these audiovisuals and accompanying printed materials range from $50 to $350.

6. National Center for Health Statistics
Division of Epidemiology and Health Promotion
6525 Belcrest Road, Room 1064
Hyattsville, MD 20782

This agency provides informational assistance in the development of health measures for health researchers, administrators, and planners.

7. Division of Cancer Prevention and Control
National Cancer Institute
National Institutes of Health
Bethesda, MD 20892-4200
(301) 496-6616

The Division of Cancer Prevention and Control (DCPC) plans and conducts basic and applied research programs aimed at reducing cancer incidence, morbidity, and mortality. Activities are carried out across five phases of research: hypothesis development, methods testing, controlled intervention trials, defined population studies, and demonstrations relevant to the prevention and management of cancer. DCPC plans, directs, and coordinates the support of basic and applied research on cancer prevention and control at cancer centers and community hospitals. It also coordinates program activities with federal and state agencies and establishes liaisons with professional and voluntary health agencies, labor organizations, cancer organizations, and trade associations.

8. Office of Cancer Communications
National Cancer Institute
National Institutes of Health
Bethesda, MD 20892
(301) 496-5583

The Office of Cancer Communications provides information on all aspects of the cancer problem to physicians, scientists, educators, Congress, the Executive Branch, the media, and the public. It fosters and coordinates a national cancer communications program designed to provide the public and health care professionals with information they need to take more responsible health actions. The CIS (800-4-CANCER) is located within this office, with a network of locations across the country.

9. National Health Information Center
Office of Disease Prevention and Health Promotion
P.O. Box 1133
Washington, DC 20013-1133
(301) 565-4167

The National Health Information Center, a service of the Office of Disease Prevention and Health Promotion, is a central source of information and referral for health questions from the public and health care professionals. It maintains a computer database of government agencies, support groups, professional societies, and other organizations that can answer questions on specific health care topics. In addition, the Center offers a library containing medical and health reference books, directories, information files, and periodicals; database development on organizations that provide health information; and a number of publications including resource guides and bibliographies.

Some publications prepared by this office are the Department of Health and Human Services (DHHS) *Prevention Reports,* which summarizes prevention-oriented findings in the scientific literature in abstract form; the *Healthfinder Series,* which provides resource lists on specific health topics and events; and *Healthy People 2000,* the National Health Promotion and Disease Prevention's objectives and health goals for the year 2000. Included are over 300 objectives in 22 priority areas, such as nutrition, tobacco use, environmental health, cancer, and HIV infections.

10. National Heart, Lung, and Blood Institute Information Center
National Institutes of Health
P.O. Box 30105
Bethesda, MD 20824-0105
(301) 951-3260

The information center is a service of the NHLBI that provides health professionals and the general public with the most current information available about high blood pressure, cholesterol, smoking, asthma, blood resources, obesity, heart attack, and heart disease. The Information Center disseminates educational, programmatic, and scientific materials and responds to inquiries. The Information Center database is also part of the Combined Health Information Database (CHID) available through BRS Information Technologies. Series publications include *Heart Memo, Lung Memo,* and *Blood Memo.*

11. Office for Substance Abuse Prevention
National Clearinghouse for Alcohol and Drug Information
P.O. Box 2345
11426 Rockville Pike, Suite 200
Rockville, MD 20852
(301) 468-2600; (800) 729-6686; TDD: (800) 487-4889

The ONCADI, a service of the Office for Substance Abuse and Prevention, provides information on the latest research results, popular press and scholarly journal articles, videos, public service announcements, prevention curricula, print material, and program descriptions on alcohol and other drugs. ONCADI publishes the bimonthly *Prevention Pipeline* and a quarterly catalogue.

12. National Institute for Occupational Safety and Health
Technical Information Branch
4676 Columbia Parkway
Cincinnati, OH 45226-1998
(513) 684-8326; (800) 35-NIOSH

The NIOSH provides technical information to the National Institute for Occupational Safety and Health research programs and supplies information to others on request.

13. National Library of Medicine
National Institutes of Health
8600 Rockville Pike
Bethesda, MD 20894
(301) 496-6308 Public Information Office
(301) 496-6095 Reference Section

The National Library of Medicine collects, organizes, and disseminates both printed and audiovisual materials. The collection, technical and scientific in nature, is primarily for medical professionals. The Library offers an extensive computerized literature retrieval service. A list of bibliographies, catalogues, and indexes with specific ordering instructions is available from the Public Information Office.

14. National Maternal and Child Health Clearinghouse
38th and R Streets NW
Washington, DC 20057
(202) 625-8410

The National Maternal and Child Health Clearinghouse provides information and publications on maternal and child health and genetics to consumers and health professionals. Materials cover such topics as smoking and pregnancy and nutrition and pregnancy.

15. National Toxicology Program
National Institute of Environmental Health Sciences
M.D. B2-04, Box 12233
Research Triangle Park, NC 27709
(919) 541-3991

The NTP coordinates and conducts toxicology and test method development research and provides information about potentially hazardous chemicals, including those that cause cancer. Information in the form of technical reports on particular chemicals, as well as the annual report on carcinogens, is available free of charge until supplies are exhausted.

16. Office of Consumer Affairs
Food and Drug Administration
5600 Fishers Lane
Rockville, MD 20857
(301) 443-3170

The Office of Consumer Affairs, Food and Drug Administration, responds to consumer inquiries and serves as a clearinghouse for consumer publications on a variety of topics including pregnancy, mammography, food and nutrition, proper use of drugs, and health fraud. Over 250 pamphlets are available free of charge; requests should be made in writing.

17. Office on Smoking and Health
Centers for Disease Control
Mailstop K-12
1600 Clifton Road, NE
Atlanta, GA 30333
(404) 448-5708

The Office on Smoking and Health produces and distributes a number of informational and educational materials. It also offers bibliographic and reference services to researchers and others. The materials and services are available free of charge. In addition, the Office produces pamphlets, posters, and public service announcements that contain various health messages.

18. Publication Distribution Office
Occupational Safety and Health Administration
US Department of Labor
200 Constitution Ave., NW—Room s4203
Washington, DC 20210
(202) 523-9667

The Publication Distribution Office responds to inquiries from the general public, health care professionals, industry, educational institutions, and other sources about a limited number of job-related carcinogens and toxic substances. The Regulatory Text of OSHA's Final Standard for Occupational Exposure to Bloodborne Pathogens is available through this office.

19. National Institute on Aging
Public Information Office
9000 Rockville Pike
Bldg. 31, Room 5C27
Bethesda, MD 20892
(301) 496-1752

The National Institute on Aging's Public Information Office carries out a legislatively mandated information and education program for the general public, mass media, physicians, health care workers, other government agencies, and service organizations. Free consumer materials are available on many topics pertaining to older adults, including cancer and smoking.

20. Office of Minority Health Resource Center
P.O. Box 37337
Washington, DC 20013-7337
(800) 444-MHRC

The MHRC is a division of the Public Health Service, Department of Health and Human Services. Its activities include a bilingually staffed toll-free number to provide minority health information and referrals to health professionals; a computerized database of materials, organizations, and programs; and a resource persons network of professionals active in the field.

Other Government Offices Related to Oncology

1. Cancer Nursing Service
National Institutes of Health
Bldg 10, Room 7D 37
9000 Rockville Pike
Bethesda, MD 20892
(301) 496-3101

Nurses from the Cancer Nursing Service provide care to patients entered on intramural clinical research trials evaluating cancer therapies.

2. Patient Referral Service
Clinical Center of the National Institutes of Health
Building 10, Room 1C 255
9000 Rockville Pike
Bethesda, MD
(301) 496-4891

COMPREHENSIVE, CLINICAL, AND CONSORTIUM CANCER CENTERS

The National Cancer Act of 1971 authorized the development of new comprehensive research and demonstration centers known as comprehensive cancer centers and specialized cancer centers. Through community outreach activities, comprehensive cancer centers are to provide coordination and leadership within their geographic regions to ensure the availability of complete care for patients with cancer.

At present, there are 28 comprehensive (*) cancer centers and 12 clinical (**) cancer centers designated by the NCI. A treatment center must meet rigorous criteria set by the NCI, including the ability to perform advanced diagnostic and treatment methods; support a strong research program; and participate in an integrated nationwide system in prevention, diagnosis, and treatment. Information about referral procedures, treatment costs, and services available to patients can be obtained from the individual cancer centers listed below (as of March 1992):

Alabama
*University of Alabama at Birmingham
Comprehensive Cancer Center
Basic Health Sciences Building, Rm 108
1918 University Boulevard
Birmingham, AL 35294
(205) 934-6612

Arizona
*University of Arizona Cancer Center
1501 North Campbell Avenue
Tucson, AZ 85724
(602) 626-6372

California
*Kenneth Norris Jr. Comprehensive Cancer Center
University of Southern California
1441 Eastlake Avenue
Los Angeles, CA 90033-0804
(213) 226-2370

*Jonsson Comprehensive Cancer Center
University of California at Los Angeles
200 Medical Plaza
Los Angeles, CA 90027
(213) 206-0278

**City of Hope National Medical Center
Beckman Research Institute
1500 East Duarte Road
Duarte, CA 91010
(818) 359-8111, ext. 2292

**University of California at San Diego Cancer Center
225 Dickinson Street
San Diego, CA 92103
(619) 543-6178

Colorado
**University of Colorado Cancer Center
4200 East 9th Avenue, Box B190
Denver, CO 80262
(303) 270-7235

Connecticut
*Yale University Comprehensive Cancer Center
333 Cedar Street
New Haven, CT 06510
(203) 785-6338

District of Columbia
*Lombardi Cancer Research Center
Georgetown University Medical Center
3800 Reservoir Road, N.W.
Washington, DC 20007
(202) 687-2192

Florida
*Sylvester Comprehensive Cancer Center
University of Miami Medical School
1475 Northwest 12th Avenue
Miami, FL 33136
(305) 548-4800

Illinois
**University of Chicago Cancer Research Center
5841 S. Maryland Avenue
Chicago, IL 60637
(312) 702-9200

Maryland
*The Johns Hopkins Oncology Center
600 North Wolfe Street
Baltimore, MD 21205
(301) 955-8638

Massachusetts
*Dana-Farber Cancer Institute
44 Binney Street
Boston, MA 02115
(617) 732-3214

Michigan
*Meyer L. Prentis Comprehensive Cancer Center of Metropolitan Detroit
110 East Warren Avenue
Detroit, MI 48201
(313) 745-4329

*University of Michigan Cancer Center
101 Simpson Drive
Ann Arbor, MI 48109-0752
(313) 936-9583

Minnesota
*Mayo Comprehensive Cancer Center
200 First Street Southwest
Rochester, MN 55905
(507) 284-3413

New Hampshire
*Norris Cotton Cancer Center
Dartmouth-Hitchcock Medical Center
One Medical Center Drive
Lebanon, NH 03756
(603) 646-5505

New York
*Memorial Sloan-Kettering Cancer Center
1275 York Avenue
New York, NY 10021
(800) 525-2225

*Columbia University Comprehensive Cancer Center
College of Physicians and Surgeons
630 West 168th Street
New York, NY 10032
(212) 305-6905

*Roswell Park Cancer Institute
Elm and Carlton Streets
Buffalo, NY 14263
(716) 845-4400

**Albert Einstein College of Medicine
1300 Morris Park Avenue
Bronx, NY 10461
(212) 920-4826

*Kaplan Cancer Center
New York University Medical Center
462 First Avenue
New York, NY 10016-9103
(212) 263-6485

**University of Rochester Cancer Center
601 Elmwood Avenue, Box 704
Rochester, NY 14642
(716) 275-4911

North Carolina
*Duke Comprehensive Cancer Center
P.O. Box 3814
Durham, NC 27710
(919) 286-5515

*Lineberger Comprehensive Cancer Center
University of North Carolina
School of Medicine
Chapel Hill, NC 27599
(919) 966-4431

*Cancer Center of Wake Forest University at the Bowman Gray School of Medicine
300 South Hawthorn Road
Winston-Salem, NC 27103
(919) 748-4354

Ohio
*Ohio State University Comprehensive Cancer Center
410 West 10th Avenue
Columbia, OH 43210
(614) 293-8619

**Case Western Reserve University
University Hospitals of Cleveland
Ireland Cancer Center
2074 Abington Road
Cleveland, OH 44106
(216) 844-5432

Pennsylvania
*Fox Chase Cancer Center
7701 Burholme Avenue
Philadelphia, PA 19111
(215) 728-2570

*University of Pennsylvania Cancer Center
3400 Spruce Street
Philadelphia, PA 19104
(215) 662-6364

*Pittsburgh Cancer Institute
200 Meyran Avenue
Pittsburgh, PA 15213-2592
(800) 537-4063

Rhode Island
**Roger Williams Cancer Center
825 Chalkstone Avenue
Providence, RI 02908
(401) 456-2071

Tennessee
**St. Jude Children's Research Hospital
322 North Lauderdale Street
Memphis, TN 38101-0318
(901) 522-0306

Texas
**Institute for Cancer Research and Care
4450 Medical Drive
San Antonio, TX 78229
(512) 616-5580

*University of Texas
M.D. Anderson Cancer Center
1515 Holcombe Boulevard
Houston, TX 77030
(713) 792-3245

Utah
**Utah Regional Cancer Center
University of Utah Medical Center
50 North Medical Drive, Room 2C10
Salt Lake City, UT 84132
(801) 581-5052

Vermont
*Vermont Cancer Center
University of Vermont
1 South Prospect Street
Burlington, VT 05401
(802) 656-4580

Virginia
**Massey Cancer Center
Medical College of Virginia
Virginia Commonwealth University
1200 East Broad Street
Richmond, VA 23298
(804) 786-9641

Washington
*Fred Hutchinson Cancer Research Center
1124 Columbia Street
Seattle, WA 98104
(206) 467-4675

Wisconsin
*Wisconsin Clinical Cancer Center
University of Wisconsin
600 Highland Avenue
Madison, WI 53792
(608) 263-8090

COOPERATIVE CLINICAL TRIAL GROUPS IN THE UNITED STATES

Following are the U.S. Clinical Trials Cooperative Groups and telephone numbers from which information can be obtained on clinical trials being conducted, eligibility criteria, treatment plan of the clinical trial, and how to refer a patient to one of these trials. Currently in the United States, fewer than 10% of eligible adult patients are entered on clinical trials. The result of this low percentage of patients is a delay in answering important therapeutic and scientific questions and in disseminating therapeutic advances to the general oncology community. There are multiple clinical trials conducted within each of the Cooperative Groups.

1. BTCG
Brain Tumor Cooperative Group
William R. Shapiro, MD
(602) 285-3895
Barrow Neurological Institute
St. Joseph's Hospital
350 West Thomas Road
Phoenix, AZ 85013
2. CALGB
Cancer and Leukemia Group B
Priscilla Stoner
(603) 646-6701
CALGB Central Office
Suite 2
444 Mount Support Road
Lebanon, NH 03766
Affiliation(s):

   Cancer Therapy Evaluation Program
   Eastern Main Medical Center
   Hematology Oncology Associates of Central New York Community Clinical
   North Shore University Hospital Community Clinical Oncology Program
   Southeast Cancer Control Consortium Community Clinical Oncology Program
   Southern Nevada Cancer Research Foundation Community Clinical Oncology
   Medical Center of Delaware Community Clinical Oncology Program
   San Diego Kaiser Permanente Community Clinical Oncology Program
   Milwaukee Community Clinical Oncology Program
   Mount Sinai Community Clinical Oncology Program
   National Surgical Adjuvant Project for Breast and Bowel Cancers
3. CCSG
Children's Cancer Study Group
Sally Boynton
(818) 447-0064
440 East Huntington Drive
Suite 300
P.O. Box 60012
Arcadia, CA 91066-6012
Affiliation(s):

   Cancer Therapy Evaluation Program
   Duluth Clinic Community Clinical Oncology Program
   Geisinger Clinical Oncology program

Iowa Oncology Research Association Community Clinical Oncology Program
Marshfield Medical Foundation Community Clinical Oncology Program
North Shore University Hospital Community Clinical Oncology Program
Sioux Community Cancer Consortium Community Clinical Oncology Program
St. Luke's Hospitals Community Clinical Oncology Program
Medical Center of Delaware Community Clinical Oncology Program
Bay Area Tumor Institute Community Clinical Oncology Program
Southern Nevada Cancer Research Foundation Community Clinical Oncology
Methodist Hospital of Indiana, Inc. Community Clinical Oncology Program
Grand Rapids Community Clinical Oncology Program

4. ECOG
Eastern Cooperative Oncology Group
AMC Cancer Research Center
1600 Pierce Street
Denver, CO 80214
(303) 293-3070
Affiliation(s):

Cancer Therapy Evaluation Program
Bergen-Passaic Community Clinical Oncology Program
Duluth Clinic Community Clinical Oncology Program
Kellogg Cancer Care Center Community Clinical Oncology Program
Geisinger Clinical Oncology Program
Green Mountain Oncology Group
Illinois Oncology Research Association Community Clinical Oncology Program
Marshfield Medical Foundation Community Clinical Oncology Program
Natalie Warren Bryant Community Clinical Oncology Program
Ochsner Community Clinical Oncology Program
Veterans Administration Cooperative Studies Program Coordinating Center
Sioux Community Cancer Consortium Community Clinical Oncology Program
St. Luke's Hospitals Community Clinical Oncology Program
Toledo Community Clinical Oncology Program
Twin Tiers Community Clinical Oncology Program
West Metro-Minneapolis Community Clinical Oncology Program
Carle Cancer Center Community Clinical Oncology Program
Iowa Oncology Research Association Community Clinical Oncology Program
Kalamazoo Community Clinical Oncology Program
Bay Area Tumor Institute Community Clinical Oncology Program
Northern California Cancer Center
Rapid City Regional Oncology Group Community Clinical Oncology Program
Methodist Hospital of Indiana, Inc. Community Clinical Oncology Program
Indiana Regional Cancer Center Community Clinical Oncology Program
Cedar Rapids Oncology Project Community Clinical Oncology Program
Mercy Hospital Community Clinical Oncology Program
San Joaquin Valley Community Cancer Program
Brooklyn Community Clinical Oncology Program

5. EORTC
European Organization for Research and Treatment of Cancer
Celestina Arrigo
Francoise Meunier, MD
32-2-774-16-11
32-2-774-16-30
Avenue Mounier 83—B11
B-1200 Brussels (Bruxelles), Belgium

6. GOG
Gynecologic Oncology Group
John R. Kellner
(215) 854-0770
Suite 1945
1234 Market Street
Philadelphia, PA 19107
Affiliation(s):
Cancer Therapy Evaluation Program

7. Intergroup Rhabdomyosarcoma Study
Jean Johnston
(804) 786-9602
Department of Pediatrics
Medical College of Virginia
Box 646
Richmond, VA 23298
Affiliation(s):
Cancer Therapy Evaluation Program

8. NSABP
National Surgical Adjuvant Project for Breast and Bowel Cancers
Mary Ketner, RN
(412) 648-9720
Scaife Hall, Room 914
3550 Terrace Street
Pittsburgh, PA 15261
Affiliation(s):

Cancer Therapy Evaluation Program
Allegheny Community Clinical Oncology Program
Central Illinois Community Clinical Oncology Program
Central Los Angeles Community Clinical Oncology Program
Columbia River Community Clinical Oncology Program
Columbus Community Clinical Oncology Program
Dayton Clinical Oncology Program
Eastern Maine Medical Center
Grand Rapids Community Clinical Oncology Program
Green Mountain Oncology Group
Hematology Oncology Associates of Central New York Community Clinical
Marshfield Medical Foundation Community Clinical Oncology Program
Ochsner Community Clinical Oncology Program
Sacramento Community Clinical Oncology Program
Southeast Cancer Control Consortium Community Clinical Oncology Program

Southern Nevada Cancer Research Foundation Community Clinical Oncology
Spartanburg Community Clinical Oncology Program
Natalie Warren Bryant Community Clinical Oncology Program
West Metro-Minneapolis Community Clinical Oncology Program
Duluth Clinic Community Clinical Oncology Program
Atlanta Regional Community Clinical Oncology Program
Kansas City Clinical Oncology Program
Medical Center of Delaware Community Clinical Oncology Program
Twin Tiers Community Clinical Oncology Program
San Diego Kaiser Permanente Community Clinical Oncology Program
Bay Area Tumor Institute Community Clinical Oncology Program
Milwaukee Community Clinical Oncology Program
St. Louis-Cape Girardeau Community Clinical Oncology Program
Wichita Community Clinical Oncology Program
Greater Phoenix Community Clinical Oncology Program
Kalamazoo Community Clinical Oncology Program
Ozark Regional Community Clinical Oncology Program
Mount Sinai Community Clinical Oncology Program
Methodist Hospital of Indiana, Inc. Community Clinical Oncology Program
California Healthcare System Community Clinical Oncology Program
Indiana Regional Cancer Center Community Clinical Oncology Program
Billings Interhospital Oncology Project
Mercy Hospital Community Clinical Oncology Program
San Joaquin Valley Community Cancer Program
Grady Hospital Minority Based Community Clinical Oncology Program
Minority-Based Community Clinical Oncology Program of Metropolitan Detroit
Kings County Minority-Based Community Clinical Oncology Program
Sioux Community Cancer Consortium Community Clinical Oncology Program
Carle Cancer Center Community Clinical Oncology Program
Toledo Community Clinical Oncology Program
San Antonio Minority-Based Community Clinical Oncology Program

9. NWTSG
National Wilms' Tumor Study Group
Daniel M. Green, MD
(716) 845-2334
Roswell Park Cancer Institute
Pediatric Division
666 Elm Street
Buffalo, NY 14263
Affiliation(s):
Cancer Therapy Evaluation Program

10. NCCTG
North Central Cancer Treatment Group
Patricia Koenig, RN
(507) 284-4642
200 First Street SW
Rochester, MN 55905
Affiliation(s):

Mayo Clinic
Cancer Therapy Evaluation Program
Duluth Clinic Community Clinical Oncology Program
Geisinger Clinical Oncology Program
Illinois Oncology Research Association Community Clinical Oncology Program
Iowa Oncology Research Association Community Clinical Oncology Program
Ochsner Community Clinical Oncology Program
Sioux Community Cancer Consortium Community Clinical Oncology Program
St. Luke's Hospitals Community Clinical Oncology Program
Carle Cancer Center Community Clinical Oncology Program
Toledo Community Clinical Oncology Program
Rapid City Regional Oncology Group Community Clinical Oncology Program
Cedar Rapids Oncology Project Community Clinical Oncology Program

11. POG
Pediatric Oncology Group
Patricia H. Gensel
(314) 367-3446
Del Coronado, Suite 2A
4949 West Pine Boulevard
Saint Louis, MO 63108
Affiliation(s):

Cancer Therapy Evaluation Program
Bergen-Passaic Community Clinical Oncology Program
Florida Pediatric Community Clinical Oncology Program
Wichita Community Clinical Oncology Program
Ochsner Community Clinical Oncology Program

12. RTOG
Radiation Therapy Oncology Group
Elaine Pakuris
(215) 574-3195
14th Floor
1101 Market Street
Philadelphia, PA 19107
Affiliation(s):

Cancer Therapy Evaluation Program
Veterans Administration Cooperative Studies Program Coordinating Center

13. SWOG
Southwest Oncology Group
Operations Office
14980 Omicron Drive
San Antonio, TX 78245-3217
(210) 677-8808
Affiliation(s):

Cancer Therapy Evaluation Program
Allegheny Community Clinical Oncology Program
Atlanta Regional Community Clinical Oncology Program
Central Illinois Community Clinical Oncology Program
Columbia River Community Clinical Oncology Program
Columbus Community Clinical Oncology Program
Dayton Clinical Oncology Program
Grand Rapids Community Clinical Oncology Program
Greater Phoenix Community Clinical Oncology Program

Kansas City Clinical Oncology Program
Northwest Community Clinical Oncology Program
Ozark Regional Community Clinical Oncology Program
Sacramento Community Clinical Oncology Program
Spartanburg Community Clinical Oncology Program
St. Louis-Cape Girardeau Community Clinical Oncology Program
Virginia Mason Medical Center Community Clinical Oncology Program
Wichita Community Clinical Oncology Program
Central Los Angeles Community Clinical Oncology Program
California Healthcare System Community Clinical Oncology Program
Billings Interhospital Oncology Project
San Joaquin Valley Community Cancer Program

Index